Oxford Textbook of
Medicine

Project Administrator Anna McNeil
Project Editor Dr Irene Butcher
Indexer Caroline Sheard
Production Manager Kate Martin
Production Editor Anna Campbell
Design Manager Andrew Meaden
Typographer Jonathan Coleclough
Illustrations Touch Media, Abingdon
Publisher Alison Langton

volume **2**

Oxford Textbook of
Medicine

Fourth Edition
Volume 2: Sections 11–17

Edited by

David A. Warrell
Professor of Tropical Medicine and Infectious Diseases and Head, Nuffield Department of Clinical Medicine, University of Oxford; Honorary Consultant Physician, Oxford Radcliffe NHS Trust, UK

Timothy M. Cox
Professor of Medicine, University of Cambridge; Honorary Consultant Physician, Addenbrooke's Hospital, Cambridge, UK
and

John D. Firth
Consultant Physician and Nephrologist, Addenbrooke's Hospital, Cambridge, UK
with

Edward J. Benz Jr
President and CEO, Dana Farber Cancer Institute; Richard and Susan Smith Professor of Medicine, Professor of Pediatrics and Professor of Pathology, Harvard Medical School, Boston, USA

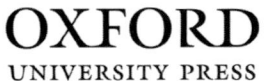

OXFORD
UNIVERSITY PRESS

OXFORD
UNIVERSITY PRESS

Great Clarendon Street, Oxford OX2 6DP

Oxford University Press is a department of the University of Oxford.
It furthers the University's objective of excellence in research, scholarship,
and education by publishing worldwide in

Oxford New York

Auckland Bangkok Buenos Aires Cape Town Chennai
Dar es Salaam Delhi Hong Kong Istanbul Karachi Kolkata
Kuala Lumpur Madrid Melbourne Mexico City Mumbai Nairobi
São Paulo Shanghai Singapore Taipei Tokyo Toronto

Oxford is a registered trade mark of Oxford University Press
in the UK and in certain other countries

Published in the United States
by Oxford University Press Inc., New York

First published 1983
Second edition published 1987
Third edition published 1996
Fourth edition published 2003

British Library Cataloguing in Publication Data
Data available

Library of Congress Cataloging in Publication Data
Data available

ISBN 0–19–262922–0 (Three volume set)
0–19–852787–X (volume 1)
0–19–852788–8 (volume 2)
0–19–852789–6 (volume 3)
Available as a three-volume set only

10 9 8 7 6 5 4 3 2 1

Typeset by Interactive Sciences Ltd, Gloucester, England
Printed in Italy
on acid-free paper by LegoPrint

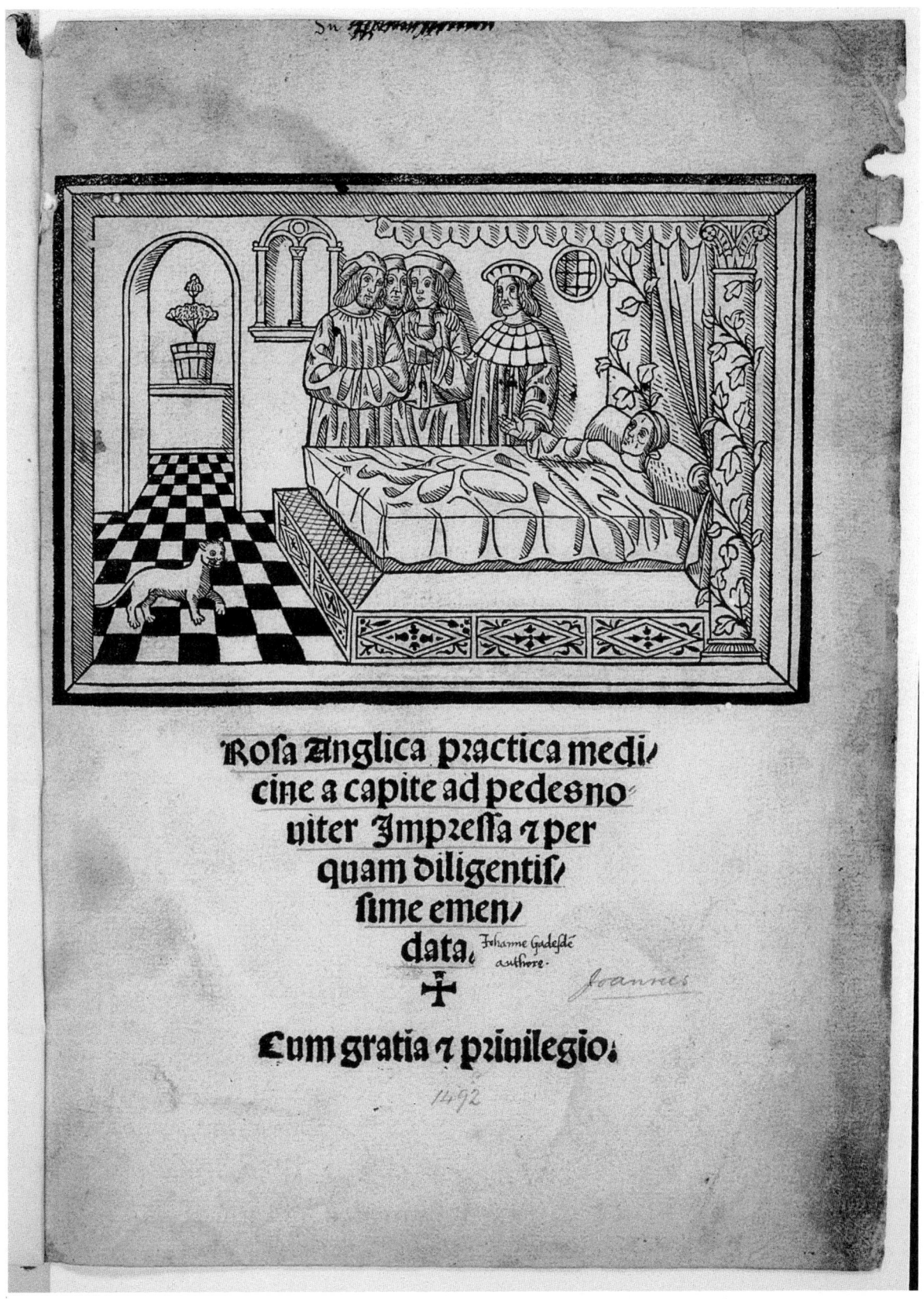

The title page of the 1492 edition of *Rosa Anglica* by John of Gaddesden (1280–1361), which was probably written in 1314. The author was a well known physician attached to Merton College, Oxford in the early part of the 14th century. His famous book was probably the first 'Oxford Textbook of Medicine'. The author was the model for the unsavoury Doctor of Physick in Chaucer's *Canterbury Tales*.

Foreword

by Professor Sir David Weatherall, FRS

It is now 20 years since the first edition of the *Oxford Textbook of Medicine* appeared on the scene, a time when the concept of the all-encompassing textbook of medicine was being questioned. Its predecessor, *Price's Textbook of the Practice of Medicine*, first published in 1922 and by then in its twelfth edition, had come under considerable criticism. One of its most voluble critics, the late J.R.A. Mitchell, had even gone to the trouble of weighing the book, after which he suggested that, because dinosaurs became extinct because of their sheer bulk, medical textbooks would suffer the same fate. In addition, he and many other reviewers suggested that large textbooks are out of date before they are published and hence are of extremely limited value. Notwithstanding Professor Mitchell's outdated views on the extinction of dinosaurs, we thought that he had a point.

After considering these arguments carefully we came to the conclusion that there was still a place for at least one major British work of reference which attempted to cover the whole field of internal medicine. This decision was based largely on the view that, because of the enormous breadth of the subject and the increasing tendency to overspecialization, very few students and practitioners could have immediate access to smaller monographs on every branch of the field; even when they are available they are not always written by those who evaluate their patients in a general medical setting. And if this is true of clinicians in the richer countries, it must apply even more to those in the developing world, where access to libraries and review articles may be limited. Furthermore, although we were well aware that textbooks rapidly become out of date, few advances in medicine lead to major changes in patient care, and those that do often require many years of critical evaluation before they become an integral part of routine clinical practice. For this reason we decided to try to produce a wide-ranging medical textbook which would have a particular emphasis on the global aspects of disease, rather than focus simply on the day-to-day medical problems of the developed world.

Since the *Oxford Textbook of Medicine* first appeared there have been profound changes, both in the practice of medicine and in the problems of the provision of medical care. None of the richer countries has been able to solve the problem of the spiralling costs of health care, which have resulted in part from the introduction of new technology but, even more importantly, from the remarkable increase in the age of their patient populations. If anything, the gap between the quality of the provision of health care between the richer and poorer countries has widened, and although some of the poorer countries have made the epidemiological transition from high death rates due to infection and malnutrition towards a more westernized pattern of illness, particularly in sub-Saharan Africa infectious disease, notably respiratory infection, AIDS, tuberculosis, and malaria, remain the major causes of death; a review of over 11 million childhood deaths in 1998 disclosed, disgracefully, that over 4 million were due to diseases for which adequate vaccines or other forms of prevention already exist. The phenomena of 'globalization', and increasing corporate dominance, are also tending to exacerbate the divide between the rich and poor nations.

Another profound change which has occurred over the last 20 years is the emphasis on the study of disease at the molecular and cellular levels and the increasing role of what is still rather optimistically called 'molecular medicine'. But while this remarkable field promises much for the health of mankind for the future, so far it has had little place in day-to-day clinical practice. Thus, while the fruits of the human genome project offer enormous potential for the better understanding, prevention, and management of the common killers of middle life and old age in richer societies, and the pathogen genome projects offer equal hope for controlling the infectious killers of the developing countries, it is still far from clear when the rich promises of these fields will come to fruition for preventative medicine and clinical care. And there is the danger that when they do, because many of them are likely to be expensive, the gap between the provision of health care in the poorer and richer countries will become even wider. Although many of the solutions to these problems depend on a complete change of attitude of governments and industry in the richer countries, there is no doubt that there will be a rapidly increasing role for their medical schools and doctors to develop collaborative programmes with those of the developing countries and, in general, to take a much more global view of disease, both in medical education and research.

The other major change in the medical field over the last 20 years has been the increasing disquiet about the pattern of medical practice. In many countries doctors have come under increasing criticism for their lack of ability to communicate adequately with patients, for their quality of patient care and, overall, for their lack of humanity. The patient community has become much more sophisticated and demanding, and in most countries there has been a rapid increase in the number of medico-legal actions taken against doctors. This trend has already had wide-ranging repercussions. There has been a major rethink about the pattern of medical education, placing less emphasis on its scientific basis and more on communication skills, ethics, and the social aspects of medicine. The remarkable revolution in the basic biological sciences that underlie medical practice, particularly in the field of genomics, is also raising new ethical issues which would have been undreamed of at the time of the first edition of this book.

In short, medical practice has entered the new millennium in a state of considerable uncertainty. The whole ethos of clinical practice is being questioned, none of the richer countries has got to grips with how to finance the increasing demands of medical care, and many of the poorer countries still have completely dysfunctional health care systems. It is very pleasing therefore to see that the new edition of the *Oxford Textbook of Medicine* reflects so many of these changing issues, as they affect internal medicine. In particular, the textbook has maintained and expanded the aspirations of its original editors towards providing a genuinely global picture of disease, not just as it affects the populations of the richer countries but as it involves the lives of all of those in the poorer countries of the world. As well as continuing to describe the major causes of ill-health and death in the populations of the poorer countries, it includes new sections on screening and the costs of health care, and has greatly increased its coverage of some of the major infectious killers, particularly HIV/AIDS. At the other end of the spectrum it has expanded its sections on the molecular mechanisms of disease and tried to put molecular medicine into perspective by defining its limits. And it has not ignored the remarkable advances in medicine which relate to the richer countries, particularly in its coverage of the problems of the aged. In doing so it has focused on the major killers of Western society, notably cancer, heart disease, and stroke, and has greatly increased the coverage of critical care and emergency medicine. This extensive revision has required the recruitment of many new authors, reflecting a change of over one-third of those from the last edition.

After the publication of the last edition of the *Oxford Textbook of Medicine* my colleague John Ledingham and I decided that it was time to stand aside and pass on our editorial roles to a younger team of editors who are still very active in the fields of medical research and practice. We are delighted to see that our younger colleagues have maintained the tradition of producing a broad-ranging medical textbook which emphasizes the pastoral, scientific, and global aspects of medical care. Despite all its problems medical practice is entering the most exciting and challenging period of its development, and we believe that it still offers the most exciting and enriching of careers for its practitioners. We trust that the 'OTM' will remain their guide and friend for many years to come.

Preface

Textbooks of medicine: *raison d'etre*

Now, in the third millennium, is there any need for a textbook of medicine? Never before has so much information on medical matters been so readily available to so many: physicians are inundated, as are their patients and everyone else. The media seem to carry more and more medical stories in more and more detail every day. The genome has been sequenced. Articulate teenagers speak of stem cells. The internet brings widespread and virtually unlimited access to biomedical information (and misinformation) of a sort: one click of a mouse, and it's all anyone's. A plethora of organizations besieges physicians with guidelines and protocols on every aspect of the practice of medicine. Traditional values are being challenged in all facets of life, including medicine, and there is an unprecedented and entirely appropriate demand for supportive evidence, not just weight of experience, to justify medical interventions.

In these circumstances, some might argue that textbooks of medicine were irrelevant, inappropriate, or even redundant. We strongly refute this. Amidst the maelstrom of 'information' in which physicians now work there is, more than ever, a need for a fixed point of reference, something by which the new, the exciting, and the fashionable can be judged. We make the bold claim that the *Oxford Textbook of Medicine* is just such a fixed point. We argue, unashamedly, that a clinical textbook in the Oslerian tradition is not only required but is essential, to provide expert review, evaluation, and recommendation.

Clinical medicine: changes, challenges, and reconsiderations

This fourth edition of the *Oxford Textbook of Medicine* emerges at a time when discoveries in molecular sciences and advances in technology provide an unprecedented range of diagnostic reagents, drugs, and bioinformatics. Yet, at the same time, there is a widespread recognition that the outcome of treatment for many patients falls short of ideal standards. Microbial resistance to antibiotics, adverse consequences of drugs, and the fallibility of doctors all contribute to failures; and we now realize how dangerous hospitals and clinics can be. Besides this, many contemporary high-tech procedures cannot cure chronic illnesses, and we lack effective weapons to influence the powerful social and behavioural factors that underlie so much illness. The advent of predictive DNA testing also poses complex ethical questions for practitioners, for which few answers are available.

Advances in biomedical science crucially drive innovation and improvement in medical practice. These are not neglected in this book, but the practice of medicine (except in dire emergency) is initiated by a patient talking with a physician and proceeds (as appropriate) through physical examination and investigation to discussion of diagnosis, prognosis, and treatment. These are the core issues of clinical medicine which form the bulk of this textbook.

A culture of public mistrust: the physician–patient relationship

Our political masters in much of the developed world, long tired of being marginalized by old-established networks within the professions, have introduced a new accountability distilled from the concept of audit. This has been exported from the world of finance to embrace the scrutiny of non-financial processes in health care and has created a political climate obsessed with cost effectiveness. The degree of central control often leads to impossible conflicts in the expectations of the public and those entrusted with provision of health care. Baroness O'Neil in her BBC Reith Lectures of 2002* has pointed out that there is often an inconsistency in the demands raised by such control, providing, as it does, perverse incentives for the specious goals and 'output measures' determined by central bodies. While it is true that much better standards of health care delivery are required and careful surveillance of clinical activities is desirable, the *Oxford Textbook of Medicine* presents an affirmation of the physician–patient relationship in the fight against illness, debility, and suffering: for this relationship should remain sacrosanct, based on professional integrity, knowledge, and human feeling.

Aims and emphases: Sir Archibald Garrod's legacy

Garrod first understood the unique interactions between heredity and environment in the genesis of human disease and asked the question: 'Why did this particular person develop this particular illness in this particular environment?' – a question that we are only just beginning to answer in an era of almost naïve enthusiasm for genetics. While the study of the invariant factors in human genetics is almost intoxicating in its simplicity, we now face the formidable challenge of identifying the contribution of the environment, with all its attendant variables, to the generation of the clinical phenotype we define as illness.

This is the background to this edition of the *Oxford Textbook of Medicine*: its remit stretches from disease as it presents to physicians at the bedside, to the attendant disturbances of cellular, tissue, and organ function, all occurring within an individual, inevitably a part of the turmoil of society. To have a complete description of all these aspects of any medical complaint would not be possible, but we recognize that many readers will not have ready access to the latest sources of scientific information. The book is therefore designed to be a proper reference point for both scientific and clinical aspects of medical practice and bears the fingerprints of Osler, Garrod, Doll, and Weatherall, all Regius Professors of Medicine in Oxford.

Limitations and strengths

The bitter practicalities of writing, editing, and producing any book, especially a work of this size, prevent its referring to the last edition of *The*

---

* *A Question of Trust.* Cambridge University Press 2002.

Lancet, Quarterly Journal of Medicine, New England Journal of Medicine, or any other periodical. But this book can and does provide the medical background against which new information should be assessed and understood. Grounded in the principles that have made the first three editions standard reference textbooks, the new edition has, like medicine itself, evolved to bring all contemporary resources to focus on the teaching and interpretation of medicine. Many new approaches and topics are included and we have incorporated the skill, experience, and perspectives of a truly international complement of highly distinguished authors, including the recently honoured Nobel Laureate in Medicine, Dr Sydney Brenner.

This fourth edition includes, for the first time, an editorial adviser based in the United States (EJB) and a greatly increased and broadened representation of North American authors. By adopting this approach, we hope we have been able to integrate and synthesize in this edition the perspectives on shared medical issues as they confront physicians and medical scientists in different countries.

At a time when there is a tendency for physicians in some parts of the world to be more and more proficient about less and less, this book is a means of their grasping what is happening and what is important in all areas of medical practice. When the movement of people, diseases, and doctors around the world is greater than ever, there is a need for a truly global perspective, which this book provides.

Acknowledgements

This edition contains much that is entirely new, but we wish here to acknowledge that it is built on the firm foundations established by the distinguished co-editors of the previous editions, Professor Sir David Weatherall and Professor John Ledingham. No work of this kind can be produced without the engagement of dedicated professionals who believe in publishing and commit themselves way beyond healthy expectations to see the task through. Mrs Alison Langton has provided guidance and discipline throughout the production and we are enormously grateful to her and her staff at Oxford University Press for their confidence, commitment, and friendship. We are particularly indebted to Dr Irene Butcher who has worked indefatigably to help us realize our aims and at every level has contributed to the organization of the final text and its complex illustrative material. Her experience, knowledge, and uncompromising attention to detail must surely be unique; her forbearance with the editors and, on rare occasions, errant contributors, has been nothing short of miraculous. We thank our contributors for their patience in delivering their sections and review of proofs for which they are responsible. Ultimately, however, the book and any errors it might contain remain the responsibility of the editors.

Finally we thank Mary, Sue, Helen, and Peggy, our constant, supportive, and forgiving wives; Professor Sir David Weatherall, Professor Alastair Compston, Dr Graham Neale, Professor Michael de Swiet, and Dr Michael Sharpe our section advisers; Professor David Lomas, Professor Julian Hopkin, Professor Michael Doherty, Professor David Isenberg, and Dr Christopher Winearls who gave advice and comment for which the editors are very grateful; and our personal secretaries, Eunice Berry (a veteran of four editions), Joan Grantham, Janet Cameron, Naoe Suzuki, and Beverly Comegys for their exceptional dedication.

Oxford, Cambridge, and Boston   DAW, TMC, JDF, EJB
January 2003

Contents

20 Nephrology

25 The eye

26 Psychiatry and drug related problems

Contributors

P. Aaby Research Professor (Novo Nordisk Foundation), Bandim Health Project, Bissau, Guinea-Bissau.
7.10.6 Measles

J. P. Ackers Professor of Postgraduate Education in Public Health, London School of Hygiene and Tropical Medicine, UK.
7.13.13 Trichomoniasis

M. W. Adler Professor of Genitourinary Medicine, Department of Sexually Transmitted Diseases, Royal Free and University College Medical School, London, UK.
21.1 Epidemiology

D. Adu Consultant Nephrologist, Queen Elizabeth Hospital, Birmingham, UK.
20.7.4 Minimal-change nephropathy, focal segmental glomerulosclerosis, and membranous nephtopathy. 20.10.4 The kidney in rheumatological disorders

Graeme J. M. Alexander University Lecturer in Medicine and Honorary Consultant Physician/Hepatologist, University of Cambridge School of Clinical Medicine, Addenbrooke's Hospital, Cambridge, UK.
14.21.4 Liver transplantation

M. Allison Consultant Hepatologist, Hepatobiliary and Transplant Unit, Addenbrooke's Hospital, Cambridge, UK.
5.5 Innate immune system. 14.21.4 Liver transplantation

Chris Andrews Registrar in Anaesthesia, Mater Misericordiae Hospitals, South Brisbane, Queensland, Australia.
8.5.7 Lightning and electrical injuries

Philip Anslow Consultant Neuroradiologist, Radcliffe Infirmary, Oxford, UK.
24.5 Imaging in neurological diseases

Mark J. Arends Senior Lecturer and Honorary Consultant, Pathology Department, University of Cambridge, UK.
4.6 Apoptosis in health and disease

James O. Armitage Dean, College of Medicine, University of Nebraska Medical Center, Omaha, Nebraska, USA.
22.4.3 Lymphoma

J. K. Aronson Reader in Clinical Pharmacology, Radcliffe Infirmary, Oxford, UK.
15.5.1 Pharmacological management of heart failure

Frances M. Ashcroft Royal Society GlaxoSmithKline Research Professor, University Laboratory of Physiology, Oxford, UK.
4.5 Ion channels and disease

T. C. Aw Professor and Head of Division of Occupational Health, Kent Institute of Medicine and Health Sciences, University of Kent at Canterbury, UK.
8.4.1 Occupational and environmental health and safety. 8.5.10 Noise. 8.5.11 Vibration

M. Bagshaw Head of Occupational and Aviation Medicine, British Airways, Harmondsworth, UK.
8.5.5 Aerospace medicine

E. L. Baker Decatur, Georgia, UK.
8.4.1 Occupational and environmental health and safety

L. R. I. Baker Consultant Physician and Nephrologist, London Clinic, London, UK.
20.14 Urinary tract obstruction

C. R. M. Bangham Professor of Immunology, Imperial College Faculty of Medicine, London, UK.
7.10.23 HTLV-I and II and associated diseases

A. P. Banning Consultant Cardiologist, John Radcliffe Hospital, Oxford, UK.
15.3.3 Echocardiography. 15.14.1 Thoracic aortic dissection

D. J. P. Barker Director, MRC Environmental Epidemiology Unit, University of Southampton, UK.
15.4.1.1 Influences acting in utero and early childhood

Roger Barker University Lecturer and Honorary Consultant in Neurology, Department of Neurology, Addenbrooke's Hospital, Cambridge, UK.
24.13.11 Disorders of movement (excluding Parkinson's disease)

D. Barlow Consultant Physician, Department of Genitourinary Medicine, St Thomas's Hospital, London, UK.
7.11.6 Neisseria gonorrhoeae

M. P. Barnes Professor of Neurological Rehabilitation, Hunters Moor Regional Rehabilitation Centre, Newcastle upon Tyne, UK.
24.13.17 Spinal cord injury and its management

John G. Bartlett Chief, Division of Infectious Diseases, Johns Hopkins University School of Medicine, Baltimore, Maryland, USA.
17.5.2.1 Pneumonia—normal host. 17.5.2.2 Nosocomial pneumonia

Christopher Bass Consultant in Liaison Psychiatry, Department of Psychological Medicine, John Radcliffe Hospital, Oxford, UK.
26.5.3 Medically unexplained symptoms in patients attending medical clinics

M. F. Bassendine Professor of Hepatology, Centre for Liver Research, The Medical School, University of Newcastle upon Tyne, UK.
14.20.2.2 Primary biliary cirrhosis

David Bates Professor of Clinical Neurology, Department of Neurology, University of Newcastle upon Tyne, UK.
24.9 Brainstem syndromes. 24.13.1 The unconscious patient

Robert P. Baughman University of Cincinnati Medical Centre, Ohio, USA.
17.11.6 Sarcoidosis

Peter J. Baxter Consultant Physician, Occupational and Environmental Medicine, University of Cambridge, UK.
8.5.12 Disasters: earthquakes, volcanic eruptions, hurricanes, and floods

Peter H. Baylis Provost and Dean of Faculty of Medical Sciences, University of Newcastle upon Tyne, UK.
20.2.1 Water and sodium homeostasis and their disorders

D. Gareth Beevers Professor of Medicine, City Hospital, Birmingham, UK.
15.16.3 Hypertensive emergencies and urgencies

Michael L. Bennish Director, Africa Centre for Health and Population Studies, Mtubatuba, South Africa.
7.11.11 Cholera

M. K. Benson Consultant Physician, Oxford Centre for Respiratory Medicine, Churchill Hospital, Oxford, UK.
17.12 Pleural disease. 17.14.2 Pleural tumours. 17.14.3 Mediastinal tumours and cysts

V. Beral Head, Cancer Research UK Epidemiology Unit, Radcliffe Infirmary, Oxford, UK.
21.6 Cervical cancer and other cancers caused by sexually tramsmitted infections

Anthony R. Berendt Consultant Physician-in-Charge, Bone Infection Unit, Nuffield Orthopaedic Centre, Oxford, UK.
18.7.1 Pyogenic arthritis. 19.3 Osteomyelitis

Nancy Berliner Professor of Medicine and Genetics, Yale School of Medicine, New Haven, Connecticut, USA.
22.4.1 Leucocytes in health and disease. 22.4.2 Introduction to the lymphoproliferative disorders

Michael Besser Professor of Medicine Emeritus, Bart's and The London School of Medicine and Dentistry, Queen Mary College, London, UK.
12.2 Disorders of the anterior pituitary. 12.3 Disorders of the posterior pituitary

Delia B. Bethell Specialist Registrar in Paediatrics, Department of Paediatrics, John Radcliffe Hospital, Oxford, UK.
7.11.1 Diphtheria

Ernest Beutler Chairman, Department of Molecular and Experimental Medicine, The Scripps Research Institute, La Jolla, California, USA.
22.5.11 Erythrocyte enzymopathies

P. C. L. Beverley Professor and Scientific Head, Edward Jenner Institute for Vaccine Research, Compton, Berkshire, UK.
6.5 Tumour immunology

R. W. Bilous Professor of Clinical Medicine, James Cook University Hospital, Middlesbrough, Cleveland, UK.
20.10.1 Diabetes mellitus and the kidney

D. Bilton Consultant in Respiratory Medicine, Papworth Hospital, Cambridge, UK.
17.9 Bronchiectasis

A. E. Bishop Senior Lecturer, Tissue Engineering and Regenerative Medicine Centre, Chelsea and Westminster Hospital, London, UK.
14.8 Hormones and the gastrointestinal tract

Carol M. Black President of the Royal College of Physicians of London and Professor of Rheumatology, Royal Free and University College Medical School, Royal Free Campus, London, UK.
18.10.3 Systemic sclerosis

S. R. Bloom Professor of Medicine and Head, Division of Investigative Science, Imperial College Faculty of Medicine, Hammersmith Campus, London, UK.
12.10 Non-diabetic pancreatic endocrine disorders and multiple endocrine neoplasia. 14.8 Hormones and the gastrointestinal tract

L. D. Blumhardt Emeritus Professor of Clinical Neurology, University of Nottingham, UK.
24.13.5 Syncope. 24.13.16 Diseases of the spinal cord

N. Boon Consultant Cardiologist, Royal Infirmary of Edinburgh, UK.
15.10.4 Cardiac disease in HIV infection

D. R. Booth Senior Hospital Scientist, Institute for Immunology and Allergy Research, Westmead Millennium Institute, Sydney, New South Wales, Australia.
11.12.3 Familial Mediterranean fever and other inherited periodic fever syndromes

Richard T. Booth Professor, Health and Safety Unit, Aston University, Birmingham, UK.
8.4.2 Occupational safety

Leszek K. Borysiewicz Professor and Principal of the Faculty of Medicine, University of Wales, Cardiff, UK.
7.4 The host response to infection

I. C. J. W. Bowler Consultant Microbiologist, Department of Microbiology, John Radcliffe Hospital, Oxford, UK.
7.9 Nosocomial infections

D. J. Bradley Ross Professor of Tropical Hygiene, London School of Hygiene and Tropical Medicine, UK.
7.13.2 Malaria

Thomas Brandt Klinikum Groshadern, Munich, Germany.
24.12.1 Eye movements and balance

P. Brandtzaeg Professor of Paediatrics, Ullevål University Hospital, University of Oslo, Norway.
7.11.5 Meningococcal infections

P. Brasseur Professor and Head of Department of Parasitology, Faculty of Medicine, Rouen, France.
7.13.3 Babesia

J. Braun Professor and Medical Director, Rheumazentrum Ruhrgebiet, Herne, Germany.
18.6 Spondyloarthritides and related arthritides

Sydney Brenner Research Professor, Salk Institute, La Jolla, California, USA, and Honorary Professor of Genetic Medicine, University of Cambridge, UK.
4.2 The human genome sequence

D. P. Brenton Sub Dean (Curriculum), Royal Free and University College Medical School, London, UK.
11.2 Inborn errors of amino acid and organic acid metabolism

Paul H. Brion Rheumatologist in Private Practice, Vista, California, USA.
18.8 Osteoarthritis

Julian Britton Consultant Surgeon, John Radcliffe Hospital, Oxford, UK.
14.3.1 The acute abdomen. 14.18.3.3 Tumours of the pancreas

Anthony F. T. Brown Associate Professor and Senior Staff Specialist, Department of Emergency Medicine, Royal Brisbane Hospital, Queensland, Australia.
16.4 Anaphylaxis

M. J. Brown Professor of Clinical Pharmacology, University of Cambridge and Honorary Consultant Physician, Addenbrooke's Hospital NHS Trust, Cambridge, UK.
15.16.2.3 Primary hyperaldosteronism (Conn's syndrome). 15.16.2.4 Phaeochromocytoma

A. D. M. Bryceson Emeritus Professor of Tropical Medicine, London School of Hygiene and Tropical Medicine, UK.
7.13.12 Leishmaniasis

Philip J. Burke Johns Hopkins Oncology Center, Baltimore, Maryland, USA.
22.3.3 Acute lymphoblastic leukaemia. 22.3.4 Acute myeloblastic leukaemia

G. M. Burnham Associate Professor of International Health, Johns Hopkins Bloomberg School of Public Health, Baltimore, Maryland, USA.
7.14.1 Cutaneous filariasis

Jacky Burrin Professor of Experimental Endocrinology, Bart's and The London School of Medicine and Dentistry, St Bartholomew's Hospital, London, UK.
12.1 Principles of hormone action

Andy Bush Reader in Paediatric Respirology, London, UK.
17.10 Cystic fibrosis

K. Bushby Professor of Neuromuscular Genetics, Institute of Human Genetics, Newcastle upon Tyne, UK.
24.22.2 Muscular dystrophy

Anthony Busuttil Regius Professor of Forensic Medicine, Forensic Medicine Section, Edinburgh University Medical School, UK.
27 Forensic medicine and the practising doctor

T. Butler Professor of Internal Medicine and Chief of Infectious Diseases, Texas Technical University Health Sciences Center, Lubbock, Texas, USA.
7.11.16 Plague

W. F. Bynum Professor of History of Medicine, Wellcome Trust Centre for the History of Medicine at University College London, UK.
2.1 Science in medicine: when, how, and what

I. Byren Consultant in Infectious Diseases and Genito-Urinary Medicine, John Radcliffe Hospital, Oxford, UK.
15.10.3 Cardiovascular syphilis

John Calam* Professor of Medicine, Imperial College London, UK.
14.7 Peptic ulcer diseases

Donald B. Calne Professor Emeritus, University of British Columbia, Vancouver, Canada.
24.13.10 Parkinsonism and other extrapyramidal diseases

P. M. A. Calverley Professor of Medicine (Pulmonary and Rehabilitation), Clinical Science Centre, University Hospital Aintree, Liverpool, UK.
17.7 Chronic respiratory failure

Giovambattista Capasso Professor of Nephrology, Second University of Naples, Italy.
20.13 Urinary stones, nephrocalcinosis, and renal tubular acidosis

* It is with regret that we report the death of Professor John Calam during the preparation of this edition of the textbook.

Jonathan R. Carapetis Senior Lecturer, Research Fellow, and Consultant in Infectious Diseases, Centre for International Child Health, University of Melbourne Department of Paediatrics, Royal Children's Hospital, Melbourne, Australia.
15.10.1 Acute rheumatic fever

Simon Carette Head, Division of Rheumatology, Toronto Western Hospital, Ontario, Canada.
18.4 Back pain and regional disorders

D. J. S. Carmichael Consultant Renal Physician, Southend Hospital, Westcliffe-on-Sea, Essex, UK.
20.16 Drugs and the kidney

D. P. Casemore Senior Research Fellow, CREH, University of Wales, St Asaph, Denbighshire, UK.
7.13.5 Cryptosporidium and cryptosporidiosis. 7.13.6 Cyclospora

D. Catovsky Professor of Haematology, Royal Marsden Hospital and Institute of Cancer Research, London, UK.
22.3.2 The classification of leukaemia. 22.3.5 Chronic lymphocytic leukaemia and other leukaemias of mature B and T cells

Bruce A. Chabner Professor of Medicine, Harvard Medical School and Massachusetts General Hospital, Boston, USA.
6.7 Cancer chemotherapy and radiation therapy

Richard E. Chaisson Professor of Medicine, Epidemiology and International Health, Johns Hopkins University Schools of Medicine and Public Health, Baltimore, Maryland, USA.
7.11.22 Tuberculosis

R. W. Chapman Consultant Gastroenterologist/Hepatologist, John Radcliffe Hospital, Oxford, UK.
14.20.2.3 Primary sclerosing cholangitis

V. Krishna K. Chatterjee Professor of Endocrinology, University of Cambridge, Addenbrooke's Hospital, Cambridge, UK.
12.1 Principles of hormone action

Dominique Chauveau Consultant Nephrologist, Department of Nephrology, Hôpital Necker, Paris, France.
20.9.1 Acute interstitial nephritis

P. F. Chinnery Senior Lecturer in Neurogenetics and Honorary Consultant Neurologist, University of Newcastle upon Tyne and Newcastle upon Tyne Hospitals NHS Trust, UK.
24.22.5 Mitochondrial encephalomyopathies

Seung-Yull Cho Professor, Section of Molecular Parasitology, Sungkyunkwan University School of Medicine, Suwon, Korea.
7.15.4 Pseudophyllidean tapeworms: diphyllobothriasis and sparganosis

Kirpal S. Chugh Professor Emeritus, Department of Nephrology, Postgraduate Institute of Medical Education and Research, Chandigarh, India.
20.7.10 Glomerular disease in the tropics

L. Chwastiak Acting Assistant Professor, Department of Psychiatry, University of Washington, Seattle, USA.
26.5.4 Anxiety and depression

C. M. Clothier Queen's Counsel (retired), London, UK.
1 On being a patient

Andrew J. S. Coats Viscount Royston Professor of Cardiology, Imperial College London and Honorary Consultant Cardiologist, Royal Brompton Hospital, London, UK.
15.2.2 The syndrome of heart failure. 15.5.3 Cardiac rehabilitation

S. M. Cobbe Walton Professor of Medical Cardiology, University of Glasgow, Glasgow Royal Infirmary, UK.
15.2.3 Syncope and palpitation. 15.6 Cardiac arrhythmias

B. J. Cohen Clinical Scientist, Central Public Health Laboratory, London, UK.
7.10.18 Parvovirus B19

J. Cohen Dean and Professor of Infectious Diseases, Brighton and Sussex Medical School, UK.
7.20 Infection in the immunocompromised host

R. D. Cohen Emeritus Professor of Medicine, Bart's and The London School of Medicine and Dentistry, Queen Mary College, University of London, UK.
11.11 Disturbances of acid-base homeostasis

Francis S. Collins Director, National Human Genome Research Institute, Bethesda, Maryland, USA.
4.1 The genomic basis of medicine

R. Collins British Heart Foundation Professor of Medicine and Epidemiology, Clinical Trial Service Unit and Epidemiological Studies Unit, University of Oxford, UK.
2.4.3 Large-scale randomized evidence: trials and overviews

Alastair Compston Professor of Neurology, University of Cambridge, UK.
24.1 Introduction and approach to the patient with neurological disease.
24.16 Demyelinating disorders of the central nervous system

Juliet Compston Reader in Metabolic Bone Diseases and Honorary Consultant Physician, Addenbrooke's Hospital, Cambridge, UK.
19.4 Osteoporosis

C. P. Conlon Consultant Physician in Infectious Diseases, Nuffield Department of Medicine, John Radcliffe Hospital, Oxford, UK.
7.8 Travel and expedition medicine. 7.10.21 HIV and AIDS

Andrew Coop Duke University Medical Center, Durham, North Carolina, USA.
6.2 The nature and development of cancer. 6.3 The genetics of inherited cancers

M. R. Cooper Freelance Science Writer, CAB International, Wallingford, Oxfordshire, UK.
8.3 Poisonous plants and fungi

Susan Copley Consultant Radiologist, Hammersmith Hospital, London, UK.
17.3.1 Thoracic imaging

Fernando F. Costa Professor of Haematology, School of Medical Sciences, Unicamp, Campinas, Brazil.
22.5.10 Disorders of the red cell membrane

J. Couvreur Professeur Associé, Laboratoire de la Toxoplasmose, Institut de Puericulture, Paris, France.
7.13.4 Toxoplasmosis

P. J. Cowen Professor of Psychopharmacology, Warneford Hospital, Oxford, UK.
26.6.1 Psychopharmacology in medical practice

T. M. Cox Professor of Medicine, University of Cambridge, and Honorary Consultant Physician, Addenbrooke's Hospital, Cambridge, UK.
11.3.1 Glycogen storage diseases. 11.3.2 Inborn errors of fructose metabolism. 11.3.3 Disorders of galactose, pentose, and pyruvate metabolism. 11.5 The porphyrias. 11.7.1 Hereditary haemochromatosis. 11.8 Lysosomal storage diseases. 12.13 The pineal gland and melatonin. 14.9.5 Disaccharidase deficiency. 22.5.4 Iron metabolism and its disorders. 33 Emergency medicine

Dorothy H. Crawford Professor of Medical Microbiology, Centre for Infectious Diseases, University of Edinburgh, UK.
7.10.3 The Epstein–Barr virus

Robin A. F. Crawford Consultant Gynaecological Oncologist, Addenbrooke's Hospital, Cambridge, UK.
13.17 Malignant disease in pregnancy

A. J. Crisp Consultant Rheumatologist, Addenbrooke's Hospital, Cambridge, UK.
19.5 Avascular necrosis and related topics

D. W. M. Crook Consultant Microbiologist/Infectious Diseases, John Radcliffe Hospital, Oxford, UK.
24.14.1 Bacterial meningitis

J. Cunningham Professor of Renal and Metabolic Medicine, The Royal London Hospital and Queen Mary's School of Medicine and Dentistry, London, UK.
20.8 Renal tubular disorders

Patrick C. D'Haese Associate Professor, Department of Nephrology and Hypertension, University of Antwerp, Belgium.
20.9.2 Chronic tubulointerstitial nephritis

Tim Dalgleish Research Scientist, MRC Cognitions and Brain Sciences Unit, Cambridge, UK.
26.5.1 Grief, stress, and post-traumatic stress disorder

D. A. B. Dance Director/Consultant Microbiologist, Public Health Laboratory, Derriford Hospital, Plymouth, UK.
7.11.15 Melioidosis and glanders

Chi V. Dang Professor of Medicine and Chief, Hematology Division, Johns Hopkins University School of Medicine, Baltimore, Maryland, USA.
22.3.7 Myelodysplasia

C. J. Danpure Professor of Molecular Cell Biology, Department of Biology, University College London, UK.
11.10 Disorders of oxalate metabolism

John H. Dark Professor of Cardiothoracic Surgery, Freeman Hospital, Newcastle upon Tyne, UK.
15.5.4 Cardiac transplantation and mechanical circulatory support

A. Davenport Consultant Renal Physician/Honorary Senior Lecturer, Centre for Nephrology, Royal Free Hospital, London, UK.
20.3.2 Clinical investigation of renal disease

G. Davey Smith Professor of Clinical Epidemiology, University of Bristol, UK.
15.4.1.2 The epidemiology of ischaemic heart disease

Alun Davies Reader and Honorary Consultant Surgeon, Department of Vascular Surgery, Faculty of Medicine, Imperial College School of Medicine, Charing Cross Hospital, London, UK.
15.14.2 Peripheral arterial disease

P. D. O. Davies Consultant Physician, Fazakerley Hospital, Liverpool, UK.
7.11.23 Disease caused by environmental mycobacteria

Alex M. Davison Professor and Consultant Renal Physician, St James's University Hospital, Leeds, UK.
20.3.1 The clinical presentation of renal disease

Marc E. De Broe Professor in Medicine, Department of Nephrology, University of Antwerp, Belgium.
20.9.2 Chronic tubulointerstitial nephritis

P. de la Motte Hall Professor, Division of Anatomical Pathology, Faculty of Health Sciences, University of Cape Town, South Africa.
14.21.6 Hepatic granulomas

M. de Swiet Professor of Obstetric Medicine, Queen Charlotte's and Chelsea Hospital, London, UK.
13.7 Thromboembolism in pregnancy. 13.8 Chest diseases in pregnancy

Barbara A. Degar Yale School of Medicine, New Haven, Connecticut, USA.
22.4.2 Introduction to the lymphoproliferative disorders

Eric Demoncheaux Research Associate, Medical School, University of Sheffield, UK.
15.15.1 The pulmonary circulation and its influence on gas exchange

D. M. Denison Emeritus Professor of Clinical Physiology, Royal Brompton Hospital, London, UK.
8.5.5 Aerospace medicine. 8.5.6 Diving medicine

John Dent Director, Department of Gastroenterology, Hepatology and General Medicine and Clinical Professor of Medicine, Royal Adelaide Hospital/Adelaide University, Australia.
14.6 Diseases of the oesophagus

Christopher P. Denton Senior Lecturer/Consultant Rheumatologist, Centre for Rheumatology, Royal Free Hospital, London, UK.
18.10.3 Systemic sclerosis

Ulrich Desselberger Consultant Virologist and Director, Clinical Microbiology and Public Health Laboratory, Addenbrooke's Hospital, Cambridge, UK.
7.10.7 Enterovirus infections. 7.10.8 Virus infections causing diarrhoea and vomiting

Charles A. Dinarello Professor of Medicine, University of Colorado, Denver, Colorado, USA.
4.4 Cytokines: interleukin-1 and tumour necrosis factor in inflammation

A. K. Dixon Professor of Radiology and Honorary Consultant Radiologist, University of Cambridge and Addenbrooke's Hospital, Cambridge, UK.
14.18.2 Computed tomography and magnetic resonance imaging of the liver and pancreas

Michael Doherty Professor of Rheumatology, University of Nottingham Medical School, UK.
18.3 Clinical investigation. 18.9 Crystal-related arthropathies

R. Doll Emeritus Professor of Medicine and Honorary Member, Cancer Studies Unit, Nuffield Department of Medicine, Radcliffe Infirmary, Oxford, UK.
6.1 Epidemiology of cancer

Michael Donaghy Reader in Clinical Neurology, University of Oxford, Honorary Consultant Neurologist, Radcliffe Infirmary, and Honorary Civilian Consultant in Neurology to the Army, Oxford, UK.
24.13.13 The motor neurone diseases

Dominique Droz Unite de Pathologie Renale, Hôpital Necker, Paris, France.
20.9.1 Acute interstitial nephritis

R. M. du Bois Professor of Respiratory Medicine, National Heart and Lung Institute, University College London and Consultant Physician, Royal Brompton Hospital, London, UK.
17.11.1 Diffuse parenchymal lung disease: an introduction. 17.11.2 Cryptogenic fibrosing alveolitis. 17.11.3 Bronchiolitis obliterans and organizing pneumonia. 17.11.4 The lungs and rheumatological diseases. 17.11.5 The lung in vasculitis

C. R. K. Dudley Consultant Renal Physician, The Richard Bright Renal Unit Southmead Hospital, North Bristol NHS Trust, Bristol, UK.
15.14.3 Cholesterol embolism

D. W. Dunne Reader in Immunoparasitology, Department of Pathology, University of Cambridge, UK.
7.16.1 Schistosomiasis

David T. Durack Consulting Professor of Medicine, Duke University, Durham, North Carolina and Vice-President, Corporate Medical Affairs, Becton Dickinson & Co., Franklin Lakes, New Jersey, USA.
7.2 Fever of unknown origin

S. R. Durham Professor of Allergy and Respiratory Medicine, Imperial College Faculty of Medicine, National Heart and Lung Hospital, and Royal Brompton Hospital, London, UK.
17.4.2 Allergic rhinitis ('hay fever')

P. N. Durrington Professor of Medicine, University of Manchester Department of Medicine, Manchester Royal Infirmary, UK.
11.6 Lipid and lipoprotein disorders

M. Eastwood Post-Retirement Honorary Fellow, Department of Medical Sciences, Western General Hospital, Edinburgh, UK.
10.3 Vitamins and trace elements

Jonathan C. W. Edwards Professor in Connective Tissue Medicine, University College London, UK.
18.1 Joints and connective tissue: introduction

Richard Edwards Emeritus Professor of Medicine, University of Liverpool, UK.
24.22.4 Metabolic and endocrine disorders

M. Elia Professor of Clinical Nutrition and Metabolism, Institute of Human Nutrition, University of Southampton, UK.
10.6 Special nutritional problems and the use of enteral and parenteral nutrition

Matthew J. Ellis Associate Professor of Medicine and Director, Breast Cancer Program, Duke University Medical Center, Durham, North Carolina, USA.
6.2 The nature and development of cancer. 6.3 The genetics of inherited cancers

Monique M. Elseviers Department of Nephrology-Hypertension, University Hospital Antwerp, Belgium.
20.9.2 Chronic tubulointerstitial nephritis

M. A. Epstein Emeritus Professor of Pathology, University of Bristol, UK.
7.10.3 The Epstein–Barr virus

E. Ernst Professor and Director, Department of Complementary Medicine, University of Exeter, UK.
2.5 Complementary and alternative medicine

David Eschenbach Professor, Department of Obstetrics and Gynecology, University of Washington, Seattle, USA.
21.4 Pelvic inflammatory disease

S. M. Evans Specialist Registrar in Gastroenterology, Royal Sussex County Hospital, Brighton, UK.
8.5.8 Podoconiosis

S. J. Eykyn Professor (and Honorary Consultant) in Clinical Microbiology, St Thomas' Hospital, London, UK.
7.11.2 Streptococci and enterococci. 7.11.4 Staphylococci. 7.11.10 Anaerobic bacteria. 15.10.2 Infective endocarditis

C. A. Eynon Director of Neurosciences Intensive Care, Southampton University Hospital NHS Trust, UK.
16.3 Cardiac arrest. 33 Emergency medicine

Christopher G. Fairburn Wellcome Principal Research Fellow and Professor of Psychiatry, Oxford University Department of Psychiatry, Warneford Hospital, Oxford, UK.
26.5.5 Eating disorders

CONTRIBUTORS

J. J. Farrar Senior Fellow, Wellcome Trust, University of Oxford Clinical Research Unit, The Hospital for Tropical Diseases, Ho Chi Minh, Vietnam.
24.14.1 Bacterial meningitis. 24.14.2 Viral infections of the central nervous system

Ken Farrington Consultant Nephrologist, Lister Hospital, Stevenage, Hertfordshire, UK.
20.6.1 Haemodialysis

D. T. Fearon Wellcome Trust Professor of Medicine, University of Cambridge, UK.
5.5 Innate immune system

John Feehally Professor of Renal Medicine, Leicester General Hospital, UK.
20.7.2 IgA nephropathy and Henoch-Schönlein purpura. 20.7.3 Thin membrane nephropathy

Alvan R. Feinstein* Professor, Yale University School of Medicine, New Haven, Connecticut, USA.
2.4.2 Evidence-based medicine

Eleanor Feldman Consultant Liaison Psychiatrist and Honorary Senior Lecturer, University of Oxford, John Radcliffe Hospital, Oxford, UK.
26.2 Taking a psychiatric history from a medical patient. 26.4 Acute behavioural emergencies

Peter J. Fenner Associate Professor, Schools of Medicine and Health Sciences, James Cook University and National Medical Officer, Surf Life Saving Association of Australia, Mackay, North Queensland, Australia.
8.5.3 Drowning

Robert Ferrari Clinical Assistant Professor, University of Alberta Hospital, Edmonton, Canada.
18.2 Clinical presentation and diagnosis of rheumatic disease

C. ffrench-Constant Professor of Neurological Genetics, University of Cambridge, UK.
24.21 Developmental abnormalities of the central nervous system

R. G. Finch Professor of Infectious Diseases, City Hospital and University of Nottingham, UK.
7.6 Antimicrobial chemotherapy

H. Firth Consultant in Medical Genetics, Department of Medical Genetics, Addenbrooke's Hospital, Cambridge, UK.
24.21 Developmental abnormalities of the central nervous system

J. Firth Consultant Physician and Nephrologist, Addenbrooke's Hospital, Cambridge, UK.
13.5 Renal disease in pregnancy. 15.15.2.2 Pulmonary oedema. 15.15.3.1 Deep venous thrombosis and pulmonary embolism. 15.18 Idiopathic oedema of women. 16.1 The clinical approach to the patient who is very ill. 20.2.2 Disorders of potassium homeostasis. 20.4 Acute renal failure. 33 Emergency medicine

Susan Fisher-Hoch Professor, University of Texas School of Public Health at Brownsville, USA.
7.10.15 Arenaviruses. 7.10.16 Filoviruses

Robert A. Fishman Professor of Neurology Emeritus, University of California San Francisco School of Medicine, USA.
24.7 Lumbar puncture

Edward D. Folland Associate Director of Cardiology and Professor of Medicine, UMass Memorial Medical Center/University of Massachusetts Medical School, Worcester, Maryland, USA.
15.3.6 Cardiac catheterization and angiography. 15.4.2.4 Percutaneous interventional cardiac procedures

J. C. Forfar Consultant Cardiologist, John Radcliffe Hospital, Oxford and Honorary Senior Lecturer, University of Oxford, UK.
13.6 Heart disease in pregnancy

I. S. Foulds Consultant Dermatologist, City Hospital, Birmingham, UK.
8.4.1 Occupational and environmental health and safety

Keith A. A. Fox Professor of Cardiology, Royal Infirmary and University of Edinburgh, UK.
15.4.2.3 Management of acute coronary syndromes: unstable angina and myocardial infarction

Richard Frackowiak Vice Provost (Biomedicine), University College London, Institute of Neurology, London, UK.
24.3 Brain and mind: functional neuroimaging

T. J. R. Francis Consultant in Diving Medicine, Tintagel, Cornwall, UK.
8.5.6 Diving medicine

Keith N. Frayn Professor of Human Metabolism, Oxford Centre for Diabetes, Endocrinology and Metabolism, University of Oxford, UK.
10.2 Nutrition: biochemical background

Alan Freeman Consultant Radiologist, Addenbrooke's Hospital, Cambridge, UK.
14.2.3 Radiology of the gastrointestinal tract

Peggy Frith Consultant Ophthalmic Physician, The Eye Hospital, Radcliffe Infirmary, Oxford and University College London Hospital, UK.
25 The eye in general medicine

Patrick G. Gallagher Associate Professor, Department of Pediatrics, Yale University School of Medicine, New Haven, Connecticut, USA.
22.5.10 Disorders of the red cell membrane

Clare J. Galton Specialist Registrar in Neurology, Neurology Department, Addenbrooke's Hospital, Cambridge, UK.
24.13.8 Alzheimer's disease and other dementias

Hector H. Garcia Associate Professor, Department of Microbiology, Universidad Peruana Cayetano Heredia and Head, Cysticercosis Unit, Department of Transmissible Diseases, Instituto de Ciencias Neurologicas, Lima, Peru.
7.15.1 Cystic hydatid disease (Echinococcus granulosus). 7.15.3 Cysticercosis

K. Gardiner Professor and Managing Director, International Occupational Health Ltd., Birmingham, UK.
8.4.1 Occupational and environmental health and safety

Lawrence B. Gardner Assistant Professor of Medicine, Johns Hopkins University school of Medicine, Baltimore, Maryland, USA.
22.3.7 Myelodysplasia

Christopher S. Garrard Consultant Physician in Intensive Care, John Radcliffe Hospital, Oxford, UK.
16.5.2 The management of respiratory failure

J. S. H. Gaston Professor of Rheumatology, University of Cambridge School of Medicine, Addenbrooke's Hospital, Cambridge, UK.
18.7.2 Reactive arthritis

Duncan Geddes Professor of Respiratory Medicine, Royal Brompton Hospital, London, UK.
17.10 Cystic fibrosis

D. G. Gibson Consultant Cardiologist, Royal Brompton Hospital, London, UK.
15.7 Valve disease. 15.9 Pericardial disease

G. J. Gibson Professor of Respiratory Medicine/Consultant Physician, Freeman Hospital, Newcastle upon Tyne, UK.
17.3.2 Respiratory function tests

A. M. Giles Scientific Officer, Health Systems, Oxford, UK.
32 Reference intervals for biochemical data

I. P. Giles ARC Research Fellow, Bloomsbury Rheumatology Unit, London, UK.
18.10.1 Autoimmune rheumatic disorders and vasculitis

Charles F. Gilks Professor of Tropical Medicine and Senior Adviser on Care, HIV/AIDS Department, World Health Organization, Geneva, Switzerland.
7.10.22 HIV in the developing world

Michael D. J. Gillmer Consultant Obstetrician and Gynaecologist, Women's Centre, John Radcliffe Hospital, Oxford, UK.
13.10 Diabetes in pregnancy

Robert H. Gilman Professor, Department of International Health, Johns Hopkins School of Public Health, Baltimore, Maryland, USA and Research Professor, Universidad Peruana Cayetano Heredia, Lima, Peru.
7.15.3 Cysticercosis

A. E. S. Gimson Consultant Physician and Hepatologist, Cambridge Liver Transplantation Unit, Addenbrooke's Hospital, Cambridge, UK.
13.9 Liver and gastrointestinal diseases during pregnancy. 14.18.1 The structure and function of the liver, biliary tract, and pancreas

P. Glasziou Huntington Centre for Risk Analysis, Boston, Massachusetts, USA.
2.4.1 Bringing the best evidence to the point of care

* It is with regret that we report the death of Professor Alvan R. Feinstein during the preparation of this edition of the textbook.

Peter J. Goadsby Professor of Clinical Neurology, Institute of Neurology, University College and The National Hospital for Neurology and Neurosurgery, London, UK.
24.13.2 Headache

D. Goldblatt Reader in Immunology and Consultant Paediatric Immunologist, Institute of Child Health, Great Ormond Hospital for Children NHS Trust, London, UK.
7.7 Immunization

John M. Goldman Professor of Leukaemia Biology and Chairman, Department of Haematology, Imperial College School of Medicine, London, UK.
22.3.6 Chronic myeloid leukaemia

Irwin Goldstein Director, Institute for Sexual Medicine and Professor of Urology and Gynecology, Boston University School of Medicine, Massachusetts, USA.
12.8.4 Sexual dysfunction

Armando E. Gonzalez Department of Public Health, School of Veterinary Medicine, Universidad Nacional Mayor de San Marcos, Lima, Peru.
7.15.1 Cystic hydatid disease (Echinococcus granulosus)

Timothy H. J. Goodship Reader in Nephrology, University of Newcastle upon Tyne and Consultant Nephrologist, Royal Victoria Infirmary, Newcastle upon Tyne, UK.
20.10.6 Haemolytic uraemic syndrome

Sherwood L. Gorbach Department of Community Health and Medicine, TUFTS University School of Medicine, Boston, Massachusetts, USA.
14.17 Gastrointestinal infections

E. C. Gordon-Smith Professor of Haematology, St George's Hospital Medical School, London, UK.
22.3.11 Aplastic anaemia and other causes of bone marrow failure. 22.8.2 Haemopoietic stem cell transplantation

J. M. Grange Visiting Professor, University College London, Centre for Infectious Diseases and International Health, Royal Free and University College Medical School, London, UK.
7.11.23 Disease caused by environmental mycobacteria

R. Gray Professor of Medical Statistics and Director, University of Birmingham Clinical Trials Unit, UK.
2.4.3 Large-scale randomized evidence: trials and overviews

John R. Graybill Professor, University of Texas Health Science Center, San Antonio, Texas, USA.
7.12.3 Coccidioidomycosis

Jackie Green Director, Centre for Health Promotion Research, Leeds Metropolitan University, Leeds, UK.
3.5 Health promotion

Brian M. Greenwood Professor of Clinical Tropical Medicine, London School of Hygiene and Tropical Medicine, London, UK.
7.11.3 Pneumococcal diseases

Roger Greenwood Consultant Nephrologist and Lead Clinician, Lister Hospital, Stevenage, Hertfordshire, UK.
20.6.1 Haemodialysis

B. Gribbin Honorary Consultant Cardiologist, John Radcliffe Hospital, Oxford, UK.
15.10.3 Cardiovascular syphilis. 15.14.1 Thoracic aortic dissection

John Grimley Evans Professor Emeritus of Clinical Geratology, Green College, Oxford, UK.
30.1 Medicine in old age

Michael L. Grossbard Chief, Hematology/Oncology, St Luke's-Roosevelt Hospital and Beth Israel Medical Center, New York, USA.
6.7 Cancer chemotherapy and radiation therapy

David I. Grove Professor and Director, Clinical Microbiology and Infectious Diseases, The Queen Elizabeth Hospital, Adelaide, Australia.
7.14.5 Nematode infections of lesser importance. 7.16.2 Liver fluke infections. 7.16.4 Intestinal trematode infections

J. P. Grünfeld Professor of Nephrology, Université Paris V - René Descartes and Head of Nephrology, Hôpital Necker, Paris, France.
20.11 Renal involvement in genetic disease

D. J. Gubler Director, Division of Vector-Borne Infectious Diseases, Centers for Disease Control and Prevention, Fort Collins, Colorado, USA.
7.10.11 Alphaviruses. 7.10.13 Flaviviruses

Mark Gurnell Specialist Registrar and Research Fellow, Department of Medicine, Division of Endocrinology and Metabolism, Addenbrooke's Hospital, Cambridge, UK.
12.1 Principles of hormone action

David M. Gustin Section of Hematology–Oncology, University of Chicago, Illinois, USA.
22.3.8 The polycythaemias. 22.3.10 Thrombocytosis

M. R. Haeney Consultant Immunologist, Salford Royal Hospitals NHS Trust, Salford, Manchester, UK.
14.4 Immune disorders of the gastrointestinal tract

Davidson H. Hamer Director, Traveler's Health Service, Tufts-New England Medical Center and Assistant Professor of Medicine and Nutrition, Tufts University, Boston, Massachusetts, USA.
14.17 Gastrointestinal infections

P. J. Hammond Consultant Physician and Endocrinologist, Harrogate District Hospital, Yorkshire, UK.
12.10 Non-diabetic pancreatic endocrine disorders and multiple endocrine neoplasia. 14.8 Hormones and the gastrointestinal tract

J. R. Hampton Professor of Cardiology, Queen's Medical Centre, Nottingham, UK.
15.2.1 Chest pain. 15.2.4 Physical examination of the cardiovascular system

M. Hanna Consultant Neurologist and Reader in Clinical Neurology, National Hospital for Neurology and Neurosurgery and Institute of Neurology, University College London, UK.
24.22.1 Introduction: structure and function

David M. Hansell Professor of Thoracic Imaging, Royal Brompton Hospital, London, UK.
17.3.1 Thoracic imaging

P. Harnden Consultant Urological Pathologist, Cancer Research UK Clinical Centre, St James's University Hospital, Leeds, UK.
20.15 Tumours of the urinary tract

J. M. Harrington Emeritus Professor of Occupational Health, University of Birmingham, UK.
8.4.1 Occupational and environmental health and safety

Anthony Harrison Fellow in Health Systems, King's Fund, London, UK.
3.3 The pattern of care: hospital and community

J. R. Harrison Force Medical Adviser, Sussex Police Authority, Lewes, UK.
8.5.9 Radiation

C. Haslett Professor of Respiratory Medicine, Royal Infirmary, Edinburgh, UK.
16.5.1 Pathophysiology and pathogenesis of acute respiratory distress syndrome. 17.1.3 'First line' defence mechanisms of the lung

Adrian R. W. Hatfield Consultant Gastroenterologist, The Middlesex Hospital, London, UK.
14.2.2 Upper gastrointestinal endoscopy

P. N. Hawkins Professor of Medicine, Royal Free and University College Medical School, London, UK.
11.12.3 Familial Mediterranean fever and other inherited periodic fever syndromes. 11.12.4 Amyloidosis

Keith Hawton Professor of Psychiatry, University Department of Psychiatry and Director and Consultant Psychiatrist, Centre for Suicide Research, Warneford Hospital, Oxford, UK.
26.5.2 The patient who has attempted suicide

R. J. Hay Professor and Dean, Faculty of Medicine and Health Sciences, Queens University, Belfast, UK.
7.11.27 Nocardiosis. 7.12.1 Fungal infections

B. Hazleman Consultant Rheumatologist, Rheumatology Department, Addenbrooke's Hospital, Cambridge, UK.
18.11 Miscellaneous conditions presenting to the rheumatologist

Nick Heather Consultant Clinical Psychologist and Director, Centre for Alcohol and Drug Studies, Newcastle, North Tyneside, and Northumberland Mental Health NHS Trust, Newcastle upon Tyne, UK.
26.7.2 Brief interventions against excessive alcohol consumption

David B. Hellmann Professor, Johns Hopkins University School of Medicine, Baltimore, Maryland, USA.
18.10.7 Polymyositis and dermatomyositis

D. J. Hendrick Consultant Physician and Professor of Occupational Respiratory Medicine, Royal Victoria Infirmary, University of Newcastle upon Tyne, UK.
17.11.8 Pulmonary haemorrhagic disorders. 17.11.9 Eosinophilic pneumonia. 17.11.10 Lymphocytic infiltrations of the lung. 17.11.11 Extrinsic allergic alveolitis. 17.11.12 Eosinophilic granuloma of the lung and pulmonary lymphangiomyomatosis. 17.11.13 Pulmonary alveolar proteinosis. 17.11.14 Pulmonary amyloidosis. 17.11.15 Lipoid (lipid) pneumonia. 17.11.16 Pulmonary alveolar microlithiasis. 17.11.17 Toxic gases and fumes. 17.11.18 Radiation pneumonitis. 17.11.19 Drug-induced lung disease

Mark Herbert Clinical Lecturer in Neonatal Paediatrics, Department of Paediatrics, University of Oxford, UK.
13.15 Infections in pregnancy

Andrew Herxheimer Emeritus Fellow, UK Cochrane Centre, London, UK.
9 Principles of clinical pharmacology and drug therapy

Martin F. Heyworth Chief of Staff and Clinical Professor of Medicine, VA Medical Center and University of Pennsylvania, Philadelphia, USA.
7.13.8 Giardiasis, balantidiasis, isosporiasis, and microsporidiosis

Tim Higenbottam Global Clinical Expert, Astra-Zeneca, Charnwood, Leicestershire and Visiting Professor of Medicine, University of Sheffield, UK.
15.15.1 The pulmonary circulation and its influence on gas exchange. 15.15.2.1 Primary pulmonary hypertension

Katherine A. High William H. Bennett Professor of Pediatrics, University of Pennsylvania School of Medicine and The Children's Hospital of Philadelphia, Pennsylvania, USA.
22.6.4 Genetic disorders of coagulation

S. L. Hillier Research Associate Professor of Obstetrics and Gynecology, University of Washington, Seattle, USA.
21.3 Vaginal discharge

David Hilton-Jones Clinical Director, Oxford MDC Muscle and Nerve Centre, Radcliffe Infirmary, Oxford, UK.
24.17 Disorders of the neuromuscular junction. 24.22.3 Myotonia. 24.22.4 Metabolic and endocrine disorders

John R. Hodges Professor of Behavioural Neurology, MRC Cognition and Brain Sciences Unit and Department of Neurology, Addenbrooke's Hospital, Cambridge, UK.
24.8 Disturbances of higher cerebral function. 24.13.8 Alzheimer's disease and other dementias

H. J. F. Hodgson Sheila Sherlock Professor of Medicine and Director, Centre for Hepatology, Royal Free and University College Medical School, London, UK.
14.9.6 Whipple's disease. 14.20.1 Viral hepatitis—clinical aspects. 14.20.2.1 Autoimmune hepatitis

A. V. Hoffbrand Emeritus Professor of Haematology, Royal Free and University College School of Medicine, London, UK.
22.5.6 Megaloblastic anaemia and miscellaneous deficiency anaemias

Ronald Hoffman Professor, Hematology-Oncology Section University of Illinois College of Medicine, Chicago, USA.
22.3.8 The polycythaemias. 22.3.10 Thrombocytosis

P. A. H. Holloway Consultant Chemical Pathologist in Intensive Care and Honorary Reader in Medicine, John Radcliffe Hospital, Oxford, UK.
32 Reference intervals for biochemical data

Richard H. Holloway Associate Professor of Medicine and Senior Consultant Gastroenterologist, Department of Gastroenterology, Hepatology and General Medicine, Royal Adelaide Hospital, Australia.
14.6 Diseases of the oesophagus

J. M. Hopkin Professor, Experimental Medicine Unit, Swansea Clinical School, University of Wales, Swansea, UK.
17.4.1 Asthma: genetic effects. 17.15 The genetics of lung diseases

Carol Ann Huff Assistant Professor of Oncology, Sidney Kimmel Comprehensive Cancer Care at Johns Hopkins, Baltimore, Maryland, USA.
26.7.3 Problems of alcohol and drug users in the hospital

I. A. Hughes Professor of Paediatrics and Honorary Consultant Paediatric Enterologist, Department of Paediatrics, University of Cambridge, UK.
12.7.2 Congenital adrenal hyperplasia

Lawrence Impey Consultant in Fetal Medicine, The Women's Centre, John Radcliffe Hospital, Oxford, UK.
13.15 Infections in pregnancy

C. W. Imrie Consultant Surgeon and Honorary Professor, Lister Department of Surgery, Royal Infirmary, Glasgow, UK.
14.18.3.1 Acute pancreatitis

H. Irving Consultant Radiologist, St James's University Hospital, Leeds, UK.
20.15 Tumours of the urinary tract

P. G. Isaacson Professor of Histopathology, Royal Free and University College Medical School, London, UK.
14.9.4 Gastrointestinal lymphoma

D. A. Isenberg The Arthritis Research Campaign Professor of Rheumatology at University College London, Centre for Rheumatology, London, UK.
18.10.1 Autoimmune rheumatic disorders and vasculitis. 18.10.2 Systemic lupus erythematosus and related disorders

C. G. Isles Consultant Physician, Medical Unit, Dumfries and Galloway Royal Infirmary, Dumfries, UK.
15.16.1.1 Prevalence, epidemiology, and pathophysiology of hypertension

C. Ison Reader in Medical Microbiology, Department of Infectious Diseases and Microbiology, Faculty of Medicine, Imperial College, St Mary's Campus, London, UK.
7.11.6 Neisseria gonorrhoeae

Alan A. Jackson Professor and Director, Institute of Human Nutrition, University of Southampton, UK.
10.4 Severe malnutrition

H. S. Jacobs Emeritus Professor of Reproductive Endocrinology, University College London Medical School, UK.
12.8.1 Ovarian disorders. 12.8.3 The breast

Robin Jacoby Professor of Old Age Psychiatry, University of Oxford Department of Psychiatry, Warneford Hospital, Oxford, UK.
30.2 Mental disorders of old age

O. F. W. James Head of Clinical Medical Sciences, Medical School, University of Newcastle upon Tyne, UK.
14.21.1 Alcoholic liver disease and non-alcoholic steatosis hepatitis

Paul J. Jenkins Senior Lecturer in Endocrinology, St Bartholomew's Hospital, London, UK.
12.2 Disorders of the anterior pituitary

B. Jennett Emeritus Professor of Neurosurgery, Institute of Neurological Sciences, University of Glasgow, UK.
24.13.6 Brain death and the vegetative state

D. P. Jewell Professor of Gastroenterology, John Radcliffe Hospital, Oxford, UK.
14.9.3 Coeliac disease. 14.10 Crohn's disease. 14.11 Ulcerative colitis. 14.22 Miscellaneous disorders of the gastrointestinal tract and liver

Vivekanand Jha Associate Professor of Nephrology, Postgraduate Institute of Medical Education and Research, Chandigarh, India.
20.7.10 Glomerular disease in the tropics

Anne M. Johnson Professor of Infectious Disease Epidemiology and Head, Department of Primary Care and Population Sciences, University College London, UK.
21.2 Sexual behaviour

A. W. Johnson CAB International, Wallingford, Oxfordshire, UK.
8.3 Poisonous plants and fungi

E. Anthony Jones Chief of Hepatology, Academic Medical Centre, Amsterdam, The Netherlands.
14.21.3 Hepatocellular failure

N. Jones Department of Virology, John Radcliffe Hospital, Oxford, UK.
7.10.25 Orf. 7.10.26 Molluscum contagiosum

S. E. Jones Research Associate, Department of Biology, Imperial College of Science, Technology and Medicine, London, UK.
7.11.33 Syphilis

Kenneth C. Kalunian Professor of Medicine, UCLA School of Medicine, Los Angeles, California, USA.
18.8 Osteoarthritis

Eileen Kaner NHS Primary Care Career Scientist, School of Population and Health Sciences, University of Newcastle upon Tyne, UK.
26.7.2 Brief interventions against excessive alcohol consumption

W. Katon Professor and Vice Chair, Director of Division of Health Services and Psychiatric Epidemiology, University of Washington, Seattle, Washington, USA.
26.5.4 Anxiety and depression

Tomisaku Kawasaki Professor and Director, Japan Kawasaki Disease Research Center, Tokyo, Japan.
18.10.8 Kawasaki syndrome

David Keeling Consultant Haematologist and Director, Oxford Haemophilia Centre and Thrombosis Unit, Churchill Hospital, Oxford, UK.
15.5.2 Therapeutic anticoagulation in atrial fibrillation and heart failure.
15.15.3.2 Therapeutic anticoagulation in deep venous thrombosis and pulmonary embolism

David P. Kelsell Non-Clinical Senior Lecturer, Centre for Cutaneous Research, Barts and The London, Queen Mary's School of Medicine and Dentistry, London, UK.
23.2 Molecular basis of inherited skin disease

John G. Kelton Dean and Vice-President, Faculty of Health Sciences, McMaster University, Hamilton, Ontario, Canada.
22.6.3 Disorders of platelet number and function

Christopher Kennard Professor and Head, Division of Neuroscience and Psychological Medicine, Imperial College London, Charing Cross Campus, London, UK.
24.11 Visual pathways

Rose Anne Kenny Professor of Cardiovascular Research, Institute of Ageing and Health, University of Newcastle upon Tyne, UK.
24.13.5.1 Head-up tilt-table testing in the diagnosis of vasovagal syncope and related disorders

M. G. W. Kettlewell Consultant Surgeon, Oxford Radcliffe Trust, UK.
14.13 Colonic diverticular disease

G. T. Keusch Associate Director for International Research, National Institutes of Health, Bethesda, Maryland, and Professor of Medicine, Tufts-New England Medical Center, Boston, Massachusetts, USA.
7.11.7 Enterobacteria, campylobacter, and miscellaneous food-poisoning bacteria

Munther A. Khamashta Senior Lecturer and Consultant Physician, Lupus Research Unit, The Rayne Institute, St Thomas' Hospital, London, UK.
13.14 Autoimmune rheumatic disorders and vasculitis in pregnancy

Maurice King Honorary Research Fellow, University of Leeds, UK.
3.7.2 Health in a fragile future

Keith P. Klugman Professor of International Health, Rollins School of Public Health and Division of Infectious Diseases, School of Medicine, Emory University, Atlanta, Georgia, USA.
7.11.3 Pneumococcal diseases

R. Knight Associate Specialist in General Medicine, Royal Sussex County Hospital, Brighton, UK.
7.13.1 Amoebic infections. 7.13.9 Blastocystis hominis infection. 7.14.2 Lymphatic filariasis. 7.14.3 Guinea-worm disease: dracunculiasis. 7.14.4 Strongyloidiasis, hookworm, and other gut strongyloid nematodes. 7.14.8 Angiostrongyliasis. 7.15.2 Gut cestodes

Michael D. Kopelman Professor of Clinical Medicine and Deputy Warden, Bart's and The London, Queen Mary's School of Medicine and Dentistry, University of London, UK.
26.3 Neuropsychiatric disorders

Peter G. Kopelman Professor of Clinical Medicine, Bart's and The London Queen Mary's School of Medicine and Dentistry, London, UK.
10.5 Obesity

Christian Krarup Professor, Department of Clinical Neurophysiology, Rigshospitalet, Copenhagen, Denmark.
24.2 Electrophysiology of the central and peripheral nervous systems

J. B. Kurtz Consultant Virologist (retired), Public Health Laboratory, Birmingham Heartlands Hospital, UK.
7.11.35 Legionellosis and legionnaires' disease

Robert A. Kyle Professor of Medicine and Laboratory Medicine, Mayo Clinic, Rochester, Minnesota, USA.
22.4.5 Myeloma and paraproteinaemias

David Lalloo Senior Lecturer in Tropical Medicine, Liverpool School of Tropical Medicine, UK.
7.11.17 Yersinia, Pasteurella, and Francisella

D. J. Lane Consultant Chest Physician (Retired), Oxford Radcliffe Hospital, UK.
17.2 The clinical presentation of chest diseases

Peter Lanyon Consultant Rheumatologist, University Hospital, Queen's Medical Centre, Nottingham, UK.
18.3 Clinical investigation

H. E. Larson Private Practice in Infectious Diseases, Marlborough, Massachusetts, USA.
7.11.21 Botulism, gas gangrene, and clostridial gastrointestinal infections

S. Lawrie Senior Clinical Research Fellow, University Department of Psychiatry, Royal Edinburgh Hospital, UK.
26.5.6 Schizophrenia, bipolar disorder, obsessive–compulsive disorder, and personality disorder

N. F. Lawton Consultant Neurologist, Wessex Neurological Centre, Southampton General Hospital and Honorary Senior Lecturer, University of Southampton, UK.
24.13.19 Benign intracranial hypertension

John H, Lazarus Professor of Clinical Endocrinology, University of Wales College of Medicine, Cardiff, UK.
13.11 Endocrine disease in pregnancy

J. W. LeDuc Director, Division of Viral and Rickettsial Diseases, Centers for Disease Control and Prevention, Atlanta, Georgia, USA.
7.10.14 Bunyaviridae

P. J. Lee Consultant in Metabolic Medicine, Metabolic Unit, National Hospital for Neurology and Neurosurgery, London, UK.
11.2 Inborn errors of amino acid and organic acid metabolism

Tak H. Lee Professor of Allergy and Respiratory Medicine, Guy's, King's and St Thomas' School of Medicine, Guy's Hospital, London, UK.
17.4.3 Basic mechanisms and pathophysiology of asthma

William M. F. Lee Department of Medicine, School of Medicine, University of Pennsylvania, Philadelphia, USA.
4.3 Molecular cell biology

T. Lehner Professor of Basic and Applied Immunology, Department of Immunobiology, Guy's, King's and St Thomas' School of Medicine, London, UK.
14.5 The mouth and salivary glands. 18.10.5 Behçet's disease

Irene M. Leigh Professor of Cellular and Molecular Medicine, Bart's and The London Queen Mary's School of Medicine and Dentistry, University of London, UK.
23.2 Molecular basis of inherited skin disease

G. G. Lennox Consultant Neurologist, Addenbrooke's Hospital, Cambridge, UK.
13.12 Neurological disease in pregnancy

E. A. Letsky Consultant Perinatal Haematologist, Queen Charlotte's and Chelsea Hospital, London, UK.
13.16 Blood disorders in pregnancy

Jeremy Levy Consultant Nephrologist, Imperial College, Hammersmith Hospital, London, UK.
20.7.7 Antiglomerular basement membrane disease

L. M. Lichtenstein Professor of Medicine and Director, Asthma and Allergy Center, Johns Hopkins University School of Medicine, Baltimore, Maryland, USA.
5.2 Allergy

D. C. Linch Professor and Head of Haematology, University College London, UK.
22.2.2 Stem-cell disorders

M. J. Lindop Consultant, Anaesthesia/Intensive Care, Addenbrooke's Hospital, Cambridge, UK.
16.6.3 Brainstem death and organ donation. 16.6.4 The patient without hope

Calvin C. Linnemann, Jr Professor and Director, Infectious Diseases Division, University of Cincinnati Medical Center, Ohio, USA.
7.11.14 Bordetella

Gregory Y. H. Lip Professor of Cardiovascular Medicine, University Department of Medicine, City Hospital, Birmingham, UK.
15.16.3 Hypertensive emergencies and urgencies

P. Little Professor of Primary Care Research, Community Clinical Sciences Division, University of Southampton, UK.
17.5.1 Upper respiratory tract infections

Roderick A. Little Honorary Professor of Surgical Science, University of Manchester, UK.
11.12.2 Metabolic responses to accidental and surgical injury

W. Littler Medical Director, University Hospital NHS Trust, Birmingham, UK.
15.10.2 Infective endocarditis

A. Llanos Cuentas Principal Professor, Facultad de Salud Publica y Administracion, Universidad Peruana Cayetano Heredia, Lima, Peru.
7.11.39.1 Bartonella bacilliformis infection

Diana N. J. Lockwood Consultant Leprologist and Senior Lecturer, Hospital for Tropical Diseases and London School of Hygiene and Tropical Medicine, UK.
7.11.24 Leprosy (Hansen's disease)

S. Logan Senior Lecturer in Paediatric Epidemiology, Institute of Child Health, London, UK.
7.10.12 Rubella

D. J. Lomas Professor of Clinical MRI, University Department of Radiology, Addenbrooke's Hospital, Cambridge, UK.
14.18.2 Computed tomography and magnetic resonance imaging of the liver and pancreas

David A. Lomas Professor of Respiratory Biology and Honorary Consultant Physician, Department of Medicine, University of Cambridge Institute for Medical Research, UK.
11.13 α_1-Antitrypsin deficiency and the serpinopathies

Thomas Look Professor of Pediatrics, Harvard Medical School and Vice-Chair for Research, Pediatric Oncology Department, Dana-Farber Institute, Boston, Massachusetts, USA.
22.3.1 Cell and molecular biology of human leukaemias

A. D. Lopez Senior Science Adviser, World Health Organization, Geneva, Switzerland.
3.1 The Global Burden of Disease Study

Elyse E. Lower Professor of Medicine, University of Cincinnati, Ohio, USA.
17.11.6 Sarcoidosis

Linda M. Luxon Professor of Audiological Medicine, University of London, Institute of Child Health, London, UK and Director, National Institute for Cancer Research, Genova, Italy.
24.12.2 Disorders of hearing

Lucio Luzzatto Professor, Department of Human Genetics, Memorial Sloan-Kettering Cancer Center, New York, USA.
22.3.12 Paroxysmal nocturnal haemoglobinuria. 22.5.12 Glucose-6-phosphate dehydrogenase (G6PD) deficiency

G. A. Luzzi Consultant in Genitourinary/HIV Medicine, South Buckinghamshire NHS Trust, Wycombe Hospital, High Wycombe, Buckinghamshire, UK.
7.10.21 HIV and AIDS

D. C. W. Mabey Professor of Communicable Diseases, London School of Hygiene and Tropical Medicine, London, UK.
7.11.40 Chlamydial infections including lymphogranuloma venerum

P. K. MacCallum Senior Lecturer in Haematology, Barts and The London, Queen Mary's School of Medicine and Dentistry, London, UK.
15.1.2.2 The haemostatic system in arterial disease

J. T. Macfarlane Consultant Physician, Nottingham City Hospital, UK.
7.11.35 Legionellosis and legionnaires' disease

K. T. MacLeod Reader in Cardiac Physiology, Cardiac Medicine, NHLI, Faculty of Medicine, Imperial College London, UK.
15.1.3.1 Physical considerations: biochemistry and cellular physiology of heart muscle

William MacNee Professor of Respiratory and Environmental Medicine, University of Edinburgh, and Honorary Consultant Physician, Lothian University NHS Trust, Edinburgh, UK.
17.6 Chronic obstructive pulmonary disease

M. Monir Madkour Consultant Physician, Military Hospital, Riyadh, Saudi Arabia.
7.11.19 Brucellosis

R. N. Maini Professor of Rheumatology in the University of London, Head of the Kennedy Institute of Rheumatology Division, Faculty of Medicine, Imperial College London, and Honorary Consultant Physician, Charing Cross Hospital, London, UK.
18.5 Rheumatoid arthritis

Hadi Manji Consultant Neurologist, National Hospital for Neurology, London and Ipswich Hospital, Suffolk, UK.
24.14.4 Neurosyphilis and neuroAIDS

J. I. Mann Professor in Human Nutrition and Medicine, University of Otago, Dunedin, New Zealand.
10.1 Diseases of overnourished societies and the need for dietary change

D. Mant Professor of General Practice, Department of Primary Health Care, University of Oxford, UK.
3.4 Preventive medicine

Victor J. Marder Orthopedic Hospital/UCLA Vascular Medicine Program, Los Angeles, California, USA.
22.6.2 Evaluation of the patient with a bleeding diathesis

A. F. Markham Professor of Medicine, St James's University Hospital, Leeds, UK.
14.15 Tumours of the gastrointestinal tract

V. Marks Professor of Clinical Biochemistry Emeritus, Post-Graduate Medical School, University of Surrey, Guildford, UK.
12.11.3 Hypoglycaemia

T. J. Marrie Professor and Chair, Department of Medicine, University of Alberta, Edmonton, Canada.
7.11.38 Coxiella burnetii infections (Q fever)

Helen Marriott Research Associate, Department of Respiratory Medicine, University of Sheffffield, UK.
15.15.2.1 Primary pulmonary hypertension

C. D. Marsden* Professor of Neurology, National Hospital for Neurology and Neurosurgery, London, UK.
24.15 Metabolic disorders and the nervous system

Jay W. Mason Professor and Chair, Department of Medicine, University of Kentucky College of Medicine, Lexington, USA.
15.8.1 Myocarditis

V. I. Mathan Professor, ICDDR, Dhaka, Bangladesh.
14.9.8 Malabsorption syndromes in the tropics

Christopher J. Mathias Professor of Neurovascular Medicine and Consultant Physician, Imperial College of Science, Technology and Medicine at St Mary's and National Hospital for Neurology and Neurosurgery, Institute of Neurology, University College London, UK.
24.13.14 Diseases of the autonomic nervous system

Peter W. Mathiesen Professor of Renal Medicine, Academic Renal Unit, University of Bristol, Southmead Hospital, Bristol, UK.
20.7.5 Proliferative glomerulonephritis. 20.7.6 Mesangiocapillary glomerulonephritis

R. McCaig Head, Human Factors Unit, Health Directorate, Health and Safety Executive, Bootle, UK.
8.5.10 Noise. 8.5.11 Vibration

Mary E. McCaul Professor, Department of Psychiatry and Behavioral Sciences, Johns Hopkins University School of Medicine, Baltimore, Maryland, USA.
26.7.1 Alcohol and drug dependence

Joseph McCormick Regional Dean, University of Texas School of Public Health at Brownsville, USA.
7.10.15 Arenaviruses. 7.10.16 Filoviruses

William J. McKenna BHF Professor of Molecular Cardiovascular Sciences, Department of Cardiological Sciences, St George's Hospital Medical School, London, UK.
15.8.2 The cardiomyopathies: hypertrophic, dilated, restrictive, and right ventricular. 15.8.3 Specific heart muscle disorders

---

* It is with regret that we report the death of Professor C. D. Marsden.

A. J. McMichael Professor and Director, Weatherall Institute of Molecular Medicine, John Radcliffe Hospital, Oxford, UK.
5.1 Principles of immunology.

A. J. McMichael Professor and Director, National Centre for Epidemiology and Population Health, Australian National University, Canberra, Australia.
3.2 Human population size, environment, and health

A. McMillan Consultant Physician, Department of Genito-urinary Medicine, Edinburgh Royal Infirmary, UK.
21.5 Infections and other medical problems in homosexual men

Martin McNally Consultant in Limb Reconstruction and Honorary Senior Lecturer in Orthopaedic Surgery, Bone Infection Unit, Nuffield Orthopaedic Centre, Oxford, UK.
19.3 Osteomyelitis

K. McNeil Director of Transplant Services, The Prince Charles Hospital, Brisbane, Australia.
17.16 Lung and heart–lung transplantation

T. W. Meade Emeritus Professor of Epidemiology, London School of Hygiene and Tropical Medicine, UK.
15.1.2.2 The haemostatic system in arterial disease

A. Meheus Professor, University of Antwerp, Belgium.
21.1 Epidemiology

David K. Menon Professor of Anaesthesia, University of Cambridge, Addenbrooke's Hospital, Cambridge, UK.
16.6.2 Management of raised intracranial pressure

Wayne M. Meyers Chief, Mycobacteriology, Armed Forces Institute of Pathology, Washington DC, USA.
7.11.25 Buruli ulcer: Mycobacterium ulcerans infection

Anna Rita Migliaccio Dirigente de Ricerca in Transfusion Medicine, Laboratory of Clinical Biochemistry, Istituto Superiore dei Sanità, Rome, Italy.
22.5.1 Erythropoiesis and the normal red cell

M. A. Miles Professor, London School of Hygiene and Tropical Medicine, UK.
7.13.11 Chagas' disease

G. J. Miller Professor of Epidemiology, Barts and The London, Queen Mary's School of Medicine and Dentistry, London, UK.
15.1.2.2 The haemostatic system in arterial disease

Mary Miller Consultant in Palliative Medicine, Sir Michael Sobell House, Churchill Hospital, Oxford, UK.
31 Palliative care

Robert F. Miller Reader in Clinical Infection and Consultant Physician, Royal Free and University College Medical School, London, UK.
7.12.5 Pneumocystis carinii

K. R. Mills Professor of Clinical Neurophysiology, King's College Hospital, London, UK.
24.4 Investigation of central motor pathways: magnetic brain stimulation

Philip Minor Public Health and Clinical Microbiology Laboratory, Addenbrooke's Hospital, Cambridge, UK.
7.10.7 Enterovirus infections

Raad H. Mohiaddin Consultant and Honorary Senior Lecturer, Royal Brompton and Harefield NHS Trust, London, JK.
15.3.5 Cardiovascular magnetic resonance and computed X-ray tomography

Andrew J. Molyneux Consultant Neuroradiologist, Radcliffe Infirmary, Oxford, UK.
24.5 Imaging in neurological diseases

Kevin Moore Senior Lecturer, Centre for Hepatology, Royal Free Hospital and University College Medical School, London, UK.
14.21.2 Cirrhosis, portal hypertension, and ascites

Pedro L. Moro Fellow, Vaccine Safety Division, National Immunization Program, Centers for Disease Control and Prevention, Baltimore, Maryland, USA.
7.15.1 Cystic hydatid disease (Echinococcus granulosus)

N. J. McC. Mortensen Professor of Colorectal Surgery, Department of Colorectal Surgery, John Radcliffe Hospital, Oxford, UK.
14.13 Colonic diverticular disease

Peter S. Mortimer Professor of Dermatological Medicine and Consultant Skin Physician, St George's Hospital Medical School, Division of Physiological Medicine, London, UK.
15.17 Lymphoedema

Alastair G. Mowat Clinical Lecturer in Rheumatology, Department of Rheumatology, Nuffield Orthopaedic Centre, Oxford, UK.
18.10.4 Polymyalgia rheumatica and giant-cell arteritis

E. R. Moxon Head, Oxford University Department of Paediatrics, John Radcliffe Hospital, Oxford, UK.
7.11.12 Haemophilus influenzae

M. F. Muers Consultant Physician, Respiratory Medicine, The General Infirmary at Leeds, UK.
17.3.4 Diagnostic bronchoscopy, thoracoscopy, and tissue biopsy

Tariq I. Mughal Consultant Haematologist and Medical Oncologist and Senior Lecturer in Oncology, Lancashire Teaching Hospitals NHS Trust and Preston and Christie Hospital NHS Trust, Manchester, UK.
22.3.6 Chronic myeloid leukaemia

J. A. Muir Gray Director of the UK National Screening Committee, Institute of Health Sciences, Oxford, UK.
3.6 Screening

P. A. Murphy Professor of Medicine and Microbiology, Johns Hopkins University and Chief, Infectious Diseases Division, Johns Hopkins Bayview Hospital, Baltimore, Maryland, USA.
7.5 Physiological changes in infected patients

C. J. L. Murray Global Programme on Evidence for Health Policy, World Health Organization, Geneva, Switzerland.
3.1 The Global Burden of Disease Study

Iain M. Murray-Lyon Consultant Physician and Gastroenterologist, Charing Cross Hospital and Chelsea and Westminster Hospital, London, UK.
14.21.5 Primary and secondary liver tumours

Jean Nachega Assistant Scientist, Johns Hopkins University, Baltimore, Maryland, USA.
7.11.22 Tuberculosis

Robert B. Nadelman Professor of Medicine, Division of Infectious Diseases, New York Medical College, USA.
7.11.29 Lyme borreliosis

N. V. Naoumov Reader in Hepatology/Honorary Consultant Physician, Institute of Hepatology, University College London, UK.
7.10.19 Hepatitis viruses (including TTV)

R. P. Naoumova MRC Senior Clinical Scientist/Honorary Consultant Physician, MRC Clinical Sciences Centre, Hammersmith Hospital, London, UK.
15.1.2.1 The pathogenesis of atherosclerosis

D. G. Nathan President, Dana-Farber Cancer Institute, Boston, Massachusetts, USA.
22.2.1 Stem cells and haemopoiesis

Graham Neale Research Fellow, Clinical Risk Unit, University College London, UK.
14.1 Introduction to gastroenterology. 14.1.1.2 Symptomatology of gastrointestinal disease. 14.16 Vascular and collagen disorders

Catherine Nelson-Piercy Consultant Obstetric Physician, Guy's and St Thomas' Hospitals Trust, London, UK.
13.14 Autoimmune rheumatic disorders and vasculitis in pregnancy

A. R. Ness Senior Lecturer in Epidemiology, Department of Social Medicine, University of Bristol, UK.
15.4.1.2 The epidemiology of ischaemic heart disease

Peter Nestor Neurologist, University of Cambridge Neurology Unit, UK.
24.8 Disturbances of higher cerebral function

J. Neuberger Professor of Hepatology and Consultant Physician, Queen Elizabeth Hospital, Birmingham, UK.
14.21.7 Drugs and liver damage. 14.21.8 The liver in systemic disease

John Newell-Price Senior Lecturer in Endocrinology, Division of Clinical Sciences, Sheffield University, Northern General Hospital, Sheffield, UK.
12.3 Disorders of the posterior pituitary

A. J. Newman Taylor Consultant Physician and Head, Department of Occupational and Environmental Medicine, Royal Brompton Harefield NHS Trust, Faculty of Medicine, Imperial College London, UK.
17.4.4 Asthma. 17.4.5 Occupational asthma

C. S. Ng Assistant Professor, Department of Radiology, University of Texas M. D. Anderson Cancer Center, Houston, USA.
14.18.2 Computed tomography and magnetic resonance imaging of the liver and pancreas

S. Nightingale Consultant Neurologist and Honorary Senior Clinical Lecturer, Royal Shrewsbury Hospital and Birmingham University, Shrewsbury, UK.
7.10.23 HTLV-I and II and associated diseases

T. Northfield Professor Emeritus, Department of Biochemical Medicine, St George's Hospital, London, UK.
14.3.2 Gastrointestinal bleeding

John Nowakowski Assistant Professor of Medicine, Department of Medicine, Division of Infectious Diseases, Westchester Medical Center, Valhalla, New York, USA.
7.11.29 Lyme borreliosis

Fujio Numano Director, Tokyo Vascular Disease Institute, Tokyo, Japan.
15.14.4 Takayasu arteritis

D. O'Gradaigh Research Registrar, Department of Medicine, Addenbrooke's Hospital, Cambridge, UK.
18.11 Miscellaneous conditions presenting to the rheumatologist. 19.5 Avascular necrosis and related topics

Stephen O'Rahilly Professor of Clinical Biochemistry, University of Cambridge, and Honorary Consultant Physician, UK.
10.5 Obesity

S. C. O'Reilly Consultant Rheumatologist, Rheumatology Department, Derbyshire Royal Infirmary, Derby, UK.
18.9 Crystal-related arthropathies

P. J. Oldershaw Consultant Cardiologist, Royal Brompton Hospital, London, UK.
15.13 Congenital heart disease in adolescents and adults

James G. Olson Head, Department of Virology, U. S. Navy Medical Research Center Detachment, Lima, Peru.
7.10.6.1 Nipah and Hendra viruses. 7.11.39 Bartonelloses, excluding Bartonella bacilliformis infections

M. Osame Professor, Third Department of Internal Medicine, Faculty of Medicine, Kagoshima University, Japan.
7.10.23 HTLV-I and II and associated diseases

Jackie Palace Consultant Neurologist, Radcliffe Infirmary, Oxford, UK.
24.17 Disorders of the neuromuscular junction

Thalia Papayannopoulou Professor of Medicine (Hematology), University of Washington, Division of Hematology, Seattle, USA.
22.5.1 Erythropoiesis and the normal red cell

S. Parish Senior Research Fellow, Clinical Trial Service Unit, Nuffield Department of Clinical Medicine, University of Oxford, UK.
2.4.3 Large-scale randomized evidence: trials and overviews

G. R. Park Director of Intensive Care Research, John Farman Intensive Care Unit, Addenbrooke's Hospital, Cambridge, UK.
16.6.1 Sedation and analgesia in the critically ill

David Parkes Professor of Clinical Neurology, King's College Hospital, London, UK.
24.13.4 Narcolepsy

C. Parry University of Oxford–Wellcome Trust Clinical Research Unit, Centre for Tropical Diseases, Ho Chi Minh City, Vietnam.
7.11.8 Typhoid and paratyphoid fevers

Steve W. Parry Consultant Physician and Honorary Senior Lecturer, Freeman Hospital and University of Newcastle upon Tyne, UK.
24.13.5.1 Head-up tilt-table testing in the diagnosis of vasovagal syncope and related disorders

J. Paul Consultant Microbiologist and Director, Brighton Public Health Laboratory, Royal Sussex County Hospital, Brighton, UK.
7.11.42 Newly identified and lesser-known bacteria. 7.17 Non-venomous arthropods

Malik Peiris Professor, Department of Microbiology, University of Hong Kong.
7.10.1 Respiratory tract viruses

Edmund D. Pellegrino Emeritus Professor of Medicine and Medical Ethics, Georgetown University Medical Center, Washington DC, USA.
2.3 Medical ethics

T. H. Pennington Professor of Bacteriology, University of Aberdeen Medical School, UK.
7.3 Biology of pathogenic micro-organisms

M. B. Pepys Professor and Head of Medicine, Department of Medicine, Royal Free Campus, Royal Free and University College Medical School, London, UK.
11.12.1 The acute phase response and C reactive protein. 11.12.4 Amyloidosis

P. L. Perine Professor of Epidemiology, School of Public and Community Medicine, University of Washington, Seattle, USA.
7.11.32 Non-venereal treponematoses: yaws, endemic syphilis (bejel), and pinta

G. D. Perkin Consultant Neurologist, Department of Neurology, Charing Cross Hospital, London, UK.
24.13.3 Epilepsy in later childhood and adults

P. L. Perrotta Assistant Professor, Pathology, Stony Brook University Hospital, New York, USA.
22.8.1 Blood transfusion

H. Persson Medical Director and Consultant Physician, Swedish Poisons Information Centre, Stockholm, Sweden.
8.3 Poisonous plants and fungi

M. C. Petch Consultant Cardiologist, Papworth Hospital, Cambridge, UK.
15.4.2.6 The impact of coronary heart disease on life and work

L. R. Petersen Deputy Director for Science, Centers for Disease Control, Division of Vector-borne Infectious Diseases, Fort Collins, Colorado, USA.
7.10.11 Alphaviruses. 7.10.13 Flaviviruses

R. Peto Professor of Epidemiology and Medical Statistics, University of Oxford, UK.
2.4.3 Large-scale randomized evidence: trials and overviews. 6.1 Epidemiology of cancer

T. E. A. Peto Consultant Physician in Infectious Diseases, Nuffield Department of Medicine, John Radcliffe Hospital, Oxford, UK.
7.10.21 HIV and AIDS

A. Phillips Senior Lecturer, Institute of Nephrology, University of Wales College of Medicine, Cardiff, UK.
20.1 Structure and function of the kidney

R. J. Playford Professor, Imperial College School of Medicine, Hammersmith Hospital, London, UK.
14.9.7 Effects of massive small bowel resection

J. M. Polak Professor and Director, Tissue Engineering and Regenerative Medicine Centre, Imperial College School of Medicine, London, UK.
14.8 Hormones and the gastrointestinal tract

Eleanor S. Pollak Associate Director, Clinical Coagulation Laboratory, Hospital of the University of Pennysylvania, University of Pennsylvania Medical Center, Philadelphia, USA.
22.6.4 Genetic disorders of coagulation

P. A. Poole-Wilson Professor of Cardiology and Cardiac Medicine, National Heart and Lung Institute, Faculty of Medicine, Imperial College London, UK.
15.1.3.1 Physical considerations: biochemistry and cellular physiology of heart muscle

F. M. Pope Consultant Dermatologist, West Middlesex University Hospital, London, UK.
19.2 Inherited defects of connective tissue: Ehlers–Danlos syndrome, Marfan's syndrome, and pseudoxanthoma elasticum

Françoise Portaels Professor and Head, Mycobacteriology Unit, Institute of Tropical Medicine, Antwerp, Belgium.
7.11.25 Buruli ulcer: Mycobacterium ulcerans infection

J. S. Porterfield Formerly Reader in Bacteriology, Sir William Dunn School of Pathology, University of Oxford, UK.
7.10.14 Bunyaviridae

Jerome B. Posner Attending Neurologist, Memorial Sloan-Kettering Cancer Center, New York, USA.
24.18 Paraneoplastic syndromes

William G. Powderly Professor of Medicine, Washington University School of Medicine, St Louis, Missouri, USA.
7.12.2 Cryptococcosis

J. J. Powell Senior Lecturer - Nutrition and Medicine, GI Laboratory, Rayne Institute, St Thomas' Hospital, London, UK.
8.5.8 Podoconiosis

Janet Powell Medical Director, University Hospitals, Coventry and Warwickshire NHS Trust, Coventry, Warwickshire, UK.
15.14.2 Peripheral arterial disease

J. W. Powles University Lecturer in Public Health Medicine, Institute of Public Health, Cambridge, UK.
3.2 Human population size, environment, and health

M. A. Preece Professor of Child Health and Growth, Institute of Child Health, University College London, UK.
12.9.2 Normal growth and its disorders

J. S. Prichard* Professor of Medicine, St James's Hospital, Dublin, Eire.
15.15.2.2 Pulmonary oedema

A. T. Proudfoot Consulting Clinical Toxicologist, National Poisons Information Service, City Hospital, Birmingham, UK.
8.1 Poisoning by drugs and chemicals

Charles Pusey Professor of Renal Medicine, Faculty of Medicine, Imperial College, Hammersmith Hospital, London, UK.
20.7.7 Antiglomerular basement membrane disease

N. P. Quinn Professor of Clinical Neurology, Institute of Neurology and Honorary Consultant Neurologist, The National Hospital for Neurology and Neurosurgery, London, UK.
24.10 Subcortical structures—the cerebellum, thalamus, and basal ganglia

Anisur Rahman Senior Lecturer in Rheumatology, Centre for Rheumatology, Department of Medicine, University College London, UK.
18.10.2 Systemic lupus erythematosus and related disorders

Lawrence E. Ramsay Professor of Clinical Pharmacology and Therapeutics, University of Sheffield and Consultant Physician, Royal Hallamshire Hospital, Sheffield, UK.
15.16.2.1 Hypertension—indications for investigation. 15.16.2.2 Renal and renovascular hypertension. 15.16.2.5 Aortic coarctation. 15.16.2.6 Other rare causes of hypertension. 20.10.2 Hypertension and the kidney

M. Ramsay Consultant Epidemiologist, Immunisation Division, PHLS Communicable Disease Surveillance Centre, London, UK.
7.7 Immunization

A. C. Rankin Reader in Cardiology, Glasgow Royal Infirmary, UK.
15.2.3 Syncope and palpitation. 15.6 Cardiac arrhythmias

C. W. G. Redman Professor of Obstetric Medicine, John Radcliffe Hospital, Oxford, UK.
13.4 Hypertension in pregnancy

Laurence John Reed Academic Unit of Psychiatry, St Thomas' Hospital, London, UK.
26.3 Neuropsychiatric disorders

A. J. Rees Regius Professor of Medicine, Institute of Medical Sciences, University of Aberdeen, UK.
20.10.3 Vasculitis and the kidney

Jeremy Rees Clinical Senior Lecturer in Neuro-oncology, National Hospital for Neurology and Neurosurgery, London, UK.
24.13.18.1 Intracranial tumours

D. Rennie Adjunct Professor of Medicine, Institute for Health Policy Studies, University of California, San Francisco, USA.
8.5.4 Diseases of high terrestrial altitudes

J. Richens Clinical Lecturer, Department of Sexually Transmitted Diseases, Royal Free and University College Medical School, London, UK.
7.11.8 Typhoid and paratyphoid fevers. 7.11.9 Intracellular Klebsiella infections

B. K. Rima Professor of Molecular Biology, Medical Biology Centre, Queen's University of Belfast, UK.
7.10.5 Mumps: epidemic parotitis

A. J. Ritchie Consultant Cardiothoracic Surgeon, Papworth NHS Trust, Cambridge, UK.
15.4.2.5 Coronary artery bypass grafting

Eberhard Ritz Professor and Head, Department of Nephrology, University of Heidelberg, Germany.
20.5.2 Bone disease in chronic renal failure

Harold R. Roberts Sarah Graham Kenan Professor of Medicine and Attending Physician, UNC Hospitals, Chapel Hill, North Carolina, USA.
22.6.1 The biology of haemostasis and thrombosis. 22.6.2 Evaluation of the patient with a bleeding diathesis

William G. Robertson Clinical Scientist, Institute of Urology and Nephrology, University College London, UK.
20.13 Urinary stones, nephrocalcinosis, and renal tubular acidosis

T. A. Rockall Senior Lecturer/Honorary Consultant, St Mary's Hospital, London, UK.
14.3.2 Gastrointestinal bleeding

Allan R. Ronald Professor Emeritus, University of Manitoba, Winnipeg, Canada.
7.11.13 Haemophilus ducreyi and chancroid

P. Ronco Professor of Renal Medicine, Université Pierre et Marie Curie (Paris 6) and Director, Renal Division and INSERM Unit 489, Tenon Hospital (Assistance Publique-Hôpitaux de Paris), Paris, France.
20.10.5 Renal involvement in plasma cell dyscrasias, immunoglobulin-based amyloidoses, and fibrillary glomerulopathies, lymphomas, and leukaemias

Antony Rosen Professor and Director, Division of Rheumatology, Johns Hopkins University School of Medicine, Baltimore, Maryland, USA.
5.3 Autoimmunity

Mark J. Rosen Chief, Division of Pulmonary and Critical Care Medicine, Beth Israel Medical Center, New York, USA.
17.5.2.3 Pulmonary complications of HIV infection

Raymond C. Rosen Professor of Psychiatry, UMDNJ-Robert Wood Johnson Medical School, Department of Psychiatry, Piscataway, New Jersey, USA.
12.8.4 Sexual dysfunction

R. J. M. Ross Professor of Endocrinology, Northern General Hospital, University of Sheffield, UK.
12.9.3 Puberty

D. J. Rowlands Honorary Consultant Cardiologist, Manchester Heart Centre, Manchester Royal Infirmary, UK.
15.3.2 Electrocardiography. 15.3.4 Nuclear techniques

M. B. Rubens Director of Imaging and Consultant Radiologist, Royal Brompton and Harefield NHS Trust, London, UK.
15.3.1 Chest radiography in heart disease. 15.3.5 Cardiovascular magnetic resonance and computed X-ray tomography

David Rubenstein Consultant Physician, Addenbrooke's Hospital, Cambridge, UK.
7.1 The clinical approach to the patient with suspected infection

P. C. Rubin Professor and Dean of Medicine, University of Nottingham, UK.
13.18 Prescribing in pregnancy

Anthony S. Russell Professor of Medicine, University of Alberta, Edmonton, Canada.
18.2 Clinical presentation and diagnosis of rheumatic disease

T. J. Ryan Emeritus Professor of Dermatology, University of Oxford, UK.
23.1 Diseases of the skin

Sara S. T. O. Saad Professor and Haematologist, Department of Internal Medicine, Hematology-Hemotherapy Division, Medical Science Faculty, State University of Campinas, Brazil.
22.5.10 Disorders of the red cell membrane

N. J. Samani Professor of Cardiology, Division of Cardiology, Department of Medicine, University of Leicester, UK.
15.16.1.2 Genetics of hypertension

Brian P. Saunders Senior Lecturer in Endoscopy, St Mark's Hospital, Northwick Park, Harrow, Middlesex, UK.
14.2.1 Colonoscopy and flexible sigmoidoscopy

S. J. Saunders Emeritus Professor, Liver Clinic, Groote Schuur Hospital and Medical Research Council/University of Cape Town Liver Research Centre, Cape Town, South Africa.
14.21.6 Hepatic granulomas

M. O. Savage Professor of Paediatric Endocrinology, St Bartholomew's and The Royal London School of Medicine and Dentistry, London, UK.
12.9.1 Normal and abnormal sexual differentiation. 12.9.3 Puberty

John Savill Professor of Medicine, Royal Infirmary, Edinburgh, UK.
20.7.1 The glomerulus and glomerular injury

---

* It is with regret that we report the death of Professor J. S. Prichard.

K. P. Schaal Professor and Director, Institute for Medical Microbiology and Immunology, Faculty of Medicine, Rheinische Friedrich-Wilhelms-Universität, Bonn, Germany.
7.11.26 Actinomycosis

Michael Schömig Physician in Charge, Division of Nephrology, Ruperto-Carola-University of Heidelberg, Germany.
20.5.2 Bone disease in chronic renal failure

Ruud B. H. Schutgens Head of Department of Clinical Chemistry, Vrije Universiteit Medical Centre (VUMC), Amsterdam, The Netherlands.
11.9 Peroxisomal diseases

J. Schwebke Associate Professor of Medicine, University of Alabama at Birmingham, USA.
21.3 Vaginal discharge

Neil Scolding Burden Professor of Clinical Neurosciences, University of Bristol Institute of Clinical Neurosciences, Frenchay Hospital, Bristol, UK.
24.15 Metabolic disorders and the nervous system. 24.20 Neurological complications of systemic autoimmune and inflammatory diseases

J. Scott Professor of Medicine, Imperial College Faculty of Medicine, Hammersmith Campus, London, UK.
15.1.2.1 The pathogenesis of atherosclerosis

A. Seaton Professor and Head of Department of Environmental and Occupational Medicine, University of Aberdeen, UK.
17.11.7 Pneumoconioses

G. R. Serjeant Professor Emeritus and Chairman, Sickle Cell Trust, Kingston, Jamaica, West Indies.
20.10.7 Sickle-cell disease and the kidney

N. J. Severs Professor of Cell Biology, National Heart and Lung Institute, Faculty of Medicine, Imperial College London, UK.
15.1.3.1 Physical considerations: biochemistry and cellular physiology of heart muscle

C. A. Seymour Professor of Clinical Biochemistry and Metabolic Medicine and Director for Clinical Advice to The Health Service Ombudsman, St George's Hospital Medical School and Office of Health Service Commissioner, London, UK.
11.7.2 Wilson's disease, Menke's disease: inherited disorders of copper metabolism

K. V. Shah Professor, Johns Hopkins Bloomberg School of Public Health, Baltimore, Maryland, USA.
7.10.17 Papoviruses

L. M. Shapiro Consultant Cardiologist, Papworth Hospital, Cambridge, UK.
15.4.2.2 Management of stable angina. 15.4.2.5 Coronary artery bypass grafting

Michael Sharpe Reader in Psychological Medicine, University of Edinburgh, Royal Edinburgh Hospital, UK.
7.19 Chronic fatigue syndrome (postviral fatigue syndrome, neurasthenia, and myalgic encephalomyelitis). 26.1 General introduction. 26.5.3 Medically unexplained symptoms in patients attending medical clinics. 26.6.2 Psychological treatment in medical practice

J. M. Shneerson Director, Respiratory Support and Sleep Centre, Papworth Hospital, Cambridge, UK.
17.13 Disorders of the thoracic cage and diaphragm

Tom Siddons Clinical Research Assistant, Pfizer Research and Development (UK), Maidstone, Kent, UK.
15.15.1 The pulmonary circulation and its influence on gas exchange

C. A. Sieff Associate Professor in Pediatrics, Dana Farber Cancer Institute, Boston, Massachusetts, USA.
22.2.1 Stem cells and haemopoiesis

J. Sieper Head of Rheumatology, Department of Medicine, University Hospital Benjamin Franklin, Berlin, Germany.
18.6 Spondyloarthritides and related arthritides

Leslie Silberstein Professor, University of Pennsylvania School of Medicine, Philadelphia, Pennsylvania, USA.
22.5.9 Haemolytic anaemia—congenital and acquired

R. Sinclair Senior Lecturer, Department of Dermatology, University of Melbourne, St Vincent's Hospital, Fitzroy, Victoria, Australia.
23.1 Diseases of the skin

Joseph Sinning Yale School of Medicine, New Haven, Connecticut, USA.
22.4.1 Leucocytes in health and disease

Thira Sirisanthana Professor of Medicine and Director, Research Institute for Health Sciences, Chiang Mai University, Thailand.
7.11.18 Anthrax. 7.12.6 Infection due to Penicillium marneffei

J. G. P. Sissons Professor of Medicine, University of Cambridge and Honorary Consultant Physician, Addenbrooke's Hospital, Cambridge, UK.
7.10.2 Herpesviruses (excluding Epstein–Barr virus)

M. B. Skirrow Honorary Emeritus Consultant Microbiologist, Public Health Laboratory, Gloucester Royal Hospital, UK.
7.11.7 Enterobacteria, campylobacter, and miscellaneous food-poisoning bacteria

Geoffrey L. Smith Professor of Virology and Wellcome Trust Principal Research Fellow, The Wright–Fleming Institute, Faculty of Medicine, Imperial College of Science, Technology and Medicine, St Mary's Campus, London, UK.
7.10.4 Poxviruses

P. H. Smith Department of Urology, St James' University Hospital, Leeds, UK.
20.15 Tumours of the urinary tract

R. Smith Consultant Physician, Nuffield Orthopaedic Centre, Oxford, UK.
19.1 Disorders of the skeleton

E. L. Snyder Professor of Laboratory Medicine, Yale University School of Medicine, New Haven, Connecticut, USA.
22.8.1 Blood transfusion

R. L. Souhami Director of Clinical Research, Cancer Research UK and Emeritus Professor of Medicine, University College London, London, UK.
6.6 Cancer: clinical features and management

C. W. N. Spearman Senior Specialist and Co-Head of Liver Clinic, Groote Schuur Hospital, Cape Town, South Africa.
14.21.6 Hepatic granulomas

C. A. Speed Honorary Consultant Rheumatologist, Addenbrooke's Hospital, Cambridge, UK.
19.5 Avascular necrosis and related topics

G. P. Spickett Consultant Clinical Immunologist, Regional Department of Immunology, Royal Victoria Infirmary, Newcastle upon Tyne, UK.
17.11.8 Pulmonary haemorrhagic disorders. 17.11.9 Eosinophilic pneumonia. 17.11.11 Extrinsic allergic alveolitis. 17.11.19 Drug-induced lung disease

S. G. Spiro Professor of Respiratory Medicine and Medical Director, Medicine, University College London Hospitals NHS Trust, Middlesex Hospital, London, UK.
17.14.1.1 Lung cancer. 17.14.1.2 Pulmonary metastases

Jerry L. Spivak Professor of Medicine and Oncology, Johns Hopkins School of Medicine, Baltimore, Maryland, USA.
22.3.9 Idiopathic myelofibrosis

A. Spurgeon Senior Lecturer, Institute of Occupational Health, University of Birmingham, UK.
8.4.1 Occupational and environmental health and safety

Paul D. Stein Director of Research, St Joseph Mercy-Oakland, Pontiac, Michigan, USA.
15.15.3.1 Deep venous thrombosis and pulmonary embolism

Tom Stevens Consultant Psychiatrist, St Thomas' Hospital and Maudsley NHS Trust, London, UK.
26.3 Neuropsychiatric disorders

J. C. Stevenson Reader and Consultant Physician, Endocrinology and Metabolic Medicine, Faculty of Medicine, Imperial College London, UK.
13.20 Benefits and risks of hormone replacement therapy

P. M. Stewart Professor of Medicine, University of Birmingham and Consultant Physician, Queen Elizabeth Hospital, Birmingham, UK.
12.7.1 Disorders of the adrenal cortex

August Stich Consultant in Tropical Medicine, Medical Mission Institute, Unit of Tropical Medicine and Epidemic Control, Wurzburg, Germany.
7.13.10 Human African trypanosomiasis

John H. Stone Associate Professor of Medicine, Johns Hopkins University, Baltimore, Maryland, USA.
18.10.7 Polymyositis and dermatomyositis

J. R. Stradling Consultant Physician and Professor of Respiratory Medicine, Churchill Hospital, Oxford, UK.
17.1.1 The upper respiratory tract. 17.8.1 Upper airways obstruction. 17.8.2 Sleep-related disorders of breathing

Frank J. Strobl Director, Scientific Affairs, Therakos Inc., Exton, Pennsylvania, USA.
22.5.9 Haemolytic anaemia—congenital and acquired

M. A. Stroud Senior Lecturer in Medicine, Southampton University Hospitals Trust, UK.
8.5.1 Environmental extremes—heat. 8.5.2 Environmental extremes—cold

Michael Strupp Associate Professor of Neurology, Department of Neurology, Klinikum Grosshadern, University of Munich, Germany.
24.12.1 Eye movements and balance

P. H. Sugden Professor of Cellular Biochemistry, Imperial College of Science, Technology and Medicine, London, UK.
15.1.3.1 Physical considerations: biochemistry and cellular physiology of heart muscle

Daniel P. Sulmasy Sisters of Charity Chair in Ethics, St Vincent's Manhattan and New York Medical College, New York, USA.
2.3 Medical ethics

J. A. Summerfield Professor of Experimental Medicine, Faculty of Medicine, Imperial College London, UK.
14.19.1 Congenital disorders of the liver, biliary tract, and pancreas. 14.19.2 Diseases of the gallbladder and biliary tree

Pravan Suntharasamai Emeritus Professor of Tropical Medicine, Faculty of Tropical Medicine, Mahidol University, Bangkok, Thailand.
7.14.9 Gnathostomiasis

J. Swales* Professor of Medicine, University of Leicester, UK.
15.16.1.3 Essential hypertension

P. Sweny Consultant Nephrologist, Royal Free Hospital, London, UK.
20.6.3 Renal transplantation

D. Swirsky Consultant Haematologist, Leeds General Infirmary, UK.
22.4.4 The spleen and its disorders

I. C. Talbot Professor of Histopathology, St Mark's Hospital for Colorectal Disorders, London, UK.
14.15 Tumours of the gastrointestinal tract

D. Tarin Director, UCSD Cancer Center, University of California at San Diego, La Jolla, USA.
6.4 Tumour metastasis

D. Taylor-Robinson Emeritus Professor of Genitourinary Microbiology and Medicine, Division of Medicine, Imperial College of Science, Technology and Medicine, St Mary's Hospital, London, UK.
7.11.40 Chlamydial infections including lymphogranuloma venerum. 7.11.41 Mycoplasmas

P. J. Teddy Consultant Neurosurgeon/Clinical Director, Department of Neurological Surgery, Radcliffe Infirmary, Oxford, UK.
24.14.3 Intracranial abscess

H. J. Testa Professor and Consultant (retired), Royal Infirmary, Manchester, UK.
15.3.4 Nuclear techniques

R. V. Thakker May Professor of Medicine, Nuffield Department of Medicine, University of Oxford, UK.
12.6 Parathyroid disorders and diseases altering calcium metabolism

David G. T. Thomas Professor of Neurological Surgery, National Hospital for Neurology and Neurosurgery, London, UK.
24.13.18.2 Traumatic injuries of the head

D. L. Thomas Associate Professor of Medicine, Johns Hopkins School of Medicine, Baltimore, Maryland, USA.
7.10.20 Hepatitis C virus

P. K. Thomas Emeritus Professor of Neurology, Royal Free Hospital School of Medicine and Institute of Neurology, London, UK.
24.6.1 Inherited disorders. 24.13.15 Disorders of cranial nerves. 24.19 Diseases of the peripheral nerves

D. G. Thompson Professor of Gastroenterology, University of Manchester, UK.
14.1.1.1 Structure and function of the gut. 14.12 Functional bowel disorders and irritable bowel syndrome

R. P. H. Thompson Consultant Physician, St Thomas' Hospital, London, UK.
8.5.8 Podoconiosis. 14.19.3 Jaundice

S. A. Thorne Royal Brompton and Harefield NHS Trust, London, UK.
15.13 Congenital heart disease in adolescents and adults

Ph. Thulliez Head, Laboratoire de la Toxoplasmose, Institut de Puericulture, Paris, France.
7.13.4 Toxoplasmosis

Tran Tin Hien Vice Director, Centre for Tropical Diseases (Cho Quan Hospital), Ho Chi Minh City, Vietnam.
7.11.1 Diphtheria

J. A. Todd Professor of Medical Genetics, University of Cambridge, UK.
12.11.2 The genetics of diabetes melllitus

C. Tomson Consultant Nephrologist, Southmead Hospital, Bristol, UK.
20.12 Urinary tract infection

Keith Tones Professor of Health Education (Emeritus), Leeds Metropolitan University, UK.
3.5 Health promotion

P. A. Tookey Lecturer, Centre for Epidemiology and Biostatistics, Institute of Child Health, London, UK.
7.10.12 Rubella

P. P. Toskes Professor of Medicine, Division of Gastroenterology, Hepatology, and Nutrition, Department of Medicine, University of Florida College of Medicine, Gainsville, USA.
14.9.2 Small bowel bacterial overgrowth. 14.18.3.2 Chronic pancreatitis

Thomas A. Traill Professor of Medicine, Johns Hopkins Hospital, Baltimore, Maryland, USA.
15.11.1 Cardiac myxoma. 15.11.2 Other tumours of the heart. 15.12 Cardiac involvement in genetic disease

David F. Treacher Consultant Physician in Intensive Care, St Thomas' Hospital, Guy's and St Thomas' NHS Trust, London, UK.
16.2 The circulation and circulatory support of the critically ill

A. S. Truswell Emeritus Professor of Human Nutrition, University of Sydney, New South Wales, Australia.
10.1 Diseases of overnourished societies and the need for dietary change

D. M. Turnbull Professor of Neurology, The Medical School, University of Newcastle upon Tyne, UK.
24.22.5 Mitochondrial encephalomyopathies

H. E. Turner Consultant Physician, Radcliffe Infirmary, Oxford, UK.
12.12 Hormonal manifestations of non-endocrine disease

A. Neil Turner Professor of Nephrology, Royal Infirmary, Edinburgh, UK.
20.7.8 Infection-associated nephropathies. 20.7.9 Malignancy-associated renal disease

Robert Twycross Emeritus Clinical Reader in Palliative Medicine, Oxford University, Sir Michael Sobell House, Churchill Hospital, Oxford, UK.
31 Palliative care

F. E. Udwadia Emeritus Professor of Medicine, Grant Medical College and J. J. Hospital, Bombay; Consultant Physician and Director-in-charge of ICU, Breach Candy Hospital; Consultant Physician, Parsee General hospital, Bombay, India.
7.11.20 Tetanus

S. Richard Underwood Professor of Cardiac Imaging, Imperial College of Science, Technology and Medicine, National Heart and Lung Institute, and Royal Brompton Hospital, London, UK.
15.3.5 Cardiovascular magnetic resonance and computed X-ray tomography

Robert J. Unwin Professor of Nephrology and Physiology, Centre for Nephrology, The Middlesex Hospital, London, UK.
20.13 Urinary stones, nephrocalcinosis, and renal tubular acidosis

V. Urquidi Assistant Professor, University of California San Diego Cancer Center and Department of Pathology, La Jolla, California, USA.
6.4 Tumour metastasis

J. A. Vale Director, National Poisons Information Service and West Midlands Poisons Unit, City Hospital, Birmingham, UK.
8.1 Poisoning by drugs and chemicals

* It is with regret that we report the death of Professor J. Swales during the preparation of this edition of the textbook.

P. Vallance Professor of Clinical Pharmacology and Therapeutics, Centre for Clinical Pharmacology, University College London, UK.
15.1.1.2 Vascular endothelium, its physiology and pathophysiology

J. van Gijn Professor and Chairman, Department of Neurology, University Medical Centre, Utrecht, The Netherlands.
24.13.7 Stroke: cerebrovascular disease

Sirivan Vanijanonta Emeritus Professor of Tropical Medicine, Faculty of Tropical Medicine, Mahidol University, Bangkok, Thailand.
7.16.3 Lung flukes (paragonimiasis)

Patrick J. W. Venables Professor and Honorary Consultant, Kennedy Institute Division, Imperial College London, UK.
18.10.6 Sjögren's syndrome

B. J. Vennervald Senior Research Scientist, Danish Bilharziasis Laboratory, Charlottenlund, Denmark.
7.16.1 Schistosomiasis

C. M. Verity Consultant Paediatric Neurologist and Associate Lecturer, Faculty of Medicine, University of Cambridge, Addenbrooke's Hospital, Cambridge, UK.
24.21 Developmental abnormalities of the central nervous system

M. P. Vessey Emeritus Professor of Public Health, Unit of Health Care Epidemiology, Department of Public Health, Oxford University, UK.
13.19 Benefits and risks of oral contraceptives

R. Viner Consultant in Adolescent Medicine and Endocrinology, University College London Hospitals and Great Ormond Street Hospital, UK.
29 Adolescent medicine

Peter D. Wagner Professor of Medicine and Bioengineering, University of California, San Diego, USA.
17.1.2 Structure and function of the airways and alveoli

Ann E. Wakefield* Professor of Paediatric Infectious Diseases, Department of Paediatrics, Institute of Molecular Medicine, University of Oxford, UK.
7.12.5 Pneumocystis carinii

D. H. Walker The Carmage and Martha Walls Distinguished Chair in Tropical Diseases, Professor and Chairman, Department of Pathology, and Director, WHO Collaborating Center for Tropical Diseases, Galveston, Texas, USA.
7.11.36 Rickettsial diseases including ehrlichiosis

J. A. Walker-Smith Emeritus Professor of Paediatric Gastroenterology, Royal Free and University College Medical School, London, UK.
14.14 Congenital abnormalities of the gastrointestinal tract

Mark J. Walport Professor of Medicine and Head, Division of Medicine, Faculty of Medicine, Imperial College London, Hammersmith Hospital, London, UK.
5.4 Complement

Julian R. F. Walters Reader in Gastroenterology, Imperial College of Science, Technology and Medicine, Hammersmith Campus, London, UK.
14.2.4 Investigation of gastrointestinal function. 14.9.1 Differential diagnosis and investigation of malabsorption

Gary S. Wand Professor of Medicine, Johns Hopkins University School of Medicine, Baltimore, Maryland, USA.
26.7.1 Alcohol and drug dependence

Ronald J. A. Wanders Professor of Inborn Errors and Metabolism and Deputy Head of the Laboratory for Metabolic Diseases, Academic Medical Centre, Amsterdam, The Netherlands.
11.9 Peroxisomal diseases

B. Ward Anaesthetic Registrar, Coventry School of Anaesthetics, UK.
16.6.1 Sedation and analgesia in the critically ill

T. E. Warkentin Professor, Department of Pathology and Molcular Medicine and Department of Medicine, McMaster University, Hamilton, Ontario, Canada.
22.6.5 Acquired coagulation disorders

D. A. Warrell Professor of Tropical Medicine and Infectious Diseases and Head, Nuffield Department of Clinical Medicine, University of Oxford, UK.
7.8 Travel and expedition medicine. 7.10.9 Rhabdoviruses: rabies and rabies-related viruses. 7.10.10 Colorado tick fever and other arthropod-borne reoviruses. 7.11.28 Rat-bite fevers. 7.11.30 Other borrelia infections. 7.11.32 Non-venereal treponematoses: yaws, endemic syphilis (bejel), and pinta. 7.13.2 Malaria. 7.13.5 Cryptosporidium and cryptosporidiosis. 7.18 Pentostomiasis (porocephalosis). 8.2 Injuries, envenoming, poisoning, and allergic reactions caused by animals. 24.14.1 Bacterial meningitis. 24.14.2 Viral infections of the central nervous system. 24.22.6 Tropical pyomyositis (tropical myositis). 33 Emergency medicine

M. J. Warrell Clinical Virologist, Centre for Tropical Medicine, John Radcliffe Hospital, Oxford, UK.
7.10.9 Rhabdoviruses: rabies and rabies-related viruses. 7.10.10 Colorado tick fever and other arthropod-borne reoviruses

Paul Warwicker Consultant Nephrologist, Renal Unit, Lister Hospital, Stevenage, Hertfordshire, UK.
20.10.6 Haemolytic uraemic syndrome

J. A. H. Wass Professor of Endocrinology and Consultant Physician, Radcliffe Infirmary, Oxford, UK.
12.12 Hormonal manifestations of non-endocrine disease

Laurence Watkins Consultant Neurosurgeon and Senior Lecturer, Institute of Neurology, London, UK.
24.13.18.2 Traumatic injuries of the head

George Watt Department of Medicine, AFRIMS, Bangkok, Thailand.
7.11.31 Leptospirosis. 7.11.37 Scrub typhus

Richard W. E. Watts Visiting Professor and Honorary Consultant Physician, Imperial College School of Medicine, Hammersmith Hospital, London, UK.
11.1 The inborn errors of metabolism: general aspects. 11.4 Disorders of purine and pyrimidine metabolism. 11.10 Disorders of oxalate metabolism

D. J. Weatherall Regius Professor of Medicine Emeritus, University of Oxford, Weatherall Institute of Molecular Medicine, John Radcliffe Hospital, Oxford, UK.
2.2 Scientific method and the art of healing. 22.1 Introduction. 22.5.2 Anaemia: pathophysiology, classification, and clinical features. 22.5.3 Anaemia as a world health problem. 22.5.5 Normochromic, normocytic anaemia. 22.5.7 Disorders of the synthesis or function of haemoglobin. 22.7 The blood in systemic disease

D. K. H. Webb Consultant Paediatric Haematologist, Great Ormond Street Hospital for Children, London, UK.
22.4.7 Histiocytoses

Kathryn E. Webert Clinical Scholar, Hematology and Fellow in Transfusion Medicine, Canadian Blood Services, McMaster University, Hamilton, Ontario, Canada.
22.6.3 Disorders of platelet number and function

A. D. B. Webster Consultant Immunologist, Department of Immunology, Royal Free Hospital, London, UK.
5.6 Immunodeficiency

Anthony P. Weetman Professor of Medicine and Dean, University of Sheffield Medical School, UK.
12.4 The thyroid gland and disorders of thyroid function. 12.5 Thyroid cancer

R. A. Weiss Professor, University College London, UK.
7.10.21 HIV and AIDS. 7.10.24 Viruses and cancer

Peter L. Weissberg BHF Professor of Cardiovascular Medicine, University of Cambridge, UK.
15.1.1.1 Introduction. 15.1.1.3 Vascular smooth muscle cells. 15.4.2.1 The pathophysiology of acute coronary syndromes

Peter F. Weller Professor of Medicine, Harvard Medical School; Chief of Allergy and Inflammation and Co-Chief, Infectious Diseases Division, Beth Israel Deaconess Medical Center, Boston, Massachusetts, USA.
22.4.6 Eosinophilia

A. K. Wells Consultant Respiratory Physician, Royal Brompton Hospital, London, UK.
17.11.4 The lungs and rheumatological diseases

Simon Wessely Professor of Epidemiological Psychiatry, Guy's, King's and St Thomas' School of Medicine and Institute of Psychiatry, London, UK.
26.6.2 Psychological treatment in medical practice

* It is with regret that we report the death of Professor Ann E. Wakefield during the preparation of this edition of the textbook.

Gilbert C. White, II John C. Parker Professor of Medicine and Pharmacology and Director, Center for Thrombosis and Hemostasis, University of North Carolina School of Medicine, Chapel Hill, North Carolina, USA.
22.6.1 The biology of haemostasis and thrombosis. 22.6.2 Evaluation of the patient with a bleeding diathesis

Joseph White SPHTM at TUMC, New Orleans, Louisiana, USA.
3.7.1 The cost of health care in Western countries

H. C. Whittle Visiting Professor, London School of Hygiene and Tropical Medicine and Deputy Director, MRC Laboratories, Banjul, The Gambia.
7.10.6 Measles

D. E. L. Wilcken Professor Emeritus of Medicine and Head, Cardiovascular Research Laboratory, University of New South Wales and Prince of Wales Hospital, Sydney, Australia.
15.1.3.2 Clinical physiology of the normal heart

James S. Wiley Professor and Head of Haematology, Nepean Hospital, Penrith, New South Wales, Australia.
22.5.8 Anaemias resulting from defective red cell maturation

P. J. Wilkinson Consultant Medical Microbiologist, University Hospital, Queen's Medical Centre, Nottingham, UK.
7.11.34 Listeriosis

R. G. Will Professor of Clinical Neurology, Western General Hospital, Edinburgh, UK.
24.13.9 Human prion disease

C. B. Williams Consultant Physician in Endoscopy, St Mark's Hospital for Colorectal Disorders, UK.
14.2.1 Colonoscopy and flexible sigmoidoscopy. 14.15 Tumours of the gastrointestinal tract

D. J. Williams Senior Lecturer/Honorary Consultant in Obstetric Medicine, Division of Paediatrics, Obstetrics and Gynaecology, Imperial College of Science, Technology and Medicine, Chelsea and Westminster Hospital, London, UK.
13.1 Physiological changes of normal pregnancy. 13.2 Nutrition in pregnancy. 13.3 Medical management of normal pregnancy

Gareth Williams Professor of Medicine, Department of Medicine, Clinical Sciences Centre, University Hospital Aintree, Liverpool, UK.
12.11.1 Diabetes

J. D. Williams Professor of Nephrology and Consultant Physician, Institute of Nephrology, University of Wales College of Medicine, Cardiff, UK.
20.1 Structure and function of the kidney

Paul F. Williams Consultant Nephrologist, The Ipswich Hospital NHS Trust, UK.
20.6.2 The treatment of endstage renal disease by peritoneal dialysis

Robert Wilson Consultant Physician and Reader, Royal Brompton Hospital and National Heart and Lung Institute, Imperial College of Science, Technology and Medicine, London, UK.
17.3.3 Microbiological methods in the diagnosis of respiratory infections

C. G. Winearls Consultant Nephrologist, Oxford Kidney Unit, Churchill Hospital, Oxford, UK.
20.5.1 Chronic renal failure

F. Wojnarowska Professor of Dermatology and Consultant Dermatologist, Oxford Radcliffe Hospital, Oxford, UK.
13.13 The skin in pregnancy

R. Wolman Consultant in Rheumatology and Sports Medicine, Royal National Orthopaedic Hospital, Stanmore, Middlesex, UK.
28 Sports and exercise medicine

Kathryn J. Wood Professor of Immunology, Nuffield Department of Surgery, University of Oxford, UK.
5.7 Principles of transplantation immunology

Nicholas Wood Professor of Clinical Neurology, Institute of Neurology, London, UK.
24.6.2 Neurogenetics. 24.13.12 Ataxic disorders

Trevor Woodage Clinical Investigator, Celera Genomics, Rockville, Maryland, USA.
4.1 The genomic basis of medicine

H. F. Woods Professor of Medicine, University of Sheffield, UK.
11.11 Disturbances of acid-base homeostasis

Gary P. Wormser Vice Chairman, Department of Medicine, and Chief, Division of Infectious Diseases, New York Medical College, Valhalla, New York, USA.
7.11.29 Lyme borreliosis

D. J. M. Wright Emeritus Reader in Medical Microbiology, Cell and Molecular Biology Section, Imperial College School of Medicine, London, UK.
7.11.33 Syphilis

V. M. Wright Consultant Paediatric Surgeon, Barts and The London NHS Trust, London, UK.
14.14 Congenital abnormalities of the gastrointestinal tract

F. C. W. Wu Senior Lecturer (Endocrinology), Royal Infirmary and University of Manchester, UK.
12.8.2 Disorders of male reproduction

Andrew H. Wyllie Professor and Head of Department of Pathology, University of Cambridge, UK.
4.6 Apoptosis in health and disease

M. A. S. Yasuda Professor, Department of Infectious and Parasitic Diseases, University of São Paulo Medical School, Brazil.
7.12.4 Paracoccidioidomycosis

Newman M. Yeilding Assistant Professor, University of Pennsylvania, Philadelphia, USA.
4.3 Molecular cell biology

Jenny Yiend Postdoctoral Research Assistant, MRC Cognition and Brain Science Unit, Cambridge, UK.
26.5.1 Grief, stress, and post-traumatic stress disorder

V. Zaman Professor, Department of Microbiology, The Aga Khan University, Karachi, Pakistan.
7.13.7 Sarcocystosis. 7.14.6 Other gut nematodes. 7.14.7 Toxocariasis and visceral larva migrans

11

Metabolic disorders

11.1 The inborn errors of metabolism: general aspects

Richard W. E. Watts

There are around three to four thousand known unifactorially inherited diseases, that is familial diseases, the inheritance of which can be described as being autosomal recessive, autosomal dominant, sex-linked recessive, or sex-linked dominant (Mendelian inheritance). The inborn errors of metabolism are those inherited diseases in which the phenotype includes a characteristic constellation of chemical abnormalities that can be ascribed to an alteration in the catalytic activity of a single specific enzyme. There are unifactorially inherited diseases in which the current techniques are too insensitive for a chemical abnormality to be identified, so that the syndrome has to be defined in clinical, gross structural, and/or pathological terms; further study may bring these into the category of inborn errors of metabolism.

Almost all the unifactorially inherited diseases arise from mutations in the nuclear genome which spans about three billion base pairs of deoxyribonucleic acid (**DNA**). A few mitochondrial proteins have their structures encoded in the mitochondrial DNA (**mtDNA**). This genetic information is transmitted only through the female line and the category of inborn errors of metabolism includes this group. Both the nuclear and the mitochondrially inherited diseases stem from single mutations within a cistron (the functional unit of DNA) which directs the synthesis of a single specific polypeptide chain. The molecular changes in the enzyme protein may affect the primary, secondary, tertiary, or quaternary structure, decreasing, increasing, or abolishing its catalytic activity. Some mutations affect the function of an activator protein, others reduce the binding of hormones and paracrine factors to cell surfaces and/or subcellular structures, and some derange the migration of proteins within cells; another group impairs the transport of metabolites across cellular and subcellular membranes (Table 1). Most intracellular enzymes are located in the cytosol where they are correctly orientated in relation to one another, sometimes as macromolecular complexes, and to their substrates. Some are bound to cellular and subcellular membranes and a minority are located in anatomically defined subcellular structures or organelles: the mitochondria, lysosomes, and peroxisomes.

Mitochondrial diseases

The mitochondrial genome is a circular double strand containing 16.5 kilobases of DNA. It encodes 13 of the respiratory chain enzymes the remainder of which, about 60, are encoded in the nuclear DNA. Abnormal mitochondrial function impairs the supply of energy for biochemical work in all tissues and therefore has wide-ranging effects. Each mitochondrion also contains 24 RNA genes that participate in intramitochondrial protein synthesis. Transcription and translation of mtDNA are regulated by the nucleus through the non-coding D-loop region of the mitochondrial genome. Human cells contain about a thousand copies of mtDNA, but the individual mitochondria in a cell may not all carry a given specific mutation and different cells carry different proportions of mutated mitochondria (heteroplasmy). The proportion of mutant mtDNA must exceed a critical level before the mitochondrial respiratory chain disease declares itself. This variability, as well as tissue-specific differences in dependence on oxidative metabolism, explains, at least partially, why some tissues are preferentially affected in patients with mtDNA diseases. Postmitotic tissues (e.g. neurones, muscle, endocrine tissues) have high levels of mutated mtDNA and are often clinically affected, whereas rapidly dividing tissues (e.g. bone marrow) are less often clinically affected. Differences in the proportions of mutated and non-mutated mtDNA between and within family members also contribute to the wide phenotypic range encountered in the mitochondrial diseases. The spermatozoal cytoplasm, including its mitochondria, is entirely lost at fertilization and, for this reason, mitochondrial diseases are only transmitted through the female line. Clinically affected women rarely transmit a mtDNA deletion to their children. However, a woman with a heteroplasmic mtDNA point mutation or duplication may

Table 1 Examples of diseases in which there is defective transport of an enzyme or metabolite within cells or across cell membranes

Disease	Metabolic abnormality
Cystinuria	Failure to transport cystine, lysine, ornithine, arginine, and homoarginine across the plasma membrane of the proximal renal tubular epithelium and the small intestinal mucosa
Cystinosis (cystine storage disease, Lignac's disease)	Failure to transport cystine produced by intralysosomal proteolysis across the lysosomal membrane and into the cytosol
Salla disease	Failure to transport N-acetylneuraminic acid (sialic acid) across the lysosomal membrane and into the cytosol
The mucopolysacchridoses	Failure to degrade glycosaminolycans (mucopolysaccharides), the undegraded mucopolysaccharides being neither transportable across lysosomal membranes nor capable of being removed from the lysosomes by exocytosis
Tay–Sachs disease	Defective post-translational processing of the alpha chain of β-N-acetylhexosaminidase (hexosaminidase A). This prevents the enzyme from migrating from the endoplasmic reticulum, where it is glycosylated, to the Golgi apparatus for phosphorylation of its mannosyl residues and hence to lysosomes and the exterior of the cell
Primary hyperoxaluria type 1 (some cases)	Mislocation of alanine: glyoxylate aminotransferase in mitochondria as opposed to its normal location in peroxisomes. This arises because a rare mutation (Gly 170 → Arg) is present simultaneously with the common polymorphism (Pro 11 → Leu). The mutation (Gly 170 → Arg) prevents dimerization of the molecule which, in turn, allows the weak mitochondrial targeting sequence generated by the polymorphism (Pro 11 → Leu) to direct the molecule to mitochondria instead of peroxisomes

Table 2 The main clinical manifestations of diseases due to mitochondrial dysfunction

Disease group	Clinical manifestations
Defects of fatty acid oxidation	Hypoglycaemia
	Hepatic dysfunction
	Cardiac failure
	Myopathy
	Sudden infant death
Respiratory chain disorders	Lactic acidosis
	Encephalopathy
	Hypotonia
	Poor feeding
	Failure to thrive
	Convulsions

transmit a variable amount of mutated mtDNA to her progeny. The number of mtDNA molecules in each oocyte is reduced and then amplified to a total of about 10^5 during early development of the oocyte; this, presumably random, process contributes to the different amounts of mutated mtDNA in different children in the same family. Women whose gametes contain high concentrations of mtDNA are more likely to have clinically affected children than mothers with lower levels of mtDNA. The general clinical manifestations of the mitochondrial diseases are shown in Table 2 and specific examples of mitochondrial diseases are given in Table 3.

Table 3 Some mitochondrial diseases. (Data from Chinnery PF and Turnbull DM (1999) *The Lancet* **354** (supplement 1), S17–S21)

Mitochondrial DNA defects

Rearrangements (deletions and duplications)
- Chronic progressive external ophthalmoplegia
- Kearns Sayre syndrome (hypoparathyroidism with deafness)
- Diabetes and deafness

Point mutations in protein encoding genes
- Leber's hereditary optic neuropathy
- Leber's hereditary optic neuropathy/dystonia
- Neurogenic weakness, ataxia, and retinitis pigmentosa
- Leigh's syndrome*

Point mutations in tRNA genes
- Mitochondrial encephalopathy with lactic acidosis and stroke-like episodes
- Myoclonic epilepsy with ragged-red fibres
- Myopathy
- Cardiomyopathy
- Diabetes and deafness
- Encephalomyopathy
- Leigh's syndrome*

Point mutations in rRNA genes
- Non-syndromic sensorineural deafness
- Aminoglycoside-induced non-syndromic deafness

Nuclear DNA defects

Nuclear genetic disorders with a mitochondrial basis
- Friedreich's ataxia (frataxin)
- Autosomal recessive hereditary spastic paraplegia

Nuclear genetic disorders of the mitochondrial respiratory chain
- Leigh's syndrome (complex I deficiency)*
- Optic atrophy and ataxia
- Leigh's syndrome (complex IV deficiency)*

Nuclear genetic disorders associated with multiple mtDNA deletions
- Autosomal dominant external ophthalmoplegia
- Mitochondrial neurogastrointestinal encephalomyopathy (thymidine phosphorylase deficiency)

*An example of different mutations providing the same clinical syndrome (phenocopies).
Abbreviations: tRNA = transfer RNA; rRNA = ribosomal RNA; mtDNA = mitochondrial DNA.

Table 4 Peroxisomal diseases

Zellweger syndrome (absent peroxisomal membranes)
Pseudo-Zellweger syndrome
Adrenoleucodystrophy
Pseudo-neonatal adrenoleucodystrophy
Acatalasia
Infantile Refsum's disease
Refsum's disease (classical form)
Hyperpipecolic acidaemia
X-linked adrenoleucodystrophy
Chondrodysplasia punctatum rhizomelia
Primary hyperoxaluria type 1

Peroxisomal diseases

Some enzymes that are encoded in the nuclear DNA are specifically expressed in peroxisomes, to which they are imported soon after translation. Mutations in the relevant genes result in the diseases listed in Table 4.

Lysosomal storage diseases

Lysosomes are subcellular organelles containing hydrolases with low optimum pH values ('acid hydrolases') which catalyse the degradation of macromolecules. The macromolecules are either derived from the metabolic turnover of structural cellular components or have entered the cell by endocytosis. The products of this macromolecular degradation process leave the lysosomes by specific efflux processes.

In most of the lysosomal storage diseases an inborn error of metabolism affects a specific lysosomal enzyme so that either undegraded or partially degraded macromolecules accumulate in the lysosomes. The engorged lysosomes distort the internal architecture of the cell, disturb its function, and inhibit the activities of other lysosomal enzymes so that macromolecules other than those related to the primary enzyme deficiency also accumulate.

Cystinosis (cystine storage disease) and Salla disease (*N*-acetylneuraminic (sialic) acid storage disease) are due to metabolic lesions involving the specific efflux processes whereby these two low molecular weight products of macromolecule metabolism (cystine and sialic acid respectively) leave the lysosome (Table 1).

Lysosomal enzymes are glycoproteins which are subject to exocytosis and re-uptake by endocytosis. Their protein moieties are synthesized on the rough endoplasmic reticulum and the oligosaccharide side chains are added in the Golgi apparatus. The addition of a terminal mannose-6-phosphate residue recognition marker is necessary if the enzyme molecule is to be correctly routed into the lysosomes, and if it is to be available for receptor mediated re-uptake from the interstitial fluids. The types of lysosomal storage diseases and the nature of their metabolic defects together with examples of each group are presented in Table 5.

Heterogeneity in the inborn errors of metabolism

The individual inborn errors of metabolism are defined on the basis of the phenotype, including the specific enzyme lesion, and by their pattern of inheritance. Close study of any particular inborn error of metabolism reveals unexpected heterogeneity. This is due to:

- Multiple allelism.
- Mutations at different gene loci affecting the structure of different polypeptide chains in a single enzyme protein.
- Mutations at different gene loci affecting different proteins with similar catalytic functions.

Table 5 Lysosomal storage diseases other than cystinosis and Salla disease (a complete listing of these diseases and their biochemistry is given in Watts and Gibbs (1986))

Name	Defect	Example
Sphingolipidoses	Failure to degrade compounds containing a sphingoid [sphinoglipids, ceramides, sphingomyelins and glycosphingolipids including the gangliosides (sialoglycosphingolipids)]	Tay-Sachs disease (GM2-gangliosidosis) Gaucher disease (glucocerebrosidosis)
Mucopolysaccharidoses	Failure to degrade the glycosaminoglycans: dermatan, heparan, and keratan sulphates. Incompletely degraded glycosaminoglycan fragments accumulate in the lysosomes as well as extracellularly. This causes secondary deficiencies of other lysosomal enzymes and other undegraded macromolecules, particularly sphingolipids, accumulate	Hurler disease Hunter disease Morquio disease
Glycoproteinoses	A group of enzyme defects in the catabolism of glycoproteins in which characteristic abnormal macromolecules accumulate	Fucisidosis Mannosidosis
Acid lipase deficiency	Two clinically distinct variants. Cholesteryl esters and triglycerides accumulate in most tissues due to deficiency of lysosomal acid lipase	Wohlman's disease Cholesteryl ester storage disease
Glycogenosis II	Lack of intralysosomal hydrolysis of glycogen	Glycogenosis type II (only member of this group)
Mucolipidoses	Originally defined as being clinically intermediate between the sphingolipidoses and mucopolysaccharidoses but without mucopolysacchariduria (abnormal glycosaminoglycan excretion). Subsequently shown to include patients with (i) deficient neuraminidase activities with respect to either glycoprotein substrates (mucolipidosis I, also classified as a glycoproteinosis and termed sialidosis) or ganglioside substrates (mucolipidosis IV); (ii) clinically mild and severe variants of uridine-diphosphate-N-acetylglucosamine: lysosomal enzyme precursor N-acetylglucosamine phosphate transferase (mucolipidoses II (I-cell disease) and III (pseudo-Hurler polydystrophy) respectively)	See opposite

- Differences in the overall genetic background against which the single mutation acts.
- Environmental factors.

Clinical pointers towards a diagnosis of an inborn error of metabolism

Although the symptoms of metabolic disease may appear vague and protean, and an inherited disease cannot be diagnosed in the absence of an appropriate family history, some clinical settings suggest the presence of an inborn error of metabolism (Table 6). In taking the family history special inquiries should be made about affected siblings, possible parental consanguinity, paternity, miscarriages, perinatal deaths, abortions, about the sexes of possibly affected relatives and their placement on the maternal or paternal side of the family, the ages at death of relatives, as well as the ethnic and geographical origins of the parents.

General approaches to the treatment of inborn errors of metabolism

The treatments available for the individual inborn errors of metabolism cover a wide range and may need to be specially developed for individual patients. However, the principles involved can be broadly classified as in Table 7. Palliative surgical and other measures may be needed to deal with specific complications (for example corneal grafting to restore vision in patients with corneal clouding due to one of the mucopolysacchridoses). Consideration should also be given to meeting the educational and social needs of these patients as well as to optimizing their overall clinical state and correcting the biochemical parameters. The successful management of patients with inborn errors of metabolism requires a multidisciplinary approach which utilizes the special skills of dieticians, social workers, educationalists, and occupational therapists as well as those of physicians, sur-

Table 6 Clinical presentation which, in the absence of acquired or other congenital causes, suggest an inborn error or metabolism

- Unexplained acute neonatal illness and/or failure to thrive in early infancy. (Marked muscle hypotonia, recurrent fits, comas, acidosis, and vomiting, especially if withholding milk feeds causes temporary improvement, are especially suggestive)
- Developmental slowing and arrest followed by retrogression
- Developmental slowing and arrest leading to unexplained mental handicap
- Unusual physiognomy, multiple skeletal deformities with developmental delay and retrogression
- Multiple skeletal deformities alone (dysostosis multiplex especially suggests a lysosomal storage disease)
- Gross visceromegaly
- Specific dietary intolerances
- Haemolytic anaemia
- Unusual body odour*
- Urolithiasis
- Cataracts in early life†
- Dislocation of the optic lens‡
- Persistent jaundice and hepatic cirrhosis in infancy.
- Abnormal cutaneous photosensitivity
- Hypopigmentation
- Abnormal drug sensitivity
- A history of recurrent perinatal deaths and/or stillbirths
- Hydrops fetalis in the absence of blood group incompatibility between mother and fetus (red cell enzyme defects)

*Examples are: phenylketonuria (mousy, musty) branched chain ketoacidosis (maple syrup), methionine malabsorption (oast house, dry celery), isovaleric acidaemia (sweaty feet), methylaminuria (stale fish), multiple carboxylase deficiency (tom cat's urine), Hawkinsinuria (swimming pool).

†Examples are: Fabry's disease, galactosaemia, galactokinase deficiency, Lowe's syndrome, mannosidosis, osteogenesis imperfecta, Refsum's disease, Wilson's disease.

‡Examples are: Ehler's–Danlos syndrome, homocystinuria, hyperlysinuria, Marfan's syndrome, sulphite oxidase deficiency.

geons, biochemists, and geneticists. It is particularly important to plan for the handover of specialist care from the paediatrician to the most appropriate adult physician when follow-up in a paediatric department becomes inappropriate. The perfect outcome is to achieve a physically and mentally normal adult who is capable of begetting normal children. Unfortunately the nature of many of the inborn errors of metabolism mitigates against the attainment of this ideal so that treatment has to aim at optimizing the child's potential in all its physical, mental, and social aspects. Treatment

Table 7 General approaches to the treatment of inborn errors of metabolism

Method	Examples
Restriction of a dietary substrate which cannot be metabolized	Phenylalanine restriction in phenylketonuria
	Protein restriction in the hyperamonaemias
	Elimination of galactose in galactosaemia
	Ultraviolet radiation (congenital erythropoietic and variegate porphyrias, and in albinism)
	Ionizing radiation in the DNA repair enzyme defects (xeroderma pigmentosum, ataxia telangiectasia)
	Infections (agammaglobinaemia).
	Medications (oestrogens, barbiturates etc. in acute intermittent porphyria)
Replacement of a missing metabolic product	Orotic aciduria: treatment by uridine which is metabolized to uridylic acid
	Hartnup disease: nicotinic acid to control skin manifestations
Removal of toxic metabolite	Haemodialysis and peritoneal dialysis as temporary treatment of an acute metabolic crisis due to a diffusible toxic metabolite, and to correct certain secondary biochemical abnormalities quickly
	Either specific chemical detoxication (e.g. penicillamine in Wilson's disease) or solubilization (e.g. penicillamine in cystinuria)
Pharmacological doses of a cofactor (only some cases of each disease respond)	Propionic acidaemia: biotin
	Ubidecarenone (respiratory chain disorders due to coenzyme Q_{10} deficiency
	Homocystinuria: pyridoxine
	Primary hyperoxaluria (type I): pyridoxine
	Methylmalonic acidaemia: vitamin B_{12}
Replacement of a missing gene product	Adenosine diaminase deficiency
	Gaucher disease: β-glucocerebosidase
	Haemophilia: clotting factor VIII
Bone marrow transplantation	Adenosine deaminase deficiency
Haematopoeitic stem cell transplantation	Adenosine deaminase deficiency
Liver transplantation	Hereditary tyrosinaemia (type I)
	Antitrypsin deficiency
	Primary hyperoxaluria (type I)
	Urea cycle disorders
	Criglar Najjar syndrome (type I)
Gene replacement	None so far (this is currently a very active research area)

The examples chosen are situations in which either the proposed treatment is established or in which it can be recommended as elective therapy even though the results of prolonged evaluation are still awaited.

and support also have to be extended to the parents and siblings who, if not overtly affected themselves, may be carriers of the abnormal gene concerned and require appropriate advice about the genetic and other aspects of the disease.

The ability to clone human genes into bacteria and yeasts which can then produce large amounts of the human gene product is widening the horizons for future treatment by enzyme administration. The development of macrophage-targeted β-glucocerebosidase enzyme replacement therapy for Gaucher disease (glucosylceramidase deficiency) type I is a notable recent development in this field and is now regarded as the definitive line of treatment. Attempts to utilize transplanted fibroblasts and amniotic cells as a source for enzyme replacement therapy have not been successful. Bone marrow transplantation has been used for the treatment of two groups of inherited metabolic disorders: those in which it is desired to replace a particular type of non-functioning bone marrow cell by its normally functioning counterpart and those in which an attempt has been made to utilize the fact that the bone marrow produces 50 to 100 g of polymorphonuclear leucocytes per day and that these cells exocytose (release) their lysosomal enzymes for endocytic uptake by enzyme-deficient cells in the body tissues generally. This strategy has been more successful with the first group of diseases, which includes disorders of neutrophil function (e.g. cyclic neutropenia), functional abnormalities of lymphocytes, and osteopetrosis. The beneficial effect on the last disease is due to the introduction of normal osteoclast precursors. The results in the second group of diseases, namely those in which the white cell lineage derived from the transplanted bone marrow is used to supply normal enzyme to enzyme-deficient tissues, for example Hurler disease (mucopolysaccharidosis IH) and metachromatic leucodystrophy, have been less successful particularly in terms of neurological function. Haemopoietic stem cells have been implanted into the fetus *in utero* to correct severe congenital immunodeficiency but this has not, so far, been applied to diseases without immunodeficiency. This procedure takes advantage of the immunological tolerance of the fetus. The possibility of using liposomes and resealed erythrocyte envelopes as carriers of therapeutic enzymes is also being explored.

Liver transplantation is used as a sophisticated form of enzyme replacement therapy in some inborn errors of metabolism where this organ is the specific site of the metabolic lesion. Liver transplantation has the advantage that the enzyme is introduced in the correct organ, the correct cell with its correct subcellular location, and correctly orientated with respect to its substrate and other enzymes with which it must act in concert. Liver transplantation can also be regarded as a form of gene replacement therapy in that the donor liver contains the normal gene which will direct the synthesis of a normal enzyme protein. Prenatal transplantation of fetal liver stem cells has potential in the treatment of some inborn errors of metabolism. Successful engraftment at the 12th to 24th week postfertilization with partial correction of the metabolic defect has been demonstrated in β-thalassemia. Treatment by gene replacement, using retroviral vectors and gene constructs to introduce the desired DNA sequence into the patient's explanted haemopoietic stem cell genome, these genetically corrected cells being cultured and then returned to the patient's circulation, may have some potential in diseases where expression of the metabolic lesion in the haemopoietic system determines the phenotype, or in those situations where genetically corrected migratory cells of haemopoietic origin can deliver normal enzyme to the enzyme-deficient tissues. Although somatic cell gene therapy possibly using viral vectors and/or gene constructs to introduce the desired DNA sequences into other cell types is currently being investigated extensively in *in vitro* model systems and in animal models of some human inborn errors of metabolism using, for example, hepatocytes, none of these have reached application in clinical practice. For example, the possibility of using herpes simplex virus type 1 as a means of introducing corrected genes into the nervous system is being explored. Another approach is to use either resealed erythrocyte cell membranes or liposomes as carriers of therapeutic enzymes. Thus, although there are some prospects of correcting some enzyme defects in the somatic cell genome, the correction of defects in the germline seems remote although the development of advanced *in vitro* fertilization techniques, preimplantation DNA analysis, gene transfer, insertion or conversion, and embryo implantation procedures may render this judgement premature. Ethical objections to human germline modifications are also being raised, and could lead to this work being discontinued.

Screening for inborn errors of metabolism

The realization that very early diagnosis is essential in order to achieve good results in the treatment of some inborn errors of metabolism, such as phenylketonuria and galactosaemia, has stimulated interest in the possibility of examining either whole populations or selected groups of predisposed individuals for the biochemical differences which characterize particular inherited metabolic diseases. Diagnosis is needed at a stage which is not only presymptomatic but which precedes the onset of self-perpetuating secondary pathological changes.

Screening for inborn errors of metabolism may be either non-selective (whole population) or selective. The latter, which includes carrier detection studies, aims to cover a part of the population. This may be defined on clinical, genetic, ethnic, or geographical grounds. Phenylketonuria and congenital hypothyroidism are the only members of this group of disorders for which neonatal whole-population screening is generally practised, although the inclusion of galactosaemia, cystic fibrosis, and congenital adrenal hyperplasia (21-hydroxylase deficiency) has been proposed. Whole-population screening should only be established for treatable or preventable diseases, and the consistency of the association of the proposed biochemical or other marker and the serious clinical phenotype must have been proved beyond any doubt. There must be a reliable and robust analytical method suitable for use with a sample of blood or urine which can be obtained without distressing either the parents or the baby. The possibility that metabolic screening will bring to light previously unrecognized variants, which are either mild and do not require treatment, or which by virtue of a fundamentally different biochemical lesion will resist the currently established therapies, has to be borne in mind. Phenylketonuria illustrates these problems. Here, beside classical phenylketonuria, whole-population screening has identified both the clinically unimportant essential (mild) hyperphenylalaninaemia, and the devastatingly serious, but treatable, inborn errors of tetrahydrobiopterin synthesis which produce the 'malignant' hyperphenylalaninaemia syndrome. It is also possible that in some cases immediate postnatal screening and treatment may be too late to prevent minor manifestations of the disease, (e.g. in congenital hypothyroidism).

The incidence of disease which merits whole-population screening should be at least similar to that of phenylketonuria in Caucasians (between 1 in 6000 and 1 in 12 000). Cystic fibrosis has an incidence of 1 in 2500 (gene frequency 1 in 25) in Caucasians and would merit neonatal whole-population screening on this basis. Molecular genetic approaches are potentially useful. If the disease is not too genetically heterogeneous and when the full range of possible causative mutations is known the specific mutation could be sought directly. Otherwise, after DNA amplification the mutational change in the DNA structure could be detected either by the presence of a restriction endonuclease site or by probing with another primer that hybridizes with only one of the alleles. An appreciable proportion of individuals classified as being homozygotes on the basis of classical genetic analysis prove to be double heterozygotes, that is they carry two different mutations in the same gene. The number of inborn metabolic errors in which the affected individuals and the heterozygous carriers can be identified by molecular genetic analysis is increasing rapidly. It includes such numerically important diseases as sickle cell anaemia, β-thalassaemia, haemophilia, Duchenne muscular dystrophy, cystic fibrosis, and phenylketonuria, as well as rarer but devastating conditions such as the Lesch–Nyhan syndrome.

Prenatal diagnosis

The procedures used in prenatal diagnosis are:

- Direct examination of the fetus by ultrasonography and fetoscopy.
- Chemical analysis of amniotic fluid.
- Biochemical and cytological analysis of cultured amniotic cells (amniocytes) obtained by amniocentesis at the fifteenth to sixteenth week of pregnancy.
- DNA analysis on uncultured amniocytes.
- Karyotypic enzymological and DNA analysis of chorionic villi obtained by biopsy at the eighth to tenth week of pregnancy.
- Biochemical studies on tissue obtained by biopsying the fetus *in utero*.

Carrier state diagnosis

Carriers are either individuals carrying the gene for a recessive disorder, which does not express itself in the heterozygous state (e.g. phenylketonuria), or those who carry the gene for a dominant disorder, that is one which does express itself in the heterozygous state, but in which symptoms occur in later life (e.g. Huntington's chorea (Huntington's disease)).

The general approaches to carrier state diagnosis are:

- The detection of minor clinical, radiological, and clinicopathological abnormalities.
- The demonstration of levels of enzyme activity in tissue (e.g. leucocytes or cultured fibroblasts) which are intermediate between those observed in individuals homozygous for the abnormal and the normal forms of the enzyme respectively (the observed level of activity may not be exactly 50 per cent of the normal value).
- The demonstration of intermediate levels of a characteristic metabolite in an accessible body fluid.
- The demonstration of mosaicism with respect to the product of the mutant gene on the X chromosome in the case of sex-linked recessive disorders.
- Direct gene analysis using either a specific gene probe or a linked restriction fragment length polymorphism.

The ability to recognize asymptomatic carriers of serious recessive diseases and presymptomatic individuals in the case of dominant disorders raises major ethical and social issues with respect to the psychological impact that this information will have on the affected individuals and their families. This is especially so with the clinically normal carriers of a crippling, lethal, and untreatable disease such as Huntington's chorea.

In vitro fertilization and the inborn errors of metabolism

The human embryo produced by *in vitro* fertilization can be biopsied at a very early stage of development (i.e. at the eight-cell stage). A single cell is removed and examined for the DNA mutation responsible for the disease which the parents are known to be carrying. This enables only fertilized ova which do not carry the mutant gene to be implanted.

Animal genetic models of inborn errors of metabolism in man

Animal genetic models of the inborn errors of metabolism can be useful in the early stages of investigating new approaches to treatment before attempting to transfer these to man. It is also possible to investigate the pathophysiology of the diseases at different stages of their evolution more easily, rapidly, and predictably than if one has to rely entirely on the *ad hoc* availability of clinical and pathological material. However, there are obvious limitations when cognitive and behavioural abnormalities are part of the clinical phenotype.

Further reading

Bax BE *et al.* (1999). Survival of human carrier erythrocytes *in vivo*. *Clinical Science* **96**, 171–8 [Important advance in method for possible enzyme replacement.]

Billings PR, Hubbard R, Newman SA (1999). Human germ line modification: a dissent. *Lancet* **353**, 1873–5. [A critical review.]

Brooks DA (1997). Protein processing: a role in the pathophysiology of genetic disease. *FEBS Letters* **409**, 115–20. [A full review of the field.]

Chan L, Teng BB, Lau P (1996). Apolipoprotein B mRNA editing protein: a tool for dissecting lipoprotein metabolism and a potential therapeutic gene for hypercholesterolaemia. *Zeitschrift für Gastroenterologie* **34** (Suppl. 3), 31–2. [Example of a current tool.]

Chinnery PF, Turnbull DM (1999). Mitochondrial DNA and disease. *Lancet* **354** (Suppl. 1), S17–S21. [Comprehensive review.]

Cox TM (2001). Gaucher's disease – an exemplary monogenic disorder. *Quarterly Journal of Medicine* **94**, 399–402. [A fully up-to-date review of clinical, biochemical, and therapeutic aspects.]

Eisensmith RC, Woo SLC (1996). Gene therapy for phenylketonuria. *European Journal of Pediatrics* **155** (Suppl. I), S16–S19. [Review of situation in a disease which is a prototype for future research.]

Graeber MB, Muller U (1998). Recent developments in the molecular genetics of mitochondrial disorders. *Journal of the Neurological Sciences* **153**, 251–63. [Review of a currently expanding field.]

Haskins M (1996). Bone marrow transplantation therapy for metabolic diseases: animal models as predictors of success in *in utero* approaches. *Bone Marrow Transplantation* **18** (Suppl. 3), S25–S27. [A short review.]

Hegele RA (1997). Small genetic effects in complex diseases: a review of regulatory sequence variants in dyslipoproteinemia and atherosclerosis. *Clinical Biochemistry* **30**, 183–8.

Khanna A *et al.* (1999). Liver transplantation for metabolic liver disease. *Surgical Clinics of North America* **79**, 153–62. [Review concentrating on general principles as exemplified by hereditary haemochromatosis and Wilson's disease.]

Lachmann RH, Efstathiou S (1999). Use of herpes simplex virus type I for transgene expression within the nervous system. *Clinical Science* **96**, 533–41. [An example of a modern approach.]

Leonard JV, Schapira AHV (2000). Mitochondrial respiratory chain disorders. *Lancet* **355**, 299–304 and 389–94.

Leonard JV, Grünewald B, Clayton P (2001). Diversity of congenital disorders of glycosylation. *Lancet* **357**, 1382–3.

Lowenstein PR *et al.* (1998). Gene therapy for inherited neurological disorders: towards therapeutic intervention in the Lesch–Nyham syndrome. *Progress in Brain Research* **117**, 485–501. [Reviews strategies for gene therapy in neurological diseases as exemplified by work on the Lesch–Nyhan syndrome.]

Sandig V, Strauss M (1996). Liver-directed gene transfer and application to therapy. *Journal of Molecular Medicine* **74**, 205–12. [Review article.]

Smith AE (1999). Gene therapy—where are we? *Lancet* **354** (Suppl. I), S1–S3. [Critical appraisal of the subject.]

Surbek DV *et al.* (1997). Intrauterine transplantation of hematopoietic stem cells for therapy of genetic diseases. *Zeitschrift für Geburtshilfe und Neonatologie* **201**, 158–70. [Report of position at time of writing.]

Touraine JL (1996). *In utero* transplantation of fetal liver stem cells into human fetuses. *Journal of Haematotherapy* **5**, 195–9. [A potentially important therapeutic area.]

Vogler C *et al.* (1998). Murine mucopolysaccharidosis VII: the impact of therapies on the clinical course and pathology in a murine model of lysosomal disease. *Journal of Inherited Metabolic Disease* **21**, 575–86.

Watts RWE, Gibbs DA (1986). Animal genetic models of some inborn errors of metabolism which occur in man. In: Watts RWE, Gibbs DA, eds. *Lysosomal storage diseases: biochemical and clinical aspects*, pp.235-6. Taylor and Francis, London.

Winchester B (1999). Outlook for screening for sphingolipidoses. *Lancet* **354**, 879–88.

11.2 Inborn errors of amino acid and organic acid metabolism

P. J. Lee and D. P. Brenton

History

Following the early insights of Garrod and pioneers such as Følling, it was the use of paper chromatography by Dent and the automated column chromatography of Moore and Stein which led to modern developments in the field of inborn errors of metabolism. The laboratory contributed more discoveries with the advent of gas–liquid chromatography and later mass spectroscopy. More recently the rise of genetics and molecular biology have revolutionized the field and now tandem mass spectroscopy is proving a powerful tool in screening and diagnosis. The inborn errors of metabolism has been a spectacularly developing field for several decades and provides vivid examples of the successful application of molecular cell biology to the diagnosis and treatment of human disease.

Introduction

An overview of amino acid metabolism and genetic defects

Humans depend upon dietary protein as a source of amino acids; some amino acids cannot be synthesized in the human body, and all are used very economically. Stool nitrogen losses are only about 1 g/day and bacterial protein accounts for much of this. Renal conservation of amino acids is extremely effective, with low clearance values (Table 1). Amino acids taken in excess of requirement are not stored but are used for energy. After the removal of the amino group for conversion to ammonia and urea (Fig. 1), the carbon skeletons degrade to major metabolic intermediates such as acetyl coenzyme A, acetoacetyl coenzyme A, pyruvate, or to citric acid cycle intermediates (Fig. 2) via individual amino acid pathways. Amino acids are referred to as glucogenic when their carbon skeletons degrade to intermediates used in gluconeogenesis and ketogenic when their degradation products can form ketone bodies. Degradative enzymes frequently have important coenzymes and inherited defects of catabolism may be due to defects of the apoenzymes or their vitamin coenzymes. Table 2 shows one biochemical classification of the genetic defects of amino acid metabolism. A clinical classification would be more practical but is difficult because of the non-specific nature of many clinical features, for example mental retardation.

Nitrogen balance and dietary treatment

Some biochemical defects such as homocystinuria respond well to vitamin (coenzyme) supplementation and others are treated by diet. Generalized moderate protein restriction is a usual approach to urea cycle defects and one or two other diseases, but very specific restriction of one or two amino acids applies crucially to a small number of essential amino acid disorders. Thirty years ago Rose and colleagues defined the eight essential amino acids in adults (Table 3) and the minimum daily requirements for sustaining nitrogen balance. This also requires an additional intake of 'non-essential' amino acid nitrogen and an adequate calorie intake. Histidine and taurine may be essential in the neonate. Dietary restriction can be used to treat specific metabolic defects of essential amino acids but is unlikely to be successful for disorders of non-essential amino acid metabolism.

Almost all ingested protein in the infant (recommended intake about 2 g/kg/day) is utilized in the synthesis of new protein for growth. This persistent anabolic state, however, is easily upset by intercurrent infection, starvation, trauma, or surgery, with a rapid swing to a catabolic state and negative nitrogen balance. The amino acids released from protein hydrolysis increase the load on urea formation and their normal pathways of intermediary metabolism. This renders infants and young children prone to frequent clinical illness with some amino acid disorders. In adults an intake of natural protein of 60 to 80 g/day is probably about twice that needed to maintain nitrogen balance and health. Adults are less prone to become catabolic than infants but the same circumstances may nevertheless precipitate it. In addition periods of particular risk include late adolescence when the growth spurt ceases and the postpartum period. Insulin and glucose can be used to reverse a catabolic state and produce positive nitrogen balance in some inborn errors.

Amino acid transport defects

General pathophysiology

Historically, the renal tubular aspects of amino acid transport have been of major importance following Dent's (1948) successful introduction into

Table 1 Plasma amino acid values, excretion, and clearances in young adult males and females (authors' data). Cystine expressed as 0.5 mol (molecular weight = 120)

Amino acid (mean) (ml/min/1.73 m²)	Plasma range (mmol/l)	Mean	Excretion (mean) (mmol/min)	Clearance
Taurine	65–179	100	0.54	5.8
Aspartic	17–51	36	0.04	1.3
Threonine	111–236	143	0.09	0.7
Serine	114–210	159	020	1.4
Glutamic	73–296	182	0.29	0.1
Glutamine	332–652	441	0.02	0.7
Glycine	180–311	246	0.64	2.6
Alanine	212–407	325	0.16	0.5
½ Cystine	14–38	26	0.04	2.0
Valine	152–270	217	0.03	0.2
Methionine	13–41	24	0.01	0.5
Isoleucine	47–58	66	0.01	0.5
Leucine	83–163	129	0.05	0.04
Tyrosine	33–79	62	0.05	0.9
Phenylalanine	54–78	64	0.05	0.8
Histidine	88–128	92	0.44	4.2
Ornithine	92–194	130	0.02	0.1
Lysine	91–170	122	0.05	0.4
Arginine	27–91	57	0.05	0.9

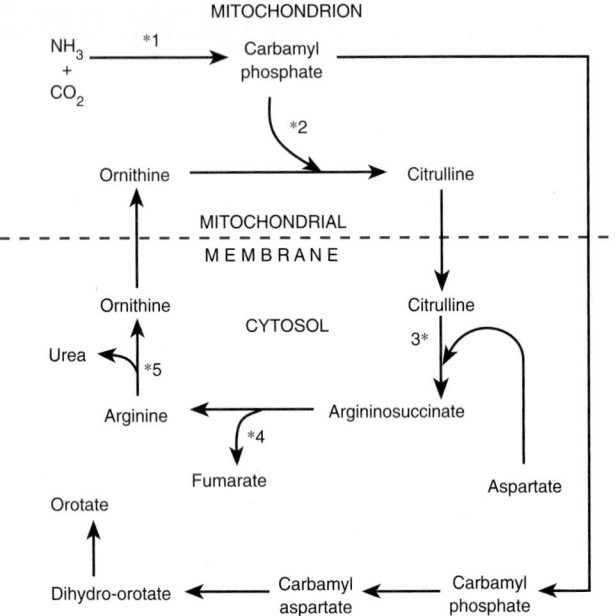

Fig. 1 The urea cycle functions partly in the mitochondrion and partly in the cytosol. Carbamyl phosphate, if it accumulates, may be diverted to orotic acid synthesis. Asterisked enzymes are: 1, carbamyl phosphate synthetase; 2, ornithine transcarbamylase; 3, argininosuccinate synthetase; 4, argininosuccinate lyase; and 5, arginase.

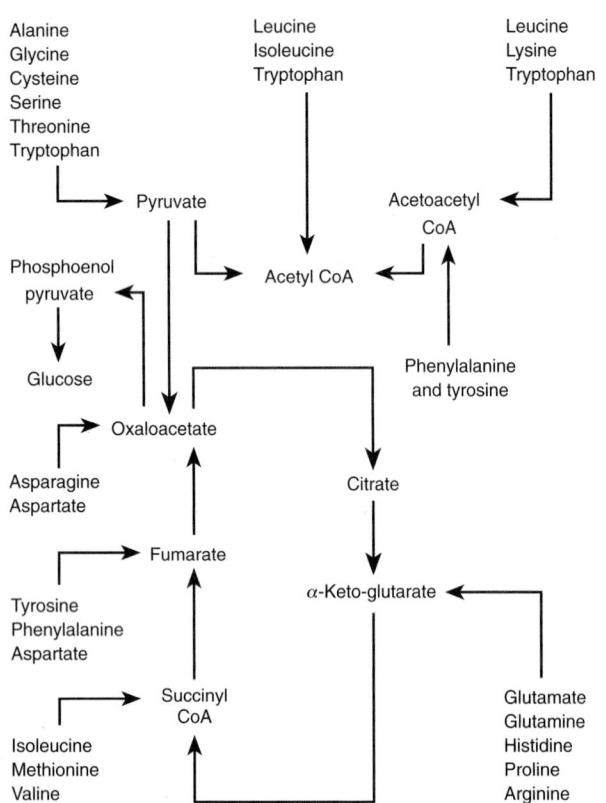

Fig. 2 Amino acids as a source of energy. The multiple entry points to the citric acid cycle for the metabolites of carbon chain catabolism.

Table 2 A biochemical classification of amino acid disorders

Defects of amino acid transport	Intestinal and renal
	Across cellular membranes
Defects of the amino group metabolism	Primary urea cycle defects
	Secondary interference of urea cycle function
Defects of carbon chain metabolism	Those close to the parent amino acid with raised amino acid concentrations but mild or no acidosis
	Those further down the pathway with organic acid accumulation and acidosis
	Those at the end of the degradative pathways which may also involve catabolism of carbohydrates or fats
Defects primarily of major vitamin coenzymes	Pyridoxine
	Vitamin B_{12}
	Biotin
	Biopterins

clinical practice of paper chromatography for the analysis of urinary amino acids. Table 4 sets out a classification of amino aciduria. Normal renal clearance values for the amino acids are given in Table 1. A general account of amino acid transport would need to cover not only the renal tubule but the intestinal mucosa, the placenta, the blood–brain barrier, cell membranes in a host of tissues, and intracellular membranes. No attempt is made here to address the generality of transport issues.

The generalized amino acidurias

The Fanconi syndrome

General aspects

There are four components to the Fanconi syndrome:

(1) characteristic low-molecular-weight proteinuria, e.g. α_1-microglobulin, β_2-microglobulin, β_1-glycoprotein, and retinol binding protein;

(2) tubular transport defects;

(3) metabolic bone disease, rickets, or osteomalacia;

(4) slow loss of glomerular function.

Glycosuria, generalized amino aciduria, and phosphaturia are a classic triad. The conservation of sodium, potassium, bicarbonate, and urate is impaired and the plasma concentrations of the last three decreased. Many examples of the Fanconi syndrome are not primarily disorders of amino acid metabolism (cystinosis is an exception) but the effects of exogenous or endogenous toxins (e.g. galactose-1-phosphate) which accumulate in other

Table 3 The essential amino acids in humans with recommended dietary intakes

	Infants (mg/kg/day)	Adults (mg/kg/day)
Leucine	161	14.0
Isoleucine	70	10.0
Valine	93	10.0
Methionine*	58	13.0
Phenylalanine*	125	14.0
Threonine	87	7.0
Lysine	103	12.0
Tryptophan	17	3.5
Histidine	28	Not essential

*Requirements are lowered by the inclusion in the diet of cystine or tyrosine, respectively.

Table 4 A classification of aminoaciduria

Overflow aminoaciduria (secondary to high plasma amino acid concentrations)	Generalized	Increased plasma concentrations of many amino acids, e.g. acute liver necrosis or amino acid infusions
	Specific	Increased plasma concentration of one or a few amino acids
Renal aminoaciduria (with normal plasma amino acid concentrations)	Generalized	The Fanconi syndrome; early premature infants
	Specific	i. Basic aminoaciduria with or without cystine; lysinuric protein intolerance; cystinuria
		ii. Neutral aminoaciduria; the Hartnup syndrome
		iii. Glycine iminoaciduria; the normal neonatal pattern; genetic iminoglycinuria

genetic defects (Table 5). The Fanconi–Bickel syndrome is a distinct genetic entity.

Maleic acid (maleate) has been used to produce experimental models of the Fanconi syndrome, as have 4-pentenoate and succinyl acetone (see below). Experimentally, maleate lowers intracellular concentrations of amino acids and sugars predominantly by increasing efflux. Maleate affects mitochondrial oxidation processes, impairs 1α-hydroxylation of 25-hydroxycholecalciferol and may directly affect cell membranes. It has still not proved possible to be sure whether the Fanconi syndrome should be regarded as a disorder of proximal or distal tubules, or both, whether efflux from cell to lumen is more important than reabsorption defects, and whether all causes of the syndrome act through a final undefined common mechanism. A central role for impaired energy production is suggested by new reports of tubular defects in mitochondrial disorders, for example cytochrome c oxidase deficiency and the Kearns–Sayre syndrome.

The Fanconi–Bickel syndrome

This is a rare autosomal recessive disorder caused by mutations in a glucose transporter gene expressed in kidney, liver, intestine, and pancreas. It is associated with hepatomegaly, glycogen storage, fasting hypoglycaemia, short stature, and proximal tubular nephropathy.

The dominantly inherited Fanconi syndrome

This disorder, of unknown cause, characteristically presents in the second to fourth decade and slowly evolves into late adult life when renal failure may be advanced (Fig. 3). The clinical presentation is commonly with rickets or osteomalacia, which require treatment with calcitriol. Potassium, sodium bicarbonate, and phosphate supplements may also be needed.

The oculocerebrorenal syndrome of Lowe

This is an X-linked disease characterized by dwarfism, severe mental retardation, and blindness secondary to cataracts, microphthalmos, and glaucoma. The tubular defect includes proteinuria, rickets but not usually glycosuria, and an amino aciduria with relative sparing of the branched chain amino acids. The *OCRC1* gene is on the long arm of the X chromosome and codes for inositol polyphosphate-5-phosphatase.

Table 5 The inherited causes of the Fanconi syndrome. Acquired causes are due to heavy metals, drugs, dysproteinaemias, and some immunological disorders of the kidney

Idiopathic
Cystinosis
Hereditary fructose intolerance
Tyrosinaemia type I
Galactosaemia
Glycogen storage disease type I
Fanconi–Bickel syndrome
Oculocerebrorenal syndrome of Lowe
Wilson's disease
Cytochrome c oxidase deficiency

Cystinosis

Clinical

Cystinosis results from defective carrier-mediated transport of cystine through the lysosomal membrane, which may rupture due to cystine crystallization in hexagonal or rectangular forms causing cell damage. In the proximal renal tubule this leads to the Fanconi syndrome. In the severe infantile form clinical presentation occurs after a few months of life with polyuria, thirst, salt and water depletion, hypokalaemia, and proximal renal tubular acidosis. Poor feeding and failure to thrive are characteristic. Hypophosphataemia and impaired 1-hydroxylation of 25-hydroxycholecalciferol contribute to florid rickets.

Photophobia develops with the accumulation of cystine crystals in the cornea and retinopathy. Hypothyroidism is common and renal failure develops leading to death by 10 years of age. Growth is invariably impaired even before kidney transplantation and the concomitant steroid immunosuppression. Sexual development is late. Intelligence is normal in early life. In transplanted patients retinopathy and visual loss may progress and central nervous system changes may occur. Cystine crystals are not seen here, but tissue cystine concentrations are very elevated. Cortical atrophy and memory defects occur in some older patients. frank neurological features are now more commonly described in survivors after renal transplantation, and may respond to treatment. The spectrum of organ defects is likely to widen in long-term postrenal transplant survivors.

Variant forms

A benign adult form presents with photophobia due to corneal crystals. There may also be crystals in the bone marrow and leucocytes but the kidney is spared and life expectancy is normal. An intermediate form is like the classic infantile form but presents in late childhood or early adult life. Renal involvement and renal failure occur.

Biochemistry

It is probable that all tissues accumulate cystine, but not equally, and some (e.g. muscle and brain) never seem to develop crystals. Crystals occur in the

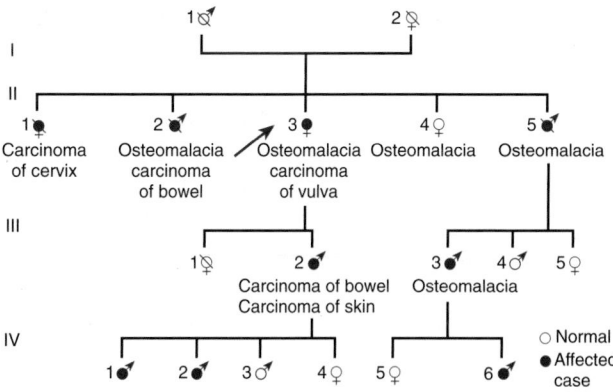

Fig. 3 Pedigree of dominantly inherited Fanconi syndrome. (From Brenton *et al.* (1981) with permission.)

tissues with the highest cystine concentrations, increasing with age to values several hundred times normal. Cultured fibroblasts and leucocytes have values of 50 to 100 times normal, but cultured lymphoid cells are only four to five times normal. Leucocyte cystine content is higher in the intermediate than the benign form, and highest in the severe classic infantile form. The intralysosomal cystine originates from proteins catabolized within the lysosome and extracellular cystine transported into the cell. Cystine egress from the lysosome is defective. The carrier is not shared by other amino acids, which have other lysosomal transport systems. Cystine loaded renal tubules have severely compromised ATP production due to a deficient intracellular phosphate concentration.

Diagnosis
This is based on the clinical features, features of the Fanconi syndrome, and the presence of cystine crystals. In the cornea these can be seen with a hand lens or a slit lamp in an older child but in infancy they are best seen in bone marrow aspirates (Fig. 4) fixed in alcohol and examined under polarized light. Analysis of peripheral leucocytes for their cystine content is possible in only a few laboratories.

Genetics
The disease is autosomal recessive. The incidence is about 1 in 200 000 live births. A higher incidence has been reported from parts of France. Heterozygotes are clinically normal but have raised leucocyte cystine concentrations. Patients have mutations in a gene (*CTNS*) on the short arm of chromosome 17 encoding a lysosomal membrane protein cystinosin. Over 30 mutations in the *CTNS* gene have been recognized in nephropathic cystinosis and others in variant forms.

Prenatal diagnosis
This has been successfully achieved using cultured amniocytes and measuring ^{35}S cystine uptake, or by direct analysis of chorionic villus samples for cystine content. Mutation analysis is now possible.

Treatment
Renal losses of salt, bicarbonate, and potassium may require initial intravenous replacement, but oral supplements including phosphate suffice later although the need for them may be substantial. Phosphate alone may not heal the rickets without the addition of calcitriol. Oral cysteamine, or phosphocysteamine, given in divided doses, depletes leucocyte cystine and gives improved growth and preservation of renal function. Cysteamine eye drops have been used in very young children to clear corneal crystals. The role of cysteamine in preventing the consequences of cystine accumulation in non-

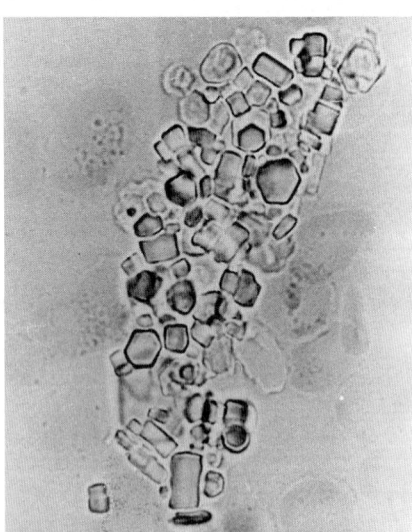

Fig. 4 Cystine crystals in the marrow of a child with cystinosis (× 2200, partially polarized light). (By courtesy of Dr B. Lake, The Hospital for Sick Children, Great Ormond Street, London and with the permission of Heinemann Medical Books.)

renal tissues after transplantation is under study. Dialysis and/or renal transplantation are required for renal failure. Transplanted kidneys do not accumulate cystine. Thyroxine is needed for hypothyroidism. Growth hormone treatment increases height but has been reported to hasten the need for renal replacement. others have not found this, and cysteamine treatment in early childhood improves growth anyway. Plasma carnitine concentrations are often low and can be increased to normal by the use of supplements but this may not help any muscular weakness.

Specific amino acidurias
The recognition of genetic disorders characterized by the excretion of a specific group of amino acids has stimulated research into amino acid transport. Major clinical problems are found in cystinuria and lysinuric protein intolerance.

Cystinuria
Clinical
Cystine stone formation in the kidneys and its attendant complications of pain, haematuria, renal obstruction, and infection is the classic clinical presentation. Only 1 to 2 per cent of all renal stones in adult life are cystine stones but the proportion is higher in childhood. The stones may have grown to large staghorn calculi before diagnosis. They are radio-opaque.

Biochemistry
Cystine has a solubility of 400 mg/litre at neutral pH and excretion varies from 400 to 1200 mg/day in affected individuals, with increased excretion of lysine (up to 2 g/day), ornithine, and arginine, and impaired intestinal absorption of the free amino acids. All are absorbed as dipeptides in combination with another amino acid outside the group. There is no deficiency of any amino acid and no urea cycle defect. The faecal and urinary excretion of diamines such as putrescine and cadaverine result from the action of intestinal bacteria on unabsorbed lysine and arginine. Experimental work indicates that one renal transport defect in cystinuria affects a low-K_m system in the brush border shared by the four amino acids. Other transport systems for cystine and the dibasic amino acids exist. Cystine excretion can exceed the glomerular filtration rate, implying the possibility of tubular secretion.

Diagnosis
Diagnosis requires an amino acid chromatogram and quantitation of cystine excretion. Calcium-containing stones have been observed in cystinuria—possibly because infection predisposes to deposition of calcium salts on small cystine deposits. Confusion is most likely when stone analysis is used for diagnosis without a chromatogram.

Genetics
Three subtypes of cystinuria were identified 30 years ago from studies of amino acid excretion and intestinal absorption. A gene on chromosome 2p with over 20 described mutations probably provides the basis for type I cystinuria with high cystine excretion and a high risk of stone formation. A second cystinuria locus on chromosome 19q may be responsible for types II and III cystinuria. Combinations of alleles at these loci probably explain the different subtypes of cystinuria and the confusing family histories. For example type I cystinuria heterozygotes have normal cystine excretion and the disease is always clearly recessive. However, type II heterozygotes excrete substantial amounts of cystine and the pedigrees can appear dominant.

Prenatal diagnosis
This has not been described.

Treatment
As the relationships between genotype, cystine excretion, and risk of stone formation especially in childhood become clearer so will the recommendations become clearer. The daily fluid intake must not be less than 3 litre/day in adults and this must include 500 ml before retiring to bed with a nocturnal rise to pass urine and drink a further 500 ml. Keeping the urine

dilute over the 24-h period is the difficult part, but may be sufficient treatment for those without stones.

Reduced protein intake diminishes cystine excretion but this is not much used in treatment. Cystine is much more soluble at alkaline pH (> 7.5). Use of sodium bicarbonate is limited by the large doses (6 g/day or more) needed to raise urine pH significantly. High sodium intakes are contraindicated in hypertension or renal failure. In addition, alkaline urine may dispose to the precipitation of calcium salts. However, high fluid intake with potassium citrate supplements is recommended by some in childhood if cystine excretion is high.

Penicillamine treatment produces the much more soluble disulphide—half cystine and half penicillamine and an overall reduction of cystine excretion greater than can be accounted for by disulphide formation. The effective dose (1 to 3 g/day) should reduce the free cystine excretion to around 200 mg/day if stones are to dissolve. It is usual to start at a dose of 125 mg/day and increase over several weeks to full dose. The unwanted side-effects include blood dyscrasias, rash with arthralgia, fever, and lymphadenopathy. A syndrome with skin lesions resembling pseudoxanthoma elasticum, elastosis perforans serpinginosa, may complicate long-term penicillamine use, as may pyridoxine deficiency. This latter effect is prevented by coadministration of 25 to 50 mg pyridoxine daily. Patients on penicillamine need blood counts every 2 weeks initially and then monthly. Regular urinalysis is needed. Proteinuria is common and above 2 g/day may necessitate stopping penicillamine, as do blood dyscrasias or other severe reactions. Penicillamine is a helpful preventive treatment in patients with recurrent stone formation at lower doses. Large doses are reserved for trying to dissolve large calculi, which may take 1 to 2 years. It is usually well tolerated in cystinuria.

α-mercaptopropionylglycine is an alternative to penicillamine to which it has structural similiarities. It has been used less than penicillamine but should be considered in patients showing the serious toxic effects of penicillamine. Captopril is a sulphydryl compound which forms a disulphide with cystine. decreased cystine excretion related to treatment with captopril does occur but no therapeutic use has yet been established for it. Similarly, decreasing sodium intake and excretion reduces cystine excretion but a therapeutic role has not been accepted.

Cystine stones are not easily broken by lithotripsy, but it may still be helpful. Percutaneous removal may have its place for smaller stones, particularly in those who cannot take penicillamine and who are unable to regulate their drinking adequately.

Lysinuric protein intolerance

Clinical

Defective ornithine, lysine, and arginine transport affect the renal tubule and intestine with only minor defects of cystine transport. Stones do not form. At weaning, vomiting and diarrhoea begin. There is nutritional deficiency. failure to thrive, poor appetite, and poor growth are common. Occasional intermittent hyperammonaemic encephalopathy occurs. Osteoporosis is an important part of the clinical picture, with vertebral collapse. Interstitial lung disease causes breathlessness, cough, fever, and reduced arterial Po_2. Intellect is normal or mildly impaired. Pregnancy is associated with haemorrhage during labour. Immunological abnormalities have been reported.

Biochemistry

Plasma concentrations of arginine, ornithine, and lysine are low but citrulline, alanine, and glutamine are increased. Renal clearance values for lysine are 20 to 30 times normal and renal losses may be up to 1 g/day. Less marked increases of orthinine and arginine excretion are found but cystine increases are minor.

Plasma lysine values fail to rise after oral lysine loads or the ingestion of lysyl peptides. Intracellular peptide hydrolysis liberates lysine, which cannot be transported across the basolateral membrane, the site of the transport defect. There is also evidence of a transport defect in cultured fibroblasts but not in red cells. A deficiency of intramitochondrial ornithine due to a transport defect across the mitochondrial membrane may impair the urea cycle, causing hyperammonaemia and orotic aciduria (see below).

Genetics

The disease is an autosomal recessive with a relatively high incidence in Finland (1 in 60 000) compared with the rest of the world. The gene has been localized to chromosome 14q coding for a permease-related protein.

Prenatal diagnosis

This is possible with molecular techniques.

Treatment

Hyperammonaemia can be largely prevented by a low-protein diet. However, adequate calorie intake is difficult to sustain in infancy and appetite often remains poor. Protein restriction does not correct lysine deficiency and oral lysine supplementation causes diarrhoea. Oral citrulline (2.5 to 8.5 g/day), absorbed via a different transport system, corrects ornithine and arginine deficiency and lowers plasma ammonia by priming the urea cycle. Acute hyperammonaemic crises are managed with intravenous glucose and intravenous or oral sodium benzoate or phenylbutyrate (see below). Citrulline treatment should be maintained but intravenous citrulline is not readily available. Intravenous ornithine and arginine have been tried.

ε-N-acetyl lysine has been used in the attempt to overcome lysine deficiency, which may be a factor in the osteoporosis and other problems. Plasma lysine concentrations rise but there is no agreement on its use, and cost and availability are a problem.

The cause of the serious interstitial pneumonia is not clear. It has not apparently responded to antibiotics given for the possibility of pneumocystis infection. Successful treatment with prednisolone has been reported.

Neutral amino aciduria: the Hartnup syndrome

This is an autosomal recessive disorder of neutral amino acid transport across the luminal brush border membrane of kidney and intestine. It does not involve cystine and the basic amino acids, the acidic acids, glycine, or the iminoacids (see Fig. 3). Clinical effects may include a light-sensitive rash on exposed skin, cerebellar ataxia, and mental disturbance, but patients with this disorder frequently remain normal. Affected individuals may respond to nicotinamide, but this does not change the amino acid transport defect. The relative deficiency of nicotinamide is attributed to the losses of the precursor amino acid tryptophan and its impaired intestinal absorption. Bacterial action on unabsorbed tryptophan generates indoles, which appear in the stools and urine and are characteristic of the disorder.

Familial renal iminoglycinuria

The excretion of glycine, proline, and hydroxyproline is raised in the Fanconi syndrome and in the inborn errors of proline or hydroxyproline metabolism when plasma concentrations of these amino acids are raised. Transient raised excretion of the three amino acids is usual in neonates, which reflects the ontogeny of one shared transport system. Genetic iminoglycinuria is an autosomal recessive defect of another transport system. The evidence supports several allelic mutations in the genetic defect with some heterozygotes having raised glycine excretion and some normal amino acid excretion. Familial iminoglycinuria is the consequence of a well worked out transport defect which is clinically harmless.

The γ-glutamyl cycle

A possible amino acid transport system

Six enzyme-catalysed reactions link the steps for the synthesis of glutathione and its metabolism (Fig. 5). Glutathione is believed to be transported to the cell membrane, where its antioxidant properties may be

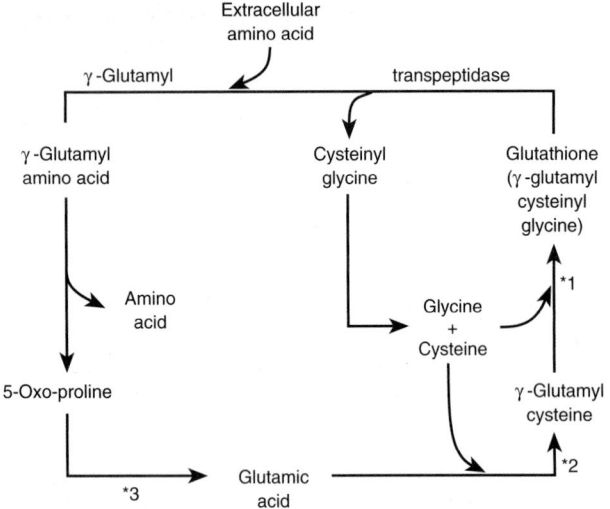

Fig. 5 The γ-glutamyl cycle synthesizes glutathione and may play a role in amino acid transport. Asterisked enzymes are: 1, glutathione synthetase; 2, γ-glutamyl cysteine synthetase; and 3, 5-oxoprolinase.

important in preventing lipid peroxidation. Tissues with low γ-glutamyl transpeptidase levels in the cell membrane transport glutathione into the body fluids and circulation. Some is filtered at the glomerulus. γ-glutamyl transpeptidase, bound to the cell membrane of transport epithelia such as the choroid plexus, ciliary body, nephron, and jejunum, has been assigned a role in the membrane transport of amino acids via the formation of γ-glutamyl amino acid peptides, which is quite different from free amino acid transport. The peptides are cleaved by γ-glutamyl cyclotransferase to free the transported amino acid and the γ-glutamyl moiety, which cyclizes to 5-oxoproline (pyroglutamic acid). Cystine is among the amino acids transported in this way and one function of the cycle may be to conserve cystine and, indirectly, cysteine. There is no suggestion of any defect in the cycle in cystinuria. The inherited defects of the γ-glutamyl cycle are summarized in Table 6. Some of the links between biochemical defects and clinical manifestations are tentative.

Defects of the urea cycle

Amino acids taken in excess of synthetic need are catabolized and the amino group converted to urea. Hyperammonaemia is one of the major metabolic abnormalities in urea cycle defects but is not unique to them (Table 7).

The formation of urea

Nearly all waste nitrogen disposal—10 to 12 g/day—is in the form of urea synthesized in the liver from ammonium ions (NH_4^+) and the α-amino nitrogen of aspartic acid (see Fig. 1). The ammonium nitrogen is incorporated into the first committed synthetic step to urea formation—the production of carbamyl phosphate for which N-acetyl glutamine is believed to be regulatory. The α-amino nitrogen of aspartic acid comes from many

amino acids during their transamination reactions with oxaloacetic acid. It is incorporated during the formation of argininosuccinic acid. Ornithine nitrogen is not incorporated into urea. Bicarbonate provides the carbon moiety of urea but this is not generally regarded as important in acid–base balance.

The source of ammonium ions (NH_4^+) for the generation of carbamyl phosphate is less clear. Glutamine synthesized in skeletal muscle is extensively taken up by the intestine. Glutamine nitrogen is released into the portal blood as alanine, ammonium ions, and citrulline. Apart from these urea precursors, ammonium ions are released into the renal vein by the action of renal glutaminase on glutamine. The generation of ammonium ions within the liver had been attributed to the deamination of glutamate by glutamate dehydrogenase. Transamination reactions involving glutamate are probably more important in linking glutamate to the urea cycle. Within the liver a number of other amino acids are deaminated and may be a source of ammonium for urea synthesis.

The extrahepatic urea cycle enzymes

The urea cycle synthesizes arginine but it has been noted that hepatic transplantation for urea cycle defects does not correct previously low plasma concentrations of citrulline and arginine. The intestine can also synthesize citrulline with the mitochondrial parts of the cycle. Other tissues contain only some of the urea cycle enzymes. Citrulline transported to a variety of tissues with the cytosolic components of the cycle can be used to synthesize arginine via argininosuccinic acid. This extrahepatic synthesis of arginine may be crucial to the body's needs.

The inherited defects of the urea cycle

Four of five inherited defects of the urea cycle (see Fig. 1) have common clinical features but arginase deficiency is different. Quite separately the activity of carbamyl phosphate synthetase can be impaired by a rare genetic defect in N-acetylglutamine formation which is not considered here. Ornithine transcarbamylase deficiency is the most common of the defects.

Clinical features of carbamyl phosphate synthetase deficiency, ornithine transcarbamylase deficiency, argininosuccinic acid synthetase deficiency, and argininosuccinic acid lyase deficiency

The neonatal presentation of these conditions is identical. After a brief normal period of 24 to 72 h, poor feeding, lethargy, and vomiting precede the descent to unresponsiveness and hyperammonaemic coma. Argininosuccinic acid lyase deficiency may be less acute and severe than carbamyl phosphate synthetase deficiency, ornithine transcarbamylase deficiency, or argininosuccinic acid synthetase deficiency because argininosuccinic acid excreted at the glomerular filtration rate (there being no tubular reabsorption) is a means of nitrogen excretion, and hyperammonaemia tends to be less severe. In males, ornithine transcarbamylase deficiency is usually fatal, but survival in the other conditions is more likely. Survivors may suffer intellectual impairment and other neurological damage. Only one of the four is X linked (ornithine transcarbamylase deficiency) and female carriers may sometimes present clinically in the neonatal period, presumably because of preponderant inactivation of the X chromosome with a normal gene.

Table 6 Genetic defects of the γ-glutamyl cycle

Enzyme deficiency	Clinical effects	Biochemical abnormalities
Glutathione synthetase	Mental retardation	Large excretion of 5-oxoproline (pyroglutamic aciduria)
Generalized deficiency	Variable central nervous system effects. Neonatal acidosis. Haemolysis	
Red cell deficiency	Haemolysis only. No urinary defect	
γ-glutamylcysteine synthetase	Haemolysis, spinocerebellar degeneration, myopathy	Generalized aminoaciduria
γ-glutamyl transpeptidase	Mental retardation	Raised plasma concentration and urine excretion of glutathione
5-oxoprolinase	Variable from no effect to enterocolitis and renal stones	Moderate increases of 5-oxoproline excretion

Table 7 Causes of hyperammonaemia

Urea cycle defects	
Transport defects of intermediates of the urea cycle	Lysinuric protein intolerance
	Hyperornithinaemia–hyperammonaemia– homocitrillinuria syndrome
Organic acidurias	Branched chain organic acid defects
	Propionic acidaemia and methylmalonic acidaemia
	Pyruvate carboxylase or dehyrogenase deficiencies
	Multiple carboxylase deficiencies
	Glutaric aciduria type II
	Acyl coenzyme A dehydrogenase deficiencies
Drugs	Valproate encephalopathy
	Reye's syndrome
Liver disorders	Cirrhosis of variable aetiology
	Portal systemic shunts
Transient neonatal hyperammonaemia	

Later presentations come in two broad clinical forms. Mental retardation and epilepsy without any clear neonatal history are well described in argininosuccinic acid lyase deficiency and also in carbamyl phosphate synthetase deficiency, ornithine transcarbamylase deficiency, and argininosuccinic acid synthetase deficiency. Children with argininosuccinic acid lyase deficiency may also show the hair defect of trichorrhexis nodosa, which is not shared by the other urea cycle defects. Another late presentation is with intermittent encephalopathy. This is seen in females who are carriers for ornithine transcarbamylase deficiency, including presentation in the puerperium after a symptomless pregnancy, and males hemizygous for ornithine transcarbamylase deficiency with less severe mutations who have presented in late childhood or the teenage years. Death has been recorded in these late onset encephalopathies. Carbamyl phosphate synthetase deficiency and argininosuccinic acid synthetase deficiency may also present in this way.

Clinical features of arginase deficiency

There is a progressive spastic quadriparesis, most marked in the legs, with psychomotor retardation, epilepsy, and poor growth. Obvious manifestations present in early childhood. Hyperammonaemic coma occurs but hyperammonaemia is less marked than in the other disorders.

Biochemistry

These defects are summarized in Table 8. Hyperammonaemia is preceded by raised plasma alanine and glutamine concentrations and may be accompanied by a rise in transaminases and prolongation of the prothrombin time. The raised excretion of orotic acid in some defects is caused by the accumulation of carbamyl phosphate, which is directed to pyrimidine synthesis (see Fig. 1).

Experimental hyperammonaemia in primates initially causes decreased activity, lethargy, and vomiting, and then hyperventilation and respiratory alkalosis, which have also been recorded in humans. Seizures and coma follow with progressive rise of intracranial pressure and cerebral oedema. The astrocytes, which occupy one-quarter to one-third of brain volume, exhibit marked swelling and mitochondrial change. High astrocyte glutamine concentrations may act osmotically to cause cerebral oedema. Many metabolic changes in hyperammonaemia are secondary to cerebral oedema. Glutamine concentrations ten times normal have been recorded in the cerebrospinal fluid in ornithine transcarbamylase deficiency and argininosuccinic acid lyase deficiency. Other amino acid abnormalities in the cerebrospinal fluid have been described in arginase deficiency. An early effect of hyperammonaemia on amino acid transport across the blood–brain barrier has been described, with tryptophan transport being regarded as particularly important.

Diagnosis

The biochemical defects are diagnostically important (see Table 8). Carbamyl phosphate synthetase deficiency can only be diagnosed when hyperammonaemia is not associated with the biochemical changes of the other urea cycle defects, although a low plasma citrulline value gives a clue. Other causes of hyperammonaemia must be excluded (see Table 7), which requires urinary organic acid analysis, consideration of Reye's syndrome, and acute valproate encephalopathy. Confirmatory enzyme assays on liver biopsy samples may be needed in carbamyl phosphate synthetase deficiency and ornithine transcarbamylase deficiency. Liver function and clotting tests should be checked.

Genetics

With the exception of ornithine transcarbamylase deficiency, the diseases are autosomal recessive. The gene for carbamyl phosphate synthetase is on the short arm of chromosome 2. Inherited deficiency is rare, with 14 mutations described. The enzyme protein may be targeted to the mitochondria by a leader peptide and the mature enzyme constitutes a relatively high proportion of mitochondrial protein. The gene for ornithine transcarbamylase is on the short arm of the X chromosome and its product targeted to mitochondria in a manner similar to carbamyl phosphate synthetase. Functional catalytic trimers form within the mitochondrial matrix. Ornithine transcarbamylase deficiency is associated with a variety of gene defects— insertions, deletions, and point mutations; about 140 have been described.

Argininosuccinic acid synthetase, argininosuccinic acid lyase, and arginase are cytoplasmic enzymes. Argininosuccinic acid synthetase catalyses the synthesis of argininosuccinic acid from citrulline and aspartic acid, requires adenosine triphosphate and magnesium ions, and functions as a tetramer of about 185 000 Da. The gene is on the long arm of chromosome 9. Argininosuccinic acid lyase, which cleaves argininosuccinic acid, functions as a tetramer of about 173 000 Da and the coding gene is on the short arm of chromosome 7. About 12 mutations have been described.

Table 8 A general approach to the biochemical disturbances in the urea cycle defects

	Normal	CPSD	OTCD	ASD	ACD	AD
Plasma ammonia	15–40	Up to 25×	Up to 25×	Up to 10–15×	Up to 10×	Up to 2–3×
Glutamine	350–650	2–3×	2–3×	2–3×	2–3×	2×
Alanine	200–400	2–3×	2–3×	2–3×	2–3×	2×
Citrulline	10–30	Low	Low	up to 200×	Increased	Normal
Arginine	30–90	Low	Low	Low	Low	Up to 15×
Argininosuccinate	Not detectable	None	None	None	400–600	None
Urine orotic acid*	2–6	Not increased	Increased	Increased	Increased	Increased
Urine amino acids	–	–	–	Citrulline	ASA	Arginine/cystine lysine

Abbreviations: AD, arginase deficiency; ALD, argininosuccinic acid lyase deficiency; ASD, argininosuccinic acid synthetase deficiency; CPSD, carbamyl phosphate synthetase deficiency; OTCD, ornithine transcarbamylase deficiency.

*Urine orotic acid in mg/day.

Normal plasma values in μmol/litre.

Fibroblast studies of argininosuccinic acid lyase indicate that crossreacting material is usually present and correlates poorly with residual enzyme activity. There are multiple complementation groups and, by implication, multiple alleles at the structural gene locus.

Hepatic arginase, a trimer of submit size around 35 000 Da, cleaving arginine to urea and ornithine, has a locus on the long arm of chromosome 6. A separate mitochondrial arginase is present in kidney.

Antenatal diagnosis

A restriction fragment length polymorphism has been helpful in diagnosis of carbamyl phosphate synthetase deficiency, with fetal liver biopsy and enzyme assay the only alternatives. Antenatal diagnosis in ornithine transcarbamylase deficiency is complex. If the mother is known to be a carrier from pedigree analysis or biochemical testing, three approaches are possible:

1. If the mutation is known within the family then direct examination of the fetal genotype is possible using appropriate probes, but this occurs in a minority of cases.
2. If a restriction fragment polymorphism is linked to the mutant gene in the family then this approach may be possible.
3. If no such information is available then sexing the fetus followed by fetal liver biopsy and enzyme assay in the male is the only approach left.

Antenatal diagnosis for argininosuccinic acid synthetase deficiency is also difficult. The enzyme can be assayed in amniocytes and placental villus material, but it is more reliable to culture amniocytes with radioactive citrulline and measure the incorporation of the radioactive products into cell protein. Amniotic fluid citrulline concentrations may help. Molecular analysis is possible in argininosuccinic acid lyase deficiency. analysis of amniotic fluid for argininosuccinic acid or enzyme assay on cultured amniocytes have been used successfully. Arginase deficiency has been detected on fetal red cells and a number of mutations have now been identified.

Heterozygote detection in ornithine transcarbamylase deficiency

Because of its X-linked inheritance carrier detection is particularly important. Pedigree analysis including DNA studies where necessary, or investigation of frank symptomatic episodes may settle the issue. The symptomless female can be a problem, however. Protein loading with serial measurements of plasma ammonia and urinary orotic acid may reveal the biochemical defect but may also cause serious symptoms. Allopurinol causes a greater excretion of orotic acid and orotidine in carrier females than in normals and forms the basis of an acceptable safe test of heterozygosity. It may fail to identify some carriers.

Treatment and prognosis

The management of acute encephalopathy involves reducing the need to synthesize urea. Dietary protein is stopped and endogenous protein breakdown suppressed by a high oral carbohydrate intake or using intravenous 10 to 20 per cent dextrose and insulin if needed to control blood glucose concentrations. The blood ammonia is lowered in the neonatal period by peritoneal dialysis or haemodialysis (more effective). Slower methods useful in carbamyl phosphate synthetase deficiency and ornithine transcarbamylase deficiency include the use of intravenous or oral sodium benzoate, which is excreted as its glycine conjugate hippuric acid, so raising nitrogen excretion. The use of sodium phenylbutyrate, which is excreted as phenyl acetylglutamine, is more effective. Serious toxicity from either benzoate or phenylbutyrate overdose is possible. in argininosuccinic acid synthetase and argininosuccinic acid lyase deficiencies, oral or intravenous arginine is an urgent and important therapy to remedy deficiency. In argininosuccinic acid lyase deficiency in particular, plasma ammonia levels fall when arginine is administered. The prognosis for severe neonatal illness is poor (see above) especially if plasma ammonia concentrations are over 1000 μmol/litre.

Maintenance treatment of all urea cycle defects (including arginase deficiency) between encephalopathic episodes involves protein restriction to the minimum required for growth and development and supplementation with arginine in argininosuccinic acid synthetase deficiency and argininosuccinic acid lyase deficiency. The continuous use of oral sodium benzoate or sodium phenylbutyrate in carbamyl phosphate synthetase deficiency and ornithine transcarbamylase deficiency may be needed to maintain low plasma ammonia concentrations. Late onset forms of the urea cycle diseases carry a better prognosis, but arginase deficiency seems relentlessly progressive. Babies with argininosuccinic acid lyase deficiency picked up by neonatal screening but who have not developed early clinical illness are reported to develop with normal IQ on large arginine supplements and a low protein intake. Others do less well and urea cycle defects generally have a poor prognosis.

Valproate should be avoided in the treatment of seizures in urea cycle defects and ornithine transcarbamylase carriers because it may precipitate coma.

Liver transplantation has sometimes been carried out for urea cycle defects. Selecting patients and balancing the risks is extremely difficult. Gene transfer therapy has been attempted but the problems of suitably safe vectors and stable expression remain.

The disorders of carbon chain metabolism

The classification in Table 2 is a useful approach, but many different catabolic pathways and associated clinical abnormalities necessitate separate consideration of individual amino acids (or groups of them) with their relevant vitamin coenzymes. Pyridoxine, because of its central and varied roles, is considered separately below. The relatively 'non-specific' nature of some biochemical abnormalities is stressed again.

Pyridoxine

Pyridoxal phosphate is the coenzyme in amino acid transaminations, decarboxylations, and deaminations. Considerable molecular detail of its role in transamination has been worked out. It is also the coenzyme in the synthesis and breakdown of cystathionine in the trans-sulphuration pathway. The normal dietary pyridoxine intake is 2 to 3 mg/day but a number of diseases respond to doses of 10 to 500 mg/day. These include deficiencies of ornithine aminotransferase, cystathionine β synthase, cystathionase, hyperoxaluria due to peroxisomal glyoxylate aminotransferase deficiency, and some neonates with seizures considered due to defective glutamine decarboxylase, the enzyme which generates γ-aminobutyric acid (see later).

'Non-specific' biochemical defects

The multiple causes of hyperammonaemia have been listed (see Table 7). Elevations of plasma glycine may also be non-specific and not necessarily a result of primary enzyme defects in glycine metabolism. Increases of glutamine and alanine in plasma are common in the early stages of ammonia accumulation. Hypoglycaemia is frequent in the organic acidurias as well as in specific defects of gluconeogenesis or glycogen metabolism. Alanine concentrations rise in lactic acidosis.

Defects of ornithine metabolism

Ornithine is a non-protein amino acid upon which the synthesis of urea takes place (see Fig. 1) and which is regenerated once the urea moiety is split off. It is also produced when arginine reacts with glycine to produce guanidinoacetate, the precursor of creatine. Ornithine-δ-amino transferase produces glutamic semialdehyde, which cyclizes to pyrroline-5-carboxyllic acid, and is also produced from proline. The decarboxylation of ornithine produces the diamine putrescine.

Deficiency of ornithine-δ-aminotransferase: gyrate atrophy

Clinical

The major abnormality is an atrophy of choroid and retina, beginning as a small yellowish spot and increasing to a circular lesion edged with pigment giving an 'atypical retinitis pigmentosa' appearance. Children present with myopia and decreased night vision progressing to blindness in middle life. Cataracts also develop but optic discs, cornea, and iris remain normal. A few patients develop mild proximal muscle weakness. Microscopic abnormalities of skeletal muscle fibres are found. Magnetic resonance imaging shows changes in the central nervous system, but the longer-term clinical implications are uncertain.

Biochemistry

Plasma ornithine values range from 400 to 1000 µmol/litre (normal 75 µmol/litre) with high concentrations in cerebrospinal fluid and aqueous humour. 400 to 900 mg/day is excreted with increased amounts of arginine and lysine (competitive inhibition of reabsorption).

The activity of ornithine-δ-aminotransferase is low in liver and skeletal muscle. Most affected patients have less than 1 per cent of normal activity in fibroblasts. Some have values up to 5 to 6 per cent and some enzyme-deficient lines show marked increase of activity with very high concentrations of pyridoxal phosphate.

Diagnosis

The clinical picture and the amino acid defects are adequate means of diagnosis. Enzyme assays can be used to confirm it.

Genetics

It is an autosomal recessive with the highest incidence in Finland, (where it may be as high as 1 in 50 000). There are several mutants, as evidenced by complementation studies. The gene has been mapped to chromosome 10q. Two pseudogenes exist on the X chromosome. Different mis-sense mutations have been described in pyridoxine responsive and non-responsive forms. Splicing defects have also been described. Over 50 mutations have been described in gyrate atrophy.

Treatment

Despite encouraging therapeutic studies on a mouse model there are no reports of clinical improvement in humans but deterioration may be slower in patients whose plasma ornithine levels fall with pyridoxine treatment (500 mg/day or less). Low-arginine diets may reduce plasma ornithine concentrations as do large doses of lysine given to augment renal ornithine excretion. Creatine has been given and has been reported to improve muscle histology, but ocular deterioration continues. Local proline deficiency in the retina has been suggested as a cause of the retinal degeneration. Proline supplementation does not stop disease progression. The best approach if patients do not respond to pyridoxine maybe a combination of diet and high lysine doses. Studies on siblings in affected families indicate that the development of retinal changes is at least delayed by control of the plasma ornithine concentration.

Hyperornithinaemia with hyperammonaemia and homocitrillinuria

Clinical

Hyperornithinaemia with hyperammonaemia and homocitrillinuria is referred to as the **HHH** syndrome. Intermittent hyperammonaemic encephalopathy with vomiting, drowsiness, and coma may date back to infancy, or patients may present much later. Impairment of IQ from low normal to more severe retardation, with epilepsy and frank neurological features, is another form of presentation. Growth tends to be poor. Chor-

ioretinal atrophy has been reported in one patient but to date has not been commonly seen.

Biochemistry

Intermittent hyperammonaemia, with plasma ornithine values three to ten times normal and increased excretion of orotic acid are believed to result from impaired transport of ornithine into the mitochondria which leads to the accumulation of carbamylphosphate. This increases orotic acid formation and the production of homocitrulline by the transcarbamoylation of lysine.

Genetics

It is an autosomal recessive. A gene for an ornithine transporter across the mitochondial membrane (*ORNT1*) has been mapped to chromosome 13q. It has been reported that three mutant alleles in this gene account for a high proportion of HHH patients in North America.

Treatment

Moderate protein reduction (1 g/kg/day) reduces plasma ammonia and ornithine concentration. Ornithine supplementation may then lower plasma ammonia further by raising intracellular ornithine concentrations, which may induce entry of more ornithine into the mitochondria. In siblings presenting as adults, treatment with citrulline and sodium phenylbutyrate has decreased plasma ammonia, increased plasma ornithine, and relieved episodic confusional episodes. The outcome of treatment in the longer term is not known.

Defects of phenylalanine metabolism
The importance of tetrahydrobiopterin

The hyperphenylalaninaemias are a group of disorders characterized by defective hydroxylation of phenylalanine to tyrosine and plasma phenylalanine values above the normal fasting range of 40 to 80 µmol/litre. Tetrahydrobiopterin is the required coenzyme for this hydroxylation and high phenylalanine values may be due to defects in the apoenzyme or the generation of tetrahydrobiopterin.

An adult phenylalanine intake is about 3 to 4 g/day, one-quarter of which is incorporated into protein and three-quarters hydroxylated to tyrosine (Fig. 6). Adults need about 1 g/day, but in classic severe phenylketonuria health is maintained on half this. Transamination to phenylpyruvic acid and decarboxylation to phenylethylamine assume much greater importance in phenylketonuria because they occur only at elevated phenylalanine concentrations.

Classic phenylketonuria
Clinical

Phenylalanine values are higher than 1200 µmol/litre (sometimes much higher). Untreated, phenylketonuria almost invariably causes severe mental retardation, with IQ values only occasionally above 60, and most often well below. a few patients have normal IQ values despite the biochemical defect; some female patients have been discovered only because of abnormalities in their offspring (see below). Brain phenylalanine concentrations measured by magnetic resonance spectroscopy have been lower than expected in some of these patients probably accounting for the preservation of IQ. Both microcephaly and epilepsy are common. About one in 20 untreated patients develop neurological problems in adult life, usually spastic paraparesis but sometimes extrapyramidal features. Pigmentary deficiency in the iris and hair are features of the untreated disease and so is eczema.

Milder variants

Mutations with greater residual enzyme activity produce phenylalanine values of 300 to 1200 µmol/litre. Those over 480 µmol/litre should be treated: some were not with variable outcome for IQ.

Biochemistry

Plasma phenylalanine concentrations are elevated to 20 to 60 times, being highest in babies. Phenyl pyruvic acid which is converted to phenyl lactic acid, phenylacetic acid, and phenylacetyl glutamine accumulates with phenylethylamine. The ketone phenylpyruvic acid in the urine gives the disease its name and a green colour in the ferric chloride test. The defective enzyme phenylalanine hydroxylase, which requires tetrahydrobiopterin as a cofactor, has been found only in the liver in humans. It has never been found in the brain of any species. Phenylalanine hydroxylase may be tetrameric or trimeric with units of molecular weight between 50 000 and 60 000.

Pathology

The pathology of phenylketonuria is not clear. Phenylalanine itself is probably the damaging agent but there is controversy about the mechanism: relative tyrosine deficiency may also be important, reflected in the pigment deficiency and changes in neurotransmitters. High phenylalanine concentrations are associated with impaired brain growth and probably fewer nerve cells. Phenylalanine inhibits an enzyme important in sulphation of myelin intermediates and myelin formation is abnormal. In animal experiments high phenylalanine concentrations reduce transport of other amino acids at the blood–brain barrier and at the placenta. In addition, many *in vitro* biochemical processes (e.g. protein synthesis) are impaired by high phenylalanine concentrations. Patients with classic phenylketonuria also have low concentrations of homovanillic acid and 5-hydroxyindoleacetic acid in the cerebrospinal fluid, indicative of possible deficiency of the neurotransmitters dopamine, noradrenaline, and 5-hydroxytryptophan.

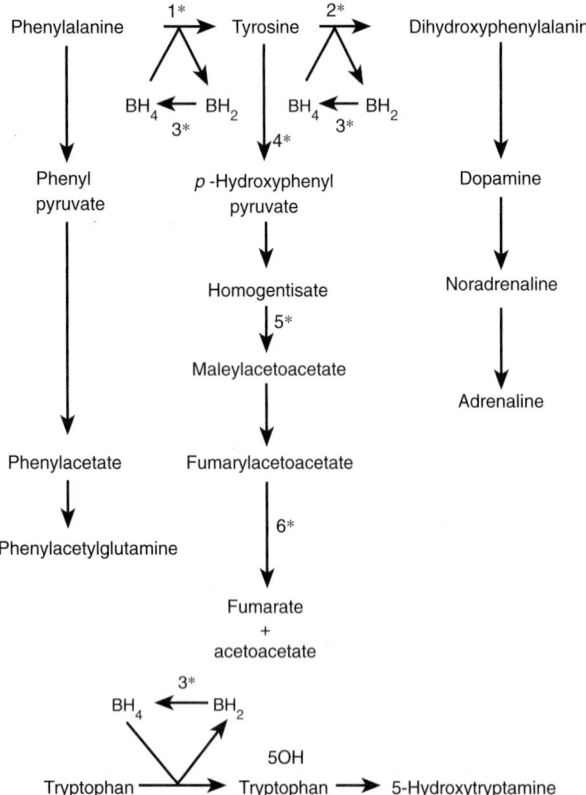

Fig. 6 The metabolism of phenylalanine and tyrosine and the role of tetrahydrobiopterin. The asterisked enzymes are: 1, phenylalanine hydroxylase; 2, tyrosine hydroxylase; 3, dihydrobiopterin reductase; 4, tyrosine aminotransferase; 5, homogentisic acid oxidase; 6, fumaryl acetoacetate hydrolase; and 7, tryptophan hydroxylase.

Dietary treatment restores normal concentrations in the cerebrospinal fluid.

Diagnosis

All newborns in the United Kingdom should be screened for raised phenylalanine values between the sixth and tenth day of life, either by Guthrie's bacterial inhibition assay, chromatography, or tandem mass spectometry. Phenylalanine values greater than 240 μmol/litre are rechecked and, if confirmed, are investigated. Raised phenylalanine values are seen in the important variants due to defects in tetrahydrobiopterin synthesis and these must be excluded as they require specific treatment. Transient neonatal hyperphenylalaninaemia is probably less common now that cows' milk, with its relatively high protein content, is used less in infancy, but it must be distinguished from permanent forms. Liver disease must be excluded.

Genetics

The disease is autosomal recessive, with an incidence in Western countries of 1 in 8000 to 12 000 live births. It is rare in Finland and Japan. One in 50 people carry a mutant gene. These include splicing mutations, deletions, and mis-sense mutations. The location on chromosome 12 has been confirmed. The majority of patients are compound heterozygotes rather than being homozygous for a single mutation. Residual enzyme activity in liver biopsies has correlated fairly well with *in vivo* studies on the conversion of deuterated phenylalanine to tyrosine and there is growing information on which genotypes cause the most severe functional defects in the enzyme. Over 400 mutations have been described. The contribution which other genes (e.g. for amino acid transport into the central nervous system) may make to the disease manifestations may, however, become clearer.

Antenatal diagnosis

Restriction fragment polymorphisms in linkage disequilibrium with these mutations have been useful in some families for antenatal diagnosis. Patient demand for antenatal diagnosis has been relatively low.

Treatment

Natural protein intake is reduced to provide just what is necessary for growth and development while keeping the plasma phenylalanine between 120 and 360 μmol/litre using the Guthrie test or other technique for regular monitoring. These are lower phenylalanine values than were once recommended because outcome in terms of IQ is closely related to the control of abnormally high values. Persistently low values may also adversely affect outcome. Despite normal or near normal IQ results, more subtle neuropsychological defects have been described in well-treated phenylketonuria patients and may be very important scholastically.

In infancy, milk restriction with supplements is relatively easy. Later it is necessary to introduce other foods on an exchange basis using tables that define the weight of the food containing 1 g of protein (roughly 50 mg phenylalanine). Fruits and some vegetables very low in protein are allowed freely. Adults with classic phenylketonuria tolerate only three to four exchanges, which provide about the same amount of phenylalanine as the free foods. These diets are supplemented with phenylalanine-free amino acid mixtures, minerals, and vitamins. Specially produced low-protein products make the diet more palatable.

Regression of IQ when diets were stopped in later childhood has led to continuation of dietary treatment into the teenage years. Patients generally have not suffered when diets have stopped at 15 or 16 years of age. However, there is no follow-up of a substantial number with respect to IQ change who have been off diet for 20 years or more, and there is concern about possible neurological deterioration.

High plasma phenylalanine concentrations may produce a pharmacological impairment of mental function revealed by psychological tests in short-term studies, which improve when concentrations fall. Long-term damage to intellect or neurological function is another issue. A small number of patients who were not on diet in adult life have developed spastic paraparesis, epilepsy, or extrapyramidal features. These may improve on diet. All these have cerebral changes on magnetic resonance imaging, as do an appreciable proportion of those off diet without neurological manifestations. The imaging changes also improve on diet regardless of whether there were clinical manifestations or not. Together with the known neurotransmitter defects there is a genuine concern for the long-term welfare of patients. Diet for life is restricting and costs £7000 to £8000 annually for the diet alone. There is an urgent need for more information.

Maternal phenylketonuria

The retrospective review of Lenke and Levy in 1980 did much to emphasize the adverse fetal effects of maternal hyperphenylalaninaemia (Table 9). Experience in other centres with large clinics broadly supports these figures. Microcephaly and congenital heart disease in the offspring of mothers returning to diet at the seventh or eighth week emphasizes the need for preconception diet. This is the best policy. Starting dietary measures very early in the first trimester (5 to 6 weeks) lowers the incidence of impaired brain development, but an increased risk certainly remains to the face and heart.

The ratio of fetal to maternal phenylalanine plasma levels is around 1.5 to 1.7 because of active placental transport. Maternal values should be controlled at between 100 and 250 μmol/litre, which requires very careful monitoring twice weekly. Some values will rise above this in the critical first trimester when tolerance is very low and nausea restricts calorie intake. Dietary tolerance in the mother increases from about week 18 due to increased requirement for growth by the fetus and uterus, but also probably because phenylalanine hydroxylase in the fetal liver can be detected early in the second trimester (Fig. 7). There is already clear evidence that lower maternal phenylalanine values result in neonates of higher birth weight and larger head circumference. Dietary control before conception prevents congenital heart disease.

Defects of biopterin metabolism

In the hydroxylation of phenylalanine the cofactor tetrahydrobiopterin is consumed and must be regenerated. A deficiency of tetrahydrobiopterin adversely affects the function not only of phenylalanine hydroxylase, but also of tyrosine hydroxylase and tryptophan hydroxylase (Fig. 7). Tyrosine hydroxylation is needed for the synthesis of noradrenaline and dopamine, and tryptophan hydroxylation for the production of 5-hydroxytryptophan. Tetrahydrobiopterin is therefore crucial to the production of neurotransmitters. The supply of this coenzyme is impaired in several enzyme defects. All produce hyperphenylalaninaemia, which may not be marked, and all produce progressive neurological disability despite a low-phenylalanine diet. About 1 to 2 per cent of newborns with abnormally raised phenylalanine values have a deficiency of tetrahydrobiopterin.

Table 9 The incidence of abnormalities in the offspring of phenylketonuric mothers

Abnormality	Maternal phenylalanine concentration (mg/100 ml) (×60 = mmol/l)			
	> 20	16–19	11–15	3–10
Mental retardation	92 (172)	73 (37)	22 (23	21 (29)
Microcephaly	73 (138)	68 (44)	35 (23)	24 (21)
Congenital heart disease	12 (225)	15 (46)	6 (33)	0 (44)
Birth weight < 2500 g	40 (89)	52 (33)	56 (9)	13 (16)

Percentage figures with sample size in parentheses (from Lenke and Levy (1980) with permission from the *New England Journal of Medicine*)

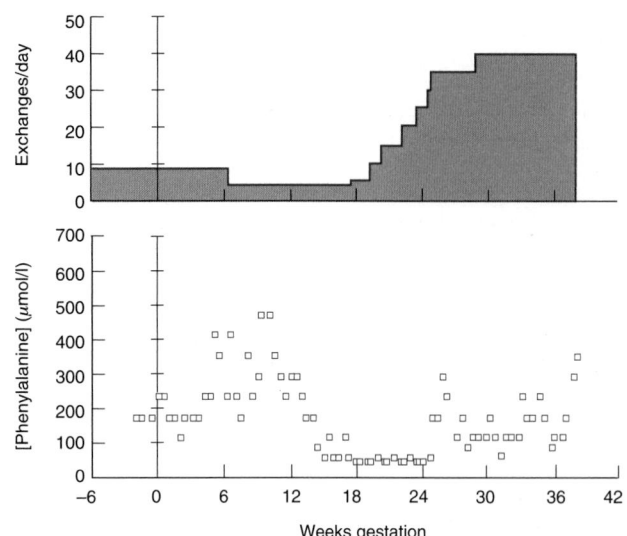

Fig. 7 Diet for a phenylketonuric mother illustrating the marked rise in phenylalanine tolerance in the second half of the pregnancy. (From Fernandes *et al.* (1990) with permission of Springer.)

Dihydropteridine reductase deficiency

Clinical
Progressive neurological deterioration occurs with psychomotor retardation, epilepsy, pyramidal, and extrapyramidal features, especially the latter. Calcification occurs in the cerebral hemispheres.

Biochemistry
Plasma phenylalanine values are elevated. The enzyme dihydropteridine reductase is a dimer or tetramer of four units, each 25 000 Da. It has a wide tissue distribution.

Diagnosis
The most reliable test is an enzyme assay on red cells. It can be carried out on dried blood spots. Oral loading tests with tetrahydrobiopterin may be useful as the plasma phenylalanine may then fall, but as it is not regenerated when the enzyme is deficient the results may be equivocal. Urinary biopterin analyses are needed in the differential diagnosis of these defects.

Genetics and prenatal diagnosis
The disease is an autosomal recessive and the enzyme assay can be carried out on cultured anmiocytes. There are crossreacting material-positive and -negative forms. The gene is on chromosome 4p encoding a protein of 244 amino acids functioning as a homodimer with over 20 described mutations.

Treatment
A low-phenylalanine diet is combined with the administration of L-dopa, 5-hydroxytryptophan, and, in some cases, folinic acid. Early treatment has been reported to give good results. Monitoring of neurotransmitters and folate in the cerebrospinal fluid may help treatment.

Guanosine triphosphate cyclohydrolase deficiency and 6-pyruvoyltetrahydrobiopterin synthase deficiency

The clinical features are similar to those of dihydropteridine reductase deficiency. Intermittent hyperthermia has been described. All urinary biopterin and neopterin values are low in the cyclohydrolase deficiency whereas 6-pyruvoyltetrahydrobiopterin deficiency has high neopterin values and low biopterin values. Tetrahydrobiopterin is used in treatment because, in the presence of dihydropteridine reductase, it can be regenerated from dihydrobiopterin. However, the clinical outcome is not assured and there is concern that tetrahydrobiopterin does not easily enter the central nervous system. Treatment, therefore, is also being attempted with low-phenylalanine diet, L-dopa, and in addition, 5-hydroxytryptophan. From reports on Saudi Arabian families with a high incidence of 6-pyruvoyltetrahydrobiopterin synthase deficiency, tetrahydrobiopterin is said to produce a good outcome if started very early in life.

Disorders of tyrosine metabolism

The steps in tyrosine metabolism starting with the rate-limiting step—the conversion to p-hydroxyphenyl pyruvic acid by tyrosine aminotransferase—are outlined in Fig. 6. They are the means of production of the catecholamines, dopamine, and the principal pigments of hair and skin. Diagnosing a specific disorder of tyrosine metabolism needs consideration of the non-specific elevations of plasma tyrosine and methionine seen in liver disorders of various aetiologies and the frequency of transient neonatal tyrosinaemia.

Neonatal tyrosinaemia

An increase of plasma tyrosine concentration and excretion of tyrosine and phenolic acids was commonly seen in premature infants given cows' milk feeds. Lower-protein infant feeds approximating to breast milk have reduced the incidence greatly. Transient deficiency of p-hydroxyphenylpyruvate oxidase is considered the unproven cause and appears to be harmless. It responds to reducing any high protein intake and sometimes to ascorbic acid. A repeat tyrosine measurement is indicated to exclude other persistent causes of a raised tyrosine.

Tyrosinaemia type I

Clinical

An acute presentation occurs in the early weeks of life with failure to thrive, vomiting, hepatomegaly, fever, oedema, and epistaxis. Death from hepatic failure occurs within the first year. A milder more chronic presentation is compatible with survival for several years with chronic liver disease, a renal tubular Fanconi syndrome with hypophosphataemic rickets, and sometimes abdominal pain and neuropathy suggestive of acute porphyria (see below). Hypertrophic obstructive cardiomyopathy has been described. One-third of patients progress to hepatocellular carcinoma of the liver.

Biochemistry

Deficiency of fumarylacetoacetate hydrolyase (see Fig. 6) is the cause. A raised plasma tyrosine (and often a raised methionine) result. Succinyl acetone is excreted, formed from fumarylacetoacetate, which also inhibits porphobilinogen synthesis so that δ-amino laevulinic acid increases in the urine. Human fumarylacetoacetate hydrolyase is a dimer with a monomer molecular weight of 43 000. Activity is found in liver, kidney, fibroblasts, lymphocytes, and amniocytes.

Diagnosis

Raised plasma tyrosine, succinyl acetone, and δ-aminolaevulinic acid excretion and a Fanconi syndrome are the biochemical markers. Fumarylacetoacetate hydrolyase can be assayed in lymphocytes or fibroblasts. It is non-specifically depressed in the liver in a variety of liver diseases. A pseudodeficiency gene in the general population causes low 'in vitro' assay results for fumarylacetoacetate hydrolyase but no clinical illness. Untreated plasma tyrosine values in proven tyrosinaemia type I may be normal, creating another diagnostic problem. Liver function tests are abnormal.

Genetics

The disease is an autosomal recessive. The acute neonatal form lacks immunologically detectable enzyme protein in contrast to the more chronic form. The fumarylacetoacetate hydrolyase gene has been localized to chromosome 15 and a variety of mutations identified.

Prenatal diagnosis and carrier detection

The measurement of succinyl acetone in amniotic fluid and fumarylacetoacetate hydrolyase in cultured amniocytes or chorionic villus samples forms the basis of prenatal diagnosis. In approximately 5 per cent of families one parent carries both a true mutant allele and the pseudogene, which lowers the parental enzyme activity into the homozygous disease state and causes confusion in prenatal diagnosis. The pseudogene also makes the detection of carriers less certain. Where the mutation is known molecular prenatal diagnosis should be possible and preferable.

Treatment

Restricted intake of tyrosine and phenylalanine may reduce the excretion of succinyl acetone and produce regression of the Fanconi tubular defects. Rickets may require treatment however. The liver disease is not cured. The risk of hepatocellular carcinoma remains. Therapeutic trials are in progress using a metabolic inhibitor, NTBC, which blocks the pathway before homogentisic acid thus reducing the production of toxic metabolites. The results are encouraging, with over 200 patients under follow-up and a greatly reduced incidence of liver damage and hepatic carcinoma since NTBC was introduced in 1991.

Liver transplantation remains the treatment of choice for some who do not respond to NTBC which may also improve renal function, although some succinyl acetone continues to be excreted. transplant timing is immensely problematic. Neither α-fetoprotein nor ultrasound are totally reliable at detecting early malignant change. After liver transplantation the future is uncertain. Chronic renal failure has occurred.

Tyrosinaemia type II

Clinical

Corneal erosions and dendritric ulcers may form within a few months of birth with later scarring, nystagmus, and glaucoma. Corneal transplants can be valuable. The skin lesions may begin after the eye lesions with blistering, painful palms and soles, and hyperkeratosis. Tongue changes have been described. Mental retardation is an inconstant feature but language defects may be more common with possible impaired co-ordination and self-mutilation. The pathology is considered secondary to the deposition of tyrosine crystals in cells precipitating an inflammatory response.

Biochemistry

Tyrosine aminotransferase, which is deficient, catalyses the formation of p-hydroxyphenylpyruvic acid (see Fig. 8) and requires pyridoxal phosphate and α-ketobutyrate. It is a liver enzyme, absent from brain, heart, and kidney, with a subunit size of 49 000 which forms dimers. The enzyme is synthesized rapidly, induced by steroids, and has a short half-life. The gene has been mapped to chromosome 16.

Plasma tyrosine values reach 20 times normal (normal 40 to 100 μmol/litre) in younger patients and 10 times normal in others. There is increased excretion of tyrosine, N-acetyl tyrosine, and tyramine; there is no Fanconi syndrome. Excreted phenolic acids come from phenylalanine or tyrosine metabolized at high concentrations by other enzymes.

Diagnosis

The clinical features and amino acid analyses are usually sufficient.

Treatment

A low-tyrosine, low-phenylalanine diet has been used to produce rapid improvement of skin and eye manifestations. There is little information on

Table 10 A classification of albinism according to whether the hair bulbs have tyrosinase activity (positive) or not (negative)

	Oculocutaneous tyrosinase −ve	Oculocutaneous tyrosinase +ve	Ocular
Hair colour	White	White Yellow tan	Normal
Skin colour	Pink	White No tan	Normal
Pigmented naevi	0	+	+
Risk of skin cancer	+++	+++	Normal
Eye colour	Grey to blue	Blue to yellow-brown	Normal range
Fundal pigment	0	0, +	0, +
Photophobia	+++	++	+++
Nystagmus	+++	++	+++
Visual acuity	Severely impaired	Impaired	Impaired
Genetics	Autosomal recessive	Autosomal recessive	X-linked or autosomal recessive

the neurological results of treatment and little on the degree of dietary control needed to sustain clinical improvement.

Alcaptonuria

Clinical

Presentation in infancy occurs only if discoloration of the urine is noticed. It is usually normal when passed, but darkens on standing (more rapidly at alkaline pH) to deep brown or almost black. Back pain begins in the second and third decade with increasing stiffness due to intervertebral disc degeneration. Involvement of the hips, knees, and shoulders follows. Greyish discoloration of cartilage is seen in the pinna, and pigment is deposited in the sclera. Abnormal pigmentation is seen in the heart valves and pigmented stones are common in the prostate. Discoloration of cartilage, tendons, and ligaments is more orange when seen microscopically (ochronosis). The prognosis for the joints is poor. By the fifth decade the lumbar spine is likely to be rigid and other joints will be seriously affected.

Pathology

The pigment is assumed to be a polymer derived from homogentisic acid after enzymatic conversion to the corresponding quinone (homogentisic acid polyphenol oxidase). Virchow described the internally pigmented cartilages including the larynx, tracheal rings, and ribs. The joint cartilages become thinned and fragmented. The intervertebral discs calcify.

Biochemistry

Homogentisic acid oxidase contains ferrous iron and several −SH groups. Molecular oxygen is consumed in splitting the ring to convert homogentisic acid to maleylacetoacetic acid. Homogentisic acid produces a false positive for glucose in the 'Clinitest' reaction but the reaction mixture quickly darkens because of the alkaline pH. There is no reaction with glucose in standard dipstick tests for glucose. Affected individuals excrete 4 to 8 g of homogentisic acid per day.

Diagnosis

In the presence of the clinical symptoms simple urine tests virtually make the diagnosis secure. The homogentisic acid can be demonstrated on thin-layer chromatography and quantitated by gas–liquid chromatography or high-pressure liquid chromatography.

Genetics

It is an autosomal recessive with an incidence of only 1 in 200 000 but small populations of very high incidence exist, especially in the former Czechoslovakia and the Dominican Republic. The gene has been localized to chromosome 3q and a variety of mutations described.

Antenatal diagnosis

This has not been required but is theoretically possible.

Treatment

The amount of homogentisic acid produced is decreased by a low-protein diet. It is very probable that specifically designed low-phenylalanine and low-tyrosine diets would lower the production still further. There seems to be no demand for such a restricting diet to deal with an arthritis which begins only in adult life and progresses slowly over many years. Ascorbic acid may slow the rate of oxidation of homogentisic acid to pigment precursors but there are no data on its clinical usefulness. Theoretically NTBC may be beneficial, but its current high cost would discourage trials and the longer-term toxicity not known.

Albinism

Tyrosinase deficiency in melanocytes prevents the conversion of *p*-hydroxyphenylalanine to dihydroxyphenylalanine and thence to dopaquinone, the precursor for pigment formation in the skin, the iris, the fundus, and the inner ear. The absence of pigment is the characteristic of the group of disorders referred to together as albinism. It is a complex group of ten or more types. The manifestations are primarily in the skin and eye.

The three main types are compared in Table 10. However, two points worth noting are: oculocutaneous albinism may also occur in association with a bleeding tendency—the Hermansky Pudlak syndrome—and in association with the leucocyte killing defect—the Chédiak–Higashi syndrome. Ocular albinism, too, in some genetic forms, occurs in association with nerve deafness.

Oculocutaneous albinism is characterized by structural optic tract defects. All the fibres at the optic chiasma cross over so there are no ipsilateral fibres and no binocular vision. The geniculate bodies and the radiation onwards to the cortex are also structurally abnormal. The inner ear lacks pigment that is normally said to be protective against noise trauma. The predisposition to squamous carcinoma of the skin is important. Further details are given in Table 10.

Disorders of sulphur amino acid metabolism

The trans-sulphuration pathway transfers the sulphur of methionine to serine to produce cysteine (Fig. 8). Methionine adenosyltransferase, with widely distributed isoenzyme forms, produces *S*-adenosylmethionine, the donor in a variety of methylation reactions. In creatine formation alone adult males may utilize more methyl groups than provided by dietary

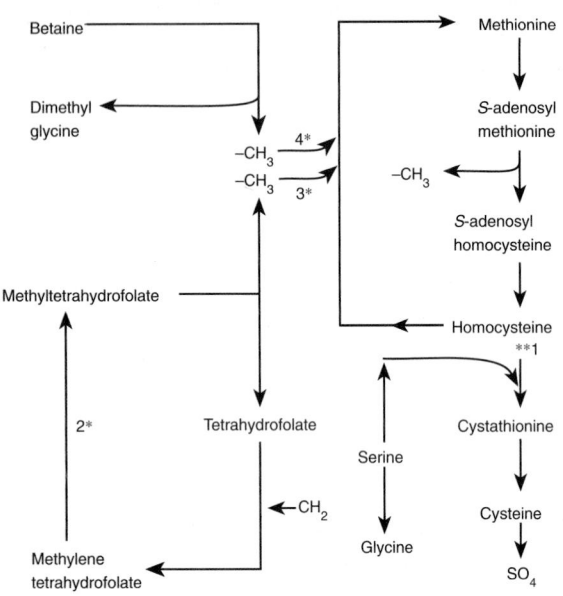

Fig. 8 The trans-sulphuration pathway from methionine to cysteine is shown on the right and the remethylation of homocysteine on the left. Asterisked enzymes are: 1, cystathionine synthase; 2, methylene tetrahydrofolate reductase, 3, methionine synthase; and 4, betaine methyltransferase.

methionine. *S*-adenosyl homocysteine is cleaved to homocysteine, the sulphhydryl compound which exists in reversible equilibrium with its disulphide homocystine. Half of the homocysteine formed goes through the trans-sulphuration pathway and the other half takes a methyl group from betaine (betaine methyltransferase) or 5-methyltetrahydrofolic acid (methionine synthase). The latter is a cobalamin-dependent enzyme which is functionally impaired in defects of vitamin B₁₂ metabolism. The remethylation of homocysteine is also impaired if the activity of the reductase that generates 5-methyltetrahydrofolate is inadequate.

When accumulation of homocystine results from defects of homocysteine remethylation plasma methionine concentrations are low. They are high when homocystine accumulates from impaired activity of cystathionine synthase, which forms the thioether cystathionine, an intermediate subsequently cleaved to produce the sulphydryl compound cysteine. Further metabolism of cysteine produces inorganic sulphate for excretion.

Cystathionine β synthase deficiency (homocystinuria)

Clinical

The classic clinical features in the older child and adult are mental retardation, lens dislocation, a thrombotic tendency, and skeletal abnormalities. Mental retardation, affecting two-thirds of patients, is sometimes gross but more commonly IQ values are around 65. Others are in the normal range with a few high values. Patients responsive to pyridoxine (vitamin B₆) (see below) have generally higher IQ values than non-responsive patients. Seizures affect about one-fifth and a few patients show extrapyramidal features, sometimes with severe involuntary movements. Psychiatric disturbances have been described but an increased frequency of schizophrenia is unproven.

Lens dislocation is acquired, usually in the preschool years, but later dislocation is well recognized especially in pyridoxine-responsive patients, and a few have not developed it even in adult life. Monocular and binocular blindness has been relatively frequent due to secondary glaucoma, staphyloma formation, buphthalmos, and retinal detachment.

The skeletal abnormalities include osteoporosis and spontaneous crush vertebral fractures. The common abnormalities seen in Marfan's syndrome—high arched palate, pectus excavatum or carinatum, genu valgum, pes cavus or planus, scoliosis—are all well recognized in homocystinuria. Arachnodactyly is less common and the fingers not infrequently (and elbows occasionally) show mild flexion contractures. Skeletal disproportion with a crown pubis length less than the pubis heel length is usual (Fig. 9).

Pathology

Thromboembolism is a major cause of morbidity and the main cause of the relatively high premature mortality. Thromboses have been described in a wide variety of arteries and veins: cerebral, coronary, mesenteric, renal, and peripheral. About 50 per cent are in peripheral veins with associated pulmonary emboli in many. Postoperative and postpartum thrombotic risks are high. Premature atheromatous vascular degeneration has been described, as has arterial aneurysm formation.

Homocysteine may interfere with crosslinking in collagen. Degeneration of zonular fibres around the lens causes the lens dislocation but these fibres are not collagen. Recent work on fibrillin in Marfan's syndrome suggests that defects in this protein may be important in cystathionine β synthase deficiency. There is still no accepted explanation for the relationship of homocystine/homocysteine to endothelial damage, platelet abnormalities, thromboses, and vascular change. Heterozygotes for the enzyme defect may be disposed to premature vascular disease and thrombosis. Finally, although the cerebral hemispheres normally have a high concentration of cystathionine, which is reduced in cystathionine β synthase deficiency, this is not considered a cause of the mental deficiency, and neither does diffuse vascular disease seem relevant to this problem.

Biochemistry

Elevated plasma methionine values between 100 and 500 μmol/litre (sometimes higher) are seen with plasma homocystine values of 50 to 200 μmol/litre (Fig. 8). A mixed disulphide (half homocysteine, half cysteine) is always present at concentrations somewhat below homocystine. Total homocysteine measured by high-performance liquid chromatography is used by some laboratories for diagnosis and monitoring treatment. This includes

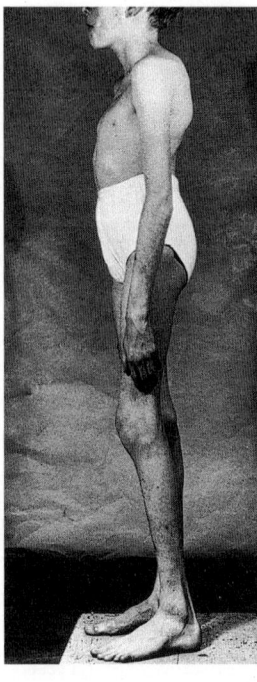

Fig. 9 Child with cystathionine synthase deficiency. Note the kyphosis and short trunk.

both homocysteine moieties of homocystine, the homocysteine moiety of the mixed disulphide, and the homocysteine bound to plasma proteins. The urinary excretion of homocystine is usually 250 to 1000 µmol/day, which accounts for only about 10 to 20 per cent of ingested methionine sulphur. The active cystathionine β synthase apoenzyme, which requires pyridoxal phosphate, is a tetramer of 63 kDa units found predominantly in liver but also in brain and intestinal mucosa. Much lower levels of activity can be found in cultured fibroblasts and stimulated lymphocytes. Residual hepatic activity of 1 to 2 per cent occurs in affected patients, this may increase two- to fourfold in pyridoxine-responsive cases. In some patients higher residual activities up to 9 to 10 per cent have been found. Heterozygotes have 25 to 45 per cent of normal activity. *In vitro* responsiveness to pyridoxal phosphate can also be detected in cultured fibroblasts.

Diagnosis

The urine gives a positive nitroprusside test (it is also positive in cystinuria). The amino acid defects are diagnostic if the plasma is deproteinized promptly to minimize binding of homocystine to protein. Plasma methionine concentrations are usually well above the normal values of 15 to 30 µmol/litre and homocystine is present in plasma and urine.

Genetics

The disease is an autosomal recessive with a birth incidence of about 1 in 40 000. The gene is on chromosome 21 with over 50 mutations already described.

Antenatal diagnosis

This has so far rested on enzyme assays on cultured amniotic cells. It is likely that work on the mutant gene will supersede this.

Treatment

Oral pyridoxine may rapidly reduce methionine and homocystine to near normal values. It should be the first treatment to try using 150 to 300 mg/day in the older child or adult and reducing the dose if a response is achieved. Very large sustained doses (1000 mg/day or more) in adults cause peripheral neuropathy. A very low-protein diet with a system of exchanges is appropriate for those not responding to pyridoxine and requires a methionine-free amino acid supplement, minerals, and vitamins. Biochemical control may only be achieved in older children and adults on natural protein intakes of 5 to 10 g/day. Cystine supplementation of diets should be considered in patients partially responsive to pyridoxine. Both folic acid (5 to 10 mg/day) and betaine (up to 12 g/day) can further reduce plasma homocystine levels but may produce large elevations of plasma methionine. Low red cell folate values occur and even megaloblastic anaemia. Low serum vitamin B_{12} values have also been found. The relationships between homocystine, the mixed disulphide, and total homocyteine values are not linear, making target values for treatment difficult to establish. Effective treatment lowers the incidence of vascular events.

Defects of homocysteine remethylation

Two defects have been described: a deficiency of methylene tetrahydrofolate reductase and a deficiency of methionine synthase (methyltetrahydrofolate homocysteine methyltransferase). The latter requires methylcobalamin as coenzyme.

Methylene tetrahydrofolate reductase deficiency

Clinical

Neurological features predominate with psychomotor retardation, seizures, abnormalities of gait, and psychiatric disturbance. Presentation occurs from early to late childhood. The risk of vascular disease is high.

Pathology

At autopsy dilated ventricles and low brain weight have been seen; thromboses may be present in arteries and veins. Demyelination occurs and the changes may resemble the classic findings of subacute combined degeneration seen in vitamin B_{12} deficiency. Calcification of the basal ganglia occurs.

Biochemistry

Plasma methionine concentrations are below normal and plasma homocystine concentrations in the range 20 to 200 µmol/litre with an excretion of 15 to 600 µmol/day.

Diagnosis

Homocystine is easily missed at low concentrations but is the important clue. The enzyme can be assayed in liver or fibroblasts.

Genetics and prenatal diagnosis

It is an autosomal recessive and enzyme assays on cultured amniocytes have been used for prenatal diagnosis. Several mutations have already been described.

Treatment

Betaine in large doses lowers plasma homocystine and raises plasma methionine. Other treatments tried alone or in combination include folinic acid, vitamin B_{12}, pyridoxine, and methionine. Some have suggested a 'cocktail' of all these treatments. It is difficult to be sure of clinical success.

Methionine synthase deficiency

The enzyme transfers a methyl group from methyltetrahydrofolate to homocysteine. Methyl cobalamin is the required coenzyme. This metabolic step may be impaired by an apoenzyme defect or defects in cobalamin metabolism, some of which limit only the formation of methyl cobalamin. Other cobalamin defects are considered under methyl malonic acidaemia.

Clinical

The characteristic findings are developmental delay and megaloblastic anaemia, but the onset may be in later in childhood with dementia and spasticity. Retinal degeneration, cardiac defects, and haemolysis have been described.

Biochemistry and diagnosis

The findings include low plasma methionine and raised homocystine in plasma and urine. Methylmalonic acid should be measured in urine to exclude other cobalamin defects (see methylmalonic aciduria). Methione synthase can be assayed in liver or fibroblasts and antenatal diagnosis has been carried out on cultured amniocytes.

Treatment

This may involve large doses of hydroxocobalamin with betaine and possibly folinic acid.

Other defects of sulphur amino acid metabolism

Among several known defects, cystathioninuria due to cystathionase deficiency is probably clinically harmless. Cystathionine in excess of 1 g/day may be excreted at clearance values close to the glomerular filtration rate.

Methionine adenosyl transferase deficiency causes raised plasma methionine levels (up to 1200 µmol/litre; normal 15 to 30 µmol/litre) which seems to be harmless. The enzyme defect is partial.

Neither of these defects is considered further but sulphite oxidase deficiency is clinically important.

Sulphite oxidase deficiency

Most cases are due to abnormalities of the molybdenum cofactor, which therefore also affects the action of xanthine oxidase and aldehyde oxidase.

Clinical

Lens dislocation occurs, with severe neurological abnormalities, delayed psychomotor development, and xanthinuria. The neurological defects include seizures and axial hypotonia with increased limb tone. The disease is fatal.

Biochemistry

Sulphite concentrations are raised and sulphite is excreted in the urine. Direct reaction in the body between sulphite and cysteine yields sulphocysteine. Plasma urate levels are low and urine xanthine is increased when the disease is due to cofactor abnormalities but not if the defect is in the apoenzyme of sulphite oxidase.

Diagnosis

There is a dipstick test for sulphite which must be applied to fresh urine. *S*-sulphocysteine can be detected on an amino acid analyser. Sulphite oxidase can be measured in fibroblasts or liver.

Genetics and prenatal diagnosis

It is an autosomal recessive disorder. Prenatal diagnosis has been carried out on cultured amniocytes by enzyme assay.

Treatment

No effective treatment is known. Some damage may be prenatal. Measures that could be considered include diets low in methionine and cystine. Penicillamine might lower sulphite concentrations by binding with it. The nature of the molybdenum-containing cofactor is not well enough understood to be a useful therapeutic approach.

Defects of glycine metabolism

Folate and activated 1-carbon units

Tetrahydrofolate carries 1-carbon units—methyl, methylene, methenyl, formyl, or forminino—bonded to the N-5 or N-10 nitrogen atoms and the units are interconvertible. One-carbon units are donated from the tetrahydrofolate derivatives in a variety of syntheses. New 1-carbon units are accepted by tetrahydrofolate in degradative reactions, of which the most important is the conversion of serine to glycine. As serine can be formed from 3-phosphoglycerate, carbohydrates are the ultimate source of 1-carbon units (Fig. 10).

The glycine cleavage system

This system, which generates methylene tetrahydrofolate from carbon-2 of glycine, and carbon dioxide from carbon-1, consists of four mitochondrial proteins. The P protein is a decarboxylase requiring pyridoxal phosphate. The heat-resistant H protein contains lipoic acid and carries the aminomethyl moiety. Both proteins are needed to generate carbon dioxide from the carbon-1 of glycine. The T protein requires tetrahydrofolate and produces methylene tetrahydrofolate from carbon-2 of glycine. The fourth protein (L protein) is needed to transfer hydrogen from the lipoic acid moiety of the H protein to nictotinamide adenine diphosphate. Reversal of the sequence synthesizes glycine. Glycine can be converted to glyoxylate and to δ-aminolaevulinic acid for porphyrin synthesis.

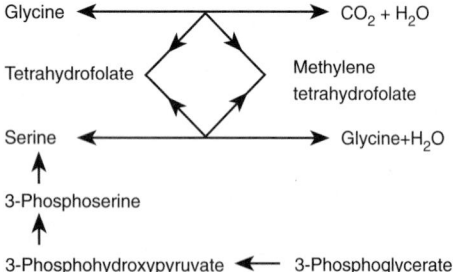

Fig. 10 Reversible glycine cleavage to carbon dioxide and water is illustrated together with reversible interconversion of serine and glycine. These reactions also serve to generate 1-carbon units. 3-phosphoglycerate (glycolysis) is the ultimate source.

Non-ketotic hyperglycinaemia

Clinical

Twenty four to 48 h after birth, lethargy, convulsions, anorexia, poor feeding, and vomiting progress to coma and unresponsiveness. Apnoea may require ventilation at least temporarily. The mortality at this stage is high. Intellectual development does not occur in survivors, seizures persist, and tendon reflexes are increased. Microcephaly, poor head control, profound retardation, and a picture of spastic cerebral palsy result. Hiccupping *in utero* maybe recognized retrospectively.

There is a later childhood form presenting with spastic paraparesis, clonus, and extensor plantar responses with modestly raised plasma and cerebrospinal fluid glycine values. Optic atrophy with cerebellar signs has also been described.

Biochemistry

The defect is in the glycine cleavage system with plasma glycine values of 600 to 1200 μmol/litre. Normal values for cerebrospinal fluid levels of glycine are around 4 to 5 μmol/litre, the cerebrospinal fluid plasma ratio being around 0.02. Cerebrospinal fluid values are greatly increased in patients, raising the cerebrospinal fluid:plasma ratio to between 0.07 and 0.30. Large quantities of glycine appear in the urine, but this is not accompanied by proline or hydroxyproline.

Diagnosis

This rests on the analysis of glycine concentrations in plasma and cerebrospinal fluid. Activity of the glycine cleavage system can be measured on liver biopsies and in a few laboratories in leucocytes.

Genetics

The variant forms are autosomal recessives. The P protein is absent in classic phenotypes. T protein defects have been found in different phenotypes and H protein defects in later onset degenerative forms. Hyperglycinaemia seems to be commoner in Japan and Finland. Different mutations in these two populations affect the P protein.

Antenatal diagnosis

The enzyme system is unstable and not present in fibroblasts or cultured amniotic cells. Chorionic villi are being used for enzyme assay in prenatal diagnosis combined with amniotic fluid glycine:serine ratios. Increasing information on causative mutations will facilitate antenatal diagnosis.

Treatment

This is very unsatisfactory. Some damage to the central nervous system may be prenatal. Plasma glycine levels can be lowered by exchange transfusion or peritoneal dialysis but without clinical improvement. Low-protein diets have only a limited effect on decreasing plasma glycine concentrations. Supplying 1-carbon units in the form of methionine or *N*-formyltetrahydrofolate has not helped. The combination of sodium benzoate to increase glycine excretion and diazepines, which compete for inhibitoryglycine receptors in the central nervous system, has lowered plasma and cerebrospinal fluid levels of glycine and reduced seizures without clearly improving prognosis. Glycine is also a coagonist at the excitatory *N*-methyl-D-aspartate (NMDA) receptor blockage which has been attempted with several agents. Success has been absent or very limited. Imipramine may warrant further trial.

Defects in branched chain amino acid (leucine, isoleucine, and valine) metabolism

These essential amino acids, with a branched carbon chain structure, collectively make up 10 to 15 per cent of animal protein and are catabolized by

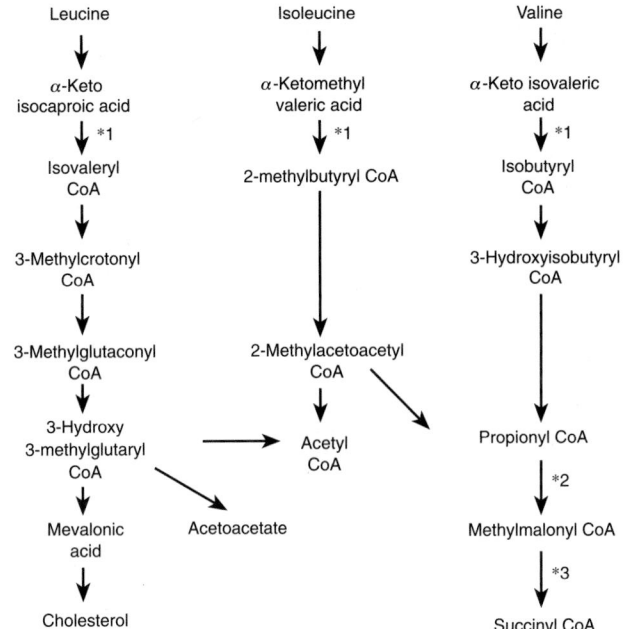

Fig. 11 Branched chain amino acid metabolism. Transamination produces the keto acids (top) all of which are metabolized by the branched chain α-ketodehydrogenase complex (asterisked) 1. 2, Propionyl coenzyme A carboxylase; and 3, methylmalonyl coenzyme A mutase.

transamination to the corresponding keto acids, 2-keto-isocaproic, 2-keto-3-methylvaleric, and 2-keto-isovaleric acids (Fig. 11). In all tissues except the liver aminotransferase activity exceeds α-ketodehydrogenase activity. Peripheral tissues, notably muscle, predominantly transaminate but the keto acids are largely transported back to the liver for subsequent metabolism.

Branched chain α-ketodehydrogenase: the role of thiamine

The oxidative decarboxylation of branched chain keto acids is analogous to the oxidative decarboxylation of pyruvate and α-ketoglutarate to acetyl coenzyme A and succinyl coenzyme A, respectively. All are three-subunit mitochondrial enzymes, the first part of which, E_1, uses thiamine pyrophosphate as a coenzyme. The thiamine moiety is crucial to the decarboxylase function of branched chain α-ketodehydrogenase (E_1) and the release of carbon dioxide. Branched chain α-ketodehydrogenase (E_2) is the core protein of the complex, the acyl transferase that generates acyl coenzyme A while its lipoate moiety is reduced. The third part (E_3) regenerates the oxidized lipoate and is actually shared by all three dehydrogenase complexes. Branched chain α-ketodehydrogenase (E_1) is active in a dephosphorylated form and inactivated by phosphorylation, which provides a control mechanism. Branched chain ketoaciduria (maple syrup urine disease) arises from defects in the branched chain α-ketodehydrogenase complex. Some patients have a thiamine responsive form of this disease (see below).

Branched chain ketoaciduria

Clinical

In the classic disease the baby is well for 2 to 3 days and then poor feeding and sleepiness progress to coma and apnoea. Vomiting is inconstant. The mortality is high and survivors show dystonia, psychomotor retardation, spastic quadriplegia, and other neurological abnormalities.

Milder forms of the disease are described, sometimes with later presentation and intermittent forms where patients may be biochemically normal between attacks but succumb during intercurrent infection or illness or excessive protein intake.

Pathology

Myelin abnormalities that occur in patients dying of branched chain ketoaciduria are also found in Poll-Hereford calves with the same genetic defect, and in other experimental animal models.

Biochemistry

In the acute stage, hypoglycaemia and hyperammonaemia may occur. Leucine values may be as high as 4000 to 5000 μmol/litre. Isoleucine and valine are also much increased in plasma and urine (see Table 1 for normal values.) The three keto acids cause mild metabolic acidosis and the sweetish smell of maple syrup in urine. Residual enzyme activity in fibroblasts is 1 to 2 per cent for the classic severe disease but 20 to 40 per cent of normal in mild variants.

Diagnosis

The plasma amino acids and urine keto acids are diagnostic. Diagnosis before 6 days of age carries a better prognosis than later diagnosis with patients discovered by neonatal screening doing best of all.

Genetics

This is an autosomal recessive disorder. Screening is possible by bacterial assay but the disease is too rare to justify the cost. The incidence is about 1 in 120 000 in Europe but 1 in 200 000 in most of the United States, although an incidence of more than 1 in 1000 has been recorded in a Mennonite community. As the E_1 component of the branched chain α-ketodehydrogenase is subdivided further into $E_{1\alpha}$ and $E_{1\beta}$ at least four genes code for the complex, plus two genes for the controlling phosphatase and kinase. Enzyme assays and immunological and complementation studies have already revealed genetic defects in $E_{1\alpha}$, $E_{1\beta}$ and E_2 in different families. The Mennonite mutation is an asparagine substitution for tyrosine in the $E_{1\alpha}$ subunit.

Prenatal diagnosis

This has been based on enzyme assays in cultured amniocytes or chorionic villus samples.

Treatment

A high calorie intake, given parenterally as 10 to 20 per cent dextrose if necessary, is needed to suppress nitrogen catabolism in the acutely ill. An amino acid mixture excluding leucine, isoleucine, and valine can be introduced by nasogastric tube to provide 2 g protein/kg/day. Normal protein sources (milk, etc.) are omitted until the branched chain amino acid concentrations fall towards normal. Both exchange transfusion and peritoneal dialysis have been used to speed biochemical recovery but haemofiltration is thought to be better. Hypoglycaemia, sepsis, and hypotension need intensive care and monitoring. Dietary treatment is lifelong but needs frequent adjustments. The aim is to keep plasma leucine, isoleucine, and valine concentrations close to their normal values (see Table 1). Coma carries a poor prognosis for subsequent development and function of the central nervous system. The incidence of impaired intellect and neurological handicap is high and special schooling will be necessary.

Responsiveness to thiamine(10 to 20 mg/day) has also been described in a few patients. It is claimed that large doses up to 500 mg/day improve some cases of classic branched chain ketoaciduria. *In vitro* evidence indicates that the $E_{1\alpha}$ subunit is stabilized by thiamine supplements, which may saturate all subunits. An increase in enzyme activity has even been described in normal subjects on thiamine treatment.

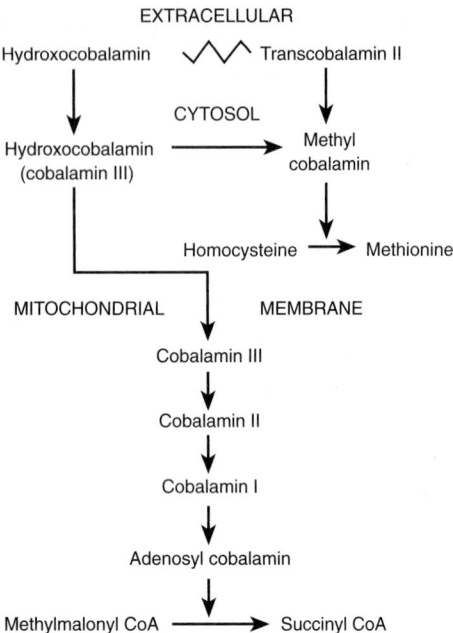

Fig. 12 Naturally occurring cobalamin is converted in the cytosol to methyl cobalamin, or adenosyl cobalamin is eventually formed by successive valency reductions of the cobalt moiety within the mitchondria.

Other defects of branched chain amino acid metabolism

Rare cases of defective deamination have been described causing isolated hypervalinaemia or hyperleucinaemia–isoleucinaemia, indicating either separate amino transferases in humans or different mutations affecting different substrate binding sites in a common enzyme.

The organic acidaemias in branched chain amino acid metabolism

The catabolic steps outlined in Fig. 11 illustrate the formation of isovaleric acid, propionic acid, and methylmalonic acid, each of which accumulates in one of the three more common organic acidaemias. In the further metabolism of two of these acids there are important vitamin coenzymes—biotin for priopionyl coenzyme A carboxylase and cobalamin for methylmalonyl coenzyme A mutase. Biotin metabolism is considered under multiple carboxylase deficiency later and cobalamin metabolism immediately below. A range of other organic acidaemias have been described after discovery by gas–liquid chromatography with mass spectroscopy; their diagnosis may beome more frequent with the wider diagnostic use of tandem mass spectroscopy. They have been reported only rarely to date and are not considered further.

Vitamin B$_{12}$ metabolism

Vitamin B$_{12}$ has a complex metabolism but is required in only two metabolic steps—the remethylation of homocysteine to methionine and the conversion of methylmalonyl coenzyme A to succinyl coenzyme A. An outline of cobalamin metabolism in the body is shown in Fig. 12. In the cytosol hydroxocobalamin may become the coenzyme methyl cobalamin, which is required by methionine synthase, or be transported into the mitochondria to be metabolized to adenosyl cobalamin, the coenzyme of methylmalonyl coenzyme A mutase.

Isovaleric, propionic, and methylmalonic acidaemias

Clinical

One to several days after a normal pregnancy and delivery the child stops feeding. Respiratory problems ensue with varying tonal change, both axial

hypotonia and episodes of generalized hypertonia and myoclonic jerking. Apnoea, coma, and death supervene. Characteristically the child is acidotic, possibly ketotic, and non-specific increases of ammonia and glycine may occur. Both hypoglycaemia and hyperglycaemia have been described, the latter causing confusion with diabetic ketoacidosis. Hypocalcaemia is also found. Early mortality is high and patients are often difficult to treat. Survivors have recurrent episodes of decompensation. There is an abnormal body odour likened to sweaty feet in isovaleric aciduria.

A more chronic form of these diseases is recognized, with anorexia, failure to thrive, psychomotor retardation, hypotonia, and weakness. Cardiomyopathy has been reported as a late complication. Damage to the basal ganglia with movement disorders is common and chronic renal failure may develop in survivors with methylmalonic aciduria.

The intermittent clinical forms present as recurrent attacks of encephalopathy and ataxia with normality between attacks. Changes in blood glucose may again be confusing (see above). Acute attacks may be followed by neurological abnormalities of a pyramidal or extrapyramidal nature. Leucopenia and thrombocytopenia sometimes occur.

Biochemistry

Isovaleric acidaemia is due to a deficiency of isovaleryl coenzyme A dehydrogenase and is characterized by the excretion in the urine of isovaleric acid, isovalerylglycine, 3-hydroxy isovaleric acid, and isovalerylcarnitine.

Isolated propionic acidaemia is due to a deficiency of the apoenzyme for propionyl coenzyme A carboxylase, a biotin-requiring enzyme. The enzyme converts proprionyl coenzyme A to methylmalonyl coenzyme A. Characteristically, plasma and urine propionate values are raised with the formation of methylcitrate from the condensation of propionyl coenzyme A with oxaloacetate (Fig. 13). Propionylcarnitine excretion is increased.

Methylmalonic acidaemia is due to deficient activity of methylmalonyl coenzyme A mutase, the enzyme converting methylmalonyl coenzyme A to

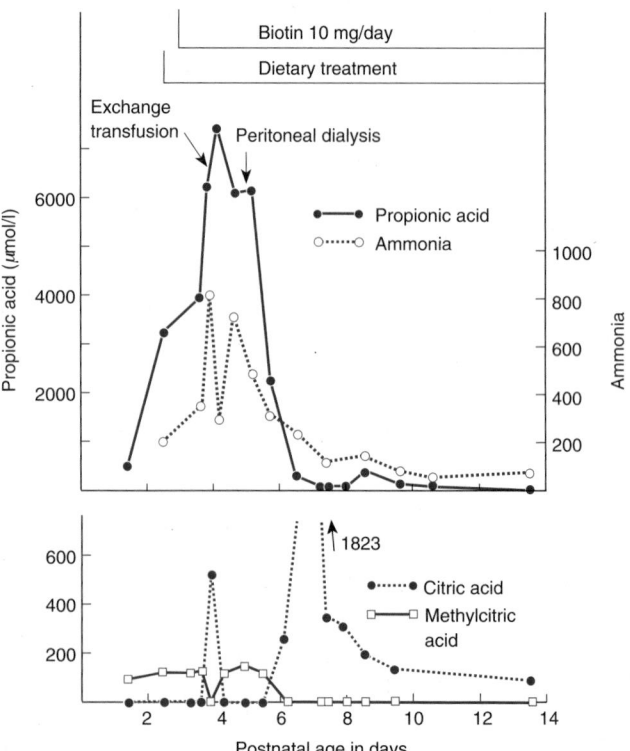

Fig. 13 Neonatal propionic acidaemia with hyperammonaemia, raised plasma methylcitrate levels, and low levels of citrate (μmol/litre). Treated by diet, exchange transfusion, and peritoneal dialysis. (From Brenton and Krywawych, unpublished data.)

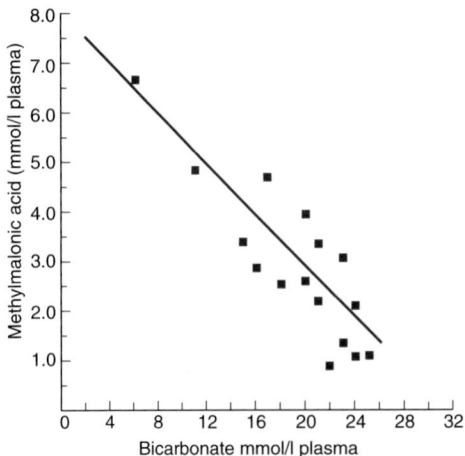

Fig. 14 Plasma concentrations of methylmalonate (a dicarboxylic acid) and bicarbonate in an affected teenage girl indicating that the acidosis is due almost entirely to the methymalonate. (From Brenton and Krywawych, unpublished data.)

succinyl coenzyme A, which requires adenosyl cobalamin. Two apoenzyme defects are described, one with virtually zero activity and one with residual activity of 2 to 75 per cent of normal. Two genetic defects in the formation of adenosyl cobalamin have been described. One affects the formation of both adenosyl and methyl cobalamin, resulting in methylmalonic aciduria and homocystinuria. The other affects only adenosyl cobalamin, and only methylmalonic aciduria occurs. Patients with severe apoenzyme defects excrete up to 5 to 6 g/day of methylmalonic acid with high blood concentrations up to 6 mmol/litre (Fig. 14). Propionate also accumulates in the blood and is excreted together with methylcitrate.

Diagnosis
Diagnosis rests upon the detection of the relevant organic acids, their conjugates, or their carnitine esters in blood and urine.

Genetics
All three diseases are autosomal recessive. Isovaleryl coenzyme A dehydrogenase is a four-unit homopolymer with a single locus on the long arm of chromosome 15. Different enzyme variants cause phenotypic variation but severe neonatal and intermittent forms have been described in the same family.

Propionyl coenzyme A carboxylase has the subunit structure α_6/β_6. The α subunit gene is on chromosome 13 and the β subunit gene is on chromosome 3. Defects in the α chain (which binds the biotin) are associated with 50 per cent enzyme activity in heterozygotes and 1 to 5 per cent activity in homozygotes. Homozygous β-chain defects are similarly severe but heterozygotes have near normal activity. β chains are produced in half-normal amounts. β chains are normally produced in excess of α chains.

Methyl malonyl coenzyme A mutase is a dimer of subunit size 75 000 with adenosyl cobalamin bound to each subunit. The gene locus is on chromosome 6. The mutant mutase with no residual enzyme activity has no detectable enzyme protein, either because none is made or because it is highly unstable.

There is now considerable information on the causal mutations in all three diseases.

Prenatal diagnosis
Isovaleric acid in amniotic fluid is measured reliably by stable isotope dilution analysis, and isovaleryl coenzyme A dehydrogenase can be measured in cultured amniocytes. The measurement of methylcitrate in amniotic fluid and enzyme assay in cultured amniocytes has been used for diagnosis of propionic acidaemia. Similar approaches to prenatal diagnosis in isolated methylmalonic aciduria have used the measurement of methylmalonate

acid in amniotic fluid and enzyme assays or studies of adenosyl vitamin B_{12} metabolism in cultured amniocytes. Molecular prenatal diagnosis will be increasingly used in families where the genotype is known.

Treatment
In the severe neonatal form of these diseases the initial treatment is concerned with removal of toxic organic acids by exchange transfusion (as urinary excretion of propionate is poor this may be followed in propionic acidaemia by peritoneal dialysis) and encouraging anabolism by the provision of calories as 10 to 20 per cent glucose and electrolyte solutions intravenously with or without insulin. Enteral feeding should be started by nasogastric tube as soon as possible (after 24 to 48 h); initially this should be with protein-free feeds, but soon changing to a low-protein feed (0.5 g/kg/day) and later increasing to tolerance and supplemented with amino acid mixtures that omit the amino acids whose metabolism is impaired. The requirements of these amino acids for growth are provided by the natural protein, whose intake must be adjusted accordingly. L-glycine supplements of 0.25 to 0.5 g/kg/day are helpful in isovaleric acidaemia because it increases the formation of the non-toxic isovalerylglycine. L-carnitine 100 mg/kg/day may help in all three diseases by replenishing carnitine and increasing the excretion of non-toxic carnitine acyl esters. Both insulin and growth hormone have been used to try and produce positive nitrogen balance and hasten recovery in catabolic states.

No true *in vivo* responsiveness to biotin has been demonstrated in isolated propionic acidaemia. However, *in vivo* response to hydroxocobalamin therapy in methylmalonic acidaemia occurs and should be tested in all such patients and continued long term if response occurs. Diet is needed long term in all three disorders; this is relatively easy in isovaleric acidaemia where a low-protein diet may suffice. A low-protein diet may also suffice in some patients with methylmalonic acidaemia, combined with regular oral sodium bicarbonate to control residual acidosis. Patients with propionic acidaemia are more difficult to manage and require a low-protein diet with more frequent supplements of amino acids. Chronic nasogastric feeding may be needed for anorexia. Oral metronizanole may reduce propionate production by gut bacteria in the intestine in propionic and methylmalonic acidaemia but therapeutic usefulness is not yet clear. Similarly, the use of L-carnitine on a chronic basis may help in all diseases but it is not proven. Patients with methyl malonic aciduria and renal failure may require renal transplantation. combined hepatic and renal transplantation carried out to cure the underlying metabolic defect has also had very variable outcome.

Disorders of γ-aminobutyric acid metabolism
γ-aminobutyric acid is formed from glutamate in the brain by the cytosolic enzyme glutamate decarboxylase, which requires pyridoxal phosphate. Pyridoxine-dependent seizures in neonates are postulated to be due to a deficiency of this enzyme, which is difficult to prove because other tissues have a genetically different mitochondrial glutamate decarboxylase. Glutamate can be regenerated from γ-aminobutyric acid by transamination with ketoglutarate (γ-aminobutyric acid transaminase), which is also pyridoxal phosphate dependent. The other product is succinic semialdehyde, which is dehydrogenated to succinate, which enters the citric acid cycle. Deficiency of succinic semialdehyde dehydrogenase leads to the excretion of 4-hydroxybutyric acid. Some more details of disordered γ-aminobutyric acid metabolism are given in Table 11.

Defects of lysine metabolism

Lysine catabolism
The main pathway is via saccharopine to acetyl coenzyme A (Fig. 15); there are other less important pathways. Glutaryl coenzyme A dehydrogenase catalyses the conversion of glutaryl coenzyme A to crotonyl coenzyme A. Deficiency of this enzyme causes glutaric aciduria type I, a serious disorder. Other lysine degradation defects are of uncertain clinical consequence.

Table 11 Defects of γ-aminobutyric acid metabolism. The asterisk indicates that deficiency of glutamic acid decarboxylase has not been proven

Deficient enzyme	Clinical	Blood/urine metabolites	Treatment
Glutamic acid decarboxylase*	Seizures	No abnormality	Pyridoxine 10–100 mg/day
GABA transaminase	Psychomotor retardation, increased growth	Increased plasma and CSF GABA	No pyridoxine response reported
Succinic semialdehyde dehydrogenase	Mental retardation, cerebellar dysfunction	Increased 4-hydroxybutyrate in blood, urine, and CSF	None but ?neurology improves with age

GABA, γ-aminobutyric acid; CSF, cerebrospinal fluid.

Glutaric aciduria type I

Clinical

Abnormalities of development of the central nervous system begin before birth with macrocephaly and defective frontal and temporal lobe development, although early clinical development is often considered normal. Delayed motor development in the early years of life with hypotonia is followed by encephalopathic episodes precipitated by intercurrent illness with ataxia, athetosis, and other involuntary movements. Severe dystonia, pyramidal defects with extensor or flexor spasms, and severe dysarthria may follow. Intercurrent infection can also precipitate acidosis, seizures, coma, and paralysis, from which recovery is incomplete. The overall picture then resembles dystonic cerebral palsy. Computed tomography and magnetic resonance imaging have revealed progressive cerebral atrophy and hyperlucency of the caudate nucleus due to striatal necrosis. Even if the diagnosis is made in asymptomatic patients, acquired motor skills such as walking and writing may be slowly lost in the childhood years.

Biochemistry

Glutaryl coenzyme A dehydrogenase deficiency causes an accumulation of glutaryl coenzyme A (also derived from tryotophan degradation), increasing glutaric acid concentrations in plasma and urine, and increasing concentrations of 3-hydroxyglutarate and glutaconic acid. These are all inhibitors of glutamic acid decarboxylase, which may explain the low γ-aminobutyric acid concentrations in the central nervous system. Neurodegeneration probably results from excessive stimulation of NMDA receptors by 3-hydroxyglutaric acid. Glutaryl carnitine is excreted in the urine even when free glutaric acid is absent. Systemic acidosis occurs in acute attacks with ketosis and hypoglycaemia.

Diagnosis

This cause of progressive dystonic cerebral palsy is usually indicated by the organic acids in plasma and urine. Sometimes the organic acids have not been detected, particularly between acute attacks. Enzyme assays on leucocytes or fibroblasts are then indicated.

Prenatal diagnosis

This has been carried out by finding glutaric acid in the amniotic fluid and enzyme assay on cultured amniocytes. Where the mutation in the family is known molecular prenatal diagnosis would be more accurate.

Genetics

The disease is an autosomal recessive. The glutaryl coenzyme A dehydrogenase gene is on chromosome 19p and over 70 mutations have been described.

Treatment

Low-protein diets reduce glutaric acid excretion. Carnitine supplementation corrects low plasma levels which are secondary to losses from glutaryl carnitine excretion. Riboflavin has been reported to diminish glutaric acid excretion in some patients, the treatment rationale being that increased flavine adenine dinucleotide might stabilize the enzyme. Baclofen has also been studied because it activates γ-aminobutyric acid receptors. When treatment is started very early in life brain degeneration may be preventable. Delay results in irreversible damage to the caudate and putamen.

Defects in the final stages of carbon chain metabolism

Biotin-dependent carboxylation

Biotin is important in transferring a 1-carbon unit (carbon dioxide) to acceptor molecules. Defects in biotin metabolism disturb the function of four enzymes—pyruvate carboxylase, acetyl coenzyme A carboxylase, propionyl coenzyme A carboxylase, and 3-methylcrotonyl coenzyme A carboxylase (Fig. 16). These apoenzymes are converted to holoenzymes by the attachment of biotin, which needs the catalytic activity of an enzyme, holocarboxylase synthetase (Fig. 17). When the holoenzymes are themselves biologically degraded the biotin is initially released still attached to lysine peptides. The enzyme biotinidase frees biotin from these peptides. It also liberates dietary biotin from proteins in the gastrointestinal tract. In its absence biotin peptides are excreted, dietary biotin is not absorbed, and biotin deficiency occurs. Biotinidase is widely distributed throughout the body.

Electron transport and the acyl coenzyme A dehydrogenases

The electrons accumulating during oxidation in the citric acid cycle are carried by reduced nicotinamide adenine dinucleotide and reduced flavine

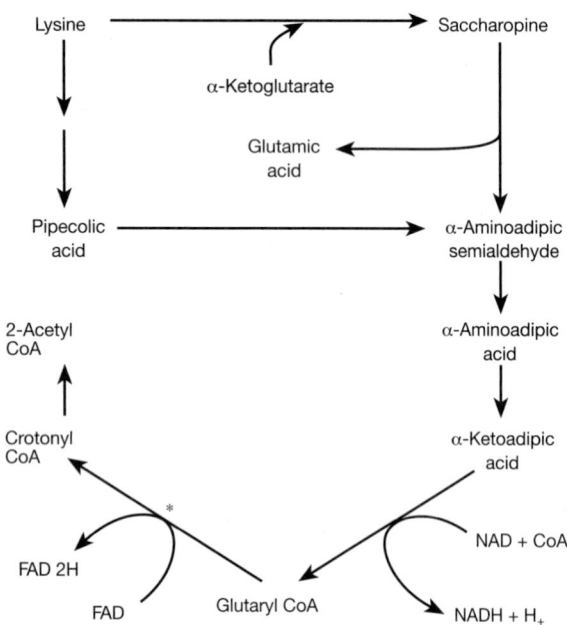

Fig. 15 The metabolism of lysine. The enzyme glutaryl coenzyme A dehydrogenase is asterisked.

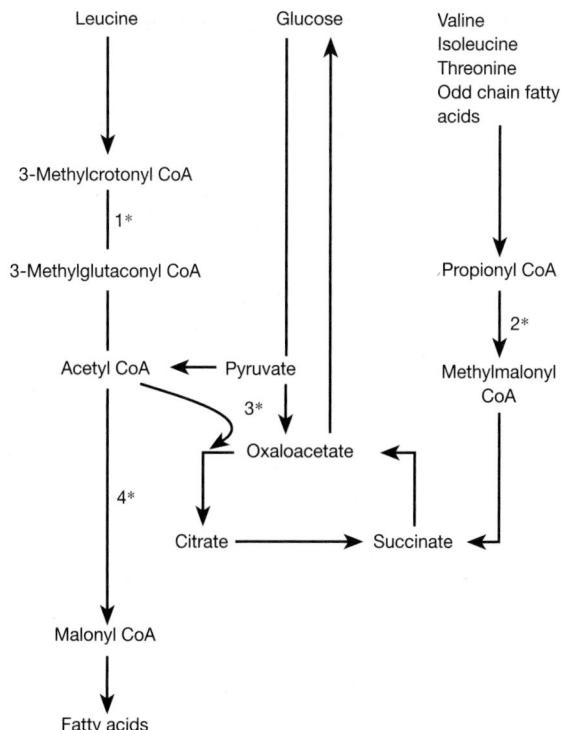

Fig. 16 Important carboxylases in amino acid metabolism. Asterisked enzymes are: 1, 3-methylcrotonyl coenzyme A carboxylase; 2, propionyl coenzyme A carboxylase; 3, pyruvate carboxylase; and 4, acetyl coenzyme A carboxylase.

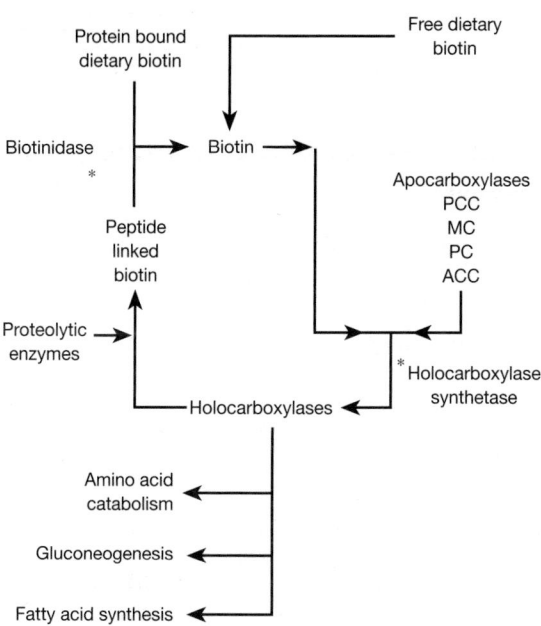

Fig. 17 The metabolism of biotin. MCC (3-methylcrotonyl coenzyme A) and PCC (propionyl coenzyme A carboxylase) are important in amino acid catabolism, PC (pyruvate carboxylase) is important in gluconeogenesis, and ACC (acetyl coenzyme A carboxylase) in fatty acid synthesis. Important enzymes are asterisked.

adenine dinucleotide to be transferred along the electron transporting chain to molecular oxygen, with the generation of adenosine triphosphate and water. Transfer from reduced nicotinamide adenine dinucleotide takes place sequentially across four multienzyme complexes (I to IV), which are part of the structure of the inner mitochondrial membrane. The flavin-containing acyl coenzyme A dehydrogenases transfer electrons differently to an intermediate electron transferring flavoprotein and from there to ubiquinone catalysed by the enzyme electron transferring flavoprotein ubiquinone oxidoreductase (Fig. 18).

Defects at this level affect not only amino acid catabolism but fatty acid oxidation, and the organic acid defects are complex. The affected acyl coenzyme A dehydrogenases include glutaryl coenzyme A dehydrogenase and defects in electron transport at this point in metabolism are labelled glutaric aciduria type II.

Multiple carboxylase deficiency

Clinical

Holocarboxylase synthetase deficiency causes neonatal acidosis with seizures, skin rash, and alopecia; it progresses to coma and death. Vomiting and ketosis are present. Biotinidase deficiency has a more variable clinical picture with progressive neurological deterioration including ataxia and seizures, developmental delay, and hypotonia. Other features of the neonatal form such as skin rash, alopecia, acidosis, and organic aciduria may not be

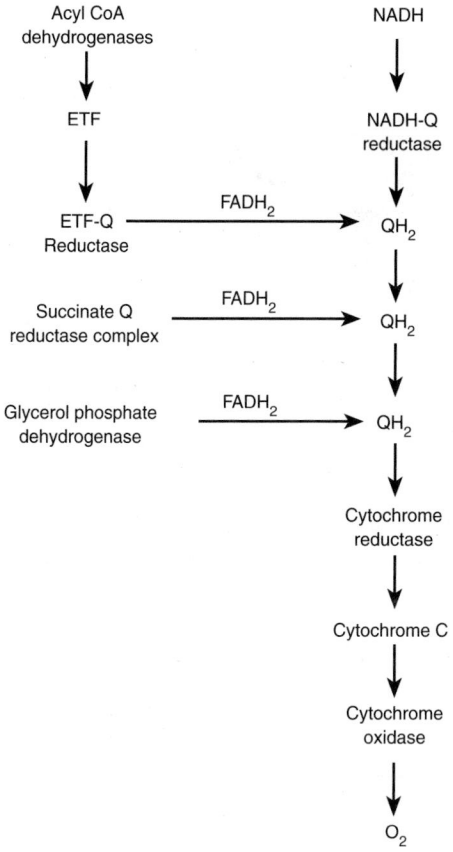

Fig. 18 The main electron transporting chain from reduced nicotinamide adenine dinucleotide (NADH) to oxygen is shown on the right, with other entry points for the flow of electrons coming from the left. ETF, electron transporting flavoprotein; $FADH_2$, reduced flavin adenine dinucleotide; QH_2, reduced ubiquinone.

prominent. Hearing loss and optic atrophy have been described. Kerato-conjunctivitis occurs.

Biochemistry

The carboxylase deficiencies cause a complex organic aciduria. Isovaleric acid (which imparts an unpleasant odour to the patient), 3-hydroxyisovaleric acid, methylcrotonic acid, and methylcrotonyl glycine result from the impaired activity of 3-methylcrotonyl coenzyme A carboxylase. Lactic acidosis, with more marked increases in cerebrospinal fluid levels of lactate, reflects defective pyruvate carboxylase activity. Impaired propionate metabolism also increases 3-hydroxypropionate and propionylglycine excretion. The accumulating acetyl coenzyme A results in ketosis.

Diagnosis

Apart from organic acid analyses biotinidase activity in plasma is reduced to 0 to 5 per cent of normal in genetic deficiency. Biotin itself can be measured in plasma and urine. The assay of holocarboxylase synthetase is difficult and possible in only a few places. The therapeutic response to biotin does not distinguish between the two defects.

Genetics

Both are recessive disorders and biotinidase deficiency seems to be more common than holocarboxylase synthetase deficiency. The gene for the latter has been assigned to chromosone 21 and several mutations described.

Prenatal diagnosis

This is only required in holocarboxylase synthetase deficiency and depends on amniotic fluid analysis for organic acids and enzyme assay in cultured amniotic cells.

Treatment

Biotinidase deficiency responds well, often dramatically, to 5 to 10 mg/day of oral biotin. Deficiency develops in a few days if biotin is stopped. Pre-existing neurological damage may not reverse. Most patients with holocarboxylase deficiency respond well to 10 mg daily, but larger doses may be needed and some have not fully responded to doses as high as 100 mg/day.

Glutaric acidaemia type II

Clinical

The most severe neonatal presentation, with associated congenital abnormalities, often leads to premature birth, metabolic acidosis, hypoglycaemia, hepatomegaly, and hypotonia. Severe cystic dysplasia of the kidneys is common; the kidneys may be palpable. Other defects include facial dysmorphism, 'rocker-bottom' feet, anterior abdominal wall defects, and defects of the external genitalia. Death usually occurs in the first week of life. Some affected neonates, without congenital defects, have the other clinical abnormalities of metabolic acidosis, hypoglycaemia, hypotonia, and hepatomegaly. The prognosis remains poor, with death in the early days or weeks of life, often with severe cardiomyopathy.

Milder forms presenting after the neonatal period, or survivors of early illness, may suffer recurrent encephalopathic episodes similar to Reye's syndrome. Cases with a predominantly late clinical presentation of lipid storage myopathy have been described. Adult presentation has been recorded. From their predominant organic acid pattern, some of these clinically milder patients are given the diagnosis of ethylmalonic-adipicaciduria.

Biochemistry

Glutaric aciduria type II is due to deficiency of electron transferring flavoprotein or electron transferring flavoprotein–ubiquinone oxidoreductase, the latter causing the severest neonatal form with congenital defects. The flavin-containing acyl coenzyme A dehydrogenases affected include glutaryl coenzyme A dehydrogenase, isovaleryl coenzyme A dehydrogenase, the long, medium, and short chain dehydrogenases used in fatty acid oxi-dation, and the dehydrogenases involved in sarcosine synthesis and breakdown. The organic acids found in urine as a consequence include short chain acids—isovaleric, 3-hydroxy isovaleric, glutaric, 2-hydroxyglutaric—the oxidation products of medium chain fatty acids—adipic, suberic and sebacic acids—ethylmalonic acid, 5-hydroxy hexanoic acid, and glycine conjugates of a variety of these. Carnitine concentrations in plasma are low and a range of acyl carnitines are found in urine and increased by carnitine therapy. Hypoglycaemia is very common.

Diagnosis

The florid organic acid pattern in severe patients is characteristic but in those more mildly affected it is less marked. Acyl carnitines are now well demonstrated by tandem mass spectrometry. Hepatomegaly and hypoglycaemia in older patients raise the diagnosis of glycogen storage diseases, but ketonaemia does not occur in glutaric aciduria type II. Electron transferring flavoprotein and electron transferring flavoprotein–ubiquinone oxidoreductase can be assayed in some centres using cultured fibroblasts.

Genetics

Both of the basic defects are autosomal recessive with assays of electron transferring flavoprotein and the electron transferring flavoprotein–ubiquinone oxidoreductase showing variable residual activity. The electron transferring flavoprotein protein has α and β subunits. The relevant genes have been localized to chromosomes 15 and 19 and mutations in both have been described.

Prenatal diagnosis

This has been carried out using amniotic fluid analysis and cultured amniocytes for electron transferring flavoprotein and oxidoreductase assays.

Treatment

Nothing has influenced severe early cases. Diets low in fats and protein reduce organic acid accumulation in milder cases and carnitine supplements increase the formation of the less toxic carnitine acyl esters. Oral riboflavin 100 to 300 mg/day has apparently been beneficial in some older patients, perhaps by stabilizing electron transferring flavoprotein or the oxidoreductase. Milder cases are helped by a high energy intake during intercurrent illness, which may need to to be intravenous.

Other defects of amino acid and organic acid metabolism

Many are not covered in the text because their rarity does not really justify it. Information is available in specialized texts.

Further reading

Adamson MD, Andersson HC, Gahl WA (1989). Cystinosis. *Seminars in Nephrology* 9, 147–61.

Anikster Y, Shotelersuk V, Gahl WA (1999). CNS mutations in patients with cystinosis. *Human Mutations* 14, 454–8.

Attree O *et al.* (1992). The Lowe's oculocerebrorenal gene encodes a protein highly homologous to inositol polyphosphate-5-phosphatase. *Nature* 358, 239–42.

Batshaw ML, Bachmann C, Luckman M (1998). Advances in inherited urea cycle disorders. *Journal of Inherited Metabolic Disease* 21, Supplement 1.

Blau N, Duran M, Blaskorvics ME (1996). *Physician's guide to the laboratory diagnosis of metabolic diseases.* Chapman and Hall, London.

Brenton DP *et al.* (1981). The adult presenting idiopathic Fanconi syndrome. *Journal of Inherited Metabolic Diseases* 4, 211–15.

Brody LC *et al.* (1992). Ornithine delta amino transferase mutations in gyrate atrophy, allelic heterogeneity and functional consequences. *Journal of Biological Chemistry* 267, 3302–7.

Burgard P, Link R, Schweltzer-Krantz S (2000). Phenylketonouria: Evidence-based clinical practice. *European Journal of Pediatrics* **159**, Supplement 2.

Camacho JA *et al.* (1999). Hyperornithinaemia–hyperammonaemia–homocitrillinuria syndrome is caused by mutations in a gene encoding a mitochondirial ornithine transporter. *Nature Genetics* **22**, 151–8.

Charnos LR *et al.* (1991). Clinical and laboratory findings in the oculo-cerebro-renal syndrome of Lowe with special reference to growth and function. *New England Journal of Medicine* **324**, 1318–25.

Chesney RW (1998). Mutational analysis of patients with cystinuria detected by a genetic screening network: Poweful tools in understanding the several forms of the disorder [editorial]. *Kidney International* **54**, 279–80.

Dent CE (1948). A study of the behaviour of some sixty amino acids and other ninhydrin-reacting substances on phenol-collidine filter paper chromatograms with notes as to the occurrence of some of them in biological fluids. *Biochemical Journal* **43**, 169–80.

Dhondt JL (1991). Strategy for the screening of tetrahydrobiopterin deficiency among hyperphenylalaninaemic patients: 15 years experience. *Journal of Inherited Metabolic Disease* **14**, 117–27.

Fernandes J, Saudubray J-M, van den Berghe G (1990). *Inborn metabolic diseases. Diagnosis and treatment*, 1st edn. Springer, Berlin.

Fowler B (1997). Disorders of homocysteine metabolism. *Journal of Inherited Metabolic Disease* **20**, 270–85.

Goodyer P *et al.* (1998). Cystinuria subtype and the risk of nephrolithiasis. *Kidney International* **54**, 56–61.

Haworth JC *et al.* (1991). Phenotypic variability in glutaric aciduria type I: report of 14 cases in five Canadian Indian kindreds. *Journal of Pediatrics* **118**, 52–8.

Holme E and Lindstedt S (1998). Tyrosinaemia Type I and NTBC. *Journal of Inherited Metabolic Disease* **21**, 507–17.

Kaplan P *et al.* (1991). Intellectual outcome in children with maple syrup urine disease. *Journal of Pediatrics* **119**, 46–50.

Lenke RL, Levy HL (1980). Maternal phenylketonuria and hyperphenylalaninemia. *New England Journal of Medicine* **303**, 1202–8.

Maestri NE *et al.* (1991). Prospective treatment of urea cycle disorders. *Journal of Pediatrics* **119**, 923–8.

Milliner DA (1990). Cystinuria. *Endocrinology and Metabolism Clinics of North America* **19**, 889–907.

Morton DH (1994). Through my window—remarks at the 125th year celebration of the Children's Hospital of Boston. *Pediatrics* **94**, 785–91.

Norden AG *et al.* (1991). Excretion of β_2 glycoprotein (apolipoprotein H) in renal tubular disease. *Clinical Chemistry* **37**, 74–7.

Paradis K *et al.* (1990). Liver transplantation for hereditary tyrosinaemia: the Quebec experience. *American Journal of Human Genetics* **47**, 338–42.

Rose WC *et al.* (1955). The amino acid requirements of man. XV The valine requirement. Summary and final observations. *Journal of Biological Chemistry* **217**, 987.

Rutchick SD, Resnick MI (1997). Cystine calculi: diagnosis and management. *The Urologic Clinics of North America* **24**, 163–72.

Santer R *et al.* (1998). Fanconi–Bickel syndrome—the original patient and his natural history; historical steps leading to the primary defect and a review of the literature. *European Journal of Pediatrics* **157**, 783–97.

Saudubray J-M *et al.* (1989). Clinical approach to inherited metabolic disease in the neonatal period: a 20-year survey. *Journal of Inherited Metabolic Disease* **12**, Supplement 1, 25–42.

Schneider JA *et al.* (1995). Recent advances in the treatment of cystinosis. *Journal of Inherited Metabolic Disease* **18**, 387–97.

Smith I (1993). Phenylketonuria due to phenyalanine hydroxylase deficiency: an unfolding story. Report of the MRC Working Party on P.K.U. *British Medical Journal* **306**, 115–19.

Smith I (1993). Recommendations on the dietary management of phenylketonuria. Report of the MRC Working Party on PKU. *Archives of Diseases in Childhood* **68**, 426–7.

Stephens AD (1989). Cystinuria and its treatment, 25 years experience at St Bartholomew's Hospital. *Journal of Inherited Metabolic Disease* **12**, 197–209.

Tada K, Kure S (1993). Non-ketotic hyperglycinaemia: molecular lesions, diagnosis and pathophysiology. *Journal of Inherited Metabolic Disease* **16**, 691–703.

Tuchman M, Holzknecht RA (1991). Heterogeneity of patients with late onset ornithine transcarbamylase deficiency. *Clinical and Investigative Medicine* **14**, 320–4.

Tuchman M, Knopman DS, Shih VE (1990). Episodic hyperammonaemia in adult siblings with hyperornithinaemia, hyperammonaemia and homocitrillinuria syndrome. *Archives of Neurology* **47**, 1134–7.

Van'T Hoff WG (2000). Molecular developments in renal tubulopathies. *Archives of Diseases in Childhood* **83**, 189–91.

Widhalm K *et al.* (1992). Long term follow up of 12 patients with the late onset variant of argininosuccinic acid lyase deficiency. *Pediatrics* **89**, 1182–4.

Wilcken DEL, Wilcken B (1997). The natural history of vascular disease in homocystinuria and the effects of treatment. *Journal of Inherited Metabolic Disease* **20**, 295–300.

Wolf B, Heard GS (1991). Biotinidase deficiency. *Advances in Pediatrics* **38**, 1–21.

11.3 Disorders of carbohydrate metabolism

11.3.1 Glycogen storage diseases

T. M. Cox

Glycogen, the main energy store in liver and muscle, is configured for the compact storage of glucose in a form that has a minimal osmotic effect but which is readily accessible and metabolically active. The molecule contains polymerized α-D-glucose units anchored covalently at their reducing termini to a small protein, glycogenin. The structure of glycogen is elaborate: its extensively arborized macromolecular arrangement is linked by α-1,4 glycosidic bonds with α-1,6 bonds at the branch points. These branch points are arranged in several tiers with increasingly long outer chains that terminate in non-reducing glucose residues. Thus the complex branched structure of glycogen also promotes its ready access to the enzymes of biosynthesis and degradation.

The liver and muscles contain between 200 and 300 g of glycogen and its polymerized structure can be seen with the electron microscope: liver glycogen consists mainly of α-aggregates or rosettes of smaller particles (β-particles) that are principally found in muscle cytoplasm. The molecular weight of glycogen in these tissues is several million daltons. Each β-particle contains up to 60 000 glucose residues, but despite its size the glycogen molecule undergoes remodelling as a result of constant breakdown and synthesis. Defects in the enzymatic steps for the synthesis, utilization, or degradation of glycogen lead to its pathological storage. Accumulation of glycogen may be generalized or involve certain tissues selectively; the stored glycogen may have a normal or aberrant structure.

Glycogen metabolism

The individual enzymatic steps for the formation and breakdown of glycogen are summarized in Fig. 1.

Glycogen biosynthesis

The immediate precursor for glycogen synthesis is uridine diphosphoglucose (**UDPG**), which is formed from glucose 1-phosphate by UDPG pyrophosphorylase. This enzyme has a high affinity for its substrates and is abundant—no deficiencies have been recorded. In contrast, glycogen synthase is a highly regulated enzyme complex that exists in distinct isoforms in muscle and liver: the enzyme catalyses the transfer of UDP glucose units to glucose residues already covalently attached to a tyrosine residue of glycogenin, which acts as a primer. The tyrosine glucosyltransferase activity has not been identified but the glycogenin adduct possesses an intrinsic glucosyltransferase activity. Initially, one molecule each of glycogen synthase and glycogenin occur as a complex in each β-glycogen particle. After

elongation, branching of the molecule is catalysed by amylo (1,4 → 1,6) transglucosidase, 'branching enzyme'.

Glycogen synthase is subject to phosphorylation control that inhibits its activity: this inhibition is overcome by the allosteric activator, glucose 6-phosphate. The phosphorylation of at least nine serine residues is brought about by protein kinases. Glucagon and adrenaline, while stimulating phosphorylase via phosphorylase kinase, indirectly inhibit glycogen synthase by maintaining protein phosphatase I in its inactive configuration. Insulin stimulates glycogen synthase by promoting its dephosphorylation through the action of this same phosphatase: protein phosphatase I is activated by a cascade of protein kinases whose phosphorylation is initiated by the insulin receptor tyrosine kinase. Inherited deficiency of glycogen synthase activity is associated with reduced storage of liver glycogen and fasting hypoglycaemia. Branching-enzyme activity is essential for the formation of the compact spherical molecules of glycogen, especially in liver. It transfers a minimum of six α-1,4-linked glucose units from the distal ends of glycogen chains to a 1,6 position on the same or a neighbouring chain. Deficiency of branching enzyme leads to the accumulation of abnormal molecules that are partially resistant to degradation.

Glycogen breakdown

Glycogen is degraded by three enzymes: phosphorylase, debranching enzyme and acid α-glucosidase. Phosphorylase brings about the sequential release of glucose units from the α-1,4-linked chains of glycogen to liberate glucose 1-phosphate. After conversion to glucose 6-phosphate by phosphoglucomutase, free glucose is formed by the action of glucose 6-phosphatase. Debranching enzyme possesses transferase and α-1,6-glucosidase activities. When phosphorylase has degraded glycogen chains to within four α-1,4-glucosyl units of an α-1,6 linkage, three glucose residues are transferred to the end of another chain by the glycosyltransferase activity. Debranching enzyme then hydrolyses the remaining α-1,6 bond to release free glucose using its amylo-1,6-glucosidase activity. Debranching enzyme also cleaves the unique glucosyl–tyrosine linkage that anchors the terminal reducing glucose unit to glycogenin. Deficiency of debranching enzyme leads to the storage of glycogen that possesses short outer chains, 'limit dextrin'.

The main product of glycogen breakdown in muscle and liver is glucose 1-phosphate, which is produced by the sequential action of phosphorylase on α-1,4 glycosidic bonds. Glucose 1-phosphate is a key intermediate of glycolysis, gluconeogenesis, glycogenolysis, and the pentose-phosphate pathway, but, by virtue of phosphoglucomutase, the hepatic glucose 6-phosphatase system is the predominant metabolic source of blood glucose. Glucose 6-phosphatase exists as a multicomponent complex in the endoplasmic reticulum of hepatocytes and, to a lesser extent, in renal tubular cells—it is not found in muscle. The system contains glucose 6-phosphatase, several proteins that facilitate the transport of glucose, glucose 6-phosphate, and phosphate, as well as other stabilizing and regulatory moieties. Several genetic defects in this compartmentalized system are recognized to affect overall glucose 6-phosphatase activity: they are associated with severe hypoglycaemia, metabolic acidosis, and hepatic disease.

Glucose 6-phosphate obtained from the breakdown of glycogen in skeletal muscle is used directly in glycolysis. Defects of muscle phosphorylase lead to a defective supply of adenosine triphosphate (**ATP**), especially during ischaemic exercise. There is a failure of conversion of glycogen to lactate, and exercise-induced muscle cramps reflect mild muscle necrosis with increased accumulation of glycogen. Phosphofructokinase-1 catalyses an irreversible step in the glycolytic pathway and is a key regulatory enzyme. Inherited defects that render it inactive or affect its positive allosteric regulation by the effectors adenosine monophosphate (**AMP**) and fructose 2,6-diphosphate resemble muscle phosphorylase deficiency. Because deficiency of phosphofructokinase affects the metabolism of endogenous glycogen as well as carbon units derived from extracellular glucose, the symptoms of phosphofructokinase-1 deficiency are more severe and of earlier onset than muscle phosphorylase deficiency. As expected, glucose 6-phosphate, fructose 6-phosphate, and glycogen, accumulate in the muscle cells.

Breakdown of glycogen in liver and skeletal muscle is brought about by the concerted activities of phosphorylase and debranching enzyme in the cytoplasm. Phosphorylase, which requires pyridoxal-5-phosphate, is activated by phosphorylation in response to hormonal or neural stimulation—a complex process that is mediated by phosphorylase kinases. Phosphorylase kinase is a multisubunit protein with regulatory, catalytic, and calcium-binding subunits that are encoded on separate genes. Separate isoforms are found in liver and muscle. The final common pathways for the

regulation of phosphorylase kinase involve protein kinase A (cAMP-dependent protein kinase), calcium and kinase activation of calmodulin, and protein phosphatases 1 and 2A.

Another enzyme, acid α-1,4-glucosidase (otherwise known as acid maltase), has an important role in the metabolism of glycogen. This lysosomal hydrolase is present in all cells except erythrocytes and, although it has no relation to glycolysis, its deficiency causes a generalized disorder in which muscle disease, especially of the heart, is usually severe. Deficiency of acid α-glucosidase is associated with rapidly progressive cardiac hypertrophy with hepatic enlargement and generalized muscle weakness. Skeletal muscle symptoms may be prominent in patients with the infantile or late-onset forms of this condition but disease progression is usually rapid. Acid α-1,4-glucosidase deficiency was the first inborn lysosomal disease to be clearly recognized and represents a prototype for the other storage diseases: intracellular vesicles containing glycogen represent lysosomes distended by an undegradable substrate that accumulates as a result of autophagy. The accumulation of glycogen in lysosomes indicates that glycogen fragments are constantly being taken up for partial degradation and macromolecular remodelling.

Clinical features

The principal features of the different glycogen storage diseases are set out in Table 1, which also gives the primary enzymatic (or translocator) defect and chromosomal locus of the cognate human gene in each case.

Many of the manifestations of the glycogen storage disorders are common to several of these diseases and correlate with the main site of storage. However, in those disorders that affect the liver, the consequential effects of

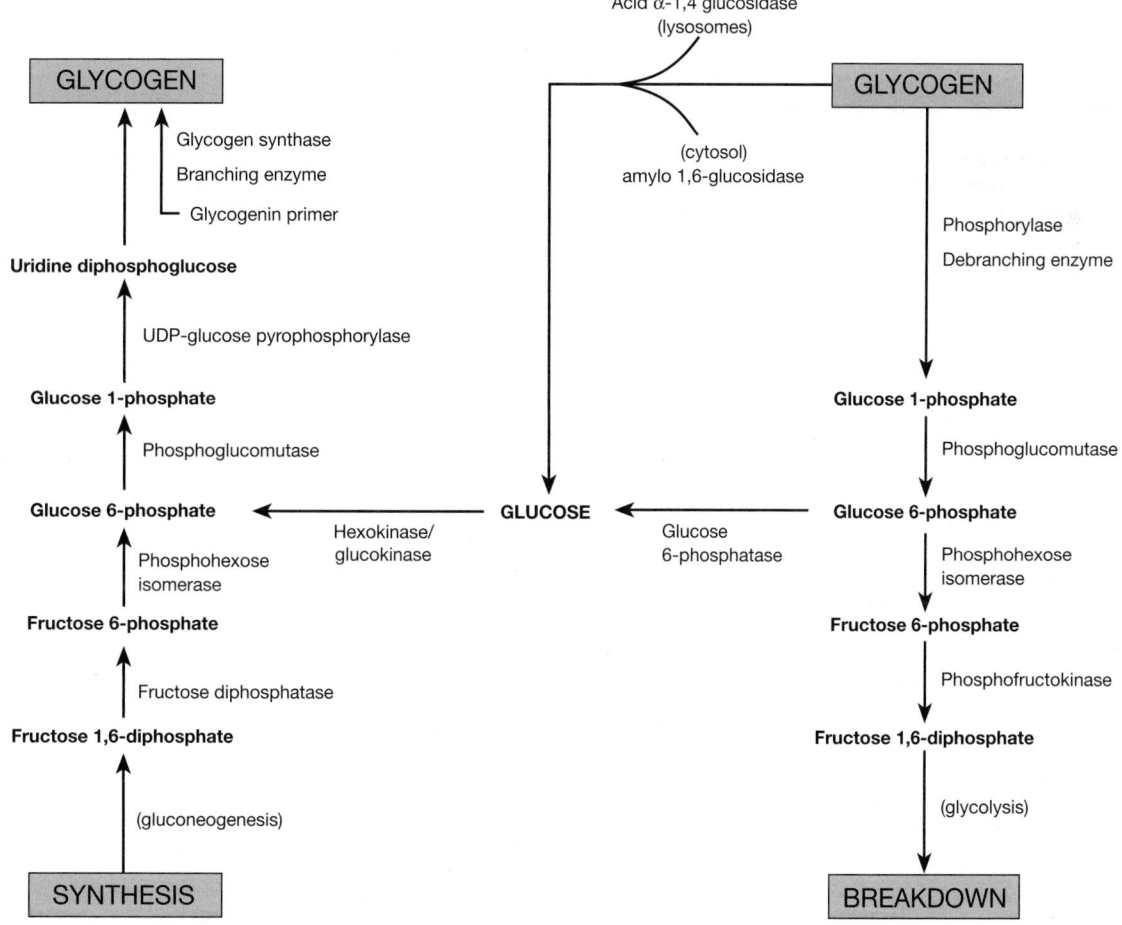

Fig. 1 The synthesis and degradation of glycogen.

Table 1 Diseases of glycogen storage

Designation number [OMIM catalogue]	Enzymatic defect and locus	Affected tissues	Principal manifestations	Diagnostic tissue
von Gierke's disease (Cori type I) [232200 232220 232240]	Glucose 6-phosphatase[a] 17q21 11q23 11q23	Liver, kidney	Usually severe: liver and kidney enlargement. Hypoglycaemia, acidosis, bleeding tendency, growth failure, hyperlipidaemia, hyperuricaemia	Liver, intestinal mucosa
Pompe's disease (type IIA) [232300]	Acid α-1,4-glucosidase (lysosomal) 17q25.2	Generalized, especially heart, muscles, and liver	Usually severe: adult cases recognized, hypotonia, cardiomegaly, weakness, and arrhythmias. Mild cases respond to a high-protein diet	Liver, muscle, myocardium, fibroblasts, leucocytes, amniotic-fluid cells
Danon's disease (type IIB) [300257]	LAMP2 (lysosomal membrane protein) Xq24	Generalized, especially heart, muscles, and liver	Usually severe: adult cases recognized, hypotonia, cardiomegaly, weakness, and arrhythmias. Mild cases respond to a high-protein diet	Liver, muscle, myocardium, fibroblasts, leucocytes, amniotic-fluid cells
Forbes–Cori disease or limit dextrinosis (type III) [232400]	Debranching enzyme 1p21	Liver and usually muscle[b]	Often mild: hepatomegaly, hypoglycaemia, progressive muscle weakness in adults. Ketosis—lactic acidosis and hyperuricaemia absent	Liver, (muscle), fibroblasts, amniotic-fluid cells
Andersen's disease or amylopectinosis (type IV) [232500]	Branching enzyme 3p12	Liver.[b] Rare variant, polyglucosan disease, affects peripheral nerves[b]	Severe: hepatosplenomegaly in infancy; death from cirrhosis and portal hypertension. Polyglucosan variant affects adults	Liver, leucocytes, (peripheral nerves)
McArdle's disease (type V) [232600]	Muscle phosphorylase 11 q 13	Skeletal muscle	Exercise-induced muscle cramps	Muscle (lactate production absent)
Hers' disease (type VI) [232700]	Liver phosphorylase 14q21–22	Liver	Moderate to severe hepatomegaly with hypoglycaemia in childhood	Liver, leucocytes
Tarui's disease (type VII) [232800]	Muscle phosphofructokinase 12q13.3	Muscle, red cells	Marked weakness and stiffness after exertion, haemolytic anaemia (Glucose 6-phosphate and fructose 6-phosphate also accumulate)	Erythrocyte, muscle (Lactate production absent)
Type VIII [306000]	Phosphorylase b kinase Xp22.2–22.1	Liver	Mild hepatomegaly. Variable hypoglycaemia. Sex-linked and autosomal recessive forms	Liver, leucocytes
Type O [240600]	Glycogen synthase 12 p 12.2	Liver	Very rare. Severe fasting hypoglycaemia: seizures before feeds. Failure of glucagon response. Reduced or absent glycogen	Liver

Table 1 *Continued*

Phospho-glucoisomerase	Red cells	Very rare. Haemolytic anaemia. Excess glycogen in liver and erythrocytes	Red cells
Lactate dehydrogenase	Muscle	Resembles McArdle's disease. Very rare	Muscle
Phosphoglycerate kinase	Muscle	Resembles McArdle's disease. Very rare	Muscle
Lactate dehydrogenase	Muscle	Resembles McArdle's disease. Very rare	Muscle

[a] Designations beyond type V are extensions of Cori's classification; beyond type VII they are controversial.

[b] Several defects described in components of the glucose 6-phosphatase system (see text). NB: Enzyme activity may be normal in tissue after freeze–thawing.

[c] Abnormal glycogen structure—total glycogen concentration may be normal.

the primary metabolic lesions are often far-reaching and the function of many different tissues may be impaired as part of a pleiotropic disturbance of biochemical homeostasis. In several instances, for example glycogen storage diseases types III and IV, pathological storage affects both liver and muscle tissue (including cardiac muscle) (Table 2).

An additional set of clinical features is observed in the enzymatic defects that affect glycolysis: typically, these are associated with acute exercise-induced muscle symptoms and signs of rhabdomyolysis. These defects are usually restricted to those tissues with a high glycolytic capacity or dependence, such as muscle and red cells; mild haemolysis results from the impaired supply of ATP to the membrane sodium–potassium ATPase of the erythrocyte.

Several unusual features of the glycogen storage diseases have been reported that remain unexplained. These include the development of hepatic adenomas (which presage malignant transformation); leucocytes and macrophages in the translocator deficiencies (types 1b, c, and d) that predispose to microbial infections and granulomatous colitis, and vasoconstrictive pulmonary hypertension. Typically, the renal disease is preceded by a hyperfiltration syndrome and mild proteinuria. An unusual feature of late-onset glycogen storage disease type II due to acid maltase deficiency, has been the association with intracerebral arterial aneurysms; glycogen storage in arterial smooth muscle with prominent vacuolation has been documented.

Table 2 Common effects of pathological glycogen storage

In liver
Hepatology
Cirrhosis
Hepatic tumours
Glomerulosclerosis
Renal calculi
Impaired somatic growth
Bleeding tendency
Hypoglycaemia
Ketosis, lactic acidosis
Hyperuricaemia (gout)
Hyperlipidaemia (xanthomas, pancreatitis)

In muscle
Skeletal muscle weakness (proximal/limb-girdle, diaphragm)
Muscle wasting
Hypertrophic cardiomyopathy
Cardiac conduction defects

(Glycolytic defects)
Exercise-induced pain and rhabdomyolysis
Haemolysis

Clinical genetics of the glycogenoses

The genes encoding the human enzymes that are defective in the individual glycogen storage diseases have been identified and mapped to their respective chromosomal loci, as indicated in Table 1. The individual disorders are inherited as autosomal recessive traits, with the exception of liver phosphorylase b kinase deficiency (type VIII) and Danon's disease (type IIb) which are X-linked diseases.

Diagnosis of glycogen storage diseases

Affecting the liver

The diagnosis may be suspected in infants and children with hepatomegaly, growth retardation, and hypoglycaemia, which is not invariable. Review of a previous biopsy may indicate glycogen deposition; glycogen deposits stain strongly within hepatocytes with the Periodic acid–Schiff reagent and the reaction characteristically is abolished by prior treatment with diastase. In many cases, a glucagon stimulation test (20 µg/kg intramuscularly) fails to induce the normal (>2 mmol/l) rise in blood glucose; however, definitive diagnosis by biopsy is warranted for prognosis, future antenatal diagnosis, and to direct treatment. Direct assay of liver tissue for glycogen and fat content as well as enzymatic analysis is desirable. Histochemical and electron microscopic study of glycogen structure provides useful additional information. Where possible, open wedge-biopsy of the liver should be carried out to obtain sufficient material for diagnosis and ensure haemostasis under direct vision; appropriate provision of platelets and blood coagulation factors should be made to correct the haemorrhagic diathesis before biopsy is carried out. However, the procedure is hazardous for young infants with acidosis or a bleeding tendency and close attention should be given to prevention of hypoglycaemia.

A particular difficulty arises in the diagnosis of certain variants of type I glycogen storage disease. The glucose 6-phosphatase system is uniquely incorporated into the endoplasmic reticulum: latency of its membrane-bound components renders diagnosis of specific lesions affecting the transport of substrates or products impossible when frozen tissue is thawed for analysis. Types 1B and 1C glycogen storage disease (in which glucose 6-phosphate translocation is defective) is an example where the study of fresh tissue is essential for establishing a diagnosis, since analysis of freeze–thawed material disrupts the integrity of the microsomal enzyme system and—by rendering it permeable to phosphate, pyrophosphate, and glucose 6-phosphate—overcomes the transport defect. Thus, where defects of glycogen storage are suspected, it is essential to seek the prior advice of a laboratory that is competent to carry out the appropriate investigations using fresh and deep-frozen biopsy material.

In muscle

Forearm exercise tests are useful for detecting defects in skeletal muscles that interfere with the supply of chemical energy in the form of ATP by the metabolic pathway that breaks down glucose and glycogen to lactate. In the absence of oxygen, glycolysis is the sole means by which ATP may be generated: the preferred energy source being glucosyl units derived from glycogen, rather than glucose obtained from the plasma. Defects in glycolysis (glycogenesis type VII and other enzyme deficiencies) cause similar symptoms. Exercise-induced cramps may occur in patients with the purine pathway disorder, myoadenylate deaminase deficiency, which may also be safely diagnosed by exercise testing. Unlike the earlier test devised by McArdle (1951), these provocative tests do not induce rhabdomyolysis accompanied by raised creatine kinase activity in the serum with acute myoglobinuric renal failure—features in the history that may indicate muscle glycogenosis.

After a 30-min rest, blood is taken from the antecubital vein of the non-exercising arm and a small sphygmomanometer cuff placed around the other wrist is inflated to 200 mmHg. A second standard cuff around the upper arm to be tested is inflated to mean arterial pressure and the patient squeezes as powerfully as possible 120 times over 2 min. Immediately afterwards, the second cuff is inflated to 200 mmHg. Blood is drawn through a needle placed in the antecubital vein of the exercising arm 2 min after completing the exercise and the upper cuff is released. To complete the test, five further samples are drawn at 1-min intervals. The samples are transported rapidly to the laboratory for analysis of lactate and ammonia. Reduced or absent generation of lactate is characteristic of glycogenolytic and glycolytic defects that affect muscle; in contrast, plasma levels of ammonia (as well as inosine and hypoxanthine) increase greatly in patients with glycogenosis types III, V, and VIII. These abnormalities reflect the excessive degradation of purines that occurs in the exercising muscles of patients in whom there is a disturbance of ATP generation. Measurement of ammonia release as well as lactate production also adds discriminatory value to the exercise test, as it controls for low levels of lactate release that result merely from inadequate exercise during performance of the test. The test may also identify myoadenylate kinase deficiency: in such patients lactate production is normal, but the failure to utilize the purine cycle to conserve intracellular nucleotides and provide alternative substrates for energy production is shown by the failure of venous ammonia concentrations to rise.

Pompe's disease due to acid maltase deficiency is a generalized disorder that predominantly affects skeletal and cardiac muscle. Carbohydrate metabolism is otherwise normal, and phosphorylysis of cytosolic glycogen in the liver is sufficient to maintain euglycaemia. The diagnosis of infantile disease may be suspected on the basis of cardiac and liver enlargement in an infant with respiratory distress and hypotonia. Macroglossia is frequent and the electrocardiogram shows left axis deviation, a short P–R interval and broad QRS complexes. In the juvenile- and adult-onset forms of acid maltase deficiency the disease resembles limb-girdle and other myopathies as well as polymyositis; some patients have been reported with myotonic features. The activity of skeletal muscle creatine kinase (**CK**) in this variant (non-CK MB fraction) is elevated in the serum and may be the first sign of intrinsic muscle disease, especially in adult patients complaining of non-specific fatiguability and weakness. Myopathic changes—occasionally with pseudomyotonic discharges—are observed on electromyography and the diagnosis is revealed by biopsy, which shows vacuolar myopathy: massive deposits of glycogen in and between myofibrils. Under the electron microscope, free and lysosomal α-glycogen particles are observed. Enzymatic deficiency of acid α-1,4-glucosidase is readily confirmed in cultured amniocytes and all tissues except erythrocytes.

Recently, the molecular basis for an unusually perplexing vacuolar cardiomyopathy associated with glycogen storage has been identified (Danon's disease). This X-linked disorder has been principally reported in male infants, boys, and men with proximal muscle weakness and prominent hypertrophic cardiomyopathy including cardiac conduction defects. Although the ultrastructural studies revealed membrane-bound inclusions of glycogen resembling Pompe's disease, acid maltase (α-1,4-glucosidase) activity was normal. In those cases with normal phosphorylase kinase activity (an enzyme that also maps to the X-chromosome), no cause for the severe cardioskeletal myopathy was apparent until it was shown to be associated with mutations in the lysosomal membrane protein, LAMP2. Families with probable Danon's disease have been reported with mild mental intellectual impairment and systemic manifestations. Clinical expression has been reported in obligate carrier female subjects in affected pedigrees showing inheritance patterns typical of an X-linked trait; the severity of the storage disease appears to be highly variable in female heterozygotes, consistent with patterns of random X-inactivation. Danon's disease can be diagnosed by molecular analysis of the *LAMP-2* gene that maps to human chromosome Xq24, and thus represents the first example of a disease due to a structural protein of the lysosomal membrane.

Definitive diagnosis of muscle glycogenoses depends on biopsy with histochemical, ultrastructural, and biochemical analyses. Biopsy should be carried out after liaison with the laboratory so that, if necessary, tissue can be stored frozen for further study and enzymatic analysis. Biopsy and electromyography may be needed to differentiate suspected glycogen storage diseases from other myopathies, including Duchenne's dystrophy, Kugelberg–Welander disease, dystrophia myotonica, and mitochondrial and secondary disorders of muscle such as polymyositis.

Individual glycogen storage diseases

The main features of these disorders are surveyed and summarized in Table 1. Brief accounts of selected conditions are set out below.

Classical type I glycogen storage disease (von Gierke's disease)

In this disease, glucose formation from glycogen and gluconeogenesis is defective and affected infants develop hypoglycaemia on fasting or as a result of intercurrent infection or other stress. The liver is enlarged at birth. It contains excess glycogen and shows gross infiltration with fat but cirrhosis and portal hypertension are rare. In contrast, growth retardation, often combined with obesity, is common. The kidneys are enlarged by glycogen deposition. Progressive focal glomerulosclerosis and proximal tubular failure with a secondary Fanconi syndrome may also occur. Stress and starvation provoke acidotic attacks with marked lactic acidaemia. Poor metabolic control causes: growth arrest; hyperuricaemia and gout; marked hypertriglyceridaemia and hypercholesterolaemia with raised very low-density lipoprotein (**VLDL**) and normal low-density lipoprotein (**LDL**) cholesterol concentrations in the plasma (skin and retinal xanthomas accompany these findings); and prolonged bleeding time related to an acquired von Willebrand-like defect affecting the platelet. Patients with defects of the glucose 6-phosphate translocase system (type 1B) are prone to bacterial infection: there is neutropenia, and neutrophil migration and chemotaxis are impaired. These patients may develop episodes of severe diarrhoea in association with granulomatous infiltration of the colonic mucosa. Partial deficiencies of the glucose 6-phosphatase system lead to variable clinical expression, and subtypes of type I glycogen storage disease have been convincingly demonstrated in patients presenting with glucagon-unresponsive hypoglycaemia with or without liver enlargement in adult life. Adult patients or children with uncontrolled disease develop hepatic adenomas; frank hepatocellular carcinomas occur.

Metabolic disturbance

The metabolic disturbance in classical type I glycogen storage serves as a paradigm for the hepatic glycogenoses.

Hypoglycaemia in von Gierke's disease is often asymptomatic and tolerance of it improves with increasing age. The primary defect leads to a profound reduction in the supply of glucose from glucose 6-phosphate in the liver leading to marked substrate-cycling. Lactate delivered from extrahepatic sources is converted to glucose 6-phosphate, which is metabolized by the pentose-phosphate shunt or transferred back into glycogen. The pentose pathway supplies precursors for purine synthesis and reducing equivalents. Residual production of glucose probably occurs by lysosomal hydrolysis of glycogen and recycling through the glycogen synthase-debranching enzyme pathway, but metabolic adaptation of the brain, which can use lactate as an alternative substrate, is very important.

Failure to dephosphorylate glucose 6-phosphate stimulates substrate cycling and increases the activity of the pentose-phosphate pathway, with enhanced production of reduced NADP (**NADPH**, reduced form of nicotinamide-adenine dinucleotide phosphate), ribose 5-phosphate, and purines—this latter ultimately leads to the overproduction of uric acid through the action of xanthine oxidase. Increased delivery of fructose 6-phosphate from the pentose-phosphate pathway leads to the excess formation of lactate as a result of phosphohexosisomerase activity. Enhanced cycling of UDPG and the glycogen synthase reaction promotes glycogen accumulation. However, small quantities of free glucose can be liberated by the α-1,6-glucosidase activity of the secondary action of debranching enzyme but the co-ordinated action of glucosyltransferase and phosphorylase releases additional glucose 1-phosphate residues for recycling. An additional (fractional) degradation of the intracellular glycogen store is probably contributed by the α-1,4-glucosidase activity of lysosomal acid maltase.

Hypertriglyceridaemia is induced by the increased provision of reduced nicotinamide-adenine dinucleotide (**NADH**) and NADPH, glycerol, and acetyl-coenzyme A (**acetyl-CoA**) because of enhanced flux through glycolysis and underutilization of gluconeogenic precursors. Malonyl-coenzyme A, derived from acetyl-CoA, inhibits the carnitine acyltransferase system and blocks the oxidation of fatty acids; thus marked ketosis does not usually develop. Lactic acidaemia results from stimulation of glycolysis at the level of phosphofructokinase by high concentrations of glucose 6-phosphate (and hence fructose 6-phosphate); lactate cannot be recycled in the liver to form new glucose and lactic acidosis results. Lactate competes with urate for excretory pathways in the kidney and thus contributes to the hyperuricaemia. Uric acid is also overproduced in the liver: it arises from the degradation of purine nucleotides by AMP-deaminase and the co-ordinated action of xanthine oxidase on inosine phosphate and hypoxanthine. The deaminase is activated when the concentration of free phosphate falls as a result of sequestration in sugar phosphate esters.

Treatment
The main objective is to maintain euglycaemia: most of the other metabolic abnormalities are thereby corrected and the prognosis improves.

In infants, normoglycaemia is maintained throughout 24 h by intravenous alimentation at 0.25 to 0.5 g/kg per hour and, later by continuous nasogastric administration at night together with glucose supplements at intervals of 1 to 2 h during the day. These intensive regimens correct acidosis, hyperuricaemia, and hyperlipidaemia; they also promote normal development and allow catch-up growth to occur in stunted infants and children. After growth in later childhood and in adult patients, metabolic control can be maintained by the use of raw cornstarch, which serves as a source of glucose that is slowly released by hydrolysis: 1 to 2 g/kg is given orally every 4 to 6 h as a suspension in water.

In type Ib glycogen storage disease it is vital to avoid intercurrent infection, and prophylactic antimicrobial drugs may therefore be necessary. In several instances, infusions of granulocyte-colony-stimulating factor has been strikingly effective in reducing the rate of infection and controlling granulomatous colitis. Patients with type Ia disease may also require treatment for their bleeding tendency. The bleeding diathesis is associated with a qualitative defect of platelet function, prolonged bleeding time, and reduced factor VIIIc and von Willebrand factor activities. These abnormalities and the haemorrhagic tendency respond to the administration of 1-deamino-8-D-arginine vasopressin (**DDAVP**) at 0.3 μg/kg infused in 50 ml of saline over 30 min intravenously. Correction of the bleeding disorder lasts for several hours and is useful for the treatment of bleeding after trauma or surgery.

Failure of metabolic control in type I glycogen storage disease appears to be associated with tissue complications: hepatic adenomas or malignant transformation, renal disease due to hyperfiltration, focal glomerulosclerosis, and postinfective scarring. Lately, an inflammatory disorder of the colon, resembling granulomatous colitis, has been recognized in type Ib disease. Type Ic disease, characterized by the increased latency of hepatic microsomal inorganic pyrophosphatase activity has now been reported. Phagocytic defects are not prominent in this disease subtype. Defective function of the microsomal glucose transporter has been reported and is designated type Id glycogen storage disease. Long-term, follow-up care with monitoring of biochemical parameters of kidney function and periodic ultrasonic examination of the liver is necessary. Continuing failure of growth, enlarging hepatic adenomas or progressive renal failure raise the question of organ transplantation. Transportal hepatocyte transplantation has been successfully achieved in this disease with correction of hypoglycaemia and lactic acidosis. Several successful renal, as well as hepatic, allografts have been carried out in patients with this condition using DDVAP infusions to control haemorrhagic manifestations. However, as regression of most complications, including hepatic adenomas, can be achieved by strict dietary measures, transplantation should be reserved for patients in whom nutritional treatment has failed. Survival into adult life (and parenthood) can be now expected.

Type II glycogen storage disease
Pompe's disease caused by acid maltase deficiency is usually a rapidly progressive disorder with effects on the heart, skeletal muscle, and nervous system. Affected children usually die within the first year or two of life, and until recently no measures other than supportive therapy and ventilatory assistance have been beneficial. Late-onset disease, usually without cardiomyopathy, occurs in juvenile and adult patients in whom it typically presents with skeletal myopathy affecting the proximal muscles. Ultimately, respiratory failure results from paralysis of the muscles of ventilation, including the diaphragm; voluntary muscles of deglutition may also be paralysed. Occasionally the disease resembles polymyositis or limb-girdle muscular dystrophy. Given that enzyme-replacement therapy is theoretically possible for lysosomal storage diseases, administration of purified acid α-1,4-glucosidase (acid maltase) has been attempted. Early trials of recombinant human acid maltase harbouring mannose 6-phosphate residues, to mediate targeting to cell-surface receptors for lysosomal uptake by skeletal myocytes, have been reported in infants with classical Pompe's disease. Two preparations (from the milk of lactating rabbits and from genetically engineered rodent cells) have been studied. Limited success was obtained in both trials, with improved muscle strength and transient mobility as well as delayed progression of myopathy. The long-term outcome is rendered uncertain by the development of neutralizing antibodies in many recipients and by the ability to manufacture sufficient enzyme. Bone marrow transplantation does not appear to be beneficial. In juvenile and adult acid maltase deficiency, muscle wasting may be arrested with improved or maintained function by institution of a high-protein, restricted-carbohydrate diet. Enzyme-replacement trials using recombinant human acid maltase have yet to be conducted in late-onset type II disease, although this treatment is likely to be more successful than in infantile disease where enzyme antigen is usually completely absent.

Type III glycogen storage disease
The clinical manifestations of Forbes–Cori's disease resemble those of type I glycogenosis, especially in infants, who present with hypoglycaemia, short stature, and hepatomegaly. Mild progressive myopathy, occasionally with signs of hypertrophic cardiomyopathy, may occur. The disorder is characterized by marked clinical variability. Generally the signs of liver disease regress during maturation and myopathy also improves with nutritional therapy as outlined for von Gierke's disease. Protein supplements, which

may provide additional sources of energy, appear to benefit the muscle disorder.

Type IV glycogen storage disease

This disorder is one of the more severe glycogenoses because the deficiency of branching enzyme in Anderson's disease gives rise to the deposition of an abnormal glycogen in many tissues. Severe inflammation occurs in the liver, resulting in early cirrhosis, with splenomegaly due to portal hypertension. This fatal disorder is characterized by failure to thrive, hepatosplenomegaly, jaundice, and hypotonia. The myopathy is often prominent with a lordotic posture and waddling gait due to limb-girdle weakness. Cardiomyopathy leading to cardiac failure develops in severely affected infants and children. Diagnosis is based on the appearances of the liver biopsy and abnormal glycogen structure shown by histochemical and biochemical analysis. Deficiency of branching enzyme is demonstrable in leucocytes. No definitive therapy is available, but a few patients have survived hepatic transplantation without the development of neuromuscular or cardiac complications up to 7 years after the procedure. Generally the prognosis is poor: without transplantation most patients die before the age of 4 years with liver failure, variceal bleeding, and intercurrent infection. Prenatal diagnosis of branching enzyme can be conducted by enzymatic analysis of amniotic cells or chorionic villi; DNA analysis of the human branching enzyme on chromosome 3p12 may also be possible for at-risk families.

Type V glycogen storage disease (McArdle's disease)

This disorder is characterized by the late onset of muscle fatigue and cramps during adolescence or early adult life. Hepatomegaly is absent. Strenuous exercise may induce episodic myoglobinuria and biochemical evidence of rhabdomyolysis. A characteristic feature is the occurrence of the 'second wind' phenomenon: progressive weakness and fatigue develop during the first 10 to 15 min of exercise, with a rapid recovery that is complete on resting; after this adaptation phase, patients are often able to continue exercise without difficulty. The mechanisms involved in this adaptive phenomenon are not clear but include increased cardiac output, blood flow to the muscles, and metabolic changes, probably including different patterns of fibre recruitment and the use of oxidative pathways. Occasionally, acute myoglobinuric renal failure may result. Muscle biopsy may show abnormal muscle fibres with necrosis, atrophy, and hypertrophied fibres alongside. The course of this disease is benign; ingestion of glucose or pre-exercise administration of glucagon may partially ameliorate the symptoms but avoidance of strenuous exercise is advisable. The muscle phosphorylase gene maps to chromosome 11q13 and sequence analysis has identified common mutations in this glycogenosis; one mutation, involving formation of a stop codon within exon 1 at position 49 (arginine) is sufficiently common to be of diagnostic value.

Type VI glycogen storage disease and phosphorylase b kinase deficiency

These disorders cause hepatomegaly, intermittent hypoglycaemia, and markedly increased liver glycogen content. Although many polypeptides constitute the intact phosphorylase b kinase complex (encoded on autosomes and the X-chromosome), glycogen mobilization is usually only partially defective. X-linked phosphorylase b kinase deficiency is the most frequent variant and is associated with growth retardation, mild ketosis, and hyperlipidaemia in childhood. The symptoms improve with age and the disorder is compatible with a normal life expectancy. Cirrhosis of the liver is very rare, and the incompleteness of the defect is shown by almost normal hyperglycaemic responses to glucagon administration. Rare autosomal variants of phosphorylase kinase deficiency affecting liver and muscle or restricted to skeletal or cardiac muscle have been documented. These subtypes are associated with hypotonia or cardiac failure, respectively. Treatment of liver phosphorylase or kinase deficiency with frequent feeding to avoid hypoglycaemia may be needed, but intensive nutritional

therapy is rarely indicated since the general prognosis is good. No specific treatment for the isolated cardiac form of kinase deficiency is known but cardiac transplantation could be considered if the diagnosis can be established.

Type VII glycogen storage disease (Tarui's disease)

This disorder, which is most frequent in patients of Japanese or Russian Ashkenazi ancestry, closely resembles type V muscle glycogenosis but severe symptoms usually come to light in childhood. There may be hyperuricaemia which is aggravated by exercise. Deficiency of red cell phosphofructokinase leads to chronic haemolysis; there is mild jaundice and a strong association with pigment-type gallstones. Decreased 2,3-diphosphoglycerate synthesis resulting from the metabolic block has been noted and probably contributes to exercise-induced symptoms by reducing oxygen delivery. Phosphofructokinase I catalyses an irreversible step in glycolysis and is an important regulatory enzyme, especially in muscle. Deficiency of phosphofructokinase I renders the pathway insensitive to positive allosteric regulation by the key effector molecules, fructose 2,6-diphosphate and AMP; hence myophosphorylase activity remains depressed. For this reason, Tarui's disease resembles a severe form of McCardle's disease. No specific therapy for this disorder is known—in contrast to McArdle's disease, neither glucagon nor glucose infusions improve exercise tolerance. Indeed, carbohydrate-rich meals aggravate the symptoms, presumably by diminishing the concentration of non-esterified fatty acids in the plasma, which serve as the alternative source of muscle energy production. Several very rare variants of phosphofructokinase deficiency are known: a severe infantile form with progressive and fatal myopathy and a late-onset form that causes fixed muscle weakness in middle-aged subjects are both clearly recognized. Approximately 15 mutations have been identified in the human muscle phosphofructokinase gene in patients with Tarui's disease; the three subunits encoding this isozyme originate from a locus on chromosome 12q13.3.

Glycogen synthase deficiency

Although glycogen synthase deficiency is very rare, it causes deficiency of glycogen formation in the liver. Most cases have been reported in infants and young children. It is, therefore, a disorder of storage rather than a true glycogenosis. The condition causes severe interprandial hypoglycaemia and marked ketosis; a notable feature is the rapid development of hyperglycaemia and lactic acidaemia on feeding. The disorder resembles fructose 1,6-bisphosphatase deficiency, but mutations in the liver glycogen synthetase gene II on chromosome 12p12.2 have been identified. Biopsy examination of the liver shows fatty infiltration and depletion of glycogen: uridine diphosphate-pyrophosphorylase, phosphorylase, glucose 6-phosphatase activities are normal but glycogen synthase is absent. Glucose polymers and uncooked cornstarch are effective therapy.

Further reading

Amalfitano A, *et al.* (2001). Recombinant human acid alpha-glucosidase enzyme therapy for infantile glycogen storage disease type II: results of a phase I/II clinical trial. *Genetic Medicine* **3**, 132–8.

Ambruso DR, *et al.* (1985). Infectious and bleeding complications in patients with glycogenosis Ib. *American Journal of Diseases of Children* **139**, 691–7.

Bao Y, *et al.* (1996). Hepatic and neuromuscular forms of glycogen storage disease type IV caused by mutations in the same glycogen-branching enzyme. *Journal of Clinical Investigation* **97**, 941–8.

Bianchi L (1993). Glycogen storage disease I and hepatocellular tumours. *European Journal of Pediatrics* **152**(Suppl 1), 563–70.

Braakhekke JP, *et al.* (1986). The second wind phenomenon in McCardle's disease. *Brain* **109**, 1087–101.

Burchell A (1992). The molecular basis of the type I glycogen storage diseases. *BioEssays*, **14**, 395–400.

Cabello A, *et al.* (1981). Glycogen storage disease in skeletal muscle. Morphological, ultrastructural and biochemical aspects in 10 cases. *Acta Neuropathologica (Basel)*, **Suppl VII**, 297–300.

Chen Y-T (2001). Glycogen storage disease. In: Scriver CR, *et al.*, eds. *The metabolic and molecular basis of inherited disease*, 8th edn, pp 1521–51. McGraw-Hill, New York.

Chen Y-T, Cornblath M, Sidbury JB (1984). Cornstarch therapy in type I glycogen-storage disease. *New England Journal of Medicine*, **310**, 171–5.

Chen Y-T, *et al.* (1988). Renal disease in type I glycogen storage disease. *New England Journal of Medicine*, **318**, 7–11.

Chou JY and Mansfield BC (1999). Molecular genetics of type 1 glycogen storage diseases. *Trends in Endocrinology and Metabolism* **10**, 104–13.

Danon MJ, *et al.* (1981). Lysosomal glycogen storage disease with normal acid maltase. *Neurology* **31**, 51–7.

de Barsy T, Hers H-G (1990). Normal metabolism and disorders of carbohydrate metabolism. *Baillière's Clinical Endocrinology and Metabolism* **4**, 499–522.

Engel AG (1970). Acid maltase deficiency in adults: studies in four cases of a syndrome which may mimic muscular dystrophy or other myopathies *Brain* **93**, 599–616.

Faivre L, *et al.* (1999). Long-term outcome of liver transplantation in patients with glycogen storage disease type 1A. *Journal of Inherited Metabolic Disease* **22**, 723–32.

Fernandes J, *et al.* (1988). Glycogen storage disease: recommendations for treatment. *European Journal of Paediatrics* **147**, 226–8.

Furakawa N, *et al.* (1990). Type I glycogen storage disease with vasoconstrictive pulmonary hypertension. *Journal of Inherited Metabolic Disease* **13**, 102–7.

Gitzelmann R, *et al.* (1996). Liver glycogen synthase deficiency: a rarely diagnosed entity. *European Journal of Paediatrics* **155**, 561–7.

Haller RG and Lewis SF (1991). Glucose-induced exertional fatigue in muscle phosphofructokinase deficiency. *New England Journal of Medicine* **324**, 364–9.

Hendrickx J, *et al.* (1995). Mutations in the phosphorylase kinase gene PHKA2 are responsible for X-linked liver glycogen storage disease. *Human Molecular Genetics* **4**, 77–83.

Janecke AR, *et al.* (1999). Molecular diagnosis of type Ic glycogen storage disease *Human Genetics* **105**, 515–17.

Kroos MA, *et al.* (1995). Glycogen storage disease type II: frequency of three common mutant alleles and their associated clinical phenotypes studied in 121 patients. *Journal of Medical Genetics* **32**, 836–7.

Lee PJ, Dixon MA, Leonard JV (1996). Uncooked cornstarch—efficacy in type I glycogenosis. *Archives of Diseases of Children* **74**, 546–7.

Marti GE, *et al.* (1986). DDAVP infusion in five patients with type Ia glycogen storage disease and associated correction of prolonged bleeding times. *Blood* **68**, 180–4.

Muraca M, *et al* (2002). Hepatocyte transplantation as a treatment for glycogen storage disease type 1a. *Lancet* **359**, 317–18.

Nishino I, *et al* (2000). Primary LAMP-2 deficiency causes X-linked vacuolar cardiomyopathy and myopathy (Danon disease). *Nature* **406**, 906–10.

Pears JS, *et al.* (1992). Glycogen storage disease diagnosed in adults. *Quarterly Journal of Medicine* **82**, 207–2.

Raben N, Sherman JB (1995). Mutations in muscle phosphofructokinase gene. *Human Mutation* **6**, 1–6.

Roe TF, *et al.* (1992). Treatment of chronic inflammatory bowel disease in glycogen storage disease type Ib with colony-stimulating factors. *New England Journal of Medicine* **326**, 1666–9.

Shaiu W-L, *et al.* (2000). Genotype–phenotype correlation in two frequent mutations and mutation update in type III glycogen storage disease. *Molecular Genetics in Metabolism* **69**, 16–23.

Shin YS (1990). Diagnosis of glycogen storage disease. *Journal Inherited Metabolic Disease* **13**, 419–34.

Slonim AE, Goans PJ (1985). Myopathy in McArdle's syndrome: improvement with a high-protein diet. *New England Journal of Medicine* **312**, 355–9.

Slonim AE, *et al.* (1983). Improvement of muscle function in acid maltase deficiency by high-protein therapy. *Neurology* **33**, 34–8.

Talente, *et al* (1994). Glycogen storage disease in adults. *Annals of Internal Medicine* **120**, 218–26.

Van den Hout JM, *et al.* (2001). Enzyme therapy for Pompe disease with recombinant human α-glucosidase from rabbit milk. *Journal of Inherited Metabolic Disease* **24**, 266–74.

Vogerd M, *et al* (1998). Mutation analysis in myophosphorylase deficiency (McArdle's disease). *Annals of Neurology* **43**, 326–31.

Willems PJ, *et al.* (1990). The natural history of liver glycogenosis due to phosphorylase kinase deficiency: a longitudinal study of 41 patients. *European Journal of Pediatrics* **149**, 268–71.

Williams JC (1986). Nutritional goals in glycogen storage disease. *New England Journal of Medicine* **314**, 709–10.

Wolfsdorf JI, Rudlin CR, Cirgler JF (1990). Physical growth and development of children with type I glycogen-storage disease: comparison of the effects of long-term use of dextrose and uncooked cornstarch. *American Journal of Clinical Nutrition* **52**, 1051–7.

11.3.2 Inborn errors of fructose metabolism

T. M. Cox

There are three inborn errors of fructose metabolism recognized: (1) essential or benign fructosuria due to fructokinase deficiency; (2) fructose 1,6-diphosphatase deficiency; and (3) hereditary fructose intolerance (fructosaemia). There are discussed in relation to the overall metabolism of fructose, a major nutrient.

Metabolism of fructose

Phosphorylated forms of fructose are critical intermediates in the glycolytic and gluconeogenic metabolic pathways in all cells. Fructose is also an important component of the diet: it occurs as a free monosaccharide in fruit, nuts, honey, and some vegetables. Free fructose is released from sucrose in the gut lumen by sucrase–isomaltase in the brush-border membrane of the mucosal epithelium. Finally, the sugar alcohol, sorbitol (a constituent of medicines and tablets, as well as some foods for diabetics), is converted quantitatively to fructose in the liver and intestine. Most individuals in developed countries ingest 50 to 150 g fructose equivalents daily in the diet.

The pathways of fructose metabolism are summarized in Fig. 1. Fructose is absorbed rapidly by a carrier mechanism that facilitates transport across the intestinal epithelium; this process is mediated by the glucose transporter isoforms, GLUT5 and GLUT2, the latter probably contributing to efflux across the basolateral membrane of the enterocyte.

It is then conveyed via the portal bloodstream to the liver, where it is assimilated. The jejunal mucosa and proximal tubule of the kidney are subsidiary sites of fructose metabolism. Assimilation of fructose depends on the concerted activities of the enzymes ketohexokinase (fructokinase), aldolase B, and triokinase, which are expressed specifically in these tissues. Uptake of fructose occurs independently of insulin and its incorporation into intermediary metabolism bypasses the regulation of glycolysis at the level of phosphofructokinase-1. For these reasons, solutions of fructose or sorbitol were advocated and, in the past, extensively used for parenteral nutrition. However, the occurrence of lactic acidosis, hyperuricaemia and other serious consequences have led to their withdrawal from hyperalimentation regimens in most, if not all, countries.

Fructokinase rapidly phosphorylates fructose at the 1-carbon position. This enzyme has a high affinity for its substrates and the intestinal mucosa and liver rapidly convert fructose to fructose 1-phosphate: in other tissues,

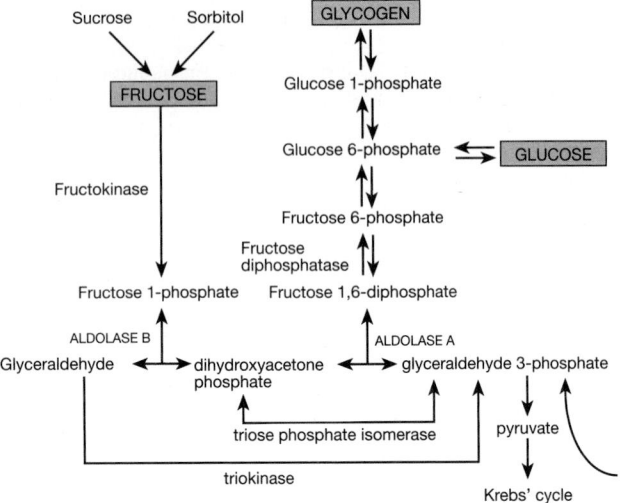

Fig. 1 Fructose metabolism.

the capacity of hexokinase to phosphorylate fructose at the 6-carbon position is limited. Similarly, the fate of fructose 1-phosphate in the fructose-metabolizing tissues is dependent on a specific isozyme of aldolase, aldolase B. This has greater activity towards fructose 1-phosphate than does its ubiquitous counterpart, aldolase A, the natural substrate of which is fructose 1,6-diphosphate. Cleavage of fructose 1-phosphate generates glyceraldehyde and dihydroxyacetone phosphate. These trioses enter the intermediary pools of carbohydrate metabolism, and, as a result of triokinase activity, glyceraldehyde is phosphorylated so that the two triose phosphates may be condensed by aldolase A to form the glycolytic and gluconeogenic intermediate, fructose 1,6-diphosphate.

Gluconeogenesis from triose phosphates, lactate, glycerol, amino acids, and Krebs cycle intermediates such as oxaloacetate, requires reversal of the committed reactions of glycolysis. It is the enzyme fructose 1,6-diphosphatase that releases the glucose precursor fructose 6-phosphate from fructose 1,6-diphosphate. Thus, when the remaining reactions of glycolysis are reversed, exogenous fructose provides a source of glucose or glycogen. Fructose 1,6-diphosphatase is active in the liver, kidney, and intestine; it is a key enzyme of gluconeogenesis.

Fructose malabsorption

Incomplete absorption of fructose with abdominal symptoms and diarrhoea reminiscent of intestinal disaccharidase deficiency is well recognized by gastroenterologists. The symptoms occur in adults and children after ingestion of fructose- or sorbitol-rich foods and drinks such as apple juice, and usually recede when these sugars are excluded from the diet. Many such individuals, as well as a high proportion of healthy control subjects, have suggestive evidence of fructose malabsorption based on breath-hydrogen tests. Unfortunately, the molecular basis of this syndrome and of the wide variation of tolerance to dietary fructose and its congeners is not known. Moreover, molecular analysis of the human *GLUT5* gene in several patients complaining of fructose-related intestinal symptoms, has hitherto failed to implicate this candidate sugar transporter. Preliminary studies suggest that lower intestines and colons of many patients who experience abdominal flatulence and diarrhoea after ingesting fructose-containing foods contain a bacterial population showing enhanced uptake and anaerobic metabolism of fructose. No conclusive evidence has yet been provided to support these observations and more fructose transport studies are needed on the mucosal epithelium of patients who complain of symptoms that indicate an intestinal malabsorption of this sugar.

Essential (benign) fructosuria (Mendelian inheritance in man (MIM) 229800)

This is a rare disorder (estimated frequency 1 in 130 000) of little clinical consequence. The abnormality is transmitted as an autosomal recessive condition and manifests itself by the presence of a reducing sugar in the blood and urine, especially after meals rich in fructose. The abnormality results from the deficiency of fructokinase activity in the liver and intestine, significantly reducing the capacity to assimilate this sugar. Mutations in the human ketohexokinase gene on chromosome 2p23.3–p23.2 have been identified in patients with essential fructosuria, thus confirming the suspected molecular defect in this condition. Fructose metabolism occurs slowly in essential fructosuria as a result of conversion to fructose 6-phosphate by hexokinase in adipose tissue and muscle, but, while plasma concentrations remain high postprandially, large amounts of fructose appear in the urine. Essential fructosuria may be confused with diabetes mellitus if the nature of the mellituria is not defined with the use of glucose oxidase strips in preference to the older chemical methods for urinalysis, such confusion is now unlikely. No treatment beyond recognition and explanation appears to be necessary.

Fructose diphosphatase deficiency (MIM 229700)

Description

This very rare, recessively inherited disorder presents with hypoglycaemia, ketosis, and lactic acidosis in early infancy. Fewer than 30 cases have been reported since its original description in 1970. Severe, sometimes fatal, acidosis is associated with infection and starvation and most cases have presented within the first few days of life or in the neonatal period. Onset during the first year of life is the rule.

In newborn infants, the severe metabolic disturbance shows itself by acidotic hyperventilation, which may be accompanied by irritability, disturbed consciousness, seizures, or coma. The unusual combination of ketonaemia, lactic acidaemia, and hypoglycaemia is induced by fasting, the administration of fructose, sorbitol, and glycerol, and by ingestion of a diet rich in fat. Episodes in the neonatal period respond well to infusions of glucose and bicarbonate but, after an interval, further attacks occur, often provoked by intercurrent infection. Lethargy accompanied by hyperventilation is followed abruptly by prostration, coma, and seizures. Investigations reveal hypoglycaemia, ketosis, and profound lactic acidosis; there is hyperuricaemia, amino aciduria, and ketonuria. If the infant survives, hepatomegaly due to fatty infiltration may be detected but overt clinical disturbances of hepatic or renal tubular function are not seen. The untreated disease is associated with growth retardation.

The first infant to be affected by fructose diphosphatase deficiency in a given family may succumb before the diagnosis is established and in any case fares worse than siblings for whom the appropriate diet and prompt control of the condition are instituted. The response to treatment is favourable, however, and fructose diphosphatase deficiency is ultimately compatible with a benign course and with normal growth and development.

Metabolic defect

Deficiency of fructose 1,6-diphosphatase causes failure of gluconeogenesis in the liver—although the abnormality may be detected in intestinal mucosa, kidney, and in cultured mononuclear cells from peripheral blood. The muscle isozyme of fructose 1,6-diphosphatase is not affected.

Between meals, blood glucose is maintained by glucogenolysis and hence the onset of disturbed metabolism in fructose diphosphatase deficiency depends on the availability of hepatic glycogen. Since febrile illnesses accelerate the consumption of liver glycogen, the accompanying anorexia with or without vomiting may deplete glycogen stores critically. Acidosis results from the accumulation of gluconeogenic precursors including lactate, pyruvate, and alanine as well as ketone bodies, which cannot be utilized. Hypoglycaemia, which is unresponsive to glucagon and associated with exhaustion of glycogen stores, occurs: this does not respond to normal gluconeogenic substrates (for example, glycerol, amino acid solutions, dihydroxyacetone, sorbitol, or fructose), indeed administration of these aggravates the metabolic disturbance.

The pathogenesis of hypoglycaemia and accompanying disturbances in fructose diphosphatase deficiency is complex and not completely explained by exhaustion of hepatic glycogen stores. Well-fed patients have a normal response to glucagon but are intolerant of high-fat diets, as well as of fructose, sorbitol, alanine, glycerol, and dihydroxyacetone administration. Challenge with these nutrients induces hypoglycaemia, hyperuricaemia, and hypophosphataemia, accompanied by an exaggerated rise in blood lactate levels. The hypoglycaemia is then unresponsive to glucagon, indicating a secondary inhibition of phosphorylase activity in the liver, which results from the build-up of phosphorylated sugar intermediates that cannot be further metabolized in the context of reduced intracellular free inorganic phosphate. Adenosine deaminase is activated primarily because of reduced phosphate concentrations, so that purine nucleotides are broken down to uric acid. Failure to utilize glucogenic amino acids and metabolites such as dihydroxyacetone and glycerol appears to stimulate triglyceride formation in the liver, which induces steatosis. Unlike hereditary fructose intolerance (see below), high concentrations of hepatic fructose 1-phosphate do not occur, and profound disturbances of blood coagulation or hepatic or renal tubule function with progressive structural damage are absent in fructose diphosphatase deficiency. Similarly, aversion to foods that aggravate the disorder does not develop in affected infants and children; this may be explained by the absence of pain and abdominal symptoms in the condition.

Diagnosis

The importance of establishing the diagnosis of fructose diphosphatase deficiency cannot be overemphasized: proper dietary control and protocols for the institution of appropriate therapy depend upon recognizing the complex disturbance that underlies this disease.

Fructose diphosphatase deficiency should be considered in otherwise normal infants who develop unexplained severe acidosis or hypoglycaemia associated with episodes of infection. The combination of ketosis and lactic acidosis with hypoglycaemia is highly suggestive of a disorder affecting the gluconeogenic pathway, including deficiency of glucose 6-phosphatase, pyruvate carboxylase, pyruvate dehydrogenase, and phosphoenolpyruvate carboxykinase. The absence of abdominal distress, haemolysis, jaundice, coagulopathy, and disturbances of the proximal renal tubule differentiate the condition from hereditary fructose intolerance, tyrosinosis, and Wilson's disease. Confusion may arise with disorders associated with secondary defects in gluconeogenesis, especially the Reye-like syndrome caused by deficiencies of long-, medium- and short-chain acyl coenzyme A dehydrogenase activities, as well as defects of carnitine metabolism. Organic acidaemias are also readily distinguished by biochemical screening methods.

Provocative tests using food deprivation and the administration of infusions of fructose, sorbitol, or glycerol should be avoided in the acutely ill infant or child with suspected deficiency of fructose 1,6-diphosphatase (or fructose intolerance). The definitive diagnosis depends on the demonstration of selectively decreased fructose diphosphatase activity in tissue samples. Most frequently, the enzymatic defect will be identified by biochemical assay of a freshly obtained liver biopsy specimen, which allows other metabolic disorders and gluconeogenic defects to be confidently excluded. The defect may also be demonstrated in biopsy samples of jejunal mucosa and in cultured monocyte-derived macrophages obtained from peripheral blood. However, the presence of fructose 1,6-diphosphatase in these tissues is metabolically inconsequential and, although useful for confirmation of the diagnosis where it is strongly suspected, in practice decisive identification of this disorder normally depends on a systematic biochem-

ical analysis of liver tissue in an experienced laboratory. The human fructose 1,6-diphosphatase (**FBP1**) gene maps to chromosome 9q22.2–q22.3 and inactivating mutations have been identified in the disease. Unlike fructose intolerance however, these mutations tend to be private and thus individually of less diagnostic significance for routine laboratory use in this disorder since mutational heterogeneity appears to be the rule. However, a minor exception to this occurs in the Japanese population, where one mutation (960–961 ins G) appears to account for almost one-half of mutant *FBPI* alleles.

Treatment

Dietary control and avoidance of starvation with rapid control of febrile illnesses is the mainstay of treatment. Minor infections and injuries require prompt attention, and intravenous glucose therapy should be instituted early in acute episodes to avoid hypoglycaemia and acidosis. Fasting should be avoided as far as possible, while night-time feeding may be needed in infants during recovery from injuries or infections and after strenuous exercise in older children. The habit of taking meals at regular 4-hourly intervals is best inculcated when the patient is young. The diet should exclude excess fat; sorbitol, sucrose, and fructose must be strictly avoided. Breast milk is rich in lactose, which is readily assimilated, but difficulties arise on transfer to artificial feeds during weaning. In addition, medications and syrups containing fructose, sucrose, or sorbitol present a special danger to patients with deficiency of fructose diphosphatase activity. A diet excluding these sugars but containing 56 per cent calories as carbohydrate with 32 per cent calories as fat and 12 per cent as protein has produced normal growth and development. Acute episodes of acidosis or hypoglycaemia are controlled rapidly by intravenous administration of glucose with or without bicarbonate as required.

Hereditary fructose intolerance (fructosaemia) (MIM 229600)

This disorder, first recognized in 1956, is the most common inherited defect of fructose metabolism with an estimated frequency of 1 in 20 000 births. The condition is transmitted as an autosomal recessive abnormality and, although it manifests itself first in early infancy, the effects of clinical disease may not be recognized until late childhood or adult life. Provided the diagnosis is made before visceral damage occurs, hereditary fructose intolerance responds completely to an exclusion diet.

The cardinal features of the illness are vomiting, diarrhoea, abdominal pain, and hypoglycaemia, which are induced by the consumption of foods, drinks, or medicines that contain fructose seizures, or the related sugars, sucrose or sorbitol. There is a generalized metabolic disturbance with lactic acidosis, hyperuricaemia, and hyperphosphataemia. Hypoglycaemia causes trembling, irritability, and cognitive impairment. Attacks are associated with pallor, sweating, and, when severe, loss of consciousness—sometimes accompanied by generalized seizures. These episodes usually occur within 30 min of feeds that contain large quantities of fructose or sucrose. Continued ingestion of noxious sugars is associated with renal tubular disease, liver damage with jaundice, and defective blood coagulation. There is failure to thrive and growth retardation. Persistent exposure to fructose in infants leads to structural liver injury with cirrhosis, amino aciduria, coagulopathy, and coma leading to death. The infant is first exposed to the offending sugars at weaning or upon transfer from breast milk to artificial feeds: survival is dependent on recognition of the effects of fruit and sugar by the mother or, especially in older infants, by vomiting or forcible rejection of food.

Infants who survive the stormy period of weaning, develop a strong aversion to sweet-tasting foods, vegetables, and fruits. This usually affords protection against the worst effects of fructose and sucrose, but abdominal symptoms with bouts of tremulousness, irritability, and altered consciousness due to hypoglycaemia usually continue. It has become clear that many cases escape diagnosis in infancy and childhood, but that the risk of illness, related to dietary indiscretion, remains throughout life. Characteristically, children and adults with hereditary fructose intolerance show a striking reduction in, or absence of dental caries.

Recently, a syndrome of chronic sugar intoxication has been recognized in older children and adolescents with hereditary fructose intolerance. General lack of vigour and developmental retardation are prominent features. Hypoglycaemia, though obvious after heavy fructose loading, may be insignificant after chronic low-level exposure in older children. Similarly, tests of hepatic and renal function may be only mildly abnormal. Persistent ingestion of fructose and sucrose is toxic to the kidney and liver, so that renal tubular acidosis (occasionally with calculi) as well as hepatospleno-megaly are frequently detectable in the younger patients. Severe growth retardation may be accompanied by rachitic bone disease that complicates the Fanconi-like syndrome of proximal renal tubular disturbance. Growth retardation responds to dietary treatment and is usually accompanied by regression of the other disease manifestations.

Provided that organ failure and serious tissue injury do not supervene, patients with hereditary fructose intolerance recover rapidly when the offending sugars are withdrawn. Children who survive by acquiring the protective eating-behaviour pattern avoid foods that they associate with abdominal symptoms. The aversion extends to most sweet-tasting items of food and drink as well as fruits and vegetables—it remains lifelong and consumption of fructose is usually reduced to less than 5 g daily. It has been shown that normal growth and development can be secured in children if less than 40 mg/kg fructose equivalents are ingested daily.

Metabolic defect

Hereditary fructose intolerance is caused by a deficiency of aldolase B in the liver, small intestine, and proximal renal tubule. These tissues suffer injury as a result of persistent exposure to fructose in patients affected by the disorder. In the absence of the fructose 1-phosphate splitting activity of aldolase B, the intracellular pool of inorganic phosphate is depleted. Studies *in vivo* by ^{31}P magnetic resonance spectroscopy show that 80 per cent of hepatic free phosphate is sequestered as sugar phosphates after the infusion of small quantities of fructose (250 mg/kg body weight). The secondary metabolic disturbances are initiated by the accumulation of fructose 1-phosphate in a milieu where free inorganic phosphate is reduced: there is competitive inhibition of aldolase A and inhibition of phosphorylase activity so that glycogenolysis and gluconeogenesis are impaired. Thus challenge with fructose leads to hypophosphataemia and hypoglycaemia that is refractory to glucagon or the infusion of gluconeogenic metabolites such as glycerol or dihydroxyacetone. During challenge with fructose, high concentrations of fructose 1-phosphate cause feedback inhibition of fructokinase, thereby limiting the incorporation of fructose in the liver. As a result, fructosaemia occurs and when the concentration exceeds about 2 mmol/l in peripheral blood, fructosuria becomes apparent. Although the assimilation of fructose by the specialized pathway is blocked, only a small fraction of the fructose load is recovered in the urine. Studies show that 80 to 90 per cent of the fructose is taken up under these circumstances by adipose tissue and muscle, where it can be alternatively metabolized by phosphorylation to fructose 6-phosphate.

Electrolytic disturbances occur during challenge with fructose. Hypokalaemia results from acute renal impairment with defective urinary acidification. There is a defect of proximal tubule function with bicarbonate wasting and acidosis. Occasionally, acute flaccid weakness due to hypokalaemia accompanies the other effects of fructose exposure. In patients with hereditary fructose intolerance, the administration of fructose reproducibly increases serum magnesium concentrations. This is probably explained by the breakdown of magnesium–adenosine triphosphate (**ATP**) complexes, releasing intracellular magnesium ions as a result of nucleotide degradation by adenosine deaminase. Significant ingestion of fructose is thus also accompanied by marked hyperuricaemia in patients with hereditary fructose intolerance.

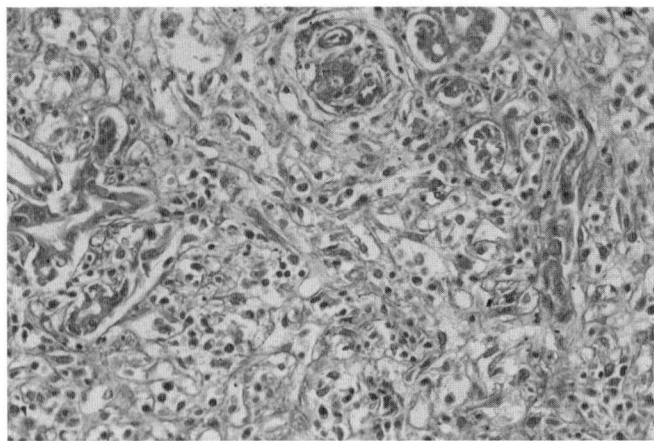

Fig. 2 The effects of fatal infusions of fructose in a young Italian girl.

Pathology and molecular genetics

Chronic ingestion of fructose in hereditary fructose intolerance causes hepatic injury: there is diffuse fatty change and increased glycogen deposition. Hepatocyte necrosis with intralobular and periportal fibrosis occurs and fully developed cirrhosis results from continued exposure to fructose. After acute experimental challenge, electron microscopy has shown irregular electron-dense material surrounded by membranous structures, suggesting a florid lysosomal reaction to intracellular deposits of fructose 1-phosphate. Fatal administration of fructose or sorbitol parenterally is associated with the abrupt onset of hepatorenal failure associated with bleeding. Histological examination shows hepatic necrosis in these cases (Fig. 2). Loss of cellular functions, for example in the proximal renal tubule, is probably caused by depletion of ATP resulting from the arrested metabolism of fructose by the specialized pathway. The source of the severe abdominal pain that follows ingestion of fructose is unknown, but stimulation of visceral afferent nerves by the local release of purine nucleotides or lactate may be responsible.

The genetic basis of aldolase B deficiency has been studied intensively. The human aldolase B gene maps to chromosome 9q22.3. Several point mutations affecting the function of the enzyme are sufficiently widespread in patients of European origin to merit diagnostic investigation. One particular mutation, Ala^{149}→Pro, which disrupts residues in a substrate-binding domain of aldolase B, is prevalent in Europe. This mutation accounts for most alleles responsible for fructose intolerance, but others, including Ala^{174}→Asp, Asn^{334}→Lys and a four-base deletion in exon 4, are sufficiently frequent and widespread to merit examination in the diagnostic laboratory (see below).

Diagnosis

In infancy and childhood, hereditary fructose intolerance most characteristically causes persistent vomiting, with failure to thrive, acidosis, hypoglycaemia, and jaundice. Clearly in very young infants there is a wide differential diagnosis, but fructose intolerance may be indicated by the nutritional history and feeding difficulties. The presence of reducing sugar in the urine may indicate that fructosuria and amino acids may also be present. Older children and adults report food aversion and may show a striking absence of dental caries. If fructose intolerance is considered, then sucrose, sorbitol, and fructose should be excluded completely before definitive tests can be carried out. Striking improvement, suggestive of hereditary fructose intolerance, may be seen within a few days. The differential diagnosis includes pyloric stenosis, galactosaemia, hepatitis, renal tubular disease, Wilson's disease, and tyrosinosis.

Since the prompt institution of strict dietary treatment has beneficial and, in infants and children, life-saving effects in those with fructose intolerance, every reasonable effort should be undertaken to make a definitive diagnosis. This will have important consequences for relatives of the propositus and will provide information critical for the introduction of a rigorous and life-long exclusion diet.

The intravenous fructose tolerance test is often useful for diagnosis, particularly in adults: 0.25 g/kg (0.2 g/kg in infants) of D(+)-fructose is infused as a 20 per cent solution over a few minutes and blood samples for potassium ions, magnesium ions, phosphate ions, and glucose are taken at regular intervals over a 2-h period. Epigastric and loin pain accompany the infusion, and hypoglycaemic coma may occur. The hypoglycaemia does not respond to glucagon, therefore glucose for parenteral injection must be available. The test should be carried out under controlled conditions with medical personnel at hand: oral challenge with fructose or sucrose may produce severe pain and shock and is best avoided. Responses differ between individuals and hypoglycaemia is usually milder in adults, but typical responses in hereditary fructose intolerance and a control subject are depicted in Fig. 3. The tolerance test should not be carried out in patients with overt signs of liver disease where it may occasionally yield misleading results, particularly in infants and children.

Aldolase B deficiency is demonstrated definitively by enzymatic analysis of biopsy samples obtained from the liver or small intestinal mucosa. Biochemical assay of fructaldolases characteristically demonstrates reduced or absent fructose 1-phosphate cleavage activity with a partial deficiency of fructose 1,6-diphosphate aldolase. Since fructaldolase deficiency may accompany other parenchymal disease of the liver, these assays are of limited value in the acutely ill or jaundiced patient.

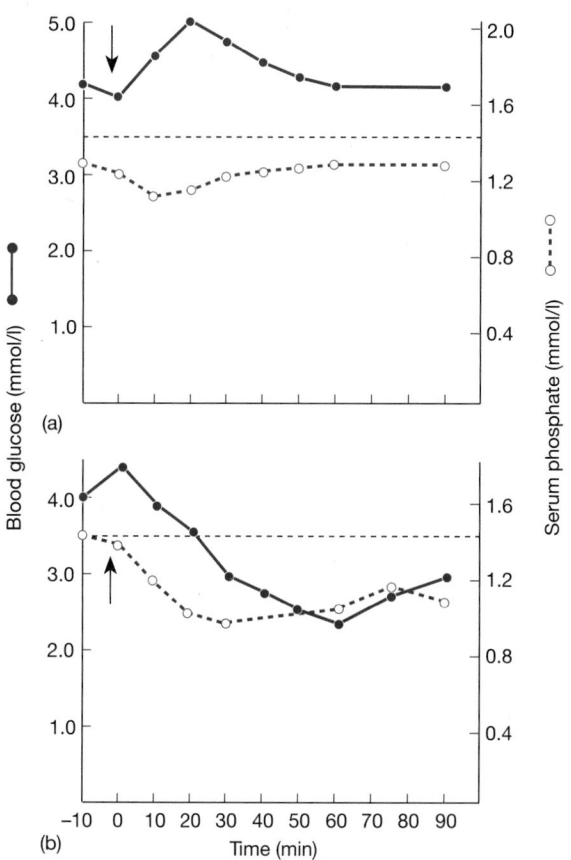

(a)

(b)

Blood glucose (mmol/l)

Serum phosphate (mmol/l)

Time (min)

Fig. 3 (a) Intravenous fructose tolerance tests in a 39-year-old woman with hereditary fructose intolerance proven by fructaldolase essay and DNA analysis. (b) An age- and sex-matched control subject with alcohol-related episodic hypoglycaemia.

Recently, a direct diagnosis of hereditary fructose intolerance has been possible, particularly in patients of European ancestry: examination of aldolase B genes for the presence of common mutations responsible for the disease can be carried out by laboratories that specialize in the molecular analysis of genomic DNA. The ability to identify disease alleles by analysing tiny samples of blood or tissue may be beneficial for the investigation of infants with this disorder and, eventually, for postnatal screening before dietary exposure occurs. Tests for fructose intolerance based on the analysis of DNA may avoid the need for invasive or hazardous investigations using tissue biopsy procedures or challenge with parenteral sugar solutions.

Treatment

Dietary treatment of fructose intolerance alleviates the disorder but requires the almost complete exclusion of sucrose, fructose, and sorbitol. The daily consumption of sugar should be reduced to less than 40 mg of fructose equivalents per kilogram body weight (that is, 2–3 g for an adult) in order to reverse the disease manifestations and establish normal development in affected infants and children. The ubiquity of fructose and its congeners in the Western diet presents serious difficulties. Adult patients have usually restricted their consumption of fructose to less than 20 g daily and the source of the residual sugar may be difficult to establish. For this reason, the advice of an experienced dietitian should be sought (Table 1). Particular care needs to be taken with sugar-coated pills and, especially, liquid medications for paediatric use, as large amounts of fructose, sucrose, and sorbitol are frequently present. Children and adults with hereditary fructose intolerance may tolerate the taste of confectionery that contains large quantities of noxious sugars but in which the sweetness is masked by other flavours such as peppermint, which they enjoy. This behaviour may lead to unexplained hypoglycaemic symptoms and other signs of sugar toxicity. Occasionally, patients are unable to tolerate certain foods that are permitted on their diet sheets—in doubtful cases it is advisable to avoid the offending item or to have it analysed. Patients with hereditary fructose intolerance may lack folic acid and vitamin C. Supplements of these vitamins in particular are recommended, especially during pregnancy, but, as with other medicines, care has to be taken to avoid harmful sugars contained in the preparation: Ketovite®; (Paines and Byrne, Ltd, Surrey, England) is a satisfactory source of these vitamins.

Prognosis

Untreated hereditary fructose intolerance is a fatal disease in infants and young children in whom it generally causes irreversible liver disease and

Table 1 Food items not allowed for patients with hereditary fructose intolerance and fructose diphosphatase deficiency[a]

Table sugar
Fruit sugar, all fruit and fruit products, including tomatoes
Sorbitol
Honey, syrup, treacle, molasses
Diabetic foods
Chocolate, sherbet
Preserves, jams, and marmalade
Frankfurters, honey-roast, and sweet-cured ham
Processed cheese spreads
Cream and cottage cheese with chives, pineapple, etc.
Flavoured milks and yoghurts
Wheatgerm, brown rice, bran
Breakfast cereals
Coffee essence, powdered milk
Carbonated sweet drinks
Allspice, nuts, coconut, carob, peanut butter
Mayonnaise, pickles, salad dressings, sauces
Some potatoes (especially stored, new potatoes)
Most legumes

[a] Further information is provided in the Further reading list.

episodic, life-threatening, hypoglycaemia. Occasionally, adolescents and adult patients may succumb to the inadvertent use of parenteral fructose or sorbitol but, except in Germany, this practice is now obsolete. With the introduction of a strict exclusion diet, the disorder is compatible with a normal life expectancy.

Further reading

Ali M, Rellos P, and Cox TM (1998) Hereditary fructose intolerance. *Journal of Medical Genetics* **35**, 353–65.

Baker L, Wingrad AI (1970). Fasting hypoglycaemia and metabolic acidosis associated with deficiency of fructose-1,6-diphosphatase deficiency. *Lancet* **ii**, 13–16.

Boesinger P, *et al.* (1994). Changes of liver metabolite concentrations in adults with disorders of fructose metabolism after intravenous fructose by ^{31}P magnetic resonance spectroscopy. *Pediatric Research* **36**, 436–40.

Bell L and Sherwood WG (1987). Current practices and improved recommendations for treating hereditary fructose intolerance. *Journal of the American Dietetic Association* **87**, 721–8.

Chambers RA and Pratt RTC (1956). Idiosyncrasy to fructose. *Lancet* **ii**, 340.

Cox TM (1993). Iatrogenic deaths in hereditary fructose intolerance. *Archives of Diseases in Childhood* **69**, 413–15.

Cox TM (1994). Aldolase B and fructose intolerance. *Journal of the Federation of American Societies for Experimental Biology* **8**, 62–71.

Greenwood J (1989). Sugar content of liquid prescription medicines. *Pharmaceutical Journal* **243**, 553–7.

Kikawa Y, *et al.* (2002). Diagnosis of fructose 1,6-bisphosphatase deficiency using cultured lymphocyte fraction: a secure and noninvasive alternative to liver biopsy. *Journal of Inherited Metabolic Disease* **25**, 41–6.

Odièvre M, *et al.* (1978). Hereditary fructose intolerance in childhood. Diagnosis, management and course in 55 patients. *American Journal of Diseases of Childhood* **132**, 605–8.

Pagliara AS, *et al.* (1972). Hepatic fructose-1,6-diphosphatase deficiency. A cause of lactic acidosis and hypoglycaemia in infancy. *Journal of Clinical Investigation* **51**, 2115–23.

Sachs B, Sternfeld L, Kraus G (1942). Essential fructosuria: its pathophysiology. *American Journal of Diseases of Childhood* **63**, 252.

Steinmann B, Gitzelmann R, Van den Berghe G (2001). Disorders of fructose metabolism. In: Scriver CR, *et al.*, eds. *The metabolic and molecular bases of inherited disease*, 8th edn, Vol II, pp 1489–520. McGraw-Hill, New York.

Wasserman D, *et al.* (1996). Molecular analysis of the fructose transporter gene (GLUT 5) in isolated fructose malabsorption. *Journal of Clinical Investigation* **98**, 2398–402.

11.3.3 Disorders of galactose, pentose, and pyruvate metabolism

T. M. Cox

Inborn errors of galactose metabolism

Galactose is derived principally from the milk sugar, lactose, in the diet by the action of mucosal lactase in the small intestine. The concentration of lactose in human breast milk is approximately 200 millimoles per litre. Newborn infants normally receive about one-fifth of their dietary energy supply in the form of galactose, which is derived from the breakdown of this lactose to galactose and glucose in equimolar amounts. After absorp-

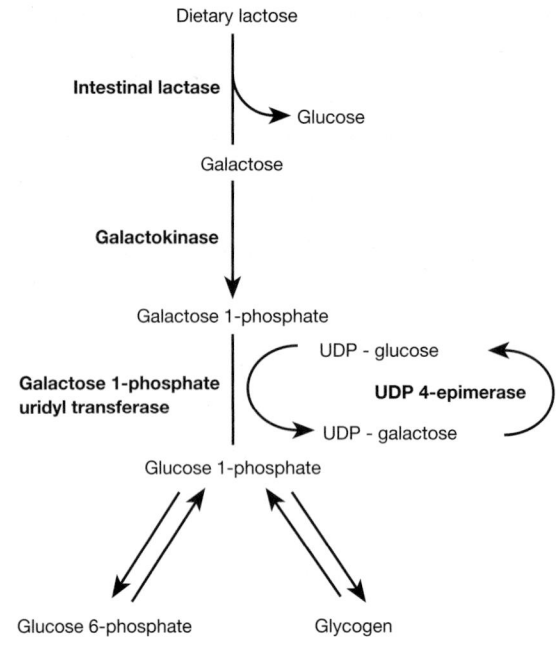

Fig. 1 Galactose metabolism.

tion, galactose serves as a source of glucose. Galactose is a component of many membrane glycoproteins and glycolipids; galactosylated lipids are abundant in nervous tissue.

The conversion of galactose to glucose involves reactions that lead to the formation of glucose 1-phosphate, which can enter the main pathways of carbohydrate metabolism, directly (Fig. 1). The first step involves phosphorylation to form galactose 1-phosphate, which is converted to glucose 1-phosphate and uridine diphosphate-galactose after reaction with the nucleoside diphosphate sugar, uridine diphosphoglucose. Uridine diphosphoglucose is regenerated by the action of uridine diphosphate-galactose-4-epimerase. The presence of this epimerase enables galactose to be produced from glucose for the synthesis of complex glycoconjugates and renders the individual potentially independent of exogenous galactose. Enzymatic defects in the interconversion of these metabolites lead to increased blood and tissue concentrations of galactose, especially after meals containing milk or dairy products. There are three inborn errors of galactose metabolism recognized: (1) galactokinase deficiency; (2) galactose 1-phosphate uridylyltransferase deficiency; and (3) uridine diphosphate-4-epimerase deficiency.

Galactokinase deficiency: 'galactose diabetes'

Failure to phosphorylate galactose in the liver and other tissues impairs its clearance from the blood so that the free sugar and its metabolites, galactonic acid and galactitol, appear in the urine. Homozygous deficiency of galactokinase occurs with an approximate frequency of 1 in 100 000 live births.

Clinical features

Precocious formation of cataracts in infants and children is characteristic, with some heterozygotes developing cataracts before the age of 40 years. When blood concentrations are high, galactose is taken up by the lens and converted to the end-product galactitol by the action of aldose reductase: subsequent toxic or osmotic effects lead to swelling and irreversible damage to lens fibres. Patients with galactokinase deficiency persistently excrete reducing sugar in their urine but, apart from possible confusion with diabetes mellitus, this has no apparent significance.

Diagnosis and treatment

Galactokinase deficiency should be suspected in infants or children with cataracts and reducing sugar should be sought in the urine. This sugar will not react with glucose oxidase test strips. Definitive diagnosis by enzymatic assay of galactokinase in erythrocytes or cultured fibroblasts differentiates the disorder from classic galactosaemia and hypergalactosaemia due to vascular disease in the liver. Treatment with a strict lactose and galactose exclusion diet prevents cataract formation. The human gene for galactokinase maps to chromosome 17q24, with a putative second locus on chromosome 15. Several mutations responsible for galactokinase deficiency have been identified in the *GALK1* gene at the chromosome 17 locus.

Galactose 1-phosphate uridylyltransferase deficiency: galactosaemia

Unlike individuals in whom galactokinase is deficient, when patients who lack uridylyltransferase activity ingest lactose, there is a significant rise in intracellular galactose 1-phosphate as well as in the blood galactose concentration. The severe consequences of classical galactosaemia thus result from the toxic effects of galactose 1-phosphate principally in cells of the liver, proximal renal tubule, and brain. Although the exact mechanism of toxicity is unknown, as in hereditary fructose intolerance, the accumulated metabolite probably inhibits other enzymatic reactions involving phosphorylated intermediates and may lead to purine nucleotide depletion.

Recognition of galactosaemia in early infancy is of paramount importance since the acute effects of galactose poisoning may be reversed by institution of a lactose exclusion diet. However, the ability of dietary therapy to promote a completely healthy long-term outcome has now been questioned by follow-up studies in large cohorts of patients with classical galactosaemia and therefore more research is needed to improve our understanding about the pathogenesis of tissue injury in this nutritional disease.

Clinical and pathological features

The affected infant appears normal at birth, but vomiting or diarrhoea, jaundice, and hepatomegaly usually occur in the first few weeks. There is failure to gain weight, subcutaneous bruising, and progressive enlargement of the liver. Cataracts may be apparent at 1 month of age, by which time abdominal distension with ascites has developed. Mental retardation does not become manifest until later in the first year of life and varies greatly in severity. Many patients suffering from galactosaemia develop severe infections with *Escherichia coli* during the neonatal period, and Gram-negative bacterial sepsis may be the first indication of this disorder in young infants. A bactericidal defect in circulating leucocytes has been postulated. In adult patients after reversal of the acute galactose toxicity syndrome, the most obvious sequelae are growth failure, neurological deficit, and primary ovarian failure with infertility.

Occasional patients with galactosaemia remain asymptomatic while ingesting milk but gradually fail to gain weight. Such patients may come to light during childhood or even adult life, because of varying degrees of mental retardation and cataracts. Hepatomegaly and intermittent galactosuria are usually present, and often there is a history of feeding difficulties on institution of modified formula feeds during the neonatal period.

The neurological manifestations of classical galactosaemia are highly variable but, despite prompt institution of dietary therapy, a degree of mental retardation is common in affected children and adults. Characteristic learning difficulties in mathematics and spatial relationships with behavioural deficits have been observed. It appears that the galactose-free diet fails to confer benefit on mental development when instituted beyond the age of 2 years. In follow-up studies of galactosaemic children and adults, a range of neurological deficits, including seizures, apraxia, extra-pyramidal disorders, and cerebellar signs, have been documented despite strict dietary measures.

Serum tests of liver function are non-specifically deranged: histological examination shows lobular fibrosis, fatty change, bile ductular proliferation and progression to frank cirrhosis. A haemorrhagic tendency is an early feature of galactosaemia and the diagnosis should be considered in jaundiced infants with signs of a bleeding diathesis. Involvement of the proximal renal tubule is shown by generalized aminoaciduria and occasionally a full-blown Fanconi syndrome with vacuolation of tubular epithelial cells. Histological examination of the brain shows non-specific signs of injury with gliosis and Purkinje cell loss in the cerebellum. Follow-up studies of female patients with galactosaemia has shown a high incidence of gonadal failure with ovarian atrophy: although this complication appears to be more common in patients in whom dietary therapy was delayed, no clear cause-and-effect relationship has been established. A toxic effect on the fetal ovary due to maternal hypergalactosaemia has been postulated to account for the hypergonadotrophic hypogonadism in affected women and girls. No evidence of gonadal failure has been found in male patients.

Genetic studies

Galactosaemia is transmitted as an autosomal recessive trait with an overall estimated frequency of 1 in 62 000. Classical galactosaemia is rare in Japan but frequent in some isolated groups, most notably in the modern Traveller population of Ireland. In this group, screening methods indicate a birth frequency of 1 in 480 compared with 1 in 30 000 in the non-Traveller Irish population. In Black patients from the United States a relatively mild disorder has been reported that is probably due to an unstable enzyme variant; uridylyltransferase activity is absent from their red cells but amounts to some 10 per cent of normal in samples of liver and small intestinal tissue. Individuals with the so-called 'Duarte variant' possess about half the normal enzyme activity in erythrocytes but remain asymptomatic.

The human galactosyl-1-phosphate uridylyltransferase gene maps to human chromosome 9p13 and encodes a protein of molecular weight 43 000 Da, which exists as a functional homodimer. Molecular analysis of the transferase gene indicates that most patients with classical galactosaemia harbour missense-type mutations and are compound heterozygotes. Several variant transferase enzymes have been described. Molecular analysis of the transferase gene has identified several widespread mutations; for example one mutant allele (Q188R) is in linkage disequilibrium with a restriction fragment-length polymorphism flanking exon 6 of the gene sequence in multiple populations worldwide, including the Irish Travellers – galactosaemic patients amongst whom, are all homozygous for Q188R. A less frequent mutation of diagnostic significance in White populations is designated R333W; the Duarte transferase mutation has been identified as N314D. Molecular analysis of the transferase gene now renders prenatal diagnosis of at-risk pregnancies possible.

Diagnosis

Galactosaemia may be suspected in an infant with growth failure, cataracts, liver disease, aminoaciduria, mental retardation, and especially where reducing sugar is present in the urine. The occurrence of unexplained bacterial sepsis, especially if due to *E. coli* infection in a newborn infant, may indicate galactosaemia. Cataracts may be detected by slit-lamp examination in the first few days of life.

The finding of hypergalactosaemia is not specific for those hereditary galactosaemias due to inherited deficiencies of galactose-metabolizing enzymes. Recent studies show that persistent hypergalactosaemia may be commonly due to portosystemic venous shunts in infants that are often associated with patent ductus venosus or other congenital vascular abnormalities in the liver. Doppler ultrasonography is a convenient non-invasive investigation to search for such shunts in young infants.

Definitive diagnosis of hereditary galactosaemia is mandatory, and relies on the determination of galactose 1-phosphate uridylyltransferase activity and other galactose-metabolizing enzymes in red cells or leucocytes by means of a specific enzymatic assay. Reliable enzymatic or genetic testing for heterozygotes can be carried out in the parents of a child who died before the diagnosis was confirmed. In particular populations, neonatal screening for elevated blood galactose and galactose 1-phosphate concentrations is carried out routinely. Molecular analysis of the gene for galactose 1-phosphate uridylyltransferase deficiency in at-risk pregnancies has been requested by some affected families.

Treatment

Without strict dietary treatment, most patients with galactosaemia die in early infancy, although some may survive with liver disease and mental retardation beyond childhood. The course of galactosaemia is altered strikingly upon withdrawal of lactose (and galactose), although the outcome of neurological disease is often disappointing. However, lactose is present in many non-dairy foods and advice from an experienced dietician, as well as meticulous attention to detail, is required to eliminate it completely. In infants, soybean milks or commercial casein hydrolysates, 'Nutramigen', are used as milk substitutes and therapy is monitored by periodic assay of red cell galactose 1-phosphate concentrations. Despite reports that galactose may be reintroduced as the patient develops, lifelong strict adherence to the exclusion diet should be advocated. In subsequent pregnancies of heterozygous mothers who have had affected children, there is evidence that premature cataracts can be avoided in the fetus if the maternal intake of lactose is restricted. In late pregnancy, lactosaemia and lactosuria are common findings and result from the physiological induction of lactose biosynthesis in mammary tissue. In rare cases (see below) there is a risk of self-intoxication when women with homozygous deficiency of the transferase become pregnant and breast feed, so that additional dietary precautions are needed to maintain metabolic control during lactation.

Prognosis

The acute manifestations of galactosaemia and growth failure respond quickly to dietary therapy and cataract formation is prevented. Unfortunately, a proportion of patients have significant neurological deficits despite prompt and conscientious treatment. An international survey of the long-term outcome in 350 patients receiving dietary therapy has been published by Waggoner and colleagues. The presence of ovarian failure and elevated galactose 1-phosphate concentrations in patients apparently ingesting no lactose or galactose raises the possibility that an endogenous pathway of galactose 1-phosphate formation from the pyrophosphorylysis of uridine diphosphate-galactose may occur. This may also explain the late emergence of neurological disease in treated patients. Long-term follow-up and periodic neuropsychiatric, as well as physical, monitoring is recommended. Recently, several pregnancies have been reported in women suffering from classical galactosaemia, including subjects homozygous for the *Q188R* mutation. In such pregnancies, high concentrations of galactitol are found in amniotic fluid but cord blood values have been determined to be within the range found in galactosaemic patients receiving strict dietary therapy. Thus, although maternal galactitol traverses the placenta, it probably does not harm the heterozygous fetus.

Uridine diphosphate-4-epimerase deficiency

Epimerase deficiency is very rare but may be identified during screening for classic galactosaemia. In most cases no symptoms attributable to galactosaemia are apparent and follow-up studies have confirmed the usually benign nature of this anomaly. However, a few cases of marked deficiency of uridine diphosphate-4-epimerase have been discovered in patients otherwise manifesting the classic features of galactosaemia. In the absence of epimerase activity, the individual is dependent on exogenous sources of galactose, since this cannot be derived from glucose. The autosomal recessive nature of this inherited disorder has been confirmed by demonstrating a partial epimerase deficiency in the healthy parents of an affected infant. As a complete deficiency of the epimerase would lead to an absolute lack of uridine diphosphate (**UDP**)-galactose for glycosphingolipid synthesis, the ingestion of very small quantities of galactose has been recommended in

this unusual disorder so that brain development and biosynthesis of essential galactosides can proceed. Because of the dual activity of the epimerase towards UDP-acetyl glucosamine as well as UDP-glucose, it has been suggested that small supplements of the aminoacetyl galactosamine should also be provided in the diets of patients with UDP galactose-4-epimerase deficiency. This condition may be contrasted with the transferase deficiency that allows the formation of small amounts of endogenous galactose in the presence of an intact epimerase. The gene for human UDP-galactose-4-epimerase has been mapped to chromosome 1p36–p35, and several mutant alleles has been identified.

Pentosuria

Pentosuria is caused by the excessive renal excretion of L-xylulose: this has no clinical significance, except that it may lead to the incorrect diagnosis of diabetes mellitus should tests for reducing sugar be carried out on the urine. Xylulose does not react with urinary test strips based on the glucose oxidase method.

Although pentosuria is a rare autosomal recessive trait, its frequency in Ashkenazi Jews may be as high as 0.05 per cent. It is caused by enzymatic deficiency of L-xylulose reductase in the oxidative pathway of glucuronate metabolism, which results in 1 to 4 g of xylulose and L-arabitol continuously appearing in the urine: output is greatly enhanced by the ingestion of glucuronic acid or drugs that are excreted as glucuronides.

Inborn errors of pyruvate metabolism

Pyruvate dehydrogenase

Deficiency of pyruvate dehydrogenase is the most common cause of lactic acidosis in newborn infants and children, but it is also associated with neurodegenerative syndromes in later life. Pyruvate dehydrogenase exists as a multienzyme complex representing the products of 10 distinct genes. However, defects in one subunit of pyruvate dehydrogenase itself (E1α) account for most patients so far investigated, although defects in dihydrolipoyl dehydrogenase (E3) are also described.

Biochemical defect

The pyruvate dehydrogenase (**PDH**) complex catalyses the conversion of pyruvate to acetyl-coenzyme A within mitochondria and operates at about 10, 40, and 70 per cent of capacity in the liver, heart, and brain, respectively. The PDH complex is critical for brain metabolism since this is normally entirely dependent on the oxidative breakdown of glucose. There are three main activities associated with the complex: (1) pyruvate dehydrogenase, a thiamine-dependent moiety (E1); (2) dihydrolipoyl transacetylase (E2); and (3) dihydrolipoyl dehydrogenase (E3). Also associated are a pyruvate dehydrogenase-specific kinase and phosphatase (both involved in overall metabolic regulation of the complex) as well as an essential lipoic acid moiety.

The accumulated pyruvate may either be reduced to lactate or transaminated to alanine, so that hyperalaninaemia and varying degrees of lactic acidaemia occur. Very rare defects in dihydrolipoyl dehydrogenase are associated with deficiency of branched-chain keto-acid dehydrogenase. Failure to carry out oxidative reactions in regions of the cortex and midbrain causes neuronal death, and deficiency of 4-carbon intermediates may critically impair neurotransmitter synthesis.

Clinical features and prognosis

Severe deficiency of pyruvate dehydrogenase affects intrauterine development and causes marked acidosis (blood lactate >10 mmol/l) at birth with early death. The clinical presentation of pyruvate dehydrogenase deficiency is strikingly heterogeneous. Many victims do not show clinically significant metabolic acidosis and come to light because of intrauterine growth failure, neonatal hypotonia asphyxia, and feeding difficulty. In some affected individuals the enzyme deficiency is responsible for a slowly progressive neurodegeneration associated with dysgenesis and other structural abnormalities in the olivopontocerebellar tract and periventricular grey matter. Cortical atrophy and agenesis of the corpus callosum have also been reported in association with spastic quadriplegia. In those with neurological manifestations, blood lactate concentrations do not exceed 10 mmol/l. Should feeding by gavage be instituted, there is a protracted course with failure of neurological development, microcephaly, quadriplegia, seizures, and blindness. Intermittent cerebellar ataxia or torsion dystonia has been recorded and choreoathetoid movements occur. Involuntary eye movements in children are associated with a progressively deteriorating course. In a few patients with intermittent cerebellar ataxia, hereditary spinocerebellar degeneration appearing in early adult life has been attributed to the deficiency of pyruvate dehydrogenase but there is no direct relationship to Friedreich's ataxia. In patients who present with severe acidosis at birth, subacute necrotizing encephalomyelopathy of the Leigh's type has been confirmed at necropsy and deficiency of pyruvate dehydrogenase activity has been demonstrated.

Genetics

The most common cause of pyruvate dehydrogenase deficiency is due to a defect in the E1α subunit—a protein encoded on the X chromosome. Although the disease is characteristically more severe in males, manifestations in the heterozygous female are unusually frequent for an X-linked disease and probably reflect the low functional reserve of the enzyme complex in the brain. Neonatal lactic acidosis is more frequent in males. An auxiliary gene for the E1α subunit is localized as a result of retroposition from the X-chromosome to the long arm of chromosome 4, but is expressed only during spermatogenesis; its presence, however, indicates the critical need for activity of the complex in nearly all tissues. Causal mutations in the E1α gene on the X chromosome have been described—most appear to be short deletions or duplications and, at present, are not generally applicable for diagnosis. However, analysis of X-chromosome inactivation patterns, by determination of methylation status, has proved useful for the evaluation of enzymatic assays of fibroblasts obtained from obligate carriers or female patients in whom the diagnosis is suspected.

Diagnosis and treatment

The diagnosis is suspected from the presence of severe acidosis at birth. It may also emerge during the investigation of neurological deficits, especially where they are associated with intrauterine growth failure. Routine screening of urine samples for organic acids may identify excessive pyruvate, lactate, and alanine excretion. In patients without clinically evident acidosis, cerebral disease is accompanied by striking elevations of lactate and pyruvate in the cerebrospinal fluid. Mutation analysis of the X-linked *PDH* gene and determination of the abundance of immunoreactive PDH protein now permits decisive diagnosis of this disease.

Neuroradiological procedures, including cerebral ultrasonography and computed tomography, reveal ventricular dilatation and cerebral atrophy. In several infant girls with PDH deficiency, magnetic resonance imaging showed hypoplasia of the corpus callosum as well as loss of normal white matter signal intensity. Proton magnetic resonance spectroscopy (**MRS**) revealed high-abundance signals for brain lactate with decreased intensity of *N*-acetylaspartate, while phosphorus MRS of skeletal muscle showed abnormally low muscle phosphorylation potentials, in keeping with the predicted biochemical disturbance. Pathological examination of previously affected siblings shows shrinkage of gyri, with involvement of the medulla shown by loss or hypoplasia of the pyramids. The pathological features of Wernicke's encephalopathy may be present. The corpus callosum may be absent. Definitive diagnosis, however, depends on genetic and enzymatic studies in skin fibroblasts or blood leucocyte samples.

Institution of a high-fat, low-carbohydrate, ketogenic diet may ameliorate the biochemical abnormalities but, given the degree of neurological impairment that is normally present at diagnosis, little clinical improvement can be expected. Therapeutic responses to the administration of high-dose thiamine have been reported in patients with partial enzymatic deficiency, notably where ataxia and abnormal eye movements reminiscent of Wernicke's encephalopathy were conspicuous. In rare patients with the autosomally recessive condition due to dihydrolipoyl dehydrogenase deficiency, oral administration of lipoic acid has been reported to correct the organic acidaemia with clinical improvement.

Pyruvate carboxylase deficiency

Inborn defects in pyruvate carboxylase, a key gluconeogeneic enzyme, cause hypoglycaemia or profound metabolic acidosis with neurological disease. The manifestations of this latter syndrome closely resemble those caused by deficiencies of pyruvate dehydrogenase activity. A severe form associated with hyperammonaemia and citrullinaemia is also recognized, particularly in patients of French descent.

Metabolic defect

Pyruvate decarboxylase is a biotin-dependent enzyme that catalyses the first step in the formation of oxaloacetate from pyruvate and is activated allosterically by acetyl-coenzyme A. Thus, hypoglycaemia would be expected only after glycogen stores had been depleted. Krebs cycle intermediates may become depleted so that there is an insufficient synthesis of neurotransmitters. There may also be a reduced supply of aspartate for the arginosuccinate synthase reaction of the urea cycle.

Clinical features

Patients with severe deficiency of pyruvate carboxylase may present with the Leigh syndrome (necrotizing encephalomyopathy with lactate/pyruvate acidosis) or hypotonia and neurological retardation. The presence of ataxia and abnormal ocular movements in life suggest the occurrence of midbrain disease resembling Wernicke's encephalopathy. Hypoglycaemia frequently occurs during intercurrent infection or during starvation and acidosis, requiring bicarbonate therapy. The most severe form, originally reported from France, progresses rapidly with evidence of liver damage, hyperammonaemia, and citrullinaemia.

Genetics

This disorder is transmitted as an autosomal recessive trait. In severely affected patients with hyperammonaemia, pyruvate carboxylase protein and its mRNA are absent in the liver. A partially inactive variant enzyme is detectable in other patients.

Diagnosis and treatment

The condition is suspected when acidosis and neurological disease occur in infants, especially in the presence of hypoglycaemia. Specific diagnosis requires enzymatic assay in fibroblasts, which can also be used for carrier detection. Disorders of pyruvate metabolism may be mimicked biochemically by mitochondrial diseases and acquired deficiencies of thiamine or biotin. Although biotin therapy has been disappointing in pyruvate carboxylase deficiency, occasional responses to high-dose lipoic acid and thiamine treatment, which may stimulate the pyruvate metabolism by the dehydrogenase complex, have been recorded.

Therapy

Episodes of acidosis are treated with intravenous sodium bicarbonate, and glucose may be required for hypoglycaemia. There is evidence that ketogenic diets containing 50 per cent fat and 20 per cent carbohydrate ameliorate the biochemical disturbance and delay the onset of neurological disease: the administration of glutamate and aspartate, which may act as a source of oxaloacetate, appear to have been beneficial in some patients.

Further reading

Inborn errors of galactose metabolism

Bowring FG, Brown ARD (1986). Development of a protocol for newborn screening for disorders of the galactose metabolic pathway. *Journal of Inherited Metabolic Disease* **9**, 99–104.

Cornblath M, Schwartz R (1991). Disorders of galactose: metabolism. In: Cornblath M, Schwartz R, eds. *Disorders of carbohydrate metabolism in infancy*, 3rd edn, pp 295–324. Blackwell Scientific, Boston.

Elsas LJ, Lai K (1998). The molecular biology of galactosemia. *Genetic Medicine* **1**, 40–8.

Gitzelmann R (1967). Hereditary galactokinase deficiency; a newly-recognized cause of juvenile cataracts. *Pediatric Research* **1**, 14–23.

Holton JB, Walter JH, Tyfield LA (2001). Galactosemia. In: Scriver CR, *et al.*, eds. *The metabolic and molecular bases of inherited disease*, 8th edn, Vol 1, pp 1553–85. McGraw-Hill, New York.

Holton JB, *et al.* (1981). Galactosaemia. A new severe variant due to uridine diphosphate galactose-4-epimerase deficiency. *Archives of Diseases in Childhood* **56**, 885–7.

Kaufman FR, *et al.* (1986). Gonadal function in patients with galactosaemia. *Journal of Inherited Metabolic Disease* **9**, 140–6.

Mizoguchi N, *et al.* (2001). Congenital porto-left renal venous shunt as a cause of galactosaemia. *Journal of Inherited Metabolic Disease* **24**, 72–8.

Murphy M, *et al.* (1999). Genetic basis of transferase-deficient galactosaemia in Ireland and the population history of Irish Travellers. *European Journal of Human Genetics* **7**, 549–54.

Schweitzer S, *et al.* (1993). Long-term outcome in 134 patients with galactosaemia. *European Journal of Paediatrics* **152**, 36–43.

Waggoner DD, Buist NRM, Donnell GN (1990). Long-term prognosis in galactosaemia: results of a survey of 350 cases. *Journal of Inherited Metabolic Disease* **13**, 802–18.

Pentosuria

Hiatt HH (2001). Pentosuria. In: Scriver CR, *et al.*, eds. *The metabolic and molecular bases of inherited disease*, 8th edn, Vol 1, pp 1590–9. McGraw-Hill, New York.

Inborn errors of pyruvate metabolism

Brown GK, *et al.* (1988). Cerebral lactic acidosis: defects in pyruvate metabolism with profound brain damage and minimal systemic acidosis. *European Journal of Pediatrics* **147**, 10–14.

Brown RM, Otero LJ, Brown GK (1997). Transfection screening for primary defects in the pyruvate E1-alpha subunit gene. *Human Molecular Genetics* **6**, 1361–7.

Brown GK, *et al.* (1994). Pyruvate dehydrogenase deficiency. *Journal of Medical Genetics* **31**, 875–9.

Dahl H-M, *et al.* (1992). X-linked pyruvate dehydrogenase E1-alpha subunit deficiency in heterozygous females: variable manifestation of the same. *Journal of Inherited Metabolic Disease* **15**, 835–47.

Hinman LM, *et al.* (1989). Deficiency of pyruvate dehydrogenase complex in Leigh's disease fibroblasts: an abnormality in lipoamide dehydrogenase affecting PDHC activation. *Neurology* **39**, 70–5.

Lissens W, *et al.* (2000). Mutations in the X-linked pyruvate dehydrogenase (E1) alpha subunit gene (PDHA1) in patients with a pyruvate dehydrogenase complex deficiency. *Human Mutation* **15**, 209–19.

Robinson BH, *et al.* (1987). The French and North American phenotypes of pyruvate carboxylase deficiency. *American Journal of Human Genetics* **40**, 50–9.

Shevell MI, *et al.* (1994). Cerebral dysgenesis and lactic acidemia: an MRI/MRS phenotype associated with pyruvate dehydrogenase deficiency. *Pediatric Neurology* **II**, 224–9.

11.4 Disorders of purine and pyrimidine metabolism

*Richard W. E. Watts**

These disorders are due to abnormalities in the biosynthesis, interconversion, and degradation of the purines, adenine and guanine and of the pyrimidines, cytosine, thymine, and uracil. All these compounds are heterocyclic bases which exist as tri-, di-, and monophosphorylated either deoxyribosylated or ribosylated derivatives (deoxyribose and ribose are pentose carbohydrates). The phosphorylated deoxyribosylated and ribosylated derivatives are termed 'nucleotides', while the purely ribosylated derivatives, which lack the phosphate group, are termed 'nucleosides'.

The polynucleotide deoxyribonucleic acid (**DNA**) contains equimolar amounts of adenylic acid (adenosine monophosphate, **AMP**), guanylic acid (guanosine monophosphate, **GMP**), thymidylic acid (thymidine monophosphate, **TMP**), and cytidylic acid (cytidine monophosphate, **CMP**). Uridylic acid (uridine monophosphate, **UMP**) replaces TMP in the polynucleotide ribonucleic acid (**RNA**).

DNA encodes, stores, and ultimately hands on genetic information. RNA transcribes and translates the genetic information so that the corresponding polypeptide strand emerges from its site of synthesis on the ribosome.

The purine nucleotides, their cyclic derivatives (CAMP and CGMP), and their more highly phosphorylated derivatives have functions in many aspects of intermediary metabolism. Purine compounds also function as signal transducers, neurotransmitters, vasodilators, and mediators of platelet aggregation.

Disorders of purine metabolism

The purine nucleotides are built up in a step-wise manner (*de novo* synthesis), undergo a series of interconversion and salvage reactions, and a final degradative process to yield uric acid, as shown in Fig. 1. Most human morbidity connected with diseases of purine metabolism is due to sodium urate monohydrate and to uric acid. The dietary intake of nucleoproteins is also an important factor in diseases due to sodium urate and uric acid. Ingested adenine and guanine nucleotides are degraded to free purine bases and, hence, to uric acid by enzymes in the intestinal juices and small-intestine mucosa so that the products of their metabolism do not mix with the corresponding endogenous metabolic pools except at the final uric acid stage.

De novo synthesis contributes about 300 to 600 mg (1.8–3.6 mmol/day) and dietary purines about 600 to 700 mg (3.6–4.2 mmol/day) to the dynamic urate metabolic pool of about 1200 mg (7.2 mmol) expressed as uric acid. Each day, about two-thirds of uric acid are excreted in the urine and about one-third is destroyed, mainly by bacterial uricolysis in the gut.

The urate anion is freely filterable at the renal glomerulus, only 5 to 10 per cent being very loosely bound to the plasma proteins (α_{1-2}-globulin fraction). The physiologically important pKa value of uric acid is 5.75, so that it exists mainly as the monovalent urate anion in plasma (pH 7.4) and

assumes more of the free acid form when it passes into regions of the renal tubule, the contents of which are at lower pH values.

The kidney handles urate by:

(1) glomerular filtration of virtually 100 per cent of the filtered load;

(2) proximal tubular reabsorption by a urate/chloride exchanger in the endothelial brush border (99 per cent of the filtered load);

(3) tubular secretion (equivalent to about 50 per cent of the filtered load);

(4) postsecretory reabsorption (equivalent to about 40 per cent of the filtered load).

Thus, the net renal clearance of uric acid is approximately 10 per cent of the filtered load and is in the range of 6 to 11 ml/min per $1.73m^2$ ($1.73m^2$ = average body surface area of an adult). The exact location of the reabsorptive, secretory, and postsecretory reabsorptive processes within the distal nephron is unclear.

Plasma urate levels

The currently quoted overall reference range for plasma urate (expressed as uric acid) in adults is 3.5 to 8.1 mg/dl (210–480 µmol/l) for men and 2.5 to 6.5 mg/dl (150–390 µmol/l) for women. The corresponding value for children is 1.0 to 4.0 mg/dl (60–240 µmol/l). It rises at puberty with female values being lower than those in men until the menopause, after which it gradually rises to the male value. Extrinsic factors, particularly diet, plumbism, the prevalence of a high ethanol intake in the community, and the prevalence of diseases such as malaria and thalassaemia, which lead indirectly to either increased purine biosynthesis or decreased excretion (Table 1), affect the plasma urate distribution in different populations.

The plasma urate concentration decreases during pregnancy, the reference range being 1.7 to 4.5 mg/dl (100–270 µmol/l). Hyperuricaemia is a characteristic and often an early feature of pre-eclampsia, preceding the proteinuria and hypertension, and is a diagnostically valuable parameter. It results from a reduced renal urate clearance and tends to be associated with hypocalciuria.

Epidemiological studies show significant variations in plasma urate concentrations between different ethnic groups: for example, Maoris and Polynesians have higher values than Western Europeans and Americans. This illustrates the genetic, presumably, polygenic aspects in the control of serum uric acid. Other epidemiological studies emphasize the importance of the environmental factors of purine, protein, and alcohol intake. For example, Gresser and Zöllner showed that the cumulated frequency of plasma urate, expressed as uric acid, rose from approximately 6.2 mg/dl (370 µmol/l) to about 9.0 mg/dl (536 µmol/l) between 1962 and 1971 in association with the improved nutritional state of the Bavarian population from the near-starvation conditions following the Second World War (Fig. 2).

Similarly, the plasma urate levels in immigrant communities with low values in their home lands, move towards the values prevailing in the host country as they adopt the lifestyle and dietary habits of that country: for example, Filipinos migrating to the United States. Similarly, migrants with

---

* We are indebted to Professor George Nuki, who wrote on this subject in the third edition of the textbook, for permission to use Fig. 4 and 7 of that contribution in this chapter.

genetically determined high urate levels become even more hyperuricaemic.

The frequency distribution of plasma urate values based on asymptomatic populations is only approximately Gaussian, with an excess of higher values due to the inclusion of some asymptomatic hyperuricaemic subjects. Although plasma is saturated with monosodium urate at a concentration of 7.0 mg/dl (420 µmol/l), higher concentrations of urate can remain in a stable supersaturated solution in plasma without producing any symptoms. Ignoring the slight asymmetry of the frequency distribution and defining normality as the mean value ± 2 standard deviations about the mean, normal values of 7.0 mg/dl (420 µmol/l) for men and 6.0 mg/dl (360 µmol/l) for women have been widely adopted. This has led to considerable overtreatment of patients who have quite innocuous plasma urate concentrations.

Gout and hyperuricaemia

Gout is a classic example of a multifactorial disease in which there is an interplay of genetic and environmental factors. The overall effects of this interplay are wide, extending from cases where there is a clear-cut family history with autosomal dominant inheritance (Fig. 3) to those where environmental factors are the determinants, although often against a genetic background that may be either unifactorial or multifactorial. Gout *per se*, does not shorten life, although some of its complications may do so in the absence of treatment.

Gout is defined as a syndrome brought about by the crystallization of monosodium urate monohydrate *in vivo* from body fluids supersaturated with this salt. The supersaturation results from either the overproduction or underexcretion of urate, or from a combination of these defects. The underlying causes of hyperuricaemia and gout are:

1. *Decreased net tubular urate secretion*: this is the major factor in the aetiology of the majority of those cases of gout previously described as being idiopathic (or primary), the hereditary predisposition to which is often compounded by environmental factors (e.g. high dietary purine intake and alcoholism).

2. *Identifiable enzymatic defects that accelerate urate* de novo *synthesis*: these are a hypoxanthine–guanine phosphoribosyltransferase (**HPRT**) deficiency which causes the Lesch–Nyhan syndrome and, in milder degrees of HPRT deficiency, some cases of the X-linked recessive hyperuricaemia, gout, and uric acid stone syndrome;

3. *Phosphoribosyl pyrophosphate (PRPPS) synthetase superactivity*: this also presents as X-linked recessive hyperuricaemia, gout, and uric acid stones and, in some cases, neurological manifestations (e.g. deafness and autism).

Secondary causes of hyperuricaemia and gout are shown in Table 1.

The following abnormalities are commonly associated with, but not causally related to hyperuricaemia and gout:

(1) obesity;

(2) dyslipidaemia (usually type 4) with raised very low-density (**VLD**) lipoproteins and normal cholesterol levels, and sometimes hypercholesterolaemia with elevated low-density lipoprotein (**LDL**)-cholesterol and low high-density lipoprotein (**HDL**)-cholesterol levels;

(3) hypertension;

(4) insulin resistance with hyperinsulinaemia and impaired glucose tolerance;

(5) ischaemic heart disease.

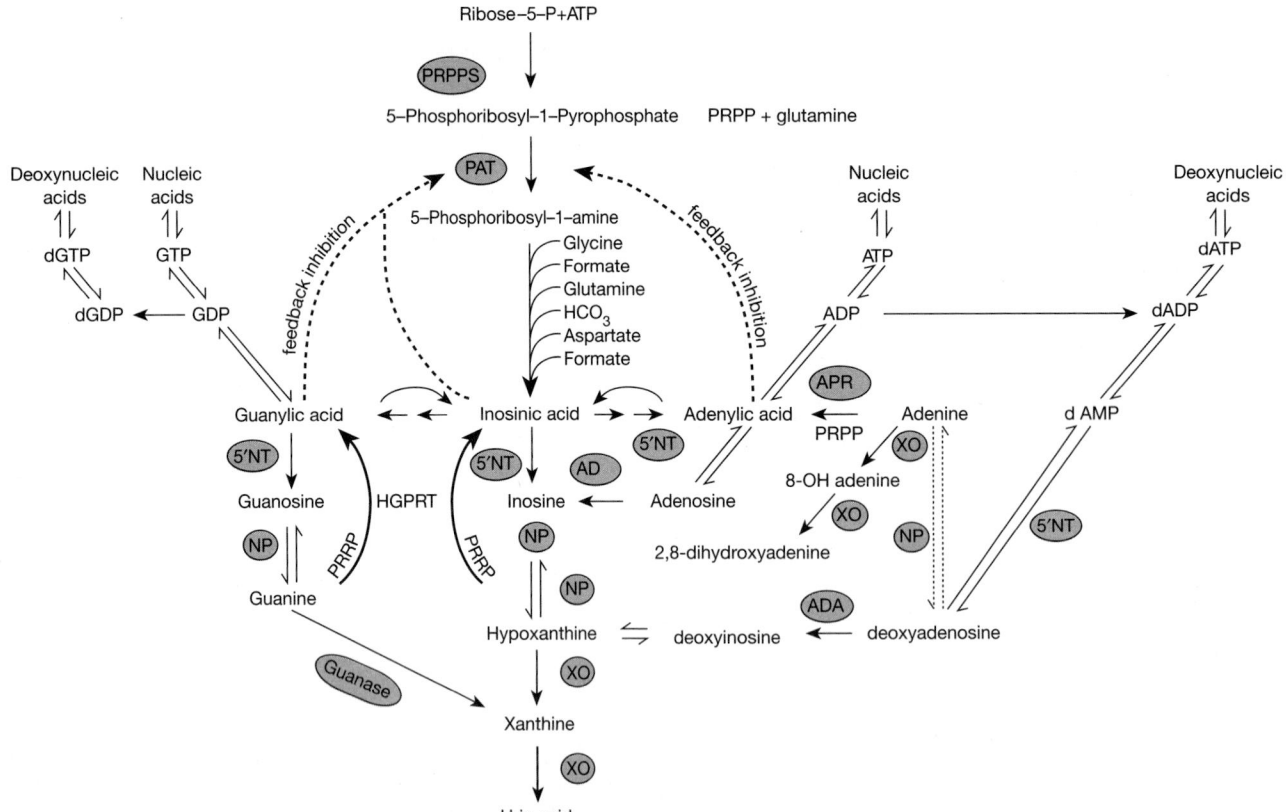

Fig. 1 Pathways of purine metabolism in humans. **ADA**, adenosine deaminase; **APRT**, adenine phosphoribosyltransferase; **HPRT**, hypoxanthine–guanine phosphoribosyltransferase; **5-NP**, nucleoside phosphorylase; **5'-NP**, 5'-nucleotidase; **PAT**, phosphoribosyl pyrophosphate amidotransferase; **PRPPS**, phosphoribosyl pyrophosphate synthetase; **XO**, xanthine oxidase.

Thus, these patients may display the features of the 'metabolic syndrome X'.

There is no evidence that uric acid is toxic to the myocardium. Hyperuricaemia may be a marker of coincident cardiac disease, but **not** a causal risk factor. The elevated plasma uric acid concentrations observed in patients with ischaemic heart disease could arise from upregulated vascular adenosine synthesis associated with ischaemia and the subsequent degradation of adenosine to uric acid. However, the relationship of urate to endothelial function is complex. Plasma uric acid accounts for 60 per cent of the free-radical scavenging activity in human plasma: it interacts with peroxynitrile to form a stable nitric oxide donor, so promoting vasodilatation and reducing the potential for peroxynitrile-induced oxidative damage. Conversely, it could have an adverse effect on endothelial function by promoting leucocyte adhesion to the endothelium. However, there is no clear evidence that these actions are significant at the clinical level.

The fractional excretion of urate is the ratio of urate clearance to the glomerular filtration rate (**GFR**). In the presence of normal overall renal function, this can be measured on a random urine sample and a simultaneous plasma sample. The equation simplifies to:

Table 1 Causes of hyperuricaemia and gout

Reduced renal excretion of uric acid

1. An inherited defect in the renal handling of urate. This summates with environmental factors in most cases of gout previously called 'primary' or 'idiopathic'. It is the sole determinant in familial autosomal dominant hyperuricaemia and gout

2. Renal glomerular disease

3. Renal tubule dysfunction:
    - (a) Tubulointerstitial nephritis
    - (b) Competition for tubule excretory mechanisms (e.g. hyperlactic acidosis and ketoacidosis from any cause)
    - (c) Drug administration (e.g. diuretics, pyrazinamide, ethambutol, ciclosporin)

4. Other conditions in which renal tubule dysfunction has been proposed
    - (a) Hypertension
    - (b) Sickle-cell anaemia (there will also be increased metabolic turnover of purines)
    - (c) Myxoedema
    - (d) Bartter's syndrome
    - (e) Down's syndrome
    - (f) Lead nephropathy
    - (g) Sarcoidosis

Increased uric acid production
Dietary sources
HPRT deficiency
PRPP-synthetase superactivity
Ribose 5'-phosphate overproduction
AMP deaminase deficiency
Glycogen storage disease type I
Glycogen storage diseases types III, V, and VII
Hereditary fructose intolerance
Myeloproliferative diseases (NB polycythaemia rubra vera)
Secondary polycythaemia
Lymphoproliferative diseases
Waldenstrom's macroglobulinaemia
Chronic haemolytic anaemia of any cause
Carcinomatosis
Extensive psoriasis
Gaucher's disease

HPRT, hypoxanthine phosphoribosyltransferase (hypoxanthine–guanine phosphoribosyltransferase); PRPP, *phosphoribosylpyrophosphate*; AMP, adenosine monophosphate (adenylic acid).

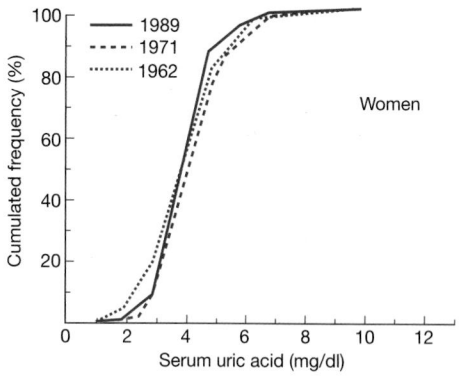

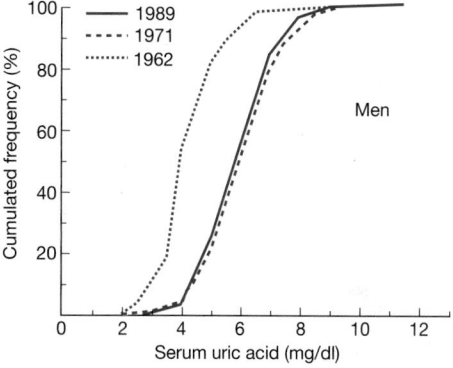

Fig. 2 Differences in the cumulated frequencies in urate levels in female and male blood donors in Bavaria between 1962 and 1989. (Reproduced with permission from Gresser and Zollner 1991.)

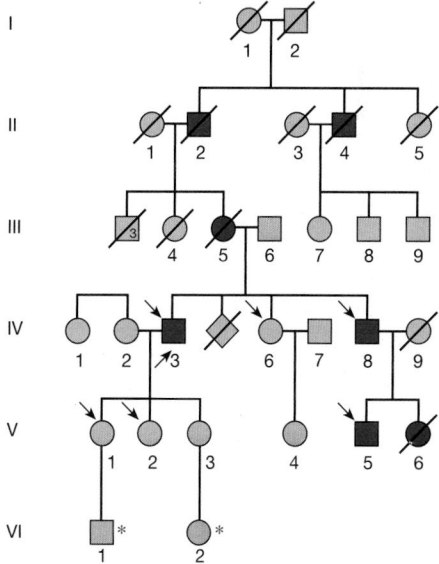

Fig. 3 Pedigree chart of a family showing autosomal dominant inheritance of gout complicated in some cases by renal failure (hyperuricaemia nephropathy). ■ ● male and female subjects, respectively, with hyperuricaemia and renal failure; □ ○ male and female subjects not known to be affected; ⌀ ⌀ deceased male and female subjects, ╱ propositus; ╲ subjects whose rates of mononuclear cell *de novo* purine synthesis was measured and shown to be normal; * babies who were examined clinically but not further investigated. (Reproduced with permission from McDermott, *et al.* (1984). *Clinical Science* **67**, 249-58. ©Biochemical Society and Medical Research Society.)

Table 2 American College of Rheumatology criteria for the diagnosis of acute gouty arthritis

1.	More than one attack of acute arthritis
2.	Maximum inflammation developing within 1 day
3.	Monoarthritis
4.	Redness over the affected joint
5.	The first metatarsophalangeal joint painful and swollen
6.	Unilateral first metatarsophalangeal joint involved
7.	Unilateral tarsal joint attack
8.	Tophus (proven or suspected)
9.	Hyperuricaemia
10.	Asymmetrical swelling within a joint on radiography
11.	Subcortical cysts without erosions seen on radiography
12.	Joint fluid culture negative for micro-organisms during an attack

The patient must have at least 6 of the above criteria, or have either proven sodium urate monohydrate crystals in the joint fluid or a proven tophus

Taken with permission from Hochberg MC (2001).

$$\text{Fractional clearance of urate} = U_{urate} \times P_{creatinine}/P_{urate} \times U_{creatinine}$$

where 'U' and 'P' represent the urine and plasma concentrations. The fractional clearance can be used to assess the role of renal tubular dysfunction in the production of hyperuricaemia, provided that the overall renal function is normal.

Acute gouty arthritis

Acute gout is a sodium urate monohydrate-induced crystal inflammation of joints, bursas, and tendon sheaths. Clinically, the affected structures—classically, the first metatarsophalangeal joint is the first joint affected—become acutely inflamed, exquisitely tender, warm to the touch, and the overlying skin becomes red, shiny, and itchy and may desquamate as the inflammation subsides spontaneously over 5 to 15 days in the absence of treatment. Inflammation is usually maximal within 24 h of onset and is accompanied by pyrexia and malaise.

Joint aspiration yields a fluid containing polymorphonuclear leucocytes and negatively birefringent sodium urate monohydrate crystals. The attacks occur most frequently when the plasma urate level is rising or falling. Monosodium urate crystals may be found within monocytes in asymptomatic joints; it has recently been proposed that the inflammatory response to monosodium urate is influenced by the state of monocyte to macrophage differentiation, the balance being tipped towards acute inflammation by the recruitment of undifferentiated monocytes and neutrophils from the bloodstream by one of the precipitants for acute gout. At the beginning of an acute gouty attack, monocyte/macrophage activation leads to the production of inflammatory cytokines (interleukins, tumour necrosis factor (TNF-α)) and the activation of cyclo-oxygenase (**Cox**)-2. Apoptotic neutrophils and crystals are removed by activated macrophages as the inflammation subsides spontaneously.

The American College of Rheumatology criteria for the clinical diagnosis of acute gout are shown in Table 2. The presence of 6 of the 11 criteria has a 95 per cent specificity in differentiating gout from pseudogout (calcium pyrophosphate gout) and an overall sensitivity of 85 per cent. The final confirmation is the demonstration of negatively birefringent sodium urate monohydrate crystals as opposed to the positively birefringent crystals of calcium pyrophosphate.

Although acute gouty arthritis is typically a monoarthritis, some patients have short, recurrent, mild attacks of discomfort and swelling of affected joints. Some 10 per cent of attacks affect more than one joint and typical attacks may provoke migratory attacks in other joints. Multiple, simultaneous attacks are rare. Some attacks are triggered by trauma, intercurrent illness, surgery, alcohol, dietary excess, diuretics, and other medications (see Table 1). An acute septic arthritis is the most important differential diagnosis of acute gouty arthritis.

Chronic tophaceous gout

Large deposits (tophi) containing monosodium urate monohydrate crystals produce firm nodules over affected joints on the extensor surfaces of the fingers, hands, olecranon bursas (commonly bilateral), extensor surfaces of the forearm, Achilles tendon, the helix of the ear, and in the renal parenchyma. Tophi may discharge white chalky material, containing sodium urate monohydrate. They cause the bone erosions and joint destruction with secondary degenerative arthritis seen on radiographs. Tophus formation can be regarded as an attempted, but disordered, healing process in response to the presence of sodium urate monohydrate crystals in tissues.

Treatment of gout

The acute attack

Full doses of any of the non-steroidal anti-inflammatory drugs are effective in terminating attacks of acute gout. Indomethacin is particularly favoured by some clinicians. Colchicine remains a very effective remedy—an initial dose of 1.0 mg followed by 0.5 mg every 6 hours until either the attack subsides or a total dose of 6.0 mg has been achieved, or symptoms of toxicity (nausea, vomiting, and diarrhoea) occur. More frequent doses of colchicine, 0.5 mg every 2 to 3 h, deliberately inducing symptoms of toxicity was previously recommended. This is unnecessary now that the non-steroidal anti-inflammatory drugs are available. Heavy dosage with colchicine can also cause gastrointestinal haemorrhage and favour the development of other severe side-effects, including profuse diarrhoea, rashes, renal and hepatic damage, more rarely peripheral neuropathy, myopathy, and alopecia in the long-term. Intravenous colchicine is no longer recommended.

An attack of acute gout can be effectively terminated by the adrenocorticotropin analogue, tetracosactrin, or by a single intravenous dose of hydrocortisone. Rebound attacks of acute gout tend to occur unless the situation is covered by either colchicine or a non-steroidal anti-inflammatory drug.

Pharmacologically, colchicine disrupts the cellular microtubular architecture in the inflammatory cells. This mode of action gives it the potential to do more widespread damage and presumably underlies its inhibitory effects on mitosis, neutrophil migration, and phagocytosis. Short intensive courses of colchicine should not be repeated at less than 3-day intervals, although lower doses (0.5 mg-2 mg per day) can be used for longer periods, as in the treatment of familial Mediterranean fever.

Interval treatment

Asymptomatic hyperuricaemia should not be treated with urate-lowering drugs unless the patient experiences more than one acute attack of gout per year (Table 3). Allopurinol, a xanthine oxidate inhibitor, is effective in preventing acute gout; it acts by reducing the serum urate concentration to a

Table 3 Hyperuricaemia detected on routine biochemical screening

1.	Search for an identifiable cause (e.g. dietary factors, myeloproliferative disease, medications)	
2.	Check renal function	
3.	Imaging to detect the presence of uric acid urinary calculi	
4.	Measure uric acid excretion after eliminating dietary and medication factors	
5.	Treat if:	
	(a)	More than one attack of acute gouty arthritis per year
	(b)	Chronic joint damage attributed to gout
	(c)	Tophi
	(d)	Hyperuricaemic nephropathy
	(e)	Uric acid urolithiasis
	(f)	*Serum urate concentration:
		>800 µmol/l (13 mg/dl in men)
		>600 µmol/l (10 mg/dl in women)

* This criterion is not universally accepted.

value below the solubility of sodium urate monohydrate in plasma so that tophaceous deposits are mobilized and healing occurs. This applies to the tophi in bones as well as elsewhere. The drug should be introduced at a low level (e.g. 100–200 mg daily) and increased under cover of either colchicine or a non-steroidal anti-inflammatory drug, which should be continued until the serum urate concentration has stabilized at a normal level. Allopurinol is then continued indefinitely.

Initiating allopurinol without cover may cause attacks of acute gout as the serum urate concentration falls. Moderately severe gout may require as much as 300 to 600 mg of allopurinol daily, and occasionally as much as 700 to 900 mg per day given in divided doses. Between 10 and 20 mg/kg body weight per day is an appropriate dose for children.

The incidence of adverse reactions to allopurinol is low but they can be severe and occasionally fatal. Reactions include erythema multiforme progressing to the Stevens–Johnson syndrome and toxic epidermal necrolysis, exfoliative dermatitis, vasculitis, interstitial nephritis, eosinophilia, hepatocellular damage, polyneuropathy, bone marrow depression, disturbances of vision and taste, as well as gastroenteropathy. Allopurinol potentiates the effect of coumarin anticoagulants (for example, warfarin), azathioprine, and 6-mercaptopurine, and predisposes to an ampicillin or amoxicillin rash. At high dosage and in the presence of greatly increased purine synthesis it may cause xanthine and oxipurinol urinary stones. There is also increased risk of toxicity with captopril (especially in the presence of renal failure) and with ciclosporin.

Much of the overall toxicity of allopurinol is due to the metabolite oxipurinol, which has a much longer half-life *in vivo* than the parent compound. Special care is necessary in the presence of renal failure, when a dose of 100 to 150 mg is usually sufficient. Patients with hyperuricaemia due to renal failure rarely develop gout, possibly due to immunoparesis.

Patients in whom allopurinol produces adverse reactions

Patients for whom the treatment of hyperuricaemia and gout is essential and who have developed severe adverse reactions to allopurinol present a special problem, especially if they have impaired overall renal function. The uricosuric drugs sulfinpyrazone, probenecid, and benzbromarone, together with a sufficiently high fluid intake to provide a measured urine output of at least 3 litres per 24 h and alkalization of the urine with sodium or potassium bicarbonate or sodium or potassium citrate, represent an approach to this problem, but may be inappropriate in the overall clinical context, for example in patients with cardiac or renal failure. Only sulfinpyrazone is readily available in the United Kingdom. Uricosuric drugs may be inefficient in the presence of renal failure and are contraindicated in the presence of uric acid urinary stones.

The use of recombinant uricase—either in its unmodified form or linked to polyethylene glycol (PEG) in order to reduce its immunogenicity—remains experimental, and is unlikely to be applied except in patients at risk of developing acute hyperuricaemic nephropathy and who cannot be given allopurinol.

The uricosuric agent benzbromarone is sometimes effective in patients with renal failure when other uricosuric agents have lost their efficacy. The use of oxipurinol (in low dosage) has also been proposed. Protocols are also available for the desensitization of patients who have experienced adverse reactions to allopurinol, and in whom the risk of uric acid stone formation with the potential for further reduction of renal function presents a problem.

Asymptomatic hyperuricaemia

Routine biochemical screening frequently identifies patients with hyperuricaemia. Guidance on their management is given in Table 3.

Acute uric acid nephropathy

This complicates the treatment of widespread malignant disease, particularly chemo- and/or radiotherapy of leukaemias and lymphomas. The nephropathy is of multifactorial origin and may form part of the acute tumour-lysis syndrome with accompanying tubular necrosis. These patients are usually underhydrated and acidotic and have high rates of uric acid production from nucleoprotein degradation in the apoptotic tumours. Acute uric acid nephropathy has occasionally been reported after extremely severe muscular exercise, after severe epileptic seizures, and in patients with gout and grossly increased rates of *de novo* purine synthesis.

The renal lesion is the intratubular precipitation of uric acid crystals. In addition, the renal pelvis and ureters may also be blocked by crystal aggregates and/or uric acid stones. Acute uric acid nephropathy can be avoided by giving allopurinol for several days before starting chemotherapy or radiotherapy. The condition presents as acute oliguric renal failure. Imaging techniques should be used to exclude the presence of bilateral ureteric obstruction by radiotranslucent uric acid stones. Treatment is by:

(1) induction of an alkaline diuresis;

(2) haemo- or peritoneal dialysis or haemofiltration;

(3) percutaneous nephrostomy and/or ureteric catheterization may be needed if there is an element of postrenal obstruction due to impacted aggregates of sodium urate crystals or uric acid stones;

(4) disruption or removal of impacted stones.

Chronic sodium urate nephropathy

Between 20 and 30 per cent of patients with untreated chronic tophaceous gout die from renal failure. These patients form an identifiable subgroup of the gouty population and an autosomal dominant inheritance is sometimes clearly apparent (Fig. 3). The term 'familial juvenile gouty nephropathy' is sometimes used for patients presenting in early life. Environmental factors exacerbate this hereditary predisposition. Such patients must be differentiated from another group of gout patients (20–30 per cent) with mild intermittent proteinuria and a good prognosis. Significant renal disease due to sodium urate deposition is very rare in asymptomatic hyperuricaemia. Patients with chronic sodium urate nephropathy have shrunken kidneys containing interstitial monosodium urate microtophi and show segmental destruction of the renal parenchyma due to tubular blockage by aggregates of uric acid crystals (microcalculi). These areas of segmental destruction have been referred to, inappropriately, as 'uric acid infarcts'.

Polycystic renal disease

Hyperuricaemia and gout may precede the onset of renal failure in patients with polycystic renal disease and about one-third of patients with polycystic renal disease develop gouty arthritis. This may be due to abnormal renal tubular handling of urate. A similar mechanism may operate in patients with medullary sponge kidney disease.

Ethanol and hyperuricaemia

Ethanol is oxidized to acetaldehyde by the liver. This raises the ratio of **NADH:NAD** (reduced nicotinamide–adenine dinucleotide:nicotinamide–adenine dinucleotide), which in turn promotes the reduction of pyruvate to lactate in the hepatocytes. Lactate competes with urate in the renal tubular excretory mechanisms and thereby promotes urate retention. There is also an element of starvation ketoacidosis in chronic alcoholics, with acetoacetate and betahydroxybutyrate also competing for the renal tubular excretory mechanisms which subserve urate tubular secretion. In addition, there is increased urate production associated with ethanol intake: first due to the high purine content of some alcoholic beverages (for example, beer) and second, the metabolism of alcohol involves increased dephosphorylation and degradation of adenine nucleotides in the liver. The free adenine produced is further metabolized to urate.

Uric acid urolithiasis

Pure uric acid stones account for 5 per cent of all urinary stones in patients in the United Kingdom. There is a much higher incidence elsewhere, for example in the Middle East. Uric acid urolithiasis occurs in 10 per cent of patients with gout. In Israel, about 40 per cent urinary calculi are composed of uric acid and 75 per cent of patients with primary gout develop renal calculus disease. Uric acid stones are more common in secondary than in primary gout and are sometimes associated with an impaired ability to alkalinize the urine. Ileostomy predisposes to uric acid urolithiasis because of (1) chronic bicarbonate loss, which leads to a persistent acidification of the urine and (2) a concentrated urine due to excessive water loss. Urinary uric acid concentrations close to, or greater than, those at which spontaneous crystallization begins are frequent in these circumstances. The genetic causes of uric acid urolithiasis are rare: (1) **HPRT** deficiency; (2) phosphoribosylpyrophosphate synthetase (**PRPPS**) superactivity; and (3) congenital renal hypouricaemia (congenital failure of the renal tubular reabsorption of urate). Renal hypouricaemia may be due to renal tubular damage by other genetic diseases or by toxic damage (Table 4) and this may be associated with other features of the Fanconi syndrome.

Table 4 Causes of hypouricaemia

Inherited disorders of uric acid and pyrimidine biosynthesis
Genetic defects in the molybdoflavoprotein enzymes:
–xanthinuria type I (xanthine oxidase deficiency only)
–xanthinuria type II (combined xanthine oxidase and aldehyde oxidase deficiencies)
–sulphite oxidase deficiency (combined xanthine oxidase, aldehyde oxidase, and sulphite oxidase deficiency)
Purine nucleoside phosphorylase deficiency
Phosphoribosylpyrophosphate synthetase deficiency

Secondary reduction in uric acid biosynthesis
Allopurinol and oxipurinol medication
Hepatic failure
Acute intermittent porphyria

Inherited renal hypouricaemia (isolated renal tubule reabsorption defect)

Inherited causes of the Fanconi syndrome and its variants (the syndrome of multiple renal tubule reabsorption defects)
Cystinosis (accumulation of intralysosomal cystine)
Galactosaemia (galactose 1-phosphate toxicity)
Hereditary fructose intolerance (fructose 1-phosphate toxicity)
Glycogen storage disease type I (glucose-1-phosphate toxicity; hypoglycaemia may prevent the glycosuria which is part of the syndrome)
Wilson's disease (copper toxicity)
Cytochrome c deficiency

Acquired causes of the Fanconi syndrome and its variants
Metal poisoning (Cd, Zn, Cu, Pb, Hg, Ur)
Multiple myelomatosis
Nephrotic syndrome
Malignant disease (paraneoplastic syndrome)
Autoimmune disease (e.g. Sjögren's syndrome)
Thermal burns
Primary hyperparathyroidism
Acute renal tubular necrosis
Renal transplant rejection

Drugs
Drugs used either as uricosuric agents or to block other aspects of renal tubule excretion (sulfinpyrazone, probenicid, benzbromazone)
Non-steroidal anti-inflammatory drugs with uricosuric properties:
–phenylbutazone
–azapropazone
–aspirin, dosage >4 g/day
Coumarin anticoagulants (e.g. warfarin)
Outdated tetracycline (5α-6-anhydro-4-epitetracycline)

Nutritional deficiencies
Vitamins B_{12}, C, D
Kwashiorkor

The urinary uric acid concentration is the main determinant of uric acid stone formation. The concentration depends on the state of hydration, the rate of purine de novo synthesis, the rate of metabolic turnover of purine compounds, the dietary intake of purines and alcohol, and the action of uricosuric drugs (for example, sulfinpyrazone). Calcium oxalate stone formation is increased 30-fold in patients with gout and hyperuricosuria is common in non-gouty stone formers. Uric acid micro crystals may act as epitaxial nucleation sites for calcium oxalate crystallization. It is also possible that colloidal uric acid adsorbs urinary glycosaminoglycan inhibitors of crystallization and crystal growth.

Uric acid stone disease is treated by hydration to maintain a urine volume of at least 3 litres per 24 h, alkalization of the urine, and allopurinol if there is hyperuricosuria. The use of sodium and potassium salts for alkalization has to be carefully reviewed in the light of concurrent diseases, particularly impaired renal and cardiac function. The standard imaging techniques (particularly ultrasonography) are required for the diagnosis of these radiotranslucent stones. They can be fragmented or removed by standard procedures.

Congenital renal hypouricaemia and uric acid stones

Reduced net tubular reabsorption of urate occurs either as an isolated renal tubular reabsorption defect due to mutations in the gene directing the synthesis of the putative urate carrier protein, or in association with other inherited and acquired renal tubule transport defects (Table 4).

Isolated reduced net tubular reabsorption of urate (hereditary renal hypouricaemia) is inherited in an autosomal recessive manner. The hyperuricosuria may amount to 1000 mg (5.9 mmol) per 24 h in the homozygote. Lesser degrees of hyperuricosuria occur in heterozygotes. About 30 per cent of the homozygotes have an associated hypercalciuria. Uric acid urolithiasis occurs in about 25 per cent of the homozygotes, most commonly in patients with combined hyperuricosuria and hypercalciuria. Only two patients with hereditary renal hypouricaemia were found by searching the clinical biochemical data on 47 420 patients in a general hospital. The causes of hypouricaemia are summarized in Table 4.

The Lesch–Nyhan syndrome and variants

The Lesch–Nyhan syndrome results from mutations in the gene that directs the synthesis of hypoxanthine–guanine phosphoribosyltransferase (**HPRT**), an enzyme which normally catalyses the salvage of hypoxanthine and guanine to inosinic and guanylic acids (inosine monophosphate, **IMP**; and guanosine monophosphate, **GMP**), respectively, as shown in Fig. 1. The clinical spectrum extends from hyperuricaemia alone to hyperuricaemia with profound neurological and behavioural dysfunction. The biochemistry and molecular genetics of this disorder have been studied extensively. A recent survey of a database of 271 cases showed that mutation analysis does not provide precise information for predicting disease severity, but that it is a valuable tool for genetic counselling in terms of confirming diagnosis, the identification of carriers, and for prenatal diagnosis.

The clinical features of the most severely affected patients who are correctly referred to as having the 'Lesch–Nyhan syndrome' or as having 'complete or virtually complete HPRT deficiency', are summarized in Table 5.

Infants affected by HRPT deficiency have a lower than average birth weight, indicating some degree of intrauterine growth retardation (Fig. 4). The first clinical sign may be the presence of red grit (uric acid crystals with adsorbed urinary pigments) on the nappy. Affected infants are hypotonic from birth, although this is frequently not remarked upon before poor head control becomes apparent at the age of about 3 months.

Postnatal growth, which becomes more marked after the second year of life, is also subnormal (Fig. 5) as indicated by sequential measurement of body weight, accurate assessment of body length being impossible due to the dystonic posturing. The overall pattern of weight growth follows centile lines for the first 2 years of life and thereafter slows to about 1 kg per year, or about half normal, a pubertal growth spurt is not observed. Head growth

Table 5 Clinical manifestations of the Lesch–Nyhan syndrome (complete or virtually complete absence of hypoxanthine phosphoribosyltransferase (HPRT) deficiency)

1.	Sex-linked recessive inheritance
2.	Failure of overall growth
3.	Muscle hypotonia
4.	Delayed motor development
5.	Torsion dystonia
6.	Aggressive behaviour
7.	Dysarthia
8.	Variable degree of intellectual deterioration, especially in later childhood
9.	Megaloblastic anaemia (in some cases only)
10.	Hyperuricaemia and hyperuric aciduria with gout and tophus development after puberty and urolithiasis (during the first decade of life)
11.	Failure of pubertal development and testicular atrophy at the age when puberty would be expected to occur

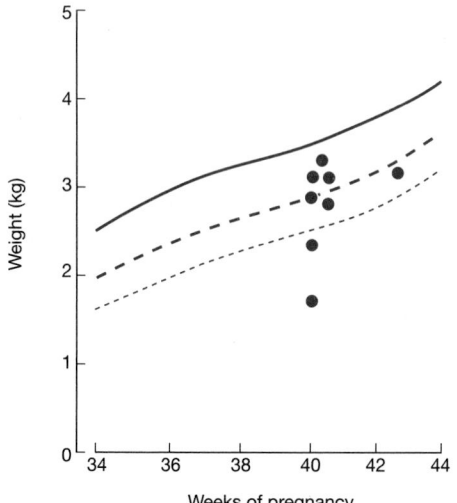

Fig. 4 Birth weight in eight boys who later developed the Lesch–Nyhan syndrome: the 50th (bold), 10th, and 3rd (interrupted) centiles are shown as lines. (Reproduced from Watts *et al.* 1987, with kind permission from Kluwer Academic Publishers.)

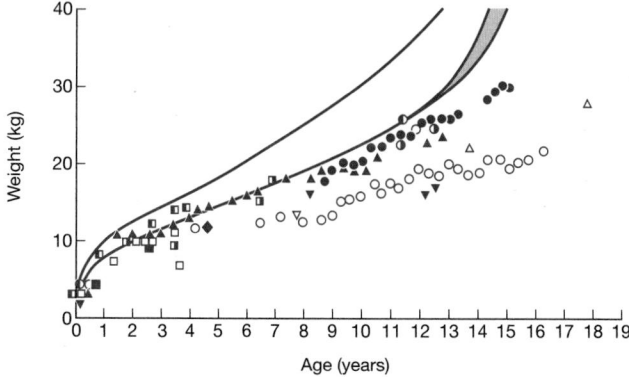

Fig. 5 Patterns of growth in weight of 13 boys with the Lesch–Nyhan syndrome: each patient is shown by a different symbol. The 50th and 3rd centiles are shown. (Reproduced from Watts, *et al.* 1987, with kind permission from Kluwer Academic Publishers.)

and bone development are less affected than weight. The poor weight gain cannot be attributed to either renal failure or malnutrition.

Torsion dystonia, with its two components of abnormal posturing and episodic rigidity, is superimposed on the basic hypotonia that is present between the dystonic episodes. Severe dysarthria is associated with dyskinesia of the face, mouth, pharynx, and the larynx, which greatly limits communication and even the ability to point accurately, thus leading to great frustration. The self-injurious behaviour and dyskinesia are eliminated or much reduced when the child is concentrating on a self-selected activity, such as watching an interesting television programme. Self-injury and dyskinesia are exacerbated by excitement such as the arrival of a visitor, fear, frustration, and unsuccessful attempts at volitional motor activity. The children also appear to be aware of the value of this behaviour as an attention-seeking manoeuvre, and sometimes appear to use it in a manipulative manner. This mixture of involuntary and volitional involuntary abnormal motor activity with an apparent interplay of unconscious and consciously mediated behaviour patterns should be common ground for behavioural scientists, neurochemists, and neuropharmacologists.

Although mental handicap has been stressed as a feature of the Lesch–Nyhan syndrome, it is of inconstant severity, and is neither marked nor specific. The apparent degree of mental handicap may be affected by the extensive disorder of expressive motor functions that exceeds the comprehension defect, by the lack of basic social and educational opportunities, and by the lack of intelligence tests for older children who have lacked these opportunities. However, for whatever combination of reasons, there does appear to be a decline of intellect from the age of 8 to 10 years.

Self-injurious behaviour usually begins at about 2 years of age. Its severity and the ingenuity with which the patients exploit new ways of self-injury exceeds that encountered in any other clinical situation. It is not a constant feature and some patients never show it; in the majority its severity waxes and wanes. Self-injury can produce very severe damage, such as complete destruction of the lower lip or traumatic amputation of a fingertip. The patients feel pain normally and are aware of their compulsion; they are afraid of it but are unable to control it. Nyhan and his colleagues consider it to be the hallmark of complete HPRT deficiency, as opposed to those patients with some residual enzyme activity (which may or may not be measurable in erythrocyte lysates).

There are no structural or ultrastructural changes in the brain as judged by light and electron microscopy. Computed tomography and electroencephalography also show no abnormality during life. MRI and PET scanning have not yet been applied to this problem.

Both the purine *de novo* synthesis and the HPRT-catalysed purine salvage pathways are present in all parts of the normal brain. HPRT activity is absent, but the *de novo* synthesis pathway remains active in patients with the Lesch–Nyhan syndrome. It has been suggested that the bone marrow and brain have particular requirements for the purine salvage pathway and that HPRT deficiency might constrain brain development. If this is so, it is not explained by particularly low activity of purine *de novo* synthesis activity in the brain. Indeed, demonstrable structural and ultrastructural changes in patients with the Lesch–Nyhan syndrome are also lacking, suggesting that the inability to salvage hypoxanthine and guanine in the Lesch–Nyhan syndrome causes a 'functional' aberration. Such a derangement could derive from either a postulated postsynaptic transmitter function for cyclic GMP (**cGMP**), or a related compound, or a consequential effect on the availability of synaptic neurotransmitters. So far, further studies have not supported the cGMP postsynaptic neurotransmitter hypothesis. The levels of HPRT activities are approximately uniform in a normal human brain. Purine salvage as well as purine *de novo* synthesis activity is also uniformly distributed in the different gross anatomical regions of the rat brain.

Evidence has been advanced for some aspects of the Lesch–Nyhan phenotype being related to dysfunction of the small central, but widely projecting, aminergic pathways involved in learning. Thus it has been suggested that self-injurious behaviour in the Lesch–Nyhan syndrome is due to an imbalance between the activities of catecholaminergic neurones and

5-hydroxytryptaminergic neurones. The catecholaminergic neurones are largely concerned with learning by reward, and the 5-hydroxytryptaminergic pathways with learning by punishment. Patients with the Lesch–Nyhan syndrome are insensitive to punishing stimuli and do not learn when such stimuli are used to reinforce the desired behaviour, which in this case is non-self injury. The ability to learn from rewarding stimuli is impaired. Psychotherapeutic techniques that are effective in eliminating self-injurious behaviour in other situations fail in patients with the Lesch–Nyhan syndrome. Thus, although the self-injurious behaviour in the Lesch–Nyhan syndrome could be modified by a programme of positive reinforcement of non-self injury and 'time out', this has proved difficult to achieve in the long term. The reinforcement strategy was found to be unsuitable for use at home because it involved apparently ignoring the self-injury and only paying attention to the child during periods of non-self injury. This was misinterpreted by friends and relations as unkindness or indifference.

The present view is that the neurological manifestations are brought about by a neurotransmitter imbalance (probably mainly in the basal ganglia). This imbalance is possibly due to a deficient supply of metabolic energy resulting from the non-salvage of hypoxanthine and guanine, thus causing a deficiency of adenine nucleotides that provide energy for short bursts of neurotransmitter synthesis.

Failure of pubertal development and testicular atrophy in HPRT deficiency are attributed to an inadequate supply of purine nucleotides to meet the increased metabolic energy requirement in the testis at this time. A similar inability to meet energy requirements may underlie the neurological manifestations. A partial defect in adrenocortical 11β-hydroxylation of steroids is demonstrable in patients with the Lesch–Nyhan syndrome after ACTH stimulation, and is thought to be linked with a failure to modulate mitochondrial function for this hydroxylation due to a deficiency of purine nucleotides.

Patients with Lesch–Nyhan syndrome whose hyperuricaemia has been controlled and who have not suffered renal damage, die in their teenage years, often with postmortem evidence of gastric aspiration during sleep. Less severe degrees of HPRT deficiency lead to the X-linked recessive hyperuricaemia gout and urolithiasis syndrome, which may also be associated with minor neurological abnormalities.

Treatment

Sufficient allopurinol should be administered to reduce the plasma urate and urine uric acid concentrations to normal in order to prevent gouty arthritis, urate nephropathy, and renal calculi. Relatively large doses of allopurinol are needed and the patient should be kept well hydrated to minimize the risk of xanthine and/or oxipurinol (the metabolic oxidation product of allopurinol) stones developing. Both types of stone are, like uric acid stones, radiotranslucent. Allopurinol treatment from birth does not prevent the behavioural phenotype. All therapeutic attempts at neuropharmacological manipulation have been unsuccessful.

Dental extraction, physical restraints with splints and bandages, and strapping the patient into a specially designed padded wheelchair fitted with a padded firm head support to prevent cervical spine injury during violent opisthotonic spasms, are usually needed to limit the effects of compulsive self-mutilation.

Children whose restraints have been temporarily released ask or indicate their wish for the bandages, straps, etc. to be replaced so that they are less able to damage themselves. Every effort should be made to exploit these patients' intellect and to keep them in a stimulating environment.

Clinical genetic aspects

The Lesch–Nyhan syndrome and its variants are inherited in a sex-linked recessive manner with no clinical manifestations in the female carriers. However, subtle alterations in purine metabolism, with small increases in the rates of *de novo* purine synthesis and increased uric acid excretion and occasionally mild asymptomatic hyperuricaemia, have been reported in females. Affected male hemizygotes are identified biochemically by HPRT assays on red cell haemolysates, the lack of HPRT being accompanied by an elevated level of phosphoribosylpyrophosphate. Genomic analysis is also possible. Carrier females are identified by the demonstration of mosaicism with respect to *HPRT+* and *HPRT–* hair roots due to random inactivation of the X-chromosome, the hair roots being clonal in origin. Autoradiographic techniques can be used to demonstrate two cell populations (*HPRT+* and *HPRT−*) in fibroblast cultures.

Early prenatal diagnosis is possible using chorionic villus samples obtained during the ninth week of pregnancy, this permits elective abortion of an affected fetus before the end of the first trimester of pregnancy. *In vitro* fertilization with enzymatic assay on a cell removed at the four-cell stage to ensure that only unaffected embryos are implanted is theoretically possible.

Phosphoribosylpyrophosphate synthetase superactivity

This enzyme catalyses the production of phosphoribosylpyrophosphate, which is required for the first specific and rate-limiting reaction on the *de novo* pathway of purine synthesis. It is subject to feedback inhibition by purine nucleotides. The known mutations in the gene regulating the synthesis of phosphoribosylpyrophosphate synthetase diminish its sensitivity to this feedback inhibition, thereby leading to hyperuricaemia, hyperuricosuria, and gout. The condition is inherited in an X-linked recessive fashion.

Affected males develop uric acid lithiasis or gouty arthritis in childhood or early adult life. Hyperuricaemia is often severe and in the range 0.5 to 1 mmol/l, with uric acid excretion of 5 to 15 mmol/24 h. Heterozygotes remain asymptomatic, although some degree of increased purine synthesis *de novo* has been demonstrated.

In some families, the disorder presents in childhood with associated neurological features such as motor and mental retardation, ataxia, deafness, hypotonia, disturbed speech, and the development of polyneuropathy, intracerebral calcifications, and dysmorphic facial features. The constellation of associated disorders varies in different families.

Heterozygotes can be identified by studies in cultured skin fibroblasts. Amniocentesis, prenatal diagnosis, and preventive abortion are not justified in this condition unless one of the unusually severe phenotypes is known to be segregating in the family. The hyperuricaemia, primary purine overproduction, and uricosuria can be well controlled with allopurinol.

2,8-Dihydroxyadeninuria

These patients lack adenine phosphoribosyltransferase activity, adenine accumulates behind the metabolic block and is oxidized under the catalytic influence of xanthine oxidase to the very insoluble compound, 2,8-dihydroxyadenine. This compound is excreted in the urine along with adenine itself, where it forms radiotranslucent stones that are white or pale fawn in colour. These rough and friable calculi have, in the past, been widely misdiagnosed as uric acid stones because 2,8-dihydroxyadenine reacts as if it were uric acid in colorimetric assays. The use of enzymatic uric acid assays has obviated this confusion.

Adenine phosphoribosyltransferase deficiency has an autosomal recessive pattern of inheritance and is clinically silent in heterozygotes. There are two subtypes (I and II). Type I patients have no detectable enzyme activity, being homozygotes or compound heterozygotes for null alleles. Type II patients have between 5 and 25 per cent residual enzyme activity. Whereas type I patients are encountered in many racial groups, the type II subtype has so far only been identified in the Japanese population. Heterozygotes for type I and type II can only be distinguished from one another by enzyme assays on extracts from cultured peripheral blood lymphocytes, both types show no activity in the red cell lysates that are generally used diagnostically.

Because of the extremely low solubility of 2,8-dihydroxyadenine in renal tubule fluid and urine, this condition often presents in early life. Severe obstructive uropathy and renal failure may occur in infancy.

Treatment is by hydration and xanthine oxidase inhibition with allopurinol, and with standard measures to disrupt or remove the stones and to manage urinary infections and renal failure.

Type I glycogenosis

Type I glycogenosis (hereditary glucose 6-phosphatase deficiency) is associated with hyperuricaemia. This is due to chronic hyperlacticacidaemia which leads to urate retention, and to increased urate production due to reduced serum phosphate concentrations. The phosphate ion inhibits AMP deaminase: the enzyme that catalyses the rate-limiting step in the metabolic pathway for the conversion of adenine nucleotides to uric acid. Thus, hypophosphataemia increases adenine nucleotide degradation to uric acid and adds to the accumulating urate burden; gouty arthritis may develop in childhood.

Treatment is by maintaining the blood glucose level in the normal range with frequent small meals and intragastric glucose infusion at night. Gout is treated in the standard manner with colchicine and/or non-steroidal anti-inflammatory drugs for the acute attacks, and with long-term allopurinol.

Xanthinuria

Xanthine stones occur in patients with xanthinuria (congenital xanthine oxidase/reductase deficiency) and occasionally in those who are being treated with the xanthine oxidase inhibitor, allopurinol. The latter is particularly likely in patients with accelerated purine *de novo* synthesis (for example, in patients with the Lesch–Nyhan syndrome). Xanthinuria is inherited in an autosomal recessive manner, and hypoxanthine and xanthine accumulate behind the metabolic block. The plasma urate concentration and urine uric acid excretion are less than about 0.06 mmol/l (1.0 mg/dl) and 0.30 mmol/24 h (50 mg/24 h), respectively, when the patient is taking an unrestricted diet. A search of general hospital clinical data on 47 420 unselected patients yielded no cases of xanthinuria. The plasma and urine 'oxypurines' (hypoxanthine plus xanthine) concentrations are characteristically elevated. Normal subjects have plasma levels between 0.00 and 0.15 mmol/l (0.00–0.25 mg/dl) and urine levels of 0.07 to 0.13 mmol/24h (11–22 mg/24 h); patients with xanthinuria have plasma levels between 0.03 and 0.05 mmol/l (0.05–0.9 mg/dl) and urine levels of 0.60 to 3.5 mmol/24 h (100–600 mg/24 h). Xanthine accounts for 60 to 90 per cent of the total xanthine plus hypoxanthine excreted, presumably reflecting the more active metabolic turnover of hypoxanthine and its efficient salvage by hypoxanthine phosphoribosyltransferase. Hypoxanthine and xanthine are mainly derived from adenine and guanine nucleotides, respectively (see Fig. 1). Hypoxanthine has a relatively high solubility and causes no problems.

At any age, about one-third of cases present with radiotranslucent xanthine stones. These stones are usually smooth, soft, and yellow–brown. Xanthinuric myopathy is a rare complication.

Xanthine stones also occur when there is a combined deficiency of the three molybdoflavoprotein enzymes—xanthine oxidase, sulphite oxidase, and aldehyde oxidase—because of defective molybdopterin cofactor synthesis. The clinical picture in these patients is overshadowed by the sulphite oxidase deficiency that produces severe brain damage and dislocation of the ocular lenses. Another subgoup of patients with xanthinuria only lack xanthine oxidase and aldehyde oxidase activity. These patients present with xanthine stones and are detected by their inability to convert allopurinol to oxipurinol, a reaction normally catalysed by aldehyde oxidase.

Adenylosuccinase deficiency

Adenylosuccinase (adenylate succinate lyase) catalyses the eighth step on the 10-step *de novo* purine synthesis pathway and the second step on one of the purine nucleotide interconversion pathways, the formation of ATP from IMP.

The patients present in infancy with severe psychomotor retardation, autism, and axial hypotonia with normal tendon reflexes. Self-mutilation has been recorded in some cases and cerebellar hypoplasia is present on computed tomographic (**CT**) scanning.

The presence of aspartic acid and glycine in body fluids suggests the diagnosis, and this is confirmed by finding succinyladenosine and succinylaminoimidazole carboxamide riboside in plasma, cerebrospinal fluid, and urine. There is gross purine overproduction with high levels of nucleosides in the urine. Urine and plasma uric acid levels are normal. Partial enzyme deficiencies have been demonstrated in liver, kidney, muscle, lymphocytes, and fibroblasts.

Adenylosuccinase deficiency is inherited as an autosomal recessive. The growth retardation has been improved by adenine (10 mg/day) and allopurinol. The latter promotes purine conservation by blocking hypoxanthine oxidation to xanthine and uric acid, and prevents the oxidation of administered adenine to 2,8-dihydroxyadenine.

Myoadenylate deaminase deficiency

Myoadenylate deaminase is the muscle-specific isoenzyme of adenylate deaminase which catalyses the deamination of adenylic acid to inosinic acid during muscle contraction. This reaction is necessary for normal muscle function. Myoadenylate deaminase deficiency may be congenital, due to a mutation in the gene directing the synthesis of the protein, or associated with a wide range of muscle diseases including the muscular dystrophies, polymyositis, and dermatomyositis.

Patients with congenital myoadenylate deaminase deficiency present at any age, including early childhood, with a syndrome of muscle weakness and muscle cramps during and after exertion. There is some decrease in muscle mass, some hypotonia, and a little muscle weakness. There may be a modest rise in plasma creatine phosphokinase levels and non-specific electromyographic changes. The lack of ammonia in the venous outflow from the affected muscles during exercise and the enzyme deficiency can be demonstrated histochemically. The pattern of inheritance is autosomal recessive, not all homozygotes have clinical symptoms and heterozygous carriers are clinically silent. A single mutant allele contains a non-sense mutation that leads to the production of a severely truncated enzyme. The acquired disorder may be due to the coincidental disease arising in a patient whose inherited myoadenylate deaminase deficiency would be otherwise silent. Genetic testing for the mutant allele can be utilized to determine whether congenital myoadenylate deaminase could be contributing to the patient's clinical presentation.

Oral ribose (2–60 g/day, or taking a dose before vigorous exercise) has been reported to produce symptomatic improvement. The risk of rhabdomyolysis has led some authors to recommend the avoidance of vigorous exercise, myoglobinuria following strenuous exercise having been reported in a few cases. Such advice is appropriate if exertion-related myoglobinuria has occurred or been suspected.

Inborn errors of purine metabolism and immunodeficiency

Adenosine deaminase (**ADA**) and purine nucleoside phosphorylase (**PNP**) catalyse sequential steps in the metabolism of purine ribonucleosides and deoxyribonucleosides (Fig. 6). These enzymes are highly expressed in lymphoid cells and their deficiency, which causes the lymphotoxic substrates 2'-deoxyadenosine (**dAdo**) and 2'-deoxyguanosine (**dGuo**) to accumulate (see Fig. 6), leads to lymphopenia and immunodeficiency.

Most patients with ADA deficiency lack both cell- (T cell) and humoral (B cell)-mediated immunity, resulting in severe combined immunodeficiency disease (**SCID**). Although PNP deficiency causes defective T-cell mediated immunity, these patients may possess either normal, hyperactive,

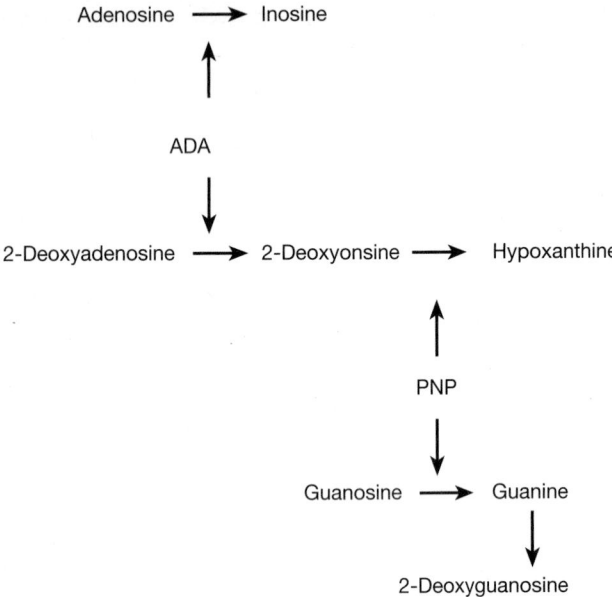

Fig. 6 Metabolic steps catalysed by adenosine deaminase (ADA) and by purine nucleoside phosphorylase (PNA).

or reduced humoral immunity. Most patients with these enzyme deficiencies present in infancy or early childhood with severe infections caused by pathogens or opportunistic organisms. About 50 per cent of patients with SCID have X-linked agammaglobulinaemia (Bruton's disease), a disease that is unrelated to ADA and PNP deficiencies and which displays an autosomal recessive pattern of inheritance.

Adenosine deaminase deficiency

About 85 per cent of patients with ADA deficiency are infants with SCID. In all patients with SCID, ADA deficiency accounts for a minority, possibly about 15 per cent. Although adenosine deaminase deficiency classically presents during infancy, a minority of patients have a clinically less severe variant and are diagnosed later. The prevalence of ADA deficiency has been estimated at between less than 1 in 10^6 and 1 in 2×10^5 live births.

ADA deficiency is inherited in an autosomal recessive fashion, the gene having been mapped to chromosome 20q13.11. The diagnosis is made by measuring ADA activity in erythrocytes. Heterozygote detection and prenatal diagnosis are best done using molecular probes for the ADA gene.

In addition to immunoparesis, about one-third of cases have multiple skeletal abnormalities, including fraying of the long bones, abnormally thick growth-arrest lines, and chondro-osseous dysphasia at the costochondral junctions. Other occasionally reported comorbidities are renal tubular acidosis, choreoathetosis, spasticity, and fine sparse hair.

The prognosis for patients with untreated adenosine deaminase-deficient SCID is very poor, with death due to multiple recurrent infections during the first year of life.

Adenosine and dAdo, derived from the breakdown of DNA due to cell death, accumulate proximal to the metabolic block—dAdo is the primary lymphotoxic precursor in adenosine deaminase deficiency, elevated levels of which are present in plasma and urine. Erythrocytes contain markedly raised levels of deoxyadenosine triphosphate (**dATP**) and reduced S-adenosylhomocysteine (**AdoHcy**) hydrolase activity due to inactivation by dAdo; erythrocyte ATP is reduced. The level of dATP in erythrocytes correlates with clinical expression and with the level of ADA activity expressed in *Escherichia coli* by mutant ADA alleles.

There are several mechanisms by which adenosine deaminase deficiency can impair immune function. Thus, accumulation of dATP can induce apoptosis in lymphoid cells, which may be related to dATP-induced inhibition of ribonucleotide reductase blocking DNA replication in dividing cells, and to dATP-induced DNA strand breaks in non-dividing lymphocytes. dATP also activates the protease (caspase 9) involved in apoptosis. AdoHcy also blocks S-adenosylmethionine (**AdoMet**)-mediated transmethylation reactions. The formation of dATP from dAdo activates IMP dephosphorylation, thereby leading to the depletion of cellular ATP. It has also been suggested that lymphocyte function may be impaired by aberrant signal transduction mediated by Ado acting through G-protein-associated receptors, or from an altered co-stimulatory function of T-cell associated ADA-complexing protein CD26/dipeptidyl peptidase IV.

Treatment

This is by bone marrow transplantation from a histocompatible donor. Repeated blood transfusions can provide temporary benefit, although repeated transfusion leads to iron overload. More sustained clinical improvement follows the weekly or twice-weekly administration of polyethylene glycol-modified bovine adenosine deaminase. The use of ADA-loaded erythrocytes membranes is also being explored.

Transplantation of T-cell-depleted marrow from an HLA-haploidentical donor has been tried, but it is associated with greater morbidity and is less effective than bone marrow transplantation in restoring immune function.

The *ex vivo* retrovirus-mediated transfer of ADA cDNA is the first attempt at somatic-cell gene therapy in humans. The efficacy of transducing stem cells has been low, but persistence of the vector myeloid cells and T lymphocytes has been demonstrated. The long-term evaluation of this approach is still awaited.

Purine nucleoside phosphorylase deficiency

PNP deficiency occurs less frequently than ADA deficiency. In addition to the clinical results of immunoparesis, more than 50 per cent of these patients have neurological abnormalities including disorders of muscle tone, delayed motor and intellectual development, ataxias, tremors, spastic tetraparesis, behavioural difficulties, and varying degrees of mental handicap. Autoimmune haemolytic anaemia and megaloblastic bone marrow have been occasional associations.

There appears to be a particular susceptibility to virus infections such as varicella, vaccinia, and cytomegalovirus. The tonsils and the thymus are small or absent and the lymph nodes are deficient in the thymus-dependent areas. Circulating lymphocyte counts are usually very low, with a low percentage of T lymphocytes and depressed or absent responsiveness to mitogen-induced transformation. Serum immunoglobulin levels and antibody responses to pneumococcal polysaccharide and keyhole limpet haemocyanin are typically increased in children with PNP deficiency, and the occasional finding of monoclonal IgG paraprotein strongly suggests that the changes in antibody production are the result of T-cell defects.

PNP deficiency is associated with the accumulation and excretion of dGuo and deoxyinosine, as well as guanosine and inosine. Paradoxically, there is massive purine overproduction and excretion, although all patients are severely hypouricaemic. Erythrocyte concentrations of dGTP are markedly raised in PNP-deficient cells. T cells, but not B cells, appear to be particularly susceptible to dGuo toxicity, probably as a result of the accumulation of dGTP, inhibition of ribonucleotide reductase, impairment of DNA synthesis, and, eventually, cell death.

The prognosis in children with PNP deficiency is often much better than that in adenosine deaminase deficiency. Since some children have remained healthy and free from viral infection until the age of 6 years, high-risk procedures such as bone marrow transplantation are currently not thought to be justified in all cases. Conservative treatment with gammaglobulin replacement and attempts at enzyme replacement with red cell transfusions in children with recurrent infections are the current approach to management.

Purine 5′-nucleotidase deficiency

Deficiency of the ecto enzyme 5′-nucleotidase is found in some patients with X-linked and 'acquired' adult-onset hypogammaglobulinaemia. There is no evidence that the enzyme deficiency causes the immunodeficiency in either case. It is currently thought much more likely to simply reflect an arrested stage of lymphocyte development in these patients.

Other disorders of purine metabolism

There are two unrelated conditions: (1) a regulatory mutation in liver adenylic deaminase as a cause of uric acid overproduction and gout in a single patient; and (2) erythrocyte adenylic acid deaminase deficiency in Japanese and Chinese peoples, which has no clinical phenotype.

Disorders of pyrimidine metabolism

The pathways of pyrimidine biosynthesis interconversion and degradation are shown in Fig. 7.

The *de novo* synthesis of pyrimidine nucleotides involves a series of six reactions beginning with the formation of carbamyl phosphate and concluding with orotidylic acid (**OMP**), which then undergoes a series of inter-conversion and salvage reactions as summarized in Fig. 7. The first three steps on the *de novo* synthesis pathway are catalysed by the multifunctional protein that encompasses carbamyl phosphate synthetase, aspartate transaminase, and dihydro-orotase. The fourth step is catalysed by dihydro-orotate dehydrogenase. The fifth and sixth steps are catalysed by the bifunctional protein encoding orotate phosphoribosyltransferase (**ORPT**) and orotidine-5′-monophosphate dehydrogenase (**OMPD**) activities. The pyrimidines are degraded to β-alanine and β-aminobutyrate (Fig. 7).

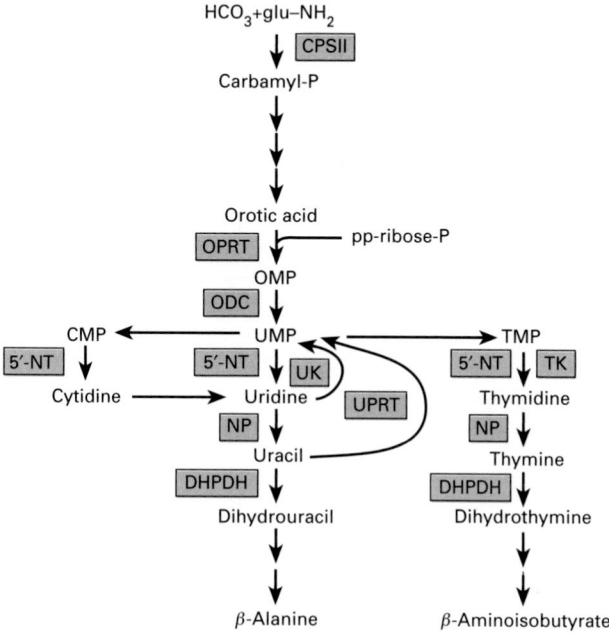

Fig. 7 Pathways of pyrimidine metabolism in humans. CPSH, carbamyl phosphate synthetase II; OPRT, orotate phosphoribosyltransferase; ODC, orotidine decarboxylase (OPRT + ODC from UMP synthase; 5′-NT, pyrimidine 5′-nucleotidase; NP, pyrimidine nucleoside phosphorylase; DHPD, dihydropyrimidine dehydrogenase; UK, uridine kinase; UPRT, uracil phosphoribosyltransferase; TK, thymidine kinase.

The inherited disorders of pyrimidine metabolism are much less common, or possibly much less easily recognized, than disorders of purine metabolism.

Orotic aciduria

Orotic aciduria is due to a deficiency of the bifunctional protein that encodes both OMP dehydrogenase and OPRT activities. There is massive overproduction of orotic acid due to loss of feed-back inhibition of carbamyl phosphate synthase, which is the first and rate-limiting step on the metabolic pathway.

Orotic aciduria presents during infancy with severe megaloblastic anaemia, orotic acid crystalluria, and, occasionally, radiotranslucent orotic acid urinary stones. Cardiac malformations, mild intellectual impairment, and strabismus have been reported. Orotic aciduria is inherited as an autosomal recessive.

Enzyme assays on erythrocyte lysates show either low levels of OPRT and OMPD (type 1 orotic aciduria) or a deficiency of ODC only (type 2 orotic aciduria). Administration of uridine (100–150 mg/kg per day), which is converted to UMP (Fig. 7), produces a prompt haematological response. Treatment needs to be started as soon as the diagnosis is made during infancy in order to minimize the possibility of persistent neurological deficits.

Some degree of orotic aciduria has been found in urea cycle defects, lysinuric protein intolerance, PNP-deficiency, normal pregnancy, and during allopurinol administration.

Pyrimidine 5′-nucleotidase deficiency

This autosomal recessive disorder leads to non-spherocytic haemolytic anaemia. Uridine triphosphate (**UTP**) and cytidine triphosphate (**CTP**) accumulate in the red cells, which show basophilic stippling. The enzyme is assayed in erythrocytes and activities between 0 and 30 per cent of normal have been reported. There is no effective treatment. Lead poisoning can also be associated with acquired erythrocyte pyrimidine 5_-nucleotidase deficiency.

Pyrimidine 5′-nucleotidase superactivity

Pyrimidine 5′-nucleotidase superactivity has been reported in four unrelated families with developmental delay and neurological abnormalities. Treatment with uridine is said to have been beneficial.

Deficiency of dihydropyrimidine dehydrogenase (DHPDH)

This autosomal recessive disorder presents with variable degrees of hypertonia, epilepsy, and autism. Some cases have only presented during adult life, when they have developed severe adverse side-effects following cancer chemotherapy with 5-fluorouracil. Uracil and thymine are elevated in the body fluids, including urine. Absent enzyme activities have been demonstrated in blood, cerebrospinal fluid, leucocytes, liver, and fibroblasts. There is no effective treatment for this condition and the prognosis for life is very variable.

N-Carbamyl-β-aminoaciduria

To date, just one patient has been detected with ureidopropionase deficiency causing N-carbamyl-β-aminoaciduria. This patient presented with choreoathetosis, hypotonia, and microcephaly.

Further reading

Ahota AS, *et al.* (2001). Adenine phosphoribosyltransferase deficiency and 2,8-dihydroxyadenine lithiasis. In: Scriver CS, *et al.*, eds. *The metabolic and molecular basis of inherited disease*, 8th edn, pp 2571–662. McGraw-Hill, New York.

Bax BE, *et al.* (2000). *In vitro* and *in vivo* studies with human carrier erythrocytes loaded with polyethylene glycol-conjugated and native adenosine deaminase. *British Journal of Haematology* **109**, 549–54.

Becker MA (2001). Hyperuricaemia and gout. In: Scriver CS, *et al.*, eds. *The metabolic and molecular basis of inherited disease*, 8th edn, pp 2513–35. McGraw-Hill, New York.

De Ruiter CJ, *et al.* (2002). Muscle function during repetitive moderate-intensity muscle contractions in myoadenylate deaminase-deficient Dutch subjects. *Clinical Science* **102**, 531–39.

Desaulniers P, *et al.* (2001). Crystal induced neutrophil activation. VII: Involvement of Syk in the responses to monosodium urate crystals. *Journal of Leukocyte Biology* **70**, 659–68.

Fam AG (2001). Difficult gout and new approaches for control of hyperuricaemia in the allopurinol-allergic patient. *Current Rheumatology Reports* **3**, 29–35.

Gresser U, Zöllner N (1991). *Urate deposition in man and its clinical consequences.* Springer-Verlag, Berlin.

Harkness, *et al.* (1988). Lesch-Nyhan syndrome and its pathogenesis: purine concentrations in plasma and urine with metabolite profiles in CSF. *Journal of Inherited Metabolic Diseases* **11**, 239–52.

Hershfield MS, Mitchell BS (2001). Immunodeficiency diseases caused by adenosine deaminase deficiency and purine nucleoside phosphorylase deficiency. In: Scriver CS, *et al.*, eds. *The metabolic and molecular basis of inherited disease*, 8th edn, pp 2585–625. McGraw-Hill, New York.

Hochberg MC (2001). Gout. In: Silman AJ and Hochberg MC, eds. *Epidemiology of the rheumatic diseases*, 2nd edn, pp 230–42. Oxford University Press, Oxford.

Jinnah HA, Friedmann T (2001). Lesch–Nyhan disease and its variants In: Scriver CS, *et al.*, eds. *The metabolic and molecular basis of inherited disease*, 8th edn, pp 2537–70. McGraw-Hill, New York.

Jinnah HA, *et al.* (2000). The spectrum of inherited mutations causing HPRT deficiency. 75 new cases and a review of 196 previously reported cases. *Mutation Research* **46**, 309–26.

Landis RC, Haskard DO (2001). Pathogenesis of crystal induced inflammation. *Current Rheumatology Reports* **3**, 36–41.

Lipkowitz MS, *et al.* (2001). Functional reconstitution, membrane targeting, genomic structure and chromosomal localisation of a human urate transporter. *Journal of Clinical Investigation* **107**, 1103–15.

Liu R, *et al.* (2000). Extracellular signal-regulated kinase[1]/extracellular signal regulated kinase 2 mitogen-activated protein kinase signalling and activation of activator protein 1 and nuclear factor kappa β transcription factors play central roles in interleukin-8 expression stimulated by monosodium urate monohydrate and calcium pyrophosphate crystals in monocytic cells. *Arthritis and Rheumatism* **43**, 1145–55.

Liu R, *et al.* (2001). Src family protein tyrosine kinase signalling mediates monosodium urate crystal-induced IL-8 expression by monocyte THP-1 cells. *Journal of Leukocyte Biology* **70**, 961–8.

MacDermott K, Allsop J, Watts RWE (1984). The rate of purine synthesis *de novo* in blood mononuclear cells *in vitro* in patients with familial hyperuricaemic nephropathy. *Clinical Science* **67**, 249–58.

Schreiner O, *et al.* (2000). Reduced secretion of pro-inflammatory cytokines of monosodium urate crystal stimulated monocytes in chronic renal failure: an explanation for infrequent gout episodes in chronic renal failure patients? *Nephropathy, Dialysis and Transplantation* **15**, 644–9.

Stone TW, Simmonds HA (1991). *Purines: basic and clinical aspects.* Kluwer Academic, Dordrecht.

Van den Berghe G, Jacken J (2001). Adenylosuccinate lyase deficiency. In: Scriver CS, *et al.*, eds. *The metabolic and molecular basis of inherited disease*, 8th edn, pp 2653–62. McGraw-Hill, New York.

Waring WS, Webb DJ, Maxwell SRJ (2000). Uric acid as a risk factor for cardiovascular disease. *Quarterly Journal of Medicine* **93**, 707–13.

Watts RWE (1985). Defects of tetrahydrobiopterin synthesis and their possible relationship to a disorder of purine metabolism (the Lesch–Nyhan syndrome). In: Weber G, ed. *Advances in enzyme regulation*, Vol 23, pp 25–58. Pergamon Press, Oxford.

Watts RWE, *et al.*(1987). Lesch–Nyhan syndrome; growth delay, testicular atrophy and a partial failure of 11β-hydroxylation of steroids. *Journal of Inherited Metabolic Diseases* **10**, 210–23.

Yakink DR, *et al.* (2000). Non-inflammatory phagocytosis of monosodium urate monohydrate crystals by mouse macrophages. *Arthritis and Rheumatism* **43**, 1779–89.

11.5 The porphyrias

T. M. Cox

The haem biosynthetic pathway holds great fascination for biochemists who marvel at the evolution of ancient enzymes which interact to bring about the formation of the pigments of life—haemoglobin, the cytochromes, chlorophyll, and the cobalamins (vitamin B_{12}). It is unfortunate that, because of complexities in their chemical structure and ambiguities in their technical nomenclature, the terminology of the porphyrin pigments and the diseases associated with their disturbed metabolism are perceived to be confusing and intimidating. These considerations apply particularly to the acute porphyrias which are rare but distressing syndromes that mimic other acute illnesses but for which recognition may be critical for the patient's survival; too often the diagnosis is not established until permanent disability or even death supervenes.

The porphyrias are caused by disturbances in the multistep pathway for the formation of haem—a pigment essential for oxygen transfer and the energy-yielding reactions of electron transport. The formation of haem is tightly regulated so that acquired or hereditary defects of any of its component reactions lead to the overproduction of haem precursors. Potentially photoactive macrocyclic compounds and toxic precursors of pyrroles thus accumulate. Most of the human porphyria syndromes result from uncommon genetically determined deficiencies of unitary enzymes of the haem biosynthetic pathway; but certain toxins including lead, iron, and hydrocarbons influence the pathway and cause porphyria in susceptible individuals. Similarly the metabolism of endogenous molecules, including steroid hormones, and xenobiotics such as alcohol and many therapeutic drugs, may disturb the delicate equilibrium that is achieved in asymptomatic patients with latent porphyria. Thus gene–environment interactions in previously fit individuals may precipitate sporadic attacks of acute porphyria.

Classification: types of porphyria

The porphyrias are disorders of metabolism characterized by overproduction of the precursors of haem synthesized principally in the liver and bone marrow. About 15 per cent of *de novo* haem biosynthesis occurs in the liver and about 80 per cent in the erythroid marrow. Hepatic synthesis of haem is subject to rapid and wide oscillations in flux; haem biosynthesis in the erythropoietic bone marrow is under most circumstances constitutive and stable. However, haem synthesis may be increased as the erythron expands and proliferates to meet the demands of blood loss or haemolysis, including ineffective erythropoiesis.

Hitherto the porphyrias have been classified into the hepatic and erythropoietic types depending on the principal location at which overproduction of haem precursors occurs. For clinical purposes, however, an operational definition of the porphyric syndromes is more usefully presented as the acute and the non-acute porphyrias. The acute porphyrias cause life-threatening neurovisceral manifestations typically precipitated by environmental factors that occur sporadically. The non-acute porphyrias are characterized by photosensitivity syndromes resulting from the overproduction of macrocyclic porphyrins which cause light-induced skin injury. Several of the acute porphyrias may be associated also with the over-

production of porphyrin intermediates and so may be accompanied at times by long-term photosensitivity which is often exacerbated during the acute attacks. In all instances it is the overproduction of haem precursors that characterizes the condition biochemically: this is the principal means by which a diagnosis can be made of the underlying enzymatic defect during the acute attack. Tables 1, 2, and 3 set out the individual defects that characterize the clinical porphyrias and summarize the clinical features of these hereditary syndromes.

Formation of haem

Haem biosynthesis is catalysed by eight enzymes and is co-ordinated between mitochondrial and cytoplasmic compartments in the cell (Fig. 1). The first committed precursor, 5-aminolaevulinate, is formed in the mitochondria from glycine and the Krebs' cycle intermediate, succinyl-CoA, by one or other of the two isozymes of 5-aminolaevulinate synthetase. Precursor 5-aminolaevulinate is then exported to the cytoplasm where it undergoes condensation to form the monopyrrole, porphobilinogen, four molecules of which are then condensed to yield the macrocyclic tetrapyrrole, uroporphyrinogen III. This reaction is brought about by porphobilinogen deaminase and uroporphyrinogen III synthetase acting co-ordinately to reverse the orientation of one porphobilinogen molecule to yield the uroporphyrinogen III isoform that is the sole precursor of biological haem. Porphyrins of the I series do not serve as biological intermediates in the formation of protoporphyrin IX or haem.

The cytoplasmic enzyme, uroporphyrinogen III decarboxylase decarboxylates the four acetate substituent side-chains to yield coproporphyrinogen III, which is then reimported into the mitochondrion for further oxidative decarboxylation. Coproporphyrinogen III oxidase modifies the

Table 1 The porphyria syndromes

Hereditary porphyria
Acute porphyrias:
Acute intermittent porphyria
Variegate porphyria[a]
Hereditary coproporphyria[a]
Doss porphyria—aminolaevulinate dehydratase deficiency
Non-acute porphyrias:
Congenital erythropoietic porphyria—Gunther's disease
Protoporphyria
Porphyria cutanea tarda[b]—sporadic or familial
Hepatoerythropoietic porphyria[c]
Acquired porphyria
Hexachlorobenzene porphyria
Lead poisoning (plumboporphyria)
Hereditary tyrosinaemia

[a] Acute syndromes also accompanied by long-term skin photosensitivity.

[b] Porphyria cutanea tarda is not a simple monogenic disorder; it is almost always provoked by environmental agents such as hepatitis C, oestrogens, iron excess, or alcohol.

[c] Homozygous uroporphyrinogen III decarboxylase deficiency.

Table 2 Main biochemical abnormalities in the porphyrias

Disorder	Enzyme defect	Biochemical abnormality
Acute intermittent porphyria	Porphobilinogen deaminase	Increased urinary porphobilinogen and 5-aminolaevulinate
Variegate porphyria	Protoporphyinogen IX oxidase	Increased urine 5-aminolaevulinate and porphobilinogen (especially acute attacks)
		Increased stool coproporphyrin III and protoporphyrin
Hereditary coproporphyria	Coproporphyinogen III oxidase	Increased urine 5-aminolaevulinate and porphobilinogen (especially acute attacks)
		Increased stool coproporphyrin III more than protoporphyrin
Doss porphyria	Aminolaevulinate dehydratase	Increased urinary 5-aminolaevulinate
		Faecal porphyrins normal
Porphyria cutanea tarda	Uroporphyrinogen III decarboxylase[a]	Increased urine uroporphyrin I and III
		Increased faecal hepatacarboxylic porphyrin and isocoproporphyrin
Congenital erythropoietic porphyria	Uroporphyrinogen III synthase	Increased urine, plasma, and red cell uroporphyrin I and coproporphyrin I Normal 5-aminolaevulinate and porphobilinogen
		Increased faecal coproporphyrin I
Protoporphyria	Ferrochelatase	Increased protoporphyrin in stool and red cells
Hexachlorabenzene porphyria	Uroporphyrinogen III decarboxylase	Increased urinary uroporphyrin I and III Hepatocarboxylic and other acetic acid substituents
Hereditary tyrosinaemia I	Aminolaevulinate dehydratase[b] (acquired deficiency)	Increased urinary 5-aminolaevulinate and succinylacetone (toxic metabolite)
Lead poisoning	Aminolaevulinate dehydratase, Ferrochelatase ± impaired iron delivery from transferrin	Increased urinary 5-aminolaevulinate raised red-cell protoporphyrin and zinc protoporphyrin

[a] Homozygous deficiency also responsible for hepatoerythropoietic porphyria.

[b] Inborn deficiency of fumarylacetoacetate hydrolase leads to excess formation of the 5-aminolaevulinate hydratase inhibitor, succinyl acetone (4,6-dioxoheptanoate).

Reference ranges: Urine—total porphyrins 20 to 320 nmol/l; 5-aminolaevulinate < 52 µmol/l (urine: creatinine porphobilinogen ratio < 1.5); porphobilinogen < 10.7 µmol/l.

Faeces—total porphyrins 10 to 200 nmol/g dry weight.

Red cell—total porphyrins 0.4 to 1.7 µmol/litre.

Laboratory ranges supplied by Porphyria Service, Department of Medical Biochemistry, University Hospital of Wales NHS Trust, Heath Park, Cardiff CF4 4XW (Professor G.H. Elder).

two propionate side-chains to vinyl groups yielding protoporphyrinogen IX, the penultimate precursor of haem. Protoporphyrinogen oxidase removes six hydrogen atoms to yield protoporphyrin IX, which is the substrate for the final step in haem biosynthesis. The insertion of ferrous ions into the porphyrin macrocycle to form ferroprotohaem (haem) is catalysed by the mitochondrial enzyme ferrochelatase.

Haem serves as a key prosthetic group in haem proteins including cytochromes, myoglobin, and haemoglobin by which it fulfills its essential biological roles as a transporter of oxygen and electrons in the respiratory chain and in the metabolism of xenobiotics. The two isozymes (constitutive erythroid and the inducible hepatic isozyme) of 5-aminolaevulinate synthetase catalyse the rate-limiting step of haem biosynthesis. The hepatic isozyme maps to the autosome, chromosome 3, but the erythroid isozyme of 5-aminolaevulinate synthetase (ALAS-2) maps to the X chromosome. These enzymes are subject to differential regulation principally involving transcriptional control in the liver and translational and post-translational control mechanisms in the erythroid cell by the end product, haem. These mechanisms regulate the activity of the whole biosynthetic pathway. Pyridoxal 5-phosphate (derived from vitamin B$_6$) is an essential cofactor for 5-aminolaevulinate synthetase isozymes. Deficiency of pyridoxine or interference with its metabolism leads to sideroblastic anaemia.

The second enzyme of the haem biosynthetic pathway, 5-aminolaevulinate dehydratase, is a multimeric enzyme with reactive sulphydryl groups that are particularly sensitive to the toxic effects of heavy metals, especially lead, so that 5-aminolaevulinate dehydratase activity is a sensitive measure of environmental and industrial toxicity. Moreover, 5-aminolaevulinate dehydratase is inhibited competitively by the metabolite succinyl acetone, concentrations of which rise to inhibitory levels in patients suffering from the defect of aromatic amino-acid degradation, tyrosinaemia type I. Patients with tyrosinaemia type I and lead poisoning suffer neurovisceral manifestations that resemble the acute porphyrias and it

appears likely that overproduction of aminolaevulinate, as a result of arrest at the 5-aminolaevulinate dehydratase reaction, contributes to this effect.

In living cells most of the macrocyclic precursors of the haem biosynthetic pathway are present as their reduced porphyrinogen precursors which are not themselves photoreactive. However, when these tetrapyrroles (uroporphyrinogen, coproporphyrinogen, and protoporphyrinogen) are produced in excess, they diffuse into plasma and tissues where they react with ambient oxygen to form their parent porphyrins, which are spectacularly fluorescent. The double-bond resonance structure of these macrocyclic compounds promotes the formation of singlet oxygen by the transfer of absorbed energy to ground-state oxygen through light activation. It appears that generation of singlet oxygen brings about the photodermatoses associated with the porphyrias; these are characterized by photosensitization of the skin and tissues exposed to light in a broad region of the spectrum including the visible range (350 to 430 nm). Porphyrias associated with overproduction of formed macocyclic haem precursors are thus associated with photosensitivity; the particular skin reactions that develop differ between the particular enzyme defects. This may be explained principally by the degree of hydrophobicity of the overproduced porphyrins and their solubility in cellular membranes.

The first tetrapyrrole that serves as an immediate precursor to haem is uroporphyrinogen III, formation of which requires co-ordinated action of the two cytoplasmic enzymes, uroporphyrinogen I synthase (porphobilinogen deaminase) and uroporphyrinogen III cosynthase. In the absence of adequate cosynthase activity, there is a marked overproduction of porphyrins of the I series, which do not form biologically active ferroprotohaem. Deficiency of uroporphyrinogen III cosynthase leads to the very rare but disabling syndrome of Gunther's disease (congenital erythropoietic porphyria). This disorder is characterized by extreme photosensitivity, haemolysis, and the passage of pink urine containing abundant porphyrins of the I isoform. Persistently high concentrations of these toxic molecules in body

Table 3 Principal manifestations of the porphyrias

Acute intermittent porphyria	Acute neurovisceral attacks
Variegate porphyria	Acute neurovisceral attacks
	Skin photosensitivity with scarring, hairiness, and pigment changes
Hereditary coproporphyria	Acute neurovisceral attacks, blistering skin lesions, photosensitivity
Doss porphyria	Acute neurovisceral attacks, susceptibility to lead exposure
Porphyria cutanea tarda	Blistering skin lesions on light exposure, pigment changes, atrophy and scarring— also may be associated with manifestations of iron storage disease
Congenital erythropoietic porphyria	Haemolytic anaemia, hypersplenism, porphyrinuria, extreme photosensitivity with skin ulceration and injury; adult- or late-onset reported
Hepatoerythropoietic porphyria	Resembles congenital erythropoietic porphyria: blisters, photosensitive skin with scar formation, haemolysis, red urine
Protoporphyria	Photosensitivity; early-onset, characterized by burning pain, oedema—scarring rare
	Occasional cholestatic liver disease, protoporphyrin gallstones—fulminant or subfulminant hepatic failure complicated by neurovisceral syndrome, especially in perioperative state
Hexachlorobenzene porphyria	Resembles sporadic porphyria cutanea tarda
Lead poisoining	Neurovisceral manifestations with signs of disordered red-cell haemoglobinization
Hereditary tyrosinaemia I	Toxic neurovisceral disease

fluids leads to staining of the teeth and bones and extreme photosensitive damage, often with cruel and painful skin disfigurement and hair loss.

Porphyria cutanea tarda is caused by deficiency of uroporphyrinogen decarboxylase, defects of which involve complex interactions between heredity and environmental factors. The enzyme activity is markedly decreased in the presence of excess tissue iron and, although rare familial cases of porphyria cutanea tarda occur, most patients have a sporadic disease which is provoked by exposure to environmental toxins such as alcohol, oestrogens, hydrocarbons, iron (often associated with mutations in the haemochromatosis gene, *HFE*), and hepatitis C. At the time of writing, the

pathogenic relationship between these external factors and the manifestations of uroporphyrinogen decarboxylase deficiency is unclear.

The final step in the haem biosynthetic pathway involves insertion of ferrous iron into the protoporphyrin nucleus generated enzymatically from protoporphyrinogen IX by protoporphyrinogen IX oxidase. This latter step occurs in the mitochondrion. Ferrochelatase depends on the iron–transferrin cycle for the delivery of iron from plasma transferrin. In the bone marrow, when the iron supply is deficient, freely available zinc may be preferentially converted to zinc protoporphyrin rather than ferroprotohaem thus offering a convenient means to monitor iron-deficient erythropoiesis. Similarly, industrial lead exposure that inhibits both iron delivery and the activity of the sulphydryl enzyme ferrochelatase causes accumulation of zinc protoporphyrin and free protoporphyrin in erythroid precursors and reticulocytes. Deficiency of ferrochelatase leads to the accumulation of free protoporphyrin in liver tissue, plasma, and the skin, where it induces marked photosensitivity. The accumulation of excess protoporphyrin in red cell precursors leads to the characteristic fluorocytes (young red cells containing excess free protoporphyrin) that are the easily recognized hallmark of patients with burning photosensitivity caused by protoporphyria.

The highly regulated control mechanism of haem biosynthesis ensures that the free concentrations of the toxic intermediates involved in the pathway are kept low unless there is a metabolic arrest at one of the biosynthetic reactions; under these circumstances an overproduction of the intermediate compounds occurs which can be used for diagnosis. This overproduction predisposes to the development of the particular clinical porphyric syndrome. A knowledge of the enzymatic steps and of the differential solubility of the haem precursors facilitates appropriate diagnostic testing for the precise identification of suspected porphyria. In principle, overproduction of the early precursors such as aminolaevulinic acid is a common feature of those syndromes associated with neurovisceral manifestations or acute attacks of porphyria. Aminolaevulinate, in particular, represents a common biochemical marker of such attacks and those syndromes that mimic the porphyrias such as hereditary tyrosinaemia type I and lead poisoning. In patients with cutaneous photosensitivity, overproduction of the formed porphyrin macrocycles can be detected also in plasma, urine, and faeces in which they are distributed according to their aqueous solubility (Table 4).

The profile of molecules that are overproduced in a given syndrome may be predicted from the level at which the enzymatic arrest occurs as flux through the pathway is stimulated by diminished negative feedback. In those porphyrias where the principal site of production appears to be in the liver, including the acute porphyrias and porphyria cutanea tarda, oscillations in the flux through the biosynthetic pathway as a result of regulatory effects from environmental or endogenous factors can occur very rapidly; indeed minute-to-minute oscillations in biosynthetic haem fluxes have been recorded in the liver. Thus in starvation and on challenge with xenobiotic reagents (which place a demand for the production of haem to meet the needs for new cytochrome formation), as well as with endogenous hormonal changes, enhanced flux through the pathway leads to toxic overproduction of 5-aminolaevulinic acid. By the same token, rapid repression of the haem biosynthetic pathway in the liver can be induced by the administration of exogenous haem—a useful agent in the control of acute attacks and which rapidly corrects the disturbed metabolism (see below).

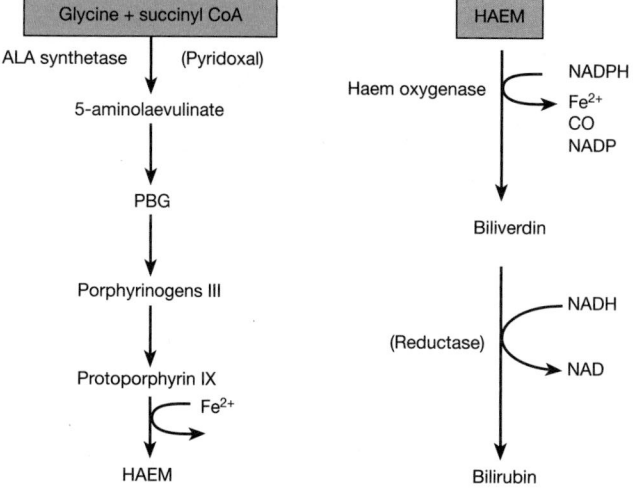

Fig. 1 Main pathways for haem biosynthesis and degradation in humans.

Table 4 Solubility and routes of excretion of haem precursors

	Plasma	Urine	Faeces
5-Aminolaevulinate	++	+++	−
Porphobilinogen	++	+++	−
Uroporphyrins I and III	+	++	+
Coproporphyrins I and III	+	+	+++
Protoporphyrin IX	+	−	+++

Haem formation in the erythron is more rapid than that in the liver but is not subject to sudden oscillations in synthetic rates. Nonetheless in patients with erythropoietic porphyrias, such as congenital porphyria, enhanced rates of red cell destruction when hypersplenism supervenes or in response to light exposure greatly exacerbate the overproduction of porphyrin intermediates and aggravate photosensitivity due to increased porphyrin release. Short-term experiments indicate that exogenous haem may partially repress the endogenous haem biosynthetic pathway in erythroid tissue but this has not proved to be useful for long-term relief in the erythropoietic porphyrias. Blood transfusion to suppress erythropoiesis or definitive replacement of bone marrow by transplantation has, however, proved to be successful in controlling the devastating manifestations of congenital erythropoietic porphyria.

Pathogenesis

The individual porphyria syndromes are described briefly below but the main manifestations (neurovisceral or phototoxic) remain the subject of further clinical research.

Acute neurovisceral attacks

These attacks occur in four of the porphyrias indicated in Tables 1 to 3. In all but one, Doss porphyria (aminolaevulinate dehydratase deficiency), the inheritance is as an autosomal dominant disease. 5-Aminolaevulinate dehydratase deficiency is inherited as an extremely rare recessive condition. Clinical expression is characterized by acute, life-threatening attacks of neuropathy that include abdominal pain, psychiatric symptoms, signs of sympathetic and hypothalamic autonomic overactivity, sometimes accompanied by convulsions and motor and sensory deficits. The syndrome is characteristically precipitated by drugs that induce hepatic haem formation and are metabolized by the hepatic cytochrome P-450 system. Neuropathological examination shows axonal degeneration and central chromatolysis in anterior horn cells and in the brain. Electromyography may reveal denervation compatible with a primary axonal neuropathy of peripheral nerves.

Although this acute porphyria is associated with lone overproduction of 5-aminolaevulinic acid, common to all those associated with acute manifestations, a toxic effect of this precursor is not the only potential mechanism of injury. The structure of aminolaevulinate is analogous to the inhibitory neurotransmitters γ-aminobutyric acid and L-glutamate. It seems likely that 5-aminolaevulinate may interfere with the action of the GABA-ergic system—the best evidence for which appears to be its ability to inhibit melatonin production in the rat pineal gland *in vivo*, as has been described in patients with recurrent acute porphyric attacks. It has been further postulated that under the conditions of the acute attack there may be a deficiency of essential haem proteins, such as the cytochrome P-450 isozymes in the liver, with further disturbances in secondary metabolism; other possibilities include a decrease in the activity of hepatic tryptophan dioxygenase, leading to increased formation of 5-hydroxytryptamine (serotonin).

At present there is no clear resolution between combined or individual effects of acute porphyria on the production of neurotoxic pseudotransmitters (aminolaevulinate) or secondary local deficiency of haem. However, early unpublished but apparently beneficial results of liver transplantation in patients with disabling recurrent attacks of acute intermittent porphyria indicate that the principal cause of the acute syndrome is the hepatic overproduction of toxic haem precursors. In any event, there is convincing evidence of abnormal neurotransmitter function and increased serotonin production—as well as direct interference of GABA receptors by toxic concentrations of 5-aminolaevulinate. Supplying exogenous haem during the acute attack, however, would be expected to correct both arms of this disturbed metabolism, which may account for the beneficial biochemical and clinical effects observed with its use. The recent development of a mouse model of porphyrinogen deaminase deficiency showing sensitivity to barbiturates serves as an authentic model of the biochemical and neuropatho-

logical manifestations of acute porphyria and may clarify much about the pathogenesis of this disturbing clinical syndrome. Detailed observations of the effects of hepatic transplantation in acute human porphyrias are also eagerly awaited.

Photosensitivity

Porphyrins absorb light maximally in the Soret region (400 to 420 nm) and in the visible wavelength region (between 500 and 600 nm); they re-emit this light energy at lower wavelengths to give pink, orange, or red fluorescence. This fluorescence is associated with the photodynamic effects and excitation to form triplet states; in the presence of oxygen in biological tissues, transfer of electronic energy leads to the generation of reactive oxygen species, including singlet oxygen, leading to complement activation and cutaneous toxicity. Careful studies examining the photoactive spectrum of skin from patients with various porphyrias has confirmed a cause-and-effect relationship between irradiance within the absorbing wavelength range of the given porphyrin and the development of weal-and-flare and other cutaneous phototoxic responses.

Distinct porphyric syndromes are associated with the accumulation of a particular formed macrocyclic porphyrin, each with its particular solubility properties in plasma and in cell membranes. In porphyria cutanea tarda, skin biopsies show subepidermal bullas and electron microscopy reveals vacuoles in the cells of the superficial dermal epithelium. In this disease, as in protoporphyria, the endothelium of the dermal capillary is thickened and the vessels are surrounded by complement and mucopolysaccharide deposits. In protoporphyria, an adequate oxygen supply has been shown to be critical for the development of experimental phototoxicity *in vivo*. Singlet oxygen and other radicals may lead to lipid peroxidation and cross-linking of membrane proteins with activation of late complement components. In the more severe disease, congenital erythropoietic porphyria, egress of uroporphyrin I from circulating erythrocytes, which may be destroyed within capillaries, leads to gross accumulation of porphyrin in dermal tissue and juxtaposed epithelium. Exposure to light is known to promote photohaemolysis indicating that light of the visible wavelength can penetrate the skin sufficiently to induce porphyrin photoactivation *in situ*.

Induction of acute porphyric attacks

Acute attacks of porphyria may be life-threatening illnesses which occur in genetically predisposed individuals who usually remain asymptomatic. The acute episodes develop on exposure to environmental or endogenous factors that place a demand for hepatic haem biosynthesis which leads to the overproduction of porphyrin intermediates and pyrrole precursors. The most frequent precipitating factors are changes in reproductive steroid hormones either due to natural hormone cycles or the administration of exogenous gonadal steroids. Starvation, including that associated with surgical procedures and anaesthesia, intercurrent infections, and many xenobiotics including alcohol as well as prescription drugs, over-the-counter agents, and chemicals present in health foods can precipitate acute porphyria.

Tables 5 and 6 list drugs that have been classified as unsafe in the porphyrias either because they have been shown to be porphyrinogenic in animals or *in vitro* studies, or have been associated with acute attacks in patients with porphyria. The table is taken from the British National Formulary published by the British Medical Association and the Royal Pharmaceutical Society of Great Britain. It is pointed out in this publication that slight changes in the chemical structure can lead to marked differences in the ability of the drug to induce attacks of porphyria. A more complete list of drugs is provided in a review by Anderson *et al.* (2001) in the Further reading section.

Acute attacks of porphyria occur in the four conditions known as the hepatic porphyrias and particularly occur for the first time in latent carriers who are aged between 15 and 40 years. Attacks have been recorded in children before puberty but are extremely rare and usually occur during febrile

Table 5 Drug classes unsafe in acute porphyrias (some class members may be used)

Amphetamines
Anabolic steroids
Antidepressants (tricyclic and monoamine oxidase inhibitors)
Antihistamines
Barbiturates
Benzodiazepines
Cephalosporins
Steroid contraceptives
Diuretics
Ergot derivatives
Gold salts
Hormone replacement therapy
Progestagens
Sulphonamides
Sulphonylureas

For individually unsafe drugs see Table 6.
From the British National Formulary (2001).
Published by the British Medical Association and Royal Pharmaceutical Society of Great Britain.

illnesses precipitated by the use of porphyrinogenic cough medicines. Although the porphyrias occur in a latent state in men with a frequency that is equal to that in women, women suffering from acute porphyria outnumber men by at least 2:1.

Clinical features of acute porphyria

The clinical manifestations of an acute attack are very diverse and the condition may be indistinguishable from many other disorders. In Table 7 are listed common neurovisceral symptoms of acute porphyric attacks and of these abdominal pain is the most common, but not invariable, presenting symptom. The pain itself may be difficult to identify since it is usually constant but poorly localized and usually unassociated with tenderness. There may be an associated colicky component and later ileus with abdominal distension which may mimic a surgical emergency. Characteristically, constipation occurs but diarrhoea with increased borborygmi may develop. The patient often becomes very distressed and tachycardia is common.

A frequent feature is the development of pain in the limbs, particularly in the upper thighs, but also in any of the somatic muscles of the chest, lumbar region, shoulders, and neck. Ultimately, muscle weakness and respiratory paralysis may occur. The patient becomes restless or frankly disturbed and deluded as in a toxic confusional state. The inability of

Table 6 Individual drugs unsafe in acute porphyria

Alcohol	Erythromycin	Nifedipine
Aluminium-containg antacids	Ethamsylate	Nitrofurantoin
Aminoglutethimide	Ethionamide	Orphenadrine
Amiodarone	Ethosuximide	Oxybutynin
Azopropazone	Etomidate	Oxycodone
Baclofen	Fenfluramine	Oxymetazoline
Bromocriptine	Flucloxacillin	Oxytetracycline
Busulphan	Flupenthixol	Pentazocine
Captopril	Griseofulvin	Phenoxybenzamine
Carbamazepine	Halothane	Phenylbutazone
Carisoprodol	Hydralazine	Phenytoin
Chloral hydrate	Hyoscine	Piroxicam
Chlorambucil	Isometheptene mucate	Prilocaine
Chloramphenicol	Isoniazid	Pyrazinamide
Chloroform	Ketoconazole	Ranitidine
Clonidine	Lignocaine	Rifabutin
Cocaine	Lisinopril[a]	Rifampicin
Colistin	Loxapine	Simvastatin
Cyclophosphamide	Mebeverine	Sulphinpyrazone
Cycloserine	Mefenamic acid	Sulpiride
Cyclosporin	Meprobamate	Tamoxifen
Danazol	Methotrexate	Theophylline
Dapsone	Methyldopa	Thioridazine
Dexfenfluramine	Metoclopramide	Tinidazole
Dextropropoxyphene	Metyrapone	Triclofos
Diclofenac	Miconazole	Trimethoprim
Doxycycline	Mifepristone	Valproate
Enconazole	Minoxidil	Verapamil
Enflurane	Nalidixic acid	Zuclopenthixol

From the British National Formulary (2001).
Published by the British Medical Association and Royal Pharmaceutical Society of Great Britain.
[a] In previous editions. This author has associated the agent with induction of porphyria.
The following drugs are thought to be safe in acute porphyrias:
Antihistamines: cetirizine, chlorpheniramine, cyclizine.
Diuretics: acetazolamide, amiloride, bumetanide, cyclopenthiazide, triamterene.
Ergot derivatives: oxytocin is probably safe.
Sulphonylureas: glipizide.
Analgesics: morphine, diamorphine, codeine, dihydrocodeine, fentanyl, and pethidine are safe.
Tranquillizers: chlorpromazine, haloperidol.
Local anaesthetics: bupivacaine, lignocaine can be used with caution.
Antimicrobials: rifamycins have been used without ill effect in some patients.

Table 7 Clinical manifestations of acute
porphyria

Abdominal pain
Vomiting
Constipation
Limb, head, neck, and chest pain
Muscle weakness
Sensory loss
Hypertension
Tachycardia
Convulsions
Respiratory paralysis
Fever
Psychiatric symptoms

attending medical personnel to identify the cause of the pain and the distress associated with it often leads to alienation and an exaggeration of the
patient's complaints which may be difficult to diagnose: often a suggestion
of hysterical conversion syndrome or worse, malingering, is made by
attending staff. Hypertension, sweating, and tremor together with tachycardia indicate marked sympathetic overactivity and cardiac arrythmias
may ensue. In about 10 per cent of severe attacks, grand mal seizures
develop; treatment of which may prolong the attack, since many anticonvulsants are porphyrinogenic. With sustained attacks there may be signs of
a peripheral neuropathy which is related to axonal degeneration, principally affecting motor nerves. Peripheral neuropathy in its early stages may
not affect the limb and tendon reflexes but with time these will be decreased
or absent. Ultimately, progressive muscle weakness affecting the respiratory
muscles, diaphragm, and swallowing may lead to paralysis and death in
prolonged attacks in which the institution of lifesaving cardiorespiratory
resuscitation measures and intensive care assessment is delayed.

In a full-blown attack, mental symptoms including anxiety, sleeplessness, and depression may be prominent. If the porphyric attack is sustained
as a result of inadequate management or diagnosis, progressive alienation,
visual and auditory hallucinations, and frank paranoia with progressive
and homicidal outbursts may occur. These are extremely difficult to contain within the routine environment of the busy acute hospital. Although
seizures may be a presenting sign of the acute attack, they are commonly
attributable to marked hyponatraemia resulting from the inappropriate
secretion of antidiuretic hormone that itself originates from hypothalamic
sympathetic overactivity. Treatment of hyponatraemia due to this cause in
the acute attack poses special difficulties (see below). The use of large volumes of hypotonic dextrose has in the past often aggravated the hyponatraemia and seizures—as well as cerebral odema.

Diagnosis of the acute attack is suspected on the basis of the past history
including photosensitivity or the intermittent discoloration of urine. There
may be a history of abdominal pain in first-degree family members, with or
without photosensitivity. Confirmation of an acute attack of porphyria
requires the demonstration of increased porphyrin precursors in the urine.
Most commonly, increased excretion of the monopyrrole, porphobilinogen, is accompanied by increased excretion of urinary 5-aminolaevulinate.
However, porphobilinogen excretion is not increased in the rare aminolaevulinate dehydratase deficiency nor in the pseudoporphyria of lead poisoning.

Acute attacks of porphyria appear to be more common in women as a
result of changes in reproductive steroid hormones and many women who
suffer from periodic attacks do so in the 1 or 2 days before onset of menstrual bleeding; usually as the menopause approaches, the pattern of these
attacks may change or worsen, but with the onset of amenorrhoea, severe
attacks of porphyria almost invariably cease. Sometimes, acute attacks lasting a day or two may have their onset in the mid-menstrual period around
the time of ovulation. Many mild attacks of porphyria resolve spontaneously within a few days, either as a result of withdrawal of the precipitating
factor or of natural hormonal rhythms. Prolonged attacks usually result

from the interaction of adverse exogenous and endogenous cofactors and
may last for many weeks or even months. The ensuing neurological injury,
accompanied in severe attacks by bulbar and respiratory paralysis, may lead
to prolonged or even permanent disability. Experience shows that in many
such cases inappropriate drugs have been given to counter the early manifestations of the condition, for example analgesics, psychotropic drugs, and
anticonvulsants. Thus the initiating medical interventions ultimately prove
to be critical determinants of outcome where the diagnosis is not suspected
or, if known, is ignored.

Outcome

An early series showed that during the first acute attack of porphyria half
the patients died. However, perhaps as a result of better hospital facilities to
deal with severe or adverse outcomes, the mortality and effects of the disease in patients with acute attacks has improved. Reports from a single
centre reported that about three-quarters of patients with acute intermittent porphyria or variegate porphyria were able to lead normal lives after an
acute attack. Recurrent attacks of pain occurred only in a minority during a
period of prolonged follow-up; these recurrent attacks were most likely to
occur in the first 3 years.

The development of national centres for the treatment of porphyria, the
early detection of genetic predisposition in at-risk first-degree relatives, and
the dramatic reduction in prescriptions of porphyrinogenic drugs such as
barbiturates and sulphonamides, together with better treatment of acute
attack, are all responsible for the improved outcome. Nonetheless, acute
porphyria remains life-threatening and deaths or marked disability due to
prolonged, mismanaged, or undiagnosed attacks are all too frequent. Rapidly recurrent attacks of porphyria may be associated with severe motor
neuropathy and sustained hypertension; postural hypotension may result
from autonomic neuropathy. In severe cases, cranial nerve palsies, typically
affecting the facial nerve and the vagus nerve, occur. Ischaemia of the
occipital cortex during acute attacks has been associated in a number of
instances with failed recognition of colours or of human faces (aprosopag-
nosis) and cortical blindness.

Although it appears that progestogens are principally responsible for
cyclical or periodic attacks in women because they are more porphyrinogenic than oestrogens, pregnancy itself is not usually associated with
adverse outcomes in women at risk from acute attacks. However, drugs
such as metoclopramide that provoke attacks may be used mistakenly to
control gastrointestinal symptoms in pregnancy and thus place the woman
and her unborn infant at risk.

Individual porphyrias

Acute porphyrias

These are, in a descending order of frequency: acute intermittent porphyria, variegate porphyria, hereditary coproporphyria, and Doss porphyria
(aminolaevulinate dehydratase deficiency). The first three of these disorders occur in at-risk heterozygotes for a single mutant allele in the cognate gene as autosomal dominant traits; 5-aminolaevulinate dehydratase
deficiency is inherited as a very rare autosomal recessive trait.

The overall frequency of heterozygosity for acute porphyrias is estimated
to be 1 in 10 000 of the population, of whom only 1 in 5 to 10 will develop
an acute attack. In certain populations (South Africa and in the Lapps of
Northern Sweden) the frequency rises to 1 in 1000 of the population. In
South Africa, a high gene frequency results from the founder effects of the
migration of a Dutch settler in the seventeenth century. Variegate porphyria
has thus spread to all ethnic groups within the South African population,
molecular analysis of which confirms the presence of a single dominant
mutant allele of the protoporphyrinogen IX oxidase gene.

In the last decade or so there has been much interest in the identification
of very rare homozygous forms of porphyria where the presence of two

mutant alleles of the causative gene are generally responsible for severe clinical disease. In most instances, the condition is not truly homozygous since those individuals affected prove to be compound heterozygotes for two mutant alleles of the cognate gene rather than true homozygotes for the many discrete but rare mutations that occur in porphyria but which would only be expected to occur in consanguineous pedigrees.

Acute intermittent porphyria

This, the most frequent of the acute porphyrias, is caused by mutations in the porphobilinogen deaminase gene that maps to human chromosome 11q23 in which well over 100 mutations have been identified. Several widespread mutations have been identified in certain populations but the majority are reported in only one or two pedigrees.

Two isozymes of the human porphobilinogen deaminase enzyme occur in the tissues: an erythroid mRNA variant and a non-erythroid transcript that encodes 17 additional amino-acid residues in its N-terminus lead to synthesis of housekeeping ubiquitous isozyme and an erythroid-specific isozyme. Most mutations cause a decrease in the abundance as well as the activity of the porphobilinogen deaminase enzyme in all tissues. A small proportion of mutations associated with lack of the detectable protein product from the mutant allele are associated with reduction of the housekeeping isozyme but normal enzymatic activity of the erythroid-specific isozyme. Thus in such patients hepatic porphobilinogen deaminase activity may be reduced to approximately half normal values while the activity of the easily accessed red-cell enzyme is within the normal range.

A few mutations lead to the synthesis of a catalytically impaired but stable porphobilinogen deaminase protein from the cognate mutant allele but these appear to be in a minority. Molecular analysis of the porphobilinogen deaminase gene in patients with acute intermittent porphyria has been very valuable in establishing diagnosis of latent heterozygotes at risk in the affected family, for the provision of appropriate counselling and for the introduction of preventative strategies (see below).

Acute intermittent porphyria is characterized solely by acute porphyric attacks and cutaneous photosensitivity does not occur. In most instances the patients do not notice any change in their urine, although on standing, the increased excretion of pyrroles leads to the formation of coloured oxidation products of porphobilinogen (loosely called porphobilin) which may lead to obvious discoloration (Fig. 2 and Plate 1). During the increased excretion of porphyrin precursors, water-soluble porphyrins form as a result of non-enzymatic photochemical reactions induce a pink discoloration. During acute attacks, copious excretion of pyrrole precursors, including porphobilin, may occasionally give the urine a striking appear-

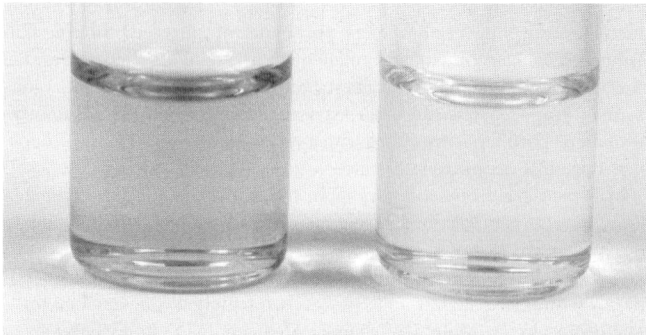

Fig. 2 Urine from a patient with acute intermittent porphyria around the time of an acute attack (left); control urine (right). A positive reaction with Ehrlich's diazo reagent is shown in the patient following the addition of 50 µl of urine to 1 ml of 2 per cent acidic dimethyl benzaldehyde. Subsequent tests showed that the pink diazo adduct was insoluble in chloroform and other organic solvents indicating the presence of excess porphobilinogen. (Urobilinogen in excess may give a positive reaction with the diazo reagent but the product is readily extracted into organic solvents.) (See also Plate 1.)

ance resembling blackcurrant juice or strong solutions of potassium permanganate.

The incidence and severity of acute attacks in acute intermittent porphyria and variegate porphyria are generally greater than in hereditary coproporphyria. Various estimates indicate between 1 in 10 to 1 in 5 of heterozygotes experience acute attacks of porphyria during their lifetime. However, increasing use of molecular diagnostic methods for screening at-risk families, institution of appropriate avoidance, and the careful dissemination of information to family members and their medical advisers will further reduce the likelihood of disease in latent gene carriers. Latent carriers of acute intermittent porphyria have a high frequency of hypertension and although this should be treated, the potential for inducing attacks is increased by the uninformed prescription of antihypertensive drugs. A proportion of subjects appear to suffer depression and other chronic mental symptoms and at least one survey has reported an increased prevalence of acute intermittent porphyria in patients attending long-stay psychiatric facilities—again putting them at risk from the ill-considered use of porphyrinogenic neuroleptic and other psychoactive drugs.

Variegate porphyria

Variegate porphyria is particularly frequent amongst South African white people and other ethnic groups within that country. The condition is associated with typical acute attacks of porphyria as well as skin manifestations (the van Rooten skin). Acute attacks of porphyria occur very much as in acute intermittent porphyria. More than half the patients come to medical attention with skin lesions alone; in the same series only one-fifth of patients had acute neurovisceral disease and a similar proportion had acute attacks as well as cutaneous disease.

Cutaneous photosensitivity resembles that seen in porphyria cutanea tarda and hereditary coproporphyria (see below) with fragility, milia, hyperpigmentation, and hairiness of light-exposed skin. During acute sunlight exposure, vesicles and even large bullas may form. Microscopic examination of the affected skin shows deposits of immunoglobulin and hyaline material that stains positively with the periodic acid–Schiff reagent in the dermal capillaries with proliferation of the basal lamina. As with porphyria cutanea tarda, ingestion of reproductive steroid, for example the oral contraceptive pill, may induce the cutaneous manifestations of variegate porphyria in otherwise latent heterozygotes.

A few severely affected patients with variegate porphyria have inherited mutations of the protoporphyrinogen oxidase gene (that maps to chromosome 1q22 to 1q23) from each parent, leading to homozygous 'dominant' variegate porphyria. These individuals present in childhood with a severe phenotype associated with marked photosensitivity, convulsions, and developmental delay; they have several skeletal abnormalities including medially deviated and shortened fifth digits. Developmental retardation is prominent, but surprisingly such patients appear to have few if any attacks of acute porphyria.

Hereditary coproporphyria

This condition is an infrequent and often mild form of acute porphyria which may be associated with cutaneous manifestations. It is due to mutations in the coproporphyrinogen III oxidase gene that maps to chromosome 3q12 and is transmitted as an autosomal dominant trait of low penetrance. The condition usually presents with acute attacks of abdominal pain as with the other acute porphyrias and about 30 per cent of patients develop cutaneous photosensitivity. As with several other porphyrias, several children presenting with marked photosensitivity in childhood have been shown to have inherited a mutant allele of the coproporphyrinogen III oxidase gene from each parent giving rise to so-called homozygous dominant hereditary coproporphyria. Particular mutations in the gene are usually restricted to individually infected pedigrees. As with the other acute porphyrias, molecular analysis of the coproporphyrinogen III oxidase gene may be of value in identifying at-risk heterozygotes for genetic counselling and provision of appropriate advice about the prevention and management of symptomatic disease.

5-Aminolaevulinate dehydratase deficiency (Doss porphyria)

Only a few affected homozygotes for this condition have been identified. Molecular analysis of the cognate gene has revealed the presence of compound heterozygosity and homozygosity for point mutations in the gene which maps to chromosome 9q34. As with the porphobilinogen deaminase gene, there are two promoter regions and alternative non-coding exons that allow for the synthesis of housekeeping and erythroid-specific transcripts. Less than 10 cases of this porphyria have been reported but it seems likely from the individual case histories of those identified that the disease will be underrecognized as the cause of acute abdominal crises usually presenting shortly after puberty and associated with neurological symptoms, including respiratory paralysis. The condition resembles acute lead poisoning. The urine contains an excess of 5-aminolaevulinate but excretion of porphobilinogen and tetrapyrrolic haem precursors is normal. Heterozygotes for aminolaevulinate dehydratase deficiency have been reported in at least one lead worker in whom peripheral neuropathy was ascribed to simple lead poisoning but it may have resulted from the susceptibility of the residual 5-aminolaevulinate dehydratase to inhibition by environmental lead.

Cutaneous porphyrias

Congenital erythropoietic porphyria is a classic but very rare syndrome now known to have an astonishing range of presentation from severe haemolytic anaemia *in utero*, severe photosensitivity presenting soon after birth (with excess porphyrins staining the teeth and urine), to mild late-onset forms presenting with skin lesions in adult life. Most patients have a mild to severe haemolysis with increased reticulocytosis, circulating normoblasts, decreased serum haptoglobin, and increased unconjugated bilirubin concentrations. Inclusion bodies are often seen in marrow, erythroid cells, and circulating normoblasts. Splenomegaly develops in childhood, thereby causing pancytopenia as a result of hypersplenism; this accelerates the haemolysis and leads to compensatory erythropoiesis in the bone marrow. Under these circumstances, splenectomy may help to control the condition.

The classic skin manifestations are of severe blistering lesions on sun-exposed skin, particularly of the hands and face, with the formation of vesicles and bullas that may become infected. There are pigmentary changes with greatly increased skin fragility. Healing of the lesions with or without consequential infection often leads to cutaneous deformities with loss of digits, scarring of the eyelids, nose, lips, scalp, and occasionally blindness due to corneal scarring. Examination of the teeth shows erythrodontia and deformities; exposure to ultraviolet light may reveal striking dental fluorescence. The condition is associated with osteoporosis and resorption of long bones as a result of gross expansion of the erythroid bone marrow.

Mutations in the uroporphyrinogen III synthase gene that maps to chromosome 10q25.3 to q26.3 have been shown to be responsible for this disease and thus may assist in the prenatal diagnosis of mothers harbouring an at-risk pregnancy and who have previously given birth to an affected infant. Constitutive activation of the haem biosynthetic pathway in erythroid cells leads to persistent overproduction of uroporphyrinogen I and coproporphyrinogen I as byproducts of the defective synthesis of uroporphyrinogen III, the sole precursor of protoporphyrin IX and haem. These reduced and colourless metabolites become oxidized to the fluorescent tissue and urinary porphyrins associated with the passage of pink urine that characterizes this often devastating disease.

Porphyria cutanea tarda

This disease is the most common of the cutaneous porphyrias and, unlike other hepatic porphyrias, is never associated with acute porphyric crises. The disease is characterized by skin blistering which is related to sunlight exposure. It occurs in several forms. Porphyria cutanea tarda may result from environmental exposure to dioxin or to hexachlorobenzene, particularly after industrial accidents such as that which occurred in Turkey in the

1960s. Occasional cases have been reported after exposure to other halogenated phenols but under these circumstances it appears simply to be an environmental toxic syndrome. Toxic cutaneous porphyria appears to be separate from the sporadic porphyria cutanea tarda which is precipitated by other specific environmental factors: increased hepatic storage iron, excess ethanol consumption, administration of oestrogens, hepatitis C virus infection, human immunodeficiency virus infection and possibly, nutritional deficiencies including antioxidants such as vitamin C.

Most individuals who develop sporadic porphyria cutanea tarda prove to have increased iron stores in association with the presence of one or more mutant alleles for the *HFE* gene that also predispose to the development of hereditary adult haemochromatosis. In addition, many patients with sporadic porphyria cutanea tarda consume excess alcohol and smoke. There is a clear association between porphyria cutanea tarda and renal impairment in which the development of disease can be explained by the presence of iron overload (as a result of defective iron utilization with or without routine iron supplementation, particularly in patients on haemodialysis) and failure to excrete excess plasma porphyrins that do not readily diffuse through the peritoneal cavity or haemodialysis membranes. In sporadic porphyria cutanea tarda there is a partial deficiency of uroporphyrinogen III decarboxylase activity in the liver and no family history of the condition. The sequencing of the human uroporphyrinogen decarboxylase gene that maps to human chromosome 1p34 has not provided any evidence of mutations to account for the tissue-specific enzyme deficiency and no isoforms of the enzyme have yet been identified. At the time of writing the molecular pathogenesis of sporadic porphyria cutanea tarda is unknown, but it is also clear that iron and other environmental influences inactivate hepatic uroporphyrinogen decarboxylase. The relationship between regulators of iron homeostasis and the demand for haem biosynthesis in the hepatocytes of affected individuals is not understood but it appears likely from studies in experimental animals that genetic variation in the expression and activity of cytochrome isozymes such as P-450 IA2 may be critical for disease expression. Irreversible inhibition of hepatic uroporphyrinogen decarboxylase may also explain the occurrence of toxic porphyria cutanea tarda after exposure to halogenated hydrocarbons, metabolites of which cause experimental uroporphyria in animals.

Less than one-quarter of patients who suffer from porphyria cutanea tarda show a familial susceptibility to the condition. In these cases, mutations occur in one allele of the human uroporphyrinogen decarboxylase gene leading to catalytic deficiency of the enzyme in all cells, including erythrocytes. In most instances the genetic defect leads to partial reduction of the enzyme protein encoded by the mutant allele. Studies of pedigrees affected by familial porphyria cutanea tarda indicate that expressivity of the trait is very low: less than 10 per cent of heterozygotes develop clinical disease. Conversely, a very few patients present with a syndrome that closely resembles congenital erythropoietic porphyria with marked blistering skin lesions, excess hair growth, and cutaneous scarring in association with the excretion of pink or red urine. These individuals represent a homozygous form of uroporphyrinogen decarboxylase deficiency, termed hepato-erythropoietic porphyria, associated with a variety of mutations in the uroporphyrinogen III decarboxylase gene.

In hepato-erythropoietic porphyria, the activity of uroporphyrinogen decarboxylase is markedly deficient although residual activity remains to preserve essential haem biosynthesis in the erythron and liver. Most patients with hepato-erythropoietic porphyria ultimately develop splenomegaly with accelerated haemolysis closely resembling congenital erythropoietic porphyria. Molecular analysis of the human uroporphyrinogen decarboxylase gene may assist the prenatal diagnosis of at-risk pregnancies in women who have already given birth to an affected infant.

The clinical features of porphyria cutanea tarda of whatever form are very characteristic and are confined to light-exposed skin (Fig. 3 and Plate 2). Most often, the only signs are of erosions resulting from minor trauma in skin with increased fragility as a result of light exposure, typically on the dorsum of the hands. Other changes include the development of large subepidermal bullae after exposure to light, which may burst leaving ulcerated

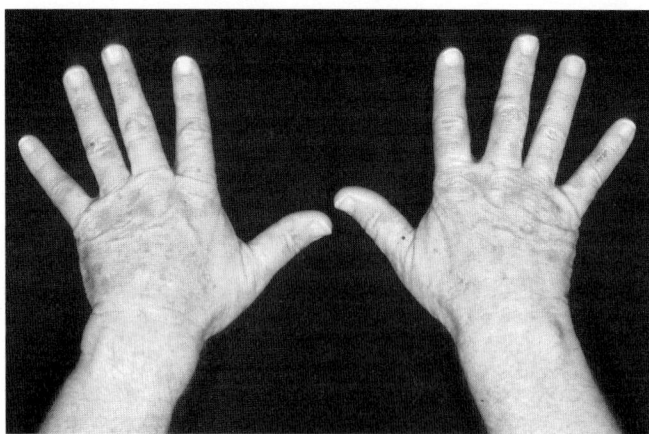

Fig. 3 Porphyria cutanea tarda in a 60-year-old heterozygote for the *HFE* C282Y mutation. This man, a taxi driver, had noticed irritation after exposure of his hands to light transmitted through the windscreen. He had noticed fragility and blistering combined with pigmentary changes typical of this disorder. After treatment by controlled phlebotomy his skin complaint has regressed. (See also Plate 2.)

lesions that are slow to heal. Increased, often accompanied by areas of decreased, pigmentation is a common feature combined with increased hair growth, particularly on the face.

Patients with porphyria cutanea tarda do not always notice the photosensitivity and rarely experience marked pain unless exposed to brilliant sunlight. Occasionally there is evidence of dermal injury and loss of nails, damage to the conjunctivae, and hair loss. Careful examination of the affected areas shows small depigmented cutaneous scars and the formation of milia. If bacterial infection occurs and there is repeated exposure to sunlight, then severe and permanent scarring may result. Typically, porphyria cutanea occurs in middle-aged men with a history of alcohol use and in women after institution of oestrogen replacement therapy: in young persons, infection with hepatitis C or the immunodeficiency virus may precipitate the disease expression. Frank signs of hepatomegaly or iron overload are rare in porphyria cutanea tarda but have been noted; as with adult haemochromatosis, there is a significantly increased frequency of hepatocellular carcinoma.

Occasional patients with porphyria cutanea tarda may notice an increase in urine excretion of formed porphyrins which, especially after concentration overnight, may resemble the colour of tea or cola. The stool and urine contains large quantities of copro-and uroporphyrins that fluoresce intensely on exposure to long-wavelength ultraviolet light when placed in a suitable vessel for its transmission (namely silica rather than standard glass). Similarly, examination of liver biopsy specimens under ultraviolet light reveals bright red/orange fluorescence; microscopical examination may also show coincidental hepatitis with or without excess deposits of stainable tissue iron reflecting the increased iron storage of this disease. In sporadic porphyria cutanea tarda, increased storage iron is reflected by modest elevations of serum ferritin that often occur in association with the presence of one or more copies of the C282Y allele of the *HFE* gene that maps to human chromosome 6 and which is associated with adult haemochromatosis.

Treatment

Sunlight exposure should be avoided as much as possible until the porphyrin abnormality is corrected. Care is needed to protect fragile skin from mechanical injury and from infection; sunblock creams may also be useful until the metabolic disturbance is controlled.

Patients with porphyria cutanea tarda should moderate or stop their intake of alcohol and avoid the use of iron tonics and sex hormones, especially oestrogens. Screening should be undertaken for chronic infection with human immunodeficiency virus and hepatitis viruses, especially hepatitis C. Management should include imaging or biopsy of the liver if serum

liver-related tests are abnormal as well as measurement of α-fetoprotein, since there is a risk of hepatocellular carcinoma in this disease.

Most patients with porphyria cutanea tarda respond to iron depletion by phlebotomy and initial iron status should be determined by measuring serum ferritin concentrations. Weekly or fortnightly removal of 500 ml of blood will usually correct the abnormal urine and plasma porphyrin profile within a few months but maintenance phlebotomy will be required, usually amounting to the removal of 2 to 4 units of blood at intervals each year. Successful therapy reduces the urinary excretion of porphyrins to normal. Patients with porphyria complicating renal failure should be treated with recombinant human erythropoietin and depleted of iron by gentle phlebotomy or parenteral desferrioxamine, if necessary.

The cutaneous manifestations of porphyria cutanea tarda respond rapidly to low-dose chloroquine treatment, which should be considered in patients with persistent symptoms or at the outset before iron storage has been fully corrected. This action of chloroquine was discovered empirically but the agent forms complexes with uroporphyrin deposits and promotes their external cellular disposal. Chloroquine promotes excretion of uroporphyrin from the liver and induces marked, but transient, porphyrinuria. Although chloroquine usually provides rapid relief from the cutaneous disease and photosensitivity, it does not correct the underlying metabolic defect in the liver; its long-term use is not recommended unless the other provocative factors in porphyria cutanea tarda have been removed. The usual effective dose of chloroquine is 100 to 200 mg once or twice weekly; larger doses are associated with marked hepatic toxicity in porphyria cutanea tarda. The drug is reported to have no therapeutic effect on other photosensitive porphyrias.

(Erythropoietic) protoporphyria

Protoporphyria is caused by the overproduction of the immediate precursor of haem, protoporphyrin IX, principally in the bone marrow. Protoporphyria causes an unusual cutaneous photosensitivity syndrome that presents in infancy. Protoporphyria is also a neglected cause of fatal hepatobiliary disease in about 5 per cent of those affected.

Recent studies indicate that protoporphyria is inherited as a recessive condition. Inheritance of mutations in the coding region of the ferrochelatase gene that partially inactivate the enzyme are coinherited in *trans* with a low-expression allele that occurs at polymorphic frequency in the population. Parent-to-offspring transmission of protoporphyria occurs in less than 10 per cent of cases but in all instances of the disease there is a marked deficiency of the enzyme ferrochelatase (less than 50 per cent of control values). The asymptomatic carrier parent shows only mild ferrochelatase deficiency. The gene for human ferrochelatase maps to chromosome 18q.

Protoporphyria characteristically presents with severe burning pain and cutaneous irritation on exposure to visible light and is usually obvious in infancy or early childhood. Erythema and diffuse oedema may follow marked light exposure but vesicles, blistering, and altered skin fragility are most unusual. After several years, increased pigmentation and thickening of the skin (lichenification) occur, especially over the knuckles. A typical feature is of shallow scarring in the malar regions of the cheeks and at the angle of the lips, where scarring is termed ragades. Overt scarring is unusual. There are no changes in urine colour. Protoporphyria is often the subject of delayed diagnosis because of the marked disparity between the severity of the symptoms and the development of physical signs in the skin.

The cutaneous pathology results from photoactivation of red-cell and plasma-derived protoporphyrin IX in skin capillaries (Figs 4, 5 and Plates 3 and 4). Protoporphyrin IX is a hydrophobic molecule that dissolves in cell membranes; it has a photoactivation spectrum in the Soret region with subsidiary activation by green and yellow light. Photoinjury is associated with complement activation and release of vasoactive factors; there is intracellular epidermal oedema accompanied by acute inflammatory changes and extravasated red cells. Deposits of hyaline material are found in superficial capillaries with thickening of the basement membranes. A supply of

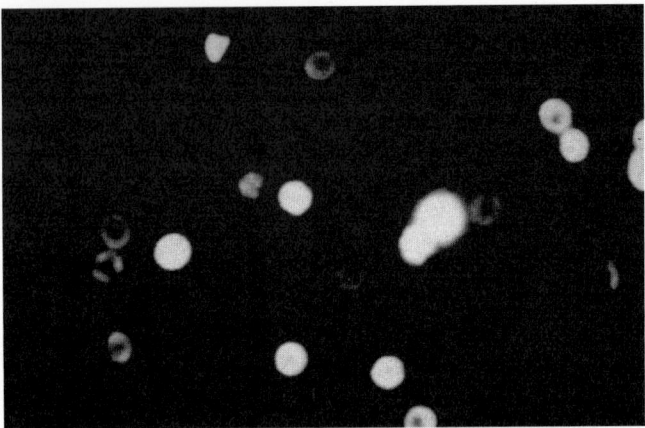

Fig. 4 Fluorescent microscopy of an unstained blood film from a patient with erythropoietic protoporphyria. Note the fluorescence of increased free protoporphyrin within individual young erythrocytes and reticulocytes. (See also Plate 3.)

oxygenated blood appears to be essential for the development of photosensitive damage in protoporphyria.

Mild hypochromic microcytic changes with mild anaemia are usually the only manifestation of disturbed haem biosynthesis and iron metabolism in the bone marrow, although examination of the marrow may reveal occasional sideroblasts with intramitochondrial iron deposits. Haemolysis is usually clinically insignificant until severe cholestatic hepatic disease occurs when splenomegaly and hypersplenism aggravate haemolysis. The photosensitivity worsens under these circumstances and there is upper abdominal pain with splenic enlargement, jaundice, and extreme photosensitivity as concentrations of free protoporphyrin in the plasma rise (Fig.

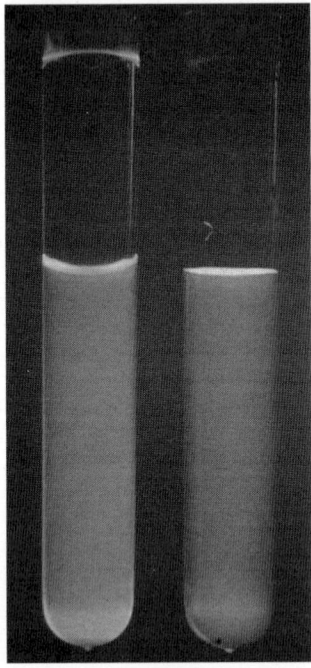

Fig. 5 Examination of human plasma under long-wave ultraviolet light. Plasma on the left was obtained from a patient with protoporphyrin hepatopathy and greatly increased photosensitivity and is compared with plasma obtained from a healthy subject on the right. Note the bright red fluorescence due to the presence of high concentrations of free protoporphyrin. Maximum fluorescence was obtained by exposure to visible light in the violet and green–yellow spectral regions corresponding to the absorbance bands of protoporphyrin.

5). A vicious cycle of decompensation is established with either fulminant hepatic failure associated with cholestasis due to protoporphyrin deposits within biliary radicals, or the development of cirrhosis. Without treatment, the prognosis is dismal and hepatic transplantation is required (see below).

Protoporphyric hepatic disease

Protoporphyria is normally associated with trivial abnormalities of serum liver-related tests but in a small proportion of patients micronodular cirrhosis with pigment deposition occurs. Examination of the liver under polarized light shows birefringent crystals with a characteristic Maltese cross appearance and examination under long-wave ultraviolet light reveals bright fluorescence. Gallstones containing precipitated protoporphyrin occur frequently in protoporphyria but cholestasis results principally from intracellular and cannalicular precipitation of protoporphyrin.

The principal source of protoporphyrin in protoporphyria is the erythron and although under emergency conditions hepatic transplantation may be effective, recurrence of protoporphyrin deposition with injury to the hepatic graft has been reported. The occurrence of this phenomenon, however, is not a contraindication to the use of hepatic transplantation when the illness requires it. Deteriorating hepatic disease is heralded by generalized abdominal pain, splenic enlargement, worsening jaundice, and haemolysis. Interruption of the enterohepatic circulation of protoporphyrin with charcoal or polymeric cationic resins such as cholestyramine may arrest the early downhill course by binding protoporphyrin or promoting hepatic bile acid secretion. However, once established, hepatic decompensation and accelerating photosensitivity is rapid.

Surgical management

Severe protoporphyrin hepatotoxicity is an indication for liver transplantation, preferably carried out by an experienced surgical team with the assistance of an informed anaesthetist and expert physicians in attendance. Consideration should be given to the simultaneous removal of the enlarged spleen at the time of the transplant procedure; there is evidence that splenectomy may reduced the haemolytic component of endstage protoporphyria.

In some patients with endstage liver disease due to protoporphyria, a bizarre neurological syndrome has been identified. In the perioperative period, axonal neuropathies requiring mechanical ventilation and cranial nerve palsies have been reported. Under these circumstances, coproporphyrin and uroporphyrins appear in the urine and may account for a blistering photosensitivity in endstage protoporphyric liver disease.

Operative treatment in patients with protoporphyria can be very dangerous as a result of phototoxic injury to visceral tissues and mucous membranes exposed to brilliant vertical lighting in the operating theatre. Surgical lights are best attenuated by the use of filters that reduce spectral power output below 530 nm; such precautions should be used throughout the perioperative period to reduce overall phototoxicity in the clinical environment. Theoretically, the definitive therapy of protoporphyria will require restoration of erythroid cell ferrocheletase activity in bone marrow. There is a single report of successful marrow transplantation in protoporphyria with coincidental myeloid leukaemia. This procedure cured the symptomatic protoporphyria. In future, either bone marrow transplantation or erythroid progenitor gene therapy will be used to correct this disease in patients suffering from life-threatening liver sequelae. Ancillary treatment by blood transfusion or red cell exchange transfusion will reduce the immediate source of plasma and red cell protoporphyrin, and in the immediate preoperative period plasmapheresis may also reduce phototoxicity. Neurological complications of fulminant protoporphyria may necessitate prolonged ventilatory support in the postoperative period.

Treatment of photosensitivity

Photosensitivity is managed by avoiding excessive light exposure, remembering that visible light of exciting green and violet wavelengths traverses ordinary window glass. Effective sunscreen preparations may assist management, especially in young children at risk. For many years β-carotene has been given to patients with protoporphyria. β-Carotene may absorb light energy at the appropriate wavelengths and also serve as a free-radical quenching agent. The preparation Lumitene (Hoffmann-LaRoche) at a dose of 120 to 180 mg/day is normally used. This causes orange staining of the skin due to carotenaemia but is otherwise well tolerated. It may improve tolerance to sunlight when plasma carotene concentrations between 10 and 15 μmol/l are achieved.

Treatment of an acute porphyric attack

It is essential to establish that the symptoms complained of are caused by an acute attack of porphyria. Of key importance is the careful laboratory analysis of urine and blood early in the course of the illness. This demonstrates elevated concentrations of porphyrins and haem precursors typified by elevated urinary 5-aminolaevulinate and porphobilinogen, which should be high in an attack of acute porphyria. The urine sample should be taken freshly from the patient and protected from light before analysis to avoid non-enzymatic conversion of the porphyrin precursors to porphyrins and hence misdiagnosis.

The immediate management of the acute attack of porphyria

This should involve scrupulous review of avoidable factors recently introduced that would have precipitated an attack. The precipitating factors are usually drugs, alcohol, exogenous or endogenous hormonal changes, fasting (including that due to dieting), or recent surgical procedures. More than 100 drugs may induce attacks of porphyria. Particular care should be taken to exclude agents that are obtained over the counter as tonics or herbal remedies, some of which may induce attacks. Tolerance of alcohol varies greatly in patients with porphyria, many of whom appear to tolerate modest amounts of alcohol. Alcohol is, however, best avoided. At the same time it is wise not to implicate alcohol in an acute attack, unless other causes have been excluded.

Abdominal pain and distress, together with anxiety, require prompt treatment: opiates which are safe in porphyria may be useful, although they often exacerbate constipation. Opiates may be combined with the phenothiazine tranquillizers, such as chlorpromazine, which may potentiate their action usefully.

Since starvation induces attacks of porphyria and haem biosynthesis may be suppressed by the ingestion of carbohydrate, it is advised that patients with minor attacks should eat regular meals containing carbohydrate in a complex form such as starch for its slow release. One-half to two-thirds of the energy intake should be derived from ingested carbohydrate. The management of an acute attack should involve repeated monitoring for the development of hyponatraemia, which may be very severe as a result of inappropriate secretion of antidiuretic hormone. In the past, intravenous glucose or fructose solutions have been advocated as a means to suppress haem biosynthesis in the liver. Great caution is needed in the use of these agents either as 5 or 20 per cent solutions since they exacerbate hyponatraemia and may cause fatal cerebral oedema. In the author's view, if the patient is sufficiently unwell not to be able to control the attack with oral carbohydrate-rich food, parenteral preparations of haem, such as haem arginate, rather than glucose or other sugar solutions, should be administered.

Haem therapy

Haem arginate is administered by a short intravenous infusion in porphyric crises of sufficient severity to merit hospital admission or those associated with limiting pain or metabolic disturbance. Haem arginate (Normosang) supplied by Orphan Europe (see below) is provided as a stable 25 mg/ml concentrate and should be administered at a dose of 3 mg/kg body weight once daily for up to 4 days to a maximum dose of 250 mg in 100 ml of physiological saline infused through a large antebrachial vein over at least 30 min. Haem arginate, like all preparations of haem, tends to polymerize and is unstable; thus the administration should be completed within 1 h after diluting the concentrate. The shelf-life of the concentrate is about 2 years. In the United States, haematin is supplied by Abbott Laboratories and appears to be a comparable preparation for suppressing hepatic haem synthesis and correcting the metabolic disturbance of the acute attack. Haem arginate and a preparation of haem albumin are apparently somewhat more stable than haematin, which tends to produce phlebitis or interfere with the action of coagulant proteins.

Recovery from an acute attack depends on the degree of damage to the nervous system and may occur within 1 or 2 days if haem therapy is introduced at the outset. Cast-iron proof of clinical benefit of haem treatment is lacking, but there is sufficient evidence for the beneficial use of therapy for it to be licensed in 19 countries, including the United Kingdom. Haem arginate therapy has a rapid effect on the excretion of aminolaevulinate and porphobilinogen in acute porphyria and retrospective studies suggest that the outcome of this treatment is better than that in patients previously documented before the use of the agent. Moreover, the results of a double-blind study comparing placebo and haem therapy showed a trend in favour of haem arginate in terms of duration of hospital stay and the requirement for pain relief but the differences did not quite reach statistical significance in the limited study of 12 patients. On the balance of probabilities, however, the evidence for a beneficial effect of haem arginate therapy, particularly at the onset of a porphyric attack, is very strong.

Haem therapy should be used in any patient with significant hyponatraemia, incipient neuropathy, seizures, or bulbar paralysis and in any patient with severe symptoms, particularly of abdominal pain. It must be recognized that patients with established neuropathy may take many months or even years to recover from an attack and, if it is to be effective, haem therapy should be introduced sufficiently early to halt its progress. Where haem therapy is not available, parenteral carbohydrate loading is the only alternative treatment for the acute attack: 2 litres of a 20 per cent w/v glucose solution is recommended over a 24-h period administered through a central venous catheter. There are risks from giving such therapy as outlined above and in the author's opinion the treatment has been superceded by the introduction of stable preparations of haem. Hypersensitivity reactions to haem arginate are rare and the drug has been used during attacks in pregnant women without injury to either the mother or child. Haem contains 10 per cent by weight of iron and the maximum daily dose of haem arginate would contain only 23 mg of elemental iron; the development of iron storage disease is therefore unlikely, except in very rare instances where the patient receives numerous infusions of haematin over prolonged periods.

Occasional patients, usually women, are seen in whom repeated acute attacks occur irrespective of the use of one or two courses of haem arginate. The reason for this is unknown but it is possible that haem arginate therapy induces tachyphylaxis as a result of exaggerated oscillation of haem catabolism by the induction of haem oxygenase in the liver. For this reason tin-protoporphyrin, an inhibitor of haem oxygenase, has been considered. This agent is only available in specialist centres and, because it contains toxic heavy metal and itself may induce photosensitivity, is currently not recommended for routine use. Recently, the combination of recurrent life-threatening porphyric attacks and poor venous access for administration of therapeutic haem preparations has led to the use of liver transplantation in a few young women stricken by this disease. Early (unpublished) reports indicate that this approach may, under exceptional circumstances, be successful.

Young women with cyclical porphyric attacks may require hormonal intervention by the use of gonadotrophin-releasing hormone analogues such as goserelin or buserelin for the release of gonadotrophins. These agents inhibit androgen, oestrogen, and progestogen production—as a result they induce menopausal-like symptoms and depression, as well as rapid decreases in trabecular bone density. Doses sufficient to suppress luteinizing and follicle-stimulating hormone concentrations in serum are required. Their prolonged use for more than a few months is not recommended but buserelin may be used intranasally and may be more convenient. To avoid the worse aspects of hypogonadism in women, low-dose oestrogen therapy under appropriate gynaecological supervision may be coadministered, once cyclic porphyric attacks have come under control. Hypertension is frequent in porphyric attacks and may be very severe as a result of sympathetic overactivity; during the attack, sinus tachycardia is frequent. β-Blockers are effective in the control of the hypertension and propanolol is safe; it also provides effective relief of sinus tachycardia.

Hyponatraemia may be very severe and in acute porphyria progresses on a daily basis during the course of the acute attack in most patients. Its management is critical and the rapid onset of severe hyponatraemia clearly contributes to the confusion and other mental symptoms associated with a porphyric attack. Prompt treatment by careful adjustment of fluid balance and fluid restriction is needed. Great care should be exercised in the presence of hyponatraemia with the use of intravenous solutions whose prescription should be reviewed frequently. The temptation to place a patient with abdominal pain on a surgical ward and administer a dilute solution of glucose is very great in current hospital practice: in the porphyric attack such management may contribute to death as a result of cerebral oedema or the complications of rapid-onset hyponatraemia. Where hyponatraemia progresses rapidly despite fluid restriction, once the diagnosis of inappropriate secretion of antidiuretic hormone is confirmed by determining urine and plasma osmolalities, hypertonic saline solutions or fluid restriction may be required for its correction.

Grand mal seizures in acute porphyric attacks pose a particular problem for management; they are often precipitated by hyponatraemia that frequently complicates the acute attack. Clearly appropriate management of the electrolytic abnormality (with the potential for life-threatening cerebral oedema) is an essential element of treatment. Status epilepticus poses special difficulties but has been treated successfully with parenteral diazepam or the related benzodiazepine, temazepam. Carbamazepine, lorazepam, and midazolam are probably (but not definitely) safe in acute porphyria. Clonazepam or valproate have been used for seizure prevention; the generally outmoded therapy of bromide may also have a role. Acetazolamide, which has been used as a minor agent in seizure prophylaxis, has been used safely in acute porphyria but many first-line drugs such as carbamazepine, sodium valproate, phenytoin, and chloral hydrate have been classified as unsafe or are frankly porphyrinogenic. Primidone and phenobarbitone are absolutely forbidden.

Further problems arise in the management of acutely disturbed patients who are not responsive to the safe phenothiazine, chlorpromazine. Thioridazine is categorized as unsafe but parenteral haloperidol has been used with good effect in occasional patients with uncontrollable or life-threatening manic aggression and paranoid disturbance. In all instances, prescription of any agent to a patient who has suffered from or is suffering from an acute porphyric crisis must involve consultation with a reliable pharmacopoea with individual drugs categorized for safety.

The ability of most drugs to initiate attacks of porphyria appears in many instances to be related to their effects on the induction of haem biosynthesis in the liver and specifically for the formation of the relevant P-450 xenobiotic metabolizing isoforms. One key isoform involved in the induction of porphyria is inhibited, at least *in vitro*, by the H_2-antagonist, cimetidine. It has been reported that cimetidine at 400 to 800 mg daily is sufficient to inhibit induction of this P-450 isozyme in adult humans. Cimetidine has been administered with occasional success as a means to inhibit or control spontaneous porphyric crises and as a last resort it might be considered in patients with life-threatening, otherwise uncontrollable, disease.

There is particular difficulty in young or middle-aged women with cyclical premenstrual attacks. Treatment with high-dose gonadotrophins continued for 1 to 2 years is likely to abort the attacks, but given alone will cause distressing symptoms of hypogonadism with depression and osteoporosis. The worst symptoms of hypogonadism can be overcome by the use of low-dose oestrogen replacement, for example with oestrogen patches, which have a significantly lower risk of provoking an attack of porphyria than progestagen-only hormone preparations. Clearly there is a risk of unopposed oestrogen therapy in patients with an intact endometrium and monitoring for the effects in those receiving oestrogen will be needed.

Acute perimenstrual attacks can be controlled by the prompt administration of haem arginate for 1 to 2 days at the predicted time of susceptibility. Although tachyphylaxis has not been recorded, there may be difficulties in withdrawing the haem arginate because of its effect on inducing haem oxygenase and hence amplifying the potential oscillations of haem biosynthesis in the liver once the haem arginate is withdrawn. The potential for iron overload developing as a result of haem arginate is most unlikely owing to its low content of iron at the doses recommended. Some authors have suggested the use of the haem oxygenase inhibitor, tin-protoporphyrin as an adjunct to the use of haem arginate. Although this may induce a more prolonged biochemical remission of the abnormalities of an acute porphyric attack, it does not induce a more rapid depression of the biochemical abnormality. Experience with tin-protoporphyrin where tachyphylaxis of haem arginate is suspected has been favourable in a few patients, but the drug itself induces photosensitivity. Tin is also potentially toxic as a heavy metal of which only limited excretion occurs. At present the use of tin protoporphyrin or its cogener, zinc deuteroporphyrin must remain speculative and more experience is necessary before these agents can be recommended for safe use in the long-term management of patients with current porphyric crises. The role of liver transplantation and, ultimately corrective gene therapy directed to the liver in acute porphyrias, awaits fuller evaluation in animal models of these diseases and in the few porphyric recipients of hepatic allografts so far recorded.

Sources of information and addresses

British National Formulary, British Medical Association, Tavistock Square, London WC1H 9JP.

United Kingdom and Royal Pharmaceutical Society of Great Britain, 1 Lambeth High Street, London SE1 7JN.

The United Kingdom Drug Information Pharmacists Group website: http://www.ukdipg.org.uk

Haem arginate (Normosang) is manufactured by Leiras Medica, PO Box 415, SF 20101, Turku, Finland supplied in the United Kingdom by Orphan Europe (UK) Ltd, 32 Bell Street, Henley-on-Thames, Oxon RG9 2BH. Telephone: 44-(0)1491 414 333; Fax: 44-(0)1491 414 443; email: info.uk@orphan-europe.com

Patient associations

The British Porphyria Association, 14 Mollison Rise, Gravesend, Kent DA12 4QJ UK. Telephone: 44-(0)1474 350390.

The American Porphyria and Canadian Porphyria Foundations may also be accessed by the internet websites.

Additional information with emphasis on the molecular genetics of individual porphyrias may be found on the Online Mendelian Inheritance in Man (OMIM) website at ww.ncbi.nlm.gov/omim.

Warning jewellery: it is often valuable in patients with acute porphyrias for them to have a wrist bracelet or neck pendant that provides information about diagnosis in medical emergencies. Details in the United Kingdom can be obtained from The MedicAlert Foundation, 12 Bridge Wharf, 156 Caledonian Road, N1 9UU. Telephone: 44-(0)207 833 3034.

Further reading

Anderson KE *et al.* (1990). A gonadotrophin releasing hormone analogue prevents cyclical attacks of porphyria. *Archives of Internal Medicine* **150**, 1469–74.

Anderson KE *et al.* (2001). Disorders of heme biosynthesis: X-linked sideroblastic anemia and the porphyrias. In: Scriver CR *et al.*, eds. *The metabolic and molecular bases of inherited disease*, 8th edn, Vol II, pp

2991–3062. McGraw-Hill, New York. [This is a most comprehensive and up-to-date account of the human biosynthetic pathway in relation to the porphyrias, a large section within a four-volume treatise on inborn errors of metabolism.]

Elder GH, Smith SG, Smyth SJ (1990). Laboratory investigation of the porphyrias. *Annals of Clinical Biochemistry* **27**, 395–412.

Elder GH, Hift RJ, Meissner PN (1997). The acute porphyrias. *Lancet* **349**, 1613–17.

Gorchein A (1997). Drug treatment in acute porphyrias *British Journal of Clinical Pharmacology* **44**, 427–34.

Kauppinen, R, Mustajoki P (1992). Prognosis of acute porphyrias: occurrence of acute attacks, precipitating factors, and associated diseases. *Medicine (Baltimore)***71**, 1–13.

Mustajoki P, Nordmann Y (1993). Early administration of heme arginate for acute porphyric attacks. *Archives of Internal Medicine* **153**, 2004–8.

Poh-Fitzpatrick MB (1985). Porphyrin-sensitized cutaneous photosensitivity: pathogenesis and treatment. *Clinics in Dermatology* **3**, 41–82.

Schmid R, ed. (1998). The porphyrias. *Seminars in Liver Disease* **18**, 1–101. [An accessible and comprehensive review of the molecular genetics, biochemistry, clinical features, and treatment of human porphyria.]

11.6 Lipid and lipoprotein disorders

P. N. Durrington

Lipids are a heterogeneous group of substances, including oils and fats, that are distinguished by their low solubility in water and their high solubility in non-polar (organic) solvents. The difference between an oil and a fat lies in its melting point. Lipids are essential as energy stores and respiratory substrates, as structural components of cells, as vitamins, as hormones, for the protection of internal organs, for heat conservation, for digestion, and for lactation. Lipoproteins are macromolecular complexes of lipid and protein; their principal function is to transport lipids through the vascular and extravascular body fluids and they are also found as components of milk. Lipoproteins include apolipoproteins and enzymes. Increased concentration of a circulating lipoprotein is termed hyperlipoproteinaemia and a decreased concentration is termed hypolipoproteinaemia. Disturbed composition of circulating lipoproteins is termed dyslipoproteinaemia.

Atherosclerosis is the context in which lipid disorders most commonly present to clinicians and this will be the principal focus of this chapter; undoubtedly lipoproteins will ultimately be implicated in many pathological processes.

Lipid physiology

Triglycerides (triacylglycerols)

These are formed by the esterification of glycerol with fatty acids, which have a hydrocarbon group attached to a carboxyl group. Generally the hydrocarbon moiety is present in a long chain. Naturally occurring fatty acids usually have even numbers of carbon atoms, most of them linked by single bonds, but some contain double bonds. Those with double bonds are termed unsaturated, whereas those with only single bonds are the saturated fatty acids. Fatty acids with one double bond are termed monounsaturated and those with more, polyunsaturated. Each double bond creates the possibility of two stereoisomers according to whether the hydrogen atoms of the –CH=CH– are both on the same side of the double bond (*cis*) or on the opposite sides (*trans*). Naturally occurring fatty acids are mostly *cis* isomers. *Trans* isomers are, however, present in the milk of ruminants, such as the cow, and in margarines.

Triglycerides in adipose tissue provide our principal energy store. The body of a 70 kg man contains some 15 kg of stored triglycerides, representing 135 000 kcal (560 000 J) of energy, which would permit survival during total starvation for up to 3 months (compare this with the 225 g of stored glycogen, representing only 900 kcal (3800 J)). Obesity represents an excess of stored fat, and it is unfortunate for those wishing to slim that considerable and very prolonged dietary energy restriction is necessary to lose weight, given the large amount of energy stored in fat. Each gram of triglyceride produces 9 cal (38 J) of energy, whereas the same mass of carbohydrate or protein only produces 4 cal (17 J), and the latter are more difficult to store because they require an aqueous environment. Thus a muscle or liver cell can only store a minimal amount of glycogen. The adipocyte, on the other hand, contains a droplet of hydrophobic triglyceride surrounded by only a tiny rim of cytoplasm: about 85 per cent of the adipocyte is triglyceride. Thus each gram of adipose tissue yields almost 8 cal (33 J) of energy, whereas tissues containing cells packed to capacity with glycogen would not even approach a yield of 1 cal (4.2 J) for each gram.

For other organs to utilize the energy in adipose tissue the stored triglyceride must first be hydrolysed to its constituent glycerol and non-esterified fatty acids, a process known as lipolysis. This is accomplished by adipose tissue lipase, an intracellular enzyme which is inhibited by insulin (not to be confused with lipoprotein lipase, an extracellular enzyme located on the vascular endothelium of fat and muscle and which is activated by insulin (see below)).

The products of lipolysis are released into the circulation and non-esterified fatty acids bind to albumin. The normally circulating concentration of non-esterified fatty acids is 300 to 800 μmol/litre (8–23 mg/dl), but this falls when insulin is secreted following a meal and rises in starvation when insulin secretion is low. Their importance as a system for transporting lipid energy should not be underestimated, even at low concentrations, since their half-life in the circulation is only 2 to 3 min and their turnover is thus 100 to 200 g/day, and even more in starvation or uncontrolled diabetes.

Non-esterified fatty acids can be oxidized to acetyl-CoA by some tissues, such as muscle and liver, and then entered into the Krebs (carboxylic acid) cycle. Other tissues, which in the fed state rely on glucose as an oxidative substrate, cannot directly utilize non-esterified fatty acids. During starvation these tissues are supplied with water-soluble ketone bodies (acetone, acetoacetate, β-hydroxybutyrate), which the liver produces by partial oxidization (β-oxidation) of non-esterified fatty acids transported to it from adipose tissue. These ketone bodies, which can readily be entered into the Krebs cycle by tissues lacking the ability to oxidize fatty acids, constitute the second system for the transport of lipid energy. They are vital for survival when dietary energy is at a premium, but are also the cause of diabetic ketoacidosis when insulin production is insufficient to suppress the flux of non-esterified fatty acids from adipose tissue, so that the production of ketone bodies takes place at a faster rate than they can be respired. The amount of insulin required to decrease blood glucose increases in the presence of high levels of circulating non-esterified fatty acids. The higher flux of non-esterified fatty acids out of adipose tissue in diabetes thus contributes to insulin resistance. In the case of non-insulin-dependent diabetes a high rate of release of non-esterified fatty acids may have pre-dated the development of hyperglycaemia by many years because obesity, which is a common antecedent of this type of diabetes, is itself associated with an increased flux of non-esterified fatty acids through the circulation and with insulin resistance.

Phospholipids

These also have at least one fatty acyl group esterified to an alcohol and one phosphate group linked both to the alcohol and to another organic compound. The glycerolipids have glycerol as the alcohol. Examples of these are phosphatidylcholine (lecithin) and lysophosphatidylcholine (lysolecithin). Another abundant class of phospholipids are the sphingolipids, such as

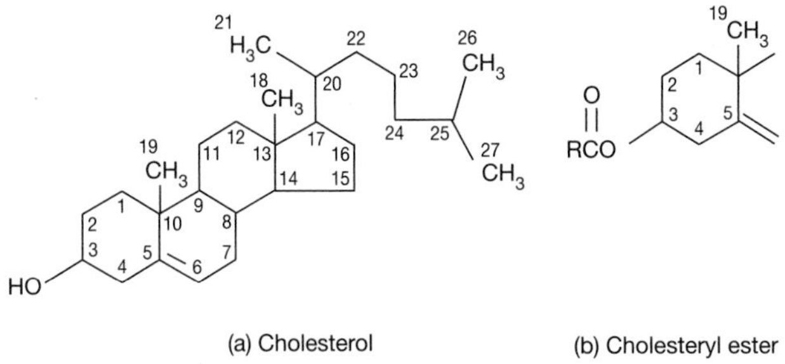

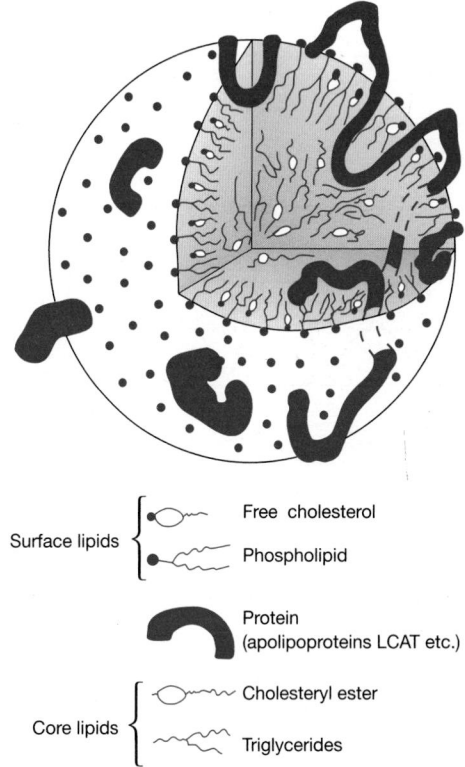

Fig. 1 The structure of free cholesterol and cholesteryl ester.

(a) Cholesterol   (b) Cholesteryl ester

sphingyomyelin. Phospholipids are essential components of cell membranes and, because of the great diversity of physical properties permitted by their structure, are responsible for much of the variation in membrane structure.

Cholesterol

Cholesterol is also an essential component of cell membranes, where it allows the phospholipid molecules to pack more closely, increasing membrane rigidity. It is also a precursor for the synthesis of steroid hormones, vitamin D, and bile acids. It is present in arterial fatty streaks and in atheromatous plaques (see below).

Cholesterol is an alcohol and may be unesterified as free cholesterol or esterified with a fatty acyl group (Fig. 1).

Lipoprotein physiology

Lipoprotein structure

The general structure of lipoprotein molecules is globular (Fig. 2). The physicochemical considerations, which govern the arrangement of their constituents, are similar to those involved in the formation of mixed micelles in the lumen of the intestine. Thus, within the outer part of the lipoprotein are found the more polar lipids, namely the phospholipids and free cholesterol, with their charged groups pointing out towards the water molecules. In physical terms, however, the role of bile salts, which are also in the outer layer in the mixed micelle, is assumed by proteins, so that the surface structure of a lipoprotein resembles the outer half of a cell membrane. Within the core of the lipoprotein particle are the more hydrophobic lipids, the esterified cholesterol and triglycerides. These form a central droplet to which are anchored, by their hydrophobic regions, the surface-coating molecules, phospholipids, free cholesterol, and proteins. The exception to this general structure is the newly formed or nascent high-density lipoprotein (**HDL**), which lacks the central lipid droplet and appears to exist as a disc-like bilayer consisting largely of phospholipids and proteins.

The protein components of lipoproteins are the apolipoproteins, a group of proteins of immense structural diversity, some of which have a largely structural role and others of which are important metabolic regulators. In addition, enzymes are found as components of lipoproteins. One example is lecithin:cholesterol acyltransferase which is located on HDLs, which are also its site of action.

Lipid transport from liver and gut to peripheral tissues

The products of fat digestion (fatty acids, monoglycerides, lysolecithin, and free cholesterol) enter the enterocytes from the mixed micelles. They are re-esterified in the smooth endoplasmic reticulum of these cells. Long-chain fatty acids (those with more than 14 carbon atoms) are esterified with monoglycerides to form triglycerides and with lysolecithin to form lecithin.

Free cholesterol is esterified by the enzyme acyl-CoA:cholesterol O-acyltransferase.

The triglycerides, phospholipids, and cholesteryl esters are then combined with an apolipoprotein, known as apoB$_{48}$, in the enterocyte. The lipoproteins thus formed are secreted into the lymph (chyle) as chylomicrons. These are large (diameter > 75 nm; density < 950 g/litre) and are rich in triglycerides but contain only relatively small amounts of protein (Fig. 3). They travel through the lacteals to join lymph from other parts of the body and enter the blood circulation via the thoracic duct. In addition to cholesterol absorbed from the diet, the chylomicrons may also receive cholesterol that has been newly synthesized in the gut or transferred from other lipoproteins present in the lymph and plasma. The newly secreted, or nascent, chylomicrons receive C apolipoproteins from HDL, which in that respect appears to act as a circulating reservoir, since later in the course of the metabolism of the chylomicron, the C apolipoproteins are transferred back to the HDL pool. The chylomicrons also receive apolipoprotein E (**apoE**), although the manner in which they do so is unclear. Unlike other apolipoproteins, which are synthesized either in the liver or the gut or both, apoE is exceptional in that it is synthesized (and perhaps secreted) by a large number of tissues: liver, brain, spleen, kidney, lungs, and adrenal gland.

Once the chylomicron has acquired the apolipoprotein, apoC-II, it is capable of activating lipoprotein lipase (Fig. 4(a)). This enzyme is located on the vascular endothelium of tissues with a high requirement for triglycerides, such as skeletal and cardiac muscle (for energy), adipose tissue (for storage), and lactating mammary gland (for milk). Lipoprotein lipase releases triglycerides from the core of the chylomicron by hydrolysing them to fatty acids and glycerol, which are taken up by the tissues locally. In this

Surface lipids
- Free cholesterol
- Phospholipid

Protein
(apolipoproteins LCAT etc.)

Core lipids
- Cholesteryl ester
- Triglycerides

Fig. 2 Lipoprotein structure. The most hydrophobic lipids (triglycerides, cholesteryl esters) form a central droplet-like core, which is surrounded by more polar lipids (phospholipids, free cholesterol) at the water interface. Apolipoproteins are anchored by their more hydrophobic regions, with their more polar regions often exposed to the surface. (Reproduced from Durrington (2002) with permission.)

way the circulating chylomicron becomes progressively smaller. Its trigly-ceride content decreases and it becomes relatively richer in cholesterol and protein. As the core shrinks, its surface materials (phospholipids, free chol-esterol, C apolipoproteins) become too crowded and they are transferred to HDL. The cholesteryl ester-enriched, triglyceride-depleted product of chy-lomicron metabolism is known as the chylomicron remnant. The $apoB_{48}$, present from the time of assembly, remains tightly anchored to the core throughout. The apoE also remains and regions of its structure are exposed, permitting chylomicron remnant catabolism via the 'remnant receptor' of the liver and also the low-density lipoprotein (**LDL**) receptors (also called $apoB_{100}$/E receptors), which can be expressed by virtually every cell in the body including the liver. Unlike the LDL receptor, which is dis-cussed in more detail later, the 'remnant receptor' is not downregulated by intrahepatic cholesterol and involves the LDL receptor-related protein, LRP, which in addition to its binding site for apoB also has receptor sites for other proteins. ApoE is inhibited from binding to its receptors earlier in the metabolism of chylomicrons because its receptor-binding domain is blocked by the apolipoprotein, apoC-III. Remnants are largely removed from the circulation by the liver. Although the clearance of these particles by the LDL receptor is theoretically possible, this route is not likely to con-tribute greatly to remnant uptake in the adult, since the binding of remnant particles to the LRP is enhanced by a trapping mechanism in the space of Disse and elsewhere the remnant particles must compete for binding to the

LDL receptor with LDL, the particle concentration of which is much higher than that of the chylomicron remnants (even more so in the tissue fluid than in the plasma). Also the LDL receptor is rapidly downregulated by the lysosomal release of free cholesterol into the cell, which follows the entry of lipoprotein–receptor complexes into the cell, whereas expression of the remnant clearance pathway is unaffected by entry of cholesterol into the liver.

The liver itself secretes a triglyceride-rich lipoprotein known as very low-density lipoprotein (**VLDL**) which allows the supply of triglycerides to tis-sues in the fasting state as well as postprandially. Very low-density lipoprotein particles are somewhat smaller than the chylomicrons (diam-eter 30–75 nm, density < 1006 g/litre). Once secreted, they undergo exactly the same sequence of changes as chylomicrons; that is the acquisition of apolipoproteins and the progressive removal of triglycerides from their core by the enzyme, lipoprotein lipase. However, some additional transform-ations are involved in their metabolism in the human. In man, the liver, unlike the gut, does not esterify cholesterol before its secretion. This pro-cess differs in species such as the rat. In the human, most of the cholesterol released from the liver each day into the circulation is secreted in the VLDL as free cholesterol, and it undergoes esterification in the circulation. Free cholesterol is transferred to HDL along a concentration gradient. There it is esterified by the action of lecithin:cholesterol acyltransferase, which esteri-fies the hydroxyl group in the 3-position of cholesterol to a fatty acyl group. This it selectively removes from the 2-position of lecithin to give lysoleci-thin. The fatty acyl group in this position is generally unsaturated and the cholesteryl esters thus formed are frequently cholesteryl oleate or choles-teryl linoleate. Familial lecithin:cholesterol acyltransferase deficiency is a very rare disorder, in which HDL fails to mature and circulating free choles-terol levels increase. It leads to anaemia, corneal opacities, proteinuria, and renal failure.

Esterified cholesterol on HDL is transferred back to VLDL. This cannot take place by simple diffusion, because cholesteryl ester is intensely hydro-phobic and because the concentration gradient is unfavourable. A special plasma protein, cholesteryl ester transfer protein or lipid transfer protein, transports cholesteryl ester from HDL to VLDL. It does this in exchange for triglycerides in VLDL and thus also contributes to the removal of core triglycerides from VLDL. The principal mechanism for the removal of tri-glycerides from VLDL is, however, lipolysis catalysed by lipoprotein lip-ase.

Another major difference between VLDL and chylomicrons is that the apolipoprotein B produced by the liver in man is not $apoB_{48}$ but is almost entirely $apoB_{100}$. As in the case of chylomicrons, the quantum of apoB packaged in the VLDL remains tightly associated with the particle until its final catabolism; its amount does not vary after secretion. It is probable that each molecule of VLDL contains one molecule of $apoB_{100}$. The $apoB_{100}$ produced in the liver contains the protein sequence necessary to bind to the LDL receptors, whereas that produced by the gut, although derived from the same gene, does not: a process of 'gene editing', which stops the ribo-some translating the messenger RNA before the receptor-binding sequence, leads to an apoB with 48 per cent of the molecular mass of that from the liver. Microsomal triglyceride transfer protein is essential for the process by which both $apoB_{48}$ and $apoB_{100}$ are packaged with triglyceride in the enter-ocyte and hepatocyte to form chylomicrons or VLDL respectively; this is defective in abetalipoproteinaemia (see below).

The circulating VLDL particles become progressively smaller as their core is removed by lipolysis and surface materials are transferred to HDL. In normal man most of the VLDL is converted to smaller LDL particles through the intermediary of a lipoprotein known as intermediate density lipoprotein (**IDL**). This has a density of 1006 to 1019 g/litre and contains apoE. In this latter respect it is similar to chylomicron remnants. In some species, such as the rat, it is largely removed by the hepatic receptors, and LDL formation is thus bypassed. The enzyme hepatic lipase may be important in the conversion of IDL to LDL.

In man, LDL particles, which are relatively enriched in cholesterol but are small enough (diameter 18–25 nm, density 1019–1063 g/litre) to cross

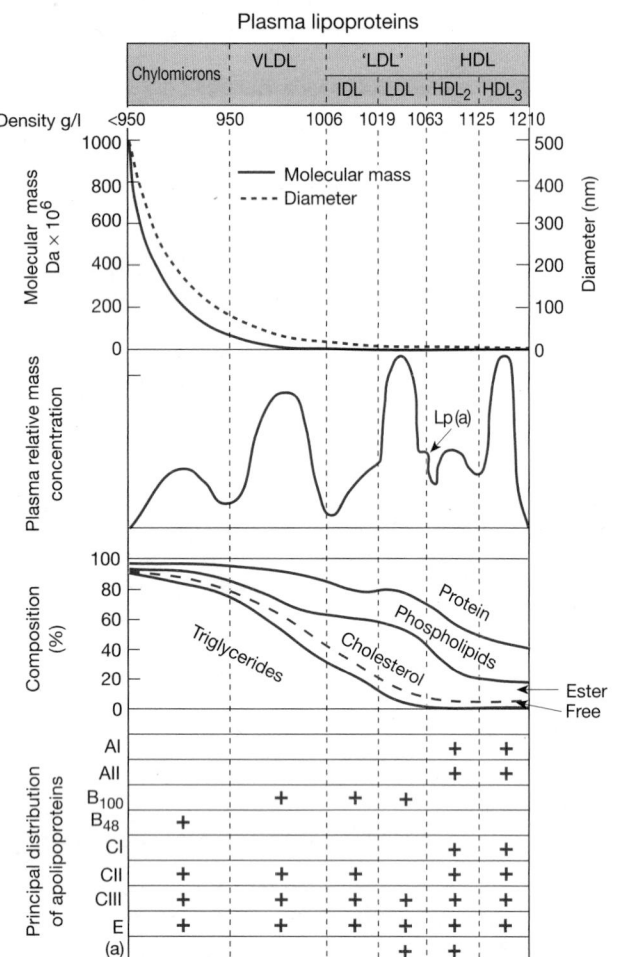

Fig. 3 The spectrum of plasma lipoprotein particles according to their hydrated density, molecular mass, molecular diameter, relative concentration, lipid composition, and apolipoprotein composition. (Reproduced from Durrington (2002) with permission.)

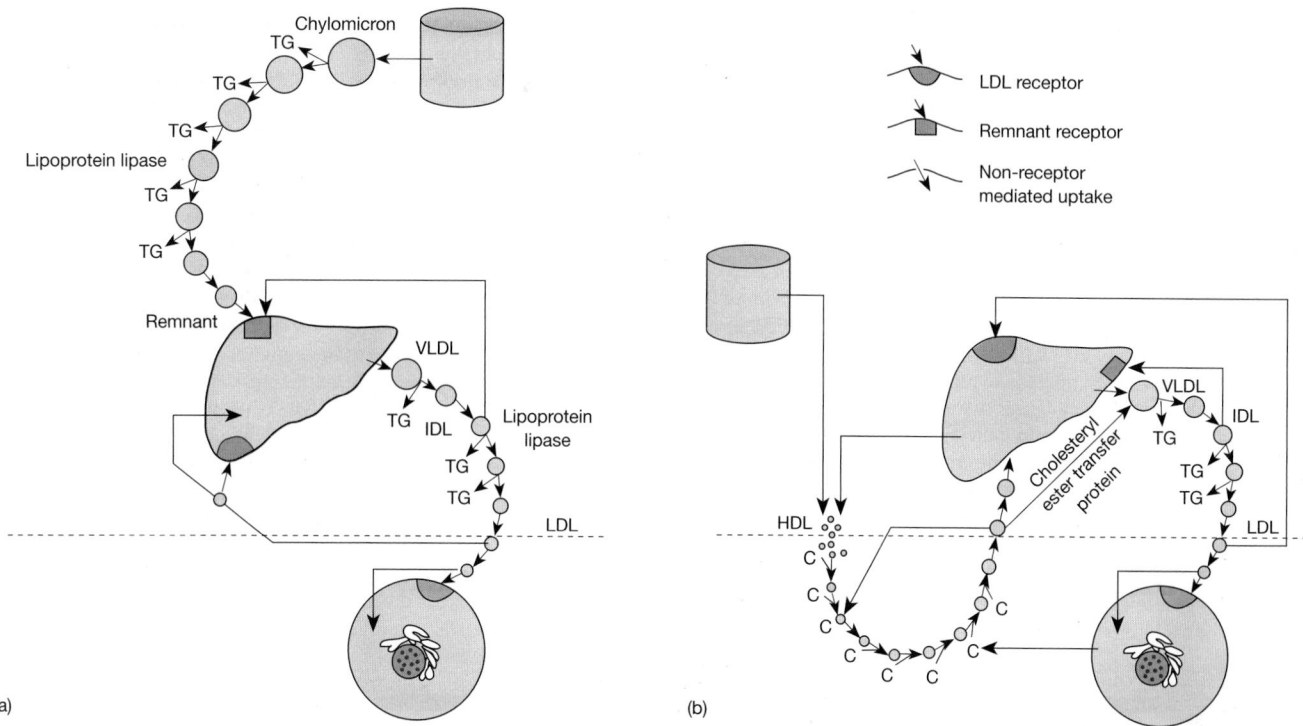

Fig. 4 Metabolism of (a) triglyceride-rich lipoproteins secreted by the gut and liver and (b) hepatic triglyceride-rich lipoproteins and lipoproteins transporting cholesterol to and from the tissues.

the vascular endothelium and enter the tissue fluid, serve to deliver cholesterol to the tissues. Their concentration in the extracellular fluid is probably about 10 per cent of that in the plasma. Cells require cholesterol for membrane repair and growth and, in the case of specialized tissues such as the adrenal gland, gonads, and skin, as a precursor for the syntheses of steroid hormones and vitamin D. Low-density lipoprotein is able to enter cells by two routes making a major contribution to its catabolism: one which is regulated according to the cholesterol requirement of each individual cell and one which appears to depend almost entirely on the extracellular concentrations of LDL.

The first of these two routes is by a cell-surface receptor, which specifically binds lipoproteins that contain apoB$_{100}$ or apoE. This is the LDL receptor. As mentioned previously, the receptor, although capable of binding apoE-containing lipoproteins, in practice binds mainly to the apoB$_{100}$-containing lipoproteins, of which LDL is the most widely distributed. After binding, the LDL–receptor complex is internalized and undergoes intracellular lysosomal degradation. The apoB moiety is hydrolysed to its constituent amino acids, and the cholesteryl ester is hydrolysed to free cholesterol. The release of this free cholesterol is the signal which regulates the cellular cholesterol content by three co-ordinated reactions. First the enzyme which is rate-limiting for cholesterol biosynthesis (3-hydroxy,3-methyl-glutaryl CoA reductase) is repressed, thus effectively centralizing cholesterol biosynthesis to organs such as the liver and gut. Secondly, the synthesis of the LDL receptor itself is suppressed. Thirdly, acyl-CoA:cholesterol O-acyltransferase is activated so that any cholesterol that is surplus to immediate requirements can be converted to cholesteryl ester, which, because of its hydrophobic nature, forms into droplets within the cytoplasm and is thus conveniently stored. The effect of the lysosomal release of free cholesterol on the expression of the LDL receptor contrasts with its effect on the hepatic remnant receptor, which is not subject to any similar downregulatory process. Free cholesterol released by lysosomal digestion of cholesteryl ester-rich, apoE-containing lipoproteins entering the hepatocyte via the 'remnant receptor' does not influence expression of this receptor mechanism; it will, nevertheless, downregulate the hepatic LDL

receptors. Defective uptake of LDL by the LDL receptor is the basis of familial hypercholesterolaemia (see below).

The other quantitatively important mechanism by which LDL cholesterol may enter cells is by a non-receptor-mediated pathway: LDL binds to cell membranes at sites other than the LDL receptors and some of it passes through the membrane by pinocytosis. High-density lipoprotein is able to compete with LDL for this type of cell membrane association. The absence of a receptor means that the 'binding' is of low affinity and thus, at low concentrations, LDL entry by this route may have little significance. However, unlike receptor-mediated entry, non-receptor-mediated LDL uptake, is not saturable, but continues to increase with increasing extracellular LDL concentrations. When LDL levels are relatively high, entry of cholesterol into the cells by this route may thus assume greater quantitative importance than that via the LDL receptor, which will be both saturated and downregulated. This appears to be the situation in the typical adult consuming a high-fat diet whose LDL cholesterol is high compared with most animals and in whom only about one-third of LDL is catabolized by receptors and two-thirds by non-receptor-mediated pathways. In hypercholesterolaemia, an even greater proportion of LDL is catabolized via the non-receptor pathway (four-fifths in patients heterozygous for familial hypercholesterolaemia, virtually all in homozygotes; see below).

Low-density lipoprotein may also be removed from the circulation by receptors other than the classical LDL receptor. These are probably responsible for the catabolism of only relatively minor amounts of LDL, but two groups of receptors present on the macrophage have excited considerable interest, because they are pertinent to atherogenesis. They are the β-VLDL receptor, a modified LDL receptor which allows the uptake of the β-VLDL from patients with type III hyperlipoproteinaemia (see below), and the scavenger receptors and oxidized LDL (**ox-LDL**) receptors, which permit the uptake of oxidized LDL by macrophages. Uptake by these receptors is so rapid that foam cells resembling those in arterial fatty streaks and atheromatous lesions are formed *in vitro*. On the other hand, uptake of unmodified LDL by the macrophage via the LDL receptor is too slow to allow foam cells to be formed. Oxidation of LDL may occur *in vivo* and is of potential relevance to atherogenesis (see below).

Lipoprotein (a)

Lipoprotein (a) (**Lp(a)**) is a lipoprotein first identified as a result of blood transfusion reactions occurring due to allotypic variation. Its exact location in the LDL and HDL$_2$ also varies from individual to individual, as does its serum concentration. It may be undetectable in some people or present at concentrations equalling those of LDL in others. The protein moiety of Lp(a), like that of LDL, contains apoB$_{100}$, but in addition apolipoprotein (a) (**apo(a)**) is also present. This contains homologous sequences of plasminogen, in which part of the plasminogen protein sequence (the kringle 4 domain) is repeated many times. The number of these repeats, which is determined at a genetic locus adjacent to the plasminogen gene, determines the molecular mass of apo(a), and individuals expressing polymorphisms with fewer kringle 4 repeats have the highest serum concentrations of Lp(a). Lp(a) is associated with the risk of coronary heart disease in people of European origin, particularly when serum cholesterol levels are also raised and when there is a family history of premature coronary heart disease. Lipoprotein (a) does not give rise to fibrinolytic activity because of a mutation in its activation site, and it may interfere with thrombolysis. Furthermore because Lp(a) binds to many different cells and connective tissue matrices, it is retained in the arterial wall longer than LDL and is thus more likely to be oxidized and taken up by macrophages, leading to atheroma (see below).

Transport of cholesterol from tissues back to liver

Cholesterol is exported by the gut and liver in quantities which greatly exceed its peripheral catabolism (largely conversion to steroid hormones and sebum). Therefore, except when the requirement for membrane synthesis is high, for example during growth or active tissue repair, the greater part of the cholesterol transported to the tissues (if it is not to accumulate there) must be returned to the liver for elimination in the bile, as bile acids and faecal sterols, or for reassembly into lipoproteins. The return of cholesterol from the tissues to the liver is termed 'reverse cholesterol transport'. It is less well understood than the pathways by which cholesterol reaches the tissues but it may well be critical to the development of atheroma. High-density lipoprotein has many features that make it very likely that it is directly involved in the reverse transport process.

The precursors of plasma HDL (nascent HDL) are disc-shaped bilayers composed largely of protein and phospholipid secreted mainly by the gut and liver (Fig. 4(b)). These are converted to the spherical, mature form of HDL by the action of lecithin:cholesterol acyltransferase. High-density lipoprotein components are also derived from surplus material (phospholipids, free cholesterol, and apoproteins) of triglyceride-rich lipoproteins released during lipolysis. ApoA-I and apoA-II, the major apolipoproteins of HDL, and apoE have been identified in nascent HDL. Other apolipoproteins and the bulk of its lipid are acquired as it circulates through the vascular and other extracellular fluids. In this respect the transformation of HDL from its lipid-depleted precursor to a relatively lipid-rich molecule is the inverse of that undergone by the other lipoproteins following their secretion.

High-density lipoprotein is a small particle compared with the other lipoproteins (diameter 5–12 nm, density 1063–1210 g/litre) and easily crosses the vascular endothelium, so that its concentration in the tissue fluids is much closer to its intravascular concentration than is the case for LDL. Because the serum HDL cholesterol concentration is only about one-quarter that of the LDL, it is often wrongly assumed that its particle concentration is lower. In fact, the particle concentrations of HDL and LDL in human plasma are often similar, and in the tissue fluids there are several times as many HDL molecules as those of other lipoproteins unless the capillary endothelium is fenestrated. Generally, therefore, cells are in contact with higher concentrations of HDL molecules than of any other lipo-

protein. In man, unlike the rat, HDL serves no function in transporting cholesterol to cells.

Recently it has been suggested that cells express receptors for HDL, particularly HDL$_3$, which might permit the transfer of cholesterol out of the cell. Passage across the cell membrane depends on an ATP-binding cassette transporter, ABCA1, which has recently been identified as the cholesterol efflux regulatory protein. Homozygosity for mutations in the *ABCA1* gene cause analphalipoproteinaemia (Tangier disease, see below) in which nascent HDL disappears rapidly from the circulation without acquiring cholesterol. Heterozygotes for *ABCA1* mutations have low levels of HDL cholesterol and accelerated atherogenesis. Factors regulating the balance between intracellular cholesterol ester and free cholesterol (activities of acyl-CoA:cholesterol *O*-acyltransferase and cholesterol esterase) may also be important. Apolipoprotein E synthesized within certain cells may also mediate the egress of cholesterol to HDL. Once outside the cell, free cholesterol must be re-esterified in order that it can be transported in any quantity in the core of lipoproteins. Therefore, whether or not HDL is involved as the initial acceptor molecule, cholesterol must at some stage on its return journey to the liver reside on HDL, because it is the site of lecithin:cholesterol acyltransferase activity. However, once cholesterol has been esterified and packed into the core of HDL, simple clearance of the whole lipoprotein particle by the liver is not the route by which most cholesterol is returned to it. This is because LDL equivalent to 1500 mg of cholesterol is produced each day, whereas the rate of catabolism of the HDL apolipoproteins A-I and A-II would permit less than 200 mg of HDL cholesterol to be returned each day. Therefore:

(1) the liver must be capable of selectively removing cholesterol from HDL and then returning the particle to the circulation with most of its apolipoproteins intact, or

(2) the cholesterol in HDL must be transferred to another lipoprotein class which is capable of being cleared in quantity by the liver, or

(3) a class of HDL, which contains little apoA-I or apoA-II, must be cleared by the liver at a much greater rate than the bulk of HDL.

In support of pathway (1), there is some evidence that hepatic lipase might act on the phospholipid envelope of HDL during its passage through hepatic sinusoids, and release the cholesteryl ester contained in its core, and that some hepatic trapping or even a receptor-mediated mechanism might enhance the process. On the other hand, in support of pathway (2) there is a well-established mechanism for the transfer of cholesteryl ester from HDL to VLDL through the agency of cholesteryl ester transfer protein. Once on VLDL, the conversion of this lipoprotein to IDL and then LDL means that the cholesteryl ester can then arrive at the liver via remnant receptors, LDL receptors, or by the non-receptor-mediated route for LDL uptake. Evidence for pathway (3), the return of cholesterol to the liver from HDL by a rapidly metabolized form of HDL present at low concentration in serum, is at present lacking in man, although it is possible that binding of the subclass of HDL containing apoE to hepatic remnant receptors permits the return of some cholesterol to the liver.

It is incorrect to regard HDL as a single homogeneous species, since it is known to be a mixture of particles differing in size, in lipid and apolipoprotein composition, and in function. Two main species can be resolved by ultracentrifugation, the less dense of which is designated HDL$_2$ (density 1063–1125 g/litre) and the more dense HDL$_3$ (density 1125–1210 g/litre). HDL$_3$ may be converted to HDL$_2$ by the acquisition of cholesterol, HDL$_3$ thus being a precursor of HDL$_2$. Whereas antisera to apoA-I precipitate virtually all of HDL, antisera to apoA-II do not, suggesting that some molecules of HDL contain apoA-I and apoA-II, whereas others contain only apoA-I. The apoA-I-only HDL molecules, which predominate in HDL$_2$, may arise from different metabolic channels than do the apoA-I/A-II particles. High-density lipoprotein containing apoE, as has previously been mentioned, may also have a different metabolic fate. Furthermore, HDL may contain other molecular species with overlapping density ranges, such as Lp(a); it is thus a highly diverse lipoprotein class.

Disorders produced by raised concentrations of lipoproteins

The incidence of coronary heart disease varies greatly in different parts of the world. Those countries with a Northern European culture (and in particular diet) have the highest rates, and places such as China, Japan, and rural Africa the lowest. Mediterranean countries are intermediate. There are, of course, many differences between these countries, but the variable that relates most closely to coronary heart disease is the median serum cholesterol of the middle-aged male population. It is of considerable interest that in a country such as Japan, where the average serum cholesterol is low, other coronary risk factors do not seem to operate. Thus in Japan coronary heart disease is comparatively uncommon, even in cigarette smokers and people with diabetes and hypertension.

Within populations there is an exponential relationship between serum cholesterol and the incidence of coronary heart disease (Fig. 5). This depends on the LDL cholesterol which comprises some 70 to 80 per cent of the total cholesterol in men and a little less in women. The greater part of the residual cholesterol in serum is on HDL, and the concentration of this HDL cholesterol is inversely related to the likelihood of developing coronary heart disease.

In populations in which death from coronary heart disease is common, fatty streaks are evident in the arteries, such as the aorta, of men dying in their late teens of causes unrelated to cardiovascular disease. This was noted in American casualties of the Korean and Vietnam wars. The fatty streak is the precursor of atheroma (see Section 15). The epidemiological and histopatholgical evidence implicating LDL in atherogenesis seems overwhelming. Yet in tissue culture, LDL uptake by macrophages or smooth muscle cells proved disappointingly slow and foam cells were not formed. Subsequently, it was found that the macrophage has receptors which will allow the rapid uptake of LDL to form foam cells if the LDL has undergone some chemical modification. Initially these receptors were known as the acetyl-LDL receptors (after the first experimental chemical modification leading to their identification), but now scavenger receptors and another class of receptors, the ox-LDL receptors, are known to be responsible for the uptake of modified LDL by macrophages. It is likely that the chemical modification leading to LDL uptake in human atherogenesis is oxidation of the polyunsaturated fatty acyl groups of phospholipids of LDL which have crossed the arterial endothelium to enter the subintimal space. The lipid peroxides so formed break down to lysophospholipids and aldehydes, which directly damage the apoB of the LDL, which then binds to the scavenger and ox-LDL receptors. The same substances are directly cytotoxic and may further damage the overlying arterial endothelium, increasing its permeability. The oxidized LDL itself and the release of the cytokines it stimulates are chemotactic to blood monocytes (from which arterial wall macrophages are derived) and may thus recruit more inflammatory cells into the lesion. HDL may protect LDL against oxidative modification by a process which involves the enzyme paraoxonase, which is tightly bound to HDL. In addition to uptake of LDL through scavenger and ox-LDL receptors, macrophages phagocytose aggregated LDL to become foam cells and take up LDL–antibody complexes via Fc (immunoglobulin crystallizable fragment) receptors. Other lipoproteins can be taken up to form foam cells. In particular, the β-VLDL (a mixture of chylomicron remnants and IDL), which accumulates in the circulation in type III hyperlipoproteinaemias (see below), is rapidly taken up by a macrophage receptor.

Triglyceride-rich lipoproteins can also be taken up by macrophages by phagocytosis to form foam cells, although these large particles would not be expected to cross the vascular endothelium unless it is fenestrated. Thus in extreme hypertriglyceridaemia, lipid-engorged macrophages are present in the mononuclear phagocyte system. They may be observed on bone marrow biopsy, and are the cause of the hepatosplenomegaly associated with extreme hypertriglyceridaemia. When hypertriglyceridaemia occurs in association with elevated levels of LDL cholesterol, it increases the likelihood of atheroma developing still further, perhaps because this combination is associated with low serum HDL cholesterol, perhaps because of an increase in circulating IDL and delayed clearance of chylomicron remnants, perhaps because it is associated with smaller LDL particles, which are more readily oxidized, or perhaps because there are associated increases in the coagulability of blood due to increased plasma fibrinogen levels and factor VII activity. When, however, triglyceride-rich lipoproteins are increased without any increase in LDL, as in familial lipoprotein lipase deficiency (see below), there appears to be only a modest risk of atheroma. There is, however, an increased likelihood of acute pancreatitis in all types of severe hypertriglyceridaemia, both primary and secondary, particularly when serum triglyceride levels exceed 20 to 30 mmol/litre (2000–3000 mg/dl). The cause of this is not known for certain, but may be attributed to the release of fatty acids by lipolysis *in situ* due to pancreatic lipase.

Normal serum lipid concentrations

Whereas the average serum concentrations of most substances, for example sodium or fasting glucose, are much the same in all parts of the world, cholesterol displays considerable variation. In Britain the median serum cholesterol for a middle-aged man is 5.8 mmol/litre and deaths from coronary heart disease comprise around 40 per cent of total mortality at this age. In China the average for men of middle age is 2 mmol/litre less, and coronary heart disease accounts for less than 5 per cent of their deaths.

Conventionally, the normal range for a variable in a particular population is chosen to include values between the 2.5 and 97.5 percentiles, or sometimes the 1 and 99 percentiles, on the assumption that 19 out of 20 of the population, or 49 out of 50 respectively, are normal. To be rational, the

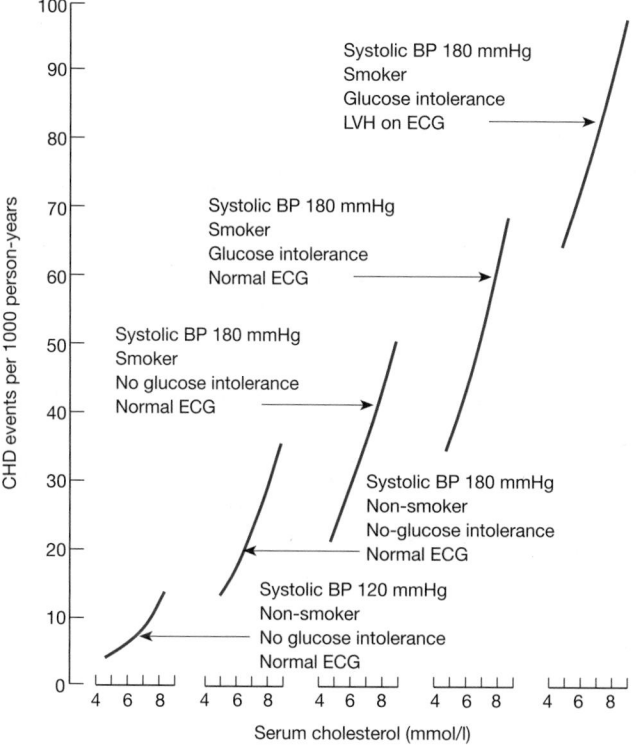

Fig. 5 The probability of 50-year-old men developing coronary heart disease each year as a function of serum cholesterol concentration, in the absence and in the presence of increasing numbers of risk factors. (Data from Kannel WB *et al.* (1973). The Framingham Study. An epidemiological investigation of cardiovascular disease. Section 28: the probability of developing certain cardiovascular diseases in eight years at specific values of some characteristis. Publication 74-618, US Department of Health Education and Welfare. Government Printing Office, Washington DC.)

implication in a medical context must also be that those people in the normal range are healthy. In the case of cholesterol, which is clearly linked to coronary heart disease, the healthy range would be more representative were it to include values from societies in which coronary heart disease is uncommon, such as China or Japan. This has led the National Institute of Health in the United States and the European Atherosclerosis Society to define healthy limits for serum cholesterol based on the risk of coronary heart disease. Thus an optimal serum cholesterol is 5.0 mmol/litre (200 mg/dl) or less. A level of 6.3 mmol/litre (250 mg/dl) (at the 75th percentile in the United States) is considered to indicate 'moderate risk' and 6.7 mmol/litre (270 mg/dl), which is the 90th percentile in the United States, 'high risk'. Some caution is required in using this concept. The risk of fatal coronary heart disease in an American middle-aged male population whose serum cholesterol is 5 mmol/litre (200 mg/dl) over the next 6 years is about 6 in 1000. At 6 mmol/litre (250 mg/dl) it is almost doubled, but that is only 10 in 1000, and at 7 mmol/litre (270 mg/dl) it is still less than 15 in 1000. Thus although these levels may be of great importance for public health initiatives aimed at reducing the cholesterol level in societies in which the risk of coronary heart disease is high, the clinician must be wary about overtreating men with cholesterol at these levels, if it is their only risk factor for coronary heart disease. The risk conferred by a particular level of cholesterol increases considerably when it is combined with another risk factor and this may considerably increase the benefits of treatment (Fig. 5). This is why there can be no single cholesterol level which demands a particular therapeutic response: the cholesterol value must always be viewed in the context of an individual's overall cardiovascular risk (see below).

An upper limit of normality for fasting serum triglycerides is often regarded as 2.2 mmol/litre (200 mg/dl). This is close to the 90th percentile for men and the 95th percentile for women. For serum HDL cholesterol a lower limit of normality of 0.9 mmol/litre (35 mg/dl) is frequently quoted, which is close to the 10th percentile for men and between the 5th and the 10th percentiles for women.

The Fredrickson/WHO classification

The concentration of four classes of serum lipoproteins when elevated can be regarded as pathological. These are chylomicrons, VLDL, LDL, and β-VLDL. The hyperlipoproteinaemias can be classified according to which of them is increased (Table 1).

The Fredrickson/WHO classification causes great confusion, largely because it is difficult to remember and is frequently wrongly regarded as a diagnostic classification when it is simply a way of reporting which of the serum lipoproteins is elevated. It is usually sufficient to remember that when cholesterol alone is elevated there is a type IIa hyperlipoproteinaemia. When both cholesterol and triglycerides are elevated the hyperlipoproteinaemia is generally type IIb, but occasionally it is type V (the serum will look milky if it is) and rarely type III. Type I is extraordinarily rare. An isolated increase in fasting serum triglycerides almost invariably signifies type IV hyperlipoproteinaemia.

All hospital laboratories, in addition to measuring cholesterol and triglyceride levels, should also measure HDL cholesterol in patients whose

overall cardiovascular risk is being critically assessed when treatment of their hyperlipoproteinaemia with drugs is under consideration. Particularly in women, an elevated level of cholesterol may result from a relatively high HDL cholesterol concentration and thus not signify any increased risk of coronary heart disease. High serum HDL cholesterol does not have a Fredrickson/WHO class, but as evidence suggests it is associated with longevity, it cannot be regarded as hyperlipoproteinaemia in the pathological sense. It is low HDL cholesterol which is associated with an increased cardiovascular risk, particularly if total serum cholesterol and triglycerides are also elevated.

Primary hyperlipoproteinaemias

Primary hyperlipoproteinaemias in which there is hypercholesterolaemia (type IIa)

Serum cholesterol levels exceeding 5 mmol/litre are common in adults in Britain and much of Europe, the United States, Australia, and New Zealand. In Britain, for example, 80 per cent of middle-aged people have levels exceeding this, and the proportion in the United States is at least 50 per cent. Most of this hypercholesterolaemia does not represent the effect of any single cause, but is due to some combination of dietary fat, obesity, and individual susceptibility to develop hypercholesterolaemia. This susceptibility is partly genetic, probably involving more than one gene, and this common type of hypercholesterolaemia is usually referred to as polygenic hypercholesterolaemia. At the very top end of the cholesterol distribution are to be found individuals who have the less common monogenic condition, familial hypercholesterolaemia.

Familial hypercholesterolaemia

Heterozygous familial hypercholesterolaemia
Familial hypercholesterolaemia is dominantly inherited. The heterozygous form of the condition affects about 1 in 500 people in Britain and the United States, making it one of the most common genetic disorders in these countries. In some populations, such as the Lebanese Christians, the Afrikaner and Cape Coloured peoples of South Africa, and French Canadians, it is considerably more common. This is because such people have descended from a relatively small number of early settlers, a few of whom by chance had familial hypercholesterolaemia. This is known as a founder effect. In yet other populations, such as Africans who have not intermingled with Europeans, familial hypercholesterolaemia appears to be rare.

Typically, the serum cholesterol in adult heterozygotes is 9 to 11 mmol/litre (350–450 mg/dl). The condition is expressed regardless of diet or age, and elevated cholesterol levels are present throughout childhood. The lipoprotein phenotype is usually IIa, but occasionally there is a moderate increase in fasting serum triglycerides to produce a IIb pattern. There is a tendency for HDL cholesterol to be at the lower end of the range, particularly if triglycerides are elevated.

The clinical hallmark of familial hypercholesterolaemia is the presence of tendon xanthomas. These appear in heterozygotes from the age of 20 onwards. The most common sites for tendon xanthomas are in the tendons overlying the knuckles and in the Achilles tendons (Plates 1 and 2). Less commonly, they may also be found in the extensor hallucis longus and triceps tendons, and occasionally other sites. It is also common to find subperiosteal xanthomas on the upper tibia where the patellar tendon inserts. The skin overlying tendon xanthomas is of normal colour and they do not appear yellow. The cholesteryl ester deposits are deep within the tendons. Tendon xanthomas feel hard because they are fibrotic. Indeed, it is not uncommon for those in the Achilles tendons to become inflamed from time to time, sometimes presenting as chronic Achilles tenosynovitis. More generalized tendinitis may follow rapid therapeutic reduction in serum cholesterol levels. Tendon xanthomas occur in only two disorders apart from familial hypercholesterolaemia, and these are so rare as not to pose any diagnostic difficulty. They are cerebrotendinous xanthomatosis, in which

Table 1 The Fredrickson/WHO classification of hyperlipoproteinaemia

Type	Lipoprotein increased	Lipids increased
I	Chylomicrons	Triglycerides
IIa	LDL	Cholesterol
IIb	LDL and VLDL	Cholesterol and triglycerides
III	β-VLDL (=IDL+chylomicron remnants)	Cholesterol and triglycerides
IV	VLDL	Triglycerides
V	Chylomicrons and VLDL	Cholesterol and triglycerides

Abbreviations: LDL, low-density lipoprotein; VLDL, very low-density lipoprotein; IDL, intermediate density lipoprotein.

plasma cholestanol is elevated and deposited in tendons, and phytosterolaemia (β-sitosterolaemia), in which there is abnormal intestinal absorption of plant sterols, which are then deposited in tendons.

Corneal arcus is also a frequent occurrence in familial hypercholesterolaemia. When it occurs in adolescence or early adulthood it is more likely to be associated with familial hypercholesterolaemia than corneal arcus occurring in middle age or later. It is, however, not uncommon to encounter patients with familial hypercholesterolaemia who have florid tendon xanthomas but no arcus. It is thus not a very valuable physical sign. Xanthelasmata palpebrarum, although occurring with greater frequency and at a younger age in familial hypercholesterolaemia, affect only a minority of heterozygotes. Xanthelasmas are not specific for any particular type of hypercholesterolaemia and occur in polygenic hypercholesterolaemia, pregnancy, primary bilary cirrhosis, and hypothyroidism. They are also common in middle-aged women, often overweight, with no very marked increase in serum cholesterol, if any. They may run in families apparently independently of hypercholesterolaemia.

Identifying those heterozygous for familial hypercholesterolaemia as early as possible is important, because of their risk of coronary heart disease. Untreated, over half of affected men die before the age of 60 years. It is not uncommon for men to have their first myocardial infarction or develop angina in their thirties and occasionally even earlier. Some 15 per cent of women with familial hypercholesterolaemia die of coronary heart disease before the age of 60 years and the majority have symptomatic coronary disease by that age. Perhaps as many as 10 per cent of women have some evidence of cardiac ischaemia before their menopause. However, whereas it is exceptional for a man with familial hypercholesterolaemia to live to 70 without symptomatic coronary heart disease, almost a quarter of women do so. This largely explains why a family history of premature coronary heart disease is absent in as many as one-quarter of patients discovered to have familial hypercholesterolaemia on screening, or in men who are discovered to have familial hypercholesterolaemia when they present with a heart attack in early life: the condition has been inherited from their mother, who has herself not yet developed coronary symptoms. Most people with familial hypercholesterolaemia are not overweight and do not have risk factors for coronary heart disease other than hypercholesterolaemia and a family history of the premature disease. Those without a family history of premature coronary heart disease (approximately 25 per cent) will be missed in screening programmes for risk factors for coronary heart disease, in which cholesterol is only measured selectively.

Those patients with familial hypercholesterolaemia who develop coronary heart disease particularly early often come from families in which the affected members have all tended to develop coronary heart disease early. This may be because other genetic factors in the family predispose to coronary heart disease. Thus low serum HDL cholesterol and increased fasting triglycerides are associated with a worse prognosis. Serum lipoprotein (a) is increased in familial hypercholesterolaemia and any familial tendency to run a high level of Lp(a) is exacerbated in those members who also have familial hypercholesterolaemia. The apoE$_4$ genotype (see below) is also associated with more aggressive atheroma in familial hypercholesterolaemia. A knowledge of the average age at which affected members of a family developed coronary heart disease may be helpful in planning how actively to treat boys and young adult women.

There is an increased risk of atheroma in other parts of the arterial tree in heterozygous familial hypercholesterolaemia, but this is strikingly less so than in the coronary arteries. Some heterozygotes have aortic systolic cardiac murmurs due to deposits of atheroma in the aortic root, sometimes involving the aortic cusps.

Homozygous familial hypercholesterolaemia

Most cases of homozygous familial hypercholesterolaemia occur in societes in which consanguineous marriages and heterozygous familial hypercholesterolaemia are frequent. The chance of marriage between unrelated heterozygotes meeting by chance in countries such as the United Kingdom or United States is 1 in 500^2, and each of their children would stand a 1 in 4 chance of being homozygotes. Assuming no adverse effect on the survival of the conceptus, an incidence of homozygous familial hypercholesterolaemia of 1 in 10^6 births would be predicted—a rare disorder.

Clinically, homozygous familial hypercholesterolaemia is characterized by the development of cutaneous xanthomas in childhood. These may be present in the first year of life or may not develop until late childhood. They are typically orange-yellow, subcutaneous, planar xanthomas, occurring on the buttocks, antecubital fossae, and the hands, frequently in the webs between the fingers. Tuberose subcutaneous xanthomas on the knees, elbows, and knuckles are also a feature. Serum cholesterol is typically greater than 15 mmol/litre (600 mg/dl). Myocardial infarction and angina frequently occur in childhood, sometimes even in infancy. Atheromatous deposits at the aortic root, invariably present by puberty, are so marked as to produce significant aortic stenosis, which contributes to the risk of sudden death. Death before the age of 30, and often considerably younger, was the rule before the advent of plasmapheresis and similar techniques for the extracorporeal removal of LDL (see below).

Polyarthritis, predominantly affecting the ankles, knees, wrists, and proximal interphalangeal joints, is common in homozygotes for familial hypercholesterolaemia.

The metabolic defect in familial hypercholesterolaemia

In familial hypercholesterolaemia there is decreased catabolism of LDL so that it remains for longer in the circulation. Normally the plasma half-life of LDL is 2.5 to 3 days, whereas in familial hypercholesterolaemia heterozygotes it is 4.5 to 5 days, and even longer in homozygotes. The molecular defect which causes this has been elucidated following the discovery of the LDL receptor (see above) by Goldstein and Brown, for which they received the Nobel prize for medicine in 1985. The gene encoding the LDL receptor protein is located on chromosome 19. Heterozygotes express only about half the LDL receptors of a normal person. Homozygotes have between none and 25 per cent of normal receptor activity. The mutations in the LDL receptor gene produce either receptors with no binding activity (receptor negative; because the receptor is not synthesized, is not transported to the cell surface, or, if it gets there, cannot be internalized after binding to LDL) or because, although the mutation allows some LDL to be bound and to enter the cell, this occurs only slowly because the binding site is abnormal (receptor defective). Some 200 mutations have been described and undoubtedly more exist. In Afrikaners or French Canadians far fewer mutations are associated with familial hypercholesterolaemia. For example, three mutations account for 90 per cent of familial hypercholesterolaemia in Afrikaners. In societies such as Britain and the United States, however, the most frequent of these mutations is likely to occur in no more than 3 to 4 per cent of patients with familial hypercholesterolaemia. This means that the prospect of developing a DNA test for this condition in most countries is unrealistic. It also means that only patients in populations with a small number of mutations, or where intermarriage is common, are homozygous in the sense that both their LDL gene mutations are identical. Most will be compound heterozygotes. For clinical purposes it is reasonable to label as homozygotes patients who have the clinical syndrome. However, it is instructive to realize that some of the heterogeneity of the severity of the syndrome relates to the nature of the two LDL mutations present. Thus the worst prognosis is associated with inheritance of two receptor-negative mutations, and the best is with two receptor-defective mutations. The type of receptor mutation in heterozygotes is also probably of some importance, but here it is blurred against a background of other acquired or genetic factors, which can find expression over a much longer time than in homozygotes.

A small proportion (3 per cent) of patients who have the same clinical features as heterozygotes for familial hypercholesterolaemia do not have an LDL receptor defect but a mutation of apoB in which glutamine is substituted for arginine at amino acid residue 3500, which is part of the LDL receptor binding domain. This disorder has been termed familial defective apoB$_{100}$, and probably has a frequency of 1 in 500 to 600 in Britain and the

United States. Only a minority of affected individuals have tendon xanthomas and typically the serum cholesterol associated with it is around 8.0 mmol/litre (310 mg/dl), which is less than in most heterozygotes for familial hypercholesterolaemia.

Common or polygenic hypercholesterolaemia

When a diagnosis of familial hypercholesterolaemia can be made, either because hypercholesterolaemia is present in childhood or an adult has the clinical features of the syndrome, a reasonably accurate estimate of clinical risk can be made and appropriate therapy given. In Britain, however, familial hypercholesterolaemia probably accounts for no more than 3 per cent of men dying of coronary heart disease before the age of 60. There is overlap between the range of LDL cholesterol levels encountered in familial hypercholesterolaemia and those due to the more common polygenic hypercholesterolaemia. Epidemiological studies have not included sufficient numbers of people with particularly high cholesterol levels to be certain, but it is probable that the risk in familial hypercholesterolaemia is greater than in polygenic hypercholesterolaemia. This may be because in the familial condition the hypercholesterolaemia has been present since birth, whereas polygenic hypercholesterolaemia is frequently not fully developed until the third or fourth decade. Furthermore familial hypercholesterolaemia, unlike many other types of hypercholesterolaemia, is associated with increased serum concentrations of Lp(a).

Estimates of how much different levels of cholesterol contribute to the overall cumulative male mortality from coronary heart disease by the age of 60 years are given in Table 2. The majority of such premature deaths come from the middle part of the cholesterol distribution, and therefore it has been argued that if a significant reduction in the incidence of coronary heart disease is to be achieved in countries such as the United Kingdom, efforts to lower cholesterol cannot simply be confined to those individuals whose plasma cholesterols lie at the upper end of the distribution. Nevertheless because the number of people in the middle range is so large (the vast majority of whom are not at increased risk of premature coronary heart disease), a different strategy must be applied to reducing their cholesterol from that applied to those in the upper part of the cholesterol distribution. This is the 'low-risk' or 'population' strategy, which aims to lower serum cholesterol by public health measures aimed at encouraging the adoption of a lower-fat diet and avoidance of obesity. Some patients from

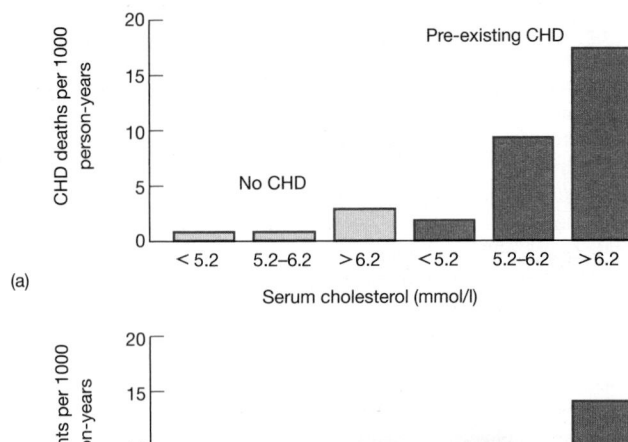

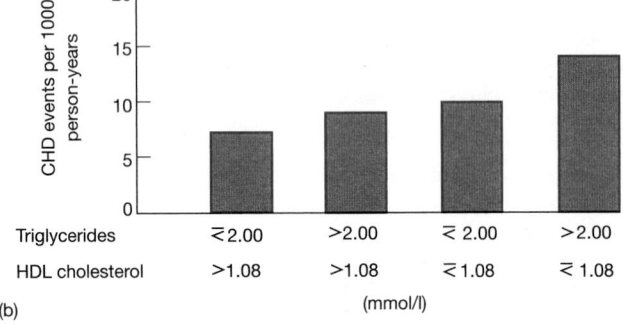

Fig. 6 (a) The risk of subsequent fatal myocardial infarction in survivors of myocardial infarction according to their serum cholesterol concentration. (Data from Pekkanan J et al. (1990) *New England Journal of Medicine* **322**, 1700–7.) (b) The likelihood of developing coronary heart disease in patients with moderately raised serum cholesterol concentrations (on average 6.9 mmol/litre) is increased when serum triglyceride levels are also raised and HDL cholesterol concentrations decreased. (Data from Manninen V et al. (1989).)

the middle range of serum cholesterol are, however, at much greater individual risk from their cholesterol level than the majority, because they have other risk factors for coronary heart disease which combine to increase their susceptibility. Probably the most potent of these is that the individual already has coronary heart disease.

In middle-aged survivors of myocardial infarction, serum cholesterol is an important indicator of cardiac prognosis (Fig. 6(a)), ranking after left ventricular function, but ahead of most of the other risk factors for coronary heart disease. Lipoproteins are also the most important risk factors for occlusion of coronary artery bypass grafts after the initial postoperative period. In people who have not yet developed coronary heart disease, the effect of risk factors such as cigarette smoking, hypertension, and diabetes synergizes with the risk from any given level of cholesterol (Fig. 5). A family history of coronary heart disease at an early age in a first-degree relative also increases the likelihood of coronary heart disease, and part of this effect is independent of other risk factors for coronary heart disease. The combination of all these factors with a relatively modestly increased serum cholesterol level can increase individual risk substantially to a level where clinical intervention is as justified as it is with more marked elevations in serum cholesterol. This is the 'high-risk' or clinical approach to prevention of coronary heart disease.

Metabolic defect in polygenic hypercholesterolaemia

In polygenic hypercholesterolaemia there is overproduction of VLDL by the liver. If this is rapidly converted to LDL there is no increase in serum triglyceride levels. The LDL receptor mechanism is probably overloaded in many individuals and in any case appears to catabolize only about one-third of LDL, so that the build-up of cholesterol in most patients is not due to any defect in the LDL receptor, but the inability of non-receptor-mediated catabolism to cope without a rise in the serum cholesterol concentration. Obesity and a high-fat diet (particularly saturated fat) are probably

Table 2 Estimates of the proportion of men in the United Kingdom dying before the age of 60 years from coronary heart disease according to their serum cholesterol and whether they have the familial hypercholesterolaemia clinical syndrome (from Durrington 2002)

Serum cholesterol (mmol/litre)	Risk of death before the age of 60 (per 1000)	Percentage of UK male population with these cholesterol levels	Percentage of UK male population dying before the age of 60 from CHD with these cholesterol levels
< 5	25	10	0.25
5–6	30	35	1.05
6–7	43	40	1.72
7–8	55	10	0.55
8–9	74	4	0.30
> 9	130	1	0.13
Heterozygous FH	500	0.2	0.1
Total			4.1

Abbreviations: CHD, coronary heart disease; FH, familial hypercholesterolaemia.

Death up to 60 in men is chosen because of limited data about cholesterol in older age groups and in women and about morbidity. The combined CHD death and non-fatal symptomatic CHD rate is probably two to three times that of CHD death.

the major reasons for the enormous differences in the prevalence of polygenic hypercholesterolaemia in different parts of the world. Undoubtedly, however, individual responses to diet vary greatly and there is a complex interplay between dietetic and genetic factors in the genesis of polygenic hypercholesterolaemia. The rise in cholesterol with age, which occurs in both men and women until the climacteric, seems less evident in societies where the cholesterol level is, for nutritional reasons, lower. There is an impression that dietary modification aimed at lowering cholesterol in middle age in societies where serum cholesterol is high does not reduce it to the extent that might be anticipated from populations habitually consuming such a diet. Whether this is simply a matter of non-compliance with diet or represents some imprinted change in metabolism caused by a high-fat diet in early life is, at present, uncertain.

Primary hyperlipoproteinaemias in which there is hypercholesterolaemia combined with hypertriglyceridaemia

Type III hyperlipoproteinaemia

Type III hyperlipoproteinaemia has several synonyms: broad beta disease, floating beta disease, dysbetalipoproteinaemia, and remnant removal disease. It is rare, probably occurring in fewer than 1 in 5000 people. Type III hyperlipoproteinaemia has the distinction of being the first clinical syndrome associated with hyperlipoproteinaemia to be described (by Addison and Gull in 1851).

Type III hyperlipoproteinaemia is due to the presence in the circulation of increased amounts of chylomicron remnants and IDL, often collectively termed β-VLDL. This is the result of decreased clearance of these lipoproteins at the hepatic 'remnant' (or apoE) receptor. There is an increase in both the serum cholesterol and fasting triglyceride concentrations. Typical levels are 7 to 12 mmol/litre (270–470 mg/dl) for cholesterol and 5 to 20 mmol/l (450–1800 mg/dl) for triglycerides. Often the molar concentrations of cholesterol and triglycerides are similar, and this may be a clue that a patient has type III hyperlipoproteinaemia. Occasionally the condition is associated with marked hypertriglyceridaemia due to overwhelming chylomicronaemia.

Xanthomas are present in more than half of the patients who have the type III lipoprotein phenotype. Characteristic of the condition are striate palmar xanthomas and tuberoeruptive xanthomas. Striate palmar xanthomas may simply be an orange-yellow discoloration within the creases of the skin of the palms of the hands. They may, however, be more florid and appear as raised, seed-like lesions (sometimes even larger) in the skin creases of the palms, fingers, and flexor surfaces of the wrists. Tuberoeruptive xanthomas are raised yellow lesions, usually on the elbows and knees (Plate 3). They may be nodular or cauliflower like, often surrounded by smaller satellites. Sometimes they may be found over other tuberosities, such as the heels and dorsum of the interphalangeal joints of the fingers. They resolve entirely with successful treatment of the hyperlipidaemia.

Type III hyperlipoproteinaemia is rare in women before the menopause, perhaps because uptake of hepatic remnant particles is enhanced by oestrogen. It is also rare in childhood, but has a definite incidence in men by early adulthood. Type III hyperlipoproteinaemia is generally an autosomal recessive condition with variable penetrance. In all cases there appears to be a mutation or polymorphism of the apoE gene, which impairs the receptor binding of apoE. The most frequent is a polymorphism, called apoE₂, in which cysteine is substituted for arginine at position 158 of the amino acid sequence. At least 90 per cent of patients with type III hyperlipoproteinaemia are homozygous for apoE₂. More often than not, however, apoE₂ homozygosity, which is present in around 1 per cent of the population, does not itself impose such a severe strain on lipoprotein metabolism that hyperlipoproteinaemia develops: its combination with some other disorder, leading to overproduction of VLDL or some additional catabolic defect, is required. This explains the association of type III hyperlipoproteinaemia with diabetes and hypothyroidism. More often, however, the additional

stimulus to hyperlipoproteinaemia is obesity or the coinheritance of a polygenic tendency to hypertriglyceridaemia. Rarer mutations of apoE have been described, which behave clinically similarly to apoE₂ homozygosity. More severe is a mutation leading to apoE deficiency, which in homozygotes does not require other factors for the expression of the type III phenotype. Heterozygous apoE deficiency finds little clinical expression, but, interestingly, mutations directly involving the receptor-binding domain of apoE (amino acids 124 to 150) produce the type III phenotype even in heterozygotes (dominant expression), implying that such mutations are a greater handicap to receptor clearance than mutations in which one gene is not producing apoE.

Type III hyperlipoproteinaemia undoubtedly causes accelerated atherosclerosis in the coronary, femoral, and tibial arteries. Intermittent claudication occurs at least as frequently as coronary heart disease and the incidence of the latter is about the same as that in familial hypercholesterolaemia. It is noteworthy that in familial hypercholesterolaemia peripheral arterial disease is uncommon relative to coronary heart disease, indicating that the leg arteries are much more susceptible to the larger lipoprotein particles in type III hyperlipoproteinaemia.

In the presence of typical xanthomas, the diagnosis of type III hyperlipoproteinaemia is not difficult. When these are absent the diagnosis must be made in the laboratory. Type IIb or V hyperlipoproteinaemia can give similar serum lipid levels. Lipoprotein electrophoresis is still available in some hospital laboratories and, when it clearly shows separate pre-beta (VLDL) and beta (LDL) bands, is useful in establishing type IIb rather than III hyperlipoproteinaemia. Frequently, however, the classical broad beta band associated with type III hyperlipoproteinaemia cannot be distinguished from a smear stretching from the origin into the pre-beta and sometimes beta region in the more severe IIb or type V phenotype. However, polyacrylamide isoelectric focusing or genotyping, available in many specialized centres, can identify apoE₂ homozygosity and this, in the presence of hyperlipidaemia, makes type III virtually certain. Rarely, the apoE mutation does not affect the electrical charge of apoE, or affects only one gene so that apoE₂ homozygosity is not found. The only way then to confirm the diagnosis is to send plasma to a centre that can provide ultracentrifugation to identify the cholesterol-rich VLDL (β-VLDL) typical of type III hyperlipoproteinaemia. It is also important in these circumstances to exclude paraproteinaemia, which can produce both hyper- and hypolipoproteinaemia and can mimic typical type III hyperlipoproteinaemia.

Type IIB hyperlipoproteinaemia

The common lipoprotein phenotype associated with a combined increase in serum cholesterol and triglycerides is IIb. In the majority of people with this, in whom it is primary, the cause is probably best regarded as a polygenic tendency exacerbated by acquired nutritional factors, such as obesity. A few patients will have tendon xanthomas, indicating familial hypercholesterolaemia (see above) but the great majority will not. Cardiovascular risk is greater for any given level of cholesterol when the serum triglyceride concentration is also elevated (Fig. 6(b)). Often the HDL is low, which further compounds the risk. In addition patients with hypertriglyceridaemia frequently have increased levels of a cholesterol-depleted small, dense LDL which contributes little to the total serum cholesterol concentration, but which is susceptible to oxidation and to which increasing attention is being paid because it may be highly atherogenic. Some authorities also believe that there is a specific syndrome in which there is a combined increase in serum cholesterol and triglycerides and a greatly increased coronary risk. They term this familial combined hyperlipidaemia. In this, multiple lipoprotein phenotypes occur in different family members: some IIa, some IIb, some IV, or occasionally even V. It is more than probable that what is being observed is the genetic tendency for hypercholesterolaemia and hypertriglyceridaemia running in the same family to combine in some members and not in others, and that when this occurs in a family susceptible to coronary disease, a particularly high premature mortality ensues. However, until the arguments about whether familial combined hyperlipidaemia is a distinct genetic entity are resolved, for practical purposes hypertriglyceridaemia (especially when HDL cholesterol is low) should be considered as an additional factor increasing the risk of hypercholesterolaemia. When these abnormalities are combined with a family history of premature coronary heart disease, there is a greatly increased risk of cardiovascular disease unless the condition is detected and treated.

Primary hyperlipidaemias in which hypertriglyceridaemia predominates

Severe hypertriglyceridaemia (types I and V)

Diagnosis and underlying mechanism

In any circumstance in which the serum triglycerides exceed 11 mmol/litre (1000 mg/dl) chylomicrons in addition to VLDL will be major contributors to the hyperlipidaemia, even when the patient is fasting. This is because in the circulation both chylomicrons and VLDL compete for the same clearance mechanism (lipoprotein lipase). The lipoprotein phenotype is usually type V. This severe hypertriglyceridaemia generally ensues when an increase in hepatic VLDL production, either familial or secondary to, for example, obesity, diabetes, alcohol, or oestrogen administration, is associated with decreased triglyceride clearance, which again may be genetic or acquired, for example hypothyroidism, beta blockade, or diabetes mellitus (diabetes can cause both an overproduction of VLDL and decreased lipoprotein lipase activity). With the clearance mechanism already overloaded with VLDL, the postprandial elevation in serum triglyceride concentrations when chylomicrons enter the circulation may be astronomical and they may spend days rather than hours in the circulation. The plasma takes on the appearance of milk and triglycerides may exceed 100 mmol/litre (9000 mg/dl) (Plate 4). Thus a patient, who might otherwise have a fasting serum triglyceride level of 5 mmol/l, can, with the injudicious use of alcohol or the development of intercurrent diabetes, achieve extraordinarily high serum triglyceride levels. Overall the frequency of severe hypertriglyceridaemia (> 11 mmol/litre (1000 mg/dl)) is probably no more than 1 in 1000 in adults and less in children.

Rarely, severe hypertriglyceridaemia is caused by familial lipoprotein lipase deficiency, a genetic deficiency in lipoprotein lipase activity. This is inherited as an autosomal recessive trait. Usually it is due to mutation in the lipoprotein lipase gene, leading to defective function or production, but occasionally it is due to a genetic deficiency of apoC-II, the activator of lipoprotein lipase. In familial lipoprotein lipase deficiency, severe hypertriglyceridaemia may be encountered in childhood. Occasionally, in children and young adults presenting for the first time, it produces type I hyperlipoproteinaemia, in which only serum chylomicron levels are elevated. It is not known why the VLDL is not also raised, but with advancing age the increase in both VLDL and chylomicrons, which might be expected if lipoprotein lipase is ineffective, becomes the rule.

Physical signs in severe hypertriglyceridaemia

Tuberoeruptive xanthomas are characteristic of extreme hypertriglyceridaemia. These appear as yellow papules on the extensor surfaces of the arms and legs, buttocks, and back. Often there is hepatosplenomegaly. Liver imaging shows the liver to be fatty, and bone marrow biopsy may reveal macrophages engorged with lipid droplets (foam cells). Because the triglyceride-rich lipoprotein may interfere with the determination of transaminases, giving spuriously high values, liver disease, in particular alcoholic liver disease, may be difficult to exclude, other than by the prompt resolution of the syndrome when a low-fat diet is instituted. Other features include lipaemia retinalis (pallor of the optic fundus, with both the retinal veins and arteries appearing white).

Complications of severe hypertriglyceridaemia

Atheroma is not a prominent complication of familial lipoprotein lipase deficiency, but it does complicate severe hypertriglyceridaemia in which there is residual lipoprotein lipase activity. It is difficult to make a precise estimate of the risk from the hyperlipidaemia *per se* because it is so frequently associated with insulin resistance or frank diabetes, which are

themselves risk factors for atherosclerosis. If these are included as part of the syndrome, both coronary heart disease and peripheral arterial disease are common. The explanation for the only modest risk of atheroma in patients lacking lipoprotein lipase is not understood but it may be because the incidence of diabetes is not increased in familial lipoprotein lipase deficiency. Also fibrinogen and factor VII activity are not increased; it is also notable that the conversion of VLDL and chylomicrons to the atherogenic IDL and remnant lipoproteins, respectively, is impaired in the absence of lipoprotein lipase.

Although atheroma may not be directly due to the high levels of triglyceride-rich lipoproteins, other complications are: acute pancreatitis may occur when serum triglyceride levels exceed 20 to 30 mmol/litre (2000–3000 mg/dl) (see above). The presentation of acute pancreatitis is similar to that from other causes (see Chapter 14.18.3.1). However, the diagnosis may not be confirmed by detecting increased serum amylase activity, because falsely low values may be encountered due to interference by triglyceride-rich lipoproteins in the laboratory method. All laboratories should inspect plasma or serum samples for milkiness before reporting normal or only moderately raised serum amylase activity in patients with severe abdominal pain (Plate 4). Clinicians may otherwise wrongly exclude the diagnosis of acute pancreatitis in favour, for example, of perforated peptic ulcer. Some patients do not develop acute pancreatitis, even when serum triglyceride levels exceed 100 mmol/litre (9000 mg/dl). Others, who are more susceptible, experience recurring acute episodes. Generally the pain subsides within a few hours or days of commencing nasogastric aspiration and intravenous fluids with nothing taken by mouth. Occasionally, if such treatment is delayed, pancreatic pseudocysts or abscesses may develop. Recurrent abdominal pain, not typical of pancreatitis, sometimes occurs in patients prone to marked hypertriglyceridaemia. It may mimic irritable bowel syndrome. Severe abdominal pain may also sometimes be the result of splenic infarction.

Pseudohyponatraemia is another consequence of extreme hypertriglyceridaemia, which may lead to serious misdiagnosis if the artefact is unrecognized. Spuriously low serum sodium values are reported, because much of the volume of the serum aliquot on which the sodium measurement is made is occupied by lipoproteins rather than water. When the serum triglycerides exceed 40 to 50 mmol/litre (3500–4500 mg/dl) the concentration of sodium in the aqueous phase (and thus the serum osmolality) may be normal while spurious serum sodium levels of 120 to 130 mmol/litre are being reported. The hazard is that these will be misinterpreted by the clinician and a patient already seriously ill with pancreatitis, or occasionally uncontrolled diabetes, will be made worse by restricting fluid intake or the infusion of hypertonic saline.

Focal neurological syndromes such as loss of vision, hemiparesis, memory loss, and loss of mental concentration may complicate extreme hypertriglyceridaemia, perhaps because of ischaemia due to sluggish microcirculation caused by the high concentrations of chylomicrons in the blood. Uniocular visual loss due to occlusion of the retinal microcirculation may likewise complicate hypertriglyceridaemia and is an indication for rapid institution of lipid-lowering therapy, and possibly antiplatelet agents. Paraesthesiae, especially in the feet, may also be an occasional feature, even in the absence of diabetes. Sicca syndrome and polyarthritis have also been described, but undoubtedly the commonest articular association is gout (see below).

Moderate hypertriglyceridaemia (type IV)

Raised fasting serum triglyceride levels in the range 2.2 to 10.0 mmol/litre (200–900 mg/dl) in the absence of a cholesterol level exceeding 5.0 mmol/litre (200 mg/dl) are occasionally discovered. Diabetes and excess ingestion of alcohol are important causes. Sometimes marked hypertriglyceridaemia is present in a fit, non-obese person with none of these factors. Family studies may then reveal similar increases in relatives, when the condition is called familial as opposed to sporadic hypertriglyceridaemia. Epidemiological studies show a univariate association between plasma triglyceride concentration and the risk of coronary heart disease, but there is little evidence that triglycerides are directly causal. Hypertriglyceridaemia is associated with low levels of HDL and glucose intolerance. When patients with established coronary disease and hypertriglyceridaemia whose serum cholesterol does not exceed 5.0 mmol/litre (200 mg/dl), are encountered they generally have low levels of HDL cholesterol and may have an increased level of cholesterol-depleted, small, dense LDL which is not evident from their cholesterol level. Such patients are likely to benefit from lipid-lowering therapy. They also have a greatly increased risk of developing diabetes mellitus over the next few years.

Hypertriglyceridaemia increases the risk of any associated increase in serum cholesterol (Fig. 6(b)), but present evidence would not favour its treatment in the absence of hypercholesterolaemia as a means of primary prevention of coronary heart disease. Occasionally, triglyceride concentrations of 5 mmol/litre (450 mg/dl) or less must be treated if they occur in patients prone to periodic exacerbations of more severe hypertriglyceridaemia associated with acute pancreatitis. Generally, levels exceeding 10 mmol/litre justify therapy, but for levels between 5 and 10 mmol/litre individual judgement should apply. In diabetes, evidence that serum triglycerides are an independent risk factor for coronary heart disease has been considered by some authorities to justify lipid-lowering therapy at lower levels than in non-diabetics when improvements in diet and glycaemic control have failed to decrease hypertriglyceridaemia.

Secondary hyperlipoproteinaemias

Secondary hyperlipoproteinaemias are those which are caused by another primary disorder (Table 3). When a disease that has hyperlipidaemia as a complication occurs in an individual who has a primary hyperlipoproteinaemia, the two frequently synergize to produce marked hyperlipoproteinaemia. This means that in societies in which polygenic hyperlipoproteinaemia is prevalent, secondary hyperlipoproteinaemia will have most impact. The best-known example of this is diabetes mellitus, which in Japan is only rarely complicated by coronary heart disease, whereas in the United Kingdom and the United States, coronary heart disease is the most common cause of premature death in diabetics.

Diabetes mellitus

The dominant hyperlipidaemia in diabetes is hypertriglyceridaemia. This is more likely to be associated with hypercholesterolaemia and with decreased HDL cholesterol in type 2 diabetes. Despite this, the risks of coronary heart disease and peripheral arterial disease are increased in both types 1 and 2 diabetes. This may be because in both disorders the hypertriglyceridaemia results not simply in an increase in VLDL, but also from an increase in IDL

Table 3 The more common causes of secondary hyperlipoproteinaemia

Endocrine	Diabetes mellitus
	Thyroid disease
	Pregnancy
Nutritional	Obesity
	Alcohol excess
	Anorexia nervosa
Renal disease	Nephrotic syndrome
	Chronic renal failure
Drugs	β-adrenoreceptor blockers
	Thiazide diuretics
	Steroid hormones
	Microsomal enzyme-inducing agents
	Retinoic acid derivatives
Hepatic disease	Cholestasis
	Hepatocellular dysfunction
	Cholelithiasis
Immunoglobulin excess	Paraproteinaemia
Hyperuricaemia	

and a small triglyceride-rich, cholesterol-depleted LDL particle. Since neither of these may contribute greatly to an increase in lipids, the term dyslipoproteinaemia is particularly aptly applied in diabetes. Also, plasma fibrinogen levels, which are increased in both types of diabetes, relate to serum triglyceride levels. Although lipoprotein abnormalities in type 1 diabetes may be less frequent than in type 2, the risk of coronary heart disease in type 1 is more often compounded by the presence of proteinuria. In diabetes uncomplicated by proteinuria, the risk of coronary heart disease is about two to three times (Fig. 5) that of non-diabetic people of a similar age. Proteinuria increases the risk by as much as 40 times. This may stem partly from hypertension and an exacerbation of the dyslipoproteinaemia, both of which may reflect the development of proteinuria. However, the increase in risk is greater than can be explained in this way (see Chapter 11.11) and may result because the proteinuria reflects a generalized increase in the permeability of arterial endothelium, enhancing the entry of macromolecules into the subintima and thus accelerating atherogenesis (see above).

The increased blood glucose in diabetes mellitus results from insulin resistance, insulin deficiency, or both. Insulin resistance may be present in non-diabetic, usually obese, people who are still able to secrete sufficient insulin to maintain control of blood sugar, but in such people there is often hypertriglyceridaemia with low HDL cholesterol and hypercholesterolaemia, hypertension, and increased risk of coronary heart disease. This syndrome is often referred to as the insulin resistance syndrome (syndrome X) or chronic cardiovascular risk syndrome. Clearly it has features in common with familial combined hyperlipidaemia and also with diabetes. Indeed, a proportion of people with syndrome X ultimately develop diabetes, sometimes not until after they have already developed coronary heart disease. This may explain in part why glycaemic control in diabetes seems to have little impact in preventing its atheromatous complications.

Diabetic women, particularly those with type 2 disease, tend to have a distribution of adipose tissue resembling that of obese men, being mostly around the abdomen and waist rather than the more female pattern which involves the buttocks and thighs, but leaves the waist relatively small. The relative protection from coronary heart disease which most women have, even those with familial hypercholesterolaemia, is largely lost by diabetic women, and it has been suggested that this may result from this androgenization. Many women with a similar body habitus, but who have not yet developed diabetes, are insulin resistant, hypertensive, have hyperlipidaemia, and have an associated increased risk of coronary heart disease.

Other secondary hyperlipoproteinaemias

Obesity

Obesity is a potent cause of hyperlipidaemia and has most impact in people with glucose intolerance. In its own right, obesity predominantly causes hypertriglyceridaemia (usually type IV), but, there is no form of primary hyperlipidaemia that it will not exacerbate. It therefore frequently accompanies hypercholesterolaemia as well as hypertriglyceridaemia. The exception appears to be familial hypercholesterolaemia, which is not associated with obesity. Alcoholic beverages, particularly wine and beer, are energy rich and may be a cause of obesity. Alcohol itself also induces hypertriglyceridaemia. Weight loss is generally associated with decreases in serum cholesterol and triglyceride levels. Anorexia nervosa is paradoxical in that it may be associated with quite marked elevations of serum cholesterol.

Thyroid failure

In hypothyroidism, serum LDL cholesterol and, less frequently, serum triglycerides are raised. Levels of HDL tend to be increased. There is decreased receptor-mediated LDL catabolism and lipoprotein lipase activity may be decreased. Hypothyroidism should always be considered in the diagnosis of hyperlipidaemia, and it is particularly important to exclude it when marked hyperlipidaemia occurs in women and in diabetic patients.

Renal disease

Renal disease is becoming an important cause of secondary hyperlipid-aemia in clinical practice, because improvements in long-term renal man-agement are now exposing coronary heart disease as the major cause of premature death in many renal disorders. In nephrotic syndrome the major lipoprotein disorder is a rise in serum LDL cholesterol. In chronic renal failure hypertriglyceridaemia is produced by an increase in both VLDL and in LDL triglycerides. Haemodialysis, chronic ambulatory peritoneal dialy-sis, and high-energy diets exacerbate the hyperlipidaemia. Following renal transplantation, many of the lipoprotein abnormalities resolve if good renal function is established, but corticosteroid therapy, weight gain, antihyper-tensive therapy, and perhaps cyclosporin treatment mean that even then hyperlipidaemia persists in about one-quarter of patients. Lipoprotein (a) is markedly elevated in renal disease, even after transplantation.

Drugs

Drugs are a common cause of hyperlipidaemia. β-adrenergic antagonists without intrinsic sympathomimetic activity raise triglycerides and lower HDL cholesterol. Thiazide diuretics tend to increase both cholesterol and triglycerides. These effects may be relatively small in people whose serum lipids are not elevated at the outset, but in patients with hypertriglycer-idaemia or with diabetes they may be substantial. Oestrogens tend to raise serum triglycerides, but will often lower LDL cholesterol after the meno-pause. They also raise serum HDL. Androgens have the opposite effect, decreasing triglycerides, raising LDL cholesterol, and lowering HDL. They may contribute to premature cardiac death in athletes unwise enough to use them in training. Glucocorticoids increase serum LDL cholesterol and triglycerides and often HDL cholesterol. Retinoic acid derivatives used in the management of skin disorders cause hypertriglyceridaemia. Phenytoin and phenobarbitone raise serum HDL cholesterol.

Liver disease

Cholestatic liver diseases, such as primary biliary cirrhosis, produce hyper-cholesterolaemia. This is not due to an increase in apolipoprotein B-containing LDL, but to an abnormal lipoprotein, designated lipoprotein X (**LpX**), produced largely as the result of reflux of biliary phospholipids into the circulation. Xanthelasmas are common in biliary obstruction and other xanthomas occasionally develop. In the later phase of chronic biliary obstruction, when secondary biliary cirrhosis and hepatocellular disease sets in, hepatic lipid biosynthesis plummets and the hyperlipidaemia of biliary obstruction resolves. Hepatocellular diseases may be associated with moderate hypertriglyceridaemia, probably because of impaired hepatic lipoprotein clearance. Concentrations of HDL are markedly decreased and lecithin:cholesterol acyltransferase activity is low. Some authorities believe that this defect in cholesterol esterification contributes to the complications of liver failure.

Hyperuricaemia

Hyperuricaemia is present in as many as half the men with hypertriglycer-idaemia. It may lead to gout, particularly if such patients are receiving diur-etic therapy. The association of hypertriglyceridaemia and hyperuricaemia appears to be more common than can be entirely explained by the coinci-dence of common aetiological factors, such as obesity and high alcohol consumption. Yet they are not causally related, because specifically lower-ing one does not usually decrease the other. They must therefore have some unknown antecedent in common.

Management of hyperlipoproteinaemia

Clinical trials have established beyond all question of doubt that reduction of serum cholesterol decreases both coronary morbidity and mortality and can prolong survival. The risk of coronary heart disease ascribable to a particular cholesterol level does, however, vary widely in different individ-uals depending on the presence of other risk factors for coronary heart disease. Thus a serum cholesterol of 6.0 mmol/litre (230 mg/dl) in a

50-year-old woman with an HDL cholesterol level of 1.9 mmol/litre (75 mg/dl) who does not smoke and is neither hypertensive nor diabetic will carry a risk of a coronary event of 1 in 40 over the next 10 years, whereas in a man of similar age the same serum cholesterol associated with an HDL cholesterol value of 0.9 mmol/litre (35 mg/dl) who is hypertensive, smokes and has diabetes the risk will be 1 in 3 over the same time interval. His likelihood of benefit from a given reduction in cholesterol will thus be much greater than hers, although both have the same concentration of serum cholesterol. The coronary risk attaching to the cholesterol level in individual patients could, were it known with reasonable accuracy, thus guide the clinician in deciding how rigorously treatment should be given. Below a certain level of risk, treatment may be more trouble than it is worth for the patient's lifestyle, presence of mind, or pocket. For a state healthcare system too there will also be a level of risk below which the cost-effective-ness of cholesterol lowering may mean that resources should be directed to some more cost-effective clinical practice.

Another consideration, as with any therapeutic intervention, is that there may be side-effects of treatment which should limit it to those patients whose risk of the disease it is intended to prevent (in this case primarily coronary heart disease) is substantially higher than the potential risk of serious side-effects. Dietary management is generally viewed as safe, and meta-analyses of dietary trials show no increase in non-cardiac mortal-ity. Until recently, however, cholesterol-lowering drugs were often viewed with suspicion. Since 1994, however, results from six clinical trials of statin drugs have established that these drugs are safe with adequate medical supervision during the 5 to 6 years of the trials. In that time the risk of coronary heart disease was decreased by one-third, the decrease becoming greater with more prolonged therapy. The lowest average annual coronary risk of participants in these trials was 1 per cent (one event per 100 people per year) and the highest 4.5 per cent. The relative reduction in risk of one-third was similar regardless of the level of risk, so a greater number of cor-onary events was prevented when the risk was highest. Other cholesterol-lowering drug therapies such as fibrates and bile acid seques-trating agents decrease coronary risk, but their safety and the magnitude of their overall benefit is not as clear as with statins, partly because design and analysis of clinical trials were better in the more recent statin trials. In a recently reported trial of men with established coronary disease and rela-tively low levels of serum cholesterol and HDL cholesterol, gemfibrozil was found to be both safe and effective. Other fibrate trials are under way.

The essential point to grasp is that the decision to treat hyperlipidaemia is not based simply on any particular cholesterol value, but on an assess-ment of individual risk of coronary heart disease. It is sensible to select for treatment those patients with a high overall probability of dying prema-turely of coronary disease. If the balance of risk suggests that they are not, they will be exposed to any possible ill-effects of such treatment with no likelihood of benefit. The identification of patients with established coron-ary heart disease, familial hypercholesterolaemia, or with more modest increases in serum cholesterol combined with multiple risk factors, includ-ing a bad family history (Figs. 5 and 6 ((a) and (b)) allows the targeting of cholesterol-lowering management to high-risk individuals, who can benefit most. Charts which can assist in the assessment of coronary risk are to be found in Section 15.16.1.

Dietary management

It is generally agreed that dietary advice should be given to people whose serum cholesterol exceeds a concentration of 5.0 mmol/litre (200 mg/dl). In a country such as the United Kingdom, however, two-thirds of men and women between the ages of 18 and 69 years have cholesterol concentrations exceeding this value. Thus, except in the case of the patients considered to be at high coronary risk, individual dietetic supervision beyond the pro-vision of a diet sheet is not reasonable. It is particularly important to remember that cigarette smoking is a greater cause of ill-health than are minor elevations of serum cholesterol, and advice to stop smoking should be reiterated whenever a medical consultation occurs.

Table 4 Dietary fatty acids and their sources

Type	Fatty acid	Source
Saturated	Myristic, palmitic, stearic	Pork, beef, sheep fat, dairy products
Mono-unsaturated	Oleic	Olive oil, rapeseed oil
Poly-unsaturated	Linoleic	Sunflower, safflower, corn, soyabean oil
	Eicosapentaenoic, docosahexaenoic	Fish oil

All can contribute to obesity. Saturated fats lead to raised cholesterol and triglyceride levels. Oleic acid and linoleic acid decrease LDL cholesterol and often triglycerides. Oleic acid is widely distributed in foods rich in saturated fats, but these sources are not helpful in a diet designed to decrease saturated fat intake. Fish oil decreases triglycerides, but does not decrease LDL cholesterol.

The principal aims of a cholesterol-lowering diet are to reduce obesity by a decrease in dietary energy intake and to decrease saturated fat consumption. Fat is a major source of dietary energy and the reduction in its intake should be the main objective of any weight-reducing diet. In the non-obese, dietary advice should focus on decreasing saturated fat to below 10 per cent of dietary energy intake and substituting it with a mixture of unrefined carbohydrate and monounsaturated and polyunsaturated fats (Table 4). Polyunsaturates in the form of linoleic acid (corn oil, sunflower oil) should not be the only fats to replace saturated fat, because it is not certain that in large amounts they do not have harmful long-term effects. In patients with established coronary disease there is increasing interest in the long-chain omega-3 fatty acids such as those found in fish oil (Table 4) which are more unsaturated and reduce sudden cardiac death, probably by suppressing ventricular arrhythmias. Eating fatty fish twice a week is thus recommended. Increasingly, too, oils rich in monounsaturated oleic acid such as olive oil, present in the diet of Mediterranean people since time immemorial, are being encouraged by nutritionists as substitutes for saturated fat. Rapeseed oil, which is much cheaper, contains almost as much oleic acid as olive oil. Dietary cholesterol itself, although featuring prominently on food labels, usually has a smaller effect on serum cholesterol concentrations than saturated fat. Decreasing its absorption with foods enriched in plant sterol or stanol esters has a small hypocholesterolaemic effect, as also does mucilaginous fibre in fruit, vegetables, and oats. Avoiding coffee is probably pointless. Some authorities believe that the epidemiological evidence indicating that alcohol is protective against coronary heart disease is strong enough to justify encouraging moderate indulgence (red wine finds particular favour in view of the lower risk of coronary heart disease in southern as opposed to northern Europe). However, alcoholic beverages in excess can lead to obesity, hypertension, atrial fibrillation, and to exacerbation of hypertriglyceridaemia (see above), and a trial of abstinence should be considered in the patient with hyperlipidaemia suspected of overindulgence.

These dietary aims do not need to be modified for the treatment of moderate hypertriglyceridaemia and are also suitable for the management of diabetes. Carbohydrate-restricted diets are no longer in general use for either of these purposes. In patients with severe hypertriglyceridaemia it is necessary to limit the production of chylomicrons and so any fat in the diet must be avoided. Often a 25 to 30 g low-fat diet (in which, if the patient is not obese, carbohydrate is substituted to maintain dietary energy intake) can be employed, but occasionally even lower fat intakes must be achieved. Lipid-lowering drugs are frequently ineffective in patients with severe hypertriglyceridaemia, whereas dietary treatment can be particularly effective. Admission to a specialized centre with experienced dietetic services is often desirable.

Drug therapy of hyperlipidaemia

The indication for drug therapy is not the failure of serum cholesterol concentration to decrease below some arbitrary level despite dietary treatment in all patients. There are people with serum cholesterol concentrations as high as 8 mmol/litre (310 mg/dl) whose risk of coronary heart disease is not sufficiently high to justify the use of lipid-lowering drugs. However, when coronary risk is high there is no scientific basis for choosing different cholesterol (or LDL cholesterol) concentrations as thresholds for intervention or as therapeutic targets. Generally if the patient is in one of the following high-risk categories lipid-lowering therapy should be instituted if the serum cholesterol persists about 5.0 mmol/litre (200 mg/dl) (LDL cholesterol > 3.0 mmol/litre (> 120 mg/dl) and the aim of treatment should be to decrease serum cholesterol to less than 5.0 mmol/litre (200 mg/dl) (LDL cholesterol < 3.0 mmol/litre (< 120 mg/dl) or by 25 per cent (LDL by 30 per cent), whichever is the lowest. Whether dietary management should be instituted at the same time as lipid-lowering drug therapy or before in order to establish whether it alone will suffice is determined by the degree of risk and the degree to which the serum cholesterol is elevated. Dietary management does not typically decrease serum cholesterol by more than 0.5 mmol/litre (20 mg/dl). Certainly in patients with established CHD, statin treatment should be introduced without delay. The high risk categories are discussed in the subsections below.

Patients with established coronary heart disease or other significant atherosclerotic disease

Secondary prevention trials of cholesterol lowering using statin drugs provide strong evidence of prolonged survival due to a decrease in coronary events and strokes. Coronary angiography also provides evidence of regression of atheroma with lipid-lowering therapy. Lipid-lowering drugs are therefore indicated in patients with coronary heart disease (including those who have undergone coronary surgery or angioplasty). It is probably reasonable to extend this policy to patients with peripheral arterial, aortic, or significant carotid atherosclerosis, because there are angiographic studies to demonstrate favourable effects of lipid-lowering therapy on femoral and carotid atheroma and because this type of disease is closely associated with risk of coronary heart disease.

Familial hypercholesterolaemia and type III hyperlipoproteinaemia

The high risk of coronary heart disease and the known metabolic defects in these conditions justifies the use of lipid-lowering drug therapy. Familial hypercholesterolaemia should, if possible, be detected in childhood or early adulthood, and the age at which statin therapy should be commenced has therefore to be considered. Generally in boys a statin should be prescribed by the age of 20 years whereas in many women it can be left until the age of 30 years (discontinuing it temporarily if there is any possibility of conception). Some authorities advocate the earlier use of statins and this should certainly be considered if the family history of coronary disease is particularly adverse.

Patients with type III hyperlipoproteinaemia are generally encountered in adulthood and treatment should be initiated with a fibrate drug in all save the minority who respond to dietary management alone. It should not be assumed that dietary control is adequate if any degree of hypertriglyceridaemia persists, because this generally indicates that significant β-VLDL is still present in the circulation.

Multiple risk factors

The risk of coronary heart disease in some patients with additional adverse factors, whose serum cholesterol remains elevated despite diet, justifies the use of lipid-lowering drugs. Just how high the risk needs to be, and how it can be determined with any degree of exactitude, is a persisting problem for the clinician. Most national and international recommendations for primary prevention of coronary heart disease provide a means of assessing an individual patient's risk (usually based on the equation derived from the Framingham study by Anderson and colleagues) to assist in the clinical decision as to when to introduce lipid-lowering medication and increasingly when to treat mild hypertension. The National Cholesterol Education Program recommends an algorithm and recommends treatment at lower levels of risk than in Europe. The Joint European Guidelines recommend 20 per cent over 10 years as an appropriate threshold of coronary risk for statin therapy. In the Joint British Guidelines the minimum level of care is considered to be treatment when coronary risk is 30 per cent or more over

10 years, but that ideally a 10-year risk of 15 per cent or more should be targeted. A computer program is available from the British Hypertension Society website (www.hyp.ac.uk/bhs/management.html) and the Family Heart Association website (www.familyheart.org) for the prediction of both coronary and stroke risk. The author's own practice is to target 20 per cent and above. It is always important to seek evidence of existing coronary heart disease, since, if present, this clarifies the decision to start lipid-lowering therapy, and justifies investigation in its own right.

Diabetes mellitus

The relative reduction in coronary risk in patients with diabetes thus far included in statin trials is at least as great as in the non-diabetic participants. Because of the higher coronary risk in diabetes this means that even greater benefit, in terms of new events prevented, accrues from statin treatment than in non-diabetics. Results of statin and fibrate trials specifically conducted in diabetes are awaited. However, current evidence strongly supports the use of statin therapy in diabetic patients with coronary heart disease or any other atherosclerotic complication. What is uncertain is whether in the primary prevention of coronary disease diabetic patients should be stratified according to risk to determine when they receive lipid-lowering drug treatment as in non-diabetics or whether they should be a special category who are all treated in the same way as patients with established coronary heart disease. The latter approach, which has been adopted by the American Diabetic Association, would mean that most patients with serum cholesterol exceeding 5.0 mmol/litre (200 mg/dl) should receive statin therapy. In favour of this approach is the knowledge that coronary risk is substantially higher in diabetics for any given concentration of cholesterol than in non-diabetics, that prediction methods are likely to underestimate risk in non-insulin-dependent diabetes, and that there is no reliable method for predicting risk in insulin-dependent diabetes.

Markedly elevated cholesterol with no other risk factors and no clearly identifiable genetic syndrome

Many people fall into this category. Some will have familial hypercholesterolaemia but have not yet developed tendon xanthomas. Knowledge that a relative has these should weigh heavily in the decision to introduce therapy. The combination of high cholesterol with raised triglycerides and low HDL and an adverse family history also favours the introduction of lipid-lowering drug therapy even in the absence of other risk factors (see above). The risk will be underestimated from coronary risk prediction charts or computer programs when there is an adverse family history or hypertriglyceridaemia. If the risk cannot be read from the charts because the ratio of serum to HDL cholesterol is too high, treatment may in any case be justified.

In women with isolated hypercholesterolaemia who are peri- or postmenopausal, the possibility of prescribing hormone replacement therapy can be considered, particularly if the menopause is surgical or spontaneously premature, or if there are also menopausal symptoms. Hormone replacement therapy often decreases LDL cholesterol and may increase HDL cholesterol. However, at present there is no randomized, placebo-controlled clinical trial evidence that this therapy is beneficial in preventing coronary heart disease. Care should be exercised in patients with hypertension (because of the salt-retaining effects of progestogen), in patients with established coronary heart disease (because of its possible thrombogenic effects), and in patients with hypertriglyceridaemia (which sex steroids exacerbate). In women at high risk of coronary disease the quality of evidence in favour of statin therapy means that reliance should not be placed on hormone replacement therapy as a means of coronary prevention.

Lipid-modifying drugs

No major therapeutic decision, such as the introduction of a particularly restrictive diet or of lipid-modifying drug therapy, should be taken as the result of a single cholesterol determination, because this will be influenced both by biological and by laboratory variation. A laboratory result for cholesterol concentration is generally within ± 10 per cent of the true mean value, but may occasionally fluctuate more widely. Increasingly, portable or 'on-site' cholesterol analysers are being used in an attempt to make cholesterol measurement as immediate for the clinician as that of blood pressure. This has some advantages, but it must be remembered that such tests may be more expensive than those performed in the laboratory, they are generally less accurate unless performed by someone who is trained and regularly uses the instrument, and the calibrations usually differ from those employed in hospital laboratories.

Non-fasting cholesterol concentrations are satisfactory for the management of patients responding to simple dietary measures, but for those in whom drug therapy is under consideration, two fasting determinations of cholesterol, triglycerides, and HDL cholesterol are generally necessary (serum cholesterol and HDL cholesterol concentrations are not affected by meals, but serum triglyceride levels are). Knowledge of the HDL and triglyceride levels is essential at this stage because abnormal values for these would be an additional factor in favour of lipid-lowering drug therapy, and because their concentration may influence the choice of drug. Fasting blood glucose and serum creatinine and transaminases should also be measured, and urine should be tested for protein. Serum thyroxine should be measured if there is any suspicion of hypothyroidism, and some authorities advocate its measurement in all patients whose serum cholesterol exceeds 8 mmol/litre (310 mg/dl) even if hypothyroidism is not clinically evident.

The first-line therapy in all forms of hypercholesterolaemia, except that associated with triglyceride levels exceeding 5 mmol/litre (200 mg/dl), are the statin drugs (3-hydroxy-3-methylglutaryl CoA reductase inhibitors)—atorvastatin, fluvastatin, lovastatin, pravastatin, rosuvastatin, and simvastatin. These agents are often effective, even in marked hypercholesterolaemia, as monotherapy. They also have a triglyceride-lowering effect, which tends to be related to the extent to which they lower cholesterol but which is generally less than with a fibrate drug. Evidence that statins decrease coronary events is provided by three large secondary prevention trials using simvastatin or pravastatin, two primary prevention trials which employed pravastatin or lovastatin, and one trial which combined primary and secondary prevention patients and involved simvastation. Advantage may be taken of the synergism of statins with bile acid sequestrating agents (cholestyramine and colestipol), by prescribing two sachets in the morning with an evening dose of statin, in patients resistant to statins alone. Their use in combination with fibrate drugs requires strict clinical supervision, because there is an increased risk that myositis may ensue. There is a small incidence of this occurring spontaneously in patients on statins, and creatine kinase levels should be monitored. Erythromycin and cyclosporin also increase the risk of myositis, and care must be taken if statins are used after cardiac or renal transplantation. Statins may be particularly valuable in patients with renal disease in whom fibrates are contraindicated and in whom bile acid sequestrating agents may exacerbate hypertriglyceridaemia; these latter agents are particularly poorly tolerated in patients already receiving multiple drug regimes.

Bile acid sequestrating agents can be used in the treatment of hypercholesterolaemia in the absence of hypertriglyceridaemia, which they may exacerbate. A dose (two sachets) is best taken well soaked in fruit juice before breakfast. In larger more frequent doses these agents often cause nausea, heartburn, and constipation. Generally for this reason they have been increasingly relegated to the sidelines since the introduction of statins. In children and women of child-bearing potential, who have heterozygous familial hypercholesterolaemia and in whom drug therapy is justified because of a particularly adverse family history, the author remains reluctant to turn to other agents, although it is often better to wait until it is safe to commence statin treatment (which is better tolerated) than to alienate the patient from the clinic with unpalatable treatment earlier. If they are prescribed, folate and vitamin D supplementation should be considered, particularly in women who may become pregnant.

In patients whose hypercholesterolaemia is combined with more marked hypertriglyceridaemia, the fibrate drugs (bezafibrate, ciprofibrate, fenofibrate, gemfibrozil) are first-line therapy. They are also often highly effective in type III hyperlipoproteinaemia and useful in primary type V hyperlipoproteinaemia and in the dyslipoproteinaemia of diabetes mellitus. Fibrates are less effective in lowering LDL cholesterol than are statins. Most of their cholesterol-lowering effect is due to a decrease in VLDL cholesterol. They do, however, decrease small dense LDL levels. This is not readily evident from routine laboratory tests, because it is unaccompanied by any substantial reduction in cholesterol. In some particularly high-risk patients with combined hyperlipidaemia statin therapy may be added to fibrate therapy in order to satisfactorily lower LDL cholesterol. The fibrate drugs raise HDL cholesterol by more than statins. They must be avoided in patients with disturbed hepatic or renal function. They potentiate anticoagulants. The mode of action of fibrate drugs, which diminish serum triglyceride levels by stimulating lipoprotein lipase and decreasing circulating non-esterified fatty acids (NEFA), probably involves stimulation of the nuclear peroxisome proliferator-activated receptor α.

Nicotinic acid (niacin) can be used to lower serum cholesterol and triglyceride levels. The effective dose is usually associated with unpleasant flushing. This can be minimized if aspirin is taken before the nicotinic acid. There are also many other side-effects, and liver function must be monitored. Nicotinic acid has not found great therapeutic favour outside the United States. Unlike other lipid-lowering drugs, it is effective in lowering serum Lp(a). Acipimox, a niacin analogue, has a similar spectrum of action to the fibrate drugs and causes less flushing. Probucol is a cholesterol-lowering drug, which lowers HDL cholesterol relatively more than LDL. Despite its undoubted antioxidant properties, it requires further clinical evaluation before it can be regarded as beneficial in its overall action and is now of limited availability. Fish oil pharmacological preparations have triglyceride-lowering properties in daily doses of several millilitres, but do not lower LDL cholesterol and may even exacerbate diabetic hyperlipidaemia. Preparations which concentrate the omega-3 long-chain fatty acids, eicosapentaenoic and docosahexaenoic acid (Table 4), may have greater therapeutic potential. Fish oil improves survival after myocardial infarction in doses which have little effect on serum triglycerides and may relate to a decreased likelihood of ventricular arrhythmias.

Non-pharmacological lipid-lowering treatment

In addition to pharmacological agents and diet, extracorporeal removal of LDL is available in many centres for severe hypercholesterolaemia, usually homozygous familial hypercholesterolaemia in which it improves survival. Plasmapheresis or LDL apheresis, using systems that absorb LDL, are the two methods employed. Plasmapheresis and most methods of LDL apheresis also lower serum Lp(a). They must be repeated every 2 to 4 weeks. Occasionally, patients with homozygous familial hypercholesterolaemia have also been treated with liver transplantation to provide an organ with normally functioning LDL receptors. Partial ileal bypass surgery has been used to treat heterozygous familial hypercholesterolaemia (it is ineffective in homozygotes), but with the advent of more effective lipid-lowering drugs this is now very rarely necessary.

Hypolipoproteinaemia

Hypolipoproteinaemia is increasing as a clinical problem, because more cases are being discovered as a result of population screening for high cholesterol. People who have had a low serum cholesterol level all their lives do not seem to be at any disadvantage unless the decrease is profound, as in abetalipoproteinaemia. Indeed, their relative freedom from cardiovascular disease may lead to longevity. When the condition is discovered for the first time it is often difficult, however, to be sure that the low cholesterol is not due to an acquired disease, such as malignancy (for example colonic or prostatic neoplasms, leukaemia, reticulosis, or myeloma) or malabsorption (due, for example, to a short bowel, blind-loop syndrome, coeliac disease, pancreatic exocrine insufficiency, or giardiasis).

Some people with serum cholesterol levels around 1.0 to 3.5 mmol/litre (40 to 140 mg/dl) will have heterozygous familial hypobetalipoproteinaemia, an autosomal dominant condition in which truncated apoB mutations have been described. The condition is benign. However, homozygous hypoapobetalipoproteinaemia and another condition, abetalipoproteinaemia (inherited as an autosomal recessive), which produce more profound hypocholesterolaemia, are associated with retinitis pigmentosa, unusually shaped erythrocytes (acanthocytes), a syndrome resembling Friedreich's ataxia (preventable with administration fat-soluble vitamins), steatorrhoea (which can create diagnostic confusion with other causes of malabsorption leading to secondary hypocholesterolaemia), and fatty liver. Mutation of the *MTP* gene rather than of the apoB gene is associated with apobetalipoproteinaemia.

Analphalipoproteinaemia (Tangier disease) is a very rare autosomal recessive disorder with virtually absent HDL, reduced LDL cholesteryl ester, and cholesteryl ester deposition throughout the body, leading to enlarged orange-yellow tonsils and adenoids, lymph node enlargement, hepatosplenomegaly, bone marrow infiltration (thrombocytopenia), orange-brown spots on the rectal mucosa, neuropathy, and corneal cloudiness. Heterozygotes for this condition are at increased risk of premature coronary artery disease. A less severe form of this disorder (fish-eye disease) has been described. In another disorder, combined deficiency of apoA-I and apoC-III due to a rearrangement of DNA affecting the transcription of both their genes, which are clustered together on chromosome 11, leads to markedly decreased serum HDL levels, accelerated atherosclerosis, and corneal opacities. Some authorities believe that a much more common genetic HDL deficiency is the cause of HDL cholesterol levels in the lower 10 per cent of the frequency distribution. Evidence for this contention is incomplete.

Further reading

Anderson KM *et al.* (1990). Cardiovascular disease risk profiles. *American Heart Journal* **121**, 293–8.

Assmann G, van Eckardstein A, Brewer HB (1995). Familial high density lipoprotein deficiency: Tangier disease. In: Scriver CR *et al.*, eds. *The metabolic and molecular bases of inherited disease*, 7th edn, pp 2053–72. McGraw-Hill, New York.

Björkhem I, Boberg KM (1995). Inborn errors in bile acid biosynthesis and storage of sterols other than cholesterol. In: Scriver CR *et al.*, eds. *The metabolic and molecular bases of inherited disease*, 7th edn, pp 2073–99. McGraw-Hill, New York.

Breslow JL (1995). Familial disorders of high-density lipoprotein metabolism. In: Scriver CR *et al.*, eds. *The metabolic and molecular bases of inherited disease*, 7th edn, pp 2031–52 McGraw-Hill, New York.

Brooks-Wilson A *et al.* (1999). Mutations in *ABC 1* in Tangier disease and familiar high-density lipoprotein deficiency. *Nature Genetics* **22**, 336–45.

Brunzell JD (1995). Familial lipoprotein lipase deficiency and other causes of the chylomicronemia syndrome. In: Scriver CR *et al.*, eds. *The metabolic and molecular bases of inherited disease*, 7th edn, pp 1913–32 McGraw-Hill, New York.

Davies MJ, Woolf N (1993). Atherosclerosis: what is it and why does it occur? *British Heart Journal* **69** (Suppl.), S3–S11.

Downs GR *et al.* (1998). Primary prevention of acute coronary events with lovastatin in men and women with average cholesterol levels: results of the AFCAPS/TEXCAPS (Air Force/Texas Coronary Atherosclerosis Prevention Study). *Journal of the American Medical Association* **279**, 1615–22.

Durrington PN (1995). Lipoprotein (a). *Baillière's Clinical Endocrinology and Metabolism* **9**, 773–95.

Durrington PN (1998). Triglycerides are more important in atherosclerosis than epidemiology has suggested. *Atherosclerosis* **141** (Suppl. 1), S57–S62.

Durrington PN (2000). Diabetic dyslipidaemia. *Baillière's Clinical Endocrinology and Metabolism* 13, 265–78.

Durrington PN (2002). *Hyperlipidaemia diagnosis and management*, 3rd edn. Butterworth Heinemann, Oxford.

Expert Panel on Detection, Evaluation and Treatment of High Blood Cholesterol in Adults (2001). Executive summary of the third report of the National Cholesterol Education Program (NCEP) Expert Panel on detection, evaluation and treatment of high blood cholesterol in adults (Adult Treatment Panel III). *Journal of the American Medical Association* 285, 2486–97.

Gaw A, Shepherd J (1999). Fibric acid derivatives. In: Betteridge DJ, Illingworth DR, Shepherd J, eds. *Lipoproteins in health and disease*, pp 1145–60. Arnold, London.

Glomset JA *et al.* (1995). Lecithin:cholesterol acyltransferase deficiency and fish eye disease. In: In: Scriver CR *et al.*, eds. *The metabolic and molecular bases of inherited disease*, 7th edn, pp 1933–51 McGraw-Hill, New York.

Goldstein JL, Hobbs HH, Brown MS (1995). Familial hypercholesterolaemia. In: Scriver CR *et al.*, eds. *The metabolic and molecular bases of inherited disease*, 7th edn, pp 1981–2030 McGraw-Hill, New York.

Gould AL *et al.* (1995). Cholesterol reduction yields clinical benefits. A new look at old data. *Circulation* 91, 2274–82.

Grundy SM (1987). Dietary therapy of hyperlipidaemia. *Baillière's Clinical Endocrinology and Metabolism* 1, 667–98.

Heart Protection Study, http://www.ctsu.ox.ac.uk

Herz J (1999). Low-density lipoprotein receptor-related protein. In: Betteridge DJ, Illingworth DR, Shepherd J, eds. *Lipoproteins in health and disease*, pp 333–59. Arnold, London.

Illingworth DR (1999). 3-Hydroxy-3-methylglutaryl-coenzyme A reductase inhibitors. In: Betteridge DJ, Illingworth DR, Shepherd J., eds. *Lipoproteins in health and disease*, pp 1161–79: Arnold, London.

Kane JP, Havel RJ (1995). Disorders of the biogenesis and secretion of lipoproteins containing the B apolipoproteins. In: Scriver CR *et al.*, eds. *The metabolic and molecular bases of inherited disease*, 7th edn, pp 1853–85 McGraw-Hill, New York.

Karathanasis SK (1992). Lipoprotein metabolism: high-density lipoproteins. In: Lusis AJ, Rotter JI, Sparkes RS, eds. *Molecular genetics of coronary artery disease*, pp 140–71. Karger, Basel.

Law MR, Thompson SG, Wald NJ (1994). Assessing possible hazards of reducing serum cholesterol. *British Medical Journal* 308, 373–9.

Law MR, Wald NJ, Thompson SG (1994). By how much and how quickly does reduction in serum cholesterol concentration lower risk of ischaemic heart disease? *British Medical Journal* 308, 367–73.

Mahley RW, Rall SC (1995). Type III hyperlipoproteinemia (dysbetalipoproteinemia): the role of apolipoprotein E in normal and abnormal lipoporotein metabolism. In: Scriver CR *et al.*, eds. *The metabolic and molecular bases of inherited disease*, 7th edn, pp 1953–80. McGraw-Hill, New York.

Manninen V *et al.* (1989). High density lipoprotein cholesterol as a risk factor for coronary heart disease in the Helsinki Heart Study. In: Miller NE, ed. *High density lipoproteins and atherosclerosis II*, pp.35–42. Excerpta Medica, Amsterdam.

Pekkanan J *et al.* (1990). Ten-year mortality from cardiovascular disease in relation to cholesterol level among men with and without preexisting cardiovascular disease. *New England Journal of Medicine* 322, 1700–7.

Rubins HB *et al.* for the Veterans Affairs High-Density Lipoprotein Cholesterol Intervention Trial Study Group (1999). Gemfibrozil for the secondary prevention of coronary heart disease in men with low levels of high-density lipoprotein cholesterol. *New England Journal of Medicine* 341, 410–18.

Sacks FM *et al.* (1996). The effect of pravastatin on coronary events after myocardial infarction in patients with average cholesterol levels. *New England Journal of Medicine* 335, 1001–9.

Sampson MJ, Betteridge DJ (1999). Hyperlipidaemia and combination drug therapy. In: Betteridge, DJ, Illingworth DR, Shepherd J, eds. *Lipoproteins in health and disease*, pp 1213–29. Arnold, London

Scandinavian Simvastatin Survival Study Group (1994). Randomised trial of cholesterol lowering in 4444 patients with coronary heart disease: the Scandinavian Simvastatin Survival Study (4S). *The Lancet* 344, 1383–9.

Schumaker V, Lambertas A (1992). Lipoprotein metabolism: chylomicrons, very-low density lipoproteins and low density lipoproteins. In: Lusis AJ, Rotter JI, Sparkes RS, eds. *Molecular genetics of coronary artery disease*, pp 98–139. Karger, Basel.

West of Scotland Coronary Prevention Group (1996). West of Scotland Coronary Prevention Study: identification of high-risk groups and comparison with other cardiovascular intervention trials. *The Lancet* 348, 1339–42.

Witztum JL, Steinberg D (1991). Role of oxidized low density lipoprotein in atherogenesis. *Journal of Clinical Investigation* 88, 1785–92.

Wood D *et al.* (1998). Joint British recommendations on prevention of coronary heart disease in clinical practice. *Heart* 80 (Suppl. 2), S1–S29.

Wood D *et al.* with members of the Task Force (1998). Prevention of coronary heart disease in clinical practice: recommendations of the Second Joint Task Force of European and other societies on coronary prevention. *Atherosclerosis* 140, 199–270.

11.7 Trace metal disorders

11.7.1 Hereditary haemochromatosis

T. M. Cox

Definition

Haemochromatosis is an hereditary disorder generally caused by inappropriate absorption of iron by the small intestine that leads to iron deposition in the viscera, in endocrine organs, and at other sites. The toxic effects of iron impair the function of these organs and cause structural injury. Haemochromatosis cannot be diagnosed in the absence of excess tissue iron, and there is strong evidence for a cause-and-effect relationship between tissue iron storage and parenchymal injury. Several genetic syndromes associated with iron storage have been identified (Table 1); these may rarely involve specific tissues selectively, such as the lens of the eye or basal ganglia of the brain, or a characteristic range of tissues including the liver, heart, and endocrine system. By common agreement, the term 'hereditary haemochromatosis' refers to a group of inherited iron-storage diseases that affect diverse tissues and cause a multisystem disorder.

Pathological storage of iron

The body contains about 4 g of iron, 3 g of which is complexed with haem to form haemoglobin, myoglobin, and the cytochromes. The non-haem storage compartment, which consists of ferritin and its proteolytic degradation product, haemosiderin, represents up to 0.5 g of elemental iron in adult women and slightly more than 1 g in adult men. Excess storage of

Table 1 Inherited disorders of iron storage

Disorder	OMIM no.	Locus	Gene/protein
Atransferrinaemia	209300	3q21	transferrin
Acaeruloplasminaemia	604290	3q23–q25	caeruloplasmin
Haemochromatosis (HFE 1) (adult)	235200	6p21.3	HFE
Haemochromatosis (HFE 2) (juvenile)	602390	1q	unknown
Haemochromatosis (HFE 3) (adult)	604250	7q22	transferrin receptor 2
Haemochromatosis (HFE 4) (adult, dominant)	606069	2q32	ferroportin
Haemochromatosis (neonatal)	231100	unknown	unknown[†]

† Autosomal recessively inherited in only a few families.

body iron (iron overload) is associated with an increase in hepatic iron concentrations and of the surrogate biomarker, serum ferritin. Minimal iron storage occurs when more than 1.5 g of total body iron is present; this is reflected in a hepatic iron concentration of approximately 30 μg atoms/g of tissue with a serum ferritin level of usually less than 250 μg/litre. Moderate iron-storage disease is reflected by a serum ferritin of approximately 500 μg/litre; under these circumstances the hepatic iron concentration rises to 100 μg atoms/g. Severe iron-storage disease (more than 5 g of storage iron) is shown by a hepatic iron concentration over 200 μg atoms/g liver tissue, with a serum ferritin level of at least 750 μg/litre—under these circumstances, tissue injury with impaired function is almost invariably present.

Clinical subtypes of haemochromatosis

Adult haemochromatosis

The familiar form of haemochromatosis is the classical adult type, which typically presents in middle age and is usually expressed in men. The disorder is inherited as a recessive trait and is due to mutations in a gene, *HFE*, that maps to the short arm of chromosome 6 in close apposition to the HLA class I loci of the human major histocompatibility complex (MHC). Expression of iron-storage disease in individuals carrying mutations in the *HFE* gene is very variable and is influenced by several environmental and sexual factors. Mutant alleles of the *HFE* gene that predispose to adult-type haemochromatosis are widespread and frequent in populations of North European origin. There is evidence from haplotype analysis that a single mutation arose on an ancestral chromosome 6 and spread throughout this population, probably as a result of the migration of the Vikings from Scandinavia. The disease occurs throughout the world as a result of intermarriage but is at its highest frequency in France, Germany, Great Britain, Scandinavia, Ireland, Northern Italy, Spain, and Eastern Europe as far as European Russia. Colonization has led to its appearance in all populations of the United States and in Australasia; for this reason hereditary adult-type haemochromatosis also occurs in South America.

Classical adult-type haemochromatosis is a slowly progressive disease affecting the liver, endocrine system, heart, and joints; it is often only diagnosed when irreversible tissue injury has occurred. The condition predisposes to the development of primary carcinomas of the liver. Other, rare, genetic forms of adult haemochromatosis occur in patients homozygous for mutations in the transferrin receptor gene type 2 (*TFR 2*) and in those heterozygous for mutant alleles of the human ferroportin gene.

Juvenile haemochromatosis

Since the identification of adult iron-storage disease by several European physicians during the nineteenth century, a similar disease has been recognized in children and young adults who may develop iron-storage disease of a more severe character, and which is now designated 'juvenile haemochromatosis'. Juvenile haemochromatosis is defined as iron-storage disease occurring before the age of 35 years; it evolves rapidly, typically affects the heart and endocrine system, and causes infantilism and hypogonadism as well as life-threatening cardiac arrhythmias. Juvenile haemochromatosis is inherited as a very rare recessive trait in which there is an increased frequency of consanguinity amongst the parents of affected subjects. Juvenile haemochromatosis resembles the severe iron-storage disease associated with the iron-loading anaemias, such as β-thalassaemia. Juvenile haemochromatosis affects males and females equally—an observation that reflects the overwhelming nature of the iron homeostatic defect: iron overload develops before the modifying effects of menstruation and dietary factors supervene. Recent studies have mapped at least one form of juvenile haemochromatosis to the long arm of chromosome 1. At the time of writing, the nature of the product of this gene is unknown.

Neonatal haemochromatosis

Neonatal haemochromatosis is a newly identified syndrome of uncertain cause, characterized by congenital cirrhosis or fulminant hepatitis associated with the widespread deposition of iron in hepatic and extrahepatic tissues. Approximately 100 cases of neonatal haemochromatosis have been reported. Neonatal haemochromatosis occurs in the context of maternal disease—including viral infection, as a complication of metabolic disease in the fetus, and sporadically or recurrently, without overt cause, in siblings. In some families, although neonatal haemochromatosis appears to have an hereditary basis, no predictive genetic test is available to inform the outcome of at-risk pregnancies.

Prevalence and epidemiology

Juvenile and neonatal haemochromatosis are rare disorders that occur sporadically, but hereditary adult haemochromatosis is widely disseminated and of global importance. Removal of toxic iron by repeated venesection improves the outcome for adult haemochromatosis. If this treatment is instituted before irreversible tissue injury occurs, venesection may restore health and a normal life expectancy. For these reasons, there has been much discussion about the early recognition of iron-storage disease by the introduction of population-based screening programmes (using genetic testing or phenotypic biochemical screening methods) that can be applied to communities at risk.

In European populations, about 1 in 10 individuals carries one copy of an allele of the *HFE* gene that predisposes to iron-storage disease, and between 1 in 100 and 1 in 400 persons in these populations are homozygotes or compound heterozygotes with biochemical abnormalities of iron storage that may lead to full-blown clinical haemochromatosis. Thus the mutant allele, designated *C282Y* of *HFE*, which is the principal determinant of iron-storage disease, occurs at polymorphic frequency and is one of the most common genetic abnormalities leading to an autosomal recessive disease in populations of North-European origin. In European patients with iron-storage disease due to hereditary haemochromatosis, the frequency of homozygosity for the *C282Y HFE* allele ranges from about 35 per cent in Southern Italy to more than 90 per cent in the British Isles, including Ireland; in Australia, homozygosity for *C282Y* occurs in almost 100 per cent of patients with hereditary haemochromatosis. However, as discussed later, although useful for diagnosis, homozygosity for the *C282Y* mutation of *HFE* is **not** tantamount to a diagnosis of established iron-storage disease nor, therefore, of clinical haemochromatosis.

Clinical expression of haemochromatosis is highly dependent on age and it is very rare for there to be detectable disease in adults below the age of 20 years. As clinical disease is much more common in men than women, it is likely to reflect environmental factors and the modification of disease expression due to blood loss associated with menstruation and the investment in pregnancies, as well as the comparatively reduced dietary complement of iron in women. Other environmental factors, particularly the consumption of alcohol, appear to interact with predisposing genetic factors to induce the clinical expression of iron-storage disease in *C282Y* homozygotes. Most patients with the disease develop symptoms at, or above, the age of 40 years. However, studies of iron metabolism by bio-

chemical measurements or tissue biopsy may reveal early evidence of iron storage in the long presymptomatic phase of this condition. With greater awareness of the diverse clinical manifestations of adult-type hereditary haemochromatosis, detection on the basis of early symptoms, for example arthritis or endocrine disease, may be possible. Thus, although the mutations that predispose to the development of haemochromatosis as a clinical entity are frequent in populations of European ancestry, there is a marked disparity in populations in which *C282Y* homozygosity is prevalent and the frequency with which symptomatic haemochromatosis is diagnosed.

Phenotypic expression of disease

For epidemiological purposes, since there is no internationally agreed case definition of haemochromatosis, caution is needed in interpreting claims that haemochromatosis is the most common inherited disorder affecting European peoples. Phenotypic expression of disease may range from the established clinical syndrome (cutaneous pigmentation, cardiomyopathy, endocrine failure—especially diabetes mellitus and hypogonadism, arthritis, and pigment cirrhosis) to a slight abnormality of blood parameters that reflect iron metabolism—elevated serum transferrin iron saturation and serum ferritin measurements. Such studies that are available to determine the penetrance and expressivity of the haemochromatosis gene have provided widely varying results in different populations: in Australia, where the mean intake of iron in the diet appears to be much greater than in the average European population today, most middle-aged male *C282Y* homozygotes appear to express at least one clinical manifestation of iron-storage disease. Similarly, a study of homozygous relatives (principally siblings) within pedigrees known to have haemochromatosis suggest that about half the men over 40 years of age, and about 1 in 6 of the women over 50 years of age, have at least one haemochromatosis-related clinical disorder. This latter survey, conducted in the United States, suggests that an important proportion of homozygous relatives of patients with established haemochromatosis, especially men, have conditions such as cirrhosis and arthropathy as well as abnormalities of serum liver-related tests that are not detected by spontaneous clinical referral.

Many reports of disease expression in haemochromatosis may, however, be questioned because of the prevalence of co-segregating genes within affected pedigrees, as well as early household environmental factors common to siblings that may predispose to disease expression. Studies in mice support this explanation, since it has been shown that several independent genetic determinants control the extent of iron-loading observed in mouse models of iron-storage disease generated by targeted disruption of the murine homologue of the *HFE* gene. In contrast, surveys conducted in outbred populations, for example in Jersey, show a great disparity between the predicted frequency of homozygosity for *C282Y* and the number of recorded cases with the disease attending local hospitals. These latter studies may reflect the widely suspected inability of clinicians to diagnose haemochromatosis, and an inability to bring together the unitary clinical manifestations of the disease into a unifying diagnostic category. However, widely differing degrees of disease penetrance almost certainly account for the apparent shortfall of diagnosed cases in populations at risk.

At present, no clear data in large unbiased population surveys are available to assess disease penetrance and the modifying effects of lifestyle factors (including alcohol, nutrition, diet) as well as pregnancy and menstruation that are likely to influence the effects and rate of iron storage in human *C282Y* homozygotes. Mortality figures show that death is rarely attributed to hereditary haemochromatosis in populations at risk. This fact contrasts starkly with the well-established known complications of the fully penetrant clinical syndrome, in which early death results from cirrhosis of the liver, hepatocellular carcinoma, endocrine failure or cardiac complications.

A contemporary study that examined the frequency of the most common symptoms of haemochromatosis in *C282Y* homozygotes, *C282Y/H63D* compound heterozygotes, and persons wild-type at these loci has been reported from California. In more than 41 000 individuals attending a health appraisal clinic, no evidence of an increased frequency of symptoms was identified in those genetically predisposed to iron-storage disease. The only significant clinical history identified in the at-risk group was that of 'hepatitis' or prior 'liver complaints'; only one of the 152 identified *C282Y* homozygotes had signs and symptoms of adult haemochromatosis. This provocative report, indicating a very low clinical penetrance (less than 1 per cent) of the haemochromatosis genotype in an unusual group of adults over the age of 26 years, raises important questions about the introduction of mass population screening for this potentially treatable iron-storage disease by genetic or even biochemical methods. However, the high prevalence of impotence, joint symptoms, chronic fatigue, and other complaints such as cardiac arrhythmias in the study group as a whole, raises disturbing questions about the valid application of this report to other populations. It is perhaps not surprising that in a group where, on average, more than 40 per cent complained of a general limitation of their health and/or joint symptoms, and in which more than 35 per cent of the male participants scored positively on symptom enquiry about impotence, a significant contribution from predisposing haemochromatosis alleles could not be identified. Nonetheless, this large study raises key questions about the utility of screening for adult haemochromatosis as a genetic disease. Before screening for haemochromatosis is introduced, there is clearly a need for other population surveys to be carried out in which the morbidity and mortality of individuals with the wild-type genotype as well as those harbouring disease alleles are investigated.

Pathophysiology and pathogenesis

Young patients with haemochromatosis absorb an increased amount of dietary iron in their upper intestine compared with normal control subjects. In established iron-storage disease, iron absorption continues at a rate that is inappropriate for the level of iron stores as reflected by serum ferritin and tissue iron determinations.

In the absence of an effective excretory pathway, the increased absorption of iron by the intestine leads to a progressive accumulation of the metal in the parenchymal cells of the liver, heart, endocrine glands, and specialized B-type synoviocytes. Excess iron accumulates in the pancreas where it is found in both acinar and endocrine cells of the islet, although there is a particular predisposition in the early phases of iron loading to the islet beta-cell. Iron also accumulates to toxic levels in the gonadotrophs of the anterior hypophysis, leading to hypogonadotrophic hypogonadism. Iron may accumulate in the adrenal gland, where it is concentrated particularly in those cells that secrete aldosterone, in the zona glomerulosa. Iron accumulates in the cardiac myocytes and conducting tissue of the heart, in the chief cells of the parathyroid, and in parenchymal cells throughout the body. The consequences of toxic iron storage include diabetes mellitus, cirrhosis of the liver, cardiomyopathy with or without conduction defects, hypogonadism, arthritis with chondrocalcinosis, adrenocortical deficiency, and, rarely, hypoparathyroidism. Evidence for the intrinsic toxicity of iron in haemochromatosis is provided by the regression of the pathological changes following measures taken to reduce iron, for example the use of iron chelators and removal of body iron by venesection. Venesection stimulates the mobilization and removal of iron from the storage compartment by increasing the demand for red cell production in the bone marrow.

Mechanism of iron toxicity

High concentrations of iron salts are toxic to cultured cells. The administration of iron chelates to experimental animals has induced diabetes with iron loading in the liver and pancreas as well as the generation of (renal) carcinomas. Injections of iron salts induce local sarcomas in experimental animals, with evidence of species susceptibility. In humans, sarcomas or carcinomas have arisen, albeit rarely, at sites of therapeutic injections of iron, and it is possible that the complications of silicosis and asbestos exposure result from the complement of iron associated with these particu-

lates. A wealth of indirect but corroborative evidence indicates that the primary effect of excess free iron is to promote the formation of oxygen free radicals, which mediate the damage to cells and tissues that is observed in iron-storage disease. In established haemochromatosis, the iron-binding capacity of plasma transferrin may be exceeded so that a proportion of the iron present in the blood remains reactive as a low-molecular-weight species only loosely attached to plasma proteins. Non-transferrin iron in human plasma stimulates the peroxidation of unsaturated lipids and can form reactive complexes that react with DNA—thus suggesting a mechanism for genome toxicity and carcinogenesis related to iron overload. Iron is highly electroreactive, and coupling of the Fenton and Harber–Weiss reactions leads to the formation of hydroxyl radicals as a result of the catalytic interactions between superoxide and ferric ions. Tissues with significant iron storage show peroxidative injury in membrane lipid fractions.

The lysosomal compartment appears to be particularly susceptible to iron-mediated damage, since iron in the form of ferritin and its degradation product, haemosiderin, accumulates within lysosomes to form the particulate ferruginous granules known as 'siderosomes'. In haemochromatosis, there is an increased activity of lysosomal enzymes with biochemical evidence of increased lysosomal fragility indicating disruption of the integrity of the lysosomal membrane by iron; these changes revert to normal when the tissue iron is removed by venesection or by the use of specific iron chelators. It seems likely that the electrochemical reactivity of iron and its particular propensity to accelerate the formation of oxygen free radicals mediate its injurious effects on cell membranes, as well as the nuclear genome leading to cancerous change. However, despite great advances in the understanding of free-radical chemistry, the cause-and-effect relationship between iron storage and tissue injury is difficult to prove unequivocally. Nonetheless, much experimental evidence points to the development of iron-mediated peroxidative injury of cellular membranes including the lysosome, as well as iron-mediated genotoxicity. Whatever their physicochemical basis might be, common mechanisms of iron toxicity clearly exist, since the pathological and clinical manifestations of all iron-storage syndromes, including secondary haemochromatosis associated with blood transfusion and the iron-loading anaemias, are almost identical.

Pathology of iron storage

Heavy deposits of iron in the tissues are associated with fibrosis and cell loss. Simple inspection reveals an overt rust-like discoloration of the liver, spleen, pancreas, heart, and lymph nodes. The liver is usually enlarged; haemosiderin is found in all cell types with the formation of fibrous septa and hyperplastic nodules. These nodules, which may be the forerunners of adenomas and hepatocellular carcinomas, contain little stainable iron—unlike the adjacent parenchyma.

The dominant site of iron deposition during the early phases is within hepatocytes but soon iron loading may be observed in all cell types, including the lining cells of biliary canaliculi, Kupffer cells, and stellate cells (Figs 1 and 2 and Plates 1 and 2).

Similarly, in the pancreas there is fibrosis and iron deposition in the acini, ducts, and islets of Langerhans. Staining with Perls' reagent reveals marked haemosiderin deposition in the exocrine and endocrine glands, including many cell types in the testes. Haemosiderin is also markedly increased in the chief cells of the parathyroid, the adenohypophysis, the zona glomerulosa of the adrenal, and the thyroid.

In the joints, there is loss of the intra-articular space with chondrocalcinosis and deposits of haemosiderin in the synovium; electron microscopy shows selective deposits of ferritin and haemosiderin within type B synoviocytes. Radiological examination of the joints shows collapse of articular surfaces, subchondral cyst formation, and prominent formation of periarticular osteophytes. In the heart, pericardial constriction with fibrosis may occasionally be observed, but the principal abnormality is seen in the myocardium with degeneration and vacuolation of cardiac myocytes and intermyocyte fibrosis that involves conducting tissue in the septa. Surviving myocytes show eosinophilic degeneration and evidence of hypertrophy.

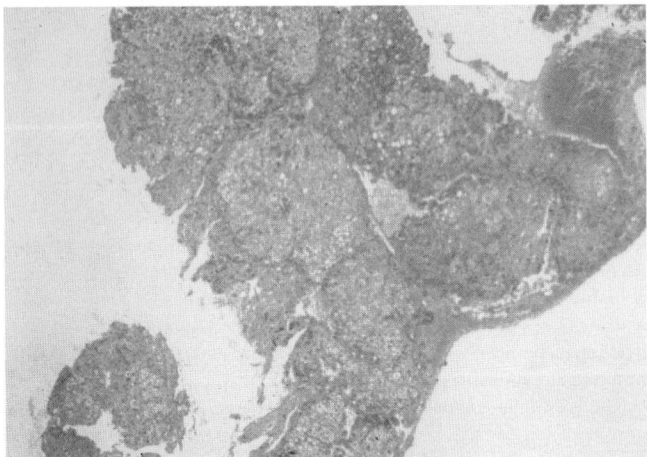

Fig. 1 Low-power, needle-biopsy appearance of liver specimen stained with haematoxylin and eosin from a 67-year-old man with adult haemochromatosis due to homozygosity for the *C282Y* mutation. Note the large hyperplastic nodules and fibrosis. (See also Plate 1.)

Microscopical examination shows that in established cases of haemochromatosis, all tissues (except the choroid plexus) are affected by the iron-storage process. In the past, it was considered that transfusional and other types of secondary iron-storage disease predominantly affected the cells of the mononuclear macrophage system, such as the Kupffer cells of the liver, rather than the parenchymal cells. Iron deposits in the macrophage system may be less damaging than in other cell types, but it is difficult at present to relate evidence of iron-mediated injury to its cellular distribution. Progressive tissue injury follows the long-term cumulative toxicity of iron storage and its consequential effects on organ structure and cellular function. A striking, but unexplained, feature of iron-storage disease in the liver and other tissues is the absence of overt necrosis; careful study of the cellular effects of iron storage on apoptotic mechanisms in diseased tissues is clearly warranted.

Quantitative aspects of iron-storage disease

Chemical determination of tissue iron content yields useful information about the severity of iron loading in haemochromatosis, and may also provide a means to judge local responses to iron-depletion therapy, such as venesection. In normal individuals, the total concentrations of liver iron do

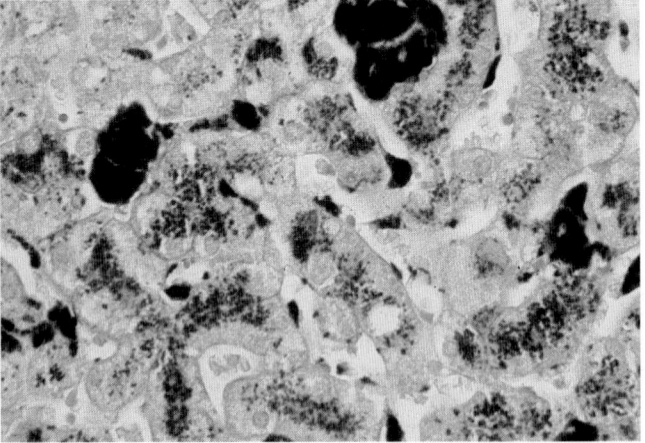

Fig. 2 High-power micrograph of the liver biopsy specimen shown in Fig. 1 stained with Perls' reagent. Note extensive deposits of ferric iron in all cell types including Kupffer cells, cells lining small biliary radicles, and in a punctate distribution within parenchymal hepatocytes. Liver cells are hyperplastic. (See also Plate 2.)

not exceed 0.15 per cent by dry weight, but in established haemochromatosis the value is usually 1 per cent or more; in severely affected patients with untreated hereditary haemochromatosis or secondary haemochromatosis the amount of iron may exceed 5 per cent of the dry weight of tissue. The overall burden of body iron in patients with haemochromatosis is usually in excess of 5 g in hereditary disease, a figure that rises with age. Estimates indicate that the total burden in patients with advanced haemochromatosis can be as much as 40 to 60 g—most of this accumulating in the liver—the pancreas and other organs such as the lymph, thyroid, pituitary, and salivary glands typically show an increase of more than 10 times the normal iron content.

Nature of the metabolic defect

In established haemochromatosis, where the burden of iron may increase body iron stores by at least tenfold, measurements usually show that iron absorption is within the normal range. Studies in young patients with rapidly progressive disease show a markedly increased absorption of iron, and all the evidence points to an increase in iron absorption to 2 to 3 mg daily throughout the lifetime of patients with haemochromatosis. After depletion therapy, the rate of recovery of iron stores is greatly enhanced for many years in patients with haemochromatosis, reflecting a persistent homeostatic abnormality in the retention of dietary iron. The daily absorption of between 2 and 4 mg of iron over a period of 30 to 40 years accounts for the degree of iron loading that occurs at presentation in patients with haemochromatosis, and compares with the normal absorption of 0.8 to 1.0 mg in men and in women, up to 2 mg daily. In effect, the abnormal absorption of iron represents a disturbed regulation of the final common pathway for the acquisition of iron from the environment by the small intestinal mucosa.

Iron absorption in hereditary haemochromatosis

A recent report, describing the transplantation of intestine and liver from an *HFE C282Y* homozygote into a recipient without haemochromatosis, has provided evidence that the small intestine is the principal site of expression of the hereditary defect in adult haemochromatosis. The transplantation was associated with early iron overloading in the recipient, together with raised serum transferrin iron saturations—a phenomenon not observed in recipients of hepatic allografts obtained from donors later found to be homozygous for the haemochromatosis gene. Studies *in vitro* and *in vivo* have suggested that there is a qualitative abnormality of the uptake and transfer of iron from the intestinal lumen in patients with hereditary haemochromatosis, although, until recently, the nature of this abnormality was unclear.

Latterly, genetic studies of mutant strains of mice with abnormalities of iron metabolism have shed light on the iron-absorption mechanism. The identification of a single gene encoding the divalent metal transporter protein, DMT 1, which is expressed in the upper small intestine and cells of the erythron, provides a molecular understanding of the iron deficiency—and the microcytic anaemia that occurs in the *mk/mk* mouse strain. A single point mutation in the *DMT1* gene interferes with the uptake of ferrous iron, since it disrupts the cognate transmembrane carrier protein mainly expressed in the mucosa of the proximal small intestine at the site of iron absorption and in the erythroid precursor cells. Since *in vitro* studies of the expressed protein DMT 1 show that it serves only as a carrier of divalent cations, and that interference with this pathway is sufficient to induce iron deficiency in a mammalian species, ferrous iron uptake is probably the main pathway by which inorganic iron is acquired by the intestine. Human *DMT1* maps to the long arm of chromosome 12 and encodes a 12 membrane-spanning protein that is expressed in the apical membrane of the upper intestine and in the apical membrane of differentiated human CaCo-2 cells of small intestinal phenotype. DMT 1 is also expressed in developing erythroid cells in which it is responsible for the intracellular delivery of iron derived from transferrin for haemoglobin synthesis.

The discovery of DMT 1 immediately indicated a possible role for this important protein in human haemochromatosis. Overexpression of *DMT1* mRNA has been identified in the intestinal mucosa of patients homozygous for the *C282Y* mutation with hereditary haemochromatosis, as well as in mice with iron-storage disease due to targeted disruption of the *HFE* gene. At the same time, studies in experimental animals have identified a cyto-chrome-containing ferrireductase that is also localized to the intestinal brush-border membrane; this reductase has been cloned from murine intestine and its human homologue has been identified. Expression of mucosal ferrireductase is specific to the apical microvillous membrane of mammalian intestinal mucosa and appears to be induced in response to nutritional iron deficiency. Mucosal ferrireductase reduces ferric irons derived from the diet in the lumen for delivery to the DMT 1 carrier protein, the final divalent pathway for inorganic iron uptake by intestinal mucosa. The mRNA species encoding murine *DMT1* exist in two isoforms, one of which contains an iron-response element (**IRE**) 3′ region—which would allow for the post-transcriptional regulation of protein expression controlled by intracellular iron status. A similar translational control of transferrin receptor expression has been described with the 3′ IRE in the mRNA encoding the human transferrin receptor. Since the IRE-containing isoform of DMT 1 is preferentially expressed in the duodenum, it seems likely that changes in intracellular iron status regulate the expression of this carrier protein in iron deficiency and haemochromatosis. Studies in *HFE* knockout mice indicate that the functional expression of the DMT1 protein is enhanced in the murine model of haemochromatosis, leading to increased iron uptake across the brush-border membrane of iron presented in the ferrous form; the action of non-rate-limiting ferrireductases at the brush-border membrane functionally coupled to DMT 1 activity appears to explain the enhanced isotopic uptake of ferrous iron in this model of haemochromatosis.

At present, our molecular understanding of transepithelial iron uptake in haemochromatosis and in health is somewhat rudimentary. A novel gene termed 'ferroportin', encoding a multitransmembrane domain protein, has been identified. The cognate protein may function as an exporter of iron across the brush-border membrane at the basal surface of the intestine as well as in placental syncytotrophoblasts. Ferrroportin appears also to be responsible for the export of iron retrieved by erythrophagocytosis by macrophages. After initial uptake, the enhanced transfer of iron across the mucosal epithelium in haemochromatosis and iron deficiency is mediated by, as yet, unknown iron-binding proteins. Delivery of the iron to the systemic circulation is mediated by the regulated downstream coexpression of the membrane protein, ferroportin. It seems likely that, in hereditary haemochromatosis and physiological iron deficiency, post-transcriptional control of carrier proteins responsible for the uptake and transfer of iron occurs in the absorptive epithelium on the tips of the intestinal villi. Thus homeostatic mechanisms in the proximal intestine operate to bring about the co-ordinated transfer of iron presented in the intestinal lumen specifically to meet body requirements. Proteins including hephaestin encoded on the X- chromosome, which is mutated in the sex-linked anaemic mouse *sla*, also mediates the transfer of iron across the intestinal mucosa.

The signal for regulating the absorptive activity of the ferrous ion transport pathway is not known. However, it seems likely that interactions between the wild-type HFE protein and transferrin receptors, including the newly described transferrin receptor 2 isoform that may be expressed in intestinal crypts, in some way instruct the developing epithelial cells within the intestinal crypt about body iron requirements. Although functional interactions of HFE molecules with the identified components of the absorptive pathway have yet to be clarified, the HFE protein probably influences iron status in intestinal stem cells within the crypt. By these means, the expression of key transport proteins such as DMT 1 and ferroportin may be imprinted, thus influencing their subsequent functional activity during ascent up the villus. At present, however, much more experimental work will be required to further our understanding of the signalling path-

ways by which the body iron status regulates the avidity of the proximal small intestine for nutritional iron presented within the lumen.

A variable but often substantial, component of dietary iron is present in the organic form as haem; a full molecular understanding of the uptake and transfer pathways for the absorption of iron complexes to the porphyrias is also needed. Whole-body studies show that the absorption of the radiolabelled iron moiety of haemoglobin is enhanced in patients with adult-type haemochromatosis. Early studies in dogs have shown that, in the presence of proteolytic digestion products of globin, the haem complex is taken up intact by mucosal epithelial cells; free iron is then released by the action of intracellular haem oxygenases. The contribution of haemoglobin, myoglobin, and cytochromes to the iron overload in patients with haemochromatosis has not been quantified but iron complexed to haem may well represent an important component of the total burden of body iron in symptomatic haemochromatosis.

Genetics and molecular biology of haemochromatosis

The principal determinant of adult haemochromatosis has long been known to be tightly linked to the human MHC loci on the short arm of chromosome 6. In 1996, mutations in the HLA class I-linked haemochromatosis gene, *HFE*, were shown to predispose to the adult form of the disease. The most common mutation in the non-classical MHC class I HFE protein affects a key cysteine residue, which contributes to the formation of the conserved α-3 helix that interacts co-translationally with the β2-microglobulin protein. This association is required for the cell-surface expression of all class I MHC molecules. Most patients with haemochromatosis are thus homozygous for a cysteine-to-tyrosine mutation at codon 282 (*C282Y*) of the nascent HFE protein; an increased frequency of this mutation, in association with the more common *H63D* missense mutation, also occurs in adult haemochromatosis (Fig. 3). A minor variant, affecting the same region in the α-1 helix, *S65C*, is also occasionally associated with the *C282Y* allele in compound heterozygotes with adult iron-storage disease.

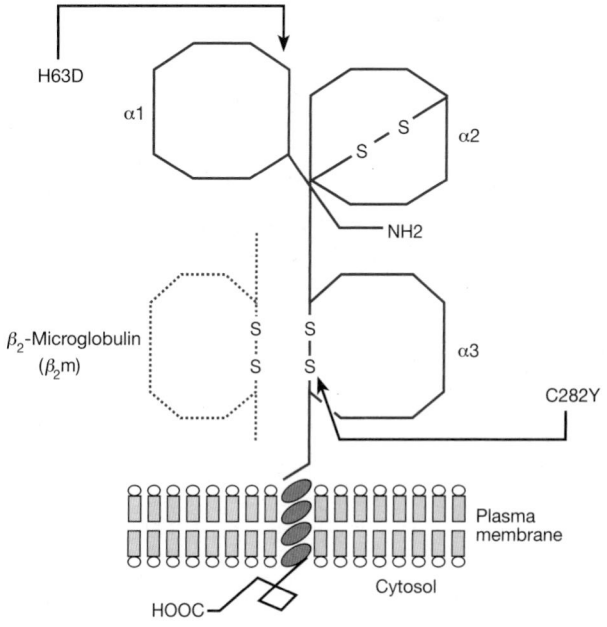

Fig. 3 Diagram of non-classical MHC class I-like HFE molecule shown in juxtaposition with the β2-microglobulin. The location of the two frequent amino-acid substitutions (*C282Y* and H63D) that predispose to the development of adult haemochromatosis is indicated by the arrows.

These missense mutations in HFE occur at a much lower frequency in control populations without iron overload. Apart from reducing cell-surface expression of the mutant C282Y polypeptide, and thus the abundance of this protein within a population of cytoplasmic vesicles, a functional explanation for the qualitative abnormality of iron metabolism that characterizes haemochromatosis is not available. Recent unsubstantiated experiments have indicated the coexpression of HFE with transferrin receptor isoforms within a vesicular intracellular compartment. Structural studies have provided a molecular basis for this interaction based on the expression of truncated soluble HFE and transferrin receptor protein *in vitro*, combined with elegant structural studies using X-ray diffraction. Latterly, a novel isoform of the transferrin receptor, transferrin receptor type 2, has been identified in intestinal crypt cells where it may colocalize with the HFE protein within intracellular vesicles. Since rare cases of adult haemochromatosis have been reported with nonsense and inactivating (null) mutations in the *TfR2* (transferrin receptor 2) gene, it seems likely that the HFE protein participates in the regulation of iron delivery to cells through the transferrin ligand. HFE may affect the delivery of transferrin-bound iron by way of the transferrin receptor, or, also plausibly, by the transferrin isoform *TfR2* in intestinal crypt cells, thereby influencing their subsequent absorptive behaviour.

Mutations in *HFE* can be easily detected by the use of restriction enzymes and analysis of amplified *HFE* gene sequences obtained from genomic DNA. Point mutations in rare cases of non-HFE-associated haemochromatosis have been identified in the *ferroportin* and in the *TfR2* genes. Patients harbouring inactivating mutations in the gene encoding the iron-transfer ligand, serum transferrin, are also reported in association with severe iron-storage disease. This finding, together with the iron-storage disease associated with enhanced iron absorption in hypotransferrinaemic mice (*hpx*), implicates this transferrin-receptor subtype in the physiological regulation of iron homeostasis.

Clinical features

Adult haemochromatosis.

The clinical features of adult haemochromatosis include skin pigmentation. The pigment may be manifest as a generalized slate-grey coloration, due principally to melanin, or localized bronzed pigmentation particularly of the lower limbs, associated with iron deposits in adnexal dermal structures as well as melanin. Histological examination of the skin reveals increased melanocyte activity in conjunction with iron deposits, particularly in cutaneous sweat and apocrine glands. Increased skin pigmentation is a common but not invariable manifestation of haemochromatosis. It increases as the disease progresses and may be a late manifestation of the condition; absence of pigmentation should never, as a consequence, be regarded as a contraindication to the diagnosis of iron-storage disease.

Iron-storage disease invariably affects the liver. The liver is usually enlarged and may be cirrhotic, but portal hypertension and splenomegaly are rare endstage features of haemochromatosis. The enlarged liver, even in the absence of cirrhosis, may contain single or multifocal hepatocellular carcinomas. Hypogonadism is often present; it is typically preceded by a long history of fatigue, sexual asthenia, and impotence, as well as premature menopause and loss of libido in women. In men, there is gynaecomastia, circumoral vertical skin wrinkling, and loss of body hair; the genitalia show premature atrophy.

Many patients with haemochromatosis suffer from arthritis at an early phase in the illness and this may indeed be the sole manifestation of the condition for many years. The arthritis typically affects the second and third metacarpophalangeal joints of the hands and feet (Fig. 4 and Plate 3). These joints show painful swelling without obvious inflammatory changes. Distal interphalangeal joint disease is also recorded and is usually considered to be typical of osteoarthritis. Many joints, including the wrist, elbow, shoulder, and knee, may be affected and the changes in these joints are typically associated with chondrocalcinosis that is detected radiolog-

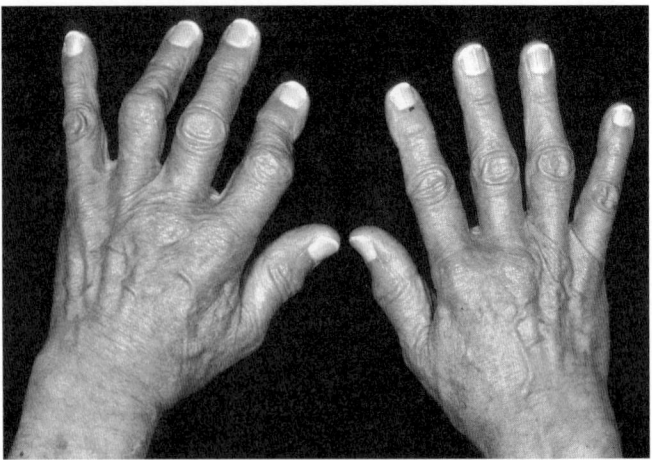

Fig. 4 Arthropathy in a man with adult haemochromatosis forced to stop manual work because of painful arthritis especially in the second and third metacarpophalangeal joints; note increased skin pigmentation. (See also Plate 3.)

ically. The affected joints show loss of joint space, subchondral cysts, and, especially in the digits, prominent osteophyte formation (Fig. 5). Recent studies show that premature and disabling arthritis in the hip and other large joints is a characteristic feature of haemochromatosis.

The symptoms of haemochromatosis are notoriously non-specific and slow in their progression. Fatigue is often reported and may be a manifestation of hypogonadism and the onset of diabetes mellitus. Atrial fibrillation may be an early manifestation of cardiomyopathy. Later, paroxysmal arrhythmias and cardiac failure supervene, leading to shortness of breath and fatigue. Occasional patients with haemochromatosis present with isolated features, such as abnormal liver-related tests detected during routine examination for health insurance, or with arthralgia and signs of arthropathy in association with either diabetes, impaired libido, or sexual failure. Cardiomyopathy with heart failure or isolated arrhythmias is an unusual lone presentation of the disease.

The differential diagnosis of haemochromatosis is very wide, but the presence of diabetes with abnormal liver function or hepatomegaly, or an association with endocrine failure or arthropathy, should prompt consideration of iron-storage disease. Likewise, the presence of seronegative polyarthropathy with pigmentation, hepatomegaly, or any of the associated endocrinological changes should initiate immediate testing for evidence of iron-storage disease.

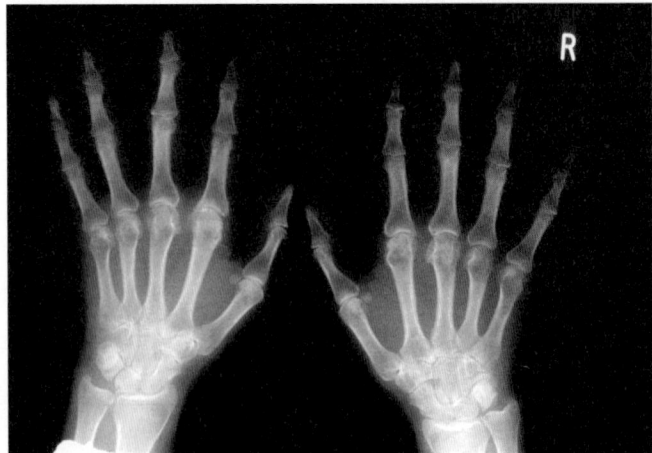

Fig. 5 Radiograph of hands in a 51-year-old woman with haemochromatotic arthropathy of the hands for many years. Note loss of joint space especially in metacarpophalangeal joints with subchondral cyst formation and osteophyte growth. Chondrocalcinosis is present in the ulnar fibro-cartilage at the wrist.

In young patients with hypogonadism or cardiomyopathy, iron-storage disease should be considered; juvenile haemochromatosis is often neglected by endocrinologists investigating young patients for infantilism or hypogonadotrophic hypogonadism. The condition may be responsible for cases of undiagnosed seronegative polyarthropathy. Iron-storage disease should be considered in any patient with signs and symptoms of chronic liver disease, including those with sustained mild elevation of serum transaminase activities, particularly since the liver is affected early in the course of the iron overload.

In fully established cases, skin pigmentation which may either be of a grey colour as a result of increased melanin, or, especially on the shins, a yellow-brown 'bronze' colour. Pigmentation in association with diabetes with or without arthropathy and hepatomegaly almost always signifies established iron-storage disease.

Diagnosis

It is critically important to make a diagnosis of haemochromatosis at the earliest opportunity. There is strong evidence that if treatment to remove iron before established structural injury occurs, then tissue function and symptoms improve. Several surveys indicate that removal of iron from patients diagnosed in the precirrhotic phase of adult haemochromatosis is associated with a normal or near-normal life expectancy.

Laboratory investigations

In adult haemochromatosis, the diagnosis can be usually established by demonstrating abnormalities of iron metabolism (fasting serum transferrin saturation with iron greater than 60 per cent), together with a measurement of serum ferritin concentration that provides evidence of increased iron stores. In most, but not all, untreated patients with pathological iron-storage disease due to haemochromatosis, the serum concentration of ferritin is elevated. Molecular analysis of the *HFE* gene for homozygosity for the common (*C282Y*) predisposing allele to the development of adult haemochromatosis may be very useful in patients of European ancestry. There is an increased frequency of compound heterozygotes for the *C282Y/H63D* or, more rarely, *C282Y/S65C* genotypes in patients with evidence of iron-storage disease.

Not all patients with adult haemochromatosis have mutations in the *HFE* gene; moreover, genetic tests are not at present available for the diagnosis of juvenile haemochromatosis or of neonatal haemochromatosis. In some patients with adult iron-storage disease, mutations have been identified in a newly identified gene that encodes a variant of the transferrin receptor—transferrin receptor type 2 (*TfR2*). Homozygosity for mutations in *TfR2* are found in some Southern European patients with adult haemochromatosis. Adult haemochromatosis due to mutations in the *HFE* gene is now known as HFE 1; juvenile haemochromatosis due to lesions in an, as yet, uncharacterized locus on chromosome 1q are now designated HFE 2, and mutations in the type 2 transferrin receptor gene cause HFE 3—another adult variant of hereditary haemochromatosis. As indicated above, HFE 2 (juvenile haemochromatosis) is a much more severe disease than either HFE 1 or HFE 3—although hypogonadism can be a presenting symptom in both HFE 1 and HFE 3 (see Table 1). A rare form of adult haemochromatosis, principally transmitted as a dominant trait, appears to be associated with point mutations in the newly described *ferroportin* gene (see above). It is believed that ferroportin is involved in the transport of iron from the intestinal epithelial cells to the body as well as to the liver. This type of haemochromatosis, now designated HFE 4, appears, if anything, to be slightly milder than haemochromatosis in the homozygous recessive forms of HFE 1, 2, and 3. HFE 4 responds poorly to iron-depletion therapy by venesection; histological examination reveals prominent iron storage within Kupffer cells.

Given the genetic variants that are now recognized as causes of haemochromatosis, it is clear that if any doubt exists as to the diagnosis, or molecular analysis of the *HFE* gene fails to identify known pathogenic

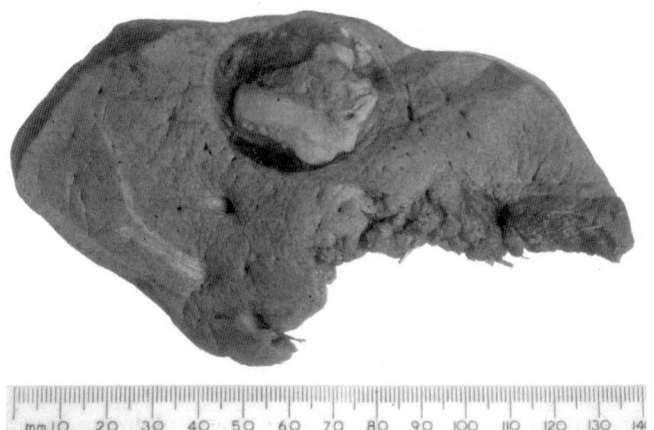

Fig. 6 Adult haemochromatosis. Section of liver lobe after surgical resection to remove a primary hepatocellular carcinoma arising in an iron-loaded but, unusually, non-cirrhotic liver in this disorder. The patient, aged 62 years, had been partially treated by venesection but recently noticed increasing lethargy: a raised serum α-fetoprotein concentration led to the diagnosis; moderate histochemical evidence of iron storage was found in the non-malignant tissue excised at surgery. (See also Plate 4.)

mutations, then tissue diagnosis is indicated. This is usually carried out by liver biopsy with histochemical determination, and preferably chemical quantification, of tissue iron content. Although a liver biopsy is associated with small but definable risks, it does offer a key opportunity for the evaluation of liver structure and of the injury consequent upon iron deposition. The finding of cirrhotic change carries with it a poor prognosis; cirrhotic change is also a major predictor of the occurrence of hepatocellular carcinoma, which occurs rarely in non-cirrhotic subjects with iron-storage disease (Fig. 6 and Plate 4).

Serum iron-saturation determinations, and particularly serum ferritin concentrations, may signify conditions other than iron-storage disease. Serum ferritin is elevated in inflammatory states, certain malignancies such as Hodgkin's disease and in any condition associated with significant necrosis of parenchymal liver cells. Under these circumstances liver biopsy is recommended, since it is most likely to provide a definitive diagnosis of iron-storage disease. Sometimes, however, liver biopsy is not possible—either because the patient will not consent to it, or because of the presence of ascites and a bleeding disorder (especially thrombocytopenia). Under these circumstances, magnetic resonance imaging (**MRI**) may provide additional information but it is an insensitive test for the presence of iron-storage disease. If a liver biopsy is not possible and MRI of the liver does not reveal increased ferromagnetic signals indicative of iron storage, there are two further options: measurement of urinary iron excretion after parenteral administration of desferrioxamine, and, where the patient will tolerate it, quantitative phlebotomy. Injection of 500 mg of desferrioxamine intramuscularly in a patient with iron overload will usually induce the daily excretion of more than 2 mg of iron as the ferrioxamine complex in the urine. Ferrioxamine excretion may be increased in patients with haemolytic anaemia but when elevated is generally indicative of iron-storage disease. Weekly phlebotomy of 500 ml will remove approximately 225 mg of iron, and thus provides a means of estimating the amount of iron removed from the storage compartment when undertaken to induce a mild hypochromic anaemia of approximately 10.5 to 11.0 g of haemoglobin/dl or a serum ferritin concentration of less than 30 μg/l. Iron overload exists when the estimated iron removed by this method exceeds 1.5 g; unfortunately quantitative phlebotomy is cumbersome and may not be possible in patients with severe liver disease associated with hypoalbuminaemia.

Diagnosis in family members

The diagnosis of haemochromatosis, whether it be of adult or juvenile form, in an individual has immediate implications for first-degree relatives. All forms of haemochromatosis have a strong hereditary basis; and even some forms of neonatal haemochromatosis may, in some families, be inherited as an autosomal recessive trait. A dominant transmission pattern has been established in the case of HFE 4.

Although the penetrance and expressivity of homozygosity for the various alleles that predispose to haemochromatosis is not yet established, the risks of the disease in first-degree family members is sufficiently high to warrant systematic study. Clearly, the implications for asymptomatic or undiagnosed relatives of the propositus are potentially very large. Hence, considerable care and sensitivity are needed in the means of informing them about the condition through the identified index case. In large families there may be formidable difficulties, so that the help of genetic counselling services as well as formal assistance from physicians practised in medical genetics may be needed. There can be little doubt, however, that at-risk relatives should be offered the opportunity for further diagnostic and clinical evaluation in relation to iron-storage disease. The condition is readily susceptible to iron-depletion therapy in its early stages; moreover, there may be additional considerations for patients who will wish to make reproductive choices and who will need to be reassured that appropriate testing can be carried out on their future offspring.

In HFE haemochromatosis, molecular analysis of the HFE gene (and, formerly, the tightly linked class I HLA class typing) may assist in assessing the risk of disease, particularly in asymptomatic siblings. Phenotypic screening, however, is useful at the level of clinical evaluation for evidence of liver disease, hypogonadism, arthritis, pigmentation, and diabetes. Determining the biochemical phenotype first involves assay of the serum parameters of disordered iron metabolism. Since the serum parameters may be abnormal before iron-mediated tissue injury has occurred, tissue biopsy should be offered to patients with serum ferritin concentrations in excess of 500 µg/l who are at risk from the liver disease.

In first-degree relatives, in whom HLA typing or molecular analysis of the HFE or TfR2 genes indicates a genetic predisposition to the disease, periodic re-evaluation is needed by clinical and biochemical testing at intervals of not more than 5 years. In members of families affected by haemochromatosis due to mutations in the HFE or TfR2 gene who were not found to carry the predisposing mutations and whose ferritin and iron parameters are normal, liver biopsy is not mandatory and the risk of the development of significant iron-storage disease in less than 5 or 10 years is extremely low. In patients with no known pregenetic disposition and normal tissue-biopsy findings, further follow-up screening is not indicated.

From the foregoing it can be seen that there is an urgent need to identify the gene responsible for juvenile haemochromatosis, accompanied by a complete genotype/phenotype evaluation for other forms of haemochromatosis. Unfortunately, no genetic locus has yet been identified for neonatal haemochromatosis, although this is a subject of continuing research. In at-risk pregnancies, neonatal haemochromatosis may be occasionally recognized by MRI during the third trimester, which may show increased iron signals in the fetal liver. After birth, biopsy of the oral mucosa on the gums or inner lip may reveal histological evidence of iron storage in minor salivary glands of affected infants.

Environmental cofactors and disease expression

Many patients with adult haemochromatosis give a history of excessive current or prior alcohol consumption. In the past, physicians have been tempted to attribute evidence of excess tissue iron in these individuals solely to the consumption of alcohol. In practice, however, it appears that those individuals who have biopsy-proven evidence of hepatic iron storage usually prove to carry two predisposing alleles of the HFE gene and therefore have true haemochromatosis. Although no clear predictors for the expression of disease in first-degree relatives at risk are available, disease expression is reduced in women of reproductive age; most practising clinicians consider that age and alcohol consumption are the main identifiable environmental factors that contribute to disease expression in predisposed homozygotes. Other comorbid factors, including heritable factors, that may influence the expression of HFE mutations in homozygous subjects, include the presence of adult coeliac disease. There are few data that define the relationship between haemochromatosis and coeliac disease but subclinical coeliac disease may ameliorate the long-standing effects of iron loading in C282Y homozygotes. Co-segregation of haemochromatosis and coeliac disease has not hitherto been reported.

Treatment

Since it is the toxicity of iron that is responsible for the manifestations of all forms of haemochromatosis, treatment is directed to the removal of iron at the earliest possible stage.

Venesection

In adult and juvenile haemochromatosis the preferred method of treatment is iron depletion by means of phlebotomy. This is best instituted by the removal of approximately 500 ml of venous blood each week by needle puncture of peripheral veins in the antecubital fossa. In young patients it may be possible to increase the frequency of venesection to twice per week after several once-weekly procedures. In elderly patients and those with hypoalbuminaemia as well as end-organ failure and heart disease, the frequency of venesection should be commuted to within the rate tolerated. Coincidental inflammatory disease may impede the erythropoietin-mediated drive to haemopoiesis, and, particularly in the early phases of treatment, mild haemorrhagic anaemia may ensure. Thus adjustments need to be made according to the early responses to venesection therapy, and regular monitoring of the haemoglobin concentration or haematocrit is advisable.

Difficulties may arise in delivering this deceptively simple treatment as a result of poor organization of health service provision and of the availability of suitable healthcare personnel to carry out the venesection procedure. Venesection should not be carried out by naïve or incompetent medical and nursing staff. Every practical effort should be made to ensure that the procedure is convenient for the patient—who is often a young or middle-aged person in full-time employment and who may find regular access to the treatment centre problematic. In cold weather, or in patients with poor circulation or inconspicuous superficial venous access, the use of local anaesthetic creams (such as EMLA cream™) or even local diffusable preparations of glyceryl trinitrate, applied 30 to 60 min before the venesection procedure may greatly improve venous access. Likewise, the simple technique of immersing the arm in warm water to improve peripheral blood flow may be critical for establishing confidence in treating staff. Since patients with haemochromatosis usually harbour a large burden of iron requiring repeated phlebotomy over a period of several years, every effort should be made to preserve the integrity of their peripheral veins. In the author's view, the use of a local anaesthetic is usually unwarranted since it involves further tissue invasion in the region of the antecubital fossa with needles; moreover, repeated injections of the irritant fluid often leads to sclerosis around the venous access site.

Duration of venesection therapy

One 500-ml unit of peripheral blood contains approximately 225 mg of elemental iron. Thus most patients with established haemochromatosis will require weekly phlebotomy for a period of 2 to 3 years. The objective of this treatment is to restore serum ferritin concentrations to within the low normal range and, if possible, to induce a mild iron-deficiency anaemia of approximately 11.5 g haemoglobin/dl. Having thus achieved a satisfactory depletion of body iron stores, interval maintenance phlebotomy, carried out according to ferritin measurements, four to six times per year is usually sufficient to maintain normal iron stores with a serum ferritin concentration less than 100 µg/l. Some authorities suggest that serum ferritin values below 30 µg/l should ideally be achieved. In patients with juvenile haemochromatosis, who have a higher than normal intestinal iron absorption, more frequent phlebotomy may be needed to maintain a healthy iron balance.

Iron chelation therapy

Alternative methods of iron removal are needed for patients with severe clinical manifestations of haemochromatosis, such as life-threatening cardiac arrhythmias and those with severe liver disease and hypoalbuminaemia, who are incapable of withstanding frequent phlebotomy. The preferred alternative involves chelation therapy with the parenteral agent, desferrioxamine. As indicated in Chapter 22.4.4, the subcutaneous administration of desferrioxamine brings about the removal of a maximum of 20 to 25 mg of iron daily and is thus generally less efficient than vigorous weekly phlebotomy. However, desferrioxamine may gain access to cellular pools of iron that are important in the pathogenesis of tissue injury in established iron-storage disease, and therefore may offer particular benefit in patients critically ill with arrhythmias due to haemochromatotic cardiomyopathy. Although the nature of this so-called 'chelatable iron pool' is unknown, there is strong circumstantial evidence that its depletion by means of intravenous desferrioxamine treatment may reverse the life-threatening consequences of terminal iron-storage disease in patients with haemochromatosis. Moreover, the removal of 140 mg of chelatable iron per week represents about two-thirds of the amount that can be removed by weekly phlebotomy. A biological advantage may also be gained by therapeutic access to a reactive low-molecular weight chelatable fraction responsible for the injurious effects of cellular iron overload.

Parenteral desferrioxamine may be given intravenously for life-threatening cardiac disease, as described in Chapter 22.4.4, or, in the non-emergent situation, by subcutaneous infusion using portable infusion pumps for 12 to 14 h five or six times per week. It must be stressed, however, that chelation therapy is not the preferred option for the treatment of established haemochromatosis and should be restricted to those patients unable to tolerate phlebotomy as a result of anaemia or hypoalbuminaemia, or in whom life-threatening cardiomyopathy or liver disease is present.

General measures

Attention should be given in patients with haemochromatosis to the diagnosis and treatment of end-organ failure. This particularly applies to the management of diabetes mellitus by diet and insulin where necessary, as well as hormone-replacement therapy for hypogonadism. (See Chapter 12.8.2.) In men, intramuscular depôt injections of testosterone enantate (250 mg every 2–3 weeks) are recommended to improve libido and inhibit the development of premature osteoporosis; similarly, conventional sex hormone-replacement therapy should be used in women with premature gonadal failure as a result of haemochromatosis. Cardiac failure in patients with haemochromatosis due to cardiomyopathy and hepatic failure consequential upon pigmentary cirrhosis should be treated by standard methods; organ transplantation may be used successfully but correction of systemic iron overload should be undertaken as soon as practicable to restore normal function in all organ systems. Rarely, end-organ hormone deficiencies result from thyroid infiltration and parathyroid and adreno-cortical disease. These deficiencies should be vigorously sought for in the clinical evaluation of the patient at presentation. The appearance of lethargy, faintness due to postural hypotension, or symptomatic hypocalcaemia demands immediate investigation and institution of appropriate replacement therapy.

Prognosis

The main causes of death in untreated patients with haemochromatosis are hepatocellular failure, primary carcinoma of the liver (including hepatocellular carcinoma), and, rarely, cholangiocarcinomas. Cardiac failure due to haemochromatotic cardiomyopathy and untreated diabetes also contribute to death. Although not categorically proven, evidence from retrospective surveys suggest that life expectancy is improved by removing iron from patients with haemochromatosis of whatever cause and the subsequent maintenance of normal iron homeostasis. Most patients experience an improvement in well being on iron-depletion therapy and, during its early phases, there is evidence that hypogonadotrophic hypogonadism may improve with this therapy. Similarly, the manifestations of cardiomyopathy with intractable cardiac failure or tachyarrhythmias can improve after the removal of iron.

The cirrhosis of haemochromatosis appears not to be reversible, although the earlier precirrhotic manifestations of hepatic disease improve greatly on the removal of iron with an apparent restoration of normal life-expectancy. In all patients there is at least a twofold increase in the survival rate at 5 years from the point of diagnosis with the introduction of phlebotomy. In patients studied during the 1950s and 1960s, the 5-year survival rate improved from 18 per cent to more than 65 per cent in all haemochromatosis subjects treated.

In patients diagnosed with haemochromatosis but without cirrhosis, iron-depletion therapy is associated with a near-normal or normal life expectancy compared with a sex- and age-matched control cohort derived from the same population. It is notable, however, that the indolent nature of this storage disorder and the long-term survival of patients who are affected by it has so far rendered long-term controlled studies of the effects of phlebotomy on eventual outcome almost impossible to achieve. However, a wealth of evidence, based on the understanding of the pathogenesis and documented responses to iron depletion in individual patient cohorts, indicates that early removal of iron is highly desirable: indeed it may be decisive in determining a good outcome from all forms of human iron-storage disease—including all subtypes of hereditary haemochromatosis so far established.

Hepatocellular carcinoma occurs mostly in patients with iron-storage disease who have established cirrhosis (which is irreversible). Although hepatocellular carcinoma and cholangiocarcinoma have been reported in non-cirrhotic patients with haemochromatosis, these are rare phenomena. Moreover, since all the evidence suggests that patients with haemochromatosis are more likely to have diabetes mellitus and other manifestations of the disease, every encouragement should be given to the prompt diagnosis of the condition and early institution of iron-depletion therapy.

Increasingly, it has been recognized that the arthropathy of haemochromatosis can be disabling whether or not it is associated simply with joint pain (arthralgia) or progressive and non-inflammatory joint destruction. The disease is associated with a loss of cartilage and, in many large joints, chondrocalcinosis. Although the response of the arthropathy to iron-depletion therapy is controversial, the weight of observation indicates that, once established, the arthropathy of haemochromatosis progresses independently of body iron status and of iron-depletion treatment. It seems intrinsically likely that effective removal of excess body iron stores before the development of joint symptoms will prevent their onset and progression. However, at present only cross-sectional data are available to support this contention.

In summary, observations in adult haemochromatosis suggest that once the disease is established in association with cirrhosis or diabetes mellitus, it diminishes life expectancy. The prognosis for cardiomyopathy in juvenile haemochromatosis is very poor but it may be improved by early diagnosis and the early institution of vigorous iron-depletion therapy. In several cases, the outcome has been improved by allogeneic cardiac transplantation. In adult patients with established pigment cirrhosis, hepatic transplantation has been undertaken and, provided the other systemic manifestations of haemochromatosis have been adequately treated, the procedure is associated with a good overall prognosis.

Prevention and control

The importance of early recognition and the institution of iron-depletion therapy in all forms of haemochromatosis cannot be overemphasized. Molecular analysis of the *HFE* gene or HLA class I haplotype screening, together with biochemical characterization using serum transferrin iron saturation estimations and serum ferritin concentrations, has the power greatly to assist in the detection of presymptomatic first-degree relatives of patients with haemochromatosis.

In relation to whole populations in which mutations in the *HFE* gene are frequent, the health implications based on mass screening remain contentious. Superficially, adult hereditary haemochromatosis due to mutations in the *HFE* gene appears to be an ideal condition for DNA-based mass-population screening. The condition is attributable to a single gene, and a single mutation of diagnostic significance is prevalent (gene frequency 5–10 per cent). Disease-related mutations in *HFE* (especially *C282Y*) are easily tested for by means of polymerase chain reaction-based techniques. At the same time, HFE-mediated haemochromatosis has a long incubation period without symptoms—and all the evidence suggests that the institution of treatment for presymptomatic disease is cheap, simple, and effective.

On the other hand, however, genetic identification of at-risk individuals is associated with problems of stigmatization, increased anxiety, and potential life-insurance weighting—all of which are familiar aspects in well-rehearsed debates about genetic testing in the general population. These aspects must be considered, together with the age-related penetrance of the homozygous state for *HFE C282Y* variants and, as yet, unknown combined genetic and environmental influences on disease expression. Uncertainty as to the significance of these factors has held back the introduction of mass-population screening by DNA-based methods. In light of the present state of knowledge, it is clear that homozygosity for the *C282Y* allele of *HFE* cannot be considered to be tantamount to a diagnosis of hereditary haemochromatosis.

More information is needed from outbred populations, rather than from homozygotes identified as a result of screening family members of index cases having full-blown clinical disease. Family studies provide a false measure of disease expressivity, presumably as a result of shared environments and of the co-segregation of potential disease-modifying genes within defined pedigrees. Finally, it must be emphasized that difficulties also occur for the evaluation of the burden of haemochromatosis in the population at large: although there are definitions of iron-storage disease that reflect the abnormal biochemical genotype, the manifestations of the clinical disease are variable and protean. Moreover, as pointed out earlier, no internationally agreed case definition of haemochromatosis exists, which creates additional difficulties for the introduction of public health measures and appropriate policy review of nationwide screening procedures.

Future directions

Although startling progress has been made in the discovery of many components that serve to regulate iron homeostasis in humans, more information is needed before a full molecular understanding of the mechanisms of iron homeostasis can be achieved. The genes responsible for severe juvenile neonatal and variant forms of adult haemochromatosis are yet to be characterized. At the same time, the functional interactions of the HFE molecule with the two transferrin receptor isoforms requires more study. An even more challenging task will be the identification of the environmental cofactors that determine the expression of iron-storage disease in genetically predisposed individuals; alcohol is a long-standing candidate

but the mechanism by which it leads to increased delivery of toxic iron to the tissues is, at present, completely unknown.

Newly identified iron-storage diseases

By general agreement, the term 'haemochromatosis' is used to describe systemic syndromes of pathological iron storage that affects many tissue and disturbs the function of diverse organ systems. Conversely, several distinct clinical syndromes of local iron toxicity have been identified, especially in the eye and brain. Although these syndromes are individually rare, they are important because they are potentially accessible to measures that reduce cellular free iron (for example, metal chelation (see above)), and because they demonstrate the central importance of metabolic iron in selected tissues. A fuller understanding of these disorders and the cognate cell metabolic pathways they affect, may well shed light on ill-understood aspects of tissue iron physiology. Additional information is available by reference to the online Mendelian Inheritance in Man (OMIM) website at www.ncbi.nlm.nih.gov/omim.

Hereditary hyperferritinaemia cataract syndrome (OMIM 600886)

The sole clinical manifestation of this condition is of congenital bilateral ferrugineous nuclear cataracts due to the disposition of excess ferritin light-chain polypeptide in the ocular lenses. The serum ferritin concentrations are moderately elevated but no evidence of systemic iron storage is found. The disorder is caused by mutations in the non-coding 5′ IRE of the ferritin L-chain gene that leads to unregulated translational overexpression of ferritin light chains. These polypeptides accumulate in the lenses and disturb their tissue organization and refractile properties. The hyperferritinaemia cataract syndrome is, as expected for an overexpression disease, inherited as a dominant trait; measurement of serum ferritin concentrations may identify at-risk family members. The gene encoding ferritin light-chain polypeptide maps to chromosome 19q3.3-qter.

Adult-onset basal ganglia disease (OMIM 606159)

A single pedigree has been identified with a dominantly inherited disorder showing features of late-onset extrapyramidal dysfunction resembling parkinsonism or Huntington's disease. Imaging and autopsy studies revealed cavitation of the basal ganglia with deposition of iron and ferritin protein in adjacent tissue, especially in the putamen and the globus pallidus; the macroscopic appearances showed widespread reddish discoloration of affected tissues. This disorder was mapped to chromosome 19q13.3 and a single mutation, a point insertion of a single adenine at nucleotide 461, was identified in exon 4 of the ferritin L-chain gene. The mutation is predicted to disrupt the carboxyterminal sequence of the ferritin light-chain molecule and disturb the iron-binding core of the hetero- or homomeric protein. Serum ferritin concentrations were found to be abnormally low in affected heterozygotes. Although this disorder has so far only been identified in a single large pedigree, it further illustrates the importance of ferritin in tissue iron metabolism and, especially, in selective regions of the brain. This disorder has been termed a 'neuroferritinopathy' and may be the first of several diseases affecting cellular iron pathways in iron-rich brain tissue.

Acaeruloplasminaemia with iron deposition (haemosiderosis) in basal ganglia (OMIM 277900)

This disorder is associated with mild systemic iron deposition and deficiency of the plasma copper-binding protein, caeruloplasmin. Caeruloplasmin has long been known to possess ferroxidase activity, and that it enhances the mobilization and delivery of iron to and from macrophages and hepatocytes: caeruloplasmin promotes iron loading of intact ferritin micelles. Acaeruloplasminaemia, due to mutations in the gene encoding caeruloplasmin on chromosome 3q21–24, is an autosomal recessive trait. The deficiency is associated with diabetes mellitus, dementia, and extrapyramidal features including parkinsonism, with choreoathetosis as well as cerebellar ataxia. MRI shows altered signals in the basal ganglia, and retinal degeneration may be apparent by fundoscopy. Excess systemic iron is demonstrable by examination of liver tissue and the serum ferritin concentration is moderately elevated; however, low serum iron transferrin saturations with hypochromic microcytic anaemia, reminiscent of copper deficiency, are usually present.

Infusions of plasma or purified caeruloplasmin may correct the systemic abnormalities of iron metabolism, but probably do not influence the dementia or the other neurological deficits—at least once these are established. The role of caeruloplasmin replacement or indeed parenteral chelation therapy with desferrioxamine or trientine, especially in the early evolution of the neurological syndrome, has not yet been established. The interplay between copper and iron metabolism is well illustrated by this severely disabling illness. Acaeruloplasminaemia illustrates the particular sensitivity of the basal ganglia to disturbances of iron metabolism. In this context, it is notable that caeruloplasmin expression is abundant in glia in the brain microvasculature juxtaposed to the pigment-containing dopaminergic neurones of the substantia nigra and inner layer of the retina.

Hallervorden–Spatz disease: pantothenate kinase-associated neurodegeneration—OMIM 234200

This disease has been familiar to neurologists and neuropathologists since its original description by two now discredited German neuroscientists of the Nazi period. The clinical features indicate basal ganglia disease and dementia with retinal degeneration leading to optic atrophy. The disorder often presents with equinovarus deformity in children and adolescents; extrapyramidal rigidity preceded by choreoathetosis usually follows rapidly. Dementia, optic atrophy, and generalized seizures occur in the latter stages, and death usually ensues by the age of 30 years. Although late-onset forms of the disease are known, a striking feature is the presence of iron pigment in the basal ganglia and substantia nigra, now easily recognized by MRI. The heredofamilial nature of this syndrome has been known since its first description. Hallervorden–Spatz disease is now known to be an autosomal recessive trait due to mutations in the pantothenate kinase 2 (**PANK2**) gene that maps to chromosome 20p13.

Pantothenate kinase-2 is abundant in the retina and target regions of the brain; it regulates the formation of coenzyme A. Deficiency of PANK-2 would deplete sensitive neural tissues with a high metabolic rate of coenzyme A; the defect may also lead to a consequential accumulation of cysteine, which normally condenses with the enzyme product, phosphopantothenate. In the presence of high concentrations of free iron, excess cysteine may accelerate the formation of cytotoxic oxygen free radicals. For some years, cysteine accumulation has been independently observed in the iron-rich nigrostriatal regions of the brain affected by this disorder. Identification of *PANK2* mutations offers the hope of improved diagnosis of this neurodegenerative disorder, and, more importantly, the prospect of specific therapy using supplementation to enhance local coenzyme A activity and phosphopantothenate concentrations in affected neural tissue.

Further practical information

Many patients' associations and societies exist to serve the needs of patients in their respective countries: International Association of Haemochromatosis Societies.

In the United Kingdom, useful information can be obtained from: The Haemochromatosis Society, Hollybush House, Hadley Green Road, Barnet, EN5 5PR. Fax: 44 (0) 208 449 1363; Email: info@ghsoc.org; Website: www.ghsoc.org

Further reading

Adams PC, Speechley M, Kertesz, AE (1991). Long-term survival analysis in hereditary haemochromatosis. *Gastroenterology* **101**, 368–72.

Beutler E, *et al.* (2002). Penetrance of 845G->A (C282Y). *HFE* hereditary haemochromatosis mutation in the USA. *Lancet* **359**, 211–18.

Bomford A, Williams R (1976). Long-term results of venesection therapy in idiopathic haemochromatosis. *Quarterly Journal of Medicine* (New Series) **XLV(95)** 611–23.

Bulaj ZJ, *et al.* (2000). Disease-related conditions in relatives of patients with hemochromatosis. *New England Journal of Medicine* **343**, 1529–35.

Burke W, *et al.* (1998). Hereditary hemochromatosis. Gene discovery and its implications for population-based screening. *Journal of the American Medical Association* **280**, 172–8.

Camaschella C, *et al.* (2000). The gene TfR2 is mutated in a new type of haemochromatosis mapping to 7q22. *Nature Genetics* **25**, 14–15.

De Gobbi M, *et al.* (2002). Clinical expression of juvenile haemochromatosis compared with HFE C282Y and HFE3 haemochromatosis. *British Journal of Haematology* (In press)

Fargion S, *et al.* (1992). Survival and prognostic factors in 212 Italian patients with genetic haemochromatosis. *Hepatology* **15**, 655–9.

Feder JN, *et al.* (1996). A novel MHC class I-like gene is mutated in patients with haemochromatosis. *Nature Genetics*, **13**, 399–408.

Finch SC, Finch CA (1955). Idiopathic hemochromatosis, an iron storage disease. Iron metabolism in hemochromatosis. *Medicine (Baltimore)* **34**, 381–430.

Fleming ME, *et al.* (1999). Mechanism of increased iron absorption in murine model of hereditary haemochromatosis: increased duodenal expression of the iron transporter, DMT-1. *Proceedings of the National Academy of Sciences, USA*, **96**, 3143–8.

Griffiths W, Cox T (2000). Haemochromatosis: novel gene discovery and the molecular pathophysiology of iron metabolism. *Human Molecular Genetics* **9**, 2377–88.

Kelly AL, *et al.* (1998). Hereditary juvenile haemochromatosis: a genetically heterogenous life-threatening iron storage disease. *Quarterly Journal of Medicine* **91**, 607–18.

Kelly AL, *et al.* (2001). Classification and genetic features of neonatal haemochromatosis: a study of twenty-seven affected pedigrees and molecular analysis of genes implicated in iron metabolism. *Journal of Medical Genetics* **38**, 599–610.

McCance RA, Widdowson EM (1937). Absorption and excretion of iron. *Lancet* **233**, 680–4.

McKie AT, *et al.* (2000). A novel duodenal iron-regulated transporter, IREG1, implicated in baso-lateral transfer of iron to the circulation. *Molecular Cell* **5**, 299–309.

McKie AT, *et al.* (2001). An iron-regulated ferric reductase associated with the absorption of dietary iron. *Science* **291**, 1755–9.

Merryweather-Clarke AT, *et al.* (1998). The effect of HFE mutations on serum ferritin and transferrin saturation in the Jersey population. *British Journal of Haematology* **101**, 369–73.

Niederau C, *et al.* (1996). Long-term survival in patients with hereditary haemochromatosis. *Gastroenterology* **110**, 1107–19.

Roetto A, *et al.* (1999). Juvenile hemochromatosis locus maps to chromosome 1q. *American Journal of Human Genetics* **64**, 1388–93.

Sheldon JH (1935). *Haemochromatosis*. Oxford University Press, London.

Simon M, Bourel M, Genetet B (1977). Idiopathic hemochromatosis: demonstration of recessive transmission and early detection by family HLA typing. *New England Journal of Medicine* **297**, 1017–21.

11.7.2 Wilson's disease, Menkes' disease: inherited disorders of copper metabolism

C. A. Seymour

Copper

Copper is ubiquitous and is present in relative excess in most diets. It is a prosthetic element of many metalloenzymes, playing a vital role in mitochondrial energy generation, melanin formation, and cross-linking of collagen and elastin. Since the liver efficiently maintains copper homeostasis by regulating excretion of copper into the bile, acquired copper deficiency is rare. Excretion of copper is dependent on its incorporation into caeruloplasmin (the major copper-binding protein in plasma, normally 20–40 mg/dl); and defects in this homeostatic mechanism lead to toxic accumulation (Fig. 1).

Copper homeostasis

Total body copper is in the range of 50 to 150 mg, of which some 8 per cent is found in the liver. Relatively high concentrations are also found in the brain, kidney, heart, and bone. Neonatal and fetal liver tissue tolerate much higher quantities than does the adult liver, where copper is stored within lysosomes in association with metallothionein.

Copper (2–5 mg daily) absorbed from the diet is transported loosely bound to albumin. This accounts for about 10 per cent of circulating copper. Net uptake of copper (around 40–60 per cent) reflects its differential binding to low molecular weight ligands present in saliva, gastric and duodenal juice, and high molecular weight ligands present in bile. The regulatory mechanisms involved in intestinal copper transport are still unknown, although binding occurs to two cytosolic proteins, one similar to superoxide dismutase and metallothionein. Metallothionein and active transport of copper–amino acid complexes are involved in absorption but maintenance of copper homeostasis depends uniquely on its excretion in

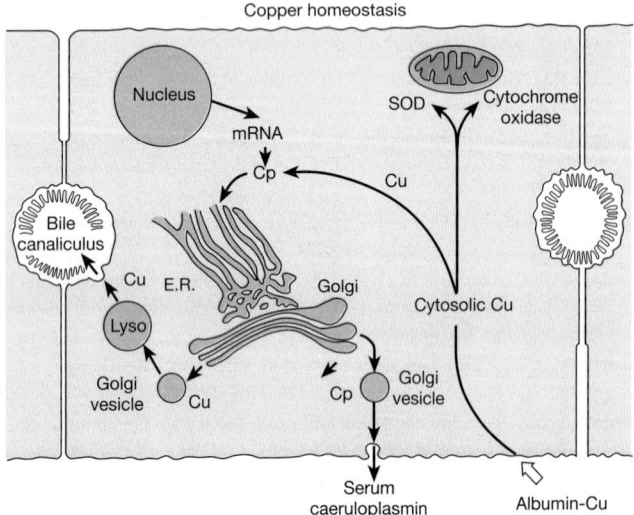

Copper homeostasis

Fig. 1 Hepatic caeruloplasmin isoforms—copper transport in the liver.

bile (1.5–1.7 mg/day); only about 0.7 μg/day is normally excreted in the urine. Any interruption in the secretion of bile leads to accumulation of copper in the liver.

Copper overload or toxicity

Copper toxicity occurs naturally in animals: the Bedlington terrier, Dominican toad (*Bufo marinus*), the mute swan (*Cygnus olor*), Long-Evans cinnamon rat, and in experimental animals given copper or in acquired copper toxicity in sheep. The Long-Evans cinnamon rat, an inbred mutant strain with autosomal recessive inheritance, most closely mimics Wilson's disease. In all these models, copper accumulates in the liver and not in the nervous system—as it does in man.

Chronic copper toxicity in man occurs in two major forms:

1. A primary (inherited) form, where copper accumulates in and damages the liver initially, and later the nervous system and other tissues, giving rise to hepatolenticular degeneration or Wilson's disease.

2. A secondary (acquired) form, where copper accumulates in similar amounts to Wilson's disease as a consequence of cholestasis, due either to biliary atresia or Indian childhood cirrhosis (congenital) or primary biliary cirrhosis (acquired). In chronic active hepatitis, lesser amounts of accumulated copper exacerbate pre-existing hepatocyte injury.

Wilson's disease

In 1912, Samuel Kinnier-Wilson, described a neurological condition with severe motor (movement) and mental disturbance due to a disorder of the basal ganglia; this was associated with cirrhosis of the liver. Perceptively, Wilson developed the hypothesis that abnormalities in the liver might be caused by 'a morbid agent' (toxin) generated within a cirrhotic liver.

Definition

Wilson's disease or hepatolenticular degeneration is an autosomal, recessively inherited disorder arising from an abnormal gene located on chromosome 13. Pathognomonic features of the disease are inadequate biliary excretion of copper (less than 1.5 mg/day), reduction in plasma caeruloplasmin (less than 200 mg/l), the major copper-carrying protein in plasma, with reduction in incorporation of copper, and consequent hepatic accumulation of copper (more than 25 μg/g dry weight). The genetic defect results in copper accumulation, initially within hepatocytes, with damage leading to cirrhosis, portal hypertension, and then as the liver is bypassed, to increased copper in the circulation which deposits in the central nervous system, cornea, kidneys, and other organs. Undiagnosed or untreated, the disorder has a fatal outcome within a few years of the onset of symptoms. Removal of copper (e.g. by chelation therapy) prevents progression of the disease, and may reverse some neurological and the corneal abnormalities. Regression of the neurological signs has also occurred after liver transplantation.

Incidence

The Wilson's disease gene is distributed world-wide and is present in all racial groups. Although generally considered a rare inborn error of metabolism, it has a prevalence of 1 in 30 000 live births, with an incidence of 15 to 30 per million live births, although this may be a low estimate as some patients are still undiagnosed when they die. Carrier frequency is about 1 per cent. There is no HLA association. A higher incidence has been noted in Jews of Eastern Europe, inhabitants of Southern Italy, Arabs, Japanese, Chinese, and Indians, and populations with high consanguinity, where the frequency may increase to 60 per million births. Because there is a high mortality associated with failure to diagnose the disease, point prevalence rates are lower than frequency at birth.

Genetics and molecular biology

Extended family studies confirmed an autosomal recessive mode of inheritance. Genetic studies of an Israeli-Arab kindred mapped the Wilson's disease gene to chromosome 13 by demonstrating a linkage between the Wilson's disease locus and the red cell enzyme, esterase D. Multipoint linkage techniques using highly variable markers in many families further localized the gene to 13q14–q21. By 1993, a candidate gene for Wilson's disease was identified by several groups, using different positional cloning strategies. The Wilson's disease gene is expressed predominantly in liver (in the transGolgi network), kidney, and placenta and less in brain, heart, lung, and pancreas. It shows functional homology with the Menkes' disease gene. Both genes are predicted to encode copper-transporting membrane p-type ATPases, with characteristic motifs and homology with the heavy-metal transporting ATPases found in bacteria and yeast. Sequence analysis of cDNA predicts that the Wilson's disease protein (ATP7B) has specific metal-binding domains, an ATP-binding domain, a cation channel, and a phosphorylation region which is involved in energy transduction from ATP hydrolysis to copper (cation) transport. Table 1 compares Wilson's with Menkes' disease.

About 70 mutations have been identified in patients with Wilson's disease. Gene deletions, nonsense and splice site mutations, likely to represent null alleles, are associated with a more severe form of the disease. A common mutation in European populations arises from substitution of histidine for glutamine (H1069Q) in the highly conserved ATP-binding region. This is associated with hepatic and neurological disease, and onset at around 20 years. Many other mutations have been reported in various ethnic groups, but none has yet clearly identified particular phenotypes. Detailed genetic and epidemiological studies have suggested that allelic heterogeneity may not be the sole cause of clinical variability of the disease; different ages of onset and disease course have been found in family members with identical mutant alleles. In the United Kingdom, a total of 37 different mutations, including H1069Q, have been reported in 52 British patients, which included 10 patients of mixed ethnic groups; 70 per cent of the mutations corresponded to those described in other Europeans. Thirty per cent of the mutations are not detectable by single mutation tests.

Clinical features (Table 1)

Wilson's disease may present in childhood, adolescence, or early adulthood. Symptoms and signs may be clinically undetectable under 5 years of age, and few present after the age of 35 years, although diagnosis over 55 years has been reported. In 90 per cent of patients, the disease presents with juvenile hepatic disease or with neurological/psychiatric manifestations. In large studies of Wilson's disease patients, initial manifestations were hepatic (40 per cent); neurological (30 per cent); psychiatric (10 per cent); haematological (12 per cent); and renal (1 per cent). 25 per cent of patients have

Table 1 Comparison of genetic copper disorders

	Wilson's disease	Menkes' disease
Clinical aspects		
Definition	Reduced/ absent biliary copper excretion leading to body copper toxicosis Hepatolenticular degeneration	Reduced intestinal copper absorption leading to copper enzyme deficiency Severe neurological disorder
Incidence	1:100 000	1:300 000
Clinical features	Kayser–Fleischer corneal ring	'Kinky' hair
	Hepatic disease	Facial dysmorphism
	Basal ganglia dysfunction	Connective tissue disorder
		Neurological impairment
Diagnosis	Serum copper low	Serum copper low
	Serum caeruloplasmin low/absent	Serum caeruloplasmin low
	Liver copper increased	Intracellular copper increased
	Urinary copper increased	
Treatment	Chelating agents: penicillamine, trientine	Copper histidinate
	Zinc sulphate	
	Thiomolybdate	
	Liver transplantation (rare)	
Prognosis	Good if early diagnosis	Fatal in severe cases
	Poor if diagnosed late or non-compliant patient	Prolongation of life with treatment
	Refractory to restarting chelating therapy	Neurological signs irreversible
Molecular aspects		
Inheritance	Autosomal recessive	X-linked recessive
Location	13q14.3	Xq13.3
Genome	22 exons, 80 kb	23 exons, 150 kb
Gene defect	Point mutations	1% cytogenetic abnormalities
	Rearrangements	28% gross rearrangement
	70 mutations described to date	80 per cent small base pair changes
	His1069Gln (H1069Q)—European	60 mutations described to date
	Arg778leu (R778L)—Oriental	
Predicted abnormal protein	1411 amino acid	1500 amino acid
	Copper-binding protein	Copper-binding protein
	p-type ATPase—ATP7B	p-type ATPase—ATP7A
Animal model	Bedlington terrier	Mottled mouse
	Long Evans cinnamon rat	

Adapted from Tümer and Horn (1997). *Medical Genetics* **34**, 265.

two or more organs involved (usually liver and brain) at the initial assessment.

Clinical presentations

Haemolytic

During the early period (neonatal to under 5 years of age), copper may accumulate in the liver without clinical signs and excess copper in red cells may present as acute haemolysis or as chronic haemolytic anaemia.

Hepatic

Hepatic presentation of Wilson's disease usually occurs at 8 to 12 years. Acute hepatitis, chronic hepatitis/cirrhosis, and fulminant hepatic failure are the three principal patterns of liver disease. Before puberty, symptoms and signs of hepatic dysfunction are common and may mimic acute hepatitis. A diagnosis of Wilson's disease should be considered if these features coincide with abdominal pain and haemolysis, or in children with hepatomegaly, increased serum transaminases, and a fatty liver.

Five to thirty per cent of patients with Wilson's disease present with chronic liver damage which progresses to cirrhosis. In the early stages, patients are vaguely unwell but later develop more specific features of liver dysfunction such as nausea, easy bruising/bleeding, fluid retention, and jaundice. Portal hypertension develops with progressive hepatic insufficiency, splenomegaly, gastro-oesophageal varices, and ascites. In adolescents and older patients, splenomegaly should always raise the diagnosis of portal hypertension and liver disease. A minority of patients present with fulminant hepatitis, encephalopathy, and coagulopathy. Hepatocellular carcinoma is rare in the cirrhosis of Wilson's disease, unlike haemochromatosis.

Neurological

Neurological presentation usually occurs in older patients, between ages 14 and 40 years and are of two general patterns, movement disorders or rigid dystonia. Symptoms may be acute or chronic in onset and rapidly progressive. In all patients there is some degree of liver damage or cirrhosis.

A common presentation in adolescence is with the insidious onset of dysarthria, deteriorating physical performance at school, with clumsiness in using a knife and fork or chopsticks, deterioration in handwriting, and in physical performance at sport. Early physical signs include flexion–extension tremor of the hands, becoming a parkinsonian 'bat's wing' or intention type; abnormal movements become more obvious, with grimacing and choreiform movements. Orolaryngeal dysphagia and sialorrhoea are associated with hypokinesia. Later features include spasticity, rigidity of limbs and neck muscles, and convulsions, which may occur as a presenting sign or on commencement of treatment. Involuntary movement disorders respond to treatment, unlike the spastic-tonic features which mimic Parkinson's disease. Cognitive and sensory functions are usually preserved until a late stage.

Psychiatric

About 60 per cent of patients with neurological features also show evidence of behavioural or psychiatric disorders caused by excess cerebral copper. Adolescents may present with a fall off in intellectual ability at school and/or with truancy. About 20 per cent of patients present with early psychiatric symptoms. Presentations vary from depression, phobias, and compulsive disorders to aggressive and antisocial behaviour. In older patients, anxiety states, intellectual deterioration, and memory loss are more common. These are important to recognize since otherwise the patient may be placed solely in mental health care rather than in the joint care of a neurologist, psychiatrist, and physician who will offer specific therapy.

Ophthalmic

Kayser–Fleischer rings (Fig. 2 and Plate 1) are almost pathognomonic of Wilson's disease. They are due to the deposition of copper in the limbus of the cornea and appear brown in a grey-blue iris, or grey in a brown eye; they are best seen by slit lamp examination. Similar appearances have been noticed in cryptogenic cirrhosis and with prolonged cholestasis. Rarely, the posterior membrane of the lens is involved, producing the appearance of a sunflower cataract.

Renal

Renal tubular acidosis due to damage by copper in the proximal and/or distal tubules is not uncommon. Aminoaciduria and nephrolithiasis may also occur. Osteomalacia and vitamin D-resistant rickets may result from tubular loss of phosphate.

Joints

Skeletal abnormalities, particularly early osteoarthritis of the spine (Scheuermann's disease), polyarthritis, hypermobile joints, and chondromalacia patellae are recognized features. In the very disabled patient with neurological disease, hypokinesia may lead to flexion contractures.

Dermatological

Rarely, the skin may be hyperpigmented, appearing slightly grey with a bluish appearance of the lunulae of the nails. Long-standing copper excess may increase skin elasticity.

Cardiac/skeletal muscle

Cardiac abnormalities occur rarely, with cardiac hypertrophy associated with interstitial fibrosis, small vessel sclerosis and perivascular myocarditis, and rarely cardiomyopathy, which may lead to congestive cardiac failure. Copper-induced rhabdomyolysis has also been described.

Endocrine disturbances

Endocrine disturbances occur as a result of liver dysfunction (for example, gynaecomastia in men). Women with cirrhosis and copper toxicity have an

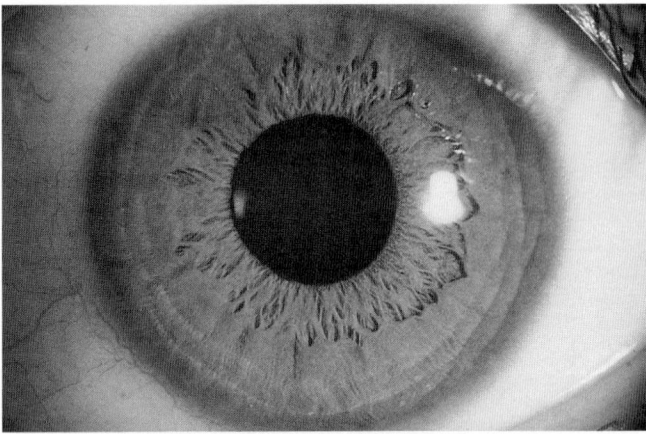

(a)

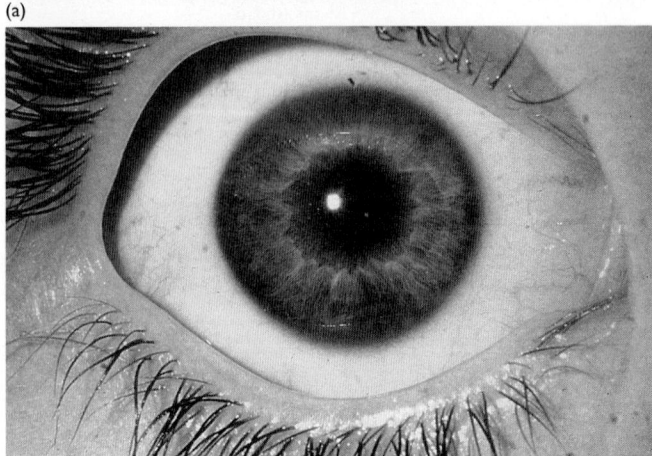

(b)

Fig. 2 Kayser–Fleischer ring in Wilson's disease. (See also Plate 1.)

increased frequency of abortion, stillbirth, premature delivery, and menstrual disturbance. Once chelation therapy has reduced the copper overload, successful pregnancies occur and chelating agents do not appear to harm the fetus or cause fetal copper deficiency. Copper may also injure other endocrine organs (e.g. causing hypoparathyroidism).

Pathology

In Wilson's disease the liver is almost invariably damaged and the histological changes vary with the amount of copper accumulated. The neonatal liver tolerates concentrations of copper that are six to eight times greater than those which injure the adult liver. The evolution of hepatocyte changes after the neonatal period is uncertain. There may be few changes in the liver lobular structure in the asymptomatic patient. Early changes evident on the liver biopsy are pericellular fatty droplet infiltration of the cytoplasm, 'glycogen' degeneration of the nuclei, and copper distributed diffusely in the cytoplasm. Other pathological changes are summarized in Table 2.

Diagnosis

General investigations

Most patients with Wilson's disease have Kayser–Fleischer rings (Fig. 2) and low plasma caeruloplasmin concentrations. Haematological investigations, such as a full blood count and haptoglobin, detect anaemia and haemolysis; mean corpuscular volume, prothrombin time, and clotting studies detect malfunction of the liver. Biochemical investigations will provide additional information. These include increased serum transaminases (altered liver cell turnover) and reduced albumin and urea (disturbed hepatocellular function). Measurement of autoantibody titres (e.g. antimitochondrial antibody) are important to exclude primary biliary cirrhosis.

Specific investigations

These are necessary to confirm the diagnosis of suspected Wilson's disease, and to monitor the efficacy and side-effects of treatment.

Serum caeruloplasmin

This can be measured enzymatically (copper oxidase), by radial immunodiffusion, or by reverse passive haemagglutination. The activity and concentration of this glycoprotein is reduced or absent (less than 200 mg/l) in

Table 2 Pathological changes in Wilson's disease

Liver	
Early changes	fat infiltration (non-specific)
	pericellular fat globules (specific)
	glycogen-containing nuclei (specific)
Intermediate changes	piecemeal necrosis, with histiocytes, lymphocytes
Late changes	cirrhosis
	nodular hyperplasia Mallory bodies
Increased apoptosis, increased apoptosis receptor APO-1	
Histochemical stains for copper (not diagnostic)	
Electron microscopy	increased hepatic lysosomes containing lipid droplets
	abnormal mitochondria, matrix replaced by vacuoles
Neuropathology	
Macroscopic	atrophy of basal ganglia
Microscopic	changes in basal ganglia, cortex, and subcortical white matter in dentate nuclei and cerebellum
	abnormal protoplasmic astrocytes and fibrillary astrocytes
	abnormal glial cells, increased astrocytic nuclei in putamen
	patchy degeneration of swollen glia
	central pontine myelinolysis (rare)

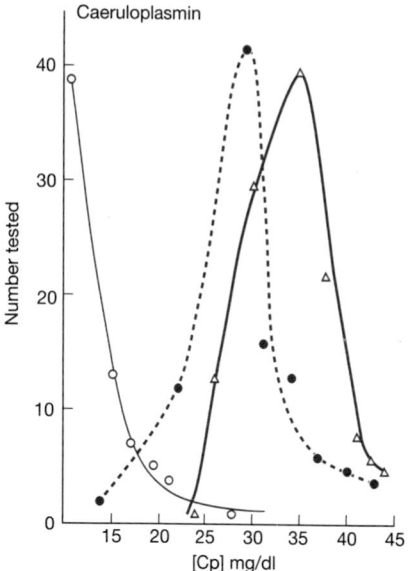

Fig. 3 Serum caeruloplasmin concentrations in controls, heterozygotes, and Wilson's disease.

95 per cent of patients with Wilson's disease. Some patients have caeruloplasmin levels in the lower range of the normal distribution which overlap with obligate heterozygotes and normal subjects (Fig. 3). Hypocaeruloplasminaemia and acaeruloplasminaemia do not always indicate Wilson's disease. The normal neonatal liver mimics the Wilson's disease patient, with low or absent plasma caeruloplasmin and high hepatic copper concentration; synthesis and secretion of caeruloplasmin to the plasma start during the first 3 to 6 months of life and hepatic copper concentrations decrease within the first 2 years of life.

Caeruloplasmin will also be reduced in protein malnourished states, reduced protein synthesis due to liver disease, protein loss due to the nephrotic syndrome, or a protein-losing enteropathy. Conversely hypercaeruloplasminaemia occurs as an acute phase protein reactant in acute inflammation, infection, pregnancy, and after oestrogen administration. This may increase previously low plasma caeruloplasmin concentrations to within the normal range.

Serum copper

Total serum copper will be reduced or low in Wilson's disease. However, non-caeruloplasmin-bound copper concentrations (loosely bound to albumin or amino acids; normally 50–100 μg/l) will be increased (more than 200 μg/l) in the untreated patient.

Urine copper

Urine excretion of copper is always increased in untreated Wilson's disease (more than 70–100 μg/24 h; normally less than 40 μg/24 h). Increased urinary copper may also occur in other liver diseases such as chronic active hepatitis and primary biliary cirrhosis. However, an increased urine copper in association with a low caeruloplasmin indicates Wilson's disease; the presymptomatic patient may still have a normal urinary copper excretion. Measurement of urine copper excretion is also important in monitoring the effects of chelating therapy where, early in treatment, urine levels may rise to 2000 μg/24 h and fall to less than 100 μg/24 h as the copper overload is reduced. Special care is needed when collecting urine samples to avoid contamination, and copper-free containers are required for the collection.

Provocation of urine copper excretion by giving penicillamine (500 mg orally) may be helpful in patients where the basal urinary copper is equivocal, and to assess the response of the Wilson's disease patient to treatment with chelating agents.

Liver copper concentration

Normal hepatic copper concentrations (15–55 µg/g dry weight of liver) can be measured by spectrophotometric assay, by atomic absorption spectrophotometry, or by neutron activation analysis. Liver biopsy allows measurement of liver copper concentration as well as histological assessment. In children or in the presence of significant liver disease (for example associated with coagulopathy), a transjugular liver biopsy may need to be considered.

In untreated Wilson's disease patients, the hepatic copper concentration is greater than 250 µg/g dry weight, and in heterozygotes, the concentration range is between 55 and 250 µg/g dry weight. Increased hepatic copper concentrations also occur in secondary copper overload conditions such as Indian childhood cirrhosis, primary biliary cirrhosis, sclerosing cholangitis, and chronic active hepatitis. These can be readily distinguished from Wilson's disease on clinical, biochemical, and histological grounds. Normal hepatic copper concentration excludes Wilson's disease in an untreated patient.

Radiocopper studies

Incorporation of orally administered radiocopper (^{64}Cu, ^{67}Cu, or ^{65}Cu) into caeruloplasmin at 1, 2, 3, and 48 h distinguishes clearly between normal patients and those with Wilson's disease, where little or no radiocopper is incorporated into the newly-synthesized caeruloplasmin.

Radiological imaging

Computer-assisted tomography and magnetic resonance imaging of the liver do not help in the specific diagnosis of Wilson's disease, although these imaging techniques will also detect non-specific associations of Wilson's disease such as splenomegaly and abnormalities in hepatic parenchyma. Central nervous system imaging with computer-assisted tomography or MRI demonstrate generalized cerebral atrophy and abnormalities in the basal ganglia.

Screening of family members

It is important that all first-degree relatives are screened for Wilson's disease once the diagnosis has been confirmed in the index patient. This is an essential part of the management of any patient with Wilson's disease. Screening of children should be after 3 years of age. It should include a history, clinical examination, slit-lamp examination of the eyes, liver enzyme and function tests, and serum caeruloplasmin concentration. If the results are suggestive of Wilson's disease, liver biopsy and a quantitative measurement of hepatic copper should follow (or radiocopper studies where liver biopsy is contraindicated).

Molecular tests

The diagnosis of Wilson's disease should be made on the basis of the clinical presentation, biochemical tests, and confirmed by DNA testing in patients with a high index of suspicion of the disease. Analysis of DNA from whole blood may be carried out to detect the common mutation H1069Q or, in Oriental populations, mutation H714Q. Most patients are compound heterozygotes carrying two mutations for the Wilson's disease gene. If the common mutations are not present, each of 21 exons in the gene must be screened by single strand conformational polymorphism (SSCP) or complete sequencing. Currently, this can only be undertaken in genetic units interested in Wilson's disease, and is not available for screening the general population. As methods for mutation detection improve, screening for this disease may become more practical.

Western blotting of caeruloplasmin isoforms obtained from whole blood or dried blood spots may be another, more simple, way of screening for Wilson's disease in the neonate and children over the age of 2 years.

Pathogenesis of the liver lesion

Copper, in free ionic form, is toxic to hepatocytes in man and in animals. Although the retained copper accumulates in lysosomes, there is no evidence that copper-filled lysosomes are more fragile, as is the case in haemochromatosis. Increased numbers of hepatic lysosomes and mitochondria have been described in untreated Wilson's disease, and lysosomes participate in excretion of copper into bile. Copper-containing mitochondria are more fragile, and it is likely that copper-induced hepatocyte damage results from impaired oxidative phosphorylation due to mitochondrial damage.

Several hypotheses have been advanced to explain the primary defect of failure in biliary excretion of copper. A link has been postulated between this gene defect and reduced plasma caeruloplasmin (Fig. 1). The liver in Wilson's disease does produce caeruloplasmin even when it is undetectable in plasma. Thus defects in this glycoprotein are likely to reflect abnormalities of processing or secretion. Evidence of reduced amounts of hepatic mRNA for caeruloplasmin has not yet been linked to the underlying metabolic defect. Two major molecular forms of caeruloplasmin are changed in Wilson's disease. The 132 kDa (plasma form) is reduced and the 125 kDa (biliary form) is absent, giving further support for a post-translational abnormality. It also suggests that caeruloplasmin may play more than a bystander role in the underlying metabolic defect. It is well established that reabsorption of biliary copper from the intestine in Wilson's disease is not increased. Characterization of the Wilson's disease gene suggests that the abnormality may be caused by an alteration in a specific membrane copper transporter (ATP7B) which may fail to bind copper and caeruloplasmin.

Management

The management of Wilson's disease involves the general care of any patient with liver disease and anaemia, and investigation of the family and siblings of the propositus, as well as specific therapy.

Diet

Strict dietary restriction of copper is not practical, but Wilson's disease patients should know which foods are high in copper. These include chocolate, liver, nuts, mushrooms, legumes, and shellfish. In addition, many Chinese dishes are high in copper and Oriental Wilson's disease patients and vegetarians will need special dietary advice. However, reducing copper in the diet is only an adjunct to the main pharmacological therapy.

Specific therapy

Walsh (1956) was the first to show how effective D-penicillamine was in removing copper from patients with Wilson's disease. The optimum time for treatment is in the early stages, and all patients with Wilson's disease should be treated, even if asymptomatic. Treatment is lifelong, unless the patient undergoes liver transplantation. The aim of treating a patient with Wilson's disease is to reduce toxic copper levels in the body tissues. This can be achieved by increasing the urinary excretion of copper. A negative copper balance should be monitored carefully since, with an increase in urine and faecal copper excretion which exceeds copper intake, increased urinary copper may reflect increased plasma non-caeruloplasmin copper (copper in its most damaging form). The effect of any therapy should be regularly monitored by clinical and radiological assessment, and by biochemical monitoring of abnormal liver enzymes and liver function. The agents commonly used in treatment of Wilson's disease, together with mechanisms of action and side-effects, are summarized in Table 3 and Fig. 4. (See also Plate 2).

Prognosis

Early diagnosis and chelation therapy is the only way to ensure a good outcome in Wilson's disease. Most symptomatic patients improve and have an almost complete resolution of their symptoms. The prognosis is best in the asymptomatic individuals who are detected early, often by meticulous screening of families of index cases. A poor prognosis is more likely in patients with severe liver damage, acute fulminant hepatic failure, acute neurological disease, and dystonia. In addition, in the presence of cirrhosis, even when copper-depleted, the risk of variceal bleeding and intercurrent infections remains.

Non-compliant patients who discontinue treatment may relapse rapidly and die; they are refractory to reversal of copper overload on restarting chelation therapy. In these patients, only liver transplantation would improve their prognosis.

Copper deficiency

Copper deficiency disorders in man are rare, occur in two forms, and have different clinical features:

1. Genetic: Menkes' disease ('steely' or 'kinky' hair syndrome) due to an X-linked recessive defect of intestinal absorption leading to defective synthesis of important copper-containing enzymes, and typical clinical features with damage to the brain and arteries. The occipital horn syndrome is a milder form of Menkes' disease.

2. Acquired: this may occur in malnourished children, adults with severe malabsorption syndromes, in patients taking regular total parenteral nutrition, or in patients regularly taking chelating agents (penicillamine) as treatment for rheumatoid arthritis. The diagnosis rests on low serum copper measurements, hypochromic microcytic anaemia, and evidence of bone demineralization.

Table 3 Treatment of Wilson's disease

Pharmacological therapy	Indication	Mechanism of action	Dose	Efficacy	Side-effects
Penicillamine (dimethyl cysteine)	First line Chelator All patients	Formation of Cu-penicillamine complexes induce cupriuresis Induction of hepatic metallothionein, copper uptake in non-toxic form	500 mg–2 g in divided doses daily before meals Maintenance dose: 1 g daily in divided doses Reduce dose to 250 mg daily if neurological symptoms worsen Add pyridoxine 25 mg daily	Improvement of clinical features May worsen neurological signs Monitor (6-monthly): Serum copper 24-h urinary copper Urine protein Aminoaciduria	Early: Worsen neurological disease (dystonia, tremor) Hypersensitivity (fever, rash) Leucopenia Thrombocytopenia Gastrointestinal symptoms Late: Systemic lupus erythematosus Nephrotic syndrome Nephritis Dermatopathy (elastosis perforans serpiginosa, Fig. 5) Arthropathy Pyridoxine deficiency
Trientine (Trien) (triethylene tetramine dihydrochloride)	Second line Chelator Wilson's disease with penicillamine intolerance Penicillamine side-effects Neurological signs worsen with penicillamine	Forms stable complexes with copper inducing cupriuresis Reduces intestinal copper absorption Increased serum free copper during cupriuresis	1–2 g in 3 divided doses daily post cibum	As for penicillamine Diminution in corneal Kayser–Fleischer ring	Early: As for penicillamine but less toxic Gastritis Late: Iron deficiency (chelates iron) Sideroblastic anaemia Bone marrow suppression (rare) Neurological worsening (much less than penicillamine)
Zinc sulphate (also as acetate, lactate, or gluconate)	Third line Wilson's disease: presymptomatic pregnancy Maintenance therapy in all Wilson's disease	Competitively inhibits intestinal copper absorption Induction of enterocyte metallothionein to increase faecal copper excretion Mobilizes endogenous copper	50–200 mg, 2–3 times daily as zinc salt 100–150 mg elemental zinc in divided doses daily (250 mg salt ≡ 45 mg elemental zinc) Given before meals Maintenance dose 300 mg three times per day	Slower onset of action than chelating agents Clinical improvement in weeks to months Claims to equal efficacy in copper depletion to chelating agents Measurement of urinary zinc indicates patient compliance	Fewer side-effects than chelating agents Minor gastrointestinal irritation (acetate<sulphate) Copper deficiency (rare) Leucopenia Anaemia (microcytic) Risk of teratogenicity (rare)
Ammonium tetrathiomolybdate	Fourth line May be used as initial treatment in severe neurological Wilson's disease Not used in hepatological Wilson's disease or childhood	Forms complexes with copper and albumin, blocking intestinal copper absorption Total plasma copper increases, plasma free copper falls, increased cupriuresis	40 mg twice daily Initiating treatment: 20 mg 6 times daily then change to zinc	Reversal of dystonia Improvement in penicillamine-induced neurological deterioration	Increase in liver transaminases Worsens hepatological Wilson's disease Reversible anaemia Bone marrow suppression Interferes with bone development

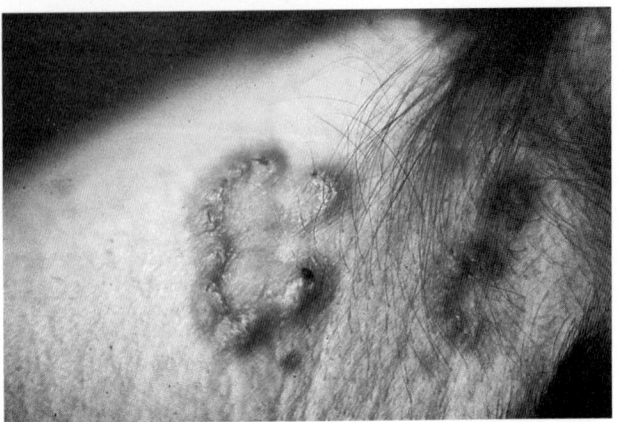

Fig. 4 Penicillamine dermatopathy—elastosis perfringens serpiginosa. (See also Plate 2.)

Menkes' disease

Menkes first described the disease in 1962, noting the X-linked recessive inheritance in a family of English–Irish descent. Subsequently, a number of case reports defined the clinical features of this disorder, and pattern of inheritance. Danks (1972) described the defect in intestinal absorption of copper which caused serum copper deficiency and which explained the diverse clinical features.

In 1982, the gene for Menkes' disease was isolated by three different groups. The gene maps to human Xq13 and encodes a p-type copper trans-porting ATPase (ATP7A). In 1983, Peltonen described abnormalities of copper and collagen metabolism in cultured fibroblasts as a feature of Menkes' disease; an increased rate of copper incorporation and accumulation of metallothionein was shown. The occipital horn syndrome, with survival to adult life, was described in 1983. Prenatal diagnosis for Menkes' disease was commenced in 1974 by measuring ^{64}Cu accumulation in cultured amniotic cells. Treatment of Menkes' disease with copper histidine commenced in 1989, with some improvement in the neurological symptoms and survival (Table 1).

Definition

Menkes' disease is a multisystem, lethal disorder of intracellular copper metabolism. It presents with the symptoms of neurodegeneration and connective tissue manifestations in skin, hair, and bone. A pathognomonic feature is the sparse, coarse, depigmented hair termed 'kinky' or 'steely' hair syndrome (Fig. 5 and Plate 3). A defect in intestinal copper absorption is associated with defective synthesis of copper enzymes and tissue copper accumulation, and this explains the changes in hair, characteristic facies, skin, and other changes. Importantly, fibroblasts in this disease contain five times the copper of normal cells. The untreated condition results in death, usually under 2 years of age. A milder form of the disease, a possible allelic mutation, is the occipital horn syndrome.

Incidence

The population frequency has been suggested by Danks to be around 1 in 40 000 per live births in Australia, but, as with Wilson's disease, this may be higher because some patients may remain undiagnosed even at death. More recent estimates suggest an incidence of 1 in about 300 000 live births in European countries, with an estimated mutation rate around 1.96×10^{-6} based on isolated Menkes' disease cases born during 1976 to 1987.

Clinical features

The first symptoms occur between 6 weeks and 6 months of age; major signs are poor growth, mental retardation, and hair abnormality. The disorder can present as a premature birth, and episodes of hypothermia may occur within the first few days or weeks of life. Some babies develop normally until 3 months of age, but many are ill from birth. The disease is progressive, culminating in death by the age of 3 years.

Classical characteristics are an abnormal facial appearance (Fig. 5) with flaccid skin, typical of cutis laxa, defective grey pigmentation of the skin, and lightly pigmented hair. Typically, the hair shaft is twisted to give pili torti, which is termed 'steely' or 'kinky' hair syndrome. Abnormalities of major arteries occur, giving thickened, tortuous vessels due to abnormal elastin fibres. Vascular complications, particularly subdural haematoma, can occur. Abnormalities in bone include Wormian bones in the skull and osteoporosis with widened metaphyses, which may fracture. Child abuse may be wrongly considered in these patients.

Progressive focal cerebral and cerebellar degeneration are also typical of the disorder, with associated convulsions and mental retardation. In the milder case of Menkes' disease, the occipital horn syndrome, ataxia and the complications of bladder or urinary diverticulae, hernias, and skin or joint laxity are prominent.

Genetics

Pedigree studies have confirmed Menkes as an X-linked recessive disease. The gene has now been mapped to Xq13.3 (Table 1).

Pathogenesis

Defective intestinal copper absorption leading to a copper deficiency and defective activity of copper-containing enzymes explain the clinical features of connective tissue and arterial abnormalities: tyrosinase (depigmentation and skin pallor); lysyl oxidase (abnormalities in arterial intima due to lack of formation of cross-links in elastin and collagen); monoamine oxidase ('kinky' hair); cytochrome c oxidase (hypothermia); and ascorbate oxidase (skeletal demineralization). The diagnostic hair abnormality probably arises from defective formation of disulphide bonds in keratin, another copper-dependent process. In Menkes' disease, most tissues including intestinal mucosa, kidney, placenta, and testis, with the exception of the

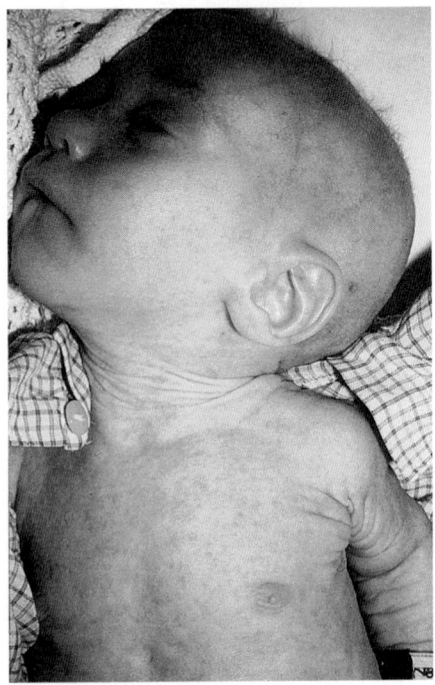

Fig. 5 Appearance in Menkes' disease. (See also Plate 3.)

liver, have an increased copper concentration. ^{64}Cu studies have demonstrated defective cellular efflux of copper.

Pathology

Major changes are in the arteries and central nervous system. In arteries, degenerative changes lead to aneurysmal dilatation, rupture or stenosis, and areas of intimal proliferation and thrombosis. In the larger arteries, fragmentation of the internal elastic lamina occurs, probably secondary to defective elastin formation. In the later stages of the disease, brain infarcts and haemorrhage occur.

Neuronal destruction and gliosis are found in the cerebral cortex. In the cerebellum, Purkinje cells are destroyed. Myelin is also defective. Changes in skeletal muscle, the iris, and retina have also been noted.

Diagnosis

Although hair changes may not be evident in the first few months of life, the initial diagnosis is based on the principal clinical features of Menkes' disease.

Biochemical tests

Reduced concentrations of serum copper and caeruloplasmin with reduction in gut mucosal and hepatic copper in association with the clinical features are diagnostic. Liver histology is normal but reduced concentrations of liver cuproenzymes, such as cytochrome oxidase and superoxide dismutase, are found in infants over 3 months of age. Accumulation of ^{64}Cu in cultured skin fibroblasts after a 20-h pulse and impaired efflux after a 24-h pulse confirms the diagnosis. Laboratories need to be skilled in radiocopper assays.

Molecular tests

Following identification of the Menkes' disease gene (MNK), fluorescence in situ hybridization, Southern blot hybridization, or PCR-based mutation analysis may detect various mutations. Chromosomal aberrations can be investigated by standard chromosome banding techniques and confirmed by in situ hybridization.

Prenatal diagnosis in the first trimester by measuring the copper content of chorionic villi using neutron activation analysis is unreliable. Contamination of samples gave false-positive results, as did intracellular copper analysis of cultured amniotic fluid cells. DNA analysis can now be carried out, but mutations must first be identified in the family and the mother's carrier status should be known. However, mutation analysis is a difficult undertaking because of the large size of MNK. Carrier detection may be possible by ^{64}Cu uptake in cultured fibroblasts, but, because of random activation of the X chromosome, may also be unreliable.

Management

Only administration of copper as copper histidinate has been shown to be successful in correcting skin, hair, and pigmentation abnormalities. The neurological damage appears to be irreversible unless treatment is started very early, as it is likely that copper damage to neurones is well established in utero. Thus, treatment should be commenced as early as possible before irreversible neuronal damage occurs. Late diagnosis treatment may prolong survival in patients up to 10 or 20 years but without significant improvement in the clinical features. Treatment with monoamine oxidase inhibitors, with the aim of correcting defective catecholamine synthesis due to deficiency of monoamine oxidase, has not been successful. What is now required is the means to deliver amounts of copper in an appropriate form, sufficient to replace tissue deficiency, but avoiding copper toxicity.

Prognosis

Prognosis varies with the mutations and clinical severity of the disease. Untreated, patients are unlikely to survive beyond 2 to 3 years of age. Use of copper histidine, particularly when commenced early, has prolonged survival to 20 years, with improvement in most of the clinical features except those due to neurological damage. In the occipital horn syndrome survival is longer.

Further reading

Wilson's disease

Brewer GJ et al. (1998). Treatment of Wilson's disease with zinc: XV long term follow-up studies. Journal of Laboratory and Clinical Medicine 132, 264–78. [Review of zinc therapy.]

Gollan JL, Gollan TJ (1998). Wilson's disease in 1998: genetic diagnostic and therapeutic aspects. Journal of Hepatology 28, 28–36. [Review of diagnostic aspects of Wilson's disease in relation to clinical presentation and monitoring of treatment.]

Gow PJ et al. (2000). Diagnosis of Wilson's disease: an experience over three decades. Gut 46, 415–9. [Clinical experience of Wilson's disease.]

Hoogengraad T (1996). Wilson's disease. Saunders, Philadelphia. [Good general clinical and historical review of all aspects of Wilson's disease.]

Roberts EA, Cox DW (1998). Wilson's disease. Baillère's Clinical Gastroenterology 12, 237–56. [Recent update on Wilson's disease.]

Menkes' disease

Christodoulou J et al. (1998). Early treatment of Menkes disease with parenteral copper (sic)-histidine: long term follow-up of four treated patients. American Journal of Medical Genetics 76, 154–64.

Danks D (1995). Disorders of copper transport. In: Scriver CR, Beaudet AL, Sly WS, Valle D, et al. eds. The metabolic basis of inherited disease, Vol. 2, pp. 2212–35. McGraw-Hill, New York.

Menkes JH (1999). Menkes disease and Wilson's disease: two sides of the same coin. European Journal of Paediatric Neurology 3, 243–53. [Comparison of the two diseases.]

Tanner MS (1999). Disorders of copper metabolism. In: Kelly DA, ed. Disease of the liver and biliary system in children, pp. 167–85. Blackwell Science, Oxford.

Tümer Z and Horn N (1997). Menkes disease: recent advances and new aspects. Medical Genetics 34, 265–74.

11.8 Lysosomal storage diseases

T. M. Cox

Definition

Lysosomal storage diseases represent the consequences of disordered lysosomal digestive function. The lysosome is an intracellular organelle that serves to degrade biological macromolecules derived either endogenously, from metabolism or cell structures, or from the breakdown of exogenous material incorporated by endocytosis.

Since lysosomes are found in most cells, disruption of their function leading to the storage of undegraded macromolecules usually affects many tissues. More than 40 lysosomal disorders are now recognized; they represent single or multiple defects in the organellar complement of specific acid hydrolases, their activator proteins, membrane proteins, or the intrinsic carrier proteins that transport the substrates or products of lysosomal digestion.

Lysosomal diseases, though often considered to be very rare, occur with a surprisingly high birth frequency. About one in 5000 live-born infants have a lysosomal storage disorder; many of these are disabling conditions: Gaucher's disease and Fabry's disease—which are glycosphingolipidoses—are possibly the most frequent. The recent addition of Batten's disease and other ceroid neuronal lipofuscinoses to this burgeoning family of disorders emphasizes the importance of the lysosomal diseases in biology and in medicine: they represent a large and disproportionate burden of illness in the population and for clinical services.

Biological importance of lysosomes

Since their discovery nearly 50 years ago by the medically qualified biologist Christian de Duve, lysosomes and their associated endosomal structures have been at the focus of an impressive body of research into molecular cell biology. De Duve recognized that, with their ready access to extracellular fluid, lysosomes could be used to deliver therapeutic proteins and other agents to the heart of the cell—a prophecy well rewarded with the development of targeted enzyme-replacement therapy for several lysosomal diseases today. The success of these treatments is predicated on detailed knowledge about the delivery of nascent lysosomal proteins to the organelle during its biogenesis, the definition of inherited defects in lysosomal function—and of the development of recombinant DNA technology for the manufacture and the post-translational modification of human proteins for therapeutic use. Greater understanding of lysosomal storage diseases has emanated from research into the metabolism of particular cellular macromolecules that accumulate in lysosomal storage diseases, and into the ebb-and-flow of substrates and products as they pass through lysosomal compartments.

Structure and function of lysosomes

Lysosomes are strikingly diverse in shape and size, but all belong to a single class of ubiquitous organelles containing numerous acid hydrolases (around 40 of which are known) with optimum activity in the pH range, 5 to 6. The matrix space of these organelles is surrounded by a single unit membrane containing transport proteins that facilitate the export of digestion products. Specialized carrier components use energy derived from ATP to maintain the optimal intraorganellar acid pH for enzymatic hydrolysis. The integrity of the lysosome membrane is maintained by highly glycosylated membrane proteins that offer protection from the activated luminal proteases with which they are in contact. Histochemical stains can identify pathological lysosomes in tissue preparations; together with electron microscopy, these methods can be used to detect abnormal lysosomes engorged with storage material in diseased tissues.

Delivery of macromolecules for lysosomal digestion

The lysosome is an intracellular digestive system but acquires complex macromolecules for breakdown by three main pathways: (1) receptor-mediated endocytosis; (2) engulfment and fusion; (3) autophagy. Receptor-mediated endocytosis occurs by means of clathrin-coated pits, a process in which molecules are delivered after internalization to a peripheral, and later to a perinuclear endosomal compartment, 'the endolysosome'. The endolysosome undergoes maturation to form a lysosome after the loss of certain membrane components and further acidification. Some molecules acquired by receptor-mediated endocytosis (for example, low-density lipoproteins) are specifically retrieved and ultimately returned to the cell surface having delivered their cargo of cholesterol within the lysosome. Other molecules that are not retrieved are ultimately degraded by fusion with mature lysosomes and enzymatic hydrolysis (for example, the epidermal growth factor (**EGF**) receptor system).

Lysosomes are also involved in a specialized process for the degradation of exogenous particulates and proteins, including microbes and effete cells such as erythrocytes and neutrophils. Although this engulfment and fusion process involving phagolysosomes is distributed throughout nature, it is particularly active in macrophages and dendritic cells that exhibit active phagocytosis. A specialized phagolysosome variant occurs in osteoclasts that are derived from myeloid cells of mononuclear phagocyte origin. The osteoclastic resorptive vacuole serves as a large exteriorized lysosomal compartment which is independently acidified for the process of bone resorption. In macrophages, cell-surface components that occur on bacteria and yeast, as well as exogenous cells, are recognized and bound by specific receptors on the plasma membrane. The phagocytes engulf foreign material to form large vesicles in which acidification and proteolysis, as well as the secretion of degradative molecules (including reactive oxygen and nitrogen species), is initiated. The phagolysosome fuses with lysosomes and further acidification occurs, so that the acid hydrolases are activated to bring about the breakdown of the ingested material.

Autophagy occurs within cells. It appears that, in a constant process of membrane fusion and flow, organelles (including the endoplasmic reticulum, mitochondria, peroxisomes, and other lysosomes) fuse with lysosomes, by which they are engulfed before breakdown. This process retrieves the basic building blocks of cellular components and proceeds hand-in-hand with *de novo* synthesis and the renewal of intracellular compartments throughout the life of all cells. When lysosomal function is impeded, the breakdown of endogenous organelle-derived macromolecules is impaired; this, together with a failure to breakdown exogenous macromolecules, results in the pathological storage of partially degraded and undegraded material.

Enzyme-replacement therapy for lysosomal storage diseases

Early experiments using fibroblasts obtained from patients suffering from mucopolysaccharidoses such as Hurler's disease and Hunter's syndrome, showed that the rate of degradation—rather than the rates of synthesis or secretion of radiolabelled glycosaminoglycans that accumulate in these diseases—is severely disrupted. In experiments in which fibroblasts obtained from genetically distinct storage disorders were co-cultured, the progressive accumulation of glycosaminoglycan that occurs when the fibroblasts are cultured separately, was prevented. Biosynthetic labelling experiments showed that degradation of the previously accumulating substrates was restored to normal in these co-culture experiments.

An investigation of this phenomenon by Elizabeth Neufeld and colleagues later showed that each of the fibroblast cultures elaborated and delivered a specific corrective factor to the medium, which ultimately proved to be a high molecular weight form of the specific hydrolases that were lacking in each of the pathological fibroblasts. These corrective factors, when taken up from the medium, restore the normal intracellular degradation of glycosaminoglycans. This secretion–recapture process was shown to be mediated by an unusual carbohydrate component, the so-called 'recognition marker', mannose-6-phosphate. This sugar is found as a terminal moiety derived by post-translational modification and during the secretion of lysosomal enzymes. Neufeld's findings led to the identification of specific receptor pathways for the biosynthesis and uptake of nascent lysosomal proteins by the organelle during the course of organellar formation—and have subtended a great deal of productive biological research. From the therapeutic aspect, however, the experiments immediately raised the possibility of functional complementation of lysosomal storage disorders by supplying particular molecular isoforms of the enzymes that are deficient in the individual storage disorders.

Characterization of lysosomal recognition markers occurred at a time when other cell-surface glycoprotein recognition systems were being identified: for example, the asialoglycoprotein receptor which was implicated by Ashwell and colleagues in the uptake of plasma proteins by parenchymal liver cells *in vivo*. Thus the concept of enzyme replacement for lysosomal storage disorders was established but it was many years before an effective treatment based on glycoprotein targeting was brought into clinical practice. Indeed, the successful use of enzyme replacement was dependent on an understanding of glycoprotein chemistry, receptor-mediated endocytosis, and the molecular cell biology of lysosomal biogenesis—all subjects that themselves depended on a detailed molecular understanding of human lysosomal storage diseases. Identification of the secretion–recapture process in the lysosomal diseases provided the key theoretical underpinning to empirical complementation studies that preceded successful enzyme-replacement therapy. Cellular complementation, by providing a source of wild-type enzyme delivered from allogeneic bone marrow transplantation, has also had spectacular successes in several lysosomal disorders.

Alternative treatments for the glycolipid disorders

For many years it has been recognized that the accumulation of storage material within lysosomes is the precipitating factor for the development of tissue injury and the inflammatory response that accompanies the lysosomal storage disorders. Although it is principally a failure of degradation or export from the lysosome that leads to the excess storage, the concept of depleting the supply of macromolecular substrate to prevent the accumulation of storage material has been developed experimentally and brought to human clinical trials.

Of particular interest has been the discovery that certain iminosugars related to deoxynojirimycin selectively inhibit the glucosyltransferase step as the first committed reaction in the biosynthesis of glycosphingolipids. Experimental studies in cultured cells with pathological storage of glycolipids in lysosomes showed regression of the intralysosomal material after exposure to low concentrations of these natural product derivatives. Later studies demonstrated the reduced storage and delayed symptom onset in experimental animal models of debilitating human glycosphingolipidoses such as Tay–Sachs disease and Sandhoff disease (see Chapter 24.6.1). *N*-butyldeoxynojirimycin, a particular analogue of these iminosugars, has previously been used in clinical trials in an attempt to inhibit the replication of human immunodeficiency virus (**HIV**), as a result of its related inhibitory activity towards α-glucosidases; in these trials, such drugs appear to be relatively non-toxic in large doses. With these data in mind, studies were undertaken to investigate the concept of substrate depletion as a treatment for established glycosphingolipidoses. Evidence of disease regression was obtained in an open-labelled trial of *N*-butyldeoxynojirimycin in patients with Gaucher's disease, as shown by the reduction in visceral enlargement, enzymatic markers of Gaucher's disease activity (plasma chitotriosidase activity), and a slow improvement in haematological parameters. In Gaucher's disease, it was anticipated that the beneficial effects of substrate depletion would be indirect, since they would result from the decrease in the delivery to the macrophage system of glycolipid substrates on the membrane of blood cells. In any event, since the iminosugars are small molecules that penetrate the blood–brain barrier, the possibility of their use (either as a monotherapy or as a synergistic treatment with enzyme therapy) for neuronopathic Gaucher's disease has been raised, as well as for the treatment of the otherwise intractable glycosphingolipidoses that cause severe neurological disease. No effective treatment is currently available for Tay–Sachs disease, Sandhoff disease, and GM1 gangliosidosis, and the juvenile and late-onset variants are thus potential targets for substrate depletion with the iminosugars.

Substrate-depletion therapy depends upon the presence of residual enzymatic activity in the lysosomes. Disturbances of the dynamic equilibrium in the supply and handling of macromolecular lysosomal substrates occur, but most, if not all, patients with glycosphingolipid disorders express residual enzymatic function. At present, clinical trials are underway not only in Gaucher's disease but in patients suffering from severe neuronopathic glycolipidoses such as late-onset GM2 gangliosidosis as well as Niemann–Pick-disease type C. This latter disorder is itself associated with a secondary accumulation of toxic glycolipids within neuronal lysosomes (see below).

The iminosugars appear to be relatively well tolerated apart from causing diarrhoea, probably as a result of impaired biosynthesis of intestinal disaccharidases as a subsidiary effect on oligosaccharide processing. Indeed, experience shows that they appear to be well-tolerated once appropriate dietary restrictions are introduced. However, several cases of peripheral neuropathy have been reported in long-term studies of patients with Gaucher's disease. The sugars are absorbed after oral ingestion and offer the hope of a therapy to arrest the progression of several severe neurological sphingolipidoses that are otherwise beyond therapeutic correction. At present, the outcome of the clinical trials based on promising animal experiments with the iminosugars and other inhibitors of glycolipid biosynthesis derivatives is urgently awaited but few better general strategic options than substrate deletion appear to be available for exploration in patients who might otherwise be without hope.

Pharmaceutical development

Lysosomal storage diseases have been a focus for several prominent therapeutic discoveries. The cooperation of informed patient groups, applied medical research funded by government organizations, and the commercial interest of medium-sized pharmaceutical companies has been promoted by recently introduced Orphan Drug legislation. This legislation has facilitated the early exclusive licensing of products for rare diseases—and has greatly enhanced corporate pharmaceutical investment.

At present, at least six recombinant human enzyme preparations are in clinical use or late stages of development. Indeed, several companies continue to express interest in this area with gene therapy, recombinant proteins, and small-molecule products in active competitive development. There can be little doubt that industry has drawn encouragement from the commercial success of recombinant human products such as erythropoietin, human insulin, and interferon-β and -γ. These are top-selling agents that have brought handsome rewards for their parent companies, whose manufacturing patents have several times been vigorously defended. At the time of writing, Genzyme Therapeutics, the United States-based company first involved in the development of targeted enzyme-replacement therapy for Gaucher's disease, is providing treatment to about 3000 patients worldwide. The company reports an annual operating profit of more than $500000000. As described here, many of the 40 or so known human lysosomal disorders are disabling and distressing conditions that cause pain and disability in infants, children and adults of all ages, and for which, until recently, no definitive treatments have been available. The unpredicted magnification of interest that has accompanied successful medical research into this area over a period of less than 50 years has been a model of utility and progress; it continues to provide for many patients the hope that, at last, definitive relief may be forthcoming.

Pathology

Although lysosomal defects occur in all tissues, the principal focus of each disease is observed in those tissues where turnover of the parent macromolecule with impaired degradation is greatest. For example, in Gaucher's disease, the turnover of parent glycolipids appears to be greatest in the mononuclear phagocytes. Here the accumulation of glycolipids derived from the breakdown of membranes present in the formed blood elements occurs; with mild or moderate impairment of the responsible enzyme, glucocerebrosidase, the pathology is restricted to the macrophage-containing tissues of the liver, spleen, bone marrow, and, occasionally, the lung. When inherited defects further impair the activity of glucocerebrosidase, additional pathology is seen in the nervous system where the accumulating glycolipid is derived from the turnover of endogenous neural sphingolipids.

Microscopic pathology shows storage within dilated vesicular spaces, which represent diseased lysosomes. Sphingolipids, being hydrophobic molecules, tend to accumulate in whorls known as 'membranous cytoplasmic bodies' where they assume a lamellar structure within lysosomal spaces. Paracrystalline and crystalline material in distended lysosomes may also be seen under electron microscopy, for example in the accumulation of the charged glycolipid sulphatide that occurs in metachromatic leucodystrophy (arylsulphatase A deficiency). With more water-soluble substrates, granular material accumulates within the vesicular spaces. These spaces represent distended and often fused lysosomes, filled for example with undegraded glycogen macromolecular complexes in acid maltase deficiency (Pompe's disease, glycogen storage disease type II, see Chapter 11.3.1). Pompe's disease was the first lysosomal storage disease to be identified. Its recognition by Henri-Gery Hers (a colleague of de Duve) led to the concept of 'autophagy' and of the rapid turnover of normal macromolecular components of the cell—including glycogen—by the lysosomal compartment. Pompe's disease has also been the subject of intensive clinical

research and early successes have been reported in trials of enzyme-replacement therapy (see the Further reading list).

Although the amount of storage material that accumulates within lysosomes in the lysosomal diseases is several hundred- or thousand-fold greater than normal, the absolute amount of material may amount to only a few grams or so. The quantity of storage material, however, bears no relationship to its pathophysiological effects. In some instances, the presence of a few grams of, for example, the sphingolipid sphingomyelin in Niemann–Pick disease, is associated with massive visceral enlargement with accompanying inflammatory ischaemic and other destructive changes due to the presence of storage cells. Similarly, marked pathological injury occurs: in the viscera and bone marrow spaces of patients with Gaucher's disease; in the heart and skeletal muscles of patients with α-glucosidase deficiency, due to modest glycogen accumulation in the sarcoplasm of striated and cardiac myocytes; and, in the form of neuronophagia, in the brain of patients with Tay–Sachs disease and GM_1 gangliosidosis. Microscopic examination of diseased tissues may also reveal pathognomic storage cells, for example the modified macrophage-derived microglia ('globoid cells') in Krabbe's disease, the striking pathological macrophages of Gaucher's disease, and the foam cells of Niemann–Pick disease types A, B, and C.

Pathogenesis

At present, there is only rudimentary knowledge about the pathological link between lysosomal storage, tissue injury, and the diverse clinical manifestations that accompany lysosomal storage diseases. In the case of the sphingolipidoses, sphingolipids participate in cell-recognition events and receptor biology; sphingolipid metabolic intermediates (lysosphingolipids) also function as signalling molecules in apoptotic and proliferative responses. However, the precise relationship between the storage material and the development of overt clinical disease is not fully understood. In one striking instance (Krabbe's disease due to β-galactosidase deficiency), however, it has been found that the unusual globoid cell can be induced *in vitro* by the pathological lysosphingolipid, psychosine, that accumulates in the diseased tissues. Psychosine and related glycolipids are thus implicated in the final pathological pathway that leads to the disease phenotype. Psychosine itself interacts with a G-protein-coupled receptor on human monocytic-lineage cells. This finding may have profound implications for other lysosomal disorders associated with cell loss and apoptotic as well as inflammatory fibrotic responses. Several indirect studies have indicated the release of inflammatory cytokines in at least one lysosomal storage disease (Gaucher's disease), which may explain the metabolic and plasma protein abnormalities associated with a sustained inflammatory response that characterizes the clinical syndrome.

In a scientific era in which the combined study of gene and protein expression offers a powerful means to understand complex functional networks that lead to tissue pathology, the lysosomal storage diseases represent a promising field for exploration using large-scale, high-throughput methods to investigate altered cell metabolism and signalling responses. An early potential application of this work has been the use of authentic experimental models of some of the more severe storage diseases generated by gene knockout technology; these models facilitate research on otherwise inaccessible tissues such as the brain during the development of the storage phenotype. Gene-expression profiling experiments conducted during periods of neuronal cell death have shown upregulation of genes related to the inflammatory process in the nervous system of mice that serve as a model of GM_2 gangliosidosis. The activation of local microglia is shown by the signature of upregulated macrophage expression markers and lymphocyte chemoattractants, as well as genes encoding antigen-presenting MHC class II molecules. Since this particular GM_2 gangliosidosis is partially ameliorated by bone marrow transplantation that supplies a population of genetically competent immune cells (and which is accompanied by the use of powerful immunosuppressant agents), it seems probable that the altered immunity accompanying bone marrow transplantation may itself modify the clinical expression of lysosomal storage diseases affecting the brain. This may occur without directly affecting the storage material.

Biochemical classification of the lysosomal storage diseases (Table 1)

Lysosomal diseases result from inherited defects in lysosomal hydrolases and the mechanisms for delivering them to the organelle; lysosomal enzyme activators and cofactors; lysosomal membrane proteins; and carrier systems for the transport of the substrates and products of lysosomal digestion between the organelle and the cytoplasm. Most of the enzymatic defects are restricted to the activity of a single hydrolase but defects of activators and cofactors, as well as proteins involved in the processing of nascent lysosomal enzymes for organellar delivery, can lead to generalized defects of lysosome function.

As the clinical manifestations for the 40 or more diseases associated with disturbed lysosomal function are very diverse, the reader is referred to specialized literature including the paediatric literature for further information (see Further reading). Broadly, the lysosomal diseases may be associated with: slowly progressive, connective-tissue disease with skeletal abnormalities; neurological symptoms that include deafness and progressive mental deterioration; and visceral syndromes affecting the spleen, liver, lung, kidney, and heart. Ocular disease occurs particularly in the mucopolysaccharidoses and in the neurosphingolipidoses: this may cause corneal opacities or severe retinal changes, including a macular cherry-red spot. Neurological symptoms may have their onset from early infancy to adulthood, beyond even 60 years. In the past, patients with Tay–Sachs disease and other late-onset gangliosidoses were misdiagnosed as having demyelinating disease, Parkinson's disease, or even hereditary ataxia.

Diagnostic features

All lysosomal diseases disturb the catabolism of complex molecules in several tissues. Thus the symptoms are usually permanent and progressive; they show no relationship to food intake and are generally independent of intercurrent illness. Those disorders that affect metabolically active organs, such as the liver and kidney, often cause functional impairment, including the manifestations of liver failure, portal hypertension, and, in the case of the kidney, rickets, metabolic acidosis, and the effects of the renal Fanconi syndrome.

The occurrence of coarse facies, joint stiffness, vacuolation in circulating lymphocytes or neutrophils, with or without associated bone changes and hepatosplenomegaly, suggests the presence of one of the mucopolysaccharidoses or glycosphingolipidoses. Disorders associated with progressive neurological and mental deterioration with visceral and skeletal changes or other somatic disturbances strongly suggest the presence of a glycoproteinosis, such as mannosidosis or fucosidosis, or one of the mucopolysaccharidoses (MPS) including Hurler's, Hunter's, or Sanfilippo's disease (MPS I–III, respectively). Skin signs are unusual in lysosomal diseases, but the presence of small angiokeratomas, particularly in the region of the buttocks and genitals, strongly suggests the diagnosis of the sphingolipidosis, Fabry disease (see below), or fucosidosis or the rare condition, Schindler's disease (acetylgalactosaminidase deficiency).

Prominent bone necrotic lesions in association with the early onset of visceral disease, with or without supranuclear ophthalmoplegias, suggest either Niemann–Pick disease type A and C or neuronopathic Gaucher's disease (type III). Ataxia is a feature of GM_1 and GM_2 gangliosidoses, and a flaccid paraparesis in young children might suggest metachromatic leucodystrophy; widespread white-matter disease in association with a frontal dementia is a characteristic presentation of juvenile and adult forms of metachromatic leucodystrophy. Early-onset leucodystrophy is often caused by metachromatic leucodystrophy and Krabbe disease is a rare but important diagnostic entity in this group since the disease may be arrested by allogeneic marrow transplantation in the first 2 months of life. Lysosomal diseases with prominent neurological manifestations are often associated with progressive mental deterioration, with or without the onset of spasticity, myoclonic seizures, and optic atrophy. Extrapyramidal signs including parkinsonism, athetoid movements, and dystonia are frequent in this group of disorders.

Lysosomal diseases are a prominent cause of progressive neurological and mental deterioration in patients whose disease starts during adolescence up to mature adult life, and should always be considered in the diagnostic examination. Corneal opacities suggest cystinosis, I-cell disease, mucopolysaccharidoses, mannosidosis, Fabry disease, and galactosialidosis, as well as one form of Gaucher's disease with neuronopathic features (the D409H type IIIc variant). Specific syndromes are described below.

Diagnostic pathology

As described earlier, the pathological manifestations of the lysosomal diseases are diverse. They may range from enlargement of viscera with infiltration by abnormal macrophages containing storage material (foam cells of Niemann–Pick disease or Gaucher's cells) to bone infarction, neuronophagia, vacuolation of renal tubular cells, and diverse tissue infiltrates. Inclusion bodies may be observed in metachromatic-stained cells of the urine deposit or in circulating neutrophils and lymphocytes (Maroteaux–Lamy disease); staining with a periodic acid–Schiff reagent may reveal diastase-resistant glycolipid storage in the kidney and other organs in Fabry disease and other glycosphingolipidoses. The presence of metachromatic storage material in nervous tissue, including peripheral nerves, is characteristic of the sphingolipidosis, metachromatic leucodystrophy (Fig. 1 and Plate 1).

Ultrastructural examination is often diagnostic for lysosomal diseases: membrane-bound vesicles containing storage material that may show a crystalline or concentric appearance, or, in the case of glycogen in Pompe's disease, a granular appearance. The presence of concentric arrays of material strongly suggest a sphingolipidosis. Amorphous material accumulates within the lysosomal vacuoles in the mucopolysaccharidoses and glycoproteinoses. The secondary effects of lysosomal hypertrophy include increased staining for tartrate-resistant acid phosphatase and other lysosomal markers, including intrinsic lysosomal membrane proteins, for example LAMP-1.

Radiology

Ultrasonography, magnetic resonance imaging (MRI), and computed tomography (CT) may reveal visceral enlargement and infiltration, for example Niemann–Pick disease, mucopolysaccharidoses, Gaucher's disease. Skeletal radiographs may reveal bone expansion in vertebrae and in the phalangeal and long bones, sometimes associated with infarction and collapse, particularly in Niemann–Pick disease type B and Gaucher's disease. Echocardiography may reveal thickening and calcification of the cardiac valves (particularly of the aortic ring), infiltration of cardiac muscle causing ventricular hypertrophy in Pompe's disease, Fabry's disease, and, especially, in mucopolysaccharidoses I, IV, and VI.

Neuroradiology is of value—particularly in patients with mucopolysaccharidoses, and in Morquio's syndrome as well as MPS syndromes I, II, and VI where instability of the atlantoaxial joint may cause fatal subluxation in relation to increased soft tissue surrounding the dens. MRI of the cervical spine in MPS is critical in judging the need for joint stabilization by posterior fusion. Similarly, investigations of the lower spine may determine the cause of progressive spinal deformity due to lumbar kyphosis, and assist in the evaluation of the need for surgical intervention. MRI of the brain is invaluable in the assessment of dementing illnesses: cortical and/or white-matter disease may be delineated. Magnetic resonance imaging is often critical for diagnosing the striking white-matter changes that occur in patients with metachromatic leucodystrophy (Fig. 2).

Table 1 Lysosomal diseases

Name	Primary defect	Principal storage
A. Generalized defects I-cell disease (mucolipidosis II)	N-acetylglucosamine-1-phosphotransferase (with hypersecretion of numerous lysosomal hydrolases)	Lipids, oligosaccharides, mucopolysaccharides
Pseudo-Hurler polydystrophy (mucolipidosis III)	N-acetylglucosamine-1-phosphotransferase (with hypersecretion of numerous lysosomal hydrolases)	Lipids, oligosaccharides, mucopolysaccharides
Multiple sulphatase deficiency (Austin's disease)	Failure to modify key cysteine residue in common active site of sulphatase enzymes (with deficiency of arylsulphatases A–C)	Mucopolysaccharides, sulphatide, and other sulphated lipids including steroid sulphates
Sphingolipid activator protein (Saposin) deficiency (a)　sap precursor (b)　sap-A (c)　sap-B (d)　sap-C (e)　GM$_2$ activator	(a)　absent saposins A–D (b)　impaired glucosyl and galactosylceramidase (c)　impaired arylsulphatase A, sphingomyelinase, β-galactosidase (d)　impaired glucosylceramidase (e)　impaired hexosaminidase A activity	(a)　ceramide, glucosylceramide, galactosyl ceramide, sulphatide gangliosides (b)　glucosyl and galactosyl ceramidase (c)　predominantly sulphatide MLD* (d)　Gaucher-like storage (e)　GM2 GA2 gangliosides
Galactosialidosis	Protective protein deficiency causing combined degradation of β-galactosidase and neuraminidase-cathepsin A	Sialyloligosaccharides
Chediak–Higashi syndrome	Impaired function of lysosomal trafficking regulator, LYST	Defective targeting of secretory lysosomal proteins including melanosome proteins, giant granules in leucocytes
Hermansky–Pudlak syndrome	HPS 1-β-3A subunit of adaptin	Defective platelets (no dense granules), melanosomes, lysosomes contain ceroid storage material
B. Transport defects Cystinosis	Cystine transporter (integral lysosomal membrane protein)	Reduced cystine efflux
Niemann–Pick diseases type C1 and 2 (distinct complementation groups)	Lysosomal membrane proteins	Impaired cholesterol and sphingolipid trafficking
Salla disease	Sialic acid transporter, sialin (AST)	Free sialic acid
Cobalamin deficiency (*Cb1F*)	Unknown cobalamin transporter	Reduced free cobalamin efflux
C. Sphingolipidoses GM$_1$ gangliosidosis (see Morquio B)	β-Galactosidase	Ganglioside GM$_1$ and asialoganglioside A
GM$_2$ gangliosidoses (a) Tay–Sachs disease (b) Sandhoff disease	 β-Hexosaminidase A β-Hexosaminidase A and B	 GM$_2$ gangliosides GM$_2$ gangliosides oligosaccharides
Anderson–Fabry disease	α-Galactosidase A	Trihexosylceramide
Gaucher's disease	Glucocerebrosidase	Glucosylceramide
Niemann–Pick disease A and B	Acid sphingomyelinase	Sphingomyelin
Krabbe's disease	β-Galactocerebrosidase	Psychosine, galactosylceramide
Metachromatic leucodystrophy	Arylsulphatase A	Sulphatide
D. Mucopolysaccharidoses (MPS) MPS I (Hurler)	α-L-Iduronidase	Dermatan sulphate, heparan sulphate
MPS I S (Scheie)	α-L-Iduronidase	Dermatan sulphate, heparan sulphate
MPS I H/S (Hurler–Scheie)	α-L-Iduronidase	Dermatan sulphate, heparan sulphate
MPS II (Hunter)	Iduronate sulphatase	Dermatan sulphate, heparan sulphate
MPS IIIA (Sanfilippo A)	Heparan N-sulphatase	Heparan sulphate
MPS IIIB (Sanfilippo B)	α-N-acetylglucosaminidase	Heparan sulphate
MPS IIIC (Sanfilippo C)	Acetyl CoA: α-glucosaminide acetyl transferase	Heparan sulphate

Table 1 *Continued*

MPS IIID (Sanfilippo D)	N-acetylglucosamine 6-sulphatase	Heparan sulphate
MPS IVA (Morquio A)	Galactose 6-sulphatase	Keratan sulphate, chondroitin 6-sulphate
MPS IVB (Morquio B) (see GM₁ gangliosidosis)	β-Galactosidase	Keratan sulphate, β-galactosyl oligosaccharides
MPS VI (Maroteaux-Lamy)	Arylsulphatase B	Dermatan sulphate
MPS VII (Sly)	β-Glucuronidase	Dermatan sulphate, heparan sulphate, chondroitin 4- and 6-sulphates
E. Glycoproteinases		
Schindler disease	α-N-acetylgalactosaminidase	N-acetylgalactosaminyl peptides and oligosaccharides
α-Mannosidosis	α-Mannosidase	Oligosaccharides
β-Mannosidosis	β-Mannosidase	β-Mannosyl glycoconjugate
Fucosidosis	α-Fucosidase	Glycopeptides, oligosaccharides
Sialidosis	Neuraminidase	Sialylated oligosaccharides
Aspartylglucosaminuria	Aspartylglucosaminidase	Aspartylglucosamine
F. Lipid disorders Farber's disease	Acid ceramidase	Ceramide
Cholesterol ester storage disease	Acid lipase	Cholesterol, cholesterol esters
Wolman's disease	Acid lipase	Cholesterol, cholesteryl esters
G. Miscellaneous defects Neuronal ceroid lipofuscinosis (CLN) (Batten's disease)		
CLN1 CLN2 CLN3 CLN8	Palmitoyl-protein thioesterase Tripeptidyl-peptidase I Lysosomal pH control Cathepsin D	Ceroid autofluorescent lysosomal storage of cytochrome C peptide and other polypeptide and lipid remnants
Papillon–Lefèvre syndrome (keratopalmar periodontitis)	Cathepsin C deficiency	No storage—neutrophil phagocytic defect
Pycnodysostosis	Cathepsin K	Type I collagen fragments

*MLD, metachromatic leucodystrophy-like material.

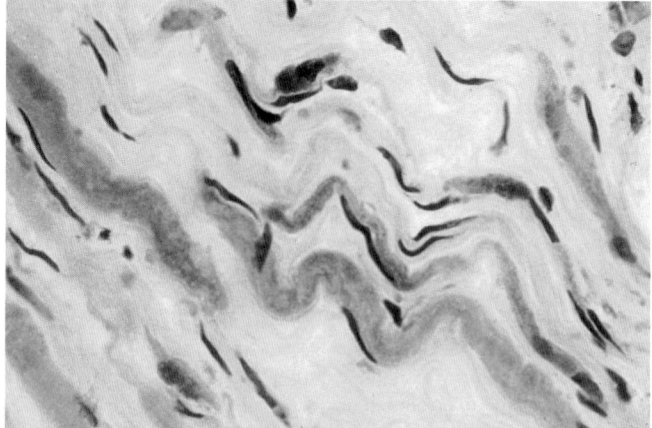

Fig. 1 Sural nerve biopsy stained with toluidine blue from the patient shown in Fig. 2 with metachromatic leucodystrophy. Note the brown-staining granular material within Schwann cells and perineurial macrophages typical of this disorder due to the deposition of the glycolipid sulphatide. (By courtesy of Dr. J. Xuereb, Addenbrooke's Hospital). (See also Plate 1.)

Diagnosis of lysosomal diseases

It is critical to establish a definitive diagnosis of a suspected lysosomal disease, even in critically ill patients, for two reasons: these disorders are inherited either as X-linked or as autosomal recessive traits, and the diagnosis may have important consequences for reproductive choice in other family members and for clarifying unexplained symptoms in at-risk relatives. Increasingly, enzyme-replacement therapy, bone marrow transplantation, or even substrate-reduction therapies may be available for their definitive treatment. Furthermore, several disorders respond well to palliative measures including renal transplantation and hepatic transplantation. Finally, a great deal of expertise is available from specialist groups with experience of treating these conditions.

Charitable associations now exist in many countries for members to share their experiences and provide advice and counselling. Above all, invaluable information about available medical services for specific conditions can be obtained through patient organizations. The Worldwide Web provides a useful entry into this, often untapped, resource where key information of importance to both patients and their doctors—and other relevant healthcare personnel—can be obtained.

The key to making the diagnosis of a lysosomal disease is enthusiastic and curious suspicion. In most circumstances, once suspected, the diagnosis can be made with relative ease by referral to a specialized regional

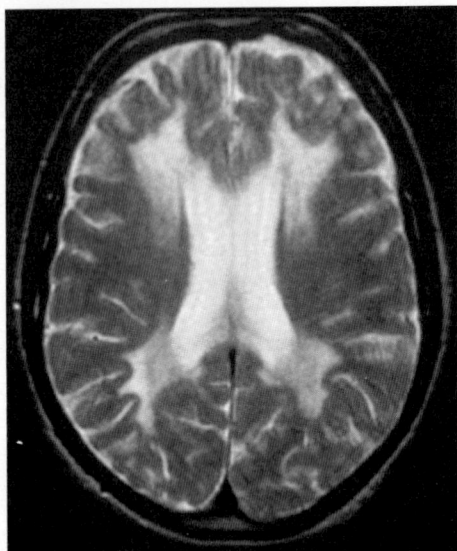

Fig. 2 Magnetic resonance imaging of the brain of a young woman with adult-onset metachromatic leucodystrophy. Notice the high signal intensity especially in the frontal white matter and periventricular regions. This patient presented with bizarre behaviour due to a frontal-type dementia; there are no neurological signs or symptoms. Short-term memory loss and lack of planning and higher executive functions are prominent features of her illness.

reference laboratory for the diagnosis of metabolic disorders; senior laboratory staff will usually advise about the handling of appropriate tissue material for diagnostic studies. In the first instance, simple histochemical stains of existing biopsy material and examination of urine metabolites, including lipids and oligosaccharides, may narrow down the diagnosis. More commonly, specific enzymatic assays are used—generally carried out on leucocytes isolated from fresh heparinized blood samples, or on fibroblasts cultured from small skin biopsies.

Molecular analysis of genes encoding lysosomal enzymes may often support the enzymatic diagnosis, and may, on occasion, provide rough guidance as to the expected phenotype of the disease. DNA-based studies are of particular value for future prenatal diagnosis in a particular pedigree, and for the diagnosis of carrier status in at-risk females for heterozygosity in the X-linked diseases such as Hunter's and Fabry's disease. Lately, there has been a strong and justified trend in favour of specific enzymatic and genetic diagnoses, rather than for diagnoses based on the examination of biopsy material by light microscopy with or without the additional use of special histochemical stains. However, electron microscopy of biopsy material may be of particular value in recognizing the type of disorder but it is rarely essential for a specific diagnosis. Hitherto, histochemical and histopathological methods have led to diagnostic inaccuracies, but it must be admitted that many cases of lysosomal disease, particularly as they affect adults, have come to light as a result in the past of bone marrow examinations, liver biopsies, and other procedures carried out in an attempt to arrive at a diagnosis in an otherwise puzzling condition.

Fabry's disease, Niemann–Pick disease type B and C, as well as Gaucher's disease, have often been diagnosed as a result in young or adult patients who have presented with particular symptoms. General physicians, haematologists, nephrologists, neurologists, gastroenterologists and hepatologists, dermatologists, and even orthopaedic surgeons may be the first to evaluate the patient—all of whom identify the condition by following diagnostic pathways appropriate to their specialty. In any event, the diagnosis of lysosomal storage diseases is rarely difficult, provided the expertise of a trusted laboratory service is available for performing biochemical assays, diagnostic DNA studies, and wide-ranging histopathological examination. The value of good communications between laboratory staff and clinical

investigators to whom these patients are referred cannot be overestimated.

Specific lysosomal diseases

Gaucher's disease

This disorder may occur at any age and is the most frequent of the lysosomal storage diseases. The condition is usually due to a catalytic deficiency of glucocerebrosidase, although rare cases of deficiency of its cognate sphingolipid activator protein (**SAP-C**) may cause a severe disease intermediate between Gaucher's disease and metachromatic leucodystrophy. Numerous mutations responsible for the enzymatic deficiency have been identified in the human glucocerebrosidase gene and the reader is referred to the specialist literature for those genotype/phenotype correlations that broadly apply to this protean disorder.

Rarely, infants are born with an almost complete lack of glucocerebrosidase activity: they die within a few days of birth or are stillborn due to skeletal deformities and/or dehydration as a result of loss of skin integrity (collodion babies). Infantile Gaucher's disease is a rare condition that is associated with death in the first 2 years of life: there is neuronopathic disease with bulbar palsy, opisthotonus, and minor visceral enlargement. This disease is invariably fatal and does not respond to either systemic or intrathecal enzyme-replacement therapy. While neurological disease may occur in children, adolescents, and young adults with Gaucher's disease, it is less severe than in the infantile variant. This clinical variant is associated with supranuclear gaze palsies, myoclonus, ataxia, and, occasionally, seizures. The neurological condition usually deteriorates slowly but is exacerbated if splenectomy is performed for the accompanying splenomegaly and associated pancytopenia.

Where possible, and with vigorous enzyme therapy, splenectomy is best avoided—a partial splenectomy may be carried out to ameliorate pressure effects and life-threatening thrombocytopenia. Subacute neuronopathic disease is not always fatal and often improves with combined bone marrow transplantation and enzyme-replacement therapy (see below). Affected children may show striking visceromegaly, with the associated gaze palsies often playing a small part in the clinical presentation. Although juvenile ('neuronopathic') Gaucher's disease (type III) occurs sporadically in all populations, there is a small isolate in Northern Sweden where all individuals are homozygous for a single point mutation in the glucocerebrosidase gene (*L444P*) that has arisen by descent from a common ancestor.

The most frequent form of Gaucher's disease is the so-called 'adult nonneuronopathic form' (type I). This disease is found in all populations, but is over-represented in Jews of Ashkenazi origin. Although the condition does not affect the nervous system, visceral and skeletal manifestations are prominent. The pathognomic abnormality is the presence of large storage cells, which are activated macrophages (Gaucher's cells), typically found in the splenic sinusoids. The Gaucher's cells (Figs 3, 4, and Plate 2) replace the Kupffer cells of the liver, alveolar macrophages of the lung and in the bone marrow.

Characteristically, Gaucher's disease presents with pancytopenia, with bleeding due to thrombocytopenia and splenic enlargement. Acutely painful episodes also occur in the bones, particularly during growth; these episodes are followed by avascular necrosis of the bone with consequential effects on the integrity of large joints, including the hip, knee, and shoulder (Fig. 5). In the era before enzyme-replacement therapy, splenectomy was often carried out during childhood to relieve the pressure effects of the enlarged organ and to ameliorate the effects of accompanying cytopenias. Although there appears to be an association between splenectomy and the development of severe bone disease, it is unclear as to whether this is directly due to the effects of the splenectomy or the consequential manifestations of disease severity. For this reason, splenectomy is avoided where at all possible. Splenectomy in Gaucher's disease carries a greatly enhanced risk of overwhelming infection; this includes infection with protozoa, such

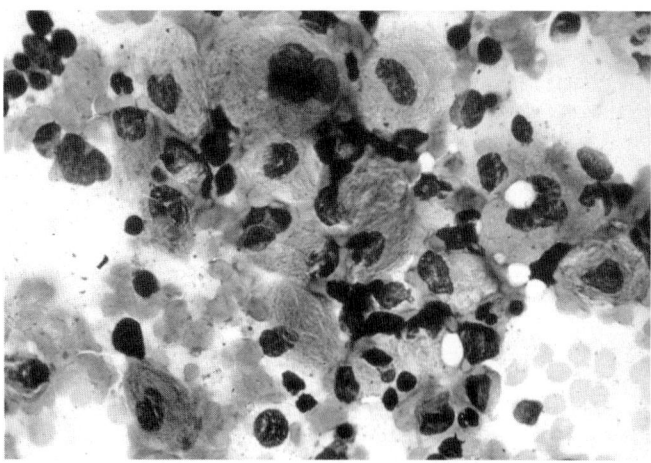

Fig. 3 Light micrograph of a Leishmann-stained bone marrow biopsy obtained from a 23-year-old man with type 1 Gaucher's disease. Note that the large, pale-blue staining Gaucher's cells with striated cytoplasm replace the Kupffer cells of the liver, alveolar macrophages of the lung and of the bone marrow. (See also Plate 2.)

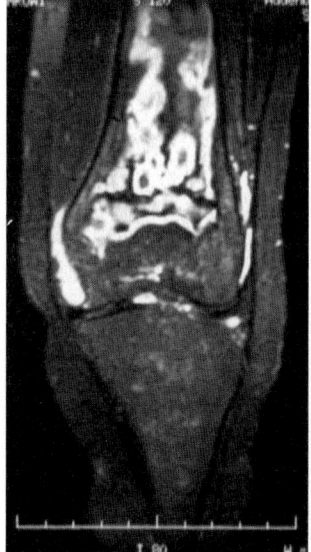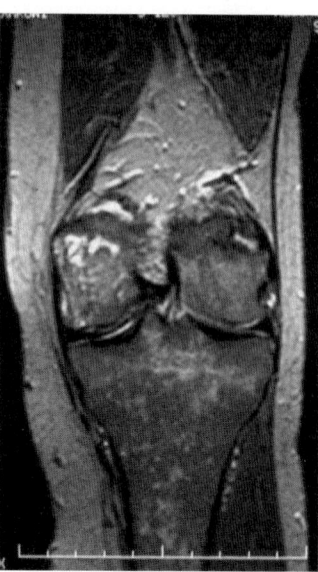

Fig. 5 T_1 (left)- and T_2 (right)-weighted magnetic resonance images obtained from the lower femur and upper tibia of a 30-year-old woman with non-neuronopathic Gaucher's disease experiencing pain due to acute avascular necrosis of bone. Note the geographical areas of increased signal intensity on the T_2-weighted image due to increased tissue water representing oedema surrounding the necrotic tissue. (By courtesy of Professor D. Lomas, Addenbrooke's Hospital.)

as babesia and malaria, as well as capsulated bacteria, for example the pneumococcus, *Haemophilus influenzae*, and *Neisseria meningitidis*.

Painful episodes may occur in patients with Gaucher's disease either due to infarction of the liver and spleen or to the so-called 'bone crises'. These latter episodes represent acute bone necrosis due to infarction. The increased frequency of infarction events is an important aspect of Gaucher's disease that, as yet, has not been explained. Bone necrosis remains an aspect of the condition that often persists despite enzyme therapy and presents a significant challenge for clinical research.

Gaucher's disease is a truly multisystem disorder, which is accompanied by many ill-understood plasma and metabolic abnormalities. These include a polyclonal immunoglobulin response that may progress to monoclonal gammopathy, amyloidosis, or even frank myeloma. Low-density lipoprotein (LDL) and high-density lipoprotein (**HDL**) cholesterol fractions are abnormal in the plasma. Some lysosomal enzymes are elevated, including tartrate-resistant acid phosphatase, hexosaminidase, and a human chitinase, chitotriosidase. This latter enzyme has proved to be very useful for monitoring Gaucher's disease activity in response to treatment, and may reflect the severity of the disease. The enzyme is elevated sometimes several hundred-fold above normal in untreated Gaucher's disease.

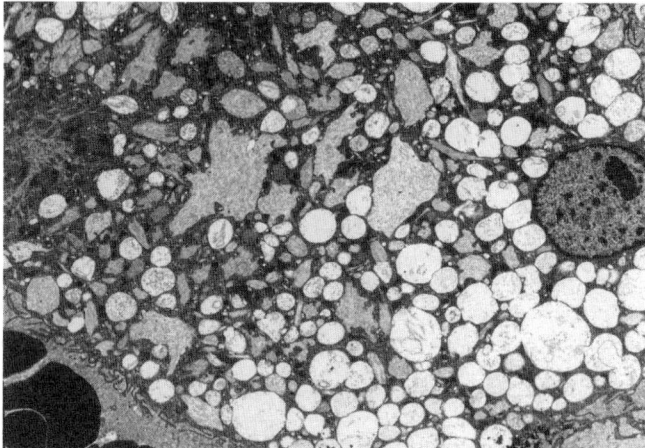

Fig. 4 Electron micrograph showing the cytoplasm of a Gaucher's cell in the spleen of a 56-year-old man removed because of life-threatening thrombocytopenia and pain due to a recent splenic infarct. Note the vesicular spaces filled with fibrillary glycolipid storage material.

Gaucher's disease may rarely be associated with pulmonary infiltrates, including reticulonodular opacities, restrictive lung defects, and various abnormalities of the pulmonary circulation causing pulmonary hypertension. The hepatopulmonary syndrome, accompanied by platypnoea and associated with severe scarring liver disease or cirrhosis and portal venous hypertension, has also been reported in severely affected adults. The osseous manifestations of Gaucher's disease are very diverse and include the presence of expanded bone lesions (Fig. 6) with surrounding cortical thinning related to Gaucher's cell infiltrates within the bone marrow ('Gauchomas'). Diffuse osteoporosis accompanied by pathological fractures may also compound the skeletal manifestations of Gaucher's disease. Kyphoscoliotic deformity due to crush fractures and vertebral avascular necrosis are common in untreated adults, particularly in postmenopausal women.

In its untreated state, Gaucher's disease is a miserable condition leading to progressive skeletal deformity, pancytopenia, and visceral enlargement with failing organ function punctuated by painful visceral bone crises. The mean age of death in a single large series reported from Pittsburgh, Pennsylvania, was 60 years during the pretreatment era but this does not take into account the poor quality of life of most affected individuals. Some homozygotes for 'mild' missense mutations in the glucocerebrosidase gene (especially the widespread mutation, N370S) may escape detection and remain asymptomatic throughout a long adult life. Detailed investigation reveals only a mild thrombocytopenia and trivial splenomegaly in some cases. However, monoclonal gammopathy is frequently present after the age of 45 years. It is uncertain as to what extent the presence of such mutations in the population at large (homozygosity for N370S occurs in about 1 in 960 Ashkenazi Jews) contributes to the development of B-cell lymphoproliferative disorders, such as B-cell lymphoma and myeloma, in this at-risk group.

The diagnosis of Gaucher's disease is based on white-cell acid β-glucosidase activity, which may be accompanied by the elevation of one or more related marker enzymes such as chitotriosidase or tartrate-resistant acid phosphatase in the serum. Spleen tissue, liver biopsy material, or bone marrow aspirates may show the characteristic oligonucleate storage cells demonstrating striated cytoplasm on Leishmann staining (see Fig. 3), but which appear as pink sheets in tissue sections stained with haematoxylin and eosin. Molecular analysis of the glucocerebrosidase gene may identify widespread mutant glucocerebrosidase alleles that cause this disease and may assist in the diagnosis and investigation of family members at risk for this recessive disorder.

Treatment

Until recently, the treatment for Gaucher's disease was palliative. Bone marrow transplantation has been undertaken in a few infants and children with rapidly progressive disease, including those with the subacute neuronopathic form type III. When successful, this may correct most of the systemic manifestations of the condition and restore growth. It may arrest further neurological deterioration. However, bone marrow transplantation is no longer in routine use because of the accompanying severe risk resulting from the procedures and constraints in the supply of donors, especially MHC-matched, first-degree relatives.

Enzyme-replacement therapy was introduced during the early 1990s in the form of a natural product extracted from the human placenta, alglucerase, 'Ceredase'. A recombinant glycoform, imiglucerase, 'Cerezyme', is now available that, like alglucerase, is modified to reveal terminal mannose residues. The recombinant protein is supplied as a lyophilized powder which is reconstituted for intravenous infusion; the preparation is given at variable frequencies, from three times a week to once every 2 weeks, and infused over approximately 60 min. Modification of the sugar residues on this protein facilitates targeting to macrophage-containing organs, in which it complements the enzyme deficiency in the pathological storage cells. After a few weeks of enzyme administration, most patients show an improvement in the blood parameters of disease activity and a reduction of the chronic

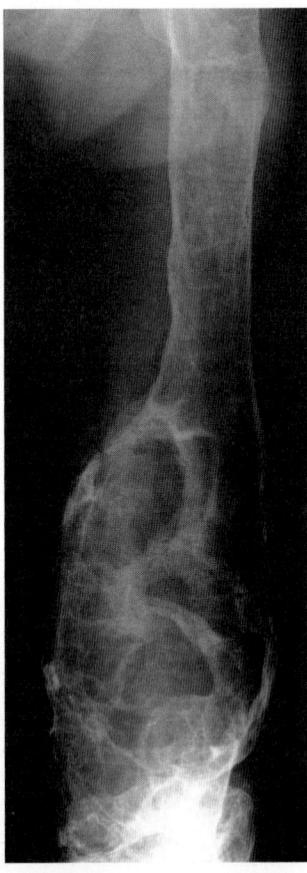

Fig. 6 Expanded lytic lesion at the distal end of the femur in a 44-year-old woman with severe Gaucher's disease complicated by osteoporosis, avascular necrosis, and, as shown, expansile lytic lesions in long bones leading to local infiltration of the marrow space by Gaucher's tissue.

inflammatory response that accompanies Gaucher's disease: the platelet count rises; and there is a correction of the hypersplenic picture, with a reduction in hepatosplenomegaly and an improvement in the asthenia that complicates Gaucher's disease. Quality-of-life measures also show clear improvement.

Controversy remains as to the appropriate dose of imiglucerase; however, most authorities agree that the administration of the enzyme should be a lifelong therapy. There are two schools of thought as to whether enzyme therapy should be administered at a high dose to start with and then reduced as evidence of disease regression becomes clear, or whether a stepwise increase in this expensive agent can be undertaken in patients with long-standing disease until evidence of disease regression can be established. Disease activity is assessed by objective parameters, including visceral enlargement, and by determination of surrogate biomarkers such as chitotriosidase and blood counts. At present, there is no agreed protocol for therapy in adults with Gaucher's disease; but in patients with the subacute neuronopathic form of the condition, international guidelines suggest that a dose of at least 120 units of enzyme per kilogram bodyweight per month is necessary to secure disease regression.

Although it would not be expected that enzyme-replacement therapy would improve the neuronopathic aspects of Gaucher's disease, there is emerging evidence that clinical improvement may be induced by enzyme-replacement therapy given at this high dosage. Enzyme-replacement therapy for Gaucher's disease is very expensive and the doses recommended range from below 5 to at least 60 IU/kg per month. Thus for an adult, this may cost as much as £200 000 per year, so placing enormous demands on healthcare provision in the long-term. In response to these pressures, there have been initiatives to develop alternative methods to treat the condition—including the use of an oral agent that inhibits the formation of the substrate delivered to macrophages. When taken for several months, the trial agent, N-butyldeoxynojirimycin reduces glycolipid storage and clinical as well as laboratory parameters of Gaucher's disease activity.

Enzyme-replacement therapy, although very expensive, is a successful treatment for Gaucher's disease, and, since most patients do express the protein antigen endogenously, hypersensitivity and immune reactions are very rare. Apart from the inconvenience of periodic intravenous infusions, treatment is well tolerated and many patients in Europe and the United Kingdom choose to take their treatment as self-administered infusions at home. In relation to treatment with iminosugars, short-duration unwanted effects (including diarrhoea due to inhibition of intestinal disaccharidases) are frequent, although they usually respond well to dietary adjustments. However, at the time of writing it is unclear as to whether or not N-butyldeoxynojirimycin will be licensed as an Orphan drug, although clearly there is an international demand for a more readily available treatment for Gaucher's disease. The occurrence of peripheral neuropathy after long-term administration in a few patients with non-neuronopathic Gaucher's disease may indicate a neurotoxicity, and restrict the indications for use of N-butyl deoxynojirimycin. Substrate-reduction therapy may, however, have wider applications in the treatment of certain sphingolipidoses, including late-onset Tay–Sachs disease, GM1 gangliosidosis, and Niemann–Pick disease type C, which affect the brain and for which no other therapy is currently available. Moreover, since the iminosugars may penetrate the brain and are orally active, they may also be of value as an adjunctive therapy in type III Gaucher's disease. Several agents of this class have been found to be effective in animal models of glycosphingolipidoses and successors to N-butyl deoxynojirimycin are actively undergoing preclinical study.

Treatment for Gaucher's disease should include appropriate immunization and antimicrobial prophylaxis in patients who have undergone splenectomy. The widespread osseous manifestations, including osteoporosis, may respond to therapy with bisphosphonate drugs, including pamidronate. Patients may require joint-replacement surgery to ameliorate the effects of bone infarction crises and, in rare instances, liver transplantation for endstage liver disease. Bone marrow transplantation probably does not have a role today, except in rare circumstances. Evidence of metabolic bone disease complicating the disorder should be always sought and osteoporosis should be treated promptly with hormone-replacement therapy, with the additional consideration of oral active or parenteral bisphosphonates. Where present, a deficiency of 25-hydroxyvitamin D should probably be treated with appropriate supplements. Because of the increased risk of infection due to intrinsic chemotactic and phagocytic defects as well as splenectomy, patients with Gaucher's disease undergoing surgery or with systemic infection should be promptly treated—preferably with parenteral antimicrobial agents.

Niemann–Pick disease

Niemann–Pick disease A and B are, respectively, neuronopathic and non-neuronopathic variants of acid sphingomyelinase deficiency, a sphingolipid disorder leading to the accumulation of sphingomyelin. Niemann–Pick disease resembles many of the manifestations of Gaucher's disease with a characteristic secondary storage cell which is also a macrophage. The Niemann–Pick cell has a foamy appearance rather than the characteristic striated cytoplasm of the Gaucher's cell. In Niemann–Pick disease, there is prominent infiltration of the lungs as well as the marrow cavity. At present, no specific treatments are available, apart from the prompt treatment of pulmonary infection and the management of the consequences of skeletal infiltrates and episodes of avascular necrosis. Some patients, including those previously misdiagnosed as having Gaucher's disease, may have undergone splenectomy to relieve pressure symptoms or the haematological effects of hypersplenism.

Niemann–Pick disease type A is associated with disabling neuronopathic features and dementia. At the present time no specific therapy for it exists. Niemann–Pick disease type B may occur in adults who have only trivial splenomegaly and minor pulmonary infiltrates that are only exacerbated at times of intercurrent pneumonic infection; they are at risk from osseous disease related to marrow infiltration, as with Gaucher's disease. Since this disease is primarily a disorder of macrophages, it should be susceptible to enzymatic complementation using the mannose receptor. At the time of writing, clinical research to develop macrophage-targeted, recombinant, human acid sphingomyelinase is well advanced. Unfortunately, no imino-sugar derivatives are available for substrate-reduction therapy for the neuronopathic manifestations of Niemann–Pick disease type A, since the biosynthesis of sphingomyelin is not regulated by the uridine diphosphate-glucosylceramide synthase reaction.

Niemann–Pick disease type C (NPC) may present with jaundice in infants or children, but the initial hepatitic illness usually resolves. Later evidence of neuronopathic disease occurs, with ataxia, seizures, supranuclear palsy, and progressive diffuse cortical injury. NPC is not due to a primary defect of acid sphingomyelinase but to mutations in two distinct lysosomal membrane proteins. These are responsible for the NPC-1 and NPC-2 subtypes of disease. Although the function of the NPC-1 and NPC-2 proteins is not fully understood, they are implicated in the intracellular transport of cholesterol and cholesterol esters to and from the lysosomal compartment. NPC is also associated with the appearance of foam cells in the macrophages; the Kupffer cells of the liver may be enlarged and a cholesterol trafficking defect is apparent in most cells. Thus the defect, though not manifest in the skin, may be detected in skin and fibroblasts after culture and exposure to low-density lipoprotein-cholesterol: in NPC, cholesterol is taken up and accumulates in intracellular droplets that stain positively with the fluorescent dye filipin. Within the brain, NPC causes neuronophagia and the accumulation of gangliosides and other complex sphingolipid storage products that may induce neuronal injury. Clinical trials are under way with the use of the iminosugar *N*-butyldeoxynojirimycin. These trials follow on from the successful arrest of the disease in mice homozygous for a spontaneous mutation in the *NPC-1* gene that provide a convincing model of the human disease. The outcome of further investigations of these mice and of the trial of this therapy in patients with NPC is urgently awaited. Niemann–Pick disease type C is an intractable condition associated with progressive neurological disease in

childhood and early adult life. Biological deterioration progresses inexorably and death usually occurs in the third or fourth decade. The use of statins and other agents that interfere with cholesterol metabolism has not been effective in arresting the course of this cruel illness.

Anderson–Fabry disease (usually shortened to Fabry's disease)

This disease is an X-linked disorder, unlike many of the lysosomal diseases, apart from Hunter's disease (MPS II). An unusual feature of Fabry's disease, is the presence of clinical signs and symptoms in the majority of heterozygous female carriers of the condition. Although these manifestations are usually less severe and of later onset than in affected hemizygous males, florid and life-shortening clinical disease has often been observed (and ignored) in affected women. Deficiency of α-galactosidase causes the accumulation of ceramidetrihexoside (otherwise known as globotriaosylceramide), which principally derives from the breakdown of lipids present in senescent red cells. Affected male hemizygotes have small, raised, red vascular skin lesions (angiokeratomas) particularly around the buttocks and genital region. These lesions are often detected in limited areas of affected heterozygous females and reflect X-chromosome inactivation patterns in the skin. With increasing age, impaired capillary circulation and progressive tubular, interstitial, and glomerular disease in the kidney leads to proteinuria and renal failure. Many patients require renal support, including haemodialysis, peritoneal dialysis, or kidney transplantation. Patients with Fabry's disease have disturbing gastrointestinal symptoms, characterized by diarrhoea shortly after eating and often abdominal pain associated with febrile attacks that are otherwise unexplained.

The most characteristic symptoms of the disease are the onset in early childhood of lancinating pain with background burning sensations in the extremities that are worse with exercise and with extremes of temperature. These attacks can be very disabling and represent neuropathic pain, which is notoriously difficult to control. The acroparasthesias are frequently attributed to Raynaud's phenomenon but this relationship is unclear, although many of the symptoms of Fabry's disease can be explained by neuropathy affecting autonomic nervous tone. Most men with established disease notice a striking absence of peripheral sweating, and impotence is very common. The abdominal symptoms may also result from autonomic neuropathy. High-tone loss of hearing is also a frequent feature of Fabry's disease, which appears to reflect a selective loss of functioning cochlear neurones. Cardiac hypertrophy occurs, especially of the left ventricle, with conduction defects leading to a shortened PR interval and a prolonged QRS complex—later accompanied by tachyarrhythmias and complete heart block. Left ventricular hypertrophy may or may not be associated with hypertension and cardiac embolic disease; disease of capillaries and medium-sized vessels in the brain associated with unusual microvascular changes, particularly in the posterior cerebral circulation, also causes stroke.

Stroke and renal failure are the most common causes of death in patients with Fabry's disease; in men, death occurs at a median age of 48 to 49 years, with a greatly reduced quality of life during the antecedent symptomatic period. Life expectancy in affected heterozygous women is also shortened. Sometimes the lancinating acroparasthesias are sufficient to cause severe depression and even suicide. Disease expression in many carrier females, who may develop renal failure, is accompanied by angiokeratomas restricted to certain dermatomes on careful examination and asymptomatic corneal opacification with whorl-like cataracts on slit-lamp examination.

Diagnosis is made by demonstrating the abnormal glycolipid in urine or plasma, as well as by assay of α-galactosidase in tears, plasma, white cells, or other tissue material. Molecular analysis of the α-galactosidase gene on the long arm of the X chromosome is worthwhile because it allows the unambiguous detection of female heterozygotes and may thus be useful during the reproductive period, particularly for antenatal diagnosis. Despite the presence of active disease, ceramide trihexoside concentrations and α-galactosidase assays are often within normal limits in affected female heterozygotes.

Hitherto, the treatment for Fabry's disease has been palliative, involving the use of anticonvulsants (including gabapentin) for the acroparasthesiae and neuropathic pain. Gastrointestinal symptoms sometimes respond to antimotility agents or to pancreatic enzyme supplements but these agents have not been subjected to control trials. Renal failure is managed by dialysis or by renal transplantation; occasionally, cardiac transplantation has been required for cardiomyopathy; pacemakers and antiarrhythmic drugs may also be needed. There is a rare cardiac variant in this disease, which appears to be predominantly manifested by restrictive cardiomyopathy in elderly patients who have a small amount of residual α-galactosidase activity in their tissues. In one remarkable instance, therapy with galactose infusions appears to have ameliorated this condition by stabilizing the nascent mutant enzyme, thereby enhancing residual α-galactosidase activity with slow clearance of cardiac glycolipid storage.

Recently, enzyme replacement using recombinant human α-galactosidase has been developed as a more definitive treatment. To date, two preparations—which may differ slightly in their post-translational glycosylation status for delivery to endothelial, epithelial, and other cells that represent the pathological focus of this disease—have been licensed: agalsidase-α (Replagal) and agalsidase-β (Fabrazyme). Administration of these preparations to male hemizygotes has improved lipid accumulation in the plasma and in renal biopsy samples from male hemizygotes with this disease. Agalsidase-α has also been shown in double-blind, crossover, placebo-controlled trials to improve clinical endpoints of the disease, including neuropathic pain, stabilization of renal function, and ventricular mass as well as conduction defects that represent infiltrative cardiomyopathy. Further clinical observations continue to be made but it is now clear that enzyme therapy is likely to be a safe and effective long-term treatment for Fabry's disease. Unlike Gaucher's disease, targeting to the affected cells and tissues in Fabry's disease probably results from uptake by the common lysosomal recognition marker, mannose-6 phosphate, as the principal ligand for protein delivery to this organelle.

The glycoproteinoses

These disorders fall into a group of lysosomal diseases associated with impaired degradation of glycoproteins. The most frequent of these disorders include fucosidosis and mannosidosis, which are inherited as autosomal recessive traits. Glycoproteinoses show some of the manifestations of the sphingolipidoses and the mucopolysaccharidoses: they are almost invariably associated with neurological disease and variable systemic manifestations. An unusual clinical feature of these conditions, which are associated with visceral enlargement (particularly hepatomegaly) and mental retardation occurring in childhood, is the appearance of angiokeratomas that are otherwise characteristic of Fabry's disease.

In a few patients, bone marrow transplantation has improved some of the systemic manifestations of mannosidosis and fucosidosis. However, trials of enzyme-replacement therapy have yet to be published beyond the study of experimental models, such as those that occur spontaneously in cattle, dogs, and other large animals. Diagnosis of the glycoproteinoses is usually prompted by the finding of increased excretion of oligosaccharides in the urine and by clinical suspicion of the diagnosis in patients with a multisystem disease that may have an obvious hereditary component. Definitive diagnosis is dependent on enzymatic studies in leucocytes or cultured skin fibroblasts. As with other lysosomal diseases, prenatal diagnosis using cultured amniocytes and chorionic villus cells may be offered by specialized laboratories.

Mucopolysaccharidoses (MPS)

These disorders are caused by a deficiency of lysosomal hydrolases that catalyse the cleavage of complex glycosaminoglycans—macromolecular components of connective tissues including joints, bones, heart, and the major arteries. Clinical manifestations of each of these disorders reflect an individual enzymatic deficiency and the resulting accumulation of mucopolysaccharide derivatives, of which dermatan, keratan, and chondroitin sulphate as well as heparan sulphate are the principal components. In general, the accumulation of the complex substrates that are normally linked to proteins to form proteoglycans is associated with visceral enlargement, as well as bony abnormalities, joint stiffness, corneal clouding, and short stature; the accumulation of heparan sulphate may particularly be associated with the development of brain disease, including thickening of the leptomeninges. Thus hydrocephalus is an often-neglected factor in cerebral impairment that may also be attributed to lysosomal storage affecting neurones of the brain and peripheral ganglia—as well as the retina.

Clinical features and pathology

Typically, these disorders are associated with coarse facial features, bone shortening, and skeletal abnormalities, as well as disturbances of dentition, the gums, and auditory canal. Abnormalities of the tracheobronchial cartilages and upper airways may be associated with respiratory infections. In the heart, the coronary arteries and valves may be infiltrated by glycosaminoglycans, leading to nodular thickening of aortic and mitral valves with clinical evidence of valvular disease malfunction. In some cases, accumulation of glycosaminoglycan occurs in the coronary arteries, which may be occluded. Similar changes may occur in peripheral arteries—particularly those supplying the viscera. In the eye, the basal layers of the cornea show swelling, cytoplasmic vacuolization, and storage granules leading to opacification.

Excess urinary excretion of glycosaminoglycan products, including dermatan sulphate and heparan sulphate, characteristically occur in the mucopolysaccharidoses. This abnormality should immediately prompt further investigations by enzymatic and genetic studies in blood leucocytes and/or fibroblasts obtained from cultured skin-biopsy samples. The inheritance pattern of the mucopolysaccharidoses is typical of autosomal recessive traits—with the exception of Hunter's disease (MPS II, which is due to iduronate sulphatase deficiency) that maps to the X chromosome and, unlike Fabry's disease, is expressed predominantly in boys and men. Female heterozygotes for Hunter's disease only very rarely show evidence of neurological impairment or connective tissue abnormalities.

Treatment of the mucopolysaccharidoses

Palliative treatment is a very important aspect of the management of these diseases, and should include the provision of multidisciplinary support for children and young adults with the accompanying developmental disabilities. Sustained provision for the long-term management of the condition in affected families is desirable.

Surgical procedures

Corneal transplantation may be required to improve vision where retinal degeneration is not dominant. Carpel tunnel syndrome with compression neuropathy of the median nerve is very common in the mucopolysaccharidoses and, when indicated, surgical treatment is often beneficial. Particular care is required in patients with mucopolysaccharidoses such as Hurler's syndrome when surgical procedures under general anaesthetic are required for relief of hydrocephalus, myringotomy, hernia repair, relief of airways obstruction due to laryngeal disease, and corrective spinal or joint surgery. Infiltration of the soft tissues of the upper and lower airways, as well as the heart and cervical spine (which may include subluxation of the atlanto-occipital joint) is associated with high perioperative mortality. Complications thus arise with the administration of a general anaesthetic beyond that of difficulties with endotracheal intubation. In particular, a tracheostomy may be required to avoid life-threatening complications of intubation. An extensive preoperative examination should be conducted when an anaesthetic is required for any procedure, particularly to assess the stability of the atlantoaxial joint, the airway, and the presence of coronary artery disease (that may predispose to perioperative myocardial infarction).

Specific treatment

Bone marrow transplantation using HLA-identical sibling and HLA-matched non-sibling donors has been extensively investigated in the mucopolysaccharidoses. Long-term clinical trials have confirmed the beneficial effects of successful transplantation with reversal of hepatosplenomegaly and obstructive airways disease. In some cases there is improved longevity, with a possible reduction also in the incidence of secondary hydrocephalus. However, at present, transplantation does not cure the condition and is unable to reverse established brain injury and most of the crippling skeletal manifestations of the mucopolysaccharidoses. If it is to be considered, bone marrow transplantation should thus be carried out early in the course of these diseases.

Enzyme-replacement therapy has long been under investigation in MPS I (Hurler's syndrome, Hurler–Scheie syndrome, and Scheie's syndrome), which was one of the first of such disorders to be subjected to intensive laboratory study. Recent studies with recombinant human α-L-iduronidase, given by weekly infusion intravenously, after 1 year clearly show a reduction in lysosomal storage: liver volume decreased; there was an improved rate of growth as well as improvement in the range of joint movements at sites characteristic of connective tissue infiltration in this condition. With a reduction in the storage material in the upper airways, there was also an improvement in episodes of hypoventilation during sleep. After a few weeks of enzyme treatment, urinary glycosaminoglycans abnormalities were corrected. Although a few patients developed serum antibodies, only transient immune reactions, including urticaria, occurred during the infusions. It appears that in patients with this disease, the first to be shown by experiments with fibroblasts *in vitro* to be corrected by enzymatic complementation, treatment with a recombinant human product reduces lysosomal storage and ameliorates several of the important clinical manifestations. Enzyme-replacement therapy is currently under clinical evaluation for patients suffering from MPS II (Hunter's syndrome with iduronate sulphatase deficiency) and MPS VI (Maroteaux–Lamy due to arylsulphatase B deficiency). Favourable responses to enzyme-replacement therapy have also been reported in animal models of related disorders, including the cone head mouse that represents a faithful model of MPS VII (Sly disease), due to deficiency of acid β-glucuronidase.

Although enzyme therapy is in an early clinical phase of application in the mucopolysaccharidoses, there has been a remarkable response from the pharmaceutical industry for the therapeutic development of enzyme-replacement therapy for lysosomal diseases. With the present state of knowledge, bone marrow transplantation seems to be ineffective for many patients with MPS; if it is to be restricted to use before the development of mental decline, the risks associated with the procedure and the need for matched donors to provide competent marrow cells limit its acceptability. Questions still arise of how clinical benefits and an improved quality of life can be best assessed. However, encouraging results showing an improved quality of life, mobility, nutrition, and educational achievements have already been documented in several MPS disorders in response to enzyme therapy—even where pre-existing developmental effects and mental retardation are established. The combined effects of marrow transplantation and enzyme replacement have yet to be systematically evaluated in clinical trials for evidence of therapeutic synergy. At the time of writing, the whole field of the lysosomal diseases such as MPS is attracting much attention as a promising area of clinical and pharmaceutical research. The earlier definition of Orphan diseases 'as those in which treatments offer little or no financial incentive for commercial development' has been abandoned: Orphan diseases are now conveniently defined 'as those which individually affect less than 1 per cent of the population'.

Recently characterized lysosomal diseases

The characterization of lysosomal defects in several ill-understood disorders with diverse clinical manifestations continues to reveal much about the role of the lysosome in cellular functions of significance in medicine and molecular physiology. Several recently studied lysosomal diseases in this category are briefly described here.

Neuronal ceroid lipofuscinoses

The neuronal ceroid lipofuscinoses (**CLN**) represent the most common group of progressive brain diseases that affect children and young adults. Childhood forms of these disorders are inherited as recessive traits and result in a progressive dementia combined with epilepsy, blindness, and an early death. The most familiar form of these diseases was previously known as Batten's disease. Pathological studies of affected patients show the characteristic accumulation of an autofluorescent storage material within neuronal lysosomes and lysosomes in other cells. The storage of this material occurs preferentially in the nervous system and is associated with progressive neuronal death leading to a marked atrophy of the brain; cerebral atrophy is particularly obvious in the early-onset forms of the neuronal lipofuscinoses. Although this complex of neurodegenerative conditions associated with lipofuscin pigments has long been recognized, the diseases were previously thought to represent disorders of other organelles. Mitochondria were implicated because degraded fragments of mitochondrial cytochrome C polypeptide were found to be one of the prominent storage molecules in neuronal tissue from patients with Batten's disease. Latterly, advances in molecular genetics have allowed the identification of defective genes and their protein products in several distinct clinical phenotypes of the neuronal ceroid lipofuscinoses.

Typical clinical forms of the neuronal ceroid lipofuscinoses include late infantile and juvenile neurodegenerative disorders; at least eight genetic loci, which encode proteins implicated in different aspects of lysosomal metabolism, have been assigned to distinct CLN phenotypes. Neuronal ceroid lipofuscinosis type I (CLN 1) is due to mutations in a gene encoding palmitoyl: protein thioesterase 1. CLN 2 is due to defects in the gene encoding tripeptidyl-peptidase, and CLN 8 is due to defects in the gene encoding human cathepsin D. To date, two lysosomal proteins of membrane location, CLN 4 and CLN 5, have also been identified. No specific therapy for Batten's disease yet exists, but the discovery of the basis of the condition and the genes involved allows for prenatal and postnatal diagnosis in affected pedigrees by molecular analysis of the implicated cognate genes. In most instances, neuronal ceroid lipofuscinoses represents defects in elements of intralysosomal protein catabolism, indicating that the turnover of the cognate proteins is very high in cortical neurones. Very recent *in vitro* studies have suggested that the use of the thiol agent, cysteamine, which is used with benefit in patients with cystinosis, may activate residual palmitoyl-protein phytoesterase activity in patients with ceroid lipofuscinosis type 1.

The realization that the neuronal ceroid lipofuscinoses in fact represent intrinsic disorders of lysosomal protein metabolism is very recent. The discovery clearly has important consequences for understanding the pathology of this family of diseases and for developing better diagnostic tools (especially for prenatal application) as well as new treatments.

Papillon–Lefèvre syndrome

This is an unusual syndrome resulting in periodontal disease with tooth loss and palmoplantar keratosis. Papillon–Lefèvre syndrome is associated with a selective deficiency of cathepsin C activity within the specific granules of neutrophilic polymorphonuclear leucocytes. It appears that the enzyme deficiency leads to the failure of bacterial clearance in the gums, thereby causing destructive periodontitis and tooth loss. The corresponding role of cathepsin C within the dermal epithelium is not known, but a failure of cathepsin C activity reproducibly leads to epithelial abnormalities and thickening of the skin, particularly on the soles of the feet. Papillon–Lefèvre syndrome is inherited as an autosomal recessive trait and several mutations have been identified within the gene encoding the cathepsin C polypeptide. Some patients with disabling skin manifestations have obtained benefit with the use of retinoids. These agents are, however, unlikely to improve early-onset destructive periodontal disease.

The importance of the Papillon–Lefèvre syndrome rests not only on the identification of lysosomal cathepsin C as an important component of immune defences against bacteria that specifically invade the privileged periodontal site, but also on the involvement of this enzyme in the normal turnover of keratinized skin. The molecular characterization of this disorder illustrates the protean manifestations of lysosomal defects and of the ubiquitous importance of lysosomes in the destruction and recycling of exogenous microbial, as well as endogenous cellular components.

Defects of organellar assembly: Chediak–Higashi (CHS) and Hermansky–Pudlak (HPS) syndromes

These rare disorders are inherited as autosomal recessive traits. Both cause oculocutaneous albinism in association with abnormal platelet granules and melanosomes in the skin and eyes. CHS predisposes to microbial infection and there are giant lysosomal granules in peripheral blood granulocytes; ceroid storage occurs in the nervous system and lungs. Although very rare, HPS occurs at a high frequency in the Swiss Alps and the Puerto-Rican population where it is the most common single gene defect. HPS causes a mild bleeding diathesis and platelet dense bodies are absent. Granulomatous colitis occurs and pulmonary changes lead to interstitial lung fibrosis; unexplained cardiomyopathy has been reported.

The Hermansky–Pudlak syndrome is caused by mutations in the adaptin, β-3A gene which is associated with altered trafficking of lysosomal proteins in melanosomes, lysosomes, and platelet-dense granules leading to storage pool deficiency. The gene maps to chromosome 10q. Chediak–Higashi syndrome has a clinical phenotype with a complex set of immune defects affecting natural killer cells and neutrophic leucocytes. Recurrent cutaneous and systemic pyogenic infections occur with defective neutrophil and monocyte migration; natural killer-cell cytotoxicity is absent. Neutrophils, melanocytes, neurones, muscle cells, and Schwann cells show giant inclusion bodies. Neurodegeneration is a prominent feature of the disease in young adults, but death often results from a rapidly progressive lymphoproliferative disorder. CHS is caused by mutations in the lysosomal trafficking regulator gene located on chromosome 1q44.

There are clear similarities between HPS and CHS, and further functional studies of their respective cognate proteins should reveal important information about the synthesis and assembly of lysosomes and related organelles.

Defects of lysosomal membrane function

In 1981 two cases of cardiomyopathy in male infants with skeletal myopathy and mental retardation were reported by Danon and colleagues. The skeletal pathology sugguested type II glycogenosis but no deficiency of acid maltase activity was present. Defects in LAMP–2, a major lysosomal membrane protein, have subsequently been identified in Danon's disease due to mutations in the gene encoding LAMP–2, located on the X-chromosome. The disease is responsible for rare forms of cardiomyopathy in adults and may also occur in heterozygous females.

Pycnodysostosis

Pycnodysostosis is a unique disorder of the skeleton caused by an inherited deficiency of another lysosomal-type acid hydrolase, cathepsin K. Cathepsin K is expressed prominently in osteoclasts, in which it is the most abundant secreted protein.

The clinical features of pycnodysostosis includes skull deformity, bone fragility with short stature, and mild osteopetrosis. Delayed fusion of the membrane bones of the skull leads to persistence of the anterior fontanelle; modelling deformities occur with micrognathia, as well as disordered eruption of the primary and secondary teeth. The dwarfed artist, Henri Toulouse-Lautrec—the product of a highly consanguineous marriage—exhibited many features of pycnodysostosis and was disabled by multiple pathological fractures that typically complicate the dense osteopetrotic bones.

A characteristic radiological feature of this disorder is the presence of short, resorbed terminal phalanges with shortened fingers; acro-osteolysis also occurs at the acromial end of the clavicle. Histological examination of affected bone reveals abnormal osteoclasts containing undigested type I collagen fragments within vacuolar spaces. Linkage studies mapped pycnodystostosis to the long arm of chromosome 1 in the same region on 1q21 as cathepsin K: multiple mutations in the cathepsin K gene have now been shown to segregate with the disease in affected pedigrees.

Thus cathepsin K, a cysteine-proteinase expressed in the lysosomes of the pathological macrophages in Gaucher's disease, is particularly abundant in the secretory products of the subosteoclastic resorptive vacuole and is critical for bone modelling and development. Defective digestion of the principal collagen in bone leads to a diffuse skeletal phenotype with clear applications for furthering our knowledge of bone physiology: at least one pharmaceutical company is currently exploring this system as a therapeutic target in osteoporosis.

Further reading

A key reference source for these and other inherited disorders is Victor McKusick's *Mendelian inheritance in man*, published by The Johns Hopkins University Press, Baltimore, MD. This catalogue of human autosomal, X-linked, and mitochondrial phenotypes contains invaluable information that is continually updated in the online version (OMIM) available through the worldwide web at: http://www.ncbi.nlm.nih.gov/htbit-post/omim

Detailed descriptions of all aspects of individual disorders are provided in the acclaimed reference book: *The metabolic and molecular bases of inherited disease*, 8th edition (2001), edited by CR Scriver, AL Beaudet, WS Sly, and D Valle, and published by McGraw-Hill, New York. The lysosomal diseases are principally described in Part 16, pp 3371–894 in the third volume of this large, four-volume work.

Additional references of relevance to particular disorders and new aspects of treatment include:

Amalfitano A, *et al.* (2001). Recombinant human acid alpha-glucosidase enzyme therapy for infantile glycogen storage disease type II: results of a phase I/II clinical trial. *Genetics in Medicine* 3, 132–8.

Barton NW, *et al.* (1991). Replacement therapy for inherited enzyme deficiency: macrophage-targeted glucocerebrosidase for Gaucher's disease. *New England Journal of Medicine* 324, 1464–70.

Cox T, *et al.* (2000). Novel oral treatment of Gaucher's disease with *N*-butyl deoxynojirimycin (OGT 918) to decrease substrate biosynthesis. *Lancet* 355, 1481–5.

Cox TM (2001). Gaucher's disease: understanding the molecular pathogenesis of sphingolipidosis. *Journal of Inherited Metabolic Diseases* 24(Suppl 2), 106–21.

Frustaci A, *et al.* (2001). Improvement in cardiac function in the cardiac variant of Fabry's disease with galactose-infusion therapy. *New England Journal of Medicine* 345, 25–32.

Gahl WA, Thoene JG, Scheider JA (2001). Cystinosis: a disorder of lysosomal membrane transport. In: Scriver CR, *et al.*, eds. *Metabolic and molecular bases of inherited disease*, 8th edn, vol III, pp 5085–108. McGraw-Hill, New York.

Gelb BD, *et al.* (1996). Pyknodysostosis, a lysosomal disease caused by cathepsin K deficiency. *Science* 273, 1236–8.

Kakkis ED, *et al.* (2001). Enzyme replacement therapy in mucopolysaccharidosis I. *New England Journal of Medicine* 344, 182–8.

MacDermot KD, Holmes A, Miners AH (2001). Anderson–Fabry disease: clinical manifestations and impact of disease in a cohort of 98 hemizygous males. *Journal of Medical Genetics* 38, 750–60.

MacDermot KD, Holmes A, Miners AH (2001). Anderson–Fabry disease: chemical manifestations and impact of disease in a cohort of 60 obligate carrier females. *Journal of Medical Genetics* 38, 769–807.

Peters C, *et al.* (1998). Hurler's syndrome II. Outcome of HLA-genotypically identical and HLA-haploidentical related donor bone marrow transplantation in fifty-four children. *Blood* **91**, 2601–8.

Schiffman R, *et al.* (2001). Enzyme-replacement therapy in Fabry disease: a randomized control trial. *Journal of the American Medical Association* **285**, 2743–9.

Spritz RA (1999) Multi-organellar disorders of pigmentation: tied up in traffic. *Clinical Genetics* **55**, 309–17.

Toomes C, *et al.* (1999). Loss-of-function mutations in the cathepsin C gene result in periodontal disease and palmoplantar keratosis. *Nature Genetics* **23**, 421–4.

Whitley CB (1993). The mucopolysaccharidoses. In: Beighton P, ed. *McKusick's heritable disorders of connective tissue*, 5th edn, pp 367–499. Mosby Year Book, Inc, St Louis, MO.

Zimran A, ed. (1997). Gaucher's disease. *Clinical haematology*, pp 621–846. Baillière Tindall, London.

11.9 Peroxisomal diseases

Ronald J. A. Wanders and Ruud B. H. Schutgens

Introduction

The peroxisomal disorders are relative newcomers to the field of inherited diseases in humans. The reason for this is that peroxisomes were the last true subcellular organelles to be discovered and were long thought to play only a minor role in cellular metabolism. Two key observations in patients suffering from a rare disease, the cerebrohepatorenal syndrome of Zellweger, changed this view completely.

A major hallmark in studies of Zellweger syndrome was the finding by Goldfischer and colleagues in 1973 that peroxisomes were completely absent in the hepatocytes and renal tubule cells of Zellweger patients. In 1982 the accumulation of certain saturated very long-chain fatty acids, notably hexacosanoic (cerotic) acid (C26:0), was reported in plasma from Zellweger patients whereas other fatty acids like palmitate, oleate, and linoleate were normal. At the same time our group reported that plasmalogens, a specific type of phospholipid, were deficient in tissues and erythrocytes from Zellweger patients. Subsequent studies soon resolved that these abnormalities were a direct consequence of the absence of peroxisomes in these patients.

Since then much has happened and it is now clear that Zellweger syndrome is the prototype of an expanding group of genetic diseases all caused by an impairment in one or more peroxisomal functions.

To provide the necessary background we will briefly describe the main functions of peroxisomes in humans as well as their biogenesis.

Functions of peroxisomes

Peroxisomes play an essential role in a range of cellular activities, which mainly have to do with lipid metabolism (see Table 1). The following functions are essential and are directly linked to certain peroxisomal disorders.

β-Oxidation of fatty acids and fatty acid derivatives

Just like mitochondria, peroxisomes are capable of oxidizing fatty acids by both α- and β-oxidation. The mechanism whereby fatty acids are β-oxidized in peroxisomes is the same as in mitochondria, involving four sequential steps of oxidation, hydration, dehydrogenation, and thiolytic cleavage.

Table 1 Functions of peroxisomes in humans

Ether-phospholid biosynthesis
Fatty acid β-oxidation
Fatty acid α-oxidation
Glyoxylate detoxification
Biosynthesis of cholesterol and dolichol
Pipecolic acid degradation
Biosynthesis of docosahaxaenoic acid
Hydrogen peroxide metabolism
Amino acid metabolism

It is well established now that there are major differences between the mitochondrial and peroxisomal β-oxidation systems, each catalysing the oxidation of a distinct set of substrates. Indeed, mitochondria take care of the oxidation of the vast majority of dietary fatty acids including oleate, palmitate, and linoleate whereas peroxisomes catalyse the β-oxidation of a range of fatty acids which are not so important for energy purposes but which do require breakdown.

These include (see Fig. 1):

1. Very long-chain fatty acids: fatty acids like tetracosanoic (lignoceric) acid (C24:0) and hexacosanoic (cerotic) acid (C26:0) cannot be β-oxidized by mitochondria but are good substrates for peroxisomal β-oxidation. Peroxisomes are not capable of fully degrading C26:0 and

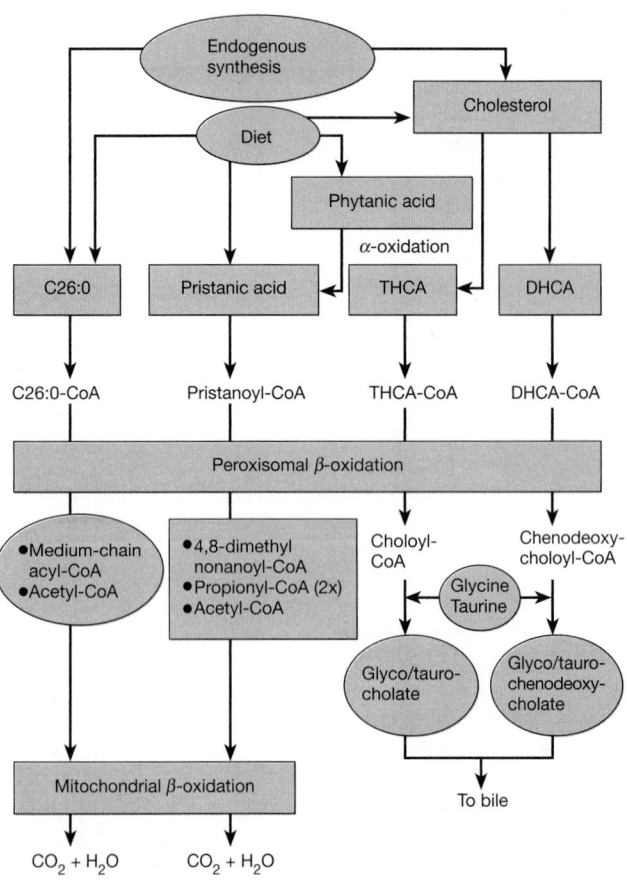

Fig. 1 Involvement of peroxisomes and mitochondria in the β-oxidation of hexacosanoic acid (C26:0), pristanic acid, and di- and trihydroxycholestanoic acid. See text for details.

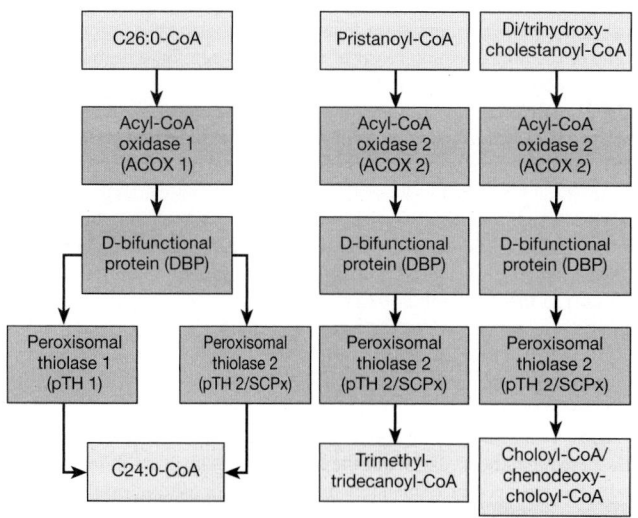

Fig. 2 Enzymology of the peroxisomal fatty acid β-oxidation machinery. See text for details.

C24:0 to acetyl coenzyme A (**CoA**) units. Instead only a few cycles occur in peroxisomes after which the chain-shortened acyl CoA units move to the mitochondria for further oxidation.

2. Pristanic acid (2,6,10,14-tetramethylpentadecanoic acid): this branched-chain fatty acid is in part derived directly from dietary sources but is also formed from phytanic acid by a process called α-oxidation (see later). Pristanic acid undergoes three cycles of β-oxidation in the peroxisome to produce 4,8-dimethylnonanoyl-CoA which is then transported to the mitochondrion for full oxidation to CO_2 and H_2O (Fig. 1).

3. Di- and trihydroxycholestanoic acid: the CoA esters of di- and trihydroxycholestanoic acid undergo one cycle of β-oxidation in the peroxisome, giving rise to the CoA esters of chenodeoxycholic acid and cholic acid respectively, which are then converted into the corresponding taurine or glycine conjugates (tauro/glycochenodeoxycholate and tauro/glycocholate respectively). This is followed by transport into bile. This implies that peroxisomes play an indispensable role in bile acid formation.

It is now clear that peroxisomes contain multiple enzymes involved in β-oxidation. These include (see Fig. 2):

1. Two acyl-CoA oxidases: both these oxidases (acyl-CoA oxidase 1 and 2) react with a variety of straight-chain acyl-CoAs whereas only acyl-CoA oxidase 2 is reactive with branched-chain acyl-CoAs. This implies that acyl-CoA oxidase 2 is involved in the oxidation of pristanoyl CoA as well as dihydroxycholestanoic acid CoA and trihydroxycholestanoic acid CoA whereas acyl-CoA oxidase 1 is not. Acyl-CoA oxidase 1 is probably the major enzyme involved in C26:0 β-oxidation.

2. Two bifunctional proteins with both enoyl-CoA hydratase and 3-hydroxyacyl-CoA dehydrogenase activity: a major difference between the two proteins is that the first bifunctional protein forms and dehydrogenates L-3-hydroxyacyl-CoA in contrast to the second enzyme, which forms and dehydrogenates D-3-hydroxyacyl-CoA. Hence the names L-bifunctional protein and D-bifunctional protein.

3. Two peroxisomal thiolases: recent studies have led to the identification of a new thiolase called SCP$_x$ or peroxisomal thiolase 2 which is the main if not exclusive enzyme involved in β-oxidation of pristanic acid as well as dihydroxycholestanoic acid and trihydroxycholestanoic acid, whereas the original thiolase (peroxisomal thiolase 1) is the main enzyme in C26:0 β-oxidation (see Fig. 2).

Ether-phospholipid biosynthesis

A second major function of peroxisomes concerns their role in the synthesis of ether-phospholipids. Indeed, the two enzyme activities responsible for the introduction of the characteristic ether linkage in ether-linked phospholipids (i.e. dihydroxyacetonephosphate acyltransferase (**DHAPAT**) and alkyldihydroxyacetonephosphate synthase (**alkyl-DHAP synthase**)), are both localized in peroxisomes. The next enzyme, acyl/alkyl-DHAP:NAD(P) oxidoreductase, is localized in both peroxisomes and the endoplasmic reticulum so that the product of the alkyl-DHAP synthase reaction, (i.e. alkyl-DHAP), is converted into alkylglycerol-3-phosphate in the peroxisome or endoplasmic reticulum (Fig. 3). All subsequent reactions involved in ether-phospholipid synthesis take place in the endoplasmic reticulum.

The functional role of plasmalogens has remained enigmatic until now. However, the identification of an isolated deficiency of either DHAPAT or alkyl-DHAP synthase in patients with severe clinical abnormalities comparable to rhizomelic chondrodysplasia punctata clearly shows that ether-phospholipids are of central importance in humans.

Phytanic acid α-oxidation

The pathway of phytanic acid α-oxidation has long remained an enigma but has recently been resolved. Phytanic acid first undergoes activation to phytanoyl-CoA after which a hydroxylation reaction takes place to generate 2-hydroxyphytanoyl-CoA as catalysed by the enzyme phytanoyl-CoA hydroxylase, which is deficient in Refsum disease (discussed later). Subsequently 2-hydroxyphytanoyl-CoA undergoes cleavage to produce formyl-CoA and pristanal, which is then dehydrogenated to pristanic acid. Activation of pristanic acid produces pristanoyl CoA, which can be degraded via β-oxidation in the peroxisome.

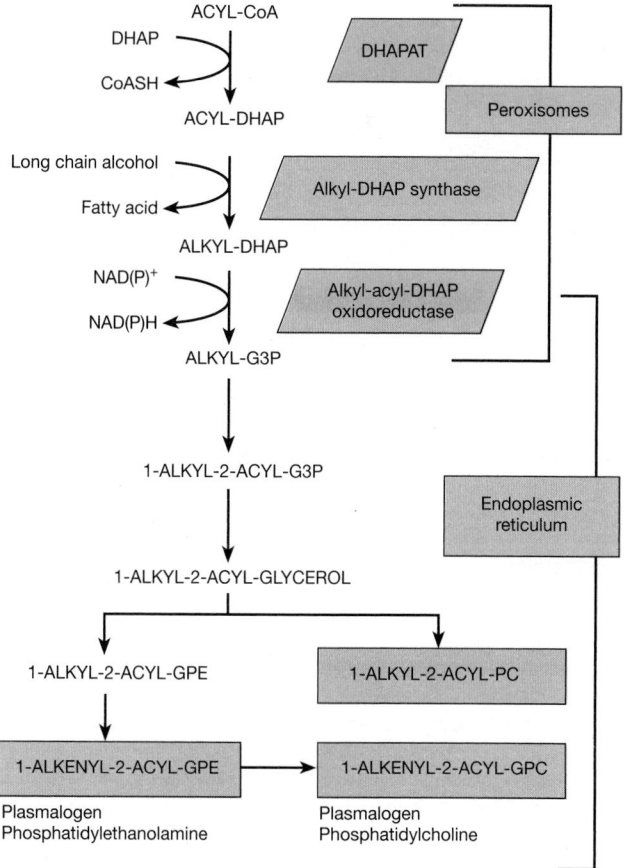

Fig. 3 Enzymology of ether–phospholipid biosynthesis. See text for details.

L-pipecolic acid oxidation

L-lysine is normally degraded by the saccharopine pathway involving the sequential action of L-lysine:2-oxoglutarate reductase and saccharopine dehydrogenase. However, L-lysine may also be degraded via the L-pipecolic acid pathway, which may especially be important in the brain. In the L-pipecolic acid pathway, L-pipecolic acid is produced from L-lysine via two enzymatic steps. L-pipecolic acid is then oxidized by L-pipecolate oxidase, a peroxisomal enzyme, at least in humans.

The function of the L-pipecolic acid pathway remains incompletely understood.

Biosynthesis of polyunsaturated fatty acids such as docosahexaenoic acid

In tissues and erythrocytes from patients with Zellweger syndrome there is a profound deficiency of docosahexaenoic acid (C22:6ω3) suggesting the involvement of peroxisomes in the formation of docosahexaenoic acid. Subsequent studies have not only established the role of peroxisomes in docosahexaenoic acid formation but have also revealed that the last step involved in formation of docosahexaenoic acid, the desaturation of clupanodonic acid (C22:5ω3) to docosahexaenoic acid, is not catalysed by a presumed Δ4-desaturase but involves a three-step pathway. In this pathway C22:5ω3 is first elongated to C24:5ω3, followed by Δ6-desaturation to C24:6ω3. The latter compound is then chain-shortened to C22:6ω3 (docosahexaenoic acid) via β-oxidation in peroxisomes.

This latter finding explains the deficiency of docosahexaenoic acid in patients with Zellweger syndrome.

Biogenesis of peroxisomes

In recent years much has been learned about peroxisome biogenesis, and many of the genes involved in peroxisome biogenesis, called *PEX* genes, are known. Although there is still discussion about the possible involvement of the endoplasmic reticulum, the model proposed by Lazarow and Fujiki is still generally accepted. The principal features of this model are:

1. Peroxisomal membrane and matrix proteins are synthesized on free polyribosomes.

2. The newly synthesized proteins are post-translationally imported from the cytosol into pre-existing peroxisomes.

3. Import of new polypeptides expands the peroxisomal compartment, making them grow until they reach a critical size which results either in division of peroxisomes into two daughter peroxisomes or in budding from the peroxisomal reticulum followed by subsequent growth.

The fact that proteins destined for peroxisomes are synthesized on free polyribosomes implies that these proteins must have specific signals which direct them to peroxisomes.

Studies, notably by Subramani and colleagues, have shown the existence of two such peroxisome targeting signals (**PTS**). Most of the peroxisomal matrix proteins are equipped with a PTS1 signal which involves a C-terminal tripeptide of the sequence serine–lysine–leucine or a conserved variant thereof. The second peroxisome targeting signal (PTS2) has been found in far fewer peroxisomal proteins and involves a stretch of nine amino acids of which amino acids numbers one, two, eight, and nine are essential with the following consensus: (arginine/lysine)–(leucine/valine/isoleucine)–XXXXX–(histidine/glutamine)–(leucine/alanine) in which X may be any amino acid. In mammals, the PTS2 signal has only been identified in peroxisomal thiolase 1, alkyl-DHAP synthase, and phytanoyl-CoA hydroxylase. Peroxisomal membrane proteins lack either a PTS1 a PTS2 signal which implies that there must be separate signals directing membrane proteins to peroxisomes.

The identification of the PTS1 and PTS2 targeting signals was soon followed by discovery of a growing number of so-called *PEX* genes required for peroxisome biogenesis. Most of these genes were first identified in the yeast *Saccharomyces cerevisiae*. Making use of databases of expressed sequence the human counterparts of these yeast genes have been identified in recent years, notably by Gould and colleagues. Most of these *PEX* genes code for peroxisomal membrane proteins with the exception of PEX5p and PEX7p. These two proteins are predominantly cytosolic and recognize the PTS1 and PTS2 signals respectively on peroxisomal proteins in the cytosol. In humans at least, the two loaded receptors functionally interact to form a complex which subsequently docks at the peroxisomal membrane. The proteins PEX13p and PEX14p play a central role in this docking process.

The following step involves dissociation of the complex followed by transport of the PTS1 and PTS2 proteins across the membrane and recycling of the receptors back to the cytosol for another round (Fig. 4). In this process multiple PEX proteins are involved, all of which essential since disruption of each single *PEX* gene is associated with a full block in peroxisome biogenesis.

Figure 4 shows a current model for peroxisome biogenesis in humans. Our increasing knowledge about the human genes involved in peroxisome biogenesis has been of tremendous importance for studies on the genetic basis of Zellweger syndrome and the other disorders of peroxisome biogenesis. Indeed, at present, 11 of the 12 *PEX* genes which underlie the 12 complementation groups which have been identified so far are now known.

The peroxisomal disorders

Table 2 lists the peroxisomal disorders identified so far. Throughout the years several classifications have been proposed for the different peroxisomal disorders. The first proposed classifying the peroxisomal disorders into three groups reflecting the extent of peroxisomal dysfunction with a generalized (group A), multiple (group B), and single (group C) loss of peroxisomal function. A second classification divided the peroxisomal disorders into two groups with the disorders of peroxisome biogenesis in group 1 and

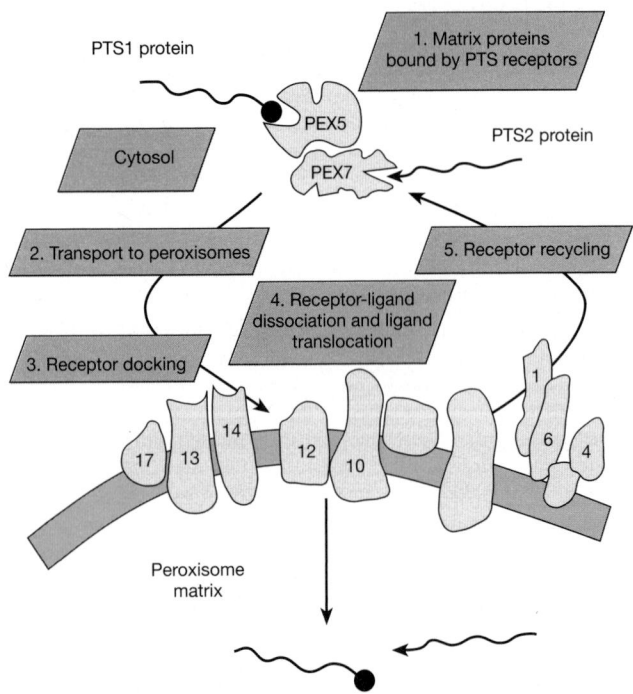

Fig. 4 Overview of the steps involved in peroxisome biogenesis including: (1) binding of ligands in the cytosol by PEX5p and PEX7p, the PTS1 and PTS2 receptors; (2) transport to and docking of PEX5p–ligand and PEX7p–ligand complexes with the peroxisomal membrane; (3) translocation of ligands into the peroxisome; and (4) recycling of the receptors back to the cytoplasm.

Table 2 The peroxisomal disorders and their enzymatic and genetic basis

Peroxisomal disorder	Enzyme deficiency established	Gene involved
Cerebrohepatorenal syndrome (Zellweger syndrome)	Generalized peroxisomal enzyme deficiency	*PEX* genes
Neonatal adrenoleucodystrophy	Generalized peroxisomal enzyme deficiency	*PEX* genes
Infantile Refsum disease	Generalized peroxisomal enzyme deficiency	*PEX* genes
Hyperpipecolic acidaemia	Generalized peroxisomal enzyme deficiency	*PEX* genes
Rhizomelic chondrodysplasia punctata type 1	Multiple peroxisomal enzyme deficiency	*PEX7*
Rhizomelic chondrodysplasia punctata type 2	DHAPAT	*DHAPAT*
Rhizomelic chondrodysplasia punctata type 3	Alkyl-DHAP synthase	Alkyl-DHAP synthase
X-linked adrenoleucodystrophy	ALD protein	*ALD*
Acyl CoA oxidase 1 deficiency	Straight-chain acyl CoA oxidase	*ACOX1*
D-bifunctional protein deficiency	D-bifunctional enzyme	*D-BP*
Peroxisomal thiolase 1 deficiency	Peroxisomal thiolase 1	
2-methylacyl CoA racemase deficiency	2-methylacyl CoA racemase	*AMACR*
Hyperoxaluria type 1	Alanine glyoxylate aminotransferase	*AGT*
Refsum disease	Phytanoyl CoA hydroxylase	*PHYH*
Glutaric aciduria type 3	Glutaryl CoA oxidase	Not known
Mevalonate kinase deficiency	Mevalonate kinase	*MK*
Acatalasaemia	Catalase	Catalase

Abbreviations: DHAPAT, dihydroxyacetonephosphate acyltransferase; alkyl-DHAP, alkyldihydroxyacetonephosphate.

the peroxisomal disorders in which a single peroxisomal function has been lost in group 2.

Below we will describe the characteristics of the individual peroxisomal disorders followed by the laboratory diagnosis of these disorders making use of a new classification based on the concept of diagnostic groups.

Cerebrohepatorenal (Zellweger) syndrome

The clinical presentation of Zellweger syndrome is dominated by craniofacial dysmorphia and profound neurological abnormalities. The craniofacial dysmorphia includes a high forehead, flat occiput, wide open sutures, large fontanelle, hypoplastic orbital ridges, epicanthus, high arched palate, external ear deformities, micrognathia, and redundant skin folds of the neck. Neurological abnormalities include severe hypo/areflexia, poor sucking, epileptic seizures, severe neonatal hypotonia, nystagmus, and sensorineural hearing loss. Furthermore, there is profound psychomotor retardation. There are also ocular abnormalities including cataracts, glaucoma, corneal clouding, Brushfield spots, pigmentary retinopathy, and optic nerve dysplasia. Because of the hypotonia and mongoloid appearance, Zellweger patients are sometimes wrongly suspected of suffering from Down's syndrome.

Pathological studies in Zellweger patients have shown a great number of abnormalities in various organs including the brain. Macroscopic abnormalities include deviant sulci and gyri with almost vertical parietal clefts and pachymicrogyria. The most striking and intriguing neuropathological abnormality is the impaired neuronal migration which leads to characteristic and unique cytoarchitectural abnormalities involving the cerebral hemispheres, the cerebellum, and the inferior olivary complex.

Patients with Zellweger syndrome usually die early in life with an average lifespan of a few months.

Neonatal adrenoleucodystrophy

The first case of neonatal adrenoleucodystrophy was described in 1978 in a boy with hypotonia, convulsions, absent grasp reflexes, slight Moro response, and little spontaneous movement at birth. Characteristic signs of adrenoleucodystrophy were found in this patient which included demyelination of the central nervous system white matter, atrophy of the adrenal cortex, ballooned adrenocortical cells, and the presence of lamellar inclusions of electrondense leaflets separated by a clear space. However, there were also a number of additional central nervous abnormalities not described for X-linked adrenoleucodystrophy and it was noted that this new type of leucodystrophy resembled Zellweger syndrome in several respects, suggesting a common aetiology. This was soon found to be true

when multiple peroxisomal abnormalities resulting from a defect in peroxisome biogenesis were described in patients with neonatal adrenoleucodystrophy.

Infantile Refsum disease

Infantile phytanic acid storage disease was first described in 1982 in three unrelated patients showing hepatomegaly, mental retardation, (minor) facial dysmorphia, retinopathy, neurosensory deafness, osteopenia, growth retardation, and elevated plasma phytanic acid levels. Because phytanic acid was known to accumulate in Refsum disease, the name infantile Refsum disease was coined. Since this initial report many additional patients have been described.

As with neonatal adrenoleucodystrophy it was soon realized that there were certain similarities between infantile Refsum disease and Zellweger syndrome, and we now know that infantile Refsum disease is also a disorder of peroxisome biogenesis which explains the multiple peroxisomal abnormalities observed in patients with infantile Refsum disease.

Hyperpipecolic acidaemia

Several cases have been reported in the literature of hyperpipecolic acidaemia. It is now clear that not all of these patients are true cases of isolated hyperpipecolic acidaemia. This implies that hyperpipecolic acidaemia has become obsolete in the classification of peroxisomal disorders. On the other hand, recent reports document the existence of apparently true cases of hyperpipecolic acidaemia although the underlying defect remains to be established.

Biochemistry of Zellweger syndrome, neonatal adrenoleucodystrophy, and infantile Refsum disease

In Zellweger syndrome, neonatal adrenoleucodystrophy, and infantile Refsum disease peroxisome biogenesis is defective resulting in the virtual absence of morphologically distinguishable peroxisomes in all the patient's cells. This has been demonstrated most convincingly in liver biopsy specimens from patients, notably by Roels and colleagues. The deficiency of peroxisomes can also be demonstrated in cultured fibroblasts from patients using immunofluorescence microscopy.

The absence of peroxisomes in patients with Zellweger syndrome, neonatal adrenoleucodystrophy, and infantile Refsum disease explains the multiplicity of biochemical abnormalities observed in these patients which are summarized in Table 3.

Table 3 Biochemical characteristics of the disorders of peroxisome biogenesis and the peroxisomal β-oxidation disorders

	Zellweger syndrome	NALD	Infantile Refsum disease	Acyl CoA oxidase deficiency	d-BP deficiency	Thiolase deficiency
Plasma						
VLCFAs	↑	↑	↑	↑	↑	↑
DHCA and THCA	↑	↑	↑	N	↑	↑
Phytanic acid	↑*	↑*	↑*	N	↑*	ND
Pristanic acid	↑†	↑†	↑†	N	↑†	ND
Erythrocytes						
Plasmalogens	↓	↓ to N	N	N	N	N
Liver						
Peroxisomes	Deficient	Deficient	Deficient	Present but enlarged	Present but enlarged	Present but enlarged
Peroxisomal enzymology						
Enzyme deficiency	Generalized	Generalized	Generalized	Acyl CoA oxidase 1	d-BP	Peroxisomal thiolase

Abbreviations: NALD, neonatal adrenoleucodystrophy; d-BP, d-bifunctional protein; VLCFAs, very long-chain fatty acids; DHCA, dihydroxycholestanoic acid; THCA, trihydroxycholestanoic acid; N, Normal; ND, not done.

*Phytanic acid is solely derived from dietary sources and may be normal in young patients not exposed to foods containing phytanic acid despite the deficiency in phytanic acid α-oxidation.

†Pristanic acid is derived from dietary sources and from phytanic acid via α-oxidation and may be normal in young patients despite the deficient capacity to β-oxidize pristanic acid.

Molecular basis of the peroxisome deficiency disorders

The genetic basis of the different disorders of peroxisome biogenesis has been elucidated. Earlier studies had already shown that the genetic basis of Zellweger syndrome, neonatal adrenoleucodystrophy, and infantile Refsum disease is very heterogeneous. This was concluded from complementation studies, which involved fusion of fibroblasts of two different patients with the same abnormality such as a defect in peroxisome biogenesis so that hybrid cells (heterokaryons) are generated containing nuclei from each patient's fibroblasts. If the defective genes in the two patients' cell lines were different, one would expect restoration of peroxisome formation, whereas in the case when the mutant genes are identical, no complementation would occur. This is most easily done using catalase immunofluorescence. Large-scale complementation studies have now shown that there are at least 12 different complementation groups representing 12 different *PEX* genes. Interestingly, there is strong over-representation of one particular group, occurring in 60 to 70 per cent of all patients with a disorder of peroxisome biogenesis. The gene defective in this group is the *PEX1* gene which codes for a protein (PEX1p) belonging to the family of ATPases associated with diverse cellular activities which obviously plays an indispensable role in peroxisome biogenesis, although its precise mode of action is unknown. Eleven of the 12 genes which underlie the different complementation groups have now been identified. We have applied complementation analysis on a systematic basis to more than 200 patients with disorders of peroxisome biogenesis: most patients belong to the PEX1 group (63 per cent), followed by PEX6 (10 per cent), and PEX12 (5.4 per cent).

The identification of the mutant *PEX* genes is important for carrier detection and prenatal diagnosis in families at risk. On the other hand current prenatal diagnostic procedures which involve analyses at the enzyme (activity measurements) and protein (immunoblotting) level are very reliable.

Rhizomelic chondrodysplasia punctata type 1

Chondrodysplasia punctata represents a genetically heterogeneous group of bone dysplasias with stippling of the epiphyses as a common feature. The rhizomelic form is characterized by the presence of stippled foci of calcification within the hyaline cartilage with coronal clefts in the vertebral bodies associated with dwarfing, cataracts, multiple malformations due to contractures, and mental retardation in virtually all patients. Ichthyosis is frequent. Inheritance is autosomal recessive. Rhizomelic chondrodysplasia punctata must be distinguished from the milder autosomal dominant form of chondrodysplasia punctata (Conradi–Hunermann syndrome) with

longer survival, absence of severe limb shortening, and usually intact intellect.

Apart from the classic presentation of rhizomelic chondrodysplasia punctata, a number of patients have now been described in the literature with a much milder presentation lacking the characteristic stigmata of rhizomelic chondrodysplasia punctata. Indeed, one such patient is still alive now at 16 years of age, has no rhizomelia, and only mild mental retardation. As we will describe below, there is not only clinical variability within rhizomelic chondrodysplasia punctata but also genetic diversity with two additional genetic types of rhizomelic chondrodysplasia punctata named types 2 and 3.

Biochemistry of rhizomelic chondrodysplasia punctata type 1 and molecular basis

Rhizomelic chondrodysplasia punctata is a true peroxisomal disorder, with the original description being of deficiency of plasmalogens in tissues and erythrocytes from patients and elevated phytanic acid levels in plasma. Subsequent studies have led to the remarkable finding of four distinct peroxisomal enzyme deficiencies at the level of:

(1) dihydroxyacetonephosphate acyltransferase (DHAPAT)

(2) alkyldihydroxyacetonephosphate synthase (alkyl-DHAP synthase)

(3) phytanoyl-CoA hydroxylase, and

(4) 41 kDa peroxisomal thiolase.

The underlying basis for this peculiar observation came when it was discovered that alkyl-DHAP synthase, phytanoyl-CoA hydroxylase, and peroxisomal thiolase all turned out to be PTS2 proteins, suggesting that the defect in rhizomelic chondrodysplasia punctata had to be in the PTS2 receptor. The gene coding for the PTS2 receptor was identified in 1997 and mutations were found in patients with rhizomelic chondrodysplasia punctata, thus establishing its molecular basis. Although many different mutations have been identified there is one frequent mutation, the Leu292Stop mutation, which occurs in more than 50 per cent of the mutant alleles.

Rhizomelic chondrodysplasia punctata type 2 (DHAPAT deficiency)

In 1992 the first patient was described with classic rhizomelic chondrodysplasia punctata but lacking the characteristic set of four peroxisomal abnormalities. Instead an isolated deficiency of only a single enzyme (DHAPAT) was found (Table 4). This enzyme catalyses the first committed step in plasmalogen synthesis and its deficiency is associated with the inability to synthesize plasmalogens.

Table 4 Biochemical abnormalities in rhizomelic chondrodysplasia types 1 (PEX7 deficiency), 2 (DHAPAT deficiency), and 3 (alkyl-DHAP synthase deficiency)

	RCDP type 1	RCDP type 2	RCDP type 3
Plasma			
Very long-chain fatty acids	N	N	N
Di- and trihydroxycholestanoicacid	N	N	N
Phytanic acid	N to ↑*	N	N
Pristanic acid	N	N	N
Pipecolic acid	N	N	N
Erythrocytes			
Plasmalogen	↓	↓	↓
Liver			
Peroxisomes	Present but abnormal	Normal	Unknown
Fibroblasts			
De novo plasmalogen synthesis	↓	↓	↓
DHAPAT	↓	↓↓	↓ to N
Alkyl-DHAP synthase	↓↓	N	↓↓
C26:0 β-oxidation	N	N	N
Pristanic acid β-oxidation	N	N	N
Phytanic acid α-oxidation	↓	N	N
Catalase immunofluorescence	N	N	N
Acyl-CoA oxidase (blot)	N	N	N
D-bifunctional protein (blot)	N	N	N
41 kDa thiolase (blot)	↓↓	N	N

Abbreviations: RCDP, rhizomelic chondrodysplasia; DHAPAT, dihydroxyacetonephosphate acyltransferase; alkyl-DHAP, alkyldihydroxyacetonephosphate; N, normal.

*Phytanic acid is derived from dietary sources and may therefore vary from normal to elevated if phytanic acid α-oxidation is deficient.

At present several cases of rhizomelic chondrodysplasia punctata type 2 have been described. Most cases had a severe clinical presentation resembling classic rhizomelic chondrodysplasia punctata type 1. As could be expected, there is also clinical heterogeneity within rhizomelic chondrodysplasia punctata type 2. In all patients identified so far, the deficiency of DHAPAT is the single abnormality due to mutations in the structural gene coding for DHAPAT.

Rhizomelic chondrodysplasia punctata type 3 (alkyl-DHAP synthase deficiency)

The first case of rhizomelic chondrodysplasia punctata type 3 in a patient showing all the clinical stigmata of classic rhizomelic chondrodysplasia punctata was identified in 1994. In this patient plasmalogen biosynthesis was found to be blocked due to the deficient activity of the second enzyme involved in plasmalogen biosynthesis, i.e. alkyl-DHAP synthase. The least affected of those patients so far identified is alive at 7½ years with mild to moderate rhizomelia, generalized flexion contractures, inability to sit, roll, or crawl, cataract, continued seizures, and profound developmental delay. The deficient activity of alkyl-DHAP synthase in these patients has been found to result from different mutations in the structural gene coding for alkyl-DHAP synthase.

X-linked adrenoleucodystrophy

There is considerable clinical heterogeneity within X-linked adrenoleucodystrophy with at least six phenotypic variants. The classification of the different phenotypes of X-linked adrenoleucodystrophy is somewhat arbitrary and is based upon the age of onset and the organs principally affected. It should be noted that there are also patients not easily assignable to either phenotype, emphasizing the variable clinical expression of X-linked adrenoleucodystrophy. The two most frequently observed phenotypes, accounting for approximately 80 per cent of all cases, are childhood adrenoleucodystrophy and adrenomyeloneuropathy.

Childhood cerebral adrenoleucodystrophy

Childhood cerebral adrenoleucodystrophy is characterized by rapidly progressive cerebral demyelination. The onset is between 3 and 10 years of age. Frequent early neurological symptoms are behavioural disturbances, a decline in school performance, deterioration of vision, and impaired auditory discrimination. The course is relentlessly progressive, and seizures, spastic tetraplegia, and dementia develop within months. Most patients die within 2 to 3 years of the onset of neurological symptoms. Some patients survive longer, albeit in a persistent vegetative state.

In most patients with childhood cerebral adrenoleucodystrophy, cerebral magnetic resonance imaging typically reveals extensive demyelination in the occipital periventricular white matter, with sparing of the U fibres. Much less frequently, the frontal lobes are affected first. The early symptoms of childhood cerebral adrenoleucodystrophy are frequently attributed to an attention deficit disorder or hyperactivity. Before the advent of reliable diagnostic tests and magnetic resonance imaging, metachromatic leucodystrophy, ceroid lipofuscinosis, globoid cell leucodystrophy (Krabbe disease), and subacute sclerosing panencephalitis were sometimes diagnosed instead of childhood cerebral adrenoleucodystrophy.

Adrenomyeloneuropathy

Adrenomyeloneuropathy is the most frequent phenotype of X-linked adrenoleucodystrophy. The onset of neurological symptoms in this phenotype usually occurs in the third and fourth decade. Neurological deficits are primarily due to myelopathy and to a lesser extent to neuropathy. Patients gradually develop a spastic paraparesis, often in combination with a disturbed vibration sense in the legs and sphincter dysfunction. Approximately 50 per cent of men with adrenomyeloneuropathy show mild to moderate cerebral involvement on magnetic resonance imaging, and in some the abnormalities of white matter may resemble the demyelination seen in childhood cerebral adrenoleucodystrophy; the spinal cord is frequently atrophic. Nerve conduction studies and electromyography are compatible with a predominantly axonal, sensorimotor polyneuropathy. Life expectancy is probably normal, unless patients develop cerebral demyelination, or when adrenocortical insufficiency is not recognized and remains untreated. Many patients with adrenomyeloneuropathy were initially diagnosed with neurological diseases such as chronic progressive multiple sclerosis and hereditary spastic paraparesis.

Biochemistry and molecular basis of X-linked adrenoleucodystrophy

The biochemical hallmark of X-linked adrenoleucodystrophy is the accumulation of very long-chain fatty acids in plasma, fibroblasts, and other cell types. Analysis of plasma very long-chain fatty acids has turned out to be an extremely powerful diagnostic method with only a few if any false negatives, at least when analysed in experienced laboratories.

The accumulation of very long-chain fatty acids, notably C26:0, is due to their impaired oxidation in peroxisomes. It was initially thought that this was due to the deficient activity of a peroxisomal enzyme catalysing the activation of very long-chain fatty acids to their CoA esters which is the first obligatory step in fatty acid β-oxidation. The *X-ALD* gene was identified using a positional cloning strategy. Remarkably the deduced ALD protein did not appear to be an acyl-CoA synthetase but instead turned out to belong to the family of ABC proteins which also includes the CFTR protein involved in cystic fibrosis and the MDR protein involved in multidrug resistance. The ALD protein is a so-called halftransporter with six transmembrane spanning elements, and probably functions as a transporter of very long-chain fatty acid CoA esters across the peroxisomal membrane either as homo- or heterodimers localized in the peroxisomal membrane. The identification of the *X-ALD* gene has allowed molecular studies in X-linked adrenoleucodystrophy patients, which have shown diverse often unique mutations.

Acyl CoA oxidase deficiency (pseudoneonatal adrenoleucodystrophy)

In 1988 Poll-The and colleagues described patients with neonatal onset hypotonia together with delayed motor development, sensory deafness, and retinopathy with extinguished electroretinograms. There was no craniofacial dysmorphia in any of the patients. Psychomotor development was severely delayed, and after the first 2 years of life a progressive neurological regression set in. Computed tomography with contrast enhancement revealed bilateral enhancing lesions and a generally hypodense cerebral white matter which led to the diagnosis of neonatal adrenoleucodystrophy. The finding of elevated levels of very long-chain fatty acids in the plasma of these patients supported this conclusion. In contrast to the findings in other patients with neonatal adrenoleucodystrophy, however, these patients had peroxisomes normally present, albeit of enlarged size, and biochemical abnormalities were restricted to the accumulation of very long-chain fatty acids. The defect in these patients was at the level of acyl-CoA oxidase, the first obligatory enzyme involved in the peroxisomal β-oxidation of very long-chain fatty acids (see Fig. 2).

All patients identified so far have severe neurological abnormalities, mild to absent craniofacial dysmorphia, and failure to thrive. In patients with acyl-CoA oxidase deficiency, plasma abnormalities are restricted to the accumulation of very long-chain fatty acids which follows logically from the role of acyl-CoA oxidase in very long-chain fatty acid β-oxidation (see Fig. 2). A large deletion in the acyl-CoA oxidase gene in the two original patients has been reported.

D-Bifunctional protein deficiency

Bifunctional protein deficiency was first described in 1989 in a patient with severe hypotonia and seizures of neonatal onset. An electroencephalogram revealed multifocal spikes. No developmental progress was observed. There was no dysmorphia and no hepatomegaly. Fontanelles were open with open metopic sutures. Visual evoked responses and brainstem auditory evoked responses were grossly abnormal. A brain biopsy at 6 weeks revealed polymicrogyria. The patient died at 5 months of age after a clinical course marked by absent developmental progress and seizures refractory to treat-

ment. Neuropathological studies revealed a polymicrogyric neocortex and focal areas of cortical heterotopia.

Laboratory analysis revealed elevated very long-chain fatty acids but liver morphology revealed the normal presence of peroxisomes. Subsequent immunoblot experiments revealed the absence of one of the peroxisomal β-oxidation enzyme proteins, i.e. bifunctional protein.

Many additional patients with bifunctional protein deficiency have since been described. Identification of such cases usually starts in a patient with a Zellweger-like phenotype in which subsequent laboratory studies reveal an isolated defect in peroxisomal β-oxidation with no abnormalities in other peroxisomal functions like plasmalogen biosyntheses and the normal presence of peroxisomes, although they are usually enlarged in both liver and in fibroblasts. Such data clearly point to a disorder of peroxisomal β-oxidation. Complementation studies have led to the identification of four groups with group 1 representing acyl-CoA oxidase deficiency, group 2 bifunctional protein deficiency, and groups 3 and 4 involving unknown defects.

Most patients turned out to belong to group 2. Remarkably, molecular studies in fibroblasts from patients belonging to group 2 failed to identify any mutations in the gene for L-bifunctional protein. This puzzling situation was resolved when a new bifunctional protein called D-bifunctional protein or multifunctional enzyme 2 was discovered which turned out to be the enzyme deficient in group 2. Molecular studies clearly identified mutations in the gene for D-bifunctional protein, thus resolving the true molecular basis of bifunctional protein deficiency. Recent studies have shown that there are three subgroups within the bifunctional protein deficiency group, which finds its basis in the fact that bifunctional protein is a single protein with two catalytic activities.

The clinical presentation of patients affected by D-bifunctional protein deficiency is usually very severe and resembles that of Zellweger syndrome in many respects. Indeed, in a recent series neonatal hypotonia (94 per cent), dysmorphic features (80 per cent), neonatal seizures (92 per cent), hepatomegaly (43 per cent), developmental delay (100 per cent), poor feeding (86 per cent), and a disordered neuronal migration (88 per cent) were found.

Biochemistry of D-bifunctional protein deficiency

In patients suffering from D-bifunctional protein deficiency there is accumulation of very long-chain fatty acids, pristanic acid, and di- and trihydroxycholestanoic acid which follows logically from the scheme of Fig. 2. This is true for most cases, but in one form of D-bifunctional protein deficiency (type B) in which the enoyl-CoA hydratase component of D-bifunctional protein is functionally inactive there is no accumulation of bile acid intermediates although the underlying basis is unclear.

Peroxisomal thiolase-1 deficiency (pseudo-Zellweger syndrome)

In 1986 a girl from consanguineous parents showing marked facial dysmorphia, muscle weakness, and hypotonia at birth was described. The patient showed no psychomotor development during her 11-month life. At autopsy the patient had renal cysts, atrophic adrenals with striated cells, minimal liver fibrosis, hypomyelination in the cerebral white matter, foci of neuronal heterotopia, and a sudanophilic leucodystophy. Taken together, these clinical findings suggested that the patient was affected by Zellweger syndrome. Morphological analysis of the liver, however, revealed abundant peroxisomes. The subsequent finding that very long-chain fatty acids in plasma were clearly elevated did suggest a peroxisomal defect possibly restricted to the peroxisomal β-oxidation system. Further proof came when elevated levels of di- and trihydroxycholestanoic acid were found in a duodenal aspirate. Immunoblot studies revealed that both the 44 kDa precursor form of peroxisomal thiolase-1 as well as the mature 41 kDa form were completely missing, indicating peroxisomal thiolase deficiency. No additional patients have been described in the literature.

Peroxisomal 2-methylacyl-CoA racemase deficiency associated with a late onset motor neuropathy: a newly identified peroxisomal disorder

A new defect in the peroxisomal fatty acid β-oxidation pathway in a number of patients suffering from an adult onset sensory motor neuropathy has been described. Sensory motor neuropathy is associated with inherited disorders including Charcot–Marie–Tooth disease, X-linked adrenoleucodystrophy/adrenomyeloneuropathy, and Refsum disease. In the latter two, the neuropathy is thought to result from the accumulation of very long-chain fatty acids and phytanic acid respectively. The plasma of two patients with adult onset sensory motor neuropathy and additional signs suggesting Refsum disease (patient 1) and X-linked adrenoleucodystrophy (patient 2) had a similar profile: normal very long-chain fatty acids, marginally elevated phytanic acid, and definitely increased levels of the 2-methyl branched-chain fatty acids pristanic acid and di- and trihydroxycholestanoic acid. This suggested a specific defect in the peroxisomal β-oxidation of branched-chain fatty acids and not in the α-oxidation system, the first enzyme step of which is defective in Refsum disease. Studies in fibroblasts revealed normal values for all parameters measured except for pristanic acid β-oxidation, which was reduced to 20 to 30 per cent of control. The activities of the enzymes directly involved in the β-oxidation of branched-chain fatty acids, which includes branched-chain acyl-CoA oxidase, D-bifunctional protein, and peroxisomal thiolase 2 (pTH2/SCPx), were all normal.

Attention was focused on 2-methylacyl-CoA racemase. As described before, this enzyme is not directly involved in the β-oxidation process itself but is important in the β-oxidation of both pristanic acid and di- and trihydroxycholestanoic acid (Fig. 2) since the enzyme catalyses the interconversion of ($2R$) and ($2S$) stereoisomers of 2-methyl branched-chain fatty acyl-CoA esters. Measurement of racemase activity in fibroblasts using ($25S$)-2,5,5-trihydroxycholestanoyl-CoA as substrate revealed a complete deficiency of the enzyme.

The finding of defined abnormalities in patients with late onset motor neuropathy resulting from a defect in the peroxisomal oxidation of 2-methyl branched-chain fatty acids at the level of 2-methylacyl-CoA racemase may have implications for the diagnosis of adult onset neuropathies of unknown aetiology.

Hyperoxaluria type 1 (alanine glyoxylate aminotransferase deficiency)

See Chapter 11.10 for further discussion.

Refsum disease

Refsum disease was first delineated as a distinct disease entity on a clinical basis by Sigvald Refsum in the 1940s under the name heredopathia atactica polyneuritiformis. Cardinal manifestations of the disease include retinitis pigmentosa, cerebellar ataxia, chronic polyneuropathy, and an elevated protein level in the cerebrospinal fluid with a normal cell count. Less constant features include sensorineural hearing loss, anosmia, ichthyosis, skeletal malformations, and cardiac abnormalities. The clinical picture of Refsum disease is often that of a slowly developing, progressive peripheral neuropathy manifested by severe motor weakness and muscular wasting, especially of the lower extremities.

Patients in whom Refsum disease is destined to develop appear to be perfectly normal as infants and do not show any obvious defects in growth and development. Onset has occasionally been detected in early childhood but not until the fifth decade in others. Most patients have clear-cut manifestations before the age of 20.

Biochemistry of Refsum disease

Studies in the early 1960s led to the identification of phytanic acid in tissues and plasma samples of Refsum patients. The enzyme defect in Refsum disease was identified at the level of phytanoyl-CoA hydroxylase.

Molecular basis of Refsum disease

The identification of the phytanoyl-CoA hydroxylase complementary DNA and gene structure has allowed molecular studies which show a variety of often unique mutations.

Glutaric aciduria type 3

In 1991 Bennett and colleagues described a patient who was investigated at 11 months of age because of failure to thrive and postprandial vomiting. Two abnormalities were found. First, she was shown to be homozygous for β-thalassaemia and second, significant glutaric aciduria was found. Studies in fibroblasts revealed normal glutaryl-CoA dehydrogenase activity whereas glutaryl-CoA oxidase activity was not detectable. This study has not been followed up at the enzyme protein and/or DNA level. No additional cases have been identified so far.

Mevalonate kinase deficiency (see Chapter 11.12.3)

Mevalonate kinase deficiency is the only disorder involving the peroxisomal part of isoprenoid biosynthesis. Interestingly, apart from the classical form of mevalonate kinase deficiency which is associated with severe abnormalities early in life including profound developmental delay, facial dysmorphia, cataract, hepatosplenomegaly, lymphadenopathy, and early death, mevalonate kinase deficiency has also been observed in hyperimmunoglobulinaemia D and periodic fever syndrome. This syndrome is an autosomal recessive disorder characterized by recurrent episodes of fever associated with lymphadenopathy, arthralgia, gastrointestinal dismay, and skin rash. In patients with hyperimmunoglobulinaemia D/periodic fever syndrome mevalonate kinase was found to be strongly reduced (1.2 to 3.4 per cent of normal) but not fully deficient as in classical mevalonate kinase deficiency.

Acatalasaemia

Acatalasaemia is a rare disease which has mainly been described in Japan and Switzerland. In Japan, acatalasemia is associated with ulcerating, often gangrenous, oral lesions whereas these abnormalities were not seen in Swiss patients.

Laboratory diagnosis of peroxisomal disorders: postnatal diagnosis

Although discussed in this chapter as a single group, the peroxisomal disorders comprise a heterogeneous group of disorders with a large spectrum of clinical signs and symptoms. Furthermore, different biochemical abnormalities are found in the various peroxisomal disorders reflecting the peroxisomal pathway(s) primarily affected. This immediately explains why there is not a single laboratory method allowing diagnosis of all peroxisomal disorders.

Earlier we introduced the concept of diagnostic groups in order to develop logical guidelines for the laboratory diagnosis of the various peroxisomal disorders. These diagnostic groups are:

I. The disorders of peroxisome biogenesis plus the disorders of peroxisomal β-oxidation with the exception of X-linked adrenoleucodystrophy which forms a distinct diagnostic group (group III). This group includes Zellweger syndrome, neonatal adrenoleucodystrophy, infantile Refsum disease, acyl-CoA oxidase deficiency, D-bifunctional protein deficiency, and peroxisomal thiolase deficiency.

II. Rhizomelic chondrodysplasia punctata complex. This includes: rhizomelic chondrodysplasia types 1, 2, and 3.

III. X-linked adrenoleucodystrophy complex. This includes all forms of X-linked adrenoleucodystrophy.

IV. The remaining peroxisomal disorders. This includes: racemase deficiency, hyperoxaluria type 1, Refsum disease, glutaryl-CoA oxidase deficiency, mevalonate kinase deficiency, and acatalasaemia.

Laboratory diagnosis of the disorders of diagnostic group I

As described earlier, the clinical presentation of the disorders of peroxisomal β-oxidation resembles that of the disorders of peroxisome biogenesis in many respects. This is immediately clear if is realized that the first cases of acyl-CoA oxidase deficiency were described under the name pseudoneonatal adrenoleucodystrophy and peroxisomal thiolase deficiency as pseudo-Zellweger syndrome. The similarity between the disorders of peroxisome biogenesis and peroxisomal β-oxidation is also clear in the case of D-bifunctional protein deficiency: patients with this defect show severe neurological abnormalities including hypotonia, seizures, and psychomotor retardation as well as craniofacial dysmorphia as discussed before.

The biochemical abnormalities of the different disorders belonging to diagnostic group I are listed in Table 3. Inspection of these data shows that very long-chain fatty acids are abnormal in all these disorders making very long-chain fatty acid analysis a reliable first-line diagnostic test to verify whether a patient with the clinical signs and symptoms of a disorder of peroxisome biogenesis or peroxisomal β-oxidation is truely affected by such a peroxisomal disorder. If abnormal, additional tests have to be performed to discriminate between either a disorder of peroxisome biogenesis or peroxisomal β-oxidation. This includes analyses in erythrocytes (plasmalogens) and plasma (bile acid intermediates, pristanic acid, and phytanic acid).

If plasmalogen levels are deficient, the diagnosis 'disorder of peroxisome biogenesis' is established. This should be followed by detailed studies in fibroblasts, to establish whether the defect is truely expressed in fibroblasts and to establish the gene defective in this patient. If plasmalogen levels are normal this usually, but not invariably, points to a disorder of peroxisomal β-oxidation thus emphasizing the value of examining fibroblasts.

Laboratory diagnosis of the disorders of diagnostic group II

Since the clinical characteristics of rhizomelic chondrodysplasia punctata type 1 (PTS2 receptor deficiency), type 2 (DHAPAT deficiency), and type 3 (alkyl-DHAP synthase deficiency) are very similar, it makes sense to include these three forms of chondrodysplasia punctata in a single diagnostic group.

The biochemical characteristics of these disorders are listed in Table 4. The fact that erythrocyte plasmalogens are deficient in all three types indicates that analysis of erythrocyte plasmalogens is a reliable initial laboratory test to establish whether one is dealing with rhizomelic chondrodysplasia punctata type 1, 2, or 3. Erythrocyte plasmalogens have always been found to be deficient, even in more mildly affected cases. This implies that if erythrocyte plasmalogens have been found to be normal, rhizomelic chondrodysplasia punctata type 1, 2, or 3 is excluded whereas the finding of deficient plasmalogen levels is diagnostic for all types of rhizomelic chondrodysplasia punctata. Detailed studies of fibroblasts are required to discriminate between types 1, 2, and 3.

Laboratory diagnosis of X-linked adrenoleucodystrophy complex (diagnostic group III)

As described above, there is great heterogeneity within X-linked adrenoleucodystrophy with childhood cerebral adrenoleucodystrophy and adrenomyeloneuropathy as the most frequent phenotypes. Studies in hundreds of patients have shown that analysis of plasma very long-chain fatty acids is a reliable initial test to verify whether a certain patient is affected by X-linked adrenoleucodystrophy. If abnormal, we usually proceed by doing a full study in fibroblasts followed by molecular analyses in blood cells of fibroblasts.

Fibroblast studies are not obligatory and it may be advisable to perform direct molecular studies in blood cells of the patient as soon as plasma very long-chain fatty acids have been found to be abnormal. Heterozygote detection is not so straightforward as for hemizygotes. Indeed, plasma very long-chain fatty acids levels have been found to be normal in about 15 per cent of obligate heterozygotes making such analysis unreliable for the detection of heterozygotes. For this reason we advocate molecular studies and omit very long-chain fatty acids analysis in families in which the molecular defect has been established. In case the family history is negative, we usually start by doing plasma very long-chain fatty acid analysis followed by detailed studies in fibroblasts including measurements of C26:0 β-oxidation activity, very long-chain fatty acid analysis, and analysis of the ALD protein by means of immunofluorescence microscopy. The latter method may be especially rewarding since it is a general feature of X-linked adrenoleucodystrophy that in many instances the product of the mutant X-ALD allele produces an unstable protein so that in cells from heterozygotes a mosaic pattern is observed with positive and negative cells upon immunofluorescence.

Laboratory diagnosis of the disorders of group IV

The disorders of group IV share no similarities and all require separate laboratory tests for diagnosis as described below.

Peroxisomal 2-methylacyl-CoA racemase deficiency

Patients with a deficiency of 2-methylacyl-CoA racemase are unable to degrade pristanic acid and the bile acid intermediates di- and trihydroxycholestanoic acid. For this reason pristanic acid and di- and trihydroxycholestanoic acid are elevated in patients whereas very long-chain fatty acids are normal. Although experience is limited, it is probably safe to say that postnatal diagnosis of such patients may either be based on analysis of pristanic acid by gas chromatography or mass spectrometry or bile acid intermediates preferably by tandem mass spectrometry. Definitive diagnosis of racemase deficiency requires detailed studies in fibroblasts including measurement of racemase activity making use of specifically synthesized substrates.

Primary hyperoxaluria type 1

In patients with hyperoxaluria type 1 alanine glyoxylate aminotransferase is deficient which leads to a block in glyoxylate detoxification. Glyoxylate may either be oxidized to oxalate or reduced to glycolate which explains why in most patients with primary hyperoxaluria type 1 there is increased urinary excretion of all three acids. Definitive diagnosis of primary hyperoxaluria type 1 requires a liver biopsy for assessment of alanine glyoxylate aminotransferase activity.

Refsum disease

In Refsum disease phytanoyl-CoA hydroxylase is deficient, leading to the impaired degradation of phytanic acid. Since phytanic acid is solely derived from exogenous sources, plasma phytanic acid levels may vary widely. Definitive diagnosis requires measurement of phytanoyl-CoA hydroxylase in fibroblasts followed by molecular analysis at the complementary DNA or preferably the genomic level.

Glutaryl-CoA oxidase deficiency (glutaric aciduria type 3).

Only a single patient with this defect has been described in the literature. In this patient there was increased urinary excretion of glutaric acid not due to glutaric aciduria type 1 (glutaryl-CoA dehydrogenase deficiency) or glutaric aciduria type 2 (electron transfer flavoprotein (ETF)/ETF dehydrogenase deficiency). Glutaryl CoA oxidase was deficient.

Mevalonate kinase deficiency

In the classic form of mevalonate kinase deficiency, urinary mevalonic acid is extremely high in all patients studied making urinary analysis of mevalonic acid a reliable method for identification. If abnormal, mevalonate kinase activity should be measured in various types of blood cell (except erythrocytes) and/or in fibroblasts followed by molecular studies.

In hyperimmunoglobulinaemia D/periodic fever syndrome mevalonate kinase is also deficient, although to a lesser extent compared with the classic type of mevalonate kinase deficiency. Importantly, urinary mevalonic acid may be completely normal in these patients, which implies that diagnosis should be based on direct enzyme analysis in white blood cells, platelets, and/or fibroblasts.

Acatalasaemia

The diagnosis of acatalasaemia is not discussed here.

Laboratory diagnosis of peroxisomal disorders: prenatal diagnosis

In recent years reliable methods for the prenatal diagnosis of virtually all peroxisomal disorders have become available, in most cases employing cultured chorionic villus samples. For this specialized area, the reader is referred to the literature listed below.

Further reading

Aubourg P et al. (1986). Neonatal adrenoleukodystrophy. Journal of Neurology, Neurosurgery and Psychiatry 49, 77–86.

Elias ER et al. (1998). Developmental delay and growth failure caused by a peroxisomal disorder, dihydroxyacetonephosphate acyltransferase (DHAP-AT) deficiency. American Journal of Medical Genetics 80, 223–6.

Ferdinandusse S et al. (2000). Mutations in the gene encoding peroxisomal alpha-methylacyl-CoA racemase cause adult-onset sensory motor neuropathy. Nature Genetics 24, 188–91.

Goldfischer S et al. (1973). Peroxisomal and mitochondrial defects in the cerebro-hepato-renal syndrome. Science 182, 62–4.

Gould SJ, Valle D (2000). Peroxisome biogenesis disorders: genetics and cell biology. Trends in Genetics 16, 340–5.

Heymans HSA et al. (1985). Rhizomelic chondrodysplasia punctata: another peroxisomal disorder. New England Journal of Medicine 313, 187–8.

Houten SM et al. (1999). Mutations in MVK, encoding mevalonate kinase, cause hyperimmunoglobulinaemia D and periodic fever syndrome. Nature Genetics 22, 175–7.

Jansen GA et al. (2000). Human phytanoyl-CoA hydroxylase: resolution of the gene structure and the molecular basis of Refsum's disease. Human Molecular Genetics 9, 1195–200.

Kelley RI et al. (1986). Neonatal adrenoleukodystrophy: new cases, biochemical studies, and differentiation from Zellweger and related peroxisomal polydystrophy syndromes. American Journal of Medical Genetics 23, 869–901.

Lazarow PB, Moser HW (1995). Disorders of peroxisome biogenesis. In: Scriver CR et al., eds. The metabolic and molecular bases of inherited disease, 7th edn, pp 2287–324. McGraw-Hill, New York.

Martinez, M et al. (1994). Blood polyunsaturated fatty acids in patients with peroxisomal disorders. A multicenter study. Lipids 29, 273–80.

Moser HW, Smith KD, Moser AB (1995). X-linked adrenoleukodystrophy. In: Scriver CR et al., eds. The metabolic and molecular bases of inherited disease, 7th edn, pp 2325–49. McGraw-Hill, New York.

Ofman R et al. (1998). Acyl-CoA-dihydroxyacetonephosphate acyltransferase—cloning of the human cDNA and resolution of the molecular basis in rhizomelic chondrodysplasia punctata type 2. Human Molecular Genetics 7, 847–53.

Poll-The BT et al. (1987). Infantile Refsum disease: an inherited peroxisomal disorder. Comparison with Zellweger syndrome and neonatal adrenoleukodystrophy. European Journal of Pediatrics 146, 477–83.

Poll-The BT et al. (1988). A new peroxisomal disorder with enlarged peroxisomes and a specific deficiency of acyl-CoA oxidase (pseudo-neonatal adrenoleukodystrophy). American Journal of Human Genetics 42, 422–34.

Roels F, Espeel M, De Craemer D (1991). Liver pathology and immunocytochemistry in congenital peroxisomal diseases: a review. Journal of Inherited Metabolic Diseases 14, 853–75.

Schram AW et al. (1987). Human peroxisomal 3-oxoacyl-coenzyme A thiolase deficiency. Proceedings of the National Academy of Sciences of the USA 84, 2494–6.

Smith KD et al. (1999). X-linked adrenoleukodystrophy: genes, mutations, and phenotypes. Neurochemical Research 24, 521–35.

Spranger JW, Opitz JM, Bidder U (1971). Heterogeneity of chondrodysplasia punctata. Humangenetik 11, 190–212.

van Grunsven EG et al. (1999). Peroxisomal bifunctional protein deficiency revisited: resolution of its true enzymatic and molecular basis. American Journal of Human Genetics 64, 99–107.

Wanders RJA, Schutgens RBH, Barth PG (1995). Peroxisomal disorders: a review. Journal of Neuropathology and Experimental Neurology 54, 726–39.

Wanders RJA, Tager JM (1998). Lipid metabolism in peroxisomes in relation to human disease. Molecular Aspects of Medicine 19, 69–154.

Wanders RJA, van Grunsven EG, Jansen GA (2000). Lipid metabolism in peroxisomes: enzymology, functions and dysfunctions of the fatty acid alpha- and beta-oxidation systems in humans. Biochemical Society Transactions 28, 141–9.

Wanders RJA et al. (1988). Peroxisomal disorders in neurology. Journal of Neurological Sciences 88, 1–39.

Wanders RJA et al. (1992). Human dihydroxyacetonephosphate acyltransferase deficiency: a new peroxisomal disorder. Journal of Inherited Metabolic Diseases 15, 389–91.

Wanders RJA et al. (1994). Human alkyldihydroxyacetonephosphate synthase deficiency: a new peroxisomal disorder. Journal of Inherited Metabolic Diseases 17, 315–18.

Watkins PA et al. Peroxisomal bifunctional enzyme deficiency. Journal of Clinical Investigations 83, 771–7.

Wilson GN, Holmes RD, Custer J (1986). Zellweger syndrome: diagnostic assays, syndrome delineation and potential therapy. American Journal of Medical Genetics 24, 69–82.

11.10 Disorders of oxalate metabolism

Richard W. E. Watts and C. J. Danpure

Introduction—oxalate, hyperoxaluria, oxalosis

The oxalate anion is metabolically inert in humans and its overall metabolism can be represented by a single-compartment model in which the oxalate metabolic pool is a little larger than the extracellular fluid volume and contains approximately 10 to 30 µmol of oxalate. The system is normally in equilibrium but expansion of the oxalate metabolic pool occurs in renal failure and when there is either overproduction or overabsorption of oxalate. Tissue deposition of calcium oxalate (oxalosis) only occurs when renal failure is combined with one of these other factors. The normal plasma oxalate concentration is 1 to 3 µmol/l and shows a circadian rhythm, being lowest in the morning and highest in the evening with superimposed postprandial rises. The urinary excretion of oxalate does not normally exceed 450 µmol/24 h in adults. The results in children are similar if they are adjusted to a standard body surface area (1.73 m²), and adult levels are reached by about 14 years of age. The urinary excretion of oxalate also increases during the waking hours and shows seasonal variations related to dietary oxalate and calcium intakes; vitamin D supply also affects calcium absorption. The oxalate in the plasma and tissues is of dietary and biosynthetic origin. The following foods and beverages have particularly high oxalate contents: beets, beetroot, celery, chocolate, cocoa, nuts, rhubarb, strawberries, spinach, and tea. They provide about 0.8 to 1.7 mmol per day, of which, only about 5 per cent is absorbed depending upon the proportion that is in soluble form and the calcium content of the diet. Some dietary oxalate is degraded by gut commensal bacteria, for example *Oxalatobacter formigenes*. The main biosynthetic source of oxalate in humans is glycine; oxalate accounts for only about 1 per cent of the total glycine metabolic turnover, via the glyoxylate anion and the C_1–C_2 fragment of ascorbate.

Glycolate, hydroxyproline, serine and the sidechains of the aromatic amino acids have been shown to be minor metabolic precursors of oxalate in experimental animals. Negligible amounts of oxalate appear to be derived from carbohydrate and polyols (for example xylitol) under normal dietary conditions. The claim that the artificial sweetening agent diethylene glycol is converted to oxalate in humans has not been confirmed. The absorption of oxalate from the small intestine involves both an active carrier mediated transport system with oxalate–chloride exchange as well as passive diffusion.

The kidney handles the oxalate ion by 100 per cent filtration at the glomerulus, tubular secretion involving active tubular transport into the lumen, and passive backdiffusion into the peritubular capillaries. The ratio (oxalate clearance)/(glomerular filtration rate) is normally about 1.2, indicating net tubular secretion. Apart from acute oxalic acid poisoning, diseases attributable to oxalate present when calcium oxalate stones form in the urinary tract and when this salt crystallizes in either the renal parenchyma (calcium oxalate nephrocalcinosis) or in other tissues (oxalosis). The disorders of oxalate metabolism are due to either overproduction or excessive absorption of oxalate, although hyperoxaluria could, at least theoretically, arise from a renal tubular abnormality causing increased net renal tubular secretion of oxalate. Impaired renal function causes oxalate retention, and there is a linear relationship between the plasma oxalate and creatinine concentrations. However, the plasma oxalate concentration does not exceed the critical value (48.5 µmol/l) at which the solubility product of calcium oxalate in plasma is exceeded and oxalosis develops before endstage renal failure supervenes, unless there is also either oxalate overproduction, as in primary hyperoxalurias I and II, or oxalate hyperabsorption. Conversely, increased oxalate biosynthesis and hyperabsorption do not cause oxalosis unless recurrent oxalate urolithiasis and nephrocalcinosis have impaired renal function. The risk of oxalosis developing, as judged by rapidly rising plasma oxalate concentration and expansion of the oxalate metabolic pool, is greatly increased when the glomerular filtration rate decreases to about 25 ml/min/1.73 m². Hyperoxaluria is the hallmark of the disorders of oxalate metabolism and Table 1 lists its causes.

Primary hyperoxaluria type I
Epidemiology
The estimated prevalence of primary hyperoxaluria type I is about 10.5 per million inhabitants with an incidence of about 1 in 120 000 live births in

Table 1 The hyperoxalurias

Primary	
Type I	Hyperoxaluria due to hepatic peroxisomal alanine:glyoxylate aminotransferase (EC 2.6.1.44) deficiency. Associated with hyperglycolic aciduria in about 75 per cent of cases
Type II	Hyperoxaluria due to glyoxylate reductase (D-glycerate dehydrogenase, EC1.1.1.29) deficiency. Associated with L-glyceric aciduria in most cases
Type III	Hyperoxaluria not associated with any other abnormal organic aciduria. Possibly a heterogeneous group, some being due to intestinal hyperabsorption (primary absorptive hyperoxaluria) others may be due to as yet unidentified defects of renal tubule function or unidentified disorders of intermediary metabolism
Secondary	
Enteric	Jejunoileal ileal bypass
	Small intestine resection
	Blind loops
	Diffuse disease of the small intestine (e.g. Crohn's disease)
	Chronic pancreatic and biliary tract disease
Other	Oxalate ingestion (acute poisoning)
	Excessive intake of ascorbic acid
	Ethylene glycol (antifreeze) poisoning
	Adverse reaction of methoxyfluorane inhalation
	Adverse reaction to xylitol infusion
	Glycine irrigation (after transurethral prostatectomy)
	Aspergillus infection
	Cystic fibrosis (absence of *Oxalatobacter formigenes* from gut flora)
	Pyridoxine (vitamin B₆) deficiency

European countries. The prevalence and incidence are greater in countries with a higher consanguinity rate.

Biochemistry and molecular biology

Primary hyperoxaluria type I is an autosomal recessive disorder of glyoxylate metabolism caused by deficiency of the liver-specific peroxisomal pyridoxal phosphate-dependent enzyme alanine:glyoxylate aminotransferase (EC 2.6.1.44). In some cases the deficient alanine:glyoxylate aminotransferase activity can be augmented by administration of pyridoxine. Alanine:glyoxylate aminotransferase normally catalyses the conversion of the intermediary metabolite glyoxylate to glycine, but its absence in primary hyperoxaluria type I allows glyoxylate to be oxidized to oxalate and reduced to glycolate instead (Fig. 1). The elevated synthesis of oxalate and glycolate leads to the hyperoxaluria and hyperglycolic aciduria characteristic of primary hyperoxaluria type I. In some families, a pseudodominant pattern of inheritance is apparent due to the segregation of three, rather than two, mutant alleles. Primary hyperoxaluria type I is phenotypically heterogeneous at both the enzymic and clinical levels. Three major enzymic categories are recognized, characterized by:

(1) The absence of both alanine:glyoxylate aminotransferase catalytic activity and alanine:glyoxylate aminotransferase immunoreactive protein (ENZ–/CRM–).

(2) The absence of alanine:glyoxylate aminotransferase catalytic activity but the presence of alanine:glyoxylate aminotransferase immunoreactive protein (ENZ–/CRM+).

(3) The presence of both alanine:glyoxylate aminotransferase catalytic activity and alanine:glyoxylate aminotransferase immunoreactive protein (ENZ+/CRM+).

Many patients in the last category can have alanine:glyoxylate aminotransferase activities similar to those found in asymptomatic heterozygotes (Fig. 2). In most of these patients disease is caused by an unparalleled protein trafficking defect in which alanine:glyoxylate aminotransferase is mistargeted to the mitochondria, where it is unable to fulfil its metabolic function (i.e. glyoxylate transamination) properly.

Alanine:glyoxylate aminotransferase is encoded by the *AGXT* gene located on chromosome 2q37.3, where it spans about 10 kbases and consists of 11 exons and 10 introns. Numerous polymorphisms and mutations

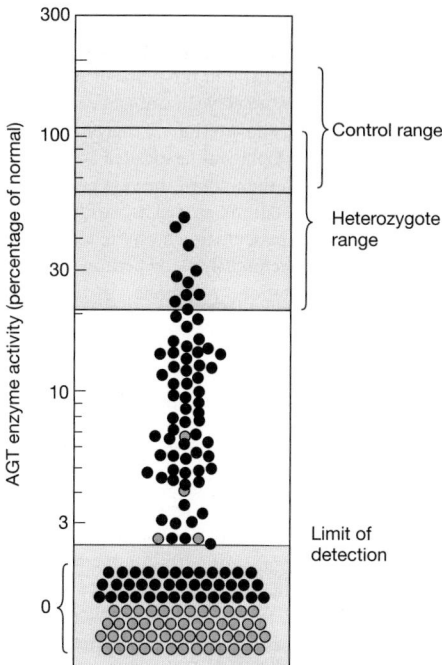

Fig. 2 Hepatic alanine:glyoxylate aminotransferase heterogeneity in patients with primary hyperoxaluria type I. Alanine:glyoxylate aminotransferase activity, expressed as a percentage of the mean normal control value, is shown for 162 patients with primary hyperoxaluria type I. Black circles, CRM+; grey circles, CRM–. Almost all patients with significant alanine:glyoxylate aminotransferase activity express the peroxisome-to-mitochondrion mistargeting phenotype.

have been identified at the *AGXT* locus; more details can be found in the review by Danpure (2001) listed in Further reading. The most common mutation found in primary hyperoxaluria type I, with an allelic frequency of 30 per cent, leads to a substitution of arginine for glycine at residue 170 and, in combination with a proline→leucine polymorphism at residue 11, is responsible for the peroxisome-to-mitochondrion mistargeting of alanine:glyoxylate aminotransferase.

Pathology

In the early stages, the pathological findings are confined to the kidney, which shows a variable degree of hydrocalycosis and hydronephrosis with multiple calculi. Nephrocalcinosis forms later, causing severe renal fibrosis and shrinkage, and the kidney feels tough and gritty when incised. Changes due to renal hypertension and recurrent pyelonephritis are often present, and the renal tubules may be blocked by aggregates of calcium oxalate crystals, particularly if the terminal illness has been associated with a hypotensive oliguric episode. The characteristic rosette-like calcium oxalate monohydrate crystals are highly birefringent and easily recognized under a polarizing microscope. Their full extent will only be observed if either unfixed tissues are examined or if non-aqueous fixatives are used, but they are usually sufficiently insoluble for some to remain and be apparent after routine fixation in formal saline. They are found most extensively in the myocardium, the tunica media of muscular arteries and arterioles, the rete testes, and at sites of rapid bone turnover. Careful examination reveals a few crystals associated with the arterial supply of all organs and tissues. Similar deposits have been found intra-axonally in peripheral nerves.

Clinical aspects

Patients usually present with recurrent urolithiasis in childhood, and if untreated die from renal failure before they are 20 years old. The terminal phase of rapidly progressing oliguric renal failure usually lasts, at most,

Hepatocyte

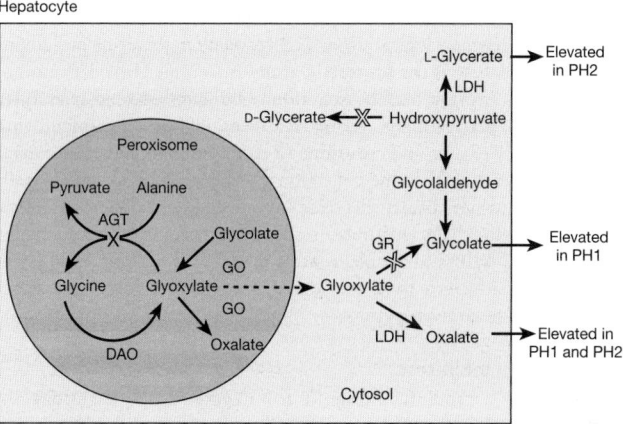

Fig. 1 Main pathways of glyoxylate metabolism in human liver cells. The black 'X' indicates the location of the defect in primary hyperoxaluria type I and the white 'X' indicates the same in primary hyperoxaluria type II: AGT, alanine:glyoxylate aminotransferase; GO, glycolate oxidase; DAO, D-amino acid oxidase; GR, glyoxylate reductase; LDH, lactate dehydrogenase. The peroxisomal membrane could be permeable to most or all of the metabolites shown. However, only the peroxisomal efflux of glyoxylate (dotted line) is shown to highlight the relationship between alanine:glyoxylate aminotransferase deficiency and the hyperoxaluria and hyperglycolic aciduria characteristic of primary hyperoxaluria type I.

only a few months and is associated with dense calcium oxalate nephrocalcinosis and with the development of systemic oxalosis. Ischaemic lesions occur on the extremities, particularly in the pulps of the fingers and toes, and are attributable to the extensive crystallization of calcium oxalate in the walls of small muscular arteries and arterioles. Progressive peripheral neuropathy and mononeuritis multiplex are associated with calcium oxalate deposition within axons and in the walls of the vasa nervorum. These vascular and neurological manifestations, as well as a wider range of oxalotic features, occur particularly in patients in whom the terminal renal failure has been treated by standard haemodialysis, by peritoneal dialysis, or by an unsuccessful renal transplantation. Additional manifestations include livedo reticularis, subcutaneous calcinosis which may ulcerate, retinal changes (white flecks, exudates, infarcts, yellow crystalline deposits, especially along the courses of the ophthalmic arteries, black 'geographic' lesions at the macula), dilated cardiomyopathy, cardiac conduction defects, synovitis, a painful osteodystrophy with dense osteosclerosis and skeletal deformation, stress fractures (especially in the vertebrae), and the changes of coincidental secondary and tertiary hyperparathyroidism.

Hyperoxaluria may present during the first months of life with seizures, advanced renal failure, and dense nephrocalcinosis but few if any calculi (the infantile type). Another small group (the adult type) follows a benign course, presenting in adult life and surviving into the fourth and fifth decade with only occasional stone formation. This latter type shows less elevation of urinary oxalate excretion than is usual in the group (juvenile type) which follows the typical clinical pattern. However, the amount of oxalate excreted and the age at which renal failure develops are not very closely correlated.

Although the usual clinical pattern is one of recurrent stones, with or without nephrocalcinosis leading inexorably to renal failure, a few patients present with severe uraemia and may give no history of urolithiasis. A few present with symptoms arising from oxalosis involving principally the heart, arteries, bones, and peripheral nerves. Considering this clinical grouping in relation to the patient's age, pyridoxine responsiveness, and the plasma and urine oxalate concentrations gives a clinical guide to prognosis.

Although the 'metabolic lesion' of primary hyperoxaluria type I is located in the peroxisome, it does not share any of the features of the other peroxisomal diseases. Similarly, patients in whom alanine:glyoxylate aminotransferase has been misrouted into mitochondria do not show evidence of mitochondrial disease (impaired fatty acid oxidation and disorders of function of the respiratory chain).

Diagnosis

Primary hyperoxaluria type I should be considered in any child with urinary stones or nephrocalcinosis and in adults with recurrent calcium oxalate stones for which no alternative explanation has been found, especially if the clinical history extends back into childhood. The presence of calcium oxalate crystals in the urinary centrifuged deposit is not a specific diagnostic sign; the 24-h urinary oxalate excretion must be measured chemically and related to the creatinine excretion. The urinary oxalate excretion can be misleadingly low in patients in advanced renal failure. About 75 per cent of patients have an associated hyperglycolic aciduria. The definitive diagnosis is made by assaying alanine:glyoxylate aminotransferase activity on a percutaneous needle biopsy of the liver, which can also be examined by immunoelectron microscopy to establish whether the enzyme protein is present and its intracellular location. It is now possible to combine this with an assay for hydroxypyruvate/glyoxylate reductase, which is essential for the diagnosis of primary hyperoxaluria type II, on the same biopsy tissue. Figure 2 shows the results of enzyme assays on patients, compared with the ranges obtained from carriers and other normals. The plasma oxalate concentration is determined when the patient is first evaluated and subsequently as a guide to prognosis and management. A progressively increasing plasma oxalate concentration indicates an increasing risk of oxalosis developing. A plasma oxalate value that is high relative to the corres-

Table 2 Diagnosis of oxalosis

Skeletal muscle biopsy: small arteries and arterioles
Bone marrow biopsy: sternal aspiration, iliac crest trephine
Soft tissue radiographs of hands
Skeleton:
    Radiographs
    $^{99}Tc^m$ hydroxymethylene diphosphonate
    Computed tomography scanning
    Bone density measurement
Joint aspiration
Arteriography
Peripheral nerve conduction
Heart:
    Electrocardiography
    Ambulatory monitoring
    Myocardial perfusion scanning (scintigraphy)
    Cardiac muscle biopsy

ponding creatinine is a valuable pointer to either oxalate overproduction or overabsorption. Early oxalosis is usually clinically silent. Some procedures that may be used to detect and evaluate it are listed in Table 2.

Prenatal diagnosis

Until a few years ago, prenatal diagnosis of primary hyperoxaluria type I was only possible by measuring alanine:glyoxylate aminotransferase activity in fetal liver biopsies in the second trimester. However, it is now possible to carry out the procedure in the first trimester by DNA (either mutation or polymorphism) analysis of material obtained from chorionic villi.

Treatment

Fluid and diet

Like all patients suffering from urinary stone disease those with primary hyperoxaluria type I should drink sufficient fluid to maintain a measured urine volume of 3 litres every 24 h with proportionately less in children. The diet should be low in oxalate and have minimum intakes of vitamins C and D, although this may need modification in children to meet the needs of growth and development.

Pyridoxine

The effect of pharmacological doses (150 to 1000 mg/day) of pyridoxine (pyridoxal phosphate is the prosthetic group in alanine:glyoxylate aminotransferase) on urinary oxalate excretion should be assessed over three 1-week periods, pretreatment, during treatment, and post-treatment, with assays of urinary oxalate and creatinine (a check for completeness of urine collection) on each 24-h urine collection . Smaller doses are occasionally effective. If the urinary oxalate decreases appreciably, pyridoxine should be continued indefinitely. A favourable response can probably be anticipated in between about 10 and 30 per cent of cases. The risks of pyridoxine-induced neuropathy have to be considered. Patients presenting in endstage renal disease may be given pyridoxine blindly.

Crystallization inhibitors

Citrates, either as sodium citrate (0.1–0.15 g/kg body weight/day) or equivalent doses of either sodium–potassium citrate (urolyte U Madaus®) or effervescent anhydrous sodium acid phosphate (phosphate Sandoz®) reduce the degree of urine calcium oxalate saturation. Neutral orthophosphates (equivalent to 2 g of elemental phosphorus per day) increase the excretion of pyrophosphate ions which inhibit heterogeneous calcium oxalate crystal nucleation, seeded growth, and aggregation. It also reduces calcium absorption. Magnesium supplements (for example 200 mg of magnesium oxide per day) also inhibit crystal growth and aggregation. The doses used should be sufficient to produce a material increase in either the urinary excretion of phosphate or magnesium. Phosphate and magnesium should be avoided if there is renal insufficiency. They may also produce diarrhoea.

Associated abnormalities

Coincidental urinary tract infections, hypercalciuria, and any urinary acidification defect should be treated vigorously on their merits. Excessive alkalization of the urine should be avoided because it may predispose to urinary tract infections and to the superimposition of phosphatic stones.

Treatment of urinary stones

Obstructive uropathy requires an immediate percutaneous nephrostomy to relieve the obstruction. Nephroscopic lithotomy, endoscopic lithotripsy with ultrasonic, electrohydraulic, and laser techniques, as well as extracorporeal shockwave lithotripsy, which produce relatively little damage to functioning kidney tissue, can be used to deal with asymptomatic stones. The kidneys should be kept as free from stones as possible and open lithotomy for large calculi should now rarely be needed. Stone debris may require either external drainage via a nephrostomy or internal drainage via a stent. However, stents and other foreign bodies in the urinary tract rapidly become encrusted with calcium oxalate deposits. Close follow-up is essential with regular radiological and/or ultrasonographic assessment. Patients who have previously passed stones often do so with little pain and unsuspected collections of stones may be found in the lower ureter on a routine abdominal radiograph. Acute hypotensive episodes are particularly dangerous causing intrarenal precipitation of calcium oxalate with acute and irreversible loss of renal function.

Transplantation

The oxalate ion has low dialysance and low filterability in the clinical context, and none of the currently available methods of replacing renal function can keep up indefinitely with the rate of oxalate overproduction once renal failure has occurred. Thus, almost all pyridoxine-resistant patients ultimately require orthotopic liver transplantation to correct the metabolic and genetic lesion together with a simultaneous renal transplant if they are approaching endstage renal disease. A small group of patients with relatively large amounts of residual catalytic enzyme activity may be suitable for an isolated renal graft. A renal transplant while the glomerular filtration rate is in the 15 to 20 ml/min/1.73 m^2 range may also be used to 'buy time' during which liver transplantation can be organized. The patient should be either haemodialysed or haemofiltered as vigorously as possible before, during, and after any grafting procedure in order to deplete the oxalate metabolic pool, minimize oxalosis, and reduce the risk to the grafted kidney.

Ideally, planning for liver and/or renal transplantation should begin when the glomerular filtration rate falls below 25 ml/min/1.73 m^2 (or 20 per cent of the mean predicted normal value) to minimize oxalosis and reduce the risk of oxalate deposits in the grafted kidney.

After a successful liver transplant the hyperglycolic aciduria returns to normal immediately. The plasma oxalate value normalizes over the course of a few weeks or months, and the urinary oxalate excretion returns to normal over the course of one or more years depending on the size of the oxalate deposits that are gradually mobilized from the tissues.

The plasma oxalate concentration should be followed sequentially before and after operation in these patients. Preoperatively, it is a guide to the extent to which the superimposition of oxalate retention on oxalate overproduction is occurring and hence to the rate at which the risk of oxalosis is increasing. Values approaching 35 µmol/l indicate that measures to reduce it are very urgently needed. Postoperatively, it is an indication of the risk of calcium oxalate damage to the grafted kidney.

Pre-emptive liver transplantation before renal failure has decreased to 25 ml/min/1.73 m^2 is an option if the disease is diagnosed early and is following an aggressive course. Partial orthotopic hepatic transplantation using tissue from a live related histocompatible donor has been proposed, but it is uncertain whether this would produce a clinically useful degree of metabolic correction. Heteroptic auxiliary liver transplantation is theoretically unsound. Although primary hyperoxaluria type I presents certain advantages as a candidate for gene therapy using retrovirus- or adenovirus-based constructs there has, as yet, been no definitive work in this area.

Primary hyperoxaluria type II

Primary hyperoxaluria type II is significantly rarer than primary hyperoxaluria type I and, as such, has been much less studied. Primary hyperoxaluria type II is caused by a deficiency of the widely-distributed enzyme glyoxylate reductase (EC 1.1.1.26/79, also known as hydroxypyruvate reductase and D-glycerate dehydrogenase, EC 1.1.1.29). Glyoxylate reductase catalyses a number of reactions, including the reduction of glyoxylate to glycolate and the reduction of hydroxypyruvate to D-glycerate (Fig. 1). Its absence in primary hyperoxaluria type II, however, allows glyoxylate to be oxidized to oxalate and hydroxypyruvate to be reduced to L-glycerate. The resulting increased synthesis of oxalate and L-glycerate, which leads to hyperoxaluria and hyper L-glyceric aciduria, is characteristic of primary hyperoxaluria type II.

Glyoxylate reductase is encoded by the GRHPR gene, which contains nine exons and eight introns, and spans about 9 kbases in the pericentromeric region of chromosome 9. A series of mutations in the GRHPR gene has been found in patients with primary hyperoxaluria type II. One case without hyper L-glyceric aciduria has been identified on the basis of immunoelectrophoresis. The clinical features, complications, and pathological findings are similar to those of primary hyperoxaluria type I. There have been no reports of possible biochemical and genetic heterogeniety of this disease. Enzyme replacement by organ transplantation has not been attempted in the type II disease, although if the liver proved to contain most of the complement of glyoxylate reductase activity, liver transplantation might be beneficial. The expression of the enzyme in leucocytes suggests that bone marrow transplantation from a fully histocompatible sibling might also be a therapeutic option.

Primary hyperoxaluria type III

Patients with primary hyperoxaluria type III, which has been attributed to oxalate hyperabsorption, do not have an associated hyperglycolic or L-glyceric aciduria and have, therefore, to be distinguished from the approximately 25 per cent of patients with primary hyperoxaluria type I with isolated hyperoxaluria. The diagnosis of primary hyperoxaluria type III rests on: firm evidence of normal intestinal anatomy, histology, and absorptive function; the demonstration of excessive oxalate absorption (this may be difficult to establish by the available ^{14}C-labelled oxalate absorption and/or oxalate loading tests); normal hepatic alanine:glyoxylate aminotransferase and glyoxylate reductase levels. The urinary oxalate excretion (usually 1–2 mmol/24 h) is similar to that in some patients with the other types of primary hyperoxaluria, and type III patients are at risk of urinary stones, renal failure, and oxalosis. The metabolic lesion has not been identified but it might involve an oxalate–chloride exchanger in the small intestine. It has been reported that thiazides reduce urinary oxalate excretion in primary hyperoxaluria type III. As in secondary hyperoxaluria due to diffuse small intestinal disease, treatment is by a low-oxalate diet with oxalate binding agents such a cholestyramine and calcium ions (given as calcium carbonate). A marine hydrocolloid preparation (ox-absorb®) has recently been developed as an intestinal oxalate binding therapeutic agent. Patients with primary hyperoxaluria type III may not be a homogeneous group and some may represent an as yet unidentified disorder of either glyoxylate or glycolate metabolism. Others may be due to deficient colonization of the gut by *Oxalatobacter formigenes*. Disorders of renal tubular function are also a theoretical possibility.

Enteric hyperoxaluria

Enteric hyperoxaluria is an uncommon but potentially serious complication of the diseases listed under this heading in Table 1. It can cause extensive urolithiasis with nephrocalcinosis and renal failure. Expansion of the oxalate pool has been demonstrated and there is the same potential for oxalosis developing as in the primary hyperoxalurias. Treatment depends upon reducing dietary oxalate intake, the use of oxalate binding agents, and correcting the steatorrhoea or abnormal gut flora in the case of cystic fibrosis.

Further reading

Allan AR *et al.* (1996). Selective renal transplantation in primary hyperoxaluria type I. *American Journal of Kidney Diseases* 27, 891–5.

Barratt TM, Danpure CJ (1996). Hyperoxaluria. In: Barratt TM, Avner ED, Harmon WE, eds. *Paediatric nephrology*, 4th edn, pp 609–24. Useful review with emphasis on paediatrics.

Cramer SD *et al.* (1999). The gene encoding hydroxypyruvate reductase (GRHPR) is mutated in patients with primary hyperoxaluria type II. *Human Molecular Genetics* 8, 2063–9. Report of new findings.

Danpure CJ, Jennings PR (1986). Peroxisomal alanine: glyoxylate aminotransferase deficiency in primary hyperoxaluria type I. *FEBS Lett.* 201, 20–4. First report of enzyme defect in primary hyperoxaluria type I.

Danpure CJ (2001). Primary hyperoxaluria. In: Scriver CR *et al*, eds. *The metabolic and molecular basis of inherited disease*, 8th edn, vol.II, ch. 133, pp 3323–67. McGraw-Hill, New York.

Danpure CJ, Rumsby G (1995). Enzymology and molecular genetics of primary hyperoxaluria type I. Consequences for clinical management. In: SR Khan, ed. *Calcium oxalate in biological systems*, pp 189–205 CRC, Boca Raton, FL.

Danpure CJ, Rumsby G (1996). Strategies for the prenatal diagnosis of primary hyperoxaluria type I. *Prenatal Diagnosis* 16, 587–98.

Danpure CJ, Smith LH (1996). The primary hyperoxalurias. In: Coe FL *et al.*, eds. *Kidney stones: medical and surgical management*, pp 859–81. Lippincott-Raven, Philadelphia. Review.

Danpure CJ *et al.* (1989). An enzyme trafficking defect in two patients with primary hyperoxaluria type I: peroxisomal alanine/glyoxylate aminotransferase re-routed to mitochondria. *Journal of Cell Biology* 108, 1345–52. Report of new findings.

Danpure CJ *et al.* (1989). Fetal liver alanine:glyoxylate aminotransferase and the prenatal diagnosis of primary hyperoxaluria type I. *Prenatal Diagnosis* 9, 271–81.

Danpure CJ *et al.* (1994). Primary hyperoxaluria type I: genotypic and phenotypic herogeneity. *Journal of Inherited Metabolic Disease* 17, 487–99. Review.

Danpure CJ *et al.* (1994). Molecular characterisation and clinical use of a polymorphic tandem repeat in an intron of the human alanine: glyoxylate aminotransferase gene. *Human Genetics* 94 55–64. Report of new findings.

Hoppe B *et al.* (1997). A vertical (pseudo-dominant) pattern of inheritance in the autosomal recessive disease primary hyperoxaluria type I. Lack of relationship between genotype, enzymic phenotype and disease severity. *American Journal of Kidney Disease* 29, 36–44.

Latta K *et al.* (1995). Selection of transplantation procedures and perioperative management in primary hyperoxaluria type I. *Nephrology, Dialysis and Transplantation* 10: [Supplement 8]: 53–57

McKusick VA. OMIMTM. Online Mendelian Inheritance in Man. wep//http://www.ncbi.nlm.nih.gov/Onim/

Purdue PE *et al.* (1991). An intronic duplication in the alanine: glyoxylate aminotransferase gene facilitates identification of mutations in compound heterozygote patients with primary hyperoxaluria type I. *Human Genetics* 87, 394–6.

Purdue PE *et al.* (1991). Characterization and chromosomal mapping of a genomic clone encoding human alanine: glyoxylate aminotransferase. *Genomics* 10, 34–42.

Purdue PE, Takada Y, Danpure CJ. (1990). Identification of mutations associated with peroxisome-to-mitochondrion mistargeting of alanine/glyoxylate aminotransferase in primary hyperoxaluria type I. *Journal of Cell Biology* 111, 2341–51.

Rumsby G, Creegeen D (1999). Identification and expression of a cDNA for human hydroxypyruvate/glyoxylate reductase. *Biochimica et Biophysica Acta* 1446, 383–8.

von Schnakenburg C, Rumsby G (1997). Primary hyperoxaluria type I: a cluster of new mutations in exon7 of the *AGXT* gene. *Journal of Medical Genetics* 34, 489–92.

Watts RWE (1994). Treatment of primary hyperoxaluria type I. *Journal of Nephrology* 7, 208–14.

Watts RWE (1997). Primary hyperoxaluria: In: Sessa A *et al.*, eds. *Contributions to nephrology*, Vol. 122, pp 143–59. Karger, Basel.

Watts RWE, Veall N, Purkiss P (1983). Sequential studies of oxalate dynamics in primary hyperoxaluria. *Clinical Science* 65, 627–33.

Williams HE, Smith LH Jr (1968). L-glyceric aciduria. A new genetic variant of primary hyperoxaluria. *New England Journal of Medicine* 278, 233–8.

Yent ER, Cahanim M (1983). Absorptive hyperoxaluria: a new clinical entity-successful treatment with hydrochlorathiazide. *Clinical and Investigative Medicine* 9, 44–50.

11.11 Disturbances of acid–base homeostasis

R. D. Cohen and H. F. Woods

In resting humans arterial blood, pH (pH_a) is normally maintained between 7.36 and 7.42, by control of the arterial partial pressure of CO_2 ($Paco_2$) and plasma bicarbonate, between the limits 4.7 to 5.8 kPa and 24 to 30 mmol/l, respectively. Intracellular pH is also controlled, but varies substantially between organs within the range 6.3 to 7.4, depending on prevailing physiological or pathological circumstances. Some intracellular organelles are particularly acid, notably lysosomes. There is a substantial daily burden of hydrogen ions (protons) derived principally from metabolism (Table 1), and disordered neutralization or elimination of this burden shifts pH in the acid direction. Inappropriate loss of protons or proton-generating substrates, or excessive input of alkali, shifts pH in the alkaline direction.

Extra- and intracellular buffers, notably haemoglobin, other proteins, bicarbonate, and phosphate, play a transient role in countering acute pH changes but normally the acid burdens listed in Table 1 are ultimately eliminated quantitatively or neutralized. These burdens have been grouped into three classes according to their mode of disposal. Carbon dioxide derived from cellular respiration is much the largest potential generator of protons, the burden in the resting subject being an order of magnitude greater than that resulting from lactic and other organic acid production as well as from urea synthesis. Protons derived from the metabolism of sulphur- and phosphorus-containing compounds constitute the smallest source and represent a burden that is about one-hundredth of that derived from carbon dioxide. Disposal of carbon dioxide is dependent on adequate respiratory function. The metabolism of sulphur-containing amino acids in the diet eventually results in the production of so-called fixed acids, namely sulphuric acid and phosphoric acid, which may originate from many sources. Neither of these acids is volatile and they are thus excreted by the kidney.

The organic acids listed in Table 1 have pK values much below that of blood pH. They are therefore present in the blood as acid anions, rather than as the undissociated acids. The equivalent amount of hydrogen ions, generated at the site of production of these acids, titrate with local tissue and blood bicarbonate and other buffers. The organic acid anions (lactate, 3-hydroxybutyrate, acetoacetate, and fatty acids) are non-volatile but, unlike the fixed acids, may be eliminated by metabolism. Figure 1 shows an example of the important principle that when these organic acid anions are metabolized to electroneutral products (e.g. glucose, or carbon dioxide and water) protons are consumed and the bicarbonate consumed at their site of production is regenerated. Protons from organic acids can also be eliminated in the urine, but normally this is a much slower process than the metabolic route. Particularly in the case of the ketone bodies, for which the renal threshold is relatively low, substantial amounts can be lost in the urine when their plasma concentration is elevated. Although in maximally acidified urine (pH 4.5) about half of the urinary ketone bodies are in the form of the undissociated acid, the remaining free anion moiety represents loss of potential alkali, since it eludes metabolism to bicarbonate.

Despite the large quantitative differences in the burden due to the three classes of acid shown in Fig. 1, their correct elimination is, in a sense, equally important, for no class is able substantially to be disposed of by a route normally used to eliminate another class. Normally, the rates of production and elimination of each class of acid are matched in a long-term steady state. The homeostasis of arterial blood pH thus provided is given quantitative expression in the Henderson–Hasselbalch equation:

$$pH_a = 6.1 + \log_{10}\{[HCO_3^-]_a/(0.225 \times Paco_2)\}$$

The constancy of arterial plasma bicarbonate concentration ($[HCO_3^-]_a$) is maintained by the removal of class I and II acids and by proton generation

Table 1 Production and elimination of hydrogen ions

Class	Daily production (mol)	Source	Excreted by lungs	Metabolic removal possible	Normal main organs of elimination
I CO_2	15	Tissue	Yes	Very minor	Lungs
II Organic acids and urea synthesis					
Lactate	1.2	Many tissues	No	Yes	Liver (50–70%), kidneys
Ketoacids[a]	0.6	Liver	No	Yes	Most tissues, urine
Free fatty acids	0.7	Adipose tissue	No	Yes	Most tissues
H^+ generated during urea synthesis	1.1[b]	Liver	No	Yes	Liver and other tissues
III 'Fixed' acids					
Sulphuric	0.1	Dietary sulphur-containing amino acids	No	No	Urinary excretion
Phosphoric		Organic phosphate metabolism	No	No	

The daily production rates for the organic acids are calculated from data in resting, 70-kg men after an overnight fast, and are proportioned up to 24 h.
[a]Because of food ingestion during the daytime, the values for the ketoacids (3-hydroxybutyric and acetoacetic) may be overestimates.
[b]On a 100g protein diet.

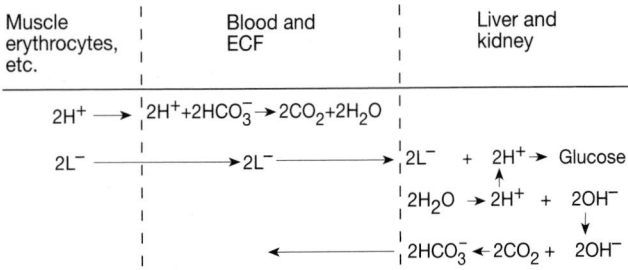

Fig. 1 A scheme, using lactate (L⁻) conversion to glucose as an example, showing how conversion of the anion of an organic acid of low pK to an electroneutral substance consumes H⁺ and regenerates HCO_3^-.

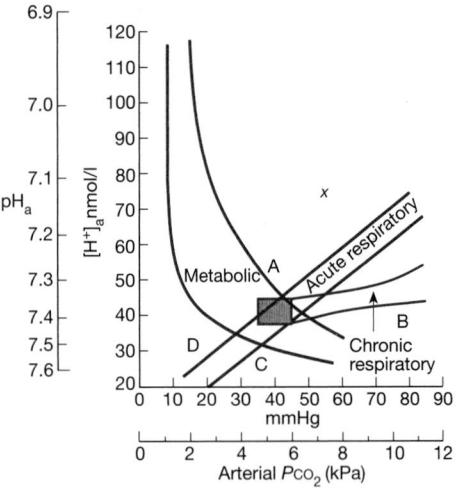

Fig. 2 A practical acid–base diagram. For explanation see text.

during ureagenesis (see below) and that of Pa_{CO_2} by the lungs, thereby fixing pH_a within a narrow range.

The roles of the kidneys and liver in acid–base homeostasis

The interplay of these organs in acid–base homeostasis has been a matter of controversy. The authors' view is that the contribution of the kidneys is not entirely what it has appeared to be, and that the role of the liver requires emphasis. Classical descriptions are based on the kidneys as the principal controllers of $[HCO_3^-]$. Yet, as may be seen in Table 1, the liver is responsible for the major part of lactate disposal and consequent bicarbonate regeneration as well as the generation of ketoacids, with the opposite acid–base consequence. There is, however evidence that both these hepatic functions are normally controlled in an attempt to preserve acid–base homeostasis. Thus at normal concentrations of blood lactate, deviations in the acid direction enhance hepatic lactate disposal. As will be seen in the case of lactate, the homeostasis may be lost at higher concentrations of lactate. Ketogenesis is itself suppressed by increasing acidosis.

Urea production is another important feature of hepatic metabolism. The production of each molecule of urea (ultimately from ammonium and carbon dioxide) is accompanied by the generation of two protons. Ureagenesis is therefore a potential acidifying mechanism. Most of the protons produced in ureagenesis are neutralized by the bicarbonate generated during the oxidation of the carbon skeleton of amino acids, but normally there is a slight excess of protons produced, which have to be eliminated by the kidneys. Urea synthesis and accompanying proton production are negatively regulated by acidosis, which constitute another acid–base regulatory system intrinsic to the liver.

The renal tubules secrete protons and those not involved in the process of bicarbonate reabsorption are buffered by urinary phosphate. Under normal conditions, about 30 mmol/day of protons are excreted in this way. Classically, urinary ammonia (NH_3) is regarded as another buffer for hydrogen ions, which are therefore removed as ammonium (NH_4^+); normally the excretion of hydrogen ions in the supposed NH_4^+ buffer amounts to about 70 mmol/day, but may increase to 500 mmol/day under severe acidifying stress in maximally acidified urine. It is, however, not possible to reconcile this view with the physicochemical fact that the ammonia/ammonium equilibrium is almost entirely in the form of ammonium at the time of generation from glutamine, and is therefore not available for buffering further protons. A more plausible explanation of the role of the kidneys is that the increase in ammonium excretion during acidosis serves to divert nitrogen from hepatic urea synthesis and consequent proton production, thus countering the acidosis.

These considerations provide a background to the interpretation of many acid–base syndromes described below.

Acid–base disorders

Definitions

The terminology of acid–base disturbances has always been confused. The terms acidaemia and alkalaemia simply indicate that pH_a is lower or higher than the normal range. Here we use the term acidosis to encompass both the situation where pH_a is low, and also that in which, although pH_a is normal, it would have been lowered if compensatory mechanisms had not occurred; an equivalent definition applies to alkalosis. When the primary disturbance is related to abnormal carbon dioxide elimination, the disturbance is referred to as 'respiratory'. All other primary disturbances, that is those related to disturbances of class II or III acid production or removal, are referred to as 'metabolic' or 'non-respiratory'. The term 'primary' is used to distinguish these processes from those which are compensatory in nature. Thus primary metabolic acidosis, lowering $[HCO_3^-]_a$, is compensated for by hyperventilation, which decreases Pa_{CO_2}; respiratory acidosis, driven by elevation of Pa_{CO_2}, is compensated for by metabolic events which result in an elevation of $[HCO_3^-]_a$.

The diagnosis of acid–base disturbances

Since the clinical manifestations of acid–base disturbances, described later, are frequently non-specific and may not be apparent until the disturbance is quite severe, laboratory investigation is indispensable. Measurement of pH_a, Pa_{CO_2}, and $[HCO_3^-]_a$ on arterial blood is the primary investigation. Estimation of plasma urea, creatinine, sodium, potassium, and chloride, and, when appropriate, lactate, ketoacids, and salicylate provides further important information.

Measurement of pH_a and Pa_{CO_2}—acid–base diagram

Blood gas analysers measure pH and P_{CO_2} and calculate plasma bicarbonate from the Henderson–Hasselbalch equation. Interpretation of results is best achieved by the use of an acid–base diagram which has pH_a and Pa_{CO_2} as its axes. Diagrams which use $[HCO_3^-]_a$ on one of the axes are less suitable, since $[HCO_3^-]_a$ is calculated from pH_a and Pa_{CO_2} and is not only subject to compounding errors in those measurements, but is affected by some poorly understood variations in pK_a in the Henderson–Hasselbalch equation in blood from severely ill patients.

The acid–base diagram in Fig. 2 has bands drawn in to show the ranges of data expected in uncomplicated acid–base disorders. It not only aids the diagnosis of acid–base disorders, but in addition the course of an individual patients disturbance and its response to treatment can be followed by serial plotting of data. The shaded square represents the approximate limits of pH$_a$ and Paco$_2$ in normal individuals. Thus a patient with uncomplicated metabolic acidosis will have values lying in the band marked 'metabolic' in the region above and to the left of the normal zone; the 'metabolic' band is the envelope of measurements of pH$_a$ and Paco$_2$ in patients with uncomplicated metabolic acidosis and alkalosis. The metabolic band is rather restricted on the alkalotic side, below and to the right of the normal zone. This is because compensation by hypoventilation for metabolic alkalosis is often poor; hypoxia may limit the degree of hypoventilation and metabolic alkaloses may be associated with intracellular acidosis, which could stimulate the respiratory centre. Marked hypocapnia is, however, occasionally seen in metabolic alkalosis.

The band marked 'acute respiratory' is the 95 per cent confidence range of values obtained in normal individuals voluntarily hyperventilating or breathing air carbon dioxide mixtures for short periods. After a few days of carbon dioxide retention, an increase in plasma bicarbonate produces substantial or complete compensation for the respiratory acidosis; the band in chronic respiratory acidosis is therefore different from the acute response, the presence of the extra bicarbonate decreasing the fall in pH$_a$ expected for a given rise in Paco$_2$.

pH$_a$ and Paco$_2$ measurements in some patients will not fall within any of the defined bands in Fig. 2. Such patients have a mixture of acid–base disorders. Thus a patient whose pH$_a$ and Paco$_2$ are represented by the point '×' has mixed respiratory and metabolic acidosis, for example a patient with uraemic acidosis and an exacerbation of chronic bronchitis with respiratory failure. pH$_a$ and Paco$_2$ values lying in sectors A and C result from a combination of two primary acid–base conditions; in sectors B and D one of the two disturbances might be compensatory for the other.

Acid–base analytical equipment usually also provides at least two additional derived acid–base variables—the standard bicarbonate and base excess or deficit. The standard bicarbonate represents what the plasma bicarbonate would be if the blood had the normal Paco$_2$ of 5.33 kPa (40 mmHg) rather than its actual value. Standard bicarbonate was introduced in an attempt to provide a measurement which was independent of respiratory disturbance and thus indicative of the underlying pure metabolic disturbance. Base deficit represents the amount of alkali in mmol needed to restore the pH of 1 litre of the patient's blood *in vitro* to normal (pH 7.4) at a Pco$_2$ of 5.33 kPa, and might at first sight be considered a quantitative measure of metabolic acidosis. Unfortunately the titration curve of blood *in vitro* is different from when it is circulating *in vivo*, since in the latter situation the interstitial and intracellular fluids also interact in the titration and may gain or lose bicarbonate from it; in addition, their buffering capacity differs from that of blood. These considerations detract from the usefulness of base excess/deficit as a guide either to diagnosis or therapy.

Further difficulties arise from ambiguities in the interpretation of base excess/deficit. Thus a patient with chronic respiratory acidosis will have a high standard bicarbonate and a base excess due to compensatory increase of plasma bicarbonate. It could be said, therefore, that this patient has simultaneously a respiratory acidosis and a metabolic alkalosis, as a base excess indicates the latter. This way of regarding the situation seems to us confusing and is incompatible with the definitions of acidosis and alkalosis we have given, which are intended to indicate the direction of the primary disturbance.

Use of the anion gap

In measurements of plasma electrolytes, the sum of the cations ($Na^+ + K^+$) normally exceeds that of the anions ($Cl^- + HCO_3^-$) by about 14 mmol/l (reference range 10–18 mmol/l). This difference is known as the anion gap and in health is attributable largely to the net negative charge on plasma proteins, but also to phosphate, sulphate, and several organic acids. Calculation of the anion gap is of great value in the differential diagnosis of metabolic acidosis, but the regrettably increasingly common practice of omitting chloride estimation from sets of plasma electrolytes frequently deprives the clinician of this important diagnostic tool.

Metabolic acidoses may be divided broadly into those with high and those with normal anion gap. Metabolic acidoses with high anion gap are due to the ingestion or endogenous generation of acids, usually organic, whose anions are not measured in routine sets of plasma electrolytes. Plasma bicarbonate is titrated by these acids and therefore decreases; the anion gap is thus widened by the presence of these unmeasured anions. The most frequent organic acids concerned are lactic and ketoacids. In uraemic acidosis, the anion gap seldom exceeds 28 mmol/l. but considerably higher values may be found in severe lactic acidosis and ketoacidosis. It should be noted that there are causes of raised anion gap other than metabolic acidosis, for example therapy with sodium salts of relatively strong acids (e.g. lactate, acetate) and high-dose sodium carbenicillin treatment.

Metabolic acidoses with normal anion gap are due to the direct loss of bicarbonate from the body, either through the gut or fistulae, through the kidney, or, rarely, to the ingestion or infusion of acid or acidifying substances. When bicarbonate is lost, more chloride is retained by the renal tubules; thus low plasma bicarbonate is accompanied by hyperchloraemia and the anion gap remains unchanged.

Causes of acid–base disturbance

Table 2 classifies those conditions associated with high anion gap metabolic acidosis by the principal organic acid involved. Often a mixture of acids is involved but where possible the predominant acid has been shown in italics. Normal anion gap metabolic acidoses are shown in Table 3, classified according to whether they are due to gut or renal bicarbonate loss, or to ingestion or infusion of acidifying agents. Metabolic alkalosis (Table 4) is due either to ingestion or infusion of excessive alkali in circumstances when it cannot be excreted (e.g. poor renal function), or to the secretion of urine which is inappropriate both in its acidity and in its ammonium content. Most of the causes of the latter occurrence are related to the complex events in potassium and chloride deficiency and are dealt with later, as is the pathogenesis of the metabolic alkalosis of acute hepatic failure. Table 5 classifies respiratory acidosis according to the level of the problem, namely, the lungs and airways, the neuromuscular and mechanical aspects of respiration, and the central nervous system. Except in the case of deliberate or inadvertent external hyperventilation, respiratory alkalosis is always due to some form of stimulus to the respiratory centre, as classified in Table 6.

The effects of acid–base disturbances

These are widespread and we limit ourselves here to a brief description of those with known clinical consequences.

Respiratory effects

Both metabolic acidosis and acute respiratory acidosis induced by breathing high Pco$_2$ gas mixtures result in hyperventilation. Deep sighing respiration (Kussmaul breathing) is a familiar sign of metabolic acidosis. pH control of ventilation is determined by the pH perceived by the carotid and aortic body chemoreceptors and by receptors in the medulla, which appear to monitor the pH of brain extracellular fluid. In the steady state, brain extracellular fluid pH is closely similar to that of cerebrospinal fluid. Sudden development of metabolic acidosis, resulting in low pH$_a$ and arterial bicarbonate, induces hyperventilation by stimulating the carotid body and aortic chemoreceptors and Paco$_2$ is thus lowered. However, the first effect on brain extracellular fluid pH is to raise it. This is because brain extracellular fluid Pco$_2$ is lowered since carbon dioxide is rapidly equilibrated across the blood–brain barrier. However, it takes many hours for the brain extracellular fluid bicarbonate to fall in response to the lowering of plasma bicarbonate, because movement of bicarbonate across the barrier is much slower than that of carbon dioxide. The temporary alkalinization of brain extracellular fluid somewhat offsets the extra ventilatory drive from the carotid and aortic chemoreceptors, so the hyperventilatory compensatory response takes some hours to reach its maximum. Though clinical circumstances usually prevent the observation of this sequence of events, the opposite, namely persistence of hyperventilation after restoration of nor-

Table 2 High anion gap metabolic acidoses

Condition	Associated plasma anions[a]
Predominant ketoacidosis	
Diabetic ketoacidosis	*3-hydroxybutyrate*, acetoacetate, lactate
Starvation ketoacidosis	*3-hydroxybutyrate*, acetoacetate
Alcoholic ketoacidosis	*3-hydroxybutyrate*, acetoacetate, lactate
Ketotic hypoglycaemia of childhood	*3-hydroxybutyrate*, acetoacetate, lactate
Predominant lactic acidosis	
Type A lactic acidosis	
Exercise	*Lactate*
Postepileptic	*Lactate*
Shock (traumatic, haemorraghic, cardiogenic, septic)	*Lactate*
Severe hypoxia, including acute pulmonary oedema	*Lactate*
Type B lactic acidosis	
Biguanide associated (phenformin, metformin, buform)	*Lactate*
Ethanol-associated	*Lactate*
Following recovery from diabetic ketoacidosis	*Lactate*
Fructose, sorbitol, or xylitol infusion	*Lactate*
Severe *P. falciparum* malaria	*Lactate*
Fulminant hepatic necrosis, severe liver disease	*Lactate*
Leukaemia and reticuloses	*Lactate*
Paracetamol poisoning	*Lactate*
Associated with sodium nitroprusside therapy	*Lactate*
Thiamine deficiency, acute beri-beri	Lactate
D(-)-lactic acidosis	*D(-)-lactate*
Short gut syndromes, jejunoileal bypass	
Lactobacillus ingestion	
Type 1 glycogenosis (hepatic glucose 6-phosphatase deficiency)	*Lactate*
Hepatic fructose 1,6-bisphosphatase deficiency	*Lactate*
Associated with mitochondrial myopathies and encephalomyopathies	*Lactate*
Treatment with nucleoside reverse transcriptase inhibitors	
Inherited syndromes e.g. MELAS	
Inherited or acquired single or multiple carboxylase deficiencies	*Lactate*, other organic acid anions
Conditions with mixed or ill-defined source of acidosis	
Uraemic acidosis	Phosphate, sulphate, etc.
Salicylate poisoning (acidotic phase)	Salicylate, ketoacids, lactate
Methanol poisoning	Formate, lactate
Ethylene glycol poisoning	Lactate, glycolate, oxalate
Paraldehyde poisoning	?
Reye's syndrome	Lactate, ?
Jamaican vomiting sickness	?
Numerous inherited organic acidurias	Various

[a]The predominant anion is shown in italics.

Except when otherwise stated, lactate refers to the L(+)-isomer

Table 3 Normal anion gap metabolic acidoses

Gastrointestinal bicarbonate loss
Diarrhoea
Pancreatic fistula
Ureteroenterostomy
Renal causes
Renal tubular acidosis type 1(gradient type)
   primary
      transient infantile type
      permanent (childhood or adult)
   secondary
      hypergammaglobulinaemia, amphotericin B therapy, autoimmune states
      vitamin D intoxication, hyperthyroidism, carnitine palmitoyl transferase
      I deficiency
Renal tubular acidosis type 2 (bicarbonate wastage)
   primary
      isolated, idiopathic Fanconi's syndrome
   secondary
      hyperthyroidism, vitamin D deficiency, outdated tetracycline, uraemia
      (occasionally), myeloma, Sjögren's syndrome, heavy metal poisoning
      hereditary disorders—cystinosis, Wilson's disease, fructose intolerance,
      galactosaemia, Lowe's syndrome
      treatment with carbonic anhydrase inhibitors
Renal tubular acidosis type 4
   hypoaldosteronism, aldosterone insensitivity, hyporeninaemia, diabetes
   mellitus, pyelonephritis, pseudohypoaldosteronism (Types I and II), non-
   steroidal anti-inflammatory agents, angiotensin converting enzyme
   inhibitors
   moderate renal insufficiency
Ingestion or infusion of acidifying agents
ammonium chloride, arginine hydrochloride, hydrochloric acid, intravenous
feeding with solutions containing excess basic amino acids
Rapid intravenous hydration (dilutional acidosis)

mal pH during therapy of metabolic acidosis is commonly seen, and may last for over 24 h.

In chronic respiratory failure, with high $Pa{CO_2}$, direct depression of the respiratory centre occurs; the respiratory response to increments of $Pa{CO_2}$ is progressively lost and ventilation becomes increasingly dependent on hypoxic drive. Alkalosis also may depress respiration and increases the difficulties of weaning artificially ventilated patients from the respirator.

Cardiovascular effects

Acidosis decreases cardiac contractility (negative inotropism) and alkalosis has smaller but opposite effects. Acidosis and alkalosis both predispose to cardiac arrythmias. The negative inotropic effects are particularly related to changes in myocardial intracellular pH and are experimentally found to

Table 4 Causes of metabolic alkaloses

Ingestion or infusion of alkali in excess of excretion
Milk-alkali syndrome
Alkaline overshoot during therapy of lactic acidosis or diabetic ketoacidosis

Loss of acid inappropriately (gastric or renal routes)
Pyloric stenosis, self-induced persistent vomiting
Potassium depletion other than in renal tubular acidosis or laxative abuse
Chloride depletion
Hyperaldosteronism, primary or secondary

Contraction alkalosis
Rapid diuresis
Other causes of mild extracellular fluid depletion

Failure of ureagenesis
Fulminant hepatic failure

Table 5 Causes of respiratory acidosis

Structural and mechanical pulmonary disease
Chronic obstructive pulmonary disease
Severe asthma
Large airway obstruction

Neuromuscular and mechanical problems
Acute ascending polyneuritis (Guillain–Barre)
Poliomyelitis
Acute porphyria
Myasthenia gravis
Motor neurone disease
Muscular dystrophies
Traumatic flail chest
Ankylosing spondylitis
Severe kyphoscoliosis
Gross obesity, sleep apnoea syndromes
Muscle relaxant drugs

Respiratory centre disorders
Organic disease affecting respiratory centre
Respiratory depressant drugs
Respiratory arrest

be rather greater in acute respiratory than in acute metabolic acidosis. In the rat, progressive metabolic acidosis reduces cardiac output as a result of bradycardia and negative inotropy; there is consequent hypotension and decreased renal and hepatic blood flow. This sequence of events may provide a model for the circulatory collapse which often occurs in patients after some hours of metabolic acidosis not originally attributable to shock. Mild to moderate metabolic acidosis has not often been associated with negative inotropic effects in the intact animal; this appears to be due to the protective effects of catecholamine release, which is increased in acidosis. In more severe acidosis, this protection breaks down. Patients receiving β-blockers may be more susceptible to the negative inotropic effects of acidosis.

Cerebral arterioles are very sensitive to the pH of brain extracellular fluid; they dilate when this falls and constrict when the pH rises. The cerebrovascular resistance is thus subject to the same type of phased responses to acid–base disturbances as described above for ventilation. Dilatation is also the response of most systemic arterioles to acidosis, although this response may be modified by catecholamine effects. The peripheral veins, however, constrict in acidosis, resulting in a shift of blood from the peripheral capacitance vessels to the central circulation. This effect has been

Table 6 Causes of respiratory alkalosis

Spontaneous or psychogenic hyperventilation
Reflex hyperventilation (e.g. pulmonary embolism)
Other stimuli to respiratory centre
    Via chemoreceptors
        low inspired oxygen concentration (e.g. high altitude)
        alveolo-capillary diffusion block (e.g. fibrosing alveolitis)
        right-to-left shunt
        carbon monoxide poisoning
    Via drugs or metabolites
        salicylate poisoning
        acute liver failure, chronic liver disease
    Persistent hyperventilation after recovery from metabolic
        acidosis
    Local lesion affecting respiratory centre
Overventilation during anaesthesia or assisted ventilation

shown to have important clinical consequences during treatment (see below).

Effects on intermediary carbohydrate metabolism

In all tissues in which observations have been made, glycolysis is inhibited by acidosis and stimulated by alkalosis, due to the effects of intracellular pH on phosphofructokinase, a rate-limiting enzyme of glycolysis. Respiratory alkalosis might therefore be expected to raise blood lactate but this effect is usually small, probably due to removal of lactate by the liver. However, in the presence of severe liver disease, gross elevation of blood lactate may be seen in association with respiratory alkalosis, and the increased production of lactate may partially compensate for the alkalosis.

Animal studies have shown that hepatic gluconeogenesis from lactate is inhibited by acidosis due to an effect on the metabolic step between pyruvate and oxaloacetate. This phenomenon may override the stimulatory effect on hepatic lactate disposal described earlier and may be responsible for perpetuating and worsening lactic acidosis.

Effects on nitrogen balance

Chronic acidosis produces negative nitrogen balance, mainly due to accelerated proteolysis in skeletal muscle. This effect is mediated through increased expression of the genes coding for ubiquitin and proteasome subunits.

Effects on blood oxygen uptake and delivery to the tissues

One of the factors determining blood uptake of oxygen during passage through the lungs, and subsequent delivery of oxygen to the tissues, is the position of the blood oxygen dissociation curve with respect to the abscissa (P_{O_2}). Right shifts of this curve improve unloading of oxygen in the tissues, but under some circumstances may impair oxygen uptake in the lungs. Left shifts have the opposite effect. The position of the curve is determined by three haemoglobin ligands, namely hydrogen ions, carbon dioxide, and 2,3-bisphosphoglycerate (2,3-BPG). Increases in all of these shift the curve to the right. Changes in intraerythrocytic pH and P_{CO_2} are often rapid, but those of 2,3-BPG are much slower. In chronic acidosis, the synthesis of 2,3-BPG is inhibited and marked reductions in the erythrocyte content of this metabolite may occur, with opposite effects in alkalosis. These changes are, however, slow in comparison with the immediate effects of changes in pH and P_{CO_2} (the Bohr effect).

The effect of these differences in time scale on oxygen delivery gives rise to a characteristic sequence of events during the development and treatment of acute metabolic acidosis. Initially, the acute acidosis causes a right shift of the curve, and thus improved oxygen release to the tissues. After several hours, erythrocyte 2,3-BPG falls, thus restoring the position of the curve towards normal. If the patient is now rapidly treated with alkali, the Bohr effect results in rapid shift to a position to the left of normal, because of the low level of 2,3-BPG. The resulting sudden deterioration of oxygen release may have adverse clinical effects unless the consequences of left shift are ameliorated by other factors, such as an increase in tissue blood flow. It may be many hours or days before erythrocyte 2,3-BPG concentrations are restored to normal.

Effects on the nervous system

Severe acidosis is frequently associated with impairment of consciousness, varying from mild drowsiness to coma. This effect is not closely related to systemic pH, and the mechanism is poorly understood. The effects on the respiratory and cardiovascular centres have been discussed above. The excitability of neural and muscular tissues is increased by alkalosis and diminished by acidosis. Tetany is a common feature of respiratory alkalosis, and may also be seen when chronic metabolic acidosis is corrected in patients with hypocalcaemia, a sequence of events which may occur in chronic renal failure. Epileptic attacks in susceptible individuals may be precipitated by alkalosis and suppressed by acidosis.

Effects on potassium homeostasis

Acute acidosis results in a shift of potassium out of the intracellular compartment into the extracellular fluid. Hyperkalaemia is thus often seen in the acidosis of renal failure, untreated diabetic ketoacidosis, and in acute respiratory failure; its mechanism is not entirely clear, factors other than extracellular pH being implicated. Alkali therapy in such patients causes a shift of potassium back into cells. As substantial amounts of potassium may be lost in the urine during the period of hyperkalaemia, overall depletion of body potassium occurs; thus alkali therapy may result in a rapid fall of plasma potassium to dangerous levels. This is a well-known hazard in the treatment of diabetic ketoacidosis and is even more dangerous in types 1 and 2 renal tubular acidosis in which plasma potassium is frequently low in the presence of acidosis (see also under Treatment below).

Chronic metabolic alkalosis is also frequently accompanied by potassium depletion, which results from distal tubular potassium secretion uninhibited by competition with hydrogen ions for secretion.

Effects on the kidney

The kidney is a major organ of acid–base regulation and many of its responses are therefore geared to acid–base homeostasis. Proton secretion is a principal function of tubular cells and in the proximal tubule is a crucial part of the mechanism for the apparent reabsorption of the large quantities of bicarbonate filtered at the glomerulus. In the cortical and medullary collecting tubules, where the main acidification of the urine takes place, the intercalated cell is equipped with the H^+-ATPase, residing in the apical (luminal) membrane, and the band 3 general anion exchanger, in the basolateral membrane. Under acid conditions H^+ and bicarbonate are generated by carbonic anhydrase within these intercalated cells. The protons are secreted into the lumen, where they titrate the phosphate buffer, or convert any bicarbonate present into carbon dioxide and water; the bicarbonate is transported by the anion exchanger in the opposite direction into the blood stream. There is now evidence of considerable plasticity of function of these cells so that in alkaline conditions the polarity of transporter expression is reversed, with the H^+-ATPase now predominating in the basolateral membrane and the anion exchanger in the luminal membrane, secreting bicarbonate into the urine. The maximum urinary pH thereby achieved is about 8.0.

As indicated earlier, there is a large increase in renal ammonium production and excretion in the urine in acidosis. The ammonium ions are derived from glutamine by the action of glutaminase in the proximal tubule; they are mainly secreted by pH-dependent non-ionic diffusion into the collecting tubule lumen, where the blood-lumen pH gradient is the greatest in acidosis. Chronic acidosis results in an increased expression of glutaminase and phosphoenolpyruvate carboxykinase. The latter enzyme is rate-limiting for gluconeogenesis, and an increase in renal gluconeogenesis is thought to play a crucial role in the high rate of ammonium production. A reinterpretation of the role of increased ammonium excretion in acidosis has been discussed above.

Effects on the distribution of metabolites and drugs

Many weak acids and bases are distributed between body compartments by the simple physicochemical process of pH-dependent non-ionic diffusion, which is based on movement of the non-dissociated hydrophobic moiety across the lipid membranes separating compartments, quite independently of any transporter. The pH differences between the compartments will determine the relative concentrations in the two spaces at equilibrium. Weak acids accumulate in the more alkaline compartment and weak alkalis in the more acid compartment. Examples of physiological metabolites distributed by this mechanism include ammonia/ammonium (weak base) and urobilinogen (weak acid). The distribution of ammonium and other amines present in advanced liver disease between blood and cerebrospinal fluid is partly determined in this way. Examples of drugs exhibiting this behaviour are salicylates and phenobarbitone (weak acids); use of their

pH-dependent distribution is made in the treatment of poisoning with these drugs by forced alkaline diuresis.

Effects on bone

Bone acts as a buffer in chronic metabolic acidosis. Leaching out of bone calcium carbonate and exchange of extracellular phosphate for carbonate within the apatite crytal result in the neutralization of protons. The first of these mechanisms causes a negative calcium balance in chronic metabolic acidosis and in chronic uraemic acidotic subjects it has been shown that calcium balance can be restored by treatment with sodium bicarbonate. Although chronic metabolic acidosis in rats results in osteoporosis, renal tubular acidosis and the acidosis associated with ureterosigmoidostomy may lead to osteomalacia, which can be corrected by alkali therapy alone.

Effects on leucocytes

Severe acidosis is often associated with marked leucocytosis, unrelated to the presence of infection. Blood leucocyte counts of up to 60 000/mm^3 have been recorded in lactic acidosis and high values are also common in diabetic ketoacidosis. This phenomenon may be partly a specific reaction to acidosis and not merely a general manifestation of stress or dehydration.

Major acid–base syndromes

Lactic acidosis

In normal resting individuals, venous blood lactate concentration is in the range 0.6 to 1.0 mmol/l. In extreme exercise this may rise to 20 mmol/l or more. Lactate is the end-product of anaerobic glycolysis. Its production by many tissues, even at rest, is accompanied by equal amounts of hydrogen ions, since its pK is low (3.8) and the undissociated acid is therefore present only in minute amounts. These protons react with blood and tissue bicarbonate to form carbon dioxide and water, but the lost bicarbonate is quantitatively restored when the lactate is converted to glucose (see Fig. 1), mainly in the liver, or oxidized in many tissues to carbon dioxide and water. When lactate is produced at a rate which exceeds the disposal rate, the regeneration of bicarbonate is incomplete and acidosis results. The pathological mechanisms leading to lactic acidosis are therefore excess production, defective disposal, or, commonly, a mixture of both. As the acidosis develops, hepatic disposal of lactate by gluconeogenesis may become further inhibited (see above), leading to a vicious circle which provides a model for the often fulminating course of lactic acidosis.

Clinically, lactic acidosis falls into two main categories. In type A lactic acidosis, much the more common, there is clinical evidence of shock, poor tissue perfusion, or hypoxia. Though increased peripheral glycolysis is an important contributor, associated poor hepatic and renal perfusion limit the lactate disposal mechanisms. Indeed in circulatory failure, the liver and kidneys may produce lactate rather than dispose of it. In type B lactic acidosis, there is no evidence at the outset of circulatory insufficiency or hypoxia, though after many hours of increasing acidosis these may supervene. The original diagnosis and cause of acidosis may be obscured if the patient does not present until this late stage. Type A lactic acidosis is a frequent manifestation of haemorrhagic, septic, cardiogenic, or traumatic shock and there is a direct relationship between the concentration of blood lactate and poor prognosis. The causes of type B lactic acidosis (Table 2) are varied and some of the mechanisms will be described below.

The initial clinical presentation in type B lactic acidosis is fairly uniform and consists of hyperventilation or dyspnoea, drowsiness or coma, vomiting, and abdominal pain, in approximately that order of frequency. The condition usually develops over a few hours, but may be more chronic, for example in the mitochondrial myopathies. Although by definition there is initially no clinical evidence of poor tissue perfusion or hypoxia, patients with severe type B lactic acidosis commonly become shocked after a few hours.

The diagnosis of lactic acidosis is based on the clinical circumstances, including the presence of a known aetiological factor, the presence of a high anion gap acidosis, and the measurement of blood lactate, for which automated apparatus is now widely available.

Biguanide-induced lactic acidosis

This class of oral hypoglycaemic agent has widespread metabolic effects, including inhibition of gluconeogenesis and the monocarboxylate transporter responsible for movement of lactate ions across cell membranes, and stimulation of glycolysis. The lactic acidosis is of the type B variety though, as indicated above, circulatory insufficiency may eventually supervene. The principal culprits were phenformin and buformin and the mortality was about 50 per cent; these biguanides are no longer used. Metformin is, however, widely used; the incidence of lactic acidosis with metformin is less than one-tenth of that with phenformin. Since metformin is almost entirely excreted in the urine, lactic acidosis may be largely avoided by care not to prescribe this drug in patients with even mild degrees of renal insufficiency, or conditions such as uncontrolled heart failure which might be expected to diminish renal function. Attempts have been made to show that the risk of lactic acidosis in diabetics taking metformin is no greater than in diabetics not receiving the drug. There have, however, been serious criticisms of those studies, and since the use of metformin is likely to increase because of its value in the prevention of diabetic microvascular complications, we strongly advise that the above precautions for its use continue to be followed.

Postictal lactic acidosis

The severe muscular contractions during convulsions may produce severe lactic acidosis in the same way as vigorous exercise. The finding of lactic acidosis in these circumstances occasionally gives rise to confusion but may be distinguished from other causes of lactic acidosis by the rapid decline of blood lactate after the cessation of convulsions, with a half-life of approximately 20 min.

Lactic acidosis in liver disease

Though impaired disposal of an administered lactate load is readily demonstrable in chronic liver disease, clinical lactic acidosis is uncommon. However, in the later stages of fulminant hepatic necrosis it may be an important part of the clinical picture. Acid–base disturbances in the earlier stages are discussed below.

Lactic acidosis in severe falciparum malaria

Lactic acidosis is a common feature of severe malaria due to *P. falciparum*, particularly in children, where it is the strongest predictor of poor prognosis. Although shock may be a factor, the lactic acidosis is frequently of the type B variety, and is attributable to many factors, including production of lactate by the parasite itself, occlusion of the microcirculation by parasites, the direct effects of high circulating levels of certain cytokines, notably tumour necrosis factor, inhibition of gluconeogenesis from lactate because of decrease in hepatic blood flow, and overproduction of lactate during the convulsions which are a common feature of cerebral malaria. Hypoglycaemia in severe malaria may be linked with lactic acidosis; it may be a manifestation of decreased gluconeogenesis or of insulin release due to quinine therapy. Acidosis appears to increase the attachment of infected erythrocytes to capillary walls, perhaps thus worsening the capillary blockage seen in the cerebral circulation and other sites. It may also inhibit the uptake of antimalarial drugs into erythrocytes.

Lactic acidosis associated with treatment with nucleoside reverse transcriptase inhibitors

There have been reports of lactic acidosis, which may be severe, associated with AIDS therapy with nucleoside reverse transcriptase inhibitors. Two mechanisms have been described—riboflavine deficiency and a mitochondrial disorder, with myopathy associated with the characteristic ragged red fibres seen in inherited mitochondrial myopathies. In the former type, the lactic acidosis rapidly responds to the administration of riboflavine.

Ethanol and methanol-induced lactic acidosis

Ingestion of ethanol after a period of fasting is a well-known cause of hypoglycaemia, which may be severe. The phenomenon is due to inhibition of gluconeogenesis, which is the sole source of endogenous glucose output when glycogen stores have been depleted. The defect in gluconeogenesis may result in moderate lactic acidosis, because ethanol diverts some of the NAD^+ needed for the oxidation of lactate to pyruvate, the first step in lactate disposal, for its own oxidation, catalysed by alcohol dehydrogenase. With withdrawal of ethanol, administration of glucose, and refeeding, the condition is normally self-limiting.

In methanol poisoning, the main contributor to the acidosis is formic acid, but lactic acidosis also plays a part, due to inhibition of gluconeogenesis by similar mechanisms to those in ethanol-induced lactic acidosis.

Salicylate and ethylene glycol poisoning

See Chapter 8.1.

D(–) lactic acidosis

In all the lactic acidoses described above, the stereoisomer involved is L(+)lactate, the end product of mammalian glycolysis. However, a few cases have been described in which the acidosis has been due to D(–)lactate. There is a very minor pathway of D(–)lactate production in mammalian tissues, but in D(–)lactic acidosis the D(–)lactate arises as a product of glycolysis in bacteria in the gut, and all cases have been associated with short gut or jejunal–ileal bypass syndromes or the therapeutic ingestion of large quantities of *Lactobacillus acidophilus*. The lactic acidosis may be severe and is often associated with disturbances of consciousness; it is presumably due to absorption of large quantities of D(–)lactate from the gut, since it may be treated by appropriate oral antibiotics. In healthy individuals, infused D(–)lactate is cleared at approximately 70 per cent of the rate for L(+)lactate, but by the non-specific 2-hydroxybutyrate dehydrogenase rather than L(+)lactate dehydrogenase. The main problem in diagnosing D(–)lactate acidosis is that D(–)lactate is not detectable by the routine blood lactate assay which employs the enzyme L(+)lactate dehydrogenase. If the condition is suspected because of unexplained high anion gap metabolic acidosis in a patient with a predisposing condition, then D(–) lactate should be assayed either by gas chromatography or using a bacterial D(–)lactate dehydrogenase.

Diabetic ketoacidosis

The pathogenesis and clinical features of diabetic ketoacidosis are described elsewhere (Chapter 12.11). Only the acid–base disturbance will be discussed here. Though the acidosis is conventionally regarded as being due mainly to overproduction of ketoacids by the liver, recent evidence has suggested that the hydrogen ions are wholly or partly derived from other tissues, though the liver is, of course, the source of ketoacid anions. Hepatic gluconeogenesis, a major source of the hyperglycaemia of diabetic ketoacidosis, proceeds at increased rates, in spite of potential inhibition by systemic acidosis. This is because, unlike in acidoses of other origins, hepatic intracellular pH does not fall in diabetic ketoacidosis.

Diabetic ketoacidosis has usually been regarded as a typical high anion gap metabolic acidosis in which extracellular bicarbonate has simply been titrated by the ketoacids. If this were the case, the fall in plasma bicarbonate should roughly equal the rise in anion gap and the plasma concentration of ketoacids. However, Adrogué and colleagues have shown that, whilst in some cases this is true, the situation is frequently more complex. Patients who present in ketoacidosis with relatively well-preserved renal function tend to have a rise in anion gap which is much less than the fall in bicarbonate. This is due to the loss of large quantities of ketoacid anions in the urine, with concomitant tubular reabsorption of chloride to maintain electroneutrality. Hyperchloraemia develops, which, together with the urinary loss of ketoacids, results in a relatively small elevation of anion gap compared with the bicarbonate deficit. In contrast, patients who have relatively poor renal function on presentation, for example because of dehydration, have much smaller urinary losses of ketoacids and present with a more classical high anion gap metabolic acidosis.

The total blood ketone body concentration in the well-controlled diabetic is about 0.1 mmol/l. In diabetic ketoacidosis, the concentration is often above 10 mmol/l and can rise as high as 30 mmol/l. Some of the most severe acidoses seen in clinical practice occur in diabetic ketoacidosis, some with pH_a values as low as 6.8. Urinary pH reaches its minimum possible value (4.5–5.3). At the lower of these values, about half the urinary ketocids are undissociated and some hydrogen ions are lost in this way. Severe depletion of erythrocyte 2,3-BPG occurs, leading to left shift of the oxygen dissociation curve, especially during treatment, and with potentially adverse consequences (see below).

In 5 to 10 per cent of patients with diabetic ketoacidosis, there is an accompanying element of lactic acidosis, with blood lactate greater than 5 mmol/l. Lactic acidosis occurs particularly when the patient is shocked, but there are rare instances of lactic acidosis supervening when treatment of the initial ketoacidosis is well advanced. There are also occasional ketotic diabetics in whom the blood lactate is low. This effect is readily reproducible in experimental animals and is thought to be related to increased hepatic disposal of lactate and suppression of peripheral glycolysis by the acidosis.

The acidosis of renal failure

Metabolic acidosis of varying degree is a classical feature of acute and chronic renal failure. It has been traditionally attributed to failure of the kidneys to excrete protons derived from 'fixed acids'—the class III acids of Table 1. In chronic renal failure the remaining functional nephrons are usually able to lower the urinary pH to the normal minimum. However, failure of proximal tubular bicarbonate reabsorption may occasionally occur and leads to a bicarbonate leak, as in type 2 renal tubular acidosis (see Chapter 20.8); in this case urinary pH does not fall to its minimum until the filtered load of bicarbonate has been substantially reduced by the fall in plasma bicarbonate. In some conditions, for example chronic pyelonephritis and chronic obstructive uropathy, the renal medulla is particularly affected, and acidification of the urine may be impaired. Nevertheless, the usually normal acidification in chronic renal failure means that the phosphate buffers in the tubular lumen are titrated by protons to the same extent as is possible in normal kidneys. However, the excretion of ammonium ions is lower than normal in chronic renal failure because of the loss of glutaminase-containing proximal tubules and reduced renal blood flow decreases the supply of glutamine. The conventional explanation of the acidosis of renal failure has been that the diminished supply of ammonia from the glutaminase reaction lowers the ability of the luminal contents to buffer secreted protons, with the result that the minimum urinary pH is attained with less protons in the ammonia/ammonium buffer system, and thus disposing of fewer protons in the urine.

However, as indicated above, the ammonia/ammonium buffer system is already virtually entirely in the protonated form (i.e. ammonium) at the time of its generation in the glutaminase reaction, so there is no capacity remaining for this system to act as a urinary buffer, either in health or in renal failure. An alternative explanation is therefore required for the acidosis of renal failure. Atkinson and Camien have suggested that the nitrogen which would in health be excreted as ammonium ions in the urine is, in chronic renal failure, effectively diverted to the liver, where it is converted to

urea with accompanying generation of protons (see above); the acidosis of renal failure is therefore due to relative overproduction of urea, rather than to failure of excretion of protons in the urine as ammonium ions.

The anion gap in uraemic acidosis seldom exceeds 28 to 30 mmol/l. The elevation is due to the accumulation of a relatively small quantities of several acid anions, including phosphate, sulphate, citrate, and other less well characterized contributions. When there is an element of proximal bicarbonate wastage, the anion gap may not be grossly raised; chloride may be reabsorbed instead of bicarbonate, leading to moderate hyperchloraemia.

The renal tubular acidoses, which are tubular disorders not, in the first instance, accompanied by glomerular failure, are discussed in Chapter 20.8.

Metabolic alkaloses associated with potassium and chloride deficiency

The most common cause of metabolic alkalosis is that associated with the use of potassium-losing diuretics; pyloric stenosis and Bartter's syndrome provide further examples of a complex aetiology. Chloride deficiency, indicated by low plasma chloride, may be due to a direct action of the diuretics, to loss from the gastrointestinal tract, as in pyloric stenosis, or to potassium deficiency itself, which has been shown experimentally to impair renal retention of chloride. Normally, most renal sodium reabsorption takes place in the proximal tubule, and it has to be accompanied by a readily reabsorbable anion to maintain electroneutrality. The most readily reabsorbable anion is chloride, and if the filtered load of chloride is low, due to hypochloraemia, some of the sodium which normally would have been reabsorbed proximally, passes to the distal segment of the nephron. Here sodium is reabsorbed by exchange with cations, principally potassium and protons, rather than accompanied by an anion. Since priority over acid–base regulation is accorded to the demands of extracellular volume control, the sodium reabsorption thus dictated causes further loss of potassium and protons into the urine, when the homeostatic response would have been to retain these latter ions. This accounts for the observation that the urine in these circumstances is acid when it should be alkaline ('paradoxical aciduria') and contains substantial quantities of potassium. Potassium loss in the urine is the principal cause of potassium depletion in pyloric stenosis, not loss in the vomit. The hypokalaemia is exacerbated by the fact that extracellular fluid volume is depleted in both diuretic therapy and in pyloric stenosis, leading to activation of the renin/angiotensin/aldosterone system, with further potassium loss. These considerations have important implications for therapy (see below).

An important cause of hypokalaemic hypochloraemic alkalosis, which is often marked, is deliberate overuse by patients of diuretics, notably frusemide, for reasons which may be related to psychological disturbances of the body image. Many of these patients are secretive about their use of diuretics; measurement of plasma frusemide is one way of diagnosing this dangerous condition.

Acid–base disturbances in fulminant hepatic failure

The most frequent acid–base disturbance in the earlier stages of fulminant hepatic failure is respiratory alkalosis, presumably due to the effects of ammonium and other amines on the respiratory centre. Metabolic alkalosis is also frequent, probably due to the failure of ureagenesis and its accompanying proton generation, but in some cases could be contributed to by potassium deficiency. Whatever the mechanism of the alkalosis, blood lactate concentration is frequently elevated, even in the absence of circulatory insufficiency. This phenomenon has been attributed to stimulation of peripheral glycolysis by alkalosis and to impairment of hepatic lactate disposal. Lactic acidosis may be a major feature in the later stages when the circulation is compromised, but is also occasionally seen in the very early stages. This early lactic acidosis is observed in paracetamol poisoning, a common cause of fulminant hepatic failure; it is associated with hypoglycaemia and may be largely related to a direct effect of paracetamol metabolites on hepatic gluconeogenesis from lactate; however, mild hypotension and dehydration also occurs.

Principles of treatment of acid–base disorders

The mainstay of treatment of acid–base disorders is to eliminate the cause of the disorder, the acid–base control mechanisms then restoring the normal situation in due course. However, it may be necessary to make a direct attempt to restore or partly restore normal acid–base status.

The treatment of respiratory acidosis is discussed in Chapter 17.11.

Acute metabolic acidosis

Major controversies still exist as to the advantages of treatment, especially with sodium bicarbonate. Randomized, controlled trials have not resolved these issues completely, largely because of the great variation of the physiological state of patients on presentation and the difficulty in establishing adequate sized, matching groups for trial purposes. Here we attempt to distinguish between conditions in which there is general consensus as to the best therapeutic approach and those in which there is less agreement. This is not an ideal approach, but is unavoidable at present.

The potential advantages of treating severe acidosis directly are improvement in cardiac performance, reduced risk of cardiac arrhythmia, redistribution of the blood volume away from the central circulation, correction of hyperkalaemia, and restoration of hepatic lactate disposal. Disadvantages lie in adverse effects on the oxygen dissociation curve, circulatory overload, especially if isotonic solutions have to be used, alkaline 'overshoot' when the acidosis is due to organic acids such as lactic acid and ketone bodies, and, allegedly, if bicarbonate is used, paradoxical intracellular acidification.

Paradoxical intracellular acidification is a concept arising from the observation that when sodium bicarbonate is infused, a significant rise in Pa_{CO_2} is observed, due to the titration of bicarbonate by hydrogen ions. Since there is an expectation that carbon dioxide will diffuse into cells much more rapidly than bicarbonate is translocated, it would be expected that intracellular pH would fall at the same time as pH_a rises; since many of the adverse effects of acidosis are directly related to effects on intracellular pH, this would be undesirable. A related observation is that in circulatory insufficiency, P_{CO_2} in mixed venous blood may be much greater than in arterial blood, where it is often normal. On occasion, bicarbonate therapy may exaggerate this difference and it has been inferred that bicarbonate must be acidifying the intracellular compartment by the mechanisms outlined above. However, considerations of the mechanisms responsible for the mixed venous hypercapnia suggest that only if arterial P_{CO_2} is raised after passage of the blood through the lungs is bicarbonate therapy likely to cause intracellular acidification. Whether Pa_{CO_2} is indeed elevated by intravenous bicarbonate therapy is dependent on numerous factors, including cardiac output, ventilation, the pulmonary dead space to total volume ratio, and, in particular, the rate of administration of bicarbonate.

Paradoxical intracellular acidification can indeed be demonstrated in closed systems such as platelets in which the carbon dioxide is not removed, and has been the reason for the development of alternative therapies such as an equimolar mixture of sodium bicarbonate and carbonate, for which the rise in Pa_{CO_2} during administration is substantially attenuated. However, it is difficult to demonstrate such an effect *in vivo*, when carbon dioxide is removed by the lungs, and in experimental animals either no change or actual elevation in intracellular pH in heart, liver, and skeletal muscle may be observed during bicarbonate administration, despite elevation of mixed venous P_{CO_2}. In any case, if doubts remain concerning this issue, the problem may be avoided by the simple expedient of administering bicarbonate slowly. Hindman has made useful calculations of the rates of bicar-

bonate administration which avoid rises in Pa_{CO_2} under a range of circumstances.

The situations in which sodium bicarbonate therapy is generally agreed to be advantageous are as follows:

1. Metabolic acidosis in severe renal failure—in acute renal failure, sodium bicarbonate treatment may correct hyperkalaemia by shifting potassium into the intracellular compartment. It may also relieve distressing hyperventilation and make time for definitive renal support therapy to be introduced. If the patient is already fluid overloaded, the bicarbonate may be administered as a hypertonic solution (e.g. 8.4 per cent; 1 mmol/ml). If the patient is dehydrated then the isotonic solution (1.4 per cent; 0.163 mmol/ml) may be given. During haemofiltration for acute renal failure in the presence of lactic acidosis, there is little doubt that the use of bicarbonate rather than lactate-containing replacement fluid is preferable, because of failure of metabolism of lactate to bicarbonate in this situation (see below). In chronically uraemic patients, the use of oral bicarbonate to treat the acidosis may improve well-being, nitrogen balance, and the osteomalacic component of renal osteodystrophy.

2. In the acidosis of severe diarrhoea it has been shown, in the specific instance of cholera, where circulatory insufficiency and loss of alkali are prominent factors, that treatment with bicarbonate is superior to that with sodium chloride solutions. These patients have severe peripheral venoconstriction, displacing their blood volume towards the lungs. The administration of saline solutions may thus induce pulmonary oedema before the volume deficit has been replaced. Sodium bicarbonate appears to relieve the peripheral venoconstriction and full replacement is therefore less hazardous.

3. In renal tubular acidosis, both chronically and in exacerbations—this subject is discussed elsewhere (Chapter 20.8) but it is necessary to re-emphasize here that in types 1 and 2 renal tubular acidosis, where hypokalaemia is a prominent feature, it is mandatory to deal with the hypokalaemia either before or at least simultaneously with the acidosis. Treatment of the acidosis first will result in a further fall in plasma potassium, by driving potassium into the cells, with potentially fatal consequences.

It is in the treatment of lactic acidosis, particularly type A, and in diabetic ketoacidosis that the uncertainty of the value of bicarbonate therapy principally lies. In animal models of lactic acidosis, treatment with bicarbonate has been shown to produce less favourable or no better haemodynamic and metabolic results than with sodium chloride. Interestingly, in an acute model of haemorrhagic shock there was little difference between bicarbonate and saline therapies; in these experiments, there had been no time for erythrocyte 2,3-BPG to fall. In contrast, in a model of diabetic ketoacidosis, developing over 48 h, in which 2,3-BPG was now virtually undetectable, treatment with bicarbonate produced a fall in blood pressure and evidence of tissue hypoxia, despite intracellular alkalinization. This suggests that acute acidoses of more than a few hour's duration may become increasingly susceptible to the adverse effects of bicarbonate. In a prospective, randomized trial of bicarbonate compared with saline in critically ill patients with lactic acidosis due to shock, there was no advantage of one therapy over the other, but this trial was not exempt from the general difficulties in mounting such trials.

The following practical guidance is therefore empirical, and largely based on current practice rather than formal trials:

1. Lactic acidosis—of paramount importance in type A lactic acidosis is the correction of hypovolaemic, cardiogenic, and other factors which are the primary cause of the condition. Such correction will promote aerobic metabolism and promote intracellular metabolism of lactate with consequent regeneration of bicarbonate (Fig. 1). Whether administration of exogenous bicarbonate can hasten this process or confer

other benefit is uncertain. In short-duration lactic acidosis, there may be less concern about effects on oxygen dissociation related to 2,3-BPG levels, but it should be remembered that unless therapy directed at the primary cause has improved the circulation, alkalinization itself may produce an unfavourable effect on oxygen release from haemoglobin. Nevertheless, the possibility of bicarbonate helping in some circumstances cannot be ruled out. If it is given, this should be relatively slowly, as the isotonic solution, unless there is a circulatory overload problem, and only in amounts sufficient to raise pH_a to a relatively 'safe' level. In the special case of the acidosis of cardiac arrest, the previous priority given to bicarbonate administration has disappeared, because of lack of evidence of efficacy and the risk of alkaline overshoot when the high levels of lactate are metabolized on restoration of cardiac output. Hypertonic sodium bicarbonate is only now recommended as a secondary treatment after prolonged arrest. In type B lactic acidosis due to biguanides, it has been conventional to use bicarbonate therapy at least to bring pH_a to 7.2 to 7.4 over several hours and survival has been linked to the achievement of that goal. However, an alternative interpretation of the data is that those patients in whom acid–base status was restored to normal would have achieved this without the aid of bicarbonate, or with the use of saline instead. Other therapies for type B lactic acidoses of different causes are discussed below.

2. Diabetic ketoacidosis—it is generally accepted that provided pH_a is not below 7.0, bicarbonate treatment is not indicated. Rehydration and insulin therapy result in improved renal function, a fall in ketone body production and an increase in ketone body metabolism, all of which contribute to correction of the acidosis. When pH_a is below 7.0 many give just sufficient bicarbonate (isotonic) to bring pH_a just above 7.0, with careful attention to changes in plasma potassium. There is, however, no evidence that this regimen is better than rehydration (with saline), insulin and potassium replacement alone, and there are data showing that such therapy delays fall in ketone body levels and lactate (if raised). The delayed fall in lactate is consistent with tissue hypoxia related to low erythrocyte 2,3-BPG as discussed above. It is therefore common practice not to give bicarbonate even at low pH_a levels. If bicarbonate is given, then it must be isotonic (1.4 per cent,163 mmol/l); to give hypertonic bicarbonate would merely exacerbate the already present hyperosmolality. The amount required seldom exceeds 0.5 to 1 litre.

The amount of alkali therapy, if given, should be determined by an iterative process of administration of a relatively small amount (e.g. 80 mmol), followed by reassessment of the clinical state, pH_a and $Paco_2$, with the aid of serial plots on the acid–base diagram in Fig. 2 before repeating the cycle.

Alkalinizing agents other than bicarbonate have been considered. Sodium lactate has the disadvantage that it has to be metabolized to neutral products plus bicarbonate before it has an alkalinizing effect (Fig. 1) and if lactate metabolism is impaired, as in shock and hypoxia in particular, it has no effect. Lactate is not a buffer in its own right at pH values encountered in health or disease. The mixture of bicarbonate and carbonate referred to above ('Carbicarb') has not been shown to have clinical advantages and is less effective than saline in animal models of diabetic ketoacidosis. THAM (trishydroxyaminomethane buffer) has the theoretical advantage of producing intracellular as well as extracellular alkalinization, but is seldom used because of unwanted effects. Sodium dichloroacetate increases lactate disposal via oxidation by activation of pyruvate dehydrogenase, and markedly lowers blood lactate in critically ill patients with lactic acidosis. However, in a multicentre trial it did not improve survival over that in a saline control group, possibly because of the severity of the associated pathologies and the diverse clinical state of the patients. However, it is of proven value in the treatment of some congenital lactic acidoses. Thiamine produces dramatic resolution of the severe lactic acidosis sometimes seen in beri-

beri. Riboflavine has produced similar results in nucleoside reverse transcriptase inhibitor-associated lactic acidosis.

Treatment of metabolic alkalosis

The first imperative is to identify the primary cause and if possible eliminate it. Where potassium-losing diuretics are responsible, they can be replaced by potassium-sparing preparations. In the most common form of chronic metabolic alkalosis, namely that associated with potassium and chloride deficiency, the primary therapies are potassium and chloride replacement. It has been shown that the potassium deficiency and alkalosis cannot be fully corrected unless there is also replenishment of chloride. Potassium supplements, whether oral or intravenous, should therefore be in the form of potassium chloride or contain other sources of chloride. It is also necessary to deal with any element of extracellular fluid volume contraction to switch off the drive to the renin–aldosterone system. It is seldom necessary to resort to administration of acid.

Further reading

Adrogué HJ, Wilson H, Boyd AE, Suki WN, Eknoyan G (1982). Plasma acid-base patterns in diabetic ketoacidosis. *New England Journal of Medicine* **307**, 1603–10.

Alberti KGMM, Darley JH, Emerson PM, Hockaday TDR (1972). 2,3-bisphosphoglycerate and tissue oxygenation in uncontrolled diabetes mellitus. *Lancet* **3**, 391–5.

Atkinson DE, Camien MN (1982). The role of urea synthesis in the removal of metabolic bicarbonate and the regulation of blood pH. *Current Topics in Cellular Regulation* **21**, 261–302.

Bellingham A, Detter JC, Lenfant C (1971). Regulatory mechanisms of hemoglobin oxygen affinity in acidosis and alkalosis. *Journal of Clinical Investigation* **50**, 700–6.

Chariot P, Drogou I, de Lacroix-Szmania I, *et al.* (1999). Zidovudine-induced mitochondrial disorder with massive steatosis, myopathy, lactic acidosis, and mitochondrial myopathy. *Journal of Hepatology* **30**, 156–60.

Cohen RD (1990). The metabolic background to acid-base homeostasis and some of its disorders. In: Cohen RD, Lewis B, Alberti KGMM, Denman AM, eds. *The Metabolic and molecular basis of acquired disease*, pp. 962–1001. Balliere Tindall, London.

Cohen RD (1991). Roles of the liver and kidney in acid-base regulation and its disorders. *British Journal of Anaesthesia* **67**, 154–64.

Cohen RD (1994). Lactic acidosis—new perspectives on origins and treatment. *Diabetes Reviews* **2**, 86–97.

Cohen RD, Woods HF (1976). *Clinical and Biochemical Aspects of Lactic Acidosis*. Blackwell, Oxford.

Cohen RD, Woods HF (1983). Lactic acidosis revisited. *Diabetes* **32**, 181–91.

Cohen RD, Woods HF (1999). Metformin and lactic acidosis. *Diabetes Care* **22**, 1010.

Cooper DJ, Walley KR, Wiggs BR, Russell JA (1990). Bicarbonate does not improve hemodynamics in critically ill patients who have lactic acidosis. *Annals of Internal Medicine* **112**, 492–8.

Emmett M, Narins RG (1977). Clinical use of the anion gap. *Medicine, Baltimore* **56**, 38–54.

Goldsmith DJA, Forni LG, Hilton PJ (1997). Bicarbonate therapy and intracellular acidosis. *Clinical Science* **93**, 593–8.

Hale PJ, Crase J, Nattrass M (1984). Metabolic effects of bicarbonate in the treatment of diabetic ketoacidosis. *British Medical Journal* **289**, 1035–8.

Hilton PJ, Taylor J, Forni LG, Treacher DF (1998). Bicarbonate-based haemofiltration in the management of acute renal failure with lactic acidosis. *Quarterly Journal of Medicine* **91**, 279–83.

Hindman BJ (1990). Sodium bicarbonate in the treatment of subtypes of acute lactic acidosis: physiologic considerations. *Anesthesiology* **72**, 1064–76.

Hood VL, Tannen RL (1998). Protection of acid-base balance by pH regulation of acid production. *New England Journal of Medicine* **339**, 819–26.

Kassirer JP, Berkman PM, Laurenz DR, Schwartz WB (1965). The critical role of chloride in the correction of hypokalaemic alkalosis in man. *American Journal of Medicine* **209**, 655–8.

Krishna S, Waller DW, ter Kuile F, *et al.* (1994). Lactic acidosis and hypoglycaemia in children with severe malaria: pathophysiological and prognostic significance. *Transactions of the Royal Society of Tropical Medicine and Hygiene* **88**, 67–73.

Luzatti R, Del Bravo P, Di Perri G, Luzzani A, Concia E (1999). Riboflavine and severe lactic acidosis. *Lancet* **353**, 901–2.

Mitchell JH, Wildenthal K, Johnson RL (1972). The effects of acid-base disturbances on cardiovascular and pulmonary function. *Kidney International* **1**, 375–89.

Oh MS, Phelps KR, Traube M, *et al.* (1979). D-lactic acidosis in a man with the short bowel syndrome. *New England Journal of Medicine* **301**, 249–52.

Orringer CE, Eustace JC, Wunsch CD, Gardner LB (1977). Natural history of lactic acidosis after grand mal seizures. *New England Journal of Medicine* **297**, 796–9.

Record CO, Iles RA, Cohen RD, Williams R (1975). Acid-base and metabolic disturbances in fulminant hepatic failure. *Gut* **16**, 144–9.

Stacpoole PW, Barnes CL, Hurbanis MD, Cannon SL, Kerr DS (1999). Treatment of congenital lactic acidosis with dichloroacetate. *Archives of Diseases in Childhood* **77**, 535–41.

Weil MH, Rackow EC, Trevino R, Grundler W, Falk JL, Griffel MI (1986). Difference in acid-base state between venous and arterial blood during cardiopulmonary resuscitation. *New England Journal of Medicine* **315**, 153–6.

11.12 Amyloid, familial Mediterranean fever, and acute phase response

11.12.1 The acute phase response and C-reactive protein

M. B. Pepys

The acute phase response

Trauma, tissue necrosis, infection, inflammation, and malignant neoplasia induce a complex series of non-specific, systemic, physiological and metabolic responses including fever, leucocytosis, catabolism of muscle proteins, and the greatly increased *de novo* synthesis and secretion of a number of plasma proteins. The synthesis of albumin, transthyretin, and high and low density lipoproteins is correspondingly decreased, and the altered plasma protein concentration profile is called the acute phase response (Table 1). Most acute phase proteins are synthesized by hepatocytes, in which transcription is controlled by cytokines including, interleukin 1 (IL-1), interleukin 6 (IL-6), and tumour necrosis factor (TNFα). The circulating concentrations of complement proteins and clotting factors increase by up to 50 to 100 per cent whereas some of the proteinase inhibitors and α1-acid glycoprotein can increase three to five fold. C-reactive protein (CRP) and serum amyloid A protein (SAA) are unique in that their concentrations can

Table 1 Plasma proteins in the acute phase response

Protein	Increased	Decreased
Proteinase inhibitors	α1-antitrypsin α1-antichymotrypsin	Inter α-antitrypsin
Coagulation proteins	Fibrinogen Prothrombin Factor VIII Plasminogen	
Complement proteins	C1s C2, B C3,C4,C5 C56 C1INH	Properdin
Transport proteins	Haptoglobin Haemopexin Caeruloplasmin	
Miscellaneous	C-reactive protein Serum amyloid A protein Fibronectin α1-acid glycoprotein Gc globulin	Albumin Transthyretin (prealbumin) High density lipoprotein Low density lipoprotein

change by more than one-thousand fold. The response persists in individuals with chronic infections, chronic inflammation, or invasive or metastatic neoplasms, and is sustained, unless there is complete hepatocellular failure, until death. All endothermic animals mount a similar response, suggesting that it may have survival value, and increased availability of proteinase inhibitors, complement, clotting, and transport proteins presumably enhances host resistance, minimizes tissue injury, and promotes regeneration and repair. However, some acute phase proteins may be harmful. For example sustained, increased production of SAA can lead to the deposition of AA-type, reactive systemic amyloid, a serious and usually fatal condition that complicates chronic infective and inflammatory diseases. CRP, through its capacity to activate complement, can exacerbate ischaemic, and possibly also other forms, of tissue damage.

C-reactive protein

CRP was the first protein to be discovered which behaves as an acute phase reactant, and was named for its calcium-dependent interaction with the somatic C-polysaccharide of pneumococci, in which CRP recognizes phosphocholine residues. CRP also binds to other substances which contain phosphocholine, including phospholipids, some plasma lipoproteins, and the plasma membranes of damaged or apoptotic but not intact cells. In addition, CRP binds specifically to small nuclear ribonucleoprotein particles when these are exposed in dead or damaged cells.

Ligand-bound CRP activates the classical complement pathway via C1, and can trigger the inflammatory, opsonizing, and complex-solubilizing activities of the complement system. A significant biological function of CRP may thus be to recognize and 'scavenge' cellular debris, promoting its safe clearance and helping to maintain tolerance to potential autoantigens. CRP may also protect against infection with pneumococci and *Haemophilus influenzae*, organisms that can express phosphocholine, and may thus contribute to innate immunity. On the other hand, CRP can also have tissue-damaging effects. Complement activation by CRP exacerbates ischaemic injury, the proinflammatory actions of CRP and its binding to phospholipids and lipoproteins may be proatherogenic, and the capacity of CRP to stimulate tissue factor production by macrophages may be prothrombotic. In contrast, CRP can suppress polymorph migration and infiltration *in vivo* and this may be anti-inflammatory.

The CRP molecule consists of five identical, non-glycosylated, non-covalently-associated polypeptide subunits, each of mass 23 027 Da, and containing 206 amino acid residues. The subunits have a flattened β-jellyroll fold with a single intrachain disulphide bond, and are arranged in an annular configuration with cyclic pentameric symmetry. There is a single calcium-dependent ligand binding site on the medial aspect of each subunit, all located on the same planar face of the molecule. A distinct but closely related plasma protein, serum amyloid P component (SAP), which is not an acute phase protein in man, has a very similar molecular structure with the same fold, characteristic of the 'lectin fold' superfamily. CRP and

SAP belong to the pentraxin family that has been highly conserved in evolution and no structural polymorphism of CRP has been observed nor has any case of CRP deficiency been described.

Serum concentration of CRP

CRP is a trace protein in overtly normal, healthy individuals, the median value being 0.8 mg/l, with an interquartile range of 0.3 to 1.7 mg/l. Ninety per cent of apparently healthy subjects have levels of less than 3 mg/l and 99 per cent less than 10 mg/l. Serial studies of normal subjects and of monozygotic and dizygotic twins show that each individual's baseline CRP value is rather constant and is substantially genetically determined. Occasional higher values of CRP seen in ostensibly healthy people almost certainly reflect intercurrent subclinical pathology, and it is clear both that values greater than 3 mg/l are not normal and that, if they persist, they may have considerable clinical significance. In large surveys of the unscreened general population, there is a trend towards higher values with increasing age, with the median value rising to about 2 mg/l, and this probably reflects the higher incidence of pathological processes, such as atherosclerosis, osteoarthritis, and other diseases. Serum CRP concentrations are lower in healthy newborns but reach adult values within a few days.

Serum CRP concentration rises rapidly in the acute phase response and can exceed 300 mg/l by 48 h after a severe stimulus such as myocardial infarction, acute systemic bacterial infection, major trauma, or surgery. With uncomplicated resolution of injury or effective treatment of infection the circulating CRP concentration generally falls equally rapidly.

The speed of change and incremental range of CRP concentration are exceptional among all the acute phase proteins, apart from serum amyloid A protein which behaves in a similar fashion. The half-life of CRP in the circulation is 19 h and is constant in all conditions regardless of the presence of an acute phase response or its cause. In contrast to other acute phase proteins, such as clotting factors, complement proteins, transport proteins, and proteinase inhibitors, CRP does not undergo significant local sequestration or consumption, fragmentation, or complex formation. This means that, unlike most of the other acute phase reactants, the single major determinant of the circulating concentration of CRP is its rate of synthesis. Since this in turn is dependent on the intensity of the acute phase stimulus, the serum CRP level usually closely reflects the extent and activity of disease. These properties underlie the value in clinical practice of precise measurement of the serum CRP concentration. Drug or other treatments do not affect CRP production unless they also affect the disease process which is responsible for induction of CRP synthesis. The only exception is combined cyclosporin and steroid treatment given after renal transplantation. This suppresses the CRP response to renal allograft rejection, though not that provoked by infection. The only physical condition which seriously interferes with the capacity to interpret CRP levels is serious hepatocellular impairment, since CRP is made exclusively in the liver.

Clinical measurement of serum CRP concentration

Conditions associated with major elevation of serum CRP concentration

Most tissue-damaging processes, infections, inflammatory diseases of unknown aetiology, and malignant neoplasms are associated with a major acute phase response of CRP. CRP production is thus a non-specific response to disease and it can never, on its own, be used as a diagnostic test. However, if the CRP result is interpreted in the light of full clinical information about the patient it can provide exceptionally useful information for clinical management. Thus in nearly all the conditions listed in Table 2 the CRP level reflects quite precisely the extent and activity of disease. With deterioration the CRP value rises, whilst with spontaneous or therapeutic-

Table 2 Conditions associated with major elevation of serum CRP concentration

Infections
Allergic complications of infection
rheumatic fever
erythema nodosum leprosum
Inflammatory disease
rheumatoid arthritis
juvenile chronic (rheumatoid) arthritis
ankylosing spondylitis
psoriatic arthritis
systemic vasculitis
polymyalgia rheumatica
Reiter's disease
Crohn's disease
familial Mediterranean fever
Necrosis
myocardial infarction
tumour embolization
acute pancreatitis
Trauma
surgery
burns
fractures
Malignant neoplasia
lymphoma, Hodgkin's disease,
carcinoma, sarcoma

ally induced remission the CRP level falls, and it thereby supplies an objective index of progress which is rarely available in any other way.

Infection

Most forms of systemic microbial infection are associated with high levels of serum CRP and, although the peak values attained in different patients cover a wide range, serial assays in individual subjects usually show an excellent correlation between the serum CRP concentration and the severity of disease and its response to treatment. Acute, systemic, Gram-positive and Gram-negative bacterial infections are among the most potent stimuli for CRP production. Systemic fungal infections occurring in immunodeficient hosts are also associated with high CRP values, whereas the levels in chronic bacterial infections such as tuberculosis and leprosy are usually rather lower, though nevertheless still markedly raised. Uncomplicated viral infections, particularly meningitis, may induce only a very modest response or none at all. Clinical rhinovirus infection (common cold) or influenza are associated with minor CRP elevation in a proportion of individuals, though this may reflect secondary bacterial infection. However, systemic cytomegalovirus or *Herpes simplex* infection of immunosuppressed patients does cause a major CRP response. Little is known about the CRP response to metazoan parasitic infestation in otherwise healthy subjects but malaria, especially *P. falciparum* infection, is associated with high CRP values as are *Pneumocystis* and *Toxoplasma* infections in immunodeficient patients.

Minor or localized, low-grade infection may not stimulate CRP production appreciably but the major CRP response in acute, serious bacterial infection is almost invariable and is present at all ages from premature neonates to the elderly. It also occurs in patients who are immunosuppressed or immunocomprised whether by a primary disease such as leukaemia, lymphoma or other malignancy, or AIDS, or by treatment with cytotoxic drugs, corticosteroids, or irradiation. This is of particular importance in the very young, in the old, in compromised hosts, and in any other patient in whom the usual clinical signs and symptoms of infection, including fever and neutrophil leucocytosis, may be masked or lacking (Figs 1 and 2). Furthermore, at the onset of bacterial infection, especially in patients who are otherwise well following elective surgery or myocardial infarction, the CRP response frequently precedes clinical symptoms, including fever, by up to 24 to 48 h.

Once infection is diagnosed or suspected and antimicrobial treatment has been commenced, frequent monitoring of the serum CRP concentration provides an objective means of assessing the response which is often not available. Effective therapy is associated with a rapid, exponential fall in CRP level, with a half-time of about 24 h, and occurrence of this pattern is an encouraging prognostic sign (Fig. 2). Normalization of the CRP usually corresponds to clinical cure of the infection and may thus be used to determine the necessary duration of antimicrobial therapy. On the other hand, especially in neutropenic or immunodeficient patients, persistent elevation of CRP at the end of a course of antibiotics often presages relapse or recurrence of infection.

When bacterial infection is complicated by abscess formation or for any other reason is less readily eradicated by antimicrobial drugs, the serum CRP concentration may remain elevated or may fall linearly rather than exponentially during treatment. Such a pattern should raise questions regarding dosage of the drugs, sensitivity of the organism, and/or stimulate a diagnostic search both for localized pus and for other underlying, non-infective pathology such as malignancy. Indeed, in the absence of one of the chronic idiopathic inflammatory conditions which are known to be associated with high CRP levels (see below), the persistence of a raised serum CRP concentration is usually a grave prognostic sign, indicating the presence of either uncontrolled infection and/or other serious pathology likely to cause death. However, with alteration in antimicrobial drug regimen or the evacuation of pus or elimination of other pathology, the rapid fall in CRP which may then be observed is a most encouraging objective sign of clinical improvement.

These considerations apply at all ages and regardless of intercurrent pathology, with the exception of severe hepatocellular impairment. In view

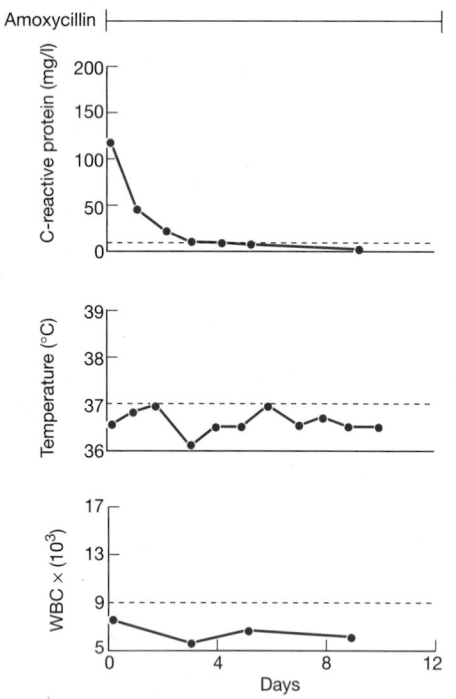

Fig. 1 A 69-year-old diabetic man was admitted with a 3-day history of confusion, cough, and incontinence of urine. There was clinical and radiological evidence of a left-sided pneumonia and although both the temperature and white cell count remained normal, the serum C-reactive protein was high (119 mg/l), confirming the suspicion of infection. Following treatment with amoxicillin, 250 mg thrice daily, the C-reactive protein level fell rapidly, in a characteristic exponential manner, and he made a speedy recovery with return of continence and improved mental state.

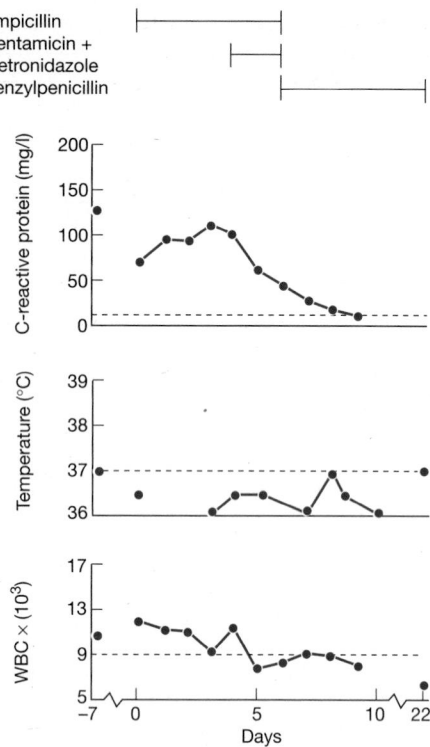

Fig. 2 An 86-year-old woman had been refusing food and drink for 6 weeks. She was dehydrated but rehydration in hospital failed to improve her mental state. She was paranoid and refused nursing and medical care. Paraphrenia was diagnosed and deterioration continued. A C-reactive protein of 130 mg/l and a white cell count of 13.5 × 10⁹/l were then found. Chest radiograph, normal on admission, now showed a cavitating lesion from which 150 ml of pus was aspirated. Intravenous ampicillin reduced neither the C-reactive protein nor white cell count prompting a change of therapy to gentamicin and metronidazole. *Strep. equinus* was finally identified in the pus and treatment was changed to benzylpenicillin alone. The C-reactive protein then fell exponentially but rather slowly. The patient's clinical and mental state gradually improved and she was eventually discharged.

of the very small amount of serum required for the assay and the speed and precision of automated CRP immunoassays it is apparent that routine monitoring of serum CRP makes a valuable contribution to the recognition and management of infectious diseases. Situations in which these applications have been well documented are listed in Table 3.

Meningitis is of particular interest in view of its potential severity and the importance of rapid diagnosis and appropriate treatment. Bacterial

Table 3 Applications of serum CRP measurement in infectious disease

Bacteraemia and septicaemia in children and adults
Bacteraemia and septicaemia in neonates
Bacterial and other infections in immunosuppressed patients
Deep fungal infections
Meningitis: viral < TB < bacterial
Bacterial infections after major elective surgery or other invasive procedures
Infective relapse after abdominal surgery for sepsis
Peritonitis in patients on chronic ambulatory peritoneal dialysis
Acute appendicitis (differential diagnosis)
Evaluation of antibiotic therapy for female pelvic infection
Laryngotracheitis/ pharyngitis/ epiglottitis in children
Chorioamnionitis after premature rupture of membranes
Disseminated versus localized gonococcal infection
Infection precipitating sickle cell crisis

meningitis is associated with much higher serum CRP levels at presentation than cases of aseptic or proven viral meningitis. The latter frequently have CRP concentrations within the normal range or which are only very slightly raised, unless they develop secondary bacterial infective complications, whilst patients with tuberculous have intermediate values. Appropriate therapy for either bacterial or tuberculous meningitis causes the CRP level to fall and this can be used to monitor objectively the response to treatment.

Baseline CRP values are much lower at birth and for the first few days than in older children or adults. Also, neonatal infections progress much more rapidly and can have a fatal outcome before the CRP response has produced concentrations detectable in routine assays. It is therefore essential to use high sensitivity methods capable of detecting and precisely measuring CRP in the range 0.05 to 5.0 mg/l, otherwise the critical initial acute phase response to infection will be missed.

Inflammatory disease

Most of the chronic inflammatory diseases of unknown aetiology (Table 2), with some notable exceptions described below, are associated with high CRP values when they are active. Serial measurements of CRP in individuals with any of these diseases generally reflect the extent and activity of their condition as determined by clinical examination and other laboratory tests. Rheumatoid arthritis is the most common and important disease in this group and the correlation between CRP values in individual patients and the extent and activity of arthritis is very well established. Importantly, there are appreciable differences between the CRP levels attained in different subjects with apparently similar severity of arthritis, but in each case the CRP value always reflects current disease activity. Furthermore, CRP values precisely predict future progression of bone erosion and joint damage. Left unchecked, high CRP levels are inevitably followed by progressive erosive disease, whilst treatments that lower CRP retard or arrest this process.

In some of the inflammatory disorders, for example systemic vasculitis or Crohn's disease (Fig. 3), unlike rheumatoid arthritis, the pathology is relatively inaccessible to direct examination and serum CRP measurement provides the best available, objective index of disease activity. Furthermore, the presence or absence of a CRP response can distinguish between symptoms or organ dysfunction which are due to currently active inflammation or which are the consequence of fibrosis and scarring from previous episodes. This can be very important when treatments include steroids and other powerful and potentially hazardous immunosuppressive, anti-inflammatory, and cytotoxic drugs. It permits precise titration of dosages and may help to avoid excessive or unnecessary use.

Induction of clinical remission and control of the underlying disease process is associated with prompt normalization of the CRP. However, CRP also becomes abnormal with intercurrent infection, a common complication of some of these disorders and their treatments, and this serves to focus diagnostic attention often before the infection has become too severe or even before it is clinically evident. Monitoring the CRP response to antimicrobial therapy can then help to confirm the diagnosis and the efficacy of therapy. Persistent elevation of the CRP after eradication of infection may indicate relapse of the underlying inflammatory disease, requiring additional anti-inflammatory treatment.

Necrosis

Myocardial infarction is invariably associated with a major CRP response, as is elective embolization leading to necrosis of tumours in the liver and elsewhere. The peak level of CRP occurs about 50 h after the onset of pain in myocardial infarction and correlates in magnitude, though not in timing, with the peak serum level of cardiac isoenzymes such as creatine kinase MB. In patients who recover uneventfully, the CRP falls rapidly towards normal in the usual exponential fashion. However, complications such as persistent cardiac dysfunction, further infarction, aneurysm formation, intercurrent infection, thromboembolism, or postinfarction syndrome are associated with either persistently raised CRP levels or secondary elevation after the initial decrease. Myocardial rupture is seen only in patients with

high peak CRP values, greater than 200 mg/l, and the peak CRP concentration after acute myocardial infarction is inversely correlated with overall outcome, including survival, in the short, medium, and long term.

Stable angina and invasive investigation, such as coronary arteriography, do not stimulate CRP production, whereas some other causes of chest pain, such as pulmonary embolism, pleurisy, or pericarditis, are usually associated with raised CRP levels. Routine assays of CRP after infarction or in patients with chest pain may thus assist in diagnosis and in the recognition and management of complications, including iatrogenic infection associated with invasive cardiovascular monitoring. The role of high-sensitivity measurements of CRP in prediction of coronary heart disease is discussed below.

Serum CRP levels closely reflect the severity and progress of acute pancreatitis, providing a better guide to intra-abdominal events than other markers such as leucocyte counts, erythrocyte sedimentation rate (ESR), temperature, and the plasma concentrations of antiproteinase. A CRP concentration greater than 100 mg/1 at the end of the first week of illness is associated with a more prolonged subsequent course and a higher risk of the development of a pancreatic collection. Serial CRP measurements can therefore guide the use of appropriate imaging techniques and help to confirm resolution before discharge from hospital.

Trauma

The CRP concentration always rises after significant trauma, surgery, or burns, peaking after about 2 days and then falling towards normal with

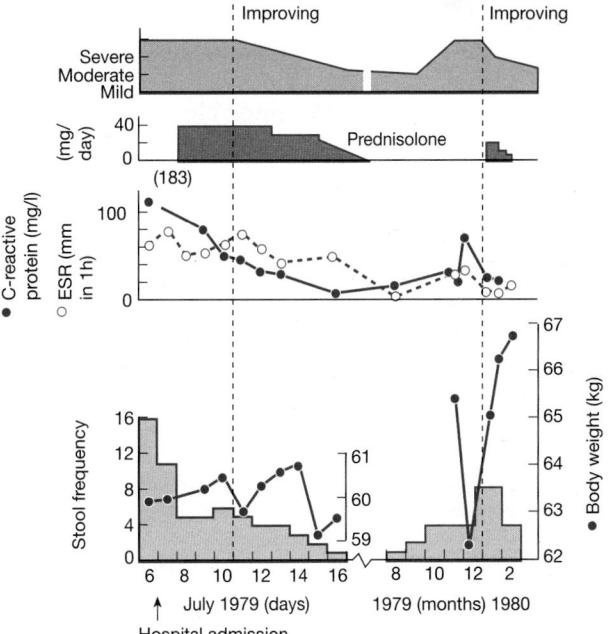

Fig. 3 A 26-year-old man with pancolonic Crohn's disease. He was admitted with severe exacerbation; temperature 38°C; pulse, 110 beats/min; 16 stools per day; haematocrit, 41.5 per cent, leucocytes 13.8 × 10⁹/l. Rectal mucosa severely inflamed with histiocytic granulomata on biopsy. Rapid improvement occurred with oral and rectal prednisolone, ampicillin, and metronidazole, with complete clinical and histological remission on day 11. Relapse 5 months later responded promptly to a short course of oral and rectal prednisolone. C-reactive protein and ESR were both high during the initial exacerbation. The rapid response to treatment was paralleled by a prompt fall in C-reactive protein, whereas the ESR responded more slowly. Despite clinical remission and a normal ESR, the C-reactive protein remained slightly elevated, suggesting persistent low-grade inflammatory activity, and it rose further during a subsequent relapse when the ESR did not change. (Reproduced from Fagan A *et al.* (1982). Serum levels of C-reactive protein in Crohn's disease and ulcerative colitis. *European Journal of Clinical Investigation* **12**, 351–9, with permission.)

recovery and healing. Infections or other tissue-damaging complications alter this 'normal' pattern of CRP response and the failure of the CRP to continue falling or the appearance of a second peak may precede clinical evidence of intercurrent infection by 1 to 2 days.

Malignancy

Most malignant tumours, especially when they are extensive and metastatic, induce an acute phase response. This is particularly so with those neoplasms which cause systemic symptoms such as fever and weight loss, for example Hodgkin's disease (stage B), and renal carcinoma, but raised CRP levels are seen with many others. In some studies, notably of prostatic carcinoma and bladder carcinoma, the CRP level at presentation has been found to correlate with the overall tumour load and also with the prognosis, being higher for a given mass of tumour in those patients who subsequently fare worse. The CRP may also correlate better with progress and regression of tumour than other, more specific, tumour markers. However, given the non-specific nature of the acute phase response and the limited number of studies performed so far, a definite role for CRP measurements in the management of cancer patients, other than in cases of intercurrent infection, has not yet been established.

Allograft rejection

In the era before routine immunosuppression with combined cyclosporin and steroid treatment, rejection episodes following renal allografting were generally associated with increased production of CRP. However, such treatment almost completely suppresses the CRP response in this situation. In contrast, the acute phase response of SAA is unaffected, and importantly, intercurrent infection still stimulates high levels of both CRP and SAA.

Conditions associated with minor elevation of serum CRP concentrations

Despite unequivocal evidence of active inflammation and/or tissue damage, the conditions listed in Table 4 are usually associated with only minor elevations of the serum CRP concentration, and in many cases it may even remain normal in the face of severe disease. The contrasts between systemic lupus erythematosus (SLE) and rheumatoid and other arthritides shown in Table 2, and between ulcerative colitis and Crohn's disease, are very striking. However, intercurrent microbial infection does provoke a major CRP response in all the conditions shown in Table 4, and this is of great value in diagnosis and management, especially in SLE and leukaemia. The basis of the apparently selective failure of the acute phase response of CRP (which is also shown by SAA) is not known, but presumably involves defect(s) in the pathways which mediate the acute phase response to autologous inflammation and tissue damage. The inbred mouse strain NZB/W, which spontaneously develops antinuclear autoimmune disease, behaves just like human SLE patients with respect to its acute phase responses and the phenomenon may thus be genetically determined. SAP knockout mice also spontaneously develop antinuclear autoimmune disease and do not handle chromatin degradation normally, indicating that pentraxins have a key role in these processes.

Pyrexia is common in SLE and may be caused by microbial infection or by activity of the lupus itself. Both SLE and its treatment predispose to infection, and steroids and immunosuppressives can mask the usual symp-

Table 4 Conditions associated with minor elevation of serum CRP concentration

Systemic lupus erythematosus
Scleroderma
Dermatomyositis
Ulcerative colitis
Leukaemia
Graft-versus-host disease

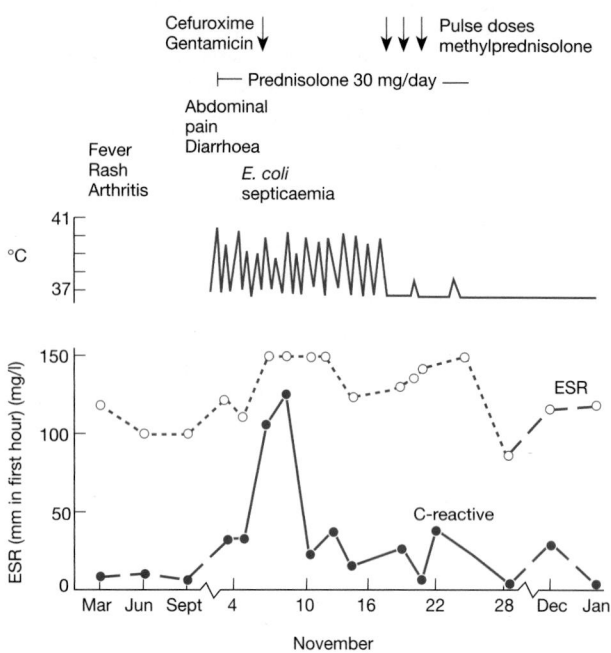

Fig. 4 A 12-year-old girl with a 3-year history of SLE; recurrent febrile episodes, polyarthritis, cutaneous vasculitis, and episodes of asymptomatic bacteriuria. Intermittent treatment was with prednisolone, azathioprine, and plasma exchange. Serum C-reactive protein was only marginally elevated throughout but ESR was persistently raised. Fever recurred with diarrhoea and abdominal pain. All microbial cultures were negative except for growth of E. coli from the urine. Despite oral cephalexin and prednisolone, her condition deteriorated with severe neutropenia, probably due to azathioprine. C-reactive protein rose from 36 to 101 and then 137 mg/l, and at this stage her blood culture grew E. coli. Intravenous antibiotics were given and the serum C-reactive protein level fell rapidly, but there was little clinical improvement. Active SLE appeared then to be the sole cause of the fever and this was confirmed by the development of a diffuse vasculitic rash and polyarthritis. Three pulse doses of methylprednisolone were given intravenously on successive days and produced a dramatic improvement in her clinical state with resolution of the fever. This case illustrates: (1) the differential response of the C-reactive protein to fever resulting from activity of SLE alone and fever due to bacterial infection; (2) the rapid response of the C-reactive protein both to the onset and to the effective treatment of serious bacterial infection; (3) the failure of ESR measurements to provide any useful information in this complex and rapidly evolving clinical situation. (Reproduced from Pepys MB, Langham JG, de Beer FC (1982). C-reactive protein in SLE. *Clinics in Rheumatic Diseases* **8**, 91–103, with permission.)

toms and signs of infection. Furthermore, infection can trigger exacerbations of SLE. This is a serious clinical situation and infection remains one of the most common causes of death in patients with SLE. CRP values of 60 mg/1 or more are very rare in SLE in the absence of infection whilst levels below 60 mg/1 are seen in patients with documented infection only when it is rather mild and often localized, for example to the skin or lower urinary tract. Differential diagnosis and management of fever in SLE are thus considerably improved by the measurement of serum CRP concentration (Fig. 4).

The reason why leukaemia patients fail to mount more than a modest CRP response, even during induction therapy when there is massive death of leukaemia cells, is not known, However, they do respond to infection. Since all febrile episodes in leukaemia must initially be treated as infective, the main value of CRP monitoring is to determine the response to therapy and assist in decisions about its duration. Acute or chronic graft-versus-host disease after bone marrow transplantion is usually associated with only a modest CRP response, if any. However, the immunosuppressive treatments used to prevent bone marrow rejection and to control graft-versus-host disease render the patients susceptible to intercurrent infections, often with unusual micro-organisms, and these are always associated with high levels of CRP. CRP monitoring therefore plays a valuable role in management in the post-transplant period.

Interpretation of clinical serum CRP measurements

Clinical measurements of serum CRP fall into two categories. First, routine measurements over the range 3 mg/l upwards in adult and general paediatric medicine. Secondly, high sensitivity measurements including the range up to 3 mg/l that are essential in neonatal medicine and for screening and prognostic investigation in adults with respect to atherothrombotic disease and osteoarthritis. The CRP response is not specific and CRP measurements on their own can never, therefore, be diagnostic of any particular condition. The CRP value can only be interpreted in the light of all other available clinical and laboratory information. Provided this is done it can make a most useful contribution to overall assessment of the patient and determination of the best management.

Routine CRP measurement

The applications fall into three main categories:

- Screening for organic disease
- Monitoring of extent and activity of disease:

infection

inflammation

malignancy

necrosis

- Detection and management of intercurrent infection.

Screening for organic disease

CRP production is a very sensitive response to organic disease. A normal CRP therefore eliminates many possible types of pathology and is a reassuring finding. Those serious conditions which only stimulate CRP production weakly if at all, for example SLE, ulcerative colitis, or leukaemia, are all readily recognized by clinical examination and other simple tests such as blood counts, rectal biopsy, or serology. The presence of a raised CRP is unequivocal evidence of active pathology though this may not necessarily be the cause of the complaint for which the patient presented. Such a finding, in the absence of other obvious abnormality, warrants a repeat CRP assay after a few days when a trivial cause such as upper respiratory tract infection will have resolved. Further investigation of a persistently raised CRP level will then depend on the severity of the complaint and other clinical findings.

Monitoring extent and activity of disease

Once the diagnosis is established, in those diseases which cause major elevation of the CRP, serial measurements reflect activity and response to treatment and can be used for monitoring. However, they can only be interpreted provided other possible intercurrent causes of an acute phase response, particularly infections, are excluded.

Detection and management of intercurrent infection

CRP production is a very sensitive response to most forms of infection and a raised level is thus a useful guide to the possible presence of infection in otherwise normal subjects or individuals with a primary condition which predisposes to infection. In disorders which themselves elevate the CRP concentration the decision as to whether infection is present or not must depend on clinical examination and other laboratory tests and the role of CRP testing is then to demonstrate rapidly and objectively whether there is a response to whatever treatment is used. Effective antimicrobial therapy of infection is always associated with a prompt fall in the CRP whilst persistent CRP elevation indicates continuing infection and/or activity of the underlying disease. There is no other objective test which yields this sort of information so accurately. Changes in results of clinical examination and tests of organ function usually lag hours or days behind the CRP response.

CRP and body temperature

The acute phase response, which is best measured clinically by quantification of the serum CRP, is part of the systemic response of the body to disease. Monitoring of this same response by measurement of body temperature is an integral part of the physical examination and of patient management. CRP production is triggered by the same cytokines which cause fever, and the serum CRP concentration therefore may be considered in part to be a biochemical measurement of the body temperature. However, the CRP response is not susceptible to the many vagaries of thermoregulation itself and routine clinical measurement of body temperature. The precise numerical value of the CRP concentration and its changes over time reflect much more accurately than the temperature the intensity of the underlying stimulus. Furthermore there is often a CRP response in the absence of fever, especially in neonates and the elderly, though also at any age in many chronic inflammatory conditions, and a case therefore exists for the inclusion of a regular serum CRP chart together with the standard temperature chart in appropriate patients.

CRP or ESR?

The only other comparable, non-specific index of the presence of disease which is routinely measured is the erythrocyte sedimentation rate (ESR). The ESR reflects, in part, the intensity of the acute phase response, especially that of fibrinogen and the α-globulins, but is also largely determined by the concentration of immunoglobulins, which are not acute phase reactants. These proteins all have half-lives of days to weeks. The rate of change of the ESR is thus very much slower than that of the CRP level and it rarely reflects precisely the clinical status of the patient at the actual time of testing. ESR is also dependent on the number and morphology of the red cells, which bear no relation to the acute phase response. Finally, there is a significant diurnal variation in ESR, depending on food intake, which is not seen in the CRP. The ESR is therefore of limited use as an objective index of disease activity on which management decisions can be based. The dynamic range of the ESR is also much less than that of CRP and the precision and reproducibility of ESR measurements is poor compared to robust immunoassays for CRP. Thus, in all clinical situations which have been carefully evaluated, ranging from acute bacterial infections to the chronic remittent inflammatory diseases, such as Crohn's disease, rheumatoid arthritis and other inflammatory arthropathies, and systemic vasculitis in its various forms, frequent prospective measurements of CRP reflect disease activity very much more closely than measurements of the ESR. Finally, ESR does not provide the information given by the high sensitivity measurement of CRP, described below. However, the ESR remains a useful screening test for the detection of paraproteinaemias, especially multiple myeloma, which do not necessarily provoke an acute phase response.

High sensitivity CRP measurements

The limitations of conventional immunoassay technology for quantifying serum proteins imposed, until recently, a lower detection limit of about 5 mg/l in most routinely available methods. The advent of more sensitive assays has revealed important new indications for CRP measurement.

Neonatal medicine

Although newborns mount just as rapid and vigorous CRP responses as adults, their baseline values are lower; the median and range in normal cord blood are only 0.04 mg/l and 0.01 to 0.49 mg/l. Since infants can succumb to infection so rapidly, high sensitivity measurements are mandatory.

Atherosclerosis and coronary heart disease

In patients with severe, unstable angina admitted urgently to hospital, CRP values above 3 mg/l are significantly predictive of poor outcome, including death, acute myocardial infarction, or the need for urgent revascularization intervention. In patients undergoing coronary angioplasty, only those with raised CRP values mount an acute phase response to the procedure and the magnitude of this response predicts early reocclusion. Among outpatients with angina and also, remarkably, among healthy normal adult populations, those in the top quintile of the CRP distribution, that is with values above about 2.5 mg/l, have a two to five-fold increased risk of suffering a coronary event in future. Increased CRP production also predicts progression and atherothrombotic events in cerebrovascular and peripheral vascular disease, although the numbers of cases studied have been smaller.

The mechanisms underlying the relationship between even modestly increased CRP production and atherothrombotic events are not known. The CRP response may reflect the inflammation that is a major feature of atherosclerotic plaques, or it may be stimulated by low grade inflammation or infection elsewhere in the body, processes that are known to be associated with atherogenesis. Although CRP levels are associated with smoking, body mass index, hyperlipidaemia, and insulin resistance, all of which are risk factors for atherosclerosis and coronary heart disease, CRP values remain significantly prognostic of coronary events even after adjustment for these variables. It is therefore possible that, in addition to being a marker of inflammation, CRP itself may contribute to pathogenesis, perhaps through its interactions with lipids, lipoproteins, complement, and coagulation. Indeed CRP is detectable within atherosclerotic plaques. There is clearly much work to be done in this exciting new field but, regardless of the underlying mechanisms, the empirical results, from many large-scale independent studies in Europe and the United States, robustly show that high-sensitivity CRP measurements provide important prognostic information.

Osteoarthritis

Modest acute phase responses of CRP, within what was previously considered the normal range, are significantly associated with the presence and extent of osteoarthritis in middle-aged populations. Among affected subjects, the CRP values also predict future progression of the disease.

Serum amyloid A protein

SAA, an apolipoprotein of high-density lipoprotein particles, is a marked acute phase reactant, its concentration rising from normal levels of about 2 mg/l by as much as 1000 times. It is essential to monitor and control SAA levels in patients with reactive systemic, AA type amyloidosis (see Chapter 11.12.4). The other indication for routine SAA measurement is in renal allograft recipients, in whom the SAA response is the most sensitive marker of rejection episodes, despite suppression of the CRP response by immunosuppression with cyclosporin and steroids.

Further reading

Boralessa H *et al.* (1986). C-reactive protein in patients undergoing cardiac surgery. *Anaesthesia* **41**, 11–15.

Danesh J, *et al.* (2000). Low grade inflammation and coronary heart disease: prospective study and updated meta-analyses. *British Medical Journal* **321**, 199–204.

Fagan EA *et al.* (1982). Serum levels of C-reactive protein in Crohn's disease and ulcerative colitis. *European Journal of Clinical Investigation* **12**, 351–60.

Griselli M *et al.* (1999). C-reactive protein and complement are important mediators of tissue damage in acute myocardial infarction. *Journal of Experimental Medicine* **190**, 1733–9.

Hartmann A *et al.* (1997). Serum amyloid A protein is a clinically useful indicator of acute renal allograft rejection. *Nephrology Dialysis, Transplantation* **12**, 161–6.

Haverkate F *et al.* (1997). Production of C-reactive protein and risk of coronary events in stable and unstable angina. *Lancet* **349**, 462–6.

Koenig W *et al.* (1999). C-reactive protein, a sensitive marker of inflammation, predicts future risk of coronary heart disease in initially healthy middle-aged men. Results from the MONICA (Monitoring Trends and Determinants in Cardiovascular Disease) Augsburg Cohort Study 1984 to 1992. *Circulation* **99**, 237–42.

Liuzzo G *et al.* (1994). The prognostic value of C-reactive protein and serum amyloid A protein in severe unstable angina. *New England Journal of Medicine* **331**, 417–24.

Pepys MB, Lanham JG, de Beer FC (1982). C-reactive protein in systemic lupus erythematosus. *Clinics in Rheumatic Diseases* **8**, 91–103.

Ridker PM *et al.* (1997). Inflammation, aspirin, and the risk of cardiovascular disease in apparently healthy men. *New England Journal of Medicine* **336**, 973–9.

Spector TD *et al.* (1997). Low level increases in serum C-reactive protein are present in early osteoarthritis of the knee and predict progressive disease. *Arthritis and Rheumatism* **40**, 723–7.

Starke ID *et al.* (1984). Serum C-reactive protein levels in the management of infection in acute leukaemia. *European Journal of Cancer* **20**, 319–25.

Wasunna A *et al.* (1990). C-reactive protein and bacterial infection in preterm infants. *European Journal of Pediatrics* **149**, 424–7.

van Leeuwen MA *et al.* (1997). Individual relationship between progression of radiological damage and the acute phase response in early rheumatoid arthritis. Towards development of a decision support system. *Journal of Rheumatology* **24**, 20–7.

11.12.2 Metabolic responses to accidental and surgical injury

Roderick A. Little

Introduction

Accidental injury remains the principal cause of death and disability in those aged less than 45 years of age in the developed world. Also, as the threats of infectious disease and starvation have been reduced in parts of the 'third world', they have been replaced by injury; at the same time, motor vehicle and interpersonal violence have increased. Since such injuries involve predominantly the young, it can be calculated that in the loss to society of productive years of life, injury presents more of a challenge than cancer and cardiovascular disease.

Humans are also subjected to the planned injury of surgery, recovery from which may be prolonged. This consumes health service resources within and outside hospital and also delays return to employment and/or independence.

Attempts to reduce the burden of injury should emphasize prevention but it is also important to lessen its biological effects. A full description and explanation of the biological responses to injury is needed so that treatment can be properly directed. For example now that the metabolic responses to major injury, surgery, and infection have been shown to be very similar, 'generic' scientifically based measures rather than empirical *ad hoc* interventions are used in treatment.

The most important advance in the description of the metabolic response to injury was the recognition, by Sir David Cuthbertson in 1932, that the response did not involve unconnected reactions but rather followed an ordered pattern. He divided the response into an initial transient 'ebb', followed by a prolonged 'flow' phase.

Table 1 Principle features of the acute (ebb phase) response to injury

Initiation of defence reaction (preparation for fight or flight)
Increased secretion of counter-regulatory hormones
Activation of sympathetic nervous system
Mobilization of energy stores
Inhibition of cardiovascular and thermoregulatory reflexes

Ebb phase

This was first described as a period of depressed vitality or metabolism and anuria which occurred during the first 1 to 2 days after injury. Subsequent analysis of the data from Cuthbertson's four patients reveals little evidence for a reduction in energy metabolism. However, his interpretation may have been influenced by previous experiments which showed an acute depression of metabolism after hind-limb muscle injury in anaesthetized cats. In these animals, the depression in metabolism was caused by a failure of tissue oxygen delivery—an unlikely occurrence in Cuthbertson's patients with single, lower-limb fractures.

It now seems that the ebb phase can be redefined as the early stage after trauma during which tissue energy production is not limited by a failure of oxygen delivery (Table 1). It is a complex neuroendocrine response, the magnitude of which depends on the generation of somatic afferent nociceptive stimuli arising from damaged tissues and the loss of intravascular volume. As well as eliciting a neurohumoral response, the nociceptive stimuli also inhibit central thermoregulation and cardiovascular reflex activity. Many aspects of this early response are reminiscent of the alerting response of the defence reaction or preparation for fight or flight. Thus, the arterial baroreceptor reflex is inhibited allowing concomitant increases in arterial blood pressure and heart rate.

In this initial phase, there is also mobilization of energy stores to fuel the anticipated increase in activity. The increases in plasma glucose concentration, which are directly related to the severity of injury, arise from the breakdown of glycogen stores in the liver and skeletal muscle. This breakdown is mediated by rises in the counter-regulatory hormones (the catecholamines, especially adrenaline, cortisol, and glucagon) which occur at this time, together with increases in antidiuretic hormone. The catecholamines may also be sufficient in the severely injured to inhibit intracellular glucose uptake and oxidation by suppressing the release of insulin. The increased activity of the sympathetic nervous system also stimulates lipolysis but the relationship between plasma concentrations of non-esterified fatty acids and severity of injury is complex. In particular, there may be stimulation of fatty acid re-esterification within adipose tissue by the raised plasma lactate that is associated with severe injury or impaired perfusion of the fat depots.

Although the main changes in protein metabolism are associated with the 'flow' phase, the acute phase plasma protein response is initiated early after injury. Hence, 6 h or so after tissue damage, plasma concentrations of the acute phase reactants (e.g. C-reactive protein and fibrinogen) rise. These rises are due to an increase in their hepatic synthesis, probably induced by interleukin-6 (IL-6). Plasma albumin concentrations often fall rapidly after injury, as a result of increased microvascular permeability rather than to a reduction in synthesis.

The role of the cytokines in mediation of the acute responses to injury remains controversial. While cytokines have been shown to mimic some of these responses, levels of plasma cytokines are not universally elevated immediately after injury. This may, of course, reflect their autocrine/paracrine rather than endocrine function. However, elevated plasma concentrations of the proinflammatory cytokines tumour necrosis factor-α (TNF-α), IL-β, IL-2, IL-6, and IL-8 occur after accidental injury. Also IL-6 levels have been directly related both to the severity of multiple trauma and to the magnitude of surgical trauma. IL-6 may also be involved in the activation of the hypothalamo–pituitary–adrenal axis by peripheral tissue injury, probably by means of the induction of cyclo-oxygenase products at the blood–brain interface (e.g. the circumventricular organs).

If the injury is not overwhelming, and with appropriate control of the airway, breathing, and circulation, the 'ebb' phase gives way to the 'flow' phase.

Flow phase

The main metabolic features of the flow phase are an increase in metabolic rate (hypermetabolism), due to catabolism (especially of skeletal muscle) and resistance to the anabolic effects of insulin (Table 2).

Hypermetabolism

There is said to be an increase in metabolic rate which is directly related to the severity of injury. Although such a relationship has been described for burned patients treated by exposure, it is not so clear after other injuries. One of the problems is that to describe a patient as hypermetabolic it is necessary that we define a normal metabolic rate for that individual; but what is a normal rate for someone who might be paralysed and ventilated, bedridden for a considerable time, receiving inadequate nutrition, and has suffered an acute reduction in body mass? All of these factors can reduce metabolic rate and thereby counteract any hypermetabolic stimuli associated with injury. It is also possible that in the most critically ill, energy expenditure may be limited by a failure of oxygen delivery. This may be the explanation for the finding of 'normal' metabolic rates in critically ill, septic patients.

What are the hypermetabolic stimuli alluded to above? There is an upward resetting of metabolic rate, perhaps triggered by a cytokine/prostanoid cascade, and there are increases in efferent sympathetic activity and substrate cycling (a process in which ATP is consumed without concomitant change in the amount of substrate or its metabolic products). Also, there is an extra organ—the wound—which contributes to whole body energy metabolism in two main ways. First, it can be the site of origin of the cytokine/prostanoid cascade mentioned above and, second, the wound is a consumer of glucose which it converts to lactate by aerobic glycolysis (an inefficient producer of ATP). The lactate produced is reconverted to glucose in the liver in an energy consuming process, thereby increasing hepatic oxygen consumption and blood flow. The evaporation of water from a burn wound or from an area of granulation tissue will also increase energy expenditure. The catabolism of lean tissue protein can also increase energy expenditure, but only in those with severe head injuries or very extensive burns is it likely to contribute more than 20 per cent to the total expenditure.

Protein metabolism

Whole body protein turnover is increased after injury with the balance between synthesis and breakdown being modified by the severity of injury and the influence of nutritional intake on synthesis. Thus, the severity of the injury increases both protein synthesis and breakdown. However, after the most severe injuries, the increase in breakdown predominates and cannot be counteracted by even the most aggressive nutritional support. It is now recognized that the increase in proteolysis in such catabolic conditions involves the ubiquitin–proteasome pathway. The increase in muscle protein

Table 2 Principle features of the flow phase response to injury

Increased metabolic rate
Increased urinary nitrogen excretion
Catabolism of skeletal muscle
Reduction in intracellular glutamine concentrations
Insulin resistance
    impaired glucose uptake into insulin dependant tissues
    impaired glucose storage
    increased hepatic gluconeogenesis
    increased lipolysis

catabolism is reflected by concomitant increases in the urinary excretion of nitrogen, 3-methylhistidine and, creatinine.

The most obvious site of net protein catabolism is skeletal muscle—although it also occurs in the respiratory muscles, the wall of the gut, and possibly the heart. Thus, in addition to problems with mobility, ventilation and the maintenance/restoration of enteral nutrition can also be compromised.

The increase in proteolysis provides amino acids as precursors for hepatic gluconeogenesis. The persistence of this glucose production at a time when plasma glucose and insulin concentrations are normal or raised can be considered as another facet of insulin resistance (see below). Plasma concentrations of several amino acids can fall at this time although their hepatic uptake is maintained by the increase in hepatic blood flow (see above). One amino acid that has received a lot of attention is glutamine, the intracellular concentration of which falls in skeletal muscle in response to injury. Glutamine is an important fuel for cells of the immune system, it is a precursor for the synthesis of glutathione (a free radical scavenger), has a role in nitric oxide metabolism, and has also been implicated in the maintenance of the integrity of the gut mucosal barrier, which may be compromised after injury.

Insulin resistance

Resistance to the 'anabolic' effects of insulin after injury is manifest in a several ways. For example hepatic glucose production, lipolysis, and net efflux of amino acids from skeletal muscle persist at plasma glucose and insulin concentrations which are inhibitory in uninjured subjects. Also the uptake of glucose into skeletal muscle is reduced, an impairment which involves glucose storage rather than oxidation.

The cause of injury-induced insulin resistance is unclear, although a role for the counter-regulatory hormones (cortisol, adrenaline, and glucagon) has been suggested. Whilst infusion of these hormones can induce insulin resistance in healthy individuals, the plasma concentrations needed are higher than those in injured/septic patients who are known to be insulin resistant. In this respect, the proinflammatory cytokines may have a role in modulating insulin sensitivity.

Plasma IL-6 concentrations in patients with cancer are positively correlated with the degree of insulin resistance and TNF-α has been implicated in the insulin resistance of diabetes and obesity. A role for IL-1 in the insulin resistance associated with endotoxaemia has also been suggested. The nature of the intracellular defect underlying insulin resistance remains to be elucidated but it may involve serine phosphorylation of insulin receptor substrate-1.

Manipulation of the metabolic response

Most efforts have been focused on trying to attenuate or reverse the loss of muscle mass. The administration of glutamine and anabolic agents such as growth hormone, insulin like growth factor (IGF), and oxandrolone have all been investigated.

Since glutamine plays such a central role in host defence mechanisms, there have been several studies of glutamine supplementation in, for example, surgical patients. These have shown preservation of intestinal mucosal integrity, enhanced immune function, and attenuation of the decrease in muscle intracellular glutamine concentration and protein synthesis. There have been fewer studies in critically ill patients, although one trial has shown that glutamine-supplemented parenteral nutrition improved 6-month survival.

The use of recombinant human growth hormone (rhGH) has produced conflicting results. Improvements in nitrogen balance have been reported in surgical, burned, and injured patients, and in the surgical group the improvement was accompanied by preservation of handgrip strength. In burned children, rhGH reduced the length of hospital stay, probably reflecting improved wound healing. However, other studies have failed to demonstrate an improvement in nitrogen balance and attenuation of muscle breakdown. The administration of IGF-1 in studies in animals and

human volunteers were encouraging, but several randomized, controlled studies in catabolic patients have failed to demonstrate any protein-sparing effect.

Oxandrolone is a testosterone analogue with anabolic activity that has been shown to be of benefit to patients with severe malnutrition and alcoholic hepatitis. A trial in patients with severe burns has shown that oxandrolone combined with an increased protein intake significantly increased the rate of weight gain and improved subjective measures of muscle strength.

Further reading

Aub JC (1920). Studies in experimental traumatic shock I. The basal metabolism. *American Journal of Physiology* **54**, 388–407.

Barton RN, Frayn KN, Little R A (1990). Trauma, burns and surgery. In: Cohen RD *et al.*, eds. *The metabolic and molecular basis of acquired disease*, pp. 684–717. Bailliere Tindall, London.

Cuthbertson DP (1942). Post-shock metabolic response. *Lancet* **1**, 433–7.

Frayn KN *et al.* (1985). The relationship of plasma catecholamines to acute metabolic and hormonal responses to injury in man. *Circulatory Shock* **16**, 229–40.

Garlick PJ, Wernerman J (1997). Protein metabolism in injury. In: Cooper GJ *et al.*, eds. *Scientific foundations of trauma*, pp. 690–728. Butterworth-Heinemann, Oxford.

Girolami A, Foex BA, Little RA (1999). Changes in the causes of trauma in the last 20 years. *Trauma* **1**, 3–11.

Griffiths RD, Hinds CJ, Little RA (1999). Manipulating the metabolic response to injury. *British Medical Bulletin* **55**, 181–95.

Little RA (1985). Heat production after injury. *British Medical Bulletin* **41**, 226–31.

Little RA, Kirkman E (1997). Cardiovascular control after injury. In: Cooper GJ *et al.*, eds. *Scientific foundations of trauma*, pp. 551–63. Butterworth-Heinemann, Oxford.

Turnbull AV, Rivier CL (1999). Regulation of the hypothalamic-pituitary-adrenal axis by cytokines: Actions and mechanisms of action. *Physiological Reviews* **70**, 1–71.

Wilmore DW, Stoner HB (1997). The wound-organ. In: Cooper GJ *et al.*, eds. *Scientific foundations of trauma*, pp. 524–9. Butterworth-Heinemann, Oxford.

11.12.3 Familial Mediterranean fever and other inherited periodic fever syndromes

P. N. Hawkins and D. R. Booth

The hereditary periodic fever syndromes are a group of multisystem disorders characterized by recurrent episodes of fever in association with inflammation that variably affects serosal linings, joints, and skin. They include familial Mediterranean fever, which is by far the most common, familial Hibernian fever, the hyperimmunoglobulin D syndrome, the Muckle–Wells syndrome, and familial cold urticaria. Although some of the individual features of these diseases overlap, there are distinctions in their mode of inheritance, their clinical features, and the frequency of symptoms. There has been substantial progress in elucidating the molecular basis of the hereditary periodic fever syndromes, which has proved to be surprisingly diverse and has opened several new avenues in inflammation research. Molecular analysis has already had a major impact on clinical diagnosis and the genetic defect in familial Hibernian fever has suggested a specific form of treatment. All of these disorders are compatible with normal life expectancy but since each of them is associated with a prominent, acute phase plasma protein response, potentially fatal systemic AA amyloidosis may develop unless the underlying inflammatory condition can be suppressed.

Familial Mediterranean fever

Familial Mediterranean fever (FMF) is an inherited, inflammatory disease that occurs most commonly in Jewish, Armenian, Turkish, and Middle Eastern Arab populations but also rarely in individuals of any ancestry. It is characterized by recurrent, acute attacks of fever, sterile peritonitis and pleurisy, arthritis, and erysipelas-like rashes lasting from 12 h to about 3 days, which in most cases can be prevented by regular prophylactic therapy with colchicine. The disorder is also known as recurrent polyserositis, periodic disease, Armenian disease, and other names besides, but the term familial Mediterranean fever is most commonly used. The recently identified gene responsible has been called *MEFV*, (Mediterranean fever), is located on chromosome 16 and appears to be expressed only in neutrophils. It encodes a hitherto uncharacterized protein called pyrin or marenostrin, and its discovery should enable the molecular basis of the disease to be unravelled. Analysis of *MEFV* has already revolutionized the diagnosis of FMF. About 30 mutations in *MEFV* have now been associated with FMF, and pairs of *MEFV* mutations, presumed to involve both alleles, can be found in most FMF patients. These findings accord with the autosomal recessive mode of inheritance that is usually evident clinically and which has long been recognized in population studies.

Pathogenesis and genetics

Pyrin, the uncharacterized protein product of *MEFV*, consists of 781 amino acids with a molecular weight of about 90 kDa. Messenger RNA for pyrin is found exclusively in neutrophils and their precursor cells. The amino acid sequence of pyrin contains zinc finger motifs, potential phosphorylation sites, and a B30.2 domain, all typical of several other proteins that act within the nucleus. Pyrin could therefore be a transcription factor and, if so, it could suppress the production of a proinflammatory molecule, or upregulate the transcription of an anti-inflammatory one. However, the same features are also found in some proteins acting outside the nucleus and which are involved in protein–protein interactions. It is likely that the *MEFV* mutations which cause FMF disrupt the structure of pyrin sufficiently to reduce its function, leading to inappropriate neutrophil activation and migration. The recurrent, acute clinical attacks, along with massive influx of neutrophils into serosal and synovial linings, would be consistent with bursts of relatively uncontrolled neutrophil activity. Patients with FMF often have prolonged periods of apparently normal health between their attacks, suggesting that reduced pyrin function has clinical consequences only in certain circumstances. Physical and emotional stress, menstruation, and diet have been reported to increase susceptibility to FMF attacks and the irregular nature of symptoms supports the notion that clinical attacks of FMF may be triggered by exogenous factors. The characteristic pattern of inflammation in serosal and synovial membranes, and the paucity of evidence in patients with FMF for exacerbation of other inflammatory processes in which neutrophils are involved, suggest that pyrin may regulate a rather specific facet of neutrophil behaviour.

The 30 or so *MEFV* mutations that are associated with FMF encode either single amino acid substitutions or deletions in the pyrin molecule. The mutations that commonly cause FMF are in exon 10 of the pyrin gene, and in exon 5 in some populations. Although a polymorphism in exon 2 encoding the pyrin variant E148Q may contribute to FMF in some cases, homozygosity for E148Q does not seem to be sufficient to cause FMF. Whilst it is inherently likely that different mutations will impair the func-

tion of a protein to differing extents, several findings indicate that the methionine residue at position 694 may be critical for the normal function of pyrin. Three different pathogenic exon 10 mutations involving M694 have been identified (M694V, M694I, and deletion M694) and individuals who are homozygous for M694V are reported to have particularly severe and early-onset FMF disease, as well as a greater propensity to develop AA amyloidosis. It is also noteworthy that simple heterozygous deletion of residue M694, which is likely to produce more severe structural disruption than an amino acid substitution, has been reported, by itself, to cause typical FMF in several British families. Recognition that *MEFV* mutations affecting a single allele may give rise to FMF suggests that a 50 per cent complement of normally functioning pyrin is not sufficient to prevent susceptibility to the disease. Severe disruption of a single *MEFV* allele by one or more mutations may therefore account for the rare reports of autosomal dominant FMF. However, transmission of FMF is pseudodominant in most families in which more than one successive generation is affected by the disease and this usually reflects consanguinity or a high incidence of the FMF trait in the population at risk. Up to one individual in seven in some Mediterranean regions is an FMF carrier, and the apparently 'mild' pyrin variant E148Q occurs very widely indeed. Pyrin E148Q has been identified in European whites, black Africans, Punjabi Indians, and Chinese populations, with an allele frequency of about 20 per cent in the latter two groups. The remarkable global prevalence of pyrin E148Q supports the hypothesis that the FMF trait conferred a survival benefit during evolution. Possible mechanisms for this include enhanced resistance to microbial infection mediated by non-specific upregulation of the inflammatory response. It is worth considering that the same process may have the potential to exacerbate chronic inflammatory disorders.

Clinical features

Patients with FMF typically present with acute attacks of fever, peritonitic abdominal pain, pleuritic chest pain, arthralgia, and rash in approximately this order of frequency. However, the pattern of tissue involvement varies substantially between patients, and even in the same patient on different occasions. Other features occasionally include myalgia, headache, orchitis, and cutaneous and renal vasculitis. The symptoms of FMF usually start in the first decade of life, and only five per cent of patients develop symptoms after 30 years of age, although the frequency and severity of attacks can alter substantially during the course of a patient's life.

A brief prodrome may occur after which the temperature rises to 38 to 40°C in almost every case. Peritonitis occurs in more than 90 per cent of cases and evolves over a few hours. It is readily misdiagnosed as acute appendicitis or some other surgical crisis. Many patients become confined to bed with severe pain and vomiting but these features can be quite mild or absent in other cases. Diarrhoea is unusual. Pleurisy occurs in about 50 per cent of patients, is typically unilateral, and can be associated with atelectasis or a small effusion. Involvement of joints also occurs in about half of the patients, and can range from polyarthralgia without overt soft tissue swelling to a more classical monoarticular synovitis affecting the knees or hips. The rash of FMF is less common but comprises very characteristic 10 to 15-cm, erysipelas-like, warm swollen lesions on the lower leg. Pericarditis, perhaps curiously, is rare. The acute crisis of FMF usually resolves in less than 3 days, and attacks tend to recur at irregular intervals of weeks or months. Direct long-term sequelae of FMF, such as serosal fibrosis and adhesions, occur rarely although a small proportion of patients do develop a chronic inflammatory arthritis that can lead to severe joint destruction. The most important and life-threatening long term consequence of FMF is AA amyloidosis (see below).

Investigations

No laboratory test is specific for FMF. The identification of *MEFV* clearly represents a major advance both in elucidating the molecular basis of the disease and for its diagnosis but the results of genetic testing in any individual must be interpreted with care. This is essential because individuals with *MEFV* mutations seem to differ greatly in their susceptibility to developing FMF and many have subclinical inflammatory disease. They may also have some other, unrelated inflammatory disease that show symptom overlaps with FMF. Another practical problem is that *MEFV* is a relatively large gene spanning 10 exons, and limited screening for common mutations will fail to identify abnormalities in many patients, particularly in those with atypical ethnic backgrounds in whom rare or new mutations are more likely. Certainly, in the absence of an exon 10 mutation, the diagnosis of FMF is unlikely in patients from ethnic groups in which FMF typically occurs. However, even the most comprehensive analysis of the *MEFV* coding region has identified only single allele mutations in some patients with classical FMF and no mutations at all in a few cases. Thus, mutations in regulatory regions of *MEFV*, or indeed mutations in other genes, might contribute to the pathogenesis of the disease in some patients; alternatively, certain heterozygotes may be unusually susceptible to FMF. The results of *MEFV* genotyping should therefore be interpreted in light of each clinical presentation and ethnic origin.

Diagnostic clinical criteria for the evaluation of patients with features suggestive of FMF are well developed. During the clinical attacks of FMF, the number of neutrophils in peripheral blood may rise from normal levels by several fold. Some patients have a mild normochromic anaemia and polyclonal hyperglobulinaemia but the most striking serological feature of the disease is the magnitude of the acute phase plasma protein response that is evoked. During a typical clinical attack, the concentration of C-reactive protein generally exceeds 100 mg/l and may be greater than 250 mg/l; the plasma concentration of serum amyloid A protein often attains even higher levels, frequently exceeding 500 mg/l (normal less than 3 mg/l). Both C-reactive protein and serum amyloid A protein have half-lives in the circulation of less than 24 h, and their concentrations fall to healthy baseline values within several days of resolution of an acute episode. Serial monitoring of these sensitive and dynamic markers has shown that bursts of inflammation occur frequently in patients with FMF in the absence of symptoms, and even, to a lesser extent, among those taking regular colchicine therapy. Our own practice in a patient with suspected FMF is to measure the concentration of C-reactive protein and serum amyloid A protein on four or five occasions at 2-weekly intervals. In many cases, this will objectively document self-limiting 'periodic' bursts of inflammation. It is often useful to repeat this type of analysis during a therapeutic trial of colchicine.

Amyloidosis

AA amyloidosis is the most significant complication of FMF since it is unpredictable, progressive and potentially fatal. AA amyloid fibrils are derived from a 76 amino acid N-terminal cleavage fragment of the 104 residue serum amyloid A protein. Before the beneficial effect of colchicine in FMF was known, the lifetime incidence of AA amyloidosis was reported to be up to 30 per cent or more. The risk of developing amyloidosis appears to be greater among Sephardic Jews and Turks than among non-Sephardic Jews and Armenians. Some patients with FMF present with AA amyloidosis before they have experienced symptoms of the inflammatory disease, a situation often referred to as (pheno)type II FMF. The lack of a clear association between the severity of symptoms in FMF and the likelihood of developing AA amyloidosis, and the different incidence of amyloidosis among various ethnic groups has led some investigators to question the nature of the relationship. However, the features of AA amyloid in patients with FMF are identical to those in patients with every other type of chronic inflammatory disease, ranging from the composition of the amyloid fibril protein to the distribution and clinical consequences of the amyloid deposits. Although there are evidently unknown genetic or environmental factors that influence susceptibility to AA amyloidosis generally, acute phase production of serum amyloid A protein is the only absolute prerequisite for AA amyloid deposition. Systematic serial monitoring of serum amyloid A protein has confirmed that a major acute phase response frequently occurs in patients with FMF in the absence of symptoms, and the magnitude and

duration of this is probably a very substantial determinant of the risk of developing amyloidosis. Evaluation of this risk is likely to become more refined when the significance of different *MEFV* mutations, serum amyloid A protein isotypes, and other factors is better understood, but for the time being all patients with FMF who have had uncontrolled inflammation, with or without symptoms, must be regarded as susceptible. *MEFV* analysis in patients with FMF complicated by AA amyloidosis, who have been evaluated in our own clinic, has demonstrated a wide spectrum and combination of mutations suggesting that amyloidosis is not restricted to any particular genotype.

AA amyloid deposition may be extensive without causing symptoms and can develop at any time from early childhood to late adult life. AA amyloid initially accumulates in the spleen, and functional hyposplenism may eventually develop. However, the most common mode of presentation is with non-selective proteinuria, nephrotic syndrome, and/or renal insufficiency. Acute renal failure may be precipitated by minor insults, and end-stage renal failure and its complications are the most frequent cause of death. Patients sometimes present with hepatosplenomegaly, occasionally without overt renal dysfunction, but renal deposits are nevertheless always present in such cases. The adrenal glands are involved in at least one-third of cases and the liver in a quarter. Although the function of these latter organs is often well preserved, hepatic amyloidosis is a sign of advanced and extensive disease and has a poor prognosis. Histological involvement of the gut is common, but tends only to cause symptoms in patients whose disease is generally very advanced. AA amyloidosis rarely ever causes overt cardiac disease. The prognosis is chiefly determined by the extent of amyloid at diagnosis and the effectiveness with which production of serum amyloid A protein can be suppressed by colchicine therapy. Proteinuria should be sought routinely in patients with FMF, and the suspicion of amyloid followed-up by renal or rectal biopsy and Congo-red staining. Serum amyloid P component scintigraphy is a sensitive and specific non-invasive method for imaging amyloid in visceral organs and can be used serially to monitor the deposits in a quantitative manner. Scintigraphic follow-up studies in more than 100 patients with AA amyloidosis, some of whom had FMF, have confirmed the findings of numerous clinical and histological case reports by demonstrating that the amyloid deposits frequently regress when production of serum amyloid A protein is reduced to normal healthy baseline levels. Routine monitoring of serum amyloid A protein should be an integral part of the management of all patients with AA amyloid and automated immunoassay systems for serum amyloid A protein are available, standardized on a World Health Organization International Reference Standard.

Treatment

The only effective treatment for FMF is colchicine, a serendipitous discovery made by Goldfinger in 1972. Regular prophylactic treatment with colchicine at a dose of 1 to 2 mg daily prevents or substantially reduces the clinical manifestations of FMF in at least 95 per cent of cases. A proportion of the remainder are poorly compliant or intolerant of the drug. Studies in which serum amyloid A protein has been monitored in FMF patients who have been rendered free of symptoms by colchicine therapy show that the subclinical inflammation is also substantially, but often not completely, prevented. Colchicine modulates neutrophil function by binding to tubulin in microtubules which inhibits motility and exocytosis of the intracellular granules and diminishes neutrophil chemotaxis *in vitro* and *in vivo*. However, colchicine is not generally effective in other acute or chronic inflammatory diseases, even in those in which neutrophils are recognized to have an important role. The mechanism by which colchicine exerts its beneficial effect in FMF, and how, if at all, it influences the pyrin pathway are not yet known.

Regular, long-term use of colchicine is advisable in every patient with FMF and mandatory in those with AA amyloidosis. Not only does this prevent amyloidosis from developing in the first place but established amyloid deposition will usually be halted by an adequate dose of the drug. Existing amyloid deposits may gradually regress. The clinical effects of amyloid may also resolve, particularly proteinuria in patients whose glomerular filtration is well preserved. FMF patients with end-stage renal failure due to AA amyloidosis are often excellent candidates for renal transplantation, since graft amyloid can also be prevented by colchicine prophylaxis. Although colchicine is an extremely toxic agent in large quantities, the small regular dose required for the treatment of FMF is generally well tolerated. The most frequent adverse effect of low-dose colchicine is diarrhoea, but this seldom prevents its use and sometimes responds to a lactose-free diet. Despite concerns about the antimitotic potential of colchicine, the drug does not appear to cause infertility or lead to birth defects, even when used throughout pregnancy, or have any other long-term adverse effect. The concentration of colchicine in breast milk is sufficiently low to permit breast feeding.

Colchicine is largely ineffective in the acute management of FMF attacks. Analgesics and intravenous fluid replacement are required in some patients but a low threshold for intravenous fluids should be the policy for FMF patients with AA amyloidosis since hypovolaemia can precipitate irreversible renal failure in these patients.

Familial Hibernian fever (tumour necrosis factor receptor associated periodic syndrome—TRAPS)

The term familial Hibernian fever was coined by Williamson in 1982, who described a large Irish family with a periodic fever syndrome inherited in an autosomal dominant manner. Affected individuals had intermittent bouts of fever, abdominal pain, painful erythematous rashes, arthralgia, and myalgia. Flares of the disease are very much less distinct than in FMF and patients frequently remain symptomatic for weeks or sometimes months on end. The clinical manifestations of inflammation are associated with a very intense acute phase response which can be sustained even when symptoms abate. Several affected individuals have developed AA amyloidosis. Only a handful of other families, most of Northern European ancestry, have been reported with similar syndromes but its genetic basis has recently been discovered. This is not only of major diagnostic value in autosomal dominant periodic fever syndromes, but it has also identified a novel mechanism of inflammation that suggests a specific therapeutic approach.

The disease is caused by at least 16 different missense mutations in the gene on chromosome 12 which encodes tumour necrosis factor receptor 1 (TNFRSF1A). Tumour necrosis factor (TNF) is a potent proinflammatory cytokine that is implicated very widely in inflammation. TNFRSF1A is expressed on the outer membrane of most cells in the body where it acts closely with TNF receptor 2 to bind TNF and lymphotoxin cytokines and signal the activation of a complex inflammatory pathway. This signalling can be turned off by enzymatic cleavage and shedding of the soluble, extracellular portion of TNFRSF1A from the cell surface into the blood. This has a dual effect since it disrupts the signalling mechanism and the soluble TNFRSF1A that is released can bind and neutralize TNF in the circulation. Many of the mutations that have been identified in autosomal dominant periodic fever syndromes are thought to disrupt conserved disulphide bonds in the extracellular TNFRSF1A domain and interfere with the physiological negative feedback control mechanism. The plasma concentration of soluble TNFRSF1A is abnormally low in many patients with these diseases, and measurement of soluble TNFRSF1A (also known as p55 protein) may be a useful way of screening for the disorder. It is now widely accepted that the dominantly inherited fever syndromes associated with TNF receptor mutations should be classified as tumour necrosis factor receptor associated periodic syndromes (TRAPS).

This disorder responds partially to colchicine in some cases but can usually be suppressed by high doses of corticosteroids and other immunosuppressive agents. The genetic basis of the disorder suggests that specific blockade of TNF might be beneficial, and early experience with this approach has been promising.

Hyperimmunoglobulinaemia D periodic fever syndrome

The hyperimmunoglobulinaemia D periodic fever syndrome (HIDS) was first described in the Netherlands in 1984. It is inherited in an autosomal recessive manner and is characterized by intermittent, irregular attacks of abdominal pain and fever in association with an acute phase response and persistent elevation of the plasma concentration of immunoglobulin D. Attacks characteristically occur every 1 or 2 months and last for 3 to 7 days, but with considerable individual variation. Unlike FMF, the abdominal pain does not usually have the overt features of peritonitis, and is frequently associated with diarrhoea as well as vomiting. Lymphadenopathy occurs in most patients and arthralgia affecting the knees and ankles is present in about two-thirds of cases. Most families are of western European origin. The acute phase response in HIDS tends to be less intense than in the other inherited periodic fever syndromes described here, and this is likely to be the reason for an apparently very low risk of developing AA amyloidosis.

HIDS has lately been attributed to several mutations affecting both alleles of the gene on chromosome 12 encoding mevalonate kinase, MVK. This enzyme is involved in isoprenoid synthesis and catalyses the phosphorylation of mevalonate to 5-phosphomevalonate. The identified mutations have been shown to reduce its enzymatic activity. Different mutations in MVK are the cause of mevalonic aciduria, another inherited and much more severe multisystem disease. Excretion of mevalonic acid in the urine is increased constitutively in mevalonic aciduria, but only during the febrile episodes, if at all, in HIDS. The pathogenesis of these disorders, including the dysregulation of immunoglobulin D production, is not understood and, as in FMF, a previously unknown pathway that can profoundly regulate an aspect of the inflammatory response may be involved.

Muckle–Wells syndrome and familial cold urticaria

Muckle–Wells syndrome and familial cold urticaria are very rare, dominantly inherited, periodic fever syndromes. Fever and rash are prominent features of both conditions, and both can be complicated by AA amyloidosis. The original family described by Muckle and Wells in 1962 had progressive sensorineural deafness, although this does not occur in other cases. Arthralgia and poorly characterized limb pain occur in both disorders, and both conditions tend to start in early childhood. The skin rash, fever, and other symptoms in familial cold urticaria are triggered by exposure to cold. The frequency and pattern of symptoms is extremely variable but they can be present for very prolonged periods in both disorders. The search for the genetic basis of these two disorders, which evidently have a number of overlapping clinical features, has lately linked both of them to chromosome 1q44. It is therefore possible that Muckle–Wells syndrome and familial cold urticaria represent different phenotypic manifestations of the same mutation, or that they might be due to different mutations in the same gene. Phenotypic expression of familial cold urticaria can presumably be influenced by climatic conditions. We have lately evaluated a family with this syndrome that resides in a warm part of India, perhaps accounting for the very mild symptoms in most of the affected members. Treatment for these disorders centres mainly on corticosteroids and immunosuppressive drugs. A therapeutic trial of colchicine is, however, worthwhile, since it seems to be quite effective in a proportion of cases. Most patients with these syndromes have a normal life expectancy, although in the absence of a generally effective treatment, the outlook is poor for individuals who develop AA amyloidosis.

Further reading

Drenth JPH *et al.* (1999). Mutations in the gene encoding mevalonate kinase cause hyper-IgD and periodic fever syndrome. *Nature Genetics* **22**, 178–81.

McDermott MF (1999). Autosomal dominant recurrent fevers. Clinical and genetic aspects. *Revue du Rheumatisme* **66**, 484–91.

Samuels J *et al.* (1998). Familial Mediterranean fever at the millennium. Clinical spectrum, ancient mutations, and a survey of 100 American referrals to the National Institutes of Health. *Medicine* **77**, 268–97.

11.12.4 Amyloidosis

M. B. Pepys and P. N. Hawkins

Introduction

Amyloidosis is a disorder of protein folding, characterized by extracellular deposition of abnormal protein fibrils. The underlying molecular abnormalities may be either acquired or hereditary and about 20 different proteins can form clinically or pathologically significant amyloid fibrils *in vivo* (Tables 1 and 2). Amyloid deposits also contain glycosaminoglycans, some of which are tightly associated with the fibrils, and also a non-fibrillar plasma glycoprotein, amyloid P component. Small, focal, clinically silent amyloid deposits in the brain, heart, seminal vesicles, and joints are a universal accompaniment of ageing. However, clinically important amyloid deposits usually accumulate progressively, disrupting the structure and function of affected tissues and leading inexorably to organ failure and death. No treatment yet exists which can specifically cause resolution, but intervention which reduces the availability of the amyloid fibril precursor proteins may lead to regression.

Clinical amyloidosis

Introduction

Amyloidosis occurs in many clinical disorders. Amyloid deposits in the brain and cerebral blood vessels are a central part of the pathology of Alzheimer's disease, which is the fourth most common cause of death in the Western world, whilst amyloid is present in the islets of Langerhans of the pancreas in all patients with type 2, maturity onset, diabetes mellitus. Amyloid deposition in the bones, joints, and periarticular structures eventually affects most patients who are on long-term haemodialysis for end-stage renal failure and is the most frequent cause of serious morbidity among the approximately 800 000 such individuals worldwide. Systemic amyloidosis complicating myeloma and other B-cell dyscrasias, or chronic infections and inflammatory diseases, is very important because diagnosis is often difficult and the prognosis is poor, but effective treatments are increasingly available. Hereditary amyloidosis is very rare, except in a few geographic foci, but its diversity is remarkable. It is important because of its poor prognosis, the complexity of clinical management, the difficult genetic issues involved, and its considerable value as a model for understanding the pathogenesis of amyloid deposition.

Although there are some correlations between fibril protein type and clinical manifestations, there are also many forms of acquired and hereditary amyloidosis in which there is little or no concordance between the fibril protein, or the genotype of its precursor, and the clinical phenotype. There are evidently genetic and/or environmental factors, which are distinct from the amyloid fibril protein itself, which determine whether, when, and where clinically significant amyloid deposits form. The nature of these

important determinants of amyloidogenesis is obscure. Furthermore, the mechanisms by which amyloid deposition causes disease are poorly understood. Whilst a heavy amyloid load is invariably a bad sign, there is often a poor correlation between the local amount of amyloid and the level of organ dysfunction. Active deposition of new amyloid is often associated with enhanced deterioration compared with stable long-standing deposits. Nascent or newly formed amyloid fibrils, generated *in vitro*, are also cytotoxic to cultured cells, whilst aged or *ex vivo* fibrils are generally inert, although it is not known how this relates to effects *in vivo*.

Reactive systemic (AA) amyloidosis

Associated conditions

AA amyloidosis occurs in association with chronic inflammatory disorders, chronic local or systemic microbial infections, and occasionally malignant neoplasms. In Western Europe and the United States the most frequent

Table 1 Acquired amyloidosis syndromes

Clinical syndrome	Fibril protein
Systemic AL amyloidosis, associated with immunocyte dyscrasia, myeloma, monoclonal gammopathy, occult dyscrasia	AL derived from monoclonal immunoglobulin light chains
Local nodular AL amyloidosis (skin, respiratory tract, urogenital tract, etc.) associated with focal immunocyte dyscrasia	AL derived from monoclonal immunoglobulin light chains
Reactive systemic AA amyloidosis, associated with chronic active diseases	AA derived from SAA
Senile systemic amyloidosis	Transthyretin derived from plasma transthyretin
Focal senile amyloidosis:	
Atria of the heart	Atrial natriuretic peptide
Brain	$A\beta$
Joints	Not known
Seminal vesicles	Seminal vesicle exocrine protein
Prostrate	β_2-Microglobulin
Atheromatous plaques	Apolipoprotein A-I N-terminal fragment
Non-familial Alzheimer's disease, Down's syndrome	$A\beta$ derived from APP
Sporadic cerebral amyloid angiopathy	$A\beta$ derived from APP
Inclusion body myositis	$A\beta$ derived from APP
Sporadic Creutzfeldt–Jacob disease, kuru (transmissible spongiform encephalopathies, prion diseases)	PrP^{Sc} derived from PrP^C
Type 2 diabetes mellitus	IAPP (amylin) derived from its precursor protein
Endocrine amyloidosis, associated with apudomas	Peptide hormones or fragments thereof (e.g. precalcitonin in medullary carcinoma of thyroid)
Haemodialysis-associated amyloidosis; localized to osteoarticular tissues or systemic	β_2-microglobulin derived from high plasma levels
Primary localized cutaneous amyloid (macular, papular)	? Keratin-derived
Ocular amyloid (cornea, conjunctiva)	Not known
Orbital amyloid	AL or AH derived from monoclonal Ig

Abbreviations: AL, monoclonal immunoglobulin light chain; AA, amyloid A; SAA, serum amyloid A protein; APP, amyloid precursor protein; IAPP, islet amyloid polypeptide; AH, monoclonal immunoglobulin heavy chain fragment; Ig, immunoglobulin.

predisposing conditions are idiopathic rheumatic diseases (Table 3). Amyloidosis complicates up to 10 per cent of cases of rheumatoid arthritis and juvenile inflammatory arthritis, although for reasons that are not clear the incidence is lower in the United States than in Europe. Amyloidosis is exceptionally rare in systemic lupus erythematosus and related connective tissue diseases and in ulcerative colitis, in contrast to Crohn's disease. Tuberculosis and leprosy are important causes of AA amyloidosis, particularly where these infections are endemic. Chronic osteomyelitis, bronchiectasis, chronically infected burns, and decubitus ulcers as well as the chronic

Table 2 Hereditary amyloidosis syndromes

Clinical syndrome	Fibril protein
Predominant peripheral nerve involvement, familial amyloid polyneuropathy. Autosomal dominant	Transthyretin variants (commonly Met30, over 60 described)
	Apolipoprotein A-I N-terminal fragment of variant Arg26
Predominant cranial nerve involvement with lattice corneal dystrophy. Autosomal dominant	Gelsolin, fragment of variants Asn187 or Tyr187
Oculoleptomeningeal amyloidosis. Autosomal dominant	Transthyretin variants
Non-neuropathic, prominent visceral involvement (Ostertag-type). Autosomal dominant	Apolipoprotein A-I N-terminal fragment of variants (nine described)
	Lysozyme variants Thr56 or His67
	Fibrinogen α-chain variants Val526 or Leu554
Predominant cardiac involvement, no clinical neuropathy. Autosomal dominant	Transthyretin genetic variants Thr45, Ala60, Ser84, Met111, Ile122
Hereditary cerebral haemorrhage with amyloidosis (cerebral amyloid angiopathy). Autosomal dominant:	
Icelandic type (major asymptomatic systemic amyloid also present)	Cystatin C, fragment of variant Glu68
Dutch type	Aβ derived from APP variant Gln693
Familial Alzheimer's disease. Autosomal dominant	Aβ derived from APP variants Ile717, Phe717 or Gly717, etc
	Aβ derived from wild type APP due to presenilin mutations
Familial dementia — probable Alzheimer's disease	Aβ derived from variant APP Asn670, Leu671
Familial Creutzfeldt–Jacob disease, GSS syndrome (hereditary spongiform encephalopathies, prion diseases). Autosomal dominant	PrP^{Sc} derived from PrP^{C} variants 51–91 insert, Leu102, Val117, Asn178, Lys200
Familial Mediterranean fever, prominent renal involvement. Autosomal recessive	AA derived from SAA
Muckle–Well's syndrome, nephropathy, deafness, urticaria, limb pain. Autosomal recessive	AA derived from SAA
Cardiomyopathy with persistent atrial standstill	Not known
Cutaneous deposits (bullous, papular, pustulodermal)	Not known

Amino acids: Met, methionine; Arg, arginine; Asn, asparagine; Tyr, tyrosine; Thr, threonine; His, histidine; Val, valine; Leu, leucine; Ala, alanine; Ser, serine; Ile, isoleucine; Glu, glutamic acid; Phe, phenylalanine; Gly, glycine; Gln, glutamine; Lys, lysine.
Abbreviations: Aβ, amyloid β; APP, amyloid precursor protein; SAA, serum amyloid A protein; PrP, prion protein; GSS, Gerstmann–Sträussler–Scheinker.

Table 3 Conditions associated with reactive systemic amyloid A amyloidosis

Chronic inflammatory disorders
  Rheumatoid arthritis
  Juvenile inflammatory arthritis
  Ankylosing spondylitis
  Psoriasis and psoriatic arthropathy
  Reiter's syndrome
  Adult Still's disease
  Behçet's syndrome
  Crohn's disease
Chronic microbial infections
  Leprosy
  Tuberculosis
  Bronchiectasis
  Decubitus ulcers
  Chronic pyelonephritis in paraplegics
  Osteomyelitis
  Whipple's disease
Malignant neoplasms
  Hodgkin's disease
  Renal carcinoma
  Carcinomas of gut, lung, urogenital tract
  Basal cell carcinoma
  Hairy cell leukaemia

pyelonephritis of paraplegic patients are other well-recognized associations (Table 3). Hodgkin's disease and renal carcinoma, which often cause fever, other systemic symptoms, and a major acute phase response, are the malignancies most commonly associated with systemic AA amyloidosis.

Clinical features

AA amyloid involves the viscera but may be widely distributed without causing clinical symptoms. More than 90 per cent of patients present with non-selective proteinuria due to glomerular deposition, and nephrotic syndrome may develop before progression to endstage renal failure. Haematuria, isolated tubular defects, nephrogenic diabetes insipidus, and diffuse renal calcification occur rarely. Kidney size is usually normal, but may be enlarged, or, in advanced cases, reduced. Endstage chronic renal failure is the cause of death in 40 to 60 per cent of cases but acute renal failure may be precipitated by hypotension and/or salt and water depletion following surgery, excessive use of diuretics, or intercurrent infection, and may be associated with renal vein thrombosis. The second most common presentation is with organ enlargement, such as hepatosplenomegaly or thyroid goitre, with or without overt renal abnormality, but in any case amyloid deposits are almost always widespread at the time of presentation. Involvement of the heart and gastrointestinal tract is frequent, but rarely causes functional impairment.

AA amyloidosis may become clinically evident early in the course of associated disease, but the incidence increases with duration of the primary condition. The mean duration of chronic rheumatic diseases such as rheumatoid arthritis, ankylosing spondylitis, or juvenile rheumatoid arthritis before amyloid is diagnosed is 12 to 14 years, although it can present much sooner. For most patients the prognosis is closely related to the degree of renal involvement and the effectiveness of treatment of the underlying inflammatory condition. In the presence of persistent, uncontrolled inflammation, 50 per cent of patients with AA amyloid die within 5 years of the amyloid being diagnosed; however, if the acute phase response can be consistently suppressed proteinuria can cease, renal function is retained, and the prognosis is much better. Availability of chronic haemodialysis and transplantation prevents early death from uraemia *per se*, but amyloid deposition in extrarenal tissues is responsible for a less favourable prognosis than for other causes of endstage renal failure.

Amyloidosis associated with immunocyte dyscrasia: monoclonal immunoglobulin light chain (AL) amyloidosis

Associated conditions

Almost any dyscrasia of cells of the B-lymphocyte lineage, including multiple myeloma, malignant lymphomas, and macroglobulinaemia, may be complicated by AL amyloidosis but most cases are associated with otherwise 'benign' monoclonal gammopathy. Amyloid occurs in up to 15 per cent of cases of myeloma, in a lower proportion of other malignant B-cell disorders, and probably in fewer than 5 per cent of patients with a 'benign' monoclonal gammopathy. In some cases deposition of AL amyloid may be the only evidence of the dyscrasia. A monoclonal paraprotein or free light chains can be detected in the serum or urine of only about 90 per cent of patients with AL amyloid, but detection of immunoglobulin gene rearrangement in the bone marrow or peripheral blood sometimes confirms a monoclonal gammopathy in the remaining cases. The paraprotein may also appear after presentation and diagnosis of the amyloid, and subnormal levels of some or all serum immunoglobulins or increased numbers of marrow plasma cells may provide less direct clues to the underlying aetiology. Until recently it has been the practice to diagnose apparently 'primary' cases of amyloidosis, with no previous predisposing inflammatory condition or family history of amyloidosis, as AL type by exclusion. However, it has lately been recognized that autosomal dominant hereditary non-neuropathic amyloidosis, particularly that caused by variant fibrinogen α-chain, may be poorly penetrant and of late onset, so that there may be no family history. The coincident occurrence of a monoclonal gammopathy may then be gravely misleading and it is essential to exclude by genotyping all known amyloidogenic mutations, and to seek positive immunohistochemical or biochemical identification of the amyloid fibril protein in all cases.

Clinical features

AL amyloid occurs equally in men and women, usually over the age of 50 but occasionally in young adults. It has a lifetime incidence, and is the cause of death, of between 0.5 and 1 per thousand individuals in the United Kingdom. The clinical manifestations are protean, as virtually any tissue other than the brain may be directly involved. Uraemia, heart failure, or other effects of the amyloid usually cause death within a year of diagnosis, unless the underlying B-cell clone is effectively suppressed.

The heart is affected in 90 per cent of patients with AL amyloid, in 30 per cent of whom restrictive cardiomyopathy is the presenting feature and in up to 50 per cent of whom it is fatal. Other cardiac presentations include arrhythmias and angina. Renal AL amyloid has the same manifestations as renal AA amyloid, but the prognosis is worse. Gut involvement may cause disturbances of motility (often secondary to autonomic neuropathy), malabsorption, perforation, haemorrhage, or obstruction. Macroglossia occurs rarely but is almost pathognomonic. Hyposplenism sometimes occurs in both AA and AL amyloidosis. Painful sensory polyneuropathy with early loss of pain and temperature sensation followed later by motor deficits is seen in 10 to 20 per cent of cases and carpal tunnel syndrome in 20 per cent. Autonomic neuropathy leading to orthostatic hypotension, impotence, and gastrointestinal disturbances may occur alone or together with the peripheral neuropathy, and has a very poor prognosis. Skin involvement takes the form of papules, nodules, and plaques usually on the face and upper trunk, and involvement of dermal blood vessels results in purpura occurring either spontaneously or after minimal trauma and is very common. Articular amyloid is rare but may mimic acute polyarticular rheumatoid arthritis, or it may present as asymmetrical arthritis affecting the hip or shoulder. Infiltration of the glenohumeral joint and surrounding soft tissues occasionally produces the characteristic 'shoulder pad' sign. A rare but serious manifestation of AL amyloid is an acquired bleeding diathesis that may be associated with deficiency of factor X and sometimes also factor IX, or with increased fibrinolysis. It does not occur in AA amyloidosis, although in both AL and AA disease there may be serious bleeding in the absence of any identifiable factor deficiency.

Senile amyloidosis

Some amyloid is present in all autopsies on individuals over 80 years of age but it is not known whether this contributes to the ageing process or whether it is an epiphenomenon that becomes clinically important only when it is extensive.

Senile systemic amyloidosis

Up to 25 per cent of old people have microscopic, clinically silent systemic deposits of transthyretin amyloid involving the walls of the heart and blood vessels, smooth and striated muscle, fat tissue, renal papillae, and alveolar walls. In contrast to most other forms of systemic amyloidosis, including hereditary transthyretin amyloid caused by point mutations in the transthyretin gene, the spleen and renal glomeruli are rarely affected. The brain is not involved. Occasionally more extensive deposits in the heart, affecting the ventricles and atria and situated in the interstitium and vessel walls, cause significant impairment of cardiac function and may be fatal. The transthyretin involved is probably usually of the normal wild type but cases with transthyretin variants have been described which may be hereditary.

Senile focal amyloidosis

Microscopic and clinically silent amyloid deposits of different fibril types, localized to particular tissues, are very commonly present in old people. Deposits of β-protein (see below) as amyloid in cerebral blood vessels and intracerebral plaques seen in 'normal' elderly brains may or may not be the harbinger of Alzheimer's disease had the patient survived long enough. Amyloid deposits are present in most osteoarthritic joints at surgery or autopsy, usually in close association with calcium pyrophosphate deposits, affecting the articular cartilage and joint capsule. However, neither the clinical significance of this age-associated articular amyloid nor its biochemical nature are known. The corpora amylacea of the prostate are composed of $β_2$-microglobulin amyloid fibrils. Amyloid in the seminal vesicles is derived from an as yet unidentified exocrine secretory product of the vesicle cells. Isolated deposits of cardiac atrial amyloid consist of atrial natriuretic peptide. Focal amyloid deposits commonly present in atheromatous plaques of elderly subjects contain fibrils composed of the N-terminal fragment of apolipoprotein A-I.

Cerebral amyloidosis

Introduction

The brain is a very common and important site of amyloid deposition (Table 4), although possibly because of the blood–brain barrier there are never any deposits in the cerebral parenchyma itself in any form of acquired

Table 4 Cerebral amyloidosis

Age-related amyloid angiopathy with or without intracerebral deposits
Hereditary amyloid angiopathy of meningeal and cortical vessels associated
    with cerebral haemorrhage:
        Icelandic type
        Dutch type
Hereditary amyloid angiopathy affecting the entire central nervous system
Alzheimer's disease: sporadic, familial, or associated with Down's syndrome
Cerebral amyloid associated with prion disease:
        Sporadic spongiform encephalopathy, Creutzfeldt–Jakob disease, variant
            Creutzfeldt–Jakob disease
        Familial prion disease, familial Creutzfeldt–Jakob disease, GSS syndrome,
            atypical familial prion disease
Familial oculoleptomeningeal amyloidosis

systemic visceral amyloidosis. However, cerebrovascular transthyretin amyloid may occur in familial amyloid polyneuropathy due to the most common transthyretin variant (methionine for valine at residue 30), and oculoleptomeningeal amyloidosis is caused by other very rare transthyretin variants. The common and major forms of brain amyloid are confined to the brain and cerebral blood vessels with the single exception of cystatin C amyloid in hereditary cerebral haemorrhage with amyloidosis, Icelandic type, in which there are major though clinically silent systemic deposits.

Alzheimer's disease

By far the most frequent and important type of amyloid in the brain is that related to Alzheimer's disease, which is the most common cause of dementia and affects over 3 million individuals in the United States and a corresponding proportion of other Western populations. It is generally a disease of the elderly and its prevalence is therefore increasing. The clinical differential diagnosis of senile dementia and the positive identification of Alzheimer's disease are difficult and often of limited precision in life. However, intracerebral and cerebrovascular amyloid deposits are hallmarks of the neuropathological diagnosis. The amyloid fibrils are composed of β-protein (Aβ), a 39- to 43-residue cleavage product of the large amyloid precursor protein. The vast majority of cases of Alzheimer's disease are sporadic but there are also families with an autosomal dominant pattern of inheritance and usually early onset. In about 20 families there are causative mutations in the APP gene for amyloid precursor protein on chromosome 21, and most other kindreds have mutations in the genes for presenilin 1 (chromosome 14) and presenilin 2 (chromosome 1). All these mutations are associated with increased production from amyloid precursor protein of Aβ1–42, the most amyloidogenic form of Aβ. Since all individuals with Down's syndrome, that is trisomy 21, develop Alzheimer's disease if they survive into their forties, there is evidently a close link between amyloid precursor protein, Aβ overproduction, Aβ amyloidosis, and the pathogenesis of Alzheimer's disease, although it remains unclear whether or how Aβ per se, or the amyloid fibrils that it forms, contribute to the neuronal loss which underlies the dementia. Synthetic amyloid β fibrils formed in vitro are markedly cytotoxic and cause the death of cultured cells by apoptosis and necrosis, but it is not clear to what extent these findings reflect phenomena that may be responsible for neurodegeneration in vivo. There is controversy about the correlation between the severity of dementia in Alzheimer's disease and the extent of amyloid angiopathy and plaques. Nevertheless the fact that patients with Alzheimer's disease caused by amyloid precursor protein and presenilin mutations have exactly the same neuropathology as sporadic cases, including tangles, argues strongly that the amyloid precursor protein and β-protein pathway can be of primary pathogenetic significance.

In addition to the Aβ amyloid deposits in the brains of patients with Alzheimer's disease and Down's syndrome, there are also extensive 'amorphous' deposits of amyloid β throughout the brain. These do not stain with Congo red, and are detectable only by immunohistochemical staining. Their significance is unknown. They apparently precede the appearance of histochemically identifiable amyloid but are not necessarily the precursor of it because they are present in areas such as the cerebellum in which Aβ amyloid is never seen. The non-fibrillar, non-amyloid protein apolipoprotein E is demonstrable in many amyloid deposits, including those of Alzheimer's disease. The ApoE4 gene (chromosome 19), encoding one of the three isoforms of this apolipoprotein, is strongly associated with predisposition to develop Alzheimer's disease and with increased amounts of amyloid in the brain, but the underlying mechanisms are unknown.

Another neuropathological feature of Alzheimer's disease, and some other neurodegenerative conditions, is the neurofibrillary tangle located intracellularly within neuronal cell bodies and processes. These tangles have a characteristic ultrastructural morphology of paired helical filaments, and although they bind Congo red and then give the pathognomonic green birefringence of amyloid when viewed in polarized light, they are completely different structurally from amyloid fibrils. They are composed of an abnormally phosphorylated form of the normal neurofilament protein, tau.

Senile cerebral amyloidosis and amyloid angiopathy

The cerebral blood vessels contain Aβ amyloid in up to 60 per cent of aged brains of non-demented individuals and there may also be focal intracerebral Aβ amyloid plaques. These deposits are usually clinically silent and may or may not be harbingers of Alzheimer's disease, had the patients survived long enough. Sometimes the amyloid angiopathy is more extensive and it is a rare but important cause of cerebral haemorrhage and stroke, to be distinguished from atherosclerotic cerebrovascular disease.

Hereditary cerebral haemorrhage with amyloidosis: hereditary cerebral amyloid angiopathy

Icelandic type

Cerebrovascular amyloid deposits composed of a fragment of a genetic variant of cystatin C are responsible for recurrent major cerebral haemorrhages starting in early adult life in members of families originating in western Iceland. There is autosomal dominant inheritance and appreciable but clinically silent amyloid deposits are present in the spleen, lymph nodes, and skin. There is no extravascular amyloid in the brain and the neurological deficits, often including dementia, of surviving patients are compatible with their cerebrovascular pathology.

Dutch type

In families originating in a small region on the Dutch coast the autosomal dominant inheritance of recurrent normotensive cerebral hemorrhages starting in middle age is due to deposition of a genetic variant of Aβ as cerebrovascular amyloid. There are also 'amorphous' Aβ deposits in the brain and early senile plaques, without congophilic amyloid cores. Multi-infarct dementia occurs in survivors but some patients become demented in the absence of stroke. Amyloid outside the brain has not been reported.

Cerebral amyloid associated with prion disease

The neuropathology of a group of progressive, invariably fatal spongiform encephalopathies which are transmissible and in some cases are hereditary, sometimes includes intracerebral amyloid plaques and amyloid cerebral angiopathy. These diseases, sporadic and familial Creutzfeldt–Jacob disease, the familial Gerstmann–Sträussler–Scheinker syndrome, and kuru are caused by prions (PrP^{Sc}), conformational isoforms of the normal physiological cellular prion protein (PrP^C). The human diseases are closely related to the animal diseases scrapie of sheep and goats, transmissible encephalopathy of mink, elk, and male deer, and bovine spongiform encephalopathy. Variant Creutzfeldt–Jacob disease is apparently the result of transmission of bovine spongiform encephalopathy to humans. The significance of amyloid per se in these disorders is not clear, because it is not always detectable histologically and is not seen, for example, in fatal familial insomnia or in bovine spongiform encephalopathy, which is apparently a result of the transmission of ovine scrapie to cattle. When scrapie or its human counterparts are transmitted to experimental animals by inoculation of affected brain tissue the development of intracerebral amyloid depends on the strain of infectious agent and the genetic background of the recipient. Even when amyloid is present in the brain it is not seen elsewhere, for example in the spleen, although the latter is a rich source of the infective agent. However, when the infective agent is exhaustively and highly purified from brain or spleen it forms typical congophilic amyloid fibrils, composed of the proteinase-resistant subunit which is the prion, PrP^{Sc}, and when amyloid deposits are present in affected brains they immunostain with antiprion antibodies. The amyloid fibril protein is thus directly related to the cause of the encephalopathy but gross amyloid deposition is evidently not necessary for expression of disease. Neuronal damage may perhaps be caused by cytotoxic prefibrillar PrP^{Sc} aggregates, or indeed by other mechanisms entirely. This is a different situation from the extracerebral amyloidoses and from cystatin C and non-hereditary cerebral amyloid angiopathies, in which amyloid deposition is invariably present when there is clinical disease.

Hereditary systemic amyloidosis

Familial amyloid polyneuropathy

Familial amyloid polyneuropathy is an autosomal dominant syndrome with onset at any time from the second decade onwards, characterized by progressive peripheral and autonomic neuropathy and varying degrees of visceral involvement affecting especially the vitreous of the eye, the heart, kidneys, thyroid, and adrenals. There are usually amyloid deposits throughout the body involving the walls of blood vessels as well as the connective tissue matrix, and the pathology is due to these deposits. Apart from major foci in Portugal, Japan, and Sweden, familial amyloid polyneuropathy has been reported in most ethnic groups throughout the world. There is considerable variation in the age of onset, rate of progression, and involvement of different systems, although within families the pattern is usually quite consistent. There is remorseless progression and the disorder is invariably fatal. Death results from the effects and complications of peripheral and/or autonomic neuropathy, or from cardiac or renal failure.

Familial amyloid polyneuropathy is caused by mutations in the gene for the plasma protein transthyretin, formerly known as prealbumin, the most frequent of which causes a methionine for valine substitution at position 30 in the mature protein, but over 60 amyloidogenic mutations have been described. There is often little correlation between the underlying mutation and the clinical phenotype, which is evidently determined by other genetic and possibly also environmental factors, although in a few cases certain mutations are uniquely associated with particularly aggressive or relatively organ-limited disease. The amyloidogenic transthyretin mutations are not always penetrant, and asymptomatic methionine 30 homozygotes over the age of 60 have been reported. Rare kindreds with the apolipoprotein A-I arginine 26 variant, which usually causes non-neuropathic amyloidosis, may present with prominent peripheral neuropathy resembling transthyretin familial amyloid polyneuropathy.

Familial amyloid polyneuropathy with predominant cranial neuropathy

Originally described in Finland but now reported in other ethnic groups, this autosomal dominant hereditary amyloidosis presents in adult life with cranial neuropathy, lattice corneal dystrophy, and distal peripheral neuropathy. There may be skin, renal, and cardiac manifestations and microscopic amyloid deposits are widely distributed in connective tissue and blood vessel walls, although life expectancy approaches normal. The amyloid fibrils are derived from variants of the actin-modulating protein gelsolin, encoded by point mutations. Individuals homozygous for these mutations have severe renal amyloidosis in addition to the usual neuropathy.

Non-neuropathic systemic amyloidosis

In this rare autosomal dominant syndrome of major systemic amyloidosis without clinical evidence of neuropathy, the patterns of organ involvement and overall clinical phenotype vary between families. The kidneys are often most severely affected leading to hypertension and renal failure, but the heart, spleen, liver, bowel, connective tissue, and exocrine glands may all be involved. Following clinical presentation, usually from the second decade onwards, there is inexorable progression to death or organ failure requiring transplantation. Clinical presentation is usually in early adulthood, although in a few kindreds it may be as late as the sixth decade. The amyloid proteins identified so far are genetic variants of apolipoprotein A-I, lysozyme, and the α-chain of fibrinogen.

Cardiac amyloidosis

Cardiac amyloidosis, without overt involvement of other viscera or neuropathy, progressing inexorably to death, is associated with certain transthyretin gene mutations and is inherited as an autosomal dominant with variable penetrance (see Table 2). By far the most common variant is isoleucine 122 transthyretin which occurs in 4 per cent of African-Americans and frequently causes cardiac amyloidosis from the sixth decade onwards.

Familial Mediterranean fever

Familial Mediterranean fever is an autosomal recessive disorder caused by mutations in the gene on chromosome 16 that encodes a neutrophil-specific protein of unknown function, called pyrin or marenostrin. The disease is characterized by recurrent episodes of fever, abdominal pain, pleurisy, or arthritis, and predominantly occurs in non-Ashkenazi Jews, Armenians, Anatolian Turks, and Levantine Arabs. In Sephardi Jews of North African origin, and in the other ethnic groups except Armenians and to a lesser extent Ashkenazi Jews, untreated familial Mediterranean fever is eventually complicated in a high proportion of cases by typical systemic AA amyloidosis. Furthermore, some patients with familial Mediterranean fever present with AA amyloidosis before they have experienced any symptoms, and this is consistent with the recent finding that a substantial acute phase plasma protein response is frequently present even in asymptomatic individuals. The different incidence of amyloid in patients with familial Mediterranean fever from different ethnic groups is not wholly explained by their specific pyrin gene mutations, and is another illustration of the unknown genetic determinants of clinical amyloidosis.

Haemodialysis-associated amyloidosis

Almost all patients with endstage renal failure who are maintained on haemodialysis for more than 5 years develop amyloid deposits composed of β_2-microglobulin. These deposits are predominantly osteoarticular and are associated with carpal tunnel syndrome, large joint pain and stiffness, soft tissue masses, bone cysts, and pathological fractures. Renal tubular amyloid concretions may also form. The serious clinical problems associated with β_2-microglobulin amyloidosis constitute the major cause of morbidity in patients on long-term dialysis. Furthermore, in some such patients more extensive deposition occurs, most commonly in the spleen but also in other organs, and a few cases of death associated with systemic β_2-microglobulin amyloid have been reported. The β_2-microglobulin is derived from the high plasma concentrations which develop in renal insufficiency and which are not cleared by dialysis. This type of amyloid also occurs in patients on continuous ambulatory peritoneal dialysis and has even been reported in a few patients with chronic renal failure who had never been dialysed.

Endocrine amyloidosis

Many tumours of APUD cells which produce peptide hormones have amyloid deposits in their stroma. These are probably composed of the hormone peptides, and in the case of medullary carcinoma of the thyroid the fibril subunits are derived from procalcitonin. In insulinomas the amyloid fibril protein is a novel peptide first identified in that site and subsequently shown to be the fibril protein in the amyloid of the islets of Langerhans in type II, maturity onset, diabetes. This peptide is called islet amyloid polypeptide (and also amylin) and shows appreciable homology with calcitonin gene-related peptide. Islet amyloid polypeptide amyloid is an almost universal feature of the pancreatic islets in type II diabetes and becomes more extensive with increasing duration and severity of the disease. Although the amyloid itself is probably not initially responsible for the metabolic defect in this form of diabetes, it is likely that progressive amyloid deposition leading to islet destruction subsequently does contribute to the pathogenesis. The possible hormonal or other role of islet amyloid polypeptide itself, which is produced by the islet B cells, is also not yet clear.

Rare localized amyloidosis syndromes

Amyloid deposits localized to the skin occur in both acquired and hereditary forms. Primary localized cutaneous amyloidosis presents in adult life as macular or papular lesions, the fibrils of which may be derived from keratin. Hereditary cutaneous amyloid lesions are rare, of unknown fibril type, and are sometimes associated with other, non-amyloid, multisystem disorders. Amyloid deposits in the eye cause local problems in the cornea (corneal lattice dystrophy) or conjunctiva, whilst orbital amyloid presents as mass lesions which can disrupt eye movement and the structure of the orbit. In one such case the fibril protein has been identified as a fragment of immunoglobulin G heavy chain.

Localized foci of AL amyloid can occur anywhere in the body in the absence of systemic AL amyloidosis, the most common sites being the skin, upper airways and respiratory tract, and the urogenital tract. They may be associated with a local plasmacytoma or B-cell lymphoma producing a monoclonal immunoglobulin, but often the cells, which must be present to produce the amyloidogenic protein, are scattered inconspicuously in the affected tissue. The clinical problems caused by these space-occupying amyloidomas are usually cured by surgical resection, but this is not always possible.

Amyloid fibrils

Regardless of their very diverse protein subunits, amyloid fibrils of different types are remarkably similar: straight, rigid, non-branching, of indeterminate length, and 10 to 15 nm in diameter. They are insoluble in physiological solutions, relatively resistant to proteolysis, and bind Congo red dye producing pathognomonic green birefringence when viewed in polarized light. Electron microscopy reveals that each fibril consists of two or more protofilaments, the precise number varying with the fibril type. The X-ray diffraction patterns of all the different *ex vivo* amyloid fibrils, and of synthetic fibrils formed *in vitro*, that have been studied demonstrate the presence of a common core structure within the filaments, in which the subunit proteins are arranged in a stack of twisted antiparallel β-pleated sheets lying with their long axes perpendicular to the long axis of the fibril. Recent observations show that many different proteins, including molecules totally unrelated to amyloidosis *in vivo*, can be refolded after denaturation *in vitro* to form typical, stable, congophilic cross β fibrils. Although it is not clear why only the 20 or so known amyloidogenic proteins adopt the amyloid fold and persist as fibrils *in vivo*, a major unifying theme that is currently emerging is that in all cases studied the precursors are relatively destabilized. Even under physiological or other conditions they may encounter *in vivo*, they populate partly unfolded states, involving loss of tertiary or higher-order structure, that readily aggregate with retention of β-sheet secondary structure into protofilaments and fibrils. Once the process has started, seeding may also play an important facilitating role, so that amyloid deposition may progress exponentially as expansion of the amyloid template 'captures' further precursor molecules.

Amyloid fibril proteins and their precursors

Immunoglobulin light chain

AL proteins are derived from the N-terminal region of monoclonal immunoglobulin light chains and consist of all or part of the variable (V_L) domain. Intact light chains may occasionally be found, and the molecular weight therefore varies between about 8000 and 30 000 Da. The light chain of the monoclonal paraprotein is either identical to, or clearly the precursor of, AL isolated from the amyloid deposits.

AL is more commonly derived from λ chains than from κ chains, despite the fact that κ chains predominate among both normal immunoglobulins and the paraprotein products of immunocyte dyscrasias. A new λ-chain subgroup, $λ_{VI}$, was identified first as an AL protein in two cases of immunocyte dyscrasia-associated amyloidosis before it had been recognized in any other form, and it has subsequently been observed in many more cases of AL amyloidosis. Furthermore, there is increasing evidence from sequence analyses of Bence Jones proteins of both κ and λ type from patients with AL amyloidosis, and of AL proteins themselves, that these polypeptides contain

unique amino acid replacements or insertions compared with non-amyloid monoclonal light chains. In some cases these changes involve replacement of hydrophilic framework residues by hydrophobic residues, changes likely to promote aggregation and insolubilization, and in others the monoclonal light chains from amyloid patients have been demonstrated directly to have decreased solubility and a greater propensity for precipitation than control non-amyloid proteins. The inherent 'amyloidogenicity' of particular monoclonal light chains has been elegantly confirmed in an *in vivo* model in which isolated Bence Jones proteins were injected into mice. Animals receiving light chains from AL amyloid patients developed typical amyloid deposits composed of the human protein whereas animals receiving light chains from myeloma patients without amyloid did not.

AA

The AA protein is a single non-glycosylated polypeptide chain usually of mass 8000 Da and containing 76 residues corresponding to the N-terminal portion of the 104-residue serum amyloid A protein (SAA). Smaller and larger AA fragments, even some whole SAA molecules, have also been reported in AA fibrils. Serum amyloid A is an apolipoprotein of high-density lipoprotein particles and is the polymorphic product of a set of genes located on the short arm of chromosome 11. Serum amyloid A is highly conserved in evolution and is a major acute phase reactant in all species in which it has been studied. Most of the SAA in plasma is produced by hepatocytes in which the synthesis is under transcriptional regulation by cytokines, especially interleukin 1, interleukin 6, and tumour necrosis factor, acting via nuclear factor κB-like and possibly other transcription factors. After secretion it is rapidly associated with high-density lipoproteins from which it displaces apolipoprotein A-I. The circulating concentration can rise from normal levels of up to 3 mg/l to over 1000 mg/l within 24 to 48 h of an acute stimulus, whilst with ongoing chronic inflammation the level may remain persistently high. Certain isoforms of SAA, the products of different genes, are predominantly synthesized elsewhere in the body by macrophages, adipocytes, and certain other cells. Although they also associate with high-density lipoproteins, their acute phase synthesis is stimulated differently and they presumably have different functions. There is also a closely related family of high-density lipoprotein trace apoproteins which are not acute phase reactants and which have been designated 'constitutive SAAs', although they do not form amyloid.

Circulating SAA is the precursor of amyloid fibril AA protein, from which it is derived by proteolytic cleavage. Such cleavage can be produced by macrophages and by a variety of proteinases but since further cleavage of AA is readily demonstrable *in vitro* it is not clear why the AA peptide persists in amyloid. Furthermore, it is not known whether in the process of AA fibrillogenesis, cleavage of SAA occurs before and/or after aggregation of monomers. Persistent overproduction of SAA causing sustained high circulating levels is a necessary condition for deposition of AA amyloid but it is not known why only some individuals in this state get amyloid. In mice, only SAA2, one of the three major isoforms of murine SAA, is the precursor of AA in amyloid fibrils. Human SAA isoforms are more complex but homozygosity for particular types seems to favour amyloidogenesis, although there may also be ethnic differences.

The normal functions of SAA are not known, although modulating effects on reverse cholesterol transport and on lipid functions in the microenvironment of inflammatory foci have been proposed. A protein, homologous with SAA, produced by rabbit fibroblasts has been reported to act as an autocrine stimulator of collagenase production *in vitro*. Other reports of potent cell regulatory functions of isolated denatured delipidated SAA have yet to be confirmed with physiological preparations of SAA-rich high-density lipoproteins. Regardless of its physiological role, the behaviour of SAA as an exquisitely sensitive acute phase protein with an enormous dynamic range makes it an extremely valuable empirical clinical marker. It can be used to monitor objectively the extent and activity of infective, inflammatory, necrotic, and neoplastic disease. Furthermore, routine monitoring of SAA should be an integral part of the management of all patients with AA amyloid or disorders predisposing to it, as control of the primary inflammatory process in order to reduce SAA production is essential if amyloidosis is to be halted, enabled to regress, or prevented. Automated immunoassay systems for SAA are available standardized to a World Health Organization international reference standard.

Transthyretin

Transthyretin, formerly known as prealbumin, is a normal non-glycosylated plasma protein, with a relative molecular mass of 54 980. It is composed of four identical non-covalently associated subunits each of 127 amino acids. It is produced by hepatocytes and the choroid plexus and is a significant negative acute phase protein. Each tetrameric molecule is able to bind a single thyroxine or triodothyronine molecule and up to 15 per cent of circulating thyroid hormone is transported in this way. Transthyretin also forms a 1:1 molecular complex with retinol-binding protein, which transports vitamin A.

Transthyretin is encoded by a single copy gene but is appreciably polymorphic and about 70 different point mutations encoding single-residue substitutions have been identified so far. Normal wild type transthyretin is an inherently amyloidogenic protein which forms the fibrils in senile systemic amyloidosis, and *in vitro* exposure to reduced pH is sufficient to generate transthyretin amyloid fibrils from the pure protein. Most of the variant forms of transthyretin have been associated with hereditary amyloidosis, and show decreased stability *in vitro* compared with the wild type. Transgenic mice expressing variant human transthyretin with a methionine 30 substitution develop extensive systemic amyloidosis, but no amyloid deposits have yet been reported in the peripheral nerves even when the transgene is expressed in the choroid plexus and transthyretin amyloid is deposited in the meninges and choroid plexus. This is another example of the important, unknown, factors, other than the presence of an amyloidogenic protein itself, that determine where and when clinical amyloidosis develops.

Individuals heterozygous for transthyretin mutations have a mixture of wild type and variant transthyretin monomers in their circulating transthyretin, and if they develop amyloidosis both forms are often present although the variant may predominate in the amyloid fibrils. Although cleavage fragments of transthyretin are commonly present, intact transthyretin subunits are also found and fibrillogenesis does not depend on an initial proteolytic step.

Aβ

The fibril protein in the intracerebral and cerebrovascular amyloid of Alzheimer's disease, Down's syndrome, and hereditary amyloid angiopathy of the Dutch type is a 39- to 43-residue sequence derived by proteolysis from a high molecular weight precursor protein, the so-called amyloid precursor protein, encoded on the long arm of chromosome 21. Several isoforms of amyloid precursor protein (APP) are generated by alternative splicing of transcripts from the 19 exon gene, and yielding major forms: APP695, APP751, and APP770. These are each single-chain, multidomain glycoproteins with the 47 residues of the carboxy terminal within the cytoplasm, a 25-residue membrane-spanning region, and the rest of the molecule lying extracellularly. APP751 and APP770 contain a 56-residue Kunitz type serine proteinase inhibitor domain encoded by exon 7. Following glycosylation and membrane insertion, APPs are cleaved extracellularly by so-called APP secretase activity, close to the transmembrane sequence, releasing, in the case of the isoforms containing the proteinase inhibitor domain, a molecule known as proteinase nexin II, which avidly binds factor XIa, trypsin, and chymotrypsin as well as epidermal growth factor-binding protein and the γ subunit of nerve growth factor. Although mRNA encoding APP695, which lacks the proteinase inhibitor domain, is the predominant species found in brain, whereas mRNA for APP751 is the most abundant in other tissues, 85 per cent of secreted APP in the brain is proteinase nexin II. Interestingly, APP secreted by a glial cell line is substantially glycosylated with chondroitin sulphate glycosaminoglycan chains. APP also undergoes high-affinity interactions with heparan sulphate. These observations suggest that APP may have important functions in cell adhesion, cell migration, and modulation of growth factor activities. APP proteinase nexin II is present in and released by platelets and probably functions in the clotting cascade.

The amyloidogenic amyloid β, encoded by parts of exons 16 and 17, corresponds to the part of the APP sequence which extends from within the cell membrane into the extracellular space. Secretase cleavage of APP to release the soluble form cannot therefore generate intact amyloid β itself, or larger fragments containing it. However, there is an alternative processing pathway for APP, in which it is taken up whole by lysosomes and cleaved to yield fragments that do contain the whole amyloid β sequence. Furthermore, APP cleaved at the *N*-terminus of amyloid β, and also free soluble amyloid β itself, are normally produced by cell lines and by mixed brain cells in culture and are present in the cerebrospinal fluid. However, the source of the amyloid β in the intracerebral amorphous deposits and of that which aggregates as amyloid fibrils in the brain and cerebral blood vessels is still not known. The 42-residue form of amyloid β is markedly the most amyloidogenic, and all the mutations in the APP and presenilin genes that are associated with hereditary Alzheimer's disease result in increased production of this amyloid β1–42. Increased availability of the precursor is thus responsible for amyloidogenesis, but the pathogenesis of neuronal damage and dementia remain unclear.

Cystatin C

Cystatin C (formerly called γ-trace) is an inhibitor of cysteine proteinases, including cathepsins B, H, and L. It is encoded by a gene on chromosome 20 and consists of a single non-glycosylated polypeptide chain of 120 residues. It is present in all major human biological fluids at concentrations compatible with a significant physiological role in proteinase inhibition. The normal concentration in cerebrospinal fluid is 6.5 mg/l (range 2.7 to 13.7, $n = 34$), but is much lower (2.7 mg/l, range 1.0 to 4.7, $n = 9$) in patients with the Icelandic type of hereditary cerebral amyloid angiopathy in whom fragments of the glutamine 68 genetic variant of cystatin C form the amyloid fibrils. This reduced concentration is useful diagnostically and is evident even in presymptomatic carriers of the cystatin C gene mutation. The point mutation that causes the disease encodes a glutamine for leucine substitution in the mature protein and the amyloid fibril protein consists of the C-terminal 110 residues of the variant. This amino-terminally truncated form is not detectable in the cerebrospinal fluid of affected patients, suggesting that cleavage takes place either in close proximity to fibril deposition or is a postfibrillogenic event. The variant cystatin C is less stable than wild type and readily forms fibrils *in vitro*. It is not known whether cerebral haemorrhage in cystatin C amyloidosis is caused simply by the damaging effects of vascular amyloid deposition or whether deficiency in inhibitory capacity for cysteinase proteinases also plays a part.

Gelsolin

Gelsolin (mass 90 000 Da) is a widely distributed cytoplasmic protein which binds actin monomers, nucleates actin filament growth, and severs actin filaments. Alternative transcriptional initiation and message processing from a single gene on chromosome 9 are responsible for synthesis of a secreted form of gelsolin (mass 93 000 Da), which circulates in the plasma at a concentration of about 200 mg/l. Its function in the blood is not known but may be related to clearance of actin filaments released by dying cells. In the Finnish type of hereditary amyloidosis the amyloid fibril protein is a 71-residue fragment of variant gelsolin with asparagine substituted for aspartic acid at position 15, corresponding to residue 187 of the mature molecule, and the same mutation has been discovered in affected kindreds from different ethnic backgrounds. In one Danish family with the same phenotype there is a different mutation at the same nucleotide, predicting a tyrosine for aspartic acid substitution at residue 187. Synthetic and recombinant peptides including the asparagine for aspartic acid substitution at residue 187 are less soluble than the wild type sequence and readily form amyloid fibrils *in vitro*.

Apolipoprotein A-I

Apolipoprotein A-I is the most abundant apolipoprotein amongst the high-density lipoprotein particles and participates in their central function of reverse cholesterol transport from the periphery to the liver. Apolipoprotein A-I variants are extremely rare and may be phenotypically silent or may affect lipid metabolism. However, nine different variants of apolipoprotein A-I, including single- and multiple-residue substitutions and deletions, have been associated with amyloidosis. Although inherited as an autosomal dominant, and usually highly penetrant, there are marked variations in age and manner of presentation even in the same family and in different kindreds with the same mutation. The amyloid fibril protein consists, in all cases studied, of the first 90 or so N-terminal residues even when the causative variant residue(s) are more distal. Wild type apolipoprotein A-I is also amyloidogenic, forming the deposits associated with atheromatous plaques in the elderly, and the various amyloidogenic mutations presumably encode sequence changes that render apolipoprotein A-I less stable and/or more liable to cleavage to yield the fibrillogenic N-terminal fragment.

Lysozyme

Lysozyme is the classic bacteriolytic enzyme of external secretions, discovered by Fleming in 1922. It is also present at high concentration within articular cartilage and in the granules of polymorphs, and is the major secreted product of macrophages. Lysozymes are present in most organisms in which they have been sought, although their physiological role is not always clear. The complete structures of hen egg white and human lysozymes are known to atomic resolution and their catalytic mechanism, epitopes, folding, and other aspects of their structure–function relationship have been analysed exhaustively. This contrasts with the absence of detailed three-dimensional structural information on all other amyloid fibril proteins and their precursors except transthyretin and β_2-microglobulin. Lysozyme, unlike transthyretin and β_2-microglobulin, is not inherently amyloidogenic, and is therefore a valuable model for investigation of amyloid fibrillogenesis. There is only one copy of the lysozyme gene in the human genome and no disease is associated with lysozyme other than amyloidosis. The mutations which cause amyloid produce substitution of threonine for isoleucine at residue 56 in one family and histidine for aspartic acid at residue 67 in others. These dramatic changes in residues which are extremely conserved throughout the lysozyme and related α-lactalbumin protein families, destabilize the native fold so that the variants readily populate partly unfolded states even under physiological conditions and spontaneously aggregate *in vitro*, and evidently also *in vivo*, into amyloid fibrils.

Islet amyloid polypeptide

Islet amyloid polypeptide (amylin) is a 37-residue molecule encoded by a gene on chromosome 12 and with 46 per cent sequence homology to the neuropeptide calcitonin gene-related peptide. Islet amyloid polypeptide is produced in the β cells of the pancreatic islets of Langerhans and is stored in and released from their secretory granules together with insulin. It has been reported to modulate insulin release, and to induce peripheral insulin resistance, vasodilatation, and lowering of plasma calcium but neither its physiological role nor its contribution to diabetes are yet known.

Amyloidogenicity of islet amyloid polypeptide depends on the amino acid sequence between residues 20 and 29, as shown by *in vitro* fibrillogenesis with synthetic peptides. The synthetic decapeptide IAPP20–29 and even the hexapeptide IAPP25–29, glycine–alanine–isoleucine–leucine–serine–serine, form amyloid-like fibrils *in vitro*, whereas other islet amyloid polypeptide fragments do not. There is also a correlation between conservation of this sequence and deposition of islet amyloid polypeptide amyloid in the islets of diabetic animals of different species. However, the role of the amyloid in diabetogenesis remains to be established. In the degu, a South American rodent, spontaneous diabetes is associated with islet amyloid composed of insulin, and xenogeneic insulin can also form amyloid in humans at sites of repeated therapeutic insulin injections.

β_2-Microglobulin

β_2-Microglobulin is a non-glycosylated, non-polymorphic single-chain protein of 99 residues with a single intrachain disulphide bridge (relative molecular mass 11 815) encoded by a single gene on chromosome 15. It becomes non-covalently associated with the heavy chain of major histocompatibility class I antigens and is required for transport and expression of the complex at the cell surface. Amino acid sequence homology places β_2-microglobulin in the superfamily including immunoglobulins, T-cell receptor α- and β-chains, Thy 1, major histocompatibility class I and II molecules, secretory component, etc. Its three-dimensional structure is a typical β-barrel with two antiparallel pleated sheets comprising three and four strands respectively, and closely resembles an immunoglobulin domain.

β_2-microglobulin is produced by lymphoid and a variety of other cells in which it stabilizes the structure and function of class I antigens at the cell surface. When these complexes are shed by cleavage of the heavy chain at the cell surface, free β_2-microglobulin is released. The circulating concentration of β_2-microglobulin is 1 to 2 mg/l and the protein is rapidly cleared by glomerular filtration and then catabolized in the proximal renal tubule. Impairment of renal function is associated with retention of β_2-microglobulin and increased circulating levels because there is no other site for its catabolism. Daily production of β_2-microglobulin is about 200 mg and in patients in endstage renal failure on haemodialysis, plasma β_2-microglobulin levels rise to and remain at levels of about 40 to 70 mg/l. Isolated unaltered β_2-microglobulin can form amyloid-like fibrils itself *in vitro*, and most studies of *ex vivo* β_2-microglobulin fibrils show the whole intact molecule to be the major subunit, although fragments and altered forms of β_2-microglobulin have also been reported.

Glycosaminoglycans

Amyloidotic organs contain more glycosaminoglycans than normal tissues and at least some of this is a tightly bound integral part of the amyloid fibrils. These fibril-associated glycosaminoglycans are heparan sulphate and dermatan sulphate in all forms of amyloid which have been investigated. Fibrils isolated by water extraction and separated from other tissue components contain 1 to 2 per cent by weight of glycosaminoglycan, none of which is covalently associated with the fibril protein. Interestingly, in systemic AA and AL amyloidosis, the only forms in which this has been studied so far, there is marked restriction of the heterogeneity of the glycosaminoglycan chains, suggesting that particular subclasses of heparan and dermatan sulphates are involved. Immunohistochemical studies demonstrate the presence of proteoglycan core proteins in all amyloid deposits, and that these are closely related to fibrils at the ultrastructural level. However, in isolated fibril preparations much of the glycosaminoglycan material is free carbohydrate chains and it is not yet clear whether this represents aberrant glycosaminoglycan metabolism related to amyloidosis or is just an artefact of postmortem degradation of core protein.

The significance of glycosaminoglycans in amyloid remains unclear, but their universal presence, intimate relationship with the fibrils, and restricted heterogeneity all suggest that they may be important. Glycosaminoglycans are known to participate in the organization of some normal structural proteins into fibrils and they may have comparable fibrillogenic effects on certain amyloid fibril precursor proteins. Furthermore the glycosaminoglycans on amyloid fibrils may be ligands to which serum amyloid P component, another universal constituent of amyloid deposits, binds.

Amyloid P component and serum amyloid P component

Amyloid deposits in all different forms of the disease, both in humans and in animals, contain the non-fibrillar glycoprotein amyloid P component. Amyloid P component is identical to and derived from the normal circulating plasma protein, serum amyloid P component, a member of the pentraxin protein family which includes C-reactive protein. Human serum amyloid P component is secreted only by hepatocytes, is a trace constituent of plasma (women: mean 24 mg/l, SD 8, range 8 to 55, $n = 274$; men: mean 32 mg/l, SD 7, range 12 to 50, $n = 226$), and is not an acute phase reactant. Nevertheless, apart from the fibrils themselves, amyloid P component is always by far the most abundant protein in all amyloid deposits.

Serum amyloid P component consists of five identical non-covalently associated subunits, each with a molecular mass of 25 462 Da, which are non-covalently associated in a pentameric disc-like ring. The tertiary fold of the subunit is dominated by antiparallel β-sheets, forming a flattened β-barrel with jellyroll topology and a core of hydrophobic sidechains. This is the so-called 'lectin fold', shared with a variety of other animal, plant, and bacterial carbohydrate-binding proteins (lectins). Serum amyloid P component is a calcium-dependent ligand-binding protein, the best defined specificity of which is for the 4,6-cyclic pyruvate acetal of β-D-galactose, but it also binds avidly and specifically to DNA, to chromatin, to glycosaminoglycans, particularly heparan and dermatan sulphates, and to all known types of amyloid fibrils. This last is the interaction responsible for the unique, specific accumulation of serum amyloid P component in amyloid deposits. Aggregated, but not native, serum amyloid P component also binds specifically to C4-binding protein and fibronectin from plasma, although serum amyloid P component is not complexed with any other protein in the circulation. In addition to being a plasma protein, serum amyloid P component is also a normal constituent of certain extracellular matrix structures. It is covalently associated with collagen and/or other matrix components in the lamina rara interna of the human glomerular basement membrane and is present on the microfibrillar mantle of elastin fibres throughout the body.

No deficiency of serum amyloid P component has been described and it has been stably conserved in evolution. There is a single copy of its gene on chromosome 1, no polymorphism of the amino acid sequence, and the single biantennary oligosaccharide chain attached to asparagine at residue 32 is the most invariant glycan of any known glycoprotein. These indications that serum amyloid P component is likely to have important physiological function(s) have lately been confirmed by the finding that mice with targeted deletion of the gene for serum amyloid P component spontaneously develop marked antinuclear autoimmunity and immune complex glomerulonephritis. Studies of these serum amyloid P component knockout mice also show that serum amyloid P component is involved in host resistance to some infections and contributes to pathogenesis of others.

The serum amyloid P component molecule is highly resistant to proteolysis and, although not itself a proteinase inhibitor, its binding to amyloid fibrils *in vitro* protects them against proteolysis. Once bound to amyloid fibrils *in vivo*, serum amyloid P component persists for very prolonged periods and is not catabolized at all, in contrast to its rapid clearance from the plasma (half-life 24 h) and prompt catabolism in the liver. These observations suggest that serum amyloid P component may contribute to the persistence of amyloid deposits *in vivo*, and indeed serum amyloid P component knockout mice show retarded and reduced induction of experimental AA amyloidosis, confirming that serum amyloid P component is significantly involved in pathogenesis of amyloidosis.

Other proteins in amyloid deposits

A number of plasma proteins, other than the fibril proteins themselves and serum amyloid P component, have been detected immunohistochemically in some amyloid deposits. These include α_1-antichymotrypsin, some complement components, apolipoprotein E, and various extracellular matrix or basement membrane proteins. None of these match the universality, quantitative, or selective importance of serum amyloid P component, and their role, if any, in pathogenesis of amyloid deposition or its effects is not known.

Diagnosis and monitoring of amyloidosis

Introduction

Until recently amyloidosis was an exclusively histological diagnosis, and green birefringence of deposits stained with Congo red and viewed in polarized light remains the gold standard. Furthermore, immunohistochemical staining of amyloid-containing tissue is the simplest method for identifying the type of amyloid fibril present. However, biopsies provide extremely small samples and therefore can never provide information on the extent, localization, progression, or regression of amyloid deposits. A major advance in clinical amyloidosis has been the development of radiolabelled serum amyloid P component as a specific tracer for amyloid. Combined scintigraphic imaging and metabolic analysis using labelled serum amyloid P component have provided a wealth of new information on the natural history of many different forms of amyloid and their response to treatment.

Histochemical diagnosis of amyloid

Biopsy

Amyloid may be an incidental finding on biopsy of the kidneys, liver, heart, bowel, peripheral nerve, lymph node, skin, thyroid, or bone marrow. When amyloidosis is suspected clinically, biopsy of the rectum or subcutaneous fat is the least invasive. Amyloid is present in these sites in more than 90 per cent of cases of systemic AA or AL amyloidosis. Alternatively, a clinically affected tissue may be biopsied directly.

Congo red and other histochemical stains

Many cotton dyes, fluorochromes, and metachromatic stains have been used, but Congo red staining, and its resultant green birefringence when viewed with high-intensity polarized light, is the pathognomonic histochemical test for amyloidosis. The stain is unstable and must be freshly prepared every 2 months or less. A section thickness of 5 to 10 μm and inclusion in every staining run of a positive control tissue containing modest amounts of amyloid are critical.

Immunohistochemistry

Although many amyloid fibril proteins can be identified immunohistochemically, the demonstration of amyloidogenic proteins in tissues does not, on its own, establish the presence of amyloid. Congo red staining and green birefringence are always required and immunostaining may then enable the amyloid to be classified. Antibodies to serum amyloid A protein are commercially available and always stain AA deposits, similarly with anti-β₂-microglobulin antisera and haemodialysis-associated amyloid. In AL amyloid the deposits are stainable with standard antisera to κ or λ in only about half of all cases, probably because the light chain fragment in the fibrils is usually the N-terminal variable domain, which is largely unique for each monoclonal protein. Immunohistochemical staining of transthyretin, Aβ, and prion protein amyloid may require pretreatment of sections with formic acid or alkaline guanidine or deglycosylation.

Electron microscopy

Amyloid fibrils cannot always be convincingly identified ultrastructurally, and electron microscopy alone is not sufficient to confirm the diagnosis of amyloidosis.

Problems of histological diagnosis

The tissue sample must be adequate (for example, the inclusion of sub-mucosal vessels in a rectal biopsy specimen), and failure to find amyloid does not exclude the diagnosis. The unavoidable sampling problem means that biopsy cannot reveal the extent or distribution of amyloid. Experience with Congo red staining is required if clinically important false negative and false positive results are to be avoided. Immunohistochemical staining requires positive and negative controls, including demonstration of specificity of staining by absorption of positive antisera with isolated pure antigens.

Non-histological investigations

Two-dimensional echocardiography showing small, concentrically hypertrophied ventricles, generally impaired contraction, dilated atria, homogeneously echogenic valves, and 'sparkling' echodensity of ventricular walls is virtually diagnostic of cardiac amyloidosis. However, clinically significant restrictive diastolic impairment may be difficult to detect even by comprehensive Doppler and other functional studies. Imaging after injection of isotope-labelled calcium-seeking tracers has poor sensitivity and specificity and is of no clinical use.

In cases of known or suspected hereditary amyloidosis the gene defect must be characterized. If amyloidotic tissue is available the fibril protein may be known and the corresponding gene can then be studied, but if no tissue containing amyloid is available, screening of the genes for known amyloidogenic proteins must be undertaken.

Biochemical and immunochemical screening tests for the presence in the plasma of amyloidogenic variant protein products of mutant genes also exist, for example for transthyretin and apolipoprotein A-I variants, but molecular genetic analysis of DNA is easier to perform and is the most direct approach. However, regardless of the DNA results, it is desirable, if possible, to also directly identify the respective protein in the amyloid.

Serum amyloid P component as a specific tracer in amyloidosis

The universal presence in amyloid deposits of amyloid P component, derived from circulating serum amyloid P component, is the basis for use of radioisotope-labelled serum amyloid P component as a diagnostic tracer in amyloidosis. No localization or retention of labelled serum amyloid P component occurs in healthy subjects or in patients with diseases other than amyloidosis (Fig. 1(a)). Radio-iodinated serum amyloid P component has a short half-life (24 h) in the plasma and is rapidly catabolized with complete excretion of the iodinated breakdown products in the urine. However, in patients with systemic or localized extracerebral amyloidosis, the tracer rapidly and specifically localizes to the deposits, in proportion to the quantity of amyloid present, and persists there without breakdown or modification (Fig. 1(b, c)). For clinical purposes, highly purified serum amyloid P component is isolated from the plasma of single accredited donors and is oxidatively iodinated under conditions that preserve its function intact. The medium-energy, short half-life, pure gamma emitter ^{123}I is used for scintigraphic imaging, and the long half-life isotope ^{125}I is used for metabolic studies. The dose of radioactivity administered (less than 4 mSv) is well within accepted safety limits and more than 3000 studies have been completed without any adverse effects. In addition to high-resolution scintigraphs, the uptake of tracer into various organs can be precisely quantified and, together with highly reproducible metabolic data on the plasma clearance and whole body retention of activity, the progression or regression of amyloid can be monitored serially and quantitatively.

Important observations regarding amyloid (which have been made for the first time *in vivo*) include the following: the different distribution of amyloid in different forms of the disease; amyloid in anatomical sites not available for biopsy (adrenals, spleen); major systemic deposits in forms of amyloid previously thought to be organ-limited; a poor correlation between the quantity of amyloid present in a given organ and the level of

organ dysfunction; a non-homogeneous distribution of amyloid within individual organs; and evidence for rapid progression and sometimes regression of amyloid deposits with different rates in different organs (Fig. 2). Examples of major regression of amyloidosis, when it has been possible to reduce or eliminate the supply of fibril precursor, are very encouraging. Studies with labelled serum amyloid P component thus make a valuable contribution to the diagnosis and management of patients with systemic amyloidosis, and these are available routinely for all known or suspected cases of amyloidosis in the National Health Service National Amyloidosis Centre at the Royal Free Hospital, London.

Management of amyloidosis

Although no treatments yet exist that specifically promote the mobilization of amyloid, there have been substantial recent advances in the management of systemic amyloidosis, in particular active measures to support failing organ function whilst attempts are made to reduce the supply of the amyloid fibril precursor protein. Serial serum amyloid P component scintigraphy in more than 1000 patients with various forms of amyloid has confirmed that control of the primary disease process, or removal of the source of the amyloidogenic precursor, usually results in regression of existing deposits and recovery or preservation of organ function. This strongly supports aggressive intervention, and relatively toxic drug regimes or other

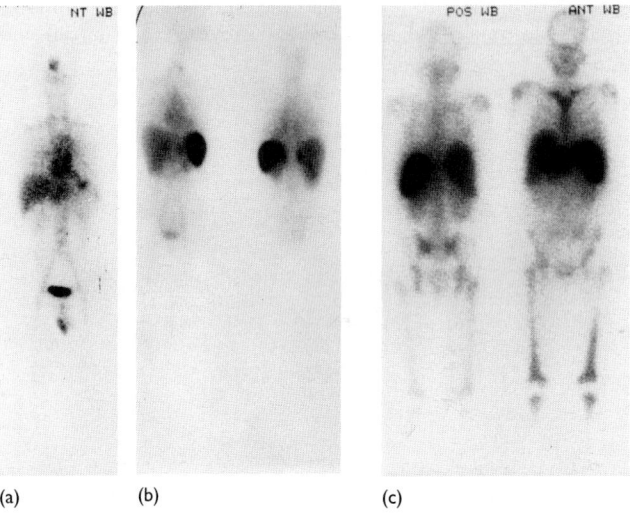

(a)   (b)   (c)

Fig. 1 Whole body scintigraphs 24 h after intravenous injection of ^{123}I-labelled human serum amyloid P component. (a) Anterior view of a normal control subject showing the distribution of residual tracer in the blood pool and radioactive breakdown products in urine in the bladder; note the absence of localization or retention of tracer anywhere in the body. (b) Posterior (left) and anterior (right) views of a patient with juvenile chronic arthritis complicated by AA amyloidosis. There is uptake of tracer in the spleen, kidneys, and adrenal glands, a typical distribution of AA amyloid in which the spleen is involved in 100 per cent of cases, kidneys in 75 per cent, and adrenals in 40 per cent. Note the reduced blood pool and bladder signal compared with (a). This patient, whose amyloid was diagnosed by renal biopsy 15 years ago when nephrotic syndrome developed, and who was then treated with chlorambucil, had been in complete remission for 10 years during which there had been no acute phase response. At the time of this scan there was no biochemical abnormality in blood or urine, despite the very appreciable amyloid deposits, illustrating the discordance between the presence of amyloid and clinical effects. (c) Posterior (left) and anterior (right) views of a patient with monoclonal gammopathy complicated by extensive AL amyloidosis. There is uptake and retention of tracer in the liver, spleen, kidneys, bone marrow, and soft tissues around the shoulder. This scintigraphic pattern of amyloid distribution is pathognomonic for AL amyloidosis; bone marrow uptake has not been seen in any other type. Note the complete absence of blood pool or bladder signal resulting from complete uptake of the tracer dose into the substantial amyloid deposits.

radical approaches can be justified by the poor prognosis. Such an approach, leading to reduced morbidity and improved survival, was the basis for the establishment of the National Health Service National Amyloid Centre. However, clinical improvement in amyloidosis is often delayed long after the underlying disorder has remitted, reflecting the very gradual regression of the deposits that is now recognized to occur in most patients. Continuing production of the amyloid precursor protein should be monitored as closely as possible long term, to determine the requirement for and intensity of treatment for the underlying primary condition. In AA amyloidosis this involves frequent estimation of the plasma SAA level, and in AL amyloidosis requires monitoring of proliferation of monoclonal plasma cells and immunoglobulin light chain production.

The treatment of AA amyloidosis ranges from potent anti-inflammatory and immunosuppressive drugs in patients with rheumatoid arthritis, to life-long prophylactic colchicine in familial Mediterranean fever, and surgery in conditions such as refractory osteomyelitis and the tumours of Castleman's disease. The alkylating agent chlorambucil can induce rapid and complete remission of inflammatory activity in many patients with rheumatoid and juvenile chronic arthritis, but its use must be considered very carefully since it is not licensed for this indication, it is potentially carcinogenic, and it causes infertility.

Treatment of AL amyloidosis is based on that for myeloma, although the plasma cell dyscrasias in AL amyloidosis are often very subtle. Prolonged low-intensity cytotoxic regimes such as oral melphalan and prednisolone are beneficial in about 20 per cent of patients. Dose-intensive infusional chemotherapy regimes such as vincristine, doxorubicin (Adriamycin), and

dexamethasone ('VAD'), and autologous peripheral blood stem cell transplantation are currently being evaluated with far more promising early results. However, very rigorous patient selection for transplantation is essential as the procedural mortality is high in individuals with multiple amyloidotic organ involvement, especially patients with autonomic neuropathy, severe cardiac amyloidosis, or a history of gastrointestinal bleeding, and in those aged over 55 years.

The disabling arthralgia of β_2-microglobulin amyloidosis may respond partially to non-steroidal anti-inflammatory drugs or corticosteroids, but even the most severe symptoms usually vanish rapidly following renal transplantation. The basis for this remarkable clinical response is unclear since although transplantation rapidly restores normal β_2-microglobulin metabolism, regression of β_2-microglobulin amyloid may not be evident for many years.

Hepatic transplantation is effective in familial amyloid polyneuropathy associated with transthyretin gene mutations since the variant amyloidogenic protein is produced mainly in the liver. Successful liver transplantation has now been reported in hundreds of patients with this condition and although the peripheral neuropathy usually only stabilizes, autonomic function can improve substantially and the associated visceral amyloid deposits have been shown to regress in most cases. Important questions remain about the timing of the procedure but, so far, early intervention seems advisable.

Supportive therapy remains critical in systemic amyloidosis, with the potential for delaying target organ failure, maintaining quality of life, and prolonging survival whilst the underlying process can be treated. Rigorous control of hypertension is vital in renal amyloidosis. Surgical resection of amyloidotic tissue is occasionally beneficial but, in general, a conservative approach to surgery, anaesthesia, and other invasive procedures is advisable. Should any such procedure be undertaken, meticulous attention to blood pressure and fluid balance is essential. Amyloidotic tissues may heal poorly and are liable to bleed. Diuretics and vasoactive drugs should be used cautiously in cardiac amyloidosis because they can reduce cardiac output substantially. Dysrhythmias may respond to conventional pharmacological therapy or to pacing. Replacement of vital organ function, notably dialysis, may be necessary and cardiac, renal, and liver transplant procedures have a role in selected cases.

Finally, a number of different therapies aimed specifically at inhibiting the formation of amyloid fibrils or promoting fibril regression are currently under development and will be evaluated clinically within the next few years. These approaches, directed at the generation of precursor proteins, the protein folding process, formed fibrils, glycosaminglycans, and serum amyloid P component, offer hope that in future amyloidosis may become a treatable condition.

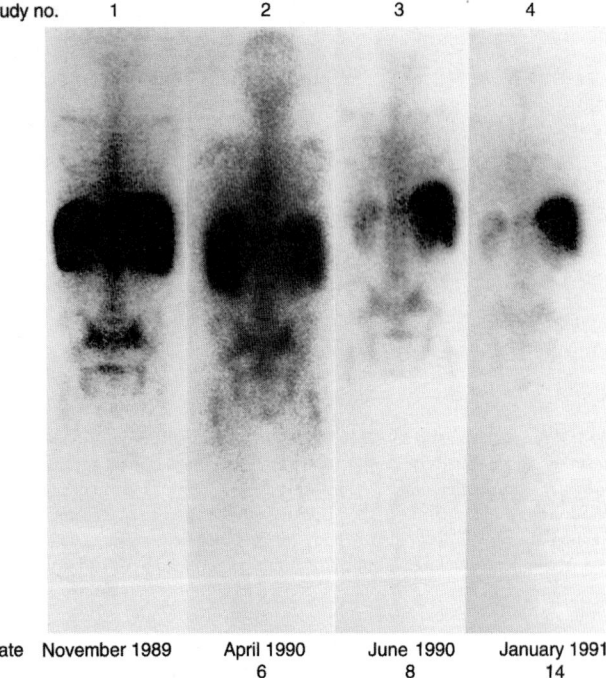

Study no.	1	2	3	4
Date	November 1989	April 1990 6	June 1990 8	January 1991 14

Fig. 2 Serial posterior whole body ^{123}I-serum amyloid P component scintigraphs of a man with AL amyloidosis complicating benign monoclonal gammopathy. At presentation, scan 1, there was uptake in the spleen, liver, and bone marrow, obscuring any possible renal signal. Chemotherapy was given before the second scan, which shows increased spleen uptake, reduced liver uptake, and some renal uptake, but no change in total amyloid load determined by measurements of the clearance and retention of the tracer (not shown). Subsequently he suffered from recurrent splenic infarction and splenectomy was performed. Thereafter, in scan 3, there was increased tracer uptake in liver, although a notably lower total amyloid load. Six months later, in scan 4, liver and kidney uptake, plasma clearance, and whole body retention of tracer were all reduced, indicating regression of amyloid. Clinically he was much improved and still remains well.

Further reading

Booth DR *et al.* (1997). Instability, unfolding and aggregation of human lysozyme variants underlying amyloid fibrillogenesis. *Nature* **385**, 787–93.

Botto M *et al.* (1997). Amyloid deposition is delayed in mice with targeted deletion of the serum amyloid P component gene. *Nature Medicine* **3**, 855–9.

Drüeke TB (1998). Dialysis-related amyloidosis. *Nephrology Dialysis Transplantation* **13** (Suppl. 1), 58–64.

Gillmore J *et al.* (2001). Amyloid load and clinical outcome in AA amyloidosis in relation to circulating concentration of serum amyloid A protein. *Lancet* **358**, 24–9.

Hardy J (1997) Amyloid, the presenilins and Alzheimer's disease. *Trends in Neurosciences* **20**, 154–9.

Hawkins PN, Lavender JP, Pepys MB (1990). Evaluation of systemic amyloidosis by scintigraphy with ^{123}I-labeled serum amyloid P component. *New England Journal of Medicine* **323**, 508–13.

Hawkins PN *et al.* (1993). Serum amyloid P component scintigraphy and turnover studies for diagnosis and quantitative monitoring of AA amyloidosis in juvenile rheumatoid arthritis. *Arthritis and Rheumatism* **36**, 842–51.

Kyle RA, Gertz MA (1995). Primary systemic amyloidosis: clinical and laboratory features in 474 cases. *Seminars in Hematology* **32**, 45–9.

Kyle RA, Gertz MA, eds (1999). *Amyloid and amyloidosis 1998*. Parthenon Publishing, Pearl River, NY.

11.13 α_1-Antitrypsin deficiency and the serpinopathies

David A. Lomas

Introduction

People of European descent are susceptible to disease arising from a genetic deficiency of the plasma protein α_1-antitrypsin. This is a 394 amino-acid, 52-kDa, acute-phase glycoprotein synthesized by the liver and macrophages and present in the plasma at a concentration of between 1.5 and 3.5 g/l. It functions as an inhibitor of a range of proteolytic enzymes but its primary role is to inhibit the enzyme neutrophil elastase. Activated neutrophil leucocytes release elastase to break down connective tissue at sites of inflammation. This breakdown is limited by the antielastase activity of α_1-antitrypsin, but if the plasma concentration of this protein falls below 40 per cent then unimpeded tissue destruction may ensue.

Genetic deficiency

α_1-Antitrypsin is subject to genetic variation resulting from mutations in the 12.2-kilobase (**kb**), 7-exon gene on the long arm of chromosome 14. Over 90 allelic variants have been reported and classified using the **Pi** (protease inhibitor) nomenclature that assesses α_1-antitrypsin mobility in isoelectric focusing analysis. Normal α_1-antitrypsin migrates in the middle (M) and variants are designated A to L if they migrate faster than M, and N to Z if they migrate more slowly. Many of these variants have been sequenced at the DNA level and shown to result from point mutations in the α_1-antitrypsin gene. For example, the Z allele results from the substitution of a positively charged lysine for a negative glutamic acid at position 342. The S allele results from the substitution of a neutral valine for a glutamic acid at position 264. It is clear that such mutations alter the overall charge of the protein and explain the changes in mobility seen on isoelectric focusing. Point mutations are inherited by simple Mendelian trait; the normal genotype is designated *PiMM* or *PiM*, a heterozygote for the Z gene is *PiMZ*, and a homozygote is *PiZZ* or *PiZ*.

The most clinically relevant variants are the S and Z alleles and the uncommon *Null* (non-production) gene. Approximately 8 per cent of people of Northern European descent are heterozygotes for the S variant (*PiMS*), although this can be as high as 28 per cent in parts of Southern Europe. The Z variant is less common and is found in 4 per cent of Northern Europeans (*PiMZ*), with 1 in 1700 being homozygotes (*PiZ*). α_1-Antitrypsin alleles are co-dominantly expressed, with each allele contributing to the plasma level of protein. Moreover, each of the deficiency alleles results in a characteristic decrease in the plasma concentration of α_1-antitrypsin; the S variant forms 60 per cent of the normal M concentration and the Z variant 10 to 15 per cent. Thus combinations of alleles have predictable effects, the MZ heterozygote has an α_1-antitrypsin plasma level of 60 per cent (50 per cent from the normal M allele and 10 per cent from the Z allele), the MS heterozygote 80 per cent, and the SZ heterozygote 40 per cent.

Molecular basis of α_1-antitrypsin deficiency

α_1-Antitrypsin functions by presenting its reactive-centre methionine residue on an exposed loop of the molecule such that it forms an ideal substrate for the enzyme neutrophil elastase (Fig. 1). The exact fit between enzyme and inhibitor causes them to form a tightly bound 1:1 complex that inhibits the enzyme and allows it to be eliminated from sites of inflammation. The Z mutation (342glutamic acid→lysine) results in normal translation of the gene, but 85 per cent of the Z α_1-antitrypsin is retained within the endoplasmic reticulum with only 10 to 15 per cent entering the circulation. The Z mutation distorts the relationship between the loop and the β-pleated A sheet that forms the major feature of the molecule (Fig. 1(a)). The consequent perturbation in structure allows the reactive-centre loop of one α_1-molecule to lock into the A sheet of a second (Fig. 1(b)) to form a dimer which then extends to form chains of loop-sheet polymers (Fig. 1(c)). The formation of these polymers is temperature- and concentration-dependent and is localized in the endoplasmic reticulum of the hepatocyte. These chains of polymers become interwoven to form the insoluble aggregates that are the hallmark of α_1-antitrypsin liver disease (Fig. 2 and Plate 1). S α_1-antitrypsin (342glutamic acid→lysine) and the rare I variant (39arginine→cysteine) also result in the formation of polymers but at a much slower rate than Z. Therefore these variants do not accumulate in the liver and cause only mild plasma deficiency.

Clinical features

α_1-Antitrypsin deficiency and emphysema

The association between α_1-antitrypsin deficiency and the development of premature panlobular emphysema was first described by Laurell and Eriksson in 1963. Patients usually present with increasing dyspnoea and weight loss, with cor pulmonale and polycythaemia occurring late in the course of the disease. Chest radiographs typically show bilateral basal emphysema with paucity and pruning of the basal pulmonary vessels. Upper lobe vascularization is relatively normal. Ventilation–perfusion radioisotope scans and angiography also show abnormalities with a lower zone distribution. High-resolution computed tomography scans with 1 to 2 mm collimation are the most accurate method of assessing the distribution of panlobular emphysema and for monitoring the progress of the pulmonary disease, although this currently has little value outside clinical trials. Lung function tests are typical for emphysema with a reduced **FEV1/FVC** ratio (forced expiratory volume in 1 second/forced vital capacity), gas trapping (raised residual volume/total lung capacity ratio), and a low gas-transfer factor.

The association of α_1-antitrypsin with the development of premature emphysema has led to the wider conclusion that emphysema results from an imbalance between proteases and antiproteases within the lung.

Undoubtedly the situation is more complex than a simple balance between elastase and α₁-antitrypsin, both in terms of the numbers of enzymes and inhibitors involved and the contribution of other mechanisms. Neverthe- less, the elastase and α₁-antitrypsin balance clearly illustrates the processes involved in the development of emphysema and the interplay between the environmental and genetic factors that determine its onset.

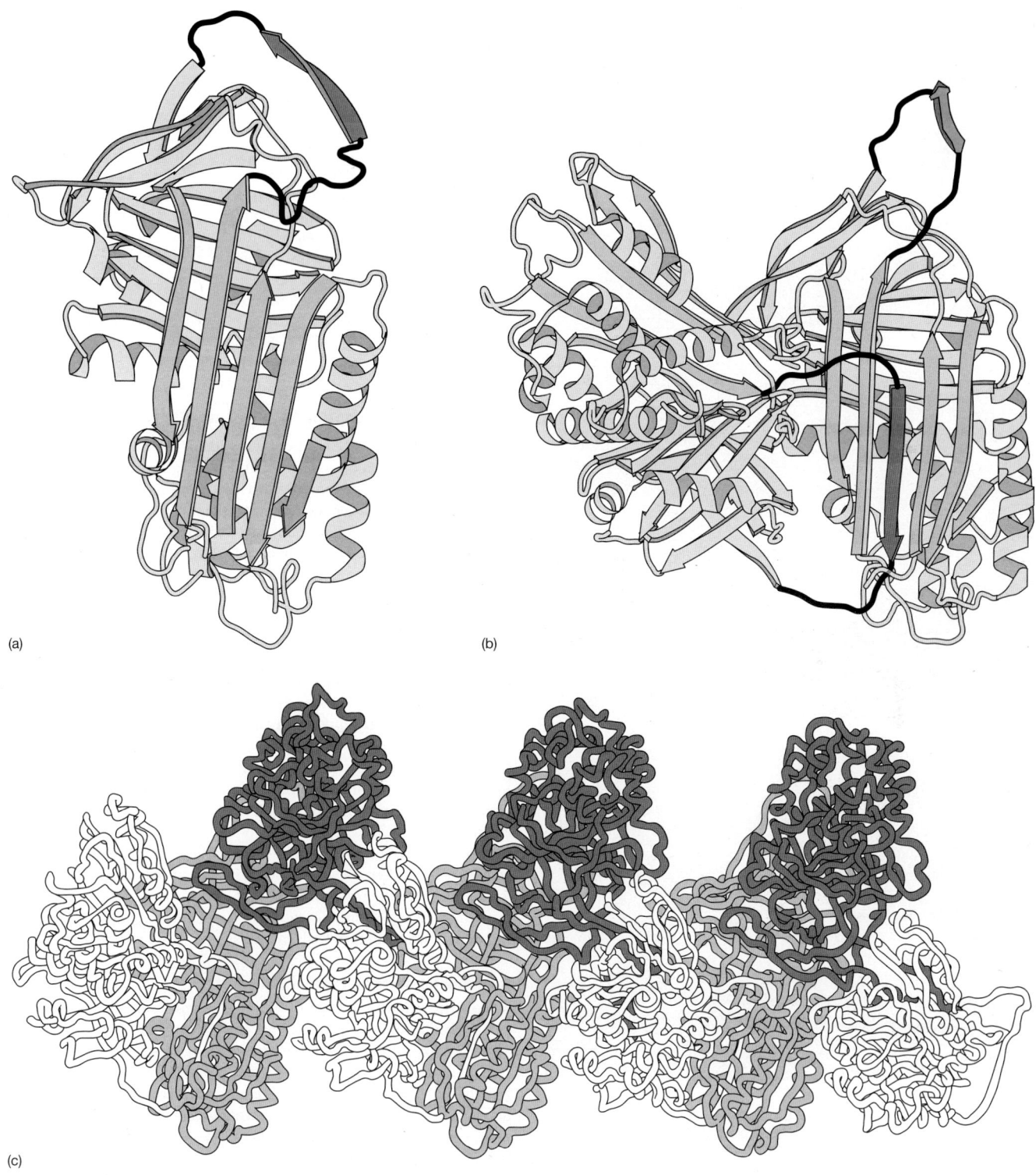

(a)

(b)

(c)

Fig. 1 The crystal structure of α₁-antitrypsin shows the reactive-centre loop (purple) held at the apex of the protein as a β-strand depicted as an arrow (a) The Z mutation opens the β-sheet A (pink) to allow the reactive loop of another molecule to insert to form a dimer (b) which can then extend to form long chains of polymers (c). In (c) white, pink, and purple represent different α₁-antitrypsin molecules linked together to form a polymer. (Figure prepared by Dr T. Dafforn, Cambridge Institute for Medical Research, and reproduced from *Nature Structure Biology* with permission.)

Decline in lung function in individuals with α₁-antitrypsin deficiency

As with other tissues, there is a decline in the elasticity of the lungs with increasing age. Clinically, the most convenient measure of lung function is the FEV₁, which is approximately 3500 ml in young adults. After the age of

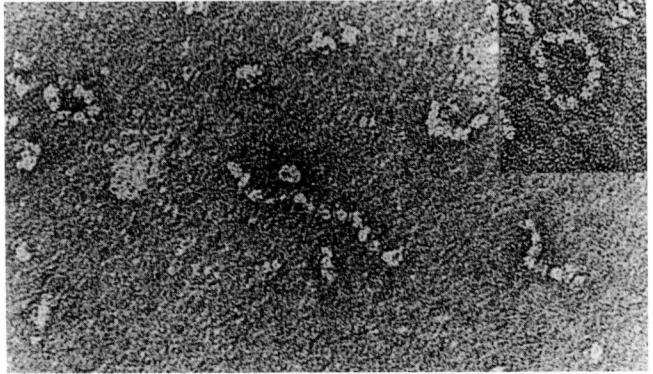

(a)

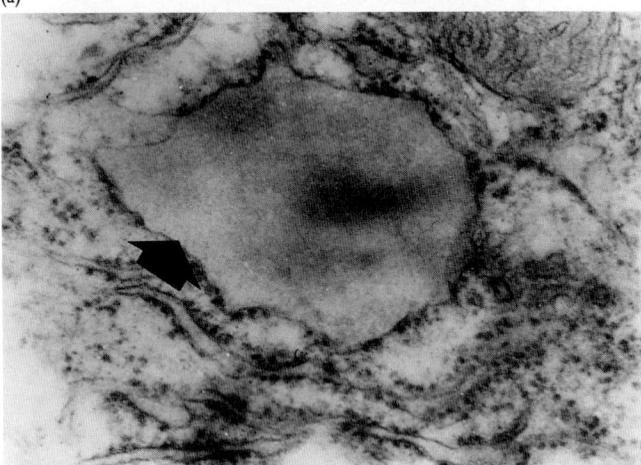

(b)

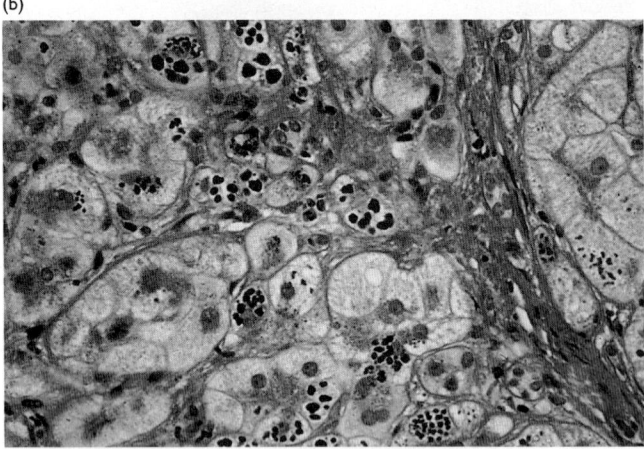

(c)

Fig. 2 (a) Electron microscopy of a chain of loop-sheet polymers isolated from a patient with α₁-antitrypsin deficiency. These polymers can form filaments or circlets (inset) that tangle within the endoplasmic reticulum of the hepatocyte (b) to form the inclusions (arrowed) which are the hallmark of the disease. These intrahepatic inclusions are characteristically Periodic acid–Schiff (**PAS**)-positive and diastase-resistant (c) (see also Plate 1) and stain positive for α₁-antitrypsin on immunohistochemistry. ((a) and (b) reproduced from the *Journal of Biological Chemistry* and *Nature*, respectively, with permission.)

30 years in healthy non-smokers, the FEV₁ decreases by 35 ml/year, although there is considerable individual variation. By old age, most people will have an appreciable loss of lung function, but only occasionally in the non-smoker will this be clinically apparent. The assessment of symptomatic hospital patients has shown that the loss of FEV₁ may be accelerated to 80 ml/year in a Z α₁-antitrypsin homozygote. As a consequence there is a hastened but still variable onset of emphysema. In this study *PiZ* non-smokers were free from dyspnoea up to the age of 50 years, with the average age of death from respiratory disease being 67 years. Again there was considerable individual variation and, particularly in women, there was a good likelihood of a full lifespan without significant respiratory impairment. The outlook, however, was poor for the *PiZ* α₁-antitrypsin homozygote who was a heavy smoker, as the loss in FEV₁ increased to 300 ml/year. The onset of dyspnoea was approximately 30 years, with death from respiratory disease by the age of 50 years. More recently the Swedish, Danish, and NIH registries have reported a more favourable outcome. These registries include individuals identified by screening and family studies and are more representative of the disease process. They show a slower rate of decline in lung function in *PiZ* homozygotes who are non- or ex-smokers (approximately 50 ml/year). However, the studies reinforce the accelerated rate of decline in lung function in *PiZ* homozygotes who continue to smoke (70–132 ml/year).

α₁-Antitrypsin deficiency and liver disease

Z α₁-antitrypsin liver disease is characterized by the accumulation of diastase-resistant, Periodic acid–Schiff (**PAS**)-positive inclusions of α₁-antitrypsin in the periportal cells (Fig. 2(c)). This insoluble material accumulates within the endoplasmic reticulum of hepatocytes stimulating a massive increase in cellular degradative activity. The *PiMZ* individuals are able to degrade much of the abnormal α₁-antitrypsin, but not the *PiZ* homozygote in whom aggregation overwhelms the degradative process resulting in α₁-antitrypsin accumulation, hepatocellular damage, and cell death. The accumulation of α₁-antitrypsin within hepatocytes is also seen with two other rare mutations, S*ᵢᵢyama* (53phenylalanine→serine), which is the commonest cause of α₁-antitrypsin deficiency in Japan, and M*malton* (52phenylalanine deletion), which is the commonest cause of α₁-antitrypsin deficiency in Sardinia. Both of these point mutations result in perturbations of α₁-antitrypsin and the ready formation of loop-sheet polymers. Cirrhosis has also been reported sporadically in *SZ* and *IZ* heterozygotes in whom the 'polymerogenic' Z and S or I α₁-antitrypsin can interlink to form chains of mixed SZ or IZ heteropolymers. The observation that polymer formation is temperature- and concentration-dependent may account for the variation in the number and density of liver inclusions between individuals. α₁-Antitrypsin is an acute-phase protein and, as such, undergoes a manifold increase in production in association with temperature increases of up to 41 °C. The increase in protein concentration and temperature during the inflammatory response favour polymerization, which in turn leads to inclusion formation and liver disease.

Neonatal jaundice and juvenile cirrhosis

Some 73 per cent of Z α₁-antitrypsin homozygote infants have a raised serum alanine aminotransferase level in the first year of life, but in only 15 per cent of people is it still abnormal by the age of 12 years. Similarly, the serum bilirubin level is raised in 11 per cent of *PiZ* infants in the first 2 to 4 months but falls to normal by 6 months of age. Cholestatic jaundice develops in 1 in 10 infants and 6 per cent develop clinical evidence of liver disease without jaundice. These symptoms usually resolve by the second year of life, but approximately 15 per cent of patients with cholestatic jaundice progress to juvenile cirrhosis. The reasons for this variable progression are unknown, but intercurrent illness and hormonal and genetic factors are likely to be involved. Indeed cholestatic jaundice in infancy is twice as common in boys than girls. The overall risk of death from liver disease in *PiZ* children during childhood is between 2 and 3 per cent.

Adult liver disease

All *PiZ* individuals have slowly progressive hepatic damage that is often subclinical and only evident as a minor degree of portal fibrosis. However, up to 50 per cent of Z α₁-antitrypsin homozygotes present with clinically evident cirrhosis and occasionally with hepatocellular carcinoma. The presence of Z α₁-antitrypsin deficiency, including the heterozygous *PiMZ* and *PiSZ* forms, should always be considered before making the diagnosis of cryptogenic cirrhosis.

Associated conditions

α₁-Antitrypsin deficiency is associated with an increased prevalence of asthma, panniculitis, Wegener's granulomatosis, pancreatitis, gallstones, and possibly bronchiectasis. There appears to be a reduced risk of cerebrovascular disease.

Diagnosis

The severe genetic deficiency of α₁-antitrypsin is readily diagnosed by low plasma levels and the virtual absence of the α₁-band on protein electrophoresis. As α₁-antitrypsin is an acute-phase protein, most laboratories will report levels with another acute-phase reactant, such as α₁-antitchymotrypsin, which allows the clinician to assess the likelihood of deficiency in the context of the inflammatory response. The acute-phase response raises the plasma level of α₁-antitrypsin, but never can the plasma level of the *PiZ* heterozygote reach the normal range. The deficiency variant is then assigned a Pi phenotype according to the migration of the protein on an isoelectric focusing gel.

Treatment

The treatment of α₁-antitrypsin deficiency depends largely on the avoidance of stimuli causing repeated pulmonary inflammation—primarily smoking. Patients with α₁-antitrypsin deficiency-related emphysema should receive conventional therapy with trials of bronchodilators and inhaled corticosteroids, pulmonary rehabilitation and, where appropriate, assessment for long-term oxygen therapy and lung transplantation. The role of lung volume-reduction surgery in this group is unclear as the disease is basal rather than apical and resections of this region are technically more difficult. Mixed results have been reported in uncontrolled trials.

The lung disease results from a deficiency in the antielastase screen. This may be rectified biochemically by intravenous infusions of α₁-antitrypsin. Registry data suggest that individuals with α₁-antitrypsin deficiency and an FEV_1 of 35–49 per cent predicted may derive benefit from replacement therapy. The only controlled trial showed a non-significant trend towards reduced progression of emphysema in individuals receiving intravenous α₁-antitrypsin. α₁-Antitrypsin replacement therapy is currently unavailable in many European countries, including the United Kingdom. It is widely used in North America.

All Z homozygotes have some liver damage and, as such, would be wise to avoid alcohol abuse. The deduction that loop-sheet polymerization of α₁-antitrypsin complicates the acute-phase response highlights the importance of antipyretic agents in *PiZ* infants with antitrypsin deficiency. Although this has yet to be proven by clinical trials, there is anecdotal evidence that these intercurrent illnesses account for the variation in progression of liver disease in infants. Moreover, there is good reason to believe that conservative treatments to lessen pyrexia and the inflammatory response will be of value in reducing α₁-antitrypsin aggregation within hepatocytes and hence liver disease. *PiZ* homozygotes should be monitored for the persistence of hyperbilirubinaemia as this, along with deteriorating results of coagulation studies, indicates the need for liver transplantation. Parents with a child with severe Z α₁-antitrypsin liver disease may require genetic counselling. The likelihood of similar severe liver damage in a subsequent Z homozygote sibling is approximately 20 per cent.

The uncommon α₁-antitrypsin deficiency-associated panniculitis usually responds to dapsone, 100 to 150 mg daily, for 2 to 4 weeks, but occasionally it necessitates the administration of intravenous α₁-antitrypsin replacement therapy.

Other 'serpinopathies'

α₁-Antitrypsin is the archetypal member of a superfamily of proteins termed the *se*rine *p*rotease *in*hibitors, or serpins, that have closely related structures and functions. These inhibitors control various inflammatory cascades, including coagulation (antithrombin), complement activation (C1-inhibitor), and fibrinolysis (α₂-antiplasmin). Pathological processes that underlie the deficiency of one member may account for deficiency of others. Indeed the process of polymer formation has also been reported in deficiency-mutants of antithrombin, C1-inhibitor, and α₁-antichymotrypsin. These polymers are inactive as proteinase inhibitors and so predispose the individual to thrombosis, angio-oedema, and chronic airflow obstruction disease, respectively. Moreover, polymerization also underlies a novel inclusion-body dementia that results from point mutations in a neurone-specific serpin, neuroserpin. The dementia, termed familial encephalopathy with neuroserpin inclusion bodies or FENIB, is inherited as an autosomal dominant trait with the inclusions of neuroserpin in the brain being PAS-positive and diastase-resistant, identical to those of Z α₁-antitrypsin in the liver. Heterozygotes with critical mutations develop early-onset dementia as the accumulated protein causes neuronal cell death. The recognition that serpin polymerization underlies all these disorders may allow the development of a common therapy.

Further reading

Davis RL *et al.* (1999). Familial dementia caused by polymerisation of mutant neuroserpin. *Nature* **401**, 376–9. [Description of two families with mutations in the serpin, neuroserpin, that form polymers *in vivo* and an inclusion-body dementia.]

Dirksen A, *et al.* (1999). A randomised clinical trial of α₁-antitrypsin augmentation therapy. *American Journal of Respiratory and Critical Care Medicine*, **160**, 1468–72. [The only randomised controlled trial of α₁-antitrypsin replacement therapy in patients with α₁-antitrypsin deficiency. The study showed a trend towards a reduced rate of progression of emphysema in patients receiving replacement therapy.]

Eriksson S, Carlson J, Velez R. (1986). Risk of cirrhosis and primary liver cancer in alpha₁-antitrypsin deficiency. *New England Journal of Medicine* **314**, 736–9. [Postmortem study demonstrating a high prevalence of liver disease in adults with PiZ α1-antitrypsin deficiency.]

Larsson C (1978). Natural history and life expectancy in severe α₁-antitrypsin PiZ. *Acta Medica Scandinavica* **204**, 345–52. [Report of 246 patients with PiZ α1-antitrypsin deficiency detailing age of onset of breathlessness. The subjects were largely ascertained from hospital populations.]

Mahadeva R, Lomas DA (1998). Alpha₁-antitrypsin deficiency, cirrhosis and emphysema. *Thorax* **53**, 501–5. [A review of the structural basis of α1-antitrypsin deficiency.]

Mahadeva R, *et al.* (1999). Heteropolymerisation of S, I and Z α₁-antitrypsin and liver cirrhosis. *Journal of Clinical Investigation* **103**, 999–1006. [Demonstration that different α1-antitrypsin variants can interlink to form polymers that are associated with cirrhosis.]

Piitulainen E, Eriksson S (1999). Decline in FEV₁ related to smoking status in individuals with severe alpha1-antitrypsin deficiency. *European Respiratory Journal* **13**, 247–51. [Report of rate of decline in lung function of 608 patients followed for 1–31 years. Current smokers have an accelerated rate of decline in lung function but ex-smokers have the same rate as non-smokers. The values are likely to be more representative than other reports as many subjects were ascertained from screening and family studies.]

Sveger T, Piitulainen E, Arborelius Jr M (1995). Clinical features and lung function in 18-year-old adolescents with α_1-antitrypsin deficiency. *Acta Pædiatrica* **84**, 815–16. [Report on the follow up of 127 subjects with PiZ α1-antitrypsin deficiency from birth to 18 years. This is the only long-term prospective study of patients with α1-antitrypsin deficiency and the only study that is free from selection bias.]

The alpha-1-antitrypsin deficiency registry study group (1998). Survival and FEV_1 decline in individuals with severe deficiency of α_1-antitrypsin. *American Journal of Respiratory and Critical Care Medicine* **158**, 49–59. [Report from the registry of 1129 patients with α1-antitrypsin deficiency who did or did not receive α1-antitrypsin replacement therapy. Replacement therapy may slow down the decline in lung function in patients with a predicted FEV1 of 35–49 per cent. This is not a randomized controlled trial and therefore the conclusions must be interpreted with caution.]

Useful web sites:

http://www-structmed.cimr.cam.ac.uk/serpins.html [An updated list of α1-antitrypsin mutants, their clinical effects, and their effect on the structure of the protein.]

http://www.alpha-1.priv.at/supportg.html [A list of international α1-antitrypsin support groups and other related web sites.]

12

Endocrine disorders

12.1 Principles of hormone action

Mark Gurnell, Jacky Burrin, and V. Krishna K. Chatterjee

Definition

Endocrinology is the study of hormones secreted by glands or cells which, acting locally or at a distance, facilitate communication between cells and different organs thus co-ordinating their activities.

Classically, the production of hormones has been associated with specialized glands or tissues including the hypothalamus, pituitary, thyroid, parathyroids, gonads, pancreatic islet cells, adrenal glands, and placenta. It is now recognized that hormones are also produced by a range of other organs and tissues which are not considered to be classical endocrine glands. The heart is the primary source of atrial natriuretic peptide factor, which controls blood pressure and intravascular volume; endothelin and nitric oxide are derived from vascular endothelium and regulate vascular tone. Endocrine cells are distributed throughout the gastrointestinal tract and are a rich source of hormones such as cholecystokinin, gastrin, secretin, vasoactive intestinal peptide; many of these gastrointestinal hormones are also produced in the brain and central nervous system, where their role is less well understood. Erythropoietin, a circulating factor that stimulates erythropoiesis, is derived from the kidney. Adipose tissue has recently been shown to produce leptin, a circulating hormone which acts centrally to control appetite.

However, as understanding of intercellular communication has advanced, the lines of division that separate different physiological systems have become blurred. For example, neuroendocrinology represents intimate connections between the nervous and endocrine systems: peptide hormones produced in the brain exert effects via the hypothalamus to control hormone secretion from the pituitary gland; in the periphery, the sympathetic nervous system modulates hormone production by the adrenal medulla and pancreatic islets. Similarly, there are complex inter-relationships between the immune and endocrine systems: for example, glucocorticoid hormones exert powerful immunosuppressive effects; conversely, cytokines (for example, tumour necrosis factor-α and interleukin-6) produced by cells of the immune system markedly influence hormone secretion by glands such as the pituitary and adrenal.

Nature of hormones

In general, hormones can be classified into those that are based on proteins or peptides and those which are chemically derived. Small peptides include hypothalamic releasing factors produced by neuroendocrine cells, which act locally on the pituitary; larger polypeptides such as insulin or growth hormone are characteristically circulating hormones that act on more distant targets. Biogenic amines including catecholamines, dopamine, and serotonin (5-hydroxytryptamine) are derived from amino acids. The majority of protein and peptide hormones interact with membrane receptors located on the cell surface. Binding to membrane receptors activates downstream signalling pathways, leading to changes in cellular function which mediate responses to hormones.

A second class of hormones includes steroids and other lipophilic substances, which act by crossing the plasma membrane to interact with intracellular receptors. Steroid hormones are derived from cholesterol and include cortisol, progesterone, testosterone, and oestradiol. Vitamin D and retinoic acid, which are synthesized from dietary sources, and thyroid hormone produced by the modification of tyrosines in thyroglobulin, are structurally dissimilar to steroids but also act via nuclear receptors.

Development of endocrine glands

The hypothalamus develops from forebrain tissue adjacent to the third ventricle. Neurones secreting releasing factors send cellular processes which terminate in portal capillaries that perfuse the pituitary gland. The latter develops from ectoderm to form the adenohypophysis or anterior pituitary; the posterior pituitary or neurohypophysis is formed directly from axonal terminals of hypothalamic neurones that grow downward. The thyroid gland develops from endoderm in the floor of the oropharynx with the migration of cells caudally to its final position in the neck. During its descent, parafollicular C cells, derived from neural crest tissue within the ultimobranchial body and parathyroid glands from the third and fourth pharyngeal pouches, become incorporated into the thyroid gland. The adrenal glands comprise a steroid-secreting cortex developed from mesoderm, together with a catecholamine-producing medulla composed of chromaffin cells derived from neural crest. Germ cells within indifferent gonadal primordia differentiate to form the ovary, or in the presence of the Y chromosome-encoded sex determining gene (*SRY*), develop into testes. Endocrine cells of the pancreas are derived from endoderm and differentiate to form the islets of Langerhans. Various transcription factors that control the development of cells within endocrine glands and their differentiation to hormone biosynthesis are listed in Table 1.

Hormone synthesis, processing, and secretion

The organization of endocrine genes is homologous to those encoding many other proteins, although there are some characteristic features. Gene

Table 1 Transcription factors involved in endocrine gland development

Gland	Transcription factor(s)
Pituitary	HESX-1, Pit-1, PROP-1
Thyroid	TTF-1, TTF-2, PAX-8
Adrenal cortex	SF-1, DAX-1
Pancreatic islet cells	IPF-1
Testis	SRY, SF-1
Ovary	SF-1, DAX-1

HESX-1, homeobox gene expressed in embryonic stem cells 1; Pit-1, pituitary transcription factor 1; PROP-1, prophet of Pit-1; TTF-1, thyroid transcription factor 1; TTF-2, thyroid transcription factor 2; PAX-8, paired box gene 8; SF-1, steroidogenic factor 1; DAX-1, Dosage-sensitive sex reversal Adrenal hypoplasia critical region on the X-chromosome 1; IPF-1, insulin promoter factor 1; SRY, sex-determining region of the Y chromosome.

transcription is usually regulated by the promoter located in the upstream 5′-flanking region of the gene (Fig. 1). Typically, the promoter may contain three types of regulatory DNA which are recognized by specific transcription factors: a hormone-response element (**HRE**) is recognized by nuclear receptors; a tissue-specific element (**TSE**) binds cell-specific transcription factors (see Table 1) which enhance the transcription of the hormone gene in a tissue-specific manner; a third class of response element mediates transcriptional activation in response to second messenger signalling pathways. A rise in intracellular cyclic AMP concentration leads to the phosphorylation of cyclic AMP response-element binding proteins (**CREBs**) which interact with CREs; cell-signalling pathways that activate protein kinase C induce the phosphorylation of the Fos–Jun (AP-1) transcription-factor complex which binds its cognate DNA regulatory sequence. Binding of transcription factors to regulatory DNA response elements, activates and stabilizes basal transcription factors (**BTFs**), promoting gene transcription and mRNA synthesis (Fig. 1).

Transcription of the gene generates mRNA, which undergoes translation in ribosomes leading to polypeptide synthesis. In some endocrine genes, alternate exon splicing allows the substitution or removal of particular exons, such that peptides of differing sequence can be produced. For example, alternate splicing of the calcitonin gene in a tissue-specific manner directs the production of calcitonin in the C cells of the thyroid, whereas calcitonin gene-related peptide (**CGRP**) is produced preferentially in the brain.

Secreted polypeptide hormones incorporate a signal sequence at the amino terminus of the protein that directs its translocation across the endoplasmic reticulum where this sequence is cleaved (see Fig. 1). Many hormones are synthesized as larger polypeptides (prohormones) which undergo proteolytic cleavage to generate smaller functional peptides. Such proteolytic processing is mediated by specific proteases (prohormone convertase 1 and 2 (**PC1**, **PC2**)) which are highly expressed in cells of neuroendocrine lineage. Examples of hormone processing include the cleavage of proinsulin with removal of an internal C peptide to yield insulin, the active hormone. However, processing of the polypeptide precursor can also yield multiple functioning products. For example, pro-opiomelanocortin is cleaved by endopeptidases to yield adrenocorticotrophin (**ACTH**), melanocyte-stimulating hormone (**MSH**-α, -β, -γ), β-endorphin, and lipocortin.

Hormones may also undergo post-translational modification such as amidation of neuropeptides or glycosylation. Modification of amino acids by the addition of carbohydrate side chains is a particular characteristic of the glycoprotein hormones (luteinizing hormone, follicle-stimulating hormone, thyroid-stimulating hormone, and human chorionic gonadotrophin) and such glycosylation affects both their biological activity as well as their half-life in the circulation (see Fig. 1).

Hormones such as growth factors and cytokines are not significantly concentrated within cells, but are released via small, clear, Golgi-derived transport vesicles that fuse with the plasma membrane, representing a 'constitutive' pathway of secretion. In contrast, many endocrine cells contain an additional 'regulated' secretory pathway, which allows the export of high concentrations of hormone stored in cytoplasmic dense-core vesicles. Chromogranin B, an acidic protein, and polypeptide proteases are additional constituents of secretory vesicles. Adrenal cells secreting catecholamine hormones contain chromaffin granules which include enzymes (for example, dopamine β-hydroxylase) that catalyse catecholamine biosynthesis. Dense-core vesicle exocytosis is mediated by a rise in intracellular calcium levels, which activates the cytoskeletal machinery, promoting vesicle translocation and docking with the plasma membrane (see Fig. 1). Cells secreting steroid hormones contain abundant mitochondrial and smooth endoplasmic reticulum which contain enzymes that mediate steroid biosynthesis. Mitochondrial side-chain cleavage enzyme converts cholesterol to pregnenolone. The latter is then converted to glucocorticoid, mineralocorticoid, or sex steroids dependent on the cell-specific expression of steroidogenic enzymes. Steroid hormones are not stored to any extent and are secreted constitutively.

Control of hormone production

The classical mechanism by which hormone-producing glands communicate is via **endocrine** pathways, whereby the products from one gland are secreted into the circulation (and exert effects on a different, distant target gland). Such endocrine pathways integrate the hypothalamus, pituitary, and various end-organs to control the production of major hormones (Fig. 2). Thus, peptide-releasing factors (for example, gonadotrophin-releasing hormone (**GnRH**), thyrotrophin-releasing hormone (**TRH**), growth-hormone releasing hormone (**GHRH**), and corticotrophin-releasing hormone (**CRH**)) from the hypothalamus, stimulate the production of trophic hormones from specific pituitary cell types; exceptions to this are somatostatin, which inhibits pituitary growth-hormone release, and dopamine, which is secreted continuously to inhibit prolactin secretion. The pituitary hormones act on end-organs to generate products, which, in turn, exert a negative feedback effect at both hypothalamic and pituitary levels to regulate their own synthesis. Tri-iodothyronine (T3) inhibits TRH and thyroid-stimulating hormone (**TSH**) production; gonadal steroids and inhibin negatively regulate hypothalamic GnRH and pituitary gonadotrophins; cortisol suppresses CRH and ACTH generation; circulating insulin-like growth factor-1 (**IGF-1**) inhibits GHRH and growth-hormone secretion (Fig. 2). Osmoreceptors in the hypothalamus sense changes in serum osmolality to control the release of vasopressin from the posterior pituitary.

In addition to these endocrine control mechanisms, other types of local regulatory pathways are recognized. **Paracrine** regulation refers to factors

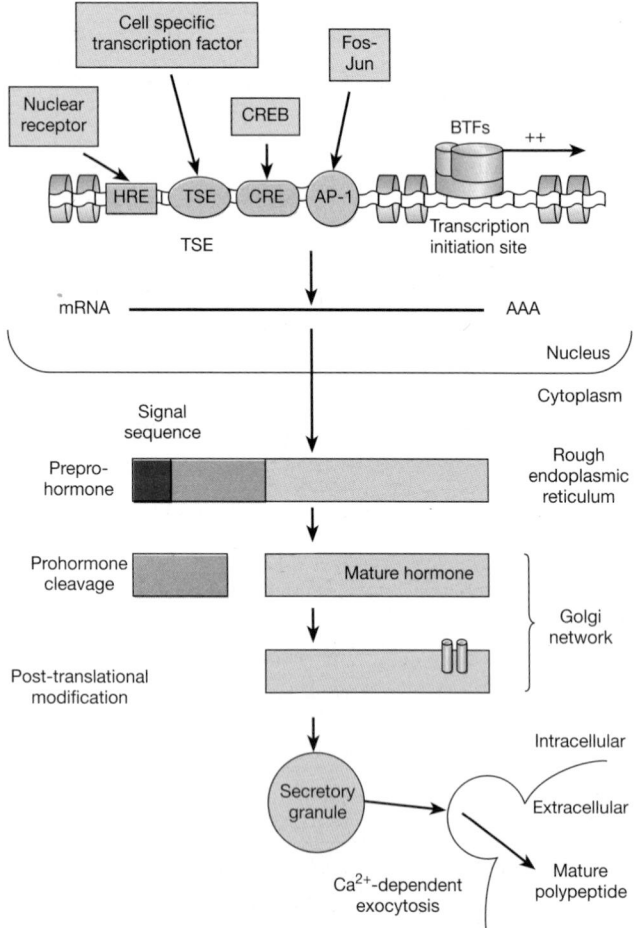

Fig. 1 Pathway of hormone synthesis, processing, and secretion.

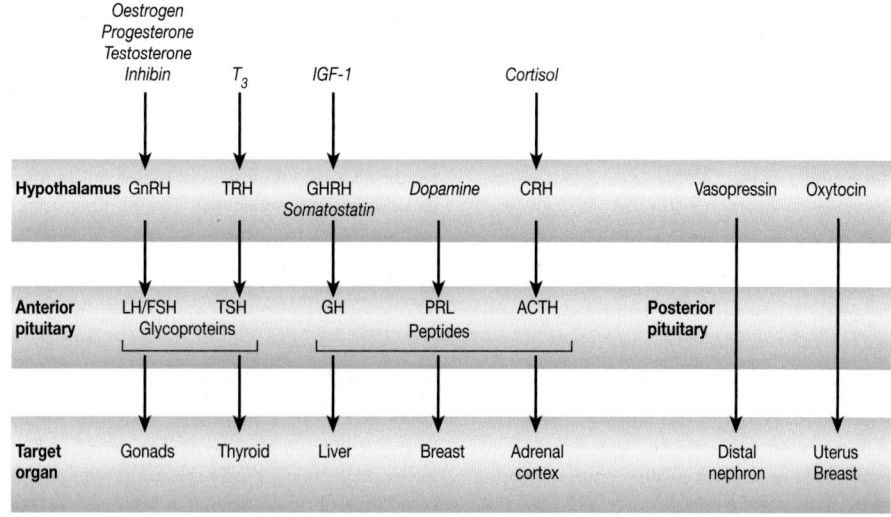

Fig. 2 Control of hormone production. Regulatory pathways integrating the hypothalamus, pituitary, and various end-organs. Hormones shown in italics exert inhibitory effects. Negative feedback regulation occurs at both hypothalamic and pituitary levels.

that are released by one cell and act upon a nearby cell in the same tissue. For example, somatostatin produced by δ cells in pancreatic islets inhibits the local production of insulin from β cells; in the testis, testosterone produced from Leydig cells exerts an effect on nearby Sertoli cells to enhance spermatogenesis. **Autocrine** control refers to a factor that acts upon the same cell in which it is produced. Examples include gonadotroph secretion of activin which stimulates the production of follicle-stimulating hormone (**FSH**) from the same cell; similarly, T cells produce interleukin-2 which acts to promote their own proliferation.

In addition to discrete hormonal responses, endocrine systems can respond to environmental stimuli by the integrated production of multiple hormones. For example, stress activates an array of pathways, with sympathetic activation mediating catecholamine release from the adrenals, and stimulation of the hypothalamus inducing multiple axes, resulting in the production of cortisol, growth hormone, prolactin, and vasopressin. The hormonal responses to starvation are also integrated by the hypothalamus. Here, diminished production of leptin from adipose tissue inhibits hypothalamic GnRH and TRH secretion, with a consequent reduction in the production of both gonadal steroids and thyroid hormone to limit reproduction and energy expenditure.

In addition to the feedback regulatory mechanisms outlined above, many hormones are released in a rhythmic or pulsatile manner. Insulin is secreted in rapid (about every 10 min) pulses in response to changes in glucose concentration in the pancreatic β cell. Gonadotrophin-releasing hormone is secreted from the hypothalamus at a lower pulse frequency of every 1.5 to 3 h, stimulating similar pulses of pituitary luteinizing hormone (**LH**) and FSH release. This hormonal rhythm controls ovarian folliculogenesis and steroid production to establish the female reproductive and menstrual cycle. Pituitary growth-hormone secretion is regulated by pulses of stimulatory GHRH and inhibitory somatostatin from the hypothalamus that are out of phase with each other, corresponding to peaks and troughs of circulating growth hormone.

Many hormonal pathways are influenced by the light–dark cycle, with circadian variation in their circulating levels. For example, the hypothalamic–pituitary–adrenal axis exhibits most activity in the early morning with peak cortisol production, followed by a nadir in glucocorticoid levels in the evening. Sleep is another environmental regulator: puberty is associated with nocturnal surges of LH; growth-hormone secretion is also enhanced nocturnally and the release of vasopressin during sleep inhibits renal diuresis.

Hormone-binding proteins

Thyroid hormones and many steroids are transported in the circulation with serum-binding proteins. Thus, thyroxine (**T4**) and tri-iodothyronine (**T3**) are bound to thyroxine-binding globulin (**TBG**), albumin, and thyroxine-binding prealbumin. Cortisol and progesterone are bound to cortisol-binding globulin (**CBG**), while oestrogens and androgens are bound to sex-hormone-binding globulin (**SHBG**). The role of serum-binding proteins is to provide a reservoir of circulating hormone. The interaction of hormones with binding proteins is relatively weak compared to their affinity for receptors, enabling them to dissociate easily. Only free hormone interacts with its receptor to elicit a biological response. Hormone-binding proteins are produced by the liver, and their synthesis can be increased (for example, by oestrogens or in pregnancy) or decreased (for example, in liver disease) thereby affecting the circulating concentration of total hormones. Accordingly, wherever possible, the concentration of free hormones in the circulation (for instance, T4, T3) or urine (cortisol) should be measured. Some protein hormones also circulate associated with binding proteins, which may modulate their action. A range of insulin-like growth-factor binding proteins (**IGFBPs**) bind to IGF-1, with some inhibiting and others facilitating the action of this peptide on target-tissue receptors. Growth hormone circulates bound to the extracellular domain of its receptor derived by cleavage from the membrane, with the complex prolonging the circulating half-life of the hormone.

Functions of hormones

The physiological roles of the major hormones can be broadly classified into three areas: control of growth and differentiation; maintenance of homeostasis; and regulation of reproduction. Some hormones have multiple functions and play a role in more than one area. In addition, some biological effects are mediated by the combined action of several different hormonal pathways. The principal actions of the major hormones are outlined in Table 2.

Linear growth is dependent on a complex interplay of many hormones and growth factors. Growth hormone plays a key role and exerts many of its effects by stimulating the hepatic production of IGF-1. Thyroid hormone also stimulates the epiphyseal growth plate in childhood, whereas production of sex steroids at puberty leads to epiphyseal closure. Other important actions of thyroid hormone include regulation of the basal metabolic rate, enhancement of myocardial contractility, and differentiation of the central nervous system.

The maintenance of homeostasis includes the control of metabolic pathways, fluid, electrolyte, and calcium balance, and regulation of blood pressure. Metabolic effects are mediated by several hormones: insulin lowers blood glucose by enhancing its cellular uptake and promotes glycogen synthesis; conversely, growth hormone, cortisol, glucagon, and adrenaline (epinephrine) act as counter-regulatory hormones to raise blood glucose. Glucagon and adrenaline stimulate glycogenolysis and, together with cortisol, promote gluconeogenesis. Other metabolic pathways are also influenced by these hormones: growth hormone and cortisol are lipolytic, whereas insulin mediates lipogenesis; insulin and growth hormone are also anabolic by promoting protein biosynthesis, whereas cortisol increases protein breakdown.

Circulating concentrations of ions and water balance are also under hormonal control. Vasopressin promotes water reabsorption via membrane channels (aquaporins) in the distal collecting ducts of the kidney; aldosterone acts at the renal distal convoluted tubule to stimulate sodium reabsorption and potassium excretion. Both parathyroid hormone (**PTH**) and vitamin D increase serum calcium levels; PTH mediates Ca^{2+} resorption from bone and kidney, whereas vitamin D acts on the gastrointestinal tract as well as these sites. Catecholamines and angiotensin-2 are potent vasoconstrictors and, together with cortisol, control blood pressure.

Hormones involved in reproduction exert effects from early in development. During embryogenesis, Müllerian-inhibiting substance (**MIS**) from the testis causes regression of female structures (uterus, fallopian tube), and testosterone promotes the development of the male structures (vas deferens, epididymis, seminal vesicles) derived from the Wolffian duct. Dihy-

drotestosterone promotes the development of male external genitalia. In both sexes, the gonadal axes are quiescent in childhood and become reactivated at puberty. Testosterone mediates virilization, secondary sexual characteristics, and spermatogenesis in the male; in females, ovarian production of oestrogen and progesterone induce secondary sexual features and control the menstrual cycle. In both sexes, gonadal steroids are required for the attainment of peak bone density at the end of puberty and its subsequent maintenance. During pregnancy, prolactin acts in concert with oestrogen to promote lactation; oxytocin stimulates uterine contraction at parturition and smooth muscle contraction in the mammary gland during suckling.

Hormone action

Hormones induce biological responses by interacting with receptors located either on the membrane or intracellularly in the cytoplasm or nucleus. Hormones bind to receptors with high affinity, such that low concentrations of free hormone associate and dissociate from receptors rapidly in a dynamic equilibrium. The interaction of hormones with receptors is usually highly specific, with individual receptors being highly selective for a single hormone even within a class of structurally related molecules (for example, steroid hormones). However, there are exceptions to this: parathyroid hormone (**PTH**) and parathyroid hormone-related peptide (**PTHRP**) share a common receptor and luteinizing hormone and chorionic gonadotrophin share another, generating similar biological responses; insulin and IGF-1 exhibit some degree of crossreactivity with their respective receptors; the mineralocorticoid receptor binds cortisol with equal or higher affinity than aldosterone.

Hormones that bind to membrane receptors act via effector proteins to activate second messenger signalling pathways. In turn, the second messengers stimulate a cascade of kinases, which then act upon target substrates in the cell membrane, the cytoplasm, or nucleus, to alter gene transcription or modulate a biochemical pathway, leading to a physiological response. Hormones that act through nuclear receptors are transported passively, or pumped actively, across the plasma membrane to interact with their targets. The hormone–receptor complex interacts with DNA sequences in target genes to either stimulate or repress their expression. The cellular actions of nuclear receptors are mediated by changes in target-gene transcription, altering mRNA synthesis, and in turn, the levels of protein product.

Signalling by membrane receptors

Membrane receptors can be divided into several groups (Table 3) depending on the signalling pathways that they utilize. The largest group consists of receptors with multiple transmembrane domains which are coupled to G-proteins; a second class of receptor contains an intracellular domain with tyrosine kinase activity; a number of hormones signal via membrane proteins that are homologous to cytokine receptors; a fourth class of hormone receptor contains an intracellular domain with serine or threonine kinase activity.

G-protein-coupled receptors (**GPCRs**) are characterized by seven separate hydrophobic domains that traverse the membrane phospholipid bilayer (Fig. 3(a)). They possess an extracellular domain of variable size, enabling further subclassification of these receptors: glycoprotein hormones or small molecule ligands (for example, calcium, γ-aminobutyric acid (**GABA**)) interact with large amino-terminal extracellular domains; biogenic amines (for example, catecholamines, serotonin (5-hydroxytryptamine)) bind to residues that lie within the transmembrane domain; other polypeptide hormones interact with residues in both the extracellular and transmembrane domains. The intracellular domains of the receptor enable interaction with G-proteins.

G-proteins typically form a heterotrimeric complex of α-, β-, and γ-subunits that bind the guanine nucleotides GTP and GDP. The complex

Table 2 Major actions of hormones

Hormone	Action
Homeostasis	
Fluid and electrolyte balance	
Aldosterone	Renal Na^+/K^+ exchange
Vasopressin	↓Renal free-water clearance
Metabolism	
Insulin	↑Cell glucose uptake; ↑glycogen synthesis; lipogenic; ↑protein synthesis
Glucagon	Glycogenolysis; gluconeogenic
Cortisol	Gluconeogenic; lipolysis; ↑protein breakdown
Growth hormone	Lipolysis; ↑protein synthesis
Testosterone	↑Protein synthesis
Calcium	
Parathyroid hormone	↑Ca^{2+} resorption from bone and kidney
	↑Renal 1α-hydroxylation of vitamin D
Vitamin D	↑Ca^{2+} absorption from gastrointestinal tract
	↑Ca^{2+} resorption from bone and kidney
Growth and development	
Growth hormone	Growth
Thyroid hormone	Growth, regulation of BMR, CNS development
Retinoic acid	Embryonic development; morphogenesis
Reproduction	
Testosterone	Sexual differentiation, virilization, spermatogenesis
Dihydro-testosterone	Male external genitalia
Oestradiol	Female external genitalia; mammary gland development
Progesterone	Uterotrophic
Prolactin	Lactation
Oxytocin	Uterine contraction; milk reflex

BMR, basal metabolic rate; CNS, central nervous system.

Table 3 Membrane-receptor families

G-protein-coupled

Glycoprotein hormones
FSH, TSH, LH/CG

Biogenic amines
Adrenaline, noradrenaline, serotonin, histamine, dopamine

Peptides
Calcitonin, PTH/PTHRP
GHRH, CRH, GnRH, SRIF, TRH
Vasopressin, oxytocin
Angiotensin
Glucagon, secretin, VIP, gastrin

Small molecules
Calcium, GABA

Tyrosine kinase
Insulin, IGF-1

Cytokine
GH, PRL, EPO, leptin

Serine/threonine kinase
Activin, inhibin, MIS

FSH, follicle-stimulating hormone; TSH, thyroid-stimulating hormone; LH, luteinizing hormone; CG, chorionic gonadotrophin; PTH, parathyroid hormone; PTHRP, parathyroid hormone-related peptide; GHRH, growth hormone-releasing hormone; CRH, corticotrophin-releasing hormone; GnRH, gonadotrophin-releasing hormone; SRIF, somatostatin; TRH, thyrotrophin-releasing hormone; VIP, vasoactive intestinal polypeptide; GABA, γ-aminobutyric acid; IGF-1, insulin-like growth factor 1; GH, growth hormone; PRL, prolactin; EPO, erythropoietin; MIS, Müllerian-inhibiting substance.

Table 4 Signalling pathways of membrane receptors

Signalling pathway	Hormone/receptor
$Gs\alpha$/cAMP↑	β-Adrenergic receptor CRH, GHRH ACTH
$Gi\alpha$/cAMP↓	Somatostatin, dopamine α-adrenergic receptor
$Gq\alpha$/IP3 and DAG	TRH, GnRH
$Gs\alpha$/cAMP↑ and $Gq\alpha$/IP3 and DAG	LH, FSH, TSH, PTH, calcitonin
JAK/STAT	GH, PRL, EPO, leptin
Tyrosine kinase/MAP kinase	Insulin, IGF-1
Ser/Thr kinase/SMAD	Activin, inhibin, MIS

$Gs\alpha$, α-subunit of G_s; $Gi\alpha$, α-subunit of G_i; $Gq\alpha$, α-subunit of G_q; DAG, 1,2-diacylglycerol; IP3, inositol 1,4,5-triphosphate; JAK, Janus kinase; STAT, signal transducer and activator of transcription; MAP, mitogen-activated protein kinase; Ser, serine; Thr, threonine; SMADs denote a contraction of 'Sma' (from *C. elegans*) and 'Mad' (from *D. melanogaster*) signalling proteins; see Table 3 for other abbreviations.

transduces signals from the receptor to downstream effectors such as adenylate cyclase, phospholipase C, or membrane voltage-dependent calcium channels. A family of different G-proteins (G_s, G_i, G_q, and others) exists with the ability to couple to different receptors and effectors, allowing a large array of potential receptor–G-protein–effector complexes, leading to diversity of cellular signalling.

A number of hormones signal via the cyclic AMP pathway (Table 4) and this mechanism is considered in further detail (Fig. 4). In the resting state, the G-protein complex is inactive and bound to GDP (Fig. 4(a)). Following hormone-binding to the receptor (Fig. 4(b)), the Gα-subunit binds GTP, becomes activated, and dissociates from the βγ complex, to interact with adenylate cyclase (Fig. 4(c)). The latter converts ATP to the second messenger, cyclic AMP. This rise in the intracellular cyclic AMP level activates protein kinase A (**PKA**) which can phosphorylate a number of cellular targets: phosphorylation of a transcription factor, the cyclic AMP response-element binding protein (CREB), stimulates the transcription of genes containing CREs; other targets for PKA include enzymes in biochemical pathways or membrane ion channels.

At least two mechanisms serve to terminate signalling via a hormone–receptor complex. First, hydrolysis of GTP to GDP by the Gα-subunit promotes its reassociation with βγ-subunits to reform an inactive complex; second, following hormone-binding, the G-protein-coupled receptors undergo phosphorylation of their intracellular domains by either PKA or other specific G-protein-coupled receptor kinases (**GRKs**). Such phosphorylation prevents further coupling to G-proteins and promotes receptor internalization. This receptor downregulation desensitizes the cell to hormone action, until further surface receptor is expressed.

Activation of their receptors by hormones such as somatostatin or dopamine is known to decrease intracellular cyclic AMP levels. Here, the hormone–receptor complex associates with a G-protein (Gi), whose α-subunit inhibits adenylate cyclase. Although many GPCRs signal via cyclic AMP, some receptors (for example, receptors for thyrotrophin-releasing hormone, gonadotrophin-releasing hormone, Table 4) are linked to different pathways. These receptors are coupled to G_q, whose α-subunit activates membrane phospholipase C (**PLC**) (Fig. 5). This enzyme catalyses the hydrolysis of phosphotidylinositol 4,5-bisphosphate (**PIP2**) to generate the second messengers inositol 1,4,5-triphosphate (**IP3**) and 1,2-diacylglycerol (**DAG**). IP3 interacts with a specific receptor located on smooth endoplasmic reticulum, inducing the opening of intracellular channels and leading to a rise in cytoplasmic calcium levels (Fig. 5). Interaction of calcium with calmodulin (**CAM**), a cytoplasmic calcium-binding protein, activates a specific kinase (CAM kinase), which regulates a number of processes including hormone secretion, gene transcription, and metabolic enzymes. The rise in cellular calcium also facilitates DAG activation of protein kinase C (**PKC**), leading to phosphorylation of the Fos–Jun transcription-factor complex, inducing target-gene expression (Fig. 5). Hormones do not signal exclusively via a single pathway, with glycoprotein hormones and some peptides, for example, activating both cyclic AMP and phosphoinositide signalling (Table 4).

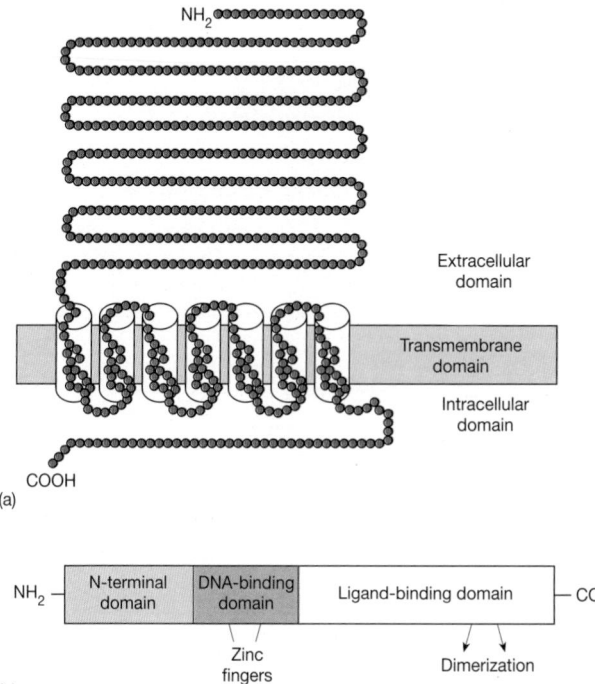

(a)

(b)

Fig. 3 Schematic representations of (a) G-protein-coupled receptor and (b) nuclear receptor illustrating their functional domains.

The tyrosine kinase class of receptors is a diverse family that transduces signalling by insulin and IGF-1 as well as by epidermal, nerve, fibroblast, and platelet-derived growth factors. Growth-factor signalling differs from that of insulin, and the latter pathway will now be considered (Fig. 6). The interaction of insulin with its receptor promotes autophosphorylation of tyrosine residues in its cytoplasmic domains. In turn, this promotes the phosphorylation of substrates (for example, Shc and insulin-receptor substrate-1 (**IRS-1**)), followed by recruitment of adaptor proteins (Grb2/SOS). The Grb2/SOS complex recruits Ras, a GTP-binding protein. Ras activation induces signalling via a series of kinases (Raf, Mek, MAP kinase),

culminating in the phosphorylation and activation of transcription factors that regulate target genes involved in mitogenesis or cellular differentiation. On the other hand, IRS-1 recruits phosphatidylinositol-3'-OH-kinase (PI3-kinase), which in turn activates protein kinase B. The latter mediates a number of the metabolic effects of insulin, enhancing translocation of a glucose transporter to the membrane to promote cellular glucose uptake, and activating enzymes involved in glycogen synthesis.

Hormones such as prolactin and GH interact uniquely with their receptors; a single polypeptide interacts simultaneously with two receptors promoting their dimerization (Fig. 7). The hormone–receptor complex

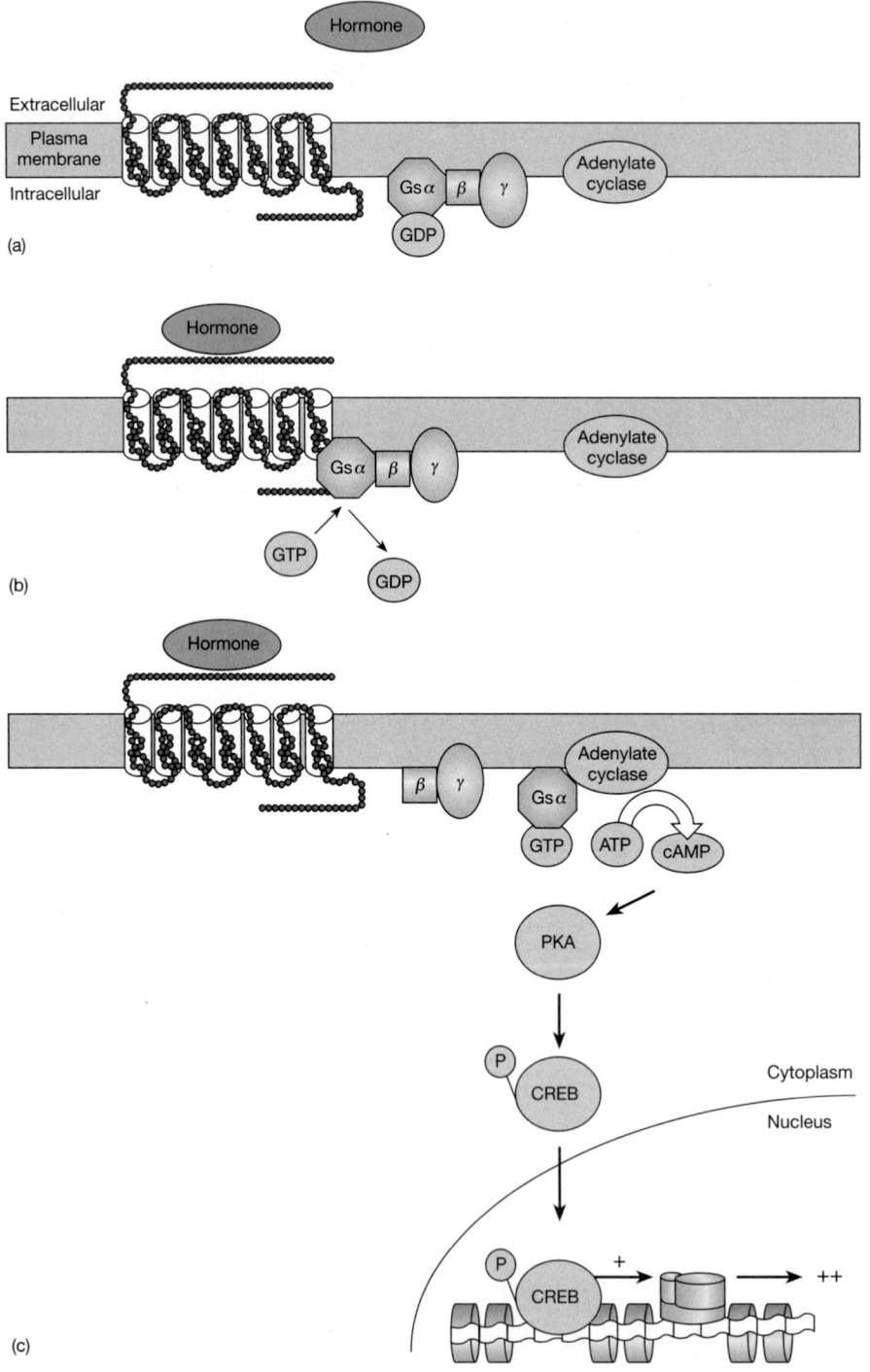

Fig. 4 G-protein-coupled receptor signalling via the cyclic AMP pathway.

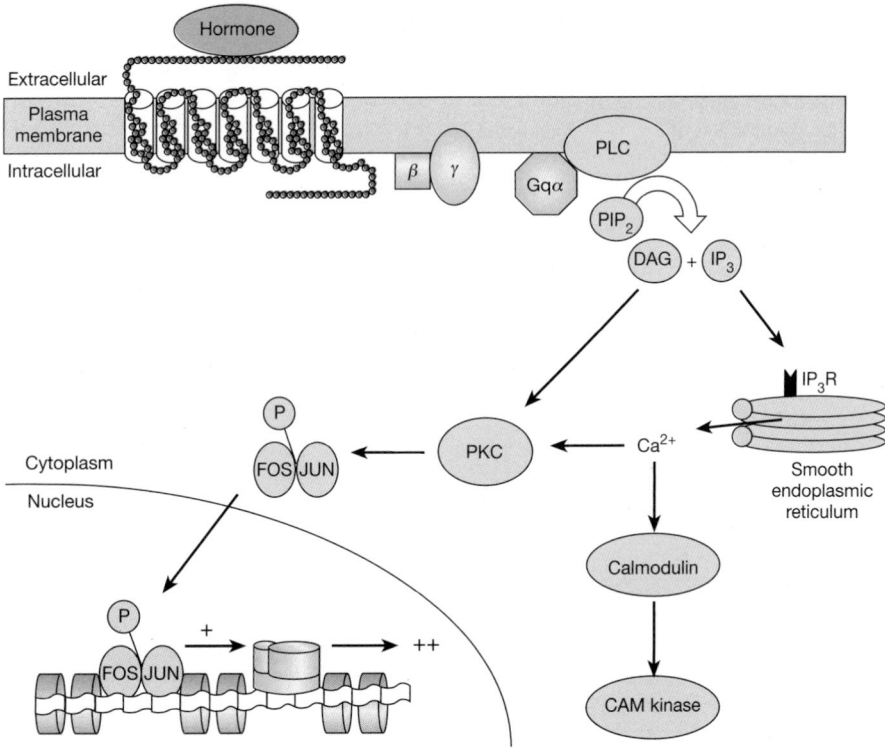

Fig. 5 G-protein-coupled receptor signalling via the phosphoinositide pathway.

recruits Janus kinases (**JAKs**) which phosphorylate **STATs** (signal transducers and activators of transcription). STATs translocate to the nucleus, interact with regulatory DNA elements, and promote target-gene transcription.

Activin and inhibin belong to the transforming growth-factor (**TGF**) class of peptides, which signal via a heterodimeric transmembrane-receptor complex with intrinsic protein serine/threonine kinase activity (Fig. 8). Here, hormone-binding promotes the association of two (type I, type II)

surface receptors with differing properties. Subsequent transphosphorylation of the type I receptor by the intracellular kinase domain of the type II receptor leads to phosphorylation and dimerization of cytoplasmic Smad proteins. The Smad complex translocates to the nucleus to activate target-gene expression (Fig. 8).

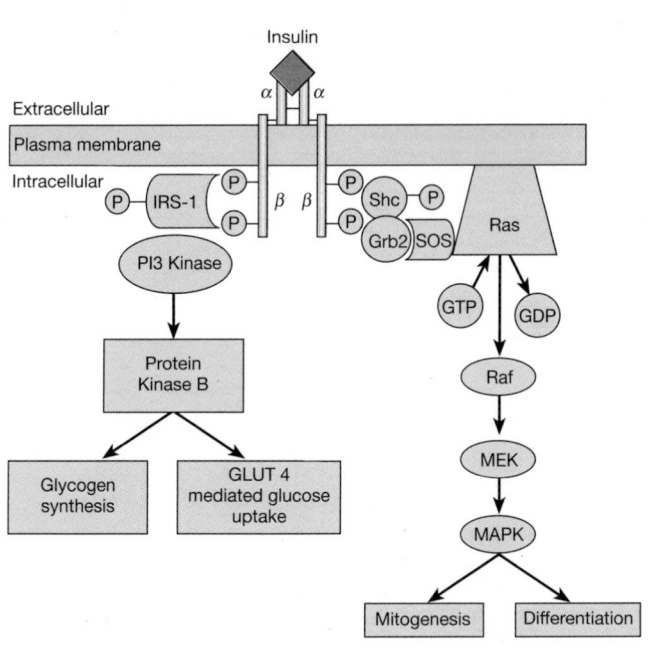

Fig. 6 Insulin action via its tyrosine kinase receptor and signalling cascade.

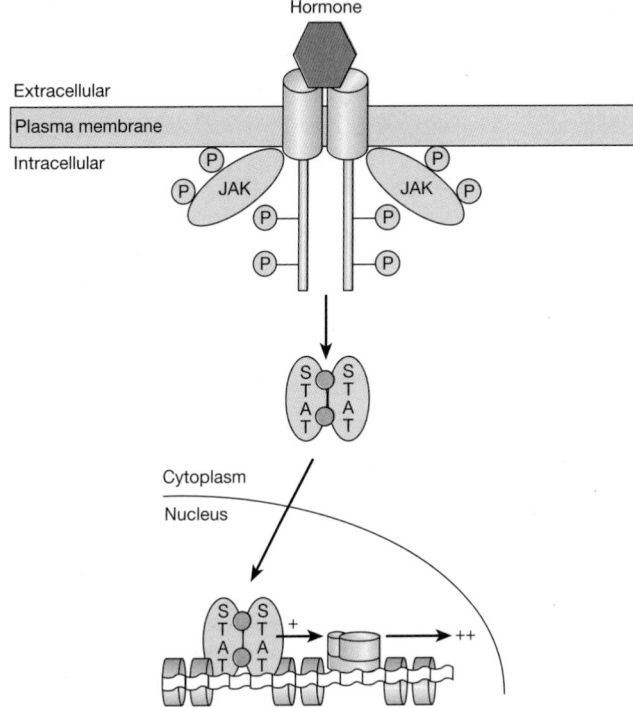

Fig. 7 Hormone signalling via the JAK–STAT pathway.

As described above, GPCR signalling is usually coupled to responses (for example, hormone secretion) by the Gα-subunit activation of cyclic AMP or phosphoinositide pathways. However, following receptor activation in some cellular contexts, the dissociated Gβ/γ-dimer subunit complex is also capable of stimulating effectors (for example, Ras, PI3-kinase), to enhance MAP kinase activity and elicit a mitogenic response.

Nuclear-receptor signalling

The nuclear receptors are a family of transcription factors that mediate the action of steroid and other lipophilic hormones. The human genome encodes approximately 60 to 70 different receptors, and it is clear that only a minority of these are targets for the action of major hormones (Table 5). The remainder comprise a large group classified as 'orphan receptors', reflecting the fact that either their ligands and/or physiological roles are still to be elucidated.

Based on homologies in their primary amino-acid sequence, nuclear receptors can be divided into distinct domains that mediate specific functions (Fig. 3(b)). A central DNA-binding domain contains cysteine-rich peptide motifs that chelate zinc to form two zinc fingers. The latter mediate receptor-binding to specific DNA sequences or hormone-response elements, usually located in target-gene promoters. The carboxy-terminal region of receptors encompasses their hormone-binding function as well as

Table 5 Hormone signalling via nuclear receptors

Nuclear receptor	Hormone
Homodimeric	
GR	Cortisol
MR	Aldosterone
ERα/β	Oestradiol
PR	Progesterone
AR	Testosterone, dihydrotestosterone
Heterodimeric	
TRα/β	Tri-iodothyronine
RARα/β/γ	all-*trans* Retinoic acid
RXRα/β/γ	9-*cis* Retinoic acid
VDR	1,25-Dihydroxy vitamin D3

GR, glucocorticoid receptor; MR, mineralocorticoid receptor; ER, [o]estrogen receptor-α or -β subtypes; PR, progesterone receptor; AR, androgen receptor; TR, thyroid hormone receptor-α or -β subtypes; RAR, retinoic acid receptor-α, -β, or -γ subtypes; RXR, retinoid X receptor-α, -β, or -γ subtypes; VDR, vitamin D receptor.

their ability to dimerize. Nuclear receptors can be divided into two major subclasses—the steroid receptors (homodimeric) and heterodimeric receptors—which differ in their mode of action.

Steroid receptors (for example, glucocorticoid, mineralocorticoid, [o]estrogen, progesterone, and androgen receptors (GR, MR, ER, PR, AR, respectively)) bind to hormone-response elements as homodimers (Fig. 9(b)). Some receptors (for example, GR, PR, AR) are bound to cytosolic heat-shock proteins. Hormone-binding to receptors promotes their dissociation from these, enabling translocation to the nucleus, dimerization, and interaction with DNA. In contrast, the thyroid, retinoic acid, and vitamin D receptors are constitutively nuclear and form heterodimers with a common partner (retinoid X receptor or **RXR**), to interact with DNA

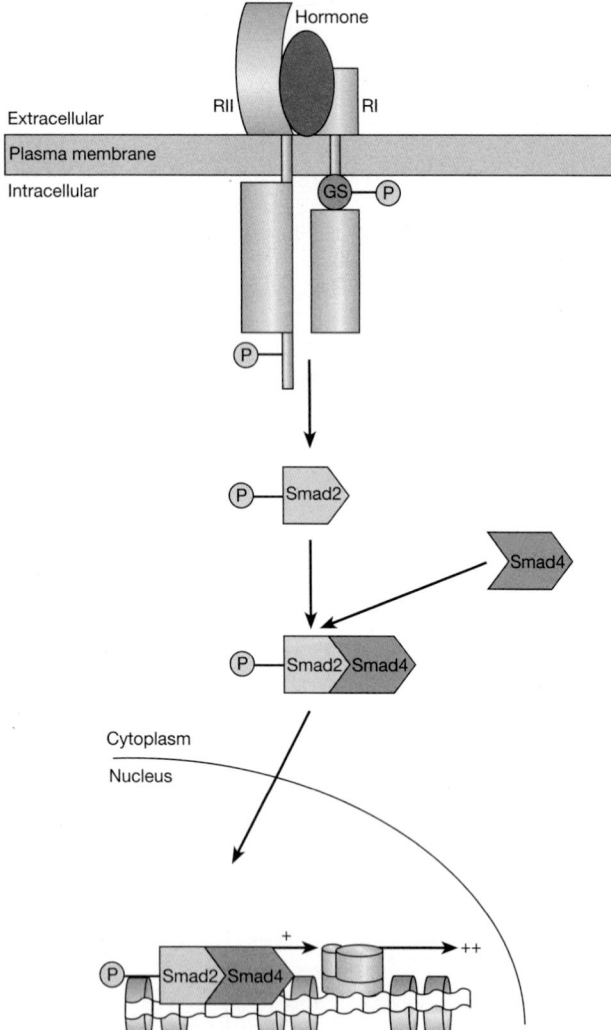

Fig. 8 Hormone signalling by the transforming growth-factor peptide family.

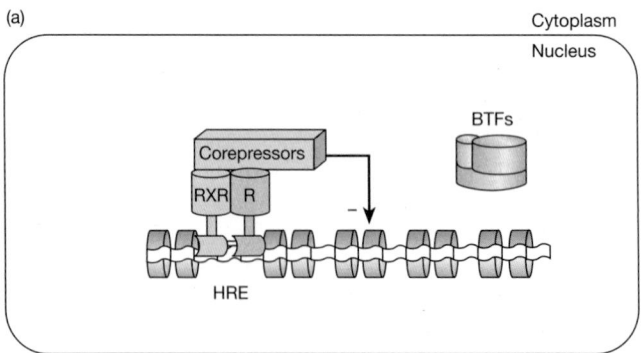

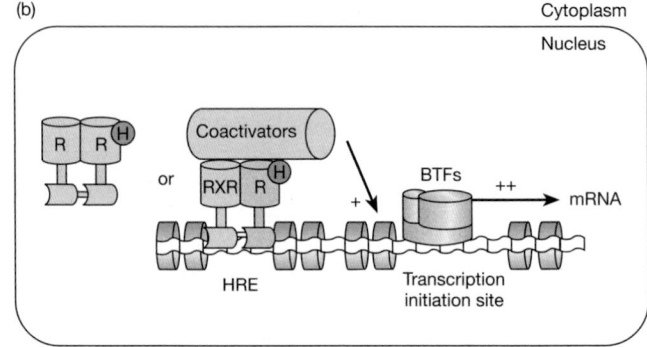

Fig. 9 Transcriptional regulation by nuclear receptors (a) In the absence of hormone, a subset of heterodimeric nuclear receptors (thyroid, retinoic acid) recruit co-repressors to inhibit gene transcription. (b) Hormone occupancy of homodimeric or heterodimeric receptors promotes their association with coactivators, leading to transcriptional activation.

even in the absence of hormone or ligand (Fig. 9(a)). In some target-gene contexts, RXR can also form homodimers to mediate retinoid signalling.

In contrast to other transcription factors whose activity is controlled by post-translational modification (for example, phosphorylation), the hallmark of nuclear receptors is their ability to modulate gene expression in a hormone-dependent manner. Thus, in the absence of ligand, the thyroid and retinoic acid receptors actively silence target-gene transcription by recruiting a co-repressor complex of cofactors (Fig. 9(a)). For all nuclear receptors, hormone-binding induces a conformational change with dissociation of co-repressors and recruitment of coactivator proteins (Fig. 9(b)). This latter complex acts to relax the interaction between histone proteins and DNA in chromatin, thereby facilitating the access of basal transcription factors and RNA polymerase which induce gene transcription.

A further mechanism that controls signalling via nuclear receptors is regulation of the supply of their ligands to cells and tissues. Tri-iodothyronine, the ligand for the thyroid-hormone receptor (**TR**), is generated from circulating thyroxine by the action of type-1 or type-2 deiodinase enzymes expressed in the liver and central nervous system, respectively; the enzyme 5α-reductase converts testosterone to dihydrotestosterone in tissues of the male external genitalia. In contrast, the enzyme 11β-hydroxysteroid dehydrogenase type 2 catabolizes cortisol in renal cells, thereby enabling the mineralocorticoid receptor to respond selectively to aldosterone rather than to glucocorticoid, which it is also capable of binding to with high affinity.

Finally, in contrast to the classical effects of steroid hormones in modulating gene expression, recent evidence indicates that they can also modulate cellular functions such as hormone secretion or neuronal excitability within seconds or minutes. These rapid effects of steroid hormones occur independently of the genome, and are probably transduced by the same signalling pathways (for example, voltage-sensitive calcium channels) that mediate rapid responses to neurotransmitter hormones.

Genetic defects and endocrine disease

The majority of endocrine diseases can be divided into conditions of hormone excess, hormone deficiency, and hormone resistance. Defects in genes involved in hormone synthesis and action give rise to a spectrum of disorders (Tables 6 and 7). Both germline gene defects causing inherited

Table 6 Genetic defects in transcription factors or nuclear receptors and endocrine disorders

Gene	Disorder or phenotype
Transcription factors	
HESX-1	Septo-optic dysplasia
Pit-1/PROP-1	GH, PRL, TSH deficiencies
TTF-1/TTF-2/PAX-8	Thyroid dysgenesis
SRY	XY female
Nuclear receptors	
DAX-1/SF-1	Adrenal insufficiency and hypogonadism
VDR	Hereditary vitamin D-resistant rickets
AR	Androgen insensitivity syndrome or spinal and bulbar muscular atrophy
ERα	Tall stature and osteoporosis
GR	Glucocorticoid resistance
TRβ	Resistance to thyroid hormone

See Tables 1 and 5 for abbreviations.

syndromes and somatic mutations leading to acquired endocrine cellular dysfunction have been described.

Defects in developmental transcription factors are usually associated with endocrine gland hypoplasia: mutations in *HESX-1* cause optic and pituitary hypoplasia with agenesis of the corpus callosum; both *Pit-1* and *PROP-1* mutations disrupt the development of multiple pituitary cell types, resulting in a combination of hormone deficiencies; defects in *TTF-1*, *TTF-2*, and *PAX-8* result in thyroid dysgenesis manifesting as neonatal hypothyroidism; mutations in the *SRY* gene lead to failure of testis development and sex reversal in XY males.

Mutations in *DAX-1* or *SF-1*, orphan members of the nuclear-receptor family, disrupt both adrenal and gonadal development. Defects in other nuclear receptors (for example, VDR, TR, GR) are characterized by tissue resistance to their respective hormone ligands. Vitamin D resistance leads to rickets, together with abnormalities of skin differentiation, hair growth, and lymphocyte function, emphasizing its important extraskeletal actions. Point mutations in the androgen receptor are associated with a spectrum of phenotypes, ranging from complete feminization of XY individuals to

Table 7 Genetic defects in membrane receptors or signalling and endocrine disorders

Gene	Loss-of-function mutation	Gain-of-function mutation
G protein-coupled receptor		
Vasopressin V2	Nephrogenic diabetes insipidus	–
ACTH	Isolated cortisol deficiency	–
Ca^{2+}	Hypocalciuric hypercalcaemia	Hypercalciuric hypocalcaemia
TSH	TSH resistance	Thyroid adenomas or non-autoimmune hyperthyroidism
LH	Leydig cell hypoplasia	Male-limited precocious puberty
FSH	Ovarian dysgenesis	FSH-independent spermatogenesis
Tyrosine kinase receptor		
RET	Hirschprung's disease	MEN type II: parathyroid neoplasia, phaeochromocytoma, medullary thyroid carcinoma
Insulin	Insulin resistance	–
Cytokine receptors		
GH	Laron dwarfism	
Signalling pathway		
Gsα	PTH, TSH, LH resistance and Albright's hereditary osteodystrophy	Somatotroph adenomas, thyroid adenomas, McCune-Albright syndrome
Giα	Ovary, adrenal, thyroid tumours	–

RET, receptor-type [tyrosine kinase]; MEN, multiple endocrine neoplasia; see Tables 3 and 4 for other abbreviations.

mildly impaired virilization in men. In addition, expansion of a polyglutamine repeat sequence in the amino-terminal domain of AR is associated
with adult-onset neuronal degeneration, leading to spinal and bulbar muscular atrophy. A homozygous defect in the oestrogen receptor in a male, led
to failure of epiphyseal closure, resulting in tall stature together with severe
osteoporosis. These manifestations suggest that testosterone effects on the
male skeleton are, in part, mediated by its enzymatic conversion to oestrogens.

A growing number of disorders associated with defects in transmembrane receptors or their signalling intermediates have been described
(Table 7). However, in addition to mutations that disrupt protein function,
gain-of-function mutations causing constitutive activation of the receptor
or signalling protein also occur. With G-protein-coupled receptors
(GPCRs), diverse loss-of-function mutations, occurring most frequently in
the extracellular domain, block hormone-binding or signalling, leading to
insensitivity to hormone action. Such hormone resistance can lead to both
hypofunction (for example, ACTH, TSH receptors) or hypoplasia (for
example, LH, FSH receptors) of target glands expressing the receptor. Conversely, gain-of-function mutations in GPCRs typically occur in the third
intracellular loop, causing constitutive activation of the receptor in the
absence of hormonal ligand. Again, the functional consequence is either
autonomous hyperfunction (for example, calcium, LH, FSH receptors) or
excessive neoplastic proliferation (for example, TSH receptor, RET tyro-
sine-kinase receptor) of the target tissues in which the receptor is expressed
(see Table 7). Constitutive activation of signal transduction may also result
from G-protein mutations. Here, specific amino-acid substitutions in Gsα
inhibit its intrinsic GTPase activity, and the GTP-bound protein constitutively activates adenylate cyclase leading to cyclic AMP accumulation.
Somatic Gsα mutations occur in a proportion of pituitary growth-hormone secreting and thyroid adenomas; more widespread expression of a
somatic Gsα mutation occurring early in development leads to polyostotic
fibrous dysplasia, café-au-lait skin pigmentation, and hyperfunction of
multiple endocrine glands, constituting the McCune–Albright syndrome.
Similarly, germline, loss-of-function mutations which reduce cellular Gsα
activity, are associated with resistance to multiple hormones, together with
characteristic bone anomalies (Albright's hereditary osteodystrophy).

Further reading

Braverman LE, Utiger RD, eds. (2000). *Werner and Ingbar's the thyroid; a fundamental and clinical text*, 8th edn. Lippincott, Williams and Wilkins, Philadelphia.

DeGroot LJ Jameson JL, eds. (2001). *Endocrinology*, 4th edn. WB Saunders, Philadelphia.

Grossman A (1998). *Clinical endocrinology*, 2nd edn. Blackwell Science, Oxford.

Lodish H, *et al.*, eds. (1999). *Molecular cell biology*, 4th edn. WH Freeman, New York.

Yen SSC, Jaffe RB, Barbieri RL, eds. (1999). *Reproductive endocrinology*, 4th edn. WB Saunders, London.

12.2 Disorders of the anterior pituitary

Paul J. Jenkins and Michael Besser

Historical introduction

The anterior pituitary gland, often termed the 'conductor of the endocrine orchestra' secretes six hormones of known function. These control many of the peripheral endocrine organs, between them regulating growth and development, sexual behaviour and the menstrual cycle, lactation, as well as the thyroid and adrenal glands. Hippocrates in 400 BC gave the first description of a prolactinoma in stating that 'if a woman who is neither pregnant nor has given birth produces milk, and menstruation has stopped...'. There are several descriptions of giants in the Old Testament, both as individuals and also as families, (Joshua XIV: 'Arba was a great man amongst the Anakim'); it is possible that Goliath was slain by David because of his bitemporal hemianopia resulting from a suprasellar growth hormone-secreting pituitary adenoma. However, despite these early descriptions, detailed knowledge of the physiology and pathophysiology of the anterior pituitary gland has only become apparent over the last 60 or 70 years and is continuing to expand.

The first major advance was the ability to purify pituitary hormones, detect their actions by bioassay, and then synthesize them. The development of radioimmunoassay in the 1960s allowed for their rapid and more precise measurement and the elucidation of their physiological role. In Oxford in the 1950s Harris demonstrated the control of anterior pituitary function by hypothalamic factors; these were later extracted from several hundred tons of porcine pituitaries, principally by Schally and Guillemin in the 1970s, leading to their being awarded the Nobel prize. The availability of these hypothalamic factors facilitated studies of their physiological effects in both normal subjects and patients with endocrine disorders. The development of modern imaging techniques such as computed tomography (**CT**) and magnetic resonance imaging (**MRI**) has greatly enhanced our ability to visualize the anatomy of the hypothalamic–pituitary region and allow the precise localization of pituitary lesions. In the 1980s the advent of molecular biological techniques allowed greater understanding of the control mechanisms at a molecular level as well as fuelling interest in potential treatments. In experienced hands, trans-sphenoidal surgery has become a safe and effective firstline treatment for most pituitary tumours thus avoiding the morbidity associated with craniotomy.

Anatomy and development

The hypothalamus is the true conductor of the endocrine orchestra since it controls the pituitary gland. It is derived from forebrain tissue on either side of the lower parts of the third ventricle. The floor comprises the optic chiasm and tracts, the pituitary stalk, and mamilliary bodies; anteriorly it is limited by the lamina terminalis and the anterior commissure, whilst posteriorly it blends with the midbrain. The pituitary gland (sometimes called the hypophysis) lies within the pituitary fossa of the sphenoid bone above the sphenoid sinus. On either side are the cavernous sinuses containing the internal carotid artery, the third, fourth, fifth (first, and second divisions), and sixth cranial nerves. Superiorly, the gland is covered by a layer of dura through which the stalk passes. Occasionally congenital enlargement of this

gap allows the usual pulsations of cerebrospinal fluid to be transmitted through into the fossa compressing the pituitary and ballooning the fossa and giving rise to the 'empty sella syndrome'. The normal pituitary is approximately the size of a large pea and weighs 100 mg; its dimensions are approximately 10 mm transversely, 9 mm anteroposteriorly, and 6 mm vertically. During pregnancy it undergoes enlargement up to almost twice its normal size as it becomes engorged with prolactin-secreting mammotroph cells under the influence of oestrogen. (Fig. 1).

Embryologically and functionally the pituitary comprises two distinct parts. The epithelial portion which forms the anterior pituitary consists of the pars distalis and intermediate lobe; this originates from the stomodeal ectoderm of Rathke's pouch, which forms a vesicle that separates from the roof of the developing mouth. The neural portion which forms the posterior lobe, pituitary stalk, and infundibulum arises along with the rest of the hypothalamus from the diencephalic forebrain. Anterior pituitary cells

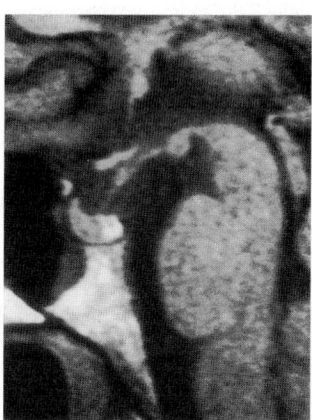

(a)

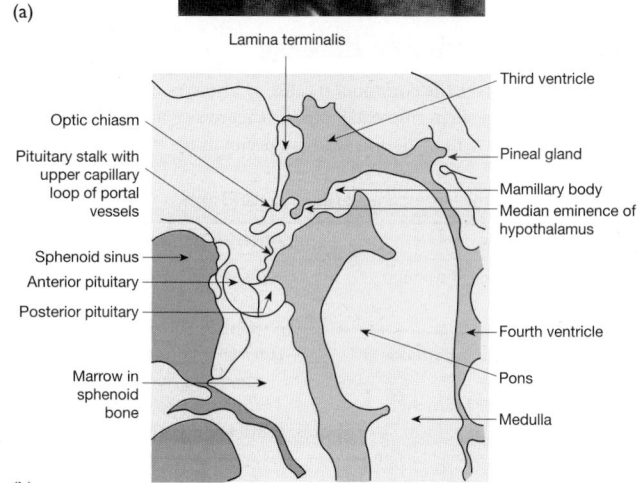

(b)

Fig. 1 Sagittal MRI scan of normal pituitary gland and an anatomical line drawing.

also extend upwards to surround the neural tissue of the pituitary stalk forming the pars tuberalis.

The blood supply to the pituitary is in keeping with this dual origin. The anterior gland receives 80 to 90 per cent of its blood supply from the hypothalamo-hypophyseal portal veins which start as a plexus of capillaries in the median eminence/infundibulum of the hypothalamus, carrying blood and hypophyseotropic hormones down the stalk to bathe the cells of the anterior pituitary. The remaining blood supply is via the pituitary capsular vessels derived from the superior hypophyseal arteries. The neurohypophysis receives its blood supply from the inferior hypophyseal branches of the internal carotid artery. Venous drainage from the anterior pituitary is via the cavernous sinuses, principally into the petrosal sinuses and thence into the internal jugular veins.

Anterior pituitary differentiation and ontogeny is now known to be carefully regulated by tissue-specific transcription factors. The first marker of anterior pituitary differentiation is expression of the α subunit. Expression of prolactin, growth hormone, and thyroid-stimulating hormones in specific cells is controlled by the POU domain transcription factors Pit-I and Prop-I. Humans with mutations of Pit-I have a syndrome of short stature, congenital hypothyroidism, and prolactin deficiency.

General physiology and regulation

In common with all endocrine glands, secretion of anterior pituitary hormones is not autonomous. Each is subject to regulation by hypothalamic peptides and, with the possible exception of prolactin, subject to the fundamental endocrine regulatory mechanism of negative feedback by hormone from the target gland (Fig. 2; Table 1). This negative feedback control is at both the hypothalamic and pituitary levels and ensures precise homeostatic maintenance of physiologically appropriate hormonal secretion. Thus, failure of the primary gland results in reduced negative feedback and consequent increased hypothalamic and pituitary stimulation and secretion. Conversely, primary overactivity of the target gland results in increased negative feedback and diminished hypothalamic and/or pituitary stimulation. This central tenet is fundamental to the laboratory interpretation of circulating hormonal levels and to the investigation of pituitary target gland disorders by means of either stimulatory or suppressive tests. In addition to this long-loop negative feedback, additional 'short-loop' feedback mechanisms exist between the pituitary and the hypothalamus.

Pituitary hormones are synthesized as part of large precursor molecules; they are then cleaved into fragments which are secreted into the circulation. One fragment is the hormone concerned and the other cosecreted fragments have no known function as endocrine factors.

Causes of pituitary disease

Pituitary adenomas are the commonest cause of pituitary disease (Table 2); they can range from silent microadenomas to aggressive invasive tumours. Autopsy data suggest that the former may occur in up to 20 per cent of

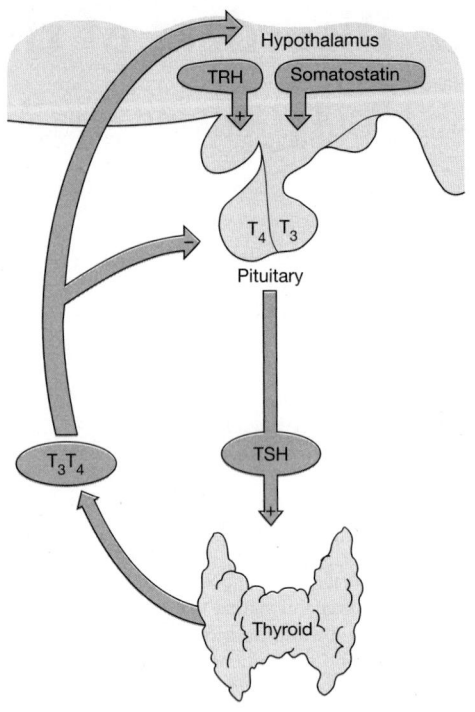

Fig. 2 Diagram of the hypothalamo-pituitary–thyroid axis showing negative feedback loops. TRH, thyrotrophin-releasing hormone; TSH, thyroid-stimulating hormone.

apparently normal people. Overall, clinically apparent pituitary tumours account for some 10 to 20 per cent of all intracranial tumours.

Pituitary tumours

With the advent of modern immunohistochemical techniques, the classification of pituitary adenomas has been simplified into that of the secreted hormone rather than the staining patterns of chromophobe, basophil, or acidophil adenomas resulting from periodic acid-Schiff staining (Table 2). Occasionally, despite these techniques, no tumour is visualized after transsphenoidal surgery even when the hormonal hypersecretion is cured postoperatively. Reasons for this may be that the tumour was so small it was missed on histological sectioning, the tumour was so small that it was not collected by the sucker during surgery, or the primary pathology was hypothalamic in origin.

Epidemiology of pituitary tumours

The annual incidence of clinically functioning pituitary tumours is estimated to be approximately 1 to 2 per 100 000 of the population. However,

Table 1 Hypothalamic–pituitary–peripheral gland axes

Hypothalamic factor	Anterior pituitary hormone	Target gland/organ	Target gland hormone
Corticotrophin-releasing hormone	Adrenocorticotrophic hormone	Cortex of the adrenal glands	Glucocorticoids (cortisol), androgens, androstenedione, dehydroepiandrostenedione
Gonadotrophin-releasing hormone	Luteinizing hormone and follicle-stimulating hormone	Ovary, testes	Oestradiol, progesterone, testosterone
Thyrotrophin-releasing hormone	Thyroid-stimulating hormone	Thyroid	Thyroxine, liothyronine
Dopamine	Prolactin	Breast	
Growth hormone releasing hormone—stimulating somatostatin—inhibitory	Growth hormone	All tissues (blood IGF-I predominantly from the liver)	IGF-I

IGF-I, insulin-like growth factor I.

it is likely that this is an underestimate for two reasons: these are rare conditions which tend to be underdiagnosed and the incidence figures depend upon cancer registrations and not mortality data, which tend to be incomplete and are not universal. Despite these reservations, the following pituitary adenomas occur in decreasing order of frequency: non-functioning adenomas, prolactinomas, growth hormone-secreting, adrenocortico-trophic hormone (**ACTH**) secreting, thyroid-stimulating hormone secreting, and luteinizing hormone/follicle-stimulating hormone (**LH/FSH**) secreting tumours.

Clinical features of pituitary disease

The clinical features of pituitary dysfunction, usually resulting from a space occupying lesion, can be divided into local effects resulting from an expanding pituitary mass, anterior pituitary hormonal deficiency, and symptoms and signs of hormonal excess from hypersecretion of a pituitary hormone.

Local mass effects

An expanding mass within the pituitary fossa may give rise to headache, neuro-ophthalmological defects or facial pain according to the size and direction of expansion. Headaches usually result from dural stretching and are classically retro-orbital or bitemporal. They tend to be worse on waking and are relieved by analgesics; the somatostatin analogue octreotide may provide striking relief beyond any effect on hormone secretion, as it may have direct analgesic effects. Sudden catastrophic headaches may result from pituitary apoplexy. Very large pituitary masses may cause obstruction of the fourth ventricle or foramen of Munro resulting in hydrocephalus and expansion of the lateral ventricles. Rarely, inferior invasion and erosion of

Table 2 Causes of pituitary disease

Hypothalamic diseases
Tumours
    Craniopharyngioma
    Hamartoma
    Germinoma
    Chordoma
    Optic glioma
    Sphenoidal ridge meningioma
    Metastases (especially breast and bronchus)
Granulomatous diseases
    Sarcoidosis
    Tuberculosis
    Langerhans' cell histiocytosis
Cranial irradiation
Head injury and surgery
Vascular malformations, e.g. haemangiomas and haemangioblastomas
Pituitary disease
Tumours
    Prolactin secreting
    Growth hormone secreting
    ACTH secreting
    Thyroid-stimulating hormone secreting
    Gonadotrophin secreting
    Functionless tumours
    Metastases (especially breast and bronchus)
    Primary pituitary carcinoma
Granulomatous diseases
    Sarcoidosis
    Tuberculosis
    Langerhans cell histiocytosis
Lymphocytic hypophysitis
Haemochromatosis
Vascular
    Apoplexy
    Sheehan's syndrome

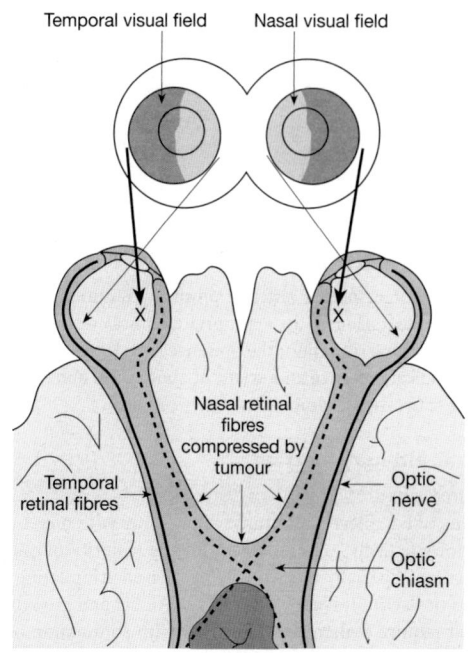

Fig. 3 Neuro-ophthalmological pathways and the classical bitemporal hemianopia that results from compression of the central optic chiasm by a pituitary tumour. However, any degree of unilateral or bilateral visual deficit can occur depending on the anatomical site of the lesion.

the sella floor may cause recurrent sinusitis or cerebrospinal fluid rhinorrhoea (confirmed by the presence of glucose in the fluid) and the risk of recurrent meningitis. Neuro-ophthalmological defects are common, particularly with macroadenomas, occurring in up to 60 per cent of such cases, although they are often asymptomatic. Although bitemporal hemianopia is the classic abnormality, any unilateral or bilateral visual field defect can occur depending on the site of impingement on the pathway of the optic nerve (Fig. 3). Lateral extension results in a squint from ocular nerve palsies. Extensive lateral invasion into the temporal lobe may result in temporal lobe epilepsy, whereas extensive superior extension may impinge upon the hypothalamus resulting in disorders of appetite, thirst, temperature regulation, and consciousness.

Hormonal deficiencies

Panhypopituitarism or varying degrees of loss of any of the six hormones may occur. Hypopituitarism resulting from a pituitary adenoma tends to occur in the sequential loss of LH, growth hormone, thyroid-stimulating hormone, and lastly ACTH and FSH. Thus, in adults the presenting clinical symptoms tend to be infertility, oligo/amenorrhoea, decreased libido, and erectile dysfunction. The clinical signs and phenotypic appearance reflect the loss of LH and growth hormone: there may be reduction of muscle bulk, decreased body hair, increased central adiposity, and small, soft testes. The facial appearance is almost pathognomonic—smooth skin with fine wrinkles, exaggerated by the loss of facial hair. Pallor may accompany ACTH deficiency. In children, hypopituitarism commonly presents with delayed puberty or impairment of growth. LH deficiency with preservation of growth hormone results in delayed fusion of the epiphyses of the long bones giving rise to a eunuchoid appearance, the span being greater than the height. Testicular size will depend on the stage of puberty prior to gonadotrophin failure and whether adrenarche, influenced by ACTH-controlled adrenal androgen secretion, is maintained. Diabetes insipidus is almost never a presenting feature of primary pituitary tumours in either childhood or adults—it occurs most commonly in association with surgical treatment of pituitary adenoma.

Hormonal excess

If the pituitary adenoma is functioning, clinical symptoms and signs will also result from excess levels of either the secreted pituitary hormone itself, for example acromegaly (growth hormone), prolactin excess (prolactinoma), or from increased stimulation and secretion of the target gland hormone, for example Cushing's disease (ACTH), thyrotoxicosis (thyroid-stimulating hormone).

Evaluation of pituitary disease

The investigation of suspected anterior pituitary dysfunction requires the evaluation and integration in an appropriate clinical setting of: the presence of endocrine hyperfunction; the presence and degree of hypopituitarism; the radiological presence and extent of anatomical abnormalities; and assessment of neuro-ophthalmological function.

Hypothalamic pituitary function

Basal measurements

Measurements of basal levels of pituitary hormones with target gland hormone secretion are likely to be sufficient for the majority of cases of pituitary dysfunction, especially those involving thyroid-stimulating hormone, LH/FSH, and prolactin. It is only disorders of ACTH and growth hormone secretion that require dynamic investigation with stimulation or suppression tests according to the clinical scenario. Although the introduction of radioimmunoassays and then immunoradiometric assays revolutionized endocrine assessment, these have now largely been superseded by modern chemiluminescent assays which have the advantages of increased automation and sensitivity, avoidance of radioisotopes, and shorter assay time.

When interpreting any basal measurement of pituitary hormone, one needs to be aware of certain caveats:

1. Interpretation of all anterior pituitary hormonal levels, with the exception of prolactin, can only be made in the knowledge of the level of the primary target gland hormone.

2. The pulsatile nature of secretion of anterior pituitary hormones, especially ACTH, growth hormone, and LH/FSH, means that random isolated single levels may not be representative of overall secretion.

3. Specific factors such as time of day, stress, fed or fasting, asleep or awake, and stage of growth and pubertal development can all influence levels.

ACTH Rapid proteolytic degradation in whole blood or frozen then thawed plasma, pulsatile secretion, and diurnal rhythm all need to be taken into account when measuring basal ACTH levels. In order to prevent degradation and thus uninterpretable results, plasma samples must be taken in an EDTA tube at 4 °C and immediately frozen. The time of day should be recorded (preferably 09.00) and samples should be taken from an in-dwelling cannula that has been *in situ* for at least 30 min in order to avoid the influence of stress. As ACTH is the prime regulator of cortisol secretion, a serum cortisol level (which does not require these logistical precautions) is a pragmatic measure of ACTH secretion; a 09.00 hour level of more than 200 nmol/l effectively excludes adrenal insufficiency under basal conditions, although it does not assess ACTH reserve (see later), whilst a 09.00 hour level of more than 550 nmol/l obviates the need for dynamic testing since the response to stress will be adequate.

Growth hormone The markedly pulsatile secretion of growth hormone means that random levels of growth hormone are of very limited use. Furthermore, secretion is affected by nutritional status, being increased by amino acids. As it is a counter-regulatory hormone to insulin, levels are increased by hypoglycaemia and decreased by hyperglycaemia (the basis for its dynamic testing in situations of suspected oversecretion). There is also increased secretion during sleep (stages 3 and 4) and in response to stress. As a result of these factors, any meaningful assessment of growth hormone secretion requires dynamic testing. The action of growth hormone on tissues is classically mediated in an endocrine manner via hepatically derived circulating insulin-like growth factor I, although there is increasing evidence that most of its actions are effected through secretion of insulin-like growth factor I locally in the target tissues acting on cells adjacent to or the same as the cell of origin of insulin-like growth factor I (so-called paracrine or autocrine actions). Insulin-like growth factor II is not growth hormone dependent. A single serum level of insulin-like growth factor I has been claimed to represent an integrated index of growth hormone secretion, but it too is subject to separate influences and is discordant in up to 25 per cent of cases, particularly in adults. Thus, levels of insulin-like growth factor I in serum may be within the lower part of the normal range even though the patient has mild growth hormone deficiency. Growth hormone levels are markedly increased during puberty but decreased in pregnancy, due to the negative feedback on the pituitary by placental growth hormone, a variant of growth hormone produced by the placenta.

LH/FSH More than for any other pituitary hormone, assays of LH/FSH must be interpreted with the simultaneous level of target gland hormone and the clinical scenario. In men a low testosterone in conjunction with low LH/FSH confirms the diagnosis of hypogonadotrophic hypogonadism rather than primary hypogonadism when LH/FSH levels would be high. In women the occurrence of the menstrual cycle is the definitive biological assay and excludes any deficiency. The occurrence of oligo/amenorrhoea requires measurement of gonadotrophins together with oestradiol, prolactin, and human chorionic gonadotrophin-β. Dynamic testing is very rarely required.

Prolactin In the absence of pregnancy (during which levels rise markedly due to the action of increased oestrogen on the pituitary) a serum prolactin level of more than 4500 mU/l is almost always indicative of a prolactinoma. Mild elevations may be in response to stress and as such require repeated measurements. The large variety of causes of hyperprolactinaemia need to be considered (see later), particularly that due to coexisting drug therapy.

Thyroid-stimulating hormone New ultrasensitive assays for thyroid-stimulating hormone have largely avoided the need for dynamic testing. A normal level of thyroid-stimulating hormone with a free thyroxine level in the normal range is indicative of euthyroidism. A subnormal level of thyroxine in conjunction with a normal or low thyroid-stimulating hormone (indicative of inadequate negative feedback) is strongly suggestive of secondary hypothyroidism. The commonly encountered low T_4 with an elevated thyroid-stimulating hormone is almost always indicative of primarily hypothyroidism, whilst conversely an elevated thyroxine or liothyronine level with a subnormal or undetectable thyroid-stimulating hormone confirms thyrotoxicosis. Secondary thyrotoxicosis as indicated by both an elevated thyroid-stimulating hormone and thyroxine level is very rare.

Dynamic endocrine testing

Where basal levels are inadequate or equivocal, dynamic endocrine tests will be required. The use of the combined anterior pituitary function test comprising LH-releasing hormone and thyrotrophin-releasing hormone is now no longer routinely used as it does not add to the clinical information obtained by basal hormone measurement. It is usually only disorders of the growth hormone and/or the ACTH axis that require either stimulatory or suppressive testing.

Insulin tolerance test The insulin tolerance test remains the gold standard for assessing the AGTH/cortisol and growth hormone reserve. Its rationale is that insulin-induced hypoglycaemia is a marked stressor to hypothalamic neurones. A fall in blood glucose below 2.2 mmol/l invokes neuroglycopenic sympathetic stimulation, a stress reaction leading to ACTH and cortisol release, which with catecholamines, glucagon, and growth hormone, act as counter-regulatory hormones liberating glucose from glycogen stores in the liver and returning blood glucose levels towards normal. Growth hormone is also released not only as a result of glucose levels falling below the neuroglycopenic threshold for stress induced release, but also in response to the subsequent stress.

Test procedure The test must be performed in a properly equipped unit by well trained experienced personnel. In these circumstances it is an extremely safe and effective test. Contraindications are the presence of ischaemic heart disease, epilepsy or unexplained blackouts, a basal 09.00 cortisol level of less than 50 nmol/l (unless receiving exogenous glucocorticoids), and untreated hypothyroidism.

The patient should be fasted from midnight and the test performed at 09.00 hours. At least 30 min prior to this, an intravenous cannula is inserted. Blood is drawn for cortisol, growth hormone, and glucose analysis at 0, 30, 45, 60, 90 and 120 min. At 0 min 0.15 U/kg of soluble human insulin is injected intravenously (0.3 U/kg in insulin-resistant states such as acromegaly or Cushing's syndrome). Pulse rate and blood pressure along with the times of the characteristic features associated with hypoglycaemia are recorded with the blood samples. Symptoms and signs of hypoglycaemia usually occur between 30 and 45 min and comprise sweating, tachycardia, drowsiness, and hunger. Blood glucose must fall to less than 2.2 mmol/l and symptoms must be evident to be regarded as sufficient hypoglycaemic stress and to interpret the cortisol and growth hormone levels. A normal cortisol response is a rise to 580 nmol/l or more and growth hormone should increase to more than 20 mU/l. Failure to reach these levels indicates deficiency of ACTH and/or growth hormone. If the cortisol response is just subnormal, ACTH reserve may be adequate for day-to-day living but inadequate to cope with stresses such as illness or surgery and exogenous corticosteroid cover would be needed. A response to less than 450 nmol/l requires hydrocortisone replacement. Additionally all subnormal responses require a patient to carry a steroid card and MedicAlert bracelet.

An alternative to the insulin tolerance test to establish adequacy of ACTH/cortisol and growth hormone secretion in the presence of contraindications is the glucagon stimulation test (1 mg glucagon is given subcutaneously and sampling performed over 4 h) but the results are less consistent than with the insulin tolerance test.

The **oral glucose tolerance test** As growth hormone secretion is inhibited by a rise in circulating glucose, the administration of exogenous oral glucose is used to confirm or exclude the diagnosis of acromegaly and remains the gold standard test for confirmation of this condition. The test is performed at 09.00 hours with the patient fasted from midnight. An intravenous cannula is inserted 30 min prior to the test and blood samples are drawn for analysis of glucose and serum growth hormone at −30, 0, 30, 60, 90 and 120 min. Glucose (75 g) dissolved in flavoured water (conveniently given as 370 ml 'Lucozade') is given to the patient immediately after the 0 min blood sample. In normal subjects, after oral glucose, serum growth hormone should be suppressed to undetectable levels (less than 0.5 mU/l). Failure to suppress is consistent with acromegaly, although it may also occur in diabetes mellitus, obesity, liver disease, and opiate dependence; in approximately 30 per cent of cases of acromegaly growth hormone levels paradoxically increase in response to glucose in this condition.

Pituitary imaging

The development of CT and subsequently MRI has revolutionized imaging of the pituitary gland, rendering the previous modalities of air encephalography and metrizamide cysternography obsolete. With their increasing availability, even the time-honoured skull radiograph has a limited role. These new techniques allow accurate visualization of the pituitary gland and, in the case of MRI, precisely delineates the extent of the surrounding invasion. If CT is used, imaging sections need to be thin (1.5 mm) and of high quality with multiplanar reconstructions; contrast should be given. Although CT is far more sensitive in demonstrating any calcification, as occurs commonly in craniopharyngiomas, MRI is nowadays the method of choice for delineating pituitary lesions. Its advantages are that it does not require ionizing radiation, it has the ability to image in any desired plane, and it shows the inherent contrast between tissues. Not only is it able to determine accurately the shape and dimensions of the anterior and posterior pituitary lobes (the latter has a high signal on T_1-weighted images in

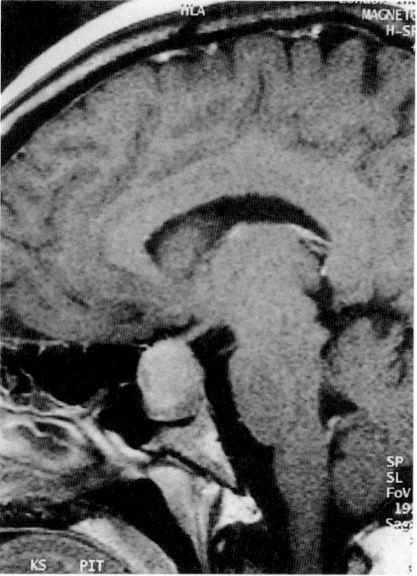

Fig. 4 MRI of a pituitary adenoma showing suprasellar extension and compression of the optic chiasm.

over 90 per cent of normal subjects) but it also delineates the hypothalamic region and optic chiasm. MRI allows accurate assessment of the size of pituitary adenomas, detecting lesions as small as 2 mm. It also determines the extent of any invasion superiorly, inferiorly, or laterally into the cavernous sinuses. On T_1-weighted images pituitary adenomas tend to be of lower signal intensity than the surrounding normal gland and enhance less briskly than the normal gland after injection with intravenous gadolinium contrast (Fig. 4).

Neuro-opthalmological assessment

Neuro-ophthalmological assessment is mandatory in all cases of pituitary dysfunction. At the initial consultation visual acuity should be assessed with the use of Snellen charts and fundoscopy performed to exclude optic atrophy, retinal vein engorgement, or papilloedema from pressure on the visual pathways. Visual fields may be assessed by confrontation using a red pin. Patients with any clinical symptoms or evidence of compression of the optic chiasm from imaging studies require formal assessment of visual fields with Goldmann perimetery or visual evoked responses, stimulating each half-field in turn.

Although permanent loss of vision and/or visual field defects usually result from long-standing compression of the optic chiasm, the shorter the time of compression the easier and more complete is the reversal of any visual field deficit. Surgical decompression or shrinkage of prolactin-secreting tumours by medical therapy often results in rapid improvement in visual fields within hours or days, although the presence of optic atrophy reduces the likelihood of this occurring. Because onset is often insidious, patients may be unaware of any alteration in their vision, although once documented its presence requires them to inform the vehicle licensing authority as driving ability may be impaired. An exception to this usual gradual deterioration is pituitary haemorrhage when visual loss may be sudden with a loss of central vision and development of bitemporal field defects and possible ophthalmoplegia often accompanied by changes in mental function.

Pituitary surgery

With the exception of prolactinomas, for which medical therapy should be preferred as the primary therapy, trans-sphenoidal surgery is now regarded as the firstline treatment for pituitary adenomas. Originally performed by Harvey Cushing around 1910, the lack of adequate visualization prevented its reintroduction for routine use until the mid-1970s. In addition to its curative aim in pituitary adenomas, trans-sphenoidal surgery is also used where other treatments have failed, for example medical therapy in prolactinomas, and for debulking large tumours prior to irradiation. Pituitary apoplexy caused by significant haemorrhage into an adenoma is a neurosurgical emergency requiring prompt intervention. The most commonly used approach is with the patient in a semireclining position via a midline nasal route. Using a sublabial or direct nasal approach, the mucosa is cleaved off the nasal septum providing access to the sphenoid sinus with subsequent removal of the sellar floor. An endoscope is now in use. A less satisfactory alternative approach is via the ethmoidal sinus. Pituitary adenomas are usually soft and easily removed with curettes, although firmer and larger tumours may require piecemeal removal. The success of trans-sphenoidal surgery depends on a number of factors:

(1) the size of the pituitary adenoma;

(2) the degree of invasion into surrounding tissues, especially into the normal remaining pituitary gland, bone, meninges, and lateral extension into the cavernous sinuses;

(3) the skill and experience of the surgeon; and

(4) any previous therapy.

The aim is for selective adenectomy leaving sufficient functioning normal gland; in cases of microadenoma cure rates as high as 90 per cent can be achieved, although rates are usually much lower (in the region of 40 to 50 per cent) for macroadenomas. Visual field defects improve in approximately 80 per cent of patients.

Complications

In experienced hands, mortality is less than 1 per cent and is related to vascular complications, hypothalamic damage, or meningitis. Morbidity relates to local complications or endocrine dysfunction. Cerebrospinal fluid rhinorrhoea may occur and if persistent will require reoperation and sealing of the leak with autologous material such as fascia lata. The risk of meningitis can be minimized by the use of prophylactic antibiotics. Postoperative worsening of endocrine deficiency tends to increase with the size of the lesion and pre-existing hormonal deficiencies. Diabetes insipidus occurs in approximately 5 per cent of cases, though it is usually minor and transient; the exact prevalence depends on the stringency of the diagnostic criteria. The syndrome of inappropriate secretion of antidiuretic hormone is common, typically occurring transiently between the fifth and eighth postoperative days; it usually responds to fluid restriction.

While most macroadenomas, even those with a suprasellar extension of 2 or 3 cm, can often be substantially removed trans-sphenoidally, extremely large and more invasive pituitary tumours may require transfrontal removal. This approach is associated with additional risks of intracranial oedema/haemorrhage or damage to the optic nerve, frontal lobe, or hypothalamus.

Pituitary irradiation

With the advent of modern trans-sphenoidal techniques, pituitary irradiation tends to be reserved for patients who are either not fit enough to undergo surgery or in whom surgery is incompletely successful. In addition to so-called conventional megavoltage irradiation which has been in routine use since the mid-1960s, newer techniques of stereotactic or focused irradiation using one or a few large doses of irradiation have been introduced more recently.

Conventional irradiation uses a linear accelerator as the source; a cobalt source is less satisfactory. It is administered in a fractionated manner over 5 to 6 weeks with a total dose of 4500 cGy given in daily doses not exceeding 200 cGy. Irradiation should be via at least three portals (two temporal and one frontal) to prevent damage to the brain or optic chiasm. Modern CT techniques allow accurate planning and minimal variation in the daily dosage to surrounding structures. Widespread longstanding experience in this technique has revealed it to be both safe and effective. Hormone hypersecretion begins to decrease within 3 to 6 months with a rapid fall occur-

ring within the first 2 years; thereafter there is a progressive exponential decline for up to 20 years. Thus most patients will be cured of their disease, although the time to achieve this varies. The use of this technique also dramatically reduces the risk of recurrence of both functioning and nonfunctioning adenomas. The major side-effect relates to the onset of hypopituitarism. In patients without preceding pituitary hypofunction, approximately 50 per cent will become deficient in growth hormone secretion after 5 years with slightly fewer becoming hypogonadal, followed much later (10 to 15 years) by deficiencies of ACTH and thyroid-stimulating hormone. These proportions increase with prior surgery. Thus any patient who has received pituitary irradiation requires lifelong careful follow-up. The other principal potential side-effect relates to damage to the optic chiasm, although this can be avoided by careful planning and keeping the daily fractionated dose to less than 200 cGy. Loss of cognitive function has been claimed to occur after irradiation, but does not occur if proper field planning and fractionated dosage is applied. The influence of prior surgery is also uncertain. Similarly there are reports of an increased incidence of secondary brain malignancies with a risk of perhaps 1 per cent at 20 years' post-irradiation. However, comparable control groups are difficult to obtain and it is likely that the predisposition to pituitary adenomas also predisposes to other cerebral tumours. The overall impression is that with careful radiotherapy the incidence of peripituitary second tumours is no greater in irradiated than non-irradiated patients with pituitary adenomas.

Stereotactic single high-dose pituitary irradiation using either the Gamma Knife (radiosurgery) or stereotactic multiple arc radiotherapy has received increasing attention in recent years, although long-term efficacy and safety data are not yet available. Care needs to be taken with tumours close to the optic chiasm. Initial impressions suggest that hypersecretory states fall to normal much earlier than after conventional radiotherapy but that hypopituitarism occurs just as often.

Individual pituitary hormones

ACTH

ACTH (adrenocorticotrophic hormone) is a 39-amino-acid peptide that is synthesized in the pituitary initially as part of a 231-residue peptide, pro-opiomelanocortin peptide. This then undergoes post-translational cleavage and modification before secretion. In the pituitary, pro-opiomelanocortin peptide is cleaved to β-lipotrophin, ACTH, a joining peptide, and an amino terminal fragment (Fig. 5). The biological activity of ACTH resides within its first 24 amino acids which are identical across species; synthetic ACTH$_{1-24}$ is used for clinical investigations. Pituitary secretion of melanocyte-

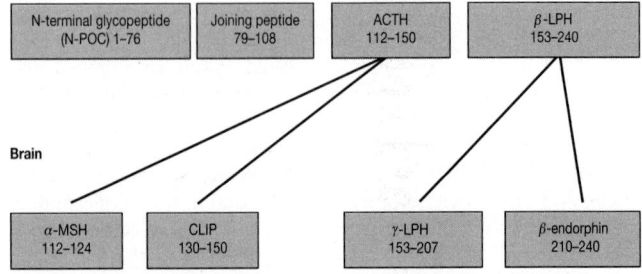

Fig. 5 Schematic representation of the pro-opiomelanocortin precursor protein and its subsequent tissue-specific cleavage products. LPH, lipotrophin; MSH, melanocyte-stimulating hormone; CLIP, coiticotrophinlike intermediate peptide.

stimulating hormone does not occur in humans; the increased pigmentation that is observed in conditions of ACTH excess is due rather to the melanocyte receptor stimulating properties of ACTH itself. ACTH G-protein coupled receptors are widely distributed in the adrenal cortex, predominantly in the zono fasiculata and reticularis. Upon binding of ACTH, cyclic AMP is generated which stimulates the synthesis and secretion of the glucocorticoid cortisol and the androgens androstenedione and dehydroepiandrostenedione. Mineralocorticoid secretion is largely controlled by the renin–angiotensin system. Long-term stimulation by ACTH acts to maintain adrenal size and growth, but there may be an additional, so far uncharacterized, hypothalamic–pituitary adrenocortical growth factors.

Secretion of ACTH is tonically controlled by hypothalamic corticotrophin-releasing hormone, although arginine vasopressin also stimulates its release, particularly in response to stress. Cortisol feeds back negatively on the hypothalamus to inhibit the secretion of both of these factors, but also inhibits their actions at the pituitary directly; ACTH itself exerts negative feedback effects on the hypothalamus via a short loop. There are probably other physiologically important, as yet unidentified, ACTH-releasing hypothalamic hormones.

The secretion of ACTH is pulsatile but with a marked circadian rhythm. Secretory bursts start around 03.00 hours, are most frequent in the one to two hours before waking and the hour thereafter before declining progressively throughout the day to reach a nadir in the late evening, just before the normal time of sleeping. Secretion is predominantly controlled by the light–dark and sleep–wake cycles and is thus altered by time shifts—this accounts for at least some of the symptoms of jet lag. Secretion is also increased by major physical and psychological stress.

Conditions of ACTH deficiency

Isolated ACTH deficiency is rare; it more commonly occurs as a late component of the panhypopituitarism associated with pituitary adenomas, trans-sphenoidal surgery, or pituitary irradiation. Its symptoms are similar to those of Addison's disease but with two important differences: there is no pigmentation—indeed patients are usually pale—and there is less risk of adrenal crises due to mineralocorticoid secretion being largely preserved. Patients typically complain of anorexia, malaise, loss of energy, and weight loss all of which contribute to them frequently being termed 'malingerers'. Severe cortisol deficiency may result in hypoglycaemia and predispose to circulatory collapse particularly during a supraimposed illness.

Conditions of ACTH excess

ACTH secretion is increased in both Addison's and Cushing's diseases (dealt with in other sections). It is also dramatically increased in the rare condition of Nelson's syndrome. This occurs in patients with Cushing's disease who have been treated by bilateral adrenalectomy. The loss of all negative feedback inhibition by cortisol can result in increasing growth of the pituitary adenoma with not only local invasion and mass effects, but also very high circulating ACTH levels which result in marked hyperpigmentation. Its incidence may be reduced by pituitary irradiation prior to adrenalectomy.

Treatment of ACTH deficiency

ACTH deficiency is best treated by glucocorticoid replacement. The standard regimen is 10 mg hydrocortisone on waking with a further 5 mg at lunchtime and 18.00 although this may need modifying according to the profile of measured serum cortisol throughout the day. Alternative regimes are prednisolone (5 and 2.5 mg) or dexamethasone (0.5 and 0.25 mg) although levels of either of these cannot be assayed in blood. It is essential that patients are educated to increase their dosage during illnesses or stress with at least a doubling of their oral medication. If vomiting occurs or during a perioperative period parenteral therapy will be required. Aldosterone production almost always remains adequate with ACTH deficiency unlike in primary adrenal insufficiency and fludrocortisone therapy is not needed.

Thyroid-stimulating hormone

The glycoprotein thyroid-stimulating hormone belongs in the same family as LH and FSH. Like other anterior pituitary hormones it is secreted in a pulsatile manner but with its effects mediated by circulating thyroxine and liothyronine from the thyroid gland. It is itself controlled by hypothalamic thyrotrophin-releasing hormone. Deficiency of thyroid-stimulating hormone almost never occurs in an isolated manner but occurs in conjunction with other pituitary hormone deficiencies.

Thyrotrophinomas

Thyrotrophin-secreting tumours (also known as TSHomas) are rare, comprising only 1 per cent of all pituitary tumours. Unlike primary thyroid gland diseases they have an equal sex incidence, with the majority presenting between the third and sixth decades of life, although cases at all ages have been recorded. Symptoms and signs result from the ensuing excess of thyroid hormone. As more than 90 per cent of the tumours are macroadenomas, visual field defects are common. Coexistant oversecretion of other pituitary hormones occurs in about 20 per cent of cases and is usually of growth hormone. Diagnosis is made on the basis of elevated circulating thyroxine with detectable or increased thyroid-stimulating hormone. The major differential diagnosis in such cases is the condition of resistance to thyroid hormone; distinguishing between the two requires both laboratory and radiological data. Generalized resistance to thyroid hormone is usually an autosomal dominant condition; however, when resistance to thyroid hormone is restricted to the pituitary it is often sporadic and patients are clinically hyperthyroid. In neither instance is a pituitary tumour present. Further differentiation is available with measurement of the α subunit of thyroid-stimulating hormone (and other glycoprotein pituitary hormones) and calculation of the α subunit/thyroid-stimulating hormone molar ratio; a ratio greater than 1.0, indicating oversecretion of the uncombined α subunit, is present in more than 90 per cent of thyrotrophin-secreting tumours, whilst a ratio of less than 1.0 is indicative of resistance to thyroid hormone.

Treatment Surgery remains the initial treatment for the majority of cases of TSHomas, although the frequency of macroadenomas means that biochemical cure rates are only about 40 per cent. As almost all of these tumours express somatostatin receptors, the use of somatostatin analogues, for example octreotide, usually enables medical control of hypersecretion of thyroid-stimulating hormone to be achieved. This is often accompanied by a reduction in tumour size.

Gonadotrophins

The gonadotrophins LH (luteinizing hormone) and FSH (follicle stimulating hormone), together with thyroid-stimulating hormone and human chorionic gonadotrophin β comprise the family of glycoprotein anterior pituitary hormones. Whilst the α subunit is common to all these hormones, it is the β subunit that is unique to each and gives biological and immunological specificity. The actions of both LH and FSH are intimately involved with maintenance of libido and fertility; in women their secretion, subject to positive and negative feedback, controls ovarian gonadal secretion and the menstrual cycle. In men, LH controls testosterone production by the Leydig cells whilst FSH stimulates Sertoli cell spermatogenesis. Deficiency of gonadotrophin secretion is usually one of the earliest occurrences in pituitary tumours.

Gonadotrophinomas

Anterior pituitary tumours that secrete intact LH and/or FSH are termed gonadotrophinomas. Tumours secreting α subunit are more common, but as this is without biological effect and rarely measured in routine clinical settings these tumours are usually classified as non-functioning adenomas. Clinically both gonadotrophinomas and non-functioning adenomas usually tend to present in a similar manner with symptoms relating to a pituitary mass. In men, FSH-secreting tumours (known as FSHomas) cause testicular enlargement due to FSH-induced hypertrophy of the seminifer-ous tubules; as such the development of bilateral testicular enlargement should prompt investigation of a possible pituitary tumour.

The diagnosis of gonadotrophinomas is controversial; most clinicians require inappropriate elevation of serum LH and/or FSH. However, immunostaining of many clinically non-functioning adenomas will frequently demonstrate staining of either gonadotrophin or α subunit.

Treatment Surgery is the main treatment for these tumours with adjunctive radiotherapy advocated by many clinicians to reduce the risk of recurrence. Medical therapy with long-acting gonadotrophin-releasing hormone agonists may reduce hormonal secretion, as may the use of somatostatin analogues, which may also result in tumour shrinkage.

Prolactin

Prolactin is a 199-amino-acid residue peptide that belongs to the same family as growth hormone with 16 per cent homology. Prolactin-secreting cells comprise approximately 10 per cent of the anterior pituitary cells in men but up to 30 per cent in multiparous women. Like other anterior pituitary hormones, prolactin is under the control of hypothalamic factors but is unique in that this comprises tonic inhibition by dopamine from the tuberoinfundibular neurones. Release also occurs after administration of thyrotrophin-releasing hormone and vasoactive intestinal peptide, which also occurs in the hypothalamus; although their physiological significance is clear in rodents it remains uncertain in humans. Prolactin synthesis is also strongly influenced by oestrogen which acts as a transcription factor for prolactin gene expression. Under this influence, concentrations are higher in premenopausal women than in men and increase during menarche and especially during pregnancy, when the gland may double in size and weight because of the increase in number of mammotroph cells. The causes of physiological and abnormal increased prolactin secretion are shown in Table 3. Following delivery, maternal levels decrease if breast feeding does not occur but remain elevated in response to suckling. Outside of lactation, nipple stimulation reflexly increases levels as does stress. Levels also increase in response to any disruption of the hypothalamic pituitary stalk or on administration of drugs that interfere with the synthesis or action of dopamine. Primary hypothyroidism may also cause levels to rise, falling again with thyroxine treatment (Table 3).

Action

Prolactin receptors, members of the cytokine superfamily, are widely distributed. Their predominant location is the mammary gland where their activation results in initiation and maintenance of lactation. During pregnancy, additional hormones are required for the development of the synthetic and secretory breast apparatus including oestrogen, insulin, cortisol, and placental mammotrophic hormones. However, the elevated oestrogen levels during pregnancy also inhibit lactation from the prepared prepuerperal breast, which occurs with their precipitous fall after delivery of the placenta. The actions of prolactin receptors at other sites is less clear. Direct effects on the hypothalamus inhibit pulsatile release of gonadotrophin-releasing hormone and thus gonadotrophin secretion, probably by increasing the inhibitory opiate (endorphin) tone in the hypothalamus, resulting in impaired gonadal function. This is the basis for the contraceptive effect of lactation, which persists as long as prolactin levels are sufficiently high, maintained by the intensive reflex of breast feeding as the sole source of feeding the baby. It is also becoming increasingly clear that prolactin has widespread effects on immune functions as well as perhaps antiapoptotic actions in several tissues including the prostate.

Disorders of secretion

Absence of prolactin secretion rarely occurs on its own and is of unknown physiological significance other than precluding lactation. However, the usual coexistent loss of gonadotrophins and resultant infertility tends to precede this clinical effect.

Prolactinomas

Prolactinomas are the most common functioning anterior pituitary tumour encountered in clinical practice. They account for 25 to 30 per cent of pituitary adenomas and are much more common in women. The majority are sporadic, although occasionally they may be part of the multiple endocrine neoplasia type 1 syndrome. They may be either pure prolactin secreting or mixed somatomammotroph (growth hormone) tumours. They are of monoclonal origin. The clinical features can be divided into local mass effects or the effects of hyperprolactinaemia either on the breast or on the gonadotrophin-releasing hormone pulse generator. In premenopausal women the commonest symptoms are secondary oligo/amenorrhoea (in up to 95 per cent of patients), galactorrhoea (20 per cent), or infertility with regular cycles. Due to these symptoms, women tend to present earlier and thus the tumours are usually microadenomas. Although increased prolactin causes decreased libido and erectile dysfunction in men, these symptoms may be ignored and male patients, like postmenopausal women, present late with mass effects such as headaches, visual field defects, or involvement of other cranial nerves from cavernous sinus extension. Galactorrhoea is rare in men.

Treatment In common with other pituitary tumours the aims of treatment are to reduce hormone secretion to normal, to reduce tumour size correcting visual field defects, and to restore normal anterior pituitary function.

Left untreated, the majority of microprolactinomas do not appear to undergo progressive enlargement. As such the need for treatment depends on the clinical situation and the patient's wishes. The introduction of the ergot-related synthetic dopamine agonist bromocriptine in 1971 revolutionized the treatment of prolactinomas. A variety of other dopamine agonists are now available, the only one with advantages being the long-

Table 3 Causes of hyperprolactinaemia

Physiological
Pregnancy
Nipple stimulation/suckling
Neonatal
Coitus
Sleep
Stress (hypoglycaemia, surgery, psychological)
Hypothalamic disease
Tumour
Granulomatous disease (sarcoidosis, tuberculosis, Langerhans' cell histiocytosis)
Cranial irradiation
Pituitary stalk section (trauma, postsurgery)
Pituitary disease
Prolactinoma
Mixed growth hormone/prolactin-secreting adenoma
Other intrasellar tumour causing stalk compression
Empty sella
Drugs
Dopamine receptor antagonists (neuroleptics, metoclopramide)
Antihypertensives (reserpine, methyldopa)
Antidepressants (tricyclics, monoamine oxidase inhibitors, 5-hydroxytryptamine reuptake blockers)
Oestrogens
Opiates
Cimetidine (parenteral)
Verapamil
Miscellaneous
Pregnancy
Polycystic ovary syndrome
Hypothyroidism
Chronic renal failure
Cirrhosis
Chest wall lesions (herpes zoster, injury)
Ectopic secretion of prolactin (bronchogenic carcinoma, hypernephroma)
Idiopathic

acting cabergoline. All of these directly activate pituitary D_2 receptors, thereby mimicking endogenous hypothalamic dopaminergic action. They are highly effective in lowering prolactin levels, stopping galactorrhoea, and restoring normal gonadal function including fertility. They also have dramatic effects producing shrinkage of the tumour in 85 per cent of patients and improvement in visual fields. Disappearance of headaches is seen within days, and if imaging is repeated, shrinkage is confirmed within 4 to 6 weeks in most cases. Given these effects, it is mandatory that a serum prolactin level should be measured in all patients presenting with a visual field defect and a pituitary mass prior to surgery (normal levels are less than 400 mU/l or 20 ng/ml). A serum level of greater than 4000 mU/l (200 ng/ml) is indicative of a prolactinoma and introduction of dopamine agonist therapy will usually avoid the need for pituitary surgery. The usual starting dose for bromocriptine is 2.5 mg once daily taken during the main course of a bulk meal. This slows absorption and will minimize the side-effects of nausea and dizziness, although most patients experience tachyphylaxis and symptoms tend to settle with repeated dosages. An initial dose of cabergoline is 0.5 mg once weekly. Other side-effects include fatigue, headache, and nasal stuffiness. Most serious is psychosis which has been reported in approximately 1 to 2 per cent of patients, although more subtle psychiatric disturbances probably occur more often. A previous psychiatric history is therefore a contraindication to the use of this class of drugs. Most patients will require long-term therapy, although a significant proportion of microadenomas undergo spontaneous resolution/infarction and it is worthwhile having an intermittent trial off therapy from time to time. In the case of macroadenomas, pituitary irradiation is often advocated after initial shrinkage with dopamine agonists, in order to prevent recurrence. Occasional resistance to medical therapy may necessitate surgical intervention. While elevated levels lower than 4000 mU/l (200 ng/ml) may be found in patients with true prolactinomas, such levels may also be found in patients with pseudoprolactinomas. The term 'pseudoprolactinoma' is used for any peripituitary mass which interrupts delivery of dopamine to the normal pituitary via the pituitary stalk, i.e. a functional pituitary stalk section results and prolactin secretion from the normal gland is disinhibited. While prolactin levels as high as 6000 mU/l (300 ng/ml) have been described in association with prolactinoma, they are usually less than 2000 mU/l (100 ng/ml). While the clinical features in patients with pseudo-prolactinomas may be identical, and are reversible with dopamine agonists, as in true prolactinomas, but pseudoprolactinomas do not shrink with medical therapy. Thus careful clinical supervision is needed during a trial of medical therapy for large tumours when prolactin levels are less than 6000 mU/l(300 ng/ml).

Hyperprolactinaema and pregnancy

As infertility is a common symptom of hyperprolactinaemia, it is likely that many women with prolactinomas will be trying to conceive whilst on dopamine agonists. Patients should be warned that they are likely to become fertile on treatment and the drug is usually stopped after confirmation of pregnancy. However, having been in use for nearly 30 years, it is clear that continued use of bromocriptine during pregnancy does not result in any adverse effects. Although there is less experience of cabergoline, there is no evidence to suggest that this should be any different.

During pregnancy, under the influence of increasing oestrogen levels, prolactinomas may enlarge like many peripituitary masses, especially meningiomas. Although the risk of this is small for microadenomas, there may be considerable expansion of macroadenomas. Such patients need very careful sequential monitoring for signs of chiasmal compression. In this event, reintroduction of medical therapy will shrink the mass and surgical intervention is rarely required. For patients with a macroadenoma, irradiation or trans-sphenoidal surgery has been advocated prior to attempting to conceive. Whilst this will reduce the risk of expansion during pregnancy, it may lead to growth hormone deficiency after some 5 years and gonadotrophin deficiency in about 50 per cent after 8 to 10 years.

Table 4 Physiological factors increasing secretion of growth hormone

Sleep (slow waves)
Malnutrition and fasting (IGF-I is low)
Stress
Exercise
Fall in blood glucose
Type I diabetes mellitus, if uncontrolled (IGF-I is low)
Cirrhosis of the liver

IGF-I, insulin-like growth factor I.

Growth hormone

Human growth hormone is a 191-amino-acid single-chain protein containing two disulphide bonds. It is synthesized by cells located largely in the lateral part of the pituitary. Some 75 per cent circulates as a 22 kDa protein and 5 to 10 per cent as a smaller 20 kDa isoform with the remainder consisting of glycosylated and sulphated isoforms. Growth hormone is secreted in a marked pulsatile manner which is due to the integrated and co-ordinated effects of both stimulatory and inhibitory controlling hypothalamic hormones. Growth hormone-releasing hormone is a positive regulator of its synthesis whilst somatostatin (a 14-amino-acid peptide) is a potent inhibitor of both the frequency and amplitude of its secretory pulses. An additional positive regulator is the newly cloned growth hormone secretagogue 'ghrelin' which acts through a receptor which is distinct from that of growth hormone-releasing hormone. These regulatory peptides are themselves under numerous extrahypothalamic influences. Amino acids, sleep, stress, and a fall in blood glucose increase secretion of growth hormone; β antagonists are able to augment other stimulatory stimuli as do dopamine and cholinergic agonists, both of which are blocked by the cholinergic blockers. Oestrogen enhances the pulse amplitude of growth hormone. Thus secretion of growth hormone is subject to complex neuroregulatory control with levels increasing in response to several physiological stimuli (Table 4).

Overall growth hormone secretion is greater in females, with middle-aged women secreting approximately 45 μg in 24 h compared with 15 μg in men of equivalent age. Secretion increases from the time of puberty, peaking between 18 and 25 years, then inexorably falling to reach low levels after 60 years.

The growth hormone receptor

The growth hormone receptor is a 638-amino-acid receptor which is widely distributed throughout the body, being most abundant in the liver. It consists of extra- and intracellular domains; signal transduction requires dimerization of the receptor, which is facilitated by growth hormone binding. The identification of the specific high-affinity binding sites of the growth hormone molecule to the receptor has allowed their modification to provide specific modified growth hormone antagonists (see below). Signal transduction is via a number of pathways including activation of the JAK/STAT proteins, the insulin receptor substrate pathway and the MAP (mitogen-activated protein) kinase pathway. The complexity and variety of these pathways allows for the different anabolic/differentiative and proliferative effects of growth hormone in different tissues. Abnormalities of the growth hormone receptor occur in Laron's syndrome characterized by failure of growth and a distinct phenotypic appearance and high levels of growth hormone but low levels of insulin-like growth factor I.

Approximately 50 per cent of secreted growth hormone circulates bound to a growth hormone binding protein which consists of the cleaved extracellular domain of the transmembrane growth hormone receptor. Binding to this receptor fragment reduces the clearance rate of growth hormone thus prolonging its bioactivity. Growth hormone binding protein is absent, or abnormal, in Laron's syndrome and reduced or abnormal in other causes of insensitivity to growth hormone.

Actions of growth hormone

The actions of growth hormone can be divided into direct metabolic effects which act in the short term to increase glucose availability, regulate free fatty acids, and increase amino acid uptake, and powerful long-term effects on skeletal and soft tissue growth mediated via insulin-like growth factor I. Insulin-like growth factor I is a basic polypeptide of 70 amino acids (molecular weight 7.5 kDa) which was until recently thought to be synthesized almost solely by the liver. However, it is also synthesized by most tissues in response to growth hormone acting in a paracrine, autocrine, or juxtacrine manner. The circulating insulin-like growth factor I derived from the liver has little importance in determining the growth effects of growth hormone but is measured to reflect the overall functional status of growth hormone since tissue levels cannot be assayed. In the serum insulin-like growth factor I circulates bound to a group of binding proteins which also occur in tissue fluids; six have so far been identified. Insulin-like growth factor binding protein 3 is the predominant carrier of insulin-like growth factor I and its concentration is dependent on growth hormone itself; it thus plays a major role in regulating the bioactivity of insulin-like growth factor I. Insulin-like growth factor I acts via two specific receptors: type I, with a similar structure to that of the insulin receptor, has the greatest affinity for insulin-like growth factor I, whilst the structurally distinct type II receptor has the greatest affinity for insulin-like growth factor II. Insulin-like growth factor II is more important in the fetus and is not growth hormone dependent.

Disorders of growth hormone secretion

Acromegaly The term acromegaly is derived from the Greek word summarizing its clinical manifestations: *akron*, extremity; *megas*, great. First described by Pierre Marie in 1886 it has an annual incidence of approximately 3 per million although this is almost certainly an underestimate. It is almost invariably due to a growth hormone-secreting pituitary tumour although very rare cases of ectopic secretion of growth hormone-releasing hormone from carcinoid tumours have been recorded. Approximately 5 per cent of cases are associated with multiple endocrine neoplasia type 1. Molecular analysis has revealed that approximately 50 per cent of cases are due to an activating mutation of the α subunit of the G-protein coupled receptor for growth hormone-releasing hormone.

Clinical features Acromegaly affects both sexes equally, although its insidious onset means that the majority of patients are not diagnosed until the age of 40 to 60 years. Younger patients tend to have more aggressive disease and are detected earlier, although gigantism, occurring before fusion of the bony epiphyses, is a rare occurrence. In common with other pituitary tumours, the clinical manifestations can be related to the neighbouring effects of a local mass or to hypopituitarism, and to specific symptoms and signs relating to excessive secretion of growth hormone and insulin-like growth factor I (Table 5). The insidious onset means that the mean delay in diagnosis is about 7 years, although diagnosis may often take 10 to 20 years. In adults, the increase in soft tissue mass and skeletal effects are responsible for the clinical features including the classical coarse facial features, broad nose, and thick lips. Increase in the size of the mandible results in prognathism and interdental separation. Frontal bossing causes prominent supraorbital ridges. Sweating is one of the most prominent symptoms and the one most sensitive to growth hormone excess. Musculoskeletal symptoms are common, consisting of increased size and breadth of hands ('spade-like' hands) and feet; increasing ring size is common and is a sensitive index of excessive secretion of growth hormone. Degenerative arthropathy of the weight-bearing hips and knees is common, often necessitating joint replacement, and of the spine with pain and neurological pressure effects. Symptomatic carpal tunnel syndrome occurs in approximately half of patients and up to 80 per cent will have subclinical abnormalities. Thyroid enlargement is common resulting in a nodular goitre. Despite these signs the diagnosis is often overlooked.

Complications of acromegaly Although originally regarded as a predominantly cosmetic disease, several epidemiological reviews have established

Table 5 Clinical symptoms and signs of acromegaly

Symptoms and signs at presentation	Overall prevalence (%)
Facial change, acral enlargement, and soft tissue swelling	100
Excessive sweating	83
Acroparaesthesial carpal tunnel syndrome	68
Tiredness and lethargy	53
Headaches	53
Oligo- or amenorrhoea, infertility	55*
Erectile dysfunction and/or decreased libido	42†
Arthropathy	37
Impaired glucose tolerance/diabetes	37
Goitre	35
Ear, nose, throat, and dental problems	32
Congestive cardiac failure/arhythmia	25
Hypertension	23
Visual field defects	17

*Percentage of female patients.
†Percentage of male patients.

that acromegaly is associated with significant morbidity and mortality. Early surveys revealed that over 50 per cent of patients died before the age of 60 years, principally due to cardiovascular and metabolic complications. With improved management of both these and the underlying disease, patients are now surviving longer. Reduction of mean serum levels of growth hormone to less than 5 mU/l (2 ng/ml) and/or a normal serum level of insulin-like growth factor I appear to be associated with a normal life expectancy.

Cardiovascular complications are a major source of morbidity and mortality. Although growth hormone in low doses may have a beneficial cardiac action, excessive amounts result in cardiomyopathy and increased left ventricular mass. Many patients develop arrythmias. Hypertension is a frequent complication requiring aggressive monitoring and management; it may persist despite lowering the levels of growth hormone. The increased cardiovascular risk factors also predispose to cerebral vascular ischaemic events. Due to the counter-regulatory properties of growth hormone on insulin, insulin resistance and impaired glucose tolerance is common often resulting in frank diabetes. This may be accompanied by a hypertriglyceridaemia. Increase in the soft tissues of the larynx and tongue can result in obstructive sleep apnoea which often requires domiciliary nocturnal continuous positive pressure airway ventilation. Anaesthetic intubation for any surgical intervention is more difficult (Table 6).

Table 6 Complications of acromegaly

Local
Headache
Visual field loss
Cranial nerve lesions
Systemic
Cardiovascular
  Cardiomyopathy
  Hypertension
Respiratory
  Kyphosis
  Obstructive sleep apnoea
Central nervous system
  Stroke
Metabolic
  Diabetes mellitus, impaired glucose tolerance (insulin resistance)
  Hyperlipidaemia (triglycerides)
Neoplastic
  Colorectal
Breast and prostate (uncertain)

The question of increased risk of malignancy in acromegaly has been controversial for many years, but recent studies have confirmed that there is an increased risk of premalignant colonic tubulovillous adenomas and colorectal carcinoma. Although comparison with comparable control groups is difficult, this increased risk of colorectal cancer appears to be at least threefold. It appears to be an age-related complication with adenomas occurring after the age of 40 years and carcinomas occurring in or after the sixth decade. Although the precise mechanisms remain uncertain it is associated with elevated levels of insulin-like growth factor I which might both increase proliferation of epithelial cells and inhibit their apoptotic response to local environmental factors such as bile salts. These patients require regular colonoscopic screening, although their associated colonomegaly makes this technically challenging. There is a suggestion that acromegaly also predisposes to breast cancer and some circumstantial evidence indicates that elderly male patients should also be screened for prostatic neoplasia.

Aims of treatment Although the aims of treatment are the same as those for any pituitary tumour, there has been controversy as to the level of reduction of growth hormone that should be considered as a satisfactory therapeutic aim. Epidemological surveys suggest that a normal life expectancy is associated with a mean serum growth hormone level of less than 5 mU/l (2 ng/ml) and/or a normal level of insulin-like growth factor I, although reference tends to be made to a 'safe' level of growth hormone rather than a cure, since physiological responses to growth hormone rarely return to normal. Larger epidemiological studies are required to confirm and refine these findings.

Treatment of acromegaly Surgery: Trans-sphenoidal surgery remains the firstline therapy for the majority of patients. It is a safe operation with low morbidity. Its success rate depends on the size of the pituitary tumour, the presurgical levels of growth hormone, and the experience of the surgeon. Safe levels of growth hormone are achieved in 60 to 80 per cent of patients with microadenomas and 30 to 40 per cent of patients with macroadenomas.

Radiotherapy: Pituitary irradiation is a very effective means of reducing secretion of growth hormone. It tends to be reserved for patients in whom levels of growth hormone remain elevated after surgery. Its efficacy depends on the preirradiation level with approximately a 50 per cent fall occurring in the first 2 years but with an exponential decline thereafter which may continue for 15 to 20 years. The majority of patients therefore eventually achieve safe levels of growth hormone with a mean interval of 5 to 7 years being required. Normalization of insulin-like growth factor I occurs in over 50 per cent of patients by 10 years. Focused radiotherapy probably results in a more rapid fall. Medical therapy is required during the interim period.

Medical therapy: For many years dopamine agonists provided the only medical therapy for acromegaly. However, unlike in prolactinomas, the response rate is relatively poor with less than 10 per cent of patients achieving safe levels of growth hormone. Furthermore, the doses required are usually very much higher than in prolactinomas with a consequent increased frequency of side-effects. The introduction of the synthetic somatostatin analogue octreotide in the early 1980s provided an enormous advance in medical therapy. Natural somatostatin has a half-life of approximately 80 s and thus cannot be used therapeutically unless by continuous intravenous infusion. Octreotide by contrast has a prolonged effect lasting 6 to 8 h and thus thrice daily subcutaneous injections provide reasonably stable concentrations of drug in the plasma. Using this regimen, growth hormone is suppressed in more than 90 per cent of patients, but only approximately 60 per cent achieve safe levels and 50 per cent a normal level of insulin-like growth factor I. The usual total daily dose ranges from 150 to 600 μg, although occasional patients may require higher doses. There is evidence that octreotide may also shrink the adenoma in many patients, although this effect is not nearly as dramatic or complete as that seen in prolactinomas following therapy with a dopamine agonist. There is no consistent evidence that such shrinkage may aid subsequent surgery. Although

generally well tolerated, the predominant side-effects are local pain at the site of injection and gastrointestinal—abdominal cramps, flatulence, and bulky or fluid stools are common although they tend to resolve with time. In the longer term, there is an increased frequency of gallstones which is due to both an inhibition of gall bladder contractility and increased bacterial deconjugation of bile acids as a result of prolonged intestinal transit time. Atrophic gastritis is another long-term complication. More recently, subcutaneous octreotide has been superseded by the development of somatostatin analogue depot formulations, of which there are currently two, octreotide LAR and lanreotide SR, both of which are administered intramuscularly. The former is available at variable doses of 10, 20, or 30 mg and is administered every 4 or 6 weeks, whilst lanreotide SR is available as a 30 mg dose administered every 14 days or less. Their efficacy is similar to subcutaneous octreotide but with the obvious advantage of increased convenience for the patient. Pegvisomant is an entirely new medical therapy for acromegaly. It is a recombinant modified growth hormone molecule that has increased affinity to one receptor binding site but with a different modification of the other binding site that prevents receptor dimerization. Its conjugation to polyethylene glycol increases its molecular size and prolongs its half-life; it is given as a subcutaneous daily injection. Phase 3 clinical trials have shown it to be extremely effective, with over 90 per cent of patients achieving a normal level of insulin-like growth factor I. The fact that it is a modified growth hormone molecule means that it interferes with most growth hormone assays and thus this measurement cannot be used as a marker of efficacy. Indeed, growth hormone levels actually rise with this medication but to date there is no evidence of pituitary tumour growth. Whether pegvisomant will become a firstline treatment in acromegaly remains to be determined.

Growth hormone deficiency Although long realized to be vitally important in children, the role and widespread influence of growth hormone in adult physiology has only become apparent over the last decade. It is now clear that not only does growth hormone have widespread functions, but its deficiency in the adult is associated with significant morbidity and mortality. Based on indirect evidence of the frequency of pituitary disease, the annual incidence of adult onset growth hormone deficiency is estimated to approximately 10 per million. In adults, pituitary adenomas remain the commonest cause, although iatrogenic causes, especially irradiation, are also common. In children, approximately 70 per cent of cases are idiopathic. As many of these children have a normal growth hormone axis on subsequent retesting in their teens and adulthood, the pathogenesis might be due to deficiency of hypothalamic growth hormone-releasing hormone or failure or delayed maturation of the hypothalamic–pituitary axis.

Clinical features Growth hormone does not appear to be necessary for intrauterine growth and most children with congenital or childhood onset growth hormone deficiency tend to present with a falling off of growth velocity and failure to grow, which if unchecked leads to short stature. Bone age is delayed but with a normal weight for height. Thus, early detection requires accurate growth and weight charts.

Over the last 10 years, there have been a large number of studies detailing the effects of growth hormone deficiency, and in the case of adults it is now clear that these patients have a distinct phenotype (Table 7).

The impairment of psychological well-being and quality of life is probably the most important symptom of growth hormone deficiency. Its occurrence has been validated by a variety of questionnaires including the Nottingham Health Profile, the Psychological and General Well-Being Schedule, and the General Health Questionnaire, as well as a specific assessment of growth hormone deficiency. Consistent findings using these measures are decreased energy and mood, increased emotional lability and social isolation, increased anxiety, and reduced overall energy levels and vitality. These measures show significant improvement with administration of growth hormone in about 85 per cent of cases, which in some patients is dramatic. Lack of effect may reflect psychological dysfunction related to previous surgery or irradiation.

Table 7 Signs, symptoms, and findings associated with adult onset growth hormone deficiency

Symptoms
Impaired psychological well-being
    Decreased mood
    Emotional ability
    Impaired self-control
    Anxiety
    Reduced vitality and energy
    Increased social isolation
Abnormal body composition
    Increased abdominal adiposity
    Reduced lean body mass
Reduced muscle strength and exercise ability

Signs
Increased body weight with increased waist–hip fat ratio
Decreased muscle strength
Reduced exercise capability
Reduced affect

Findings
Impaired cardiac function
Increased cholesterol and low-density lipoprotein
Reduced high-density lipoprotein
Reduced lean body mass and increased fat mass
Insulin resistance
Increased fibrinogen and plasminogen activator inhibitor level
Increased mortality from vascular events

Growth hormone deficiency is associated with a reduction of lean body mass of approximately 7 to 8 per cent and an increase in fat mass of the same amount. This tends to be in a central distribution resulting in increased waist–hip ratio. There is decreased fluid volume comprising total body water. Administration of growth hormone will reverse all of these changes with an increase in lean body mass of up to 5 kg, predominantly skeletal muscle, and a corresponding reduction of fat mass with a consequent decreased waist–hip ratio. There is an increase in total body water. One of the most important effects of growth hormone appears to be a significant reduction in bone mineral density, with several studies showing an increase in osteoporotic fractures. Although recombinant growth hormone increases bone mineral density, it takes a minimum of 12 months for the effect to be measurable (using dual-energy X-ray absorptiometry scanning) and as yet there are no studies showing a consequent reduction in the rate of osteoporotic fractures. Impaired muscle strength and exercise performance is a frequent symptom and sign of growth hormone deficiency. Maximum oxygen uptake is reduced to approximately 80 per cent of that of age-, sex-, and height-matched controls. Whilst it improves with administration of growth hormone, not all measures of strength and muscle function are restored to normal and several years of treatment may be required.

Growth hormone deficiency has been associated with a two- to threefold increased mortality relating to vascular disease. Possible mechanisms might be related to the demonstrated increased thickness of the arterial intima and atherosclerotic plaques of carotid arteries, as well as the increased risk factors for ischaemic heart disease such as body mass, total cholesterol and low-density lipoprotein, and reduction in high-density lipoprotein. Metabolic effects of insulin resistance and hyperinsulinaemia with decreased carbohydrate metabolism might also be important. The abnormal lipid profile improves with growth hormone treatment, although an associated increase in lipoprotein (a), which is proposed to be an independent risk factor for atherosclerosis, remains of some concern.

Growth hormone deficiency is associated with impaired cardiac function comprising decreased left ventricular mass, impaired systolic function, and reduced ejection fraction. Whilst there is anecdotal evidence of dramatic increases in cardiac performance, the majority of studies have shown con-siderably milder effects on increased ventricular mass, stroke volume, and cardiac output.

Treatment of adult growth hormone deficiency The aims of treatment are to improve and normalize the abnormalities associated with growth hormone deficiency. At present, most endocrine units only offer growth hormone replacement to patients who have a severe growth hormone deficiency (i.e. a peak growth hormone response of less than 9 mU/l after insulin-induced hypoglycaemia) and who are symptomatic or have abnormal metabolic/bone investigations. It is not yet routinely administered to all patients with growth hormone deficiency. In part this is due to its cost (in 2000 approximately £5000 per annum). There is, however, growing interest in the role of recombinant growth hormone therapy in the frail elderly with a view to improving their functional capacity, as it is suggested that the physiological decrease in growth hormone secretion in the elderly might be responsible for the associated changes in body composition. At present, however, trials of growth hormone administration in these patients are limited and there is obvious concern about the long-term safety issues (see below). Amongst patients in whom growth hormone treatment is indicated, the development and widespread availability of recombinant growth hormone has avoided the risk of transmission of Creutzfeldt–Jacob disease which was associated with the use of pituitary-derived natural growth hormone before 1985. The development of modern cartridge pens has also facilitated its administration, which is usually as a once daily subcutaneous injection in a manner similar to insulin. Currently, childhood doses are calculated according to body weight with the end point being growth velocity. Early studies in adults also used a weight-based regimen but the doses tended to be supraphysiological with an increased incidence of side-effects. It is now clear that individual dose titration should be performed with an initial daily dose of 0.8 U (0.3 mg). which is subsequently titrated according to the serum values of insulin-like growth factor I. The aim is to restore serum insulin-like growth factor I to the upper half of the age-matched normal range. This gradual titration ensures a more physiological replacement and minimizes the side-effects. The average maintenance dose in men is 0.8 U (0.3 mg) whilst in women it is higher at 1.2 U (0.4 mg). Regardless of the final dose, it has become clear that a minimum of 6 months' treatment is required to establish whether or not benefit has occurred.

Side-effects Too large an initial dose, or too rapid an increase, results in sodium and water retention and thus oedema, weight gain, and carpal tunnel syndrome. There may be changes in glucose metabolism and alterations in cortisol metabolism such that hypopituitary patients taking hydrocortisone may need adjustment of their dose. Hypopituitarism seems to be associated with a reduced incidence of malignancy and there is a theoretical possibility that this might be increased back to normal, particularly as several epidemiological studies have demonstrated serum insulin-like growth factor I to be a risk factor for prostate, breast, and colorectal cancer. These safety issues will be clarified by continual analysis of the on-going long-term surveillance programmes that have been established, although there is no current evidence supporting this theoretical concern.

Craniopharyngiomas

Craniopharyngiomas are rare tumours with an incidence of approximately 1 to 2 per million population, but constitute the commonest intracranial tumour of childhood. They are derived from remnants of Rathke's pouch and as such arise within or above the pituitary fossa. They usually contain both cystic and solid components with the cyst containing oily fluid that is rich in human chorionic gonadotrophin β. Although histologically these tumours are benign, they are often locally invasive with a strong tendency to recur. Their frequent involvement of the hypothalamus, pituitary, and optic pathways means that the clinical symptoms may be severe. Over half the cases occur in childhood when growth failure is the predominant complaint; presenting symptoms in adults include amenorrhoea and decreased libido. Hypothalamic symptoms, which are often most disabling, include obesity, hyperphagia, diabetes insipidus, and disturbances of sleep. In addition, as the tumours tend to be large, symptoms of a space occupying lesion and visual symptoms are common.

A unique feature is the frequent presence of calcification within the tumour, which aids in its diagnosis as it is visible on both skull radiographs and CT scans. MRI is optimal for visualizing the cystic components and for determining the extent of local invasion but does not show the calcification. There exists considerable controversy about the optimal treatment of these tumours. Early series tended to favour radical resection in order to reduce the chances of recurrence. However, such an approach, particularly in childhood, results in considerable damage to the optic apparatus and hypothalamus with an increased mortality and morbidity. Many units now favour the subtotal removal with postoperative irradiation. Recurrence of cysts is often dealt with by drainage and the insertion of yttrium-90 seeds into the cyst cavity.

Lymphocytic hypophysitis

Although not described until 1962, lymphocytic hypophysitis is increasingly recognized as a cause of pituitary dysfunction. It is an autoimmune disease with more than 90 per cent of cases occurring in women, often in relation to pregnancy when it occurs in the late third trimester or puerperium. However, men and patients of any age can be affected. Histologically, the disease is characterized by infiltration of the pituitary by lymphocytes and plasma cells with the formation of follicles containing germinal centres. There is subsequent destruction of the gland and fibrosis. Lymphocytic hypophysitis tends to present in either of two ways. In pregnancy, there is often a rapidly expanding pituitary mass presenting with headaches and visual failure. Alternatively, outside of pregnancy there may be an insidious onset of hypopituitarism. Diabetes insipidus occurs in approximately 10 per cent of cases. The major differential diagnosis is that of Sheehan's syndrome, although it is highly likely that many cases previously ascribed to Sheehan's syndrome were due to hypophysitis. Unlike pituitary adenomas, the destruction of pituitary cells in hypophysitis tends to affect corticotrophs and thyrotrophs predominantly, with deficiency of ACTH and/or thyroid-stimulating hormone occurring in approximately 80 per cent of patients. There are no specific radiological features, with both CT and MRI showing a varying appearance: the pituitary mass may appear hypo- or isointense with variable enhancement. More than 50 per cent show suprasellar extension.

The treatment for this condition is controversial. As there have been numerous reports of spontaneous resolution, particularly during pregnancy, the development of a pituitary mass in the third trimester or puerperium may warrant a conservative approach, although careful monitoring of visual fields is essential. Some endocrinologists familiar with this condition advocate a trial of steroids, although evidence of their efficacy remains anecdotal. Outside of pregnancy, the differential diagnosis of a pituitary mass is broad and trans-sphenoidal surgery is indicated both to remove the mass and to obtain a histological diagnosis. Although it is an autoimmune disease, there are no specific antibodies available for its diagnosis; however, the presence of antithyroid or other organ-specific antibodies is frequent.

Further reading

Carroll PV *et al.* (1998). Growth hormone deficiency in adulthood and the effects of growth hormone replacement: a review. Growth Hormone Research Society Scientific Committee. *Journal of Clinical Endocrinology and Metabolism* **83**, 382–95.

Ezzat S *et al.* (1994). Acromegaly. Clinical and biochemical features in 500 patients. *Medicine (Baltimore)* **73**, 233–40.

Ho KKY (2000). Growth hormone replacement therapy in adults. *Current Opinion in Endocrinology and Diabetes* **7**, 89–95.

Jenkins PJ *et al.* (1995). Lymphocytic hypophysitis: unusual features of a rare disorder. *Clinical Endocrinology* **42**, 529–34.

Jenkins PJ *et al.* (1997). Acromegaly, colonic polyps and carcinoma. *Clinical Endocrinology* **47**, 17–22.

Jenkins PJ *et al.* (2000). IGF-1 and the development of colorectal neoplasia in acromegaly. *Journal of Clinical Endocrinology and Metabolism* **85**, 3218–21.

Orme SM *et al.* (1998). Mortality and cancer incidence in acromegaly: a retrospective cohort study. *Journal of Clinical Endocrinology and Metabolism* **83**, 2730–4.

Trainer PJ, Besser M, eds (1995). *The Bart's endocrine protocols.* Churchill Livingstone, Edinburgh.

Trainer PJ *et al.* (2000). Treatment of acromegaly with the growth hormone-receptor antagonist pegvisomant. *New England Journal of Medicine* **342**, 171–7.

12.3 Disorders of the posterior pituitary

John Newell-Price and Michael Besser

Anatomy

The posterior pituitary lies immediately dorsal and caudal to the anterior pituitary gland and is an extension of the ventral hypothalamus. The major function of the posterior pituitary is the release of the nonapeptide peptide hormones arginine vasopressin (AVP) and oxytocin. These are synthesized in the magnocellular neurones of the supraoptic and paraventricular nuclei of the hypothalamus, and pass by axonal transport, to be stored in nerve endings in the posterior pituitary (Fig. 1). Efferent fibres from these nuclei also project to the median eminence, the brainstem, the floor of the third ventricle, and the spinal cord. Afferent fibres arise from osmoreceptors adjacent to, but separate from, the supraoptic and paraventricular nuclei, probably in the organum vasculosum of the lamina terminalis or subfornicial organ rostrally in the hypothalamus; signals are also received from the brainstem, and from the vagus and glossopharyngeal nerves that receive input from the pharynx and baroreceptors of the heart and great vessels. All these fibres carry the sensory signals modulating AVP and oxytocin release.

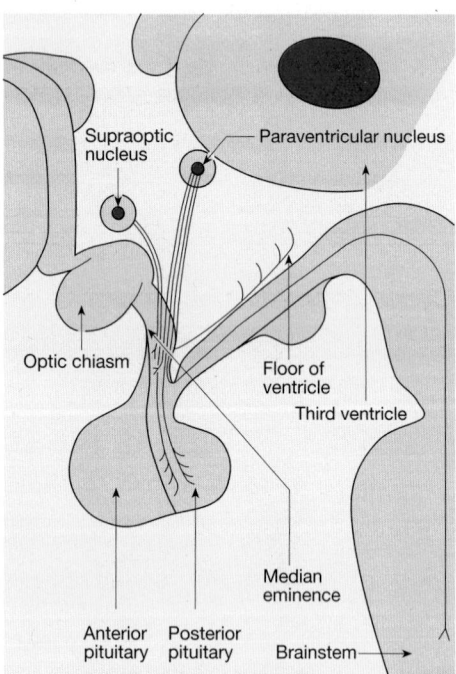

Fig. 1 Schematic representation of the neuronal pathways from the paraventricular and supraoptic nuclei. The nerves project to the posterior pituitary, the median eminence, the floor of the third ventricle, and the brainstem. Afferent fibres from the osmoreceptors and thirst centre are shown. (Reproduced from Besser GM and Thorner MO, 1994, with permission.)

Vasopressin and oxytocin

Vasopressin and oxytocin have molecular weights of 1087 Da and 1007 Da, respectively. The genes for both these hormones are located on chromosome 20q13 in close physical proximity. Each peptide is synthesized as a 145-amino acid precursor comprising a signal peptide, the peptide hormone AVP or oxytocin, and their specific neurophysin—I for oxytocin and II for AVP. The AVP precursor has, in addition, a glycoprotein at the C-terminus. AVP and oxytocin are composed of a six-member disulphide ring with a three-amino acid tail (Fig. 2). The differing amino acids at positions 3 and 8 have a profound effect on the biological action. In the synthesizing nuclei, granules are formed containing the precursor complex of neurophysin and oxytocin or vasopressin. During axonal transport processing cleaves off the active hormone from the neurophysin, and the products are stored in the nerve termini in the posterior pituitary. On firing of the nerves, AVP or oxytocin together with the relevant neurophysin are released into the systemic circulation. Most AVP circulates as free hormone and has a half-life of approximately 10 min. AVP is principally cleared by the liver and kidneys, whilst oxytocin is cleared in these sites and in the uterus.

Arginine vasopressin

Physiology

Actions of arginine vasopressin

At least three distinct receptors, V1a, V1b, and V2, mediate the actions of AVP. Each of these is a member of the superfamily of seven-transmembrane-domain, G-protein-coupled receptors. The first two signal by inositol-phosphate pathways, whilst the V2 receptor activates adenylate cyclase

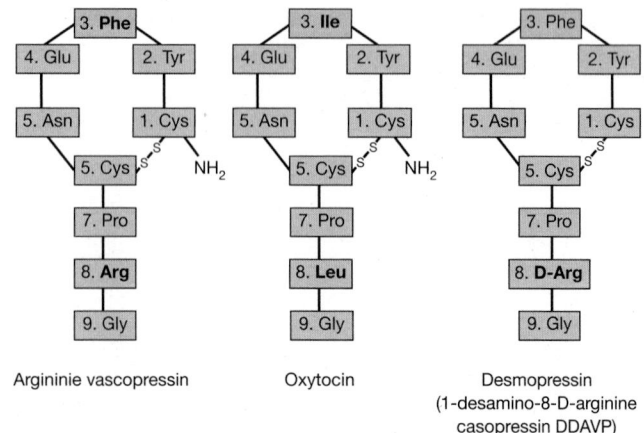

Fig. 2 The structure of vasopressin, oxytocin, and desmopressin. Amino acid differences are highlighted in bold.

with an increase in intracellular cAMP. The V2 receptor is expressed almost exclusively in the collecting tubules of the kidney. When AVP binds to the receptor, an increase in intracellular cAMP results in the insertion of a water-conducting channel (aquaporin 2) into the apical membrane of the collecting duct. This allows water to pass from the lumen of the tubule along a concentration gradient into the cell, and then into the renal interstitium, via the AVP-independent aquaporin channels that are constitutionally active in the basolateral cell membrane, thus accounting for the antidiuretic action of AVP. Activation of the V1a receptor in vascular smooth muscle results in vasoconstriction and increases blood pressure but at much higher blood concentrations. Activation of the V1b receptor in the anterior pituitary, in synergy with corticotropin-releasing hormone (**CRH**), is involved in the release of ACTH, but the vasopressin involved in ACTH release derives predominantly from the paraventricular nuclei and represents a separate neuroanatomical system.

Control of arginine vasopressin secretion
There are three principal stimuli to AVP release—a rise in circulating osmolality, a drop in blood pressure, and a stressful event. An increase in plasma osmolality is sensed in the osmoreceptor cells, and this is the major physiological stimulus to the secretion of AVP. There is a tight linear positive correlation between the plasma osmolality and the release of AVP, and a similar relationship holds between osmolality and thirst, which is probably sensed in a centre distinct from, but adjacent to, the osmoreceptor. A loss of extracellular water will stimulate vasopressin secretion to conserve water, accompanied by thirst and a drive to drink. In combination, these processes maintain the plasma osmolality within the narrow range of 285 to 295 mOsmol/kg (Fig. 3). An increase in the plasma sodium concentration is a greater stimulus to AVP secretion than other solutes, and in humans maximum antidiuresis is achieved at plasma vasopressin concentrations between 2 and 4 pmol/l. After ingestion of fluid, there is a fall in the plasma vasopressin levels before a change in the osmolality, which is presumed to occur via a pharyngeal reflex that inhibits AVP release.

AVP release after a fall in blood pressure, as after haemorrhage, is sensed by baroreceptors in the heart, aorta, and the great vessels. The accompanying water retention helps, together with the sodium retention that follows aldosterone release, to restore the blood volume. AVP is also released under non-specific stress, particularly if associated with nausea or vomiting.

Disorders of arginine vasopressin secretion

Diabetes insipidus
Polyuria with dilute urine may result from vasopressin deficiency (cranial diabetes insipidus, **DI**), resistance to the actions of AVP (nephrogenic DI), and excessive fluid drinking (primary polydipsia). The causes of diabetes insipidus are shown in Table 1. Simple destruction or removal of the posterior pituitary gland, or damage to the distal part of the pituitary stalk, usually results in a temporary DI lasting for 6 weeks to 6 months, since the proximal nerve endings grow out to find systemic capillaries in any scar formed and begin direct secretion again. Upper stalk, median eminence, or more extreme hypothalamic damage results in permanent diabetes insipidus.

An individual deficient in AVP will pass approximately 40 ml/kg of urine in 24 h (between 3 and 20 litres), leading to the clinical features of polyuria, polydipsia, nocturia, and in children nocturnal enuresis. In the complete absence of AVP the maximally dilute urine has an osmolality of approximately 50 mOsmol/kg. As long as there is free access to water, normovolaemia and normonatraemia are maintained by an intact thirst centre. Glucocorticoids are necessary for adequate free-water clearance by the kidneys. Thus if there is a coexistent ACTH deficiency because of a hypothalamic or pituitary lesion, diabetes insipidus may not become manifest until the institution of corticosteroid replacement therapy. It the thirst centre is destroyed as part of the hypothalamic lesion, dangerous dehydration may ensue.

Familial causes are very rare and have been documented as being due to mutations in either the gene encoding the signal peptide or neurophysin molecule, but not of the gene for the AVP peptide itself. Interestingly, symptoms are not usually present at birth but gradually develop between 1 and 6 years of age. It is hypothesized that the changes resulting from such mutations interfere with correct protein folding, and cause retention of a mutant peptide within the neurones which then undergo degeneration, with diabetes insipidus becoming manifest when approximately 80 per cent have been destroyed. Diabetes insipidus is very rarely a presenting feature of an anterior pituitary tumour, although it is frequent after surgical treatment. Therefore, if DI is present at diagnosis of a pituitary mass lesion this should alert the clinician to possible primary hypothalamic lesions such as craniopharyngioma or germinoma.

Differential diagnosis of diabetes insipidus
In a normal individual the plasma osmolality will range from 285 to 295 mOsmol/kg, but urine can be concentrated to more than twice the concentration of plasma. Significant diabetes insipidus is excluded if the urine to plasma (U:P) osmolality ratio is more than 2 to 1, provided that the plasma osmolality is no greater than 295 mOsmol/kg. In diabetes insipidus, despite

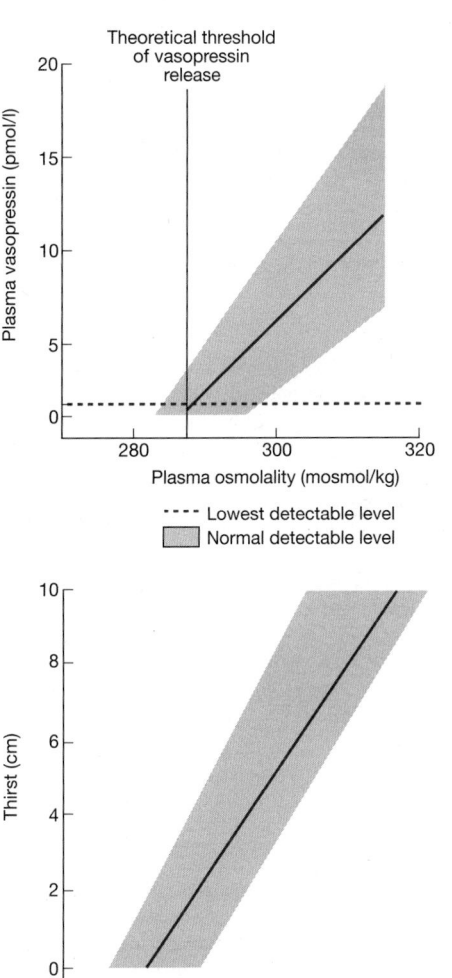

Fig. 3 The relationship between plasma osmolality and plasma arginine vasopressin concentration, and between plasma osmolality and thirst. AVP concentrations and thirst sensation rise in a linear fashion in relation to plasma osmolality. (Reproduced from Besser GM and Thorner MO, 1994, with permission.)

Table 1 Causes of diabetes insipidus

Cranial diabetes insipidus

Acquired

Idiopathic (30 per cent of all cases of cranial diabetes insipidus)
Tumours (craniopharyngioma, germinoma, metastases to pituitary and
 hypothalamus)
Trauma
Cerebral hypoxia
Infections (bacterial and tuberculous meningitis, encephalitis, congenital
 cytomegalovirus, toxoplasmosis)
Vascular (aneurysm, arteriovenous malformations, infarction)
Granuloma (neurosarcoid, Langerhan's histiocytosis)
Lymphocytic hypophysitis

Familial

Autosomal dominant
Rarely autosomal recessive
DIDMOAD* syndrome

Nephrogenic diabetes insipidus

Acquired

Osmotic diuresis (diabetes mellitus)
Drugs (lithium, demeclocycline, tetracycline)
Chronic renal failure
Postobstructive uropathy
Metabolic (hypercalcaemia, hypokalaemia)
Infiltrative (amyloid)

Familial

X-linked (V2-receptor defect)
Autosomal recessive (aquaporin-2 defect)

*DIDMOAD; diabetes insipidus, diabetes mellitus, optic atrophy, deafness.

the raised plasma osmolality, the urine is inappropriately dilute with a U:P ratio below 2. Any cause of polyuria will give a relative resistance to the actions of AVP since the renal medullary concentrating gradient will be washed out. Furthermore, hypercalcaemia or hypokalaemia cause resistance to the actions of vasopressin, possibly by decreasing the level of cAMP within renal tubular cells. The commonest investigation used to discriminate normality from the various causes of diabetes insipidus is the water-deprivation test (Table 2).

There are no contraindications to this test in the fully hydrated patient. Before the test can be performed and adequately interpreted both the thy-

Table 2 Water-deprivation test

Preparation
- Fluids given freely until 07.30 h on the morning of the test
- Light breakfast at 06.30 h, no tea, coffee, or smoking

Fluid deprivation
- No fluid for 8 h from 07.30 h (dry snacks allowed)
- Weigh the patient at 0, 4, 6, 7, 8 h
- Plasma and urine osmolality measured on an hourly basis
- If >3 per cent of body weight lost, immediately measure plasma osmolality, and if this is >305 mOsmol/kg then give desmopressin 2 µg intramuscularly and allow the patient to drink
- At 8-h fluid deprivation: if urine output is not decreased, the U:P ratio <2, and plasma osmolality is not concentrated, continue water deprivation for a further 1 h

Response to desmopressin
- At the end of the water-deprivation period give desmopressin 2 µg intramuscularly
- Collect urine samples hourly for 4 h, but allow free fluids

roid function and adrenal reserve must be normal, or the patient must be on replacement therapy. Impaired renal function, hypercalcaemia, and hypokalaemia need to be excluded. It is important that covert drinking is avoided and that the individual is continuously monitored to prevent severe dehydration. The patient is allowed free access to water overnight to avoid dehydration and the test is started in the morning. Drinking is not allowed for 8 h. Urine and plasma osmolality are followed and close adherence to a defined protocol is essential for safety (Table 2).

Interpretation of the water-deprivation test A normal response is for the urine volume to gradually fall with fluid deprivation, with a increase in osmolality and a U:P osmolality ratio above 2 towards the end of the test; but the plasma osmolality should remain below 295 mOsmol/kg. In cranial diabetes insipidus there is little rise in urine osmolality, the U:P ratio is less than 2, and frequently the plasma osmolality rises above 295 mOsmol/kg. However, following desmopressin the urine concentrates normally, whereas in nephrogenic diabetes insipidus there is no rise in urine osmolality following desmopressin. Primary polydipsia often gives results that are difficult to interpret since the patient may be water-overloaded at the start of the test, and in addition has a decreased medullary concentrating gradient in the kidney. The combination of these two factors often results in U:P ratios of less than 2 at the end of the test and with a plasma osmolality of less than 285 mOsmol/kg, the threshold for AVP secretion.

In circumstances where the plasma osmolality does not rise above 295 mOsmol/kg, it is still possible that vasopressin secretion is abnormal despite a U:P ratio above 2. Unfortunately this may occur in mild cases of cranial and nephrogenic diabetes insipidus (DI), and in primary polydipsia causing diagnostic confusion. One excellent means to further investigate these patients is to give a 5 per cent hypertonic saline infusion and then measure plasma AVP levels; patients with cranial DI will demonstrate low levels of AVP, whilst the levels of AVP will be increased in those with nephrogenic DI. However, AVP is only measured in a few centres and an alternative is an extended water-deprivation test.

The extended water-deprivation test may be performed in mild cases and if the results from the standard water-deprivation test are equivocal. This is similar to the standard test except that the patient starts somewhat dehydrated, avoiding drinking from 18.00 h the day before the test, which is then started the next morning. Water deprivation is continued until the urine osmolality reaches a plateau (less than 30 mOsmol/kg increase between three consecutive samples), and then desmopressin 2 µg intramuscular is given and the patient allowed to drink. In normal subjects, endogenous AVP secretion under these circumstances is sufficient to maximally concentrate the urine so that no further increase in osmolality is seen after desmopressin. A urine osmolality rise of 9 per cent or more after desmopressin suggests partial cranial DI. Primary polydipsia is suggested when urine concentrates normally if the plasma osmolality rises above 290 mOsmol/kg before desmopressin, with no further rise following desmopressin in the presence of polydipsia and polyuria.

Treatment of cranial diabetes insipidus

Desmopressin is a synthetic analogue of AVP with high selectivity for the V2 receptor and a prolonged half-life, giving it profound antidiuretic properties and, at antidiuretic doses, little pressor activity. In adults the normal daily dose by intranasal spray is between 10 and 40 µg in divided doses. It is essential to instruct the patient carefully in the administration of the spray so that it may be adequately absorbed from the olfactory mucosa. Oral preparations allow for easier administration, but variability in the bioavailability between patients means that the oral dose may range between 100 and 600 µg daily (and occasionally more) in divided doses. In the perioperative period, or in critically ill patients, it may be necessary to administer desmopressin parenterally at doses of between 1 and 4 µg daily. The main side-effect is hyponatraemia if excess fluid is ingested or administered. Patients should be encouraged to drink only in response to their thirst to avoid water intoxication. All other pharmaceutical treatments are inferior.

Individuals with cranial diabetes insipidus and an intact thirst centre usually do not present particular management problems. However, in the presence of destructive hypothalamic lesions the thirst centre may also be damaged and management of water balance is frequently difficult. In adipsic patients this is best achieved by setting a fixed dose of desmopressin and weighing them when they are normovolaemic. These individuals will then need to be instructed to maintain their daily weight by drinking, taking into account insensible losses, and in hotter climates this may involve twice-daily weighing. In some circumstances, an automated audible reminder to drink may be necessary if hypothalamic damage has affected the patient's memory.

Nephrogenic diabetes insipidus

Nephrogenic diabetes insipidus has diverse causes (Table 1). Congenital nephrogenic diabetes insipidus typically presents with profound polyuria and hypernatraemia from birth, in contrast to congenital cranial diabetes insipidus. The condition needs urgent recognition since repeated episodes of hypernatraemia with polyuria, vomiting, constipation, fever, irritability, and a failure to thrive may result in long-term cognitive impairment. The drive to drink may impair eating and lead to delayed growth. The X-linked condition is associated with mutations of the V2 receptor, whilst in autosomal recessive disease there is deficiency of aquaporin. Other than direct mutational analysis, infusion of desmopressin may allow discrimination between the two types: in the autosomal recessive condition there will be an increase in blood pressure, and in circulating Von Willebrand factor and factor 8 to two to threefold the basal level. As these effects are dependent on intact V2 receptor signalling they will not be seen in the X-linked form.

Treatment of nephrogenic diabetes insipidus Drugs such as lithium should be withdrawn if possible. Thiazide diuretics reduce the urine output by enhancing sodium excretion to the expense of water and decreasing glomerular filtration rate. Amiloride may need to be coadministered to avoid hypokalaemia. Cyclo-oxgenase inhibitors such as indometacin may also be of benefit.

Syndrome of inappropriate antidiuresis (SIADH)

Excessive and inappropriate secretion of vasopressin either from the posterior pituitary or from ectopic sources, such as small-cell lung cancer, results in inappropriately concentrated urine, dilute plasma, and hyponatraemia with continuing renal sodium excretion. Since there are many causes of hyponatraemia the diagnosis of SIADH should only be entertained in the absence of oedema-forming states, hypovolaemia, or hypotension, and when renal and adrenal function are normal (Table 3). Typically, the condition is asymptomatic during the initial stages, especially if the fall in the serum sodium level is slow. Rapid onset of hyponatraemia is associated with confusion, drowsiness, convulsions, coma, and death. Symptoms are uncommon until the serum sodium falls to 120 mmol/l or less, or the plasma osmolality drops below 268 mOsmol/kg. In cases where vasopressin is secreted from an ectopic source, such as small-cell lung cancer, there is a complete disassociation of the concentration of plasma vasopressin from plasma osmolality. In contrast, in certain central nervous system conditions vasopressin is secreted in a regulated fashion but inappropriately at a low plasma osmolality. This is in keeping with an osmostat that is set at a lower level. Pragmatically, however, the management of the metabolic disturbance is the same whatever the cause. States associated with sodium depletion must be excluded. The urinary sodium concentration will be very low in patients with a low body sodium concentration, unless they are on diuretics, whereas it will be normal or high in those with SIADH.

Table 3 Causes of the syndrome of inappropriate antidiuresis (SIADH)

Central nervous system disorders	Tumours
Head injury	Carcinoma (especially
Meningitis	lung)
Encephalitis	Lymphoma
Brain tumour	Leukaemia
Brain abscess	Thymoma
Cerebral haemorrhage/thrombosis	Sarcoma
Guillain–Barré syndrome	Mesothelioma
Acute intermittent porphyria	
Respiratory causes	**Drugs**
Pneumonia	Carbamazepine, clofibrate,
Tuberculosis	chlorpropamide,
Emphysema	thiazides, phenothiazines,
Severe asthma	monoamine
Pneumothorax	oxidase inhibitors
Positive-pressure ventilation	(MAOIs), selective
	serotonin-reuptake
Miscellaneous	inhibitors (SSRIs),
Idiopathic	cytotoxics, desmopressin,
Acute psychosis	vasopressin, oxytocin,
	lansoprazole

Management of the syndrome of inappropriate antidiuresis

It is clear that the underlying cause will require treatment on its own merits. Fluid restriction is the cornerstone of treatment: Fluid restriction to between 500 and 750 ml/24h usually reverses any adverse clinical features and restores the circulating sodium level and osmolality to normal. The use of hypertonic saline infusions is very rarely required and only if severe drowsiness or convulsions are experienced, which are unresponsive to fluid restriction and if the serum sodium is around 100 mmol/l. Hypertonic saline should only be administered under close supervision to avoid rapid increases in the plasma sodium concentration and the risk of central pontine myelinolysis. The plasma sodium concentration should rise by no more than 0.5 mmol/l per hour. Drugs such as demeclocycline, which induce nephrogenic diabetes insipidus, may be helpful but the effects are often short lasting.

Oxytocin

Actions of oxytocin

Oxytocin binds to its specific cell-surface receptor expressed predominantly in the myometrial cells of the uterus and breast, and the ductal and epithelial cells of the breast. Expression of the receptor is increased by oestrogen, and receptor numbers increase during pregnancy. In the gravid uterus the myometrial cells are probably maintained in a tonic state of relaxation by the levels of cAMP induced by the actions of placental corticotropin-releasing hormone (CRH). The oxytocin receptor signals via phospholipase C; an increase in intracellular calcium causes phosphorylation of the CRH receptor, resulting in its desensitization and decoupling of CRH receptor signalling. The combined effect of these processes is to stimulate myometrial contraction. This is utilized in obstetric practice where infusions of synthetic oxytocin are used to initiate and sustain labour.

Control of oxytocin secretion

Cervical distension causes the release of oxytocin, which may be involved in the onset of parturition in the human as it is in lower species. In lactating women the release of oxytocin is stimulated by suckling, which then causes contraction of the myoepithelial cells within the breast alveoli and milk ejection.

Further reading

Baylis PH, Thompson CJ (1988). Osmoregulation of vasopressin secretion and thirst in health and disease. *Clinical Endocrinology (Oxford)* **29**, 549–76.

Baylis PH (1994). The posterior pituitary. In: Besser GM, Thorner MO, eds. *Clinical Endocrinology*, pp 5.1–5.14. Mosby-Wolfe, London.

Fujiwara TM, Morgan K, Bichet DG (1995). Molecular biology of diabetes insipidus. *Annual Review of Medicine* **46**, 331–43.

Moses AM, Notman DD (1982). Diabetes insipidus and syndrome of inappropriate antidiuretic hormone secretion (SIADH). *Advances in Internal Medicine* **27**, 73–100.

Oksche A, Rosenthal W (1998). The molecular basis of nephrogenic diabetes insipidus. *Journal of Molecular Medicine* **76**, 326–37.

Thompson CJ, *et al.* (1986). The osmotic thresholds for thirst and vasopressin release are similar in healthy man. *Clinical Science* **71**, 651–6.

Trainer PJ, Besser GM (1995). *The Barts endocrine protocols*. Churchill Livingstone, London.

12.4 The thyroid gland and disorders of thyroid function

Anthony P. Weetman

Structure of the thyroid gland

Development

The human thyroid develops as a diverticulum in the pharyngeal floor around 3 weeks of gestation. This median anlage moves caudally, remaining connected to the pharynx via the thyroglossal duct, which subsequently is obliterated when the thyroid begins to expand as two distinct lobes, around 2 months of gestation. The foramen caecum marks the point in the tongue where the thyroid develops and there is sometimes an upward extension of thyroid tissue from the isthmus, the pyramidal lobe, arising from the lower part of the thyroglossal duct. At the same time, the lateral anlage ultimobranchial bodies, derived from the fifth branchial pouches, fuse with the developing thyroid to which they contribute the parafollicular calcitonin-secreting clear (C) cells. Synthesis of thyroid hormone begins at week 11, at the same time as thyroid stimulating hormone (TSH) production by the pituitary. There is significant maternal-to-fetal thyroxine (T4) transfer so that babies with no endogenous thyroid hormone production are nonetheless largely protected from the adverse effects of fetal hypothyroidism on development of the brain, lung, and skeleton. Preterm infants of less than 27 weeks gestation have immature thyroid function and their neurological development may be improved by temporary thyroxine supplementation.

Anatomy and histology

The adult thyroid weighs 15 to 20 g and each lobe is around 4 cm in length and 2 cm in width, although the right lobe is often larger than the left. The isthmus connecting the two lobes lies just below the cricoid cartilage. The blood supply on each side is derived from the external carotid artery via the superior thyroid artery and from the subclavian artery via the inferior thyroid artery. There is adrenergic and cholinergic innervation which regulates blood flow. The thyroid is attached to the trachea by connective tissue and the recurrent laryngeal nerves lie between the trachea and the posterior aspect of the lobes.

The gland is made up of lobules, each comprising 20 to 40 spherical follicles. The follicles vary considerably in size, but average 200 μm in diameter, and are made up of a single layer of thyroid follicular epithelial cells (Fig. 1). The cells are cuboidal when quiescent and columnar when active, and have a microvillous apical membrane. The follicular lumen contains colloid, the principal constituent of which is the glycoprotein thyroglobulin, secreted by the thyroid cells. Each follicle is surrounded by a rich capillary network. C cells lie scattered between follicular epithelial cells or in the interstitium, and account for around 1 per cent of the epithelial mass.

Thyroid hormone synthesis and metabolism

Synthesis and secretion

Thyroid hormone synthesis requires iodide uptake and oxidation, iodination of certain tyrosine molecules on thyroglobulin, and coupling of the iodotyrosines to form the thyroid hormones triiodothyronine (T3) and T4 (Fig. 2). Iodide is actively transported into the thyroid cell by the Na$^+$/I$^-$ symporter, which is also expressed in breast tissue and the salivary glands. Perchlorate, thiocyanate, and pertechnetate are also transported by the same symporter and these anions can competitively inhibit iodide uptake. The recommended daily intake of iodine is 150 μg for adults (200 μg during pregnancy) but there is wide variation in actual intake, with many countries having borderline or frankly deficient intakes of less than 50 to 100 μg, while in Western Europe and North America intake is excessive (up to 750 μg/day).

Iodide is oxidized by thyroid peroxidase, a haem-containing enzyme located at the apical border of the thyroid cell, and is rapidly incorporated into tyrosine residues to form monoiodotyrosine and diiodotyrosine. Thyroid peroxidase is also responsible for the coupling of these iodotyrosines, with different sites in the thyroglobulin molecule being responsible for the formation of T3 or T4. Normally, each thyroglobulin molecule contains 3 to 4 T4 molecules, but only 20 per cent of thyroglobulin molecules contain a T3 molecule. Thyroglobulin acts as slow turnover reservoir for thyroid hormone, thus ensuring maximum use is made of often scarce dietary iodine. Around a 7-week supply of T4 is contained in the normal thyroid. Thyroid hormone is released from the gland after endocytosis of colloid and lysosomal hydrolysis of the thyroglobulin to yield T4 and T3, which are secreted from the basal membrane into the capillaries in a ratio of 10:1. Released iodotyrosines are deiodinated for iodide recycling.

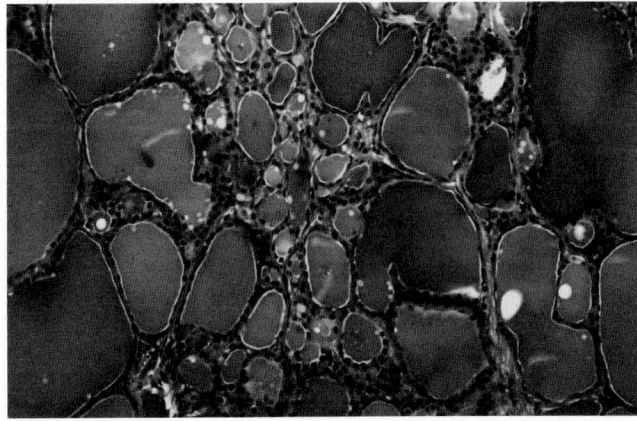

Fig. 1 Photomicrograph showing the histology of a normal thyroid. Thyroid epithelial cells are arranged in follicles containing colloid. (Original magnification ×200; photomicrograph by courtesy of Dr K. Suvarna.)

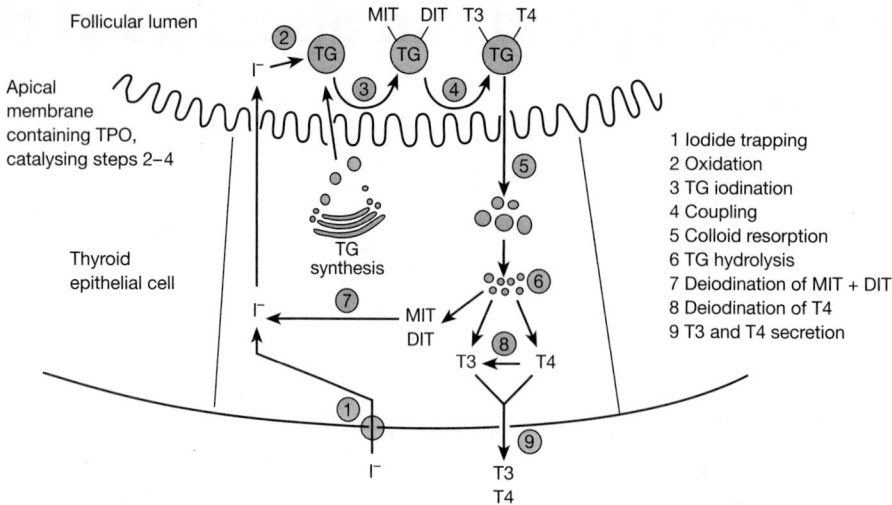

Fig. 2 Steps in the synthesis of thyroid hormones. TG = thyroglobulin, TPO = thyroid peroxidase, MIT = monoiodotyrosine, DIT = diiodotyrosine.

Thyroid hormone transport

Up to 90 per cent of the total T3 in the circulation is derived from peripheral conversion of T4 to T3 by deiodinase enzymes (see below) rather than thyroid secretion. Only 0.03 per cent of T4 and 0.3 per cent of T3 in the circulation exist as free hormone, able to diffuse into tissues. The remainder is protein bound. T4 binds predominantly to thyroxine-binding globulin, and to a lesser extent to transthyretin (or prealbumin); a little is bound to albumin. T3 binds to thyroxine-binding globulin and albumin, with little bound to transthyretin. Alteration in the concentration or binding capacity of thyroid hormone binding proteins can produce major changes in total but not free thyroid hormone levels (Table 1).

Metabolism of thyroid hormone

The half-life of T4 in the circulation is 7 days, contrasting with the much shorter half-life of T3 (24 h). The most important metabolic pathway for T4 is outer ring (5') deiodination to T3 (Fig. 3). This is catalysed by type 1 and 2 deiodinase, while type 3 deiodinase catalyses inner ring (5) deiodination leading to hormone inactivation. Type 1 deiodinase can also catalyse inner ring deiodination of T3 and T4. All three enzymes have a selenocysteine moiety as the active catalytic site. Type 1 deiodinase is expressed predominantly in the liver, kidney, thyroid, and brain, type 2 in the pituitary, brain, placenta, skeletal muscle, and heart (tissues critically dependent on thyroid hormone for development or function), and type 3 in the brain,

Table 1 Conditions in which there is altered binding of thyroid hormones to binding proteins

Thyroxine-binding globulin (TBG)	
Increased binding	Genetic variation in TBG
	Oestrogens (pregnancy, oral contraception, hormone replacement therapy, tamoxifen)
	Other drugs (perphenazine, opiates, 5-fluorouracil, clofibrate, mitotane)
	Hepatitis, cirrhosis
	Acute intermittent porphyria
Decreased binding	Genetic variation in TBG
	Steroids (testosterone, anabolic steroids, glucocorticoids)
	Acromegaly
	Nephrotic syndrome
	Protein malnutrition
	Acute severe illness
	L-Asparaginase
Albumin	
Decreased binding	Any cause of hypoalbuminaemia
Increased binding	Genetic variation
Tranthyretin	
Increased binding	Genetic variation
Competition for binding sites	
Drugs	Phenytoin
	Carbamazepine
	Salicylates and non-steroidal anti-inflammatory drugs
Non-esterified fatty acids	

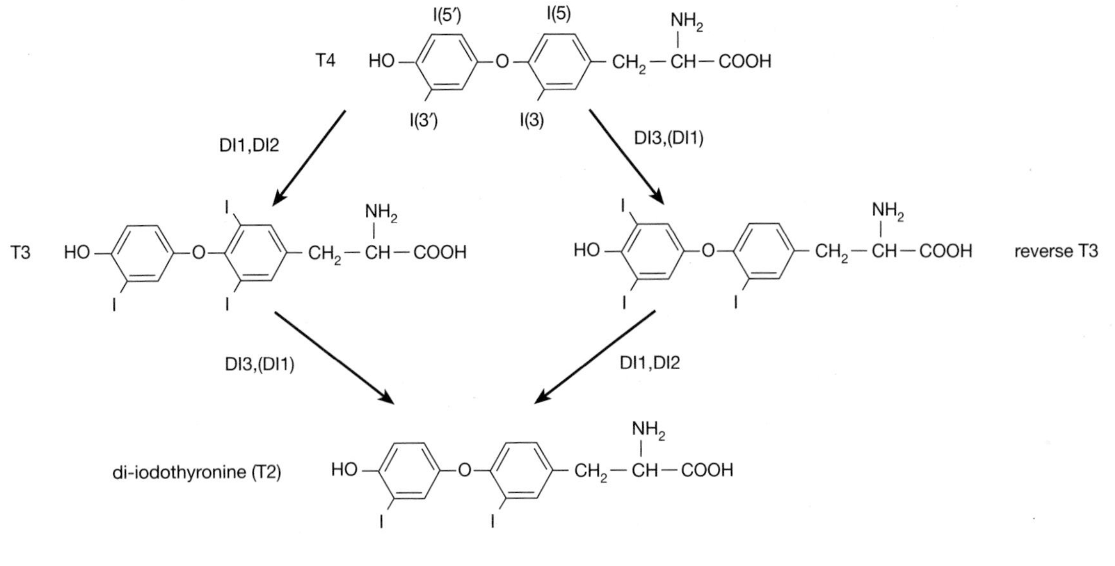

Fig. 3 Main deiodination pathway for thyroid hormones. DI = deiodinase enzyme; parentheses denote a minor contribution. Deiodination of T3 also yields 3,5-T2 and deiodination of reverse T3 also yields 3',5'-T2. T2 is further deiodinated to monoiodothyronine and thyronine.

placenta, and skin. The type 1 deiodinase is largely responsible for the generation of circulating T3 from T4, whereas T3 generated by the type 2 enzyme mainly provides intracellular T3 at specific sites.

Around 40 per cent of T4 is metabolized to T3 and 40 per cent is converted to reverse T3 by the type 3 deiodinase. This same enzyme is responsible for the main metabolic pathway for T3 which is converted to 3,3'-dioiodothyronine. Starvation, trauma, and drugs (propylthiouracil, amiodarone, glucocorticoids, propranolol) impair T4 to T3 conversion and must be borne in mind in interpreting tests of thyroid function (see below). In addition to deiodination, a small proportion of thyroid hormone is metabolized by conjugation of the phenolic hydroxyl group with sulphate or glucuronic acid, which increases water solubility and allows urinary and biliary excretion. Biliary iodothyronine glucuronides can be reabsorbed, constituting an enterohepatic cycle.

Thyroid hormone action

Thyroid hormone acts as a transcription regulatory factor, mediated by T3 binding to nuclear receptor isoforms which belong to the same superfamily as steroid and retinoic acid receptors. All such receptors possess a conserved DNA-binding domain, containing two zinc fingers which interact with specific DNA response elements, and a hormone-binding domain. Alternative splicing results in two pairs of thyroid hormone receptor (Fig. 4) whose tissue expression varies during development. Thyroid hormone receptors bind to DNA as homodimers or heterodimers (with the retinoid X receptor). Without ligand, basal gene transcription is inhibited by a corepressor. When T3 binds, homodimers dissociate, releasing corepressor and allowing gene transcription; the stable heterodimer binds coactivators in the presence of T3 with the same outcome. The α2 thyroid hormone receptor does not bind T3 and may act as a natural inhibitor of receptor activity. Knockout mice devoid of all known thyroid hormone receptors have an abnormal pituitary–thyroid axis and impaired growth and bone maturation, but not the severe manifestations of complete hypothyroidism, indicating the potential for other mechanisms of thyroid hormone action.

Regulation of thyroid function

The main regulator of thyroid function is TSH (thyrotropin), secreted by thyrotrophs in the anterior pituitary in response to the tripeptide thyrotropin-releasing hormone (TRH), derived from the hypothalamic supraoptic and paraventricular nuclei. Thyroid hormones exert a classical negative feedback effect on thyrotrophs; the acute effect is mediated by T3 in the

pituitary which is derived from T4 by type 2 deiodination. Thyroid hormones also inhibit hypothalamic TRH synthesis. TRH-stimulated TSH secretion is inhibited by dopamine and somatostatin, while α-adrenergic activation stimulates TSH release. Cytokines, particularly interleukin-1, interleukin-6, and tumour necrosis factor, inhibit TSH synthesis and may be responsible for the suppression of TSH seen in severe illness.

Within the thyroid, TSH binds to the G protein-coupled TSH receptor, leading to intracellular signalling predominantly via cyclic AMP. TSH increases iodide transport and organification, endocytosis of colloid and thyroid hormone secretion, as well as thyroid follicular epithelial cell division. Autoregulatory mechanisms can modulate thyroid function when TSH levels are constant. The most important is iodine intake. Increased iodide transport transiently decreases organification and reduces thyroid hormone synthesis (the Wolff–Chaikoff effect); after several weeks under normal conditions, the thyroid escapes and resumes hormone production. Sudden increases in iodine intake can also block thyroid hormone release acutely. In iodine deficiency, thyroid hormone production is switched to preferential T3 synthesis, but this effect is largely TSH-mediated rather than autoregulatory.

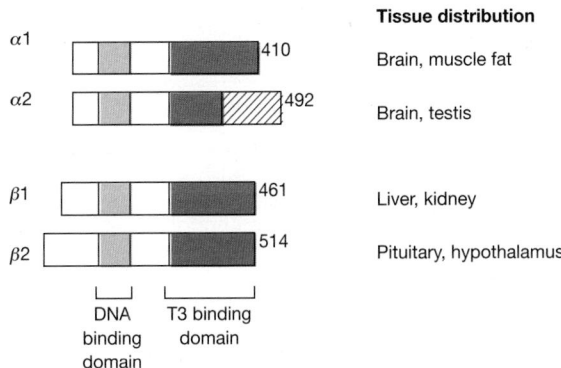

Fig. 4 Structure of the thyroid hormone receptors. The numbers indicate the amino acid content. Homologous areas are shaded; the lack of homology in the T3-binding domain of the α2 receptor (hatched area) prevents T3 binding and the function of this receptor is unknown.

Laboratory investigation of thyroid function

Determining thyroid status

The introduction of sensitive immunoradiometric assays for circulating TSH, with a detection level of 0.1 mU/l or less, has transformed the evaluation of thyroid status. A normal TSH level rules out primary thyroid dysfunction. Low levels of thyroid hormones elevate TSH as a result of negative feedback, while excessive thyroid hormone suppresses TSH. The TRH test for detecting low TSH levels is now redundant. Besides primary thyroid disorders, other conditions may alter TSH levels and must be borne in mind when using TSH as a screening test for thyroid dysfunction (Table 2), as must the possibility of secondary (pituitary or hypothalamic) disturbances of thyroid function.

It is therefore essential to confirm thyroid status when TSH levels are abnormal, or when pituitary or hypothalamic abnormalities are possible, by measuring circulating thyroid hormone levels. Methods which measure total T3 or T4 are prone to artefacts caused by abnormal thyroid hormone binding (Table 1), although in the absence of such abnormalities these tests are reliable. When altered binding is suspected or found, compensation can be made by calculation of the free T3 or free T4 index. These indices are derived from the total hormone levels and measurement of the differential distribution of radiolabelled T3 between unoccupied protein binding sites in the sample and an absorbent resin (hence the term resin uptake test). Thyroxine-binding globulin levels can also be measured directly.

However, the ready availability of immunoassays for free T3 and free T4 has generally supplanted these methods. The immunoassays rely on the ability of a radiolabelled thyroid hormone analogue to bind to thyroid hormone antibody but not to plasma binding proteins. The analogue then competes for antibody binding with the free thyroid hormone in the sample. Despite initial concerns about the theoretical basis and performance of such assays, recent improvements allow generally reliable estimation of free thyroid hormones. In cases of doubt, free hormone levels can be measured by physical separation from bound hormone, using ultracentrifugation or equilibrium dialysis.

Several indirect methods can be used to determine thyroid status. The thyroidal uptake of radioiodine (^{123}I, ^{131}I) or ^{99m}Tc-pertechnetate is increased in hyperthyroidism and decreased in hypothyroidism, but can be affected by excessive dietary iodine and destructive processes in the thyroid,

so that uptake is low when the patient is thyrotoxic (see Destructive thyroiditis below). Serum thyroglobulin is raised in hyperthyroidism of all types but is also raised in destructive thyroiditis and thyroid cancer. Its main role in investigation is follow-up of treated thyroid cancer (see Chapter 12.5). A number of non-specific tests have also been used to determine end organ responses to thyroid hormones, including basal metabolic rate, tendon relaxation time, and serum levels of cholesterol, ferritin, sex hormone-binding globulin, and liver enzymes.

Thyroid function in non-thyroidal illness and pregnancy

Assessing thyroid function in severely ill patients often reveals abnormalities termed the sick euthyroid syndrome. Many of the changes are due to cytokine release, but therapeutic agents such as dopamine and glucocorticoids also contribute, as do unknown factors. Any major, acute illness or starvation can result in a decrease in circulating T3 (total and free) with normal levels of T4 and TSH. Reverse T3 levels rise. The severity of the illness correlates with the magnitude of the fall in T3, and in very sick patients total T4 levels also fall. Analogue-based free T4 assays generally produce normal results but sometimes high or low values occur. In 10 to 15 per cent of sick individuals, TSH levels are abnormal (raised or lowered). Psychiatric illness can be associated with raised total and free T4 levels with normal T3.

There is no proven benefit from thyroid hormone administration in the sick euthyroid syndrome and the hormone changes may be protective, limiting catabolism (although this view is regularly challenged). The importance of these alterations lies in their potential to cause diagnostic confusion. Thyroid function tests should only be requested in ill patients when thyroid disease is genuinely suspected. Abnormal thyroid function tests due to the sick euthyroid syndrome return to normal after recovery and therefore repetition of testing is the simplest way to confirm the reason for unusual results.

Pregnancy also affects thyroid function testing. The most obvious change is the rise in thyroxine binding globulin, which elevates total but not free T3 and T4 levels. In addition, the reference ranges for free T3 and T4 are higher than normal in the first half of pregnancy, because placental human chorionic gonadotropin (hCG), at high levels, acts as a weak stimulator of the TSH receptor. There is a reciprocal fall in TSH levels during the first trimester, but TSH returns to normal in the second trimester as hCG

Table 2 Causes of abnormal serum TSH concentrations

Raised TSH	Free thyroid hormone levels
Overt hypothyroidism	↓
Subclinical hypothyroidism	N
Sick euthyroid syndrome	↓ or N
Dopamine antagonists (acute effect)	N
TSH-secreting pituitary adenoma	↑
Thyroid hormone resistance syndrome	↑
Adrenal insufficiency	↓ or N
Lowered TSH	
Overt thyrotoxicosis	↑
Subclinical thyrotoxicosis	N
Recently treated hyperthyroidism	N
Thyroid-associated ophthalmopathy without Graves' disease	N
Excessive thyroxine treatment	N or ↑
Sick euthyroid syndrome	↓ or N
First trimester of pregnancy	N or ↑
Pituitary or hypothalamic disease	N or ↓
Anorexia nervosa	N or ↓
Dopamine, somatostatin (acute effect)	N
Glucocorticoids	N

N = normal, ↑ = increased, ↓ = decreased.

levels decline. Occasionally, these changes are sufficient to cause transient 'gestational' hyperthyroidism, associated with hyperemesis gravidarum. Antithyroid drugs are usually unnecessary in this condition, and attention should be directed to controlling the vomiting and giving parenteral fluids. Renal clearance of iodine is increased in pregnancy, leading to maternal and neonatal goitre and mild hypothyroidism in areas where iodine intake is marginal (50 µg/day). These complications can be prevented by supplemental iodine, 150 to 200 µg/day.

Determining the cause of thyroid dysfunction

The most frequent cause of thyroid dysfunction in iodine-sufficient areas is autoimmunity and the simplest test for this is measurement of thyroid autoantibodies, particularly those directed against thyroid peroxidase (the 'microsomal' antigen). Antibodies against thyroglobulin are also easily measured but are almost always accompanied by thyroid peroxidase antibodies, so testing for the latter alone is usually adequate. Different methods, including haemagglutination, immunofluorescence, radioimmunoassay, and enzyme-linked immunosorbent assay, give different prevalence rates for thyroid autoantibodies. Almost all patients with autoimmune hypothyroidism, and around 75 per cent with Graves' disease, have thyroid peroxidase antibodies. Generally lower levels are found in 5 to 15 per cent of healthy women and 2 per cent of men, and in slightly higher proportions of patients with nodular goitre and thyroid cancer, and results therefore need to be interpreted carefully. Individuals with positive thyroid autoantibodies but normal thyroid function are at increased risk of developing autoimmune hypothyroidism (around 2 per cent per year).

Thyroid imaging by scintiscanning is useful in determining the aetiology of thyroid disease when this is not obvious clinically, particularly in hyperthyroidism and ectopic thyroid tissue. Its role in the evaluation of a solitary thyroid nodule is considered in Chapter 12.5. ⁹⁹ᵐTc is usually used as it has a short half life (6 h) which allows safe administration of high activity and rapid scanning. ¹²³I is not as readily available but is also preferable to ¹³¹I, especially in children, as it too has a short half life and does not emit beta radiation. ¹³¹I imaging is particularly useful in planning treatment of thyroid cancer and localization of metastases. The place of ultrasound imaging is less clear. The technique allows accurate determination of thyroid size, which may be useful in follow-up of goitre, and can help to determine the nature of an atypical neck mass. Its role in evaluating nodular thyroid disease is considered in Chapter 12.5. CT scanning is particularly valuable in determining the extent of a retrosternal goitre and assessing tracheal compression (Fig. 5). In contrast, a standard chest radiograph can be misleading in evaluating tracheal compression, particularly in the anterior–posterior plane.

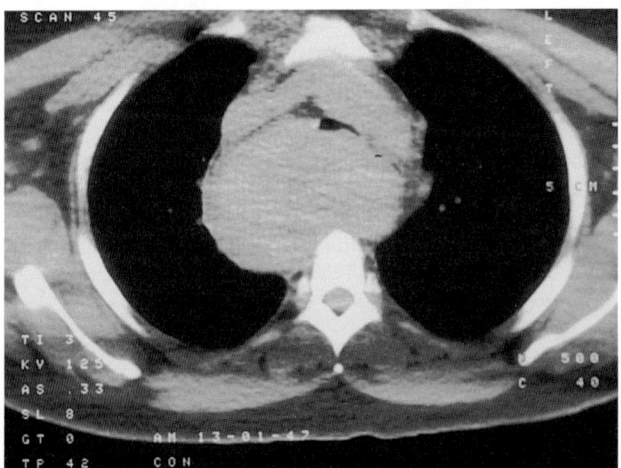

Fig. 5 CT scan of the chest in a patient with a large retrosternal goitre causing tracheal compression.

Goitre

The distribution of thyroid size in any population forms a continuous, positively skewed curve, whose shape depends on the age, sex, and country of residence of the individuals assessed. Hence a precise definition of goitre is impossible. Ultrasound is the most accurate method to assess thyroid size and estimates of goitre prevalence based on inspection and palpation underestimate the true frequency. However, simple schemes, such as that used by WHO/UNICEF, are useful in field studies of goitre prevalence:

Grade 0 = no visible or palpable thyroid

Grade 1 = thyroid enlargement that is palpable but not visible when the neck is in the neutral position

Grade 2 = thyroid enlargement which is both visible and palpable with the neck is in the neutral position

Grade 3 = goitre visible at a considerable distance

Of the many causes of goitre (Table 3), those associated with disturbances of thyroid function are considered later. The remainder can be classified broadly as endemic and sporadic non-toxic goitres.

Endemic goitre

Prevalence

Goitre is said to be endemic when the prevalence exceeds 10 per cent in children aged 6 to 12 years, although this figure is arbitrary and it has recently been suggested that a prevalence of more than 5 per cent should be used.. Over 200 million people are affected world-wide, especially in the Himalayas, Andes, and parts of Africa, although Eastern and Southern Europe are also involved.

Aetiology

The main cause is iodine deficiency, with goitre prevalence exceeding 30 per cent in areas with very low iodine intakes (<30 µg/day). However, endemic goitre is not exclusively related to iodine deficiency. Naturally occurring goitrogens, such as those in vegetables of the cabbage family and in cassava, exaggerate the effects of iodine deficiency by the action of thiocyanates and cyanoglucosides, respectively, on iodine transport. Where selenium and iodine deficiency coincide, thyroid cell destruction and gland fibrosis minimize goitre formation. In Japan, endemic goitre actually results from iodine excess, as well as goitrogens in seaweed, and in Kentucky, chemical pollution of water is goitrogenic.

Clinical presentation

Diffuse goitre is more frequent in girls, and gradually becomes nodular with age and increasing iodine deficiency. Endemic goitres can be massive but give few compressive symptoms. In areas of marginal iodine deficiency, such as Belgium, goitre only appears, and is then modest, when demands on thyroidal iodide metabolism are increased during puberty or in pregnancy.

The major impact of endemic goitre and iodine deficiency on health is the association with endemic cretinism. Two forms of cretinism can be delineated in separate geographical areas, but there is considerable overlap. Firstly, when maternal iodine intake is severely reduced, causing hypothyroidism, there is reduced placental transfer of T4 to the fetus, resulting in a profound neurological deficit in the infant, with mental deficiency, deafness, speech defects, and spastic gait. Secondly, hypothyroidism in the infant after birth produces the typical cretin features, in particular stunted growth. The thyroid in cretins may be enlarged or atrophic and it is clear from field studies that iodine deficiency alone cannot account for the multiple forms of endemic cretinism.

Management

Iodine supplementation is perhaps the simplest and cheapest of remedies and the condition it prevents has devastating consequences; it is sobering

Table 3 Causes of goitre

Endemic goitre
Iodine deficiency
Goitrogens

Sporadic goitre

Simple, non-toxic goitre: diffuse or multinodular (colloid goitre)	
Toxic multinodular goitre	
Hashimoto's thyroiditis	
Graves' disease	
Destructive thyroiditis	Postpartum thyroiditis
	Silent thyroiditis
	Subacute thyroiditis
	Amiodarone
Goitrogens, including drugs with an antithyroid action	
Genetic disorders	Dyshormonogenesis
	Thyroid hormone resistance syndrome
	McCune–Albright syndrome
	TSH receptor mutation
Infiltration	Riedel's thyroiditis
	Amyloidosis
	Sarcoidosis
Secondary	TSH-secreting pituitary tumour
	Excessive stimulation from human chorionic gonadotrophin in pregnancy or choriocarcinoma

that iodine deficiency still persists. There are few complications from iodine supplementation, although thyrotoxicosis may result in a variable proportion of individuals (the Jod–Basedow phenomenon), some of whom have avoided this previously through lack of sufficient iodine. It is political, social, and economic inertia which are at the heart of continuing iodine deficiency. Effective programmes are best targeted at women intending pregnancy and children. Iodization of salt or bread is widely used in developed nations, but intramuscular or oral iodized oil as a single annual dose, or iodination of drinking water, is preferable in areas where distribution of iodized foodstuffs is a problem.

Sporadic goitre

Prevalence

Goitre occurs in around 5 per cent of the iodine-sufficient population and is four times more common in women. However, the prevalence varies with area and generally declines with age; over 60 per cent of goitres found in adolescents regress over the next 20 years. The character also changes over time, from a diffuse (sometimes called simple) goitre to a multinodular goitre. The presentation of single thyroid nodules is dealt with in Chapter 12.5, but it is worth mentioning here that solitary thyroid nodules increase in frequency with age.

Aetiology

The aetiology of sporadic goitre is largely unknown. Unidentified goitrogens may be responsible in a few patients, and in others, mild iodine deficiency in infancy may initiate goitrogenesis which persists despite a subsequently normal iodine intake. A large proportion are probably the result of mild defects in hormone synthesis; compensatory growth ensures normal thyroid function and current tests cannot identify the nature of the defect. Familial clustering of sporadic goitre supports this idea. Although TSH is the most obvious thyroid growth factor, TSH levels by definition are normal in sporadic goitre, which may therefore be the result of other autocrine and paracrine growth factors (e.g. insulin-like growth factor-1, epidermal growth factor, fibroblast growth factor). A role for growth stimulating autoantibodies has also been suggested, but remains controversial.

Progression to a multinodular goitre occurs when unencapsulated nodules form in a long-standing diffuse goitre. These nodules contain colloid-rich, polyclonal follicles, and are usually distinct from adenomas, which are encapsulated and derived from a single thyroid follicular cell with a somatic mutation conferring growth advantage. However, some goitres contain both nodules and adenomas, suggesting a spectrum of pathological changes. Because thyroid follicular cells are heterogeneous, nodules generally develop with varying degrees of function, giving rise to 'hot' and 'cold' areas on scintiscanning with radioiodine. Some nodules develop autonomy and may eventually cause hyperthyroidism, completing the evolution from non-toxic to toxic multinodular goitre (see below). Other nodules undergo degeneration with haemorrhage, fibrosis, and cyst formation.

Clinical presentation

Patients usually seek attention because of the appearance of the neck or a sensation of pressure or discomfort. Equally, they may be unaware of a long standing small goitre which is noticed on examination. Careful palpation is sufficient to distinguish true goitre, which moves on swallowing, from a prominent pad of fat over the front of the neck. Very large goitres can cause dysphagia or even stridor when the trachea is compressed, but these symptoms are uncommon. Venous compression at the thoracic inlet is even rarer; this sign is exacerbated by asking the patient to raise her arms (Pemberton's sign). Pain in the thyroid, which radiates to the jaw, is uncommon and suggests either destructive thyroiditis (see below) or haemorrhage into a cyst in a multinodular goitre. In the latter, the pain is usually unilateral, acute, and associated with a rapid change in thyroid size; symptoms resolve spontaneously in a few days.

Investigations

Thyroid function should be assessed by checking TSH levels, and then free T3 and T4 levels if the TSH is abnormal, to rule out goitre associated with thyroid dysfunction. The presence of thyroid peroxidase antibodies is also useful as a marker of an underlying autoimmune thyroiditis, which occurs in 10 to 20 per cent of multinodular goitres. Imaging, in my view, has only a limited place in the investigation of sporadic goitre, although in many centres, scintiscans and ultrasound are widely used. Ultrasound is useful in determining thyroid size accurately and may reassure an anxious patient that the thyroid is not enlarging. In most cases it is not necessary. Thyroidal uptake of radioisotopes (especially ^{99m}Tc) is indicated if destructive thyroiditis is suspected as a cause of goitre. Otherwise, the major role for imaging is to ensure there is no tracheal compression or intrathoracic/retrosternal component in a patient with suggestive symptoms, and a CT scan is then the preferred investigation (Fig. 5).

Treatment

Most patients with euthyroid sporadic goitre do not require treatment. Neck discomfort or cosmetic concerns may prompt intervention but it is necessary to take a careful history to ensure that discomfort or difficulty swallowing is indeed caused by the goitre. There is no cost–benefit analysis which shows the superiority of any single treatment. Thyroxine, given at doses to maintain slightly suppressed TSH levels (0.1 to 0.3 mU/l), leads to a reduction in goitre size in up to 60 per cent of patients but is unlikely to have any effect on a very nodular goitre or when the TSH level is already low (so-called subclinical hyperthyroidism, discussed below). There are concerns about the long-term effects of suppressive doses of thyroxine on the heart and skeleton, and treatment must be continued long-term to maintain any improvement.

Radioiodine has recently been used in some centres, with doses of ^{131}I ranging from 600 to 3400 MBq (hospitalization is required for doses greater than 800 MBq). Goitre size is usually reduced by more than 50 per cent at 2 years, and most of the improvement occurs within 2 to 3 months. Tracheal compression by a goitre can be treated with ^{131}I, despite theoretical concerns over acute worsening due to a radiation thyroiditis. However, there are as yet no long-term follow-up data on such patients, although hypothyroidism certainly occurs in 20 to 40 per cent by 5 years.

Surgery is used in other centres, and is particularly indicated for severe tracheal compression or retrosternal goitres, and if there is any suspicion of malignancy. Subtotal thyroidectomy is undoubtedly effective, but goitre may recur in around 20 per cent of patients within 10 years and does not seem avoidable by giving thyroxine replacement. Complications, including recurrent laryngeal nerve damage, hypoparathyroidism, and hypothyroidism, are more likely with the biggest goitres, near total thyroidectomy, and reoperation.

Hypothyroidism

Introduction

Impaired production of thyroid hormones is usually due to a primary abnormality of thyroid gland or iodine deficiency; occasionally it is secondary to pituitary or hypothalamic disorders, dealt with in Chapters 12.2 and 12.3. The onset of primary hypothyroidism is gradual and may be detected when the TSH is elevated (to compensate for impaired thyroid output) but the free thyroid hormone levels are normal. This state is subclinical hypothyroidism. As thyroid damage continues, TSH levels rise further but free T4 levels fall. The TSH at this stage is usually greater than 10 mU/l, symptoms become apparent, and the patient is said to have overt or clinical hypothyroidism.

Aetiology

The causes of hypothyroidism are listed in Table 4. The commonest cause world-wide is iodine deficiency, discussed in the preceding section. In iodine sufficient areas, autoimmune hypothyroidism and thyroid damage after radioiodine or surgical treatment for hyperthyroidism are the major causes.

Table 4 Causes of hypothyroidism

Primary

Iodine deficiency

Autoimmune hypothyroidism: Hashimoto's thyroiditis, primary myxoedema

Iatrogenic: ^{131}I treatment, subtotal or total thyroidectomy, external irradiation for lymphoma or cancer involving the neck

Drugs: iodine-containing contrast media, amiodarone, lithium, antithyroid drugs, p-aminosalicyclic acid, interferon-α and other cytokines, aminoglutethimide

Congenital hypothyroidism: absent or ectopic thyroid gland, dyshormonogenesis[1], TSH receptor mutation

Destructive thyroiditis: postpartum thyroiditis, silent thyroiditis, subacute thyroiditis

Infiltrative disorders: amyloidosis, sarcoidosis, haemochromatosis, scleroderma, cystinosis, Riedel's thyroiditis

Secondary

Hypopituitarism: tumours, trauma, pituitary surgery or irradiation, infiltrative disorders, infarction

Isolated TSH deficiency or inactivity

Hypothalamic disease: tumours, trauma, infiltrative disorders, idiopathic

Drugs: bexarotene

[1]The following types of dyshormonogenesis are due to mutations in the genes given in parentheses: iodide transport defect (Na$^+$/I$^-$ symporter), defective iodide organification (thyroid peroxidase, pendrin), loss of iodide reutilization (dehalogenase), deficient thyroid hormone synthesis (thyroglobulin). Defects in monoiodotyrosine coupling also occur but are as yet poorly characterized.

Epidemiology

The prevalence of overt hypothyroidism in Caucasians is around 2 per cent in women and 0.2 per cent in men, with a mean age of 60 at diagnosis. Subclinical hypothyroidism is even more common (6 to 8 per cent of women and 3 per cent of men). Around 4 per cent of these individuals progress to overt hypothyroidism annually if thyroid peroxidase antibodies accompany the elevated TSH. Half this number progress in the absence of thyroid peroxidase antibodies. Focal lymphocytic infiltration of thyroid, associated with thyroid autoantibody positivity, occurs in up to 15 per cent of healthy women and 2 per cent of men without an elevated TSH, representing the earliest manifestation of thyroid autoimmunity; 2 per cent of these people progress to overt hypothyroidism annually. Congenital hypothyroidism occurs in about 1 in 4000 births and this high frequency has led to the widespread introduction of neonatal screening.

Pathogenesis

Autoimmune hypothyroidism is primarily the result of autoreactive T-cell-mediated cytotoxicity directed against thyroid follicular cells. Cytokines derived from the locally infiltrating T cells, macrophages, and dendritic cells impair thyroid cell function and enhance T-cell-mediated cytotoxicity. The role of thyroid autoantibodies in thyroid cell destruction is unclear, but thyroid peroxidase antibodies fix complement and may cause secondary damage. In 10 to 20 per cent of patients, antibodies which block the TSH receptor are partially or wholly responsible for hypothyroidism and transplacental passage of these antibodies (but not thyroid peroxidase antibodies) occasionally causes transient neonatal hypothyroidism. Genetic and environmental factors are involved in the aetiology but, as with most autoimmune disorders, the complex interaction of these factors has so far prevented a full understanding. Polymorphisms in the HLA-DR and CTLA-4 genes are associated with autoimmune hypothyroidism, and a high iodine intake may be an important environmental factor in some cases.

Congenital hypothyroidism is caused by thyroid aplasia or hypoplasia in 60 per cent of cases and in 30 per cent there is an ectopic gland. Mutations in thyroid-specific transcription factors have been found in some of these cases. In the remaining 10 per cent, hypothyroidism is due to dyshormono-genesis (Table 4).

Clinical features

The cardinal features in adults with hypothyroidism are shown in Table 5. However, the ready availability of reliable screening tests for hypothyroidism, especially TSH assays, has led to the recognition of many patients in whom there are only vague or non-specific symptoms, such as tiredness, weight gain, and poor concentration. The differential diagnosis is accordingly vast but the high frequency of hypothyroidism should prompt its exclusion when any suggestive features are present, particular in middle aged women with chronic fatigue or depression.

Autoimmune hypothyroidism may present with a goitre (Hashimoto's thyroiditis) or without (atrophic thyroiditis or primary myxoedema). When present, the goitre is of variable size but is often hard and irregular, sometimes giving rise to suspicion of a malignancy, which then requires exclusion by fine needle aspiration biopsy. Primary lymphoma of the thyroid is a rare but important association (Chapter 12.5). Thyroid pain due to autoimmune thyroiditis is also a rare complication. Patients may notice a Hashimoto goitre before any thyroid dysfunction has developed and annual follow-up is then needed.

The most dramatic presentation of hypothyroidism is myxoedema coma, which is fortunately rare. In addition to the usual features, there is hypothermia (as low as 23°C) and coma, sometimes with seizures. Mortality is 50 per cent even with intensive treatment. Patients are typically elderly and either previously undiagnosed or poorly compliant with medication. There is generally an additional precipitant, such as respiratory depression due to drugs, chest infection, heart failure, stroke, blood loss, or exposure to cold.

Autoimmune hypothyroidism is frequently associated with other autoimmune conditions. In the type 2 autoimmune polyglandular syndrome, autoimmune thyroid disease (hypothyroidism or Graves' disease) is associated with type 1 diabetes mellitus and/or Addison's disease. This syndrome is autosomal dominant with variable penetrance. In the rare, autosomal recessive type 1 autoimmune polyglandular syndrome (chronic mucocutaneous candidiasis, Addison's disease, and hypoparathyroidism), autoimmune hypothyroidism is found in 5 to 10 per cent of patients. Other common associations include pernicious anaemia, vitiligo, and alopecia areata and there is a significant excess of autoimmune hypothyroidism in coeliac disease, dermatitis herpetiformis, chronic active hepatitis, rheumatoid arthritis, systemic lupus erythematosus, and Sjögren's syndrome. Breast cancer patients and individuals with Down's and Turner's syndromes have a higher than expected frequency of thyroid autoimmunity. Around 5 per cent of patients with thyroid-associated ophthalmopathy, discussed later in this chapter, have autoimmune hypothyroidism and 15 per cent of patients with Graves' disease successfully treated with antithyroid drugs develop hypothyroidism 10 to 20 years later. This relationship with Graves' disease is further emphasized by rare patients who oscillate between hyper- and hypothyroidism over a period of months. The likely explanation is fluctuation in the relative levels of TSH receptor stimulating and blocking antibodies, but the cause of these changes is unknown.

Juvenile hypothyroidism is uncommon. The features of adult hypothyroidism (Table 5) may be present, but the diagnosis is usually suggested by retarded growth and dentition, and an infantile face. Myopathy with muscle enlargement is common. Puberty is usually delayed, yet sometimes is precocious. Congenital hypothyroidism is typically unrecognizable at birth but, if not identified by screening, gives rise to prolonged jaundice, failure to thrive, impaired growth, feeding difficulties, constipation, and hypotonia. Left untreated, even for a few weeks after birth, there is permanent neurological damage, resulting in intellectual impairment.

Pathology

In Hashimoto's thyroiditis there is a prominent diffuse and focal lymphocytic infiltrate with germinal centre formation. The thyroid follicles show varying degrees of destruction and little or no colloid. The remaining thyroid follicular cells have an increased number of mitochondria, giving rise to oxyphil metaplasia (Askanazy or Hürthle cells). There is a variable degree of fibrosis. In atrophic thyroiditis, fibrosis is the most prominent feature, with a less obvious lymphocytic infiltrate than in Hashimoto's thyroiditis. Thyroid follicles are usually sparse, reflecting the later stage at which this form of autoimmune hypothyroidism is diagnosed. Whether there is a natural progression from Hashimoto's to atrophic thyroiditis is unclear, although the goitre usually decreases with thyroxine replacement.

Laboratory diagnosis

Measuring the serum TSH is the first step in diagnosing hypothyroidism, with the important caveat that this approach will miss most cases of secondary hypothyroidism in which the serum TSH measured by immunoassays may be low, normal, or even slightly raised, due to the secretion of bioactive forms of the hormone. If secondary hypothyroidism is suspected, for instance in the follow-up of a patient with treated pituitary disease, it is essential to check the free T4 level. The TSH is elevated in other settings besides primary overt hypothyroidism (Table 2). It is therefore important to confirm the diagnosis by measuring the free T4 in all samples in which the TSH is elevated. Measurement of free T3 adds nothing to the diagnosis, especially as values may be within the reference range in a quarter of hypothyroid patients, due to extrathyroidal conversion of T4.

If myxoedema coma is expected, it is essential that treatment is initiated immediately without awaiting confirmation of the diagnosis. These patients often have dilutional hyponatraemia, hypoglycaemia, and electrocardiography changes (low voltage, prolonged QT interval, flat or inverted T waves, and heart block). Other non-specific features which may be found in any patient with hypothyroidism are elevation in serum liver and muscle enzymes (the raised creatine phosphokinase particularly may cause unnecessary concern), raised cholesterol, and anaemia. The anaemia is

Table 5 Clinical features of hypothyroidism

Symptoms
- Tiredness, weakness
- Dry skin
- Altered facial appearance
- Feeling cold
- Hair dry, unmanageable and thinning
- Poor memory and concentration
- Constipation
- Weight gain with poor appetite
- Dyspnoea
- Hoarse voice
- Menorrhagia (later, oligomenorrhoea or amenorrhoea), decreased libido
- Paraesthesiae
- Deafness

Signs
- Dry coarse skin
- Cool peripheries
- Puffy face, hands, and feet
- Yellow skin due to carotene accumulation
- Diffuse alopecia
- Bradycardia
- Peripheral oedema
- Slow relaxing tendon reflexes
- Carpal tunnel syndrome
- Serous cavity effusions
- Galactorrhoea (raised prolactin)
- Enlarged salivary glands
- Rarely: ataxia, dementia, psychosis, steroid-responsive encephalopathy[1], coma

[1]Associated specifically with Hashimoto's thyroiditis; may occur with positive thyroid antibodies in the absence of overt thyroid dysfunction.

usually normocytic or macrocytic, but microcytosis occurs when hypothyroidism is accompanied by menorrhagia.

The aetiology is usually easily established. In the absence of a history of treated hyperthyroidism or iodine exposure, the majority of juvenile or adult onset primary hypothyroidism in iodine-sufficient countries is due to autoimmune hypothyroidism. Transient hypothyroidism due to destructive thyroiditis is considered later. The diagnosis of autoimmune hypothyroidism is confirmed by the presence of thyroid peroxidase antibodies, usually at high levels, although occasionally these antibodies are absent. Cytological diagnosis of Hashimoto's thyroiditis is possible using fine needle aspiration biopsy, but is only necessary if there is uncertainty over the cause of a nodular goitre.

Once congenital hypothyroidism is diagnosed by routine testing after birth, it is usual to initiate thyroxine immediately. Treatment can then be stopped without neurological consequences at age 3 to 4 years to establish that life-long thyroxine replacement is necessary. At this time, the aetiology can be established by scintiscanning and/or ultrasound. Dyshormonogenesis, suspected when there is detectable thyroid tissue and a family history, requires specialized investigation to establish the diagnosis and increasingly this is possible by direct analysis of gene mutations. The commonest of these defects is Pendred's syndrome in which there are mutations in the pendrin gene encoding a chloride/iodide transporter present in the thyroid and cochlea, leading to goitre, mild hypothyroidism, and deafness. The thyroid abnormalities usually appear in the second or third decade, rather than at birth. The diagnosis can be made easily by the perchlorate discharge test, which shows an excessive decline of radioactivity in the thyroid when potassium perchlorate is given 2 to 3 h after allowing the thyroid to take up a tracer dose of radioiodine.

Treatment

In adult patients without heart disease and below the age of 60, treatment can begin with the estimated replacement dose of thyroxine. If there is no remaining thyroid tissue (indicated by a very high TSH and very low or undetectable free T4), the full replacement dose is 1.6 µg thyroxine/kg body weight, which is around 100 to 150 µg/day. In practice, the typical starting dose is 50 to 100 µg thyroxine daily, the lower dose being reserved for patients with mild to moderate biochemical abnormalities. Dosage changes should be based on TSH levels measured 2 to 3 months after starting treatment, the main goal of treatment being to normalize the TSH. A similar period is required to assess the effect of any change to the dosage, made as 25 or 50 µg increments or decrements depending on how abnormal the TSH is. Treatment is usually straightforward, although if there is only partial thyroid failure when treatment is begun, the dose of thyroxine may require adjustment over many months.

Once on a full replacement dose, TSH levels should be checked at intervals of 1 to 3 years, depending on their stability. Fluctuating or elevated TSH levels in a previously stable patient, or thyroxine requirements in excess of 200 µg/day, usually indicate compliance problems. It is important to rule out malabsorption or abnormal thyroxine kinetics caused by drugs: cholestyramine, ferrous sulphate, lovastatin, aluminium hydroxide, rifampicin, amiodarone, carbamazepine, and phenytoin all alter the absorption or clearance of T4. A common cause for poor compliance is worsening angina. Optimization of antianginal treatment is then required, although some patients may simply prove intolerant of full thyroxine replacement if their coronary artery disease is extensive and irremediable. It is important to remind poorly compliant patients that, because of the long half-life of thyroxine, missed tablets should always be taken and that this is safe.

In the elderly, or in individuals with heart disease, the usual starting dose is 25 µg thyroxine daily (or on alternate days when there is severe angina). Dosage should be increased slowly with increments of 12.5 to 25 µg thyroxine. Proportionately higher doses of thyroxine are needed during the first year of life than in adults, and the starting daily dose of thyroxine for congenital hypothyroidism is 10 µg/kg body weight. There is a continuing debate on the benefit of thyroxine in subclinical hypothyroidism. It is rea-sonable to commence thyroxine when subclinical hypothyroidism is coupled with the presence of thyroid peroxidase antibodies, as there is a high risk of progression to overt hypothyroidism. Modest improvements in mental function and lipid levels occur when thyroxine is given to some patients with subclinical hypothyroidism, but long-term studies on the benefits of treatment have not been conducted. At present, it seems reasonable to offer a 3-month trial of thyroxine to thyroid peroxidase antibody-negative patients with subclinical hypothyroidism. If the patient notices an improvement in the symptoms which prompted thyroid function testing, thyroxine is continued, but is stopped if there is no benefit. All patients with subclinical hypothyroidism or positive thyroid peroxidase antibodies should be offered annual testing for the development of overt hypothyroidism.

Another problem is posed by the occasional patient with overt hypothyroidism who continues to feel unwell or who fails to lose weight after the TSH is normalized with thyroxine replacement. It can take around 3 months from achieving full replacement for all symptoms to disappear, and weight gained during hypothyroidism will generally only be lost by following an appropriate diet. It is sensible to ensure that the TSH level is in the lower half of the reference range and sometimes a small increment of thyroxine can achieve this, improving symptoms but not suppressing the TSH. More controversial is the treatment of such patients with higher doses of thyroxine which suppress the TSH. This approach may resolve symptoms but at the risk of atrial fibrillation due to subclinical thyrotoxicosis. The other recognized adverse effect of excessive thyroxine is a decrease in bone mineral density, particularly in postmenopausal women who have previously had hyperthyroidism and therefore already have a low skeletal mass. However, the changes in bone mineral density are modest and no increase in fracture rate has been reported as a result of thyroxine given at supraphysiological doses. It should be emphasized that, in the absence of coronary artery disease, thyroxine has no adverse effects when given at doses which return TSH levels to normal.

Treatment of myxoedema coma consists of thyroid hormone replacement, treatment of any precipitating factor, and supportive therapy. If an intravenous preparation is available, 500 µg thyroxine is given as a single intravenous bolus; the same dose can be given by a nasogastric tube but absorption may be slow. Thereafter, 50 to 100 µg thyroxine is given daily. An alternative is to use triiodothyronine, which has the theoretical benefit of not needing conversion for its activity, but the potential disadvantage of excessive doses causing cardiac arrhythmias. The usual dose is 10 µg triiodothyronine every 4 to 6 h, and it can be given intravenously or by nasogastric tube. Some centres combine thyroxine (200 µg) with triiodothyronine (25 µg) as a single bolus. Patients usually require ventilation initially but external warming should be avoided as it may provoke cardiac failure through peripheral vasodilation and increased oxygen consumption. Instead, space blankets are used. Intravenous infusion of hypertonic saline or glucose may be required to correct metabolic problems. Parenteral hydrocortisone is given at doses of 50 mg every 6 h to treat the reversible decline in adrenal reserve which occurs in marked hypothyroidism. If infection is suspected as a precipitant, broad spectrum antibiotics should be used early.

Prognosis

Thyroxine treatment is usually life-long and, properly taken, restores normal health and lifespan. Occasional patients may discontinue thyroxine and remain euthyroid. Errors in initial diagnosis account for some of these; in others, a spontaneous decline in TSH receptor blocking antibody levels may be responsible. There is no easy means of ascertaining whether a patient continues to need thyroxine, short of stopping it and measuring the TSH 6 weeks later. As remission is uncommon, and of uncertain duration, few endocrinologists at present attempt withdrawal.

Special problems in pregnant women

Untreated hypothyroidism impairs fertility and increases the risk of miscarriage. Children born to such mothers have varying degrees of intellectual impairment. It is therefore essential that thyroxine replacement is monitored closely in women with hypothyroidism who intend to become or who are pregnant. Ideally the TSH and free T4 should be checked prior to conception, once pregnancy is confirmed, and at the beginning of the second and third trimesters. The requirement for thyroxine can increase by 50 to 100 per cent during pregnancy but reverts to normal after delivery. There are no implications for breast feeding.

Areas of uncertainty or needing further research

There has been a recent revival of the concept that thyroid hormone replacement should consist of both thyroxine and triiodothyronine, based on the observation that deiodinase activity varies between tissues, suggesting that in some organs the level of the active thyroid hormone, T3, is insufficient when only thyroxine is given. The short half-life of triiodothyronine makes it alone unsuitable for replacement. Improvements in mental function in a trial of 50 µg of the daily dose of thyroxine with 12.5 µg triiodothyronine have been modest and short-term, and further work is needed. Because hypothyroidism is frequent, routine screening of certain groups or even the entire population has been advocated (Table 6) but the cost–benefit of setting up new screening programmes is unclear. If widely adopted, screening will turn up many individuals with subclinical hypothyroidism, for whom the benefits of early treatment with thyroxine have not yet been fully established.

Thyrotoxicosis

Introduction

Thyrotoxicosis is defined as the state produced by excessive thyroid hormone. Hyperthyroidism exists when thyrotoxicosis is caused by thyroid overactivity but there are several types of thyrotoxicosis which are not due to hyperthyroidism, the most obvious being administration of excessive thyroxine.

Table 6 Indications for screening for hypothyroidism

Established
Congenital hypothyroidism
Previous treatment for hyperthyroidism
Previous neck irradiation (e.g. for lymphoma)
Pituitary tumours, including follow-up after surgery or irradiation
Treatment with lithium or amiodarone
Subclinical hypothyroidism

Worthwhile
Antepartum[1] in type 1 diabetes mellitus
3 months postpartum after a prior episode of postpartum thyroiditis
Unexplained infertility
Non-specific complaints in women >40 years old
Refractory depression or bipolar affective disorder with rapid cycling
Turner's syndrome
Down's syndrome
Autoimmune Addison's disease

Uncertain
Patients with a family history of thyroid autoimmunity
Dementia or obesity without other evidence of thyroid disease
Antepartum to detect unsuspected hypothyroidism[2]
Breast cancer

[1]Measure thyroid peroxidase antibodies also; screen euthyroid antibody-positive women 3 months postpartum for postpartum thyroiditis.

[2]It is also uncertain whether all pregnant women should be checked for thyroid peroxidase antibodies as predictors of postpartum thyroiditis.

Table 7 Causes of thyrotoxicosis

Primary hyperthyroidism
Graves' disease
Toxic multinodular goitre
Toxic adenoma
Drugs: iodine excess (Jod–Basedow phenomenon), lithium, amiodarone
Thyroid carcinoma or functioning metastases
Activating mutation of the TSH receptor
Activating mutation of the Gsα protein (McCune–Albright syndrome)
Struma ovarii (ectopic thyroid tissue)

Thyrotoxicosis without hyperthyroidism
Ingestion of excess thyroid hormone (thyrotoxicosis factitia)
Subacute thyroiditis
Silent thyroiditis
Other causes of thyroid destruction: amiodarone, ^{131}I or external irradiation (acute effect), infarction of an adenoma

Secondary hyperthyroidism
TSH-secreting pituitary tumour
Chorionic gonadotrophin-secreting tumours
Gestational thyrotoxicosis
Thyroid hormone resistance (usually euthyroid)

Aetiology

The causes of thyrotoxicosis are shown in Table 7. Graves' disease is responsible for 60 to 80 per cent of cases and nodular thyroid disease (toxic multinodular goitre and toxic adenoma) accounts for most of the rest. Destructive thyrotoxicosis is dealt with in the next section.

Epidemiology

The prevalence of thyrotoxicosis is Caucasians is 2 to 3 per cent in women and 0.2 to 0.3 per cent in men. The peak age of onset for Graves' disease is between 20 to 50, whereas toxic multinodular goitre occurs more often in later life.

Pathogenesis

Graves' disease is caused by TSH receptor stimulating antibodies, clearly demonstrated by the occurrence of transient, neonatal thyrotoxicosis in babies born to mothers with Graves' disease whose antibody levels are high enough for transplacental transfer to affect the fetus. As with autoimmune hypothyroidism, genetic factors, including HLA-DR and CTLA-4 gene polymorphisms, are associated with the disease; the concordance rate in monozygotic twins is about 20 per cent and much less in dizygotic twins. A high iodine intake, smoking, and stress have all been identified as environmental factors, but in many patients the genetic and environmental triggers remain elusive. Smoking is a major risk factor for the development of thyroid-associated ophthalmopathy. These eye signs are due primarily to swelling of the extraocular muscles, the result of fibroblast activation by cytokines released by infiltrating T cells and macrophages, leading to glycosaminoglycan accumulation, oedema, and fibrosis. The close correlation between ophthalmopathy and thyroid disease is best explained by an unidentified, shared orbital and thyroid autoantigen.

Toxic multinodular goitre evolves from a non-toxic sporadic goitre (see above) and is particularly likely when iodine intake increases, either gradually as a result of changes in the diet, or acutely when iodine-containing agents (amiodarone, some contrast media) are given. More than 50 per cent of toxic adenomas are due to a somatic activating mutation in the genes encoding the TSH receptor or the associated Gsα protein, and a similar but unknown mechanism leading to constitutive activation of a clone of thyroid cells must underlie the remainder.

Clinical features

The typical features of thyrotoxicosis from any cause are shown in Table 8, but their presence and severity depend on the duration of disease and the age of the patient. Occasionally there are paradoxial manifestations, such as the weight gain which can occur in up to 10 per cent of patients when the increase in appetite exceeds the effects of increased metabolism, and apathetic or masked thyrotoxicosis in the elderly which mimics depression. The most dramatic but rare presentation is thyrotoxic crisis or storm, with a mortality of 20 to 30 per cent even with treatment. Patients typically are previously undiagnosed or partially treated, and have an acute exacerbation of thyrotoxicosis precipitated by acute illness (infection, stroke, diabetic ketoacidosis) or trauma, especially directly to the thyroid (surgery or radioiodine). Exact diagnostic criteria for thyrotoxic crisis are not agreed and its frequency is sometimes exaggerated. There is marked fever (>38.5°C), delirium or coma, seizures, vomiting, diarrhoea, and jaundice, death being caused by arrhythmias, heart failure, or hyperthermia.

The differential diagnosis of thyrotoxicosis includes any cause of weight loss, anxiety, and phaeochromocytoma, but simple biochemical testing can readily distinguish thyrotoxicosis from these conditions. Once the diagnosis of thyrotoxicosis is made, it is essential to determine the cause (Table 7), as this determines treatment. Graves' disease is usually clinically distinctive; there is a small to moderate, diffuse, firm goitre and around a half of these patients have signs of thyroid-associated ophthalmopathy (Table 9, Fig. 6). There may be evidence of another autoimmune disorder, in the patient or her family, with the same associations as autoimmune hypothyroidism described above. Less than 5 per cent of patients have pretibial myxoedema,

Table 8 Clinical features of thyrotoxicosis of any cause

Symptoms
  Hyperactivity, irritability, altered mood
  Heat intolerance, sweating
  Palpitations
  Fatigue, weakness
  Weight loss with increased appetite
  Diarrhoea, steatorrhoea
  Polyuria
  Oligomenorrhoea, amenorrhoea, loss of libido

Signs
  Sinus tachycardia, atrial fibrillation in the elderly
  Fine tremor
  Warm, moist skin
  Goitre
  Palmar erythema, onycholysis, pruritus, urticaria, diffuse pigmentation
  Diffuse alopecia
  Muscle weakness and wasting, proximal myopathy, hyper-reflexia
  Eyelid retraction or lag
  Gynaecomastia
  Rarely: chorea, periodic paralysis (in Asian males), psychosis, impaired consciousness

which is better called thyroid dermopathy as it can occur anywhere, especially after trauma (Fig. 7 and Plate 1). These patients almost always have moderate to severe ophthalmopathy and 10 to 20 per cent have clubbing (thyroid acropachy). Thyroid dermopathy most commonly occurs as non-pitting plaques with a pink or purple colour but no inflammatory signs. Nodular and generalized forms, the latter mimicking elephantiasis, also occur. Hyperplasia of lymphoid tissue, including splenomegaly and thymic enlargement, is sometimes found in Graves' disease.

The absence of these features of Graves' disease and the presence of a multinodular goitre strongly suggest toxic multinodular goitre, although nodular thyroid disease is so common that occasional patients with Graves' disease may cause confusion when their thyrotoxicosis arises in a pre-existing multinodular gland. In toxic adenoma, the solitary thyroid nodule is usually readily palpable. Other, rare causes of thyrotoxicosis can usually be easily identified from the history and biochemical investigations.

Pathology

In Graves' disease, there is thyroid hypertrophy and hyperplasia. The follicles show considerable folding, contain little colloid, and are composed of tall columnar cells. Gland vascularity increases. There is a focal and diffuse lymphocytic infiltrate and lymphoid hyperplasia may occur in the lymph nodes, spleen, and thymus. These changes are all reversed by antithyroid drugs. Toxic multinodular goitre comprises a mixture of areas of follicular hyperplasia and nodules filled with colloid. There is a variable degree of fibrosis, haemorrhage, and calcification. Toxic adenomas are encapsulated and cellular, sometimes with little evidence of follicle formation, and occasionally containing unusual cell forms suggesting malignant change. However, capsular invasion is absent and this is the cardinal feature which distinguishes a follicular adenoma from carcinoma.

Laboratory diagnosis

Measuring the serum TSH is the simplest way to exclude primary thyrotoxicosis. A normal or slightly raised TSH level can rarely be associated with hyperthyroidism in the case of a TSH-secreting pituitary adenoma. A low TSH level is not always the result of thyrotoxicosis (Table 2). Therefore the diagnosis of thyrotoxicosis must be confirmed by measuring thyroid hormone levels. Free hormone assays are preferable to those for total hormone, to eliminate binding protein effects (Table 1). Measuring only free T4 alone is adequate in most cases of thyrotoxicosis, which can be confirmed by the presence of a suppressed TSH and elevated free T4 level. However, in up to 5 per cent of patients, only free T3 levels are elevated (T3 toxicosis), especially during the earliest phase of the disorder. Therefore, if both free T3 and T4 are not measured routinely by a laboratory, it is essential to request free T3 analysis in any sample showing a suppressed TSH but normal free T4 level. Rarely, the free T4 is elevated but the free T3 is normal. This arises when Graves' disease or nodular thyroid disease is precipitated by the administration of excess iodine (the Jod–Basedow phenomenon).

Although it is possible to measure TSH receptor stimulating antibodies and thus prove the existence of Graves' disease in a thyrotoxic patient, these assays are cumbersome or expensive, and at present therefore are not

Table 9 Clinical features of thyroid-associated ophthalmopathy

Signs and symptoms	Assessment	Approximate frequency[1]
Lid lag, lid retraction	Measure lid fissure width	50–60%
Grittiness, discomfort, excessive tearing, retrobulbar pain, periorbital oedema	Self assessment score by patient; activity score by clinician	40%
Proptosis	Exophthalmometry or CT/MR-based measurement	20%
Extraocular muscle dysfunction (typically causing diplopia looking up and out)	Hess chart or similar; CT/MR scan to detect muscle size	10%
Corneal involvement, causing exposure keratitis	Rose Bengal or fluorescein staining	<5%
Loss of sight due to optic nerve compression	Visual acuity and fields, colour vision; CT/MR scan	<1%

[1] In patients with Graves' disease. Patients often have multiple signs and in 5–10 per cent, signs are unilateral.

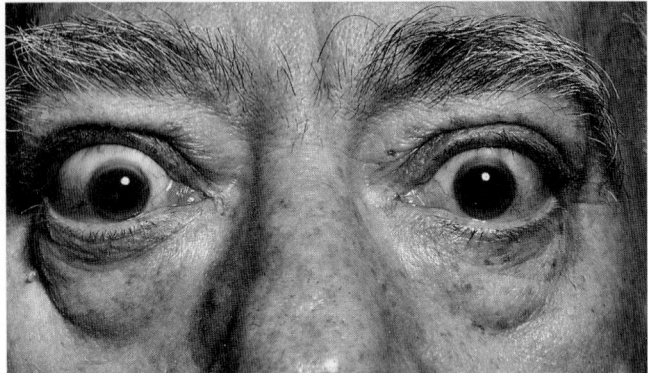

(a)

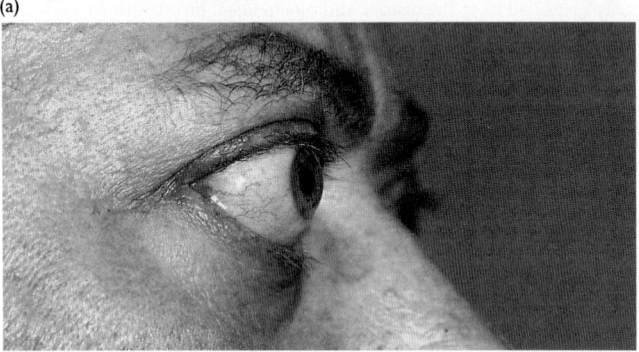

(b)

Fig. 6 Thyroid-associated ophthalmopathy (a) upper lid retraction, periorbital oedema, and scleral injection; (b) chemosis (conjunctival oedema) and proptosis.

widely used. Almost as much information can be gained by measuring thyroid peroxidase antibodies which are present in around 75 per cent of patients with Graves' disease. In cases of diagnostic uncertainty, a thyroid scintiscan will demonstrate a diffuse goitre with high isotope intake in Graves' disease and reveal nodular thyroid disease as well as ectopic thyroid

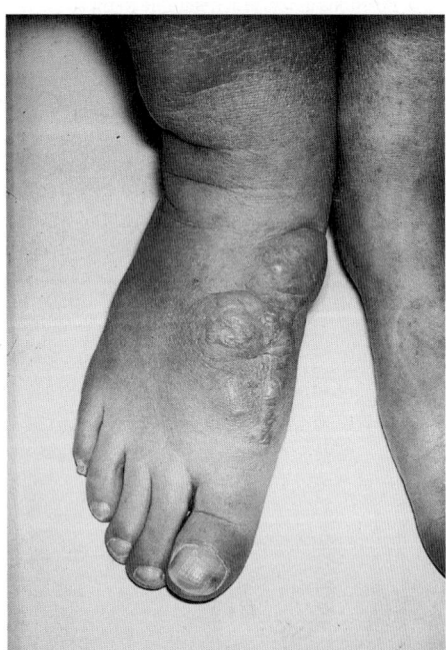

Fig. 7 Thyroid dermopathy (pretibial myxoedema) affecting the lateral aspect of the shin and the dorsum of the foot; the patient also had thyroid acropachy. (See also Plate 1.)

tissue in the extremely rare struma ovarii. In destructive and factitious thyrotoxicosis, the thyroid scan shows virtually no isotope uptake and the diagnosis of factitious thyrotoxicosis can be confirmed by measuring serum thyroglobulin levels, which are suppressed in contrast to the raised levels in all other causes of thyrotoxicosis. When a TSH-secreting pituitary adenoma is suggested biochemically, the diagnosis is made by demonstrating both an elevated level of the α-subunit common to glycoprotein hormones including TSH and a pituitary tumour on CT, or preferably MR, imaging. Prolonged thyrotoxicosis can cause a number of non-specific biochemical abnormalities, especially abnormal liver function tests, hypercalcuria, and elevated serum levels of ferritin. Less commonly, serum calcium and phosphate may be raised, glucose intolerance or diabetes may occur, and rarely there may be a microcytic anaemia or thrombocytopenia.

Treatment

Definitive diagnosis is the most important determinant of treatment selection for thyrotoxicosis. In particular, antithyroid drugs only achieve a cure in Graves' disease. When due to a subacute or silent thyroiditis, discussed below, spontaneous resolution of thyrotoxicosis is expected and symptomatic treatment with β-blockers such as propranolol, 20 to 80 mg three times daily, is indicated. Although β-blockers will rapidly alleviate symptoms in all types of hyperthyroidism, definitive treatment is also necessary, and when euthyroidism is restored, β-blockers can be gradually withdrawn.

There are three types of treatment for Graves' disease: antithyroid drugs, radioiodine (^{131}I), and surgery. Local policy and patient age dictate the order of their use. For young or middle aged adults, antithyroid drugs are generally used initially in Europe and Japan, whereas radioiodine is preferred in North America. Surgery is particularly useful in patients with a large goitre, but is less frequently used in North America than elsewhere. The local availability of an experienced surgeon is crucial. There is more international agreement over the preferential use of radioiodine for a recurrence after antithyroid drugs and as first line treatment in the elderly with Graves' disease.

The main antithyroid drugs used in Europe are carbimazole and its active metabolite methimazole, whereas propylthiouracil is preferred in North America. There is little to choose between them in normal practice, as all exert their principal action by inhibiting iodide oxidation and organification by thyroid peroxidase. Propylthiouracil additionally inhibits the activity of type 1 deiodinase, reducing T3 formation in many tissues, but this activity is only of clinical importance in very severe hyperthyroidism, and more frequent dosing is necessary with this drug.

Two regimens are used to avoid antithyroid drug-induced hypothyroidism and achieve the best chance of remission, which occurs in 40 to 60 per cent of patients and is inversely proportional to dietary iodine intake. The first method is to titrate the dose of antithyroid drug, giving carbimazole (or methimazole) 20 mg two or three times daily, and then lowering the dose every 3 to 4 weeks or so, based on free T4 measurements, until a maintenance dose of 5 to 10 mg once daily is achieved. Equivalent starting and maintenance doses of propylthiouracil are 100 to 200 mg three times daily and 50 mg once or twice daily. Maximum remission rates occur after 18 to 24 months of treatment.

The second regimen is to start with the same dose of antithyroid drug but then to add thyroxine 100 µg daily after 3 to 4 weeks when free T4 levels are usually becoming normal, rather than lowering the dose of drug. Thereafter the patient is maintained on 40 mg carbimazole or methimazole once daily (alternatively, 100 to 150 mg propylthiouracil three times daily) and thyroxine, the latter being adjusted if necessary 4 weeks after starting to achieve normal free T4 levels. The block–replace regimen achieves the same remission rate as the titration regimen within 6 months; continuation beyond this time is not necessary but can be used if a patient wishes to ensure euthyroidism for a particular period of time. Patients with the biggest goitres almost always relapse after antithyroid drug treatment, but unfortunately there are no reliable predictors of which other patients will relapse, and therefore it is usual practice to follow patients closely (for

Table 10 Side-effects of antithyroid drugs

Common
Rash (typically maculopapular)
Urticaria
Arthralgia
Fever, sometimes with malaise

Rare
Gastrointestinal symptoms
Abnormal taste and smell
Arthritis
Agranulocytosis[1]

Very rare
Thrombocytopenia
Aplastic anaemia
Hepatitis
Lupus-like syndrome, vasculitis
Hypoglycaemia due to the insulin autoimmune syndrome

[1]All patients must be warned in writing, before treatment commences, to seek medical advice and stop medication if features suggesting agranulocytosis (fever, mouth ulcers, sore throat) develop.

example every 3 months) in the first year after stopping treatment. Thereafter, an annual check of thyroid function is warranted as recurrence occurs in 10 to 20 per cent 1 to 5 years after treatment, and autoimmune hypothyroidism may supervene in around 15 per cent.

The side-effects of antithyroid drugs are shown in Table 10; most occur in the first 3 months of treatment and there is a moderate dose dependency. Substituting propylthiouracil for carbimazole or vice versa usually reverses the common side-effects but further antithyroid drugs should be avoided if bone marrow disturbance develops. Lower doses of antithyroid drugs can be used in areas of low iodine intake. Lithium and potassium perchlorate have antithyroid actions and are alternatives when antithyroid drugs are not tolerated but these drugs are difficult to use, their side-effects are serious and they are given as a last resort. Anticoagulation with warfarin should be considered in all patients with atrial fibrillation; only 50 per cent of patients revert to sinus rhythm when euthyroidism is restored. In the remainder, attempts at cardioversion should be made, ideally when hyperthyroidism has been definitively treated with radioiodine. Digoxin is useful to control atrial fibrillation acutely but higher doses than normal are needed in the thyrotoxic state.

There are several dosage methods for radioiodine administration, which aim to achieve maximum cure rates with the minimum of subsequent hypothyroidism. Accurate dosimetry based on uptake tests has now largely fallen out of favour, as the results have been little or no better than more empirical methods of dose calculation. A simple formula is to give 200 MBq ^{131}I for a small goitre, 400 MBq for a large goitre, and 600 MBq for Graves' disease complicated by heart failure, but local policies vary, not least because less ^{131}I is needed when iodine intake is low. Around 5 to 10 per cent of patients treated this way require a second dose of ^{131}I, while hypothyroidism rates are 10 to 20 per cent after one year and 5 to 10 per cent annually thereafter. An alternative approach, based on the premise that hyperthyroidism is much more serious than predictable hypothyroidism, has been to attempt deliberate ablation of the thyroid with a fixed dose of 600 MBq ^{131}I. Even with this dose, some patients require a second treatment. Close follow-up is needed in the first year after treatment, and an annual test of thyroid function thereafter is recommended. Transient cytoplasmic, rather than nuclear, damage may cause hypothyroidism in the first 2 to 3 months after ^{131}I treatment, which then resolves. It is usual to delay a second dose of ^{131}I for at least 4 to 6 months after the first, as hyperthyroidism is controlled only slowly by radiation-induced nuclear damage. Antithyroid drugs or β-blockers are useful in the interim.

Radioiodine is contraindicated in pregnancy and breast feeding. There are no teratogenic risks if men or women attempt conception 4 months or more after treatment. Overall mortality rates from cancer are not increased by radioiodine, although there is a theoretical risk of an increase in the frequency and aggressiveness of thyroid cancer in children and adolescents, which makes many endocrinologists reluctant to use ^{131}I in this group, unless other treatments fail or are rejected. Another concern is the precipitation of thyrotoxic crisis by ^{131}I, but in practice this must be rare. To minimize the risk, antithyroid drugs can be given for up to 4 or more weeks prior to radioiodine, particularly in the elderly who are at special risk. Thyroid-associated ophthalmopathy may appear or worsen after radioiodine, especially if the patient smokes. A 3-month tapering course of prednisolone, starting with 40 mg daily at the time of ^{131}I administration, will prevent such worsening but an extended course of antithyroid drugs, with scrupulous maintenance of euthyroidism, may well be preferable until the orbital disease becomes inactive.

Surgery for Graves' disease consists of subtotal or near total thyroidectomy, and in the best centres achieves cure in more than 98 per cent of patients but with a hypothyroidism rate similar to radioiodine. Lower rates of hypothyroidism are inevitably associated with a higher recurrence rate. Patient preference is the main determinant of when surgical treatment is used to treat relapses after antithyroid drugs. Euthyroidism must be achieved with a further course of these drugs prior to surgery to avoid thyrotoxic crisis. Stable iodine (e.g. Lugol's iodine three drops three times daily) is often also given for 7 to 10 days prior to surgery, to block hormone synthesis acutely. Specific complications of surgery include haemorrhage leading to laryngeal oedema, damage to the recurrent laryngeal nerves, and hypoparathyroidism. These problems occur in less than 1 per cent of cases in experienced hands and the last two are often transient.

The management of thyroid-associated ophthalmopathy is summarized in Table 11. Symptoms and signs are usually mild to moderate, although still capable of creating considerable anxiety and disturbance of social function. Severe ophthalmopathy is fortunately rare (1 to 5 per cent of cases) and requires specialist ophthalmological management. Signs usually stabilize 12 to 18 months after onset, and may improve thereafter in 30 to 50 per cent of patients, although improvement is less likely for marked proptosis or diplopia. Corrective surgery for diplopia or cosmetic problems should only be considered in this stable phase. Thyroid dermopathy is left untreated and may resolve spontaneously. Surgical removal usually worsens the situation and, when troublesome, the best treatment is topical, high potency corticosteroids. Octreotide may also be beneficial.

Toxic multinodular goitre is usually managed by radioiodine treatment. Antithyroid drugs will control the hyperthyroidism but relapse is inevitable

Table 11 Treatment of thyroid-associated ophthalmopathy

Mild to moderate disease
Reassurance and explanation
Avoid hypo- and hyperthyroidism
Stop smoking
Protect eyes from dust and bright light
Artificial tears; simple eye ointment at night
Sleep with more pillows or the head of the bed elevated
Diuretics
Stick-on prisms

Severe disease (worsening diplopia, exposure keratitis, sight loss)
Corticosteroids (e.g. prednisolone 40–80 mg daily, tapered over >3 months)
Radiotherapy (10 fractionated doses of 2 Gy)
Immunosuppressive agents (azathioprine, cyclosporin A)
Intravenous immunoglobulin
Octreotide
Orbital decompression (usually transantral)

Stable, burnt out disease
Prisms
Surgery to extraocular muscle
Cosmetic eyelid surgery

when the drugs are stopped. Long-term use of antithyroid drugs may be indicated in the very old or frail, or when incontinence poses an insuperable problem for the safe disposal of excreta after [131]I. The therapeutic dose of ^{131}I used for toxic multinodular goitre is generally higher than for Graves' disease (600 to 800 MBq) because there is uneven uptake of the isotope and usually a large goitre. Surgery is sometimes used as an alternative in patients with a retrosternal goitre or if there is any suspicion of a malignancy. Toxic adenoma is also usually treated with ^{131}I and the rate of subsequent hypothyroidism is low because the function of the normal thyroid tissue is suppressed at the time the patient is hyperthyroid and therefore receives little irradiation. When there is a large (>5 cm) nodule or in young patients (<20 years) surgical excision is preferable and subsequent hypothyroidism is uncommon. Treatment of rare forms of primary hyperthyroidism is by surgical removal of the source of thyroid hormone or radioiodine. TSH-secreting pituitary adenomas causing secondary hyperthyroidism are usually treated by transphenoidal surgery, with radiotherapy for any residual tumour. Octreotide can also be used to lower TSH secretion.

Thyrotoxic crisis is a medical emergency whose management consists of antithyroid treatment, identification and treatment of any underlying precipitant, and supportive measures. Propylthiouracil is given as a loading dose of 600 mg and then 250 mg four times daily, either orally, by stomach tube, or per rectum. Carbimazole or methimazole are less effective alternatives, as they do not reduce T4 deiodination. Stable iodine blocks thyroid hormone synthesis and release but is safe to give only when iodine organification is arrested by propylthiouracil. Lugol's iodine, 5 drops four times daily, is given orally or by stomach tube 1 h after the first dose of propylthiouracil; ipodate 500 mg twice a day is an alternative. Control of the heart rate is central to managing the heart failure which frequently occurs, and in all but the most severe cases propranolol should be given (40 mg orally or 2 mg intravenously every 4 h), with careful monitoring of ventricular function. Diuretics and digoxin are used as needed. Plasmapheresis, dialysis, or cholestyramine (to interrupt the enterohepatic circulation of thyroid hormones) may be useful in extreme cases. Supportive measures include dexamethasone 2 mg four times daily, which also inhibits T4 to T3 conversion, oxygen, cooling, and intravenous fluids.

Prognosis

Although spontaneous remission occurs in Graves' disease, its exact frequency is unknown and is unlikely to be more than 10 per cent, with no guarantee of persistence. Remission does not occur in other types of hyperthyroidism. Mortality rates in untreated hyperthyroidism are also uncertain but are probably around 30 per cent. Even after successful treatment, there is a three-fold increased risk of death from osteoporotic fracture and a 1.3-fold increased risk of death from cardiovascular disease and stroke. It is important that the patient with Graves' disease understands that the course of ophthalmopathy is independent of the thyroid disorder; eye signs appear one or more years before or after the onset of hyperthyroidism in a quarter of patients and progression of the orbital disease frequently occurs despite restoration of euthyroidism.

Special problems in pregnant women

Graves' disease during pregnancy is often treated with propylthiouracil, as carbimazole and methimazole have been associated with fetal aplasia cutis, but some dispute the significance of this association. The block–replace regimen is contraindicated in pregnancy, as preferential placental transfer of antithyroid drug will cause fetal hypothyroidism. Instead, the dose of antithyroid drug should be titrated to the lowest dose which results in maternal free T4 levels in the upper part of the reference range. TSH receptor stimulating antibodies decline during pregnancy and it is usually possible to stop treatment at the beginning of the third trimester. Subtotal thyroidectomy can be performed in the second trimester for women intolerant of antithyroid drugs.

Transplacental passage of TSH receptor antibodies causes fetal and neonatal thyrotoxicosis in 1 to 5 per cent of mothers with Graves' disease and can be predicted by demonstrating a high level of these antibodies in the maternal circulation at the beginning of the third trimester. Poor intrauterine growth and a high fetal heart rate also suggest this diagnosis. Fetal thyrotoxicosis is treated by giving the mother antithyroid drugs and the neonate requires treatment for 1 to 3 months after delivery. Failure to treat untrauterine and neonatal thyrotoxicosis causes low birth weight, premature closure of the sutures, and intellectual impairment. Breast feeding is safe with low doses of antithyroid drugs, but when high doses are needed (e.g. 20 mg or more carbimazole daily), thyroid function should be checked every 1 to 2 weeks in the baby. Patients with Graves' disease who have entered remission prior to or during pregnancy have an increased risk of relapse around 3 to 6 months after delivery, and should be offered thyroid function testing at this time.

Areas of uncertainty or needing further research

The pathogenesis of thyroid-associated ophthalmopathy is poorly understood, and remains an obstacle to developing better treatments. Outcome after antithyroid drug treatment in Graves' disease cannot yet be predicted but improved assays for TSH receptor antibodies may permit better assessment in the near future. Antithyroid drugs modulate the autoimmune response favourably in those patients whose Graves' disease remits, indicating the potential for more specific immunotherapy aimed at the cause of the disease, that would be preferential to present treatments which merely block or destroy the thyroid.

The evolution of hyperthyroidism is gradual and patients with multinodular goitre in particular are now recognized at the stage of subclinical hyperthyroidism, that is with a low or suppressed TSH but normal free T3 and T4 levels. Their optimum management is uncertain. There is a two to three-fold increased risk of atrial fibrillation over 10 years in subclinical thyrotoxicosis, as well as deleterious effects on bone mineral density, but no clinical trials have been performed to show a clear benefit from early intervention. Many endocrinologists simply follow such patients carefully, electing to treat when overt hyperthyroidism is shown by an abnormal free T3 level (T3 usually increases before T4). However, in the elderly with known cardiac disease, there is an increasing tendency to use radioiodine for sustained subclinical hyperthyroidism.

Destructive thyroiditis

Acute thyroiditis is rare and usually caused by bacterial infection of the thyroid via a pyriform sinus connecting the gland with the oropharynx. There is severe thyroid pain with fever and malaise, but thyroid function is rarely disturbed. Diagnosis is made by fine needle aspiration biopsy, with culture of the specimen, and treatment consists of antibiotics, surgical drainage of any abscess, and excision of the sinus which is identified by barium swallow.

Subacute (or de Quervain's) thyroiditis is due to thyroid infection by any of a number of viruses, especially mumps, Coxsackie, influenza, adenoviruses, and echoviruses. The most prominent symptom is pain in the thyroid, often radiating to the ears. A small, tender goitre can be palpated which is usually diffuse, but there can be asymmetrical involvement. Systemic upset with fever is variable but sometimes profound, and symptoms of a prodromal viral infection several weeks earlier may be recalled. There is a granulomatous thyroid inflammation with follicular destruction and the release of thyroid hormones often results in a transient thyrotoxicosis, lasting 1 to 4 weeks. Continuing thyroid destruction then leads to a phase of hypothyroidism once stored hormone is depleted. This lasts 4 to 12 weeks before euthyroidism is restored, but relapses occur in 10 to 20 per cent of cases. Sometimes only one phase of thyroid disturbance is seen. Confirmation of the clinical diagnosis is made by finding an elevated erythrocyte sedimentation rate (ESR) and low or absent radioiodine uptake by the thyroid. Thyroid function requires continuous monitoring as the disease evolves. Mild cases may resolve spontaneously with aspirin as symptomatic treatment, but most patients benefit from prednisolone 40 to 60 mg daily, which rapidly alleviates the pain. The dose is tapered over 6 to 8 weeks, depending largely on symptoms. Propranolol may be useful for thyrotoxic symptoms, and temporary thyroxine replacement is sometimes needed during the hypothyroid phase.

Silent thyroiditis is an autoimmune disorder in which there is a transient but painless thyroid destruction, giving rise to the same kind of thyroid function disturbances as subacute thyroiditis. As well as the absence of thyroid pain, there is no sign of a systemic inflammatory response (including a normal ESR) and the two conditions are therefore readily distinguished. The commonest setting for silent thyroiditis is in the postpartum period in a women with positive thyroid peroxidase antibodies and a mild underlying autoimmune thyroiditis, exacerbated for unknown reasons at this time. Such postpartum thyroiditis is common, being detectable in up to 5 per cent of women 3 to 6 months after delivery when repeated biochemical testing is done, although in many of these women the changes in thyroid function are mild and asymptomatic. Postpartum thyroiditis is three times more common in type 1 diabetes mellitus. Thyroid uptake tests are useful in the postpartum period to distinguish thyrotoxicosis due to postpartum thyroiditis from Graves' disease. ^{99m}Tc is used in preference to ^{131}I and only requires cessation of breast feeding for a day. Treatment is with propranolol for thyrotoxic symptoms and thyroxine for hypothyroidism. Thyroxine should be withdrawn 1 year after delivery and thyroid function tested 6 weeks later, as 90 per cent of women recover normal thyroid function. However, annual follow-up is needed as around 20 per cent of these women have permanent hypothyroidism 5 years later. The condition usually recurs in subsequent pregnancies.

Amiodarone inhibits T4 deiodination, and in all amiodarone-treated patients free T4 levels are in the upper half of the reference range or mildly elevated. Several months to years after starting amiodarone, however, effects on the thyroid may become manifest. In patients with mild thyroid dysfunction, especially autoimmune thyroiditis and positive thyroid peroxidase antibodies, the excessive iodine released from the drug causes hypothyroidism. This is treated as usual with thyroxine. Paradoxically, the high level of iodine causes hyperthyroidism in other subjects who are predisposed to this because of an underlying multinodular goitre or incipient Graves' disease (Jod–Basedow phenomenon). This is called type 1 amiodarone-induced thyrotoxicosis (AIT); type 2 AIT is due to thyroid destruction via drug-induced lysosomal activation. Colour-flow Doppler thyroid scanning shows an increase in vascularity in type 1 but not type 2 AIT, while serum IL-6 levels may be elevated in type 2 but not type 1 AIT. Mixed forms sometimes make an exact diagnosis impossible.

Treatment of AIT can be difficult and biochemical changes are often out of proportion to the symptoms. Amiodarone should be stopped if possible but often this cannot be done and in any case the drug has a very long half-life. Antithyroid drugs are often ineffective in type 1 AIT and potassium perchlorate may need to be added, 200 mg four or five times daily. There is a high frequency of agranulocytosis (up to 1 per cent) with this drug. Prednisolone is also used at doses of 40 to 60 mg daily, and is particularly helpful in type 2 AIT. Thyroidectomy is another alternative in severe cases.

Thyroid hormone resistance syndrome

Mutations in one allele of the β thyroid hormone receptor gene (Fig. 4) cause thyroid hormone resistance (homozygous mutation is lethal). The mutations affect the hormone binding domain and the mutant receptor inhibits the activity of normally encoded receptors, so called dominant negative inhibition, resulting in an autosomal dominant pattern of inheritance. The condition is usually discovered during screening for a goitre but children may sometimes present with short stature, hyperactivity, or mild learning difficulties. Thyrotoxic features in some patients were originally ascribed to selective pituitary resistance to thyroid hormone, leading to

increased thyroid hormone secretion and therefore thyrotoxicosis in the peripheral tissues. However, the same receptor mutations occur in generalized and pituitary resistance syndromes, and although differential tissue expression of receptor subtypes presumably underlies the occasional expression of thyrotoxic signs and symptoms, the exact molecular basis is unknown.

The diagnosis is suggested by the presence of a normal or elevated TSH with elevated free T3 and T4 levels. Non-specific biochemical changes of thyrotoxicosis, such as elevated ferritin, sex hormone binding globulin, and liver enzymes, are absent. The main differential diagnosis is a TSH-secreting adenoma. Thyroid hormone resistance can be confirmed by direct mutational analysis. Treatment is usually not required as reducing thyroid hormone levels to normal causes hypothyroidism. If thyrotoxic symptoms do occur, treatment is with β-blockers or thyroid hormone analogues (e.g. triac) aimed at lowering TSH secretion.

Further reading

Abramowicz MJ, Vassart G, Refetoff S (1997). Probing the cause of thyroid dysgenesis. *Thyroid* **7**, 325–6.

Amino N, *et al.* (1999). Screening for postpartum thyroiditis. *Journal of Clinical Endocrinology and Metabolism* **84**, 1813–21.

Arbelle JE, Porath A (1999). Practice guidelines for the detection and management of thyroid dysfunction. A comparative review of the recommendations. *Clinical Endocrinology* **51**, 11–18.

Bartalena L, Pinchera A, Marcocci C (2000). Management of Graves' opthalmopathy. *Endocrine Reviews*, **21**, 168–99.

Beck-Peccoz P, *et al.* (1996). Thyrotropin-secreting pituitary tumors. *Endocrine Reviews* **17**, 610–38.

Bodenner DL, Lash RW (1998). Thyroid disease mediated by molecular defects in cell surface and nuclear receptors. *American Journal of Medicine* **105**, 524–38.

Braverman LE, Utiger RD, eds (1996). *Werner and Ingbar's The Thyroid*, 7th edn. Lippincott-Raven, Philadelphia.

Brix TH, Kyvik KO, Hegedüs L (1998). What is the evidence of genetic factors in the etiology of Graves' disease? A brief review. *Thyroid* **8**, 727–32.

Burrow GN, *et al.* (1994). Maternal and fetal thyroid function. *New England Journal of Medicine* **20**, 1072–8.

Comtois R, Faucher L, Laflèche L (1995). Outcome of hypothyroidism caused by Hashimoto's thyroiditis. *Archives of Internal Medicine* **155**, 1404–8.

Davies TF, ed (1997). Newer aspects of clinical Graves' disease. *Baillière's Clinical Endocrinology and Metabolism* **11**, 431–601.

DeGroot LJ, *et al.* (1999). *Thyroid disease manager.* http://www.thyroidmanager.org.

Delange F (1994). The disorders induced by iodine deficiency. *Thyroid* **4**, 107–28.

Dumont JE, *et al.* (1995). Large goitre as a maladaptation to iodine deficiency. *Clinical Endocrinology* **43**, 1–10.

Ferretti E, *et al.* (1999). Evaluation of the adequacy of levothyroxine replacement therapy in patients with central hypothyroidism. *Journal of Clinical Endocrinology and Metabolism* **84**, 924–9.

Franklyn JA, *et al.* (1998). Mortality after the treatment of hyperthyroidism with radioactive iodine. *New England Journal of Medicine* **338**, 712–8.

Gharib H and Mazzaferri EL (1998). Thyroxine suppressive therapy in patients with nodular thyroid disease. *Annals of Internal Medicine* **128**, 386–94.

Glinoer D (1997). The regulation of thyroid function in pregnancy: Pathways of endocrine adaption from physiology to pathology. *Endocrine Reviews* **18**, 404–33.

Göthe S, *et al.* (1999). Mice devoid of all known thyroid hormone receptors are viable but exhibit disorders of the pituitary-thyroid axis, growth and bone maturation. *Genes and Development* **15**, 1329–41.

Haddow JE, *et al.* (1999). Maternal thyroid deficiency during pregnancy and subsequent neurophysiological development of the child. *New England Journal of Medicine* **341**, 549–55.

Hermus AR, Huysmans DA (1998). Treatment of benign nodular thyroid disease. *New England Journal of Medicine* **338**, 1438–47.

Houghton DJ, Gray HW, MacKenzie K (1998). The tender neck: thyroiditis or thyroid abscess? *Clinical Endocrinology* **48**, 521–4.

Jarlev AE, *et al.* (1995). Is calculation of the dose in radioiodine therapy of hyperthyroidism worthwhile? *Clinical Endocrinology* **43**, 325–9.

Ko GTC, *et al.* (1996) Thyrotoxic periodic paralysis in a Chinese population. *Quarterly Journal of Medicine* **89**, 461–8.

Koutras DA (1999). Subclinical hyperthyroidism. *Thyroid* **9**, 311–5.

Laurberg P, *et al.* (1998) Guidelines for TSH receptor antibody measurements in pregnancy: Results of an evidence-based symposium organized by the European Thyroid Association. *European Journal of Endocrinology* **139**, 584–6.

Le Moli R, *et al.* (1999). Determinants of longterm outcome of radioiodine therapy of sporadic non-toxic goitre. *Clinical Endocrinology* **50**, 783–9.

Mandel SJ, Brent GA, Larsen PR (1993). Levothyroxine therapy in patients with thyroid disease. *Annals of Internal Medicine* **119**, 492–502.

Newman CM, *et al.* (1998). Amiodarone and the thyroid: A practical guide to the management of thyroid dysfunction induced by amiodarone therapy. *Heart* **79**, 121–7.

Nicoloff JT, LoPresti JS (1993). Myxedema coma: A form of decompensated hypothyroidism. *Endocrinology and Metabolism Clinics of North America* **22**, 279–90.

Radioiodine Audit Subcommittee of the Royal College of Physicians Committee on Diabetes and Endocrinology and The Research Unit of the Royal College of Physicians (1995). *Guidelines: The use of radioiodine in the management of hyperthyroidism*, 26 pp. Royal College of Physicians of London.

Rapoport B, *et al.* (1998). The thyrotropin (TSH)-releasing hormone receptor: Interaction with TSH and autoantibodies. *Endocrine Reviews* **19**, 673–716.

Rivkees SA, *et al.* (1998). The management of Graves' disease in children, with special emphasis on radioiodine treatment. *Journal of Clinical Endocrinology and Metabolism* **83**, 3767–76.

Schwartz AE, *et al.* (1998). Thyroid surgery—the choice. *Journal of Clinical Endocrinology and Metabolism* **83**, 1097–105.

Singer PA, *et al.* (1995). Treatment guidelines for patients with hyperthyroidism and hypothyroidism. *Journal of the American Medical Association* **273**, 806–12.

Toft AD (1999). Thyroid hormone replacement—one hormone or two? *New England Journal of Medicine* **340**, 469–70.

Vanderpump MPJ, *et al.* (1995). The incidence of thyroid disorders in the community: A twenty-year follow-up of the Whickham Survey. *Clinical Endocrinology* **43**, 55–68.

Van Sande J, *et al.* (1995). Somatic and germline mutations of the TSH receptor gene in thyroid diseases. *Journal of Clinical Endocrinology and Metabolism* **80**, 2577–85.

Van Wassenaer AG, *et al.* (1997). Effects of thyroxine supplementation on neurologic development in infants born at less than 30 weeks gestation. *New England Journal of Medicine* **336**, 21–6.

Volpé R (1993). The management of subacute (DeQuervain's) thyroiditis. *Thyroid* **3**, 253–5.

Weetman AP (1997). Hypothyroidism: Screening and subclinical disease. *British Medical Journal* **314**, 1175–8.

Weetman AP (2000). Medical progress: Graves' disease. *New England Journal of Medicine*, **343**, 1236–48.

12.5 Thyroid cancer

Anthony P. Weetman

Thyroid cancer is by far the most common endocrine malignancy but it constitutes less than 1 per cent of all cancers. Most thyroid cancers arise in the follicular epithelial cells of the thyroid and may be differentiated or undifferentiated (Table 1). Tumours of the parafollicular C cells (medullary carcinoma) and other malignancies such as lymphoma and sarcoma behave in a different fashion from thyroid follicular epithelial cancers and are dealt with at the end of this chapter.

Primary thyroid follicular epithelial tumours

Aetiology

Excessive stimulation of the thyroid by thyroid-stimulating hormone accounts for the higher proportion of follicular carcinomas compared with papillary carcinomas in iodine-deficient areas. The thyroid-stimulating antibodies of Graves' disease do not increase the risk of developing thyroid cancer, but incidental thyroid tumours that arise in this disorder may behave more aggressively because of activation of thyroid-stimulating hormone receptors. Low-dose external beam radiation (10–1500 cGy) to the head and neck increases the risk of papillary thyroid cancer over 10 to 30 years. Higher thyroid radiation doses, including those arising from radio-iodine given for treatment of hyperthyroidism, are not associated with an increased risk of malignancy because thyroid cells are destroyed rather than transformed. However, death from thyroid cancer, which is an unusual outcome, may be slightly increased by radio-iodine treatment, suggesting an effect of radiation on tumour dedifferentiation. In Belarus and Ukraine, the incidence of papillary carcinomas in children and young adults has increased 5 to 10 years after the disastrous release of radio-iodine and other radionuclides from the Chernobyl nuclear reactor. This is ascribed to the potent mutagenic effects of radio-iodine on the growing thyroid gland.

Familial forms of papillary and follicular carcinomas exist but are unusual (less than 5 per cent of cases). There are associations with familial adenomatosis polyposis, including the Gardner's syndrome variant, Cowden's disease (multiple hamartoma syndrome), Peutz–Jehgers syndrome, and ataxia-telangiectasia.

Papillary carcinomas do not arise from hyperplastic nodules or adenomas. In about one-third of these tumours one of five distinct rearrangements of the *ret* proto-oncogene, a member of the receptor tyrosine kinase family, occurs. The resulting chimaeric oncogenes are termed *ret/PTC* (for papillary thyroid carcinoma). *ret/PTC3* is particularly linked to radiation. In 10 to 20 per cent of papillary cancers there is oncogenic activation of the *trk* gene.

Follicular carcinomas probably arise, at least in some cases, from follicular adenomas. Activation of the *ras* oncogene occurs in both these tumours (and in some papillary thyroid cancers) and they share cytogenetic abnormalities, especially on chromosome 3. Rarely follicular carcinomas are associated with activating mutations of the thyroid-stimulating hormone receptor and Gsα protein (encoded by the *gsp* gene), similar to those found in toxic adenoma. Anaplastic carcinoma may arise in a papillary or follicular carcinoma and is associated with inactivating mutations of the p53 tumour suppressor gene.

Epidemiology

Papillary microcarcinomas are less than 1 cm in diameter and occur in 4 to 36 per cent of autopsy specimens; they are more frequent in areas of high iodine intake. Clearly most of these do not become malignant. Excluding tumours which are found coincidentally, the annual incidence of thyroid follicular epithelial cancer is around 4 per 100 000. In iodine-sufficient countries, papillary carcinoma accounts for more than 80 per cent of these; follicular carcinoma constitutes about 10 per cent, and anaplastic carcinoma 5 to 10 per cent. Women are two to four times more likely to develop thyroid cancer than men; the peak incidence is between 30 and 50 years of age.

Table 1 Classification of thyroid malignancies

Primary thyroid follicular epithelial tumours	Differentiated	Papillary
		Follicular
	Poorly differentiated	Insular
		Other
	Undifferentiated (anaplastic)	
C cell epithelial tumours (medullary carcinoma)		
Primary non-epithelial tumours	Lymphoid origin (lymphoma, plasmacytoma)	
	Mesenchymal cell origin (sarcoma)	
	Other (teratoma)	
Secondary non-thyroidal tumours	Metastases	
	Extension of tumour from adjacent structures	

Clinical features

Most patients present with an asymptomatic thyroid nodule: this may be noticed by themselves or relatives—sometimes the nodule is detected during physical examination for another complaint. The difficulty for diagnosis arises because thyroid nodules are frequent and only about 5 per cent of palpable thyroid nodules are malignant. Diffuse or multinodular thyroid enlargement occurs in around 10 per cent of the population, and is four times more common in women than men. Solitary thyroid nodules occur in up to 5 per cent of the population and are usually hyperplastic or colloid nodules. The remaining 5 to 20 per cent of nodules are neoplastic but this figure includes follicular adenomas as well as malignant tumours.

It can be seen that determining which thyroid nodules are malignant poses a great difficulty, which has been exacerbated by the widespread use of ultrasound examination of the neck. Up to 60 per cent of adult thyroids have nodules detectable by high-resolution ultrasound scanning. If these nodules are impalpable and there are no other associated features, such ultrasound findings can be ignored. However, a palpable thyroid nodule should always be properly evaluated. Another problem is determining which, if any, nodules warrant investigation in a multinodular goitre. It seems reasonable to investigate further if there have been any new symptoms (see below) or if one nodule is larger than the others.

There are usually no symptoms or signs to indicate that a solitary thyroid nodule is malignant because most tumours progress slowly and present before disease is advanced. Age and sex are important considerations, since a malignancy is more likely in a solitary nodule when the patient is a child or adolescent, is over 60 years old, or is a man between the ages of 20 and 60 years. Previous exposure to radiation and a family history of thyroid cancer should also arouse suspicion. A carcinoma is more likely if the nodule has grown recently or is hard, irregular, or fixed on palpation. Clinical assessment should include careful examination of the cervical, submental, and supraclavicular lymph nodes. Late-presenting features include hoarseness, dysphagia, or dyspnoea which may indicate local invasion, but these symptoms can occasionally occur with an enlarging benign goitre. Rarely the diagnosis only becomes apparent when metastatic disease is detected in bone or lung.

The relatively indolent presentation of papillary and follicular thyroid carcinoma contrasts with that of anaplastic carcinoma in which a rapidly enlarging and fixed thyroid mass occurs, sometimes with local pain. Extension to the oesophagus, trachea, and/or recurrent laryngeal nerves is frequent and the overlying skin may also be infiltrated.

Pathology

There are several variants of papillary thyroid carcinoma united by their characteristic cytological features. The nuclei are large, clear ('Orphan Annie', after the eyes of the cartoon character), and have longitudinal grooves and invaginations of cytoplasm (Fig. 1). Two-thirds of tumours are unencapsulated and display papillary and follicular structures, the remainder comprise the encapsulated, follicular, tall cell, sclerosing, and clear cell variants.

The encapsulated variant has a better prognosis than average and the tall cell variant a worse prognosis. Half of papillary carcinomas contain degenerate calcified papillae, termed psammoma bodies. The tumour is multicentric in up to 80 per cent of cases if the resected thyroid is examined carefully. Metastasis is via the lymphatics and local lymph nodes are infiltrated in 40 to 50 per cent of cases (more in young patients). Distant metastases are found in less than 5 per cent of patients at presentation: the lung is the most common site.

Follicular carcinoma is characterized by follicular differentiation with a solid growth pattern and without the nuclear features of papillary carcinoma. The tumour is encapsulated but there is invasion of the capsule and vessels (Fig. 1). This invasion is the crucial feature which distinguishes follicular carcinoma from follicular adenoma, self-evidently a distinction only possible by histological examination. Minimally and widely invasive sub-

types are recognized, the latter having a worse prognosis. When 75 per cent or more of the tumour cells exhibit oxyphilic staining due to mitochondrial accumulation, this is termed a Hürthle cell carcinoma, which probably also has a worse prognosis. Lymph node metastases are unusual, as is multicentricity in the thyroid. Metastasis occurs via the bloodstream, typically to bone and lungs.

When follicular differentiation is poor or absent, the tumour is classified as an insular carcinoma with a poor prognosis. In anaplastic carcinoma

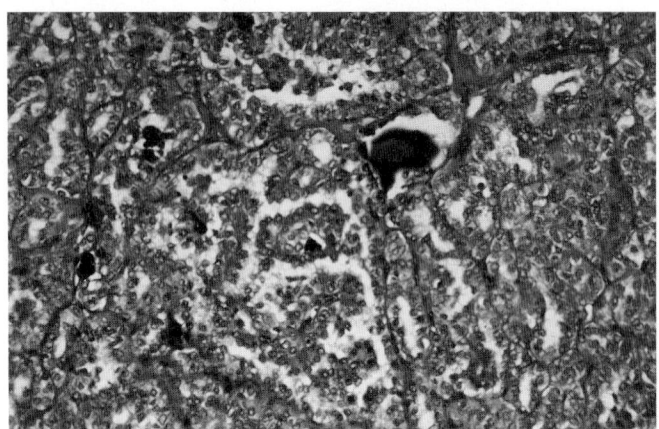

(a)

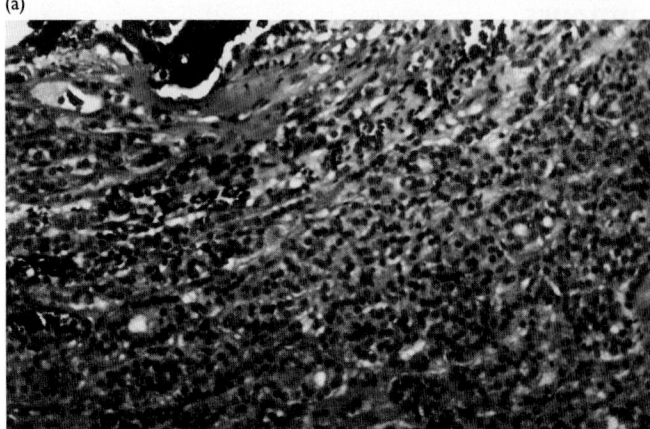

(b)

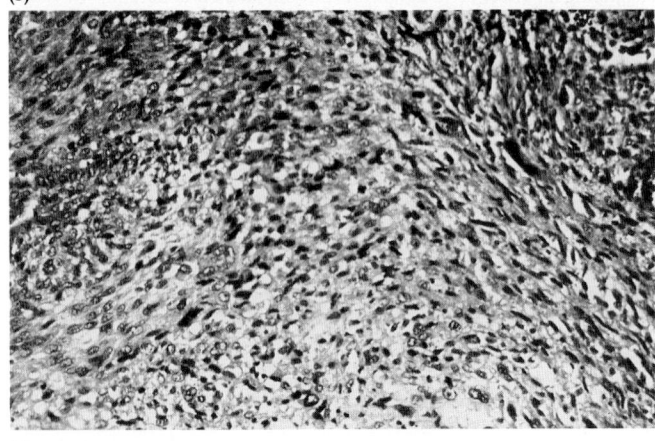

(c)

Fig. 1 Histopathological features of thyroid follicular epithelial carcinoma: (a) papillary carcinoma, with psammoma bodies and typical nuclear appearance; (b) metastatic follicular carcinoma, eroding vertebral bone; (c) anaplastic carcinoma showing pleomorphic spindle cells. (All sections, original magnification ×200; photomicrographs by courtesy of Dr K. Suvarna.)

there is no capsule, the cells are atypical, including spindle, multinuclear, and squamoid forms, and mitoses are frequent (Fig. 1).

Diagnosis

Thyroid epithelial cancers generally fail to affect thyroid function. However, this should be evaluated in all patients presenting with a thyroid nodule: a low circulating level of thyroid-stimulating hormone strongly suggests an autonomous benign nodule. Anaplastic carcinoma may occasionally cause hypothyroidism, but the most frequent cause of an elevated level of thyroid-stimulating hormone with a hard, nodular thyroid is Hashimoto's thyroiditis. Some Hashimoto glands are so irregular that a malignancy may be suspected. There is no increased or decreased risk of thyroid epithelial carcinoma in Hashimoto's thyroiditis, but thyroid lymphoma almost always occurs in association with autoimmune thyroiditis. Therefore any dominant or atypical area in a Hashimoto goitre requires careful evaluation. Thyroid peroxidase and/or thyroglobulin antibodies occur in about one-quarter of patients with thyroid follicular epithelial carcinoma, coincident with the presence of a lymphocytic infiltrate which, in turn, is associated with a more favourable prognosis. Although the serum thyroglobulin concentration is extremely useful in follow-up, as discussed below, this investigation is useless in diagnosis: levels may not be elevated with some cancers and, even when elevated, cannot be causally distinguished from those which occur in benign adenoma, multinodular goitre, Graves' disease, or destructive thyroiditis.

In the past solitary thyroid nodules were investigated by radionuclide and/or ultrasound imaging but neither technique is able to diagnose malignancy accurately. Radionuclide scanning can be performed with $^{99}Tc^m$ pertechnetate or radio-iodine (^{123}I or ^{131}I), with similar information being obtained from either nuclide. Most thyroid cancers fail to take up radionuclide ('cold' nodules), but the more frequent benign lesions such as colloid nodules, cysts, adenomas, and thyroiditis behave similarly. About 20 per cent of nodules have normal or increased radionuclide uptake. Malignancy cannot be excluded with these appearances, however. The only exception is when the nodule is 'hot' and the surrounding thyroid tissue fails to take up radionuclide, indicating the presence of a toxic adenoma which is almost invariably benign. This type of nodule will cause suppression of thyroid-stimulating hormone and will be suspected from routine testing of thyroid function. In summary, radionuclide scanning adds little to diagnosis.

The use of ultrasound is more controversial. Cystic nodules have a lower risk of malignancy than those which are solid, but thyroid cancer cannot be reliably excluded by ultrasound. Predicting the presence of malignancy based on the echo pattern of the tumour, and more recently using colour-flow Doppler, may be successful in up to 80 per cent of cases but this depends on considerable experience. As well as the poor specificity of ultrasound, the technique is so sensitive that many small unsuspected nodules will be uncovered, complicating the evaluation. Ultrasound is useful for accurate measurement of thyroid and nodule size, which can be helpful in monitoring patients and in guiding biopsy, although this procedure is usually performed without imaging.

Fine needle aspiration biopsy is undoubtedly the current technique of choice for investigation of a thyroid nodule. Local anaesthetic is not needed because the procedure causes little discomfort. It is usual to take two to six biopsies to increase the sample yield. Essentially three diagnoses are possible: benign (65–75 per cent of specimens), malignant (5 per cent), and indeterminate (20–30 per cent), but an experienced cytopathologist is needed to obtain reliable results. Papillary carcinoma is readily diagnosed by fine needle aspiration biopsy, and medullary carcinoma and lymphoma can also be detected by use of immunohistochemical staining.

Follicular carcinomas cannot be distinguished cytologically from a follicular adenoma, and these tumours account for the bulk of needle aspiration specimens labelled indeterminate (or suspicious). Open biopsy and histological examination is the only secure diagnostic method in this set-

ting. About 15 per cent of biopsies reported in experienced centres are considered unsuitable for diagnosis. It is relatively simple to repeat the biopsy but a persistently equivocal biopsy should be grounds for considering surgery, since malignant tumours will be found in about half of the cases. A cyst may be aspirated during biopsy. If this fails to reaccumulate and no lesion remains palpable, a malignancy is highly unlikely, but recurrence of a cyst may indicate malignant disease and require surgery for definitive diagnosis. Overall, the sensitivity and specificity of fine needle aspiration biopsy is greater than 90 per cent.

Treatment

Surgical excision

A total or near total thyroidectomy should be performed since papillary carcinomas are often bilateral and removal of thyroid tissue facilitates subsequent ablation by radio-iodine. There is controversy regarding surgery for low-risk unifocal papillary carcinomas (those less than 5 cm in diameter, especially in young patients) but bilateral resection is associated with a lower rate of local recurrence than unilateral total lobectomy. In papillary carcinoma, the ipsilateral central lymph nodes should be dissected, as should all palpable nodes.

After surgery, radio-iodine is usually administered to remove any remaining thyroid tissue, which then allows thyroglobulin or ^{131}I total body scanning to be used in follow-up to detect metastases. This treatment also destroys occult carcinoma and, by scanning after ablation, metastatic disease is revealed. Local policies vary, but in most centres an ^{131}I scan is performed 1 to 2 months after surgery and an ablation dose of 1100 to 3700 MBq ^{131}I is given, depending on the size of the remnant. In 15 to 30 per cent of patients a second treatment dose of ^{131}I is necessary to achieve ablation. Iodine exposure, including iodine-containing contrast media, may prevent accumulation of ^{131}I during treatment.

In patients whose tumour is less than 1.5 cm in diameter, excision alone without radio-iodine ablation is indicated. Whether all other patients require ablation is controversial. Clinical staging scores (see below) may help to identify other low-risk patients who do not require ablation excision.

Radio-iodine therapy

High levels of stimulation by thyroid-stimulating hormone are required to produce maximum uptake of ^{131}I; this is achieved by a period of 30 to 45 days without thyroxine replacement and can thus lead to the development of severe hypothyroid symptoms. The short action of tri-iodothyronine, 20 μg three times daily, as a replacement is therefore preferable in the weeks before scanning and ^{131}I treatment, because only 2 weeks are needed when this is stopped to increase endogenous thyroid-stimulating hormone. Even this short period without thyroid hormone may be troublesome for the patient and recombinant thyroid-stimulating hormone suitable for intramuscular administration is now available and can be given without cessation of thyroid hormone replacement.

Long-term thyroid replacement therapy

The third aspect of treatment is to maintain the patient for life on thyroxine at doses sufficient to suppress levels of thyroid-stimulating hormone to 0.1 mU/litre or less, because thyroid-stimulating hormone is a growth factor for thyroid carcinoma. The optimum level of thyroid-stimulating hormone is unknown, but higher levels can be accepted in those patients known to be disease-free for several years, compared with newly treated patients. In almost all patients, satisfactory suppression of thyroid-stimulating hormone can be achieved without inducing thyrotoxic symptoms. The effective thyroxine dosage is 2.2 to 2.8 μg/kg body weight.

Anaplastic carcinoma is rapidly fatal. The tumour does not take up radio-iodine. Surgery has a limited role in relieving obstructive symptoms and external beam radiotherapy is useful in palliation. The place of chemotherapy (usually doxorubicin combined with other drugs) is unclear.

Follow-up

Lifelong follow-up is necessary for papillary and follicular cancer because recurrence may occur many years after apparent cure. As well as monitoring the concentration of thyroid-stimulating hormone and performing careful neck palpation, serum thyroglobulin should be measured. Detectable levels of thyroglobulin after thyroid ablation indicate persistent or recurrent disease. In many centres, thyroglobulin levels are checked when the patient is not taking thyroxine replacement, as the rise in thyroid-stimulating hormone will stimulate thyroglobulin production and exaggerate any increase. This is particularly useful in high-risk patients: in those at low risk (see next section), it is reasonable to measure thyroglobulin without withdrawing thyroxine.

If thyroglobulin is detectable, the patient should have a total body ^{131}I scan and any recurrent disease can then be treated with a therapeutic dose of 3700 MBq ^{131}I. Many centres also perform a total body scan at 6 to 12 months after initial ablation, but repeated routine scans thereafter have now been superceded by measurement of thyroglobulin. The only exception is in the patient with thyroglobulin antibodies which interfere with many assays for thyroglobulin. If this is the case, repeated scans are the only way to ensure that the patient remains free of disease.

For metastatic disease, usually in the lung, treatment with radio-iodine can be repeated every 4 to 6 months, but there is little benefit above a cumulative dose of 18 500 MBq. Bone metastases may respond to ^{131}I or external beam radiotherapy. The best survival in metastatic thyroid cancer occurs in young patients with small metastases, indicating the overall value of early treatment for this disease.

Prognosis

At least seven scoring systems have been advocated to assess prognosis in papillary and follicular carcinoma. These take into account the age and sex of the patient, tumour characteristics (especially size, extension, and metastases), and completeness of excision. An example of the predictive power of such scoring is shown in Table 2. The risk of death increases with age, especially after 60, while tumour recurrence is commonest in those aged under 20 and over 60. Men have a worse prognosis than women, but the difference is small.

With proper treatment the rate of recurrence of papillary carcinoma is about 15 per cent, and the cause-specific death rate is approximately 5 per cent at 20 years. In other words, 85 per cent of these patients present with features of the group with the best prognosis, for instance achieving a score of less than 6 in the system described in Table 2. In follicular carcinoma, the cause-specific survival rate is 80 per cent at 20 years after treatment and 70 per cent at 30 years. However, in the subgroup with metastases at presentation the 10-year survival is only 20 per cent. The median survival time for anaplastic carcinoma is 4 to 12 months and those with distant metastases at presentation have a median survival time of only 3 months.

Table 2 An example of the predictive value of a scoring system (used to divide patients into four prognostic groups) in determining outcome in papillary carcinoma.

The overall score is the sum of the following:
  3.1 (if ≤ 39 years old) or 0.08 × patient age (if ≥ 40 years old)
  0.3 × size of tumour in centimetres
  1, if resection is incomplete
  1, if there is extrathyroidal extension
  3, if there are metastases

Score	20-year survival (%)
< 6	99
6–6.99	89
7–7.99	56
≥ 8	24

Data from Hay ID et al. (1993) Surgery **114**, 050–8.

Prevention

In the event of a nuclear accident, prompt administration of stable iodine prevents the uptake of inhaled and ingested radioactive iodine isotopes. Emergency arrangements should be in place close to nuclear installations to provide for distribution of potassium iodate tablets, and arrangements for the United Kingdom are detailed in the Department of Health document PL/CMO (93) 1.

Special problems in pregnancy

A solitary nodule in a pregnant woman should be evaluated by fine needle aspiration biopsy. If the biopsy suggests malignancy, surgery can be undertaken in the second or third trimester, but if the nodule is discovered late in the third trimester, it is probably best to defer surgery until after delivery.

Medullary carcinoma of the thyroid

This accounts for 5 to 10 per cent of all thyroid cancers. About 80 per cent are sporadic with a peak incidence at 40 to 50 years of age. Hereditary autosomal dominant forms occur as part of multiple endocrine neoplasia type 2A or 2B or as isolated familial medullary carcinoma. These forms are associated with germline point mutations in the *ret* proto-oncogene and preneoplastic C cell hyperplasia (Table 3).

The pathological findings are of an encapsulated tumour with round, spindle shaped, or polyhedral cells arranged in a variety of patterns that have no prognostic significance. There is variable fibrosis and three-quarters of tumours show marked deposition of amyloid—a feature associated with a good prognosis. Heterogeneous staining for calcitonin, a hormone of C cells, is associated with a poorer outcome, reflecting dedifferentiation. Even the smallest medullary tumours may be associated with local lymph node metastases.

The presentation of sporadic medullary carcinoma is typically with a solitary thyroid nodule, accompanied by cervical lymphadenopathy in 50 per cent of cases. Lung, liver, or bone metastases are present at diagnosis

Table 3 Types of medullary carcinoma of the thyroid

Type	Frequency	Associated lesions	*ret* gene mutation
Sporadic	80%	None	Occasional somatic mutations in tumour tissue
Multiple endocrine neoplasia type 2A	10%	Phaeochromocytoma, hyperparathyroidism	Germline: codon 634, less commonly 609, 611, 618, 620
Multiple endocrine neoplasia type 2B	3%	Phaeochromocytoma, mucosal neuromas, Marfanoid habitus	Germline: codon 918
Familial medullary thyroid carcinoma	7%	None	Usually germline mutation in codons 609, 611, 618, 620 or 634

in 10 per cent of cases. Symptoms due to local invasion or the paraneo-plastic production of polypeptides and prostaglandins (flushing, diarrhoea, and Cushing's syndrome) are less common presenting features.

The diagnosis is often apparent from fine needle aspiration biopsy. Basal serum calcitonin concentrations are almost invariably elevated and confirm the diagnosis. There is controversy over the utility of routine serum calcitonin measurement in the work-up of all thyroid nodules: most centres perform aspiration biopsy initially. Newly diagnosed patients should be screened for other evidence of multiple endocrine neoplasia and a careful family history is also essential. In particular, phaeochromocytoma occurring as part of an inherited cancer syndrome must be excluded before surgery.

Testing genomic DNA for *ret* mutations in the germline is now widely available and should ideally be carried out on leucocyte DNA from all new patients. The absence of the most common mutations, coupled with a negative family history and the absence of C-cell hyperplasia or multicentric tumours in the resected thyroid, indicates that further family testing is not warranted. When a *ret* mutation is detected, there is a clear benefit from family testing, as prophylactic thyroidectomy in affected individuals improves outcome. However, there are some kindreds in whom familial medullary carcinoma occurs without a recognizable *ret* mutation and family screening must then be undertaken annually, up to the age of 35 to 40 years, using pentagastrin-stimulated serum calcitonin measurements as a guide to the presence of the inherited abnormality.

Medullary carcinoma should be treated by total thyroidectomy, with dissection of the central and other involved lymph nodes; this may require a second completion operation if the diagnosis is not made at the outset. Thyroxine replacement is needed at physiological doses rather than doses which suppress thyroid-stimulating hormone. After surgery the patient should be monitored by measurement of serum calcitonin concentration. Cure, defined as a persistently normal calcitonin level, occurs in only about one-third of patients, but 80 to 90 per cent of patients in whom there is an elevated calcitonin level and only nodal disease survive for 10 years. The best management of persistent disease is unclear, but local recurrence with identifiable lymph node involvement should be dealt with surgically. Radiotherapy and chemotherapy have a variable and at best partial effect. Profuse (secretory) watery diarrhoea is frequently a troublesome feature of extensive disease; this may respond to treatment with loperamide, but somatostatin analogues, for example octreotide, may be needed.

Age, stage and size of tumour, and completeness of surgical removal are important prognostic features. Familial medullary carcinoma has the best outcome; in contrast, the tumour associated with multiple endocrine neoplasia type 2B is very aggressive. The overall 10-year survival is 70 to 80 per cent.

Primary thyroid lymphoma

Less than 5 per cent of thyroid malignancies are non-Hodgkin's B-cell lymphoma. The peak incidence is between 50 and 80 years of age, and women are affected three times more frequently than men. The typical presentation is a rapidly enlarging thyroid mass in a patient with Hashimoto's thyroiditis. The clinical features may suggest anaplastic carcinoma. The diagnosis can be made by fine needle aspiration biopsy and confirmed by large needle or open biopsy. Accurate staging is then necessary to plan treatment, which is with external beam radiotherapy and anthracycline-based chemotherapy. Intensive treatment has produced 8-year survival rates approaching 100 per cent.

Further reading

Ain KB (1998). Anaplastic thyroid carcinoma: behavior, biology, and therapeutic approaches. *Thyroid* **8**, 715–26.

Dulgeroff AJ and Hershman JM (1994). Medical therapy for differentiated thyroid carcinoma. *Endocrine Reviews* **15**, 500–15.

Fagin JA (1997). Editorial: familial nonmedullary thyroid carcinoma—the case for genetic susceptibility. *Journal of Clinical Endocrinology and Metabolism* **82**, 342–4.

Hay ID *et al.* (1993). Predicting outcome in papillary thyroid carcinoma: development of a reliable prognostic scoring system in a cohort of 1779 patients surgically treated at one institution during 1940 through 1989. *Surgery* **114**, 1050–8.

Hay ID *et al.* (1998). Unilateral total lobectomy: is it sufficient surgical treatment for patients with AMES low-risk papillary thyroid carcinoma? *Surgery* **124**, 958–66.

Hesmati HM *et al.* (1997). Advances and controversies in the diagnosis and management of medullary thyroid carcinoma. *American Journal of Medicine* **103**, 60–9.

Ladenson PW (1999). Strategies for thyrotropin use to monitor patients with treated thyroid carcinoma. *Thyroid* **9**, 429–33.

Matsuzuka F *et al.* (1993). Clinical aspects of primary thyroid lymphoma: diagnosis and treatment based on our experience of 119 cases. *Thyroid* **3**, 93–9.

Schlumberger MJ (1998). Papillary and follicular thyroid carcinoma. *New England Journal of Medicine* **338**, 297–306.

Schlumberger M, Baudin E (1998). Serum thyroglobulin determination in the follow-up of patients with differentiated thyroid carcinoma. *European Journal of Endocrinology* **138**, 249–52.

Suárez HG (1998). Genetic alterations in human epithelial thyroid tumours. *Clinical Endocrinology* **48**, 531–46.

Taylor T *et al.* (1998). Outcome after treatment of high-risk papillary and non-Hürthle-cell follicular thyroid carcinoma. *Annals of Internal Medicine* **129**, 622–7.

Wartofsky L *et al.* (1998). The use of radioactive iodine in patients with papillary and follicular thyroid cancer. *Journal of Clinical Endocrinology and Metabolism* **83**, 4195–200.

12.6 Parathyroid disorders and diseases altering calcium metabolism

R. V. Thakker

Calcium homeostasis

Most of the total of 1 kg of calcium in the healthy adult is present within the crystal structure of bone mineral and less than 1 per cent is in soluble form in the extracellular and intracellular fluid compartments. In the extracellular fluid compartment about half of the total calcium is ionized and the rest is principally bound to albumin or complexed with counter-ions. Ionized calcium concentrations range from 1.17 to 1.33 mmol/l, and the total serum calcium concentration ranges from 2.12 to 2.62 mmol/l. Measurements of free ionized calcium are not often undertaken because they are difficult; most laboratories report total serum calcium concentration for routine clinical use. However, the usual 2:1 ratio of total to ionized calcium may be disturbed by disorders such as metabolic acidosis, which reduces calcium binding by proteins, or by changes in protein concentration, caused by cirrhosis, dehydration, venous stasis, or multiple myeloma. In view of this, total serum concentrations are adjusted, or 'corrected', to a reference albumin concentration; thus, the corrected serum calcium may be related to a reference albumin concentration of 41 g/l and, for every 1 g/l of albumin above or below the reference value, the calcium is adjusted by 0.016 mmol/l, respectively. For example a total serum calcium of 2.70 mol/l with an albumin concentration of 47 g/l would be equivalent to a corrected serum calcium of 2.60 mmol/l, thereby correcting the initial apparent hypercalcaemic value to a normal value.

The extracellular concentration of calcium is closely regulated (Fig. 1) within the narrow physiological range that is optimal for those cellular functions that are affected by calcium. Indeed both hypercalcaemia and hypocalcaemia impair the function of many different organ systems. Regulation of extracellular calcium takes place through complex interactions (Fig. 2) at the target organs of the major calcium regulating hormone, parathyroid hormone (PTH), and vitamin D and its active metabolites, 1,25-dihydroxy $(1,25(OH)_2)$ vitamin D. The parathyroid glands secrete PTH at a rate that is appropriate to, and depending upon the prevailing extracellular calcium ion concentration. Parathyroid gland disorders cause either hypercalcaemia or hypocalcaemia and these can be classified according to whether they arise from an excess of PTH, its deficiency, or insensitivity to its effects (Table 1, Fig. 2).

The *PTH* gene is located on chromosome 11p15 and consists of three exons (transcribed regions) which are separated by two introns. Exon 1 of the *PTH* gene is 85 bp in length and is untranslated whereas exons 2 and 3 code for the 115 amino acid pre-proPTH peptide. Exon 2 is 90 bp in length and encodes the initiation (ATG) codon, the prehormone sequence and part of the prohormone sequence. Exon 3 is 612 bp and encodes the remainder of the prohormone sequence, the mature PTH peptide, and the 3′ untranslated region. The 5′ regulatory sequence of the human *PTH* gene contains a vitamin D response element 125 bp upstream of the transcription start site, which down-regulates *PTH* mRNA transcription in response to vitamin D receptor binding. *PTH* gene transcription (as well as PTH peptide secretion) is also dependent upon the extracellular calcium concentration, although the presence of a specific upstream 'calcium response element' has not yet been demonstrated.

The mature PTH peptide is secreted from the parathyroid chief cell as an 84 amino acid peptide; however, when the *PTH* mRNA is first translated it is as pre-proPTH peptide. The 'pre' sequence consists of a 25 amino acid signal peptide (leader sequence) which is responsible for directing the nascent peptide into the endoplasmic reticulum to be packaged for secretion from the cell. The 'pro' sequence is six amino acids in length and, although its function is less well defined than that of the 'pre' sequence, it is also essential for correct PTH processing and secretion. After the 84 amino acid mature PTH peptide is secreted from the parathyroid cell, it is cleared from

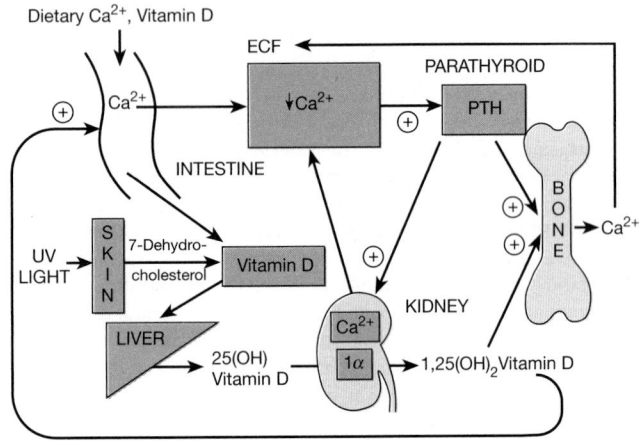

Fig. 1 Regulation of extracellular fluid (ECF) calcium (Ca^{2+}) by parathyroid hormone (PTH) action on kidney, bone, and intestine. A decrease in ECF Ca^{2+} is sensed by the calcium-sensing receptor (Fig. 2), and this leads to an increase in PTH secretion which predominantly acts directly on kidney and bone that possess the PTH-receptor (PTHR, Fig. 2). The skeletal effects of PTH are to increase (+) osteoclastic bone reabsorption but as osteoclasts do not have PTHRs, this action is mediated via the osteoblasts, which do have PTHRs and in response release cytokines and factors that activate osteoclasts. In the kidney, PTH stimulates (+) the 1α hydroxylase (1α) to increase the conversion of 25-hydroxy vitamin D (25(OH)D) to the active metabolite 1,25-dihydroxy vitamin D ($1,25(OH)_2D$). In addition, PTH, increases (+) the reabsorption of Ca^{2+} from the renal distal tubule and inhibits the reabsorption of phosphate from the proximal tubule, thereby leading to hypercalcaemia and hypophosphataemia. PTH also inhibits Na^+–H^+ antiporter activity and bicarbonate reabsorption, thereby causing a mild hyperchloraemic acidosis. The elevated $1,25(OH)_2D$ acts on the intestine to increase (+) absorption of dietary calcium and phosphate, and it is important to note that PTH does not appear to have a direct action on the gut. Thus, in response to hypocalcaemia and the increase in PTH secretion, all of these direct and indirect actions of PTH on the kidney, bone, and intestine will help to increase ECF Ca^{2+}, which in turn will act via the calcium-sensing receptor to decrease PTH secretion.

the circulation with a short half-life of about 2 min, via non-saturable hepatic uptake and renal excretion.

PTH shares a receptor with PTH-related peptide (PTHrP); this PTH/PTHrP receptor (Fig. 1) is a member of a subgroup of the G protein-coupled receptor family. The PTH/PTHrP receptor gene is located on chromosome 3p21–p24 and is expressed in kidney and bone, where PTH is its predominant agonist. Expression of the PTH/PTHrP receptor also occurs in the brain, heart, skin, lung, liver, and testis where is mediates the actions of PTHrP. Mutations involving the genes that encode these proteins

and receptors in this calcium regulating pathway (Fig. 2) are associated with hypercalcaemic and hypocalcaemic disorders (Table 1).

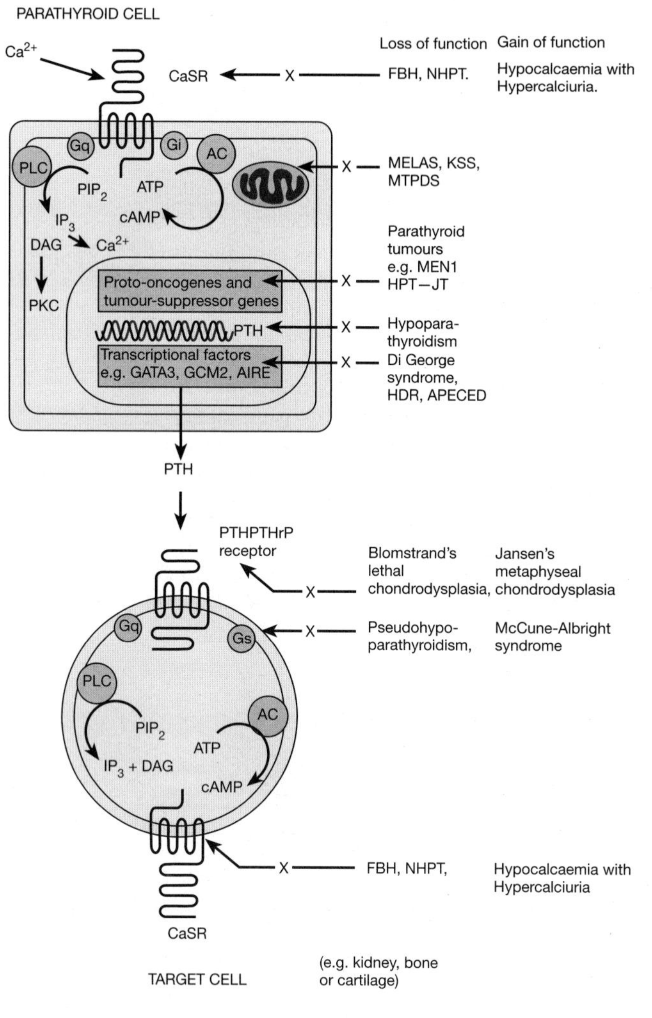

Hypercalcaemia

Clinical features and investigations

The clinical presentation of hypercalcaemia varies from a mild, asymptomatic, biochemical abnormality detected during routine screening to a life-threatening medical emergency. In general, the presence or absence of symptoms correlates with the severity and rapidity of onset of the hypercalcaemia. Thus, symptoms do not usually develop when serum calcium is below 3.00 mmol/l and are invariably present when the hypercalcaemia exceeds 3.50 mmol/l. However, there is a considerable variability and some patients may be symptomatic with mild hypercalcaemia (2.65–2.90 mmol/l). Although there are many causes of hypercalcaemia (Table 2), the signs and symptoms of hypercalcaemia are similar, regardless of aetiology. Indeed the clinical manifestations of hypercalcaemia involve several organ systems that include the renal, musculoskeletal, gastrointestinal, neurological, and cardiac systems (Table 3), and many of these have been referred to as 'moans, groans, pains, and stones'. Investigations should be directed at confirming the presence of hypercalcaemia and establishing the cause (Table 2).

The causes of hypercalcaemia can be classified according to whether serum PTH concentrations are elevated (i.e. primary hyperparathyroidism) or low (i.e. not due to a parathyroid tumour). Primary hyperparathyroidism and malignancy are the most common causes and account for more than 90 per cent of patients with hypercalcaemia. Detailed clinical history and examination will usually help to differentiate between these two diagnoses. In primary hyperparathyroidism, the hypercalcaemia is often less than 3.00 mmol/l, asymptomatic, and may have been present for months or years. If symptoms, for example nephrolithiasis, are present then they have usually been present for several months. However, in malignancy, the patients are usually acutely ill, often with neurological symptoms, the hypercalcaemia is more than 3.00 mmol/l, and the cancer (e.g. lung, breast, or myeloma) is often readily apparent. Hypercalcaemia from causes other than primary hyperparathyroidism or malignancy may also occur (Table 2) and a careful history (e.g. for vitamin D ingestion, drugs, renal disease) and examination (e.g. for thyrotoxicosis, adrenal disease, granulomatosis diseases), together with appropriate investigations (Table 4) are essential for establishing the diagnosis.

Management of hypercalaemia

The management of hypercalcaemia depends on the severity of the hypercalcaemia and the presence of symptoms. Thus, asymptomatic patients with mild hypercalcaemia, that is serum calcium below 3.00 mmol/l, do not usually need urgent treatment. However, a patient with severe hypercalcaemia, that is a serum calcium above 3.50 mmol/l, would require treatment regardless of symptoms, whilst a patient with moderate hypercalcaemia, that is a serum calcium in the range 3.00 to 3.50 mmol/l, would require urgent treatment if symptomatic. Before instituting treatment, it is always important to consider the underlying causes (Table 2) and to initiate investigations (Table 4).

The acute management of hypercalcaemia involves general measures to enhance hydration and diuresis, and specific measures using drugs to lower serum calcium. Dehydration due to hypercalcaemic symptoms, for example anorexia, nausea, vomiting and polyuria because of defective urinary concentration, is very common and patients may require 5 to 10 l of 0.9 per cent sodium chloride over a 24 to 48-h period. This vigorous hydration with normal saline may lower serum calcium by 0.25 to 0.75 mmol/l; it enhances urinary calcium excretion by increasing glomerular filtration and reducing proximal and distal renal tubular reabsorption of calcium and sodium. This saline diuresis may need adjuvant therapy with a loop diuretic, for example frusemide 20 to 100 mg to control complications due to

Fig. 2 Schematic representation of some of the components involved in calcium homeostasis. Alterations in extracellular calcium are detected by the calcium-sensing receptor (CaSR), which is a 1078 amino acid G-protein coupled receptor. The PTH/PTHrP-receptor, which mediates the actions of PTH and PTHrP, is also a G-protein coupled receptor. Thus, Ca^{2+} and PTH and PTHrP involve G protein-coupled signalling pathways and interaction with their specific receptors can lead to activation of Gs, Gi, and Gq, respectively. Gs stimulates adenylcyclase (AC) which catalyses the formation of cAMP from ATP. Gi inhibits AC activity. cAMP stimulates PKA which phosphorylates cell-specific substrates. Activation of Gq stimulates PLC, which catalyses the hydrolysis of the phosphoinositide (PIP_2) to inositol triphosphate (IP_3), which increases intracellular calcium, and diacylglycerol (DAG), which activates PKC. These proximal signals modulate downstream pathways, which result in specific physiological effects. Abnormalities in several genes, which lead to mutations in proteins in these pathways, have been identified in specific disorders of calcium homeostasis (Table 1). Adapted from Thakker RV, (2000). Parathyroid disorders. Molecular genetics and physiology. In: Morris PJ, Wood WC, eds. *Oxford Textbook of Surgery*, 2nd edn, pp. 1121–9. Oxford University Press, Oxford.

volume overload, especially in the elderly and those with impaired cardio-vascular and renal function. Saline diuresis may lead to hypokalaemia, hypomagnesaemia, and electrolyte imbalance, which will need correction.

If saline diuresis is not successful, and particularly if the hypercalcaemia is very severe, then more specific measures, for example dialysis and/or

drugs, will be required. The drug of choice is pamidronate, which is a potent bisphosphonate that is administered parenterally. A recommended regimen is to administer 60 to 90 mg intravenously as a single infusion. Other bisphosphonates, for example etidronate and clodronate and other agents such as mithramycin, calcitonin, and gallium nitrate, have also been

Table 1 Parathyroid diseases and their chromosomal locations

Metabolic abnormality	Disease	Inheritance	Gene/gene product	Chromosomal location
Hypercalcaemia	Multiple endocrine neoplasia type 1	Autosomal dominant	MENIN	11q13
	Multiple endocrine neoplasia type 2	Autosomal dominant	RET	10q11.2
	Hereditary hyperparathyroidism and jaw tumours (HPT-JT)	Autosomal dominant	Unknown	1q21–31
	Sporadic hyperparathyroidism	Sporadic	PRAD1/CCND1	11q13
			Retinoblastoma	13q14
			Unknown	1p32-pter
	Familial benign hypercalcaemia (FBH)			
	FBH3q	Autosomal dominant	CaSR	3q13–21
	FBH19p	Autosomal dominant	Unknown	19p13
	FBHOk	Autosomal dominant	Unknown	19q13
	Neonatal hyperparathyrodism (NHPT)	Autosomal recessive	CaSR	3q13–21
		Autosomal dominant		
	Jansen's disease	Autosomal dominant	PTHR/PTHrPR	3p21.1–p22
	William's syndrome	Autosomal dominant	Elastin, LIMK (and other genes)	7q11.23
	McCune–Albright syndrome	Mutations during early embryonic development?	Gsα	20q13.2–13.3
Hypocalcaemia	Isolated hypoparathyroidism	Autosomal dominant	PTH	11p15 [a]
		Autosomal recessive	PTH	11p15 [a]
		X-linked recessive	Unknown	Xq26–27
	Hypocalcaemic hypercalciuria	Autosomal dominant	CaSR	3q13–21
	Hypoparathyroidism associated with polyglandular autoimmune syndrome (APECED)	Autosomal recessive	AIRE-1	21q22.3
	Hypoparathyroidism associated with Kearns–Sayre and MELAS	Maternal	Mitochondrial genome	
	Hypoparathyroidism associated with complex congenital syndromes			
	DiGeorge	Autosomal dominant	RNEX40[c]	22q11/10p
			NEX2.2-NEX3[c]	
			UDF1L[c]	
	HDR syndrome	Autosomal dominant	GATA3	10p
	Blomstrand lethal chondrodysplasia	Autosomal recessive	PTHR/PTHrPR	3p21.1–p22
	Kenney–Caffey	Autosomal dominant[b]	Unknown	?
	Barakat	Autosomal recessive[b]	Unknown	?
	Lymphoedema	Autosomal recessive	Unknown	?
	Nephropathy, nerve deafness	Autosomal dominant[b]	Unknown	?
	Nerve deafness without renal dysplasia	Autosomal dominant	Unknown	?
	Dysmorphology, growth failure	Autosomal recessive	Unknown	1q42–43
	Pseudohypoparathyroidism (type Ia)	Autosomal dominant parentally imprinted	Gsα	20q13.2–13.3
	Pseudohypoparathyroidism (type Ib)	Autosomal dominant parentally imprinted	Unknown	20q13.3

MELAS = mitochondrial encephalopathy, stroke-like episodes, and lactic acidosis; HDR = hypoparathyroidism, deafness, and renal dysplasia; ? = location not known.

[a]Mutations of PTH gene identified only in some families.

[b]Most likely inheritance.

[c]Most likely candidate genes.

Table 2 Causes of hypercalcaemia

High parathyroid hormone (PTH) levels

Primary hyperparathyroidism[a] (adenoma, hyperplasia, or carcinoma): non-familial or familial, e.g. MEN1, MEN2, HPT-JT, FIHP

Tertiary hyperparathyroidism (hyperplasia or adenoma in chronic renal failure)

Low parathyroid hormone (PTH) levels

Malignancy[a]

    Primary

        Parathyroid hormone related protein, PTHrP (carcinoma of lung, oesophagus, renal cell, ovary, and bladder)

        Excess production of 1,25 dihydroxy vitamin D (lymphoma)

    Secondary

        Lytic bone metastases[a] (multiple myeloma[a] and breast carcinoma[a])

        Other location, ectopic factors (e.g. cytokines)

Excess Vitamin D

    Exogenous vitamin D toxicity by parent D compound, 25 (OH) vitamin D_3, or 1,25 $(OH)_2$ Vitamin D_3 in vitamin preparations, cod-liver oil, herbal medicines

    Endogenous production of 25 (OH) vitamin D_3—William's syndrome

    Endogenous production of 1,25 $(OH)_2$ vitamin D_3, e.g. granulomatous disorders (sarcoidosis, TB, histoplasmosis, coccidiomycosis, leprosy) and lymphoma

Drugs

    Thiazide diuretics

    Lithium

    Total parenteral nutrition

    Oestrogens/antioestrogens, testosterone

    Milk-alkali syndrome

    Vitamin A toxicity

    Foscarnet

    Aluminium intoxication (in chronic renal failure)

Non-parathyroid endocrine disorders

    Thyrotoxicosis

    Phaeochromocytoma

    Acute adrenal insufficiency

    Vasoactive intestinal polypeptide hormone producing tumour (VIPoma)

    Immobilization

Inappropriate parathyroid hormone (PTH) levels due to altered set point

Familial benign hypocalciuric hypercalcaemia (FBH or FHH)

[a]Most common causes

used in the past. Glucocorticoid therapy (e.g. hydrocortisone 120 mg/day in three divided doses) is particularly effective when the hypercalcaemia is mediated by the actions of 1,25-dihydroxy vitamin D, for example in granulomatosis disease or lymphoma (Table 2), or myeloma. Once the acute management of hypercalcaemia has been completed, then appropriate treatment for the underlying cause, for example parathyroidectomy for primary hyperparathyroidism, needs to be undertaken.

Table 3 Clinical features of hypercalcaemia

Renal

Stones (nephrolithasis) and neprhocalcinosis, polyuria

Musculoskeletal

Bone pain, osteopenia, fractures, muscular weakness, especially proximal myopathy

Gastrointestinal

Nausea, vomiting, lack of appetite, constipation, peptic ulcers, and pancreatitis

Neurological

Tiredness, lethargy, inability to concentrate, increased sleepiness, depression, confusion, coma

Cardiac

Bradycardia, first-degree A-V block, arrhythmias, shortened QT interval

Table 4 Preliminary investigations for hypercalcaemia

Blood

× 2–3 estimations of serum calcium, phosphate, albumin, urea and electrolytes, creatinine, alkaline phosphatase, liver function tests

PTH

Hb, FBC, ESR

Electrophoretic protein strip

25-OH Vitamin D_3 (and if indicated, 1,25 $(OH)_2$ Vitamin D_3)

Thyroid function tests

Magnesium

Urine

× 2–3 estimations of 24-h urinary calcium and creatinine, and clearance ratios

Imaging

Chest radiograph

Radiograph of hands

Ultrasound of kidneys

Hypercalcaemic diseases

Hypercalcaemia may arise through one more of three mechanisms: increased bone resorption, increased gastrointestinal absorption of calcium, and decreased renal calcium excretion. For example: lytic bone metastases cause increased bone resorption; thiazide diuretics lead to a decrease in calcium excretion; and excessive PTH will either directly or indirectly, by increasing 1,25-dihydroxy vitamin D production, stimulate bone resorption and calcium absorption from the gut and renal tubules. The hypercalcaemic diseases may be classified according to whether serum PTH concentrations are elevated or reduced (Table 2). In addition, hypercalcaemia may also be classified as being due to: an excess of PTH (e.g. primary or tertiary hyperparathyroidism) from parathyroid tumours; an excessive production of PTHrP; a defect in the PTH receptor (i.e. the PTH/PTHrP receptor); an excess production of down-stream mediators, for example 1,25-dihydroxy vitamin D; or an altered set point in the calcium-sensing receptor (Fig. 2).

Hyperparathyroidism

Hyperparathyroidism is characterized by high concentrations of serum immunoreactive PTH, and three types, referred to as primary, secondary, and tertiary, are recognized. Primary and tertiary hyperparathyroidism are associated with hypercalcaemia (Table 2), whereas secondary hyperparathyroidism is associated with hypocalcaemia (see below). Primary hyperparathyroidism may arise as an isolated endocrinopathy or as part of a multiple endocrine neoplasia (MEN) syndrome, and tertiary hyperparathyroidism usually arises in association with chronic renal failure.

Primary hyperparathyroidism

Primary hyperparathyroidism, which affects 1 in 1000 adults, is one of the two most common causes of hypercalcaemia and is due to an excessive secretion of PTH from one or more parathyroid tumours. In 80 per cent of patients this tumour is a solitary parathyroid adenoma, and in 15 per cent to 20 per cent of patients hyperplasia involving all four parathyroids is present. Parathyroid carcinoma accounts for less than 0.5 per cent of patients with primary hyperparathyroidism. Primary hyperparathyroidism usually occurs between the ages of 40 to 65 years, and is three times more common in females than males. The underlying causes of primary hyperparathyroidism are largely unknown, but abnormalities of several genes have been identified. Thus, abnormalities of the *cyclin D1* (*CCNDI*), *retinoblastoma*, *calcium-sensing receptor* (*CaSR*), *MEN type 1* (*MEN1*), and *type 2* (*MEN2*) genes together with other genes, yet to be identified, on chromosomes 1p and 1q (Table 1) are associated with the development of some parathyroid tumours.

Clinical features Many patients with primary hyperparathyroidism will be asymptomatic and the hypercalcaemia, which is usually mild, will have been detected by chance at the time of biochemical screening for other reasons. However, it is important to note that nearly half the patients will

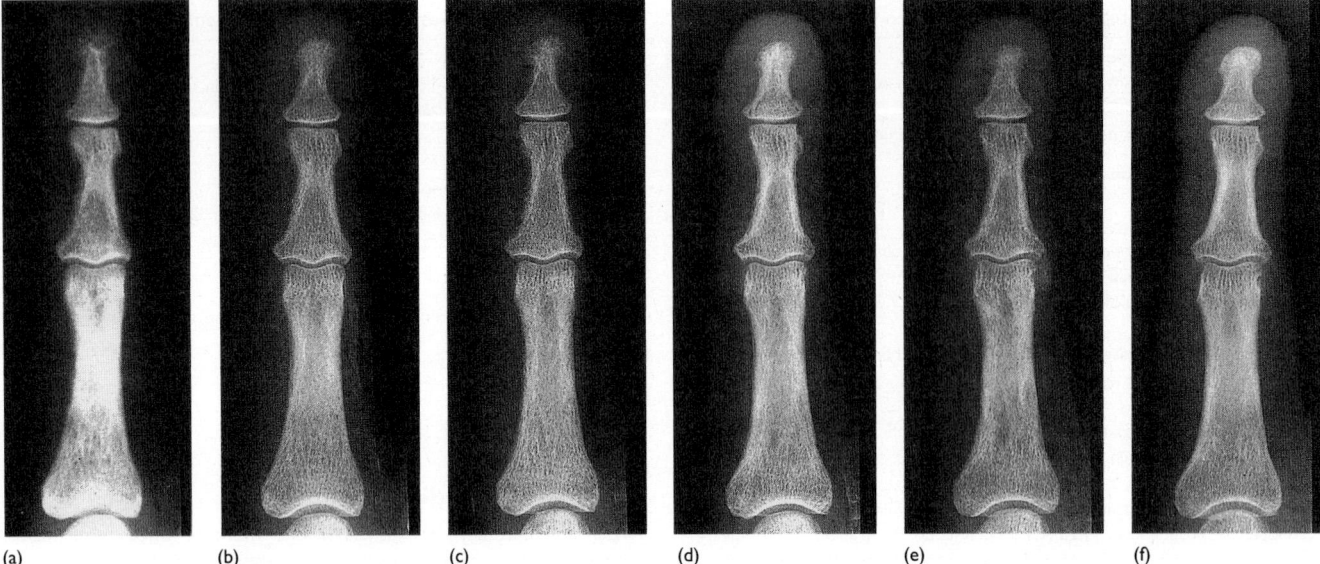

(a)   (b)   (c)   (d)   (e)   (f)

Fig. 3 Renal osteodystrophy over a 9-year period in a patient with chronic renal failure. Marked periosteal erosions were seen (a) despite treatment with 1α-hydroxy cholecaliferol, and a resolution was observed following dialysis (b). Note the vascular calcification. One year later a relapse was noted with periosteal erosions (c) and the use of calcitriol resolved these (d). Unfortunately, a relapse occurred 2 years later (e), and following renal transplantation a marked resolution was observed (f).

have subtle neuromuscular symptoms such as fatigue and weakness and this becomes apparent only in retrospect after a successful parathyroidectomy.

Symptomatic hypercalcaemia (Table 3) predominantly affects the skeletal, renal, and gastrointestinal systems; peptic ulcers and pancreatitis may develop. The skeletal changes of osteitis fibrosa cystica due to subperiosteal resorption of the distal phalanges (Fig. 3), tapering of the distal clavicles, a 'salt and pepper' appearance of the skull, bone cysts, and brown tumours of the long bones are now identified in less than 5 per cent of patients. However, osteopenia, as assessed by bone mineral density, occurs in 25 per cent of patients. Renal stone disease (nephrolithiasis and nephrocalcinosis) occurs in 20 per cent of patients and hypercalciuria occurs in 30 per cent of patients; renal impairment may complicate this disease.

Investigations In the presence of hypercalcaemia, the finding of elevated circulating PTH concentrations establishes the diagnosis, as the PTH will be elevated in approximately 90 per cent of patients with primary hyperparathyroidism, who will invariably have hypercalcaemia. However, it is important to make sure that the immunoradiometric (IRMA) and immunochemiluminometric (ICMA) assays for PTH are being used to measure the intact molecule, rather than the older radioimmunoassays which were not as reliable. The only other hypercalcaemic disorders in which PTH may occasionally be elevated are those related to familial benign hypocalciuric hypercalcaemia (FBH or FHH), immobilization, or lithium or thiazide use (Table 2), and a careful history and a cessation of drug use will help to exclude these possibilities. About one-third of patients with primary hyperparathyroidism will have a low serum phosphate and in the others it will be in the lower range of normal. In addition, some patients will have a small increase in serum chloride concentration and a concomitant decrease in bicarbonate concentration. Serum alkaline phosphatase activity may be elevated in some patients, and urinary calcium excretion is increased in 30 per cent of patients. The circulating 1,25-dihydroxy vitamin D concentration is elevated in some patients with primary hyperparathyroidism although it is not of diagnostic value as it is also elevated in other hypercalcaemic disorders such as sarcoidosis and lymphomas. The serum 25-hydroxy vitamin D concentration is within the normal range. Densitometric scanning is of use in detecting early skeletal changes. Patients with primary hyperparathyroidism develop reduced bone mineral densities (osteopenia) primarily of the cortical bone (e.g. distal third of forearm) rather than the cancellous

bone (e.g. lumbar spine). The hip bones, which are an equal mixture of cortical and cancellous bone, show intermediate reductions in bone mineral density. Overall, the risk of bone fractures in patients with mild primary hyperparathyroidism is similar to those in matched, normal controls. However, successful parathyoidectomy does lead to an increase in bone mineral density over a 6 to 12-month period and this continues for up to 10 years. Indeed, bone mineral density measurements are used in the evaluation of patients with primary hyperparathyroidism and in deciding conservative as opposed to surgical management (Table 5).

Preoperative localization to define the site(s) of the parathyroid tumours may be undertaken. The non-invasive tests consist of ultrasonography, computed tomography (CT), magnetic resonance imaging (MRI), and scintigraphy with technetium-99m sestamibi. Sestamibi scintigraphy has now become established as the best and most convenient localization test; this can be performed with computed tomographic techniques (SPECT) to give a three-dimensional image with greater anatomical resolution. It is important to note that there is an appreciable incidence of false positive rates with all the non-invasive localization procedures and so a confirmation using two methods is preferable. Invasive localization tests consist of arteriography and selective venous sampling for PTH in the veins draining the thyroidal region. These tests are time-consuming, expensive, difficult, and dependent on the skill of the radiologist. It is generally accepted that these preoperative localization tests are indicated in those patients who have had previous neck surgery. However, their role in patients who have

Table 5 Guidelines for the management of primary hyperparathyroidism, recommended by NIH consensus conference

Surgery recommended if patient meets any one of the following criteria:

- Serum calcium >3.00 mmol/l (>12 mg/dl)
- Any complication of primary hyperparathyroidism e.g. nephrolithiasis, bone erosions of osteitis fibrosa cystica
- An episode of acute primary hyperparathyroidism with life-threatening hypercalcaemia
- Marked hypercalciuria (>9 mmol/l per 24 h or >400 mg/24 h)
- Reduction in bone mass at the distal radius as determined by bone densitometry; >2 standard deviations below age and sex-matched controls
- Age <50 years old

not had prior surgery remains to be established and at present the preferences and expertise of the local medical, radiology, and surgery teams usually determine the use of venous sampling procedures.

Management and treatment Parathyroidectomy, which is the definitive cure, is a generally successful and safe procedure if undertaken by an experienced surgeon. Thus surgery is recommended for symptomatic patients and for those who have skeletal and renal complications. However, the decision to recommend surgery, which does have a small risk, may be difficult in asymptomatic patients, who may constitute over 50 per cent of patients with primary hyperparathyroidism. The natural history of primary hyperparathyroidism in most patients is to progress slowly or not at all. For example amongst asymptomatic patients, only 25 per cent will have progressive disease, which is usually manifested as a decrease in bone mineral density during a 10-year period. This has lead to a controversy regarding the indications for surgery, and guidelines have been provided by the Consensus Development Conference on the Management of Asymptomatic Primary Hyperparathyroidism (Table 5). However, these guidelines may not exclusively influence the decision for or against surgery and a careful evaluation and assessment of the risks and benefits is considered by most medical and surgical teams in conjunction with the patient. Clearly, some patients will not wish to continue living with a curable disease and will prefer surgery despite the guidelines (Table 5), whilst other patients will decline surgery, despite having guideline indications for surgery, because they may have coexisting medical conditions that make them feel that the risks of surgery are too great.

Patients who do not undergo parathyroidectomy should be evaluated clinically, and also monitored for serum calcium, creatinine, and PTH at 6 to 12-monthly intervals, and for bone mineral density and nephrolithiasis at 12-monthly intervals. In addition, the following medical guidelines are recommended. First, they should avoid dehydration and remain ambulant. Second, the dietary intake of calcium should be moderate, that is at or below 1000 mg/day, and thiazide diuretics should be avoided. Finally, they should avoid herbal and tonic remedies that may contain Vitamin D or A. These measures may help and at present an effective and safe drug for the treatment of primary hyperparathyroidism is not available. Drugs that have been used include oral phosphate, oestrogens in postmenopausal women, and the bisphosphonates—alendronate and clodronate. Phosphate is not used because of concerns related to soft tissue ectopic calcification, and although oestrogen does increase bone density in postmenopausal women, it has little effect on the serum calcium and PTH concentrations. The bisphosphonates inhibit bone resorption and do reduce serum calcium. However, these effects are not sustained. A more targeted approach using drugs that alter the function of the calcium sensing receptor, CaSR (see below), is being evaluated, and these calcimimetic agents may provide a medical therapy; for example use of such an agent has been shown to reduce serum calcium and PTH in postmenopausal women with asymptomatic primary hyperparathyroidism.

Uraemic hyperparathyroidism

Serum PTH levels rise in response to hypocalcaemia and this secondary hyperparathyroidism usually resolves with treatment of the underlying cause of hypocalcaemia (Table 6). However, in chronic renal failure the secondary hyperparathyroidism may persist for a longer time, and eventually the parathyroid cells gain an autonomous function, secreting excessive PTH despite hypercalcaemia; this state is referred to as tertiary hyperparathyroidism (Table 2). The cause of progression from the early, presumably polyclonal, secondary hyperplasia of the parathryoids to the later, presumably monoclonal, tumours is not understood and appears to involve genes other than those involved in the aetiologies of the sporadic and familial forms of primary hyperparathyroidism (Table 1).

Clinical features and treatment In chronic renal failure, the ensuing phosphate retention and decreased production of 1,25-dihydroxy vitamin D result in hypocalcaemia and secondary hyperparathyroidism. This combination of biochemical abnormalities results in a severe bone disease that shows combined features of hyperparathyroidism and vitamin D deficiency (i.e. osteomalacia). Thus in renal osteodystrophy, bone erosions (Fig. 3) and osteomalacia are simultaneously observed. Treatment is based on correcting the hypocalcaemia, for example with oral administration of calcium salts, which also ameliorates the hyperphosphataemia by chelating phosphate in the intestines, and with calcitriol (1,25-dihydroxy vitamin D). The use of the most appropriate phosphate binder is not well established but it is clear that aluminium-containing compounds are to be avoided. Aluminium in these preparations and as a contaminant of dialysis solutions contributed in the recent past to the osteomalacic osseous disease and other aspects of metal toxicity in patients with renal failure (e.g. hypochromic anaemia and encephalopathy). Early treatment of the metabolic disturbance will prevent or delay the onset of severe secondary hyperparathyroidism and tertiary hyperparathyroidism, which requires parathyroidectomy.

Familial primary hyperparathyroidism

Primary hyperparathyroidism is most frequently encountered as a non-familial disorder. However, approximately 10 per cent of patients with primary hyperparathyroidism will have a hereditary form which may either be part of the multiple endocrine neoplasia type 1 (MEN1) and type 2 (MEN2) syndromes, or part of the hereditary hyperparathyroidism–jaw

---

Table 6 Causes of hypocalcaemia

Low parathyroid hormone levels (hypoparathyroidism)
Parathyroid agenesis
    Isolated or part of complex developmental anomaly (e.g. Di George syndrome)
Parathyroid destruction
    Surgery[a]
    Radiation
    Infiltration by metastases or systemic disease (e.g. haemochromatosis, amyloidosis, sarcoidosis, Wilson's disease, thalassaemia)
Autoimmune
    Isolated
    Polyglandular (type 1) [a]
Reduced parathyroid function (i.e. parathyroid hormone secretion)
    Parathyroid hormone gene defects
    Hypomagnesaemia[a]
    Neonatal hypocalcaemia (may be associated with maternal hypercalcaemia)
    Hungry bone disease (postparathyroidectomy)
    Calcium-sensing receptor mutations

High parathyroid hormone levels (secondary hyperparathyroidism)
Vitamin D deficiency[a]
    As a result of nutritional lack[a], malabsorption[a], liver disease, or Vitamin D receptor defects
Vitamin D resistance (rickets)
    As a result of renal tubular dysfunction (Fanconi's syndrome) or Vitamin D receptor defects
Parathyroid hormone resistance
    (e.g. pseudohypoparathyroidism, hypomagnesaemia)
Drugs
    Calcium chelators (e.g. cirated blood transfusions, phosphate; cow's milk is rich in phosphate)
    Inhibitors of bone resorption (e.g. bisphosphonates, calcitonin, plicamycin)
    Altered vitamin D metabolism (e.g. phenytoin, ketaconazole)
    Foscarnet
Miscellaneous
    Acute pancreatitis
    Acute rhabdomyolysis
    Massive tumour lysis
    Osteoblastic metastases (e.g. from prostate or breast carcinoma)
    Toxic shock syndrome
    Hyperventilation

[a]Most common causes.

tumour (HPT-JT) syndrome. In addition, hereditary primary hyperparathyroidism may develop as a solitary endocrinopathy and this has also been referred to as familial isolated hyperparathyroidism (FIHP). Investigations of these hereditary and sporadic forms of primary HPT have helped to identify some of the genes and chromosomal regions that are involved in the aetiology of parathyroid tumours (Table 1). FIHP has been reported in several kindreds, and some have been shown to harbour mutations of the MEN1 gene whilst in other families linkage to polymorphic loci from chromosome 1q21–q31, the region of the HPT-JT syndrome, has been shown. In addition, analysis of parathyroid tumours from FIHP patients has revealed loss of heterozygosity (LOH) involving chromosome 1q21–q31 loci. FIHP located on chromosome 1q21–q31 has been reported to be associated with a high incidence of early-onset parathyroid carcinomas. These familial syndromes associated with parathyroid tumours will be briefly reviewed.

Multiple endocrine neoplasia type 1 (MEN 1) MEN1 is characterized by the combined occurrence of tumours of the parathyroids, pancreatic islet cells, and anterior pituitary. Parathyroid tumours occur in 95 per cent of MEN1 patients, and the resulting hypercalcaemia is the first manifestation of MEN1 in about 90 per cent of patients. Pancreatic islet cell tumours occur in 40 per cent of MEN1 patients and gastrinomas, leading to the Zollinger–Ellison syndrome, are the most common type and also the important cause of morbidity and mortality in MEN1 patients. Anterior pituitary tumours occur in 30 per cent of MEN1 patients, with prolactinomas representing the most common type. Associated tumours, which may also occur in MEN1, include adrenal cortical tumours, carcinoid tumours, lipomas, angiofibromas, and collagenomas. The gene causing MEN1, which is located on chromosome 11q13 and represents a putative tumour suppressor gene, consists of 10 exons that encode a 610 amino acid protein, referred to as 'MENIN'. The majority (>80 per cent) of the germ line *MEN1* mutations in families are inactivating. MENIN has been shown to be located in the nucleus, where it directly interacts with the N-terminus of the AP1 transcriptional factor JunD. MENIN suppresses JunD-activated transcription and thus MENIN acts via the transcriptional regulation pathway to control cell proliferation.

Multiple endocrine neoplasia type 2 (MEN2) MEN2 describes the association of medullary thyroid carcinoma (MTC), phaeochromocytomas, and parathyroid tumours. Three clinical variants of MEN2 are recognized—MEN2a, MEN2b, and MTC-only. MEN2a is the most common variant, where the development of MTC is associated with phaeochromocytomas (50 per cent of patients), which may be bilateral, and parathyroid tumours (20 per cent of patients). MEN2b, which represents 5 per cent of all MEN2 cases, is characterized by the occurrence of MTC and phaeochromocytoma in association with a Marfanoid habitus, mucosal neuromas, medullated corneal fibres, and intestinal autonomic ganglion dysfunction leading to multiple diverticulae and megacolon. Parathyroid tumours do not usually occur in MEN2b. MTC-only is a variant in which medullary thyroid carcinoma is the sole manifestation of the syndrome. The gene causing all three MEN2 variants was mapped to chromosome 10cen–10q11.2, a region containing the c-*RET* proto-oncogene which encodes a tyrosine kinase receptor with cadherin-like and cysteine-rich extracellular domains and a tyrosine kinase intracellular domain. Specific mutations of c-*RET* have been identified for each of the three MEN2 variants. Thus in 95 per cent of patients, MEN2a is associated with mutations of the cysteine-rich extracellular domain and mutations in codon 634 (Cys→Arg) account for 85 per cent of MEN2a mutations. MTC-only is also associated with missense mutations in the cysteine-rich extracellular domain and most mutations are at codon 618. MEN2b is associated with mutations in codon 918 (Met→Thr) of the intracellular tyrosine kinase domain in 95 per cent of patients. Mutational analysis of c-*RET* to detect mutations in codons 609, 611, 618, 634, 768, and 804 in MEN2a and MTC-only, and codon 918 in MEN2b, has been used in the diagnosis and management of patients and families with these disorders.

Hyperparathyroidism–jaw tumour (HPT-JT) syndrome The HPT-JT syndrome is an autosomal dominant disorder characterized by the development of parathyroid tumours and fibro-osseous jaw tumours. In addition, some patients may also develop Wilms' tumours, renal cysts, renal hamartomas, renal cortical adenomas, papillary renal cell carcinomas, pancreatic adenocarcinomas, testicular mixed germ cell tumours with a major seminoma component, and Hurthle cell thyroid adenomas. It is important to note that the parathyroid tumours may occur in isolation and without any evidence of jaw tumours, and this may cause confusion with other hereditary hypercalcaemic disorders such as MEN1, familial benign hypercalcaemia (FBH), which is also referred to as familial hypocalciuric hypercalcaemia (FHH), and FIHP. HPT-JT can be distinguished from FBH, as in FBH serum calcium concentrations are elevated from the early neonatal or infantile period whereas in HPT-JT such elevations are uncommon in the first decade. In addition, HPT-JT patients, unlike in FBH, will have associated hypercalciuria. The distinction between HPT-JT patients and MEN1 patients, who have only developed the usual first manifestation of hypercalcaemia (>90 per cent of patients), is more difficult and is likely to be influenced by the operative and histological findings and the occurrence of other characteristic lesions in each disorder. It is noteworthy that HPT-JT patients will usually have single adenomas or a carcinoma, whilst MEN1 patients will often have multiglandular parathyroid disease. The distinction between FIHP and HPT-JT in the absence of jaw tumours is difficult but important as HPT-JT patients may be at a higher risk of developing parathyroid carcinomas. These distinctions may be helped by the identification of additional features, and a search for jaw tumours, renal, pancreatic, thyroid, and testicular abnormalities may help to identify HPT-JT patients. The jaw tumours in HPT-JT are different from the brown tumours observed in some patients with primary hyperparathyroidism, and do not resolve after parathyroidectomy. Indeed ossifying fibromas of the jaw are an important distinguishing feature of HPT-JT from FIHP, and the occurrence of these may occasionally precede the development of hypercalcaemia in HPT-JT patients by several decades. The gene causing HPT-JT has been mapped to chromosome 1q25–q31.

Malignancy

The hypercalcaemia of malignancy is usually due to increased bone resorption, which may either be directly due to skeletal metastases or indirectly due to tumour-production of a humoral factor that stimulates osteoclastic bone resorption. The cancers that typically metastasize to produce lytic bone lesions are from the breast, lymphomas, or multiple myeloma (Table 2). The cancers that are typically associated with the humoral hypercalcaemia of malignancy (HHM) are squamous carcinomas of the lung, oesophagus, cervix, vulva, skin, head, or neck, but other types from the kidney, bladder, ovary, and breast may also occur. HHM accounts for up to 80 per cent of patients with malignancy-associated hypercalcaemia. The most common factor causing HHM is parathyroid hormone related peptide (PTHrP), which can be measured in the serum by immunoassay. However, these assays are relatively insensitive and the failure to detect serum PTHrP does not exclude the diagnosis of HHM. Patients with HHM generally have hypercalcaemia associated with lower or undetectable serum PTH levels, marked hypercalcaemia, and a reduced plasma 1,25-dihydroxy vitamin D level. Therapy of HHM is aimed at: (1) reducing the tumour load by surgery, radiotherapy, and/or chemotherapy; (2) reducing osteoclastic bone resorption by use of bisphosphonates or calcitonin; and (3) increasing renal calcium clearance by a saline diuresis.

Granulomatous disorders

Several granulomatous disorders are associated with hypercalcaemia (Table 2) and this is invariably associated with elevated circulating concentrations of 1,25-dihydroxy vitamin D, which is due to extrarenal synthesis. Sarcoidosis is the most frequently encountered granulomatous disorder associated with hypercalcaemia and 10 per cent of patients with sarcoidosis will have hypercalcaemia and about one-half will become hypercalciuric. The finding of raised serum angiotensin converting enzyme (ACE) activity may help in confirming the diagnosis. Glucocorticoids (e.g. 40 to 60 mg of prednisolone) decrease 1,25-dihydroxy vitamin D production and restore the calcium concentration to normal. Failure to achieve normal serum calcium concentrations within 10 days of glucocorticoid therapy (e.g. hydrocortisone 40 mg, three times per day), which is referred to as the steroid suppression test, should suggest the coexistence of another cause for the hypercalcaemia, for example primary hyperparathyroidism or malignancy.

Endocrine causes of hypercalcaemia other than hyperparathyoidism

Several non-parathyroid disorders (Table 2) are associated with hypercalcaemia and these include thyrotoxicosis, phaeochromocytoma, Addison's disease, VIPomas, familial benign hypocalciuric hypercalcaemia, Jansen's disease, and William's syndrome.

Thyrotoxicosis

Mild hypercalcaemia (<3.00 mmol/l) frequently accompanies thyrotoxicosis, which leads to increased bone turnover and resorption. The hypercalcaemia may respond to treatment with β-adrenergic blockers.

Familial benign hypocalciuric hypercalcaemia and neonatal primary hyperparathyroidism

Familial benign hypercalcaemia (FBH), which is also referred to as familial hypocalciuric hypercalcaemia (FHH), is an autosomal dominant disorder with a high degree of penetrance, that is characterized by lifelong asymptomatic hypercalcaemia in association with an inappropriately low urinary calcium excretion (i.e. calcium clearance to creatinine clearance ratio <0.01). A normal circulating parathyroid hormone (PTH) concentration and mild hypermagnesaemia are also typically present. Although most patients with FBH are asymptomatic, chondrocalcinosis and acute pancreatitis have occasionally been observed. In addition, children of consanguineous marriages within FBH kindreds have been observed to have life-threatening hypercalcaemia due to neonatal primary hyperparathyroidism (NHPT). NHPT is defined as symptomatic hypercalcaemia with skeletal manifestations of hyperparathyroidism in the first 6 months of life. NHPT children often present in the first few days or weeks of life with failure to thrive, dehydration, hypotonia, constipation, rib cage deformities, and multiple fractures due to bony undermineralization. Children with NHPT often require urgent parathyroidectomy, which corrects the PTH-dependent hypercalcaemia and bone demineralization. FBH is due to heterozygous inactivating mutations of the calcium sensing receptor (CaSR) and NHPT is often associated with inactivating homozygous CaSR mutations (Fig. 2). However, NHPT has also been observed in children where only one parent had clinically apparent FBH, and many other NHPT patients appear to be sporadic, that is both parents have normal serum calcium concentrations. In such NHPT patients with heterozygous CaSR mutations, the mutant CaSR may exert a dominant negative action on the normal CaSR. The human CaSR is a 1078 amino acid cell surface protein which is expressed in parathyroids, thyroid cells, and kidney, and is a member of the family of G-protein coupled receptors. The *CaSR* gene is located on chromosome 3q21–q24.

Jansen's disease

Jansen's disease is an autosomal dominant disease that is characterized by short-limbed dwarfism, due to metaphyseal chondrodysplasia, and severe hypercalcaemia and hypophosphataemia, despite normal or undetectable serum levels of PTH. These abnormalities are associated with activating mutations of the PTH receptor (Fig. 2) and thus this represents a PTH-independent activation of the PTH receptor (PTHR). Two different mutations of the PTHR have been identified, and these involve codon 223 (His→Arg) and codon 410 (Thr→Pro). Expression of the mutant receptors in COS-7 cells resulted in constitutive, ligand-independent accumulation of cAMP, while the basal accumulation of inositol phosphates was not increased. These findings provide a likely explanation for the abnormalities

observed in mineral homeostasis and growth plate development in this disorder.

William's syndrome

William's syndrome is an autosomal dominant disorder characterized by supravalvular aortic stenosis, elfin-like facies, psychomotor retardation, and infantile hypercalcaemia. The underlying abnormality of calcium metabolism remains unknown but abnormal 1,25-dihydroxy vitamin D₃ metabolism or decreased calcitonin production have been implicated, although no abnormality has been consistently demonstrated. Hemizygosity due to a microdeletion at the *ELASTIN* locus on chromosome 7q11.23 in over 90 per cent of patients with the classical William's phenotype has been demonstrated. This microdeletion has been reported to involve another gene, designated *LIM-KINASE*, that is expressed in the central nervous system. The calcitonin receptor gene has been localized to chromosome 7q21 and close to the region deleted in William's syndrome. However, the calcitonin receptor gene was not involved in the deletion found in four patients with William's syndrome, indicating that it is unlikely to be implicated in the hypercalcaemia of such children. While the involvement of the *ELASTIN* and *LIM-KINASE* genes in the deletions of William's syndrome patients can explain the respective cardiovascular and neurological features of this disorder, it seems possible that another, as yet uncharacterized, gene that is within this contiguously deleted region is likely to be involved to explain the abnormalities of calcium metabolism.

Drugs

Several drugs (Table 2) can cause hypercalcaemia by different mechanisms. Compounds containing vitamins D and A are common and frequently associated with hypercalcaemia. The use of thiazide diuretics is often associated with hypercalcaemia. The hypercalcaemia appears to be largely renal in origin, as thiazides enhance distal renal tubular calcium reabsorption. Hypercalcaemia reverses rapidly with discontinuation of the drug.

The milk-alkali syndrome was first described in the 1930s, generally in the context of ulcer treatment with large quantities of milk together with sodium bicarbonate. Today, the responsible agent is usually calcium carbonate, although consumption of large quantities of dairy products (milk, cheese, and yoghurt) may still contribute. Classical features include moderate to severe hypercalcaemia with alkalosis and renal impairment. The amount of calcium ingested by patients with this syndrome is usually 5 to 15 g/day. Treatment consists of: (1) discontinuing the ingestion of the calcium containing compounds(s) and antacids; (2) rehydration; and (3) saline diuresis.

Hypocalcaemia

Clinical features and investigations

The clinical presentation of hypocalcaemia (serum calcium <2.12 mmol/l) ranges from an asymptomatic biochemical abnormality to a severe, life-threatening condition. In mild hypocalcaemia (serum calcium 2.00–2.12 mmol/l), patients may be asymptomatic. Those with more severe (serum calcium <1.9 mmol/l) and long-term hypocalcaemia may develop: acute symptoms of neuromuscular irritability (Table 7); ectopic calcification (e.g. in the basal ganglia, which may be associated with extrapyramidal neurological symptoms); subcapsular cataract; papilloedema; and abnormal dentition. Investigations should be directed at confirming the presence of hypocalcaemia and establishing the cause. Hypocalcaemia (Table 6) can be classified by cause, according to whether serum parathyroid hormone (PTH) concentrations are low (i.e. hypoparathyroid disorders) or high (i.e. disorders associated with secondary hyperparathyroidism). Hypocalcaemia is most commonly caused by hypoparathyroidism, a deficiency or abnormal metabolism of vitamin D, acute or chronic renal failure, or hypomagnesaemia. In hypoparathyroidism, serum calcium is low, phosphate is high, and PTH is undetectable; renal function and concentrations of the

Table 7 Hypocalcaemic clinical features of neuromuscular irritability

Paraesthesia, usually of fingers, toes, and circumoral regions
Tetany, carpopedal spasm, muscle cramps
Chvostek's sign[a]
Trousseau's sign[b]
Seizures of all types (i.e. focal or petit mal, grand mal or syncope)
Prolonged QT interval on ECG
Laryngospasm
Bronchospasm

[a]Chvostek's sign is twitching of the circumoral muscles in response to gentle tapping of the facial nerve just anterior to the ear; it may be present in 10 per cent of normal individuals.
[b]Trousseau's sign is carpal spasm elicited by inflation of a blood pressure cuff to 20 mmHg above the patient's systolic blood pressure for 3 min.

25-hydroxy and 1,25-dihydroxy metabolites of vitamin D are usually normal. The features of pseudohypoparathyroidism are similar to those of hypoparathyroidism except for PTH, which is markedly increased. In chronic renal failure, which is the most common cause of hypocalcaemia, phosphate is high and alkaline phosphatase, creatinine, and PTH are elevated; 25-hydroxy vitamin D_3 is normal and 1,25-dihydroxy vitamin D_3 is low. In vitamin D deficiency osteomalacia, serum calcium and phosphate are low, alkaline phosphatase and PTH are elevated, renal function is normal, and 25-hydroxy vitamin D_3 is low. The most frequent artifactual cause of hypocalcaemia is hypoalbuminaemia, such as occurs in liver disease or the nephrotic syndrome.

Management of acute hypocalcaemia

The management of acute hypocalcaemia depends on the severity of the hypocalcaemia, the rapidity with which it developed, and the degree of neuromuscular irritability (Table 7). Treatment should be given to symptomatic patients (e.g. with seizures or tetany) and asymptomatic patients with a serum calcium of less than 1.90 mmol/l who are at high risk of developing complications. The preferred treatment for acute symptomatic hypocalcaemia is calcium gluconate, 10 ml 10 per cent w/v (2.20 mmol of calcium) intravenous, diluted in 50 ml of 5 per cent dextrose or 0.9 per cent sodium chloride and given by slow injection (>5 min); this can be repeated as required to control symptoms. Serum calcium concentrations should be assessed regularly. Persistent hypocalcaemia may be managed acutely by administration of a calcium gluconate infusion; for example, dilute 10 ampoules of calcium gluconate, 10 ml 10 per cent w/v (22.0 mmol of calcium), in 1 litre of 5 per cent dextrose or 0.9 per cent sodium chloride, start infusion at 50 ml/h and titrate to maintain serum calcium concentrations in the normal range. Generally, 0.3 to 0.4 mmol/kg of elemental calcium infused over 4 to 6 h increases serum calcium by 0.5 to 0.75 mmol/l. If hypocalcaemia is likely to persist, oral vitamin D therapy (see below) should also be administered. In hypocalcaemic patients who are also hypomagnesaemic, the hypomagnesaemia must be corrected before the hypocalcaemia will resolve. This may occur in the postparathyroidectomy period or in patients with severe malabsorption, for example those with established coeliac disease.

Management of persistent hypocalcaemia

The two main agents available for the treatment of hypocalcaemia are supplemental calcium, about 10 to 20 mmol calcium 6 to 12 hourly, and vitamin D preparations. Patients with hypoparathyroidism seldom require calcium supplements after the early stages of stabilization with vitamin D. A variety of vitamin D preparations have been used. These include: vitamin D_3 (cholecalciferol) or vitamin D_2 (ergocalciferol), 25 000 to 100 000 units (1.25–5 mg/day); dihydrotachysterol (now seldom used), 0.25 to 1.25 mg/day; alfacalcidol (1α-hydroxycholecalciferol), 0.25 to 1.0 μg/day; and calcitriol (1,25-dihydroxy cholecalciferol), 0.25 to 2.0 μg/day. In children, these preparations are prescribed in doses based on body weight. Cholecalciferol and ergocalciferol are the least expensive preparations but

have the longest durations of action and may result in prolonged toxicity. The other preparations, which do not require renal 1α-hydroxylation, have the advantage of shorter half-lives and thereby minimize the risk of prolonged toxicity. Calcitriol is probably the drug of choice because it is the active metabolite and, unlike alfacalcidol, does not require hepatic 25-hydroxylation. Close monitoring (at about 1–2-week intervals) of the patient's serum and urine calcium concentrations are required initially, and at 3 to 6-monthly intervals once stabilization is achieved. The aim is to avoid hypercalcaemia, hypercalciuria, nephrolithiasis, and renal failure. It should be noted that hypercalciuria may occur in the absence of hypercalcaemia.

Hypocalcaemic diseases

Hypocalcaemic diseases (Table 6) may arise because of a destruction of the parathyroid glands, failure of parathyroid gland development, or reduced PTH secretion or PTH-mediated actions in target tissues. Thus, these diseases may be classified as being due to a deficiency of PTH, a defect in the PTH-receptor (i.e. the PTH/PTHrP receptor), or an insensitivity to PTH caused by defects down-stream of the PTH/PTHrP receptor (Fig. 2). The diseases may also be classified as being part of the hypoparathyroid disorders, of the calcium sensing receptor abnormalities, or of the pseudohypoparathyroid disorders.

Hypoparathyroidism

Hypoparathyroidism is characterized by hypocalcaemia and hyperphosphataemia, which are the result of a deficiency in parathyroid hormone (PTH) secretion or action. Serum concentrations of immunoreactive PTH are low or undetectable and the concentrations of 1,25-dihydroxy vitamin D_3 are usually in the low normal to low range but alkaline phosphatase activity is unchanged. The daily urinary excretion of calcium is reduced, although the fractional excretion of calcium is increased. Nephrogenous cyclic adenosine monophosphate (cAMP) excretion is low and renal tubular reabsorption of phosphate is elevated. Urinary cAMP, plasma cAMP, and urinary phosphate excretion increase markedly after administration of exogenous bioactive PTH (Chase–Aurbach and Ellsworth–Howard tests). Hypoparathyroidism may result from agenesis (e.g. the DiGeorge syndrome) or destruction of the parathyroid glands (e.g. following neck surgery, in autoimmune diseases), from reduced secretion of PTH (e.g. neonatal hypocalcaemia or hypomagnesaemia), or resistance to PTH (which may occur as a primary disorder (e.g. pseudohypoparathyroidism or secondary to hypomagnesaemia). In addition, hypoparathyroidism may occur as an inherited disorder (Table 1) that may either be part of a complex congenital defect (e.g. DiGeorge syndrome), or as part of a pluriglandular autoimmune disorder, or as a solitary endocrinopathy, which has been referred to as isolated or idiopathic hypoparathyroidism. Hypoparathyroidism may also complicate iron storage disease, especially secondary haemochromatosis in children and adolescents. In thalassaemic children, destruction of the parathyroids is associated with ill health and frank tetany, which may elude diagnosis and effective treatment unless hypoparathyroidism is suspected.

Isolated hypoparathyroidism

Isolated hypoparathyroidism may either be inherited or it may be acquired by damage to the parathyroids at surgery, by infiltrating metastases, or systemic disease (Table 6).

Inherited hypoparathyroidism Patients with inherited forms of hypoparathyroidism may develop hypocalcaemic seizures in the neonatal or infantile periods and require life-long treatment with oral vitamin D preparations, for example calcitriol. Autosomal dominant, autosomal recessive, and X-linked recessive inheritances for hypoparathyroidism have been observed (Table 1). Some of the autosomal forms are due to mutations of the *PTH* gene, the calcium sensing receptor (see below), and the transcriptional factor *GCM2* (glial cells missing 2).

Acquired forms of hypoparathyroidism Hypoparathyroidism may occur after neck surgery, irradiation, or because of infiltration by metastases or systemic disease, for example haemochromatosis, amyloidosis, sarcoidosis, Wilson's disease, or thalassaemia (Table 6). Surgical damage to the parathyroids occurs most commonly after a radical neck dissection, for example laryngeal or oesophageal carcinoma treatment, a total thyroid resection, or after repeated parathyroidectomies for multigland disease (e.g. in MEN1 or MEN2, see above). Hypocalcaemic symptoms begin 12 to 24 h postoperatively and may need treatment with oral or intravenous calcium. Parathyroid function often returns, but persistent hypocalcaemia requires treatment with vitamin D preparations.

Neonatal hypoparathyroidism resulting in hypocalcaemia may occur in the baby of a mother with hypercalcaemia caused by primary hyperparathyroidism. Maternal hypercalcaemia results in increased calcium delivery to the fetus, and this fetal hypercalcaemia suppresses fetal PTH secretion. Postpartum, the infant's suppressed parathyroids are unable to maintain normocalcaemia. The disorder is usually self-limiting, but occasionally therapy may be required. In addition, the feeding of cow's milk, which has a high phosphate content, to babies may also result in hypocalcaemia in some children.

Functional hypoparathyroidism may result from severe hypomagnesaemia (<0.40 mmol/l), which may be due to a severe intestinal malabsorption disorder (e.g. Crohn's disease) or a renal tubular disorder. It is associated with hypoparathyroidism because magnesium is required for the release of PTH from the parathyroid gland and also for PTH action via adenyl cyclase. Magnesium chloride, 35 to 50 mmol intravenously in 1 litre of 5 per cent glucose or other isotonic solution given over 12 to 24 h may be repeatedly required to restore normomagnesaemia.

Complex syndromes associated with hypoparathyroidism
Hypoparathyroidism may occur as part of a complex syndrome which may either be associated with a congenital developmental anomaly or with an autoimmune syndrome. The congenital developmental anomalies associated with hypoparathyroidism include the DiGeorge, the HDR (hypoparathyroidism, deafness, and renal anomalies), the Kenney–Caffey and Barakat syndromes, and also syndromes associated with either lymphoedema or dysmorphic features and growth failure (Table 1).

DiGeorge syndrome Patients with the DiGeorge syndrome (DGS) suffer from neonatal hypoparathyroidism, T-cell immunodeficiency, congenital heart defects, and deformities of the ear, nose, and mouth (e.g. cleft lip and/or palate). Children with DGS often die from infections related to the immunodeficiency. The disorder arises from a congenital failure in the development of the derivatives of the third and fourth pharyngeal pouches with resulting absence or hypoplasia of the parathyroids and thymus. Most cases of DGS are sporadic but an autosomal dominant inheritance of DGS has been observed and an association between the syndrome and an unbalanced translocation and deletions involving chromosome 22q11.2 have also been reported. In some patients, deletions of another locus on chromosome 10p13–p14 have been observed in association with DGS and this is referred to as DGS type 2 (DGS2), whilst patients with the 22q11.2 deletions are referred to as DGS type 1 (DGS1). Studies of the DGS1 deleted region on chromosome 22q11.2 have revealed three genes (referred to as *RNEX40*, *NEX2.2-NEX3*, and *UDFIL* to be involved). However, although these are involved in the chromosomal deletions, the mechanisms by which they lead to the varied manifestations of DGS remain to be elucidated.

Hypoparathyroidism, deafness, and renal anomalies (HDR) syndrome HDR is an autosomal dominant disorder in which patients often have asymptomatic hypocalcaemia with undetectable or inappropriately normal serum concentrations of PTH, and normal brisk increases in plasma cAMP in response to the infusion of PTH. Bilateral, symmetrical, sensorineural deafness involving all frequencies occurs, and the renal abnormalities consist mainly of bilateral cysts that compress the glomeruli and tubules and

lead to renal impairment. Cytogenetic abnormalities involving chromosome 10p14–10pter have been identified in HDR patients. HDR patients do not have immunodeficiency or heart defects, which are key features of DGS2, and indeed there are two non-overlapping regions; thus, the DGS2 region is located on 10p13–14 and HDR on 10p14–10pter. HDR patients have a haploinsufficiency of the zinc finger transcription factor GATA3.

Mitochondrial disorders associated with hypoparathyroidism Hypoparathyroidism has been reported to occur in three disorders associated with mitochondrial dysfunction: the Kearns–Sayre syndrome (KSS), the MELAS syndrome, and a mitochondrial trifunctional protein deficiency syndrome (MTPOS). Kearns–Sayre syndrome is characterized by progressive external ophthalmoplegia and pigmentary retinopathy before the age of 20 years, and is often associated with heart block or cardiomyopathy. The MELAS syndrome consists of a childhood onset of mitochondrial encephalopathy, lactic acidosis, and stroke-like episodes. In addition, varying degrees of proximal myopathy can be seen in both conditions. Both the Kearns–Sayre and MELAS syndromes have been reported to occur with insulin dependent diabetes mellitus and hypoparathyroidism, and mitochondrial gene abnormalities have been identified in some patients. Mitochondrial trifunctional protein deficiency is a disorder of fatty acid oxidation that is associated with peripherial neuropathy, pigmentary retinopathy, and acute fatty liver degeneration in pregnant women who carry an affected fetus. Hypoparathyroidism has been observed in one patient with trifunctional protein deficiency.

Kenney–Caffey syndrome Hypoparathyroidism has been reported to occur in over 50 per cent of patients with the Kenney–Caffey syndrome, which is associated with short stature, osteosclerosis, and cortical thickening of the long bones, delayed closure of the anterior fontanel, basal ganglia calcification, nanophthalmos, and hyperopia. Parathyroid tissue could not be found in a detailed post mortem examination of one patient and this suggests that hypoparathyroidism may be due to an embryological defect of parathyroid development. The molecular genetic defect has not been identified.

Additional familial syndromes Single familial syndromes in which hypoparathyroidism is a component have been reported (Table 1). Thus, an association of hypoparathyroidism, renal insufficiency, and developmental delay has been reported in one Asian family in whom autosomal recessive inheritance of the disorder was established. The occurrence of hypoparathyroidism, nerve deafness, and a steroid-resistant nephrosis leading to renal failure, which has been referred to as the Barakat syndrome, has been reported in four brothers from one family, and an association of hypoparathyroidism with congenital lymphoedema, nephropathy, mitral valve prolapse, and brachytelephalangy has been observed in two brothers from another family. Molecular genetic studies have not been reported from these two families. A syndrome in which hypoparathyroidism was associated with severe growth failure and dysmorphic features has been reported in twelve patients from Saudi Arabia. Consanguinity was noted in 11 of the 12 patients' families, the majority of which originated from the Western province of Saudi Arabia. This syndrome, which is inherited as an autosomal recessive disorder, has also been identified in families of Bedouin origin and homozygosity and linkage disequilibrium studies have located this gene to chromosome 1q42–q43.

Blomstrand's disease Blomstrand's chondrodysplasia is an autosomal recessive disorder characterized by early lethality, dramatically advanced bone maturation, and accelerated chondrocyte differentiation. Affected infants, who usually have consanguineous unaffected parents, develop pronounced hyperdensity of the entire skeleton with markedly advanced ossification, that results in extremely short and poorly modelled long bones. Mutations of the PTH/PTHrP receptor that impair its function are associated with Blomstrand's disease. Thus, it seems likely that affected infants will, in addition to the skeletal defects, have abnormalities in other organs, including secondary hyperplasia of the parathyroid glands, presumably due to hypocalcaemia.

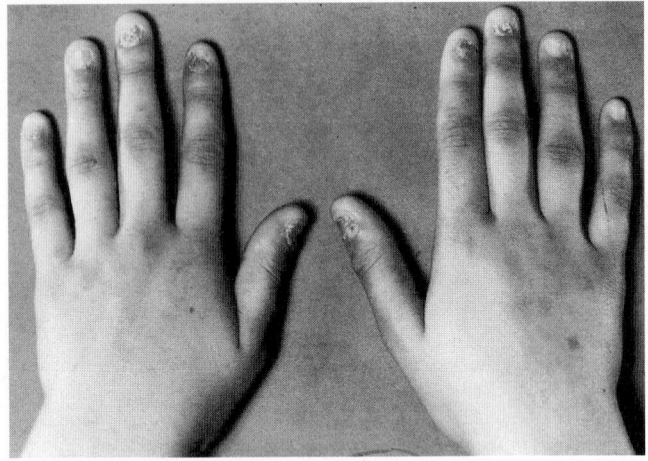

Fig. 4 Moniliasis and hyperpigmentation of the hands, particularly over the knuckles, is seen in this 8-year-old patient with hypoparathyroidism and Addison's disease. The patient also had vitiligo, and thus had some of the features of the polyglandular autoimmune syndrome type 1. Reproduced with permission from Thakker RV. Hypocalcaemic disorders. In: Thakker RV, Wass JAH, eds (1997). *Endocrine Disorders, Medicine,* vol. 25, pp. 68–70. The Medicine Group (Journals) Ltd, Abingdon, Oxon.

Pluriglandular autoimmune hypoparathyroidism This syndrome (Fig. 4) comprises of hypoparathyroidism, Addison's disease, candidasis, and two or three of the following: insulin-dependent diabetes mellitus, primary hypogonadism, autoimmune thyroid disease, pernicious anaemia, chronic active hepatitis, steatorrhoea (malabsorption), alopecia (totalis or areata), and vitiligo. The disorder has also been referred to as either the autoimmune polyendocrinopathy candidasis ectodermal dystrophy (APECED) syndrome or the polyglandular autoimmune type 1 syndrome. Antibodies directed against the adrenal, thyroid, and parathyroid glands are detected in the sera of some patients. The polyglandular autoimmune type 2 syndrome is characterized by adrenal insufficiency, insulin-dependent diabetes mellitus, and thyroid disease, and does not involve hypoparathyroidism. APECED, which has an autosomal recessive inheritance, has a high incidence in Finland and amongst Iranian Jews. The *APECED* gene, which has been located to chromosome 21q22.3, encodes a 545 amino acid protein that contains motifs suggestive of a transcriptional factor and includes a nuclear localization signal, two zinc-finger motifs, a proline-rich region, and three LXXLL motifs. The gene is referred to as *AIRE* (autoimmune

regulator); six *AIRE* mutations have been reported in APECED families and a codon 257 (Arg→Stop) mutation was the predominant abnormality in 82 per cent of the Finnish families.

Calcium-sensing receptor (CaSR) abnormalities

The CaSR, which is located in the plasma membrane of the cell (Fig. 2), is at a critical site to enable the cell to recognize changes in extracellular calcium concentration. Thus, an increase in extracellular calcium leads to CaSR activation of the G-protein signalling pathway, which in turn increases the free intracellular calcium concentration and leads to a reduction in transcription of the *PTH* gene. CaSR mutations that result in a loss of function are associated with familial hypocalciuric hypercalcaemia (see above). However, CaSR missense mutations that result in a gain of function (or added sensitivity to extracellular calcium) lead to hypocalcaemia with hypercalciuria. These hypocalcaemic individuals are generally asymptomatic and have serum PTH concentrations that are in the low–normal range, and because of the insensitivities of previous PTH assays in this range such patients have often been diagnosed to be hypoparathyroid. In addition, such patients may have hypomagnesaemia. Treatment with vitamin D or its active metabolites to correct the hypocalcaemia in these patients results in marked hypercalciuria, nephrocalcinosis, nephrolithiasis, and renal impairment. Thus, these patients need to be distinguished from those with hypoparathyroidism.

Pseudohypoparathyroidism (PHP)

Patients with pseudohypoparathyroidism (PHP), which may be inherited as an autosomal dominant disorder, are characterized by hypocalcaemia and hyperphosphataemia due to PTH resistance rather than PTH deficiency. Five variants are recognized on the basis of biochemical and somatic features (Table 8) and three of these—PHP type Ia (PHPIa), PHP type 1b (PHPIb), and pseudopseudohypoparathyroidism (PPHP)—will be reviewed in further detail. Patients with PHPIa exhibit PTH resistance (hypocalcaemia, hyperphosphataemia, elevated serum PTH, and an absence of an increase in serum and urinary cyclic AMP and urinary phosphate following intravenous human PTH infusion), together with the features of Albright's hereditary osteodystrophy (AHO), which includes short stature, obesity, subcutaneous calcification, mental retardation, round facies, dental hypoplasia, and brachydactyly (i.e. shortening of the metacarpals (Fig. 5), particularly the third, fourth, and fifth). In addition to brachydactyly, other skeletal abnormalities of the long bones and shortening of the metatarsals may also occur. Patients with PHPIb exhibit PTH resistance only and do not have the somatic features of AHO, whilst patients with PPHP exhibit the somatic features of AHO in the absence of

Table 8 Clinical, biochemical and genetic features of hypoparathyroid and pseudohypoparathyroid disorders

	Hypoparathyroidism	Pseudohypoparathyroidism (PHP)				
		PHPIa	PPHP	PHPIb	PHPIc	PHPII
AHO manifestations	No	Yes	Yes	No	Yes	No
Serum calcium	↓	↓	N	↓	↓	↓
Serum PO₄	↑	↑	N	↑	↑	↑
Serum PTH	↓	↑	N	↑	↑	↑
Response to PTH:						
Urinary cAMPᵃ (Chase–Aurbach test)	↑	↓	↑	↓	↓	↑
Urinary PO₄ (Ellsworth–Howard test)	↑	↓	↑	↓	↓	↓
Gsα activity	N	↓	↓	N	N	N
Inheritance	AD/AR/X	AD	AD	AD	AD	Sporadic
Molecular defect	PTH/CaSR/ GATA3/Gcm2/ others	GNAS1	GNAS1	?GNAS1	?adenyl cyclase	?cAMP targets
Other hormonal resistance	No	Yes	No	No	Yes	No

↓ = decreased, ↑ = increased, N = normal, AD = autosomal dominant, AR = autosomal recessive, X = X-linked, AHO = Albright's hereditary osteodystrophy, ? = presumed, but not proven.

ᵃplasma cAMP responses are similar to those of urinary cAMP.

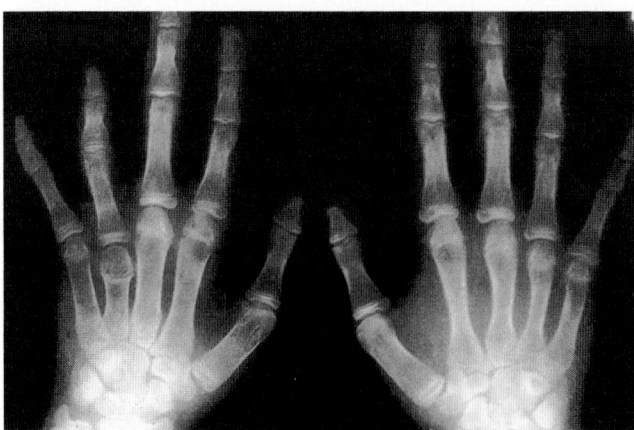

Fig. 5 Radiograph of both hands of a patient with pseudohypoparathyroidism type 1a. The patient has a normal right hand, but there is shortening of the left fourth metacarpal (brachydactyly). Metatarsals may be similarly shortened. Reproduced with permission from Thakker RV. Hypocalcaemic disorders. In: Thakker RV, Wass JAH, eds (1997). *Endocrine Disorders, Medicine*, vol. 25, pp. 68–70. The Medicine Group (Journals) Ltd, Abingdon, Oxon.

PTH resistance. The absence of a normal rise in urinary excretion of cyclic AMP excretion after an infusion of PTH in PHPIa indicated a defect at some site of the PTH receptor–adenyl cyclase system (Fig. 2). This receptor system is regulated by at least two G proteins, one of which stimulates (Gsα) and another which inhibits (Giα) the activity of the membrane-bound enzyme that catalyses the formation of the intracellular second messenger cyclic AMP. Interestingly, patients with PHPIa may also show resistance to other hormones, for example thyroid-stimulating hormone (TSH), follicle-stimulating hormone (FSH), and luteinizing hormone (LH), that act via G-protein coupled receptors. Inactivating mutations of the Gsα gene (referred to as *GNAS1*), which is located on chromosome 20q13.2, have been identified in PHPIa and PPHP patients. However, *GNAS1* mutations do not fully explain the PHPIa or PPHP phenotypes, and studies of PHPIa and PPHP that occurred within the same kindred revealed that the hormonal resistance is parentally imprinted. Thus, PHPIa occurs in a child only when the mutation is inherited from a mother affected with either PHPIa or PPHP; and PPHP occurs in a child only when the mutation is inherited from a father affected with either PHPIa or PPHP. *GNAS1* mutations have not been detected in PHPIb, which has been considered to be due to a defect of the PTH/PTHrP receptor. However, studies of the PTH/PTHrP receptor gene and mRNA in PHPIb patients have not identified mutations, and linkage studies in four unrelated kindreds have mapped the PHPIb locus to chromosome 20q13.3, a location that also contains the *GNAS1* gene. In addition, parental imprinting of the genetic defect was observed and this is similar to the findings in kindreds with PHP-type Ia and/or PPHP. Two possible explanations for these observations have been proposed. First, PHPIb maybe due to a defect in a tissue- or cell-specific enhancer, or promoter, of the *GNAS1* gene and this may affect, directly or indirectly, the expression levels of the Gsα-specific transcripts. Or, second, PHPIb may be caused by a defect in a gene close to the *GNAS1* gene which is transcribed only from the maternal allele and affects PTH/PTHrP receptor or Gsα expression and/or function in some renal cells.

Further reading

Bilezikian JP (1999). Primary hyperparathyroidism. In: Favus MJ, ed. *Primer on the metabolic bone diseases and disorders of mineral metabolism*, 4th edn, pp. 187–92. Lippincott–Raven, Philadelphia.

Bilezikian J, Thakker RV (1998). Hypoparathyroidism. *Current Opinion in Endocrinology and Diabetes* **4**, 427–32.

Bouillon R (2001). Vitamin D: from photosynthesis, metabolism, and action to clinical applications. In: DeGroot LJ, Jameson JL, eds. *Endocrinology*, 4th edn, pp. 1009–28. WB Saunders, Philadelphia.

Bringhurst FR (2001). Regulation of calcium and phosphate homeostasis. In: DeGroot LJ, Jameson JL, eds. *Endocrinology*, 4th edn, pp. 1029–52. WB Saunders, Philadelphia.

Deftos LJ (1998). *Clinical essentials of calcium and skeletal disorders*, 1st edn. Professional Communications, Oklahoma.

Goltzman D, Cole EC (1999). Hypoparathyroidism. In: Favus MJ, ed. *Primer on the metabolic bone diseases and disorders of mineral metabolism*, 4th edn, pp. 226–30. Lippincott-Raven, Philadelphia.

Indridason OS, Quarles LD (1999). Tertiary hyperparathyroidism and refractory secondary hyperparathyroidism. In: Favus MJ, ed. *Primer on the metabolic bone diseases and disorders of mineral metabolism*, 4th edn, pp. 198–202. Lippincott-Raven, Philadelphia.

Levine MA (1999). Parathyroid hormone resistance syndromes. In: Favus MJ, ed. *Primer on the metabolic bone diseases and disorders of mineral metabolism*, 4th edn, pp. 230–5. Lippincott-Raven, Philadelphia.

Marx SJ (2000). Hyperparathyroid and hypoparathyroid disorders. *New England Journal of Medicine* **343**, 1803–75.

Roberts MM, Stewart AF (1999). Humoral hypercalcaemia of malignancy. In Favus MJ, ed. *Primer on metabolic bone diseases and disorders of mineral metabolism*, 4th edn, pp. 203–7. Lippincott-Raven, Philadelphia.

Shane E (1999). Hypercalcaemia: pathogenesis, clinical manifestations, differential diagnosis and management. In: Favus MJ, ed. *Primer on the metabolic diseases and disorders of mineral metabolism*, 4th edn, pp. 183–7. Lippincott-Raven, Philadelphia.

Shane E (1999). Hypocalcaemia: pathogenesis, differential diagnosis and management. In: Favus MJ, ed. *Primer on the metabolic bone diseases and disorders of mineral metabolism*, 4th edn, pp. 223–6. Lippincott-Raven, Philadelphia.

Stewart AF (1999). Miscellaneous causes of hypercalcaemia. In: Favus MJ, ed. *Primer on the metabolic bone diseases and disorders of mineral metabolism*, 4th edn, pp. 215–19. Lippincott-Raven, Philadelphia.

Thakker RV (1998). Disorders of the calcium sensing receptor. *Biochemica et Biophysica Acta* **1448**, 166–70.

Thakker RV (1998). Multiple endocrine neoplasia–syndromes of the twentieth century. *Journal of Clinical Endocrinology and Metabolism* **83**, 2617–20.

Thakker RV (2000). Parathyroid disorders. Molecular genetics and physiology. In: Morris PJ, Wood WC, eds. *Oxford textbook of surgery*, pp. 1121–9. Oxford University Press, Oxford.

Thakker RV (2001). Multiple endocrine neoplasia type 1. In: DeGroot LJ, Jameson JL, eds. *Endocrinology*, pp. 2503–17. WB Saunders, Philadelphia.

Thakker RV, Juppner H (2001). Genetic disorders of calcium homeostasis caused by abnormal regulation of parathyroid hormone secretion or responsiveness. In: DeGroot LJ, Jameson JL, eds. *Endocrinology*, pp. 1062–74. WB Saunders, Philadelphia.

12.7 The adrenal

12.7.1 Disorders of the adrenal cortex

P. M. Stewart

Introduction

Three main types of hormone are produced by the adrenal cortex—glucocorticoids (cortisol, corticosterone), mineralocorticoids (aldosterone, deoxycorticosterone), and sex steroids (mainly androgens). The biochemical pathways involved in their synthesis are shown in Fig. 1. Glucocorticoids are secreted in relatively high amounts (cortisol 10 to 20 mg/day) from the zona fasciculata under the control of ACTH, whilst mineralocorticoids are secreted in low amounts (aldosterone 100 to 150 μg/day) from the zona glomerulosa under the principal control of angiotensin II. Classic endocrine feedback loops are in place to control the secretion of both hormones—cortisol inhibits the secretion of both corticotrophin-releasing factor and ACTH from the hypothalamus and pituitary, respectively, and the aldosterone-induced sodium retention inhibits renal renin secretion.

Within the adrenal cortex, cholesterol is taken up from circulating cholesterol bound to low-density lipoprotein and an initial, rate-limiting step in adrenal steroidogenesis is the uptake of cholesterol by mitochondria dependent upon a recently characterized protein, steroidogenic acute regulatory protein (or StAR). Thereafter, the functional zonation of the adrenal cortex is achieved in part through the discrete expression and regulation of the final steroidogenic enzymes—aldosterone synthase, expressed in the glomerulosa, and 11β-hydroxylase in the fasciculata (Fig. 1).

Aldosterone acts physiologically to stimulate sodium transport across epithelial cells in the distal nephron, colon, and salivary gland. This involves the interaction of aldosterone with the mineralocorticoid receptor and the induction of the basolateral sodium–potassium ATPase pump and the apical sodium channel. This is mediated through the induction of a novel gene, serum- and glucocorticoid-induced kinase (sgk). The mineralocorticoid receptor, however, is non-selective *in vitro*; paradoxically cortisol and aldosterone have the same intrinsic affinity for this receptor, raising the question as to how aldosterone is the preferred mineralocorticoid *in vivo*. This selectivity is achieved at a prereceptor level through the expression of an enzyme, 11β-hydroxysteroid dehydrogenase type 2 (**11β-HSD2**), which efficiently inactivates cortisol to cortisone allowing aldosterone to occupy the mineralocorticoid receptor. Inhibition of 11β-HSD2 results in cortisol, conventionally regarded as a glucocorticoid, acting as a potent mineralocorticoid.

Glucocorticoids have more diverse and extensive roles than mineralocorticoids, regulating sodium and water homeostasis, glucose and carbohydrate metabolism, inflammation, and stress. These effects are mediated by the interaction of cortisol with the ubiquitous glucocorticoid receptors and the induction or repression of target gene transcription.

Adrenocortical diseases are relatively rare, but part of their importance lies in their relative ease of diagnosis and the availability of effective therapy. The diseases are most readily classified on the basis of whether there is hormone excess or deficiency (Table 1). In most instances this excess or deficiency arises from abnormal secretion of hormones. However, the defect may also relate to a change in corticosteroid metabolism (for example glucocorticoid-suppressible hyperaldosteronism, liquorice ingestion) or to defective receptors (for example glucocorticoid resistance).

Glucocorticoid excess—Cushing's syndrome

Harvey Cushing first described a case of the 'polyglandular syndrome' secondary to pituitary basophilia in 1912 and linked this to bilateral adrenal hyperplasia several years later. The first case of an adrenal adenoma was probably reported by H.G. Turney in 1913 (Fig. 2).

Definition

Cushing's syndrome comprises the symptoms and signs associated with prolonged exposure to inappropriately elevated levels of free plasma glucocorticoid (Fig. 2). This definition thus takes into account the elevated corticosteroid levels that may be found in severely depressed patients but which appear to be appropriate to the condition and also the increased total (but normal free) glucocorticoid levels found when there is an increase in circulating cortisol-binding globulin (for example in patients on oestrogen therapy). The use of the term glucocorticoid in the definition covers both

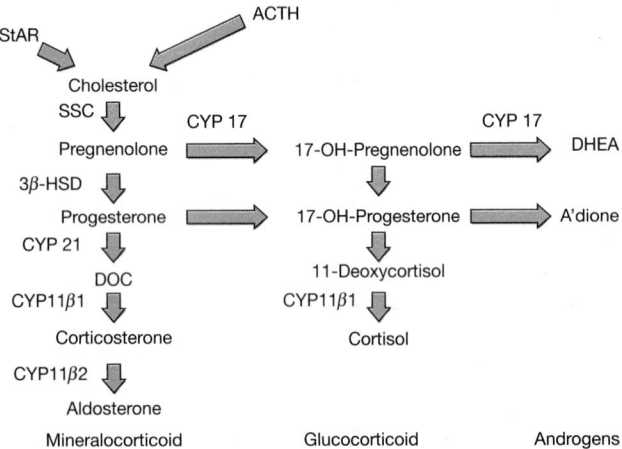

Fig. 1 Pathways of adrenocortical steroid biosynthesis.

endogenous (cortisol) and exogenous (such as prednisolone, dexamethasone) excess.

Classification of Cushing's syndrome

The condition is most readily classified into ACTH-dependent and ACTH-independent causes (Table 2). The term Cushing's syndrome is used to describe all causes whilst that of Cushing's disease is reserved for cases of pituitary-dependent Cushing's syndrome.

ACTH-dependent causes

Cushing's disease

When iatrogenic causes are excluded, the most frequent cause of Cushing's syndrome is Cushing's disease, which accounts for approximately 70 per cent of cases. The adrenal glands show bilateral adrenocortical hyperplasia with widening of the zona fasciculata and reticularis.

Cushing himself raised the question as to whether his disease was a primary pituitary condition or secondary to an abnormality in the hypothalamus. The release of ACTH from the pituitary is controlled by corticotrophin-releasing factor (**CRF**) acting synergistically with arginine vasopressin. If there was hypothalamic dysfunction in Cushing's disease, it might be expected that one or other of these would be produced in excess, yet measurement of CRF in both the circulation and cerebrospinal fluid has shown that the levels are low. This would suggest that CRF is not involved, but patients with Cushing's disease show an exaggerated ACTH response to CRF, suggesting that there may be an enhanced sensitivity of corticotrophs to this factor. However, *in vitro* experiments with microadenomas from patients with Cushing's disease have not confirmed this. By contrast there is some evidence for enhanced arginine vasopressin production in Cushing's disease and this might interact with CRF to promote tumour growth and ACTH release.

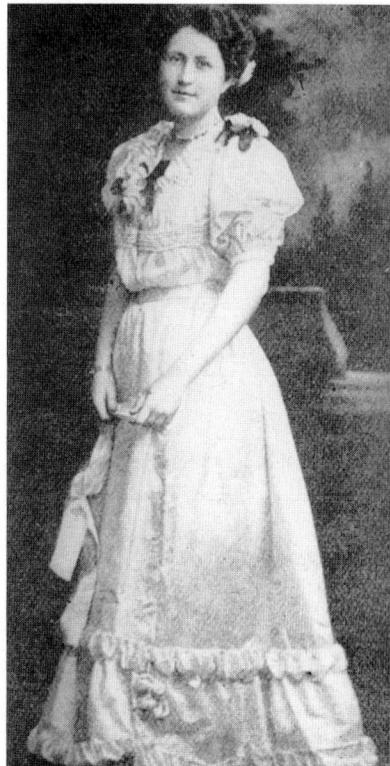
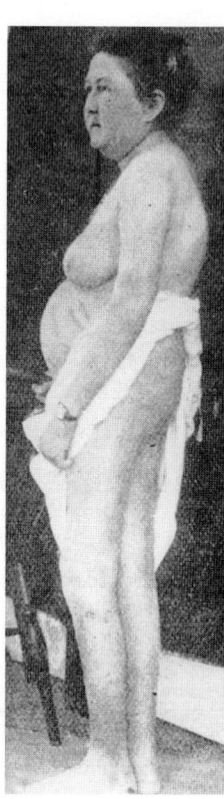

Fig. 2 H. G. Turney's case of Cushing's syndrome before and after developing the condition.

Whether or not the hypothalamus has an initiating role, there is abundant evidence that at presentation the condition is pituitary, rather than hypothalamus, dependent. In over 90 per cent of cases the disease is due to a pituitary adenoma of monoclonal origin; basophil hyperplasia is very uncommon. Selective surgical removal of the microadenoma usually results in cure with a very low recurrence rate.

Ectopic corticotrophin-releasing factor (CRF) production

This is a very rare cause of pituitary-dependent Cushing's disease. However, cases have been described in which a tumour (for example medullary thyroid, prostate carcinoma) has been shown to contain CRF but not ACTH. It has been suggested that ectopic CRF production may explain the metyrapone responsiveness and suppression with high-dose dexamethasone found in some patients with the ectopic ACTH syndrome.

Table 1 Adrenocortical diseases

Glucocorticoid excess
Cushing's syndrome
Glucocorticoid deficiency
Primary:
    Congenital adrenal hyperplasia (21 hydroxylase, 3β-hydroxysteroid
        dehydrogenase, 17-hydroxylase, 11β-hydroxylase, and StAR
        deficiencies)
    Addison's disease
    Hereditary adrenocortical unresponsiveness to ACTH
Secondary:
    Post-corticosteroid therapy
    Hypothalamic/pituitary disease
Mineralocorticoid excess
Aldosteronism
Other mineralocorticoids—monogenic forms of hypertension
Glucocorticoid resistance
Mineralocorticoid deficiency
Congenital adrenal hyperplasia
Congenital adrenal hypoplasia
Disorders of terminal part of aldosterone biosynthetic pathway
Pseudohypoaldosteronism
Hyporeninaemia
Addison's disease
Adrenal androgens
Excess:
    Congenital adrenal hyperplasia (21-hydroxylase, 11β-hydroxylase
        deficiency)
    Polycystic ovary syndrome (PCOS), tumours
Deficiency:
    Congenital adrenal hyperplasia (17-hydroxylase, 3β-hydroxysteroid
        dehydrogenase deficiency)
Adrenal incidentalomas and carcinomas

Table 2 Classification of causes of Cushing's syndrome

ACTH-dependent
Iatrogenic (treatment with ACTH$_{1-39}$ or Synacthen®, ACTH$_{1-24}$)
Cushing's disease (pituitary-dependent)
Ectopic ACTH syndrome
Ectopic corticotrophin-releasing factor syndrome
?Macroscopic nodular adrenal hyperplasia
ACTH-independent
Iatrogenic (such as pharmacological doses of prednisolone or dexamethasone)
Adrenal adenoma
Adrenal carcinoma
Carney's syndrome
McCune–Albright syndrome
Aberrant receptor expression (gastric inhibitory polypeptide, interleukin 1β).
Alcohol

ACTH, adrenocorticotrophic hormone.

Table 3 Tumours associated with the ectopic ACTH syndrome

Tumour type	Approximate incidence (%)
Small-cell lung carcinoma	50
Non-small-cell lung carcinoma	5
Pancreatic tumours (including carcinoids)	10
Thymic tumours (including carcinoids)	5
Lung carcinoids	10
Other carcinoids	2
Medullary carcinoma of thyroid	5
Phaeochromocytoma and related tumours	3
Rare carcinomas of prostate, breast, ovary, gallbladder, colon	10

Ectopic ACTH syndrome

Cushing's syndrome may be associated with non-pituitary tumours producing ACTH, most commonly a small-cell carcinoma of the bronchus (Table 3). These conditions are described further in Chapter 12.11.

Macroscopic nodular adrenal hyperplasia

In about 20 to 40 per cent of patients with Cushing's disease there is bilateral adrenocortical hyperplasia associated with one or more nodules. These may be up to several centimetres in diameter. Such nodules are a trap for the unwary (see below) as they may be mistaken for primary adrenal tumours.

ACTH-independent causes

Adrenal adenoma and carcinoma

With the exclusion of iatrogenic Cushing's syndrome, adrenal adenomas are responsible for about 10 per cent of cases and carcinomas for about the same. Carcinomas are the most common cause of Cushing's syndrome in children. The aetiology of these tumours is unknown.

Carney's syndrome

This is an autosomal dominant condition comprising mesenchymal tumours (especially atrial myxomas), spotty skin pigmentation, peripheral nerve tumours, and various endocrine tumours, one of which may lead to Cushing's syndrome. The adrenals then contain multiple, small, pigmented nodules. The condition has been described as pigmented multinodular adrenocortical dysplasia. It does not appear to be ACTH dependent and recent evidence suggests that the condition results because of mutations in the regulatory subunit R1A of protein kinase A.

McCune–Albright syndrome

In this condition fibrous dysplasia and cutaneous pigmentation may be associated with pituitary, thyroid, adrenal, and gonadal hyperfunction. The adrenal hypersecretion may produce Cushing's syndrome. The underlying abnormality is a somatic mutation in the α-subunit of the stimulatory G protein which is linked to adenyl cyclase. The mutation results in the G protein being constitutively activated (that is, in the adrenal mimics constant ACTH stimulation). Adrenal nodular formation may occur.

Aberrant receptor expression

Recently patients have been described with nodular hyperplasia, ACTH-independent Cushing's syndrome, and enhanced adrenal responsiveness to gastric inhibitory polypeptide (**GIP**). The biochemical clues were the presence of subnormal morning levels of plasma cortisol and a rise in cortisol after food. This food-dependent form of Cushing's syndrome resulted from the normal increase in GIP after eating. The adrenocortical tissue of these patients responded *in vitro* to low doses of GIP, whereas there was no such effect in normal adrenal cortex, suggesting that in some unknown manner adrenal GIP receptors are linked to steroidogenesis in these patients. Not surprisingly, the clinical syndrome is related to food intake. Fasting can produce adrenal insufficiency. It remains to be seen whether abnormalities of adrenal sensitivity to GIP play a subtle role in other types of Cushing's

syndrome. Similarly Cushing's syndrome due to a cortisol-secreting adrenal adenoma has recently been attributed to aberrant expression of receptors for interleukin 1.

Alcohol-associated pseudo-Cushing's syndrome

In the original description of this syndrome, urinary and plasma cortisol levels were elevated and were not suppressed with dexamethasone. Plasma ACTH has been found to be normal or suppressed. The frequency and pathogenesis of this condition remain unknown but a 'two-hit' hypothesis has been put forward to explain its aetiology. Chronic liver disease irrespective of the cause is associated with impaired cortisol metabolism, but in alcoholics this is associated with an increase in cortisol secretion rate, rather than concomitant suppression in the face of impaired metabolism. With abstinence from alcohol the biochemical abnormalities rapidly revert to normal.

Clinical features of Cushing's syndrome

The classic features of Cushing's syndrome with centripetal obesity, moon face, hirsutism, and plethora are well known following Cushing's initial description in 1912 (Figs 2 and 3). However, this gross clinical picture is not always present. The signs and symptoms in patients with Cushing's syndrome are listed in Table 4 together with the most discriminatory features distinguishing Cushing's from simple obesity. Weight gain and obesity were the commonest symptom and sign, but the distribution of fat was not invariably centripetal; a 'buffalo hump' was present in about half the patients.

Gonadal dysfunction is very common, with menstrual irregularity in females and loss of libido in males. Hirsutism is frequently found in female patients, as is acne.

Psychiatric abnormalities have been reported in all series of patients with Cushing's syndrome regardless of cause. Depression and lethargy are among the commonest problems, but poor concentration, paranoia, and overt psychosis are also well recognized. Lowering of plasma cortisol by medical or surgical therapy usually results in a rapid improvement in the psychiatric state.

Most patients with long-standing Cushing's syndrome have lost height because of osteoporotic vertebral collapse. This can be assessed by measuring the patient's height and comparing it with their span; in normal subjects these measurements should be equal. Pathological fractures, either spontaneous or after minor trauma, are not uncommon. Rib fractures, in contrast to those of the vertebrae, are often painless. The radiograph appearances are typical, with exuberant callus formation at the site of the healing fracture.

The plethoric appearance of the patient with Cushing's syndrome is caused by thinning of the skin and is not due to true polycythaemia. In

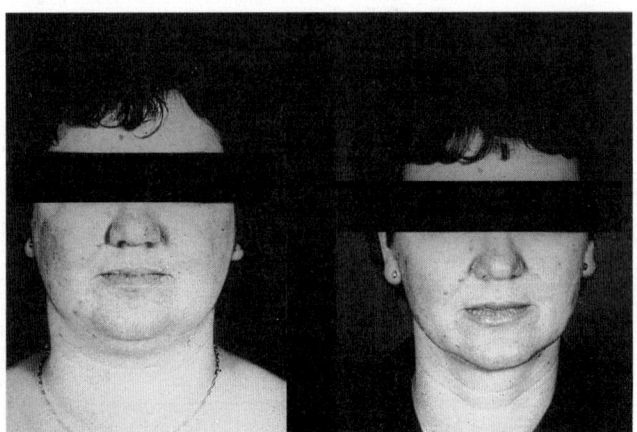

Fig. 3 Typical facies of a patient with Cushing's syndrome before and after treatment.

those with a high concentration of haemoglobin, the red cell mass is usually normal and the polycythaemia due to a reduced plasma volume.

The typical red-purple livid striae of the syndrome are found most frequently on the abdomen but may also be present on the upper thighs and arms. They are very common in younger patients and less so in those over 50.

Myopathy and bruising are two of the most discriminatory features of the syndrome. The myopathy involves the proximal muscles of lower limb and shoulder girdle. Complaints of weakness such as inability to climb stairs or get up from a deep chair are relatively uncommon, but observation of whether the patient can rise from a crouching position often reveals the problem. Bruising of the skin is often extensive and occurs with unknown or trivial trauma.

Hypertension is another prominent feature; even though epidemiological data show a strong association between blood pressure and obesity, hypertension is much more common in patients with Cushing's syndrome than in those with simple obesity.

Pigmentation is rare in Cushing's disease but common in the ectopic ACTH syndrome. However, in some pituitary tumours there is abnormal processing of the pro-opiomelanocortin (POMC) precursor molecule, with resulting pigmentation.

Infections are more common in patients with Cushing's syndrome. In many instances these are asymptomatic as the normal inflammatory response may be suppressed. Reactivation of tuberculosis has been reported. In the skin, fungal infection is frequently found. Glucose intolerance may be a predisposing factor, with overt diabetes being present in up to one-third of patients in some series.

Ocular effects may include raised intraocular pressure, chemosis, and exophthalmos (present in up to one-third of patients in Cushing's original series). Cataracts, a well-recognized complication of corticosteroid therapy, seem to be uncommon, except as a complication of diabetes.

Special features of Cushing's syndrome
Cyclical cushing's syndrome

Of particular clinical interest has been a group of patients with cyclical Cushing's syndrome, characterized by periods of excess cortisol production (for example, 40 days) followed by intervals of normal cortisol production (for example, 60 to 70 days). Some of these patients demonstrate a paradoxical rise in plasma ACTH and cortisol when treated with dexamethasone, and occasional patients show benefit with dopamine agonist (bromocriptine) or serotonin antagonist (cyproheptadine) therapy. Most patients have been thought to have pituitary-dependent disease and in many of these patients basophil adenomas have been removed, some with long-term cure. However, cortisol secretion may show some evidence of cyclicity in other causes of Cushing's syndrome, notably the ectopic ACTH syndrome.

Children

In children all the above features occur, but growth arrest is almost invariable. The dissociation between height and weight on the growth chart is obvious. It is important to try to obtain previous growth data so as to be able to calculate growth velocity. If the patient is growing along the same centile line, then the diagnosis of Cushing's syndrome is highly unlikely. In addition to glucocorticoid-induced growth arrest, androgen excess may result in precocious puberty.

Pregnancy

Pregnancy is rare in women with Cushing's syndrome because of associated amenorrhoea due to androgen excess or hypercortisolism. However, approximately 100 such cases have been reported, 50 per cent of which are due to adrenal adenomas. A few cases of true pregnancy-induced Cushing's syndrome have been reported with regression postpartum. In these cases the aetiology is unknown. Establishing a diagnosis and cause can be difficult; normal pregnancy is associated with a threefold increase in plasma cortisol due to increased production rates and increases in cortisol-binding globulin. Urinary free cortisol also rises and dexamethasone does not suppress plasma cortisol to the same degree as the non-pregnant state. Untreated the condition has a high maternal and fetal morbidity and mortality. Adrenal and/or pituitary adenomas should be excised. Metyrapone, which is not teratogenic, has been effective in many cases in controlling the hypercortisolism.

Adrenal carcinomas

In addition to the normal features resulting from glucocorticoid excess, the patient may present with other problems relating to (i) the tumour, for instance abdominal pain from the primary tumour or with secondary deposits, or (ii) the secretion of other steroids, such as androgens or mineralocorticoids. Thus, in females, in addition to hirsutism, there may be other features of virilization, with clitoromegaly, breast atrophy, deepening of the voice, temporal recession, and severe acne.

Ectopic ACTH syndrome

If this is due to a small-cell lung carcinoma, the clinical presentation more commonly resembles Addison's disease than Cushing's syndrome. The patients are very commonly pigmented and have lost weight, but the association of this with hypokalaemic alkalosis and glucose intolerance should alert the clinician. Patients with benign tumours, such as bronchial carcinoids which produce ACTH, present with the typical features of Cushing's syndrome.

Table 4 Prevalence of symptoms and signs in Cushing's syndrome and discriminant index compared with prevalence of features in patients with simple obesity

	%	Discriminant index
Symptoms		
Weight gain	91	
Menstrual irregularity	84	1.6
Hirsutism	81	2.8
Psychiatric	62	
Backache	43	
Muscle weakness	29	8.0
Fractures	19	
Loss of scalp hair	13	
Signs		
Obesity	97	
Truncal	46	1.6
Generalized	55	0.8
Plethora	94	3.0
Moon face	88	
Hypertension	74	4.4
Bruising	62	10.3
Red/purple striae	56	2.5
Muscle weakness	56	
Ankle oedema	50	
Pigmentation	4	
Other findings		
Hypertension	74	
Diabetes	50	
Overt	13	
Impaired GTT	37	
Osteoporosis	50	
Renal calculi	15	

Data from Ross and Linch (1982).
GTT, glucose tolerance test.

Table 5 Tests used in the diagnosis and differential diagnosis of Cushing's syndrome

---

Diagnosis
—does the patient have Cushing's syndrome?
Circadian rhythm of plasma cortisol
Urinary free cortisol excretion*
Low-dose dexamethasone suppression test*
Insulin tolerance test
Differential diagnosis
—what is the cause of the Cushing's syndrome?
Plasma ACTH
Plasma potassium
High-dose dexamethasone suppression test
Metyrapone test
Corticotrophin-releasing factor
Inferior petrosal sinus ± selective venous sampling for ACTH
MRI/CT scanning of pituitary/adrenals
Scintigraphy
Tumour markers

---

* Valuable outpatient screening tests (see text).

Investigation of patients with suspected Cushing's syndrome

There are two stages in the investigation of a patient with suspected Cushing's syndrome: (1) Does the patient have Cushing's syndrome? (2) If the answer to (1) is yes, then what is the cause? Unfortunately many investigators fail to make this distinction and ill-advisedly use tests that are relevant to question (2) to try to answer question (1). In particular it is essential that radiological investigations are not undertaken until Cushing's syndrome has been confirmed biochemically. The principal diagnostic tests are listed in Table 5.

Diagnostic tests

Circadian rhythm of plasma cortisol

In normal subjects, plasma cortisol concentrations are at their highest first thing in the morning and reach a nadir at around midnight (less than 100 nmol/l). This circadian rhythm is lost in patients with Cushing's syndrome such that in the majority of patients the 09.00 h level of plasma cortisol is normal but nocturnal levels are raised. Random morning levels of plasma cortisol are therefore of little value in making the diagnosis. In addition, various factors such as stress of venepuncture, intercurrent illness, and admission to hospital may result in normal subjects losing their circadian rhythm. It is therefore good practice not to measure plasma cortisol until the patient has been in hospital for 48 h.

Very few laboratories have developed methods for the measurement of free levels of plasma cortisol. As more than 90 per cent of plasma cortisol is protein bound, the results of the conventional assay will be affected by drugs or conditions which alter levels of cortisol-binding globulin. Thus oestrogen therapy or pregnancy may elevate cortisol-binding globulin and hence total plasma cortisol. In practice, therefore, circadian rhythm is not a widely used screening test.

Urinary free cortisol excretion

For many years the diagnosis of Cushing's syndrome was based on the measurement of urinary metabolites of cortisol (24-h urinary 17-hydroxycorticosteroid or 17-oxogenic steroid excretion, depending on the method used). However, the sensitivity and specificity of these methods is poor and most investigators have replaced these assays with the much more sensitive measurement of urinary free cortisol excretion. Urinary free cortisol is an integrated measure of plasma free cortisol. As cortisol secretion increases, the binding capacity of cortisol-binding globulin is exceeded and results in a disproportionate rise in urinary free cortisol. This is a useful screening test, but even so, it is accepted that urinary free cortisol may be normal in up to 8 to 15 per cent of patients with Cushing's syndrome.

Measurement of the cortisol–creatinine ratio on the first urine specimen passed on waking obviates the need for a timed collection and has been used by some as a sensitive screening test, particularly if cyclical Cushing's syndrome is suspected. Urine aliquots are stable when left at room temperature for up to 7 days and can then be sent by post to the local endocrine laboratory.

Low-dose/overnight dexamethasone suppression tests

In normal subjects, administration of a supraphysiological dose of glucocorticoid results in suppression of ACTH and hence of cortisol secretion. In Cushing's syndrome of whatever cause there is a failure of this suppression when low doses of the synthetic glucocorticoid dexamethasone are given.

The overnight test is often used as an outpatient screening test. Various doses of dexamethasone have been used, usually given at midnight. A normal response is a plasma cortisol of less than 50 nmol/l between 08.00 and 09.00 h the following morning. A dose of 1.5 or 2 mg gives a 30 per cent false-positive rate, whereas after 1 mg this is reduced to 12.5 per cent with a false-negative rate of less than 2 per cent. Thus, the outpatient overnight test has high sensitivity but low specificity, and further investigation is often required.

In the 48-h test, plasma cortisol is measured at 09.00 h on day 0 and 48 h later following dexamethasone given in a dose of 0.5 mg every 6 h for 48 h. This test is reported as having a 97 to 100 per cent true-positive rate and a false-positive of less than 1 per cent.

Certain drugs (phenytoin, rifampicin) may increase the metabolic clearance rate of dexamethasone thereby giving false-positive results.

Insulin tolerance test

Patients with severe depression may show many of the biochemical features of Cushing's syndrome (loss of circadian rhythm of plasma cortisol, increased urinary free cortisol, failure of cortisol suppression with low-dose dexamethasone). Patients with Cushing's syndrome are also frequently depressed. It is thus important in a depressed patient to take particular care in distinguishing the two conditions. In normal subjects and patients with severe endogenous depression, insulin-induced hypoglycaemia results in a rise in ACTH and cortisol levels, a response which does not usually occur in Cushing's syndrome.

Differential diagnostic tests

Once the biochemical diagnosis has been made, a series of investigations is required to determine the cause of the Cushing's syndrome.

Plasma ACTH at 09.00h

This will differentiate ACTH-dependent from ACTH-independent causes. ACTH is either within the normal reference range (50 per cent of cases) or elevated in patients with Cushing's disease. ACTH levels in the ectopic ACTH syndrome are high but overlap values seen in Cushing's disease in 30 per cent of cases and cannot therefore be used to differentiate these two conditions (Fig. 4). The measurement of ACTH precursors (pro-ACTH, POMC) is not routinely available but may be more useful in detecting an ectopic source of ACTH.

In patients with adrenal tumours, plasma ACTH is invariably undetectable. This can also occur with degradation of ACTH; consequently, non-haemolysed blood samples should be taken on ice and immediately separated.

Diagnosis is a problem in those patients whose plasma ACTH levels are low normal or intermittently detectable. This may occur in macronodular hyperplasia. The danger is that in some patients the asymmetry of the nodular hyperplasia may lead to a diagnosis of adrenal adenoma, the plasma ACTH is ignored, and an inappropriate adrenalectomy is performed. Conversely, in some patients with this syndrome an autonomous adrenal tumour develops and, despite detectable ACTH, unilateral adrenalectomy is required.

Plasma potassium (see also Chapter 20.2.2)
Hypokalaemic alkalosis is present in more than 95 per cent of patients with the ectopic ACTH syndrome, but is present in fewer than 10 per cent of patients with Cushing's disease. The aetiology of this is now becoming clearer. Patients with the ectopic syndrome usually have higher cortisol secretion rates that saturate the renal protective 11β-hydroxysteroid dehydrogenase type 2 enzyme resulting in cortisol-induced, mineralocorticoid hypertension (see apparent mineralocorticoid excess syndrome, below). In addition, these patients have higher levels of the ACTH-dependent mineralocorticoid, deoxycorticosterone.

High-dose dexamethasone suppression test
The rationale for this test is that in Cushing's disease there is negative feedback control of ACTH but it is set at a higher level than normal. Thus in this disease cortisol levels are not suppressed with a low dose of dexamethasone but are with a high dose. The original test introduced by Liddle was based on giving dexamethasone at a dose of 2 mg every 6 h for 48 h and measuring urinary 17-oxogenic steroids. Suppression was defined as a greater than 50 per cent fall in 24-h urinary 17-oxogenic steroids. In the

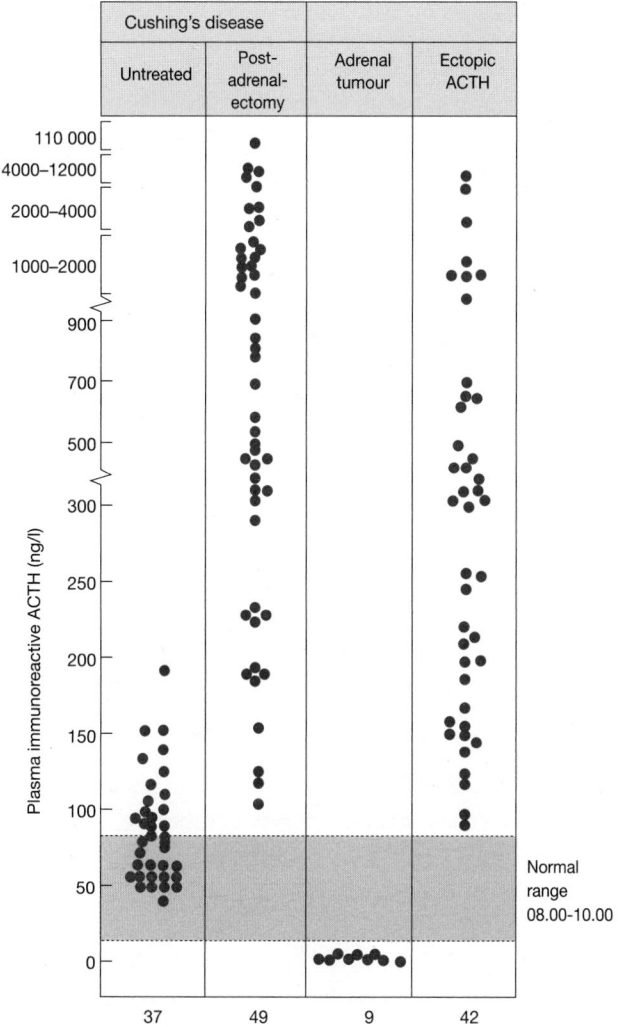

Fig. 4 Immunoreactive N-terminal ACTH levels in plasma samples taken between 08.00 and 10.00 h in normal subjects (hatched area), and patients with Cushing's disease either untreated or postadrenalectomy, patients with adrenal tumours, and in the ectopic ACTH syndrome (by courtesy of Professor Lesley Rees).

modern test, plasma cortisol is measured at 0 and after 48 h or, less commonly, 8 mg of dexamethasone is given orally at 23.00 h and plasma cortisol taken at 08.00 h on the same day (basal sample) and at 08.00 h on the following morning. In both these tests greater than 50 per cent suppression of plasma cortisol in comparison with the basal sample has been used to define a positive response. In Cushing's disease about 90 per cent of patients have a positive 48-h test in comparison with 10 per cent with the ectopic ACTH syndrome. With overnight high-dose testing, 89 per cent sensitivity and 100 per cent specificity has been reported for Cushing's disease. A further variation on this test is the 5-h infusion of dexamethasone (1 mg/h).

Metyrapone test
Metyrapone is an 11β-hydroxylase inhibitor which blocks the conversion of 11-deoxycortisol to cortisol and deoxycorticosterone to corticosterone (Fig. 1). This lowers plasma cortisol and, via negative feedback control, increases plasma ACTH. This in turn stimulates an increase in the secretion of adrenal steroids proximal to the block. Given in doses of 750 mg every 4 h for 24 h, patients with Cushing's disease exhibit an exaggerated rise in plasma ACTH with 11-deoxycortisol levels at 24 h exceeding 1000 nmol/l. In most patients with the ectopic ACTH syndrome there is little or no response, but occasional patients (possibly those producing both ACTH and CRF) have an 11-deoxycortisol response which may be similar to that in Cushing's disease.

The metyrapone test was originally used to distinguish patients with Cushing's disease from those with a primary adrenal cause. However, these can be more reliably distinguished by measuring plasma ACTH and CT scanning of the adrenals. As indicated, the test does not reliably distinguish between Cushing's disease and the ectopic ACTH syndrome and the value of this test has been questioned. It should be reserved for patients when the results of other tests are equivocal.

Corticotrophin-releasing factor (CRF) test
CRF is a 41 amino acid peptide, identified by Vale in 1981 from ovine hypothalami. The ovine sequence differs by seven amino acid residues from that of the human, but despite this, stimulates the release of ACTH in humans. The test involves the intravenous injection of either ovine or human CRF in a dose of 1 µg/kg body weight or a single dose of 100 µg. The test can be performed in the morning or afternoon, and after basal sampling, blood samples for ACTH and cortisol are taken every 15 min for 1 to 2 h after administering CRF.

In normal subjects, CRF produces a rise in ACTH and cortisol, and this response is exaggerated in Cushing's disease. It is typically absent in the ectopic ACTH syndrome and in patients with adrenal tumours. In distinguishing pituitary-dependent Cushing's from the ectopic ACTH syndrome the response of ACTH to CRF has a specificity of 90 per cent, and with cortisol as the end-point, 95 per cent. Using an ACTH increase of 100 per cent over basal or a cortisol rise of 50 per cent as an end-point, this positive response eliminates a possible diagnosis of the ectopic ACTH syndrome.

As with the other tests, patients with macronodular hyperplasia may present a problem in diagnosis and show no response to CRF. The test is valuable in distinguishing patients who are obese and depressed from those with Cushing's disease; in the former the CRF response is either normal or reduced.

Inferior petrosal sinus sampling/selective venous catheterization
To distinguish Cushing's disease from the ectopic ACTH syndrome it may be necessary to identify the source of ACTH secretion. As blood from each half of the pituitary drains into the ipsilateral inferior petrosal sinus, catheterization of both sinuses with simultaneous sampling of venous blood can distinguish a pituitary from an ectopic source and aid in the lateralization of a pituitary microadenoma (Fig. 5). In patients with the ectopic ACTH syndrome, there is usually no ACTH gradient between the inferior petrosal sinus samples and simultaneously drawn peripheral venous levels. In Cushing's disease the ipsilateral:contralateral ACTH ratio is usually greater than 1.4. However, because of the problem of intermittent ACTH

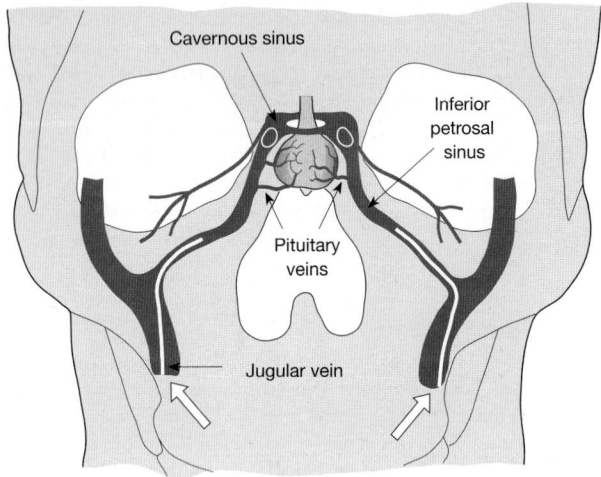

Fig. 5 Positions of bilateral catheters in inferior petrosal sinus sampling.

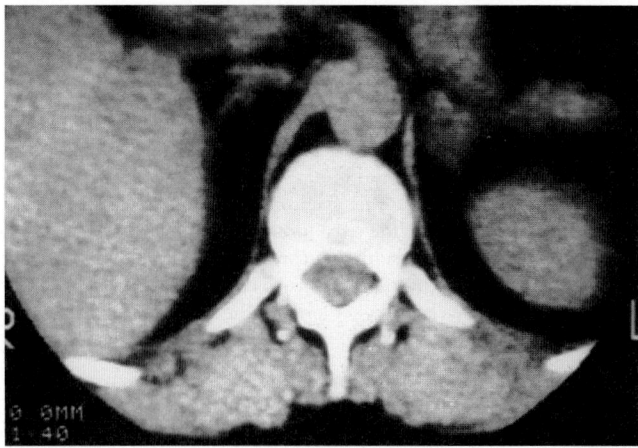

Fig. 6 CT scan of adrenals in patient with asymmetrical nodular hyperplasia. The macronodule on the left was initially thought to be an adrenal tumour. The biochemistry indicating ACTH-dependent Cushing's syndrome was ignored and a unilateral adrenalectomy performed without cure of the hypercortisolism. Further investigation confirmed Cushing's disease and a selective pituitary microadenomectomy resulted in cure.

secretion, it is useful to make measurements before and at intervals (for example, 2, 5, and 15 min) after intravenous injection of 100 μg of synthetic ovine CRF. Using this approach, patients with Cushing's disease and bilateral inferior petrosal sinus ratios of less than 1.4 can be readily distinguished from those with the ectopic syndrome. The precise ratio that distinguishes Cushing's disease from the ectopic syndrome has been debated. Some authors use 2 rather than 1.4.

It is clear that inferior petrosal sinus sampling is a useful technique for making the differential diagnosis in ACTH-dependent Cushing's syndrome. However, it should be reserved for those cases where the differential diagnosis is still in doubt after high-dose dexamethasone and peripheral CRF testing. Inferior petrosal sinus catheterization may also be of value to the surgeon who is planning to explore the pituitary in a patient with Cushing's disease in whom imaging techniques have failed to demonstrate a microadenoma.

Rarely, selective catheterization of vascular beds may be required to identify the source of ectopic ACTH secretion, for example from a small pulmonary carcinoid or thymic tumour.

Tumour markers
Many tumours responsible for the ectopic ACTH syndrome also produce peptide hormones other than ACTH or its precursors.

Imaging
MRI/CT scanning of pituitary and adrenals There is no doubt that high-resolution, thin-section, contrast-enhanced imaging using either CT or MRI has revolutionized the investigation of Cushing's syndrome. However, it is essential that the results of any imaging technique must always be interpreted in the light of the biochemical results if mistakes are to be avoided. In imaging the adrenals, asymmetrical nodular hyperplasia may lead to a false diagnosis of adrenal adenoma (Fig. 6). Owing to the presence of 'pituitary incidentalomas', pituitary MRI/CT scanning may produce false-positive results, particularly for lesions of less than 5 mm in diameter.

Pituitary MRI is the investigation of choice if the biochemical tests suggest Cushing's disease, with a sensitivity of 70 per cent and specificity of 87 per cent (Figs 7 and 8). About 90 per cent of ACTH-secreting pituitary tumours are microadenomas (that is, less than 10 mm in diameter). The classic features of a pituitary microadenoma are a hypodense lesion after contrast, associated with deviation of the pituitary stalk and a convex upper surface of the pituitary gland (Fig. 7). With such small tumours it is not surprising that the sensitivity of CT scanning is relatively low (20 to 60 per cent) with a similar specificity.

By contrast, for adrenal imaging, CT scanning rather than MRI is the investigation of choice offering better spatial resolution (Fig. 9). Once again, it is stressed that 'adrenal incidentalomas' are present in up to 5 per

cent of normal subjects, and thus adrenal imaging should not be performed unless biochemical investigation suggests a primary adrenal cause. Adrenal carcinomas are large and often associated with metastatic spread at presentation (Fig. 10).

In patients with 'occult' ectopic ACTH syndrome, high-definition MRI/CT scanning with images every 0.5 cm may be required to detect small ACTH-secreting carcinoid tumours.

Adrenal scintigraphy This is of value in certain patients with primary adrenal pathology. The most commonly used agent is ^{131}I-6β-iodomethyl-19-norcholesterol. This is a marker of adrenocortical cholesterol uptake. In patients with adrenal adenomas the isotope is taken up by the adenoma but not by the contralateral suppressed adrenal. Adrenal scintigraphy is useful in patients with suspected adrenocortical macronodular hyperplasia, in which CT scanning may be misleading by suggesting unilateral pathology,

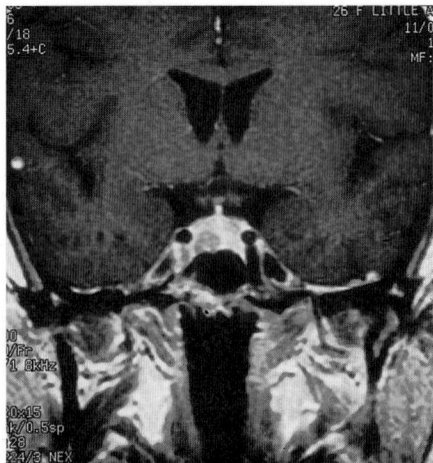

Fig. 7 MRI scan of pituitary demonstrating the typical appearance of a pituitary microadenoma. A hypodense lesion is seen in the left side of the gland with deviation of the pituitary stalk away from the lesion. Following a biochemical diagnosis of Cushing's disease, this patient was cured following trans-sphenoidal hypophysectomy.

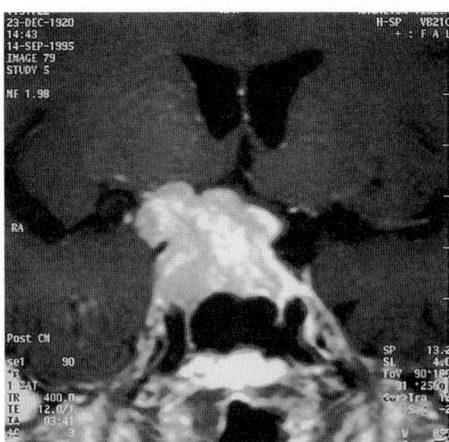

Fig. 8 MRI scan of the pituitary gland demonstrating a large macroadenoma in a patient with Cushing's disease. In contrast to smaller tumours, these tumours are invariably invasive and recur following surgery.

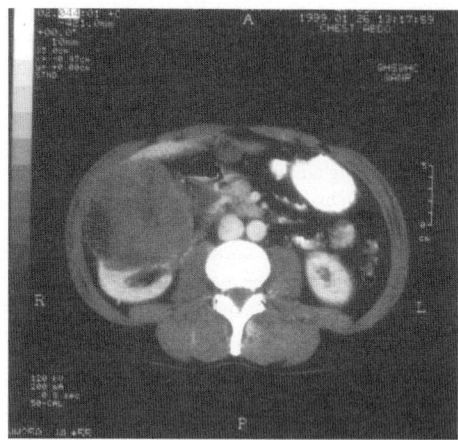

(a)

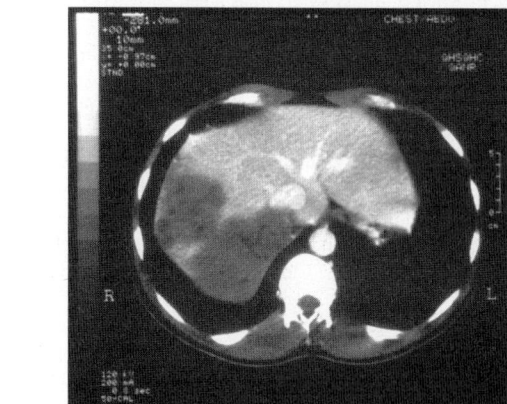

(b)

Fig. 10 CT scan of a patient with rapidly progressing Cushing's syndrome due to a right-sided adrenal carcinoma. An irregular right adrenal mass is shown (a) with a large liver metastasis (b).

whereas with isotope scanning the bilateral adrenal involvement is identified (Fig. 11).

Prognosis of untreated Cushing's syndrome

Studies carried out prior to the introduction of effective therapy suggested that 50 per cent of patients with untreated Cushing's syndrome died within 5 years. Even with modern management, an increased prevalence of cardiovascular risk factors persists for many years after an apparent 'cure'. Close follow-up of all patients is recommended.

Treatment of Cushing's syndrome

Adrenal causes

Adrenal adenomas should be removed by unilateral adrenalectomy, with 100 per cent cure rate. With the increasing experience of laparascopic adrenalectomy in most tertiary centres, this has now become the surgical treatment of choice for unilateral tumours, reducing surgical morbidity and postoperative hospital stay compared with traditional open approaches. After surgery it may take many months or even years for the suppressed adrenal to recover. It is wise therefore to give slightly suboptimal replacement therapy with dexamethasone at a dose of 0.5 mg in the morning, with intermittent measurement of the 08.00 h level of plasma cortisol prior to taking dexamethasone. When the morning plasma cortisol is above 180 nmol/l, dexamethasone can be stopped. A subsequent insulin tolerance test may then demonstrate whether the response to stress is normal.

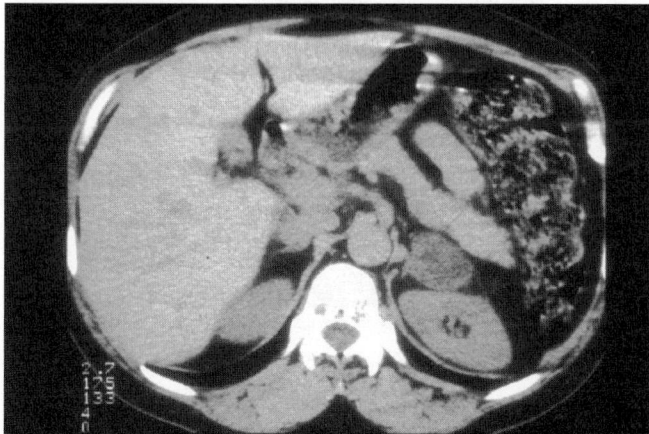

Fig. 9 Typical solitary left-sided adrenal adenoma on adrenal CT scanning.

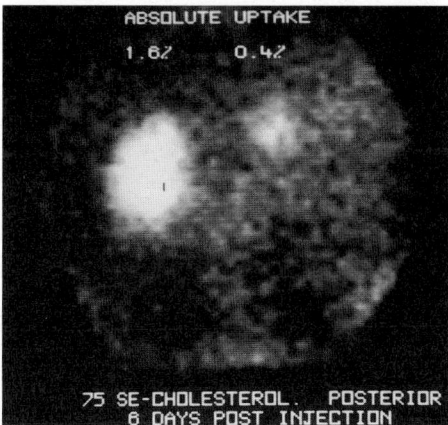

Fig. 11 Adrenal scintigraphy in a patient with Cushing's syndrome and macronodular hyperplasia. Note asymmetrical uptake in the adrenals, with 1.6 per cent uptake on the left and 0.4 per cent on the right.

Adrenal carcinomas have a very poor prognosis and most patients are dead within 2 years. It is usual practice to try to remove the primary tumour, even though metastases may be present, so as to enhance the response to the adrenolytic agent o,p'-DDD (Mitotane, see below). Radiotherapy to the tumour bed and to some metastases, such as those in the spine, may be of limited value.

Pituitary-dependent Cushing's disease

The treatment of Cushing's disease has been improved by trans-sphenoidal surgery conducted by an experienced surgeon. Before the selective removal of a pituitary microadenoma the treatment of choice was bilateral adrenalectomy. This had an appreciable mortality even in the best centres (about 4 per cent) as well as morbidity. The main risk was the subsequent development of Nelson's syndrome (postadrenalectomy hyperpigmentation with locally aggressive pituitary tumour) (Fig. 12 and Plate 1). To avoid this, pituitary irradiation was often carried out following bilateral adrenalectomy. These patients required lifelong replacement therapy with hydrocortisone and fludrocortisone. Nowadays bilateral adrenalectomy is reserved for the occasional patient with Cushing's disease in whom no pituitary tumour can be found, or when pituitary surgery has failed, or where the condition has recurred.

After selective removal of a microadenoma, the surrounding corticotrophs are normally suppressed (Fig. 13). In these cases plasma cortisol concentrations are also suppressed postoperatively and glucocorticoid replacement therapy is required. Using the dexamethasone regime described above after removal of an adrenal adenoma, there is usually (but not invariably) gradual recovery of the hypothalamic–pituitary–adrenal axis (Fig. 14). A non-suppressed plasma cortisol postoperatively suggests that the patient is not 'cured', even though cortisol secretion may have fallen to normal or subnormal values. Close follow-up of such individuals is required.

In the past, pituitary irradiation was often used in the treatment of Cushing's disease. However, the improvements in pituitary surgery have resulted in far fewer patients being so treated. In children pituitary irradiation appears to be effective. Radiotherapy is not recommended as a primary treatment but is reserved for patients not responding to pituitary microsurgery or when bilateral adrenalectomy has been performed, or in those with established Nelson's syndrome.

Ectopic ACTH syndrome

Treatment of the ectopic ACTH syndrome depends on the cause. If the tumour can be found and has not spread, then its removal can lead to cure (for example bronchial carcinoid or thymoma). However, the prognosis for small-cell lung cancer associated with the ectopic ACTH syndrome is poor. The cortisol excess and associated hypokalaemic alkalosis and diabetes mellitus can be ameliorated by medical therapy (see below). Treatment of the small-cell tumour itself will also, at least initially, produce improvement (see Chapter 17.13). Sometimes, if the ectopic source of ACTH cannot be found, it may be necessary to perform bilateral adrenalectomy and then follow the patient carefully (sometimes for several years) to find the primary tumour.

Medical treatment of Cushing's syndrome

Several drugs have been used in the treatment of Cushing's syndrome. Their site of action is shown in Fig. 15. Most commonly, metyrapone has been given, often to lower cortisol concentrations prior to definitive therapy, or while awaiting benefit from pituitary irradiation. The daily dose has to be determined by measuring either plasma or urinary free cortisol. The aim should be to achieve a mean plasma cortisol of about 300 nmol/l during the day or a normal urinary free cortisol. The drug is usually given in doses ranging from 250 mg twice daily to 1.5 g every 6 h. Nausea may be produced and can be alleviated (if not due to adrenal insufficiency) by giving the drug with milk.

Aminoglutethimide is a more toxic drug which in high dose blocks initial steps in the biosynthetic pathway and thus affects the secretion of ster-

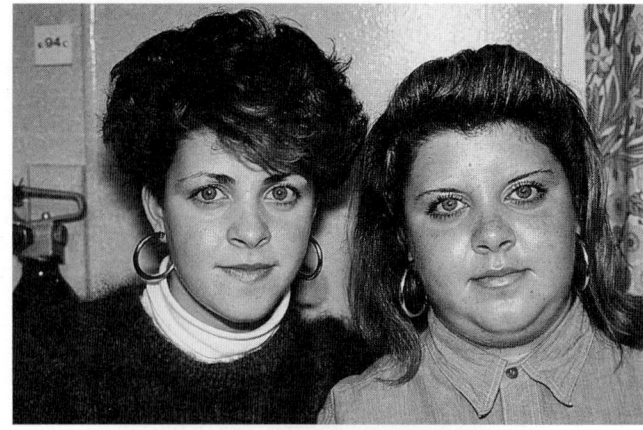

(a)

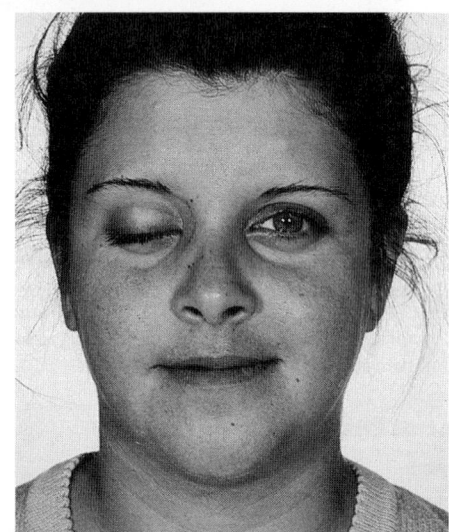

(b)

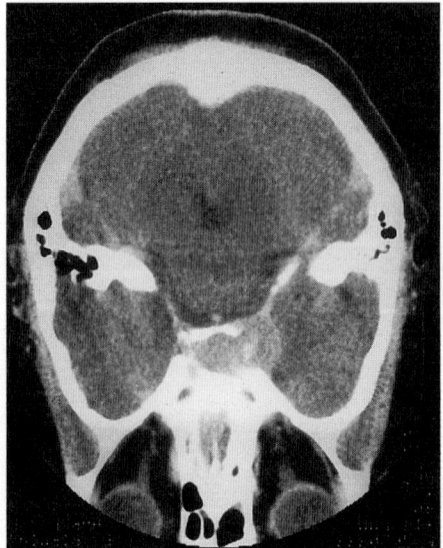

(c)

Fig. 12 A young woman with Cushing's disease, photographed initially alongside her identical twin sister (a). In this case treatment with bilateral adrenalectomy was undertaken and several years later the patient re-presents with Nelson's syndrome and a right III cranial nerve palsy due to cavernous sinus infiltration from a locally invasive corticotrophinoma. (See also Plate 1.)

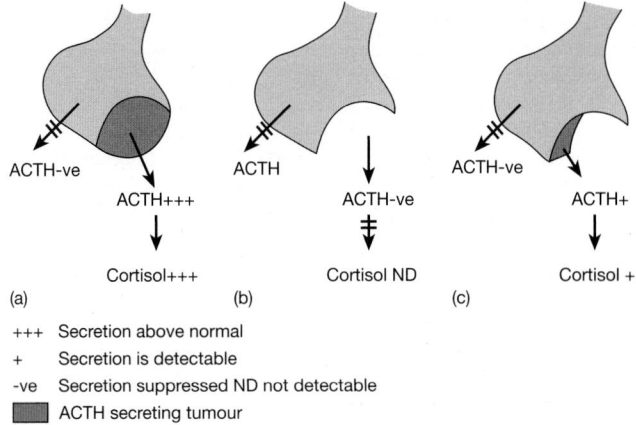

+++ Secretion above normal
+ Secretion is detectable
-ve Secretion suppressed ND not detectable
▨ ACTH secreting tumour

Fig. 13 Selective removal of a microadenoma and its effect on the hypothalamic–pituitary–adrenal axis. Because the surrounding normal pituitary corticotrophs are suppressed in a patient with an ACTH-secreting pituitary adenoma, successful removal of the tumour results in ACTH and hence adrenocortical deficiency with an undetectable (less than 50 nmol/l) level of plasma cortisol. A plasma cortisol of more than 50 nmol/l postoperatively implies that the patient is not cured. (Figure by courtesy of Dr Peter Trainer.)

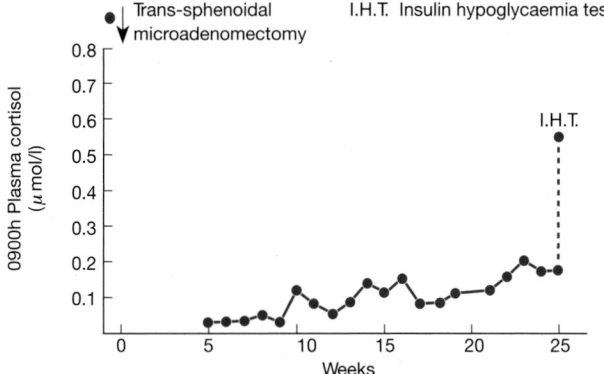

Fig. 14 Gradual recovery of function of the hypothalamic–pituitary–adrenal axis after removal of a pituitary ACTH-secreting microadenoma. The insulin hypoglycaemia test eventually demonstrated the return of a normal stress response.

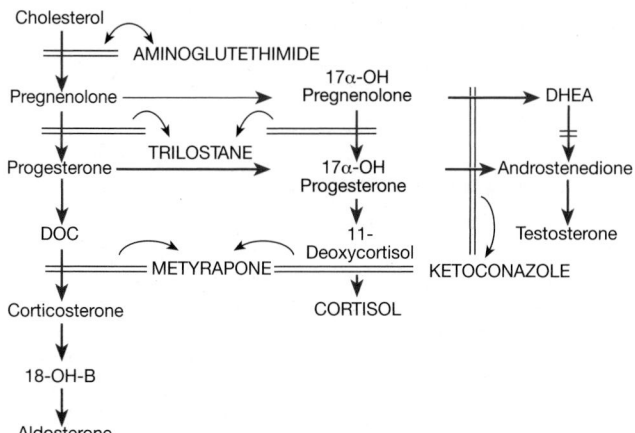

Fig. 15 Medical treatment of Cushing's syndrome: site of action of various drugs.

oids other than cortisol. In doses of 1.5 to 3 g daily (start with 250 mg every 8 h) it commonly produces nausea, marked lethargy, and a skin rash.

Trilostane, a 3β-hydroxysteroid dehydrogenase inhibitor, is ineffective in Cushing's disease, since the block in steroidogenesis is overcome by the rise in ACTH. However, it can be effective in patients with adrenal adenomas.

Ketoconazole is an imidazole which has been widely used as an antifungal agent; it produces abnormal liver function tests signifying hepatitis in about 14 per cent of patients. Ketoconazole blocks a variety of steroidogenic cytochrome P450-dependent enzymes and thus lowers plasma cortisol levels. For effective control of Cushing's syndrome, 400 to 800 mg of ketoconazole daily have been required.

o,p'-DDD, or Mitotane, is an adrenolytic drug which is taken up by both normal and malignant adrenal tissue causing adrenal atrophy and necrosis. Because of its toxicity, Mitotane has been used mainly in the management of adrenal carcinoma. Doses of up to 8 g/day are required to control glucocorticoid excess, though evidence that it causes tumour shrinkage or improves long-term survival is scant. The drug will also produce mineralocorticoid deficiency and both glucocorticoid and mineralocorticoid replacement therapy may be required. Side-effects are common and include fatigue, skin rashes, and gastrointestinal disturbance.

Glucocorticoid deficiency—primary and secondary hypoadrenalism

Primary hypoadrenalism refers to glucocorticoid deficiency occurring in the setting of adrenal disease, whilst secondary hypoadrenalism arises because of deficiency of ACTH, the major trophic hormone controlling cortisol secretion. The principal distinction between these two conditions is that mineralocorticoid deficiency invariably accompanies primary hypoadrenalism but this does not occur in secondary hypoadrenalism because only ACTH is deficient; the renin–angiotensin–aldosterone axis is intact.

Primary hypoadrenalism

Congenital adrenal hyperplasia

Various inherited enzyme defects in the synthesis of adrenocortical hormones have been identified and this group of conditions is addressed in Chapter 12.7.2.

Addison's disease

Thomas Addison described this condition in his classic monograph published in 1855. Addison worked with Bateman, a dermatologist who produced one of the first classifications of skin disease. It seems likely that this stimulated Addison's interest in the skin pigmentation which is so characteristic of this disease.

Aetiology

This is a rare condition with an estimated incidence in the developed world of 0.8 cases per 100 000 population. The causes of Addison's disease are listed in Table 6.

Worldwide, infectious diseases are the most common cause of primary adrenal insufficiency. Leading causes include tuberculosis, fungal infections (histoplasmosis, crytococcus), and cytomegalovirus. Adrenal failure may occur in the acquired immunodeficiency syndrome. In tuberculous Addison's disease, the adrenals are initially enlarged with extensive epithelioid granulomas and caseation. Calcification eventually ensues in most cases (Fig. 16). Both the cortex and the medulla are affected.

In the Western world, autoimmune adrenalitis accounts for over 70 per cent of all cases of Addison's disease. Pathologically, the adrenal glands are atrophic with loss of most of the cortical cells, but the medulla is usually intact. Adrenal autoantibodies can be detected in up to 75 per cent of newly diagnosed cases and have recently been characterized. The major autoantigen is the adrenal enzyme, 21-hydroxylase, but antibodies directed against cholesterol side-chain cleavage and 17α-hydroxylase may rarely be detected. Fifty per cent of patients with Addison's disease have an associated autoimmune disease and these 'polyglandular autoimmune syndromes' have been classified into two distinct variants. Type I is inherited as an autosomal recessive condition and comprises Addison's disease, chronic mucocutaneous candidiasis, and hypoparathyroidism. The condition is rare and usually presents in childhood with either candidiasis or hypoparathyroidism. Other autoimmune conditions such as pernicious anaemia, thyroid disease, chronic active hepatitis, and gondal failure may occur but are rare. Autoantibodies to 21-hydroxylase are not normally present.

Type II polyglandular autoimmune syndrome is more common and may comprise Addison's disease, autoimmune thyroid disease, diabetes mellitus, and hypogonadism. The condition has an inherited basis with linkage to

Table 6 Aetiology of adrenocortical insufficiency

Primary: Addison's disease
Tuberculosis
Autoimmune:
  Sporadic
  Polyglandular deficiency type I
  (Addison's disease, chronic mucocutaneous candidiasis,
    hypoparathyroidism, dental enamel hypoplasia, alopecia, primary
    gonadal failure)
  Polyglandular deficiency type II (Schmidt's syndrome)
  (Addison's disease, primary hypothyroidism, primary hypogonadism,
    insulin-dependent diabetes, pernicious anaemia, vitiligo)
Metastatic tumour
Lymphoma
Amyloid
Intra-adrenal haemorrhage (Waterhouse–Friderichsen syndrome) following
  meningococcal septicaemia
Haemochromatosis
Adrenal infarction or infection other than tuberculosis (especially AIDS)
Adrenoleucodystrophies
Congenital adrenal hypoplasia (DAX-1 mutations)
Hereditary adrenocortical unresponsiveness to ACTH
Bilateral adrenalectomy
Secondary
Exogenous glucocorticoid therapy
Hypopituitarism:
  Selective removal of ACTH-secreting pituitary adenoma
  Pituitary tumours and pituitary surgery, craniopharyngiomas
  Pituitary apoplexy
  Granulomatous disease (tuberculosis, sarcoid, eosinophilic granuloma)
  Secondary tumour deposits (breast, bronchus)
  Postpartum pituitary infarction (Sheehan's syndrome)
  Pituitary irradiation (effect usually delayed for several years)
  Isolated ACTH deficiency

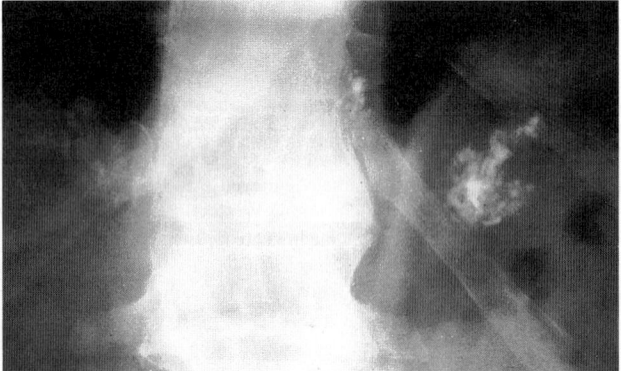

Fig. 16 Plain radiograph of the abdomen showing adrenal calcification in a patient with tuberculous Addison's disease.

the HLA major histocompatibility complex, notably HLA DR3 and DR4. Autoantibodies to 21-hydroxylase are usually present and are predictive for the development of adrenal destruction.

With the exception of tuberculosis and autoimmune adrenal failure, other causes of Addison's disease are rare (Table 6). Adrenal metastases (commonest primary lung, breast) are often found at postmortem examinations but adrenal insufficiency from these is uncommon. Necrosis of the adrenals due to intra-adrenal haemorrhage should be considered in any severely sick patient and this may be due to infection, trauma, or hypercoagulability. Intra-adrenal bleeding may be found in any cause of severe septicaemia, particularly in children. When this is due to meningococcus, the association with adrenal insufficiency is known as the Waterhouse–Friderichsen syndrome. Adrenal replacement leading to glandular failure may also occur with amyloidosis and haemochromatosis. Adrenal hypoplasia congenita is an X-linked disorder comprising congenital adrenal insufficiency and hypogonadotrophic hypogonadism. The condition is caused by mutations in the DAX-1 gene, a known member of the nuclear receptor family which is expressed in the adrenal cortex, gonads, and hypothalamus.

X-linked adrenoleucodystrophy is a cause of adrenal insufficiency in association with demyelination within the nervous system due to a failure of β-oxidation of fatty acids within peroxisomes. Increased accumulation of very long-chain fatty acids occurs in many tissues and serum assays can be used diagnostically. Only males have the fully expressed condition and carrier females are usually normal. Two forms are recognized. Adrenoleucodystrophy presents at 5 to 10 years of age with progression eventually to a blind, mute, and severely spastic tetraplegic state. Adrenal insufficiency is usually present but does not appear to correlate with the neurological deficit. X-linked adrenoleucodystrophy accounts for about 10 per cent of cases of adrenocortical failure in boys and men. Adrenomyeloneuropathy, by contrast, presents later in life with the gradual development of spastic paresis and peripheral neuropathy. As both the childhood and the adult condition result from the same mutant gene (recently mapped to chromosome Xq28), it has been suggested that there is an additional autosomal modifier gene. Monounsaturated fatty acids which block the synthesis of the saturated very long-chain fatty acids have been used for treatment. A combination of erucic acid and oleic acid (Lorenzo's oil) has led to normal levels of very long-chain fatty acids, but this has not altered the rate of neurological deterioration; bone marrow transplantation appears to be more effective if undertaken in the early stages of the disease.

Familial glucocorticoid deficiency is a rare, autosomal recessive cause of hypoadrenalism which usually presents in childhood. The renin–angiotensin–aldosterone axis is intact and children usually present either with neonatal hypoglycaemia or later with increasing pigmentation, often with enhanced growth velocity. Patients have glucocorticoid deficiency with very high plasma ACTH levels—this occurs because of mutations in the melanocortin-2 or ACTH receptor. A variant syndrome is called the triple A or Allgrove's syndrome and refers to the triad of adrenal insufficiency due to ACTH resistance, achalasia, and alachrima. Mutations have not been found in the ACTH receptor and the molecular basis for this inherited syndrome is unknown.

Secondary hypoadrenalism (ACTH deficiency)

This is a common clinical problem and is most often due to a sudden cessation of exogenous glucocorticoid therapy or a failure to give glucocorticoid cover for intercurrent stress in a patient who has been on long-term glucocorticoid therapy. Such therapy suppresses the hypothalamic–pituitary–adrenal axis, with consequent adrenal atrophy and this may last for months after stopping glucocorticoid treatment. Adrenal atrophy and subsequent deficiency should be anticipated in any subject who has taken more than the equivalent of 30 mg of oral hydrocortisone per day (approximately 7.5 mg/day of prednisolone or 0.75 mg/day of dexamethasone) for longer than 1 month. In addition to the magnitude of the dose of glucocorticoid, the timing of administration of the dose may affect the degree of adrenal suppression. Thus prednisolone in a dose of 5 mg given last thing at night and 2.5 mg in the morning will produce more marked suppression of the hypothalamic–pituitary–adrenal axis compared with 2.5 mg at night and 5 mg in the morning because the larger evening dose blocks the early morning surge of ACTH.

Other causes of secondary adrenal insufficiency are rare (Table 6) and reflect inadequate ACTH production from the anterior pituitary gland. In many of these, other pituitary hormones are deficient in addition to ACTH, so that the patient presents with partial or complete hypopituitarism. The clinical features of hypopituitarism make this a relatively easy diagnosis to make (see Chapter 12.4). However, if there is isolated ACTH deficiency, this diagnosis may be readily missed.

Clinical features of adrenal insufficiency

The most obvious feature which differentiates primary from secondary hypoadrenalism is skin pigmentation (Fig. 17), which is nearly always present in primary adrenal insufficiency (unless of short duration) and absent in secondary. The pigmentation is seen in sun-exposed areas, recent rather than old scars, axillas, nipples, palmar creases, pressure points, and in mucous membranes (buccal, vaginal, vulval, anal). The cause of the pigmentation has long been debated but probably reflects increased melanocyte activity induced by POMC-related peptides including melanocyte stimulating hormone (MSH). In autoimmune Addison's disease there may be associated vitiligo (Fig. 17).

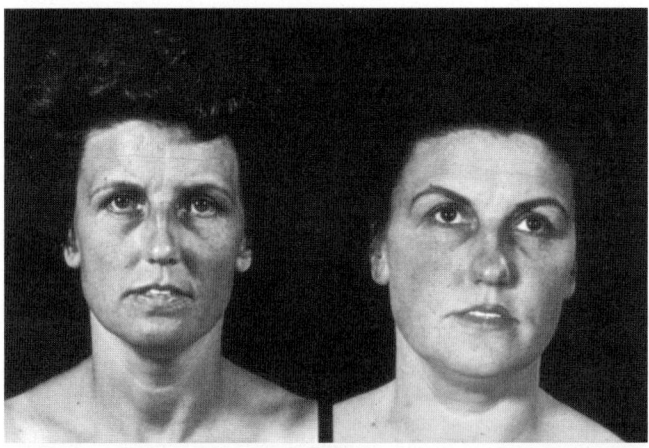

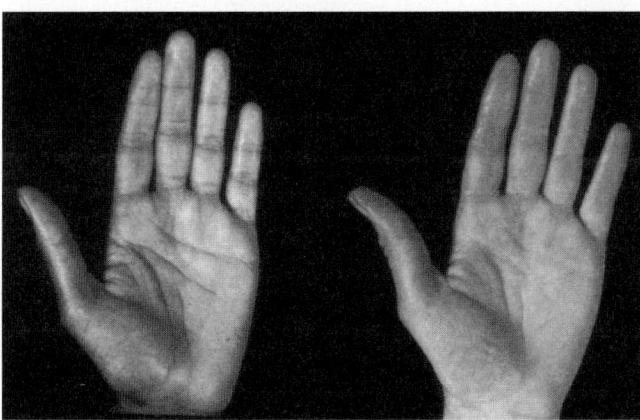

Fig. 17 Pigmentation in a patient with Addison's disease before and after treatment with hydrocortisone and fludrocortisone (by courtesy of Professor C.R.W. Edwards).

Patients with primary adrenal failure usually have both glucocorticoid and mineralocorticoid deficiency. In contrast, those with secondary adrenal insufficiency have an intact renin–angiotensin–aldosterone system. This accounts for differences in salt and water balance in the two groups of patients, which in turn result in different clinical presentations.

Primary adrenal failure may present with hypotension and acute circulatory failure (addisonian crisis). Anorexia may be an early feature, which progresses to nausea, vomiting, diarrhoea, and sometimes, abdominal pain. These crises may be precipitated by intercurrent infection or by stress, such as a surgical operation. Alternatively, the patient may present with vague features of chronic adrenal insufficiency—weakness, tiredness, weight loss, nausea, intermittent vomiting, abdominal pain, diarrhoea or constipation, general malaise, muscle cramps, and symptoms suggestive of postural hypotension. Salt-craving may be a feature and there may be a low-grade fever. The lying blood pressure is usually normal but almost invariably there is a fall in blood pressure on standing.

In secondary adrenal insufficiency due to hypopituitarism, the presentation may relate to deficiency of hormones other than ACTH, notably luteinizing hormone/follicle-stimulating hormone (infertility, oligo-/amenorrhoea, poor libido), thyroid-stimulating hormone (weight gain, cold intolerance), and growth hormone (hypoglycaemia). Patients with isolated ACTH deficiency present with malaise, weight loss, and other features of chronic adrenal insufficiency.

Laboratory investigation of hypoadrenalism

Routine biochemical profile

In established primary adrenal insufficiency, hyonatraemia is present in about 90 per cent of cases and hyperkalaemia in 65 per cent. The blood urea concentration is usually elevated. In secondary adrenal failure there may be a dilutional hyponatraemia with normal or low blood urea because glucocorticoids are required to maintain glomerular filtration rate and excrete a water load. Hypoglycaemia has been found in up to 50 per cent of patients with chronic adrenal insufficiency.

Plasma cortisol/ACTH

Clinical suspicion of the diagnosis should be confirmed with definitive diagnostic tests. Basal plasma cortisol and urinary free cortisol levels are often in the low normal range and cannot be used to exclude the diagnosis. In primary adrenal insufficiency the simultaneous measurement of plasma cortisol and plasma ACTH reveals an ACTH level which is disproportionately elevated in comparison with plasma cortisol (Fig. 18).

Mineralocorticoid status

Another difference between primary and secondary hypoadrenalism is in the renin–angiotensin–aldosterone axis. In primary hypoadrenalism there is normally mineralocorticoid deficiency with elevated plasma renin activity and either low or low normal plasma aldosterone. It is remarkable how frequently the investigation of zona glomerulosa activity is ignored in Addison's disease compared with the assessment of zona fasciculata function.

Stimulation tests

In practice all patients suspected of having adrenal insufficiency should have an ACTH stimulation test. This involves the intramuscular or intravenous administration of 250 µg of tetracosactrin (Synacthen ®), comprising the first 24 amino acids of normally secreted 1–39 ACTH. Plasma cortisol levels are measured at 0 and 30 min after ACTH administration and a normal response is defined by a peak plasma cortisol of more than 550 nmol/l. Levels of less than 550 nmol/l in response to Synacthen are found in both primary and secondary adrenal insufficiency, though rarely false-positive results have been reported, particularly in cases of secondary hypoadrenalism. A low-dose ACTH stimulation test giving only 1 µg ACTH has been proposed to screen for adequacy of function of the hypothalamo–pituitary–adrenal axis with the suggestion that it may be

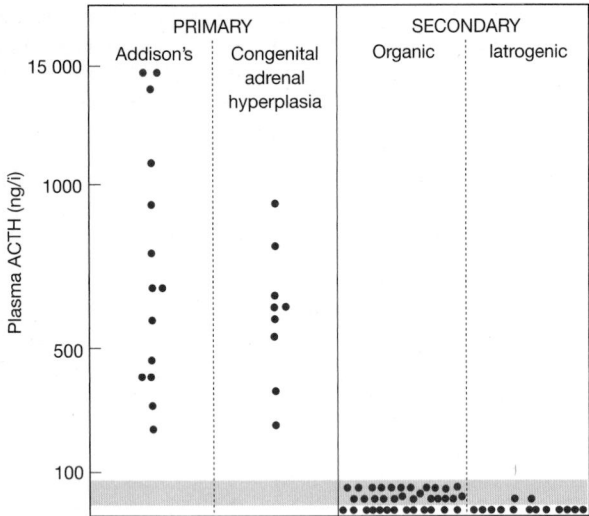

Fig. 18 Morning immunoreactive ACTH values in patients with hypoadrenalism. The reference range is indicated by the horizontal lines (by courtesy of Professor L. H. Rees.)

more sensitive than the conventional 250 µg test. At present there are insufficient data to support such a concept.

A prolonged ACTH stimulation test, involving the administration of depot tetracosactrin in a dose of 1 mg by intramuscular injection, with measurement of plasma cortisol at 0, 4, and 24 h will differentiate primary from secondary hypoadrenalism. In normal subjects the plasma cortisol at 4 h is more than 1000 nmol/l and the value at 24 h shows little further increase. Patients with secondary hypoadrenalism show a delayed response with usually a much higher value at 24 than at 4 h, but in primary hypoadrenalism there is no response at either time. However, the test is now rarely required if plasma ACTH has been appropriately measured at baseline.

The insulin-induced hypoglycaemia or insulin tolerance test remains one of the most useful in assessing ACTH and growth hormone reserves. It should not be performed in patients with ischaemic heart disease (check ECG before test), epilepsy, or severe hypopituitarism (that is plasma cortisol at 09.00 h less than 180 nmol/l). The test involves the intravenous administration of soluble insulin in a dose of 0.1 to 0.15 U/kg body weight, with measurement of plasma cortisol at 0, 30, 45, 60, 90, and 120 min. Adequate hypoglycaemia (blood glucose less than 2.2 mmol/l with signs of neuroglycopenia—sweating and tachycardia) is essential. In normal subjects the peak plasma cortisol exceeds 500 nmol/l. However, the response to hypoglycaemia can be reliably predicted by the response to acute ACTH stimulation (see above); a safer, cheaper, and quicker test. If the ACTH test is normal, insulin-induced hypoglycaemia testing is not necessary in the vast majority of cases unless there is a need to document endogenous growth hormone reserve in a patient with pituitary disease. An insulin tolerance test is only required if, in a patient with suspected hypopituitarism, there is a subnormal response to ACTH. Some patients have an inadequate response to ACTH but then respond normally to hypoglycaemia. They do not require corticosteroid replacement therapy.

Other tests

Radioimmunoassays to detect autoantibodies such as those against the 21-hydroxylase antigen are now available and should be undertaken in patients with primary adrenal failure. In autoimmune Addison's disease it is also important to look for evidence of other organ-specific autoimmune disease. In long-standing tuberculous adrenal disease there may be adrenal atrophy with calcification on plain radiographs or CT scanning. Early morning urine samples should be cultured for mycobacteria if tuberculosis is suspected.

Treatment of acute adrenal insufficiency

This is an emergency, and treatment should not be delayed while waiting for definitive proof of diagnosis. However, in addition to measurement of plasma electrolytes and blood glucose, appropriate samples for ACTH and cortisol should be taken before giving corticosteroid therapy. If the patient is not critically ill, an acute ACTH stimulation test can be performed. However, if necessary, this can be delayed and carried out with the patient on corticosteroid therapy, provided the drug used does not interfere with the plasma cortisol assay (for example, change from hydrocortisone to dexamethasone).

Intravenous hydrocortisone should be given in a dose of 100 mg every 6 h. If this is not possible, then the intramuscular route should be used. In the shocked patient, 1 litre of normal saline should be given intravenously over the first hour. Because of possible hypoglycaemia, it is normal to give 5 per cent dextrose saline. The subsequent saline and dextrose therapy will depend on biochemical monitoring and the patient's condition. Clinical improvement, especially in the blood pressure, should be seen within 4 to 6 h if the diagnosis is correct. It is important to recognize and treat any associated condition, such as an infection, which may have precipitated the acute adrenal crisis.

After the first 24 h the dose of hydrocortisone can be reduced, usually to 50 mg intramuscularly every 6 h for the second 24 h and then, if the patient can take by mouth, to oral hydrocortisone, 40 mg in the morning and 20 mg at 18.00 h. This can then be rapidly reduced to the normal replacement dose of 20 mg on wakening and 10 mg at 18.00 h. Some patients will require more than 30 mg/day, but increasingly most patients can cope with less than this dose (usually 15 to 25 mg/day in divided doses). In primary adrenal failure, cortisol day curves with simultaneous ACTH measurements may provide some insight into adequacy of replacement therapy, but unfortunately there are no good objective tests in secondary adrenal failure. Nevertheless, crude objectives such as weight, well being, and blood pressure are important in this regard.

In primary adrenal failure, mineralocorticoid replacement is usually also required in the form of fludrocortisone (or 9α-fluorinated hydrocortisone) in a dose of 0.05 to 0.1 mg/day. The mineralocorticoid activity of this is about 125 times that of hydrocortisone. After the acute phase has passed, the adequacy of mineralocorticoid replacement can be assessed by measuring electrolytes, supine and erect blood pressure, and plasma renin activity; too little fludrocortisone may cause postural hypotension with elevated plasma renin activity, whilst too much causes the converse.

Patients receiving glucocorticoid replacement therapy should be advised to double the dose in the event of intercurrent febrile illness, accident, or mental stress such as an important examination. If the patient is vomiting and cannot take by mouth, parenteral hydrocortisone must be given urgently, as indicated above. For minor surgery, 50 to 100 mg of hydrocortisone hemisuccinate is given with the premedication. For major procedures this is then followed by the same regimen as for acute adrenal insufficiency.

Every patient on glucocorticoid therapy should be advised to register for a MedicAlert bracelet or necklace and must carry a 'Steroid card'.

Mineralocorticoid excess

Hypertension affects 10 to 25 per cent of the population. In most cases, no underlying cause for the patient's raised blood pressure is apparent, and they are labelled as having 'essential' hypertension. Mineralocorticoid-based hypertension may account for secondary causes of hypertension, and classically refers to hypertension caused by increased sodium and water retention by the kidney and expansion of the extracellular fluid compartment resulting in suppression of endogenous plasma renin activity. Unlike the majority of cases of secondary aldosteronism which arise either in the setting of reduced oncotic pressure (nephrosis, cirrhosis) or in patients with cardiac failure, oedema is not a feature of primary aldosteronism, probably because of the 'escape' phenomenon. Nevertheless, in the short term, intravascular volume is reset at a higher level and this leads to increased cardiac output and blood pressure. In the chronic state, hypervolaemia cannot be consistently demonstrated and other mechanisms may be equally important in raising blood pressure. Mineralocorticoid receptors have been characterized in the vasculature and heart, and depending upon the activity of local 11β-HSD, either glucocorticoids or mineralocorticoids may increase vascular tone, by potentiating catecholamine and angiotensin II-induced vasoconstriction, or by inhibiting endothelial relaxation. Mineralocorticoids can also modulate blood pressure centrally, independent of changes in renal electrolyte transport or vascular reactivity.

Mineralocorticoid hypertension: differential diagnosis

A comprehensive list of the causes of mineralocorticoid hypertension is given in Table 7.

Primary aldosteronism

First described by Conn in 1955, this is the commonest cause of mineralocorticoid hypertension. Prevalence rates of 0.5 to 2 per cent have been widely reported in the literature in unselected patients with 'essential' hypertension, but many of these studies relied on detecting hypokalaemia and, in the light of recent observations, will have underestimated true prevalence rates. By contrast, studies suggesting much higher prevalence rates of 5 to 12 per cent in hypertensive populations have been conducted in specialist centres and are therefore subject to selection bias.

Symptoms are often absent or non-specific but include tiredness, muscle weakness, thirst, polyuria, and nocturia due to hypokalaemia. Spontaneous hypokalaemia (less than 3.5 mmol/l) is rare in untreated hypertension; when found in a patient on diuretics these should be withdrawn, and potassium stores replenished and remeasured 2 weeks later. Despite this, it is now accepted that up to 40 per cent of patients with surgically confirmed primary aldosteronism will have normal serum potassium concentrations.

In approximately two-thirds of patients, primary aldosteronism is due to a small (0.5 to 2 cm), solitary aldosterone-producing adenoma of the adrenal which is commoner in women than men (male:female ratio 1:3). One-third of cases are caused by bilateral adrenal hyperplasia, and the remaining few (less than 2 per cent) by glucocorticoid-suppressible hyperaldosteronism or adrenal carcinomas. The aetiology of aldosterone-producing adenoma is unknown, although rarely it may have a genetic basis and can occur as a component of multiple endocrine neoplasia type I.

Primary aldosteronism is confirmed by demonstrating subnormal supine and erect plasma renin activity and an elevated plasma aldosterone concentration in a patient with no antihypertensive treatment for at least 3 weeks. However, primary aldosteronism may also occur with suppressed plasma renin activity and normal plasma aldosterone concentration, and some investigators advocate measures of aldosterone secretion over a 24-h period or salt suppression studies to further confirm the diagnosis. If severe hypertension prevents complete cessation of antihypertensive therapy during this diagnostic period, α-blockers such as prazosin or doxazosin interfere least with the renin–angiotensin–aldosterone axis. A single ratio of plasma renin activity/plasma aldosterone concentration may be a sensitive screening test, even in patients still taking antihypertensive medication, but depending upon the assays used and population salt intake, this requires validation in each centre.

The differential diagnosis of aldosterone-producing adenoma, bilateral adrenal hyperplasia, and glucocorticoid-suppressible hyperaldosteronism requires an understanding of the control of aldosterone secretion in each condition. In normal physiology, aldosterone secretion is under the control of angiotensin II through the renin–angiotensin system; ACTH and potassium are less important chronic secretogogues. Aldosterone-producing adenoma represents an autonomous source of aldosterone production which is not regulated by angiotensin II (ACTH assumes more importance in the control of aldosterone secretion in aldosterone-producing adenoma). By contrast, the zona glomerulosa in bilateral adrenal hyperplasia is more sensitive to angiotensin II; for a given angiotensin II infusion there is a much greater aldosterone response than normal. Finally, in glucocorticoid-suppressible hyperaldosteronism, aldosterone secretion and the secretion of intermediary metabolites (18-hydroxy and oxo-metabolites of cortisol and corticosterone) are under the control of ACTH. The optimal method(s) of establishing the differential diagnosis of primary aldosteronism is complicated and still controversial. In our clinical practice this is undertaken as a day case admission as illustrated in Fig. 19, measuring the response of aldosterone to erect posture (high in bilateral adrenal hyperplasia, absent in aldosterone-producing adenoma), to ACTH (absent in bilateral adrenal hyperplasia, increased in aldosterone-producing adenoma, exaggerated in glucocorticoid-suppressible hyperaldosteronism), and 18-hydroxy- or 18-oxo-cortisol/corticosterone in the plasma or urine. This study is only valid if plasma renin activity is seen to rise on adopting the erect posture and cortisol (reflecting underlying ACTH secretion) to fall between 08.00 h and 12.00 h.

Adrenal MRI/CT scanning should not be performed until a biochemical diagnosis has been made because of the high incidence of non-functioning adrenal incidentalomas. Thereafter, an MRI/CT scan should be the first localization procedure; CT has a better spatial resolution and may be more sensitive in detecting smaller aldosterone-producing adenomas (Fig. 20 and Plate 2). Adrenal scintigraphy studies (iodocholesterol scanning) have been found useful in some centres. Adopting the approach outlined in Fig. 19, few patients need invasive adrenal vein cannulation, although this may be required to make a diagnosis or to assist in the lateralization of a lesion if the posture and/or imaging studies are inconclusive. In particular, angiotensin II-responsive aldosterone-producing adenomas have been reported,

Table 7 Differential diagnosis of mineralocorticoid excess

Cause	Offending mineralocorticoid
Primary aldosteronism	Aldosterone
Congenital adrenal hyperplasia	Deoxycorticosterone
11β-Hydroxylase deficiency	
17α-Hydroxylase deficiency	
Glucocorticoid receptor resistance	Deoxycorticosterone
Glucocorticoid receptor mutations	
Metyrapone, RU486 ingestion	
Deoxycorticosterone-secreting adrenal	Deoxycorticosterone
tumour	
Liddle's syndrome	None
11β-Hydroxysteroid dehydrogenase	Cortisol
deficiency	
Apparent mineralocorticoid excess	
Liquorice and carbenoxolone ingestion	
Ectopic ACTH syndrome	

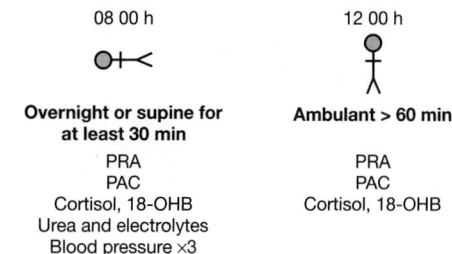

Fig. 19 Day case investigation of a patient suspected of having primary aldosteronism. Supine and erect plasma renin activity (PRA), plasma aldosterone concentration (PAC), cortisol (F), 18-hydroxycorticosterone (18-OHB) (or 18-OHF), electrolytes, and blood pressure are measured as shown. The posture study is only valid if there is a rise in PRA on adopting the erect posture and a fall in F concentrations between 08.00 h and 12.00 h (reflecting a circadian fall in ACTH levels). (Reproduced with permission of the author and *The Lancet*.)

and this may explain why the overall accuracy of posture studies in primary aldosteronism is only 70 to 80 per cent. Although technically difficult and not without risk, the demonstration of an aldosterone ratio of greater than 10:1 in one adrenal vein compared with the other remains the most sensitive diagnostic test. Simultaneous cortisol measurements ensure adrenal vein cannulation and, when expressed as an aldosterone/cortisol ratio, improve diagnostic accuracy.

One reason for establishing a definitive diagnosis is that treatment is surgical excision in the case of aldosterone-producing adenoma, but strictly medical for bilateral adrenal hyperplasia and glucocorticoid-suppressible hyperaldosteronism. The last responds well to dexamethasone at 0.25 to 0.5 mg/day. Patients with aldosterone-producing adenoma who are not suitable for surgery or decline operation and patients with bilateral adrenal hyperplasia should be treated with amiloride (starting dose 5 to 10 mg/day increasing to 30 mg/day depending upon blood pressure, urea, and electrolyte response). Spironolactone is as effective but in high doses frequently causes painful gynaecomastia and menstrual irregularity. In aldosterone-producing adenoma, normokalaemia is restored in 100 per cent of patients postoperatively and blood pressure falls to normal values in 70 per cent. With the ever increasing experience of laparascopic adrenalectomy, surgical morbidity can be kept to a minimum. Pre- and perioperative treatment should involve the co-ordinated management of surgeon and endocrinologist. Aldosterone secretion from the contralateral normal adrenal gland may be suppressed and hypoaldosteronism postoperatively should be anticipated and treated appropriately by increasing sodium intake and/or transient fludrocortisone therapy.

Monogenic hypertension

Hypertension is known to be a phenotype of some well-documented gene mutations; 17α-hydroxylase deficiency and 11β-hydroxylase deficiency are forms of congenital adrenal hyperplasia in which mineralocorticoid excess occurs because of ACTH-driven deoxycorticosterone excess. A similar process is thought to explain the hypertension seen in patients with glucocorticoid resistance due to mutations in the glucocorticoid receptor (GR) gene (Table 1). More recently, a significant advance in our understanding of the molecular basis of cardiovascular disease has been the elucidation of other single gene defects causing mineralocorticoid hypertension (Fig. 21).

Glucocorticoid-suppressible hyperaldosteronism

Glucocorticoid-suppressible hyperaldosteronism was first reported in 1966 and is an autosomal dominant form of low-renin hypertension characterized by aldosterone excess under the control of ACTH rather than the normal principal secretogogue, angiotensin II. There are two important consequences of this; first, there is dysregulation of aldosterone secretion because of loss of the negative feedback loop (aldosterone does not suppress ACTH secretion), and second, the exogenous administration of a glucocorticoid such as dexamethasone, by decreasing ACTH secretion, results in suppression of aldosterone secretion and can be used therapeutically.

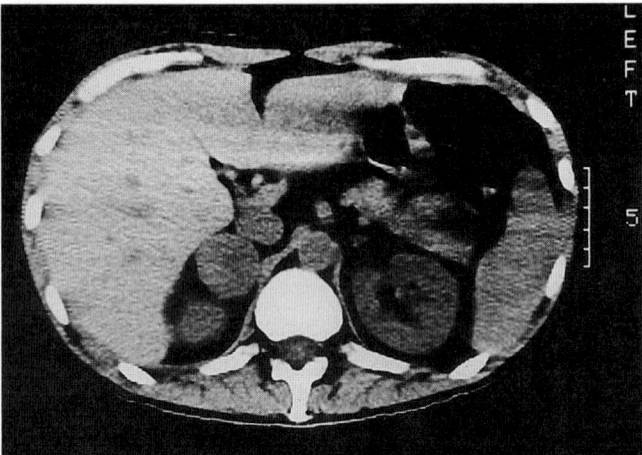

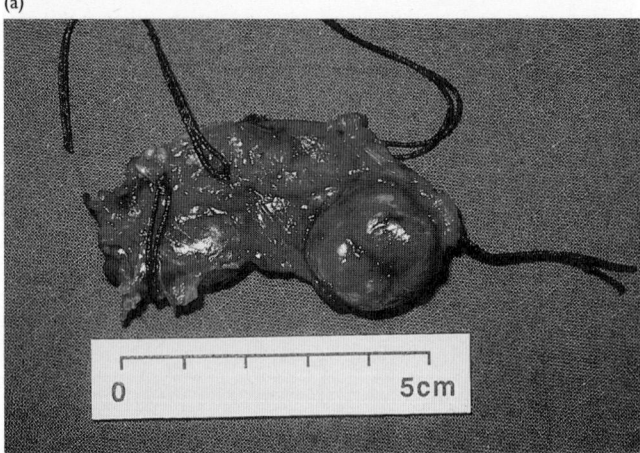

Fig. 20 (a) Adrenal CT scan demonstrating a solitary adrenal adenoma in a patients with Conn's syndrome. (b) The characteristic yellow appearance of the cut surface of the excised tumour reflects the high cholesterol content of these tumours. (See also Plate 2.)

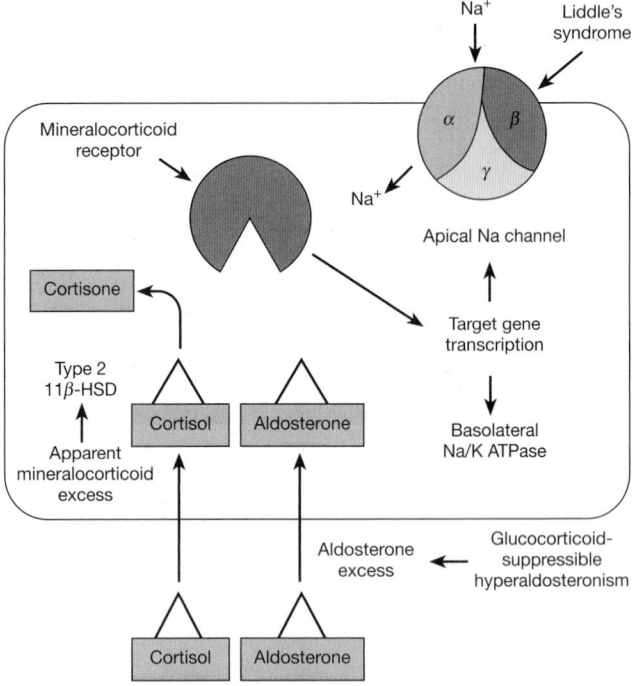

Fig. 21 Three causes of monogenic mineralocorticoid hypertension are detailed. A schematic diagram representing an epithelial cell in the distal colon or distal nephron is shown. In normal physiology, aldosterone interacts with the mineralocorticoid receptor (MR) to stimulate sodium reabsorption via induction of the apical sodium channel and serosal Na+/K+-ATPase pump. GSH (glucocorticoid-suppressible hyperaldosteronism) is a cause of aldosterone excess due to the production of a chimeric gene, 11β-hydroxylase/aldosterone synthase, within the adrenal cortex. Apparent mineralocorticoid excess results because cortisol cannot be inactivated to cortisone by the type 2 isoform of 11β-hydroxysteroid dehydrogenase (11β-HSD2); cortisol can then act as a potent mineralocorticoid. Liddle's syndrome occurs because of constitutively active mutations in the β- or γ-subunits of the apical sodium channel.

Long-term glucocorticoid therapy leads to reactivation and normal regulation of the renin–angiotensin–aldosterone axis. A further characteristic of glucocorticoid-suppressible hyperaldosteronism is the secretion of large quantities of 18-hydroxy- and 18-oxo-corticosterone/cortisol metabolites, again under the control of ACTH, and while there is some overlap with levels seen in aldosterone-producing adenoma, these provide a diagnostic marker for the condition.

The molecular basis for glucocorticoid-suppressible hyperaldosteronism was described by Lifton and colleagues following the cloning and characterization of the two final enzymes in cortisol and aldosterone synthesis, 11β-hydroxylase and aldosterone synthase, respectively. 11β-Hydroxylase converts 11-deoxycortisol to cortisol in the zona fasciculata, and aldosterone synthase converts corticosterone to aldosterone through an enzymatic step involving 11β-hydroxylation and 18-hydroxylation and oxidation. These enzymes are encoded by two genes, *CYP11B1* and *CYP11B2*, lying in tandem on chromosome 8. Despite the similarity in the coding sequences of 11β-hydroxylase and aldosterone synthase (more than 95 per cent), their 5' sequences differ, permitting regulation of 11β-hydroxylase by ACTH through cAMP and aldosterone synthase by angiotensin II through intracellular calcium ions, thereby establishing functional zonation of the adrenal cortex. In glucocorticoid-suppressible hyperaldosteronism a hybrid gene is formed at meiosis from unequal cross-over of the *CYP11B1* and *CYP11B2* genes and this contains proximal components of *CYP11B1* and distal components of *CYP11B2*. As long as the breakpoint of the hybrid gene is in or 5' to exon IV of the *CYP11B1* gene, the product of this gene can synthesize aldosterone, but is now under the control of ACTH (Fig. 22). The chimeric gene can be detected by Southern blotting or by long poly-merase chain reaction, providing a screening test for glucocorticoid-suppressible hyperaldosteronism and the facility for prenatal diagnosis.

In the wake of such advances, numerous kindreds have been reported with glucocorticoid-suppressible hyperaldosteronism and an international register for such cases has been established, which to date comprises 167 cases from 27 genetically proven pedigrees. Interesting observations to come from these larger cohorts are that potassium may be normal in up to 50 per cent of cases and there is poor correlation between genotype and phenotype (potassium, blood pressure) both between and within families. Severe mineralocorticoid excess has been reported in some individuals with this gene defect, but in other members of the same family, the gene defect has caused no abnormal phenotype. Patients with glucocorticoid-suppressible hyperaldosteronism are more susceptible to cerebrovascular haemorrhage.

Liddle's syndrome

In 1963, Grant Liddle described a family with several siblings affected by early-onset hypertension and hypokalaemia associated with low renin and low aldosterone levels. The condition responded well to inhibitors of epithelial sodium transport such as triamterene, but not to mineralocorticoid receptor antagonists such as spironolactone, and studies on erythrocytes suggested a generalized defect in sodium transport. Furthermore, in the proband of one of Liddle's original patients, renal transplantation resulted in blood pressure and potassium returning to normal levels, arguing against a circulating mineralocorticoid.

Mineralocorticoid-dependent epithelial sodium transport requires the activation of the apical sodium channel. Three subunits of this channel, α, β, and γ, have been cloned and characterized. Full sodium conductance requires the concerted action of α/β or α/γ subunits and cannot be sustained by any subunit in isolation. The β and γ subunits lie in close proximity on chromosome 16 and mutations in these subunits have been described in kindreds affected with Liddle's syndrome. In each case these cause deletions of the C-terminus part of the protein (45 to 75 amino acids) producing a sodium channel which is constitutively active. Liddle's syndrome is inherited as an autosomal dominant trait and several other kindreds have been reported following the description of the genetic basis for the condition. As is the case with glucocorticoid-suppressible hyperaldosteronism, potassium has been reported to be normal in several patients.

Apparent mineralocorticoid excess and abnormalities of 11β-hydroxysteroid dehydrogenase type 2

Apparent mineralocorticoid excess was first described in detail by Ulick and New in the late 1970s. This is an autosomal recessive form of low renin, low aldosterone hypertension in which cortisol, conventionally regarded as a glucocorticoid, is able to act as a potent mineralocorticoid. The condition can be diagnosed from a 24-h urine collection analysed for cortisol metabolites using gas chromatography. Affected individuals have a characteristic increase in urinary cortisol compared with cortisone metabolites (tetrahydrocortisols/tetrahydrocortisone ratio or urinary free cortisol/urinary free cortisone ratio). Serum cortisol levels are unhelpful because although patients with apparent mineralocorticoid excess have a prolonged plasma cortisol half-life, a reduction in cortisol secretion rate mediated by the negative feedback mechanism ensures normal circulating concentrations. This defect in cortisol metabolism occurs because of loss of 11β-hydroxysteroid dehydrogenase (11β-HSD) activity.

Two isozymes of 11β-HSD catalyse the interconversion of hormonally active cortisol (**F**) to inactive cortisone (**E**). 11β-HSD1 is predominantly found in the liver, adipose tissue, and gonad and acts principally as an oxo-reductase generating F from E, but it is the 11β-HSD2 isoform, acting as an efficient dehydrogenase inactivating F to E which is expressed in the mineralocorticoid target tissues, kidney, colon, and salivary gland, that is more important in modulating corticosteroid control of blood pressure. Aldosterone gains access to the mineralocorticoid receptor *in vivo* only when 11β-HSD2 activity is intact and F can be inactivated to E at a prereceptor level (Fig. 23). Homozygous inactivating mutations in the human

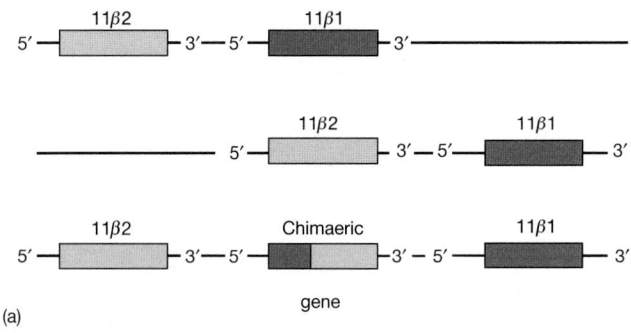

(a)

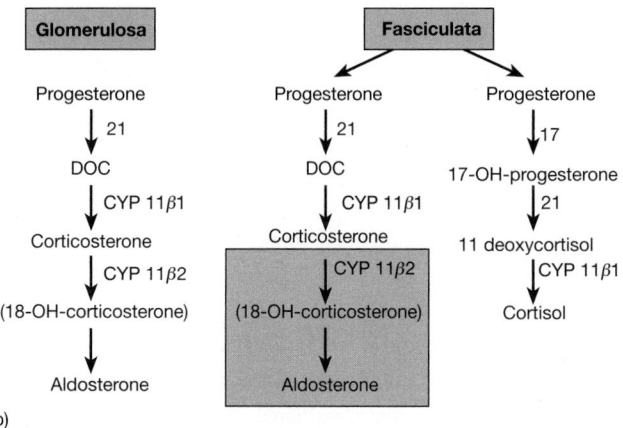

(b)

Fig. 22 (a) Chimeric gene responsible for glucocorticoid-remediable hyperaldosteronism and its impact upon adrenal steroid secretion. (b) The chimeric gene is expressed in the zona fasiculata (boxed area) and can synthesize aldosterone but is under the regulatory control of ACTH.

11β-HSD2 gene have been identified in over 20 patients with apparent mineralocorticoid excess and result in cortisol-mediated, mineralocorticoid hypertension. The condition is inherited as an autosomal recessive trait and the majority of heterozygotes, with a few notable exceptions, have a normal phenotype. Milder forms of apparent mineralocorticoid excess have been described and there appears to be a close correlation between genotype and phenotype. Spironolactone or amiloride (often in higher doses than those used to treat primary aldosteronism) can be used therapeutically, as can dexamethasone, which suppresses endogenous cortisol secretion, but itself is not a good substrate for 11β-HSD2.

Liquorice has been associated with a mineralocorticoid excess state since the late 1940s when Reevers, a Dutch Physician, used a liquorice preparation, 'succus liquoritiae', to treat patients with dyspepsia. This was the origin of the antiulcer drug, carbenoxolone, which also resulted in mineralocorticoid side-effects in up to 50 per cent of patients. The active 'mineralocorticoids' in both cases are glycyrrhizic acid and its hydrolytic product, glycyrrhetinic acid, which themselves have little inherent mineralocorticoid activity, but cause hypertension and hypokalaemia by inhibiting 11β-HSD2. Such patients will also have an increase in the urinary ratio of cortisol to cortisone metabolites (THF+allo-THF/THE), although not to the same degree as patients with apparent mineralocorticoid excess.

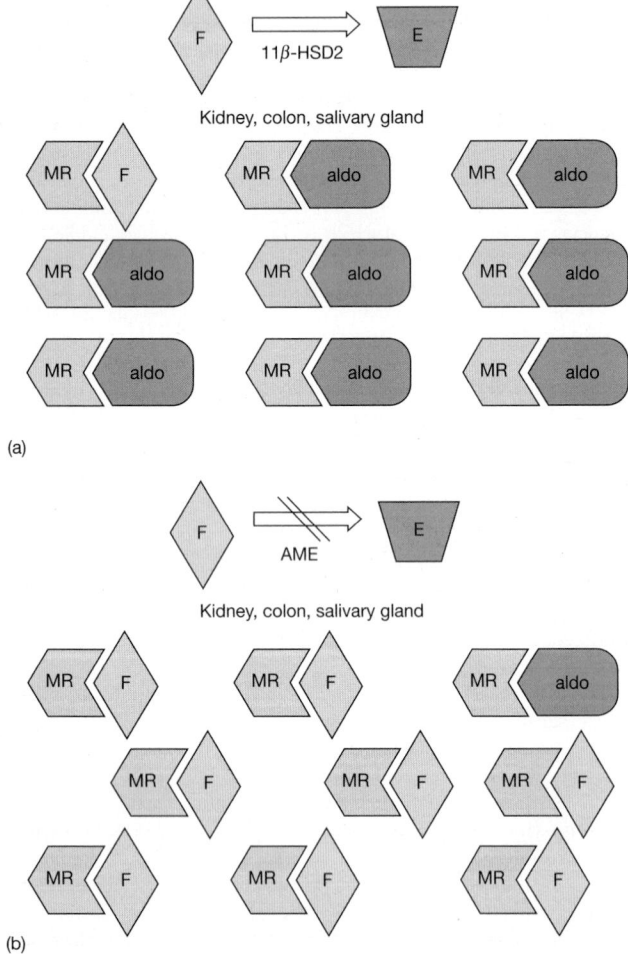

(a)

(b)

Fig. 23 (a) The role of 11β-hydroxysteroid dehydrogenase (11β-HSD2) in protecting the non-specific mineralocorticoid receptor from cortisol. (b) With congenital or acquired deficiency of the enzyme, F (cortisol) cannot be inactivated to E (cortisone) and acts as a potent mineralocorticoid.

Cortisol is also the offending mineralocorticoid in patients with some forms of Cushing's syndrome. In ectopic ACTH syndrome, for example, the high cortisol secretion rate overwhelms renal 11β-HSD2, resulting in spill over on to the mineralocorticoid receptor. A high THF+allo-THF/THE ratio is also observed in some patients with pituitary-dependent Cushing's syndrome and this may explain the hypertension in these cases.

These unusual causes of mineralocorticoid hypertension have significantly enhanced our understanding of corticosteroid biosynthesis and hormone action. In addition they raise new questions as to the role of adrenal steroids in wider populations of patients with hypertension. Defects in the activity of 11β-HSD have been reported in patients with 'essential hypertension', but have not consistently been associated with mineralocorticoid excess. Endogenous circulating inhibitors of 11β-HSD2 have also been described, so-called 'glycyrrhetinic acid-like factors' or GALFs. Levels are higher in pregnancy, and some studies, but not others, report increased levels in patients with hypertension. At present, however, the identity of such GALFs is unknown.

Who should we suspect as having mineralocorticoid-based hypertension?

All patients with hypertension should have serum electrolytes measured and those with hypokalaemia must be investigated (Fig. 24). Because hypokalaemia may be absent in many cases of proven mineralocorticoid hypertension, patients with severe hypertension (for example those on triple antihypertensive therapy) and those with a family history of hypertension or cerebrovascular disease should also be screened. At present the incidence of primary aldosteronism, glucocorticoid-suppressible hyperaldosteronism, Liddle's syndrome, and apparent mineralocorticoid excess in unselected (that is, community rather than hospital-based) populations with 'essential' hypertension is unknown. Until this is defined, one cannot be more dogmatic in deciding who should and should not be screened for mineralocorticoid-based hypertension. In the interim these diagnoses will not be made unless they are considered. Wherever possible the elucidation of the underlying basis of a patient's hypertension should be sought so that appropriate therapy can be targeted to the patient.

Glucocorticoid resistance

A small number of patients have been described who have increased cortisol secretion but with none of the stigmas of Cushing's syndrome. These patients are resistant to suppression of cortisol with low-dose dexamethasone but respond to high doses. ACTH levels are elevated and lead to increased adrenal production of androgens and deoxycorticosterone. Thus the patients may present with the features of androgen and/or mineralocorticoid excess. Treatment with a dose of dexamethasone adequate to suppress ACTH (usually 3 mg/day) results in a fall in adrenal androgens and often return of plasma potassium and blood pressure to normal levels. Many of these patients have been found to have point mutations in the steroid-binding domain of the glucocorticoid receptor, with consequent reduction of glucocorticoid-binding affinity.

Mineralocorticoid deficiency

These syndromes are listed in Table 8. They can be divided into those that are congenital and others that are acquired.

Adrenal insufficiency

Mineralocorticoid deficiency may occur in some forms of congenital adrenal hyperplasia and these are discussed elsewhere (see Chapter 12.7.2).

Similarly, other causes of adrenal insufficiency (for example Addison's disease and congenital adrenal hypoplasia) are discussed above.

Primary defects in aldosterone biosynthesis

Failure of conversion of corticosterone to 18-hydroxycorticosterone or of 18-hydroxycorticosterone to aldosterone usually presents as a salt-wasting crisis in neonatal life (Fig. 1). Hyperkalaemia, metabolic acidosis, dehydration, and hyponatraemia are found. The condition has been called corticosterone methyl oxidase (**CMO**) deficiency, but this was before the final

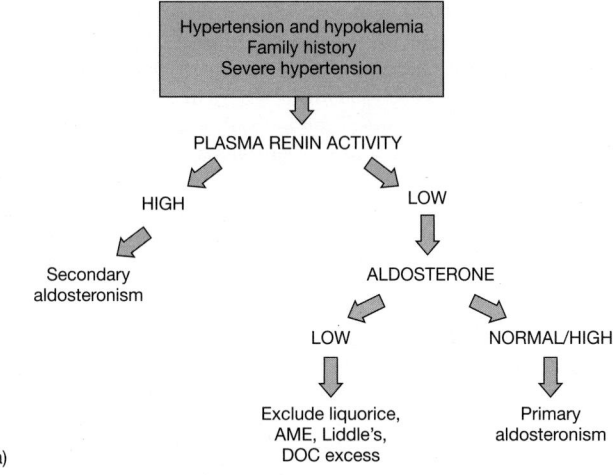

(a)

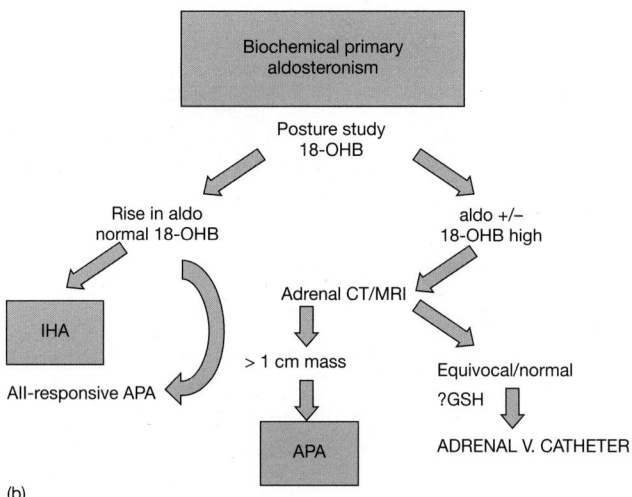

(b)

Fig. 24 Proposed algorithm for investigating mineralocorticoid-based hypertension. In practice the posture study (Fig. 19) can be included when the initial biochemical confirmation studies are performed.

Table 8 Causes of mineralocorticoid deficiency

Addison's disease
Adrenal hypoplasia
Congenital adrenal hyperplasia (17-hydroxylase and 3β-hydroxysteroid
   dehydrogenase deficiencies)
Pseudohypoaldosteronism types I and II
Hyporeninaemic hypoaldosteronism
Aldosterone biosynthetic defects
Drug induced

enzyme(s) involved in the conversion of deoxycorticosterone to aldosterone were characterized and cloned. In fact a single enzyme, aldosterone synthase carries a multistep reaction involving 11-hydroxylation of deoxycorticosterone to corticosterone, 18-hydroxylation of corticosterone to 18-hydroxycorticosterone, followed by 18-dehydrogenation to aldosterone. Two variants of CMO deficiency are described; CMO I is characterized by low 18-hydroxycorticosterone and aldosterone levels, whereas patients with CMO II deficiency have hypoaldosteronism but high 18-hydroxycorticosterone concentrations. In both cases, mutations in the gene encoding aldosterone synthase have been described and the discrepant 18-hydroxycorticosterone levels seem likely to be explained on the basis of variable 18-hydroxylase activity of the related CYP45011β-hydroxylase 1 enzyme. CMO II is much more common in Iranian Jews than in the Caucasian population.

Defects in aldosterone action: pseudohypoaldosteronism

Pseudohypoaldosteronism type I presents in infancy with severe salt-wasting and failure to thrive but with very high plasma aldosterone, and plasma renin activity levels with inappropriate urinary sodium loss. The mineralocorticoid receptor appears to be defective, as judged by studies looking at the binding of aldosterone to monocytes, but molecular studies have failed to show any abnormality in the mineralocorticoid receptor itself. Recently, inactivating mutations in the α, β, and γ subunits of the epithelial sodium channel have been shown to explain the condition, that is, exactly the opposite phenotype of Liddle's syndrome. Acquired forms of pseudohypoaldosteronism can occur in patients after renal transplantation, following obstructive uropathy, and in premature infants.

Pseudohypoaldosteronism type II or Gordon's syndrome is an autosomal dominant disorder characterized by hyperkalaemia but not salt-wasting in contrast to the type I condition. Patients have resistance to the mineralocorticoid effects of aldosterone on tubular potassium transport, but not to those of sodium and chloride transport. As a result, affected individuals have hyperchloraemia, hypertension, and suppression of plasma renin activity. Recent intronic deletions in the gene encoding a serine-threonine kinase, WNK, have been described in affected cases.

Hyporeninaemic hypoaldosteronism

Angiotensin II is a key stimulus to aldosterone secretion, and thus damage or blockade of the renin–angiotensin system may result in mineralocorticoid deficiency. Various renal diseases have been associated with damage to the juxtaglomerular apparatus and hence renin deficiency. Of these the most common (more than 75 per cent of cases) is diabetic nephropathy.

The usual picture is of an elderly patient with hyperkalaemia, acidosis, and mild to moderate impairment of renal function. Plasma renin activity and aldosterone are low and fail to respond to sodium depletion, the erect posture, or frusemide administration. Unlike those with adrenal insufficiency, patients with hyporeninaemic hypoaldosteronism have normal or elevated blood pressure but no postural hypotension. Muscle weakness and cardiac arrythmias may also occur. Other factors may also contribute to the hyperkalaemia, including the use of potassium-sparing diuretics, potassium supplementation, insulin deficiency, and β-adrenoceptor blocking drugs, and prostaglandin synthetase inhibitors which inhibit renin release.

Treatment of primary renin deficiency is with fludrocortisone in the first instance together with dietary potassium restriction. However, these patients are not salt depleted and may become hypertensive with fludrocortisone. In such a setting, the addition of a loop-acting diuretic such as frusemide is appropriate. This will also increase the excretion of acid and thus improves the metabolic acidosis.

Adrenal 'incidentalomas'

With the more widespread use of high-resolution imaging procedures (CT, MRI), incidentally discovered adrenal masses have become a common problem. An adrenal mass will be uncovered in up to 4 per cent of patients imaged for non-adrenal pathology. Over 80 per cent of cases are non-functioning with phaeochromocytomas and cortisol- or aldosterone-secreting adenomas comprising the remainder. As a result, all patients with incidentally discovered adrenal masses should undergo appropriate endocrine screening tests (24-hour urinary catecholamines, urinary free cortisol and overnight dexamethasone suppression tests, plasma renin activity/aldosterone, adrenal androgens) to exclude a functional lesion. The possibility of malignancy should be considered in each case. In patients with a known extra-adrenal primary, the incidence of malignancy is obviously much higher (up to 20 per cent of patients with lung cancer, for example, have adrenal metastases on CT scanning). Primary adrenal carcinoma is rare—in one study only 26 of 630 incidentalomas were found to be adrenal carcinomas. In true incidentalomas, size appears to be predictive of malignancy—a lesion of less than 5 cm in diameter is most unlikely to be malignant. Non-functioning lesions of less than 5 cm can therefore be treated conservatively and patients followed with annual imaging. Functional lesions, or tumours larger than 5 cm in diameter should be removed by laparascopic adrenalectomy.

Further reading

Cushing's syndrome

Atkinson AB et al. (1985). Five cases of cyclical Cushing's syndrome. British Medical Journal 291, 1453–7.

Kirschner LS et al. (2000). Mutations of the gene encoding the protein kinase A type I-alpha regulatory subunit in patients with the Carney complex. Nature Genetics 26, 89–92.

Lacroix A et al. (1992). Gastric-inhibitory polypeptide-dependent cortisol hypersecretion—a new cause of Cushing's syndrome. New England Journal of Medicine 327, 974–80.

Mampalam TJ, Tyrell B, Wilson CB (1988). Transsphenoidal microsurgery for Cushing's disease. A report of 216 cases. Annals of Internal Medicine 109, 487–93.

Newell-Price J et al. (1998). The diagnosis and differential diagnosis of Cushing's syndrome and pseudo-Cushing's states. Endocrine Reviews 19, 647–72.

Plotz CM, Knowlton AI, Ragan C (1952). The natural history of Cushing's syndrome. American Journal of Medicine 13, 597–614.

Ross EJ, Linch DC (1982). Cushing's syndrome—killing disease: discriminatory value of signs and symptoms aiding early diagnosis. Lancet ii, 646–9.

Wallace C et al. (1996). Pregnancy-induced Cushing's syndrome in multiple pregnancies. Journal of Clinical Endocrinology and Metabolism 81, 15–21.

Willenberg HS et al. (1998). Aberrant interleukin-1 receptors in a cortisol-secreting adrenal adenoma causing Cushing's syndrome. New England Journal of Medicine 339, 27–31.

Zovickian J et al. (1988). Usefulness of inferior petrosal sinus venous endocrine markers in Cushing's disease. Journal of Neurosurgery 68, 205–10.

Mineralocorticoids

Botero-Valez M, Curtis JJ, Warnock DG (1994). Brief report: Liddle's syndrome revisited—a disorder of sodium reabsorption in the distal tubule. New England Journal of Medicine 330, 178–81.

Conn JW (1955). Primary aldosteronism: a new clinical syndrome. Journal of Laboratory and Clinical Medicine 45, 6–17.

Edwards CRW et al. (1988). Tissue localisation of 11β-hydroxysteroid dehydrogenase-tissue specific protector of the mineralocorticoid receptor. Lancet ii, 986–9.

Fraser R, Davies DL, Connell JMC (1989). Hormones and hypertension. Clinical Endocrinology 31, 701–46.

Gagner M et al. (1997). Laparoscopic adrenalectomy: lessons learned from 100 consecutive procedures. Annals of Surgery 226, 238–46.

Gittler RD, Fajans SS (1995). Primary aldosteronism (Conn's syndrome). Journal of Clinical Endocrinology and Metabolism 80, 3438–41.

Gordon RD et al. (1992). Primary aldosteronism: hypertension with a genetic basis. Lancet 340, 159–61.

Hansson JH et al. (1995). Hypertension caused by a truncated epithelial sodium channel γ subunit: genetic heterogeneity of Liddle syndrome. Nature Genetics 11, 76–82.

Lamberts SWJ et al. (1992). Cortisol receptor resistance. The variability of its clinical presentation and response to treatment. Journal of Clinical Endocrinology and Metabolism 74, 313–21.

Lifton RP et al. (1992). A chimaeric 11β-hydroxylase/aldosterone synthase gene causes glucocorticoid remediable aldosteronism and human hypertension. Nature 355, 262–5.

Pascoe L et al. (1992). Glucocorticoid-suppressible hyperaldosteronism results from hybrid genes created by unequal crossovers between CYP11B1 and CYP11B2. Proceedings of the National Academy of Sciences, USA 89, 8327–31.

Rich GM et al. (1992). Glucocorticoid-remediable aldosteronism in a large kindred: Clinical spectrum and diagnosis using a characteristic biochemical phenotype. Annals of Internal Medicine 116, 813–20.

Shimkets RA et al. (1994). Liddle's syndrome: heritable human hypertension caused by mutations in the α-subunit of the epithelial sodium channel. Cell 79, 407–14.

Stewart PM et al. (1987). Mineralocorticoid activity of liquorice: 11β-hydroxysteroid dehydrogenase deficiency comes of age. Lancet ii, 821–4.

Stewart PM et al. (1995). 11β-Hydroxysteroid dehydrogenase activity in Cushing's syndrome: Explaining the mineralocorticoid excess state of the ectopic ACTH syndrome. Journal of Clinical Endocrinology and Metabolism 80, 3617–20.

White PC, Curnow KM, Pascoe L (1994). Disorders of steroid 11β-hydroxylase isozymes. Endocrine Reviews 15, 421–38.

White PC, Mune T, Agarwal AK (1997). 11β-Hydroxysteroid dehydrogenase and the syndrome of apparent mineralocorticoid excess. Endocrine Reviews 18, 135–56.

Wilson FH et al. (2001). Human hypertension caused by mutations in WNK kinases. Science 293, 1030.

Young WF et al. (1996). Primary aldosteronism: adrenal venous sampling. Surgery 120, 919–20.

Addison's disease

Addison T (1855). On the constitutional and local effects of disease of the suprarenal capsules. S. Highley, London.

Betterle C, Greggio NA, Volpato M (1998). Clinical review 93: Autoimmune polyglandular syndrome type 1. Journal of Clinical Endocrinology and Metabolism 83, 1049–55.

Erturk E, Jaffe CA, Barkan AL (1998). Evaluation of the integrity of the hypothalamo-pituitary adrenal axis by insulin hypoglycaemia test. Journal of Clinical Endocrinology and Metabolism 83, 2350–4.

Oelkers W (1996). Adrenal insufficiency. New England Journal of Medicine 335, 1206–12.

Stewart PM et al. (1988). A rational approach for assessing the hypothalamo-pituitary adrenal axis. Lancet i, 1208–10.

Miscellaneous

Kloos RT et al. (1995). Incidentally discovered adrenal masses. Endocrine Reviews 16, 460–84.

12.7.2 Congenital adrenal hyperplasia

I. A. Hughes

Congenital adrenal hyperplasia comprises a family of inherited disorders of adrenal steroidogenesis, characterized by deficiency of cortisol and an accumulation of substrate precursors. A pathophysiological consequence of inadequate cortisol and aldosterone production is ACTH hypersecretion and hyperplastic adrenals. Genital abnormalities are not a universal feature of all forms of congenital adrenal hyperplasia and the original adrenogenital syndrome nomenclature is now seldom used. Figure 1 shows the pathways of adrenal steroidogenesis. The rate-limiting step is the delivery of cholesterol from the outer to the inner mitochondrial membrane to act as substrate for the action of P450scc, a mixed-function oxidase side-chain cleavage enzyme. The intracellular transport of cholesterol is controlled by a number of proteins, including steroid acute regulatory (StAR) protein. The synthesis of cortisol is predominantly controlled by ACTH acting via a G protein-coupled receptor activation of cyclic AMP. Table 1 is a summary of the types of enzymes involved in adrenal steroidogenesis and the known localization of the genes that encode each enzyme. Deficiency of 21-hydroxylase activity is the cause for congenital adrenal hyperplasia in more than 90 per cent of cases.

21-Hydroxylase deficiency

Clinical presentation

Congenital adrenal hyperlasia due to 21-hydroxylase deficiency is a continuum of disorders which can manifest from birth to adult life (Table 2).

The classical form of this enzyme deficiency presents in infancy in one of two forms. The most dramatic is with ambiguous genitalia of the newborn, whereby a female fetus becomes virilized *in utero* due to the effect of excess adrenal androgen converted peripherally to testosterone and masculinizing the external genital anlagen. Milder forms of virilization manifest either as isolated clitoromegaly or as isolated labial fusion. There is evidence that aldosterone biosynthesis is deficient in up to 75 per cent of cases; in affected males, salt loss is initially the sole manifestation as the onset of virilization in males is delayed beyond infancy.

Late-onset or non-classical forms of congenital adrenal hyperplasia are also recognized. There may be delay in the onset of virilization in the non-salt-losing male. The signs of precocious sexual development are also accompanied by tall stature, due to the growth-promoting effect of androgens. The testes remain prepubertal in size (less than 4 ml in volume), which is a useful distinguishing feature from other causes of precocious puberty associated with increased gonadotrophin secretion. The non-classical form of congenital adrenal hyperplasia in females may present with early onset of pubic hair growth or later after puberty with signs of hirsutism and symptoms of menstrual dysfunction. It is important to exclude an adrenal tumour as the cause of late-onset signs of virilization. In adult females, the symptoms and signs are similar to those associated with polycystic ovarian syndrome. Male infertility has also been ascribed to 21-hydroxylase deficiency. Tumours arising from testicular adrenal rests are a complication generally, but not exclusively, in inadequately treated males.

Tests to establish a diagnosis

The characteristic biochemical hallmark is an elevated plasma concentration of 17OH-progesterone, generally greater than 300 nmol/l (normal less than 10 nmol/l). Newborn screening for congenital adrenal hyperplasia is established in several countries in an effort to identify affected males before

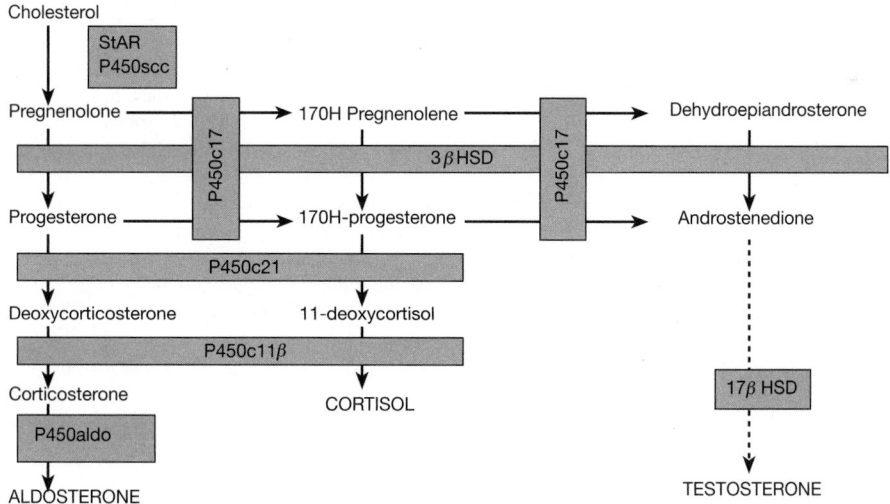

Fig. 1 Pathways of adrenal steroidogenesis. Enzymes involved as defined in the text are represented within the boxes. The dashed line denotes extra-adrenal synthesis of testosterone, catalysed by 17β-hydroxysteroid dehydrogenase. StAR, steroid acute regulatory protein.

Table 1 Genes and enzymes involved in adrenal steroidogenesis

Enzyme activity	Site of enzyme	Gene/chromosome
Cholesterol side-chain cleavage (P450scc)	Mitochondrion	*CYP11A/15q23-q24*
3β-hydroxysteroid dehydrogenase/isomerase (3βHSD)	Endoplasmic reticidium	*HSD3B1, HSD3B2/1p11-p13*
17α-hydroxylase (P450c17)	Endoplasmic reticulum	*CYP17/10q24-q25*
21-hydroxylase (P450c21)	Endoplasmic reticulum	*CYP21, CYP21P/6p21.3*
11β-hydroxylase (P450c11)	Mitochondrion	*CYP11B1, CYP11B2/8q21-q22*

Table 2 Clinical manifestations of 21-hydroxylase deficiency from birth to adulthood

Type	Female		Male	
	Age	**Clinical signs**	**Age**	**Clinical signs**
Classic	Neonatal	Ambiguous genitalia, occasional male phenotype, salt loss in 75%	Late neonatal	Occasional pigmented scrotum, salt loss in 75%, unexpected death
			Early childhood	Penile growth, pubic hair, rapid linear growth, increased musculature
			Adult	Testicular adrenal rest tumour, oligospermia
Non-classic (late-onset)	Late infancy	Clitoromegaly	Late infancy	Occasional delayed salt loss
	Childhood	Pubic hair, rapid growth	Childhood	Pubic hair, tall stature
	Adolescence	Abnormal menses, hirsutism, acne	Adolescence	Not known
	Adult	Hirsutism, oligomenorrhoea, infertility	Adult	

the onset of life-threatening salt loss. The world-wide incidence of 21-hydroxylase deficiency is approximately 1 in 14 000 births.

The diagnosis of late-onset 21-hydroxylase deficiency requires an ACTH stimulation test. Studies of women with signs of hyperandrogenism show only about 5 per cent of hormone profiles consistent with late-onset congenital adrenal hyperlasia. Polycystic ovarian syndrome is a well recognized and more frequent cause of hirsutism and infertility, although ultrasonographic evidence of polycystic ovaries is common in congenital adrenal hyperplasia. The disease frequency for the late-onset form is estimated as 0.1 per cent of the general population, but as high as 3 to 4 per cent of Ashkenazi Jews.

Treatment in early infancy, childhood, and adolescence

Glucocorticoid replacement in the form of hydrocortisone should be started; if the infant is in salt-losing crisis, parenteral hydrocortisone with intravenous saline and dextrose is needed. Hypoglycaemia may be a problem. The cortisol secretion rate is about 6 to 8 mg/m^2 per day so that an oral hydrocortisone dose no more than 15 to 20 mg/m^2 per day should be used initially. For salt-losers, aldosterone replacement is given in the form of 9α-fludrocortisone (florinef), 100 to 150 µg daily. Salt added to the feeds is sometimes needed during the first few months of life.

Surgical reconstruction of the external genitalia is required for the virilized female infant at 6 to 12 months of age. The procedure involves reducing the size of the clitoris and exposing the opening of the vagina on to the perineum. Further assessment of the vaginal opening is undertaken around puberty to determine whether treatment with dilators is required. Ongoing medical treatment is adjusted according to body surface area. The hydrocortisone dose should be trebled in times of stress, and parenteral steroids given to cover surgical procedures. Other glucocorticoid preparations used include cortisone acetate, prednisolone, and dexamethasone. Prednisolone and dexamethasone are both longer-acting glucocorticoids which appear to be useful for treatment in the postpubertal age group. Dexamethasone can be used as a single daily dose and appears to regulate menses more efficiently in the young adult female patient. Some girls, however, develop side-effects, such as excessive weight gain and striae formation on quite small doses of dexamethasone. Dexamethasone is 80 to 100 times more potent than hydrocortisone in suppressing 17OH-progesterone levels.

Monitoring treatment

The rate of linear growth is the main clinical yardstick of control before puberty (Table 3). Growth is normally rapid during infancy; over-treatment during this period may be a factor leading to reduced final height and to obesity in childhood. Growth monitoring is supplemented by bone age measurements. Androgens stimulate epiphyseal maturation through local conversion to oestrogens so that advanced skeletal maturation inevitably reduces the length of growing time and leads to short adult stature. The onset of the pubertal growth spurt is a milestone to monitor in both sexes, while delayed menarche in girls indicates inadequate control and increased

plasma testosterone concentrations. In adults, regular menses and ovulation in the female and normal spermatogenesis in the male are reliable clinical indicators of adequate control.

Some of the tests listed in Table 3 are used as additional markers of control. There is a marked diurnal rhythm in 17OH-progesterone so that single random measurements are inadequate to monitor control. A daily profile is a useful measure of control, especially as capillary blood spot and saliva assays are available. Androstenedione can also be used as a marker of control. Random plasma testosterone measurements are useful to monitor control in infants, children, and adult females, but not in pubertal boys and adult males because of testosterone secretion by the testis. Serum electrolytes are an insensitive index of the adequacy of mineralocorticoid replacement, but renin measurement and blood pressure recordings should be undertaken routinely after infancy. An elevated plasma renin indicates the need for 9α-fludrocortisone treatment even if there has been no overt salt loss. Salt losers invariably like a salty diet even when adequately replaced with mineralocorticoid.

Outcome in treated 21-hydroxylase deficiency

The survival rate for the salt-wasting form of 21-hydroxylase deficiency has improved in recent years. However, an unequal sex incidence suggests that male infants still die in infancy from an unrecognized adrenal crisis. Achieving normal growth is a problem in management and patients rarely reach their predicted adult height. A recent clinical trial of lowering the glucocorticoid dose by blocking the action of androgen with an antiandrogen and the conversion of androgen to oestrogen with an aromatase inhibitor is showing promising results for improved growth.

Fertility is reduced in adult females. Contributory factors include inadequate vaginal introitus, and anovulatory cycles from increased progesterone concentrations acting as a 'mini-pill'. These problems are remediable and pregnancy rates are now improving. Nevertheless, there is evidence of lower maternalism and heterosexuality in adult females. Those who do

Table 3 Parameters to monitor treatment in congenital adrenal hyperplasia

Clinical
Infancy and childhood growth rates
Weight gain
Striae formation
Signs of puberty
Blood pressure
Regularity of menses
Skeletal age
Bone density scan
Biochemical
Profile of 17OH-progesterone (saliva, blood spots)
Plasma androstenedione
Plasma testosterone
Plasma renin activity
Urinary steroid metabolite excretion

become pregnant need careful monitoring to maintain steroid levels within the pregnancy-related range. Delivery is usually by caesarean section, and the offspring are normal even if testosterone levels increase slightly during pregnancy. Adult males who stop taking glucocorticoid replacement may develop oligospermia; this is usually reversible if treatment is restarted. Testicular tumours may also occur from ACTH hyperstimulation of testicular adrenal-rest cells. Laparoscopic adrenalectomy is a radical form of treatment in patients recalcitrant to medical management, particularly females with persistent signs of virilization.

Genetics of 21-hydroxylase deficiency

Congenital adrenal hyperplasia is an autosomal recessive condition; the CYP21 gene is closely linked to the major histocompatibility complex on the short arm of chromosome 6. Studies of HLA haplotypes show an association between the uncommon A3, Bw47, DR7 haplotype in the classical salt-losing form, whereas in the non-classical late-onset form, there is a strong association with HLA-B14, DR1.

Two genes, CYP21 and a pseudogene, CYP21P, were identified within the class III region of the HLA complex on chromosome 6p21.3 and are approximately 30 kb apart. They are adjacent to, and in tandem repeat with C4A and C4B genes which encode for the fourth component of serum complement (Fig. 2). CYP21P is functionally inactive because of a series of deleterious mutations, but is 97 per cent homologous with the active gene. Each gene comprises 10 exons. Misalignment and unequal crossing over between sister chromatids during meiosis leads to a major gene deletion. This is always associated with the severe, salt-losing form of congenital adrenal hyperplasia. The frequency of gene deletions as a cause of 21-hydroxylase deficiency is about 25 per cent and is highest in northern European populations. Another frequent genotype is associated with gene conversion events in which there is non-reciprocal transfer of multiple mutations from CYP21P to the active CYP21 gene. Such large-scale conversions may account for a further 10 to 15 per cent of cases, all manifesting with the severe, salt-losing form. The majority of gene conversion events are small scale in nature. Several point mutations have now been identified while linked microsatellites are useful for prenatal diagnosis when the family genotype has previously been ascertained.

A sufficient number of alleles have now been studied to indicate general concordance between genotype and phenotype. The mutations which cause more than 90 per cent of cases of 21-hydroxylase deficiency are shown in Fig. 3 in relation to the expected phenotype. The most common mutation in classic 21-hydroxylase deficiency affects mRNA splicing due to a nucleotide base change (A/C to G) in the second intron. A stretch of nucleotides which is normally spliced out is retained, so that the translational reading frame is altered and an inactive protein synthesized. Most patients with this mutation have the salt-losing form of congenital adrenal hyperplasia, but some patients who are homozygous for this mutation are salt replete. Presumably, enough normally spliced mRNA is generated to

produce some enzyme activity. Other examples leading to salt loss are shown in Fig. 3. In vitro functional assays of wild type and mutant CYP21 enzymes using progesterone and 17OH-progesterone as substrate show total absence of enzyme activity for mutations leading to salt loss. A specific mutation associated with non-salt-wasting occurs in exon 4, changing isoleucine to an asparagine (Ile172Asn). This mutation results in an enzyme with about 1 per cent of normal activity, sufficient for adequate aldosterone production.

The non-classical or late-onset form of 21-hydroxylase deficiency is associated with a mutant enzyme which has 50 per cent and 20 per cent of normal activity in vitro with substrates 17OH-progesterone and progesterone, respectively. An example is Val251Leu in exon 7 which is associated with the haplotype HLA-B14, DR1. This single mutation accounts for the majority of non-classical cases of congenital adrenal hyperplasia, and is most frequently found in East European Jews. Genetic studies in 21-hydroxylase deficiency show that many patients are compound heterozygotes. In general, the phenotype reflects the less deleterious mutation.

Prenatal diagnosis and treatment

Chorionic villus sampling and molecular analysis of the CYP21 gene has enabled an earlier and more reliable diagnosis to be made. Furthermore, there is the option of offering prenatal treatment to prevent virilization of an affected female fetus. Figure 4 outlines the current protocol used for the prenatal diagnosis and treatment of 21-hydroxylase deficiency.

Maternal dexamethasone treatment is started early as fetal adrenal steroidogenesis is established by the eighth week of gestation. CYP21 genotyping of the index case, parents, and unaffected siblings should have been performed previously. DNA analysis is then more reliable, especially if the straightforward technique of linked microsatellite markers is used. Dexamethasone is chosen as the glucocorticoid since, unlike hydrocortisone and prednisolone, this steroid is not inactivated by placental 11β-hydroxy-

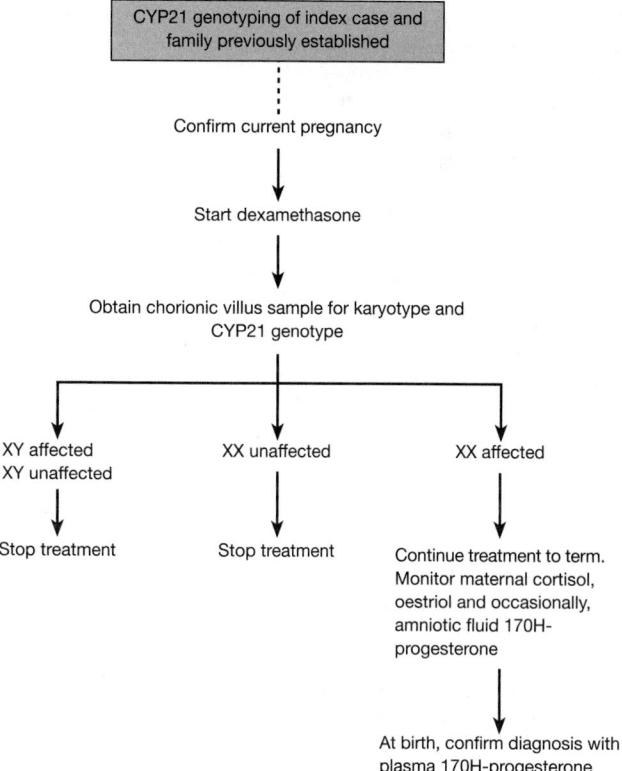

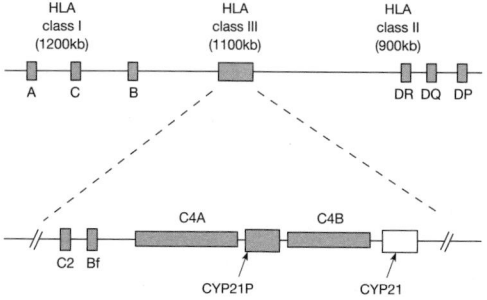

Fig. 2 Schema of the HLA gene region on chromosome 21p. The active 21-hydroxylase gene is CYP21, the inactive pseudogene, CYP21P. The two genes are in tandem repeat with complement C4A and C4B genes.

Fig. 3 Genotype: phenotype correlations for the 10 most frequent causes of 21-hydroxylase deficiency. E6 cluster refers to three mutations (Ile 236 Asp, Val 237 Glu, Met 239 Lys) in exon 6.

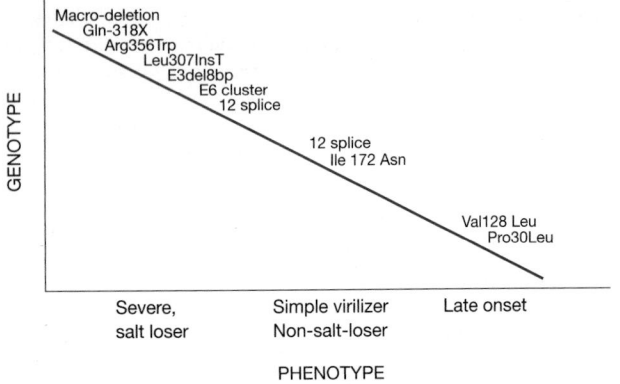

Fig. 4 Outline protocol for prenatal management of 21-hydroxylase deficiency.

steroid dehydrogenase. The conventional starting dose is 20 μg/kg per day based on prepregnancy bodyweight, administered in three divided doses. Once the diagnosis has been confirmed by molecular genetic analysis, treatment is only continued to term in the case of an affected female fetus. Thus, seven out of eight fetuses will be exposed unnecessarily to dexamethasone for about 6 weeks during early gestation. Fetal adrenal suppression is monitored by serial measurements of maternal plasma or urinary oestriol concentrations. This steroid metabolite is formed as a result of placental aromatization of weak androgen substrates produced uniquely by the fetal adrenal gland. More direct evidence of adrenal suppression can be obtained by collecting amniotic fluid for measurement of 17OH-progesterone and testosterone.

The outcome of prenatal treatment is satisfactory in the majority of cases when treatment is started early and continues uninterrupted to term. Thus, the external genitalia in affected females are completely normal or so mildly affected that surgery is not required. There have been isolated reports of other abnormalities in treated infants but no specific pattern is emerging to suggest that prenatal dexamethasone treatment is detrimental to postnatal growth and development. This treatment to prevent a congenital malformation is still experimental and should be undertaken as part of a clinical trial which includes long-term outcome surveillance. Maternal side-effects of the treatment include excessive weight gain, striae formation, hypertension, and glucose intolerance.

Other forms of congenital adrenal hyperplasia

P450scc deficiency

This extremely rare form of the condition has also been variously called cholesterol desmolase deficiency and lipoid adrenal hyperplasia. The production of all classes of steroid hormones is deficient in gonadal as well as in adrenal tissue. Affected males have female external genitalia because of failure to synthesize testosterone. Affected 46XX females have developed puberty spontaneously suggesting the enzyme deficiency is less severe in the ovary compared with the testis.

The gene encoding P450scc is designated *CYP11A* and it was assumed that mutations in this gene caused lipoid adrenal hyperplasia. However, no mutations were found in several cases studied. Furthermore, adrenal tissue studied from an affected patient showed normal P450scc cDNA. When the human StAR gene was cloned, subsequent studies identified deleterious StAR mutations in patients with this form of congenital adrenal hyperplasia. The disorder is most common in the Japanese population; a premature stop codon at amino acid 258 substituting for glutamine is a frequently reported mutation. The StAR gene is expressed in the adrenals and gonads, but not the placenta, explaining why congenital lipoid adrenal hyperplasia is not a lethal disorder. Further analysis of the P450scc gene in

a patient with lipoid adrenal hyperplasia who had a normal StAR gene, revealed a heterozygous mutation. The child had survived 4 years before developing an acute adrenal crisis.

3β-Hydroxysteroid dehydrogenase deficiency

3β-Hydroxysteroid dehydrogenase/isomerase (3βHSD) is a non-P450 membrane-bound enzyme which converts Δ^5 to Δ^4 steroids in the adrenals and gonads. Hence it is needed for the synthesis of glucocorticoids, mineralocorticoids, progesterone, androgens, and oestrogens. Two highly homologous genes, *HSD3B1* and *HSD382*, control the expression of two human isoenzymes. Type I enzyme is expressed predominantly in the placenta and peripheral tissues, whereas type II is expressed in the adrenals and gonads. Deficiency of 3βHSD activity also causes severe glucocorticoid and mineralocorticoid deficiency. Genital abnormalities occur, mainly in males because of the production of weak androgens by the testis. Diagnosis is confirmed by an elevated ratio of Δ^5 (170H-pregnenolone) to Δ^4 (170H-progesterone) steroids and analysis of urinary steroid metabolites.

Molecular studies show the majority of patients have missense mutations in the *HSD3B2* gene. Nevertheless, there is significant conversion of Δ^5 to Δ^4 steroids in peripheral tissues through the action of type I 3βHSD . Consequently, some patients have elevated levels of Δ^4 steroids (17OH-progesterone, androstenedione), which has led to a mistaken diagnosis of 21-hydroxylase deficiency. Extraglandular steroid synthesis accounts for 40 per cent of androgen production in adult males and most oestrogen production in prepubertal and postmenopausal females. Spontaneous onset of puberty and menarche are reported in females with 3βHSD deficiency.

17α-Hydroxylase deficiency

A single P450c17 enzyme catalyses 17α-hydroxylase and 17,20-lyase reactions. Both are required for the synthesis of sex hormones (C19 steroids), whereas only 17α-hydroxylase activity is required to synthesize cortisol (C21, 17-hydroxysteroids). Mineralocorticoid biosynthesis is not dependent on the presence of the P45017α enzyme, so that ACTH-stimulated, low renin hypertension is a typical feature of P45017α hydroxylase deficiency due to excess production of C21, 17-deoxysteroids such as aldosterone. There is an accompanying hypokalaemic, metabolic alkalosis. Inadequate androgen in affected males causes a phenotype ranging from female genitalia to an ambiguous appearance or features of a hypospadic male. Females lack breast development and have primary amenorrhoea. The P450c17 enzyme operates as a qualitative regulator of steroidogenesis using pregnenolone as substrate.

Increased corticosterone, deoxycorticosterone, and progesterone and decreased levels of testosterone, oestradiol, and renin characterize this enzyme defect. Measurements of steroid metabolites delineate patterns indicative of 17α-hydroxylase or 17,20-lyase deficiency alone, or combined. Most patients have a mutant P450c17 which leads to loss of both enzyme activities.

The 6.5-kb human *CYP17* gene comprises eight exons. A frequent mutation is a 4-bp duplication in exon 8 which, as a result of altering the reading frame, leads to a shortened carboxy-terminal sequence. Expression studies of the mutant protein show absence of both 17α-hydroxylase and 17,20-lyase activities. This is consistent with biochemical findings and a clinical female phenotype in affected males and females. The differential catalytic activity of this enzyme is manifest at adrenarche with the development of the zona reticularis and increased 17,20-lyase activity. This causes increased concentrations of dehydroepiandrosterone (DHEA) and its sulphate (DHEAS), independent of any change either in ACTH or cortisol levels. The increase in adrenal androgens may lead to early onset of pubic and axillary hair, body odour, and a moderate advance in skeletal maturation. Premature adrenarche must be differentiated from late-onset congenital adrenal hyperplasia or an adrenal tumour. Studies on the regulation of 17,20-lyase activity suggests a role for P450c17 phosphorylation in mediating the increased differential enzyme activity occurring at the time of adrenarche.

11β-Hydroxylase deficiency

Deficiency of 11β-hydroxylase activity accounts for about 5 per cent of cases of congenital adrenal hyperplasia. The enzyme is required for the terminal conversion of 11-deoxycortisol to cortisol and deoxycorticosterone to corticosterone. Consequences of increased ACTH stimulation are salt and water retention, low-renin hypertension, and virilization secondary to the increased production of deoxycorticosterone and adrenal androgens. Newborn females and infant males are more profoundly virilized than is the case with 21-hydroxylase deficiency. Prepubertal breast development is another specific and unexplained feature. Hypertension can develop in early childhood, the severity not necessarily correlating with plasma levels of deoxycorticosterone.

The diagnosis is confirmed by elevated concentrations of 11-deoxycortisol and deoxycorticosterone in plasma and their tetrahydro metabolites in urine. Plasma concentrations of androstenedione and testosterone are increased. Moderately elevated levels of 17OH-progesterone may lead to an erroneous diagnosis of 21-hydroxylase deficiency. Treatment requires only glucocorticoid replacement, although transient salt-wasting may follow an initial fall in levels of the potent mineralocorticoid, deoxycorticosterone. Antihypertensive treatment may be necessary if hypertension has been long-standing. Milder or late-onset deficiency occurs and manifests similar features to the late-onset form of 21-hydroxylase deficiency.

11β-Hydoxylase activity is a function of the *CYP11B1* gene which comprises nine exons and is located on chromosome 8q22. The gene is highly expressed in the adrenals; transcripts are controlled by ACTH and to a lesser extent, by angiotensin II. Located on the same chromosome, at a distance of about 40 kb, is the highly homologous *CYP11B2* gene which encodes aldosterone synthase (also referred to as corticosterone methyloxidase II) which catalyses the conversion of corticosterone via 18OH-corticosterone to aldosterone.

Mutations throughout the *CYP11B1* gene cause 11β-hydroxylase deficiency. The majority are missense mutations with some clustering occurring in exons 2, 6, 7, and 8. The highest incidence of this form of congenital adrenal hyperplasia occurs in an inbred population of Sephardic Jews in Morocco. A single amino acid substitution (Arg448His) is the cause. This alters the haeme-binding sequence which is a unique and conserved feature of all cytochrome P450 enzymes. Prenatal treatment with dexamethasone has also been used successfully in this form of congenital adrenal hyperplasia to prevent virilization of an affected female fetus. The late-onset or non-classic form of 11β-hydroxylase deficiency has been found in one study to be associated with compound heterozygote mutations of the *CYP11B1* gene. Studies of hirsute women with marginally elevated levels of 11-deoxycortisol have not revealed mutations in the *CYP11B1* gene.

Further reading

Acerini CL, Hughes IA (2000). 21-Hydroxylase deficiency defects and their phenotype. In: Hughes IA, Clark AJL, eds. *Adrenal disease in childhood. Clinical and molecular aspects*, pp. 93–111. Karger, Basel.

Alizai NK, Thomas DF, Lilford RJ, Batchelor AG, Johnson N (1999). Feminizing genitoplasty for congenital adrenal hyperplasia: what happens at puberty? *Journal of Urology* 161, 1588–91.

Bose HS, Sugarawa T, Strauss JF III, Miller WL (1996). The pathophysiology and genetics of congenital lipoid adrenal hyperplasia. *New England Journal of Medicine* 335, 1870–8.

Cerame BL, Newfield RS, Pascoe L, et al. (1999). Prenatal diagnosis and treatment of 11β-hydroxylase deficiency congenital adrenal hyperplasia resulting in normal female genitalia. *Journal of Clinical Endocrinology and Metabolism* 84, 3129–34.

Forest MG, Morel Y, David M (1998). Prenatal treatment of congenital adrenal hyperplasia. *Trends in Endocrinology and Metabolism* 9, 284–9.

Hughes IA (1998). Congenital adrenal hyperplasia—a continuum of disorders. *Lancet* 352, 752–4.

Jaaskelainen J, Vouitilainen R (1997). Growth of patients with 21-hydroxylase deficiency: an analysis of the factors influencing adult height. *Pediatrc Research* 41, 30–3.

Jaaskelainen J, Lavo A, Voutilainen R, Partanen J (1997). Population-wide evaluation of disease manifestation in relation to molecular phenotype in steroid 21-hydroxylase (CYP21) deficiency: good correlation in a well defined mutation. *Journal of Clinical Endocrinology and Metabolism* 8, 3293–7.

Lajic S, Wedell A, Biu T-H, Ritzen EM, Holst M (1998). Long-term somatic follow-up of prenatally treated children with congenital adrenal hyperplasia. *Journal of Clinical Endocrinology and Metabolism* 83, 3872–80.

Lo JC, Schwitzgebel VM, Tyrrell JB, et al. (1999). Normal female infants born of mothers with classic congenital adrenal hyperplasia due to 21-hydroxylase deficiency. *Journal of Clinical Endocrinology and Metabolism* 84, 930–6.

Meyer-Bahlburg HFL (1999). What causes low rates of child-bearing in congenital adrenal hyperplasia? *Journal of Clinical Endocrinology and Metablism* 84, 1844–7.

Miller WL (1998). Prenatal treatment of congenital adrenal hyperplasia: a promising experimental therapy of unproven safety. *Trends in Endocrinology and Metabolism* 9, 290–2.

Miller WL, Auchus RJ (2000). Biochemistry and genetics of human P450c17. In, Hughes IA, Clark AJL, eds. *Adrenal disease in childhood. Clinical and molecular aspects*, pp. 63–92. Karger, Basel.

Moisan AM, Ricketts ML, Tardy V, et al. (1999). New insight into the molecular basis of 3β-hydroxysteroid dehydrogenase deficiency: identification of eight mutations in the HSD3B2 gene in eleven patients from seven new families and comparison of the functional properties of twenty-five mutant enzymes. *Journal of Clinical Endocrinology and Metabolism* 84, 4410–25.

Pang S, Wallace AM, Hofman L, et al. (1998). Worldwide experience in newborn screening for classical congenital adrenal hyperplasia due to 21-hydroxylase deficiency. *Pediatrics* 81, 866–74.

Premawardhana LDKE, Hughes IA, Read GF, Scanlon MF (1997). Longer term outcome in females with congenital adrenal hyperplasia (CAH): the Cardiff experience. *Clinical Endocrinology* 46, 327–32.

Tajima T, Fujieda K, Kouda N, Nakae J, Miller WL (2001) Heterozygous mutation in the cholesterol side chain cleavage enzyme (p450scc) gene in a patient with 46,XY sex reversal and adrenal insufficiency. *Journal of Clinical Endocrinology and Metabolism* 86, 2820-5..

Van Wyk JJ, Gunther DF, Ritzen EM, et al. (1997). The use of adrenalectomy as a treatment for congenital adrenal hyperplasia. *Journal of Clinical Endocrinology and Metabolism* 81, 3180–9.

White PC, Speiser PW (2000). Congenital adrenal hyperplasia due to 21-hydroxylase deficiency. *Endocrine Reviews* 21, 245–91.

White PC, Curnow KM, Pascoe I (1994). Disorders of steroid 11β hydroxylase enzymes. *Endocrine Reviews* 15, 421–38.

Zucker KJ, Bradley SJ, Oliver G, Blake J, Fleming S, Hood J (1996). Psychosexual development of women with congenital adrenal hyperplasia. *Hormones and Behaviour* 30, 300–18.

12.8 The reproductive system

12.8.1 Ovarian disorders

H. S. Jacobs

Approach to the patient with ovarian disorders

Synchronization of the changes in the ovary and uterus and the hypothalamic–pituitary unit is complex and, not surprisingly, the ovulatory cycle is vulnerable to disturbances at any of the levels of endocrine organization. Ovarian cyclicity may also be disrupted by a deterioration in general health, a protective mechanism that avoids reproduction occurring in circumstances adverse to fetal development.

In obtaining the history, information about the regularity of the menstrual cycle is relevant in women concerned about fertility because the chance of conception is directly related to the rate of ovulation. If a woman ovulates only six rather than the usual 12 to 13 times a year, it will take her twice as long to conceive as a woman of the same age with a regular monthly cycle. Oligomenorrhea (interval between menstrual periods of more than 6 weeks but less than 6 months) is usually a consequence of the polycystic ovary syndrome (see later); amenorrhoea (no periods for more than 6 months) has a broader spectrum of causes (Tables 1 and 2). The

Table 1 Causes of primary amenorrhoea in 90 consecutive cases seen in the author's clinics

Cause	Percentage
Premature (primary) ovarian failure	36
Hypogonadotrophic hypogonadism	34
Polycystic ovary syndrome	17
Hypopituitarism	4
Congenital anomalies	4
Hyperprolactinaemia	3
Weight-related amenorrhoea	2

Table 2 Causes of secondary amenorrhoea in 570 consecutive cases seen in the author's clinics

Cause	Percentage
Polycystic ovary syndrome	36
Premature (primary) ovarian failure	24
Hyperprolactinaemia	17
Weight-related amenorrhoea	10
Hypogonadotrophic hypogonadism	6
Hypopituitarism	4
Exercise-related amenorrhoea	3

duration of a menstrual disturbance is relevant both to its cause and its consequences. For example, a history of delayed menarche implies that the disturbance was present from the age of 12, a common finding in women with polycystic ovary syndrome. A history of weight fluctuation is important because weight loss, often in the context of mild (and denied) anorexia nervosa, is a common cause of amenorrhoea and weight increase a common precipitant of the clinical expression of polycystic ovary syndrome. Bulimia may complicate either of the above conditions and, like anorexia nervosa, requires specialist management in its own right. It is always relevant to inquire about a family history of the patient's complaint since an increasing number of mono- and polygenic causes of reproductive disturbance are now recognized.

The association of amenorrhoea with galactorrhoea implies hyperprolactinaemia and an association with symptoms of oestrogen deficiency (flushing and sweating attacks and/or vaginal dryness and discomfort during intercourse) implies an increased risk of osteoporosis. Symptoms of hyperandrogenism (seborrhoea, acne, and excessive hair growth) imply increased production of androgens, which, in most cases, is caused by polycystic ovary syndrome. It is preferable to use the term 'unwanted hair' rather than 'hirsutism' to avoid provoking a debate with the patient about what is and what is not excessive. On the other hand, whether the unwanted hair is severe enough to be helped by present methods of treatment is a matter for the physician's judgement. Some women express a concern, which should not be trivialized, that the development of unwanted hair means they are turning into a man. They need a clear explanation of the underlying disorder and reassurance that treatment is available.

If the patient has previously used an oral contraceptive, one should determine whether it was primarily for contraception or had been prescribed to correct a menstrual disturbance. In the latter case, it is important to appreciate that treatment with an oral contraceptive does not cure such problems, which are therefore likely to recur when it is stopped. Oral contraceptives do not cause amenorrhoea after discontinuation. Amenorrhoea occurring after discontinuation of an oral contraceptive therefore needs the same investigation as amenorrhoea temporally unrelated to previous use of an oral contraceptive.

Most women with menstrual disturbances want reassurance about their present or future fertility. Their age is clearly of great importance in this evaluation which will also have to determine the extent to which failure to ovulate is an adequate explanation of the failure to conceive. Many older women need advice about the long-term effects of oestrogen deficiency and the wisdom of hormone replacement therapy.

Amenorrhoea

While the classification is usually into primary (the patient has never had a menstrual period) or secondary amenorrhoea (interval between periods exceeds 6 months) most of the common causes can present as either, as seen in Tables 1 and 2. With the exception of structural abnormalities, such as an absent uterus, differences between primary and secondary amenorrhoea are outweighed by similarities so here they are considered primarily in terms of their aetiology.

In young women with primary amenorrhoea there may have been congenital abnormalities in the development of the ovaries, genital tract, or external genitalia or a perturbation of the normal process of puberty (Chapter 12.9.3). Investigation is appropriate when menstruation has not occurred by the age of 16 in the presence of normal secondary sexual development or by the age of 14 in its absence.

Developmental abnormalities

Developmental abnormalities of the mullerian duct, external genitalia, and the problems of intersexual abnormalities are dealt with elsewhere.

Gonadal dysgenesis

The commonest cause of gonadal dysgenesis is Turner's syndrome, in the severest form of which a 45XO karyotype is associated with a characteristic phenotypic appearance. Typically patients are of short stature, with cubitus valgus, webbed neck, low hairline, shield chest, and widely spaced nipples. The palate is often arched and the fourth metacarpal short. Lymphoedema, multiple pigmented naevei, and hearing loss are common. Coarctation of the aorta occurs in 10 to 20 per cent and hypertension independent of that abnormality occurs more commonly than in the normal population. The condition occurs in about 1 in 2500 female births. Spontaneous and, indeed, ovulatory cycles occasionally occur, particularly if there is chromosomal mosaicism, but in the long term premature ovarian failure is inevitable. It is important to determine the karyotype as the presence of a Y chromosome in an individual with gonadal dysgenesis means residual gonadal tissue must be removed because of an increased risk of malignancy.

Serum gonadotrophin concentrations are elevated compared with those of normal girls of the same age and may approach the menopausal range. Oestrogen levels are low, the uterus is small and bone densitometry shows skeletal decalcification; a history of spontaneous fracture is common. In addition to cardiovascular and renal assessment, autoimmune thyroiditis and diabetes mellitus should be excluded.

Management includes initiation of low-dose oestrogen therapy (starting with no more than 5 μg of ethinyl oestradiol per day) to promote breast development without prejudicing linear growth. The dose is gradually raised over 12 to 18 months. Maintenance therapy is with a cyclical oestrogen–progestogen preparation (such as an oral contraceptive), as regular withdrawal bleeding is necessary to prevent endometrial hyperplasia and the risk of malignancy. While it is now possible to provide fertility to women with Turner's syndrome through ovum donation, shortage of oocytes remains an important and usually critically limiting factor. Given the prevalence of hypertension and cardiovascular disorder, careful medical assessment before referral is required.

Hypothalamic causes of amenorrhoea

Hypothalamic hypogonadotrophic hypogonadism may be functional or organic and can occur in an isolated form or in association with more widespread endocrine disorders, as in patients with infiltrating (sarcoidosis, tuberculosis), expanding (craniopharyngioma), or traumatic (head injury) lesions of the hypothalamus. Hypogonadotrophic hypogonadism that is potentially reversible occurs in primary and secondary iron overload syndromes and is a frequent presenting feature of juvenile haemochromatosis. Lesions of the pituitary stalk are increasingly recognized.

Idiopathic hypogonadotrophic hypogonadism is characterized by low serum levels of gonadotrophins and gonadal steroids in the absence of structural defects of the hypothalamic–pituitary axis. Idiopathic hypogonadotrophic hypogonadism usually results from a congenital defect of secretion of gonadotrophin-releasing hormone, although mutations of the gene encoding the gonadotrophin-releasing hormone receptor have also been described.

Hypogonadism with anosmia. In a number of idiopathic hypogonadotrophic hypogonadism pedigrees mis- and non-sense mutations and partial and complete deletions have been identified in a gene located in the distal part of the short arm of the X chromosome (Xp22.3). These mutations are associated with hypogonadotrophic hypogonadism and anosmia, as features of Kallman's syndrome in boys and men. This (*KAL*) gene lies next to the steroid sulphatase locus, so patients may exhibit a contiguous gene syndrome comprising complete X-linked Kallman's syndrome and ichthyosis. The *KAL* gene encodes a molecule with similarities to proteins involved in neural cell adhesion and axonal pathfinding. X-linked Kallman's syndrome arises from a defect of embryonic migration of olfactory and gonadotrophin-releasing hormone producing neurones from the anlage of the olfactory lobes into the hypothalamus. In affected females the disorder is usually inherited as an autosomal recessive or dominant trait, generally with incomplete penetrance. The molecular cause in these cases is not known.

In women Kallman's syndrome presents with delayed puberty and primary amenorrhoea. Characteristically the patient cannot smell curry or the difference between tea and coffee. There are signs of marked oestrogen deficiency, usually amounting to sexual infantilism. Adult stature is normal. Mirror movements, in which voluntary movements of one limb are associated with involuntary, non suppressible and homologous mirror movements of the contralateral limb, occur in 85 per cent and unilateral renal agenesis in 31 per cent of X-linked cases.

Investigations reveal subnormal serum gonadotrophin and oestradiol concentrations, on pelvic ultrasound the uterus and ovaries are small, and bone densitometry reveals skeletal demineralization (Fig. 1). Renal imaging may show an absent kidney; MRI of the brain shows absent or abnormal olfactory bulbs and sulci, with a normal pituitary gland.

Management of idiopathic hypogonadotrophic hypogonadism involves induction of pubertal maturation, initially with small doses of oestrogen (not more than 5 μg/day of ethinyl oestradiol) to optimize breast development. Delay in recognition and treatment impairs full development and so has important psychosocial implications. Surgical referral for breast augmentation is appropriate if development remains inadequate after a year's

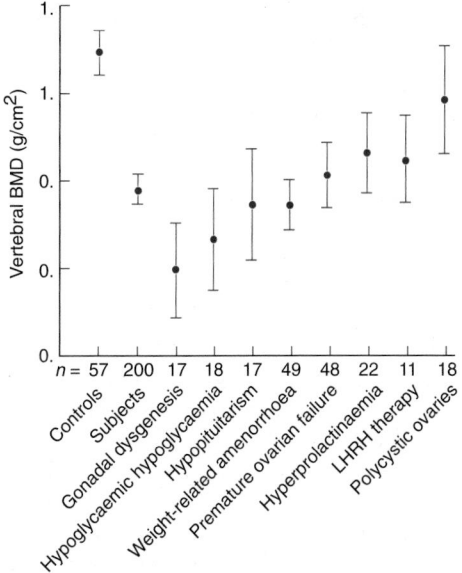

Fig. 1 Vertebral bone mineral density measurements in 200 young women with amenorrhoea, arranged by diagnosis. With the exception of the bone mineral density measurements in the women with polycystic ovary syndrome, the bone mineral density measurements of all other groups were significantly below those of the controls.

treatment with gradually increasing doses of oestrogen. Maintenance hormone treatment is with an oral contraceptive preparation. Bone densitometry should be repeated to ensure that the dose of oestrogen is adequate. While an increase of 5 to 6 per cent per year for 2 to 3 years is expected, delay in diagnosis may result in failure to attain normal peak bone mass. Treatment with pulsatile gonadotrophin-releasing hormone or gonadotrophin injections allows an excellent prognosis for fertility.

Functional hypogonadotrophic hypogonadism

Weight-related amenorrhoea

Amenorrhoea is usual when the body fat content falls below 17 per cent or the body mass index falls below 19 kg/m^2. The latter figure assumes an average amount of exercise; for competitive athletes, particularly those in track events, the figure would be higher. Depending on the age of onset, the patient may present with primary or secondary amenorrhoea.

The neuroendocrine mechanisms that signal this critical level of nutritional reserve are uncertain but centre on reduced secretion of leptin which results in impaired secretion of gonadotrophins, particularly luteinizing hormone. Serum insulin and insulin-like growth factor 1 levels are low so there is also reduced insulin drive to the ovaries. The consequent anovulation is protective because it avoids reproduction occurring in adverse circumstances. Quite apart from the obstetric evidence of premature delivery of immature babies to women who are underweight, there is also a link between deficient fetal nutrition and an increased prevalence in adults of cardiovascular and pulmonary disease.

Self-imposed starvation

The cause is often anorexia nervosa (Chapter 26.5.5). In patients presenting with amenorrhoea, loss of appetite is usually denied and the patient often draws attention to what she regards as a normal pattern of eating. These women characteristically maintain a good appetite which they have to suppress. In contrast, some women lose weight as a feature of the anorexia of depression, occasioned perhaps by the breakup of a relationship; in this condition the patient does lose her appetite. The prognosis for a return of normal weight and spontaneous menstrual cycles is much better than that in women with anorexia nervosa.

Exercise-related amenorrhoea

Amenorrhoea is common in ballet dancers and high-performance athletes, particularly during phases of intensive training and performance. The amenorrhoea is associated with reduced body weight and body fat content. Psychological stress is unlikely to be a major determinant because amenorrhoea is not common in Olympic swimmers, who, though as competitive as track athletes, have a normal body fat content.

Involuntary starvation

Worldwide, the most important causes of starvation are social disintegration, famine, and war. Increasingly we recognize that the deleterious physical effects of starvation are passed to the next generation, inter alia, through the adverse effects of fetal malnutrition on adult health.

Altered absorption

In patients with malabsorption, for instance in women with cystic fibrosis, amenorrhoea is associated with reduced body mass index and body fat content and resolves when nutrition improves.

Investigation of weight-related amenorrhoea

The diagnosis is made in part by identifying that the patient's weight is subnormal for her height, bearing in mind the effect of high-performance training on replacing body fat with more dense muscle. It is also made by exclusion, because self-imposed weight loss is common in young women and may coexist with other conditions.

Women with weight-related amenorrhoea have subnormal serum gonadotrophin (particularly luteinizing hormone) and oestradiol concentrations, with small ovaries and a small uterus on ultrasound scanning. Skeletal demineralization is the rule, except in those with coexisting poly-

cystic ovaries (see later). Serum markers of bone resorbtion are low, indicating that, in contrast to the osteoporosis of oestrogen deficiency, this is a 'low-turnover' osteoporosis. The most likely cause is reduced osteotrophic stimulation by insulin-like growth factor 1 and leptin.

Management involves explanation, identification of psychiatric conditions for which specialist advice is needed, and correction of oestrogen deficiency. Optimally the latter is achieved through weight gain. Oestrogen deficiency may, however, be so severe that if the patient is unable to put on weight, it may be preferable for her to take oestrogen rather than have the clinician adopt a purist position. Bone mineral density, however, only improves when the patient gains weight: oestrogen treatment is ineffective. So far as fertility is concerned, medical induction of ovulation should be eschewed until the patient's weight has returned to normal so that nutritional risks to the unborn child (and adult) have been minimized. In the event, when the body mass index returns to normal, induction of ovulation is rarely required.

Pituitary causes of amenorrhoea

While a non-functioning pituitary tumour sometimes causes amenorrhoea, the commonest pituitary cause is hypersecretion of prolactin. The subject is discussed further in Chapter 12.2.

Ovarian causes of amenorrhoea

Primary ovarian failure

Primary ovarian failure occurs normally at the menopause ('age appropriate primary ovarian failure') because of the process of atresia (Fig. 2) that results in almost complete depletion of oocytes and follicles by about the age of 50. If the rate of atresia is faster than normal, the causes of which are discussed below, depletion of oocytes and follicles occurs prematurely and 'age inappropriate' or 'premature' ovarian failure develops.

Oocytes do not divide once they have been laid down in the ovary. Thus unlike the testis, the ovary has a finite complement of germ cells. Oocytes 'used' in the process of ovulation account for a minute proportion of those that are lost, and it can be seen from Fig. 2 that most atresia occurs during intrauterine life when endocrine influences are least important. The apoptotic process of atresia is controlled genetically. Loss of the second X chromosome, as in 45XO Turner's syndrome, accelerates the rate. This observation, together with the occurrence of familial cases of premature ovarian failure, has prompted the search for genes critical for normal ovarian development. Three loci on the X chromosome appear to be vital: the first is Xp22, which contains a series of genes that escape X inactivation, among which is the ZFX gene. Premature ovarian failure is one of the features of the transgenic mouse with this gene 'knocked out'. The SOX3 gene (mapped to Xq26–27.2), the homologue of the SRY gene on the Y chromosome that determines testicular development, also escapes X inactivation and fulfils several of the criteria for a candidate gene. The third region of interest is Xq13–22 because several women with premature ovarian failure and break points in this region have been described. Familial premature ovarian failure also occurs without cytogenetic abnormality and autosomal dominant, autosomal recessive, and X-linked patterns of inheritance have been described. The condition may be present in families with galactosaemia, blepharophimosis, and fragile X syndrome. The presentation is particularly intriguing in the last case because the association is specifically with the premutation, until recently thought not to have a phenotype other than the risk of transmitting fragile X syndrome.

Destruction of genetic material by ionizing irradiation, anticancer chemotherapy, and viral infections, such as mumps oophoritis, can cause premature ovarian failure (Table 3). The association of premature ovarian failure with thyroiditis, adrenalitis, and diabetes mellitus has led to the hypothesis that in many cases the cause is autoimmune. While reliable tests are not widely available, autoantibodies to ovarian cells, oocytes, or gonadotrophin receptors have been reported in up to 80 per cent of cases, a

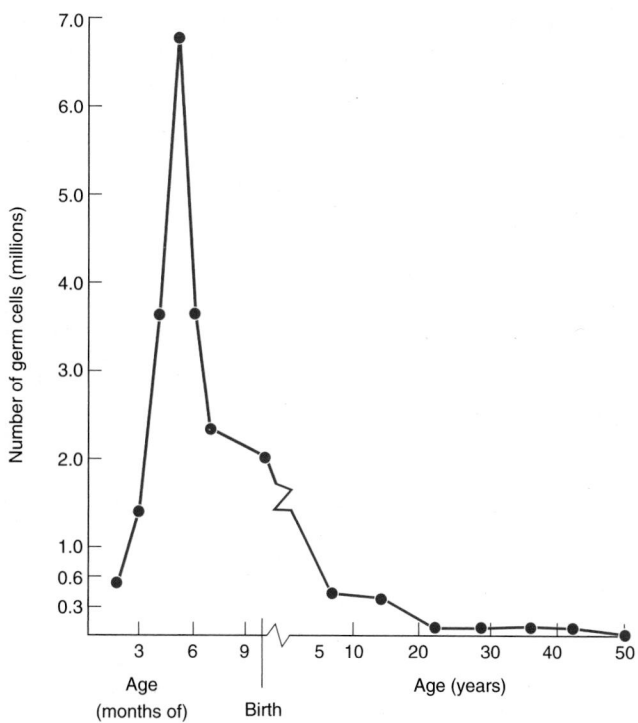

Fig. 2 The number of oocytes in the gonads in relation to age. Note that the maximum rate of atresia occurs before birth. (After Baker TG (1963). *Proceedings of the Royal Society (Biology)* **158**, 417)

result consistent with the author's finding of thyroid and adrenal autoantibodies in more than half of the patients remaining after those with chromosomal causes had been excluded. Finally, the presence in follicular fluid of toxic pollutants from tobacco smoke, such as cotinine, a congener of nicotine, may account for the earlier menopause that occurs in women who smoke cigarettes.

The symptoms of primary ovarian failure are those of oestrogen deficiency, together with infertility. Investigation reveals subnormal oestradiol and raised serum gonadotrophin concentrations. While the serum luteinizing hormone is often elevated in patients with polycystic ovary syndrome, a rise in the concentration of follicle-stimulating hormone always suggests primary ovarian failure. Autoantibodies should be sought because their presence alerts the clinician to the possible development of pluriglandular endocrine failure. Pelvic ultrasound shows undetectable or small ovaries and a small uterus. Bone densitometry usually reveals significant demineralization.

Table 3 Causes of primary ovarian failure in 320 cases seen in the author's clinics

Cause	Number	Percentage
Idiopathic	169	52.6
Turner's syndrome	73	22.7
Autoimmune disease*	22	6.9
Anticancer chemotherapy	21	6.5
'Resistant ovaries'	10	3.1
Surgery	7	2.2
Radiotherapy	6	1.9
Galactosaemia	6	1.9
Familial	3	0.9
Miscellaneous	4	1.2

* Sixteen had primary hypothyroidism and six had Addison's disease. Three of these patients had diabetes mellitus.

Patients with premature ovarian failure usually require hormone replacement therapy, the indications, precautions, etc. being the same as those for women in whom the menopause has occurred at a normal age. In some women there may be a spontaneous return of ovulatory menstrual cycles, albeit usually temporary, and therefore pregnancies do sometimes occur. Treatment with glucocorticoids or immunolytic drugs for women with autoimmune ovarian failure has occasionally proven successful but formal controlled trials are lacking and these treatments are not recommended. The ovaries do not respond to further stimulation with gonadotrophins so the only chance of childbearing for most women is through ovum donation. The problems of supplies of donor oocytes are formidable.

Resistant ovary syndrome

This ill-defined syndrome refers to women with amenorrhoea and elevated serum gonadotrophin concentrations in whom, paradoxically, oestrogen levels are well maintained. The persistent secretion of oestradiol suggests persistence of ovarian follicular activity, an implication occasionally confirmed histologically or by ultrasound assessment of the ovaries and by the occasional and unpredictable occurrence of pregnancy. The ovaries do not respond to further stimulation with exogenous gonadotrophins. While both cause and prognosis remain obscure the condition is most easily understood as a transitional phase on the way to primary ovarian failure.

Polycystic ovary syndrome

A full description of polycystic ovary syndrome is given later. Its clinical expression, typically dating from the time of puberty, involves a menstrual disorder (usually oligomenorrhoea but amenorrhoea in 26 per cent of cases) hyperandrogenization, and weight increase.

The indications for treatment of amenorrhoea in women with polycystic ovary syndrome depend upon the patient's needs. For women who wish to conceive, induction of ovulation is required, combined with attempts to reduce insulin drive to the ovaries by diet, exercise, and insulin-sensitizing drugs such as metformin (see later). For women needing contraception, an oral contraceptive is appropriate, the choice of preparation depending on the degree of associated unwanted hair. An oral contraceptive is also appropriate for women troubled by the lack or unpredictability of menstruation. For the remainder, it is acceptable to remain amenorrhoeic, provided annual ultrasound scans of the endometrium shows that overstimulation has not occurred.

Investigation of amenorrhoea

The patient's stature, nutritional status, the presence of unwanted hair (male pattern or the lanugo of anorexia nervosa) or acanthosis nigricans, and the physical stigmata of oestrogen deficiency are important parts of the physical examination. Pelvic ultrasound reveals the ovarian dimensions and whether they have the characteristic internal echoes of polycystic ovaries and the size of the uterus and degree of endometrial thickening. Hormone assays reveal subnormal serum oestradiol levels associated with elevated (primary ovarian failure) or subnormal (hypogonadotrophic hypogonadism) gonadotrophin concentrations. Serum ferritin measurements are conducted to screen for excessive iron storage in patients with low gonadotrophin concentrations. Assessment of white blood cell karyotype and measurement of autoantibodies is undertaken in patients with primary ovarian failure. Bone densitometry may reveal demineralization of spine and hips. Radiological assessment of the pituitary is undertaken in patients with hyperprolactinaemia.

Treatment of amenorrhoea

In addition to correcting the cause whenever possible, management is directed at minimizing the long-term complications of oestrogen deficiency. When the cause cannot be corrected oestrogen replacement therapy, usually in the form of an oral contraceptive, is appropriate. Outcome should be monitored by ensuring that sufficient oestrogen is administered to cause withdrawal bleeds and that there is an improvement in bone density if skeletal demineralization has been demonstrated.

Hyperandrogenization

Normal hair growth and androgen production in women

At birth the fetus is covered in lanugo hair which rapidly disappears and is not seen again unless anorexia nervosa develops, although very rarely such hair appears as a non-metastatic complication of malignancy. The follicles in the skin of prepubertal children grow soft, short, and fair vellus hair, which, together with scalp, eyebrow, and eyelash hair, is known as nonsexual hair. In response to the secretion of adrenal androgens at puberty, both boys and girls develop terminal hair in the axillae and lower pubic triangle (ambosexual hair). Terminal hair is long, pigmented and coarse. In boys the further increase of (testicular) androgen secretion leads to the development of terminal hair in the upper pubic triangle and on the face, chest, abdomen, and arms and legs—that is, male pattern hair.

Perception of hairiness depends in part on its distribution and in part on its character and pigmentation. While there is racial variation in the density of hair follicles (Native Americans and Orientals having few and women from the Mediterranean littoral having many follicles per unit area of skin) it is the development of male pattern hair in women which constitutes hirsutism.

The sources of androgens in normal women are shown in Fig. 3 from which it can be seen that 50 per cent of directly secreted and 75 per cent of peripherally derived testosterone normally originates from the adrenal cortex. Testosterone circulates specifically bound to sex hormone binding globulin, from which it disassociates and diffuses into target tissues where it is either 5α reduced to a more powerful androgen, dihydrotestosterone, or aromatized to oestradiol. The dihydrotestosterone–nuclear protein receptor

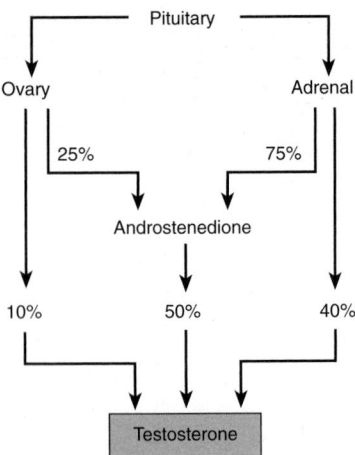

Fig. 3 Sources of androgens in normal women.

complex associates with the specific DNA receptor to cause androgen-specific protein synthesis and the expression of androgen action.

Synthesis of sex hormone binding globulin, whose concentration largely determines the total serum testosterone concentration, takes place in the liver, stimulated by thyroxine and inhibited by insulin and to a lesser extent by androgens. The rate of clearance of sex hormone binding globulin is reduced by oestrogen.

Clinical hyperandrogenization

Hyperandrogenization in women is manifest as seborrhoea, persistent acne, and the development of a male pattern of distribution and quality of hair. Male pattern hair loss may also occur, particularly in women with male family members who are bald. Clitoromegaly and increased muscle bulk are signs of severe and usually long-standing overexposure to androgens.

Although defects in adrenal steroid biosynthesis (congenital and late onset adrenal hyperplasia), Cushing's syndrome, and adrenal androgen secreting tumours may all cause oversecretion of androgens and therefore present with hirsutism, the commonest cause by far is polycystic ovary syndrome, in which condition there is an increase in the direct ovarian secretion of androgens.

Polycystic ovary syndrome

Polycystic ovaries are readily identified by pelvic ultrasound, because they are larger than normal (average volume three times that in normal women) and have a highly echodense central stroma in which cysts of 2 to 6 mm diameter are arranged around the circumference (Fig. 4). When ovaries with this appearance are detected in women complaining of specific symptoms, the term polycystic ovary syndrome is used (Table 4). Defined in this way, the polycystic ovary syndrome corresponds to the condition described over 50 years ago by Stein and Leventhal.

Patients with this condition commonly present in their late teens or early twenties, complaining of the consequences of hyperandrogenization or of a menstrual disturbance (Table 4). There is often a family history of similar complaints but even when that is absent an ultrasound scan usually reveals polycystic ovaries in first-degree relatives. Infertility is caused by failure of ovulation, although hypersecretion of luteinizing hormone is also important in this regard. Obesity, often associated with an increase in the ratio of waist to hip circumference, is the third classical feature.

Endocrine features

The classical profile is of hypersecretion of luteinizing hormone and androgens with normal circulating follicle-stimulating hormone, prolactin, and

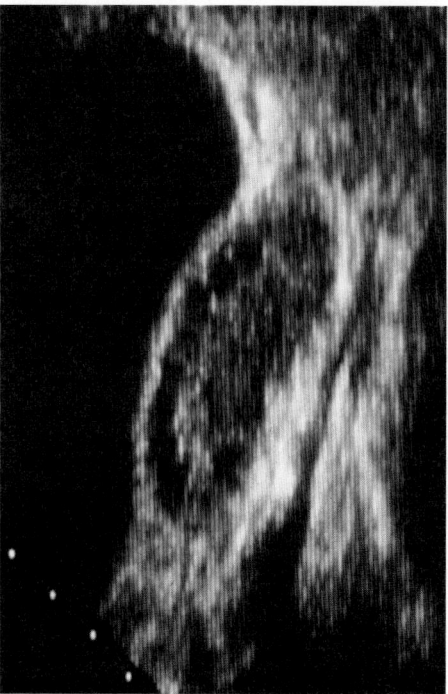

Fig. 4 Transabdominal ultrasound image of a polycystic ovary. Note the enlarged ovary with the echodense central stroma and the necklace of cysts around the circumference.

thyroxine concentrations. In fact a spectrum of endocrine findings occurs, reflecting the phenotypic heterogeneity of the polycystic ovary syndrome. In a study of more than 1500 cases, 44 per cent had an elevated serum luteinizing hormone and 22 per cent an elevated serum total testosterone concentration. Levels of luteinizing hormone were raised most commonly in the women complaining of infertility and of testosterone in those complaining of hirsutism.

The nature of the primary disturbance underlying these findings is uncertain. A central problem is failure of the polycystic ovary to convert androgens, made in excessive amounts by the abundant theca and interstitial cells of the hyperplastic ovarian stroma, into oestrogens. The androgens (predominantly androstenedione and testosterone) are released into the circulation and converted in the skin to dihydrotestosterone. In liver and fat tissue, they are converted into oestrogens at a rate which increases with the degree of obesity. The high levels of oestrogen (predominantly oestrone) inhibit secretion of follicle-stimulating hormone and may stimulate secretion of luteinizing hormone. The former effect contributes to persistent anovulation and the consequent lack of progesterone (which in the normal luteal phase limits the proliferative action of oestradiol) means that the action on the uterus of the normally weak oestrogen oestrone is unopposed. These patients are consequently at risk from endometrial hyperplasia and neoplasia. The raised levels of luteinizing hormone stimu-

Table 4 Diagnosis of polycystic ovary syndrome

Ultrasound	Presence of polycystic ovaries
	Enlarged ovaries
	Ten or more cysts (6–8 mm) arranged around the periphery
	Echodense central stroma
Clinical	Presence of polycystic ovaries together with characteristic symptomatology
	Menstrual disturbance
	Hyperandrogenization
	Obesity

late the excessive numbers of theca and interstitial cells to oversecrete androgens. Exposure of the ovaries to high levels of luteinizing hormone at inappropriate times of the cycle may also impair fertility through an action on the developing oocyte.

The above model does not explain the variable clinical presentation of polycystic ovary syndrome. It is likely that environmental factors lead to expression of the underlying, probably inherited, condition.

Many patients with polycystic ovary syndrome, particularly those who are anovulatory, are resistant to the action of insulin. While several types of insulin resistance are currently recognized (Chapter 12.11), in women with polycystic ovary syndrome the resistance is specifically to insulin-mediated extrasplanchnic disposal of glucose. As a consequence, euglycaemia can only be maintained through compensatory hypersecretion of insulin, the clinical clue to which is the development of acanthosis nigricans (see Plate 1). The insulin resistance spares the liver (the fasting glucose concentration is normal, serum sex hormone binding globulin and high-density lipoprotein concentrations are suppressed), the skin, and the ovary. Ovarian dysfunction results, in direct proportion to the intensity of compensatory hyperinsulinism.

A specific defect in transduction of the insulin signal has been described in women with polycystic ovary syndrome. In addition, as children enter puberty, insulin resistance develops in response to the increase of growth hormone secretion that underlies the acceleration in growth at this age. Obesity itself, present in some 40 per cent of women with polycystic ovary syndrome, worsens insulin resistance and so causes further deterioration of ovarian function. Should the patient come from a family with diabetes mellitus, there is the added risk of developing the insulin resistance of non-insulin-dependent diabetes mellitus.

Hypersecretion of insulin inhibits hepatic synthesis of sex hormone binding globulin which, particularly in obese patients, results in an apparent disparity between circulating testosterone concentrations and the degree of hirsutism. In these women the concentration of unbound testosterone, and by implication the rate of production of testosterone, is very high despite serum total testosterone concentrations which may be within the normal range. Hypersecretion of insulin also has non-reproductive adverse effects in patients with polycystic ovary syndrome. Thus an inverse relation of the cardioprotective high-density lipoprotein to cholesterol concentration and the fasting serum insulin concentration has been demonstrated, together with subnormal total high-density lipoprotein concentrations (Fig. 5). These data, together with reports of an increased incidence of coronary heart disease, hypertension, and diabetes in follow-up studies of patients with histologically verified polycystic ovaries, indicate

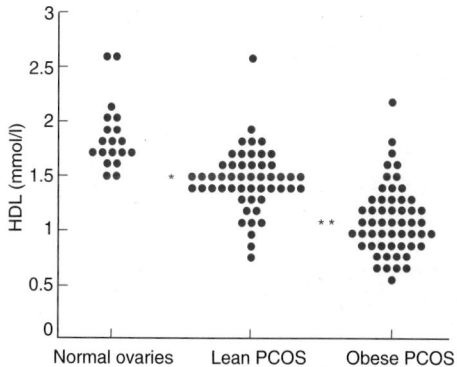

Fig. 5 Serum high-density lipoprotein concentrations in lean and obese women with polycystic ovary syndrome. Note that despite maintaining a normal body mass index, slim women with polycystic ovary syndrome have a statistically significant depression of their fasting high-density lipoprotein cholesterol concentration. The high-density lipoprotein falls even further in women with polycystic ovary syndrome who are obese.

the clinical importance of hypersecretion of insulin and its control in patients with polycystic ovary syndrome.

The familial nature of polycystic ovary syndrome has led to extensive investigation of its genetics. Thus far linkage with genes involved in the steroid biosynthetic pathway (*CYP11A*) and the control of insulin secretion have been identified and confirmed. *CYP11A* encodes the side chain cleavage enzyme which converts cholesterol to pregnenolone, a rate limiting step in steroid biosynthesis. Presumably a mutation causing upregulation of this enzyme could result in an increase in androgen secretion, a cardinal feature of the syndrome. The linkage described with the large class III alleles of the insulin gene variable number tandem repeats (*INS VNTR*) also occurs with type 2 diabetes mellitus. Class III *INS VNTR* promotes insulin secretion, perhaps resulting in insulin resistance as a secondary event. The effects of these and other candidate genes may be expressed in fetal development or through obesity in later life.

Other ovarian causes of hirsutism

Hyperthecosis

Characterized pathologically by the presence of islands of luteinized theca cells within the ovarian stroma at a distance from follicles, the clinical features include very marked hypersecretion of androgens and of insulin. The condition is probably most easily regarded as a severe form of the polycystic ovary syndrome.

Ovarian tumours

Androgen secreting tumours of the ovary are derived from sex cord or stromal cells and include Sertoli–Leydig cell tumours (arrhenoblastomas), hilar cell tumours, lipoid cell tumours, and adrenal rest tumours. Other non-hormone secreting tumours (Brenner, cystadenoma, and cystadenocarcinoma) have been reported to stimulate androgen secretion by the surrounding ovarian stroma. These conditions are all very rare causes of hirsutism.

Diagnosis of hyperandrogenism

Adrenal causes of hyperandrogenism are discussed in Section 12.7 but hypersecretion of androgens by polycystic ovaries is much more common. While an ovarian tumour is suggested by a short history of rapidly advancing hirsutism, amenorrhoea, and a serum testosterone concentration in the male range, such lesions are in fact rare. A serum testosterone exceeding 10 nmol/litre is more commonly associated with polycystic ovary syndrome and severe insulin resistance, as suggested clinically by the presence of acanthosis nigricans, than with the development of an ovarian tumour.

Pelvic ultrasound will detect polycystic ovaries or an ovarian tumour. The serum total testosterone concentration reflects in part the rate of production of testosterone and in part the serum concentration of sex hormone binding globulin; it should be interpreted in the light of the patient's body weight and a concentration within the normal range should not therefore be dismissed in women who are overweight. Serum luteinizing hormone concentrations are often raised but with a normal level of follicle-stimulating hormone. Serum prolactin concentrations are modestly elevated (up to 2500 mu/litre) in 15 per cent of patients with polycystic ovary syndrome. About half of these cases have a microadenoma detected by MRI scan.

A small number of patients with hirsutism have no diagnosable cause for their cutaneous virilism. Labelled 'idiopathic hirsutism', these patients may have enhanced sensitivity of androgen-dependent tissues, perhaps caused by increased dermal activity of the 5α reductase enzyme.

Management of hirsutism

Medication reduces the rate of hair growth but cosmetic treatment is required to remove existing unwanted hair. Hair can be camouflaged by bleaching and removed by plucking, waxing, electrolysis, or laser. The latter two methods offer the possibility of long-term hair removal. Laser treatment works by selective thermolysis and, with present equipment, is only suitable for removal of dark hair from a fair skin.

In the United Kingdom the preferred drug for treatment of hyperandrogenization is cyproterone acetate. This steroid is a peripheral antiandrogen, a progestogen, and a mild glucocorticoid. In combination with oestrogen, it suppresses secretion of gonadotrophin and so reduces the secretion of ovarian androgens. It is also contraceptive. Its glucocorticoid activity may reduce secretion of adrenal androgens. Finally, it blocks uptake of the dihydrotestosterone–protein complex by the DNA acceptor protein in the nucleus of androgen sensitive cells, so acting as a peripheral antiandrogen.

Treatment is administered cyclically, together with oestrogen, given most conveniently in the form of Dianette (Fig. 6). Seborrhoea and acne usually clear up in about 6 weeks but it takes 12 to 18 months to realize the maximum improvement of unwanted hair. Cosmetic treatment is continued while on the medication, the impact of therapy being indexed by a reduction in the number of treatments required.

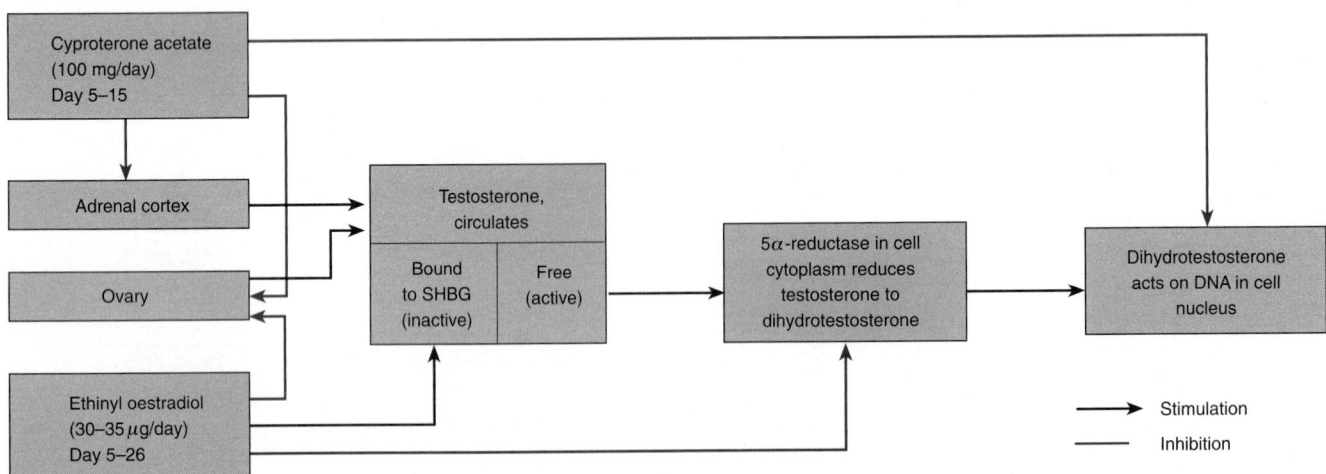

Fig. 6 The use of cyproterone acetate and ethinyloestradiol in the treatment of hirsutism. In the author's practice, ethinyloestradiol is usually replaced with Dianette®, a conveniently packaged formulation of ethinyloestradiol (35 µg) and cyproterone acetate (2 mg). (After *Medicine International* (1989))

Adverse reactions, contraindications, and surveillance are essentially those advised for treatment with the oral contraceptive pill. As symptoms remit, the dose of cyproterone acetate is reduced until the patient is taking the lowest dose compatible with symptomatic relief. Eventually treatment with Dianette alone is usually sufficient for maintenance. In patients not responding to this regimen, other antiandrogens, such as aldactone and flutamide, may be tried. Inhibition of the type II 5α reductase enzyme with finasteride has similar efficacy. Indeed the major difference between the available medications is in the pattern of adverse effects rather than in efficacy. Since these drugs are not contraceptive the patient must be warned of possible feminizing effects on a male fetus if they are taken inadvertently during pregnancy. They are therefore optimally prescribed with an oral contraceptive.

Infertility

Infertility can be defined as absence of conception after a year of unprotected intercourse, but it is most logically evaluated in relation to normal fertility. The maximum conception rate per ovulation is 25 to 30 per cent, so that the best cumulative conception rates are about 60 per cent after 6 months and 85 per cent after a year. Other than mechanical bars to conception (for example gynaecological problems such as occluded fallopian tubes) the important factors that reduce a woman's fertility are her age and any process that reduces the number of ovulations per unit time. The central strategy of medical management of female infertility is therefore the diagnosis and treatment of the causes of anovulation. An additional strategy is to ensure that ovulation, and thus conception, occurs in as favourable an environment as possible.

Ovulation is only proven by the occurrence of pregnancy, so indirect methods of detection are required. In practice, ovulation is usually inferred retrospectively by detection of a corpus luteum, indexed endocrinologically either by measurement of serum progesterone concentrations or indirectly by the effects of progesterone on basal body temperature or endometrial histology. Ovulation can be predicted ultrasonically by detecting the development of a preovulatory follicle of average diameter 20 to 22 mm, followed by its collapse and replacement by a solid structure, i.e. visualization of a corpus luteum. The preovulatory surge of luteinizing hormone can be detected by the patient herself using one of a number of commercially available immunological urine tests. These methods are used to determine whether anovulation can account for a couple's infertility and whether treatment has actually resulted in ovulation; prediction of ovulation is helpful for timing investigations and maximizing the chance of conception by ensuring intercourse around the time of ovulation.

Conception rates after the age of 35 are only half of those before the age of 25. Demographic changes in northern Europe (median maternal age at first birth in the United Kingdom is now 27 years) have resulted in a steady increase in the number of couples requesting consultations for infertility.

The causes of amenorrhoea are discussed above. All except primary ovarian failure are correctable (and that condition is treatable by oocyte donation) so the fertility prognosis for this group of patients is excellent. The commonest cause of oligomenorrhoea is polycystic ovary syndrome and while patients with this condition usually ovulate readily in response to treatment, in about 40 per cent hypersecretion of luteinizing hormone impairs fertility, despite the occurrence (spontaneously or as a result of treatment) of otherwise normal ovulation. The mechanism is uncertain but may involve an adverse effect of the high levels of luteinizing hormone on completion of the final stages of oocyte maturation.

Failure to ovulate despite (more or less) regular menstrual cycles is an unusual but recognized cause of infertility.

Infertility not explained by ovulatory failure is usually treated by *in vitro* fertilization and embryo transfer.

Table 5 Induction of ovulation

Hypothalamic level:
    Enchance secretion of GnRH
    Weight increase
    Suppression of hyperprolactinaemia—bromocriptine, pituitary surgery
    Anti-oestrogens—clomiphene citrate, tamoxifen
    Replace secretion of GnRH
    Pulsatile GnRH therapy
Pituitary level:
    Enhance secretion of gonadotrophins
    Pulsatile GnRH therapy
    Replace gonadotrophins*
    Human menopausal gonadotrophin: 75 IU of FSH and 75 IU of LH per ampoule
    Follitropin: 75 IU FSH, less than 0.4 IU LH per ampoule
    Human chorionic gonadotrophin: ampoule size varies

Abbreviations: FSH, follicle-stimulating hormone; GnRH, gonadotrophin releasing hormone; LH, luteinizing hormone.
* More purified urinary extracts and recombinant versions of FSH and LH are now available.

Induction of ovulation

Table 5 shows the agents commonly used and the endocrine level at which they exert their actions. Anti-oestrogens enhance hypothalamic secretion of gonadotrophin releasing hormone by competing with oestrogen receptors, thus simulating oestrogen deficiency. The drug is taken for 5 days and provokes gonadotrophin secretion and thence follicular development. The most commonly used preparation is clomiphene, which is a racemic mixture, one isomer having oestrogenic and the other anti-oestrogenic activity. Most slim patients with polycystic ovary syndrome ovulate in response to clomiphene. Obese patients, who are usually hyperinsulinaemic, can be treated with metformin, which in a dose of 500 mg three times per day will often result in ovulation or enhance the response to treatment with clomiphene.

In patients not responding to the above treatments, pituitary secretion of gonadotrophins can be enhanced by injection of gonadotrophin releasing hormone. It is administered in a pulsatile fashion, usually by the subcutaneous route, the injections being given at 90 min intervals by a portable miniaturized pump.

For patients with structural lesions of the pituitary, gonadotrophin secretion can be replaced by injections of gonadotrophins. The preferred preparations are those synthesized by recombinant technology. Follicular development is induced by the injection of follicle-stimulating hormone (together with luteinizing hormone in those patients with hypogonadotrophic hypogonadism); ovulation is triggered and the corpus luteum maintained by a single injection of human chorionic gonadotrophin which has luteinizing hormone-like bioactivity and a very long half-life.

The objective of treatment is unifollicular ovulation with full-term delivery of a single infant. The response is monitored by ultrasound assessment of the ovaries and uterus and by measurement of plasma oestradiol concentrations. Human chorionic gonadotrophin is administered according to strict criteria (not more than three follicles of diameter equal to or greater than 16 mm, or six follicles equal to or greater than 14 mm diameter).

Complications of ovulation induction include multiple births (the perinatal mortality of twins is three times that of singletons) and the ovarian hyperstimulation syndrome. The latter condition occurs almost entirely in women with polycystic ovary syndrome who have received high-dose and inadequately monitored gonadotrophin therapy. It results from massive follicular luteinization and so only occurs after ovulation has been triggered by human chorionic gonadotrophin or, very rarely, by a spontaneous surge of luteinizing hormone. Symptoms usually appear 5 to 10 days after administration of human chorionic gonadotrophin. In its mildest form it consists of ovarian enlargement and discomfort but in the more severe forms abdominal distension, nausea, vomiting, and diarrhoea develop. As a result of increased vascular permeability, protein-rich fluid accumulates in the peritoneal and sometimes the thoracic cavity; hypovolaemia develops, associated with haemoconcentration, decreased central venous pressure, low blood pressure, and tachycardia. The patient develops a tense ascites, respiration is embarrassed, and urine formation is suppressed. A hypercoagulable state may develop with the risk of cerebral and peripheral venous thrombosis and embolism.

In managing this syndrome, its self-limiting nature should be borne in mind. Treatment is designed first to maintain blood volume while correcting fluid and electrolyte balance, second to avoid thromboembolic phenomena (by full heparinization if severe hypercoagulability is detected), and third to relieve abdominal and pulmonary symptoms (by paracentesis under ultrasound control).

Further reading

Berchuk A, *et al.* (1996). Role of BRCA1 mutation screening in the management of familial ovarian cancer. *American Journal of Obstetrics and Gynecology* **175**, 738–46.

Dunaif A (1997). Insulin resistance and the polycystic ovary syndrome: mechanism and implications for pathogenesis. *Endocrine Reviews* **18**, 774–800.

Kalantaridou SN, Davis SR, Nelson LM (1998). Premature ovarian failure. *Endocrinology and Metabolism Clinics of North America* **27**, 989–1006.

Sourander L, *et al.* (1998). Cardiovascular and cancer morbidity and mortality and sudden cardiac death in postmenopausal women on oestrogen replacement therapy (ERT). *Lancet* **352**, 1965–9.

12.8.2 Disorders of male reproduction

F. C. W. Wu

Physiology of the hypothalamic–pituitary–testicular axis

The adult testis performs two functions—the production of androgens and spermatozoa (Fig. 1). These functions are dependent on trophic hormones from the hypothalamus and anterior pituitary which are responsive to the negative feedback action of testicular hormones, thus forming a closed-loop functional axis (Fig. 2).

Gonadotrophin releasing hormone (GnRH) is synthesized in neurosecretory neurones in the hypothalamus and then released episodically into the pituitary portal circulation at a frequency of 1 to 2 hourly. GnRH stimulates synthesis and secretion of both luteinizing hormone (LH) and follicle stimulating hormone (FSH) in the gonadotrophs of the anterior pituitary gland. Each episode of GnRH secretion elicits an immediate release of gonadotrophins into the systemic circulation. The pulsatile pattern of LH secretion is more clearly defined, with its rapid release and shorter circulating half-life than FSH (Fig. 2). This intermittent mode of GnRH stimulation avoids desensitization of the pituitary gonadotrophs by continuous GnRH exposure, and is therefore obligatory for maintaining normal gonadotrophin secretion. Pituitary FSH secretion can also be modulated by locally produced activin, a peptide hormone of the inhibin family which stimulates FSH.

LH stimulates biosynthesis of androgenic steroids by binding to specific surface membrane receptors on the Leydig cells. This activates the cyclic AMP/ protein kinase and the steroidogenic acute regulatory protein which mobilizes cholesterol substrate, transfers cholesterol from the outer to

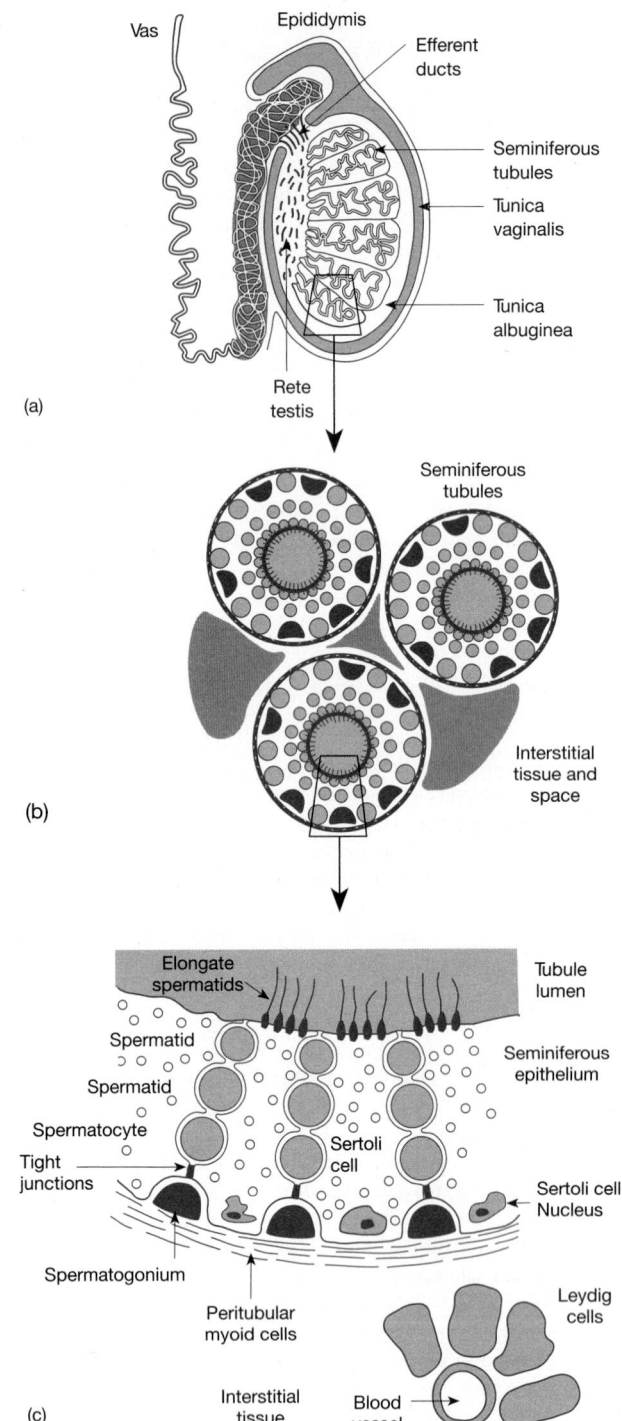

Fig. 1 (a) Human testis, epididymis, and vas deferens showing efferent ducts leading from the rete testis to the caput epididymis and the cauda epididymis continuing to become the vas deferens. (b) Cross-section through a seminiferous tubule showing central lumen, seminiferous epithelium, and interstitial space containing Leydig cells. (c) Anatomical relationships in the seminiferous epithelium between germ cells (spermatogonia, spermatocytes, and spermatids), Sertoli cells, peritubular myoid cells, and Leydig cells.

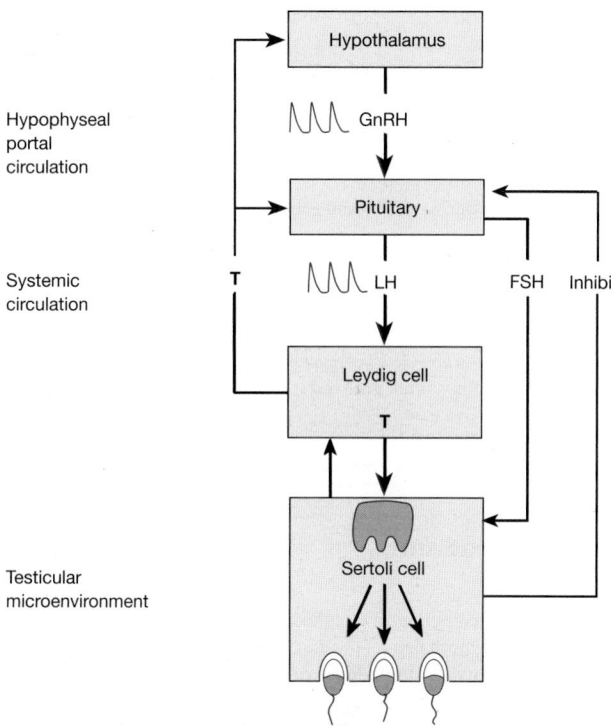

Fig. 2 Functional relationships in the hypothalamic–pituitary–testicular axis and testicular microenvironment. Gonadotrophin releasing hormone (GnRH) is secreted into the hypophysial circulation in an episodic manner which is reflected by an luteinizing hormone (LH) pulse in the systemic circulation. Open arrows represent positive stimulation and closed arrows negative feedback.

include pubertal growth spurt, skeletal maturation, fusion of epiphyses at the end of puberty, bone mass accrual and maintenance, some aspects of male-specific behaviour (in mouse models), fluid resorption from the testicular efferent ducts, and FSH feedback regulation. Much of the action of circulating testosterone is therefore regulated or refined locally at many different target tissues by 5α-reductase and aromatase expression. The relative contribution of circulating (endocrine action) compared with locally-produced (paracrine or intracrine action) hormones and the balance between androgen and oestrogen receptor activation are crucial to the physiological effects of androgens in man.

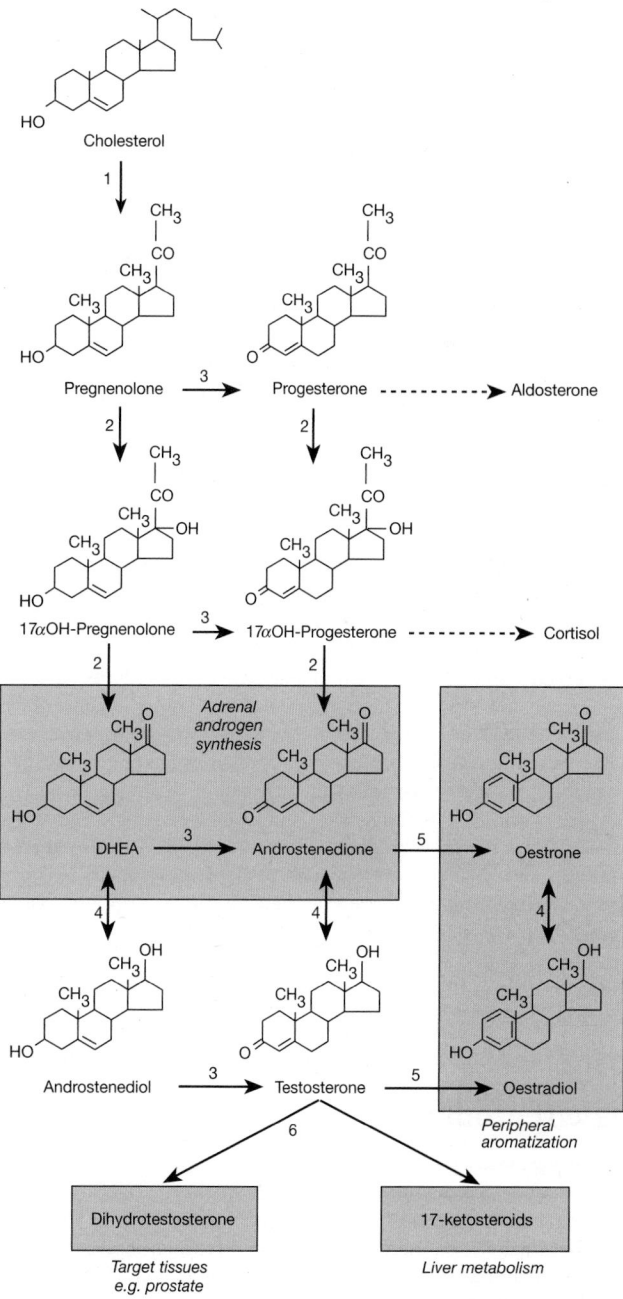

Fig. 3 Steroidogenic pathway from cholesterol to testosterone and further conversion of testosterone: (1) cholesterol side-chain cleavage; (2) 17α-hydroxylase/17,20-lyase; (3) 3β-hydroxysteroid dehydrogenase; (4) 17β-hydroxysteroid dehydrogenase; (5) aromatase; (6) 5α-reductase.

inner mitochondrial membrane where it is converted to pregnenolone by splitting the side-chain at position C21. Figure 3 shows the principal steps in the steroidogenic pathway in which the carbon skeleton of the parent compound, cholesterol, is progressively hydrolysed to form various androgenic steroids. Testosterone is the main end product of the biosynthetic pathway in adult Leydig cells. The daily testicular production rate of testosterone is between 3 and 10 mg. As the principal circulating androgen secreted by the adult testes, testosterone exerts the major negative feedback action on gonadotrophin secretion by restricting the frequency of GnRH release from the hypothalamus and by reducing the amplitude of LH response to GnRH. Androgens are essential for the differentiation, growth, and function of the male genital ducts (epididymis) and accessory glands (seminal vesicles and prostate), male secondary sexual characteristics, and sexual potency (Table 1). Testosterone circulates in plasma bound to sex hormone binding globulin (SHBG) and albumin. In man, 60 per cent of circulating testosterone is bound to SHBG, 38 per cent to albumin, and 2 per cent is free. Free and albumin-bound testosterone constitute the bioavailable fractions of circulating testosterone. Androgen action is mediated through specific binding to intranuclear androgen receptors which increase transcription of specific androgen-responsive genes in target cells. In target organs, such as the fetal external genitalia, prostate, and facial hair follicles, full activation requires the local metabolism of testosterone by the enzyme 5α-reductase to 5α-dihydrotestosterone, an androgen which is several-fold more potent than testosterone (Fig. 3).

Recently described males with mutant oestrogen receptor (oestrogen resistance) and *CYP19* gene encoding aromatase (oestrogen deficiency), and the corresponding gene-knockout mouse models, have revolutionized our understanding of the role of oestrogens in men. An increasing variety of androgen-dependent functions in males are now known to be mediated by the oestrogen receptors α and β via conversion of testosterone to oestradiol by the widely distributed P450 aromatase in target tissues. These

Table 1 Physiological action of androgens and clinical features of androgen deficiency

Physiological action	Onset before puberty	Onset after puberty
Increase bone mass and density	Osteoporosis	Osteoporosis, female fat distribution
Fusion of long bone epiphyses	Tall, eunuchoidal habitus	
Decrease subcutaneous/ visceral fat	Female fat distribution	Female fat distribution
Laryngeal enlargement	Unbroken, high-pitched voice	
Secondary sexual hair development	Lack of pubic, axillary, and facial hair, no temporal recession	Decrease facial and pubic hair, no temporal recession
Increase pilosebaceous activity	Lack of sebum, pale, smooth	Atrophy, fine wrinkles, pale
Stimulation of erythropoiesis	Moderate anaemia	Moderate anaemia
Increase muscle mass	Underdeveloped, poor physical stamina	Decrease strength and physical stamina
Penile growth	Infantile	
Prostate and seminal vesicle growth	Underdeveloped, no ejaculate	Atrophy, low volume or absence of ejaculate
Stimulation of spermatogenesis	Not initiated, very small testes	Regression, small testes
Stimulation of sexual interest	Not developed	Decrease
Stimulate erectile function	Low/ absent spontaneous erection	Decrease erection
Effects on mood and behaviour	Placid	Low moods, unassertive, tiredness

The endocrine (androgen synthesis) and gametogenic (spermatogenesis) functions of the testis are closely interlinked. Although testosterone is important as the principal circulating androgen, its local (paracrine) action within the testis is crucial, together with FSH, for the initiation and maintenance of normal spermatogenesis and hence fertility (Figs 1 and 2). Since germ cells do not possess receptors for FSH or testosterone, these hormone signals are transduced through the Sertoli and peritubular cells. Sertoli cells create an insular microenvironment in the seminiferous tubules by providing the physical framework and elaborating an ever-changing chemical myriad of growth factors and cytokines for the developing germ cells enmeshed in their cytoplasm (Fig. 1). Sertoli cells also secrete inhibin B, a glycoprotein hormone, which inhibits FSH secretion by the pituitary (Fig. 2).

Spermatogenesis is a complex, repetitive series of cytodifferentiation processes in the seminiferous epithelium whereby cohorts of undifferentiated diploid germ cells (spermatogonia) proliferate and transform into greatly expanded populations of haploid spermatozoa (Fig. 1). The human testes produce around 200 million spermatozoa per day. Mitotic divisions of spermatogonial stem cells form subpopulations of spermatogonia which, at regular intervals of 16 days, differentiate into primary preleptotene spermatocytes to initiate meiosis. Meiotic reduction divisions of spermatocytes generate round spermatids which then transform (spermiogenesis) into compact, virtually cytoplasm-free, elongated spermatids. Condensed nuclear DNA forms the sperm head with an overlying Golgi-derived acrosome cap and a tail (containing nine pairs of microtubules arranged around a central pair) capable of propelling, flagellar movements. Mature spermatozoa are released from Sertoli cell cytoplasm into the tubular lumen some 74 days after their initial development from spermatogonia. The control systems regulating germ cell divisions and development remain poorly understood.

Male reproductive disorders

Male hypogonadism is a descriptive term for the clinical complex associated with androgen deficiency due to the failure of Leydig cell function. Concomitant impairment of spermatogenesis is likely since the seminiferous tubules will also be androgen deficient or directly involved by the same pathological process. However, infertility is usually an isolated abnormality of spermatogenesis where patients seldom show any clinical evidence of androgen deficiency. In the last 10 years, an increasing number of specific genetic defects have been identified, by genomic DNA mapping, to be associated with abnormal gonadal function and development. This has greatly improved our understanding of the pathogenesis of these conditions.

Male hypogonadism
Aetiology

A large number of pathological conditions can lead to destruction or malfunction of the hypothalamic–pituitary–testicular axis (Table 2). It is important to identify the underlying cause of hypogonadism and distinguish between pituitary-hypothalamic (secondary or hypogonadotrophic hypogonadism) and testicular (primary or hypergonadotrophic hypogonadism) disorders. The causal lesion may require specific treatment e.g. pituitary tumour, haemochromatosis. Hypogonadotrophic conditions are amenable to treatment aimed at inducing or restoring spermatogenesis while primary testicular failure, which is usually irreversible, is not.

Diagnosis
General clinical features of hypogonadism

The age of onset of androgen deficiency critically influences the manifestation of hypogonadism (Table 1). Prepubertal onset of testosterone deficiency gives rise to sexual infantilism and patients will present with delayed puberty. Eunuchoidal body proportions (arm span greater than height and heel–pubis exceeding crown–pubis lengths by at least 5 cm; Fig. 2) develop due to the continued growth of long bones (growth hormone-mediated) allowed by the delayed closure of their epiphyses and lack of the testosterone/oestradiol-induced spinal growth in late puberty.

Postpubertal onset of testosterone deficiency leads to regression of spermatogenesis, diminished sex drive and erection, loss of ejaculation, muscle atrophy, poor stamina, and decreased secondary sexual hair and shaving frequency. However, no change is observed in body and penile proportions or voice (Table 1). Symptoms and signs of hypogonadism usually develop and progress insidiously. It is therefore common for patients to present only after many years following the onset of hypogonadism. Furthermore, young patients who has never been adequately androgenized may not be aware, or even deny, that secondary sexual function is subnormal. In contrast, after surgical or traumatic/inflammatory castration, adults may experience hot flushes from acute withdrawal of androgens. Fetal onset of defective androgen action due to androgen receptor abnormalities or steroidogenic enzyme deficiency cause failure of masculinization of the genitalia resulting in intersexual states (Table 2).

Clinical findings associated with hypogonadism

Hypothalamic–pituitary tumours are suggested by headache, impairment of visual acuity or visual field loss, polyuria and polydipsia, or evidence of pituitary hormone excess such as Cushing's disease, acromegaly, and hyperprolactinaemia. Hyperprolactinaemia causes loss of sex drive even in the presence of normal testosterone. Primary testicular failure is suggested by a history of orchitis, testicular trauma, surgery, torsion, irradiation, or chemotherapy. An increasing number of chronic systemic diseases (Table 2) are associated compromised hypothalamic–pituitary–testicular function. With improved survival resulting from specific treatment, the role of gonadal dysfunction in the quality of life of these patients is increasingly important.

Table 2 Classification and aetiologies of male reproductive disorders

Condition	Cause/ pathogenesis	Hypogonadism	Infertility
Hypothalamic/pituitary			
Isolated GnRH deficiency	Congenital GnRH deficiency	+	+
Kallmann's syndrome	Xp22.3 *KAL-1* gene mutation, Congenital GnRH deficiency	+	+
GnRH insensitivity	4q13.1 GnRH receptor gene mutation	+	+
Fertile eunuch (Pasqualini syndrome)	Partial GnRH deficiency, low LH		
Hypogonadotrophic hypogonadism/ adrenal hypoplasia	Xp21.2–3 DAX1 gene mutation	+	+
Constitutional delayed puberty	Functional GnRH deficiency—self limiting	+	+
Male anorexia nervosa	Weight-related, reversible, functional GnRH deficiency	+	+
Hyperprolactinaemia	Pituitary adenoma, drug-induced (see below)	+	+
Congenital hypopituitarism	*PROP1* gene mutation, hypogonadotrophic, GH, prolactin, TSH, ACTH combined deficiency	+	+
Acquired hypopituitarism	Pituitary adenoma, craniopharygioma, haemochromatosis, irradiation, transfusion siderosis, sarcoidosis, tuberculosis, histiocytosis X	+	+
Biologically inactive LH	LHβ gene mutation	+	+
Isolated FSH deficiency	FSHβ gene mutation	?	+
Testicular			
Klinefelter's syndrome	47XXY, 48XXXY, 47XXY/46XY, mosaic, etc.	+	+
46 XX male	Translocation of SRY to X chromosome	+	+
Sex chromosome or autosome abnormalities	Translocation, deletion	+	–
Mixed gonadal dysgenesis	XY/XO mosaic, true hermaphroditism	+	+
Testicular agenesis (congenital anorchia)	Absence of testicular tissues postnatally	+	+
Testicular torsion	Destruction of testicular tissue	+	+
Surgical orchidectomy	Destruction of testicular tissue	+	+
Testicular trauma	Destruction of testicular tissue	+	+
Testicular tumour	Destruction of testicular tissue	+	+
Orchitis	Destruction of testicular tissue	+	+
Sickle cell disease	Microinfarcts in testis from vascular occlusion	+	+
Noonan–Leopard syndrome	12q22 gene defect in autosomal dominant form, cryptorchidism, Turner's stigmata, e.g. short stature, webbed neck, pectus excavatum, hypertelorism, ptosis, right-sided congenital heart disease	+	+
Persistent mullerian duct syndrome	AMH gene or AMH type II receptor gene mutation, fallopian tubes and uterus present with cryptorchidism	±	+
Congenital steroidogenic enzyme deficiencies	10q24.3CYP17 17,20-desmolase;	+	+
	9q22 HSD17b3 17-OH-steroid dehydrogenase gene mutation	+	+
LH insensitivity	LH receptor gene mutation, pseudohermaphroditism	+	+
Idiopathic infertility	Defective spermatogenesis of uncertain aetiology	–	+
Varicocele	Reflux in spermatic vein	–	+
Microdeletions Yq chromosome	Deletion of azoospermic factor (AZFs)	–	+
Cryptorchidism	Congenital deficiency of testosterone or AMH action, dysgenetic gonads	±	+
Immotile cilia syndrome	Absent dynein arms of sperm tail microtubules	–	+
Globozoospermia	Absence of acrosome cap on sperm head	–	+
FSH insensitivity	2p21 FSH receptor gene mutation	?	+
Post-testicular			
Immunological infertility	Sperm antibodies	–	+
Immotile cilia (Kartargener's syndrome)	Dynein arms absent in sperm tail	–	+
Young's syndrome	Mercury poisoning ?	–	+
Congenital bilateral absence of vas deferens	*CFTR* gene mutation and intronic variant	–	+
Genital tract obstruction	Postinfection, postvasectomy, herniorrhaphy	–	+
Accessory gland/ prostate infection	Bacterial, chlamydia, abnormal seminal fluid	–	+
Retrograde ejaculation	Autonomic neuropathy, postprostatectomy	–	+
Coital insufficiency	Defective vaginal insemination	–	+

Table 2 Continued

Condition	Cause/ pathogenesis	Hypogonadism	Infertility
Target tissues			
Androgen insensitivity syndromes	Xq11–12 androgen receptor gene mutation	+	+
Androgen receptor defects	Xq11–12 androgen receptor gene CAG repeats expansion		
5α-reductase deficiency	2p23 5α-reductase2 gene mutation	+	+
Oestrogen insensitivity	ERα gene mutation	–	?
Aromatase deficiency	CYP19 gene mutation	–	?
Systemic diseases			
Acute critical illnesses	Cytokine or cortisol-induced multilevel dysfunction in HPT axis	+	–
Chronic debilitating illnesses including cardiac failure, neoplasia, uncontrolled diabetes	Cytokine or caloric deprivation-induced multilevel dysfunction in HPT axis	+	+
Liver cirrhosis	Primary testicular failure followed by gonadotrophin deficiency	+	+
Chronic renal failure	Hypogonadotrophic	+	+
Thyrotoxicosis	Increase SHBG, gonadotrophins and oestradiol	+	+
Cushing's syndrome	Multilevel dysfunction in HPT axis	+	+
Haemochromatosis	Hypogonadotrophic	+	+
HIV infection	Hypogonadotrophic	+	+
Morbid obesity	Hypogonadotrophic, low SHBG, total, and free testosterone	+	+
Obstructive sleep apnoea	Hypogonadotrophic	+	+
Rheumatoid arthritis	Suppression of testosterone during flare-up	+	?
Acute febrile illness	Temporary suppression of spermatogenesis	–	+
Cystic fibrosis	CFTR gene mutation	–	+
Untreated congenital adrenal hyperplasia	Suppression of gonadotrophins	–	+
Neurological diseases			
Dystrophia myotonica	Myotonin protein kinase (MT-PK) gene CTG repeats expansion	+	+
Prader–Willi syndrome (hypothalamic)	Deletion/ mutation of imprinting centre in paternal 15q11–13, hypogonadotrophic, mental retardation, hypotonia, hyperphagia, obesity, short stature	+	+
Laurence–Moon syndrome	Hypogonadotrophic, retinitis pigmentosa, mental retardation, obesity, paraplegia	+	+
Bardet–Biedl syndrome	Defects in BBS loci 16q21, 15q22.3, or 3p12, hypogonadotrophic, retinitis pigmentosa, mental retardation, obesity, polydactyly	+	+
Familial cerebellar degeneration (Friedrich's)	9p frataxin gene GAA repeats expansion, hypogonadotrophic, progressive ataxia	+	+
Kennedy's syndrome	Xq11–12 androgen receptor gene CAG repeats expansion, late onset androgen resistance, progressive spinobulbar muscle atrophy	+	+
Temporal lobe epilepsy	Unknown	+	–
Spinal cord injury	Abnormal thermoregulation or neuroregulation of testis	–	+
Fragile X syndrome	FMR1 gene CCG repeats expansion—mental retardation, macro-orchidism	–	–
Drugs/ chemical or physical agents			
Digitalis, spironolactone, cyproterone acetate flutamide, bicalutamide, cimetidine	Antiandrogenic	+	+
Corticosteroids	Multilevel dysfunction in HPT axis	+	+
Ketoconazole, aminoglutethimide	Inhibits steroidogenesis	+	+
Antipsychotics, sedatives	Hyperprolactinaemia, gonadotrophin suppression	+	+
Anticonvulsants	Increase SHBG and decrease free testosterone	+	+
Ethanol	Direct suppression of testicular functions, hepatotoxic	+	+
Opiate, cocaine, cannabis abuse	Suppression of gonadotrophins	+	+
Cytotoxic chemotherapy	Agent-specific, dose-related germ cell loss	–	+
Ionising irradiation	Dose-dependent loss of spermatogonia, spermatocytes	–	+
Sulfasalazine	Abnormal sperm morphology and motility	–	+
Nitrofuratoin	Direct suppression of spermatogenesis	–	+
Anabolic steroids, oestrogens, progestins	Gonadotrophin suppression or antiandrogenic	(+)	+
Lead, mercury, cadmium	Implicated adverse effects on spermatogenesis		+
Pesticides, fungicides, amoebicides	Direct toxic action on spermatogonia	–	+

HPT = hypothalamic–pituitary–testicular; FSH = follicle stimulating hormone; TSH = thyroid-stimulating hormone; ACTH = adenocorticotrophic hormone; SHBG = sex hormone binding globulin; AMH= antimullerian hormone.

The use of recreational drugs and medications which interfere with pituitary–testicular function or androgen action should be sought (Table 2). Evidence of alcohol abuse should be noted. Ethanol causes a lowering of plasma testosterone through a direct toxic effect on Leydig cell steroidogenesis. Testicular atrophy and gynaecomastia, found in 50 per cent of men with hepatic cirrhosis, are due to altered androgen steroid metabolism, increased sex-hormone-binding globulin, and increased oestrogen production. These changes are usually irreversible.

Neurological diseases can be associated with hypogonadism. Postpubertal atrophy of the seminiferous tubules occurs in 80 per cent of patients with dystrophia myotonica, an autosomal dominant disorder characterized by myotonia, distal muscle atrophy, lens opacities, and premature frontal balding. Variable degrees of androgen deficiency also exist. Hypogonadotrophic hypogonadism is associated with familial cerebellar ataxia, Laurence–Moon, Bardet–Biedl, and Prader–Willi syndromes. Defective spermatogenesis is common in paraplegia or quadraplegia following spinal injury because of the inability to maintain a low scrotal temperature.

Specific condition

Klinefelter's syndrome is the commonest cause of male hypogonadism with an incidence of 2 per 1000 live births. It is a developmental disorder of the testis resulting from the presence of an extra X chromosome derived from the non-disjunction of parental (maternal origin in two-thirds of cases) germ cells during meiosis. The most common karyotype is 47 XXY (80–90 per cent) but rarer variants include 46 XY/47 XXY mosaic, multiple X + Y, and the so-called XX male syndrome. Accelerated atrophy of germ cells before puberty and hyalinization of the seminiferous tubules gives rise to sterility and small, firm testes. Leydig cells appear relatively hyperplastic but cell mass is in fact normal. The degree of Leydig cell steroidogenic defect (mechanism of which remains uncertain) is very variable ranging from the virilized, adult male presenting with infertility (see below) to the eunuchoidal youth who fails to complete sexual maturation. In midadulthood, 80 per cent of patients have reduced testosterone with elevated LH, FSH, and oestradiol. Other features include gynaecomastia, reduced body hair, long legs, tall stature, learning (verbal and cognitive) difficulties, poor school performance, behavioural disturbances, and autoimmune endocrinopathies including diabetes mellitus. There is also an increased incidence of osteopenia, breast tumour, testicular and extratesticular (especially mediastinal and retroperitoneal) germ cell tumours, varicose veins, and leg ulcers. Mental retardation is associated with higher order X chromosome polysomy.

Kallmann's syndrome, with an incidence of 1 in 7500 males, is a sporadic or familial (X-linked or autosomal) form of congenital hypogonadotrophic hypogonadism associated with a number of somatic congenital abnormalities including anosmia or hyposmia (defective smell sense), red–green colour blindness, synkinesis, nerve deafness, cleft-lip or palate, and renal malformations. The X-linked variety is caused by deletion or mutation in the KAL-1 gene in Xp22.3 encoding an cell adhesion protein. Faulty embryonic migration of GnRH-secreting neurones from their site of origin in the nose to the hypothalamus prevents normal axonal secretion into the pituitary portal circulation in the median eminence. GnRH is thus unable to target the gonadotrophs in the anterior pituitary. The same migratory defect affects the olfactory neurones in the nose, resulting in aplasia of the olfactory bulb and anosmia.

Total and free testosterone declines gradually but variably with age in men from the age of 40 years onwards. This is amplified by the age-related increase in SHBG and exacerbated by concomitant non-gonadal diseases and medications. In some elderly men, testosterone may fall below the young adult physiological range. Differentiation of non-specific symptoms of ageing, such as frailty, decreased muscle strength, lack of stamina, and decline in libido, from those of mild hypogonadism is difficult. Whether these functional changes, normally accepted as part of healthy ageing, are causally related to alterations in circulating testosterone is unclear. The existence and prevalence of a male climacteric remains controversial.

Investigation

Confirmation of hypogonadism

The clinical suspicion or diagnosis of hypogonadism must be confirmed by demonstration of low circulating testosterone before replacement therapy is commenced. Samples obtained between 8 and 9 a.m. avoid the physiological, diurnal trough levels of testosterone later in the day. In the presence of background changes in SHBG, such as in ageing, obesity, anticonvulsant medications, diabetes, thyrotoxicosis, and liver disease, free testosterone can be calculated from the total testosterone and SHBG concentrations. Free testosterone assays are technically demanding and result obtained by commercial kits can be misleading.

Assessment of the hypothalamic–pituitary–testicular axis and target tissue resistance

Measurement of LH, FSH, and prolactin is required to differentiate between primary and secondary hypogonadism. The physiological basis for differentiating between hypogonadotrophic and hypergonadotrophic hypogonadism is illustrated in Fig. 1. Pathologies in the hypothalamus and pituitary will give rise to low or low–normal gonadotrophins and low testosterone, that is a state of hypogonadotrophic hypogonadism or secondary testicular failure where the potential for stimulating testicular function by exogenous gonadotrophin or GnRH replacement is maintained. Conditions affecting the testes will interrupt normal testicular negative feedback. This results in elevated gonadotrophin levels with low testosterone, characteristic of hypergonadotrophic hypogonadism or primary testicular failure. Failure of spermatogenesis with reduced testicular size is commonly associated with a rise in FSH alone. The value of circulating inhibin B and mullerian inhibiting hormone for diagnostic purposes is currently being assessed. Patients with androgen insensitivity syndromes have elevated testosterone with high LH but normal to low FSH. Increased LH or FSH is associated with the very rare LH and FSH resistance syndromes.

Human chorionic gonadotrophin (hCG) stimulates Leydig cell steroidogenesis and plasma testosterone increases over 4 to 7 days. It is useful for detecting the presence of functional testicular tissue in patients with impalpable testes, assessing functional reserve of the testes prior to treatment with exogenous gonadotrophin or GnRH, and in differentiating hypergonadotrophic hypogonadism from rare cases who produce immunologically detectable, but biologically inactive, LH in excess.

Stimulation tests of gonadotrophin secretory reserve using clomiphene and GnRH seldom give additional information and has become largely obsolete, especially with the improved sensitivity and range of modern gonadotrophin immunoassays.

Assessment of the pituitary

Patients with hypogonadotrophic hypogonadism without the stigmata of Kallmann's syndrome should undergo full pituitary functional and anatomical assessment to exclude an underlying pituitary tumour. They require pharmacological tests of growth hormone and ACTH reserve, thyroid function tests, visual field charting, and MR or CT scanning of the pituitary and hypothalamus.

Other investigations

Suspected Klinefelter's syndrome should be confirmed by chromosome karyotyping on peripheral blood lymphocytes. Ultrasound and MR scan are useful in locating ectopic or intra-abdominal testes. DNA analysis can help confirm the diagnosis of androgen resistance syndromes and an increasing number of rare causes of hypogonadism (Table 2) such as haemochromatosis.

Treatment objectives

Treatment objectives are to:

(1) relieve the symptoms of androgen deficiency;

(2) prevent the long-term consequences of androgen deficiency such as osteopenia;

(3) reproduce physiological, circulating, and tissue levels of plasma testosterone, dihydrotestoerone, and oestradiol;

(4) induce fertility, if required, in hypogonadotrophic patients;

(5) treat any specific underlying diseases.

The mainstay of treatment of the hypogonadal male is androgen replacement. Although hypogonadotrophic patients have the potential for fertility, gonadotrophin and pulsatile GnRH therapy should only be employed when there is a requirement for fertility because of the expense and complexity of these regimens. Previous testosterone treatment does not jeopardize subsequent response to gonadotrophin so that younger hypogonadotrophic subjects should be treated by testosterone in the same manner as hypergonadotrophic patients to initiate and maintain virilization and sexual function.

Androgen replacement

The circulating half-life of free testosterone is short (10 min) due to rapid degradation by the liver. To achieve sustained physiological circulating concentrations, testosterone has to be administered in a modified form or by a parenteral route so that its rate of metabolism or absorption is retarded.

Injectable testosterone esters are the commonest first-line androgen preparations. A mixture of four different testosterone esters (propionate, phenylpropionate, isocaproate, and decanoate) (Sustanon, Organon, Oss, the Netherlands), 250 mg 2 to 3-weekly, and testosterone enanthate (Primoteston depot, Schering, Berlin, Germany), 200 mg 2-weekly, are the most popular. Whilst undoubtedly effective, these preparations inevitably give rise to high supraphysiological peak testosterone levels within the first week which then fall sharply to lower limits of normal before the next dose. Some patients are disturbed by fluctuations in libido, mood, and stamina associated with the repeated rise and fall of testosterone levels as well as the painful, deep, intramuscular injections.

Crystalline testosterone compressed into cylindrical pellets, surgically implanted subcutaneously under local anaesthesia, provide a depot source of testosterone for several months. Peak testosterone levels are achieved after 2 to 4 weeks, followed by a gradual decline over subsequent months. A total dose of 800 mg (4 × 200 mg implants) can maintain physiological concentrations of testosterone over 6 months, which some patients find more convenient than more frequent injections. The implantation procedure can be complicated, though rarely, by haemorrhage and infection. Even in experienced hands, 10 per cent of implanted pellets are extruded. Implants should only be used as maintenance therapy for patients who have already shown satisfactory tolerance to androgen effects of shorter-acting preparations.

Testosterone undecanoate is administered orally and absorbed from the gut through intestinal lymphatics. Low bioavailability (<0.5 per cent), variable absorption, multiple daily dosing, and higher costs has restricted the use of testosterone undecanoate despite the obvious appeal of oral administration. To maintain testosterone consistently within the physiological range, two to three times daily administration of 80 mg (2 × 40 mg capsules) of testosterone undecanoate is required. Intestinal 5α-reductase action gives rise to a disproportionate and unphysiological increase in dihydrotestosterone relative to testosterone. Oral testosterone undecanoate is useful in the induction of puberty in adolescents where lower doses are preferable, and as second line treatment in adults who are intolerant of injections or implants.

17α-alkylated androgens are relatively weak androgens but some may have more potent anabolic effects. 17α-alkylated compounds cause cholestatic jaundice in a reversible and dose-related manner while long-term treatment is associated with peliosis hepatis (haemorrhagic cysts in the liver) and liver tumours. Consequently, 17α-methyl testosterone, oxymetholone, and fluoxymesterone have now been withdrawn from the market in many countries. As a group, 17α-alkylated androgens are not recommended for clinical use but they are the most commonly abused anabolic steroids. Mesterolone, which is not hepatotoxic, is a weak androgen with low clinical efficacy but remains commercially available.

Transdermal testosterone preparations offer the advantages of stable physiological levels of testosterone without peaks and troughs, painless self-administration, minimal risk of overdosing and low potential for abuse. A 60 cm² translucent membrane (Testoderm™, ALZA, Palo Alto, United States) applied to the scrotum delivers testosterone at a rate of 4 or 6 mg per day. Daily renewal of Testoderm™ in the morning maintains plasma testosterone within the adult physiological range with a normal diurnal profile. 5α-Dihydrotestosterone levels are elevated because of abundant 5α-reductase activity in genital skin. This does not seem to have any adverse consequences even after several years of treatment. Local skin irritation is negligible. A non-scrotal transdermal system (Androderm™ or Andropatch™ SmithKline Beecham, Welwyn Garden City, United Kingdom) delivers testosterone at 2.5 mg (6.5 cm diameter) or 5 mg (13 cm diameter) daily. At a dose of 5 mg daily applied at bedtime, plasma testosterone, dihydrotestosterone, and oestradiol are maintained within the physiological range throughout 24 h with a small diurnal variation. While clinical efficacy is satisfactory, the major drawback of Andropatch™ is skin reaction at the application sites, which occurs in 60 to 70 per cent of cases. A new, non-scrotal testosterone (Testoderm TTS™, ALZA, Palo Alto, United States) has recently become available and is said to have a lower incidence of skin irritation.

Many novel androgen preparations are currently under clinical investigation or being developed. Most promising are testosterone gel, cyclodextrins, buccal preparations, and esters with long half-lives (testosterone undecanoate or decanoate in castor oil for intramuscular injection 2 to 3-monthly) and selective androgen receptor modulators such as 7α-methy-19-nortestosterone (MENT).

The choice of preparations depends on age of the patient, the patient's own preference, facilities for injections, and available experience for surgical implants. Many boys with constitutional delayed puberty will spontaneously enter or progress in puberty after short courses of testosterone, for example intramuscular testosterone enanthate 50 mg monthly or oral testosterone undecanoate 40 mg daily for 3 to 6 months. The low doses of testosterone will stimulate linear growth and promote virilization without premature epiphyseal fusion. In patients with no evidence of spontaneous progression, gradually increasing doses of testosterone over 3 to 4 years will ensure full virilization except for testicular growth. They can be maintained on adult replacement doses subsequently if hypogoandotrophic hypogonadism appears to be permanent. Testosterone treatment can be safely started after the age of 14. Indeed, delayed treatment can be associated with permanently impaired peak bone mass.

The invasive nature of the implantation procedure and the long duration of action make them less than ideal for the induction of puberty in adolescents and the initiation of treatment in androgen-naive young adults where a more gradual and flexible increase in dose is desirable. For these reasons, testosterone implant is usually reserved for maintenance treatment in young adults, replacement having been initiated with intramuscular or oral preparations. Almost all adult patients respond well to testosterone enanthate 200 mg 2-weekly, 300 mg 3-weekly or Sustanon 250 mg 2 to 3-weekly. In the absence of a satisfactory biological marker for androgen action, monitoring of treatment is best gauged by clinical response and documenting plasma testosterone within the low–normal range immediately before the next dose so that appropriate adjustments of dosing intervals can be made.

Hypogonadal patients over the age of 50 starting testosterone for the first time should be checked for pre-existing, occult prostatic cancer with digital rectal examination and prostate-specific antigen (PSA) measurement. These should also be repeated in the first 3 to 6 months after initiating treatment to ensure that there is no deterioration. Subsequent monitoring for prostatic disease should not differ from eugonadal men of comparable age since there is no increased relative risk in hypogonadal patients on long-term testosterone replacement.

Testosterone replacement therapy is safe and side-effects are rare. They may include acne, transient priapism, gynaecomastia, fluid retention, increase in haematocrit, obstructive sleep apnoea, and exacerbation of pre-existing behavioural disturbances. Testosterone is contraindicated in patients with known prostatic cancer and breast cancer. In older patients with benign prostatic hyperplasia, sleep apnoea, polycythaemia, dyslipidaemia, cardiac failure, liver disease, and renal failure, a cautious approach with reduced doses of testosterone, careful dose titration, and close supervision or specific management of the coexisting problems usually allow patients to benefit from androgen replacement.

Infertility

Infertility is defined as the inability of a couple to initiate a pregnancy after 12 months of unprotected intercourse. Some 8 to 15 per cent of married couples experience involuntary infertility. Of these, male factors alone are estimated to be responsible in 30 per cent and contributory in a further 20 per cent of subfertile couples. Thus, male infertility may affect 5 per cent of men of reproductive age. A secular trend of declining semen quality (sperm density) in men over the last 50 years has been reported in some but not other regions of Europe. This, together with a concurrent increase in incidence of testicular cancer, hypospadias, and cryptorchidism, has raised the question of possible environmental endocrine disruptors with oestrogenic or antiandrogenic actions influencing prenatal or neonatal testicular and genital tract development. The concern prompted the recent development of sensitive techniques for monitoring potential deleterious reproductive effects of environmental chemicals. However, there is currently no evidence that the incidence of male infertility is increasing.

Aetiologies

Male infertility, comprising a heterogeneous group of disorders (Table 2), represents the male partner's contribution to a couple's failure to conceive. This implied failure to fertilize normal ova is usually associated with defective spermatogenesis giving rise to absent (azoospermia) or low sperm output (oligozoospermia: <20 million/ml) and/or abnormal spermiogenesis giving rise to spermatozoa with poor motility (asthenozoospermia:<50 per cent of spermatozoa showing progressive motility) and abnormal morphology (teratozoospermia: <15 per cent normal forms). The pathogenic basis of defective spermaotgenesis or spermiogenesis remains poorly understood. Testicular histology may show quantitative reduction in all germ cell types (hypospermatogenesis), Sertoli cells only, or maturation arrest at the primary spermatocyte (premeiotic) or spermatid (postmeiotic) stage.

Idiopathic azoospermia/ oligozoospermia

By far the commonest form of male infertility (60 per cent) is idiopathic azoo/oligozoospermia, usually associated with asthenozooopermia and teratozoospermia. This probably represents the end result of a multitude of ill-defined pathologies which disrupt normal seminiferous tubular functions. However, recent molecular analyses have revealed that a substantial proportion of these cases hitherto classified as idiopathic have discrete gene defects associated with impaired spermatogenesis (see below).

Asthenozoospermia

Reduced velocity or vigour of sperm motility may be due to metabolic/functional defects or ultrastructural malformations in the axonemal complex of the sperm tail usually associated with oligozoospermia or a high percentage of dead and abnormally-shaped sperm. The latter finding may indicate a recently-recognized condition, epididymal necro/asthenozoospermia. Testicular spermatozoa are normal, the defects occurring during epididymal transit. Rarely, complete asthenozoospermia (with normal sperm density) may result from absence of dynein arms (sites of Na/K ATPase activity) linking individual microtubules. This is associated with similar defects in respiratory cilia and a history of chronic respiratory infection, bronchiectasis, and sinusitis (immotile cilia syndrome). In addition, some of these patients have situs inversus (Kartagener's syndrome). Absence of the central pair of microtubules in the sperm tail is an even rarer cause of complete asthenozoospermia—the 9+0 syndrome.

Teratozoospermia

An extreme example of abnormal sperm morphology is the failure of acrosome cap development in the sperm head leading to formation of round-headed spermatozoa (globozoospermia) which are unable to bind to the zona pellucida of ova, a prerequisite for fertilization.

Chromosome disorders

Chromosome abnormalities identified by cytogenetic studies of blood lymphocyte are found in 15 per cent of azoospermic patients; 90 per cent of these have Klinefelter's syndrome. Other chromosomal abnormalities encountered include reciprocal X or Y autosomal translocations, XYY and XX males, reciprocal and robertsonian autosomal translocations, supernumerary autosomes, and inversion of autosomes.

Klinefelter's (47XXY) patients are azoospermic. Spontaneous pregnancies have been reported in Klinefelter's patients with 46XY/47XXY mosaicim. The mechanism by which an extra X chromosome gives rise to spermatogenic failure is not known. Inactivation of the X chromosome in primary spermatocytes is necessary for spermatogenesis to proceed normally through meiosis. Hyalinized seminiferous tubules devoid of germ cells are pervasive in the atrophic testes. Occasionally, isolated foci of tubules with preserved spermatogenesis can be identified in testicular biopsy of 47 XXY patients.

Y chromosome microdeletions

A major breakthrough in the understanding of the molecular genetics of male infertility is the recent characterization of three non-overlapping regions (designated azoospermic factors AZFa, ASFb, and AZFc) on the long arm of the Y chromosomes (Yq11) which contain multiple genes involved in spermatogenesis. Microdeletions in these AZF loci, identifiable only by PCR amplification of DNA but not routine karyotyping, have been found in 3 to 37.5 per cent of patients previously considered to have idiopathic azoospermia and severe oligozoospermia but not in fertile control populations. Larger deletions (involving more than one AZF locus) are associated with more severe testicular phenotypes and the incidence of microdeletions is highest amongst azoospermic patients with Sertoli cell-only histology. AZFc is by far the most frequently encountered deletion. Y chromosome microdeletions are emerging as the second most common specific aetiology of male infertility (after varicoceles).

Several cloned genes have been mapped to each of the AZF intervals. At least one strong candidate gene is associated with each deletion cluster—DFFRY in AZFa, RBMY in AZFb, and DAZ in AZFc. These are multicopy gene families scattered in both arms of the Y chromosome with the latter two being expressed only in the testis. The specific products of these candidate genes and their functional significance remain unclear. Male infertility associated with microdeletions of Y chromatin is probably attributable to reduced copy number of more than one of these gene families. Other, as yet unidentified, genes important in spermatogenesis within or outside the AZF loci of the Y chromosome are highly likely. A significant proportion of patients with microdeletions of the Y chromosome is oligozoospermic and not azoospermic. Transmission of specific Y chromosome microdeletions to male offspring by assisted conception techniques has been clearly documented.

Defects in target tissue

Mutations in the ligand binding or DNA binding domains of the androgen receptor cause defects in androgen action and varying degrees of failure of masculinization during primary sexual development (androgen insensitivity syndromes) despite raised levels of testosterone being produced by inguinal or intra-abdominal testes. These defects are, in descending order of severity:

- Complete testicular feminization—female phenotype and female external genitalia with absent uterus and Fallopian tubes. Presents with primary amenorrhoea.

- Incomplete testicular feminization—female phenotype and female external genitalia with minimal virilization such as clitoral hypertrophy and partial fusion.
- Reifenstein's syndrome—ambiguous genitalia with perineoscrotal hypospadias, poor penile development, bifid scrotum, and gynaecomastia at puberty.

In contrast to the above, expansion of CAG polyglutamine repeats to greater than 40 in the N-termial domain of the androgen receptor causes X-linked spinal bulbar muscular atrophy (Kennedy's disease) associated with gynaecomastia, poor virilization, and azoospermia due to 'late-onset' androgen resistance. Expansion of CAG glutamine repeats to between 25 to 40 is associated with a four-fold increased risk of oligozoospermia or azoospermia without clinical evidence of neuromuscular degeneration. This may represent a exclusively testicular form of androgen insensitivity.

5α-reductase-2 deficiency–deficient 5α-dihydrotestosterone action in the genital tract causes clitoral hypertrophy with perineoscrotal hypospadias and blind-ending pseudovagina, inguinal testes with epididymis and vas. Usually raised as girls, these patients dramatically virilize at puberty without gynaecomasita.

Males with oestrogen resistance and aromatase deficiency are normally virilized at birth and have normal pubertal development except for non-fusion of epiphyses resulting in extreme tall stature and osteoporosis in adulthood. Effects on spermatogenesis and fertility are currently unclear.

Cryptorchidism

Cryptorchidism has a prevalence of 2.5 to 5 per cent at birth which declines to 1 per cent by 1 year. Spontaneous descent rarely occurs after this age. Undescended testes can be a feature of many hypogonadotrophic conditions, and intersexual and dysgenetic states such as androgen insensitivity syndromes and Noonan's syndrome. The persistent mullerian duct syndrome is caused by defects in antimullerian hormone (AMH) production or action during fetal development. The presence of Fallopian tubes and uterus obstructs testicular descent. The lower temperature in the scrotum is a prerequisite for normal spermatogenesis. Undescended testes are therefore exposed to the harmful effects of the higher temperature in the abdomen and inguinal region. The testis which is not permanently in a low scrotal position by the age of 2 years will have sustained permanent damage to the seminiferous epithelium. Orchidopexy after 2 years of age for undescended testes does not improve fertility. For these reasons, treatment should ideally be undertaken between 1 and 2 years of age. hCG or intranasal GnRH are currently being increasingly used for early initial treatment of cryptorchidism. If hormonal treatment is unsuccessful, orchidopexy can be carried out by the age of 2 years. The risk of testicular tumour in a patient with a history of undescended testis, whether successfully treated by orchidopexy or not, is four to five-fold higher than the general population.

Testicular tumours

It is important to remember that infertility can be a presenting symptom of testicular tumours, the commonest malignancy in young adult men. With increasing use of testicular ultrasound, it has become clear that there is a significantly higher risk of testicular tumours in infertile men (in the absence of cryptorchidism) compared to the general population. Carcinoma *in situ*, an obligatory precancerous state, is occasionally encountered incidentally in diagnostic testicular biopsies. Without treatment, 50 per cent of carcinomata *in situ* progress to malignant seminoma or non-seminomatous germ cell tumours.

Varicocele

Varicocele is a dilatation of the scrotal portion of the pampiniform plexus due to reflux of blood in the internal spermatic veins, usually involving the left side from the renal vein. It usually gives rise to a reduction in ipsilateral testicular volume but varying degrees of hypospermatogenesis are often seen in both testes. Although a varicocele is clinically detectable in up to 40 per cent of male partners of infertile couples, its significance in male infertility remains controversial. Increased scrotal temperature, hypoxia, and exposure of the testes to adrenal metabolites have been postulated as possible mechanisms by which spermatic vein reflux can induce seminiferous tubular damage. Since varicoceles can be detected clinically in 15 per cent of fertile young men, it must not be assumed that this condition is invariably or solely responsible for infertility without actively excluding other possible aetiologies including those in the female partner.

Sperm autoimmunity

Immunological infertility is a specific disorder caused by sperm membrane-bound IgA antibodies found in around 5 per cent of men presenting with infertility. Conditions predisposing to sperm autoimmunity include vasectomy, testicular injury/inflammation, genital tract infection/obstruction, and family history of autoimmune disease. Male patients with significant antisperm antibody titres usually have severely suppressed fertility potential due to sperm agglutination, poor sperm transit through cervical mucus, and blocked sperm–oocyte fusion.

Genital tract infection

Infection in the lower genital tract is a major cause of male infertility in the global context. Chlamydia, gonococcus, Gram-negative enterococci, and tubercle bacillus are the usual pathogens. If not treated by appropriate antibiotics promptly, inflammation of the accessory glands and excurrent ducts may give rise to disturbed function, formation of sperm antibody, and permanent structural damage with obstruction in the outflow tract. Asymptomatic prostatitis due to occult and usually focal infection is best diagnosed by transrectal ultrasound examination of the prostate.

Excurrent duct obstruction

Vasectomy and previous genitourinary infections, usually sexually transmitted or tuberculous, are the most common causes of obstructive azoospermia. Congenital bilateral agenesis of the wolffian duct-derived structures, corpus/cauda epididymis, vas deferens and seminal vesicles (CBAVD) characterized by impalpable scrotal vasa, distended caput epididymis, acidic non-coagulating semen of reduced volume (<2 ml) devoid of fructose and sperm is present in 95 per cent of males with cystic fibrosis. They carry homozygous or compound heterozygous mutations in the cystic fibrosis transmembrane regulator (*CFTR*) gene. More commonly (6 per cent of azoospermic men and 1–2 per cent of infertile males), patients present with CBAVD without frank respiratory tract disease or pancreatic insufficiency. They have milder heterozygous mutations and/or the 5T variant in intron 8 of the *CFTR* gene, giving rise to a predominantly genital phenotype of cystic fibrosis. Renal and urinary tract abnormalities are common in these patients. In Young's syndrome, progressive epididymal obstruction is due to progressive inspissation of amorphous secretion in the lumen. In these patients, the high incidence of chronic sinopulmonary infection from childhood and bronchiectasis is presumably the consequence of the same abnormality in the respiratory tract. Epidemiological data has recently raised the possibility of mercury poisoning in this condition.

Coital disorders

Inadequate coital frequency, technique (including the use of vaginal lubricants with spermicidal properties), and faulty timing of intercourse may contribute to continuing infertility but are rarely the only aetiological factor in the infertile couple.

Diagnosis

History

Particular attention should be paid to the following aspects. Previous surgery such as herniorrhaphy in childhood, trauma, or torsion suggests possible damage to the vas or testis. History of cryptorchidism and genitourinary infections are important aetiological factors. Delayed onset of puberty may suggest the possibility of gonadotrophin deficiency. A history of recurrent chest infection, sinusitis, or bronchiectasis may be obtained in patients with epididymal obstruction (Young's syndrome), immotile cilia syndrome, and CBAVD associated with cystic fibrosis. Chronic disorders such as renal failure, liver disease, malignancy, diabetes, and multiple sclerosis are associated with a variety of testicular and sexual dysfunctions. Each patient should be asked about episodes of pyrexia within the past 12 weeks because of transient suppression of spermatogenesis. Careful enquiry should also be made about occupational or environmental exposure to testicular toxins, radiation, current medications, previous treatment, or recreational drugs. Painful ejaculation, haemotospermia, and pain in the perineum are symptoms suggestive of chronic infection in the prostate and seminal vesicles. It is important to establish that vaginal intercourse takes place with appropriate frequency and timing without the use of vaginal lubricants.

Examination

Assessment of height, weight, body habitus, and secondary sexual development should be carried out in all patients. Measurement of testicular volumes by comparison with Prader's orchidometer provide a convenient clinical index of seminiferous tubular mass. Normal adult testicular volume is between 15 and 35 ml. Testicular volume is a key finding in differentiating between azoospermia due to seminiferous tubular failure (reduced volumes) and that arising from excurrent duct obstruction (normal volume). Testicular size is also a useful indicator of the degree of testicular development in hypogonadotrophic patients. If not in the scrotum, the lowest position of the testes should be defined with the patient upright. Irregular contour, induration, or abnormal consistency of the testis suggest previous orchitis, surgery, or malignancy. Special attention should also be paid to the palpation of the epididymis and scrotal vas. An enlarged and tense caput epididymis may be palpable in cases of obstructive azoospermia. Irregularity and induration of the epididymis and vas suggest previous infection. In congenital agenesis of wolffian duct-derived structures, the scrotal vasa are either impalpable or extremely thin. The patient should be examined standing so that varicoceles can become visible (grade 3) or palpable (grade 2), or detected as a venous impulse in the spermatic cord during valsalva manoeuvre (grade 1). Rectal examination may reveal irregular contour or abnormal consistency and tenderness in the prostate in the presence of chronic prostatitis and enlarged seminal vesicles due to ejaculatory duct obstruction.

Investigations

Conventional parameters of the semen analysis such as sperm density, percentage of motile sperm, quality of sperm movements, and sperm morphology provide a semiquantitative index of fertility potential. Although a variety of tests of sperm function, such as computer-aided sperm movement analyses, cervical mucus penetration, acrosome reaction, sperm-zona binding, and hamster oocyte penetration, have been devised, none are sufficiently reliable and accurate to be used routinely in clinical practice. Infertile men with oligozoospermia produce spermatozoa harbouring abnormal DNA with strand breaks and redundant cytoplasm which may produce excessive reactive oxygen species. Chromatin structure and cytoplasmic enzyme (LDH-X or CK-M) assays are being applied to assess functional integrity of spermatozoa. They may provide more reliable quantitative biochemical measures of male fertility to guide management in the future.

Measurement of plasma FSH is useful in distinguishing primary from secondary testicular failure and in identifying patients with obstructive azoospermia. In the presence of azoospermia or oligozoospermia, an elevated FSH, particularly with reduced testicular volume, is presumptive evidence of severe and usually irreversible seminiferous tubular damage. Low or undetectable FSH (usually associated with low LH and testosterone with clinical evidence of androgen deficiency) is suggestive of hypogonadotrophism. Conversely, azoospermia with normal FSH and normal testicular volume usually indicates the presence of bilateral genital tract obstruction. The potential role of inhibin B measurement as a circulating marker of Sertoli cell function in routine diagnostic workup of male infertility is currently being evaluated. Testosterone and LH measurements are only indicated in the assessment of the infertile male when there is clinical suspicion

of androgen deficiency, Klinefelter's syndrome, or sex steroid abuse. A high LH and testosterone should raise the possibility of abnormalities in androgen receptors while low LH and testosterone suggest gonadotrophin deficiency. Hyperprolactinaemia is not a recognized cause of male infertility but prolactin measurement should be undertaken if there is clinical evidence of sexual dysfunction (particularly diminished libido) or pituitary disease leading to secondary testicular failure. Oestradiol measurement is rarely indicated except in the presence of gynaecomastia.

Chromosome analysis by karyotyping or fluorescent in situ hybridization (FISH) should be carried out in patients with azoospermia, testicular atrophy, and elevated FSH, primarily to confirm the diagnosis of Klinefelter's syndrome. Screening for Y chromosome microdeletions should be considered in all patients with sperm density less than 5 million/ml by an appropriate number of PCR-based DNA markers and confirmed by Southern blotting. The need for testicular biopsy has largely been superseded by the use of plasma FSH in recent years to differentiate between primary testicular failure and obstructive lesions. Undetectable or very low levels of seminal fructose is used to confirm the clinical diagnosis of vasal and seminal vesicle agenesis or blocked ejaculatory ducts in the presence of obstructive azoospermia. An increase in number (more than 1 million/ml) of peroxidase-positive or monoclonal antibody-detected leucocytes in the semen may indicate genital tract infection. Semen culture for pathogens are difficult because of the bactericidal properties of seminal plasma and urethral and skin commensals. Antisperm antibodies are detected by the mixed agglutination reaction where sheep red blood cells or polyacrylamide beads are coated with rabbit antibodies to specific classes of human Igs. These will attach to motile spermatozoa carrying specific IgA on the surface of the sperm head or tail. Ultrasound examination of the testis has become a routine investigation for infertile males with non-obstructive azoospermia or severe oligospermia to detect occult testicular tumours. In patients with persistent or treated cryptorchidism, testicular ultrasound should be carried out annually. Ultrasound of the urinary tract is indicated in patients with CBAVD. Transrectal ultrasound can aid the diagnosis of asymptomatic chronic prostatitis.

Management

Pregnancies can occur in subfertile couples without treatment albeit with a much reduced probability depending on the duration of infertility, age, and coexisting subtle abnormalities in the female partner in addition to the defects in sperm quality. Since the majority of patients with male infertility present no recognizable or reversible aetiologies, management remains largely empirical.

Subfertility due to idiopathic hypospermatogenesis

Although a wide variety of empirical medical treatments, including gonadotrophins, androgens, and antioestrogens, have been tried in attempts to improve fertility in subfertile men, none have been shown to be effective when assessed in randomized, controlled therapeutic trials and are therefore not recommended. Instead, assisted conception techniques are increasingly applied to overcome idiopathic male infertility. This is based on the premise that placing a large number of 'prepared' motile spermatozoa in close proximity to ovulated or retrieved oocytes in vivo or in vitro can enhance the probability of fertilization. Intrauterine insemination (IUI) of more than 1 million washed, motile spermatozoa (freed of seminal plasma, leucocytes, and abnormal/ dead spermatozoa) is a relatively simple and inexpensive technique with few complications. Pregnancy rates of 5 to 10 per cent per cycle can be expected. This can be combined with controlled ovarian stimulation of the female using gonadotrophins but the risk of multiple pregnancies increases. In vitro fertilization (IVF) involves more intensive gonadotrophin stimulation of the female, suppression of spontaneous ovulation, and collection of multiple oocytes by laparoscopy or transvaginal-ultrasound-guided ovarian puncture which are then coincubated with prepared spermatozoa in culture medium. In patients with moderate oligozoospermia, average fertilization rates of 30 per cent and live birth rates of 5 to 12 per cent per treatment cycle can be expected. In those with severe and multiple defects in semen parameters, standard IVF is less effective. For these cases, microinjection of single live spermatozoon directly into harvested oocytes (intracytoplasmic sperm injection, ICSI) has become the treatment of choice. This bypasses the sperm–oocyte interactions normally required for fertilization in natural conception or IVF and can achieve a remarkably high fertilization and live birth rates ((55 and 26 per cent per cycle respectively) even with the most severely abnormal samples. Since only a few spermatozoa are required, ICSI has revolutionized management of extreme oligozoospermia and azoospermia irrespective of aetiology. Non-obstructive azoospermia is often intermittent and careful examination of centrifuged deposits of semen to detect and harvest occasional ejaculated spermatozoa for ICSI should be attempted repeatedly before resorting to alternatives. Even in patients with persistent azoospermia, isolated foci of spermatogenesis may be preserved so that testicular sperm extraction via multiple biopsies can often yield viable testicular spermatozoa (including several patients with Klinefelter's syndrome) for ICSI.

In obstructive azoospermia, epididymal spermatozoa can be aspirated by an open procedure or percutaneous needle puncture of the proximal epididymis. In these circumstances, cryostorage of harvested spermatozoa for subsequent ICSI is required; this does not appear to compromise efficacy. In children born after successful ICSI treatment, the incidence of major congenital abnormalities is not increased compared to natural pregnancies but there is a small increase in sex chromosome aneuploidy in some series. Concern regarding the developmental potential of children born after ICSI has been raised. Long-term follow-up of children from ICSI births is indicated.

Specific treatable conditions

Removal or withdrawal from antispermatogenic agent or drug exposure may lead to improvement in fertility. This is most commonly seen in patients with inflammatory bowel diseases changing treatment from sulfasalazine to 5-aminosalicylic acid which removes the offending moiety, sulfapyridine. Withdrawal from anabolic steroid abuse invariably leads to recovery of spermatogenesis although this may take many months because of the long half-lives of some preparations. Cryopreservation of semen should be offered to all male patients of reproductive ageing before commencing anticancer chemotherapy or testicular irradiation.

When patients with hypogonadotrophic hypogonadism desire fertility, they can discontinue exogenous androgen replacement and start on human chorionic gonadotrophin (hCG 2000 IU, subcutaneous, twice weekly) for 6 to 12 months. This should maintain normal testosterone levels. Patients with postpubertally-acquired gonadotrophin deficiency (e.g. from pituitary tumour) where spermatogenesis has previously been established, usually respond to hCG treatment alone to reinitiate germ cell development. If there is no spermatozoa in the ejaculate at the end of 12 months, human menopausal gonadotrophin (hMG), which contain both FSH and LH, or recombinant FSH should be added at 75 to 150 IU, subcutaneous, thrice weekly. Combined treatment may be required for a further 12 months. Most patients with congenital forms of hypogonadotrophic hypogonadism will require FSH to stimulate Sertoli cell division and initiate spermatogenesis. In general, around 70 per cent should show active spermatogenesis and 50 per cent could be expected to achieve spontaneous pregnancies even if sperm densities remain in the oligozoospermic range. Patients with hypothalamic GnRH deficiency, can be treated by pulsatile GnRH delivered 2-hourly by a battery-driven portable infusion minipump. Many find this form of chronic therapy impractical and too demanding. The outcome of treatment is similar to that obtained with exogenous gonadotrophin therapy.

Active infection in the genital tract should be treated by appropriate antibiotics (erythromycin, doxycycline, or norfloxacin) for 4 weeks for the patient and his partner.

Obstructive azoospermia due to epididymal obstruction can be treated by microsurgical epididymovasostomy. High pregnancy rates can only be achieved by a few experienced microsurgeon. A more feasible alternative is to obtain spermatozoa from the caput epididymis or efferent ducts proximal to the site of obstruction by direct needle aspiration (microepididymal sperm aspiration or percutaneous epididymal sperm aspiration) for use in assisted fertilization procedures (usually ICSI). In patients with CBAVD, *CFTR* mutation screening of the partner and genetic counselling should be undertaken beforehand because of the risk of cystic fibrosis in offspring.

Sperm antibody can be treated by immunosuppression with high-dose prednisolone 0.75 mg/kg per day or prednisolone 20 mg twice daily on days 1 to 10 and 5 mg on days 11 and 12 of the partner's cycle for three to six cycles. Side-effects are common, including irritability, sleeplessness, arthralgia, muscle weakness, peptic ulceration, glucose intolerance, and bilateral aseptic necrosis of femoral heads. Results of controlled trials of glucocorticoid treatment are conflicting. IVF and ICSI are increasingly being applied to manage immunological male infertility.

Varicocele can be treated either by open surgical ligation or transfemoral embolization of the internal spermatic veins. Results of treatment of varicocele from eight prospective, controlled therapeutic trials are confusing. Coexisting female factors contributing to infertility, insufficient samples size, high dropout rates, and lack of randomization/ blinding or sham procedures are some of the more important confounding variables which typify difficulties of treatment trials in male infertility. Nevertheless, the Royal College of Obstetricians and Gynaecologists recently concluded that treatment of varicocele in oligozoospermic, but not normospermic, subfertile men can significantly improve semen quality and pregnancy rate. The cost of varicocele treatment per live birth is less with surgical ligation (and embolization) than for assisted conception techniques.

Retrograde ejaculation can be treated medically with α-adrenergic, anticholinergic agents or imipramine. If unsuccessful, spermatozoa can be recovered from bladder catheterization and irrigation with culture medium for artificial insemination or IVF. Semen can be obtained by masturbation, vibrators, or electroejaculation from patients with various coital dysfunctions.

Untreatable sterility

Patients with persistent, non-obstructive azoospermia without retrievable postmeiotic germ cells, unable to undergo or failed to be helped by ICSI should be counselled regarding the options of continuing childlessness, adoption, and donor insemination.

Genetic screening and counselling

This has become important with the realization that genetic disorders could account for an increasing proportion of infertility previously believed to be idiopathic and that there is a high probability of transmitting infertility to male offspring if assisted reproductive treatment is successful. Furthermore, the long-term health of the ICSI offspring remains an unsettled question. Counselling should therefore be carried out in all couples considering microassisted fertilization techniques. It is also recommended that chromosome karyotyping and Y chromosome screening be performed in patients with azoospermia and severe oligozoospermia (less than 5 million/ml) regardless of the coexistence of other clinical abnormalities such as varicocele or cryptorchidism. This not only allows a firm diagnosis to be made but also encourages the clinician to forego empirical treatment and couples who conceived by assisted reproduction techniques may inform their son at a suitable age that he is likely to have fertility problems. Patients with obstructive azoopsermia due to CBAVD and their partners should undergo *CFTR* gene screening followed by genetic counselling if positive.

Erectile impotence

Erectile failure may be caused by neurological disorders such as autonomic neuropathy (usually complicating diabetes), multiple sclerosis and spinal injuries, vascular disease involving pelvic vessels, retroperitoneal and bladder neck surgery, medications (commonly α and β-adrenergic antagonists, psychotropic agents), alcohol abuse, severe systemic disease, psychological dysfunctions (including depression), relationship problems, androgen deficiency, and hyperprolactinaemia. Loss of libido characterizes androgen deficiency and hyperprolactinaemia, while normal spontaneous morning erection is suggestive of psychogenic impotence. Testosterone deficiency is uncommon (less than 5 per cent) in patients who present with erectile dysfunction without loss of libido. Management should aim to correct any reversible underlying disease (e.g. prolactinoma) or substitute offending medications. Androgen replacement is only indicated in patients with total or free plasma testosterone in the hypogonadal range. The use of phosphodiesterase inhibitor (PGE5 inhibitors), such as sildenafil, to enhance the neurovascular cGMP-mediated nitric oxide synthesis in penile vasculature has been remarkably successful in a treating a wide variety of erectile dysfunction. This has largely superseded the use of vacuum devices and intracavernosal injection of vasodilator agents such as papaverine or prostaglandin E1. These are reserved for cases with severe neurogenic impotence unresponsive to PGE5 inhibitors.

Further reading

Bhasin S, ed. (1998). The therapeutic role of androgens. *Balliere's Clinical Endocrinology and Metabolism* **12**.

Griffen JE (1992). Androgen resistance—the clinical and molecular spectrum. *New England Journal of Medicine* **326**, 611–18.

Hargreave TB, ed. (1994). *Male Infertility*, 2nd edn. Springer-Verlag, Berlin.

Mooradian AD, Morley JE, Korenman SG (1987). Biological actions of androgens. *Endocrine Reviews* **8**, 1–27.

Nieschlag E, Behre HM, eds (1997). *Andrology Male Reproductive Health and Dysfunction.* Springer-Verlag, Berlin.

Nieschlag E and Behre HM, eds (1998). *Testosterone action. Deficiency. Substitution*, 2nd edn. Springer-Verlag, Berlin.

Royal College of Obstetricians and Gynaecologists (1998). *The Management of Infertility in Secondary Care—Evidence-based Clinical Guidelines no.3.* Royal College of Obstetricians and Gynaecologists Press, London.

Royal College of Obstetricians and Gynaecologists (1998). *The Management of Infertility in Tertiary Care—Evidence-based Clinical Guidelines no.6.* Royal College of Obstetricians and Gynaecologists Press, London.

Templeton A, Cooke I, O'Brien PMS, eds (1998). *Evidence-based Fertility Treatment.* Royal College of Obstetricians and Gynaecologists Press, London.

Wang C, ed. (1999). *Male Reproductive Function.* Endocrine Updates. Kluwer Academic Publishers, Boston.

World Health Organization (1992). *Guidelines for the Use of Androgens in Men.* WHO, Geneva.

Wu FCW, ed. (2000). Male fertility and infertility. *Balliere's Best Practice in Clinical Endocrinology.*

12.8.3 The breast

H. S. Jacobs

Gynaecomastia

Gynaecomastia is defined as benign enlargement of the male breast caused by proliferation of the glandular components. Clinically the distinction from enlargement by fat tissue is made by examining the patient in the supine position, the breast being held between thumb and forefinger and the fingers gently moved towards the nipple. A firm or rubbery mobile disc-like mound of tissue arising concentrically from beneath the nipple and areola indicates the presence of gynaecomastia. The most important condition that needs to be excluded is carcinoma of the male breast. Cancer usually presents as a unilateral eccentric mass that is hard and fixed to underlying tissue; it may be associated with skin tethering, nipple discharge, or axillary lymphadenopathy. Mammography and fine needle aspiration are helpful in the differential diagnosis but if doubt remains

biopsy is appropriate. While cancer of the male breast is rare, it has to be recognized that it is 16 times more common in Klinefelter's syndrome than in other men. Other causes of gynaecomastia are not, however, associated with an increased risk of breast cancer.

Pathogenesis

Microscopically breast tissue in both sexes appears identical at birth. It remains quiescent until puberty when, in boys, the ducts and surrounding mesenchymal tissue transiently proliferate, only to involute and ultimately to atrophy. Gynaecomastia is characterized by initial proliferation of the fibroblastic stroma and ductal system. Progressive fibrosis and hyalinization then occur in association with regression of the epithelial components. These regressive changes occur even if the stimulus (for example oestrogen treatment) continues. When gynaecomastia has been present for more than a year, clinical regression is rarely complete because the fibrosis persists even when the cause has been removed.

Since oestrogens stimulate and androgens inhibit development of breast tissue, gynaecomastia arises whenever there is an imbalance between these hormones. An alteration in the ratio of free androgen to free oestrogen, rather than a specific concentration of either, is thought to underlie most cases of gynaecomastia.

In men 98 per cent of testosterone is directly secreted by the testes, whereas the origin of oestrogen is more complex (Fig. 1): thus only about 15 per cent of oestradiol and less than 5 per cent of oestrone are directly secreted. In both cases the remainder is produced by extraglandular conversion (aromatization) of androgenic precursors in peripheral tissues such as adipose tissue, liver, and muscle. There is also substantial interconversion of oestrone and oestradiol. Treatment of normal men with human chorionic gonadotrophin results in an increase of directly secreted oestradiol in proportion to the increase of testosterone, so that while directly secreted oestradiol in normal men rarely amounts to more than 6 μg/day, when levels of luteinizing hormones are persistently high substantial amounts of oestradiol may be directly secreted by the testis.

Causes

Gynaecomastia may be physiological or pathological. Physiologically it occurs at three times of life: the first is neonatally in response to transplacental passage of oestrogens, the second is during puberty for reasons that are not at all clear, and the third is in elderly men, probably because of the decline in Leydig cell function that occurs normally with age.

Pathological gynaecomastia is caused by a deficiency of testosterone formation or action, enhanced production of oestrogen, drugs, and unknown causes.

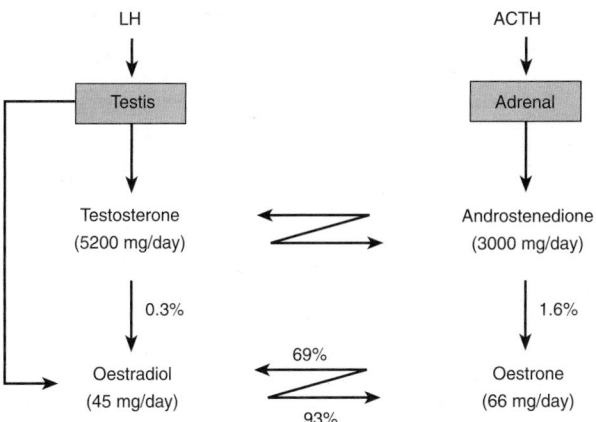

Fig. 1 Sources of oestrogen in men.

Testosterone deficiency

The commonest cause is Klinefelter's syndrome, about half the cases of which develop gynaecomastia at the time of puberty. The serum testosterone is usually about 50 per cent of normal, the gonadotrophin concentrations are raised, and the serum oestradiol is above normal. The diagnosis is suspected clinically and confirmed by white blood cell karyotype. Congenital causes of testosterone deficiency include defects in testosterone biosynthesis and congenital anorchia. Acquired causes include viral orchitis (usually mumps), trauma, neurological disease (myotonia dystrophica and spinal cord lesions), and renal failure. Androgen resistance syndromes are associated with high rates of secretion of testosterone and oestradiol; because of the large amounts of precursor (testosterone) there is also excessive extragonadal conversion of androgens to oestrogens.

Increased secretion of oestrogen

Testicular tumours, such as Leydig and Sertoli cell tumours, may secrete androgens and oestrogens autonomously; gonadotrophin secretion is therefore suppressed and azoospermia is common. They may be too small to be detected clinically but ultrasound can be very helpful. Some testicular tumours, for example choriocarcinomas, secrete human choionic gonadotrophin which then stimulates oestrogen secretion by the contralateral testis. Human choionic gonadotrophin may also be secreted by non-testicular tumours such as a bronchogenic carcinoma.

True hermaphroditism may be associated with gynaecomastia because of oestrogen secretion by the ovotestis.

Increased extragonadal production of oestrogens

Adrenal disease

Congenital adrenal hyperplasia caused by 2,1-hydroxylase or 3β or 17β steroid dehydrogenase deficiencies results in increased availability of adrenal androgen for peripheral aromatization. Adrenal carcinoma may be associated with massive oestrogen production, usually caused by extraglandular aromatization of the enormous amounts of androgen secreted by the tumour but occasionally directly secreted.

Liver disease

Cirrhosis, particularly alcoholic cirrhosis, is typically associated with gynaecomastia, testicular atrophy, and impotence. Plasma and urinary excretion of oestrogen is increased. The mechanism is in part decreased hepatic extraction of androstenedione and consequently an increase in its extrasplanchnic aromatization and partly reduced testosterone secretion by the testes. The gynaecomastia of starvation and refeeding may also be related to disturbed liver function.

Drugs

Oestrogens and oestrogen-like drugs

The most familiar use of oestrogen is in the treatment of advanced carcinoma of the prostate, indeed it is the development of gynaecomastia in this situation that has provided the model for most of our understanding of the evolution of the histological changes in the breast in gynaecomastia. Oestrogen residues in food (via injected animals) and cosmetic products have been reported as a cause of gynaecomastia.

Treatment with digitalis glycosides may cause gynaecomastia, the drug acting either as an oestrogen or as an oestrogen precursor.

Drugs that enhance oestrogen secretion

Treatment with human chorionic gonadotrophin and clomiphene can cause increased oestrogen secretion. The development of gynaecomastia in men treated with human chorionic gonadotrophin usually means that the dose used has been too high.

Drugs that inhibit testosterone secretion

Ketoconazole, an antifungal agent that is also used in the management of certain forms of Cushing's syndrome, blocks steroid synthesis in Leydig cells and, if a high dose is maintained, gynaecomastia may result.

Spironolactone causes gynaecomastia in as many as 50 per cent of men treated with 150 mg/day. The drug suppresses testosterone synthesis (by inhibiting 17,20-desmolase) but it also acts as a peripheral antiandrogen.

Drugs that block testosterone action

Cyproterone acetate and flutamide are two antiandrogens used in the management of advanced prostatic disease which usually produce gynaecomastia. Cimetidine, but not ranitidine, is antiandrogenic and is associated with a significant risk of gynaecomastia.

Whereas in most series between 50 and 75 per cent of cases of gynaecomastia are labelled idiopathic because no endocrinopathy can be identified, there are increasing reasons to suspect that environmental pollution, either with oestrogens or antiandrogens, is responsible for many of the cases.

Diagnosis

The history should include enquiry about drugs as well as possible environmental exposure to oestrogens and antiandrogens. Examination should include the testes. While small firm testes are characteristic of Klinefelter's syndrome, asymmetrical enlargement suggests a Leydig cell tumour (most readily diagnosed by ultrasound). Evaluation of alcohol intake and liver function is appropriate. Endocrine assessment should include measurement of testosterone, oestradiol, gonadotrophins, and dehydroepiandrosterone sulphate (high levels suggest adrenal disease) concentrations.

Treatment

Once gynaecomastia has been present for about a year medical treatment is unlikely to lead to a reduction in breast size because of the fibrosis which usually develops by this time. Consequently surgery is the mainstay of treatment. The psychological effects of persistent breast development in adolescent boys may be severe and surgery should be considered at an early stage: temporizing rarely produces resolution. Medical therapy with androgens or anti-oestrogens produces uncertain effects and can only be expected to have much benefit if administered early in the course of the disorder. Gynaecomastia caused by oestrogen treatment, as in the treatment of prostatic disease, can be prevented by pretreatment with low-dose irradiation of the breasts.

Galactorrhoea

Galactorrhoea is defined as a persistent discharge of milk or milk like secretion in the absence of parturition or beyond 6 months postpartum in a non-nursing mother. Galactorrhoea is not a sign of breast cancer and not a risk factor for it.

There are essentially two types of galactorrhoea—spontaneous galactorrhoea or galactorrhoea present on expression only. In the latter case the menstrual cycle is usually intact and an endocrine cause is rarely found. It is spontaneous galactorrhoea that is significant in endocrine terms and which is usually associated with amenorrhoea. It is in this situation that hyperprolactinaemia occurs.

In the puerperium there is a clear correlation between the amount of prolactin released in response to suckling and the volume of milk secreted. In contrast, in inappropriate lactation, that is, in galactorrhoea, no such relation exists, presumably because the breasts have not been prepared for lactation by the oestrogen- and progesterone-rich environment of pregnancy. When this observation is considered in relation to the ease and widespread availability of prolactin measurements, one can readily appreciate that the physical sign of galactorrhoea has ceased to have much diagnostic significance. In women with amenorrhoea caused by hyperprolactinaemia, for example, only about 20 per cent have galactorrhoea. Thus the evaluation of galactorrhoea nowadays is essentially the evaluation of hyperprolactinaemia.

Management

The essential investigation is the measurement of serum prolactin. The management of hyperprolactinaemia is outlined in Chapter 12.2. For women with non-hyperprolactinaemic galactorrhoea the important advice is first to stop expressing the milk, the second is the reassurance that it is not a sign of cancer, or a risk factor for it, and third is a trial of drug therapy with bromocriptine. In the author's experience, after they have received appropriate reassurance, patients with non-hyperprolactinaemic galactorrhoea rarely need drug therapy. Such patients are, however, very sensitive to the adverse effects of the drug and side-effects are common, even with low doses.

Further reading

Berchuck A, *et al.* (1998). Familial breast-ovarian cancer syndromes: BRCA1 and BRCA2. *Clinical Obstetrics and Gynecology* **41**, 157–66.

Haney AF (1997). Galactorrhea. *Current Therapy in Endocrinology and Metabolism* **6**, 393–6.

12.8.4 Sexual dysfunction

Raymond C. Rosen and Irwin Goldstein

Introduction

Sexual dysfunction is a common complaint in men and women and is associated with a broad range of medical, psychological, and interpersonal causes. Despite significant progress in basic research and clinical therapeutics in recent years, sexual problems remain among the most frequently overlooked and mismanaged patient complaints. Patient–physician communication difficulties, lack of knowledge, and inadequate reimbursement are frequently cited reasons for these shortcomings. Few physicians are adequately trained in the diagnosis and treatment of sexual dysfunction, and many patients seek assistance from inappropriate or unqualified providers. This trend is particularly unfortunate, since sexual problems frequently impact on patients' interpersonal functioning and quality of life. Moreover, new treatment options are available which offer significant therapeutic potential for many individuals.

Sexual problems are generally classified according to the four-phase model of sexual response originally proposed by Masters and Johnson. These include: (i) sexual desire disorders (hypoactive sexual desire disorder, sexual aversion disorder); (ii) sexual arousal disorders (erectile dysfunction, female arousal disorder); (iii) orgasmic disorders (female orgasmic disorder, premature or delayed ejaculation); and (iv) sexual pain disorders (dyspareunia, vaginismus). The specific dysfunctions and corresponding phases of the sexual response cycle are shown in Table 1.

Although public and professional attention has focused predominantly on erectile dysfunction, other sexual problems (e.g. hypoactive sexual desire, premature ejaculation) are more commonly reported in community-based surveys. Sexual dysfunction is more prevalent in women than men; recent British and American studies have found that about 40 per cent of women and 30 per cent of men have had one or more sexual problems in the past. Less than 10 per cent of these problems are typically brought to the attention of a physician or other health-care provider.

Medical management of sexual dysfunction should always begin with a thorough history and physical examination. In appropriate clinical contexts, at least one question regarding sexual function ought to be included in the initial examination of every patient, regardless of age or gender (such as 'Are you satisfied with your current sexual functioning or relationship?'). A physical examination and laboratory testing are important, since sexual problems are frequently associated with underlying medical illnesses or risk factors (such as diabetes, cardiovascular disease). The role of depression or other psychiatric disorders should also be considered, as well as possible iatrogenic effects of prescription or non-prescription drugs. It is also important to evaluate relationship and lifestyle factors in all cases. Finally, the patient's needs and expectations, as well as cultural or family issues should be taken into account.

Male sexual dysfunction

Male sexual dysfunction may be divided into erectile dysfunction, premature ejaculation, hypoactive sexual desire, and priapism.

Erectile dysfunction

Epidemiology

Erectile dysfunction is a significant and common medical problem, with recent epidemiological studies suggesting that approximately 10 per cent of men aged 40 to 70 have severe or complete erectile dysfunction, defined as the total inability to achieve or maintain erections sufficient for sexual performance. An additional 25 per cent of men in this age category have moderate or intermittent erectile difficulties. The disorder is highly age-dependent, as the combined prevalence of moderate to complete erectile dysfunction rises from approximately 22 per cent at age 40 to 49 per cent by age 70 (Fig. 1). Although less common in younger men, erectile dysfunction still affects 5 to 10 per cent of men below the age of 40. Findings

Table 1 Sexual response phases and associated dysfunctions

Phase	Characteristics	Dysfunctions
Desire	First phase of sexual response Characterized by subjective feelings of sexual interest or appetite, sexual urges, or fantasies. No identifiable physiological correlates	Hypoactive sexual desire disorder; sexual aversion disorder
Excitement	Second phase of sexual response Includes both subjective and physiological concomitants of sexual arousal. Penile erection in males; vaginal engorgement and lubrication in females	Female sexual arousal disorder; male erectile disorder
Orgasm	Third phase of sexual response Includes climax or peaking of sexual tension, rhythmic contractions of the genital musculature, and intense subjective involvement	Female orgasmic disorder; male orgasmic disorder; premature ejaculation
Resolution	Final phase of sexual response Includes a physical release of tension and subjective sense of well being. Most men have a refractory period for further sexual stimulation	Sexual pain disorders; dyspareunia; vaginismus

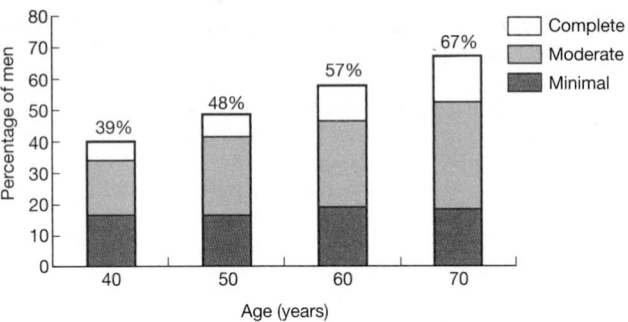

Fig. 1 Prevalence of erectile dysfunction (Feldman HA *et al.*, 1994).

from these studies show that erectile dysfunction impacts significantly on mood state, interpersonal functioning, and overall quality of life.

Clinical context

Erectile dysfunction is strongly related to both physical and psychological health. Among the major risk factors are diabetes mellitus, heart disease, hypertension, and decreased high-density lipoprotein levels. Medications for diabetes, hypertension, cardiovascular disease, and depression may also cause erectile difficulties. In addition, there is a higher prevalence of erectile dysfunction among men who have undergone radiation or surgery for prostate cancer, or who have a lower spinal cord injury or other neurological diseases (such as Parkinson's disease, multiple sclerosis). Lifestyle factors, including smoking, alcohol consumption, and sedentary behaviour are additional risk factors. The psychological correlates of erectile dysfunction include anxiety, depression, and anger. Despite its increasing prevalence among older men, erectile dysfunction is not considered a normal or inevitable part of the ageing process. It is rarely (in fewer than 5 per cent of cases) due to ageing-related hypogonadism, although the relationship between erectile dysfunction and age-related declines in androgen remains controversial.

Pathophysiology

Basic research on neurovascular mechanisms has contributed greatly to our understanding of normal and pathological processes of erection. There is increasing evidence that the state of trabecular smooth muscle contractility is regulated by a delicate balance between neurotransmitter and vasoactive substances mediating erectile tissue contraction (consistent with flaccidity) and relaxation (consistent with erection). The neurotransmitter nitric oxide (NO) has been found to play a major role in inducing trabecular smooth muscle relaxation, as shown in Fig. 2: cGMP binds to cGMP-dependent protein kinases (PKG) and to cGMP-dependent ion channels, leading to lowering of intracellular calcium concentration and activation of myosin light-chain phosphatases, resulting in inhibition of smooth muscle contractility and enhancement of penile erection (Fig. 2).

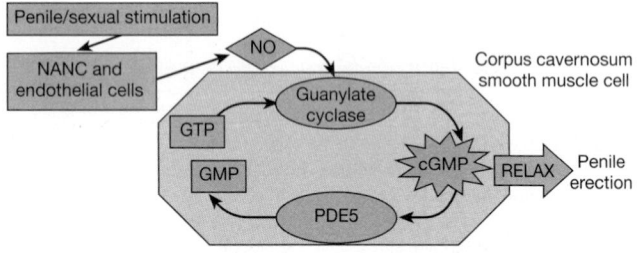

Fig. 2 Penile erection: the nitric oxide–cGMP mechanism. cGMP, cyclic guanosine monophosphate; GTP, guanosine triphosphate; NANC, non-adrenergic non-cholinergic neurones; NO, nitric oxide; PDE5, phosphodiesterase type 5.

Multiple vasoactive agents, including vasoactive intestinal polypeptide, prostaglandin E_1, forskolin, phosphodiesterase inhibitors, and α-adrenergic receptor antagonists affect smooth muscle contractility, each via a specific mechanism. Ultimately, all act by changes in intracellular calcium and modulation of specific smooth muscle myosin light-chain kinases and myosin light-chain phosphatases. These enzymes rapidly change the state of myosin phosphorylation and result in either smooth muscle contraction (flaccidity) or relaxation (erection). The role of central nervous system and spinal mechanisms has also been elucidated in recent studies. Understanding of these biochemical and neural mechanisms regulating erection has permitted the rational development of new pharmacological strategies for the management of erectile dysfunction.

Diagnosis and evaluation

Guidelines for diagnosis and evaluation were recently established by the 1st International Consultation on Erectile Dysfunction (Table 2). According to these guidelines, the first step in the process is the taking of a comprehensive sexual, medical, and psychosocial history. In obtaining a sexual history, special attention should be paid to personal or cultural sensitivities. History taking should be aimed at characterizing the severity, onset, and duration of the problem, and evaluating the need for specialized testing. A physical examination and selected laboratory testing should be performed on all patients with complaints of erectile dysfunction. Although not different from a routine physical examination, special emphasis is placed on review of genitourinary, endocrine, vascular, and neurological systems. The physical examination may corroborate aspects of the medical history (such as poor peripheral circulation), and may occasionally reveal unsuspected physical findings (such as Peyronie's plaques, small testes, prostate cancer). The physical examination also provides an opportunity for patient education and reassurance regarding normal genital anatomy.

Selective laboratory testing should be performed in all cases. This includes investigation of the hypothalamic–pituitary–gonadal axis via assessment of androgenic status, particularly if sexual desire is reduced. There is disagreement about the relative value of the various testosterone assays, including total, free, and bioavailable testosterone. However, strong consensus exists that at least one of these assays should be performed. A serum prolactin determination may be obtained in selected cases. Standard serum chemistries, full blood count, and lipid profiles may be of value and should be obtained, if not performed in the past year. Determination of serum thyroid-stimulating hormone may also be of value, as both hyper- and hypothyroidism are associated with erectile difficulties. Finally, measurement of serum prostatic specific antigen may be indicated based upon the patient's age and relative risk status.

Specialized diagnostic procedures, such as nocturnal penile tumescence and rigidity testing or other specialized vascular or neurological techniques, may play a role in selected cases. For example, CT and MR imaging, penile Doppler ultrasound, penile arteriography, cavernosal/pudendal/sphincter electromyography, or other tests may be of value in evaluating young patients with pelvic or penile trauma who may be candidates for reconstructive vascular surgery. Patients with complicated diabetes or other endocrinopathies may benefit from further endocrinological studies. Similarly, patients with complicated psychological or relationship problems may be suitably referred to a mental health or sex therapy specialist. Finally, patients with a history of cardiac disease or significant cardiovascular risk factors should be evaluated for potential cardiac risk associated with sexual activity: consensus guidelines have recently been established (Table 3).

Treatment

Results of the initial evaluation and specialized testing should be carefully reviewed with the patient and (if possible) their partner prior to initiating therapy. Potentially modifiable risk factors, such as cigarette smoking or alcohol abuse, should be addressed. Prescription drugs such as antihypertensives or antidepressants may be implicated in the patient's erectile difficulties, and should be altered when medically possible. Patients with

Table 2 Summary, diagnosis, and evaluation of erectile dysfunction

I. Highly recommended evaluation and tests
1. Comprehensive sexual, medical, and psychosocial history
    (a) Medical and sexual history
    (b) Erectile dysfunction intensity and impact scales
2. Focused physical examination

II. Recommended diagnostic tests
1. Fasting glucose or glycosylated haaemoglobin (HbA1C) and lipid profile
2. Evaluation of the hypothalamic–pituitary–gonadal axis with a testosterone assay

III. Optional diagnostic tests
1. Psychological and/or psychiatric consultation
2. Laboratory investigations
(Serum prolactin, luteinizing hormone, thyroid-stimulating hormone, complete blood count, urinalysis)

IV. Specialized evaluation and diagnostic tests
1. In depth psychosexual and relationship evaluation
2. Psychiatric evaluation
3. Nocturnal penile tumescence and rigidity (NPTR) assessment
4. Vascular diagnostics
5. Specialized endocrinological testing
6. Neurophysiological testing

specific endocrine deficiencies such as hypogonadism should be placed on hormone replacement therapy prior to initiation of direct therapies for erectile dysfunction. Sexual problems in the partner, such as a lack of lubrication, hypoactive sexual desire, or dyspareunia (painful intercourse) should also be addressed. Patients and partners should be fully informed about the range of treatment options available and the risks and benefits associated with each.

Direct therapies for erectile dysfunction can be stratified according to the mechanism of action, degree of invasiveness, ease of administration, reversibility, and relative costs associated with each (Table 4).

Sexual counselling and education

First-line options include sexual counselling or education, and oral agents (such as sildenafil). These options can be used alone or in combination. Brief sexual or couple's counselling is aimed at resolving specific psychological or interpersonal causes, such as relationship distress, sexual performance concerns, dysfunctional communication patterns, and comorbid sexual dysfunctions (such as hypoactive sexual desire). Advantages of sexual counselling include its non-invasiveness and relatively broad applicability. The major disadvantages are the lack of acceptability for many patients and uncertain efficacy.

Oral therapies

Sildenafil citrate (Viagra) is the first oral drug to be widely approved for the treatment of erectile dysfunction. It is a potent and selective inhibitor of type 5 phosphodiesterase, the primary form of the enzyme found in human penile erectile tissue (Fig. 2), thereby preventing the breakdown of cyclic guanosine monophosphate (cGMP), the intracellular second messenger of nitric oxide. Because nitric oxide is released following sexual stimulation, sildenafil only works when a man is sexually stimulated. Its mechanism of action is entirely peripheral and includes direct effects on smooth muscle relaxation and vasodilation of the penile arterioles. Sildenafil is administered 'on demand' in dosages of 25, 50, or 100 mg, and is effective in approximately 30 to 60 min, requiring ongoing sexual stimulation to be effective. Cardiac safety does not appear to be a major concern, except for patients receiving nitrates in any form, or those who have other cardiac risk factors associated with sexual activity itself (Princeton Consensus). Sildenafil is contraindicated for men receiving nitrate therapy, including short- or long-acting agents delivered by oral, sublingual, transnasal, or topical administration. Efficacy has been reported at 43 to 82 per cent, depending upon aetiology and severity of erectile dysfunction. The drug's side-effects include headaches, flushing, dyspepsia, and nasal congestion. A small percentage of men (2 to 3 per cent) may also experience mild alterations in

Table 3 Sexual activity/cardiac risk (Princeton Guidelines)

Grade of risk	Categories of cardiovascular disease	Management recommendations
Low risk	Asymptomatic, < 3 major risk factors for coronary artery disease Controlled hypertension Mild, stable angina Post-successsful coronary revascularization Uncomplicated past myocardial infarction (> 6–8 weeks) Mild vascular disease Left ventricular dysfunction/congestive heart failure (NYHA class I)	Primary care management Consider all first-line therapies Reassess at regular intervals (6–12 months)
Intermediate risk	≥3 Major risk factors for coronary artery disese, excluding gender Moderate, stable angina Recent myocardial infarction (2–6 weeks) Left ventricular dysfunction/congestive heart failure (NYHA class II) Non-cardiac sequelae of atherosclerotic disease (e.g. stroke, peripheral vascular disease)	Specialized cardiovascular testing (e.g. exercise tolerance test, echocardiogram) Restratification into high risk or low risk based on the results of cardiovascular assessment
High risk	Unstable or refractory angina Uncontrolled hypertension Left ventricular dysfunction/congestive heart failure (NYHA class III/IV) Recent myocardial infarction (< 2 weeks), stroke High-risk arrhythmias Hypertrophic obstructive and other cardiomyopathies Moderate/severe valvular disease	Priority referral for specialized cardiovascular management Treatment for sexual dysfunction to be deferred until cardiac condition stabilized and dependent on specialist recommendations

NYHA, New York Heart Association.

Table 4 Direct treatment interventions for erectile dysfunction

Sexual counselling and education
Oral agents
Sildenafil—selective inhibitor of phosphodiesterase type 5
Apomorphine—centrally acting dopaminergic agonist (taken sublingually)
Phentolamine—α-adrenergic blocking agent with central and peripheral activity
Other drugs under investigation include vardenafil and tadalafil
  (phosphodiesterase type 5 inhibitor), melanotan II (α- melanocyte-
  stimulating hormone analogue), L-arginine/yohimbine combination
Local therapies
Intracavernosal injection therapies
    Papaverine
    Phentolamine
    Alprostadil (prostaglandin E₁)
    Combinations of agents
Intraurethral therapy
    Alprostadil
Vacuum constriction devices
Surgical therapy
Vascular surgery
    Microvascular arterial bypass
    Venous ligation
Penile implants

colour vision (blue hue), visual brightness or sensitivity, or blurred vision.

Other oral agents are in development at the time of writing: some of these are based on a similar mechanism of action to sildenafil (i.e. PDE-5 inhibition), whereas others depend upon central dopaminergic activity, the dopamine–oxytocin pathway that originates from the hypothalamus and pituitary areas in the brain, or peripheral and/or central sympathetic inhibition. Some of these agents are in advanced clinical trials, but none has received regulatory approval yet in the United States or Europe. Combination oral agents are also being evaluated in some trials, and may play an important role in the future.

Local therapies

Injectable, intraurethral, or topical agents are classified as second-line therapies for erectile dysfunction according to recent guidelines. These should be selected based upon: (i) failure, insufficient response, or adverse side-effects associated with one or more of the first-line therapies, or (ii) patient/partner preferences. These interventions consist of intraurethral administration or intracavernosal injection of alprostadil. Vacuum pump devices can also be included in this category. Although widely utilized, these treatments are associated with variable efficacy, a high patient discontinuation rate, possible risk of side-effects, and moderately high costs.

Intracavernosal injection therapy

Prior to the approval of sildenafil, intracavernosal self-injection was the most common medical therapy for erectile dysfunction. Different forms of prostaglandin are used primarily for this purpose: alprostadil sterile powder and alprostadil alfadex are both synthetic formulations of prostaglandin E₁. Injection therapy is effective in most cases of erectile dysfunction, regardless of aetiology. It is contraindicated in men with a history of hypersensitivity to the drug employed, in those at risk for priapism (e.g. sickle-cell disease, hypercoagulable states), and in men receiving monoamine oxidase inhibitors. The effective therapeutic range is between 1 and 60 μg with the majority of responders (85 per cent) requiring less than 20 μg. In general, intracavernosal injection therapy with alprostadil is effective in 70 to 80 per cent of patients, although discontinuation rates are high in most studies. Side-effects include prolonged erections or priapism, penile pain, and fibrosis with chronic use. In addition to single-agent injection therapy, various combinations of alprostadil, phentolamine, and/or papaverine are widely employed in urological practice. Intracavernosal

injections have been shown to be effective in about 70 to 80 per cent of men who fail first-line therapy with sildenafil.

Intraurethral alprostadil

Alprostadil may be administered intraurethrally in the form of a semi-solid pellet inserted by means of a special applicator. To obtain an effective concentration of alprostadil in the corpora cavernosa, 125 to 1000 μg of the drug are required. In a mixed group of patients with organic erectile dysfunction, 65 per cent of men receiving intraurethral alprostadil responded with a firm erection when tested in the office, and 50 per cent of administrations to that subset resulted in at least one episode of successful intercourse in the home setting. Side-effects associated with the intraurethral administration of alprostadil include penile pain and hypotension. Prolonged erections and penile fibrosis are rare, although the clinical success rate is low.

Vacuum constriction device therapy

The use of vacuum constriction device (**VCD**) therapy is a well-established, non-invasive treatment that has recently been approved by the United States Food and Drug Administration for over-the-counter distribution. It provides a useful treatment alternative for patients for whom pharmacological therapies are contraindicated, or who do not desire other interventions. Vacuum constriction devices apply a negative pressure to the flaccid penis, thus drawing venous blood into the penis, which is then retained by the application of an elastic constriction band at the base of the penis. Efficacy rates of 60 to 80 per cent have been reported in most studies. Like intracorporal injection therapy, VCD treatment is associated with a high rate of patient discontinuation. The adverse events occasionally associated with VCD therapy include penile pain, numbness, bruising, and delayed ejaculation.

Surgical treatments

Surgical implantation of a penile prosthesis, which was at one time the mainstay of treatment for erectile dysfunction, is now performed only in rare or special cases. For select cases of severe, treatment-refractory erectile dysfunction, for patients who fail pharmacological therapy or who prefer a permanent solution for the problem, surgical implantation of a semi-rigid or inflatable penile prosthesis is available. Various types of surgical prostheses have been described in the literature. The inflatable penile prosthesis provides a more aesthetic erection and better concealment than semi-rigid prostheses, although there is an increased rate of mechanical failure and complications (5 to 20 per cent) with the former. Despite the cost, invasiveness, and potential medical complications involved, penile implant surgery has been associated with high rates of patient satisfaction in previous studies. It should be noted, however, that these studies were conducted prior to the advent of newer forms of therapy (e.g. sildenafil).

Premature ejaculation

Definition and epidemiology

Premature ejaculation is difficult to define precisely. In part, it depends on the timing or speed of the partner's response, and whether satisfactory intercourse has been achieved. The preferred definition currently is that offered by DSM-IV: 'Persistent or recurrent ejaculation with minimal sexual stimulation or before, upon, or shortly after penetration and before the person wishes it'. In making the diagnosis, clinicians should consider the circumstances of the problem, including the degree of associated distress in the male and his partner. Some authors distinguish between primary or life-long premature ejaculation, and secondary or situational forms of the disorder. Other aspects of sexual functioning should be carefully evaluated, particularly since premature ejaculation can develop as a secondary reaction to erectile dysfunction. Otherwise, little is known about either the pathophysiology or aetiology of the disorder.

Premature ejaculation is a common disorder, affecting approximately 25 to 40 per cent of adult men at some time. In the National Health and Social Life Survey, approximately one-third of men in each age cohort reported problems with ejaculating too rapidly. Despite its greater prevalence, premature ejaculation has attracted less attention among health professionals and the lay public than erectile dysfunction. This may be due, in part, to the fact that men are able to function sexually (i.e. to perform intercourse) despite a mild or moderate degree of premature ejaculation. In the most severe cases, however, the male ejaculates before penetration is achieved. Far fewer men with premature ejaculation seek professional help for their problem, including those with the most severe forms of the disorder. This is unfortunate, since simple and effective therapies are widely available.

Treatment

Treatment of premature ejaculation consists of either behavioural/sex therapy training or pharmacological treatment. Masters and Johnson popularized the most widely used 'Stop–Start' technique in the 1970s. The method involves direct stimulation of the male until premonitory sensations are experienced just prior to orgasm. All stimulation is stopped at this point. After repeated practices over 4 to 8 weeks, the male becomes more aware of these anticipatory sensations and is able to delay or control his ejaculation to a much greater degree. This conditioning technique is often effective when practiced regularly by the male and his partner. However, it demands significant motivation on the part of the couple, and treatment efficacy is not always maintained over time.

The use of new pharmacological treatments, particularly the serotonin-uptake inhibiting drugs (**SSRIs**), has grown considerably in recent years. Among the specific drugs used for this purpose, sertraline and paroxetine have been most extensively studied. Clomipramine, which is not a true serotonin-uptake inhibitor, although highly serotonergic, appears the most potent inhibitor of ejaculation to date, but can cause unpleasant side-effects, such as drowsiness or light-headedness, and may also cause decreased sexual desire or loss of erectile ability in some patients. Some authors recommend initial use of one of these agents on a daily basis, and then as needed during subsequent weeks. In one study, rapid ejaculation resumed shortly after withdrawal of clomipramine therapy that had been administered for the previous 8 weeks. To guard against this, patients should be encouraged to practice conditioning exercises along with use of the medication, and a combination of drug and non-drug therapies for premature ejaculation are currently recommended by most authors, although no controlled studies have been performed.

Hypoactive sexual desire

Hypoactive or low sexual desire is reported by about 10 to 15 per cent of men in population-based or community studies. It may be due to a variety of causes, including endocrine disorders (such as hypogonadism), other medical conditions (such as renal insufficiency), psychiatric illnesses (such as depression), or psychological factors. Various prescription (such as SSRIs) and non-prescription drugs (such as alcohol) can temporarily suppress sexual desire, as can partner conflicts or other sexual problems (such as erectile dysfunction).

Men with chronic low desire should receive a thorough medical and endocrine examination, including evaluation of the hypothalamic–pituitary–gonadal axis. Treatment should be based on identification of the relevant aetiological cause, wherever possible. Currently, there are no pharmacological agents which are safe and effective for treatment of hypoactive desire disorders in men.

Priapism

Priapism is a pathological condition defined by a persistent penile erection, greater than 4 to 6 h in duration, which persists after the cessation of sexual stimulation. Priapism is distinguished from prolonged erection, defined by a penile erection lasting up to 4 h, that spontaneously undergoes detumescence. There are two forms of priapism, veno-occlusive priapism, also referred to as low-flow or ischaemic priapism, and arterial priapism. It is essential to distinguish veno-occlusive from arterial priapism since the former is an emergency urological condition.

Veno-occlusive priapism
Introduction
Veno-occlusive priapism, the more common form of the disorder, typically presents as painful, tender, and persistent penile erection. Unless treated, it may cause irreversible damage to the erectile tissue, corporal fibrosis, and permanent erectile dysfunction. Veno-occlusive priapism is the consequence of a failure to regulate corporal veno-occlusion and is a 'closed-compartment syndrome' associated with absent cavernosal arterial inflow. The pathophysiology is based on unremitting corporal venous outflow obstruction, similar to other closed-compartment syndromes in the arms and legs.

Veno-occlusive priapism typically develops in stages. At first, in the presence of complete corporal veno-occlusion, cavernosal arterial inflow persists while intracavernosal pressures are lower than cavernosal artery systolic perfusion pressures. The presence of persistent cavernosal arterial inflow without corporal venous outflow results in intracavernosal pressure and volume increasing until maximal values of each are achieved.

In the next stage, intracavernosal pressure approximates cavernosal artery systolic pressure, thereby preventing further cavernosal arterial inflow. The consequences of absent cavernosal arterial inflow over time include: (i) an increase in corporal P_{CO_2}, (ii) a decrease in corporal pH, and (iii) a decrease in corporal P_{O_2}. The development of corporal tissue acidosis and hypoxia in this stage of veno-occlusive priapism results in adverse biochemical and cellular changes in the corporal tissue, which act to perpetuate the completeness of corporal veno-occlusion. A partial reversal of this process may occur during this phase with pharmacological or surgical intervention, when intracavernosal pressure lower than the cavernosal artery systolic pressure is transiently achieved. However, unless the primary aetiological cause is addressed, veno-occlusion and prolonged erection will probably recur. Over time, the intracavernosal blood will again become acidotic and hypoxic. Individuals in the intermediary second stage will either resolve the veno-occlusive priapism or progress to the third and final stage.

In the final stage of veno-occlusive priapism, irreversible changes to erectile tissue result from persistent exposure to acidotic and hypoxic corporal blood, which is clinically described as black, crankcase oil in appearance. It is not yet known when irreversible erectile tissue changes occur in an individual patient. It is likely that many factors contribute to the conversion from reversible stage II to irreversible stage III veno-occlusive priapism.

Aetiology
The main causes of venous priapism are listed in Table 5. Failure to regulate corporal veno-occlusion may be secondary to extraluminal or intraluminal obstructive pathophysiologies of the subtunical venules. Classic extraluminal obstructive mechanisms include pharmacological agents that induce persistent corporal smooth muscle relaxation, such as α-blockers and drugs with α-adrenergic effects (trazodone, clozapine), or intracavernosal/intraurethral agents (papaverine, prostaglandin E_1). Androgen administration may also cause priapism, perhaps related to facilitation of nitric oxide synthase (NOS) enzyme activity. Other extraluminal obstructive pathophysiologies are related to persistent neurological stimuli from central nervous system disorders such as spinal stenosis, as well as from erectile tissue infiltration with metastatic or local invasive tumours. Common intraluminal obstructive mechanisms include hyperviscosity, haematological disorders (sickle-cell disease, leukaemia), 20 per cent lipid administration in total parenteral nutrition, or fat embolism (pelvic fractures).

Management

A precise diagnosis should be established in all cases of priapism prior to therapeutic intervention. Veno-occlusive priapism can be diagnosed either by obtaining blood gas values (Po_2, pH, Pco_2) or determining cavernosal artery Doppler flow (absent in veno-occlusive priapism; present and bounding in arterial priapism). Aspects of the patient's history, particularly the presence or absence of penile pain, may also be of value in distinguishing veno-occlusive from arterial priapism. In patients with intact sensory nerves (i.e. excluding spinal cord injury, diabetes, etc.) veno-occlusive priapism is inevitably painful because of absent arterial inflow and resulting ischaemia. Arterial priapism is rarely associated with significant penile pain, although discomfort may be reported, particularly in the perineum—often the site of trauma. Since priapism may result in irreversible erectile dysfunction, it is important to establish the premorbid erectile function of the patient.

Other important aspects of the history include the occurrence and duration of previous episodes of prolonged erection or priapism, and response to previous therapies. Individuals with previous episodes of prolonged erection, often referred to clinically as 'stuttering' priapism, should be assessed for the presence of haematological conditions, such as sickle-cell disease or trait. Past or current use of intracorporal vasorelaxants (papaverine, prostaglandin E_1), psychotropic agents (trazodone, clozapine), α-blockers (prazosin), anticoagulants (heparin, coumarin), recreational drugs (cocaine), and over-the-counter adrenergic agonists (phenylephrine) should also be carefully assessed. Other aetiological factors include: penile or perineal trauma, such as falling on to a bicycle bar; haematological neoplasms such as leukaemia; metastatic or locally infiltrating neoplasms such as renal, bladder, or prostate carcinoma; neurological conditions such as

Table 5 Main causes of venous priapism

Haematological causes
   Haematological disorders
      Sickle-cell disease
      Thrombocythaemia
      Leukaemia
      Erythrocytosis
      Thalassaemia
Fat emboli
   Hyperlipidic parenteral nutrition
Iatrogenic
Miscellaneous
   Inflammation, infection, haemodialysis
   Metabolic causes
Pathological prolonged relaxation of cavernous smooth muscle
   Drugs
      Anticoagulant
      Antihypertensive
      Antidepressive
      Psychotrophic
      Androgen (testosterone)
      Erectogenic (intracavernous injections and oral)
      α-Blocker
      Parasympathometics
      Cocaine, alcohol
   Neurological disorders
      Spinal cord lesions
      Cauda equina compression
      Autonomic neuropathy
      Spinal stenosis
   Infection or toxic
      Rabies, scorpion sting
      Malaria

spinal cord compression or acute lumbosacral disc prolapse; coagulopathy, such as disseminated intravascular coagulopathy; and elevated intravascular fat levels such as during total parenteral nutrition or following a fat embolism.

The goal of treatment for veno-occlusive priapism is to restore normal cavernosal arterial inflow. When appropriate, based on the duration and severity of the priapism, initial treatment may consist of non-specific medical management. This will involve aspiration of intracavernosal blood and/or interval saline lavage of the corpora cavernosa with large-bore butterfly needles (bilateral if indicated), with or without a penile block (1 per cent lidocaine without adrenaline). If cavernosal arterial blood flow is not re-established, intracavernosal adrenergic agonist therapy may be initiated to induce corporal smooth muscle contraction pharmacologically and thus initiate detumescence. Interval intracavernosal irrigation with large-bore butterfly needles may also be used. When administering intracavernosal adrenergic therapy, consideration for cardiovascular monitoring should be considered, especially if the agent selected has significant $β_1$-activity and the patient has a history of cardiovascular disease.

When veno-occlusive priapism is related to a specific aetiology, full resolution typically requires specific medical management. Such patients include those who have utilized pharmacological agents which have induced persistent corporal smooth muscle relaxation, who have a neurogenic pathophysiology, erectile tissue infiltration, or intraluminal obstructive mechanisms such as sickle-cell disease, leukaemia, or 20 per cent lipid administration in total parenteral nutrition. All remediable causes of priapism should be managed with disease-specific therapy. This may include discontinuation of the drug causing the persistent smooth muscle relaxation (cocaine, trazodone, etc.), irradiation (leukaemia), hydration and exchange transfusion (sickle-cell disease), appropriate therapy for any neurological condition, or substituting 10 per cent for 20 per cent lipids in total parenteral nutrition.

Surgical treatment should be considered if the erection recurs despite repeated adrenergic agonist administration, thereby resulting in loss of cavernosal arterial inflow. This may consist of a Winter's procedure, which involves the development of percutaneous shunts between the corpus spongiosum and the corpora cavernosa. Should a percutaneous shunt not restore arterial inflow in the cavernosal arteries, an Al Ghorab (distal) shunt is indicated. A transverse incision is fashioned in the glans penis 1 cm proximal to the corona. Blunt dissection allows exposure and excision of the distal portions of the corpora cavernosa. The glans is then closed, creating an open fistula between the corpora cavernosa and corpus spongiosum. Several proximal shunting procedures have been described for the management of recalcitrant veno-occlusive priapism, including cavernovenous (cavernosaphenous and cavernodorsal vein) and proximal cavernosal–spongiosal (Quackles). The role of these procedures and their indications are not clearly defined.

Arterial priapism

Arterial priapism is a rare condition involving the inability to regulate arterial inflow, the usual cause being trauma to the perineum or penis. Such trauma can result in a lacerated cavernosal artery that sends arterial blood directly to the lacunar spaces, bypassing physiological helicine arteriolar resistance mechanisms. An arterial–lacunar fistula can often be identified on duplex Doppler ultrasonography (usually located in the perineum) and selective internal pudendal arteriography. Clinical presentation is with a painless, non-tender, moderately (not fully) rigid penile erection.

Arterial priapism is not a medical emergency since the condition does not involve absent cavernosal arterial inflow with resultant erectile tissue ischaemia. Management involves 'watchful waiting'. For patients who wish to undergo treatment, surgical ligation of the cavernosal artery fistula or arterial embolization is typically performed.

Table 6 Female sexual dysfunctions as defined by the International Consensus Development Conference on Female Sexual Dysfunction

I.	Sexual desire disorders
IA	Hypoactive sexual desire disorder—the persistent or recurrent deficiency (or absence) of sexual fantasies/thoughts, and/or desire for, or receptivity to, sexual activity, which causes personal distress
IB	Sexual aversion disorder—the persistent or recurrent phobic aversion to and avoidance of sexual contact with a sexual partner, which causes personal distress
II	Sexual arousal disorder—the persistent or recurrent inability to attain or maintain sufficient sexual excitement, causing personal distress. It may be expressed as a lack of subjective excitement or a lack of genital (lubrication/swelling) or other somatic responses
III	Orgasmic disorder—the persistent or recurrent difficulty, delay in, or absence of attaining orgasm following sufficient sexual stimulation and arousal, which causes personal distress
IV	Sexual pain disorders
IVA	Dyspareunia—recurrent or persistent genital pain associated with sexual intercourse
IVB	Vaginismus—recurrent or persistent involuntary spasm of the musculature of the outer third of the vagina that interferes with vaginal penetration, which causes personal distress
IVC	Non-coital sexual pain disorder—recurrent or persistent genital pain induced by non-coital sexual stimulation

Female sexual dysfunction

Introduction

Female sexual dysfunctions are broadly defined as alterations or disturbances in sexual functioning in women that are associated with subjective dissatisfaction or distress. These consist primarily of disorders of sexual desire, arousal, orgasm, and/or sexual pain (Table 6). While each of these disorders is uniquely defined, there is often significant overlap in affected patients. As noted above, about 40 per cent of adult women in community-based studies complain of one or more sexual dysfunctions in the past year. There has been limited investigation of the anatomy, physiology, and molecular biology of female sexual response, and the aetiology and pathophysiologies of specific sexual dysfunctions in women are not well understood. Stimulated in part by advances in male sexual dysfunction, there is increasing interest in basic science and clinical management aspects of female sexual dysfunction.

Anatomy and physiology

There are multiple anatomical structures which comprise the internal and external female genital tract, including the clitoris, labia minora, and corpus spongiosum (vestibular) erectile tissue, periurethral glans, urethra, anterior fornix, pubococcygeus muscle, and cervix. There are also multiple non-genital peripheral anatomical structures involved in female sexual response, such as salivary and sweat glands, cutaneous blood vessels, and nipples.

Internal and external genitalia

The vagina consists of a cyclindrical sheath of autonomically innervated smooth muscle (longitudinal outer, inner circular layer) lined by stratified squamous epithelium and a subdermal layer rich in capillaries. The vaginal wall consists of an inner glandular mucous-type stratified squamous cell epithelium supported by a thick lamina propia. This epithelium undergoes hormone-related cyclical changes, including slight keratinization of the superficial cells during the menstrual cycle. Deep to the epithelium lies the smooth muscle of the muscularis. There is a surrounding deeper fibrous layer above the muscularis, which provides structural support to the vagina and is rich is collagen and elastin, to allow for expansion of the vagina during sexual stimulation. Three sets of skeletal muscles surround the vagina, including the ischiocavernosum, bulbocavernosus, transverse perinei and levator ani, and pubococcygeus muscles.

The main arterial supply to the vagina flows to its superior aspect and arises from vaginal branches of the uterine artery. The middle portion of the vagina receives blood from the inferior vaginal artery, a branch of the hypogastric artery. The middle haemorrhoidal and the clitoral arteries send branches to the distal aspect of the vagina.

Autonomic efferent innervation of the vagina originates from the hypogastric plexus and the sacral plexus. These give rise to the uterovaginal nerves that contain both parasympathetic and sympathetic fibres, travelling within the uterosacral and cardinal ligaments to supply the proximal two-thirds of the vagina and the corporal bodies of the clitoris. Somatic afferent innervation is provided by the pudendal nerve, which reaches the perineum through Alcock's canal. There is an abundance of nerve fibres in the distal and anterior aspect of the vagina: these play a major role in sexual function and can easily be injured during pelvic surgery, or from blunt perineal trauma.

The vulva includes the labia minora, labia majora, the clitoris, the urinary meatus, the vaginal opening, and the corpus spongiosum erectile tissue (vestibular bulbs) of the labia minora. The labia majora are fatty folds covered by hair-bearing skin that fuses anteriorly with the mons veneris, or anterior prominence of the symphysis pubis, and posteriorly with the perineal body or posterior commissure. The labia minora are smaller folds covered by hairless skin laterally and by vaginal mucosa medially, and which fuse anteriorly to forms the prepuce of the clitoris, and posteriorly in the fossa navicularis. The perineal branch of the pudendal nerve innervates the labia. The main arterial supply arises from the inferior perineal branch of the internal pudendal, and by branches of the femoral artery.

The corpus spongiosum erectile tissues are paired structures located beneath the skin of the labia minora. The arterial supply is by the bulbar and posterior labial branches of the internal pudendal artery. The corpus spongiosum terminates in the glans clitoris. The corpora cavernosa of the clitoris measure up to 13 cm in length. The body of the clitoris consists of two paired erectile chambers composed of endothelial-lined lacunar spaces, trabecular smooth muscle, and trabecular connective tissue (collagen and elastin) surrounded by a fibrous sheath, the tunica albuginea. The arteries include the dorsal and clitoral cavernosal arteries, which arise from the iliohypogastric pudendal bed. The autonomic efferent motor innervation occurs via the cavernosal nerve of the clitoris, arising from the pelvic and hypogastric plexus.

As described above, the sexual response cycle in both men and women occurs in four stages: desire, arousal, orgasm, and resolution. The mechanisms underlying sexual response are less well understood in women than in men, particularly the role of central nervous system and hormonal processes. Sexual arousal responses in the genital and non-genital peripheral anatomical structures are largely the product of spinal cord reflex mechanisms. The spinal segments are under descending excitatory and inhibitory control from multiple supraspinal sites. The afferent reflex arm is primarily via the pudendal nerve; the efferent reflex arm consists of co-ordinated somatic and autonomic activity. One spinal sexual reflex is the bulbocavernosus reflex involving sacral cord segments S2, 3, and 4 in which pudendal nerve stimulation results in pelvic floor muscle contraction. Another spinal sexual reflex involves vaginal and clitoral cavernosal autonomic nerve stimulation and results in clitoral, labial, and vaginal engorgement.

In the unstimulated state, clitoral corporal and vaginal smooth muscles are under contractile tone. Following sexual stimulation, neurogenic- and endothelial-mediated release of nitric oxide (NO) plays a key role in clitoral cavernosal artery and helicine arteriolar smooth muscle relaxation. This leads to clitoral engorgement, a rise in clitoral cavernosal artery inflow, and an increase in clitoral intracavernosal pressure. The result is extrusion of the glans clitoris and enhanced sensitivity.

In the basal state the vaginal epithelium reabsorbs sodium from the submucosal capillary plasma transudate. Following sexual stimulation, neurotransmitters including NO and vasoactive intestinal peptide modulate vaginal and vaginal arteriolar smooth muscle relaxation. A dramatic increase in capillary inflow in the submucosa overwhelms sodium reabsorption leading to 3 to 5 ml of vaginal transudate, enhancing lubrication essential for pleasurable coitus. Vaginal smooth muscle relaxation results in increased vaginal length and luminal diameter, especially in the distal two-thirds. Vasoactive intestinal polypeptide is a non-adrenergic non-cholinergic neurotransmitter that plays a key role in enhancing vaginal blood flow, lubrication, and secretions.

Hormones

Steroid hormones play an important role in the regulation of female sexual function. Symptoms associated with diminished oestrogen include vaginal dryness, irritation, and pain, as well as causing complaints regarding sexual function such as decreased sexual arousal, decreased genital sensation, and difficulty achieving orgasm. Oestrogen replacement in postmenopausal or surgically menopausal women restores clitoral and vaginal pressure thresholds to premenopausal levels. Oestrogens have also vasoprotective and vasodilatory effects, which result in increased vaginal and clitoral blood flow, preventing atherosclerotic compromise of the iliohypogastric arterial bed. Thickness and rugae of the vaginal wall, as well as vaginal lubrication, are both oestrogen dependent. Oestrogen also improves integrity of vaginal mucosal tissue and has beneficial effects on vaginal sensation, vasocongestion, and secretions. By contrast, oestrogen deprivation leads to decreased pelvic blood flow resulting in clitoral fibrosis, thinned vaginal epithelial layers, and decreased vaginal submucosal vasculature.

In addition to conventional hormone replacement therapy and topical oestrogen creams, exogenous water- and oil-based lubricants have been used for alleviating symptoms of vaginal irritation and dryness. Although some of these agents have properties similar to vaginal fluid, they are limited by application time and duration of effectiveness. Oestrogen replacement therapy and oestrogen creams are effective for relieving symptoms of vaginal dryness in many women, but they are not a viable alternative for all women.

Low testosterone levels are often associated with a decline in sexual arousal, genital sensation, libido, and orgasm. Testosterone administration in women with decreased desire has been successful, although there are no currently approved testosterone preparations for this purpose. It has also been shown that menopausal women respond better to parental oestrogen–androgen than oestrogen alone in restoring sexual desire, energy, and sense of well being.

Specific sexual dysfunctions in women

Hypoactive sexual desire disorder

Hypoactive sexual desire disorder is defined as chronic or persistent deficiency of sexual interest or desire. It is distinguished from sexual aversion disorder, which is characterized by persistent or recurrent phobic aversion to, and avoidance of, sexual contact with a partner. Hypoactive sexual desire disorder is the most commonly reported sexual problem in women, affecting approximately 20 to 30 per cent of those aged 30 to 70 years. It is age-related and strongly associated with other medical and psychiatric disorders, particularly chronic illnesses and depression. It may be related to the use of prescription drugs, particularly antidepressants (e.g. SSRIs), alcohol abuse, or hormonal changes. Low sexual desire in women is also frequently associated with partner conflicts or the presence of other sexual dysfunctions (such as erectile dysfunction, anorgasmia). The degree of personal distress associated with the disorder varies widely and should be taken into account in making the diagnosis.

Female sexual arousal disorder

Female sexual arousal disorder refers to a chronic or persistent lack of subjective or physical arousal during sexual stimulation. This is characterized by an inability to achieve an adequate lubrication–swelling response of the vagina and labia for the completion of sexual activity, or a lack of subjective arousal during sexual activity. Although women with sexual arousal disorder may perform intercourse, the lack of adequate lubrication may result in pain or vaginal irritation. Findings from the National Health and Social Life Survey in the United States showed that approximately 20 per cent of women aged 18 to 59 reported difficulty in lubrication during sexual stimulation. Similar prevalence estimates were reported in a large-scale British study, which also found that sexual arousal difficulties became commoner with agieng, and that marital difficulties, anxiety, and depression were all significant risk factors.

Orgasmic disorder

Orgasmic disorder in women is a persistent or recurrent difficulty, delay in, or absence of orgasmic attainment despite adequate sexual stimulation and arousal. Primary anorgasmia refers to the woman who has never experienced orgasm through any means, whereas secondary orgasmic dysfunction occurs when a woman is unable to have orgasm with a particular partner or by means of specific stimulation (i.e. sexual intercourse). Both types of orgasmic dysfunction are common, affecting 10 to 20 per cent of women in population-based studies and associated with medical or psychiatric illnesses, use of prescription or non-prescription drugs, and specific neurological disorders (such as spinal cord injury). Relationship conflicts were also found to be significantly associated with the occurrence of orgasmic difficulties in women in a recent British study.

Dyspareunia

Dyspareunia, or pain associated with sexual intercourse, is common in women. The pain may occur before, during, or after intercourse. In most cases it is caused by a lack of lubrication or other physical cause. According to the National Health and Social Life Survey, about 15 per cent of women have experienced pain during sexual activity during the past year. In postmenopausal women, the prevalence of dyspareunia may be even higher. A wide variety of medical or organic conditions are associated, including hymenal scarring, pelvic inflammatory disease, and vulvar vestibulitis. However, dyspareunia is not reliably associated with any particular medical disorder. Moreover, anatomical or physiological factors that may have caused the original pain may not be the same factors responsible for maintaining it. Accordingly, some authors have recommended an interactive or multidimensional model of physical and psychological determinants of dyspareunia.

Vaginismus

Vaginismus, or involuntary spasms of the musculature of the outer third of the vagina, is a significant cause of penetration difficulties in women. The disorder is often seen in sex therapy clinics, occurring in approximately 15 to 17 per cent of women presenting for treatment who often complain of secondary dyspareunia in addition to other sexual dysfunctions. Women with primary or generalized vaginismus typically avoid gynaecological examinations and tampon use, in addition to sexual intercourse. Vaginismus can occur in association with vaginal pain due to various medical conditions, although it is more frequently related to psychological or interpersonal factors.

Management of female sexual dysfunction

Diagnostic assessment

There is no consensus on the routine diagnostic assessment of the woman with sexual dysfunction. Common features of the work-up typically include history (sexual, psychosocial, and medical), physical examination (external genitalia, internal genitalia), and laboratory testing (oestrogen, testosterone, glucose, full blood count, creatinine, liver function tests, cholesterol, urine analysis, vaginal cultures as appropriate). Specialized tests, such as vaginal photoplethysmography, have been reported in the literature, but are not used in routine clinical practice. Other specialized investigations may include: (i) neurological (somatosensory evoked potential, electromyography), (ii) hormonal, and (iii) psychological (depression, anxiety).

Treatment

There are limited data on safety and efficacy of the various primary psychological and hormonal treatments that have been used for female sexual dysfunction.

Psychological therapy has demonstrated efficacy in sexual desire, orgasmic disorders, vaginismus, and sexual pain disorders. Oestrogen and/or androgen replacement hormonal therapy may be useful in sexual desire, arousal, orgasmic, and dyspareunia sexual pain disorders. Oestrogen replacement is indicated in menopausal women to relieve hot flushes, prevent osteoporosis, lower the risk of cardiovascular disease, improve clitoral sensitivity, and decrease pain and burning during intercourse. In combination with oestrogen, methyl testosterone is used to treat symptoms of inhibited desire, dyspareunia, and lack of vaginal lubrication, as well as for its vasoprotective effects.

Other treatment options with scant efficacy and safety evaluations include vaginal lubricants, vasodilator agents such as sildenafil citrate, vaginal dilators, pelvic floor rehabilitation using biofeedback electromyography, and Kegel exercises.

Patient and partner education is an essential component in the management of female sexual dysfunction and should be a continuous element at each phase in the process of care. Modification of known risk factors (hypertension, hyperlipidaemia, prescription drugs, cigarette smoking, and alcohol abuse) and self-destructive behaviours is part of good clinical practice.

Summary

Female sexual dysfunction is age-related and common, affecting 30 to 50 per cent of women. Improved understanding of both normal and dysfunctional sexual response in women is the keystone to enhanced management. A collaborative and comprehensive evaluation, patient and partner education, modification of reversible causes, and an individualized treatment plan should be the standard management of women with sexual dysfunction.

Basic science and clinical research in female sexual function and dysfunction are needed to overcome the gender gap, achieve a more balanced therapeutic perspective between psychological and physiological factors, and offer female patients enhanced opportunity for relief of a persistent or recurrent sexual condition that causes significant personal distress.

Further reading

Bastuba MD *et al.* (1994). Arterial priapism: Diagnosis, treatment and long term follow up. *Journal of Urology* **151**, 1231–7.

Cooper AJ, Cernovsky ZZ, Colussi K (1993). Clinical and psychometric characteristics of primary and secondary premature ejaculators. *Journal of Sex and Marital Therapy* **19**, 276–88.

DeBusk R *et al.* (2000). Management of sexual dysfunction in patients with cardiovascular disease: Recommendations of the Princeton Panel. *American Journal of Cardiology* **86**, 175–81.

Dunn KM, Croft PR, Hackett GI (1998). Sexual problems: a study of the prevalence and need for health care in the general population. *Family Practice* **15**, 519–24.

Feldman HA *et al.* (1994). Impotence and its medical and psychosocial correlates: Results of the Massachusetts Male Aging Study. *Journal of Urology* **151**, 54–61.

Goldstein I *et al.* (1998). Oral sildenafil in the treatment of erectile dysfunction. *New England Journal of Medicine* **338**, 1397–404.

Hakim LS *et al.* (1996). Evolving concepts in the diagnosis and management of high flow priapism. *Journal of Urology* **155**, 541–8.

Jardin A *et al.* eds (2000). *Erectile dysfunction: 1st International Consultation on Erectile Dysfunction. Plymouth, U.K.* Health Publications, United Kingdom.

Kulmala RV, Lehtonen TA, Tammela TLJ (1996). Preservation of potency after treatment of priapism. *Scandinavian Journal of Urology and Nephrology* **30**, 313–16.

Lauman EO, Paik A, Rosen RC (1999). Sexual dysfunction in the United States: Prevalence and predictors. *Journal of the American Medical Association* **281**, 537–44.

Lue TF (2000). Erectile dysfunction. *New England Journal of Medicine* **342**, 1802–13.

Masters WH, Johnson VE (1970). *Human sexual inadequacy.* Little, Brown, Boston.

Rosen RC, Lane RM, Menza M (1999). Effects of SSRIs on sexual function: A critical review. *Journal of Clinical Psychopharmacology* **19**, 67–85.

Spector IP, Carey MP (1990). Incidence and prevalence of the sexual dysfunctions: A critical review. *Archives of Sexual Behavior* **19**, 389–409.

Spycher MA, Hauri D (1986). The ultrastructure of the erectile tissue in priapism. *Journal of Urology* **135**, 142–7.

12.9 Disorders of development

12.9.1 Normal and abnormal sexual differentiation

M. O. Savage

Introduction

Disorders of sexual differentiation are characterized by an abnormality in the formation of the internal or external genital structures. Most are genetically determined and are associated with an ambiguous appearance of the external genitalia. During the past three decades, the study of intersex disorders has changed in orientation. The emphasis has moved away from descriptive clinical syndromes towards the biochemical and molecular nature of the defects that cause them. If such an aetiological approach is to be used, a fundamental understanding of normal sexual differentiation is required. This provides the basis for the classification, investigation, and management of patients with abnormal sexual differentiation.

Physiology of fetal sexual differentiation

In the male, it is established that the castrated embryo develops as a female, indicating that the fetal testis is essential for male development. The chromosomal sex of the embryo, established at conception, directs the development of either ovaries or testes. In the male, specific genes on the short arm of the Y chromosome, known as the sex-determining region of the Y chromosome, code for testis determination, and hence contribute to testicular differentiation. Testicular Leydig cells synthesize and secrete testosterone from 8 weeks of gestation, aided by stimulation with placental human chorionic gonadotrophin (hCG). Testosterone diffuses locally to maintain and virilize the wolffian ducts which become the vas deferens, seminal vesicles, and epididymis. Antimüllerian hormone, or müllerian-inhibitory factor, is a glycoprotein which is secreted during the same time period by testicular Sertoli cells to inhibit the formation of the uterus, fallopian tubes, and upper vagina from the müllerian structures.

In androgen-dependent tissues, testosterone is converted to dihydrotestosterone which virilizes the external genitalia. Peripheral androgen action depends on the binding of the androgen in the target tissues to a receptor coded by an X chromosome.

In the female, ovarian development occurs in the presence of two X chromosomes and external gonadal development occurs spontaneously. Genital development in both sexes is completed by 20 weeks of fetal life. In the male, growth of the formed penis is dependent upon continued testicular testosterone secretion under stimulation by pituitary gonadotrophins.

Table 1 Classification of intersex states

Female pseudohermaphrodite: virilization of genetic female with ovaries
Male pseudohermaphrodite: incomplete virilization of genetic male with testes
True hermaphrodite: individual with ovarian and testicular tissue

Classification of intersex states

The classification that forms the basis of clinical assessment and management depends on gonadal morphology (Table 1). Female pseudohermaphroditism describes genital ambiguity resulting from abnormal virilization of a female with normal ovaries. The male counterpart—male pseudohermaphroditism—is the result of incomplete virilization of a male with differentiated testes. Thirdly, the true hermaphrodite possesses both ovarian and testicular tissue.

Female pseudohermaphroditism

Female pseudohermaphrodites have 46 XX karyotypes with normal ovaries and müllerian structures, but the external genitalia are virilized. The aetiology of female pseudohermaphroditism is given in Table 2. The degree of genital ambiguity can range from enlargement of the clitoris or fusion of the posterior labia to a completely male appearance, depending on the timing of androgen production and the concentration of androgens in the fetal circulation. Virilization may be caused by excessive production of either fetal or maternal androgens.

Virilization by fetal androgens

Congenital adrenal hyperplasia (see also Chapter 12.7.2)
The commonest cause of ambiguous genitalia in the newborn female is a recessively inherited enzyme defect of cortisol synthesis, with diversion of

Table 2 Aetiology of female pseudohermaphroditism

Virilization by fetal androgens
Congenital adrenal hyperplasia
    21-Hydroxylase deficiency
    11β-Hydroxylase deficiency
    3β-Hydroxysteroid dehydrogenase deficiency
Other causes of fetal androgen overproduction
    Fetal adrenal adenoma
    Nodular adrenal hyperplasia
    Persistent fetal adrenal (preterm infants)
Fetal virilization by maternal androgens
Ovarian tumours
Adrenal tumours
Iatrogenic fetal virilization
Testosterone and progestins
Female pseudohermaphroditism with associated congenital malformations

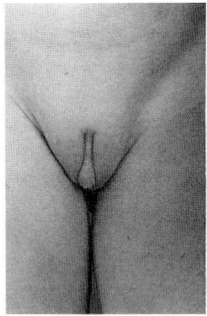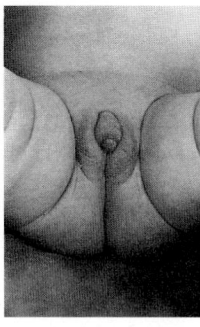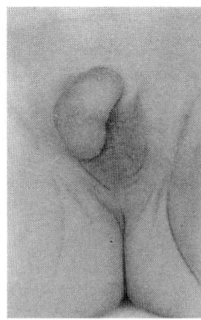

Fig. 1 Variation in degree of virilization in three female infants with 21-hydroxylase deficiency.

intermediates to androgen production. A reduction in steroid 21-hydroxylase or absence of 11β-hydroxylase or 3β-hydroxysteroid dehydrogenase can be the cause of this condition. These enzymes are part of the steroid biosynthetic pathways which link cholesterol with cortisol, aldosterone, and androgens. In the absence of, or lowered potential for, cortisol production, there are high adrenocorticotrophic hormone (ACTH) levels leading to adrenal hyperplasia and excess androgen production.

21-hydroxylase deficiency This form of congenital adrenal hyperplasia accounts for 90 per cent of cases of female pseudohermaphroditism, and should be excluded before proceeding to assign other causes for ambiguous genitalia. The degree of virilization can be variable (Fig. 1). In Europe, 60 per cent of all cases will develop salt depletion due to decreased production of aldosterone in the first 2 weeks of life. Usually, there is enlargement of the clitoris associated with a degree of posterior labial fusion and the formation of a hypoplastic lower vagina which may open into the urethra.

17-Hydroxyprogesterone is a biosynthetic precursor of cortisol, and plasma levels are elevated in 21-hydroxylase deficiency. After the third day of life, there is good discrimination between plasma levels of 17-hydroxyprogesterone in affected cases (100–800 nmol/l) and those of normal infants (less than 15 nmol/l). Measurement of plasma renin activity and aldosterone help to define the extent of mineralocorticoid deficiency. Analysis of urine steroid excretion using chromatography and mass spectrometry can provide a reliable diagnostic profile from day 3 after birth. A variant of 21-hydroxylase deficiency, due to a milder defect, is the non-classical form of the disease, characterized by absence of neonatal genital ambiguity but development of other signs of androgen excess such as hirsutism.

11β-hydroxylase deficiency This defect probably accounts for about 5 per cent of all cases of congenital adrenal hyperplasia. The disorder is caused by mutations of the *CYP11B1* gene which abolish enzyme activity. The virilization may be severe, with affected females sometimes raised as males. The plasma concentration of 11-deoxycortisol (compound S) is elevated, and may exceed 1000 nmol/l. The urine steroid pattern will show high excretion of 6-hydroxytetrahydro-11-deoxycortisol as well as of tetrahydro-S.

3β-hydroxysteroid dehydrogenase deficiency This rare defect was originally described in male infants with incomplete virilization. However, a paradoxical androgen affect may be seen in female infants due to a very high level of dehydroepiandrosterone, the steroid precursor immediately proximal to the enzyme block. A non-classical or attenuated form of 3β-hydroxysteroid dehydrogenase deficiency has been described which presents with virilization in postadrenarchal or peripubertal females.

Virilization by maternal androgens
Virilization of the external genitalia by a maternal ovarian or adrenal androgen-secreting tumour is a rare but well-recognized cause of female pseudohermaphroditism. The degree of virilization may be striking.

Other causes of fetal virilization
Female pseudohermaphroditism due to maternal administration of progestogen preparations became recognized about 30 years ago. A number of dysmorphic childhood syndromes may also be associated with virilized female genitalia.

Male pseudohermaphroditism
Male pseudohermaphroditism arises as a result of a disturbance of male genital development in patients with testes and a 46 XY karyotype. The genital anomaly can vary from apparently female to male external genitalia with a small penis or perineal hypospadias. The three main aetiological groups (Table 3) are impaired Leydig cell activity, peripheral androgen insensitivity, and deficient testosterone and antimüllerian hormone production by incompletely differentiated testes.

Impaired testicular secretion of testosterone
Inborn errors of testosterone biosynthesis
These rare disorders (Fig. 2) lead to defective testosterone synthesis during the critical period of fetal sexual differentiation. The result is inadequate

Table 3 Aetiology of male pseudohermaphroditism

Impaired Leydig cell activity
Inborn errors of testosterone biosynthesis
    Deficient formation of pregnenolone
    3β-Hydroxysteroid dehydrogenase deficiency
    17α-Hydroxylase deficiency
    17,20-Desmolase deficiency
    17β-Hydroxysteroid dehydrogenase deficiency
Leydig cell hypoplasia: luteinizing hormone receptor defect
Androgen insensitivity syndromes
Androgen receptor defects
    Complete androgen insensitivity
    Incomplete androgen insensitivity
5α-Reductase deficiency
Incomplete differentiation of testes with deficient testosterone and antimüllerian hormone production
Mixed gonadal dysgenesis
Dysgenetic male pseudohermaphroditism
XY pure gonadal dysgenesis
Drash syndrome
Other forms
Iatrogenic male pseudohermaphroditism
Associated with other congenital anomalies
Persistent müllerian structures

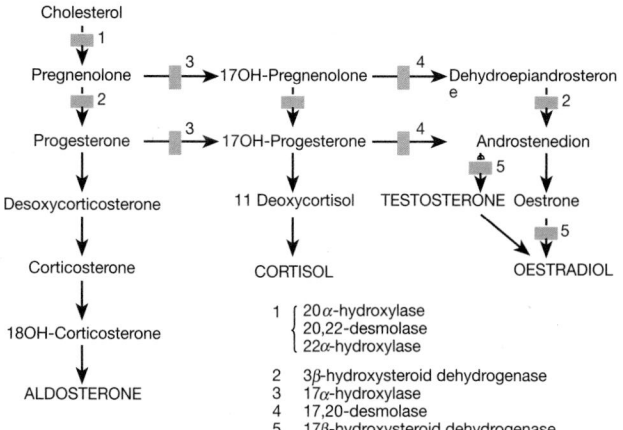

Fig. 2 Enzyme defects in testosterone biosynthesis.

testosterone secretion, either locally to virilize the wolffian ducts to form the vas deferens, seminal vesicles, or epididimis, or peripherally to virilize the external genitalia. Synthesis of antimüllerian hormone, being a glycoprotein rather than a steroid, is unaffected. When the enzyme deficiency, inherited as an autosomal recessive trait, is situated early in the biosynthetic pathway, adrenal steroid synthesis may also be affected.

Deficient formation of pregnenolone Three closely related microsomal enzymes (20α-hydroxylase, 20,22-desmolase, and 22α-hydroxylase) are necessary for the conversion of cholesterol to pregnenolone. Deficiency of one of these enzymes leads to impaired synthesis of cortisol, aldosterone, and testosterone. Accumulation of cholesterol has been demonstrated in the hyperplastic adrenal leading to the term congenital lipoid adrenal hyperplasia. Recently, the gene responsible for the disorder has been cloned and validated by the demonstration of a non-sense mutation. The gene encodes for a protein named StAR (steroidogenic acute regulatory protein).

Deficiency of 3β-hydroxysteroid dehydrogenase Male patients with this enzyme deficiency are poorly virilized and usually develop salt loss and adrenal failure in infancy. Some subjects have survived puberty, which has been characterized by virilization and gynaecomastia. Urinary pregnenetriol and plasma dehydroepiandrosterone are elevated, as is plasma renin activity. Several mutations of the type II 3β-hydroxysteroid dehydrogenase enzyme have been reported.

Deficiency of 17α-hydroxylase This defect in cytochrome P450c17 results in decreased cortisol synthesis by the adrenal cortex and testosterone by the fetal testes, resulting usually in a complete lack of virilization. Several different mutations of the *CYP17* gene have been reported. The disorder is identified biochemically by demonstrating high serum and urinary levels of progesterone and corticosterone. A compensatory increase in ACTH leads to excess mineralocorticoid secretion, causing hypertension, hypokalaemia, and low plasma renin activity.

Deficiency of 17,20-desmolase This rare defect is related to 17-hydroxylase deficiency as both enzyme activities are coded by the same gene. Impaired virilization may be variable in degree. Biochemically, identification of the defect relies on elevation of plasma 17-hydroxyprogesterone, 17-hydroxypregnenolone, and urinary pregnanetriolone.

Deficiency of 17-ketosteroid reductase (17β-hydroxysteroid dehydrogenase) Patients with this defect are born with female-looking external genitalia and a phallus closely resembling a normal clitoris. There are three types of 17β-hydroxysteroid dehydrogenase enzyme. Abnormalities of the type 3 enzyme, which has specific testicular expression, causes this disorder and several different mutations of the respective gene have been described. There is a high prevalence of this disorder within the Arab population of the Gaza Strip. The enzyme defect interferes with conversion of androstenedione to testosterone, adrenal steroid synthesis being unaffected. There is elevation of the androstenedione to testosterone ratio, particularly after hCG stimulation. Subjects are usually raised as girls; however, gender conversion to male has been described, coinciding with the marked virilization which occurs at puberty.

Androgen insensitivity syndromes

Mechanisms of androgen action

Testosterone, the principal androgen secreted by the testis, circulates bound to two proteins, sex hormone binding globulin and albumin. The protein-bound steroid is in dynamic equilibrium with the free hormone. Free testosterone enters the target cell by a passive mechanism (Fig. 3). Inside the cell, testosterone can be reduced to dihydrotestosterone by the enzyme 5α-reductase. Testosterone or dihydrotestosterone binds with high affinity to specific receptor proteins to form an androgen–receptor complex. This complex enters the cell nucleus and, after transformation into a DNA binding state, binds to specific nucleotide sequences which promote transcrip-

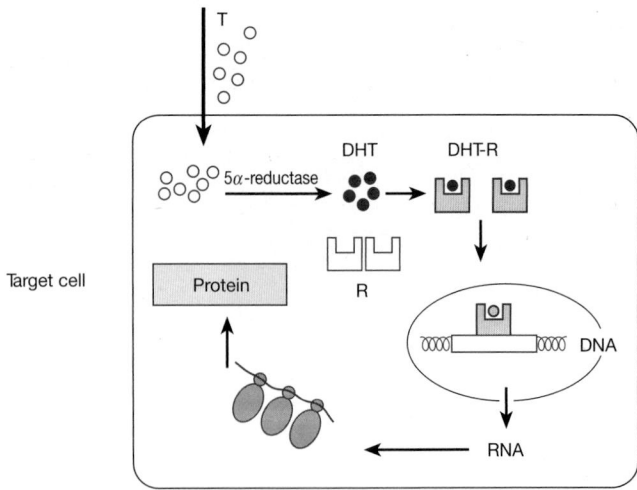

Fig. 3 Scheme of intracellular androgen action (adapted from Hughes and Pinsky, 1989). T, testosterone; DHT, dihydrotestosterone; R, receptor.

tion of messenger RNA, resulting in clinical virilization. The gene encoding the human androgen receptor has recently been cloned.

Although testosterone and dihydrotestosterone bind to the same receptor, the two hormones perform different roles in androgen physiology (Fig. 4). Testosterone regulates secretion of luteinizing hormone, virilizes the wolffian ducts during fetal life, and may be essential for spermatogenesis. Dihydrotestosterone is responsible for formation of the external genitalia and prostate, and for most secondary sexual effects, such as hair growth and enlargement of the genitalia.

Clinical features of androgen insensitivity

Abnormalities of androgen action may have a severe effect on male sexual differentiation, resulting in incomplete virilization during fetal life and at puberty. The syndromes of androgen insensitivity probably account for the majority of cases of male pseudohermaphroditism. There are three main forms. The most important numerically is an X-linked cystolic androgen receptor defect. This may be manifested by a broad clinical spectrum from complete androgen insensitivity to a virtually normally formed male with infertility. The second form is known as receptor-positive resistance, where a similar spectrum of clinical defects is associated with apparently normal receptor function. Thirdly, 5α-reductase deficiency is an autosomally inherited enzyme defect resulting in impaired conversion of testosterone to dihydrotestosterone in the target cell.

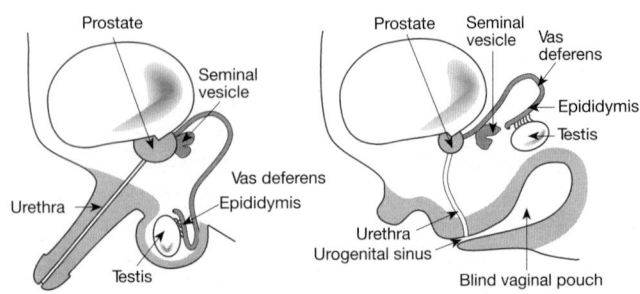

Fig. 4 Roles of testosterone and dihydrotestosterone in male sexual differentiation in the normal male (left) and the patient with 5α-reductase deficiency (right). Testosterone, heavy shading; dihydrotestosterone, light shading.

Androgen receptor defects

These defects may be expressed clinically as a spectrum of deficient formation of the male internal and external genitalia.

Complete androgen insensitivity The typical patient with presents after puberty with primary amenorrhoea, or before puberty with inguinal hernias and palpable testes. The phenotype and psychosexual orientation is female. Breasts develop as in a normal woman, but pubic and axillary hair is scanty and the vagina is blind-ending due to regression of müllerian structures, which are virtually always absent. Wolffian structures are usually absent and the gonads show Leydig cell hyperplasia with no spermatogenesis. There is a significant risk of gonadal malignancy occurring after puberty, when gonadectomy is recommended.

Incomplete androgen insensitivity Here there is a range of impaired virilization from clitoral enlargement and labial fusion to small external genitalia, usually with hypospadias. At puberty, feminization may be dominant, with gynaecomastia a feature in some patients.

The endocrine features of androgen insensitivity are essentially similar in the range of clinical defects. Testicular androgen secretion is normal or increased. Plasma testosterone may be elevated in infancy but is normal during the remainder of the prepubertal period. At puberty, plasma testosterone, oestradiol, and sex hormone binding globulin levels are elevated. Plasma gonadotrophins are normal in childhood but both luteinizing hormone and follicle stimulating hormone levels are consistently elevated during and after puberty, due to insensitivity of the hypothalamic androgen receptor. Patients are usually infertile.

5α-Reductase deficiency

This autosomal recessive disorder is characterized by impaired conversion of testosterone to dihydrotestosterone in androgen-dependent target cells. It was first described in the Dominican Republic, and occurs principally in areas of high consanguinity. The clinical features can be summarized as showing male internal genital structures and female external genitalia (Fig. 4). Fetal dihydrotestosterone-dependent development is abnormal, resulting in a rudimentary phallus and absent prostate. The wolffian structures develop normally, and the testes differentiate with spermatogenesis capable of progressing to the spermatozoa stage. Most subjects are raised as females but gender conversion to male occurs at puberty, coinciding with striking virilization of body habitus (Fig. 5) and male psychosexual orientation. Virilization during and after puberty, however, is incomplete, as the penis remains small and body and facial hair is sparse.

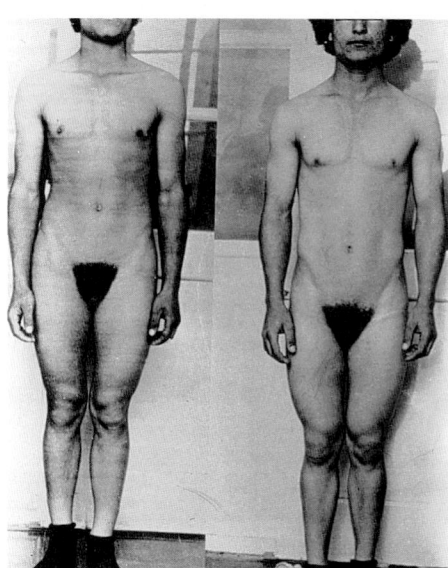

Fig. 5 Two Greek Cypriot brothers with 5α-reductase deficiency.

The endocrine features comprise low plasma dihydrotestosterone with normal testosterone and an elevated testosterone to dihydrotestosterone ratio. This abnormal ratio is the cardinal diagnostic feature. There is also elevation of the ratio of 5β : 5α androgen metabolites (i.e. aetiocholanolone to androsterone) in urine.

Male pseudohermaphroditism related to abnormal testicular differentiation

Incomplete differentiation of the fetal testes due to a defect of the Y-chromosomal genes responsible for testicular determination may cause genital ambiguity. Incompletely formed or dysgenetic testes secrete insufficient testosterone and antimüllerian hormone for normal male development. A number of clinical syndromes exist in this category.

Dysgenetic male pseudohermaphroditism

In this syndrome there are bilateral dysgenetic testes, persistent müllerian structures, cryptorchidism, and poorly virilized external genitalia.

Mixed gonadal dysgenesis

Here there is asymmetrical gonadal differentiation with a testis present on one side and a streak gonad on the other. The internal structures are also asymmetrical, reflecting the endocrine function of the ipsilateral gonad. Many patients have a mosaic XO/XY karyotype and features of Turner's syndrome.

Drash syndrome

This syndrome combines dysgenetic testes, genital ambiguity, glomerulonephritis, and Wilms' tumour.

True hermaphroditism

The diagnosis of true hermaphroditism is made when ovarian as well as testicular tissue is present in the same individual. Van Niekerk has published an extensive review of the literature, including a large personal series. The most common presenting symptoms are abnormal appearance of the external genitalia. Most patients have a 46 XX karyotype: about half are pure 46 XX and about a third are mosaics or chimeras with 46 XX cell lines, that is 46 XX/46 XY. A few patients with a pure 46 XY karyotype have been reported. Occasional familial cases of true hermaphroditism have been described in the literature.

Other 46 XX intersex states

Pure gonadal dysgenesis

This disorder, which may be familial, is usually associated with female external genitalia. Clitoromegaly is sometimes present. The gonads are streaks and the karyotype may be 46 XX or XY. 46 XY gonadal dysgenesis, inherited as an X-linked recessive or male-limited autosomal dominant condition, has also been described.

XX male

A number of XX males have been described. These are normal-appearing males with normal intelligence and male psychosexual orientation. Gynaecomastia, sparse facial hair, small genitalia, and hypospadias may occur in this syndrome. The testes are small and resemble Klinefelter testes histologically. There is absence of spermatogenesis, leading to sterility. Families have been reported containing both an XX male and a 46 XX true hermaphrodite.

Gonadal neoplasia and intersex states

It is now established that a number of intersex disorders carry an increased risk of gonadal tumours. Two important risk factors are the presence of dysgenetic gonadal tissue and a Y chromosome. Intra-abdominal gonads are more susceptible than scrotal glands. The commonest tumour is a gonadoblastoma which is a premalignant lesion but can progress to an invasive tumour.

Table 4 Patient with intersex state: clinical assessment

Family history, general examination for dysmorphic features
Examination of external genitalia
No gonads palpable
  Female pseudohermaphrodite: congenital adrenal hyperplasia
    (21-hydroxylase deficiency)
  Male pseudohermaphrodite
One gonad palpable
  Abnormal gonadal differentiation
  Mixed gonadal dysgenesis (XO/XY)
  True hermaphroditism
Two gonads palpable
  Male pseudohermaphrodite
  Impaired testosterone biosynthesis
  Androgen receptor defect
  5α-Reductase deficiency
  True hermaphroditism

Table 5 Patient with intersex state: laboratory assessment

No gonads palpable
Karyotype, plasma 17-hydroxyprogesterone, 11-deoxycortisol
One gonad palpable
Karyotype, hCG test, gonadal biopsy, pelvic ultrasonography, laparotomy
Two gonads palpable
Karyotype, hCG test (hCG 1000 units daily×3), plasma testosterone,
  dihydrotestosterone, dehydroepiandrosterone, androstenedione on days 0
  and 4
In vitro androgen binding studies
Sinogram
DNA analysis

Clinical and laboratory assessment of patients with intersex states

The assessment of patients with intersex states may be considered from the point of view of the paediatrician assessing an infant with ambiguous genitalia. The same principles apply to the older child or adult. It must be emphasized that the general appearance of the external genitalia, while important in deciding the appropriate gender for the child, is of very little help in defining the aetiology of the disorder.

Clinical assessment

The principles of clinical assessment are shown in Table 4. A history of a similar disorder in other family members may shed light on the likely diagnosis. Many of these conditions are genetically determined. Examination for other anomalies which could point to a dysmorphic syndrome known to be associated with abnormal genital development is also relevant. The most important aspect of the examination, however, is careful palpation of the gonads.

If no gonads are palpable, the most likely diagnosis is female pseudohermaphroditism due to congenital adrenal hyperplasia, and this is virtually certain if symptoms of salt loss develop. Other possible disorders are true hermaphroditism or male pseudohermaphroditism with intra-abdominal gonads. When both gonads are palpable in the scrotum or labial folds, the patient is likely to be a male pseudohermaphrodite, and measurement of plasma androgens will indicate whether the aetiology is a testicular or peripheral defect. A true hermaphrodite with bilateral ovotestes may also present in this way. The presence of only one palpable gonad or asymmetry of the perineum is suggestive of mixed gonadal dysgenesis; true hermaphroditism with asymmetrical gonads is the other differential diagnosis.

Laboratory assessment

A similar scheme may be devised as a guide to confirming the aetiology biochemically (Table 5). In all intersex patients a karyotype is indicated. If no gonads are palpable, determination of plasma 17-hydroxyprogesterone will confirm or exclude 21-hydroxylase deficiency. In 11β-hydroxylase deficiency the plasma 11-deoxycortisol concentration is elevated. The infant with two palpable gonads needs an hCG stimulation test to assess testicular androgen secretion. Numerous hCG regimens exist, of which two examples are 1000 IU daily for 3 days or a single injection of 1500 IU/m² body surface area. Basal and poststimulatory concentrations of testosterone, dihydrotestosterone, and androstenedione should distinguish a disorder of testosterone biosynthesis from a syndrome of androgen insensitivity.

If one gonad is palpable, gonadal biopsy may be helpful, particularly if ovarian tissue is suspected. Pelvic ultrasonography or exploratory laparotomy for identification of internal genital structures may also be indicated.

In any patient with incomplete virilization, urethrography should be performed to identify a vaginal cavity communicating posteriorly with the urethra.

Medical management

Choice of gender

Parents are usually shocked to learn that there is doubt as to the sex of their child; they are often under the impression that the child may grow up to be neither male nor female. Temptation to give a provisional opinion should be avoided until the nature of the disorder is known and an informed answer can be given. The decision as to the appropriate sex-of-rearing is based mainly on the appearance of the external genitalia and on the likely pattern of secondary sexual development at puberty. This decision should be taken jointly by the endocrinologist, urologist, and the parents. The gender should be assigned as soon as possible; however, in some cases of severe ambiguity, there is a case for waiting to assess the effect of early treatment with depot testosterone (25–50 mg at monthly intervals) on phallic growth as a guide to androgen responsiveness.

The concept that, once established, gender identity and role are more or less fixed has now been questioned. Although change of gender may be extremely difficult, the possibility of gender conversion should be viewed with an open mind in the individual subject who, because of spontaneous virilization or feminization at puberty, finds existence in their original gender intolerable.

Sex hormone therapy

Long-term treatment with androgens to promote phallic growth in early childhood has rightly fallen into disrepute because of the acceleration of bone maturation, which leads to loss of ultimate growth potential. While standard testosterone treatment is effective for inducing pubertal development in males with androgen-responsive syndromes, it is of limited value in patients with androgen insensitivity. Induction of full masculization in these patients is still very unsatisfactory. It has, however, been demonstrated that some further virilization in adult patients may be effectively induced using supraphysiological doses of depot testosterone (500 mg weekly). Effects, albeit slow to appear, were seen specifically in penile length and facial and body hair growth.

Further reading

Eckstein B, Cohen S, Farkas A, Rosler A (1989). The nature of the defect in familial male pseudohermaphroditism in Arabs of Gaza. *Journal of Clinical Endocrinology and Metabolism* **68,** 477–85.

Forest MG (1981). Inborn errors of testosterone biosynthesis. *Pediatric and Adolescent Endocrinology* **8,** 133–55.

Hughes IA, Pinsky L (1989). Sexual differentiation. In: Collu R, Ducharne JR, Guyda HS, eds. *Paediatric endocrinology*, pp. 251–93. Raven Press, New York.

Imperato-McGinley J *et al.* (1982). Hormonal evaluation of a large kindred with complete androgen insensitivity: evidence for secondary 5-alpha-reductase deficiency. *Journal of Clinical Endocrinology and Metabolism* **54**, 931–41.

Kirk JMW, Perry LA, Shand WS, Kirby RS, Besser GM, Savage MO (1990). Female pseudohermaphroditism due to a maternal adreno-cortical tumour. *Journal of Clinical Endocrinology and Metabolism* **70**, 1280–4.

Pang S, Lerner AJ, Stoner LS (1985). Late onset adrenal steroid 3β-hydroxysteroid dehydrogenase deficiency: A cause of hirsutism in pubertal and post-pubertal women. *Journal of Clinical Endocrinology and Metabolism* **60**, 428–35.

Price P *et al.* (1984). High dose androgen therapy in male pseudohermaphroditism due to 5-alpha reductase deficiency and disorders of the androgen receptor. *Journal of Clinical Investigation* **74**, 1496–508.

Savage MO, Lowe DG (1990). Gonadal neoplasia and abnormal sexual differentiation. *Clinical Endocrinology* **32**, 519–33.

Savage MO, Sultan C (1999). Intersex. In: Mundy AR, Fitzpatrick JM, Neal DE, George NJR, eds. *Scientific basis of urology*, pp. 421–37. Isis Medical Media, Oxford.

van Niekerk WA (1981). True hermaphroditism. *Pediatric and Adolescent Endocrinology* **8**, 80–99.

Williams DM, Patterson MN, Hughes IA (1993). Androgen insensitivity syndrome. *Archives of Disease in Childhood* **68**, 343–4.

Wilson JD, Griffin JE, Leshin M, MacDonald PC (1983). The androgen resistance syndromes. In: Stanbury JB, Wyngaarden JB, Fredridison DS, Goldstein JL, Brown MS, eds. *The metabolic basis of inherited disease*, pp. 1001–26. McGraw-Hill, New York.

12.9.2 Normal growth and its disorders

M. A. Preece

The normal curve of growth

The upper panel of Fig. 1 shows the curve of height attained (or distance) for a typical male from birth to 18 years of age. It contains all the relevant information about growth in height of an individual child. In the lower panel the growth data have been converted to height velocity in cm/year. This is calculated from the distance data by dividing the difference between two height measurements (as close to 1 year apart as possible) by the exact time elapsed between them. The calculated velocity is plotted at the mid-point of the time interval over which it is measured. This representation of growth is particularly useful as it emphasizes the dynamic nature of the growth process.

The growth velocity in any one year is a more sensitive measure of events occurring in that year than is the coincident height distance datum, which is a measurement summating all previous growth. Thus, the more sensitive measures of the velocity curve may show rather dramatic change in growth during disease or during treatment, where the simpler distance curve would be less sensitive.

There are three epochs of growth: early, rather fast growth before the age of 2 years; relatively slow steady growth during the preschool and primary

school years; and then the period around puberty when the adolescent growth spurt dominates the growth pattern.

Epochs of growth

Infancy

During the first year of life the infant has an average height velocity of about 25 cm/year. However, since this is a time when the velocity is changing dramatically, measurement over shorter time periods should be considered. The velocity during the first 3 months is equivalent to 3.3 cm/month in boys and 3.0 cm/month in girls, dropping to 1.2 cm/month and 1.3 cm/month respectively by the last 3 months of that year. During the next 3 years there is a further deceleration to a velocity of 0.5 cm/month, or 6 cm/year, which is the average through much of middle childhood. This continues with gentle slowing until puberty.

The first 3 years are also the time of increased channelling of the growth curve. At birth, the length of the baby is determined mostly by the fetal environment which, in turn, is much dependent on maternal size; the father's height is poorly correlated with the child's. During the next 2 to 3 years, the influence of the father's genetic make-up increases progressively until there is equal influence from both parents. This phenomenon can result in some rather bizarre growth patterns where mother and father have very different heights. For example, when the child is born to a tall mother but short father, the initially rather large baby will tend to grow unusually slowly until the genetically expected channel is achieved.

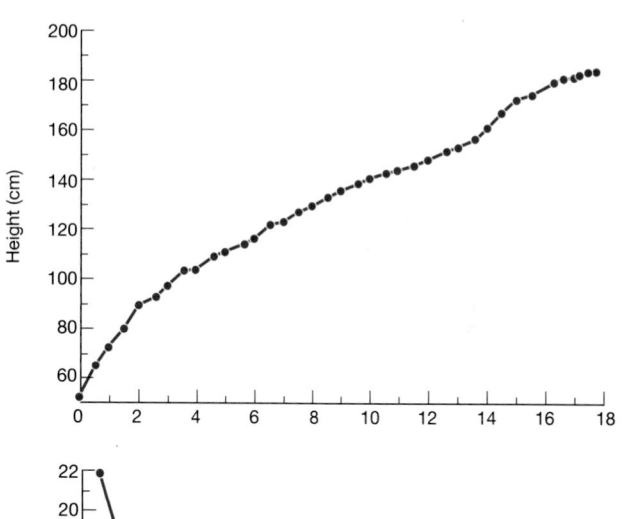

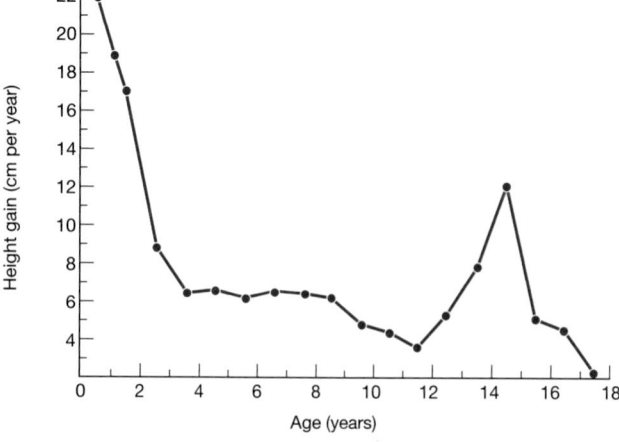

Fig. 1 The growth in height of an individual boy from birth to 18 years of age. The top panel shows the height attained or distance curve and the lower panel shows the data replotted as height gain or growth velocity. (Reproduced from Tanner JM (1962). *Growth at adolescence*, Blackwell, Oxford, with permission.)

Middle childhood

Although in healthy children growth is a moderately steady process, there are fluctuations that occur in the short and middle term, the most striking of which are related to seasonal changes. Most children grow faster in spring and summer, with relatively slow periods in the autumn and winter; a few children show a reversed pattern, and others no regular pattern at all. There is a rather constant, but small, growth spurt at 6 to 7 years of age in both boys and girls, with no sexual dimorphism; it has been attributed to the onset of adrenal androgen secretion that occurs at about that age.

Puberty

There is little difference in growth rates between males and females before 10 years of age. Then the typical female starts her adolescent growth spurt and, for a few years, is taller than a male of the same age. About 2 years later the male starts his spurt and by the age of 14 is the taller. The major difference in adult height between males and females (14 cm in the United Kingdom) is established at puberty. About 11 cm comes from the extra 2 years of prepubertal growth of boys and 3 cm from their more intense growth spurt.

Sexual dimorphism in height during puberty is reflected in many other body dimensions. At this time there is a more dramatic growth spurt in males for most body dimensions, occurring about 2 years later than in females. A major exception is the more dramatic and sustained growth spurt of the female pelvis. There are also associated changes in soft tissues, leading to the greater muscularity of the male.

Metabolic and endocrine factors controlling growth

Each of the epochs of growth described above is associated with particular metabolic or hormonal factors which exert their effects in an almost sequential manner. These distinctions should not be overstated, however, and are only useful as a general guide to the most important factors at a given age. In essence, infant growth is dominated by nutritional considerations, the childhood period by growth hormone, and puberty by the sex hormones, but nutrition has an important role throughout and growth hormone is important in early infant growth, as shown by the reduced size at birth of children with congenital growth hormone deficiency. Thyroid hormone is also important throughout the growing period. Throughout growth the actions of growth hormone and possibly other hormonal and nutritional factors are in part mediated by the insulin-like growth factors and their binding proteins.

Disorders of growth

Growth disorders are predominantly problems of childhood, and patients seen by the adult physician are inevitably left with a legacy of events which have occurred before maturity. In many cases where the condition was successfully treated during childhood there may be no residual problem with stature in adult life. In contrast, there are many situations when this happy outcome is not achieved and there is still a persistent problem requiring attention in the adult clinic. Thus the importance of the various disorders is different and what follows reflects this.

Short stature

Definition

What is considered as short (or for that matter tall) stature is essentially arbitrary. It is usually considered as a height that falls below the second centile for the relevant population; these values for adults are given in Table 1. This is easy when the discrepancy is severe but difficulties arise with patients whose height lies close to this limit. In this situation the per-

Table 1 Critical heights (in cm) for male and female adults in the United Kingdom

	2nd centile	50th centile	98th centile
Females	152	164	176
Males	164	178	192

ceptions of the patient may greatly colour the situation and its management. The most important decision is whether the apparent short stature is a symptom of a disorder that requires attention, and therefore most stress is placed upon diagnosis.

Classification of short stature

The major categories of short stature are shown in Table 2. The process of attributing such labels to an individual patient is largely one of clinical assessment, including critical appraisal of the pattern of growth combined with appropriate confirmatory investigations.

Familial short stature

This relatively common condition is among the most difficult to manage. It is sometimes referred to as normal or idiopathic short stature. Patients usually present in childhood with heights clustered around the second centile. The parents are usually of comparable size and the child's stature is simply reflecting the genetic inheritance. This apparently straightforward situation is made difficult because of the considerable social pressures that now exist; parents and their children simply find it hard to accept the situation and want it changed.

Diagnosis The clinical picture is clear: the child will be at or below the second centile for height with a normal growth velocity measured over 1 year. The height will be appropriate for the family and it is critical that parental heights are properly taken into account. The simplest way to do this is to measure both parents and then determine their height centiles. The child's predicted adult height is calculated by an appropriate method that takes into account skeletal maturity; this predicted adult height should lie within a range of 10 cm above or below the midparental height centile, which represents the 2nd to 98th centiles for that family.

The general medical picture is of good health, apart from the usual childhood illnesses. Similarly, apart from short stature, no abnormalities are found on general examination. In this situation no investigations are necessary other than the assessment of skeletal maturity for the prediction of adult height.

Management The main problem is to persuade the patient and the family that there is no medical problem. Even when this is achieved, there is often a wish to change the prognosis for height. In recent years there have been many clinical trials of human growth hormone in this situation. While definitive data are still scarce, there is increasing evidence that although a short-term acceleration of height velocity is almost always achieved, this is not maintained, and adult height is relatively unchanged. When such treatment is started after the age of 11 years this is moderately certain, but there remains some uncertainty if the human growth hormone is started at younger ages (6 to 8 years). Even if this is more successful, there remains a

Table 2 Major groups of disease processes leading to short stature

Familial short stature
Constitutional delay of growth and/or puberty
Intrauterine growth retardation
Environmental short stature
Chronic paediatric disease
Endocrine disease
Genetic/chromosomal disorders
Dysmorphic syndromes
Bone dysplasias

considerable debate about the ethics and cost-effectiveness of such treatment of normal healthy children.

Constitutional delay of growth and/or puberty

This problem is largely covered elsewhere (see Chapter 12.9.3). Here comment is restricted to noting that in many cases the delay in maturation is evident well before puberty when the presentation is purely of short stature associated with delayed skeletal maturation. There is often an associated element of familial short stature; the delay is amenable to treatment with anabolic steroids or androgens, whereas the familial element is unaffected.

Intrauterine growth retardation

This comprises a relatively large group of children who share the common feature of being born inappropriately small for gestational age, usually assessed in terms of birth weight. Many show a sustained period of accelerated or 'catch-up' growth and reach the normal centiles for height and weight. However, a significant number fail to do this and remain below the 2nd centile although growing at a normal velocity. In some cases this clinical picture is part of a more general dysmorphic or genetic syndrome, but it may occur alone.

Diagnosis Traditionally intrauterine growth retardation is diagnosed when a baby is born with a birth weight more than two standard deviations below the mean for gestational age, maternal height, and parity. However, this criterion is changing to reflect intrauterine diagnosis by fetal ultrasound measurements.

In addition to the birth characteristics, the growth curve is typical and there are a number of other clinical features. The facies are small and triangular with a normal sized cranium which, compared with the small face, can give the impression of hydrocephalus. The general habitus is very lean and there may be a degree of limb asymmetry in about 50 per cent of cases. There are often other minor dysmorphic features.

Many children have severe feeding problems in the first few years of life, which may compound the lean appearance and create further anxieties for the families. There may be a degree of delayed skeletal maturation, but this is very variable. General and endocrine investigations are unhelpful.

Management In all but the most severely affected children growth velocity is normal as long as the intrauterine growth retardation is not part of a more generalized dysmorphic syndrome. However, the long-term prognosis for height is usually rather worse than appears in childhood. This is because puberty tends to be prompt and the adolescent growth spurt attenuated, so that less growth is achieved in the teenage years than might be expected.

The only active treatment that is being pursued at present is the use of human growth hormone, but this is still under clinical trial. Early results suggest short-term benefit, but predicted mature height is little changed, as in the case of familial short stature.

Environmental short stature

Over the past 30 years it has become clear that children's growth may be adversely affected by their environment other than by malnutrition or infection. This effect may be due to emotional or physical abuse or neglect and may sometimes present in the most bizarre of ways, often imitating other organic disorders such as growth hormone insufficiency. It is most common in young children but may rarely present in young teenagers and, strikingly, may present in a single child in a family where the other children thrive.

Diagnosis This is a diagnosis which is notoriously easy to miss. In its most classical form it presents as an apparently straightforward diagnosis of growth hormone insufficiency although there will often be additional features of bizarre eating habits, behavioural abnormalities, or other evidence of abnormal family dynamics. In many cases where an initial diagnosis of growth hormone insufficiency is made, treatment with human growth hormone is started, often with early success. However, the accelerated growth soon falters and during the subsequent reappraisal the real diagnosis is uncovered.

As the above suggests, endocrine investigations are often misleading. Once the suspicion is raised the only way to confirm the diagnosis is a period of time away from the family environment, either by a hospital admission or by short-term fostering. A period of accelerated growth (initially weight gain followed by increase in height) makes the diagnosis. There is then the need for a detailed social and psychiatric appraisal of the family.

Management Once the diagnosis is made the management is predominantly that of manipulation of the family circumstances, either by extensive social and psychiatric support for the family with the child *in situ*, or more commonly by removing the child from the family and placement elsewhere by fostering or adoption.

With proper management in childhood those who have suffered from environmental short stature should not present medical problems in adult life. However, it is highly likely that there may be continuing psychological problems and particularly the possibility of subsequent abuse of one or more of their own children.

Chronic paediatric disease

Any child with a longstanding chronic disease will show some degree of growth disorder if the primary activity of the underlying condition is less than optimally controlled. This may be due to the disease itself or to its treatment; the use of high doses of systemic corticosteroids is a particularly important example of the latter. However, it is very unusual for such a child to present with short stature as the primary symptom because the underlying disease is usually evident at an earlier stage. Notable exceptions to this rule are some gastrointestinal diseases, especially coeliac and inflammatory bowel disease. Irrespective of the primary disease, a degree of delayed skeletal maturation is prominent and may be the first feature of disordered growth to appear.

Management is targeted at the primary disease wherever possible. Adjunctive therapies, such as human growth hormone in chronic renal failure, are being studied within clinical trials. The long-term benefits of such treatments remain unclear at the present time.

Endocrine disease

The endocrine causes of short stature form the main group of readily treated growth disorders. Many of the details will have already been covered in the chapters on the relevant endocrine glands and only a brief summary is given here.

Hypothyroidism Inadequately treated congenital or acquired juvenile hypothyroidism is always associated with marked growth failure. Congenital disease ought to be diagnosed by neonatal screening programmes, such that growth is never a problem, although some delay in initiating thyroid replacement may lead to the more serious problems of intellectual impairment. On the other hand, juvenile hypothyroidism, usually due to autoimmune thyroiditis, can be far more insidious and often presents with growth failure as the sole symptom.

Diagnosis In any undiagnosed short child consideration should always be given to the possibility of juvenile hypothyroidism. The classical features of adult disease such as constipation and intellectual impairment are usually absent and poor growth may be the only abnormality. Most typically the child grows with a very low velocity, rapidly crossing centiles downwards. General medical examination may be quite normal unless the disease is long established and severe; such symptoms and signs as may be present are no different from those in adults. A goitre may be present, depending upon the stage of the disease.

A striking delay in skeletal maturation is often seen; to the unwary this may lead to an incorrect diagnosis of constitutional delay of growth and/or puberty, as the degree of maturational delay will usually be sufficient to apparently explain the height deficit. For this reason thyroid function tests should be undertaken early and will confirm or deny the diagnosis without

Table 3 The causes of growth hormone insufficiency

Congenital
Genetic
Sporadic, usually with multiple pituitary hormone deficiencies, with
    hypoglycaemia and giant cell hepatitis
Perinatal associations, e.g. breech delivery
Midline defect including septo-optic dysplasia, cleft-lip and palate, and pituitary
    aplasia

Acquired
Tumours of the pituitary or hypothalamus, particularly craniopharyngioma
Cranial irradiation, either as treatment for solid tumours or prophylaxis for
    childhood leukaemia
Head injury or surgery to the hypothalamopituitary region
Langerhans cell histiocytosis
After meningitis, particularly tuberculous
Temporarily as part of environmental short stature

ambiguity. Serum T_3 or T_4 will be low, with an elevated serum concentration of thyroid-stimulating hormone.

Management Thyroid replacement with L-thyroxine is relatively straightforward, with an initial dose of 100 µg/m²/day; this is fine-tuned according to growth response, clinical examination, and maintenance of a suppressed thyroid-stimulating hormone concentration with either a normal serum T_3 concentration or serum T_4 in the upper normal range. The prognosis for height is generally very good, except in those diagnosed and treated well into puberty, when the outcome is less satisfactory.

Growth hormone insufficiency Growth hormone insufficiency may occur as an isolated disorder of uncertain aetiology, as part of more complex diseases and developmental anomalies, or as part of more extensive hypothalamopituitary disease. A list of such conditions is given in Table 3. Recently, it has become clear that there are a number of genetic causes of growth hormone insufficiency and wider pituitary malfunction. Deletions or mutations of the structural growth hormone gene on chromosome 17 is now well recognized as are the cascade of homeobox genes responsible for pituitary development including *PIT1*, *PROP1* and *HESX1*.

The principal differences between the congenital and acquired forms are that the onset of the growth failure occurs differently. In the first case there is failure of normal growth from a very early age which can usually be detected within the first year of life. In contrast, acquired growth hormone insufficiency can lead to abnormally slow growth at any age before maturity. In the latter situation the assessment of height velocity assumes far greater importance as height may remain within the normal centiles for several years before the child becomes overtly short and below the third centile.

Particularly noteworthy is the pattern of growth in children receiving cranial or craniospinal irradiation as this may be rather different from other causes of growth hormone insufficiency. In both cases there may be associated early puberty, particularly with radiation doses below 2400 cGy, leading to a rather confusing picture as the early but rather attenuated adolescent growth spurt may mask the onset of growth hormone insufficiency. When the spine is involved in the radiation field there may be a combination of growth hormone insufficiency and direct damage to the spinal epiphyses, with subsequent failure of spinal growth which is not due to the endocrine abnormalities and is not responsive to endocrine replacement.

Diagnosis Children with growth hormone insufficiency grow with a slow height velocity and, depending on whether the insufficiency is congenital or acquired later, fall progressively further below the second centile or cross height centiles downwards. The degree of short stature can range from relatively mild to very severe, depending on the degree of insufficiency, the age of onset, and parental heights. As in many short stature disorders, the parents' heights still modify the expression of the disorder such that children with growth hormone insufficiency born to tall parents will tend to be more normal in height for longer than those with equivalent disease born to shorter parents.

Other clinical features include a rather young appearance, with immature facies and sometimes a quite striking degree of frontal bossing. There is usually an excess of subcutaneous fat, giving a rather cherubic appearance, and in boys there may be hypoplastic genitalia not necessarily due to associated gonadotrophin deficiency but caused by a severe growth hormone insufficiency in the intrauterine or neonatal perod.

The diagnosis is confirmed by a variety of endocrine measurements (see Chapter 12.2). Growth hormone is secreted in an episodic manner such that measurement in single serum samples is valueless. It is most commonly measured in several samples following pituitary stimulation by a provocative agent, of which the most important are listed in Table 4. The definition of a normal response is still rather arbitrary, but is usually set at a peak of more than 7 mg/l at some point following the administration of the provocative agent. It is important that the characteristics of different growth hormone assays are taken into account and centres carrying out these tests should establish their own cutoff values. The place of growth hormone releasing hormone is uncertain; it tests the integrity of the hypothalamopituitary axis but does not detect primary hypothalamic disease, which is probably the most important cause of growth hormone insufficiency.

Additional aids to diagnosis are the measurement of growth hormone concentrations in serial blood samples taken frequently (every 15 to 20 min) over 24 h, or the measurement of basal serum concentrations of insulin-like growth factor I together with insulin-like growth factor binding protein 3. The former approach is laborious and labour intensive and is probably unhelpful except in some rare situations where an assessment of physiological growth hormone secretion is required. Measurement of insulin-like growth factor I and its binding protein is rather too insensitive for routine clinical use.

Growth hormone insufficiency may be isolated or part of a wider constellation of pituitary hormone deficiencies, and it is important to check thyroid and adrenal function at an early stage. Gonadotrophin deficiency is relatively common but difficult to confirm prior to the age of puberty, and it may not be until puberty fails to occur spontaneously that suspicion is raised (see Chapter 12.9.3).

Having confirmed the diagnosis of growth hormone insufficiency, isolated or otherwise, it is important to determine the underlying aetiology and, in particular, seek an intracranial space-occupying lesion. Craniopharyngioma is the most important lesion and the use of modern imaging techniques, cranial computed tomography or magnetic resonance imaging, is mandatory. These lesions are most commonly associated with multiple pituitary hormone deficiencies, although these may take some years to become manifest (see Chapter 12.2).

Management The treatment of growth hormone insufficiency is the same whatever the underlying aetiology: human growth hormone, 5 to 10 mg/m²/week (0.2–0.4 mg/kg/week; 1 mg pure protein = 3 IU), by daily subcutaneous injection. The growth velocity is the best indicator of response and it should show a clear acceleration, usually to 10 cm/year or more. A poor response indicates the need to review the diagnosis. It is essential that any coexisting pituitary hormone deficiencies (such as deficiency of thyroid-stimulating hormone leading to secondary hypothyroidism) are adequately treated with appropriate replacement.

Treatment is continued until growth is complete and may therefore last for many years. For this reason it is particularly important to review dosage as growth occurs and ensure that injection sites are cared for adequately.

Growth hormone receptor deficiency This is a very rare disorder whose importance lies in the ability to mimic the much more common severe growth hormone insufficiency. The clinical phenotypes may be indistinguishable but in the case of growth hormone receptor deficiency there is excessive secretion of growth hormone by the pituitary gland; the fault lies

Table 4 Provocative tests for growth hormone insufficiency

Provocative agent	Route	Dose	Mechanism of action
Insulin	Intravenous	0.05–0.15 IU/kg	Neurohypoglycaemia
Glucagon	Intramuscular	0.1 mg/kg	Neurohypoglycaemia
Clonidine	Oral	0.15 mg/m²	β-Agonist
Arginine	Intravenous	500 mg/kg	Uncertain (basic amino acid)
Growth hormone releasing hormone	Intravenous	1 µg/kg	Physiological

in the growth hormone receptor, which is either absent or non-functioning, leading to a deficiency of insulin-like growth factor I. The abnormality is due to one of several mutations in the receptor gene, which is inherited according to an autosomal recessive pattern. Until now it has been untreatable but clinical trials of recombinant insulin-like growth factor I look promising.

Adrenocortical excess (see also Chapter 12.7.1) An excess of circulating corticosteroids is a potent cause of growth failure, whether due to endogenous overproduction or exogenous medication. In the former case, the aetiology may be hypothalamopituitary or adrenal in origin, as in adults. The diagnosis of Cushing's disease in childhood is rare and taxing to make, although once considered, the approach does not differ from that in adults. Iatrogenic glucocorticoid excess is much more common and is most often related to overuse of topical steroids for atopic disease; inhaled steroids for asthma and powerful dermatological preparations for eczema are particularly important. The management of the growth failure is entirely dependent on reducing the glucocorticoid load usually by the introduction of an alternative non-steroidal treatment for the underlying condition.

Genetic/chromosomal disorders, dysmorphic syndromes, and bone dysplasias

For the purposes of this book these last three categories can be considered together. For the main part they are individually rare, but are so many and varied that together they make a significant contribution to the causes of short stature. The approach to diagnosis depends heavily on clinical suspicion backed up by chromosomal and radiological investigation.

Turner syndrome This is the only condition that will be discussed in any detail as it is relatively common (about 1 in 2500 to 3500 female births), surprisingly easy to miss, and amenable to useful treatment. Turner syndrome tends to present in two distinct age groups: birth or infancy and mid childhood. The young girls usually have a number of the classical features, including coarctation of the aorta leading to early clinical suspicion. However, a large number of affected girls only have subtle clinical signs, and in these patients short stature is virtually the only significant feature. Diagnosis is confirmed by chromosomal analysis, which may reveal a 45X karyotype with complete absence of one X chromosome, a more subtle structural abnormality of one X, such as an isochromosome, or a mosaic combination of cells with different chromosomal complements.

Untreated girls with Turner's syndrome reach adult heights of between 134 and 156 cm but this is dependent on their parents' heights; girls from tall families will be relatively tall for the diagnosis, even reaching into the lower part of the normal range. Puberty is usually, but not always, absent.

Treatment for both the short stature and the lack of puberty is possible. The latter requires the use of oestrogen and progestogens. A typical regimen would be the slow introduction of ethinyl oestradiol at about 12 to 13 years of age in a dose of 1 µg/day increasing to doses of 20 to 30 µg/day over 2 years. It should be given continuously at first but when adult doses are reached it should be omitted for one week in every four, when a withdrawal bleed will occur, mimicking menstruation. At the same time it is important that a progestogen, such as norethisterone 5 mg/day, is introduced for the last week of the cycle. More recently, clinical trials have shown that moderate growth benefit can be achieved by the combined use of

human growth hormone (7–10 mg/m²) and the mild anabolic steroid, oxandrolone (1.25–2.5 mg/day).

Tall stature

The causes of excessive growth are far fewer than those of short stature. Most common are variants of normal, usually with tall parents; pathological causes of tall stature are very rare.

Definition

This can be defined in a complementary way to short stature (see above); it is equally arbitrary. In practical terms, boys find difficulty in accepting heights above 200 cm, whereas most girls find 185 cm the limit.

Classification

The principal causes of tall stature are familial tall stature, pituitary gigantism, Sotos syndrome, Marfan syndrome, and homocystinuria; only the first will be discussed in any detail.

Familial tall stature

This is more or less the mirror image of familial short stature which is discussed above. There is often an element of advanced maturation with a skeletal age that exceeds chronological age by several years and early pubertal development. The diagnosis is made by clinical appraisal, including knowledge of parental heights and the demonstration that predicted adult height is appropriate for the family. Exclusion of other potential causes is often possible on clinical grounds, but the exclusion of excessive growth hormone secretion may be necessary.

Management The calculation of a predicted adult height, which because of the advanced skeletal maturation is often less than the family fears, may be all that is necessary as the expected height is then acceptable. If this is not the case, then other pharmacological treatments may need discussion. At present these are unsatisfactory, although in girls it may be possible to curtail final height by induction of puberty early using physiological doses of ethinyl oestradiol, if they present early enough. In the past high-dose ethinyl oestradiol (100–300 µg/day) has been advocated in an attempt to accelerate skeletal maturation. However, the benefits are far from certain, there may be quite unpleasant side-effects, and the long-term safety is unclear.

The use of testosterone in boys, in an analogous manner to the use of oestrogen in girls, is of even less value and is probably contraindicated.

Other causes of tall stature

Pituitary gigantism with excessive growth hormone secretion is extremely rare but does occasionally require specific exclusion, usually by demonstration of normal suppression of growth hormone secretion to undetectable levels by oral glucose (1.75 g/kg). Serum concentrations of insulin-like growth factor I will usually be high but may overlap the normal range.

Marfan syndrome is characterized by disproportionately long limbs and digits (arachnodactyly), and is usually associated with a high-arched palate and pectus excavatum. It is an important diagnosis to make because of the risk of eye problems and dissection of the aortic root and arch. Ultrasound examination of the heart and aorta should be a regular routine.

Sotos syndrome and the other dysmorphic causes of tall stature are even rarer and can usually be diagnosed on other criteria. They are not considered further here.

Further reading

Dattani MT, Robinson IC (2000). The molecular basis for developmental disorders of the pituitary gland in man. *Clinical Genetics* **57**, 337–46.

Massoud AF, Hindmarsh PC, Brook CGD (1992) Disorders of stature. In: Grossman A, ed. *Clinical endocrinology*, 2nd edn, pp 855–84. Blackwell Scientific, Oxford.

Preece MA (1992). Principles of normal growth: auxology and endocrinology. In: Grossman A, ed. *Clinical endocrinology*, 2nd edn, pp 845–54. Blackwell Scientific, Oxford.

Preece MA (1999). Evaluation of growth and development. In: Barratt TM, Avner ED, Harmon WE, eds. *Pediatric nephrology*, 4th edn, pp 329–41. Lippincott, Williams and Wilkins, Baltimore.

Tanner JM (1962). *Growth at adolescence*. Blackwell, Oxford.

Woods KA *et al.* (1997). Phenotype–genotype relationships in growth hormone insensitivity syndrome. *Journal of Clinical Endocrinology and Metabolism* **82**, 3529–35.

12.9.3 Puberty

R. J. M. Ross and M. O. Savage

Introduction

Puberty, as defined by the *Concise Oxford dictionary*, is 'the state of being functionally capable of procreation' through the natural development of reproductive organs. The word is derived from '*puber*' meaning adult, and not 'pubic', which refers to the lower part of the abdomen, the pubes. There is a popular misconception that the onset of puberty is heralded by the development of pubic hair, but breast budding is usually the first sign of puberty in girls and an enlargement in testicular size in boys. A clear understanding of normal pubertal development is essential for the management of patients with disordered puberty, as in many cases counselling and reassurance is all that is required.

Sexual differentiation takes place at two stages of life: the first *in utero* extending to the perinatal period, and the second occurring at puberty. Between these two stages is the 'quiescent period'. The physiological changes that accompany sexual differentiation and the hormonal factors that control these changes are well defined, but what determines the duration of the 'quiescent period' and the onset of puberty remains to be established. What is known is that puberty is centrally driven, and this is well illustrated by the failure of pubertal development in children with Kallmann's syndrome and the changes that occur in anorexia nervosa. In Kallmann's syndrome there is a failure in the migration of gonadotrophin-releasing hormone (**GnRH**) neurones to the hypothalamus during fetal life. Affected patients present with hypogonadotrophic hypogonadism associated with anosmia. When puberty is delayed or arrested by anorexia nervosa it may be induced by the pulsatile administration of GnRH. The GnRH pulse generator is therefore essential for normal puberty, and the cues that switch it to pubertal mode include, most importantly, age and maturation of the central nervous system, environmental factors such as stress, social factors (probably the reason for an earlier onset of puberty in Western countries), and metabolic factors such as nutrition, body composition, and leptin.

The onset of puberty is characterized by an increase in basal luteinizing-hormone (**LH**) levels and in the amplitude and frequency of LH pulses independent of gonadal changes. Gonadal activation stimulated by the rise

in gonadotrophin (LH and follicle-stimulating hormone (**FSH**)) secretion results in rising levels of the sex steroids. Apart from their action on sexual maturation, gonadal steroids have a direct effect in stimulating skeletal growth and also a central action in stimulating increased growth-hormone (**GH**) production. A consistent pattern of hormonal changes results in a relatively constant pattern of growth and pubertal development, characterized in girls by the development of breasts, pubic hair, and the onset of menstruation, and in boys by an increase in testicular volume, genitalia size, and the appearance of pubic hair. This is best appreciated by plotting a child's development on growth and development records. A loss of the normal pattern of development suggests pathology. For instance, a boy who at 8 years has a height above the 97th centile, stage 3 genitalia, and pubic hair, but testes less than 4 ml is likely to have an abnormal source of androgens, such as an androgen-secreting tumour or congenital adrenal hyperplasia.

Timing of puberty

Disorders of puberty can be classified by the timing of the onset of sexual characteristics into either precocious or delayed puberty. Precocious puberty is characterized by signs of sexual maturation appearing less than 2.5 standard deviations (**SD**) from the mean: before 8 years of age in a girl and before 9 years in a boy. In Western society puberty is considered delayed when there are no signs of pubertal maturation in a girl aged 13.4 years (2 SD) or a boy aged 13.8 years. As a simple working rule, investigation should be considered if there are no signs of puberty at 14 years of age. These ages are guidelines as they vary between populations and over time.

Precocious puberty

Precocious puberty can be classified into true (pituitary gonadotrophin-dependent) or pseudo (pituitary gonadotrophin-independent) precocious puberty (Table 1). In true precocious puberty, as in normal puberty, there is activation of the hypothalamopituitary axis and thus the normal pattern of puberty is preserved (complete precocious puberty). In pseudo precocious puberty, for example that caused by an adrenal adenoma, the normal pattern of puberty is lost (incomplete precocious puberty). Pseudo precocious

Table 1 Causes of precocious puberty

Isolated thelarche and isolated pubarche
True precocious puberty (pituitary gonadotrophin-dependent)
Idiopathic
sporadic
familial
CNS abnormalities
congenital (e.g. hydrocephalus)
acquired (e.g. irradiation, surgery, and infection)
tumours, including hypothalamic hamartomas, gliomas, and pineal tumours
Hypothyroidism
Pseudo precocious puberty (pituitary gonadotrophin-independent)
McCune–Albright syndrome (polyostotic fibrous dysplasia)
Adrenal disorders
adenomas and carcinomas
congenital adrenal hyperplasia
Gonadal disorders
ovarian cyst
ovarian tumours
testotoxicosis
Leydig-cell tumour
Ectopic gonadotrophin-producing tumours
dysgerminoma, hepatoblastoma, teratoma, chorionepithelioma
Exogenous sex steroids

puberty may be isosexual, with appropriate male or female puberty, or heterosexual, when there is virilization of a girl (as in congenital adrenal hyperplasia), or feminization of a boy (as in an oestrogen-producing Leydig cell tumour). Two conditions do not fit clearly into this classification: isolated thelarche and isolated pubarche.

Isolated thelarche and isolated pubarche

Breast enlargement in the absence of other signs of puberty is called premature thelarche. It is most common under the age of 2 years and may persist from neonatal breast enlargement. There is usually spontaneous regression and later a normally timed puberty. Isolated pubarche is the early appearance of pubic hair with or without axillary hair. It is more commonly seen in girls than boys and characteristically between 4 and 6 years of age. It is associated with adrenarche, an increase in adrenal androgen secretion seen in middle childhood. There can be a slight growth spurt and advance in bone age, but this is part of normal development. It can be differentiated from abnormal forms of virilization, including adrenal tumours and congenital adrenal hyperplasia, by measuring the sex steroid hormone profile, including dehydroepiandrosterone-sulphate (**DHEA-S**), and demonstrating normal suppression of adrenal androgens by dexamethasone. It has been suggested that premature adrenarche may be a precursor of the polycystic ovarian syndrome in girls, and some clinicians advocate long-term follow up for these patients.

Precocious puberty

Precocious puberty presents much more commonly in girls than boys, and in the majority of girls no organic cause is found and it is idiopathic and sporadic. In contrast, in boys idiopathic precocious puberty is rare and, although there are families with familial true precocious puberty, most commonly it is due to CNS tumours, either hypothalamic hamartomas or gliomas, or dysgerminomas (Table 1).

The clinical investigation of precocious puberty is first directed towards distinguishing between a true, pseudo, isosexual, or heterosexual condition. History and examination will help to establish whether there is a normal pattern of pubertal development, as in true precocious puberty, or an abnormal pattern as seen in pseudo precocious puberty. In girls, ultrasound of the pelvis will demonstrate the effect of oestrogens on uterine size and define the appearance of the ovaries. Measurement of the gonadotrophin response to GnRH should be made, as should basal measurements of β-human chorionic gonadotrophin, adrenocorticotrophic hormone, adrenal steroids (including cortisol, 17-hydroxyprogesterone, DHEA-S, and androstenedione), testosterone, oestrogen, and thyroid hormones. Steroid profiles may also be made on urine collections. Skeletal maturation should be determined by measuring bone age.

True precocious puberty

In true precocious puberty the gonadotrophins will show a pubertal response to GnRH with a greater rise of LH than FSH. In the normal prepubertal child there is only a small rise in the gonadotrophins and the response of FSH is greater than that of LH. In pseudo precocious puberty the gonadotrophins are usually suppressed unless true puberty has also been initiated, which may occur due to excessive sex-steroid secretion from any cause. Acquired hypothyroidism is associated with increased levels of FSH and may result in breast development and menstruation in girls and testicular enlargement in boys. These patients usually have stunted growth and the diagnosis is easily made by the measurement of thyroid stimulating hormone levels. Once a diagnosis of true precocious puberty is made, appropriate scanning of the hypothalamopituitary axis should be performed using magnetic resonance imaging (**MRI**).

Pseudo precocious puberty

The further investigation of pseudo precocious puberty depends on the findings of the original screening tests. Adrenal tumours will be associated with an increased production of adrenal steroids which is not suppressed by a low-dose dexamethasone suppression test. Imaging will pick up adrenal carcinomas (usually greater than 6 cm in diameter) and most adenomas, although on occasion venous catheter sampling is required. Congenital adrenal hyperplasia in girls usually presents early with virilization and ambiguous genitalia; however, it may present later in boys with virilization and tall stature, but prepubertal testes. There is a typical urinary steroid profile, and in the commonest form there is 21-hydroxylase deficiency, with levels of ACTH and 17-hydroxyprogesterone raised, and low levels of cortisol. Ovarian tumours are best detected by ultrasound scanning, as are testicular tumours. The McCune–Albright syndrome (polyostotic fibrous dysplasia) is an unusual cause of precocious puberty due to postzygotic activating mutations in the gene encoding the G protein, G alpha s, resulting in activation of the signal-transduction pathway generating cyclic AMP. Girls usually present with autonomous ovarian activity, but this may be succeeded by true precocious puberty. Patients have patches of *café-au-lait* pigmentation with a ragged border and fibrous dysplasia of the bones. Testotoxicosis is an unusual inherited disorder due to activating mutations of the gene for the LH receptor. It is characterized by pubertal levels of testosterone, pubertal-sized testes, and a suppressed hypothalamogonadal axis. Tumours producing human chorionic gonadotrophin (**hCG**) can be detected by measuring hCG and scanning appropriate sites, including the gonads, liver, and pineal gland.

Treatment

There are four aims in the treatment of precocious puberty:

(1) to remove the primary cause;

(2) to treat the psychosocial consequences;

(3) to allow a normal puberty; and

(4) to promote normal growth.

Children with precocious puberty appear much older than they are, and this can result in considerable psychological difficulties and behavioural problems. Growth is stimulated both by a direct action of sex steroids on skeletal maturation and by the induction of GH secretion. This early maturation of the skeleton results in early fusion of the epiphysis, and although the child is initially tall, his or her ultimate height may be very short.

Girls with only slightly advanced pubertal development often require no treatment because puberty only advances slowly, and they do not have a significant loss in their height potential. GnRH analogues are now the treatment of choice in true precocious puberty. They act by downregulating the GnRH receptor and switching off the secretion of LH and FSH. GnRH analogues have been produced as nasal sprays, daily injections, and monthly depot injections. In our experience, depot injections have proved the most effective (goserelin 3.6 mg/month). GnRH may produce an initial period of stimulation, which can be prevented by giving concomitant treatment with cyproterone acetate (100 mg/m^2 once a day for the first 6 weeks). Occasionally the acute suppression of oestrogen production at the start of treatment will precipitate an oestrogen-withdrawal bleed.

In pseudo precocious puberty removal of the primary cause is the mainstay of treatment for patients with tumours, and treatment with glucocorticoids for patients with congenital adrenal hyperplasia. In patients with congenital activating mutations of receptors or residual disease after treatment of tumours, cyproterone acetate, a peripherally acting antiandrogen, at a dose of 50 to 100 mg daily is effective in halting the progress of the physical features of puberty, and is useful in suppressing menstruation. Cyproterone acetate is a weak glucocorticoid and may suppress ACTH and the adrenal glands. Testolactone, and a combination of this with spironolactone and GnRH analogues, has proven effective in improving height prediction.

Any effective treatment of precocious puberty will slow the growth rate through the consequent reduced secretion of sex steroids and GH. Patients treated to arrest puberty will have longer to grow, but their reduced growth rate and already reduced growth potential mean that, despite the use of

GnRH analogues, they will not achieve the height of which they were originally capable. The addition of GH treatment for 2 to 3 years during conventional therapy with GnRH analogues may improve the height prognosis in children with a low growth velocity.

Delayed puberty

The causes are summarized in Table 2. The individual conditions which may cause it are discussed in other parts of this book. Here, discussion is limited to the management of constitutional delay of growth and adolescence.

Constitutional delay of growth and adolescence (CDGA)

CDGA occurs in otherwise normal adolescents who have relatively short stature, delayed puberty and bone age, and a height prognosis appropriate

Table 2 Causes of pubertal delay

Hypogonadotrophic hypogonadism (low LH and FSH)
Constitutional delay in growth and adolescence (CDGA)
  sporadic
  familial
Chronic diseases
  Crohn's, renal failure, thalassaemia
Malnutrition
  coeliac disease, cystic fibrosis, anorexia nervosa
Hypothalamopituitary
  hypopituitarism (idiopathic, tumours, craniopharyngiomas)
  isolated LH and FSH deficiency (Kallmann's, Prader–Willi, and
    fertile eunuch syndromes)
  isolated GH deficiency
  hyperprolactinaemia
  leptin deficiency or resistance
  polycystic ovarian disease
  exercise (gymnasts)
Hormonal
  hypothyroidism, Cushing's syndrome

Hypergonatrophic hypogonadism (high LH and FSH)
Congenital
  chromosome abnormalities (Turner's and Klinefelter's syndromes)
  gonadal dysgenesis/agenesis
  steroid hormone or receptor deficiency (5α-reductase deficiency
    and testicular feminization)
Acquired
  radiotherapy, surgery, chemotherapy, trauma, torsion,
    autoimmunity

in relation to their parents. It presents far more commonly in boys than girls and is the commonest cause of delayed puberty in boys, with Turner's syndrome being the commonest in girls. CDGA needs to be distinguished from isolated gonadotrophin deficiency, but this is rarely easy as gonadotrophin levels are low, with a low or prepubertal response to GnRH in both conditions. A positive family history may indicate CDGA, and associated anosmia suggests Kallmann's syndrome. If in doubt and if treatment is indicated, then the patient should be reassessed after therapy (see below) to see if puberty then progresses without treatment.

Psychological problems are common in children with delayed puberty and short stature. Recent studies have suggested that delayed puberty may be associated with a reduced spinal bone density, putting adults at risk of bone fracture later in life. Thus, there are good reasons for treating this condition, which may be considered as a variant of normal growth.

Intervention with sex steroids or anabolic steroids is a safe treatment that brings forward the timing of the growth spurt without reducing the height potential. The object of treatment is to stimulate normal puberty and maximize linear growth. In boys a reasonable starting dose of testosterone esters is 25 to 50 mg monthly, increasing gradually to 250 mg every 4 weeks, although puberty may be induced more rapidly over a 6-month period and the course of treatment may be as short as 3 months. Oral Oxandralone (unlicensed, but available on a named-patient basis from Searle, UK), 2.5 mg daily, will similarly increase growth velocity.

In girls, ethinyloestradiol at an initial dose of 2 to 10 μg daily can later be increased to between 10 and 20 μg daily, with the addition of progesterone when the oestrogen dose has reached 20 μg (for example, medroxyprogesterone acetate 5 mg on days 1–14 of the calendar month).

Further reading

Klien KO (1999). Editorial: Precocious puberty: who has it? Who should be treated. *Journal of Clinical Endocrinology and Metabolism* **84**, 411–14.

Leschek EW, *et al.* (1999). Six-year results of spironolactone and testolactone treatment of familial male-limited precocious puberty with addition of deslorelin after central puberty onset. *Journal of Clinical Endocrinology and Metabolism* **84**, 175–8.

Pasquino AM, *et al.* (1999). Adult height in girls with central precocious puberty treated with gonadotropin-releasing hormone analogues and growth hormone. *Journal of Clinical Endocrinology and Metabolism* **84**, 449–52.

Saenger P (1992). Editorial: Premature adrenarche: a normal variant of puberty? *Journal of Clinical Endocrinology and Metabolism* **74**, 236–8.

Stanhope R, Albanese A, Shalet S. (1992). Delayed puberty. *British Medical Journal* **305**, 790.

12.10 Non-diabetic pancreatic endocrine disorders and multiple endocrine neoplasia

P. J. Hammond and S. R. Bloom

Pancreatic endocrine tumours

Pancreatic endocrine tumours (islet cell tumours, gastroenteropancreatic tumours) are rare, the most frequent, insulinomas and gastrinomas, occurring with an annual incidence of 1 per million, with others having an incidence of less than 1 per 10 million. Functioning tumours usually present with the symptoms of hormone excess. They may secrete the pancreatic hormones insulin, glucagon, and somatostatin, or ectopic hormones such as gastrin, vasoactive intestinal polypeptide (VIP), or parathyroid hormone related peptide (PTHrP) (see Chapter 12.6). Non-functioning tumours can reach a large size in an apparently well patient, as characteristically these tumours cause little non-endocrine systemic upset. They were once often mistakenly identified as adenocarcinomas, but are now increasingly diagnosed as a result of detection of their secretion of functionally inactive peptides, such as pancreatic polypeptide and neurotensin, or immunohistochemical staining for neuroendocrine markers, such as chromogranin and neurone-specific enolase. They probably account for 50 per cent of all pancreatic endocrine tumours. This section will initially consider aspects of tumour biology, diagnosis, and management common to all tumours, before describing each syndrome.

Natural history

These tumours were originally described as APUDomas because it was thought that they had a common origin from neural crest cells with the ability to perform amine precursor uptake and decarboxylation (APUD). However, this theory has since been disproved, and it has been proposed that the neuroendocrine and mucosal endocrine cells of the gastroenteropancreatic axis are derived from a common, bipotential endoplacal stem cell.

The genetic basis for the development of sporadic pancreatic endocrine tumours is largely unknown. However, about 25 per cent of them, particularly gastrinomas and insulinomas, occur as part of the familial autosomal dominant multiple endocrine neoplasia type 1 (MEN1) syndrome (see below), in which there is a mutation in the *menin* gene in the q13 region of chromosome 11, and loss of heterozygosity for this region has been demonstrated in some patients with sporadic gastrinoma and insulinoma.

Islet cells are pluripotential with respect to peptide production. Thus 70 per cent of tumours are associated with elevated pancreatic polypeptide levels, and in a small proportion of cases other hormones, particularly gastrin, may become elevated and cause secondary syndromes during the course of the disease. Altered processing of peptide precursor molecules may result in a variety of molecular weight forms of the same peptide being secreted, and not all the immunoreactive peptide is bioactive. This can have clinical implications; for example large molecular forms of glucagon (enteroglucagon) can cause villous hypertrophy and slowed intestinal transit, and large forms of somatostatin have been reported to cause hypoglycaemia, rather than the hyperglycaemia usually associated with the somatostatinoma syndrome.

Most pancreatic endocrine tumours are slow-growing and prolonged survival is often possible, even in the presence of metastatic spread, the median survival being about 5 years. However, some patients have aggressive, rapidly spreading disease, particularly those with non-functioning tumours, whose median survival is little over 2 years. Early in the disease, morbidity and mortality result from the effects of peptide hypersecretion rather than tumour bulk. The unpredictable nature of these tumours makes it difficult to give an accurate prognosis, occasional patients surviving for decades, and, combined with their rarity, this has made it difficult to assess the efficacy of different therapeutic strategies.

Diagnosis

Pancreatic endocrine tumours can usually be diagnosed by hormonal radioimmunoassay of a single fasting plasma sample, and for certain syndromes a small number of confirmatory tests. Several conditions other than tumour are associated with increased circulating gut hormone levels (Table 1), particularly renal failure, but the elevations are usually more modest than those associated with tumour syndromes. Gut hormone radioimmunoassays are not well standardized, and the use of different antibodies and assay techniques in different laboratories can give different values on the same sample. However, concentrations are usually of the same order of magnitude in all assays and show a similar percentage increase above normal.

Most glucagonomas, non-functioning tumours, and pancreatic VIPomas and somatostatinomas are large (greater than 2 cm) tumours, which may be calcified and have metastasized to the liver in the majority of cases. Such tumours are easily localized by abdominal computed tomography

Table 1 Causes of elevated gut hormones other than pancreatic endocrine tumours

All hormones
Non-fasting sample
Chronic renal failure
Gastrin
Hypercalcaemia
Achlorhydria
G-cell hyperplasia
Vasoactive intestinal polypeptide
Hepatic cirrhosis
Bowel ischaemia
Glucagon
Hepatic failure
Oral contraceptives and danazol
Stress
Prolonged fast
Familial hyperglucagonaemia
Pancreatic polypeptide
Elderly
Pernicious anaemia
Hypercalcaemia
Neurotensin
Fibrolamellar hepatoma

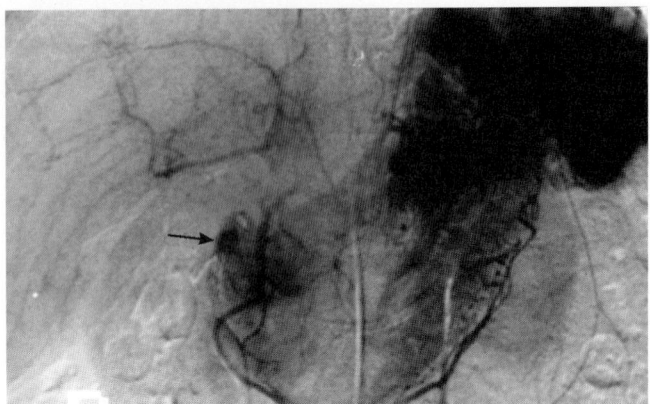

Fig. 1 Venous phase of coeliac axis angiogram demonstrating gastrinoma blush in duodenal wall (arrowed).

(CT) scanning and ultrasonography. However, localization of tumours producing more active hormones, which are therefore detected earlier in their lifecycle, may be very difficult; for example 40 per cent of gastrinomas and insulinomas are microadenomas, less than 1 cm in diameter. Insulinomas often occur in the distal two-thirds of the pancreas, and over 90 per cent of gastrinomas are found in the gastrinoma triangle, bounded by the third part of the duodenum, the neck of the pancreas, and the porta hepatis, about 20 per cent of these being in the duodenum. CT scanning and meticulous, highly selective angiography (Fig. 1) will localize 70 per cent of these microadenomas. Magnetic resonance imaging (MRI) may be more sensitive at detecting small pancreatic lesions than CT scanning, but this method requires further evaluation. Transhepatic percutaneous portal venous sampling is a sensitive method of detecting hormone gradients, but cannot give accurate enough resolution to assist the surgeon in most cases, and is an expensive procedure not without risk. In experienced hands, endoscopic ultrasonography may be more sensitive than conventional imaging, with a resolution of 2 mm and a detection rate of over 75 per cent for tumours in the pancreatic head (Fig. 2), but visualization is poorer for lesions of the pancreatic tail and duodenum. Intraoperative ultrasonography has a sensitivity of over 90 per cent for pancreatic tumours, and endoscopic transillumination of the duodenum may allow the surgeon to detect an occult gastrinoma. Functional radiological localization has been described for both insulinomas and gastrinomas. Injection of calcium or secretin into the artery supplying the tumour causes a marked rise in insulin or gastrin levels, respectively, in the hepatic vein, and allows equivocal lesions to be verified, or the site of unlocalized lesions to be more accurately predicted, and can be used to confirm tumour resection intraoperatively.

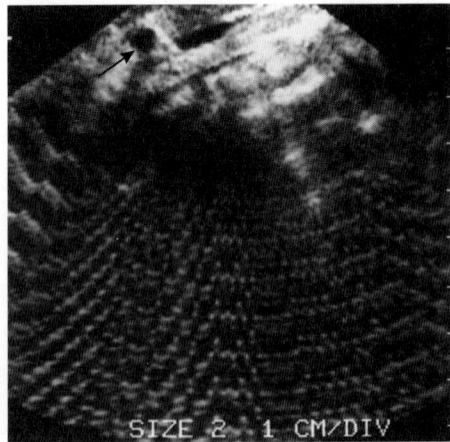

Fig. 2 Endoscopic ultrasound showing a 0.7 cm insulinoma in the head of the pancreas (arrowed).

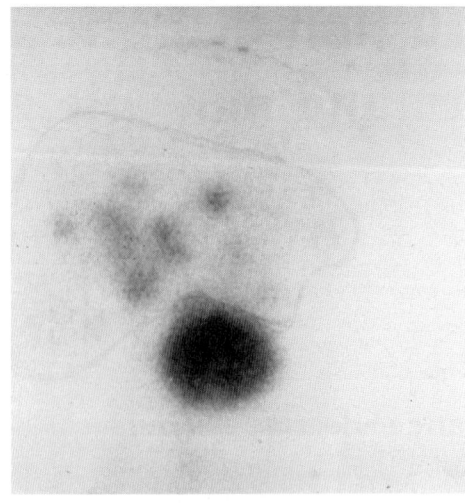

Fig. 3 ^{111}Indium-labelled somatostatin analogue scan showing the large primary tumour and diffuse hepatic metastases in a patient with a pancreatic glucagonoma.

Somatostatin receptor scintigraphy with radiolabelled somatostatin analogues has proved useful in demonstrating the extent of metastatic disease (Fig. 3), and may assist in the localization of extrapancreatic VIPomas, but is less effective in detecting microadenomas. There is controversy as to whether invasive imaging, usually angiography with provocative testing, or non-invasive imaging, principally endoscopic ultrasonography and somatostatin receptor scintigraphy, is the preferred option for localization of small tumours, but the choice will probably be determined by local expertise.

Confirmation of the diagnosis can be made by immunocytochemical analysis of resection specimens or liver biopsies, in addition to conventional histology. Antisera against non-specific markers, such as chromogranins, provide evidence for a neuroendocrine origin, while antisera to different peptides identify the specific tumour type.

Treatment

Surgery offers the only hope of cure for pancreatic endocrine tumours, and all sporadic tumours without evidence of metastatic spread should be resected if possible. Surgical cures have been reported for a few patients with hepatic metastases amenable to enucleation, and, recently, liver transplantation has been successfully performed in patients with metastatic disease confined to the liver.

In the majority of patients, surgical cure is not possible and the aim of treatment in these cases is symptomatic palliation. Until the terminal stages of the disease, this is directed at reducing the symptoms of hormone excess in those with functional tumours. This can be achieved by reducing tumour bulk or inhibiting hormone secretion or action. Reduction of tumour bulk surgically is usually precluded by the operative morbidity. A variety of chemotherapy regimens have been reported as effective, although it is difficult to demonstrate that a particular regimen prolongs survival due to the small numbers of patients for analysis and the unpredictable nature of the tumours. The standard regimen consists of streptozotocin and 5-fluorouracil, with response rates of 80 per cent for functioning tumours, VIPomas responding particularly well, and about 50 per cent for non-functioning tumours. The combination of doxorubicin and streptozotocin has been reported to be more effective, preventing progression of disease for long periods and probably prolonging survival, and other studies have combined doxorubicin, streptozotocin, and 5-fluorouracil. Other agents advocated are dacarbazine for glucagonomas, and cisplatin and etoposide for anaplastic tumours. Another effective means of reducing tumour load in patients with extensive hepatic disease is embolization of the hepatic arterial supply to the metastases, a patent portal vein being needed to support the normal liver parenchyma. Response rates with this procedure are between 60 and 80 per cent. Additional benefit may be gained by chemoembolization, where chemotherapy is delivered via the catheter during the procedure.

Inhibition of hormone release and action is achieved by using the subcutaneous somatostatin analogue, octreotide. Native somatostatin inhibits multiple endocrine functions, acting particularly by blocking hormone effects on the target tissue, but has a half-life in circulation of only 3 min. Octreotide has a half-life of 2 h in the circulation and can be given in three doses daily. The clinical sequelae of peptide hypersecretion are often greatly diminished 24 h after the first injection, although patients become progressively resistant to its effects over many months or years, in part due to continued tumour growth. Recently, long-acting formulations of octreotide have become available, meaning that injections need only be given every 2 to 6 weeks, depending on the response.

Tumour syndromes

Gastrinoma

Gastrinomas are the commonest pancreatic endocrine tumour. Sixty per cent are malignant, 50 per cent of patients having metastases at the time of diagnosis, and up to 30 per cent of patients have the multiple endocrine neoplasia type 1 (MEN1) syndrome. The majority of tumours are pancreatic, but between 20 and 40 per cent are duodenal, and these are usually microadenomas, as little as 1 mm in diameter. Sporadic duodenal microgastrinomas are solitary, but in those patients with MEN1 they are usually multiple and associated with pancreatic microadenomas. Primary lymph node gastrinomas have been described but may represent metastases from duodenal microgastrinomas.

The gastrinoma syndrome was first described in 1955 by Zollinger and Ellison, who reported the triad of fulminating ulcer diathesis, recurrent ulceration with a poor response to therapy, and pancreatic non-β-cell islet tumours. The syndrome is the result of excess gastrin-stimulated gastric acid secretion. This causes severe, multiple peptic ulcers, which are usually duodenal, but may occur in the oesophagus and jejunum, and are often associated with complications such as haemorrhage, perforation, and stricture formation. Diarrhoea and steatorrhoea, due to acid inactivation of small bowel enzymes and mucosal damage, may be prominent features, frequently preceding ulcer disease by 12 months or more.

The diagnosis of the gastrinoma syndrome requires the demonstration of a raised fasting gastrin concentration, associated with increased basal gastric acid secretion. The patient should, ideally, not take H_2 blockers for 3 days or omeprazole for 2 weeks before the test. Hypergastrinaemia and raised acid output may also arise from retained antrum following partial gastrectomy or the rare condition of G-cell hyperplasia. The intravenous secretin test distinguishes these conditions from gastrinoma and can aid diagnosis when other investigations are equivocal. In the presence of a gastrinoma, gastrin levels are elevated by at least 50 per cent following secretin, while there is no such increase in association with G-cell hyperplasia or retained antrum. Furthermore, gastrin levels are increased in response to a test meal in the latter conditions but not in association with a gastrinoma. Endoscopy may be valuable in demonstrating oesophageal and duodenal ulceration and hypertrophy of the gastric mucosa, while immunocytochemical analysis of antral biopsies may demonstrate G-cell hyperplasia. Localization of microgastrinomas may be aided preoperatively by endoscopic ultrasound or selective arterial secretin injection, or intraoperatively by ultrasonography or duodenotomy with transillumination and careful palpation. Small tumours often secrete gastrin rapidly and store little peptide so that histological diagnosis may only be possible by *in situ* hybridization to demonstrate synthesis of gastrin messenger RNA.

Since all gastrinomas may have the potential to metastasize, localized non-metastatic tumours should be resected, and regular attempts at localization should be made for occult tumours. In the past, the morbidity and mortality of the gastrinoma syndrome resulted from the severe peptic ulceration and associated complications. The best treatment for this was total gastrectomy to remove the source of acid hypersecretion. The H2-blockers provided relief of symptoms for many patients but often failed to suppress acid secretion adequately. The introduction of proton-pump inhibitors, which almost completely inhibits gastric acid production in all cases, has transformed the management of these patients, and offers the best palliation for those with metastatic disease. Most experience has been gained with omeprazole, but there is evidence that the newer agents are equally effective. Omeprazole is acid-labile and so initially should be administered with an H2-blocker. Since the introduction of proton-pump inhibitors, morbidity and mortality now occur much later and result from tumour bulk. Chemotherapy is effective in less than 50 per cent of cases, but hepatic embolization may be beneficial in the remainder.

VIPoma

VIPomas arise in the pancreas in 90 per cent of cases. The remaining tumours are mainly gangliomas or ganglioneuroblastomas originating in the sympathetic chain or adrenal medulla, and these tumours are especially common in children. Most extrapancreatic tumours are benign, but 50 per cent of pancreatic VIPomas have metastasized at the time of diagnosis, usually to local lymph nodes and the liver.

The features of the VIPoma (Verner–Morrison, pancreatic cholera) syndrome (Table 2) reflect the known biological actions of VIP. Large-volume diarrhoea without steatorrhoea is the cardinal symptom, most patients excreting more than 3 litres daily, with volumes of over 20 litres described. It is often intermittent at first, but in severe crises the volume loss coupled with the vasodilatory effects of VIP and the associated hypokalaemia may precipitate cardiovascular collapse.

Hypokalaemia results from loss in stools and activation of the renin–angiotensin system, and may be profound. The loss of bicarbonate in the stool leads to acidosis, which may mask the true potassium deficit. Achlorhydria or hypochlorhydria occurs in over 50 per cent of patients and distinguishes this diarrhoeal syndrome from that associated with gastrinoma, but its absence in a proportion of patients makes the acronym WDHA (watery diarrhoea, hypokalaemia, and achlorhydria) syndrome inappropriate. In up to 50 per cent of cases there is glucose intolerance as a result of the glucagon-like actions of VIP. Other features include: hypercalcaemia, probably due to PTHrP secretion and exacerbated by the dehydration; hypomagnesaemia due to loss in stools; and flushing of the head and neck, which can occur on tumour palpation and may be associated with a marked fall in systemic blood pressure. In advanced cases, extreme weight loss may occur.

VIPomas are usually associated with markedly raised plasma VIP concentrations, but because the half-life of VIP in circulation is only 2 min, the diagnosis is best confirmed by the finding of elevated circulating peptide histidine–methionine, which is produced from the prepro-VIP molecule, is more stable in plasma, and is cosecreted by VIPomas. Pancreatic polypeptide levels are elevated in 75 per cent of cases and neurotensin in 10 per cent. Ganglioneuroblastomas may secrete noradrenaline and adrenaline and so be associated with elevated urinary catecholamines and catecholamine metabolites.

VIPomas are usually large and so localization is rarely a problem. Occasionally, angiography may be necessary to detect small pancreatic lesions,

Table 2 Features of the VIPoma syndrome

Clinical features	Biochemical features
Secretory diarrhoea	Raised plasma VIP
Severe dehydration and weakness	Hypokalaemic acidosis
Hypotension and cardiac standstill	Hypochlorhydria
Abdominal colic	Hypercalcaemia—probably due to PTHrP
Flushing	Hypomagnesaemia
Weight loss	Glucose intolerance

PTHrP, parathyroid hormone related peptide.

or radiolabelled somatostatin or *m*-iodobenzylguanidine (MIBG) scanning to identify extrapancreatic tumours.

Resection specimens from pancreatic tumours show the structural and secretory patterns of epithelial endocrine tumours, while those from ganglioneuroblastomas show neurones and nerve fibres, together with Schwann cells. Immunocytochemistry detects VIP and peptide histidine–methionine, and electron microscopy shows poorly granulated tumours, with characteristic, small secretory granules.

Patients with non-metastatic disease should have surgical resections, and this is feasible in the majority of ganglioneuroblastomas. Chemotherapy provides very effective palliation for those with metastatic disease, and the excellent response to the comparatively non-toxic regimen of streptozotocin and 5-fluorouracil makes the use of other advocated agents, particularly α-interferon, unnecessary. Similarly, hepatic embolization is not usually indicated for metastatic VIPomas. Acute VIPoma crises should be managed with fluid and electrolyte support, and monitoring of central venous pressure is usually required. A number of drugs, including prednisolone, indomethacin, metoclopramide, lithium carbonate, and opiates, have been used with varying degrees of success to treat the diarrhoea. These have now been superseded by the somatostatin analogue, octreotide. Ninety per cent of patients respond to octreotide, with reduction of diarrhoea almost to normal and resolution of the electrolyte imbalance within 48 h, and it may be life-saving in an acute crisis. Unfortunately, the median duration of response to octreotide alone is less than 1 year, and so its use is probably best combined with chemotherapy.

Glucagonoma

Glucagonomas are α-cell tumours of the pancreas which secrete various forms of glucagon and other peptides derived from the preproglucagon molecule. They have an estimated annual incidence of 1 in 20 million, with a marginal female preponderance, and invariably present in adulthood. Over 70 per cent of patients have metastases at the time of diagnosis.

The characteristic feature of the glucagonoma syndrome is the rash of necrolytic migratory erythema, which occurs in almost all patients, although it often remains undiagnosed for many years (Plate 1). It usually starts in the groins and perineum, migrating to the distal extremities. The initial lesions are erythematous patches, which become raised and may be associated with bullae. These lesions break down and gradually heal, often leaving an area of hyperpigmentation, only to recur in another site. All mucous membranes may be involved, commonly leading to angular stomatitis, cheilitis, and glossitis. The cause of the rash is unknown. A direct effect of glucagon on the skin, glucagon-induced prostaglandin release, amino acid or free fatty acid deficiency, or zinc deficiency, due to the similarity with acrodermatitis enteropathica, have all been proposed as the underlying mechanism. The rash has been reported in a few patients without glucagonomas, who either had coeliac disease or cirrhosis, both of which may have led to elevation in glucagon and glucagon-like peptides. Other common features of glucagonomas include: impaired glucose tolerance, and occasionally mild diabetes requiring insulin therapy; progressive weight loss, which is occasionally severe enough to be fatal; venous thrombosis, which may be life-threatening; normochromic normocytic anaemia, probably as a result of direct bone marrow suppression by glucagon; bowel disturbance and nail dystrophy. Mental slowness, depression, and paraneoplastic neurological syndromes have also been described.

The diagnosis of glucagonoma is confirmed by demonstrating raised fasting plasma glucagon concentrations by radioimmunoassay; the elevation is usually 10- to 20-fold. Localization is almost never a problem, since tumours are invariably large and pancreatic, with metastases in the majority of cases. Barium studies often show thickened jejunal and ileal mucosa due to the trophic effects of large forms of glucagon on the small bowel. The tumour tissue contains large quantities of extractable glucagon which is localized to a-cells. Electron microscopy shows dense-core secretory granules and the core is often eccentric. Fifty per cent of tumours produce pancreatic polypeptide and coproduction of gastrin and insulin has been described. Skin biopsies show necrolysis of the stratum Malpighi of the epidermis in early lesions, but only a non-specific dermatitis at later stages.

Surgical cure of glucagonomas is rarely possible, although it has been claimed for patients with resectable metastatic disease; recently, successful liver transplantation for patients with metastatic glucagonomas has been reported. Surgery is complicated by the tendency to venous thrombosis, the catabolic effects of glucagon, and anaemia. A significant proportion of glucagonomas fail to respond to the combination of streptozotocin and 5-fluorouracil, and in these cases dacarbazine or hepatic embolization may be necessary. Octreotide is particularly effective in treating the rash, with resolution usually occurring within the first month of treatment and persisting for at least 6 months, but it has little impact on the other features of the syndrome. Other simple treatments for the rash which are worth using in all cases are topical or oral zinc and a high-protein diet. Amino acid infusions and blood transfusion may also be effective, but the tendency of the rash to spontaneous remission, often following hospitalization, throws doubt on the value of such procedures. The thrombotic tendency, which can result in fatal pulmonary emboli, is refractory to conventional anticoagulation, but aspirin or dipyridamole may be of benefit.

Somatostatinoma

Somatostatinomas are extremely rare, with an estimated annual incidence of about 1 in 40 million. Fifty per cent of these tumours are pancreatic, the remainder arising in the duodenum. Approximately 50 per cent of duodenal somatostatinomas occur in association with neurofibromatosis type I (von Recklinghausen's disease) and these tumours are usually periampullary. Pancreatic tumours usually present late with hepatic metastases, but duodenal tumours are frequently identified earlier as a result of local effects.

The somatostatinoma syndrome is characterized by the triad of cholelithiasis, diabetes mellitus, and steatorrhoea, the latter occurring in almost all patients with pancreatic tumours. These features result from the inhibitory actions of somatostatin on gallbladder contraction and secretion, insulin secretion, and pancreatic exocrine secretions. Hypoglycaemia has occasionally been described, possibly due to larger molecular forms of somatostatin having a greater inhibitory effect on counter-regulatory hormones than on insulin. Other features of the syndrome include hypochlorhydria, anaemia, postprandial fullness, and weight loss. The full syndrome is rarely seen in association with duodenal somatostatinoma, gallbladder disease being the only common manifestation. These tumours usually present as a result of effects on local structures, such as obstruction of the ampulla of Vater causing jaundice or pancreatitis, or intestinal obstruction or haemorrhage.

Circulating levels of somatostatin are usually elevated greater than 10-fold in association with pancreatic tumours, but duodenal tumours are associated with much lower levels, probably because they are usually about one-tenth the size of the pancreatic lesions. Multiple molecular weight forms of somatostatin may be demonstrated by column chromatography of plasma or tumour extracts, and these may explain unusual clinical features. Localization is rarely a problem as barium examinations or endoscopy will identify duodenal lesions. Duodenal somatostatinomas are classified histologically as duodenal carcinoids. Duodenal carcinoids have the usual features of neuroendocrine tumours but often contain psammoma bodies. Those associated with neurofibromatosis type I are more likely to be pure somatostatinomas and to contain psammoma bodies.

Surgical resection of duodenal somatostatinomas is usually curative, although a Whipple's procedure may be needed to ensure clearance of periampullary tumours. Pancreatic tumours have almost always metastasized by the time of diagnosis and so palliation with chemotherapy or hepatic embolization are the only therapeutic options.

Pancreatic polypeptide, neurotensin, and other hormones

Pancreatic polypeptide (PP) can be extracted from almost all pancreatic endocrine tumours and is secreted by up to 75 per cent of them. The finding of elevated circulating pancreatic polypeptide in association with other tumour syndromes indicates a pancreatic tumour source. However, pancreatic polypeptide itself has no recognized physiological role and no associated tumour syndrome, and pure PPomas can be regarded effectively as non-functioning tumours. Similarly neurotensin, which is elevated in 10 per cent of VIPomas, does not cause a characteristic syndrome. Interestingly, neurotensin is produced by fibrolamellar hepatomas.

Hypercalcaemia is a feature of the VIPoma syndrome and may also occur in association with pancreatic endocrine tumours without other hormone syndromes. Secretion of parathyroid hormone related peptide (PTHrP) by pancreatic endocrine tumours has now been reported in a number of cases, and synthesis of PTHrP messenger RNA in normal and tumorous islets has been described. It is highly probable, therefore, that almost all cases of hypercalcaemia in association with pancreatic endocrine tumours are mediated by PTHrP. In these patients the hypercalcaemia responds to both octreotide and bisphosphonates.

The hypothalamic hormone, growth hormone releasing hormone (GHRH), was originally isolated from a pancreatic endocrine tumour, and there have been subsequent reports of patients with acromegaly and gigantism as a result of GHRH secretion by pancreatic endocrine tumours. Treatment options for these patients have included surgical resection, octreotide therapy, and liver transplantation.

Another hypothalamic releasing factor, corticotrophin releasing hormone, may be produced by pancreatic endocrine tumours, but this only causes Cushing's syndrome when the tumour also secretes corticotrophin. One patient with an enteroglucagon-secreting tumour of the right kidney, causing villous hypertrophy and slowed intestinal transit, steatorrhoea, and mild diabetes, has been reported, and there has been one case of acromegaly due to a growth hormone secreting pancreatic endocrine tumour. Other peptides produced by islet-cell tumours include neuropeptide Y, neuromedin B, calcitonin gene-related peptide, bombesin, and motilin, but these are not associated with recognized clinical syndromes.

Non-functioning tumours

Tumours not associated with a recognized hormonal syndrome may account for half of all pancreatic endocrine tumours. They usually present late with symptoms attributable to tumour bulk, such as anorexia and weight loss, or to effects on local structures, such as obstructive jaundice or intestinal obstruction or haemorrhage. They are often mistakenly diagnosed as adenocarcinomas, but the presence of elevated circulating gut hormones, such as pancreatic polypeptide or neurotensin, and the use of immunocytochemical analysis, can point to the correct diagnosis. Non-functioning tumours usually respond poorly to chemotherapy, but hepatic embolization may be beneficial. They have a poor prognosis as a result of their late presentation and lack of response to therapy.

Multiple endocrine neoplasia

The multiple endocrine neoplasia syndromes (MEN1 and MEN2) are familial conditions with an autosomal dominant pattern of inheritance and a high degree of penetrance. The genetic defect has been identified for both types of MEN—the MEN1 gene, menin, on chromosome region 11q13, and the MEN2 gene, ret, on chromosome region 10q11.2. In MEN2 there have been few mutations identified, so that rapid mutation screening is possible, and genotype–phenotype correlations have been identified. In MEN1 many different mutations have been identified, often occurring in only one kindred, and mutation detection can only be done by formal gene sequencing. Identification of specific gene defects in these syndromes may provide novel therapeutic options for tumour prevention in affected individuals.

Multiple endocrine neoplasia type 1 (MEN1)

MEN1 is characterized by the association of parathyroid hyperplasia, pancreatic endocrine tumours, and pituitary adenomas. This association was first described by Underdahl in 1953, and the autosomal dominant inheritance was first proposed in 1954 by Wermer, whose name provided the eponym for the syndrome. The prevalence of the condition has been estimated at about 1 in 10 000. The affected gene has been termed menin and is found on the 11q13 region of the long arm of chromosome 11. It encodes a nuclear protein which interacts with the JunD component of the transcription factor AP-1. The development of tumours fits the 'two-hit' model proposed by Knudson and demonstrated by familial retinoblastoma, whereby there is a germline mutation of the MEN1 gene on one chromosome 11, followed by a somatic deletion of the same region on the other chromosome, leading to loss of heterozygosity for that allele and subsequent tumour formation. A substantial proportion of MEN1 cases arise through sporadic mutations, and these patients present between the third and fifth decades, while familial cases can be identified earlier through screening, usually biochemical but increasingly genetic once the mutation affecting a kindred has been sequenced.

Parathyroid hyperplasia and adenomas

Hyperparathyroidism is the presenting feature of MEN1 in the majority of patients, and occurs in almost all cases. Patients present either with asymptomatic hypercalcaemia on biochemical screening or with the features of sporadic hyperparathyroidism. All four glands are diffusely hyperplastic and there may be nodule formation. Whether true adenomas develop remains controversial, but it is assumed that the presence of a capsule indicates adenomatous change. All patients should be operated on to prevent later morbidity from hypercalcaemia and there are two surgical approaches. Subtotal parathyroidectomy may be performed, but hyperparathyroidism will almost always recur, necessitating excision of the remaining parathyroid tissue. However, most surgeons would perform total parathyroidectomy, either with autotransplantation of one gland to the forearm, which can later be removed if hyperparathyroidism recurs, or with immediate replacement therapy with 1α-hydroxycholecalciferol.

Pancreatic endocrine tumours

Pancreatic endocrine tumours occur in about 70 per cent of patients with MEN1, and usually present between the ages of 15 and 50 if not identified by screening. They account for most of the morbidity and mortality of the MEN1 syndrome. Over 60 per cent of tumours are gastrinomas and about 30 per cent are insulinomas, the two coexisting in about 10 per cent of cases. VIPomas have rarely been described and there are only isolated reports of glucagonomas, but non-functioning tumours may occur frequently. Diffuse hyperplasia of the pancreas is usually seen, similar to the parathyroid, and in the majority of cases there are multiple adenomas, most of which are less than 1 cm in diameter. Duodenal microgastrinomas are very common, probably accounting for almost half of all MEN1-associated gastrinomas, and are usually multiple, with up to 15 separate tumours described.

The surgical approach to pancreatic endocrine tumours in MEN1 is controversial. Surgical cure is best achieved by removing the pancreas and duodenum with adjacent lymph nodes, but such an aggressive approach is only justified in families in which the pancreatic disease has been extremely malignant, and in these kindreds it should be performed only when pancreatic disease is biochemically apparent. An alternative, potentially curative, approach is to perform a subtotal pancreatectomy with enucleation of palpable tumours in the head and careful exploration for duodenal lesions, which should also be resected. A more conservative strategy is to enucleate gross lesions to reduce the risk of developing metastatic disease, although size dose not necessarily correlate with metastatic potential, and then control hormonal syndromes with appropriate medical therapy. The latter approach may be appropriate for gastrinomas because proton-pump inhibitors are such an effective treatment, but for insulinomas, where medical therapy is often unsuccessful and symptoms usually recur after enucleation alone, more aggressive surgical management may be the best option. The treatment of metastatic disease is the same as in sporadic cases.

Pancreatic endocrine tumours associated with MEN1 are less malignant than sporadic tumours and carry a better prognosis, with a median survival of 15 years compared to 5 years for patients with sporadic tumours. This may reflect more indolent disease or earlier diagnosis.

Pituitary adenomas

The true incidence of pituitary adenomas in MEN1 is disputed. They are detected by screening in 30 per cent of patients, but are found at autopsy in over 50 per cent of patients. Unlike the pancreas and parathyroid, there does not appear to be diffuse pituitary hyperplasia, and loss of heterozygosity for the MEN1 locus is much less common in pituitary tumours than in parathyroid and pancreatic lesions.

Prolactinomas are the commonest tumours, occurring in about two-thirds of cases, with acromegaly accounting for about 30 per cent, and other functioning tumours being rare. Treatment is the same as for sporadic pituitary tumours (see Chapter 12.6).

Other lesions

Lesions in other tissues have been reported in association with MEN1, but their relationship to the syndrome remains controversial. Carcinoid tumours of the foregut, midgut, and thymuta occur in about 10 per cent of cases, and are often found in the pancreas, but are rarely symptomatic. Lipomas occur in a significant proportion of patients and act as a marker for affected individuals. Adrenal lesions are common autopsy findings in normal individuals, but do appear to occur more frequently in MEN1, with an incidence of up to 40 per cent. Furthermore, *menin* gene mutations have been demonstrated in individuals with atypical familial endocrine syndromes including phaeochromocytoma. Histology of adrenal lesions associated with MEN1 usually demonstrates nodular hyperplasia and there is no associated excess hormone secretion. Loss of heterozygosity of the MEN1 locus is not found in these lesions and it has been proposed that there may be a circulating adrenal growth factor, possibly secreted by the pancreas, since there is a strong correlation with pancreatic tumours, particularly insulinomas. MEN1-associated adrenal tumours showing loss of heterozygosity for 11q13 have been reported but are very rare. Thyroid disease has been reported in association with MEN1, but does not appear to occur more frequently than in the normal population.

Screening

The screening of first- and second-degree relatives of patients with MEN1 is aimed at early detection of parathyroid, pancreatic, or pituitary lesions in gene carriers, to reduce the associated morbidity. There is no evidence that screening reduces mortality, although the identification of affected individuals in 'malignant' kindreds with aggressive pancreatic disease may allow curative surgery which would be expected to prolong survival. Screening lowers the age of detection of the syndrome by about 20 years.

The most useful screening investigations are a serum calcium, fasting gastrin, and prolactin, although in practice a full gut hormone screen is usually performed. It has been suggested that the most sensitive markers of pancreatic disease are basal and test-meal-stimulated pancreatic polypeptide and gastrin, and basal insulin and proinsulin, identifying lesions at least 3 years before there are any radiological abnormalities. Since pancreatic tumours are the only life-threatening manifestation of the syndrome, such a screening protocol may be warranted. The MEN1 syndrome rarely develops before the age of 5 or after the age of 70, and so screening should be performed annually from 5 to 65, and at longer intervals thereafter. Eighty per cent of affected individuals will have been identified by the fifth decade. Screening of patients with apparently sporadic pancreatic endocrine tumours for evidence of MEN1 is probably justified, especially in those with gastrinomas or insulinomas. There is little evidence to support screening in those with sporadic pituitary tumours. MEN1 is present in 15 per cent of all patients with hyperparathyroidism, but hypercalcaemia

may be associated with elevated fasting gastrin and pancreatic polypeptide, and, whereas in those at risk of MEN1 this finding would be highly significant, in those with sporadic hyperparathyroidism this very rarely indicates pancreatic disease, so screening of all patients is not warranted.

Genetic mutation analysis can be used to screen for affected individuals in kindreds where the gene mutation has been identified, but if this is not the case biochemical screening is still needed.

Multiple endocrine neoplasia type 2 (MEN2)

Multiple endocrine neoplasia type 2 is the association of medullary cell carcinoma of the thyroid (MTC) and phaeochromocytoma. The association was first recognized in 1932, but it was not until 1961 that it was noted that the risk of phaeochromocytoma in patients with MTC was increased 14-fold. MEN2 has since been subdivided: in MEN2A, or Sipple's syndrome, parathyroid hyperplasia may occur; MEN2B is associated with mucosal neuromas and marfanoid habitus. In addition, there is a familial form of MTC without other features. Germ line mutations of the *ret* proto-oncogene, a receptor tyrosine kinase, have been identified in all three syndromes. In MEN2A and familial MTC, mutations occur in the extracellular domain, whilst in MEN2B mutation in the tyrosine kinase domain has been demonstrated. The MEN2 phenotypes reflect the expression of *ret* in different tissues. Tumours in affected individuals are heterozygous for the *ret* mutation, and so it is the only known dominantly inherited proto-oncogene. It is likely that activation of *ret* leads to hyperplasia in affected tissues and that a somatic mutation in another oncogene is required for carcinogenesis. Thus loss of heterozygosity for the short arm of chromosome 1 has been described in phaeochromocytomas and MTC associated with MEN2. New mutations are uncommon in MEN2A, and probably account for less than 10 per cent of cases, whereas new mutations account for about 50 per cent of cases with MEN2B. Those patients with MEN2A not identified by screening usually present in the fourth and fifth decades, while those with MEN2B present much earlier due to their characteristic phenotype.

Medullary cell carcinoma of the thyroid (MTC)

MTC is a tumour of the C cells of the thyroid (see Chapters 12.4 and 12.5), which secrete calcitonin, and this acts as a tumour marker. Twenty-five per cent of cases are familial. The incidence of MTC in MEN2 is probably 100 per cent. Familial MTC alone is the most benign form of MTC, while MTC in association with MEN2B is the most malignant form of the disease. In MEN2, the initial thyroid lesion is C-cell hyperplasia, which has been found as early as the age of 3 years in MEN2A and may be present at birth in MEN2B. Over the subsequent 5 to 10 years, microscopic MTC develops and finally gross tumours become apparent. Metastases are invariably present when tumours are already palpable, but there is speculation that they may occur with clinically occult disease. All forms of hereditary MTC are bilateral, with multifocal tumours, usually occurring at the junction of the upper third and lower two-thirds of the thyroid.

In MEN2A, MEN2B, and familial MTC genotype screening has largely replaced biochemical screening for MTC using pentagastrin-stimulated calcitonin, with over 95 per cent of kindreds with MEN2 and over 80 per cent of those with familial MTC having germline mutations of the *ret* gene, 99 per cent of MEN2 kindreds having a mutation in codon 918. In families with a known *ret* mutation it has been recommended that a positive genotype should result in a total thyroidectomy with lymph node clearance by the age of 2 years in MEN2B kindreds and at age 3 in MEN2A and familial MTC kindreds. In MEN2B MTC has been reported as early as 15 months of age with metastases by the age of 3 years. Prior to thyroidectomy those with a positive genotype should be screened biochemically for phaeochromocytoma, which, if confirmed, should be resected first. In those patients with MTC not identified by screening, thyroidectomy should still be performed, unless distant metastases, usually to lung or liver, are present. It is probable that in all patients with palpable disease, metastases to local lymph nodes will be present, so a central lymph node dissection should also be performed, probably with lateral node sampling to look for further spread. The prognosis is poor in this group, with recurrent disease in about 20 per cent of patients with clinically occult but macroscopic MTC and in over 60 per cent of those with palpable MTC. It is particularly poor in individuals with MEN2B who present with clinically apparent MTC. Their 10-year survival is about 50 per cent, and death from metastatic disease in the mid-twenties is common.

Phaeochromocytoma

Phaeochromocytoma is familial in 5 per cent of cases, 20 per cent of whom have MEN2. Fifty per cent of individuals with MEN2 develop phaeochromocytoma. About 70 per cent are bilateral, almost all are benign, and they are rarely extra-adrenal. The initial lesion, similar to that in the thyroid, is adrenal medullary hyperplasia, followed by nodule formation and, subsequently, development of multiple, multifocal phaeochromocytomas (see Chapter 15.16.2.4).

Symptoms and biochemical abnormalities are rare during the stage of medullary hyperplasia. MEN2-associated phaeochromocytomas are characterized by excessive adrenaline secretion, so that palpitation and other β-adrenergic symptoms predominate initially, with hypertension a late feature, although often present by the time of diagnosis. A urine adrenaline: noradrenaline ratio of greater than 0.15 in a patient with MEN2 indicates medullary hyperplasia or phaeochromocytoma. The treatment for adrenal medullary hyperplasia or phaeochromocytoma is bilateral adrenalectomy, since the incidence of bilateral disease is high, and the mortality from phaeochromocytoma in MEN2 about 15 per cent, usually due to sudden death. If an adrenal lesion is identified at the same time as MTC, the adrenalectomy should be performed first.

Other features of MEN2A

Parathyroid hyperplasia occurs in up to 80 per cent of patients with MEN2A, but less than 20 per cent have hypercalcaemia, the remainder being identified at the time of thyroidectomy. Parathyroidectomy should be performed in those with hypercalcaemia and in the remaining patients grossly enlarged glands should be removed at the time of thyroidectomy.

Cutaneous lichen amyloidosis, often preceded by intense pruritus, has been described in two kindreds with MEN2A and provides a phenotypic marker for the syndrome.

Other features of MEN2B

The characteristic phenotype of marfanoid habitus and mucosal neuromas (Fig. 4) identifies affected individuals with MEN2B and allows early intervention, since these features usually predate MTC and phaeochromocytoma. Neuromas are commonly ocular and oral, causing whitish-yellow or pink nodules on the anterior aspect of the tongue, lips, and eyelids, with thickening of the mucosa and often eversion of the lower lids. The nasal bridge may be broadened, pedunculated neuromas are found on cheek mucosa, and the corneal nerves are thickened and medullated. Involvement of peripheral motor and sensory nerves can cause a peroneal muscular atrophy type picture. Intestinal ganglioneuromatosis affects about 75 per cent of cases. Neuromas involve the autonomic nerves of both the myenteric and submucosal plexi and can cause poor suckling with failure to thrive, altered bowel habit, recurrent pseudo-obstruction, toxic megacolon, and occasionally dysphagia and vomiting, possibly due to achalasia. Almost all patients have a marfanoid habitus, usually associated with skeletal abnormalities, particularly slipped femoral epiphyses. Delayed puberty is another common feature of the syndrome.

Screening

Screening to identify affected individuals by genotyping and for early biochemical detection of adrenal disease reduces both morbidity and mortality in MEN2. A positive genotype identifies individuals for thyroidectomy. If a kindred's genotype has not been identified an elevated pentagastrin-stimulated calcitonin but normal basal calcitonin identifies individuals at the stage of C-cell hyperplasia or microscopic MTC. Where it is indicated biochemical screening in MEN2A or familial MTC should commence at age 3 and be performed annually. In MEN2B individuals with the phenotype do not need screening, as they should have a thyroidectomy before the age of

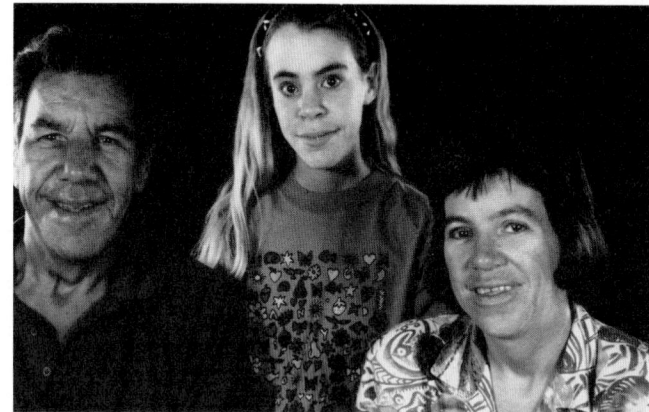

(a)

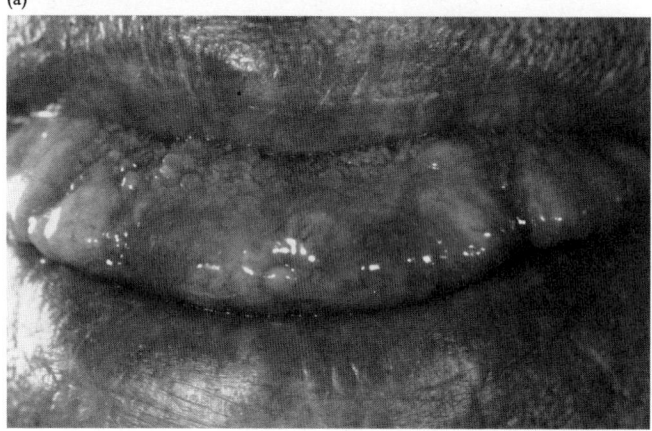

(b)

Fig. 4 (a) Characteristic phenotype of MEN2B showing facial appearance. (b) Characteristic phenotype of MEN2B showing mucosal neuromas on tongue.

2 years. Urinary metanephrines and catecholamines identify at least 95 per cent of phaeochromocytomas. Urinary vanillylmandelic acid levels are less useful, being associated with a high number of false positives and negatives. MIBG and/or CT scanning or measurement of plasma catecholamines may identify phaeochromocytomas missed by urinary assays. Serum calcium should be measured at the annual screening to identify overt hyperparathyroidism. In families where a mutation has been characterized, affected individuals can be identified by mutation screening.

Other syndromes associated with endocrine neoplasia

There are other syndromes which overlap with the multiple endocrine neoplasia syndromes and gene mutation analysis can identify those which are true variants of MEN1 or MEN2. Phaeochromocytomas may be associated with pancreatic islet-cell tumours alone, or in combination with other syndromes: von Hippel–Lindau syndrome is associated with a high incidence of phaeochromocytomas, islet-cell tumours, cerebellar haemangioblastomas, retinal angiomas, and renal cell carcinoma; neurofibromatosis type I (von Recklinghausen's syndrome) is often associated with phaeochromocytoma and, rarely, with duodenal somatostatinoma and medullary thyroid carcinoma; and phaeochromocytoma may be associated with prolactinoma as a mixed MEN syndrome.

Further reading

Ajani JA, Carrasco CH, Charnsangavej C, Samaan NA, Levin B, Wallace S (1988). Islet cell tumors metastatic to the liver: effective palliation by sequential hepatic artery embolization. *Annals of Internal Medicine* **108**, 340–4.

Arnold J, O'Grady J, Bird G, Calne R, Williams R (1989). Liver transplantation for primary and secondary hepatic apudomas. *British Journal of Surgery* **76**, 248–9.

Chandrasekharappa SC *et al.* (1997). Positional cloning of the gene for multiple endocrine neoplasia-type 1. *Science* **276**, 404–7.

Gorden P, Comi RJ, Maton PN, Go VL (1989). NIH conference. Somatostatin and somatostatin analogue (SMS 201–995) in treatment of hormone-secreting tumors of the pituitary and gastrointestinal tract and non-neoplastic diseases of the gut. *Annals of Internal Medicine* **110**, 35–50.

Grauer A, Raue F, Gagel RF (1990). Changing concepts in the management of hereditary and sporadic medullary thyroid carcinoma. *Endocrinology and Metabolism Clinics of North America* **19**, 613–35.

Hofstra RM *et al.* (1994). A mutation in the RET proto-oncogene associated with multiple endocrine neoplasia type 2B and sporadic medullary thyroid carcinoma. *Nature* **367**, 375–6.

Jensen RT, ed. (1989). Gastrointestinal endocrinology. *Gastroenterology Clinics of North America* **18**, 671–931.

Krejs G, ed. (1987). Gastrointestinal endocrine tumours. *American Journal of Medicine* **82** (Suppl. 5B), 1–3.

Moertel CG, Lefkopoulo M, Lipsitz S, Hahn RG, Klaassen D (1992). Streptozocin-doxorubicin, streptozocin-fluorouracil or chlorozotocin in the treatment of advanced islet-cell carcinoma. *New England Journal of Medicine* **326**, 519–23.

Mulligan LM *et al.* (1993). Germ-line mutations of the RET proto-oncogene in multiple endocrine neoplasia type 2A. *Nature* **363**, 458–60.

Oberg K, ed. (1991). Recent advances in diagnosis and treatment of neuroendocrine gut and pancreatic tumours. *Acta Oncologica* **28**, 301–449.

Rosch T *et al.* (1992). Localization of pancreatic endocrine tumors by endoscopic ultrasonography. *New England Journal of Medicine* **326**, 1721–6.

Rossi P *et al.* (1989). Endocrine tumors of the pancreas. *Radiologic Clinics of North America* **27**, 129–61.

Sheppard BC, Norton JA, Doppman JL, Maton PN, Gardner JD, Jensen RT (1989). Management of islet cell tumors in patients with multiple endocrine neoplasia: a prospective study. *Surgery* **106**, 1108–17.

Skogseid B *et al.* (1991). Multiple endocrine neoplasia type 1: a 10-year prospective screening study in four kindreds. *Journal of Clinical Endocrinology and Metabolism* **73**, 281–7.

Thakker RV and Ponder BA (1988). Multiple endocrine neoplasia. *Baillières Clinical Endocrinology and Metabolism* **2**, 1031–67.

Vasen HF *et al.* (1992). The natural course of multiple endocrine neoplasia type IIb. A study of 18 cases. *Archives of Internal Medicine* **152**, 1250–2.

Vinayek R, Frucht H, Chiang HC, Maton PN, Gardner JD, Jensen RT (1990). Zollinger-Ellison syndrome. Recent advances in the management of the gastrinoma. *Gastroenterology Clinics of North America* **19**, 197–217.

Wynick D and Bloom SR (1991). The use of the long-acting somatostatin analog octreotide in the treatment of gut neuroendocrine tumors. *Journal of Clinical Endocrinology and Metabolism* **73**, 1–3.

12.11 Disorders of glucose homeostasis

12.11.1 Diabetes

Gareth Williams

Diabetes mellitus can be defined as a state of chronic hyperglycaemia sufficient to cause long-term damage to specific tissues, notably the retina, kidney, nerves, and arteries.

This functional label gives little insight into the long and colourful history of this disease, its clinical and scientific importance, or its immense personal and socio-economic impact. Diabetes was recognized in antiquity, and its clinical features (with empirical treatment guidelines) were recorded over 3500 years ago in the Egyptian 'Ebers' papyrus. Our understanding of the disease has advanced greatly, especially during the last two decades, but many aspects of its management remain imperfect.

Diabetes is and will remain a threat to global health. In the United Kingdom, at least 2 per cent of the population (over 1 million people) are diabetic and the disease absorbs 5 to 10 per cent of the total health budget. Worldwide, diabetes probably affects 150 million people and its prevalence is predicted to double by 2015.

Diagnosis of diabetes

Blood glucose concentrations are is normally tightly regulated: fasting values lie between 3.5 and 5.5 mmol/l and even large carbohydrate loads do not raise the concentration above 8 mmol/l. It is logical to define diabetes by the blood glucose concentrations which cause the chronic complications of the disease but the choice of the diagnostic glucose levels has been contentious (and has stirred up much passion among epidemiologists). One difficulty is that some diabetic complications show a 'threshold' effect with the risk rising above a cutoff level (for example fasting plasma glucose of 6 to 7 mmol/l for retinopathy), whereas macrovascular disease (atheroma) does not (see later). Another problem is that even the current criteria are not self-consistent: for example, 30 per cent of newly diagnosed type 2 diabetic patients will have a 'normal' fasting plasma glucose, while another 30 per cent will have a 'normal' value 2 h after an oral glucose tolerance test.

The current diagnostic criteria for diabetes and other hyperglycaemic states (Fig. 1) have been approved by the World Health Organization and most national diabetes associations. All values refer to venous plasma glucose concentrations:

1. Diabetes mellitus: fasting glucose more than 7.0 mmol/l and/or a value exceeding 11.1 mmol/l, either at 2 h during an oral glucose tolerance test or in a random sample. The corresponding levels in non-SI units are 126 and 200 mg/dl respectively. The diagnostic fasting glucose level was lowered from the previous value of 7.8 mmol/l to reflect more accurately the risk of developing diabetic retinopathy.

2. Impaired glucose tolerance: fasting glucose less than 7.0 mmol/l and 2-h oral glucose tolerance test value between 7.8 and 11.1 mmol/l.

3. Impaired fasting glucose: fasting glucose 6.1 to 6.9 mmol/l (110 to 124 mg/dl).

Impaired glucose tolerance (**IGT**) and the recently distinguished impaired fasting glucose (**IFG**) are intermediate categories of hyperglycaemia that carry definite risks and so require follow-up and risk-factor management (see below). They are often transient stages and overlap to some extent: about one-third of subjects with impaired fasting glucose also have impaired glucose tolerance, while one-quarter of those with impaired glucose tolerance also show impaired fasting glucose.

The new criteria put much emphasis on the fasting plasma glucose concentration. However, the time-consuming oral glucose tolerance test is still required in some cases with borderline fasting hyperglycaemia, because the 2-h oral glucose tolerance test value in such patients may be high enough to put them at risk of microvascular complications. Moreover, the oral glucose tolerance test remains the only way to define impaired glucose tolerance.

Practical screening and diagnostic procedures

Figure 2 shows an algorithmic approach to screening for and diagnosis of diabetes and its associated hyperglycaemic states. Certain high-risk groups need to be actively screened for type 2 diabetes, which may be present (and causing complications) for several years before it is noticed. These include subjects predisposed to develop type 2 diabetes through genotype and/or phenotype, those affected by diabetogenic conditions such as pregnancy,

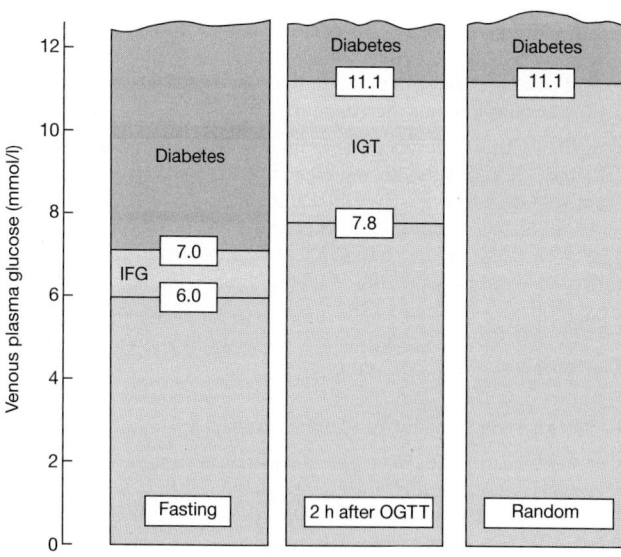

Fig. 1 Diagnostic thresholds for diabetes, impaired glucose tolerance (IGT), and impaired fasting glucose (IFG). From the Expert Committee on the Diagnosis and classification of diabetes mellitus (1997). *Diabetes Care* **20**, 1183–97. For conversion to mg/dl, multiply values in mmol/l by 18.

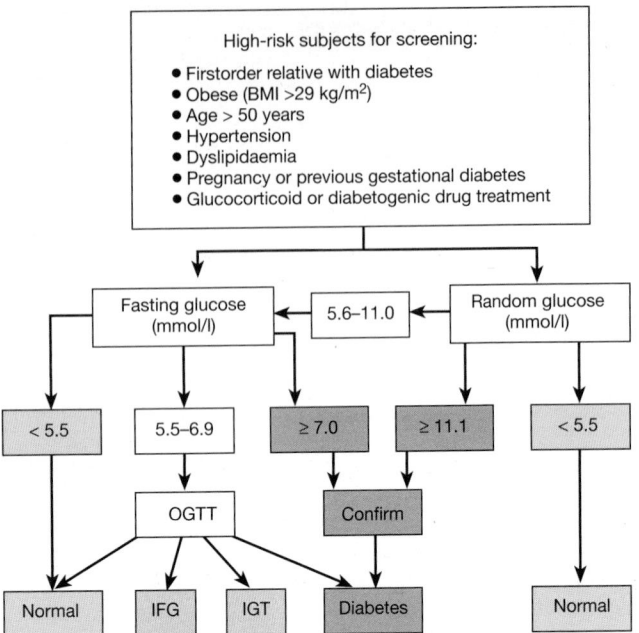

Fig. 2 Screening algorithm for diagnosing diabetes, impaired glucose tolerance, and impaired fasting glucose. All glucose values relate to venous plasma (mmol/l). Adapted from data in Shaw JE and Zimmet P (2000). Do we know how to diagnose diabetes and do we need to screen for the disease? In: Gill GV, Pickup JC, Williams G, eds. *Difficult diabetes*, pp 3–21. Blackwell Science, Oxford.

endocrine disorders or certain drugs, and those with other cardiovascular risk factors in whom hyperglycaemia must not be missed.

Diabetes is not a trivial diagnosis, and certain practical points must be carefully observed:

1. Glucose should be measured in venous plasma using a quality-controlled laboratory method. Capillary (finger-prick) samples contain higher glucose levels than venous blood, from which glucose has been extracted by the tissue bed; whole-blood glucose levels are lower than in plasma, because red cells actively metabolize glucose and so contain only low concentrations. These differences may reach 0.5 to 1.0 mmol/l. Portable glucose meters correlate well with laboratory glucose methods, but because of potential technical errors they should not be used to make or refute the diagnosis.

2. An oral glucose tolerance test is indicated for borderline hyperglycaemia (Fig. 2). After an overnight fast, the subject drinks 75 g of anhydrous glucose dissolved in 250 ml water (or 394 ml Lucozade); venous blood is sampled at baseline and 2 h later. Food intake should be normal during the preceding few days: poor nutrition can cause delayed hyperglycaemia with a raised 2-h value (the 'lag' curve).

3. Abnormal values need confirmation. Postchallenge glucose levels in particular can vary considerably. Because of this and possible laboratory error, the diagnosis of diabetes should ideally be verified using a further sample on another day. Obvious exceptions are grossly raised values in seriously ill patients, especially children.

4. Diabetes must not be diagnosed from indirect measures of hyperglycaemia such as raised glycated haemoglobin (HbA_{1c}) or fructosamine levels in blood, or glycosuria. HbA_{1c} and fructosamine reflect average blood glucose concentrations, but the measurements are not sufficiently sensitive or standardized (several different methods are in use) to be used diagnostically. Glycosuria depends on the renal threshold for glucose reabsorption and its presence does not necessarily indicate hyperglycaemia; conversely, glucose may be absent from the urine in diabetic subjects who also have a high renal threshold. However,

abnormal results with any of these tests suggest diabetes and indicate the need for formal blood glucose screening.

Impaired glucose tolerance (IGT)

Impaired glucose tolerance is a metastable state: within 5 years, about 25 per cent of subjects with impaired glucose tolerance deteriorate into type 2 diabetes, while a further 25 per cent revert to normoglycaemia. The degree of hyperglycaemia in impaired glucose tolerance falls, by definition, below the threshold for microvascular complications but is enough to predispose to cardiovascular disease (see later).

Subjects found to have impaired glucose tolerance must be followed up because of the hazards of both diabetes and macrovascular disease. An oral glucose tolerance test should be repeated at least annually, and dietary and lifestyle advice given to decrease metabolic and cardiovascular risks; increased physical activity, a low-fat diet and weight loss convincingly reduce both the progression to type 2 diabetes and cardiovascular events. Risk factors such as smoking, hypertension, dyslipidaemia, and obesity should be managed actively. Specific antihyperglycaemic treatments (with metformin or thiazolidinediones, to improve insulin sensitivity) are currently being evaluated.

Impaired fasting glucose (IFG)

As with impaired glucose tolerance, the 5-year risk of progressing to type 2 diabetes appears to be about 25 per cent, and IFG predisposes to cardiovascular disease. Long-term monitoring and management should therefore be as for impaired glucose tolerance.

Metabolic basis of diabetes

Diabetes is due to inadequate production of insulin and/or 'resistance' to the glucose-lowering and other actions of insulin. To put this in context, key aspects of normal metabolism will be briefly reviewed.

The islets of Langerhans

There are about 1 million islets of Langerhans in the normal adult: insulin is produced by the β (B) cells, which make up the bulky core of each islet; β cells also synthesize the peptide known as amylin or islet-associated polypeptide. The other islet cell types, mostly surrounding the β-cell core, are the α (A) cells that produce glucagon, the δ (D) cells that produce somatostatin, and the PP cells that synthesize pancreatic polypeptide. All islet cells are derived embryologically from the buds of gut endoderm which also give rise to the exocrine pancreatic tissue.

The various islet cell types communicate with each other through the hormones they secrete into the islet's rich capillary plexus and probably by paracrine effects on adjacent cells; these interactions presumably regulate hormone secretion. Insulin inhibits release of glucagon, while glucagon powerfully stimulates insulin secretion—an action exploited in the testing of β-cell reserve (see below). Somatostatin suppresses the secretion of insulin and glucagon. Amylin can inhibit insulin secretion under experimental conditions but its physiological role is uncertain. Amylin also polymerizes outside the β cell to produce fibrils of amyloid material, which have been implicated in the progressive β-cell damage of type 2 diabetes.

Insulin

Insulin has a molecular weight of 5800 Da; it is made up of an A chain (21 amino acid residues) and a B chain (30 residues), joined covalently by two disulphide bridges. The precursor molecule, proinsulin, consists of the A and B chains linked end-to-end through a connecting (C) peptide which is cleaved off during insulin processing. In the circulation, insulin is monomeric but in crystals and more concentrated solutions (for example in the insulin vial and the subcutaneous injection site), six insulin molecules self-associate around a central Zn^{2+} ion. Self-association influences the pharmacokinetic properties of subcutaneously injected insulin: the rate-limiting dissociation of hexamers into monomers slows the absorption of even 'fast-acting' insulin.

Insulin regulates metabolism in birds, fish, and reptiles as well as mammals, and its structure is remarkably well conserved across the phyla. Three species of insulin are used therapeutically; the human sequence differs from porcine at a single residue (B30) and from bovine at two others. These differences affect the pharmacokinetic and immunogenic characteristics of the insulins (see below). The physicochemical behaviour of insulin has been successfully manipulated in synthetic 'designer' insulins that have improved absorption profiles: modification of the C terminus of the B chain, a region crucial for self-association, produces analogues that remain in the monomeric state and are therefore absorbed faster than the native soluble insulin (see below).

Insulin biosynthesis and processing

Insulin is a product of the preproinsulin (*INS*) gene, located on the short arm of chromosome 11, whose coding region contains three exons. Translation of *INS* mRNA in the rough endoplasmic reticulum produces preproinsulin, which is successively cleaved during its passage through the Golgi vesicles and secretory vesicles to yield first proinsulin and finally insulin and C peptide. Proinsulin is converted into insulin by the proteolytic excision of the C-peptide chain; the two intermediate cleavage products (with either end of the C peptide remaining attached to insulin) are called 'split products' of proinsulin. Normally, almost all proinsulin is processed through this 'regulated' pathway to yield equimolar amounts of insulin and C peptide. However, a 'constitutive' pathway may predominate in dysfunctional β cells (for example in type 2 diabetes and insulinoma), when processing is not complete and large quantities of proinsulin and split products may be released into the circulation.

C peptide is generally regarded as an inert byproduct of insulin production. However, its structure is also conserved across species and it may have vasoactive and other properties.

Insulinopathies are point mutations in the *INS* gene which either produce a mutant insulin (for example, insulin Chicago: a phenylalanine for leucine substitution at residue B25) or interfere with one of the cleavage sites of proinsulin so that the mutant split product cannot be further processed (for example, proinsulin Tokyo). These conditions are inherited as autosomal dominant traits; circulating insulin-like or proinsulin-like immunoreactivities may be extremely high but glucose intolerance is often surprisingly mild.

Insulin secretion

Glucose is the main insulin secretagogue; this action of glucose is modulated by other ingested nutrients, by hormones released by the islets and the gut, and by the autonomic innervation of the islet. The process gives insight into the mode of action of the sulphonylureas and related drugs, and the cause of maturity onset diabetes of the young (see below).

Glucose-stimulated insulin secretion

The amount of insulin released by the normal β cell is tightly coupled to blood glucose levels and begins to increase immediately when blood glucose rises. The ability of the β cell to sense ambient glucose levels accurately and rapidly depends on the glucose transporter isoform GLUT-2 and the glucose metabolizing enzyme glucokinase, while insulin release hinges on depolarization of the β-cell membrane which is controlled by a specific ion channel, the ATP-sensitive K⁺ channel. The characteristics of GLUT-2 allow glucose at physiological concentrations to freely enter the β cell, where it is immediately converted by glucokinase into glucose-6-phosphate—the point of entry into the glycolytic pathway which ultimately yields ATP; ATP production within the β cell is therefore proportionate to extracellular glucose.

ATP binds to and closes the ATP-dependent K⁺ channel; when open, this channel allows K⁺ ions to leave the β cell along their concentration gradient and thus helps to maintain the negative charge inside the β-cell membrane. ATP-induced closure of the channel therefore causes K⁺ ions to accumulate

within the cell and the membrane to depolarize, which triggers the opening of specific (voltage-gated) Ca^{2+} channels in the membrane. Ca^{2+} ions then flood into the β cell from the outside and activate the contractile proteins which drag the secretory vesicles containing insulin and C peptide to the cell surface. Here, the vesicles fuse with the cell membrane and release their contents into the extracellular space (exocytosis), from where insulin and C peptide enter the islet capillaries.

Other factors affecting insulin secretion

Sulphonylureas induce insulin secretion by closing the same ATP-sensitive K⁺ channel as glucose: they bind to a specific sulphonylurea receptor (SUR-1) linked to the K⁺ channel protein (called Kir 6.2). Repaglinide also closes this K⁺ channel, but binds to a different site from the sulphonylureas. By contrast, diazoxide locks the channel open, hyperpolarizing the β-cell membrane and inhibiting insulin secretion—hence its use in treating insulinoma.

Glucagon and glucagon-like peptide-1 7–36 amide (**GLP-1**; a gut peptide with insulin secretagogue (incretin) actions), both stimulate insulin secretion by raising cytosolic Ca^{2+} concentrations; binding to their receptors increases generation of cyclic AMP which blocks removal of Ca^{2+} into intracellular organelles. Conversely, somatostatin and possibly amylin act to decrease production of cyclic AMP and inhibit insulin secretion. Arginine stimulates insulin secretion, possibly by depolarizing the β-cell membrane as it enters the cell (it is cationic).

The autonomic nervous system is an important modulator of insulin secretion; it is stimulated by the parasympathetic (vagal) outflow and inhibited by the sympathetic. Vagal stimulation is mediated by acetylcholine acting via muscarinic receptors, while the inhibitory sympathetic neurotransmitter is noradrenaline, interacting with α_2 adrenoceptors.

Diseases due to defects in insulin secretion in perhaps 10 per cent of pedigrees is due to mutations affecting glucokinase (glucokinase-dependent maturity onset diabetes of the young). These impair ATP production from glucose, blunting the insulin response of the β cell to rising glucose and resulting in variable hyperglycaemia (see below). By contrast, familial neonatal hyperinsulinism is caused by mutations in *SUR-1* that close the ATP-sensitive K⁺ channel, leading to sustained insulin secretion and severe hypoglycaemia soon after birth.

Normal pattern of insulin secretion

Insulin concentrations in peripheral blood show basal levels of about 10 mU/l that tend to fall overnight, on which are superimposed prandial peaks reaching 80 to 100 mU/l, roughly proportionate to the amount eaten. The prandial peaks are elicited by the insulin secretagogue effects of glucose and other nutrients, augmented by incretin gut peptides (such as GLP-1) and the vagal outflow (the early cephalic phase of insulin release).

Very frequent sampling (every minute) shows that 'basal' insulin secretion is in fact pulsatile, with clear but low-amplitude peaks every 9 to 13 min. This may help to keep the target tissues sensitive to insulin; loss of this pulsatility is an early sign of β-cell dysfunction in type 2 diabetes. An acute insulin secretagogue challenge (for example an intravenous glucose bolus) induces a sharp 'first-phase' insulin peak, loss of which is another early abnormality in type 2 diabetes.

The insulin response elicited by eating is larger than when an equivalent nutrient load is given intravenously. This is because glucose entering the gut stimulates neuroendocrine cells in the gut wall to release 'incretin' hormones which act on the β cell to enhance insulin secretion (the 'enteroinsular axis': see Chapter 14.8). An important incretin appears to be GLP-1, a product of alternative processing of the preproglucagon gene (glucagon itself is not produced, in contrast to the islet α cell). GLP-1 released from the small intestine augments insulin release in the presence of glucose, an effect being explored in the treatment of type 2 diabetes.

Peripheral insulin levels are lower than those in the portal vein, into which the islets drain, because up to 30 per cent of insulin is removed on its first pass through the liver—one of the main targets for insulin action. The kidney also actively clears and degrades insulin; the circulating half-life is only a few minutes.

C peptide provides a robust measure of residual β-cell function, because it is cleared more slowly than insulin and its plasma concentrations are therefore more stable. C peptide is generally measured after intense β-cell stimulation with the powerful insulin secretagogue glucagon; alternatives are a heavy oral load of carbohydrate, or simply the measurement of 24-h secretion of C peptide in urine (it is cleared largely intact through the kidneys). In normal subjects and most with type 2 diabetes, peak C-peptide concentrations at 6 min after 1 mg of intravenous glucagon are 1 to 4 nmol/l, whereas type 1 diabetic individuals are typically 'C-peptide negative', with peak levels less than 0.6 nmol/l.

The insulin receptor and signal transduction

The insulin receptor belongs to the family that also includes the insulin-like growth factor 1 receptor. Insulin receptors are found in the obvious insulin target tissues (fat, liver, and skeletal muscle) but also in unexpected sites, such as the brain and gonads, in which glucose uptake does not depend on insulin.

The insulin receptor is a 400-kDa heterotetramer composed of two α and two β glycoprotein subunits, interconnected by disulphide bridges (Fig. 3). Both α and β subunits are encoded within a complex gene (22 exons) on chromosome 19q. The α subunit (135 kDa) lies entirely extracellularly, while the β subunit (95 kDa) spans the cell membrane and extends into the cytoplasm. Part of the intracytoplasmic tail functions as a

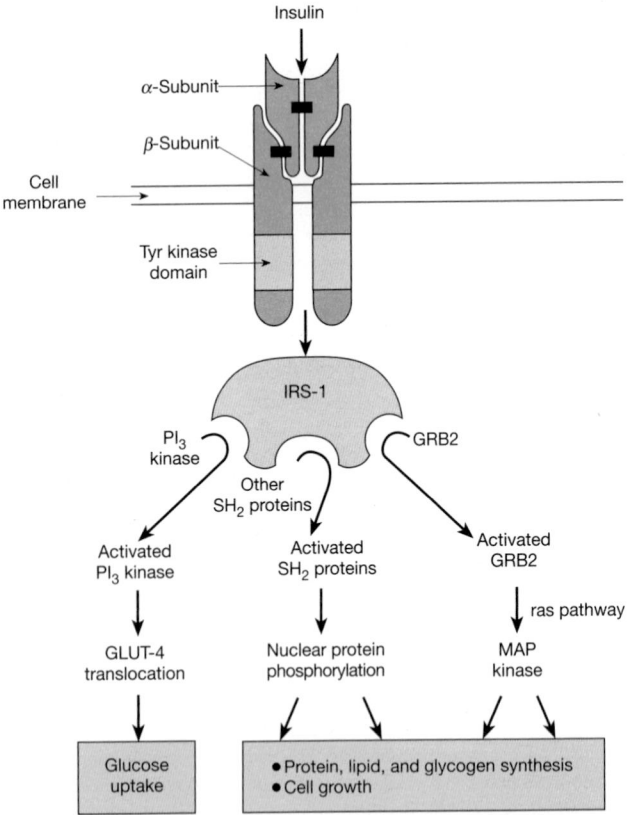

Fig. 3 The insulin receptor and signal transduction pathways within insulin's target cells. Binding of insulin to the extracellular α subunits of the receptor activates the tyrosine (Tyr) kinase domain of the intracellular β subunit. This phosphorylates insulin receptor substrate 1 (IRS-1) and the related IRS-2, which in turn phosphorylate other signalling proteins. These activated proteins then trigger other reactions that result in the biological actions of insulin, including enhanced glucose uptake, anabolic effects, and cell growth. PI₃ kinase, phosphatidylinositol 3 kinase; MAP kinase, mitogen-activated protein kinase.

tyrosine kinase, attaching phosphate groups from ATP to tyrosine residues elsewhere on the receptor (autophosphorylation) and on other intracellular proteins. This tyrosine kinase activity is essential for insulin signalling and for insulin to exert its many effects on its target tissues. Insulin binds to a site on the extracellular α subunits, and binding triggers a conformational change in the receptor which activates the tyrosine kinase domain of the β subunits.

Postreceptor mechanisms

The activated receptor phosphorylates tyrosine residues on specific intracellular proteins which initiate the signal transduction pathway within the target cell. One protein is the large (130 kDa) insulin receptor substrate 1, which has numerous phosphorylation sites that can accept other proteins possessing specific 'SH2' domains. 'Docking' and activation (phosphorylation) of these proteins by insulin receptor substrate 1 begins a cascade of intracellular reactions that lead ultimately to the effects of insulin on glucose, lipid, and protein metabolism and its many other actions. The details remain elusive, but the mitogen-activated protein kinase pathway is involved in glycogen synthesis, while the phosphatidylinositol 3 kinase pathway mediates glucose transporter translocation (see Fig. 3).

Receptor turnover

Receptors that bind insulin are 'internalized', i.e. taken up into the target cell by an invagination of the cell membrane that is coated with the protein clathrin. Bound insulin is degraded in the lysosomes, while most of the insulin receptors are carried back to the cell surface and reinserted into the membrane. The density of receptors on the cell surface is therefore a dynamic quantity, regulated partly by new receptor synthesis and partly by receptor recycling, which in turn is determined by insulin binding. Prolonged exposure to high insulin concentrations increases the proportion of internalized receptors and so decreases the density of receptors available on the cell surface. This 'downregulation' of receptors reduces the sensitivity of the target tissue to insulin.

Disorders due to insulin receptor defects

Many mutations have now been described in the insulin receptor, including point mutations that cause single-residue substitutions or truncation of the α or β subunits. Mutations affecting the tyrosine kinase domain interfere with insulin signalling and can lead to severe insulin resistance and glucose intolerance, sometimes with serious mental and physical abnormalities (for example in 'leprechaunism') which confirm the importance of insulin in fetal development.

Antibodies may develop against the insulin receptor and usually cause insulin resistance with variable hyperglycaemia (the 'type B' insulin resistance syndrome); rarely, hypoglycaemia results from antibodies that activate the receptor (analogous to thyrotoxicosis induced by antibodies to the thyroid-stimulating hormone receptor in Graves' disease).

Metabolic actions of insulin

Insulin functions as an anabolic hormone, favouring the uptake, utilization, and storage of glucose, the storage of lipids as triglyceride, and preventing the breakdown of protein.

Effects on carbohydrate metabolism

Insulin lowers blood glucose in two main ways (Fig. 4). At low basal concentrations (overnight and between meals) it shuts off the production of glucose by the liver, which is the main determinant of fasting glycaemia. Hepatic glucose output is fuelled by both glycogen breakdown (glycogenolysis) and gluconeogenesis (i.e. glucose synthesis from substrates including lactate, glycerol, and alanine and other amino acids); the rate-limiting enzymes for these processes are powerfully inhibited by insulin. Conversely, insulin stimulates glycogen synthesis.

At higher concentrations, such as after meals, insulin also stimulates glucose transport into skeletal muscle (where it is utilized to provide energy via glycolysis, or stored as glycogen) and into fat (where it is used to synthesize triglycerides). In both these tissues, insulin enhances glucose uptake

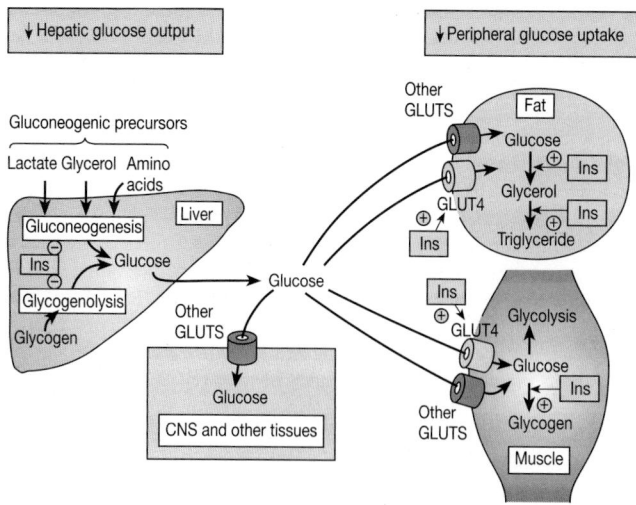

Fig. 4 Effects of insulin on glucose homeostasis. Insulin inhibits gluconeogenesis and glycogen breakdown in the liver, thus decreasing hepatic glucose output. Blood glucose is also lowered by increased glucose uptake into fat and skeletal muscle, mediated by the insulin-stimulated glucose transporter, GLUT-4. (Non-insulin mediated glucose uptake is effected by other GLUT proteins.)

through a specific glucose transporter protein, GLUT-4 (Fig. 4). Insulin causes GLUT-4 units to be translocated rapidly to the cell surface and inserted into the membrane: there, GLUT-4 units act as hydrophilic pores through which glucose can cross the otherwise impermeable membrane into the cell, following its concentration gradient. Insulin also stimulates GLUT-4 synthesis. Overall, insulin acting via GLUT-4 can increase glucose uptake into muscle and fat by up to 40-fold over the basal 'non-insulin mediated' glucose uptake. Non-insulin mediated glucose uptake occurs through other glucose transporter isoforms that operate in the absence of insulin, notably GLUT-1 in peripheral tissues and erythrocytes and GLUT-3 in brain.

Effects on lipid metabolism

Insulin inhibits triglyceride breakdown (lipolysis), while promoting its synthesis (lipogenesis). Lipolytic enzymes that split triglyceride into glycerol and free fatty acids are powerfully inhibited by insulin, even at low basal insulin concentrations. Profound insulin deficiency, such as in untreated type 1 diabetes, is therefore required before uncontrolled lipolysis occurs and generates enough free fatty acids to cause ketoacidosis (see below).

Effects on protein metabolism

Insulin inhibits protein catabolism and thus reduces the generation of amino acids which can act as gluconeogenic precursors to enhance glucose production by the liver and kidney. Insulin also promotes protein synthesis and cellular and tissue growth.

Other actions of insulin

These include vasodilatation, mediated by endothelial production of nitric oxide; growth and differentiation of the fetal nervous system; and enhanced tubular reabsorption of Na+ ions by the kidneys.

Measurements of insulin action

Glucose lowering is the most easily tested biological action of insulin, and forms the basis for most measurements of 'insulin resistance'. Several methods are used in the research setting; theoretically, the simplest could be used in clinical diabetes care, to identify patients with marked insulin resistance who might benefit particularly from insulin-sensitizing drugs such as the thiazolidinediones.

1. *Homeostatic model assessment* (HOMA) is an index derived by mathematical modelling of the relationship between the fasting glucose and insulin concentrations: with decreasing insulin sensitivity, insulin

secretion increases in an attempt to maintain euglycaemia, resulting in compensatory hyperinsulinaemia. Homeostatic model assessment can be performed on a single fasting blood sample and compares well with the insulin–glucose clamp.

2. *Insulin–glucose (hyperinsulinaemic–euglycaemic) clamp.* Insulin is infused intravenously to achieve constant high concentrations and a separate infusion of glucose is adjusted to maintain blood glucose 'clamped' at a normal value. The more glucose required, the greater is the insulin sensitivity. The clamp is generally regarded as the 'gold standard' method but demands blood glucose measurements every few minutes and takes some hours to perform.

3. *Intravenous glucose tolerance test.* An intravenous glucose bolus stimulates insulin release, and mathematical modelling of the relationship between the insulin peak and the decay in blood glucose levels can yield indices of both insulin secretion and insulin sensitivity.

Insulin resistance

Insulin resistance (or insensitivity) is a poorly defined term signifying decreased biological activity of insulin, and which is usually equated with impaired glucose-lowering.

There is no universal normal range for insulin sensitivity, because the ability of insulin to lower glucose varies considerably between and within individuals—it is influenced, for example, by levels of physical activity and fitness. Subjects with 'insulin-resistant' conditions such as type 2 diabetes or essential hypertension commonly show reductions of 40 to 60 per cent in glucose disposal (measured by the clamp technique), as compared with matched healthy controls, yet many apparently normal subjects also have comparable decreases in insulin sensitivity. There is no argument about extreme examples of insulin resistance: in some patients with so-called 'leprechaunism', over 20 000 U/day of insulin have failed to control hyperglycaemia and ketosis. A working definition of clinically relevant insulin resistance in insulin-treated diabetic patients is a daily requirement of more than 1.5 U/kg.

Causes of insulin resistance

Inherited causes

Inherited causes include the very rare mutations affecting the insulin receptor or postreceptor signalling pathways which can lead to extreme insulin resistance; milder polygenic defects contribute to the insulin resistance of type 2 diabetes (see below). Insulin receptor mutations cause clinically distinct syndromes, often with acanthosis nigricans and, in women, features of polycystic ovary disease and masculinization; hyperglycaemia is variable. Specific syndromes include the speculatively named 'leprechaunism' and various inherited lipodystrophies in which fat is lost from subcutaneous and other depots in defined but unexplained anatomical patterns (see Chapter 10.5). Recently, mutations affecting the *PPAR-γ* gene (the target for the thiazolidinedione drugs; see below) have been shown to modify insulin sensitivity.

Obesity

Obesity induces insulin resistance, especially in skeletal muscle, while weight loss can improve insulin sensitivity in the obese. Insulin resistance is particularly associated with truncal (central) obesity, where fat is deposited in and around the abdomen; both the subcutaneous and intra-abdominal (visceral) fat depots have been implicated to various degrees that may reflect ethnic and other differences.

It is still not clear how an increased fat mass can decrease whole-body insulin sensitivity, but circulating fat-derived products are presumed to be responsible. Intra-abdominal fat depots would secrete potentially diabetogenic mediators into the portal circulation—where they would be delivered directly to the liver—and this may explain the association of visceral adiposity with insulin resistance. Possible candidates include free fatty acids and the cytokine tumour necrosis factor-α; both are secreted by adipocytes and, under experimental conditions at least, interfere with aspects of insulin action. Levels of free fatty acids are raised in obese subjects, apparently because lipolysis is enhanced, and free fatty acids may cause hyperglycaemia by competing with glucose metabolism in liver and muscle. In liver, free fatty acids enhance gluconeogenesis by stimulating the rate-limiting enzyme pyruvate carboxylase and so increase hepatic glucose production. In muscle, free fatty acids inhibit glycolysis at the level of phosphofructokinase and glucose oxidation via pyruvate dehydrogenase, causing a decrease in glucose utilization and a secondary reduction in glucose uptake (the 'glucose–fatty acid' or Randle cycle). *In vitro*, tumour necrosis factor-α inhibits the tyrosine kinase activity of the insulin receptor that is crucial for insulin signalling. Production of tumour necrosis factor-α by adipose tissue is increased in obesity but its role as a mediator of insulin resistance in human obesity is uncertain. Recently, a novel adipocyte product, adiponectin, has been shown to enhance insulin sensitivity in rodents; intriguingly, circulating adiponectin concentrations are decreased in human obesity.

Physical inactivity strongly predisposes to obesity and also promotes insulin resistance which can be reversed by regular exercise. The mechanism is unknown but physical training is known to stimulate translocation of GLUT-4 glucose transporters to the surface of muscle cells independently of insulin.

Other acquired causes

There are several other acquired causes of insulin resistance. Intrauterine growth retardation may contribute (see the 'Barker–Hales' hypothesis below). Physiological states of insulin resistance, due to the appropriate oversecretion of the counter-regulatory hormones whose metabolic actions oppose those of insulin, are puberty and pregnancy (see gestational diabetes, Chapter 13.10). Endocrine diseases that induce insulin resistance and can cause glucose intolerance and overt diabetes through excessive production of anti-insulin hormones include acromegaly (prevalence of diabetes and impaired glucose tolerance each around 25 per cent), Cushing's disease (diabetes around 30 per cent), thyrotoxicosis, and the very rare glucagonoma (diabetes in more than 90 per cent of cases). In these disorders, diabetes is mostly non-ketotic, although insulin may be needed to control hyperglycaemia.

Intercurrent illnesses, for example myocardial infarction, stroke, or severe infections, induce the secretion of counter-regulatory stress hormones that can cause marked insulin resistance—insulin-treated diabetic patients may need twice their usual insulin dosages during such episodes. Many drugs decrease insulin sensitivity, including glucocorticoids, β₂ adrenoceptor agonists (ritodrine, salbutamol), and certain oral contraceptive pills containing high-dose oestrogen or levonorgestrel; glucocorticoid-induced hyperglycaemia commonly requires insulin treatment.

The 'type B' insulin resistance syndrome is due to the development of autoantibodies against the insulin receptor which interfere with insulin binding and/or signalling. Most patients are young women, usually with pre-existing autoimmune diseases such as lupus erythematosus, and masculinization often occurs. Acquired lipodystrophies are also associated with insulin resistance, sometimes severe. 'Immune insulin resistance' describes insulin-treated patients with very high insulin requirements (sometimes several thousand U/day) because of high titres of insulin-binding antibodies that bind and inactivate administered insulin. This has become very rare since the introduction of highly purified human-sequence insulin preparations with low immunogenicity (see below).

Metabolic and clinical features of insulin resistance

The metabolic disturbance due to insulin-resistant syndromes ranges from subclinical glucose intolerance to severely symptomatic hyperglycaemia, sometimes with ketosis. A crucial determinant is the capacity of the individual's β cells to secrete insulin in response to the rises in blood glucose that are due to impaired insulin action. The resulting hyperinsulinaemia is extremely variable, with plasma insulin levels ranging from twice normal in many obese subjects to 500 times normal in patients with defects of insulin

receptors. Near-normoglycaemia can be maintained as long as hyperinsulinaemia can compensate for the underlying defect in insulin signalling; diabetes occurs when β-cell failure supervenes and insulin secretion falls below a critical level. In the total absence of functional insulin receptors (for example in 'leprechaunism'), massive endogenous hyperinsulinaemia or administration of industrial insulin dosages cannot prevent severe diabetes, although very high insulin concentrations may exert some metabolic actions through 'cross-talk' with the insulin-like growth factor-1 receptor.

Acanthosis nigricans, a characteristic skin manifestation of severe insulin resistance, may be due to high insulin concentrations activating growth factor receptors (perhaps the insulin-like growth factor-1 receptor) that drive the proliferation of keratinocytes and melanocytes. Hyperplasia of these cells leads to a velvety thickening and variable darkening of the skin, especially in the axillae, groin, and nape of the neck (see Chapter 23.1). Widespread acanthosis nigricans can also accompany gut tumours, which may also secrete dermal growth factors.

Increased androgen concentrations may lead to hirsutism and occasionally virilization in women with severe insulin resistance; high insulin concentrations may stimulate androgen production by the ovaries, which often show a polycystic appearance. Insulin resistance is a feature of polycystic ovary syndrome, especially in obese patients (Chapter 12.8.1). Enhancing insulin sensitivity through weight loss or treatment with metformin or the thiazolidinediones can decrease androgen levels and improve hirsutism and menstrual dysfunction.

The 'insulin resistance syndrome', or 'metabolic syndrome X'

This term identifies the co-occurrence of insulin resistance and glucose intolerance (ranging from mild to overt type 2 diabetes), with truncal obesity, dyslipidaemia (raised triglycerides and a high low density lipoprotein:high-density lipoprotein ratio), and hypertension (see Fig. 5).

These abnormalities are all common in most westernized populations, and it is still not clear whether or not this constellation of cardiovascular risk factors represents a genuine syndrome with a common underlying cause. Reaven and others have argued that insulin resistance is the central abnormality, and that the key features can be explained either by loss of specific actions of insulin or by the effects of the compensatory hyperinsulinaemia on organs that remain relatively insulin sensitive. For example, raised insulin levels could contribute to hypertension by enhancing retention of Na⁺ by the kidney; conversely, blood pressure could also be raised through loss of the direct vasodilator action of insulin. The pattern of abnormalities would therefore require 'insulin resistance' to affect certain tissues and specific actions of insulin but not others. Other proatherogenic defects identified in subjects with various features of syndrome X include increased coagulability of the blood (for example increased levels of plasminogen activator inhibitor 1) and impaired endothelial-mediated vasodilatation. The relationship of these abnormalities to insulin resistance is

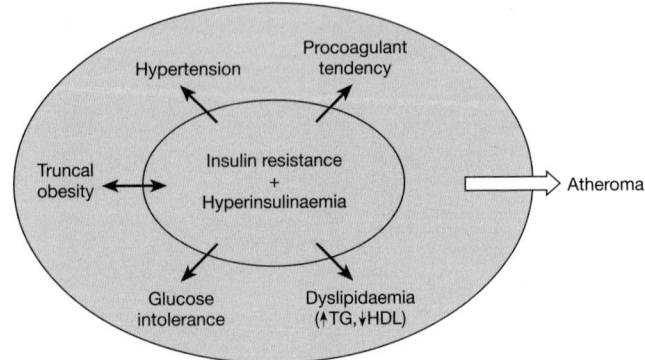

Fig. 5 Syndrome X, a constellation of atherogenic risk factors which may each be related to insulin resistance and/or the hyperinsulinaemia that accompanies insulin-resistant states. ↑TG, hypertriglyceridaemia; ↓HDL, reduced high-density lipoprotein cholesterol.

uncertain. Obesity, dyslipidaemia, hypertension, and glucose intolerance are all independent cardiovascular risk factors; any possible proatherogenic role of hyperinsulinaemia *per se* remains controversial.

The aetiology of syndrome X is unresolved. Adiposity, insulin sensitivity, and blood pressure show variable strengths of familial transmission that differ between populations and generally suggest polygenic inheritance of minor genes. On the other hand, Barker and Hales have suggested that fetal malnutrition programmes insulin resistance, hypertension, and dyslipidaemia in middle to late adult life. The underlying mechanisms remain elusive. Because obesity leads to insulin resistance and glucose intolerance, dyslipidaemia, hypertension, and atheroma, weight gain in middle age may be particularly hazardous in subjects who were underweight at birth.

Syndrome X is important clinically because it predisposes to atheroma formation and substantially increases the risk of dying prematurely from myocardial infarction or stroke. Treatment of syndrome X is currently based on correcting any factors (for example type 2 diabetes, hypertension, and dyslipidaemia) present in the individual patient. Lifestyle and dietary modification that achieves weight loss can improve most aspects of the syndrome, and specific insulin-sensitizing drugs such as the thiazolidinediones (see later) may prove beneficial.

Types and classification of diabetes mellitus

The current World Health Organization classification is based on aetiology (Table 1). Type 1 and type 2 diabetes together account for 90 to 95 per cent of cases and will be described in detail.

Type 1 diabetes

'Type 1' diabetes—now preferred to 'insulin-dependent' diabetes—is due to autoimmune killing of the β cells (the so-called 'type-1 process'). A similar clinical picture of insulin dependence can be caused by other forms of severe pancreatic damage.

Epidemiology and demographic features

Type 1 diabetes is considerably rarer than type 2, accounting for between 5 and 15 per cent of all diabetes and 30 to 50 per cent of insulin-treated cases in various populations. It appears predominantly in childhood, with a peak age at presentation of about 11 years in girls and 14 years in boys—hence the old description of 'juvenile-onset'. However, it can develop at any age, and about 5 per cent of newly diagnosed Caucasian diabetic patients over 65 years have type 1 diabetes.

The prevalence of type 1 diabetes varies considerably throughout the world. Incidence is highest in northern European countries (about 30 to 35 cases per 100 000 children per year in Scotland and Finland) and declines progressively towards the equator; there are some isolated 'hot spots' such as Sardinia, where the incidence is as high as in Finland. High susceptibility is found in European populations throughout the world, while African and Oriental populations are relatively spared (incidences of less than 1 per 100 000 per year). Superimposed on this geographical variation are time-related changes in incidence that hint at the importance of the environment in causing the disease. Type 1 diabetes presents more frequently during the winter months, particularly in children aged 10 to 14 years. In several countries (for example Sweden, Scotland, and Poland), there have been sharp 30 to 50 per cent increases in incidence over 10- to 20-year periods, although the explanation and significance of these secular trends are not clear.

Susceptibility to type 1 diabetes shows no gender bias.

Aetiology

Type 1 diabetes is an autoimmune, predominantly T-cell-mediated process that selectively destroys the β cells. Susceptibility is multifactorial, resulting from the impact of environmental agents in a genetically disadvantaged subject. Of these two components, the environment appears more import-

ant; genetic factors explain only 30 to 40 per cent of total susceptibility. Immunogenetic aspects are discussed in detail in Chapter 12.11.2.

Genetic factors

Over 20 genetic loci are associated with type 1 diabetes, although only two (*IDDM1* and *IDDM2*) account for most of the genetic predisposition.

IDDM1 lies within the major histocompatibility complex region on chromosome 6, that encodes several proteins intimately involved in immune responses. Of particular importance is the *DQB1* gene; this encodes the DQB1 peptide chain, which forms part of the cleft in the surface of the HLA class II molecule that is crucial in presenting peptide fragments of antigen to the T-helper lymphocyte. Changes in the structure of the DQB1 peptide could therefore influence the coupling between the class II molecule–peptide complex and the T-lymphocyte receptor, and thus

Table 1 Classification of diabetes mellitus according to aetiology (World Health Organization 1998)

Type 1 diabetes	β-Cell destruction, usually leading to absolute insulin deficiency (15–20% of cases in Europe and the United States)
Type 2 diabetes	Some degree of insulin resistance, with relative insulin deficiency (75–80% of cases in Europe and the United States)
Type 3 diabetes:	Other types with specific causes (5% of cases in Europe and the United States)
3A Genetic defects of β-cell function	MODY: MODY1 (HNF-4α mutations), MODY2 (glucokinase mutations), MODY3 (HNF-1α mutations) Others, including mitochondrial DNA defects (MELAS)
3B Genetic defects of insulin action	'Type A' insulin resistance syndrome 'Leprechaunism' Rabson–Mendenhall syndrome Congenital lipodystrophies
3C Diseases of the pancreas	Pancreatitis, chronic and acute Carcinoma of the pancreas Haemochromatosis, cystic fibrosis Pancreatectomy, trauma
3D Endocrino-pathies	Acromegaly Cushing's disease and syndrome Phaeochromocytoma Glucagonoma
3E Drug- or chemical-induced	Glucocorticoids β-Blockers Thiazides Diazoxide
3F Infections	Congenital rubella Cytomegalovirus
3G Uncommon forms of immune-mediated diabetes	'Type B' insulin resistance (insulin receptor antibodies) 'Stiff man' syndrome
3H Other genetic syndromes	Prader–Willi syndrome DIDMOAD Down's syndrome Turner's syndrome Klinefelter's syndrome
Type 4 diabetes	Gestational diabetes or glucose intolerance

Abbreviations: MODY, maturity onset diabetes of the young; HNF, hepatic nuclear factor; MELAS, myopathy, encephalopathy, lactic acidosis, and stroke-like episodes (associated with type 1 or type 2 diabetes); DIDMOAD, diabetes insipidus, diabetes mellitus, optic atrophy, and deafness modulate the immune response against the (auto)antigenic peptide. Specific *DQB1* polymorphisms have been shown to predispose to type 1 diabetes (for example DQB1*0302), whereas others (such as DQB1*0602) are protective—at least in certain racial groups. The relationships of these polymorphisms to the long-recognized influences of the DR3 and DR4 class II antigens (which increase several-fold the risk of type 1 diabetes) and of the protective DR2 are discussed further in Chapter 12.11.2.

IDDM2 corresponds to the insulin gene (*INS*), whose uniqueness as a β-cell product makes it an obvious candidate gene. As the insulin coding sequence is unchanged in type 1 diabetes, diabetogenic polymorphisms might affect the level of expression of the *INS* gene: variants which enhanced insulin expression could promote β-cell damage, because 'resting' the β cell (for example by giving exogenous insulin) in type 1 diabetic animals improves β-cell survival, in parallel with reduced expression of the putative autoantigen GAD65 (a specific isoform of the enzyme glutamic acid decarboxylase (**GAD**), expressed in the β-cell membrane).

Environmental factors

Viruses have long been popular candidates as a 'trigger' for diabetes. Some (for example mumps, coxsackie, cytomegalovirus, and rubella) infect the pancreas but normally damage the entire gland, particularly the exocrine tissue, rather than causing selective β-cell injury. Certain viruses target the β cell in animals (for example the Kilham rat virus) and can cause insulin-dependent diabetes, either though their direct cytolytic effects or by provoking a type 1-like autoimmune process. Important contenders in humans are coxsackie viruses (especially B4), rubella, and retroviruses.

Serological studies indicate that recent coxsackie B infections are relatively common among newly diagnosed patients with type 1 diabetes; these could represent the final insult in the disease's long natural history. Coxsackie viruses capable of damaging rodent β cells have also been isolated post-mortem from the islets of type 1 diabetic subjects. About 20 per cent of children who survive intrauterine rubella infection develop type 1 diabetes, with typical autoimmune markers. Retrovirus particles and RNA have recently been identified in β cells from type 1 diabetic patients, and two-thirds of newly diagnosed cases are reported to have antibodies against the protein encoded by the retroviral RNA.

Viruses could trigger or maintain autoimmune β-cell damage in various ways. Acute or persistent viral infection of β cells could release β-cell antigens that are normally sequestered beyond the reach of the immune cells. Certain viral proteins may elicit an immune response which crossreacts with specific β-cell antigens that happen to be similar ('molecular mimicry'): for example, peptide sequences of the P2-C capsid protein of coxsackie B viruses may crossreact with GAD65 in the β-cell membrane.

Other environmental factors are suggested to include bovine serum albumin from cows' milk and various toxins. Bovine serum albumin contains a peptide sequence that may crossreact with a β-cell surface protein (see below); this was suggested as an explaination for an apparent excess risk of type 1 diabetes among children fed with cows' milk in the neonatal period, although a protective effect for breast feeding remains controversial. Various toxins selectively damage β cells, including streptozotocin, a nitrosourea used to induce experimental diabetes in rodents. Related nitrosamine compounds have been blamed for the higher risk of type 1 diabetes in the children of women who eat fermented smoked mutton (a traditional delicacy in Iceland).

Autoimmune features

Type 1 diabetes has strong associations with endocrine and other autoimmune diseases, including Schmidt's syndrome (with hypothyroidism and adrenocortical failure) and the polyglandular autoimmune deficiency syndromes.

Most β-cell damage is probably inflicted by T lymphocytes. 'Insulitis'—infiltration of the islets with immune cells, mostly cytotoxic/suppressor (CD8+) T lymphocytes—is a pathognomic feature of the disease, and circulating T-helper lymphocytes can be identified that react against β-cell antigens including GAD65.

Various circulating autoantibodies also occur. Some target antigens unique to the β cell, while other autoantigens are shared by other islet cell types. Notable β-cell selective autoantibodies are those that recognize GAD65, a heat-shock protein (hsp60), and insulin itself. GAD catalyses the conversion of glutamic acid to γ-aminobutyric acid (**GABA**), whose role in the β cell is uncertain. Studies in rodents with type 1 diabetes suggest that the level of GAD65 expression influences the intensity of the autoimmune attack on the β cells. The GAD67 isoform of the enzyme is also expressed in the central nervous system, and autoimmune damage of GABAergic neurones is presumed to explain the association of type 1 diabetes with the rare 'stiff man' syndrome (Section 24).

GAD65 antibodies are present in 70 to 90 per cent of newly diagnosed type 1 patients, and insulin autoantibodies in 40 to 70 per cent. Islet cell antibodies and islet cell surface antibodies are present in 80 to 90 per cent and 30 to 60 per cent respectively of newly diagnosed patients. Islet cell antibodies and islet cell surface antibodies recognize uncharacterized antigens that are common to β and non-β cells in the islets (which share the same embryological origin). These antibodies cannot explain the selective destruction of β cells, although some islet cell surface antibodies are complement-fixing and may target the β cell preferentially; islet cell antibodies and islet cell surface antibodies could be raised secondarily to β-cell damage.

High titres of each of these classes of antibodies have some value in predicting diabetes in high-risk individuals—a risk of about 50 per cent for GAD65 antibodies in first-order relatives of subjects with type 1 diabetes. However, they are clearly not the immediate cause of the disease: they are found in many subjects who do not go on to develop it, including a few per cent of the normal population. These antibodies are therefore general markers of autoimmunity against the β cell, rather than evidence of β-cell destruction, which is primarily cell mediated. Titres of all these antibodies tend to be high at presentation and (according to prospective studies of high-risk subjects) during the months leading up to this. Thereafter, antibody levels decline progressively and may even become undetectable, possibly through dwindling of the antigen load that perpetuates autoimmunity as any remaining β cells disappear.

Natural history of type 1 diabetes

β-cell damage might be initiated by direct viral attack, environmental toxins, and/or a primary immune attack against specific β-cell antigens such as GAD65, perhaps via molecular mimicry. T-helper lymphocytes (CD4+) are activated by β-cell antigens presented together with diabetogenic class II antigens by antigen-presenting cells (macrophages) and perhaps by β cells themselves ('aberrant' class II antigen expression may be induced in β cells by certain cytokines generated during the autoimmune process). Activated T-helper cells produce cytokines that attract T and B lymphocytes and encourage them to proliferate in the islet, leading to insulitis. B lymphocytes might then damage β cells by producing antibodies against released β-cell antigens, while cytotoxic (CD8+) T lymphocytes directly attack β cells carrying the target autoantigens. Insulitis is a patchy and unpredictable process that might flare up after encounters with new environmental triggers such as viral infections, but which can also fade and abort for unknown reasons.

Several years of progressive autoimmune damage usually precede the clinical onset of diabetes. This long prediabetic phase is asymptomatic, although careful testing (for example with the intravenous glucose tolerance test) reveals loss of the first phase, then increasingly obvious disturbances of insulin and C-peptide secretion, and eventually glucose intolerance. Finally, when the β-cell mass has been eroded to a critical level (probably 5 to 10 per cent of normal), falling insulin secretion can no longer restrain hyperglycaemia and clinical diabetes develops.

Residual β-cell mass is variable at presentation of type 1 diabetes: some newly diagnosed type 1 patients are C-peptide positive, and β-cell secretion may improve temporarily during the 'honeymoon period' that can follow the lowering of blood glucose when insulin treatment is started (see below). With continuing β-cell destruction, endogenous insulin production declines progressively, and more than 90 per cent of type 1 patients become permanently C-peptide negative within 5 years of presentation. Ultimately, insulitis burns itself out and the immune cells retreat, leaving islet remnants that are devoid of β cells but which still contain intact α, δ, and PP cells.

The protracted prediabetic phase provides an opportunity to prevent subjects with active insulitis from developing clinical disease. A combination of autoantibody titres and genetic markers (HLA haplotypes) can be used to predict the chances of the disease developing in high-risk subjects, such as the siblings of children with type 1 diabetes; various immunosuppressive and immunomodulatory treatments are currently undergoing clinical trials.

Metabolic disturbances of type 1 diabetes

In untreated type 1 diabetes, insulin concentrations are generally 10 to 50 per cent of non-diabetic levels in the face of hyperglycaemia which would normally greatly increase insulin secretion. Such severe deficiency cannot sustain the normal anabolic effects of insulin and leads to runaway catabolism in carbohydrate, fat, and protein metabolism. Each of these processes accelerates hyperglycaemia, while the oxidation of excess free fatty acids generated by triglyceride breakdown can result in diabetic ketoacidosis.

Carbohydrate metabolism

Basal hyperglycaemia is due mainly to unrestrained production of glucose by the liver and is accentuated after eating by the failure of glucose to be cleared peripherally (see Fig. 4). Hepatic glucose output is boosted, especially by increased gluconeogenesis: the normal inhibition of the process by insulin is lost, while the supply of gluconeogenic precursors (glycerol from lipolysis, amino acids such as alanine from protein breakdown) is increased. Increased gluconeogenesis in the kidney may also contribute. Postprandial glucose uptake into muscle and fat, mediated by insulin and GLUT-4, is greatly decreased; this is partly offset by increased non-insulin dependent glucose uptake into peripheral tissues, via glucose transporters that do not require insulin.

The overall result is hyperglycaemia, commonly in the range of 15 to 25 mmol/l and higher after meals. Glucose concentrations of over 40 mmol/l are not uncommon during intercurrent illness and especially when insulin treatment is omitted or not increased sufficiently.

Fat metabolism

Lipolysis is stimulated by severe insulin deficiency, generating glycerol (a gluconeogenic precursor) and free fatty acids, the substrate for ketone formation. Ketogenesis is particularly enhanced by concomitant glucagon excess (see below). Mobilization of body fat contributes to weight loss in untreated type 1 diabetes.

Protein metabolism

Loss of the net anabolic effect of insulin encourages catabolism of proteins (primarily through the proteasome-mediated pathway), thus generating amino acids including gluconeogenic precursors such as alanine and glutamine. Muscle wasting may be prominent.

Role of counter-regulatory hormones

The effects of hypoinsulinaemia are compounded by the counter-regulatory hormones which are secreted in excess in response to stress (for example infections, myocardial infarction, trauma, surgery) and when circulating volume falls (for example in hyperglycaemic dehydrated patients). Insulin deficiency also leads to increased glucagon secretion because insulin normally inhibits the α cells.

Glucagon increases hepatic glucose production, both by driving glycogen breakdown and by increasing uptake of glucogenic amino acids by the liver and enhancing gluconeogenesis. It also stimulates ketogenesis by increasing entry of free fatty acids (as their fatty acyl-CoA derivatives) into liver mitochondria (see Fig. 8 below). Glucagon excess is an important fac-tor that promotes diabetic ketoacidosis, acting synergistically with insulin deficiency (see below).

Cortisol and catecholamines enhance gluconeogenesis. Cortisol, catecholamines, and growth hormone oppose the lipogenic action of insulin and favour lipolysis, in the presence of hypoinsulinaemia. Cortisol is a powerful inducer of proteolysis, whereas growth hormone co-operates with insulin to stimulate protein synthesis.

Clinical features of type 1 diabetes

The classical presentation of untreated or poorly controlled type 1 diabetes reflects the consequences of catabolism and hyperglycaemia (Table 2). These features usually develop progressively and quite rapidly over a period of a few days to a few weeks.

Diuresis is due mainly to the osmotic effect of glucose remaining in the renal tubule, when its concentration exceeds the reabsorption threshold for glucose (corresponding generally to plasma glucose levels of about 10 mmol/l). The osmotic loads of urinary ketones and of electrolytes that are obligatorily lost with glucose also contribute. Urine output may reach several litres per day, causing polyuria, nocturia, and in children, enuresis.

Thirst generally parallels urine output and can be very intense; it is characteristically made worse by sugar-rich drinks. Taking water to bed at night is a useful sign of pathological thirst. A high fluid intake is an important homeostatic response to diuresis, and patients unable to drink (for example through nausea in ketoacidosis) can rapidly become dehydrated and hypovolaemic.

Weight loss, due to loss of fat and muscle and later to dehydration, can be dramatic and reach several kilograms over a few weeks. The energy deficit caused by catabolism and urinary losses of glucose can amount to several hundred calories per day. Appetite is often increased; the mechanism in humans is not known; falls in circulating leptin and insulin, both of which act on the central nervous system to inhibit feeding, are probably responsible for hyperphagia in diabetic rodents.

Table 2 Typical features of type 1 and type 2 diabetes, with some distinguishing characteristics

	Type 1 diabetes	Type 2 diabetes
Osmotic and glycosuric symptoms: polyuria, nocturia, enuresis; thirst, polydipsia; blurred vision; genital candidias (pruritus vulvae, balanitis)	+ → ++	± → ++
Systemic symptoms: malaise, tiredness, lack of energy	+ → ++	0 → ++
Catabolic features: recent weight loss; muscle wasting and weakness	+ → ++	0 → +
Ketoacidosis	Spontaneous	Rare; mostly precipitated by intercurrent illness
Diabetic microvascular complications at presentation	–	±
Age at presentation	Young > old	Old > young
Obesity	±	± (most)
Family history	±	±
Clinical insulin dependence (weight loss and hyperglycaemia without insulin replacement)	+	–
Special investigations:		
C peptide	Positive	Negative
Type 1 HLA haplotype	±	–
Islet cell antibodies: ICA, ICSA, GAD	±	–

Abbreviations: ICA, islet cell antibodies; ICSA, islet cell surface antibodies; GAD, glutamic acid decarboxylase.

Systemic symptoms include tiredness, malaise, lack of energy, and muscular weakness.

Blurred vision is commonly due to changes in the shape of the lens due to osmotic shifts, typically causing longsightedness. Rarely, acute 'snowflake' cataracts develop because of reversible refractile changes, rather than the permanent denaturation of lens proteins in senile cataract.

Infections are often present because hyperglycaemia predisposes to infections and also because infections stimulate the secretion of stress hormones. Genital candida infections, causing recurrent pruritus vulvae in women and balanitis in men, are frequent and should always prompt testing for diabetes. Pyogenic skin infections and urinary tract infections, sometimes complicated by severe renal damage, are also common, and certain rare infections have a particular predilection for diabetic people (see below).

Diabetic ketoacidosis presents with hyperglycaemic symptoms, which are usually severe, together with nausea and vomiting, acidotic (Kussmaul) breathing, the smell of acetone on the breath, and, especially in children, altered mood and clouding of consciousness that may progress to coma. Diabetic ketoacidosis is described in detail later.

Unlike type 2 diabetes, which is often present for several years before diagnosis, hyperglycaemia in newly presenting type 1 patients develops too acutely for chronic diabetic complications to appear. Because obvious symptoms appear quickly, very few cases are picked up fortuitously, although doctors who have forgotten to think of diabetes in their differential diagnosis of weight loss or hyperventilation may be surprised when hyperglycaemia is detected by routine screening.

Prognosis of type 1 diabetes

Before the introduction of insulin during the early 1920s, type 1 diabetes was invariably fatal, usually within months. With various semistarvation diets, hyperglycaemic symptoms could be improved somewhat and life extended by a few miserable months.

With modern insulin treatment, type 1 diabetic patients can be rescued from diabetic ketoacidosis, although one-third of deaths in diabetic children and young adults are still due to metabolic emergencies, notably ketoacidosis. The main threat to survival with type 1 diabetes is now chronic tissue damage, particularly renal failure from nephropathy, and vascular disease, notably myocardial infarction and stroke. Throughout adult life, the overall risk of dying within 10 years is about fourfold higher for patients with type 1 diabetes than for their non-diabetic peers.

There is encouraging evidence from Europe and the United States that the outlook for type 1 diabetes has improved over the last 10 to 20 years, with definite declines in the incidence of microvascular complications and extended survival—at least in countries able to afford effective diabetes care. This is partly attributable to tighter control of hyperglycaemia, which can reduce by 30 to 40 per cent the risks of nephropathy and retinopathy developing or progressing to a clinically significant degree (see below). Other measures have undoubtedly contributed, including better treatment of raised blood pressure and blood lipids.

Tragically, however, in many parts of the world patients with type 1 diabetes still die today as they did a century ago, simply because insulin is not available.

Type 2 diabetes

Type 2 diabetes is a heterogeneous condition, diagnosed empirically by the absence of features suggesting type 1 diabetes (Table 2) and of the many other conditions that cause hyperglycaemia (Table 1). Diagnostic accuracy may depend on the thoroughness of investigation: for example, up to 10 per cent of subjects with late onset diabetes show evidence of autoimmune β-cell damage and thus probably have slowly evolving type 1 diabetes.

The term 'type 2' replaces 'non-insulin dependent' which was both clumsy and confusing: many type 2 patients require insulin to control hyperglycaemia.

Epidemiology and demographic features

Type 2 diabetes accounts for 85 to 90 per cent of diabetes worldwide and is very common. It affects about 2 per cent of the Caucasian populations in most westernized countries, the prevalence rising with age to 10 per cent of those over 70 years. It is substantially commoner in certain immigrant populations in more affluent countries, for example 5 per cent or more of young and middle-aged adults in some Asian or Afro-Caribbean groups in the United Kingdom.

Type 2 diabetes is most commonly diagnosed in those over 40 years of age and the incidence rises to a peak at 60 to 65 years. However, much younger people are now presenting with type 2 diabetes, following the rapid rise in childhood obesity. Up to one-third of North Americans diagnosed as diabetic under 20 years of age have type 2 diabetes, Afro-Caribbeans and Mexicans being at particular risk. Maturity onset diabetes of the young, which commonly presents before 25 years of age, is now classified separately (see below for more details).

The prevalence of type 2 diabetes shows striking geographical variation—entirely different from that of type 1—and ranges from less than 1 per cent in rural China to 50 per cent in the Pima Indians of New Mexico. Prevalence is also rising rapidly and, worldwide, will double within 10 to 15 years. This pandemic is largely explicable by westernization (so-called 'Cocacolonization'), and is following in the wake of the obesity that is spreading throughout the world. The Pima Indians illustrate this process especially vividly, although most developed and developing countries are showing the same phenomenon albeit more slowly. Diabetes was rare while the Pimas led a frugal existence in desert conditions and were lean and physically active. Following urban resettlement and exposure to overnutrition and inactivity, there were rapid increases in the prevalence of obesity (currently 80 per cent of adult Pimas have a body mass index of over 30 kg/m^2) and later of type 2 diabetes. The Pimas' spectacular susceptibility to obesity and diabetes may be explained by the selection of 'thrifty' genes, i.e. those encouraging the storage of excess energy as fat, which would favour survival in their original harsh environment. In a setting of readily available food, cars, and television, the same thrifty genes would lead to obesity and ultimately diabetes (see below).

There is a 3:2 male preponderance among subjects with type 2 diabetes.

Aetiology

Type 2 diabetes is due to the combination of insulin resistance and β-cell failure, the latter preventing sufficient insulin secretion to overcome the insulin resistance. These two components vary in importance between different individuals, who may be clinically quite similar, and each has numerous possible causes. Susceptibility is determined by the interactions between genes and environment. The steeply rising prevalence of type 2 diabetes suggests that diabetogenic genes are common and are now enjoying an unparalleled opportunity to express themselves through the global spread of 'Cocacolonization' and obesity.

Genetic factors

Overall genetic susceptibility to type 2 diabetes is probably 60 to 90 per cent, rather less than was previously deduced from twin studies. Generally, transmission does not follow simple mendelian rules, and this polygenic pattern presumably reflects the inheritance of a critical mass of minor diabetogenic minor polymorphisms which interfere with insulin action and/or insulin secretion. Having a first-order relative with the disease increases by fivefold an individual's chances of developing it, representing a lifetime risk in Caucasians of about 40 per cent.

Genetic factors may partly determine both insulin resistance and β-cell failure, although to different degrees in different individuals. Insulin sensitivity appears to be largely genetically determined, at least in some populations. Genes leading to insulin resistance could encode regulators of energy balance, metabolic enzymes, or the proteins that signal insulin action, and presumably include 'thrifty' genes favouring fat deposition.

Specific genes have not been firmly incriminated: particular polymorphisms associated with type 2 diabetes have been reported (for example the β_3 adrenoceptor implicated in lipolysis and energy expenditure, the insulin signalling protein insulin receptor substrate-1, and glycogen synthetase) but subsequently questioned. Mutations affecting the insulin receptor and glucose transporters do not appear to cause common type 2 diabetes, although mutations of insulin receptors can lead to severe insulin resistance (see above).

Diabetogenic genes leading to inadequate production of insulin could decrease insulin secretion in response to glucose, or impair β-cell viability. Mutations affecting glucokinase cause maturity onset diabetes of the young 2 (see below) and rare cases (less than 1 per cent) of apparently typical type 2 diabetes; otherwise, mutations in the known components of the β cell's glucose-sensing or insulin-secreting machinery are not responsible for common type 2 diabetes.

Environmental factors

These clearly play a critical part, because obesity and type 2 diabetes are spreading too rapidly to be explicable by changes in the genome; environmental factors are also important in practice because they may be modified to treat and prevent the disease. Known environmental diabetogenic factors mostly induce insulin resistance (for example obesity, pregnancy, intercurrent illness, certain drugs). Hyperglycaemia *per se* can both impair insulin sensitivity and inhibit insulin secretion (so-called 'glucotoxicity').

Specific risk factors for type 2 diabetes

Obesity, itself determined by both genes and environment, is one of the most important risk factors, apparently due to aggravation of insulin resistance (see above). The diabetogenic properties of excess fat depend not only on its bulk but also on its anatomical distribution and the time of life at which it is laid down. The risks of developing type 2 diabetes begin to increase steeply once the body mass index exceeds 28 kg/m²; some studies estimate the risk at a body mass index over 35 kg/m² to be 80-fold higher than for individuals with a body mass index of less than 22 kg/m²—a lifetime risk of about 50 per cent. Fat in the truncal (central) distribution is more diabetogenic than that deposited around the hips and thighs, and the visceral (intra-abdominal) depot is strongly associated with insulin resistance. Increasing adiposity after the early twenties, especially around the waist, aggravates the risk of high body mass index.

Physical inactivity, especially from the twenties onwards, is an independent predictor of diabetes in middle age, the risk increasing by about threefold for sedentary people as compared with regular athletes. This is due to worsening insulin resistance, which can be improved by physical training.

The still controversial Barker and Hales hypothesis suggests that poor fetal growth can 'programme' enduring metabolic and vascular abnormalities that are manifested in adult life, especially in people who were underweight at birth but then become obese. These abnormalities include key features of 'syndrome X' (hyperglycaemia, hypertension, dyslipidaemia), resulting in atheroma formation, myocardial infarction and stroke (see above). Evidence, mainly from animals, suggests that maternal and therefore fetal malnutrition during a critical early phase of fetal development can reduce β-cell mass and permanently impair insulin secretory reserve; deficiencies of sulphur-containing amino acids may be responsible in experimental animals but the relevance to humans is unknown. Other studies suggest that insulin sensitivity may also be reduced into adult life.

β-Cell failure in type 2 diabetes

β-Cell failure is an obligatory defect in the pathogenesis of type 2 diabetes: near normoglycaemia can be maintained even in severe insulin resistance (due for example to mutations in the insulin receptor), as long as the β cell can respond to the challenge and secrete enough insulin to overcome the resistance.

Subtle abnormalities of insulin secretion, including loss of the physiological pulses and of the first-phase response to intravenous glucose injection, are seen in normoglycaemic subjects who later develop the disease. These defects presumably indicate that the β cell is already stressed in trying to produce enough insulin to overcome insulin resistance. Normoglycaemic first-order relatives of type 2 diabetic subjects also show loss of pulsatility of insulin secretion which might indicate an inherited tendency to β-cell failure.

The mechanism of β-cell failure in human type 2 diabetes is not known. Histologically, the islets in type 2 diabetes show no features of type 1 autoimmune insulitis, and β-cell mass is not so dramatically reduced. Animal models of the disease suggest various causes, including synchronized β-cell apoptosis (possibly mediated by nitric oxide) in the Zucker diabetic fatty rat, and the deposition of amyloid fibrils (see above) in the rhesus monkey. Amyloid deposits are also prominent in the islets of some type 2 diabetic patients but may merely be due to dysfunctional β-cell hypersecretion rather than the cause of β-cell damage. Once hyperglycaemia is established, 'glucotoxicity' *per se* may further worsen both insulin secretion and insulin resistance.

In established type 2 diabetes, insulin secretion is unequivocally subnormal and tends to decline progressively with time, as illustrated by the long-term follow-up data from the United Kingdom Prospective Diabetes Study. Initially, plasma insulin levels may be higher than in non-diabetic subjects but are still inappropriately low, as the normal pancreas would produce much higher insulin concentrations in response to diabetic levels of blood glucose. Conventional radioimmunoassays may overestimate insulin levels in type 2 diabetic patients because of crossreaction with incompletely processed insulin precursors (proinsulin and its split products) released by the 'constitutive' pathway which operates in the malfunctioning β cell (see above). Many type 2 patients ultimately need insulin replacement; this indicates relatively severe insulin deficiency, although still not as profound as in type 1 diabetes. Some type 2 patients who require insulin early have autoimmune markers characteristic of type 1 diabetes, suggesting that they in fact have an indolent variant of type 1 diabetes.

Natural history

Longitudinal and cross-sectional studies indicate that insulin resistance develops first and that compensatory increases in insulin secretion can initially maintain near-normoglycaemia. Worsening insulin resistance is thought to drive the β cells towards maximal insulin output, a metastable stage that probably corresponds to impaired glucose tolerance (see above). Rescue is still possible if insulin resistance is decreased, for example through weight loss or insulin-sensitizing drugs: about 25 per cent of subjects with impaired glucose tolerance return to normoglycaemia within 5 years. However, if insulin resistance persists or worsens, the β cells fail and insulin production falls. At this point, the brake limiting hyperglycaemia is released and blood glucose rises into the diabetic range. The bell-shaped response of insulin secretion, initially increasing to compensate but ultimately failing, has been termed the 'Starling curve' of the β cells because it recalls the classical plot of cardiac output against preload in heart failure.

In common type 2 diabetes, these events usually take many years, and significant hyperglycaemia may have been present for several years at the time of diagnosis. The whole process can be greatly accelerated by acute increases in insulin resistance induced, for example, by steroid treatment or pregnancy.

Metabolic disturbances in type 2 diabetes

Hyperglycaemia is the most obvious abnormality, the extreme case being the hyperosmolar non-ketotic state. Lipid metabolism is also disturbed but true ketoacidosis occurs only exceptionally and is usually provoked by intercurrent events such as infections or myocardial infarction.

Blood glucose concentrations are raised both in the basal (fasting) state and after eating. This reflects the impairment of insulin action in both liver and skeletal muscle, where insulin respectively shuts off hepatic glucose production and stimulates glucose uptake after meals. Hepatic glucose output is increased, due mainly to unsuppressed gluconeogenesis, and this is largely responsible for hyperglycaemia overnight and before meals. In muscle, GLUT-4 activity and glycogen synthesis are especially decreased; this reduces insulin-stimulated glucose uptake into muscle after meals, although basal glucose uptake (non-insulin mediated glucose uptake; see above) is higher than in normal subjects because of the mass-action effect of hyperglycaemia. The degree of hyperglycaemia varies widely: many patients have fasting plasma glucose levels of 8 to 13 mmol/l with post-prandial peaks of up to 20 mmol/l, while values exceeding 60 mmol/l are not uncommon in the hyperosmolar non-ketotic state.

Insulin deficiency is less profound than in type 1 diabetes, so mobilization of triglyceride (loss of body fat, ketoacidosis) and catabolism of protein (muscle breakdown) are not usually pronounced. Diabetic ketoacidosis may develop in patients with apparently typical type 2 diabetes who can subsequently be controlled by oral hypoglycaemic agents rather than insulin. Diabetic ketoacidosis is usually precipitated by severe intercurrent illness (for example myocardial infarction, stroke, or pneumonia) in which excessive secretion of counter-regulatory stress hormones exacerbates the metabolic disturbance caused by relative insulin deficiency.

Clinical features

Many cases present with classical symptoms of osmotic diuresis, blurred vision due to hyperglycaemia-related refractive changes in the lens, and genital candidiasis (Table 2).

Weight loss may occur but is generally less dramatic than with newly presenting type 1 diabetes, and may not be obvious because many type 2 patients—over two-thirds in the United Kingdom—are obese. Rapid or severe weight loss in patients who otherwise appear to have type 2 diabetes should be regarded with suspicion as it may point to an early need for insulin replacement (and possibly type 1 diabetes itself) or to coexisting illness: a well-recognized but unexplained association with recent onset type 2 diabetes is carcinoma of the pancreas.

The hyperosmolar non-ketotic state can present with confusion or coma (see below); as mentioned above, diabetic ketoacidosis is rare.

Chronic diabetic complications may be a presenting feature, because hyperglycaemia severe enough to cause tissue damage may already have been present for several years. Extrapolating the numbers of microaneurysms (which only develop at diabetic glucose concentrations) in type 2 patients at various intervals after diagnosis suggests that significant hyper-

glycaemia is present for an average of 5 to 7 years before diagnosis. Common problems are arterial disease (myocardial infarction, stroke, and peripheral vascular disease), cataract—which are common in the older population—and retinopathy, especially maculopathy, which can damage central vision.

Increasing numbers of diabetics are detected by screening, either in high-risk groups such as the obese and those with cardiovascular disease, or at routine health checks. Many of these are nominally asymptomatic but will admit to symptoms such as nocturia or perineal irritation if asked directly.

Prognosis of type 2 diabetes

A long-held and prevalent misconception is that type 2 diabetes is 'mild'. Some patients do have relatively unexciting or asymptomatic hyperglycaemia but this can still be enough to cause complications which wreck the patient's life just as much as in type 1 diabetes. Moreover, hyperglycaemia can be as hard to control (even with insulin) as in type 1 patients.

Overall, life expectancy is shortened by up to a quarter in patients with type 2 diabetes presenting in their forties, with vascular disease (myocardial infarction and stroke) being the main cause of premature death. Renal failure from diabetic nephropathy is becoming more common in type 2 patients as their survival from vascular complications improves, and the disease is now the most frequent pathology among people waiting for renal replacement therapy in the United States and some European countries.

Type 2 diabetes is therefore an important threat to the patient's health and survival, and must be taken seriously by patients and their medical attendants, even if the blood glucose concentrations are not dramatically raised. Accordingly, treatment guidelines for the disease are rigorous (Table 3).

Maturity onset diabetes of the young (MODY)

In 1974, Tattersall described a rare familial form of non-insulin dependent diabetes that he distinguished from the generality of cases by its early age of onset, autosomal dominant inheritance, and apparently low risk of microvascular complications. MODY is now known to differ fundamentally from

Table 3 Treatment targets for diabetic patients

	Glycaemic control		
	Low risk	Arterial risk	Microvascular risk
Fasting blood glucose (mmol/l)	< 5.5	> 6.5	> 6.0
Post-prandial peak glucose (mmol/l)	< 7.5	≥ 7.5	> 9.0
HbA$_{1c}$ (DCCT aligned)	≤ 6.5	> 6.5	> 7.5
	Serum lipids (mmol/l)		
	Low risk	Arterial risk	High arterial risk
Total cholesterol	< 4.8	4.8–6.0	> 6.0
HDL cholesterol	> 1.2	1.0–1.2	< 1.0
LDL cholesterol	< 3.0	3.0–4.0	> 4.0
Fasting triglycerides	< 1.7	1.7–2.2	> 2.2
	Blood pressure (mm Hg)		
	Low risk	Unacceptable	
General	< 130/80	> 140/90	
Patients with microalbuminuria	< 125/75		
	Body-mass index (kg/m^2)		
	Low risk	Acceptable	Increased risk
Men	< 25	25–27	> 27
Women	< 24	24–26	> 26

DCCT, Diabetic Control and Complications Trial.

'Ideal' treatment targets ('low-risk' values) may not be appropriate for some patients. Risks are stratified for arterial disease and/or microvascular complications. Collated from various sources including: European Diabetes Policy Group (1999) *Diabetic Medicine* **16**, 716–30; American Diabetes Association (2002) *Diabetes Care* **25** (Suppl. 1); and Ramsay LE *et al.* (1999) *British Medical Journal* **319**, 630–5.

type 2 diabetes in its aetiology and is classified separately as type 3A. It probably accounts for about 1 per cent of non-insulin dependent diabetes and is diagnosed strictly by:

1. Early onset: diabetes is diagnosed before 25 years in the subject and in at least one other family member. Some cases with glucokinase mutations present before 5 years of age.
2. Absence of features of type 1 diabetes, with C-peptide positivity and no requirement for insulin within 5 years of diagnosis.
3. Autosomal dominant inheritance across at least three generations.

MODY is due to failure of the β cell to secrete enough insulin to maintain normoglycaemia: insulin is released in response to glucose but in amounts consistently lower than in non-diabetic subjects. This is explained by failure of the β-cell's glucose-sensing apparatus, which depends on the integrated operation of GLUT-2, glucokinase, and the downstream enzymes that generate ATP from glycolysis of glucose. In contrast to common type 2 diabetes, insulin sensitivity is normal.

Various molecular lesions have now been identified. The first were mutations in the glucokinase gene (on chromosome 7p), which interfere with the enzyme's ability to phosphorylate glucose—the first and rate-limiting step in glycolysis. Glucokinase-dependent MODY (now termed MODY 2) only accounts for about 10 per cent of cases. It is characterized by very early onset hyperglycaemia which is mild and worsens slowly, taking decades to reach truly diabetic levels; it follows that microvascular complications are late to develop.

Other forms of maturity onset diabetes of the young are MODY 1, due to mutations in hepatic nuclear factor 4α (on chromosome 20q) and accounting for only 5 per cent of cases, and the most frequent (65 per cent of cases), termed MODY 3 and caused by hepatic nuclear factor-1α mutations (chromosome 12q). The hepatic nuclear factors are a family of transcription factors that regulate the expression of various genes, but their pathological relevance here is not clear.

Management of MODY is as for type 2 diabetes and using the same treatment targets, because it is now clear that patients with MODY are not protected against chronic complications. Diet and oral hypoglycaemic agents are often effective, especially in the milder MODY 2, but insulin may ultimately be needed.

Other types of diabetes (see Table 1)

Diabetes in pancreatic disease
Chronic pancreatitis, most commonly due to alcohol abuse, causes diabetes that needs insulin in about one-third of cases. Widespread flecks of fine to medium calcification are often scattered through the pancreas, outlining it on a plain abdominal radiograph. Concomitant destruction of the islet α cells means that glucagon secretion is lost as well as insulin; diabetic ketoacidosis is therefore rare, while hypoglycaemia can be profound and prolonged—a particular hazard in those who continue to drink alcohol. Acute pancreatitis causes acute hyperglycaemia in 50 per cent of cases but few develop permanent diabetes.

Carcinoma of the pancreas is associated with newly presenting type 2 diabetes, and should be suspected in older patients with weight loss (especially when accompanied by abdominal or back pain and jaundice). The mechanism is unknown but appears to be due to tumour products that cause insulin resistance rather than to β-cell loss.

Genetic diseases that cause diabetes through pancreatic damage include haemochromatosis and cystic fibrosis. In one-half of cases of haemochromatosis, heavy deposition of haemosiderin in the islets causes diabetes, usually requiring insulin; associated features are slate-grey skin pigmentation due to deposition of iron in the dermis ('bronze diabetes'), cirrhosis, secondary gonadal failure, and pyrophosphate arthropathy. Magnetic resonance imaging shows abnormal signals in liver and pancreas, while serum ferritin concentrations are greatly elevated; diagnosis is usually possible by means of molecular analysis of the HFE gene but Perl's stain for iron deposition in a liver biopsy may be necessary (see Chapter 11.7.1). Cystic fibrosis

causes pancreatic exocrine failure, with an increasing risk of diabetes (often requiring insulin) that approaches 25 per cent in subjects who survive beyond 20 years of age.

Gestational diabetes
This includes all degrees of hyperglycaemia (impaired glucose tolerance as well as overt diabetes) diagnosed during pregnancy in previously normoglycaemic women. It is covered in Chapter 13.10.

Malnutrition-related diabetes
This controversial diagnostic category was omitted from the most recent World Health Organization classification. It included 'fibrocalculous pancreatic diabetes' and 'protein-deficient diabetes mellitus'. Fibrocalculous pancreatic diabetes was identified by dense pancreatic fibrosis, the formation of discrete and often spectacularly large stones in the dilated pancreatic ducts, and recurrent abdominal pain; protein-deficient diabetes mellitus was a vaguer entity that lacked the pancreatic stones. Patients conforming to these 'syndromes' were rare even in the tropical zones where they were described (less than 5 per cent of all diabetes), and the current consensus is that they represent type 2 diabetes or chronic pancreatitis superimposed on malnutrition.

Management of diabetes

The treatment of diabetes has traditionally concentrated on correcting hyperglycaemia, the most obvious and easily monitored biochemical abnormality and the cause of troublesome symptoms as well as specific chronic diabetic complications. This approach has not been entirely successful, partly because it is difficult to normalize blood glucose but also because macrovascular disease—the principal cause of morbidity and premature death—is heavily dependent on other factors, notably hypertension and dyslipidaemia. The current treatment targets for both type 1 and type 2 diabetes (Table 3) are therefore more holistic, tackling cardiovascular risk factors and obesity in addition to hyperglycaemia.

This section describes the roles of lifestyle modification and antidiabetic drugs, followed by specific treatment strategies for type 1 and type 2 diabetes.

Diet and lifestyle modification and management of obesity

About 80 per cent of patients with type 2 diabetes are obese, as are at least 30 per cent of those with type 1 disease. Obesity is arguably one of the greatest obstacles to successful management of diabetes: it worsens insulin resistance, dyslipidaemia, and hypertension and is now recognized in its own right as a risk factor for coronary-heart disease. Proven benefits of 10 per cent weight loss in type 2 patients with a body mass index of 30 to 40 kg/m² include falls in fasting glucose of 2 to 4 mmol/l and a 1 per cent decrease in HbA₁c—comparable with sulphonylureas or metformin—and reduced dosages of antidiabetic drugs, including insulin. There may also be variable improvements in blood pressure and dyslipidaemia (decreased triglycerides and low-density lipoprotein cholesterol, increased high-density lipoprotein). The traditional focus on obesity has been in type 2 diabetes, but there is no reason to assume that the cardiovascular hazards of obesity do not also apply to type 1 diabetes.

Weight reduction is regarded as the 'cornerstone' for treating obese type 2 diabetics but is often undermined by a lack of determination. Accordingly, doctors have little confidence in its efficacy and tend to assume that most obese patients will be 'dietary failures'. However, with clear advice, better understanding of the causes of obesity, and the use of realistic targets, the currently poor track record of diet and lifestyle therapy can be greatly improved. All members of the diabetes team must understand the principles (but not the detail) of lifestyle management so that a strong and unified message can be given to the patient.

The notion of the 'diabetic diet' must now finally be laid to rest. Traditionally, carbohydrate intake was restricted because of the simplistic assumptions that sugar alone raised blood glucose and might even be diabetogenic; this strategy favoured a high fat intake that undoubtedly helped to sustain obesity and probably predisposed to atheroma. Current advice is close to the 'healthy eating' recommendations for the whole population and can therefore be suggested for all the patient's family, which will greatly increase the chances of compliance.

The following diet and activity recommendations apply to both type 1 and type 2 diabetes. The aims are to:

1. Correct obesity, which worsens insulin resistance, reduces the efficacy of glucose-lowering, antihypertensive, and lipid-modifying drugs, and is an independent risk factor for macrovascular disease. Management of obesity is discussed in detail in Chapter 10.5.

2. Reduce cardiovascular risk, by limiting fat, cholesterol, sodium, and alcohol intakes.

3. Avoid hypoglycaemia in patients receiving insulin or sulphonylureas by optimizing the timing and content of meals.

The steps in designing dietary advice for the individual patient are shown in Fig. 6.

Reducing total energy intake

This should be reduced by 500 to 600 cal/day (2100 to 2520 J/day) in patients who are overweight (body mass index over 28 kg/m^2). This energy deficit mobilizes fat preferentially, whereas protein, glycogen, and water are also lost with more aggressive energy restriction; initially, the rate of weight loss will be 0.5 to 1.0 kg/week (adipose tissue contains around 7000 cal/kg (29 400 J/kg).

The desired energy intake should be calculated from standard formulae that employ the subject's age, sex, weight, and level of physical activity to estimate energy expenditure, which must equal energy intake under steady-state conditions. The standard dietary history is a waste of time for trying to assess energy intake, because overweight subjects consistently under-report how much they eat. Specific advice about how to cut energy intake is best left to the dietician, but hinges on reducing fat intake—a simple message that can be reinforced by the entire diabetes care team. Fat-rich foods not only have the highest energy density (9 cal/g (38 J/g) compared with 4 cal/g (17 J/g) for carbohydrate and protein), but also have poor satiating effects and so tend to encourage overeating.

The initial target should be 10 per cent loss of starting weight, not the 'ideal' body weight or body mass index, which is only rarely attained by obese diabetic patients. When energy intake is cut acutely, type 2 patients

often show an immediate fall in blood glucose, due to a drop in hepatic glucose output, even before weight loss begins.

Weight loss during an energy deficit of 500 to 600 cal/day (2100 to 2520 J/day) is a slow process: for a 100 kg patient, 10 per cent weight loss may take several months. Frequent contact and encouragement are the best predictors of success, and the patient should be reassured that weight loss by a small but tolerable change in lifestyle is much more likely to be maintained than weight lost by a crash diet. As weight falls, resting energy expenditure also declines: it is proportional to lean body mass, which also decreases, although at a slower rate than fat. This means that greater reductions in energy intake (more than 600 cal/day (2520 J/day) will be needed to maintain the same rate of weight loss. If the 10 per cent target is met, further loss towards an 'ideal' body mass index of around 23 kg/m^2 may be feasible.

Weight loss is harder to achieve in diabetic patients than in their non-diabetic counterparts; possible reasons include fears about sugar rather than fat, and the adipogenic effects of insulin, sulphonylureas, and thiazolidinediones. In practice, weight loss of even 10 per cent is not commonly achieved by diet and lifestyle modification alone; only 15 to 30 per cent of newly diagnosed type 2 diabetic patients can normalize glycaemia initially by this means, and fewer than 10 per cent can sustain this for 5 years or more. The progressive β-cell dysfunction in type 2 diabetes (see above) makes it inevitable that the proportion of 'dietary failures' will increase steadily.

Improving dietary composition

Intakes of fat, salt, and refined sugar are generally too high in westernized populations. Current recommendations for healthy eating are based on evidence of beneficial effects on body weight, glycaemic control, lipids, and blood pressure (Fig. 6).

Fat should provide less than 30 per cent of total energy intake (in most industrialized countries, it accounts for 40 per cent). Polyunsaturated or monounsaturated fats (for example sunflower or olive oils respectively) are preferred to saturated animal fats, which should comprise less than 10 per cent of total energy intake. Patients may need to be reminded that 'good' unsaturated fats still contain 9 cal/g (38 J/g) and therefore sustain obesity just as effectively as the others. Cholesterol should be limited to less than 250 mg/day (less if dyslipidaemia is present).

Carbohydrates should account for more than 55 per cent of total energy intake, preferably in the form of foods rich in soluble fibre (such as pulses, root and leaf vegetables, and fruit); the current World Health Organization recommendation for the general population is for the consumption of at least four portions of fruit or vegetables per day. Sugary drinks (especially fizzy glucose solutions that are supposed to give energy) should be avoided, except to treat hypoglycaemia. The present recommendation, which seems reasonable but is not based on evidence, is to limit added sucrose to less than 25 g/day and total sucrose intake to less than 50 g/day.

Protein should contribute 10 to 15 per cent of total energy—close to current levels in the general population. (For patients with renal impairment, see Chapter 20.10.1.)

Sodium intake should be less than 6 g/day, and less in patients with hypertension.

Alcohol contains 7 cal/g (29 J/g), and beers and wines in particular can be fattening. Intake should not exceed three units (30 g) per day in men and two units (20 g) per day in women, and should be further limited or avoided in those with hypertension or obesity. Alcohol can delay recovery from hypoglycaemia (see below); 'diabetic' beers (low sugar, but strong in alcohol) and spirits with sugar-free mixers are especially likely to provoke hypoglycaemia.

Moderate amounts of sucrose are acceptable (see above), while non-caloric sweeteners (such as aspartame) have no adverse metabolic effects. So-called 'diabetic' sweets and foods contain sorbitol or fructose instead of glucose, and are an expensive way to get diarrhoea; they should be avoided by patients, and withdrawn by the manufacturers.

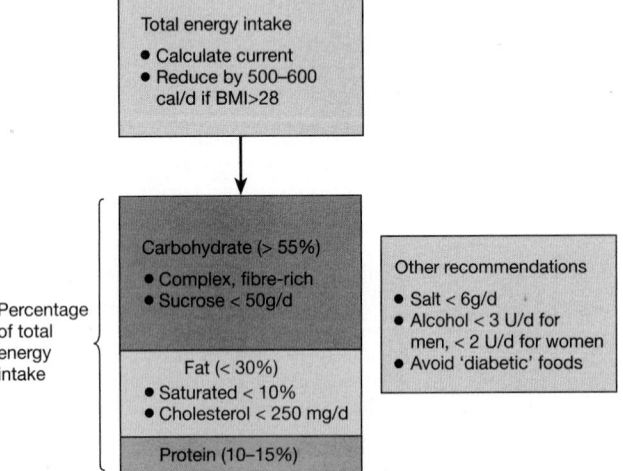

Fig. 6 Dietary recommendations for diabetic people. These guidelines now reflect 'healthy eating' for the general population, rather than a 'diabetic diet'.

Optimizing meal patterns

Judging the size and content of meals so as to limit glycaemic excursions remains an art rather than a science, and a skill which some patients develop with experience. Dosages of glucose-lowering drugs that act acutely to cover meals (short-acting insulin and sulphonylureas) can be tailored reasonably accurately to meals of similar composition but may not be matched to other meals, even when the total weights of carbohydrate, fat, and protein are similar.

There has been much interest in the ability of various foods to raise blood glucose, usually measured as the 'glycaemic index', i.e. the area under the curve of the rise in plasma glucose after eating a standardized load (50 g) of the food, expressed as a percentage of the area under the glucose curve after ingesting 50 g of glucose. Foods with a low glycaemic index include pulses and cereals, probably because of their high fibre and complex carbohydrate contents, while bread has a surprisingly high index. The glycaemic index of many foods such as potatoes and pasta varies widely according to the method of cooking (and even the shape of the pasta), and mixing different foods in a real-life meal has unpredictable effects on the overall postprandial glucose rise. It may be sensible to base meals around components with a low glycaemic index but it is clearly not feasible to use the index to adjust dosages of antidiabetic medication.

Increasing physical activity

Short-term exercise and improved physical fitness both increase insulin sensitivity, partly through increased translocation of GLUT-4 units to the surface of skeletal muscle cells; this effect is independent of insulin, and can enhance glucose uptake (under clamp conditions) better than metformin or the thiazolidinediones. Several studies, notably that conducted in Malmö, Sweden, have demonstrated that regular physical exercise reduces by 50 per cent the risk of impaired glucose tolerance progressing to type 2 diabetes, and also significantly decreases cardiovascular events. Exercise must therefore be encouraged in all diabetic patients, but the advice must be realistic, achievable, and safe. Brisk walking for 30 to 40 min every day is better physiologically than a hectic workout in the gym once or twice a week and is within almost everyone's reach.

Potential hazards of exercise are hypoglycaemia, which may be delayed by several hours (see below), and cardiac disease. Patients at risk should have an ECG, with consideration for an exercise tolerance test and echocardiography, and appropriate treatment for ischaemic heart disease or heart failure. Exercise remains beneficial and important in these cases but should be built up gradually.

Antiobesity drugs and bariatric surgery in diabetes

Antiobesity drugs may be indicated in selected obese diabetic patients with a body mass index over 28 kg/m^2 and who have demonstrated by losing weight beforehand through diet and exercise alone that they are prepared to make long-term changes in their lifestyle. Without this commitment, clinically useful weight loss is unlikely to be achieved or maintained beyond the period of drug prescription (currently 2 years for orlistat and 1 year for sibutramine); the medical and pharmacoeconomic benefits of modest weight loss for a couple of years in the obese patient's middle age are not known but are probably not dramatic.

Drugs currently available in many countries are orlistat, a gastrointestinal lipase inhibitor, and sibutramine, a combined serotonin/noradrenaline reuptake inhibitor. With each of these, up to 30 per cent of obese type 2 patients lose 10 per cent or more of body weight within 6 to 12 months, HbA$_{1c}$ can fall by 1 per cent or more, and dosages of glucose-lowering drugs, including insulin, may be decreased.

Surgical treatment with gastric banding or gastric bypass operations is indicated in selected patients with a body mass index over 40 kg/m^2 (Chapter 10.5). This approach can achieve dramatic weight loss (up to 70 per cent of excess fat, maintained for several years), often with an impressive reversal of glucose intolerance: about 90 per cent of cases with type 2 diabetes or impaired glucose tolerance are returned to normoglycaemia.

Smoking

Smoking is at least as common among diabetic patients as in the general population. Smoking greatly amplifies macrovascular risk in diabetic subjects: 10-year mortality (mainly from myocardial infarction) is about 50 per cent higher than in diabetic non-smokers and twice as high as in non-diabetic non-smokers. Smoking may also accelerate the progression of nephropathy and possibly retinopathy.

Many diabetic people, especially young women, continue to smoke as a means of keeping thin, and because they fear gaining weight if they stop. Nicotine reduces fondness for sweet energy-dense foods and may also be mildly thermogenic. Weight gain after stopping smoking averages 3 kg but about 20 per cent of cases gain more than 6 kg; much of this weight is often lost within the following 1 to 2 years, and it can be limited or prevented by careful dietetic support beforehand and in the months after cessation. Moreover, the risks of continuing to smoke are much greater than this degree of weight gain, especially in diabetic people. Nicotine chewing gum may help patients to give up the habit.

Glucose-lowering drugs

Insulin

Insulin is the rational treatment for type 1 diabetes and the only drug that can normalize blood glucose in many type 2 diabetic patients. Unfortunately, subcutaneously injected insulin cannot match the physiological profile of normal insulin secretion (Fig. 7) and is a poor substitute for the finely tuned β cell with its nearly instantaneous capacity for 'in-flight' adjustment. Moreover, insulin given subcutaneously is absorbed into the systemic circulation rather than secreted into the portal system where an immediate effect on the liver, and first-pass clearance by that organ, are important in regulating the metabolic actions of insulin.

Insulin manufacture

Insulin was traditionally extracted from pork and beef pancreases in acid ethanol and purified by precipitation and recrystallization. Soluble (or

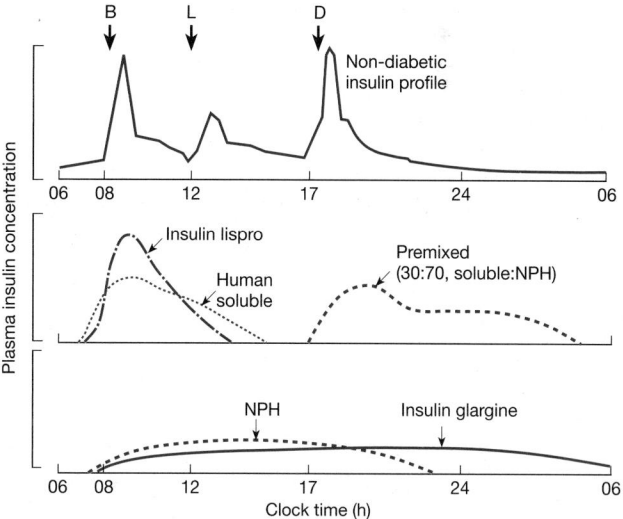

Fig. 7 Time course of insulin preparations, compared with the normal diurnal profile of plasma insulin concentrations in non-diabetic subjects (top). Breakfast (B), lunch (L), and dinner (D) were given as shown. Fast-acting analogues (such as lispro) act more rapidly than conventional soluble ones but are still sluggish compared with normal prandial insulin release. Premixed insulins injected in the early evening cover the evening meal adequately, but the long-acting component can cause hyperinsulinaemia and troublesome hypoglycaemia in the small hours. None of the conventional 'long-acting' insulins reliably lasts 24 h; new long-acting analogues such as insulin glargine may provide adequate background insulin levels with once-daily injections.

'crystalline') insulin prepared in this way was contaminated with other islet proteins, including glucagon and pancreatic polypeptide, which had an adjuvant-like effect and enhanced the immunogenicity of the injected insulin; immune reactions were relatively common with the 'dirty' animal insulins in use until the 1970s (see below). More sophisticated purification techniques including gel filtration yield 'highly purified' or 'monocomponent' insulins which only rarely provoke immune reactions.

Biosynthetic human-sequence insulin, produced by recombinant DNA technology, entered clinical practice in the early 1980s and was the first genetically engineered protein to be used therapeutically. The current approach is to introduce a synthetic gene for recombinant proinsulin or a novel insulin precursor into yeast; the secreted product is then cleaved enzymatically to yield insulin and C peptide.

There are some clinically relevant differences between the three species used therapeutically, although the shortcomings of insulin therapy relate mainly to the general pharmacokinetic misbehaviour of injected insulin. Human insulin is more lipophilic than porcine and bovine insulins and is slightly more rapidly absorbed: human soluble especially may lower glucose faster and patients being transferred from other species should be warned of this and prandial doses reduced initially by one-third. Human ultralente has a shorter and steeper action profile than its animal counterparts, particularly the bovine preparation; in real life, human ultralente behaves similarly to lente or isophane insulins and does not provide adequate basal levels for a full 24 h. Human insulin has been suggested to interfere with awareness of hypoglycaemia but the balance of evidence does not support this view (see below). Early beef insulins were especially prone to cause immune reactions (see below), although highly purified preparations do not appear to be particularly immunogenic.

Most insulin manufacturers are now turning to biosynthetic production of human-sequence insulin. Some patients prefer to continue using animal insulins—for reasons that may or may not appear scientifically sound—and these wishes should be respected by both clinicians and the pharmaceutical industry.

Insulin absorption

Absorption of insulin injected subcutaneously is slow and unpredictable. Individual day-to-day variability in the amount absorbed within a few hours can exceed 50 per cent. This means that small changes (less than 10 per cent) in insulin dosage are unlikely to influence glycaemic control, and that insulin treatment should generally not be adjusted on a daily basis.

Insulin absorption is influenced by the physical state of the insulin (soluble or delayed action), its speed of dissociation into monomers, the lipophilicity of the insulin species, and by blood flow and other characteristics of the injection site. Absorption is accelerated, and may lead to noticeably faster falls in blood glucose, by stimulating general or local blood flow through exercise, hot climate, saunas, and/or massaging the injection site. Conversely, absorption is slowed when subcutaneous blood flow is reduced, for example in cold conditions or hypovolaemic states. Lipohypertrophy, which may develop at frequently used injection sites, can significantly delay absorption—another reason for avoiding such areas.

The anatomical site of injection also influences the rate of subcutaneous absorption. It is fastest in the abdomen (also a good site to limit any effects of exercise) and arm, and slower in the leg. These differences are often eclipsed by the overall variability in absorption. Absorption from muscle is faster, presumably because of its higher blood flow, and this route is preferred for the emergency treatment of hyperglycaemia or ketoacidosis if the best option, controlled intravenous infusion, is not practicable.

Insulin preparations

Soluble (regular, or short-acting) insulin injected subcutaneously begins to lower glucose within 30 min, has a peak effect between 1 and 2 h and lasts 3 to 5 h (Fig. 7). This action profile is suitable for covering meals or hyperglycaemic emergencies and for use in insulin pumps or infusions. However, it would have to be injected several times per day to control hyperglycaemia

around the clock, at the cost of frequent hypoglycaemia. Long-acting preparations are therefore used to cover basal insulin requirements.

Various approaches have been used to slow and prolong insulin absorption, especially the chemical combination of insulin into complexes that release it slowly. More recently, synthetic analogues have been designed whose structure promotes precipitation when injected subcutaneously (see Fig. 7).

Isophane insulins are also known as 'NPH' ('neutral protamine Hagedorn', from the director of the Danish laboratory where they were developed). They consist of a microcrystalline complex of insulin and the highly basic protein protamine (intriguingly isolated from fish sperm), together with trace amounts of Zn^{2+}. Isophanes were derived from protamine-zinc insulin which has a longer but highly unpredictable action profile. Isophanes produce peak plasma insulin levels at variable intervals between 4 and 8 h after injection, and their glucose-lowering action wears off rapidly after 10 to 12 h.

Insulin-zinc suspensions (lente insulins) employ higher Zn^{2+} concentrations which encourage insulin to form crystalline lattices. Varying the reaction pH can produce either larger crystals which are particularly slow to dissolve ('ultralente') or the amorphous 'semilente' which releases insulin faster; the familiar 'lente' is a 70:30 mixture of ultralente and semilente. Ultralente made with bovine insulin has a long, relatively flat action profile that can last 24 h or more, while human ultralente and the lente insulins of all three species have glucose-lowering profiles similar to that of isophane. These long-acting insulins have a cloudy appearance and need to be shaken before use to bring the insulin into suspension; visibly large particles or discoloration indicates that the insulin has become denatured and will have lost activity. Both lente and isophane insulins can be injected alone or mixed with soluble insulin.

Premixed insulins contain a short-acting soluble component together with a longer-acting lente or isophane. The aim is to provide prandial cover and then basal levels for several hours thereafter. Many preparations are available, with the proportion of short-acting insulin varying from 10 to 50 per cent. 30:70 mixtures are popular.

All these insulin types have been produced with porcine-, bovine- and human-sequence insulins, and are available in vials for pen injection devices.

Insulin analogues

The pharmacokinetic properties of native insulins of any species are poorly suited to subcutaneous injection: soluble insulins (despite their high-speed trade names) are too slow and prolonged in duration, while long-acting insulins do not provide reliable enough 24-h basal levels to be given once daily. Various synthetic insulin analogues, designed by molecular modelling, have improved physicochemical characteristics.

Fast-acting analogues are modified at the C-terminal end of the B chain, an area crucial in the self-association of insulin molecules, so as to resist dimerization and hexamerization. Insulin hexamers formed in the subcutaneous injection site, dissociate slowly into absorbable monomers, and this is a rate-limiting step in insulin absorption. Faster-acting analogues include insulin lispro (interchanging the B28 lysine and B29 proline residues of the normal human sequence) and insulin aspart, which carries aspartic acid at position B28 instead of the usual proline. They have an appreciably faster and shorter action profile (Fig. 7), and day-to-day variability in absorption and glycaemic responses may also be decreased. They can therefore reduce both prandial hyperglycaemia and the risk of postprandial hypoglycaemia. Overall, HbA_{1c} falls, with a reduced frequency of hypoglycaemia, when a fast-acting analogue is substituted for soluble insulin.

Long-acting insulin analogues are clear but precipitate when injected subcutaneously. Dissociation into monomers is at least as slow as with conventional long-acting insulins and can provide basal levels for 24 h with a single daily injection, perhaps with less variability. An example currently entering clinical practice is insulin glargine (A21glycine, with two extra arginine residues extending the C terminus of the B chain).

Side-effects of insulin

Hypoglycaemia is the most common complication of insulin treatment and can be unpleasant, debilitating, and occasionally life-threatening.

Mild hypoglycaemia is common—many insulin-treated patients have at least one episode most weeks—but serious attacks causing unconsciousness or requiring the assistance of others are rare, about once every three patient years. Predictably, the frequency of both mild and severe attacks rises progressively when mean blood glucose levels are lowered by intensive insulin therapy; hypoglycaemia was three times more frequent in the tightly controlled group of the Diabetic Control and Complications Trial than in conventionally treated patients (see below).

The manifestations and treatment of hypoglycaemia are covered in detail later. As discussed there, there is no convincing evidence that the use of human as opposed to animal insulins specifically interferes with awareness of hypoglycaemic symptoms.

Weight gain is due to the anabolic effects of insulin, compounded by energy saved from glycosuria and sometimes by overeating after hypoglycaemia. Fear of weight gain discourages some patients, especially young women, from taking their full insulin dosages; deliberate omission or underdosing of insulin may be used surprisingly often to stay thin.

Lipohypertrophy is local thickening of subcutaneous tissue at frequently used injection sites, and is probably due to the lipogenic effects of high local insulin concentrations. Lipohypertrophy can be unsightly and can significantly delay insulin absorption. It can be prevented by rotating injections around several sites, and large lesions can be removed by liposuction.

Insulin allergy, now very rare with highly purified (especially human) insulins, can include local IgE-mediated erythematous reactions or even anaphylaxis. Lipoatrophy (localized pitting of the skin due to loss of subcutaneous fat) is apparently related to a chronic immune response generated around insulin crystals. 'Immune insulin resistance' was seen with impure animal and especially bovine insulins; high titres of insulin-binding antibodies mop up free insulin from the circulation, resulting in very high insulin requirements (occasionally more than 10 000 U/day), sometimes with unpredictable hypoglycaemia following release of antibody-bound insulin.

Insulin oedema is rare, and is usually seen in patients recovering from ketoacidosis who have been deprived of insulin for long periods. Fluid retention is probably due to the sodium-conserving effects of insulin on the renal tubule, and may cause ankle or generalized oedema. It usually resolves within a few days, although treatment with diuretics or ephedrine may be required.

Insulin regimens

Different individuals may need quite different insulin regimens, depending on their residual insulin reserve and severity of insulin resistance, as well as the desired tightness of control and the inconvenience that the patient will accept. Specific insulin schedules used in type 1 and type 2 diabetes are described later.

Insulin dosage The healthy pancreas secretes about 40 to 60 U of insulin daily. Therapeutic insulin requirements range from less than this in thin type 1 patients (notably during the 'honeymoon period') to more than 200 U/day in very obese, insulin-resistant type 2 patients. High insulin requirements are often due to insulin resistance (see above), whereas low or falling dosages may be caused by weight loss (including anorexia nervosa), coeliac disease, or loss of counter-regulatory hormones in Addison's disease or hypothyroidism—all these conditions being associated with type 1 diabetes. Changing dosages, especially in previously stable subjects, should prompt investigation of these possibilities. Some patients with 'brittle' diabetes or psychological maladaptation to life with diabetes may pretend to take very high or very low dosages (see later).

Types of insulin Formularies contain a bewildering assortment of insulins, many distinguished by imaginative claims about their action profile. Practically, prescribers should become familiar with regimens based on one or two preparations from the following broad classes:

1. Fast-acting insulin: either a soluble (regular) insulin such as Humulin S or Actrapid, injected 30 to 40 min before eating, or a faster-acting analogue (for example lispro or aspart) which can be given immediately before or even shortly after eating.

2. Long-acting insulin: either a lente insulin (for example Humulin Zn or Insulatard) or an isophane (for example Humulin I or Monotard). With either, circulating insulin falls to below useful levels after 10 to 14 h; they therefore need to be given twice daily in C-peptide negative patients, although those with residual insulin secretion (or who are given three premeal injections of soluble insulin) may be able to maintain good glycaemic control with a single bedtime injection. Bovine (but not human) ultralente can last a full 24 h, but its absorption is erratic. The long-acting analogues currently being introduced (such as insulin glargine) have flat, steady action profiles that may provide basal insulin levels with a single daily injection.

The timing of long-acting insulin injections does not have to be yoked to mealtimes as tightly as for soluble insulin but it is convenient to inject the morning dose at the same time as the prebreakfast soluble, either separately or mixed in the same syringe (glargine cannot be mixed with other insulins). When a second long-acting injection is needed, this is best given at bedtime, rather than together with the presupper soluble dose. This is because the action profile of long-acting insulin clashes with the physiological changes in insulin sensitivity that occur overnight. Growth hormone is normally secreted in large spikes on entering deep sleep, typically between 24.00 and 02.00 hours; this induces delayed insulin resistance which raises blood glucose during the hours leading up to breakfast. This 'dawn phenomenon' is accentuated if insulin levels are falling simultaneously—as happens if long-acting insulin is injected in the early evening. Another hazard with this timing is potentially dangerous nocturnal hypoglycaemia when insulin levels peak during the early morning (typically 02.00 to 04.00). Both problems can be reduced by delaying the long-acting injection to bedtime (22.00 to 23.00), when the risk of nocturnal hypoglycaemia is lower, and insulin levels generally persist long enough to counteract the insulin resistance of the dawn phenomenon.

3. Premixed insulins (for example 30 per cent short-acting with 70 per cent long-acting) are obviously more convenient than giving short- and long-acting insulins separately, but they lack flexibility. Premixed insulin injected 30 to 40 min before breakfast can achieve good glycaemic control through the morning and afternoon, but timing the evening dose is problematic: giving it before supper will tend to cause both early-morning hypoglycaemia and fasting hyperglycaemia because of the time course of the long-acting component, and simply increasing the evening dosage often makes nocturnal hypoglycaemia worse while failing to lower the prebreakfast glucose.

Insulin injections

Most insulin formulations are now available for both conventional syringes or pen injection devices. Pen injectors are compact, convenient, and easy to use: the required dose is 'dialled up' and injected by pressing the plunger; the ratchet mechanism of most pens gives an audible click that can help blind patients to count dosages.

Syringes and pens carry very fine (28 to 31 gauge) needles that allow insulin to be injected almost painlessly. The needle should be pushed in vertically and the insulin injected over a few seconds. 'Backtracking' of insulin to the skin surface, which can occasionally cause loss of several units of insulin, may be reduced by leaving the needle in place for a short while. A spot of bleeding may occur; very rarely, sudden hypoglycaemia may be due to direct injection of insulin into a subcutaneous vein.

Injections can be given into any site that is accessible and well upholstered with adipose tissue, especially the abdomen, thighs, buttocks, and upper arms. The abdomen has the advantage (theoretically at least) of relatively faster absorption that is less influenced by exercise, as compared with the limbs. Rotating injection sites, for example between the abdomen and leg, or around the quadrants of the abdomen, helps to avoid local reactions, especially lipohypertrophy which can make insulin absorption slow and erratic.

Jet injectors fire a metered dose of insulin as a high-pressure aerosol that penetrates the skin. These have is obvious appeal to patients with needle phobia, although there may be bruising and delayed discomfort at the injection site. Jet injectors are bulky and expensive and do not offer any pharmacokinetic advantages over conventional injections.

Insulin pumps

Portable insulin pumps that administer continuous subcutaneous insulin infusion were developed by Pickup and colleagues in the late 1970s. Modern pumps are compact and light and worn in a belt or holster. Soluble insulin in a special cartridge is delivered through a fine-bore cannula and a butterfly-type cannula, which is inserted subcutaneously in the anterior abdominal wall and generally left in place for 1 to 2 days; the pump can be safely removed for 30 to 40 min for bathing or other activities. Different basal rates can be preprogrammed, and mealtime boluses are selected and given by pressing a button. Typical basal rates are 1 to 2 U/h during the day and 0.5 to 1 U/h overnight, with mealtime boluses (given 30 min before the main meals) amounting to about 50 per cent of the total daily dose. Insulin lispro has been used in pumps and may slightly improve control compared with conventional soluble insulin.

Continuous subcutaneous insulin infusion can achieve relatively steady insulin levels under laboratory conditions but cannot overcome the fundamental variability of subcutaneous insulin absorption. When used carefully by highly motivated patients who are supported by an experienced diabetes care team, continuous subcutaneous insulin infusion can achieve glycaemic control which is at least as good as that achieved with multiple injections; the two were used side by side in the Diabetic Control and Complications Trial. Insulin pumps are expensive (£1000 to £1500 (US$1500 to 2300)) as are consumables (another £1000 per year); medical backup can also be costly to provide. Continuous subcutaneous insulin infusion is only indicated for well-informed patients who are prepared to monitor their blood glucose frequently and take some responsibility for adjusting the pump. It is widely used in the United States and some European countries but less in the United Kingdom.

Infections at the infusion site with pyogenic skin commensals or unusual organisms (for example atypical mycobacteria) are uncommon but can be troublesome and cause rapid deterioration in glycaemic control. An increased rate of diabetic ketoacidosis was reported with earlier and less reliable pumps. With continuous subcutaneous insulin infusion, the subcutaneous insulin depot is only a few units, and any interruption of insulin delivery (such as with pump failure or cannula blockage) can lead to rapid rises in blood glucose and especially ketone levels. However, modern pumps carry no excess risk of diabetic ketoacidosis as compared with intensified injection therapy. Similarly, the risk of hypoglycaemia due to the pump over-running is now very low.

Continuous intraperitoneal infusion The peritoneum is a good route for insulin administration: absorption is very rapid across its large surface area and insulin enters the portal circulation. Continuous intraperitoneal insulin infusion has been used in some cases, mostly employing a pump and reservoir implanted subcutaneously in the abdomen and delivering insulin through a flexible cannula sewn into the peritoneal cavity. The reservoir is filled with soluble insulin through an injection port lying just beneath the skin and is emptied by a liquid gas compression system at a rate that can be varied by an external electromagnetic control. Continuous intraperitoneal insulin infusion can provide basal insulin; meals need to be covered by additional insulin, usually injected subcutaneously.

Intraperitoneal pumps are expensive and convincing indications for their use are rare. They have been successful in some patients with apparently very high subcutaneous insulin dosages but surprisingly normal intravenous requirements. It is now clear that this situation is not due to a mysterious syndrome of 'subcutaneous insulin resistance', and that most of not all of these patients are interfering with their own treatment (see

below). In this setting, continuous intraperitoneal insulin infusion is probably effective because these pumps are difficult to sabotage.

Oral hypoglycaemic agents

Sulphonylureas and repaglinide

The sulphonylureas were the first orally active glucose-lowering drugs to be used and were discovered in the 1930s when early sulphonamide antibiotics were found to cause hypoglycaemia. The 'first generation' (chlorpropamide, tolbutamide) have since been superseded by the 'second generation' (for example gliclazide and glibenclamide) and by newer agents such as glimepiride. Repaglinide acts in a similar way to the sulphonylureas.

Mode of action Sulphonylureas are insulin secretagogues but insulin synthesis is not stimulated. Insulin levels peak within 1 to 2 h and decline within 4 to 6 h for the short-acting drugs (such as gliclazide) but may remain elevated for much longer with chlorpropamide and glibenclamide, which therefore carry a greater risk of hypoglycaemia. An 'extrapancreatic' action has also been attributed to sulphonylureas, i.e. improving insulin sensitivity. This effect is small and is probably explained by the non-specific decrease in insulin resistance ('glucotoxicity') when hyperglycaemia is corrected by any means.

Repaglinide acts in a similar way to the sulphonylureas but is structurally different. It is derived from the non-sulphonylurea part of the glibenclamide molecule (called meglitinide), which was found fortuitously to have glucose-lowering activity of its own.

Efficacy and potency The ability of these agents to lower glycaemia depends on how much insulin is available for release from the β cells (which are already stimulated by hyperglycaemia) and by the severity of insulin resistance. In practice, all sulphonylureas lower basal and postprandial glucose levels by no more than 2 to 4 mmol/l and HbA$_{1c}$ by 1 to 2 per cent; mild hyperglycaemia may therefore be corrected but patients with fasting glucose in excess of 13 mmol/l are very unlikely to achieve normoglycaemia (so-called 'primary failure'). Moreover, as β-cell function declines progressively in type 2 diabetes, many patients who initially respond well to sulphonylureas will subsequently need additional glucose-lowering drugs; this 'secondary failure' overtakes 5 to 10 per cent of patients per year, in a cumulative fashion. These limitations apply to all sulphonylureas and repaglinide: the more potent drugs have lower therapeutic dosages than the earlier agents but cannot lower glycaemia any further.

Pharmacokinetics Most are taken twice daily with meals; glimepiride is taken once daily and repaglinide with each meal. Chlorpropamide has a very long action profile, while glibenclamide shows variable and sometimes prolonged hypoglycaemic activity. Sulphonylureas and repaglinide bind to circulating proteins and may be displaced by other strongly protein-bound drugs, causing hypoglycaemia (see below). All these drugs are cleared through the kidneys and can accumulate in renal failure, causing frequent hypoglycaemia and other side-effects. Gliquidone is metabolized mainly in the liver and may be slightly less hazardous in patients with renal impairment, although insulin is usually indicated in these cases.

Side-effects Weight gain is due to the anabolic effects of hyperinsulinaemia, compounded by reduced losses of energy through glycosuria. Weight gain is typically 2 to 3 kg greater than with diet alone or metformin.

Hypoglycaemia is rarer than with insulin, but the risk is greater with longer-acting sulphonylureas (glibenclamide, chloropropamide), in renal failure, and in the elderly.

Sulphonylureas can cause allergic reactions including skin rashes (notably Stevens–Johnson syndrome) and marrow dyscrasias, and can precipitate acute intermittent porphyria. Side-effects exclusive to chlorpropamide include the syndrome of inappropriate secretion of antidiuretic hormone (see Chapter 20.2.1) and acetaldehyde-mediated facial flushing on drinking alcohol.

The cardiovascular safety of sulphonylureas has remained under a cloud since tolbutamide was associated with an excess of cardiovascular deaths during an essentially uninterpretable study (the UGDP) conducted in the

1970s; the presence of the SUR-2 receptor on cardiomyocytes has recently reinforced suspicions that these drugs may trigger ischaemia and arrhythmias (by preventing preconditioning). However, the recent United Kingdom Prospective Diabetes Study found no evidence that patients treated with sulphonylureas suffered cardiovascular events more often than those treated with insulin. Glimepiride is highly selective for SUR-1.

Indications and contraindications These drugs are first-line therapy for type 2 patients in whom lifestyle and dietetic measures have failed to control hyperglycaemia. Because of their tendency to increase weight, they are best suited to non-obese patients. They can be usefully combined with metformin, which may partly offset weight gain, or insulin.

Insulin secretagogues are inappropriate for severely insulin deficient patients or during intercurrent illness, when insulin is needed, and are unlikely to be effective if fasting glucose exceeds 13 mmol/l. Sulphonylureas are contraindicated in renal failure: all should be stopped and insulin started if serum creatinine exceeds 250 μmol/l. Pregnancy has been viewed as a contraindication, because sulphonylureas cross the placenta and could cause fetal hyperinsulinaemia and perhaps teratogenesis; however, a recent study did not substantiate these concerns (see Chapter 13.10).

Many drugs interact with sulphonylureas, the most common interaction being hypoglycaemia due to displacement and/or decreased clearance of protein-bound sulphonylureas (for example by sulphonamides, fibrates, salicylates, and probenecid). Potential interactions must always be checked for any drug being contemplated in patients receiving sulphonylureas.

Choice of drug There is little to choose between the newer agents; chlorpropamide is now obsolete. Glibenclamide should be avoided in the elderly because of its unpredictable tendency to cause hypoglycaemia.

Metformin

Metformin and phenformin are biguanides, the class of compounds responsible for the mild hypoglycaemic action of goat's rue (an otherwise undistinguished weed). Phenformin is no longer available in many countries because it carries a 10-fold greater risk of lactic acidosis, while metformin only recently entered clinical use in the United States.

Mode of action Metformin acts primarily by inhibiting gluconeogenesis in the liver, thus reducing the raised hepatic glucose output which underpins basal and overnight hyperglycaemia; this effectively enhances the action of insulin on the liver. Peripheral glucose uptake may also be increased, while gastrointestinal side-effects may help to reduce fondness for food. Metformin does not stimulate insulin secretion.

Overall, metformin lowers blood glucose (especially postprandial) by 2 to 4 mmol/l and HbA$_{1c}$ by 1 to 2 per cent, which is comparable to the effect of sulphonylureas. On its own, metformin does not cause hypoglycaemia, although this can obviously occur when it is combined with either a sulphonylurea or insulin. Weight does not usually increase with metformin, and may fall.

Metformin may have beneficial cardiovascular effects, as the United Kingdom Prospective Diabetes Study found a reduction in vascular events in the metformin-treated group only (see below). It is not clear whether this is related to specific metabolic effects of metformin (improved insulin sensitivity), to its antiobesity properties, or to other actions such as reported reductions in blood pressure and coagulability.

Pharmacokinetics Metformin is given twice or thrice daily with meals. It is cleared mainly through the kidneys, and the increase in plasma levels in renal failure is a major risk factor for lactic acidosis.

Side-effects Gastrointestinal symptoms (30 per cent of cases) include altered taste, loss of appetite, heartburn, abdominal discomfort and bloating, and diarrhoea (metformin is the commonest cause of this in the diabetic clinic). These problems are mostly mild, but may discourage the patient from taking the drug; they can be reduced by starting with a low dosage and increasing it slowly.

Lactic acidosis is very rare with metformin (about 3 cases per 100 000 patient-years) if it is carefully prescribed. This stems from the mode of action of metformin, namely the inhibition of hepatic gluconeogenesis—a process that constantly consumes the lactate produced by glycolysis. Blood lactate levels are modestly raised in patients receiving biguanides, and can escalate rapidly and cause life-threatening acidosis if lactate is overproduced (for example in respiratory or cardiac failure), or is not cleared by the liver (hepatic failure), or if metformin accumulates in renal failure. Lactic acidosis is described in detail later.

Megaloblastic anaemia can occur due to impaired absorption of vitamin B$_{12}$.

Indications and contraindications Metformin is a first-line alternative to sulphonylureas in type 2 patients whose hyperglycaemia does not respond adequately to modification of diet and lifestyle; as it does not tend to cause weight gain, and may even reduce weight, it is often used in obese patients. Its addition can also be helpful in obese patients who are poorly controlled by sulphonylureas or insulin. Metformin is being evaluated in insulin-resistant conditions such as polycystic ovary syndrome and in impaired glucose tolerance.

Contraindications include all the major organ failures— renal, hepatic, cardiac, and respiratory. It should not be used when serum creatinine concentration exceeds 125 μmol/l.

Thiazolidinediones

Thiazolidinediones are a novel class of glucose-lowering drugs which improve insulin sensitivity. There are distinct differences between individual thiazolidinediones which influence their therapeutic spectrum and safety. Rosiglitazone and pioglitazone are currently available in many countries; troglitazone has been withdrawn because it caused rare but life-threatening hepatic damage.

Mode of action and pharmacokinetics Thiazolidinediones bind to specific receptors in the nucleus which have the cumbersome title 'peroxisome proliferator activating receptor-γ' (PPAR-γ). PPAR-γ and the related peroxisome proliferator activating receptor-α (the target for the fibrate class of lipid-lowering drugs) are ligand-activated transcription factors whose natural ligands appear to be fatty acid derivatives. PPAR-γ that has bound a thiazolidinedione forms a heterodimeric complex with another nuclear receptor, RXR, bound to its own endogenous ligand, retinoic acid. The heterodimer then binds to specific recognition motifs found in the promoter sequences upstream of many genes, notably those involved in adipocyte and lipid metabolism.

The affinity of individual thiazolidinediones at PPAR-γ parallels their glucose-lowering ability in animal models of type 2 diabetes, but their precise mode of action remains uncertain. Thiazolidinediones exert concerted effects that encourage the storage of triglyceride in mature adipocytes, including the differentiation of preadipocytes into adipocytes and enhanced expression of lipogenic enzymes; overall, circulating levels of free fatty acids fall and this may reduce hepatic glucose production and increase glucose uptake into muscle as described earlier. The net effect is to enhance the action of insulin—hence their description as 'insulin sensitizers'. Thiazolidinediones have negligible glucose-lowering action unless insulin resistance and hyperglycaemia are present. As with metformin, they do not cause hypoglycaemia when used alone, but can exaggerate the hypoglycaemic effects of insulin or sulphonylureas.

Efficacy and potency Alone, all thiazolidinediones lower glucose by 2 to 3 mmol/l and HbA$_{1c}$ by 1 per cent, somewhat less than the sulphonylureas. For unknown reasons, blood glucose declines slowly during thiazolidinedione treatment, and a maximal effect may not be reached for several weeks. Rosiglitazone is the most potent thiazolidinedione to date but, as with the more potent sulphonylureas, cannot lower blood glucose further than the other thiazolidinediones.

Pharmacokinetics All are metabolized in the liver and cleared chiefly through the kidney. They are highly protein bound.

Side-effects Weight gain, averaging 1 to 4 kg, is due mainly to fat deposition. This appears to spare the visceral depot associated with insulin resistance and does not negate the glucose-lowering action.

Fluid retention of unknown aetiology may cause a mild dilutional anaemia (haemoglobin typically falls by 1 to 2 g/dl) and ankle oedema (in 5 to 10 per cent of cases); rarely, heart failure may be precipitated in patients with pre-existing myocardial dysfunction, especially if they are also treated with insulin.

Hepatic damage, ranging from subclinical elevations of hepatic enzymes to fulminant and fatal hepatic necrosis (about one case per 1000 patient-years), has been reported with troglitazone but does not appear to be a risk with rosiglitazone or pioglitazone.

Indications and contraindications Thiazolidinediones are currently regarded as second-line drugs for treating type 2 diabetes when sulphonylureas or metformin are ineffective or insuitable. They can be combined with either a sulphonylurea or metformin, when HbA$_{1c}$ may fall by more than 1 per cent; if HbA$_{1c}$ has not fallen by more than 1 per cent within 6 months of adding a thiazolidinedione, it should be discontinued. When pioglitazone is used with insulin, insulin dosage can be reduced but weight gain may be problematic; rarely, heart failure may be precipitated (the combination of rosiglitazone with insulin is currently contraindicated). Subjects with impaired glucose tolerance treated with a thiazolidinedione have a lower risk of progressing to overt type 2 diabetes, and the drugs can improve hirsutism and menstrual dysfunction (sometimes inducing ovulation) in women with polycystic ovary syndrome.

Contraindications include hepatic dysfunction and congestive heart failure. Although these is no evidence of hepatotoxicity with thiazolidinediones other than troglitazone, it seems prudent to monitor liver enzymes periodically and to stop the drug if transaminases rise to more than 1.5 times the upper limit of normal, or if any other signs of hepatic dysfunction appear.

α-Glucosidase inhibitors

Acarbose (and the related miglitol and voglibose) are inhibitors of α-glucosidase, an enzyme of the brush border of the small intestine essential for the breakdown of dietary starch to disaccharides, which are then hydrolysed to the absorbable monosaccharides. Their rationale is to block digestion of complex carbohydrates and so damp post-prandial glycaemic rises. The therapeutic effect is small: post-prandial glucose may fall by 1 to 2 mmol/l, with predictably little impact on overnight glucose, and HbA$_{1c}$ by 0.5 per cent or less. Side-effects due to carbohydrate malabsorption (flatus, abdominal bloating, gassy diarrhoea) are common and probably damage compliance. Despite its poor efficacy and low tolerability, acarbose is still widely prescribed and in some countries is regarded as a first-line drug.

Practical management of hyperglycaemia

Most newly diagnosed diabetic patients are easily allocated to either type 1 or 2 on clinical criteria (Table 2) and treatment is started accordingly. However, initial impressions may be misleading: a thin young patient may not need insulin because he has MODY, whereas a classical maturity-onset subject may lose weight rapidly and develop ketoacidosis because he has type 1 diabetes. Continuing monitoring and vigilance are therefore essential.

Type 1 diabetes

These patients must be given insulin immediately and for life. The insulin regimen will depend particularly on any remaining endogenous insulin, the patient's body weight, lifestyle, and motivation. Patients with residual insulin secretion, especially newly presenting and particularly during the 'honeymoon period'(see below), can often fill in gaps in insulin replacement and enjoy good glycaemic control with few injections and low insulin dosages. However, C-peptide negative patients will require exogenous insulin to cover both basal and prandial needs (Fig. 7) to achieve good control. Regimens include:

1. Twice daily long-acting insulin with preprandial short-acting insulin. Lente or isophane is injected before breakfast (and can be mixed with prebreakfast short-acting insulin) and at bedtime (see above). Soluble insulin is injected 30 min before breakfast and the evening meal, or a fast-acting analogue (such as lispro or aspart) given with food. Midday meals, unless large, are usually covered satisfactorily by the morning's long-acting dose and do not need separate short-acting insulin.

2. Once daily long-acting insulin with preprandial short-acting insulin is currently unsatisfactory because both lente and isophane run out too quickly, but longer-lasting analogues such as glargine may be effective when injected once daily at bedtime or breakfast. Short-acting insulin is given separately to cover meals, as above.

3. Premixed insulins injected before breakfast and before the evening meal suit some patients and many doctors, but often fail to control overnight and/or fasting glucose levels (see above).

Insulin dosages should be titrated according to blood glucose and HbA$_{1c}$ monitoring (Table 3). Highly motivated patients may be suitable for continuous subcutaneous insulin infusion treatment as discussed above.

Starting insulin therapy

Patients at risk of ketoacidosis need hospital admission, while those who are clinically well can start insulin at home, supervised by a specialist diabetes nurse. Good control can often be achieved with long-acting insulin injected at breakfast and bedtime, starting with low dosages (for example 8–12 U in the morning and 4–6 U at night) to avoid potentially demoralizing hypoglycaemia. Short-acting insulin can then be added to cover excessive prandial hyperglycaemia. Wherever practicable, patients should be encouraged to give their own injections as soon as possible.

Newly diagnosed patients starting insulin need to be warned about a possible 'honeymoon period' of good glycaemic control, when the fall in glucose levels allows partial recovery of the remaining β cells. Blood glucose can often be easily controlled with low insulin dosages (and exceptionally, without exogenous insulin) but the honeymoon ultimately ends within a few months: blood sugar levels and insulin requirements then escalate, because of the progressive loss of remaining β cells.

Poor diabetic control and 'brittle' diabetes

In real life, relatively few type 1 patients approach the high-quality glycaemic control aspired to in Table 3. This largely reflects the pharmacokinetic shortcomings of current insulin preparations and the unpredictable nature of subcutaneous absorption. The patient's compliance is a crucial determinant of overall diabetic control; teenagers are notoriously resistant to advice abut diabetes, as with other matters, and many have markedly elevated HbA$_{1c}$ concentrations. This clearly increases the risk of future diabetic complications.

A few patients have such poor metabolic control that they cannot live a normal life. Most have chronically high blood glucose and suffer recurrent hospital admissions with ketoacidosis; some suffer frequent hypoglycaemia, while others have an unstable or 'brittle' blood glucose profile that can swing rapidly between hyper- and hypoglycaemia. Occasionally, endocrine or intercurrent illnesses are found to be responsible (Table 4), but most cases remain 'idiopathic' after even intensive investigation. It is now clear that poor compliance, often with deliberate interference with treatment, is responsible in many of these patients. Most are young women who tend to be obese and are generally hyperglycaemic despite apparently high insulin dosages; when tested under controlled conditions, however, their intravenous and subcutaneous insulin requirements are unremarkable. Many are probably omitting insulin or taking only small doses: common motives include escape from difficulties at school or home, or wanting to stay thin (disturbances of body image are common in this group). Initially, such patients may appear to lead charmed lives despite frequent hospital admissions but many die prematurely (especially from ketoacidosis or hypoglycaemia); significant diabetic complications frequently develop during their twenties or thirties.

Table 4 Causes of poor glycaemic control in type 1 diabetic patients

Characteristics	Cause
1. High insulin requirements, chronic hyperglycaemia ± recurrent ketoacidosis	Obesity
	Puberty
	Endocrine diseases: Cushing's syndrome, thyrotoxicosis
	Drugs: especially glucocorticoids
	Immune insulin resistance
2. Low insulin requirements, recurrent hypoglycaemia	Weight loss
	Loss of hypoglycaemia awareness
	Endocrine diseases: adrenocortical failure, hypothyroidism, growth hormone deficiency, hypopituitarism
	Gastroparesis
	Coeliac disease
	Liver disease
3. Erratic glycaemic profile, frequent hyper- and hypoglycaemia ('brittle' diabetes)	Pancreatic damage
	Overtreating hypoglycaemia
	Gastroparesis
	Recurrent or chronic infections: tuberculosis, sinusitis

For 1, 2, and 3 always consider:
Unsuitable insulin regime
Poor diabetes education
Deliberate non-compliance
Appetite disorders: anorexia nervosa, food bingeing

Management can be extremely difficult. Patients with sustained poor control should be admitted selectively for intensive education, observation, and exclusion of other possible causes (Table 4). In some cases, it may be necessary to confirm that insulin is effective at conventional doses (for more information see the paper by Schade and Duckworth in Further reading). Even close supervision in hospital does not exclude ingenious interference with insulin treatment or glucose monitoring. Intensified insulin schedules or continuous subcutaneous insulin infusion may help in some cases but the key is more likely to be sympathetic counselling (perhaps with psychotherapy) of the patient and his or her family.

Experimental and future treatments for type 1 diabetes
Pancreatic transplantation, usually performed in conjunction with renal transplantation for patients with diabetic nephropathy, can achieve good results including long-term withdrawal of exogenous insulin in 10 per cent of cases. The whole gland or a segment is transplanted into the pelvis and anastomosed to the iliac vessels; to avoid damage from pancreatic exocrine secretions, the duct is either occluded or drained into the bladder (when urinary amylase excretion can indicate the health of the graft). Problems are the need for lifelong immunosuppression (required anyway for renal transplantation) and the global shortage of donor organs.

Pancreatic islet transplantation is gaining ground, especially transcutaneous injection into the portal vein of islets isolated from a donor pancreas; these colonize and function well in the liver, the first stop for insulin secreted physiologically. A novel immunosuppressive regimen without glucocorticoids can improve the outcome (most cases become insulin independent), but two or three donor pancreases are currently needed for each recipient.

Prevention of type 1 diabetes by aborting insulitis during the long prediabetic phase has been achieved by immunosuppression in some high-risk subjects, especially the siblings of type 1 patients who have diabetogenic HLA class II antigens and high titres of GAD and islet cell antibodies. Better immunosuppressive regimens may improve the results.

Antidiabetic drugs under development include aerosolized insulin that exploits the lung's large absorptive area and enters the bloodstream rapidly,

and various low molecular weight insulin mimetics that either bind to the insulin receptor or enhance postreceptor signalling.

Management of type 2 diabetes
Dietary and lifestyle measures form an essential foundation for management of type 2 diabetes and must be maintained throughout, even though fewer than 10 per cent of patients can be controlled satisfactorily for more than a year by these means alone.

Patients who fail to meet the glycaemic targets in Table 3 should generally follow the steps outlined below, although compromises may be more appropriate in the elderly or those at risk of hypoglycaemia. Progress should be reviewed every 3 months or so if blood glucose is unacceptably high; the inexorable deterioration of β-cell function in type 2 diabetes means that there is no point in delaying decisions to increase drug doses or add insulin.

First-line oral hypoglycaemic agents for so-called 'dietary failure' are a sulphonylurea (or repaglinide) or, particularly for obese patients (those with a body mass index in excess of 30 kg/m²), metformin. Dosages can be increased to a maximum over a few weeks. Should one class fail, the other can be tried but a dramatic improvement is unlikely.

Combination oral therapy: two of sulphonylurea (or repaglinide), metformin, or a thiazolidinedione can be used together. Some diabetologists would try adding acarbose at this stage. Triple therapy is generally not worth trying.

Long-acting insulin with a first-line oral agent: although seemingly illogical, a bedtime injection of isophane can control blood glucose overnight and before breakfast, and this apparently helps oral hypoglycaemic agents to act more effectively during the day. The combination of metformin (thrice daily with meals) with bedtime isophane often achieves good glycaemic control, while limiting the weight gain that commonly follows the introduction of insulin in type 2 patients. Isophane with a sulphonylurea or pioglitazone may increase weight; rosiglitazone is contraindicated in combination with insulin.

Insulin therapy can range from once- or twice-daily long-acting insulin in subjects with residual insulin, to the more intensified basal and prandial regimens used in type 1 diabetes. Large dosages (100 to 150 U/day) may be needed to achieve good glycaemic control in obese, highly insulin-resistant subjects. As in type 1 diabetes, rapidly acting and very long-acting analogues may be able to improve on the currently available native insulins.

Obesity (and therefore insulin resistance) may worsen when insulin treatment is started; possible reasons include reduced losses of energy through glycosuria, a tendency to relax dietary restriction when a more effective means of lowering glycaemia is introduced, and sometimes overeating during hypoglycaemic episodes. Increasing insulin resistance may lead to escalating insulin dosages. The possible hazards of insulin-induced obesity are not clear but could theoretically include vascular disease, which may be hinted at by the lower frequency of cardiovascular events among patients treated with metformin in the United Kingdom Prospective Diabetes Study trial. At present, however, the consensus is probably to aim for the glycaemic targets in Table 3 (which will reduce the risks of microvascular complications) and to accept an increase in weight, while actively treating other cardiovascular risk factors.

Experimental and future treatments for type 2 diabetes
GLP-1 is an incretin hormone that stimulates insulin secretion and may also induce satiety, particularly by delaying gastric emptying. Blood glucose can be lowered comparably to sulphonylureas with GLP-1 infused intravenously. Buccal and orally active preparations are under development, as are inhibitors of dipeptidyl peptidase IV, the enzyme which degrades GLP-1.

Combined peroxisome proliferator activating receptor α/γ agonists have insulin-sensitizing and lipid-lowering actions in animals. Various novel insulin secretagogues and non-thiazolidinedione insulin sensitizers are in development; one agent (S15261) combines both these properties.

Antiobesity drugs could have an important impact in many type 2 patients. Agents currently in preclinical testing include neuropeptide Y receptor (Y5) antagonists, melanocortin-4 receptor agonists, and low molecular weight leptin mimetics (see Chapter 10.5).

Monitoring diabetic control

Treatment targets for blood glucose and type 1 and type 2 diabetes (Table 6) have been selected to reduce the risk of chronic diabetic complications. Avoiding acute episodes of hyper- and hypoglycaemia is also important.

Blood glucose monitoring

Blood glucose concentration can be easily and quickly measured in small drops of blood (a few microlitres or less), using various test strips; the ability to perform such measurements is an essential skill for all professionals delivering diabetes care and for most diabetic patients. Test strips contain glucose oxidase (which catalyses the oxidation of glucose to gluconic acid) together with a detection system to measure specific reaction products, either electrochemically or colorimetrically (using dyes sensitive to hydrogen peroxide). The signal is read by a reflectance meter or electrically, and converted into the glucose concentration in the sample. Colour-based test strips can also be read by eye against a printed standard scale, although this may be difficult for partially sighted or colour-blind patients.

A drop of blood is obtained by pricking the sides of the fingertip, avoiding the sensitive pads; various lancets and automatic finger-pricking devices are available. Blood must cover the reaction area completely and be left in contact for exactly the period stipulated; some meters read out automatically at this point, whereas other strips must be wiped dry and left for the colour to develop. Failure to follow the manufacturer's instructions is the main cause of inaccurate readings, which are disturbingly frequent. With attention to detail, readings correspond closely to laboratory measurements of glucose (which also employ the glucose oxidase reaction) but are not reliable enough to be used for diagnosing diabetes.

Monitoring schedules

Type 2 diabetes treated with diet and oral agents can be monitored using fasting glucose and values in the midafternoon, both of which correlate with overall glucose level, measured once or twice per week.

Insulin-treated patients may need more frequent monitoring to adjust insulin dosages. Fasting glucose is determined by the previous evening's long-acting insulin, while values before the evening meal reflect mainly the morning's long-acting dose. Prandial short-acting insulin dosages can be titrated from the glucose rise 90 to 120 min after eating. Readings can be scattered across these time points on different days; most patients can be persuaded to check their glucose levels once or twice per day.

Written records help to bring out general patterns in glucose control. Patients must also be encouraged to check their glucose if they feel unwell and, crucially, frequently during intercurrent illness. Occasional tests during the night (especially between 02.00 and 04.00) are useful in patients at risk of nocturnal hypoglycaemia, including those injecting long-acting or premixed insulins in the early evening.

Checking the self-monitoring technique and the patient's action plan when glucose levels fall outside the target range is a core part of the patient's diabetic education.

HbA₁c and fructosamine

These tests measure the non-enzymatic reaction of glucose with circulating proteins (see below), and therefore reflect longer-term blood glucose levels. Glycated (glycosylated) haemoglobin (HbA$_1$) results from the combination of glucose with the N-terminal valine residue of the B chain of adult Hb (HbA), and can be separated from unaltered HbA by electrophoretic and other methods. HbA$_1$ includes the stable HbA$_{1c}$ fraction, which is most closely related to average blood glucose levels over the preceding 6 to 8 weeks.

The various assay methods for HbA$_{1c}$ are now being standardized to match the methodology used in the Diabetic Control and Complications Trial (DCCT), which defined the long-term risks of diabetic microvascular complications (see below). For assays conforming to DCCT standards, non-diabetic HbA$_{1c}$ ranges from 3.5 to 5.5 per cent of total HbA, with 'good' control defined as less than 7 per cent and 'poor' control as more than 8 per cent; some poorly compliant patients have HbA$_{1c}$ concentrations of 14 to 16 per cent. HbA$_{1c}$ measurements are a useful index of medium-term glycaemic control, but may be invalidated by abnormal red cell turnover (values are spuriously low in haemolysis, bleeding, and pregnancy), in renal failure (carbamylated HbA coelutes with HbA$_{1c}$, falsely raising levels), and with abnormal haemoglobins (HbF also comigrates with HbA$_1$).

Serum albumin also undergoes glycation, which is measured by the fructosamine reaction. As albumin turns over faster than haemoglobin, the fructosamine concentration reflects mean blood glucose over the previous 1 to 2 weeks. Assays are cheap but not standardized between laboratories, and are generally less reliable and reproducible than measurements of HbA$_{1c}$.

Measurements of urinary glucose and ketones

Urinary glucose concentrations can be measured easily using glucose oxidase test strips, but are of limited use: urinary glucose concentration depends on the renal threshold (which can lie between 7 and 13 mmol/l), urine output, and the time since the bladder was last emptied. Crucially, hypoglycaemia cannot be detected. Urinary glucose measurements are acceptable in type 2 diabetic patients with a normal renal threshold who are not receiving hypoglycaemic medication (insulin or sulphonylureas) and in patients who decline to prick their fingers.

Urinary ketone measurements can be useful for predicting impending ketoacidosis, particularly during intercurrent illness when blood glucose is high. Moderate ketonuria can be caused by fasting or undereating, including during infections.

Structures for diabetes care

Diabetes is best managed by the combined efforts of a team of specialists with complementary and overlapping skills: physician, specialist diabetes nurse, dietician, and chiropodist. The specialist diabetes nurse has a crucial role in educating patients about diabetes and its practical management, and in starting and adjusting therapy. Many patients are more receptive and responsive to information given by specialist nurses than by doctors. There must be frequent contact with and easy access to other specialists (ophthalmologist, vascular surgeon, renal physican, obstetrician, and clinical psychologist), ideally in the setting of combined clinics. Each member of the team has a particular niche but all must agree common strategies (such as dietary advice for obesity) to avoid giving the patients conflicting or inconsistent information.

Diabetes care can be delivered effectively by hospital-based clinics, community 'miniclinics' run by well-informed general practitioners or practice nurses, or by 'shared care' schemes that involve both primary and secondary sectors. Because of the unpredictable course and potential complications of diabetes, all patients must be thoroughly reviewed each year and be rapidly referred for specialist help if the need arises.

A check list for the annual review is suggested in Table 5.

Diabetes education

Living and coping with diabetes is a considerable burden that is poorly appreciated by many doctors and nurses. Careful education about diabetes, its complications, and its practical management can provide great reassurance to patients and also reduce emergency hospital admissions and complications such as foot ulceration and amputation.

Diabetes education is most effectively provided by the specialist diabetes nurse, but all members of the diabetes care team should understand the key messages, and check and reinforce these whenever possible. These include:

• Causes of hyperglycaemia and diabetic symptoms.

- Own treatment: diet and lifestyle; drawing up and injecting insulin; oral agents; recognizing and treating hypoglycaemia.
- Self-monitoring technique; targets and danger levels; how to respond to poor control.
- 'Sick-day' rules: monitoring during intercurrent illness; how to adjust own treatment; when and how to call for help (see Table 6).

Employment, driving, and insurance

Because of the risk of hypoglycaemia, patients treated with insulin (type 1 or 2) are barred from active service in the police, fire service, or armed forces and from driving heavy-goods or public service vehicles. Specific diabetic complications, notably sight-threatening retinopathy, may preclude particular jobs or pastimes.

Patients must inform the driving licence authorities and their driving insurer that they are diabetic, and those receiving insulin or with clinically significant retinopathy may require periodic medical confirmation of fitness to drive. Frequent hypoglycaemia, especially with decreased awareness of symptoms, is a bar to driving.

Special life insurance policies are available from companies endorsed by patient-centred organizations such as Diabetes UK and the American Diabetes Association. Many patients find it valuable to join these organizations.

Intercurrent events in diabetes and their management

Infections

Diabetic patients probably have increased susceptibility to pyogenic bacterial infections, especially when diabetes is poorly controlled. Hyperglycaemia can impair the killing of micro-organisms by neutrophils and macrophages and may also interfere with the function of T lymphocytes. Some infections particularly associated with diabetes include:

- Tuberculosis, often widespread and cavitating.

Table 5 Routine annual review of a diabetic patient: key points include those specific to patients taking insulin.

	History and discussion	Examination	Investigations
Diabetic treatment	Diet, physical activity Weight and change Glucose-lowering drugs	Weight, height, BMI Waist–hip ratio Insulin injection sites	
Diabetic control	Self-monitoring results (± check technique) Hyperglycaemic symptoms Hypoglycaemia and awareness of symptoms		HbA_{1c} Liver function tests (if taking thiazolidinedione or metformin)
Diabetes education and skills (± family or associates)	General knowledge Treatment targets 'Sick day' rules Hypoglycaemia treatment Insulin injection technique		
Diabetic complications: Macrovascular	Ischaemic heart disease (angina, MI, failure, arrhythmias) Peripheral vascular disease (claudication, stroke, TIA) Smoking history Other risk factors (hypertension, dyslipidaemia, family history)	Examine heart, including signs of failure. Blood pressure, lying and standing Peripheral pulses, strength and bruits	Fasting lipid screen (total, HDL and LDL cholesterol; triglycerides). ECG (if other risk factors or age > 40)
Eyes (retinopathy and cataract)	Altered activity, loss of vision	Visual activity (± corrected). Fundoscopy (dilate pupils)	
Nephropathy			Blood electrolytes, urea, creatinine. Microalbumia screen (e.g. albumin:creatinine ratio) or timed urinary albumin excretion
Neuropathy	Altered or reduced sensation Pain Weakness in limbs Autonomic symptoms (sweating, postural dizziness, gastrointestinal)	Sensory testing screen as appropriate (feet: see below) Postural blood pressure drop	
Feet	Pain, numbness Ulceration: current and previous Footwear (sensible?) Foot care	General condition: posture, callus Pulses and perfusion Oedema Sensory deficits (light touch, pin prick, monofilament)	
Sexual function	Erectile and ejaculatory problems (men)		
Other illnesses	Other medication (possible effects on glycaemic control and interactions with antidiabetic drugs)		

Abbreviations: BMI, body mass index; MI, myocardial infarction; HDL, high-density lipoprotein; LDL, low-density lipoprotein; TIA, transient ischaemic attack.

Table 6 'Sick day' rules for patients with type 1 diabetes

If you feel unwell, and even if you think it's a minor infection:

- NEVER stop taking your insulin—you often need more when you're unwell
- Check your blood glucose every 4 h—glucose levels can rise very fast during infections
- Test your urine for ketones each time you pass some—ketones are an important warning sign
- Contact your doctor at once if you
    - start vomiting
    - get high glucose levels (over 15) that don't come down after insulin
    - get hypos (glucose under 3)
    - get ketones in the urine
    - are worried and don't know what to do

- Necrotizing fasciitis, rapidly spreading necrosis of subcutaneous tissues down to muscle, usually due to β-haemolytic streptocci with staphylococci and often anaerobes.

- Gas-forming infections with anaerobes and clostridia, including 'emphysematous' pyelonephritis, cholecystitis, cystitis, and foot infections. Plain radiography shows gas in the affected tissues.

- Diabetic foot ulcers (see below) are often infected, with the risk of osteomyelitis and deep soft-tissue spread.

- Urinary tract infections may be complicated by ascending infections with pyelonephritis and renal or perinephric abscess (sometimes with gas), and occasionally acute papillary necrosis. Severe loin pain and systemic symptoms, with deteriorating renal function, should suggest these possibilities and the need for urgent imaging.

- 'Malignant' or necrotizing otitis externa, due to pseudomonas infection, can invade the skull and facial nerve.

- Periodontal infections, sometimes causing tooth loss, are common.

- Rhinocerebral mucormycosis is a highly invasive fungal infection that originates in the sinuses but often spreads into the orbit and cranial cavity. Mortality is about 50 per cent, even with debridement and high-dose intravenous amphotericin B.

The bacterial infections often require aggressive intravenous antibiotic treatment with cover against anaerobes. Fastidious and rare organisms should be considered when standard antibiotic regimens are ineffective.

Diabetic control during infections

Minor viral infections rarely disturb diabetic control, but increased secretion of counter-regulatory stress hormones during severe infections, especially with fever, can rapidly worsen insulin resistance in both type 1 and 2 diabetes.

Type 1 patients may need twice as much insulin as usual, even if they are unable to eat. Failure to increase the insulin dosage will therefore allow glucose to rise, sometimes dramatically fast, and risk precipitating ketoacidosis. It is therefore essential to continue taking insulin, to monitor blood glucose frequently, and to increase insulin if sustained hyperglycaemia develops. A rise of 30 to 50 per cent in long-acting insulin is often enough, but requirements will be determined by blood glucose levels and should be decided in consultation with the diabetes care team. Avoidable deaths still occur every year because poorly educated patients (sometimes advised by ignorant doctors) reduce or even stop taking insulin because they feel ill, are not eating, and are worried about becoming hypoglycaemic. Clear 'sick-day' rules (Table 6) are a crucial part of diabetes education, which must be regularly checked and reinforced.

During severe infections, insulin needs may fluctuate rapidly and the safest way to give insulin is by continuous intravenous infusion, backed up by frequent (hourly) blood glucose measurements (see below).

Type 2 patients may similarly lose glycaemic control, and are often best transferred temporarily to subcutaneous or intravenous insulin.

Although not firmly evidence-based, it would seem best to maintain blood glucose between 5 and 10 mmol/l during intercurrent infections.

Myocardial infarction

This is discussed in detail later.

Surgery

Surgery can be hazardous to diabetic patients: the counter-regulatory stress response to surgical trauma can rapidly lead to hyperglycaemia and ketoacidosis, especially in insulin-deficient patients, while poorly controlled diabetes accelerates catabolism and delays wound healing. Moreover, insulin and the sulphonylureas can cause severe hypoglycaemia in fasted or anorexic patients, which can be particularly dangerous during general anaesthesia.

Glycaemic control must therefore be meticulous throughout the preoperative period. A routine management policy should be agreed between the diabetes care team, surgeons, anaesthetists, and ward staff, and this will greatly reduce the risks of operating on diabetic people. Fitness for surgery should be carefully assessed, in view of cardiovascular or other complications. Patients may need to be admitted some days before operation to optimize their treatment.

For type 2 patients who are well controlled by diet or oral agents and undergoing minor surgery only, long-acting sulphonylureas (glibenclamide) should be changed to short-acting ones (for example gliclazide) some days before surgery to reduce the risk of hypoglycaemia. Oral agents and breakfast should be omitted on the morning of operation and blood glucose should be monitored closely. Persistent hyperglycaemia should be treated with the intravenous glucose–potassium–insulin regimen described below.

For all other diabetic patients, subcutaneous insulin should be stopped on the morning of surgery, and a continuous intravenous infusion of balanced amounts of glucose, potassium, and insulin should be given (Table 7). If the patient is in steady state, the glucose–potassium–insulin (GKI) infusion will both maintain satisfactory glycaemic control (5–10 mmol/l) and prevent hypokalaemia. This regimen should be started on the morning of surgery and continued until the patient is able to eat and drink normally, when the usual treatment can be resumed. GKI bags must be changed if glucose levels are unsatisfactory. Alternatively, insulin may be

Table 7 The glucose–potassium–insulin infusion regime

Infusion (standard recipe)

500 ml of 10 per cent dextrose plus
15 U soluble insulin (e.g. Actrapid) plus
10 mmol KCl

Instructions

Infuse at 100 ml/h

Check blood glucose every hour

If blood glucose deviates outside target range of 5–10 mmol/l, then take down the bag and replace it as follows:

- if blood glucose < 5 mmol/l, put 10 U insulin in new bag with 10 mmol KCl
- if blood glucose > 10 mmol/l, put 20 U insulin in new bag with 10 mmol KCl

(Lower or higher insulin dosages are occasionally needed)

Check plasma K^+ every 6 h and adjust accordingly

Indications and contraindications

Indications: temporary measure for diabetic patients in steady state, i.e. not eating and no other antidiabetic medication

Contraindications: not for treatment of severe hyperglycaemia or ketoacidosis given as a variable-rate intravenous infusion, which provides greater flexibility.

Acute metabolic complications of diabetes and their treatment

Diabetic ketoacidosis

This is uncontrolled hyperglycaemia with hyperketonaemia severe enough to cause metabolic acidosis. It remains a major cause of death in patients with type 1 diabetes under 20 years of age, and episodes still carry an overall mortality of 5 to 10 per cent (50 per cent in elderly patients with diabetic ketoacidosis precipitated by infection or myocardial infarction). Prompt diagnosis and careful management can prevent many deaths.

Causes

Diabetic ketoacidosis only develops when severe insulin deficiency, compounded by an excess of glucagon, stimulates lipolysis and a massive increase in ketogenesis (see above). It therefore almost always occurs in untreated or poorly treated type 1 diabetes and is generally regarded as the hallmark of that disease. However, diabetic ketoacidosis can occur in subjects with type 2 diabetes who are relatively insulin deficient, especially when the secretion of counter-regulatory hormones (especially glucagon) is increased by severe intercurrent illness. Precipitating factors include:

- Newly presenting type 1 diabetes.
- Omission or underdosing of insulin by established type 1 diabetic patients, which may be deliberate in patients with disturbances of body image.
- Intercurrent illness, such as infections, myocardial infarction, stroke, trauma, surgery, and burns. Many patients (and their doctors) fail to increase insulin dosages or monitor blood glucose during such events.

About 30 to 40 per cent of episodes are unexplained; omitted or inadequate insulin treatment should always be suspected if no obvious infective or other cause is found.

Pathophysiology

Diabetic ketoacidosis is due to the accumulation of ketones, i.e. acetoacetate and its derivatives, 3-hydroxybutyrate (or β-hydroxybutyrate) and acetone (Fig. 8). They are generated by β oxidation of free fatty acids within the mitochondria of the liver. Free fatty acids enter the cytoplasm of hepatocytes and combine with coenzyme A (**CoA**) to form their fatty acyl-CoA

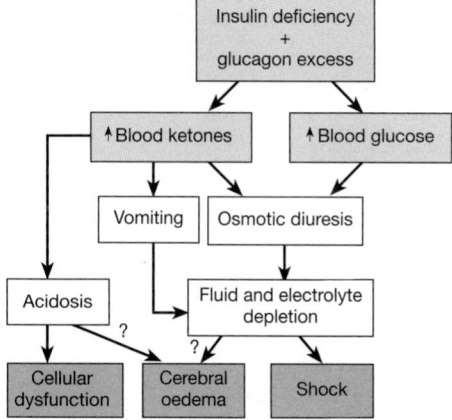

Fig. 8 Pathophysiological changes in diabetic ketoacidosis. Cellular dysfunction induced by intracellular acidosis, cerebral oedema, and shock are potentially life-threatening.

derivatives. These are then transported into the mitochondria by the 'carnitine shuttle', a complex of two linked enzymes, carnitine palmitoyl transferase I (CPT-I) on the outer mitochondrial membrane and carnitine palmitoyl transferase II (CPT-II) on the inner. CPT-I, and the overall activity of the shuttle, is powerfully inhibited by insulin and stimulated by glucagon. Once inside the mitochondria, free fatty acids undergo β oxidation to yield ATP (oxidative phosphorylation) and acetyl-CoA. The latter is converted to acetoacetate, which may be oxidized to 3-hydroxybutyrate or undergo condensation to produce acetone.

Ketones are transported out of the liver and are used as metabolic fuels by various tissues including the brain; they supply a few per cent of total energy needs after an overnight fast, but the proportion rises to over one-third during prolonged fasting. When produced in excess, they can accumulate rapidly, especially if plasma levels exceed 10 mmol/l (about 50 times normal), when tissue uptake mechanisms become saturated. Ketogenesis is greatly enhanced in uncontrolled type 1 diabetes because of the combination of low insulin with increased glucagon concentrations: lipolysis is unrestrained, and the uptake into liver mitochondria of the increased amounts of fatty acyl-CoA is stimulated by the synergistic effects on CPT-I of high glucagon and low insulin. The main consequences of raised circulating ketone levels are shown in Fig. 8 and listed below:

- Acidosis. Acetoacetate and 3-hydroxybutyrate are both moderately strong organic acids and lower the extracellular pH when the buffering capacity of plasma proteins is exceeded. Ion exchange across cell membranes leads to intracellular acidosis which compromises cellular metabolism because many crucial enzymes operate within a narrow pH range. Clinical measurements of acid–base status are confined to extracellular fluid and may underestimate the severity of intracellular acidosis.
- Diuresis. Ketones are filtered in the urine and are osmotically active. They therefore exacerbate the osmotic diuresis caused by glycosuria and the resulting polyuria, electrolyte losses, dehydration, and hypovolaemia.
- Nausea, through direct stimulation of the chemoreceptor trigger zone in the medulla.

Clinical features

Diabetic ketoacidosis usually presents with classical hyperglycaemic symptoms (Table 2), together with features of acidosis and hyperketonaemia:

- Acidotic (Kussmaul) breathing is deep, sighing hyperventilation which has been mistaken for panic attacks, pulmonary embolism, and left ventricular failure.
- Nausea and vomiting are ominous signs, because dehydration develops quickly in polyuric patients unable to drink.
- Drowsiness and coma occur late and may indicate early cerebral oedema.

The patient generally looks ill and may show postural hypotension and other signs of dehydration and hypovolaemia. Acetone (nail varnish remover) is volatile and may be smelled on the breath. Some patients are hypothermic due to heat loss from peripheral vasodilation, and this may mask the pyrexia of infection. Children with diabetic ketoacidosis often complain of abdominal pain, sometimes mimicking acute appendicitis or other surgical emergencies. A full examination is essential to identify any intercurrent illness.

Investigations and diagnosis

Once suspected, the diagnosis can be confirmed on the spot with a finger-prick blood glucose measurement and urinalysis for ketones. Treatment with intravenous saline and insulin should begin immediately, and baseline investigations carried out. Venous blood is taken for biochemical screening and arterial blood for pH and acid–base status. Additional tests to identify the cause of the episode should include a full blood count, urine and blood

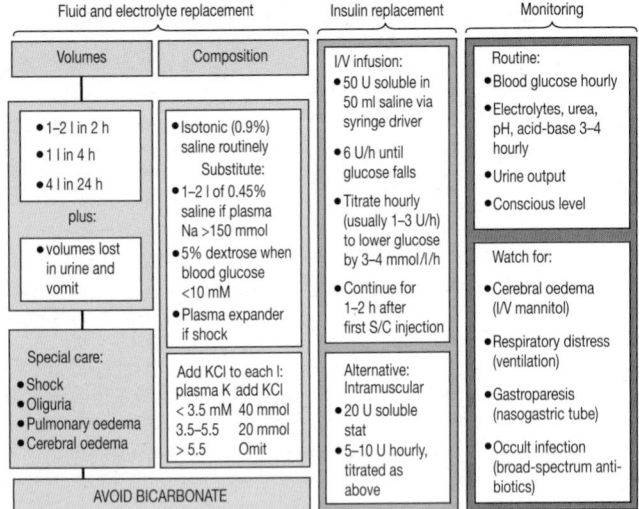

Fig. 9 Guidelines for the management of diabetic ketoacidosis.

culture, chest radiograph, and, especially in older patients, ECG and cardiac enzymes or troponin levels.

Typical values and some diagnostic pitfalls in diabetic ketoacidosis are shown in Fig. 9. Plasma ketone levels are measured by some laboratories but are not usually needed for safe management. High ketone concentrations cause a large anion gap: i.e. plasma [Na$^+$ + K$^+$] exceeds [HCO$_3^-$ + Cl$^-$] by more than 17 mmol/l.

Management

Diabetic ketoacidosis is a potentially life-threatening medical emergency that requires urgent treatment with scrupulous clinical and biochemical monitoring: many avoidable disasters still happen because the patient is abandoned once treatment has been started. Severe diabetic ketoacidosis is best managed initially on a high-dependency or intensive care unit.

The highest priority is to correct hypovolaemia and dehydration, which will often improve acidosis and hyperglycaemia. Insulin replacement must also be started urgently. However, it now appears likely that the high mortality of diabetic ketoacidosis has been partly due to overenergetic replacement of intravenous fluids (especially bicarbonate) and perhaps insulin, which may predispose to the development of cerebral oedema. The treatment guidelines below (Fig. 9) are based on large studies that have reported very low mortality and morbidity.

Fluid replacement

Good intravenous access is crucial: a large peripheral vein may be used but a central venous cannula is safest for severely hypovolaemic patients and for the elderly or those at risk of heart failure, in whom monitoring of central venous pressure is essential.

Most patients recover rapidly with slower fluid replacement than was previously recommended. For those who are not shocked give:

- 1 to 2 litres in 2 h, then
- 1 litre over the next 4 h, then
- 4 litres over the next 24 h.

Fluid losses in urine or vomit should be added to these volumes. Shocked or oliguric patients may require faster fluid repletion, possibly with plasma expanders rather than saline, while slower replacement is safer in those with signs of fluid overload, heart failure, or any suspicion of cerebral oedema. Urine output must be monitored closely, as must blood pressure, central venous filling, and signs of pulmonary or peripheral oedema.

Saline containing potassium is the logical fluid to replace the losses of Na$^+$, K$^+$, and Cl$^-$ induced by the osmotic diuresis of diabetic ketoacidosis.

The use of intravenous bicarbonate to try to correct acidosis is contentious, both biochemically and in terms of clinical outcome (see below).

Isotonic (0.9 per cent) saline is used initially. Half-isotonic (0.45 per cent) saline has been suggested to replace 1 or 2 litres of isotonic saline, if severe hyperosmolarity (> 350 mosmol/kg) and/or hypernatraemia (> 150 mmol/l) are present. However, the rationale may be flawed: 0.9 per cent ('normal') saline is already hypotonic with respect to the patient's hypertonic plasma, and the use of even more hypotonic solutions would seem likely to exacerbate the intracellular movement of water which may lead to cerebral oedema. Five per cent dextrose is generally substituted when plasma glucose has fallen to 10 to 14 mmol/l to prevent hypoglycaemia (insulin is still required to prevent ketogenesis and promote glucose utilization in the tissues).

Intravenous sodium bicarbonate was previously recommended for severe acidosis. However, the hope that adding alkali will correct acidosis may be oversimplistic. HCO$_3^-$ and H$^+$ ions (from 3-hydroxybutyric and acetoacetic acids) combine extracellularly to produce H$_2$CO$_3$, which dissociates to produce water and CO$_2$; this may reduce extracellular acidosis, but as cell membranes are impermeable to HCO$_3^-$ ions, the all-important intracellular acidosis is not improved. Indeed, CO$_2$ can enter cells where it can combine with water to produce H$_2$CO$_3$, itself a weak organic acid that can dissociate into H$^+$ and HCO$_3^-$ ions. Paradoxically, therefore, intravenous bicarbonate administration could worsen intracellular acidosis and there is evidence from animal models of acidosis that this occurs. Worryingly, a recent study identified bicarbonate administration as the most important independent predictor of cerebral oedema in children with moderately severe diabetic ketoacidosis. Another problem with high-strength (8.4 per cent) sodium bicarbonate solution is the intense thrombophlebitis it causes when given intravenously, which can obliterate even large central veins.

The current consensus is that bicarbonate is unlikely to do good but runs the risk of doing harm, and that it should not be used in the treatment of diabetic ketoacidosis

Potassium replacement

Diabetic ketoacidosis always depletes total body K$^+$ stores to a variable degree because of electrolyte losses through osmotic diuresis, but H$^+$/K$^+$ exchange across the plasma membrane encourages K$^+$ to leak out of cells in acidosis. Plasma K$^+$ levels can therefore be low, normal, or high, and dangerous hyperkalaemia can be present, especially if severe hypovolaemia causes prerenal failure. During insulin replacement, K$^+$ is carried intracellularly with glucose, and plasma K$^+$ levels can fall rapidly. Frequent monitoring of K$^+$ (every 3 to 4 h initially) is therefore essential in the safe management of diabetic ketoacidosis, and patients with marked K$^+$ disturbances should have continuous ECG monitoring.

Potassium replacement should be determined by current plasma K$^+$ levels:

- Add 20 mmol of KCl to each litre of intravenous fluid if K$^+$ is normal (3.5–5.0 mmol/l).

- Add 40 mmol/l of KCl to each litre if plasma K$^+$ is less than 3.5 mmol/l.

- Omit KCl if plasma K$^+$ is more than 5.0 mmol/l, because of the risk of precipitating arrhythmias.

Insulin replacement

Continuous intravenous infusion is the best way to give insulin in diabetic ketoacidosis; subcutaneous and intramuscular absorption are too erratic to be safe and the rate of fall of glucose (one of the factors implicated in cerebral oedema) cannot be easily controlled.

50 U soluble insulin (for example Actrapid or Humulin S) should be added to 50 ml isotonic saline (i.e. 1 U/ml) and delivered by a syringe driver pump, either into a separate vein or piggy-backed into the intravenous fluids line.

Because the half-life of insulin in the circulation is only a few minutes, blood glucose and ketone levels will rise rapidly if insulin delivery is interrupted; hourly monitoring of blood glucose is therefore mandatory during intravenous insulin. Failure of glucose to fall usually means that the pump has been turned off or that the infusion cannula is blocked. Initially, 6 U/h (i.e. 6 ml/h) should be given and once blood glucose has started to fall, the rate can then be titrated so that glucose falls by 3 to 4 mmol/l every hour. Faster rates of fall are unnecessary, commonly cause hypoglycaemia, and are thought to predispose to cerebral oedema. Most patients need 1 to 3 U of insulin per hour, and the requirement will become clear after 3 to 4 h of blood glucose monitoring.

A typical intravenous sliding scale (based on hourly glucose measurements) is:

- blood glucose less than 5 mmol/l: give 0.5U/h

- blood glucose 5 to 10 mmol/l: give 2 ml/h

- blood glucose more than 10 mmol: give 4 ml/h.

An alternative to the syringe driver is to dilute insulin into a larger volume (50 U soluble insulin into 500 ml of saline; 0.1 U/ml) and to regulate delivery (for example 20 ml/h (2 U/h)) using an electronic drip counter or a paediatric giving-set with a burette.

The GKI infusion used for perioperative management of diabetic patients is not appropriate because it assumes that the patient is in steady state (which is not the case) and because K^+ disturbances may be exacerbated; moreover, making up and changing GKI infusion bags is time-consuming and very rarely done as often as is needed to control the fall in glucose.

If it is impossible to give a controlled intravenous infusion, then intramuscular soluble insulin can be injected every 4 h or so, starting with 20 U and attempting to titrate subsequent dosages (for example 5–10 U hourly).

Other complications

Intercurrent illness must be treated energetically. Broad-spectrum antibiotics are often given prospectively. Myocardial infarction (see below) has a poor prognosis if it causes diabetic ketoacidosis.

Shock may lead to prerenal failure and sometimes acute tubular necrosis. Plasma expanders and inotropes may occasionally be required for severe hypotension, although rehydration as above is usually adequate.

Cerebral oedema still accounts for 50 per cent of fatalities in diabetic ketoacidosis, especially in children, although modern management protocols with slower fluid replacement and low-dose intravenous insulin infusion can markedly reduce its incidence. The cause is thought to be shifts of ions and water into the brain, particularly the movement of water into dehydrated, hypertonic cells when relatively hypotonic fluids reach the extracellular space. Such shifts would be predicted with isotonic and particularly with hypotonic fluids. Risk factors for cerebral oedema include over-rapid falls in blood glucose, excessive fluid replacement, and high insulin dosages. Insulin can affect various ion transport mechanisms in the brain, but its role remains mysterious and may simply reflect changes in extracellular osmolarity. Interestingly, CT scanning before fluid and insulin replacement has demonstrated subclinical cerebral oedema in children with diabetic ketoacidosis.

Swelling of the brain within the cranium causes coning, leading to cardiorespiratory arrest. It presents as a decline in consciousness, usually rapid and often when the patient's metabolic state has been stabilized. Papilloedema may be present, and CT or MR scanning will show characteristic swelling, with loss of cortical features and squashing of the ventricular system (Fig. 10). It is usually fatal (in more than 90 per cent of established cases), but intravenous mannitol (0.2 g/kg over 30 min, repeated hourly if there is no improvement) may help by raising the osmolality of extracellular fluid and drawing free water out of the brain; there is no firm evidence to support the use of dexamethasone.

Adult respiratory distress syndrome is due to accumulation of fluid in the alveoli, perhaps due to ionic and water shifts or to excessive leakiness of the pulmonary capillaries. Hypoxia is severe, and chest radiography shows an appearance like left ventricular failure but with a normal heart size. Risk factors include rapid fluid replacement. It carries a poor prognosis, but ventilation with high-concentration oxygen may be useful supportive treatment.

Acute gastric dilatation (gastroparesis) presents with vomiting and may show a succussion splash and a ground-glass appearance on abdominal radiograph. Nasogastric drainage may be needed to prevent aspiration, especially in the unconscious patient.

Hypothermia indicates a poor outcome. It may respond to rewarming with a space blanket.

Subsequent management

When the patient can eat and drink, intravenous fluids and insulin can be discontinued. There is no need for a GKI regimen; instead, the patient can be restarted on their usual insulin regimen (or on twice daily long-lasting insulin, if newly diagnosed). The intravenous insulin infusion should be maintained until the first injection has had time to act (3–4 h for long-acting insulin alone).

The causes of the episode must be determined if possible, and efforts made to prevent it from happening again. The patient's understanding of diabetes, including the 'sick-day' rules (Table 6), must be checked and reinforced if necessary. Recurrent diabetic ketoacidosis is a feature of brittle diabetes, and these patients need careful monitoring and counselling.

Hyperosmolar non-ketotic state (HONK)

Hyperosmolar non-ketotic state is distinguished from diabetic ketoacidosis by the absence of gross hyperketonaemia and metabolic acidosis. Hyperglycaemia can be greater than in diabetic ketoacidosis and, together with a rise in urea due to dehydration and prerenal failure, may elevate the plasma osmolality to well over 350 mosmol/kg.

Ketosis does not develop because circulating insulin levels are high enough to suppress lipolysis and ketogenesis; these patients are therefore C-peptide positive, with type 2 diabetes which is often previously undiagnosed. It is more common in people of Afro-Caribbean origin. Precipitating factors include myocardial infarction, stroke, infection, and diabetogenic drugs such as glucocorticoids and thiazide diuretics; fizzy glucose drinks may also contribute.

Presentation is typically with classical hyperglycaemic symptoms (polyuria, intense thirst, weight loss, blurred vision), without the features of ketoacidosis. Confusion, drowsiness, and coma are commoner than in diabetic ketoacidosis.

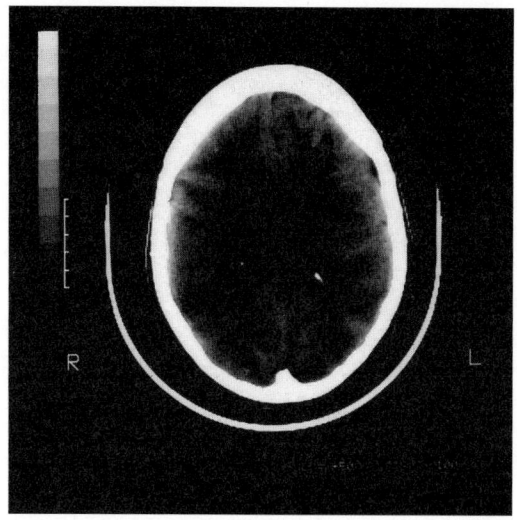

Fig. 10 Cerebral oedema in a patient recovering from diabetic ketoacidosis. The CT scan shows generalized swelling and loss of cortical detail with squashing of the cerebral ventricles.

Complications include thrombotic events such as stroke and peripheral arterial occlusion, and deep venous thrombosis and pulmonary embolism, these being due to increased blood viscosity. Mortality exceeds 30 per cent because these patients are old and often have a serious precipitating illness.

Biochemical features of hyperosmolar non-ketotic state are:

- Hyperglycaemia: often over 50 mmol/l, sometimes over 90 mmol/l.
- Hypernatraemia: often over 155 mmol/l (may be artefactually depressed by high glucose levels).
- Uraemia due to dehydration, with or without renal failure.
- Hypersmolality: over 350 mosmol/kg.
- Blood and ketone levels are normal or only slightly raised (usually through anorexia).
- Arterial pH, venous bicarbonate, and anion gap show no features of severe acidosis.

Management is largely as for diabetic ketoacidosis:

- Saline replacement must be particularly cautious in older patients, in whom cardiac disease is common. Half-isotonic (0.45 per cent) solution is often given if plasma sodium exceeds 150 mmol/l or osmolality exceeds 350 mosmol/kg; the rationale for preferring this to isotonic saline is not proven, but the risks of cerebral oedema appear to be lower than in diabetic ketoacidosis.
- Potassium levels must be carefully monitored and replaced as above.
- Intravenous insulin infusion at low doses rapidly controls hyperglycaemia in most cases.
4. Low-dose heparin (5000 U subcutaneously 8-hourly) should be given prophylactically, but full anticoagulation should be reserved for proven thromboembolism as the risks of fatal gastrointestinal bleeding are high. Intercurrent illness must be sought and treated appropriately.

After recovery, many of these patients can be successfully weaned off insulin. Drugs and other precipitating factors must be identified and avoided if possible.

Lactic acidosis

Lactate is generated by glycolysis and its levels rise rapidly during tissue anoxia (for example during shock, cardiac failure, or pneumonia) or when the liver is prevented from utilizing it as a gluconeogenic substrate (for example in hepatic impairment). Lactic acidosis is best known in diabetic patients as a rare but often fatal complication of the biguanides, phenformin and metformin, which act mainly by inhibiting hepatic gluconeogenesis. The risk is about 10 times higher with phenformin than with metformin, and it is very rare during metformin treatment as long as other predisposing factors (the major organ failures) are avoided.

Lactic acidosis presents as coma with metabolic acidosis (reduced arterial pH and venous bicarbonate) and a wide amino gap due to hyperlactataemia. Blood glucose levels are usually raised.

Treatment is still unsatisfactory. Intravenous sodium bicarbonate may paradoxically aggravate intracellular acidosis, although forced ventilation to blow off carbon dioxide may help (see above). Haemodialysis may both clear lactate and hydrogen ions, and correct any sodium overload following bicarbonate administration. Sodium dichloroacetate, which stimulates pyruvate dehydrogenase to metabolize lactate, is undergoing evaluation.

Mortality remains high (over 30 per cent), partly because of the organ failures that commonly coexist.

Hypoglycaemia

Hypoglycaemia is an inevitable side-effect of antidiabetic drugs that raise circulating insulin levels, namely insulin itself and sulphonylureas; it does not occur with metformin or thiazolidinediones alone, or with dietary restriction. Common contributory factors are:

- Accelerated insulin absorption, for example due to exercise or hot surroundings.
- Unfavourable timing of insulin injection: injecting too soon before eating can cause late postprandial hypoglycaemia, while long-acting insulins injected in the early evening often cause nocturnal hypoglycaemia.
- Too much insulin injected: dosage errors are quite common, particularly in the elderly.
- Inadequate food intake: missed, delayed, or small meals; vomiting, including gastroparesis.
- Exercise hastens insulin absorption while enhancing insulin action; delayed hypoglycaemia may occur many hours later because muscle continues to take up glucose to replenish glycogen.
- Alcohol inhibits hepatic gluconeogenesis, preventing the increase in hepatic glucose output that is crucial for restoring euglycaemia.
- Impaired awareness of early warning symptoms (see below).

Progressively more frequent or severe attacks may be caused by various conditions, which should always be sought:

- Weight loss, including anorexia nervosa and appetite disorders (relatively common in young women with type 1 diabetes).
- Loss of counter-regulatory hormones: Addison's disease, hypothyroidism, hypopituitarism, blunted glucagon secretion in long-standing type 1 diabetes.
- Intestinal malabsorption, notably coeliac disease (commoner in type 1 diabetes).
- Renal failure, which impairs the clearance of insulin.
- Deliberate inappropriate injection of insulin, often in the context of 'brittle' diabetes.

Manifestations

Clinical features of hypoglycaemia are due to an autonomic discharge, predominantly sympathetic, together with the cerebral effects of neuroglycopenia. Falling glucose levels are sensed by glucose-sensitive neurones, which are found in the periphery (vagal sensory endings in the portal vein) and medulla as well as the hypothalamus. This triggers a powerful sympathetic discharge that releases adrenaline from the adrenal medulla and noradrenaline from sympathetic nerve endings, causing the familiar 'flight or fight' response. Features include pallor (cutaneous vasoconstriction), sweating, tremor (a β_2-adrenergic effect on skeletal muscle) and tachycardia; systolic blood pressure rises due to increased cardiac output while pulse pressure widens—giving the typical bounding pulse—because β_2-mediated vasodilatation in skeletal muscle causes peripheral resistance to fall.

Hypoglycaemia also triggers the secretion of counter-regulatory hormones, namely glucagon and adrenaline (both crucial to restoring euglycaemia), growth hormone, and cortisol. Collectively, these inhibit insulin secretion and raise blood glucose by enhancing hepatic glycogenolysis and gluconeogenesis, causing glucose to pour out of the liver. Defects in glucagon or adrenaline release (which occur for example in long-standing type 1 diabetes), or in the ability of the liver to produce glucose (for example the presence of ethanol which inhibits gluconeogenesis, or a recent glucagon injection which depletes liver glycogen) will delay recovery of blood glucose.

The physiological and neurological features of hypoglycaemia usually develop in a fixed sequence when blood glucose is lowered in a controlled fashion in the laboratory. However, this hierarchy may not be apparent in real life, and some patients specifically lose their awareness of the early warning symptoms (see below). Key events as glucose falls are:

- ~3.8 mmol/l: increased glucagon and adrenaline secretion
- ~3.0 mmol/l: onset of hypoglycaemic symptoms
- ~2.8 mmol/l: neuroglycopenia and cognitive impairment

- at less than 1.0 mmol/l: coma.

Symptoms of hypoglycaemia

The symptom complex can be extremely variable, and hypoglycaemia should be suspected as the cause of any 'funny turn' in patients treated with insulin or sulphonylureas. Autonomic manifestations include sweating, tremor, tachycardia, and hunger, while neuroglycopenia can cause drowsiness, confusion, inco-ordination, dysarthria, and automatic or disinhibited behaviour; distinct neurological deficits include aphasia, diplopia, and hemiparesis. Non-specific malaise and headache afterwards are also common. Nocturnal episodes may pass completely unnoticed by the patient, or may cause sweating and restlessness (often obvious to the patient's partner), vivid nightmares, or a hung-over feeling the following morning.

Awareness of hypoglycaemic symptoms

Diabetic patients rely on the early autonomic symptoms (sweating, shaking, and hunger) to warn them of an impending hypoglycaemic attack, when corrective action can be taken. In some patients the early warning symptoms are attenuated or not noticed at all; this clumsily named 'hypoglycaemia unawareness' is potentially dangerous because severe neuroglycopenia (confusion, fitting, irrational behaviour, coma) may suddenly incapacitate the patient. Reduced awareness of hypoglycaemia occurs particularly in two settings, which may coexist:

- Long-standing type 1 diabetes. Some 30 to 50 per cent of patients with diabetes of more than 20 years' duration have decreased awareness of symptoms, and many also show a flat glucagon response to hypoglycaemia. Blunted recognition of hypoglycaemia by the central nervous system may be responsible.

- Excessively tight glycaemic control impairs awareness of hypoglycaemia; for unknown reasons, even a single episode can blunt perception of symptoms and counter-regulatory hormone responses for some days. Conversely, relaxing control and avoiding hypoglycaemia completely for several weeks can partially restore awareness of warning symptoms.

The use of human insulin has been suggested to impair awareness of hypoglycaemic symptoms. Human insulin is relatively lipophilic—hence its faster subcutaneous absorption—which could theoretically promote its entry into the brain. Insulin may act directly on the brain to affect various autonomic processes, but detailed comparisons of human and animal insulins, both in the laboratory and in real life, have not shown any species differences in counter-regulatory responses or the intensity of hypoglycaemic symptoms.

Sequelae of hypoglycaemia

Even the most dramatic neurological manifestations of acute hypoglycaemia—including aphasia, hemiparesis, fitting, and unconsciousness—usually resolve rapidly when blood glucose is normalized. Recovery from profound coma may take many hours or even days, and this is probably due to cerebral oedema. Patients who survive severe and prolonged hypoglycaemic coma may show permanent neurological damage, including memory loss, aphasia, and a vegetative state. There are concerns that repeated mild attacks, especially in children and perhaps particularly at night, can cause cumulative intellectual impairment, but this is not yet proven.

Severe hypoglycaemia has been implicated in precipitating myocardial infarction or stroke, particularly in the elderly; rises in blood pressure and increased coagulability of the blood following sympathetic stimulation may contribute. Like any convulsions, hypoglycaemic fits may cause injury, including limb and vertebral crush fractures.

Prolonged severe hypoglycaemia can be fatal and is one of the most common causes of death in young type 1 patients. Post-mortem studies show neuronal damage and necrosis in the hippocampus and cerebral cortex. Hypoglycaemia has been suspected as a cause of death in patients found unexpectedly dead in bed; arrhythmias may be responsible.

Diagnosis and detection of hypoglycaemia

Hypoglycaemia is easy to diagnose but is also easily missed; differential diagnoses include transient ischaemic attacks, psychosis, drunkenness, epilepsy, and migraine. Symptoms may be instantly recognizable to some patients, but may present atypically. If suspected, the blood glucose levels should be checked, taking care to avoid under-reading artefacts with reagent test strips. Urinalysis is obviously of no use—hence all patients receiving insulin or sulphonylureas must be able to check their blood glucose. The patient's close associates should also know how to diagnose and treat hypoglycaemia.

Various experimental hypoglycaemia detectors are undergoing development, including measurements of subcutaneous glucose by implanted sensors or transcutaneous near-infrared spectroscopy, but none is yet suitable for routine clinical use.

Prevention and treatment of hypoglycaemia

Insulin-treated patients fear hypoglycaemia as much as blindness or renal failure, and this may prevent them from tightening their diabetic control as much as their doctors would prefer. Many doctors underestimate the impact of hypoglycaemia; asking about it and trying actively to prevent it are an essential part of diabetes care.

Attention to the factors listed above should help to reduce the frequency and severity of attacks. Advice about exercise, moderating alcohol intake, and timing of insulin injections and meals are particularly important. Nocturnal hypoglycaemia can be reduced by checking the blood glucose at bedtime, and by taking long-acting carbohydrate (for example bread or cereal) if the level is less than 6 mmol/l.

Blood glucose levels of less than 3 mmol/l should be treated immediately (Table 8). Oral glucose or sucrose or other carbohydrate should be given if the patient can swallow safely. Give 20 to 30 g (e.g. six Dextrosol tablets or 150 ml Lucozade) initially; if possible, check blood glucose 15 min later and repeat if the glucose has not risen. Taking too much carbohydrate—which is understandable, given the unpleasantness of hypoglycaemia—can cause marked rebound hyperglycaemia.

If the patient is unconscious, give either:

- Glucagon 1 mg (0.5 mg in children), subcutaneously or intramuscularly; with either route glucose should rise within 10 to 15 min. Side-effects of glucagon include malaise, nausea, and abdominal discomfort and, because it acts primarily by breaking down hepatic glycogen (a limited resource), a second injection may be ineffective.

Table 8 Management of hypoglycaemia

Immediate	
Patient conscious	Oral glucose (20–30 g) or sucrose
Patient unconscious	Intravenous glucose (30–50 ml of 50 per cent solution)
	or
	Intramuscular or subcutaneous glucagon (1 mg; 0.5 mg in children)*
Then	Check blood glucose after 15–20 min
	Confirm recovery (glucose > 5 mmol/l)
On recovery	Identify cause
	Re-educate patient to avoid future episodes
If recovery is delayed	
Patient unconscious	Set up infusion of 10 per cent dextrose; transfer to hospital
Patient conscious	Take more oral glucose

*Caution with glucagon: often causes nausea and malaise; depletes liver glycogen—a second injection may therefore be ineffective; contraindicated in hypoglycaemia caused by sulphonylureas (glucagon stimulates insulin secretion).

- Intravenous glucose: 15 to 20 g intravenously, as 50 per cent or 10 per cent solution (the former may cause painful thrombophlebitis, even if given into a large vein).

Glucose gels or jam can be smeared inside the mouth and cheeks in the unconscious patient, but these alone are unlikely to correct serious hypoglycaemia.

On recovery, blood glucose should be checked and oral glucose given as above. Slow recovery from coma may be due to cerebral oedema, which has a high mortality (around 10 per cent) but may respond to intravenous mannitol and forced ventilation with high inspired oxygen concentration.

Once the episode is treated, its cause must be identified if possible and corrective action taken to prevent it from happening again.

Chronic complications of diabetes

Long-term tissue damage is now the major burden of the disease, the greatest source of fear for diabetic people, and the most expensive item in the diabetes health-care budget. The list of complications is depressingly long but fortunately at least 40 per cent of diabetic patients escape clinically significant complications, and improved diabetes care should reduce the risks even further.

Microvascular complications—retinopathy, nephropathy, and neuropathy—are specific to diabetes and reflect damage inflicted on the microcirculation throughout the body. Retinopathy and nephropathy are obviously 'microvascular' disorders; the microcirculation of nerves (vasa nervorum) is also damaged in diabetic neuropathy, although other functional and structural abnormalities in the nerves themselves probably contribute. Macrovascular disease is simply atherosclerosis. This causes typical coronary heart disease, stroke, and peripheral arterial disease, but often behaves more aggressively than in non-diabetic people.

Other complications are due to irreversible biochemical and structural changes in tissues chronically exposed to hyperglycaemia. These include cataract, whose formation during normal ageing is accelerated by diabetes, and specific soft tissue disorders such as limited joint mobility (diabetic cheiroarthropathy).

Causes of chronic diabetic complications

Role of hyperglycaemia

Tissue lesions are identical in all types of diabetes, indicating that hyperglycaemia (or a closely related metabolic abnormality) is likely to be responsible. Microvascular disease in the retina, kidneys, and nerves is generally determined by the severity and duration of hyperglycaemia, although individual susceptibility varies considerably. By contrast, macrovascular disease does not display a clear dose–response relationship with hyperglycaemia: instead, the risk is increased above glucose values that lie below the 'diabetic' range (see above).

Recent intervention studies have confirmed that improving glycaemic control is rewarded by partial protection against microvascular complications but not atheroma. This principle is valid for both type 1 and type 2 diabetes, and is now embodied in their treatment targets (Table 3). Two 'landmark' studies are generally cited, although several smaller ones have also reached the same conclusion.

Type 1 diabetes

The Diabetic Control and Complications Trial (DCCT) was a 12-year North American study of over 1400 patients that compared 'intensive' insulin treatment (aiming for an HbA$_{1c}$ of 6 per cent) with 'conventional' (i.e. bad) regimens of once or twice daily injections (HbA$_{1c}$ about 9 per cent). Intensive treatment consisted of at least three daily injections or the insulin pump (continuous subcutaneous insulin infusion), and achieved a mean HbA$_{1c}$ of 7 per cent.

The DCCT concluded that improved glycaemic control reduced the risks of microvascular complications. In subjects who were initially free of complications, intensified treatment for 9 years decreased the prevalence of a defined degree of background retinopathy by 70 per cent (i.e. from 55 per cent with conventional treatment to 15 per cent), while the risks of developing microalbuminuria or clinical neuropathy fell by 33 per cent and 70 per cent respectively (Fig. 11). In subjects who already had background retinopathy at baseline, intensified treatment reduced the overall progression of retinopathy by 50 per cent; more importantly the risks of suffering sight-threatening retinopathy or requiring laser treatment were reduced by a similar degree. The development of clinical nephropathy (overt albuminuria) and neuropathy were each decreased by about 60 per cent. By contrast, intensified insulin treatment did not reduce the prevalence of macrovascular disease.

Type 2 diabetes

The United Kingdom Prospective Diabetes Study (UKPDS) was guided through its 20-year course by the late Robert Turner, who died shortly after it was completed. This huge trial followed the outcome of over 5000 patients treated with diet and lifestyle alone (termed 'conventional' treatment), or together with sulphonylureas, metformin or insulin; confusingly, sulphonylureas and insulin treatments were both described as 'intensive' treatment. The trial confirmed the real-life difficulty of achieving good glycaemic control, especially against the progressive deterioration of type 2 diabetes: very few patients achieved and maintained the 'intensive' target fasting plasma glucose of 6 mmol/l. The trial has been criticised for its convoluted design (which diluted its statistical power) and both the lumping and splitting of data for outcome analysis. Nevertheless, it yielded useful messages about the importance of treating both hyperglycaemia and hypertension and about the natural history of the disease itself. Its conclusions

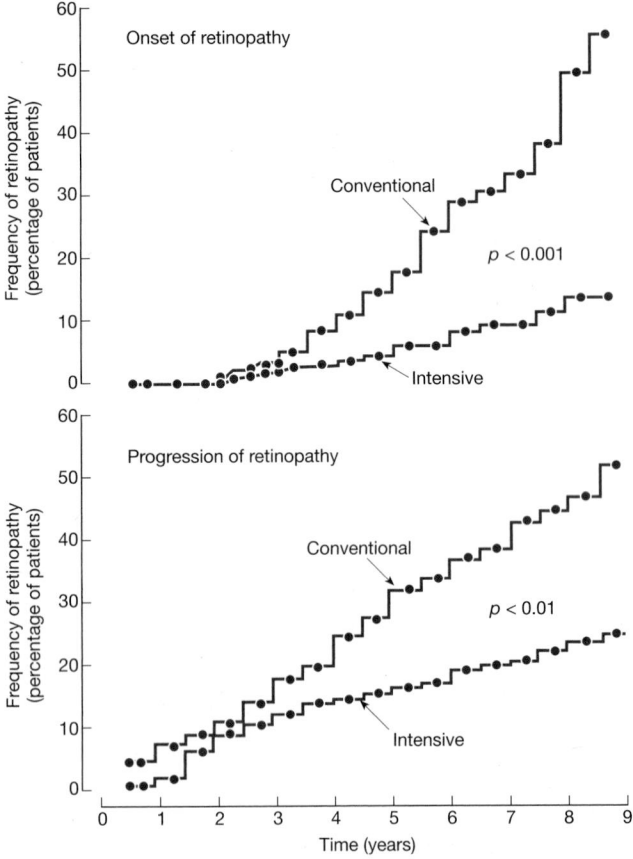

Fig. 11 Intensive insulin therapy and improved diabetic control reduces the risks of type 1 diabetic patients developing retinopathy (upper panel) and of established retinopathy progressing (lower panel). Data from the Diabetic Control and Complications Trial (DCCT).

were broadly similar to those of the DCCT: improved glycaemic control decreased the risk of microvascular complications. Lowering HbA$_{1c}$ from 7.9 per cent (conventional) to 7.0 per cent (intensive) decreased the lumped rate of microvascular events by 25 per cent (Fig. 12), including sight-threatening retinopathy (20 per cent) and development of microalbuminuria (33 per cent). Across a reasonably wide range of HbA$_{1c}$, lowering HbA$_{1c}$ by 1 per cent reduced the risk of microvascular disease by about one-third. Improved glycaemic control had no overall effect on macrovascular disease, although metformin treatment only significantly decreased cardiovascular events (see above).

Possible mechanisms of hyperglycaemic tissue damage

High glucose levels can damage the function and structure of many tissues. The mechanisms currently thought most relevant to human diabetic complications probably operate to different degrees in different tissues.

Glycation of proteins and macromolecules

Glycation begins with the non-enzymatic combination of glucose and other reactive sugars with amino groups of proteins, and with acceptor groups of other long-lived macromolecules such as nucleic acids. Glycation is initially reversible, yielding a Schiff base which undergoes molecular rearrangement to form an Amadori product. Amadori products then undergo further reactions, including covalent crosslinking with the sugar groups in other glycated proteins. These irreversibly modified molecules,

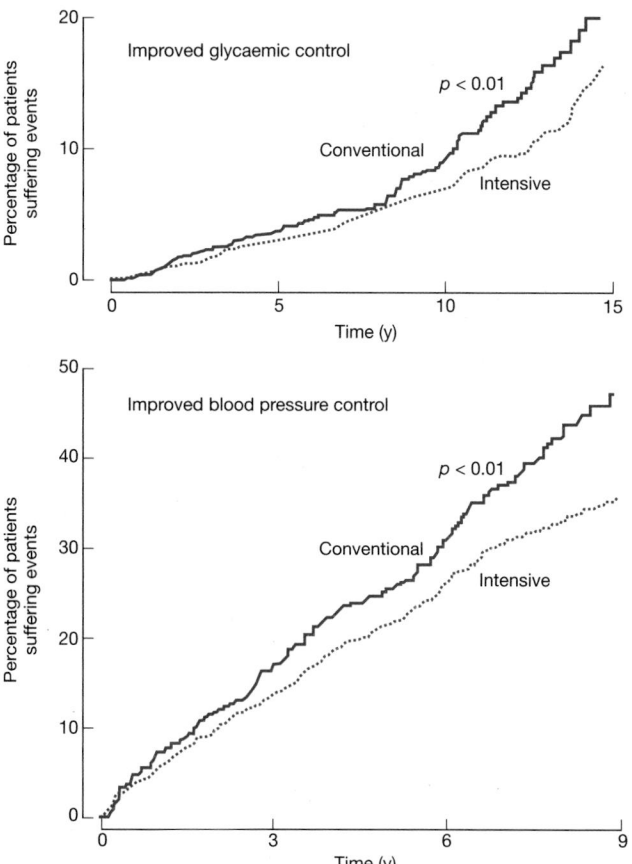

Fig. 12 Benefits of improving glycaemic and blood-pressure control in type 2 diabetic patients. Upper panel: 'intensive' treatment with glucose-lowering drugs reduces the risks of suffering any microvascular complication by about 25 per cent. Lower panel: tighter control of blood pressure reduces the risks of suffering any diabetes-related complication (including micro- and macrovascular disease) by about 24 per cent. Note the scale differences in both axes. Data from the United Kingdom Prospective Diabetes Study (UKPDS).

collectively termed 'advanced glycation endproducts', resist normal degradation mechanisms and thus accumulate.

Advanced glycation endproducts (AGE) can interfere with tissue structure and function in several ways. Stiffening of connective tissue in the limited joint mobility syndrome (see below) is related to crosslinking of collagen by AGE, while the same process in the proteins of the lens fibre (crystallins) causes cataract. AGE also damage blood vessels, and formation of AGE in the basement membrane increases vascular permeability. AGE in the arterial wall may bind low-density lipoprotein and promote atherogenesis. Curiously, endothelial cells carry specific receptors for AGE (so-called 'RAGE)', the binding of which generates oxygen free radicals that may induce oxidative damage and favour coagulation.

Overactivity of the polyol pathway

Polyols are sugar alcohols formed from their respective sugars (for example sorbitol from glucose) under the action of aldose reductase, the rate-limiting enzyme of the polyol pathway. This enzyme is expressed in various tissues susceptible to diabetic complications, notably the retina, glomerulus, lens epithelium, and Schwann cells of the nerves.

Glucose is preferentially shunted through the polyol pathway under hyperglycaemic conditions, generating sorbitol which is poorly diffusible and therefore accumulates intracellularly. This, together with reciprocal intracellular depletion of myoinositol (another polyol, involved in phosphatidylinositol metabolism) may lead to activation of protein kinase C (see below) and the production of highly reactive sugars that can glycate proteins. Increased glucose flux through the polyol pathway also generates oxygen free radicals and can deplete antioxidants which normally mop up free radicals.

At present, the importance of the polyol pathway in humans remains uncertain, and aldose reductase inhibitors (for example sorbinil and ponaltrestat) have failed to show any convincing benefits in human microvascular complications.

Protein kinase C activation

This enzyme is stimulated by diacylglycerol, which is generated intracellularly in hyperglycaemia. Protein kinase C may mediate adverse effects such as increased vascular permeability and enhanced basement membrane synthesis, although the mechanisms remain obscure.

Abnormal microvascular blood flow

Diabetes interferes with blood flow through the microcirculation, potentially impairing the supply of nutrients and oxygen to the tissues. Resting blood flow is increased in the retina, glomerulus, and other tissues, apparently in response to hyperglycaemia; this may damage the endothelium, favouring thrombogenesis (diabetes also enhances the coagulability of the blood) and perhaps the release of vasoconstrictors such as the endothelins, which may cause microvascular occlusion.

Other factors

Individual susceptibility to microvascular and macrovascular complications varies widely, to a degree that is not entirely explicable by differences in hyperglycaemia. Other risk factors include hypertension, which predisposes to atheroma and is also crucial in determining the rate of deterioration of diabetic nephropathy (see Chapter 20.10.1) and perhaps retinopathy. Smoking is implicated in retinopathy and nephropathy as well as macrovascular disease. Familial clustering of markers for nephropathy has been reported (Chapter 20.10.1), but no convincing candidate genes have yet emerged.

Diabetic eye disease

Eye complications are greatly feared by diabetic patients, with good reason: in the United Kingdom and most westernized countries, diabetes (especially diabetic retinopathy) is the most common cause of blindness in people of working age. Annual screening is advisable with prompt referral for laser treatment if appropriate.

Diabetic retinopathy

This is an easily demonstrated example of the microvascular damage that diabetes inflicts throughout the body. The retina is particularly vulnerable because of its high metabolic and oxygen demands and its dependence on an intact blood–retinal barrier; moreover, small lesions that would pass unnoticed in other vascular beds can have a devastating impact on the patient and his or her quality of life. The Plate section for Section 25 shows the stages and lesions of retinopathy.

Epidemiology

Minor 'background' changes, especially the characteristic microaneurysms, are very common in type 1 patients. Microaneurysms begin to appear after 5 years, affecting about 50 per cent of cases at 10 years and virtually all after 20 years. By contrast, the formation of new vessels that defines proliferative retinopathy emerges after 10 years, reaching a plateau at about 40 per cent of all cases after 20 years. The incidence of maculopathy follows a similar curve, ultimately affecting 10 to 20 per cent of cases (more in older subjects). These different patterns suggest that distinct processes are responsible, and that susceptibility to neovascularization and maculopathy may be determined by factors additional to hyperglycaemia.

In type 2 patients, background changes and sometimes maculopathy and proliferative retinopathy may be present at diagnosis, consistent with the generally long duration of subclinical hyperglycaemia.

All grades of retinopathy can complicate any type of diabetes of sufficiently long duration, with some provisos. Retinopathy may be slow to appear in the mildly hyperglycaemic variants of MODY, while some racial groups (for example Native Americans and Afro-Caribbeans) appear more susceptible. The sexes are equally affected.

Aetiology and pathogenesis

Progression of retinopathy is generally related to the severity and duration of hyperglycaemia, while lowering blood glucose can slow or even prevent the process (see above). Hyperglycaemia damages the retinal vessels in various ways; glycation of key proteins and overactivity of protein kinase C appear to be more important than abnormalities of the polyol pathway.

When differences in glycaemic control are allowed for, there remains considerable individual variability in susceptibility. Genetic factors appear less important than in nephropathy (see above), while hypertension and possibly cigarette smoking may accelerate progression.

Increased vascular permeability, which leads to macular oedema and hard exudates, is an early abnormality, demonstrable by fluorescein angiography. Likely causes include glycation and other changes in the basement membrane of the microvessels, abolishing the negative charge which normally repels plasma proteins such as albumin, and endothelial cell damage, which opens up the tight intercellular junctions that constitute the blood–retinal barrier. Local production of vascular endothelial growth factor, which enhances permeability, may also contribute. Fallout of pericytes, the specialized contractile cells that enclose the capillaries, may weaken the capillary wall, increasing retinal blood flow and leading to the formation of microaneurysms. Increased retinal blood flow, perhaps following pericyte loss and hyperglycaemia *per se*, may cause endothelial damage and thrombogenesis and also enhance protein extravasation. Capillary occlusion is probably due to the formation of microthrombi following endothelial damage and diabetes-related changes in coagulability. Closure produces areas of capillary non-perfusion, which can be surprisingly widespread when shown by fluorescein angiography, and ultimately foci of ischaemia where the retina may infarct (causing cotton-wool spots) and angiogenesis may be stimulated.

New vessel formation is thought to be stimulated by growth factors released by ischaemic tissues, which cause endothelial cells to proliferate. A currently favoured angiogenic factor is vascular endothelial growth factor, a 46 kDa dimeric protein which is expressed, together with its receptors, by retinal endothelial cells; its expression is enhanced by hypoxia and its effects include both increased vascular permeability and endothelial cell proliferation. New vessels sprout initially as solid buds of endothelial cells that later

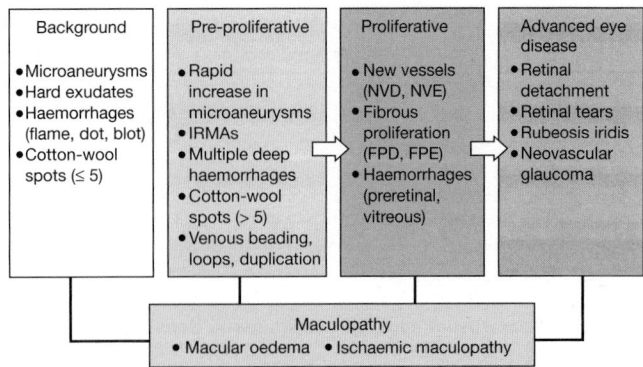

Fig. 13 Stages of diabetic retinopathy. Maculopathy may develop at any stage. IRMAs, intraretinal microvascular abnormalities; NVD/NVE, new vessels on the disc/elsewhere; FPD/FPE, fibrous proliferation on the disc/elsewhere.

canalize. They can grow within the retina, forward into the vitreous, or across the iris, and are indirectly responsible for the main vision-threatening complications of diabetic retinopathy. They are fragile and rupture easily, causing retinal, preretinal (subhyaloid), vitreous, or anterior chamber haemorrhages, while the fibrous tissue that proliferates around them can cause retinal traction and detachment and lead to glaucoma.

Lesions, clinical stages, and natural history

The stages of diabetic retinopathy are summarized in Fig. 13, and the lesions are illustrated in the Plates for Section 25.

Background retinopathy Individual lesions may appear and regress but their total density tends to increase with lengthening duration of diabetes. Vision is not damaged unless maculopathy coexists; over 50 per cent of patients do not progress beyond this stage.

Microaneurysms are outpouchings of capillaries, perhaps representing ballooning of the weakened capillary wall or endothelial buds attempting to revascularize ischaemic retina. They appear as tiny red dots. Microaneurysms are not fixed features: about 50 per cent disappear within 3 years. The sudden appearance of numerous microaneurysms often indicates worsening retinal ischaemia and can herald preproliferative and proliferative changes.

Hard exudates are due to the precipitation in the retina of lipoproteins and other circulating proteins that escape from abnormally leaky retinal vessels. They are yellow-white spots or streaks with a waxy or shiny appearance, and often form clusters or arcs (a circinate pattern) around the macula and foci of capillary leakage. Like microaneurysms, their distribution and extent can vary markedly with time.

Haemorrhages are due to the rupture of weakened capillaries, their size and shape depending on their situation. Small 'dot' and larger 'blot' haemorrhages are spheroidal because they are contained within the densely packed deeper layers of the retina, whereas 'flame' haemorrhages track along nerve fibre bundles in the more superficial layers. Haemorrhages outside the retina (preretinal or vitreous) generally originate from new vessels and therefore indicate proliferative change.

Maculopathy Disease of the macula, serious enough to affect central vision, can accompany any stage of diabetic retinopathy including background, and may be present in newly diagnosed type 2 patients.

Macular oedema is due to extravasation of plasma proteins across abnormally leaky capillaries. It may cause only retinal thickening which may be undetectable by routine fundoscopy, even when advanced enough to reduce visual acuity. Exudates, often circinate, and spotty 'cystoid' changes may occur.

Ischaemic maculopathy is the result of extensive capillary closure and can cause severe central visual loss. As with macular oedema, fundoscopy may appear deceptively normal; the macula may simply look featureless.

Maculopathy presents as progressive and painless loss of central vision. Testing of visual acuity is important in routine screening for maculopathy: poor acuity with no obvious explanation (for example cataract, vitreous haemorrhage) must always prompt further investigations for macular oedema or ischaemia. Retinal thickening can be identified easily by slit-lamp examination, while fluorescein angiography will demonstrate both ischaemic areas (hypofluorescent) and sites of vascular leakage (hyperfluorescent).

Preproliferative retinopathy This stage indicates worsening retinal ischaemia which, if left untreated, often leads to the formation of new vessels. It is defined by one or more of the following, of which intraretinal microvascular abnormalities and venous beading are the most ominous:

- Multiple deep round haemorrhages, especially when appearing over a short period.
- Multiple (more than five) cotton-wool spots, which are due to the accumulation of axoplasm at the edges of retinal infarcts. They appear as dead-white patches with vague borders.
- Intraretinal microvascular abnormalities (IRMA) are flat clusters of abnormal capillaries which, unlike new vessels, are confined to the retina and do not leak fluorescein.
- Venous abnormalities include dilatation (due to general retinal hyperaemia and the shunting of blood around infarcted or non-perfused areas), beading, looping, and reduplication. Beading probably represents the terminations of occluded capillaries, while looping and reduplication may be due to local diversion of blood flow.
- Arterial abnormalities include occlusion, when the vessel is reduced to a thin white line.

Proliferative retinopathy New vessels appear as fine fronds or arcades of abnormal structure, commonly arising on the optic nerve head ('new vessels disc' or 'NVD') or 'elsewhere' ('NVE'), especially at the bifurcation of veins. Greyish fibrous tissues and haemorrhages may be found in association.

Proliferative retinopathy threatens vision through the complications of the abnormal new vessels, namely haemorrhage, retinal detachment, and glaucoma. Overall, only 10 per cent of untreated patients retain useful vision after 10 years. New vessels on the disc (NVD) carry the worst prognosis: if left untreated, the chances of becoming blind within 5 years are over 50 per cent (compared with 30 per cent for new vessels elsewhere (NVE)). Vitreous haemorrhages tend to recur, and 30 per cent of eyes are blind within 1 year of the first bleed. Fortunately, laser photocoagulation has revolutionized the outlook for proliferative retinopathy.

Advanced diabetic eye disease This represents endstage damage that commonly leads to blindness; vitreoretinal surgery has improved the prognosis somewhat:

- Vitreous and preretinal haemorrhages develop when new vessels grow forward from the retina, cross the potential preretinal (subhyaloid) space, and enter the vitreous. These vessels rupture easily: associated fibrous tissue contracts and tears them, as does the normal shrinkage of the vitreous with age. Vitreous haemorrhages appear as reddish or dark opacities that may completely fill the eye and block the view of the retina. Preretinal (subhyaloid) haemorrhages have a flat top (if the subject has been upright), because the red cells sediment within the haemorrhage cavity.
- Retinal detachment occurs: the retina is pulled off the underlying choroid by contracting strands of fibrous tissue associated with the formation of new vessels or previous vitreous haemorrhages. The retina may appear wrinkled (traction lines) or thrown into folds or bumps, sometimes with a visible tear.
- New vessels grow on to the iris (rubeosis iridis), usually in the context of widespread proliferative retinopathy. Vessels and diffuse reddening of the iris may be seen with the ophthalmoscope. The main complication is glaucoma, caused by proliferating fibrovascular tissue

obstructing the filtration angle in the anterior chamber. Signs include circumcorneal injection, a fixed irregular pupil and corneal haze; the eye is often intensely painful.

Symptoms of diabetic retinopathy

There may be no visual symptoms, even with extensive proliferative changes, until sight-threatening complications occur:

- Vitreous haemorrhage and retinal detachment cause sudden loss of vision that is painless but often terrifying. Retinal detachment occurring behind a vitreous haemorrhage may be reported by the patient as a further deterioration in already poor vision.
- Maculopathy presents as a gradual painless decline in central vision, which may not be noticed by the patient but is picked up on routine eye screening.
- Rubeosis and particularly neovascular glaucoma cause worsening vision with pain and redness in the eye.

Other causes of visual loss need to be considered in diabetic patients, including cataract, stroke, retinal artery or vein occlusion, and hypoglycaemia and glaucoma.

Examination of the eyes in diabetic patients

This should be performed routinely on diagnosis, annually thereafter (or every 6 months if marked background or other changes are present), and immediately if the patient reports any change in vision. There should be close liaison with the ophthalmologist, and a low threshold for referral: indications for seeking expert advice are shown in Table 9.

Visual acuity must be checked with a Snellen chart, with the pupils undilated, and both uncorrected and corrected for refraction errors (with the patient's spectacles or a pinhole). Poor visual acuity (worse than 6/12) that is not correctable and has no other obvious cause (cataract, vitreous haemorrhage) is usually due to maculopathy, and this must be actively excluded (see below).

The iris and pupil are examined for evidence of rubeosis or glaucoma. Pupillary reflexes should be checked: an afferent pupillary defect (see Section 25) indicates severe retinal or optic nerve disease, such as retinal detachment.

Fundoscopy must be used to check both eyes through fully dilated pupils: peripheral new vessels may otherwise be invisible. Relative contraindications to mydriatics are intraocular lens implants; referral to the ophthalmologist is then advisable. The disc, entire retina, and macula must be carefully scanned. Binocular ophthalmoscopy provides good all-round and three-dimensional views, especially of vitreous haemorrhage and retinal detachment.

Additional specialist investigations include:

Table 9 Indications for ophthalmological referral in patients with diabetes. (From Barry PJ (1996). The management of diabetes eye disease. In: Pickup JC, Williams G, eds. *Textbook of diabetes*, 2nd edn, Ch. 47. Blackwell Science, Oxford)

Condition	Urgency
Cataract	Routine (few months)
Macular pathology (hard exudates, oedema) Increasing number of retinal haemorrhages Preproliferative changes	Soon (few weeks)
Fall in visual acuity (≥ two lines) New vessels Rubeosis iridis Advanced diabetic eye disease, including glaucoma	Urgent (1 week)
Retinal detachment Vitreous haemorrhage	Immediate (within 48 h)

- Retinal photography: including 'non-mydriatic' cameras that allow photography of most of the retina, through partly dilated pupils (in a darkened room). These are widely used in community screening for retinopathy.
- Slit-lamp microscope: useful for examining the anterior chamber (for rubeosis and glaucoma) and assessing retinal thickness (for detecting macular oedema).
- Fluorescein angiography: fluorescein injected intravenously binds to albumin and so only escapes outside abnormally permeable vessels; sites of leakage are highlighted by persistent fluorescence when the retina is photographed under ultraviolet light. This is useful for showing the foci of leakage (for example for targeting laser photocoagulation) and for the diagnosis of macular oedema.
- B-scan ultrasound provides a cross-sectional image of the eye and can show retinal detachments that are invisible on fundoscopy because of a dense vitreous haemorrhage or cataract.

Management of diabetic retinopathy

Specific treatments for sight-threatening retinopathy have improved greatly, but general preventative measures are still crucial. These include:

- Tight glycaemic control, as highlighted by the DCCT and the UKPDS. Paradoxically, a rapid reduction in hyperglycaemia can provoke a transient deterioration in retinopathy, with worsening of the background condition or the development of preproliferative changes. This is probably due to an acute fall in retinal blood flow (which is elevated by hyperglycaemia), thus worsening ischaemia in already underperfused areas. Typically, the acute lesions resolve and the overall long-term outcome is improved if good glycaemic control can be maintained.
- Control of hypertension is likely to be important; the EUCLID study of enalapril showed beneficial effects which may reflect the inhibition of angiotensin-converting enzyme as well as lowering of blood pressure.
- Stopping smoking: smoking is thought to hasten the progression of retinopathy.
- Regular eye screening is essential, because even severe diabetic retinopathy may cause few or no symptoms.

Specific treatments Laser photocoagulation can preserve useful vision in many cases of proliferative retinopathy and maculopathy. The blue-green light of the argon laser is maximally absorbed by vascular structures. It has a spot size of 50 to 500 µm and can be used to target discrete lesions such as clusters of leaking vessels identified by fluorescein angiography, but is usually employed to destroy larger areas of generally diseased retina. Panretinal photocoagulation ablates the peripheral retina with 1500 to 2000 burns that spare only a keyhole-shaped central area that includes the disc, the macula, and the maculopapillary nerve bundle running between them. Panretinal photocoagulation effectively concentrates the remaining retinal blood flow on to this crucial region which serves central, high-resolution colour vision, at the expense of the periphery. It is indicated for formation of new vessels (on the disc or elsewhere and rubeosis), and can be very effective: the chance of blindness within 5 years is reduced from 50 per cent to 25 per cent in patients at risk. It is increasingly used in the preproliferative phase to prevent the formation of new vessels. Photocoagulation is also used to treat macular oedema, in a 'grid' pattern around the central macula to destroy leaky capillaries; this reduces the 3-year risk of becoming blind from 30 per cent to 15 per cent.

Vitreoretinal surgery can now restore useful vision to some blind or severely impaired eyes. Techniques include vitrectomy (aspiration of vitreous haemorrhage and fibrovascular debris) and reattachment of detached or torn retina (using high-powered lasers to 'stitch' down the retina). Easy and rapid access to ophthalmologists and surgeons is often critical: for example, a detached retina must be repaired within a few weeks if it is to remain viable.

Practical aids for visual handicap range from pen injection devices and 'talking' blood glucose meters, to social support networks and national organizations for the visually impaired.

Cataract in diabetes

The normal lens transmits light because the fibre cells of the lens and the stacks of crystallin proteins which they contain are aligned in parallel. Normal ageing causes irreversible chemical modification ('browning') of the crystallins, with crosslinking and distortion that interrupt transmission of light and thus cause clouding of the lens. Diabetes accelerates the formation of these senile cataracts, probably through non-enzymatic glycation and crosslinking of AGE-modified crystallins.

Cataract is the most common cause of severe visual loss in diabetic patients over the age of 30, and is usually a typical 'senile' nuclear cataract with a characteristic radial spoke pattern. Much rarer is the 'snowflake' cataract with opacities scattered through the lens, which tends to occur in children presenting with severe hyperglycaemia. Here, the 'opacities' are reversible and are presumably due to local pockets of osmotic imbalance which distort the alignment of the lens crystallins.

Treatment of cataracts is conventional, usually removal and replacement by an intracapsular plastic lens. Long-term outcome is often not as good as in non-diabetic patients, because of coexisting maculopathy or proliferative retinopathy.

Gaucoma is more common in diabetics.

Other ocular problems

Cranial nerve palsies, especially of the third and sixth nerves, cause typical limitations of eye movement, often with acute onset of pain (see below and Chapter 23.13.15).

Eye infections include the rare but extremely destructive mucormycosis, which often spreads from the sinus to involve the orbit (see Chapter 7.12.1).

Diabetic neuropathies

Clinical syndromes

Diabetes damages nerves, both somatosensory and autonomic, in various ways that cause clinically distinct syndromes (Fig. 14). Subclinical nerve damage is common among diabetic patients, but significant neuropathic symptoms are fortunately unusual.

Diffuse symmetrical polyneuropathy

This is classically a distal 'glove and stocking' peripheral polyneuropathy that affects all sizes of sensory and motor fibres; a variant selectively picks

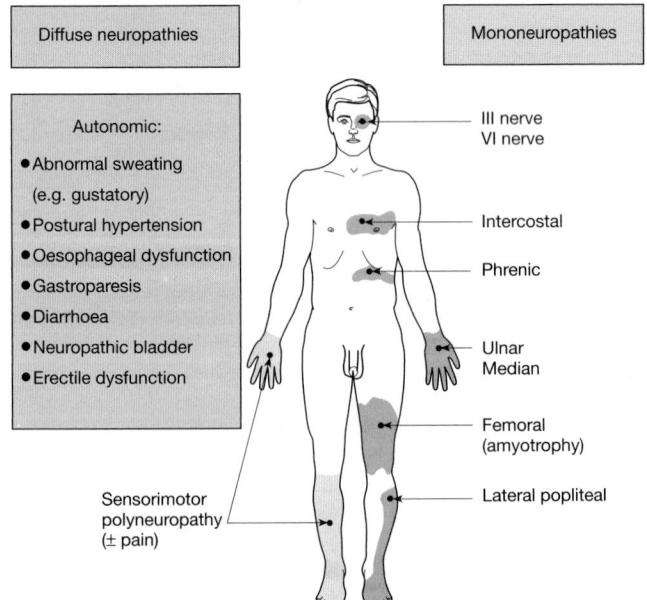

Fig. 14 Clinical manifestations of diabetic nerve damage.

off small C fibres (see below). Both forms may be accompanied by neuropathy involving the sympathetic and parasympathetic divisions of the autonomic nervous system.

Aetiology The diffuse nature of the nerve damage and its predilection for longer nerves is typical of toxic and metabolic neuropathies, and suggests cumulative damage that must reach a critical level before the function of a nerve is impaired. Both metabolic and vascular factors may contribute. The duration and severity of hyperglycaemia are generally related to the prevalence of neuropathy, while the DCCT confirmed that good glycaemic control decreased by the risks of developing neuropathy by about 70 per cent. Hyperglycaemia could damage nerves by glycation of key proteins. In the nerves of diabetic animals, polyol pathway overactivity has also been implicated (Schwann cells express aldose reductase), while myoinositol depletion may impair nerve conduction by inhibiting Na^+,K^+-ATPase activity; in human diabetic neuropathy, however, the roles of polyols are less convincing and a role for aldose reductase inhibitors has not been demonstrated. There is some evidence of blockage of the vasa nervorum by microthrombi, which could follow the formation of AGE and the other mechanisms described earlier. Microvascular occlusion could contribute to intraneural hypoxia, demonstrated in the nerves of both animal and human diabetics.

Pathological changes affect both axons and Schwann cells. Axons fall out by dying back distally, sometimes accompanied by sprouting of regenerating nerve endings. Schwann cell damage leads to segmental demyelination. Nerve conduction velocity is slowed, in proportion to structural nerve damage.

Epidemiology and natural history About 30 per cent of unselected diabetic patients have evidence of neuropathy on formal testing, but only 10 per cent suffer significant symptoms. Signs of neuropathy may be present in up to 10 per cent of newly diagnosed type 2 diabetic patients.

Nerve function generally worsens progressively over months or years, and areas of numbness may advance up the legs and occasionally involve the hands. Symptoms, including pain, may be variable; pain in particular may develop acutely, especially after weight loss or periods of poor diabetic control. Acute flareups tend to resolve after weeks or months, especially if glycaemic control is improved.

Symptoms and signs Sensory symptoms are the commonest manifestation; muscle weakness occasionally predominates. Sensory symptoms may include loss of sensation, which can be profound, as well as 'positive' symptoms of pain, paraesthesiae, and allodynia (i.e. pain provoked by a normally innocuous stimulus, such as light touch or contact with bedclothes). Loss of the sense of touch and joint position may give the sensation of walking in thick socks, and Romberg's sign may be positive. Reduced pain sensation, which paradoxically may coexist with neurogenic pain, is potentially dangerous and an important cause of damage to neuropathic feet (see below). Horrifying accounts involving neuropathic diabetic feet include full-thickness burns to the soles after crossing a hot beach, pressure ulceration from a day's walking in tight new shoes, and transfixing the foot inside the shoe by stepping on a nail.

The mechanism of neuropathic pain is unknown; spontaneous firing of unstable regenerating nerves may be responsible. Pain is typically neurogenic, usually described as burning, shooting, or electric shock-like sensations, often with unpleasant pins and needles and allodynia. The feet and legs are usually affected, and the hands only rarely; neuropathic symptoms in the hands are usually due to damage to the ulnar and/or median nerves, which can be bilateral (Fig. 15 and Plate 1). Pain is characteristically worse at night, and can severely disturb sleep and cause depression (and suicide).

Examination may reveal symmetrical 'stocking' sensory loss affecting all modalities. Sensory deficits are frequently patchy and may be much less

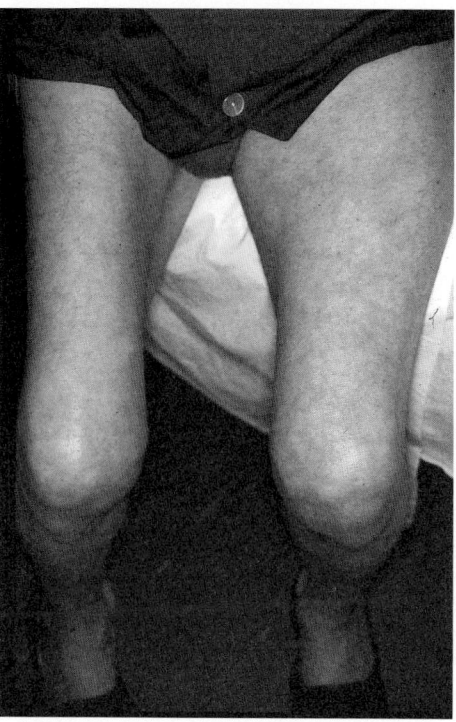

(a)

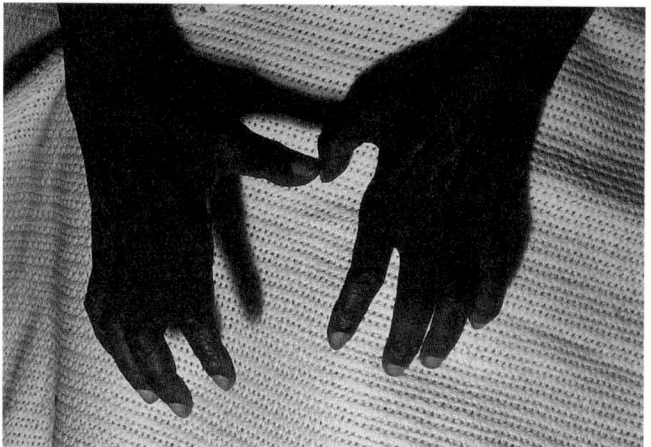

(b)

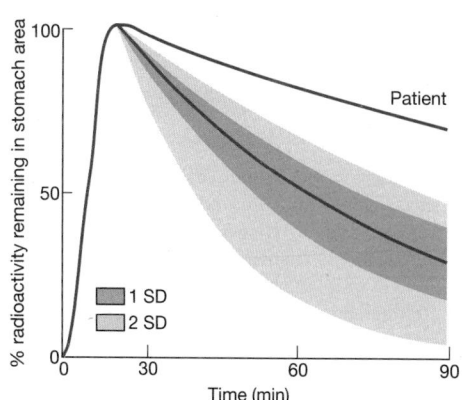

(c)

Fig. 15 (a) Diabetic amyotrophy: quadriceps right wasting due to femoral neuropathy (with thanks to Dr Geoff Gill, University Hospital Aintree, Liverpool). (b) Wasting of small muscles of the hands due to both ulnar and median nerve lesions. (See also Plate 1.) (c) Gastroparesis: grossly delayed gastric emptying. The normal range for clearance of the radiolabelled test meal from the stomach area is shown in in the darker shade (50 per cent confidence interval) and lighter shade (95 per cent confidence interval).

impressive than the symptoms suggest; clinical findings may even be normal in acute painful neuropathy. Tendon reflexes in the legs are often reduced or absent, and there may occasionally be marked muscle wasting. Neuropathic foot problems due to somatosensory and autonomic nerve damage may also be obvious, including ulceration, increased skin blood flow, and Charcot's arthropathy. The hands are less commonly involved.

Diffuse small-fibre neuropathy

This rare variant affects especially young women with type 1 diabetes, and may be autoimmune in origin. There is loss of temperature and pain sensation in a stocking distribution, other modalities remaining intact. Autonomic neuropathy is frequent, usually with postural hypertension, gustatory sweating, and diarrhoea. Ulceration and Charcot's arthropathy affecting the feet are common.

Autonomic neuropathy

Autonomic disturbances commonly accompany somatosensory neuropathy, and the autonomic nerves are presumably damaged by the same mechanisms. Up to 40 per cent of unselected diabetic people have abnormal tests of autonomic neuropathy, but only a few of these suffer major symptoms; however, these can be very debilitating and these patients have a significantly reduced life expectancy. The sympathetic and parasympathetic divisions are both affected.

Clinically apparent features are commonest in patients with long-standing diabetes and include:

- Abnormal sweating, mediated by cholinergic sympathetic nerves; this is one of the commonest autonomic symptoms. Profuse 'gustatory' sweating of the face and trunk (the area supplied by the superior cervical ganglion) may be provoked by eating, while sweating in the feet is often reduced.

- Postural hypotension, with a systolic fall exceeding 20 mmHg on standing, is due to failure of the normal sympathetically mediated increases in cardiac output and vasoconstrictor tone. This causes dizziness and blackouts, which may be mistaken for arrhythmias or myocardial ischaemia. Symptoms and the degree of postural drop may vary considerably with time. Postural hypotension may be exacerbated by the vasodilator effects of antihypertensives, nitrates, tricyclic antidepressants (used to treat neuropathic pain), and insulin.

- Disturbed gastrointestinal motility. Dysphagia may be due to oesophageal dysmotility. Gastric stasis, due to failure of the pylorus to relax when the antrum contracts, causes particular difficulties with emptying liquids and presents with recurrent vomiting. There may be obvious fullness in the epigastrium, sometimes with a succussion splash. Disturbances of motility in the colon most commonly lead to diarrhoea (characteristically but not always worse at night), which may be exacerbated by bacterial overgrowth of the relatively immotile small bowel. As with all these gastrointestinal symptoms, diarrhoea is often episodic and may alternate with constipation. Anorectal dysfunction is luckily rare, but can cause severe faecal incontinence.

- Neuropathic bladder, due to damage to the sacral nerves, prevents normal emptying and can lead to a permanently distended, sometimes palpable, bladder, with overflow incontinence. Hydroureter and hydronephrosis are other complications, and ascending urinary tract infections are common.

- Sexual difficulties include failure of erection (a parasympathetic response mediated by the sacral nerves) and sometimes failure of ejaculation (a sympathetic reflex transmitted by the lumbosacral outflow). Erectile failure is relatively common in diabetic men, affecting about 50 per cent of those over 55 years; as in the non-diabetic population, depression and anxiety (including fears about poor sexual performance) are common contributory factors. Arterial inflow to the corpora cavernosa may be compromised by atheromatous disease of the pudendal arteries or common iliac arteries, the latter causing the Leriche syndrome of impotence with claudication of the buttocks.

- Abnormal blood flow. Sympathetic denervation allows vasodilatation and relaxation of precapillary sphincters in the skin, hence the warm skin and distended veins characteristic of the neuropathic foot. Increased blood flow in bone may be an early abnormality in Charcot's arthropathy.

- Sudden unexplained death is more common in patients with severe autonomic symptoms. Possible causes include cardiorespiratory arrest and arrhythmias triggered by hypoglycaemia, awareness of which is blunted in many patients with long-standing diabetes.

Acute mononeuropathies

These syndromes are due to acute damage to isolated peripheral nerves, presumably due to a vascular event rather than metabolic damage. Limited histological studies show focal demyelination, probably consistent with this. Occasionally, two or more nerves can be affected more or less simultaneously (mononeuritis multiplex).

Diabetic amyotrophy

This is due to damage of one of the major nerve trunks or roots (radiculopathy) supplying the leg. The femoral nerve is most commonly involved, causing symptoms in the quadriceps muscle; other muscle groups are less often affected. Femoral neuropathy causes neurogenic pain of acute onset (burning or lancinating, usually severe), with weakness and often surprisingly rapid wasting in the quadriceps, and loss of the knee tendon reflex (Fig. 15). For unknown reasons, some patients have extensor plantar reflexes, in which case a spinal or cauda equina lesion must be excluded.

Amyotrophy most commonly presents in patients over 50 years of age, often following a period of poor diabetic control. Pain usually resolves spontaneously over several months, especially if diabetic control is improved, but muscle strength and tendon reflexes may take much longer to return.

Cranial and other nerve palsies

These are common, affecting the third and sixth nerves in particular. Third nerve palsy is often accompanied by pain behind the eye, and may need to be differentiated from an aneurysm of the posterior communicating artery; however, unlike in classical third nerve palsy, ptosis and pupillary dilatation are usually absent. Acute neuropathic damage may also affect the phrenic nerve (causing an elevated hemidiaphragm), and intercostal or truncal nerves, causing shingles-like pain and sometimes localized bulging of the abdominal wall. All these acute palsies tend to resolve spontaneously.

Pressure palsies

These include the median, ulnar, and occasionally lateral popliteal nerves, and are thought to be due to pressure damage superimposed on hypoxic or otherwise compromised nerves. These present in the classical way, but often recover slowly and incompletely, and respond poorly to surgical decompression (see Fig. 15).

'Insulin neuritis'

This is a transient deterioration in nerve function, often with pain and dysthaesiae affecting the legs symmetrically, which follows an acute improvement in glycaemic control, usually after starting insulin therapy. It may be due to an acute fall in nerve perfusion analogous to the decrease in retinal blood flow thought to explain a temporary deterioration in retinopathy under these circumstances (see above). Symptoms usually resolve within weeks or months.

Diagnosis of diabetic neuropathies

Peripheral sensorimotor neuropathies

A carefully taken history is usually diagnostic. The key qualities of neuropathic pain should distinguish it from claudication and night cramps.

Sensory deficits should be mapped on the legs and hands, for both large-fibre (vibration with a 128-Hz tuning fork, joint position sense, light touch, temperature, e.g. with a cold tuning fork) and small-fibre modalities (pin prick, light touch); objective losses may not match the patient's symptoms.

A useful test uses the Semmes–Weinstein nylon monofilament, which is pressed against the skin until it buckles; the patient's inability to feel the 10-g filament indicates neuropathy severe enough to predict foot ulceration. Various bedside instruments can be used to assess specific sensory modalities, such as the biothesiometer (for vibration sense) and thermal threshold testers; age-related normal ranges are available for these methods but they are quite variable and add little to routine management. Muscle wasting and weakness should be sought, and the tendon reflexes checked.

Peripheral diabetic neuropathy must be differentiated from other metabolic neuropathies, including vitamin B$_{12}$ deficiency, uraemia, and alcohol, all of which may affect diabetic patients.

Autonomic neuropathy

The most convenient tests are of cardiovascular autonomic function, which detect loss of the normal reflexes that modulate heart rate during respiration (mainly vagal) and that increase heart rate and blood pressure on standing (sympathetic). The simplest test is to measure heart rate (RR interval) from an ECG tracing during controlled deep breathing (5 s inspiration, then 5 s expiration, repeated for 1 min); the physiological bradycardia on expiration is lost, with a difference of less than 10 beats/min between inspiration and expiration. Reflex bradycardia during the Valsalva manoeuvre is similarly abolished. More sophisticated measures employing spectral analysis of variability of heart rate during normal breathing are more sensitive.

Postural hypotension is defined as a drop of more than 20 mmHg drop in systolic blood pressure, measured 30 s after standing. Postural drops often vary considerably through the day and from week to week.

Abnormalities of cardiovascular autonomic tests are common in patients with long-standing diabetes, especially type 1, and do not necessarily indicate that symptoms such as vomiting, diarrhoea, or erectile dysfunction are due to autonomic neuropathy. Other specific tests include:

- Gastroparesis: a plain abdominal radiograph may show a 'ground glass' appearance in the epigastrium, while endoscopy (always indicated to exclude pyloric obstruction) shows a dilated, poorly contracting stomach with a closed pylorus. Gastric emptying studies using radiolabelled test meals show delayed disappearance of radioactivity, particularly of a liquid test meal; however, abnormalities may not be consistent with the severity of symptoms (see Fig. 15).

- Neuropathic bladder and associated hydroureter and hydronephrosis can be confirmed by ultrasound or intravenous urography.

- Erectile failure is often multifactorial (see above). If it is due to autonomic neuropathy, other signs of autonomic dysfunction, especially neuropathic bladder, are usually prominent.

Treatment of diabetic neuropathies

General measures

Poor glycaemic control should be corrected. As well as helping to prevent the development of neuropathy, this may curtail pain in the acute syndromes; insulin neuritis is rare and usually self-limiting. Once established, chronic sensory motor neuropathy tends to progress, irrespective of glycaemic control. Specific treatments which aim to prevent or reverse diabetic nerve damage—aldose reductase inhibitors and aminoguanidine (which prevents the formation of AGE)—have so far been disappointing. Numb feet are at greatly increased risk of ulceration and require sensible shoes and good foot care (see below).

Pain may be difficult to treat; pain management programmes in specialized pain relief clinics may be helpful. The following should be tried in sequence:

- Simple analgesics (aspirin, paracetamol) are mostly unhelpful. Opiates are generally regarded as ineffective in neurogenic pain and are yet to be tested adequately in diabetic neuropathy.

- Tricyclic drugs suppress neurogenic pain, in addition to their antidepressant effects. Amitriptiline or imipramine can be started at 25 mg at bedtime (10 mg in the elderly), increasing weekly to a maximum of 75 to 150 mg. Side-effects, including postural hypotension, may limit the dosage. A phenothiazine such as fluphenazine (2.5–5 mg) is said to enhance the analgesic effect of tricyclics but its use is not evidence-based and it often exacerbates postural hypotension.

- Anticonvulsants, which stabilize the neurone membrane and may prevent spontaneous firing of C fibres, may be substituted for trycyclics or used in combination with them. Carbamazepine (initially 100 mg once or twice daily, up to 800 mg/day in divided doses) is often effective. Sodium valproate or phenytoin are alternatives. Gabapentin appears promising, but has yet to be compared adequately with tricyclics. Gabapentin has been given at doses of 900 to 3600 mg/day in divided doses—rather more than the standard antiepileptic regimen but apparently well tolerated.

Pain in the feet may respond to topical application of capsaicin ointment; capsaicin causes the burning sensaton of hot chillies, and depletes the pain-transmitting C fibres of the neurotransmitter substance P. Pain may be transiently worsened after application but relief can last for many hours. Contact hypersensitivity (allodynia) can be helped simply with a bed cradle to prevent contact with bed clothes, or by applying Opsite® adhesive plastic film to the skin.

Other drugs that have proved successful in some but not all trials include oral mexiletine (a class 1b antiarrhythmic agent that stabilizes nerve cell membranes; up to 450 mg/day in divided doses) and clonazepam (0.5–3 mg) in patients whose sleep is disturbed by 'restless legs'. Some patients unresponsive to drug therapy may benefit from implantation of a dorsal column stimulator, designed to exploit the 'gate' control of pain transmission.

Autonomic neuropathic symptoms may be treated as follows:

- Excessive sweating may be controlled by oral clonidine or topical 1 per cent glycopyrrholate ointment; systemic anticholinergics such as poldine have also been effective but have many side-effects, including urinary retention.

- Postural hypotension may be helped simply by raising the head of the bed at night. Fludrocortisone can be useful, but aggravates coexistent supine hypertension; very high doses (up to 1 mg/day) may be needed. The α_1-adrenergic agonist midodrine (2.5–10 mg daily) may also be helpful, but can also worsen hypertension.

- Vomiting due to gastroparesis often responds to metoclopramide or domperidone, and the prokinetic drug erythromycin (cisapride has been withdrawn because of arrhythmias). Some patients unresponsive to drug therapy may require intrajejunal feeding, most conveniently by percutaneous endoscopic gastrostomy; some patients benefit from surgical drainage procedures such as a roux-en-Y gastrojejunostomy.

- Diarrhoea is often improved or cured by erythromycin or tetracycline when bacterial overgrowth is a contributory factor.

- Neuropathic bladder may respond to regular bladder training, but intermittent self-catheterization may be needed.

- Erectile dysfunction can be treated with oral sildenafil 4 mg, which should be taken about 1 h before intercourse. It is effective in about 50 per cent of diabetic patients but is absolutely contraindicated in those taking nitrates in any form, because of the risk of profound hypotension and circulatory collapse. Alternatives, if sildenafil is contraindicated or ineffective, include the injection of vasodilators such as papaverine or prostaglandin E$_1$ into the corpus cavernosum, intraurethral alprostadil, or the use of vacuum tumescence devices. Coexistent contributory factors such as depression, alcohol, or drugs (including β-blockers and thiazides) should be sought and treated. Counselling of the couple is obviously important.

Diabetic nephropathy

This is covered in detail in Chapter 20.10.1.

Macrovascular disease

Diabetes of all types increases the background risk of atheroma, amplifying the hazards of additional cardiovascular risk factors such as hypercholesterolaemia, hypertension, and smoking. Atheroma appears earlier, spreads faster and more extensively, and carries greater morbidity and mortality than in non-diabetic people. Overall risks for myocardial infarction, stroke, and limb ischaemia are two to four times higher than in the general population, and diabetic women lose the premenopausal protection which their euglycaemic counterparts normally enjoy. This increased level of risk is comparable with that in non-diabetic subjects who have already suffered a myocardial infarct. Accordingly, it has been argued that primary cardiovascular prevention for diabetic patients should be as active as secondary prevention in the non-diabetic population. Macrovascular disease, especially coronary heart disease, is the main cause of premature death in type 2 diabetes.

As discussed earlier, cardiovascular risk is increased above glucose levels that lie below the 'diabetic' range: IGT also predisposes to coronary-heart disease, but not to retinopathy. This relationship probably explains why 'tight' glucose control has not yet been shown to prevent macrovascular disease, because none of the trials (for example the DCCT or the UKPDS) has managed to achieve even near normoglycaemia. There is a very strong relationship between microalbuminuria and premature death from cardiovascular disease (see Chapter 20.10.1). This presumably reflects widespread damage to the endothelium, which both predisposes to atheroma formation and enhances albumin leakage in the glomerulus.

Cardiovascular risk factors tend to cluster together with type 2 diabetes in the so-called 'metabolic syndrome X' (see above). These risk factors are also common in the type 1 diabetic and the non-diabetic populations. Because their impact is worsened by diabetes, they require active management. Treatment of obesity and smoking is discussed in Chapters 10.5 and 3.5.

Dyslipidaemia in diabetes

Type 1 and type 2 diabetes are both commonly accompanied by lipid disorders that are strongly atherogenic but may appear deceptively trivial on routine screening (Fig. 16).

In poorly controlled type 1 diabetes, the most obvious abnormality is hypertriglyceridaemia. This is due mainly to increased production of very

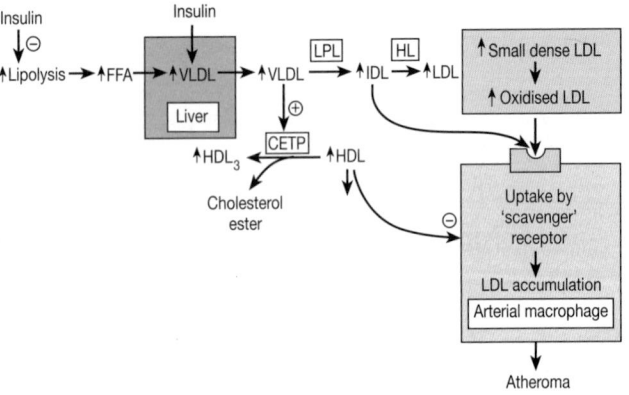

Fig. 16 Mechanisms of lipid abnormalities in diabetes. Insulin resistance or loss of insulin leads to increased lipolysis and hepatic secretion of very low-density lipoprotein (VLDL). High levels of VLDL stimulate cholesterol ester transfer protein which converts the antiatherogenic high-density lipoprotein (HDL) into HDL₃, which lacks this protective effect. VDLPs are stripped of triglyceride by lipoprotein lipase to yield atherogenic intermediate-density lipoprotein (IDL), and then by hepatic lipase to produce low-density lipoprotein (LDL), including the highly atherogenic small dense oxidized fractions. These, with IDL, are taken up by arterial wall macrophages, forming the 'foam cells' that initiate the atheromatous plaque.

low-density lipoprotein by the liver, driven by high levels of free fatty acids resulting from enhanced lipolysis in fat; triglyceride levels can be lowered by improved insulin therapy. Total cholesterol concentrations are often 'normal', while HDL may be increased, although this is predominantly the HDL₃ subclass which does not confer protection against atheroma (see Chapter 11.6). As stressed below, a 'normal' cholesterol is not necessarily reassuring because modified LDL particles in diabetes are particularly atherogenic and because cardiovascular risk in diabetic people is increased at all levels of cholesterol.

Dyslipidaemia in type 2 diabetes is also subtle, and similar to that of obesity and syndrome X. High-density lipoprotein cholesterol is reduced, increasing the ratio of LDL to HDL, while triglycerides are often modestly raised. The abnormalities are also due to excessive production of VLDL by the liver, due to insulin resistance rather than insulin deficiency: free fatty acids levels are raised by lipolysis (adipocytes are resistant to the normal antilipolytic action of insulin), while the inhibition by insulin of hepatic production of VLDL is lost. High levels of VLDL favour the production of two highly atherogenic cholesterol particles, namely IDL and small dense LDL, which is easily oxidized; both IDL and oxidized LDL are taken up, via specific receptors, by macrophages in the artery wall and are then transformed into foam cells (see Chapter 11.6). High triglyceride levels also accelerate the removal of cholesterol ester (via cholesterol ester transfer protein) from HDL, ultimately reducing levels of HDL and producing the non-protective HDL₃ fraction.

Risks of dyslipidaemia

Cardiovascular events including fatal myocardial infarction are three to four times commoner among diabetic patients than in the general population, across a wide range of cholesterol levels including 'normal' values. The risks of the slightly raised triglyceride concentrations are less obvious, and are currently the subject of large-scale trials with fibrates.

Management

This remains controversial, although the consensus is that diabetic people benefit at least as much from statin therapy as the non-diabetic population. The high background risk of diabetes is reflected in the lower treatment thresholds for hypercholesterolaemia in the various risk-factor tables (see Chapter 11.6), and lipid-lowering drugs are now used at ever lower cholesterol levels. Indeed, the American Diabetes Association recommends statin therapy for any diabetic patient with a total cholesterol of more than 5 mmol/l, aiming to maintain cholesterol below this level. It seems reasonable at present to consider adding a fibrate if triglycerides then remain in excess of 2.3 mmol/l.

Pharmacoeconomic arguments may intrude, and it is debatable whether dyslipidaemia should be treated exhaustively in patients who make no effort to stop smoking. Other factors that aggravate dyslipidaemia—obesity, poor glycaemic control, and drugs such as thiazides and β-blockers—should be tackled if possible.

Hypertension

Hypertension commonly accompanies diabetes: about 40 per cent of type 2 patients are hypertensive at diagnosis, and probably two-thirds of the diabetic population are inadequately treated with respect to current management guidelines (Table 3).

Causes

Essential hypertension is an integral feature of the metabolic syndrome X, associated with obesity and insulin resistance. Possible mechanisms include enhanced central sympathetic tone (possibly mediated in part by raised insulin levels), and increased total body sodium and extracellular fluid volume, to which the Na⁺-retaining effects of hyperinsulinaemia could contribute; loss of insulin-induced vasodilatation due to insulin resistance could also play a role. Secondary hypertension may also develop because of specific diabetic complications, notably nephropathy (loss of the normal nocturnal dip in blood pressure can be an early feature: see Chapter 20.10.1), stenosis of the renal artery due to atheroma, and stiffening of the larger conduit arteries causing isolated systolic hypertension. Supine hypertension can coexist with postural hypotension—a particularly difficult combination to treat effectively.

Treatment targets

The blood pressure thresholds for active management have fallen progressively, with wider appreciation of the damage inflicted by even modest hypertension in diabetic patients and of the benefits of control of blood pressure. The American Diabetes Association now recommends 130/80 mmHg (recorded in the clinic) as the treatment target for blood pressure, and that consistently higher values require active treatment; levels exceeding 140/90 mmHg are increasingly regarded as unacceptably poor. Ambulatory blood pressure readings are lower than those recorded in the clinic, and mean daytime levels of less than 130/75 mmHg are the current target. Target blood pressure (clinic readings) for patients with microalbuminuria is 125/75 mmHg.

Impact of hypertension in diabetes

Like all cardiovascular risk factors, the atherogenic hazards of hypertension are amplified in the diabetic population. Hypertension also plays a crucial role in accelerating the progression of diabetic nephropathy and also of retinopathy. Several studies have shown that treating hypertension reduces the risks of myocardial infarction and stroke by 30 to 70 per cent; in the UKPDS, 'tight' blood pressure control (averaging 144/82 mmHg compared with 154/87 mmHg in less tightly controlled subjects) reduced stroke by 40 per cent and the need for photocoagulation by 30 per cent, although strangely, no effect on myocardial infarction was observed (Fig. 12).

Management

This should begin with lifestyle modification, including restricting energy intake and increasing exercise in the obese, and reducing alcohol and sodium intakes. If actually carried out, these general measures can lower blood pressure at least as effectively as many antihypertensive drugs. Most patients, however, will require drugs and many need combination therapy. Antihypertensive drugs can be used in the conventional stepped approach (Chapter 15.16.1.3) to achieve the target blood pressure, ideally 130/80 mmHg; less stringent targets may be appropriate for elderly patients or those who cannot tolerate tight blood pressure control because of other problems.

The choice of hypotensive drugs is less important than the level of blood pressure achieved, although some agents have properties that are better suited to diabetes. All these drugs can worsen or precipitate postural hypotension in autonomic neuropathy.

Diuretics

High-dose thiazides (e.g. 5 mg bendrofluazide) can worsen hyperglycaemia in type 2 diabetes, apparently by impairing insulin secretion (a consequence of K^+ depletion) and possibly increasing insulin resistance. Low dosages (for example, 2.5 mg bendrofluazide) do not appear to aggravate glucose intolerance. Diuretics can precipitate hyperosmolar non-ketotic coma, while thiazides may also worsen dyslipidaemia.

β-Blockers

β-Blockers may also raise blood glucose in type 2 patients by increasing insulin resistance (possibly related to weight gain) and by interfering with insulin release (which is stimulated by β_2 adrenoceptors). β-blockers can also aggravate dyslipidaemia and impotence, while non-cardioselective agents can mask the sympathetically driven symptoms of hypoglycaemia. Low dosages of cardioselective β-blockers (for example, atenolol or metoprol) are safe, and are also indicated for treating angina and in the secondary prevention of myocardial infarction.

Angiotensin converting enzyme (ACE) inhibitors

These can effectively control blood pressure when combined with low-dose diuretics and are useful in the many diabetic patients who also have heart failure or left ventricular dysfunction, especially following a myocardial infarct. They reduce proteinuria, by relaxing the efferent arterioles in the glomerulus, and slow the development of both nephropathy and retinopathy; some evidence points to specific beneficial effects in nephropathy, in addition to the lowering of blood pressure (see Chapter 20.10.1). ACE inhibitors do not worsen blood glucose or lipids, and may even improve insulin sensitivity. They are contraindicated in renal artery stenosis, which is relatively common in arteriopathic diabetic patients, and can cause dangerous hyperkalaemia in those with hyporeninaemic hypoaldosteronism (type 4 renal tubular acidosis) which can be associated with diabetic nephropathy.

Calcium channel antagonists

These have no adverse metabolic effects and are useful in patients with angina or tachyarrhythmia.

Other drugs

Other drugs include α_1-adrenoreceptor antagonists (for example doxazosin), which may slightly improve insulin sensitivity; angiotensin II receptor antagonists (for example losartan, candesartan), which are useful alternatives when angiotensin converting enzyme inhibitors are poorly tolerated because of cough; and moxonidine, a centrally acting sympathetic drug acting on imidazoline I_1 receptors.

Coronary heart disease

Compared with their non-diabetic counterparts, clinically significant coronary heart disease is over twice as common in diabetic men and postmenopausal women and four times commoner in premenopausal women.

Angina

It is said that myocardial ischaemia can be painless in patients with long-standing diabetes and autonomic neuropathy, presumably because of sensory denervation of the heart; however, the overall prevalence of 'silent' myocardial ischaemia appears to be similar to that in the general population.

Angina should be treated first with conventional drugs, remembering the diabetogenic and other hazards of β-blockers and the potential of nitrates and calcium-channel antagonists to aggravate postural hypotension. Recent studies have confirmed that coronary artery stenting and bypass grafting markedly reduce fatal myocardial infarction in diabetic patients; it follows that exercise testing and coronary angiography should be performed sooner rather than later in those with worsening angina.

Myocardial infarction

The risk of fatal myocardial infarction is as high in diabetic people as in non-diabetics who have already suffered an infarct. Mortality from myocardial infarction is over twice as high as in matched non-diabetic controls, whether or not thrombolytic agents are used. About 75 per cent of diabetic patients are dead within 5 years of their first infarct, the main causes of death being heart failure and acute cardiogenic shock.

Primary prevention

Independent risk factors—hypertension, dyslipidaemia, smoking, and obesity—must be treated energetically in all diabetic patients, and poor glycaemic control should be tightened even though this alone is unlikely to protect against coronary heart disease. Specific prophylactic therapy, comparable to secondary prevention measures (i.e. measures given after an initial infarct) in the non-diabetic population, is increasingly recommended for diabetic people with any evidence of ischaemic heart disease, because their risk of infarction is so high. This includes a cardioselective β-blocker (for example, atenolol or metoprolol) and/or an angiotensin converting

Table 10 Prevention and treatment of myocardial infarction in diabetic patients

Primary prevention
Optimize glycaemic control
Seek and treat hypertension
Seek and treat dyslipidaemia
Stop smoking
Aspirin in patients over 40 years

Acute myocardial infarction
Thrombolytic drugs (usual indications)
Tight glycaemic control (glucose 5–10 mmol/l) for at least 48 h: low-dose intravenous insulin infusion
Aspirin
β-Blocker or ACE inhibitor (if congestive heart failure or marked left ventricular dysfunction)

Secondary prevention
Aspirin
β-Blocker or ACE inhibitor (as above)
Statin, to maintain total cholesterol < 4.8 mmol/l
Optimize glycaemic control
Tight blood pressure control
Stop smoking
Consider coronary revascularization (angioplasty plus stent, or bypass grafting)

ACE, angiotensin converting enzyme.

enzyme inhibitor if echocardiography shows left ventricular dysfunction with an ejection fraction of less than 40 per cent. β-Blockers improve survival at least as much as in the general population; the case for angiotensin converting enzyme inhibitors is not yet proven in diabetes. Some authorities recommend aspirin in all diabetic patients over 40 years of age, although the dosage (75–300 mg/day) remains undecided.

Acute myocardial infarction should be managed as follows (Table 10):

- Thrombolytic drugs should be given; survival is improved at least as much as in the non-diabetic population. Proliferative retinopathy is not a contraindication, and the risk of intraocular haemorrhage is very low.

- Glycaemic control should be optimized during the acute episode. There is evidence that long-term survival is improved if intensive insulin treatment is started on admission of a diabetic patient and continued for some months afterwards. The Diabetes Mellitus Insulin Glucose Infusion in Acute Myocardial Infarction (DIGAMI) Study showed that late (> 1 year) cardiovascular deaths were significantly reduced by one-quarter (from 44 per cent to 33 per cent after 3 years) in hyperglycaemic patients who received an insulin–glucose infusion in the coronary care unit, followed by multiple daily subcutaneous insulin injections for 3 months. Follow-up studies in progress should identify which elements conferred protection; theoretical mechanisms include lowering of free fatty acid levels, which may worsen ischaemic myocardial damage. In the meantime, it is reasonable to control hyperglycaemia (aiming for 5–10 mmol/l) during the first 48 h in all known diabetic patients, and in those diagnosed diabetic at admission (blood glucose over 11 mmol/l, with HBA$_{1c}$ in the diabetic range). This can be done most easily with a simple sliding scale continuous intravenous insulin infusion as used to treat diabetic ketoacidosis (see above). Delivering insulin as a 1 U/ml solution with a syringe driver avoids unnecessary intravenous fluids—this is an important consideration, as heart failure is a common (and often fatal) complication of myocardial infarction in diabetic people. Alternatively, the (cumbersome) DIGAMI protocol can be used (see Malmberg K *et al.* in Further reading).

- Secondary prevention must include aspirin with a β-blocker and/or angiotensin converting enzyme inhibitors, as discussed above. Total cholesterol should be reduced to less than 4.8 mmol/l with a statin,

with the option of adding a fibrate to control residual hypertriglyceridaemia. Early echocardiography and exercise testing or equivalent stress testing are needed, followed when appropriate by coronary angiography and ultimately referral for coronary angioplasty and stenting or bypass grafting.

Stress-induced hyperglycaemia and myocardial infarction

The intense sympathetic discharge triggered by an infarct can push blood glucose acutely into the diabetic range in previously normoglycaemic individuals. Stress-induced hyperglycaemia can be distinguished from previously undiagnosed diabetes because the HBA$_{1c}$ will be normal. The acute management of these individuals is uncertain; they were classified as 'diabetic' in the DIGAMI Study and also enjoyed improved survival with intensive insulin therapy. Pending further information, a pragmatic strategy would be to control glycaemia tightly during the admission with intravenous insulin for 48 h as described above, and then to monitor blood glucose closely and treat any persistent hyperglycaemia with insulin.

Heart failure

This is common in diabetic people with ischaemic heart disease and is a major cause of death in those who suffer an infarct. In addition to ischaemia from coronary artery disease, a specific diabetic cardiomyopathy may contribute to failure, as left ventricular function may be impaired in the absence of obvious atheroma on coronary angiography. Various defects in contractility and calcium flux within cardiomyocytes have been identified in diabetic animal models, but their relevance to humans is not clear. Echocardiography may show specific abnormalities early in diastole as well as areas of dyskinesia and a reduced ejection fraction. Moderate or severe left ventricular dysfunction, with an ejection fraction of less than 40 per cent, should be treated with an ACE inhibitor.

Stroke

Cerebrovascular accidents, mostly embolic, are two to five times commoner in diabetics than in the general population. They are managed conventionally. As with myocardial infarction, a stroke can acutely raise blood glucose in both diabetic and non-diabetic people. Trials are currently under way to determine whether tight glycaemic control can also improve the outcome of a stroke in hyperglycaemic individuals; for the moment it seems reasonable to keep blood glucose within the range 7 to 10 mmol/l, with the early use of insulin (probably subcutaneously) if this proves difficult.

Peripheral vascular disease

This is very common in the legs, often with diffuse disease distally as well as in the iliac and femoral arteries. Consequences include intermittent claudication, pain at rest, and gangrene which is usually dry and may lead to the loss of one or more toes. Severe atheroma in the iliac arteries can cause the Leriche syndrome, with buttock claudication and erectile failure; the latter may also be due to involvement of the pudenal arteries.

Investigation and management are conventional. Intermittent claudication may improve with the simple advice to stop smoking and keep walking, but a shortening claudication distance or pain at rest require urgent investigation. Angiography often shows widespread atheroma, and this may preclude reconstructive surgery. Otherwise, standard operations such as femoral–popliteal bypass and the use of the saphenous vein *in situ* for more distal disease can achieve good results and must not be withheld from people simply because they have diabetes. Nonetheless, diabetes still accounts for about one-half of all non-traumatic leg amputations.

Patients with diabetic renal failure or autonomic neuropathy may show calcification of the artery walls, often easily visible in the digital arteries on plain radiography of the feet (Fig. 17 and Plate 2). This medial sclerosis (Mönckeberg's) is not directly related to atheroma, although the two often coexist.

Other manifestations of peripheral vascular disease include angina-like abdominal pain after eating, which is due to narrowing of the mesenteric artery, and renal artery stenosis which can contribute to hypertension and precipitate acute renal impairment soon after starting an angiotensin converting enzyme inhibitor.

Diabetic foot disease

The feet are at the mercy of various diabetic complications and problems such as ulceration and resistant deep infections often cause long and expensive hospital admissions. Ulceration and severe ischaemia leading to gangrene of the toes or forefoot are the commonest problems.

Diabetic foot disorders are best managed in a dedicated combined clinic. Prevention is extremely important. Many problems can be avoided by teaching the patients basic foot care, by regularly checking their feet and shoes, and by providing prophylactic chiropody and special footwear as appropriate. Charcot's arthropathy most commonly affects joints in the ankle or foot.

Neuropathy damages the foot through motor, sensory and autonomic involvement. Distal motor neuropathy alters the posture of the foot by weakening its small intrinsic muscles and allowing the unopposed action of

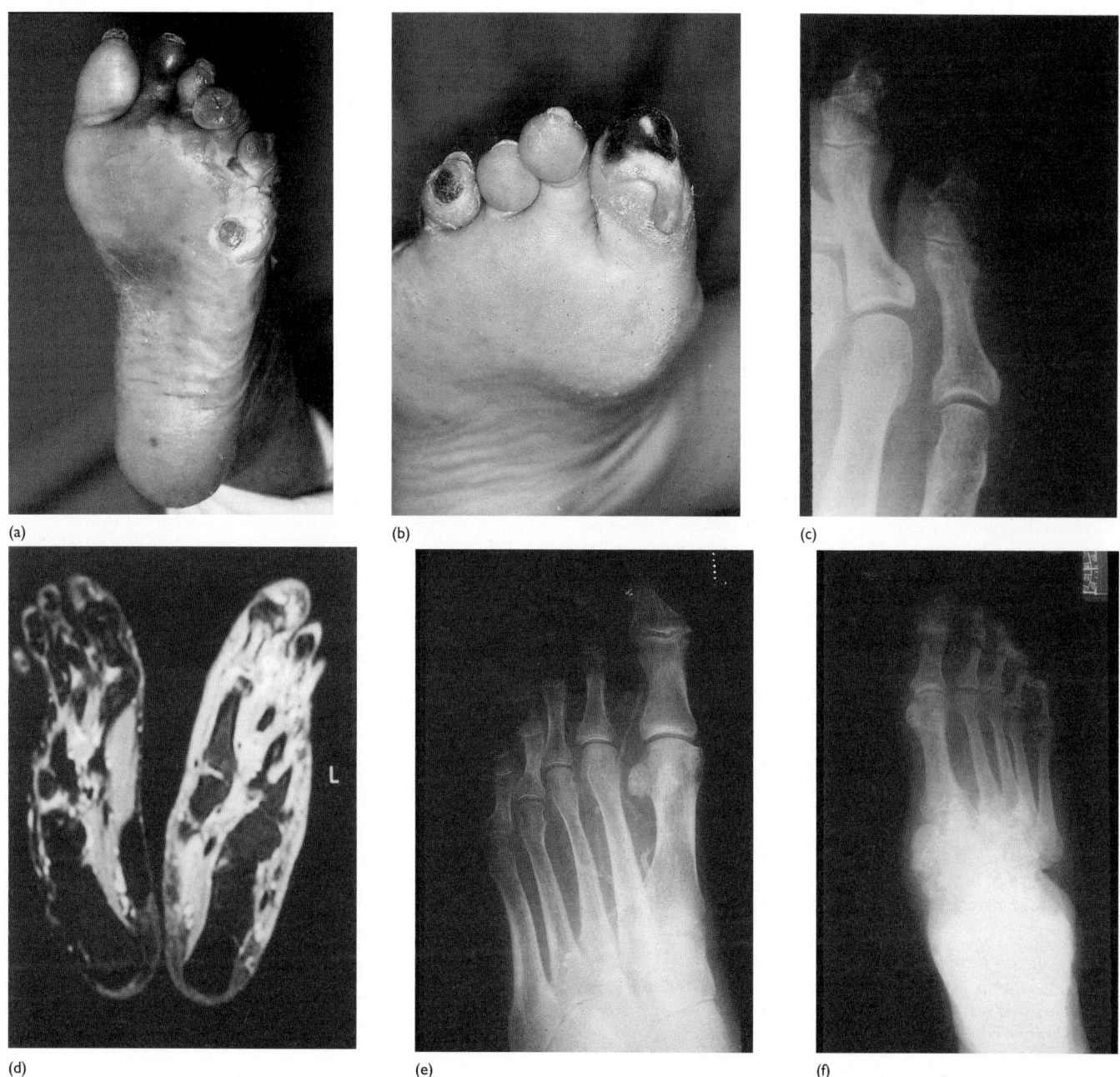

Fig. 17 The diabetic foot. (a) Typical punched-out neuropathic ulcer on the lateral aspect of the sole in an ischaemic foot with gangrene of the second, fourth, and fifth toes. (b) Ulceration and digital gangrene, caused by wearing tight shoes on a severely ischaemic foot. (c) Osteomyelitis in the diabetic foot. Early changes can be subtle: in this case, an erosion at the lateral edge of the distal end of the proximal phalanx of the fifth toe. ^{111}In-labelled white cell scanning showed an intense 'hot spot' at this site (with thanks to Dr Hans Laasch, Manchester Royal Infirmary). (d) Osteomyelitis affecting the proximal phalanx of the left big toe and the adjacent metatarsophalangeal joint, visible as an abnormally high signal on MR imaging. Associated oedema shows as a high signal in the surrounding soft tissues (with thanks to Dr King Sun Leong, Whiston Hospital). (e) Mönckeberg's medial sclerosis, outlining the digital arteries on this plain radiograph. (f) Charcot's arthropathy, showing massive destruction of the distal ankle joint. (See also Plate 2.)

the long extensors to claw the foot, concentrating pressure on the heel and the metatarsal heads. Shear forces generated by walking and shoes cause the skin over pressure points to thicken into callus; eventually, pressure damage leads to foci of liquefactive necrosis deep within the callus, and these break through to the surface to form an ulcer (Fig. 17).

Autonomic denervation opens up arteriovenous anastomoses, shunting blood to the skin—hence the warm skin and dilated veins of the neuropathic foot. Shunting may also deprive the tissue bed of oxygen and nutrients, thus worsening ischaemia from arterial disease. Increased blood flow may also be an initiating factor in Charcot's arthropathy (see below). Sensory denervation and loss of pain sensation can allow the foot to be damaged by agents such as over-tight new shoes, a drawing pin, or sharp stones in the shoe.

Ischaemia, due to peripheral vascular disease and possibly microvascular damage, can lead to ischaemic ulceration and to gangrene of the toes or forefoot (Fig. 17).

Foot ulceration

This is usually multifactorial, although one cause (for example, neuropathy) may initiate or dominate the process.

Trauma includes the normal wear and tear of walking in shoes and damage from foreign bodies, often undetected because of neuropathy. Inexpert do-it-yourself chiropody is another cause.

Infection commonly complicates diabetic foot ulcers, and often penetrates deep into the soft tissues and bone. Mixed organisms are usually responsible, including staphylococci, pseudomonas, and anaerobic organisms, sometimes gas-forming. Osteomyelitis is particularly ominous and requires urgent diagnosis and treatment (Fig. 17).

Clinical features of diabetic foot ulcers

Primary neuropathy and ischaemic ulcers can generally be distinguished as below, but careful examination of the whole foot is essential so that all the possible contributory causes can be adequately treated.

- Primarily neuropathic ulcers occur at high-pressure sites (heel, metatarsal heads) and appear cleanly punched out of the surrounding callus (Fig. 17). The foot may be numb, with or without neuropathic pain, and the ulcer is often painless and may not have been noticed by the patient. Typical neuropathic features including clawed posture of the foot, warm skin, and sensory loss.
- Ischaemic ulcers tend to affect the edges of the foot and are often painful. There may be a history of intermittent claudication, absent foot pulses, and cold skin, sometimes with obviously ischaemic toes or previous amputation (Fig. 17).
- Traumatic ulceration may hint at its causes, for example symmetrical damage across the toes and margins of the feet from tight shoes (Fig. 17).
- Infection may cause local signs of inflammation, although the skin may appear deceptively normal even over extensive and serious deep infection, and pain may be absent. Anaerobes and pseudomonas characteristically produce a foul smell, while gas formation may occasionally cause crepitus in the subcutaneous tissues.

Investigation of diabetic foot ulcers

Effective treatment depends on identifying the cause(s) of ulceration. Neuropathy and ischaemia are assessed and managed as above. Swabs or curettings from deep in the ulcer should be cultured for both aerobic and anaerobic organisms. Plain radiography of the foot may show gas in the soft tissues or osteomyelitis, which can be difficult to distinguish from Charcot's arthropathy; MRI scans and ^{111}In-labelled white cell scans are highly specific for infection (Fig. 17).

Management of diabetic foot ulcers

Predominantly neuropathic ulcers are treated by the chiropodist to remove callus, and the foot protected with a lightweight plaster cast to unload pressure from the affected area, which accelerates healing while keeping the patient mobile; this may need to be worn for several weeks. Extra-depth or custom-built shoes, or pressure-absorbing socks, will reduce pressure loading and help to prevent recurrence. Ischaemia is treated as above, aiming to avoid or limit amputation.

Infection must be treated with appropriate antibiotics and repeated cultures may be needed to ensure that mixed infections, especially including fastidious organisms and anaerobes, are completely covered. Soft-tissue infections may respond to oral broad spectrum antibiotics such as amoxicillin and flucloxacillin, or coamoxiclav, combined with metronidazole if anaerobic infection is suspected; deep infections and osteomyelitis may require some weeks of intravenous treatment with drugs such as clindamycin, and surgical debridement. Amputation may be needed in refractory cases.

Charcot's arthropathy

This is fortunately rare, affecting fewer than 0.5 per cent of diabetic patients. It usually occurs in those with dense peripheral neuropathy and profound sensory loss, often with symptomatic autonomic damage. Reduced pain sensation is assumed to favour traumatic damage, and acute flareups are often preceded by injuries, which may be apparently trivial. Interestingly, blood flow to the affected area is increased early in the Charcot process, possibly because sympathetic denervation allows dilation of arterioles supplying the bone; this may stimulate osteoclast activity and bone resorption.

The ankle and joints in the mid- and forefoot are most commonly affected; non-weight-bearing joints are very rarely involved. The natural history is variable but can lead to massive destruction of the articular surfaces and resorption of adjacent bone, often with a large effusion that can become acutely inflamed and mimic septic or inflammatory arthritis. In advanced cases, the joint degenerates into a 'bag of bones'. The process is generally painless, but acute flareups can cause discomfort. The most important differential diagnosis is from septic arthritis and osteomyelitis. Radiographic appearances are characteristic in advanced cases (Fig. 17), but may be ambiguous early on; [99]Tc[m] bone scans show increased uptake while the white cell scan is usually negative. Magnetic resonance imaging is probably best able to distinguish Charcot's arthropathy from osteomyelitis. An acutely inflamed joint may need to be aspirated to exclude infection, especially if systemic symptoms, neutrophilia, or raised erythrocyte sedimentation rate are present.

Treatment is often unsatisfactory. Non-steroidal anti-inflammatory drugs can provide symptomatic relief, while off-loading pressure with a plaster-cast boot may temporarily halt bone destruction, but neither appears to improve eventual outcome. Pamidronate may slow the disease process by inhibiting osteoclast activity. Surgery should be avoided if possible, because the Charcot process may then spread to neighbouring joints. Occasionally, amputation is the only option for a dangerously unstable or painful foot.

Other tissue complications of diabetes

Limited joint mobility, also known as the diabetic hand syndrome or cheiroarthropathy, is probably due to glycation of collagen and other connective tissue proteins. It is particularly common in type 1 diabetes, and may develop during childhood. It causes worsening flexion deformities of the fingers so that their palmar surfaces cannot be opposed when the hands are pushed together (the 'prayer sign'), often with Dupuytren's contracture. Median and ulnar nerve lesions, presumably compressive, are often associated. Rarely, thickening of skin over the metacarpophalangeal and interphalangeal joints causes Garrod's knuckle pads (Fig. 18 and Plate 3).

Necrobiosis (lipoidica diabeticorum) is strongly associated with diabetes, although 25 per cent of affected patients are normoglycaemic. Necrobiosis is the hyaline degeneration of collagen. The lesions present as trophic, non-scaling yellowish areas, often with telangiectasias (Fig. 19 and Plate 4). They are commonest on the shins but may appear elsewhere, slowly enlarge, and may perforate. Their progression is unrelated to gly-caemic control. Topical or locally injected steroids may be helpful. (The histologically similar granuloma annulare is not convincingly associated with diabetes.)

Diabetic dermopathy ('shin spots') is the commonest skin disorder in diabetic patients and is also seen in non-diabetic patients. These atrophic brownish or erythematous lesions, usually in the pretibial area, generally cause no problems and often resolve within a year or so.

Diabetic bullae (bullosis diabeticorum) are due to subepithelial splitting and present as tense and painful blisters which appear and heal within a few weeks. Differential diagnoses include pemphigoid.

Diabetic osteopenia: poorly controlled type 1 diabetes causes general loss of bone mineral, although this does not appear to increase fracture rate significantly. Plain radiographs of the feet may show low-density phalanges that taper and may be smoothly eroded— an appearance imaginatively described as resembling partly sucked candy.

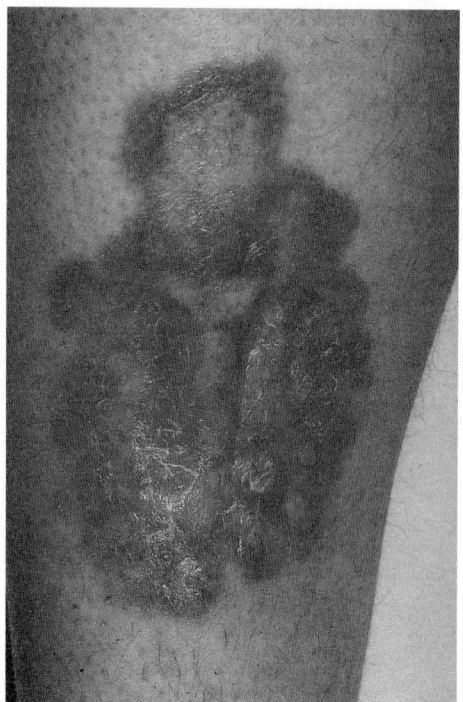

Fig. 19 Necrobiosis lipoidica diabeticorum (with thanks to Dr Geoff Gill, University Hospital, Aintree, Liverpool). (See also Plate 4.)

Further reading

American Diabetes Association (2000). Clinical practice recommendations 2000. *Diabetes Care* **23** (suppl. 1).

DeFronzo RA (1999). Pharmacologic therapy for type 2 diabetes mellitus. *Annals of Internal Medicine* **131**, 281–303.

European Diabetes Policy Group (1999). A desktop guide to type 2 diabetes mellitus. *Diabetic Medicine* **16**, 716–30.

Glaser N *et al.* (2001). Risk factors for cerebral edema in children with diabetic ketoacidosis. *New England Journal of Medicine* **344**, 264–9.

King H, Aubert RE, Hennan WH (1998). Global burden of diabetes, 1995–2025. Prevalence, numerical estimates, and projections. *Diabetes Care* **21**, 1414–31.

Malmberg K for the DIGAMI (Diabetes Mellitus Insulin Glucose Infusion in Acute Myocardial Infarction) Study Group (1997). Prospective randomized study of intensive insulin treatment on long-term survival after acute myocardial infarction in patients with diabetes mellitus. *British Medical Journal* **314**, 1512–15.

Pickup JC, Williams G, eds (2002). *Textbook of diabetes*, 3rd edn. Blackwell Science, Oxford. [Comprehensive, well-illustrated, and up to date for most clinical aspects of diabetes and its management.]

Ramsey LE *et al.* (1999). British Hypertension Society guidelines for hypertension management 1999: a summary. *British Medical Journal* **319**, 630–5.

Schade DS, Duckworth WC (1986). In search of the subcutaneous insulin resistance syndrome. *New England Journal of Medicine* **315**, 147–53.

Serup P, Madsen OD, Mandrup-Poulson T (2001). Islet and stem cell transplantation for treating diabetes. *British Medical Journal* **322**, 29–32.

Shapiro A *et al.* (2000). Islet transplantation in seven patients with type 1 diabetes mellitus using a glucocorticoid-free immunosuppressive regimen. *New England Journal of Medicine* **343**, 230–8.

The DECODE Study Group (1999). Glucose tolerance and mortality: comparison of WHO and American Diabetes Association diagnostic criteria. *Lancet* **354**, 617–21.

The Diabetes Control and Complications Trial Research Group (1993). The effect of intensive treatment of diabetes on the development and

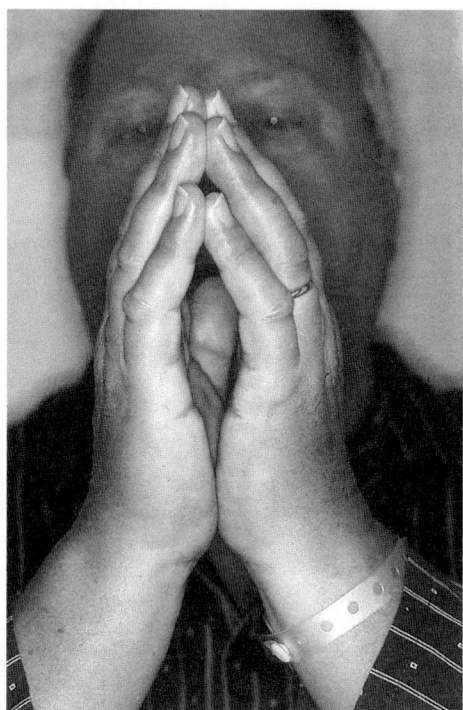

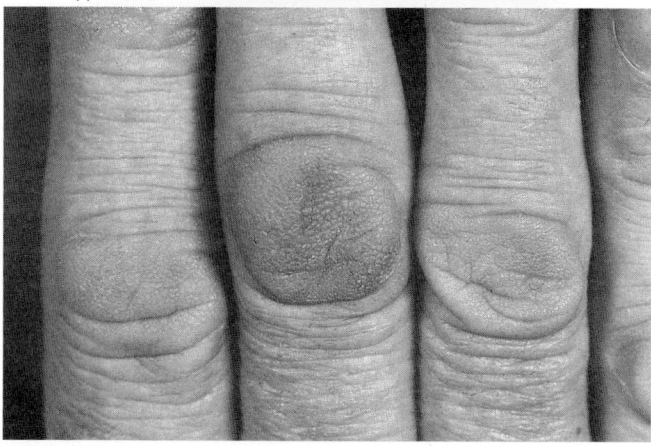

Fig. 18 The hands in long-standing diabetes. (a) Limited joint mobility (cheiroarthropathy), showing the 'prayer sign'. (b) Thickening of the skin over the knuckles and proximal interphalangeal joints (Garrod's pads). (See also Plate 3.)

progression of long-term complications in insulin-dependent diabetes mellitus. *New England Journal of Medicine* **329**, 977–86.

The Diabetes Control and Complications Trial Research Group (1995). Adverse events and their associations with treatment regimens in the Diabetes Control and Complications Trial. *Diabetes Care* **122**, 561–8.

UK Prospective Diabetes Study Group (1998). Tight blood pressure control and risk of macrovascular and microvascular complications in type 2 diabetes. *British Medical Journal* **317**, 703–13.

UK Prospective Diabetes Study Group (1998). Intensive blood glucose control with sulphonylureas or insulin compared with conventional treatment and risk of complications in patients with type 2 diabetes (UKPDS 33). *Lancet* **352**, 837–53.

Some useful websites

American Diabetes Association: www.diabetes.org

International Diabetes Federation: www.idf.org

Online Diabetes Resources: www.mendosa.com/faq.htm. Useful compendium of links covering clinical practice, research, and patient-based organizations.

Diabetes UK: www.diabetes.org.uk

United Kingdom Prospective Diabetes Study: www.drl.ox.ac.uk

12.11.2 The genetics of diabetes mellitus

J. A. Todd

Type 1 diabetes

Type 1 is the most severe form of diabetes, with acute onset, often in children. Within white European populations, incidence varies from three cases/100 000 individuals in the population per year in Romania to over 45/100 000 per year in Finland. Its main cause is a massive and irreversible destruction of the islet β cells by the body's own immune system, in an immune-mediated autoimmune response. Life-threatening insulin deficiency results. The median age at diagnosis is about 12 years. However, as many as 25 per cent of cases are now diagnosed under age 5 years and the disease can still be diagnosed over age 60 years

The immune attack of the islets probably begins, in most cases, before age 2 years, even though diagnosis may not occur until many years later. Most autopsy pancreas samples from children who died during acute onset of the disease show immune infiltration, especially cytotoxic T lymphocytes. Newly diagnosed patients and subjects in families with the disease are positive for autoantibodies against several proteins expressed in β cells. The first of these autoantibodies to appear are those against the insulin molecule itself, and current knowledge indicates that it is a primary, aetiological antigen in β-cell destruction. The immune-mediated nature of the disease is also supported by the observations that the immunosuppressant, cyclosporin, can alter the disease course and that it very strongly associated genetically with the T lymphocyte activation genes, the HLA class II genes. The disease is clustered in families, along with other immune-mediated diseases such as thyroid disease and rheumatoid arthritis. Spontaneous rodent models of type 1 diabetes also indicate that immune-mediated destruction of β cells underlies type 1 diabetes. Most importantly, the disease can be transferred from diabetic mice to healthy recipients using T lymphocytes only. It is unlikely that the β cells themselves are passive targets of a dysregulated immune system and resistance to type 1 diabetes may well involve genes expressed in β cells.

The factors that determine the initiation and duration of the, often long, prodromal phase before diagnosis are unknown. In many countries, the incidence of type 1 diabetes is increasing dramatically, two to three-fold over the last 20 to 30 years, particularly in children under age 5 years. This cannot be due a change in the gene pool and must reflect an increasingly permissive environment. Diet and infection have both been implicated, by analogy with conditions such as coeliac disease, in which gluten is the major triggering factor, but as yet no major factor has been identified. The role of the environment cannot be underestimated. Nevertheless, there can be very few cases with a purely environmental aetiology as at least 95 per cent of cases possess the known disease-associated alleles at the major locus, the HLA class II genes. The HLA genotype is a necessary factor but not a sufficient one to explain disease occurrence. Environmental factors (not best described as 'triggers') are probably not necessary and are definitely not sufficient, but because we live lifestyles with numerous diet and infection exposures they undoubtedly play a role in most cases, either in disease initiation or precipitation in individuals genetically predisposed to the disease. It is likely that no single type 1 diabetes non-HLA gene is necessary; it remains to be determined whether combinations of non-HLA alleles is necessary. Even if the genotype of individuals is identical (monozygotic twins or inbred strains of mice) and the environment shared, for example inbred diabetic mice in a animal facility with highly regulated and uniform, infection-free environment, there is a large discordance in disease occurrence owing to unknown stochastic or random developmental factors. Despite a fully disease-permissive environment and genotype, disease might still not develop.

Disease inheritance

Type 1 diabetes is classified as a multifactorial or complex disease and not a single-gene or simple mendelian disease because possession of the disease genotype does not guarantee development of the disease—the penetrance of the genotype is less than 100 per cent. Most evidently, only 25 to 70 per cent of genetically-identical twins both develop type 1 diabetes. The disease is strongly inherited but this inheritance is complex.

By analysis of the occurrence of disease in families, the mode of inheritance was modelled most parsimoniously by a single major locus in combination with many other loci but with lesser individual effect than the major locus. This is referred to as a 'polygenic background'. It has its roots in the classical theory of the genetics of continuous traits or phenotypes for which numerous alleles, each with small effect, contribute to the overall (disease) phenotype. The transmission of disease in families, measured as the risk of disease, follows a distinctive pattern: a rapid non-linear decline in risk from first-degree relatives (6 per cent) to third-degree relatives, at which point the risk is not much different from the risk in the general population (0.4 per cent). A simple, single-gene disease exhibits a linear decline in risk. The rapid decline in risk in type 1 diabetes families is explained by the need for susceptibility alleles at several loci to be present simultaneously. Hence, marriage of a susceptible family member to a carrier of a non-susceptibility allele at one of the disease-associated loci can substantially reduce risk. An analogy is the removal of one can in a pyramid of cans resulting in collapse of the entire pile. Multigenerational families with type 1 diabetes are very rare due to this polygenic inheritance.

Molecular genetics

The major locus, at the HLA region on chromosome 6p21, is not due to allelic variation in one gene, but in several genes that can be epistatic with each other. Such complexity can only be verified by finding the actual disease loci and identifying the relevant functions of their products. A necessary step in this process is to estimate how major is the major locus. These estimates, unfortunately, depend on which genetic model is assumed and include estimates of the contribution of HLA to the clustering of type 1 diabetes in families ranging from 40 to 70 per cent. In addition, HLA-identical siblings develop type 1 diabetes less frequently than identical twins, indicating the modifying effect on HLA disease genes by non-HLA genes across the genome.

Advances in technology, and painstaking collection of data from families with two or more affected siblings, the only type of multiplex families actually available, have allowed direct evaluation of the relative contributions of different regions of the genome to familial clustering. This is referred to as linkage analysis, in which the siblings share diabetes and they also share the chromosome regions that cause the diabetes more often than expected by chance (assuming random transmission of alleles under Mendel's laws). The first genome-wide searches for linkage showed conclusively that type 1 diabetes is a major locus disease because no convincing loci other than HLA were found, despite good statistical power. This is not the case for other, closely related autoimmune diseases such as rheumatoid arthritis, autoimmune thyroid disease, or multiple sclerosis in which, although the HLA region is linked to disease, its effect is not as dominating as in type 1 diabetes. In these three diseases, it appears that no single locus has a major effect. Yet, because adopted unrelated children brought up in families with multiple sclerosis have the same risk as a randomly selected member of the general population, it is certain that familial clustering is due to shared alleles. There are, however, many disease loci (with susceptibility or resistance alleles) scattered across the genome. This situation presents a practical problem in that genes of small effect require hundreds, if not thousands, of sib-pairs to achieve convincing statistical support for deviation from random allele sharing. Except in the context of international consortia combining data sets, or perhaps in certain populations such as Iceland where remarkable family records are available, this is not feasible.

Association studies

Genes for both rare, mendelian diseases and common, complex diseases can be detected and precisely mapped by analysing the sharing of alleles by unrelated cases compared to unaffected controls. This is referred to as association or linkage disequilibrium mapping. It assumes that a proportion of living cases have inherited the same mutation from the original person in whom the disease-predisposing mutation or polymorphism arose. Cases (and controls) that carry the allele of the mutation share not only this allele but also the flanking DNA. If the mutation arose very recently in the population then the amount of flanking DNA associated with the mutation will be much larger than if, for example, the mutation predated the colonization of Europe. This is because homologous recombination of chromosomes will not have had enough time to break up the physical linkage between the mutation allele and alleles of the flanking loci that were present at the time when the mutation occurred. When recombination events between nearby loci have recombined their alleles completely, such that combinations of alleles at neighbouring loci (haplotypes) occur at frequencies no different from that expected by chance (that is the product of the allele frequencies observed in the population), then the alleles are said to be in linkage equilibrium. When alleles occur together non-randomly, they are said to be in linkage disequilibrium.

Whereas 2000 evenly spaced, biallelic or single nucleotide polymorphisms are sufficient to search the genome for chromosome regions that show linkage to disease, over 100 000 are required to probe the genome for chromosome regions or markers that are so close to a disease causal variant that the marker alleles and the disease locus alleles are in association or linkage disequilibrium. The density of polymorphic markers will depend on the demographic history of the population and the particular region of the genome. Single nucleotide polymorphisms occur as frequently as 1 per 1000 base pairs of DNA, so that as many as 3 million polymorphisms occur in the genome. Technologies are being developed that are capable of carrying out hundreds of thousands of assays to identify alleles at polymorphic loci across the genome, especially those that occur in the regions of genes that either encode proteins or determine their expression. By resequencing the human genome from tens of individuals, hundreds of thousands of polymorphisms are being identified and mapped onto the first draft of the sequence.

Until the ability to generate and type dense maps of polymorphic markers from large chromosome regions is a reality, both technically and economically, geneticists are restricted to focusing efforts on candidate genes—genes for which the expression or presumed function might be of relevance to the development of the disease. This more limited approach has historically been moderately successful. The candidate gene-association approach was used to identify the only two known genes for type 1 diabetes, the HLA class II genes and the repetitive DNA polymorphism in the 5' regulatory region of the insulin gene, on chromosomes 6p21 and 11p15, respectively (designated *IDDM1* and *IDDM2*). As marker typing technology improves, candidate genes will be analysed in much larger numbers.

Linkage studies in type 1 diabetes are continuing and meta-analyses of over 1000 affected sib-pair families are underway. This number of families provides the statistical power to detect disease loci with intermediate effects. Chromosome regions that show significant evidence of linkage to disease will be subjected to a more systematic association analysis in which very dense maps of polymorphisms will be developed, in the order of several single nucleotide polymorphisms per 10 kb of DNA, and typed in cases, controls, and families to find disease-associated regions that explain the linkage of the broader chromosome region to the disease. This is still a daunting task given current technology. Disease-linked chromosome regions usually encompass 15 cM to 15 Mb of DNA, indicating that at least 1500 evenly spaced polymorphic markers might have to be typed before the disease locus is located. This assumes that the linked region contains one disease locus, which seems unlikely given data from the mouse model of type 1 diabetes, and the fact that thousands of genes function in the immune system, for which a high polymorphism is beneficial in the defence against infection. Before embarking on such studies, it will be necessary to be confident that the evidence for linkage of the chromosome region to disease is convincing (P, probability, value less than 2×10^{-5}) and that the association study has sufficient statistical power to detect the association at P values in the range of 10^{-5} to 10^{-8}. These low P values take into account the very large number of tests carried out in studies of this kind. If a linked region contains several disease genes and each has several alleles, some or all which might be rare (1–5 per cent allele frequency in the population), then the prospects for sufficiently powerful studies are not favourable. If association studies are undertaken without prior evidence of linkage then, in the absence of convincing data implicating the function of the gene in disease, P values in the order of 10^{-8} are required to achieve results significant at the 5 per cent level (P = 0.05), taking into account the hundreds of thousands of tests that would be conducted across the whole genome. This assumes that hundreds of thousands of polymorphic markers, or at least all markers required to detect all haplotypes and constitute a continuous linkage disequilibrium map across the entire genome, have been typed in the study or are anticipated to be typed in future studies worldwide. Until technology is available that can tackle a 'whole genome association analysis' studies will be restricted to candidate genes or chromosome regions linked to disease.

Type 1 diabetes genes

We know the identity of two of the genes (termed insulin-dependent diabetes mellitus, IDDM, genes): *IDDM1* is comprised of a number of genes of related function, the human leucocyte antigen (HLA) class II genes, encoded in tandem in the major histocompatibility complex on chromosome 6p21. The *HLA-DQB1*, *-DQA1*, and *-DRB1* loci act as a 'superlocus' in disease with many alleles at the three different, but adjacent and homologous, loci interacting in epistatic ways. Their products allow T lymphocytes to recognize foreign and self-proteins in the form of peptide bound to the surface-expressed HLA class II molecules. They ensure that the body's immune system can recognize self-proteins and remain tolerant to them. Certain alleles, the most potent of which are referred to collectively as DR3 and DR4, are permissive for the anti-β-cell immune response, whereas other alleles, such as DR2, are dominantly protective against type 1 diabetes. The precise mechanisms underlying HLA class II mediated susceptibility and resistance are still uncertain. Moreover, this information, concerning a necessary and key step in disease pathogenesis, has not been translated into a way of modulating disease susceptibility. Although the translation of genetic–physiological research results such as these into therapy is the main goal, early attempts to block or modify HLA class II function directly in autoimmune disease have not been successful.

The second locus is referred to as *IDDM2*, now identified as a polymorphic DNA sequence composed of repeats of short oligonucleotides embedded in the 5' regulatory region of the insulin gene on chromosome 11p15. The two main variants of this polymorphism differ in size (that is number of repeats), sequence, and in their regulation of expression of the insulin gene. This differential regulation of insulin at the transcriptional level varies according to the tissue; very low levels of insulin are expressed in the thymus, the organ in which HLA class II molecules mediate the establishment and maintenance of immune tolerance. The type 1 diabetes protective allele of the insulin gene 5' repeat polymorphism is associated with increased expression of insulin (and its precursor preproinsulin) in the thymus. Since insulin is a key autoantigen in type 1 diabetes, a plausible model for the physiological action of this polymorphism in disease protection is increased tolerance to insulin and its precursors owing to their increased expression, and consequently HLA class II molecule-mediated immune tolerance. Peptides from insulin (and/or its precursors) bind to the HLA class II molecules in the generation of a healthy, β-cell tolerant T lymphocyte repertoire. This model fits much of the available data, particularly from rodent models of the disease. There are, however, missing links; for example the precise peptides involved, the affinity with which they bind to different HLA class II allotypes, and the consequences of these events for the immune system downstream of the HLA class II peptide T lymphocyte antigen receptor are uncertain. Again, it is not clear how this presumed pathway can be modulated to restore immune function to a level at which an individual is resistant to disease. This challenge is particularly acute since the very first events in disease and in immune tolerance may occur before age 2 years.

The risk of carrying disease-susceptible HLA class II and insulin gene alleles does not exceed 30 per cent. Informing a family member or an individual of this risk is not useful, and maybe harmful, in the absence of a safe way to modulate this risk and restore normal function. In a research context, the longitudinal follow-up of children from birth who carry the HLA susceptibility alleles or have type 1 diabetic parents could provide insights into the environmental factors that determine the development of the disease. The typing of protective alleles, such as HLA DR2, or more precisely the DQB1*0602 allele, already has some diagnostic benefit in clinical trials to prevent the disease. Positivity for the protective allele provides a criterion for exclusion from a trial, since DR2/DQB1*0602 positive subjects are at least 50 times less likely to develop type 1 diabetes than a randomly selected member of the population.

Current research

The search is proceeding for other type 1 diabetes genes using the genetic approaches of linkage and association. In concert with these efforts new tools are being applied, including the mass, parallel analysis of gene transcription using microarrays, the analysis of protein expression and modification using mass spectroscopy, the analysis of events *in vivo* using imaging techniques, and the investigation of cell metabolism using nuclear magnetic resonance spectroscopy. These approaches, in combination, will provide further details of immune system and islet cell physiology in the search for pathways and pathway–environmental factor interactions that could be

manipulated to prevent the disease or rejection of transplanted islets or β cells.

Further reading

Bach JF (1994). Insulin-dependent diabetes mellitus as an autoimmune disease. *Endocrinology Reviews* 15, 516–42.

Pipeleers D, Ling Z (1992). Pancreatic beta cells in insulin-dependent diabetes. *Diabetes and Metabolism Reviews* 8, 209–27.

Risch NJ (2000). Searching for genetic determinants in the new millennium. *Nature* 405, 847–56.

Rose NR, Mackay IR, eds (1998). *The Autoimmune Diseases*, 3rd edn. Academic Press, San Diego.

Strachan T, Read AP (1999). *Human molecular genetics 2*, 2nd edn. BIOS Scientific Publishers, Oxford.

Tisch R, McDevitt H (1996). Insulin-dependent diabetes mellitus. *Cell* 85, 291–7.

Todd JA (1999). From genomics to aetiology in a multifactorial disease, type 1 diabetes. *Bioessays* 21, 164–74.

Weiss KM, Terwilliger JD (2000) How many diseases does it take to map a gene with SNPs? *Nature Genetics* 26, 151–7.

12.11.3 Hypoglycaemia
V. Marks

Introduction

Hypoglycaemia means low blood glucose concentration (<3.0 mmol/l). It is not a disease entity but a biochemical abnormality whose importance lies in its effects upon brain function. These are responsible, directly or indirectly, for the signs and symptoms produced by hypoglycaemia and often provide the first clue to the presence of curable or preventable disease.

The brain obtains glucose from the blood by means of facilitated transport and mainly utilizes the glucose-transporting protein GLUT 1. The activity of this protein is increased by hypoglycaemia and reduced by hyperglycaemia. It is not insulin-dependent. Although blood glucose concentration is the single most important factor determining glucose availability to the brain, it is not the only one. Indeed there is a poor correlation between blood glucose concentration and the severity and nature of cerebral symptoms—especially in diabetic patients. It is therefore important to distinguish hypoglycaemia, a description of blood glucose, from neuroglycopenia, which is responsible for the signs and symptoms to which hypoglycaemia gives rise.

Four distinct, but not mutually exclusive, neuroglycopenic syndromes are recognized:

1. Acute neuroglycopenia, the most common, is normally associated with iatrogenic and experimental hypoglycaemia and is characterized by profuse sweating, anxiety/nervousness, tremor, tachycardia, hunger, and paraesthesia—all of which can be attenuated by adrenergic and cholinergic blockade—and by speech and visual disturbances, unsteady gait, confusion, and a sense of fatigue, which are independent of the autonomic nervous system.

2. Subacute neuroglycopenia occurs in most varieties of spontaneous hypoglycaemia and, when it occurs in insulin-treated diabetic subjects,

363

is called hypoglycaemia unawareness. It is characterized by a reduction in spontaneous movements and speech, somnolence, inefficient cerebration and work performance, personality change, and amnesia of varying severity. Other signs and symptoms common to acute and subacute neuroglycopenia include transient hemiplegia, hypo- or hyperthermia, convulsions, diploplia, and strabismus. The symptoms of both acute and subacute neuroglycopenia are ephemeral but, unless aborted by restoration of normoglycaemia, can progress to stupor, coma, or, in exceptional cases, death from cerebral oedema.

3. Chronic neuroglycopenia is rare and virtually confined to patients with hypoglycaemia due to insulinoma or diabetic patients over-zealously treated with insulin. It is characterized by insidious changes in personality, defective memory, psychosis—often with paranoid features—or mental deterioration resembling dementia.

4. Hyperinsulin neuronopathy, the clinical features of which may be mistaken for motor neurone disease, is a form of chronic neuroglycopenia. Temporary elevation of the blood glucose level has no discernible effect on cerebral or neuronal function but removal of the causative agent often does over the course of a year or two.

Experimental and iatrogenic hypoglycaemia

There is a hierarchy in the activation of brain centres as hypoglycaemia develops which is, however, not often observed in spontaneous hypoglycaemia. The tissue most sensitive to a falling blood glucose level is the normal pancreatic β-cell which virtually ceases secreting insulin as blood glucose concentrations fall to about 4.0 to 4.2 mmol/l. The sympathetic nervous system is activated and glucagon is secreted as the blood glucose concentration reaches about 3.7 mmol/l. Stimulation of growth hormone secretion occurs at glucose levels of about 3.5 mmol/l and that of ACTH and cortisol at about 3.3 mmol/l. The threshold for vasopressin release has not been determined. Most subjects experience symptoms only after their blood glucose concentration has fallen below 3 mmol/l but objective evidence of minor cognitive impairment, of which the subject is usually completely unaware, occurs at concentrations nearer 4 mmol/l.

Patients, whether diabetic or not, with recent experience of hypoglycaemia often tolerate lower blood glucose levels before symptoms develop and counter-regulatory hormones are secreted. They remain, however, just as sensitive to the deleterious effect of hypoglycaemia on cognitive function.

Some of the cerebral symptoms of neuroglycopenia and effects upon neuronal viability are due to liberation of the excitatory amino acids, glutamate and aspartate, rather than solely to decreased intracellular energy production.

Definition

Hypoglycaemia is defined arbitrarily by the blood glucose concentration; it is not determined by whether symptoms are present or not. For most purposes, an arterial (or capillary) blood glucose concentration below 3.0 mmol/l can be considered diagnostic of hypoglycaemia and one of 2.5 mmol/l or less pathological and demanding of investigation as to cause. The possibility that a patient's symptoms are of neuroglycopenic origin should not be dismissed solely on the basis of blood glucose concentration. Normoglycaemic neuroglycopenia must be considered.

Classification

Iatrogenic hypoglycaemia as a consequence of insulin or sulphonylurea treatment for diabetes is common and accounts for most hypoglycaemia encountered in practice. It seldom presents diagnostic difficulties. There are, on the other hand some 100 or so causes of spontaneous hypogly-

caemia, all of which are rare. Collectively, they are responsible for 0.1 per cent of all patients arriving in accident and emergency or medical investigation departments.

Table 1 lists the main causes of hypoglycaemia, which vary in frequency from country to country. Although all may occur in infants and children,

Table 1 Principal causes of hypoglycaemia

Induced
Insulin: iatrogenic, accidental, factitious, felonious
Sulphonylurea: iatrogenic, accidental, factitious, felonious

Spontaneous
Pancreatic causes
  Insulinoma: benign, malignant, multiple, and microadenomatosis
  Insular hyperplasia: nesidioblastosis or functional hyperinsulinism
  Pluriglandular syndrome
  Pancreatitis
Extrapancreatic IGF-II secreting neoplasms
  Mesenchymal tumours
  Haemangiopericytoma
  Primary hepatic carcinoma
  Adrenal tumour
  Various other carcinomas
Autoimmune hypoglycaemia
  Autoimmune insulin syndrome (AIS)
  Anti-insulin receptors
  Pancreatic 'Graves' disease
Toxic hypoglycaemia
  Alcohol
  Drugs, e.g. pentamidine, quinine, paracetamol
  Poisons, e.g. mushrooms
Alimentary (reactive) hypoglycaemia
  Postgastrectomy
  Alcohol-provoked reactive hypoglycaemia
  Non-insulinoma pancreatogenic hypoglycaemia
  Idiopathic postprandial syndrome
Organ failure
  Acute and chronic hepatocellular disease
  'End-stage' kidney disease
  Congestive cardiac failure
  Acute respiratory failure
Endocrine disease
  Pituitary insufficiency: generalized or specific, e.g. selective ACTH deficiency
  Adrenocortical insufficiency: congenital or acquired
  Hypothyroidism
  Selective hypothalamic insufficiency
  Phaeochromocytoma
Inborn errors of metabolism
  Hepatic glycogen storage diseases
  Hereditary fructose intolerance (HFI) and galactosaemia
  Disorders leading to defective gluconeogenesis (e.g. fructose 1,6 bisphosphatase deficiency)
  Disorders of mitochondrial β-oxidation (e.g. medium-chain acyl CoA dehydrogenase deficiency, MCAD).
Hypoglycaemia of the newborn
  Transient hyperinsulinaemic hypoglycaemia
  Persistent hyperinsulinaemic hypoglycaemia (nesidioblastosis)
  Hypoinsulinaemic hypoglycaemia of the newborn
Miscellaneous causes
  Bacterial, viral, and parasitic infections, especially malaria
  Diseases of the nervous system
  Prolonged carbohydrate deprivation: starvation, anorexia nervosa
  Excessive exercise (especially in combination with certain drugs)
  Chronic renal dialysis

the main causes of hypoglycaemia in this age group are not usually encountered in adults.

Presentation

Patients classically present either to accident and emergency in a stuporose or comatose state with concurrent hypoglycaemia or to outpatient departments with a normal blood glucose level but a history suggestive of recurrent neuroglycopenic episodes or progressive neurological/psychological dysfunction.

Management of the stuporose/comatose hypoglycaemic patient

Hypoglycaemia should be suspected in any case of altered consciousness, coma, hemiplegia, apparent alcoholic intoxication, or epilepsy, and eliminated or supported (though not established) by a point-of-care blood glucose determination. The diagnosis is confirmed by formal laboratory glucose analysis. Hypoglycaemia may also be caused by, and contribute to the symptomatology of, congestive cardiac failure, liver or kidney disease, malaria, and other severe infections. Management falls quite clearly into two separate phases.

Emergency treatment

Glucose 25 g (50 ml of 50 per cent w/vol) should be given intravenously to alleviate hypoglycaemia after sufficient venous blood (20 to 30 ml) has been withdrawn for subsequent laboratory analysis to determine its cause. Glucagon 1 mg may be given intramuscularly if venous access is not available, especially in cases of iatrogenic hypoglycaemia (in which it is usually effective).

Recovery of consciousness ordinarily occurs within 10 min. A further injection of 25 g glucose plus 100 mg hydrocortisone is indicated if recovery is delayed beyond 20 min. Specific measures to reduce brain swelling must be introduced if recovery does not occur within a further 20 min.

Prolonged, formerly called irreversible, hypoglycaemic coma is due to cerebral oedema and a consequence of profound hypoglycaemia generally lasting 5 h or more. Its treatment includes the use of intravenous mannitol and dexamethasone. Blood glucose must be monitored constantly and sufficient glucose infused to keep it within the range 5 to 10 mmol/l until consciousness is restored or permanent brain damage established. In cases of suicidal insulin or sulphonylurea overdose, glucose in doses up to 80 g/h given as a 25 to 50 per cent solution through a central line may be required.

Investigation

The second stage and third stages are similar to those employed in investigating patients suspected of suffering from a hypoglycaemic disorder but currently asymptomatic (Fig. 1).

Management of the asymptomatic patient suspected of having a hypoglycaemic disorder

Diagnosis takes place in three sequential stages:

(1) suspicion of hypoglycaemia and its confirmation by measurement of the blood glucose concentration during a 'spontaneous' neuroglycopenic episode;

(2) determination of its aetiology on the basis of specific investigative procedures;

(3) localization of the lesion responsible if the hypoglycaemia has an anatomicopathological rather than a purely metabolic aetiology.

Confirmation of hypoglycaemia

Most patients, excepting those presenting in stupor or coma, are normoglycaemic and asymptomatic when first seen. Suspicion of hypoglycaemia is aroused by a history of subacute neuroglycopenia, that is episodes of altered behaviour or disturbed consciousness or, in a minority of cases, symptoms suggestive only of acute neuroglycopenia. Because of the nature of their illness, patients are often unable to supply a reliable history of their condition.

Exclusion or confirmation that a patient's symptoms are hypoglycaemic in origin can often be achieved by teaching them, or their relatives, to collect capillary blood during spontaneous symptomatic episodes occurring in the course of everyday life. Blood collected into specially prepared tubes or filter paper should be sent to the laboratory for glucose analysis since point-of-care monitoring systems are insufficiently reliable in the hypoglycaemic range to warrant initiation of detailed investigation and may cause confusion. A blood glucose concentration during a symptomatic episode greater than 3.5 mmol/l effectively eliminates hypoglycaemia as its cause. Glucose concentrations lower than this are unusual and require further investigation.

Hyperinsulinism

This is a misnomer for the syndrome to which insulinoma gives rise. It would better be called dysinsulinism since its hallmark is inappropriate rather than excessive secretion of insulin or proinsulin.

Insulinoma

Insulin-secreting tumours (insulinomas) are the most common type of neoplasm affecting the endocrine tissues of the pancreas. They have an incidence of one case or more per million of the population. Eighty per cent of insulinomas are benign and solitary, 7 to 10 per cent are multiple—often as part of the MEN 1 syndrome—and 8 to 10 per cent malignant. They occur at any age but are rare before the age of 10 and infrequently diagnosed after the age of 70. The lack of cases after age 70 may be due to their mode of presentation, which is often that of progressive dementia, rather than to their rarity. There is a 6:4 ratio in favour of women for benign but not for malignant tumours.

Insulinomas are composed mainly, or exclusively, of β-cells. Most are between 10 and 20 mm in diameter at diagnosis, though tumours as small as 5 mm in diameter have been associated with severe symptoms. Regardless of size, they occur at all sites in the pancreas with equal frequency.

Histological classifications, whilst valuable for the light they throw on insulin secretory mechanisms, contribute little to clinical management. Malignant insulin-secreting tumours are impossible to distinguish, clinically or histologically, from benign ones unless metastases are present. Some have the histological appearance of carcinoid tumours and both may contain and secrete other peptide hormones of which glucagon, somatostatin, ACTH, and GhRH are amongst the commonest. Only rarely, however, do these biochemical endocrinopathies manifest themselves clinically. There is no evidence that malignant tumours ever begin as benign tumours or that benign tumours ever become malignant.

The average time between the onset of symptoms and diagnosis of insulinoma is currently about a year but symptoms persisting over 30 years or more without evidence of permanent brain damage are not unknown. Diagnostic delays are usually due to reluctance by patients to seek help or failure by clinicians to suspect hypoglycaemia, rather than any difficulties in confirming the presence of an insulinoma once the possibility has been considered. Only very rarely is an insulinoma found at autopsy as the cause of unexplained death.

In a minority, probably not exceeding 1 to 2 per cent, functionally defective β-cells are distributed throughout the pancreas rather than in discrete tumours. Clinically and biochemically, such patients are indistinguishable from patients with insulinomas. Biologically, such patients resemble infants with persistent hyperinsulinaemic hypoglycaemia of infants (formerly nesidioblastosis).

Chemical pathology

Endogenous hyperinsulinism is characterized by failure of the abnormal β cells to stop secreting insulin in response to hypoglycaemia. This is ordinarily the most sensitive physiological response to a falling blood glucose concentration and becomes apparent at a level (4.2–4.0 mmol/l) well above the threshold for neuroglycopenic symptoms. A consequence of insulin secretion persisting during fasting is inhibition of hepatic glucose release and a gradual fall in blood glucose to below the level capable of sustaining normal brain function.

Paradoxically, the functionally abnormal β cells are often insensitive to hyperglycaemia *per se* and so produce glucose intolerance as well as fasting hypoglycaemia. They do, however, respond, often excessively, to other insulin secretagogues including glucagon, sulphonylureas, L-leucine, and the intestinal incretins GIP and GLP-1, and may therefore present with reactive rather than fasting hypoglycaemia.

Typically, plasma cortisol and growth hormone levels in patients with insulinomas are normal even in the presence of hypoglycaemia. This would ordinarily be considered evidence of hypothalamicopituitary insufficiency but responsiveness returns after restoration of permanent normoglycaemia. Plasma free fatty acid and β-hydroxybutyrate concentrations are typically suppressed (<600 μmol/l) but rise, though not to expected levels, during prolonged fasting.

Diagnosis

Diagnosis is made by demonstrating that the symptoms are caused by hypoglycaemia, provoked by fasting and/or rigorous exercise, relieved by intravenous glucose, and are caused by inappropriate insulin and/or proinsulin secretion. Plasma concentrations of total immunoreactive insulin, C-peptide, proinsulin, and proinsulin-like fragments are all high with regard to the prevailing blood glucose concentration but are not necessarily high in absolute (quantitative) terms.

Thus in the presence of concurrent hypoglycaemia (blood glucose less than 3 mmol/l), plasma total immunoreactive insulin concentrations of more than 30 pmol/l and C-peptide concentrations more than 100 pmol/l are inappropriately high. When both peptide levels are inappropriately high, a diagnosis of endogenous hyperinsulinism is virtually certain, providing sulphonylurea ingestion and various rare autoimmune diseases and infections, such as malaria, can be excluded. If hypoglycaemia is absent at

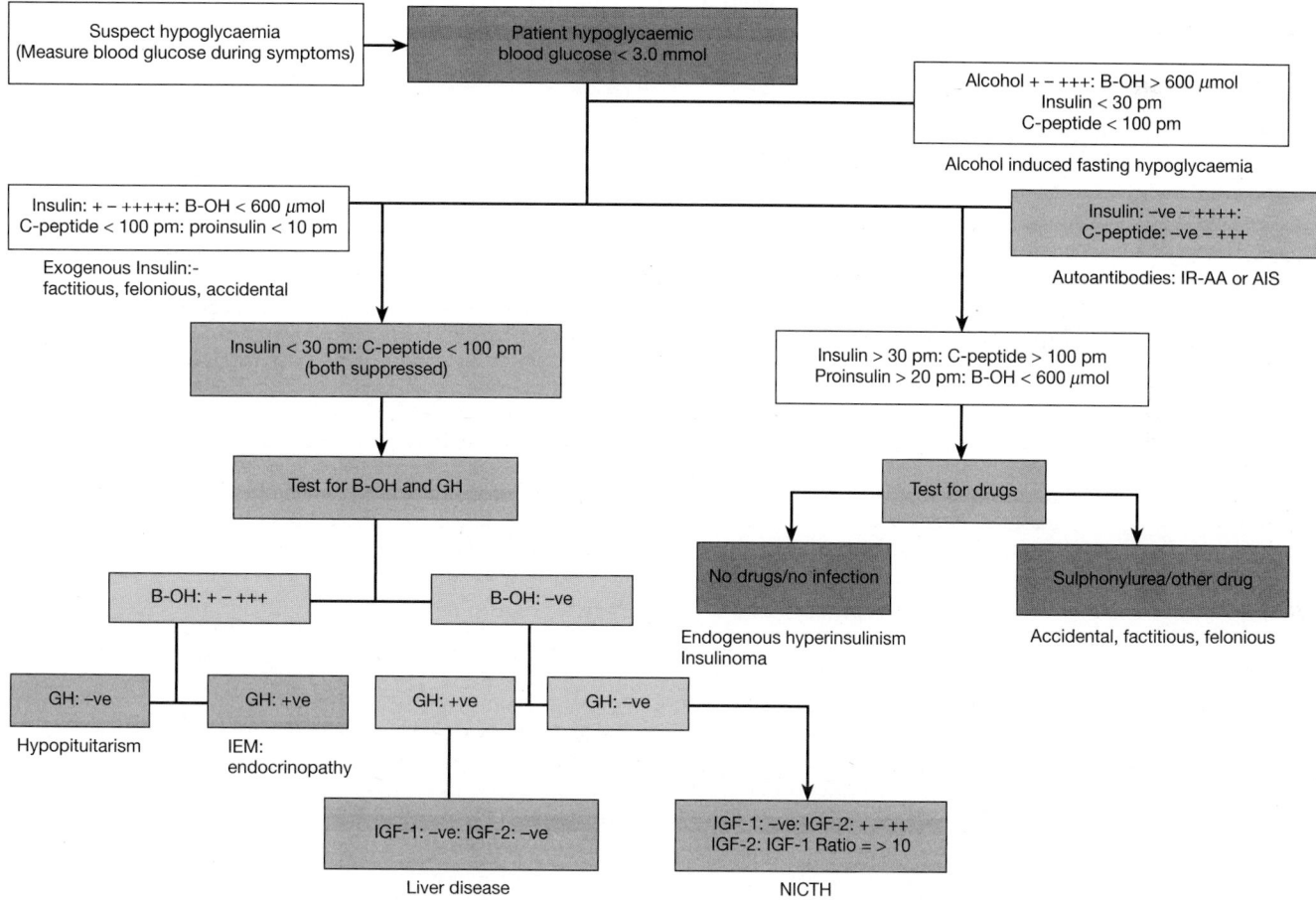

Fig. 1 Investigation of a patient suspected of suffering from hypoglycaemia who is hypoglycaemic (but not unwell from some other cause, e.g. congestive cardiac failure, septicaemia, liver or renal failure) at the time of examination. It is customary to measure plasma total insulin immunoreactivity (IRI), C-peptide, proinsulin, β-hydroxybutyrate, growth hormone, IGF-1 and IGF-2, alcohol, and sulphonyureas simultaneously or sequentially on the initial hypoglycaemic blood sample. + to ++++: insulin >30 to 300 000 pmol/l; C-peptide >150 to 10 000 pmol/l; proinsulin >20 pmol/l; GH ≥ 5 mU/l; BHB >600 μmol/l; alcohol ≥2 to 100 mmol/l. –ve: insulin <25 pmol/l; C-peptide <100 pmol/l; GH <1 mU/l; B-OH <600 μmol/l; IGF-1 < 10nmol/l; IGF-2 <45 nmol/l. Abbreviations: IEM = inborn errors of metabolism, NICTH = non-islet cell hypoglycaemia, GH = growth hormone, B-OH = β-hydroxybutyrate, IR-AA = insulin receptor autoantibodies, AIS = autoimmune insulin syndrome.

the time of sampling plasma insulin, C-peptide and proinsulin assays become uninterpretable.

Fasting under close observation for up to 72 h produces symptomatic hypoglycaemia with inappropriate hyperinsulinaemia (proinsulinaemia and C-peptidaemia) in over 98 per cent of insulinoma patients but not in healthy men and women who, if they do become hypoglycaemic, invariably have appropriately suppressed plasma insulin levels. As an alternative to prolonged fasting, the overnight fasted patient can be exercised to exhaustion on a treadmill. In insulinoma patients, this fails to produce the normal suppression of plasma insulin and C-peptide secretion. It is, however, rarely necessary to subject a patients to these tests, especially if investigations are restricted to those who have blood glucose levels below 3 mmol/l during spontaneous episodes occurring in every-day life. Dynamic function tests including oral glucose, tolbutamide, glucagon, L-leucine, and insulin–hypoglycaemia/C-peptide suppression tests are unnecessary for the diagnosis of hyperinsulinism.

Some 5 to 10 per cent of insulinomas secrete only, or mainly, proinsulin and thus the diagnosis may be missed if an insulin-specific assay, rather than one capable of detecting total immunoreactive insulin, is used. Moreover, unusually efficient extraction of insulin by the liver can lead to low plasma total immunoreactive insulin concentrations in peripheral blood in the presence of genuinely inappropriate insulin secretion. This can occur in infants with nesidioblastosis as well as in adults with endogenous hyperinsulinism in whom inappropriately high plasma C-peptide levels will confirm the diagnosis. Hyperproinsulinaemia, that is a plasma proinsulin concentration of greater than 20 pmol/l, is found in some 95 per cent of patients with endogenous hyperinsulinism; its absence should raise doubts about the accuracy of the diagnosis.

Pre- and intraoperative localization

A diagnosis of endogenous hyperinsulinism, established on the basis of inappropriate hyperinsulinaemia, is almost synonymous with one of insulinoma. The treatment of choice is surgical ablation. Localization by an experienced surgeon at laparotomy is remarkably (96 per cent) successful but can be further improved by use of intraoperative ultrasound.

Though virtually every imaging technique has been advocated for preoperative localization of insulinoma, none is sufficiently reliable to justify dismissing a diagnosis made on sound clinical and biochemical grounds. Endoscopic ultrasound, with a 90 per cent prediction rate, and pancreatic intra-arterial calcium injection with hepatic venous sampling are currently the only imaging techniques that are useful for localization prior to operation. Venous sampling is especially indicated when surgery has failed to reveal a tumour and/or diffuse islet hyperplasia is suspected. It is the only way of establishing a diagnosis of non-insulinoma pancreatogenic hypoglycaemia.

Treatment

Surgical ablation ensures an excellent prognosis with no reduction in life expectancy except when the tumour is malignant. Even then, since these tumours grow slowly and rarely spread beyond the liver, removal of the primary tumour, and as many hepatic secondaries as possible, may add years of useful life. Operative mortality for adenomas is under 2 per cent, except in the elderly. Benign tumours recur in up to 5 per cent of patients.

In patients over 70 years of age, and others in whom surgery is impracticable, treatment with diazoxide (200–600 mg/day) combined with chlorothiazide (1 g/day) to increase its effectiveness, is well tolerated. It is the treatment of choice in hyperinsulinism due to diffuse islet hyperplasia, non-insulinoma pancreatogenic hypoglycaemia, and after surgical debulking in cases of metastatic insulinoma. Only when diazoxide/chlorothiazide treatment fails to relieve hypoglycaemia are other drugs, such as octreotide, β-blockers, or calcium channel blockers worth trying. In patients with malignant insulinomas, embolization or surgical debulking of hepatic

metastases may produce remissions lasting several years—as may treatment with cytotoxic agents such as streptozotocin and 5-fluorouracil.

Non-islet cell tumour hypoglycaemia (NICTH)

The symptoms of hypoglycaemia produced by non-islet cell tumours (NICTH) may be indistinguishable from that of insulinoma. The symptoms are almost invariably those of subacute neuroglycopenia and the features of autonomic nervous activation are absent. Biochemically, NICTH is characterized by fasting hypoglycaemia, hypoketonaemia, and low plasma total immunoreactive insulin, C-peptide, and proinsulin levels. Growth hormone, ACTH, and glucagon secretion are depressed during both hypo- and normoglycaemia and plasma IGF-1 levels are always low—unlike in insulinoma when they are normal or high.

NICTH can occur with almost every histological type of malignant tumour but is rare. Although sarcomas are disproportionately well represented, less than 1 per cent of them develop hypoglycaemia. It is, however, common in patients with haemangiopericytomas, which are themselves rare. Amongst the carcinomas, no histological type is exempt from NICTH but only in primary hepatomas is it at all common.

Chemical pathology

Regardless of histological type, hypoglycaemia due to non-islet cell tumours (NICTH) results from overproduction of an abnormally large form of IGF-2. This has many of the biological and immunological properties of IGF-2 itself but binds less avidly to plasma IGF binding proteins (IGF-BP) of which there are at least six normally present in plasma.

Big IGF-2 is generated by the removal of a 24 amino acid leader sequence from the N-terminus of prepro IGF-2. Normally, it then undergoes cleavage at its carboxy terminus to produce regular IGF-2. Failure to do so leaves the E-domain intact and the secretion of big IGF-2—the cause of NICTH.

There is characteristically a marked reduction in the most plentiful of the plasma binding proteins, IGF-BP3, and a partial compensatory increase in IGF-BP2 the net effect of which is, however, to reduce IGF protein binding capacity. Consequently plasma 'free (big) IGF-2' is increased without any corresponding increase in total immunoreactive IGF-2.

The exact mechanism by which big IGF-2 produces hypoglycaemia is unknown and may involve several steps, the most important of which is activation of insulin and IGF receptors on peripheral tissues and their increased uptake of glucose. The next most important is suppression of glucagon and growth hormone secretion.

Ectopic insulin secretion

Ectopic insulinomas are confined to the duodenum and are rare (<1 per cent). Ectopic insulin production by a non-islet cell tumour is extremely rare and has been established in only one case and suggested in five others. The coincidence of an insulinoma and another type of tumour has been described rather more often.

Diagnosis

The diagnosis of NICTH is seldom in doubt once thorough investigations into the cause of hypoglycaemia have been initiated:

1. Hypoglycaemia, once it has developed, seldom remits for more than very brief periods after meals.

2. The tumours are usually, though not invariably, sufficiently large to reveal themselves either on physical examination or as a result of comparatively straightforward imaging.

In the laboratory, findings of low plasma insulin, C-peptide, and proinsulin concentrations (<30, <100, and <20 pmol/l respectively) in the presence of hypoglycaemia and hypoketonaemia are highly suggestive of

NICTH. Clinical laboratory assays typically measure both big and regular forms of IGF-2 and generally reported as normal (50–100 nmol/l) but IGF-I levels are invariably low (<10 nmol/l). Consequently, plasma IGF-2:IGF-1 ratios, expressed on a molar basis, are abnormally high (>10) and not seen in any other condition except gross undernutrition. Assays for the E-domain of proIGF-2 have been developed. Although useful for establishing recurrence, they provide less accurate initial diagnostic information than the IGF-2:IGF-1 ratio.

Treatment

Treatment of choice is surgical. In rare cases of benign tumour NICTH, the cure is permanent. In malignant cases, ablation or debulking of secondaries may produce prolonged remissions. Symptomatic relief may be obtained by the use of a combination of diazoxide and chlorothiazide but less predictably than with insulinoma. Prednisolone, in doses up to 60 mg/day, produces improvement in the biochemical profile and remissions from hypoglycaemia in many cases but has no effect upon tumour growth itself. Growth hormone and long-acting glucagon preparations also produce symptomatic relief given alone or with prednisolone.

The postprandial syndrome

The appearance of symptoms suggestive of acute neuroglycopenia in relation to the ingestion of food has been called the postprandial syndrome. It has many causes, one of the less common is hypoglycaemia.

Reactive hypoglycaemia

Following an initial rise, venous blood glucose concentrations may decrease in normal healthy volunteers as far as 2 mmol/l below fasting levels after ingestion of a liquid glucose load of 75 g or more on an empty stomach. A smaller fall in arterial blood glucose also occurs and may, in up to 50 per cent of normal healthy subjects, be accompanied by mild symptoms. This phenomenon, referred to as reactive hypoglycaemia, rarely occurs in every day life when normal mixed meals are eaten. When it does, diagnostic difficulties may arise since symptoms are usually vague, unspecific, and indistinguishable from those due to other illnesses, especially neurosis.

In the period 1950 to 80, the diagnosis of reactive hypoglycaemia, referred to by lay writers simply as 'hypoglycaemia', reached epidemic proportions in the United States. In most cases, the diagnosis was based on misattribution of the normal response to oral glucose. Whilst some patients with postprandial syndrome may have a lower threshold to neuroglycopenia, experiencing symptoms at (arterial) blood glucose levels of 3.5 to 4.0 mmol/l rather than the more customary level of 2.8 to 3.3 mmol/l, most do not. Nor do they manifest any abnormalities of glucose homeostasis.

Criteria for the recognition and diagnosis of reactive hypoglycaemia were laid down at the Third International Symposium on Hypoglycaemia, adherence to which has greatly reduced the number of persons misdiagnosed. The criteria include a history of food-stimulated autonomic symptoms appropriate to acute neuroglycopenia—a capillary blood glucose concentration measured during a spontaneous symptomatic episode below 3 mmol/l and rapid relief by oral glucose. Sometimes, when suspicion is high and blood collection during every day life proves difficult, it may be necessary to give the patient a standard meal and observe the glycaemic, symptomatic, and electroencephalographic responses over the ensuing 5 h. The oral glucose load test is not appropriate.

The term reactive hypoglycaemia is not a definitive diagnosis in its own right; it is only the first step towards determining causation. Almost every condition in which hypoglycaemia is induced by fasting, may present as reactive hypoglycaemia. Organic causes, including acquired and inherited metabolic derangements, must, therefore, be eliminated before making a diagnosis of idiopathic reactive hypoglycaemia—which is rare. Conditions in which patients experience only reactive, but not fasting, hypoglycaemia

include partial gastrectomy and jejuno–oesophageal anastamosis (also referred to as alimentary hypoglycaemia), autoimmune insulin syndrome, and, recently identified, non-insulinoma pancreatogenous hypoglycaemia. Reactive hypoglycaemia, unaccompanied by fasting hypoglycaemia, occurs in up to 2 per cent of patients harbouring insulinomas.

Clinical features

Typically, patients present with a history of transient episodes of dizziness, anxiety, palpitations, sweating, hot flushes, and even convulsions or brief periods of altered consciousness extending over a period of 1 to 30 years. Between episodes they are well and asymptomatic. Patients rarely notice any relationship of symptoms to food but may do so when prompted. Physical, including radiological, investigation is generally normal except in alimentary hypoglycaemia. In them, but few others, food-induced reactive hypoglycaemia may be of sufficient severity as to cause loss of consciousness.

Acute-neuroglycopenia-like symptoms experienced by some patients with the postprandial syndrome are rarely associated with any abnormality of glucose homeostasis or insulin secretion though exaggerated enteroglucagon, GIP, and tGLP-I response to food may occur. What role, if any, these hormones play in the aetiology of the syndrome is unknown. Some patients with these symptoms are sensitive to modest reductions in blood glucose concentration to which most healthy subjects would be oblivious and in them the possibility of non-hypoglycaemic neuroglycopenia may be entertained.

Alcohol-induced reactive hypoglycaemia

Symptomatic reactive hypoglycaemia may occur in healthy young subjects after ingesting a mixture of alcohol, sucrose, and quinine given as gin and tonic and, less commonly, with other mixtures of alcohol and carbohydrate on an empty stomach. Simultaneous ingestion of carbohydrate-rich snacks increases the severity of the hypoglycaemia; snacks rich in fat reduce it.

Diagnosis

Diagnosis of reactive hypoglycaemia is suggested by the clinical history and confirmed or refuted by glucose measurements made on capillary blood collected during spontaneous symptomatic episodes. Other laboratory tests, including measurement of plasma insulin, C-peptide, proinsulin, and β-hydroxybutyrate are used to exclude conditions such as non-insulinoma pancreatogenous hypoglycaemia, autoimmune insulin syndrome, and other conditions that do not produce hypoglycaemia during fasting but do require specific treatment.

Capillary blood glucose concentrations of less than 3.5 mmol/l, measured in an accredited laboratory on two or more occasions, establishes hypoglycaemia as a factor in the symptomatology. The oral glucose load test, formerly the lynch-pin for diagnosis, may be frankly misleading especially when conducted on individuals who have taken a self-prescribed low carbohydrate diet (<100 g/day) and should rarely be employed. A standard glucidic breakfast providing 100 g of readily assimilated starchy food has been advocated in its stead but is seldom indicated.

Treatment

Prevention of fluctuations in blood glucose is key to the management of reactive hypoglycaemia and is achieved by minimizing intake of rapidly absorbed carbohydrates such as sucrose, bread, and potato starch. Frequent small meals, rich in dietary fibre—and taken without alcohol—offer the best chance of symptomatic relief. Incorporation of soluble dietary fibre supplements, such as guar and glucomannan, in meals and taking α-glucosidase inhibitors, such as acabose and miglitol, with them reduce blood glucose excursions but their side-effects are often worse than discomfort from minimal hypoglycaemia.

Prognosis

Idiopathic postprandial syndrome is a self-limiting disorder but may be resistant to all physical treatments. Some patients respond well to psychotherapy and/or avoidance of alcohol.

Autoimmune hypoglycaemia

Autoimmune diseases are important causes of spontaneous hypoglycaemia. Three main types are recognized.

Autoimmune insulin syndrome

The autoimmune insulin syndrome occurs throughout the world but is rare outside Japan. It is due to polyclonal autoantibodies to insulin resembling those produced in response to exogenous insulin but more likely to bind proinsulin and its cleavage products including C-peptide.

Hypoglycaemia typically occurs as a late response to the ingestion of food. Insulin secreted early in response to a meal is sequestered by antibodies present in the plasma and rendered temporarily inactive. Dissociation of the insulin–antibody complex, after absorption is complete, produces an inappropriately high free plasma insulin level resulting in hypoglycaemia. This, though often profound, is of limited duration, rarely leading to coma and never to death.

There is often a history of autoimmune disease affecting other organs, especially the thyroid, and many patients have received treatment with methimazole, carbimazole, or other thiol-containing drugs.

Free plasma insulin concentrations are always inappropriately high and C-peptide usually depressed during hypoglycaemia. C-peptide concentrations may, however, be normal or high depending on the binding characteristics of the autoantibody.

Treatment is dietary and aimed at avoiding excessive insulin secretion in response to meals until spontaneous remission occurs, usually within a few years of onset. Surgery, in the mistaken belief that the patient has islet hyperplasia or insulinoma, must be avoided.

Insulin-receptor autoantibodies

Hypoglycaemia due to insulin-receptor autoantibodies is rare but may be the first indication of the causative disease. More often it develops in a patient already known to be suffering from an autoimmune disease or a neoplasm—especially lymphoma. Typically, hypoglycaemia is intractable but occasionally occurs only in response to food. Its immediate cause is binding of stimulatory autoantibodies to insulin receptors on hepatic and peripheral cell membranes, simulating the effects of insulin itself.

Clinically, the symptoms are indistinguishable from that of insulinoma though usually of shorter duration and greater severity. Plasma C-peptide and proinsulin concentrations are low (<20 pmol/l). Plasma insulin, though also often low, may be very high (>1000 pmol/l) due to its delayed clearance from the blood. Diagnosis can usually be inferred from the clinical associations and evidence suggestive of hyperinsulinism, that is coincident low blood glucose and β-hydroxybutyrate, but depressed plasma C-peptide, proinsulin (and usually insulin), concentrations rule it out. Definite diagnosis depends upon demonstrating antireceptor antibodies in the patient's plasma using *in vitro* bioassay techniques.

Treatment is that of the primary disease. Glucocorticoids and other immunosuppressants have been used with benefit in some cases but although remissions may occur, the prognosis is generally poor.

Islet-cell-stimulating antibodies

Antibodies capable of stimulating insulin release from isolated pancreatic β-cells *in vitro* have been held responsible for a form of hyperinsulinaemic hypoglycaemia analogous to Grave's disease of the thyroid. The evidence is, however, inconclusive.

Drug and toxin-induced hypoglycaemia

Medicines and toxins, such as alcohol, paracetamol, quinine, *Amanita* (toadstools), and *Blighia* (ackee) are collectively amongst the most frequent causes of non-iatrogenic hypoglycaemia. They produce their effects in various ways, mostly by interfering with hepatic glucose production, counterregulatory hormone action, or by stimulating insulin secretion.

Alcohol hypoglycaemia

Alcohol-induced hypoglycaemia is the most common cause of non-iatrogenic hypoglycaemia. The patient is usually stuporose or comatose. Sometimes they are aggressively unco-operative and their symptoms attributed to alcoholic intoxication rather than to hypoglycaemia. Characteristically, hypoglycaemia develops within 6 to 36 h of the ingestion of moderate to large amount of alcohol (>30 g) by fasting or malnourished subjects who may be, but often are not, habituated to alcohol. Hypothermia is more common than with other causes of hypoglycaemia and may provide the first clue to diagnosis. Children, in whom there is a 25 per cent mortality, are particularly susceptible to this type of hypoglycaemia.

Blood glucose is less than 2.5 mmol/l and alcohol almost always present, generally at a concentration below 20 mmol/l (100 mg/100 ml). Plasma and urinary ketones are high but often overlooked because traditional tests for ketones detect only acetone and acetoacetate rather than β-hydroxybutyrate—the redox pair member normally present in alcoholic ketoacidosis.

Once considered, the diagnosis is seldom in doubt and is due to inhibition by alcohol of hepatic gluconeogenesis from lactate and glycerol. It can be confirmed by demonstrating hypoglycaemia, raised plasma β-hydroxybutyrate, and low plasma insulin, C-peptide, and proinsulin levels together, in most cases, with measurable amounts of alcohol.

Consciousness can be restored with intravenous glucose but not glucagon—which is ineffective. Long-term treatment is avoidance of the predisposing factors.

Accidental, factitious, and felonious hypoglycaemia

In these states, although hypoglycaemia is due to exogenous hypoglycaemic agents, this fact is not revealed by the history. The correct diagnosis emerges only from critical examination of laboratory test results and other non-clinical or forensic evidence. Typically the patient is hypoglycaemic and stuporose or comatose when first seen and—unless the possibility of drug-induced hypoglycaemia is suspected from the outset, and appropriate samples of blood and urine collected for insulin, C-peptide, proinsulin, and sulphonylurea assay—the correct diagnosis may never be made.

Sulphonylureas

Dispensing or prescription errors are an important cause of hypoglycaemia—a sulphonylurea being substituted for another drug with a similar name (e.g. diabinese™ for diamox™). In hospital, victims of accidental hypoglycaemia often have received medication intended for someone else. Because patients are often elderly and slip slowly into hypoglycaemic coma without warning, the diagnosis may be delayed or missed completely.

Deliberate sulphonylurea overdose with suicidal or felonious intent is uncommon. It may be difficult to distinguish from accidental overdose in a diabetic patient unless the plasma sulphonylurea level is abnormally high or a suicide note is found. Treatment with diazoxide and intravenous glucose may be required for many days to prevent recurrent hypoglycaemia.

Insulin

Factitious insulin-induced hypoglycaemia is as common in previously healthy subjects as in insulin-dependent diabetics and is due to deliberate, but concealed, injection of insulin. The history suggest insulinoma but is eliminated by the laboratory results which reveal high plasma insulin and low C-peptide (and proinsulin) concentrations during hypoglycaemia. In long-standing factitious hypoglycaemia, and in insulin-treated diabetics, insulin antibodies may be present in the plasma. Although once considered a strong pointer to factitious hypoglycaemia, the presence of insulin antibodies should nowadays suggest autoimmune insulin syndrome.

Suicidal overdosing with insulin is not confined to diabetic patients and is usually unsuccessful. Most patients are found within 12 h of injecting themselves and are restored to consciousness by appropriate treatment. Plasma C-peptide is unrecordably low and (free) insulin concentrations generally greater than 2000 pmol/l. In factitious hypoglycaemia, a form of Munchausen syndrome, plasma insulin concentrations are generally lower than this.

Murder or attempted murder with insulin is exceedingly rare and virtually confined to infants, critically ill patients, and the elderly. The victims are often dead when first seen; if suspected, the diagnosis can be made retrospectively by demonstrating inordinately high concentrations of insulin in blood drawn from a peripheral blood vessel or in tissue removed from the putative injection site. Blood, cerebrospinal fluid, and vitreous glucose measurements are uninterpretable after death.

Organ failure

Hypoglycaemia can occur, sometimes as a dominant feature, in almost any serious and life threatening illness. Most notably are: congestive cardiac failure; acute liver failure; chronic renal failure; bacterial, viral, and parasitic infections (especially malarial); and terminal malnutrition. The cause of the hypoglycaemia is seldom in doubt but its recognition and restoration of normoglycaemia sometimes dramatically alters the course of the illness.

Endocrine hypoglycaemia

Hypoglycaemia is a rare but important presenting sign of several endocrine disorders of which Addison's disease, pan-hypopituitarism, and isolated ACTH deficiency are the most common. The typical clinical features of endocrinopathy are inconspicuous and the diagnosis may be missed unless specifically sought through appropriate laboratory testing. Paradoxically, reactive hypoglycaemia is a rare manifestation of pheochromocytoma with which its symptomatology may be confused. Primary glucagon deficiency has only once been documented as a cause of hypoglycaemia.

Inborn errors of metabolism

Many inborn errors of carbohydrate metabolism—which usually present as hypoglycaemia in childhood—can first manifest themselves in adult life. Mild variants may be responsible for obscure cases of hypoglycaemia which occur only under very stressful conditions, such as prolonged fasting or exceptionally violent exercise, and for which no endocrine or organic cause can be found.

Further reading

Auer RN (1998). Insulin, blood glucose levels, and ischemic brain damage. *Neurology* **51**, S39–43.

Boles RG *et al.* (1999). Glucose transporter type 1 deficiency: a study of two cases with video-EEG. *European Journal of Pediatrics* **158**, 978–83.

Bolli GB, Fanelli CG (1999). Physiology of glucose counterregulation to hypoglycemia.. *Endocrinology and Metabolism Clinics of North America* **28**, 467–93.

Clark PM (1999). Assays for insulin, proinsulin(s) and C-peptide. *Annals of Clinical Biochemistry* **36**, 541–64.

Cryer PE (1999). Symptoms of hypoglycemia, thresholds for their occurrence, and hypoglycemia unawareness. *Endocrinology and Metabolism Clinics of North America* **28**, 495–500.

Grant CS (1999). Surgical aspects of hyperinsulinemic hypoglycemia. *Endocrinology and Metabolism Clinics of North America* **28**, 533–54.

Koch CA, Rother KI, Roth J (1999). Tumor hypoglycemia linked to IGF-II. In: Rosenfeld R, Roberts C Jr, eds. *Contemporary endocrinology: the IGF system*, pp. 675–98. Humana Press, Totowa, New Jersey.

Lteif AN, Schwenk WF (1999). Hypoglycemia in infants and children. *Endocrinology and Metabolism Clinics of North America* **28**, 619–46.

Marks V (1999). Murder by insulin. *Medico-Legal Journal* **67**, 147–63.

Marks V, Teale JD (1998). Tumours producing hypoglycaemia. *Endocrine-Related Cancer* **5**, 111–29.

Marks V, Teale JD (1999). Drug-induced hypoglycemia. *Endocrinology and Metabolism Clinics of North America* **28**, 555–77.

Marks V, Teale JD (1999). Hypoglycemia: factitious and felonious. *Endocrinology and Metabolism Clinics of North America* **28**, 579–601.

Redmon JB, Nuttall FQ (1999). Autoimmune hypoglycemia. *Endocrinology and Metabolism Clinics of North America*, **28**, 603–18.

Seckle MJ *et al.* (1999). Hypoglycemia due to an insulin-secreting small-cell carcinoma of the cervix. *New England Journal of Medicine* **341**, 733–6.

Service FJ (1999). Diagnostic approach to adults with hypoglycemic disorders. *Endocrinology and Metabolism Clinics of North America* **28**, 519–32.

Teale JD, Marks V (1998). Glucocorticoid therapy suppresses abnormal secretion of big IGF-II by non-islet cell tumours inducing hypoglycaemia (NICTH). *Clinical Endocrinology* **48**, 491–8.

Thomson GA *et al.* (1998). A comparative study of glucose meter accuracy during biochemical hypoglycaemia in humans. *Practical Diabetes International* **15**, 135–8.

12.12 Hormonal manifestations of non-endocrine disease

H. E. Turner and J. A. H. Wass

Introduction

Several endocrine syndromes may develop in association with diseases that are not primarily disorders of an endocrine gland. In most the cause is a tumour, usually but not invariably malignant, that develops in tissue not normally looked upon as the site of the particular hormone synthesized. Other 'non-endocrine conditions' may also be associated with either hormonal excess or deficiency, for example sarcoidosis and AIDS. Certain drugs may also modify hormonal biochemistry and cause hormonal imbalance syndromes.

Syndromes of ectopic hormone secretion

In 1941, Albright suggested that the hypercalcaemia sometimes associated with malignant disease without osteolytic metastases might be due to the secretion by the tumour of a parathyroid hormone-like peptide; we now know that this is true (parathyroid hormone related protein, PTHrP). Later it was shown that hypersecretion of adrenocorticotrophin (ACTH), not from the pituitary but from an ectopic site, was the cause in about one-fifth of patients with Cushing's syndrome.

Although 'ectopic' hormone secretion has classically been recognized in the context of neoplasia, and defined as the release of a hormone from a site different from the gland that normally produces the hormone, it is increasingly being recognized that many hormones are synthesized by 'non-endocrine' tissue. Thus the syndromes of neoplastic ectopic hormone secretion are actually due to the pathological over-secretion and/or inappropriate production of hormones. Increasing recognition of the importance of paracrine secretion of hormones such as insulin-like growth factors (IGF-1), their modulation by growth factors and binding proteins, for example IGFBPs1, 2, and 3, and their role in progression of neoplasia adds greatly to these complexities.

Many different hormones are ectopically secreted by neoplasms arising in diverse organs, notably the bronchus, breast, pancreas, kidney, and ovary as well as in mesenchymal tissue. Although a particular endocrinopathy may be associated with a specific type of tumour in a particular organ, the relationship is not invariable. An example is the lung, where squamous cell carcinomas are often associated with hypercalcaemia due to parathyroid hormone related peptide, while small cell lung cancer and bronchial carcinoid tumours are both associated with ectopic ACTH secretion, but with very different clinical manifestations. Indeed, many neoplasms elaborate more than one hormonal substance at the same or at different times and thus may produce a mixed endocrine picture (for example pancreatic endocrine tumours producing ACTH and insulin). Furthermore, the amount of ectopic hormone(s) produced may fluctuate from time to time (for example cyclical Cushing's syndrome in ectopic ACTH secretion). In some instances, the changes induced by the ectopic hormone may mimic very closely, and be clinically indistinguishable, from those found in the true endocrinopathy. In others, the picture is less characteristic and domin-

ated more by abnormalities of biochemistry or hormone levels. Thus, in many cases of ectopic ACTH production by small cell lung cancer, the downhill course of the illness may be too rapid for the classical features of florid Cushing's syndrome to develop, and hypokalaemic alkalosis with diabetes predominates.

Criteria for diagnosis

The diagnosis of ectopic hormone production depends on a number of criteria, although it is seldom practicable or possible to confirm them all:

1. There is an association of the tumour with an endocrine syndrome.

2. Even though the endocrine syndrome may not be clinically florid, there is an elevated or inappropriately raised plasma level of the putative hormone.

3. Removal or suppression of the tumour induces a regression of the endocrinopathy and a fall in the hormone level.

4. The clinical picture and hormone levels are uninfluenced by removal of the gland that normally secretes the hormone.

5. The hormone level is higher in venous blood draining the tumour than in the arterial blood supplying it.

6. Extraction or immunohistochemical staining shows a higher concentration of the hormone in the tumour than in adjacent, non-involved tissue.

7. Demonstration can be made of tumour cell synthesis of identifiable hormones *in vitro* or of mRNA coding for the hormone.

Chemical structure

Most syndromes of ectopic hormone secretion are due to peptide hormones. It is rare for tumours to secrete steroid hormones because of the complexity of the enzyme cascade required for steroid biosynthesis. Tumours may, however, be associated with altered steroid metabolism—for example increased aromatase activity in hepatocellular carcinoma leads to feminization and gynaecomastia due to androgen conversion to oestrogens.

The precise amino acid sequences of hormones of ectopic origin are being increasingly defined. In general, they appear to resemble closely those of their normally occurring counterparts (except parathyroid hormone (PTH) and PTHrP). There is a tendency for a greater proportion of higher molecular weight precursors, prohormones, or subunits and fragments to be associated with an ectopic origin than with 'true' endocrinopathies but it is not always clear whether this is due to differences in biosynthesis or in intracellular or extracellular processing. Minor differences in molecular structure are sometimes reflected in disparities between bioassay and immunoassay.

Prevalence

Clinically evident syndromes are less common than biochemical or hormonal abnormalities. The prevalence of ectopic production of ACTH, corticotrophin-releasing hormone (CRH), parathyroid hormone related protein (PTHrP), calcitonin, chorionic gonadotrophin (hCG), prolactin, or growth hormone, without clinical manifestations, is high when extensive biochemical and hormonal assays are applied to patients with cancer. These assays bring closer the prospect of finding a diagnostic 'marker' for tumours in general and, in particular, as is already the case with the monitoring of hCG or its subunits, to determine the response of tumours to treatment.

Hypercalcaemia in the absence of detectable bony metastases is the most common abnormality. It occurs in about 15 per cent of patients with squamous cell carcinoma, usually of the bronchus, carcinoma of the kidney, ovary, or breast. Next most common in neoplastic diseases is the syndrome of inappropriate antidiuresis (SIAD), usually associated with a small cell lung cancer and reported in 40 per cent of such cases. Cushing's syndrome due to ectopic ACTH or CRH secretion occurs in about 5 per cent of patients with small cell lung cancer, and in association with other neoplasms. Biochemical accompaniments of Cushing's syndrome in the absence of the clinical features are much more common, occurring in 50 per cent of patients with small cell lung cancer.

Pathogenesis

As techniques for molecular analyses have evolved, it has become clear that every somatic cell is capable of synthesizing every polypeptide hormone. However, only under pathological circumstances is that capability ever likely to be expressed. A variety of hypotheses for ectopic hormone synthesis and secretion have been made. None explains all of the observed facts. Fundamentally, all cells inherit an identical complement of DNA. They are therefore totipotential and have all the coded information required for the synthesis of all proteins and peptides, including protein hormones. The normal inability of non-endocrine tissue to synthesize hormones is ascribed to 'repressors' that mask specific segments of the DNA molecule. It seems possible that when a cell becomes malignant this normal repression becomes ineffective, allowing the unmasked DNA to synthesize proteins or peptides 'foreign' to the cell concerned. Such a 'de-repression' hypothesis does not explain why certain tumours are more prone to secrete certain ectopic hormones. Neuroendocrine cells, characterized by the presence of peptide hormone granules, are likely to be the origin of some tumours associated with hormone secretion, such as small cell lung cancer and bronchial carcinoids. Another hypothesis suggests that there are a small number of special proliferative cells in normal mature tissues that have fetal characteristics with the ability to produce peptide hormones—a process of 'dysdifferentiation' rather than 'de-repression'. There is currently no unifying mechanism with supportive experimental evidence to explain ectopic hormone production. Further information on the control of gene expression and hormone production, the role of oncogenes, and paracrine growth factors may provide further insight.

Treatment

Treatment of the clinical or biochemical abnormalities associated with endocrinopathies of non-endocrine origin is best directed at the primary disorder. In neoplastic disease, this may involve surgical excision, radiotherapy, or chemotherapy. Sometimes the tumour secreting the ectopic hormone is extremely difficult to locate even with the use of sophisticated imaging techniques such as magnetic resonance imaging (MRI), radiolabelled isotope scanning (e.g. [111]Indium-penetreotide imaging), or using selective venous catheterization.

More specific therapy may be necessary to contain the metabolic abnormality until such time as the fundamental disorder can be controlled. For example immediate measures may be required to reduce hypercalcaemia with fluids and bisphosphonates, or steps taken (administration of metyr-apone) to diminish corticosteroid secretion from adrenal glands stimulated by ectopic ACTH secretion.

Ectopic secretion of calciotropic hormones

Malignancy is the most common cause of hypercalcaemia in the hospital inpatients and may be due to direct tumour spread to the bones or related to secreted calcium-releasing factors. Often several different mechanisms are involved in the same patient.

After its discovery in 1987, it was shown that PTHrP is responsible for hypercalcaemia in up to 70 per cent of patients with this tumour-associated phenomenon. PTHrP shares amino acid homology with PTH between positions 2 and 13 of the 84 residues of PTH and acts via the PTH receptor. The PTHrP gene is located on the short arm of chromosome 12; that of PTH is on chromosome 11. The PTHrP gene may be activated by transactivation, hypomethylation (renal carcinomas), or the effect of growth factors and cytokines, including IGF-1 and epidermal growth factor, while glucocorticoids and vitamin D_3 suppress PTHrP levels. Unlike PTH-mediated hypercalcaemia, dihydroxycholecalciferol is suppressed in PTHrP-mediated hypercalcaemia. PTHrP is made by squamous carcinomas as well as renal, bladder, ovary, skin, pancreas, and breast carcinomas, and lymphomas.

Other factors can be involved in hypercalcaemia unassociated with osseous metastases. 1,25-Dihydroxy vitamin D_3 is not uncommonly made by lymphoproliferative tumours, which are either high grade or widely disseminated. Transforming growth factor-α (TGFα) which stimulates osteoclastic bone resorption, is also made by squamous carcinoma, and renal and breast carcinomas. Some tumours cosecrete both TGFα and PTHrP. Interleukin-1, which is a very powerful stimulator of osteoclastic bone resorption, is also made by squamous carcinomas as well as some haematological malignancies. Tumour necrosis factor (TNF) and lymphotoxin also stimulate osteoclastic bone resorption. These related cytokines cause hypercalcaemia *in vivo*; lymphotoxin is produced by cultured myeloma cells *in vitro* and accounts for the hypercalcaemia seen in this condition. Prostaglandins of the E series may also cause hypercalcaemia.

It is important to remember that primary hyperparathyroidism itself is common, particularly in the elderly; two diseases may coexist. For this reason, primary hyperparathyroidism should always be considered when hypercalcaemia occurs, even if it is in a patient within the setting of malignant disease. It is now possible to differentiate between these two conditions by using the PTH two-site radioimmunoassay.

Paraneoplastic hypercalcaemia may be either asymptomatic or dominate the clinical picture and be life-threatening as a consequence of dehydration and renal failure. The features of hypercalcaemia and its general management are discussed elsewhere (see Chapter 12.6).

Oncogenic osteomalacia is a rare syndrome usually associated with benign mesenchymal tumours (e.g. haemangiopericytomas) where phosphaturia, hypophosphataemia, and normocalcaemia are associated with suppressed 1,25 dihydroxy vitamin D. It may be due to an unknown phosphaturic factor which also inhibits 1-α-hydroxylase.

Syndrome of inappropriate antidiuresis (SIAD)

This syndrome is usually, but not invariably, associated with high levels of circulating arginine vasopressin. Other, as yet unidentified, antidiuretic substances are sometimes involved. There is hyponatraemia and impaired water excretion in the absence of hypovolaemia, hypotension, or deficiency of cardiac, renal, thyroid, or adrenal function. Associated with hyponatraemia, there is a reduction in plasma osmolality and inappropriately normal/low urine concentration.

Bronchogenic carcinoma is the commonest malignancy associated with SIADH. Although SIADH in association with malignancy may be due to the tumour itself, it may also result from treatment (e.g. chemotherapy such as cyclophosphamide), an intercurrent illness such as pneumonia, or a complication such as hydrocephalus or cerebrovascular accident (Table 1).

Ectopic ACTH secretion

Pro-opiomelanocortin (POMC) is a 31 kDa precursor for both ACTH and β-lipotrophin as well as for other polypeptides derived from it, including γ-lipotrophin and β-endorphin. A variety of non-pituitary tumours are capable of secreting POMC-derived peptides, accounting for about 20 per cent of patients with Cushing's syndrome. Approximately 50 per cent of these ectopic ACTH-producing tumours are in the lung and the rest are present in a variety of other tissues (Table 2). Some tumours, particularly pancreatic islet cell tumours which are seldom (< 5 per cent) associated with Cushing's syndrome, can, in addition to ACTH, also secrete a number of other hormones, including insulin, gastrin, and glucagon (see Chapter

Table 1 Conditions associated with the syndrome of inappropriate antidiuresis (SIAD)

Malignancies
Carcinoma
Small cell lung
Pancreas—islet cell
Duodenum
Colon
Bladder
Prostate
Thymus
Cervix
Lymphoma

Lung diseases
Pneumonia
Viral
Bacterial
Fungal
Tuberculosis
Lung abscess
Asthma
Pneumothorax
Chest wall injury
Mechanical ventilation

Central nervous system diseases
Cerebral trauma
Cerebrovascular accident
Meningitis
Encephalitis
Brain tumours—primary or secondary (e.g. cerebellar haemangioblastoma)
Cerebral abscess
Hydrocephalus
Guillain–Barré syndrome
Delirium tremens
Acute intermittent porphyria

General surgery

Drugs
Vasopressin
Desmopressin (DDAVP)
Oxytocin
Thiazides
Vincristine, vinblastine
Cyclophosphamide
Phenothiazines
Tricyclic antidepressants
Carbamazepine
Chlorpropamide
Clofibrate

Metabolic causes
Porphyria

Table 2 Types of neoplasm causing ectopic pro-opiomelanocortin (ACTH) secretion

Small cell carcinoma of the bronchus
Bronchial carcinoid
Thymic carcinoid
Islet cell pancreatic tumour
Phaeochromocytoma
Medullary carcinoma of the thyroid
Breast carcinoma
Tracheal carcinoma
Oesophageal carcinoma
Gastric carcinoma
Ileal carcinoma
Appendicular carcinoma
Colonic carcinoma
Ovarian carcinoma
Prostatic carcinoma
Squamous carcinoma of the cervix
Adrenal medullary paraganglioma
Melanoma

12.10). This accounts for the usefulness, when screening for ectopic ACTH, of measuring other hormones (e.g. calcitonin, hCG) which may be cosecreted, the presence of which raises the suspicion of an ectopic hormone-secreting tumour. Very rarely, corticotrophin releasing hormone (CRH) is secreted ectopically in association with ACTH.

While small cell lung cancer is the most common source, carcinoids anywhere, but particularly bronchial carcinoids, phaeochromocytoma, and medullary carcinoma of the thyroid may also secrete ACTH ectopically (Table 2).

The exact mechanism of synthesis of ectopic POMC-derived peptides is still debated. POMC mRNA can be found in the majority of tumours, but ACTH secretion is much less common, probably due to the lack of the signal sequence required for translocation. Changes in promoter usage and also in POMC processing may lead to ectopic secretion of ACTH. In addition, many tumours associated with ectopic ACTH secretion are of neuroendocrine morphology and may arise from progenitor cells associated with ACTH secretion.

Presentation

The clinical picture is variable. In patients with small cell lung cancer who have a rapidly progressive tumour, the physical features of Cushing's syndrome may not have time to develop. The major features are weight loss, proximal muscular weakness, polyuria, thirst, oedema, carbohydrate intolerance with glycosuria, and sometimes pigmentation due to ACTH. Hypokalaemic alkalosis is a characteristic finding; the plasma potassium is less than 3.2 mmol/l and the bicarbonate greater than 30 mmol/l, the urine potassium loss being the direct cause of most of the symptoms. This hypokalaemia is in part due to the very high cortisol levels, which have a mineralocorticoid action, and corticosterone and 11-deoxycorticosterone which may also be produced in excess. The 11β-hydroxysteroid dehydrogenase enzyme may also function abnormally, causing decreased inactivation of cortisol and corticosterone. The serum cortisol level is usually greatly elevated (>1000 nmol/l) and the plasma ACTH level is also raised (>200 µg/l). These high levels do not usually occur in pituitary-dependent Cushing's disease.

When the ectopic sources are other than a small cell lung cancer, the clinical manifestations may be quite indistinguishable from Cushing's disease and cushingoid features may antedate by months or years any evidence of a tumour causing ectopic ACTH secretion. The degree of elevation of ACTH is less marked than with small cell lung cancer and is proportional to tumour size. Some carcinoid tumours may be small and difficult to locate. The real problem is to differentiate ectopic ACTH secretion from pituitary-dependent disease (Table 3). The presence of a hypokalaemic alkalosis

Table 3 Response to tests used to differentiate ectopic ACTH secretion from Cushing's disease (from Howlett *et al.* 1986)

	Ectopic ACTH (% of cases)	Cushing's disease (% of cases)
Hypokalaemia <3.2 mmol/l	100	10
Diabetes mellitus	78	38
Dexamethasone 8 mg/day (no suppression)	89	22
CRH test excessive response	0	>90

CRH = corticotrophin-releasing hormone.

(< 3.2 mmol/l) is very useful test in the differential diagnosis. Lack of suppression on high-dose dexamethasone testing is found in 90 per cent patients with ectopic disease, but also up to 20 per cent with pituitary disease. However, the CRH test is very useful in differentiation as patients with ectopic ACTH secretion show an absent rise in cortisol whereas pituitary dependent disease is associated with an exaggerated response in 95 per cent patients. Because most of the tumours secreting POMC are in either the chest or abdomen, MRI or computed tomography (CT) will often reveal the source of ectopic hormone secretion. In patients in whom the lesion is not readily visible by imaging techniques, selective venous catheterization and sampling may help determine a source of ACTH by comparing levels at various sites within the venous system. Such sampling should include inferior petrosal sinuses in case of pituitary-dependent disease.

Treatment

Removal of the primary growth or its control with radiotherapy or chemotherapy will relieve the endocrine manifestations. A relapse may occur if metastases develop because these, too, usually secrete ACTH. When it proves impossible to control a primary tumour, adrenocortical hypersecretion may be reduced by 'medical adrenalectomy', giving the 11β-hydroxylase inhibitor of the conversion of 11-deoxycortisol to cortisol, metyrapone (500–4000 mg/day). Aminoglutethimide (1000–1500 mg/day) may also be used but frequently causes a skin rash. Ketoconazole (400–800 mg/day), which can cause fatal liver damage, and the adrenolytic drug mitotane are also useful. RU-486, a glucocorticoid antagonist at the receptor level, has been used as palliative therapy for some patients (10–30 mg/kg per day). Lastly, the long-acting somatostatin analogue, octreotide (0.3 mg/day, subcutaneously), has also been used in the treatment of ectopic ACTH syndrome.

Bilateral adrenalectomy is an alternative approach, but frequently it is not practical for patients with rapidly progressive metastatic disease. It may be possible to embolize the arterial supply of the adrenal gland if patients are not suitable surgical candidates for adrenalectomy. Medical treatment needs to be monitored carefully so that adrenal insufficiency is avoided.

Ectopic secretion of insulin-like growth factors

The insulin-like growth factors, IGF-I and II, share some sequence homology and actions of insulin. IGF-II is important in fetal growth, whereas IGF-I, synthesized in the liver, mediates most of the actions of growth hormone. IGFs circulate bound to one of six binding proteins (IGFBPs). Of these, the most important is IGFBP3, which itself is growth hormone-dependent and binds 75 per cent of IGF-I and IGF-II.

IGF-II secretion from tumours may be associated with hypoglycaemia. Usually the tumour is large and of mesenchymal origin, arising in the abdomen or thorax. Symptoms are those of neuroglycopenia—sweating, tachycardia, disorientation, drowsiness, fits, and coma. Histology shows a mesothelioma, a fibrosarcoma, or other sarcoma such as a leiomyosarcoma. Other neoplasms associated with hypoglycaemia are haemangiopericytoma, hepatoma, adrenal carcinoma, lung carcinoma, Wilms' tumour, and colonic carcinoma.

IGF-II secretion leads to suppression of growth hormone and insulin, and reduced production of IGFBP3, IGF-I, and acid labile subunit (ALS), leading to reduced formation of the IGF–IGFBP3–ALS complex which protects the IGFs from degradation. IGF-II circulates as a smaller complex which has enhanced tissue and receptor bioavailability, allowing access to the insulin receptor. There is also an increase in the large molecular weight molecules and the increased amounts of 'big' IGF-II not detected on radioimmunoassay. Growth hormone deficiency, decreased gluconeogenesis, and increased glucose metabolism by the tumour, which is usually large, may also contribute to hypoglycaemia. Treatment of these tumours is difficult. The hypoglycaemia is often not responsive to diazoxide, glucagon, octreotide, or corticosteroids. However, administration of growth hormone may be effective—increasing IGFBP3 and IGF-I and antagonizing the effect of excess IGF-II. The underlying tumour may be resistant to radiotherapy; surgery, although effective if possible, is not always feasible.

IGF-I and IGF-11 may also play an important role in tumour progression. Studies of breast cancer cells have suggested that IGF-I may have local mitogenic effects, and a role for IGF-II has recently been proposed in hepatocellular, colorectal, and adrenocortical tumours.

Ectopic human chorionic gonadotrophin secretion

Human chorionic gonadotrophin is a glycoprotein consisting of an α- and a β-subunit. The α-subunit is species specific and is the same for all glycoprotein hormones (luteinizing hormone (LH), follicle stimulating hormone (FSH), and thyroid stimulating hormone (TSH)). The β-subunit determines receptor interaction and specific hormone activity. The β-subunit of hCG is very similar to that of LH and this can cause problems with cross-reaction in assays. Clinically silent, ectopic secretion of hCG, with or without its free α- and β-subunits, occurs in many patients (Table 4).

In the first decade of life, ectopic hCG production may cause isosexual precocious puberty in boys with hepatoblastoma. hCG, through its LH-like action, causes Leydig cell stimulation in the testes. In turn, testosterone levels reach those of a normal adult, and secondary sexual characteristics develop together with premature skeletal maturity. The testes remain small because there is no seminiferous tubule growth as this is dependent on FSH. Precocious puberty is rare in girls.

Intracranial teratoma, choriocarcinoma, and pinealoma are associated with ectopic hCG secretion. In men this may be associated with gynaecomastia. In some this is due to cosecretion of oestrogen which may, in women, be associated with dysfunctional uterine bleeding. Other tumours

Table 4 Human chorionic gonadotrophin (hCG) in sera of patients with malignant tumours (from Vaitukaitis 1991)

Tissue	Percentage of cases with ectopic secretion of hCG
Breast	21
Lung	10
Gastrointestinal tract	18
Pancreas (more commonly hCG -α)	33
Stomach	22
Liver	21
Small intestine	13
Large intestine	12
Biliary tract	11
Ovary (adenocarcinoma)	40
Testis	62
Seminoma	38
Embryonal cell carcinoma	58
Choriocarcinoma	100
Mixed	73

associated with hCG secretion are testicular tumours, ovarian adenocarcinoma, and stomach, pancreatic, and liver tumours.

hCG is a useful tumour marker in gestational trophoblastic disease (choriocarcinoma) and in some men with testicular tumours, and provides an early warning of recurrent disease. However, it is important to measure other tumour markers, for example α-fetoprotein, which may also be secreted by non-seminomatous germ cell tumours. Discordance of marker levels and tumour progress may be seen. In central nervous system disease, cerebrospinal fluid/plasma ratios may help in the correct localization of tumours, as hCG does not cross the blood–brain barrier and levels in cerebrospinal fluid remain undetectable in pregnancy. Thus, cerebrospinal fluid concentrations higher than plasma suggest primary central nervous system disease.

In some patients, most commonly with choriocarcinoma and massive elevation of hCG, the latter, through its weak TSH activity, due to its biochemical similarity to TSH, may cause goitre and hyperthyroidism. This most frequently occurs in women, is not associated with eye signs, and is usually associated with modest biochemical abnormalities. Treatment of the tumour results in a resumption of a euthyroid state but, if this is not possible, carbimazole or propylthiouracil may be required.

Ectopic human placental lactogen

Human placental lactogen (hPL), also called human chorionic somatomammotropin (hCS), is a trophoblastic hormone which may be secreted ectopically in association with lung tumours, testicular tumours, and trophoblastic disease. It is usually associated with gynaecomastia in men, and these tumours may also be associated with increased levels of oestradiol and hCG.

Ectopic growth hormone releasing hormone and growth hormone secretion

Most patients with acromegaly (98 per cent) have benign growth-hormone-producing pituitary adenomas. Less than 2 per cent of patients with acromegaly have ectopic growth hormone releasing hormone (GHRH) production. A patient with a carcinoid tumour of the pancreas producing GHRH enabled the final elucidation of the structure of this important hypothalamic peptide which stimulates anterior pituitary growth hormone secretion. Besides the pancreas, lung carcinoid tumours, small cell lung cancer, and phaeochromocytoma may produce GHRH ectopically and cause acromegaly by stimulation of the pituitary somatotrophs. Histologically, the two can be differentiated by the presence of somatotroph hyperplasia in ectopic GHRH secretion. These tumours are usually clinically apparent and GHRH levels in the circulation are elevated. GHRH can also be secreted by hypothalamic hamartomas, which also result in anterior pituitary somatotroph hyperplasia.

Ectopic growth hormone secretion has been reported in patients with bronchial, pancreatic, and gastrointestinal carcinoma, and cells cultured from an undifferentiated lung cancer have been shown to synthesize growth hormone in vitro. Breast carcinoma and ovarian tumours may also occasionally secrete growth hormone but no clinical syndrome has been clearly identified as caused by ectopic growth hormone.

Ectopic prolactin secretion

Prolactin may be secreted by bronchial carcinoma and renal cell carcinoma; the usual endocrine manifestation is galactorrhoea and there may be marked hyperprolactinaemia. These abnormalities are reversed if the tumour is controlled or removed. Difficulties in differential diagnosis may arise unless the underlying abnormality is clinically obvious or suspected, because in most instances the hyperprolactinaemia will be attributed to a prolactin-secreting adenoma. Suspicion of an ectopic source may only arise when the prolactin level is not lowered by bromocriptine treatment. An autocrine role for prolactin in breast and prostate cancer has recently been postulated.

Ectopic calcitonin secretion

Increased serum calcitonin levels are encountered in a variety of cancers apart from medullary carcinoma of the thyroid. The most common of these are small cell lung cancer, leukaemia, and neoplasms of the breast and pancreas. It is often produced as part of a multihormonal profile in conjunction with, for example, gastrin, ACTH, and somatostatin. Ectopic calcitonin may differ from the normal hormone in having more high molecular weight components; it does not cause any apparent symptoms and does not produce hypocalcaemia.

Ectopic renin secretion

Although hypertension associated with hyper-reninism and increased aldosterone production is usually due to a renal lesion, ectopic secretion of renin has also been described in association with cancer of the lung, pancreas, and ovary. The clinical picture is usually dominated by the underlying neoplasm but the patient has hypertension and the cause of this may be suspected from the associated hypokalaemia and its accompanying muscle weakness. Effective treatment of the primary lesion will reduce the increased renin and aldosterone levels and hence the raised blood pressure. When the underlying cause cannot be eradicated, the use of an angiotensin enzyme inhibitor will control the hypertension.

Ectopic aldosterone secretion

Hypertension and hypokalaemia related to ectopic secretion of aldosterone from a non-adrenal neoplasm have been described in patients with ovarian tumours. Its pathogenesis is different from the others described in this section. The aberrant production of a steroid, aldosterone, rather than a peptide, is presumably due to biochemical change in the ovarian steroidogenic cells. Attention is likely to be focused on a suspected lesion of the adrenal zona glomerulosa because the hyperaldosteronism is associated with low plasma renin activity. The ovarian lesion may initially be clinically silent and only revealed by pelvic imaging.

Endocrine manifestations of non-endocrine diseases

Systemic disease of non-endocrine glands may influence endocrine function due to a specific effect of the disease itself, due to a general response to either acute or chromic illness, or due to drug therapy used to treat the illness itself (Table 5). Often hormonal perturbations may be a complex mixture of all of these mechanisms, as may be seen for example in AIDS or critically ill patients on intensive therapy units. This section includes examples of systemic disease causing endocrine disorders.

A commonly encountered hormonal disturbance encountered in many hospital inpatients is the 'sick euthyroid syndrome'. Peripheral conversion of T_4 to T_3 is reduced, and typical thyroid function tests in this syndrome are a normal or reduced TSH in association with reduced T_3 and T_4 (and increased rT_3 if measured). Severe illness may also interfere with hypothalamopituitary function and lead to hypogonadotrophic hypogonadism. Possible mechanisms include increased cortisol levels, stress, cytokines, or opioids given as analgesia.

Disorders influencing hypothalamopituitary function

Anorexia nervosa is associated with complex changes in hypothalamopituitary function, with reduction in GnRH and gonadotrophin secretion leading to hypogonadotrophic hypogonadism but increased growth hormone secretion is associated with increased peripheral resistance to growth hormone.

Iron overload due to haematological conditions such as β thalassaemia major and to haemochromatosis may cause iron deposition in the anterior

Table 5 Hormonal abnormalities associated with non-endocrine disorders

Disease	Endocrine abnormality
Severe illness	Sick euthyroid syndrome ($\downarrow$TSH $\downarrow$T$_4$ $\downarrow$T$_3$ $\uparrow$rT$_3$)
	Hypogonadism ($\downarrow$LH $\downarrow$testosterone/oestradiol)
Anorexia nervosa	Hypogonadotrophic hypogonadism ($\downarrow$GnRH $\downarrow$LH/FSH $\uparrow$GH)
Iron overload	Hypogonadotrophic hypogonadism ($\downarrow$LH/FSH $\downarrow$T or E$_2$)
Hyperemesis gravidarum	Thyrotoxicosis ($\downarrow$TSH $\uparrow$T$_4$, $\uparrow$hCG)
HIV infection and AIDS	$\uparrow$T$_4$ $\uparrow$T$_3$ $\uparrow$TBG (HIV)
	Opportunistic infections may cause goitre, hypo- or hyperthyroidism
	Adrenal infiltration (infection, lymphoma, and Kaposi's sarcoma), however Addison's rare
	Impaired aldosterone and adrenal androgen secretion, with preferential glucocorticoid production
Cytotoxic chemotherapy and radiotherapy	Hypogonadotrophic hypogonadism ($\downarrow$ LH/FSH $\downarrow$T/E$_2$)
	Premature ovarian and testicular failure due to direct cytotoxic effect
Coeliac disease	Reversible androgen resistance ($\uparrow$FSH/LH $\downarrow$testosterone)
Alcoholic liver disease	Androgen deficiency ($\downarrow$testosterone $\uparrow$SHBG $\uparrow$E$_2$)
Sarcoidosis and other granulomatous disorders	$\uparrow$1,25 DHCC $\uparrow$calcium
HTLV-1 infection	$\uparrow$PTHrP $\uparrow$calcium

pituitary gland, and in particular in the gonadotrophs. This leads to hypogonadotrophic hypogonadism, which may be ameliorated to a degree by venesection and iron chelation therapy. Haemochromatosis may also lead to other hormonal changes due to pancreatic involvement causing diabetes mellitus, and cirrhosis associated with secondary hyperaldosteronism and hypogonadism.

Thyroid

Hyperemesis gravidarum in the first trimester of pregnancy may be associated with clinical and biochemical features of thyrotoxicosis, as the molecules hCG and TSH share very similar β subunits, allowing cross reactivity when high levels of hCG occur.

Opportunistic infections of the thyroid gland may occur, in conditions associated with immunosuppression such as AIDS. Infection with cytomegalovirus, *Cryptococcus*, and *Pneumocystis carinii* have been described. In addition, some patients with HIV infection have increased T$_4$ and T$_3$ due to increased thyroid binding globulin. As the disease progresses, T$_4$ and T$_3$ levels fall as patients develop biochemical features of sick euthyroidism.

Adrenal

Opportunistic infections (CMV, atypical mycobacteria, *Cryptococci*, *Toxoplasma*, and *Pneumocystis*), lymphoma and Kaposi's sarcoma may involve the adrenal glands in HIV and AIDS. The adrenal gland is the most commonly involved endocrine gland at autopsy. However, frank adrenal insufficiency is rare because this requires destruction of over 90 per cent of the adrenal cortex.

Gonads

Chemotherapy and irradiation may be associated with gonadal failure due to hypothalamopituitary gonadotrophin deficiency following, for example, cranial irradiation or due to testicular/ovarian damage following cytotoxic drug therapy such as cyclophosphamide, cisplatin, and busulfan.

Coeliac disease is associated with reversible male infertility due to androgen resistance, and improves on a gluten free diet. Alteration of gonadal steroid metabolism may occur in, for example, chromic liver disease, particularly if alcohol related. Elevated sex hormone binding globulin (SHBG) and oestradiol levels are associated with a reduction in bioavailable testosterone leading to testicular atrophy, gynaecomastia, and erectile impotence.

Gynaecomastia

Palpable breast glandular tissue is prevalent in population studies of men and boys. Subareolar glandular tissue more than 2 cm diameter is found in

35 to 60 per cent of men. Gynaecomastia may occur as a result of different conditions (Table 6) as well as drug therapy, and results from an alterations in the ratio of oestrogen to androgen. Gynaecomastia has been found in association with testicular and adrenal neoplasms, Klinefelter's syndrome, thyrotoxicosis, cirrhosis, primary hypogonadism, malnutrition, and ageing (Table 6). An increase in free oestrogen, a decrease in free endogenous androgens, androgen-receptor defects, and partially enhanced secretions of breast tissue may underlie these changes. Increased aromatization of oestrogen precursors occurs in patients with obesity, liver disease, and hyperthyroidism, and as a result of ageing.

Calcium

Hypercalcaemia in sarcoidosis is due to increased circulating 1,25 dihydroxy vitamin D. This is produced by alveolar macrophages in a dose-

Table 6 Non-endocrine conditions associated with gynaecomastia

Neoplasms
Ectopic production of human chorionic gonadotrophin or
   human placental lactogen
Liver disease (18%)
Starvation during recovery phase (refeeding)
Renal disease and dialysis (1%)
Drugs (10–20%)
   Antiandrogens/inhibitors of androgen synthesis
      Cyproterone
      Flutamide
      Spironolactone
   Antibiotics
      Ketoconazole
   Antiulcer medication
      Cimetidine
      Omeprazole
      Ranitidine
   Cancer chemotherapeutic agents
      Alkylating agents
   Cardiovascular drugs
      Captopril
      Digoxin
      Methyldopa
      Nifedipine
   Psychoactive drugs
      Haloperidol
      Phenothiazines
   Drugs of abuse
      Cannabis

dependent fashion stimulated by γ interferon, which is one factor responsible for the maintenance of the inflammatory process in sarcoidosis. Other granulomatous disorders (tuberculosis, histoplasmosis, coccidiomycosis, ruptured silicone breast implants) may rarely be associated with hypercalcaemia due to the same mechanism. Treatment with glucocorticoids or hydroxychloroquine are effective in lowering 1,25 dihydroxycholecalciferol and calcium.

HTLV-1 infection may be associated with hypercalcaemia, due to trans-activation of the PTHrP gene on chromosome 12.

Drug-induced endocrine manifestations

Several pharmaceutical drugs may induce manifestations of endocrine disease. More commonly they may influence the results of hormonal assays and lead to mistaken diagnosis. It may not be a major problem when it is known that the patient is taking a particular compound and, from its molecular structure, it is appreciated that such a substance could influence the endocrine system or the results of hormonal assays. The problem is greater, however, when the drug in question has no clear relationship to a hormone and the mechanism by which it induces an endocrine manifestation, or interferes with an assay procedure, is not readily apparent.

Thyroid

Abnormalities of thyroid function test measurements

Drugs can interfere with thyroid function tests. Some act by inhibiting the conversion of thyroxine (T_4) to triiodothyronine (T_3), others by increasing thyroid-binding globulin. β-Blockers with membrane stabilizing properties, such as propranolol, inhibit peripheral conversion of T_4 to T_3. Oral cholecystographic agents and amiodarone, a heavily iodinated antiarrhythmic agent, are also potent inhibitors of T_4 to T_3 conversion and produce decreased serum T_3 concentrations and an increase in reverse T_3. Oestrogen increases thyroid-binding globulin, due to an increase in the sialic acid content of thyroxine-binding globulin, which prolongs its half-life in the circulation. Thus women on oestrogens, for example the contraceptive pill, have high total T_4 concentrations but are euthyroid. Such results may also be seen on tamoxifen. Heroin and methadone addicts also have raised levels of thyroxine-binding globulin, as do patients on the lipid-lowering agent, clofibrate.

A decreased serum T_4 does not necessarily indicate the presence of hypothyroidism. Many pharmacological agents lower the total T_4 concentration by interfering with the binding of T_4 to one or more of the thyroid-binding proteins. Therapeutic levels of phenytoin lower the level of serum T_4 and high concentrations are capable of inhibiting the binding of T_4 and T_3 to thyroid-binding globulin. High doses of salicylates have the same effect. Diclofenac, a non-steroidal anti-inflammatory drug structurally similar to thyroxine, also interferes with thyroid hormone binding. Phenylbutazone, anabolic steroids, and glucocorticoids may also be associated with a low total T_4 and normal thyroid function. Measurement of free thyroxine (fT_4) will obviate the problems of misleading results from the measurement of total T_4.

Drug-induced hyperthyroidism

Amiodarone may cause hyperthyroidism due to its high iodine content, or due to a destructive thyroiditis. Biochemically, there may be a marked elevation of total thyroxine, a relatively normal level of T_3, and a suppressed TSH. Often thyrotoxicosis is masked by the β-blocking effect of the drug. Because of the large iodine load, it may be very difficult to treat with antithyroid drugs, and steroids may also be necessary to suppress thyroid hormone levels into the normal range. Even if amiodarone is stopped, its effects continue for many weeks because it is predominantly stored in adipose tissue. Contrast media and iodine-containing cough medicines may similarly induce hyperthyroidism (Jod–Basedow phenomenon).

Drug-induced hypothyroidism

Increased iodide intake may also lead to decreased iodide trapping and a decrease in synthesis of thyroid hormones, hypothyroidism, and goitre. Iodine is contained in a number of 'tonics' and cough medicines. Amiodarone, besides producing thyrotoxicosis, may cause iodine-induced hypothyroidism in patients replete with iodine. Lithium blocks iodine uptake and the release of thyroid hormones. It also interferes with cAMP formation and thus inhibits the effects of TSH stimulation and may lead to goitre, although only 2 per cent of patients on lithium actually develop clinical features of hypothyroidism.

Adrenal cortex

Abnormalities of adrenal hormone measurements

Drugs may interfere with tests of adrenal function. Thus, for example, phenytoin accelerates metabolism of dexamethasone, and patients on phenytoin may not suppress cortisol normally during dexamethasone suppression tests. Furthermore, during the assessment of adrenal reserve, chronic topical application of steroids, as well as inhalation of steroids for asthma, may suppress adrenal function. Oestrogens, by enhancing hepatic production of cortisol-binding globulin, which binds between 90 and 97 per cent of circulating cortisol, increases cortisol-binding globulin two-to threefold. Thus, assessment of glucocorticoid replacement in patients on oestrogens is influenced by this effect and oestrogens should be stopped 6 weeks prior to the test.

Drug-induced Cushing's syndrome

Chronic, excessive intake of alcohol causes alcoholic pseudo-Cushing's syndrome. These patients behave biochemically as if they have Cushing's syndrome with absent dexamethasone suppression. This occurs through a centrally mediated mechanism with hypersecretion of pituitary ACTH and secondary secretion of cortisol by the adrenals.

Drug-induced primary aldosteronism

Primary aldosteronism can be mimicked by the mineralocorticoid effect of glycyrrhizic acid contained in both carbenoxolone and liquorice. Cortisol is normally inactivated by conversion to the inactive metabolite, cortisone, by the enzyme 11β-hydroxysteroid dehydrogenase but these compounds inhibit the enzyme, which is important in the kidney because it protects renal mineralocorticoid receptors from cortisol.

Drug-induced adrenal insufficiency

The antifungal agent, ketoconazole, and the short-acting anaesthetic, etomidate, are imidazole derivatives with significant inhibitory effects on 11β-hydroxylase. While they do not usually produce clinical insufficiency, they may do so in subjects with limited pituitary or adrenal reserve. Rifampicin and phenytoin, which both accelerate the metabolism of cortisol by inducing hepatic mixed-function oxygenase enzymes, can also provoke adrenal insufficiency in similar patients with limited pituitary or adrenal reserve. In such patients, increased doses of replacement therapy are necessary.

Gonads

Several drugs can affect testicular function, leading to hypogonadism and infertility. Mechanisms include the direct inhibition of testosterone synthesis or competitive inhibition of androgen action at receptor level. Spironolactone acts as a partial androgen receptor antagonist. Alcohol reduces testosterone levels acutely and chronically, by both a central and a gonadal effect on testosterone synthesis, secretion, and metabolism. Cimetidine has antiandrogen effects due to direct interaction with the androgen receptor and it may also exert antiandrogen effects at the pituitary and hypothalamus leading to gynaecomastia and impotence in males. Anticonvulsants, for example phenytoin, increase sex hormone-binding globulin and therefore decrease free testosterone levels. They also enhance testosterone to oestradiol conversion. Sulfasalazine causes reversible male infertility associated with oligospermia.

Infertility may occur as a result of cytotoxic therapy, caused in particular by the alkylating agents such as cyclophosphamide. These produce depletion of the germinal epithelium and lead to a raised FSH level, and oligo- or azoospermia, but normal LH and testosterone levels in males, and may lead to premature ovarian failure in women.

In women, hirsutism can be caused by a number of drugs, including danazol, phenytoin, diazoxide, and minoxidil.

Pharmacological doses of glucocorticoids may lead to hypogonadism because of inhibited gonadotrophin release. Drugs such as tricyclics, benzodiazepines, antihypertensives, and antipsychotics may also lead to hypogonadotrophic hypogonadism in both sexes.

Prolactin

Prolactin is controlled predominantly by a hypothalamic inhibitory mechanism through dopamine secretion. A number of drugs can cause hyperprolactinaemia and galactorrhoea usually acting through a dopaminergic mechanism. They may elevate prolactin to a sufficient extent to cause a clinical suspicion of prolactinoma, and in such patients a careful drug history is particularly important. Metoclopramide, pimozide, and sulpiride all act as dopamine antagonists and may considerably elevate prolactin, with all the attendant effects thereof. Fluoxetine may also lead to elevated serum prolactin, although tricyclic antidepressants are not usually associated with hyperprolactinaemia.

Phenothiazines, chlorpromazine, perphenazine, and trifluoperazine also act as dopamine antagonists, as do haloperidol and butyrophenone. Reserpine and methyldopa both decrease catecholamine stores and may cause hyperprolactinaemia. Oestrogens, in high doses, may slightly elevate prolactin but normal contraceptive pills do not. Verapamil, by decreasing dopaminergic tone, may also increase prolactin levels.

Gynaecomastia

Gynaecomastia may occur due to treatment with various drugs (Table 6). Drugs such as spironolactone and ketoconazole, which can displace steroids from sex-hormone binding globulin, displace oestrogens more easily than androgens. Activation of the oestrogen receptors in breast tissue may take place with drugs that have structural homology with oestrogen, such as digoxin; griseofulvin and cannabis may have the same effect. A decrease in androgen occurs in older men and with drugs such as spironolactone and ketoconazole that inhibit the biosynthesis of testosterone. The mechanism for the induction of gynaecomastia by captopril and calcium-channel blockers (nifedipine) is unclear. With cimetidine and omeprazole, this effect may be due to a direct antiandrogen effect or the inhibition of liver cytochrome P450.

Posterior pituitary

The syndrome of inappropriate antidiuresis is characterized by normovolaemic hyponatraemia with persistent secretion of vasopressin, despite a reduced plasma osmolality. A number of drugs can cause this syndrome, including thiazide diuretics, vincristine, vinblastine, cyclophosphamide, chlorpropamide, phenothiazines, carbamazepine, clofibrate, and tricyclic antidepressants (Table 1).

Nephrogenic diabetes insipidus can be induced by lithium in the therapeutic range, and up to 20 per cent of patients receiving long-term therapy may develop this complication. Demethylchlortetracycline produces dose-dependent nephrogenic diabetes insipidus, and both the concentrating defect and the unresponsiveness to vasopressin are reversible on cessation of the drug.

Parathyroid

Lithium therapy can cause an increase in parathyroid gland size, either with hyperplasia or adenoma. This hyperparathyroidism leads to mild hypercalcaemia and sometimes osteoporosis. Thiazide diuretics, by causing haemoconcentration and hypocalciuria, may also result in mild hypercalcaemia but this is usually transient (4–6 weeks); after this time, other causes of hypercalcaemia should be sought.

Vinblastine and colchicine inhibit parathyroid hormone secretion which may result in hypocalcaemia.

Further reading

Bell NH (1991). Endocrine complications of sarcoidosis. *Endocrinology and Metabolism Clinics of North America* 20, 645–54.

Braunstein GD (1993). Current concepts: gynecomastia. *New England Journal of Medicine* 328, 490–5.

Chopra IJ (1997). Clinical review 86: Euthyroid sick syndrome: is it a misnomer? *Journal of Clinical Endocrinology and Metabolism* 82, 329–34.

Daughaday WH and Deuel TF (1991). Tumour secretion of growth factors. *Endocrinology and Metabolism Clinics of North America* 20, 539–63.

Docter R, Krenning EP, DeJong M, Hennemann G (1993). The sick euthyroid syndrome: changes in thyroid hormone serum parameters and hormone metabolism. *Clinical Endocrinology* 39, 499–510.

Grinspoon SK, Bilezikian JP (1992). HIV disease and the endocrine system. *New England Journal of Medicine* 327, 1360–5.

Guise TA, Mundy GR (1998). Cancer and bone. *Endocrine Reviews* 19, 18–54.

Howlett TA, Drury PL, Perry L, Doniach I, Rees LH, Besser GM (1986). Diagnosis and management of ACTH-dependent Cushing's syndrome: comparison of the features in ectopic and pituitary ACTH production. *Clinical Endocrinology* 24, 699–713.

Hung W, Blizzard RM, Migeon CJ, Camacho AM, Nyhan WL (1963). Precocious puberty in a boy with hepatoma and circulating gonadotropin. *Journal of Pediatrics* 63, 895–903.

Kovacs L, Robertson GL (1992). Syndrome of inappropriate antidiuresis. *Endocrinology and Metabolism Clinics of North America* 21, 859–76.

Melmed S (1991). Extrapituitary acromegaly. *Endocrinology and Metabolism Clinics of North America* 20, 507–18.

Penny E *et al.* (1984). Circulating growth hormone releasing factor concentrations in normal subjects and patients with acromegaly. *British Medical Journal* 289, 453–5.

Turner HE, Wass JAH (1997). Gonadal function in men with chronic illness. *Clinical Endocrinology* 47, 379–403.

Vaitukaitis JL (1991). Ectopic hormonal secretion and reproductive dysfunction. In: Yen SSC, Jaffe RB, eds. *Reproductive endocrinology*, 3rd edn, pp. 795–806. WB Saunders, Philadelphia.

Vanderpump MPJ and Tunbridge WMG (1993). The effects of drugs on endocrine function. *Clinical Endocrinology* 39, 389–97.

Wass JAH, Jones AE, Rees LH, Besser GM (1982). HCGB producing pineal choriocarcinoma. *Clinical Endocrinology* 17, 423–31.

White A, Clark AJL (1993). The cellular and molecular basis of the ectopic ACTH syndrome. *Clinical Endocrinology* 39, 131–41.

12.13 The pineal gland and melatonin
T. M. Cox

The pineal gland is prominent in birds, reptiles, and other vertebrates in which it responds to sunlight by the secretion of hormones that affect reproduction and thermoregulatory behaviour. In humans the gland has been known since antiquity. Although an endocrine function was considered for many years, this was only given credibility in 1958 by the pioneering work of Lerner, who isolated a small molecule from bovine pineal glands that he named melatonin because it caused blanching of melanophores in vertebrate skin. Many questions remain unanswered about the function of the human pineal gland, but its secretion of the chronobiotic molecule, melatonin, has prompted enormous interest in the fields of travel medicine, neurophysiology, and endocrine research.

Structure

The pineal is less than 1 cm in its longest diameter and weighs less than 0.2 g; it lies above the posterior aspect of the third cerebral ventricle. Normal pineal tissue contains nests of large epithelial-like cells; it also contains neuroglial components, principally of astrocytic type, which occasionally become malignant. Human pineal tissue calcifies with age but this does not necessarily diminish its secretory activity. The pineal gland is considered to reside outside the functional blood–brain barrier.

Pathology

Pineal tumours are rare and are of three types: pinealomas, which represent a neoplastic expansion of the large epithelial cells that cluster within a fibrous stroma in the adult pineal; glial tumours, that resemble astrocytomas occurring elsewhere to cause gliomas in the central nervous system; and teratomas, which arise in the midline within residual pluripotential embryonic cells. It has been known for many years that pineal tumours may disturb sexual maturation and it had been long considered that the pineal secreted a substance that inhibits gonadal function, thus explaining the precocious puberty associated with pineal disease. Treatment of pineal tumours by surgical excision or radiation appears to suppress melatonin secretion leading to sleeping difficulties; melatonin replacement therapy has been reported to benefit such patients with defective melatonin release.

Melatonin

Melatonin, like serotonin, is an endogenous indoleamine derived from tryptophan. The first step in indoleamine synthesis is the 5-hydroxylation of tryptophan by tryptophan hydroxylase—an enzyme with requirements for dioxygen, iron, and tetrahydrobiopterin. The enzyme arylalkylamine,

N-acetyl transferase, regulated by the sympathetic transmitter noradrenaline, appears to be the rate-limiting step in melatonin synthesis. The enzyme is localized principally in the pineal gland but also within specific cells in the upper gastrointestinal tract. Melatonin binds to specific receptors including the seven-transmembrane G-protein coupled receptors (Mel 1A and 1B) as well as nuclear receptors (including the transcription factor RXR/OR-α) that are associated with melatonin signalling. Membrane G-protein receptors for melatonin are principally expressed in the nervous system whereas the nuclear transcription factor is expressed in the periphery. Melatonin (formal chemical name, N-acetyl-5-methoxytryptamine) has been found within membrane-bound bodies in pinealocytes. In experimental animals these show light-dependent morphological changes associated with melatonin secretion under altered environmental light conditions. Melatonin appears to exert its main effects through MT-1 receptors in discrete regions of the hypothalamus that modulate the secretion of growth hormone-releasing hormone (GnRH). This occurs through a complex interneurone circuit which includes neurones containing serotonin, dopamine, and glutamate transmitters.

The role of melatonin and the pineal gland in photoperiodism

Exposure to light influences the secretion of melatonin, and melatonin release is suppressed particularly under illuminance with short-wavelength light. There is evidence that a photoreceptive system, which does not involve retinal rods or cones, mediates this effect. Rhythmic melatonin secretion leads to concentrations in the plasma or cerebrospinal fluid that are up to 10 times higher at night than in the daytime; maximum concentrations are observed in childhood and melatonin levels thereafter decline with age. It appears that melatonin serves as a chronobiotic molecule which acts to delay the sleep–wake cycle of the intrinsic body clock in the suprachiasmatic nucleus. There is evidence that the endogenous clock has a cycle of longer than 24 h, but becomes entrained to synchronize with daily environmental rhythms. Several syndromes associated with long-term insomnia in humans appear to result from slower or faster sleep–wake cycling. Melatonin may play a critical role in such entrainment, since synthesis of melatonin in the pineal induced at night is regulated by sympathetic outflow from the suprachiasmatic nucleus. Exposure to light at high illuminancy may improve disorders of the circadian rhythm that affect sleep. Experiments conducted in blind people have led to the use of synthetic melatonin, before the normal endogenous nocturnal peak, to re-entrain the biological clock. Melatonin-replacement therapy has thus been suggested as a means to improve sleep in night-shift workers, in elderly individuals with insomnia, in patients with pineal tumours, and in those suffering from the effects of jet lag, who have desynchronized rhythms. Careful balance studies have shown that jet lag is associated with asynchronous sleep–wake urine sodium secretion, disturbed fluid balance, and other biochemical abnormalities.

Pharmaceutical use of melatonin

Many studies have been carried out to investigate the efficacy of melatonin as a chronobiotic agent for the alleviation of symptoms associated with rapid eastward travel (jet lag). This application is based on the photoperiodism of humans and other primates and the demonstrated efficacy of melatonin in the regulation of circadian rhythm disturbances in experimental animals. The results of a recent comprehensive study by Herxheimer and Petrie to assess the effectiveness of oral melatonin, taken in different dosing regimens for alleviating jet lag after travel across several time zones, show that the agent is effective in preventing or reducing jet lag. Its short-term use appears to be safe on an occasional basis.

The review showed that in 9 out of 10 trials, melatonin taken close to the target bedtime at destination decreased jet lag in flights crossing five or more time zones. Daily doses of melatonin between 0.5 and 5.0 mg orally appeared to be similarly effective, although sleep was induced faster and better after 5 mg rather than 0.5 mg. Use of a slow-release preparation of 2 mg of melatonin was relatively ineffective in this study suggesting that a short-lived, higher peak was more effective. The drug appears to be relatively safe and side-effect reporting has been low—except in patients with epilepsy or those who are taking warfarin in whom convulsant effects or increased bleeding, respectively, have been reported. It appears possible that melatonin potentiates the action of warfarin. Given that melatonin acts physiologically to regulate the onset of puberty, excess use of melatonin may theoretically influence reproductive development in children and reduce sexual activity, if overused, in adults. No evidence of these effects has yet been reported.

In summary, the evidence is that oral ingestion of melatonin may be indicated for occasional use after transmeridian flights that would induce daytime fatigue and sleep disturbance associated with the gastrointestinal complaints, weakness, malaise, and loss of mental efficiency and other symptoms that typify with jet lag. Clearly, since the drug is not as yet licensed in all countries, routine pharmaceutical control quality must be established. Its use and safety in pregnancy has not yet been completely validated. At a time when prion-related diseases may result from the ingestion or injection of material derived from brain or other animal tissue, only pure biosynthetic melatonin should be considered for human use. Melatonin derived from bovine pineal or other biological sources should be avoided.

Melatonin is widely taken in certain communities, particularly in the United States, where it is claimed to provide indiscriminant protection against ageing, degenerative diseases, cancer, immune dysfunction, and reproductive and psychiatric illnesses. None the less it should be acknowledged that melatonin does have diverse physiological actions in humans, as in other vertebrates, which are incompletely understood. At present the principal indication for exogenous melatonin is for the control of sleep disorders and treatment of symptoms associated with jet lag, rather than the many conditions for which our scientific understanding of its proposed benefits is as yet inchoate.

Further reading

Herxheimer A, Petrie KJ (2001). Melatonin for preventing and treating jet-lag. (*Cochrane Review*), *Cochrane Database Systems Review* **1**, CD 001520 issue (1).

Karasek M (1998). Melatonin in humans—where are we 40 years after its discovery. *Neuro-endocrinological Letters* **20**, 179–88.

Lewy AJ *et al.* (1992). Melatonin shifts human circadian rhythms according to a phase–response curve. *Chronobiology International* **9**, 380–92.

Zisapel N (2001). Circadian rhythm sleep disorders: pathophysiology and potential approaches to management. *CNS Drugs* **15**, 311–28.

13

Medical disorders in pregnancy

13.1 Physiological changes of normal pregnancy

D. J. Williams

Since modern *Homo sapiens* emerged 100 000 years ago, it is estimated that the human population has increased from 50 000 to around 6000 million. Such reproductive success has defied gross reproductive inefficiency. Only 20 to 35 per cent of fertilized ova result in a successful pregnancy (10–25 per cent of *in vitro* fertilizations), most failing around the time of implantation with chromosomal abnormalities. The usual outcome of a successful pregnancy is a single offspring, produced after 9 months. Indeed, if the fetal brain was not programmed to outgrow the maternal pelvic outlet, anthropological comparisons with the great apes indicate that human pregnancy would last 16 months. The price of a relatively short pregnancy is neonatal immaturity and a prolonged period of nurture.

Preparing for pregnancy

The female body prepares for pregnancy during every menstrual cycle. It is not only the endometrium that anticipates implantation of a fertilized ovum, but the whole cardiovascular system. During the postovulatory or luteal phase of each menstrual cycle there is a decrease in systemic vascular resistance by approximately 20 per cent, leading to a 10 per cent fall in mean arterial pressure compared with the follicular phase. Cardiac output increases by almost 20 per cent, and renal vasodilatation increases both renal blood flow and glomerular filtration by approximately 10 per cent. All of these changes resolve with involution of the corpus luteum and onset of menses.

Haemodynamic changes in pregnancy

If fertilization is successful, there is progression of the haemodynamic changes established in the menstrual cycle. A progressive fall in systemic vascular resistance by up to 40 per cent creates a maximal decrease in mean arterial pressure by the end of the first trimester. Diastolic blood pressure falls between 5 and 15 mmHg, before rising to non-pregnancy levels at term, whilst systolic blood pressure remains unchanged throughout pregnancy. A gestational increase in heart rate from approximately 72 to 85 beats/min and of stroke volume by up to 30 per cent combine with the reduction in systemic vascular resistance to increase cardiac output. By 24 weeks, cardiac output reaches a maximum of 50 per cent above non-pregnant levels, which is sustained until term, except in the supine position during the third trimester when cardiac output falls as the gravid uterus compresses the inferior vena cava. Left ventricular wall thickness and left ventricular mass increase progressively throughout pregnancy, by up to 30 per cent and 50 per cent respectively. Cardiac output returns almost to prepregnancy levels within 2 weeks of delivery.

Distribution of increased cardiac output

Although it is technically difficult to measure blood flow to particular maternal viscera during pregnancy, it is clear that the timing and extent of changes to blood flow varies between organs. This is summarized in Fig. 1. Mammary artery blood flow increases early in pregnancy, breast tenderness and swelling being amongst the first symptoms.

Mechanism of haemodynamic change

The onset of physiological change during the menstrual cycle suggests that maternal rather than fetoplacental factors initiate gestational adaptation. Oestrogen, mainly in the form of 17B-oestradiol, is a potent vasodilator. It is produced by the corpus luteum during the luteal phase of each menstrual cycle and for the first 10 weeks of pregnancy. After 10 weeks, the placenta elaborates its own 17B-oestradiol, so that by term maternal oestradiol levels are approximately 250-fold higher than those found during the menstrual cycle. 17B-oestradiol relaxes vascular smooth muscle through both endothelium-dependent and independent mechanisms. All of the endothelium-derived vasodilators, nitric oxide, prostacyclin, and endothelial-derived hyperpolarizing factor have been implicated in the gestational fall of systemic vascular resistance. Much less is known about the vascular effects of progesterone. Circulating progesterone levels increase by a similar amount to 17B-oestradiol and may play a role in reducing pressor responsiveness to angiotensin II. Although the precise mechanism of maternal vasodilatation is likely to be different in different vascular beds, a healthy endothelium is essential for normal cardiovascular adaptation to pregnancy.

Fluid balance during pregnancy

Arterial dilatation creates a relatively 'under-filled' state, which stimulates the renin–angiotensin–aldosterone system. As a result, sodium and water retention throughout pregnancy leads to a 6 to 8 litre rise in total extracellular fluid volume. An increase in plasma volume is apparent by week 6

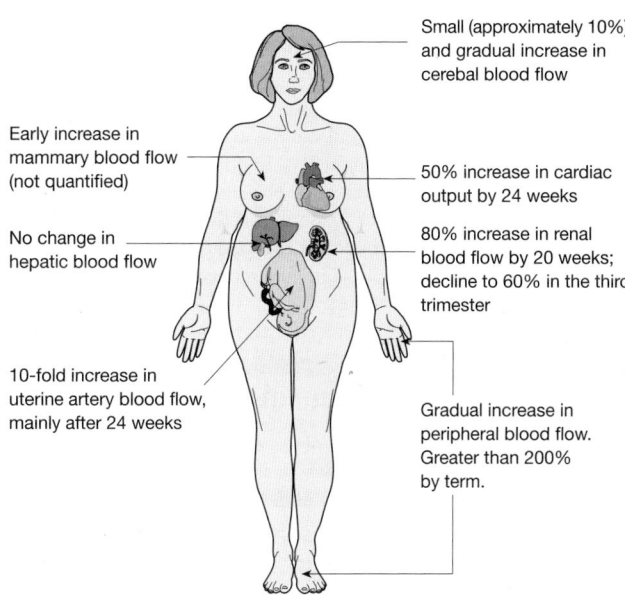

Small (approximately 10%) and gradual increase in cerebral blood flow

Early increase in mammary blood flow (not quantified)

No change in hepatic blood flow

10-fold increase in uterine artery blood flow, mainly after 24 weeks

50% increase in cardiac output by 24 weeks

80% increase in renal blood flow by 20 weeks; decline to 60% in the third trimester

Gradual increase in peripheral blood flow. Greater than 200% by term.

Fig. 1 Changes in maternal organ blood flow during healthy pregnancy.

and continues until week 32 when it is 40 per cent (approximately 1.2 l) above non-pregnant levels. Furthermore, shortly after conception the osmotic threshold for thirst falls and plasma osmolality drops by 10 mosmol/kg. A concomitant fall in the threshold for secretion of antidiuretic hormone (AVP) prevents a water diuresis and sustains low plasma osmolality until term. During the second half of pregnancy, placental production of vasopressinase increases maternal antidiuretic hormone degradation, but plasma antidiuretic hormone levels remain stable as pituitary secretion of antidiuretic hormone increases four-fold. Plasma atrial natriuretic peptide levels are normal until the second trimester, when they rise by approximately 40 per cent.

Immunological changes during pregnancy

It is often presumed that pregnant women are immunosuppressed in order that the fetal 'semiallograft' can survive. This is not true. Certain aspects of maternal immunity are modulated, but it is the placenta that deserves most credit for eluding maternal immunity. Much harm is prevented by the physical separation of maternal and fetal blood. Fetal haemolytic disease is an example of the harm that can follow a breach in this barrier, a Rhesus-negative mother becoming isoimmunized against Rhesus-positive fetal blood.

In normal pregnancy, the placenta has to invade uterine tissue and become bathed in maternal blood. To avoid a hostile immune response, the surface layers of placenta express a unique non-polymorphic HLA G, rather than classical histocompatibility antigens. It is thought that HLA-G confers resistance to lysis by maternal T cells and natural killer cells. The placenta also expresses a plethora of complement control systems to protect itself from maternal complement (serum levels of complement factors C3 and C4 are elevated during pregnancy).

The number and activity of natural killer cells in maternal peripheral blood are diminished during pregnancy, and fetal survival is further enhanced by a shift away from maternal T-helper 1 responses that promote cell-mediated immunity, towards a stronger T-helper 2 response that promotes antibody production. In consequence, pregnant women are more prone to severe infections with intracellular pathogens such as malaria and leprosy and are more likely to suffer reactivation of viruses such as Epstein–Barr. Conversely, circulating levels of maternal immunoglobulin increase and once transferred to the fetus have a role in passive immunity. The mechanism by which these immune changes take place is unclear, but increased circulating levels of metabolically active cortisol may play a role.

Healthy pregnancy is also a proinflammatory state. Neutrophils increase in number and develop a proinflammatory phenotype. Mean total white cell count increases to 9.0×10^9/l and can rise as high as 40.0×10^9/l during labour, returning to normal within 6 days. Erythrocyte sedimentation rate (ESR) rises as a consequence of increased fibrinogen and globulin. An ESR over 30 mm/h is usual and up to 70 mm/h is within normal limits. Circulating levels of C reactive protein do not change during healthy pregnancy. Anatomical changes to the maternal immune system include involution of the thymus and enlargement of the spleen.

Ventilatory changes during pregnancy

The increased metabolic demands of pregnancy lead to a progressive increase in oxygen consumption, reaching almost 20 per cent by term. To compensate, pregnant women breathe more deeply, tidal volume increasing from approximately 500 to 700 ml, whilst respiratory rate remains unchanged. Effective alveolar ventilation actually surpasses the body's demand for oxygen, creating a respiratory alkalosis with P_{CO_2} falling from 5.0 to 4.0 kPa. Over-breathing is stimulated by direct effect of progesterone on the respiratory centre, particularly increasing sensitivity to CO_2.

Renal changes during pregnancy

An 80 per cent increase in renal blood flow and 55 per cent increase in glomerular filtration rate occur by 16 weeks gestation. The rise in renal blood flow causes the kidneys to swell so that they appear approximately 1 cm longer on ultrasonography. The renal pelvis and ureters dilate, sometimes appearing obstructed to those unaware of these changes.

Serum levels of creatinine and urea fall, so that levels considered normal outside pregnancy can suggest renal impairment during pregnancy. Proteinuria increases slightly during pregnancy, but levels over 260 mg/24 h should be considered abnormal. Gestational glycosuria reflects reduced tubular glucose reabsorption and does not necessarily indicate abnormal carbohydrate metabolism. Furthermore, reduced tubular absorption of bicarbonate creates a metabolic acidosis that compensates for the respiratory alkalosis, keeping maternal pH at 7.4.

The production of all three renal hormones, erythropoietin, active vitamin D, and renin, increases during healthy pregnancy, but their effects are masked by other physiological changes. In early pregnancy, peripheral vasodilatation exceeds the renin–aldosterone mediated plasma volume expansion, so blood pressure falls by 12 weeks. The 40 per cent expansion of plasma volume exceeds the effect of a two to four-fold increase in maternal serum erythropoietin levels, which stimulates only a 25 per cent rise in red cell mass. This creates a 'physiological anaemia', which should not normally cause haemoglobin concentration to fall to less than 9.5 g/dl (see Chapter 13.3). Similarly, active vitamin D circulates at twice non-gravid levels, but concomitant halving of parathyroid hormone levels, as well as hypercalciuria and increased fetal requirements, keeps plasma ionized calcium levels unchanged.

Liver metabolism during pregnancy

The size of the liver and its blood flow appear not to change during healthy pregnancy, hence liver blood flow accounts for proportionately less of the cardiac output as pregnancy progresses. There are, however, changes to hepatic synthetic function and metabolism. Circulating concentrations of fibrinogen, ceruloplasmin, transferrin, and binding-proteins, for example thyroid-binding globulin, increase, while serum albumin levels fall by approximately 25 per cent. Serum cholesterol increases by 50 per cent and triglycerides by up to 300 per cent. The normal ranges for aspartate transaminase, alanine transaminase, gamma glutamyl transferase, and bilirubin decrease by at least 20 per cent from the first trimester until term. After the fifth month, placental production of alkaline phosphatase increases maternal plasma levels by up to four-fold. Telangiectasia and palmar erythema are common signs of healthy pregnancy that resolve postpartum.

Gastrointestinal system

Nausea and vomiting affect about 60 per cent of women during the first trimester. The rise and fall of human chorionic gonadotrophin (hCG) levels correlate chronologically with the onset and improvement of these symptoms, but the role of hCG in gestational nausea is unproven and the cause remains unknown. Relaxation of intestinal smooth muscle by progesterone creates many of the other pregnancy-induced gastrointestinal changes. Gastric motility and small bowel transit are slowed, especially during labour. The gallbladder enlarges and empties slowly in response to meals. A decrease in lower oesophageal pressure makes gastro-oesophageal reflux more common.

Endocrine changes

Thyroid function

During pregnancy, the thyroid faces three challenges. Firstly, increased renal clearance of iodide and losses to the fetus create a state of relative iodine deficiency. In geographical areas where dietary iodine intake is low, pregnancy stimulates growth of thyroid goitres. Secondly, high oestrogen levels induce hepatic synthesis of thyroid binding globulin, but free thyroxine and tri-iodothyronine levels remain within the normal range throughout pregnancy. Thirdly, placental hCG shares structural similarities with thyroid-stimulating hormone and has weak thyroid-stimulating hormone-like activity. Although hCG rarely stimulates free T4 levels into the thyrotoxic range, trophoblastic disease and hyperemesis gravidarum are often associated with high hCG levels and can lead to hyperthyroxinaemia. In these circumstances, the mother remains clinically euthyroid.

Pituitary function

Once ovulation has occurred and the uterus is prepared for implantation, the maternal pituitary makes only a small contribution to a successful pregnancy. The only pituitary hormone to increase significantly during pregnancy (by approximately 10-fold) is prolactin, which is responsible for breast development and subsequent milk production.

Pituitary secretion of growth hormone is mildly suppressed during the second half of pregnancy by placental production of a growth hormone variant. The role of the latter is unclear, but may contribute to gestational insulin resistance.

Placental production of adrenocorticotrophic hormone leads to an increase in maternal adrenocorticotrophic hormone levels, but not beyond the normal range for non-pregnant subjects. Free cortisol levels double and in the second half of pregnancy may contribute to insulin resistance and striae gravidarum.

High oestrogen levels during pregnancy stimulate lactotroph hyperplasia, resulting in pituitary enlargement. These high levels, together with those of progesterone, suppress luteinizing hormone and follicular stimulating hormone. Plasma follicular stimulating hormone levels recover within 2 weeks of delivery, but pulsatile luteinizing hormone release is only resumed in women who do not breast feed. In suckling mothers, prolactin inhibits gonadotrophin-releasing hormone and hence luteinizing hormone.

Coagulation

In anticipation of haemorrhage at childbirth, normal pregnancy is characterized by low grade, chronic intravascular coagulation within both the maternal and uteroplacental circulation. There are increased levels of clotting factors (V, VIII, and X), decreased levels of the endogenous anticoagulant protein S and decreased fibrinolytic activity. These changes lead to an acquired protein C resistance in up to 38 per cent of pregnant women. However, postpartum contraction of the uterus by oxytocin is probably more effective at preventing haemorrhage than any changes to the coagulation system.

Carbohydrate metabolism

During the first trimester, women are more sensitive to insulin than when non-pregnant. From 20 weeks onwards, insulin resistance develops, hence women in the second half of pregnancy respond to a glucose load by producing more insulin, but with less effect. Obese women, who are already insulin resistant, are more likely to develop gestational diabetes. Hormones that might mediate this insulin resistance include cortisol, progesterone, oestrogen, and human placental lactogen. Placental production of human placental lactogen, a growth hormone-like protein, coincides temporally with insulin resistance.

Skin and hair during pregnancy

Hyperpigmentation affects up to 90 per cent of pregnant women. Areas that are normally hyperpigmented, such as the areolae and vulva, become darker. This may be mediated by oestrogen and progesterone, which are powerful melanogenic stimulants. Hair growth increases during pregnancy and hair loss is accelerated postpartum. The gestational rise in corticosteroids and ovarian androgens contributes to the number of hairs in the growing phase (anagen). Postpartum, the levels of these hormones fall and hairs move back into the resting phase (telogen).

Further reading

Chamberlain G, Broughton-Pipkin F, eds (1998). *Clinical physiology in obstetrics*, 3rd edn. Blackwell Science, Oxford. [Comprehensive text on physiological changes in healthy pregnancy.]

De Swiet M, ed (1995). *Medical disorders in obstetric practice*, 3rd edn. Blackwell Science, Oxford. [Each chapter describes the physiology of a different organ system before giving details of pathophysiology.]

References

Chapman AB *et al.* (1997). Systemic and renal hemodynamic changes in the luteal phase of the menstrual cycle mimic early pregnancy. *American Journal of Physiology* **273**, F777–82. [Carefully conducted study on physiological changes during the menstrual cycle.]

Chapman AB, *et al.* (1998). Temporal relationships between hormonal and hemodynamic changes in early human pregnancy. *Kidney International* **54**, 2056–63.[Serial study correlating haemodynamic with neurohumoral changes from preconception to 36 weeks gestation.]

Gill TJ (1997). Genetic factors in reproduction and their evolutionary significance. *American Journal of Reproductive Immunology* **37**, 7–16. [Review of evolution of reproduction and development of immunity.]

Lindheimer MD, Davison JM, eds (1994). Renal disease in pregnancy. *Baillieres Clinical Obstetrics and Gynaecology* **8**, 209–527. [Several chapters on renal function and fluid balance during healthy pregnancy.]

Poston L and Williams DJ (1999). The endothelium in human pregnancy. In: Vallance P, Webb D, eds. *Vascular endothelium in human physiology and pathophysiology*, pp. 247–81. Harwood Academic Publishers, Amsterdam. [Review of role of endothelium in vascular changes of pregnancy.]

Robson SC, *et al.* (1989). Serial study of factors influencing changes in cardiac output during human pregnancy. *American Journal of Physiology* **256**, H1060–5. [Comprehensive serial study on cardiovascular haemodynamics during healthy pregnancy.]

13.2 Nutrition in pregnancy

D. J. Williams

Introduction

The ability to adapt to different environmental and nutritional conditions is a key requirement for reproductive success. In the developed world, where food is generally plentiful, dietary recommendations are based on the average food intake amongst healthy pregnant women. In nations where food is scarce, dietary recommendations are based on minimal requirements for health and fall far below the average intake of a woman who eats to satisfy her appetite. Pregnant women adapt several metabolic pathways to minimize extra nutritional requirements and optimize fetal growth. However, despite these metabolic adaptations, millions of pregnant women are unable to provide enough nutrition for their fetus to thrive. Poor prenatal nutrition not only affects perinatal outcome, but also appears to dictate susceptibility to some adult diseases and possibly the health of the next generation.

Weight gain in pregnancy

Well-nourished mothers with free access to food gain up to 30 per cent of their prepregnancy weight, of which only 25 per cent is fetal. By contrast, mothers with limited access to food gain as little as 10 per cent of their prepregnancy weight, of which up to 60 per cent is fetal. Liberal weight gain increases birth weight, but also increases the rate of caesarean section and maternal complications such as gestational diabetes and pre-eclamspia. Limiting weight gain increases the incidence of low birth weight (defined as less than 2500 g at term). In 1990 the Institute of Medicine in the United States published guidelines for weight gain in pregnancy that were adjusted according to prepregnancy maternal weight (Table 1). These recommendations, based on large observational studies, have stood the test of many subsequent analyses and minimize the overall risk of both low and high (more than 4500 g at term) birth weights.

Caucasian women who kept within the Institute of Medicine recommendations retained 1 kg postpartum, while black women retained 3 kg. Opponents of the recommendations therefore believe that they are too generous and encourage postpartum weight retention. However, only 23 per cent of obese women could keep within the guidelines, and those unable to do so doubled their risk of a poor pregnancy outcome and increased the

Table 1 Recommended weight gain in pregnancy (adapted from recommendations of the Institute of Medicine of the United States)

Maternal body mass index (kg/m2)	Recommended weight gain (kg)
Low BMI (< 19.8 kg/m²)	12.5–18
Normal BMI (19.8–26.0 kg/m²)	11.5–16
High BMI (26.1–28.9 kg/m²)	7–11.5
Obesity (> 29 kg/m²)	< 7

BMI = body mass index.

likelihood of postpartum weight retention. Unless the mother is under- or overweight (BMI less than 19.8 or more than 29 kg/m²), measurement of weight gain during pregnancy is a poor predictor of pregnancy outcome.

Pregnancy weight gain in the developing world

In developing nations more than 20 per cent of babies are of low birth weight, of which only 25 per cent are premature; in comparison, in developed nations only 6 per cent of babies are of low birth weight, of which most (55 per cent) are premature. Nutritional supplements for malnourished women during pregnancy need to be administered with care. Chronic malnutrition limits maternal stature, including pelvic size. Hence protein and energy supplements in pregnancy may disproportionately increase fetal growth and lead to obstructed labour, a major cause of maternal and perinatal death in the developing world. A pragmatic recommendation is to be particularly aware of this possibility when including primiparous women of less than 1.5 m in height in supplementary feeding programmes aimed at accelerating fetal growth. Furthermore, improved obstetric care must accompany nutritional advice.

Energy requirements during pregnancy

The rate of human fetal growth is slow and the daily incremental energy stress of human pregnancy is relatively low compared with that in other species. This allows a mother time to adapt her metabolism and energy expenditure to diverse nutritional conditions. In well-nourished societies the total energy costs of pregnancy can be as high as 520 MJ (124 000 kcal), compared with −30 MJ (−7100 kcal) in countries where food is scarce (Fig. 1).

The three major components of energy expenditure in an average well-nourished mother are growth of the fetus and reproductive tissues (about 18 per cent), new maternal fat stores (about 38 per cent), and increased maternal metabolism (about 44 per cent). Poorly nourished women try to maintain fetal growth by depressing their basal metabolic rate until late pregnancy and by laying down less fat. Although such adaptations usually result in successful reproduction, they are inevitably a compromise with regards to perinatal health. However, attempts to quantify minimal energy requirements for good perinatal health will always be confounded by huge individual variability and practical difficulties of attributing a single nutritional component to morbidity—a multifaceted problem.

In well-nourished women, the basal metabolic rate changes little until about 16 weeks' gestation, then increases rapidly until term (Fig. 2). During the middle trimester large amounts of maternal fat are laid down as energy stores. If food intake becomes limited during late pregnancy, maternal fat can be mobilized to support the period of most rapid fetal growth. This strategy of fat storage before anticipated energy demands is also used by birds before migration and hibernating mammals. Even poorly nourished

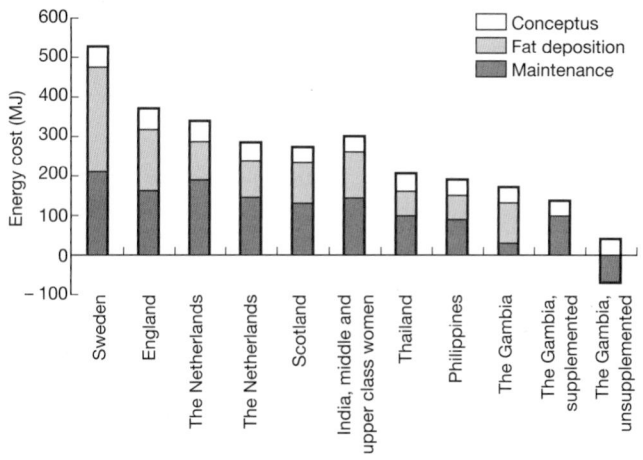

Fig. 1 Estimated total energy costs of pregnancy in different nutritional environments. The women from The Gambia were supplemented with a balanced protein-energy diet. (From Prentice and Goldberg (2000).)

women with low gestational weight gains lay down some extra fat. Conversely, well-nourished women with free access to food rarely need to utilize all their fat stores to support late fetal growth. Excess fat remains difficult to lose postpartum.

In the United Kingdom, the calculated total energy cost of pregnancy is about 70 000 kcal (Table 2). As a consequence, pregnant women have been recommended to increase energy intake by around 250 kcal/day during the

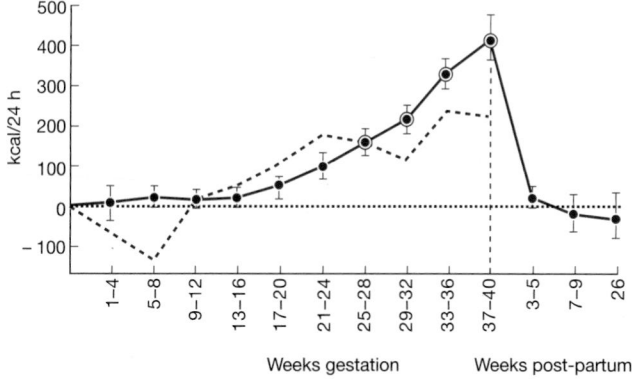

Fig. 2 The energy cost of gestational increase in basal metabolic rate in well nourished women in the United Kingdom (data derived from over 100 pregnancies). This amounts to 30 100 kcal (solid line) each pregnancy, when the total gestational energy requirement was 69 050 kcal. Total energy intake increased by only 22 000 kcal (dashed line). Maternal energy expenditure must reduce by 47 000 kcal to meet the extra demands of pregnancy. (Adapted from Durnin (1991), with permission.)

Table 2 Components of gestational weight gain and energy cost (adapted from Durnin (1991), with permission)

	Weight (g)	Energy (kcal)
Fetus	3400	8330
Placenta	640	730
Uterus, breasts, and fluids	5800	3490
Maternal fat	2400	26 400
Basal metabolic rate	–	30 100
Total	12 240	69 050

last two trimesters. However, careful studies of well-nourished women have found that maternal energy intake actually increases by little more than 100 kcal/day after the first trimester (22 000 kcal in total) (Fig. 2). The shortfall of nearly 50 000 kcal is made up by an economy of energy expenditure, including reduced physical activity and diet-induced thermogenesis.

The mechanisms that control the diverse metabolic responses to pregnancy are not understood. Leptin, a protein produced by adipose tissue and the placenta, circulates in increasing amounts during pregnancy and controls peripheral energy status and body fat. Ob/ob mice (deficient in leptin) become insensitive to exogenous leptin when pregnant, consistent with the build-up of maternal fat stores until the last trimester. Furthermore, leptin is integrated with the hypothalamo–pituitary–gonadal axis and may explain why thin women with low leptin levels remain infertile until they have adequate fat stores. A precise role for leptin during pregnancy remains to be elucidated.

Carbohydrate metabolism

During the first half of pregnancy, women produce more insulin in response to a glucose load and are more sensitive to exogenous insulin than in the non-pregnant state. These changes affect carbohydrate and lipid metabolism to favour increased fat production and storage. During the second half of pregnancy a woman becomes increasingly resistant to insulin, so that at term the action of insulin is 50 to 70 per cent lower than in the non-gravid state. As a consequence the fat stores laid down in the first half of pregnancy are mobilized and postprandial blood glucose levels remain higher for longer. Circulating levels of fatty acids and glycerol increase and are used by the mother as an energy source in preference to glucose and amino acids, which are left for the fetus. As a consequence, fasting pregnant women oxidize fat and produce ketones far sooner than they do when they are not pregnant. Women with an exaggerated peripheral resistance to insulin develop gestational diabetes mellitus.

Protein metabolism

Pregnancy is an anabolic state. Protein and nitrogen metabolism adapt early and gradually throughout healthy pregnancy to provide for tissue growth. Well-nourished women are estimated to accumulate an extra 500 g to 1 kg of protein during pregnancy. Almost half of the protein accumulates as increased maternal lean body mass, while the rest lies within the fetus and reproductive tissues.

In the United Kingdom the daily increment of dietary protein has been calculated to increase gradually throughout pregnancy to 8.5 g at term, but this does not take into account reduced hepatic metabolism of branched chain amino acids and hence reduced urea synthesis. The rate of urea synthesis declines by 30 per cent during the first trimester and by 45 per cent during the third trimester, hence serum urea concentration falls, providing more nitrogen for protein synthesis.

Vitamins and micronutrients

In some parts of the developing world micronutrient deficiencies are endemic and have serious consequences for fetal, neonatal, and maternal well-being, for example hypothyroidism due to iodine deficiency and night blindness due to vitamin A deficiency. Such deficiencies are rare in developed countries.

Calculated increments in the recommended daily allowance of specific nutrients are derived from estimates of the cost of fetal growth and increased maternal metabolism. These calculations do not usually take account of maternal metabolic adaptations that make the need for extra nutrients unnecessary, for example increased intestinal absorption of calcium offsets the need for an increase in dietary calcium. Conversely, increased folic acid excretion leads to an underestimate of folic acid requirements. Furthermore, individual micronutrients interact with each other and changes to one may have a detrimental effect on the activity of another.

It is now widely accepted that supplemental folic acid (400 μg/day) during the first trimester reduces the risk of neural tube defects. With this exception, extra vitamins and micronutrients are not necessary for healthy pregnant women who eat a balanced diet. Indeed, excessive amounts of certain micronutrients can be harmful to the fetus.

Vitamin A

Vitamin A is a lipid-soluble vitamin essential for healthy embryogenesis and fetal growth. Preformed vitamin A is found in dairy products and liver: the recommended daily allowance during pregnancy is 2000 to 2700 iu/day (670–899 retinol equivalents; RE). Vitamin A deficiency is endemic in some parts of the world: some small studies have shown a minor increase in birth weight with maternal vitamin A supplements of 6000 to 8000 iu/day (2000–2670 RE/day). Breast milk is rich in vitamin A, and is important for neonatal immunity.

Excessive doses of vitamin A in the diet (more than 15 000 iu/day (5000 RE/day)), or supplements of vitamin A (more than 10 000 iu/day), are teratogenic. Pregnant women who take vitamin A supplements of more than 10 000 iu/day (3335 RE/day) have a 1 in 57 risk of a birth defect attributable to this. Drugs that are derived from vitamin A, such as the retinoids (for example isotretinoin), are associated with an estimated 25-fold increased risk of malformation. As a consequence, the American College of Obstetricians and Gynecologists has recommend that the daily dose of vitamin A should not exceed 5000 iu/day (1665 RE/day) during pregnancy. The carotenoids (β-carotene) that are precursors to vitamin A do not appear to be teratogenic and are now being substituted for preformed vitamin A in multivitamin preparations. In general, vitamin A supplements are unnecessary for well-nourished women and potentially harmful to the fetus.

Thiamine (vitamin B₁)

Thiamine deficiency is endemic in some developing countries, but is also a global problem in women with hyperemesis gravidarum. Severe and persistent vomiting during pregnancy leads to thiamine deficiency and can cause Wernicke's encephalopathy. Thiamine replacement is therefore an essential supplement for women with hyperemesis gravidarum.

Vitamins C and E

Serum vitamin C levels fall by about 50 per cent during pregnancy, hence it is recommended that this amount is supplemented, although benefits are unproven. The antioxidant properties of vitamins C and E may reduce the risk of pre-eclampsia, but larger studies are needed to confirm this possibility.

Iodine

More than 800 million people live in iodine-deficient areas. Inadequate dietary iodine leads to maternal hypothyroidism and is detrimental to *in utero* growth and development. Supplemental iodine (usually added to salt) given to pregnant women can prevent these consequences.

Zinc

Zinc deficiency is associated with intrauterine growth restriction and teratogenesis. During pregnancy, maternal zinc levels remain stable through increased intestinal absorption. Excess iron supplements, smoking, alcohol abuse, or subsistence cereal diets high in phytate can all inhibit zinc absorption: under such conditions pregnant women may benefit from 25 mg zinc daily.

Iron

During pregnancy expansion in plasma volume exceeds the increase in red cell mass causing a fall in haemoglobin concentration. Healthy pregnant women not taking iron supplements drop their haemoglobin from 13.3 g/dl to 11.0 g/dl by 36 weeks' gestation. The minimum incidence of low birth weight (less than 2500 g at term) and preterm labour is associated with a haemoglobin of 9.5 to 10.5 g/dl. In the non-gravid state, a haemoglobin of 9.5 to 10.5 g/dl would indicate anaemia, but unless the mean corpuscular volume is less than 84 fl, supplemental iron is probably unnecessary. A meta-analysis of randomized controlled trials examining the benefit of supplemental iron found a significant reduction in women with a haemoglobin of less than 10 g/dl, but no effect, beneficial or harmful, on maternal or fetal outcome.

In the developing world, anaemia (of multiple causes) is endemic. The risk of maternal death is increased with severe anaemia (haemoglobin less than 7.0 g/dl), a condition where supplemental iron is unlikely to have much effect. Evidence that mild to moderate anaemia is associated with increased maternal and fetal risk is hard to find. Despite this, many developing countries advocate a policy of iron and folic acid supplementation for all pregnant women. More studies are necessary to monitor the effects of this policy on maternal and perinatal outcome.

Anaemia in pregnancy is discussed in more detail in Chapter 13.16.

Calcium

The growing fetus gains about 50 mg calcium per day by midpregnancy and about 300 mg/day at term. The breastfed infant receives about 250 mg of calcium in breast milk each day. The recommended daily allowance of calcium during pregnancy and lactation is 1.2 g/day, but women with much less dietary calcium undergo metabolic adaptations to meet the demands of pregnancy and lactation without any detriment to their health or that of the fetus.

During pregnancy, maternal calcium absorption increases twofold, stimulated by increased 1,25-dihydroxyvitamin D activity due to placental synthesis of 1,25-dihydroxyvitamin D and increased renal 1-α-hydroxylase activity. Although urinary calcium excretion doubles during pregnancy, fasting urinary calcium excretion, corrected for the increased creatinine clearance, is unchanged. The concentration of parathyroid hormone falls during pregnancy, suggesting that the pregnant woman receives enough calcium for her growing fetus. There are two caveats: one is the pregnant adolescent who needs to meet the demands of her own growth and that of the fetus; the other is the apparent benefit of supplemental calcium for women on a low-calcium diet, not a normal calcium diet, to prevent pre-eclampsia.

Following delivery, circulating 1,25-dihydroxyvitamin D concentrations return to non-pregnant levels. During the first 3 to 6 months of breastfeeding, mineralization of the maternal axial skeleton declines by approximately 3 to 5 per cent. After 6 months, bone demineralization recovers whether or not breastfeeding continues. Calcium supplements of 1 g/day given to lactating women do not prevent bone demineralization or improve the calcium concentration of breast milk, even if the woman is on a low-calcium diet. Furthermore, repeated long periods of breastfeeding in women with a low calcium intake do not contribute to osteoporosis in later life.

Fetal programming—the influence of fetal nutrition on adult disease

Epidemiological studies have found that low birth weight due to intrauterine growth restriction (rather than prematurity) is associated with an increased risk of cardiovascular disease in adulthood. It is hypothesized that a poorly growing fetus makes metabolic adaptations *in utero* to optimize growth and development. Despite these physiological adaptations birth weight remains low, and because of them the individual is indelibly programmed to insulin-resistant syndromes that are detrimental to long-term cardiovascular health. These issues are discussed in Chapter 15.4.1.1.

It has also been suggested that impaired insulin-mediated fetal growth and insulin resistance in later life is genetically determined. Fetal growth is partly genetically programmed, but the intrauterine environment appears to be more important: the relationship between birth weight and the body size of a surrogate mother who receives a donor egg is stronger than with the genetic mother.

Animal studies have shown that the composition of maternal diet can influence fetal growth and consequently blood pressure in her offspring. At present not enough is known about the mechanisms that control human fetal growth to give maternal nutritional advice that might eventually reduce the risk of cardiovascular disease in her children. Understanding these mechanisms may be fundamental to ameliorating the global epidemic of cardiovascular disease.

Foods to avoid during pregnancy

Food contaminated with *Listeria monocytogenes* can cause listeriosis. During pregnancy, this organism has a predilection to replicate at the uteroplacental site, leading to septic abortion in early pregnancy, or neonatal listeriosis in later pregnancy. To reduce the risk of infection with listeria, pregnant women should avoid eating soft ripened cheeses, all types of pâté, and undercooked meats. This is discussed in section 13.15.

Acute maternal infection with *Toxoplasma gondii* can cross the placenta to the fetus. Congenital infection is least likely during early pregnancy, but more severe when it occurs. The risk of congenital infection can be kept to a minimum by not eating undercooked meat, taking care while handling raw meat, and avoiding contact with cat faeces. This is discussed in Chapter 13.15.

Food cravings during pregnancy

Common food cravings during pregnancy are for dairy products and occasionally for non-organic material such as soil (pica). Common aversions are to alcohol, caffeine, and meats.

Further reading

Abrams B, Altman SL, Pickett KE (2000). Pregnancy weight gain: still controversial. *American Journal of Clinical Nutrition* **71** (suppl.), 1233S–1241S.

Atallah AN, Hofmeyr GJ, Duley L. (2000). Calcium supplementation during pregnancy for preventing hypertensive disorders and related problems. *Cochrane Database System Review.*

Butte NF (2000). Carbohydrate and lipid metabolism in pregnancy: normal compared with gestational diabetes mellitus. *American Journal of Clinical Nutrition* **71** (suppl.), 1256S–1261S.

Durnin JVGA (1991). Energy requirements of pregnancy. *Diabetes* **40** (suppl. 2), 152–6.

Campbell-Brown M, Hytten FE (1998). Nutrition. In: Chamberlain G, Broughton-Pipkin F, eds. *Clinical Physiology in Obstetrics*, 3rd edn, pp 165–91. Blackwell Science, Oxford. A thorough review of nutrition in pregnancy.

Hattersley AT, Tooke JE (1999). The fetal insulin hypothesis: an alternative explanation of the association of low birthweight with diabetes and vascular disease. *The Lancet* **353**, 1789–92.

Institute of Medicine (United States) (1990). *Nutrition during pregnancy. Report of the Committee on Nutritional Status during pregnancy and lactation, food and nutrition board.* National Academy Press, Washington, DC.

Kalhan SC (2000). Protein metabolism in pregnancy. *American Journal of Clinical Nutrition* **71** (suppl.), 1249S–1255S.

Kalkwarf HJ *et al.* (1997). The effect of calcium supplementation on bone density during lactation and after weaning. *New England Journal of Medicine* **337**, 523–8.

Koop-Hoolihan LE *et al.* (1999). Longitudinal assessment of energy balance in well-nourished, pregnant women. *American Journal of Clinical Nutrition* **69** (suppl.), 697–704.

Mahomed K (2000). Iron supplementation in pregnancy (Cochrane Review). *The Cochrane Library*, Issue 3. Update Software, Oxford.

O'Brien SPM, Wheeler T, Barker DJP, eds (1999). *Fetal programming. Influences on development and disease in later life.* RCOG Press, London. A comprehensive series of reviews and research articles on fetal programming.

Prentice A. (2000). Calcium in pregnancy and lactation. *Annual Review of Nutrition* **20**, 249–72.

Prentice AM, Goldberg GR (2000). Energy adaptations in human pregnancy: limits and long term consequences. *American Journal of Clinical Nutrition* **71** (suppl.), 1226S–1232S.

Ramakrishnan U *et al.* (1999). Micronutrients and pregnancy outcome: A review of the literature. *Nutrition Research* **19**, 103–59.

Rothman KJ *et al.* (1995). Teratogenicity of high vitamin A intake. *New England Journal of Medicine* **333**, 1369–73.

Rush D (2000). Nutrition and maternal mortality in the developing world. *American Journal of Clinical Nutrition* **72** (suppl.), 212S–240S.

13.3 Medical management of normal pregnancy

D. J. Williams

Introduction

Until very recently *Homo sapiens* thrived with nothing but the most primitive antenatal care. The introduction of hospital-based childbirth in the United Kingdom was a disaster. In the mid 1800s it became clear to some that unhygienic medical practice was responsible for puerperal sepsis and a high maternal mortality rate. From the 1930s, maternal mortality in the United Kingdom fell from 1 in 100 deliveries in the worst maternity hospitals, to 1 in 10 000 deliveries today. Globally, however, there are still 585 000 pregnancy-related maternal deaths each year, meaning that one woman dies every minute of every day as a consequence of pregnancy and childbirth.

With the exception of a high death rate from AIDS in many developing nations, the causes of maternal mortality worldwide are similar to those found in developed countries before the implementation of modern obstetric practices (Fig. 1). In the developed world, the dramatic reduction in the number of maternal deaths from obstetric complications has not been matched by a similar fall in deaths associated with pre-existing maternal disease. This latter observation is partly due to the success of modern medicine in helping more women with congenital or chronic disease to survive until reproductive age, and partly due to the inability of physicians to manage otherwise familiar medical conditions during pregnancy.

Misplaced concern about fetal welfare often denies the mother life-saving investigations and treatment. Substandard care is therefore responsible for many maternal deaths in consequence. Clinical anxiety may be amplified when a doctor is presented with a healthy woman who has everything to lose by meddlesome intervention. The general physician should therefore be aware of the symptoms and signs of normal pregnancy and familiar with advice on how women should prepare for and maintain a healthy pregnancy.

Maternal factors that influence pregnancy outcome

Maternal age

More women are having babies later in life than ever before. In the United States, between 1969 and 1994, the median age at first birth increased from 21.3 to 24.4 years and the proportion of first time mothers aged 30 years or more increased from 4 per cent to 21 per cent. The prevalence of pregnancy-induced hypertension, gestational diabetes, and thrombosis is increased in women over 35 years.

Fetal aneuploidy, most notably trisomy 21 (Down's syndrome), also increases with maternal age. At 25 years of age, the risk of a pregnancy with trisomy 21 is 1:1250, at 35 years it is 1:385, and at 45 years it is 1:30. These risks can be refined during pregnancy (from 16 weeks) by information derived from measurement of maternal serum concentrations of α-fetoprotein, human chorionic gonadotrophin, and unconjugated oes-

triol (the triple test). Some centres derive a risk of chromosomal abnormality from an ultrasound measurement of skinfold thickness at the back of the fetal neck (nuchal translucency screening, around 12 weeks). Women found to be at high risk of a chromosomal abnormality can be offered diagnostic testing with amniocentesis (which carries a 0.5 to 1.0 per cent risk of miscarriage).

Maternal weight

Maternal health is threatened by a high prepregnancy weight. Pre-eclampsia and gestational diabetes mellitus are more common in overweight women (body mass index (**BMI**) more than 26), and the risk of late fetal death is also increased. However, maternal obesity protects against the

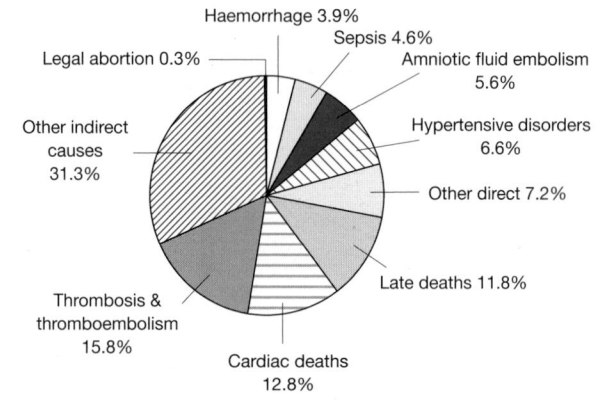

(a)

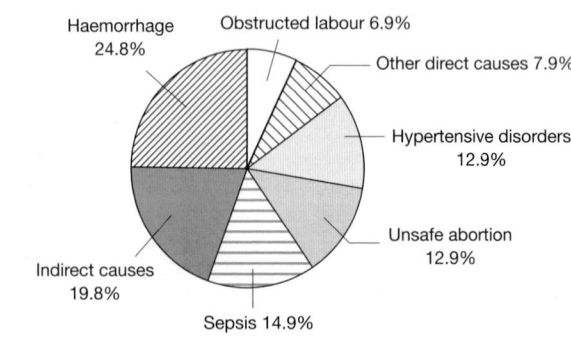

(b)

Fig. 1 (a) Causes of maternal mortality in the United Kingdom 1994–6 (adapted from Department of Health (1998)). (b) Causes of 585 000 maternal deaths worldwide in 1990. Direct deaths are a direct consequence of pregnancy; indirect deaths are due to the effects of pregnancy on pre-existing maternal disease. (Reproduced from Liljestrand (1999), with permission.)

delivery of an infant which is small for gestational age, whereas underweight women (BMI less than 19) are more prone to have babies with lower birth weights.

Weight gain during healthy pregnancy varies between 10 and 16 kg in Western societies, i.e. about 20 per cent of prepregnancy weight. Lean, nulliparous women who eat to appetite gain 0.65 to 1.1 kg during the first 10 weeks of pregnancy, about 0.45 kg per week during the second trimester, and about 0.36 kg per week during the last trimester. Maternal weight gain correlates poorly with fetal growth. Unless the mother is underweight before pregnancy (BMI less than 19), regular antenatal measurements of maternal weight are not helpful and fetal growth is most accurately assessed by serial ultrasound measurements.

Past medical history

Pregnancy is a medical stress test for the woman, which is particularly evident in those with chronic medical disorders. A diseased maternal organ may lose residual function attempting to accommodate the physiological demands of pregnancy. Furthermore, women with severe pre-existing disease are more likely to have an adverse fetal outcome.

Pregnancy can also uncover subclinical disease; for example inherited thrombophilias may lead to thrombosis only in combination with the hypercoagulable environment of healthy pregnancy. However, the physiological changes of pregnancy are not always damaging: some conditions improve, whilst others deteriorate (Table 1).

Family history

Gestational conditions tend to run in families. Pre-eclampsia, gestational diabetes mellitus, obstetric cholestasis, and probably hyperemesis gravidarum and postnatal depression have genetic components. Inherited thrombophilias may also have a direct impact on pregnancy outcome.

Infertility and multiple pregnancies

In 1978 the birth of the first baby by *in vitro* fertilization (**IVF**) gave hope to the 15 per cent of couples who are infertile. Since then over 200 000 children have been born throughout the world using IVF, and in the United Kingdom a healthy baby is born from 17.4 per cent of IVF cycles on average. The cause of infertility may itself lead to problems in pregnancy, for example women with polycystic ovary syndrome are at increased risk of pregnancy-induced hypertension and gestational diabetes.

In most cases of IVF, two embryos are returned to the woman. As a consequence, 28.9 per cent of deliveries from IVF conceptions lead to multiple births. Following natural conception, multiple births affect only 11 per 1000 pregnancies in the United States and Europe. Women with multiple pregnancies are more vulnerable to pre-eclampsia and premature delivery.

Ovarian hyperstimulation syndrome

To increase the yield of eggs, women receiving IVF undergo ovarian stimulation with gonadotrophins, following which up to 14 per cent develop an ovarian hyperstimulation syndrome, which is severe in 1 to 2 per cent of cases. In ovarian hyperstimulation syndrome, multiple follicles develop into corpus lutea that produce excessive amounts of progesterone, resulting in massive ovarian enlargement and increased vascular permeability. Protein-rich fluid shifts into serous cavities, causing ascites, and in more severe cases pleural and pericardial effusions. The fluid shift results in haemoconcentration and hypotension, increasing the risk of thrombosis and reducing renal perfusion. Most cases of ovarian hyperstimulation syndrome are mild, but death has followed acute respiratory distress, hepatorenal failure, thromboembolism, and rupture of grossly enlarged ovaries. Management is mainly supportive, including careful fluid balance, thromboprophylaxis, analgesia, and adjustment of luteal stimulation under the guidance of a specialist in assisted conception. In some cases, paracentesis relieves pressure symptoms.

Diagnosis of pregnancy

Pregnancy can be diagnosed within a day of missing a menstrual bleed by identifying a rise in concentration of urinary human chorionic gonadotrophin. At this time the embryo is 2 weeks old, but obstetric convention dictates that the gestation of pregnancy is calculated from the first day of the last menstrual period, i.e. 2 weeks earlier than embryonic age. Teratogenic drugs interfere with organ development in the 2 to 8 weeks postconception (embryonic period). After 9 weeks and until delivery, the conceptus is known as a fetus, but it is still vulnerable to the effects of drugs given to the mother.

Table 1 Effect of pregnancy on pre-existing conditions

Conditions that tend to improve during pregnancy	
	Mitral and aortic regurgitation
	Raynaud's phenomenon
	Mild hypertension (worsens towards term)
	Hyperthyroidism
	Sarcoid
	Rheumatoid arthritis
	Multiple sclerosis (relapses postpartum)
	Peptic ulceration
Conditions that are unpredictable during pregnancy	
	Asthma
	Systemic lupus erythematosus (tends to relapse postpartum)
	Inflammatory bowel disease
Conditions that tend to deteriorate during pregnancy	
Cardiovascular system	Mitral and aortic stenosis
	Pulmonary hypertension (40–50 per cent risk of maternal mortality)
	Congenital cyanotic heart disease
	Supraventricular arrhythmias
	Vascular aneurysms
	Epistaxis
	Varicose veins and piles
Respiratory system	Viral pneumonia
	Pulmonary embolus
Gastrointestinal system	Gastro-oesophageal reflux (in third trimester)
	Constipation
Genitourinary system	Urinary tract infections
	Reflux nephropathy
	Renal impairment (GFR / <30 ml/min)
	HUS/TTP
Musculoskeletal system	Osteoporosis
	Antiphospholipid syndrome (DVT and recurrent miscarriage)
Endocrine system	Diabetes mellitus and insipidus
	Hypothyroidism
	Hyperlipidaemia
	Pituitary macroadenoma
Neurological system	Epilepsy
	Cerebrovascular accidents
	Depression (postnatal)
	Headache
	Carpal tunnel syndrome
Haematological system	Anaemia and thrombocytopenia
	Sickle cell disease
	Thrombophilias
Infections	Intracellular pathogens (e.g. malaria, leprosy, listeria)
	Viral infections (e.g. varicella and influenza)

GFR, glomerular filtration rate; HUS/TTP, haemolytic-uraemic syndrome/thrombotic thrombocytopenic purpura; DVT, deep vein thrombosis.

Screening of maternal health during pregnancy

Pregnancy is an opportunity for women to be screened for occult disease. In the United Kingdom, healthy women are encouraged to register with an antenatal clinic at 12 to 14 weeks' gestation. However, by this gestation they will have missed the opportunity to take folic acid prophylaxis against neural tube defects, and may not recognize the need to adjust social behaviour (see below) or stop regular medications.

At the first antenatal visit, a medical and obstetric history is combined with cardiovascular examination, urinalysis, and laboratory tests. Identification of maternal infection with HIV, hepatitis B, or syphilis is crucial for appropriate management of the woman and her partner, and to minimize the risk of vertical transmission to the infant. Rhesus antibody screening allows prophylactic measures to prevent haemolytic disease of the fetus.

Further antenatal checks are usually performed at 20 weeks (combined with a detailed scan of the fetus), 26 to 28 weeks (combined with a glucose tolerance test and full blood count), 30, 32, 34 (full blood count), and 36 weeks, then weekly until delivery. At each visit, obstetric assessment is combined with a check of blood pressure and urinalysis.

Screening for asymptomatic bacteriuria during healthy pregnancy and subsequent treatment reduces the risk of maternal pyelonephritis and fetal morbidity. The cost-effectiveness of such screening depends on the prevalence of asymptomatic bacteriuria in the pregnant population. If the prevalence is less than 5 per cent, as in many developed nations, screening is probably not cost-effective. However, in the developing world asymptomatic bacteriuria is far more common and screening is worthwhile. As the recurrence rate of asymptomatic bacteriuria is about 30 per cent, women identified with an occult infection should be screened monthly throughout the remainder of their pregnancy. These issues are discussed in Chapter 13.5.

Symptoms and signs of healthy pregnancy

Fatigue

Fatigue is a common symptom that often begins early in healthy pregnancy. Towards term, changes in maternal size and shape as well as nocturia cause insomnia. If daily living is significantly compromised, anaemia or hypothyroidism should be excluded.

Cardiovascular system

The hyperdynamic circulation of pregnancy causes alterations to the cardiovascular system that can mimic heart disease (see Chapter 13.6). Furthermore, palpitations, dizziness, syncope, and dyspnoea are common symptoms of healthy pregnancy. Failure to distinguish between benign physiological change and significant pathology creates unnecessary anxiety and investigations.

Clinical examination

During healthy pregnancy, the peripheral pulses are full, bounding, and often collapsing, suggesting aortic regurgitation to the untutored. From mid-gestation onwards the jugular venous pressure becomes more obvious and may be raised due to increased intra-abdominal pressure. The apex beat is more forceful and because of the increase in cardiac output may suggest cardiomegaly in normal patients. However, if the apex beat is more than 2 cm outside the midclavicular line, this should be considered abnormal. On auscultation, an ejection systolic flow murmur can be heard in up to 90 per cent of healthy pregnant women. During the last trimester, increased mammary blood flow can produce a bruit that varies with the pressure of the stethoscope.

In developed countries it is very rare for new heart lesions to be identified during pregnancy: most women with heart disease are diagnosed early in life. By contrast, women from developing nations are more likely to present with previously unrecognized cardiac abnormalities.

Palpitations

Transient sinus tachycardia, up to 130 beats/min, and premature atrial and ventricular ectopic beats are common features of healthy pregnancy, especially in women who complain of palpitations. As pregnancy may expose previously asymptomatic abnormalities of cardiac conducting tissue, investigations should include a 12-lead ECG. During healthy pregnancy, the QRS axis moves to the left as the diaphragm becomes elevated and Q waves and inverted T waves are frequently seen in lead III and aVR. Pregnant women with syncope or presyncope coinciding with palpitations should have a 24-h Holter monitor. Thyrotoxicosis, anaemia, hypokalaemia, excess caffeine, or tobacco should be excluded.

Oedema

By the end of pregnancy, 80 per cent of healthy women will have some degree of oedema. This is due to a fall in plasma albumin concentration of 5 to 10 g/litre and reduced venous return. Unless peripheral oedema is very severe, or is associated with pulmonary oedema, diuretics should be avoided: they attenuate the plasma volume expansion of healthy pregnancy, which can lead to restriction of fetal growth. Severe and rapid onset of oedema, especially affecting hands and face, may herald pre-eclampsia and warrants further assessment.

Blood pressure

Peripheral vasodilatation leads to a slight fall in blood pressure by the end of the first trimester, which gradually returns to non-pregnant values during the third trimester. Systolic and diastolic readings are approximately 10 mmHg higher when measured sitting or standing as compared with the left lateral position, hence blood pressure should be measured with the mother in the same position at each antenatal visit. A blood pressure reading before 20 weeks' gestation is essential to allow later discrimination between pre-existing hypertension and pregnancy-induced hypertension.

Respiratory system

Dyspnoea

The physiological hyperventilation of pregnancy leads to a subjective feeling of breathlessness in about 70 per cent of women. The maximum incidence of breathlessness is between 28 and 31 weeks' gestation, but approximately 50 per cent of women will feel breathless before 20 weeks. The early onset of dyspnoea and improvement towards term suggests that the gravid uterus has little influence on this physiological symptom. Women with gestational dyspnoea are more sensitive to CO_2 and hypoxia than asymptomatic women and respond with excessive ventilation. However, physiological dyspnoea does not usually interfere with daily activities and further investigations are only necessary if symptoms or signs suggest cardiorespiratory disease, for example chest infection, pulmonary embolus, or heart failure.

Radiological imaging in pregnancy

In general, management of pregnant women should consider the health of the mother before that of the fetus. Nowhere is this consideration ignored more than with the use of X-rays. Although ionizing radiation is a known carcinogen, there is very little—if any—increased risk of childhood cancer following prenatal exposure to X-rays. Radiation from a chest radiograph is minimal (0.02 mSv), equivalent to 3 days of background radiation. During healthy pregnancy, chest radiographs show an increased cardiothoracic ratio and pulmonary vascular markings. Pregnant women suspected of a pulmonary embolus should not be denied a ventilation-perfusion scan (1.3 mSv).

Gastrointestinal system

Nausea and vomiting

During early pregnancy, approximately 75 per cent of all healthy women will feel nauseated and up to 50 per cent will vomit. Nausea usually begins around the fifth week; by the 14th week it will have resolved in 50 per cent of women, but 10 per cent of healthy pregnant women will still feel nauseated at 22 weeks. Contrary to popular belief, nausea is rarely confined to the mornings (less than 2 per cent), but affects 80 per cent of sufferers all day. Beneficial palliative measures include rest, eating carbohydrates, and drinking carbonated drinks.

Vomiting is severe and persistent in approximately 1.5 per cent of pregnant women. This progresses to hyperemesis gravidarum when there is dehydration, weight loss, and ketonuria (see section 13.09). Ptyalism is a frequent accompaniment, due to an inability to swallow saliva. Biochemical changes often include elevated liver transaminases, elevated free T_4, and depressed thyroid-stimulating hormone. Hyperthyroxinaemia associated with hyperemesis gravidarum coincides with the rise and fall of serum human chorionic gonadotrophin, which has thyroid-stimulating activity. Treatment of hyperemesis corrects the abnormal biochemistry.

Antiemetics have not been fully evaluated in early pregnancy. The clinician must therefore balance the potential risks of teratogenesis with the risks of leaving the mother malnourished, inadequately hydrated, and vulnerable to thrombosis. Most antiemetics, including antihistamines, phenothiazines, metoclopramide, pyridoxine (vitamin B_6), and ginger have been used to treat hyperemesis with some success and without fetal harm. More severe cases have responded to steroid treatment (prednisolone 30 mg daily) or serotonin antagonists. Intravenous rehydration and occasionally parenteral nutrition are necessary. Hyperemesis gravidarum can lead to Wernicke's encephalopathy, hence thiamine (vitamin B_1) supplementation is essential.

New onset of nausea and vomiting during the second half of pregnancy suggests pathology unrelated to hyperemesis and may herald pre-eclampsia. Gastro-oesophageal reflux is a common problem of late pregnancy that usually improves with antacids or a change in diet, but persistent symptoms during pregnancy have been safely treated with H_2 receptor antagonists or proton pump inhibitors. Increased circulating progesterone levels relax intestinal smooth muscle and commonly provoke constipation. Increased dietary fibre and avoidance of unnecessary iron supplements provide symptomatic relief.

Neurological system

Headaches are common in healthy pregnancy. Many pregnant women develop migrainous type headaches for the first time in early pregnancy: if these are recurrent or do not respond to occasional paracetamol, then regular aspirin 75 mg daily or propranolol 10 to 20 mg thrice daily are good prophylactic measures. Severe, persistent headache that presents for the first time in pregnancy, or is accompanied by focal neurological signs, requires investigation with magnetic resonance imaging (see section 13.12).

Introduction of an epidural catheter during labour can lead to accidental puncture of the dura and leak of cerebrospinal fluid, causing headache that improves when lying flat. If there is no improvement within 24 h, then an injection of 2 to 3 ml of autologous blood at the site of dural puncture (blood patch) usually resolves the headache.

Carpal tunnel syndrome affects approximately 20 per cent of healthy pregnancies. It begins during the second half of pregnancy and is associated with excessive weight gain and fluid retention. Pain and numbness of the first three fingers and wrist can be severe. Wrist splints alleviate symptoms, usually making surgical intervention inappropriate, as the majority of cases recover within a few weeks of delivery.

Musculoskeletal system

Low back and pelvic pain affect approximately 50 per cent of all pregnancies. A combination of mechanical stress on the spine and pelvis and the effects of relaxin, a hormone produced by the corpus luteum to relax ligaments in anticipation of childbirth, are believed to be responsible. Some women develop radicular symptoms as the uterus presses on nerve roots and the lumbar sacral plexus, but only 1 per cent develop true sciatica with a dermatomal distribution. Progressive neurological symptoms necessitate further investigations, often with magnetic resonance imaging. Most women will benefit from massage, exercises, or a maternity cushion. Others gain relief from transcutaneous electrical nerve stimulation or a trochanteric support belt. Non-steroidal anti-inflammatory drugs should be avoided in the third trimester, and used sparingly in early pregnancy because of fetal effects.

Skin

Pruritis is a common symptom of late pregnancy, thought to be related to increased cutaneous blood flow. If there is an associated rash, then gestational skin conditions need to be considered (see Chapter 13.13). If there is no rash, then liver function should be checked to exclude obstetric cholestasis.

Supplements for a healthy pregnancy

Folic acid and multivitamins

In the United Kingdom and United States spina bifida or anencephaly (neural tube defects) affect approximately 1 in 1000 pregnancies. The neural tube develops and then closes within 28 days of conception. Women who take 400 μg folic acid daily around the time of conception and for the first 2 months of pregnancy reduce their risk of a pregnancy complicated by neural tube defects by approximately 70 per cent. Foods fortified with folic acid provide only 100 μg folic acid and natural folate-rich foods even less: these lower doses of folic acid are of no proven benefit as prophylaxis against neural tube defects. Women who have had a baby affected by spina bifida, who are taking anticonvulsants, or who have coeliac disease, require higher doses of folic acid (5 mg daily).

Multivitamin preparations without folic acid do not reduce the risk of neural tube defects. Multivitamins taken periconceptually may reduce the risk of some congenital heart defects, but beyond the first trimester are of no proven benefit for healthy women on a balanced diet.

Iron

During healthy pregnancy the haemoglobin concentration falls as plasma volume expands. A gestational fall in haemoglobin of 3 g/dl to 9.5 to 10.5 g/dl is associated with the least incidence of small babies and premature delivery. Conversely, a haemoglobin of more than 12 g/dl at the end of the second trimester is associated with a three-fold increase in pre-eclampsia and intrauterine growth restriction (both are plasma contracted states). In the developed world, supplemental iron should be reserved for those who have a haemoglobin of less than 9.5 g/dl and a mean corpuscular volume of less than 84 fl in the third trimester. In the developing world, malnutrition and chronic infection diminish iron stores that are further exhausted during pregnancy. Under these conditions, routine supplemental iron and folate may have the potential to improve maternal and neonatal outcome (see section 13.02 for further discussion).

Prophylaxis against pre-eclampsia

Pre-eclampsia affects approximately 3 to 5 per cent of healthy nulliparous women. It is a heterogeneous, multisystem disorder to which predisposed women are vulnerable in different ways. Aetiology is uncertain, but likely to be multifactorial. It is no surprise, therefore, that none of the prophylactic measures given in an attempt to reduce the incidence of pre-eclampsia have proved to be beneficial in large randomized controlled trials. Such measures have included low-dose aspirin, dietary magnesium, zinc, and calcium, antihypertensive drugs, fish oil supplements, and antioxidant vitamins. A clearer understanding of the pathogenesis of pre-eclampsia is necessary before we can expect success from prophylactic measures, and when these are available they will probably need to be individualized.

Thyroxine and iodine

During the first trimester, neurodevelopment of the fetus depends on maternal thyroxine and subclinical hypothyroidism in the mother has been associated with impaired neurodevelopment of the infant. It has therefore been suggested that all women should be screened during early pregnancy, or before conception, for hypothyroidism. The difficulties of implementing this measure are probably outweighed by more easily applied public health measures to increase iodine intake. The benefit of thyroxine replacement in women with 'low normal' thyroxine levels has not been established.

Behavioural habits during pregnancy

Exercise

Pregnancy outcome is improved by regular exercise throughout a healthy pregnancy. The gestational increases in both cardiac output and respiratory work are enhanced further by exercise. In late pregnancy, non-weight-bearing exercises such as swimming are usually preferred. Exercise may be harmful to women with impaired cardiac or respiratory function who struggle to fulfil the physiological demands of pregnancy alone.

Alcohol

Heavy alcohol consumption during pregnancy leads to the 'fetal alcohol syndrome' in approximately one-third of offspring. The susceptibility of the fetus to alcohol depends on genetic vulnerability, nutritional status of the woman, and her abuse of other drugs. The developmental and neurological abnormalities that make up the fetal alcohol syndrome affect approximately 1 to 2 per 1000 live births. Drinking one to two units of alcohol each day has not been shown to be harmful to the fetus.

Tobacco

Women should stop smoking during pregnancy as it impairs fetal growth. Nicotine gum contains less nicotine than cigarettes and none of the other toxins, making them a preferable alternative during pregnancy. Nicotine patches provide a constant release of nicotine throughout the day that exceeds that of periodic nicotine gum. Smoking is a major source of oxidant stress, but paradoxically women who smoke before and during pregnancy suffer less pre-eclampsia than non-smokers.

Caffeine

Large quantities of caffeine (more than six cups of coffee a day) increase the risk of spontaneous abortion. Moderate caffeine consumption is unlikely to be harmful.

Travel

Aircraft are pressurized to an oxygen partial pressure equivalent to that found at 8000 ft (2440 m) above sea level. During a routine commercial flight, healthy pregnant women (32 to 38 weeks' gestation) increase their heart rate and blood pressure but drop their oxygen saturation. Despite these maternal responses, fetal heart rate remains unchanged. Airlines are reluctant to carry women after 36 weeks' gestation. Long flights also increase the risk of deep vein thrombosis.

Lactation

Breastfeeding is beneficial to the infant. However, the mother who breastfeeds for 6 months or longer transiently loses 4 to 5 per cent of bone density in her lumbar spine. Calcium supplementation does not prevent this transient loss of bone mineral density, which recovers spontaneously 6 months after delivery, whether or not the mother continues to breast feed.

Postnatal depression

Almost half of all women develop the 'maternity blues'. This is characterized by tearfulness, anxiety, and irritability, starting around the third to fifth postpartum days and usually resolving with nothing more than reassurance by the tenth day. Approximately 10 per cent of women develop non-psychotic postnatal depression 4 to 6 weeks postpartum, with a maximum incidence at 3 months postpartum. The depression is similar to that occurring at other times, but is often accompanied by thoughts of harming the baby. Although most women recover without treatment over 3 to 6 months, recovery can be hastened by counselling. Women who fail to respond to counselling or who have severe depression may benefit from antidepressant treatment. Small amounts of tricyclic antidepressants and selective serotonin reuptake inhibitors appear in breast milk, but not enough to recommend stopping breastfeeding. Nonetheless, the infant should be watched for possible unwanted effects. Women who have had postpartum depression are more likely to suffer depression in later life.

Future maternal health

'Gestational syndromes' must be monitored postpartum until they resolve or reveal occult disease. For example, proteinuria related to pre-eclampsia can take up to 12 months to disappear, but may expose the 2 to 5 per cent of women with pre-eclampsia who have occult renal impairment. Similarly, abnormal liver function that does not resolve postpartum suggests non-gestational liver disease.

Insulin resistance underlying gestational diabetes mellitus resolves immediately postpartum. However, women who have had gestational diabetes mellitus have a 20 to 60 per cent risk of developing type 2 diabetes mellitus within 5 to 16 years of pregnancy. Similarly, both pregnancy-induced hypertension and pre-eclampsia, but not eclampsia, increase the mother's risk of cardiovascular disease in later life (Fig. 2).

Despite all of the above, most women complete an uncomplicated pregnancy. This bodes well for maternal health during subsequent pregnancies.

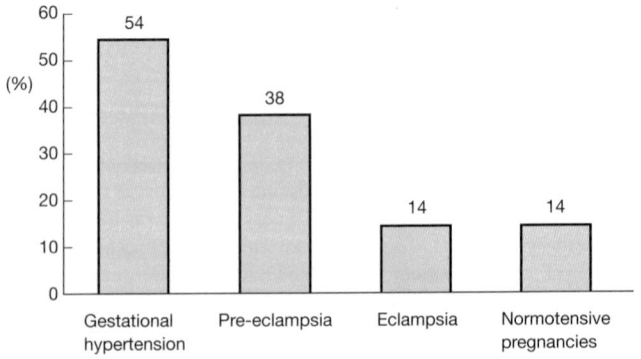

Fig. 2 Prevalence of hypertension 13.7 ± 5.1 years after pregnancy-induced hypertension (111 women), pre-eclampsia (80 women), eclampsia (14 women), and normotensive pregnancies (86 women). (Reproduced from Marin *et al.* (2000), with permission.)

Furthermore, those who were normotensive during pregnancy are less likely than the national average to have cardiovascular disease in later life.

Further reading

Botto LD *et al.* (1999). Neural-tube defects. *New England Journal of Medicine* **341**, 1485–90. Comprehensive review of neural tube defects.

Department of Health (1998). *Why mothers die. Report on confidential enquiries into maternal deaths in the United Kingdom 1994–1996.* Department of Health, London. Audit of maternal deaths in the United Kingdom with comments on management.

Garcia-Rio F *et al.* (1996). Regulation of breathing and perception of dyspnoea in healthy pregnant women. *Chest* **110**, 446–53. Thorough study of pattern and mechanism of dyspnoea during normal pregnancy.

Greer IA (1999). Thrombosis in pregnancy: maternal and fetal issues. *The Lancet* **353**, 1258–65. Review of management of thromboembolic disease in pregnancy.

Haddow JE *et al.* (1999). Maternal thyroid deficiency during pregnancy and subsequent neuropsychological development of the child. *New England Journal of Medicine* **341**, 549–55.

Human Fertilization and Embryology Authority (1999). *Eighth annual report.* HMSO, London.

James DK *et al.*, eds (1999). *High risk pregnancy*, 2nd edn. WB Saunders, London. Comprehensive review of management of normal and abnormal pregnancies.

Kalkwarf HJ *et al.* (1997). The effect of calcium supplementation on bone density during lactation and after weaning. *New England Journal of Medicine* **337**, 523–8.

Kjos SL, Buchanan TA (1999). Current concepts: gestational diabetes mellitus. *New England Journal of Medicine* **341**, 1749–56.

Lacroix R, Eason E, Melzack R (2000). Nausea and vomiting during pregnancy: a prospective study of its frequency, intensity and patterns of change. *American Journal of Obstetrics and Gynecology* **182**, 931–7.

Liljestrand J (1999). Reducing perinatal and maternal mortality in the world: the major challenges. *British Journal of Obstetrics and Gynaecology* **106**, 877–80. Commentary on global problem of perinatal and maternal mortality.

Marin R *et al.* (2000). Long-term prognosis of hypertension in pregnancy. *Hypertension in Pregnancy* **19**, 199–209. Thirteen year follow-up of women with hypertension in pregnancy.

Steer PJ (2000). Maternal hemoglobin concentration and birth weight. *American Journal of Clinical Nutrition* **71**, 1285S–1287S. Review of relationship between maternal haemoglobin and clinical outcome.

Whelan JG 3rd, Vlahos NF (2000). The ovarian hyperstimulation syndrome. *Fertility and Sterility* **73**, 883–96.

13.4 Hypertension in pregnancy

C. W. G. Redman

Cardiovascular changes in pregnancy

Cardiac output increases during the first trimester to about 1.5 l/min above the levels of non-pregnant women. No further increase occurs in the second and third trimesters. Towards full term, it declines in the supine but not lateral recumbent position, owing to the pressure of the gravid uterus on the inferior vena cava, which reduces venous return to the heart. In the third trimester, about two-thirds of the additional cardiac output is distributed to the placental circulation and to augment renal plasma flow. The increased output is the result of both a greater stroke volume and a higher pulse rate. Plasma volume increases progressively during the second and third trimesters and is significantly correlated with the birthweight of the conceptus, being higher in multiple pregnancies. Arterial pressure falls in the second half of the first trimester at about the same time as the cardiac output is increasing, meaning that peripheral resistance decreases relatively more than the cardiac output increases. The uteroplacental circulation is too small at this time to cause these changes, which must therefore result from a generalized arteriolar dilatation.

In the later weeks of pregnancy, there is a tendency for the diastolic pressure to rise slowly towards what it was before pregnancy began, the systolic pressure remaining more or less unchanged. However, in the supine position, with vena caval compression and reduced venous return, the arterial pressure may be atypically low with a narrowed pulse pressure and reflex vasoconstriction. The fall in systolic pressure may exceed 30 per cent in 10 per cent of cases and cause 'the supine hypotension syndrome'—evident as restlessness, faintness, hyperpnoea, and pallor.

Hypertension in pregnancy: definition, causes, and terminology

Definition

The average blood pressure during the first half of the second trimester is about 120/70; 140/85 and 160/95 correspond to two and three standard deviations above the mean, respectively. Hypertension in obstetric practice is conventionally recognized at or above an arbitrary threshold of 140/90. This is appropriate for the first half of pregnancy, but in the second half about one-quarter of all women will be hypertensive by this criterion, meaning that these limits are too low to define an unusual group that merits extra clinical attention. About 2.5 per cent have a maximum arterial pressure of 160/105 or more and about 1 per cent of 170/110 or more; these are more relevant limits for identifying third trimester hypertension.

Causes of hypertension in pregnancy

Hypertension in pregnancy has three possible aetiologies. Most important, it may be caused by the pregnancy as part of the syndrome of pre-eclampsia, a specific disorder of pregnancy that is common, dangerous, and poorly understood. Second, it may represent chronic hypertension, a long-term attribute of the woman. In some women chronic hypertension may be revealed for the first time during pregnancy—typically towards the end; but the condition is of the woman not of her pregnancy. Third, and much more rarely, it may be a new medical condition coinciding with pregnancy by chance.

Pre-eclampsia is a common syndrome that becomes evident in the second half of pregnancy (although its origins may lie in the first half). It is defined in terms of the transient development of new hypertension and proteinuria, these may be severe, but regress after delivery.

Terminology

Eclampsia is characterized by grand-mal convulsions. Pre-eclampsia (previously called pre-eclamptic toxaemia (PET)) is so called because it may precede eclampsia, as well as a number of other possible crises. These other crises (described below) are just as dangerous as eclampsia and occur as commonly or even more so. Not all cases of eclampsia are preceded by a prodromal illness of pre-eclampsia, so the terminology is altogether too simplistic to describe the events that can occur. Toxaemia is an obsolete expression, previously used to describe any hypertension or proteinuria in pregnancy, whether pregnancy-induced or not.

Pregnancy-induced hypertension (PIH), transient hypertension of pregnancy, or gestational hypertension are terms used to describe new hypertension, which appears after mid-term (20 weeks) and resolves after delivery. They therefore describe one of the components of the pre-eclampsia syndrome. For reasons that are historical rather than logical, and which are to some extent arbitrary, PIH is deemed to be a mandatory part of pre-eclampsia. However, PIH on its own (a common clinical presentation) is not pre-eclampsia; at least one more sign is required to make the diagnosis. The clusters of clinical features that comprise any syndrome are chosen for convenience; they describe outward appearances and embody no special truth about the underlying disease or diseases. When a syndrome such as pre-eclampsia is 'defined', rules are set that bring consistency to what is being discussed. The rules may be sensible or not, but their validity cannot be tested because there is no standard to which to refer. All the definitions of pre-eclampsia suffer from these limitations and none can be said to be the best. The conventional components of the cluster are PIH combined with new proteinuria that regresses after delivery.

Almost all hypertension presenting before mid-term (gestational age of 20 weeks) indicates pre-existing or chronic hypertension, the rare exceptions being women with atypical very early onset pre-eclampsia. However, normotension in the first half of pregnancy does not necessarily mean long-term normotension: the fall in blood pressure induced in early pregnancy may be exaggerated in some women and many with relatively severe hypertension may have normal blood pressures (without treatment) by 12 weeks; indeed, in one study as many as 60 per cent of women with chronic hypertension defined before pregnancy were normotensive by the end of the first trimester. In other words, some women enjoy the benefits of pregnancy-induced normotension just as others suffer the disadvantages of pregnancy-induced hypertension. Pregnancy-induced normotension tends

Table 1 Definition of pre-eclampsia (International Society for the Study of Hypertension in Pregnancy)

Hypertension	Diastolic pressure ≥ 90mmHg or two or more consecutive occasions ≥ 4 h apart or ≥ 110 mmHg once
Proteinuria	24 h urine collection ≥ 300 mg protein or two MSUs collected more than 4 h apart with ≥ + on stick test
Pre-eclampsia	New hypertension and new proteinuria developing after 20 weeks gestational age and regressing remotely after delivery

Table 2 Risk factors for pre-eclampsia

Maternal factors	Placental/fetal factors
Primigravidity	Advancing gestational age
Primipaternity[1]	Poor placentation[3]
Short period of cohabitation[2]	Multiple pregnancy
Increasing maternal age	Hydatidiform mole
Previous pre-eclampsia	Triploidy
Obesity (syndrome X, polycystic ovarian syndrome)	Trisomy 13
	Trisomy 16 mosaic
Medical disorders	Placental hydrops
Diabetes	
Chronic hypertension	
Chronic renal disease	
Antiphospholipid antibody syndromes	
Migraines	
Asthma	
Family history of pre-eclampsia	
Stressful job	

[1]There is a partner specificity about the occurrence of pre-eclampsia. Hence it is not simply the first pregnancy that is an important risk factor but the first by the current partner.
[2]Stable cohabitation with a single partner seems to reduce the risk of pre-eclampsia in the first pregnancy by that partner.
[3]See text for explanation of terminology.

to be lost in the third trimester. If the prepregnancy blood pressures are unknown then this may be misinterpreted as pregnancy-induced hypertension rather than recognized for what it is, namely re-establishment of the normal, long-term blood pressure.

Pregnancy-induced hypertension thus represents at least two clinical situations; early pre-eclampsia or occult, chronic hypertension. In many cases, the signs of pre-eclampsia are not confirmed, but nevertheless the blood pressure reverts to normal after delivery. It is possible that these cases represent the very early stages of pre-eclampsia, an alternative being that an innate tendency to hypertension has been revealed in pregnancy but will become overt only many years later. The studies have not been done to confirm or refute this suggestion.

Pre-eclampsia

Pre-eclampsia becomes evident in the second half of pregnancy, during labour or even, for the first time and without apparent preceding problems, in the immediate puerperium, but it always resolves more remotely after delivery. It is common, can be dangerous to both mother and baby, and of unknown cause.

A typical definition of pre-eclampsia is given in Table 1. This and other current definitions require that hypertension and proteinuria, both pregnancy-induced, should be present before the syndrome is recognized. It is now acknowledged that the disorder originates in the placenta, meaning that pre-eclampsia is probably the most common form of secondary hypertension in clinical practice. It is increasingly evident that there are related syndromes, characteristic of the end of pregnancy, which share the same placental causes but do not necessarily provoke hypertension. Hence, although hypertension is conventionally required as a defining feature of pre-eclampsia, it is better considered to be one of several useful signs, but not a central part of the pathology which is more extensive and can involve the maternal liver, clotting, and nervous systems.

The incidence of pre-eclampsia depends on how it is defined and how assiduously the signs are sought. It is possible only to estimate the size of the problem; in the United Kingdom the incidence is of the order of one in 20 to 30 maternities.

Some of the factors that affect susceptibility are listed in Table 2; these include fetal-specific as well as maternal-specific components. Primigravidae are several times more prone to the condition. In parous women, pre-eclampsia particularly affects those who have had the problem before. The predisposition to pre-eclampsia is in part familial, probably genetic, but the pattern of inheritance is not clear. Other factors must also be relevant because pre-eclampsia does not affect identical twin sisters concordantly.

Certain medical problems predispose to pre-eclampsia, including some (chronic hypertension, renal disease) that can mimic the disorder. Superimposed pre-eclampsia refers to the mixed syndrome comprising pre-eclampsia in an individual with pre-existing hypertension or renal disease. In the absence of a specific diagnostic test for pre-eclampsia it can be difficult or impossible to disentangle what elements of proteinuric hypertension are caused by a chronic medical problem or which arise from superimposed pre-eclampsia, and the conventional definitions of pre-eclampsia cease to apply. If a woman is permanently proteinuric there are,

for example, no accepted criteria for diagnosing 'proteinuric pre-eclampsia'. Nevertheless, it seems that chronically hypertensive women are three to seven times more likely to develop higher blood pressures and proteinuria ('superimposed pre-eclampsia') than normotensive women. Women with hypertension associated with chronic renal disease are particularly susceptible.

Aetiology and pathogenesis of pre-eclampsia

The primary pathology of pre-eclampsia is not known for certain, but the presence of a placenta is both necessary and sufficient to cause the disorder. A fetus is not required as pre-eclampsia can occur with hydatidiform mole. A uterus is probably not required because pre-eclampsia may develop with abdominal pregnancy (that is an ectopic pregnancy in the peritoneal cavity). Central to management is delivery, which removes the causative organ, namely the placenta. The primary involvement of the placenta explains why pre-eclampsia is associated with two syndromes not one; the fetal syndrome of nutritional and respiratory deprivation can be as important a part of the illness as the maternal syndrome, or even more so.

The placental problem appears to be a relative ischaemia secondary to deficiencies in the uteroplacental circulation or to an excessively large placenta (with multiple pregnancies for example). The uteroplacental circulation may be compromised by two lesions involving the spiral arteries, which are the end-arteries supplying the intervillous space. The first, poor placentation, is a partial lack of the structural modifications of the spiral arteries that occur between weeks 8 and 18 (before there is clinical evidence of pre-eclampsia), when the arteries become dilated in preparation for the hugely expanded uteroplacental blood flow of the second half of the pregnancy. The second is 'acute atherosis', when aggregates of fibrin, platelets, and lipid-loaded macrophages (lipophages) partially or completely block the ends of the arteries. Neither change is specific to pre-eclampsia; they can also occur with intrauterine growth retardation without a maternal syndrome. Hence the spiral artery changes may be only an associated, but not primary, feature of pre-eclampsia. The relationship of pre-eclampsia with processes that depend on placentation could mean that it originates much earlier than when the maternal syndrome becomes overt. Once pre-eclampsia is established, uteroplacental blood flow is reduced. There is no direct evidence that placental ischaemia can cause pre-eclampsia but in various animal models impeding the placental blood supply can induce a pre-eclamptic-like illness.

The secondary pathology of pre-eclampsia includes all the features of the maternal syndrome, short of decompensation. The maternal syndrome is typically variable in the time of onset, speed of progression, and the extent to which it involves different systems including arterial, coagulation, renal, central nervous, and hepatic. Until recently it was impossible to explain how a single pathological process might cause not only hypertension but also convulsions, disseminated intravascular coagulation, jaundice, hepatic dysfunction, or normotensive proteinuria (among others). However, the concept that the maternal endothelium is the target organ for the pre-eclampsia process has resolved this difficulty. In short, the maternal syndrome is not primarily a hypertensive problem, but the sum of the consequences of diffuse endothelial dysfunction, causing widespread circulatory disturbances in different organ systems as well as generalized arterial and coagulation abnormalities. Latterly, it has been shown that the endothelial dysfunction is one aspect of a more generalized, systemic maternal inflammatory response that also affects circulating leukocytes and other components of the inflammatory system (for example the clotting system). Moreover, this increased inflammatory response is well established in the third trimester of normal pregnancy, when it is not intrinsically different from that in pre-eclampsia except that it is milder. It is thought that pre-eclampsia develops when the pregnancy-induced, systemic inflammatory response causes one or other maternal system to decompensate. In other words, the disorder is not a separate condition but simply the extreme end of a range or continuum of maternal, systemic inflammatory responses engendered by pregnancy itself. This concept has profound implications for clinical practice. If true, it is unlikely that there ever will be a single cause, single diagnostic test, or single preventive measure for pre-eclampsia.

Under certain circumstances the secondary disturbances of pre-eclampsia can become so severe that they cause decompensation, and the tertiary pathology is what makes the condition so dangerous for the mother and baby. It leads to a number of crises that are listed in Table 3.

Clinical characteristics of pre-eclampsia

Usually, hypertension precedes proteinuria, although the converse can happen. Pre-eclampsia is more variable than is generally appreciated—in the time of onset for example. Thus, although pre-eclampsia is defined as presenting after 20 weeks, it may occur earlier or, at the other extreme, become evident only after delivery. The speed with which it progresses and how it involves different maternal systems is also variable.

The hypertension of pre-eclampsia appears to be caused by an increased peripheral resistance secondary to generalized, maternal endothelial dysfunction. There is no single haemodynamic pattern, both increased and decreased cardiac output having been reported. Some of the differences between studies may reflect drug use, for example treatment with vasodilators stimulates cardiac output by reducing afterload. The blood pressure is typically unstable at rest, possibly owing to reduced baroceptor sensitivity. Circadian variation is altered with, first, a loss of the normal fall in blood pressure at night then, in the worst cases, a reversed pattern with the highest readings during sleep.

Pre-eclampsia may cause arterial pressures that are well above the level (i.e. a mean pressure of about 140 mmHg) at which arterial and arteriolar damage would be expected. It is not, therefore, surprising that an important cause of maternal death from pre-eclampsia and eclampsia is cerebral haemorrhage, the pathology of which is similar to that seen in other hypertensive states. As far as it is known, cerebral haemorrhage is the only consequence of pre-eclampsia likely to be affected by antihypertensive treatment.

The involvement of the kidneys in pre-eclampsia has long been recognized. Proteinuria usually develops after the onset of hypertension, although in 10 per cent of cases it is detected first. The proteinuria is moderately selective, increases until delivery, and not uncommonly exceeds 10 g/24 h, pre-eclampsia being the commonest cause of nephrotic syndrome in pregnancy. It is associated with impaired glomerular perfusion and filtration, both reflected in a reduced creatinine clearance and increased plasma creatinine and urea concentrations. The typical renal glomerular lesion of pre-eclampsia is glomerular endotheliosis, when the endothelial cells of the glomeruli swell and block the capillary lumina so that the glomeruli appear enlarged and blood-less. The lesion, which represents direct histological confirmation of endothelial damage in pre-eclampsia, has been defined in research investigations; renal biopsy is never indicated for clinical management. Hyperuricaemia, resulting from a reduced renal urate clearance, is often an early feature of pre-eclampsia, preceding proteinuria and is useful for diagnosis at that stage. However, it is not consistently present so that its absence does not exclude the condition. It tends to be associated with hypocalciuria, another early change in renal function. As the plasma urate rises, the plasma concentrations of urea and creatinine at first remain steady, tending to increase slowly after proteinuria has become established. The tertiary pathology of renal involvement in pre-eclampsia is acute renal failure arising from either tubular or cortical necrosis.

Generalized oedema is an inconsistent feature. It may develop suddenly and is associated with accelerated weight gain. Ascites is not uncommon with severe disease. Laryngeal oedema can cause respiratory obstruction and difficulties with intubation when general anaesthesia is required. Pulmonary oedema is a dangerous complication. In association with modern methods of ventilatory support it may progress to the adult respiratory distress syndrome, which is increasingly a cause of maternal death in this condition.

The clotting system is often, but not invariably, disturbed in pre-eclampsia, with accelerated intravascular generation of thrombin and parallel reductions in the platelet count ascribed to increased consumption. The time course is variable, but a fall in the platelet count may be a relatively early sign—antedating proteinuria for example. However, even when eclampsia supervenes, the majority of women have normal platelet counts at the time of presentation. The coagulation disturbances may decompensate to give overt disseminated intravascular coagulation (DIC). A further complication is microangiopathic haemolysis that may cause a sudden drop in haemoglobin associated with haemoglobinuria, fragmented or distorted red cells (schistocytes) on the peripheral blood film, and reduced serum haptoglobin concentrations.

The severe clotting abnormalities of pre-eclampsia, particularly DIC, are often associated with liver pathology, long recognized as an important and dangerous component of the disorder. When there is also the associated complication of haemolysis, the acronym HELLP syndrome has been used to label the concurrence of haemolysis, elevated liver enzymes, and low platelet counts. This is often not associated with marked hypertension or other conventional indices of severe pre-eclampsia. Indeed, liver damage and low platelet counts have been observed in primigravidae without hypertension or proteinuria but with the typical hepatic histology of pre-eclampsia, including fibrin deposition in the sinusoids. Epigastric pain and

Table 3 Tertiary pathology of pre-eclampsia

Maternal crises
Eclampsia
HELLP syndrome
Cerebral haemorrhage
Cortical blindness
Acute renal cortical necrosis
Acute renal tubular necrosis
Pulmonary oedema and adult respiratory distress
  syndrome (ARDS)
Laryngeal oedema
Disseminated intravascular coagulation
Hepatic infarction
Hepatic rupture
Fetal (placental) crises
Intrauterine asphyxia
Intrauterine death
Placental abruption

vomiting are the typical symptoms of the HELLP syndrome, which may present so suddenly as to be misinterpreted as biliary colic or other surgical emergencies. Hepatic tenderness and raised serum liver enzymes are the signs. Serum bilirubin is usually normal, but jaundice is possible and may be a presenting feature. In certain severe cases, typically of multiparae rather than primiparae, there may be bleeding under the liver capsule which may rupture to cause massive haemoperitoneum, shock, and (usually) maternal death. These issues are discussed in Chapter 13.9.

Eclampsia is the most dramatic evidence of involvement of the nervous system. It resembles other forms of hypertensive encephalopathy, having similar symptoms and cerebral pathology. One of the complications of hypertensive encephalopathy is cortical blindness, a feature of severe pre-eclampsia and eclampsia as well. Average blood pressures in eclampsia are high (170–195/110–120), but cases with much lower blood pressures are not as rare as with non-obstetric forms of hypertensive encephalopathy. Eclampsia is not associated with gross papilloedema or retinopathy. Ten per cent of cases of eclampsia are totally unheralded, that is without a warning prodrome of hypertension and proteinuria. The name hypertensive encephalopathy is misleading in that it suggests that the syndrome is caused by hypertension. The hypertension is an associated feature; there is no good evidence that hypertension causes eclampsia or other forms of hypertensive encephalopathy, and none that adequate medical control of the blood pressure prevents eclampsia. It is now generally agreed that eclampsia results from acute cerebral circulatory disturbances secondary to endothelial dysfunction. Cerebral vasospasm with focal ischaemia and oedema are major features that have been demonstrated by magnetic resonance imaging or CT scanning.

Diagnosis of pre-eclampsia

Pre-eclampsia is usually symptomless, hence its detection depends on signs or investigations. Nonetheless, one symptom is crucially important because it is so often misinterpreted. The epigastric pain, which reflects hepatic involvement and is typical of the HELLP syndrome, may easily be confused with heartburn, a very common problem of pregnancy. However, it is not burning in quality, does not spread upwards towards the throat, is associated with hepatic tenderness, may radiate through to the back, and is not relieved by giving antacids. It is often very severe, described by sufferers as the worst pain that they have ever experienced. Affected women are not uncommonly referred to general surgeons as suffering from an acute abdomen, for example acute cholecystitis.

In general, none of the signs of pre-eclampsia is specific; even convulsions in pregnancy are more likely to have causes other than eclampsia in modern practice. Diagnosis, therefore, depends on finding a coincidence of several pre-eclamptic features, the final proof being their regression after delivery. There are two ways to make the diagnosis. For research purposes the rules have to be followed that require the presence of both pregnancy-induced hypertension (PIH) and pregnancy-induced proteinuria. However, this is too restrictive for clinical practice, where there are presentations with the broad attributes of pre-eclampsia that do not fit these strict definitions; clinicians need to take a broader view and accept a wider range of combinations of the possible features of the syndrome, some of which are listed in Table 4. As with all syndromes, the more of the features that are clustered together the more certain is the diagnosis, but the absence of any one feature does not exclude the diagnosis. For example eclampsia can occur without proteinuria, and even hypertension seems not to be an essential component. To diagnose pre-eclampsia superimposed on long-term hypertension or renal disease there are, as stated already, no clear rules. In these circumstances, the diagnosis has to be made intuitively by judging the exacerbation of the long-term hypertension or proteinuria, in association with the appearance of other associated signs.

In practical terms, hypertension, proteinuria, and excessive weight gain have to be the signs of interest for screening in routine antenatal clinics. Different definitions have been proposed as to what constitutes hypertension, but the details are less important than the principle of an increment

Table 4 The pre-eclampsia syndrome—possible features

A. Maternal syndrome
Pregnancy-induced hypertension
Excessive weight gain (>1.0 kg/week)
Generalized oedema
Evidence for haemoconcentration
    increased haematocrit
Disturbances of renal function
    hyperuricaemia
    proteinuria
    raised plasma creatinine, reduced creatinine clearance
    hypocalciuria
Increased circulating markers of endothelial dysfunction
    von Willebrand factor
    cellular fibronectin
Laboratory evidence of excessive activation of the clotting system
    reduced plasma concentration of antithrombin III
    thrombocytopenia
    increased circulating d-dimer
Increased blood concentrations of liver enzymes
    raised serum alanine aminotransferase, serum aspartate
    aminotransferase
B. Fetal syndrome
Intrauterine growth retardation
Intrauterine hypoxaemia

from a recording taken in the first half of pregnancy, which establishes the existence of pregnancy-induced hypertension (PIH). Between weeks 20 and 30 the blood pressure is normally steady so that even a small, consistent rise is clinically important. Between week 30 and term the diastolic will rise by about 10 mmHg on average. A sustained rise of at least 25 mmHg to a threshold of 90 mmHg or more is typical of pre-eclampsia. However, these are only guidelines: there is no clinical situation where rigid interpretation of the blood pressure is helpful.

The same applies to other measurements such as changes in the plasma urate. As a rough guide, abnormal levels are in excess of 0.30, 0.35, 0.40, and 0.45 mmol/l at 28, 32, 36, and 40 weeks respectively; or, if a baseline taken before 20 weeks is available, then increases of 0.10, 0.15, 0.20, and 0.25 mmol/l at 28, 32, 36, and 40 weeks respectively.

Proteinuria and evidence of reduced glomerular filtration rate are later signs. The changes in the measurements of renal function are usually within the normal range for non-pregnant individuals. In general, abnormal concentrations of plasma creatinine and urea are above 100 μmol/l and 6.0 mmol respectively. The proteinuria of pre-eclampsia ranges from 0.5 to 15 g/24 h depending on the individual and the stage of evolution of the disorder. In terms of stick testing, 0.5 g/24 h corresponds to at least + in every specimen of urine tested, and when this point is reached the disease can be said to have entered its proteinuric phase.

Thrombocytopenia ($<100 \times 10^9$/l) and increased plasma fibrin/fibrinogen degradation products (or specific fragments thereof such as the D-dimer) tend to be late developments, if they occur at all. The same is true for raised liver enzymes. In regard to the latter, it should be noted that plasma alkaline phosphatase is always elevated in late pregnancy because of the contribution from the placental isoenzyme, hence its measurement is not a useful guide to hepatic function. Serum bilirubin is rarely abnormal. Gamma-glutamyl transferase is increased only late in the evolution of the HELLP syndrome. The best simple tests are plasma aspartate amino transferase or lactate dehydrogenase.

New hypertension and the *de novo* occurrence of one other sign allows the diagnosis to be made with reasonable certainty, but PIH on its own is not pre-eclampsia, although the term is commonly, but wrongly, used to mean mild or early pre-eclampsia. It is true that PIH maybe the first indication of the onset of pre-eclampsia, but until other signs appear this

Table 5 Preterm pre-eclampsia carries the highest maternal mortality

Period of enquiry	1988–90	1991–93	1994–96
All maternal deaths attributed to hypertensive diseases	26	19	17
Delivery at or before 37 weeks (% total)	19 (73%)[1]	15 (79%)	16 (94%)[2]
Delivery after 37 weeks (% total)	7 (27%)	4 (21%)	1 (6%)

[1]One woman died undelivered.

[2]Three women died undelivered; inadequate information in three deaths (date omitted).

Derived from reports on Confidential Enquiries into Maternal Deaths in the United Kingdom.

remains unconfirmed. Often spontaneous or induced delivery prevents further developments so that a final certain diagnosis cannot be made.

Complications of pre-eclampsia

Complications of pre-eclampsia are listed in Table 3. Eclampsia complicates 1 in 2000 maternities in the United Kingdom and carries a maternal mortality of 2 per cent. The HELLP syndrome is commoner, probably about 1 in 500 maternities, but may be as dangerous as eclampsia itself. These two major maternal crises can present unheralded by prodromal signs of pre-eclampsia. In other words, our terminology is not exact in the sense that eclampsia can precede pre-eclampsia. Antepartum eclampsia is likely to occur earlier in gestation and is more dangerous than that presenting in labour or after delivery, and preterm disease is generally more dangerous than that at term (Table 5). Most postpartum crises develop in the first 12 h after delivery, but later is possible and eclampsia has been documented as late as 22 days after delivery.

Cerebral haemorrhage is a lesion that can kill women with pre-eclampsia or eclampsia. In that cerebral haemorrhage is a known complication of severe hypertension in other contexts, it must be assumed that this is a major predisposing factor in this situation, although this has not been proved. Adult respiratory distress syndrome appears to have become more common, it is not known whether this is a consequence of modern methods of respiratory support rather than of the disease itself.

Prevention of pre-eclampsia

All the evidence is that, once it becomes overt, pre-eclampsia cannot be reversed except by delivery. Reliable methods of primary prevention are therefore needed, but none that is completely effective is known. If the concepts of pathogenesis described previously are correct, it is unlikely that any single measure will be effective for all susceptible women, but specific measures of reducing the susceptibilities among subgroups of women may be identified. Measures that may be effective or are definitely not effective are summarized in Table 6.

There is no evidence that blood pressure control attenuates the progression of early pre-eclampsia, nor that it prevents superimposition of pre-eclampsia in chronically hypertensive women who otherwise are more susceptible to the disorder. The only clear advantage of antihypertensive treatment is where the hypertension is so severe that delivery is essential to preserve maternal safety. At early gestational ages antihypertensive treatment can allow prolongation of pregnancy in this context, the benefit not being from prevention but palliation. However, the extent of the presumed benefit has not been measured because severe hypertension is a reason for

Table 6 Proposed measures for the prevention of pre-eclampsia

Proven to be ineffective	May be effective for at least some women
Weight restriction	Low-dose aspirin and other antiplatelet agents
Salt restriction	
Diuretics	Antioxidant vitamins (Vitamin C and E)
Antihypertensive agents	
Calcium supplements	
Fish oil	

exclusion from randomized trials of treatment, hence in all contexts antihypertensive treatment helps to protect the mother from the consequences of her problem, but not from the problem itself.

Trials of antiplatelet agents, in particular low doses of aspirin, have given mixed results. Those which have shown antiplatelet therapy to be ineffective have tended to be the largest with the least selective recruitment. There may be a modest effect in preventing or delaying the maternal syndrome, if low-dose aspirin is started early enough, well before the onset of signs. The benefits appear to be greatest in preventing early-onset pre-eclampsia (which is relatively rare) and least in preventing the disorder presenting at term (which is common). Antiplatelet therapy does not benefit women if started after the signs of pre-eclampsia have appeared. As yet there has been no clear demonstration that perinatal survival is improved. Low dose aspirin in pregnancy seems to be safe, but there may be a slight increase in maternal bleeding problems around the time of delivery. No adverse effect on the fetus has yet been identified.

At the time of writing there is one small trial suggesting benefit from the prophylactic use of antioxident vitamins C and E started in midgestation in carefully selected groups of at-risk women. It is too soon to know if this is likely to be confirmed as a safe and effective preventive regimen.

Management of pre-eclamptic hypertension

Control of the blood pressure is only a part of patient management. The definitive treatment is always delivery, which removes the cause of the problem, that is the placenta. If the affected woman can be delivered before irreversible damage has occurred (for example cerebral haemorrhage) a complete and rapid recovery is assured. Hence the purpose of medical management is to protect the mother from the dangers of her illness during the relatively brief interval after the disease is diagnosed and before elective delivery. The main objective is to prevent extreme hypertension. The threshold at which antihypertensive treatment should be started is a matter of opinion, a conservative criterion being to begin treatment if maximum readings (systolic or diastolic) repeatedly reach or exceed 170 or 110 mmHg, respectively.

Hydralazine has been the preferred antihypertensive agent for the treatment of acute severe pre-eclampsia, given intravenously by either continuous infusion (5–10 mg/h) or intermittent boluses (of 5 mg), or by intramuscular or subcutaneous injections (of 5–10 mg). After intravenous administration there is a delay of about 20 to 30 min in the onset of action and its effect is relatively short-lived, lasting 2 to 3 h. Side effects are common and include reflex tachycardia, anxiety, restlessness, hyper-reflexia, and severe headaches. These symptoms and signs may affect 50 per cent of women and simulate the features of impending eclampsia, when the symptoms of the disease cannot be disentangled from those caused by the treatment. Labetalol, a combined α and β-adrenergic blocking agent that can be given intravenously, lowers the blood pressure smoothly but rapidly without the tachycardia characteristic of treatment with hydralazine. A typical regimen starts with 20 mg/h, which is doubled every 30 min until control has been gained, but there are no adequate trials of its parenteral use in pregnancy to show how it might affect perinatal outcome. Sodium nitroprusside and nitroglycerine are rapidly acting vasodilators that have been used to manage hypertensive emergencies in pregnancy, but both should be reserved for use by specialists, usually in the context of intensive cardio-vascular monitoring. The danger is of overdose with problems associated with extreme and sudden hypotension.

The calcium channel blocking agent, nifedipine, is an effective vasodilator that acts rapidly when given by mouth. Nifedipine capsules, which act too abruptly (within 10–15 min), should not be used. The slow-release tablets have a slower onset of action (about 60 min) but a more prolonged effect; whereas a long-acting preparation, formulated for once a day administration, is less convenient for acute control of pre-eclamptic hypertension. Nifedipine is at least as safe as hydralazine to use in pregnancy and is less likely to cause troublesome tachycardia. In theory, nifedipine could interact with parenteral magnesium sulphate given to prevent or treat eclampsia because the magnesium ion inhibits calcium channels; in practice there has been a report of two cases of profound hypotension in this context. Nimodipine, another calcium channel blocker but with a selective effect on the cerebral circulation, may have particular advantages for treating cerebral ischaemia in eclamptic women.

Diuretics are avoided because they exacerbate the hypovolaemia of pre-eclampsia, which is often severe, but they are indicated if complications such as pulmonary or laryngeal oedema occur.

Good blood pressure control in pre-eclampsia does not ameliorate its other features; the disease persists and remains relentlessly progressive until delivery. Escape from control is common. Adequate treatment does not prevent other complications such as eclampsia, the HELLP syndrome, abruption, or progressive fetal respiratory impairment. A persisting inability to control maternal arterial pressure is one of several indications for immediate delivery.

Longer-term control of pre-eclamptic hypertension

The control of pre-eclamptic hypertension must always be extended for a few days at the least, and frequently for longer. Therefore, once the blood pressure has been controlled acutely, the effects of treatment need to be prolonged. The requirements are for a drug that is safe in pregnancy, has an onset of action in 6 to 12 h, allows some titration of effect, and can safely be combined with a second drug if needed. The choice lies between methyldopa and various β adrenergic blocking agents (β-blockers).

In adequate doses, methyldopa can control the blood pressure within 6 to 12 h: a loading dose of 500 to 1000 mg is followed by 250 to 750 mg four times a day. Sedation is the rule for the first 48 h and thereafter tiredness is common. Postural hypotension is rarely a problem in the antenatal patient. Although β-blockers cause fewer subjective side-effects, their safety in pregnancy has not been so exhaustively investigated. A preparation such as atenolol, with its slow onset of action and flat dose–response curve, is not ideal for the day to day titration of blood pressure control, but its short-term safety for the fetus and neonate has been adequately demonstrated. Oxprenolol and labetalol are faster-acting alternatives; which agent is preferred depends on the clinician's familiarity with their use.

Recent evidence suggests that long-term lowering of the blood pressure has a modest but statistically significant effect in reducing the baby's birthweight. Whether this has any long-term implications is not known. However, it is a good reason for using antihypertensive agents parsimoniously and only where there is clear evidence of a maternal risk.

Prevention of eclamptic convulsions

Eclampsia is probably caused by focal cerebral vasoconstriction and ischaemia secondary to endothelial damage and therefore is neither the result of hypertension, nor prevented by antihypertensive treatment. The best mode of prevention is well-timed delivery. It is debated whether any prophylactic anticonvulsant medication needs to be offered routinely in all cases of advanced pre-eclampsia and, if so, what it should be. Intravenous diazepam (5 mg by slow intravenous injection) is preferred to stop eclamptic convulsions, although most are self limiting. Thereafter, it is reasonable to use medication to prevent recurrent convulsions. Agents that improve cerebral perfusion are more effective than those that suppress neuronal excitability.

In the former category is parenteral magnesium sulphate, widely used in the United States to prevent or treat eclampsia; in the latter is phenytoin. There is now clear evidence from a large, double-blind, controlled trial that magnesium sulphate administration is superior.

Chronic hypertension complicating pregnancy

Pregnant women with chronic hypertension tend to be older, fatter, slightly taller, and frequently with clear family histories of hypertension. Owing to the physiological changes of pregnancy, their hypertension may be ameliorated or masked by the beginning of the second trimester so that the diagnosis is missed unless prepregnancy blood pressure readings are available. As explained above, the blood pressure tends to climb back to the levels that characterize the non-pregnant state towards the end of the third trimester. If these are high this normal change can be misinterpreted as pre-eclampsia, the distinction being that the blood pressure fails to settle after delivery.

Pre-eclampsia superimposed on chronic hypertension tends to be more severe, to occur at earlier stages of pregnancy, to cause more fetal growth retardation, and to be recurrent in later pregnancies. Pre-eclampsia occurring in normotensive women tends not to recur. If a blood pressure of 140/90 in the first half pregnancy is taken as evidence of chronic hypertension, then affected individuals have an approximately five-fold increased risk of later pre-eclampsia compared to normotensive women. This close link between the two conditions led earlier clinicians to conclude that chronic hypertension is extremely dangerous when combined with pregnancy. It is now clear that the particular risks of chronic hypertension are entirely attributable to the increased chance of developing superimposed pre-eclampsia. The majority of chronically hypertensive women who do not get pre-eclampsia can expect a normal and uncomplicated perinatal outcome. In other words, the dangers of chronic hypertension in pregnancy have been over-emphasized.

Chronic hypertension can only be diagnosed with certainty during pregnancy on the basis of readings taken in the first half, preferably before 16 weeks of gestation. Without the benefit of such readings, hypertension in the second half of pregnancy cannot be interpreted because the possibility that it may represent pre-eclampsia cannot be excluded. The signs of pre-eclampsia in chronically hypertensive women are the same as in other women, except that the blood pressure increases from a higher baseline. There may be progressive hyperuricaemia, abnormal activation of the clotting system, or new proteinuria.

Treatment of chronic hypertension in pregnancy

If antihypertensive treatment has been started before conception, the patient may seek advice about the possible effects of her medication on the growth and development of her fetus. None of the commonly used antihypertensive drugs is known to be teratogenic, but this does not preclude the possibility of subtle problems that are, as yet, unknown. For this reason it is appropriate that women with no more than moderate hypertension stop treatment before conception. By the 12th week of pregnancy, the normal fall in blood pressure is such that treatment may no longer be needed, at least until the beginning of the third trimester. Although angiotensin converting enzyme (ACE) inhibitors are often considered to be teratogenic, this is not the case; there is clear evidence that they are fetotoxic (causing growth restriction, oligohydramnios, and intrauterine and postnatal renal failure in the second and third trimester) but none that they are teratogenic. After 3 months of pregnancy they are contraindicated but not before.

If chronic hypertension is diagnosed for the first time in pregnancy, it is necessary to treat those in whom it presents an immediate (as opposed to a long-term) hazard. The precise levels at which this is necessary is a matter of opinion not fact; we take a cut-off point at 170/110 mmHg. In general

Table 7 Antihypertensive drug use in pregnancy

Trimester	Drugs to avoid		Possible agents
	Relatively contraindicated	**Absolutely contraindicated**	
First	None known	None known	Avoid all if possible
Second	β-blockers Diuretics	ACE inhibitors	Methyl dopa Clonidine Prazosin (doxazosin) Nifedipine
Third	Diuretics	ACE inhibitors	Methyl dopa Clonidine Prazosin (doxazosin} Nifedipine β-blockers

medical practice, the purpose of treating less severe chronic hypertension (that is 140–169/90–109 mmHg) is to prevent long-term complications such as heart failure, aortic dissection, or coronary and cerebral vascular disease. These problems are so rare in pregnant women that in themselves they cannot justify treatment for the brief period of pregnancy. Thus, moderate hypertension *per se* carries no intrinsic maternal risk over the brief period of 9 months, except insofar as it may be the precursor of more severe hypertension. However, the higher the arterial pressure the greater the eventual perinatal mortality. The risks evolve through simple progression if the mild hypertension indicates early pre-eclampsia. By contrast, if the mild hypertension indicates a pre-existing problem, then the risk is of later superimposition of pre-eclampsia which is, as stated above, several times more likely in chronically hypertensive women. Antihypertensive treatment can only be useful if either it halts the progression of mild pre-eclampsia or prevents the superimposition of pre-eclampsia in women with long-term hypertension. There is no evidence in support of either possibility, indeed there is good evidence that control of moderate, long-term hypertension does not prevent superimposed pre-eclampsia but does cause mild fetal growth retardation. Thus, there are neither clear fetal nor maternal indications for treating moderate hypertension in pregnancy.

Oral antihypertensive agents that are used in pregnancy

The choice of oral antihypertensive agents in pregnancy is dictated by considerations of fetal safety (Table 7). Methyl dopa is the preferred agent because its fetal effects have been defined more clearly than those of other agents. Its antihypertensive action and side-effects are the same as in non-pregnant individuals. The usual treatment schedule is 1.0 to 3.0 g/day in divided doses. It can be supplemented by nifedipine.

Labetalol is a popular alternative. However, long-term β-adrenergic blockade extending throughout the second and third trimesters has been associated with significant fetal growth retardation and for this reason should be avoided. ACE inhibitors are contraindicated in the second and third trimesters.

In the unlikely event that diuretics are essential for good blood pressure control, they can be continued throughout pregnancy, but their use carries certain disadvantages if pre-eclampsia supervenes, as already discussed.

Hypertension in the puerperium

In relation to both chronic hypertension and pre-eclampsia, the highest blood pressures are often recorded in the puerperium, typically peaking at about 5 to 7 days after delivery. Antihypertensive treatment therefore has to be continued, in some women for 3 to 6 weeks or even longer after delivery. There is no clear evidence that treatment interferes with breast feeding (Table 8).

Long-term sequelae of hypertension in pregnancy

Severe pre-eclampsia and eclampsia can cause irreversible maternal complications, particularly acute renal cortical necrosis or cerebral haemorrhage. In the absence of these problems, there is no evidence that long-term health is impaired. However, in terms of life expectancy, pre-eclamptic women fall into two groups. Those who become normotensive soon after delivery have a normal life expectancy. Those who remain hypertensive not only tend to suffer recurrent pregnancy-induced hypertension but have a higher incidence of later cardiovascular disorders and reduced life expectancy, compatible with the diagnosis of underlying arterial disease.

Conclusions

A raised blood pressure is one of many secondary effects of pre-eclampsia on the mother. In pre-eclampsia the main differential diagnosis is from chronic hypertension, which in its pure form does not share the renal, coagulation, hepatic, and placental abnormalities of pre-eclampsia. The perinatal risks of chronic hypertension in pregnancy result from superimposed pre-eclampsia.

Extreme hypertension (≥170/110 mmHg) in pregnancy, whatever the underlying cause, is as dangerous as it is in any other medical situation and demands treatment. However, there is no clear reason for treating more moderate hypertension on either maternal or fetal grounds. As far as it is known, the progression of moderate pre-eclampsia is not delayed, nor is the later superimposition of pre-eclampsia on moderate chronic hypertension prevented.

Methyl dopa is the most thoroughly tested antihypertensive agent for use in pregnancy; no significant adverse reaction has been observed. Labetolol is a popular alternative. In general, β-adrenergic blocking agents are safe for short-term use but cause significant fetal growth retardation if administered over longer periods (from the second trimester), although the clinical trial data are less complete than for methyl dopa. Diuretics should primarily be reserved for the treatment of heart failure complicating pre-eclampsia. Angiotensin converting enzyme inhibitors are contraindicated for use in pregnancy because of adverse effects on fetal renal function.

Table 8 Antihypertensive drugs and breast feeding

Drug	Secretion in breast milk
Methyl dopa	Minimal secretion; too small to be harmful
Labetalol	Secreted in breast milk in small amounts
Atenolol	Secreted in breast milk in small amounts
Nifedipine	Secreted in breast milk
ACE inhibitors	Secreted in breast milk but in small amounts that are unlikely to be harmful

Further reading

Davey DA, MacGillivray I (1988). The classification and definition of the hypertensive disorders of pregnancy. *American Journal of Obstetrics and Gynecology* **158**, 892–8.

Department of Health (1998). *Why mothers die. Report on confidential enquiries into maternal deaths in the United Kingdom 1994–1996*, pp. 36–46. HM Stationery Office, London.

National High Blood Pressure Education Program (1990). National High Blood Pressure Education Program Working Group Report on high blood pressure in pregnancy. *American Journal of Obstetrics and Gynecology* **163**, 1691–712.

Redman CWG (1991). Current topic: pre-eclampsia and the placenta. *Placenta* **12**, 301–8.

Redman CWG, Roberts JM (1993). Management of pre-eclampsia. *Lancet* **341**, 1451–4.

Redman CWG, Sacks GP, Sargent IL (1999). Preeclampsia: an excessive maternal inflammatory response to pregnancy. *American Journal of Obstetrics and Gynecology* **180**, 499–506.

Roberts JM, Redman CWG (1993). Pre-eclampsia: more than pregnancy-induced hypertension. *Lancet* **341**, 1447–51.

Sibai BM, Ramadan MK, Usta I, Salama M, Mercer BM, Friedman SA (1993). Maternal morbidity and mortality in 442 pregnancies with hemolysis, elevated liver enzymes, and low platelets (HELLP syndrome). *American Journal of Obstetrics and Gynecology* **169**, 1000–6.

The Eclampsia Trial Collaborative Group (1995). Which anticonvulsant for women with eclampsia? Evidence from the Collaborative Eclampsia Trial. *Lancet* **345**, 1455–63.

von Dadelzsen P, Ornstein MP, Bull SB, Logan AG, Koren G, Magee LA (2000). Fall in mean arterial pressure and fetal growth restriction in pregnancy hypertension: a meta-analysis. *Lancet* **355**, 87–92.

13.5 Renal disease in pregnancy
J. Firth

Changes in the kidneys and urinary tract during normal pregnancy

Anatomical

The most obvious anatomical change in the urinary tract during pregnancy is dilatation of the calyces, renal pelvis, and ureter. Contrary to popular belief, the ureters are not floppy and toneless, indeed tone is increased, but urinary stasis within the ureters may nevertheless contribute to the risk of asymptomatic bacteriuria developing into acute pyelonephritis. Ureteric dilatation can persist for 3 or 4 months after pregnancy, and long term in about 10 per cent of women who have had children. The kidney enlarges by about 1 cm in length during pregnancy.

Functional

Renal blood flow increases by 70 to 80 per cent between conception and midpregnancy, falling to a value 50 to 60 per cent above the non-pregnant level during the third trimester. Between conception and 16 weeks of pregnancy the glomerular filtration rate increases about 50 per cent above baseline and remains at this elevated level until delivery. Plasma creatinine decreases from a mean non-pregnant value of 73 μmol/l to 65, 51, and 47 μmol/l in successive trimesters.

Urinary excretion of glucose increases soon after conception and may rise 10-fold above non-pregnant values, hence glycosuria is common during pregnancy. This occurs because of decreased tubular reabsorption of glucose, but the reason for this is not known. Glucose excretion returns to normal non-pregnant levels within a week of delivery.

Plasma uric acid concentration decreases by about 25 per cent during normal pregnancy because of increased urinary excretion (the precise mechanism is unknown). In pregnancies complicated by pre-eclampsia or intrauterine growth retardation, the plasma uric acid concentration is higher than normal and serial measurements can be used to monitor progress. (See Chapter 13.4 for further discussion.)

The mean albumin excretion rate in pregnancy is 12 mg/day, with 29 mg/day the upper limit of normal (no different from that in the non-pregnant state). However, slightly increased urinary protein excretion is normal in pregnancy, such that proteinuria in pregnancy should not be considered abnormal until it exceeds 500 mg/day, which is over twice the upper limit of normal outside of pregnancy.

Pregnancy in women with known renal disease

Is pregnancy advisable?

Normal pregnancy is rare in women with serum creatinine more than 250 to 300 μmol/l, but many women who have renal disease will seek medical advice regarding pregnancy, the most typical questions being 'will pregnancy make my kidneys worse or do any long-term damage?' and 'will having kidney disease affect the pregnancy or baby?' The bottom line is that there is no strong medical contraindication to pregnancy from the 'renal point of view' if kidney function is only mildly compromised, proteinuria is not in the nephrotic range, and hypertension is nothing other than mild, although no woman can be given a 100 per cent guarantee. Table 1 gives a guide to the likely outcome of pregnancy in women with renal disease.

Women with a serum creatinine of less than 125 μmol/l usually have successful obstetric outcomes and there is no evidence that pregnancy adversely affects their renal prognosis. Some would suggest that more guarded advice should be given to patients with lupus nephropathy, mesangiocapillary glomerulonephritis, focal segmental glomerulosclerosis, and (perhaps) IgA nephropathy and reflux nephropathy.

When serum creatinine is in the range 125 to 250 μmol/l there is serious concern that pregnancy may cause immediate deterioration in renal function, severe hypertension, variable obstetric outcome, and an increased rate of decline of renal function postpartum.

Most women with serum creatinine more than 250 μmol/l are not fertile. The chances of conception, a normal pregnancy, and a healthy child are low; the risks to maternal health are high and pregnancy should be strongly discouraged. Women in this situation who are desperate to conceive should be told that their best chance of becoming pregnant and having a child is 1 year after successful renal transplantation.

Monitoring and management of pregnancy in women with renal disease

The chances of a successful outcome to pregnancy in a woman with renal disease are best if there is close co-operation between the patient, obstetrician, and nephrologist. At regular visits the following should be monitored: blood pressure, 24-h urine collection for proteinuria and creatinine clearance, urinary culture (for covert bacteriuria), and fetal development. Management of difficult cases requires achieving an acceptable balance between maternal and fetal interests, which is not always easy.

It is common for proteinuria to develop or to increase substantially during pregnancy in women with renal disease. Pregnancy can be allowed to continue as long as blood pressure is normal and renal function does not deteriorate. Reversible causes, such as volume depletion or urinary infection, should be sought if renal function does decline, but significant and otherwise unexplained deterioration in renal function is reason to recommend elective delivery.

The incidence of pre-eclampsia in patients with pre-existing renal disease is not known, hypertension and proteinuria being manifestations of both. The management of hypertension is the same, whether the cause is renal disease or pre-eclampsia, and is as discussed in Chapter 13.4, although whether or not mild hypertension should be treated in pregnant women with renal disease is a contentious issue. Blood pressure above 170/110 mmHg in the third trimester would be an indication for starting

Table 1 The likely outcome of pregnancy in women with renal disease

Baseline renal function: effect on pregnancy outcome and long-term consequences of pregnancy for maternal renal function			
Baseline serum creatinine	Problems during pregnancy (%)	Successful obstetric outcome[a] (%)	Adverse long-term consequences for maternal renal function[a] (%)
<125 µmol/l	26	96	<3
125–250 µmol/l	47	89	25
>250 µmol/l	86	46	53
Hypertension: effect on pregnancy and renal function in women with chronic renal disease			
	Intrauterine growth retardation (%)	Preterm delivery (%)	Deterioration in renal function during pregnancy (%)
Normotension	2.3	11.4	3.0
Hypertension	15.6	20.0	15.0
Fetal mortality: effect of hypertension or renal deterioration during pregnancy in women with chronic renal disease			
	Hypertension (%)	Deterioration in renal function during pregnancy (%)	Hypertension + deterioration in renal function (%)
Absent throughout pregnancy	18	12	10
Present at some time during pregnancy	34	27	40
Present but controlled from first trimester	20	–	–
Present and uncontrolled from first trimester	100	–	–
Present only during third trimester	12	–	–

[a] There is less chance of a successful obstetric outcome and more chance of adverse long-term consequences for maternal renal function if complications develop before 28 weeks gestation.

This information is drawn from outcome data of over 3000 pregnancies, as described in Davison JM and Baylis C. Pregnancy in patients with underlying renal disease. In: Davison AM, Cameron JS, Grunfeld J-P, Kerr DNS, Ritz E, Winearls CG, eds. *Oxford textbook of clinical nephrology*, 2nd edn, pp. 2327–48. Oxford University Press.

antihypertensive treatment in routine obstetric practice. By contrast, treatment of blood pressure above 140/90 mmHg in a non-pregnant woman of child-bearing age would be indicated in general medical practice to prevent long-term complications, and in those with renal disease (particularly if proteinuric) most nephrologists would recommend that arterial pressure be lowered even further than this. It is not known whether or not blood pressure in pregnancy should be treated more aggressively in women with renal disease than in those without.

Women with renal transplants

Fertility returns in women of child-bearing age after successful renal transplantation and over 90 per cent of pregnancies that survive the first trimester end successfully. It is generally recommended that women should not attempt to conceive for the first year after transplantation. Thereafter the risks are similar to those suggested above for a woman with disease of her native kidneys; the risk of problems is low in the patient with good renal function, no proteinuria, and no hypertension, and there is no medical reason to dissuade such a woman from becoming pregnant. By contrast, the hypertensive woman with proteinuria and a poorly functioning graft is at high risk of adverse maternal and fetal outcome and should be strongly dissuaded from pregnancy. Prednisolone, azathioprine, and cyclosporin seem to be safe in pregnancy, there being no need for dosage adjustment in most cases. The presence of a renal transplant is not a contraindication to normal vaginal delivery and is not an indication for caesarean section. There is no increase in the incidence of congenital abnormalities in the infants of mothers with renal transplants.

Renal complications that can occur in pregnancy

Urinary tract infection

Asymptomatic bacteriuria

The incidence of asymptomatic bacteriuria is 2 to 10 per cent in pregnant and non-pregnant young women. If not treated, 40 per cent of women with asymptomatic bacteriuria will develop acute symptomatic infection during pregnancy, and treating pregnant women with asymptomatic bacteriuria should prevent approximately 70 per cent of all cases of symptomatic urinary tract infection in pregnancy. Untreated asymptomatic bacteriuria is associated with low birth weight and preterm delivery. Treatment is effective at clearing asymptomatic bacteriuria and reducing the incidence of pyelonephritis, preterm delivery, and babies with low birth weight.

E. coli is responsible for over 75 per cent of cases of bacteriuria in pregnancy. The choice of drug should be determined by the sensitivity of the organism isolated. Amoxicillin and cephalosporins are safe in pregnancy, as is nitrofurantoin, except in the last few weeks (it can produce neonatal haemolysis if used at term). Trimethoprim is contraindicated in the first trimester (folate antagonist) and quinolones should not be used at all in pregnancy (they cause arthropathy in animal studies). There is no good evidence to determine the first choice of antibiotic (pending culture results) or the duration of treatment. Use of single, high-dose therapy is controversial and some would recommend a 2-week course, with repeat urinary culture performed 1 week after treatment is stopped and monthly thereafter until delivery. About 25 per cent of patients will suffer recurrent infection and require a second course of treatment.

Symptomatic infection

Acute cystitis affects about 1 per cent of pregnant women. Treatment is as for asymptomatic bacteriuria, with the aim of abolishing symptoms and preventing acute pyelonephritis. A Cochrane review that included five studies of antibiotic treatment of symptomatic urinary infection in pregnancy concluded that there were no significant differences between any of the treatments studied and was unable to recommend any particular regimen.

Acute pyelonephritis presents with the same symptoms as it does in patients who are not pregnant (see Chapter 20.12), but the differential diagnosis in pregnancy includes uterine fibroid degeneration and abruptio placentae, and distinction from appendicitis can be particularly difficult. Preterm labour occurs in about 4 per cent of mild cases and 20 per cent of severe cases, where there is associated respiratory distress. Treatment is usually with intravenous antibiotics (typically amoxicillin or a cephalosporin) in the first instance, switching to oral therapy as the patient improves. Some advocate a 3-week course for acute pyelonephritis in pregnancy, but without firm evidence that this is necessary. However, since pyelonephritis recurs in up to 25 per cent of women during pregnancy it is important thereafter to monitor closely for evidence of recurrent urinary infection, with or without instigating prophylactic treatment with a bedtime dose of an appropriate antibiotic.

Acute renal failure specific to pregnancy

The priorities in dealing with acute renal failure in a pregnant woman are no different from those that apply to any other patient: treatment of life-threatening complications, fluid resuscitation (if necessary), establishing a precise diagnosis, treatment of any underlying condition (if possible), and timely provision of renal replacement therapy (if indicated). These issues are discussed in Section 20.5. There are, however, some causes of acute renal failure that are specific to pregnancy.

Obstetric acute renal failure

In the developed world, the incidence of obstetric acute renal failure has fallen dramatically over the last 40 years. In Leeds (United Kingdom), obstetric causes accounted for 26 per cent of cases of acute renal failure between 1956 and 1959, compared to 1.3 per cent between 1980 and 1988. A significant fall has also been seen in some parts of the developing world, where in Chandigarh (North India) obstetric causes were responsible for 25 per cent of cases of acute renal failure 30 years ago, compared with around 10 per cent today. By contrast, in a study from Turkey, the proportion of cases of acute renal failure due to obstetric causes changed only from 17 per cent to 14 per cent over the period 1980 to 1997. Where a decline in the incidence of obstetric acute renal failure has been seen, this is almost certainly attributable to improvements in perinatal care and a reduction in the numbers of septic abortions. Should acute renal failure develop in pregnancy or the puerperium then obstetric causes listed in Table 2 should be considered in addition to the conditions that can present in any patient (see Tables 1, 2, and 3 of Chapter 20.4).

In most cases of acute renal failure in pregnancy, the clinical progress of the condition is typical of acute tubular necrosis, with full recovery of renal function if the patient survives. However, for reasons that are not known, pregnant women are particularly susceptible to acute cortical necrosis. The incidence of this has fallen in the developed world, from 1 in 10 000 in the decade from 1960 to less than 1 in 80 000 pregnancies in the decade from 1970 in one large study, but it still carries the risk of permanent renal fail-

Table 2 Some obstetric causes of acute renal failure

Pathogenesis	Clinical condition
Volume depletion + Hypotension	Antepartum haemorrhage
	Postpartum haemorrhage
	Abortion
	Hyperemesis gravidarum
Volume depletion + Hypotension + Coagulopathy	Antepartum haemorrhage
	Pre-eclampsia/ eclampsia
	Amniotic fluid embolism
	Acute fatty liver of pregnancy
	Haemolytic uraemic syndrome (idiopathic postpartum renal failure)
Volume depletion + Hypotension + Coagulopathy + Infection	Septic abortion
	Chorioamnionitis
	Puerperal sepsis
	Pyelonephritis[a]
Urinary tract obstruction	Damage to ureters during caesarean section
	Haematoma in the pelvis

[a] Can cause acute renal failure outside of pregnancy, but pregnant women are at particular risk.

ure, although delayed and partial recovery is not uncommon. (See Chapter 20.4 for further discussion.)

Acute fatty liver of pregnancy

Acute fatty liver of pregnancy is a disease of the third trimester or puerperium in which there is jaundice and severe hepatic dysfunction. In early series, the incidence of acute renal failure was over 50 per cent, but this is now much reduced, both as a consequence of the recognition of milder cases and through improved management of severe cases. The explanation for acute renal failure is unknown. Renal biopsy shows non-specific changes. (See Chapter 13.9 for further discussion.)

Haemolytic uraemic syndrome (idiopathic postpartum renal failure)

The haemolytic uraemic syndrome can present peripartum or at any time in the first few weeks after delivery, when it is often termed idiopathic postpartum renal failure. This can be a devastating condition (maternal mortality 5–20 per cent, fetal mortality 30 per cent), the cause of which is not known. Blood pressure can vary from low to very high. There may be severe heart failure and also neurological manifestations such as coma or epileptic fitting. The blood film shows a microangiopathic haemolytic anaemia, sometimes with a consumption coagulopathy in addition. Treatment is primarily supportive, but some authorities also recommend plasma exchange, although in this rare condition there are no randomized, controlled trials to justify its use. If the patient survives then renal function rarely, if ever, recovers completely and many remain dependent on dialysis. (See Chapter 20.10.6 for further discussion.)

Miscellaneous conditions

Acute hydroureter and hydronephrosis and the 'overdistension syndrome'

The anatomical changes associated with pregnancy can very occasionally be exaggerated, with massive distension of the ureters and renal pelvis. This is usually asymptomatic, but can rarely have clinical consequences. The 'overdistension syndrome' varies from transient, mild loin pain to recurrent attacks of severe loin or lower abdominal pain radiating to the groin. Variation in symptoms with posture and position are typical. Urine specimens are sterile, but can show microscopic haematuria. Diagnosis is confirmed by ultrasonography. Nursing in the knee–chest position often provides relief, but very uncommonly nephrostomy and/or ureteral stenting are required.

Rupture of the urinary tract

The development of severe, persistent pain or haematuria in a pregnant patient with acute pyelonephritis or the 'overdistension syndrome' suggests the very rare complication of rupture of the urinary tract. This can be retroperitoneal or intraperitoneal and is more likely to occur in those with pre-existing disease of the kidneys or urinary tract, perhaps because mild weaknesses are exposed by the physiological changes of pregnancy. Distinction from other obstetric or abdominal catastrophes can be very difficult.

Further reading

Jones DC, Hayslett JP (1996). Outcome of pregnancy in women with moderate or severe renal insufficiency. *New England Journal of Medicine* **335**, 226–32.

Meyers SJ *et al.* (1985). Dilatation and nontraumatic rupture of the urinary tract during pregnancy: a review. *Obstetrics and Gynecology* **66**, 809–15.

Packham DK *et al.* (1989). Primary glomerulonephritis and pregnancy. *Quarterly Journal of Medicine* **71**, 537–53.

Pertuiset N, Grünfeld JP (1994). Acute renal failure in pregnancy. *Baillieres Clinical Obstetrics and Gynaecology* **8**, 333–51.

Romero R *et al.* (1989). Meta-analysis of the relationship between asymptomatic bacteriuria and preterm delivery/low birth weight. *Obstetrics and Gynecology* **73**, 576–82.

Selcuk NY *et al.* (1998). Changes in frequency and etiology of acute renal failure in pregnancy (1980–1997). *Renal Failure* **20**, 513–7.

Smaill F (2001). Antibiotics for asymptomatic bacteriuria in pregnancy (Cochrane review). *Cochrane Database Systematic Review* **2**, CD000490. http://www.update-software.com/abstracts/ab000490.htm

Vazquez JC, Villar J (2000). Treatments for symptomatic urinary tract infections during pregnancy. *Cochrane Database Systematic Review* CD002256. http://www.update-software.com/abstracts/ab002256.htm

Wolff JM *et al.* (1995). Non-traumatic rupture of the urinary tract during pregnancy. *British Journal of Urology* **76**, 645–8.

13.6 Heart disease in pregnancy

J. C. Forfar

Introduction

Up to 10 per cent of maternal deaths in the United Kingdom result from heart disease, and the proportion is higher in developing countries. Although rheumatic heart disease has declined world-wide, it remains an important and treatable condition in pregnancy. The improved survival of patients with treated complex congenital heart lesions presents difficult challenges for planning and management. Unfortunately, information on fetal and maternal risks in such situations is often inadequate, making it difficult to know what the best treatment is. Maternal involvement in the analysis of risks and benefits is of the greatest importance.

Cardiovascular changes in pregnancy

Significant circulatory changes occur during pregnancy (Table 1). Cardiac output increases by up to 50 per cent through increase in both heart rate and stroke volume secondary to a fall in systemic vascular resistance. The fall in blood pressure results from vasodilation mediated by gestational hormones, increased heat production, and the low resistance uteroplacental circulation. Pressure of the gravid uterus on the cava in the supine position can result in substantial falls in cardiac output and blood pressure in some women, causing weakness, light-headedness, dizziness, and even syncope. The supine hypotensive syndrome of pregnancy is relieved by turning to one side.

Blood volume increases early in pregnancy and more slowly from mid-pregnancy. These changes follow activation of the renin–angiotensin–aldosterone mechanism by oestrogens and secondary retention of salt and water. Increases in plasma volume (average 50 per cent) are faster and greater than red cell mass (average 25 per cent), thus accounting for the so-called 'physiological anaemia of pregnancy', when haemoglobin averages 11 g/dl.

Blood pressure, cardiac output, and oxygen consumption increase with the pain and anxiety of labour and from expansion of blood volume with uterine contraction. Despite blood loss on delivery, blood volume is effect-ively (although not actually) increased by the contracting empty uterus postpartum, and augmented preload acutely increases cardiac output. These changes return to normal over 24 h.

Cardiovascular evaluation in pregnancy

Assessment of heart disease in pregnancy is complicated by the functional changes described above, which may simulate or mask underlying heart disease. Routine investigative methods may be limited because of potential risks to the fetus.

Fatigue, reduced exercise capacity, breathlessness, and light-headedness are common symptoms during pregnancy. The increase in respiratory rate and reduced tidal volume may be perceived as breathlessness and this, combined with some peripheral oedema from increased blood volume and caval compression, with minor distension of the neck veins, may lead to an erroneous diagnosis of heart failure. The increased volume peripheral pulses, occasionally 'collapsing', and vasodilatation during later pregnancy can mimic aortic regurgitation or hyperthyroidism. The apical impulse is prominent and occasionally displaced, simulating volume loading. Heart sounds are commonly loud and may be palpable with exaggerated splitting. An apical S3 is not uncommon in pregnancy but S4 is less common and its presence should promote investigation for possible heart disease.

A soft systolic murmur at the base and lower left sternal edge occurs in most pregnancies and can radiate to the suprasternal notch and the neck. A continuous venous flow murmur may be audible in the neck along with a systolic or continuous murmur from increased flow to the breasts. Both murmurs decrease with stethoscope pressure and are less audible when the patient is upright. A diastolic murmur is rare in normal pregnancy and should prompt investigation. Murmurs associated with organic heart disease increase in intensity in pregnancy (from increased flow) and conclusions based on murmur intensity should therefore be made with caution.

Cardiovascular investigations in pregnancy

Electrocardiography (ECG)

Minor flattening of the T-waves and minor left or right QRS axis shift are common in normal pregnancy. Sinus tachycardia and atrial or ventricular premature beats are likewise frequent findings, particularly during labour and delivery. Exercise testing may confirm a clinical diagnosis of ischaemic heart disease or assess functional capacity. A low level protocol is recommended.

Chest radiography

Although the radiation dose is minimal, this test is best avoided unless there are clear indications. The uterus should be shielded. Straightening of the left heart border and prominence of the pulmonary conus are common findings, along with prominent pulmonary vascular markings. A small

Table 1 Haemodynamic changes during normal pregnancy

	Trimester		
	1st	2nd	3rd
Cardiac output	+ +	+ + +	+ + +
Heart rate	+	+ +	+ + +
Stroke volume	+	+ +	+
Systemic vascular resistance	-	−	-
Blood volume	+ +	+ + +	+ + +
Systolic blood pressure	+ -	-	+ -
Diastolic blood pressure	-	−	-

+ - = no change; +, + +, + + + = small, moderate, large increase; -, − = small, moderate decrease pleural effusion may be seen early postpartum and usually resolves quickly.

Doppler echocardiography

Cardiac ultrasound is safe and provides valuable anatomical and functional information throughout pregnancy. Late in normal pregnancy a small peri-cardial effusion can sometimes be seen. Trivial tricuspid and pulmonary regurgitation may be considered a variant of normal at this stage.

Cardiac catheterization

This should only be undertaken if an intervention is required for patient management. Balloon mitral valvuloplasty is an alternative to closed val-votomy for symptomatic severe mitral stenosis in pregnancy. Aortic and pulmonary balloon valvuloplasty have also been performed, as has coron-ary angioplasty. The brachial approach is preferable to minimize radiation exposure, and full shielding is appropriate. Radionuclide imaging tech-niques during pregnancy are best avoided because of uncertainty of the level of radiation exposure to the fetus.

Heart disease in pregnancy

Cardiac reserve (assessed by history and functional classification) is an important determinant of risk in pregnancy. Patients with heart disease and with no, or minimal, symptoms prior to pregnancy have a relatively small risk of complications. Patients with moderate or severe limitation prior to pregnancy are at much higher risk, and careful monitoring, and sometimes intervention, are required. Patients symptomatic at rest prior to pregnancy have a high maternal and even higher fetal mortality and pregnancy is con-traindicated until their functional class can be improved.

It is therefore important that accurate diagnostic and functional evalu-ation of heart disease is undertaken in all patients prior to pregnancy, aim-ing to predict maternal and fetal risk as far as possible. The issues of maternal morbidity, long-term survival, and risks of fetal heart disease need to be discussed with the patient. It is preferable, in those with complex congenital heart disease, that such discussions take place well before preg-nancy is contemplated so that appropriate action may be taken. Where pre-dicted maternal mortality is above 30 per cent, sterilization or pregnancy termination may be most appropriate. The management of anticoagulant therapy before and during pregnancy requires special consideration (see below).

Congenital heart disease

This accounts for up to one-third of heart disease in pregnancy. Maternal and hence fetal outcome is determined by the nature of the disease, previ-ous surgical repair, functional capacity, cyanosis, and the presence of pul-monary hypertension. Heart failure, arrhythmias, and systemic hypertension are more common with cyanotic congenital heart disease and

when functional status is compromised. Infective endocarditis is a risk peripartum.

Fetal mortality averages 40 per cent in maternal cyanotic congenital heart disease, over twice that for the acyanotic mother with congenital heart disease. Low birth weight for gestational age and prematurity are more common in cyanotic mothers. The risk of important congenital defects in the fetus of mothers with congenital heart disease varies between 3 and 15 per cent.

Elective induction of labour at fetal maturity often allows better plan-ning of monitoring and availability of key personnel. Caesarean section is usually performed for obstetric reasons rather than maternal status. Hae-modynamic monitoring and maintenance of filling pressures minimize maternal risk. Antibiotic chemoprophylaxis is indicated during uncompli-cated vaginal delivery in the presence of a valve prosthesis, a right to left shunt, or a surgical left to right shunt. In some centres, prophylactic anti-biotics are used more widely.

Maternal risk can be classified according to structural diagnosis (Table 2).

Acyanotic shunt lesions

Atrial septal defect

This common lesion is usually well tolerated in pregnancy, even with a substantial left to right shunt. Antibiotic prophylaxis is not indicated for an isolated secundum atrial septal defect. Elective closure should be con-sidered following delivery.

Ventricular septal defect

This lesion is well tolerated in pregnancy unless there is persistent pulmon-ary hypertension or impaired cardiac reserve.

Persistent ductus arteriosus

Percutaneous transcatheter closure of a persistent ductus arteriosus has occasionally been required during pregnancy because of the development of heart failure resistant to medical therapy, but the majority have a low risk provided pulmonary hypertension is not severe.

Acyanotic obstructive lesions

Aortic valve disease

Mild aortic stenosis can be missed in pregnancy because of the prevalence of a flow-related systolic murmur and confusion between a split first heart sound and the ejection click from a bicuspid valve. Asymptomatic patients with moderate or severe aortic stenosis may require careful haemodynamic monitoring during labour and delivery. Patients with symptomatic severe aortic stenosis should be advised against pregnancy, or should consider ter-mination. Valvotomy and percutaneous balloon valvuloplasty have been performed successfully in the second and third trimesters for severe symptoms.

Coarctation of the aorta

Pregnancy is usually uneventful, although impaired fetal development, hypertension, heart failure, and aortic dissection have all been described. If possible, aortic coarctation should be corrected prior to pregnancy.

Table 2 Congenital heart disease (CHD) and maternal risks during pregnancy

Low	Medium	High
Atrial septal defect	Cyanotic CHD without pulmonary hypertension	Eisenmenger syndrome
Small ventricular septal defect	Palliated complex CHD	Primary pulmonary hypertension
Small persistent ductus arteriosus	Hypertrophic obstructive cardiomyopathy	Symptomatic severe aortic stenosis
Mild coarctation of aorta	Symptomatic mitral stenosis	
Corrected tetralogy of Fallot	Ebstein's anomaly	

Pulmonary stenosis

The risks associated with pregnancy in this condition are low, although heart failure has been described. Balloon valvuloplasty or surgical valvotomy are intervention options, but clinical experience of these in pregnancy is small.

Cyanotic lesions

Tetralogy of Fallot

This is the commonest cyanotic congenital heart disease in adults. Pregnancy may cause major clinical deterioration because of augmented right ventricular pressure from increased blood volume and increased right to left shunting from reduced systemic vascular resistance. Reduced arterial oxygen saturation and a high haematocrit are worrying signs, and careful monitoring of labour and delivery is essential. Maternal and fetal risk are reduced where the defect has been surgically repaired, and this should be performed prior to pregnancy. Palliative aortopulmonary shunting leaves a significant risk during pregnancy.

Eisenmenger's syndrome

The high maternal mortality with this condition has been confirmed by several studies, although there are some isolated successes. One in four pregnancies reach term with a very high prevalence of growth retardation, prematurity, and perinatal death. Because of this, pregnancy is contraindicated and early termination should be considered. Thromboembolism is more common and anticoagulation should be considered in late pregnancy and postpartum. Intensive haemodynamic monitoring to avoid blood loss and blood pressure swings and to maintain filling pressures is appropriate.

Complex cyanotic congenital heart disease

The increasing success of palliative and corrective surgical procedures for complex cyanotic congenital heart disease has allowed pregnancy to be contemplated in those surviving to child-bearing age. Successful pregnancies have been reported with a single ventricle, corrected and uncorrected transposition of the great vessels, tricuspid and pulmonary atresia, but the risks are substantial and often inappropriate. Even in the absence of severe pulmonary hypertension, serious cardiovascular complications occur in one-third of pregnancies. The literature probably presents an underestimate of the risk because of a tendency to report success.

Rheumatic heart disease and other valve lesions

Rheumatic heart disease

Although rare in the United Kingdom, acute rheumatic fever may develop or recur during pregnancy and the associated carditis carries a substantial maternal risk. Antibiotic chemoprophylaxis has been advised throughout pregnancy in patients with a history of recurrent rheumatic fever.

Patients with rheumatic valvular disease should be managed according to disease site and severity. Careful haemodynamic monitoring may be necessary in late pregnancy, labour, and postpartum.

Mitral stenosis

This is the commonest cardiac lesion in pregnancy, with complications including heart failure, atrial arrhythmias (particularly fibrillation), and thromboembolism. Digoxin and β-blockade may be effective in controlling the ventricular rate and maintaining cardiac output when arrhythmias ensue. Diuretics reduce pulmonary congestion but hypovolaemia should be avoided. Asymptomatic or mildly symptomatic patients usually progress uneventfully. Severe symptomatic mitral stenosis can be successfully relieved by percutaneous balloon valvuloplasty or closed or open valvotomy. Both fetal and maternal risks appear to be modest with these procedures, although experience of balloon valvuloplasty is small. Systemic and pulmonary thromboembolism is a special complication in pregnancy

and chronic anticoagulant therapy should be considered in those at higher risk based on standard criteria (see Chapter 13.7).

Mitral regurgitation

This lesion is usually well tolerated, presumably because of reduced systemic vascular resistance. Vasodilator therapy and digoxin may be indicated.

Mitral valve prolapse

This has been recognized in up to 15 per cent of women of child-bearing age and provided mitral regurgitation is not severe, there appears to be little risk to mother or fetus.

Aortic valve disease

Severe rheumatic aortic valve disease is uncommon in pregnancy. Aortic regurgitation is more frequent, but like mitral regurgitation is fairly well tolerated, partly because of the fall in systemic vascular resistance and tachycardia, both of which reduce myocardial work.

Cardiomyopathy in pregnancy

Hypertrophic cardiomyopathy

Pregnancy appears to be well tolerated, although symptoms of heart failure can develop or worsen at any stage. It is uncertain whether the risk of sudden death is increased by pregnancy. Careful haemodynamic monitoring may be indicated during labour and delivery, and avoidance of systemic vasodilatation, blood loss, and hypotension are essential. The role of β-blockade is uncertain, but these drugs can be useful in managing symptoms related to elevated left ventricular filling pressure and where there is an obstructive element to the condition.

Peripartum cardiomyopathy

This form of dilated cardiomyopathy causes left ventricular systolic dysfunction and heart failure in the last trimester of pregnancy or within the first 6 months postpartum. Other causes of dilated cardiomyopathy presenting in pregnancy should be excluded. The disease is rare in Europe but commoner in parts of Africa, with a prevalence of up to 1 per cent. Although the cause is unknown, the age at onset, geographical frequency variation, and substantial recovery of ventricular function in the majority of individuals suggest a unique and specific syndrome. Myocarditis, nutritional deficiency, small vessel coronary disease, and maternal immunological responses to a fetal antigen have all been proposed as mechanisms. Endomyocardial biopsy reveals inconsistent changes. The role of genetic factors is poorly defined.

Clinical examination reveals cardiomegaly, a third or fourth heart sound, and commonly functional mitral and tricuspid regurgitation. ECG abnormalities are widespread and usually non-specific, and a variety of arrhythmias have been described. The haemodynamic changes are similar to other forms of dilated cardiomyopathy.

Most patients respond to conventional management with digoxin, diuretics, and vasodilators. Angiotensin converting enzyme (ACE) inhibitors may affect fetal renal function and are not recommended. The role of immunosuppresive therapy is controversial and not established.

Fifty per cent of patients show substantial or complete recovery of ventricular function within 6 months postpartum. In the remainder, there is persistent left ventricular dysfunction and chronic heart failure. Progressive clinical deterioration and early death occur in a minority. There is a significant risk of thromboembolism and anticoagulant therapy is often appropriate.

The risk or relapse in a subsequent pregnancy is substantial (up to 40 per cent) and is greater in patients with persistently abnormal ventricular function.

Ischaemic heart disease

Symptomatic coronary artery disease in pregnancy has a prevalence of around 1 in 10 000. Conventional risk factors apply: particularly smoking and previous oral contraceptive use in combination, and hypercholesterolaemia. Peripartum myocardial infarction is occasionally associated with normal epicardial coronary arteries at subsequent angiography. Spasm, *in situ* thrombosis, dissection, and plaque rupture have been proposed as mechanisms.

Myocardial infarction is associated with a maternal mortality up to 25 per cent. Low-dose aspirin is relatively safe but use of thrombolytic drugs and percutaneous coronary intervention has not been adequately evaluated. Haemodynamic monitoring may be appropriate peripartum and elective caesarean section should be considered.

The Marfan syndrome

Pregnancy in patients with the Marfan syndrome is associated with an increased incidence of aortic dissection and death, particularly if existing cardiovascular disease is identified. An aortic root diameter of less than 4.5 cm and absence of progressive aortic dilatation and aortic regurgitation suggest a better outcome. However, selective literature reporting probably overestimates the true risk. In patients with established aortic root dilatation, pregnancy is undesirable and if root enlargement is progressive during the first trimester, termination must be considered. β-Blockade may reduce the rate of aortic dilatation during pregnancy, but clinical experience is limited. Regular monitoring of aortic root diameter is recommenced. Elective caesarean section may be preferable to vaginal delivery in those with significant aortic root dilatation.

Aortic dissection in the absence of the Marfan syndrome is rare, and occurs most frequently during the third trimester of pregnancy and peripartum. Precordial and transoesophageal echocardiography is the diagnostic investigation. Emergency measures to reduce blood pressure are required, although maternal and fetal mortality is high.

Primary pulmonary hypertension

A high maternal mortality rate (up to 40 per cent) has been reported and pregnancy is contraindicated. Haemodynamic deterioration during pregnancy is not predictable on the basis of preconception haemodynamics. Anticoagulation is recommended during pregnancy and early post partum.

Cardiac arrhythmias

Atrial and ventricular premature beats occur commonly in pregnancy and appear to have no adverse consequences. Patients with a substrate for supraventricular tachycardia, such as atrioventricular nodal or atrioventricular re-entry tachycardia, may experience symptomatic deterioration in pregnancy, or may develop symptoms for the first time. Bradycardia and heart block are rare and are usually congenital. Specific causes should be sought and, if appropriate, removed. Antiarrhythmic drug therapy should be initiated only for persistent arrhythmias threatening the mother or fetus (see below). Catheter ablation procedures should be undertaken postpartum to avoid unpredictable exposure to ionizing radiation.

Cardiac surgery in pregnancy

Although many cardiac operations have been described in pregnancy, including those on cardiopulmonary bypass, detailed evaluation of the risk–benefit balance is inadequate. There have been many reports of mitral valvotomy with low maternal and fetal mortality. In general, surgery considered essential for maternal health should be performed during the middle trimester or towards the end of the third trimester when elective or emergency delivery can be planned. Sustained uterine contraction is essential postpartum to minimize the risk from systemic heparinization during cardiopulmonary bypass. In appropriate circumstances, balloon valvuloplasty or coronary angioplasty seem attractive options.

Pregnancy and valve prosthesis

Increased cardiac output, a hypercoagulable state, deterioration of the bioprosthesis, and fetal risks from anticoagulation all potentially complicate pregnancy with a valve prosthesis. However, patients with no or minimal limitation before pregnancy usually have a favourable outcome. The risk of thromboembolic events with mechanical valves appears increased, partly related to anticoagulant control and the use of fixed-dose heparin regimens in the first trimester. Tissue valves are often recommended for women who wish to have children, but the long-term durability of heterograft valves in particular is questionable and premature degeneration from progressive leaflet calcification is more common in the young.

Cardiovascular drugs in pregnancy

All drugs should be avoided where possible during pregnancy and the risk/benefit balance carefully evaluated in terms of maternal health and fetal risk. For information on prescribing in pregnancy, see Chapter 13.18. Two specific issues will be discussed here: anticoagulation and the use of prophylactic antibiotics for those at risk of endocarditis.

Anticoagulation

There is no ideal anticoagulant in pregnancy. Use must depend on individual assessment of risks and benefits. Warfarin has been most widely used but has significant maternal and fetal side-effects. The risk of haemorrhage at delivery means that it should be discontinued approaching term. Fetal risks are derived from the transplacental passage of warfarin: there is a relatively high incidence of spontaneous abortion and stillbirth, and use during the first trimester has been associated with a 'coumarin embryopathy' in 5 to 15 per cent of infants so exposed. This syndrome includes hypoplasia of the nasal bone and epiphyseal stipling (chondrodysplasia punctata). Central nervous system disease, including optic atrophy and blindness, mental retardation, cerebral palsy, and intracranial bleeding have all been described and linked to warfarin.

Heparin, because of its molecular weight, does not cross the placenta. Its use in pregnancy is not without difficulty, although recent studies have shown satisfactory outcomes. Complications of long-term subcutaneous therapy include haematoma and abscess formation in the abdominal wall, thrombocytopenia, and osteoporosis. Self-injection of an adjusted dose of heparin subcutaneously every 12 h is a satisfactory approach. Fixed-dose regimens should be avoided. There is a consensus that intravenous heparin should be substituted close to term and discontinued at the onset of labour. Low molecular weight heparins have not been adequately studied during pregnancy. When the risk of thromboembolic complications is very high, for example with a mechanical mitral valve prosthesis continuous warfarin therapy (INR 2–3.5:1) may be a reasonable strategy.

A suggested strategy for the management of anticoagulation in pregnancy is shown in Fig. 1. In patients at moderate risk this involves early substitution of heparin for warfarin (preferably prior to conception) and return to warfarin from the end of the first trimester until 2 weeks before term. Continued heparin therapy throughout the pregnancy is an alternative widely practised in North America where litigation fears limit oral anticoagulation use. With the exception of premature infants, warfarin

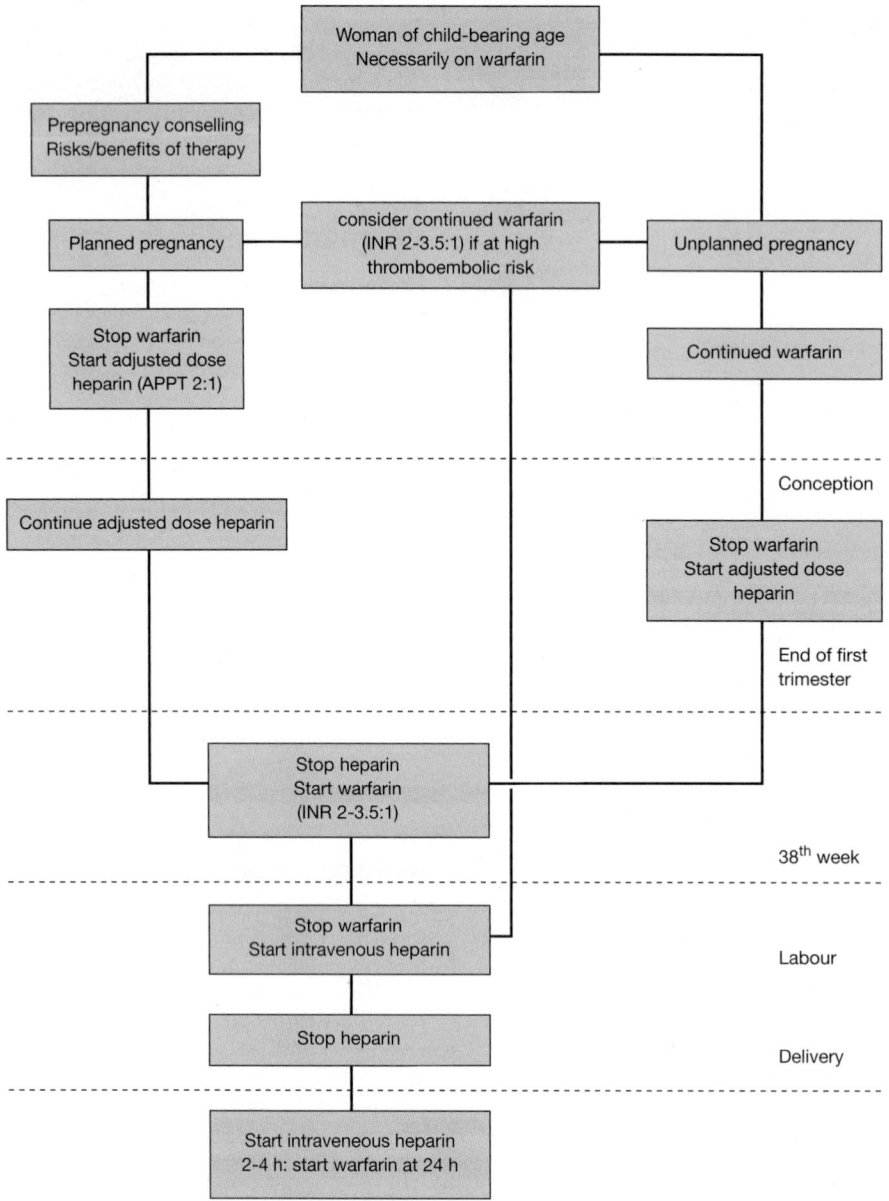

Fig. 1 A strategy for anticoagulation during pregnancy.

excretion in breast milk does not cause significant anticoagulation for the infant.

Prophylactic antibiotics

The incidence of bacteraemia associated with an uncomplicated vaginal delivery is low and thresholds for antibiotic chemoprophylaxis are uncertain. Routine prophylaxis is recommended for prosthetic heart valves, congenital heart disease with a right to left shunt, and when aortopulmonary anastomosis has been created with prosthetic material. Many physicians, however, also routinely administer prophylactic antibiotics to those at conventional risk from endocarditis, including valvular heart disease, ventricular septal defect, and hypertrophic obstructive cardiomyopathy. Treatment with intravenous ampicillin and gentamicin approximately 1 h prior to delivery is recommended with a second dose 8 h later. Slow intravenous infusion of vancomycin and gentamicin can be used in those who are aller-

gic to penicillin. For patients at low risk, conventional chemoprophylaxis with oral amoxycillin is widely practised.

Further reading

Elkayam U, Gleicher N (eds) (1990). *Cardiac problems in pregnancy—diagnosis and management of maternal and fetal disease*, 2nd edn. John Wiley, Chicester.

Perloff JK (1992). Congenital heart disease. In: Gleicher N, ed. *Principles and practice of medical therapy in pregnancy*, 2nd edn. Appleton and Lange, Norwalk, Conn.

Sullivan JM, Ramanathan KB (1985). Management of medical problems in pregnancy—severe cardiac disease. *New England Journal of Medicine* **313**, 304–9.

Weiderhorn J, Rubin JM, Frishman WH, Elkayam U (1987). Cardiovascular drugs in pregnancy. *Cardiology Clinics* **5**, 651–745.

13.7 Thromboembolism in pregnancy

M. de Swiet

This section is concerned with thromboembolism in pregnancy, specifically deep vein thrombosis and pulmonary embolism. Arterial thromboembolism, which in pregnancy usually arises because of mitral valve disease and/or atrial fibrillation, cardiomyopathy, and the presence of artificial heart valves, is considered elsewhere. Cerebral vein thrombosis is considered in Section 15.

Significance and incidence

Pulmonary embolus is a leading cause of maternal mortality in the United Kingdom, responsible for 46 deaths between 1994 and 1996 (21 deaths per million maternities). In addition, deep vein thrombosis is a major cause of morbidity: about 80 per cent of women who have deep vein thrombosis in pregnancy have symptoms in the same leg at follow-up 11 years later. Because of the difficulties in diagnosis of non-fatal cases (see below) it is difficult to obtain precise data for the incidence of non-fatal pulmonary embolus or deep vein thrombosis. However, recent figures for the incidence of venous thromboembolism in the United Kingdom (Scotland) are 1.0/1000 maternities in women under 35 years of age and 2.4/1000 in those over 35 years. About twice as many episodes occur antenatally as in the 6-week postnatal period. Pulmonary embolism contributes 10 to 20 per cent of all cases; the remainder are deep vein thromboses.

In Africa and the Far East the condition has been almost unknown, in part due to the lower prevalence of inherited thrombophilias (see below); but those countries that have become more affluent have seen a corresponding increase in the incidence of thromboembolism.

Risk factors

It is generally believed that pregnancy itself is a risk factor for venous thromboembolism, presumably because of activation of the clotting system. Venous stasis in the lower limbs caused by obstruction of the venous return by the enlarging uterus is another factor. This effect is more marked in the left leg than the right and accounts for the fact that in pregnancy deep vein thrombosis is approximately ten times more common in the left leg than the right.

Analysis of fatal cases of pulmonary embolus shows that increasing age and parity are important risk factors: the risk of dying from pulmonary embolus in a woman aged over 40 years in her fifth pregnancy is nearly 100 times greater than in a primigravid woman aged 20 to 30 years. Caesarean section (and probably other forms of complicated instrumental delivery) increases the risk about three-fold. Oestrogen therapy to suppress lactation also increases the risk of thromboembolism and should no longer be used. Women who have had thromboembolism in the past have a 1 in 10 to 1 in 20 risk of thromboembolism in pregnancy, the risk being the same whether or not the previous episode occurred whilst taking oestrogen-containing oral contraceptives. It is not known whether previous thromboembolism in pregnancy increases the risk in subsequent pregnancies above the figures given. It is likely that prolonged periods of bed rest and obesity are also predisposing factors.

The most important specific haematological risk factors for thromboembolism are the thrombophilias. Acquired thrombophilia mainly comprises the antiphospholilpid syndromes, characterized by the presence of lupus anticoagulant and anticardiolipin antibodies, considered in Chapter 13.14. Knowledge of the inherited thrombophilias is expanding rapidly. Current estimates of the pregnancy risks of thromboembolism are as follow: factor V Leiden heterozygote: 1in 437 pregnancies; protein C deficiency: 1 in 113; type 1 antithrombin deficiency 1 in 3; type 2 antithrombin deficiency 1in 42. Increased risks that have not been accurately quantified also exist for those with protein S deficiency, the prothrombin gene mutation, and hyperhomocysteinaemia. Women with thrombophilia who have a family history of thromboembolism, and particularly those who have themselves already had an episode of thromboembolism, have a further increase in risk.

It must also be remembered that the fetus is at risk in maternal thrombophilia. The risks of miscarriage, second and third trimester loss, abruption, premature rupture of membranes, and pre-eclampsia are best characterized for acquired antiphospholipd syndrome, but they are increased in varying degree for the inherited thrombophilias as well.

Patients with any of the sickling conditions (Hb SS, Hb SC, Hb S thalassaemia) are at increased risk of developing the sickle lung syndrome in pregnancy, one component of which is probably thrombosis *in situ*. Management of haemoglobinopathies in pregnancy is considered in Chapter 13.16.

Diagnosis

The clinical features of pulmonary embolus and deep vein thrombosis are considered in Chapter 15.15.3.1. These do not differ in pregnancy, but the frequent occurrence in normal pregnancy of leg oedema, breathlessness, minor degrees of pleural effusion in the puerperium, and abnormalities of the electrocardiograph, make the clinical diagnosis even more difficult in those who are pregnant than in those who are not. Furthermore, the problems of anticoagulant therapy with its associated risks to the fetus are such that every effort must be made to make the diagnosis by objective criteria. The implications of this policy are as follows.

Deep vein thrombosis

All patients who have a history compatible with deep vein thrombosis and supporting physical signs in the legs should have a real-time ultrasound examination of the leg veins with additional Doppler blood flow studies if possible. This technique has been compared with venography in the non-pregnant state and shown to have high sensitivity and specificity for symptomatic femoral vein thrombosis. The direct comparison has not been made in pregnancy. Ultrasound is not yet accurate for calf vein thrombi, but these do not cause pulmonary emboli and the ultrasound test, being non-invasive, can be repeated to ensure that a calf vein thrombosis is not extending into the thigh. Ultrasound cannot be used above the inguinal ligament, but iliofemoral thrombosis is usually clinically obvious.

Table 1 Features of some 'occult' causes of collapse in pregnancy

	Predisposing circumstances	Common presenting features	Helpful diagnostic features in acute stage	
			Clinical	Investigations
Amniotic fluid embolism	Labour, not necessarily precipitate	Respiratory distress, cyanosis		Squames in SVC or sputum
Pulmonary embolus	Increasing age, multiparity, thromboembolism, operative delivery, bedrest, oestrogens, haemoglobinopathy		Jugular venous pressure+, 3rd heart sound, parasternal heave	ECG, chest radiograph, lung scan, blood gas, pulmonary angiography
Myocardial infarction	Increasing age	Chest pain, respiratory distress, cyanosis	Pain character, jugular venous pressure +, crepitations	ECG
Dysrhythmia	Pre-existing	Tachycardia/bradycardia	Pulse	ECG
Aspiration of gastric contents	Anaethesia, not necessarily with vomiting	Respiratory distress, cyanosis	Bronchospasm	
Pneumothorax and pneumomediastinum	Previous history, labour	Chest pain	Chest signs	Chest radiograph
Intra-abdominal bleeding	Labour, though may occur spontaneously	Abdominal pain	Jugular venous pressure not elevated, signs in abdomen, laparotomy, paracentesis, culdocentesis	

Reproduced from de Swiet (1995), with permission

Pulmonary embolus

If a patient has a major pulmonary embolus, there is usually little doubt about the diagnosis. However, pulmonary embolus is often considered as a cause of collapse in pregnant women, particularly at the time of delivery, and the differential diagnosis of occult causes of collapse without obvious bleeding or inverted uterus is considered in Table 1. Perhaps the most important cause of confusion is intra-abdominal bleeding, with irritation of the diaphragm causing chest and shoulder-tip pain. Treatment of such a patient with anticoagulants would probably be fatal. The most important clinical features to note are the presence of abdominal signs and low jugular venous pressure in abdominal bleeding, and the raised jugular venous pressure and cardiac signs of pulmonary artery obstruction in pulmonary embolus. However, the problem of diagnosis usually arises in the patient who has pleuritic chest pain with, or without, physical signs, and either absent or non-specific signs on chest radiography. Arterial blood gas estimation may be helpful: blood samples should be taken with the patient sitting and, in cases of major pulmonary embolus, will show respiratory alkalosis with hypoxaemia. However, the definitive investigation is a lung scan, preferably a ventilation perfusion scan if there are any radiological signs in the lung parenchyma. The radiation exposure from the short-lived isotopes that are used (^{81}Kr^m for ventilation and ^{99}Tc^m for perfusion) is trivial. If the patient has normal blood gases and a negative lung scan, it is reasonable to exclude pulmonary embolus.

Treatment

Surgery

If the facilities and an expert team are available, the occasional patient who does not die from a massive pulmonary embolus and remains shocked and hypotensive (blood pressure less than 90 mmHg systolic, PaO_2 less than 60 mmHg, urine output less than 20 ml/h) one h after the onset of symptoms, should be considered for pulmonary embolectomy under cardiopulmonary bypass. If the patient reaches the operating theatre alive, the results are excellent. Alternatively, it may be possible to fragment the clot and improve pulmonary blood flow with a catheter introduced into the pulmonary artery. This requires only the simplest image-intensifying equipment, such as is available in most intensive care units (see Section 16).

The place of surgery (embolectomy) in massive iliofemoral thrombosis, where it might decrease the incidence of subsequent postphlebitic leg symptoms, is unclear.

Thrombolytic therapy

Streptokinase and/or urokinase treatment is probably underused for non-pregnant patients with pulmonary embolus. However, there are specific problems in pregnancy, such as bleeding, the initiation of premature labour, and the subsequent inco-ordinate uterine action associated with the release of fibrin degradation products. Therefore, in pregnancy, thrombolytic therapy should only be used in shocked patients with life threatening pulmonary embolism and as an alternative to embolectomy.

Filters

There is no substantive evidence of benefit of temporary or permanent caval interrupt devices in patients judged to be at high risk of pulmonary embolism. In pregnancy their use should be limited to those who have recurrent pulmonary embolism despite adequate anticoagulation. In practice, this happens very rarely; most recurrent pulmonary emboli occur in women who have not been adequately anticoagulated.

Anticoagulant therapy

For the reasons given above, the majority of patients will be treated with anticoagulants, the objective being to prevent further thromboembolism. As in the non-pregnant state, heparin should be used initially. Neither unfractionated heparin (UH) nor any of the low molecular weight heparins (LMWH) cross the placenta or are secreted into breast milk in significant quantities, and if heparin were to be secreted in breast milk it would not be absorbed from the infant's gastrointestinal tract, being denatured in the stomach. The only acute problem with heparin therapy is bleeding. Possible long-term problems are discussed below.

Traditionally, in the acute phase of treatment in pregnancy, heparin has been given by continuous intravenous infusion, starting at 40 000 units/24 h, adjusting the rate to double the activated partial thromboplastin time, and continuing for about 10 days. However, in the non-pregnant state clinical trials have shown that initial treatment of both deep vein thrombosis and pulmonary embolus with fixed high dose LMWH given by intermittent subcutaneous injection is as effective as intavenous infusion of UH. Typical regimens include enoxaparine 1 mg/kg 12 hourly. The advantages of LMWH regimen are considerable, in particular the lack of need for monitoring and dose adjustment, and the possibility of ambulatory treatment. It is very likely that the use of such regimen in the acute phase of thromboembolism treatment will also become standard in pregnancy, but there are concerns about this. The trials performed in the non-pregnant state have been of LMWH supported by very early additional warfarin therapy; this will not happen in pregnancy (see below), and LMWH will be used on its own for varying periods at varying intensities of therapy. Furthermore, the clotting system is activated in pregnancy, such that the doses of LMWH that have been successfully evaluated in the non-pregnant state may not be appropriate for pregnancy. Until more experience is obtained it is recommended that those using high-dose LMWH in acute phase treatment check the anti-Xa heparin assay, aiming for trough levels greater than 0.4 units/ml and peak levels less than 1.0 units/ml.

After the acute phase, the therapeutic options are oral anticoagulants, of which there is far more experience with warfarin than phenindione, and subcutaneous heparin of one sort or another. The problems with warfarin therapy in pregnancy are maternal bleeding, particularly in the puerperium, miscarriage, teratogenesis (chondrodysplasia punctata), fetal microcephaly, optic atrophy, and fetal bleeding, both retroplacental and intracerebral. The latter complications can occur with warfarin therapy at any gestational age. For these reasons warfarin should not be used in venous thromboembolism in pregnancy, although its use is necessary in those with artificial heart valves.

Once intravenous heparin has been discontinued, the patient should be given subcutaneous injections of heparin at prophylactic doses, either UH 10 000 twice daily or a LMWH such as enoxaparine 40 mg once daily. In practice, most patients receive LMWH because once daily injections are more convenient. Other possible advantages of LMWH, which remain unproven, are greater and more constant bioavailabilty, a superior risk ratio of antithrombotic activity to bleeding risk, less heparin-induced thrombocytopenia, and less bone demineralization (see below). Most patients can learn to inject themselves and administer the treatment at home. Bruising appears to be related more to the injection technique than to the type of heparin. It is not clear what degree of monitoring (if any) is necessary in this phase of heparin treatment. If the anti-Xa heparin level is less than 0.3 units/ml there should be no risk of bleeding, but the minimum heparin level for effective chronic phase or prophylactic therapy is not known. Common practice has been to check the anti-Xa heparin level at varying intervals and only adjust the dose downwards should the level be greater than 0.3 units/ml. In the absence of recurrence of thromboembolism the dose has not been increased to more than those levels recommended above. An alternative when using UH is to measure the thrombin time, which is very sensitive to excess UH (but not LMWH) activity: if it is not prolonged the patient should not be at any excess bleeding risk. In practice, when using injections of UH 10 000 twice daily or enoxaparine 40 mg once daily it is very uncommon for the anti-Xa level to be greater than 0.3 units/ml or for any of the standard clotting tests (activated partial thromboplastin time, thrombin time, INR) to be abnormal; hence the uncertainty about the need to perform these tests.

Assuming that the standard clotting tests are normal, there is no increased risk from bleeding in labour and subcutaneous heparin therapy should be continued through labour. Although there has been concern about the possibility of epidural haematoma formation in women taking subcutaneous heparin given epidural anaesthesia, this concern is not justified. Nevertheless, epidural block is often withheld until 2 h after an injection of UH or 4 h after an injection of LMWH. If an epidural catheter has been inserted similar constraints relate to its removal.

After delivery the dose of subcutaneous UH heparin is reduced to 7500 units twice daily; the dose of LMWH need not be changed. This treatment should be continued for the first week of the puerperium. After that time, the risk of secondary postpartum haemorrhage is small and patients may switch to oral warfarin therapy if that appears more desirable. Breast feeding is safe in patients taking warfarin: insignificant quantities of warfarin (though not phenindione) are secreted in the milk. Since blood-clotting parameters do not return to normal immediately after delivery, anticoagulation should be continued for some time after delivery in a patient who had thromboembolism in the antenatal period. Six weeks is often the time chosen, but the length of time is quite arbitrary.

Prophylaxis

Previous thromboembolism

Should any form of prophylactic therapy be given in pregnancy to women who have had an episode of thromboembolism in the past, granted the 5 to 10 per cent risk of recurrence? Trial data are not adequate to answer this question. Warfarin therapy is contraindicated because of the complications noted above. Some clinicians would use subcutaneous heparin throughout pregnancy, but the incidence of maternal side-effects—heparin induced thrombocytopenia (HIT) (see Chapter 13.16), alopecia, and bone demineralization—are a cause of considerable concern.

Heparin-induced thrombocytopenia is very uncommon in obstetric practice. The incidence may be less with LMWH than with UH, but patients who have had HIT with UH are certainly at risk if they take LMWH. A better alternative is the heparinoid organon. There are anecdotal reports of its use in pregnancy: it is also given parentally and does not cross the placenta. Clinical bone demineralization has been reported in patients taking as little as 10 000 units of heparin/day for 19 weeks, and there is evidence of subclinical bone demineralization in many patients taking heparin 20 000 units/day for more than 3 months.

If prophylaxis is to be given, the alternatives to 'standard dose' UH or LMWH prophylaxis are: the use of smaller quantities for shorter periods of time; low dose aspirin (75 mg/day); or no prophylaxis in the antenatal period, starting heparin in labour, continuing in the puerperium for at least 1 week, and with the option of switching to warfarin for a further 5 weeks. None of these strategies has been fully evaluated.

Given the balance of risks, most clinicians would not advise prophylaxis for the patient who has simply had a single episode of thromboembolism in the past. They would, however, suggest that the patient accept the risk of prolonged subcutaneous heparin therapy if she has had more than one well-documented episode of thromboembolism, or if she has had a single episode of thromboembolism and has a known inherited or acquired thrombophilia. Patients who have had a single episode but also have a family history of thromboembolism in a first-degree relative should also receive prophylactic heparin throughout pregnancy: they may well have thrombophilia that has not yet been detected.

Thrombophilia

As indicated above, advances are being made very rapidly in this field. The risk of thromboembolism in pregnancy depends on the manner in which the condition was detected. Those found to have thrombophilia following an episode of thromboembolism are at greatest risk; those found because of a family history are at intermediate risk; and those found through population screening are at least risk.

Patients who have the antiphospholipid syndrome and have had previous thromboembolism should take prophylactic UH or LMWH throughout pregnancy and for at least 6 weeks after delivery. They are also likely to be taking low-dose aspirin for fetal reasons. If they have a particularly bad history of thromboembolism they should take LMWH in relatively high dose, granted their need to take warfarin aiming for INR 3 to 4 when not pregnant. If they have been taking heparin and aspirin in pregnancy for fetal reasons only, and have no history of previous thromboembolism, most clinicians would discontinue thromboprophylaxis at delivery unless there were other risk factors such as delivery by emergency Caesarean section.

Type 1 antithrombin deficiency has such a high risk of thromboembolism that women should take high-dose LMWH throughout pregnancy regardless of their history of thromboembolism. Antithrombin concentrate is now available and depending on the measured level of antithrombin may be given to cover labour or if the woman has an episode of thromboembolism.

It is difficult to be dogmatic about management of other forms of thrombophilia given the lack of trial data. However, patients with Type 2 antithrombin deficiency and those with homozygous factor V Leiden should probably have prophylactic low-dose heparin throughout pregnancy, whatever their past history, and if they have had a previous clot the level of anticoagulation could be increased by increasing the dose. In the remaining thrombophilias, protein C and S deficiencies, the prothrombin gene mutation, heterozygous factor V Leiden, and hyperhomocysteinaemia, heparin prophylaxis may be withheld during pregnancy but given peripartum if there is no past history of thromboembolism. Aspirin can be given to cover the antenatal period. If there is a past history of thromboembolism, prophylactic heparin should be given throughout pregnancy. Patients with hyperhomocysteinaemia should take folic acid supplements; the optimal dose is not clear, 5 mg daily should be sufficient.

Protein S deficiency cannot be diagnosed reliably in pregnancy since the levels of both free and bound protein S decrease in normal pregnancy. Genetic tests for factor V Leiden should be performed if the activated protein C resistance is low in pregnancy. However a low activated protein C resistance in pregnancy does not necessarily indicate abnormality since the activated protein C resistance is also decreased in normal pregnancy.

If a woman considering pregnancy is known to be protein C deficient, her partner's protein C status should be checked. Protein C deficiency is usually expressed in the heterozygous form. However, homozygous protein C deficiency can occur and the individual is then dependent on lifelong infusions of protein C concentrate to prevent recurrent episodes of thromboembolism.

Further reading

Dahlman T, Lindvall N, Hellgren M (1990). Osteopenia in pregnancy during long-term heparin treatment: A radiological study post partum. *British Journal of Obstetrics and Gynaecology* 97, 221.

Department of Health (1998). *Why mothers die, report on confidential enquiries into maternal deaths in the United Kingdom 1994–96.* HMSO, London.

de Swiet M (1995). Thromboembolism. In: de Swiet M, ed. *Medical disorders in obstetrics practice*, 3rd edn, pp. 116–42. Blackwell Scientific Publications, Oxford.

de Swiet M, *et al.* (1983). Prolonged heparin therapy in pregnancy causes bone demineralization. *British Journal of Obstetrics and Gynaecology* 90, 1129–34.

Greer IA (1999). Thrombosis in pregnancy: maternal and fetal issues. *Lancet* 353, 1258–65.

Howell R, Fidler J, Letsky E, de Swiet M (1983). The risks of antenatal subcutaneous heparin prophylaxis: a controlled trial. *British Journal of Obstetrics and Gynaecology* 90, 1124–8.

Maclon NS, Greer IA (1996). Venous thromboembolic disease in obstetrics and gynaecology: the Scottish experience. *Scottish Medical Journal* 41, 83–6.

Nelson Piercy C, Letsky E, de Swiet M (1997). Low molecular weight heparin for obstetric thromboprophyllaxis: experience of 69 pregnancies in 61 women at high risk. *American Journal of Obstetrics and Gynecology* 176, 1062–8.

13.8 Chest diseases in pregnancy

M. de Swiet

Physiology

The pregnant woman at rest increases her minute volume by about 40 per cent within the first trimester of pregnancy. This is achieved by an increase in tidal volume rather than in respiratory rate, and is more than adequate to account for the increased metabolic rate of the mother and fetus, even in the later stages of pregnancy when maternal oxygen consumption increases by about 45 ml/min. The stimulus to increased ventilation is said to be increased progesterone secretion, but it is likely that this is not the only factor.

The majority view is that vital capacity and airways resistance do not change in pregnancy, although, surprisingly, transfer factor is reduced. The uterus enlarging within the abdomen partly accounts for a 20 per cent reduction in residual volume, but this reduction, together with change in the shape of the chest wall, occurs early in pregnancy, before there can be any mechanical effect due to the uterus. The reduction in residual volume is more marked when supine than sitting. Pao_2 in the sitting or erect posture is unchanged in pregnancy, but falls by up to 2 kPa (15 mmHg) in patients who are supine in late pregnancy, probably due to unequal ventilation/perfusion ratios subsequent to airways closure during tidal breathing. Therefore, where possible, blood gases for diagnostic purposes should always be taken in pregnant patients when they are sitting. $Paco_2$ falls to about 4.0 kPa (30 mmHg) and plasma bicarbonate falls proportionally to about 20 mmol/l, hence there is no change in the arterial pH.

Breathlessness is a common symptom in pregnancy, presumably associated with the 40 per cent increase in ventilation that occurs in normal women. However, this cannot be the entire explanation because ventilation increases from before 4 weeks' gestation, whereas the maximum incidence of onset of breathlessness is at 28 to 31 weeks' gestation. Breathlessness is worrying for the doctor (and for the patient) because it may also be associated with cardiopulmonary disease, particularly pulmonary embolism. In the absence of other features of cardiopulmonary disease, and with normal findings on examination, useful investigations are chest radiography, arterial blood gas estimation, oximetry to determine oxygen saturation at rest and on exercise, and full lung function testing including measurement of transfer factor.

Lung disease in pregnancy—general considerations

Although ventilation does increase by 40 per cent in pregnancy, this increase is trivial in comparison to the marked increase (perhaps ten-fold) that is possible during exercise. This considerable reserve of ventilatory capacity is not greatly challenged by pregnancy and respiratory failure due to chronic respiratory disease is uncommon in pregnancy, the major problem for women with chronic conditions such as asthma or tuberculosis being the effect of therapy on pregnancy.

By contrast, acute respiratory failure is a major cause of maternal mortality: adult respiratory distress syndrome (ARDS) is the final common pathway for many obstetric disasters, carrying a mortality of about 70 per cent. Indeed, much of the practice of modern obstetrics is directed towards the avoidance of ARDS. For example the trend towards epidural rather than general anaesthesia reduces the risk of inhalation of stomach contents, and therefore of ARDS. Epidural, rather than general anaesthesia, is specifically indicated in all patients with significant chest disease.

Adult respiratory distress syndrome

The management of this condition is described in Chapter 16.5.2. Specific obstetric causes are indicated in Table 1: of these, pre-eclampsia is probably now the most common, followed by shock with or without disseminated intravascular coagulation. Some of these obstetric causes of ARDS warrant further consideration.

Inhalation of stomach contents

This only occurs in the absence of an effective gag reflex, which in obstetric practice is almost invariably associated with general anaesthesia. Most obstetric units starve their patients once labour is established, and it is a common though declining practice to give regular antacid therapy, since it is believed that the low pH of gastric contents makes them particularly harmful to the lungs, although ARDS has developed in patients given aluminium hydroxide in labour after inhalation of stomach contents at pH 6.4. Avoidance of inhalation is the single most important preventive measure. Since the maternal mortality from inhalation has fallen from 6 per cent of all maternal deaths in England and Wales in 1976 to 1978 to only one death in the United Kingdom in 1994 to 1996, current measures are probably having some effect.

Table 1 Obstetric causes of adult respiratory distress syndrome (ARDS)

Shock:
Antepartum haemorrhage
Postpartum haemorrhage
Aspiration of stomach contents
Disseminated intravascular coagulopathy:
    Accidental haemorrhage
    Amniotic fluid embolus
    Severe pre-eclampsia/eclampsia
    Dead fetus syndrome
Infection:
    Gram-negative septicaemia
    Puerperal sepsis
    Acute pyelonephritis
Anaphylaxis
Hydatidiform mole

Amniotic fluid embolism

This catastrophe occurs because amniotic fluid and other material of fetal origin enters the maternal circulation. Usually, though not invariably, it occurs at the end of a vigorous labour with intact membranes, generally with some obstetric intervention. Important elements in the pathogenesis are widespread deposition of platelet and fibrin thrombi, and disseminated intravascular coagulation (DIC) caused by the very high thromboplastin activity of amniotic fluid. The initial presentation is with profound hypotension and cyanosis. If the patient survives this, she is at risk of dying from haemorrhage due to DIC, and if she survives the DIC she is at risk from ARDS. In the anaesthetized patient, differentiation from inhalation is important. Bronchospasm is common in inhalation, but very rare in amniotic fluid embolus. DIC is an early presenting feature in amniotic fluid embolus, but it occurs late after inhalation. The differential diagnosis of other causes of collapse in pregnancy is considered in Table 1 of Chapter 13.7.

The diagnosis of amniotic fluid embolus can only be confirmed by finding fetal material, that is squames or hairs, in the maternal blood (from central venous pressure lines), in the sputum, or in the lungs at autopsy. However, even the finding of fetal material in maternal blood is not specific, since this has been reported in some normal women having Swann Ganz catheterization in labour. There is no specific treatment.

Asthma

Bronchial asthma is the commonest chest disease in pregnancy, with prevalence of 3 to 5 per cent. In keeping with the lack of change in airways resistance in normal pregnancy, there is little evidence that pregnancy consistently affects the clinical course of asthma. Those studies that have been performed suggest that airways responsiveness to a metacholine challenge improves during pregnancy, but this beneficial effect is trivial by comparison with the inappropriate reluctance of patients and their carers to continue normal therapy for asthma in pregnancy (see below).

There has always been concern about a possible effect of asthma on the outcome of pregnancy. Large epidemiological studies do suggest increased risks of preterm delivery, low birthweight, and congenital malformations, with relative risks of 1.3 to 2.2 compared to healthy controls. These risks almost certainly relate to poor treatment, though the cause of the birth defects is not clear. Other studies have shown no excess fetal risks when asthma specialists manage asthma in pregnancy and achieve good control of symptoms.

It is unusual for patients to have acute attacks of asthma in labour. Perhaps the high circulating levels of endogenous catecholamines, corticosteroids, and prostaglandins are protective.

The treatment of patients with asthma does not require modification in pregnancy. Current management guidelines for asthma recommend a stepped care approach. Those with infrequent attacks should take inhaled betasympathomimetics as required to relieve symptoms, but if these are being used on a daily basis, additional regular inhaled glucocorticoids should be taken. The dose of inhaled glucocorticoid may be increased to for example beclomethasone 2000 µg per day. Alternatively a long acting β-agonist such as salmeterol or an anticholinergic drug (ipatropium) may be added. Oral prednisone should be used if these drugs do not achieve adequate control.

There is sufficient experience with all these classes of drug to recommend their use in pregnancy, but it seems sensible to use those with which there is most experience: namely oral salbutamol and inhaled beclomethasone, salmeterol, and ipatropium. Theophyllines can also be used in pregnancy, though their volume of distribution increases, making dosing difficult and emphasizing the need for monitoring of blood levels. Disodium cromogylcate has also been used extensively in pregnancy without problems, but little is used now because it is ineffective. There is insufficient experience to recommend the use of leukotriene antagonists in pregnancy.

The concern that oral steroids may be teratogenic and cause facial clefts is not supported by current studies. There is also no evidence of suppression of the fetal hypothalamo–pituitary–adrenal axis, at least with doses of up to 25 mg prednisone per day. Prednisone or hydrocortisone (by contrast with betamethasone or dexamethasone) are extensively metabolized by placental enzymes and little crosses the placenta. Women who have taken extended courses of oral steroids in the previous year should be given parenteral steroids to cover labour, as in any other situation where addisonian collapse is a possibility.

Of other drugs sometimes given to patients with asthma, aminoglycosides should only be given for more than 24 h in pregnancy if there is no alternative, and then with continuous monitoring of blood levels. This is because of the risk of damage to the fetal eighth nerve and kidney. Tetracycline should not be used because it causes permanent discoloration of the fetal teeth. Iodine-containing expectorants should not be used in pregnancy or in lactating women, since the iodine freely crosses the placenta, is excreted in breast milk, and may cause hypothyroidism in the infant.

It has been suggested that ergometrine can cause severe bronchospasm in patients with asthma. Syntocinon® should therefore be used for the management of the third stage of labour.

In summary, the management of patients with asthma requires little modification in pregnancy. In the unlikely event of an attack severe enough to require ventilation, maternal hypoxaemia should be avoided because of the associated severe fetal hypoxaemia; so also should hypocapnia ($P\text{co}_2$ <17 mmHg, 2.3 kPa) and alkalosis (pH > 7.6) since these have been associated with fetal hypoxaemia, probably due to impaired placental transport.

Chronic bronchitis, bronchiectasis, and emphysema

These conditions are now very uncommon in pregnancy. Since pulmonary hypertension is poorly tolerated in pregnancy, cor pulmonale is likely to be the factor limiting maternal safety. The presence of arterial hypoxaemia puts the fetus at risk from intrauterine growth restriction.

Cystic fibrosis

Better management in childhood means that more patients with cystic fibrosis are surviving and wanting to have children. Recent analysis of 20 series concerning 217 pregnancies in 162 women indicated that pregnancy did not affect mortality, when pregnant women with cystic fibrosis were compared to non-pregnant women with cystic fibrosis. However, 24 per cent of all deliveries were preterm. Poor outcomes were associated with a pregnancy weight gain of less than 4.5 kg and a prepregnancy forced vital capacity of less than 50 per cent of the predicted value. This group is likely to produce a preterm infant and to suffer increased loss of pulmonary function and increased maternal mortality. In one small study, four out of seven women with prepregnancy FEV_1 below 60 per cent predicted died within 3.2 years of delivery, whereas all 15 women with prepregnancy FEV_1 above 60 per cent predicted survived.

Apart from high quality and intensity of obstetric and medical care, no specific measures are necessary in pregnant patients with cystic fibrosis. Most of the drugs used have been considered above. Inhaled aminoglycosides are probably safe in pregnancy.

Patients may have malabsorption due to pancreatic involvement in cystic fibrosis, and an increase in pancreatic supplements may be necessary. Diabetes mellitus can also become manifest for the first time in pregnancy, and all with cystic fibrosis should be screened for diabetes early in pregnancy, and at about 28 weeks' gestation. There is also an increased risk of pneumothorax in labour (see below).

There has been concern that women with cystic fibrosis should not breast feed their infants because of the possibility of very high sodium content of their milk (up to 280 mmol/l). This risk has probably been exaggerated, since the samples of breast milk initially analysed were taken from women who were not lactating freely, a situation in which all breast milk has high sodium content. More recent studies have indicated that once lactation has been established, the breast milk has normal sodium content. Lactation should not threaten the mother's weight providing this was reasonably maintained before pregnancy.

For couples who have had one child affected by cystic fibrosis, first-trimester prenatal diagnosis is possible on genetic material prepared from chorionic villi using linked DNA probes in at least two-thirds of cases. The prevalence of the gene in the community is said to be 1 in 20, although the overall prevalence of the disease is 1 in 2500. Therefore, women with cystic fibrosis should be counselled that there is a 1 in 20 to 1 in 44 chance that their child will have the condition if the father's status is unknown. If the father is a heterozygote, the risk is 1 in 2. All the children of affected mothers will be carriers.

Kyphoscoliosis

Mild degrees of kyphoscoliosis have no effect on pregnancy, and successful pregnancy is possible in patients with severe disease and a vital capacity of as little as 1000 ml. As in the other chest diseases, hypoxaemia and pulmonary hypertension are the limiting factors, and some with severe kyphoscoliosis become exhausted and then hypoxaemic in the last trimester. Any suggestion of excessive fatigue should be an indication for hospital admission for rest and nasal intermittent positive pressure ventilation if this is not available at home. Progressive hypoxaemia, with or without evidence of fetal compromise, is an indication for delivery. Labour and/or caesarean section are best managed with the assistance of epidural anaesthesia, which reduces the risk of atelectasis. It can be given to most patients, even those with very severe spinal abnormalities.

Pneumothorax and pneumomediastinum

There are rare complications of pregnancy (incidence less than 1 in 10 000) but they probably occur more commonly in those who are pregnant than those who are not. This is particularly so in labour, when it is supposed that the raised intrathoracic pressure due to straining is a contributing factor. However, there is often some predisposing condition such as asthma, cystic fibrosis, emphysema, or lymphangioleiomyomatosis. Cocaine use has also been implicated. Both pneumothorax and pneumomediastinum present with chest pain, and if there is a substantial leak of air the patient may be hypotensive and cyanosed (tension pneumothorax, malignant pneumomediastinum). The differential diagnosis of these and other occult causes of collapse in pregnancy are considered in Chapter 13.7. The physical signs and management of the pneumothorax are no different in pregnancy from those in the non-pregnant state, and are described in Chapter 17.12. If a patient has a past history of pneumothorax or pneumomediastinum, she should have an elective forceps delivery to prevent recurrence during straining in labour.

Tuberculosis

Before the advent of antituberculous therapy, tuberculosis was the cause of many maternal deaths, particularly in the puerperium. This is no longer so, and there should be no excess mortality from tuberculosis in pregnancy. However, a high index of suspicion is necessary to make the diagnosis in pregnancy: most centres in the United Kingdom have not screened for tuberculosis in pregnancy by routine Mantoux testing and/or chest radio-graphs for many years. In the future, and in areas with high prevalence of tuberculosis in pregnancy, this policy may have to be changed.

The placenta is a very efficient filter, and intrauterine infection of the fetus almost never occurs, though neonatal infection from the mother can certainly be a problem.

None of the front line antituberculous drugs, rifampicin, pyrazinamide, isoniazid, or ethambutal, has been shown to be teratogenic despite extensive experience. However, isoniazid (and rifampicin) can cause serious hepatitis, which in the case of isoniazid seems to be a particular risk for pregnant women. Pregnant patients should therefore have regular liver function tests and receive supplementary pyridoxine when taking isonazid. A dose of 50 mg/day has been shown to give adequate blood levels in pregnancy, but the conventional dose of 10 mg/day may also be effective. Streptomycin (an aminoglycoside) should be avoided for the reasons given above. Ethionamide should not be used because of reports of multiple congenital abnormalities. Within these limitations, the pregnant patient with tuberculosis should be treated in the same manner as she would be in the non-pregnant state. In particular, patients with HIV disease or those with drug-resistant tuberculosis should be treated without regard to the pregnancy: the risk of inadequate maternal therapy is far greater than any potential risk of antituberculous treatment for the fetus.

Patients who have been adequately treated in the past for tuberculosis do not require prophylactic therapy in pregnancy. After birth, babies should only be isolated from their mothers if the mothers are still smear positive. Since modern antituberculosis regimes render the sputum sterile within 2 weeks and markedly reduce the number of organisms within 24 h, this should not occur frequently. The neonate should be treated with prophylactic isoniazid for 3 months. After this period BCG vaccination is given in the United Kingdom but not in the Unites States. It is not clear whether neonatal BCG vaccination adds any further protection to isoniazid prophylaxis. It is not without risks: skin ulceration and osteitis may occur, and occasionally disseminated disease, particularly if the mother has an immunodeficiency state. As isoniazid therapy does not affect the immunogenicity of BCG vaccine, there is no longer any rationale for the use of isoniazid-resistant BCG neonatal vaccination.

Sarcoid

This condition is rarely a problem in pregnancy. Patients who have had sarcoid in the past have no extra risk of relapse in pregnancy. Those who have active sarcoid during pregnancy tend to improve, possibly because of the increase in free as well as protein-bound cortisol levels. There is a tendency to deteriorate in the puerperium, but this should not be overemphasized. Since patients take many vitamins in pregnancy, those with sarcoid should be warned not to take vitamin D to which they may be very sensitive.

Pneumonia

Pneumonia is an uncommon complication of pregnancy, and unless the diagnosis is clear-cut, other conditions that produce chest symptoms and signs, such as pulmonary embolus, should always be considered. Bacterial pneumonia should be treated with antibiotics. For community-acquired pneumonia the antibiotics of choice in the United Kingdom are likely to be a penicillin or a macrolide such as erythromycin, both of which are suitable for use in pregnancy. Aggressive antipyretic therapy with tepid sponging, fans, and regular paracetamol should be used, because of the association between pyrexia and premature labour. During epidemics, such as the influenza epidemic in 1930, viral pneumonia has caused a high mortality in pregnancy, and clinicians should be aware that this condition should not be dismissed lightly.

Ten per cent of maternal varicella infections may be complicated by pneumonia, which has an appreciable mortality, particularly in pregnancy. All pregnant women who have close exposure to varicella-zoster virus and who have no demonstrable antibody should therefore receive zoster immune globulin. Those who develop varicella should receive acyclovir 10 to 30 mg/kg daily in three divided doses for 5 days.

Further reading

Brost BC, Newman RB (1997). The maternal and fetal effects of tuberculosis therapy. *Obstetrics and Gynecology Clinics of North America* **24,** 659–73.

Demissie K, Breckenridge MB, Rhoads GG (1998). Infant and maternal outcomes in the pregnancies of asthmatic women. *American Journal of Respiratory and Critical Care Medicine* **158,** 1091–5.

Department of Health (1998). *Why mother die, report on confidential enquiries into maternal deaths in the United Kingdom 1994–96.* HMSO, London.

de Swiet M (1995). Diseases of the respiratory system. In: de Swiet M, ed. *Medical disorders of obstetric practice*, 3rd edn, pp. 1–32. Blackwell Scientific Publications, Oxford.

de Swiet M (1998). The respiratory system. In: Chamberlain GVP, Broughton Pipkin F, eds. *Clinical physiology in obstetrics*, 3rd edn, pp. 111–28. Blackwell Science, Oxford.

Edenborough FP, Stableforth DE, Webb AK, Mackenzie WE, Smith DL (1995). Outcome of pregnancy in women with cystic fibrosis. *Thorax* **50,** 170–4.

Margono F, Mroueh J, Garely A, White D, Duerr A, Minkoff HL (1994). Resurgence of active tuberculosis among pregnant women. *Obstetrics and Gynecology* **83,** 911–14.

Milne JA, Howie AD, Pack AI (1978). Dyspnoea during normal pregnancy. *British Journal of Obstetrics and Gynaecology* **85,** 260–3.

Morgan M (1979). Amniotic fluid embolism. *Anaesthesia* **34,** 20–32.

White RJ, Coutts II, Gibbs CJ, MacIntyre C (1989). A prospective study of asthma during pregnancy and the puerperium. *Respiratory Medicine* **83,** 103–6.

13.9 Liver and gastrointestinal diseases during pregnancy

A. E. S. Gimson

Introduction

Gastrointestinal and liver disease in pregnancy includes those diseases specific to that condition, those occurring with increased frequency during pregnancy, and those already present at conception or arising coincidentally during the course of pregnancy (Table 1). Liver or gastrointestinal dysfunction is present in fewer than 5 per cent of pregnancies in Europe and the United States, but their recognition and management is important as increased maternal and fetal morbidity and mortality may result without prompt intervention.

Table 1 Liver diseases during pregnancy

Diseases specific to pregnancy	Hyperemesis gravidarum Intrahepatic cholestasis of pregnancy Acute fatty liver of pregnancy Hypertension-associated liver diseases of pregnancy
Diseases where pregnancy increases frequency or severity of presentation	Budd–Chiari syndrome—increased frequency; low antithrombin III levels Acute cholecystitis—increased risk of gallstones/complications Acute viral hepatitis E—increased frequency of acute liver failure in the third trimester Hepatic tumours—vascular hepatic tumours may enlarge and rupture Variceal haemorrhage—more common in non-cirrhotic portal hypertension
Liver diseases manifesting during but unrelated to pregnancy	Acute viral hepatitis A, B, cytomegalovirus, Epstein–Barr virus Chronic liver diseases Drug hepatotoxicity

There are significant physiological changes in hepatic function during pregnancy. Increased circulating blood volume and cardiac output are not associated with any changes in hepatic blood flow, but there is increased azygous flow, which results rarely in the formation of small oesophageal varices. Gallbladder motility is reduced and bile lithogenicity increased due to increased hepatic cholesterol synthesis and excretion into bile. Minor but important changes in laboratory blood tests occur due to haemodilution or alteration in hepatic synthesis (Table 2).

Increased gastric myoelectric activity may be manifest as nausea and vomiting, but there are few other significant changes in gastrointestinal function during normal pregnancy.

Liver disease specific to pregnancy

Hyperemesis gravidarum

Although nausea and vomiting may occur in up to 75 per cent of pregnancies, severe vomiting leading to dehydration, ketonuria, electrolyte disturbances, and nutritional deficiency is rare, developing in 2 to 16 of every 1000 pregnancies. Nutritional deficiency has been so severe as to progress to Wernicke's encephalopathy and changes in serum sodium may precipitate osmotic demyelination (central pontine myelinolysis). More common in younger women and in obesity, recent surveys do not suggest any relationship with parity or gravidity. Elevated transaminases, by two- to threefold, occur in 50 per cent of cases, with a minor rise in alkaline phosphatase and bilirubin in 10 per cent. Liver histology shows few abnormalities or hepatic steatosis only. The aetiology is unclear and may be multifactorial: positive *Helicobacter* serology has been reported in up to 90 per cent of cases, and changes in thyroid function are present in 50 per cent. An elevated free T_4 with suppressed thyroid-stimulating hormone correlates with elevated human chorionic gonadotrophin levels in these patients, raising the possibility that gestational thyrotoxicosis may also have role in pathogenesis. In some cases psychological factors are also important.

Table 2 Effects of pregnancy on laboratory blood tests

Parameter	Effect	Trimester with maximum change	Mechanism
Bilirubin	Nil	–	–
AST/ALT	Nil	–	–
Bile salts	Nil	–	–
5-Nucleotidase	Nil	–	–
γ-glutamyl transpeptidase	Nil	–	–
Alkaline phosphatase	+ 1–300%	Third	Increased bone/placental isoenzyme
Albumin	– 10–60%	Second	Dilution, reduced synthesis
Gammaglobulin	– 10%	Second	Dilution
Fibrinogen	+ 50%	Second	Increased hepatic synthesis
Cholesterol	+ 100%	Third	Increased hepatic synthesis

Management, which may include hospitalization, is symptomatic and includes rehydration and correction of nutritional deficiencies. Psychological support is crucial. Treatment of symptomatic gastro-oesophageal reflux is important and antiemetics are required, with metoclopramide and promethazine as effective as newer 5-HT₃ antagonists. There are uncontrolled reports of benefit with corticosteroids. In rare cases there may be recurrence in subsequent pregnancies.

Intrahepatic cholestasis of pregnancy

A cholestatic disorder of the second and third trimesters, this is the most common cause of jaundice during pregnancy, after acute viral hepatitis. Initially starting with pruritus, jaundice follows after 1 to 4 weeks in 20 to 60 per cent of cases, associated with pale stools and dark urine. Diagnosis is by history and the classic biochemical features of an elevated bilirubin (less than $100 \mu mol/litre$) and increased aminotransferases (rarely more than 250 iu/litre), with no significant rise in alkaline phosphatase or γ-glutamyl transpeptidase. Serum bile acids increase three- to 100-fold: those factors with the highest predictive diagnostic value being total bile acid concentration of more than $11.0 \mu mol/litre$ and a cholic/chenodeoxycholic acid ratio of more than 1.5 with a cholic acid percentage over 42. An ultrasound scan is necessary to exclude choledocholithiasis, and further imaging of the bile duct with magnetic resonance cholangiopancreatography will occasionally be needed. A liver biopsy is not required for diagnosis, but shows a canalicular cholestasis with no hepatocellular necrosis.

The epidemiology of intrahepatic cholestasis of pregnancy is interesting, with marked geographical variation. The highest incidence, over 10 per cent, has been recorded in Araunucanian Indians in Chile, with 2 to 3 per cent in Sweden and 0.1 per cent in Canada. It is reported to be rare in Afro-Caribbeans. Family studies have suggested a dominant mode of transmission in a few kindreds, and a non-sense mutation has been reported in the *MDR3* gene that encodes an ATP-dependent transporter of phosphatidylcholine across the canalicular membrane in one family. An association with *HLA-B8*, *HLA-B12*, and *DPB1* alleles is unconfirmed. It is more common in women with a history of contraceptive pill induced jaundice (50 per cent), those with benign recurrent intrahepatic cholestasis, where there are multiple gestations, and it may be more common in women who are positive for hepatitis C virus antibodies. In France it has been associated with use of progesterone in early pregnancy.

The aetiology is unknown, but one hypothesis suggests enhanced sensitivity of components of the bile salt excretion apparatus to oestrogen: pregnancy impairs sulphation of both monohydroxy bile salts and oestrogen, which may enhance the cholestatic potential of both compounds.

Intrahepatic cholestasis of pregnancy is associated with an increased incidence of fetal prematurity (fivefold increase), fetal distress, stillbirths, and meconium staining of amniotic fluid (1.5-fold increase), but perinatal mortality is normal with modern management. Reports of maternal morbidity from postpartum haemorrhage relate to vitamin K deficiency and are not a feature of recent series.

Treatment is symptomatic, with the bile salt ursodeoxycholic acid (10–15 mg/kg/day) the treatment of choice and better than *S*-adenosyl-methionine. Ursodeoxycholic acid relieves pruritus, reduces bile salt levels in maternal serum, and may reduce the frequency of fetal complications. Both bile salt sequestration with cholestyramine and dexamethasone have given variable results. Vitamin K should be given before delivery.

Most authors recommend early elective delivery at 38 weeks to prevent late fetal complications, and this policy has been shown to improve fetal outcome. More recently there have been suggestions that a policy of careful observation and induction of labour only for fetal distress may be used, but there is anxiety that classical markers of fetal distress may not be adequate in this setting.

Intrahepatic cholestasis of pregnancy recurs in up to 60 to 80 per cent of subsequent pregnancies and is associated with a late increased incidence of gallstones. Oral contraceptives should be used with caution, although early reports of liver abnormalities were predominantly with high-dose pills and combined low-dose preparations may cause fewer problems.

Acute fatty liver of pregnancy

Acute fatty liver of pregnancy, a microvesicular steatosis during the last trimester of pregnancy, was first adequately described by Sheehan in 1940. Occurring in 1 in 14 000 pregnancies between the 34th and 36th weeks, it is more common in primigravidae, with male fetuses, and with twin pregnancies. Up to 40 per cent may have associated features of pre-eclampsia, with peripheral oedema, hypertension, and proteinuria, and occasionally the **HELLP** (Haemolysis, Elevated Liver enzymes and Low Platelet count) syndrome (see below). Acute fatty liver of pregnancy occurs only rarely before the third trimester, but postpartum presentations are well recorded. Initial symptoms are of headache, fatigue, nausea, and vomiting with abdominal discomfort. In severe cases jaundice develops within 14 days. This may progress to manifest all the features of acute liver failure, including coma, renal failure, and death. However, less severe cases are now described more commonly, with recent series reporting a 10 to 20 per cent fetal and maternal mortality.

The cause of many cases of acute fatty liver of pregnancy may be a fetal–maternal interaction resulting from abnormalities of mitochondrial fatty acid oxidation. Schoeman first reported a case of acute fatty liver of pregnancy associated with a defect of fatty acid oxidation in the fetus. More recently a mutation has been identified involving substitution of glutamine for glutamic acid at amino acid residue 474 of the alpha subunit of long-chain 3-hydroxyacyl-CoA dehydrogenase, an enzyme that forms one component of a trifunctional protein catalysing the last three steps in the β-oxidation of fatty acids within mitochondria. Heterozygote mothers carrying fetuses with long-chain 3-hydroxyacyl-CoA dehydrogenase deficiency may develop either acute fatty liver of pregnancy or HELLP syndrome in up to 80 per cent of cases. Mitochondrial oxidation of fatty acids is already impaired during pregnancy, mediated by oestrogen and progesterone, and long chain 3-hydroxyacyl metabolites produced by the fetus can accumulate and be toxic to the liver. Because presentation of children with long-chain 3-hydroxyacyl-CoA dehydrogenase deficiency may occur late after birth, with non-ketotic hypoglycaemia and sudden infant death, the early identification and treatment of such cases is important. For this reason diagnostic molecular testing is recommended on all mothers and offspring of acute fatty liver of pregnancy and HELLP pregnancies.

The important differential diagnosis is between acute viral hepatitis with liver failure, acute fatty liver of pregnancy, and hypertension-associated liver dysfunction of pregnancy. The presence of features of pre-eclampsia in up to 40 per cent may make this distinction difficult. In acute fatty liver of pregnancy transaminases are elevated to less than 500 iu/litre, in contrast to viral hepatitis where values are usually higher. Hypoglycaemia is more common in acute fatty liver of pregnancy than in pre-eclampsia, and a blood film commonly showing neutrophilia, normoblasts, thrombocytopenia, target cells, and giant platelets may also help to make the diagnosis of acute fatty liver of pregnancy. Prothrombin and partial thromboplastin times are prolonged with low antithrombin III levels. Although hepatic steatosis in acute fatty liver of pregnancy may be detected by ultrasonography, CT scanning is more sensitive with attenuation values less than half normal and less than spleen, the reverse of normal. Hyperuricaemia is present in 80 per cent, but is not pathognomonic as this may also be found in pre-eclampsia.

Despite all these biochemical and radiological tests, and because differentiation of acute fatty liver of pregnancy from acute viral hepatitis and hypertension-associated liver diseases is important in assessing the prognosis for future pregnancies, a liver biopsy may be necessary to distinguish between these three diagnoses. Histology demonstrates a microvesicular fat deposition with rare hepatocyte necrosis and minimal inflammation, a pattern similar to that seen in Reye's syndrome, tetracycline and sodium valproate hepatotoxicity, Jamaican vomiting sickness due to a toxin in unripe ackee fruit, some urea cycle enzyme deficiencies, and defects in mitochondrial fatty acid oxidation.

Other obstetric causes of renal failure that are associated with minor changes in liver blood tests rarely need to be considered. These include thrombotic thrombocytopenic purpura and haemolytic uraemic syndrome. The former is particularly associated with neurological signs, including epileptic fits, without evidence of disseminated intravascular coagulation, whereas haemolytic uraemic syndrome may occur postpartum and with microangiopathic anaemia.

After the diagnosis of acute fatty liver of pregnancy has been established, the most important component of management is early delivery of the fetus. A policy of careful monitoring has been proposed for the mildest cases, but extreme caution is required as deterioration can be sudden and unpredictable. Vaginal delivery can be tried first, but caesarean section will usually require general anaesthesia as a spinal anaesthetic in the presence of coagulation deficits may be dangerous. Hypoglycaemia is prevented by intravenous dextrose infusion; aggressive correction of coagulation abnormalities with fresh frozen plasma, cryoprecipitate, and antithrombin III has also been recommended. Liver transplantation has been used (very rarely) for cases failing to respond to early delivery and intensive care.

The risk of recurrence of acute fatty liver of pregnancy is very low, the few recorded cases most probably being due to associated recurrent metabolic defects in the fetus.

Hypertension-associated liver diseases of pregnancy

Hypertension occurs in up to 8 per cent of pregnancies and is the most common cause of maternal mortality in developed countries. Abnormalities of liver blood tests have been described in three clinical syndromes associated with hypertension in pregnancy: pre-eclampsia/eclampsia, spontaneous hepatic rupture, and the HELLP syndrome.

Pre-eclampsia/eclampsia

The development of peripheral oedema, proteinuria, and hypertension (blood pressure above 140/90 mmHg or an increase of 30 mmHg systolic and 15 mmHg diastolic pressure above pre-existing levels) occurs in up to 5 per cent of all deliveries, more commonly with primigravidae, extremes of age, multiple gestations, and family history. Pre-eclampsia is discussed in detail in section 13.04, but there are abnormalities of liver biochemistry in up to 25 per cent of mild cases and up to 80 per cent of those with severe disease, i.e. those with renal impairment, visual disturbance, headache, fits, and the onset of eclampsia. The usual abnormality is a rise in transaminases, with jaundice occurring only in the most severe cases. The alanine aminotransferase levels are usually less than 150 iu/litre, lower than in acute fatty liver of pregnancy, and bilirubin is less than 100 μmol/litre. Changes in coagulation parameters, with elevated D-dimers, reflect the intravascular activation and consumption of clotting factors. Antithrombin III levels are low. Liver histology in the early stages shows few changes except for deposition of fibrinogen within sinusoids and the space of Disse. Blockage of sinusoids by fibrin may progress to frank infarction of hepatic parenchyma, when the low levels of coagulation factors may then predispose to haemorrhage into these infarcted areas. This combination of infarcts and associated haemorrhage, often covert and without apparent clinical consequence, may be demonstrated on ultrasound or CT scan of the liver.

The management of liver dysfunction in this context is that for pre-eclampsia, with correction of hypertension and coagulation defects, early delivery being the most important aspect. Anticonvulsant prophylaxis must be considered. Very close fetal monitoring is important. Liver biochemistry improves after delivery, but a late cholestatic phase with rise in alkaline phosphatase and γ-glutamyl transpeptidase is common.

Spontaneous hepatic rupture

Spontaneous rupture of the liver is fortunately rare, occurring in 1 in 100 000 deliveries. In 80 per cent of cases liver haematomas, segmental or larger infarcts, and rupture occur in patients with severe pre-eclampsia and eclampsia: the remainder occur in association with acute fatty liver of pregnancy, or underlying hepatic adenomata, hepatocellular carcinoma, haemangioma, choriocarcinoma, or liver abscess.

The classical presentation is with right upper quadrant pain, nausea, vomiting, and hypotension in an older woman with severe pre-eclampsia during the third trimester. Right upper quadrant tenderness may be associated with frank peritonism where rupture into the peritoneum has occurred. The diagnosis can be confirmed by ultrasonography or CT scanning. Current treatment is conservative if possible, starting with angiography and hepatic artery embolization, proceeding to laparotomy, use of collagen meshes, and hepatic artery ligation if necessary. Successful orthotopic liver transplantation has also been recorded, but associated coagulation abnormalities are difficult to manage. The baby should be delivered by caesarean section. Successful subsequent pregnancies are recorded, as is recurrent haemorrhage, hence careful monitoring of any future pregnancy is necessary.

Haemolysis, elevated liver enzymes, and low platelet count (HELLP syndrome)

Weinstein first described a syndrome of haemolysis, elevated liver enzymes, and a low platelet count in patients with severe pre-eclampsia or eclampsia. HELLP syndrome occurs in 10 per cent of pregnancies with severe pre-eclampsia. Strict criteria should be used for the diagnosis: haemolysis with a characteristic peripheral blood smear, serum lactate dehydrogenase greater than or equal to 600 U/litre, serum aspartate aminotransferase greater than or equal to 70 U/litre and platelet count less than 100×10^9/litre. An abnormal peripheral blood smear with fractured red blood cells (schistocytes, echinocytes, spherostomatocytes) is sensitive but not specific for HELLP, and the elevated serum lactate dehydrogenase is another indicator of haemolysis. Some cases display only one or two of the above criteria and have been labelled as having partial HELLP: these have been shown to follow a less severe clinical course. HELLP syndrome has also been classified (by Martin and colleagues) according to platelet count: class 1 platelet counts less than or equal to $50\,000 \times 10^9$/litre, class 2 more than 50 000 to less than or equal to $100\,000 \times 10^9$/litre, and class 3 more than $100\,000 \times 10^9$/litre, which is equivalent to partial HELLP.

The reason why some cases with severe pre-eclampsia progress to HELLP syndrome is not clear. Whilst the haemolysis is clearly related to intravascular deposition of thrombin and mechanical fracture of red cells, and there is fibrin deposition obstructing hepatic sinusoids, the factors causing particular damage to the hepatic microcirculation are unknown. Overt disseminated intravascular coagulation is not usually a major component; when defined as hypofibrinogenaemia (< 300 mg/dl) and elevated D-dimers (> 40 μg/ml) it occurred in 21 per cent of a series of 442 cases. Compared with other cases with severe pre-eclampsia, those with HELLP syndrome tend to be older, Caucasian, and multiparous.

Symptoms usually start in the second or third trimester, with 15 per cent starting prior to 26 weeks and 30 per cent only developing symptoms after delivery. HELLP syndrome has protean manifestations but universal early symptoms include malaise and fatigue, followed by nausea, vomiting, and headache shortly thereafter (Table 3). Epigastric and right upper quadrant pain are ominous signs, particularly when accompanied by right shoulder tip pain. Weight gain and peripheral oedema are found in 50 per cent, with diastolic blood pressure greater than or equal to 90 mmHg in all but a small minority.

The fall in platelet count and rise in transaminases usually reach their nadir in the first 2 days postpartum. Aspartate aminotransferase and lactate dehydrogenase are elevated in unison, along with other markers of hepatocellular or sinusoidal cell dysfunction, glutathione-S-transferase and hyaluronic acid.

Maternal complications associated with HELLP syndrome occur in up to 50 per cent of cases. Blood transfusion to correct hypovolaemia, anaemia, or coagulopathy is required in 50 per cent, with features of disseminated

Table 3 Clinical features and complications of hypertension-associated liver diseases

	HELLP syndrome		Pre-eclampsia	
	Martin et al. (1999)	Sibai et al. (1993)	Audibert et al. (1996)	Martin et al. (1999)
Symptoms (%)				
Nausea/vomiting	35	36	5	15
Headache	61	31	40	68
Epigastric/ abdominal pain	50	65	5	13
Maternal complications (%)				
None	51		91	89
Haematological/ DIC	32	21	0	1
Cardiopulmonary	22	6	1	10
Renal	3	8	0	0
Neurological/ ophthalmic	4.5	2	0	1
Hepatic	1.5	1	0	0
Obstetric complications (%)				
Eclampsia	13	8	9	5
Abruptio placentae	3	16	5	1
Perinatal mortality /1000 births	119	–	–	57

DIC, disseminated intravascular coagulation.

intravascular coagulation in 25 per cent, and pleural effusions or pulmonary oedema in 15 to 20 per cent. Renal failure due to acute tubular necrosis may occur in 3 to 8 per cent. Obstetric complications are also associated with the degree of fall in platelet counts, with placental abruption (16 per cent) and wound haematomas after caesarean section the most prevalent. Eclampsia is approximately two to three times more common in patients with class 1 HELLP than in those with milder varieties, and consistent with this the maternal mortality was 1.5 per cent in a large series, with a perinatal mortality in Martin *et al.*'s tertiary referral practice of 119/1000 infants. Overall perinatal mortality is strongly related to time of delivery, with rates as high as 30 per cent in some series, although this may be due to case selection. Mortality was 9.5 per cent in a large series assessing class 1, 2, and 3 cases. Preterm infants born before 32 weeks from mothers with HELLP syndrome had a higher frequency of severe intraventricular haemorrhage than other preterm infants. Birth weights tend to be lower in severe HELLP than in pre-eclampsia alone.

Preterm patients with HELLP syndrome should be treated at a referral centre with appropriate obstetric, anaesthetic, and haematological support. Management of the coexisting pre-eclampsia is crucial, with seizure prophylaxis using magnesium sulphate and blood pressure control with labetolol, ketanserin, or hydrallazine if blodd pressure is over 160/105 mmHg. Antenatal corticosteroids enhance fetal lung maturity if the pregnancy is of less than 32 weeks gestation. Careful fluid resuscitation is required to prevent volume overload, particularly in the presence of renal impairment, as is very close fetal monitoring.

Aside from signs of significant fetal distress, indications for urgent delivery include persistent severe right upper quadrant or shoulder tip pain, often associated with hypotension and thrombocytopenia, which indicate possible liver haematoma or impending rupture. Early delivery, at the safest time for mother and fetus, is strongly recommended in the absence of treatment that unequivocally improves the haematological abnormalities and both maternal and fetal outcome. Although arguments have been put forward for a more conservative approach in patients with mild disease—with careful monitoring of coagulation profiles, fetal growth and well being, and with the timing of delivery depending on clinical judgement—this management strategy is not without risk and has not been examined in a randomized controlled trial.

Attempts have been made to improve the outcome of HELLP with medical management alone in an effort to buy time to enhance fetal maturity and to improve the mother's clinical condition prior to delivery. Although plasma volume expansion, antithrombotic agents, plasma exchange, and corticosteroids have all been advocated, no therapies have been shown to allow safe deferral of delivery and improve outcome. In one study dexamethasone given predelivery resulted in a modest prolongation of pregnancy, whereas two other trials have shown significant improvements in haematological and biochemical parameters when given postpartum. In a trial of invasive haemodynamic monitoring, plasma volume expansion and afterload reduction, laboratory parameters improved with prolongation of gestation by 21 days, but no significant change in perinatal mortality.

Recurrence of HELLP syndrome in subsequent pregnancies is uncommon: it recurred in only 5 per cent of a series of 139 normotensive women after an index pregnancy with HELLP syndrome, despite 25 per cent developing pre-eclampsia. In hypertensive cases a further pregnancy was associated with pre-eclampsia in 70 per cent and HELLP syndrome in 8 per cent.

Differential dagnosis of jaundice during pregnancy

Many patients with acute fatty liver of pregnancy have signs of pre-eclampsia and such cases may be part of a clinical syndrome that includes hypertension-associated liver diseases. Evidence for this possibility includes the finding of microvesicular hepatic steatosis in cases with pre-eclampsia; indeed one study found fat deposition by special staining in all 41 cases studied. Histological evidence of both pre-eclampsia and acute fatty liver of pregnancy has also been demonstrated in some cases, and pregnancies associated with pre-eclampsia have been followed in the next by HELLP syndrome. Despite this there are usually features in the clinical history or laboratory findings (Table 4) that allow discrimination between these diagnoses. The size of the liver, degree of hyperbilirubinaemia, abnormalities on peripheral blood film, presence of hypoglycaemia, and disseminated intravascular coagulation are the most discriminatory tests. The differential diagnosis of jaundice and abnormal liver blood tests differs in the three trimesters of pregnancy (Table 5).

Liver diseases not specific to pregnancy

Budd–Chiari syndrome

Thrombosis in one or more hepatic veins has an increased prevalence during pregnancy and in those on the oral contraceptive pill. This relates to low antithrombin III levels and may be more common in those with an underlying procoagulant state or presence of antiphospholipid antibodies. Right upper quadrant pain, hepatomegaly, and maternal ascites should suggest the diagnosis, with confirmation by ultrasonography or hepatic venous angiography. Although hepatic venous balloon dilatation or insertion of a transjugular intrahepatic stent shunt has been recommended for Budd–Chiari syndrome, there are few data on their use during pregnancy. Maternal mortality remains very high.

Cholelithiasis

Gallbladder sludge and gallstones develop in 31 per cent and 9 per cent of pregnancies respectively, although most resolve thereafter. Prior use of oral contraceptives, increased cholesterol synthesis, reduced cholesterol carriage in bile, and impaired gallbladder motility all accounted for the increased lithogenicity of bile. Symptomatic gallstone disease should be managed in the usual way. Magnetic resonance cholangiopancreatography can accurately detect common bile duct stones without exposing the fetus to radiation, with endoscopic sphincterotomy and/or stent placement reserved for those in whom they are detected. In most cases surgery can be deferred until after delivery.

Table 4 Clinical features and laboratory variables in acute fatty liver of pregnancy, HELLP syndrome, and pre-eclampsia

	Acute fatty liver of pregnancy	HELLP	Severe pre-eclampsia
Frequency	1 in 13 000	4 in 1000	7 in 100
Clinical features	Nausea/vomiting (70%)	Malaise/lethargy (90%)	Oedema (80%)
Examination	RUQ pain (65%)	Nausea/vomiting (35%)	Weight gain (75%)
	Small liver	Oedema/weight gain (60%)	RUQ tenderness
	Jaundice	RUQ tenderness (80%)	Mental status changes
	Encephalopathy later	Hypertension (80%)	
	Hypertension 40%	Liver normal size	
Investigations	Leucocytosis	Bilirubin < 100 μmol/l	Bilirubin variable
	Bilirubin >100 μmol/l	ALT 150 iu/l	ALT 150–200 iu/l (unless infarction)
	ALT 300 iu/l	Hypoglycaemia rare	DIC 7%
	Hypoglycaemia	DIC 25%	
	DIC 75%		
Maternal mortality	< 20%	1.5%	<1%
Fetal mortality	15%	35%	–
Recurrence	Very rare	4–8%	25%

Abbreviations: RUQ, right upper quadrant: ALT, serum alanine aminotransferase; DIC, disseminated intravascular coagulation.

Viral hepatitis

Acute viral hepatitis is the most common cause of jaundice during pregnancy (Table 5), with no specific change to presentation, clinical course, or outcome for acute hepatitis A, B, cytomegalovirus, or Epstein–Barr virus infection.

Transmission of virus from a mother with acute hepatitis B to her offspring occurs in 50 per cent of cases, rising to 70 per cent when hepatitis starts in the third trimester. Transmission of virus from mothers with chronic hepatitis B carriage is less common, but depends on the level of viral replication. The rate is at least 90 per cent in those who are hepatitis B virus DNA positive, and who are usually hepatitis B e antigen positive, as is most common in Orientals. Following vertical transmission up to 80 per cent of offspring become chronic HBsAg carriers. Transmission of hepatitis B can be effectively interrupted by use of hepatitis B immunoglobulin at birth, with hepatitis B virus vaccination within 7 days and at 1, 2, and 12 months.

Transmission of hepatitis C from chronic carriers occurs in up to 8 per cent of cases, being higher in those with high maternal viral load. Anti-hepatitis C virus seroconversion of infants following transmission may take 6 to 12 months to appear, but detection of hepatitis C virus RNA by polymerase chaine reaction allows detection of transmission sooner.

Acute hepatitis E is due to an RNA virus and occurs, often in waterborne epidemics, predominantly in the Middle and Far East. In pregnancy it is associated with a mortality of up to 20 per cent due to development of acute liver failure during the third trimester, but transmission to offspring has not been recorded.

Variceal haemorrhage

Changes in splanchnic haemodynamics, increased cardiac output and azygous blood flow, and an increase in circulating blood volume have all been suggested as risk factors for variceal bleeding during pregnancy. Evidence for this remains controversial, although recent large series with non-cirrhotic portal hypertension report a haemorrhage rate of 13 per cent. Treatment of variceal bleeding during pregnancy should be with conventional endoscopic techniques, with use of transjugular intrahepatic stent shunts or surgical shunts reserved for rescue therapy.

Liver tumour during pregnancy

The first presentations of focal nodular hyperplasia, hepatic adenoma, hepatocellular carcinoma, and cholangiocarcinoma have all been reported during pregnancy. Adenomas, in some cases related to prior oral contraceptive use, may undergo vascular engorgement during pregnancy and rupture has been reported. Secondary tumours, including hepatic choriocarcinoma and ovarian teratomas, may also rupture.

Pregnancy following orthotopic liver transplantation

Fertility returns quickly following liver transplantation. Pregnancy does not alter the risks of cellular rejection, but immunosuppressive drug toxicity needs to be carefully monitored. Azathioprine may cause neonatal pancytopenia, and cyclosporin A is associated with a 40 per cent incidence of hypertension, which may be lower with Tacrolimus.

Pregnancy during chronic liver disease

Most patients with established cirrhosis are infertile, but a few remain fertile, although with a high rate of prematurity, low-birthweight babies, and stillbirths. There is little evidence that pregnancy results in deterioration in liver dysfunction in patients with cirrhosis, and improvement of inflammatory activity occurs in some cases of autoimmune chronic active liver disease. There is no increased rate of relapse after delivery. Patients with treated Wilson's disease are able to conceive and successful pregnancies whilst taking D-penicillamine or trientine have been reported.

Pregnancy during gastrointestinal disease

Only a few gastrointestinal diseases occur with altered frequency during pregnancy.

Gastro-oesophageal reflux

Symptomatic gastro-oesophageal reflux is present at some stage in up to 80 per cent of pregnancies. It is mainly due to a reduced lower oesophageal sphincter pressure rather than elevated intra-abdominal pressure from a gravid uterus. Treatment with antacid is recommended, with avoidance of H_2 antagonists or proton pump inhibitors unless symptoms and complications of gastro-oesophageal reflux outweigh potential drug toxicity. Acid-pepsin reflux combined with vomiting in early pregnancy may precipitate haematemesis, occasionally with a Mallory–Weiss tear, for which management should be as in the non-pregnant state. Upper gastrointestinal endoscopy is a safe procedure during pregnancy.

Inflammatory bowel disease

Stable inactive ulcerative colitis and Crohn's disease do not affect fertility, are not associated with increased fetal risk, and disease control is not impeded by pregnancy. There are few data on the effect of drug therapy on fertility, although sperm counts may be reduced in men on salazopyrine. The risk of relapse of inflammatory bowel disease during pregnancy has been assessed at between 30 and 50 per cent, but this is no higher than

Table 5 Differential diagnosis of abnormal liver blood tests during pregnancy

Diagnosis	Frequency	Clinical features, diagnostic criteria, and investigations
First trimester		
Acute viral hepatitis	As general population	IgM anti-HAV, IgM anti-HBc, IgM anti-HEV, IgM anti-CMV/CMV PCR, EBV serology, IgM anti-Herpes simplex
Cholelithiasis	Unknown	RUQ pain, fever, gallstones/dilated common bile duct on USS/MRCP for choledocholithiasis
Drug-induced hepatotoxicity	Unknown	Drug history
Hyperemesis gravidarum	0.3–1%	Young, overweight, multiple births. ALT < 200 iu/l. Low TSH in 50%
Intrahepatic cholestasis of pregnancy	0.1%	Pruritus. ALT < 300 iu/l, bilirubin < 100 µmol/l, bile acids × 30–100
Second trimester		
Acute viral hepatitis	As general population	As for first trimester
Cholelithiasis	Unknown	As for first trimester
Drug hepatotoxicity	Unknown	As for first trimester
Intrahepatic cholestasis of pregnancy	0.1%	As for first trimester
Pre-eclampsia–eclampsia*	5–10%	Lethargy (90%), weight gain, hypertension. Bilirubin < 100 µmol/l, ALT 150–300 iu/l unless infarction. Hypoglycaemia rare, DIC 7%
HELLP syndrome*	0.1%	RUQ pain, vomiting, haemolysis (LDH > 600 iu/l, blood film), ALT > 70 iu/l, platelets < 100, bilirubin < 100 µmol/l, ALT 150–300 iu/l unless infarction. Hypoglycaemia rare, DIC 25%
Third trimester		
Intrahepatic cholestasis of pregnancy	0.1%	As for first trimester
Pre-eclampsia–eclampsia	5–10%	As for second trimester
Hepatic rupture	0.0001%	RUQ/shoulder tip pain, low blood pressure/peritonism. CT scan, angiography
HELLP syndrome	0.1%	As for second trimester
Acute fatty liver of pregnancy	0.008%	Nausea/vomiting (70%), RUQ pain (65%), small liver, hypertension (40%), encephalopathy later, leucocytosis. Bilirubin > 100 µmol/l, ALT 300 iu/l. Hypoglycaemia, DIC 75%. USS
Acute viral hepatitis	As general population	As for first trimester
Cholelithiasis	Unknown	As for first trimester
Drug hepatotoxicity	Unknown	As for first trimester

*Rare in this trimester.

Abbreviations: IgM, immunglobulin M; HAV, hepatitis A virus; HEV, hepatitis E virus; CMV, cytomegalovirus; PCR, polymerase chain reaction; EBV, Epstein–Barr virus; RUQ, right upper quadrant; USS, ultrasound scan; MCRP, magnetic resonance cholangiopancreatography; ALT, serum alanine aminotransferase; TSH, thyroid-stimulating hormone; LDH, serum lactate dehydrogenase; DIC, disseminated intravascular coagulation.

comparable non-pregnant control groups. Folate and iron supplementation are recommended, with regular monitoring of nutritional status.

Active inflammatory bowel disease is associated with involuntary infertility, and when very severe it is prudent to recommend deferring any attempt to conceive. Increased fetal loss may occur when active inflammatory bowel disease is first manifest during pregnancy, with recent reports suggesting that the site of disease activity (colonic or small bowel) does not affect outcome. Most studies have demonstrated that corticosteroids, sulphasalazine, and 5-aminosalicylic acid preparations are safe to use during pregnancy. Colonoscopy, in expert hands, can be performed during pregnancy without risk, although it is often possible to defer this procedure.

Acute appendicitis

The most common non-obstetric emergency requiring surgery, acute appendicitis occurs in 1 in 2500 to 1 in 3500 pregnancies. It is not clear if reports of a more aggressive clinical course reflect delays in diagnosis or reporting bias. Clinical management is similar to that of the non-pregnant case: surgery must not be deferred as the frequency of prematurity and perinatal mortality may be increased if perforation occurs.

Coeliac disease

Women with untreated coeliac disease have a markedly increased risk of abortion and low-birthweight babies, which can be reversed following institution of a gluten-free diet. Screening for coeliac disease should be considered in women with a previous history of abortion or unfavourable pregnancy outcomes.

Further reading

Audibert *et al.* (1996). Clinical utility of strict criteria for the HELLP syndrome. *American Journal of Obstetrics and Gynecology* **175**, 460–4.

Ibdah *et al.* (1999). A fetal fatty-acid oxidation disorder as a cause of liver disease in pregnant women. *New England Journal of Medicine* **340**, 1723–31.

Knox T, Olans L (1996). Liver disease in pregnancy. *New England Journal of Medicine* **335**, 569–76.

Kochhar R *et al.* (1999). Pregnancy and its outcome in patients with noncirrhotic portal hypertension. *Digestive Disease Science* **44**, 1356–61.

Korelitz (1989). Inflammatory bowel disease and pregnancy. *Gastroenterology Clinics of North America* **27**, 213–24.

Martin JN *et al.* (1999) The spectrum of severe preeclampsia: comparative analysis by HELLP (hemolysis, elevated liver enzyme levels, and low platelet count) syndrome classification. *American Journal of Obstetrics and Gynecology* **180**, 1373–84.

Martinelli P *et al.* (2000). Coeliac disease and unfavourable outcome of pregnancy. *Gut* **46**, 332–5.

Mayberry J, Weterman IT (1986). European survey of fertility and pregnancy in women with Crohn's disease; a case control study by the European Collaborative group. *Gut* **27**, 821–5.

Modigliani R (1997) Drug therapy for ulcerative colitis during pregnancy. *European Journal of Gastroenterology and Hepatology* **9**, 854–7.

Nicastri P *et al.* (1998). A randomised placebo-controlled trial of ursodeoxycholic acid and S-adenosylmethionine in the treatment of intrahepatic cholestasis of pregnancy. *British Journal of Obstetrics and Gynaecology* **105**, 1205–7.

Palma J *et al.* (1997). Ursodeoxycholic acid in the treatment of cholestasis of pregnancy: a randomized, double-blind study controlled with placebo. *Journal of Hepatology* **27**, 1022–8.

Sibai *et al.* (1993). Maternal morbidity and mortality in 442 pregnancies with hemolysis, elevated liver enzymes, and low platelets (HELLP syndrome). *American Journal of Obstetrics and Gynecology* **169**, 1000–6.

13.10 Diabetes in pregnancy

Michael D. G. Gillmer

Prior to the introduction of insulin treatment in 1921, diabetes was a rare complication of pregnancy with near 50 per cent maternal and fetal mortality. Within a decade of the introduction of insulin therapy, maternal mortality had fallen to between 2 and 3 per cent, but fetal mortality remained above 40 per cent until the 1950s despite recognition that 'rigid control' of diabetes was vital to achieve an optimal pregnancy outcome. This concept has remained central to the management of the disease in pregnancy, with hindsight suggesting that the early poor fetal outcome was due to incomplete understanding of the pathophysiology of the condition, and to a lack of suitable technology for assessing adequate diabetic control.

Metabolic changes in pregnancy

Pregnancy induces substantial alterations in carbohydrate, lipid, and amino acid metabolism, which have been described as a combination of 'facilitated anabolism' and 'accelerated starvation'. From a teleological standpoint these changes appear to ensure the optimal availability of nutrients for both fetus and mother.

Carbohydrate metabolism

Fasting plasma glucose concentrations gradually decline during pregnancy by approximately 0.5 mmol/l, reaching a nadir in the third trimester. Postprandial glucose concentrations increase, despite a rise in both basal and stimulated insulin secretion. This appears to be due to peripheral insulin resistance induced by placental hormones, and to the effects of oestrogen and progesterone on the maternal pancreas.

Although insulin sensitivity appears to increase transiently during the first trimester of pregnancy in some women, there is thereafter a progressive decline which is reflected by an increased insulin:glucose ratio. Human placental lactogen, a polypeptide hormone, is one of the main causes of the insulin resistance that characterizes pregnancy. Other possible factors include increased fat stores, raised prolactin and free cortisol concentrations, sequestration of insulin by the placenta, and changes in insulin receptor affinity and number.

Serial glucose tolerance tests indicate a progressive decline in tolerance with advancing gestation. After an oral glucose load in late pregnancy there are higher peak plasma glucose concentrations, a delay in the rise to the peak concentration and an increase in the total area under the glucose tolerance curve compared with the non-pregnant state. Despite these changes pregnant women maintain efficient glucose homeostasis, but with slightly lower preprandial and higher postprandial plasma glucose concentrations following mixed meals than in non-pregnant women.

Although insulin does not cross the placental barrier, glucose crosses freely by a process of facilitated diffusion. Fetal exposure to maternal hyperglycaemia causes premature stimulation of the fetal β-cells of the pancreatic islets of Langerhans and results in fetal hyperinsulinaemia. This stimulates excessive fetal growth, leading to the macrosomia that characterizes the infant of the diabetic mother.

Lipid metabolism

Plasma concentrations of triglycerides, cholesterol, phospholipids, and free fatty acids all increase during pregnancy. During early pregnancy increased food intake coupled with moderate postprandial hyperinsulinism create ideal conditions for lipogenesis, so-called 'facilitated anabolism'. During late pregnancy food intake declines, insulin resistance is established, and in the presence of high circulating levels of human placental lactogen, lipolysis is enhanced during the fasting state, when there is also a significant increase in ketones, so-called 'accelerated starvation'. The increase in circulating free fatty acids concentrations is thought to have an important influence on maternal metabolism, providing an alternate source of maternal fuel at a time in pregnancy when fetal and maternal glucose needs are maximal.

Plasma cholesterol increases by approximately 25 per cent during pregnancy, a change which probably reflects increased synthesis and decreased catabolism. Lipoprotein triglyceride and cholesterol do not cross the placenta, but free fatty acids cross freely by simple diffusion.

Protein and amino acid metabolism

Amino acids are crucial for fetal development and fetal protein accumulation occurs rapidly in late pregnancy. Despite this there is an increase in maternal amino acid excretion in the third trimester, consisting mainly of the non-essential amino acids glycine, histidine, serine, and alanine. In addition, most amino acid concentrations fall in pregnancy, in particular ornithine, glycine, taurine, and proline, while the postprandial peak concentrations of leucine, isoleucine, serine, and alanine following a mixed meal in late pregnancy are lower than those observed in non-pregnant subjects. Starvation in pregnancy causes a two to three-fold rise in valine, leucine, and isoleucine, but a fall in alanine concentrations.

The concentration of most free amino acids is higher in fetal than in maternal plasma, indicating placental amino acid transfer against a concentration gradient.

Gestational diabetes

Gestational diabetes may be defined as '...carbohydrate intolerance of variable severity with onset or first recognition during the present pregnancy...' This definition includes not only those women in whom diabetes occurs transiently during pregnancy and regresses after delivery, but also those in whom type 1 diabetes arises *de novo* during pregnancy and persists long term.

Screening for gestational diabetes has traditionally involved performing glucose tolerance tests on all women with 'risk factors' or 'potential diabetic features'. However, these are present in 30 per cent or more women in most communities, but not all of those who develop significant glucose intolerance during pregnancy, meaning that many women are subjected to unnecessary tests, whilst others who develop gestational diabetes are missed. 'Risk factors' are therefore of limited value for screening purposes.

Universal screening programmes based on blood glucose measurement have become popular (although controversial) in recent years. The American Diabetes Association (ADA) and American College of Obstetricians (ACOG) have both endorsed the use of a 50-g oral glucose load at 24 to 28 weeks gestation. Venous plasma glucose is measured an hour later and a value equal to or greater than 7.8 mmol/l (140 mg/dl) is recommended as the threshold for a full diagnostic oral glucose tolerance test (GTT). This screening procedure has been shown to be the most sensitive (79 per cent) and specific (87 per cent) of the screening tests available, but is probably only appropriate in populations with a high prevalence of diabetes or for those at increased risk, such as older women and those who are grossly obese. A simpler and more cost effective protocol involves a so-called 'timed' random blood glucose measurement at antenatal booking and at 28 weeks gestation, repeated whenever glycosuria occurs. A full glucose tolerance test is indicated if the plasma glucose exceeds 6 mmol/l in the fasting state or 7 mmol/l within 2 h of a meal. Screening by means of glycosylated haemoglobin or plasma protein measurements, including fructosamine, have proved to be too insensitive for use in pregnancy.

The glucose tolerance criteria for the diagnosis of gestational diabetes are controversial and this, together with the poor reproducibility of the test, may explain some of the inconsistent results of screening programmes. The American College of Obstetricians and Gynaecologists has retained the 100-g oral glucose tolerance test, but in Europe a 75-g load is used, following the World Health Organization's recommendation. It has been suggested that the criteria for 'impaired glucose tolerance' after a 75-g glucose tolerance test should be used for the diagnosis of 'gestational diabetes', but this is not universally accepted (see below). The WHO criteria are shown in Table 1, together with the ACOG standards for a 100-g oral glucose tolerance test, Oxford data from a study of the 75-g oral glucose tolerance test in 491 women at 28 to 34 weeks gestation, and data from a multicentre study of the Diabetic Pregnancy Study Group (DPSG) of the European Association for the study of Diabetes (EASD) involving 354 women in the third trimester of pregnancy.

It is apparent from these data that if gestational diabetes is diagnosed using the WHO criteria for impaired glucose tolerance (IGT), this will lead to increased diagnosis of the condition, as a significant number of women will have a 2-h venous plasma glucose in excess of the WHO limit of 8.0 mmol/l. Widespread acceptance of the WHO criteria for IGT as diagnostic of gestational diabetes could therefore explain the continued uncertainty about the adverse clinical effects of gestational diabetes on pregnancy outcome. It is suggested that the modified WHO criteria shown in Table 2 are used in clinical practice, and that a clear distinction is made between

Table 1 Upper limits for normal glucose tolerance criteria in pregnancy (venous plasma glucose, mmol/l)

	DPSG/EASD[a] (75 g)	Oxford[b] (75 g)	ADA/ACOG[b] (100 g)	WHO (75 g) IGT diabetes
Fasting	5.2	6.0	5.8	<7 >8
1 h	10.5	12.5	10.5	–
2 h	9.0	9.5	9.2	8–11 >11
3 h	–	7.5	8.1	–

[a] Based on 95th centile limits.
[b] Based on mean +2 standard deviations.
For acronyms, see text.

Table 2 Recommended modified WHO diagnostic criteria for the diagnosis of gestational impaired glucose tolerance and diabetes

	Normal	IGT	Diabetes
Fasting	<6.0	>6.0–< 8.0	>or = 8.0
2 h	<9.0	>9.0–<11.0	>or =11.0

Table 3 Timing of blood tests in pregnant diabetic women

Before breakfast	Preprandial
Before coffee	Postprandial
Before lunch	Preprandial
Before tea	Postprandial
Before supper	Preprandial
Bed time	Postprandial

women with impaired glucose tolerance and true diabetes during pregnancy.

Medical management

In the early 1970s it was recognized that the perinatal mortality in diabetic women is positively correlated with the mean maternal blood glucose concentration during pregnancy. This finding, together with the observation that blood glucose concentrations in normal pregnant women rarely exceed 6 mmol/l, except during the hour after a meal, focused attention on the need for 'rigid control' of the maternal diabetes. Ideally, blood glucose concentrations should be measured preprandially and postprandially, as shown in Table 3, on at least 2 days each week, or more frequently if indicated, and maintained between 4 and 6 mmol/l. Measurements of glycosylated haemoglobin or fructosamine are used in many units to provide an indication of medium to long-term glycaemic control and can prove helpful, especially in non-compliant patients.

Congenital malformations

Type 1 insulin dependent diabetes preceding pregnancy is associated with a significant increase in the risk of major congenital anomalies of between 7 and 14 per cent. The precise aetiology remains obscure in most cases, but the frequency is undoubtedly increased in women with poor diabetic control preceding pregnancy and during the first trimester. The incidence also varies depending on the definitions applied in diagnosing major malformations (Table 4).

There is a three to five-fold increase in the incidence of neural tube, cardiac, and renal anomalies which account for more than a half of current perinatal deaths and are also an important cause of avoidable long-term morbidity. As the organ systems commonly affected in diabetes are all fully formed by 9 weeks gestation, that is 7 weeks after the first missed menstrual period, it is vital that all women in the reproductive age group are advised that they must make serious efforts to achieve optimal diabetic control before planning a pregnancy and that this should be maintained throughout the period of embryogenesis. In addition, all diabetic women should be advised to take folate supplements for at least 4 weeks prior to conception to reduce the risk of delivering a child with a neural tube defect.

Table 4 Congenital anomalies seen in infants of diabetic mothers

Central nervous system	Anencephaly, encephalocoele, meningomyelocele, spina bifida, holoprosencephaly
Cardiac	Transposition of great vessels, ventricular septal defect, situs inversus, single ventricle, hypoplastic left ventricle
Renal	Agenesis, multicystic dysplasia
Skeletal	Caudal regression
Gastrointestinal	Anal/rectal atresia, small left colon
Pulmonary	Hypoplasia

Team care

'Team care' is an essential part of the modern management of the pregnant diabetic woman. The most important member of the team is the woman herself: she obviously has responsibility for her diabetes on a day-to-day basis, and usually has the clearest understanding of how optimal glycaemic control can be achieved. She should ideally attend a joint diabetic–antenatal clinic where she can be seen by specialist diabetic nurses, midwives, dietitians, and medical staff including an obstetrician, a physician, and a neonatal paediatrician with a special interest in this condition.

It is important to see these patients as early as possible in pregnancy, after which the frequency of clinic visits will depend on several factors, including the blood glucose concentrations achieved and the occurrence of diabetic or obstetric complications. An average two or three-fold increase in insulin requirements occurs during pregnancy. It is therefore preferable to see all diabetic women at least every 2 weeks until 34 weeks gestation, and then weekly until delivery, as this facilitates the frequent alterations of insulin dose that need to be made as pregnancy progresses and also ensures adequate dietary advice. If control is poor and more frequent advice is required, this can usually be given by telephone contact.

Diet and insulin therapy

The management of women who are diagnosed as gestational diabetics depends on their preprandial and postprandial blood glucose concentrations. If these are 6 to 8 mmol/l, a high fibre isocaloric diet is advised initially, and the woman retested. If the preprandial plasma glucose concentrations remain above 6 mmol/l on this diet or if they initially exceed 8 mmol/l then insulin therapy is commenced, using a long-acting preparation at bedtime in the first instance. Preprandial short-acting insulin is added before meals if the postprandial values remain above 6 mmol/l. Oral hypoglycaemics are not used because they cross the placenta and stimulate the fetal pancreatic β-cells causing fetal hyperinsulinaemia, the pathological process that insulin treatment aims to avoid. Non-pregnant diabetics using oral hypoglycaemic agents should ideally be changed to insulin treatment when planning a pregnancy.

Human insulin is preferred, as this produces least antibodies and reduces the theoretical risks of fetal β-cell damage or macrosomia due to the transplacental passage of injected insulin bound to antibody.

The form of insulin therapy that is currently most widely used for the control of type 1 diabetes in pregnancy is a mixture of short-acting insulin three times daily before meals combined with an intermediate or long-acting injection at bedtime. However, twice daily injections of short and intermediate-acting insulin remain popular. Fixed ratio insulin mixtures have a limited role, but in practice the patient's prepregnancy insulin regimen should only be changed if it proves impossible to achieve the desired standard of control without doing so. The pregnant diabetic is particularly prone to overnight ketoacidosis and the continuous subcutaneous insulin infusion (CSII) pump is no longer considered appropriate in pregnancy as disruption of the infusion through pump failure, catheter blockage, or disconnection can rapidly lead to ketoacidotic coma, with the risk of fetal or even maternal death.

Pregnancy is characterized by a decline in fasting plasma glucose concentrations and a plentiful supply of alternate substrates for energy requirements, including ketones derived from the β-oxidation of free fatty acids. Hypoglycaemia is therefore rare, and unlike hyperglycaemia does not appear to have any demonstrable adverse effect on the fetus. However, because of endeavours to achieve very tight diabetic control, pregnant diabetics are at increased risk of hypoglycaemia. They should therefore be provided with glucagon that can be administered by a third party in the event of severe hypoglycaemia.

Management of diabetes during and after labour

It is important to maintain normoglycaemia during labour in order to reduce the risk of neonatal hypoglycaemia. This is most easily achieved using combined insulin and dextrose infusions. Dextrose 10 per cent solution is infused at 100 ml/h and blood glucose measurements are made every hour. Insulin (6 units in 60 ml normal saline) is administered simultaneously, at an initial rate of 1 unit (10 ml) /h using an infusion pump. The insulin infusion rate is doubled or halved as necessary to maintain the blood glucose concentration between 4 and 6 mmol/l. During labour the insulin requirement may fall dramatically, presumably because of the increased glucose demand due to uterine work, and it is frequently necessary to switch the insulin infusion off towards the end of the first stage.

After delivery the insulin infusion rate must be halved to prevent hypoglycaemia as there is a rapid increase in insulin sensitivity following the delivery of the placenta. It is also essential to return to the prepregnancy insulin dose immediately the patient resumes her normal diet: profound hypoglycaemia can occur if the dose required prior to delivery is administered at this time.

Retinopathy

Rapid reduction of blood glucose concentrations has been shown to accelerate diabetic retinopathy in both pregnant and non-pregnant subjects. There is also evidence that pregnancy and hypertension complicating pregnancy may act as independent risk factors for the progression of diabetic retinopathy. Formal retinal assessment, with dilated pupils, should therefore be performed before pregnancy so that improved diabetic control can be achieved over 3 to 9 months before a planned conception. This should avoid the need for acute improvement of the blood glucose concentrations in early pregnancy and thus minimize the risk of exacerbating proliferative retinopathy. All women should have a full ophthalmic assessment in early pregnancy to assess their retinal state and determine the possible need for laser therapy.

Nephropathy

Overt nephropathy is associated with various pregnancy complications, including pre-eclampsia, growth retardation, and fetal distress, but there is little evidence to suggest that pregnancy will hasten the progression of overt nephropathy to endstage renal failure. Patients seeking advice about pregnancy should therefore be warned that although their renal disease may have an adverse effect on pregnancy, which could necessitate prolonged hospitalization and premature delivery, possibly by caesarean section, there is usually no need to avoid or terminate pregnancy.

Obstetric management

Antenatal assessment of the fetus

Accurate information about the duration of pregnancy, fetal growth, and fetal well being are vital in the management of the pregnant diabetic. Technological developments, particularly in the use of diagnostic ultrasound, have revolutionized fetal assessment and become central to the modern obstetric management of diabetes in pregnancy.

The fetal crown–rump length should be measured during the first trimester to confirm the duration of pregnancy. In some women this technique has identified 'early growth delay' in which the fetal crown–rump length measurement is smaller than expected from the gestational age. This condition is associated with an increased rate of congenital malformations and poor fetal growth, and is thought to be due to 'less-than-optimal' metabolic compensation in early pregnancy.

A biparietal diameter measurement is also performed in the mid-trimester, ideally at 16 weeks gestation, to provide additional information about gestational age. Blood for serum α-fetoprotein should also be taken at this gestation, both to screen for neural tube defects and as part of the 'triple test' used to screen for Down's syndrome. In assessing the result of these investigations it must, however, be borne in mind that the serum α-fetoprotein and unconjugated oestriol concentrations observed in diabetic pregnancy are lower than those in non-diabetic women and a specific algorithm is required for the interpretation of these screening tests in women with type 1 diabetes.

A detailed fetal ultrasound examination to exclude congenital anomalies is performed between 18 and 20 weeks, so that termination of the pregnancy can be considered if appropriate. Further cardiac anomaly scans may be performed at 28 and 34 weeks gestation. Serial studies of growth based on measurements of the fetal head and abdominal circumferences in the second trimester provide the best means of identifying those pregnancies in which the fetus is becoming macrosomic, when it is still possible to institute optimal metabolic control and reduce the likelihood of this complication. However, although an association between birthweight and maternal blood glucose concentrations has been demonstrated during the third trimester of pregnancy, the cause of fetal macrosomia in diabetes is still uncertain and there are many examples of women who deliver infants with birthweights above the 97th centile despite excellent metabolic control in late pregnancy. However, the situation is further complicated by the finding of a two-fold increase in small-for-dates infants (birthweight below the 10th centile) in diabetics with very tight control (mean blood glucose concentration of less than 4.8 mmol/l), indicating that excessively tight blood glucose control may have a deleterious effect on the growth of the diabetic fetus, and possibly on its development.

Obstetric complications of diabetes in pregnancy

Proteinuric hypertension occurs approximately twice as often in diabetics as in normal women. Serum urate and creatinine concentrations should therefore be measured at every antenatal visit and 24-h urine protein concentrations from 24 weeks gestation. These provide the earliest biochemical evidence of proteinuric pre-eclampsia and also serve to clarify those blood pressure changes in late pregnancy which are due to pre-existing essential hypertension. Although the reason for the increased incidence of pre-eclampsia in diabetics is unknown, a link with glycaemic control has been established and the incidence of this complication is reduced with optimal diabetic control.

Polyhydramnios is one of the hallmarks of diabetic pregnancy, and occasionally the presenting feature in gestational diabetes. The cause of this complication, which has an overall incidence of approximately 15 per cent, remains uncertain, but may be due to an osmotic diuresis induced in the fetus by feto–maternal hyperglycaemia. This would be in keeping with the fact that polyhydramnios generally lessens as diabetic control improves.

Premature labour is more frequent in diabetic pregnancy and may, in some instances, be due to underlying polyhydramnios. Conventional management with intravenous β-sympathomimetic agents causes hepatic glycogenolysis and insulin resistance, predisposing to hyperglycaemic ketoacidosis. This treatment is therefore potentially hazardous in diabetic women and should be avoided whenever possible or used with extreme caution, even in non-insulin dependent patients. Use of glucocorticoids in diabetic pregnant women may necessitate the administration of very high doses (up to 30 units/h) of intravenous insulin to maintain normoglycaemia.

Fetal well being and maturity

Unexplained intrauterine death during the last 3 to 4 weeks of pregnancy has been recognized as a considerable problem in the management of diabetic pregnancy since the preinsulin era. However, the so-called 'fetal biophysical profile', a real time ultrasound technique, has revolutionized the late pregnancy management of this condition and made it unnecessary to admit diabetic women routinely for daily monitoring in late pregnancy. These assessments, which should be performed at least weekly from 36 weeks gestation, have also made it possible to prolong diabetic pregnancies to near term or beyond.

Antenatal Doppler ultrasound assessments have also been used widely in diabetic pregnancy in recent years, the results providing the reassurance necessary to prolong uncomplicated diabetic pregnancies beyond term, but unlike the biophysical profile have not proved helpful in predicting fetal demise in diabetic women, unless the pregancy is complicated by fetal growth retardation.

Timing of delivery

Poorly controlled diabetes is associated with fetal pulmonary and hepatic immaturity, predisposing to the neonatal respiratory distress syndrome and jaundice. The optimal time for delivery in uncomplicated diabetic pregnancy appears to be in the 39th week (273 days). Despite this, some authors have advocated deferring delivery until 40 weeks or later as this allows a larger number of women to enter labour spontaneously. This policy is associated with a higher incidence of macrosomic and stillborn babies and has not been shown to have any significant benefit.

Management of labour

One of the main aims in management of the pregnant diabetic woman is to achieve a spontaneous vaginal delivery. Elective caesarean section may be indicated when there is significant fetal macrosomia, with abdominal circumference greatly in excess of the head circumference, fetal malpresentation, or a history of a previous caesarean section. Continuous fetal heart rate and contraction monitoring is advised because of the increased incidence of fetal distress. Pain relief in labour is particularly important because painful uterine contractions cause catecholamine release, leading to glycogenolysis and hyperglycaemia. Epidural anaesthesia is ideal but not vital, especially in the multiparous patient who may have a rapid and uncomplicated labour. If intravenous fluids are required for 'preloading' prior to insertion of an epidural or for the administration of oxytocin, it is essential that 0.9 per cent saline or Hartmann's solutions and not dextrose are used to avoid fetal hyperglycaemia, which predisposes to neonatal hypoglycaemia.

Efforts to predict the risk of shoulder dystocia have been conspicuously unsuccessful to date. This possibility must always be considered when the abdominal circumference exceeds the head circumference, especially if the fetus is macrosomic.

The neonate

Insulin is present in the human pancreas from 11 weeks gestation, and although the pancreatic response to insulin secretogues is sluggish in normal infants, fetal exposure to high concentrations and large fluctuations of glucose and amino acids during poorly controlled diabetic pregnancy appears to produce premature maturation of the fetal β-cells. This causes hyperinsulinaemia, which predisposes to neonatal hypoglycaemia that may occur during the first 24 h after delivery, when high circulating insulin concentrations inhibit both glycogenolysis and lipolysis, thus depriving the infant of alternative energy sources.

Other neonatal problems include, the respiratory distress syndrome, polycythaemia, jaundice, renal vein thrombosis, hypocalcaemia, hypomagnesaemia, and cardiomyopathy, all of which appear to be related directly or indirectly to fetal hyperinsulinaemia. The incidence and severity of neonatal complications is closely related to diabetic control during pregnancy, and the infant of the well-controlled diabetic mother does not usually require admission to a special care nursery, unless a problem arises after delivery.

The puerperium and contraception

Diabetics are at increased risk of wound infection following surgery and prophylactic antiobiotics are therefore advised following both elective and emergency Caesarean section or operative vaginal delivery.

Breast feeding is encouraged, but as this reduces the insulin requirement by approximately 25 per cent an appropriate reduction must be made once lactation is established. Women who choose not to breast feed or in whom breast feeding is unsuccessful should resume their prepregnancy insulin dose after delivery.

All diabetic women should be seen for a 6-week postnatal examination and should be offered contraceptive advice at this time. The nature of the advice will depend on age, parity, and future reproductive plans. The progesterone only (mini-pill) has virtually no effect on carbohydrate or lipid metabolism and is therefore suitable for the breast feeding diabetic woman. Provided she is prepared to accept the slightly higher failure rate of this method when ovulation resumes, then it may also be used long term. Modern, low-dose, combined oral contraceptive preparations have little effect on high or low density lipoprotein concentrations or carbohydrate metabolism and can be used safely, especially in younger, insulin-dependent and gestational diabetics. Early concerns about the apparently high failure rates of copper-containing intrauterine devices in diabetics have been refuted in recent studies. The woman who has completed her family should be encouraged to consider a laparosopic sterilization.

Further reading

Dornhorst A and Hadden DR, eds (1996). *Diabetes and pregnancy—an international approach to diagnosis and management.* John Wiley and Sons, Chichester. A comprehensive review of the subject.

Reece EA, ed. (1996). Diabetes in pregnancy. *Obstetrics and Gynecology Clinics of North America* **23**. A further review of this subject.

Reece EA, Coustan DR, eds (1995). *Diabetes mellitus in pregnancy.* Churchill Livingstone, New York. A comprehensive textbook.

13.11 Endocrine disease in pregnancy

John H. Lazarus

Introduction

During pregnancy the physiology of the mother and fetus changes constantly. For instance, maternal oestrogen concentrations rise and affect hepatic protein synthesis and plasma volume increases by as much as 50 per cent with consequent haemodilution. Endocrine function in the developing fetus is initially almost entirely dependent on maternal function as most endocrine glands do not produce hormones until the second trimester. Thereafter the fetus becomes less reliant on maternal hormones as the fetal glands develop and mature. This section will discuss the important therapeutic aspects of endocrine disease in pregnancy.

Pituitary disease

Prolactinoma

Pituitary adenomas are the most common pituitary disorder affecting pregnancy and prolactinomas are the most common of the hormone-secreting adenomas. Prolactinomas are a common cause of reproductive and sexual dysfunction and hyperprolactinaemia must be corrected to allow ovulation and fertility. The main concern during pregnancy is of symptomatic enlargement leading to visual impairment. There is less than a 2 per cent risk of this happening with a microprolactinoma, but a greater than 15 per cent risk with a macroprolactinoma. It is safe for patients to become pregnant following bromocriptine treatment; the prolactinomas may decrease in size, remain unchanged, or in some cases achieve complete resolution. Treatment with bromocriptine is safe during gestation, but a macroadenoma may require debulking prior to pregnancy. Cabergoline has also been used during pregnancy with no deleterious effects. The concern during pregnancy is the development of visual impairment which may occur with a macro-prolactinoma but not with a microprolactinoma.

Acromegaly

Fertility is impaired in acromegaly due to concomitant hyperprolactinaemia and decreased gonadotrophin reserve. The main aims of therapy in an acromegalic woman wishing to conceive are therefore to normalize prolactin and growth hormone levels to promote fertility. With the use of surgery as well as dopamine agonists and octreotide, many women with this condition are now able to achieve pregnancy.

The pituitary gland enlarges during normal gestation and may increase by 45 per cent during the first trimester. Pituitary adenomas can also enlarge, and pregnancy exacerbates acromegaly in about 17 per cent of cases. Patients with adenomas greater than 1.2 cm are at greater risk of visual loss during pregnancy. Management can be difficult, and risks need to be judged carefully. Those with microadenomas should discontinue medical therapy (bromocriptine or somatostatin analogues) during pregnancy and be assessed at each trimester (Fig. 1). In patients with macroadenomas removal before pregnancy leads to a greater risk of infertility, but if not resected there is a greater risk of pituitary enlargement and visual impairment during gestation. More detailed assessment during pregnancy is therefore recommended including regular visual field checks and MRI examinations in those patients with significantly large tumours at the beginning of pregnancy. However, although the metabolic and cardiovascular complications of acromegaly might be expected to result in increased risk to both mother and fetus, these potential hazards do not seem to be realized.

Some women with apparent prolactinomas or non-functioning pituitary tumours will be found to have multiple endocrine neoplasia type 1 (MEN1). In this situation screening of the child should be offered.

Cushing's syndrome

Cushing's syndrome during pregnancy is associated with a high incidence of maternal and fetal complications, only about one-quarter of patients

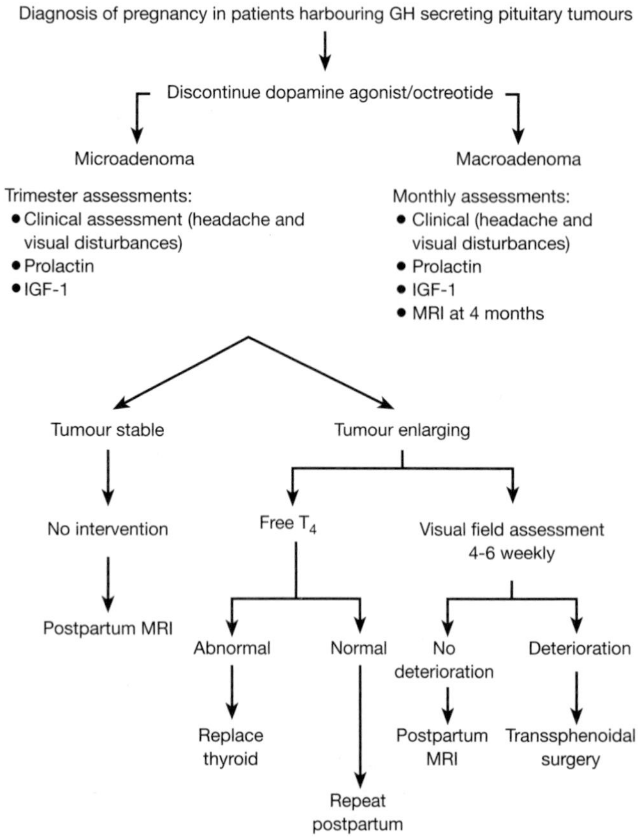

Fig. 1 Scheme for management of growth hormone secreting pituitary tumours in pregnancy (reproduced from Herman-Bonert *et al.* 1998, with permission).

having an uncomplicated pregnancy. The diagnosis of the disease during gestation is difficult because many of the biochemical features, such as elevated cortisol levels and loss of the normal glucocorticoid feedback, are present during normal pregnancy. The use of corticotrophin-releasing hormone and dexamethasone testing can be helpful and MRI is valuable. Transphenoidal surgery has been successfully performed during pregnancy. This operation should be carefully considered if any pituitary tumour enlarges during pregnancy, especially when there is evidence of increasing visual field impairment.

Diabetes insipidus

Central diabetes insipidus may present during pregnancy. It is seen in women with Sheehan's syndrome, partial postpartum hypopituitarism, and associated with infiltrative disorders such as histiocytosis X. ADH deficiency is corrected using intranasal synthetic 1-deamino-8-D-arginine-vasopressin (DDAVP). During pregnancy this seems to be safe for both mother and baby. It does not affect delivery and has no adverse effects on the neonate.

Postpartum hypopituitarism

Sheehan's syndrome is caused by pituitary infarction following significant hypotension occurring at the time of delivery. Advances in obstetric care mean that it is now uncommon in the 'developed' world. However, lymphocytic hypophysitis is now increasingly recognized as a cause of hypopituitarism occurring late in pregnancy and in the postpartum period, and around 60 per cent of cases of women found to have adenohypophysitis are pregnant or have recently been delivered. They typically present with symptoms of an expanding pituitary tumour. Headaches, visual symptoms, inability to lactate, and amenorrhoea occur. Hyperprolactinaemia and elevated growth hormone levels are found. Computed tomography or magnetic resonance imaging reveals a pituitary mass mimicking an adenoma in about four-fifths of patients. Evaluation of pituitary function shows isolated or multiple anterior pituitary deficiency. Adenocorticotrophic hormone secretion is impaired, most frequently followed by that of thyroid-stimulating hormone (TSH), gonadotrophins, growth hormone, and prolactin. Histology shows lymphocytic infiltration and this may extend up to the pituitary stalk to the infundibulum. Antibodies to pituitary tissue may be present but often are not. Other autoimmune diseases, particularly postpartum thyroiditis, may be associated. In addition to the pituitary symptoms described, patients are at risk of adrenal failure and death has been reported.

Adrenal function should therefore be assessed in all patients. The diagnosis of lymphocytic hypophysitis may only be made at surgery, but if the condition is suspected beforehand, then surgery should be avoided and corticosteroids given, since these can reduce the size of the pituitary mass.

Thyroid disease

Maternal thyroid function during pregnancy

Thyroid physiology and function alter significantly during pregnancy. Thyroid volume increases in iodine deficient areas but not in areas of iodine sufficiency. There is increased synthesis of thyroxine-binding globulin, but free thyroxine decreases during the second and third trimester. During the first trimester the maternal thyroid is to some extent controlled by placental human chorionic gonadotrophin, a weak thyroid stimulator, and during this period TSH levels are suppressed.

Hyperthyroidism

Hyperthyroidism is associated with impaired fertility and the presence of thyroid antibodies is a marker for miscarriage and recurrent abortion even in those who are euthyroid. Nevertheless, hyperthyroidism occurs in 0.2 per cent of pregnancies. This is usually due to Graves' disease, but other

causes include hydatidiform molar disease and gestational thyrotoxicosis due to high human chorionic gonadotrophin concentrations. Since the incidence of hyperthyroidism in pregnancy is low, and the symptoms of hyperthyroidism frequently overlap with those of the pregnancy itself, a high index of clinical suspicion is required to make the diagnosis. Further difficulties arise because thyroid function tests vary during normal pregnancy (see above) and each laboratory should ideally establish its own normal ranges for those who are pregnant. However, it is particularly important to consider whether a borderline test at this time really indicates thyroid dysfunction, and any result should be repeated before treatment is started. The diagnosis of hyperthyroidism is best made by noting an elevated serum free tri-iodothyronine in association with a suppressed TSH, the free thyroxine being elevated or at the upper limit of normal.

Untreated hyperthyroidism is associated with an increased risk of abortion and, if the pregnancy is completed, the baby may be of low birth weight and may show transient hyperthyroidism due to the transplacental passage of thyroid stimulating antibodies. Neonatal hyperthyroidism can also occur in babies born to euthyroid mothers who have been treated for Graves' hyperthyroidism in the past. It is therefore prudent to measure thyroid stimulating antibodies in the first trimester in any woman with active Graves' hyperthyroidism as well as those previously treated. If values are high, they should be measured again at 36 weeks and—if elevated—the obstetrician and paediatrician alerted to the possibility of a thyrotoxic infant.

Hyperthyroidism in pregnancy can be managed with either antithyroid drugs or surgery, the latter being optimally performed in the second trimester. Radioiodine therapy is completely contraindicated during pregnancy: non-pregnant women should undergo a pregnancy test 1 or 2 days before ^{131}I administration and be advised not to conceive for at least 4 months thereafter. If radioiodine has been administered after 12 weeks gestation (i.e. after the fetal thyroid is functional) there may be a case for therapeutic abortion. Propylthiouracil is the preferred antithyroid drug (Table 1) as fetal side-effects have been reported with carbimazole and methimazole. These are rare but significant, including aplasia cutis and a possible methimazole embryopathy, characterized by choanal atresia and other defects. If necessary, propylthiouracil should be continued in low dose right up to delivery and into the puerperium. An exacerbation of Graves' disease often occurs postpartum and this should be checked. Propylthiouracil does cross into breast milk but in lower concentrations than carbimazole or methimazole so that breast feeding can usually be permitted, but if breast feeding is prolonged, then thyroid function should be monitored in the neonate.

Hypothyroidism

Hypothyroidism is associated with relative infertility because of anovulation and menorrhagia. There is an increased incidence of stillbirths, congenital malformations, and maternal obstetric complications if the condition is untreated. In iodine-deficient areas the risk of neonatal brain damage is increased, resulting in cretinism in severe cases. This is due to the

Table 1 Management of Graves' hyperthyroidism in pregnancy

Confirm diagnosis

Start propylthiouracil

Render patient euthyroid—continue with low dose antithyroid drug up to and during labour

Monitor thyroid function regularly throughout gestation (4–6 weekly), adjusting antithyroid drug dosing if necessary

Check thyroid stimulating antibodies at 36 weeks gestation

Discuss treatment with patient
    effect on patient
    effect on fetus
    breast feeding

Inform obstetrician and paediatrician

Review postpartum—check for exacerbation

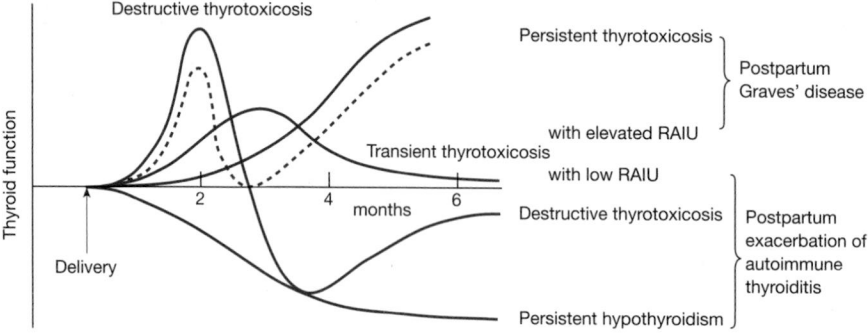

Fig. 2 Diagram to illustrate the progression to different types of thyroid dysfunction observed in the postpartum period (reproduced from Amino *et al.* 1999, with permission).

fact that the developing fetal nervous system is entirely dependent on T4 derived from the mother in the first trimester. Even in iodine-sufficient countries mild hypothyroidism during pregnancy is associated with impaired child development and a case for screening for maternal hypothyroidism in early pregnancy can be made. Pregnant patients with hypothyroidism of any degree should always be treated with thyroxine. In those already receiving T4 when found to be pregnant, the dose should be increased by at least 50 μg/day (and more if necessary) as it has been shown that dose requirements increase during gestation.

Fetal and neonatal thyroid dysfunction

The fetus of a mother with thyroid dysfunction during pregnancy should be regarded as a patient in its own right. Transplacental passage of maternal thyroid stimulating IgG immunoglobulins from a mother with Graves' disease may cause fetal hyperthyroidism as well as neonatal disease. Fetal hyperthyroidism is treated with propylthiouracil and the fetal heart rate monitored carefully to avoid hypothyroidism. If the mother is euthyroid, possibly with a history of previously treated Graves' hyperthyroidism, an hyperthyroid fetus may still occur due to thyroid stimulating IgGs. The fetal state is diagnosed by noting a high fetal heart rate and may be confirmed if necessary by the specialized procedure of fetal blood sampling. Treatment of the fetal hyperthyroidism in this situation is by maternal administration of high-dose propylthiouracil (300–450 mg/day). It is also necessary to give thyroxine during gestation to prevent maternal hypothyroidism.

In addition to transient neonatal hyperthyroidism, a hypothyroid state can also occur at birth due to maternal TSH-receptor-blocking antibodies. Both of these conditions are transient and the mother can be reassured. Other causes of transient neonatal hypothyroidism include maternal antithyroid drug administration, iodine deficiency, and ingestion of goitrogens by the mother.

Permanent neonatal hypothyroidism has an incidence of 1/4000 live births and is screened for routinely using whole blood TSH concentrations usually obtained by heel prick at 5 to 7 days. Recent advances in molecular biological diagnosis have revealed a number of specific hereditary gene defects (e.g. in the structure of thyroglobulin) which may require parental DNA analysis for appropriate genetic counselling.

Postpartum thyroid disease

Patients with hypothyroidism almost invariably have circulating antithyroid antibodies (usually antithyroid peroxidase (anti-TPO)). In euthyroid women, anti-TPO antibodies are found in 10 per cent at the routine antenatal booking clinic. These women are at risk of developing postpartum thyroid dysfunction (Fig. 2). Postpartum thyroiditis is a destructive process, not influenced by T4 or iodine treatment. It is characterized by transient hyperthyroidism followed by hypothyroidism, occurring in 5 to 9 per cent of anti-TPO positive women (Fig. 3). Although a minority of patients

have been described with this condition who have no demonstrable immune abnormalities, the great majority have anti-TPO antibodies. Their hyperthyroidism is relatively asymptomatic but may require treatment with β-adrenoreceptor-blocking agents in some cases. Carbimazole is not effective. By contrast, the hypothyroidism is often symptomatic and thyroxine should be given. It persists at 1 year in 20 to 30 per cent of cases, and those that recover from transient postpartum thyroid dysfunction should have their thyroid function measured annually as nearly 50 per cent will develop hypothyroidism in the next 7 years. Mild depressive symptomatology is more common in postpartum women with anti-TPO antibodies than those without these markers. Recurrent postpartum thyroid dysfunction will occur in up to 75 per cent of those women who have experienced a previous episode.

At present, measurement of anti-TPO antibodies is not part of the routine antenatal screening performed at around 14 weeeks gestation. Such screening would predict the development of postpartum thyroiditis. Recent data also suggests that the development of children of anti-TPO positive mothers may be impaired. A case can therefore be made to support antenatal screening for anti-TPO antibodies. Similar arguments have been put forward for antenatal screening of TSH levels.

Thyroid nodules

Thyroid nodules may be clinically detectable in up to 10 per cent of pregnant women. Most of these lesions will be benign colloid nodules but between 5 and 20 per cent are true neoplasms, either benign follicular adenomas or carcinomas of follicular or para-follicular (C-) cell origin. It is often debatable whether investigation of a thyroid nodule should actually be performed during pregnancy. Many experts would pursue matters if a

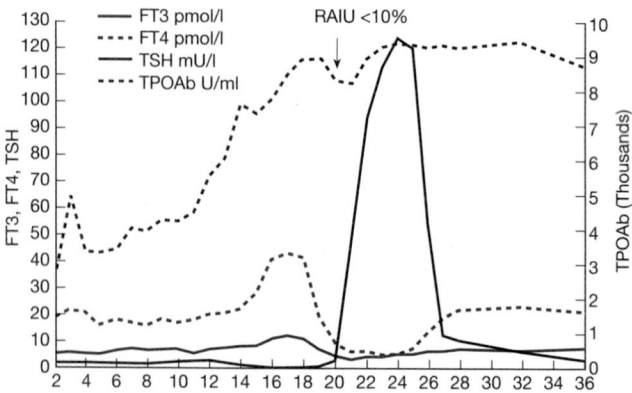

Fig. 3 Clinical chart illustrating the course of postpartum hyper- and hypothyroidism in a woman studied weekly for 36 weeks postpartum. Figures are weeks postpartum. Delivery at time 0 (reproduced from Lazarus *et al.* 1999, with permission). RAIU = radioiodine uptake.

lump was found early on, but delay until the postpartum period if a nodule presented after 5 to 6 months gestation. Fine-needle aspiration biopsy is diagnostic in about 90 per cent of cases. In the remaining 10 per cent, ultrasound-guided biopsy may produce diagnostic tissue. If neck exploration is recommended, this should preferably be performed during the second trimester to avoid abortion in the first and premature labour in the third. Pregnancy does not adversely affect the course (generally favourable) of differentiated thyroid cancer: recurrence and distant metastases occur at the same rates in pregnant and non-pregnant women. In general, differentiated thyroid cancer should not be a contraindication to pregnancy or an indication for abortion. The position for medullary cell carcinoma is less clear cut.

Parathyroid disease

Although diseases of the parathyroid glands are uncommon in women of childbearing age, hyperparathyroidism during pregnancy can lead to acute pancreatitis, hypercalcaemic crisis, and toxaemia. There is an increased incidence of prematurity and neonatal hypercalcaemia if maternal calcium levels are high. If necessary, parathyroidectomy can be undertaken safely in the second trimester. Hypoparathyroidism is treated with vitamin D analogues, the dose of which may need to be increased to maintain normocalcaemia during gestation. Calcium levels should be monitored regularly throughout pregnancy, at least in each trimester.

Adrenal disease

The diagnosis of adrenal disease is often delayed in pregnancy. Adrenal tumours are very rare, but their pathophysiological consequences for mother and fetus are dire. In patients with phaeochromocytoma, hypertension may initially be mistaken for pregnancy-associated hypertension. This should be managed medically, as should primary aldosteronism, with surgical resection considered postpartum.

Occasionally phaeochromocytoma can be familial and screening of the child and other family members for measurable calcitonin levels, evidence of neurofibromatosis, von Hippel Lindau syndrome, or thyroid enlargement should be offered. It is also important to consider screening for multiple endocrine neoplasia type 2, associated RET mutations, and mutations in the von Hippel Lindau gene.

Addison's disease

Addison's disease is rarely diagnosed during pregnancy, but can present as a postpartum addisonian crisis. Symptoms may be attributed to pregnancy or its complications, leading to delayed diagnosis. The condition is readily confirmed by measurement of plasma cortisol, the short synacthen test, and adenocorticotrophic hormone levels. Antibodies to 21-hydroxylase should be measured to confirm the autoimmune nature of the disease, and other autoimmune conditions sought.

Congenital adrenal hyperplasia

Women with severe congenital adrenal hyperplasia have decreased fertility rates because of oligo-ovulation due to elevated androgen levels. Successful conception requires careful endocrine monitoring and possibly induction of ovulation. Problems occur during pregnancy in women with 21-hydroxylase deficiency (P450c21 deficiency),11-hydroxylase deficiency (P450c11), and 3 β-hydroxysteroid dehydrogenase deficiency. Gestational management must involve adequate adrenal steroid replacement and adrenal androgen suppression. Clinical status, serum electrolytes, and androgen levels should be measured regularly and glucocorticoid and mineralocorticoid therapy adjusted or increased as necessary. As the genetic basis of 21- and 11-hydroxylase deficiency is known, prenatal diagnosis is possible. Infants should also be evaluated clinically and, in most cases, biochemically.

Miscellaneous endocrine conditions

Gonadal dysgenesis (Turner's syndrome) is characterized by streak ovaries and infertility. Advances in *in vitro* fertilization and embryo transplantation have made pregnancy possible for some of these patients.

Further reading

Badawy SZ, Marziale JC, Rosenbaum AE, Chang JK, Joy SE (1997). The long-term effects of pregnancy and bromocriptine treatment on prolactinomas—the value of radiologic studies. *Early Pregnancy* 3, 306–11. Useful clinical study.

Chittacharoen A, Phuapradit W (1997). Pheochromocytoma during pregnancy: case report. *Journal of Obstetric and Gynaecology Research* 23, 209–12. Discussion of diagnosis and treatment.

Ciccarelli E, Grottoli S, Razzore P, *et al.* (1997). Long-term treatment with cabergoline, a new long-lasting ergoline derivate, in idiopathic or tumorous hyperprolactinaemia and outcome of drug-induced pregnancy. *Journal of Endocrinological Investigation* 20, 547–51. Reviews of nearly 50 patient with hyperprolactinaemia.

Garner PR (1998). Congenital adrenal hyperplasia in pregnancy. *Seminars in Perinatology* 22, 446–56. Discussion of biochemistry and management during pregnancy.

Glinoer D (1997). The regulation of thyroid function in pregnancy: Pathways of endocrine adaptation from physiology to pathology. *Endocrine Reviews* 18, 404–33. Excellent review of this subject.

Hall R (1995). Pregnancy and autoimmune endocrine disease. *Bailliere's Clinical Endocrinology and Metabolism. Autoimmune Endocrine Disease* 9, 137–55. Detailed discussion of this subject.

Harrington JL, Farley DR, van Heerden JA, Ramin KD (1999). Adrenal tumors and pregnancy. *World Journal of Surgery* 23, 182–6. Clinical aspects of four adrenal tumours in pregnancy from the Mayo clinic.

Herman-Bonert V, Seliverstov M, Melmed S (1998). Pregnancy in acromegaly: successful therapeutic outcome. *Journal of Clinical Endocrinology and Metabolism* 83, 727–31. Review by experienced endocrinologists.

Lo JC, Schwitzebel VM, Tyrrel JB, *et al.* (1999). Normal female infants born of mothers with classic congenital adrenal hyperplasia due to 21-hydroxylase deficiency. *Journal of Clinical Endocrinology and Metabolism* 84, 930–6. Highlight key issues in management, particularly endocrine monitoring.

Maniker AH, Krieger AJ (1996). Rapid recurrence of craniopharyngioma during pregnancy with recovery of vision: a case report. *Surgical Neurology* 45, 324–7. Unusual but important case of craniopharyngioma.

Mestman JH (1998). Parathyroid disorders of pregnancy. *Seminars in Perinatology* 22, 485–96. Comprehensive review of subject.

Molitch ME (1998). Pituitary disease in pregnancy. *Seminars in Perinatology* 22, 457–70. Review of all pituitary disease with emphasis on adenomas.

Molitch ME (1999). Medical treatment of prolactinomas. *Endocrinology and Metabolism Clinics of North America* 28, 143–69. Detailed discussion of therapy of the commonest of pituitary tumours.

Ray JG (1998). DDAVP use during pregnancy: an analysis of its safety for mother and child. *Obstetrical and Gynecological Survey* 53, 450–5. Large literature review of DDAVP use during pregnancy.

Ross RJ, Chew SL, Perry L, Erskine K, Medbak S, Afshar F (1995). Diagnosis and selective cure of Cushing's disease during pregnancy by transsphenoidal surgery. *European Journal of Endocrinology* 132, 722–6. Complex case illustrates diagnosis and management of this condition.

13.12 Neurological disease in pregnancy

G. G. Lennox

Introduction

A wide range of neurological problems occasionally complicate pregnancy and the puerperium. Pre-existing neurological diseases, such as epilepsy and myasthenia gravis, sometimes become more troublesome or, like myotonic dystrophy, pose obstetric difficulties. New neurological disorders can occur, ranging from diseases of the peripheral nerves and muscles that are relatively common but generally benign, to diseases of the central nervous system that are rare but potentially life-threatening. In all these situations the presence of the fetus influences management.

Disorders of muscle and neuromuscular transmission

Muscle disorders

Muscle cramps, particularly on waking, are extremely common in the third trimester. They are almost never a symptom of serious neurological disease and often respond to calcium supplements. Restless legs syndrome, in which there is a feeling of discomfort in the legs that is relieved by movement, is also common, especially on retiring to bed. It may respond to correction of underlying anaemia (particularly if this is due to folate or iron deficiency); otherwise management in pregnancy is aimed at promoting the rapid onset of sleep, for example by reducing caffeine intake. Drug treatment (with levodopa, clonazepam, or codeine) is best avoided. Polymyositis, although rare in young women, can deteriorate during pregnancy. Treatment with corticosteroids is thought to be safe, as is azathioprine if another immunosuppressive agent is necessary.

Most of the congenital myopathies and muscular dystrophies, apart from myotonic dystrophy, cause no special problems in pregnancy unless they are of sufficient severity to compromise ventilation, either because of respiratory muscle weakness or associated scoliosis. Such cases should ideally be assessed in a specialist unit prior to pregnancy because the cardiorespiratory demands of pregnancy, combined with the splinting effect of the fetus on the diaphragm, can lead to ventilatory failure and a temporary need for mechanical ventilation.

Myotonic dystrophy

Myotonic dystrophy is an autosomal dominant disorder due to an expanded triplet repeat in the myotonin protein kinase gene. The expansion tends to increase during transmission from mother to child, so that a mildly affected or asymptomatic mother may have a severely affected fetus. This probably accounts for the excess of polyhydramnios and perinatal death. The myotonia affects the smooth muscle of the uterus, prolonging labour and increasing the risk of postpartum haemorrhage because of uterine inertia. Moderately affected mothers may also develop symptoms of cardiomyopathy during labour. (See Chapter 24.22 for further discussion.)

Myasthenia gravis

Myasthenia gravis deteriorates, improves, and remains stable during pregnancy in roughly equal proportions of patients, but the response is neither predictable nor reproducible in subsequent pregnancies. It deteriorates during the puerperium in about half of all patients, an effect that may also occur after abortion. The mechanism of these changes is not clear. Corticosteroids, oral anticholinesterases, and plasmapheresis can all be employed in the usual manner during pregnancy. It is reasonable to continue azathioprine where this has been prescribed before pregnancy for severe myasthenia, bearing in mind the risk of inducing neonatal leucopenia. Thymectomy can be performed during pregnancy (for example where a malignant thymoma is suspected) but may take up to a year to have a therapeutic effect and ideally should be performed well before any planned pregnancy. Myasthenia does not usually influence labour, although the second stage may be prolonged by fatigue and obstetric anaesthesia is complicated by the need to avoid drugs with adverse effects on neuromuscular transmission—regional anaesthesia being preferable when possible. Acetylcholine receptor antibodies can cross into the fetal circulation, giving rise to transient neonatal myasthenia in up to 20 per cent of the babies from affected mothers. Expert paediatric support must therefore be available at delivery. (See Chapter 24.17 for further discussion.)

Disorders of nerves and nerve roots

Facial palsy

The incidence of facial nerve palsy (Bell's palsy) is substantially increased during pregnancy and the puerperium (as Bell himself described). The reason for this is not known. There have been no studies of treatment in this specific context but it is reasonable to treat promptly with prednisolone, beginning at 40 mg daily and reducing over a 2-week course.

Mononeuropathies

Carpal tunnel syndrome, due to compression of the median nerve in the wrist, is very common in pregnancy, characteristically causing pain and tingling in the hands at night and after use. Most cases can be managed with nocturnal wrist splints, although steroid injections into the carpal tunnel may tide the patient over into the puerperium, when symptoms usually remit. Diuretics are of little value. Surgical decompression during pregnancy should be reserved for cases with severe pain, weakness, or wasting, when usually there have been symptoms either before pregnancy or early in the first trimester. In troublesome cases it is worth considering delayed surgery to prevent recurrence in subsequent pregnancies, which is common.

The lateral cutaneous nerve of the thigh can be compressed as it crosses the inguinal ligament. This is particularly common in the third trimester and causes tingling, hypersensitivity, or numbness in the midlateral thigh, which may be bilateral. Usually no treatment is required, but troublesome cases may respond to transcutaneous nerve stimulation or a local nerve block. Remission after delivery is the rule.

Lumbosacral root and plexus problems

Backache is very common in pregnancy, particularly in women with a past history of back pain or occupations that involve bending and lifting. It is traditionally blamed on changes in posture and hormonally mediated relaxation of spinal and sacroiliac joints. The pain is usually confined to the lumbar region but may radiate into the buttock or thigh. There may be tenderness over one or other sacroiliac joints. Radiological investigations are not needed if there are no abnormal neurological signs. Management is conservative.

Abrupt onset of pain that radiates below the knee with focal weakness, numbness, or reflex loss is most likely to be due to a prolapsed intervertebral disc. Provided that the signs are unilateral with no sphincter impairment, conservative management is again appropriate, with analgesia and advice to keep mobile. If this fails then magnetic resonance imaging is thought to be a safe method of investigation prior to consideration of lumbar microdiscectomy.

Obstetric nerve palsies are becoming less common with improvements in obstetric care, but still occur in cases of prolonged or complicated labour (for example due to cephalopelvic disproportion, dystocia, and primiparity), in difficult forceps deliveries, and as a result of traction or haematoma formation in caesarean section. Damage to the common peroneal nerve from incorrectly positioned leg holders is now rare.

The baby may compress the lower parts of the lumbosacral plexus during labour. This will typically give rise to focal neurological deficits depending on which parts of the plexus have borne the brunt of the pressure. Most commonly there is a unilateral footdrop, which may only become apparent when the mother starts to mobilize. Examination also reveals sensory loss that characteristically involves the dorsolateral foot and leg, distinguishing plexus damage from a common peroneal palsy where the sensory loss is confined to the dorsum of the foot. Compression of the upper lumbosacral plexus leads to weakness of iliopsoas as well as the quadriceps muscles, which distinguishes it from more distal damage to the femoral nerve. Both may give rise to sensory loss in the anteromedial thigh and loss or depression of the knee jerk. In most cases the prognosis is good, with spontaneous recovery over a couple of months. Particular care must be taken in subsequent deliveries to avoid further damage to the same nerve, as recovery after repeated injury will tend to be less complete.

Long, complicated, or instrumental deliveries may also damage the obturator or pudendal nerves. Obturator neuropathy leads to weakness of hip adduction and rotation, together with some sensory loss in the upper medial thigh. Pudendal nerve damage may be initially asymptomatic but probably contributes to the subsequent development of perineal descent and stress incontinence.

Generalized neuropathies

Chronic inflammatory demyelinating polyradiculoneuropathy can present or relapse during pregnancy, and can be treated with corticosteroids or (if necessary) intravenous immunoglobulin. The incidence of acute Guillain Barre syndrome is increased in the puerperium and can be managed in the usual ways.

The combination of the nutritional demands of pregnancy and hyperemesis gravidarum can lead to thiamine deficiency. This most commonly causes a subacute sensory neuropathy, but cases of acute Wernicke's encephalopathy (with any combination of altered consciousness, ataxia, and ophthalmoplegia, leading if untreated to death) have been described. Both conditions respond promptly to parenteral thiamine 100 mg daily.

Pregnancy can precipitate relapse in acute intermittent porphyria: abdominal pain typically precedes autonomic and sensory neuropathy, sometimes with seizures and psychiatric disturbance. Finally, lepromatous neuropathies may present or deteriorate during pregnancy, making careful clinical supervision advisable.

Disorders of the central nervous system

Headache

The most common form of headache during pregnancy (as at other times) is chronic daily headache of the tension type. This may be a continuation of pre-existing headaches or a new phenomenon, compounded by anxiety, depression, or poor sleep. Neurological examination is usual in such cases and the treatment should concentrate on explanation and reassurance, coupled if necessary with advice about relaxation techniques. Occasional paracetamol may be helpful; aspirin should be avoided in the third trimester.

Migraine usually improves during pregnancy, but approximately 20 per cent of sufferers get worse and occasionally migraine actually begins in pregnancy. No single hormonal change has been convincingly linked to these divergent responses. Whilst migraine can generally be identified accurately on clinical grounds, diagnosis is more difficult when it presents for the first time in pregnancy, particularly if accompanied by the transient focal deficits of migraine aura such visual disturbances or hemiplegia. Other potential causes of headache in pregnancy, such as eclampsia (Chapter 13.4), subarachnoid haemorrhage, cerebral venous thrombosis, cerebral infarction, intracranial tumour, and intracranial infection must be considered and excluded by careful neurological and general examination, supplemented if necessary by brain imaging (see below). Some women present in pregnancy with migraine aura without headache, which can also give rise to diagnostic difficulty: it may be necessary to exclude causes of transient ischaemic attack.

Acute migraine attacks should be treated promptly with rest and paracetamol; prochlorperazine is probably a safe treatment for vomiting. Ergot derivatives must be avoided in pregnancy (and breastfeeding), and the triptan drugs have not yet been shown to be safe. If attacks are frequent then attention should be paid to relevant lifestyle factors such as irregular sleep or meals and worry. Prophylactic drug treatment is occasionally necessary, and the greatest experience lies with propranolol which, in doses of 20 to 80 mg three times a day, appears to be both effective and safe, despite its effect on placental blood flow. Women with migraine commonly develop a dull non-specific headache of variable severity in the first few days after delivery. This usually responds to simple analgesia, particularly if the woman has been warned about the phenomenon.

Tumours

Although the incidence of cerebral and spinal tumours is probably no greater than at other times, some tumours expand during pregnancy and may present unusually rapidly. This probably reflects a mixture of hormonal and vascular factors; most meningiomas and some neurofibromas and gliomas express oestrogen and progesterone receptors and placental growth factor.

Neurofibromatosis type 1 presents particular problems in pregnancy. Women with this condition experience an increased rate of spontaneous first trimester abortions, perhaps also intrauterine fetal growth retardation and stillbirths, and have a high rate of caesarean section. Most women notice that cutaneous neurofibromas grow or appear *de novo* during pregnancy.

Meningiomas are particularly liable to expand in the third trimester, causing local mass effects such as headache, cranial nerve palsies, hemiparesis, or paraparesis, which may remit after delivery. Corticosteroids can be given to reduce surrounding oedema, and surgery can often be delayed until after delivery. Gliomas tend to present earlier in pregnancy and have a reputation for following an aggressive course. They may require early surgical intervention, and it is sometimes also appropriate to consider termination of the pregnancy. Women with known intracranial mass lesions require careful assessment prior to delivery: prolonged Valsalva manoeuvres can increase intracranial pressure and elective caesarean section may be necessary.

Choriocarcinoma is a tumour peculiar to pregnancy and the most common form of malignancy associated with pregnancy. It usually presents after molar pregnancy or abortion, but 15 per cent of cases occur during or after normal pregnancy. Neurological manifestations due to brain or spine metastases are common. The brain metastases have a tendency to invade blood vessels, giving rise to strokes through infarction or haemorrhage. Spinal metastases cause cord or cauda equina compression that may be rapid in onset. There are usually multiple pulmonary metastases on chest radiography and the serum chorionic gonadotrophin is greatly elevated. Early diagnosis and treatment (with chemotherapy and radiotherapy) improves survival, but the mortality rate of cases with neurological manifestations remains high.

The normal pituitary gland and some pituitary tumours such as prolactinomas expand during pregnancy. Their management, the possibility of pituitary apoplexy, and the postpartum differential diagnosis of lymphocytic hypophysitis are discussed in Chapter 13.11.

Stroke

There is probably an increased incidence of stroke during pregnancy and the puerperium, although it remains rare. There are some causes of stroke which seem to be more common in pregnancy, but most cases are due to one of the usual causes of stroke in non-pregnant young women. Cerebral infarction due to large cerebral artery occlusion may be slightly more common. Possible explanations for this include the mild hypercoagulable state that develops in the later stages of pregnancy and persists for a few weeks afterwards, also the phenomenon of paradoxical embolism from the leg or pelvic veins. Cerebral infarction may occur as a result of hypoxia–ischaemia or disseminated intravascular coagulation in the context of major obstetric emergencies such as amniotic fluid embolism. Unless the cause is obvious, ischaemic stroke in pregnancy should be investigated comprehensively in the same way that it would in a young non-pregnant woman.

There is a rare syndrome of segmental cerebral vasoconstriction in the puerperium, which usually presents with headaches, seizures, or focal deficits (especially visual field defects). It has a predilection for the posterior cerebral circulation and can give rise to multiple infarcts or haemorrhages. The condition, generally termed postpartum angiopathy, can occur spontaneously but has also been described in women taking bromocriptine. There are reports of successful treatment with corticosteroids and vasodilators, but there have been no prospective studies. The condition can recur in subsequent pregnancies.

Cerebral venous thrombosis, like deep vein thrombosis of the legs, is commoner in the puerperium, and the two conditions may coexist. Classically it gives rise to headache and neurological deficit that evolves over several hours and may become bilateral, with seizures and papilloedema; other cases present with the syndrome of benign intracranial hypertension. The diagnosis can usually be made with magnetic resonance imaging, including magnetic resonance venography. Although venous infarcts frequently undergo haemorrhagic transformation, the currently available evidence favours treatment with heparin. If the patient survives then recovery may be surprisingly complete.

The incidence of aneurysmal subarachnoid haemorrhage is not increased during pregnancy but its management is difficult. In general, neurosurgical considerations take precedence over obstetric ones and the aneurysm is treated in the usual way. If it is not technically possible to isolate the aneurysm then conventional wisdom is to deliver the baby (once it is mature) by caesarean section, although there is no definite evidence to suggest an increased risk of rebleeding during vaginal delivery. Intracranial and subarachnoid haemorrhage from arteriovenous malformations is much less common but the same principles of management apply. Women with untreatable vascular malformations (including cavernomas) should be counselled about the increased risk of bleeding (perhaps due to a mixture of hormonal and vascular factors) throughout pregnancy.

Epilepsy

Most women with pre-existing epilepsy have no change in the frequency of their seizures during pregnancy, but some 30 per cent have more frequent seizures. These are often women whose epilepsy has been hard to control at other times. Anticonvulsant plasma levels tend to fall in the later stages of pregnancy through increased volumes of distribution and rates of elimination: consensus guidelines recommend that plasma levels are monitored routinely and dosage adjusted to keep these steady. This approach is not entirely foolproof because most laboratories are unable to measure the changes in protein binding that also occur during pregnancy, increasing the availability of free drug. If the dosage is increased prophylactically during pregnancy then it is important to remember to reduce the dosage again in the postpartum period.

An equally important reason for deteriorating control of seizures is lack of adherence to anticonvulsant therapy because of fear of teratogenic effects. This is best addressed by counselling well before pregnancy, which should include a discussion of the risks of uncontrolled epilepsy to both mother and fetus, although it must be admitted that this is made difficult by the lack of quantitative data. As always, the aim of treatment is to control the epilepsy using a single anticonvulsant in the lowest effective dosage, and it is reasonable to try to reduce or withdraw anticonvulsants prior to pregnancy if there is a chance that the epilepsy may have remitted. It is unwise to attempt this during pregnancy itself.

All the anticonvulsant drugs are either known teratogens or of unknown safety in pregnancy. Epilepsy roughly doubles the risk of fetal malformation and most of this risk seems to be due to the treatment rather than the epilepsy or its cause. This translates into an absolute risk in the region of 5 to 10 per cent, although many of these malformations are minor. The risk is greatest in women taking two or more anticonvulsants. In the case of more serious abnormalities, phenytoin, barbiturates, carbamazepine, and sodium valproate all appear to be associated with facial clefts, cardiac septal defects, and a pattern of craniofacial and digital dysmorphism known as the fetal anticonvulsant syndrome. Sodium valproate and to a lesser extent carbamazepine appear to be associated with neural tube defects. Some of these defects may be secondary to drug-induced folate deficiency and it is good practice to offer folate supplements (5 mg daily) routinely to all potentially fertile women who are taking anticonvulsants, especially in the 3 months prior to and the first trimester of any planned pregnancy. Carbamazepine is traditionally regarded as the safest of the anticonvulsants for which we have reasonable data, but the teratogenic effects of sodium valproate appear to be dose dependent and dosages of less than 1 g daily may be equally safe. This is important when treating women with conditions such as juvenile myoclonic epilepsy which respond much better to valproate than carbamazepine. Several registers are currently collecting prospective data on the safety of the newer anticonvulsants (lamotrigine, gabapentin, vigabatrin, topiramate, tiagabine, etc.) but, at the time of writing, these must all be regarded as of unknown safety in pregnancy.

In addition to worries about teratogenic effects (which arise in the first 8 weeks of gestation), there are growing concerns about the potential for anticonvulsants to produce more subtle adverse effects on brain development and the subsequent behaviour and intelligence of the child. Such effects have been demonstrated in relation to anticonvulsant polytherapy including barbiturates, and it is possible that they may occur with other drugs. Prospective studies are in progress, but at the moment there is no clear guidance for women with epilepsy or their doctors in relation to the magnitude of these risks.

Carbamazepine, phenytoin, and the barbiturates accelerate vitamin K metabolism and increase haemorrhagic risks. Again it is considered to be good practice to offer the mother vitamin K supplements during the last month of pregnancy and to give the baby vitamin K at birth.

Epilepsy presenting for the first time in pregnancy requires investigation in the same way as adult-onset epilepsy in general. Idiopathic epilepsy that only occurs in pregnancy (so-called gestational epilepsy) is rare. Women presenting with serial seizures or status epilepticus are particularly likely to have an underlying secondary cause such as eclampsia, stroke, tumour, or encephalitis. Epilepsy during labour is usually either iatrogenic (for example, omission of normal anticonvulsant therapy) or again symptomatic of serious intracranial disease. Eclampsia (see Chapter 13.4) is clearly the first consideration, but other possibilities include amniotic fluid embolism and cerebral venous thrombosis.

All the anticonvulsants pass into breast milk to some extent, but this need not prevent breastfeeding. Only the barbiturates occasionally cause problems with excessive sedation, but this small risk must be balanced against the problems of effectively withdrawing barbiturates by not breast-feeding. This can lead to the baby becoming irritable and jittery; impaired suckling and withdrawal seizures have also been reported.

Multiple sclerosis

Pregnancy raises complex issues for women with multiple sclerosis. Preconceptual considerations include the small risk (approximately 3 per cent) of their child inheriting the disease and the practical burdens that child care imposes upon a mother with existing and potentially progressive disability. Several epidemiological studies have shown that the incidence of relapses of multiple sclerosis falls during pregnancy itself, with a compensatory rise in the puerperium (with between 20 and 40 per cent of women reporting an exacerbation of symptoms.) It has been suggested that this reflects the production of pregnancy-associated proteins with immunosuppressive properties, such as α-fetoprotein, and changes in T-lymphocyte subsets. There is no evidence of any long-term detrimental effect on disability, and no evidence of any adverse effect from epidural anaesthesia or breastfeeding.

Relapses in pregnancy are treated in the normal way, with rest supplemented by a short course of oral or intravenous steroid if there is serious new disability. High-dose steroids given late in pregnancy can cause neonatal adrenal suppression. The manufacturers of interferon-β advise women taking it to avoid pregnancy and discontinue it during pregnancy and breastfeeding unless there are compelling reasons to continue with therapy.

Many women with multiple sclerosis have impaired bladder emptying, which predisposes to urinary tract infection. Severe spinal cord disease is a particular risk because it may mask the usual symptoms of urinary infection; regular urine culture is a sensible precaution. Paraplegia (from any cause) otherwise has little effect on pregnancy, but can lead to premature and unheralded labour, hence regular monitoring is needed in the third trimester. High spinal cord lesions can cause autonomic instability during labour; this can be blocked by careful regional anaesthesia.

Movement disorders

Pregnancy aggravates any tendency to chorea, an effect termed chorea gravidarum. This should not be regarded as a specific diagnosis, and unless there is a definite history of previous Sydenham's chorea it should prompt a search for all the usual causes of the condition, including thyrotoxicosis and systemic lupus erythematosus. Chorea can be florid and exhausting so that treatment with a small dose of a neuroleptic such as haloperidol may be required. Recurrence in subsequent pregnancies (or with the combined oral contraceptive) is common, perhaps because of the effects of oestrogens on the sensitivity of dopamine receptors.

Parkinsonism is rare in women of child-bearing age but tends to worsen slightly during pregnancy. Preconceptual counselling is difficult because there are no useful data in relation to the teratogenicity of the drugs used in young patients; levodopa has teratogenic effects in animals. Dystonic disorders also sometimes worsen in pregnancy, the effect being especially marked in dopa-responsive dystonia where an increase in levodopa therapy may be required. Wilson's disease is an exception and sometimes improves in pregnancy. Concerns about the potential teratogenic effects of therapy with penicillamine must be balanced against the risks of catastrophic neurological deterioration if therapy is abruptly withdrawn, although in the future treatments such as zinc may turn out to be a safe alternative.

Further reading

Aube M (1999). Migraine in pregnancy (review). *Neurology* **53** (4) (suppl. 1), 26–8.

Batocchi AP *et al.* (1999). Course and treatment of myasthenia gravis during pregnancy. *Neurology* **52**, 447–52.

Confraveux C *et al.* for the Pregnancy in Multiple Sclerosis Group (1998). Rate of pregnancy-related relapse in multiple sclerosis. *New England Journal of Medicine* **339**, 285–91.

Grosset DG *et al.* (1995). Stroke in pregnancy and the puerperium: what magnitude of risk? *Journal of Neurology, Neurosurgery and Psychiatry* **58**, 129–31.

Isla A *et al.* (1997). Brain tumour and pregnancy. *Obstetrics and Gynecology* **89**, 19–23.

Koch S *et al.* (1999). Long-term neuropsychological consequences of maternal epilepsy and anticonvulsant treatment during pregnancy for school-age children and adolescents. *Epilepsia* **40**, 1237–43.

Quality Standards Subcommittee of the American Academy of Neurology (1998). Practice parameter: management issues for women with epilepsy (summary statement). *Neurology* **51**, 944–8.

Rudnick-Schoneborn S *et al.* (1998). Different patterns of obstetric complications in myotonic dystrophy in relation to the disease status of the fetus. *American Journal of Medical Genetics* **80**, 314–21.

Shneerson JM (1994). Pregnancy in neuromuscular and skeletal disorders. *Archives of Chest Disease* **49**, 227–30.

13.13 The skin in pregnancy

F. Wojnarowska

The skin undergoes profound alterations during pregnancy as a result of endocrine, metabolic, and physiological changes. Some of these are trivial and chiefly cosmetic, producing no or minor symptoms, others can be distressing and/or of major medical importance. Pregnancy will profoundly modify expression of pre-existing skin disease and there are dermatoses which are specific to pregnancy: these are described in detail below.

Common skin changes in pregnancy

Vascular changes and lesions

There is increased skin blood flow during pregnancy and this makes the skin more prone to itch and to oedema, manifest as tightening of rings and shoes. Spider naevi and palmar erythema are common, as are haemangiomas. Pyogenic granuloma may develop: this is a benign tumour with a tendency ulcerate and to bleed, and is sometimes clinically confused with melanoma. It often recurs after local destruction.

Pigmentary changes and pigmented lesions

There is darkening of the nipples, genitalia, and linea alba. The unsightly and sometimes psychologically distressing facial pigmentation of melasma (chloasma) affects many women, is worse with sunlight, and can be reduced by the use of high protection factor (SPF 25) UVB and UVA sun screens.

Pigmented naevi can increase in number, size, and pigmentation. Melanoma may occur and is associated with a poor prognosis in pregnant women (see Section 23). Any rapidly changing, irregularly shaped, or irregularly pigmented mole should be biopsied to exclude a dysplastic naevus or melanoma.

Hair changes

There is diminished shedding of hair, due to prolongation of anagen. This is perceived as thickening of the hair, which increased sebum secretion makes appear more lustrous. The synchronized shedding after parturition gives rise to the distressing postpartum telogen effluvium. Hirsutism may begin or worsen in pregnancy as there is an associated increase in androgens.

Pilosebaceous changes

The increased oestrogens of pregnancy usually improve acne, but there may be worsening of acne in some unfortunate patients, and the entire skin is usually greasier.

Striae

Striae on the breasts and abdomen are very common in pregnancy, but do not necessarily relate to either the total weight gain or the rate of weight gain. There is much individual variation.

Cutaneous infections

Candida of the vulva as well as the vagina may occur. Cutaneous and genital warts thrive in pregnancy. Treatment of genital warts is by physical destruction as podophyllin must not be used in pregnancy. Genital herpes simplex infections can pose problems as regards delivery during active infections.

The pregnancy dermatoses

There are five major dermatoses which occur in pregnancy, and some that can be precipitated by pregnancy.

Pruritus of pregnancy

Itching occurs in about 20 per cent of pregnancies. Sometimes this is in association with an inflammatory dermatosis. Often there are no physical signs, other than scratch marks, and iron deficiency must be excluded. In about 2 per cent of women itching is related to cholestasis of pregnancy, when it is termed pruritus gravidarum. The itching begins in the third trimester and affects the abdomen, palms, and soles. Liver function tests are abnormal and bile salts are raised. It resolves postpartum, but will recur in subsequent pregnancies.

Management consists of emollients and sometimes antihistamines. Chlorpheniramine is the one usually recommended for pregnancy. The non-sedating antihistamines are probably ineffective.

Polymorphic eruption of pregnancy (pruritic urticated papules and plaques of pregnancy)

This dermatosis affects 1 in 240 singleton pregnancies but is more common in multiple births, and is thus being seen more often in the context of *in vitro* fertilization. It is more common with a male foetus. The dermatosis usually begins in the third trimester and occasionally postpartum. It is most common in first pregnancies or the first multiple pregnancy.

The lesions usually begin in the striae on the abdomen and thighs, and then spread to the whole trunk and limbs, including the hands and feet. The lesions are raised red papules (Plate 1) and plaques, occasionally polycyclic, and rarely may blister on the lower legs. The itching can be very severe, preventing sleep. The histopathology shows oedema, perivascular lymphocytes, and eosinophils. Immunofluorescence does not demonstrate any circulating or bound immunoreactants.

The aetiology is unknown, but there is an association with a low serum cortisol. The increased frequency in multiple births may relate to the mechanical effect of the abdominal stretching or to an increased immune complex load.

Treatment is with reassurance and emollients, for example aqueous cream and 1 to 2 per cent menthol, is helpful, but is not always sufficient. Antihistamines and moderate to very potent topical steroids, which will have significant absorption (see Table 1), and occasionally systemic steroids or induction, may be required. The condition resolves over days to weeks

Table 1 Examples of topical steroids

Group	Generic name	Trade names
Mild	Hydrocortisone 1%	Numerous
Moderately potent	Hydrocortisone 1% with urea	Alphaderm, Calmurid HC
	Clobetasone butyrate	Eumovate
	Flurandrolone	Haelan
Potent	Betamethasone valerate	Betnovate RD, Betnovate
	Betamethasone dipropionate	Propaderm, Diprosalic, Diprosone
	Hydrocortisone 17-butyrate	Locoid
	Fluticasone propionate	Cutivate[a]
	Mometasone furoate	Elocon[a]
Very potent	Clobetasol propionate	Dermovate

[a] New topical steroids.

after delivery. It does not usually recur. The outcome of the pregnancy is not adversely affected.

Prurigo of pregnancy

This is may affect 1 in 300 pregnancies. It commences at the end of the second or beginning of the third trimester. The eruption is scattered over the abdomen and limbs, and comprises excoriated papules. There is intense pruritus. It is essential to make sure that iron deficiency is not a contributing factor.

Histopathology shows a perivascular infiltrate with thickened epidermis. Direct and indirect immunofluorescence are negative. Treatment is with reassurance and emollients, and if this is not sufficient, with antihistamines and moderate to very potent topical steroids or occlusive coal tar or icthapaste bandages, which can be applied over topical steroids to the limbs. The condition resolves in days to weeks after delivery. It does not usually recur.

Pruritic folliculitis

This is rare and most commonly affects pregnancies with a male foetus. The lesions are pruritic papules and pustules that present in the third trimester, affect the trunk, and may spread to the limbs. Topical steroids may be helpful. Pruritic folliculitis is associated with a low birth weight.

Pemphigoid gestationis (herpes gestationis)

Pemphigoid gestationis is the most severe of the pregnancy dermatoses. It occurs in 1 in 50 000 pregnancies. The name herpes gestationis is best abandoned as the herpes refers to the herpetiform grouping of the blisters rather than herpes infection. Pemphigoid gestationis commences from the second trimester onwards and quite often in the first week postpartum (range 5 weeks gestation to 4 weeks postpartum). It usually occurs in the first and subsequent pregnancies, although 8 per cent of pregnancies are skipped.

The eruption begins around the umbilicus and spreads to the whole trunk, limbs, hands, and feet, including the palms and soles, and rarely the face. The mouth and vulva may be involved. The eruption usually commences as an annular red raised plaque around the umbilicus. The lesions comprise annular lesions, papules, and plaques. Vesicles and blisters are seen (Plate 2). The mucosal lesions may be blisters or erosions. Pruritus is severe and sleep often impossible. Transplacental transmission to the fetus occurs in about 3 per cent of affected pregnancies, and the neonate develops transient self-limiting blisters (Plate 3).

Histopathology demonstrates eosinophilia, subepidermal blisters, and tear-drop vesicles within the epidermis, continuous with the subepidermal blisters. Direct immunofluorescence demonstrates that C3 component of complement and IgG1 are bound at the basement membrane zone of the dermoepidermal junction. The patient's serum has circulating IgG1 basement membrane zone antibodies that bind C3. These immunoreactants are also found at the basement membrane zone of the amnion (Plate 4). The

mothers have HLA DR 3, 4, and are C4 null, and there is an association with thyroid and less commonly other autoimmune disease.

The aetiology is only partially understood. The pathogenicity of the circulating basement membrane zone antibodies is demonstrated by transplacental transmission of the disease. The major target antigen is BP180/collagen XVII (chief epitope—the transmembrane NC16A domain) and BP230 is a further antigen. Both antigens are present in skin, mucosa, and amnion associated with the hemidesmosome and adhesion complex linking epithelium to dermis/mesenchyme, and are targets in other autoimmune blistering diseases. The placenta shows increased expression of antigen presenting cells, but it is unclear why breakdown of tolerance occurs, and why normal components of amnion and stratified squamous epithelium become antigenic.

Treatment with potent or very potent topical steroids and chlorpheniramine is sometimes successful, but usually systemic steroids, for example prednisolone 20 to 80 mg daily, are required, with the dose adjusted according to disease activity. There is usually a postpartum flare, necessitating increased steroids. The disease slowly resolves postpartum, but persists for several months. There is an increased incidence of premature births and small-for-dates babies. The classical teaching is that it recurs earlier and is more severe in subsequent pregnancies, but this has not always been our experience.

Dermatoses in response to pregnancy

Urticaria (hives) and dermographism (wealing in response to pressure, for example scratching) may be precipitated by pregnancy. Erythema multiforme due to pregnancy has been described.

Dermatoses and the effect of pregnancy

Atopic eczema

Atopic eczema is the commonest skin problem presenting in pregnancy. It can be severe and life ruining, and life threatening if secondary infection with herpes simplex (eczema herpeticum) or *Streptococcus* occurs. The effect of pregnancy on pre-existing atopic eczema is unpredictable: the immunosuppression can lead to improvement, but often there is deterioration of the eczema. The eczema becomes more widespread and may result in erythroderma in the most severe cases. Secondary infection with *Staphylococcus aureus* and *Streptococcus* is a frequent complication. The skin is red, dry, and scaly with areas of excoriation and thickening or lichenification.

Treatment is a major problem in pregnancy, as there is a dilemma in balancing the need for treatment with the wish to minimize the use of potent topical steroids which will be absorbed and may affect the foetus. The use of emollients may lessen the requirements for topical steroids, and steroids should be used in the minimum quantities and strengths necessary to control the disease (see Table 1). Many topical steroids contain anti-septics and antibiotics which will be absorbed and may be contraindicated in pregnancy. The sedating antihistamine, chlorpheniramine, may help with sleep. Secondary infection often requires systemic antibiotics such as erythromycin or flucloxacillin.

Psoriasis

Psoriasis may improve or deteriorate during pregnancy. Therapy poses special problems as all the systemic treatments are contraindicated: methotrexate is a folic acid antagonist, acitretin is teratogenic, ciclosporine results in intrauterine growth retardation, and psoralens with UVA are still not proven to be safe. Topical therapy with steroids should be avoided if possible. Coal tars and dithranol have been widely used in pregnancy but are not proven to be safe, and the new vitamin D analogues are not licensed for use in pregnancy. The ideal is minimum treatment, with emollients and if necessary UVB.

A severe form of pustular psoriasis, impetigo herpetiformis, may occur in pregnancy and is best managed with bedrest and emollients.

Autoimmune dermatoses in pregnancy

Cutaneous lupus erythematosus

Cutaneous lupus erythematosus does not seem to be adversely affected or improved by pregnancy. However such patients should be screened for anti-Ro and anticardiolipin antibodies etc. (see Chapter xxx), preferably prior to conception, to identify at-risk pregnancies.

Autoimmune bullous diseases

Linear IgA disease, an autoimmune blistering disease with IgA basement membrane zone antibodies, usually improves with pregnancy, such that some patients can discontinue their dapsone therapy. Despite the deposition of immunoreactants in the amnion basement membrane zone the fetus is not adversely affected. There is usually an exacerbation 3 months postpartum.

Pemphigus vulgaris, an autoimmune blistering disease with widespread mucosal and cutaneous erosions caused by antibodies to desmosomal components, can be transmitted across the placenta, with devastating results to the fetus. This does not occur in the related pemphigus foliaceus, which is endemic in Brazil.

Further reading

Collier P, Kelly SE, Wojnarowska F (1993). Linear IgA disease and pregnancy. *Journal of the American Academy of Dermatology* **30**, 407–12.

Holmes RC, Black MM, Dann J, *et al.* (1982). A comparative study of toxic erythema of pregnancy and herpes gestationis. *British Journal of Dermatology* **106**, 499–510.

Jenkins RE, Hern S, Black MM (1999). Clinical features and management of 87 patients with pemphigoid gestationis. *Clinical and Experimental Dermatology* **24**, 255–9.

Kelly SE, Wojnarowska F (1993). Pemphigoid gestationis. *European Journal of Dermatology* **4**, 16–20.

Muller S, Stanley JR (1990). Pemphigus: pemphigus vulgaris and pemphigus foliaceus. In: Wojnarowska F and Briggaman RA, eds. *Management of blistering disease*, pp 43–62.

Vaughan Jones SA, Hern S, Nelson-Piercy C, Seed PT, Black MM (1999). A prospective study of 200 women with dermatoses of pregnancy correlating clinical findings with hormonal and immunopathological profiles. *British Journal of Dermatology* **141**, 71–81.

13.14 Autoimmune rheumatic disorders and vasculitis in pregnancy

Catherine Nelson-Piercy and Munther A. Khamashta

Autoimmune diseases affect 5 to 7 per cent of the population, are commoner in women of child-bearing age, and are frequently encountered in pregnancy. Pregnancy is associated with suppressed cell-mediated immunity and enhancement of humoral immunity, but these changes revert postpartum accompanied by sudden reductions of oestrogen, progesterone, and cortisol levels. The postpartum period is therefore a time of susceptibility to autoimmune disorders and women who already have an autoimmune disorder may suffer disease exacerbation following pregnancy. Conversely, autoimmune diseases may remit or improve during pregnancy, but this is not a universal rule and autoimmune rheumatic/connective tissue diseases can flare or present in pregnancy with disastrous consequences. This chapter considers the relationship between pregnancy and rheumatoid arthritis, systemic lupus erythematosus (SLE), antiphospholipid syndrome (APS), vasculitides, and scleroderma, and how pregnancy affects treatment of these disorders. The management of these conditions during pregnancy provides the obstetrician and physician with particular challenges and concerns related to not only the mother but also the fetus.

Rheumatoid arthritis

The adult form of the disease is more common in women (female to male ratio = 3:1), and approximately 1 in every 1000 to 2000 pregnancies are affected.

Effect of pregnancy on rheumatoid arthritis

Up to 75 per cent of women with rheumatoid arthritis experience improvement during pregnancy. Originally it was thought that this was the result of raised cortisol levels but these do not correlate with symptoms. Another hypothesis is a maternal immune response to fetal paternally inherited HLA class II gene products, supported by the finding that maternal–fetal disparities for HLA DQA were observed in 78 per cent of women whose rheumatoid arthritis went into remission during pregnancy, but in only 25 per cent in those whose disease remained active. Other theories attribute the improvement to high oestrogen levels, although ethinyl oestradiol given to postmenopausal women with rheumatoid arthritis is not effective. Pregnancy specific proteins such as α_2-glycoprotein (PAG) have also been implicated, and in experimental models α_2-glycoprotein improves arthritis. Removal of immune complexes by the placenta is another postulated mechanism.

Improvement usually begins during the first trimester, when rheumatoid nodules may also disappear, but 90 per cent of those who experience remission suffer postpartum exacerbations. The largest study of disease activity in pregnancy in 140 women with rheumatoid arthritis confirmed improvement in joint swelling and pain in two-thirds of subjects by the third trimester. However, only a minority had no joints with active disease, disability as assessed by the Health Assessment Questionnaire changed little compared to prepregnancy, and only 16 per cent went into complete remission. Disease response in a previous pregnancy was predictive of response in the index pregnancy. An increase in the mean number of inflamed joints was seen postpartum, but this could not be predicted from previous puerperal relapse. In women without the condition, there is an increased incidence of rheumatoid arthritis onset in the postpartum period.

Effect of rheumatoid arthritis on pregnancy

Unlike SLE, there seems to be no adverse effect of rheumatoid arthritis on pregnancy, and neither the fertility rate or spontaneous abortion rate is significantly altered. However, the infants of woman who have anti-Ro antibodies are at risk of neonatal lupus (see below). Atlantoaxial subluxation is a rare complication of a general anaesthetic for a caesarean section, and very rarely limitation of hip abduction is severe enough to impede vaginal delivery. The main concerns relate to the safety during pregnancy and lactation of the medications used to treat rheumatoid arthritis, although only 20 to 30 per cent of pregnant women with rheumatoid arthritis will require medications to control flares or systemic disease.

Treatment of rheumatoid arthritis (and other rheumatic disorders) in pregnancy

Paracetemol should be the first line analgesic, and there are no known adverse effects in pregnancy. Aspirin and non-steroidal anti-inflammatory drugs (NSAIDs) are not teratogenic, but salicylates (in analgesic doses) and NSAIDs may increase the risk of neonatal haemorrhage via inhibition of platelet function. NSAIDs may also lead to oligohydramnios via effects on the fetal kidney, and as they are prostaglandin synthetase inhibitors may cause premature closure of the ductus arteriosus (because prostaglandin E_2 relaxation of pulmonary vessels is inhibited) with neonatal primary pulmonary hypertension. They are usually avoided in pregnancy, especially in the last trimester, but the risk to the ductus arteriosus may have been exaggerated since premature closure has not been encountered when indomethacin is used for the treatment of premature labour. Impairment of ductal flow is rare before 27 weeks and resolves within 24 h of NSAID discontinuation. Oligohydramios is also reversible. In occasional circumstances, and especially prior to 28 weeks gestation, NSAIDs may be used for control of arthritic pain if there are relative contraindications to steroids, for example in patients on heparin. They should be discontinued at least 6 to 8 weeks prior to delivery. The recently introduced cyclo-oxygenase type-2-selective (COX-2) NSAIDs, although currently contraindicated in pregnancy, have been reported to show only minor renal and no ductal effects on the fetus when used to prevent premature labour.

Corticosteroids may be continued during pregnancy and are preferable to NSAIDs if paracetemol is insufficient to control symptoms in the third trimester. Prednisolone is metabolized by the placenta and very little (10 per cent) active drug reaches the fetus, unlike dexamethasone and betamethasone which cross the placenta more readily. Exceedingly large doses of cortisone are associated with an increased incidence of cleft palate in rodents, and one case–control study has suggested an increased risk of cleft lip following first-trimester exposure. There are many other studies supporting no increased risk of abortion, stillbirth, congenital malformations, adverse fetal effects, or neonatal death attributable to maternal steroid therapy. However, in women with antiphospholipid syndrome, treated with high doses of prednisolone throughout pregnancy, an increased frequency of premature rupture of the membranes has been reported. Although suppression of the fetal hypothalamic–pituitary–adrenal axis is a theoretical possibility with maternal systemic steroid therapy, there is no evidence that this occurs. Corticosteroid usage in pregnancy increases the risk of gestational diabetes, infection, and osteoporosis. If a woman is on long-term maintenance steroids, parenteral steroids should be administered to cover the stress of labour and delivery. Prednisolone is safe in breast-feeding mothers since <10 per cent of active drug is secreted into breast milk.

The alkylating agents cyclophosphamide and chlorambucil, and the folic acid antagonist methotrexate, are all teratogenic and fetotoxic and are contraindicated in pregnancy and lactation. Methotrexate should be discontinued at least 3 months prior to conception and folic acid supplementation given preconceptually. Azathioprine, the commonest cytotoxic used in rheumatoid arthritis and SLE, seems safe based on its successful use in large numbers of renal transplant mothers and women with SLE. However, neonatal immunosuppression has been noted and conflicting information exists regarding breast feeding while taking azathioprine. Cyclosporin has been associated with a higher rate of intrauterine growth restriction (IUGR) than azathioprine in renal transplant patients and should be avoided if possible.

D-penicillamine, a chelating agent used particularly in the management of the extra-articular features of rheumatoid arthritis, crosses the placenta and is teratogenic, with a 5 per cent risk of congenital collagen defect. It should therefore be stopped before conception in women with rheumatic diseases, but continued use is crucial for successful outcome of pregnancy in Wilson's disease, where there are about 90 reported cases. Gold salts are teratogenic in animals, but there is no conclusive evidence for such an effect in humans. They can therefore be continued during pregnancy if they are controlling disease, although most would avoid initiation of treatment during pregnancy.

Antimalarials, such as hydroxychloroquine, used in rheumatoid arthritis and particularly in subacute cutaneous lupus, are safe in doses used for malarial prophylaxis. There has been concern over larger doses, when concentration in the fetal uveal tract may result in retinopathy. Nevertheless, in 215 pregnancies in women exposed to chloroquine the congenital abnormality rate was no higher than background. There is also increasing experience of the use of hydroxychloroquine in pregnant women with SLE. It seems to have no adverse effect on the neonate, and should be continued through pregnancy for two reasons. Firstly, cessation may precipitate a flare of lupus. Secondly, it has a very long half-life, such that discontinuation will not prevent fetal exposure.

Sulphasalazine, another second-line agent, has been used extensively in the treatment of inflammatory bowel disease in pregnancy and appears to be safe. It may be continued throughout pregnancy, although concomitant folate supplementation is recommended.

Systemic lupus erythematosus (SLE)

SLE is much more common in women than men (ratio 9:1), particularly during the child-bearing years, (ratio 15:1). The prevalence is approximately 1 per 1000 women and may be increasing. The fundamental issues concerning the effect of SLE on pregnancy are the presence or absence of anti-Ro/La and antiphospholipid antibodies (see below), the activity of the disease, and the presence or absence of hypertension and renal involvement.

Effect of pregnancy on SLE

SLE flares may be difficult to diagnose during pregnancy since many features such as hair fall, oedema, facial erythema, fatigue, anaemia, raised ESR, and musculoskeletal pain also occur in normal pregnancy. Whether pregnancy exacerbates SLE and increases the likelihood of flare postpartum is controversial. Six controlled studies have addressed this issue. These differ in the ethnicity of the populations, the criteria for flare, and the SLE activity scales employed. Three found no increased risk of deterioration in pregnancy; three, including the most recent study from St Thomas', suggested that SLE was more likely to flare during pregnancy and the puerperium. The studies are consistent in showing that 58 to 70 per cent of women flare during pregnancy. Steroids do not prevent these flares, and it is not our practice to prescribe prophylactic steroids or increase steroid dosage prophylactically during pregnancy or postpartum.

In 242 pregnancies in 156 women with lupus nephritis, kidney function was unchanged in 59 per cent, transiently impaired in 30 per cent, and permanently deteriorated in 7.1 per cent. As in all types of renal disease, there is a greater risk of deterioration in patients with hypertension, heavy proteinuria, and high baseline serum creatinine.

Effect of SLE on pregnancy

SLE is associated with increased risks of spontaneous abortion, fetal death, pre-eclampsia, preterm delivery, and IUGR. A prospective study of 108 pregnancies in 90 lupus patients showed a live birth rate of 82 per cent, a 43 per cent incidence of prematurity, and a 30 per cent incidence of IUGR. Most of the fetal losses were in association with secondary antiphospholipid syndrome. Pregnancy outcome is particularly affected by renal disease. Even quiescent renal lupus is associated with increased risk of fetal loss, pre-eclampsia, and IUGR, particularly if there is hypertension or proteinuria. For women with SLE in remission, and without hypertension, renal involvement, or the antiphospholipid syndrome, the risk of problems in pregnancy is probably no higher than in the general population.

Management of SLE in pregnancy

When possible, this should begin with preconception counselling. Knowledge of the anti-Ro/La antiphospholipid antibody, and renal and blood pressure status allows prediction of the risks to the woman and her baby (see below). The outlook is better if conception occurs during remission. Pregnancy care is best undertaken in multidisciplinary, combined clinics where physicians and obstetricians can monitor disease activity and fetal growth and uterine and umbilical artery Doppler blood flow regularly.

Disease flares must be actively managed. Corticosteroids are the drug of choice (see above for discussion of anti-inflammatory agents and immunosuppression in pregnancy). Hydroxychloroquine should be continued since stopping may precipitate flare. Azathioprine is also usually continued, since this acts as a 'steroid-sparing' agent. Differentiation of active renal lupus from pre-eclampsia is notoriously difficult and the two conditions may be superimposed. Since hypertension, proteinuria, thrombocytopenia, and renal impairment are all features of pre-eclampsia, diagnosis of lupus flare requires other features, such as a rising anti-dsDNA antibody titre, the presence of red blood cells or cellular casts in the urinary sediment, or a fall in complement levels. Elevation of complement split products, particularly Ba and Bb, often accompanies flares so high ratios of CH50/Ba may differentiate pre-eclamptics from those with active lupus. The only definitive investigation to reliably differentiate a renal lupus flare from pre-eclampsia is renal biopsy, but this is rarely undertaken in pregnancy.

For control of hypertension, the drug of choice is methyl dopa, with nifedipine or hydrallazine as second-line agents.

Neonatal lupus syndromes

These conditions are models of passively acquired autoimmunity. Autoantibodies directed against cytoplasmic ribonucleoproteins Ro and La cross the placenta causing immune damage in the fetus. Several clinical syndromes have been described, of which cutaneous neonatal lupus is the most common, and congenital heart block is the most serious. They rarely coexist. More than 90 per cent of mothers of affected offspring have anti-Ro antibodies, and 50 to 70 per cent anti-La antibodies. About 30 per cent of patients with SLE are anti-Ro positive, and in such women the risk of transient cutaneous lupus is about 5 per cent and the risk of congenital heart block about 2 per cent. The risk of neonatal lupus is increased if a previous child has been affected, rising to 16 per cent with one affected child and 50 per cent if two children are affected. It is important to recognize that not all Ro-positive mothers of neonates with congenital heart block have SLE. A large proportion are asymptomatic, but 48 per cent of these developed symptoms of connective tissue disease in a mean of 2.6 years in one study. Mothers of babies with neonatal lupus have a higher frequency of HLA-DR3, often with A1 and B8. There is no correlation between the severity of maternal disease and the incidence of neonatal lupus.

The cutaneous form of neonatal lupus usually manifests in the first 2 weeks of life. The infant develops typical geographical skin lesions similar to those of adult subacute cutaneous lupus, usually of the face and scalp, which appear after sun or UV light exposure. The rash disappears spontaneously within six months, suggesting a direct antibody-mediated mechanism. Residual hypopigmentation or telangiectasia may persist for up to 2 years, but scarring is unusual. Sunlight and phototherapy should be avoided.

Congenital heart block appears *in utero*, usually around 18 to 20 weeks, and may be fatal. The mechanism of damage is not fully understood. There is no treatment that reverses congenital heart block, although salbutamol given to the mother may be beneficial if bradycardia is causing fetal heart failure. Dexamethasone and plasmapheresis have been used to treat non-immune hydrops resulting from myocarditis and pericarditis, but have no effect on the conduction defect. Perinatal mortality is increased with one-fifth of affected children dying in the early neonatal period, but most infants who survive this period do well, although two-thirds require pacemakers.

Antiphospholipid syndrome

Anticardiolipin antibodies and lupus anticoagulant (LA) are overlapping subsets of antiphospholipid antibodies. The combination of either of these with one or more of the characteristic clinical features (thrombosis, recurrent pregnancy loss, or adverse pregnancy outcome—premature birth before 34 weeks due to pre-eclampsia or IUGR) is known as the antiphospholipid syndrome (APS). Other associated features include thrombocytopenia and haemolytic anaemia, livedo reticularis, cerebral involvement (particularly epilepsy, cerebral infarction, chorea, and migraine), heart valve disease (particularly of the mitral valve), systemic and pulmonary hypertension, and leg ulcers. APS was first described in patients with SLE, but it is now recognized both that most patients with APS do not fulfil the diagnostic criteria for SLE, and that those with primary APS do not usually progress to SLE. Although the clinical features of primary and SLE-associated APS are similar, and the antibody specificity is the same, the distinction is important, and patients with primary APS should not be labelled as 'lupus'.

Recurrent pregnancy loss, typically in the second trimester, is one of the most consistent features of APS. Fetal death is typically preceded by IUGR, oligohydramnios, and features of pre-eclampsia. Fetal loss represents one part of a spectrum of fetal compromise and a wide range of pregnancy morbidity has been reported in APS including recurrent first trimester miscarriage, second and third trimester loss, severe early-onset pre-eclampsia, IUGR, placental abruption, and prematurity. Since the classification criteria for APS have recently been amended, a patient with adverse pregnancy outcome may now be labelled as APS without a history of fetal loss. The risk of fetal loss is directly related to antibody titre, particularly the IgG anticardiolipin antibodies, although many women with a history of recurrent loss have only IgM antibodies. Quantifying the risk is difficult, and the presence of antiphospholipid antibodies does not preclude successful pregnancy. The antibodies should be regarded as markers for a high-risk pregnancy, but previous poor obstetric history remains the most important predictor of fetal loss in these women.

The prevalence of antiphospholipid antibodies in the general obstetric population is low (<2 per cent), so universal screening is not warranted. However, the prevalence of antiphospholipid antibodies is increased in women with pregnancy complications including severe early-onset pre-eclampsia, abruption, intrauterine fetal death, or IUGR without hypertension. In one study, 29 per cent of women with severe early-onset pre-eclampsia were found to have anticardiolipin antibodies compared with 2 per cent of controls.

The pathogenesis of fetal loss in these patients is not fully understood, but there is typically massive infarction and thrombosis of the placental and decidual vessels, probably secondary to spiral artery vasculopathy. One hypothesis is that anticardiolipin antibodies cause thrombosis by binding to co-factor β_2-glycoprotein, an endogenous coagulation inhibitor. Platelet deposition and prostanoid imbalance may be implicated, as they might be in pre-eclampsia.

Studies on pregnancy outcome in women known to have APS show differing rates of obstetric complications depending on their presentation. Those found to have APS as a result of recurrent miscarriage have lower rates of complications (see Table 1) than those discovered because of late losses, thrombosis, or other systemic manifestations.

Management of antiphospholipid syndrome in pregnancy

The management of pregnancy in women with APS is the subject of much debate. Aspirin inhibits thromboxane and may reduce the risk of vascular thrombosis, but its use as a single agent in APS pregnancy has only been subjected to randomized clinical trial in low-risk women. It was not found to be beneficial. There are several non-randomized studies in women with fetal loss suggesting that it is effective, and it can prevent pregnancy loss in experimental APS mice. Most centres now advocate low-dose aspirin (75 mg) for all women with APS, some even prior to conception, in the belief that the placental damage occurs early in gestation, and that aspirin prevents failure of placentation. We also advocate intra and postpartum (3–5 days) prophylaxis with heparin, especially in the event of caesarean section.

APS is the most frequent cause of acquired thrombophilia. However, unlike the congenital thrombophilias, thrombosis can be arterial or venous, and affects vessels of all sizes. The risk of recurrent thrombosis in patients with APS may reach 70 per cent, and women with APS and previous thromboembolism are at extremely high risk in pregnancy and the puerperium. Warfarin should be stopped and heparin started before 6 weeks gestation to avoid warfarin embryopathy. Subcutaneous unfractionated

Table 1 Pregnancy complications in different populations of women with antiphospholipid syndrome

	Study			
	Utah[a]	St. Thomas'[b]	Liverpool[c]	St. Mary's[d]
Pregnancies (n)	82	60	53	150
Population	Predominantly late loss/ thrombosis/SLE	Predominantly late loss/ thrombosis/ SLE	Predominantly recurrent miscarriage	All recurrent miscarriage
Pre-eclampsia (%)	51 (severe 27%)	18	3	11
IUGR (%)	31	31	11	15
Preterm delivery (%)	22	43	8	24

[a]Ware-Branch 1992; [b]Lima 1996; [c]Granger 1997; [d]Backos 1999

(10 000 u twice daily) or low-molecular weight heparin (enoxaparin 40 mg once daily; dalteparin 5000 once daily-twice daily) should be continued intrapartum and postpartum until warfarin has been reintroduced. It is occasionally necessary to use warfarin in women with previous arterial thromboses if heparin proves inadequate to prevent further transient ischaemic events.

Opinion is divided about the best antenatal therapy for those with recurrent pregnancy loss, but without a history of thromboembolism. Treatment with high-dose steroids (in the absence of active lupus) to suppress lupus anticoagulant and anticardiolipin antibodies, in combination with aspirin, was initially recommended because of improved (50 per cent) fetal survival compared to historical controls. However, high doses of prednisolone caused considerable maternal morbidity, and subsequent studies have failed to demonstrate better fetal outcome. Whether this can be improved by adding heparin to low-dose aspirin in women with recurrent miscarriage but without a history of thrombosis has been the subject of several studies, but remains controversial. Many centres have traditionally reserved the addition of heparin for those women with previous late losses or intrauterine deaths, and using such strategies live birth rates of 70 to 75 per cent can be achieved. However, two studies in different populations of women have suggested that aspirin and heparin can improve the live birth rate from about 40 per cent to about 70 to 80 per cent in woman with a history of recurrent miscarriage. In both, the excess losses in the aspirin alone group occurred prior to 13 weeks, after which outcomes were similar. This suggests that the beneficial effects of heparin occur before 13 weeks and raises the possibility that heparin may be stopped after this time if there is no history of thrombosis or a late loss. A more recent randomized controlled trial demonstrated no increase in live birth rate with aspirin and LMWH compared to aspirin alone.

Immunosuppression with azathioprine, intravenous immunoglobulin, and plasmapheresis have all been tried, but the numbers treated do not allow firm conclusions regarding efficacy. Trials of intravenous immunoglobulin in recurrent miscarriage have been stopped prematurely because of its cost and lack of obvious benefit.

Pregnancy complicated by APS requires expert care and a team approach by obstetricians, physicians, and haematologists. Close monitoring of both mother and fetus is essential. Ultrasound monitoring of fetal growth and uteroplacental blood flow is crucial, allowing for timely delivery. Uterine artery waveforms are assessed at 20 and 24 weeks gestation and those pregnancies with evidence of an early diastolic notch are monitored very closely with 2-weekly growth scans because of the high risk of IUGR. Where there are no notches, we recommend 4-weekly assessment of growth and amniotic fluid volume. Doppler flow studies of the umbilical artery may be used, as in other pregnancies at high risk of fetal compromise through uteroplacental insufficiency.

Vasculitis

Since the primary vasculitides occur principally in the post child-bearing years and are commoner in men, pregnancy is very uncommon in patients with Wegener's granulomatosis, polyarteritis nodosa (PAN), or Churg–Strauss vasculitis. Less than 50 pregnancies have been reported in total. In general, maternal and fetal outcome are dependent on disease activity. Reported cases would suggest that disease onset or flare is more likely during pregnancy or postpartum. Maternal death occurred in two of 20 pregnancies in women with Wegener's granulomatosis, none of seven pregnancies (in four women) in Churg–Strauss, and in all of seven women in whom PAN was diagnosed during pregnancy. Fetal outcome is usually successful in controlled or remitted disease, but active disease is associated with fetal demise. In the 20 pregnancies in Wegener's granulomatosis there were two intrauterine fetal deaths (both in women with active disease), four elective terminations, and the other infants survived. Despite the high maternal postpartum mortality in PAN, there were only two intrauterine deaths and nine surviving infants. Neonatal cutaneous vasculitis, resolving

with treatment, has been reported in infants of mothers with cutaneous PAN.

In view of the significant maternal and fetal morbidity and mortality associated with active disease, it is important to adopt an aggressive approach to treatment with immunosuppression in the case of flare. Azathioprine is the drug of choice in pregnancy if immunosuppression with corticosteroids is insufficient, but life-threatening disease may necessitate the use of pulsed cyclophosphamide despite the risks.

Scleroderma

Although a rare disease, scleroderma is more common in women (female to male ratio = 3:1) and this is especially so during the reproductive years (10:1). Previously it was thought that fertility may be impaired in women with or destined to develop scleroderma, but more recent studies have demonstrated normal pregnancy rates in scleroderma. Indeed pregnancy may have an aetiological role: persistent fetal microchimerism being more common in women with scleroderma than controls, leading to the hypothesis that fetal antimaternal graft–versus–host reactions may be involved in pathogenesis (see Chapter 18.11.3).

Effect of pregnancy on scleroderma

Early case reports highlighted the risk from renal crises, even in women without a prior history of renal involvement, and renal disease was the commonest cause of death in these pregnancies. However, more recent case series and case–control studies have reported far fewer renal crises. A retrospective study of 86 pregnancies found no change in symptoms in 88 per cent, improvement in 5 per cent, and deterioration in 7 per cent. Ten-year survival of women with scleroderma, with or without pregnancy, was similar. A prospective series of 89 pregnancies in 58 women found stability in 61 per cent, improvement in 20 per cent, and worsening in 19 per cent. There were only five cases of renal crisis in these two series and all occurred in women with early diffuse scleroderma—the highest risk group for renal crises even outside pregnancy. Progressive cutaneous disease is unusual during or immediately after pregnancy. Raynaud's phenomenon usually improves in pregnancy as a result of vasodilation and increased blood flow. Reflux and oesophagitis often worsen related to the decreased lower oesophageal tone of pregnancy. Arthralgias also worsen. There is no evidence that pregnancy worsens cardiac or respiratory disease, although those with severe pulmonary fibrosis and pulmonary hypertension are at extremely high risk of postpartum deterioration, as with pulmonary hypertension from any cause.

In general, women with limited scleroderma without organ involvement do better than those with diffuse disease. The extent of diffuse disease and systemic involvement (particularly lung, cardiac, and renal) influences prognosis, but there are no absolute rules. Those with early (less than 4 years) disease, diffuse disease, or antitopoisomerase (anti-ScL-70) antibodies are at greater risk of having more active aggressive disease than those with long-standing disease and anticentromere antibodies. Women with renal involvement often have associated hypertension and rapid deterioration is possible.

Effect of scleroderma on pregnancy

Although early literature suggested an increased risk of miscarriage in scleroderma, case–control studies found no increase when women with scleroderma were compared to those with rheumatoid arthritis or normal controls. A more recent, prospective study did find a 22 per cent incidence of miscarriage (compared with 13 per cent in controls) in women with diffuse disease. There is an increased risk of premature delivery (24 per cent in limited disease and 33 per cent in diffuse disease, versus 5 per cent in controls) and IUGR, but overall success is now reported to be 70 to 80 per cent. The risks of adverse outcome are highest for women with early diffuse disease. There is no increased risk of pre-eclampsia in the absence of hypertension or renal involvement.

Management

Women should be assessed prior to conception for the extent of organ involvement. Those with renal impairment, severe cardiomyopathy, severe restrictive lung disease or pulmonary hypertension should be advised against pregnancy. Those with early diffuse disease should delay pregnancy until the disease stabilizes. Disease-remitting drugs such as D-penicillamine and cyclosporin A should preferably be discontinued before conception if disease is stable, although inadvertent first trimester exposure should not cause undue concern.

High-level, joint obstetric and medical care is appropriate with frequent and regular multidisciplinary monitoring of disease activity and fetal growth. Particular attention to blood pressure monitoring is essential: hypertension may indicate a renal crisis. Coincident renal impairment or microangiopathic haemolytic anaemia should prompt the initiation of an ACE inhibitor. These drugs have revolutionized the management and survival in renal scleroderma and should not be withheld in pregnancy. They are usually contraindicated, but in scleroderma the benefit outweighs the risk of fetal renal toxicity.

Management of scleroderma during pregnancy is largely symptomatic. Calcium antagonists may be used for Raynaud's phenomenon and histamine blockers and proton-pump inhibitors for reflux. NSAIDs are best avoided, as previously discussed, and corticosteroids (more than 15 mg/day) must also be avoided in early diffuse scleroderma since they can precipitate a renal crisis. Caution is needed if β-adrenergic agonists are required for preterm labour since scleroderma patients may have silent myocardial damage making them more vulnerable to ischaemia and pulmonary oedema. Venepuncture, venous access, and blood pressure measurement may be difficult because of skin or blood vessel involvement. General anaesthesia may be complicated by difficult endotracheal intubation, and regional anaesthesia may also be difficult. Early assessment by an obstetric anaesthetist is advisable and epidural anaesthesia and analgesia is encouraged as vasodilation improves skin perfusion of the extremities. Other measures to reduce problems related to Raynaud's phenomenon include warming of the delivery room and any intravenous fluids as well as socks and gloves.

Close observation must continue in the immediate postnatal period, particularly in those with cardiac, pulmonary, or renal involvement. The most recent data, although derived from retrospective postal questionnaire, suggest that outcomes are not significantly worse than controls, provided pregnancy is well-timed and carefully monitored. Clinicians are therefore becoming more optimistic in counselling women with scleroderma considering pregnancy.

Further reading

Antirheumatic drugs and immunosuppressive agents in pregnancy

Bermas BL, Hill JA (1995). Effects of immunosuppressive drugs during pregnancy. *Arthritis and Rheumatism* 38,1722–32. [Excellent in-depth review.]

Ostenson M (1998). Nonsteroidal anti-inflammatory drugs during pregnancy. Second international conference on rheumatic diseases in pregnancy. *Scandinavian Journal of Rheumatology* 27 (Suppl 107), 128–32. [Succinct review.]

Ostenson M, Ramsey-Goldman R (1998). Treatment of inflammatory rheumatic disorders in pregnancy. *Drug Safety* 19, 389–410. [Comprehensive review.]

Ramsey-Goldman R (1998). The risk of cytotoxic drugs during pregnancy. *Scandinavian Journal of Rheumatology* 27 (Suppl 107), 133–5. [Succinct review.]

Rheumatoid arthritis

Barrett JH *et al.* (1999). Does rheumatoid arthriitis remit during pregnancy and relapse postpartum? Results from a nationwide study in the United Kingdom performed prospectively from late pregnancy. *Arthritis and Rheumatism* 42, 1219–27. [Excellent report and review of the current knowledge.]

Nelson JL, Ostensen M (1997). Pregnancy and rheumatoid arthritis. *Rheumatic Disease Clinics of North America* 23, 195–212. [Comprehensive review.]

Silman AJ (1998). Reproductive events and the risk of development of rheumatoid arthritis. Second international conference on rheumatic diseases in pregnancy. *Scandinavian Journal of Rheumatology* 27 (Suppl 107), 113–5. [Succinct review.]

Systemic lupus erythematosus

Buchanan NMM *et al.* (1996). Hydroxychloroquine and lupus pregnancy: a review of a series of 36 cases. *Annals of the Rheumatic Diseases* 55, 486–8. [Largest reported series of hydroxychloroquine use in pregnancy.]

Khamashta MA, Hughes GRV (1997). Pregnancy in systemic lupus erythematosus. *Current Opinion in Rheumatology* 8, 424–9. [Comprehensive review.]

Khamashta MA, Ruiz-Irastoza G, Hughes GRV (1997). Systemic lupus erythematosus flares during pregnancy. *Rheumatic Disease Clinics of North America* 23,15–30. [Review of studies examining frequency of lupus flares in pregnancy.]

Lima F *et al.* (1995). Obstetric outcome in systemic lupus erythematosus. *Seminars in Arthritis and Rheumatism* 25, 184–92. [Report of large series of lupus pregnancies.]

Oviasu E, Hicks J, Cameron JS (1991). The outcome of pregnancy in women with lupus nephritis. *Lupus* 1, 19–25. [Important study suggesting that women with lupus nephritis should not be discouraged from becoming pregnant.]

Parke AL (1998). Antimalarial drugs, systemic lupus erythematosus and pregnancy. *Journal of Rheumatology* 15, 607–10. [Comprehensive review.]

Neonatal lupus

Tseng CE, Buyon JP (1997). Neonatal lupus syndromes. *Rheumatic Disease Clinics of North America*, 23, 31–54.

Waltuck J, Buyon JP (1994). Autoantibody-associated congenital heart block: outcome in mothers and children. *Annals of Internal Medicine* 120, 544–51. [Largest recorded series of congenital heart block, long-term outcome.]

Antiphospholipid syndrome

Backos M *et al.* (1999). Pregnancy complications in women with recurrent miscarriage associated with antiphospholipid antibodies treated with low dose aspirin and heparin. *British Journal of Obstetrics and Gynaecology* 106, 102–7. [A study describing obstetric outcome in different populations of treated APS pregnancies.]

Cowchock S, Reece A (1997). Do low-risk pregnant women with antiphospholipid antibodies need to be treated? *American Journal of Obstetrics and Gynecology* 176, 1099–100. [Randomized controlled trial of aspirin for asymptomatic aPL positive.]

Cowchock FS, Reece EA, Balaban D, Branch DW, Plouffe L (1992). Repeated fetal losses associated with antiphospholipid antibodies: a collaborative randomized trial comparing prednisone with low-dose heparin treatment. *American Journal of Obstetrics and Gynecology* 166, 1318–23. [Important trial showing aspirin and heparin is better than aspirin and prednisolone.]

Dekker GA *et al.* (1995). Underlying disorders associated with severe early-onset pre-eclampsia. *American Journal of Obstetrics and Gynecology* 173, 1042–8. [Excellent study showing that more than one-fifth of severe early-onset PET is aPL-related.]

Gordon C, Kilby MD (1998). Use of intravenous immunoglobulin therapy in pregnancy in systemic lupus erythematosus and antiphospholipid antibody syndrome. *Lupus* 7, 429–33. [Review article.]

Granger KA, Farquharson RG (1997). Obstetric outcome in antiphospholipid syndrome. *Lupus* **6**, 509–13. [A study describing obstetric outcome in different populations of treated APS pregnancies.]

Harris EN, Spinnato JA (1991). Should anticardiolipin tests be performed in otherwise healthy pregnant women? *American Journal of Obstetrics and Gynecology* **165**, 1272–7. [Large study proving that aPL screening is not warranted in healthy pregnant women.]

Kerslake S, Morton KE, Versi E, *et al.* (1992). Early Doppler studies in lupus pregnancy. *American Journal of Reproductive Immunology* **28**, 172–5. [Succinct review.]

Khamashta MA *et al.* (1995). The management of thrombosis in the antiphospholipid-antibody syndrome. *New England Journal of Medicine* **332**, 993–7. [Seminal study highlighting need for long-term warfarin in APS.]

Kutteh WH (1996). Antiphospholipid antibody-associated recurrent pregnancy loss: treatment with heparin and low-dose aspirin is superior to low-dose aspirin alone. *American Journal of Obstetrics and Gynecology* **174**, 1574–89. [A study suggesting aspirin and heparin superior to aspirin alone for first trimester miscarriage in APS.]

Langford K, Nelson-Piercy C (1999). Antiphospholipid syndrome in pregnancy. *Contemporary Reviews in Obstetrics and Gynaecology* , 11, 93-8. [Comprehensive review.]

Lima F *et al.* (1996). A study of sixty pregnacies in patients with the antiphospholipid syndrome. *Clinical and Experimental Rheumatology* **14**, 131–6. [A study describing obstetric outcome in different populations of treated APS pregnancies.]

Lockshin MD (1993). Which patients with antiphospholipid antibody should be treated and how? *Rheumatic Disease Clinics of North America* **19**, 235–47. [Comprehensive review.]

Lubbe WF *et al.* (1983). Fetal survival after prednisone suppression of maternal lupus-anticoagulant. *Lancet* **i**, 1361–3. [Seminal study showing improved pregnancy outcome with steroids.]

Nelson-Piercy C (1997). Hazards of heparin: Bleeding, allergy, heparin-induced thrombocytopenia, osteoporosis. In: Greer I, ed. *Thromboembolic disease in obstetrics and gynaecology.* Bailliere's Clinical Obstetrics and Gynaecology 11, pp 489–509. [Review of side-effects of heparin.]

Nelson-Piercy C, Letsky EA, de Swiet M (1997). Low molecular weight heparin for obstetric thromboprophylaxis: experience of 69 pregnancies in 61 high risk women. *American Journal of Obstetrics and Gynecology* **176**, 1062–8. [Largest reported series of low molecular weight heparin use in pregnancy.]

Rai R, Cohen H, Dave M, Regan L (1997). Randomized controlled trial of aspirin and aspirin plus heparin in pregnant women with recurrent miscarriage associated with phospholipid antibodies (or antiphospholipid antibodies). *British Medical Journal* **314**, 253–7. [A study suggesting aspirin and heparin superior to aspirin alone for first trimester miscarriage in APS.]

Vianna JL *et al.* (1994). Comparison of the primary and secondary antiphospholipid syndrome: a European multicenter study of 114 patients. *American Journal of Medicine* **96**, 3–9. [First study to compare primary and secondary APS.]

Ware-Branch D (1994). Thoughts on the mechanism of pregnancy loss associated with the antiphospholipid syndrome. *Lupus* **3**, 275–80. [Review of pathophysiology.]

Ware-Branch D *et al.* (1992). Outcome of treated pregnancies in women with antiphospholipid syndrome: an update of the Utah experience. *Obstetrics and Gynecology* **80**, 614–20. [A study describing obstetric outcome in different populations of treated APS pregnancies.]

Wilson WA *et al.* (1999). International consensus statement on preliminary classification criteria for definite antiphospholipid syndrome: Report of an international workshop. *Arthritis and Rheumatism* **42**, 1309–11. [Important paper discussing updated criteria for APS.]

Vasculitides

Lima F *et al.* (1995). Pregnancy in granulomatous vasculitis. *Annals of the Rheumatic Diseases* **54**, 604–6. [Case series and literature review.]

Ramsey-Goldman R (1998). The effect of pregnancy on the vasculitides. *Scandinavian Journal of Rheumatology* **27** (Suppl. 107), 116–7. [Succinct review.]

Scleroderma

Artlett CM, Smith B, Jimenez SA (1998). Identification of fetal DNA and cells in skin lesions from women with systemic sclerosis. *New England Journal of Medicine* **338**, 1186–91. [Microchimerism as a cause of scleroderma.]

Steen VD (1997). Scleroderma and pregnancy. *Rheumatic Disease Clinics of North America* **23**, 133–47. [Comprehensive review.]

Steen VD, Medsger TA (1998). Case-control study of corticosteroids and other drugs that either precipitate or protect from the development of scleroderma renal crisis. *Arthritis and Rheumatism* **41**, 1613–9. [Important study showing steroids may precipitate renal crisis.]

Steen VD, Medsger TA (1999). Fertility and pregnancy outcome in women with systemic sclerosis. *Arthritis and Rheumatism* **42**, 763–8. [Excellent and most recent study of this issue.]

13.15 Infections in pregnancy

Mark Herbert and Lawrence Impey

Introduction

Maternal immunity is suppressed in pregnancy and the fetal immune system is developmentally immature, thus infections in pregnancy can be devastating both for the mother, as is occasionally seen with varicella, and for the fetus, as is exemplified by congenital infections such as those caused by toxoplasmosis, syphilis, rubella, and cytomegalovirus (CMV).

Infections in pregnancy can be divided into four groups:

- Maternal illness made more severe by the pregnant state;
- Congenital infections acquired transplacentally, including *Toxoplasma gondii*, *Treponema pallidum*, rubella, CMV, *Listeria monocytogenes*, *Falciparum* spp., and *Trypanosoma* spp.;
- Fetal infection arising secondary to ascending maternal infection with preceding chorioamnionitis, caused by *Streptococcus agalactiae* and *Escherichia coli*;
- Neonatal sepsis acquired perinatally, such as HIV, HBV, and *Chlamydia trachomatis*.

Preterm delivery is an important cause of long-term handicap, and clinical evidence of infection in the placenta or neonate further increases the risk. Even with term delivery, maternal infection is associated with an increased rate of neonatal encephalopathy and cerebral palsy. This association is poorly understood. Chorioamnionitis is polymicrobial, and even *Candida* spp. have been implicated. It usually presents after preterm rupture of the membranes, but subclinical infection, usually ascending, may cause cervical changes and amniotic damage. Abdominal pain, fever, maternal and fetal tachycardia, and an offensive discharge are classic presentations, but chorioamnionitis is frequently asymptomatic in the early stages. Its management involves intravenous antibiotics and delivery, whatever the gestation.

In this chapter, we list the most important infective organisms in pregnancy, describe their maternal and fetal effects, and discuss their prevention, identification, and treatment. Detailed discussion of their pathology and features in adults is described elsewhere in the book.

Human immunodeficiency virus (HIV)

In the United Kingdom, the prevalence of HIV in pregnant women in inner London has risen from 0.04 per cent in 1989 to 0.4 per cent in 2000; in the rest of the United Kingdom, it is about 0.02 per cent. In parts of Africa, the seropositive rate among pregnant women exceeds 20 per cent, and an estimated 2.4 million HIV-infected women deliver every year.

Almost all HIV in infancy is acquired intrapartum or during breast feeding. Vertical transmission is highest in underdeveloped countries, if there are concomitant sexually transmitted diseases, in preterm delivery, and where the CD4 count is low and the viral load is high, as in early and late disease. Transmission rates are 15 to 20 per cent in Europe and North America and 25 to 35 per cent in Africa, India, and Thailand. Women with HIV are at greater risk of other sexually transmitted diseases and other coexisting disease, and consequently an increased vertical transmission rate

and poorer obstetric outcomes. One-third of infected neonates die in infancy.

In the United Kingdom, viral antigen ELISA screening for HIV is offered to all pregnant women. Ideal management requires interdisciplinary co-operation, screening for other sexually transmitted diseases, and regular CD4 counts. Depending on the resources available, there are several drug regimens that are known to decrease vertical transmission, including:

- The PACTG 076 protocol: oral zidovudine 100 mg five times per day from 14 to 34 weeks gestation until labour; intravenous zidovudine in labour, 2 mg/kg intravenously over 1 h followed by 1 mg/kg per h until delivery, and oral zidovudine 2 mg/kg four times per day given to the infant for 6 weeks. Oral zidovudine given only to mother in late pregnancy, 300 mg two times per day from 36 weeks gestation, then every 3 h throughout labour.
- The HIVNET regimen of a single oral 200 mg dose of nevirapine given to mothers in labour and a single 2 mg/kg dose given to the infant at 48 to 72 h old. In sub-Saharan Africa, 110 000 HIV-positive births could be prevented over the next 5 years by this regimen.

Zidovudine and lamivudine together, from early second trimester are probably better than AZT alone. Occasional severe adverse effects in neonates have been reported. Antiretroviral therapy, elective caesarean section, and avoidance of breast feeding together reduce vertical transmission to less than 1 per cent. It is uncertain if elective caesarean section confers benefit in addition to retroviral therapy if the viral load is less than 1000 HIV copies/ml blood. Even in women on treatment there is a small but definite transmission rate with breast feeding, which should be avoided.

Rubella

A world-wide pandemic of rubella between 1962 and 1964 hastened the impetus for developing a vaccine, which has had a dramatic impact on the incidence of the congenital rubella syndrome. However, 10 to 20 per cent of the adult population in North America remain susceptible and small outbreaks still occur.

The incubation period is 16 to 18 days (range 14–21). There is a 1 to 5-day prodrome of low-grade fever, headache, malaise, anorexia, mild conjunctivitis, coryza, sore throat, cough, and lymphadenopathy (suboccipital, postauricular, and cervical) before the onset of a rash that lasts for 1 to 5 days. Arthritis and arthralgia occur in up to 70 per cent of adult women after the rash. Rare complications are thrombocytopenia, acute postinfectious encephalitis, myocarditis, Guillain–Barré syndrome, relapsing encephalitis, optic neuritis, bone marrow aplasia, and progressive panencephalitis.

The major sequelae in the fetus are cataracts, deafness, mental retardation, and heart disease, especially pulmonary arterial hypoplasia, patent ductus arteriosus, and coarctation of the aorta. The risk of the congenital rubella syndrome is greatest in early pregnancy: 90 per cent of infants will be affected before 11 weeks gestation, falling to 24 per cent at 15 to 16 weeks gestation. At 25 weeks, transmission to the fetus is approximately

25 per cent rising to 100 per cent at term, but the congenital rubella syndrome does not usually occur after the first trimester. Embryo resorption may occur in very early gestation, or abortion in later pregnancy.

Parvovirus B19

Parvovirus B19 binds to the P antigen present on erythrocytes, erythroblasts, and myocardium and can cause fetal anaemia (haemolytic and aplastic) and cardiac dysfunction. About 0.25 per cent of pregnant women are infected, but respiratory-borne epidemics, particularly in spring, may increase this fourfold. Half of adults are immune. Pregnancy does not alter the symptoms; 20 per cent are asymptomatic; the rest have a rubelliform or characteristic 'slapped cheek' rash, and 80 per cent with rash have arthralgia or arthritis.

Infection in pregnancy carries a 9 per cent fetal mortality rate, mainly arising from infection before 20 weeks gestation, and 3 per cent develop hydrops fetalis characterized by generalized fetal oedema, particularly ascites (Fig. 1). Two-thirds recover without intervention.

Maternal anti-B19 IgM antibody indicates recent infection. Ascertaining fetal involvement is more difficult because invasive sampling has a 1 per cent miscarriage risk and fetal IgM is not present before 22 weeks gestation. PCR for viral DNA can be performed on amniotic fluid, fetal blood, or other tissue. After diagnosis, regular ultrasound examination aids identification of fetal disease, and *in utero* transfusion of red cell concentrate via the umbilical vein is used to treat severe fetal hydrops. Adverse fetal effects are very rare more than 18 weeks after infection, thus regular ultrasound examinations are continued for this period.

Herpes simplex virus (HSV)

Genital herpes is predominantly caused by HSV-2, but up to 30 per cent of cases are due to HSV-1. Approximately 20 per cent of women in developed countries have been infected with HSV-2, but 90 per cent of these give no history. Primary infection in pregnancy occurs in 2 per cent of susceptible women. This is usually asymptomatic, but primary herpes may be characterized by genital pain and ulceration, discharge, dysuria, lymphoedema, and systemic symptoms. Acyclovir may be helpful in reducing the severity and frequency of recurrences. A rare but severe manifestation of HSV infection in pregnancy is disseminated disease, with necrotizing hepatitis, thrombocytopenia, leukopenia, disseminated intravascular coagulopathy, and more than 50 per cent mortality.

True congenital HSV is extremely rare in the West, but is important because of very high neonatal mortality. It occurs in an estimated 1 in 200 000 pregnancies, accounting for 3 per cent of all neonatal herpes. Neonatal infection following viral shedding in labour occurs in up to 30/100 000 in parts of North America, but is often much lower in other countries. Transmission is almost 50 per cent in active primary infection, but nearer 1 per cent with active recurrent herpes because of passive fetal immunity. Most neonatal herpes occurs in women without a history.

Caesarean section is advised for intrapartum primary herpes. If vaginal delivery is unavoidable or the membranes have been ruptured for more than 4 h, then the infant should be treated with acyclovir. With recurrent active herpes the risks of caesarean section probably outweigh the benefits. Caesarean section is not indicated if lesions are absent at the onset of labour.

Cytomegalovirus (CMV)

CMV is the commonest congenital infection in developed countries. Seventy five per cent of pregnant women are immune; less in higher socioeconomic classes or in developing countries. Around 1 to 4 per cent of women acquire primary infection in pregnancy; this may be asymptomatic, but commonly produces an infectious mononucleosis-like illness.

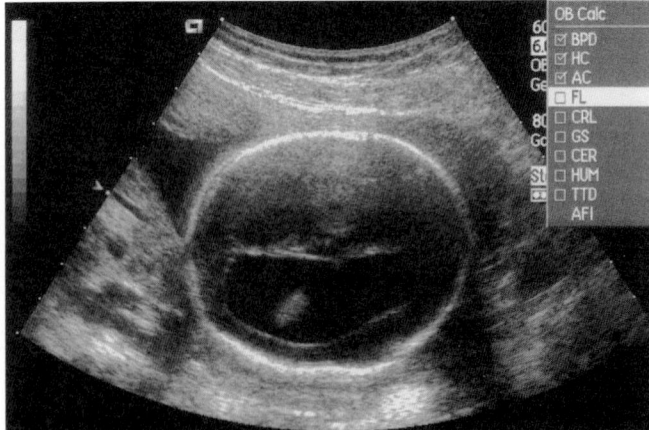

(a)

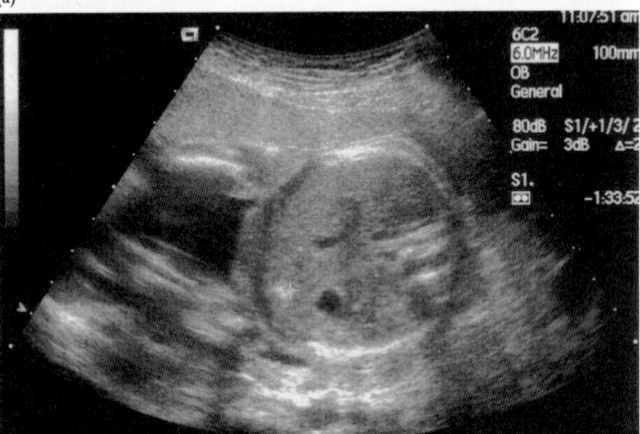

(b)

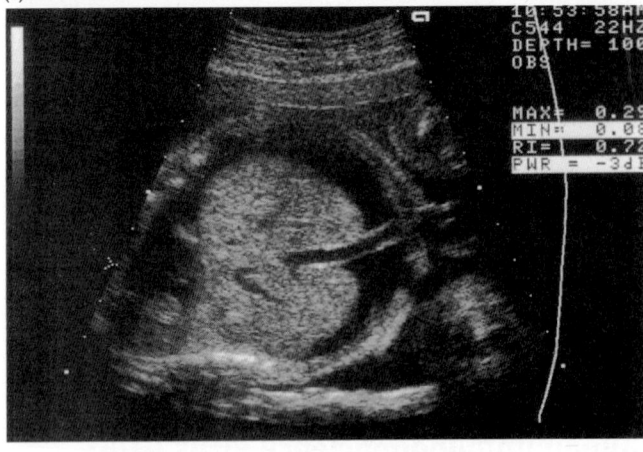

(c)

Fig. 1 Antenatal ultrasound scans: (a) fetal head showing ventriculomegaly secondary to congenital toxoplasmosis; (b) fetal abdomen showing intrahepatic calcification (marked with +) as seen in congenital varicella infection; (c) fetal abdomen showing ascites in parvovirus infection.

Transplacental transmission follows 40 per cent of primary infections and less than 1 per cent of secondary recurrences. After primary infection, 5 to 15 per cent of neonates are symptomatic, and of these more than 80 per cent develop severe neurological sequelae including mental impairment and sensorineural hearing loss. Even asymptomatic infants have a 5 to 15 per cent risk of hearing impairment. The outcomes of CMV infection in pregnancy are shown in Fig. 2.

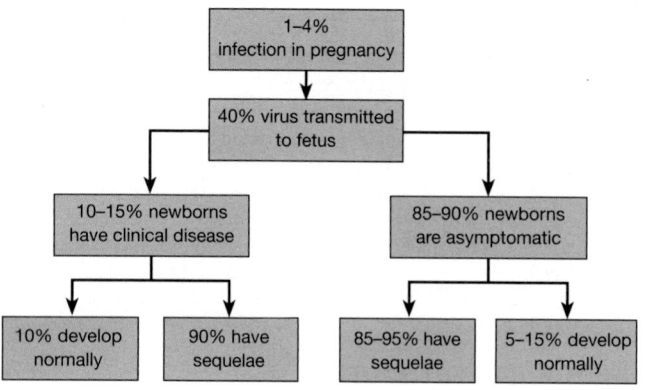

Fig. 2 The outcome from CMV infection in pregnancy.

In pregnant women, a diagnosis made by IgM or rising IgG titres can be confirmed by amniotic fluid PCR taken at least 6 weeks after maternal infection. High viral load and abnormal prenatal ultrasound findings such as intra-abdominal or cranial calcification, cerebral ventriculomegaly, and cardiomegaly, are associated with, but do not accurately predict, a poor long-term prognosis. Termination of pregnancy may be offered. There is no effective therapy. The chance of normal childhood development without evidence of fetal damage is approximately 75 per cent. Intravenous ganciclovir given to the infant reduces hearing loss in the most severely affected. CMV screening may be valuable in the future when orally available drugs are marketed.

Herpes zoster (VZV)

The varicella zoster virus incubation period is 10 to 21 days, infectivity being from 2 days before the rash appears to when all the vesicles are covered. Eighty five per cent of adults in the West are immune, infection only occurring in 1 in 2000 pregnancies. A much higher proportion of adults in developing countries are non-immune. The presence of maternal IgG indicates immunity, whilst IgM indicates primary infection. Invasive fetal testing is not often helpful.

Primary infection in pregnancy may be severe, with pneumonia in 10 per cent and occasional maternal death. Before 20 weeks, 2 per cent of fetuses develop the congenital varicella syndrome, characterized by neurological, optical, and limb anomalies. Ultrasound findings 5 weeks after infection include polyhydramnios and echogenic foci in the fetal liver (Fig. 1).

Varicella zoster immunoglobulin (**VZIG**) should be given, preferably within 72 h of contact, to pregnant women who are non-immune as determined by serology. Women who develop varicella after 12 weeks gestation should be given acyclovir, intravenously if pneumonia develops. Specialist referral is advised with respiratory symptoms, dense lesions, or if new vesicles are still appearing after 6 days. Neonatal zoster may occur if maternal infection occurs 5 days before to 2 days after delivery; this is associated with up to a 30 per cent neonatal mortality. Babies born to mothers who develop perinatal chickenpox should be given intramuscular VZIG.

Hepatitis B

Ten per cent of hepatitis B infected adults become chronic carriers, compared to 90 per cent of infants following vertical transmission. Detectable hepatitis B surface antigen (HepBsAg positive) in blood indicates infectivity and is present from 4 to about 24 weeks after infection; thereafter its presence is associated with chronic infection. Individuals with hepatitis B surface antibodies (HepBsAb positive) are immunologically cured. Detectable hepatitis B e antigen (HepBeAg positive) indicates high infectivity.

In the West, less than 1 per cent of pregnant women are HepBsAg positive, although the incidence is rising; in parts of Africa and Asia, the rate is 25 per cent. The risk of perinatal transmission relates to maternal viral antigen status. In HepBsAg positive/HepBeAg negative mothers the risk is 5 to 20 per cent, whereas in HepBsAg positive/HepBeAg positive it is 70 to 90 per cent. Targeted screening only identifies about half of chronic carriers, hence universal screening has been advocated in the West.

Vertical transmission can be reduced by more than 90 per cent by active immunization, with 0.5 ml hepatitis B vaccine, of all infants born to HepBsAg positive mothers, with additional passive immunisation (200 IU of hepatitis B immunoglobulin within 12 h of birth) for infants born to HepBeAg positive or HepBsAb negative mothers. Unfortunately, compliance with this regimen is often poor, and the WHO recommends universal vaccination in countries with high prevalence.

Hepatitis C

Approximately 3 per cent of pregnant women world-wide are infected with Hepatitis C. In inner London, the rate is 0.8 per cent, but it is 30 per cent in HIV positive women. Hepatitis C leads to chronic hepatitis in about 80 per cent. Progression is insidious and most pregnant women are asymptomatic. Liver transaminases may be normal, but if elevated, tend to reduce during pregnancy.

Vertical transmission of HCV occurs in approximately 6 per cent if HCV is detectable by PCR in the mother; otherwise the risk is negligible. Coexisting HIV infection increases the rate of vertical transmission to 23 per cent. Infected infants usually remain viraemic and prone to chronic hepatitis. Antibody levels are usually detectable within 3 months after infection. The ELISA has a sensitivity of 95 per cent, but should be supplemented by a recombinant immunoabsorbant assay (RIBA). PCR is used to confirm infection in infants.

Interferon-α reduces disease activity but is not recommended in pregnancy, although it may be used postpartum. Elective caesarean section, formula feeding, or administration of immune globulin do not reduce vertical transmission to the neonate.

Bacterial vaginosis

An overgrowth of anaerobic organisms such as *Gardnerella vaginalis* and *Mycoplasma hominis* causes this condition, which is characterized by excessive Gram-negative bacilli and cocco-bacillary organisms compared to lactobacilli on Gram staining. Bacterial vaginosis is not sexually transmitted, but is associated with sexually transmitted diseases and is rare before the onset of sexual activity. The prevalence varies from 5 to 20 per cent, depending much on the diligence with which the diagnosis is sought. Three of four Amsel's criteria are required for diagnosis: a thin white homogeneous discharge, clue cells, raised vaginal pH (>4.5), and a positive 'whiff test' (fishy odour when adding 10 per cent KOH to the discharge). At least 50 per cent of women with bacterial vaginosis have no symptoms, but an offensive, thin white discharge is often found. Its presence is strongly associated with a history of, and an increased risk for, late miscarriage and preterm birth. As prematurity is the major cause of neonatal mortality and morbidity in developed countries, the condition is extremely important. Bacterial vaginosis usually responds to metronidazole or clindamycin. Antibiotics reduce but do not eliminate the risk of prematurity. The role of screening for bacterial vaginosis in pregnancy is controversial.

Streptococci

Group A streptococci (*Streptococcus pyogenes*) remain an important cause of puerperal sepsis world-wide, but this is now rare in the West. Group B streptococci (*Streptococcus agalactiae*) usually cause less severe maternal disease. Overall, 12 to 26 per cent of pregnant women are colonized by

Group B streptococci, particularly in the urine, and its presence is associated with preterm delivery. Ascending infection with chorioamnionitis and fetal infection may occur following rupture of the membranes. Intrauterine infection may cause stillbirth.

Early-onset neonatal streptococcal sepsis has a mortality of 6 per cent and occurs in 0.5 to 3.7 per 1000 live births. Risk factors include prematurity, prolonged rupture of the membranes, intrapartum maternal fever, heavy colonization, low maternal antibody levels, and a previously affected infant. Although 70 per cent of neonates born to carriers are colonized, only 1 to 2 per cent will develop disease.

Intrapartum penicillin greatly reduces early-onset neonatal disease. Preventative strategies are based on risk factors, either alone or in conjunction with screening. With the former, women are treated if they have a previous history, intrapartum fever, are in preterm labour, or where the membranes have been ruptured for more than 18 h. By treating 18 per cent of women, 70 per cent of neonatal sepsis is prevented. In a combined screening and risk-based approach, third trimester vaginal and anal swabs are taken, and treatment of 27 per cent of all pregnant women can prevent 86 per cent of sepsis.

Listeria monocytogenes

Listeria monocytogenes is a Gram-positive bacillus that can cause serious disease in pregnant women, fetuses, and newborns. Infection is from salads contaminated with animal faeces, undercooked meats, unpasteurized milk, soft cheeses, and pates. In the United Kingdom, the incidence has been as high as 5 cases/100 000 live births, but world-wide the incidence has fallen as a result of public health campaigns about the likely source of infection.

Maternal disease manifests as bacteraemia, with fever, sore throat, headache, and chills. Diarrhoea, pyelitis, and back ache may occur. Symptoms generally recede without treatment, although a few mothers develop meningitis. Transplacental infection of the fetus is the most likely route of acquisition rather than ascending infection. Infection before 24 weeks gestation usually results in abortion; still birth or prematurity occurs after this gestation. The fetus may die, become macerated and then seed bacteraemia to the mother. Apparent meconium staining of liquor in preterm birth is highly suggestive of listeriosis. Two patterns of disease are seen, granulomatosis infantiseptica, in which the baby and the placenta are covered in miliary granulomata, and pneumonia without granulomata. Meningitis may coexist.

Listeria is resistant to all cephalosporins. The accepted treatment, based on animal model testing, is ampicillin with an aminoglycoside for synergy. There is little human data to support the view that ampicillin is better than penicillin G, but the usual practice is to change to ampicillin when listeriosis is confirmed.

Syphilis

The prevalence of *Treponema pallidum* infection in pregnancy is 0.2 per cent in London and 0.02 per cent in the rest of the United Kingdom, but in Africa, South East Asia, and Russia it is endemic. Pregnancy does not alter the clinical manifestations. Vertical transmission is predominantly transplacental, and occurs in up to 90 per cent of untreated women, particularly those with early disease. Most affected pregnancies result in congenital syphilis, miscarriage, preterm delivery, stillbirth, or neonatal death. Ultrasound appearances of the infected fetus may be normal or show hepatomegaly and other abnormalities. At birth, babies exhibit rhinitis, osteitis, and skin bullae. Hutchinson's triad of abnormal teeth, interstitial keratitis, and sensorineural deafness arise later in the untreated child.

Non-treponemal tests (e.g. VDRL) are usually employed for screening. Sensitivity is highest in secondary syphilis and lowest early in the infection, and false-positive results occur with concomitant infections or autoimmune disease. The diagnosis should be confirmed with a specific treponemal test (e.g. FTA-ABS). Screening in pregnancy is cost effective, even

where the disease is rare, and 121 women were identified by antenatal screening in the United Kingdom in 1994 to 97, meaning that 18 600 tests needed to be performed to detect one case.

Two intramuscular doses of benzyl penicillin, 2.4 MU 1 week apart, are given to treat syphilis in pregnancy. In true penicillin allergy, a 5 to 10-day regimen of high dose oral ceftriaxone is recommended. Treatment will prevent congenital infection in 98 per cent of cases. The rare Jarisch–Herxheimer reaction to treatment may precipitate preterm labour. VDRL titres should fall until undetectable or less than 1 in 4, otherwise retreatment is necessary.

Chlamydia trachomatis

The incubation period of *Chlamydia trachomatis* infection is 7 to 21 days. It is one of the commonest sexually transmitted diseases world-wide, and infects about 5 to 7 per cent of pregnant women. Endocervical swabs are best for screening, though urine testing may be easier. PCR has the highest sensitivity and specificity, followed by culture and then ELISA.

Chlamydia infection is mostly asymptomatic in pregnant women. Pelvic infection is very rare during pregnancy, but after delivery endometritis and salpingitis may lead to tubal damage and infertility, and 12 per cent of induced abortions are followed by pelvic infection. Maternal infection, particularly that which is recently acquired, is associated with prematurity, chorioamnionitis, and possibly stillbirth. Treatment reduces but does not eradicate these risks. Neonatal conjunctivitis occurs in up to 50 per cent exposed newborns and later-onset pneumonia in a smaller proportion.

Tetracyclines are contraindicated in pregnancy and erythromycin is not well tolerated. A single dose of azithromycin 1 g ensures compliance. Concerns about this drug in pregnancy remain unsubstantiated. Sexual contacts should be screened, and as reinfection rates are high, repeat testing is advised after at least 3 weeks to ensure a cure has been achieved. Screening or even prophylaxis of all mothers following abortion is cost effective.

Gonorrhoea

Neisseria gonorrhoea infection is endemic in many developing countries, but is declining in the West. Cervical culture will detect most infections, whereas PCR testing is expensive and does not enable antibiotic sensitivity testing. As with non-pregnant women, 80 per cent are asymptomatic in pregnancy. Pharyngeal and disseminated systemic infection with fever, rash, and septic arthritis are more common in pregnancy, but salpingitis is rare. Gonococcal cervicitis is associated with chorioamnionitis and a fourfold increase in prematurity. Ophthalmia neonatorum arises in 40 per cent if mothers are untreated. Gonococci have also been implicated in postpartum and postabortion endometritis and salpingitis. Penicillinase-producing strains are common, and treatment with 250 mg single dose intramuscular ceftriaxone, or 400 mg oral cefixime is recommended. Disseminated infection warrants intravenous therapy. The patient should be screened for other sexually transmitted diseases; indeed, antichlamydia therapy is often given at the same time. A test of cure should be taken at least 3 days after antibiotics.

Mycobacterium tuberculosis

In 1990, the WHO estimated that 90 million people developed tuberculosis and 30 million died from it. The highest rates of infection are in young adults, hence exposure during pregnancy must be common.

The pathogenesis and course are similar in pregnancy as in women who are not pregnant. The main additional concern is spread to the fetus, either through maternal disseminated disease and transplacental spread, or through direct extension of maternal genitourinary tuberculosis. Genital

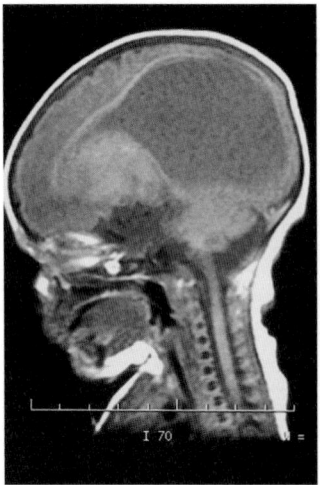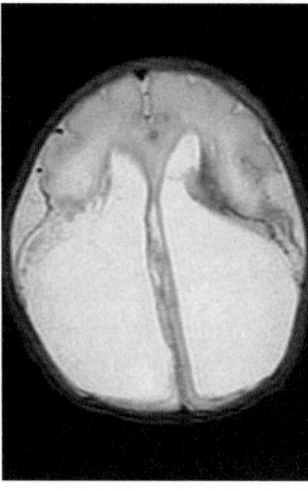

Fig. 3 MRI head of a 20-day-old baby with congenital toxoplasmosis, showing severe ventriculomegaly from hydrocephalus.

tuberculosis often has a long and indolent course with potential involvement of the fallopian tubes (90–100 per cent of women with genital infection), uterus (50–60 per cent), ovaries (20–30 per cent), and cervix (5–15 per cent). Genital infection is more likely to manifest as sterility and therefore is unusual as a cause of congenital infection.

Chemotherapy of tuberculosis during pregnancy provides the same excellent outlook as treatment in any other person. Providing proper treatment is received, there is no adverse effect of pregnancy, birth, the postpartum period, or lactation on the course of tuberculosis, and tuberculosis has little effect on the pregnancy outcome. Pregnancy is an opportunity to screen for tuberculosis. Women coinfected with HIV may have suppressed skin test reactivity and there is good argument for thoroughly investigating these women in pregnancy when they opportunistically present to health carers.

Congenital tuberculosis is very rare, but its incidence is increasing because of coinfection with HIV in pregnancy.

Toxoplasmosis

Toxoplasma gondii is a protozoan parasite acquired from eating uncooked meat or contaminated salad. The incubation period is 5 to 18 days. The prevalence of congenital toxoplasmosis is less than 0.1 per cent in most parts of the developed world.

Toxoplasmosis is frequently asymptomatic, but 10 to 20 per cent of mothers have lymphadenopathy or a flu-like episode. Microcephaly, hydrocephalus (Figs 1 and 3), cerebral cystic lesions and calcification, and chorioretinitis are the severe sequelae in the fetus, leading to mental retardation and blindness. The risk of vertical transmission increases with gestation, but the severity of disease decreases, hence the highest risk for congenital toxoplasmosis with poor outcome is when maternal infection occurs between 10 to 24 weeks gestation. Congenital toxoplasmosis may rarely result from maternal infection up to 6 months prior to conception.

Diagnosis is difficult because serological tests have poor sensitivity, so much so that in proven cases no antibody may be detectable. Conversely, IgM may persist for months after infection and its identification should prompt a repeat test 3 weeks later. Screening is not advised in low prevalence countries. Confirmation of fetal infection is best achieved using PCR of amniotic fluid.

Treatment in pregnancy is with 1 g spiramycin three times per day until the diagnosis has been definitively made, but this is not of proven benefit in established congenital toxoplasmosis. Most authorities are now using pyrimethamine (50 mg/day), sulfadiazine (1 g three times/day), and folinic acid (50 mg/week) until delivery, but not starting this regimen until the second trimester onwards.

Cerebral ventriculomegaly or intracranial calcification on antenatal ultrasound examination may predict a worse outcome, and termination of pregnancy may be offered; yet normal development, including reversion of brain calcification and hydrocephalus, are possible following treatment of the neonate with pyrimethamine and sulfadiazine for 1 year.

Malaria

Millions of women world-wide are at risk of malaria during pregnancy each year. Parasitaemia is more frequent and the parasite load is higher in pregnancy, especially in primiparous women and during the second trimester; and cerebral malaria, pulmonary oedema, and renal failure occur more

Table 1 A guide to the safety of antimicrobial agents in pregnancy

Drugs	Probably safe but limited human studies	Potential or proven risk in pregnancy, but benefits may outweigh risk	Fetal abnormalities, risk greater than benefit
β-Lactams	+		
Aminoglycosides		+	
Macrolides	+		
Sulfonamides		+	
Tetracycline			+
Antiparasitic agents, except quinine		+	
Quinine			+
Antimycobacterial agents: INH, pyrazinamide, rifampicin, dapsone, ethambutol		+	
Antimycobacterial agents: ethionamide, thalidomide, clofazimine/cycloserine			+
Acyclovir, valacyclovir, famciclovir		+	
Ribavirin			+

Adapted from: Gilbert DN, Moellering RC, Sande MA (2000). *The Sandford Guide to Antimicrobial Therapy*, 13th edn. Antimicrobial Therapy, Inc, Sandford, USA.

Table 2 Notes on other infections in pregnancy

Infection	Notes
HHV6	Transplacental transfer occurs, probably without any effect on the fetus
HPV	Vertical transmission has been reported rarely; if vaginal warts are massive they may obstruct delivery
Enteroviruses	50 per cent have a mild respiratory or gastrointestinal illness; some have severe cramping abdominal pains simulating placental abruption that can lead to unnecessary emergency caesarean section; newborns with vertically acquired echoviral infections may have fulminant hepatic necrosis, severe coagulopathy from disseminated intravascular coagulopathy, and meningitis or myocarditis
Japanese B encephalitis virus	Particularly high mortality rates with fetal death have been reported in pregnancy
Lassa fever	Increased mortality for women in pregnancy, survival is improved by abortion and ribavirin (see Table 1)
Trichomonas vaginalis	Infections are common in pregnancy, can be transmitted to the newborn around birth, but there are no adverse effects on the fetus
Mycoplasma hominis	A commensal of the lower female genital tract; controversial disease role in newborns
Ureaplasma urealyticum	As for *M. hominis*
Lyme disease	*Borrelia burgdorferi* in gestation has a good prognosis if recognized early and treated aggressively; fetal death or disease, including meningoencephalitis, occurs without maternal treatment
Schistosomiasis	Placental infection occurs in up to 25 per cent in bilharzia infested areas, but there is no effect on gestational age or birth weight
Candida spp.	The incidence of vaginal thrush increases with each trimester; rarely, vaginal thrush in pregnancy predisposes to congenital candidiasis

commonly. Severe malarial anaemia of pregnancy and placental infection cause spontaneous abortions, stillbirths, and intrauterine growth retardation. Malaria is one of the few preventable causes of low birth weight.

Congenital malaria from transplacental spread occurs in approximately 1 per cent of infected pregnancies. The newborns have fever, respiratory distress, pallor, anaemia, hepatomegaly, jaundice, and diarrhoea.

Controlled trials of antimalarial chemoprophylaxis during pregnancy demonstrate little risk and good benefit. Treatment of identified cases rather than chemoprophylaxis is not the best practice as most infected women are not diagnosed antenatally. In areas with sensitive plasmodium, chloroquine is recommended, but in many parts of the world mefloquine is preferable.

Trypanosomiasis

Trypanosoma cruzi (American trypanosomiasis; Chagas' disease) infection in pregnancy in Central and South America accounts for 1 to 10 per cent of all abortions. Infection occurs from insect bites or blood transfusions, with parasitaemia and fever occurring 2 to 3 weeks later. Congestive heart failure from myocarditis is more likely in pregnancy, and overall the disease has 10

to 20 per cent mortality; miscarriage, intrauterine growth retardation, or preterm delivery may also occur. Congenitally infected babies may have jaundice, anaemia, hepatosplenomegaly, encephalitis, pneumonitis, and hydrops fetalis from cardiac involvement. Diagnosis is through placental histology or blood smear examination for parasitaemia. There is no safe and reliable treatment in pregnancy.

T. brucei gambiense and *T. brucei rhodesiense* (African sleeping sickness) have similar adult mortality as American trypanosomiasis. Congenital trypanosomiasis is rarely described, but this is probably an under-reporting phenomenon.

A guide to the general safety of antimicrobial drugs in pregnancy is given in Table 1. The reader is advised to check current recommendations on every individual drug, for instance from the British National Formulary, before commencing any therapy in pregnancy. Table 2 gives brief notes on a few other infections in pregnancy.

Further reading

Brocklehurst P (2001). Interventions aimed at decreasing the risk of mother-to-child transmission of HIV infection (Cochrane Review). In: *The Cochrane Library*, Vol. 2. Update Software, Oxford.

Brown HL, Abernathy MP (1998). Cytomegalovirus infection. *Seminars in Perinatology*, **22**, 260–6.

Daffos F, Forestier F, Capella-Pavlovsky M, *et al.* (1988). Prenatal management of 746 pregnancies at risk for congenital toxoplasmosis. *New England Journal of Medicine* **31**, 271–5.

de March AP (1975). Tuberculosis and pregnancy: five to ten year review of 215 patients in their fertile age. *Chest* **68**, 800–5.

Grether JK, Nelson KB (1997). Maternal infection and cerebral palsy in infants of normal birth weight. *Journal of the American Medical Association* **278**, 207–11.

Hurtig A-K, Nicoll A, Carne C, *et al.* (1998). Syphilis in pregnant women and their children in the United Kingdom: results from national clinician reporting surveys 1994–7. *British Medical Journal* **317**, 1617–9.

Kenyon S, Boulvain M (2001). Antibiotics for preterm premature rupture of membranes (Cochrane Review). In: *The Cochrane Library*, Vol. 2. Update Software, Oxford.

King J, Flenady V (2001). Antibiotics for preterm labour with intact membranes (Cochrane Review). In: *The Cochrane Library*, Vol. 2. Update Software, Oxford.

Levy R, Weissman A, Blomberg G, Hagay Z (1997). Infection by parvovirus B19 during pregnancy: a review. *Obstetrics and Gynecology Survey* **55**, 254–9.

Liesnard C, Dooner C, Brancart F, Gosselin F, Delforge ML, Rodesch F (2000). Prenatal diagnosis of congenital cytomegalovirus infection: a prospective study of 237 pregnancies at risk. *Obstetrics and Gynecology* **95**, 881–8.

Marsden PD (1971). South American trypanosomiasis (Chagas' disease). *International Review of Tropical Medicine* **4**, 97–121.

McAuley J, Roizen N, Patel D, *et al.* (1994). Early and longitudinal evaluations of treated infants and children and untreated historical patients with congenital toxoplasmosis: the Chicago Collaborative Treatment Trial. *Clinical Infectious Diseases* **18**, 38–72.

Miller E, Fairley CK, Cohen BJ, Seng C (1998). Immediate and long term outcome of human parvovirus B19 infection in pregnancy. *British Journal of Obstetrics and Gynaecology* **105**, 174–8.

Mofenson LM and the Committee on Pediatric AIDS (2000). American Academy of Pediatrics. Technical report: perinatal human immunodeficiency virus testing and prevention of transmission. *Pediatrics* **106**, 1–12.

Murphy DJ, Sellers S, MacKenzie IZ, Yudkin PL, Johnson AM (1995). Case-control study of antenatal and intrapartum risk factors for cerebral palsy in very preterm singleton babies. *Lancet* **346**, 1449–54.

Ohto H, Terazawa S, Sasaki N, *et al.* (1994). Transmission of hepatitis C virus from mothers to infants. The vertical Transmission of Hepatitis C

Collaborative Strudy Group. *New England Journal of Medicine* **330**, 744–50.

Remington JS, Klein JO, eds (2001). *Infectious diseases of the fetus and newborn infant*, 5th edn. WB Saunders, Philadelphia.

Schaefer G, Zervondakis IA, Fuchs FF, *et al.* (1975). Pregnancy and pulmonary tuberculosis. *Obstetrics and Gynecology* **46**, 706–15.

Smaill F (2001). Intrapartum antibiotics for Group B streptococcal colonisation (Cochrane Review). In: *The Cochrane Library*, Vol. 2. Update Software, Oxford.

Smith JR, Cowan FM, Munday P (1998). The management of herpes simplex infection in pregnancy. *British Journal of Obstetrics and Gynaecology* **105**, 255–60.

13.16 Blood disorders in pregnancy

E. A. Letsky

The physiological changes of pregnancy result in profound changes in the maternal haematological system. Plasma volume increases progressively, reaching a peak during the third trimester that is about 45 per cent or 1250 ml above non-pregnant values. Total red cell mass increases by about 20 to 30 per cent, resulting in haemodilution and hence a decline in haemoglobin concentration, packed cell volume, and red cell count. In the absence of iron deficiency the mean cell haemoglobin concentration remains at non-pregnant values and there is a slight increase (approximately 4 fl) in mean cell volume. As a result of these changes, anaemia cannot be diagnosed in pregnancy using criteria applied to non-pregnant individuals.

The changes in blood volume and haemodilution are so variable that the normal range of haemoglobin concentration can lie between 10.0 and 14.5 g/dl in healthy pregnancy at 30 weeks' gestation in women who have received parenteral iron. However, haemoglobin values of less than 10.5 g/dl in the second and third trimesters are probably abnormal and require further investigation. The World Health Organization (WHO) recommends that the haemoglobin concentration should not fall below 11.0 g/dl at any time during pregnancy.

Iron-deficiency anaemia

Effects of iron deficiency on the blood

The expansion of red cell mass represents the largest single demand for iron in pregnancy, amounting to a net gain of about 500 to 600 mg. In addition, 250 to 350 mg is needed for transfer to the fetus by active transport across the placenta, mainly in the last 4 weeks of pregnancy. Daily requirements for iron increase three- to four-fold and are met by an increased rate of absorption from the gut, together with mobilization of maternal iron stores. The mean serum iron concentration of healthy pregnant women is about two-thirds of the levels for non-pregnant individuals. Total iron-binding capacity is increased because transferrin levels more than double as pregnancy advances. In consequence, the saturation of iron-binding capacity is, in healthy pregnancy, lower (at about 25 per cent) than is normal for other situations. Serum ferritin (reflecting iron stores) declines during the first half of pregnancy to a nadir of about 15 to 20 µg/l, where it remains until delivery. Many women enter pregnancy with low or depleted iron stores even if the haemoglobin concentration is normal, and the majority of those who do not receive supplements have no stores at all at the end of pregnancy.

The anaemia of iron deficiency is the most common haematological problem in pregnancy. The earliest effect of iron deficiency on the erythrocyte outside pregnancy is a reduction in cell size, which appears to be the most sensitive index of underlying iron deficiency. This, however, is a very poor indicator of iron deficiency during pregnancy because of the established larger population of younger red cells. A fall in red cell haemoglobin concentration (mean corpuscular haemoglobin, mean corpuscular haemoglobin concentration) or the concentration of circulating haemoglobin is also a relatively late development in iron deficiency and is preceded by depletion of iron stores followed by a reduction in serum iron levels. A state of iron deficiency can be diagnosed before anaemia has developed by finding a serum ferritin of less than 30 µg/l and a serum iron of less than 10 µmol/l, with less than 15 per cent saturation of the total iron binding capacity. In recent years, serum ferritin, uninfluenced by recently ingested iron, has largely replaced serum iron and total iron-binding capacity as a non-invasive indicator of iron status.

Serum transferrin receptor (TfR) provides a new and allegedly reliable method for assessing cellular iron status. TfR is a transmembrane protein, present in all cells, that binds transferrin iron and transports it to the cell interior. Any reduction in iron supply results in an increase in TfR synthesis and, like serum ferritin, TfR has been shown to circulate in the plasma in small amounts which reflect the total body mass of TfR. As soon as cellular iron deficiency is established, the serum TfR rises in direct proportion to the degree of iron lack. This rise precedes the reduction in mean corpuscular volume and is therefore particularly valuable in identifying tissue iron deficiency in pregnancy. In combination with serum ferritin, serum TfR will give a complete picture of iron status, the serum ferritin reflecting iron stores (in the absence of chronic inflammatory disease) and the TfR reflecting tissue iron status. A bone marrow examination is now very rarely necessary to assess iron status during pregnancy.

Non-haematological effects of iron deficiency

Iron deficiency causes more than just anaemia and treatment with oral or parenteral iron results in improved well-being long before the haemoglobin rises significantly. The various effects of iron deficiency on cellular function may be responsible for the reported association between iron deficiency during pregnancy and preterm birth, and effects on neuromuscular transmission may underlie the anecdotal reports of increased blood loss at delivery in anaemic women.

Effects of iron deficiency on the fetus

The fetus derives its iron from maternal serum by active transport across the placenta in the last 4 weeks of pregnancy. The concentration of ferritin in cord blood is substantially higher than that in the mother's circulation at term and falls within the normal adult range, whether or not the mother is iron deficient. However, babies born to iron-deficient mothers have lower cord ferritin levels that those born to iron-replete mothers, and this has an important bearing on iron stores and development of anaemia in the first year of life when iron intake is very poor.

There have also been suggestions of behavioural abnormalities in children with iron deficiency, and iron deficiency in the absence of anaemia is associated with poor performance in the Bayley Mental Developmental Indices. Moreover, poor performance of 12- to 18-month-old iron-deficient, anaemic infants in mental and motor development can be improved to the level of iron-sufficient infants by treatment with ferrous sulphate.

Even more far-reaching effects of maternal iron deficiency during pregnancy have been suggested. A correlation has been shown between maternal iron-deficiency anaemia, high placental weight, and an increased ratio of placental weight to birthweight. This suggests that maternal iron deficiency results in poor fetal growth compared to that of the placenta. High blood pressure in adult life has been linked to lower birthweight and with those whose birthweight was lower than would be expected from the weight of the placenta. Prophylaxis of iron deficiency may therefore have important implications for the prevention of adult hypertension.

Giving iron in pregnancy

Because anaemia it is a late sign of iron deficiency, pregnant women are frequently given iron supplements prophylactically. The justification for doing this is still debated, although there is no question that iron deficiency is prevented. This is likely to be more important in poor than in developed countries, where controlled trials have demonstrated the effect of routine oral iron supplements on maternal well-being and perinatal outcome.

The main argument in favour of routine iron supplementation in pregnancy is that if iron deficiency is detected in the third trimester there may not be time to correct it by either oral or parenteral supplements. There is no haematological benefit in giving parenteral as opposed to oral iron and the maximal response to be expected in pregnancy is a rise in haemoglobin of approximately 0.8 g/l weekly. The main advantage of intravenous infusion is that it ensures adequate iron for response and avoids any undesirable side-effects associated with oral preparations, but parenteral iron is not without its risks. Otherwise, blood transfusions may be needed, with their associated hazards. On balance, a small daily supplement of oral iron given routinely, from the sixteenth week of pregnancy, seems the more sensible approach. It need not be considered as mandatory, but side-effects, which are most commonly bowel upsets, particularly constipation, are usually overcome by simple nutritional measures.

In iron-deficient women it may take more than a year after delivery for the haemoglobin to return to prepregnancy levels. By contrast, if iron supplements are given the haemoglobin is in the normal prepregnancy range 5 to 7 days after delivery, providing blood loss is not excessive.

Folic acid deficiency

Effects of folate deficiency on the blood and its treatment

When the diet is inadequate, pregnancy can lead to a state of negative folate balance. The pregnant woman needs approximately twice as much folic acid, 200 to 250 μg daily, as do non-pregnant individuals. The increase meets the needs of the growing uterus and conceptus and the expanded red cell mass. As pregnancy advances, serum folate falls to about half the non-pregnant value at term. The red cell folate content shows a slight decline over the same period.

Megaloblastic anaemia in pregnancy is usually the result of dietary folate deficiency. Its incidence is therefore variable, dependent on the socio-economic status of the population and whether or not folic acid supplements are given routinely as part of antenatal care. It occurs more frequently in multiple pregnancies, with about half of cases presenting in the third trimester and the remainder after delivery.

Deficiencies of iron and folate are often combined, with folate deficiency revealed by the failure of a patient to respond to iron supplements. The diagnosis can be difficult to make. The peripheral blood film may be unhelpful because the expected macrocytosis is masked by iron deficient microcytosis. Hypersegmentation of the neutrophils can also be seen in pure iron deficiency. Measurements of serum and red cell folate concentrations, as well as the excretion of formiminoglutamic acid after a histidine load (which is increased in normal pregnancy), can all be difficult to interpret because the results need to be related to the normal range that is expected for healthy pregnant women and not those derived from non-pregnant subjects. The diagnosis can only be confirmed by examination of a bone marrow aspirate.

There is a strong case for prophylaxis during pregnancy, particularly in countries where overt megaloblastic anaemia is frequent. Women with a poor diet should be given 300 μg of folate daily. The risk of adverse effects is very small because vitamin B_{12} deficiency in pregnancy is rare (see below): subacute combined degeneration of the cord has never been reported in these circumstances. Folic acid should be given with supplemental iron. If gastrointestinal megaloblastic changes are established, oral supplements will have no effect and absorption in general will be impaired. This situation can only be reversed by administration of intramuscular folic acid.

Non-haematological effects of folate deficiency

It is still argued to what extent folate deficiency may alter the outcome of pregnancy. Claims of an association between folate deficiency and placental abruption, abortion, and pre-eclampsia have not been substantiated. It has been shown that the incidence of prematurity and low birthweight can be reduced by giving supplements in poorly nourished populations, but has no effect in well-nourished women.

Effects of folate deficiency on the fetus

There is an increased risk of megaloblastic anaemia in the neonate of a folate-deficient mother, especially if delivery is preterm. There are also data suggesting an association between periconceptional folic acid deficiency, harelip, cleft palate, and, most important of all, neural tube defects. The latter has been confirmed by a multicentre, controlled trial of prepregnancy folate supplementation by the Medical Research Council.

In the United Kingdom, it is recommended that women contemplating pregnancy should take folate supplements of 400 μg daily. It has also been shown in Hungary, in a large, randomized trial, that periconceptional supplement of 800 μg of folic acid prevented the first occurrence of neural tube defects. The prevalence of harelip with or without cleft palate was not reduced by this supplementation.

Vitamin B_{12}

Maternal vitamin B_{12} stores, which are of the order of 3000 μg, are largely unaffected by pregnancy. The stores in the new-born infant are about 50 μg. The concentration of serum B_{12} falls during pregnancy from non-pregnant levels of 205 to 1025 μg/l to 20 to 512 μg/l at term, associated with preferential transfer of plasma B_{12} to the fetus. The recommended intake of vitamin B_{12} is 2.0 μg daily in the non-pregnant and 3.0 μg/day during pregnancy. This will be met by almost any diet that contains animal products, however deficient in other essential substances. Strict vegans, who will eat no animal produce whatsoever, can have a deficient B_{12} intake and should be given oral supplements during pregnancy. Recently, B_{12} deficiency associated with megaloblastic anaemia has been found in a proportion of women in Malawi whose main diet is maize and who eat little or no animal protein.

Vitamin B_{12} deficiency in pregnancy is very rare. Addisonian pernicious anaemia does not usually occur during the reproductive years, associated as it is with infertility. Pregnancy is only likely to occur after the deficiency has been corrected.

Haemoglobinopathies

It is important to recognize the genetic defects of haemoglobin structure and synthesis early in pregnancy, or preferably before conception, because:

- the clinical effects may complicate obstetric management and appropriate precautions can be taken

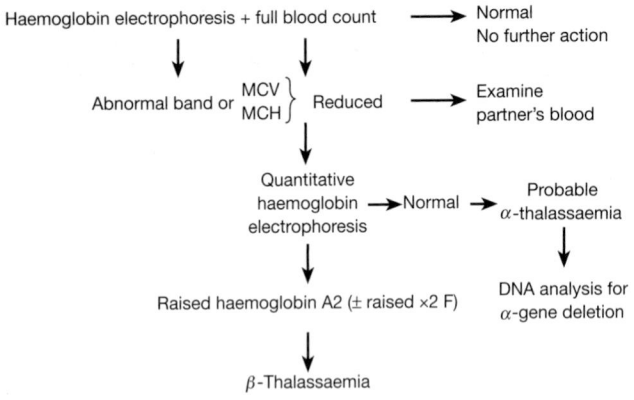

Fig. 1 Screening for haemoglobinopathies.

- it is now possible to offer prenatal diagnosis to those women carrying a fetus at risk of a serious defect of haemoglobin synthesis or structure at a time when termination of pregnancy is feasible (Fig. 1).

The two clinically significant groups of haemoglobinopathies, the sickle-cell syndromes and the thalassaemias, are described in detail in Section 22. Only special problems related to pregnancy will be discussed here.

Screening procedures vary from location to location and often only involve 'high-risk' populations. The most difficult situations arise in the United Kingdom, Europe, or the United States in antenatal obstetric units that care for a significant proportion of mothers from varying racial backgrounds. Figure 1 is a scheme that has been used with success in an obstetric unit serving a cosmopolitan population. This involves examination of red cell indices, haemoglobin electrophoresis, and, where indicated, quantitation of HbA₂ (and HbF) on every sample of blood taken at booking. If a haemoglobin variant or thalassaemic indices are found, the partner is requested to attend so that his blood can also be examined. By this means the chances of a serious haemoglobin defect can be assessed early in pregnancy, allowing counselling of the parents and the possibility of offering them prenatal diagnosis by fetal blood sampling or transabdominal chorion villus sampling, even though this will result in a late termination of pregnancy if indicated and desired. A recent audit of prenatal diagnosis, the first in 10 years in the United Kingdom, has shown that take-up is poor, particularly in Asian communities, and that at least six couples have sued their obstetrician for failure to inform them of the possibility of severe haemoglobinopathy in offspring.

Sickle-cell syndrome

It is essential to identify sickle-cell haemoglobin and the particular syndrome involved in the affected pregnant woman. The preferred procedure is to determine if there is an abnormal band on electrophoresis at booking (see above) and to perform a sickling test only on those cases where there is such a band, to confirm that this is sickle haemoglobin. The distinction between sickle-cell trait (HbA/S), sickle-cell anaemia (HbS/S), and HbS/C disease is then immediately apparent and nine out of ten unnecessary sickling tests are avoided in women of relevant racial groups.

Women with sickle-cell trait have no difficulties from overt sickling in pregnancy, but care is needed if a general anaesthetic is required during labour. There is an increased risk of pre-eclampsia, and tissue infarction can occur, even in the sickle-cell trait, if an adequate oxygen level is not maintained or if there is severe dehydration or shock.

Women with sickle-cell disease present special problems in pregnancy. Fetal loss is high, thought to be due to both impaired oxygen supply and sickling infarcts in the placental circulation. Abortion, severe pre-eclampsia, preterm labour, and other complications are more common than in women with normal haemoglobin. Although many women with sickle-cell

disease have no complications, the outcome in any individual case is always in doubt.

Increasing numbers of obstetric units have adopted prophylactic transfusion regimes designed to maintain the proportion of HbA at 60 to 70 per cent of the total, but the benefit of such prophylaxis remains to be proven by a large multicentre trial with contemporary controls. A small, controlled trial in the United States suggested that the outcome is similar in women transfused prophylactically compared to those transfused only when indications arise. Prophylactic regimens are expensive and time consuming and may not be applicable in developing countries where the problem is widespread. In addition, there can be problems of alloimmunization to minor blood group red cell antigens: these have resulted in severe, delayed, and sometimes fatal haemolysis in the mother, and haemolytic disease of the new-born in some cases, not to mention the other hazards of blood transfusion.

Against this background of uncertainty, a reasonable compromise, particularly where blood transfusion facilities are limited, is to supervise pregnant women with sickle-cell anaemia with care throughout the pregnancy and to administer regular folate supplements. If they become severely anaemic or have crises during the second half of pregnancy, an exchange transfusion is appropriate. Alternatively, if they present with haemoglobin values of less than 7 g/dl it is also acceptable to transfuse them up to a level of 12 to 14 g/dl, since this will reduce the level of HbS to a safe value without the need for exchange transfusion. During labour, management is directed towards preventing dehydration and acidosis. There is some controversy concerning the safest form of anaesthetic during labour or to cover delivery, but if regional, rather than general, anaesthesia is used, precautions must be taken to prevent venous pooling in the lower limbs. In view of the non-functioning spleen, it is also sensible to give twice daily penicillin to protect against pneumoccocal infections even if pneumovax has been administered.

Special mention should be made of the problem of HbSC disease (see Section xx) in pregnancy. Many women with this disorder go through pregnancy with no complications, but occasionally there may be severe sickling episodes, either late in pregnancy or early in the puerperium, which may lead to maternal death due to massive infarctive crises, particularly in the lungs. Any woman with this disorder who develops a painful crisis late in pregnancy, or who develops symptoms and signs suggestive of a chest infection or small pulmonary embolus, requires urgent exchange transfusion. Examination of the stained blood film in the so-called chest syndrome will show large numbers of nucleated red cells. Cerebral sickling infarcts are not unusual and if not fatal may result in long-term morbidity.

As regards the fetus or neonate, most centres have developed programmes for antenatal diagnosis of sickle cell anaemia using DNA analysis of amniotic or chorionic cells, or of fetal blood. If these are not available, it is important to identify homozygous infants by agar gel electrophoresis or isoelectric focusing immediately after birth. The first 2 years of life are particularly hazardous for an infant with sickle-cell anaemia. Death due to infection and splenic sequestration is common, hence mothers must be advised to present the infants early with any unusual symptoms.

Thalassaemia syndromes

The clinical and haematological manifestations of the α- and β-thalassaemias are described in Section 22. Only certain points relevant to pregnancy will be discussed here.

α-Thalassaemia

The homozygous state for α-thalassaemia produces Bart's haemoglobin hydrops syndrome. Pregnancy with an α-thalassaemia hydrops is associated with severe, sometimes life-threatening, hypertension and proteinuria, the so-called mirror syndrome (of severe rhesus haemolytic disease). Vaginal deliveries are associated with obstetric complications resulting from the large fetus and bulky placenta and the small stature of the mother (usually of Far-Eastern origin).

If routine screening of the parents shows that the mother is at risk of carrying such a child, then she should be referred as early as possible for prenatal diagnosis so that termination of an affected fetus can be carried out before these severe obstetric problems occur. Although this is not yet a common problem in the United Kingdom, it may well become more frequent if there is an influx of immigrants from Hong Kong and the Far East, as has already occurred in the United States and Australia. Transfusion *in utero*, which has been successful in only a handful of cases, is not recommended. The fetus is usually not viable and may have a variety of associated physical defects.

β-Thalassaemia

Pregnancy is extremely rare in transfusion-dependent homozygous β-thalassaemics but is now being seen with increasing frequency in women with β-thalassaemia intermedia. These patients may become profoundly anaemic and require regular transfusions during pregnancy.

Perhaps the most common problem associated with haemoglobinopathies and pregnancy is the anaemia developing in the antenatal period in women who have thalassaemia minor, heterozygous β-thalassaemia. They can be identified by examination of the blood sample taken at booking (see Fig. 1). The level of haemoglobin in early pregnancy may be normal or slightly below the normal range. Many women with thalassaemia minor enter pregnancy with depleted iron stores, hence they require the usual oral iron supplements in the antenatal period. Oral iron for a limited period will not result in significant iron loading, even in the presence of replete iron stores, but parenteral iron should never be given. A serum ferritin estimation can be carried out early in pregnancy, and if iron stores are found to be high then iron supplements can be withheld.

Folic acid, 5.0 mg daily, is recommended to cover the requirements of ineffective erythropoiesis. Blood transfusion may be indicated if the anaemia does not respond to oral iron and folate, the latter given parenterally as well as orally.

All women with mixed racial background should be screened for β-thalassaemia early in pregnancy. The partners of those who are found to be carriers should also be screened so that prenatal diagnosis can be offered where there is a risk of conceiving a homozygous child.

Miscellaneous anaemias specific to pregnancy

Many systemic medical conditions may further complicate the physiological haemodilution of pregnancy: these are discussed elsewhere.

A rare form of haemolytic anaemia appears to be specific to pregnancy. It remits after delivery but recurs in about half of affected women in later pregnancies. Although no autoantibody has been identified, the condition responds to corticosteroids or to infusion of human immunoglobulin (see below). The infant may be affected in about 20 per cent of cases.

There is a rare form of aplastic anaemia that occurs for the first time in pregnancy, remits after delivery, and then recurs again in subsequent pregnancies. The cause is unknown. It does not respond to any form of bone marrow stimulant or corticosteroid therapy and the management is symptomatic.

Disorders of haemostasis

Normal pregnancy is accompanied by major changes in the coagulation and fibrinolytic systems. There are significant increases in the procoagulant factors V, VIII, and X, and a very marked increase in plasma fibrinogen. In uncomplicated pregnancy, there is no change in antithrombin concentrations during the antenatal period, a fall during delivery, and then an increase 1 week postpartum. Protein C levels appear to remain constant or increase slightly, but protein S activity falls significantly during normal pregnancy.

The result of these physiological changes is to alter the usual balance between the procoagulants and anticoagulants in favour of the factors promoting blood clotting. In addition, fibrinolytic activity appears to be reduced during healthy pregnancy but returns to normal rapidly after separation of the placenta and completion of the third stage of delivery. This effect is mediated by placentally derived plasminogen activator inhibitor type II.

These changes in the haemostatic systems, together with the increase in blood volume, help to reduce the chances of abnormal haemorrhage at delivery, but they also convert pregnancy into a hypercoagulable state that may carry special hazards for both the mother and fetus. These hazards include a spectrum of haemostatic disorders, from thromboembolism through to the many conditions associated with disseminated intravascular coagulation.

Disseminated intravascular coagulation

This is associated with a wide variety of complications of pregnancy. It may be well compensated, with little change in tests of haemostatic function and no bleeding, as seen in prolonged retention of a dead fetus and mild preeclampsia, or it may result in intractable haemorrhage with gross consumption of coagulation factors and platelets and raised levels of fibrin degradation products, as seen classically in abruptio placentae (see Table 1).

Other complications of pregnancy in which disseminated intravascular coagulation may take a part include amniotic fluid embolism; septic abortion and intrauterine infection; hydatidiform mole; placenta accreta; preeclampsia and eclampsia, and prolonged shock from any cause (see Fig. 2).

Table 1 Spectrum of severity of disseminated intravascular coagulation (DIC): its relationship to specific complications in obstetrics

	Severity of DIC	*In vitro* findings	Obstetric conditions commonly associated
Stage 1	Low-grade compensated	FDPs↑ Platelets↓ Increased ratio VWF: factor VIIIC	Pre-eclampsia Retained dead fetus
Stage 2	Uncompensated but no haemostatic failure	As above plus fibrinogen↓ Platelets↓ Factors V and VIII↓	Small abruption Severe pre-eclampsia
Stage 3	Rampant with haemostatic failure	Platelets↓↓ Gross depletion of coagulation factors, particularly fibrinogen FDPs↑↑	Abruptio placentae Amniotic fluid embolism Eclampsia

Rapid progression from stage 1 to stage 3 is possible unless appropriate action is taken.

FDP, fibrin degradation products; VWF, von Willebrand factor.

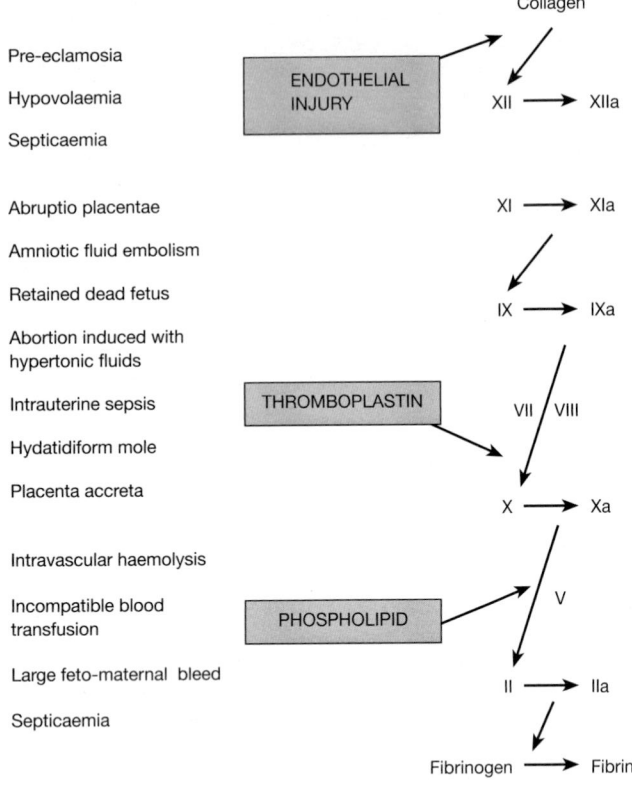

Fig. 2 Trigger mechanisms of disseminated intravascular coagulation during pregnancy. Interactions occur in many of these obstetric complications.

Disseminated intravascular coagulation in pregnancy is always a secondary process. Useful and rapid screening tests include the platelet count, partial thromboplastin time (intrinsic coagulation), prothrombin time (extrinsic coagulation), thrombin time, fibrinogen concentration, and levels of fibrin degradation products. Aside from standard supportive care (see Section 22) and removal of the triggering mechanism where this is known, management of the obstetric patient with disseminated intravascular coagulation should also seek to achieve an empty and contracted uterus.

Pre-eclampsia and haemostatic changes

Pre-eclampsia may be associated with marked changes in the normal physiological response of the haemostatic mechanisms during pregnancy (Table 2). The combination of a reduced platelet lifespan and a fall in the platelet count without platelet-associated antibodies indicates a low-grade coagulopathy. Once the disease process is established the most relevant

Table 2 Haemostatic changes in pre-eclampsia

Prostacylin generation	Decreased
Platelets	Decreased numbers[a]
	Decreased lifespan
	Decreased 5HT (serotonin)
	Increased plasma β-thromboglobulin and platelet factor IV
Factor VIII complex	Increased ratio VWF[a]/factor VIIIC
Antithrombin	Decreased
Soluble fibrinogen products	Increased, particularly fibrinopeptide-A
Fibrin degradation products	Increased in serum[a] and urine

[a]The most useful markers of severity and outcome.
VWF, von Willebrand factor.

haemostatic abnormalities appear to be the platelet count, factor VIII coagulation activity, and serum fibrin degradation products. Those women with the most marked abnormalities in these parameters suffer the greatest perinatal loss. It has been shown that if the platelet count is above $100\times10^9/l$ there are no disturbances in haemostatic function and therefore no need for coagulation screening tests.

Rarely, in very severe pre-eclampsia, the patient develops microangiopathic haemolysis. This causes profound thrombocytopenia and leads to confusion in differential diagnosis between pre-eclampsia, HELLP syndrome, haemolytic uraemic syndrome (HUS), and thrombotic thromboctyopenia (TTP). The recent identification of deficient metalloproteinase in TTP, either due to an IgG antibody in the acute form or to a genetic defect in the chronic relapsing form, will help to distinguish this condition from severe pre-eclampsia, HELLP syndrome, and HUS, which is essential if appropriate management with fresh frozen plasma is to be applied. In relation to pregnancy, haemolytic uraemic syndrome usually presents in the postpartum period with renal failure.

Platelet disorders

Thrombocytopenia is a common haematological abnormality in pregnancy and can have important implications for both mother and fetus. It may occur as part of the pathophysiology of pregnancy itself, or pregnancy may be superimposed on a background of haematological disease.

Incidental thrombocytopenia

As pregnancy advances there is a progressive small, but significant, fall in the platelet count in individual patients, probably due to haemodilution. Approximately 8 per cent of healthy pregnant women have thrombocytopenia at term, with platelet counts between 90 and $150\times10^9/l$. These women have no history of pre-eclampsia or immune thrombocytopenia and there is no increased incidence of thrombocytopenia in their offspring.

Thrombocytopenia and disseminated intravascular coagulation

Low-grade disseminated intravascular coagulation, as observed in pre-eclampsia, may be associated with further decrements but the platelet count rarely falls below $50\times10^9/l$, even in acute defibrination syndromes. Clearly, thrombocytopenia and platelet consumption represent only one aspect of this condition (see above) and will be corrected quickly when haemostatic mechanisms return to normal, usually without the use of, or need for, platelet transfusion.

Idiopathic thrombocytopenic purpura

Idiopathic thrombocytopenic purpura (ITP) is a rare condition, but relatively common in women of reproductive years. Patients in remission may still have elevated levels of platelet-associated IgG (PAIgG), especially following splenectomy. This is important in pregnancy because of the possibility of placental transfer of antibody resulting in fetal thrombocytopenia. Measurement of maternal platelet count, serum platelet antibody, and PAIgG are useful diagnostic tools but are not predictive of neonatal thrombocytopenia.

In the past, analysis of the literature gave an overall incidence of neonatal thrombocytopenia of 52 per cent with significant morbidity in 12 per cent, but we know now that this incidence was distorted because only symptomatic women were likely to have been investigated and reported. More recent analyses show an incidence of fetal thrombocytopenia of around 10 per cent, with severe thrombocytopenia (platelets fewer than $50\times10^9/l$) in less than 5 per cent overall. Fetal and neonatal morbidity and mortality is negligible even in the face of severe thrombocytopenia. Thrombocytopenia in the neonate tends to become more severe in the first few days of life and measures can be taken to correct this at birth before the nadir is reached, if indicated.

Pregnant women with ITP nearly always have the chronic form of the disease. The main clinical difficulty is that effects of treatment have to be considered in relation to the progress of pregnancy in both mother and fetus. The mild condition may require no treatment, but if the platelet count falls below 50×10^9/l, or there is clinical evidence of bleeding, then prednisolone is required (60 mg daily, reducing rapidly to the lowest possible dose that maintains the platelet count above 50×10^9/l). The prevalence of pre-eclampsia, gestational diabetes, postpartum psychosis, and osteoporosis are all increased by corticosteroids, hence the dose and duration of treatment should be the minimum needed to reduce the risk of bleeding or to raise the platelet count of any asymptomatic woman at term, allowing her to have epidural or spinal analgesia if desired or indicated.

The introduction of treatment by intravenous monomeric polyvalent human IgG has altered the management options in pregnancy dramatically. Used in the original recommended dose of 0.4 g/kg for 5 days by intravenous infusion, a persistent and predictable response is obtained in approximately 80 per cent of cases. There is no doubt about the value of this treatment in selected cases of severe symptomatic thrombocytopenia, but it cannot be advocated indiscriminately in view of its high cost and unproven benefit in milder cases. Analysis of recent reports indicates that the postulated beneficial transplacental effect on fetal platelets is unreliable and that exogenous IgG may not cross the placenta.

Splenectomy is now hardly ever indicated in the pregnant patient with ITP, but remains an option if all other attempts to increase the platelet count to safe levels fail. It is best carried out in the second trimester because surgery is best tolerated then and the size of the uterus does not make the operation technically difficult.

Mode of delivery

The most contentious problem in pregnancy associated with maternal ITP is the mode of delivery of the fetus. Even if the mother has to deliver in the face of a low platelet count, she is unlikely to bleed from the placental site once the uterus is empty, but she is at risk of bleeding from surgical incisions, soft-tissue injuries, or tears. Platelets should be available for transfusion but not given prophylactically.

The major risk at delivery is to the thrombocytopenic fetus, which as a result of birth trauma may suffer intracranial haemorrhage. Maternal platelet count, maternal platelet-associated IgG, splenectomy status, and history may give a crude indication of the likelihood of fetal thrombocytopenia but cannot be used in an individual case to predict the fetal platelet count. It is, however, unlikely for the fetus to have severe thrombocytopenia if the mother has no history of ITP before the index pregnancy and has no detectable IgG platelet antibody.

Platelet counts in blood obtained by transcervical fetal scalp sampling prior to, or early in, labour have been used to make a decision about the mode of delivery. However, this mode of sampling is not without risk of significant haemorrhage in the truly thrombocytopenic fetus, often gives false positive results, and demands urgent action to be taken on the results obtained. In addition, by the time that results are available the fetus may have already descended so far in the birth canal that caesarean section is technically difficult and traumatic for the fetus. The only way a reliable platelet count can be obtained is by a percutaneous transabdominal fetal cord blood sample, but this is not widely available and not without its difficulties, including a risk of approximately 1 per cent for the fetus. Decisions concerning the mode of delivery often have to be taken without knowledge of the fetal platelet count.

There is no good evidence that caesarean section is less traumatic than uncomplicated vaginal delivery, although this mode of delivery allows more overall control and there are usually no unpredictable complications. At the time of writing the emphasis of management is to return to a non-interventional policy of sensible monitoring, supportive therapy, and a mode delivery determined mainly by obstetric indications and not primarily by either the maternal or fetal platelet count.

Alloimmune thrombocytopenia

Fetal and neonatal alloimmune thrombocytopenia develops as a result of maternal sensitization to paternally derived fetal platelet antigen, the pathogenesis being analogous to that of Rh haemolytic disease of the new-born. The mother is not thrombocytopenic but the fetus can have a very low platelet count and is at risk of spontaneous intrauterine intracranial haemorrhage. This results from a specific antibody interfering with glycoprotein-binding sites and profoundly altering platelet function, particularly, aggregation. The most common platelet antigen involved is HPA-1, but a platelet incompatibility does not invariably result in alloimmunization. The maternal immune response appears to be restricted to those women with HLA-B8 and HLA-DR3 antigens. Thus, although 1 in 50 pregnancies are incompatible with respect to HPA-1 antigens (98 per cent prevalence of HPA-1a in the United Kingdom), only 1 in 5000 births are affected.

The children of first pregnancies (unlike rhesus disease) are often affected and the disease process can begin in early fetal life. Management is aimed at identifying the fetus at risk and correcting the thrombocytopenia *in utero*. Screening of women for HPA-1a status is not established. Investigation of neonatal intracranial haemorrhage or unexplained intrauterine death should include screening of parental blood for platelet antigens and maternal platelet antibodies. The approaches to the management of this problem are all controversial. One protocol involves fetal blood sampling at 20 to 22 weeks gestation and treating the mothers with thrombocytopenic fetuses with intravenous IgG 1 g/kg/week, with or without steroids, until delivery. This has been reported as successful in some units but others. The overall results of multicentre trials of the efficacy of maternal intravenous IgG administration are variable, with more successful reports from North America and general scepticism from European centres. Another approach is to administer weekly compatible platelet transfusions to the fetus. This has been successful in a number of cases but involves frequent hazardous procedures. Whatever approach is used, immediate predelivery administration of compatible platelets to the fetus is recommended. The accepted management when the diagnosis is established shortly after birth is to transfuse specially prepared HPA-1a negative platelets from pre-selected blood-bank donors or, if facilities are available, washed platelets from the mother.

Inherited defects of haemostasis

Von Willebrand's disease

Von Willebrand's disease is the most frequent of all inherited haemostatic abnormalities and is therefore the most likely coagulopathy to affect women in pregnancy. In normal pregnancy, a rise in both VIIIC and von Willebrand factor is observed. Patients with all but the severest forms of von Willebrand's disease show a similar but variable rise in both these factors during pregnancy, although there may not be a reduction in the bleeding time. After delivery, normal women maintain an elevated level of VIIIC for at least 5 days. In women with von Willebrand's disease the duration of this elevation seems to be related to the severity of the disorder. The general consensus is that the most important determinant for abnormal haemorrhage at delivery is a low factor VIIIC level. Appropriate factor VIII concentrates, containing von Willebrand factor activity as well as factor VIIIC, should be standing by to cover delivery but are rarely required to achieve haemostasis. Cryoprecipitate, with all the hazards of a fresh plasma product, is no longer recommended. There is virtually no place for desmopressin in obstetric practice, except perhaps in the puerperium. Any rise in factor VIII attributable to desmopressin will have been achieved under the influence of pregnancy itself. By contrast, desmopressin has a valuable place in women undergoing gynaecological or other surgery.

Haemophilia

The risks in pregnancy for the female carrier of haemophilia are two-fold:

1. She may, due to lyonization (random deletion of the X chromosome), have very low VIII or IX levels and be at risk of excessive bleeding, particularly following a surgical or traumatic delivery.

2. Fifty per cent of her male offspring will inherit haemophilia. This has important implications now that prenatal diagnosis of these conditions is possible.

It is important to identify carriers prior to pregnancy, not only to provide appropriate management for the rare case with pathologically low coagulation activity but also to provide genetic counselling. Changes in factor VIII complex may make the identification of carriers more difficult during pregnancy. Clinical problems occur more often in carriers for Christmas disease, since factor IX does not rise in response to healthy pregnancy in the same way as does factor VIII. Appropriate heat-treated concentrates are available to treat abnormal haemorrhage: cryoprecipitate and fresh frozen plasma should never be used unless heat-treated concentrates are not available.

It is possible to make an accurate prenatal diagnosis of haemostatic disorders. A fetal blood sample suitable for coagulation factor assays can be obtained from 18 weeks' gestation onwards and used to diagnose or exclude deficiencies of factors VIII and IX in male fetuses. In many cases at risk it is now possible to make rapid, early diagnosis of these conditions by DNA analysis of chorion villus samples or amniotic fluid cells obtained earlier in pregnancy. However, some few families remain where the recombinant DNA technology is not informative, so that fetal blood sample coagulation factor assays will continue to be of value.

Many women refuse prenatal diagnosis. If the fetus is male, scalp electrodes and sampling should be avoided during labour. Cord blood should be taken to establish the diagnosis to avoid haemostatic stress in the neonate.

Factor XI Deficiency (plasma thromboplastin antecedent deficiency)

This is a rare coagulation disorder, less common than the haemophilias. It has an autosomal recessive inheritance and therefore both men and women may be affected. Usually only homozygotes have clinical evidence of a coagulation disorder. Spontaneous haemorrhages and haemarthroses are rare but problems arise from the profuse bleeding which may follow major trauma or surgery if no prophylactic factor XI concentrate is given. The diagnosis is made by finding a prolonged partial thromboplastin time with a low factor XI level in an assay system in which all other coagulation tests are normal. Occasionally women with postpartum haemorrhage are found to have this abnormality. Fortunately the condition rarely causes problems either during pregnancy or delivery or in the newborn child. Prolonged bleeding at ritual circumcision is unusual. There is no justification in screening routinely for this condition either in the mother, fetus, or neonate. Women with factor XI deficiency should be given documentation of their defect so that appropriate measures can be taken to cover surgery or accidental trauma.

Genetic vascular disease

Ehlers Danlos Syndrome (EDS)

It is often forgotten that an essential part of the haemostatic system is healthy vasculature. The Ehlers Danlos syndrome may be associated with bleeding because of increased fragility of vessels due to defects in collagen synthesis. The disease has an autosomal dominant inheritance and has been subdivided into 10 subtypes of which type IV is the most severe and may have lethal complications, the most important of which is rupture of the long arteries. EDS IV is associated with an abnormality of collagen type III as a result of mutations in the corresponding gene COL3A1.

Surgical procedures should be avoided unless essential because the tissues are friable and massive bleeding may occur and healing of incisions may be delayed. Pregnancy and delivery will be involved with obvious potential hazards.

The diagnosis of this condition may be missed, especially in an obstetric gynaecological scenario, where many women complain of easy bruising,

which is one of the main presenting symptoms, but platelet function and coagulation screening tests will yield normal results. Although there is no effective treatment or prophylaxis for this potentially lethal condition, appropriate management and precautions at least can be instituted, combined with sensitive genetic counselling regarding the autosomal dominant inheritance of this disorder.

Further reading

Anaemias and related disorders

Alberman E, Noble JM (1999). Commentary: Food should be fortified with folic acid. *British Medical Journal* **319**, 93.

Bothwell TH (2000). Iron requirements in pregnancy and strategies to meet them. *American Journal of Clinical Nutrition* **72**, 257S–64S.

Carriaga MT, Skikne BS, *et al.* (1991). Serum transferrin receptor for the detection of iron deficiency in pregnancy. *American Journal of Clinical Nutrition* **54**, 1077–81.

Czeizel AE and Dudas I (1992). Prevention of the first occurrence of neural-tube defects by periconceptional vitamin supplementation. *New England Journal of Medicine* **327**, 1832–5.

Gill PS, Modell B (1998). Thalassaemia in Britain: a tale of two communities. *British Medical Journal* **317**, 761–2.

Goodall HB, Ho Yen DO, *et al.* (1979). Haemolytic anaemia of pregnancy. *Scandinavian Journal of Haematology* **22**, 185–91.

Howard RJ, Tuck SM, *et al.* (1995). Pregnancy in sickle cell disease in the UK: results of a multicentre survey of the effect of prophylactic blood transfusion on maternal and fetal outcome. *British Journal of Obstetrics and Gynaecology* **102**, 947–51.

Kadir RA, Sabin C, *et al.* (1999). Neural tube defects and periconceptional folic acid in England and Wales: retrospective study. *British Medical Journal* **319**, 92–3.

Koshy M and Burd L (1991). Management of pregnancy in sickle cell syndromes. *Hematology/Oncology Clinics of North America* **5**, 585–96.

Larrabee KD, Monga M (1997). Women with sickle cell trait are at increased risk for preeclampsia. *American Journal of Obstetrics and Gynecology* **177**, 425–8.

Letsky EA (1998). The haematological system. In: Broughton Pipkin F and Chamberlain GVP, eds. *Clinical physiology in obstetrics*, pp. 71–110. Blackwell Science, Oxford.

Letsky EA (2001). Maternal anaemia in pregnancy. Iron and pregnancy – a haematologist's view. *Fetal and Maternal Medicine Review* **12**, 159–75.

Medical Research Council (MRC) (1991). Prevention of neural tube defects: results of the Medical Research Council Vitamin Study. MRC Vitamin Study Research Group. *Lancet* **338**, 131–7.

Modell B, Petrou M, *et al.* (1997). Audit of prenatal diagnosis for haemoglobin disorders in the United Kingdom: the first 20 years. *British Medical Journal* **315**, 779–84.

Perry KG Jr and Morrison JC (1990). The diagnosis and management of hemoglobinopathies during pregnancy. *Seminars in Perinatology* **14**, 90–102.

Rushton DH, Dover R, *et al.* (2001). Why should women have lower reference limits for haemoglobin and ferritin concentrations than men? *British Medical Journal* **322**, 1355–57.

Snyder TE, Lee LP, *et al.* (1991). Pregnancy-associated hypoplastic anemia: a review. *Obstetrical and Gynecological Survey* **46**, 264–9.

Van den Broek NR, Letsky EA, *et al.* (1998). Iron status in pregnant women: which measurements are valid? *British Journal of Haematology* **103**, 817–24.

Wald N J, Bower C (1995). Folic acid and the prevention of neural tube defects. *British Medical Journal* **310**, 1019–20.

Walter T (1994). Effect of iron-deficiency anaemia on cognitive skills in infancy and childhood. *Baillieres Clinical Haematology* **7**, 815–27.

Haemostasis

Burrows RF, Kelton JG (1995). Perinatal thrombocytopenia. *Clinics in Perinatology* **22**, 779–801.

David A, Letsky EA, *et al.* (In press). Factor XI deficiency presenting in pregnancy: diagnosis and management. *British Journal of Obstetrics and Gynaecology.*

Forbes CD, Greer IA (1992). Physiology of haemostasis and the effect of pregnancy. In: Greer IA, Turpie AGG, Forbes CD, eds. *Haemostasis and thrombosis in obstetrics and gynaecology*, pp. 1–25. Chapman and Hall, London.

Furlan M, Robles R, *et al.* (1998). Von Willebrand factor-cleaving protease in thrombotic thrombocytopenic purpura and the hemolytic-uremic syndrome. *New England Journal of Medicine* **339**, 1578–84.

Hamel BCJ, Pals G, *et al.* (1998). Ehlers-Danlos syndrome and type III collagen abnormalities: a variable clinical spectrum. *Clinical Genetics* **53**, 440–46.

Kadir RA. (1999). Women and inherited bleeding disorders: Pregnancy and delivery. *Seminars in Hematology* **36**, 28–35.

Leduc L, Wheeler JM, *et al.* (1992). Coagulation profile in severe preeclampsia. *Obstetrics and Gynecology* **79**, 14–8.

Letsky EA (in press). Coagulation defects. In: de Swiet M, ed. *Medical disorders in obstetric practice*, 4th edn. Blackwell Science, Oxford.

Letsky EA, Greaves M (1996). Guidelines on the investigation and management of thrombocytopenia in pregnancy and neonatal alloimmune thrombocytopenia. *British Journal of Haematology* **95**, 21–6.

Van den Broek N, Letsky EA. (In press). Pregnancy and the Erythrocyte Sedimentation Rate. *British Journal of Obstetrics and Gynaecology.*

Weatherall DJ, Letsky EA (2000). Genetic haematological disorders. In: Wald NJ, Leck I eds. *Antenatal and neonatal screening* 2nd edn, Oxford University Press, Oxford pp. 243–81.

13.17 Malignant disease in pregnancy

Robin A. F. Crawford

Introduction

Cancer is rare during pregnancy, quoted as occurring in only about 1 per 1000 live births. Most malignancies affecting this age group have been seen during pregnancy. Tumours of the uterine cervix, ovary, breast, or thyroid can metastasize to the placenta but not the fetus. Gestational trophoblastic disease arises from fetal chorion and is a malignant transformation of the placenta. Melanoma and haematological tumours, which also can invade the placenta, may cross into the fetal circulation. Pregnancy may cause enlargement of a pituitary tumour and a previously silent tumour may present with symptoms in pregnancy. Rare cases of colonic and neurological cancers developing in pregnancy have been reported in the literature. The diagnosis and treatment of the cancer may have been made prior to the pregnancy: discussion of teratogenesis and effects of treatment are also included in this chapter.

The placenta has several crucial functions. It is a fetal respiratory organ, a sophisticated endocrine unit, and a membrane that allows preferential and selective transfer of substrates from the mother to the fetus for fetal growth and development. In addition, the placenta is largely an effective barrier between the mother and the fetus. Transfer of fetal cells into the maternal circulation is common and probably occurs throughout gestation in all pregnancies. The transfer of maternal cells to the fetus, by contrast, is a relatively rare event.

Concurrence of pregnancy and cancer does raise complex therapeutic and ethical dilemmas, because the most appropriate and timely treatment for the mother may not be in the best interests of the fetus. Extra-abdominal surgery and anaesthesia during pregnancy rarely carry any risks to the fetus, and intra-abdominal surgery may be safely carried out in the second trimester. However, fetal cells divide and differentiate rapidly during the first trimester, and radiation and chemotherapy carry well-recognized risks to the fetus, including the risk of abortion, congenital abnormalities, or preterm birth. As a result, physicians may be reluctant to treat the mother aggressively at the time of initial diagnosis. Instead, in many cases they defer treatment for several weeks or months until the fetal lungs have matured. This delay, however, may substantially reduce the mother's chance of surviving the disease.

It is impossible to establish a threshold dose of ionizing radiation below which such treatment is safe for the fetus, inasmuch as exposure during the first trimester to a dose as low as 10 cGy appears to increase the risk of fetal abnormalities and exposure to 3 to 5 cGy increases the risk of childhood cancers. The risk is negligible if exposure to the fetus is less than 1 cGy. The dose of radiation, the gestational age of the fetus, and the practicability of shielding the fetus from radiation must be balanced against potential benefits to the mother.

Chemotherapy administered to the mother during the first trimester carries well-recognized risks including abortion or congenital abnormalities. Drugs that preferentially interfere with rapidly growing tissues, such as methotrexate, can harm the fetus. Use of antagonists of folate, purine, or pyrimidine synthesis during organogenesis results in congenital malforma-tions in up to 25 per cent of fetuses, although this figure is much lower if the mother only receives therapy with a single agent. Treatment after the first trimester, when structural development is largely complete, is reasonably safe in many diseases and more appropriate than postponement of treatment. Chemotherapy after the first trimester has been associated with slight increases in the incidence of preterm birth and fetal growth retardation and, when administered shortly before delivery, with transient neonatal myelosuppression. Nevertheless, the long-term outcomes of the children of women who received chemotherapy during the second or third trimester are generally good.

In practical terms, acute leukaemia is virtually the only condition requiring immediate chemotherapy in a pregnant woman. When faced with cancer in the first trimester, the available information should be explained to the woman and her partner, who should give informed unhurried consent before treatment starts. In the majority of these situations, a consensus decision is reached between the woman, her partner, and the responsible physician to proceed with chemotherapy. However, the ethical issues are very complex and decisions have to be made on an individual basis.

As there is increasing success with the treatment of childhood cancers, more women will enter the reproductive age group having survived cancer treatment. There appears to be no overall increased risk of either congenital malformations or childhood cancers in the offspring of cancer survivors based on series of several thousand children. An increased incidence of spontaneous abortions, low-birth-weight babies, and neonatal deaths has been described for women with Wilms' tumour who had received at least 20 Gy abdominal radiation. Survivors of Hodgkin's disease who had received both radiation and chemotherapy (but not either alone) also appear to be at increased risk of spontaneous abortions.

Gestational trophoblastic disease

Gestational trophoblastic disease is a group of diseases which arise in the fetal chorion during various types of pregnancy. Histologically they are categorized as one of two types of hydatidiform mole (partial or complete), gestational choriocarcinoma or placental site trophoblastic tumour. Gestational trophoblastic disease is notable for several reasons. Firstly, the tumours are genetically different from the host, having antigens derived from the male partner. Secondly, apart from the placental site tumour, they secrete human chorionic gonadotrophin in amounts proportional to the viable tumour volume, allowing human chorionic gonadotrophin to be used as an ideal tumour marker. Thirdly, even metastatic disease can be cured with chemotherapy, the use of methotrexate in the early 1950s having shown reproducible results.

Complete and partial hydatidiform moles present as abnormal pregnancies ending in first or second trimester abortions. The complete mole is diploid (of paternal origin), is commonly diagnosed on ultrasound, and has no fetal elements present. The partial mole is triploid with paternal and maternal origin, has fetal elements present, and is usually diagnosed after the products of conception are examined pathologically. Gestational choriocarcinoma is a highly malignant tumour derived from syncytial and cytotrophoblastic cells. When villi are present in association with malignant trophoblasts, it is classified as a molar pregnancy. If there is diagnostic doubt about the possibility of combined molar pregnancy with a viable fetus, then the ultrasound scan should be repeated before intervention. If the twin pregnancy is associated with a partial mole, it should be allowed to proceed. If the twin pregnancy is associated with a complete mole, it may proceed after appropriate counselling. These pregnancies are associated with a reduced live birth rate of 25 per cent and are at risk of pre-eclampsia and haemorrhage. The subsequent need for chemotherapy in these rare cases is about 20 per cent, and is the same whether the pregnancy is terminated spontaneously or therapeutically, or allowed to proceed to term.

Gestational trophoblastic disease arises in various types of pregnancy, most of which are clinically recognized as abnormal. The incidence is 1.54 per 1000 live births. The most common are molar pregnancies, but gestational trophoblastic disease can also arise following abortions, ectopic pregnancies, or even after normal full-term pregnancies. Clinical surveillance of patients who have had a molar pregnancy is the only practical method of detecting and preventing gestational trophoblastic disease. In the United Kingdom, all patients with a histological diagnosis of a molar pregnancy are registered and followed up at one of three screening centres (Charing Cross Hospital in London, Sheffield, and Dundee). Only 7.5 per cent of women with hydatidiform mole require chemotherapy in the United Kingdom, and more than half of the patients who require chemotherapy for their gestational trophoblastic disease have a preceding molar pregnancy. Patients who develop gestational trophoblastic disease after an abortion or full-term pregnancy are more difficult to detect. They present with symptoms attributable to metastases. Sites of initial metastases (in order of frequency) are lung, vagina, brain, liver, gastrointestinal tract, and kidney. The interval between pregnancy and the development of metastatic gestational trophoblastic disease may be years. Because these tumours are rare, many clinicians do not consider gestational trophoblastic disease as part of any differential diagnosis.

Any woman of reproductive age who has an undiagnosed tumour or unexplained bleeding from any organ other than the uterus should have a human chorionic gonadotrophin estimation to exclude the highly treatable gestational trophoblastic disease.

Patients with gestational trophoblastic disease are classified as having a low or high risk depending on a scoring system devised at Charing Cross Hospital and now modified by the World Health Organization. The score relies on factors such as age, the antecedent pregnancy, the interval between presentation and the previous pregnancy, the human chorionic gonadotrophin level, the blood group, the size of the largest tumour, site and number of metastases, and whether the patient had received prior chemotherapy. In the United Kingdom the low-risk group will be offered methotrexate with folinic acid rescue. The high-risk group and those low-risk patients who have resistant or persistent disease will be offered combination chemotherapy. The initial diagnosis may be made by surgical excision or biopsy of a suspicious lesion, but surgery otherwise has little role, excepting rarely to remove a cerebral metastasis to prevent a cerebral bleed.

The overall survival for patients with gestational trophoblastic disease is now about 94 per cent. Women should be advised not to conceive for 6 months after a negative human chorionic gonadotrophin reading. The risk of further molar pregnancy is low (1:74).

Cancer of the cervix

Carcinoma of the cervix may be diagnosed during pregnancy with an incidence of approximately 1 in 2200 pregnancies. In the United Kingdom, with the recent success of the cervical screening programme, the incidence is probably lower. Pregnant women with cervical cancer generally present with early stage disease and the prognosis is similar to that of non-pregnant patients.

The presenting symptom is usually vaginal bleeding. It is therefore important to check the cervix with a visual examination when pregnant women present with irregular vaginal bleeding. There is a tendency to assume that vaginal bleeding in early pregnancy is related to miscarriage, organize an ultrasound to check for fetal viability, and forget vaginal examination. In the case of an obvious cancer, a wedge biopsy under general anaesthetic is appropriate for diagnosis and staging. If there is any doubt, colposcopy can be used to assess the cervix. There is an increased risk of bleeding when taking a biopsy from the pregnant cervix, but there is no increased rate of fetal loss.

Patients with cervical intraepithelial neoplasia can be managed expectantly until after delivery. There is no contraindication for a vaginal delivery for women with cervical intraepithelial neoplasia. Indeed, there are several series which suggest that vaginal delivery is associated with a higher rate of regression of severe dysplasia than is usually seen. Standard practice would be to review with colposcopy at approximately 3 months after delivery. Management of women with microinvasion of the cervix is usually via cone biopsy under a general anaesthetic, allowing the pregnancy to continue.

When cervical cancer is diagnosed in early pregnancy, treatment options include immediate radical hysterectomy or to delay treatment until the fetus is viable, followed by classical caesarean section (scar in the upper segment of the uterus) and radical hysterectomy. This is appropriate for stage 1B cases, where the tumour is confined to the cervix and is less than 4 cm in diameter. In one series there was no difference in survival between the two modes of treatment. Typically, women diagnosed in the first trimester will be offered immediate surgery. Women diagnosed after 24 to 28 weeks' gestation are usually managed expectantly until after 32 weeks' gestation and then delivered by caesarean radical hysterectomy. Steroids are usually given to accelerate fetal lung maturity. The outlook may be worse for patients who deliver vaginally across a cervical cancer, but this has not been substantiated.

Cancer of the ovary

The stated incidence of adnexal masses occurring in pregnant women is from as rare as 1 in 2500 to as frequent as 1 in 81 live births. With the use of routine early ultrasound, the true incidence of adnexal masses is closer to the latter figure. Most of these (more than 95 per cent) are benign. Complications of a benign adnexal mass include pain due to torsion, rupture, and haemorrhage, obstruction of the pelvic outlet, and infection. Most cysts are managed conservatively, avoiding surgery. When necessary, surgery to remove cysts is usually performed in the second trimester. The advantage of waiting until the second trimester is that most cysts resolve spontaneously and that the rate of fetal loss is reduced.

The rationale for removing persistent adnexal masses is to exclude malignancy. Ovarian cancer in pregnancy is rare, with a reported incidence of 1 case per 17 000 to 38 000. This is because the usual age of childbirth is greater than the peak incidence of germ cell tumours and substantially less than the usual age of those with epithelial cancer. In addition, pregnancy protects against ovarian cancer. Two-thirds of the cancers detected are epithelial and the remaining are germ cell (usually dysgerminoma) and stromal cell types. Cysts which are simple on ultrasound and less than 5 cm in diameter have almost no malignant potential. Larger cysts with nodules, septa, or rapid growth are more likely to be malignant. Tumour markers are not helpful in pregnancy: CA 125 can be raised by pregnancy, as can α-fetoprotein and human chorionic gonadotrophin.

The management of the ovarian cancer is similar to that in the non-pregnant woman. Appropriate surgical staging is required: the author's preference being that removal of the cyst, taking of peritoneal washings for cytology, biopsy of the contralateral ovary, and biopsies of any abnormal areas are sufficient at the primary operation. It is also preferable to wait 48 h for a definitive diagnosis from paraffin sections, rather than expect the pathologist to give an immediate result from frozen section. This delay also allows the woman and her partner to consider the implications of the diagnosis. Most of the women seen with a malignant diagnosis in pregnancy will have early stage epithelial cancer: FIGO stage 1A or B, meaning well or moderately differentiated tumour confined to one or both ovaries, or to have borderline histology. No further therapy would then be necessary. Therapeutic termination is not required and pregnancy *per se* does not worsen outcome. Fuller staging may be considered 6 to 12 weeks after delivery. The decision to use chemotherapy postoperatively depends on the stage and differentiation of the tumour, the gestational age of the fetus, and the wishes of the mother. The treatment of malignant germ cell tumours can be carried out without affecting the pregnancy in the second two trimesters, especially if alkylating agents are avoided.

Cancer of the breast

Gestational breast cancer is defined as a breast cancer presenting either during pregnancy or up to 1 year postpartum. It was originally thought that pregnancy-related cancer carried a worse prognosis, but this has not been substantiated. Although breast cancer is regarded as a hormonal-dependent tumour, termination of pregnancy and oophorectomy do not provide a better outcome for the woman. Women becoming pregnant after treatment for breast cancer have a similar or better survival when controlled for age and stage.

Breast cancer is often diagnosed at a late stage as breast lumps may be difficult to detect against a background of pregnancy-related hypertrophy. Consequently, investigation of masses is often delayed. Mammography is not harmful to the fetus with appropriate shielding. When a breast mass is found, the most important step is to make a histological diagnosis. If the diagnosis of breast cancer is made, treatment is the same as for the non-pregnant woman. Obviously, chemotherapy in the first trimester is associated with risks for the developing fetus.

Suppression of lactation as a therapeutic manoeuvre is not necessary, with two exceptions. Firstly, if breast surgery is required during the puerperium, suppression of lactation can decrease the size and vascularity of the breast, allowing for a safer surgical procedure. Secondly, suppression of lactation is recommended in women receiving chemotherapy as some of the drugs can reach the breast milk and cause neonatal neutropenia.

Melanoma

The incidence of melanoma in pregnancy is between 0.14 to 2.8 cases per 1000 deliveries. Melanoma in pregnancy is unusual in that it can metastasize to the placenta and to the fetus. As this is a rare phenomenon, therapeutic abortion is not indicated, but careful examination and follow-up of the baby is warranted. Current evidence suggests that the clinical outcome for pregnant patients is similar to that of non-pregnant patients. Early detection and biopsy are performed as usual, and the surgical management is the same. Since most recurrences of melanoma occur in the first 3 years following initial diagnosis, it may be appropriate to delay further pregnancies until this time period has elapsed.

Thyroid cancer

It is not uncommon to find thyroid nodules which require further investigation during pregnancy. Most cancers are well differentiated with a very good prognosis. When a diagnosis is made, treatment proceeds as normal, with the exception that radio-iodine is contraindicated. Cancers discovered early in the pregnancy can be treated surgically in the second trimester. Tumours discovered in later pregnancy can have their investigation and treatment delayed until after delivery. Thyroxine is given to reduce the level of thyroid-stimulating hormone. There is no evidence to suggest that pregnancy alters the outcome for thyroid cancer. Thyroid cancer is not an indication for termination of pregnancy.

Lymphoma

As Hodgkin's disease is a disease of young adults (mean age 32 years), it is not surprising that there are more cases diagnosed in pregnancy than there are of non-Hodgkin's lymphoma (mean age of diagnosis of 42 years). The reported incidence of Hodgkin's disease in pregnancy is between 1 in 1000 and 1 in 6000 deliveries.

Although historically believed to be exacerbated by pregnancy, there does not seem to be any influence of pregnancy on the outcome for Hodgkin's disease. If treatment is required, most patients can be managed without compromise to mother or fetus. Patients presenting with localized Hodgkin's disease relatively late in pregnancy may be observed with limited staging and not treated until after delivery.

By contrast, in non-Hodgkin's lymphoma, patients with Burkitt's lymphoma in pregnancy appear to have a highly aggressive disease involving the breast or ovary. The outlook for pregnant women with non-Hodgkin's lymphoma may be bleak, some dying prior to delivery.

Leukaemia

Leukaemia in pregnancy is rare, with an incidence of 1 per 100 000 pregnancies. This may be because the majority of cases of acute lymphoblastic leukaemia occur before reproductive age and the majority of cases of acute myeloid leukaemia occur afterwards. Chronic lymphocytic leukaemia is a disease of the elderly, hence chronic myeloid leukaemia constitutes 90 per cent of the cases of chronic leukaemia seen in pregnancy.

Since the introduction of intensive chemotherapy, the survival of pregnant women with leukaemia is similar to that of non-pregnant women. It does not appear that intrauterine exposure to antileukaemic chemotherapy produces detrimental late effects to the resulting children. Women treated with non-alkylating agents have no apparent decrease in fertility, although this is reduced by 33 per cent when alkylating agents are used.

Cancer of the colon

The reported incidence of colorectal cancer in pregnancy of 1 per 50 000 pregnancies may now be an underestimate as a reflection of the trend for women to delay pregnancy until later in life. A more recent study has reported an incidence of 1 per 13 000 live births. With increased awareness of inherited genetic traits and the availability of genetic testing, more and more patients at risk (for example those with familial adenomatous polyposis and hereditary non-polyposis coli) are undergoing screening. This may reduce the numbers of pregnant women diagnosed with colon cancer.

It appears that colorectal cancer in pregnancy is particularly common in the rectal region, below the peritoneal reflection. The importance of this is that 88 per cent of tumours are within reach of the flexible sigmoidoscope, allowing detection with a minimum of inconvenience to the patient and no risk to the fetus.

Presenting symptoms are similar to those in non-pregnant women. However, the combination of altered bowel habit, abdominal pain/swelling, and anaemia is common in pregnancy, such that these symptoms are frequently ascribed to the pregnancy itself. Assessment of the pregnant patient with colorectal cancer is similar to that of the non-pregnant patient. Radiological imaging is avoided in the first trimester. Carcinoembryonic antigen is not affected significantly by pregnancy and so can be used as a marker.

Patients younger than 40 years generally have a poorer prognosis due to delayed diagnosis and advanced stage at presentation. Pregnant women are no different in this respect. The overall fetal prognosis is relatively favourable as the diagnosis is usually made close to term and the fetus can be delivered coincident with the surgery for the colon cancer.

Further reading

Cappell MS (1998). Colon cancer during pregnancy. The gastroenterologist's perspective. *Gastroenterology Clinics of North America* **27**, 225–56. A good review of a rare condition.

Seminars in Oncology **16**, 335–436 (1989). This volume is dedicated to cancer in pregnancy and gives various overviews relating to gynaecological cancers, leukaemia and lymphoma, melanoma, and breast cancer. It is perhaps a little dated.

http://www.hmole-chorio.org.uk Choriocarcinoma UK Information website with up to date recommendations about management.

13.18 Prescribing in pregnancy

P. C. Rubin

Introduction

Prescribing in pregnancy is essentially about balancing risks. The damage that a drug may cause to the fetus must be weighed against the harm that may befall the mother and her unborn child if a disease goes unchecked.

While knowledge in most therapeutic areas has grown rapidly in recent decades, information on the use of drugs in pregnancy has developed sporadically, with case reports being more usual than large, prospective clinical trials. The reasons are not surprising and largely relate to concern about teratogenesis.

Thalidomide is a name inescapably associated with prescribing in pregnancy. Drug-induced fetal abnormality did not begin with thalidomide: there is an Old Testament exhortation to have 'no strong drink, neither eat any unclean thing' during pregnancy. However, the scale of the thalidomide tragedy brought to the general public for the first time the realization that drugs could harm the developing baby. Thalidomide was marketed in Germany in 1956 and subsequently in other countries as a sedative and hypnotic which had the particular attraction of being safe in overdose. Indeed, the drug was considered so safe that in some countries it was available without prescription. Then between 1960 and 1961 Germany experienced what amounted to an epidemic of phocomelia, a birth defect involving absence of the long bones with hands and feet being attached directly to the trunk. What had previously been an extremely rare condition (no cases had been reported in the 10 years to 1959) was being seen almost commonly. Various causes—viral, radioactivity, food preservatives—were considered as culprits, until one doctor retrospectively questioned his patients and found that 20 per cent had taken thalidomide in early pregnancy. On repeat questioning, asking specifically about the drug, 50 per cent admitted taking thalidomide, many having not mentioned it before since the drug was so obviously innocent. In fact, around 80 per cent of women who took thalidomide in the first trimester had a deformed baby. More than 10 000 such babies had been born before the drug was removed from the market.

The thalidomide experience had far-reaching ramifications. Drug regulation as we know it stems largely from the disaster. Doctors and their patients recognized that there is no such thing as a safe drug. In addition, the pharmaceutical industry has largely avoided obtaining systematic information on drug use in pregnancy. The reasons are obvious and understandable, but for the prescribing doctor the statement that 'the safety of this drug in pregnancy has not been established' is not helpful when faced with a woman who is, or may become, pregnant.

Identifying teratogenic drugs

Information on drug-induced fetal abnormality comes from case reports, case studies, and epidemiological studies. Case reports are a two-edged sword. Describing a single association between a drug and a fetal abnormality can be very useful in first identifying a real problem: warfarin was first linked to teratogenesis in this way. However, the problem with case reports is that they may be showing nothing more than a chance associ-ation, because fetal abnormalities occur in around 2 per cent of pregnancies, and caution must be exercised in their interpretation. This is well demonstrated by the Debendox® saga.

Most cases of morning sickness do not require treatment. However, some do, and the drug for which most information is available was withdrawn from the market in 1983 in view of mounting public concern about its safety. This drug was a mixture of doxylamine succinate and pyridoxine hydrochloride and was marketed as Debendox® or Bendectin®. Despite having been used by over 30 million pregnant women over a quarter of a century, and notwithstanding carefully designed clinical trials suggesting that the drug was not teratogenic, individual case reports linking the use of the drug to fetal abnormality were given considerable publicity and led to its withdrawal. In view of the extremely high number of exposures, many chance associations between drug use and fetal abnormality were inevitable. This episode illustrated that in an emotional area such as the use of drugs during pregnancy, well-chosen and carefully presented anecdotes can be more powerful than a substantial body of scientific data carefully accumulated over many years.

Case studies are more secure in that they describe several patients where the same drug and malformation were linked: phenytoin and the retinoids were found to be teratogenic in this way. Epidemiological studies are of two major types: cohort studies, which prospectively study exposed and unexposed groups, and case-control studies, which retrospectively compare the pregnancies of abnormal and normal offspring. So far as teratogenesis is concerned, case-control studies are the norm because of the size and expense of cohort studies. The relationship between diethylstilbestrol use in the first trimester and vaginal adenocarcinoma in teenage offspring was found in a case-control study.

The effect of drugs on the fetus

A drug can harm the fetus only if it crosses the placenta, but most drugs do. The placenta offers a lipid barrier to the transfer of drugs, and the rate at which a drug crosses from mother to baby will depend on its lipophilicity and polarity. However, with the exception of drugs administered acutely around the time of delivery, the rate of transfer is of little importance, and for any course of drug treatment it should be assumed that transfer will occur. The only notable exceptions are heparin—including low molecular weight preparations—and insulin.

Drugs can adversely affect the developing fetus in different ways depending on the gestation at which exposure occurs. For this reason it is appropriate to consider organogenesis, fetal growth and development, the breast-fed infant, and childhood growth and development separately.

Prescribing in the first trimester

Organogenesis occurs between 18 and 55 days of gestation and it is during this time that drugs can cause anatomical defects. A drug can cause a teratogenic effect only if it is present in the embryo during organogenesis, and

Table 1 Some commonly used drugs that are known to be teratogenic

Drug	Main abnormality	Approximate risk (%)
Phenytoin	Craniofacial	6
Carbamazepine	Craniofacial, limb	6
Sodium valproate	Neural tube	2
Warfarin	Chondrodysplasia punctata	Up to 25
	Facial anomalies	
	CNS anomalies	
Lithium	Cardiac (Ebstein complex)	2
Danazol	Virilization of female fetus	Uncertain
Retinoids	Multiple	High

even a definite teratogen will not cause a structural defect if it is given following this period. These seemingly obvious statements become relevant in prepregnancy counselling and in providing advice when exposure to a possible teratogen has occurred during pregnancy. Being present in the embryo during organogenesis is not necessarily synonymous with being prescribed during this period. The retinoids are stored in adipose tissue and released slowly, so a teratogenic effect can occur long after the course of treatment has been completed. It is important to recognize that teratogenic effects are not seen in all cases: on the contrary, most first trimester exposures to teratogenic drugs will not harm the baby. Clearly there is more to drug-induced fetal abnormality than simply the drug: the genetic make up of the baby is important too. Some drugs that are definitely teratogenic in the human, together with approximate risks, are listed in Table 1.

Preventing drug-induced teratogenesis—short of the obvious solution of not taking the drug—is difficult. Where there is a risk of neural tube defect, folic acid 5 mg daily should be prescribed from the time that pregnancy is planned. No direct evidence currently exists to support this approach, but the approach is logical: folic acid is known to be effective in the secondary prevention of naturally occurring neural tube defect, and anticonvulsants lower folate levels. Some reports have also claimed a direct relationship between dose and fetal abnormality. For example, one meta-analysis involving over 1000 babies exposed to sodium valproate found a higher risk of abnormality at doses above 1 g per day compared with less than 600 mg daily. In epileptic pregnancies, polypharmacy is accompanied by a greater risk of fetal abnormality, but since these women are likely to have the more severe forms of the disease, cause and effect is hard to establish. Many of the abnormalities caused by these drugs can be detected by detailed ultrasound scanning at 18 to 20 weeks' gestation. However, the defects caused by warfarin involve mainly soft tissue and do not fall into this category.

Table 1 is not comprehensive and includes only those drugs commonly encountered in general medical practice. Some drugs used in specialist areas are teratogenic, for example several drugs used in cancer chemotherapy. Many more drugs may be teratogenic in a small percentage of exposures, but definitive information is not available because both prediction and detection of human teratogens is difficult. Predicting the effect of a drug in the human usually depends on studying its pharmacology in experimental animals. This is not fruitful in the area of teratogenesis because species variation is so great. For example, thalidomide causes phocomelia only in primates, while lithium causes cardiac abnormalities in humans at doses that produce no effect in the rat. Detecting teratogenic effects is complicated by the normal occurrence of fetal abnormalities, hence if a drug is teratogenic very occasionally it can be very difficult to distinguish its effects from those arising naturally.

Even if a drug is a teratogen, the balance of benefits and risks may still be in favour of its use. For example, chloroquine and proguanil are indicated for malarial prophylaxis in areas where *Plasmodium falciparum* remains sensitive. Currently available evidence suggests that chloroquine may cause a very small increase in birth defects: in one study 169 infants whose mothers took chloroquine-base 300 mg once weekly were compared with 454 children whose mothers took no drug. Abnormal babies were born to 1.2 per cent of the treated group, compared to 0.9 per cent of the controls:

not a significant difference, but the study was too small to detect anything less than a fivefold increase in abnormality rate. By contrast to the possibility of this small increase in risk, malaria presents a major risk to the health and life of both mother and baby, particularly when an expatriate woman is travelling in an endemic area. The argument in favour of using prophylaxis is therefore overwhelming—but not so overwhelming as the advice for pregnant travellers to avoid malarial areas!

Similar arguments apply to corticosteroids, which have acquired a reputation for causing oral cleft defects. The evidence in support of this effect is at best conflicting and is easily outweighed by the benefits of steroids in conditions such as severe asthma, inflammatory bowel disease, systemic lupus erythematosus, or organ transplantation. The placenta inactivates around 90 per cent of prednisolone, whilst corticosteroids, such as betamethasone, that are used to accelerate fetal lung maturity have much greater penetration to the fetus.

Prescribing later in pregnancy

Beyond organogenesis, the fetus undergoes growth and development. The scope for producing anatomical defects has largely passed, exceptions being premature closure of the ductus arteriosus caused by indometacin and bleeding into the fetal brain produced by warfarin. Growth and function tend to be the targets of drug adverse effects for the remainder of the pregnancy.

The possible effects of some commonly used drugs later in pregnancy are shown in Table 2.

Table 2 Some drugs that can cause harm later in the pregnancy

ACE inhibitors	First trimester exposure fairly common and low risk
	Avoid in remainder of pregnancy because of fetal and neonatal renal damage
Antithyroid drugs	Fetal hypothyroidism if used in excessive dose
Aspirin	Analgesic doses associated with neonatal bleeding; not seen with low-dose aspirin
β-Agonists	Pulmonary oedema can occur in management of preterm labour, particularly when combined with excessive fluids and/or corticosteroids
β-Blockers	Use throughout pregnancy associated with around 25% risk of intrauterine growth retardation; not seen with short-term use in third trimester
Benzodiazepines	Drug dependence in the fetus
Corticosteroids	Claims that these drugs cause intrauterine growth retardation, or suppress the fetal adrenal, are not supported by the available evidence
Heparin	Maternal osteoporosis: risk increases with dose and duration of exposure
Indomethacin	Multiple neonatal morbidity; premature closure of ductus
Phenytoin	Neonatal haemorrhage accompanied by low levels of vitamin K-dependent clotting factors
Tetracyclines	Tooth discoloration. No evidence of harm following limited exposure in first trimester
Warfarin	Fetal cerebral haemorrhage—can occur with therapeutic INR in the mother

ACE, angiotensin-converting enzyme

Table 3 Some drugs that have been used in breast-feeding women without evidence of harm to the baby

β-Blockers	Metronidazole
Bronchodilators (inhaled)	Opioids (therapeutic administration)
Carbamazepine	Oral contraceptives
Carbimazole (high doses may suppress the neonatal thyroid)	Paracetamol
	Penicillins
Codeine	Phenytoin
Corticosteroids	Propylthiouracil (high dose may suppress neonatal thyroid)
Digoxin	
Heparin	Sodium valproate
H_2-antagonists	Tricyclic antidepressants
Methyldopa	Warfarin

Drugs and breast feeding

Most women now elect to breast feed their babies, and the majority will take a drug during this time. Iron, mild analgesics, antibiotics, laxatives, and hypnotics are the most commonly used. Much work has been performed on the pharmacokinetic aspects of breast feeding, but systematic studies on the effect of drug ingestion by the mother on her breast-fed baby are lacking.

Milk consists of fat globules suspended in an aqueous solution of protein and nutrients. Drugs move from plasma to milk by passive diffusion of the unionized and non-protein-bound fraction. Since breast milk has a slightly lower pH than plasma, drugs that cross most extensively into breast milk are lipid-soluble, poorly protein-bound, weak bases. However, even for drugs that do cross readily into breast milk, considerable dilution has already occurred in the mother. Thus, when the concentration of a drug in breast milk and the volume of the milk consumed by the baby are translated into a dose, it is often the case that the baby receives too little drug to have any detectable pharmacological effect.

Some of the more commonly used drugs that, on the basis of experience, have a good safety record in breast-feeding mothers are listed in Table 3. It will be seen from this that many of the drugs that would be indicated for common medical problems in this context are safe to use. However, some qualification is needed about two of the drugs listed in Table 3. Oestrogen-containing oral contraceptives may suppress lactation if they are taken before the milk supply is well established, and in some women may do so even after this time: progestogen-only contraceptives do not influence lactation at any stage. Metronidazole is not harmful to the baby but is said to make the milk taste bitter and may therefore interfere with feeding.

Some drugs have been shown to affect the baby when ingested in breast milk: these are listed in Table 4. There are several other drugs for which theoretical risks exist, or for which isolated reports of serious adverse consequences have appeared. For example, aspirin is contraindicated in young children because of the possible association with Reye's syndrome, and some authorities consider that the drug should therefore be avoided in women who are breast feeding. No evidence is available to support this view, but unless the use of aspirin is considered essential in a breast-feeding woman (and such an eventuality must be rare), then it is probably best avoided. Similarly, indometacin has been associated with one case of neonatal convulsion when used during lactation: a decision with regard to its

Table 4 Some drugs that may be harmful to the baby when used in breast-feeding women

Amiodarone:	risk from release of iodine
Barbiturates:	drowsiness
Benzodiazepines:	lethargy and weight loss
Iodine:	risk of neonatal hypothyroidism
Laxatives:	diarrhoea
Lithium:	hypotonia, lethargy, cyanosis
Phenobarbital:	drowsiness

appropriateness in any given patient would depend on the likelihood of real benefit accruing from its use.

Behavioural teratology

The most obvious consequences of a drug-induced fetal abnormality occur at or shortly after birth in the form of anatomical defects, and studies in teratology have largely concentrated on immediate pregnancy outcome. However, drugs can, on occasion, cause problems that become manifest only after several years. The most striking example is diethylstilbestrol which, when given during early pregnancy, can lead to adenocarcinoma of the vagina in teenage offspring. In addition to late morphological effects, concern has been expressed that drugs given during pregnancy can influence behavioural development, although the available evidence is to the contrary.

Anticonvulsants

Several studies have claimed that the use of anticonvulsants during pregnancy is associated with impaired intellectual development of the children, but it is difficult to carry out studies in this area and the choice of control group is crucially important. When all children of treated epileptic mothers in a single hospital in Finland were studied prospectively, using the offspring of untreated epileptic women and age-matched children of the same social class as controls, no difference was found in intellectual development at the age of 5.5 years. At present it appears likely that, in the absence of any obvious morphological abnormality at birth, anticonvulsant use during pregnancy is not associated with impairment of intellectual development but studies of sufficient statistical power have not yet been performed.

Antihypertensive drugs

One of the earliest trials on the treatment of hypertension during pregnancy involved a comparison of methyldopa with no treatment. The children underwent physical and psychomotor assessment at 4 and 7.5 years. The 4-year-old children from the treatment group had a slightly smaller head circumference than their untreated controls, but there were no other physical or psychomotor differences. The evaluation at 7.5 years revealed no differences between the two groups. The reputation of methyldopa as a safe drug in pregnancy is largely based on this very well-conducted study.

The effects on childhood development of atenolol versus placebo have similarly shown no detrimental effects, a wide range of physical and psychomotor tests being performed on the children at the age of 1 year.

Effect of pregnancy on drugs

Influence of pregnancy on dose requirements

While the emphasis on what drugs can do to the pregnancy is both understandable and appropriate, the physiological changes of pregnancy can have a clinically important influence on drug disposition and effect. The plasma concentrations of some drugs fall to an extent that is clinically important during pregnancy.

Among the many physiological changes in pregnancy, the most important from the standpoint of drugs are those that influence clearance. By the third trimester renal blood flow has nearly doubled and the activity of some, but not all, liver metabolic pathways is increased during pregnancy. A further factor tending to reduce drug concentrations is an increase in body water, with around an additional 7 litres being retained by the end of pregnancy.

The importance of these changes is well illustrated by the influence of pregnancy on anticonvulsant dose requirements. The plasma concentrations of phenytoin and carbamazepine decrease as pregnancy progresses. An increase in systemic clearance is the main reason—for example, the clearance of phenytoin increases by over 100 per cent by the third trimester—with an increased volume of distribution making a further contribution. An example of the influence of pregnancy on the concentration

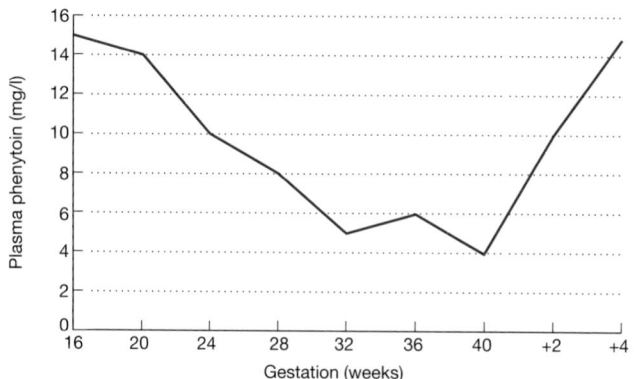

Fig. 1 Plasma phenytoin concentration during and following pregnancy in a woman who remained on a constant dose of 300 mg/day throughout. She had a seizure at 38 weeks' gestation and delivered at 40 weeks. The dose should have been increased when the phenytoin concentration began to fall.

of phenytoin is shown in Fig. 1. The reduction in anticonvulsant concentration can be substantial and, if the dose is not increased, then seizure control may be lost. The physiological changes of pregnancy resolve in the 6 weeks following delivery, and there is a progressive return to prepregnancy dose requirements during this time.

Not all drugs metabolized in the liver show reductions in plasma concentration during pregnancy. For example, the clearance of propranolol is unchanged, presumably because this is determined by liver blood flow, which is not altered by pregnancy.

Since renal blood flow increases during pregnancy, the clearance of drugs eliminated by this route can also be expected to increase. Lithium clearance doubles during pregnancy, so that dose increases, guided by drug-level monitoring, are likely to be needed. Dose requirements fall rapidly following delivery and care must be taken to avoid the development of toxicity. The clearance of ampicillin nearly doubles during pregnancy. Formal pharmacokinetic studies have not been performed with cephalosporins, but plasma levels of around 50 per cent of those found in non-pregnant subjects have been reported. By contrast to drugs with a reasonably well-

defined therapeutic range, the falling plasma levels of penicillin or cephalosporin antibiotics are of less obvious significance. However, it seems prudent to give doses at the higher end of the recommended range when using these agents to treat systemic infections during pregnancy.

Drug protein binding in pregnancy

The protein binding of drugs is also altered by pregnancy. The mechanism is not fully understood: although the concentration of albumin falls substantially in a normal pregnancy, there is no correlation between the concentration of albumin and the free fraction of the drug, at least not for all drugs. The free and pharmacologically active concentration of anticonvulsants is increased in pregnancy by 30 to 50 per cent, which has consequences for the interpretation of plasma drug levels.

Therapeutic drug monitoring during pregnancy

Epilepsy is the commonest condition for which therapeutic drug monitoring during pregnancy should be performed. This area is controversial because in non-obstetric practice therapeutic drug monitoring is considered of less value than seizure control as a guide to drug management. However, during pregnancy there is a high likelihood that drug levels will fall because of pharmacokinetic changes. In addition, measuring levels is a useful guide to poor compliance with treatment, which is a feature of the pregnant epileptic. Waiting for a seizure to occur is not without risk: women die from poorly controlled epilepsy in pregnancy. Since the free fraction of anticonvulsants increases during pregnancy, it is the unbound level that should preferably be recorded. Alternatively, saliva samples can be used to guide treatment, since these have been shown to correlate well with the plasma concentration of unbound drug.

Further reading

Briggs GG, Freeman RK, Yaffe SJ (1998). *Drugs in pregnancy and lactation*, 5th edn. Williams and Wilkins, Baltimore.
Rubin PC (2000). *Prescribing in pregnancy*, 3rd edn. British Medical Journal, London.

13.19 Benefits and risks of oral contraceptives

M. P. Vessey

Introduction

The basic physiological principles underlying a hormonal approach to contraception had already been elaborated by the mid 1930s, but the development of practical methods of hormonal birth control had to await the synthesis of potent orally active steroids some 20 years later. Much of the physiological and clinical development of the 'the pill' was done by Pincus and Rock in the United States in the 1950s; great credit must be given to these two for their contribution to one of the great medical breakthroughs of the twentieth century. Indeed, in 1999 it was estimated that about 110 million women were taking oral contraceptives, 62 million of them in developing countries.

There are several different types of oral contraceptive regimen, but the most important preparations include both an oestrogen and a progestogen. In the United Kingdom, only two oestrogens have been used, ethinylestradiol and mestranol, but seven progestogens are currently available (northisterone, norethisterone acetate, ethynodiol diacetate, levonorgestrel, desogestrel, norgestimate, gestodene) while others have been used in the past (e.g. norethynodrel, chlormadinone acetate, megestrol acetate). Since the dosage of the constituent steroids may be varied (the trend has generally been downwards over the years both for the oestrogen and progestogen components), it is not surprising that the number of different oestrogen–progestogen formulations marketed currently or in the past is very large—over 100 in the United Kingdom. This adds greatly to the difficulties confronting those trying to assess safety.

Oral contraceptives have many metabolic effects, although these are fewer with modern preparations than with earlier ones. None the less, it has been said that 'almost every metabolic parameter that is capable of laboratory investigation has been reported to be altered in one way or another by some contraceptive steroid'. This implies that the results of routine laboratory tests may be altered by oral contraceptives, a point of considerable practical importance. In this chapter, however, attention will be largely concentrated on effects of the pill on morbidity and mortality, as revealed by epidemiological studies.

Until the mid 1970s, most of the available data about the benefits and risks of the pill had been derived from uncontrolled clinical trials and from case-control studies. One large-scale randomized study, including 9757 women allocated either to an oral contraceptive or to a vaginal method of contraception, had been started in Puerto Rico in 1961 by Pincus, but it proved to have serious shortcomings and contributed little to knowledge. Since the mid 1970s, an enormous amount of epidemiological information has been obtained from two large British cohort studies, the Royal College of General Practitioners Oral Contraceptive Study and the Oxford–Family Planning Association (Oxford–FPA) Contraceptive Study. Between them, these investigations recruited 63 000 women of child-bearing age (about half of whom were users of the pill and half users of other methods or no method of contraception) who have now been carefully followed up for an average of around 25 years. Many of the findings described in this chapter are derived from these two cohort studies.

Information about the benefits and risks of oral contraception in the developing world is sparse. The reader is cautioned not to extrapolate the data summarized here to parts of the world to which they clearly do not apply.

Benefits of combined oral contraceptives

High efficacy

By far the most important beneficial effect of these preparations is their remarkable efficacy which, coupled with a high degree of acceptability (at least among the young), has given many women freedom from anxiety about pregnancy. If taken conscientiously, no more than about two to four women in every thousand using a combined preparation should become accidentally pregnant each year. In practice, pills are often missed and much less satisfactory results are then obtained.

Suppression of menstrual disorders

It has long been known that oral contraceptives suppress some menstrual disorders, notably menorrhagia and dysmenorrhoea, leading to a reduction in hospital referral for diagnosis and treatment of these conditions and to a lessened risk of iron-deficiency anaemia.

Suppression of benign breast disease

Epidemiological studies have consistently shown that use of older, higher-dose oral contraceptives seems to decrease the occurrence of benign lumps in the breast, reducing the need for hospital referral for diagnosis and treatment of such lesions by up to 50 per cent. The effect is most pronounced in long-term users, appears to wear off after discontinuation of use, and is probably attributable to the progestogen component of the pill. More recent studies considering lower-dose pills have tended to find less impressive effects on benign breast disease than did the earlier studies.

Pelvic inflammatory disease

Oestrogen–progestogen oral contraceptives reduce the risk of symptomatic pelvic inflammatory disease and probably reduce the severity of the disease as well. There is, however, evidence that the protective effect of the pill is less against pelvic inflammatory disease caused by chlamydial infection than against disease caused by other organisms.

Suppression of functional ovarian cysts

Since oral contraceptives act principally by inhibiting ovulation, it is not surprising that follicular cysts and particularly corpus luteum cysts are relatively uncommon in pill users, although this may apply less to modern, very low-dose pills than to older, high-dose ones.

Suppression of ovarian cancer and endometrial cancer

Epidemiological studies reported during the past 15 years have demonstrated that the risk of both epithelial ovarian cancer and endometrial cancer is reduced by up to 50 per cent in women who have used combined oral contraceptives for at least 5 years. Longer durations of use offer additional protection while shorter durations of use still provide some beneficial effect. The protective effect appears to persist for many years after cessation of pill use; this is important from the public health point of view since ovarian and endometrial cancer are rare in young women amongst whom oral contraceptive use is most prevalent.

Other possible beneficial effects

While the beneficial effects already described may be considered established, a number of others have been reported in some studies and deserve mention. These include a lessened risk of thyroid disease, rheumatoid arthritis, fibroids, endometriosis, and colorectal cancer. An increased peak bone mass has also been reported in long-term users. Further work is necessary before the significance of these observations can be adequately assessed.

Risks of combined oral contraceptives

Oral contraceptives are well known to cause minor side-effects such as nausea, headache, and breast tenderness. Although such symptoms are common enough and unpleasant enough to lead to discontinuation of the pill by up to 25 per cent of women, they disappear when medication is stopped and do not represent a serious threat to health.

Cardiovascular effects

The best known substantial adverse effects of oral contraceptive use are cardiovascular, comprising venous thrombosis and embolism, thrombotic stroke, and acute myocardial infarction. The evidence concerning haemorrhagic stroke is rather less convincing. All these conditions are rare in young women and the absolute risk associated with pill use is very low. The risks, in most studies, are confined to current pill users and do not depend on duration of pill use. The risk of acute myocardial infarction (and to a lesser extent stroke) in pill users seems to be concentrated in women with other risk factors for cardiovascular disease, notably cigarette smoking and hypertension.

In 1995, findings were published from a multinational study by the World Health Organization which indicated that the risk of venous thromboembolism attributable to oral contraceptive use was twice as high in women using pills containing gestodene or desogestrel as in women using pills containing older progestogens. Some additional studies have confirmed this observation while others have not, and this remains a controversial topic.

The mechanisms underlying adverse cardiovascular reactions to the pill are uncertain. However, oral contraceptives have effects on the coagulation system, on serum lipids, on carbohydrate metabolism, on blood pressure, and on the structure of vessels. Any or all of these effects might be of significance. In recent years, there has been great interest in the effect of oral contraceptive use on venous thromboembolism in women with thrombophilic disorders. Thus the risks associated with factor V Leiden and current oral contraceptive use appear to multiply, such that a woman with both these characteristics may have a risk of venous thromboembolism which is about 30 times higher than that in a woman without either of them.

Breast cancer

Large numbers of studies have been conducted on oral contraception and breast cancer, but no consensus was reached on their interpretation until a collaborative re-analysis of 54 studies was published in 1996. It was found that the relative risk of having breast cancer diagnosed in current users of combined oral contraceptives in comparison with never-users was 1.24. There was also some increase in risk in ex-users, but this was no longer apparent 10 or more years after stopping. Cancers diagnosed in women who had used combined oral contraceptives were clinically less advanced than those diagnosed in women who had never done so. It is not known whether there is an increased risk of dying from breast cancer as well as an increased risk of having breast cancer diagnosed in women using the pill.

Hepatocellular adenoma and carcinoma

Hepatocellular adenoma and carcinoma are extremely rare (but serious) conditions in women of child-bearing age. In those without exposure to the pill, the incidence might be around one per million per annum. Oral contraceptive users suffer a higher incidence than this, but there is reason to believe that the increase in risk is much less in those taking modern, low-dose pills.

Impairment of fertility

Despite a vast literature, prior use of oral contraceptives has not been incriminated either as a cause of prolonged secondary amenorrhoea (say absence of periods for more than 6 months) or of prolactinoma of the pituitary, which is sometimes associated with this condition. Many women do, however, experience some temporary impairment of fertility after stopping the pill, especially those over the age of 30 trying to have a first baby. In the majority this lasts only a month or so, but in some recovery may be much slower. It seems unlikely that oral contraceptives are ever a cause of permanent infertility.

Other possible adverse effects

A large number of studies have indicated a positive association between long-term oral contraceptive use and cervical cancer. The interpretation of this association is uncertain, mainly because cancer of the cervix is so strongly associated with sexual activity that it is extremely difficult to isolate any independent effect of the method of contraception used.

Several studies have examined the possible relationship between oral contraceptive use and malignant melanoma; they have not given consistent results. The same is true for studies of hydatidiform mole and choriocarcinoma.

In the past, there was considerable anxiety about an increase in the risk of cholelithiasis in pill users. Further work has shown the effect, if present, to be minimal. The evidence concerning chronic inflammatory bowel disease is more convincing. Many other possible adverse effects of oral contraceptives have been suggested, including depression, urinary tract infection, and fetal malformation if taken inadvertently during pregnancy. In every case, the balance of evidence is not compelling. A recent concern centres around human immunodeficiency virus (HIV) infection being commoner in pill users, with worrying findings in prostitutes in Nairobi. These results have not, in general, been replicated in other studies and there is no clear evidence of an adverse effect of pill use on the risk of HIV infection.

Progestogen-only oral contraceptives

Low doses of progestogens taken every day by mouth have been extensively investigated as contraceptives. Such preparations do not consistently inhibit ovulation and their mode of action is uncertain. Their efficacy is lower than that of the oestrogen–progestogen pill, but they can give entirely adequate protection in older women who may prefer not to use conventional pills. A major disadvantage of progestogen-only oral contraceptives is their tendency to disrupt the menstrual cycle in many women, producing irregular bleeding, whilst those who become accidentally pregnant when using them have about a 5 per cent chance of an ectopic gestation. These drawbacks probably account for the fact that progestogen-only pills represent only a small fraction of all oral contraceptives consumed. Their main advantage is that they appear to be free from the undesirable metabolic effects of combined preparations. In addition, they can be taken safely by women who are breast feeding without risking the reduction in milk production that usually occurs if combined oral contraceptives are taken.

Balance of benefits and risks

A number of authors have provided analyses of varying degrees of complexity in which they have attempted to weigh up the benefits and risks of taking the pill. Three approaches are outlined here. In the first, which uses hospital inpatient morbidity data from the Oxford–FPA study, supplemented where necessary by other epidemiological data, a comparison is made over a 1-year period of women using either oral contraceptives or a condom for contraception. The approach is fully described elsewhere (see Further reading), but Table 1 summarizes the main findings. Despite the sizeable cardiovascular risks (older 50 μg pills were used in the Oxford–FPA study) the overall results are quite favourable as far as oestrogen–progestogen oral contraceptives are concerned. Similar analyses reported from the Royal College of General Practitioners Oral Contraceptive Study have produced comparable results.

The second approach involves constructing models that consider what is known about the effects of oral contraceptives and other methods of birth control on mortality, and estimating the balance of benefit and risk over a period of many years. This approach is too complex to describe here because of space limitations, but details are available elsewhere (see Further reading). Not surprisingly, the results obtained in such analyses depend to an important extent on whether or not oral contraceptives increase the risk

Table 1 Morbidity (in terms of first hospital admissions) experienced by women aged 25 to 39 years using either combined oral contraceptives (OCs) or relying on the condom to try to prevent pregnancy for 1 year; based on data from the Oxford–FPA study, supplemented by other epidemiological data

Reason for first hospital admission	Number of first hospital admissions in one year among 100 000 women relying on	
	Combined oral contraceptives	Condom
Beneficial effects of OCs		
Menstrual problems	375	500
Anaemia	22	30
Benign breast disease	115	230
Pelvic inflammatory disease*	60	60
Functional ovarian cysts	15	60
Ovarian cancer	5	10
Endometrial cancer	2	4
Harmful effects of OCs		
Acute myocardial infarction	10	5
Thrombotic stroke	50	10
Haemorrhagic stroke	7	5
Venous thromboembolism	100	20
Breast cancer	37	30
Hepatocellular adenoma	2	0
Hepatocellular carcinoma	0	0
Accidental pregnancy†		
Term birth	300	3040
Spontaneous abortion	63	640
Extrauterine pregnancy	3	20
Induced abortion	134	1300

*These rates are equal because both OCs and a condom offer protection against pelvic inflammatory disease.

†The failure rate for OCs has been taken to be 5 per 1000 per year and for the condom to be 50 per 1000 per year. The data relate to events and not just first hospital admissions.

Older 50 μg contraceptive pills were mainly used in the Oxford-FPA study.

Table 2 Mortality in the Oxford–FPA study

Cause of death	Oral contraceptive at entry	Diaphragm/ IUD at entry
Malignant melanoma	0.7 (1)*	0.7 (1)
Breast cancer	23.1 (31)	27.1 (37)
Cervix cancer	4.4 (7)	0.9 (1)
Corpus cancer	0.0 (0)	1.4 (2)
Ovarian cancer	3.6 (5)	9.1 (12)
Other tumours	17.7 (26)	21.6 (27)
Ischaemic heart disease	9.2 (15)	2.8 (3)
Cerebrovascular disease	4.2 (7)	2.9 (3)
Other circulatory disease	2.4 (3)	4.1 (6)
Suicide and probable suicide	6.1 (10)	5.6 (6)
Other accidents, etc.	2.3 (4)	2.0 (2)
All other causes	9.9 (15)	11.7 (14)
All causes	84.3 (124)	90.9 (114)

*Rates per 100 000 woman-years with numbers of deaths in parentheses. None of the above differences reaches statistical significance.

of death from breast cancer (as opposed to merely increasing the rate of diagnosis of the disease), the length of time after discontinuation of oral contraceptive use that the protective effect against epithelial ovarian cancer and endometrial cancer persists, and the ages at which oral contraceptives are used. Considering the current pattern of oral contraceptive use in developed countries, which is predominantly by women below the age of 35 years, the balance of benefits and risks seems entirely acceptable.

The final approach is a more direct one. It involves examination of the mortality rates observed in the major cohort studies, comparing oral contraceptive users with non-users. Data published in 1989 from the Oxford–FPA study relating to the first 238 deaths are shown in Table 2. Although the numbers are small, the pattern of mortality reflects what is known about the effects of oral contraceptive use from other studies. Overall, the mortality ratio comparing users with non-users is 0.93 (95 per cent confidence interval 0.71–1.22). In a corresponding analysis from the Royal College of General Practitioners study including 1599 deaths, the overall mortality ratio was 1.02 (95 per cent confidence interval 0.92–1.13), while the large Nurses' Health cohort study in the United States reported an overall mortality ratio of 0.93 (95 per cent confidence interval 0.85–1.01) based on 2879 deaths. These data clearly offer considerable reassurance about the effects of oral contraceptives.

The pill has been studied extremely intensively over the past four decades. On the whole, it has stood up well to close scrutiny. It remains an excellent method of contraception for younger women. There remains some doubt, however, about its suitability for those aged over 40. Women in this age group are, however, usually well served by progestogen-only pills if a reversible method of contraception is required.

Further reading

Beral V *et al.* (1999). Mortality associated with oral contraceptive use: 25 year follow up of cohort of 46,000 women from Royal College of General Practitioners' Oral Contraception Study. *British Medical Journal* **318**, 96–100.

Colditz GA for the Nurses' Health Study Research Group (1994). Oral contraceptive use and mortality during 12 years of follow-up: the Nurses' Health Study. *Annals of Internal Medicine* **120**, 821–6.

Collaborative Group on Hormonal Factors in Breast Cancer (1996). Breast cancer and hormonal contraceptives: collaborative reanalysis of individual data on 53,297 women with breast cancer and 100,239 women without breast cancer from 54 epidemiological studies. *Lancet* **347**, 1713–27.

Hannaford PC, Kay CR (1998). The risk of serious illness among oral contraceptive users: evidence from the RCGP's oral contraceptive study. *British Journal of General Practice* **48**, 1657–62.

International Agency for Research on Cancer (1999). Hormonal contraception and post-menopausal hormonal therapy. In *Monographs on the evaluation of carcinogenic risks to humans*, vol. 72. WHO, IARC, Lyon.

Oldfield K, Milne R, Vessey M (1998). The effects on mortality of the use of combined oral contraceptives. *British Journal of Family Planning* 24, 2–6.

Vessey MP (1990). The Jephcott Lecture 1989. An overview of the benefits and risks of combined oral contraceptives. In: Mann RD, ed. *Oral contraceptives and breast cancer*, pp 121–32. Parthenon, Carnforth.

Vessey MP, Smith MA, Yeates D (1986). Return of fertility after discontinuation of oral contraceptives: influence of age and parity. *British Journal of Family Planning* 11, 120–4.

Vessey MP *et al.* (1989). Mortality among oral contraceptive users: 20 year follow up of women in a cohort study. *British Medical Journal* 299, 1487–91.

WHO Scientific Group (1998). Cardiovascular disease and steroid hormone contraception. *WHO Technical Report Series* no. 877. WHO, Geneva.

13.20 Benefits and risks of hormone replacement therapy

J. C. Stevenson

Introduction

The acute effects of female sex hormone deficiency such as vasomotor symptoms are well known, but the importance of the longer-term effects of ovarian failure have only been recognized recently. The menopause, the time of a woman's last menstrual period, is a useful marker for ovarian failure and occurs naturally at an average age of around 51 years, although it may occur at any time after puberty. A postmenopausal state can usually be inferred by the absence of menses for 12 months in a woman of appropriate age. The demonstration of elevated gonadotrophin levels may help to confirm the diagnosis in hysterectomized women.

Clinical features of menopause

A number of symptoms may arise soon after loss of ovarian function at the menopause. These include hot flushes and night sweats, and psychological symptoms such as mood swings, depression, anxiety and irritability, and difficulties with memory and concentration. Later there may be genitourinary problems such as vaginal dryness and dyspareunia, and increased urinary frequency and urge incontinence. However, it is the long-term consequences of hormone deficiency, particularly osteoporosis and cardiovascular disease, which pose a major health problem for women.

The menopause is recognized as a substantial risk factor for the development of osteoporosis, and perhaps one in every two women will have this disease by the end of their lives. The classical osteoporotic fractures are of the vertebrae, distal forearm, and proximal femur, but osteoporosis may also result in fractures of the ribs and pelvis, proximal humerus, ankle, and phalanges. Hip fracture is by far the most serious in terms of morbidity, mortality, and cost to the health service: one in five women die and at least 50 per cent of the remainder end up in institutionalized care, such that the health service costs of osteoporosis are now approaching a billion pounds annually in the United Kingdom.

Increased risk of cardiovascular disease is the most important consequence of ovarian failure. Coronary heart disease is the leading cause of death in women, and although it occurs at a later age than in men, overall more women than men die from the disease. The occurrence of coronary heart disease in women is frequently overlooked, and women are less likely than men to undergo both investigation and treatment for this disease.

It is now becoming apparent that oestrogen deficiency has profound neurological effects. Alzheimer's dementia is more common in elderly women than men, and the menopause has adverse effects on the central nervous system, including cognitive function.

Benefits of hormone replacement therapy

The main indications for the use of hormone replacement therapy are relief of menopausal symptoms and prevention of osteoporosis. Hormone replacement therapy will abolish vasomotor symptoms, often within days of starting treatment, whilst psychological and genitourinary symptoms may take weeks or even months to respond. It is therefore worthwhile persisting with therapy for several months in the absence of rapid symptomatic response, and treatment should be continued for at least several months after symptomatic relief has been obtained.

Hormone replacement therapy is well established for both the prevention and treatment of osteoporosis, and is as effective as any other agent currently available. It conserves, and to some extent increases, bone density and results in a reduction in the risk of fracture. Therapy should be offered to any woman considered at increased risk of osteoporosis, and particularly those with an early menopause. When the risk of osteoporosis is uncertain, bone density measurement can greatly aid clinical decision-making.

Hormone replacement needs to be given long-term when started in the early postmenopause, but few women are at immediate risk of osteoporotic fracture at this age. An alternative strategy is to commence hormone replacement in elderly women who are at a much greater risk for osteoporotic fracture. This approach results in a relatively rapid reduction in risk of fracture, and is thus more cost-effective. It also avoids the necessity of prolonged therapy. However, the elderly are less tolerant of the side-effects of treatment, particularly cyclical bleeding and mastalgia, and regimens that avoid bleeding are to be preferred for this age group. This includes those with lower doses of oestrogen than used in the early postmenopause, which are effective for bone conservation in the elderly. Cessation of hormone replacement therapy leads to a loss of bone density, but only at the usual postmenopausal rate, and the benefit gained by the skeleton from a suitable period of treatment persists into old age.

It is most likely that prevention of cardiovascular disease will become a major indication for hormone replacement therapy in the future. There are many mechanisms, both established and potential, whereby hormone replacement therapy might benefit the cardiovascular system, and these are summarized in Table 1. The effects vary depending on the type of oestrogen or progestogen and the route of administration. In general, hormone replacement produces a lowering of low-density lipoprotein cholesterol and an increase in high-density lipoprotein cholesterol, thus reversing the changes in lipids and lipoproteins brought about by the menopause. An improvement in glucose tolerance, due to enhancement of insulin secretion and elimination or a reduction in insulin resistance, may be seen. There are also direct effects of oestrogen on arteries, which improve their function by endothelium-dependent and non-endothelium-dependent mechanisms. Hormone replacement therapy should therefore be considered for use in women with increased cardiovascular risk, such as those with established coronary heart disease, diabetics, hypertensives, and cigarette smokers.

Population studies have shown that a reduction in the incidence of cardiovascular disease of around 50 per cent can be achieved with hormone replacement. However, a recent randomized prospective study of hormone replacement therapy for the secondary prevention of coronary heart disease failed to show any overall benefit in outcomes, although an eventual reduction in events by over one-third was observed by the end of the trial. Concerns have been raised about the reliability of these findings, due in part to

Table 1 Hormone replacement therapy and the cardiovascular system: possible mechanisms of action

---

Decreased total cholesterol
Decreased triglycerides
Decreased LDL cholesterol
Decreased LDL cholesterol oxidation
Increased HDL and HDL_2 cholesterol
Increased small dense LDL particle clearance
Increased postprandial lipid clearance
Decreased insulin resistance
Decreased circulating insulin concentrations
Decreased proportion of insulin propeptides
Improved glucose tolerance
Decreased proportion of android fat
Decreased NEFA flux
Decreased fibrinogen
Decreased plasminogen activator inhibitor-1
Increased tissue plasminogen activator
Increased arterial NO production
Decreased endothelin-1 release
Reduced calcium channel ion flux
Enhanced potassium channel ion flux
Decreased ACE activity
Decreased blood pressure
Increased arterial blood flow
Improved arterial remodelling

---

*Abbreviations: LDL, low-density lipoprotein; HDL, high-density lipoprotein; NEFA, non-esterified fatty acids; NO, nitric oxide; ACE, angiotensin-1-converting enzyme.

certain aspects of the trial design, and further studies are awaited to clarify the position.

Therapeutic regimens

Hormone replacement therapy consists of oestrogen, which should be given continuously, with the addition of cyclical progestogen in women who have not had a hysterectomy. Progestogens are necessary to prevent endometrial hyperplasia and neoplasia, and to regulate any uterine bleeding that may occur. Oestrogen is given as oral estradiol 17β, estrone sulphate, or conjugated equine oestrogens. Alternatively, estradiol 17β can be administered transdermally through adhesive skin patches, or implanted subcutaneously as pellets. The synthetic alkylated oestrogens, such as ethinylestradiol, are not used in hormone replacement therapy because of their potency and unwanted side-effects. The progestogens used are either derivatives of 19 nortestosterone, such as norgestrel and norethisterone, or the less androgenic C-21 steroids, such as dydrogesterone and medroxyprogesterone acetate. Natural progesterone can be used but is often poorly tolerated because of drowsiness. Progestogens are usually given in the minimal dose necessary for endometrial protection for 12 or more days per month, and result in a regular uterine bleed. The usual doses of hormones are shown in Table 2.

The main drawback to current hormone replacement therapy regimens is the necessity of uterine withdrawal bleeding, although this is often fairly light, particularly in older patients, and tends to diminish with time. With a satisfactory and regular bleeding pattern, there is usually no need for endometrial screening. However, cyclical bleeding becomes less acceptable as women get older, and thus regimens that avoid such bleeding become preferable. Preparations giving continuous progestogen with continuous oestrogen are used to induce endometrial atrophy and hence abolish uterine bleeding, resulting in amenorrhoea in up to 70 to 80 per cent of women. These therapies are less successful in younger women, where transient episodes of spontaneous ovarian activity may result in irregular bleeding.

Tibolone, a synthetic compound with oestrogenic, progestogenic, and androgenic properties, is an alternative that avoids cyclical bleeding. It relieves vasomotor symptoms and appears as effective as hormone replacement therapy for the prevention and treatment of osteoporosis, but it is not established whether it has other benefits associated with hormone replacement therapy such as desirable cardiovascular effects or effects on the central nervous system. Similarly, it is not known whether it has the same potential risks, such as for the breast.

Raloxifene is a so-called selective estradiol receptor modulator, a synthetic compound which binds to the oestrogen receptor but causes conformational changes that result in different tissue-specific actions. Thus it can act similarly to an oestrogen in the skeleton, preventing osteoporotic vertebral fractures, but like an anti-oestrogen in the breast, causing a reduction in incidence of breast cancer, at least in the short term. It does not cause uterine bleeding, but does not relieve vasomotor or genitourinary symptoms. Studies are awaited to determine what, if any, are its actions on the cardiovascular and central nervous systems.

Table 2 Usual daily doses of oestrogens and progestogens used in hormone replacement therapy. (The lowest doses are often sufficient for the elderly, whilst the higher doses may be needed for the young and acutely postmenopausal women)

	Drug	Dose
Oral preparations		
Oestrogens	Micronized oestradiol 17β	1–2 mg
	Estradiol valerate	1–2 mg
	Estrone sulphate	1.5 mg
	Conjugated equine oestrogens	0.625–1.25 mg
Progestogens	DL-norgestrel	0.15 mg
	Norethisterone acetate	0.7–1.0 mg
	Dydrogesterone	10–20 mg
	Medroxyprogesterone acetate	5–10 mg
Others	Tibolone	2.5 mg
	Raloxifene	60 mg
Other preparations		
Oestrogens	Transdermal estradiol 17β	0.025–0.1 mg
	Estradiol 17β implant	25–50 mg (6 monthly)
Progestogens	Transdermal norethisterone acetate	0.25 mg
	Transdermal levonorgestrel	0.02 mg

Side-effects of hormone replacement therapy

Oestrogenic side-effects such as breast tenderness and nausea are sometimes experienced on commencing therapy, particularly by older patients who are many years postmenopause. These side-effects are transient and usually resolve after about 3 months of therapy. More commonly, side-effects are due to the progestogen and can include breast tenderness, abdominal and pelvic pain, backache, depression, irritability, and migraine.

Risks of hormone replacement therapy

The main concern about hormone replacement therapy, particularly with prolonged treatment, is the risk of breast cancer. Epidemiological evidence remains conflicting: whilst some studies show no overall increased risk of breast cancer, others show an increase with prolonged usage. However, in studies looking at mortality from breast cancer, women taking hormone replacement therapy who develop the disease appear to have a better survival than those not on treatment. It seems prudent to avoid hormone replacement therapy where possible in women with breast cancer, but the disease need not be considered a total contraindication in all cases.

Previous endometrial hyperplasia or neoplasia is not a contraindication, provided the disease has been eradicated. Similarly, endometriosis and uterine fibroids rarely cause a problem, although they may occasionally worsen. There is growing epidemiological evidence that hormone replacement therapy may result in a decrease of around 40 per cent in the incidence of colorectal cancer.

Despite previous beliefs, hormone replacement therapy does not cause hypertension, except as a rare idiosyncratic reaction. There is a small absolute increase in the risk of venous thromboembolism, although whether this is seen with non-oral low-dose therapy is not known. It is therefore prudent to exclude a pre-existing thrombophilia in patients with a relevant past or family history.

Many women gain weight after the menopause, most commonly due to excessive calorie intake, not as a result of taking hormone replacements. Weight gain may occasionally occur due to fluid retention, particularly associated with progestogen use, but increases in body fat are not caused by hormone replacement therapy, although there is a redistribution of body fat, with a reduction in the metabolically harmful central obesity.

Most of the other reputed adverse effects of hormone replacement therapy are unsubstantiated, and have largely arisen from an inappropriate extrapolation of data obtained with oral contraceptive use.

Hormone replacement therapy is a treatment with considerable benefits for many women. The choice of therapeutic agents should be tailored to suit the individual case. There are advantages and disadvantages of certain preparations and combinations, but overall the therapy used should be the one that the patient finds most acceptable. This will encourage compliance with long-term therapy, resulting in the greatest health benefits.

Further reading

Collaborative Group on Hormonal Factors in Breast Cancer (1997). Breast cancer and HRT: collaborative reanalysis of data from 51 epidemiological studies of 52,705 women with breast cancer and 108,411 women without breast cancer. *The Lancet* **350**, 1047–59.

Ginsburg J, Prelevic GM (2000). The place of tibolone in menopausal therapy. In: Studd JWW, ed. *The management of the menopause. The millennium review 2000*, pp 59–67. Parthenon Publishing Group, Carnforth.

Grodstein F, Newcomb PA, Stampfer MJ (1999). Postmenopausal hormone replacement therapy and the risk of colorectal cancer: a review and meta-analysis. *American Journal of Medicine* **106**, 574–82.

Henderson VW (1997). Estrogen, cognition, and a woman's risk of Alzheimer's disease. *American Journal of Medicine* **103**, 11S–18S.

Hulley S *et al.* (1998). Randomized trial of estrogen plus progestin for secondary prevention of coronary heart disease in postmenopausal women. *Journal of the American Medical Association* **280**, 605–13.

Marsh MS, Stevenson JC (1997). Hormone replacement therapy and heart disease. In: Julian DG, Wenger NK, eds. *Women and heart disease*, pp 279–95. Martin Dunitz, London.

Oger E, Scarabin PY (1999). Assessment of the risk for venous thromboembolism among users of hormone replacement therapy. *Drugs Aging* **14**, 55–61.

Spencer CP, Stevenson JC (1997). Oestrogens and anti-oestrogens for the prevention and treatment of osteoporosis. In: Meunier P, ed. *Osteoporosis: diagnosis and management*, pp 111–22. Martin Dunitz, London.

Stevenson JC (1996). Metabolic effects of the menopause and oestrogen replacement. In: Barlow DH, ed. *Baillière's clinical obstetrics and gynaecology. The menopause: key issues*, pp 449–67. Ballière Tindall, London.

Stevenson JC. (1998). Various actions of oestrogens on the vascular system. *Maturitas* **30**, 5–9.

Willis DB *et al.* (1996). Estrogen replacement therapy and risk of fatal breast cancer in a prospective cohort of postmenopausal women in the United States. *Cancer Causes and Control* **7**, 449–57.

14

Gastroenterology

14.1 Introduction to gastroenterology

Graham Neale

At the end of the nineteenth century clinical science emerged in French and German universities. The concepts generated there spread to the medical schools of North America and led to the development of academic medicine. In 1897 the American Gastroenterological Association was founded. However, clinicians were slow to apply the spirit of enquiry to their practice, and well into the twentieth century static electricity or bitter tonics were used to treat 'gastric neurasthenia'; sarsparilla and dandelion were used as 'biliary stimulants'; and colonic lavage was a popular treatment for 'autointoxication'. Few advances in the understanding of gastrointestinal physiology in the first half of the twentieth century had any direct impact on clinical practice. Before the Second World War clinicians with a special interest in abdominal disease remained general physicians, few of whom thought it worthwhile learning to use the semiflexible gastroscope. Oesophagoscopy was the province of otorhinological or thoracic surgeons; and sigmoidoscopy with rigid instruments was undertaken more often in operating theatres than in medical outpatient clinics.

After the Second World War the emergence of simple methods for obtaining biopsies of the liver and small intestine and the more rational management of inflammatory bowel disease led to the rapid development of gastroenterology as a specialty. The 1960s and 1970s brought major advances in the understanding of the pathophysiology of gastrointestinal disease which have laid the principal foundation for modern clinical practice (Table 1). This was the scientific growth period of clinical gastroenterology.

Then in the 1980s and 1990s the development of endoscopic techniques based on fibre optics revolutionized practice, taking us into the technological era of clinical gastroenterology. How long this will last is uncertain. It seems likely that gastroenterologists will become less involved in routine endoscopy. The simpler procedures will probably be undertaken by certified non-physician endoscopists (possibly with robotic instruments) and diagnostic endoscopic retrograde cholepancreatography and colonoscopy will be eliminated by improved scanning procedures. The speed of change may depend on the tenacity with which specialists in gastroenterology cling on to the simpler endoscopic techniques which often provide them with substantial earnings. However, ultimately just a few interventional endoscopists may remain, concentrating on 'high-tech' therapeutic techniques.

Moreover if straightforward curative treatments emerge for inflammatory bowel disease the role of the gastroenterologist will undoubtedly change. Already in the Western world more than half the referrals to specialists in gastroenterology are for advice on managing patients with an irritable bowel. Providers of funding for health care will get an increasing grip on cost efficiency. With better organization of medical knowledge and outcomes research, general practitioners should be able to provide the majority of routine care.

For the physician-gastroenterologist there will be a renewed emphasis on the need to develop advanced interpretative and diagnostic skills. These will underpin therapeutic decision-making and the counselling of patients—who are themselves now far better informed about health and disease. It is possible that some gastroenterologists will evolve into digestive health physicians working as members of teams involving surgeons, radiologists/scanners, pathologists, microbiologists, immunologists, and geneticists. These teams will deal with structural lesions by sophisticated minimally invasive procedures; they may control disease by new techniques of immune modification; and develop methods to correct genetic defects affecting the gastrointestinal tract and adjacent organs. They will depend on the material sciences, information technology, and new means of communication, and will be advising individuals about their health profiles. They will prescribe pharmaceuticals and work with dietitians to alter health risks and to produce health benefits. As a group, digestive health physicians will need to know a great deal about the role of nutrition in health and disease.

Table 1 Landmarks in clinical gastroenterology

1895	Discovery of X-rays followed rapidly by imaging of the gastrointestinal tract (Roentgen, Wurzburg)
1902	Discovery of the first hormone—secretin (Bayliss and Starling, University College London)
1924	Development of cholecystography (Graham and Moore, St Louis)
1932	First semiflexible gastroscope (Wolf and Schindler, Munich)
1953	Recognition of gluten-induced enteropathy (Dicke, Utrecht)
1954	First successful image-transmitting fibre-optic bundle (Hopkins, Imperial College London)
1957	The flexible gastroscope developed (Hirschowicz, Ann Arbor, Michigan)
1963	First human liver transplantation (Starzl, Chicago)
1964	Recognition of the intestinal mucosal Na^+/glucose cotransport (Schultz and Zalusky, Brookes, Texas) leading to treatment of diarrhoeal disease by oral replacement fluid therapy (Phillips, Dacca, Bangladesh)
	Structure of gastrin established (Gregory *et al.* Liverpool)
1965	Australia antigen discovered (Blumberg, Philadelphia).
1969	Western diets and gastrointestinal disease (Burkitt, MRC Units, Uganda and London)
1972	Development of H_2-receptor antagonist (Black, SKF Laboratories, Welwyn Garden City)
	Development of CT scanning (Hounsfield, EMI Laboratories, Hayes, Middlesex)
1975	CT scanning first applied to the abdomen by Alfidi (Cleveland Clinic)
1981	NH^+,K^+-ATPase shown to be the proton pump for the gastric mucosa (Sachs, Birmingham, Alabama)
	Substituted imidazoles developed to inhibit gastric proton pump (Hassle Research Laboratories, Sweden)
1983	First culture of *H. pylori* (Marshall and Warren, Perth, Australia)
1988	Sequence of genetic alterations underlying the development of colorectal tumours (Vogelstein *et al.*, Johns Hopkins Hospital, Baltimore)

Other important developments including an understanding of the microbiology of the gut, techniques for biopsy of the liver and small intestine, artificial feeding (both enteral and parenteral), the discovery and use of a wide spectrum of gastrointestinal hormones and advances in gastrointestinal surgery (including laparoscopic procedures) arose from the work of several research workers often in more than one unit without landmark descriptions.

If these changes are to occur then educational policies will have to change. Most illnesses have multiple causes and management decisions will come to be made through sophisticated risk analysis. All clinicians should have a good background in clinical science in order to cope with the emerging information era. The sections on gastroenterology and clinical nutrition in the *Oxford Textbook of Medicine* provide such a background in an important segment of clinical practice.

Further reading

Booth CC (1985). What has technology done to gastroenterology? *Gut* **26**, 1088–94. An important warning that gastroenterologists should remain physicians and not become technologists.

Chen TS, Chen PS, eds (1995). *A history of gastroenterology*. Parthenon Publishing Group, New York. An interesting book of essays on key developments in gastroenterology.

14.1.1 Anatomy and clinical physiology

14.1.1.1 Structure and function of the gut

D. G. Thompson

Introduction

This chapter provides a brief overview of the structure and function of the gastrointestinal tract (excluding the liver and pancreas). For more detail readers are referred to the Further reading list. Emphasis has been placed on those aspects of gastrointestinal anatomy and physiology which help an understanding of the nature of gastrointestinal symptoms and/or guide an approach to therapy.

Anatomy

Gross anatomy

The gastrointestinal tract is a hollow tube of approximately 5 to 6 m in length, stretching from the oral cavity to anal sphincter (Fig. 1). It is arbitrarily divided into a series of organs which serve different functions, and is joined to the liver and pancreas, the major organs of digestion.

Anatomical structure

The gastrointestinal tract possess a broadly similar structure throughout its length (Fig. 2) with an innermost epithelium, a subepithelial lamina propria, and two muscle layers, an inner circular and an outer longitudinal layer, between which lies the myenteric plexus, the intrinsic neural control system of the musculature. While this description most accurately describes the small intestine, the other organs of the gastrointestinal tract differ only subtly from this stereotype.

Oesophagus

In the oesophagus, the innermost layer is a squamous rather than colomnar epithelium. The musculature in the upper third is striated and controlled directly via extrinsic neural pathways, unlike the lower two-thirds which has smooth muscle and a myenteric plexus.

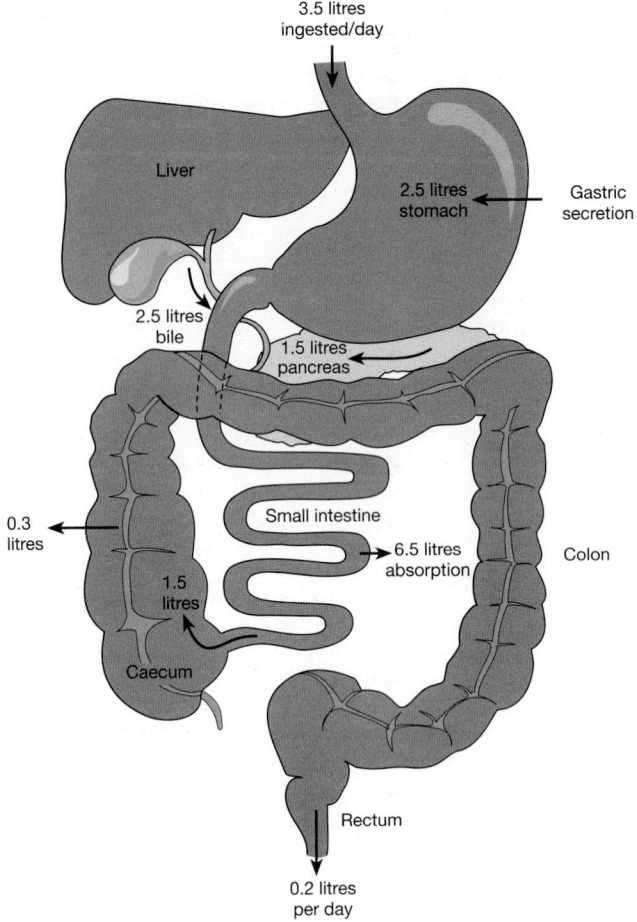

Fig. 1 Schematic diagram of the gastrointestinal tract showing the major organs of the tract and their connections. The figure also shows the average daily fluid flux across the intestinal mucosae to indicate sites and volumes of absorption and secretion in the various organs.

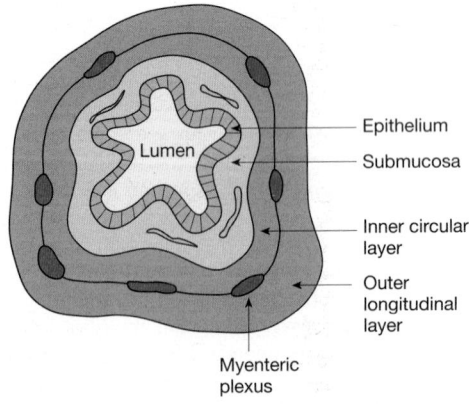

Fig. 2 A generalized structure of the intestine in cross section. A central lumen is bounded by an epithelial layer, which in turn is surrounded by a submucosal layer containing neural and vascular connections to the epithelium. Outside the submucosae lie circumferential and longitudinal muscular layers with the controlling neuronal myenteric plexus lying between.

Stomach

The anatomy of the stomach differs from the intestine, possessing an additional oblique muscular layer and at either end a sphincter—specialized musculature designed to act as a unidirectional valve to control the flow of luminal contents. The sphincter between the oesophagus and stomach (the lower oesophageal sphincter) lies at the level of the diaphragm. The sphincter between the stomach and small intestine is known as the pylorus.

Small intestine

The small intestine is arbitrarily divided into duodenum, jejunum, and ileum. The duodenum (so named because it is 12 fingers' breadth in length) is retroperitoneal, and possess on its medial aspect the ampulla of Vater which connects the pancreatic and common bile ducts to the duodenal lumen. The jejunum (Latin, empty, after death) is mobile and free on a mesentery. The ileum (Greek, twisted) begins indistinctly from the jejunum and ends at the caecum.

Colon and rectum

The colon differs from the small intestine in its muscular structure—the inner circular layer is similar but the outer longitudinal layer is condensed into three 'worm like' structures, the taeniae coli. At the proximal end of the colon, the caecum (Latin, blind ending) arises the vermiform appendix, named because of its worm like appearance. The ascending and descending colon are retroperitoneal whereas the transverse and sigmoid colon are freely mobile on a mesentery, extending to the pelvic floor following which it expands into the rectum.

Anal sphincter

The anal sphincter provides an important continence mechanism and has two parts, an internal sphincter of smooth muscle and an external sphincter of striated muscle.

Functional anatomy

The function of the gastrointestinal tract is closely associated with its structure.

The epithelial layer

The epithelium lies in contact with the luminal contents and ranges in permeability from being largely impermeable (oesophageal squamous epithelium) to highly permeable (intestinal epithelium). The absorptive function of the epithelial layer is modulated by a network of neurones, the submucous plexus, which receive input from the central nervous system. In addition, the neurones of the submucous plexus and the nerve terminals of extrinsic afferent nerves, particularly those running in the vagus trunk, are modulated by signals arising from the epithelium.

Neuromusculature of the gut

The striated muscle in the gastrointestinal tract (upper oesophagus and anus) is directly innervated by second order (lower motor) neurones (arising from the brainstem and spinal cord respectively) and therefore under direct central nervous system control whereas smooth muscle is largely autonomous, being controlled 'locally' by the enteric nervous system without direct innervation from the central nervous system. The central nervous system can, however, indirectly influence the muscular function of the gastrointestinal tract via its innervation of the myenteric plexus.

Immune system of the gastrointestinal tract

Throughout the gastrointestinal tract lie discreet clusters of immune cells which provide immunosurveillance and immune protection, that is Peyers patches in the small intestine and the appendix (see Chapter 14.4).

The function of the gastrointestinal tract

The function of the gastrointestinal tract is the transport, digestion, and elimination of ingested material to supply nutrients, vitamins, minerals, and electrolytes which are essential for life, together with the protection of the rest of the body from injurious or allergenic material.

Secretion/absorption

The gastrointestinal tract is responsible for movement of very large volumes across its lumen (Fig. 1). Overall, more than 8 litres enter the lumen per day. In contrast, only 200 to 300 ml is expelled per day as stool, the remainder being efficiently absorbed by the small intestine and proximal colon. The major digestive/absorptive organ of the gastrointestinal tract is the small intestine. Without the small intestine life is impossible whereas the possession of the small intestine without oesophagus, stomach, or colon is still compatible with reasonable nutrition. The various organs of the gastrointestinal tract subserve different functions to ensure that ingested nutrients are adequately digested or eliminated.

Oesophageal function

The oesophagus functions as a conduit to transport ingested food masticated by the mouth and salivary glands, through the thoracic cavity and into the proximal stomach.

Gastric function

The stomach acts as a storage, a sterilizing, and a digestive tank. Its receptive function enables large quantities of food to be eaten rapidly and stored and processed until adequately prepared for delivery to the small intestine. The presence of pathogens in food is reduced by the secretion of hydrochloric acid upon meal ingestion while the production of peptidases and lipase capable of operating in a low pH commence the process of digestion.

Small intestinal function

The small intestine is the major site of digestion and absorption. It regulates the speed of delivery of gastric contents via a sensing mechanism located in the epithelium, comprising endocrine cells sensitive to the pH, osmolarity, and chemical composition of the luminal contents, and signals both to intrinsic and to extrinsic neurones of the vagus to delay gastric emptying. This sensory signal also stimulates the delivery of bile and production of pancreatic secretion ensuring that these major digestive materials are delivered to the intestine only in the presence of nutrients.

The absorption of digesta is achieved through the intestinal mucosa. While some passes between the intestinal cells, most is actively transported through the epithelial cells via specific transporters (e.g. peptide, hexose transporters). The small intestinal is also a major absorptive organ, retrieving over 6 litres of fluid per day from the lumen (Fig. 1), the end result of which is the delivery of a small quantity of unabsorbed food (1.5 l) into the caecum.

Regional variation in intestinal absorption

The intestine shows regional differences in its absorptive function. The jejunum is responsible for the majority of nutrient and fluid absorption, whereas the ileum has additional, specific absorptive functions, in particular the absorption of vitamin B_{12} and the absorption of bile salts. Surgical resection of the ileum may thus be associated with development of B_{12} deficiency and of diarrhoea resulting from passage of bile salts into the colon where they induce secretion.

The colon

The colon's function is to salvage water and electrolyte from the small intestinal effluent, converting over a litre of material from the intestine into small pellets for elimination. In addition to its water and electrolyte absorptive function, the colon also salvages unabsorbed calories from the lumen, particularly undigested carbohydrate, for example starch polysaccharides. These are incompletely digested in the small intestine and thus pass to the colon where the anaerobic bacteria of the lumen ferment the carbohydrate to short chain fatty acids, which are absorbed to provide a secondary nutrient source.

The rectum

The rectum provides a storage function, enabling the elimination of colonic residue (defecation) to be restricted to times of personal convenience.

Neural control of gastrointestinal function

For the greater part of the time, the gastrointestinal tract is controlled by its own nervous system—the enteric nervous system. The enteric nervous system is not entirely autonomous however, and requires some local and central nervous system 'reflexes' for adequate co-ordination of functions along its length. For example the co-ordination of the passage of luminal contents into the small intestine from the stomach requires sophisticated control, which is provided by a vagally mediated reflex operating via the brainstem. This circuitry alters the gut from its fasted state to the fed state, that is gastric relaxation, the induction of gall bladder emptying, and pancreatic secretion, thus ensuring the provision of digestive enzymes at the appropriate time. An additional relay function is provided by prevertebral ganglia where visceral afferent neurones synapse with efferent relay neurones to integrate contractile patterns and contraction force.

The intrinsic nervous system

The intrinsic nervous system acts as a local control system with its own 'programmes', examples of which are the peristaltic reflex and the migrating motor complex.

Peristaltic reflex

This basic 'programme' responds to local luminal distension by an ascending muscular excitation pathway and descending inhibition (Fig. 3) which ensures aboral propulsion of luminal contents. This reflex is best seen in the oesophagus where it is known as secondary or non-swallow-related peristalsis. While the reflex can be induced in the small intestine or colon, it is not a major factor for luminal transit.

The migrating motor complex

This comprises a triphasic pattern of aborally propagating contractions in the distal stomach and small intestine during the fasted state which probably serve to maintain an empty lumen and reduce bacterial growth. Periods of quiescence are followed by irregular contractile activity which then terminates in a aboral migrating burst of regular contractions, which slowly migrate from the distal stomach down to the terminal ileum. This

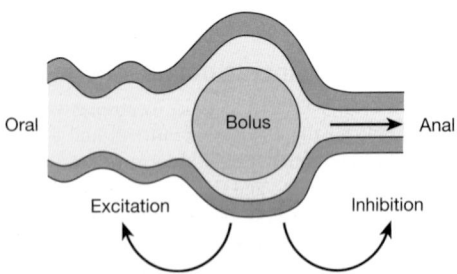

Fig. 3 Peristaltic reflex. The peristaltic reflex is the mechanical response of the intestine to the intraluminal distension. Note the presence of proximal motor excitation and distal inhibition which together propel the distending bolus from mouth to anus.

pattern, which characterizes the fasted state, is interrupted on food ingestion by a vagally mediated reflex which converts the pattern into a fed one.

The immune function of the gut

Being the major route of nutrient absorption, the gastrointestinal tract is also a potential portal for pathogen entry. The gastrointestinal tract therefore requires a sophisticated immune surveillance system together with a process for eliminating intestinal pathogens and the ability to either tolerate or eliminate ingested antigens. Details of this process are more fully dealt with in Chapter 14.4.

Disturbances of local physiological control mechanisms and origins of symptoms

Disturbances of local neuromuscular function are associated by the disturbances transit and elimination or secretion and absorption. An example of disturbed transit resulting from disturbed neuromuscular function is achalasia or slow transit constipation. Examples of disturbance of secretion and absorption are secretory diarrhoeas or the hyperacidity associated with *Helicobacter pylori* infection. Examples of symptoms which follow damage to extrinsic neural control are exemplified by the symptoms of truncal vagotomy, that is rapid transit and impaired nutrient–enzyme mixing result in poor digestion and an osmotic diarrhoea.

The relationships between gastrointestinal symptoms and the central nervous system are relevant to the understanding of functional gastrointestinal 'disorders'; it is well recognized that psychological disturbances, for example anxiety or depression combined with local disturbances of gastrointestinal physiology produce pain, nausea and vomiting, and altered bowel habit.

Further reading

Johnson LR, *et al.*, eds (1981). *Physiology of the gastrointestinal tract.* Raven Press, New York.

Schultz SG, ed. (1991). The gastrointestinal system. In: *Handbook of physiology*, Section 6, Vols I–IV. American Physiological Society, Oxford University Press, New York.

14.1.1.2 Symptomatology of gastrointestinal disease

Graham Neale

The skilful analysis of symptoms indicating disorders of the digestive system is an integral part of the practice of internal medicine. Many patients with abdominal symptoms do not have easily defined organic conditions. The traditional skills of taking a careful history and examining the patient thoroughly are invaluable in managing patients who have functional disorders such as 'irritable bowel', non-ulcer dyspepsia, non-specific diarrhoea, recurrent abdominal pain, and somatization disorder. One might suppose that the enormous advances in endoscopic, scanning, and other techniques will have made clinical diagnosis less important, but this is not so: most gastrointestinal disorders are minor self-limited disorders of uncertain cause or are functional in nature, thereby often eluding definition by these procedures. Moreover the early suspicion of life-threatening disease and prompt referral of patients for investigation depends on clinical judgement.

Disorders of swallowing

Pharyngeal disease

Difficulty in swallowing is an important symptom that requires prompt resolution. Oropharyngeal disorders cause difficulty in initiating swallowing, regurgitation through the nasopharynx, a sensation of sticking in the throat, or the feeling of a lump in the throat on or after swallowing. Coughing and choking on swallowing is usually a symptom of pharyngeal disease and indicates failure to close the larynx. More rarely it is a sign of an obstructive lesion in the lower gullet which allows food and secretions to accumulate and spill into the larynx, especially at night. This symptom needs urgent attention to reduce the risk of aspiration pneumonia. Painful lesions of the oropharynx are usually demonstrated quite easily by simple inspection.

Patients with neurological disorders such as Parkinson's disease, motor neurone disease, myaesthenia gravis, and dermatomyositis only rarely present with disorders of swallowing and the clinician has only to be aware of the way in which known illnesses may affect the swallowing process. Oropharyngeal dyskinesia is common in the early phase of recovery after a stroke and may be persistently troublesome in patients with brainstem lesions.

Patients with the sensation of a lump in the throat on or after swallowing require an imaging technique to look for a pharyngeal pouch, a postcricoid web, or carcinoma and rarely pressure from a large osteophyte as a result of cervical spondylosis. It is unwise to submit patients with suspected pharyngeal lesions to conventional fibre-optic oesophagoscopy as a first examination because of the risks of perforation. Patients with a persistent feeling of 'a lump in the throat' without any demonstrable disease ('globus hystericus') usually respond well to the taking of a careful history, a single scanning procedure, and firm reassurance. They are more often women than men and they nearly always show signs of an anxiety state.

Oesophageal pathology

Dysphagia

Oesophageal dysphagia causes a sensation of food sticking in the gullet and is nearly always due to organic disease. The symptoms vary from discomfort to severe pain and the patient is rarely able to localize the site of the obstruction accurately. Associated symptoms such as regurgitation, vomiting, and coughing or choking are common. Oesophageal dysphagia is caused by obstructive lesions or more rarely by neuromuscular disorders. The common intrinsic lesions are inflammatory strictures secondary to reflux or tumours. Extrinsic compression may occur as a result of mediastinal lesions or vascular disorders (for example an aortic aneurysm). Neuromuscular disorders such as diffuse oesophageal spasm and dystrophia myotonica are much less common than obstructive pathology. The duration, progression, and frequency of symptoms help determine the likely nature of the pathology. Steady progression of dysphagia over a few weeks suggests malignant obstruction whereas association with a long history of heartburn suggests an inflammatory stricture. The dysphagia of neuromuscular disorders is usually confined to solids, and progresses, whereas that of achalasia is initially episodic and in the early stages often wrongly attributed to a functional disorder.

Heartburn

Heartburn is an extremely common symptom. It is an episodic lower retrosternal or epigastric burning that radiates upwards. It is caused by gastro-oesophageal reflux and commonly occurs an or hour or two after meals (especially if these are fatty or spicy); it may be precipitated by heavy physical work and bending. Symptoms often occur on lying down and are characteristically relieved by the ingestion of antacids. Most pregnant women suffer heartburn.

Oesophageal pain

Odynophagia is oesophageal pain felt within 15 s of swallowing and may be associated with the impaction of a lump of food at a site of mechanical blockage or a hold-up with oesophageal spasm. Odynophagia without hold-up occurs with intrinsic inflammatory disorders (such as reflux or candidal oesophagitis) and extrinsic disorders (such as mediastinitis). Hot liquids and alcohol may cause odynophagia in a normal gullet (the so-called 'tender oesophagus').

Oesophageal pain not clearly related to swallowing is characteristically retrosternal, often has a crushing quality, and may radiate to the jaw thereby mimicking cardiac pain. Patients with these symptoms are usually investigated for angina before being referred to a gastroenterologist: some will be shown to have reflux-associated chest pain or a primary disorder of motility (e.g. diffuse oesophageal spasm). High-amplitude contractions of the distal oesophagus are often discovered in patients with attacks of chest pain of uncertain cause and these are believed to be related to psychological stress.

Dyspepsia, nausea, and vomiting

Dyspepsia, nausea, and vomiting are extremely common symptoms which can be produced by a wide range of conditions from the most serious (such as end-stage neoplastic disease) to the most trivial (such as over-indulgence in food or alcohol). Patients may speak of indigestion (to describe any low-grade upper abdominal discomfort) and sickness (to describe either nausea or vomiting).

Dyspepsia

Dyspepsia is upper abdominal or lower chest discomfort or pain related to eating which may be described by the patient as a burning, a heaviness, or an aching and is often accompanied by other symptoms such as nausea, fullness in the upper abdomen, or belching. Although the symptoms of upper gastrointestinal disease are imprecise and non-specific, care in taking the clinical history will often facilitate making the correct diagnosis quickly and limit unnecessary investigation. All too often, an over-stretched, relatively inexperienced clinician will spend a few minutes talking to the patient and then arrange a battery of blood tests, gastrointestinal endoscopy (and biopsy), ultrasonic examination of the abdomen, and some conventional radiology before telling the patient that he can find nothing wrong (and possibly implying that the patient is too ready to complain). Certain aspects of history-taking yield important clues:

- How clearcut is the patient's description of symptoms? Peptic ulcer often gives well-localized pain in the epigastrium. In about 40 per cent of patients with dyspepsia this comes on after a meal and wakes the patient at night. Attacks of central abdominal pain which cause the patient to double up may indicate gallstones although, if there is associated cholecystitis, the pain is more likely to be in the right upper quadrant (often radiating to the right shoulder).

- For how long has the patient had symptoms and how constant are they? A short history makes organic disease likely.

- Has the patient any associated diseases and what drugs are being taken? Many drugs cause upper abdominal symptoms especially aspirin and non-steroidal anti-inflammatory drugs.

- Has the patient lost significant weight? Are there associated symptoms? Vomiting suggests organic disease, alcoholism, or pregnancy.

- Has the patient any worries or anxieties that may be related to dyspepsia of recent onset (especially in women and in the young)? Sometimes patients will deliberately conceal their worries for fear that the clinician will too readily accept them as the cause of their symptoms.

- Details about dietary habits, smoking, and intake of alcohol should be obtained and it may be necessary not to take what the patient says at face value.

For the older patient (over 45 years) with dyspepsia of recent onset, gastroscopy is nearly always indicated in order to identify early gastric cancer. By the time the patient has the classical triad of symptoms of this disease—loss of appetite, loss of weight, and loss of strength—it is usually too late to achieve a surgical cure. Regrettably the early symptoms of gastric cancer are usually mild and non-specific.

The symptoms of patients known to have infection with *Heliobacter pylori* by serological testing are difficult to assess. Most infected patients are symptomless and most of those who have dyspeptic symptoms without ulceration are not cured by treatment with appropriate antibiotics.

Nausea

The term nausea should be restricted to the feeling of being about to vomit. Acute nausea is usually accompanied by hypersalivation. Nausea is caused by labyrinthine stimulation (as in motion sickness); distension of hollow viscera, or any severe somatic pain and by some drugs, especially opiates and those used in chemotherapy for malignant conditions.

Again the clinician has to define carefully what the patient means by nausea. It may be used to describe anorexia, an aversion to food, abdominal fullness, or a sinking feeling in the abdomen. In the absence of a recognizable cause persistent or frequent nausea without vomiting often proves to be psychologically determined.

Vomiting

Vomiting is the forceful ejection of gastric contents through the mouth by the co-ordinated contraction of abdominal and gastric muscles with relaxation of the lower oesophageal sphincter. Non-productive vomiting is called retching. Vomiting occurs with peptic ulceration, especially when there is delayed gastric emptying (pyloric stenosis), and with advanced gastric cancer. It occurs with disorders of the biliary tree (especially as a result of gallstones) and with acute pancreatitis (in which it is a prime symptom). It is an important symptom of intestinal obstruction, especially with lesions above the ileocaecal valve, and it may occur with any cause of peritoneal inflammation such as appendicitis. Metabolic causes of vomiting include diabetic ketoacidosis, hypoadrenalism, and uraemia. Drugs which cause vomiting include opiates, some antibiotics (for example erythromycin), and chemotherapeutic agents. Alcoholism, raised intracranial pressure, and pregnancy are important causes of early morning vomiting.

Effortless vomiting without a definable cause may be psychogenic. This is usually a disorder of young women many of whom have suffered psychological trauma (such as sexual abuse). It is not related to the vomiting of bulimia, a condition that is part of the anorexia nervosa syndrome (see Chapter 26.5.5). Rumination has to be distinguished from vomiting. Rumination is the repetitive regurgitation of gastric contents into the mouth after meals, the regurgitated material then being reswallowed. It is not associated with nausea, heartburn, or discomfort and often appears to be simply an acquired habit.

Abdominal pain

Pain in the 'acute abdomen'

Most patients with acute abdominal pain are promptly referred to a surgeon. However, this does not always happen and the end-result may be disastrous. Thus all clinicians should be able to assess a patient with acute abdominal pain. The site of the pain is usually helpful, but it is diffuse or atypical in at least 25 per cent of patients with acute gastrointestinal pathology. It is important to determine whether movement or coughing aggravate the pain as in appendicitis and generalized peritonitis (including perforated peptic ulcer and pancreatitis). Pain exacerbated by inspiration points to pathology in the upper abdomen (especially cholecystitis) or adjacent to the diaphragm. A detailed analysis of the type of pain is usually unhelpful but it is useful to know if it is intermittent, colicky, or constant. Some pain radiates in a characteristic manner—urological (loin-to-groin),

gynaecological (to the back or thigh), and cholecystitis (to the shoulder tip). In contrast, the pain of appendicitis and diverticulitis does not radiate. The pain of intestinal obstruction is colicky and often associated with vomiting. Severe pain without physical signs and with normal routine tests (laboratory and simple radiological) raises the possibility of mesenteric vascular occlusion especially in patients over the age of 50 years or those known to be at risk of thromboembolic disease. Acute porphyria is the other condition to consider. The pain is diffuse and severe and most frequently occurs in the third decade with females being much more frequently affected than males. Tenderness is almost always absent but tachycardia and anxiety are prominent. During the attack the urine will contain excess δ-aminolaevulinic acid and, usually, porphobilinogen.

Upper abdominal pain

Pain in the upper abdomen has been considered under the heading dyspepsia. Upper abdominal discomfort is so common that its presence alone is of no value in distinguishing between those patients with organic disease and those with a functional disorder. Moreover patients with an irritable bowel, diverticular disease, and occasionally with other colonic pathology may have discomfort in the centre of the abdomen which they may describe as indigestion. In such circumstances there is usually also a history of some change in bowel habit that will indicate the true nature of the condition. Disease in the small intestine is proportionately rather uncommon and is frequently misdiagnosed as an irritable bowel. Symptoms are rarely specific but should be reinterpreted in the light of screening investigations (such as the blood count, a straight radiograph of the abdomen, and assessment of serum markers of inflammatory disease).

Lower abdominal pain

With lower abdominal pain analysis of symptoms often does not help to determine the cause. Indeed inflammatory and neoplastic colonic disorders often may not give rise to pain and when pain does occur, it is usually diffuse and central. However, focal pain and tenderness in the left iliac fossa often indicates diverticulitis and, more rarely, colonic cancer. Focal pain in the right iliac fossa may be a marker of Crohn's ileocaecal disease. The passage of stool or flatus will often relieve the pain of colonic disease and an irritable bowel; in contrast it tends to exacerbate the pain of local rectal conditions. A history of recent-onset lower abdominal pain in patients over the age of 40 years is an indication for prompt investigation.

Proctalgia fugax is a very painful paroxysmal perineal pain occurring unexpectedly often at night and may last for up to half an hour. The pathogenesis is uncertain and it is unassociated with any signs of disease. The condition is often recurrent but is self-limiting.

Diarrhoea and constipation

The general public knows well what is meant by 'an attack of diarrhoea' or 'being constipated' but these conditions are not easy to define in medical terms. First one must recognize that to a lay person, constipation means passing a stool less often than normal and usually with difficulty. But 'normal' may be anything from two or three times a day to two or three times a week. Moreover the mass and consistency of a normal stool varies considerably depending on diet, gender, and individual factors. Subjects eating a Western diet pass 80 to 200 g of stool each day with more women at the lower end of this range. To add to the difficulty of assessing bowel function, the frequency of bowel habit may bear no relation to the volume of faecal material passed nor to the amount of stool in the colon. Thus care must be taken to define exactly what is happening and it is advisable to take the common-sense view that a change in normal bowel habit is significant. Two warnings are appropriate: first, most people are loath to mention incontinence (they will usually say that they have diarrhoea and will have to be

Table 1 Salt and water absorption by the gastrointestinal tract

Site	Passage of fluid in 24 h	Concentration of Na+ in the lumen (mM)	Total Na+ received in 24 h (mmol)	Mucosal characteristics with respect to salt/water
Duodenum/jejunum	7–8 litres	150	1000	Acts as semi-permeable membrane. Salt and water follows absorption of nutrients and bicarbonate
Ileum	? 2–3 litres	100–110		Active absorption of salt/water (chloride/bicarbonate exchange)
Proximal colon	1.5 litres	100	160	Decreasing permeability. Active absorption of salt and water
Distal colon/rectum	50–100 ml	40–50	3–5	Low permeability. Na/K exchange

Salt and water absorption is disturbed by: osmotic pressure from the gut (e.g. malabsorbed sugars/peptides; purgative salts); reduced mucosal permeability (mucosal enteropathies as in coeliac disease); reduced active absorption (e.g. by the small intestine in coeliac disease and by the large intestine in colitis); increased mucosal secretion (in response to bacterial toxins (e.g. cholera), inflammatory mediators (e.g. cytokines/leukotrienes), or neurohormonal mediators (as in a patient with a VIPoma); abnormal motility (e.g. diabetic autonomic neuropathy).

asked specifically about soiling); secondly in those with persistent unexplained diarrhoea, it is best to examine the stool because patients' descriptions of their faeces are often uninformative.

Diarrhoea

The clinician needs to understand some basic gastrointestinal physiology in order to understand the mechanisms of diarrhoea and to make sense of a patient's symptoms (Table 1). Most cases of diarrhoea can be diagnosed quite simply from the history, an examination of the stools, and, when appropriate, direct examination of the rectal mucosa. Acute infective diarrhoea is recognized by its recent onset, sometimes preceded by nausea or vomiting and a general systemic upset. Abdominal pain often occurs with *Campylobacter* infection, and although passage of blood and mucus can occur with any severe infection, it is more common with *Shigellosis* and infection with *E. coli* 0157.

In assessing chronic or recurrent diarrhoea, it is worth trying to distinguish diarrhoea of large bowel origin from that of the small intestine. Large bowel diarrhoea characteristically occurs on rising, may be associated with pain which is relieved by defaecation, and often contains mucus and sometimes red blood. The differential diagnosis usually rests between inflammation and neoplasm. Small bowel diarrhoea occurs at any time, and although often watery, the stool may also contain excess fat. Steatorrhoea occurs in coeliac disease, pancreatic insufficiency, stagnant loop syndromes, and massive intestinal resection. Drugs (such as beta-blockers,

diuretics, antacids, and antibiotics) as well as excess intake of beer may also cause diarrhoea.

In assessing diarrhoea that otherwise remains unexplained, it may be worth distinguishing between osmotic and secretory mechanisms. This is done by measuring the concentration of the major cations (sodium and potassium) and stool osmolality. If the measured osmolality is little more than the sum of the cations multiplied by two (to allow for the unmeasured anions), then the patient has a secretory diarrhoea. In contrast, if there is a significant osmolar gap then there must be another solute in the stool. Unfortunately this test may be unreliable if the volume of stool is less than 500 to 600 ml per day.

Constipation

Each year about 1 per cent of the population consult their family doctor complaining of constipation. The mode of presentation ranges from the acute onset of colonic obstruction to a lifelong disability. The most common causes of constipation are shown in Table 2. In taking a clinical history it is important to determine exactly what the patient means by constipation. A relatively sudden change in bowel habit without any significant change in dietary habit or medication suggests an organic disorder. A desire to defaecate, especially if associated with colicky discomfort, suggests organic obstruction. Constipation from a young age increasing slowly with time indicates a disorder of normal colonic function, a condition that is much more common in women than men. Colon physiologists distinguish between 'slow transit' and 'outlet obstruction' constipation (Fig. 1) but this

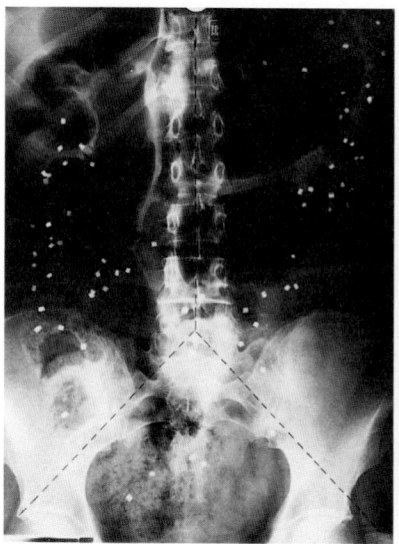

(a)

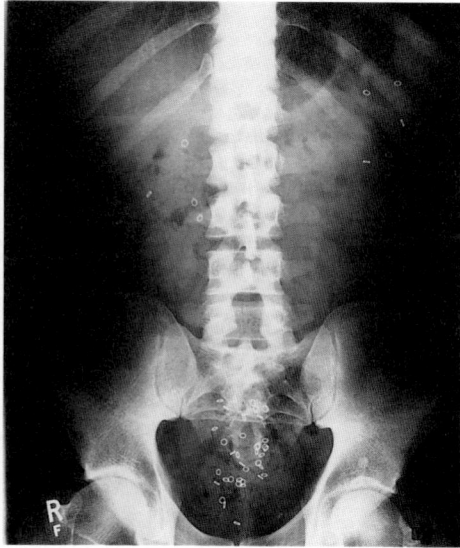

(b)

Fig. 1 Functional constipation illustrated by the use of markers (patient takes one marker capsule daily for 14 days, each capsule containing 10 radio-opaque pellets). (a) Abdominal radiograph of a 58-year-old woman with 'slow transit' constipation (colonic inertia). Seventy three pellets were retained after 14 days equally distributed between right and left colons (mean transit time 7.3 days, median normal for women 3.0 days). (b) Abdominal radiograph of a 30-year-old man who, a year previously, had an emergency laminectomy for an acute prolapsed disc. He complained of constipation since the operation and was shown to have 'outlet obstruction' presumably due to impaired rectoanal reflexes. Fifty seven pellets were retained with nine in the right colon, nine in the left colon, and 39 in the rectosigmoid segment (mean transit time 5.7 days, median normal for men 2.3 days). (By courtesy of Dr J. H. Cummings, MRC Microbiology and Gut Biology Group, University of Dundee. Figure 1(a) has been published previously in *Diseases of the gut and pancreas* ed. Misiewicz JJ, Pounder RE, and Venables CW, and is reprinted with the permission of Blackwell Scientific Publications.)

Table 2 Causes of constipation

- Poor diet (inadequate intake of poorly absorbed carbohydrate)
- Functional disorders (slow transit constipation,'outlet obstruction' constipation—see Fig. 1)
- Failure to respond to rectal distension (bed-bound patients,some psychiatric patients)
- Extrinsic disorders of colonic innervation especially to sacral outflow
- Intrinsic neurological pathology: Hirschsprung's, diabetic neuropathy
- Chronic pseudo-obstruction (neuromuscular)
- Metabolic disorders, e.g. myxoedema, hypercalcaemia
- Drugs: opiates, anticholinergics
- Obstructive: neoplasm, inflammatory (e.g. Crohn's disease)

distinction is of limited value in management. 'Low fibre' diets (as ingested by many young people living away from the family home for the first time), some drugs (especially opiates and drugs with anticholinergic activity such as antidepressants), metabolic disorders, and neurological disease must be considered—although in most cases no cause can be established. In women it is also necessary to consider the obstetric history and to consider the possibility of pelvic floor dysfunction. Straining at stool over a prolonged period may lead to rectal prolapse and incontinence and it may be necessary to ask the patient specifically about such symptoms.

Further reading

Neale G (1998). Reducing risks in gastroenterological practice. *Gut* **42**, 139–42. Describes common errors in diagnosis and the importance of taking a careful history.

Snape WT Jr, ed (1996) *Consultations in gastroenterology*, section I, pp 1–155. WB Saunders, Philadelphia. A clinical approach to the diagnosis of nutritional and gastroenterological disorders.

Yamada T, ed (1999) *Textbook of gastroenterology*, pp 637–936. Lippincott, Williams and Wilkins, Philadelphia. An exceptionally comprehensive account of how to assess the symptoms of all patients with gastrointestinal disease.

14.2 Methods for investigation of gastrointestinal disease

14.2.1 Colonoscopy and flexible sigmoidoscopy

Christopher B. Williams and Brian P. Saunders

Development

Colonoscopes are similar to gastroscopes, but with greater flexibility to pass loops in the bowel. Early instruments had limited angulation and relatively clumsy characteristics. Colonoscopy was therefore initially looked on as a second-line procedure, time-consuming and potentially traumatic. Polypectomy was introduced in 1972 and this, coupled with recognition of the accuracy of the technique and (with biopsies) in diagnosing or excluding inflammatory disease or neoplasm, started an explosion of demand. Development of video-colonoscopes in the 1980s added high quality videotaping and prints which, with improved and more agile instruments, has contributed to making colonoscopy acceptable both for routine clinical use and for well-person surveillance and screening.

Colonoscopes range from 60 to 70 cm flexible sigmoidoscopes, thin very flexible paediatric instruments also used in adults with fixation or stricturing, up to 165 cm long colonoscopes with different flexibility characteristics and instrumentation channel sizes. Further technical improvements include higher resolution and zoom-magnification, better control ergonomics, adjustable shaft flexibility and electronic means of imaging shaft loops on-screen without fluoroscopy. Ultrasound colonoscopes, thin ultrasound probes for use with conventional instruments and magnetic resonance-compatible scopes are also being evaluated.

A large range of accessories can be introduced through the suction/instrumentation channel of a colonoscope, including biopsy or grasping forceps, washing, spraying or deflation tubes, cytology brushes, and injection needles. Therapeutic accessories include insulated forceps, polypectomy snares and retrieval devices, coagulating probes and argon plasma coagulating catheters, laser light guides, haemostatic clip and nylon loop applicators, dilating balloons, and metal stent introducers. It is also possible to preload onto the tip means of applying constricting loops or bands. Use of an external 'overtube' allows a looping instrument to be stiffened or exchanged for another without having to recommence the procedure. CO_2 insufflation apparatus is available which, since the gas is exhaled within 10 to 15 min, ensures that patients are not left distended after the procedure.

Cleaning and disinfection

As for all flexible endoscopes, skilled maintenance, regular checks, and meticulous cleaning are essential. All parts, including air, water, and instrumentation channels must be accessed during cleaning. It is not possible to sterilize a colonoscope but, after scrupulous mechanical cleaning and 'high level disinfection' (usually in an automated washing machine with 2 per cent glutaraldehyde solution and subsequent rinse cycles), all viral agents (including HIV and hepatitis B) and bacteria are inactivated. It takes at least 30 min to clean and disinfect an instrument so, allowing for repairs, three or more colonoscopes are needed to provide a routine service. Mycobacterial spores require even longer (60 min) exposure; prolonged disinfection is therefore recommended before and after examination of AIDS patients, not only because of patient susceptibility to infection but also their increased likelihood of harbouring mycobacteria. Accessories may be disposable or require autoclave sterilization or high-level disinfection, as directed by the manufacturers.

Patient preparation

Flexible sigmoidoscopy preparation is normally by disposable enema (hypertonic phosphate or similar) given or self-administered 10 to 15 min before the procedure. Some patients prefer to avoid the indignity of an enema by taking full oral preparation and this is also advisable in any patient with a colon narrowed by pronounced diverticulosis or stricturing.

Full bowel preparation is usually the most unpleasant part of colonoscopy. Oral preparation must be preceded by dietary restrictions, which include stopping iron or constipating agents in the preceding days, and taking low fibre diet (with no nuts, mushrooms, or iron-containing red wine) for 24 h.

Purgative preparation is cheap and generally best tolerated, but some individuals can suffer considerable cramping, explosive incontinence, or vasovagal reaction. A senna preparation on the afternoon or evening before exam is followed 2 to 3 h later by an osmotic purge (commonly magnesium citrate, sodium phosphate, or mannitol 10 per cent). The last dose should be taken only a few hours before the procedure to avoid the solidifying action of the proximal colon. Large quantities of clear fluids (including alcohol in moderation) are encouraged up to the time of examination to avoid adherent residue, which is difficult to flush or aspirate.

Fluid overload is the alternative approach, achieved by ingestion of 3 to 4 l of isotonic solution, usually polyethylene glycol (PEG)–electrolyte solution which avoids the electrolyte losses that occur if normal saline or 5 per cent mannitol are used. This approach is ideal for patients with active inflammatory bowel disease. Commercial PEG–electrolyte preparations can be prepacked for postage and are flavoured. Around 10 per cent of patients become nauseated, vomit, or become distended and stop drinking, any of which results in poor preparation, especially in the proximal colon.

If there is any possibility that the patient is obstructed, full oral preparation is contraindicated because of the possibility of perforation; a smaller volume should be given, supplemented by enemas. In the presence of massive bleeding it may be preferable to proceed direct to colonoscopy and rely on the purgative effect of blood, rather than waste time on preparation. In extreme cases of overwhelming blood loss peroperative 'caecostomy lavage' has been described, but nasal-tube lavage is a more usual compromise before emergency colonoscopy.

Psychological preparation of the patient should not be forgotten, since most of those scheduled for colonoscopy are apprehensive, whether through embarrassment, expected discomfort, or fear of colorectal cancer. Explanatory literature and a friendly telephone manner at the time of booking the exam can help a great deal. Equally, a warm and reassuring atmosphere on reception, whilst obtaining 'informed consent' and also during the procedure, can help transform colonoscopy from an ordeal into a reasonable and well-tolerated experience.

Medication

'Conscious sedation' is offered to most patients, unless they are likely to be easy to examine (flexible sigmoidoscopy, with a previously easy examination, or sigmoid resection or stoma) or are motivated to try without medication. The unpleasant gnawing quality of 'visceral pain' caused by the inevitable stretching of colon or attachments during insertion is tolerable for a few spells of 20 to 30 s. Prolonged examinations or the lowered pain threshold of patients presenting with features of irritable bowel syndrome or diverticulosis can be made considerably more pleasant with a minimal dose of a sedative–analgesic combination. Combing a low dose of benzodiazepine (typically, midazolam 2–3 mg, intravenous), with an opiate analgesic (pethidine 25–50 mg, intravenous) reduces discomfort and anxiety and gives the patient a well-deserved feeling of euphoria. Low-level sedation of this kind does not inhibit conversation, the ability to complain of pain or to change position when necessary. Smaller doses should be given in small, elderly, and sick patients but incremental larger doses (especially opiate) can be needed in apprehensive, younger ones. Pulse oximetry monitoring is routine and nasal oxygen, resuscitation equipment, and reversal agents (flumazenil, naloxone) should be immediately accessible. Sedated patients must be accompanied home. On-demand, self-administered nitrous oxide/oxygen inhalation has been shown by some to be equally effective for skilled endoscopists, giving rapid recovery and allowing return home without escort.

General anaesthesia is rarely needed and generally best avoided, since in an unconscious patient position change is made more difficult and removal of the warning given by pain may tend to more aggressive technique. For the few patients with particular reasons for general anaesthesia and an expert encoscopist, propofol anaesthesia gives excellent results and also more rapid recovery than after high doses of conventional sedatives. In certain countries with enough anaesthetists available (France, Australia) this approach is commonly employed, whereas in others (Germany, northern Italy, Japan, China) unsedated colonoscopy is routine.

Antispasmodics are decried by many, on the basis that they are thought to elongate the colon and make insertion more difficult. In randomized trial, we have shown this to be untrue and routinely use them (hysocine-N-butyl bromide) both in order to speed insertion and to optimize the view for greater accuracy.

Antibiotics are only given to those with immunosuppression or immunodepression, previous endocarditis, heart valve prosthesis, septal defects, recent vascular prosthesis, or ascites.

Flexible sigmoidoscopy

Flexible sigmoidoscopy is the kindest and most logical means of examining proximal to the rectosigmoid junction (15 cm) whereas the rectum and the anal canal are better seen with the appropriate rigid instrument. Paradoxically the sigmoid colon, especially the sigmoid-descending colon junction, is the most difficult part of colonoscopy. In the presence of severe diverticular disease it may be impossible to reach even mid-sigmoid without expertise and a thin endoscope; after hysterectomy it may be cruel to examine without sedation. For this reason, although flexible sigmoidoscopy is both better tolerated and more accurate and effective than aggressive, rigid proctosigmoidoscopy, depth of insertion should be limited to what is tolerable by the individual patient. Some endoscopists mistakenly attempt to

'reach the splenic flexure' routinely. This is potentially unkind and also a mistaken concept. Without fluoroscopy or the use of newer means of imaging, even expert endoscopists can be completely mistaken between sigmoid-descending junction and splenic flexure. At 60 cm of insertion the 'scope tip can be anywhere between mid-sigmoid and caecum, and there are no positive localizing landmarks.

Insertion of the 'scope tip usually follows digital lubrication with jelly, the blunt tip of the instrument being gently inserted as the sphincters relax. Thereafter the 'scope is coaxed in as gently as possible, without haste or force, steering and 'cork-screwing' around bends with twisting movements. Blind insertion with 'red-out', guesswork, or 'push through' are all avoided as far as possible. Any small polyps (up to 5 mm) that may be adenomas are normally snared or destroyed at once, as they may be difficult to see on withdrawal or if left for subsequent colonoscopy. Because of the remote possibility of explosive gas concentrations after limited preparation, either repeated suction with air reinflation or use of CO_2 should precede electro-surgery; alternatively 'cold snaring' with physical removal of the polyp can be employed. If in doubt a biopsy can be taken, both to give some idea of the size of any lesion against the open forceps and to give partial histology.

Total colonoscopy

In expert hands, and in the absence of obstruction, a severely ulcerated colon, or other contraindication, total colonoscopy is possible in over 99 per cent of cases, with little sedation or suffering and virtually no complications. In less expert hands 'total colonoscopy' or 'completion' rates as low as 33 to 45 per cent have been reported and 75 per cent is common. The principle difference in technique between expert and inexpert is the ability, whilst keeping sufficient orientation for steering purposes, to pull-back and crumple the looped segment of colon already traversed, whilst simultaneously straightening the way or bend ahead. The ideal is to keep the colonoscope as straight as possible and to pleat or 'concertina' the colon over it, avoiding the unnecessary loops and pain by caused by pushing too hard or too long. The ideal is not always immediately achievable, so patience and determination—tempered by humanity—are essential qualities for the colonoscopist.

Paradoxically a freely mobile colon, without the conventionally fixed segments in the descending and ascending parts, can be as difficult to traverse as one with adhesions. This is principally because atypical loops may form, sometimes uncontrollable until the instrument tip eventually reaches a fixed point, giving a 'hold' and allowing the shaft to be straightened back. Happily, this type of long and mobile colon, whilst being a nightmare for the endoscopist, typically also has long enough attachments that the patient experiences little discomfort.

From the point of view of the patient, colonoscope stretch discomfort is frequently felt as 'wind pain', rapidly relieved as soon as the causative loop can be straightened. True over-distension is easily removed by aspiration. Further distress may be produced by the unpleasant illusion of incontinence given when the body-warmed and lubricated shaft is withdrawn through the sensitive anal canal; it is kind to prewarn the patient of this phenomenon and to preserve decorum by aspirating any fluid found during insertion through the rectosigmoid.

Once the colonoscope has successfully passed into the descending colon and has been straightened back to remove sigmoid colon looping, it is likely that the rest of the insertion phase will be considerably easier. When the 'scope shaft is straight it feels responsive and free, as do the angling controls—whereas the more looped the colonoscope is the more 'snarled up' everything becomes, and the more the patient suffers. Avoiding looping and responding to pain are the basis for successful, kind, and safe insertion. It also minimizes instrument repair bills and maximizes accuracy and ease of targeting lesions, since a straight instrument handles better.

This practical philosophy underlies the reason for simple but effective 'tricks of the trade' such as position change. It is obvious that in left lateral position there will be pooling of any fluid in the left colon; the transverse colon will also tend to sag down and so make the splenic flexure more acute. It therefore follows that, at the splenic and any flexure where there is a poor view or difficulty in insertion, position change may improve matters (to supine or right lateral at the splenic, but back to left lateral again for hepatic flexure). Adding only the simple principles of pulling back as often as possible to straighten each loop before tackling the next, avoiding over-distension to keep the bowel reasonably deflated and supple, and trying assistant hand-pressure whenever an unavoidable loop may be accessible (sigmoid and transverse colon) and the 'art of colonoscopy' is explained. Insensitivity, impatience, aggression result in the endoscopist being too muscular and tense to handle the shaft and controls sensitively, and so cause needless looping, pain, failure, and complications.

Contraindications, risks, and limitations

There are few contraindications to colonoscopy. It is, however, a relatively strong vasovagal assault with potential for arrythmias and so is contraindicated for 2 to 3 months after myocardial infarction. The tip, shaft, and air pressure involved in insertion have potential to exacerbate any existing risk of perforation. Colonoscopy is thus contraindicated in the acute phase and 2 weeks after an episode of diverticulitis, and also in severe acute or deeply ulcerated colitis of any variety (ulcerative, Crohn's, ischaemic, or infective). Patients with acute localized or rebound tenderness of the abdomen, free air, or dilated colon on radiograph should not be submitted to colonoscopy without special reason, due consultation, and by an expert endoscopist—who may decide to abandon the procedure.

The risks of diagnostic colonoscopy, as implied above, are to a great extent related to the training, personality, and handskills of the endoscopist. Regrettably large-scale audit shows figures of around 1 perforation in 1500 examinations, although this can be balanced against avoidance of the considerably worse complications of surgery. Therapy inevitably increases the likelihood of complications, principally bleeding but occasionally perforation after polypectomy or dilatation. Perforation may be actual (needing surgery) or threatened as the 'postpolypectomy syndrome' (managed conservatively with rest and antibiotics). Immediate bleeding can occur in around 1 per cent of polypectomies but is usually easily stopped by submucosal adrenaline injection (5–20 ml of 1/10 000 dilution, which is safe because of portal drainage) or by local electrocoagulation, clipping, or nylon loop application. Delayed haemorrhage can occur for up to 10 to 14 days after removal or local coagulation of even small polyps; it is usually self-limiting, but can be substantial and require admission to hospital and transfusion. Aspirin has been implicated as a risk factor in some series and should ideally be stopped for a week before and after polypectomy. Anticoagulants and other antiplatelet agents should similarly be withdrawn if possible or special measures instituted.

The greatest causes of colonoscopy-related mortality (1 in 10 000 exams) are patients referred (not always correctly) for surgery following endoscopic complications and deaths directly due to over-sedation, usually in the elderly. There have been unnecessary deaths when an internist has persisted in conservative management without involving a surgeon in management of suspected perforation. Surgical fatalities or major morbidity have resulted in others found at operation to have only a point perforation which would clearly have sealed spontaneously. In managing suspected perforation, due consultation between endoscopist and an endoscopically-aware, preferably laparoscopy-oriented, surgeon is essential. The need to modify sedation is described above and the endoscopist should also not be too proud to abandon an examination which is proving unreasonable, rather than to 'flatten' the patient. CT colography ('virtual colonoscopy') can image the proximal colon during the same visit.

The major limitations of colonoscopy relate to the fact that it is dependent on hand-skills and that tortuous, angulated, and haustrated colonic anatomy results in some 'blind spots' for the endoscopist. Areas that the endoscopist sees are extremely accurately evaluated, with a resolution of under 1 mm. The percentage of mucosa unseen is uncertain but is probably around 10 to 15 per cent overall. The likelihood of larger and 'significant' lesions being missed is much lower than this because colonic neoplasms are usually protuberant. Paradoxically, pathology can be missed in the capacious distal rectum or the anal canal, which can be avoided by retroverting the endoscope and/or examining with a rigid proctoscope as well.

Indications

The indications for colonoscopy are wide and constantly expanding, and are likely to continue to do so until alternative and less invasive techniques ('virtual colonoscopy' or genetic tests) are perfected. Where there is a shortage of endoscopic personnel, skill, or facilities it is possible to reduce the load of 'total colonoscopy' either by cross-referring for radiographs or related imaging techniques. It is also possible to combine these with prior flexible sigmoidoscopy on the same visit on the basis that limited colonoscopy covers the highest yield area, which is also the most prone to 'misses' or over-diagnosis.

High-yield indications include patients with bleeding, anaemia, or occult blood loss. Persistent bleeding, especially if dark or 'mixed-in' with the stool, is of sinister import, although it can be due only to local mucosal traumatization in diverticular disease. Good clinicians may select out for sigmoidoscopy alone patients with obviously fresh bleeding on defecation or with spotting 'on the paper'. However, the presence of blood in a patient of 50 years or more (so at-risk for colorectal neoplasia) is increasingly used as an excuse for the reassurance of a whole colon screening examination. Of all patients with blood loss referred for colonoscopy, around 10 per cent will have a 'significant' lesion, either a neoplastic polyp of 1 cm diameter or greater or malignancy. Colonoscopy is considered the investigation of choice for major bleeding, being readily available and offering immediate therapy and a high degree of diagnostic accuracy. Angiodysplasia, small ectatic vascular lesions in the proximal colon of elderly subjects with bleeding or anaemia, are relatively rare but are an example of a condition easily diagnosed and treated by colonoscopy—but by virtually no other method.

Chronic diarrhoea or known inflammatory disease is accurately and easily assessed by endoscopy and biopsy. The terminal ileum can be accessed or biopsied in over 80 per cent of cases by an experienced endoscopist. Endoscopic differential diagnosis between the focal or 'apthoid' (mouth-like) ulcers with intervening normal mucosa in Crohn's disease and the generally reddened surface of ulcerative colitis is easy and definitive in around 90 per cent of cases. A few remain as 'indeterminate colitis' and differential diagnosis can be more difficult in severe or chronic cases. The possibility of infective colitis, including tuberculous or amoebic, must be borne in mind and extra specimens taken for microscopy and culture if in doubt. Biopsies typically show somewhat greater extent of inflammation than is visible to the eye, and so must be taken at intervals around the colon in any patient with bowel frequency, to exclude 'microscopic colitis' or the related phenomenon of 'collagenous colitis'. Chronic inflammatory disease affecting more than half the colon carries an increased long-term risk of cancer or mucosal dysplastic (precancerous) change, and so indicates annual or 2-yearly surveillance from 8 to 10 years after onset of symptoms. Ischaemic colitis, typically affecting a short segment around the splenic flexure, can show changes ranging from mild reddening to marked ulceration or even near gangrene.

Polyps of almost any size can be removed endoscopically, leaving for transanal proctological management only very large, sessile rectal polyps up to 12 cm from the anal verge. Around 5 to 10 per cent of polyps will contain focal, high-grade dysplasia or invasive carcinoma. Even 'malignant polyps' or 'polypoid cancers' having no adenoma present can be managed conservatively by endoscopy alone if complete removal is confirmed histologically by a margin of 1 mm between the limit of invasion and the plane of excision, and the tumour is also well or moderately differentiated. Placing one or more India ink tattoos near the polypectomy site gives a permanent marker for endoscopic follow-up, or localizes it if surgery or laparoscopy is indicated. Lasers have been used for ablation of the post-polypectomy remnants of sessile polyps, but the newer alternative technique of argon plasma coagulation is cheaper, easier, and safer.

Cancer prevention or surveillance colonoscopy gives a strong guarantee to the patient even when negative, both because of the accuracy of colonoscopy and the generally slow time-course of development of colonic neoplasms. Follow-up at 3 to 5-year intervals after polypectomy does yield further adenomas in 30 to 50 per cent of patients, especially those with three or more or large polyps on the initial examination. A large series has suggested that the incidence of colorectal cancer is reduced by polypectomy and follow-up. Patients at genetic risk merit colonoscopic surveillance, especially those with a first-degree relative with colorectal cancer under 45 years of age, two or more affected first-degree relatives, or those assessed genetically as belonging to a 'hereditary non-polyposis colon cancer' family with autosomal dominant risk (see Chapter 14.15). Follow-up, ablating minute or 'flat' adenomas, is scheduled at 1 to 5-year intervals according to perceived individual risk.

Abnormalities on other diagnostic methods are ideally checked colonoscopically. Abnormalities seen on scanning frequently turn out to be spurious, presumably faecal, and the majority of positive occult blood tests prove to be 'false' for neoplasm. Supposed 'strictures' on barium enema often prove to be due to spasm or uncomplicated sigmoid diverticulosis. Others, such as anastomotic strictures, typically after Crohn's resection, are usually easily and effectively balloon-dilated. Even patients with typical malignant 'apple-core' strictures should ideally have preoperative total colonoscopy to exclude other synchronous neoplasms, if necessary using a small-diameter instrument (sometimes a paediatric gastroscope). If this proves impossible, endoscopy should be rescheduled within 6 months after resection. Colonoscopy has effectively supplanted 'diagnostic laparotomy'; it also avoids the numerous resections previously performed in diverticular disease when radiographs could 'not exclude the possibility of malignancy'—which the endoscopist can in a few minutes.

There are low-yield indications for colonoscopy, where alternative investigations such as flexible sigmoidoscopy, barium enema, 'virtual colonoscopy', or other approaches may be justified. These include patients with simple constipation of long standing, bloating, left iliac fossa discomfort, or combinations of these symptoms suggesting 'irritable bowel syndrome'. Where the patient is young, the extra accuracy of 'one-off' colonoscopy may be justified. In elderly patients, the greater likelihood of diverticular disease and difficult (and so more hazardous) colonoscopy may be a further disincentive, although these patients find the distension and manoeuvres of barium enema more unpleasant than sedated colonoscopy.

Cost effectiveness and relationship to other techniques

Flexible endoscopy seems superficially expensive and is demanding of professional time. However, modern colonoscopes are surprisingly robust and, properly handled and maintained, will perform thousands of examinations without expensive repairs.

Newer teaching methods, including use of computer simulation to improve handskills, should help to improve standards and speed training of doctors in colonoscopy and nurse practitioners to undertake flexible sigmoidoscopy.

Sigmoidoscopy provides rapid, unsedated examination, so allowing 'one-stop' patient management and avoiding the need to return for prepared exam–whether colonoscopy, radiography, or scanning. Flexible endoscopy has the general advantage that it leaves only gas (air or CO_2) in the colon, and so can be followed by any other modality if complete, whereas barium takes several days to clear.

Total colonoscopy, its accuracy increasing to near microscopic levels with newer and more agile instruments, is likely to remain the diagnostic 'gold standard' for the foreseeable future. Other, newer methods such as 'virtual' colonoscopy and genetic screening, may have an invaluable screening and selection role, but are unlikely to provide definitive tissue diagnosis or therapy. Endoscopy, providing that the bowel is prepared appropriately, can follow immediately to check or treat patients with a positive scan. It is therefore possible that colonoscopy will, in future, relinquish some of its present front-line role, but it is highly likely that requirements for it will increase if population screening for the prevention of colorectal cancer becomes routine.

14.2.2 Upper gastrointestinal endoscopy

Adrian R. W. Hatfield

Background

Subsequent to the pioneering work on the transmission of light down flexible optic fibres by Professor Hopkins in 1954, 'gastro-cameras' were replaced by early, flexible, fibre optic endoscopes in the mid-1960s, which led to the development of gastrointestinal endoscopy as we now know it. A major disadvantage of fibre optic endoscopes has been the deterioration of the fibre bundle with time leading to poor images. The recent availability of cheaper, miniaturized colour chips has led to the development of video endoscopes, providing an excellent, clear view which does not deteriorate with the age of the endoscope. With appropriate improvements in software, the endoscopic video image can be magnified and modern instruments will zoom up to 25 × magnification and the mucosal detail can also be enhanced electronically so that small lesions of a few mm can be seen quite clearly. The modern video endoscope image can be instantly printed out and archived digitally on a computer system.

The external specifications and handling of the new video endoscopes are similar to their previous, fibre optic counterparts and thus the techniques for disinfection and endoscopy are similar for both ranges of equipment. The disadvantage of the modern equipment is that the video endoscopy system needs considerable hardware. In most instances a video monitor, light source, and processor are located in an endoscopy unit and not easily moved to a different location such as an operating theatre for emergency endoscopy. In the acutely bleeding patient, the presence of blood in the lumen of the gastrointestinal tract diminishes the efficiency of the video chip and the image obtained is often poor. In this situation, a conventional fibre optic endoscope will often give a much better view and will be more easily taken into the operating theatre for such an emergency.

Endoscopy units and disinfection techniques

It is now well recognized that the care of the instruments and other equipment, together with the important aspects of patient safety, are greatly improved by having a purpose built endoscopy unit staffed by experienced endoscopic nursing staff who are trained in handling and disinfecting endoscopes and patient safety during and after intravenous sedation.

Most endoscopy units have a purpose built disinfecting machine which can take single or multiple instruments and, after suitable mechanical cleaning, a disinfecting agent will be automatically pumped through the channels of the instrument for a given period of time and flushed out afterwards. The choice of disinfecting agent varies between units but the trend has been away from hazardous agents such as glutaraldehyde (Cidex) to less harmful agents, such as Nu-Cidex or Tristel, that do not need sophisticated extraction and ventilation.

For routine, simple diagnostic upper gastrointestinal endoscopy many patients are now routinely endoscoped without sedation, after local anaesthesia to the throat only. 'No sedation endoscopy' is suitable for busy units with long lists of day cases. However, large numbers of endoscopies, particularly in apprehensive or sick inpatients and those needing more complicated procedures, are still performed under intravenous sedation.

There are now clear guidelines, drawn up by the British Society of Gastroenterology, as to the practice of administering intravenous sedation for endoscopic procedures. Patients are now monitored with pulse oximetry and oxygen is given routinely to the ill or elderly and to other patients if oxygen saturation falls during the procedure. The precise choice of sedation will vary between units and will depend on the patient and the type of procedure performed, however diazemuls and midazolam remain the two most common sedative agents used, often combined with pethidine for more lengthy or invasive procedures. It is not uncommon to reverse the effect of the benzodiazepine sedation with flumazenil (Anexate) and any opiate sedation with naloxone (Narcan). On rare occasions general anaesthesia will need to be used for endoscopy, usually for children or adults with ventilatory problems.

Specific risk of infection with endoscopy

Patients with heart murmurs were routinely given antibiotics to cover endoscopic procedures in the past. It is now recommended that only patients with prosthetic valves need be given routine prophylactic antibiotic cover, with a single parenteral dose of a broad-spectrum penicillin before the procedure.

Current disinfecting agents and schedules will cope with hepatitis B and C and HIV infection. All endoscopic staff wear disposable gloves and the nurse nearest the patient's mouth will usually wear a visor to cover eyes, nose, and mouth, particularly with a patient of known infective risk. As there is no effective way of sterilizing an endoscope against prions (at present thought to be the transmissible agent in Creutzfeldt–Jakob disease), the current Department of Health Guidelines make it clear that all equipment used on patients with suspected Creutzfeldt–Jakob disease should be destroyed afterwards. Patients with suspected Creutzfeldt–Jakob disease are not therefore endoscoped and alternative ways of diagnosis or treatment are usually sought.

Diagnostic endoscopy in the gastrointestinal tract

Endoscopy has now become the investigation of choice in patients with retrosternal or upper abdominal symptoms where, previously, barium radiology would have been employed. The advantages of detecting grades of inflammation and erosive change, rather than radiologically obvious ulceration, are obvious. Equally, the ability to take samples from the gastrointestinal tract with brush cytology or biopsy greatly enhances the diagnosis, not just in differentiating between benign and malignant ulcers and strictures, but also in assessing degrees of inflammatory change and in detecting dysplasia, for example in Barrett's oesophagus.

Endoscopy will detect oesophageal varices in patients with liver disease at an early stage. In the symptomatic patient with liver disease and gastrointestinal bleeding, endoscopy is particularly important as the site of bleeding may be variable and the management very different. Bleeding oesophageal varices can be managed endoscopically in a number of therapeutic ways.

In the last 10 years, it has become routine to take gastric biopsies in patients with peptic problems to detect the presence of *Helicobacter pylori*. The routine use of a simple CLO test, where mucosal biopsies are inserted into a gelatine well containing a colouring agent that turns yellow to red in the presence of *Helicobacter* urease, will be satisfactory. In some patients,

gastric biopsies are necessary in this situation for culturing the bacteria to ascertain sensitivity in patients with infection resistant to multiple eradication therapies. In younger patients where malignant disease is less of a concern, serum, faecal, or breath test analysis is an acceptable alternative to establishing *Helicobacter* infection and thus such patients could be treated initially without endoscopy and gastric biopsy.

Most gastric cancers in the United Kingdom are diagnosed when the patient is symptomatic and thus the finding of a mucosal cancer is rare. Most lesions are straightforward to diagnose endoscopically and biopsies are usually confirmatory. Cancers that infiltrate the wall of the stomach below the mucosa are difficult to diagnose endoscopically as endoscopic biopsies are usually quite superficial. In this situation a 'double punch' type technique is useful, where a second biopsy is taken from the deeper submucosa through the small defect of the first biopsy. 'Linitis plastica' is difficult to assess endoscopically, particularly where Buscopan may have been used routinely to inhibit peristalsis at the start of the endoscopy. In such patients, a barium meal may help in the diagnosis by showing the lack of gastric motility.

Small bowel endoscopy (enteroscopy)

For many years, routine upper gastrointestinal endoscopes were not of sufficient length to pass beyond the duodenojejunal flexure into the small bowel. Enteroscopes are now made that can be advanced under direct vision down the upper small intestine or, alternatively, a thinner endoscope is allowed to pass down the small bowel spontaneously and then the bowel lumen is visualized on withdrawal. Such endoscopic procedures are lengthy and difficult and will not necessarily view the entire small bowel. A more comprehensive view is sometimes obtained, particularly in the hunt for obscure bleeding lesions, by passing a standard upper gastrointestinal endoscope up and down the small intestine through small enterotomies at the time of laparotomy, with a surgeon concertinering the small bowel over the shaft of the endoscope. Recently a video capsule has been developed which, when swallowed, transmits a good view of the entire small bowel during transit through the gut.

The rather lengthy, tedious, and unpredictable techniques of small bowel biopsy using a Crosby capsule have been largely superseded by routine upper gastrointestinal endoscopy with biopsies from the distal duodenum. Such biopsies have been shown to be very representative of the upper jejunal mucosa. This technique is now used routinely in the diagnosis of coeliac disease.

Therapeutic endoscopy in the upper gastrointestinal tract

Over the last 20 years, a wide range of therapeutic manoeuvres have been developed for use in various situations in the upper gastrointestinal tract.

Gastrointestinal bleeding

Oesophageal varices can be injected through the mucosa with ethanolamine oleate under direct vision. Paravasal injection is best avoided as it can lead to secondary bleeding from mucosal ulceration and sometimes later oesophageal stricture formation. Endoscopic sclerotherapy can be repeated at weekly or monthly intervals until the varices have been obliterated. Bleeding gastric varices can also be injected but these are more difficult to obliterate. More recently, endoscopic banding techniques have been employed, both in the acutely bleeding patient and the chronic situation. Single or multiple bands could be put on varices in the oesophagus or, sometimes, in the fundus of the stomach. The addition of thrombin into gastric varices after banding may enhance successful eradication and reduce the risk of bleeding if the bands slip off too early.

Bleeding erosions and ulcers can be injected with dilute adrenaline (1:10 000). This may be satisfactorily in reducing bleeding in the short term and can always be repeated if necessary. Endoscopic laser therapy can be employed around a visible vessel in the base of an ulcer. A similar effect can be obtained by the use of multicontact diathermy probes or heater probes. Bleeding vascular abnormalities, such as angiodysplasia, can be treated with thermal probes but more satisfactorily with non-contact laser which does not pull off a coagulum and has the extra benefit of destroying vessels just below the mucosa.

Benign oesophageal strictures

Commonly, a peptic stricture above a hiatus hernia secondary to reflux will produce dysphagia but benign strictures due to other causes, such the swallowing of corrosive substances and postsurgical anastomotic strictures, can be treated by the same endoscopic techniques. In the past, bougies of increasing size were passed over a previously endoscopically placed guidewire and the stricture slowly dilated. More recently, high pressure dilating balloon catheters, passed over the wire under radiological screening or directly through the scope under direct endoscopic vision, can be used more efficiently and safely with better patient tolerance.

Achalasia of the cardia can be treated with balloon dilatation using a larger balloon of 30 to 40 mm diameter, where the aim is to rupture muscle fibres to weaken the circular muscle sphincter. Alternatively, botulinum toxin can be injected through the mucosa into the muscle sphincter circumferentially at the time of endoscopy. The improvement in swallowing after this procedure is limited and may need to be repeated every 6 months.

Malignant gastro-oesophageal strictures

Most of patients with non-operable tumours of the stomach or oesophagus producing dysphagia are palliated by the insertion of some sort of oesophageal stent. By and large, silicone rubber prostheses have been replaced by self-expanding metal stents which can be very easily and safely placed through a malignant stricture without the need for prior dilatation, thus reducing the risk of perforation. Most of these stents now have a membrane to prevent tumour ingrowth through the mesh but this will sometimes occur at one or either end. Such tumour overgrowth can be treated with endoscopic laser therapy. Brachytherapy can be given via an endoscopically sited tube through the stricture prior to stenting.

Removal of foreign objects

Most solid objects such as marbles, rings, and coins should pass spontaneously and the need for removing foreign bodies is usually because they are sharp and may cause damage if left *in situ*. Most objects can be snared or trapped in a basket and removed intact. Sharp objects can be pulled into a endoscopic overtube to protect the oesophagus during withdrawal.

Polyps and small tumours

Most gastric polyps are entirely benign and do not need removing. Leiomyomas of the stomach or duodenum can be watched if small, but if over 5 cm in size should probably be removed. Often such patients will go directly to surgery but newer endoscopic techniques using submucosal resection can tackle lesions that do not infiltrate beyond the submucosa. Careful prior assessment with endoscopic ultrasound is usually needed to make sure that a small tumour can be technically removed in this way.

Assisted nutrition

There are now many types of enteral feeding tube that can be sited in the upper gastrointestinal tract. Although most fine-bore feeding tubes can be passed on the ward or under radiological control, the prior passage of an endoscopic guidewire into the stomach which is then rerouted through the nose, can allow feeding tubes to be positioned accurately, often through an oesophageal stricture or difficult anastomosis, or positioned in the duodenum in patients with gastric stasis. The endoscopic positioning of a nasojejunal feeding tube, beyond the duodenojejunal flexure, is now becoming a common alternative to intravenous feeding in patients with complicated pancreatitis where 'pancreatic rest' is needed.

Techniques for placing a gastrostomy tube endoscopically (PEG) are now simple and straightforward. After transabdominal puncture into a distended stomach under direct endoscopic vision, a PEG tube with diameters from 8FG to 24FG can be pulled back down the oesophagus through the stomach and a flange, balloon, or button will allow the tube to be anchored firmly up against the gastric mucosa. In patients where there is gastric stasis or in pancreatitis, a small jejunal extension tube can be inserted through the PEG and positioned endoscopically into the distal duodenum or beyond the DJ flexure (PEJ).

Endoscopic ultrasound

Special endoscopes are available with a dual capability of endoscopic and ultrasound imaging. Either a rotating or a fixed linear array transducer will provide an ultrasound image at a point where the endoscopist can accurately direct the probe in the lumen of the oesophagus, stomach, or duodenum. Although CT scanning will stage most larger tumours of the upper gastrointestinal tract, pancreas, and bile duct, endoscopic ultrasound is particularly useful in staging small tumours and particularly mucosal tumours. The linear array ultrasound endoscope can be used for needle biopsy of tumours in the wall of the gastrointestinal tract or head of pancreas and sometimes adjacent lymph nodes. Although endoscopic ultrasound is still developing in the United Kingdom, it is used more commonly elsewhere in Europe where gastroenterologists are routinely trained in abdominal ultrasound.

Endoscopy and disorders of the pancreas and biliary tree

Diagnostic endoscopic retrograde cholangiopancreatography

The development of side-viewing duodenoscopes in the 1970s allowed endoscopic visualization of the papilla of Vater and cannulation of the pancreatic and biliary duct systems, endoscopic retrograde cholangiopancreatography (ERCP). For many years ERCP was the gold standard of investigating pancreatic and biliary disorders but, with the advent of CT and MR scanning, the need for diagnostic ERCP has diminished. ERCP is still extremely useful in the diagnosis of patients with gallstones, sclerosing cholangitis, and biliary tumours where scanning is normal or equivocal, in the absence of overt jaundice. A tissue diagnosis can be obtained with brush cytology and endoscopic biopsy within the bile duct, avoiding the need for percutaneous biopsy.

Diagnostic ERCP is still useful in the assessment of patients with pancreatitis, congenital abnormalities, such as pancreas divisum, and in some patients with a pancreatic mass on scanning where the diagnosis is not clear. Most patients with a carcinoma of the pancreas will present with obstructive jaundice and will need a therapeutic procedure, others without jaundice will usually be diagnosed on ultrasound or CT scanning.

In specialized centres, biliary and pancreatic manometry is performed to assess patients with pancreatobiliary pain with no apparent structural abnormalities. At ERCP, a perfused catheter can be inserted into the bile duct and into the pancreatic duct and pull-through manometry performed. This will show whether elevated basal and peak pressures indicate sphincter of Oddi dysfunction.

Therapeutic endoscopic retrograde cholangiopancreatography

Gallstones

The endoscopic removal of common bile duct stones at the time of ERCP is the treatment of choice for patients presenting with pain, abnormal liver function tests, jaundice, or cholangitis. Following previous cholecystectomy, about 10 per cent of patients will ultimately represent with bile duct stones and endoscopic management is far safer than further surgical exploration of the bile duct. Prior to laparoscopic cholecystectomy, it is particularly important to investigate and to endoscopically clear the bile duct of stones, if suspected. Failure to do so may increase the likelihood of postoperative bile duct leaks. At the time of ERCP if stones are located in the biliary tree, a small diathermy cut is made into the bile duct through the papilla and, through the sphincterotomy, stones can be extracted with a balloon or basket. If the stones are too numerous or too large to extract at the first procedure, small pigtail stents are inserted into the bile duct to guarantee good drainage without stone impaction and therefore reduce the incidence of postprocedure cholangitis.

Most large stones can ultimately be removed using a mechanical crushing basket (lithotripter) or sometimes with the help of extracorporeal shock wave lithotripsy, following which fragments can be removed from the bile duct at follow-up ERCP. In experienced hands, the technical failure rate is low and thus the need for surgical reintervention is uncommon. Only in patients with very large bile duct stones, intrahepatic stones, or stones above biliary strictures is there a need for further procedures, such as intraduct choledochoscopy, using small endoscopes with direct contact lithotripsy using a pulse dye laser or an electrohydraulic probe. Very elderly or frail patients with large bile duct stones can be managed long-term by simple placement of an endoscopic stent beside the stones for drainage to prevent jaundice and/or cholangitis. Such stents can be changed over the years as per necessary.

Benign strictures

Postoperative anastomotic strictures or those following bile duct damage at the time of cholecystectomy can initially be managed with intermittent biliary balloon dilatation at the time of ERCP or simple endoscopic stent placement. In the young patient after a trial of dilatation or stenting for a reasonable length of time, about 1 year, surgical reconstruction of the bile duct might be needed if it is clear that endoscopic treatment is not leading to resolution of the stricture. In patients with primary sclerosing cholangitis, there may be single or multiple strictures in the intrahepatic and extrahepatic biliary tree, often in association with pigment stones, which can be difficult to dilate or stent. A variable proportion of patients with primary sclerosing cholangitis develop a cholangiocarcinoma and this can be very difficult to prove even with good ERCP, biliary cytology, CT, and MR scanning.

Malignant bile duct obstruction

Pancreatic and bile duct cancer and carcinoma of the ampulla of Vater can all produce stricturing of the biliary tree at different levels. At ERCP the stricture can be dilated and then an endoscopic 10 or 12FG polyethylene stent placed to relieve jaundice. These stents are cheap and usually stay patent for 4 to 5 months. In pancreatic cancer, about one-third of patients will survive long enough to occlude their stent, in which case a further procedure is performed to remove the blocked stent and replace it with a new one. Self-expanding metal stents offer a way of palliating patients for longer as they have a lumen of 10 mm which gives excellent long-term drainage. At present, biliary metal stents have an open mesh and tumour infiltration may occur, causing recurrent jaundice and/or sepsis. In that situation, a plastic stent can be inserted through the blocked metal stent to achieve drainage. Membrane-covered metal stents are now becoming available which should avoid the problem of tumour ingrowth and hopefully remain patent for longer.

In some patients with cholangiocarcinoma at the hilum of the liver, separate obstruction to right and left main ducts or subsegments may be found. In such a situation, more than one stent may be necessary to relieve jaundice or sepsis. Brachytherapy for cholangiocarcinoma can be administered endoscopically using an iridium wire source inserted down an endoscopically placed catheter inside the stent within the cholangiocarcinoma. Photodynamic therapy (PDT) can also be administered using a diffuser laser fibre, endoscopically sited within the malignant biliary stricture(s).

Pancreatitis

In patients with acute, relapsing and chronic pancreatitis a variety of endoscopic therapies can be performed. After pancreatic sphincterotomy, stones can be removed from the pancreatic duct, strictures can be stented, and drainage of the dorsal duct in pancreas divisum can be achieved. Peripancreatic fluid collections and pseudocysts can also be managed by pancreatic duct drainage or direct endoscopic cyst puncture and stenting techniques. Pancreatic endotherapy is difficult and can be associated with complications. Nevertheless, in selected patients it may be very valuable and avoids difficult and complex pancreatic surgery.

Gastric outlet obstruction

About 10 per cent of patients with pancreatobiliary tumours will develop gastric outlet obstruction as a late complication as tumour infiltrates the duodenum. Conventionally, a surgical gastric bypass has been unavoidable and this has carried a substantial morbidity/mortality as these patients are often very frail in the latter stages of their malignant disease. A large-diameter, self-expanding metal 'enteral' stent can now be placed in the stomach and duodenum at the time of endoscopy. This rapidly relieves symptoms of gastric outlet obstruction and allows the patients to eat a reasonable diet, without vomiting, thus avoiding the need for bypass surgery.

Hazards and complications

Diagnostic endoscopy carries very few risks. With careful attention to nursing techniques and sedation protocol, cardiovascular problems during endoscopy and aspiration pneumonia after are extremely rare. Direct damage to the upper gastrointestinal tract during insertion and subsequent inspection down to the duodenum is extremely unusual but rarely the cricopharynx, lower oesophagus above the cardia, and duodenal cap are sites of direct perforation with the endoscope, more commonly with inexperienced endoscopists. An unrecognized pharyngeal pouch represents a real hazard during insertion of the endoscope and might lead to a perforation if undue force is applied.

Most complications of endoscopy occur during therapeutic procedures and are specific to the type of procedure being performed.

The perforation rate following oesophageal dilatation is extremely low now that techniques and equipment have improved. The development of self-expanding stents in the oesophagus avoids the need for forceful dilatation of malignant strictures and this has radically lowered the postprocedure complication rate of perforation. Due to the size of the balloon used in dilating achalasia of the cardia, perforations can be seen. Anybody who develops pain or discomfort after oesophageal dilatation should be assumed to have developed perforation, a chest radiograph should be obtained and if there is evidence of mediastinal air or surgical emphysema, conservative management with nil-by-mouth, parenteral antibiotics, and intravenous feeding is advocated. Many patients will settle conservatively without the need for surgical intervention.

The complications of ERCP are well known and more frequent than those of other endoscopic manoeuvres in the upper gastrointestinal tract. Even with diagnostic ERCP, up to 2 per cent of patients may develop postprocedure pancreatitis after either manipulation at the papilla or the injection of contrast into the pancreas. Such pancreatitis is usually self-limiting and mild although the serum amylase may reach extremely high levels.

Some patients have a very elevated amylase without any pain. After endoscopic sphincterotomy and any therapeutic manoeuvre in the pancreatic or biliary tree, pancreatitis and bleeding can occur. Between 2 and 5 per cent of patients may have some degree of bleeding, but only a small proportion of these will need a blood transfusion or, rarely, surgical intervention. With the use of periprocedure antibiotics and the routine use of biliary stents after incomplete gallstone clearance within the bile duct, the incidence of postprocedure cholangitis is minimal.

14.2.3 Radiology of the gastrointestinal tract

Alan Freeman

The widespread introduction of endoscopic techniques has lessened the need for radiological examination of the intestinal tract, and has completely replaced it in the examination of the stomach. There is, however, still a major radiological role in the investigation of the small and large bowel; the small bowel will be considered first.

The small intestine

The small intestine may be examined by a number of radiological means which include: plain films, barium contrast studies, ultrasound, CT, nuclear medicine, and MR. Plain film radiography performed in cases of suspected small bowel obstruction typically include films taken with both vertical and horizontal beam, the object being to demonstrate dilated loops and air–fluid levels. This role, however, is increasingly replaced by CT and apart from this, plain films have no other function. Barium studies of the small bowel have been the mainstay of examination for almost a century and, correctly performed, provide good morphological detail of the bowel. There are two types of examination; the first is the so-called barium follow through wherein the patient drinks a quantity of barium sulphate and then sequential films are taken of its passage through the small bowel. The second is the small bowel enema or enteroclysis and in this technique a tube is passed into the third part of the duodenum and barium sulphate is continuously infused, thus outlining the small intestine. This latter technique can also be used to provide a double contrast effect by infusing methyl cellulose, which provides a negative contrast against the positive contrast of barium sulphate.

Both techniques have advantages and disadvantages. The follow through is simple to perform and of course is more comfortable for the patient. However, it is imperative that fluoroscopy is performed at regular intervals together with abdominal compression so that all loops of small bowel are outlined. Enteroclysis by its very nature means that the barium column is observed in a continuous fashion and any minor obstruction or abnormality is thus more likely to be observed. Proponents of enteroclysis therefore argue that it is a more accurate test, but it is difficult to make a direct comparison as it is obviously difficult to perform both techniques on a cohort of patients. Given the relatively low incidence of disease of the small intestine, it seems reasonable in most instances to perform a follow through study in the first instance and to reserve enteroclysis for unresolved problems, subacute obstruction, etc.

Both types of contrast study suffer from the fact they only demonstrate the mucosal surface of the bowel and disease in the wall of the bowel or outside of it may be easily overlooked. In this situation, some form of cross-sectional imaging, typically ultrasound or CT, may well give more information.

Ultrasound, to date, has not found a huge role because it is highly operator dependent and requires considerable time. Its advantage of course is

that it is radiation free. Usually, a high frequency ultrasound probe, in the order of 5 mHz, is used and the whole abdomen is carefully covered quadrant by quadrant with graded compression. Dilated, fluid-filled loops of bowel are relatively easy to examine, but the presence of excess gas within bowel loops, deep pelvic loops, and patient obesity all provide major impediments to full examination by ultrasound.

These factors, however, provide no problem for CT which, despite its use of ionizing radiation, is finding an increasing role in the investigation of small bowel disease. This particularly applies to acute small bowel obstruction where it provides not only confirmation of the diagnosis but often demonstrates the site and the nature of the obstructing lesion. As the images are usually enhanced by means of intravenous contrast agents, they can provide useful information as to the viability or otherwise of the obstructed loops. Thickening and infiltration of the bowel wall is readily appreciated at CT, as is the demonstration of exophytic tumours such as leiomyomas and lymphoma.

Nuclear medicine studies, which involve the injection of a radio-labelled substance, have major roles in the demonstration of inflammatory conditions involving the small bowel and for the demonstration of potential bleeding sources from the small bowel. In the former, the patients white blood cells are extracted and then labelled with Tc 99m pertechnetate. These white cells are then reinjected into the patient. The cells concentrate at the site of inflammation and this activity is demonstrated on a gamma camera. The technique is known as labelled white cell scanning. Alternatively, indium may be used as the isotope when a longer half-life is required and this particularly applies in the diagnosis of possible intra-abdominal abscess. This does involve a higher radiation dose to the patient.

If bleeding from the small bowel is the problem, then the patient's red blood cells are extracted and again labelled with Tc 99m pertechnetate. The labelled cells are reinjected into the patient and the abdomen is scanned under a gamma camera. A bleeding source of more than approximately 0.5 ml/min, can be identified as a hotspot, indicating the probable site. A more specific bleeding source is a Meckel's diverticulum and if this is symptomatic it is likely to contain ectopic gastric cells which may be demonstrated by the simple injection by pertechnetate by itself.

Magnetic resonance imaging (MR) of the small bowel holds huge promise and is likely to become the most important technique in the future. It has major advantages in that it involves no radiation and image reconstruction can be performed in almost any plane. Indeed, image reconstruction is so fast that in effect, MR fluoroscopy of the bowel can produce images similar to those obtained at barium fluoroscopy. Because of the lack of ionizing radiation, areas of interest or difficulty can be 'revisited' time and again until fully evaluated. To obtain these images, the bowel does need to be distended which usually involves passing a nasoduodenal tube and utilizing water or methyl cellulose as the distention and contrast agents.

Anatomy of the small bowel

Strictly speaking, the small bowel commences at the pylorus and includes duodenum, jejunum, and ileum. However, the first part of duodenum, proximal to the superior duodenal flexure, is usually more closely aligned to the stomach in relation to pathology and investigation and for practical purposes, this chapter will discuss small bowel from mid-descending duodenum onwards. The third part of the duodenum commences at the inferior duodenum flexure and passes across the midline at roughly the level of L3 to ascend to the duodenal–jejunal junction. This is marked by the peritoneal ligament of Treitz. At this point, the small bowel emerges from the retroperitoneum to become an intraperitoneal structure. It is then divided roughly into equal lengths of jejunum and ileum, with jejunal loops occupying the left upper quadrant and ileal loops the right lower quadrant. The ileum terminates at the ileocaecal junction where it again becomes a retroperitoneal structure. Morphologically, jejunum can be distinguished from ileum both by its size (it is usually about 1 cm larger in diameter) and by the presence of valvulae connivente or plicae semilunaris. The latter gives it its characteristic fold pattern on contrast studies as opposed to the relatively featureless ileum.

Pathology of the small bowel

Coeliac disease and malabsorption states

Coeliac disease, caused by a sensitivity to gluten, is characterized by atrophy of the small intestinal villous pattern. The definitive diagnosis thus rests with duodenal or jejunal biopsy, but radiology retains a role in evaluating complications as well as excluding other causes or malabsorption.

Barium follow through studies have been the mainstay and demonstrate changes which include dilatation of jejunal loops (to more than 3.5 cm), flocculation of the barium suspension, thickening of the fold pattern (particularly if there is associated hypoproteinaemia), and delayed transit. Many of these features are very subjective and thus radiology cannot be used as a test to exclude coeliac disease. Marked mucosal effacement typically involving the duodenum, but sometimes the whole of the jejunum, may be a prominent feature leading to the so-called 'moulage' appearance which is specific for coeliac disease and for the rare graft-versus-host syndrome (Fig. 1). Likewise, transient intussusceptions occurring during the examination are only seen with coeliac disease.

Complications, such as the development of lymphoma, may be demonstrated by both barium studies and CT, whilst stricture formation following ulcerative jejunitis, often regarded as a prelymphomatous condition, is best assessed by barium studies.

Other causes of malabsorption include jejunal diverticulosis and short bowel syndrome, plus infiltrative causes such as intestinal lymphangectasia, Whipple's disease, eosinophilic gastroenteritis, amyloidosis, and mastocytosis:

- Jejunal diverticulosis causes malabsorption because of intestinal stasis and subsequent bacterial overgrowth. The diverticula usually protrudes through the mesenteric border of the jejunum and can be demonstrated on small bowel series as a number of sac-like structures containing barium, particularly if erect views are taken.

- Short bowel syndrome results if extensive lengths of small bowel have been resected, often either as a result of vascular accidents or following complications of Crohn's disease. The bowel will adapt by increasing its diameter, but an overall length of less than 50 cm is usually incompatible with life. This situation is particularly severe if the terminal ileum

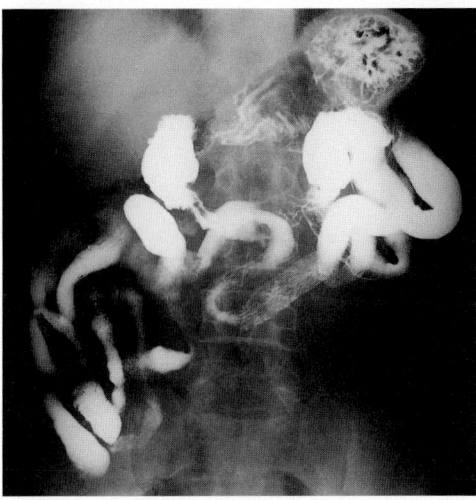

Fig. 1 Severe coeliac disease showing moulage phenomena. There has been complete obliteration of the small bowel fold pattern such that the barium follow through appearances resemble toothpaste squeezed from a tube, leading to the alternative term of 'tube of toothpaste' sign. This particular study was performed because the patient was thought to have a carcinoma of the stomach and thus illustrates one of the very varied ways in which coeliac disease can manifest.

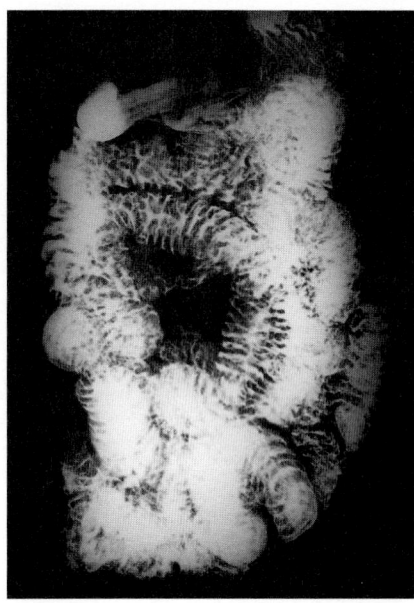

Fig. 2 Intestinal lymphangiectasia demonstrated by thickening and straightening of the fold pattern together with a faint granular background due to the dilated lymphatics. In this case lymphangiectasia was secondary to an underlying lymphoma.

has been resected because of its specialized function in the absorption of vitamin B_{12} and in the enterohepatic circulation of bile salts.

The various small bowel infiltrations are rare:

- Intestinal lymphangestasia is characterized by the presence of dilated lymph vessels in the mucosa which cause protein and lymphocytic loss into the small bowel. It may be primary or secondary, with the secondary form being caused by conditions which obstruct the bowel lymphatics, such as lymphoma, carcinoma, postradiation changes, and occasionally in association with heart failure and constrictive pericarditis. High-quality barium studies may demonstrate the dilated lymphatics as very fine, mm-size nodules, mainly in the jejunum (Fig. 2).

- Whipple's disease is caused by a bacillus resulting in a syndrome of steatorrhoea, abdominal pain, and arthralgia. It has a male predominance. Barium studies show thickened folds together with slight dilatation of the bowel lumen. In addition, CT may demonstrate bowel wall thickening together with mesenteric lymphadenopathy, the lymph nodes usually being of low attenuation.

- Eosinophilic gastroenteritis—in this condition, the wall of the bowel is infiltrated with eosinophils and there is usually a peripheral eosinophilia as well. Often, there is a history of atopy and the triad of eosinophilic gastroenteritis, asthma, and mononeuritis multiplex comprise the Churg–Strauss syndrome. Symptoms resulting from small bowel involvement depend on the major site of location of eosinophilic infiltration, which may be either mucosal or serosal. With the former diarrhoea, malabsorption, and protein loss are dominant, whereas the latter is characterized by ascites. Barium studies in cases of mainly mucosal involvement show fold thickening together with nodular filling defects, whereas serosal involvement is better assessed by CT, which shows both the bowel wall thickening and ascites.

- Amyloidosis and mastocytosis are very rare causes of malabsorption with infiltration in both cases, causing thickening of the valvulae conniventes. Amyloidosis is characterized by the deposition of amyloid fibres in the small bowel and may be primary or secondary (Fig. 3).

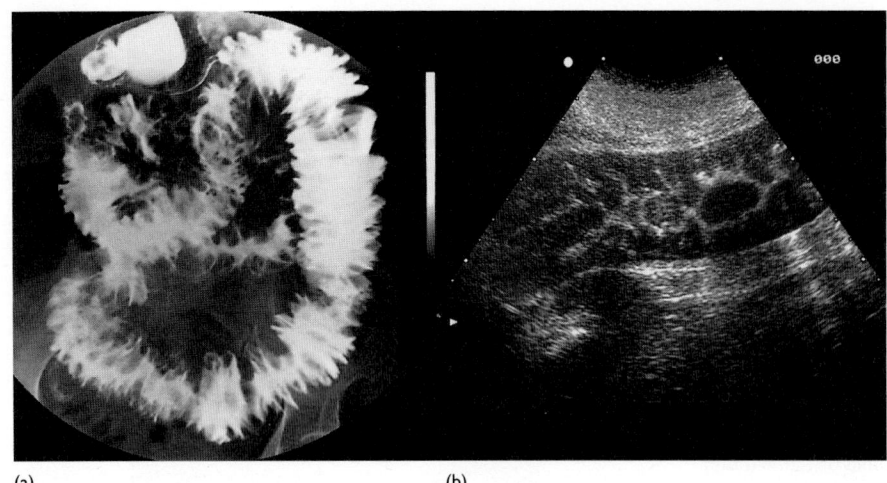

(a)   (b)

Fig. 3 Amyloidosis of the small bowel shown on a barium follow through (a) and ultrasound examination (b). There is complete disorganization of the normal small bowel fold pattern (a) and the degree of thickening of the small bowel wall is best appreciated on the ultrasound (b).

Tumours of the small intestine

These may be benign or malignant and are relatively uncommon:

- Benign tumours include leiomyomas, haemangiomas, and adenomas. Bleeding or intussusception are the commonest presentations, particularly from leiomyomas. These tumours may grow into the bowel lumen, but often have a significant exoenteric mass, in which case they can grow to a very large size without causing clinical symptoms. They may, therefore, be demonstrated on barium studies as a filling defect, sometimes with a central ulcer which results from necrosis, whereas CT is the best method for demonstrating the exocentric component. A number of syndromes include small bowel polyps as part of their features and these include Peutz–Jegher's with small bowel hamartomas, Gardener's with adenomas, and Cronkhite Canada with retention polyps. Many of these have an association with periampullary carcinoma.

Malignant tumours of the small bowel include carcinoid, carcinoma, lymphoma, and metastases:

- Carcinoid typically arises in the distal ileum and presents as a smooth, submucosal mass. At this stage, they behave like a benign tumour. Later, local infiltration occurs causing extensive tissue thickening and a desmoplastic reaction. This may be severe enough to cause bowel obstruction. Once the tumour has reached a size of 2 cm or more, it is likely to display true invasiveness, metastasizing via the portal vein to the liver. Radiological assessment is best by CT, which can show evidence of local infiltration into the mesentery typically with a central spiculated mass, and later very vascular liver metastases.

- Adenocarcinoma of the small bowel is rare with an approximate incidence of 1 in 100 000. These tumours are most commonly found in the jejunum. The usual macroscopic appearance is that of an annular, concentric tumour which gives rise to an apple-core appearance on barium studies or sometimes a large mass (Fig. 4). Prognosis is poor as the majority of tumours have metastasized at the time of surgery.

- Lymphoma may involve the gastrointestinal tract and indeed is the most common location for extra nodal disease. In contradistinction to carcinoma, the ileum is more frequently involved than the jejunum. A number of macroscopic forms are seen including: (1) multiple nodular defects; (2) diffuse infiltration (Fig. 5); (3) the infiltration may destroy the muscularis propria leading to the so-called aneurysmal form with bowel dilatation; (4) large endoexoenteric masses with excavation; (5) large extraluminal masses. The latter is a particular feature of HIV-associated Burkett's lymphoma.

- Metastatic disease to the small bowel may arrive by either transcoelomic spread or via the haematogenous route. Common tumours to seed across the peritoneal cavity are from the colon, pancreas, and

stomach with the addition of the ovary in females. The commonest source for haematogenous metastases to the small bowel is malignant melanoma which produces characteristic submucosal masses with a central umbilical-type ulcer. Carcinoma of the bronchus and breast also are major causes of haematogenous metastases.

Crohn's disease and inflammatory small bowel conditions

Crohn's disease is the commonest inflammatory condition to affect the small bowel in Western populations and is characterized by a chronic course of progression with spontaneous remission. The cause remains unknown and despite the presence of non-caseating granulomas on biopsy, extensive investigation into infectious agents has so far proved inconclusive. It may involve any part of the gastrointestinal tract, but in the great majority of cases the small bowel demonstrates most macroscopic change, and when involved the terminal ileum is the usual site.

The disease starts with mucosal ulceration which then becomes transmural with fissure ulcers. Healing is accompanied by fibrosis and stricture formation and there is considerable thickening of the bowel wall. Skip lesions may occur affecting considerable lengths of small bowel. Fistulation

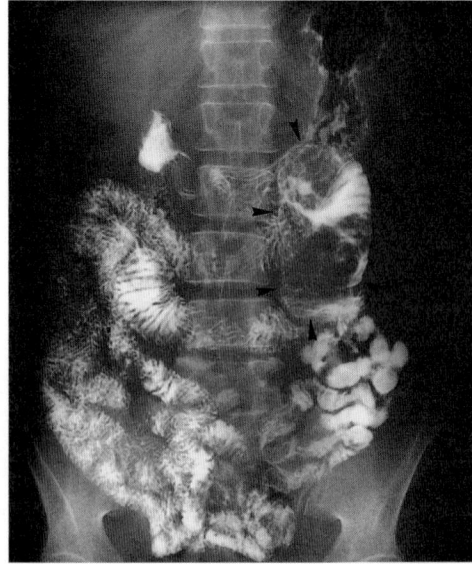

Fig. 4 Adenocarcinoma of the jejunum. This follow through examination in an anaemic patient demonstrates the large mass (arrowheads) arising from the proximal jejunum at a site just distal to the ligament of Treitz—a common position. Note also the normal small bowel pattern distal to this tumour when compared to the abnormal patterns shown on

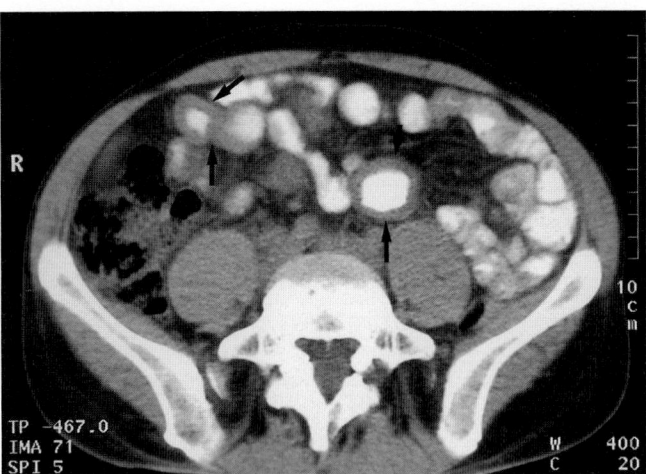

Fig. 5 Lymphoma of the small bowel as shown at CT examination. Several loops are involved demonstrating marked thickening of the bowel wall to a width of 5 to 6 mm (arrows).

is a characteristic of the disease and these may be enteric, enterocutaneous, or extend into the muscles of the abdominal wall and pelvis. Intra-abdominal abscesses also characterize severe disease. Radiological assessment is by means of Tc99m white blood cell scanning, barium follow through studies, CT, and MR. White cell scanning is used as the initial test for a patient with symptoms and signs of possible Crohn's disease (Fig. 6). It is also used to document disease activity and response to therapeutic measures. It is highly sensitive but may produce false positive results from other conditions which cause terminal ileal inflammation. Barium studies are then performed to demonstrate morphological detail. These may show the earliest change of Crohns disease which is an aphthoid ulcer resulting from ulceration on the tip of a lymphoid follicle. Next comes distortion and thickening of the fold pattern which in some instances becomes completely effaced. Finally, development of deep, interlacing, linear ulcers give rise to the characteristic cobblestone pattern due to oedema of mucosal islands between the ulcers. If stricture formation occurs, this is best appreciated by barium studies and if there is a long segment of stenosis, this is sometimes referred to as the string sign. The demonstrations of fistula is also shown by

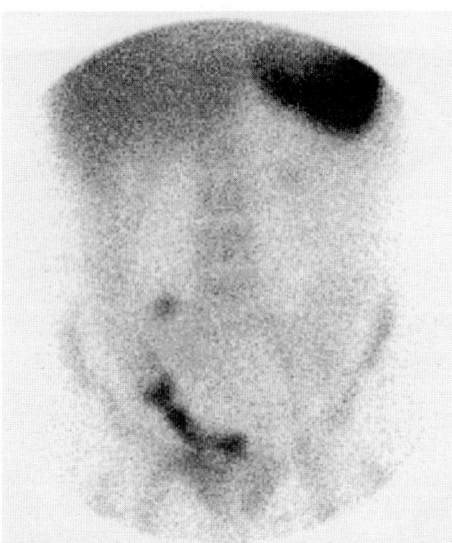

Fig. 6 Crohn's disease of the small bowel as demonstrated by a technetium 99m labelled white cell scan. There is grade III activity in the right iliac fossa indicative of highly active Crohn's disease in the terminal ileum. Note the normal accumulation of isotope in the spleen. (By courtesy of Dr Jane Dutton.)

barium studies, but this is now increasingly in the realm of spiral CT which can also demonstrates intra-abdominal abscesses and abnormal intra-abdominal fat. The role of MR imaging in Crohn's disease is also evolving rapidly because this can demonstrate the thickened bowel wall, inflammatory changes in the mesentery, and, in particular, the presence and anatomy of fistula formation.

Other inflammatory conditions of the small bowel include infection, such as *Yersinia enterocolitica* and tuberculosis. The former is associated with changes of terminal ileitis and is usually self limiting. The latter may affect any part of the gastrointestinal tract, but typically the ileocaecal region. Now that bovine tuberculosis has largely disappeared, the bacillus in most cases has arrived from swallowing infected sputum. Barium studies usually demonstrate changes in both the terminal ileum and caecum, a helpful point in distinguishing this from Crohn's disease, although the appearances can be very similar. There may be two type of appearance—the ulcerative form and the hypertrophic form. The latter is characterized by thickened and matted loops of bowel in the right iliac fossa. In addition, tuberculous enteritis may present as ascites from tuberculous peritonitis.

Postradiation enteritis and bowel ischaemia

Postradiation enteritis is considered here because the pathophysiology is one of endarteritis obliterans. This may follow any form of radiotherapy, either external beam or cavity therapy, and is most commonly encountered in female patients who have had therapy for carcinoma of the cervix. Thus, it typically involves small bowel loops which lie deep in the pelvis and these are made more susceptible if there is adhesive disease which fixes them in this position. Initial changes are of mucosal oedema but major problems from fibrosis and stricture formation occur later, in some instances after a latent period as long as 25 years. Sinuses and fistulae can be particularly problematic if there has been previous surgery to the radiation-damaged bowel. These changes are well appreciated at barium follow-through studies.

Bowel ischaemia and infarction may result from both arterial and venous occlusion. Arterial thrombosis of the superior mesenteric artery results in catastrophic infarction of most of the small bowel and carries a dismal prognosis. On the other hand, multiple, small emboli may cause episodes of non-occlusive ischaemia from which the bowel makes a good recovery. These typically are shown as areas of narrowing due to oedema with an abrupt transition to normal small bowel between the involved segments. Venous occlusion may result from volvulus of the bowel, blood dyscrasias, and malignant infiltration in the mesentery.

The colon

Colonoscopy has revolutionized imaging approaches to the colon because of its therapeutic as well as diagnostic role. However, it is not without risk, and barium enema examination still remains a much used alternative. CT is an increasingly used technique particularly since the advent of spiral CT allows three-dimensional reconstruction and thus so-called virtual colonoscopy.

For all three techniques a completely clean and empty colon is a prerequisite. This is achieved by colonic lavage, usually using an oral preparation the day before the examination, such as Picolax or Klean prep. For barium enema examination, the patient is placed on a fluoroscopic table and barium sulphate is run into the colon up to the level of the transverse colon. The excess is then drained out and air or carbon dioxide is insufflated into the colon to achieve a so-called double contrast effect, that is luminal distension with air and mucosal coating by barium sulphate. Up to 12 images are then taken of the colon with the patient in different positions so that the entire bowel is demonstrated in double contrast.

For CT examination, no positive contrast is used but the colon is simply distended with air, usually after the administration of a spasmolytic drug such as Buscopan. So-called volume rendering of the data following spiral CT examination permits a three-dimensional reconstruction of the lumen

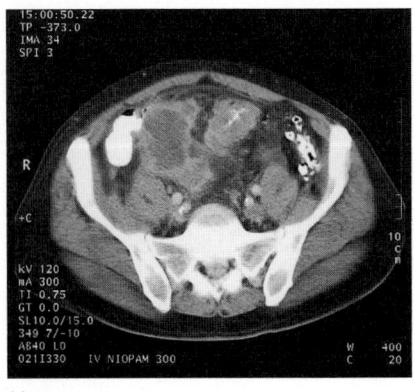
(a)

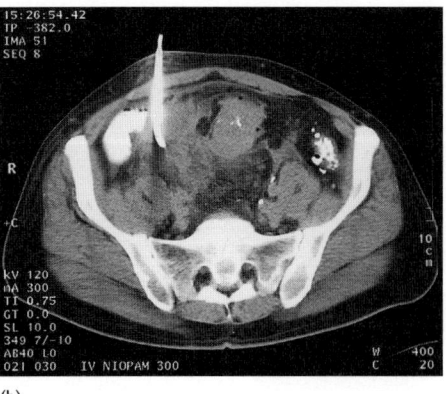
(b)

Fig. 7 Diverticular disease and its complication as shown at CT examination (a) demonstrating the marked thickening of the sigmoid wall and to the right of this is a fluid collection demonstrated by a low attenuation mass. This has been drained under CT control with the drainage catheter shown in position (b).

of the colon, thus allowing the operator to apparently 'fly' through the colon in a manner similar to colonoscopy, hence the term virtual colonoscopy.

CT without bowel preparation has also been used in the detection of gross colonic abnormalities in elderly patients, thus sparing them the discomfort of bowel preparation and a barium enema, both of which are likely to be less than optimal in this group.

Anatomy of the large bowel

The colon commences with the caecum and appendix in the right iliac fossa and these structures lead into the ascending colon which is a retroperitoneal structure. After the hepatic flexure the transverse colon is again intraperitoneal, suspended by the transverse mesocolon. The splenic flexure marks the transition to descending colon which is again retroperitoneal. Finally, the sigmoid and proximal rectum are intraperitoneal with the peritoneal reflection sited at the junction of the mid and lower third of rectum.

Pathology of the colon

Diverticular disease and irritable bowel syndrome

Diverticular disease and its complications are one of the commonest conditions to affect the colon. It results from raised intraluminal pressure causing a bleb of mucosa to herniate through the bowel wall at points of potential weakness, where the nutrient artery pierces the wall to supply the colon. This is accompanied by hypertrophy of the circular muscle fibres in the bowel wall, which is the first sign of this condition. Diverticula by themselves may not cause symptoms and indeed they are said to be present in one-third of the population over the age of 60. They may, however, become inflamed, resulting in a number of complications which include local and segmental abscess formation, perforation and fistula formation, stricture formation, and colonic bleeding. The usual location is the sigmoid colon which, with severe diverticular change, may become very distorted. A barium enema is the best technique for demonstrating the presence and extent of diverticulosis and these are shown as small barium-filled out-pouchings from the bowel wall. Most of the complications of diverticular disease, however, are best appreciated at CT. This demonstrates the marked thickening of the bowel wall as well as the presence of fistulae and abscesses. The latter are shown as soft tissue areas of fluid density either within or immediately adjacent to the wall of the bowel (Fig. 7). Stricture formation, however, is best assessed at barium enema and will usually require colonoscopy for biopsy purposes as the distinction between benign diverticular stricture and one secondary to malignancy is often difficult.

The diagnosis of irritable bowel syndrome is not radiological but clinical. However, in many instances the distinction from diverticular disease and colonic carcinoma is impossible and therefore a further examination, usually a barium enema, is indicated to exclude these diseases.

Colorectal cancer and polyp formation

Colorectal cancer is the second most common cause of death from cancer in the Western world and early detection can have a profound effect on prognosis. It is now clear that colorectal cancer arises as a result of a number of mutations resulting in a chromosome instability pathway. The first macroscopic change is the formation of an adenomatous polyp which over time, often two or three decades, will eventually become a frank carcinoma. The percentage of polyps, which, if left alone will become a carcinoma is unknown, but any attempt to reduce the mortality from colorectal cancer starts with their detection and subsequent removal. Polyp detection is achieved by both barium enema and CT colonography.

At barium enema, a polyp may be demonstrated as a filling defect in the barium column or as a ring of increased density on the air contrast views. They may be sessile or pedunculated.(Fig. 8). The size of the polyp is significant as lesions under 5 mm in size have little or no statistical association with an increased risk of cancer. Any polyp over the size of 10 mm should be removed and once they reach 20 mm they will almost certainly be malignant. For obvious reasons, their detection requires a colon that is completely clean as residual faecal material can readily be misinterpreted as polyp.

Carcinoma of the colon has several macroscopic appearances including annular stricture, a proliferative type, a large polypoid type, and schirrhous. Both barium enema and CT examinations detect of all of these.

CT colonography has two major advantages. First, if a tumour is demonstrated, then it can be formally staged at the same examination, that is by

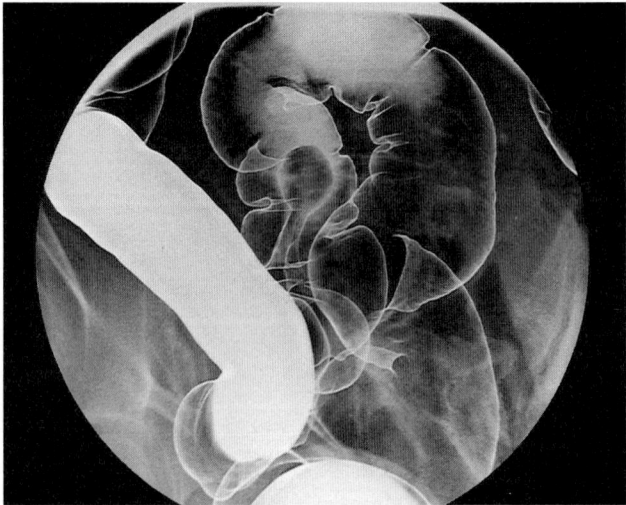

Fig. 8 Colorectal polyp in the mid sigmoid as shown on a barium enema. This is a pedunculated polyp and with the presence of a such a long stalk is likely to be benign. A sessile polyp of this size would have to be regarded as definitely suspicious and possibly malignant.

looking for involvement of the lymph nodes or the presence of liver metastases. Second, if a further clarification or a therapeutic manoeuvre is indicated, then colonoscopy may be performed immediately after the CT as only air has been insufflated into the colon.

Inflammatory bowel disease

The two main causes of idiopathic inflammatory bowel disease are ulcerative colitis and Crohn's disease with an approximate ratio of 3:1. Ulcerative colitis invariably starts in the rectum and spreads proximally, whereas Crohn's disease more commonly involves the right colon. Both conditions are best appreciated at barium enema, though the complications of Crohn's disease, that is fistulae and abscess formation, are best demonstrated by CT. The radiological appearances reflect the pathophysiology. Ulcerative colitis results in fine mucosal ulceration which always involves the rectum and then may spread proximally to involve the entire colon. There is loss of the haustral pattern and the mucosa demonstrates a fine granular appearance. Crohn's disease in contradistinction demonstrates more discreet and deep ulcers. The latter represent fissure ulcers which may extend throughout the whole thickness of the bowel wall. There is discontinuity of involvement as well as asymmetry. The picture is completed by terminal ileal involvement. An unusual feature of Crohn's disease is its earliest appearance, which is that of aphthous ulceration caused by ulcers appearing on the surface of hypertrophied lymphoid aggregates.

Other causes of colitis include pseudomembranous (caused by an overgrowth of *Clostridium difficile* often following antibiotic usage) as well as the various infective colitides, for example shigella, campylobacter, or CMV. The last named is usually only a problem in the immunocompromised patient. Postradiation colitis typically affects the sigmoid colon, for example after treatment for carcinoma of the cervix.

Further reading

Bartram CI (1999). Imaging in coloproctology. *Clinical Radiology* **54**, 413–14.

Freeman AH (2001). CT and bowel disease. *British Journal of Radiology* **74**, 4–14.

Herlinger H, Maglinte DT, Birnbaum BA, eds (1999). *Clinical imaging of the small intestine*, 2nd edn. Springer-Verlag, New York.

14.2.4 Investigation of gastrointestinal function

Julian R. F. Walters

Digestion and absorption of food by the gastrointestinal (**GI**) tract is achieved by the integration of multiple steps: the complex foods taken in through the mouth are digested into simpler molecules which can be transported across mucosal epithelial cells into the metabolic pool of the body. The contents of the gastrointestinal tract also need to be moved to regions where specialized digestive and absorptive functions can take place, and physical and immunological barriers must be maintained to prevent injury from toxic or immunologically active substances and bacteria.

These functions are assessed clinically in a variety of ways. Much can be learnt indirectly from techniques not principally aimed at defining GI function. Patients will describe appetite, dietary intake, weight changes, and the frequency and nature of their bowel movements. Clinical examination may reveal malnutrition—either generalized or specific. Many blood measurements of absorbed dietary components (such as iron, folate, vitamin B_{12}, cholesterol, and triglycerides), or their metabolic products (such as haemoglobin, albumin) can be abnormal when GI function is impaired, and their serial changes can be used to follow improvements with treatment. Radio-

logical studies (see Chapter 14.2.3) can demonstrate functional changes as well as anatomy, and physiological measurements are central to studies of motility disorders (Chapter 14.12). Tests aimed at giving specific measurements of GI function are described below.

Intake and output

Nutritional assessment

The dietary history is a critical part of the investigation of GI function. For instance, a high intake of milk in a patient of African ethnicity will suggest that diarrhoea may be due to lactase non-persistence. Vitamin B_{12} deficiency in a vegan is most likely to be due to dietary deficiency rather than malabsorption.

Patients may not accurately recall what they eat. Assessment can be improved by keeping a detailed diary with formal recording of the diet over a week, this will enable the usual intakes of a full range of nutrients to be calculated. Total calories, fat, protein and nitrogen, water, electrolytes, individual vitamins, minerals, and trace elements can all be assessed in this way.

Assessment of nutritional status can indirectly provide evidence of gastrointestinal dysfunction. Calculation of the body mass index (kg/m^2) gives a measure of obesity, and hence fat stores. More detailed estimates of body composition can be made by anthropometry, measuring skin-fold thickness, or body density. Dual-energy, X-ray absorptiometry will assess the percentage of fat, and bone mineral density as a measure of calcium stores.

These estimates of nutritional status can change over time. If the intake of any particular nutrient exceeds the losses, the body is in positive balance, as occurs during growth. If the losses are greater, the result is a negative balance. Losses from all sources must be included. Urinary loss is obvious for water, electrolytes and minerals, and nitrogenous compounds. Carbon dioxide and heat losses reflect metabolism and calorie consumption: research calorimetric techniques can estimate these accurately. Absorption by the GI tract is a major factor is determining overall balance—with unabsorbed nutrients and excreted matter being egested in faeces.

Faecal output

Stool weight and volume can vary in the healthy individual, but averages about 200 g/24 h. This volume increases in diarrhoea or other forms of malabsorption, and may be as high as several litres/24 h in patients with secretory diarrhoea, such as that due to cholera. Accurate measurements of faecal volume and electrolyte composition are then helpful in maintaining an accurate fluid balance.

Patients may complain of diarrhoea but mean urgent, frequent, or unformed stools, rather than an increase in volume. Stool charts, recording frequency and volume, help to define the change in the nature of the stools. Changes in frequency and volume with simple changes such as fasting help to differentiate osmotic diarrhoea from secretory or inflammatory causes. Stool electrolytes and osmolarity are also helpful here: a large osmotic gap suggests an unabsorbed ion from, for example, magnesium salts taken as laxatives, or the products of unabsorbed carbohydrate fermentation. Stool pH is low after carbohydrate malabsorption, as in lactase deficiency (non-persistence) or sucrase–isomaltase deficiency.

Faecal fat output is increased in most forms of generalized malabsorption and results in steatorrhoea. Patients frequently describe stools that float or are foul-smelling, but to be sure that this is due to fat, qualitative and quantitative estimations need to be performed. Fat droplets in the stool can be detected microscopically after staining with lipid-soluble dyes. Accurate estimation of the loss of fat in the faeces requires a 3-day collection of stools while the patient is on a defined fat-intake diet. An average output of more than 5 g/24 h for a 70 to 100 g daily fat intake is abnormal. Patients and clinical and laboratory staff dislike this test for obvious reasons.

Gas, wind, explosive stools, and foul odours are frequent complaints. Although volumes of flatus and the presence of various gases have been measured in research studies, these have not been adopted as routine clinical investigations.

Stool microscopy for faecal leucocytes can be helpful in diagnosing inflammatory diarrhoea. Detection of bacterial pathogens, parasites, ova, or toxins may show the cause.

Digestive secretions

In patients with possible malabsorption, who have an adequate dietary intake but large volume stools, an important clinical decision is whether digestion is at fault (such as pancreatic exocrine insufficiency) or whether absorption is the problem (as in coeliac disease). Often this is rapidly established by employing tests with high positive-predictive-values for common individual diseases, such as endomysial serology for coeliac disease or imaging studies for chronic pancreatitis (see Chapter 14.18.3.2).

Intubation of the lumen to collect the contents for measurements of secretory rates and composition is the definitive way to study digestive juices produced by the stomach, pancreas, liver, and intestine. Though necessary for basic physiological and pharmacological studies, tube tests are now rarely performed in a clinical setting. Endoscopes are generally now used, which enable direct vision and biopsy of anatomical lesions, and can, on occasions, also provide functional information.

A large number of tubeless tests have been developed to indirectly measure digestion and absorption, or to help differentiate between the two types of disorder. Many involve small doses of radionuclides. Other tests use markers of breath hydrogen or urinary excretion (Table 1). Selection of these tests in clinical practice depends on their predictive values, reliability, cost, and ease of use.

Gastric secretion

The gastric mucosa secretes acid, pepsin, and some other products such as intrinsic factor. Measurements of acid output have historically been important in diagnosing the cause and response to treatment of acid-related diseases such as duodenal ulceration. This has become less relevant with the discovery of *Helicobacter pylori* and potent acid suppression with histamine H2-receptor antagonists and proton-pump inhibitors.

Intubation of the stomach with a nasogastric tube allows the gastric contents to be sampled. Tube positioning is important. Swallowed salivary secretion will raise the pH and so will refluxing duodenal contents, common after retching. The yellow colour of bile will indicate duodenal reflux into the stomach. After an overnight fast, gastric aspiration allows the volume of resting secretions to be measured and the pH determined. Normal resting volumes are less than 50 ml. pH values above 4 suggest impaired acid secretion, as in the gastric atrophy and achlorhydria found in pernicious anaemia, or as the result of acid-suppressant drugs. Gastric pH can also easily be measured at endoscopy.

Estimation of basal and peak acid output requires continuous sampling and titration of the aspirate with sodium hydroxide. A marker can be infused to correct for loss of gastric contents into the duodenum. A basal acid output of about 5 mmol over 1 h is normal. Low values are found in achlorhydria. The detection of a high basal output is important in making

the diagnosis of Zollinger–Ellison syndrome. However, this clinical decision is now usually made after finding a high serum gastrin level in a patient treated with a proton-pump inhibitor, who because of symptoms is unable to discontinue therapy.

Peak acid output following pentagastrin stimulation quantifies the ability of the stomach to maximally produce acid. There was considerable interest in the use of this test for research purposes before the aetiology of duodenal ulcer became clear. However, it is of little clinical use now that our understanding of pathophysiology and therapeutics has advanced.

Biliary secretions

Bile samples, mixed with pancreatic secretions and other duodenal contents, can be collected from the duodenum at upper endoscopy (or after intubation). Endoscopic retrograde cholangiopancreatography (**ERCP**) allows bile to be collected from the bile ducts. Microscopy of bile can detect cholesterol crystals. The proportions of bile acids, phospholipids, and cholesterol are relevant in the study of biliary cholesterol saturation and gallstone formation, but have little clinical use.

Bile secretion by the liver is not easily measured directly. Clearance from the circulation can be determined for a number of compounds normally secreted into the bile. Apart from measurements of bilirubin, such tests have found little clinical use. The nuclear medicine **HIDA** (hepatoiminodiacetic acid; lidofenin) scan gives a measure of biliary secretion as well as helping define functional anatomy. The gallbladder function of contraction in response to a meal, or cholecystokinin (**CCK**), can be measured by imaging techniques, of which ultrasound is the most convenient.

Pancreatic secretions

Pancreatic secretion of a large number of digestive enzymes and bicarbonate is crucial for the digestive process. Duodenal intubation allows their collection for assay of the activities of some of the key enzymes such as trypsin, lipase, and amylase; however, these duodenal contents will be mixed with bile and duodenal secretions, or with those from the stomach. Pure pancreatic juice can be collected at ERCP.

Although a number of stimulation tests have been used to diagnose pancreatic exocrine insufficiency, their clinical usage is very limited: virtually all patients can be managed without the need to resort to these function tests. The duodenum is intubated, usually under fluoroscopic control. Secretin, which stimulates bicarbonate secretion, or CCK, which stimulates enzyme secretion, are given intravenously, either alone or in combination. The contents of the duodenum are then aspirated for assay of bicarbonate and enzyme concentrations. The Lundh meal is an alternative standardized stimulus to pancreatic secretion.

Several indirect, tubeless pancreatic tests have been developed and are much simpler and more convenient to perform. The pancreolauryl test relies on the hydrolysis of fluorescein dilaurate by pancreatic esterases. The fluorescein is absorbed and excreted in the urine where it can be assayed easily. The test is administered on 2 days, each time with a standard breakfast and similar urine collections. On the first day, a test capsule containing fluorescein dilaurate is given, and on the second, a control capsule of non-esterified fluorescein. To diagnose pancreatic insufficiency, the ratio of fluorescein recovered in the urine with the dilaurate test substance will be less than 20 per cent of that with the control. Another test uses *N*-benzoyl-L-tyrosyl-*p*-aminobenzoic acid (**NBT-PABA**) as an alternative substrate. Following a similar principle, pancreatic chymotrypsin activity releases *p*-aminobenzoic acid (**PABA**), which is assayed in the urine. This test seems to be less reliable than that with pancreolauryl.

A different type of indirect test for pancreatic exocrine dysfunction involves the determination of proteolytic enzymes in the faeces—these enzymes are produced by the pancreas and are stable during passage through the intestine. Chymotrypsin activity has been used as a test for many years. An improved method using an immunological assay for human-specific elastase I has recently been developed.

Table 1 Breath tests in general use for gastrointestinal diseases

Type of test	Substrate	Clinical use
Hydrogen	Lactose	For lactase deficiency
	Lactulose	For orocaecal transit
	Glucose	For small intestinal bacterial overgrowth
Carbon dioxide (^{13}C or ^{14}C)	Urea	Urease activity from gastric *Helicobacter pylori* infection

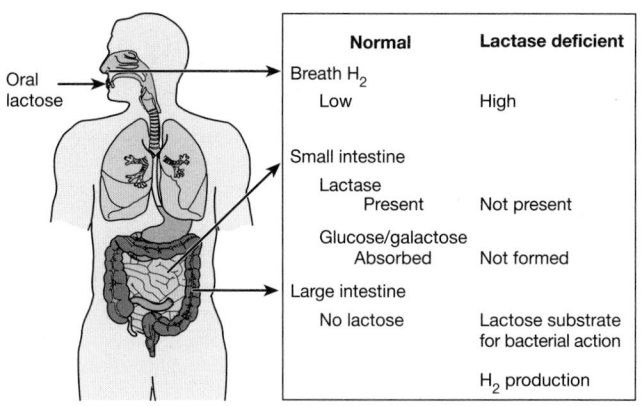

Fig. 1 Lactose-hydrogen breath test for lactase deficiency.

All these indirect tests are generally reliable in patients with severe exocrine pancreatic insufficiency causing steatorrhoea, where they can have adequate specificity for pancreatic disease if borderline test results are repeated or ignored. Many patients with severe intestinal disease will have somewhat abnormal results. The sensitivity of the tests is such that patients with lesser degrees of pancreatic functional impairment will be missed and considerable pancreatic damage may have occurred before the tests become abnormal.

Intestine

The role of brush-border enzymes in digestion is clearly important. Individual enzyme activities (e.g. sucrase–isomaltase) can be measured directly in small-bowel biopsies, obtained at endoscopy or using a capsule or biopsy tube. Indirect tests of intestinal digestive enzyme function are closely linked with those of absorption and are described below. Intestinal secretions, such as those from the Brunner's glands in the duodenum or from the crypts in secretory diarrhoea, are not directly measured.

Absorption

Carbohydrates

The xylose absorption test has been used for many years as a simple measure of absorption and malabsorption. Xylose does not need to be digested, is absorbed by the jejunum, does not undergo significant metabolism, and is excreted efficiently by the kidney. Urine is collected for 5 h after oral administration of the sugar to a fasted subject. Usually 25 g is given and more than 17 per cent should be recovered in the urine. A smaller dose of 5 g causes less diarrhoea. The test measures the area of functioning mucosa and has reasonably good sensitivity for intestinal mucosal abnormalities such as coeliac disease. The measurement of blood levels is said to improve accuracy. False-positive low levels of xylose excretion can occur with delayed gastric emptying, ascites, and with insufficient urinary output. As described elsewhere, serological tests are now available that are simpler, more specific, and more sensitive in screening for coeliac disease.

Lactose tolerance testing can be performed to diagnose lactase deficiency. This is similar to the glucose tolerance test, except that 50 g of lactose is given instead of glucose. Blood glucose levels are measured, and should increase if brush-border lactase is present to split the lactose in to glucose and galactose. In subjects without brush-border lactase, the lactose is not digested or absorbed and the blood glucose level does not rise. The lactose passes through the small bowel to the large intestine where it is then broken down by bacteria, thereby causing symptoms of gaseousness and diarrhoea.

The breath-hydrogen test for lactose intolerance is based on this principle (Fig. 1). Hydrogen is only produced in the body from the bacterial

fermentation of carbohydrates in the gut. Hydrogen diffuses into the blood and is excreted in the breath. Breath hydrogen can be measured simply and relatively cheaply to an accuracy of a few parts per million (**p.p.m**). Colonic bacteria produce a background level of breath hydrogen from the fermentation of unabsorbed colonic contents. After taking oral lactose, breath hydrogen is measured every 30 min. An increase greater than 20 p.p.m. implies that, rather than being absorbed in the small intestine, the sugar has been broken down by bacteria in the colon. As described below, bacterial overgrowth in the small intestine elevates breath hydrogen after glucose administration, and can also do this when lactose is given. Similar breath-hydrogen tests can be performed with other sugars when fructose or sucrose malabsorption is suspected.

Fat

The estimation of non-absorbed fat, that is faecal fat, is discussed above. A tubeless test, which does not require faecal collection, is the [^{14}C]triolein test. This has been advocated as a simple method to determine lipid absorption. After digestion and absorption of the labelled triglycerides, metabolism in the liver produces ^{14}C-labelled CO_2 which is detected in the breath. This test is not widely used and is only sensitive to large changes in fat absorption.

Bile salts

Bile salts, critical for lipid absorption, undergo an enterohepatic circulation where the conjugated bile salts (such as glycocholate and taurocholate) are reabsorbed in the ileum. Failure to reabsorb these salts increases their concentrations in the colon where they produce a secretory diarrhoea. Tests have been developed to look for evidence of bile salt malabsorption.

The SeHCAT test uses radiolabelled selenohomocholic acid as the taurine conjugate. This is given orally and whole-body retention is measured with a gamma camera after 7 days. Low values result from an excessive loss of bile salts. Bile salt malabsorption, often producing SeHCAT retention values of less than 5 per cent, is found after ileal resection, with ileal disease such as Crohn's, and in idiopathic bile salt malabsorption due to transporter defects. Small intestinal bacterial overgrowth results in deconjugation of the bile salts, which will also impair absorption and retention.

Vitamin B$_{12}$ and the Schilling test

Absorption of vitamin B$_{12}$ (the cobalamins) is particularly complex. Vitamin B$_{12}$ deficiency is common, and, if not nutritional, is due to one of several GI disorders. Intrinsic factor, produced by the stomach, binds cobalamins in the intestine. The intrinsic factor–vitamin B$_{12}$ complex interacts with a receptor in the brush-border membrane of the terminal ileum and is taken up by the cell. Vitamin B$_{12}$ is stored in the liver. Pancreatic enzyme activity is necessary to release dietary vitamin B$_{12}$ from R-proteins in the diet so that it can bind to intrinsic factor. Bacterial overgrowth in the small intestine can split the intrinsic factor–vitamin B$_{12}$ complex before it can be absorbed.

The Schilling test uses radioisotopes of cobalt to label cobalamin. A two-part test is usually performed, with two isotopes, ^{57}Co and ^{58}Co, simultaneously. One isotope is used to label free vitamin B$_{12}$ and the other to label a complex of intrinsic factor and vitamin B$_{12}$. After an overnight fast, both are given together by mouth, and unlabelled cobalamin is given by intramuscular injection to ensure that binding sites are occupied. Absorbed radiolabelled vitamin B$_{12}$ is excreted in the urine. This is collected for 24 h and should normally contain more than 10 per cent of the ingested dose, with an equal ratio of the two isotopes. In gastric disease, such as pernicious anaemia, or after gastrectomy, absorption is reduced when vitamin B$_{12}$ is given alone but not when it is given with intrinsic factor. In terminal ileal disease, or after resection, absorption of both forms is low. Small-bowel bacterial overgrowth mimics ileal disease, but antibiotic treatment restores vitamin B_{12} absorption to normal.

Gastrointestinal transit

Physiological function tests have been developed to measure the motility of the gut in propelling the contents of the diet through the areas involved in digestion and absorption. These are described in full in Chapter 14.12.

Oesophageal function

Peristalsis in the oesophagus, with appropriately timed relaxation of the upper and lower oesophageal sphincters, is necessary for efficient and comfortable swallowing, without symptoms of dysphagia. Gastro-oesophageal reflux through the lower sphincter will produce heartburn. Oesophageal manometry, with multiple fine tubes passed through the nose and connected to sensors, will measure the pressures in the oesophagus and at the sphincters at rest and during swallowing. Disordered peristalsis, spasm, achalasia, nutcracker oesophagus, and conditions associated with reflux can be diagnosed (see Chapter 14.6).

Monitoring gastro-oesophageal acid reflux with pH-sensitive electrodes over 24 h is useful in diagnosing the severity of gastro-oesophageal reflux disease (**GORD**), and in relating atypical symptoms to episodes of reflux. A small, portable recording device allows the times of symptoms, meals, and sleeping to be recorded, so they can be analysed together with episodes of low pH. A composite score can be calculated, reflecting the severity of reflux. A bile-sensitive electrode is also available, and may be of use in patients with adequate acid suppression but who still suffer symptoms from duodenogastric and gastro-oesophageal reflux.

Gastric emptying

This can be measured by a range of imaging tests, of which radionuclide labelling of liquid and solid food is probably the most effective technique. Tracer quantities of technetium and/or indium are incorporated into simple foods. Gamma scanning over the stomach allows the time course of gastric emptying to be determined. These measurements are useful in conditions such as diabetic gastroparesis or after gastric surgery where bloating, nausea, or vomiting are problems. Radiological measurements of barium emptying, although widely available, are less reliable unless the contrast is incorporated into food. Ultrasound and magnetic resonance imaging (**MRI**) have also been used.

Intestinal transit

Radionuclide techniques, as used to measure gastric emptying, can also determine small-bowel transit by timing the appearance of counts over the caecum. Estimates of transit times through the large intestine can be obtained with further imaging.

Mouth-to-caecum transit times can be estimated simply with breath-hydrogen testing. As described above, breath hydrogen is derived from the bacterial metabolism of unabsorbed carbohydrates. Lactulose, a non-absorbed sugar, is given by mouth and breath hydrogen sampled every 15 to 30 min. A rise in breath-hydrogen values indicates that the lactulose has reached the caecum. A rapid rise will occur if there is bacterial overgrowth in the small intestine.

Dye markers taken by mouth will give an estimate of the whole-gut transit time when they are detected in the stool.

Radiological markers, small differently shaped pieces of radio-opaque plastic, can be useful in determining transit through the large intestine. These are taken daily for several days. A plain abdominal radiograph shows the number remaining and their distribution in the parts of the colon.

Defecation and anorectal physiology can be measured with manometry in response to balloon inflation in the rectum.

Tests of gastrointestinal integrity and barrier functions

Several tests examine other aspects of GI physiology not discussed above. Evidence for infection, structural damage, or loss of barrier functions can be obtained.

Infection

Helicobacter pylori infection of the stomach is common and can be detected at endoscopy by microscopy, culture, or the biopsy urease test. The urea breath test, an indirect test, is now one of the commonest breath tests performed to look at gastric pathophysiology. Either radiolabelled [^{13}C]- or [^{14}C]urea is given by mouth to fasting subjects. The urease activity of *H. pylori* in the stomach metabolizes this to radiolabelled CO2, which is then exhaled. A standard amount of CO_2 is collected in a breath sample and the activity of the isotope determined—by mass spectrometry for ^{13}C or scintillation counting for ^{14}C. As there are no other sources of urease activity in the body, this is a very specific test. Low-level *H. pylori* infection, as can occur when acid production is suppressed with histamine H2-receptor antagonists or proton-pump inhibitors, can give negative results and reduce the sensitivity of this test.

Bacterial overgrowth in the small intestine can be detected by the glucose-hydrogen breath test (Fig. 2). Glucose given by mouth is normally fully absorbed, but some metabolism to hydrogen will occur if bacteria are present in the small intestine. This will be measurable in the exhaled breath, which is collected every 30 min for 2 h. A positive test produces a diagnostic rise of 20 p.p.m. above a low baseline. It may be necessary to give a diet low in non-absorbable polysaccharides to reduce baseline hydrogen production. This test has a sensitivity of about 80 per cent. Alternative tests, which are less popular, involve the administration of radiolabelled compounds such as the bile salt, cholyl-[^{14}C]glycine (glycocholate), and measuring ^{14}C-labelled CO_2 in the breath (Fig. 3).

Mucosal damage

Several tests will give abnormal results if the gastrointestinal mucosa is damaged. The faecal occult blood test becomes positive with a relatively small loss of blood per day. Dietary components containing blood or peroxidase can give positive tests. The presence of leucocytes in faeces suggest inflammatory causes of diarrhoea.

White-cell scanning has a role in diagnosing and assessing the activity of inflammatory bowel disease. Autologous white cells, labelled with indium or technetium, are reinjected intravenously and collect in areas of inflammation. Imaging with a gamma camera, at multiple time points, indicate white-cell accumulation at sites of diseased bowel and chemokine production. The complexity and the radiation dosage involved limits the use of this test.

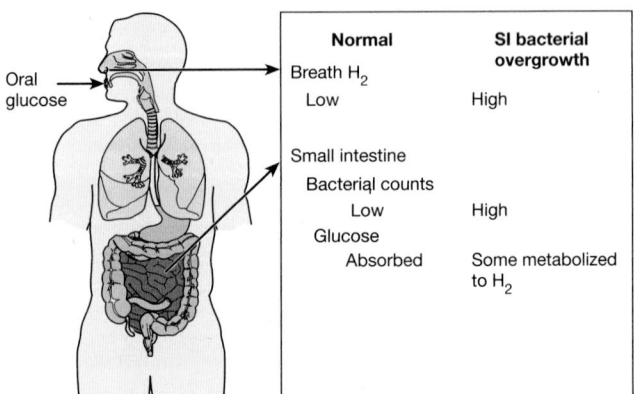

Fig. 2 Glucose-hydrogen breath test for small intestinal bacterial overgrowth.

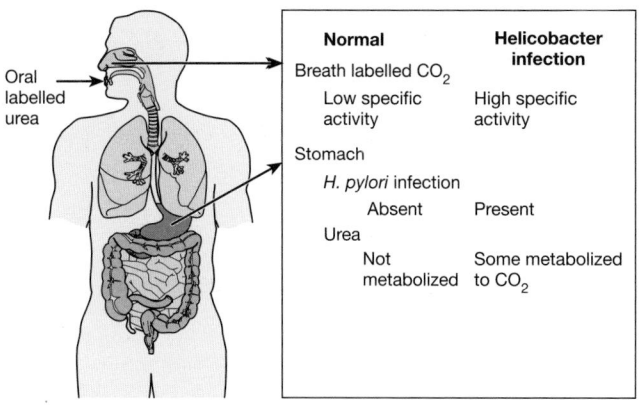

	Normal	Helicobacter infection
Breath labelled CO_2	Low specific activity	High specific activity
Stomach		
H. pylori infection	Absent	Present
Urea	Not metabolized	Some metabolized to CO_2

Fig. 3 Urea breath test (^{13}C or ^{14}C) for *H. pylori* infection.

Calprotectin is a calcium-binding protein found in leucocytes. It is stable in the gut lumen and so can be quantified in the stool. It can be detected in faeces in a variety of inflammatory conditions and its simplicity may make it suitable as a first-line screening test.

In patients with small intestinal lymphangiectasia, lymphocytes are lost into the lumen of the gut. The full blood count may then show a lymphopenia. Protein loss also occurs in this disorder. Many other inflammatory and ulcerative conditions can produce a protein-losing enteropathy, and several tests have been employed in attempts to quantify this loss. Since α1-antitrypsin is resistant to breakdown in the intestine, faecal measurements can provide an indication of the loss of serum proteins into the lumen. *In vivo*-labelled [^{51}Cr]albumin is also used to estimate GI protein loss.

The permeability of the intestine can be investigated using a number of different probes: usually sugars, which normally have little uptake in the gut but can enter the body in disease states. These probe substances will then be excreted and measured in the urine. Lactulose is one such sugar that is normally excluded. When administered together with another molecule which is taken up and excreted readily, such as rhamnose or mannitol, the ratio can correct for individual differences in gastric emptying or urine collection. Although the results of these tests are usually abnormal in coeliac disease, specific serological tests, such as endomysial IgA antibodies, are much more specific and sensitive for use in screening. Intestinal permeability changes have been described in other diseases but roles in their pathogenesis are uncertain.

Further reading

Bouchier IAD, *et al.*, eds (1993). *Gastroenterology: clinical science and practice*, 2nd edn. WB Saunders, London.

Yamada T, *et al.*, eds (1991). *Textbook of gastroenterology*. Lippincott, Philadelphia.

14.3 **Major gastrointestinal emergencies**

14.3.1 **The acute abdomen**

Julian Britton

Most patients with acute abdominal pain are treated in the community: a minority are admitted urgently to hospital and then, usually, put under the care of a surgeon. Two-thirds of such patients, wherever they live, are suffering from either abdominal pain for which no cause is found or acute appendicitis. In the remaining one-third many disorders account for the pain and, rarely, the cause lies outside the abdomen. Sometimes patients with a surgical diagnosis present to a physician because the abdominal symptoms and signs are overshadowed or suppressed by a medical condition. Occasionally patients in hospital for another reason will develop an acute abdomen.

The management of acute abdominal pain depends on clinical skill, and investigations play only a small part. Sometimes immediate treatment must take precedence over making a diagnosis. More commonly the clinician has time to take a history, to examine the patient, and to consider a differential diagnosis.

Diagnosis

The history

An accurate history is the essential foundation for the diagnosis of abdominal pain. This requires time, patience, and skill. The doctor should give the patient his or her undivided attention and take care not to interrupt the flow of words. The way patients tell their story is as important as the story itself. Any additional questions should be short, specific, and direct and must be couched in language the patient understands. Body language and sentence construction must not suggest any particular answer. Negative findings are always as useful as positive ones. It is important to obtain sufficient but no more than sufficient information. Unnecessary or irrelevant facts can be misleading and will always add to the difficulties of analysis.

Pain

The nature of the pain is the best guide to the diagnosis. The site and any radiation of the pain may suggest which intra-abdominal organ is the source of the symptom. How and when the pain started and whether it has been constant since then are useful points for consideration. Perforation of the bowel, rupture of an aneurysm, and acute ischaemia all occur suddenly and the pain is severe from the outset. Acute inflammation starts slowly and the pain is constant and increases in severity with time. Colic comes and goes and implies an origin from a viscus containing smooth muscle. Aggravation of the pain on sudden movement is equivalent to rebound tenderness on examination and suggests local peritonitis.

Other symptoms

Nausea and vomiting often accompany abdominal pain, but not necessarily together. Retching without vomiting suggests acute intestinal obstruction with impending strangulation. Anorexia is a non-specific symptom particularly in ill children. Disturbances of bowel function are always important and the complete absence of stool or flatus implies intestinal obstruction. The urinary and the genital systems are common sources of abdominal pain and patients must be asked about the associated symptoms. Complications of previous abdominal surgery cause pain and so, sometimes, do therapeutic drugs.

Examination

General observation of the patient is important. Demeanour is a good guide to the overall severity of the illness. Patients with peritonitis lie perfectly still. Patients with colic are restless. Abdominal distension can be often observed through the sheets and jaundice or the smell of melaena are also important signs.

Pulse, temperature, and blood pressure are essential measurements and changes over time are more valuable than isolated readings. Examination of the abdomen itself follows the pattern of inspection, palpation, percussion, and auscultation. It must include a rectal and vaginal examination and examination of the urine.

If palpation causes pain it is essential to decide if guarding, rigidity, and rebound tenderness are present as well. Rebound tenderness is a reliable guide to the presence of peritonitis. A silent abdomen carries the same implication, and in the context of pain is usually a clear indication that a patient requires an urgent laparotomy. Two surgical conditions which are commonly missed are a small strangulated femoral hernia in an obese patient and pelvic appendicitis. Careful examination of the groin should identify the former. In the latter case the abdominal signs are often subdued because somatic pelvic pain is not referred to the anterior abdominal wall. Tenderness on the right side of the pelvis may be the only positive physical sign and it is critically important to overcome any reluctance to perform a rectal examination.

Investigation

With one exception, simple blood tests do not help to diagnose acute abdominal pain but they are important in managing the surgical patient. The exception is the serum amylase which should be measured in every patient with abdominal pain unless the diagnosis is otherwise obvious. High levels of amylase activity are strongly suggestive of acute pancreatitis. Unfortunately serum amylase is also elevated in patients with biliary colic, perforated peptic ulcer, ischaemic bowel, or ruptured aortic aneurysm. A false negative result is found if the blood sample is taken too late after the onset of pancreatitis because amylase concentrations return to normal within about 48 h. A raised peripheral blood leucocyte count or the presence of white cells or red cells in the urine are useful pointers to intra-abdominal inflammation or disease of the urinary tract, but neither test is specific.

Radiology

Plain abdominal radiographs are helpful in confirming intestinal obstruction and may show calculi in the gall bladder or the renal tract. Air under the diaphragm on an erect chest radiograph is definite evidence of perforation of the bowel or stomach but does not identify the site of the perforation (Fig. 1). About one in ten patients with a perforated peptic ulcer does not show free intraperitoneal air.

An ultrasound examination may show a swollen tender retrocaecal appendix. Computed tomography will confirm acute pancreatitis and acute diverticulitis.

Making a diagnosis

Even experienced doctors only make a correct diagnosis in three-quarters of patients with abdominal pain, whilst junior doctors are right only about half the time. Patterns of disease provide a useful guide: all over the world acute appendicitis and non-specific abdominal pain are the most common diagnoses in a surgical setting (Table 1). Acute cholecystitis is the third most common cause of an acute abdomen in the developed world, whilst in Africa small bowel obstruction is frequent. In a medical ward it would be unusual to encounter non-specific abdominal pain: diverticulitis, a perforation, a ruptured abdominal aortic aneurysm, or mesenteric infarction from embolism secondary to atrial fibrillation or coronary thrombosis would be more likely.

Occasionally a patient presents with all the classical symptoms and signs of a condition. More commonly the clinician has to analyse the data in a number of different ways often based on anatomy, pathology, or, sometimes, by elimination. Pragmatic doctors simply decide if the abdominal symptoms and signs justify surgery. If they do then the diagnosis becomes apparent at operation. If they do not then the patient is re-examined after a few hours. If the signs worsen then surgery is required. If the patient improves then continued observation is appropriate. The only risk of active observation is that the patient deteriorates significantly in the time spent watching, with a consequent increase in the complication rate after surgery.

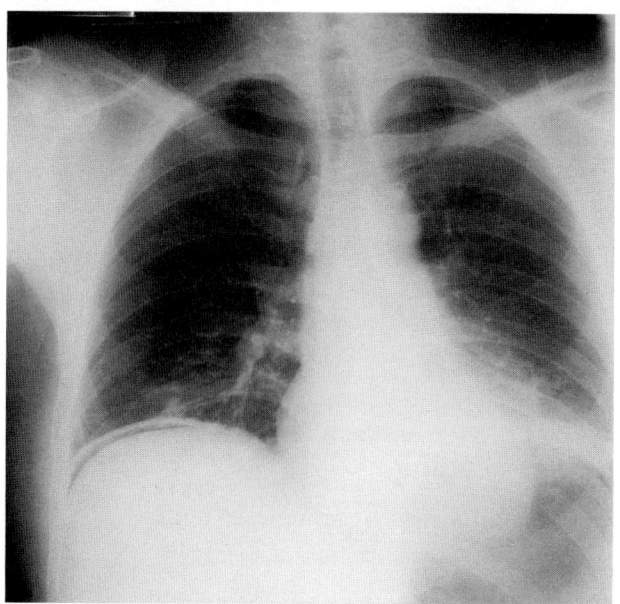

Fig. 1 An erect chest radiograph demonstrating free gas under the right diaphragm. (From Britton J (2000). The acute abdomen. In: Morris PJ, Wood WC, eds. *Oxford textbook of surgery*, 2nd edn. Oxford University Press, Oxford, 1823–42.)

Table 1 The causes of acute abdominal pain seen in hospitals in the developed world

Cause	Percentage of cases
Non-specific abdominal pain	34
Acute appendicitis	28
Acute cholecystitis	10
Small bowel obstruction	4
Acute gynaecological disease	4
Acute pancreatitis	3
Renal colic	3
Perforated peptic ulcer	2
Cancer	2
Diverticular disease	1
Miscellaneous	9

(After de Dombal FT (1991). *Diagnosis of acute abdominal pain*, 2nd edn. Churchill Livingstone, Edinburgh.)

Surgical causes of abdominal pain

Acute appendicitis

The incidence of acute appendicitis is declining, but the disease remains frequent and often eludes diagnosis. Periumbilical pain moving to the right iliac fossa over a few hours and accompanied by nausea and fever are the classical symptoms. Tenderness, guarding, and rebound tenderness which is worse in the right iliac fossa are the important physical signs. When all these symptoms and signs are present there is little need for investigation and the treatment is a prompt appendicectomy. Prophylaxis against venous thrombosis is important and appropriate antibiotics given before operation are known to reduce the incidence of subsequent septic complications.

Laparoscopy is valuable when the diagnosis is not clear, particularly in young women in whom the rate of appendicectomy with a normal appendix is high. Laparoscopic removal of the appendix is also possible. Whichever method of appendicectomy is adopted, drinking followed by eating may start in a few hours. Most patients stay in hospital for 24 or 48 h.

Non-specific abdominal pain

Three out of every ten patients admitted to a surgical ward with acute abdominal pain are discharged without a diagnosis. This does not mean that there is no pain or that there is no cause. Acute appendicitis can sometimes resolve.

Acute cholecystitis

This is easy to diagnose, particularly with the assistance of an ultrasound examination. Bed rest, intravenous fluids, and, for most patients, antibiotics will allow the inflammation to resolve. If there is no improvement, the gall bladder should be drained either percutaneously or surgically (Fig. 2). In most instances a cholecystectomy should be performed on the next available operating list.

Intestinal obstruction

Abdominal pain, abdominal distension, vomiting, and constipation are the typical symptoms and signs of obstruction. Adhesions, hernias, and cancer of the large bowel are common causes. Obstruction due to adhesions will sometimes resolve itself during treatment with intravenous fluids and nasogastric suction. Hernias can sometimes be reduced. In most other instances, surgery is required after appropriate resuscitation.

Perforated peptic ulcer

Surgery to close the perforation and to lavage the peritoneal cavity is the standard treatment. Patients benefit later from treatment to suppress acid secretion and to eliminate *Helicobacter pylori*.

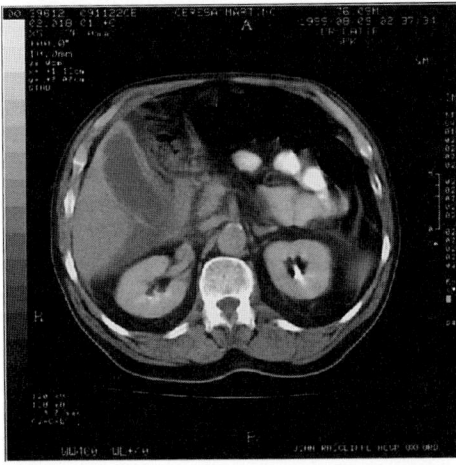

Fig. 2 This abdominal computed tomography scan shows acute cholecystitis. Fluid can be seen within the thickened wall of the gallbladder. The gall bladder was subsequently drained with a percutaneously placed pigtail catheter.

Diverticulitis

This presents with pain and tenderness in the left iliac fossa accompanied by fever. The diagnosis is easily confirmed by computed tomography if necessary. Bed rest, intravenous fluids, and antibiotics are the standard treatment. When colonic perforation occurs, and this can be surprisingly silent, resection of the bowel and a temporary colostomy will be required.

Acute pancreatitis

This is a capricious disease and may complicate other medical or surgical conditions. Treatment is with intravenous fluids and analgesia. Computed tomography will confirm the suspected diagnosis and also helps in the management of complications such as a pancreatic abscess or a pseudo-cyst.

Medical causes of abdominal pain

Pneumonia

Pneumonia may present with referred abdominal pain in the young and the old especially when complicated by diaphragmatic pleurisy. Sometimes the pneumonia results from inflammation below the diaphragm and it is important to treat both conditions.

Hepatitis

Intrahepatic cholestasis due to drugs, viral hepatitis, or alcohol is easy to confuse with cholangitis caused by extrahepatic obstruction. If the bile ducts are not dilated on ultrasound examination 1 week after the onset of jaundice then large duct obstruction is unlikely to be the cause.

Herpes zoster

Persistent severe pain precedes the rash in herpes zoster (shingles). When one of the lower thoracic or upper lumbar dermatomes is involved patients will present with abdominal pain. The diagnosis is usually impossible before the rash has appeared and is obvious once it has.

Drugs

Digoxin, non-steroidal analgesics, laxatives, and drugs which cause constipation can all cause abdominal pain. The first is notorious for causing nausea, vomiting, and abdominal pain when given to excess.

Gastroenteritis

Severe colic is sometimes a presenting feature of gastroenteritis. Diarrhoea and vomiting are not far behind and the diagnosis is rarely difficult. Patients should be isolated as soon as the diagnosis is suspected and stool cultures should be requested promptly.

Diabetes mellitus

Children with acute type 1 diabetes may complain of abdominal pain. They are always ketotic and hyperglycaemic and the diagnosis can often be made by smelling the patient's breath. A surgeon should check that some septic focus is not an underlying cause and refer the patient urgently to a physician.

Rarities

Rare causes of abdominal pain such as sickle cell crises, acute porphyria, lead poisoning, or a spinal tumour are often only made after a considerable period of time and then usually by exclusion. The diagnosis is often suggested by appropriate review of the past history and family history of the patient. Once the possibility of these rarities is considered it is a simple matter to arrange the relevant tests: since these disorders greatly aggravate the risks of exploratory surgery under general anaesthesia, prompt diagnosis and rapid referral for definitive treatment is highly desirable.

Management of the medical patient with abdominal pain

Observation

Most patients who develop acute abdominal pain on a medical ward will require the opinion of an experienced surgeon. If this is deemed unnecessary or a surgeon is not immediately available then the patient should be placed under observation and reviewed at frequent intervals.

Pain relief

Analgesia suppresses abdominal signs and is best not given until a diagnosis has been made. However, a surgeon can allow for the diagnostically confounding effects of analgesia provided it is clear which drug has been given and when; patients in pain should be given the analgesia they need.

Antibiotics

Treating undiagnosed abdominal pain with antibiotics is not recommended. They are rarely curative.

Resuscitation

Patients who may need an abdominal operation should not be given any food or drink by mouth and should be resuscitated with appropriate intravenous fluids. There will then be the minimum of delay if surgery under general anaesthesia is required.

Further reading

Britton J (2000). The acute abdomen. In: Morris PJ, Wood WC, eds. *Oxford textbook of surgery*, 2nd edn, 1823–42. Oxford University Press, Oxford. [A more detailed account of the diagnosis and treatment of acute abdominal pain.]

de Dombal FT (1991). *Diagnosis of acute abdominal pain*, 2nd edn. Churchill Livingstone, Edinburgh. [A compilation of scientific studies of abdominal pain completed over 20 years.]

Martin RF, Rossi RL, eds (1997). Abdominal emergencies. *Surgical Clinics of North America*, **77**, 1226–470. [An up-to-date series of articles on the diagnosis and management of the acute abdomen with an American perspective.]

14.3.2 Gastrointestinal bleeding

T. A. Rockall and T. Northfield

Introduction and definition

Acute gastrointestinal haemorrhage is classified by its origin, from either the upper or the lower gastrointestinal tract, anatomically demarcated by the ligament of Treitz. Only when gastrointestinal bleeding is acute does it constitute an emergency. Chronic, low-volume blood loss is usually subclinical until such time as it presents with iron deficient anaemia.

Acute upper gastrointestinal haemorrhage (AUGIH)

Epidemiology

The incidence of AUGIH in the United Kingdom is approximately 1 per 1000 adults/year, of which 15 per cent of cases occur in patients already in hospital. The male incidence is twice that of the female in all age groups except the elderly, where they are similar. The annual incidence increases dramatically with age, rising to nearly 5 per 1000/year in the over 75 age group. In the United Kingdom in 1993, about one-quarter of cases occurred over the age of 80 years.

Aetiology

Many gastrointestinal lesions may result in haemorrhage but peptic ulcer is the most frequent in the United Kingdom (Table 1). Each diagnostic group has its own aetiological factors. *Helicobacter pylori* infection and ingestion of aspirin and non-steroidal anti-inflammatory drugs (NSAID) are important for ulcer disease and erosions of the upper gastrointestinal tract. Ulceration may also occur at the site of surgical enterostomies (stomal ulcers) and in association with the Zollinger–Ellison syndrome. Peptic ulceration at specific sites is associated with major haemorrhage due to the anatomical relation of major arteries—the posterior wall of the first part of the duodenum (gastroduodenal artery), the lesser curve of the stomach (left gastric artery), and posterior wall of stomach (splenic artery).

Liver disease due to alcohol and hepatitis are the principal causes in Western countries of portal hypertension, which leads to oesophageal varices; variceal bleeding may rarely affect the stomach and the remaining gastrointestinal tract. Mallory–Weiss tears are mucosal lesions at the

Table 1 Diagnoses following acute upper gastrointestinal haemorrhage

Diagnosis	%
Not established	25
Peptic ulcer	35
Erosive disease	11
Oesophagitis	10
Mallory–Weiss tear	5
Oesophageal varices	4
Upper gastrointestinal malignancy	4
Other	6

oesophagogastric junction associated with profuse vomiting; haematemesis occurs which is usually minor and always self-limiting. The most common malignant causes of upper gastrointestinal haemorrhage are adenocarcinoma of the stomach and gastric lymphoma, but acute bleeding is an unusual presentation. Other causes include benign tumours (or those with uncertain malignant potential) such as the stromal tumours (previously described as leiomyomas) which may bleed when the mucosal surface ulcerates, angiodysplasia (and other vascular lesions), aortoduodenal fistula, haemobilia, and trauma.

Clinical features

Upper gastrointestinal haemorrhage usually presents with haematemesis or 'coffee-ground' vomiting and melaena. Frank haematemesis indicates a severe bleed. It is not always a feature but melaena will always follow a significant bleed. In rapid bleeding, symptoms of hypovolaemia may precede haematemesis or melaena. These include postural hypotension, syncope, shock, and even death. In most cases, the causative lesion will not be known until diagnostic endoscopy is undertaken. The patient should be asked about ingestion of NSAIDs and whether blood was present in the first vomit (it is usually absent in Mallory–Weiss tear). Signs of chronic liver disease may be present in patients with oesophageal varices but this does not confirm the cause of blood loss since peptic ulcer is a common synchronous lesion. Melaena is a clinical diagnosis made on the observation of black, tarry, offensive stool on rectal examination or passed spontaneously. In patients with rapid haemorrhage, usually accompanied by shock, fresh blood may be passed per rectum (haemochezia) and may thus be difficult to distinguish from lower gastrointestinal haemorrhage. A mix of fresh blood and melaena may indicate a lesion in the lower small intestine (e.g. Meckel's diverticulum).

Laboratory diagnosis

AUGIH is a clinical diagnosis. The initial haemoglobin estimation is not a useful indicator of the volume of blood lost until time for haemodilution has passed. The haemoglobin may be normal in a patient with a large, acute haemorrhage. Equally, the haemoglobin may be low in a patient with iron deficiency anaemia resulting from chronic haemorrhage who presents with a small, acute bleed. The haemoglobin and haematocrit after volume resuscitation are more useful. Platelet count and coagulation studies are important to exclude a bleeding disorder and are of particular relevance in patients receiving therapeutic anticoagulants and in those with liver disease.

Treatment

The management of acute upper gastrointestinal haemorrhage falls into four principal stages.

Assessment, resuscitation, and monitoring

Important aspects of assessment are confirmation that a bleed has occurred and the degree of hypovolaemic shock that has resulted. Resuscitation is as for any hypovolaemic patient with the immediate aim of rapidly replenishing blood. Tachycardia, vasoconstriction, sweating, hypotension (including a postural drop), tachypnoea, and a low central venous pressure all indicate hypovolaemia. Adequate resuscitation is evidenced by a normal pulse rate, blood pressure and central venous pressure, production of urine, and an improving level of consciousness. Central venous access and placement of a urinary catheter will help in the resuscitation and monitoring of the more severe cases and those with major cardiovascular and respiratory comorbidity. Once circulating blood volume has been restored, management should be aimed at monitoring the patient for continued or recurrent bleeding, replacing blood, making a diagnosis, and instituting therapy. Regular pulse, blood pressure, central venous pressure, and urine output will give a good guide. Fresh haematemesis obviously indicates further acute haemorrhage. The passage of further fresh melaena has to be interpreted in the light of the cardiovascular signs and repeated estimations of blood haemoglobin concentration.

Diagnosis and haemostasis

In most instances, the diagnosis is obscure until upper gastrointestinal endoscopy is undertaken. This diagnostic, and potentially therapeutic, procedure should be undertaken as soon as possible after resuscitation is complete. The aim of endoscopy is fourfold:

(1) to make a diagnosis;

(2) to assess the risk of further haemorrhage based upon the site, size, and nature of the lesion (including stigmata of recent haemorrhage);

(3) to apply haemostatic therapy where appropriate;

(4) to inform the surgeon as to the site of the lesion in cases requiring urgent surgery due to rapid, ongoing blood loss and to exclude varices in these cases.

Haemostasis occurs spontaneously in most cases. When bleeding continues, haemostasis can be achieved by endoscopic, surgical, or radiological means. Endoscopic haemostatic therapy may be given in the form of injection of adrenaline or sclerosants (e.g. polidocanol) either alone or in combination, or other substances such as fibrin glue. The application of heat energy in the form of laser (Argon or NdYAG), heater probe, or diathermy are also effective for peptic ulcer with active bleeding or visible vessels. There is good trial evidence that endoscopic therapy reduces the rate of rebleeding in these subgroups and one trial has shown a reduction in mortality. There is no randomized, controlled trial evidence that planned, repeated endoscopic therapy further reduces rebleeding in peptic ulcer. Repeated injection or banding have been shown to reduce rebleeding and mortality from oesophageal varices.

Surgery is indicated in massive, acute bleeding not amenable to endoscopic therapy or where endoscopic therapy fails to control active bleeding. Many units would attempt a second endoscopic therapy especially in young patients before resorting to surgery. There is some evidence that early surgical intervention in those over 60 is appropriate. There is no place for a third attempt at endoscopic therapy and surgery is indicated. In cases where endoscopic therapy has failed and surgery is deemed to be exceptionally high risk, visceral angiography may allow for embolization (e.g. the gastroduodenal artery in duodenal ulcer).

Uncontrolled variceal haemorrhage may be controlled with a Sengstaken–Blakemore tube as a temporary measure before more definitive treatment. Where endoscopic therapies subsequently fail, transjugular intrahepatic portosystemic shunt (TIPSS) is a minimally invasive method of creating a portosystemic shunt. Finally, oesophageal transection is occasionally life saving where all other attempts at haemostasis have failed.

Treatment of causative lesion

Treatment of the causative lesion should be started as soon as possible after diagnosis. There is, however, no evidence that drug therapy alters the outcome of the bleeding episode in terms of rebleeding or death. Histamine (H_2) receptor antagonists and proton pump inhibitors both heal ulcers but neither have been shown to affect the outcome of the bleeding episode. Where the causative lesion is a tumour (benign or malignant) then elective surgery may be indicated. Angiodysplasia can be treated with laser or argon beam. Specific treatments may be required for rarer causes such as tuberculosis.

Prevention of recurrence

Recurrent episodes of bleeding from peptic ulcers can be achieved by eradicating *H. pylori* infection and through the avoidance of ulcerogenic drugs. Persistent ulceration despite these measures may require long-term acid suppressive therapy and Zollinger–Ellison syndrome should be excluded. Variceal haemorrhage can be prevented through programmes of variceal eradication by injection or banding and also by TIPSS, or ultimately liver transplantation where indicated.

Prognosis

Prognosis depends on many factors including the severity of the bleed, the age of the patient, the associated comorbidity of the patient, the diagnostic category, the endoscopic features (stigmata of recent haemorrhage), and whether continued or recurrent bleeding is a feature. Overall, the crude mortality for patients presenting to emergency departments with acute upper gastrointestinal haemorrhage is about 10 per cent. Most deaths occur in the elderly and those with severe comorbidity. Death in those under the age of 60 with no comorbidity is very low (0.1 per cent) regardless of the severity of the haemorrhage. The factors that contribute to mortality have been combined in a prognostic risk score. This is represented in Table 2. The mortality associated with each risk score is represented in Table 3.

Acute lower gastrointestinal haemorrhage

Epidemiology

The incidence of lower gastrointestinal haemorrhage has not been well defined but it is common. Most (90 per cent) of acute lower gastrointestinal bleeds will stop spontaneously although 35 per cent will require blood transfusion, and 5 per cent will require urgent surgical intervention.

Table 2 Acute upper gastrointestinal haemorrhage scoring system

Variable	SCORE			
	0	1	2	3
Age	< 60 years	60–79 years	≥ 80 years	
Shock	'No shock'	'Tachycardia'	'Hypotension'	
	Systolic BP ≥ 100	Systolic BP ≥100	Systolic BP < 100	
	Pulse < 100	Pulse ≥ 100		
Comorbidity	No major comorbidity		Cardiac failure	Renal failure
			Ischaemic heart disease	Liver failure
			Any major comorbidity	Disseminated malignancy
Diagnosis	Mallory–Weiss tear	All other diagnoses	Malignancy of upper gastrointestinal tract	
	No lesion identified and no stigmata of recent haemorrhage			
Major stigmata of recent haemorrhage	None or dark spot only		Blood in upper gastrointestinal tract	
			Adherent clot	
			Visible or spurting vessel	

Table 3 Observed rebleeding and mortality by risk score

Score	0	1	2	3	4	5	6	7	8+
Rebleed (%)	4.9	3.4	5.3	11.2	14.1	24.1	32.9	43.8	41.8
Deaths no rebleed (%)	0	0	0.3	2.0	3.5	8.1	9.5	14.9	28.1
Deaths rebleed (%)	0	0	0	10.0	15.8	22.9	33.3	43.4	52.5
Deaths total (%)	0	0	0.2	2.9	5.3	10.8	17.3	27.0	41.1

Aetiology

As in upper gastrointestinal haemorrhage, several pathological causes are responsible. Most causative lesions are colonic or anorectal and only 3 per cent originate in the small bowel. In the Western world, diverticular disease represents the largest proportion of cases (40 per cent), followed by inflammatory bowel disease (20 per cent, including Crohn's, ulcerative colitis, infectious colitis, and ischaemic colitis), neoplasia (15 per cent), benign anorectal disease (10 per cent), and arteriovenous malformations (2 per cent). Other lesions are rare and include radiation injury, Meckel's diverticulum, other small bowel pathology, and varices. Bleeding is not uncommonly associated with coagulopathy but studies have shown the distribution of causative lesions in these cases to be the same. In severe cases, however, generalized mucosal bleeding may occur.

Iatrogenic causes of haemorrhage include postpolypectomy bleeding and anastomotic bleeding. The risk of haemorrhage after polypectomy is estimated to be between 0.2 per cent and 3 per cent. Haemorrhage is usually immediate but may be delayed. When identified, endoscopic haemostatic techniques are usually successful (injection of adrenaline, resnaring, recoagulating, placement of a ligature or clip).

Acute colonic diverticular bleeding is common. The estimated risk of bleeding with this disease is about 15 per cent. After a single bleed, the risk of recurrence is 25 per cent and after two bleeds it is 50 per cent. Eighty per cent of all bleeds stop spontaneously and no therapy is indicated. Operative intervention should be considered after two major bleeds because the risk of further recurrence is high. However, many of these patients are frail and elderly and continuation of conservative treatment for multiple, self-limiting episodes may be appropriate. Inflammatory bowel disease often manifests itself as bloody diarrhoea but more rarely may present with profuse haemorrhage. This is more common in Crohn's disease than in ulcerative colitis because the inflammation involves the whole thickness of the bowel wall. Up to 6 per cent of patients with this disease may sustain a major haemorrhage. About 50 per cent stop bleeding spontaneously but of these 35 per cent will rebleed. For this reason, urgent surgery is usually indicated for patients with a life-threatening haemorrhage as a result of inflammatory colitis. The operation usually required is a total colectomy. The rectum is usually preserved at this stage unless this is the site of major haemorrhage. Ischaemic colitis rarely causes severe haemorrhage. Bloody diarrhoea is more usual and may be accompanied by pain.

Benign and malignant colonic tumours may present as profuse bleeding although occult blood loss and minor fresh bleeding is more common. Rarely is urgent surgical intervention required. Vascular anomalies occur with increasing frequency with age. They may originate from chronic, partial venous obstruction of submucosal veins due to incompetence of the precapillary sphincters and arteriovenous malformations. These lesions are usually multiple and are most frequent in the caecum and ascending colon. Bleeding is usually slow, intermittent, and recurrent although once again it is occasionally massive (2–15 per cent). Most (90 per cent) stop spontaneously but 25 to 85 per cent will recur. The treatment of choice is endoscopic coagulation if the lesions can be identified. Colectomy is reserved for those with repeated major haemorrhage.

Benign anorectal disease does present as lower gastrointestinal haemorrhage and a careful examination of the anorectum is imperative before initiating more invasive examinations. However, anorectal lesions are common and complete colonic evaluation is usually required even after identifying an anorectal source such as haemorrhoids.

Diagnosis and treatment

A good history from the patient may give clues as to the cause of colorectal haemorrhage. Important points include a prior history of bleeding, the presence of liver disease, and drug usage (aspirin, non-steroidal anti-inflammatory drugs, and warfarin) as well as the exact nature of the bleeding—specifically the duration, the colour of the blood, the relationship to defaecation, whether the blood is mixed with or separate from the stool, an associated change in bowel habit, or mucus discharge. Bright red blood separate from the stool suggests an anorectal cause. Diarrhoea and mucous associated with darker blood mixed in with the stool suggests colitis or neoplasm. None of these clinical features, however, is absolutely diagnostic.

Resuscitation measures are as for bleeding from the upper gastrointestinal tract. However, since most lower gastrointestinal bleeds stop spontaneously, initial management should be conservative with transfusion and correction of clotting abnormalities. Once haemorrhage has ceased, bowel preparation and colonoscopy can be undertaken in a stable patient and with a much higher chance of detecting the pathological lesion (85–90 per cent).

In the small proportion of patients in whom active colonic bleeding continues, investigation to localize the source of the haemorrhage is indicated so that directed treatment can be administered in the form of endoscopic therapy, interventional radiology, or surgery. Colonoscopy is favoured by many clinicians but the use of bowel preparation is still debated. Some favour the use of a purgative together with distal colonic washouts before endoscopy, whilst other authors have argued that this is unnecessary because of the cathartic effect of blood in the colon. In one study, the causative lesion was identified in three-quarters of patients without preparation. This compares favourably with studies which have used mechanical preparation methods. Colonoscopy should be abandoned if massive haemorrhage obscures the diagnosis or severe mucosal or ischaemic colitis is encountered, as the risk of perforation in these cases is high.

Nuclear scintigraphy can be used to detect active haemorrhage. It is very sensitive and can detect bleeding rates of less than 1 ml/min. Tc99m labelled sulphur colloid can be used, which has the advantage of no preparation but the half-life is very short and its rapid enhancement of the liver and spleen can obscure the diagnosis. A better method is the use of Tc99m labelled red cells. Unfortunately, although sensitive, it is also very non-specific and localizes the lesion very poorly. It may be useful immediately before angiography to confirm active haemorrhage before undertaking the more invasive procedure. Whenever there is massive, active haemorrhage, however, this is unnecessary and the patient should proceed directly to visceral angiography.

Selective mesenteric angiography can also detect a rate of bleeding of 0.5 to 1.0 ml/min. The sensitivity reported in various studies ranges from 40 to 86 per cent. Once the site of haemorrhage is identified, the patient can proceed directly to surgery or there is the therapeutic possibility of arterial infusion of vasopressin or selective embolization. Vasopressin infusion has considerable side-effects including mesenteric thrombosis, intestinal infarction, myocardial ischaemia, hypertension, arrythmias, and death. Nitroglycerin may be infused simultaneously to counteract the systemic effects of the drug. There is a wide range in the reported rate of initial control of the haemorrhage, and the rebleeding rate is high (22–71 per cent).

Selective embolization using coil springs or gelfoam into the most distal vessel results in high initial rates of haemostasis and the rate of intestinal infarction is low. It is a good technique for patients with a very high predicted operative mortality.

From a practical aspect, investigation should start with examination of the abdomen and rectum, followed by proctosigmoidoscopy. If there is any suspicion of an upper gastrointestinal cause, then upper gastrointestinal endoscopy is recommended. Colonoscopy is the investigation of choice to evaluate the colon and terminal ileum. Where this fails, visceral angiography should be undertaken, which may allow the site of haemorrhage to be identified and treatment instituted.

In about 5 per cent of cases, the source of bleeding remains obscure. Additional investigations may include small bowel enteroscopy or laparotomy with on-table enteroscopy.

Further reading

Northfield TC, Smith T (1970). Central venous pressure in the clinical management of acute gastrointestinal bleeding. *Lancet* **1**, 990–1.

Palmer KR, Church NI (1999). Therapeutic endoscopy for upper gastrointestinal bleeding. *Continued Medical Education Journal Gastroenterology, Hepatology and Nutrition* **2**, 75–8.

Peterson WL, Cook DJ (1998). Antisecretory therapy for bleeding peptic ulcer. *Journal of the American Medical Association* **280**, 877–9.

Rockall TA, Logan RFA, Devlin HB, Northfield TC (1995). Incidence of and mortality from acute upper gastrointestinal haemorrhage in the United Kingdom. *British Medical Journal* **311**, 222–6.

Rockall TA, Logan RFA, Devlin HB, Northfield TC (1996). Risk assessment following acute upper gastrointestinal haemorrhage. *Gut* **38**, 316–21.

Steele RJC (1989). Endoscopic haemostasis for non-variceal upper gastrointestinal haemorrhage. *British Journal of Surgery* **76**, 219–25.

Swain CP, Kirkham JS, Salmon PR, Bown SG, Northfield TC (1986). Controlled trial of Nd-YAG laser photocoagulation in bleeding peptic ulcers. *Lancet* **i**, 1113–6.

Vernava AM, Moore BA, Longo WE, Johnson FE (1997). Lower gastrointestinal bleeding. *Diseases of the Colon and Rectum* **40**, 846–58.

Williams SG, Westaby D (1994). Management of variceal haemorrhage. *British Medical Journal* **308**, 1213–7.

14.4 Immune disorders of the gastrointestinal tract

M. R. Haeney

Introduction

The gut is protected by several mechanisms. The intercellular tight junctions of the epithelial cells form an important physical barrier; these cells turn over every 24 to 96 h. Any injury to the epithelial barrier results in rapid migration of adjacent viable epithelial cells to cover the denuded area, a process called 'restitution', while lymphocytes and macrophages migrate through pores in the basement membrane to provide temporary protection. The acid pH of the stomach and the proteolytic enzyme content of the intestine are formidable chemical barriers to many organisms. A change in the normal microflora of the intestine or impaired gut motility may allow pathogenic bacteria to flourish. Microbial antigens that resist these defences and penetrate the epithelial surface encounter the mucosal immune system.

Functional morphology of the gut-associated lymphoid tissue

Lymphocytes are found at three sites within the mucosa (Fig. 1):

(1) organized lymphoid aggregates (Peyer's patches) beneath the epithelium of the terminal small intestine;

(2) lymphocytes within the epithelial cell layer (intraepithelial lymphocytes);and

(3) lymphocytes scattered among other immunocompetent cells within the lamina propria.

Gut-associated lymphoid tissue is divided into two functional compartments: an afferent arm—Peyer's patches—where interaction occurs between luminal antigens and the immune system, and an effector arm—the lymphocytes of the intraepithelium and lamina propria.

Peyer's patches

These are covered by a specialized epithelium (follicle-associated epithelium) that has no microvilli but whose surface seems wrinkled or folded under the scanning electron microscope (Fig. 1). These microfold, or M, cells sample and transport particulate antigens from the lumen into the 'dome' area, where T and B cells mix freely with the microfolds of the M cells and priming of both types of lymphocyte occurs. Within Peyer's patches are specialized T cells that induce immature IgM-bearing B lymphocytes to switch isotype to IgA.

Lymphocytes are mobile: an array of cell surface receptors permits adhesion to endothelial cells and to components of the extracellular matrix. Primed B lymphoblasts, committed mainly to producing IgA antibody, migrate from Peyer's patches, via the lymphatics and mesenteric lymph nodes, to the thoracic duct and hence into the circulation. These cells return preferentially to the lamina propria, a process known as 'homing'. Once back in the gut, they mature into IgA plasma cells and are responsible for local and secretory antibody defences. The number of IgA-containing cells in the lamina propria far exceeds the numbers containing IgM, IgG, or IgE.

Intraepithelial lymphocytes

There is a similar migration pathway for T lymphocytes whereby T blasts from mesenteric nodes 'home' both to the epithelium and to the lamina propria. Intraepithelial lymphocytes are phenotypically and functionally distinct from peripheral blood lymphocytes. Peripheral T cells rarely express the human mucosal lymphocyte antigen (HML-1) but nearly all intraepithelial lymphocytes do. Human mucosal lymphocyte antigen CD103 is a novel $\alpha E\beta 7$ integrin which binds to its ligand, E-cadherin, expressed on gut epithelial cells. This interaction may direct homing of intraepithelial lymphocytes to the epithelium but is more likely to selectively retain intraepithelial lymphocytes within the epithelial compartment. Intraepithelial lymphocytes are not a homogeneous population: about 10 per cent do not express the CD3 antigen and therefore are not T cells. About 70 per cent are CD8+ and show increased expression of the γ/δ form of the T-cell receptor compared with peripheral blood lymphocytes (see Chapter 5.1). In experimental models, some intraepithelial lymphocytes are cytotoxic and some have natural killer activity, functions important in the control of enterovirus infection. Intraepithelial lymphocytes also seem to have a role in controlling the cell barrier function of epithelial cells, i.e. 'restitution'. However, the function of intraepithelial lymphocytes in humans is unclear.

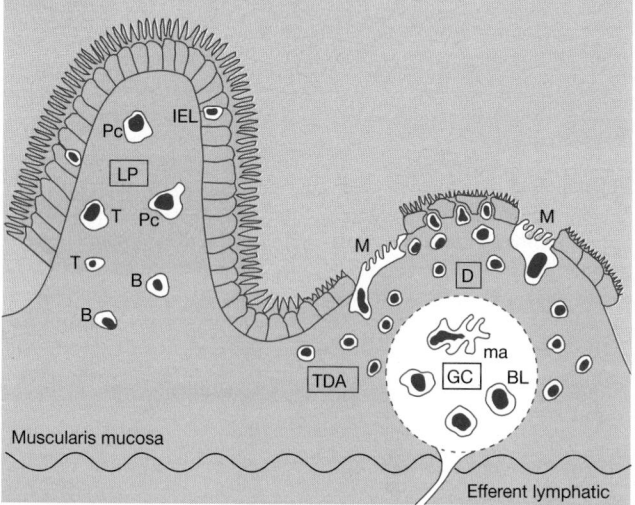

Fig. 1 Organization and structure of gut-associated lymphoid tissue. On the left, T and B lymphocytes and plasma cells (PC) can be seen in the lamina propria, with intraepithelial lymphocytes (IEL) between the columnar epithelial cells. On the right, there is a Peyer's patch covered by cuboidal epithelium with occasional 'M'cells. The Peyer's patch comprises three areas: the dome (D) of T and B lymphocytes; the thymus-dependent area (TDA); and the germinal centre (GC) containing macrophages (Ma) and B lymphoblasts (BL).

Lamina propria lymphocytes

Large numbers of lymphocytes, natural killer cells, mast cells, macrophages, and plasma cells occur in the lamina propria. T and B lymphocytes are both found, but T cells predominate in a ratio of about 4:1. In contrast to intraepithelial lymphocytes, 80 per cent of these T cells are CD4+. They do not proliferate well after stimulation of the T-cell receptor, yet produce large amounts of cytokines interleukin 2, interleukin 4, interferon-γ, and tumour necrosis factor-α. T-cell homing to the lamina propria is determined mainly by the integrin $\alpha4\beta7$ on primed cells interacting preferentially with mucosal addressin cell adhesion molecule 1 expressed on the microvascular endothelium in the lamina propria.

Secretory immunoglobulins

The plasma cells of the lamina propria secrete mainly IgA, which is specially adapted for its function. IgA is synthesized as a dimer with two IgA molecules linked by a smaller 'joining' peptide (the J chain), also produced by the plasma cells. The secretory component is a 70 kDa fragment of the polymeric immunoglobulin receptor synthesized by epithelial cells and is essential for transport of secretory IgA into the gut lumen. The polymeric Ig receptor binds the dimeric IgA; the complex is endocytosed and transported through the cytoplasm to the luminal surface of the cell where proteolysis of the receptor occurs. The IgA dimer is released into the gut attached to the proteolytic fragment of the receptor now called secretory component. Secretory component also protects the IgA molecule from degradation by proteolytic enzymes.

Secretory IgA predominates in the saliva and in gastric and intestinal secretions, where it tends to be concentrated in the mucous layer overlying epithelial cells. Secretory IgA neutralizes viruses, bacteria, and toxins and prevents the adherence of pathogenic micro-organisms to gut epithelium and so blocks the uptake of antigen into the systemic immune system.

Spectrum of intestinal immune responses

Ingestion of antigens can lead to local immunity, a systemic immune response, or a state of specific immune unresponsiveness (tolerance).

Local immune responses

These can occur independently of a systemic response. For example, immunization against poliomyelitis with oral Sabin vaccine gives better protection than the injected Salk vaccine, even though both induce serum antibodies. Local IgA antibody, produced in response to the oral vaccine, partly blocks uptake of pathogenic virus into the circulation.

Systemic immune responses

Macromolecules are absorbed by the intestine into the portal or systemic circulations, via either the glandular epithelium covering the villus or the M cells. Up to 2 per cent of a dietary protein load appears antigenically intact in the circulation. Sinusoidal phagocytes (Kupffer cells) of the liver destroy much of the antigen but enough passes through the liver to stimulate systemic antibody production, particularly in the spleen. Antibody formed in the spleen enters the portal circulation to complex with incoming antigen. Circulating immune complexes of IgA and dietary antigens are regularly found in normal people after meals.

Systemic tolerance

A unique feature of the mucosal immune system is its ability to downregulate immune responses to dietary antigens (oral tolerance). Native Americans knew that eating the leaves of poison ivy prevented contact dermatitis on subsequent exposure to the plant. This observation can be reproduced in animals by feeding them antigen; they become immunologically unresponsive (tolerant) to subsequent parenteral injections of that antigen. Oral tolerance can affect all aspects of the systemic immune response: a single feed of protein antigen suppresses systemic IgM, IgG, and IgE responses as well as T-cell mediated immunity. This has led to attempts to treat autoimmune diseases by feeding autoantigens to patients.

Immunological disorders of the gastrointestinal tract

Normally, the intestinal immune system steers a delicate course between the undesirable extremes of immunological incompetence, with resulting vulnerability to ingested pathogens (for instance, the gastrointestinal consequences of primary and secondary immunodeficiencies), and hypersensitivity to dietary antigens, with immunologically mediated reactions each time that antigen is eaten.

Primary immunodeficiency diseases

Immunocompromised patients are at risk from two sources of infection: common pathogens, which invade even the immunologically healthy, and 'opportunistic' agents that can invade and infect only those with weakened defences. In the compromised host, most infections are due to common pathogens that are readily identified and controlled. The difficult problems arise from opportunistic infections because these often elude isolation, may not respond to available drugs, and carry a high fatality. Indeed, the identification of certain opportunistic infections implies an underlying immunodeficiency that demands further investigation.

It is beyond the scope of this section to deal with all the gastrointestinal complications of every known form of primary and secondary immunodeficiency. Instead, attention will be focused on representative disorders.

Common variable immunodeficiency (CVI)

Common variable immunodeficiency is an example of one of the primary antibody deficiency syndromes described in Section 5.

Definition

Common variable immunodeficiency is a heterogeneous group of disorders characterized by low serum immunoglobulin levels, a normal or low proportion of circulating B lymphocytes and, in about one-third of patients, impaired cell-mediated immunity. It can present at any age and, in the United States and Western Europe, the prevalence is about 40 per million of the population. Most cases are sporadic, although some are inherited.

Clinical features

Patients present typically with recurrent sinopulmonary infections, most frequently caused by pneumococci, streptococci, and *Haemophilus influenzae*. Less commonly, they present with arthropathy, skin sepsis, meningitis, osteomyelitis, or other severe systemic bacterial infections (see Section 7).

With certain exceptions, these patients are not unduly susceptible to viral or fungal infections, because cell-mediated immunity is usually preserved. There are rarely any diagnostic physical signs of antibody deficiency, although examination often shows evidence of the consequences of previous infections, particularly bronchiectasis.

Between 30 and 50 per cent of patients with common variable immunodeficiency have gastrointestinal problems at some time. Virtually any part of the gastrointestinal tract may be affected (Table 1) but the most common symptoms are diarrhoea (intermittent or chronic) and weight loss. An approach to the diagnosis of these complications is shown in Fig. 2.
Stomach *Achlorhydria and pernicious anaemia* Achlorhydria is found in about 30 per cent of patients and the associated atrophic gastritis occasionally leads to a syndrome resembling pernicious anaemia except that the atrophic gastritis involves the whole stomach without antral sparing, the serum gastrin concentrations remain normal, and autoantibodies to gastric parietal cells and intrinsic factor are absent.

Table 1 Gastrointestinal disorders associated with common variable immunodeficiency and other forms of primary antibody deficiency.

Infective	Giardiasis
	Campylobacter enteritis
	Cryptosporidiosis
	Strongyloides stercoralis
	Salmonella/shigella infection
	Viral enteritis
	Bacterial overgrowth
Other	Pernicious anaemia-like syndrome
	Hypogammaglobulinaemic sprue
	Coeliac disease
	Carcinoma of the stomach
	Nodular lymphoid hyperplasia
	Inflammatory bowel disease
	Non-granulomatous jejunoileitis

Gastric cancer Patients with common variable immunodeficiency have a 47-fold increase in the incidence of carcinoma of the stomach. It is sufficiently common to warrant yearly gastroscopic examination in hypogammaglobulinaemic patients who have atrophic gastritis. The high concentrations of microbial enzymes and nitrites found in the gastric juices may lead to local production of carcinogenic *N*-nitroso compounds. Chronic active gastritis induced by *Heliobacter pylori* and overexpression of p53 may also play a role in gastric carcinogenesis.

Small intestine *Infective complications* Although infestation with *Giardia lamblia* is the most common identifiable cause of malabsorption, in many patients the cause is never found. Giardiasis is virtually confined to adults and is rarely seen in boys with X-linked hypogammaglobulinaemia. Giardiasis may also cause diarrhoea, villous abnormalities, vitamin B_{12} and folate malabsorption, steatorrhoea, disaccharidase deficiency, and protein-losing enteropathy but the pathogenetic mechanisms are poorly understood.

Examination of at least three consecutive fresh stool specimens is essential to detect the cysts of *G. lamblia* (Fig. 2). If this fails, duodenal aspiration and jejunal biopsy are needed to establish the diagnosis. In particularly difficult cases, a therapeutic trial of metronidazole can be useful, although infestation frequently recurs. Most patients show symptomatic improvement after treatment with either a 7-day course of metronidazole (2 g daily as a single dose) or mepacrin (100 mg, three times daily for 10 days). Other parasitic infestations occur. *Cryptosporidium* infection occasionally causes self-limiting diarrhoea but has a much more sinister outcome in boys with CD40 ligand deficiency (hyper IgM syndrome) and in patients with human immunodeficiency virus (**HIV**) infection.

Bacterial infections also cause diarrhoea in patients with common variable immunodeficiency and *Campylobacter jejuni* is frequently responsible. Rarely, campylobacter causes an ascending cholangitis and hepatitis. Treatment is a 2-week course of erythromycin (500 mg, four times daily) with follow-up stool culture to ensure that treatment has been effective.

Shigella or salmonella diarrhoea does not occur more commonly than normal. Similarly, while overgrowth of commensal bacteria is common, bacterial counts rarely exceed 10^5 organisms/ml, compared with counts of more than 10^6/ml in the blind-loop syndrome. Nevertheless, it is common practice to treat these patients empirically with tetracycline and metronidazole, often with symptomatic improvement.

Nodular lymphoid hyperplasia Nodular lymphoid hyperplasia describes the presence of lymphoid nodules in the lamina propria of the gut. Although described in many disorders and occasionally in healthy individuals, nodular lymphoid hyperplasia should make the clinician suspect common variable immunodeficiency. It occurs in 20 to 50 per cent of patients but is not necessarily symptomatic. The nodules, which are 1 to 3 mm in diameter, appear as protrusions on fibreoptic endoscopy (Fig. 3 and Plate 1) and as multiple filling defects on barium studies (Fig. 4). Nodular lymphoid hyperplasia restricted to the rectum or colon can present with rectal bleeding, abdominal pain and features of intestinal obstruction, but rarely with diarrhoea.

The ultrastructure of these nodules is similar to Peyer's patches, and lymphoblasts containing IgM are found in the centres of the follicles. The condition probably represents hypertrophy of the gut-associated lymphoid tissue in response to antigens in the gut lumen. In one series of nodular lymphoid hyperplasia in individuals with normal serum immunoglobulins, every patient had intestinal giardiasis, suggesting an aetiological link with persistent infestation. Although nodular lymphoid hyperplasia is not premalignant in patients with hypogammaglobulinaemia, intestinal lymphoma has been reported in apparently immunocompetent subjects with extensive small-bowel nodular lymphoid hyperplasia.

Hypogammaglobulinaemic sprue In a few patients with unexplained diarrhoea, the mucosal lesion resembles coeliac disease or tropical sprue but with reduced or undetectable plasma cells within the lamina propria. In tropical regions, about 1 per cent of patients with 'sprue' may be suffering from a primary humoral immunodeficiency syndrome. Malabsorption in patients with hypogammaglobulinaemic sprue can improve rapidly after replacement immunoglobulin therapy.

Although extremely rare, patients with common variable immunodeficiency may have concomitant gluten-sensitive coeliac disease.

Inflammatory bowel disease About 5 per cent of patients with common variable immunodeficiency have features of inflammatory bowel disease with radiological and histological findings of Crohn's disease. Others have proposed a specific common variable immunodeficiency enteropathy characterized by low-grade microscopic colitis, increased intraepithelial lymphocytes, and an intact crypt architecture with a good response to an elemental diet.

Non-granulomatous jejunoileitis This is a rare feature of common variable immunodeficiency and has a poor prognosis.

Management

The cornerstone of treatment of antibody deficiency is immunoglobulin replacement; enough must be given to prevent further infections and reduce the incidence of complications. Intravenous or subcutaneous immunoglobulin therapy is the treatment of choice and is discussed more fully in Section 5.

Antibody-deficient patients respond as promptly as others to appropriate antibiotics but longer courses of treatment are usually needed to ensure complete eradication of the micro-organism.

Selective IgA deficiency (see also Section 5)

Definition

Selective IgA deficiency refers to a serum IgA concentration below the limit of detection (< 0.01 g/l). By definition, the serum IgG and IgM concentrations are normal.

Aetiology

Selective IgA deficiency is common and occurs in about 1 in 700 of healthy adults. Most cases are sporadic, but there is an association with inheritance of the HLA B8, DW3 haplotype, and with deficiencies of IgG2 and IgG4. It is sometimes linked with defects in chromosome 18, particularly in the autosomal recessive syndrome of ataxia telangiectasia. Selective IgA deficiency may also be due to drugs such as phenytoin or penicillamine.

Clinical features

Although selective IgA deficiency is associated with a range of disorders, most IgA-deficient individuals are asymptomatic, possibly because IgM-producing cells provide high local concentrations of IgM antibody or because symptomatic individuals are those who also have deficiency of IgG2 antibodies to polysaccharide antigens.

Gastrointestinal complications (Table 2) *Pernicious anaemia* Selective IgA deficiency is associated with pernicious anaemia. Unlike common variable immunodeficiency, the anaemia conforms to the classical Addisonian type in that atrophic gastritis and raised serum gastrin levels occur.

Malabsorption and steatorrhoea IgA deficiency occurs in about 1 in 40 of patients with coeliac disease, over 15 times more frequently than in the general population. Patients with selective IgA deficiency and a flat jejunal mucosa respond to dietary gluten withdrawal in a way typical of classical coeliac disease.

Antibodies to dietary antigens Secretory IgA helps prevent absorption of food antigens through the intestinal mucosa and there is a high prevalence of serum antibodies to food proteins in patients with selective IgA deficiency. For instance, about a third of IgA-deficient blood donors have serum antibodies to milk compared with 0.3 per cent of healthy controls. IgA-deficient subjects also tend to have autoantibodies to antigens such as collagen and IgA itself (see below).

Gastrointestinal infection With the exception of *G. lamblia* infestation, other infections rarely persist. Even giardiasis is far less frequent than in common variable immunodeficiency. However, in the past, IgA-deficient patients were prone to develop chronic diarrhoea and malabsorption after

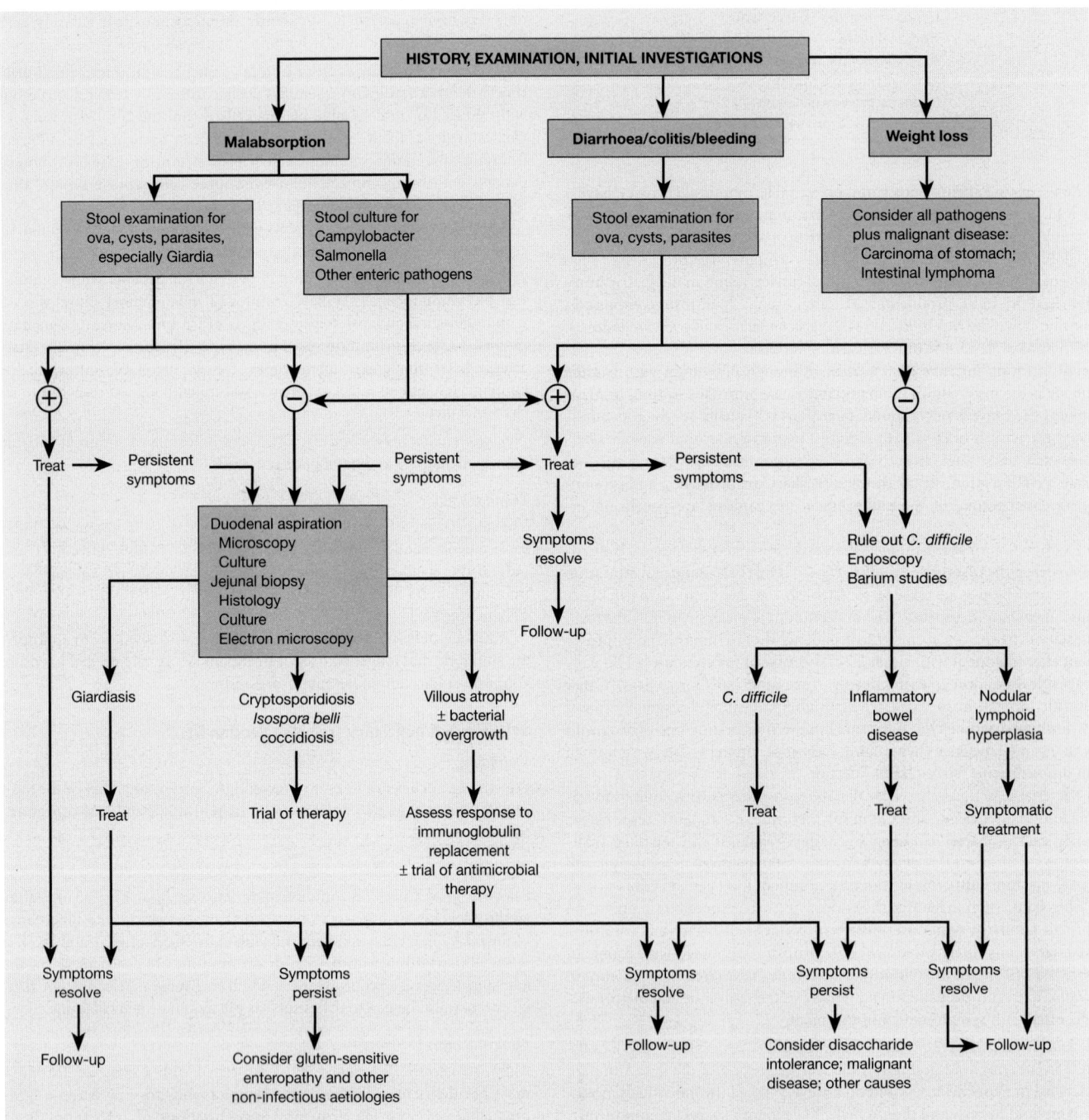

Fig. 2 A scheme for the investigation of gastrointestinal complications in patients with common variable immunodeficiency. (Reproduced from Haeney MR (1989). Gastrointestinal disease in the immunocompromised host. In: Turnberg LA, ed. *Clinical gastroenterology* by permission of Blackwell Science, Oxford.)

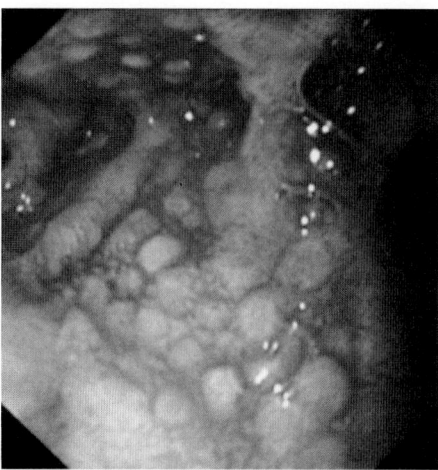

Fig. 3 The appearance of nodular lymphoid hyperplasia on upper gastrointestinal endoscopy. (See also Plate 1.)

truncal vagotomy and gastroenterostomy for duodenal ulceration. This was due to overgrowth of commensal bacteria in the upper intestinal tract, presumably because of the combined effects of deficiency of local antibody production, achlorhydria, and impaired gastrointestinal motility.

Inflammatory bowel disease Crohn's disease and ulcerative colitis occur in patients with IgA deficiency but their frequency is difficult to judge from the widely varying published reports.

Malignant disease Oesophageal, gastric, and colonic neoplasms have been reported but it is not certain whether the risk of malignancy is truly increased.

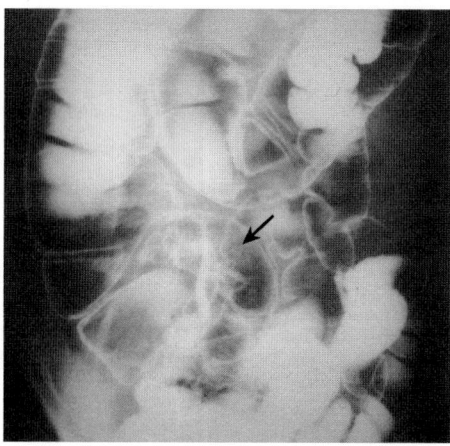

Fig. 4 A double-contrast barium enema showing nodular lymphoid hyperplasia in the terminal ileum (arrowed).

Table 2 Gastrointestinal disorders sometimes associated with selective IgA deficiency.

Infections	Giardiasis, bacterial overgrowth
Autoimmune disease	Pernicious anaemia, antiepithelial cell antibody
Hypersensitivity disorders:	Coeliac disease, cows' milk protein intolerance, inflammatory bowel disease
Neoplasia	Carcinoma of the oesophagus, stomach, colon
Other	Nodular lymphoid hyperplasia, disaccharidase deficiency.

Management

Patients with selective IgA deficiency rarely warrant immunoglobulin replacement therapy, unless IgG2 deficiency is also present. Antibodies to IgA develop in about a third of patients with selective IgA deficiency: high titres of antibodies may cause severe reactions to plasma or blood transfusions or even the trace amounts of IgA present in intravenous immunoglobulin preparations.

Other types of primary immunodeficiency

Gastrointestinal problems occur in other types of immunodeficiency (Table 3) (see Section 5). These conditions are much rarer than primary antibody deficiency. Most defects involving cell-mediated immunity present within the first 6 months of life. Infants with severe combined immunodeficiency, for example, grow and develop normally for a few months but then fail to thrive, frequently with a clinical triad of pneumonia, mucocutaneous candidiasis, and intractable diarrhoea caused by one or more of a range of micro-organisms. Some disorders are associated with unusual gastrointestinal features (Table 3).

Secondary immunodeficiency

Secondary immunodeficiency describes conditions in which the immune defect results from underlying disease and is far more common than primary immunodeficiency. In many cases, the secondary immunodeficiency is of minor relevance to the clinical picture but occasionally its severity may mask the underlying condition. AIDS is a florid example of the gastrointestinal complications seen in patients with secondary defects predominantly involving cell-mediated immunity.

HIV and the gastrointestinal tract

The gastrointestinal tract is a major target organ in HIV infection and AIDS, irrespective of the route of acquisition of the infection. Breast feeding can transmit HIV in humans, implying that the intestine is also an important portal of entry for the virus. In a simian model, severe depletion of CD4+ lymphocytes in the lamina propria and of intraepithelial lymphocytes occurs during primary infection and persists throughout the course of the infection. These dynamic changes in intestinal T lymphocytes are more severe than those seen in blood or peripheral lymph nodes. About half of patients with HIV infection will have gastrointestinal involvement at some time, and any level of the tract, from mouth to anus, can be involved (see also Section 7).

There are three main mechanisms in the pathogenesis of gastrointestinal disease: direct infection of enterocytes by HIV; opportunistic and other infections; and opportunistic tumours (Figs. 5 and 6). A major change in the small intestine is a partial villous atrophy, detectable early in the natural history of HIV infection. Enteropathogens causing intestinal infections are of the same types as in immunocompetent subjects but the infections are much more aggressive and invasive, and elicit little host immune response, so familiar symptoms and signs may be absent. A systematic and thorough search for likely pathogens is essential (Fig. 6). Multiple infections and tumours may coexist, so the organism isolated is not necessarily the cause of the symptoms. Colonic complications increase in frequency as immunodeficiency worsens. Clinically, patients experience diarrhoea, intestinal bleeding, and abdominal pain. Toxic megacolon, intussusception, idiopathic colonic ulceration, and pneumatosis intestinalis have also been described.

The clinical features of HIV infection and AIDS are discussed in detail in Chapter 7.10.21.

Immunodeficiency secondary to gastrointestinal disease

A low serum IgG concentration may be due to increased intestinal loss of immunoglobulin. A useful clue is a low serum albumin because there are no known conditions where immunoglobulin is selectively lost from the gut. The major causes of protein losing enteropathy are discussed in Chapter 14.22.

Intestinal lymphangiectasia (see also Chapter 14.15)
This immunodeficiency results from increased loss of lymphatic fluid containing immunoglobulins and lymphocytes. There is a selective loss of naive T lymphocytes expressing CD4/CD45RA. The basic defect is an abnormal dilatation of the lymphatic vessels in the intestine. There is a primary familial form in children, who present with diarrhoea, malabsorption, and growth retardation. Such children may have abnormal lymphatics elsewhere in the body causing chylous ascites, pleural effusions, and localized areas of oedema. The condition may also occur secondarily to lymphatic obstruction, for example due to intestinal lymphoma or constrictive pericarditis (see Sections 15 and 22). The diagnosis should be suspected when there is T-cell lymphopenia, hypoalbuminaemia, and hypogamma-globulinaemia. The diagnosis is confirmed by finding dilated lymphatics in a jejunal biopsy (Fig. 7). The primary form of the disease responds well to a low-fat diet with additional medium-chain triglycerides. In secondary forms, correction of the underlying disease process is needed.

Food allergy and intolerance

Introduction
Food allergy is one of the most controversial topics in medicine. It undoubtedly exists but extravagant claims that a staggering array of symptoms are due to food 'allergy' have confused the subject. Such claims are too rarely supported by objective, scientific observations and have provoked a sceptical response from many doctors. The major cause of confusion lies in the lack of agreement on definitions and diagnostic criteria.

Table 3 Gastrointestinal disease in selected types of primary immunodeficiency. (Reproduced from Haeney MR (1989). Gastrointestinal disease in the immunocompromised host. In: Turnberg LA, ed, *Clinical gastroenterology*, Ch.16, pp. 371-55, by permission of Blackwell Scientific Publications, Oxford)

Condition	Functional defect	Typical age at presentation	Major clinical features	Gastrointestinal complications
X-linked lymphoproliferative syndrome	Inherited vulnerability to infection with Epstein–Barr virus	Childhood	Fatal or chronic infectious mononucleosis. Aplastic anaemia. Hypo-gammaglobulinaemia. Malignant B-cell lymphoma	As for antibody deficiency. Malignant lymphoma of the terminal ileum
Severe combined immunodeficiency	Impairment of cell-mediated immunity and antibody production sometimes associated with inherited deficiency of the enzyme adenosine deaminase	Infancy	Wide spectrum of infection. Non-immunological features in subtypes	Chronic oral and intestinal candidiasis. Persistent diarrhoea due to rotavirus, cytomegalovirus, other viruses, cryptosporidium, *Campylobacter*, *Salmonella*
CD40 ligand deficiency (hyper IgM syndrome)	Defective interaction between T and B lymphocytes: failure to switch from IgM to IgG production. Defective interaction between T cells and macrophages	Infancy	Impaired antibody production. Neutropenia. Suspectibility to *Pneumocystis carinii* pneumonia and cryptosporidiosis	Persistent cryptosporidiosis. Ascending cholangitis and cirrhosis
Di George anomaly (a catch 22 syndrome with Chromosome 22q 11 deletions)	Impairment of cell-mediated immunity and antibody production (non-familial)	From birth	Hypoparathyroidism: tetany and convulsions. Cardiovascular defects. Immunodeficiency. Abnormal facies	Oesophageal atresia. Chronic intestinal candidiasis. Diarrhoea of uncertain aetiology
Wiskott–Aldrich syndrome	Progressive impairment of antibody production and cell-mediated immunity	Infancy or early childhood	Thrombocytopenia: bleeding. Eczema. Immunodeficiency. Malignant disease	Bloody diarrhoea. Food allergic disease. Intestinal lymphoma
Chronic granulomatous disease	Defective neutrophil killing of catalase-producing organisms (often X linked)	Infancy	Severe skin sepsis due to *Staphylococcus aureus*, fungi, Gram-negative bacilli. Lymphadenopathy. Hepatosplenomegaly. Deep abscesses	Diarrhoea and steatorrhoea with PAS-positive histiocytes in the lamina propria
Chronic mucocutaneous candidiasis	Imparied cell-mediated immunity to *Candida albicans*	Childhood	Chronic *Candida* infection of mucous membranes, nails, skin. Associated endocrinopathy: Addison's disease, hypoparathyroidism, diabetes mellitus, thyroiditis	Chronic oral and intestinal candidiasis
Defective yeast opsonization	Impaired complement function	Infancy	None	Protracted diarrhoea of uncertain cause

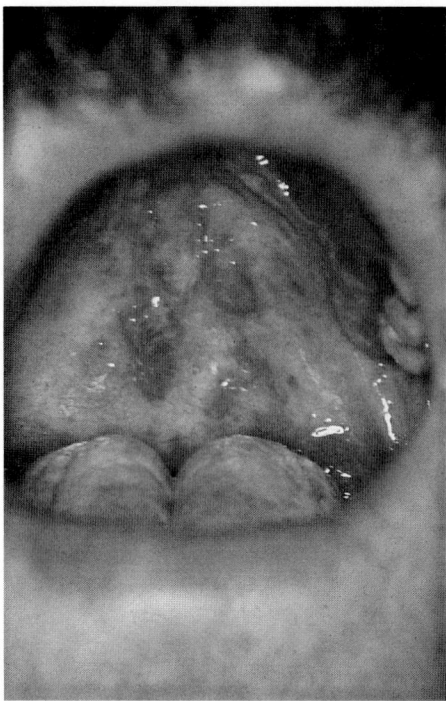

Fig. 5 Kaposi's sarcoma of the oral cavity in a patient with AIDS.

Definition

Food allergy refers to a form of exaggerated reactivity (hypersensitivity) of the immune system to an ingested antigen. The term should be used only when the abnormal reaction is proved to be immunologically mediated, either by IgE or some other immune mechanism (Table 4). The term food intolerance should be used to describe all abnormal, reproducible reactions to food when the causative mechanism is unknown or is non-immunological. Food allergy and intolerance must be distinguished from food fads and psychological aversion to foods.

Aetiology

Food allergy

Although the gut provides a physical barrier to the antigen load in the lumen, up to 2 per cent of a protein meal can appear antigenically intact in the circulation. This was shown by injecting serum from a patient with known sensitivity to fish into the skin of a normal subject. A wheal and flare response at the skin test site (positive Prausnitz–Kustner reaction) was observed shortly after the normal subject ate the appropriate antigen, showing that this must have crossed the gut and triggered IgE-sensitized mast cells at the skin test site.

Atopic individuals have a higher prevalence of food allergy. The allergic components of foods are mainly glycoproteins with molecular weights between 10 and 70 kDa and most are heat stable and resistant to proteolysis, with the exception of those causing the oral allergy syndrome (see below).

In some forms of food allergy, damage involves immune mechanisms other than IgE. For instance, in coeliac disease there is strong evidence that exaggerated local T-cell mediated reactivity to dietary gluten causes the villous atrophy.

Food intolerance

Non-immunological mechanisms of reproducible, adverse reactions to food are much more common and include irritant, toxic, pharmacological, or metabolic effects of foods, enzyme deficiencies, or even the release of substances produced by fermentation of food residues in the bowel. Some foods contain pharmacologically active substances (such as tyramine or phenylethylamine) that act directly on blood vessels in sensitive subjects to

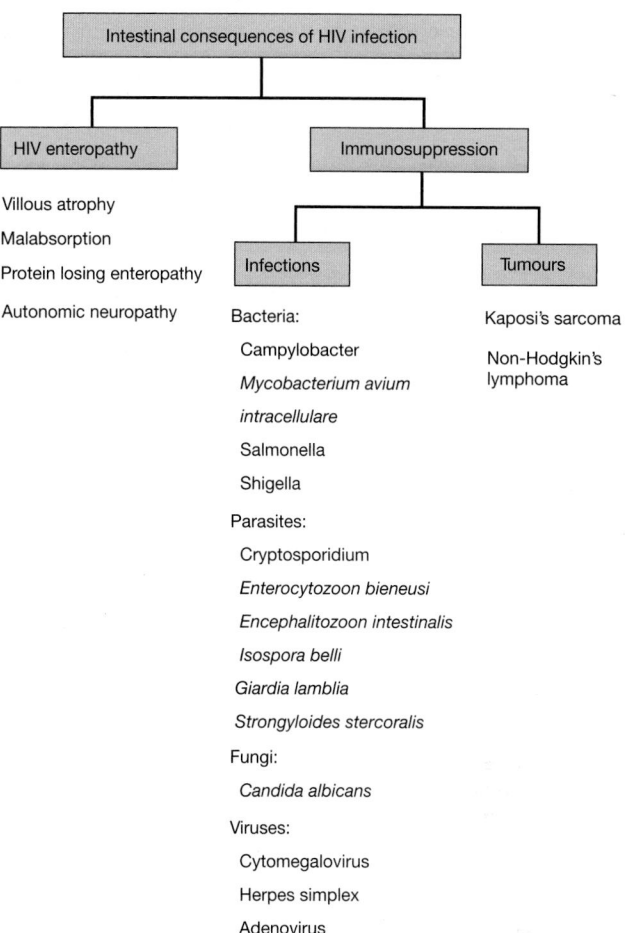

Fig. 6 Gastrointestinal consequences of HIV infection. (Redrawn from Chapel HM *et al.* (1999). *Essentials of clinical immunology*, 4th edn, by permission of the authors and Blackwell Science, Oxford.)

produce migraine. Traces of drugs, food additives (for example monosodium glutamate), colouring agents (for example tartrazine), or preservatives (for example benzoic acid) can also cause symptoms in susceptible people by mechanisms which are ill understood, but are probably due to direct effects on mast cells.

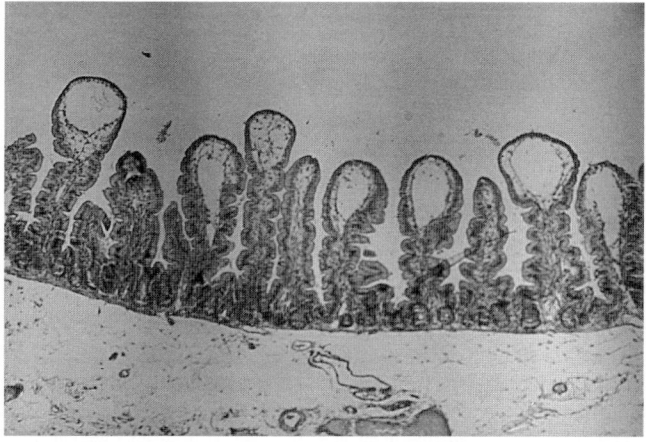

Fig. 7 A jejunal biopsy from a patient with intestinal lymphangiectasia showing dilated central lacteals.

Table 4 Classification of adverse reactions to foods

Reproducible adverse reaction on food challenge		Immune mechanism		Non-immune mechanism	
Open	Blind	IgE	Other		Examples
Food allergy					
+	+	+	–	–	Immediate reactions to nuts, eggs, milk shellfish, fish
+	+	–	+	–	Coeliac disease, cows' milk protein intolerance
Food intolerance					
+	+	–	?	+	Irritable bowel syndrome (some), food induced migraine, reactions to sulphites, nitrites, food additives
Food aversion					
+	–	–	–	–	

Prevalence

The general public perceives food allergy to be a major health problem but epidemiological studies do not support this view. Food allergy affects 2 to 5 per cent of children under 5 years but only 1 per cent of adults. In one survey of 7500 households in the United Kingdom, about 20 per cent of the sample reported a food intolerance but this was confirmed by double-blind, placebo-controlled food challenge in only 1.4 per cent. However, the prevalence of peanut allergy appears to have increased significantly over the last 20 years.

Reactions to food additives, while they exist, are also not as common as most people believe. In a second population study in the United Kingdom, 7.4 per cent had symptoms suggestive of intolerance to food additives; further clinical assessment and additive challenge showed a true prevalence of 0.01 to 0.23 per cent.

Clinical features

Food reactions can be early or late, confined to the gastrointestinal tract or occur at sites remote from the gut (Fig. 8).

Gut-related symptoms

About 75 per cent of young children, but only 10 per cent of adults, present with local gastrointestinal symptoms of food intolerance.

Early reactions These are often 'immediate' in onset, occurring within minutes or up to 2 h after ingestion, recur on challenge testing, and include, apart from gastrointestinal disturbances, such features as perioral rash, angioedema of the lips or tongue, tingling of the throat, urticaria, asthma, or even anaphylaxis. Such acute and severe allergic reactions are mostly due to IgE antibodies to foods and are the least controversial form of food allergy. They are fairly easy to diagnose and the offending food is readily identified, usually by the parent: although any food may be responsible, 90 per cent of reactions are caused by cows' milk (in infants), peanuts, tree nuts, eggs, fish, and shellfish. Peanut is the most allergenic food known and peanut allergy is lifelong.

In some cases, anaphylaxis only occurs when the food is eaten 2 to 4 h before exercise, so-called food-dependent, exercise-induced anaphylaxis.

Allergy to latex rubber is increasingly common and several high-risk groups are recognized, notably patients with spina bifida or multiple uro-logical procedures, and health care workers. Latex allergy may crossreact with plant defence proteins, called chitinases, in foods, typically melon, banana, avocado, chestnut, celery, passion fruit, or peach.

Oral allergy syndrome describes itching and lip swelling without involvement of other target organs. It occurs in patients with pollen allergy and is due to crossreactivity with epitopes in fresh (but not cooked) fruits and vegetables such as apples, carrots, hazelnuts, kiwi fruit, or raw potatoes.

Allergic eosinophilic gastroenteritis is characterized by intolerance to multiple foods, eosinophilic infiltration of the stomach and small intestine, peripheral eosinophilia, and positive skin prick tests and radioallergosorbent tests (see below) to foods.

Late reactions Symptoms occurring over 2 h after food ingestion, such as diarrhoea, bloating, or a fatty stool are suggestive of food intolerance, if not allergy. Features of the irritable bowel syndrome (see below) may be accompanied by allergic symptoms elsewhere but usually occur in isolation and without any evidence of an immunological reaction.

Remote symptoms

Some patients with acute, IgE-mediated reactions to foods also experience rhinitis, asthma, urticaria, angioedema, or eczema. However, eating the implicated foods does not always cause these remote systems. Sneezing bouts, blocked nose, or asthma can also occur after taking wine or other alcoholic drinks because of the irritant effect of sulphite preservatives or other components. This is not an immunological reaction. Many patients with atopic eczema find that certain foods provoke a transient red and blotchy rash but it is mainly in children that food makes eczema worse. Elimination diets rarely improve atopic eczema in adults.

What is more debatable is whether food intolerance plays any part in remote symptoms such as hyperactivity/attention deficit disorder, enuresis, or arthritis.

Specific syndromes of food allergy

Food allergy contributes to a number of common intestinal disorders where the immunological mechanisms are not IgE mediated.

Coeliac disease

The characteristic histological lesion in untreated cases of coeliac disease (see Chapter 14.9.4) is loss of normal villi and a marked increase in the

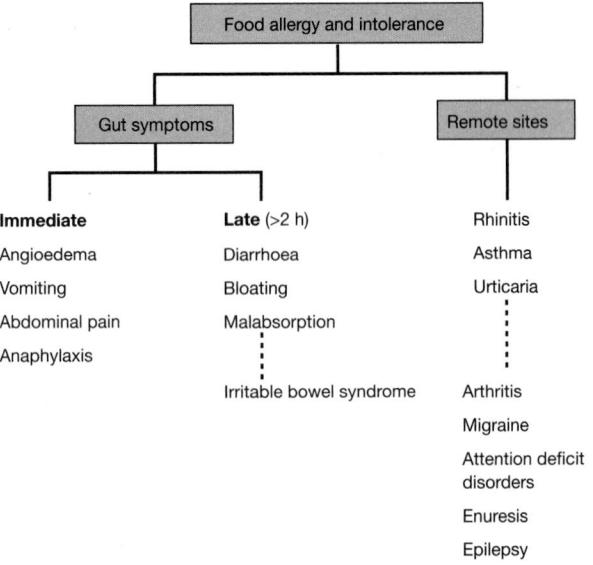

Fig. 8 Clinical spectrum of food allergy and intolerance. (Redrawn from Chapel HM *et al.* (1999). *Essentials of clinical immunology*, 4th edn, by permission of the authors and Blackwell Science, Oxford.)

numbers of CD8+ intraepithelial lymphocytes, particularly those expressing the γ/δ T-cell receptor. It is believed that HLA class II molecules on antigen-presenting cells expose processed peptides from ingested wheat gliadin to immunocompetent T cells. Gliadin-specific, HLA DQ2-restricted T cells have been isolated from small intestinal biopsies of coeliac patients. T-cell infiltration of the small bowel epithelium is seen within hours of gluten exposure and resolves on treatment with a gluten-free diet, strongly suggesting that intestinal damage is due to a T-cell mediated reaction to gluten.

Cows' milk protein enteropathy

Milk proteins can cause a malabsorption syndrome similar to coeliac disease. Cows' milk protein enteropathy in babies causes failure to thrive, diarrhoea, malabsorption, and even intestinal bleeding and colitis. Jejunal biopsies show villous atrophy and lymphocytic infiltration.

Symptoms disappear when cows' milk is removed from the diet. Reintroduction of cows' milk causes a recurrence of symptoms. After a viral gastrointestinal infection, cows' milk may also be poorly tolerated for a while because of a temporary inability to digest lactose. Thus, in babies and small children with chronic gastrointestinal symptoms and failure to gain weight, trials (under medical supervision) of milk exclusion are justified and the diagnosis can usually be confirmed by food challenge. Recovery often occurs within a few months.

Recognized syndromes of food intolerance

In some conditions, a relationship to foods can be convincingly demonstrated in a proportion of patients. Sometimes, symptoms are provoked by the known irritant, pharmacological, or metabolic effects of food.

Irritable bowel syndrome

Irritable bowel syndrome is a descriptive term for several conditions that produce a similar range of abdominal symptoms (see Chapter 14.13). Irritable bowel syndrome is characterized by alternating constipation and diarrhoea, abdominal bloating, and colicky pain. In a variant of this disorder, however, constipation predominates and gastrointestinal transit times are greatly increased. Most cases are unrelated to food intolerance but in a minority of patients—usually those with predominant diarrhoea, with some bloating and pain—a relationship to specific foods can be demonstrated. Some patients who improve on a restricted diet are able to identify certain foods, notably cereals and dairy products, that provoke symptoms when reintroduced. However, not all gastroenterologists are convinced of a causal relationship between food and irritable bowel syndrome.

Lactose intolerance (see Chapter 11.3)

Many adults cannot digest lactose because of a deficiency of the enzyme lactase. In them, undigested sugar is fermented in the lower bowel, causing diarrhoea and wind. Lactose intolerance is not common in Europeans but affects up to 90 per cent of adult Africans and Orientals. It can also occur as a transient result of gastroenteritis and even as a secondary effect of cows' milk protein intolerance. This can cause confusion in diagnosis unless a lactose challenge is performed separately from a cows' milk protein challenge.

Fructose intolerance

This is discussed in Chapter 11.3.

Miscellaneous syndromes

Migraine and headache Coffee and coffee withdrawal can provoke migraine in susceptible people. Certain cheeses cause headaches in many people, probably due to their tyramine or phenylethylamine content. Red wines, especially port, cause headaches in susceptible people because of their content of congeners.

Asthma Foods preserved by sulphites, particularly white wine, dried fruit, and fruit salads in supermarkets and restaurants, sometimes provoke asthma by the release of sulphur dioxide.

Urticaria While IgE-mediated food allergy causes acute urticaria and angioedema, allergy rarely induces chronic urticaria. However, food dyes and preservatives often trigger chronic urticaria in sensitive subjects.

Chinese restaurant syndrome Monosodium glutamate, used to enhance flavour in food and found in large amounts in Chinese food, may cause a syndrome of chest pain, sweating, nausea, dizziness, and fainting in susceptible individuals. However, double-blind studies have not convincingly demonstrated that monosodium glutamate is the culprit.

Controversial issues

Behavioural problems in children

The belief that foods and food additives can induce behavioural problems, particularly attention deficit disorder, is a controversial one. A diet free of preservatives, salicylates, and artificial flavours has been claimed to benefit up to 70 per cent of such children but most well-designed, double blind, placebo controlled challenges have failed to support a causal link. Children with behavioural disorders may improve temporarily for a few weeks when given a diet avoiding food additives but this appears to be a placebo effect. Parents who suspect food additive intolerance in their child may insist on maintaining the child on a restrictive diet, even when dietary challenges prove negative. Extreme examples have been termed 'Munchausen's syndrome by proxy'.

Psychological distress in adults

Some patients with a multiplicity of vague and variable symptoms, such as unexplained fatigue and malaise, and disturbances of sleep, appetite, or libido turn to the diagnosis of food allergy as an explanation. Only a few have clearcut psychiatric illness, others inadvertently cause symptoms by overbreathing or by somatizing their psychological distress. Having made their own diagnosis of food allergy, they have difficulty in accepting they are not allergic to foods, even though their food aversions may have resulted in a dangerously inadequate diet. They will frequently seek out practitioners who are prepared to endorse their views, whether valid or not. Early diagnosis and sympathetic management is essential if unnecessary consultations and inappropriate allergy tests are to be avoided.

Diagnosis

Food allergy should not be diagnosed without clear indications, as needless dietary restrictions can seriously disrupt not only the patient's life but also the whole family and may occasionally cause malnutrition. No test can replace a careful clinical history and thorough examination to exclude other, sometimes more likely, causes of the patient's symptoms.

Skin tests and radioallergosorbent tests

Skin prick tests and radioallergosorbent tests for detecting serum IgE antibodies are positive in about 75 per cent of patients who have IgE-mediated, acute, early reactions to foods such as nuts, egg, or fish. Usually, the offending antigen is obvious from the clinical history and confirmatory tests are needed only if there is clinical doubt. In patients with late symptoms at sites remote from the gut (Fig. 6), skin and blood tests are notoriously unreliable for many reasons:

(1) Foods, as antigen sources, are poorly standardized and contain multiple, ill-defined antigens.

(2) The antigen content of the food will depend on whether it is raw or cooked.

(3) Some foods cause non-specific ('irritant'), positive skin reactions.

(4) Patients may have IgE antibodies but no symptoms.

(5) Food reactions can be mediated by mechanisms other than IgE antibodies.

For most patients with suspected food intolerance, laboratory tests are of little diagnostic value.

Elimination diets and challenge tests

In the absence of reliable laboratory tests, elimination diets and food challenge form the basis of diagnosis. To minimize bias and suggestion, the relationship between food and symptoms should be established by a placebo controlled, double blind challenge under medical supervision. In some cases, for example in chronic urticaria or when the symptoms are mild and largely subjective, it may be necessary to repeat the challenge before accepting that the association is not simply coincidental. In several series, only a quarter of reported 'adverse reactions' can be confirmed by double blind challenge. Although these rules are simple to state, they are difficult to carry out in practice. However, the alternative is that of prolonged, unsupervised, dietary manipulation, usually self-imposed or inflicted by parents on their children, with the attendant risks.

Food challenges are not without risk: there is a danger of precipitating an anaphylactic reaction. This is well-recognized in children with relatively mild symptoms of food intolerance, who develop anaphylaxis when the food, often cows' milk, is reintroduced after a period of avoidance.

Bogus or unproven laboratory tests

The absence of reliable laboratory tests has led to the promotion of controversial 'alternative' tests: these are at best misleading and at worst dangerous. New diagnostic procedures, like new drugs, require scientific validation: they must be reliable and reproducible. When presented with coded, duplicate samples, some 'alternative' laboratories in the United Kingdom were unable reliably to identify food allergies in patients known to have them; they gave inconsistent results for paired samples from the same patient; they reported many allergies in non-allergic subjects; and they often gave dubious and risky dietary advice.

Provocation-neutralization testing This has been critically evaluated by the Royal College of Physicians of London, the American College of Physicians, and the California Medical Association: these bodies concluded that reported studies were seriously flawed and that the method lacked scientific validity. Under double blind conditions, the response of patients to active and control injections appeared to be due to suggestion and chance.

Leucocytotoxic testing This involves incubating a patient's leucocytes with various food extracts and inspecting the cells for damage. The high number of false positive and false negative results led the American Academy of Allergy to conclude that there was no evidence that the test was effective in diagnosis of food allergy.

Other tests Hair analysis, applied kinesiology, radionics, radiaesthesia, psionic medicine, and auriculocardiac reflex testing have never been objectively evaluated and are more a matter of gullibility and faith than science. Electrodermal (Vega) testing does not correlate with skin prick testing and cannot distinguish atopic from non-atopic individuals.

Treatment

Dietary management

Recognition of the offending food and its elimination from the diet is the cornerstone of treatment. In patients with acute IgE-mediated reactions to a single food, such as shellfish, this is usually straightforward. Patients with anaphylactic reactions to foods need to be careful to avoid accidental exposure. A problem for such patients is the use of a food, most notably nuts, as an undeclared or 'hidden' ingredient in manufactured foods or restaurant meals. Where there remains a risk of accidental ingestion it may be appropriate for some patients to carry a preloaded syringe of adrenaline (epinephrine) for self-injection.

In less clearcut situations, certain foods or food additives are eliminated empirically because they are frequently implicated in that form of food intolerance: for example, a diet free of cereal grains and dairy products may be beneficial in certain patients with irritable bowel syndrome, while a diet free of azodyes, preservatives, and salicylates helps a proportion of patients with chronic intractable urticaria.

Patients who seem intolerant of a wide range of foods may need a very restricted diet, sometimes called a 'few-food' diet. If symptoms are improved, then foods can be reintroduced one at a time. This is both diagnostic and therapeutic, but care is essential as anaphylaxis can occur on reintroduction, especially in children. Expert advice from specially trained dietitians is essential to avoid nutritional deficiency.

Sodium cromoglycate

Oral sodium cromoglycate has been used as an adjunct to diet in selected patients with food allergy, especially those with accompanying allergic reactions in the eyes, nose, and skin. Its effectiveness is still unproven.

Immunotherapy

Although immunotherapy (hyposensitzation) is effective in wasp or bee venom anaphylaxis and in some forms of allergy to inhaled allergens, it has never been evaluated scientifically in food intolerance. There is considerable interest in future immunization with peptides containing T-cell epitopes.

'Alternative' therapies

Provocation-neutralization therapy and enzyme-potentiated desensitization are two treatments used by 'alternative' practitioners: neither is of proven value, although both induce significant placebo responses.

Food allergy seems particularly vulnerable in inducing unorthodox treatments which have not been scientifically validated by double blind, placebo controlled trials or confirmed by independent investigators. The hazard of the unconventional approach to therapy is that potentially serious problems can be misdiagnosed and mistreated.

Further reading

Ament ME, Ochs HD, Davis SD (1973). Structure and function of the gastrointestinal tract in primary immunodeficiency syndromes. A study of 39 patients. *Medicine (Baltimore)* 52, 227–48.

Barrett S (2000). www.quackwatch.com.

Blanshard C (1999). Gastrointestinal manifestations of HIV infection. *Hospital Medicine* 60, 24–8.

Burks AW, Stanley JS (1998). Food allergy. *Current Opinion in Pediatrics* 10, 588–93.

Corley DA, Cello JP, Koch J (1999). Evaluation of upper gastrointestinal tract symptoms in patients with HIV. *American Journal of Gastroenterology* 94, 2890–6.

David TJ (1993). *Food and food additive intolerance in childhood.* Blackwell Scientific, Oxford.

Ernst PB et al. (1999). Regulation of the mucosal immune response. *American Journal of Tropical Medicine and Hygiene* 60, 2–9.

Frieri M, Kettelhutt BV, eds (1999). *Food hypersensitivity and adverse reactions.* Marcel Dekker, New York.

Haeney MR (1994). Diagnostic tests in allergic disease. In: Spickett GP, Lewin I, eds. *Current themes in allergy and immunology,* pp 1–7. Royal College of Physicians, London.

Hein WR (1999). Organization of mucosal lymphoid tissue. *Current Topics in Microbiology and Immunology* 236, 1–15.

Jewett DL, Fein G, Greenberg MH (1990). A double-blind study of symptom provocation to determine food sensitivity. *New England Journal of Medicine* 323, 429–33.

Lewith GT et al. (2001). Is electrodermal testing as efficient as skin prick tests for diagnosing allergies? A double blind, randomised block design study. *British Medical Journal* 322, 131–4.

Royal College of Physicians (1992). *Allergy. Conventional and alternative concepts.* Royal College of Physicians, London.

So ALP, Mayer L (1997). Gastrointestinal manifestations of primary immunodeficiency disorders. *Seminars in Gastrointestinal Disease* 8, 22–32.

Strobel S, Mowat AM (1998). Immune responses to dietary antigens: oral tolerance. *Immunology Today* 19, 173–81.

Teahon K *et al.* (1994). Studies on the enteropathy associated with primary hypogammaglobulinaemia. *Gut* **35**, 1244–9.

Viney JL, Fong S (1998). β7 integrins and their ligands in lymphocyte migration to the gut. *Chemical Immunology* **71**, 64–76.

Young E *et al.* (1994). A population study of food intolerance. *The Lancet* **343**, 1127–30.

Zullo A *et al.* (1999). Gastric pathology in patients with common variable immunodeficiency. *Gut* **45**, 77–81.

14.5 The mouth and salivary glands

T. Lehner

Dental caries and sequelae

Aetiology

Dental decay or caries is a very common chronic disease and causes much pain and discomfort. Caries is most frequent in children and young adults. It affects the pits and fissures of the occlusal surfaces, and the enamel of the approximal surfaces of teeth. Root caries (at the neck of the tooth) occurs later in life. Caries is an infection caused by the aggregation of bacteria on the surface of the tooth, referred to as dental plaque.

The development of dental caries requires the presence of cariogenic bacteria that produce acid below the critical pH (5.5) required for dissolving enamel and sugar in the diet that can be metabolized by bacteria. *Streptococcus mutans*, *Streptococcus sanguis*, *Lactobacillus acidophilus*, *Lactobacillus casei*, and *Actinomyces viscosus* are cariogenic. However, *S. mutans* appears to be the most efficient cariogenic organism. Germ-free studies have clearly shown that *S. mutans* induces caries rapidly in the absence of other organisms; it is a facultative anaerobic, non-haemolytic, acidogenic organism, producing extracellular and intracellular polysaccharides. The organism fulfils Koch's postulates as a cause of dental caries.

The most common carbohydrates in our diet are starch and sucrose, with smaller amounts of glucose, fructose, and lactose. However, the most important substrate in humans is sucrose. Sucrose gives rise to heavy plaque formation, with considerable amounts of extracellular polysaccharide. The most important polysaccharide is dextran (glucan), which is synthesized in large amounts by the constitutive enzyme glucosyltransferase (dextran-sucrase). Dextran allows plaque to stick to the surface of the enamel.

Streptococci do not possess a cytochrome system but contain glycolytic enzymes which will convert glucose to lactic and other organic acids. The pH inside the plaque may fall within 2 to 3 min of rinsing the mouth with glucose or sucrose from a level of about 6.5 to 5; the critical pH below which decalcification of enamel occurs is thought to be about 5.5. Caries is the end result of a complex sequence of microbial and biochemical processes terminating in acid formation.

Pathology

Caries develops as a result of acid formed by the bacterial plaque acting on sucrose. The enamel becomes demineralized and plaque bacteria penetrate along the enamel prisms. This process progresses slowly through the enamel layer, but once the dentine is reached, destruction by decalcification and proteolysis of the dentine is rapid. The pulp reacts by an acute inflammatory response that results in necrosis, as the pulp is enclosed within the rigid walls of the tooth and the exudate cannot expand to adjacent tissues. Eventually, infection and toxic materials spread from the opening of the root canal to the tissues around the apex of the tooth and induce periapical inflammatory changes, which may terminate in an acute or chronic abscess or a chronic granuloma. If epithelial proliferation takes place within the granuloma or abscess, then a cyst may develop, which will increase in size over many years before it may be revealed clinically. A dental abscess represents a mixed infection with a variety of streptococci, staphylococci, and other organisms.

The immunological changes are complex, but serum IgG, IgA, and IgM antibodies, as well as cell-mediated immunity to *S. mutans*, can be correlated with the DMF (**D**ecayed, **M**issing, and **F**illed teeth) index of caries. Salivary IgA antibodies are also found. Although humans have the potential to mount humoral and cellular immune responses to *S. mutans* under natural conditions, the immunity achieved is commonly ineffective. Immunization experiments with *S. mutans* have been successfully carried out in rats and monkeys, with a significant reduction in caries. There are two principal immunological mechanisms of protection against caries. One involves salivary IgA antibodies, which can be induced by direct immunization of the minor salivary glands or by immunization of the gut-associated lymphoid tissue, from where sensitized B cells may home to the salivary glands. Salivary antibodies may prevent *S. mutans* from adhering to the tooth surface and thereby prevent caries. The alternative mechanism involves all the humoral and cellular components elicited by systemic immunization. Antibodies, complement, polymorphonuclear leucocytes, lymphocytes, and macrophages pass from the gingival blood vessels to the gingival domain of the tooth. Bacterial colonization of the tooth can therefore be influenced by systemic immunity and an important mechanism is probably that of IgG-induced opsonization, binding, phagocytosis, and killing of *S. mutans* by phagocytes.

Clinical features

The patient complains of toothache aggravated by hot or cold drinks or food. The throbbing pain becomes progressively worse, affects the patient especially at night, and may radiate to the face and ear. If relief is not sought the pain becomes excruciating in intensity, and the tooth becomes tender to bite on. This will be followed by death of the dental pulp and the development of an acute swelling due to an abscess or cellulitis. With an acute abscess the inflammatory exudate may penetrate through the bone to the soft tissues. Whilst the pain is reduced the oedematous swelling of the face increases, and if the upper canine is involved the swelling spreads to the eyelid and may present an alarming appearance. The regional lymph nodes are tender and enlarged and there may be fever and some malaise.

Much less commonly a cellulitis or infection by β-haemolytic streptococci may give rise to a spreading infection along the fascial planes, especially of the submaxillary and sublingual spaces. The inflammatory exudate may occasionally spread along the parapharyngeal spaces into the loose connective tissue of the glottis causing oedema of the glottis and respiratory obstruction. The attendant brawny swelling of the neck and floor and the mouth, difficulty in swallowing, trismus, fever, and malaise is referred to as Ludwig's angina. An alternative chronic course is the development of a chronic pulpitis, granuloma, abscess, and eventually cyst around the apex of the offending tooth, and these may proceed without symptoms or only slight discomfort.

Although the patient may point out the painful tooth this can be misleading because the pain often radiates to adjacent teeth. The offending tooth is located by finding the caries, most commonly in the pits and fissures of the occlusal surfaces or the approximal surfaces of adjacent teeth. The tooth responds with pain on application of a hot or cold stimulus, and later is tender to percussion and may be discoloured. Dental radiographs will confirm or localize the carious tooth and, at a later stage, periapical pathological changes.

Treatment

The principles of treatment are to remove the caries, apply a non-irritant material such as zinc oxide and eugenol dressing to protect the pulp, and then restore the tooth with a filling. The most common filling material is dental amalgam which contains mercury. Public anxiety has been aroused by anecdotal evidence that amalgam fillings are toxic and can cause poor memory and lassitude or even multiple sclerosis. There is, however, no scientific evidence to justify these claims, though as a precautionary measure, the United Kingdom Department of Health recommends that mercury-containing amalgam fillings should not be used in pregnant women. The alternatives to amalgam are a number of composite filling materials. If the pulp is damaged irreversibly it will have to be extirpated and root-canal therapy instituted. The alternative to conservative treatment is extraction of the offending tooth. A dental abscess is effectively dealt with by extraction of the diseased tooth, for this removes the source of infection and drains the pus.

If the tooth is to be saved, the pus is drained by an intraoral incision and/or establishing drainage through the root canal. Antibiotics are usually given for acute abscesses and oral penicillin such as phenoxymethylpenicillin, 250 mg four times a day for about 7 days, is adequate. Cellulitis should first be treated by intramuscular penicillin in the form of benzylpenicillin, 1 megaunit (MU) four times a day. The swelling should then be incised to relieve the pressure and provide drainage; extraction of the tooth under general anaesthesia should take place as soon as the patient's condition permits.

Prevention of dental caries is best practised by careful plaque removal by the individual, and by limiting the intake of sugar, especially the frequent consumption of sweets and sweetened drinks. The type of toothpaste used matters less than the method of tooth brushing, though fluoride in toothpaste decreases the incidence of caries in children by up to 40 per cent. Water fluoridation, however, is the most effective public health preventive measure. One part per million of fluoride in the drinking water will decrease the incidence of caries in children by up to 60 per cent. There is no evidence of toxicity from water fluoridation. The ethical and scientific issues of water fluoridation are complex and have been the subject of a report by the Royal College of Physicians of London.

Differential diagnosis

Toothache occasionally needs to be carefully differentiated from sinusitis and neuralgia. Throbbing pain that is exacerbated by thermal stimuli and is more severe at night is an important diagnostic feature. An abscess or cellulitis caused by dental caries has been confused with mumps, although mumps is confined predominantly to the parotid fascia, earache may be a prominent feature, and pain is elicited by pulling on the ear lobe. A chronic granuloma or a dental cyst are usually diagnosed radiologically, unless the cyst becomes large and a swelling becomes clinically evident.

Course and prognosis

The acute sequence of events from dental caries is acute pulpitis, periodontitis, resulting in an abscess or cellulitis. If treated promptly the sequelae can be prevented, but if not treated the patient will lose the tooth and may develop facial scarring due to a discharging sinus. With slow progression of caries or incomplete removal of decay chronic pulpitis may supervene followed by chronic periadenitis, which may result in a periapical granuloma,

abscess, or cyst. Dental caries is in most instances a progressive condition and can be halted only by a dental surgeon.

Gingival and periodontal disease

Aetiology

A mild inflammation of the gingiva (gum) and slight destruction of the collagen fibres of the periodontal membrane are found in most adults. Advanced destruction of the periodontal membrane, including the supporting bone, is found in about half of the middle-aged or older population. A close association has been found between accumulation of bacterial plaque and gingivitis. During this process a change occurs from a predominantly Gram-positive coccal form of plaque to a complex population of filamentous organisms, spirochaetes, vibrios, and Gram-negative cocci. Of the Gram-positive organisms, *Actinomyces viscosus* appears to be involved in the development of gingivitis. Gram-negative organisms are thought to be essential in the development of periodontal disease. *Porphyromonas gingivalis*, *Actinobacillus actinomycetemcomitans*, *Fusobacteria* and *Capnocytophaga* spp. have been implicated in this disease. The cell walls of the Gram-negative organisms contain lipopolysaccharides and those of the Gram-positive organisms have lipoteichoic acids, dextrans or levans, which may be responsible for a variety of immunological functions.

The causative factors responsible for periodontal disease are not known, but bacterial plaque is thought to be involved. There are two views concerning the microbial aetiology: that the non-specific mixed organisms in dental plaque are responsible for the development of periodontal disease or that specific organisms are responsible. The hypothesis of specific microbial aetiology has received support from observations that *P. gingivalis* is the predominant organism isolated from periodontal disease. Furthermore, a specific but rare type of juvenile and rapidly progressing adult periodontitis is associated with *A. actinomycetemcomitans*. Invasiveness of these microorganisms probably plays an important part in their virulence, and some of the periodontopathic bacteria can be found in the gingiva of adult as well as juvenile periodontitis. However, innate and acquired host factors may be more important than bacteria in determining the development of periodontal disease.

Dental plaque may calcify, especially in adults and the elderly, to produce calculus. This is often found on the lingual surface of the lower incisors and the buccal surface of the upper molars, i.e. opposite the orifices of the major salivary glands. Chronic gingival inflammation may persist for many years and breakdown of the periodontal membrane, with loss of the supporting bone, may follow and increase in severity over the years. This is referred to as periodontitis, or 'pyorrhoea' as it used to be called, and is the most important cause of loss of teeth after the age of 40, when the incidence of dental caries has greatly diminished. An important feature of periodontitis is that it affects many teeth, and may result in complete loss of the dentition. As mentioned above, a very rare type of rapid destruction of the supporting dental tissues is found in children or young adults and is referred to as juvenile periodontitis; one or more teeth may become mobile and may be lost before 21 years of age.

Pathology

There are four immunopathological stages:

1. The initial lesion is found in the normal clinical state, with a localized inflammatory response of polymorphonuclear leucocytes; complement activation and chemotaxis generated by plaque antigens and possibly immune complexes may account for this stage.

2. The early lesion shows a localized infiltration of predominantly T with a few B lymphocytes. In the circulation, lymphocytes are sensitized at this stage to plaque antigens.

3. The established lesion is characterized by a localized plasma cell infiltration and peripheral blood lymphocytes can be stimulated to proliferate by plaque antigens. This stage can persist for years, with early pocket formation.
4. The advanced lesion marks the transition to a destructive immunopathological mechanism, with ulceration of the pocket epithelium and localized destruction of collagen and bone.

Periodontitis is a progressively destructive process leading to loss of teeth. The immunological processes are complex, and cytokines may play a significant role, especially raised levels of tumour necrosis factor-α, interleukin 1β, interferon-γ, prostaglandins, and metalloproteinases. Destruction of the periodontal ligament and bone eventually leads to loss of support of the teeth.

Clinical features (Figs 1 and 2)

The symptoms of chronic gingivitis or periodontitis are usually so mild that they go unnoticed by the patient. They may, however, complain of discomfort from their teeth, bleeding of gums and associated halitosis, difficulty on eating, looseness of teeth, and occasionally abscess formation. A lack of severe symptoms allows the disease to progress to an irreversible stage before help is sought. Periodontal disease is commonly associated with diabetes. Smoking is a well-documented risk factor. Recently a significant link has been found between periodontal disease and cardiovascular thrombosis. Surprisingly, periodontal disease in pregnant women has been associated with an increased risk of low birth weight and premature birth. It is not clear whether transient bacteraemia in the last trimester might elicit a mechanism responsible for these findings.

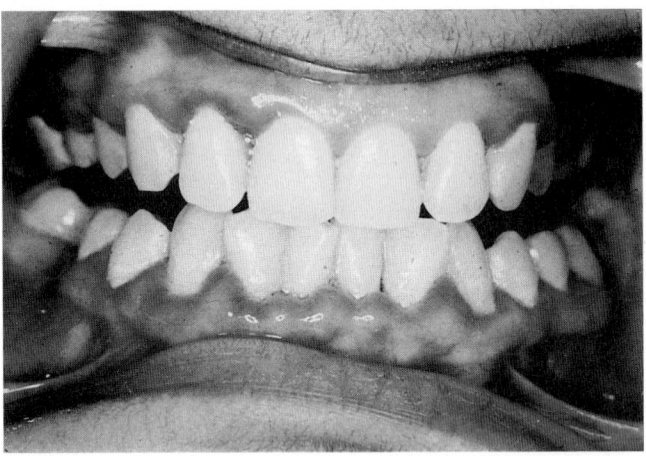

Fig. 1 Chronic gingivitis, with erythema and oedema of the gingival margin of the lower teeth and especially the upper right lateral incisor.

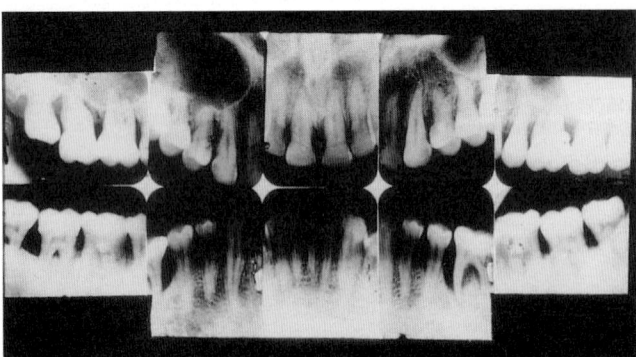

Fig. 2 Radiograph of teeth showing advanced periodontitis with loss of supporting bone of the teeth.

Differential diagnosis

Chronic gingivitis can be differentiated from acute ulcerative gingivitis by the sudden onset, malaise, characteristic halitosis, pain, and ulceration of the gingiva in the latter. Herpetic gingivostomatitis occurs predominantly in children and again the onset is acute, with fever, malaise, pain, and ulceration of the gingiva and oral mucosa (see below). Desquamative gingivitis associated with bullous lesions and lichen planus may cause difficulties in differential diagnosis and the points to bear in mind are that the attached gingiva shows diffuse erosive areas and evidence of bullous lesions may be found in the oral mucosa. Periodontitis is clinically differentiated from gingivitis by the loss of connective tissue attachment to the teeth, leading to pocket formation. There is progressive bone loss, readily diagnosed by radiographic examination of the teeth, and eventually loosening of teeth.

Treatment

The aims in the management of gingivitis and mild periodontitis are to remove dental plaque and calculus by scaling the teeth, and this can be done only by a dentist or dental hygienist. Prevention is, however, much more effective by plaque control, which involves careful tooth brushing with the aid of plaque-disclosing solutions and regular use of dental floss and wood points. Chlorhexidine rinses (0.2 per cent) twice a day prevent the accumulation of plaque and decrease gingival inflammation. In some forms of periodontitis tetracycline or metronidazole can be helpful; preparations are available that can be applied locally, but these are generally used in addition to local surgical treatment. However, once deep periodontal pockets have been formed, these are treated by root planing, gingival curettage, or surgically. It should be appreciated that the management of periodontal disease is dependent upon meticulous plaque control.

Course and prognosis

If the bacterial plaque is not removed, gingivitis may progress to periodontitis and after many years will result in increased mobility and loss of teeth. This process, however, is reversible by plaque control and, if necessary, eradication of pockets, as long as there is sufficient bone to support the teeth.

Herpes simplex and other viral infections

Herpes simplex virus type 1 is responsible for certain orofacial infections (see also Section 7).

Primary herpetic gingivostomatitis

Aetiology

Clinical or subclinical primary infections by herpes simplex virus type 1 are acquired in early childhood, probably in the second and third years of life. Primary herpetic infection in the first year is rare, because most mothers have neutralizing IgG antibodies to the virus that are transferred through the placenta to the fetus. Serum virus complement-fixing and neutralizing antibodies are found in about 50 per cent of children at 5 years of age. The disease is common in children, but is also seen, less frequently, in adults.

Pathology

Herpes simplex virus is a DNA virus and there are two types: type 1 is found predominantly in the orofacial region and type 2 in the genital region. There are three genes (α, β, γ) and the β gene codes for viral glycoproteins gB, gC, gD, and gE. These viral glycoproteins have been well characterized: gB is involved in viral penetration of the cell membrane, gC constitutes the C3b receptor (binding activated C3b), and gE is the crystallizable fragment receptor for IgG. Antibodies against gD neutralize herpes simplex virus and block its penetration. Hence this viral infection generates many significant immunological molecules in the host cell, in addition to expressing a viral antigen on the cell surface.

Infection starts with the entry of herpesvirus into epithelial cells. Viral replication takes place inside the nucleus, and this is associated with the formation of intranuclear inclusion bodies and giant cells. As more epithelial cells become infected, degenerative and oedematous changes give rise to vesicle formation. The intraepithelial vesicles contain oedema fluid, with giant cells and degenerating cells with intranuclear inclusion bodies. The vesicles rupture early, resulting in ulcers that heal rapidly.

Clinical features

The disease is recognized by an acute onset of a sore mouth and often sore throat, fever, and extensive inflammation of the gums, followed by formation of vesicles and ulcers of the oral mucosa, and regional lymphadenitis. Infants display considerable fretfulness, sleeplessness, and refusal to eat. Initially there are crops of small ulcers but these coalesce to produce large, shallow, irregular ulcers with surrounding inflammation. Herpetic keratitis is not often associated with herpetic stomatitis, and herpetic encephalitis is extremely rare but may occasionally complicate herpetic stomatitis.

Diagnosis

The early phase of infection can be confused with a cold but the development of vesicles and ulcers makes that diagnosis unlikely. Recurrent aphthous ulcers may occasionally be misdiagnosed in the adult, though the important differentiating points are the acute onset, sore throat, fever, and lymphadenitis in herpetic infection. Laboratory tests can be useful in confirming the diagnosis. Direct examination of a smear from the lesion can be helpful if intranuclear inclusion bodies or giant cells are found. Culture of the virus may assist in the diagnosis, but the herpesvirus is also found in carriers. A rise in antibody titre to the virus during an infection can be a useful aid in diagnosis.

Treatment

Patients are advised to rest for 2 to 4 days; a soft diet is indicated, and an adequate fluid intake is emphasized. The mouth is cleansed by thorough rinsing with hot salt water six times daily and the teeth are cleaned with a wet flannel. In infants, special attention must be paid to the fluid intake and sleep. A useful sedative to use is promethazine elixir, given in doses of one teaspoonful (5 mg/5 ml) at night-time.

Acyclovir tablets (200 mg), two to four times daily, can be helpful if started at an early stage of infection. However, in late onset of primary herpetic infection, tetracycline mouthwash can speed up recovery; however, this should not be used in children.

Course and prognosis

The natural course of this infection is 7 to 14 days, during the initial days of which eating is usually difficult, but healing of the ulcers occurs spontaneously. Recurrence of herpetic lesions intraorally is rather rare in otherwise healthy subjects but occurs frequently in patients with cellular immunodeficiencies.

Recurrent herpetic infection

This is also called recurrent herpes labialis or cold sores.

Aetiology

The lesion is caused by herpes simplex virus type 1 and is commonly found from childhood to past middle age in both sexes. A variety of factors may precipitate the lesions: the common cold, fever, exposure to sunlight, local trauma, emotional stress, menstruation, dental treatment, and section of the sensory root of the trigeminal ganglion are among the best known. Severe herpetic infections, affecting the lips, perioral skin, and mouth, are seen in patients receiving immunosuppressive drugs.

Pathology

Primary herpes simplex infection is followed by viral latency in the trigeminal ganglion. The relation between primary infection, latency, and recurrent infection by herpes simplex virus has not been completely elucidated. However, there is evidence that primary infection induces immune responses to the virus; antibody and cell-mediated cytotoxic mechanisms kill most of the virus-infected cells. The virus is sequestered to the nerves and will migrate along the axons to the trigeminal ganglion. Indeed, the entire herpes simplex virus genome can be found in the trigeminal ganglion, although the DNA is qualitatively different. A number of clinical precipitating factors may induce derepression of the viral genome and virus replication, which will then migrate along the axon to be shed at the nerve endings. In the presence of some defect in cell-mediated immunity acting at the neuroepithelial junction, recurrent herpetic lesions will be precipitated. Cytokine production, especially interferon-γ, may be impaired, and a decrease in cytotoxic CD8 T cells is involved in recurrent herpetic infection.

Clinical features (Fig. 3)

The lesions are usually limited to the vermilion border of the lips and adjacent skin. A single blister or a crop of blisters may develop a day after the prodromal phase. The duration of the lesion usually varies between 3 and 10 days, but secondary infection by *Staphylococcus pyogenes* commonly occurs. The lesion recurs at various intervals often at the same site for many years, and the rate of recurrence may be related to the type of precipitating factor involved. The significance of cellular immunity is highlighted by herpes simplex virus infections found in cell-mediated immunodeficiency states, such as AIDS, and in patients receiving immunosuppressive therapy.

Diagnosis

Localization to the vermilion border of the lips and the history of recurrences make this a readily recognizable condition. Laboratory assistance is rarely required but the findings are similar to those described for primary herpetic infection, except that there is an elevated initial antibody titre which does not usually increase during recurrent infection. Staphylococcal infection from the anterior nares should be excluded.

Treatment

Acyclovir (acycloguanosine) cream (5 per cent) can be effective if applied during the prodromal phase. Staphylococcal infection responds readily to mupirocin or fucidin ointment, applied three times daily. In the severe type of mucocutaneous herpetic infection in immunosuppressed patients, acyclovir tablets (200 mg) are administered two to four times daily.

Course and prognosis

The lesions heal usually within about 7 days but recurrences are difficult to prevent. If the precipitating factors are known, some preventive measures

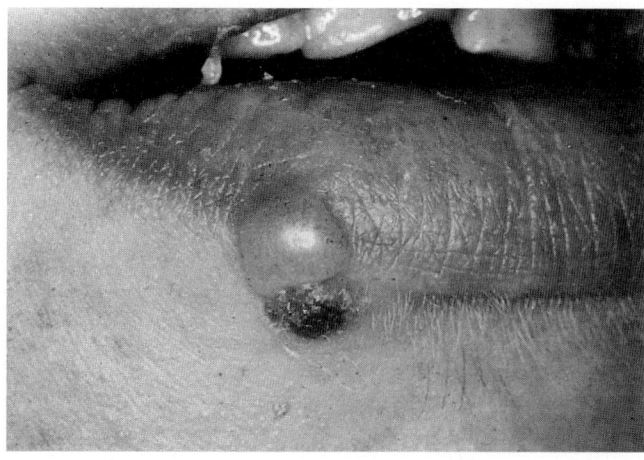

Fig. 3 Recurrent herpes labialis vesicle on the vermilion border of the lower lip.

can be taken such as applying a barrier cream to the lips before exposure to the sun.

Herpes zoster infection

Herpes zoster infection of the skin of the face, innervated by the second or third branch of the trigeminal nerve, may be associated with unilateral oral vesicles. These break down early to produce ulcers along the oral distribution of the maxillary or mandibular branches.

Herpangina

This is a rare infection by the coxsackie group A viruses, usually affecting the soft palate and the oropharyngeal region. Children tend to be affected more often than adults and the mode of presentation of the disease is similar to that in primary herpetic stomatitis. The diagnosis can be firmly established only by isolating the virus from a lesion or by showing an increase in antibody titre. The disease appears to be self-limiting and specific treatment is not necessary.

Hand, foot, and mouth disease

This is another virus infection caused by coxsackie A5, 10, and 16 (see Section 7). The mouth is sore due to multiple small vesicles or ulcers, which most commonly affect the hard palate, tongue, and buccal mucosa. There are associated vesicular lesions on the hands and feet. The diagnosis is confirmed by isolating the virus from the lesion. The disease is self-limiting within about 2 weeks and no specific treatment is necessary.

Measles

This is an acute exanthematous virus infection of children (see Chapter 7.10.6). Whitish macules on the buccal mucosa, known as Koplik's spots, may precede the development of the red macular rash by 2 to 3 days.

AIDS (see Chapter 7.10.21)

Aetiology

This is an infection by the human immunodeficiency virus (**HIV-1**) affecting primarily CD4+ T cells, macrophages, Langerhans, and dendritic cells. In addition to the CD4 receptor all HIV-1 strains require the coreceptor CCR5 or CXCR4 for viral entry.

Pathology

Entry of HIV into the host is by the interaction between gp120, CD4, and CCR5 or CXCR4 on the cell membrane. The trimolecular complex enables the viral particle to enter the cell by fusion between the viral and cell membranes. Hence, the primary target of HIV is the CD4 subset of T cells which decrease in number as the cells become infected and killed, but the CD8 subset is not affected, resulting in a decrease in the CD4:CD8 cell ratio. It is not clear whether the virus kills CD4 cells directly or indirectly by an immune mechanism.

Clinical features

There are five main populations at risk:

1. Homosexual men: those with multiple sex partners and the anal-receptive partner in anogenital intercourse are at greatest risk.

2. Transmission of HIV during vaginal intercourse is common in parts of Africa and Asia; female prostitutes may carry the virus in their genital secretions.

3. Intravenous drug abusers can spread the virus via infected needles from one person to another, directly by the vascular route.

4. Those who have received a blood transfusion with HIV-infected blood, especially haemophiliacs treated with factor VIII.

5. Perinatal HIV infection of babies from infected mothers.

There is some epidemiological evidence that oral sex might lead to HIV infection, but it is unlikely that salivary transmission of HIV can occur. Comparative isolation studies of HIV from body fluids have been made and their results suggest that whilst HIV can be cultured from whole saliva, the frequency of isolation is low (up to 9 per cent) as compared with semen (21 per cent) or plasma (55 per cent). The quantity of HIV isolated from saliva is also low. The available evidence suggests that the HIV resides in the cellular fraction of oral fluid, presumably CD4+ T cells and macrophages, and not the fluid fraction originating mostly from the salivary glands.

The special significance to dentists of oral transmission of HIV is self-evident, as they work in a pool of saliva, often mixed with gingival blood. However, seropositive conversions were not found among about 1000 dental staff in the United States and the same number tested in Germany. Only 1 out of 1309 dentists in another study in the United States was seropositive and he did not wear protective gloves. This is an almost negligible prevalence of HIV seropositivity in a population of dentists, among whom more than 90 per cent admitted to needlestick injuries. The transmission of HIV during dental procedures remains a possibility, especially since a case has been documented of a Californian dentist passing HIV to his patients. However, the details of this case are most perplexing and the route of transmission has not been established.

This section will be confined to the oral manifestations of AIDS. It is of significance that oral candidiasis and hairy leucoplakia may predict the development of AIDS. A variety of opportunistic infections may develop in the mouth. Fungal infection with candida, especially *Candida albicans*, is common. All varieties of oral candidiasis have been recorded in AIDS, but it appears that the chronic hyperplastic and atrophic varieties are more frequent than the pseudomembranous variety. Other fungal lesions may occur but are rare (for example histoplasmosis and cryptococcosis).

Viral infections with herpes simplex virus give rise to recurrent oral herpetic lesions affecting the palate or gum and present as painful vesicles that ulcerate. It should be remembered that recurrent intraoral herpetic lesions are extremely uncommon in the rest of the population (unlike recurrent herpes labialis). Orofacial lesions due to herpes zoster have also been recorded but are rather rare. Epstein–Barr virus appears to cause hairy leucoplakia, which is a raised white plaque commonly affecting the tongue and is clinically similar to chronic hyperplastic candidiasis. Similar lesions have not been recorded in the general population. Papillomavirus may induce single or multiple warts in the mouth of AIDS patients.

Kaposi's sarcoma is a neoplasm of the vascular endothelial cells. Oral lesions present as red or purple macules or papules, often affecting the palate and tongue. Other neoplasias are less common but non-Hodgkin's lymphomas and carcinomas have been recorded.

Gingivitis and periodontitis may show changes similar to those of acute necrotizing ulcerative gingivitis (see below), except that these may be superimposed on rapidly progressing periodontitis. The condition can be painful and has been associated with rapid loss of soft tissue and bone support, leading to loss of teeth.

Recurrent oral ulcers are probably more common in patients with AIDS than in the general population. Enlargement of the salivary glands, especially of the parotid glands, might be caused by a viral infection.

Differential diagnosis

As oral manifestations of AIDS may occur early in the disease, oral candidiasis, herpetic infections, leucoplakia, oral or gingival ulcers, salivary gland swellings, and oral tumours should be suspected, especially in young men (and women) falling into the population groups most at risk of HIV infection.

Treatment

In addition to the general management of AIDS, the teeth and gums should receive a great deal of attention to maintain a high standard of oral hygiene. Otherwise the lesions should be treated as for any other oral condition. Routine dental treatment can be difficult to arrange in a dental practice, but most hospitals have made special arrangements for AIDS patients.

Fungal infections (see Section 7.12)

Candidiasis

This is also called moniliasis or thrush.

Aetiology

Candida is a commensal organism in the mouth found in 20 to 40 per cent of the normal population. Most normal subjects show serum-agglutinating antibodies and a cutaneous delayed hypersensitivity reaction to candida. It is not clear whether candida infection of the oral mucosa is endogenous or exogenous, but as the organism is ubiquitous, a suitable environment and impaired immune responses are the most important conditions conducive to infection by candida. Oral candidiasis can be an early manifestation of AIDS (see above). Although most species of candida can become pathogenic, *C. albicans* is most frequently found in oral infections.

Pathology

The different varieties of candidiasis have in common a superficial invasion of epithelium by fungal hyphae; it is unusual for the hyphae to penetrate the basement membrane. However, in immunodeficient patients candida may spread by the vascular route to the heart, kidneys, and brain. Raised titres of antibodies to candida are found in serum and secretory IgA antibodies in the saliva of patients with oral candidiasis. Antibodies and complement are necessary for optimal phagocytosis of candida by polymorphonuclear leucocytes or macrophages. There is evidence that serum antibodies to the 44 to 60 kDa candida antigen prevent systemic candidiasis. In contrast, cell-mediated immunity is involved in chronic mucocutaneous candidiasis, with a spectrum of cellular immunodeficiencies.

Clinical features

Oral candidiasis develops in a variety of conditions predisposing to candidal proliferation: diabetes mellitus, anaemias, cell-mediated immunodeficiencies (such as AIDS or thymic defects), broad-spectrum antibiotics, immunosuppressive drugs, and leukaemias. Local factors commonly predisposing to oral candidiasis are dry mouth due to Sjögren's or sicca syndrome, irradiation, dentures, or steroid sprays used for asthma.

Varieties of oral candidiasis

There are four main varieties of oral candidiasis.

Acute pseudomembranous candidiasis (thrush)

This disease is commonly seen in infants as well as in debilitated adults, particularly in diabetes mellitus and malignant diseases (especially leukaemia and lymphoma). Iatrogenic agents are also important predisposing factors; systemic antibiotics, corticosteroids, and immunosuppressive drugs seem to enhance candida infection. Local antibiotic and corticosteroid treatment can enhance oral candidiasis. Clinical manifestations of thrush are usually symptomless white papules or cotton-wool-like exudates that can be rubbed off leaving an erythematous mucosa.

Acute atrophic candidiasis (Fig. 4)

This may follow acute pseudomembranous candidiasis and is usually associated with broad-spectrum antibiotic therapy; it is hence referred to as 'antibiotic sore tongue'. It is the only type of oral candidiasis that is consistently painful, showing a smooth erythematous tongue, with angular cheilitis and (less often) inflamed lips and cheeks.

Chronic atrophic candidiasis

This type of candida infection is better known as 'denture stomatitis', for it presents as a diffuse erythema of the palate limited to the denture-bearing mucosa. The denture covering the palatal mucosa predisposes to proliferation of candida. The lesion is usually symptomless but is often associated with angular cheilitis (Fig. 5).

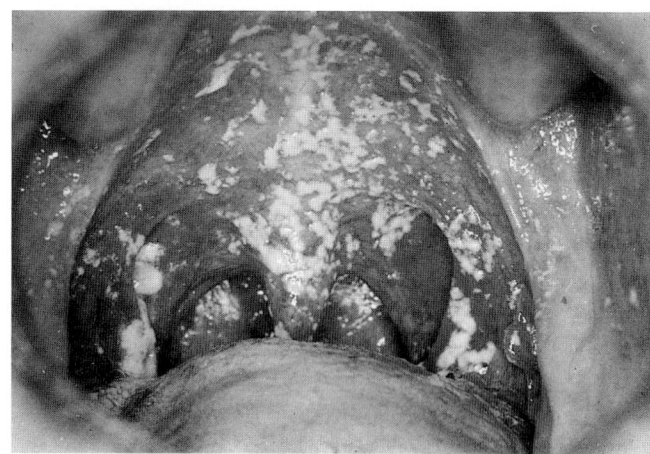

Fig. 4 Oropharyngeal thrush, following the application of a steroid spray in a patient with asthma.

Chronic hyperplastic candidiasis

This lesion presents as a firm, diffuse white patch, or as numerous white papules with intervening erythema on the tongue, cheeks, or lips. The lesion may persist for many years or for life and should be distinguished from leucoplakia. This variety of candidiasis can be associated with skin lesions and there are three clinical types of mucocutaneous candidiasis:

1. Chronic localized mucocutaneous candidiasis. This starts in childhood as an intractable oral candida infection, with involvement of nails and sometimes the adjacent skin of the hands and feet. A number of other skin sites may show persistent candida infection.

2. Chronic localized mucocutaneous candidiasis with granuloma. This condition begins in infancy and the clinical manifestations are similar to those in the previous type of candidiasis, with the important additional feature of granulomatous masses affecting the face and scalp. Recurrent respiratory tract infection has been recorded in a quarter of affected children.

3. Chronic localized mucocutaneous candidiasis with endocrine disorder. This is found in children and young adults. A strong familial incidence is often found and candidiasis commonly precedes the endocrine abnormalities. The clinical features of candida infection are similar to those seen in the localized mucocutaneous variety. The association with hypoparathyroidism and Addison's disease, and less often pernicious anaemia and hypothyroidism, illustrates the relationship

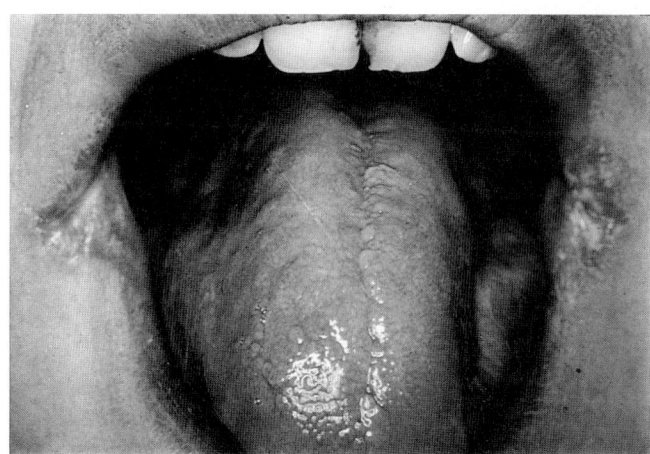

Fig. 5 Angular cheilitis caused by candidal infection.

between cell-mediated immunodeficiencies and autoimmune endocrine disorders.

Differential diagnosis

Chronic hyperplastic candidiasis can cause some difficulties in differential diagnosis from leucoplakia and the laboratory tests are useful in this, as well as in the other types of candidiasis, in establishing the diagnosis. AIDS must be considered, particularly in homosexual males. A culture from the lesion yields candida, usually *C. albicans*, and direct examination of scrapings shows the Gram-positive hyphae and yeast cells of candida. Biopsy of the lesion in chronic mucocutaneous candidiasis is helpful, as in addition to the superficial invasion of epithelium by candida hyphae, there is usually extensive epithelial hyperplasia. The dermis shows an intense mononuclear cell infiltration with a large proportion of plasma cells.

A rise in convalescent serum antibody titre to candida may assist in the diagnosis of the acute types of candidiasis, but there may be an impaired antibody titre in the chronic type of candidiasis. Chronic mucocutaneous candidiasis usually shows some defects in cell-mediated immunity and this should be determined by investigating delayed hypersensitivity, lymphocyte proliferation, and generation of interleukins on stimulation with candida. It is essential that the endocrine function should be tested in children with chronic candidiasis of the mouth and nails.

Treatment

Oral candidiasis responds readily to topical oral treatment with antifungal drugs: sucking tablets of nystatin 500 000 IU four times a day or amphotericin B 100 mg four times a day for 1 to 2 weeks is very effective. Alternative antifungal agents, such as miconazole and fluconazole, are equally effective. Chronic mucocutaneous candidiasis, however, is often unresponsive to topical oral treatment and may necessitate intravenous administration of amphotericin B. Endocrine replacement therapy is essential if there is an associated endocrine disorder. Although almost complete eradication of the lesions can be accomplished, the disease tends to return after the drug is discontinued because of the underlying immunological defect which needs to be rectified.

Bacterial infections

Acute (necrotizing) ulcerative gingivitis

This is also called Vincent's gingivitis or acute fusospirochaetal gingivitis.

Aetiology

An infective cause of acute ulcerative gingivitis has been widely accepted, although the organisms thought to be responsible are disputed. *Fusobacterium fusiformis* and *Borrelia vincenti* have been favoured on account of their presence in large numbers in direct examination of smears from the lesions. *Bacteroides melaninogenicus* has also been implicated as the causative organism, but evidence is accumulating in favour of a mixed bacterial pathogenesis of Gram-negative organisms (fusobacteria, veillonella, bacteroides, leptotrichia), which may be responsible for the lesions due to their endotoxin activity.

Whatever role micro-organisms may play, a number of predisposing factors are recognized. Of the local factors poor oral hygiene with accumulation of dental bacterial plaque, defective restorations, and pericoronitis are most important. The prevalence of acute ulcerative gingivitis is rather high and it is seen more commonly in young adults and smokers. A lowered general resistance may also predispose to the disease.

Pathology

The gum undergoes an acute inflammatory reaction, with an intense polymorphonuclear response and fibrinous exudate. This leads soon to necrosis of the epithelium and thrombosis of the small blood vessels.

Clinical features

Acute ulcerative gingivitis is readily recognized by the sudden onset of painful, bleeding gums and a characteristic foul breath. Except for primary herpetic stomatitis, this is the only other oral mucosal infection in which there is a rise in temperature, which may reach 39 °C, regional lymphadenitis, anorexia, and significant malaise. Oral examination reveals necrotic, punched-out ulcers, predominantly affecting the interdental gingiva. At times there are shallow necrotic ulcers affecting the oropharyngeal mucosa, which shows diffuse erythema; this has been referred to as Vincent's angina. In the presence of erupting wisdom teeth, the overlying gum can show ulceration and oedema causing partial trismus.

Diagnosis

This disease is often confused with primary herpetic stomatitis because of the acute onset. However, patients with primary herpetic stomatitis are usually younger and their breath is stale but lacks the distinct foul quality of that found in ulcerative gingivitis. First vesicles and then numerous well-defined ulcers are scattered over the oral mucosa, unlike the tendency for localization of necrotic sites to the gingiva in ulcerative gingivitis. Direct examination of a smear from the lesion reveals a large number of spirochaetal and fusiform organisms, with a decrease in the mixed bacterial flora.

Treatment

Metronidazole is very effective and should be taken 200 mg by mouth three times daily for 3 to 4 days. Phenoxymethyl penicillin, 250 mg taken four times daily for a week is equally effective in clearing the symptoms. Oxidizing agents, hydrogen peroxide mouthwash, and a variety of peroxyborate preparations are also useful. During the acute phase, patients are advised to use a soft toothbrush or a soft cloth to clean their teeth, and they are encouraged to rinse their mouths forcibly with warm saline every 3 h.

Although treatment with drugs is effective in clearing the acute phase, recurrences can be prevented only by careful attention to oral hygiene. The teeth have to be scaled and polished, and the patient is instructed as to the best method of tooth brushing and control of dental plaque. Frequent examinations by a dental surgeon are advisable.

Course and prognosis

In the absence of treatment the acute phase may gradually disappear leaving behind a partially necrosed gingiva and chronic inflammation. Inadequate treatment commonly leads to recurrent ulcerative gingivitis over many years, with halitosis, gingival bleeding, and recession.

Cancrum oris (noma)

This is a rapidly spreading gangrene of the lips and cheeks, mostly confined to children in parts of tropical Africa. It is thought to be an extension of acute ulcerative gingivitis when associated with other diseases, especially measles. Cancrum oris is very rare in the United Kingdom, but can be seen during the terminal stages in patients with leukaemia, especially when treated with a variety of cytotoxic, anti-inflammatory, and immunosuppressive drugs.

Tuberculosis

Oral tuberculosis is rare and usually associated with pulmonary tuberculosis. The presenting feature is usually a painful ulcer which may be single or multiple, often large, with a depressed, granulomatous floor and some induration of the base. The tongue, lips, and cheeks may be affected. Diagnosis is based on microscopical and cultural demonstration of *Mycobacterium tuberculosis* and a biopsy of the lesion, which will show a tuberculous granuloma. With the rise in the prevalence of tuberculosis, especially due to AIDS, oral tuberculous lesions may also reappear. Oral tuberculosis responds readily to specific chemotherapy.

Syphilis

Treponema pallidum may affect the mouth in all stages of syphilis but is uncommon (see also Chapter 7.11.33).

Primary stage

A chancre appears within 2 to 4 weeks of infection. The lesion presents on the lip or tongue as a painless, small, firm nodule that breaks down and forms an ulcer with raised indurated edges. The regional lymph nodes show discrete, rubbery enlargement. The diagnosis depends on direct observation of *T. pallidum* by darkground illumination. This stage is highly infective, but serological tests are usually negative during the initial 3 to 4 weeks.

Secondary stage

This develops 1 to 4 months after infection and presents as a generalized maculopapular rash and lymphadenitis. Shallow, snail-track ulcers affect the tonsils, tongue, or lips, and the saliva is highly infective. The serological tests for syphilis are positive.

Tertiary stage

This is delayed by 3 to 15 years after infection. Gumma and leucoplakia are the typical oral manifestations at this stage. A gumma starts as a swelling of the palate, tongue, or tonsils; it undergoes necrosis and results in a painless, punched-out, deep ulcer, with a 'wash-leather' floor. The lesion may heal by scarring, or give rise to perforation. Leucoplakia usually affects the dorsum of the tongue as an irregular, diffuse white patch that cannot be rubbed off.

The treatment of oral syphilis is the same as that used in other sites, but the response in the tertiary stage is rather poor.

Oral ulceration

In view of the great variety of oral ulcers a classification will be given first (Table 1). Only recurrent oral ulcers will be dealt with fully and the other types of ulcer will be considered predominantly under differential diagnosis.

Recurrent oral ulcers

Three types of ulcer will be described: minor aphthous ulcers, also known as aphthae; major aphthous ulcers, also referred to in the literature as periadenitis mucosa necrotica recurrens; and herpetiform ulcers. Aphthous stomatitis is another term used to describe these ulcers.

Aetiology

These are the most common lesions affecting the oral mucosa and the prevalence varies between 10 and 34 per cent in the population. Although a number of causes has been suggested, the aetiology of recurrent aphthous ulcers has not been fully established. Trauma is unlikely to play an essential role, though it might precipitate ulceration, as is seen following dental treatment. There is no evidence that vitamin deficiency or food allergy is involved. Infection by the herpes simplex virus has been excluded as a cause of this type of ulceration. Whilst emotional stress may often influence the pattern of the disease, it is unlikely to be the direct cause. A family history of recurrent aphthous ulcers is often present and the highest incidence of ulcers is recorded in siblings in whom both parents have recurrent aphthous ulcers. A hormonal disturbance may play a part, as in some female patients there is a relationship between the ulcers and the menstrual period; the onset of ulceration may coincide with puberty, or the ulcers may develop only after the menopause and the ulcers often disappear during pregnancy. The part that autoimmunity may play in the pathogenesis of this disease has not been fully elucidated. However, oral epithelial cells share common antigens with the 65 kDa heat shock protein that is found in Gram-positive organisms. A specific peptide of 15 amino acid residues (91–

105), derived from the sequence of the 65 kDa heat shock protein has recently been found to stimulate lymphocytes from patients with recurrent oral ulcers. The role of this peptide in the pathogenesis of oral ulceration is under investigation.

Pathology

An early intense lymphomonocytic infiltration, especially with a perivascular distribution, is a constant histological finding suggesting a delayed hypersensitivity reaction. This is followed by a polymorphonuclear infiltration. Immunohistological investigations suggest an enhanced immune response, with a significant increase in the number of CD4 and CD8 subsets of T cells, Langerhans cells, and macrophages and the expression of HLA DR in the epithelial cells.

Clinical features (Fig. 6)

Minor aphthous ulcers

About 80 per cent of recurrent oral ulcers are of this type; they are very common, especially in the 10 to 40 year age group, and they are found more frequently in females than males.

A prodromal phase is recognized by most patients 1 to 2 days before the onset of ulceration, as a soreness or burning sensation. With the breakdown of epithelium and associated inflammatory reaction the pain increases in severity, particularly on eating. The ulcers are round or oval, up to five in number, and enlarge in size, although they remain well under 1 cm. They have a yellow floor with a slightly raised margin and often marked surrounding erythema and oedema. The most common sites of involvement

Table 1 Classification of oral ulcers

Recurrent oral ulcers
Minor aphthous, major aphthous, and herpetiform
Behçet's syndrome

Microbial infection
Primary herpes simplex infection
Herpes zoster infection
Acute ulcerative gingivostomatitis
Human immunodeficiency virus
Tuberculosis
Syphilis

Neoplastic ulcers
Carcinoma
Leukaemia

Haematological disorders
Anaemia
Neutropenia, agranulocytosis

Dermatological disorders
Erosive lichen planus
Pemphigus
Benign mucous membrane pemphigoid
Erythema multiforme and Stevens–Johnson syndrome
Reiter's syndrome

Granulomatous disorders
Histiocytosis X
Wegener's granulomatosis

Iatrogenic agents
Drug allergy
Drug-induced agranulocytosis
Cytotoxic drugs
Radiotherapy

Trauma
Denture, teeth, or foreign body
Chemical

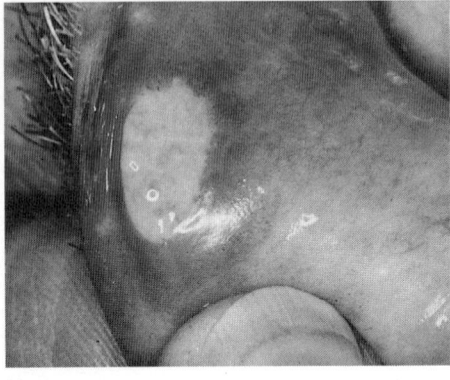

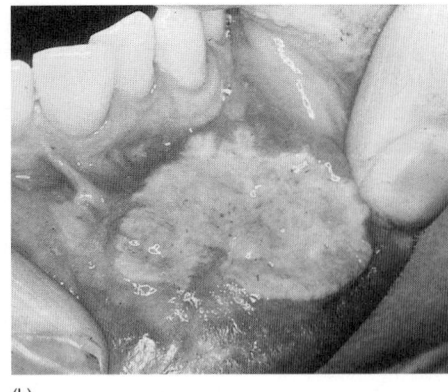

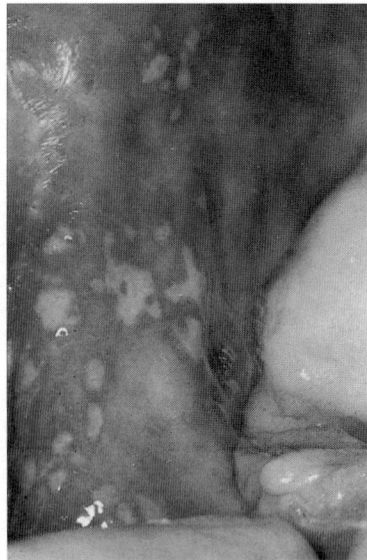

Fig. 6 The three types of recurrent oral ulcer: (a) minor aphthous ulcer; (b) major aphthous ulcer; (c) herpetiform ulcer.

are the mucosa of the lips and cheeks and margin of the tongue, and the ulcers last for 4 to 14 days. The rate of recurrence varies from 1 to 4 months and is usually irregular, though in some females ulcers may precede the menstrual period.

Major aphthous ulcers

These are severe variants of minor aphthous ulcer and fewer than 10 per cent of patients with recurrent oral ulcers have this type of ulcer. The pain that develops after the prodromal symptoms can be severe and persistent, so that patients find it difficult to eat and swallow food and often lose weight. Examination may reveal one to ten ulcers at a time and some of these may enlarge to about 3 cm. The ulcers are necrotic with a raised margin and inflammation of the adjacent tissue, so they occasionally mimic a carcinomatous ulcer. In addition to the lips, cheeks, and tongue, the soft palate and tonsillar region are commonly involved. There may be some regional lymph node enlargement. Healing of an ulcer may take 10 to 40 days and recurrences are so frequent that the patient suffers from continuous ulceration. Multiple small scars may result from large ulcers and these may assist in the diagnosis of major aphthous ulcers. The prevalence of major aphthous ulcers is raised in ulcerative colitis. A striking association has been found in smokers who give up the habit and develop recurrent aphthous ulcers.

Herpetiform ulcers

These are recurrent crops of up to a hundred minute ulcers, affecting any part of the mouth including the gum, palate, and dorsum of the tongue. They account for fewer than 10 per cent of recurrent oral ulcers and are much more common in females than males. Patients present with pain on eating and talking, and often with dysphagia; malaise and loss of weight can be prominent features. The lesions persist for 7 to 14 days and new ulcers

commonly appear before the previous crop has healed, so that ulceration becomes continuous.

Diagnosis

The differential diagnosis of the three types of recurrent oral ulcer is given in Table 2. It is important to differentiate these ulcers from those found in patients with iron, folate, or vitamin B_{12} deficiency, who constitute fewer than 5 per cent of patients with recurrent oral ulcers. About 2 per cent may suffer from coeliac disease due to gluten enteropathy, and these ulcers respond readily to a gluten-free diet.

Agranulocytosis or neutropenia may manifest as shallow necrotic ulcers, predominantly affecting the oropharyngeal region. The ulcers tend to persist, unlike major aphthous ulcers which recur at different sites. However, cyclical neutropenia can mimic minor aphthous ulcers and the diagnosis depends on serial weekly white blood cell counts.

One of the most common diagnostic errors is to confuse the effects of denture trauma with aphthous ulcers, although the former are usually localized to the mucosa covering the mandibular and maxillary alveolus and the buccal and lingual sulci. The relation between denture trauma and ulceration is usually simple to find and requires the attention of a dentist.

The differential diagnosis from pemphigus, benign mucous membrane pemphigoid, and erythema multiforme is important and will be described below.

Not infrequently, patients with major aphthous ulcers are suspected of having a carcinoma, though a careful history will make it evident that these ulcers have recurred at different sites in the mouth. Although major aphthous ulcers may have a raised margin this is due to inflammation and not invasion, so that palpation fails to elicit the induration usually detected in carcinomatous ulcers. If in doubt biopsy of the ulcer is warranted.

Table 2 Differentiating features of the three varieties of recurrent oral ulcers

	Minor aphthous ulcers	Major aphthous ulcers	Herpetiform ulcers
Sex ratio F:M	1.3:1	0.8:1	2.6:1
Age of onset	10–19 years	10–19 years	20–29 years
Number of ulcers	1–5	1–10	10–100
Size	< 10 mm	> 10 mm	1–2 mm
Duration	4–14 days	10–40 days	7–10 days
Healing with scars	8 per cent	64 per cent	32 per cent
Recurrence	1–4 months	1–4 weeks	1–4 weeks
Sites	Lips, cheeks, tongue	Lips, cheeks, tongue, pharynx, palate	Lips, cheeks, tongue, pharynx, palate, floor, gum
Treatment (local)	Corticosteroids	Corticosteroids with or without tetracycline	Tetracycline

Treatment

Topical corticosteroids are the best means to relieve aphthous ulcers. They are most effective if application is started during the prodromal phase when the mucosa has not yet ulcerated. If steroids are applied early ulceration may be prevented, but application at a later stage may still reduce the severity and duration of ulceration. The most useful preparations are triamcinolone in orabase, containing 0.1 mg triamcinolone per 100 g of an adhesive base, betamethasone, containing 0.5 mg steroid per tablet, or beclomethasone spray, up to six puffs daily. The tablets are kept in the mouth, or the ointment is applied to the ulcers, three to four times daily until the ulcer disappears. Systemic prednisolone has to be resorted to occasionally in patients with major aphthous ulcers when topical corticosteroids fail to control the ulcers.

Topical tetracycline is the drug of choice in suppressing herpetiform ulcers but is also useful in controlling some major aphthous ulcers, particularly when there is severe inflammation. Its mode of action is not clear and an effective preparation is to use capsules containing 250 mg tetracycline; the powder from a capsule is dissolved in 10 ml of water and kept in the mouth four times daily. Chlorhexidine solution (0.2 per cent) can be used as a mouthwash, which keeps the teeth free of dental plaque, and may facilitate remission of ulceration.

Course and prognosis

Minor aphthous ulcers may recur from early childhood for many years, and these ulcers may often cause only transient discomfort to which the patient becomes accustomed. However, major aphthous and herpetiform ulcers usually cause a great deal of discomfort, difficulty in eating, and loss of weight. In children, major aphthous ulcers are particularly troublesome and need careful management. In the majority of patients with recurrent oral ulceration the disease burns itself out, but this may take many years. In a very small proportion of patients extraoral sites may become involved, of which the vulvovaginal region is most common, to form part of Behçet's syndrome. There is no way of predicting the development of Behçet's syndrome in patients with recurrent oral ulcers (see Chapter 18.10.5).

Bullous lesions

These are diseases that often affect the skin and mouth, but sometimes involve only the oral mucosa. Three conditions will be discussed in this section: pemphigus vulgaris, benign mucous membrane pemphigoid, and erythema multiforme (see Chapter 23.1).

Pemphigus vulgaris

Aetiology

This is a rare disease which in many instances presents in the mouth, although oral lesions are found at some stage of the disease in all patients. Autoimmunity plays a part in the pathogenesis of pemphigus vulgaris, with IgG antibodies targeted to normal epithelial membrane glycoproteins (66, 150, and 210 kDa). Autoantibodies may bind to keratinocytes and cause a loss of interepithelial adhesion. A significant association has been established with HLA DR4 and DRW6 in patients with pemphigus and either of these gene products may confer disease susceptibility.

Pathology

This shows loss of interepithelial adhesion, intraepithelial bullae, and acantholytic cells, with a diffuse leucocytic infiltration of the lamina propria.

Clinical features (Fig. 7)

The disease affects females two to three times as often as males, usually those over the age of 30 years. Painful, fluid-filled blisters or bullae may

appear in any part of the mouth and burst within a few hours, resulting in shallow ulcers. These persist for weeks or months, but new lesions appear throughout the disease process. Oral manifestations of the disease may persist for many months, without overt ill health, but skin lesions, malaise, and loss of weight may occur at a later stage.

Differential diagnosis

Clinically the lesions are differentiated from recurrent aphthous ulcers by the presence of bullae, and when these ulcerate the edges lack the well-defined character of aphthous ulcers. Only occasionally is the Nikolsky sign helpful—rubbing the mucosa to induce a bulla. The most important diagnostic test is the presence of acantholytic cells on microscopic examination of direct scrapings from the lesion and a biopsy must always be taken. Antibodies to interepithelial antigens assist in the diagnosis. Pemphigus must be differentiated from pemphigoid and dermatitis herpetiformis (see below).

A less severe and rather rare variant of pemphigus vulgaris is pemphigus vegetans. Vegetation may be found on the oral mucosa and lips, and histological examination shows intraepithelial abscesses containing numerous eosinophils.

Treatment

Systemic corticosteroids such as prednisolone are given initially in doses of 40 to 60 mg/day and this is gradually reduced to the minimal dose that will

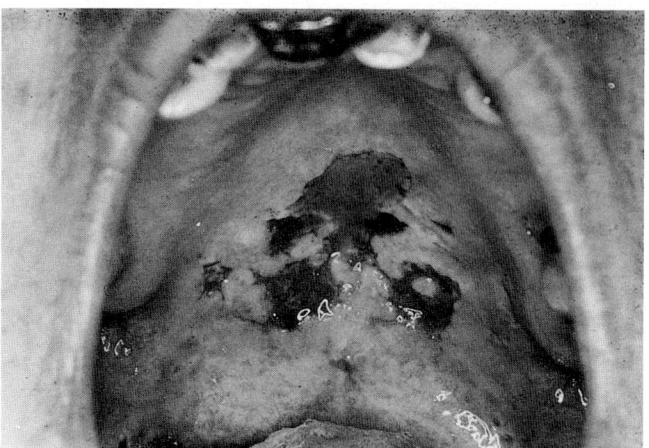

(a)

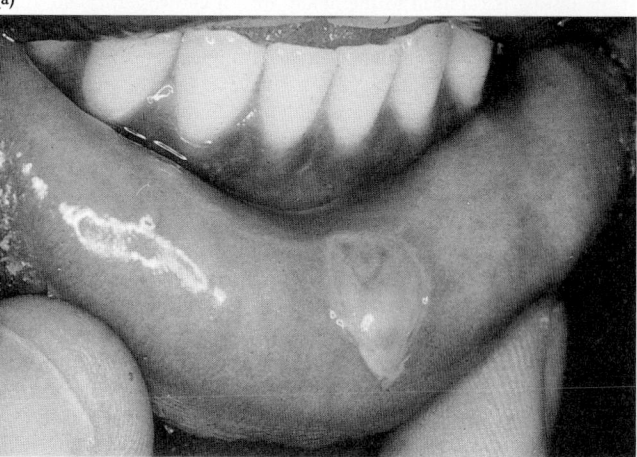

(b)

Fig. 7 (a) Bullae and erosions of pemphigus vulgaris affecting the palate. (b) Bullae and erosions of pemphigus vulgaris affecting the lower lip.

prevent formation of new lesions. In order to keep the steroid dose to a minimum azathioprine can also be used, with a dose of 200 mg/day.

Course and prognosis

Treatment with corticosteroids must be maintained for life and has completely changed the prognosis of the disease. Patients rarely die now from the disease but they may develop the side-effects of steroid therapy.

Benign mucous membrane pemphigoid

Aetiology

This is a rare disease, affecting women twice as often as men, usually those over the age of 40 years. The aetiology is ill understood but there is some evidence that autoantibodies to the epithelial basement membrane may play a part in this disease.

Pathology

This shows subepithelial bullae, and the epithelium tends to detach itself from the underlying lamina propria. IgG, IgA, or IgM, with or without complement, are found in the basement membrane.

Clinical features

Bullous lesions involve the oral mucosa, conjunctiva, and the skin around the genitals, but in some patients only the mouth is involved. The bullae rupture within a day or two leaving erosions and ulcers. The gingiva is commonly involved, giving rise to persistent pain, bleeding, and a diffuse, raw, fiery red lesion. Other mucous membranes can be involved, such as the nose, larynx, pharynx, oesophagus, vulva, vagina, penis, and anus. The oral lesions usually heal without scarring unlike those of the conjunctiva.

Differential diagnosis

Benign mucous membrane pemphigoid can be differentiated from pemphigus vulgaris on clinical grounds but only a biopsy examination will establish the diagnosis. There are no acantholytic cells and the bullae are subepithelial and not suprabasilar. Furthermore, autoantibodies can be detected, probably in fewer than half of patients, binding to the basement membrane of epithelium and not to the interepithelial substance. The disease should be differentiated from linear IgA disease, which shows linear deposition of IgA in the basement membrane, and dermatitis herpetiformis, in which IgA deposits are found in the papillae.

Treatment

If the disease is confined to the mouth topical corticosteroids are often adequate to control the lesions. However, when other sites are involved systemic corticosteroids are indicated, as in pemphigus.

Course and prognosis

This is a chronic disease which persists, often with exacerbations and remissions, over many years. The conjunctivitis may result in adhesions, corneal opacity, and blindness.

Erythema multiforme

Aetiology

Erythema multiforme may develop at any age but often occurs in young males. Many agents have been associated with this disease—drugs, such as sulphonamides and barbiturates, microbial infections, especially with herpes simplex virus—but a large proportion appears to be idiopathic.

Pathology

There is intracellular oedema with a zone of liquefaction degeneration of the upper layers of epithelium. Subepithelial bullae are often present and the lamina propria is infiltrated with lymphocytes, monocytes, neutrophils, and eosinophils.

Clinical features (Fig. 8)

Oral manifestations may not be a significant feature. However, the mouth can be affected without skin involvement and the diagnosis is then more difficult. The patient develops painful, extensive erosions and ulcers with a predilection for the palate, tongue, and cheeks. The gum may show extensive erosions, which tend to bleed. Haemorrhagic crusting of the lips is often seen. A severe variant of erythema multiforme, which affects the eyes and genitalia in addition to the skin and mouth, is referred to as Stevens–Johnson syndrome.

Differential diagnosis

The diagnosis of oral lesions without the typical skin manifestations can be difficult. The clinical features to note are the extensive erosions affecting the palate, tongue, cheeks, and gingiva, and the haemorrhagic crusting of the lips. These features should avoid confusion with aphthous ulcers. An association with drugs or microbial infection is helpful in making the diagnosis. The age and sex prevalence differs from that in benign mucous membrane pemphigoid. A biopsy examination can formally exclude pemphigus and erosive lichen planus. The differential diagnosis of Stevens–Johnson syndrome from Behçet's syndrome has been discussed and the points noted about Reiter's syndrome also apply here (see Chapter 18.6).

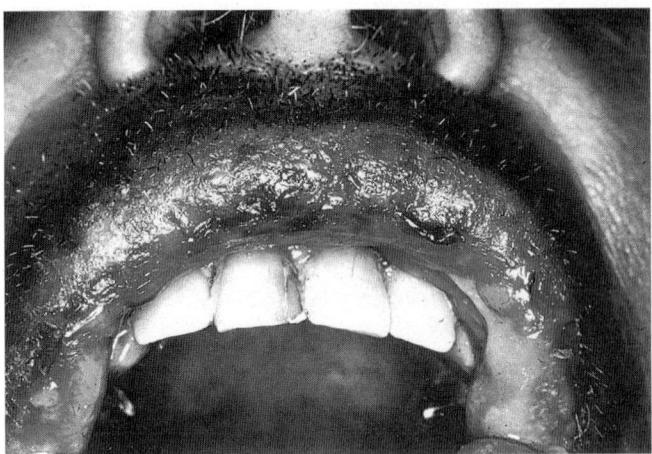
(a)

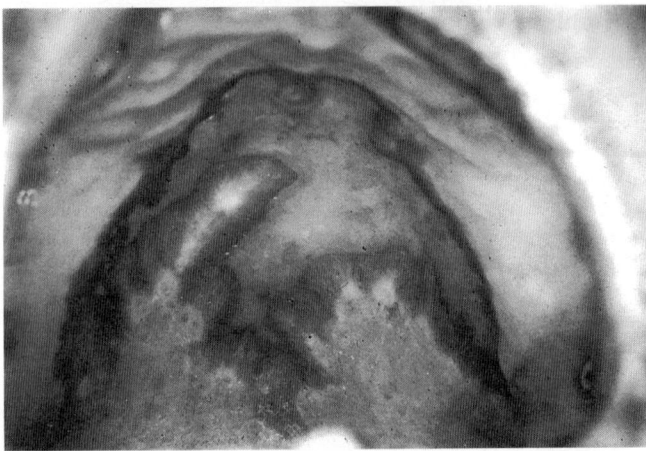
(b)

Fig. 8 Erythema multiforme: (a) haemorrhagic crusted upper lip; (b) diffuse erosion of the palate.

Treatment

Whenever possible the offending drug or infection should be eliminated. The oral lesions often respond to topical tetracycline. Treatment with systemic corticosteroids may be indicated for extraoral manifestations.

Course and prognosis

If the causative agent is not found the lesions may recur over many years and cause a great deal of discomfort. In Stevens–Johnson syndrome, blindness may result from intercurrent bacterial infection.

Lichen planus

This is a disease that may affect the skin, the mouth, or both mucocutaneous surfaces (see Chapter 23.1).

Aetiology

Although the prevalence of oral lichen planus is not known it is surprisingly common in adults. Very little is known about its aetiology, but the condition can develop in graft versus host reaction after bone marrow transplantation. Several drugs are capable of inducing lichenoid changes in the mouth (for example penicillinase, colloidal gold). It seems to be associated with emotional or psychiatric stress. However, in most patients no cause can be determined.

Pathology

The pathological changes are hyperkeratosis, hyperplasia, and a characteristic liquefaction degeneration of the basal cell layers of the epithelium. The lamina propria shows a well-defined lymphomonocytic infiltration.

Clinical features (Fig. 9)

In the mouth the lesions may remain symptomless for years and not infrequently they are first noticed by a dentist during routine examination. Some patients complain of a furry thickening of the mucosa and others of pain or bleeding from the gums on eating. There are three types of oral lichen planus: hypertrophic, erosive, and bullous. The hypertrophic variety is most common and is usually seen in all three types. There are white striae and minute papules, most commonly affecting the posterior part of the buccal mucosa, lips, and dorsum of tongue, though the palate, gum, and floor of the mouth are also involved. The striae crisscross giving rise to a fine lacy or fern-like pattern, and less commonly a honeycomb or annular patter. At times the striae may fuse together and result in a diffuse, somewhat smooth, shiny white plaque which may be difficult to differentiate from leucoplakia. Indeed, the dorsum of the tongue usually manifests diffuse white patches instead of the striated pattern.

In bullous lichen planus a bulla is rarely seen, presumably because it bursts to produce ulcers. Erosive lichen planus, however, is common, and

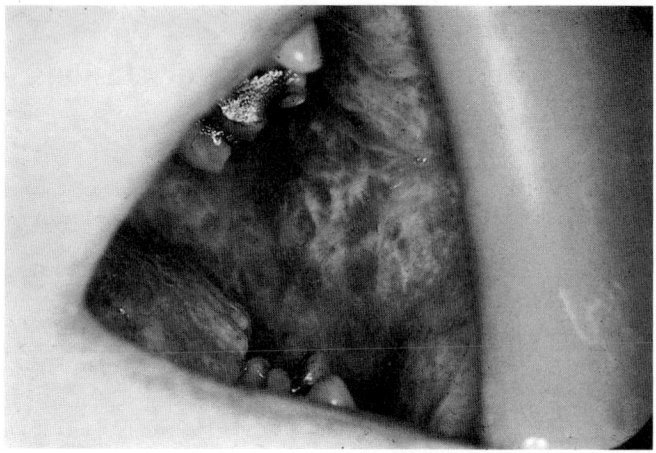

Fig. 9 Striae of lichen planus affecting the buccal mucosa and tongue.

patients complain of pain and discomfort on eating. There may be large shallow ulcers up to 3 cm in size surrounded by white striae and papules. The favoured sites are the same as in the hypertrophic variety, and whilst the latter may break down to result in erosive lichen planus, it is remarkable how often the hypertrophic variety remains unchanged. Except for discomfort, difficulties with eating, and occasionally loss of weight, there are no general manifestations and the regional lymph nodes are not enlarged, except with secondary infection. Not infrequently lichen planus may affect only the gum, inducing a diffuse, fiery red gingivitis and scattered erosions. This is a particularly troublesome type of lichen planus, referred to as desquamative gingivitis, with pain and bleeding, and tends to be resistant to treatment. It should be stressed that many patients with oral lichen planus do not have skin lesions.

A great deal of attention has been paid to the potential for carcinomatous transformation of lichen planus. Applying critical criteria, 1 to 2 per cent of oral lesions of lichen planus may transform to squamous cell carcinoma.

Differential diagnosis

The striae and papules of lichen planus are sufficiently distinctive features in the mouth to differentiate lichen planus from other lesions without the necessity for a biopsy examination. However, the diffuse hypertrophic variety can be confused with leucoplakia and then a biopsy is helpful. Erosive lichen planus may very occasionally lack the distinctive striae, and then erythema multiforme and benign mucous membrane pemphigoid should be excluded. Both systemic and discoid lupus erythematosus can present in the mouth as central erosions surrounded by a keratinized margin.

Treatment

In the absence of symptoms, hypertrophic lichen planus does not require any treatment. The patient, however, needs to be appraised as to the nature of the disease. Topical corticosteroids are usually effective in the treatment of erosive lichen planus but also suppress the striae and papules of the hypertrophic variety. Triamcinolone in orabase ointment applied three to four times a day is useful in localized lesions, but betamethasone (as sodium phosphate) is more effective and is usually used in the form of 0.5 mg tablets, kept in the mouth three times daily. An alternative is to use an aerosol inhaler containing beclomethasone, and applying four to six puffs daily. For these drugs to be helpful, they must be applied for one to several months. The lesions almost invariably recur, although the length of remissions varies greatly and corticosteroids may have to be applied with every remission.

Cleaning the teeth tends to be painful and the accumulation of a large amount of dental plaque aggravates the gingivitis. The patient should use a very soft toothbrush and needs to have the teeth scaled every 3 to 6 months. Chlorhexidine mouthwash can be helpful in controlling dental plaque.

Course and prognosis

The disease is chronic and tends to persist for years, with natural remissions and exacerbations. Topical corticosteroids prolong the remissions, and the erosions and discomfort are kept under control. Since carcinomatous transformation, especially of the erosive type of lichen planus, can take place in a small proportion of patients, they should be followed up regularly at a stomatological clinic.

Leucoplakia

White patches of the oral mucosa that cannot be removed by scraping are referred to as leucoplakia. By convention, lichen planus and lupus erythematosus are excluded from this group.

Aetiology

The prevalence of leucoplakia is not known, but it seems that during the past two decades it has become less frequent. There are many causes of leucoplakia and as these may have distinctive features they will be classified below. It should be noted, however, that in about half the leucoplakias a cause cannot be found. Syphilitic, candidal, and AIDS leucoplakias have been discussed, elsewhere. Causes include:

1. Physical and chemical agents: frictional keratosis, smoker's keratosis.
2. Microbial infection: chronic hyperplastic candidiasis, tertiary syphilis, and AIDS.
3. Congenital and hereditary leucokeratosis.
4. Idiopathic causes.

Pathology

The microscopic features of leucoplakia show a spectrum of changes; at the benign end is epithelial keratosis alone, followed by hyperplasia, and then epithelial atypia at the premalignant end. The lamina propria shows a parallel increase in mononuclear cells, especially plasma cells. Carcinoma *in situ* is the least common histological finding.

Clinical features

The white patches vary from a soft, slightly thickened mucosa, involving a small or large mucosal surface, to hard, irregular white plaques with intervening normal, erosive, or ulcerated sites. The latter is often referred to as speckled leucoplakia and must be recognized clinically because of its greater propensity to carcinomatous transformation. Any part of the oral mucosa or gum may be involved but the cheeks and tongue are most often affected.

Frictional keratosis is usually found along the occlusal line of the buccal mucosa and presents as a linear white patch of even consistency.

Smoker's keratosis (Fig. 10) shows a characteristic distribution of the soft and adjacent hard palate, as keratinized papules with central red dots. The distribution is due to involvement of the palatal mucous glands and the red dots are the openings of the ducts. It is usually caused by pipe smoking, but cigarette smoking may also lead to keratosis of a diffuse type, most commonly affecting the cheeks.

Congenital and hereditary leucokeratosis can be distinguished by the presence of diffuse, soft, white plaques, often with a folded surface. The lesions tend to be symmetrical and affect the floor of the mouth. Other members of the family may have similar lesions.

Differential diagnosis

All leucoplakias should be biopsied, except smoker's keratosis of the palate, as even small white patches have at times proved to be early carcinomas (Fig. 11). It is also essential to find out the degree, if any, of epithelial atypia as this affects the prognosis of leucoplakia. Direct examination of scrapings can be helpful in the presence of candida hyphae; cultures should also be set up for candida. Serological tests can further aid in the diagnosis of candidiasis but are essential in the diagnosis of syphilitic leucoplakia.

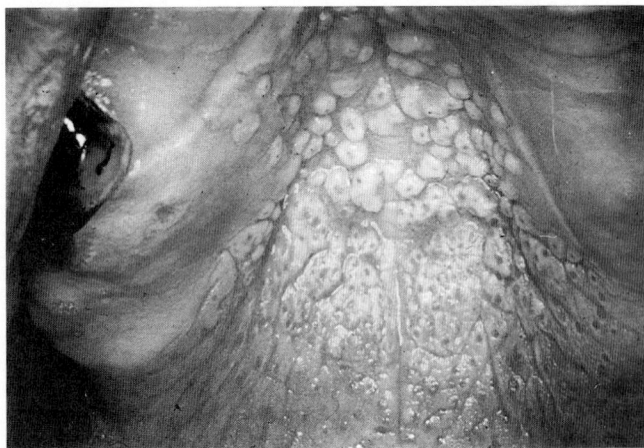

Fig. 10 Smoker's keratosis of the palate.

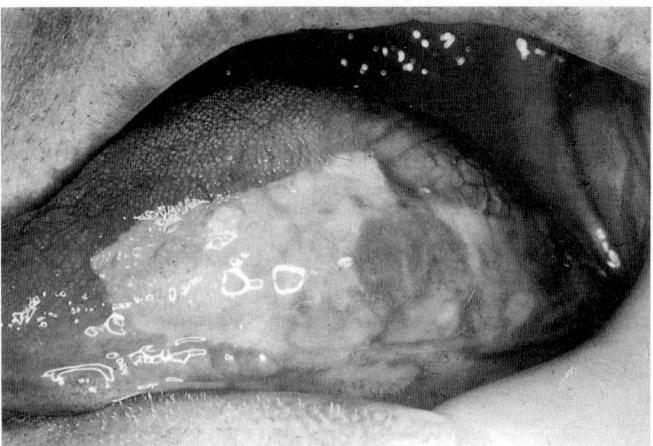

Fig. 11 Leucoplakia of the tongue, which on biopsy examination showed a well differentiated squamous cell carcinoma.

Treatment

Smoker's keratosis is reversible in many instances if the patient gives up smoking. Frictional keratosis can also be cleared if some local cause of irritation is removed. Candida leucoplakia should be treated with topical antifungal drugs, though this rarely results in permanent clearance of the lesion. Syphilis should be managed by a course of penicillin and stringent follow-up, so as to detect any carcinomatous transformation early. Leucoplakia showing evidence of epithelial atypia should be excised and if the lesion is large a skin graft may be required. However, in many cases the lesion recurs, even after repeated excision. There is no satisfactory treatment for leucoplakia and the most important point is long-term follow-up so as to detect in time the development of an incipient carcinoma.

Course and prognosis

Leucoplakia may persist for life, without any discomfort or change. However, about 5 per cent of all leucoplakias may undergo malignant changes and this figure increases to about 30 per cent in leucoplakias showing histological evidence of epithelial atypia. It seems that epithelial atypia is more commonly associated with speckled leucoplakia, and the latter as well as syphilitic leucoplakia has a worse prognosis. In contrast, smoker's keratosis and frictional keratosis have a very good prognosis if the offending cause is removed. Congenital or hereditary leucokeratosis is thought to be free of malignant changes, although recently a few cases with carcinomatous transformation have been reported.

Benign neoplasms, cysts, and developmental and inflammatory lesions of the soft tissues

There are numerous benign neoplasms and soft tissue lesions of the mouth. This section will be restricted to some essential features of the following lesions: papilloma, fibroma, lipoma, neurofibroma, hamartoma, pigmented naevus, lymphangioma, denture granuloma, giant cell reparative granuloma, fibrous polyp, pregnancy tumour, mucous retention, and extravasation cysts.

Aetiology

The cause of benign neoplasms is unknown and the parts that physical or chemical irritation and microbial infection may play are ill understood. Mucous retention or extravasation cysts are caused by trauma or obstruction of the orifices of the ducts of the minor salivary glands. Whereas true benign neoplasms are rare, inflammatory lesions and cysts are commonly found in the mouth.

Clinical features

The soft tissue tumours present as painless, slow-growing swellings affecting any part of the mouth, but if they originate from the gum they are referred to as epulides. Fibrous polyps are the most common inflammatory lesions of the oral mucosa and result from trauma or irritation from rough edges of carious teeth. Most of the tumours are sessile, some are pedunculated as with some fibromas, and others are flat and pigmented as with the naevi. They are usually symptomless except for bleeding from hamartomas and giant cell reparative granulomas.

Differential diagnosis

There are some distinguishing clinical features, but the definitive diagnosis will depend on the histological examination of the excised specimen. A papilloma can be recognized by its firm, small, keratinized, finger-like processes. Lymphangiomas are soft swellings which may cause considerable enlargement of the lip or tongue. Hamartomas are flat or nodular red lesions that may blanch when compressed; they are occasionally confused with pregnancy tumours, which are rather vascular granulomatous swellings of the gingiva found during pregnancy. Giant cell reparative granulomas are also very vascular, maroon-coloured lesions originating from the gingiva. Denture granulomas can be readily recognized from their relation to the flange of a denture; the lesion is often elongated, and can be indented or ulcerated by the denture. Mucous retention or extravasation cysts are small, often bluish, swellings affecting the lips or cheeks.

Treatment

Surgical excision, with a margin of normal tissue at the base of the lesion, is usually indicated. Pregnancy tumours, however, commonly regress spontaneously.

Course and prognosis

The soft tissue neoplasms will enlarge over the years and interfere with the normal functions of the mouth. Bleeding from any of the lesions is rarely profuse. Only the giant cell reparative granuloma has a tendency to recur after excision.

Oral carcinoma

Aetiology

Carcinoma of the mouth accounts for about 2 per cent of all cancers in Britain and the United States. The prevalence increases significantly after the age of 40 years and more than twice as many men as women are affected. The incidence of oral cancer, however, in India and Sri Lanka may account for about 40 per cent of all cancers. As in other carcinomas the cause is unknown, but smoking and alcohol have been implicated. There is some epidemiological evidence to support this, but unlike lung cancer it is pipe or cigar rather than cigarette smoking that have been associated with oral cancer. The association with chronic oral sepsis and irritation has not been critically examined. There is some evidence that microbial agents, particularly *Treponema pallidum*, *Candida albicans*, human papillomavirus, and HIV, may directly or indirectly influence the development of carcinoma.

Among the predisposing lesions, leucoplakia is the best-known; in 5 per cent of all patients and in about 30 per cent of those showing evidence of epithelial atypia the leucoplakia may undergo carcinomatous transformation (Fig. 12). Submucous fibrosis is another precancerous condition and is found predominantly in India and Sri Lanka. It seems to be related to eating chillis and possibly chewing betel nuts; it affects the palate, buccal mucosa, and tongue.

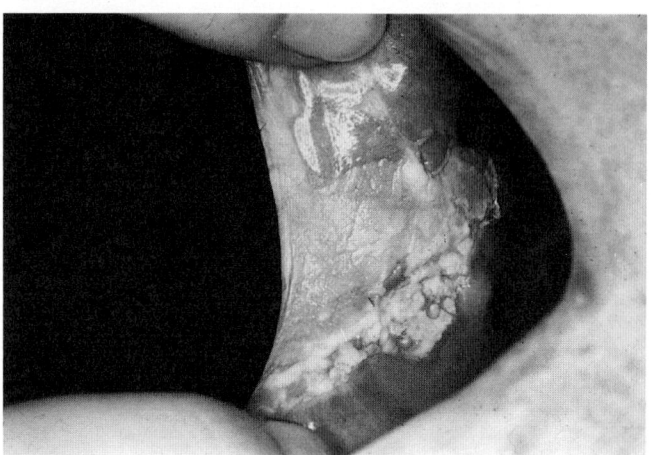

Fig. 12 Leucoplakia of the buccal mucosa, the lower edge of which is raised and on biopsy proved to be a well-differentiated squamous cell carcinoma.

Pathology

Squamous cell carcinoma in the mouth is usually a well-differentiated keratinizing neoplasm invading the surrounding tissue. Poorly differentiated, anaplastic oral carcinomas are much less frequent and are especially rare with carcinoma of the lip. Spread occurs by local invasion: lymph node metastasis is less common than is generally thought, and occurs at a late stage.

Clinical features

The presenting features of carcinoma vary with the site of involvement but there are two types, a lump or an ulcer. The patient complains of a swelling or ulcer that is resistant to healing and gradually enlarging in size. There may be little pain initially, but at a later stage discomfort and occasional bleeding may occur. Cancer of the tongue may give rise to local pain and earache. Whereas some patients complain of an excess of saliva, especially with the larger tumours, a dry mouth may be found during the early stages of malignant change and should be noted as another feature favouring malignancy. A small lump may enlarge to a hard swelling before the covering mucosa breaks down. A malignant ulcer shows a raised and often everted edge, and the most important feature is induration at the base of the lesion. Any part of the mouth can be involved but the lips (usually the lower lip) and tongue are most common, each accounting for about 25 per cent of oral carcinomas. The floor of the mouth, gingiva, cheek, hard and soft palate, and oropharynx may account for about 10 per cent of the carcinomas. In most patients there is only one lesion but some patients may have two or even multiple carcinomas. Metastasis may occur at a late stage to the submandibular or upper cervical lymph nodes, and occasionally to the submental nodes.

Differential diagnosis

Any long-standing or indurated lesion in the mouth, especially of elderly or middle-aged patients, should be queried for malignancy and biopsy examination is essential. A traumatic ulcer caused by a denture can be confused with a malignant ulcer, but it may lack induration, the offending part of the denture may fit into the ulcer, and removing the denture for about a week may bring about healing of the lesion. Major aphthous ulcers have been mentioned elsewhere (see above), but the salient differentiating features are a history of recurrent ulcers at different sites of the mouth over many years.

Adenocarcinoma of the small salivary glands may present as a lump of the soft palate, lips, or cheeks and only a biopsy will establish the diagnosis firmly. Carcinoma *in situ* is rare in the mouth, but it may present as a diffuse, erythematous, somewhat velvety lesion, affecting a part of the soft palate or cheek. Again a biopsy examination must be carried out for diagnosis.

Treatment

The principles of treatment of oral carcinomas are those applied to other carcinomas of the body. Surgical excision of the lesion and a margin of adjacent healthy tissue is the most common practice, and this may be extended if necessary to block dissection of the regional lymph nodes. Radiotherapy is an alternative approach and is commonly used in primary treatment of cancer of the lip, in inoperable cases, or with recurrent carcinoma following surgery. Chemotherapy is used less often in the management of cancer of the mouth and the results are variable. Management of oral cancer is a complex subject outside the scope of this section. It should be emphasized that oral hygiene is particularly important with any treatment so as to avoid ascending parotitis. A dry mouth usually follows radiotherapy and again meticulous oral hygiene should be advised, so as to prevent rampant caries and candida infection.

Course and prognosis

The 5-year survival rates differ considerably with the anatomical site of the cancer. Carcinoma of the lip has by far the best prognosis, irrespective of whether treatment is by surgery or radiotherapy, and the 5-year survival rate is about 80 per cent. In contrast the figures for carcinoma of the tongue range from 25 to 35 per cent, floor of the mouth 20 to 40 per cent, cheek 30 to 50 per cent, and oropharynx, palate, and gingiva at about 25 per cent. The prognosis is significantly better in the absence of lymph node involvement.

Diseases of the salivary glands

Xerostomia

Xerostomia is a term describing dryness of the mouth and can be due to a variety of conditions.

Aetiology

Dry mouth is a common manifestation, especially in middle-aged women, and can be caused by anxiety and emotional and mental stress. Iatrogenic xerostomia is secondary to a number of drugs, the most common of which are antihistamines, tricyclic and other antidepressants, phenothiazine, hypotensive agents, diuretics, and preparations containing atropine. Another common cause is secondary to radiotherapy, but the salivary flow tends to recover although it may take many months. Some diseases affect the salivary glands directly and cause dryness of the mouth, for example Sjögren's syndrome and sialadenitis. Another large group of agents cause xerostomia by inducing changes in fluid balance; diabetes, anaemia, dehydration, and oedema are common examples.

Pathology

Diseases affecting the salivary glands cause a destruction of the secretory components by mononuclear cell infiltration and fibrosis of the salivary acini.

Clinical features

The patient complains of dryness of the mouth and sometimes the eyes, soreness of the mouth, especially the tongue and throat, and discomfort on swallowing of solids and at times difficulty in speaking. The most convincing clinical evidence of xerostomia is an atrophic, dry oral mucosa, often fiery red, due to infection by candida. Inspection of the duct orifices of the major salivary glands will fail to reveal salivary flow. Whole salivary flow rates are readily determined by collecting unstimulated (resting) or lemon juice stimulated saliva. Arbitrary levels of resting saliva of less than 0.1 ml/min and stimulated saliva of less than 0.5 ml/min are indicative of impaired salivary function. The patient may develop rampant caries or if he or she wears dentures there may be difficulties with retention.

Differential diagnosis

A thorough history may establish psychogenic or iatrogenic causes and diseases affecting fluid balance. Sialography and labial gland biopsy may be necessary in the diagnosis of Sjögren's syndrome, though a raised erythrocyte sedimentation rate, rheumatoid factor, antinuclear factor, autoantibodies, and HLA typing may assist in the diagnosis. Nevertheless there will be a large proportion of patients in whom a specific cause cannot be found.

Treatment

Management of the patient is clearly directed to elimination of the cause of xerostomia but this may be difficult or at times impossible to achieve. In such cases, palliative measures are helpful and these include frequent sips of water, meticulous oral hygiene, and early treatment or preferably prevention of candidiasis by topical nystatin or amphotericin B. Each patient responds differently; some prefer glycerin as a lubricant, others carboxymethylcellulose, and the latter can be taken as a solution or spray (Glandosane). A mucin preparation can also be helpful as a spray or as a lozenge (Saliva Orthana).

Sialadenitis

Bacterial or viral infections and rarely allergic reactions may cause inflammation of the salivary glands. These agents may give rise to acute, chronic, or allergic sialadenitis, and recurrent parotitis.

Aetiology

Ascending infection of the parotid gland used to be a common complication in elderly, postoperative patients who were predisposed by dehydration, reduced salivary flow, and lack of oral hygiene. Acute parotitis may also follow the use of drugs causing xerostomia. The most common microorganisms involved are *Staphylococcus aureus*, *Streptococcus viridans*, and pneumococcus. The most common acute parotitis is mumps (see Section 7). The salivary glands are sometimes affected by HIV infection, with an enlargement of the parotid glands. Chronic sialadenitis is usually associated with duct obstruction and therefore affects the submandibular gland. Recurrent sialadenitis is a disease of unknown aetiology and may be associated with a decreased salivary flow causing retrograde infection. The disease may affect both adults and children.

Pathology

Acute sialadenitis shows an acute inflammatory reaction of the salivary tissue with a predominantly neutrophil infiltration, except in mumps in which there is an infiltration by mononuclear cells. In both chronic and recurrent sialadenitis there is a marked periductal and acinar infiltration by mononuclear cells, with some epithelial hyperplasia of the duct accompanied by acinar atrophy and fibrosis.

Clinical features

The presenting symptoms of acute sialadenitis are a painful swelling in one of the parotid glands of an elderly patient. Commonly the patient has a low-grade fever, oedema of the cheek, some trismus, and a purulent discharge may be expressed from the duct opening. In contrast, mumps affects healthy children and young adults.

In chronic sialadenitis there are usually clinical features of obstruction of the duct of one of the submandibular glands. There is pain and swelling in the submandibular or retromandibular region, with a reddened duct orifice discharging pus. Recurrent parotitis presents as an acute pain and swelling of one or both parotid glands, with erythema of the duct orifices and pus discharging from them. There may be an associated fever and malaise. Recurrences vary from weeks to months and after repeated attacks the affected gland may remain enlarged.

Differential diagnosis

There is little clinical difficulty in the differential diagnosis between acute sialadenitis of the parotid gland in the elderly patient due to ascending infection and mumps in the healthy young subject. Any discharging pus should be cultured for organisms and its antibiotic sensitivity should be determined. Recurrent parotitis, however, can cause difficulties; in addition to a history of recurrent painful swelling and discharging pus, sialography may show sialectasis and duct dilatation. In chronic sialadenitis there is usually clinical or radiological evidence of calculus and sialography may show duct dilatation.

Several granulomatous diseases may very occasionally affect the salivary glands, such as sarcoidosis, tuberculosis, syphilis, and actinomycosis. When there is bilateral salivary and lacrimal enlargement this is often referred to as Mikulicz's syndrome. Allergic sialadenitis is also rare and to determine the allergic agent can be difficult as drugs, foods, pollen, and other agents have been implicated.

Treatment

In acute, chronic, or recurrent sialadenitis the relevant antibiotics should be used to control the infection, but occasionally surgical drainage may also be necessary. Careful oral hygiene measures are important in all types of sialadenitis. In chronic sialadenitis the cause of obstruction, such as a calculus, should be removed. The treatment of recurrent parotitis is more difficult and if antibiotics do not control the disease, surgical intervention should be considered.

Course and prognosis

Acute sialadenitis will resolve with the aid of antibiotics and general management of the patient. Chronic sialadenitis may persist for many years and may lead to destruction of the gland unless the cause of duct obstruction is removed early. Recurrent parotitis in childhood may show spontaneous recovery after puberty.

Salivary duct obstruction due to calculus

Aetiology

The submandibular salivary ducts and, to a lesser extent, glands are the most common sites for the development of stones. Calcium phosphates and carbonates are deposited from the saliva round a nidus of desquamated cells or micro-organisms.

Clinical features

Salivary calculus is usually found in adults and the presenting symptoms are a sudden unilateral swelling and pain of the gland related to eating. The swelling may take minutes to appear and hours to subside. Examination reveals a soft swelling of the affected gland and careful digital palpation along the course of the salivary duct will localize the calculus. This may vary in size from a small grain to a concretion 10 to 20 mm in length. The presence and localization of a stone in a duct needs to be confirmed by radiographs, but the presence of calculi in the gland can be diagnosed only by radiography. Over 80 per cent of calculi are found in the submandibular duct or gland.

Differential diagnosis

Recurrent unilateral swelling associated with eating is characteristic of salivary gland obstruction but occasionally this may be caused by external agents. Trauma from a denture or sharp tooth may cause obstruction of the orifice of the parotid duct.

Treatment

If the calculus is near the orifice of the duct it can occasionally be teased out, otherwise surgical removal is indicated.

Course and prognosis

Single calculi do not tend to recur, but if treatment has been delayed numerous calculi may have formed inside the gland which may occasionally have to be excised.

Salivary gland tumours

A variety of epithelial tumours affect the major and minor salivary glands, of which the commonest is pleomorphic adenoma, or mixed salivary tumour (74 per cent), followed by adenocarcinoma (12 per cent), adenoma (8 per cent), mucoepidermoid tumour (3 per cent), and acinic cell tumour (2 per cent); the percentages give the prevalence in the parotid glands. Only pleomorphic adenoma will be considered in any detail and further reading should be consulted for other tumours.

Pleomorphic adenoma

Aetiology

The cause of this tumour is unknown, although salivary gland tumours can be produced in animals by carcinogenic hydrocarbons, polyomavirus, and other agents. The tumour originates from epithelial cells of the ducts, acini, or myoepithelial cells and these are thought to be capable of producing the stromal mucins of this tumour.

Pathology

The epithelial cells proliferate to form duct-like structures, sheets, and cords within a connective tissue stroma, which may show mucous, cartilaginous, or hyaline appearance. The tumour is encapsulated, although satellite tumours are often found outside the capsule.

Clinical features

The tumour is usually found in adults and the parotid salivary gland is most commonly affected, followed by the submandibular gland and rarely the sublingual gland. The minor salivary glands, however, are also affected, and the most frequent sites are the glands of the palate, lips, and cheeks. The tumour presents as a small, painless swelling, which may take years to enlarge and is not attached to the overlying skin or mucosa.

Differential diagnosis

As the tumour is slow growing it needs to be differentiated only from other tumours. Adenocarcinoma, mucoepidermoid carcinoma, and adenoid cystic carcinoma may mimic pleomorphic adenoma in its slow growth, but some may grow more rapidly, invade the adjacent skin or mucosa, and metastasize. These tumours can often be differentiated only on histopathological examination, and wherever possible an excision biopsy should be done.

Treatment

Surgical excision with a margin of normal tissue is the treatment of choice, as the tumour is radioresistant.

Course and prognosis

If left untreated the tumour may enlarge to a grotesque size. A small proportion of pleomorphic adenomas may undergo carcinomatous transformation. The tumour has a bad record for recurrences after excision and this is thought to be due to leaving behind satellite tumours outside the capsule.

Neoplasms, cysts, developmental lesions, and dystrophies of the bones and teeth

This section covers a very large number of lesions found in the jaws. Only essential features, especially of differential diagnosis, will be covered in the following disorders:

(1) benign neoplasms: osteoma, chondroma, fibroma, ossifying fibroma, and giant cell tumour;

(2) malignant neoplasms: osteosarcoma and chondrosarcoma;

(3) cysts and tumours of dental origin: periodontal and dentigenous cysts, keratocysts, and ameloblastoma;

(4) dental malformations or odontomes;

(5) osteodystrophies: giant cell reparative granuloma, brown tumour of hyperparathyroidism, fibrous dysplasia, and Paget's disease.

Aetiology

The cause of the neoplasms and osteodystrophies is not known. Periodontal cysts, which are the most common lesions in this group, develop as a consequence of chronic periapical infection.

Clinical features

The bony tumours and cysts are commonly symptomless unless they have reached a large size and the patient notices a swelling, or a denture ceases to fit. Pathological changes are often noticed by the dentist through movement of teeth or on routine radiographic examination of the teeth. Hyperparathyroidism should be excluded in cases when a giant cell granuloma is suspected. Cysts can be found at any age, but giant cell reparative granulomas, ossifying fibroma, and fibrous dysplasia are often seen in young people, unlike Paget's disease of bone which is seen only in the elderly. There is a predilection for the mandible to be involved more commonly with ossifying fibroma and giant cell reparative granuloma. Odontomes are developmental malformations of dental tissues that become calcified. This is a diverse group of disorders and varies from a simple enamel pearl, consisting of a nodule of ectopic enamel attached to a tooth, to a complex composite odontome, which is an irregular mass of calcified dental tissues. Ameloblastoma is a rare but important epithelial neoplasm of the jaws. Young adults are most often affected, the tumour is slow-growing, and affects the mandible more often than the maxilla. The neoplasm is locally invasive but does not metastasize. Osteosarcoma and chondrosarcoma are found in children or young adults but may develop in the elderly with Paget's disease. They present as fast-growing, painful, and firm swellings and they may metastasize to the lungs early.

Differential diagnosis

The diagnosis of bony lesions of the jaws is made on the basis of radiological appearances and the histological features of the biopsy. Periodontal cysts are very frequent and show a radiolucent rounded area with a sharply defined outline. If the crown of a tooth is enclosed within the cyst, it is referred to as a dentigerous cyst. The latter and keratocysts are usually found in the young, but with some keratocysts a tooth may be missing. Dental cysts must be differentiated from ameloblastomas, which tend to show multilocular and sometimes a honeycomb pattern on radiographs. These radiolucent lesions should also be differentiated from secondary carcinoma and myelomatosis. Giant cell reparative granuloma and tumour (osteoclastoma) show a radiolucent area, sometimes loculated, and the outline is not as well defined as a dental cyst. Hyperparathyroidism can be excluded by the radiographic appearance of other bones and by the calcium and phosphate levels in the blood. Ossifying fibromas are more common than fibromas and radiographs show a well-defined radiolucent area with speckled calcification. This can usually be distinguished from the 'ground glass' appearance, without a distinct border, found in fibrous dysplasia. In Paget's disease there is a distinctive 'cotton wool' appearance on radiographic examination and the alkaline phosphatase levels are high. Odontomes can be readily recognized on clinical examination, but those that are unerupted, particularly the compound and complex composite odontomes, show on radiographs a mass of overlapping denticles and an irregular radio-opaque mass respectively. Osteosarcoma and chondrosarcoma show patchy areas of bone resorption and deposition.

Treatment

The treatment of dental cysts is by enucleation of the cyst lining and usually extracting the involved tooth. The tumours and malformations are excised but some, such as giant cell reparative granuloma, can be curettaged. Brown tumours will recur unless the underlying hyperparathyroidism has been treated. Fibrous dysplasia may require removal of excessive tissue for cosmetic or functional reasons, but this should be delayed until normal bone growth has ceased. Bony changes in Paget's disease are best not interfered with, except when there are functional reasons such as inability to fit a denture. Composite odontomes should be removed surgically. The treatment of ameloblastoma is by local excision, with a generous margin of normal bone, or by hemimandibulectomy. Sarcoma of the jaw must be dealt with by early radical excision.

Course and prognosis

If the cysts or benign tumours are removed surgically they do not recur, except with keratocysts and the reparative granulomas. Ameloblastomas may recur after several excisions, without metastases, and this is why some surgeons prefer to do a hemimandibulectomy. The prognosis of the jaw sarcomas is very poor and the 5-year survival rate is between 25 and 40 per cent. Fibrous dysplasia tends to be self-limiting, but in Paget's disease there may be progressive enlargement, especially of the maxilla.

Miscellaneous disorders

In this section a brief discussion will be given on the following three topics: oral manifestations of blood disorders, halitosis, and disorders of the temporomandibular joint.

Oral manifestations of blood disorders

Mild anaemias or deficiencies of iron, folate, or vitamin B$_{12}$ may manifest themselves as glossitis (Fig. 13) with a sore tongue or mouth, angular cheilitis, or recurrent ulceration (see Section 22). The tongue is commonly depapillated, the corners of the mouth may be inflamed and fissured, and occasionally there may be small shallow ulcers affecting the lips, tongue,

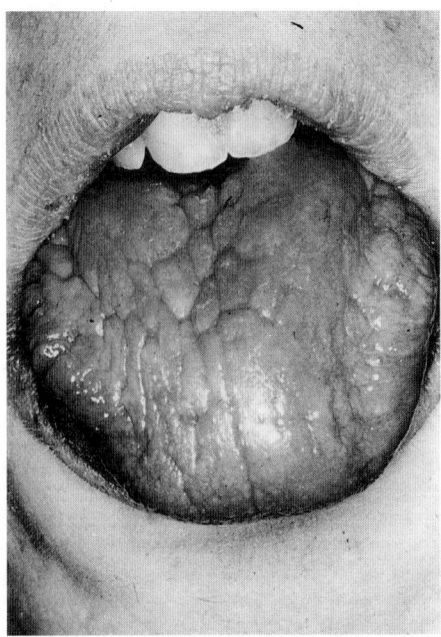

Fig. 13 Smooth, depapillated, erythematous tongue in a patient with iron deficiency anaemia.

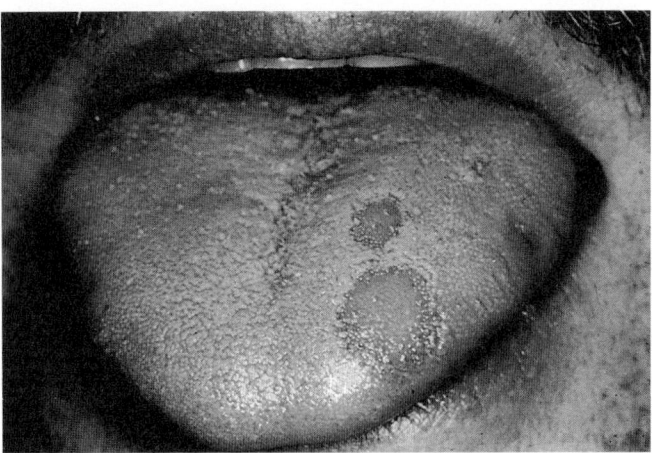

Fig. 14 Round or oval, depapillated lesions with a raised margin in a patient with erythema migrans of the tongue.

and cheeks. The cause of any haematological deficiency should be investigated and, especially with folate deficiency, coeliac disease should be excluded. Replacement therapy usually deals with the clinical features effectively. It should, however, be emphasized that the complaint of a sore tongue can be associated with many other causes, such as erythema migrans, candidiasis, lichen planus, recurrent aphthous ulceration, and black hairy tongue.

Erythema migrans (geographical tongue) is particularly common and is characterized by oval, depapillated areas with a well-defined edge affecting the dorsum of the tongue (Fig. 14). The lesions move from one site to another. The aetiology of erythema migrans is unknown and treatment is rather unsatisfactory. It is noteworthy that a sore tongue is a frequent complaint in middle-aged women, often without any demonstrable aetiological factor.

Acute leukaemia, particularly the myelomonocytic form, may occasionally present in the young in the form of sore, bleeding gums. This may vary from slight inflammation to that showing bulbous enlargement of the gingiva. There are usually inadequate local causes for such a gingivitis and anaemia may be evident; blood tests should be requested to exclude leukaemia.

Leucopenia and agranulocytosis, especially those due to drugs, may become clinically evident by ulceration of the throat or the mouth. Purpura may be associated with a deficiency of platelets, so that bleeding from the gum may also be a feature.

Many haemorrhagic disorders may become evident after extraction of a tooth, because bleeding does not stop. Less commonly, gingival bleeding may direct attention to the blood disorder.

Halitosis

Bad breath is usually a trivial complaint, though it is heightened by social pressures. There are four possible sources of halitosis: the mouth, nasopharynx, lungs, and the gastrointestinal tract. Altered blood round the gum may be the most important oral cause, and this may be associated with debris or pus from gingivitis and periodontal pockets. A characteristic halitosis is found in acute ulcerative gingivitis. It should be noted that bad taste and bad breath are subjective sensations which are often confused. Excessive bacterial plaque on the teeth is not a principal cause of halitosis; nevertheless, meticulous oral care should be advised.

Chronic tonsillitis may be responsible for halitosis but atrophic rhinitis causing ozaena is probably the most important cause to be excluded. Occasionally, respiratory tract infections may cause halitosis and a variety of gastrointestinal disorders have been associated with bad breath but there is little evidence to substantiate this. Frequently all these sources of halitosis

may be excluded without finding a cause and these patients may have a fixation about bad breath related to emotional or sexual problems.

Temporomandibular joint disorders

The patient complains of pain, clicking, or limitation of movement. It is found in young women more often than men. Examination may reveal limitations in jaw movement, tenderness of the joint, and crepitus on movement, discovered by palpating the head of the condyle through the overlying skin. The cause is difficult to establish but malocclusion might be one of several factors. The condition may clear spontaneously but in some patients the occlusion should be checked and a bite-raising appliance is often helpful. Rheumatoid arthritis and osteoarthritis of this joint are occasionally seen clinically. Dislocation of the joint, which becomes fixed in the open position, may be caused by a blow on the jaw or during dental extractions under general anaesthesia. Ankylosis of the joint is nowadays extremely rare but in the past was caused by osteomyelitis.

Further reading

Atkinson JC *et al.* (1990). Major salivary gland function in primary Sjögren's syndrome and its relationship to clinical features. *Journal of Rheumatology* **17**, 318–22.

Bouquot JE, Weiland LH, Kurland LT (1988). Leukoplakia and carcinoma *in situ* synchronously associated with invasive oral/oropharyngeal carcinoma in Rochester Minn., 1935–1984. *Oral Surgery, Oral Medicine, Oral Pathology* **65**, 199–207.

Carlsson J (1989). Microbial aspects of frequent intake of products with high sugar concentrations. *Scandinavian Journal of Dental Research* **97**, 110–14.

Chau MN, Radden BG (1989). A clinical-pathological study of 53 intra-oral pleomorphic adenomas. *International Journal of Oral and Maxillofacial Surgery* **18**, 158–62.

Dummer PMH *et al.* (1990). Factors influencing the caries experience of a group of children at the ages of 11–12 and 15–16 years: results from an ongoing study. *Journal of Dentistry* **18**, 37–48.

Eley BM (1997). The future of dental amalgam: a review of the literature. Part 3. Mercury exposure from amalgam restorations in dental patients. *British Dental Journal* **182**, 331–8.

Fox PC, Busch KA, Baum BJ (1987). Subjective reports of xerostomia and objective measures of salivary gland performance. *Journal of the American Dental Association* **115**, 581–4.

Gibbons RJ (1989). Bacterial adhesion to oral tissues: a model for infectious diseases. *Journal of Dental Research* **68**, 750–60.

Goldberg HI *et al.* (1994). Trends and differentials from cancers of the oral cavity and pharynx in the United States, 1973–1987. *Cancer* **74**, 565–72.

Greenspan D, Greenspan JS (1996). HIV-related oral disease. *Lancet* **348**, 729–33.

Hasan A *et al.* (1995). Recognition of a unique peptide epitope of the mycobacterial and human heat shock protein 65–60 antigen by T cells of patients with recurrent oral ulcers. *Clinical Experimental Immunology* **99**, 392–7.

Helander SD, Rogers RD (1994). The sensitivity and specificity of direct immunofluorescence testing in disorders of mucous membranes. *Journal of the American Academy of Dermatology* **30**, 65–75.

Herrod HG (1990). Chronic mucocutaneous candidiasis in childhood and complications of non-Candida infection. *Journal of Pediatrics* **116**, 377–82.

Hogewind WF *et al.* (1989). The association of white lesions with oral squamous cell carcinoma: A retrospective study of 212 patients. *International Journal of Oral and Maxillofacial Surgery* **18**, 163–4.

Holmstrup P *et al.* (1988). Malignant development of lichen planus-affected oral mucosa. *Journal of Oral Pathology* **17**, 219–25.

Huilgol SC, Bhogal BS, Black MM (1995). Immunofluorescence of the immunobullous disorders. *European Journal of Dermatology* **5**, 186–95.

Kashima HK *et al.* (1990). Human papilloma virus in squamous cell carcinoma, leukoplakia, lichen planus, and clinically normal epithelium of the oral cavity. *Annals of Ontology, Rhinology and Laryngology* **99**, 55–61.

Larsson KS (1995). The dissemination of false data through inadequate citation. *Journal of Internal Medicine* **238**, 445–50.

Lehner T (1992). *Immunology of oral diseases.* Blackwell, Oxford.

Lloyd RE, Ho KH (1988). Combined CT scanning and sialography in the management of parotid tumors. *Oral Surgery, Oral Medicine, Oral Pathology* **65**, 142–4.

Lozada-Nur F, Gorsky M, Silverman S (1989). Oral erythema multiforme: clinical observations and treatment of 95 patients. *Oral Surgery, Oral Medicine, Oral Surgery* **67**, 36–40.

Newbrun E (1989). Frequent sugar intake—then and now: interpretation of main results. *Scandinavian Journal of Dental Research* **97**, 103–9.

Page RC *et al.* (1997). Advances in the pathogenesis of periodontitis: summary of developments, clinical implications and future directions. *Periodontology* **14**, 216–48.

Seaman S, Thomas FD, Walker WA (1989). Differences between caries levels in 5 year old children from fluoridated Anglesey and non-fluoridated mainland Gwynedd in 1987. *Community Dental Health* **6**, 215–21.

Van der Meij EH *et al.* (1999). A review of the recent literature regarding malignant transformation of oral lichen planus. *Oral Surgery, Oral Medicine, Oral Pathology* **88**, 307–10.

Van der Waal I *et al.* (1997). Oral leukoplakia: a clinicopathologivcal review. *Oral Oncology* **33**, 291–301.

Williams DM (1989). Vesiculobullous mucocutaneous disease: pemphigus vulgaris. *Journal of Oral Pathology and Medicine* **18**, 544–53.

Williams RC (1990). Periodontal disease. *New England Journal of Medicine* **322**, 373–82.

14.6 Diseases of the oesophagus

John Dent and Richard H. Holloway

Introduction

Oesophageal function testing

Techniques are now available for the precise measurement of oesophageal function. The benefits of oesophageal function testing are most apparent when it is the only means for the accurate diagnosis of a treatable disorder. However, it is also valuable for the recognition of disorders for which there is no definitive therapy, since symptoms can be explained. Oesophageal function testing is relatively expensive and time-consuming and so should not be requested for the assessment of trivial symptoms or when the information gained will not aid management.

Barium radiology

The barium swallow is often undervalued for the diagnosis of structural abnormalities. Useful information can also be obtained about the motor function of the pharynx and oesophagus by videotaping the images and analysing, in slow-motion replay, repeated tests of standardized stimuli. The sensitivity of barium radiology is enhanced by the use of provocative solid boluses, such as bread, or barium tablets. Videofluoroscopy is essential for the proper analysis of pharyngeal motor function, and complements other tests of oesophageal motor function such as manometry. Optimal results from radiology are achieved when there is a partnership between a clinician and a radiologist who have a special interest in oesophageal motor disorders; if the particular question(s) that are being pursued by the clinician are well communicated to the radiologist the examination technique can then be tailored accordingly.

Oesophageal manometry

Oesophageal manometry provides the most direct indication of patterns of oesophageal motor function. It is most helpful in the diagnosis of dysphagia, after exclusion of fixed, structural defects. Manometry plays only a minor role in the management of reflux disease; it assists if there is no oesophagitis and mild dysphagia is present, or if surgery is planned. Prolonged, ambulatory 24-h manometry, which requires sophisticated miniaturized equipment, may be useful in patients with dysphagia or non-cardiac chest pain.

24-h ambulatory oesophageal pH monitoring

The principal value of this procedure is to determine the association between symptoms and episodes of acid reflux. Investigation of this relationship is only of importance in a minority of patients in whom the origin of troublesome symptoms is unclear (Fig. 1).

Radionuclide measurement of oesophageal transit

Computerized scintigraphic analysis of the movement of swallowed radiolabelled boluses can give quantitative information about the patterns of movement of material down the oesophagus. However, its poor spatial resolution makes it an inadequate method for the display of oesophageal anatomy. If structural abnormalities have been adequately excluded, slow or interrupted transit suggests abnormal motility, although patterns of transit are usually non-specific. If good barium radiology is available, radionuclide testing of oesophageal transit becomes redundant.

General management of oesophageal dysphagia

Symptomatic treatment of dysphagia is frequently necessary because of the limited options and efficacy of treatments for oesophageal disorders. Although these measures may appear obvious, this aspect of management is commonly neglected by both patient and physician.

Optimization of bolus consistency

Large particles of solid food may impact on strictures. Large boluses require greater propulsive force even in the absence of stricture, and may trigger oesophageal spasm. Boluses should therefore be small and, in some circumstances, reduced to semiliquid or liquid form. This can be achieved by the use of fluids in bolus preparation and avoidance of hard fibrous foods. Poor dentition should be treated. In some patients, defects of oesophageal function may be so severe that the diet should be pureed. Consultation with a dietitian will assist patients in identifying and preparing suitable food and in maintaining nutrition.

Assistance with oesophageal transit

Liquids assist transit by reducing the viscosity of food and providing a pressure head in the oesophagus. Gas generated within the oesophageal body from effervescent drinks can act as a piston which displaces oesophageal contents into the stomach in the erect position and may be sufficient to overcome an achalasic sphincter. The value of gravity in assisting transit should never be forgotten. Patients with severely impaired oesophageal transit should be advised to swallow medications in the upright position and with plenty of water so as to avoid injurious contact of the oesophagus with potentially corrosive tablets.

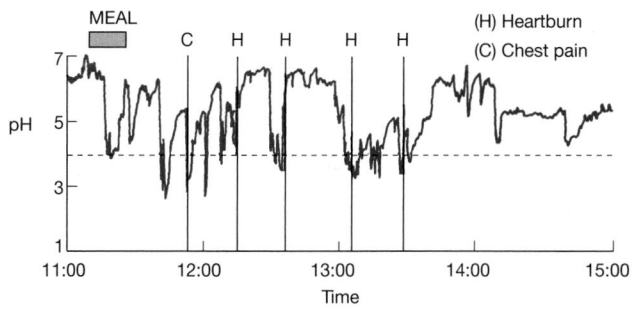

Fig. 1 Section of a 24-h oesophageal pH monitoring study showing the association of heartburn with episodes of acid reflux after a meal.

Alternative/supplementary approaches to feeding

Rarely, the above measures fail to maintain nutrition. Percutaneous endoscopic gastrostomy should then be used.

Gastro-oesophageal reflux disease

This is by far the most common oesophageal disorder. Reflux symptoms occurring at least once in 6 months are experienced in about one-third of people. Management should be tailored to the wide range of severity.

Definition

Gastro-oesophageal reflux occurs to some degree in everybody. It should only be considered a disease when it gives rise to significant symptoms or complications sufficient to impair the quality of life. The terms reflux or peptic oesophagitis should be reserved for circumstances when endoscopy shows that the oesophageal mucosa is clearly breached by the action of the refluxed gastric contents. Minor changes such as erythema, oedema, or friability have been shown to be very unreliable indicators of the presence of oesophagitis.

Aetiology

In most patients reflux disease arises from the excessive exposure of the distal oesophagus to refluxed acid, usually because of an abnormal frequency of reflux episodes. In a few patients, however, symptoms arise with relatively normal levels of acid exposure, presumably because of sensitization of the oesophageal mucosa.

In most patients reflux occurs as a result of defective neural control of the lower oesophageal sphincter. Severe reflux disease can also result from damage to the oesophagus as in scleroderma. Hiatus hernia is common in patients with reflux disease and causes displacement of the sphincter from the hiatus formed by the diaphragmatic crura. The hiatus provides important extrinsic support to the sphincter and helps to maintain gastro-oesophageal competence, particularly during straining. Hiatus hernia therefore impairs sphincter function and also acid clearance.

Most reflux occurs during the day, usually after food, but nocturnal reflux is also very important. Refluxed acid is cleared from the oesophagus by peristalsis and swallowed saliva. Slow clearance of oesophageal acidification contributes significantly to prolonged acid exposure in about 50 per cent of patients.

Consequences of excessive reflux

Symptoms

These are an important source of disability. Heartburn is most important and when it occurs on more than 2 days a week causes significant impairment of quality of life. However, presentation may be with the less specific pattern of dyspepsia, or with regurgitation, haematemesis, and dysphagia due to either stricture or motor dysfunction of the oesophageal body. Reflux may cause respiratory symptoms such as hoarseness, persistent cough, and asthma, which may predominate in some patients.

Oesophagitis

The chemical insult from excessive exposure of the mucosa to acid and pepsin leads to distal oesophageal erosion or ulceration in between 40 and 60 per cent of patients with troublesome reflux symptoms. The extent of ulceration varies greatly, from tiny patches of erosion to extensive circumferential ulceration in a small minority.

The risks of oesophagitis are not well defined. Peptic stricture and/or oesophageal columnar metaplasia (Barrett's oesophagus) are typically only associated with severe oesophagitis.

Stricturing causes dysphagia which may be debilitating and lead to malnutrition. Treatment with dilatation (bougienage) is a burden and is associated with a risk of perforation.

Columnar metaplasia (see below) is associated with the risk of developing oesophageal adenocarcinoma. It may also be associated with deep benign oesophageal ulceration within the columnar-lined segment. Occasionally such ulcers erode into mediastinal structures or the pleural space, sometimes with fatal consequences.

Bleeding from oesophagitis is relatively common, but is rarely life-threatening except when it occurs from a deep ulcer associated with columnar metaplasia..

Diagnosis and assessment of severity

History

The history is pivotal for diagnosis because of the extremely high prevalence of reflux-induced symptoms and the lack of a definitive, inexpensive diagnostic test for reflux disease. Fortunately, the specificity of patterns of symptoms of reflux disease is arguably the highest of any of the more common gastrointestinal diseases and the majority of patients can be diagnosed confidently on the basis of their history. The strategic use of history and initial empirical therapy as a means to assess diagnosis and severity is summarized in Fig. 2, and discussed in detail in the section on treatment below.

Endoscopy

When investigation is needed, endoscopy is the first choice as it is the only test that can give sensitive recognition and grading of oesophagitis and reliable diagnosis of oesophageal columnar metaplasia. Endoscopy also allows for the effective identification of significant peptic strictures, other types of oesophagitis, and other upper gastrointestinal disorders such as peptic ulcer disease and oesophageal and gastric carcinoma. As discussed above, however, most patients with reflux disease do not have endoscopically visible mucosal damage, so a negative endoscopy does not exclude the diagnosis of reflux disease. The value of endoscopy as the initial investigation is greatly enhanced by the accurate diagnosis of endoscopic biopsy and, where indicated, cytology brushings.

Oesophageal function tests

The place of these is summarized in Fig. 2. Oesophageal manometry and ambulatory pH monitoring have a limited but important role in the diagnosis of reflux disease. Oesophageal pH monitoring is most useful in patients with troublesome symptoms but without endoscopic signs of oesophagitis in whom a trial of therapy has failed, and patients with atypical symptoms that cannot be clearly related to reflux. Patients with suspected reflux symptoms but with no endoscopic evidence of oesophagitis who are being considered for antireflux surgery should also undergo oesophageal pH monitoring.

Barium swallow and meal

This is an inappropriate primary diagnostic test; it is of no value for the detection of abnormal reflux, and is insensitive for the diagnosis of oesophagitis and cannot grade it. Other pathologies such as gastric ulcer and oesophageal stricture are demonstrated with reasonable sensitivity, but adequate evaluation of these findings requires endoscopic biopsy. In contrast, barium swallow has an important secondary role in the investigation of the mechanisms of troublesome dysphagia. Barium swallow is the best method for recognizing extrinsic oesophageal compression which may be producing symptoms that could be interpreted as being due to reflux, and in the assessment of anatomically complex hiatus hernia. The mere demonstration of hiatus hernia, however, does not necessarily indicate the presence of reflux disease.

Principles of management

New treatments have transformed management in recent years. The major aims of treatment are to provide adequate symptomatic relief and control of oesophagitis. Reduction of oesophagitis to minor patchy erosions is

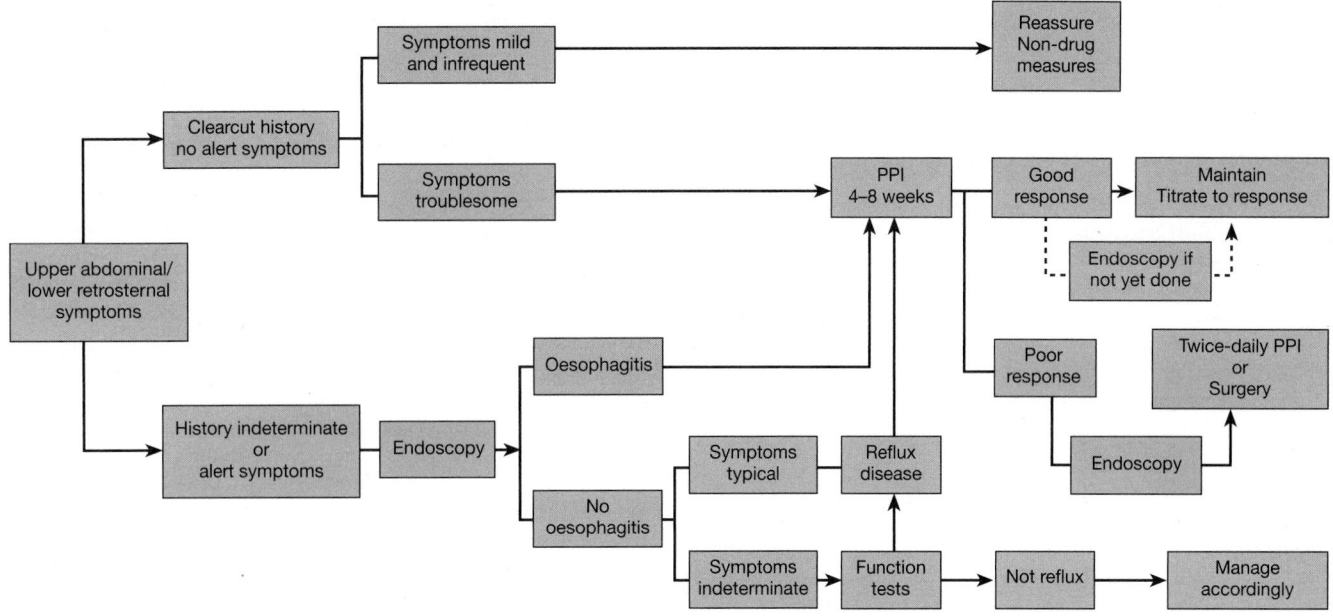

Fig. 2 Principal decision paths for management of reflux disease.

probably sufficient to prevent the complications of oesophagitis, although adequate symptomatic relief is usually achieved only when oesophagitis is completely healed. Management steps are easily confused, as endoscopy, assessment of symptoms, and treatment are used not only for diagnosis, but also assessment of severity and titration of therapy.

Cost-efficient, secure diagnosis

The steps needed for diagnosis are shown in Fig. 2. When the history is classical, the symptoms are only mild to moderate, and there are no alert symptoms, endoscopy is effectively redundant. Given the high proportion of patients who have no endoscopic abnormality, a negative endoscopy should not detract from the soundness of a diagnosis based on symptoms. When symptoms are indeterminate, or alert symptoms of dysphagia, hae-matemesis, or weight loss are present, endoscopy is the primary diagnostic approach. The place of endoscopy in patients with troublesome or severe but classical symptoms is becoming less relevant because of the advent of highly effective initial high-level medical therapy with proton pump inhibitors.

Assessment of severity

Morbidity arising from symptoms and the presence and severity of oeso-phagitis are the two most important measures of severity of reflux disease. However, they show only poor correlation. The response of symptoms to low- and medium-level therapy (see Table 1 and below) gives an indirect approximation of the severity of oesophagitis and helps to determine further action.

Tailoring and titration of therapy

Classification of therapies by level of efficacy regardless of their mechanism of action (Table 1) provides a framework for the tailoring and titration of long-term management. The lowest effective dose of any agent should be used in long-term therapy. Figure 2 and Table 2 summarize the logic of using endoscopic findings to choose an appropriate level of initial therapy. As the responsiveness of individual patients varies, therapy needs to be titrated upwards or downwards through levels of efficacy in order to find the lowest level that is effective, on the basis that this will minimize drug costs.

Most patients with reflux disease will have an initial trial of empirical therapy. There are two main options for this. Initial low- to medium-level therapy is the traditional model outlined in Fig. 2. This has the disadvantage of giving less crisp diagnostic information, and often gives only slow relief of symptoms, but will usually identify patients with severe oesophagitis since these will usually not respond adequately. Initial high-level medical therapy is now available. This is most likely to give crisp confirmation of the diagnosis and prompt relief of symptoms. For optimum cost-effectiveness,

Table 1 Levels of first-line antireflux therapy

Level of therapy	Treatment
Low	Antacids, non-drug measures
Middle	Normal dose H_2 receptor antagonists
Upper	Half-dose proton pump inhibitor
High	Once daily proton pump inhibitor
Highest	Once daily proton pump inhibitor High-quality antireflux surgery

Table 2 Efficacy of levels of antireflux therapy: estimated proportions of patients with adequate symptom control and healing of oesophagitis where applicable

Level of therapy	Grade of oesophagitis*			
	Endoscopy negative (%)	Mild (%)	Moderate (%)	Severe (%)
Low	0–20	0–20	0	0
Middle	20–50	60–80	0–20	0
High	50–70	80–100	60–80	40–60
Highest	50–70	80–100	80–100	60–90

*Mild, moderate, and severe oesophagitis correspond to Los Angeles grades A, B, and C/D respectively.

it should be followed by a step-down approach to long-term therapy as outlined in Fig. 2.

Options for treatment of oesophagitis and symptoms arising directly from reflux

Non-drug measures and antacids

The efficacy of these traditional approaches is often over-rated. The most useful measures are avoidance of large meals and provocative foods, drinks, and physical activities. The benefits to reflux disease of stopping smoking, weight loss, and elevation of the bedhead are uncertain. Antacids will not usually prevent symptoms, but may be effective in aborting episodes of heartburn. These low-cost measures are worth a trial in patients with mild intermittent symptoms (Tables 1 and 2), and should be used as maintenance therapy if they prove effective, provided that their impact on lifestyle is acceptable to the patient. They are unlikely to succeed in people with troublesome reflux symptoms.

Acid suppression

Inhibition of secretion of gastric acid makes gastric juice less injurious but does not stop reflux. This has deservedly become the most widely used drug therapy because of its high efficacy and adjustability. The more severe the oesophagitis, the higher the level of acid suppression that is needed (Table 2). Proton pump inhibitors have a special role because of their effectiveness in reduction of food-stimulated acid secretion and their greater overall efficacy in control of acid secretion compared with histamine-2 receptor antagonists.

Long-term treatment with acid suppressants maintains patients free of symptoms and oesophagitis indefinitely but withdrawal is usually associated with prompt relapse. The maintenance dose appears to be the same as the lowest effective healing dose. There have been concerns about the safety of long-term acid suppression ever since the introduction of histamine-2 receptor antagonists. To date, follow-up of patients treated continuously for 10 or more years with acid suppression has shown no evidence of any effects of significance, but in the context of patients who may require treatment with these agents for decades, more extensive follow-up is still needed. Given these theoretical safety considerations and also drug cost, long-term treatment of reflux disease with these agents should use the lowest effective dose.

Motility stimulants

Only cisapride has been adequately researched. It has medium efficacy for both short- and long-term management. It appears unlikely that much is gained from an increase in dosage. The principal effect of cisapride appears to be on oesophageal acid clearance. Unfortunately, it has been recognized recently that cisapride has effects on cardiac conductance that may rarely lead to sudden death at peak serum levels encountered during therapy in some patients, especially when various drugs are coadministered. Because of the risk of cardiac effects, cisapride must be regarded as a second- or third-line therapy that needs to be used with special precautions.

Combination medical therapy

Use of cisapride and histamine-2 receptor antagonists in combination gives moderately improved results but is less effective than monotherapy with proton pump inhibitors. Given the safety concerns described above, and its relatively high cost, such combination therapy should be reserved for special cases.

Antireflux surgery

In skilled hands, antireflux surgery is a very effective long-term therapy. Negative factors are the dependence of the results on the expertise of the surgeon and the morbidity and small (approximately 0.5 per cent) mortality associated with the surgery itself. Laparoscopic antireflux surgery is a major advance, as it achieves good control of reflux with a major reduction in the morbidity inherent in the more traditional approach. More information is needed about long-term results.

Choice between therapies

Selection of a medical or surgical therapy should take account of the severity of disease and the risks of antireflux surgery specific to the patient. It should also take account of the patient's age, both from the point of view of operative risk and the time over which the patient will need treatment for reflux disease, the cost of effective medical therapy, and, naturally, the preferences of the patient. In the United States, good open antireflux surgery becomes cost-effective compared with medical therapy after about 10 years, although this assessment does not take into account the cost of mortality. The breakeven point is likely to be shorter with laparoscopic surgery and in countries where the costs of surgery are lower than in the United States. Cost comparisons also need to take into account the decreasing price of acid suppressing agents. The choice between medical therapies should be largely governed by the local cost of the alternatives that give the necessary level of treatment, as all of the first-line options are safe and well tolerated.

Management of complications of reflux disease

Peptic stricture

Dysphagia secondary to stricture (Fig. 3) needs to be distinguished from the more common dysphagia seen in patients with reflux disease which is due to defective triggering and control of oesophageal body peristalsis (see the section on non-specific oesophageal motor disorders below). Peptic stricture is managed by a combination of peroral dilatation and healing of oesophagitis by either medical or surgical means. Provided oesophagitis is healed, stricture is usually not an ongoing problem.

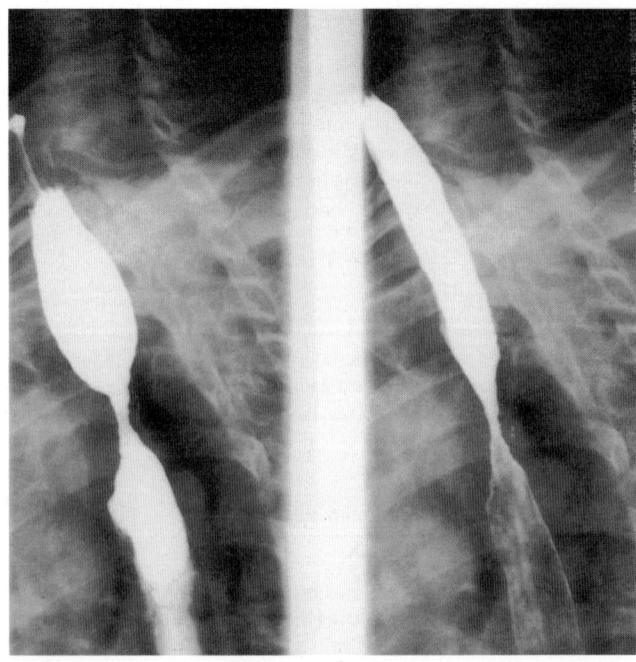

Fig. 3 Peptic stricture: asymmetrical circumferential narrowing with associated intramural diverticulosis suggests benign aetiology; the site suggests Barrett's mucosa, subsequently proven by endoscopy. (By courtesy of Dr H. Harley.)

Oesophageal columnar metaplasia (Barrett's oesophagus)

This increasingly recognized consequence of oesophagitis is dealt with in the section on oesophageal neoplasia. The association of columnar metaplasia with oesophageal adenocarcinoma contributes to the logic of vigorous treatment of severe oesophagitis.

Respiratory complications

Respiratory disease may occur as a result of either direct aspiration of refluxed gastric contents or from the reflex effects of gastro-oesophageal reflux. It is difficult to prove that reflux disease which coexists with respiratory disease is actually the cause of the respiratory problem. The best investigative approach is probably a trial of high-level acid inhibition with at least a double-dose of proton pump inhibitor for at least 2 months. Management of respiratory disease by antireflux surgery is a gamble that can only be supported primarily by clinical evaluation.

Regurgitation

Voluminous regurgitation is the main symptom in a small subgroup of patients with reflux disease. They may present complaining of vomiting, but a detailed history reveals that there is no prior nausea, and no effort involved in the appearance of the gastric content in the mouth. The determinants of high-volume reflux and regurgitation have not been defined. Treatment with proton pump inhibitors can have substantial benefits, but in more severe cases antireflux surgery is usually the only effective management.

Non-cardiac chest pain

Reflux is an important cause of non-cardiac chest pain (see below).

Primary oesophageal motor disorders

Idiopathic achalasia and achalasia-like states

Definition

These disorders are characterized by absent or incomplete relaxation of the lower oesophageal sphincter and impairment of peristalsis of the oesophageal body. Idiopathic achalasia, which was first described over 300 years ago, accounts for most cases and has an annual incidence of approximately 1 to 2 per 100 000. It affects all ages, but is diagnosed most often in early to mid adult life. The syndrome is also seen in Chagas disease and can sometimes accompany the intestinal pseudo-obstructive syndrome. Achalasia may be a manifestation of paraneoplastic neural dysfunction and may also be secondary to oesophageal amyloidosis.

Secondary or pseudoachalasia can arise from neoplastic infiltration of the gastro-oesophageal junction, and has been reported with carcinoma of the stomach, oesophagus, lung, pancreas, prostate, and with lymphoma.

Aetiology

Impairment of inhibitory neural control of the distal oesophagus is the universal abnormality. The syndrome can probably be produced by neural damage at several sites. The clearest evidence is degeneration of myenteric inhibitory neurones which, in the early stages, is associated with an inflammatory response.

Symptoms

Dysphagia with solids is almost universal. Regurgitation is also prominent. The regurgitated material tastes bland because it never enters the stomach. Cramping chest pain occurs in some patients during an early hypercontracting phase of the disorder. Weight loss is seen in patients with disabling dysphagia. The course of symptoms over time is variable. In some patients, symptoms remain static for many years but in others there is a progression with increasing problems with regurgitation over several years, as a result of development and increase of oesophageal dilatation. When this occurs, respiratory problems secondary to aspiration can become a major feature.

Diagnosis

Idiopathic achalasia is diagnosed on average 2 years after its first presentation, Delay is especially likely if oesophageal dilatation is absent. Dilatation varies in degree from a minor increase in oesophageal calibre to a grossly enlarged, colon-like oesophagus. Barium swallow shows oesophageal retention with a gastro-oesophageal junction that tapers smoothly to a closed sphincter, with occasional spurts of flow into the stomach (Fig. 4). In the absence of dilatation, a barium swallow is often reported as normal.

Oesophageal manometry is the only sensitive method for demonstration of the characteristic motor dysfunction. It is not unusual for manometry to be diagnostic of achalasia even though barium studies have been judged to be normal.

Idiopathic achalasia and achalasia-like states should be distinguished from constriction of the gastro-oesophageal junction by an infiltrating or encasing malignancy at the cardia. This diagnosis is often difficult to make. As a minimum, patients should be evaluated clinically for any symptoms or signs suggestive of malignancy, and upper gastrointestinal endoscopy should be done with mucosal biopsies. Computed tomography scanning is also of value.

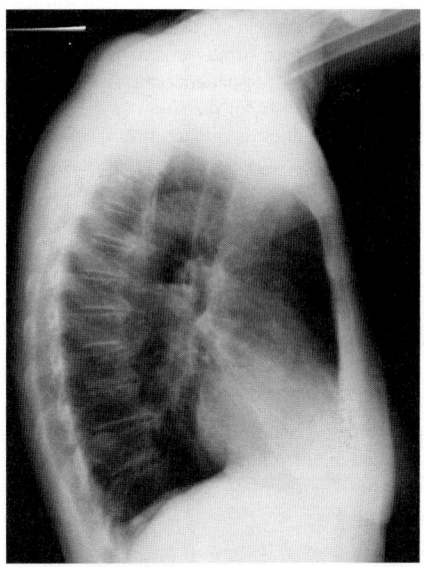

(a)

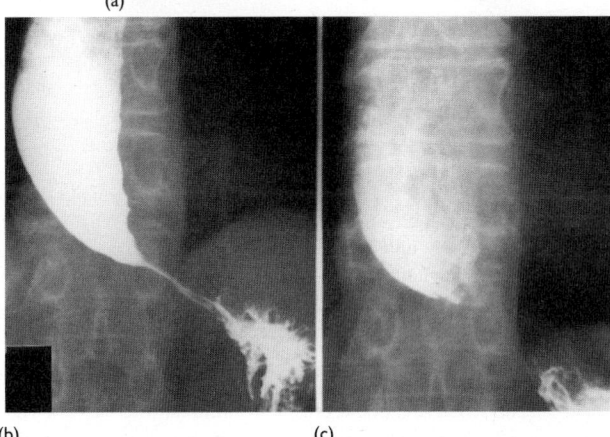

(b)　　　　　　　　(c)

Fig. 4 Achalasia. (a) A lateral chest film shows the air–fluid level in the mid oesophagus just behind the air column of the trachea. (b) On a posteroanterior view this level is almost invisible. Barium-filled dilated oesophagus; intact mucosa in distal achalasia segment.

Treatment

There are four potential approaches to treatment: drug therapy with agents that relax the lower oesophageal sphincter, mechanical disruption of the sphincter by either pneumatic dilatation or surgical myotomy, and pharmacological poisoning of the remaining excitatory nerves to the sphincter with botulinum toxin. The results of reduction of lower oesophageal sphincter pressure with drugs such as calcium antagonists and β-adrenergic agonists compare poorly with mechanical disruption of the sphincter, and by inference botulinum toxin.

Oesophagomyotomy, which is now being done increasingly as a laparoscopic or thoracoscopic procedure, is highly effective but is associated with a 5 to 10 per cent risk of troublesome gastro-oesophageal reflux. This risk can be minimized by the incorporation of an antireflux procedure.

Balloon dilatation is an attractive approach because of its simplicity and low cost, but it often needs to be repeated and in some hands fails in up to 40 per cent of patients, especially those who are young. It also carries a risk of perforation of about 5 per cent. With the development of minimally invasive surgery for oesophagomyotomy, balloon dilatation will probably be used most in older patients who have other medical problems that increase the risks of surgery.

Endoscopic injection of the sphincter with botulinum toxin is the most recent innovation. This toxin acts on residual excitatory nerves thereby lowering sphincter pressure. Short-term results are comparable to those of pneumatic dilatation but the procedure usually has to be repeated within 1 to 2 years. The toxin is also relatively expensive. It is a simple, low-risk procedure and most applicable to patients with significant coexisting morbidity which renders them unfit for dilatation or myotomy.

When oesophageal dilatation is present, prompt treatment is indicated to prevent its worsening, because of the morbidity and poor therapeutic outcome associated with gross oesophageal dilatation. Oesophageal emptying can be assisted by effervescent drinks (see above).

Prognosis

If effective treatment is applied before the development of major dilatation results are excellent, despite the persistence of major physiological abnormalities. Achalasia carries a very significantly increased risk for oesophageal carcinoma up to many years later which ranges from 2 to 7 per cent in authoritative reports. There is no apparent reduction of this risk with treatment. The average interval from diagnosis of achalasia to development of carcinoma has been estimated as 28 years. It is not usual practice to undertake surveillance for this risk, but some clinicians recommend periodic screening endoscopy.

Diffuse oesophageal spasm

Definition

Episodic chest pain and/or dysphagia resulting from spastic contractions of the distal half of the oesophageal body in the absence of any precipitating structural stenosis. There are no generally agreed criteria for diagnosis.

Aetiology

It is widely assumed that this is a dysfunction of neural control but there is a lack information that addresses this or other possibilities. What is known of the epidemiology is unhelpful with regard to aetiology. Stress is an unlikely primary precipitant but may exacerbate the problem. Good prevalence data are lacking. Diffuse spasm affects all ages and is much less common than achalasia.

Symptoms

Virtually all patients have episodic, crushing central retrosternal pain which can be excruciating; cardiac ischaemia is often the first diagnosis. Intermittent dysphagia occurs in about two-thirds of patients and leads to temporary abandonment of eating until symptoms abate—usually over about 30 min, but episodes of oesophageal obstruction can last for several hours. In most patients, symptomatic episodes occur less than once a month but in severe cases these may occur several times a week, or each time food intake is attempted.

Diagnosis

As with any intermittent fault, full-blown dysfunction is usually absent during investigation, but in a minority of patients there is asymptomatic motor dysfunction. Barium swallow then shows trapping of beads of contrast in the distal oesophagus—'the corkscrew oesophagus'—or sustained obliteration of the distal oesophageal lumen. Oesophageal manometry may show intermittent, simultaneous, prolonged, and vigorous oesophageal contractions interspersed with normal swallow-induced peristalsis. Relaxation of the lower oesophageal sphincter is normal. 24-h ambulatory manometry improves diagnostic accuracy by increasing the likelihood of capturing symptomatic episodes but is not necessary in all patients.

Most frequently the diagnosis is made on the basis of the history and the exclusion of other problems that may mimic diffuse oesophageal spasm. Most important amongst these is Schatski ring (see below). Achalasia is readily excluded by manometry. When appropriate, myocardial ischaemia should be excluded.

Treatment

There is no specific therapy. Smooth muscle relaxants such as nitrites, nitrates, and calcium antagonists may reduce symptoms but their use is often limited by side-effects. In many patients, reassurance is the most important management since the intensity and nature of symptoms gives rise to great concern. Opiate therapy is sometimes necessary. In the rare case of frequent, disabling spasm, long oesophagomyotomy can give good relief.

Prognosis

The major significance is impairment of quality of life and concern about life-threatening cardiac disease. There is no consistent progression over time. There are several reports of progression of diffuse oesophageal spasm to achalasia but in most of these it seems likely that early, spastic achalasia was initially misdiagnosed as diffuse oesophageal spasm.

Hypertensive peristalsis or nutcracker oesophagus

Definition

This is defined purely by the manometric criterion of primary peristaltic pressure waves in the oesophageal body that have peaks in excess of 250 mmHg (Fig. 5). There is preservation of the normal peristaltic pattern of a broad progression of the time of onset of the contraction wave in the oesophageal body.

Aetiology

This is not understood. It is not clear if it is a true motor disorder, and it may just represent the upper end of a continuum of peristaltic wave amplitudes. It has been shown to vary over time within individuals. There are indications that psychological factors can influence peristaltic amplitude. A minority of patients with hypertensive peristalsis also experience episodes of diffuse oesophageal spasm suggesting that the underlying dysfunction may be related to diffuse oesophageal spasm and is likely to involve neural control mechanisms.

Symptoms

The only clinical significance of hypertensive peristalsis is its relationship to non-cardiac chest pain. Hypertensive peristalsis alone does not produce dysphagia or derangement of oesophageal transit, because, by definition, peristalsis is preserved.

Treatment and prognosis

These are discussed in the section on non-cardiac chest pain.

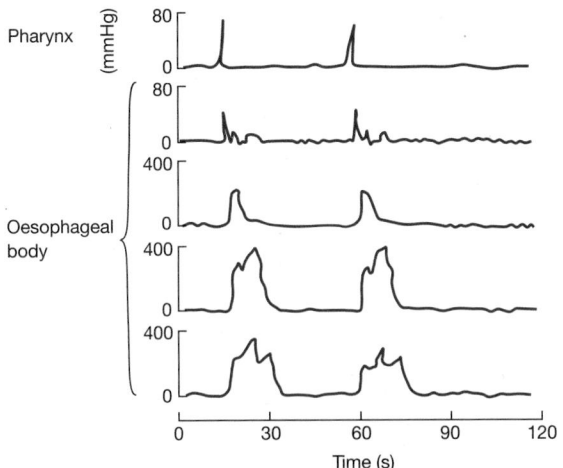

Fig. 5 Oesophageal manometric tracing made from points along the oesophagus in a patient with hypertensive peristalsis. The time of onset of the pressure waves shows a normal peristaltic gradient, but the contractions in the distal half of the oesophagus are very vigorous so that the peak pressures are abnormally high. The high-amplitude pressure waves are also somewhat prolonged and multipeaked.

Non-specific oesophageal motor disorders

Definition

This is a ragbag of manometrically defined oesophageal motor abnormalities which occur in isolation from other more clearly defined syndromes of oesophageal dysfunction, or in association with diseases such as gastro-oesophageal reflux disease, diffuse oesophageal spasm, and diabetic and other autonomic neuropathies. The pragmatic definition of these dysfunctions is that they are departures from normal patterns of oesophageal motor function which do not actually define specific diseases, but which are of clinical significance. Non-specific oesophageal motor disorder is the commonest single functional diagnosis made in most oesophageal manometric laboratories.

Aetiology

This is unknown, but it should not be assumed that only one mechanism is involved. Intermittent occurrence of dysfunctions suggests that they are due to defective neural control.

Symptoms

Multipeaked, swallow-induced distal oesophageal body contraction waves stand out from the other patterns not only functionally but also symptomatically. This pattern is loosely associated with the hypercontraction disorders of diffuse oesophageal spasm and hypertensive peristalsis, but sometimes does not appear to have any clinical significance.

Hypocontraction dysfunctions, recently termed 'ineffective' peristalsis, are associated with defective triggering and progression of both primary and secondary peristalsis. Failure to develop a propagated pressure wave of sufficient strength to maintain closure of the oesophageal lumen leads to deranged oesophageal transit. This probably explains the association of these disorders with mild intermittent dysphagia which occurs characteristically with solids. The non-obstructive dysphagia and slow oesophageal acid clearance seen in gastro-oesophageal reflux disease are due to such dysfunction. Secondary oesophageal body peristalsis has not yet been widely evaluated, but defects of this are probably an important cause of intermittent dysphagia, since, at least in patients with non-obstructive dysphagia and reflux disease, dysfunction of secondary peristalsis is substantially more common than primary peristaltic dysfunction. Oesophageal manometry with an adequate number of recording points in the oesophageal body is the only sensitive means for diagnosis.

Treatment

In most cases patients with symptoms found to be due to non-specific oesophageal motor disorders are in search of an explanation of the origin of their symptoms and reassurance rather than relief of symptoms. Cisapride may improve triggering and amplitude of peristaltic contractions and so theoretically transit. Usually, however, the symptoms arising from primary peristaltic dysfunction are not sufficiently severe to warrant continuous therapy. Secondary peristaltic dysfunction may be more troublesome, but there is no good information on the effect of prokinetic or other drugs on this.

Prognosis

These dysfunctions do not remit spontaneously. Patients are often helped by the measures outlined in the section on general management of oesophageal dysphagia, which minimize the demands on oesophageal transport mechanisms and provide propulsive forces that substitute for oesophageal contractions.

Non-cardiac chest pain

Definition

Implicit in this rather circuitous and negative label is the view that this pain has a cardiac-like quality, but there is no evidence for a cardiac origin. The oesophagus is the next most likely origin, but it is unlikely that all such pain arises from the oesophagus.

Aetiology

Long-term monitoring of oesophageal pH and motility has given us mixed messages. Evidence for triggering of pain by reflux or oesophageal motor dysfunction has been found in between one-fifth and one-half of patients evaluated. Oesophageal mucosal pain due to gastro-oesophageal reflux is the most common and rewarding positive diagnosis. Frank oesophageal spasm associated with achalasia and diffuse oesophageal spasm is an unusual but convincing cause of non-cardiac chest pain. In the majority of patients, most episodes of pain occur independently of reflux and any motor abnormality, although many of these patients have non-specific oesophageal motor disorders or hypertensive peristalsis (see above). Recently, sustained contraction of the longitudinal muscle has been identified by prolonged intraluminal ultrasonography in association with a high proportion of episodes of pain. Nevertheless, in many patients non-cardiac chest pain appears to be a primary oesophageal pain disorder and any motor disorder may be an epiphenomenon.

Symptoms

By definition, the pain resembles cardiac pain in its sensation and distribution. It can be very intense and distressing, can disturb sleep, and may be worse during periods of emotional stress. Postprandial occurrence, in association with heartburn, suggests that it may be caused by reflux. When pain is associated with dysphagia, vigorous achalasia or oesophageal spasm are very possible.

Diagnosis

Investigation is demanding and relatively unrewarding. Firstly, myocardial ischaemia should be assumed to be the cause until proven otherwise. Endoscopy should then follow. In patients who are having recurrent problems, monitoring of oesophageal pH and oesophageal motility studies are both indicated.

Treatment

If the pain is triggered by gastro-oesophageal reflux, high-level therapy should be tried (see section on gastro-oesophageal reflux disease). Achalasia and diffuse oesophageal spasm should be treated on their own merits. Half or more of patients will still have no clearcut diagnosis. In these, treatment with anxiolytics and antidepressants has been found to be moderately

Table 3 Systemic diseases associated with disturbance to oesophageal motility

Connective tissue diseases
Scleroderma
Mixed connective tissue disease
Polymyositis/dermatomyosits
Neuromuscular disorders
Myotonic dystrophy
Myasthenia gravis
Chronic intestinal pseudo-obstruction
Other disorders
Diabetes mellitus
Alcohol abuse
Amyloidosis

effective. Agents that reduce the strength of oesophageal contraction, such as calcium antagonists, appear ineffective in hypertensive peristalsis.

Prognosis

When the pain is clearly due to reflux disease, diffuse oesophageal spasm, and achalasia, the prognosis is as for these conditions. In patients in whom there is no such clear relationship, continuing anxiety about the origin of the symptoms and the fear that this might be cardiac tends to persist, with repeated admissions to hospital because of attacks of pain.

Oesophageal motor disorders secondary to systemic disease

Oesophageal motility may be affected by a number of systemic diseases (Table 3). These diseases may affect the striated or smooth muscle itself or the neural control mechanisms.

The division of the oesophageal musculature into striated and smooth muscle components is revealed clearly by the myopathic diseases that affect the oesophageal musculature. In patients with peripheral myopathy this would normally have been diagnosed. Weak or absent oesophageal contraction in the affected segment has the expected adverse impact on oesophageal transit, with a pattern of symptoms similar to the hypocontraction states of non-specific oesophageal motor disorders (see above). The management of these dysfunctions is along general lines (see section on general management of oesophageal dysphagia).

Diseases of oesophageal smooth muscle

Scleroderma

Definition and aetiology

This eventually involves the smooth muscle of the oesophagus in at least three-quarters of patients. It may be part of the CREST (**C**alcinosis, **R**aynaud's syndrome. (o)**E**sophageal dysphagia, **S**clerodactyly, **T**elangiectasia) syndrome The time of onset of symptoms from oesophageal involvement is very variable in relation to other manifestations but is sometimes the presenting symptom. Muscle atrophy and fibrosis are the cardinal features, but neuropathic abnormalities may also contribute to dysfunction. Smooth muscle peristalsis is feeble or totally absent and the tone of the lower oesophageal sphincter subnormal or absent.

Symptoms

Troublesome reflux symptoms are the most common consequence of loss of function. The pattern of dysphagia resembles that seen in non-specific oesophageal motor disorder (see above). If dysphagia is severe, peptic stricture should be excluded, as complete loss of oesophageal smooth muscle peristalsis rarely leads to disabling dysphagia.

Treatment

Reflux disease is frequently severe and should be managed by high-level medical therapy in order to prevent complications such as stricture (see above). Antireflux surgery is relatively contraindicated because of the poor propulsive function of the oesophageal body.

Other disorders

A scleroderma-like picture of oesophageal dysfunction is sometimes seen in other connective tissue disorders such as mixed connective tissue disease. The smooth muscle segment is also involved in systemic myopathies including polymyositis–dermatomyositis and myotonic dystrophy.

Abnormal oesophageal motility is common in diabetes mellitus, and may be a feature of amyloidosis, chronic alcoholism, and the pseudo-obstructive syndrome. In these disorders, the disturbance is believed to be primarily due to dysfunction of neural control mechanisms.

Disorders of striated muscle

Involvement of the striated muscle segment of the oesophagus is rare and usually present with high dysphagia, often in association with oropharyngeal dysfunction (see Chapter 14.5). The inflammatory myopathies (dermatomyositis, polymyositis, and inclusion body myositis), the muscular dystrophies (myotonia dystrophica and oculopharyngeal dystrophy), and myasthenia gravis are the most common causes.

Abnormalities of oesophageal anatomy

Non-neoplastic abnormalities which distort oesophageal anatomy may interfere with normal function or may merely pose difficulties in the interpretation of findings.

Sliding hiatus hernia

Definition

Around 90 per cent of hiatus hernias are of this type in which the gastro-oesophageal junction is displaced upwards into the thorax, giving a simple shaped pouch of intrathoracic stomach.

Aetiology

The phreno-oesophageal ligament is effaced in sliding hiatus hernia, but it is not clear whether this is a primary defect of gastric anchorage.

Symptoms

Many patients with hiatus hernia are asymptomatic. Despite this, physiological studies indicate that herniation of the gastro-oesophageal junction impairs its function as an antireflux barrier by removing the normal diaphragmatic crural compression from the lower oesophageal sphincter. Thus, hiatus hernia can be taken as a risk factor for reflux disease, but not an abnormality that makes the diagnosis.

Treatment

Symptoms of gastro-oesophageal reflux are the only ones of major significance. These should be treated along conventional lines (see gastro-oesophageal reflux disease).

Prognosis

This is essentially that of any associated reflux disease.

Rolling or para-oesophageal hiatus hernia

Definition

A variable part of the stomach herniates through the hiatus alongside a normally situated gastro-oesophageal junction. This pattern of herniation may produce a gross disturbance of gastric anatomy, usually with a narrow exit from the herniated pouch into the main stomach cavity. Some rolling hernias are also associated with displacement of the gastro-oesophageal junction above the hiatus in which case these are known as mixed hernias.

Symptoms

Obstruction and distension of the pouch causes upper abdominal discomfort and can progress to strangulation. Gastric volvulus can occur because of the laxity of the gastric anchorage and may obstruct the gastro-oesophageal junction. Both of these problems have a very high mortality and demand urgent surgery. Elective surgery is normally recommended to reduce and anchor rolling hiatus hernias in order to remove these risks.

Prognosis

Unfortunately, there are no adequate data on the degree of risk associated with rolling hiatus hernia or on any anatomical factors that are especially hazardous.

Schatzki ring (B ring)

Definition

This is a characteristic short luminal stenosis which occurs at the gastro-oesophageal junction (Fig. 6). It is made up only of mucosa and submucosa, and may narrow the lumen to a few millimetres or cause a clinically insignificant minor indentation.

Aetiology

This is unknown. There is no firm evidence that reflux oesophagitis is the cause although this is sometimes assumed to be the case.

Symptoms

With mechanically significant rings, intermittent dysphagia occurs on eating solids. Meat is often the culprit, leading to the common term of 'steakhouse syndrome'. Episodes of bolus obstruction are not unusual, with associated chest pain caused by powerful oesophageal contractions. Failure to recognize a Schatzki ring frequently leads to the incorrect diagnosis of primary diffuse oesophageal spasm. Sensitive diagnosis is only achieved by an expert radiologist who has been asked to look for this abnormality. Adequate distal oesophageal distension during the barium swallow is essential for detection and this is best achieved by prone-oblique views. A less well-tailored barium examination and endoscopy frequently fail to show a symptomatic ring.

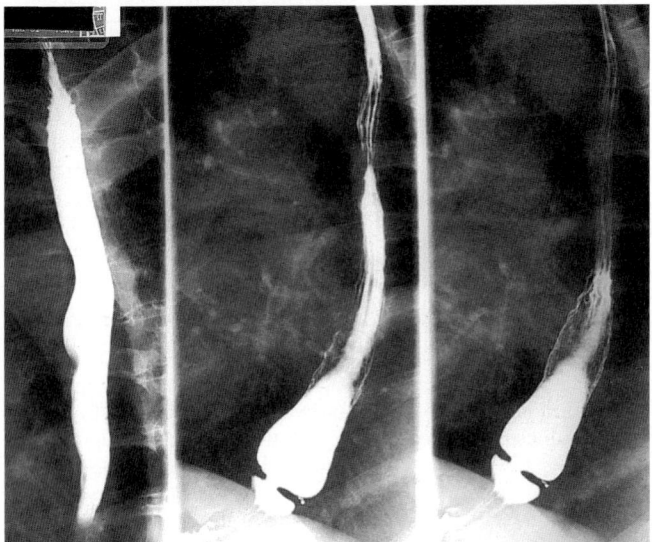

Fig. 6 Schatzki ring: a thin (2 to 4 mm in height), annular constriction at the gastro-oesophageal junction, best shown on prone-oblique views.

Treatment

Disruption of the ring by simple peroral dilatation or endoscopic diathermy or laser is very rewarding, as the dysphagia and chest pain are cured, sometimes after many years of symptoms. However, there is a significant incidence of recurrence and repeated dilatations at intervals are often needed.

Other rings and webs

Other short oesophageal stenoses may develop because of peptic stricture, muscular rings, and cervical webs with (Plummer–Vinson syndrome) or without iron-deficiency anaemia.

Oesophageal diverticula and pseudodiverticula

Wide-mouthed multiple diverticula are characteristic of scleroderma oesophagus. In the non-sclerodermatous oesophagus, diverticula occur in the mid and distal oesophagus, both types probably being 'blow-outs' secondary to hypercontraction motor disorders. These can become very large. It is rare for them to cause symptoms, but they may be associated with dysphagia and regurgitation of retained contents. Unless symptoms are disabling, they are best left undisturbed because leakage is common following surgical removal.

Multiple intramural outpouchings of barium are characteristic of intramural pseudodiverticulosis which appears to be due to dilatation of the ducts of submucosal glands by an unknown process.

Extrinsic oesophageal compression

This is a relatively common cause of dysphagia, and is most often a result of malignant mediastinal lymphadenopathy. Barium swallow or endoscopy usually show a relatively long constriction of the oesophageal lumen of variable calibre, associated with a normal mucosal appearance. Dilatation of such a compression is usually unrewarding because of its elastic recoil.

Mechanically significant extrinsic compression may also result from an enlarged heart, a dilated or unfolded aorta, or an aortic aneurysm. Kyphosis may accentuate the mechanical impact of these abnormalities. Congenital vascular abnormalities can also compress the oesophagus in adults, an aberrant right subclavian artery being by far the most common.

Mechanical, chemical, and radiation trauma

Mallory–Weiss tear

These mucosal tears extend across the gastro-oesophageal junction and are normally induced by vigorous straining associated with vomiting. Bleeding is the only consequence of significance. In 10 per cent of cases bleeding is severe enough to cause hypovolaemia. The history is usually quite characteristic, but definitive diagnosis requires endoscopy. Continued bleeding usually responds to endoscopic injection or electrocoagulation, vascular embolization, or vasopressin infusion. Very rarely, surgery is needed to underrun a persistently bleeding artery at the base of the tear.

Barogenic oesophageal rupture (Boerhaave's syndrome)

In this uncommon condition, straining and vomiting cause oesophageal rupture, most often in the left lower third of the oesophagus. High-volume spillage of the gastric contents into the pleural space causes shock and pain in the chest and upper abdomen with radiation to the back, left chest, or shoulder. The chest radiograph becomes abnormal only some hours after rupture. Surgical repair and drainage are usually necessary, and if this is delayed beyond 24 h, the mortality is very high. Unfortunately, diagnostic delay is not unusual.

Iatrogenic oesophageal perforation

Physicians encounter this problem most often as a result of their involvement in dilatation of oesophageal strictures, pneumatic bag dilatation for achalasia, or through problems with the management of oesophageal varices by balloon tamponade. Even with meticulous technique and appropriate equipment, oesophageal perforation can occur. Perforation is strongly suggested by development of chest or epigastric pain directly after instrumentation, sometimes with dyspnoea. Pneumothorax and surgical emphysema are diagnostic. Any suspicion of perforation should be acted upon by taking a chest radiograph which should be repeated in several hours if it is negative. Broad-spectrum antibiotics should be given on suspicion, as they are most effective in minimizing the risks of mediastinitis when given from the outset. Surgical consultation should occur promptly; the choice between conservative and surgical management needs to be individualized. Increasingly, instrumental perforation is being managed non-surgically with nasogastric suction, antibiotics, and intravenous nutrition with good results, primarily because instrumental injury usually occurs when the stomach is empty.

Caustic ingestion

Definition and aetiology

Strong acids and alkalis are both very damaging to the oesophagus and are found in high concentrations in many agents commonly used in the household for cleaning and maintenance. Laryngeal and gastric injuries may overshadow oesophageal injury. Because of their relative lack of taste, alkaline solutions are more likely to be swallowed accidentally in large amounts. Alkaline injury is especially deep; acid tends to form a superficial coagulant, which limits penetration.

Symptoms

The severity and extent of injury are immensely variable and cannot be predicted accurately from estimates of the volume ingested. Around half of patients with a history of caustic ingestion have no significant injury. Oropharyngeal and laryngeal injury confirm caustic ingestion and can be a major threat to the airway, but do not predict the existence and severity of oesophageal injury which causes odynophagia, dysphagia, or haematemesis. Prompt fibreoptic panendoscopy appears to be safe. This may be normal or show only patchy mucosal oedema, erythema, and small haemorrhagic ulcers, indicative of superficial damage with a good prognosis. Extensive and circumferential ulceration, and grey or brown/black ulceration suggest transmural injury.

Treatment

Patients with severe injury must be observed closely for signs of perforation. Nasogastric suction should be used with the administration of broad-spectrum antibiotics as these appear to reduce the severity of infective complications. The use of steroids is controversial, the balance of evidence tending to oppose their use. Oesophageal stricture is to be expected with severe injury and appears not to be prevented by routine dilatation in the first 2 weeks after injury. A barium study should be done at 2 to 3 weeks to screen for stricturing, and then subsequently at about 3-monthly intervals thereafter for a year, so that the development of stricturing is recognized at a stage when dilatation may have some impact.

Prognosis

The main short- to medium-term risk is the development of stricture. Caustic strictures are difficult and hazardous to treat by peroral dilatation so that about half of patients require oesophageal resection. In the long term (average onset 40 years after injury) carcinoma of the oesophagus is a major hazard, the risk being 1000 to 3000 times the expected risk.

Table 4 Common causes of medication-induced oesophagitis

Severe injury—high risk
Slow-release potassium chloride
Non-steroidal anti-inflammatory drugs
Tetracycline
Quinidine
Alendronate
Less severe injury—high risk
Many antibiotics
Iron supplements
Occasional injury
Ascorbic acid
Mexiletine
Slow-release theophylline
Captopril
Phenytoin
Zidovudin

Medication-induced oesophagitis

Definition and aetiology

This entity was only recognized in 1970. The chemical properties of medications pose hazards to the oesophageal mucosa because of the relative susceptibility of this to injury through pH-dependent and other mechanisms. This susceptibility arises in part from the high local concentrations of medications that occur in the oesophageal lumen when a tablet gets 'hung up'. Pills move surprisingly slowly through the normal oesophagus. Defective oesophageal transport, poor pill design, increased mucosal susceptibility to injury, and poor pill-taking technique contribute to the problem. Medications known to have an especially high risk for oesophageal damage are listed in Table 4.

Symptoms

Symptoms are those for any form of oesophagitis with stricturing which can be very difficult to manage. Probably, much pill-induced injury goes unrecognized. Pill-induced injury is by far the most likely cause of oesophagitis and/or benign stricture at the level of the aortic arch, where pills can lodge for prolonged periods. Injury at the distal oesophagus, the other common site of hold-up, is probably usually misdiagnosed as being due to reflux disease.

Treatment and prognosis

Medications and formulations with a high risk of injury should be identified and avoided if possible, especially in elderly patients with reflux disease or abnormal oesophageal transit. Pill transit is facilitated if pills are taken in the erect position with plenty of water. Pharmaceutical companies need to pay more attention to the use of shapes, sizes, and coatings that can assist transit of pills through the oesophagus. Stricturing may require surgery.

Chemotherapy-induced oesophageal problems

Chemotherapy causes oesophageal problems in several ways. Therapy may impair mucosal defences by affecting cell turnover leading to 'mucositis'. This in turn may reduce resistance of the mucosa to damage from other agents, and increase susceptibility to infective oesophagitis from immune suppression. Oesophageal transit and acid clearance may be impaired through the neurotoxic effects of some agents. Fistulation or perforation may occur through cytotoxic effects on a malignancy in the oesophageal wall. The striking recent observation that combination chemotherapy is associated with the development of oesophageal columnar metaplasia in women being treated for breast cancer demands further investigation.

Oesophageal neoplasms

Cure is only possible in the small minority of patients whose disease presents early. Several approaches are possible for palliation and data are somewhat conflicting about the relative merits of each. Some approaches require considerable technical skill.

Squamous cell carcinoma

Definition

This is simply defined as a squamous carcinoma arising from the squamous oesophageal mucosa. It is by far the most common oesophageal neoplasm. In some parts of the world it is the most common of all cancers, but in the Western world it accounts for approximately 4 per cent of cancer deaths and has an annual incidence in the United States of 5 per 100 000 in Whites and 17 per 100 000 in Blacks.

Aetiology

The striking geographical variation in incidence suggests a major contribution from environmental factors. There are multiple proven or putative risk factors which include heavy alcohol use and intake of carcinogens from smoking, from soil and water, and from high rates of consumption of nitrosamines and aflatoxins. Other factors implicated are vitamin A deficiency, chronic candida infection, injury to the oesophageal mucosa due to ingestion of a corrosive substance years previously, and chronic irritation from oesophageal retention in achalasia. Some hereditary conditions such as tylosis predispose to squamous carcinoma. Invasive carcinoma is preceded by mucosal dysplasia and carcinoma *in situ*.

Symptoms

Dysplasia and carcinoma *in situ* are asymptomatic, and are only recognized by screening programmes set up in very high-risk areas, usually using blind cytological sampling methods. Inexorable progression of dysphagia over a few weeks is the almost universal presentation. Dysphagia usually only occurs when the tumour has become circumferential. Rarely, malignant mucosal ulceration presents with pain of the oesophageal mucosa due to malignant oesophageal ulceration. Substantial weight loss has often occurred by the time of presentation.

Barium swallow typically reveals a stricture with an irregular, lobulated mucosal outline (Fig. 7), but occasionally the appearance mimics benign peptic stricture. The diagnosis is best proven by fibreoptic endoscopy, with mucosal biopsy and brush cytology. Occasionally, an asymptomatic oesophageal carcinoma is diagnosed when endoscopy is done for some other reason. Early lesions are often unimpressive, so that any minor mucosal irregularity should be sampled thoroughly by biopsy and cytology.

Treatment

In very early, usually asymptomatic, carcinoma, resective surgery is the treatment of choice as it achieves high rates of cure. Curative resective surgery should only be attempted after careful staging of the tumour by clinical examination, chest radiograph, thoracic and abdominal computed tomography scanning, bronchoscopy, and liver function tests. Endoscopic oesophageal ultrasound is a much needed advance in the sensitivity of definition of the local extent of the tumour, but is not yet widely available. Palliation poses many challenges. There is a sorry lack of critical comparison of options. Resective surgery is unattractive, especially in elderly patients, because of its morbidity and mortality. Radiotherapy, with or without chemotherapy, is usually the best option for management of malignant obstruction. Repeated peroral dilatation, peroral placement of stenting tubes, laser photocoagulation, and injection of sclerosants are all options for the management of recurrent malignant strictures which have potential for improving the quality of life. Oesophagopulmonary fistula is a distressing development which usually causes pneumonia and persistent cough and which can sometimes be controlled by stenting.

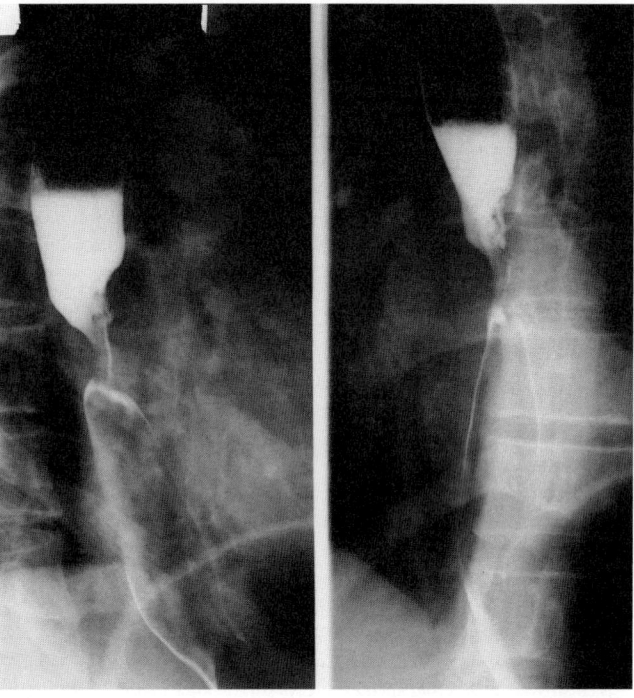

Fig. 7 Squamous carcinoma: a circumferential luminal narrowing which is asymmetrical and irregularly shouldered; the mucosal aspect is ulcerated.

Prognosis

This remains dismal except for regions where screening programmes identify early, asymptomatic cases. Only about one-quarter of patients are deemed to be potentially curable by surgery, and of these, about one-quarter will be alive and free of disease after 5 years. Thus, the overall 5-year survival rate is approximately 6 per cent. Such figures must be interpreted cautiously, because of differences between studies in the scope of presurgical staging, definitions of resectability, and criteria for exclusion of patients from consideration for surgery on the grounds of debility, old age, and other medical problems.

Adenocarcinoma and oesophageal columnar metaplasia (Barrett's oesophagus)

Definition

Between 80 and 90 per cent of adenocarcinomas arising in the oesophagus occur in association with oesophageal columnar metaplasia, or Barrett's oesophagus. In the minority of adenocarcinomas occurring in a squamous-lined oesophagus, the oesophageal mucus glands appear to be the source of malignant change.

Aetiology

Oesophageal columnar metaplasia (Barrett's oesophagus) develops as a result of the healing of severe reflux oesophagitis with metaplastic epithelium. This occurs from the gastro-oesophageal junction upwards over a distance that varies from 2 or 3 cm to the full length of the oesophagus. Oesophageal columnar metaplasia carries a 40-fold risk for development of oesophageal adenocarcinoma. Surveillance programmes in patients with oesophageal columnar metaplasia have shown a rate of development of adenocarcinoma that varies from 1 in 50 to 1 in 175 patient years. Occurrence of adenocarcinoma is very strongly associated with prior development of high-grade dysplasia in the metaplastic segment. The reasons for an apparently real increase in oesophageal adenocarcinoma are unknown. An increase in the prevalence of reflux oesophagitis, related to the reduced prevalence of *Helicobacter pylori* infection and a consequent increase in gastric acid secretion, is a plausible explanation.

Symptoms

The presentation of adenocarcinoma resembles that of squamous carcinoma (see above). Adenocarcinoma tends to be more fleshy and intraluminal but still presents at a very late stage. Metastatic disease is more common on presentation of adenocarcinoma than with squamous carcinoma.

Initial diagnosis and staging are along the same lines as for oesophageal squamous carcinoma.

Treatment of established adenocarcinoma

Careful staging is the cornerstone of appropriate management. Because of the usually distal site of occurrence of oesophageal adenocarcinoma, resection with oesophagogastrostomy is often best. Adenocarcinoma appears to respond less frequently to radiotherapy and chemotherapy than squamous carcinoma.

Management of the risk for adenocarcinoma in oesophageal columnar metaplasia

This is a very active field of research. Development of high-grade dysplasia in the columnar metaplastic segment precedes development of adenocarcinoma. This dysplasia can be recognized with sensitivity if at least four radially spaced biopsies are taken at every 2 cm of columnar-lined oesophagus. It is controversial whether such expensive surveillance methods are justified by the relatively low rate of recognition of early adenocarcinoma. There is also controversy about how a diagnosis of high-grade dysplasia should be acted upon. Some authorities recommend oesophageal resection on confirmation of this diagnosis, whilst others favour close surveillance with endoscopic ultrasound and repeated biopsies, with oesophageal resection being reserved for when there is clear evidence of disruption of the structure of the oesophageal wall, indicative of early invasive carcinoma. Others advocate perendoscopic ablation by laser or argon beam coagulation, or mucosal resection in the case of true intramucosal carcinoma. In large part, the approach to management of high-grade dysplasia is substantially moulded by the morbidity and risks of resective surgery and the availability of endoscopic ultrasound. In younger, fit patients, the balance is more strongly in favour of early resection than it is in older, less fit patients. Lack of detailed knowledge about the natural history of high-grade dysplasia makes the decision-making process especially difficult.

Failure to discuss the risk for adenocarcinoma and the option of endoscopic surveillance with a patient who has oesophageal columnar metaplasia could well be viewed as an indefensible lapse of practice, despite the uncertainties about cost-effectiveness.

Prognosis

For established symptomatic adenocarcinoma, prognosis is every bit as dismal as for squamous carcinoma. Post-mortem studies have shown that only a small proportion of patients with oesophageal columnar metaplasia are diagnosed as having this condition during life. Consequently, the impact of endoscopic surveillance can at best only be limited. For those patients in whom screening is undertaken, it has been clearly established that high-quality screening leads to diagnosis of oesophageal adenocarcinoma at a stage when it may be cured by resection.

Other oesophageal tumours

Primary malignant tumours

Primary malignant tumours other than squamous carcinoma and adenocarcinoma are rare and all have a poor prognosis. These include malignant melanoma, lymphoma, carcinoid, leiomyosarcoma, neuroendocrine carcinoma (small cell carcinoma), adenoid cystic carcinoma, and pseudosarcoma. These tumours show a mixture of polypoid and infiltrating features and are usually only clearly distinguished from the more common malignancies by histology.

Benign oesophageal tumours

Leiomyoma is a relatively common oesophageal tumour which rarely causes symptoms. It is usually intramural but can become pedunculated. Around two-thirds of benign oesophageal tumours are leiomyomas. They usually only cause symptoms if they are very large, or on a long pedicle. Other benign intramural tumours of the oesophagus include lipomas and granular cell tumours. The main risk of these is that they are mistaken for malignant tumours and operated on inappropriately.

Squamous cell papillomas of the mucosa can mimic a polypoid squamous carcinoma and so should be removed endoscopically for histological diagnosis.

Infective oesophagitis and other non-neoplastic mucosal diseases

Most of these cause symptoms because of mucosal hypersensitivity. When the course is prolonged, interference with food intake may become a dominant problem in patient management. Viral oesophagitis can sometimes cause major haemorrhage. Some disorders damage the full thickness of the oesophageal wall and so lead to stricturing. Infective oesophagitis is by far the most important of these disorders, and has become more prevalent with the increased number of people who are immunosuppressed through HIV infection or chemotherapy.

Table 5 Major causes of infective oesophagitis

Pathogen	Management	Remarks
Immunocompetent patients		
Candida albicans	Topical/oral antifungals	By far the most common
Herpes simplex	Acyclovir if severe	Unusual, may denude mucosa
Varicella zoster	Acyclovir if severe	In association with chickenpox/herpes zoster
Bacteria		Rare in well individuals
Immunocompromised patients		
Candida albicans	Systemic antifungals	Most common; oral disease almost diagnostic
Cytomegalovirus	Prophylaxis and treatment with gancyclovir or foscarnet	Serpiginous to giant ulcers in distal half
Herpes simplex	Prophylaxis and treatment with acyclovir or foscarnet	Circumscribed ulcers, raised edges to coalescence. Oral lesions
Tuberculosis	Conventional	From miliary and local spread
Gram-positive cocci, Gram-negative bacilli	Intravenous antibiotics	Often with systemic infection
Syphilis	Conventional	Associated with tertiary syphilis elsewhere. Inflammatory stricture

Diagnosis is often aided by the setting in which the oesophageal problem occurs. Cutaneous or oral disease can suggest what is happening in the oesophagus, but barium swallow adds relatively little to the assessment of mucosal hypersensitivity. Endoscopy is the diagnostic method of choice. Mucosal appearance and the distribution of oesophageal lesions can be virtually diagnostic. In addition, biopsies and brushings allow for histological diagnosis and identification of infectious agents. Endoscopy has most to offer in patients with chronic symptoms, or those who are immunosuppressed.

Infective oesophagitis

The more important causes of infective oesophagitis are summarized in Table 5. Immune status is a major determinant of the pattern of infection. Though infective oesophagitis may be severe in immunocompetent patients it is characteristically self-limited and topical therapy is normally all that is needed (Table 5).

Immunocompromised patients usually need aggressive, systemic therapy, otherwise the infection does not resolve. The infection can be difficult to eradicate, tends to recur, and can cause major disability. Two or more infections are not unusual (Table 5).

Helicobacter pylori does not appear to be of any primary significance in the pathogenesis of oesophageal mucosal disease.

Other non-neoplastic mucosal diseases

Skin and systemic diseases associated with lesions of the oropharynx may also involve the oesophagus. These include epidermolysis bullosa, Behçet's disease, lichen planus, pemphigus vulgaris, bullous pemphigoid, benign mucous membrane (cicatrial) pemphigoid, and drug-induced disease (Steven's Johnson syndrome and toxic epidermal necrolysis).

Chronic, and less frequently acute, graft versus host disease may cause severe oesophageal problems through mucosal desquamation or mural damage. Resultant stricturing shows considerable variation in appearance.

Rarely, Crohn's disease can cause indolent, craggy ulceration and/or stricturing. Oesophageal sarcoidosis can mimic Crohn's disease.

Further reading

Anand BS *et al.* (1998). A randomized comparison of dilatation alone versus dilatation plus laser in patients receiving chemotherapy and external beam radiation for esophageal carcinoma. *Digestive Diseases and Sciences* **43**, 2255–60.

Balaban DH *et al.* (1999). Sustained esophageal contraction: a marker of esophageal chest pain identified by intraluminal ultrasonography. *Gastroenterology* **116**, 29–37.

Cook IJ, Kahrilas PJ (1999). AGA technical review on management of oropharyngeal dysphagia. *Gastroenterology* **116**, 455–78.

Dent J *et al.* (1999). An evidenced-based appraisal of reflux disease management—the Genval Workshop Report. *Gut* **44** (Suppl. 2), S1–S16.

Dent J, Holloway RH (1996). Esophageal motility and reflux testing. State-of-the-art and clinical role in the twenty-first century. *Gastroenterology Clinics of North America* **25**, 51–73.

DeVault KR (1996). Lower esophageal (Schatzki's) ring: pathogenesis, diagnosis and therapy. *Digestive Diseases* **14**, 323–9.

Ellis FH Jr. (1998). Long esophagomyotomy for diffuse esophageal spasm and related disorders: an historical overview. *Diseases of the Esophagus* **11**, 210–14.

Falk GW (1999). Endoscopic surveillance of Barrett's esophagus: risk stratification and cancer risk. *Gastrointestinal Endoscopy* **49**, S29–S34.

Fennerty MB (1999). Perspectives on endoscopic eradication of Barrett's esophagus: who are appropriate candidates and what is the best method? *Gastrointestinal Endoscopy* **49**, S24–S28.

Kahrilas PJ (1997). Anatomy and physiology of the gastroesophageal junction. *Gastroenterology Clinics of North America* **26**, 467–86.

Lagergren J *et al.* (1999). Symptomatic gastroesophageal reflux as a risk factor for esophageal adenocarcinoma. *New England Journal of Medicine* **340**, 825–31.

Lundell LR *et al.* (1999). Endoscopic assessment of oesophagitis: clinical and functional correlates and further validation of the Los Angeles classification. *Gut* **45**, 172–80.

McCord GS, Staino A, Clouse RE (1991). Achalasia, diffuse spasm and non-specific motor disorders. *Bailliere's Clinical Gastroenterology* **5**, 307–35.

Roth JA and Putnam JBJ (1994). Surgery for cancer of the esophagus. *Seminars in Oncology* **21**, 453–61.

Spechler SJ (1999). AGA technical review on treatment of patients with dysphagia caused by benign disorders of the distal esophagus. *Gastroenterology* **117**, 233–54.

Tobin RW (1998). Esophageal rings, webs, and diverticula. *Journal of Clinical Gastroenterology* **27**, 285–95.

Vaezi MF (1999). Achalasia: diagnosis and management. *Seminars in Gastrointestinal Disease* **10**, 103–12.

Weston S *et al.* (1998). Clinical and upper gastrointestinal motility features in systemic sclerosis and related disorders. *American Journal of Gastroenterology* **93**, 1085–9.

Young MA, Rose S, Reynolds JC (1996). Gastrointestinal manifestations of scleroderma. *Rheumatic Diseases Clinics of North America* **22**, 797–823.

14.7 Peptic ulcer diseases

*John Calam**

Introduction

Peptic ulcers are common: individuals in Western populations have a life-time risk of 1 in 10 of developing an ulcer. They are a major cause of illness and death and are economically important. Research in the field of peptic ulcers initially focused on the elevated secretion of gastric acid in duodenal ulcer disease. Treatments to combat acid progressed from alkaline antacid preparations through histamine H_2-receptor antagonists, to proton pump inhibitors; maintenance therapy was required because ulcers recurred when the medication was stopped. Our understanding of peptic ulcer disease was radically changed in 1983 by the discovery of *Helicobacter pylori* and there-after its role in gastric and duodenal ulcers. Most patients with ulcers are infected with *H. pylori*, and eradicating the infection permanently cures the ulcers (Fig. 1). Inhabitants of developing countries are also commonly infected with *H. pylori*, but the prevalence is lower and is falling in regions where better sanitation and hygiene limit transmission.

As *Helicobacter* is controlled, another ulcerogenic factor has become important. Non-steroidal anti-inflammatory drugs (**NSAIDs**), often prescribed for musculoskeletal conditions which particularly affect the elderly, lead to ulcers in a population that is less well able to withstand the major complications of haemorrhage and perforation. The chance of dying as a result of a peptic ulcer is currently about a thousand times greater in the elderly than in the young, and peptic ulcers thus remain a challenge to modern medicine.

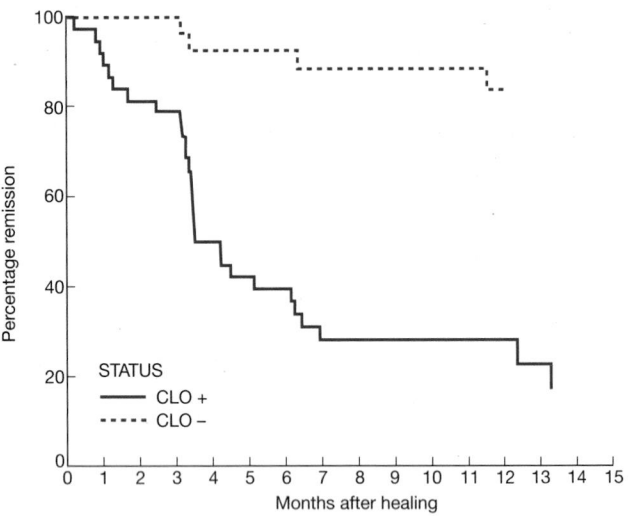

Fig. 1 Demonstration in 1988 by Marshall and colleagues that eradication *of H. pylori* greatly prolongs remission of duodenal ulcer disease. CLO+ and – refer to the diagnosis of infection after attempted eradication by the biopsy urease test, the CLO test, which Marshall also invented. (Reproduced from Marshall BJ *et al.* (1988). *Lancet* **ii**, 1437–42, with permission.)

* It is with great regret that we report the death of John Calam during the preparation of this edition.

Definition

A gastrointestinal ulcer is defined as a breach in the epithelium that penetrates the muscularis mucosae. If the muscularis is not breached it is called an erosion. Duodenal ulcers and gastric ulcers are often considered together as peptic ulcers but differ considerably with regard to epidemiology, pathogenesis, presentation, and management: they are discussed separately. This chapter will also address acute erosive gastritis and non-ulcer dyspepsia. Oesophageal ulcers are discussed with erosive oesophagitis in Chapter 14.6. The Zollinger–Ellison syndrome is discussed in Chapters 12.10 and 14.8.

The major causes of peptic ulcers are *H. pylori* infection and NSAIDs.

Helicobacter pylori

Spiral bacteria were observed by European investigators in the stomachs of animals in the nineteenth century and in humans at the beginning of the twentieth century; but interest waned when a prominent American investigator reported no such bacteria in gastric biopsies from 1000 patients. In 1981 a British study showed that duodenal ulcers remain healed for longer after administration of the antibacterial bismuth than after the H_2-antagonist drug cimetidine. In 1983, the Australians Warren and Marshall succeeded in culturing *H. pylori* (originally known as *Campylobacter pyloridis*) from human gastric biopsies. They were assisted by new selective culture media, and serendipity—growth was achieved when the culture plates were incubated for longer than planned during a holiday. Warren and Marshall soon noticed the association between *H. pylori* infection and gastritis, that almost all patients with duodenal ulcers are infected, and that eradication of infection largely prevents recurrence of ulcers.

The epidemiology of *H. pylori*

Population surveys reveal two patterns of *H. pylori* infection. In developing counties about 80 per cent of the population are infected by the time they are adults and remain infected. In the West, the prevalence rises gradually throughout life to about 60 per cent in old age (Fig. 2). But this is due to a cohort effect rather than gradual acquisition of infection throughout life. The infection is usually acquired before the age of 5 years. Older Westerners were children when infection was much more prevalent than it is now. An exception is that adults frequently acquire infection during wartime: the prevalence of *H. pylori* in the West is distinctly lower in those born after the Second World War. It remains high in the poor and in immigrants from developing countries.

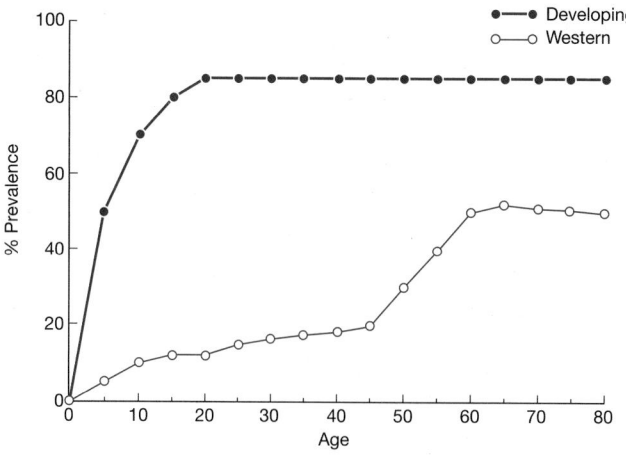

Fig. 2 *H. pylori* prevalence in Westernized versus developing countries. (Adapted from Marshall BJ (1994). *American Journal of Gastroenterology* **89**, S116–118, with permission.)

Bacteriology and transmission of *H. pylori*

Helicobacter pylori is a Gram-negative microaerophilic bacillus (Fig. 3). It uses its spiral shape and four to six flagellae, located at one end, and to move through the gastric mucus layer. It is well adapted to the gastric environment; for example its abundant urease generates alkali by splitting urea into two NH_4^+ ions and one HCO_3^- ion. Indeed *H. pylori* can only survive on gastric-type mucosa, perhaps because its adhesins bind specifically to certain motifs on gastric cells. It is readily cultured from gastric biopsies on selective media, but transport to the laboratory must be rapid. Transmission is from person to person, often within families. It is unclear whether spread is usually oral–oral or faecal–oral. Infection via drinking water occurs in developing countries. There is no significant animal reservoir. The genomes of several *H. pylori* strains have been sequenced and vary considerably. Different strains contain different lengths of 'cag pathogenicity island'. This is a cassette of genes involved in pathogenicity, plus the gene *cagA*. The presence of antibodies to cagA protein in a patient reflects the presence of the island, and is associated with ulcers and cancer. Variations

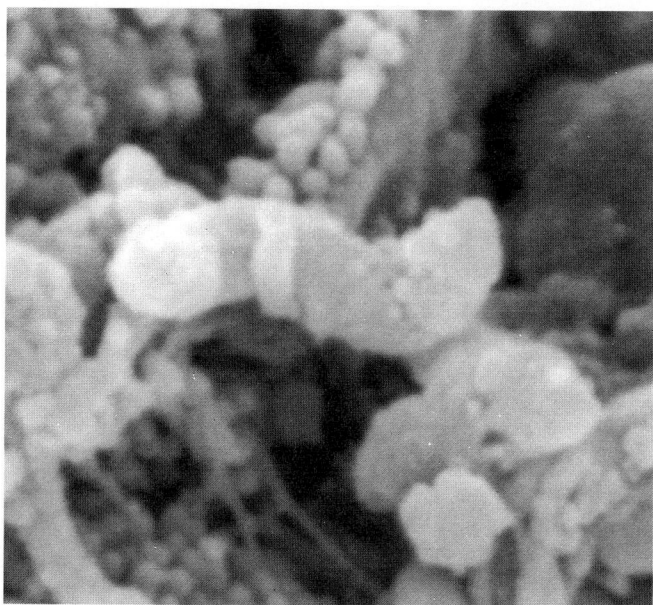

Fig. 3 Electron micrograph of *H. pylori*.

in the gene *vacA* that encodes the *H. pylori* vacuolating toxin also appear to influence the likelihood of these consequences of infection.

Diagnosis of *H. pylori* infection

Three methods can be used to detect *H. pylori* in gastric biopsies:

1. The biopsy urease test depends on the the ability of the bacterium to generate alkali.
2. *H. pylori* bacteria are readily detected histiologically using special stains.
3. Bacterial culture allows the antibiotic sensitivity of the patient's strain to be determined.

Two tests allow *H. pylori* to be diagnosed without endoscopy:

1. Serology is accurate and convenient but remains positive for several months after successful eradication, and is not useful for determining whether eradication has been successful.
2. The urea breath test. The patient drinks a solution of urea containing carbon atoms labelled with ^{13}C or ^{14}C. Labelled CO_2, generated by bacterial urease, can be detected in the breath by mass spectroscopy or radioactive counting if the infection is present (Fig. 4). This test is ideal for testing the success of eradication, if this is required (see below).

Factors that determine the accuracy of the diagnostic tests

These tests are all quite accurate but can give incorrect results under certain circumstances: all except serology can give false negative results if the patient has received antibiotics during the past month. Also, the bacterium tends to move from the antrum to the proximal stomach when proton pump inhibitors are given. Biopsies should then be taken from the proximal gastric mucosa as well as the antrum. Proton pump inhibitors can inhibit *H. pylori*'s urease, which can affect results based on this enzyme. Serological tests remain positive for up to a year after the infection has been eradicated.

Disease associations of *H. pylori* infection

Gastritis

This was noted to occur in subjects who were accidentally or experimentally infected with the bacterium. A first infection is followed by a period of low or absent acid secretion, which lasts for weeks or months and which was called 'epidemic achlorhydria' before the cause was discovered. Before

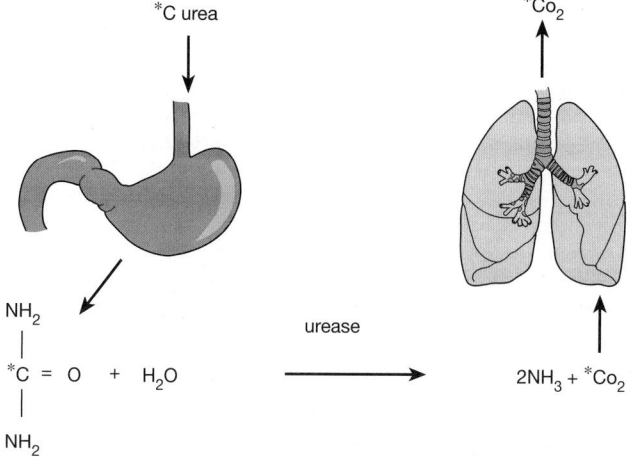

Fig. 4 Urea breath test. The patient drinks a solution of urea containing ^{13}C or ^{14}C carbon. If *H. pylori* is present then the carbon isotope appears in exhaled carbon dioxide.

H. pylori was identified, it was well known that patients with duodenal ulcers have antral gastritis, whilst those with gastric ulcers and gastric cancer have pangastritis. *H. pylori* clearly contributes to the gastritis associated with these diseases because the inflammation resolves when the infection is eradicated. *H. pylori* gastritis is typically 'chronic superficial', meaning that lymphocytes and macrophages are located superficially. Infiltration with neutrophils ('activity') is variable. Prolonged infection predisposes to mucosal atrophy in which the number of chief and parietal cells in the gastric mucosa falls. Atrophy may then proceed to intestinal metaplasia in which the gastric epithelium is replaced with one resembling small or large intestine. The inflammatory response may diminish or even eradicate the infection by reducing acid secretion and the number of gastric cells to which *H. pylori* can adhere. Inflammatory mechanisms in *H. pylori* gastritis have been studied in detail because of their role in the pathogenesis of ulcers and cancer and their relevance to vaccine development. This topic is beyond the scope of this chapter. Briefly, *H. pylori* bacteria remain extracellular but induce gastric epithelial cells to express class molecules and chemokines such as IL-8. These recruit and activate inflammatory cells that express diverse inflammatory mediators including tumour necrosis factor-α, and products such as reactive oxygen species. *H. pylori* gastritis cannot be diagnosed on the basis of endoscopic appearance alone because the mucosa usually either looks normal or mildly reddened.

Duodenitis

Some individuals develop patches of metaplastic gastric mucosa in their proximal duodenum. This change depends on the rate of gastric acid secretion, being abundant in the Zollinger–Ellison syndrome and absent in pernicious anaemia. Gastric metaplasia is important because it allows *H. pylori* to colonize the duodenum leading to duodenitis. This can be erosive and increases the risk of chronic duodenal ulceration.

Gastric cancer

The World Health Organization has classified *H. pylori* as a gastric carcinogen. Infection is associated with an approximately eightfold increased risk of gastric cancer. Eradication of *H. pylori* from Japanese patents with early gastric cancer greatly diminished the risk of recurrent cancer after endoscopic resection. Gastric cancer is beyond the scope of this chapter but bears on the question of whether to eradicate *H. pylori* from individuals without ulcers—an issue which is currently unresolved.

Gastric MALT lymphoma (see Chapter 14.9.4)

Tumours of gastric mucosa-associated lymphoid tissue (**MALT**) are much more prevalent in *H. pylori* infection. This is as expected because uninfected gastric mucosa contains hardly any lymphocytes. Lymphomas restricted to the gastric mucosa usually disappear when *H. pylori* is eradicated because *H. pylori*-specific T cells provide contact-dependent help for growth of malignant B cells. The abnormal B-cell clone often remains detectable by gene rearrangement studies, and tumours reappear if the patient is reinfected. These lesions are less likely to respond to *H. pylori* eradication alone if they extend beyond the gastric mucosa. Chemotherapy or surgical excision may then be indicated, and therefore these tumours are generally best managed in a specialist centre.

Likelihood of disease following *H. Pylori* infection

Most individuals who are infected with *H. pylori* do not develop clinical disease. The likelihood of disease depends on the nature of the infecting strain, which is highly variable. The genome of more aggressive strains contains a pathogenicity island with genes encoding proteins that stimulate cytokine production. Infection with such strains can be identified by the presence of antibodies to cagA protein which is highly antigenic. Variations in *vacA* also affect the likelihood of serious clinical outcomes of the infection. However, people from parts of the world where heavy infection is frequent often harbour infection with more than one strain of *H. pylori*, which complicates this relationship.

Treatment of *H. pylori* infection

At the time of writing the following 1-week triple therapies are recommended in the British National Formulary because they provide the best combination of efficacy and convenience:

- Proton pump inhibitor twice daily plus amoxicillin 1000 mg twice daily plus clarithromycin 500 mg twice daily.
- Proton pump inhibitor twice daily plus metronidazole 400 mg thrice daily plus clarithromycin 500 mg twice daily.

The proton pump inhibitor can be either omeprazole 20 mg twice daily, or lansoprazole 30 mg twice daily. An H_2 antagonist, such as cimetidine, or an antibacterial agent such as bismuth citrate 400 mg twice daily can be used instead of the proton pump inhibitor.

The choice between these regimens depends on the local rate of metronidazole resistance. This is increased in inner-city areas because of immigration from developing countries where metronidazole is widely used, but is lower elsewhere in the United Kingdom. Resistance to clarithromycin is currently about 5 per cent in the United Kingdom but higher in the rest of Europe. Resistance to amoxicillin is exceedingly rare. It is important to encourage each patient to comply accurately, because about 60 per cent of strains will become resistant to metronidazole or clarithromycin if they are exposed to these without being eradicated. This lessens the chance that further attempts at eradication will succeed. An effective regimen for such cases is a proton pump inhibitor given twice daily, tripotassium dicitratobismuthate (TDB, DeNol) 120 mg four times daily 30 min before meals and at night, tetracycline 500 mg four times daily, and metronidazole 400 mg thrice daily all given for 2 weeks. *H. pylori* eradication regimens are subject to continued modification and it is thus recommended that current British National Formulary or local guidelines be consulted.

Whether eradication therapy has been successful or not can be determined by the urea breath test, but this must be performed at least 4 weeks after the end of the eradication regimen to avoid false negative results. Patients must be retested if persistent infection would be hazardous, for example after haemorrhage of an ulcer, but this is unnecessary if symptoms from an uncomplicated ulcer have disappeared.

The role of non-steroidal anti-inflammatory drugs in peptic ulceration

Ingestion of NSAIDs (including aspirin) is the main cause of gastric and duodenal ulcers that are not associated with *H. pylori* infection. The ratio of *H. pylori*- to NSAID-associated ulcers is about 95:5 in the duodenum and 80:20 in the stomach because NSAIDs affect the stomach more than the duodenum. The ratio also depends on local *H. pylori* prevalence and NSAID use. In prosperous areas with low *H. pylori* prevalence and many elderly persons taking NSAIDs, the latter is now the main culprit. This is important because the elderly are less able to withstand the ulcer-related complications of haemorrhage and perforation. Use of NSAIDs greatly increases the risk of admission to hospital with an ulcer, and the chance of ulcer haemorrhage during ingestion of NSAIDs increases with the dose and duration of therapy. It also varies from drug to drug. NSAIDs act by inhibiting the enzyme cyclo-oxygenase which converts arachidonic acid to prostaglandins which normally protect gastrointestinal epithelia by increasing blood flow and secretion of mucus and bicarbonate. The isoenzymes cyclo-oxygenase-1 and cyclo-oxygenase-2 are largely responsible for the mucosal protective and anti-inflammatory effects respectively of NSAIDs (Fig. 5). Therefore newer NSAIDs, such as celecoxib and rofecoxib, that are highly selective for cyclo-oxygenase-2, control inflammation with less risk of causing ulcers.

Ingestion of NSAIDs leads to a 'chemical' gastritis that is a milder form of the gastritis produced by reflux of bile into the stomach. The mucosa shows foveolar hyperplasia, oedema, vasodilatation and congestion, and few inflammatory cells. Ingestion of NSAIDs very often causes acute erosive

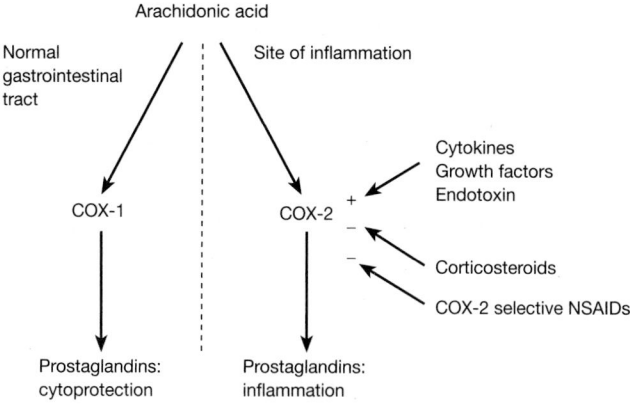

Fig. 5 The different roles of cyclo-oxygenase-1 and -2. Most existing NSAIDs inhibit both cyclo-oxygenase-1 and cyclo-oxygenase-2.

gastritis that typically goes unnoticed unless it causes frank bleeding. Erosions tend to heal by the process of mucosal adaptation when NSAIDs are taken for more than about a week. Chronic ulcers develop with more prolonged ingestion of NSAIDs.

Prevention and control

The use of alternative medications such as paracetamol is the best way to prevent NSAID-associated ulcers. NSAIDs are now generally avoided in non-inflammatory conditions such as osteoarthritis. When NSAIDs are required a cyclo-oxygenase-2-selective drug is preferred. If an ulcerogenic NSAID has to be continued in a patient at risk then ulcer prophylaxis is indicated. Proton pump inhibitors and misoprostol are both effective in healing and preventing NSAID-associated ulcers. The former are generally preferred because they have fewer side-effects: misoprostol in particular tends to cause diarrhoea (see below).

Other factors which increase the risk of peptic ulceration

Cigarette smoking strongly predisposes to peptic ulceration. This may be because nicotine stimulates acid secretion and reduces mucosal blood flow, but eradication of *H. pylori* prevents the ulcerogenic effect. A moderate alcohol intake is not harmful and might even decrease the risk of duodenal ulceration. Duodenal ulceration is considerably more common in patients with cirrhosis or chronic pancreatitis, presumably because bile and pancreatic juice normally neutralize gastric acid when it enters the duodenum. It is usual to recommend a 'bland' diet in ulcer disease but no particular food is known to increase the risk of duodenal ulcer disease. Indeed the traditional Japanese diet, high in salt, pickles, and raw fish, may contribute to the low prevalence in Japan of duodenal ulcer disease and the high prevalence of gastric ulcers and cancer by causing corpus gastritis, which diminishes acid secretion. Hyperparathyroidism increases the prevalence of duodenal ulcer disease. Elevated circulating calcium concentrations stimulate gastrin release, and parathyroid tumours are associated with gastrinomas in the multiple endocrine neoplasia-1 syndrome (see Chapter 12.10).

The epidemiology of peptic ulcers

Ulcers of the stomach and duodenum led to 4111 deaths in England and Wales in 1996. This remains a cause for concern, but most peptic ulcers do not produce life-threatening illness.

Duodenal ulcer epidemiology

Duodenal ulcers are often asymptomatic so their prevalence can only be established by investigating apparently healthy people. Such a study in Finland showed that 1.4 per cent of the entire population had a duodenal ulcer at any time. The lifetime prevalence was 10 per cent in males and 4 per cent in females. In the United Kingdom duodenal ulcers are more common in the north of the country and in urban rather than rural regions. The incidence of duodenal ulcers gradually increases with age but peaks at about 60 years of age. In most parts of the world duodenal ulcers are about three times as common as gastric ulcers, but gastric ulcers are more common in some places including Japan, Sri Lanka, and the Andean region. The epidemiology of peptic ulcers is changing quite rapidly: in late nineteenth-century England, gastric ulcers occurred in young women and were much more common than duodenal ulcers. From the turn of that century until about 1960 the incidence of duodenal ulceration rose several times to become more common than gastric ulceration, which is now uncommon under the age of 40 years. Factors that might have contributed include cigarette smoking and the spread of *H. pylori* during the Depression and wartime. Also the integrity of the acid-secreting mucosa might have improved as the increasing use of refrigeration diminished the salt content of the diet and fresh fruit and vegetables provided antioxidants. Since 1960, the incidence of duodenal ulceration has stopped rising and may even have declined. The declining prevalence of *H. pylori* and early treatment of it has further changed the situation so that it is now becoming unusual for a gastroenterologist to see active duodenal ulcer disease in some prosperous regions in the west.

Gastric ulcer epidemiology

In most parts of the world chronic gastric ulcers are less common than duodenal ulcers, but gastric ulcers are still quite common. The most accurate epidemiological studies are from Finland. At any time about 0.3 per cent of that population has a gastric ulcer. The lifetime prevalence of gastric ulceration is 4 per cent in males and 3 per cent in females and the prevalence of *H. pylori* infection is similar in males and females. Gastric ulcers are rare in people under the age of 40 years and tend to occur in the lower socio-economic groups.

Duodenal ulcers

Duodenal ulcer is a common illness with serious complications. Over 90 per cent of these ulcers are due to *H. pylori* infection and can be permanently cured by its eradication (Fig. 1) but it is not possible to achieve this worldwide. Duodenal ulceration in the absence of *H. pylori* infection is the exception and is usually due to NSAIDs, Crohn's disease, or the Zollinger–Ellison syndrome.

Pathogenesis

Duodenal ulcer disease is associated with antrum-predominant *H. pylori* gastritis: the proximal stomach that secretes acid is relatively spared. *H. pylori* antritis suppresses expression of the inhibitory peptide somatostatin and increases release of the acid-stimulating hormone gastrin. Gastrin elevates acid secretion both immediately and through the trophic effects of gastrin on the oxyntic mucosa. Eradication of *H. pylori* reverses these effects on gastric physiology. The increase in acid secretion directly damages the duodenal mucosa. Acid hypersecretion also produces gastric metaplasia in the proximal duodenum (Fig. 6). This allows *H. pylori* bacteria to colonize the duodenum and produce duodenitis that further impairs mucosal integrity and diminishes duodenal bicarbonate secretion. These changes result in duodenal ulcers.

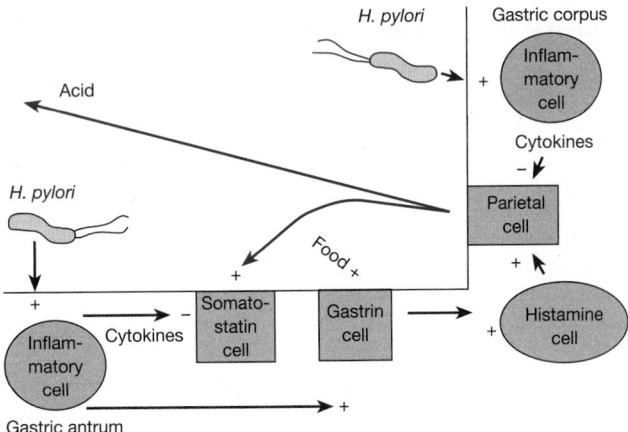

Fig. 6 Pathophysiology of *H. pylori* infection. Food stimulates gastrin cells in the gastric antrum to release gastrin. Circulating gastrin stimulates enterochromaffin-like cells in the gastric corpus to release histamine that stimulates adjacent parietal cells to secrete acid. Normally acid stimulates secretion of somatostatin that inhibits further gastrin release. Cytokines released in *H. pylori* antral gastritis suppress antral somatostatin-cells, leading to hypersecretion of gastrin and acid. But cytokines released in *H. pylori* gastritis of the gastric corpus tend to suppress parietal cells leading to diminished acid secretion.

Clinical presentation

Duodenal ulcers typically present with pain that is dull and located in the epigastrium or to the right of it over the duodenum itself. It is characteristically relieved by eating, then gets worse when the stomach empties. The pain usually wakes the patient from sleep in the middle of the night and is relieved by eating food, drinking milk, or taking an alkali preparation (antacid). Night pain is due to high nocturnal acid secretion without the buffering effect of food. The pain is also episodic with exacerbations lasting a few weeks separated by pain-free periods. These last for several weeks or months and probably reflect spontaneous healing of the ulcer. Pain radiating to the back suggests a posterior penetrating ulcer. Note that many ulcers do not cause pain and present with bleeding. This is particularly likely in the elderly, or if the patient is taking NSAIDs. Patients with duodenal ulcer often have other symptoms such as retrosternal burning and acid regurgitation. Nausea and vomiting are unusual and appetite is preserved. Persistent vomiting suggests pyloric stenosis. Symptoms resulting from other complications are described below.

Differential diagnosis

Gastro-oesophageal reflux disease also causes pain when the patient is in bed but patients usually notice an acid taste in the mouth or burning in the chest. Pancreatic pain typically radiates to the back, is exacerbated by eating, and is relieved by leaning forwards. Gallstone pain tends to be colicky and is exacerbated by eating fat. Pain due to the irritable bowel syndrome can occur in the epigastrium and be affected by eating but it usually extends to the lower abdomen and is typically affected by defaecation. Duodenal ulceration seen at endoscopy is usually due to *H. pylori* but NSAIDs, Crohn's disease, and the Zollinger–Ellison syndrome need to be considered, particularly if *H. pylori* is absent or if ulceration persists after it is eradicated.

Pathology

In duodenal ulcer disease the duodenum contains patches of gastric metaplasia colonized by *H. pylori* bacteria leading to infiltration with lymphocytes and neutrophil polymorphs. The ulcer itself consists of a breach in the epithelium with ulcer slough, inflammatory cells, and varying amounts of collagen scar in the base.

Diagnosis of duodenal ulceration

Duodenal ulcers are diagnosed most accurately by endoscopy. Antral biopsies can be tested for *H. pylori* and local treatment can be applied if the ulcer is bleeding (see below). Between episodes of ulceration the duodenum may show scarring or deformity. The presence of duodenitis also provides a clue to the diagnosis. High-quality double-contrast barium radiology is only slightly inferior. If an ulcer is seen, the likelihood of *H. pylori* infection is about 90 per cent—which is sufficient to justify treatment.

Treatment

Healing of duodenal ulcers can be accelerated by a number of acid-suppressing or mucosal protective drugs, but *H. pylori* eradication is now the mainstay of treatment (see above). Of the acid suppressors, proton pump inhibitors are more effective that histamine H_2-receptor antagonists, but the difference is not great in duodenal ulcer disease. *H. pylori* eradication should be commenced immediately. It is usually unnecessary to continue acid suppression after eradication therapy because eradication heals duodenal ulcers rapidly. However, it is sensible to continue acid suppression for about 8 weeks if the ulcer was complicated by bleeding or pyloric stenosis. *H. pylori* occasionally proves impossible to eradicate: healing may then be achieved and maintained by acid suppression. Alternatively prolonged remissions can be induced by courses of tripotassium dicitratobismuthate (DeNol).

Prognosis

Recurrence of *H. pylori*-related duodenal ulceration is uncommon after successful eradication. The rate of reinfection with *H. pylori* is about 0.7 per cent per annum in Western adults. Higher rates of reinfection have been reported in developing countries but this is not universal and the reinfection rate is 1 per cent per annum in China. Apparent reinfection in the West is often actually persistence of the initial infection. Recurrent ulceration in the absence of *H. pylori* may be due to NSAIDs, Crohn's disease, or the Zollinger–Ellison syndrome. In some patients recurrent ulceration after eradication of *H. pylori* is associated with persistent high acid output in the absence of a gastrinoma.

Gastric ulcers and erosions

Breaches in the gastric epithelium take two forms. Chronic benign gastric ulcers are relatively large and usually single. Acute erosive gastritis produces many small ulcers or erosions.

Chronic benign gastric ulcer

Gastric ulcers are important because they cause ill health, bleed and occasionally perforate, and because they are sometimes difficult to distinguish from gastric cancers. Most are associated with *H. pylori* infection and eradicating the bacterium greatly diminishes recurrence of ulcers, which demonstrates the causative role of the bacterium. Most other chronic gastric ulcers are associated with ingestion of NSAIDs . At the beginning of the twentieth century gastric ulcers were more common in the United Kingdom than duodenal ulcers and often occurred in young women. Now they are less prevalent than duodenal ulcers and typically occur in older people with low incomes. In some countries, including Japan, gastric ulcers are still more common than duodenal ulcers.

Pathogenesis

Ulceration occurs when luminal aggressive factors overcome mucosal defence. Suppression of acid accelerates healing of gastric ulcers so acid clearly contributes, but rates of acid secretion are normal or slightly below normal in these patients so acid cannot be regarded as the main cause. The duodenogastric reflux is increased in patients with gastric ulcers, and the

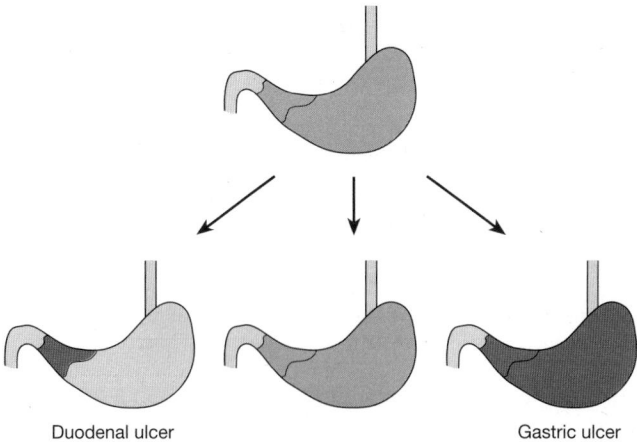

Duodenal ulcer   Gastric ulcer

Fig. 7 Relationship between the distribution of *H. pylori* gastritis and the clinical outcome of the infection. Initially the infection affects the entire stomach. Most patients then develop a mild pangastritis and no clinical disease. Patients with duodenal ulcer have antrum-predominant gastritis, a healthy corpus and high acid secretion. Marked pangastritis is associated with low acid secretion and an increased risk of gastric cancer.

refluxed fluid weakens the mucosal barrier. *H. pylori* might cause ulceration directly by releasing a toxin such as its vacuolating toxin. Alternatively products of the inflammatory cells that it attracts, such as oxygen radicals or proteolytic enzymes, might compromise mucosal integrity (Fig. 7). The hydrophobic barrier of the mucosa is impaired in *H. pylori* infection. Non-steroidal anti-inflammatory drugs cause ulceration largely through inhibiting the production by cyclo-oxygenase-1 of protective prostaglandins in the gastrointestinal tract. In future this can be avoided by using highly selective inhibitors of cyclo-oxygenase-2, such as celecoxib and refecoxib. This is the isoenzyme that is involved in the inflammatory diseases for which these drugs are used (see above).

Clinical features

Patients with chronic gastric ulcers tend to be over 40 years old and from lower socio-economic groups. Epigastric pain is the most frequent symptom. It occasionally radiates to the back if the ulcer is located posteriorly. Food or antacids usually relieve it. It typically occurs in exacerbations lasting for several weeks with symptom-free periods in between. Night pain occurs in a minority of patients with gastric ulcer compared with most of those with duodenal ulcers. Gastric ulcers quite often produce nausea, anorexia, or weight loss suggestive of gastric cancer. Some patients vomit, but many ulcers have no symptoms until the patient presents with haemorrhage, and in practice one cannot reliably distinguish between these diseases on the basis of symptoms. Most patients with epigastric pain have non-ulcer dyspepsia or gastro-oesophageal reflux disease, rather than gastric or duodenal ulcers: gallstones can also cause epigastric pain but this tends to be colicky, at the right costal margin, and is exacerbated by fatty food. Pancreatic pain tends to be more constant, radiates to the back, and may be relieved by leaning forward. The differential diagnosis of gastric ulceration includes gastric cancer, lymphoma, Crohn's disease, syphilis, tuberculosis, and sarcoidosis. Importantly, gastric cancers occasionally produce ulcers that resemble simple peptic ulcers and these can heal when acid secretion is suppressed; further confusion may arise because biopsies from the ulcer edge do not always contain malignant cells.

Pathology

Histological examination of a chronic gastric ulcer shows a breach in the gastric mucosa that penetrates the muscularis mucosae. The base is composed of chronic inflammatory cells, and slough and fibrous tissue in varying proportions. The edge of the ulcer shows evidence of increased

proliferation. The surrounding gastric epithelium may show *H. pylori* gastritis or chemical gastritis caused by NSAIDs or bile reflux.

Laboratory diagnosis

Cancer is excluded by examining multiple biopsies from the edge of the ulcer. *H. pylori* is sought as described above, but biopsy-based methods are prone to give false negative results because the stomachs of these patients typically contain areas of atrophy or intestinal metaplasia which are not colonized by the bacterium.

Treatment

Treatment of chronic gastric ulcers is by removing the cause if possible and giving ulcer healing agents if necessary. *H. pylori* is eradicated as described above. NSAIDs are discontinued if possible. In addition, administration of a proton pump inhibitor such as omeprazole accelerates healing of the ulcer. Until the ulcer heals, the patient should have an endoscopic examination every 4 to 6 weeks and multiple biopsies should be taken from the ulcer edge to exclude cancer. If NSAIDs have to be continued, the stomach can be protected against further ulceration by a proton pump inhibitor or misoprostol.

Prognosis

The immediate dangers are from complications and undiagnosed malignancy. Gastric ulcers are very likely to recur if they are healed by acid suppression alone. However, they unlikely to reappear if the cause is removed or adequate prophylaxis is given.

Acute erosive or haemorrhagic gastritis

Introduction

Acute gastric erosions are breaches in the gastric epithelium that are often multiple and small ({lt} 3 mm), reflecting an acute diffuse response to the gastric insult. If they do breach the muscularis mucosae they are called acute gastric ulcers. Cushing and Curling ulcers are historical terms used to describe ulcers in patients with head injury and burns respectively, but most acute gastric ulcers are now associated with severe illness or ingestion of NSAIDs or alcohol.

Acute gastric erosions in severe illnesses

These are common—80 per cent of patients receiving respiratory support from mechanical ventilators studied after 3 days in a British intensive care unit had erosions:

(a) Acute gastric ulcers in patients with injury to the central nervous system were described by Cushing. Ulcers that frequently bleed occur in 50 to 70 per cent of patients with head injuries. They also occur after spinal injuries and after surgery to the central nervous system. The injury might cause the ulcers by increasing the release of gastrin because these patients have elevated acid secretion and plasma gastrin levels.

(b) Curling described acute duodenal ulcers in patients with severe burns; however, acute gastric ulcers are even more common, and were present in 86 per cent of such patients in one recent study.

(c) Acute gastric ulcers occur in patients suffering from many severe illnesses, including severe trauma, sepsis, shock, and major organ failure, presumably because these diminish gastric perfusion and compromise the metabolic integrity of the gastric mucosa.

Acute gastric ulcers due to ingested substances

Non-steroidal anti-inflammatory drugs including aspirin produce acute gastric ulcers by inhibiting synthesis of protective prostaglandins by cyclo-oxygenase-1. These impair mucosal protection by diminishing mucosal blood flow and the secretion of mucus and bicarbonate. Ulceration is most extensive shortly after the start of therapy: the stomach then adapts and ulceration subsides.

Alcohol induces acute gastric ulceration by a direct toxic effect. Studies in experimental animals suggest that vascular thrombosis also contributes to alcohol-induced ulceration.

Clinical features

The patient may complain of epigastric pain, nausea, anorexia, or vomiting but symptoms are usually absent until haemorrhage occurs The bleeding may be occult, show itself as small amounts of blood or 'coffee grounds' in gastric aspirates, or occur suddenly as a substantial haemorrhage.

Diagnosis

Acute gastric ulcers and erosions are readily seen with an endoscope, but the appearance varies from multiple erosions to submucosal haemorrhages to one or more points of active bleeding. During healing the ulcer may be elevated by surrounding oedema. Endoscopy is the principal diagnostic procedure and angiography is rarely needed.

Treatment and prevention

This disease is both treated and prevented by minimizing injurious factors. This involves correction of shock, sepsis, and respiratory and renal failure and avoidance of NSAIDs and alcohol. It is also important to correct coagulopathy that is frequently present in sick patients. Suppression of acid secretion is protective. This may be achieved with a histamine H_2-receptor antagonist or a proton pump inhibitor. However, it is recognized that acid suppression allows overgrowth of bacteria in the stomach lumen. This increases the risk of sepsis, particularly through aspiration in patients with impaired consciousness or cough reflex; hence prophylaxis with the antipepsin agent sucralfate, is generally preferred in patients undergoing intensive care.

The management of patients with established acute gastric ulceration involves blood transfusion, correction of coagulopathy, and suppression of acid secretion. The benefit from acid suppression is slight once haemorrhage has occurred. Endoscopic intervention and surgery are not usually appropriate because the condition is diffuse. If an operation is required it may need to be radical to control the haemorrhage (for example total gastrectomy).

Complications of ulcer disease

Haemorrhage

Haemorrhage remains a challenging problem and is the main cause of death from peptic ulcers. Blood loss may be slow and present as unexplained anaemia but more typically presents acutely with haematemesis or melaena or both with varying degrees of hypovolaemic shock. Such cases should be managed jointly by physicians and surgeons from the outset. Older patients need particular attention because they are much more vulnerable to the effects of hypovolaemia. Immediate action should be directed to the correction of circulatory shock by blood transfusion. Further transfusion may be required to keep the patient's haemoglobin level above 10 g/dl. Disorders of coagulation, pre-existing or due to transfusion, should also be corrected. Endoscopy is performed, preferably after the patient's condition has stabilized, to define the source of bleeding and to apply endoscopic treatments. Ulcers which are actively bleeding or show stigmata, such as adherent clot or a visible vessel, which make further bleeding likely can be treated with lasers, heater probes, or local injection of adrenaline. Rebleeding is an indication for surgery. After the acute episode, it is important to attend to the cause of the ulcer. Eradication of H. pylori, if it is present, greatly diminishes the frequency of further episodes of bleeding in future, but this is a measure that is frequently overlooked. Non-invasive tests can be used to diagnose the infection if biopsies were not taken at the time of endoscopy during the acute bleeding. NSAIDs are contraindicated after haemorrhage from NSAID ulcers. It is generally unnecessary to give long-term prophylaxis if the cause of ulceration has been removed, but this

may be advisable if the patient is elderly, frail, or does not have rapid access to hospital.

Perforation

Ulcer perforation typically presents with a sudden onset or worsening of pain with considerable abdominal tenderness followed by the onset of peritonitis with board-like rigidity, rebound tenderness, and loss of bowel sounds. Gas in the peritoneum may lead to loss of liver dullness to percussion, and is usually visible beneath the diaphragm on erect chest radiograph. The patient is unwell with tachycardia, leucocytosis, and sometimes fever. The differential diagnosis includes acute pancreatitis, acute cholecystitis, and other causes of an acute abdomen such as gut infarction or perforation of other organs (see Chapter 14.3.1). The patient is resuscitated with intravenous fluids and antibiotics before transfer to theatre for repair of the perforation. Note that perforation, like other abdominal emergencies, may have a less specific presentation in the elderly, who may collapse or suffer confusion rather than the characteristic pain. Again, once the acute event has been dealt with, it is important to identify and treat the cause of the ulcer.

Pyloric stenosis

Repeated duodenal ulceration sometimes leads to stenosis of the pyloric canal or proximal duodenum. The narrowing is due to oedema as well as fibrosis so it can resolve without the need for surgery. The main symptom is vomiting which may contain food eaten the previous day. Typical symptoms of duodenal ulceration may or may not precede the onset of vomiting. Patients rapidly become dehydrated and develop hypokalaemia with a metabolic acidosis, they may also be malnourished. A succussion splash, which is normally present up to 4 h after a meal, is present at other times. Barium radiology or upper endoscopy show a distended stomach containing retained food and secretions and with a narrowed pyloric canal. The differential diagnosis includes cancer of the distal stomach. Most of these patients settle without the need for further intervention if treated by gastric aspiration, acid suppression, and intravenous fluids for a few days. If not, the stenotic region can be dilated using a balloon passed via an endoscope. A few patients require an operation, but again the cause of ulceration must be identified and appropriately treated.

Gastrinoma

The Zollinger–Ellison syndrome comprises an association of pancreatic tumour, gastric hypersecretion, and intractable ulceration. The tumour causes the syndrome by releasing gastrin so it is called a gastrinoma. This disease is discussed in Chapter 12.10.

Non-ulcer dyspepsia

Dyspepsia is upper abdominal or lower chest discomfort or pain, related to eating, which may be accompanied by other gastrointestinal symptoms such as nausea, vomiting, anorexia, or distension. Non-ulcer dyspepsia refers to cases of dyspepsia where no ulcer or other cause such as gallstones or gastro-oesophageal reflux disease is found. Historically, it was the introduction of modern investigative techniques, particularly endoscopy, which allowed these patients to be identified. Advances in clinical investigation allow some patients considered to have non-ulcer dyspepsia to be diagnosed and treated appropriately. For instance oesophageal pH studies might change the diagnosis to endoscopy-negative gastro-oesophageal reflux disease (GORD) (see Chapter 14.6). Some patients may therefore elude diagnosis because in effect they are not fully investigated. The diagnosis of non-ulcer dyspepsia is not intellectually satisfying but it is important to make. First the patient benefits from the reassurance of knowing that he or she has a recognized medical condition; secondly insight will be gained ultimately into the causes of non-ulcer dyspepsia and how it behaves in response to different treatments.

Epidemiology

Non-ulcer dyspepsia is exceedingly common. In one survey in southwest England, 38 per cent of the entire adult population had had dyspepsia during a 6-month period and a further 25 per cent gave a past history of dyspeptic symptoms. Many or even most of these individuals have non-ulcer dyspepsia.

Symptoms and their pathogenesis

Patients report a variety of symptoms. Research reveals a series of abnormalities of physiological function. Symptoms and the corresponding pathophysiology are described together below; in practice the relationship between symptoms and disorders of function remains ill defined and many patients have more than one symptom. A common theme is that irritation, mild injury, or anxiety diminish thresholds for perception of pain and discomfort in the gastrointestinal tract.

Burning

Many patients with dyspepsia report burning in the epigastrium or chest, or other symptoms suggesting gastro-oesophageal reflux. Irritation of the oesophagus, for example by alcohol or previous reflux episodes, diminishes the threshold for oesophageal pain, so that very mild reflux then causes symptoms. If studies of oesophgeal pH and manometry show definite reflux, the patient can be reclassified as having endsocopy-negative gastro-oesophgeal reflux disease. In busy clinical practice this distinction may be considered unnecessary because the treatment of the two conditions is similar and usually empirical.

Distension

A frequent complaint is that the abdomen feels distended, a symptom that also occurs in irritable bowel syndrome, but if the distension is largely felt in the upper abdomen and after meals, it is considered to be typical of non-ulcer dyspepsia. In addition, there is frequently a sensation of early statiety after meals and a proportion of non-ulcer dyspeptics show delayed gastric emptying on scintigraphy, the cause of which is unknown, although anxiety may contribute. Reflux of duodenal contents into the stomach also occurs more frequently in non-ulcer dyspeptics. The differential diagnosis includes ascites and obesity. Some patients create a bizarre appearance of distension by contracting their diaphragms and increasing their lumbar lordosis.

Pain

Pain is a frequent symptom in non-ulcer dyspepsia, although its origin is usually difficult to establish. It may be due to muscular spasm. The differential diagnosis includes diffuse oesophageal spasm and achalasia as well as other painful conditions including pancreatitis and gallstone disease.

Nausea, vomiting, and satiety

If nausea and vomiting persist in the absence of an organic lesion it is important to exclude other causes such as drugs, metabolic disease, and disorders of the inner ear or central nervous system. Otherwise it is important to consider bulimia, anorexia nervosa, and psychogenic vomiting.

Diagnosis

The physical examination is unremarkable apart from the upper abdomen which is often tender. Investigation aims to exclude other diseases. This is partly to direct treatment and partly so that the patient can be reassured. The condition is so prevalent that it is unnecessary and impractical to investigate all patients fully. Clinical judgement is required. Upper endoscopy is indicated if the picture suggests organic disease or if symptoms persist. Upper abdominal ultrasound scanning is indicated if gallstones are suspected. Whether to test all dyspeptics for *H. pylori* remains controversial (see below). The infection has proved to be no more prevalent in patients with non-ulcer dyspepsia than in the general population.

Treatment

Explanation of the diagnosis with reassurance may relieve anxiety and thus diminish symptoms. Remaining symptoms can then usually be managed with antacids without the need for further medical attention. If treatment is prescribed proton pump inhibitors are most effective but also most expensive (Fig. 8). Alkalis, histamine H_2-receptor antagonists, and prokinetics are often helpful and less expensive. Most large randomized double-blind studies show that eradication of *H. pylori* does not improve symptoms in non-ulcer dyspepsia.

Prognosis and areas of uncertainty

Non-ulcer dyspepsia is a benign condition with no complications and a good prognosis. Only a minority of patients require long-term maintenance therapy. The problem is that some of the many dyspeptics in the community will develop serious organic disease. In a recent study, Swedes who reported symptoms of reflux were eight times more likely than healthy control subjects to develop adenocarcinoma of the gastro-oesophageal junction. Refluxed acid causes Barrett's oesophagus where these cancers originate (see Chapter 14.6). Therefore we need to learn how to manage this risk in the population of patients with dyspepsia. The second area of controversy is whether to eradicate *H. pylori* if it is found in a patient with non-ulcer dyspepsia.

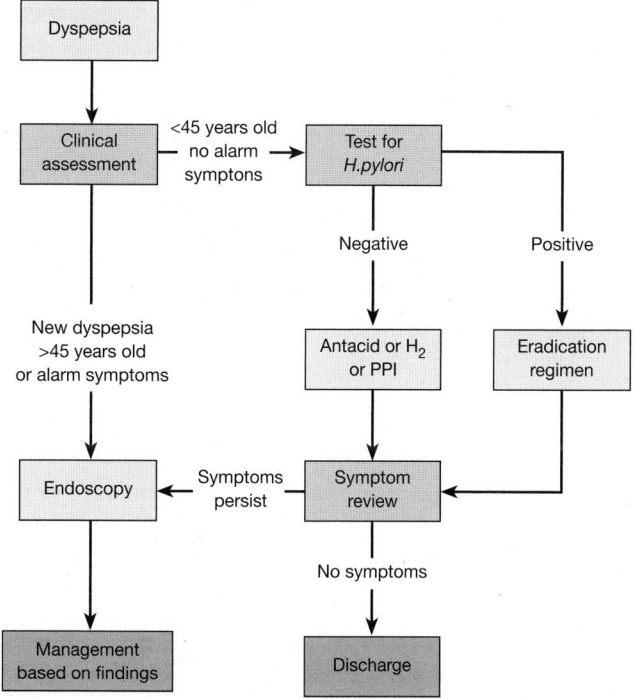

Fig. 8 Flow chart for the management of a patient presenting with dyspepsia of unknown cause that has failed to respond to lifestyle measures and antacids: H_2 = histamine H_2-receptor antagonist; PPI = proton pump inhibitor.

Strategies for management of peptic ulcers and dyspepsia: the role of tests for *H. pylori*

The investigation and treatment of these conditions consume considerable healthcare resources (Fig. 9). Appreciation of the pathogenic role of *H. pylori* has prompted debate over how dyspepsia can be managed more efficiently. All agree that patients with recent onset of dyspepsia over the age of 45 years should be endoscoped promptly to exclude early gastric cancer. Three strategies have emerged for the management of younger patients:

1. 'Treat symptomatically and endoscope those with persisting symptoms'. This is the traditional approach. Initial treatment is with alkalis and less expensive acid-suppressing drugs. Those with persisting or troublesome symptoms are referred for endoscopy. Diagnoses such as ulcer, oesophagitis, and non-ulcer dyspepsia and the *H. pylori* status can then be made precisely, and management organized accordingly. The argument against this policy is that it does not make intelligent use of testing for *H. pylori* to rationalize demand for endoscopy.

2. 'Test and investigate'. The rationale is as follows: Research shows that patients under 45 years of age who are serologically negative for *H. pylori* and not taking NSAIDs are very unlikely to have peptic ulcers or gastric cancer. Therefore if these individuals are not normally endoscoped, endoscopy waiting lists and the number of negative examinations can be reduced. Negative *Helicobacter* serology allows the patient to be reassured that they have no serious disease and can be treated symptomatically with alkalis and acid-suppressing drugs. In practice, the main issue is whether the absence of *H. pylori* is sufficiently reassuring to relieve anxiety and the pressure for further investigations.

3. 'Test and treat'. Eradication of *H. pylori* heals and prevents gastric and duodenal ulcers. The World Health Organization has declared that *H. pylori* is a class 1 carcinogen. Therefore it is proposed to test all patients

under 45 years of age with dyspeptic symptoms for *H. pylori*, and treat those who are infected. Endoscopy is reserved for patients whose symptoms persist after *H. pylori* eradication and those with new dyspepsia over the age of 45 years. The issue here is whether it is desirable to eradicate *H. pylori* from patients without ulcers. Most dyspeptics under 45 years of age do not have ulcers, even if they are infected with *H. pylori*. Overall this policy appears seems sensible. The main arguments against it are that antibiotic use will increase and that there is some controversial evidence that *H. pylori* protects against oesophageal disease. Overall, policies based on testing for *H. pylori* are less efficient in populations where the prevalence of the infection is very low, such as prosperous parts of North America, or very high, as in developing countries or in recent immigrants from them. Furthermore, in parts of the world with inadequate sanitation, reinfection rates can be as high as 30 per cent per annum, which diminishes the value of eradication.

Treatments for peptic ulcer disease and non-ulcer dyspepsia

Antacids

Alkalis provide temporary symptomatic relief of pain in peptic ulcer disease but do not accelerate healing compared with placebo unless very large quantities are given. They are more useful in GORD and non-ulcer dyspepsia than in peptic ulcer disease. They usually contain the alkaline salts or hydroxides of magnesium or aluminium. Those based on magnesium are laxative and those based on aluminium tend to cause constipation. Some preparations contain mixtures of magnesium and aluminium to overcome this. Some preparations contain alginate which forms a flocculent raft on the gastric contents to reduce the effects of bile and acid reflux and protect the oesophageal mucosa.

Bismuth preparations

Tripotassium dicitratobismuthate (bismuth chelate, DeNol)

This bismuth complex acts mainly by suppressing *H. pylori* infection. It also has a protective effect on the mucosa, probably by stimulation of the synthesis of mucosal prostaglandins. Tripotassium dicitratobismuthate heals gastric and duodenal ulcers about as effectively as histamine H_2-receptor antagonists. It produces longer remissions of duodenal ulcer disease than do H_2 antagonists. This is probably because of its effect against *H. pylori* and because it remains in the gastric mucosa for several weeks after treatment. Currently tripotassium dicitratobismuthate is chiefly used as a component of second-line *Helicobacter* eradication regimens (see above). Bismuth preparations cause black stools—not to be confused with melaena. The bismuth content of tripotassium dicitratobismuthate is quite low. In the past 'epidemics' of bismuth encephalopathy occurred in Europe after patients ingested large amounts of other preparations containing unchelated bismuth. Tripotassium dicitratobismuthate only causes this complication if patients with impaired renal function take excessive doses for long periods.

Ranitidine bismuth citrate

This complex contains bismuth and the histamine H_2-receptor antagonist ranitidine. It can be used to treat duodenal ulceration associated with *H. pylori* infection. However, its main role is as a component of some highly effective *H. pylori*-eradication regimens (see above). It is contraindicated in moderate to severe renal failure and is not used for maintenance therapy since it may cause bismuth encephalopathy. It darkens the stools and can cause a black tongue.

Sucralfate

Sucralfate is a complex of aluminium hydroxide and sulphated sucrose, the properties of which include protection of the mucosa and ulcer healing. It

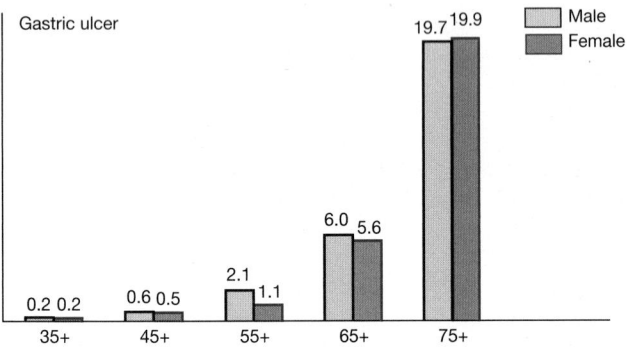

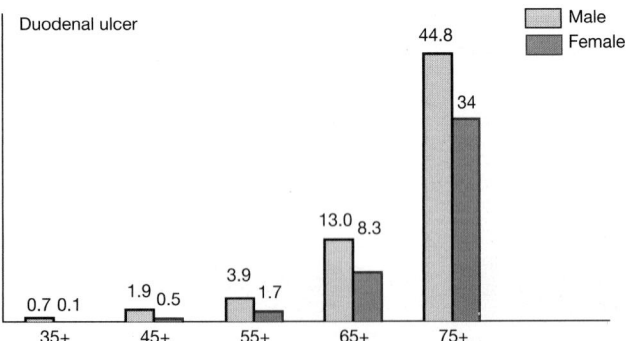

Fig. 9 (a) and (b) Age-specific death rates from peptic ulcer for England and Wales as rates per 100 000 per annum in 1998.

is a weak antacid and may act by stimulating the synthesis of mucosal prostaglandins. It also binds bile salts. It is about as effective as histamine H$_2$-receptor antagonists at healing gastric and duodenal ulcers, but this role has now largely been taken over by proton pump inhibitors and *H. pylori* eradication. Currently sucralfate is mainly used in the prophylaxis of acute erosive gastritis in severely ill patients (see above). Side-effects are few but include mild constipation. It is to be avoided in patients with renal failure who occasionally develop aluminium toxicity.

Misoprostol

Misoprostol is a synthetic prostaglandin that increases the resistance of the stomach and duodenum to damage. Mechanisms include increased blood flow and secretion of mucus and bicarbonate. Misoprostol also mildly inhibits acid secretion. It accelerates healing of gastric and duodenal ulcers but this role has largely been taken over by proton pump inhibitors which are more effective, and by *H. pylori* eradication. The main use of misoprostol is in the prevention of gastroduodenal damage by NSAIDs, when these have to be given. The idea of replacing prostaglandins, the production of which is blocked by inhibitors of cyclo-oxygenase, is elegant, but this role has largely been taken over by proton pump inhibitors that are more effective and are about equally priced. The main side-effect of misoprostol is diarrhoea. This can be severe but is less likely if single doses do not exceed 200 µg. This is taken two to four times daily for prophylaxis. Note that misoprostol can induce abortion, so it should be avoided in women of childbearing age.

Histamine H$_2$-receptor antagonists

Secretion of gastric acid is normally stimulated by histamine, released from enterchromaffin-like cells in the gastric mucosa and acting on histamine H$_2$ receptors on parietal cells. Histamine H$_2$-receptor antagonists inhibit acid secretion by blocking this receptor. Sir James Black was awarded the Nobel prize for discovering this class of drug (as well as β-adrenergic antagonists). During the 1980s these drugs provided optimal treatment of peptic ulcer disease before being superceded by proton pump inhibitors and *H. pylori* eradication in the 1990s. However, they remain useful and are currently much less expensive. They are of use in non-ulcer dyspepsia and milder cases of gastro-oesophageal reflux disease (see Chapter 14.6). They protect the duodenum, but not the stomach, from ulceration due to NSAIDs. These drugs are not effective in haematemesis and melaena. Protection against acute erosive gastritis has not been shown consistently in trials. The four H$_2$ antagonists are cimetidine, ranitidine, nizatidine, and famotidine; but only the first two of these are widely used, largely due to the effects of marketing rather than to any differences in efficacy. Compared with ranitidine, cimetidine is less expensive, but it interacts with the metabolism of warfarin and anticonvulsants; it may cause mental confusion in the elderly.

Proton pump inhibitors

These drugs act by inhibiting the hydrogen/potassium adenosine triphosphatase enzyme system (H+/K+ATPase or 'proton pump') which pumps acid into the gastric lumen. They are prodrugs which are weak bases that are taken up into the acidic spaces in parietal cells, where the low pH creates a sulphenamide that is hydrophobic and therefore cannot diffuse away. The drug then forms disulphide bonds with cystine residues in the alpha chain of the proton pump, leading to its irreversible inactivation. Acid secretion is only restored when the cell synthesizes new proton pump protein. So these drugs are longer acting than H$_2$ antagonists even though they are cleared rapidly from the circulation. Once-daily dosing is satisfactory in most cases. Proton pump inhibitors are considerably more effective at preventing and healing gastro-oesophageal reflux disease than any other class of drug.

In peptic ulcer disease their therapeutic advantage is smaller but significant. Their role in therapy is:

(a) As a component of *H. pylori* eradication regimens. In this role they act by elevating the intragastric pH so that bacterial multiplication is encouraged and bacteriocidal antibiotics can act.

(b) They accelerate healing of ulcers during and after *H. pylori* eradication. This is particularly relevant to chronic gastric ulcers that tend to be slow to heal because they are large.

(c) They prevent NSAID-related ulcers if these agents have to be given. In this respect, proton pump inhibitors are more effective at protecting the stomach and duodenum than other classes of drug.

(d) Omeprazole is the treatment of choice for the Zollinger–Ellison syndrome (see Chapter 14.8). Proton pump inhibitors are also highly effective in the treatment of non-ulcer dyspepsia, but most cases can be managed successfully with less expensive remedies.

They are currently the class of drug that is responsible for the greatest drug-expenditure in the United Kingdom and there is pressure to restrict their use. The main side-effects are diarrhoea and headache. The former may be less frequent with omeprazole than lansoprazole. Proton pump inhibitors can interact with the metabolism of other drugs including anticoagulants and anticonvulsants. Antacids and sucralfate impair absorption of lansoprazole.

Motility stimulants

Prokinetic drugs are not used to treat peptic ulcers, but are of use in non-ulcer dyspepsia as well as gastro-oesophageal reflux disease (see Chapter 14.6). Metoclopramide and domperidone are dopamine agonists that increase gastric emptying, small bowel transit, and the tone of the lower oesophageal sphincter. They can cause hyperprolactinaemia, leading to gynaecomastia, galactorrhoea, and diminished libido. Dystonias can occur, particularly in younger patients, and more often with metoclopramide than domperidone. Both are inexpensive. Cisapride is a motility stimulant that is believed to act by promoting release of acetylcholine in the gut wall. It has several side-effects and important drug interactions. In particular cisapride can cause serious arrhythmias and is contraindicated if the QT interval is prolonged. Concomitant medication with macrolide antibiotics increases the circulating concentrations of cisapride and the risk of arrhythmia.

Prevention and control

H. pylori infection will diminish worldwide if its transmission can be diminished by public health measures. Immunization has been shown to be effective in animal models but a human version is still some way off. Mass eradication is not a serious option due to the cost and the risk of generating antibiotic resistance. NSAID-associated ulceration is diminished by a policy of not using these drugs in non-inflammatory arthritis, and by using cyclo-oxygenase-2-selective drugs.

Special problems in pregnant women

Pregnancy decreases the frequency of peptic ulcers but gastro-oesophageal reflux is frequent. Treatment is largely with dietary and lifestyle changes, together with antacids or sucralfate. Persistent symptoms are treated with H$_2$-receptor antagonists. If symptoms continue and are severe despite these interventions, upper endoscopy and/or therapy with proton pump inhibitors may be considered during the second or third trimester. Misoprostol should be avoided because it can induce abortion.

Occupational, quality of life, and psychological aspects

Chronic peptic ulcer disease certainly impairs quality of life, but happily this can be improved either with acid-suppressing drugs or *H. pylori* eradication. There is no objective evidence to support the widespread belief that psychological stress predisposes to peptic ulcers. The myth is perpetuated by using the obsolete term 'stress ulcer' to describe acute erosive gastritis.

The need for further research

The main area of uncertainty is over how to apply our knowledge about *H. pylori* to the general population. It could be argued that whole populations should be tested and treated if found to be infected because the bacterium clearly plays a major causative role in important diseases including peptic ulcers and gastric cancer. Against this there is the cost, which would be considerable, and a significant risk of generating antibiotic-resistant strains of *H. pylori* and other bacteria. Some studies raise the possibility that *H. pylori* infection might protect against oesophageal diseases, but this is controversial and several studies do not support the idea. Long-term studies of the effects of eradication compared with no eradication in healthy infected patients would help to resolve this, but would be a major undertaking. At present no country is evaluating mass eradication, with the exception of Japan where *H. pylori* and gastric cancer are both unusually prevalent. Developing countries lack the resources to mount such a programme. General improvements in public health and hygiene in the west are diminishing the prevalence of *H. pylori* infection without the need for specific action against this bacterium. On the other hand it is quite usual to eradicate *H. pylori* from infected patients without ulcers, even though the overall conclusion from trials is that this does not improve symptoms. This may be irrational but it points to the difference between the science of medicine and its art. Informing the patient that a serious infection has been found and eradicated can have a very useful and reassuring effect and ultimately might even prevent late complications of persistent infection.

Further reading

Calam J (1996). *Clinician's guide to Helicobacter pylori.* Chapman and Hall Medical, London.

Farthing MG, Patchett SE, eds (1998). *Helicobacter* infection. *British Medical Bulletin* **54**, 1–263.

Hawkey CJ (199). COX-2 inhibitors. *The Lancet* **353**, 307–14.

Talley NJ, ed (1998). Dyspepsia. *Baillière's clinical gastroenterology*, vol. 12, pp 417–630. Baillière Tindall, London.

14.8 Hormones and the gastrointestinal tract

P. J. Hammond, S. R. Bloom, A. E. Bishop and J. M. Polak

Introduction

The discovery of secretin, the first recognized hormone, by Bayliss and Starling in 1902 marked the birth not only of gastrointestinal endocrinology, but of endocrinology itself. This was followed in 1905 by the identification of gastrin, but the technique of identifying hormones was, thereafter, more successfully applied to the study of secretions from the ductless glands, and gastrointestinal endocrinology languished for the next six decades. The determination of the amino acid structure of gastrin following its extraction from a solid tumour in 1964 marked a renewed interest in the field, and the introduction of techniques for large-scale chemical extraction and purification of gut peptides resulted in the discovery of further gut peptides. Most of the gut peptides, such as cholecystokinin and substance P, have been identified within the central and peripheral nervous systems, playing a neuromodulatory role in many organs. These neurocrine peptides are synthesized in nerve cells rather than endocrine cells in the gut and act locally as peptide neurotransmitters or neuromodulators.

The endocrine cells of the gastrointestinal tract are not grouped into anatomically distinct glands, like most endocrine cells, but are scattered through the length of the gastrointestinal tract. The principal role of gut peptides is in the integration of gastrointestinal function, and they regulate the actions of the epithelium, muscles, and nerves throughout the gastrointestinal tract. This local effect of peptides may be either autocrine, regulating the function of the cell secreting them, or paracrine, influencing the behaviour of neighbouring cells of different type. Thus somatostatin, originally identified as a hypothalamic inhibitor of growth hormone release, has been shown to have inhibitory effects in many different organ systems. It is locally released and its main mechanism of action is a direct one on neighbouring cells, for example to inhibit gastric acid and insulin secretion. In addition to altering gastrointestinal function many peptides, such as gastrin, secretin, and enteroglucagon, probably play an important paracrine role in controlling the growth and development of the gastrointestinal tract. In contrast, for most gut peptides there is little evidence that they act as true hormones in an endocrine fashion.

Two techniques have contributed to the increased understanding of gastrointestinal endocrinology. Molecular biology has helped identify members of peptide families by molecular cloning techniques, and has provided information about peptide processing, which has shown that different peptides may originate from a single common precursor. Sensitive peptide radioimmunoassay has allowed detection of gut peptides, which have very low concentrations in plasma and tissues. Furthermore, the specific peptide antibodies can be used for immunocytochemistry to demonstrate the cellular and neuronal localization of gut peptides (Fig. 1), and for immunoneutralization studies to elucidate the pathophysiological functions of gut peptides. Peptide localization is further defined by electron microscopy, which demonstrates specific peptide storage granules (Fig. 2), and *in situ* hybridization, which allows the sites of peptide synthesis to be identified. The most recent advance in gastrointestinal endocrinology has been the molecular characterization of hormone receptors by cloning techniques. This has demonstrated different receptors for the same ligand and provides an explanation for the diverse biological actions of many gut peptides in the same tissues. The development of agonists and antagonists to specific receptors will allow the physiological roles of the gut peptides to be fully characterized, and may be of therapeutic benefit in restoring normal gastrointestinal function in a disease.

This section describes the gut peptide hormones and neurotransmitters, classifying them by common structure or precursor peptides, and then outlines abnormalities in gastrointestinal disease. The roles of gut peptides in the syndromes associated with gastroenteropancreatic tumours are considered in detail in Chapter 14.18.3.3, while the carcinoid syndrome is described at the end of this section.

Hormones and paracrine peptides

Gastrin–cholecystokinin family

Gastrin

Gastrin occurs in a variety of molecular forms but all the biological activity resides in the four carboxy-terminal amino acids. The major molecular forms contain 17 (G17; 2098 Da), 14 (G14; pentagastrin), and 34 (G34; big

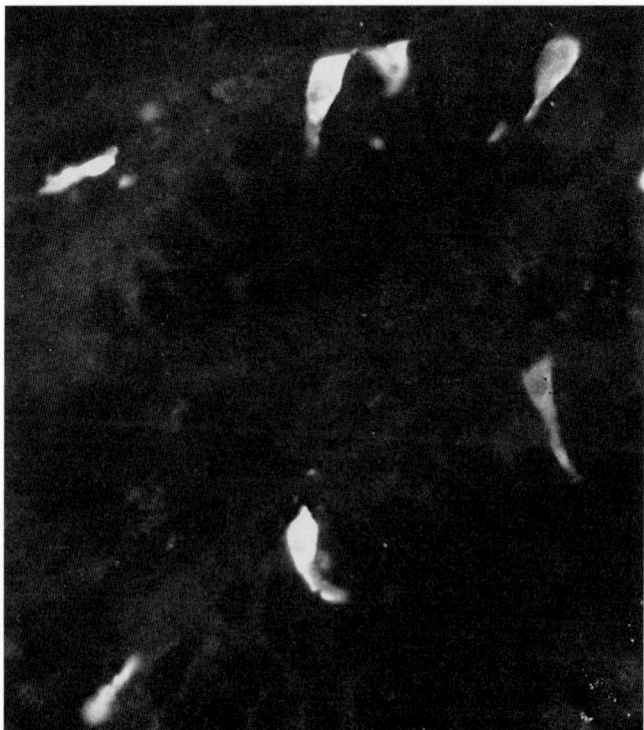

Fig. 1 Somatostatin cells, immunostained using the technique of indirect immunofluorescence, in the mucosa of human colon (×300).

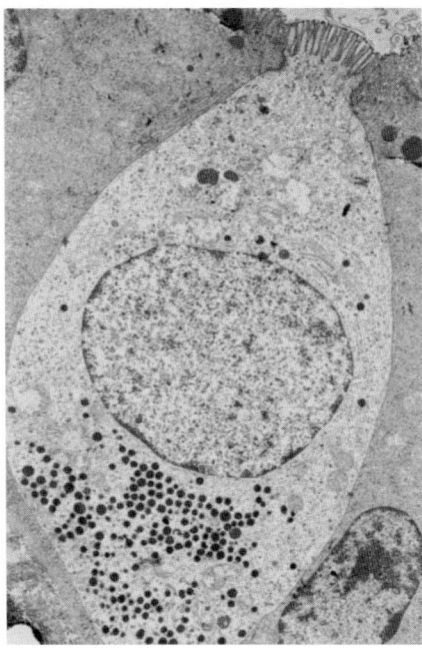

Fig. 2 Electron micrograph of a mucosal endocrine cell showing well-developed microvilli and secretory granules grouped at the basal membrane (×5500).

gastrin) amino acids. Larger molecular forms have been described but may be artefacts. In humans, gastrin is particularly localized to the gastric antrum, where G17 is the predominant form, but is also found in the upper small intestine, mainly as G34. These two are the predominant circulating forms. Gastrin is synthesized in G cells and electron microscopy shows gastrin granules to be large and electron lucent.

Gastrin release is particularly stimulated by protein ingestion and gastric distension. Its main physiological action is the stimulation of gastric acid secretion. Gastrin's other important physiological role appears to be its trophic effect on the gastric mucosa. Infusion of gastrin stimulates gastric motor activity and contraction of the lower oesophageal sphincter, but the physiological significance of this action is unclear.

Cholecystokinin

Cholecystokinin has an identical, five amino-acid, carboxy-terminal sequence to gastrin, but its specificity is conferred by the adjacent three amino acids, and this octapeptide confers its biological activity. It is found in the gut in 33, 39, or 58 amino-acid molecular forms predominantly, and is produced by the I cells of the duodenal and jejunal mucosa. The octapeptide cholecystokinin is a neurotransmitter in the central nervous system and a small amount is found in specific enteric neurones of the upper gastrointestinal tract.

Cholecystokinin secretion is stimulated by long-chain fatty acids and certain amino acids. The development of cholecystokinin antagonists specific for the two cholecystokinin receptor subtypes (cholecystokinin A, which is cholecystokinin specific, and cholecystokinin B, which appears to be also the only gastrin receptor) has allowed the important physiological roles of cholecystokinin to be characterized. The cholecystokinin A receptor appears to be involved in stimulation of gallbladder contraction and trophic effects on the duodenum and pancreas. The ability of cholecystokinin A receptor antagonists potently to inhibit meal-stimulated gallbladder contraction may be of therapeutic value in biliary colic.

The secretin family

The secretin family comprises a number of peptides with significant sequence homology. These include, in addition to secretin, glucose-dependent insulinotropic peptide, glucagon, enteroglucagon (see below),

vasoactive intestinal peptide, peptide histidine methionine, and growth hormone-releasing factor. The last is released from the hypothalamus, mainly as a 44 amino-acid peptide, to stimulate release of growth hormone, but is also found in significant concentrations, mainly in a 40 amino-acid form, in the small intestinal mucosa, where its function is unknown.

Secretin

Secretin is a 27 amino-acid peptide (3056 Da), which appears to occur in only one molecular form, the whole molecule being needed for full biological activity. Circulating concentrations of secretin are lower than those of most other gut hormones. It is produced by S cells sparsely scattered throughout the duodenal and jejunal mucosa and is stored in characteristic secretory granules.

The main stimulus to secretin secretion is a duodenal pH of less than 4.5, although this occurs rarely. It is probably also secreted late after a meal, but the timing and quantities of this secretion are uncertain. The main physiological role of secretin is stimulating production of watery, alkaline pancreatic juices in response to acid in the duodenum. It may play an important part in the developing gastrointestinal tract, concentrations of secretin being particularly high in the early postnatal period.

Glucose-dependent insulinotropic peptide

Glucose-dependent insulinotropic peptide (**GIP**) is a 42 amino-acid peptide (5105 Da) with considerable sequence homology at the amino-terminal to secretin, glucagon, and vasoactive intestinal peptide. It is produced by K cells, predominantly in the upper small intestinal mucosa, but also in the gastric antrum and ileum, and is stored in large granules.

At pharmacological doses, GIP inhibits gastric secretions, and was originally named gastric inhibitory peptide. However, its physiological role appears to be as a component of the enteroinsular axis, being released in response to a mixed meal, particularly carbohydrates and long-chain fatty acids, and stimulating insulin release. This potentiation of insulin release in response to oral as opposed to intravenous glucose is the incretin effect. GIP has recently been implicated in the stimulation of cortisol release in two patients with ACTH-independent Cushing's syndrome whose serum cortisol rose postprandially.

Vasoactive intestinal peptide

Vasoactive intestinal peptide (**VIP**) is a 28 amino-acid peptide neurotransmitter (3326 Da) widely distributed through the central and peripheral nervous systems. The highest concentrations of VIP occur in the submucosa of the intestinal tract, where it is found in postganglionic intrinsic nerves (Fig. 3). VIP is a potent stimulator of small intestinal and colonic enterocyte secretion of water and electrolytes, acting via an elevation in cAMP. Other important actions include: smooth-muscle relaxation, both in the alimentary tract and in the systemic vasculature; stimulation of insulin release, counteracted by a direct glucagon-like effect of VIP in stimulating hepatic gluconeogenesis and glycogenolysis; stimulation of pancreatic bicarbonate secretion; and relaxation of the gallbladder, pyloric sphincter, and circular muscle of the small intestine with contraction of the longitudinal muscle. VIP inhibits release of gastric acid but not at physiological concentrations in humans.

Peptide histidine methionine is a 27 amino-acid neuropeptide with considerable sequence homology to VIP and derived from the adjacent exon of the prepro-VIP gene. It mimics the actions of VIP, probably acting via the same receptor, but is less potent.

Pituitary adenylate cyclase-activating peptide is a recently identified peptide occurring in 27 and 38 amino-acid forms and with considerable sequence homology to VIP. It has a similar tissue distribution to VIP and shares the same receptor outside the central nervous system and pituitary gland. It has similar actions to VIP on intestinal secretion and motility.

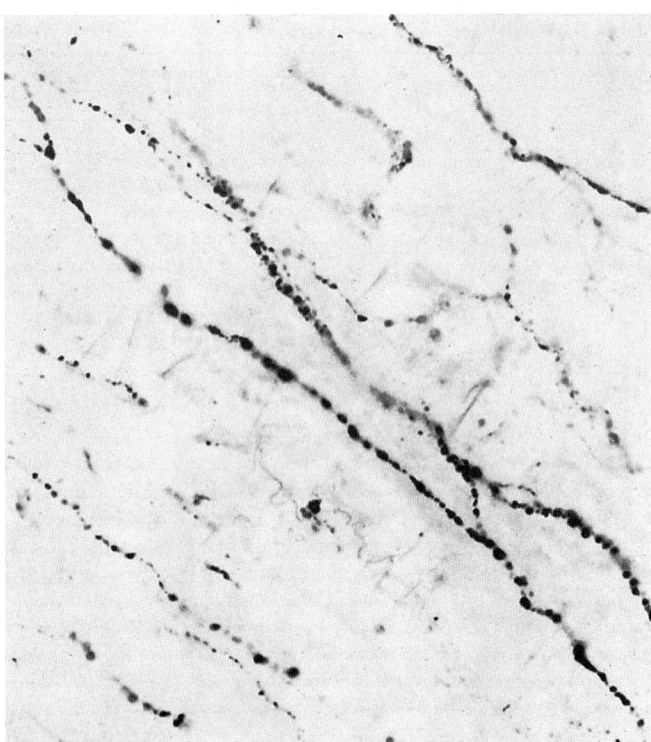

Fig. 3 Vasoactive intestinal polypeptide fibres, immunostained using the unlabelled antibody enzyme (PAP) method, in the submucosa of human colon (×500).

Peptide products of preproglucagon

In the pancreas the major product of the preproglucagon molecule is pancreatic glucagon, but in the intestinal L cells preproglucagon is cleaved into enteroglucagon, a 69 amino-acid peptide containing the entire sequence of pancreatic glucagon, and the two glucagon-like peptides (GLP-1_{7-36} NH$_2$ and GLP-2; see below).

Enteroglucagon

Enteroglucagon (also termed glicentin) is found in high concentrations in the mucosa of the ileum, colon, and rectum. It is released after a mixed meal, particularly of carbohydrate and long-chain fatty acids. Pure enteroglucagon has not become available for infusion studies and so evidence for its physiological role remains circumstantial. The amount of enteroglucagon secreted is proportional to the amount of unabsorbed food entering the colon, and high enteroglucagon concentrations are found in conditions associated with loss of the small intestinal absorptive capacity. Thus it has been postulated that enteroglucagon has a trophic effect on the small intestinal mucosa and may be important in gut adaptation. Enteroglucagon is further cleaved by the L cells to produce oxyntomodulin, a 37 amino-acid peptide released into the circulation, which is a potent inhibitor of pentagastrin-stimulated gastric acid secretion.

Glucagon-like peptide 1

Glucagon-like peptide 1 (**GLP-1**) is a 36 amino-acid peptide, which is secreted in a cleaved form containing the 30 carboxy-terminal amino acids (GLP-1_{7-36} NH$_2$). It is a more potent stimulus to insulin secretion than GIP, and appears to be the most important incretin in humans. It also inhibits secretion of glucagon and potentiates release of somatostatin. Infusion of GLP-1_{7-36} NH$_2$ greatly reduces insulin requirements following a meal in patients with type 1 or 2 diabetes, and this effect may have therapeutic potential.

Pancreatic polypeptide, neuropeptide Y, and peptide tyrosine tyrosine

Pancreatic polypeptide, neuropeptide Y, and peptide tyrosine tyrosine are peptides with structurally similar genes and propeptide molecules probably derived from a common ancestral gene.

Pancreatic polypeptide

Pancreatic polypeptide is a 36 amino-acid peptide (4226 Da) first isolated as a contaminant during the purification of insulin. It is produced by specific cells found at the periphery of the pancreatic islets, particularly those in the head of the pancreas, and scattered through the exocrine pancreas. Pancreatic polypeptide granules are small and electron dense.

Concentrations of pancreatic polypeptide rise dramatically after a meal, particularly one high in protein, and this is at least in part due to activation of cholinergic fibres from the vagus. At physiological plasma concentrations, this polypeptide inhibits pancreatic exocrine and biliary secretion, and these may represent its biological actions, although there are no obvious consequences of its deficiency or excess.

Neuropeptide Y

Neuropeptide Y is a 36 amino-acid peptide neurotransmitter, which is often colocalized with noradrenaline. It is found in both extrinsic adrenergic nerves to the myenteric plexus and in intrinsic nerves in the myenteric and submucosal plexi, and highest concentrations occur in the upper intestine and distal colon. It is a potent vasoconstrictor, inhibits intestinal secretion, and depresses colonic motility.

Peptide tyrosine tyrosine

Peptide tyrosine tyrosine (**PYY**) is a 36 amino-acid peptide found in endocrine cells of the ileum, colon, and rectum. It has a similar distribution to enteroglucagon, with which it is often colocalized. It is released after a meal, particularly one containing carbohydrates or long-chain fatty acids, and its main function appears to be to slow intestinal transit, allowing more time for absorption. Other actions include delaying gastric emptying, decreasing intestinal motility, and inhibiting gastric acid secretion.

Bombesin and the gastrin-releasing peptides

Bombesin is a 14 amino-acid peptide (1620 Da) initially isolated from amphibian skin. It was found to be a potent stimulator of gastrin, and hence of gastric acid secretion. Its mammalian counterparts have similar properties and so were named gastrin-releasing peptides. In humans, gastrin-releasing peptide is a 27 amino-acid peptide found in the gut in the intrinsic neurones of the myenteric and submucosal plexi, particularly in the stomach and pancreas. In addition to its effect on gastrin, it stimulates release of motilin and cholecystokinin, and pancreatic enzyme secretion. Gastrin-releasing peptide has been shown to be an autocrine growth factor for small-cell lung carcinomas, and probably has trophic effects on the developing gut.

Opioids

The opioid peptides leu- and met-enkephalin and dynorphin are widespread through the nerves of the myenteric and submucosal plexi of the gastrointestinal tract. Their principal actions appear to be inhibition of gastrointestinal secretion and increased smooth muscle contractility.

Tachykinins

Substance P is an 11 amino-acid peptide (1345 Da) whose existence was demonstrated in 1931 through its ability to cause smooth-muscle contraction and vasodilatation. A number of homologous peptides have now been characterized, and are collectively known as tachykinins, because of their rapid action. In humans there are two tachykinin genes, preprotachykinin

A encoding substance P and neurokinin-α, and preprotachykinin B encoding neurokinin-β. These three tachykinins are localized to neurones in the myenteric and submucosal plexi throughout the gastrointestinal tract, with high concentrations in the duodenum and jejunum. Their principal effects are smooth-muscle contraction, vasodilatation, and inhibition of intestinal absorption.

Other gut peptides

Motilin

Motilin is a 22 amino-acid peptide (2700 Da) secreted by small intestinal M cells, whose density decreases from duodenum to ileum. The biological activity resides in the 9 amino-terminal amino acids. Peaks in motilin secretion coincide with initiation of the duodenal myoelectric complex, and so motilin appears to control the reflex motor activity of the small intestine, which occurs at approximately 2-hourly intervals in the fasted state, keeping the small intestine free of debris. Circulating amounts of motilin rise after a meal or drinking water and it may have a physiological role in accelerating gastric emptying and colonic transit. The macrolide antibiotics, such as erythromycin, are motilin-receptor agonists, hence their side-effects of diarrhoea and abdominal cramps.

Neurotensin

Neurotensin is a 13 amino-acid peptide (1673 Da) present throughout the central nervous system, and in enteric neurones and N cells of the ileal mucosa. It was originally isolated from bovine hypothalamus.

Plasma neurotensin concentrations rise after a meal, particularly those with a high fat content, and the rise is proportional to the size of the meal. At physiological doses, neurotensin inhibits gastric acid secretion and gastric emptying, and stimulates pancreatic exocrine and intestinal secretion. However, as with pancreatic polypeptide, there are no obvious consequences of neurotensin excess.

Somatostatin

Somatostatin was initially isolated from the hypothalamus as a 14 amino-acid peptide (1640 Da) that inhibited the release of growth hormone. It is widely distributed throughout the central and peripheral nervous system, and is found in a variety of endocrine tissues. In the gastrointestinal tract it occurs in 14 and 28 amino-acid forms. Somatostatin is secreted by specialized (D) cells distributed throughout the gut mucosa and on the inner rim of the pancreatic islets. D cells have all the characteristics of endocrine cells, but also possess axon-like basal elongations along which the peptide can be transported and secreted directly on to local cells. Five human somatostatin receptors have now been identified and cloned, the type 1 receptor predominating in the gastrointestinal tract. As gastrointestinal and other neuroendocrine tumours often possess high-density somatostatin receptors, scintigraphy with radiolabelled somatostatin analogues has been used for tumour localization (see Carcinoid syndrome below).

Somatostatin inhibits hormone release and blocks the response of the effector tissue, and inhibits a wide range of gastrointestinal functions (Table 1). Its acts principally as a paracrine factor or neurotransmitter, although small amounts of somatostatin are released into the plasma in response to physiological stimuli, including food ingestion, and so it may have an endocrine role.

Chromogranin-derived peptides

These structurally related, acidic proteins are present in the secretory granule matrix of neuroendocrine cells and are useful markers of normal and neoplastic neuroendocrine cells. To date, this family of proteins has been shown to consist of three molecules: chromogranin A, the first to be identified and also known as (parathyroid) secretory protein I; chromogranin B, or secretogranin I; and chromogranin C, or secretogranin II. It appears that the chromogranins have dual physiological roles: they may act in the processing of some regulatory peptides and prohormones. Their latter property was suspected when the primary structures of the three proteins were

Table 1 Inhibitory actions of somatostatin

Hormone release	Physiological function
Growth hormone	Lower oesophageal sphincter contraction
Thyroid-stimulating hormone	Gastric acid secretion
Insulin	Gastric emptying and secretions
Glucagon	Absorption of nutriments
Pancreatic polypeptide	Splanchnic blood flow
Gastrin	Gallbladder contraction and secretions
Secretin	Pancreatic enzyme and bicarbonate secretion
Gastric inhibitory polypeptide	
Motilin	
Enteroglucagon	

determined. All were found to contain multiple pairs of basic amino acids, forming sites for potential proteolytic cleavage. Chromogranin A gives rise to several peptides, including catestatin, chromostatin, vasostatin, and parastatin. Another derived peptide, pancreastatin was first characterized as a potent inhibitor of insulin release and later found in mucosal cells throughout the gut, where it is often co-stored with other peptides. It is released by gastrin from enterochromaffin-like cells of the gastric fundus, fitting with its action of enhancing meal-stimulated gastric acid secretion. The chromogranin B molecule yields, amongst other peptides, GAWK (from its first four amino acids: glycine, alanine, tryptophan, and lysine), a peptide distributed abundantly throughout the gut in both mucosal endocrine cells and intramural nerves. Chromogranins are proving to be of relevance to clinical medicine as plasma concentrations of chromogranins A and B can be used to determine the presence of a neuroendocrine tumour and as a means to monitor the efficacy of treatment.

Other peptide neurotransmitters

Calcitonin gene-related peptide is a 37 amino-acid peptide produced by alternative splicing of the calcitonin gene transcript. It is a widespread neurotransmitter and in the gut occurs in both extrinsic sensory nerves and intrinsic neurones. It inhibits gastric acid and pancreatic secretion, and causes relaxation of vascular smooth muscle.

Galanin is a 29 amino-acid peptide neurotransmitter isolated from porcine intestine. It is widely distributed in enteric nerve terminals and in nerves supplying the liver and pancreatic islets. Its main actions are inhibition of intestinal smooth-muscle contraction and inhibition of postprandial insulin release.

The potent vasoconstricting peptide endothelin has been demonstrated in the plexi of the gastrointestinal tract and in mucosal epithelial cells. However, its role in the regulation of gastrointestinal function is unknown.

Gut peptides in gastrointestinal disease

Gastric pathology

The most common cause of an elevated level of gastrin is achlorhydria, which may be the result of atrophic gastritis, pernicious anaemia or uraemia, or from iatrogenic causes such as the use of H_2-receptor antagonists or the proton-pump inhibitor omeprazole, or following vagotomy. The elevation in gastrin is a consequence of the loss of negative feedback on gastrin secretion by the low stomach pH. If the antrum is mistakenly retained after gastric surgery, this similarly removes the antral G cells from exposure to gastric acid and is associated with high gastrin concentrations. Achlorhydria-related hypergastrinaemia results in hyperplasia of the gastric histamine-producing enterochromaffin (**ECL**) cells. Atrophic gastritis in humans, and prolonged achlorhydria as a result of antisecretory therapy (for example, omeprazole) in rats, are associated with gastric carcinoid tumours, and these are thought to develop as a result of the direct trophic effect of gastrin on the ECL cells. Antisecretory therapy in humans has not been associated with the development of these tumours, but recommended therapeutic doses should not be exceeded and in patients on long-term therapy, hypergastrinaemia should be avoided.

Peptic ulcer disease is not usually associated with abnormalities in gut peptide secretion, although a decrease in somatostatin release in patients infected with *Helicobacter pylori* may influence the paracrine regulation of gastric function.

After gastrectomy or truncal vagotomy, patients may develop the dumping syndrome due to accelerated gastric emptying. In these individuals there is a marked increase in the postprandial rise of VIP, neurotensin, PYY, and enteroglucagon, and a decrease in the release of motilin. VIP and neurotensin may both contribute to the postprandial hypotension associated with dumping, but neurotensin may have a beneficial effect in slowing gastric transit. The long-acting somatostatin analogue octreotide, which inhibits release of these peptides and inhibits gastric emptying, is often a very effective treatment for this condition.

Malabsorption

Malabsorptive conditions are associated with a decrease in the amount of peptides produced in the affected region, and a compensatory elevation of other peptides, particularly those trophic peptides implicated in the bowel's adaptation to loss of absorptive surface, such as enteroglucagon.

Coeliac disease is an autoimmune disease resulting from dietary gluten sensitivity and it is associated with villous atrophy of the upper small intestine (see Chapter 14.9.3). The postprandial peptide response in patients with untreated coeliac disease shows greatly reduced secretion of GIP and secretin, which originate from the affected region of bowel. In contrast, there is marked elevation of enteroglucagon, neurotensin, and PYY (Fig. 4). The decrease in secretin and increase in PYY may be responsible for the reduced pancreatic exocrine and biliary secretion found in this condition. Enteroglucagon stimulates enterocyte turnover in the affected segment, despite the villous atrophy. It may have a trophic effect on the remaining small intestinal mucosa and delay gut transit time, and neurotensin may help to improve absorption by delaying gastric emptying. In tropical sprue, a postinfective malabsorptive state usually seen in travellers to Asia and Central and South America, a different profile of postprandial peptide

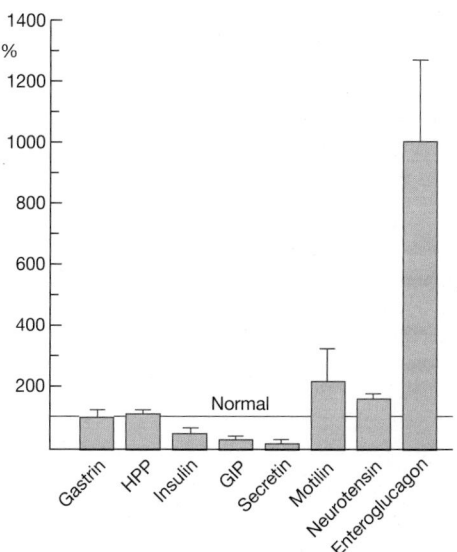

Fig. 4 The percentage incremental rise in gut hormones following a standard test breakfast in patients with coeliac disease compared with normal controls.

release is seen. There is marked elevation in enteroglucagon and PYY, as in coeliac disease, but also in motilin secretion, whilst other peptides behave normally. After successful treatment of coeliac disease or tropical sprue, peptide responses return to normal.

Chronic pancreatitis (see Chapter 14.18.3.2) results in varying degrees of pancreatic endocrine dysfunction in addition to the exocrine insufficiency. Thus patients often have insulin-dependent diabetes, and basal and arginine-stimulated glucagon concentrations may be reduced, although they are elevated in some individuals. Basal, and meal- and secretin-stimulated concentrations of pancreatic polypeptide are reduced if steatorrhoea is associated with chronic pancreatitis. The early loss of pancreatic polypeptide secretion in most individuals probably reflects the location of its secretory cells throughout the exocrine pancreas and on the periphery of the islets. However, secretion of pancreatic polypeptide is occasionally preserved and its concentration is not of diagnostic value in chronic pancreatitis.

Cystic fibrosis is often associated with diabetes mellitus and pancreatic exocrine insufficiency. Fasting and milk-stimulated concentrations of pancreatic polypeptide are usually suppressed. GIP concentrations fail to rise after a milk stimulus, implying a failure of the enteroinsular axis, and this may contribute to the associated glucose intolerance.

The malabsorption associated with pancreatic exocrine insufficiency of any cause leads to an excess of nutriments in the colon, and as a result the concentrations of enteroglucagon, PYY, and neurotensin are raised. The gut adaptation resulting from the effects of these peptides may contribute to the improvement in absorptive function with age in patients with cystic fibrosis.

Intestinal resection

Intestinal resection has profound effects on gut peptide concentrations. A jejunoileal bypass used to be constructed in patients with gross obesity. Peptide concentrations were normal preoperatively, but patients were hyperinsulinaemic and glucose intolerant. After the procedure there was an almost complete absence of the prandial GIP response and consequently a much reduced first-phase insulin response. The initial beneficial effects of the operation were ultimately negated by massive hypertrophy of the remaining bowel. The appearance of large volumes of undigested nutrients in the distal ileum is associated with a 16-fold increase in enteroglucagon responses and an eightfold increase in neurotensin secretion, and this may provide an explanation for the hypertrophy. After partial ileal resection, the concentrations of gastrin, enteroglucagon, pancreatic polypeptide, motilin, and PYY are elevated, but after colonic resection only gastrin and pancreatic polypeptide are raised, as there is a decrease in production of the other predominantly colonic peptides.

Diarrhoea

In acute infective diarrhoea, the concentrations of enteroglucagon, PYY, and motilin are increased, probably contributing to the altered gut motility and aiding mucosal repair. Patients with Crohn's disease have an elevated pancreatic polypeptide, GIP, motilin, and enteroglucagon, while in ulcerative colitis there is a modest elevation in pancreatic polypeptide, GIP, motilin, and gastrin, the last in response to the hypochlorhydria associated with the disease. Elevated levels of endothelin have been reported in ulcerative colitis and Crohn's disease and oral administration of an endothelin receptor antagonist in a model of colitis was found to ameliorate diarrhoea and tissue damage. No demonstrable abnormalities in gut peptides account for disordered motility in the irritable bowel syndrome.

Intestinal tumours

The trophic effects of gut peptides may contribute to proliferation of malignant gut tumours. In particular, colon carcinoma cells have receptors for a number of potentially mitogenic peptides, including gastrin, gastrin-releasing peptides, and VIP.

Neuropathic disease

In conditions associated with destruction of intrinsic enteric nerves there is loss of the neurocrine peptides found in the affected region. Chagas' disease (see Section 7) results from chronic infection with *Trypanosoma cruzi* and in the gastrointestinal tract can result in mega-oesophagus and megacolon. Concentrations of VIP and substance P and of their nerve fibres are greatly reduced in biopsies from affected segments. Similar changes are seen in the affected bowel from children with Hirschsprung's disease, which results from an aganglionic colonic segment. In contrast, neuropeptide Y-containing, mostly adrenergic, nerves are not reduced. Also, patients with the Shy–Drager syndrome, who have chronic autonomic failure with loss of preganglionic extrinsic nerves, have no abnormalities in neurocrine peptides or peptidergic nerve fibres on rectal biopsies (Fig. 5). Acquired immune deficiency disease is frequently accompanied by diarrhoea without evidence of secondary infection, and reduced immunostaining for substance P, VIP, and somatostatin in biopsies suggests a neuropathic process may be responsible. Alterations in neuroactive peptides have been observed in a number of inflammatory diseases. Increased density of VIP innervation has been reported in several gut diseases including reflux oesophagitis, radiation colitis, ulcerative colitis, and Crohn's disease. Calcitonin gene-related peptide has been shown to mediate the protective effect of sensory nerves in experimental colitis. It was recently reported that upregulation of the galanin-1 receptor is a mechanism for the increased colonic fluid secretion in infectious diarrhoea resulting from various pathogens.

Carcinoid syndrome

Introduction

The term *Karzinoide* was originally used by Obendorfer in 1907 to describe a carcinoma-like lesion without malignant qualities. It has now come to refer to tumours capable of producing serotonin (5-hydroxytryptamine; **5-HT**). However, several different cell types either synthesize or take up 5-HT and so the term carcinoid is applied to a variety of malignant

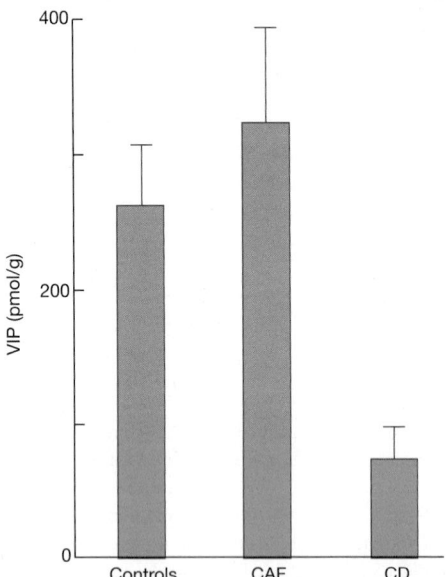

Fig. 5 Rectal vasoactive intestinal polypeptide concentrations (pmol/g wet tissue) in controls and patients with chronic autonomic failure (CAF) and Chagas' disease (CD) with gastrointestinal involvement. Reduced concentrations were seen in Chagas' specimens (reproduced from *Lancet*, 1980, **i**, 559, with permission).

tumours with different biological behaviour grouped by their similar histological appearances. This section will focus primarily on those tumours associated with the classic carcinoid syndrome.

Primary gastrointestinal carcinoid tumours are derived from the embryonic foregut (thyroid, bronchus, stomach, common bile duct, and pancreas), midgut, or hindgut. The most common sites for carcinoid tumours are the appendix and rectum, but these tumours are often found incidentally on histological examinations of appendicectomy and rectal biopsy specimens. These tumours are almost always benign. Rectal neuroendocrine tumours generally produce glucagon-like peptides and PYY rather than 5-HT and are not usually associated with a clinical syndrome, even when they metastasize.

The carcinoid syndrome occurs in about 10 per cent of patients with carcinoid tumours. It does not develop when the tumour drains through a normal liver, and so midgut tumours have almost always metastasized, usually to the liver, before symptoms develop. The carcinoid syndrome is most commonly due to a metastatic midgut tumour, about 50 per cent of which metastasize to the liver. Primary carcinoid tumours are bronchial in origin in about 10 per cent of cases, and rarely occur in the ovary and testis. Tumours in these sites may be associated with the syndrome in the absence of metastases. The annual incidence of the carcinoid syndrome is about 1 in 500 000.

Clinical manifestations

The cardinal feature of the classic carcinoid syndrome is the flush. The carcinoid flush predominantly involves the head and upper thorax, and is usually associated with a tachycardia, hypotension, and increased skin temperature. Patients may have a sensation of intense heat and wheezing may occur. Rarely, flushing extends to the trunk and limbs, and may be associated with lacrimation, facial oedema, and great distress. Attacks are paroxysmal, and usually unprovoked, although precipitating factors include alcohol or food ingestion, stress, emotion, or exertion. Flushing initially lasts for only a few minutes, but as the disease progresses may become almost continuous, and such patients often develop a chronically reddened and cyanotic facial hue, with widespread telangiectasia, the leonine facies. This fixed flush is more commonly seen with bronchial carcinoids, which are often metabolically inactive, but when associated with flushing can cause severe attacks lasting for hours or days, occasionally with profound hypotension and even anuria. Gastric carcinoids are often associated with raised, localized, wheal-like areas of flushing, which are usually pruritic and may migrate.

The other characteristic feature of the syndrome is secretory diarrhoea, which may be profuse, with passage of several litres a day occasionally accompanied by electrolyte disturbance. It may be associated with cramping abdominal pain, nausea, and vomiting. Rarely these symptoms may result from small bowel obstruction from a large ileal carcinoid tumour, but the majority of primary tumours are small, usually being less than 1 per cent of total body tumour weight. Hepatic metastases may cause right hypochondrial pain, particularly if the liver capsule is involved or stretched, and acute exacerbations may occur if metastases become ischaemic and undergo autonecrosis. Weight loss and, in the later stages, cachexia are common as a result of poor dietary intake, malabsorption, and increased catabolism. Pellagra with dermatitis of sun-exposed areas may occur, the increased conversion of 5-hydroxytryptophan into 5-HT causing nicotinamide deficiency.

Cardiac valve abnormalities affect about 50 per cent of patients. They occur as a result of endocardial fibrosis, with plaques of smooth muscle in a collagenous stroma deposited on the valves. Lesions are almost always on the right-hand side, left-sided valve damage only occurring in association with bronchial carcinoids, which drain into the left atrium, or atrioseptal defects with right to left shunting. The most common lesions are tricuspid incompetence and pulmonary stenosis, and the usual clinical outcome is oedema and breathlessness due to right ventricular failure, which can be fatal. The other causes of breathlessness in association with the carcinoid

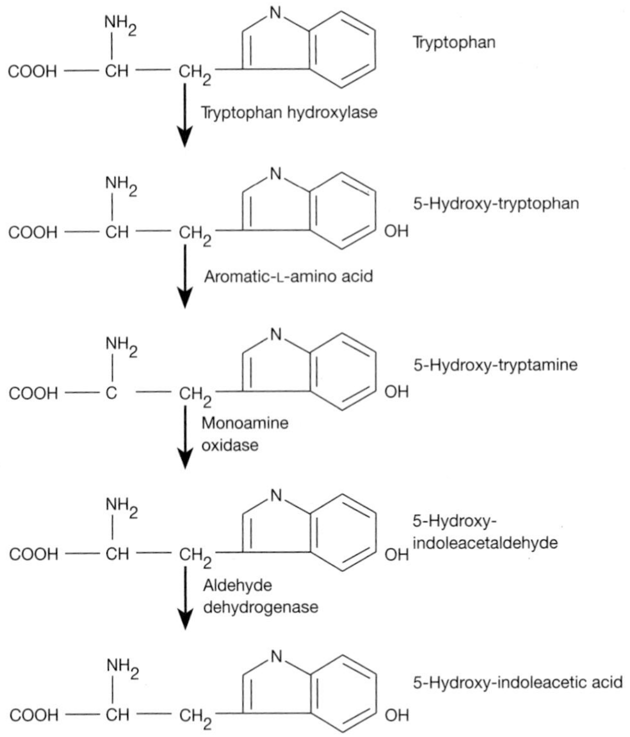

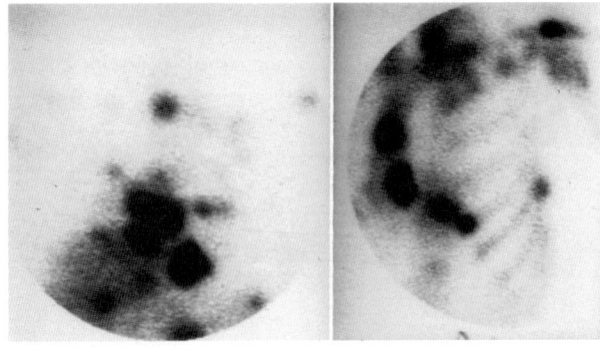

Fig. 6 Biochemical pathway for the synthesis and degradation of 5-hydroxytryptamine.

syndrome are bronchospasm, which affects a small number of patients, often occurring with flushing attacks, and metastatic involvement of the lung and pleura. Arthritis occurs in a small number of patients, and sclerotic bone metastases may be seen, usually in association with foregut tumours.

Carcinoid tumours, in common with other gastroenteropancreatic tumours, have the potential to produce a variety of peptide products and may be associated with other syndromes, with or without the carcinoid syndrome. The most common of these associated syndromes is Cushing's, due to an ectopic ACTH-secreting, bronchial or pancreatic carcinoid. Carcinoid tumours may also be a feature of multiple endocrine neoplasia type 1 (see Chapter 12.10).

Biochemistry

The biologically active metabolite characteristically produced by metastatic carcinoid tumours is 5-HT, synthesized from the amino acid tryptophan (Fig. 6). 5-HT probably plays a part in the pathogenesis of some of the symptoms of the carcinoid syndrome, particularly the diarrhoea and bronchoconstriction. It is metabolized to 5-hydroxyindole acetic acid (**5-HIAA**), which accounts for 95 per cent of the urinary excretion of 5-HT.

A variety of vasoactive substances may be secreted by carcinoid tumours and have been implicated in the pathogenesis of the flush. Flushing can be provoked by intravenous noradrenaline, which has been shown to activate kallikrein in the tumour, leading to synthesis and release of bradykinin. Other possible mediators of the flush include histamine, the tachykinins substance P and neurokinin A, and prostaglandins, although the flush is rarely affected by inhibitors of prostaglandin synthesis, such as indomethacin. Gastric carcinoids are derived from histamine-producing enterochromaffin cells and histamine is probably the cause of the characteristic wheal-like flush seen with gastric tumours.

Investigations

The diagnosis of carcinoid syndrome is made on the basis of elevated concentrations of 5-HIAA in a 24-h urine collection, and urinary 5-HIAA acts as a marker of disease progression. Various foods, including avocados, bananas, aubergines, pineapples, plums, and walnuts, should be avoided while collecting specimens to prevent false-positive results. A number of drugs and other substances interfere with the spectrophotometric assay: paracetamol, fluorouracil, methysergide, and caffeine give false-positive results, and ACTH, phenothiazines, methyldopa, monoamine oxidase inhibitors, and tricyclic antidepressants false-negatives. The other products of carcinoid tumours are not routinely assayed. Circulating markers of neuroendocrine tumours, such as pancreatic polypeptide and chromogranin, may corroborate the diagnosis, and other gut hormones are occasionally elevated in association with carcinoid tumours, most frequently gastrin.

Localization of carcinoid tumours is rarely a problem, as most have gross hepatic metastases, visible on computed tomographic (**CT**) scanning or abdominal ultrasonography, at the time of diagnosis. In those rare cases where the syndrome occurs in the absence of metastases, tumour localization may offer the prospect of cure. These tumours are unlikely to be in the gastrointestinal tract and so chest radiographs and CT scans of the chest and pelvis should be taken. The recently developed, indium-labelled, somatostatin analogue pentetreotide may prove valuable in localizing these tumours, although the resolution is only about 1 cm and bronchial carcinoids are frequently atypical and do not bear somatostatin receptors. An alternative method of isotopic localization is using 123-*m*-iodobenzylguanidine (MIBG) scanning, which may be equally effective. These scanning techniques can be useful in patients with metastatic disease to demonstrate the extent of spread (Fig. 7), particularly in those who are being considered for liver transplantation, which would be precluded by the presence of extrahepatic metastases. Angiography may be of value in assessing suitability for hepatic embolization. Carcinoid tumours have characteristic histological features being composed of regular polygonal cells arranged in nests. The capacity of 5-HT to reduce silver salts (so-called argentaffinity) led to the development of a diagnostic histochemical stain, but more recently, immunostaining for serotonin has been used to identify the tumours.

Treatment

The realistic aim of therapy in patients with the carcinoid syndrome is to relieve the symptoms. Simple treatments such as codeine phosphate, diphenoxylate, and loperamide may help to control the diarrhoea. Many of the symptoms can be controlled with the peripheral 5-HT antagonists: cyproheptadine, a 5-HT type 2 receptor blocker, often helps the diarrhoea; ketanserin may be effective in reducing flushing; and the 5-HT type 3 receptor antagonist ondansetron can alleviate nausea and anorexia. Parachlorphenylalanine, an inhibitor of tryptophan hydroxylase, and chlorpromazine block synthesis of 5-HT, but are rarely used. Histamine may mediate some

Fig. 7 Indium-111-labelled somatostatin analogue scan (left) in a patient with carcinoid syndrome showing metastases to liver, bone, and intrathoracic lymph nodes compared with a conventional base scan (right).

of the features of the syndrome, especially in patients with gastric carcinoids, and in these cases H$_1$- and H$_2$-receptor blockade may be useful. With the exception of simple antidiarrhoeal agents, these treatments have been largely superseded by the long-acting, subcutaneously administered, somatostatin analogue octreotide. This inhibits the release of the mediators of the syndrome by the tumour and antagonizes their peripheral effects. Octreotide is effective in alleviating symptoms in over 90 per cent of patients. It is rarely associated with significant side-effects: the acidic solution can cause pain at the injection site; gallstones often develop, but are rarely of clinical significance; and a few patients develop steatorrhoea, which can be prevented by giving pancreatic enzyme supplements. Octreotide is now the first-line treatment for most patients and may be lifesaving in the carcinoid crisis, when symptoms become severe and continuous. In addition to octreotide, during crises patients usually need close monitoring of fluid and electrolytes, often by measurement of central venous pressure, and appropriate replacement therapy. Minor injury including overenthusiastic clinical examination of large carcinoid masses in the liver may induce a life-threatening state akin to the tumour lysis syndrome characterized by pain, fever, shock, and renal failure compounded by hyperuricaemia and hyperphosphataemia. Allopurinol, and the judicious use of infusions of sodium bicarbonate to make the urine more alkaline, as well as antimicrobials, may reduce the threat of renal failure in this condition. Corticosteroids may improve shock.

The principal disadvantage of octreotide is that patients develop resistance with time, and most become refractory to any form of treatment after about 4 years. Vitamin supplements containing nicotinamide are necessary when patients have pellagra, and these can be given prophylactically. The treatment of cardiac manifestations is the same as for valve disease and cardiac failure of other causes. Patients with painful bony metastases may benefit from palliative radiotherapy.

In patients who fail to respond or are intolerant to octreotide, tumour debulking may provide palliative relief. Surgery is rarely indicated, although enucleation of large metastases may give some benefit. Carcinoid tumours rarely respond to chemotherapy, either with streptozotocin and 5-fluorouracil, or with a variety of other agents, including cyclophosphamide and doxorubicin, although recent evidence suggests interferon-α may be of more benefit. The most effective means of debulking is hepatic embolization, which devascularizes the tumour while the blood supply to the normal liver is maintained by the portal vein. Octreotide should be given in high dose during this intervention, as the necrotic metastases release large quantities of vasoactive mediators that can cause a severe carcinoid crisis with profound hypotension, leading to acute renal failure (see tumour lysis syndrome above).

Prognosis

Carcinoid tumours behave like other gastroenteropancreatic tumours, with the majority following an indolent course. The median survival from the time of diagnosis is about 5 years, with a range of up to 20 years. Thus palliation is very worthwhile in these patients, allowing them to lead a normal life until the terminal stages of the disease.

Multiple endocrine neoplasia and non-diabetic pancreatic endocrine disorders are described in Chapter 12.10.

Further reading

Besterman HS *et al.* (1978). Gut hormone profile in coeliac disease. *Lancet* **i**, 785–8.

Bloom SR, Long RG, eds. (1982). *Radioimmunoassay of gut regulatory peptides.* Saunders, London.

Cook GC *et al.* (1979). Gut hormone responses in tropical malabsorption. *British Medical Journal* **i**, 1252–5.

Gorden P *et al.* (1989). NIH conference. Somatostatin and somatostatin analogue (SMS 201–995) in treatment of hormone-secreting tumors of the pituitary and gastrointestinal tract and non-neoplastic diseases of the gut. *Annals of Internal Medicine* **110**, 35–50.

Gronbech JE, Soreide O, Bergan ATI (1992). The role of resective surgery in the treatment of the carcinoid syndrome. *Scandinavian Journal of Gastroenterology* **27**, 433–7.

Gutniak M *et al.* (1992). Antidiabetogenic effect of glucagon-like peptide-1 (7–36) amide in normal subjects and patients with diabetes mellitus. *New England Journal of Medicine* **326**, 1316–22.

Hodgson HJ, Maton PN (1987). Carcinoid and neuroendocrine tumours of the liver. *Baillière's Clinical Gastroenterology* **1**, 35–61.

Jensen RT, ed. (1989). Gastrointestinal endocrinology. *Gastroenterology Clinics of North America* **18**, 671–931.

Kvols LK (1989). Therapy of the malignant carcinoid syndrome. *Endocrinology and Metabolism Clinics of North America* **18**, 557–68.

Lacroix A *et al.* (1992). Gastric inhibitory polypeptide-dependent cortisol hypersecretion—a new cause of Cushing's syndrome. *New England Journal of Medicine* **327**, 974–80.

Long RG *et al.* (1980). Neural and hormonal peptides in rectal biopsy specimens from patients with Chagas' disease and chronic autonomic failure. *Lancet* **ii**, 559–62.

Long RG, Adrian TE, Bloom SR (1981). Gastrointestinal hormones in pancreatic disease. In: Mitchell CJ, Kelleher J, eds. *Pancreatic diseases in clinical medicine*, pp 223–39. Pitman Medical, Tunbridge Wells.

Maton PN, Jensen RT (1992). Use of gut peptide receptor agonists and antagonists in gastrointestinal diseases. *Gastroenterology Clinics of North America* **21**, 551–664.

Moss SF *et al.* (1992). Effect of *Helicobacter pylori* on gastric somatostatin in duodenal ulcer disease. *Lancet* **ii**, 930–2.

Oberg K, ed. (1989). Neuroendocrine gut and pancreatic tumours. *Acta Oncologica* **28**, 301–449.

Oberg K, ed. (1991). Recent advances in diagnosis and treatment of neuroendocrine gut and pancreatic tumours. *Acta Oncologica* **28**, 301–449.

Reznik Y *et al.* (1992). Food-dependent Cushing's syndrome mediated by aberrant adrenal sensitivity to gastric inhibitory polypeptide. *New England Journal of Medicine* **327**, 981–6.

Thompson JC (1991). Humoral control of gut function. *American Journal of Surgery* **161**, 6–18.

Winkler H, Fischer-Colbrie R (1992). The chromogranins A and B: the first 25 years and future perspectives. *Neuroscience* **49**, 497–528.

Wynick D, Bloom SR (1991). The use of the long-acting somatostatin analog octreotide in the treatment of gut neuroendocrine tumors. *Journal of Clinical Endocrinology and Metabolism* **73**, 1–3.

14.9 Malabsorption

14.9.1 Differential diagnosis and investigation of malabsorption

Julian R. F. Walters

Malabsorption by the gastrointestinal tract results in excess loss of dietary nutrients in the faeces and, if dietary intake does not increase to compensate, nutritional deficiency in the body. The normal physiology of nutrient absorption is complex—specific molecular mechanisms have evolved for each of the various types of nutrient. Understanding the principles involved in normal absorption enables different causes of malabsorption to be appreciated, appropriate differential diagnoses to be made, and investigations planned accordingly.

Principles of normal absorption

Absorptive capacity

For each of the classes of nutrients, the overall efficiency of intestinal absorption varies. Some compounds, such as components of dietary fibre, are not absorbed even in health. Others are normally almost completely absorbed, but in disease, absorption is insufficient to cope with the load, giving symptoms of diarrhoea from excess faecal water, or steatorrhoea from excess faecal fat.

The principal determinants of the maximum absorptive capacity are the area of the intestinal mucosa, increased by surface folding, villi, and microvilli to about 200 m², and the function of the individual cellular transporting mechanisms. As part of the total absorptive process, the intestine also has to reabsorb endogenous secretions produced to aid digestion. Approximately 7 litres of digestive fluids from salivary, gastric, biliary, pancreatic, and intestinal sources add significantly to the absorptive requirements for water, electrolytes, protein, and fat. Secretory diarrhoea and protein-losing enteropathy are conditions where endogenous output exceeds the absorptive capacity of the bowel.

Sites of absorption

Gastrointestinal motility mixes food with digestive secretions and propels them from the mouth to the anus. During this passage, nutrients are exposed to specialized areas of the gut with specific digestive or absorptive functions. The duodenum and proximal jejunum are mostly involved with digestion and fluid secretion. However, the more acidic pH in this area means the solubility and hence the absorption of polyvalent cations such as iron and calcium is high. The bulk of nutrient absorption takes place in the more distal jejunum and ileum. The terminal ileum is specialized for cobalamin (vitamin B_{12}) and bile salt absorption. The colon salvages fluid and electrolytes not absorbed by the small intestine and absorbs short-chain fatty acids produced by colonic bacteria from poorly digested carbohydrates. Loss of specialized areas by surgical resection or disease activity can produce specific patterns of malabsorption.

The intestinal epithelial cells differentiate as they move from crypt to villus tip. The older villus-tip enterocytes perform most of the absorptive functions, though some digestive enzymes are found in less mature cells. Fluid secretion probably occurs from the crypts. Goblet cells secrete mucus, trapping an unstirred water layer which is a relative barrier to the diffusion of large molecules but allows the smaller products of digestion to reach the surface of the epithelium. Other epithelial cells secrete various hormones or have immunological functions.

Mechanisms of absorption

Absorption occurs by transcellular and paracellular pathways. The paracellular pathway is through the tight junctions which link the epithelial cells. By this pathway, passive absorption of small molecules occurs by diffusion down electrical and concentration gradients. Solvent drag is the term used to describe movement down concentration gradients, which are themselves created by the movement of water. Active transport takes place through the epithelial cell against these gradients and necessitates the expenditure of energy generated within the cell.

Three steps are involved in transcellular absorption: entry to the cell at the apical (brush-border) membrane, passage through the cytoplasm, and exit from the cell at the basolateral membrane. Polarization of the enterocyte produces differences in structure and function of the apical and basolateral membranes. Specific carrier molecules are present in one of these membranes but not the other; this asymmetry generates vectorial flow in a single direction through the cell. The molecular basis for absorption of most types of nutrients has now been defined.

Diagnosis of malabsorption

The diagnosis of malabsorption is often missed until it is obvious. Diseases of the small intestine, colon, pancreas, liver, and stomach can all produce malabsorption; these may be obvious (such as the result of previous surgery) or may not be suspected until malabsorption is diagnosed.

History

Delayed growth and development, loss of weight, lassitude, and weakness may be described, but can be due to many other conditions. Changes in the nature of the stool or frequency of bowel habit suggest gastrointestinal disease but are not invariable, as apparently normal stools or constipation can also be found. In describing their faeces, patients may indicate the features of steatorrhoea, rather than watery diarrhoea. Careful questioning is needed to differentiate descriptions of changes in stool frequency or volume, and the passage of gas, liquid, oil, or grease. Bloating, borborygmi, and abdominal discomfort are often reported and seepage of oil from the anus may be described.

A previous history of abdominal surgery, radiation, and alcohol or drug usage may immediately make obvious the likely cause of malabsorption. A family history of coeliac disease or dermatitis herpetiformis makes gluten sensitivity more likely. Malabsorption of nutrients such as iron, folate and vitamin B_{12}, calcium, or vitamin K can give specific histories of anaemia, bone disease, and fractures, or bleeding and bruising.

Examination

General nutritional status can be assessed by height, weight, body mass index, and by anthropomorphic measurements such as skin fold thickness. Anaemia, bruising, petechias, ascites, oedema, glossitis, mucosal changes, and neuromuscular irritability (including positive Trousseau's or Chvosteck's signs) may be found and indicate specific deficiencies. Pigmentation and clubbing can occur. Abdominal distension, scars from previous surgery, masses, or fistulas can suggest specific diagnoses. The nature of the stools must be examined.

Evidence from routine investigations

Commonly obtained haematological and biochemical investigations can show a reduced haemoglobin concentration, microcytosis or macrocytosis, raised red cell distribution width, thrombocytopenia, and low serum iron, transferrin saturation, B_{12}, and folate. The prothrombin time or international normalized ratio (INR) may be raised. Albumin, calcium, phosphate, 25-hydroxyvitamin D, zinc, and other nutrients may be reduced. Elevated alkaline phosphatase and parathyroid hormone can suggest metabolic bone disease secondary to malabsorption.

Differential diagnosis

When malabsorption is suspected, two parallel diagnostic pathways need to be followed: first, to define the extent of the nutritional deficiency, and second, to define the cause of the malabsorption.

Generalized or isolated nutrient malabsorption?

When an isolated nutritional deficiency, such as that of B_{12} or iron, is identified, it must be remembered that this may be due to a more generalized process and evidence for malabsorption of other nutrients may be found if looked for. However, abnormalities in specific transport pathways, either genetic or acquired, account for some common types of malabsorption (Table 1).

Malnutrition, maldigestion, or malabsorption?

Evidence of deficiency of a nutrient does not necessarily imply malabsorption. In many cases, nutritional intake is impaired, or insufficient to meet increased demands. Pregnancy places additional demands on iron, calcium, and many other nutrients. Menorrhagia requires extra iron intake. Excessive loss of protein, electrolytes, and water may require increased intake, and additional calories are required in catabolic states such as infection, surgery, and critical care. Assessment of intake and requirements may determine that poor nutrition is the principal factor and dietary supplementation is required.

Impaired digestion, usually from pancreatic insufficiency, will produce a clinical state similar to malabsorption resulting from intestinal disease. Absorption of simple nutrients, as in an elemental diet, will be normal, but complex foods, particularly fats, will not be hydrolysed to forms that can be absorbed. Evidence of pancreatic disease should be looked for with imaging and function tests.

Conditions that cause malabsorption are listed in Table 2. Some such as coeliac disease are common, others such as the short bowel syndrome in patients with extensive surgery may be obvious, but other diagnoses may not be made unless specifically sought.

Investigation of malabsorption

Function tests

Tests to investigate absorptive functions are described in Chapter 14.2.4. These may be necessary to define the extent of nutrient malabsorption, but in most cases are not needed in routine clinical practice, where the emphasis is usually on defining the precise pathological cause of the malabsorption. The Schilling test for B_{12} malabsorption is particularly useful in diagnosing functional ileal disease.

Table 2 Causes of malabsorption

Common	
Coeliac disease	Gluten-sensitive enteropathy
Small bowel bacterial overgrowth	Gastric surgery and achlorhydria
	Intestinal blind loops post-surgery
	Jejunal diverticula
	Intestinal strictures
	Fistulas (as in Crohn's disease)
	Impaired peristalsis (fibrosis)
Pancreatic insufficiency	Chronic pancreatitis
	Cystic fibrosis
Less common	
Short bowel syndrome	Intestinal resection for Crohn's disease, mesenteric vascular disease, or injury
Chronic infections	Tropical sprue
	Giardiasis
	Other parasites (e.g. *Strongyloides* sp.)
	Tuberculosis
	AIDS
Lymphoma	Immunoproliferative small-intestinal disease
	Enteropathy-associated T-cell lymphoma
	Refractory sprue and ulcerative jejunoileitis
Radiation enteritis	Fibrosis
	Atrophy
	Strictures
	Lymphangiectasia
Intestinal lymphangiectasia	Congenital
	Infective
	Fibrotic
	Malignant
	Cardiac
Drugs	Orlistat
	Laxatives
	Neomycin (and many others rarely)
	Cholestyramine (and certain others with specific interactions)
Allergic	Eosinophilic enteritis
	Milk and soya enteropathy
Immunodeficiency	Autoimmune enteropathy
Rare	
Whipple's disease	
Amyloidosis	
Abetalipoproteinaemia	
Most specific transporter defects	

Table 1 Common forms of malabsorption of specific nutrients

Nutrient	Condition
Lactose	Lactase non-persistence
Vitamin B_{12}	Pernicious anaemia (loss of intrinsic factor)
Bile salts	Bile salt diarrhoea

Faecal fat measurements are often necessary to confirm that malabsorption (or maldigestion) needs to be investigated. The absorption of fat depends on a large number of different steps and is a sensitive indicator of malabsorption. Faecal collections are made over several days on a defined fat intake. Despite the unpleasantness of these collections and assays, this may be the only way of confirming that fat malabsorption is in fact occurring. A number of other tests have been developed in attempts to circumvent these problems.

The pancreolauryl test (see Chapter 14.2.4) is a simple way to look for impaired lipid digestion, and is sufficiently sensitive to diagnose pancreatic insufficiency when it is severe enough to produce steatorrhoea. False positives can occur in a range of intestinal conditions.

Xylose absorption tests have been used traditionally to help differentiate pancreatic maldigestion (when they are usually normal) from intestinal malabsorption such as coeliac disease (when they are usually abnormal). This test may give many false-positive results and has largely been superseded by tests aimed at detecting specific pathologies. Testing stools or urine for laxative abuse may be necessary, and endocrine causes of diarrhoea and malabsorption, although rare, should not be forgotten.

Serological tests for coeliac disease

IgA-class endomysial antibody serology is a highly sensitive and specific test which has simplified screening for coeliac disease in patients with any suggestion of possible malabsorption. These antibodies are detected by immunofluorescence on sections of monkey oesophagus or umbilical cord, and are a subclass of the previously used reticulin antibodies. False-negative results in coeliac disease occur in the presence of selective IgA deficiency (approximately 1 in 50 of the population), but IgG-class endomysial antibodies are detected. With effective treatment of coeliac disease with a gluten-free diet, endomysial antibodies become negative. Gliadin antibodies have much lower specificity and are not valuable in screening.

The antigen recognized by endomysial antibodies is now known to be tissue transglutaminase. More easily performed tests with this antigen, such as enzyme-linked immunoassays (ELISAs), will replace immunofluorescent testing for endomysial antibodies when they are confirmed to be as reliable.

The availability of simple blood tests, with high positive and negative predictive values for coeliac disease, means that this condition can now be strongly suspected before intestinal biopsy is performed.

Endoscopy and small bowel histology

Endoscopy is widely available and enables tissue to be taken from the small intestine to make a histological diagnosis of the pathology causing malabsorption. Oesophagogastroduodenoscopy allows biopsies from the upper duodenum. At colonoscopy, biopsies can be taken from the terminal ileum. Enteroscopy allows much more of the small bowel to be inspected and biopsies taken. Fortunately, common intestinal diseases such as coeliac disease are diffuse and diagnosis can usually be made from duodenal biopsies taken at routine upper endoscopy. Multiple biopsies reduce the likelihood of sampling error.

Biopsy of the more distal parts of the jejunum and ileum may be performed using the Crosby capsule or other similar designs. The capsule attached to a fine tube is swallowed allowing biopsies to be taken under fluoroscopic control, after which the capsule is recovered. Systems for multiple biopsies have been developed. These capsules are generally safe, but are used infrequently now that coeliac disease is usually diagnosed by endoscopic duodenal biopsies. Unfortunately, none of these methods allows reliable targeting to specific areas of small intestine seen on radiology. Laparotomy (or laparoscopy) may be needed to take full-thickness biopsies from jejunal and ileal lesions.

Mucosal appearances at endoscopy may be abnormal, suggesting histological diagnoses. With modern endoscopes, the resolution and magnification is such that villi can be detected. A smooth mucosa, with reduced folds of Kerckring, scalloped valvulae conniventes, pallor, and a mosaic appearance suggest villous atrophy, as in coeliac disease. Small white spots can indicate areas of intestinal lymphangiectasia. In the terminal ileum, ulceration can indicate Crohn's disease. Biopsies can be directed to abnormal areas.

Histology will be definitive in most small bowel diseases. Villous atrophy with crypt hyperplasia is most frequently caused by coeliac disease. Tropical sprue, allergy to cows' milk protein in children, and a range of other conditions occasionally cause a similar picture. Intestinal lymphangiectasia, lymphoma, eosinophilic enteritis, Whipple's disease, amyloid, and abetalipoproteinaemia have characteristic appearances. Parasites including *Giardia* sp. may be seen.

Radiology

Plain abdominal films may show calcification in chronic pancreatitis, faecal loading, or abnormal gas-filled loops of bowel.

Contrast studies of the small intestine will define abnormal anatomy. Small bowel enema (enteroclysis) is preferred for showing mucosal detail, although barium follow-through studies are more easily tolerated and can give better images of proximal duodenum and terminal ileum. Mass lesions or strictures from Crohn's disease, tuberculosis, lymphoma, other tumours, fibrosis, radiation, ischaemia, or drug-induced injury will be demonstrated. Enteric fistulas and diverticula are diagnosed. Post-surgical anatomy can be defined and the length of remaining intestine in the short bowel syndrome estimated.

Endoscopic retrograde cholangiopancreatography (ERCP), and increasingly magnetic resonance cholangiopancreatography (MRCP), will show pancreatic abnormalities that can cause pancreatic exocrine insufficiency. CT, ultrasound, and angiography have roles in further defining conditions associated with malabsorption.

Microbiology

Small bowel bacterial overgrowth is a common and frequently undiagnosed cause of malabsorption. Absolute bacterial counts in proximal small-intestinal fluid are hard to obtain without contamination, so diagnosis tends to be on clinical suspicion confirmed indirectly via glucose hydrogen breath testing (see Chapter 14.2.4).

Infestations causing malabsorption (including *Giardia* and *Strongyloides* spp.) will be diagnosed by demonstrating parasites in fresh stool, or duodenal aspirates.

Response to treatment

Confirmation of the diagnosis of malabsorption is often made by assessing the response to treatment. Symptomatic patients with typical villous atrophy and positive antibody tests, who respond clinically and serologically to a gluten-free diet, can be confirmed to have coeliac disease and do not routinely need further biopsies. In small intestinal bacterial overgrowth, the diagnosis is often only finally made by the response to broad-spectrum antibiotics, which will also correct the abnormal Schilling test in this condition. Pancreatic exocrine insufficiency can be confirmed with a satisfactory response to enzyme replacements.

Further reading

American Gastroenterological Association (1999). American Gastroenterological Association medical position statement: guidelines for the evaluation and management of chronic diarrhea. *Gastroenterology* **116**, 1461–3.

Booth CC, Neale G, eds (1985). *Disorders of the small intestine*. Blackwell, Oxford.

British Society of Gastroenterology. Guidelines in gastroenterology: tests for malabsorption. http://www.bsg.org.uk/guidelines/27727.html

Walker-Smith JA *et al.* (1990). Revised criteria for diagnosis of coeliac disease. *Archives of Disease in Childhood* **65**, 909–11.

Table 1 Characteristic clinical features of SBBO

Diarrhoea
Steatorrhoea
Cobalamin (vitamin B$_{12}$) malabsorption
Decreased urinary xylose excretion
Hypoalbuminaemia

14.9.2 Small bowel bacterial overgrowth

P. P. Toskes

Introduction

The occurrence of malabsorption in a patient with overgrowth of bacteria in the small intestine is known as small bowel bacterial overgrowth (**SBBO**).

Until recently, SBBO was typically associated with patients in whom disordered motility or structural abnormalities of the gastrointestinal tract were identified (Table 1). It is now recognized that SBBO occurs in a range of conditions associated with abnormal motility including gastroparesis, irritable bowel syndrome, and chronic pancreatitis—three conditions that now account for most patients in whom bacterial overgrowth is documented. Thus SBBO should be suspected in patients with these conditions whose symptoms prove resistant to conventional treatment or in whom steatorrhoea, weight loss, or flatulence develop unexpectedly. SBBO is now also recognized as the most important cause of malabsorption in elderly subjects, in whom a structurally intact small intestine becomes inhabited by colonic flora. Establishing a diagnosis of suspected SBBO by rigorous investigation is of key importance to its proper treatment.

Indigenous bacterial populations of the normal gastrointestinal tract

An understanding of SBBO is based upon a thorough knowledge of the indigenous bacterial populations of the normal gastrointestinal tract (Table 2). The proximal small intestine is normally inhabited by a few bacteria. Qualitative and quantitative changes appear at the ileum and become quite striking in the colon. Table 3 indicates the endogenous factors that prevent SBBO in humans. Of the factors listed, by far the two most important are the normal intestinal motility and an appropriate amount of gastric

Table 2 Indigenous bacterial population of the normal human gastrointestinal tract

Feature	Stomach	Jejunum	Ileum	Colon
Total bacterial counts*	0–3	0–4	5–8	10–12
Aerobes/facultative anaerobes*	0–3	0–4	2–5	2–9
Anaerobes*	0	0	3–7	9–12

* Log 10 colony-forming units (CFU) per gram of contents.

Table 3 Important endogenous factors preventing SBBO

Normal intestinal motility
Appropriate gastric acid secretion
Intact ileocaecal sphincter
Immunoglobulins within intestinal secretions

acid secretion. When either or both of these mechanisms are inhibited, SBBO may ensue.

Thus the stomach and proximal small intestine normally contain relatively few bacteria, which are usually lactobacilli, enterococci, Gram-positive aerobes, or facultative anaerobes present in concentrations of up to 10^4 viable organisms per gram of jejunal contents. Coliforms are rarely found in the healthy proximal small intestine. Anaerobic *Bacteroides* are not found in the proximal small intestine of a healthy gastrointestinal tract. The ileum represents a zone of transition from the sparse populations of the proximal small intestine and the very dense bacterial populations of the colon. In the colon the bacterial population increases up to one million times and reaches 10^9 to 10^{12} bacteria per gram of colonic content. The quality of the bacteria also change remarkably in the colon. Here there are fastidious anaerobic bacteria such as *Bacteroides*, anaerobic lactobacilli, and clostridia. These anaerobes outnumber the aerobic bacteria by as much as 10 000 to 1. The complexity of the colonic flora is such that more than 400 different species may be present in the colon of a single individual.

Bacteria normally metabolize bile acids, androgens and oestrogens, exogenous and endogenous cholesterol, unabsorbed dietary lipids, proteins, and carbohydrates as well as fibre, protein and urea, and other substances. The by-products of this metabolism may be of benefit or harm to the normal host. An exaggeration of this metabolism occurs in the presence of SBBO. It is noteworthy that the normal bacterial flora also are important in the metabolism of some drugs and other xenobiotics. Drugs metabolized by intestinal bacteria are listed in Table 4. The importance of the excessive metabolism of medications that may occur in SBBO is yet to be defined. Perhaps the relatively frequent occurrence of SBBO in the elderly may lead to ineffective medication of this age group.

Clinical conditions associated with SBBO

Table 5 lists the recognized clinical conditions associated with SBBO. In the past when much more gastrointestinal surgery was performed, the common causes of clinically significant bacterial overgrowth were structural abnormalities (for example Billroth II, anastomosis, surgery for Crohn's disease). Stagnant loops of intestine resulting from fistulas or surgical enterostomies and leading to SBBO were also common. Duodenal and jejunal diverticula can lead to SBBO, particularly if there is an associated hypo- or achlorhydria. Figure 1 depicts multiple duodenal and jejunal diverticula in a patient with cobalamin (vitamin B$_{12}$) malabsorption and steatorrhoea secondary to SBBO. Obstruction of the small intestine caused by Crohn's disease, adhesions, radiation damage, lymphoma, or tuberculosis may cause SBBO. Devastating malabsorption may occur secondary to SBBO associated with a gastrocolic or gastrojejunocolic fistula with colonic contents passing into the stomach or upper small intestine. SBBO may result from the ileal anal pouch procedure used to treat ulcerative colitis and adenomatous polyposis. The dysmotility syndrome, especially if combined with hypo- or achlorhydria, may lead to SBBO. Such motility disturbances include scleroderma, intestinal pseudo-obstruction, and diabetic autonomic neuropathy. Figure 2 demonstrates a diffusely dilated small intestine in a patient with diarrhoea, steatorrhoea, and scleroderma associated with SBBO. Antibiotic therapy completely reversed the abnormalities. Subjects

Table 4 Common drugs metabolized by intestinal bacteria

Digoxin
L-Dopa
Colchicine
Morphine
Conjugated oestrogens
Chloramphenicol
Rifampin
Sulphasalazine

Table 5 Clinical conditions associated with SBBO

Site	Associated clinical condition
Gastric proliferation	Hypochlorhydria or achlorhydria, especially when combined with motor or anatomical disturbances
	Sustained hypochlorhydria induced by proton pump inhibitor
Small intestinal stagnation:	
Anatomical	Afferent loop of Billroth II partial gastrectomy
	Duodenal–jejunal diverticulosis
	Surgical blind loop (end-to-side anastomosis)
	Surgical recirculating loop (end-to-side anastomosis)
	Ileal anal pouch
	Obstruction (stricture, adhesion, inflammation, neoplasm)
Motor	Scleroderma
	Idiopathic intestinal pseudo-obstruction
	Absent or disordered migrating motor complex
	Diabetic autonomic neuropathy
Abnormal communication between proximal and distal gastrointestinal tract	Gastrocolic or jejunocolic fistula
	Resection of diseased ileocaecal valve
Miscellaneous	Chronic pancreatitis
	Immunodeficiency syndromes
	Cirrhosis

with an absent or disordered migrating motor complex may develop SBBO. Such patients have no radiographic abnormalities and present with unexplained malabsorption. Elderly patients may develop malabsorption secondary to SBBO, and indeed it has been suggested that bacterial overgrowth may be the most common cause of clinically important malabsorption in the elderly. The elderly often have motor disorders (often induced by previous gastrointestinal tract surgery) and decreased acid secretion. The importance of both normal intestinal motility and normal gastric acid secretion in the prevention of clinically significant SBBO cannot be overemphasized. For example, patients with scleroderma and reflux oesophagitis who are well while receiving H₂ receptor antagonists may

develop marked malabsorption manifested by diarrhoea and steatorrhoea after introduction of a proton pump inhibitor.

Up to 40 per cent of patients with chronic pancreatitis may have concomitant SBBO. The management of such patients may be quite problematic unless the clinician recognizes the need to treat both the pancreatic insufficiency and the SBBO. These patients with chronic pancreatitis may develop SBBO because of a decrease in intestinal motility resulting from pain, use of narcotics, inflammatory changes or obstruction from the large inflamed pancreas, or previous pancreatic surgery.

Several other clinical entities are associated with SBBO, but the pathogenesis is ill understood. These include endstage renal disease, cirrhosis, myotonic muscular dystrophy, fibromyalgia, chronic fatigue syndrome, and

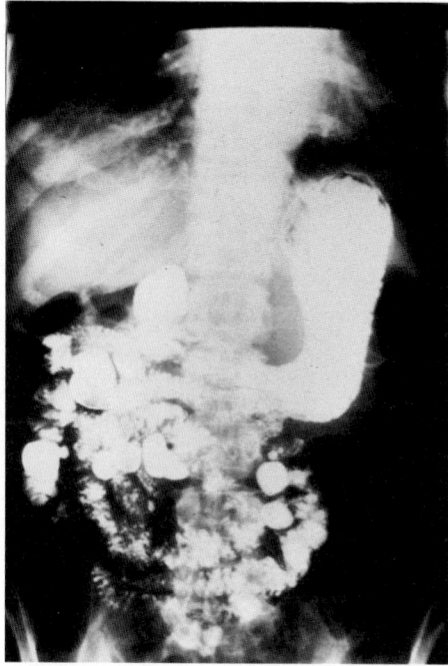

Fig. 1 Multiple duodenal and jejunal diverticula in a patient with cobalamin malabsorption and deficiency and steatorrhoea associated with SBBO.

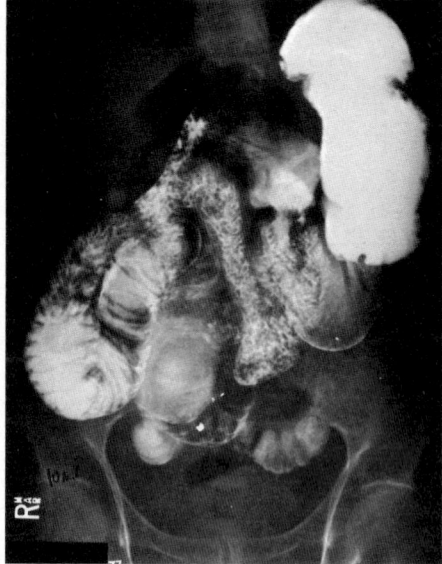

Fig. 2 An upper gastrointestinal and small bowel series in a woman with scleroderma who presented with severe weight loss, cobalamin (vitamin B₁₂) deficiency and marked steatorrhoea. These abnormalities were corrected by broad spectrum antibiotics. Note the marked dilatation of intestinal segment was seen throughout the entire small bowel.

various immunodeficiency syndromes such as chronic lymphocytic leukaemia, immunoglobulin deficiencies, and selected T-cell deficiency.

Clinical manifestations of SBBO

No matter what the clinical condition leading to SBBO may be, there are several typical features as listed in Table 1. In addition, non-specific symptoms of nausea, bloating, abdominal distention, and abdominal pain may be the presenting symptoms of SBBO.

In suspected cases, a thorough evaluation is warranted; many of these patients may have had small bowel diverticula for years before suddenly developing marked symptoms as a result of SBBO. It may be that such patients needed to have a significant reduction in their gastric acid secretion before the structural abnormality could contribute to the SBBO. It is important to realize that SBBO may be superimposed on several clinical conditions whose initial symptoms are exactly those of SBBO. Patients with Crohn's disease, radiation enteritis, short bowel syndrome, or lymphoma may have superimposed SBBO. To what extent the malabsorption is the result of the primary intestinal disease or the consequence of SBBO is often difficult to determine. Weight loss associated with clinically apparent steatorrhoea has been observed in about one-third of patients with SBBO severe enough to cause cobalamin deficiency. Osteomalacia, vitamin K deficiency, night blindness, and even hypocalcaemic tetany as well as the vitamin E deficiency syndromes (neuropathy, retinopathy, T-cell abnormalities) may result.

Mechanisms of the metabolic abnormalities associated with SBBO

The malabsorption of nutrients associated with SBBO can largely be attributed to the abnormal intraluminal effects of the overgrowth flora combined with enterocyte injury induced by the overgrowth flora. A patchy small-intestinal mucosal lesion has been identified in experimental animals with SBBO and in human subjects with the condition. Steatorrhoea associated with SBBO results from bacterial alteration or bile salts, which leads to an impairment of micelle formation. In addition, accumulation of toxic concentrations of free bile acids may also contribute to the steatorrhoea by inducing a patchy intestinal mucosal lesion, thereby impairing the transport of fat. The predominant cause of the anaemia associated with SBBO is cobalamin deficiency. The anaemia is megaloblastic and serum cobalamin levels are low. Neurological changes indistinguishable from those of pernicious anaemia may ensue. The anaemia can be corrected by physiological doses of cobalamin. Cobalamin malabsorption that cannot be corrected by exogenous intrinsic factor is a characteristic of clinically significant SBBO. Competitive uptake of cobalamin, particularly by Gram-negative anaerobes, appears to be the mechanism responsible for the cobalamin malabsorption in SBBO. Iron deficiency may also occur in association with SBBO due to blood loss through the gastrointestinal tract, perhaps resulting from patchy ulceration. These patients may have blood detected on examination of their stools together with a microcytic and hypochromic anaemia. In some patients there may be two populations of red blood cells, microcytic and macrocytic. Folate deficiency is not a common occurrence in SBBO because the overgrowth flora synthesize folate and it is available for the host to utilize; serum folate levels may be elevated.

Hypoproteinaemia is frequent is SBBO and is occasionally severe enough to lead to oedema. Its causes are multifactorial but include decreased uptake of amino acids by a damaged small intestine, intraluminal breakdown of protein and protein precursors by bacteria, and protein-losing enteropathy.

A decrease in urinary xylose excretion is frequently seen in patients with SBBO. The primary reason for the decreased urinary xylose excretion is intraluminal degradation of the sugar by the overgrowth flora. Diarrhoea has many potential causes: the overgrowth flora may produce organic acids

that increase osmolarity of the small intestine and decrease intraluminal pH. Furthermore, bacterial metabolites such as free bile acids, hydroxy fatty acids, and organic acids stimulate secretion of water and electrolytes into the lumen.

General diagnostic approach to patients suspected of having SBBO

SBBO should be considered in the differential diagnosis of any patient who presents with diarrhoea, steatorrhoea, weight loss, or macrocytic anaemia, particularly if the patient is elderly and has had previous abdominal surgery. A history of previous surgery for small intestinal obstruction should raise the question of whether the obstruction was bypassed by an end-to-side anastomosis, leaving a blind pouch, or side-to-side anastomosis, resulting in recirculation of the contents of the small intestine. The presence of dysphagia in a patient with malabsorption should suggest the diagnosis of scleroderma, and repeated bouts of intestinal obstruction without obvious organic cause should suggest intestinal pseudo-obstruction. Figure 3 suggests an algorithm for the evaluation of patients with malasorption including those with SBBO. This algorithm emphasizes the use of non-invasive, inexpensive tests. It also focuses on the fact that, in most medical centres, clinically important malabsorption is more likely to be due to pancreatic insufficiency or SBBO then coeliac disease or tropical sprue. When the history suggests that SBBO may be contributing to the malabsorption, further evaluation is necessary for optimal management. The presence of steatorrhoea should be documented. If the patient has clinically significant bacterial overgrowth, cobalamin absorption is frequently impaired, even though the patient may not yet have developed low levels of serum cobalamin. Intrinsic factor will not improve cobalamin absorption in these patients. The urinary excretion of xylose may be decreased and the serum folate level may be increased in some, but not all, patients with SBBO.

Specific diagnosis of SBBO

The definitive diagnosis of SBBO requires a properly collected and appropriately cultured aspirate from the proximal small intestine. The specimen should be obtained under anaerobic conditions, serially diluted, and cultured on several selected media. In patients with SBBO, the total concentration of bacteria generally exceeds 10^5 organisms per millilitre of jejunal secretions. *Bacteroides*, anaerobic lactobacilli, coliforms, and enterococci

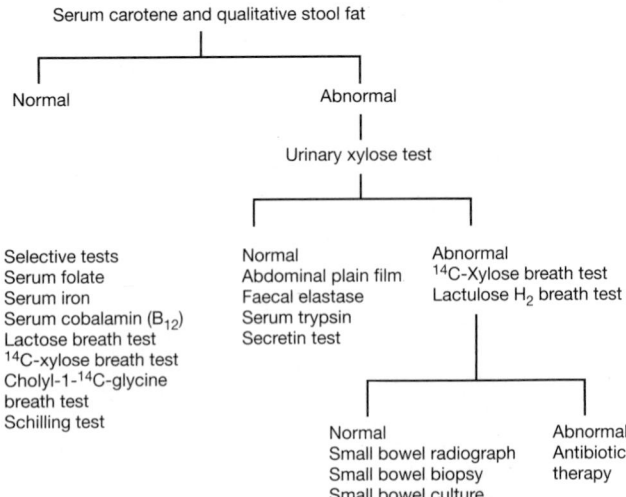

Fig. 3 Algorithm for evaluation of malabsorption. (From Toskes, 1992. Malabsorption. In: Wyngaarden JB, Smith LH, Bennett JC, eds. *Cecil's textbook of medicine*, 19th edn, pp 687–99. WB Saunders, Philadelphia, with permission.)

are all likely to be present in varying numbers. Although in most patients the intraluminal microbial proliferation can be documented in the proximal jejunum, it is important to recognize that pockets of overgrowth may be missed by a single culture and that bacterial overgrowth may occur in the more distal parts of the small intestine.

A properly collected and analysed intestinal culture requires intubation of the small intestine and it is both time-consuming and expensive. In many clinical practices today, small intestinal intubation for quantitative cultures to demonstrate SBBO is simply not performed. Consequently, a variety of surrogate tests for detecting SBBO have been devised based on the varied metabolic actions of the bacteria within the overgrowth flora. Table 6 lists these various tests and compares them in respect to sensitivity, specificity, and simplicity. Measurement of urinary excretion of indican, phenols, drug metabolites, and deconjugated para-amino benzoic acid suffer from a lack of sensitivity and specificity in distinguishing SBBO from other causes of malabsorption. The quantification of deconjugated bile acids and short-chain fatty acids in jejunal secretions requires an intubation of the intestine and thus is resisted by clinicians and patients for the same reasons that cultures of the intestine are not popular.

Another approach to diagnosing SBBO is the timed analysis of breath excretion of volitle metabolites produced by intraluminal bacteria. Both the measurement of expired, labelled carbon dioxide after oral administration of ^{14}C- or ^{13}C-labelled substrates, and breath hydrogen after administration of non-labelled fermentable substrate have been utilized.

The first breath test to be utilized clinically to detect SBBO was the bile acid or ^{14}C-cholyglycine breath test. This test, unfortunately, suffered from signfiicant false-negative and false-positive results. The bile acid breath test does not distinguish SBBO from ileal damage or resection with excessive breath $^{14}CO_2$ production resulting from bacterial deconjugation within the colon of the unabsorbed labelled bile salt. This was particularly problematic because SBBO may be superimposed on ileal damage in conditions such as Crohn's disease, lymphoma, and radiation enteritis. False-negative results have also been described with this test in 30 to 40 per cent of patients with culture-proven SBBO.

Studies in experimentally induced SBBO demonstrated that the overgrowth flora had the capacity to metabolize significant quantities of xylose and produce carbon dioxide. A 1-g ^{14}C-xylose breath test was developed and found to be sensitive and specific for detecting the presence of SBBO in patients with culture-proven SBBO. Xylose was chosen as a substrate because: (i) it is catabolized by Gram-negative aerobes which are always part of the overgrowth flora; (ii) it is predominantly absorbed in the proximal small intestine in contrast to the predominant ileal absorption of bile salts, leading to virtually 'no dumping' of xylose into the colon; and (iii) it is metabolized substantially less than other proximally absorbed substrates such as glucose. Elevated $^{14}CO_2$ levels appear in the breath of 85 per cent of patients with culture-proven SBBO within the first 60 min of the test, with the 30-min sample being the most reliable. Laboratories throughout the world have demonstrated the reliability of the ^{14}C-xylose breath test when compared with intestinal culture. In those studies that utilized intestinal culture as the gold standard and evaluated shorter sampling intervals, particularly the 30-min time point, the sensitivity and specificity approxi-

mated 90 per cent. Some recent studies have raised doubts as to the reliability of the ^{14}C-xylose breath test, but those studies evaluated patients with severe disorders of motility and it is quite possible that the xylose never left the stomach appropriately to come in contact with the overgrowth flora in the proximal small intestine. In addition, there must be an overgrowth of Gram-negative coliforms for the xylose test to be positive. In at least one of the recent studies failing to confirm the reliability of the ^{14}C-xylose breath test, the cultures also lacked Gram-negative coliforms. Others have suggested refinement of the ^{14}C-xylose breath test to include a transit marker for intestinal motility, which may enhance its specificity.

It is not recommended that ^{14}C-labelled xylose be used as a substrate in the diagnosis of SBBO in children or fertile women. Consequently, ^{13}C-labelled xylose has been developed and demonstrated to be an effective test in detecting SBBO. These ^{13}C-labelled substrates have been utilized in selected centres but are not yet in general use in clinical practice.

Breath hydrogen analysis allows a distinct separation of metabolic activities of the overgrowth flora from that of the human host because hydrogen is not produced to any significant extent in mammalian tissue. Excessive breath hydrogen production has been noted in patients with bacterial overgrowth after the administration of 50 to 80 g of glucose or 10 to 12 g of lactulose. A fasting elevation of breath hydrogen is an excellent test for detecting SBBO, but only about one-third of subjects with culture-proven SBBO will have elevated fasting levels of breath hydrogen.

There must be rigorous attention paid to methodological details when utilizing a hydrogen breath test. Certain foods that cause prolonged excretion of hydrogen must be avoided the night before the test, and 2 h must elapse after cigarette smoking or physical exercise sufficient to produce hyperventilation before taking the test. It is also recommended that a mouthwash be performed before testing to eliminate the possibility of an early hydrogen peak resulting from oral bacteria. Finally, strict interpretation criteria must be adopted. Even with careful attention to these details, the sensitivity and specificity of the hydrogen breath test is disappointing when used to detect SBBO. Recent studies have demonstrated that up to 27 per cent of normal subjects failed to show any rise in breath hydrogen following the administration of lactulose. The non-radioactive nature and the ease of performance of hydrogen breath tests make them quite attractive. However, many studies indicate that these tests have an unacceptable lack of sensitivity and specificity for clinical use and clinical laboratories do not pay attention to the critical details required for their proper conduct.

Therapeutic approach to the management of SBBO

The aim of therapy for SBBO is to correct when feasible the cause of the stasis, but surgery is often impractical (scleroderma, multiple diverticula, diabetes, intestinal pseudo-obstruction) and unacceptable to the patient. Thus, management of patients with SBBO is lifelong. Antibiotic therapy is the cornerstone of treatment and remarkable improvement in symptoms can be achieved in most patients. It is important to emphasize once again that SBBO may be a treatable component of the malabsorption seen in

Table 6 Tests for SBBO

Tests	Simplicity	Sensitivity	Specificity	Safety
Culture	Poor	Excellent	Excellent	Good
Urinary indican	Good	Poor	Poor	Excellent
Jejunal fatty acids	Poor	Fair	Excellent	Good
Jejunal bile acids	Poor	Fair	Excellent	Good
Fasting breath H_2	Excellent	Poor	Excellent	Excellent
^{14}C-bile acid breath test	Excellent	Fair	Fair	Good
^{14}C-xylose breath test	Excellent	Excellent	Excellent	Good
Lactulose-H_2 breath test	Excellent	Fair	Fair	Excellent
Glucose-H_2 breath test	Excellent	Good	Fair	Excellent

patients with conditions such as Crohn's disease, intestinal lymphoma, or radiation enteritis. The deterioration in absorption in such patients may not be caused by their primary disease process but by the associated overgrowth. Clinicians also must be aware that bacterial overgrowth may be present without causing any disease. Not all patients who have a pathological flora in the proximal small intestine develop clinically important symptoms. An abnormal breath test or a pathological culture must be put into perspective before therapeutic decisions are made.

It would seem attractive to select the appropriate antibiotic by evaluation of the sensitivity of the bacteria present in the small bowel lumen. However, this approach is very problematic because there are many different bacterial species present, often with very different antimicrobial sensitivities. Under such conditions, it may be extremely difficult to select the most appropriate agent on the basis of the sensitivity results. It is important to select an antibiotic that is effective against both aerobic and anaerobic enteric bacteria. Although most patients with clinically significant malabsorption secondary to SBBO have a flora that is largely overgrown with anaerobes, malabsorption associated predominantly with the overgrowth of Gram-negative aerobes also occurs.

Table 7 lists antimicrobial agents that have been effective in treating SBBO whether in controlled clinical trials or extensive clinical practice. Antibiotics whose activities are largely limited to anaerobes, such as metronidazole or clindamycin, are not usually effective as monotherapy. Antibiotics that are known to have poor activity against anaerobes should not be used in treating SBBO; such antibiotics include penicillin, ampicillin, the oral aminoglycosides, kanamycin, and neomycin. Historically, the treatment of first choice has been tetracycline, but recent experience in the United States suggests that up to 60 per cent of patients with SBBO do not respond to tetracycline largely because of *Bacteroides* resistance to this drug.

In most patients, a single course of therapy (7 to 10 days) markedly improves symptoms and the patient may remain symptom-free for months; in others, symptoms recur quickly and acceptable results can only be obtained with cyclic therapy (1 week out of every 4); and in still others, continuous therapy may be needed for 1 to 2 months. If the antimicrobial agent is effective there will be a resolution or marked diminution of symptoms within 1 week. Diarrhoea and steatorrhoea will decrease and cobalamin malabsorption will be corrected.

Prolonged antibiotic therapy poses potential clinical problems including diarrhoea, enterocolitis, patient intolerance, and bacterial resistance. A prokinetic agent that could help clear the small intestine of the overgrowth flora would be an attractive therapy. Experimental animal studies suggest that SBBO might be favorably influenced by prokinetic agents. There have

been two small studies of these agents in patients with SBBO, one utilizing cisapride and one using octreotide. Both agents led to positive results in respect to SBBO following the prokinetic treatment. Another study utilizing octreotide and erythromycin in patients with scleroderma and SBBO attained positive responses following prokinetic therapy. Large controlled trials of prokinetic therapy in patients with SBBO have yet to be completed. Since the days of Metchkinoff, it has been thought that one could manipulate the intestinal flora by giving live 'probiotic' microbial supplements that would change the balance in the intestinal flora. Studies to date with probiotic therapy in subjects with SBBO have been disappointing. A recent placebo-controlled, randomized cross-over trial compared norfloxacin, amoxicillin–clavulanic acid, and *Saccharomyces boulardii* in 10 symptomatic patients with SBBO. Both antibiotic treatments led to significant decreases in symptoms and a substantial improvement in the results of hydrogen breath testing. The probiotic treatment with *S. boulardii* did not result in any improvement in these parameters.

Nutritional support is an important part of treatment of SBBO and may be needed despite attempts to control the bacterial overgrowth by antimicrobial agents because there may be irreversible damage to the enterocytes. Therefore, a lactose-free diet and substitution of a large proportion of dietary fat by medium-chain triglycerides may be necessary. Patients with cobalamin malabsorption should receive monthly injections of cobalamin (1000 µg). Deficiencies of other nutrients such as calcium and vitamin K should also be corrected.

Clinicians should have a low threshold for suspecting SBBO as a cause of malabsorption. The algorithm presented in Fig. 3 emphasizes the performance of simple, outpatient testing to pinpoint the cause of the malabsorption. Therefore, an appropriate attempt should be made to document whether SBBO is present or not. The consequences of SBBO can lead to serious malabsorption that results in clinically important deficiencies of several nutrients and, moreover, can be easily diagnosed and treated.

Further reading

Attar A *et al.* (1999). Antibiotic efficacy in small intestinal bacterial overgrowth-related chronic diarrhea: a cross-over, randomized trial. *Gastroenterology* **117**, 794–7.

Bishop WP (1997). Breath hydrogen testing for small bowel bacterial overgrowth—a lot of hot air? *Journal of Pediatric Gastroenterology and Nutrition* **25**, 245–9.

Bouhnik Y *et al.* (1999). Bacterial populations contaminating the upper gut in patients with small intestinal bacterial overgrowth syndrome. *American Journal of Gastroenterology* **94**, 1327–9.

Corazza GR *et al.* (1990). The diagnosis of small bowel bacterial overgrowth. *Gastroenterology* **98**, 302–5.

DeBoissieu D *et al.* (1996). Small-bowel bacterial overgrowth in children with chronic diarrhea, abdominal pain, or both. *Journal of Pediatrics* **128**, 203.

Fried M *et al.* (1996). Duodenal bacterial overgrowth during treatment with omeprazole in outpatients. *Gut* **35**, 23–7.

King CE, Toskes PP (1986). Comparison of the 1-gram [^{14}C]xylose, 10-gram lactulose-H$_2$, and 80-gram glucose-H$_2$ breath tests in patients with small intestine bacterial overgrowth. *Gastroenterology* **91**, 1447–51.

Saltsman J *et al.* (1994). Bacterial overgrowth without clinical malabsorption in elderly hypochlorhydric subjects. *Gastroenterology* **106**, 615–18.

Soudah H, Hasler W, Owyang C (1991). Effect of octreotide on intestinal motility and bacterial overgrowth in scleroderma. *New England Journal of Medicne* **325**, 1461–7.

Toskes P, Kumar A (1998). Enteric bacterial flora and bacterial overgrowth syndrome. In: Feldman M, Scharschmidt B, Sleisenger M, eds. *Sleisenger and Fordtran's gastrointestinal and liver disease*, 1523–35. WB Saunders, Philadelphia.

Table 7 Effective antimicrobial agents for treating SBBO

Agent	Dose/day (10-day course)
Tetracycline	250 mg four times
Doxycycline	100 mg twice
Minocycline	100 mg twice
Amoxycillin–clavulanic acid	850 mg twice
Cephalexin +	250 mg four times
metronidazole	250 mg three times
Colistin +	250 000 IU/kg
metronidazole	250 mg three times
Trimethoprim–sulphamethoxazole	One double-strength tablet twice
Chloramphenicol	250 mg four times
Ciprofloxacin	500 mg twice
Norfloxacin	400 mg twice

14.9.3 Coeliac disease

D. P. Jewell

Definition

Coeliac disease is an inflammatory disorder of the small intestine induced by the prolamins of certain cereals, namely the gliadins of wheat, hordeins of barley, and secalins of rye. The inflammation is associated with loss of villous height and crypt hypertrophy and leads to malabsorption. The functional and histological abnormalities are reversed towards normal following exclusion of those cereals from the diet; they reappear on luminal challenge with the noxious prolamins.

History

Coeliac disease may well have been recognized in ancient times, as Aretaeus, the Cappadocian, wrote of the 'coeliac affection'. This was clearly a malabsorptive illness with steatorrhoea, affecting children and adults, but whether it represents a gluten-sensitive enteropathy is impossible to know. Samuel Gee of St Bartholomew's Hospital, London gave an excellent account of the disease in 1888 and concluded that 'if the patient is to be cured at all, it will be by means of a diet'. It was the Dutch paediatrician, W.K. Dicke, who finally recognized the role of wheat and his initial observations made in the 1930s were confirmed during the 'winter of starvation' in Holland in 1944. He noted that children with coeliac disease paradoxically improved as bread became virtually unobtainable. Using dietary challenge and faecal fat output as an indicator, Dicke together with J. H. van de Kamer and H. A. Weijers showed that it was gliadin, the alcohol-soluble component of gluten, that was the damaging substance. The demonstration of a flat intestinal mucosa by J. Paulley in 1954 and the development of a technique to take biopsies from the small intestine by Margot Shiner in 1956, who studied the histological findings with I. Doniach, as well as Rubin and colleagues in 1960, characterized the disease histologically and allowed easy and accurate diagnosis. The ability to follow the response of the mucosa to dietary manipulation by serial biopsy also allowed clinicians to demonstrate that coeliac disease in children was the same disease as idiopathic steatorrhoea in adults. Therefore, the disease is now referred to as coeliac disease or as a gluten-sensitive enteropathy.

Pathology

Coeliac disease affects the small intestine but the mucosal inflammation can vary in severity and in extent. Many patients have very mild proximal disease and the mucosal damage can be patchy. The characteristic, but not specific, feature is loss of villous height so that, under a dissecting microscope, the mucosa appears completely flat (Fig. 1). This is confirmed on histological examination (Fig. 2). The mucosa may be completely flat or there may be very short, broad villi—this appearance is often called subtotal villous atrophy. However, the total mucosal thickness (surface epithelium to muscularis mucosae) is usually normal or only slightly reduced because the crypts become elongated—usually referred to as crypt hypertrophy. The surface epithelial cells become flattened, the basal polarity of their nuclei is lost, and the microvilli of the brush border become short and irregular. This last change is revealed by electron microscopy.

Within the lamina propria, there is a marked infiltration of chronic inflammatory cells—plasma cells and lymphocytes. In addition, there is an increase in neutrophils, eosinophils, and mast cells. The proportion of intraepithelial lymphocytes is also increased in comparison with the number of enterocytes, although the absolute number is probably not increased.

Within the plasma cell population, there is an increase in the cells producing IgA, G, and M isotypes, although IgA cells still predominate. There is a marked increase in the proliferation rate of crypt cells, which, in a histological section, is shown by numerous mitoses at the base of the crypts. This increase in crypt cell proliferation is thought to be mediated by cytokines released by the underlying lymphocytes and macrophages and leads to elongation of the crypts and loss of villous height.

It has been proposed that three stages in the development of coeliac disease are defined—infiltrative, hyperplastic, and destructive. These stages have been identified on the basis of challenge studies as well as biopsies of asymptomatic members of coeliac families. In the infiltrative stage, the epithelium becomes infiltrated with increased numbers of lymphocytes and this is the lesion frequently seen in patients with dermatitis herpetiformis. This stage leads on to the point where there is some inflammation of the lamina propria, with elongation of crypts. Both these stages are asymptomatic and can be regarded as latent coeliac disease. The destructive stage is the full lesion with loss of villi and a marked inflammatory infiltrate. Whether this classification is helpful, or indeed representative of what actually happens, is not yet clear.

As well as these characteristic changes in the small intestine, there may be a diffuse infiltration of other mucosal surfaces with lymphocytes and plasma cells. In particular, a proctitis has been recognized recently, but this is only detected if a rectal biopsy is taken and is virtually never severe

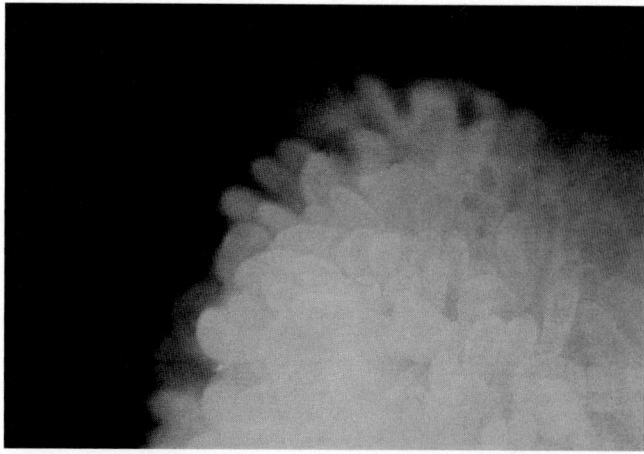

(a)

(b)

Fig. 1 (a) Dissecting microscopic appearance of a normal jejunal biopsy. (b) Dissecting microscopic appearance of coeliac disease.

enough to cause symptoms. This generalized mucosal infiltration presumably represents homing patterns of lymphocytes sensitized within the small-intestinal lamina propria.

Following a gluten-free diet, these histological changes return towards normal. For the majority of patients, a repeat biopsy after 3 months will show much less inflammation, the villous height will have increased, and the crypt elongation will have diminished. The mucosa usually returns to normal in children, but in adults, minor changes may persist with a crypt :villous ratio of 1:2 rather than the normal ratio of 1:4.

When patients in remission on a gluten-free diet are challenged with gluten, histological changes may be seen within a few days. In fact, electron microscopic changes may occur within a few hours of challenge and a fall in brush-border disaccharidase activity occurs in 24 h. However, some patients may take much longer to relapse and there have been some individuals who have virtually no histological change for up to a year.

Epidemiology

Coeliac disease is primarily a disease of Caucasians and, as it is closely associated with the extended haplotype HLA B8-DR3-DQ2, it is rare in those parts of the world where this haplotype is uncommon. Over 90 per cent of individuals with coeliac disease possess HLA DQ2, most of the remainder having HLA DQ8. The prevalence of coeliac disease in Europe and North America is about 1 in 300—much higher than was previously thought. This apparent increase has been due to more frequent diagnosis resulting from the accuracy of screening programmes that measure antiendomysial antibodies (see below).

There is little sex difference, although some studies have shown a preponderance of women. There is a familial incidence, with about 10 per cent

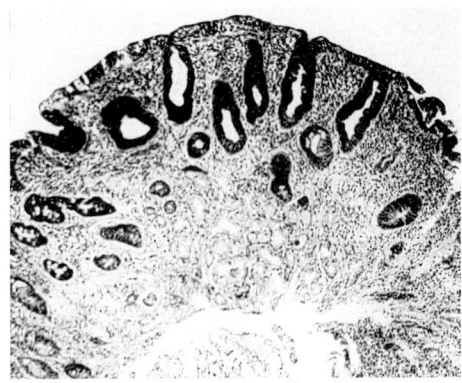

(a)

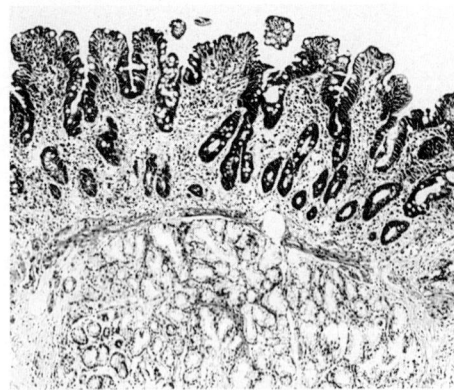

(b)

Fig. 2 Histological appearances of a distal duodenal biopsy in a patient with coeliac disease before (a) and after (b) a 3-month period on a gluten-free diet. Following treatment, there is much less inflammation and the villous pattern has begun to reappear.

of first-degree relatives being affected, and studies of monozygotic twins have shown a concordance of 70 per cent. These data indicate a strong genetic susceptibility.

Pathogenesis

There are two clear facts about the aetiopathogenesis of coeliac disease. The first is that fractions of gliadin, the alcohol-soluble component of gluten, are the toxic dietary constituent, together with similar fractions of rye and barley prolamins. The second is that there is a genetic susceptibility to gluten intolerance because of the close association with the HLA haplotype B8-DR3-DQ2 in northern Europeans and with B8-DR5/7-DQ2 in southern Europeans. This difference is due to the fact that the same DQ α–β heterodimer can be encoded on the same chromosome (*cis* position) in DR3 individuals or on opposite chromosomes (*trans* position) in DR5/DR7 individuals (see Section 5). This suggests that DQ molecules confer most of the susceptibility. What is not clear is how this particular haplotype interacts with gluten to produce mucosal inflammation in one person whereas the majority of people with this haplotype are able to ingest gluten with impunity. The other unsolved question is the exact nature of the toxic peptide.

An attractive hypothesis to explain why certain individuals lose oral tolerance to gluten is that it occurs as a result of an infection with adenovirus 12. This hypothesis was suggested by the observation that there was a dodecapeptide on the surface of α-gliadin which was similar to a peptide contained within an E1b protein of the virus. Many patients with coeliac disease demonstrate cellular and humoral immune responses to the virus, and so it is conceivable that the immune response to the virus cross-reacts with the gliadin peptide and thus induces intestinal inflammation. The gliadin dodecapeptide is now known to bind avidly to DQ2.

Some progress has been made in determining the toxic peptide, but in most studies toxicity has been assessed by *in vitro* methods rather than by direct feeding studies in patients. The amino acid sequences that seem to be shared by these toxic peptides are pro–ser–glu–glu or ser–pro–glu–glu. Two recent studies have identified an epitope (PQPQLPY) which appears to be dominant for the induction of a T-cell response. Furthermore, it requires the deamidation of a specific glutamine (at position 65) by tissue transglutaminase to elicit the response. B-cell responses also appear to depend on deamidation in this sequence. This is particularly interesting as tissue transglutaminase is now known to be the antigen to which the antiendomysial antibody is directed (see below).

The inflammatory lesion in the small intestine seems to result from an immunological reaction to the gluten peptides, with both cellular and humoral responses being involved. The mucosal abnormality is usually a proximal one and is presumably a reflection of luminal concentration of the relevant peptides. The release of cytokines and inflammatory mediators is thought to amplify the immune response and to influence epithelial stem-cell kinetics, with subsequent crypt elongation and loss of villous height. Malabsorption occurs because of loss of absorptive area and the presence of a population of immature surface epithelial cells whose absorptive and secretory function may be additionally impaired by cytokines and inflammatory mediators.

Clinical features

Coeliac disease in infants classically presents soon after weaning at the point that cereals are introduced. The babies usually fail to thrive, are miserable, refuse to eat, and lose weight. The abdomen becomes distended, there is muscle wasting, and they may have diarrhoea, which usually has the features of steatorrhoea. Abdominal pain and vomiting may be prominent symptoms and can mislead the clinician. Rectal prolapse may occur.

In older children, growth retardation is a common presentation and if the gastrointestinal symptoms are minimal, the diagnosis can be overlooked. Nutritional deficiencies can occur and may again be the reason for presentation, anaemia being the most common deficiency. Delayed puberty is another mode of presentation.

In adults, the most common presentations are anaemia and variable abdominal symptoms of discomfort, bloating, excess wind, and an altered bowel habit. Mouth ulcers are also frequent and can be the presenting symptom. The anaemia is most commonly due to iron deficiency and frequently occurs in the absence of intestinal symptoms; the macrocytic anaemias that sometimes occur in coeliac disease are described in Section 22. Many patients presenting with diarrhoea, wind, and abdominal pain are wrongly diagnosed as having an irritable bowel syndrome and there may then be a considerable delay before the true diagnosis is made. Patients suspected of having an irritable bowel syndrome should be specifically questioned about mouth ulcers and weight loss, either of which can be a pointer to organic disease. They should also be asked about feeding difficulties as a child, about growth milestones, and the age of achieving puberty. Less commonly, patients will present with a more typical history, with features of steatorrhoea, weight loss, bruising, and other symptoms of nutritional deficiencies resulting from malabsorption.

The classic findings in infants are those of an irritable child with stunted growth, muscle wasting, and a 'pot belly'. The infant usually has feeding difficulties and may show evidence of colic, and has a marked diarrhoea. However, in toddlers and older children who present with growth failure or anaemia, there may be few signs. Similarly, in adults, there may be no physical signs in those presenting with symptoms suggestive of an irritable bowel syndrome. Signs of iron deficiency may be present and there may be aphthous ulcers in the mouth, mild finger clubbing, and evidence of recent weight loss. It is very unusual, nowadays, for patients to show evidence of bleeding and osteomalacia (or rickets in children). Even less common are patients who are so malnourished that they have signs of ascites and hypoproteinaemic oedema.

Diagnosis

The crucial test to establish the diagnosis is a small-intestinal biopsy. This has traditionally been taken from the duodenal–jejunal junction (the ligament of Treitz) using a Crosby capsule. However, a distal duodenal biopsy taken at endoscopy is being used increasingly to make the diagnosis and comparative studies with a true jejunal biopsy have justified its use.

Several serological tests have been developed as screening tests which include antibodies to gliadin (IgA or IgG isotype), IgA antibodies to reticulin, and IgA antibodies to endomysium. The endomysial antibody has proved to be the most useful with a specificity and sensitivity of 90 to 95 per cent. The antibody is detected by immunofluorescence using monkey oesophagus or human umbilical vein. The antibody is directed towards tissue transglutaminase and is increasingly being detected using enzyme-linked immunosorbent assay (ELISA) with transglutaminase-coated wells. The titre falls as the disease goes into remission on a gluten-free diet, but can take 3 to 12 months to become negative. Failure of the serum to become negative for the antibody, or reappearance of the antibody suggests non-compliance with the diet. Since it is an IgA antibody that is measured, a false-negative result may occur in the 5 per cent or so of patients with coeliac disease who have a coexistent IgA deficiency. The antiendomysial antibody is useful for screening high-risk populations, such as family members of patients with coeliac disease, diabetes, or osteoporosis.

Assessment of malabsorption

Careful documentation of nutritional deficiency as a result of malabsorption must be made and should include the following.

Full blood count

The haemoglobin level may be low, but the mean corpuscular volume may be low (iron deficiency), high (vitamin B_{12} or folate deficiency), or within the normal range. This can occur either because there is no significant deficiency of a haematinic or because there is a mixed deficiency, usually a combination of iron and folate. The red cell folate is a more reliable indicator of folate deficiency than the serum concentration and if it is low, there may be a pancytopenia. Vitamin B_{12} concentrations are only low in patients with extensive involvement of the small intestine and so are usually normal. Serum iron, total binding capacity, and ferritin concentrations should be measured to record the patient's iron status.

Biochemistry

Quantitative estimations of faecal fat excretion are becoming progressively more difficult to obtain despite their obvious value in assessing small-intestinal function. Qualitative assessment of excess fat by staining faecal smears with Sudan black or oil red O can be a reasonable alternative but merely records the presence or absence of a steatorrhoea. Fat malabsorption is inevitably accompanied by malabsorption of the fat-soluble vitamins A, D, E, and K. Serum concentrations of β-carotene, calcium, alkaline phosphatase, vitamin D, and the prothrombin time (INR—international normalized ratio) should therefore be assayed. Patients with diarrhoea may become hypokalaemic. Serum magnesium concentrations may also be low in severe coeliac disease and, with hypocalcaemia, can lead to tetany. Serum albumin is often low, as is the concentration of zinc.

Immunological tests

In addition to the titres of diagnostic antibodies discussed above, serum immunoglobulin concentrations should be measured. The most common pattern of abnormality is a raised IgA with a low IgM, but virtually any pattern may be seen. However, 5 per cent of patients with coeliac disease have an associated IgA deficiency, and loss of villous height and crypt hypertrophy frequently accompany common-variable acquired immunodeficiency.

Radiology

Barium radiology cannot give a positive diagnosis of coeliac disease and is not usually necessary unless it is required to exclude other small-intestinal diseases. In patients with mild disease the appearances may be normal, but if abnormalities are present, the appearances vary according to the radiological technique used. If a barium meal and follow-through is done, the small intestine may appear dilated and the barium often segments and flocculates. The proximal loops may appear smooth with a corresponding accentuation of the valvulae conniventes in the ileum—the so-called jejunization of the ileum. If a small-bowel enema is used (enteroclysis), the features are those of dilation and oedema of the valvulae conniventes.

Differential diagnosis

Few patients present with overt malabsorption, so the diagnosis of coeliac disease requires a high index of suspicion. However, once a biopsy is obtained that shows appearances compatible with coeliac disease, the differential diagnosis is limited.

For infants, the most common differential diagnosis is cow's milk allergy. An eosinophilia in the lamina propria as well as in peripheral blood is common, but this can also occur in coeliac disease. A soya milk allergy can also cause a flat small-intestinal mucosa. The precise diagnosis is usually dependent on a dietary history and the results of dietary exclusion.

In adults, infection with giardia, common-variable hypogammaglobulinaemia, lymphoma, Crohn's disease, and other small-intestinal diseases such as radiation enteritis, amyloid, and Whipple's disease may all show villous flattening and mucosal inflammation. Tropical sprue is usually associated with less marked changes—so-called partial villous atrophy—but has to be considered in patients who have spent time in endemic areas. Rarely, patients may be seen with a flat biopsy but with crypt hypoplasia—these do not respond to a gluten-free diet. Some patients with crypt hypoplasia also have a thickened band of subepithelial collagen, so-called collagenous sprue. Systemic diseases such as the vasculitides and systemic sclerosis may also be associated with an abnormal mucosal biopsy. Bacterial overgrowth of the small intestine may be associated with some mucosal inflammation and minor villous changes but they are rarely sufficiently severe to be confused with coeliac disease.

Dermatitis herpetiformis is commonly associated with an abnormal mucosal biopsy. The mucosal inflammation can be as severe as coeliac disease and responds to gluten withdrawal. The skin lesions also respond to a gluten-free diet, albeit slowly.

Non-specific infections of the small intestine may lead to a degree of malabsorption and mucosal inflammation. In only a small proportion can giardia be detected, and the precise aetiology of the majority is never determined. The illness is usually sudden in onset and gets better spontaneously over several weeks. It has been named 'temperate sprue'. Although this entity is uncommon, it can mislead clinicians. Most patients presenting in this way are started on a gluten-free diet as soon as the result of the biopsy is known and their improvement is regarded as a dietary response. Thus a patient presenting with a very short history of symptoms and whose mucosal biopsy suggests coeliac disease must be considered carefully. HLA typing and the presence of serum endomysial antibodies may be very helpful in making the correct diagnosis. If there is still doubt, the patient should be given a gluten-free diet but when the mucosa has recovered, a gluten challenge with subsequent biopsy should be undertaken.

Associated diseases

There is an increased prevalence of autoimmune diseases in patients with coeliac disease, especially those that are associated with the HLA B8-DR3 phenotype. These include diabetes, thyroid disease, and Addison's disease. Fibrosing alveolitis, systemic lupus erythematosus, and polyarteritis have also been reported. There may be an increase in epilepsy, especially temporal-lobe epilepsy, in patients with coeliac disease.

About 5 per cent of individuals with coeliac disease have an isolated IgA deficiency but the reason for and significance of this are not clear.

Treatment

Once the diagnosis is confirmed by a small-intestinal biopsy, patients should be started on a gluten-free diet. This diet should also exclude barley and rye, but with oats the need is less clear. As the evidence for oat toxicity is confused, many clinicians allow oats and only exclude them if the repeat biopsy does not show a good histological response. However, others exclude oats as the diet is begun and then consider reintroducing them once the disease has gone into histological remission.

All patients should be advised of the diet by a dietician and should be told to keep to it strictly. For children, the parents must be well briefed, including being told of the dangers of many sweets and 'fast foods'. For all patients, the diet is a lifelong necessity. Many children inevitably ingest small amounts of gluten during adolescence and many of them remain asymptomatic and develop normally. This has given rise to the highly erroneous view that children can 'grow out' of the disease. If the diagnosis was correct in the first place, then the patient has coeliac disease for life and if the diet is not strict, it may predispose them to complications in the future.

Patients should also be given details of the national coeliac society, if there is one. Most countries in which coeliac disease occurs have such a society. They provide a considerable amount of information about the disease and update patients about the gluten contents of new products appearing in the supermarkets. They also give invaluable advice about diet and foreign travel, as well as providing a social forum for patients and opportunities for fund raising to support research.

Nutritional supplements may be necessary at the start of treatment. If there are low serum concentrations of iron and folate, or biochemical evidence of osteomalacia, appropriate supplements are clearly required. How-

ever, once a gluten-free diet has begun, mucosal recovery occurs rapidly so that long-term supplementation is rarely necessary.

Patients with extensive mucosal damage are unable to digest lactose because of lactase deficiency. These patients may need a lactose-free as well as a gluten-free diet until there is histological recovery.

Once patients have been on the diet for 3 to 4 months, a further small-intestinal biopsy must be obtained to check for histological recovery. If the mucosa is still inflamed and villous height has not returned towards normal, a thorough review of the patient's diet is needed. Hidden sources of gluten (Communion wafers being a classic example) can often be found by a skilled dietician. If oats have not been excluded, then this is worth doing. In children, additional exclusion of soya products is occasionally needed.

Long-term follow-up, preferably in specialized clinics, is desirable but need only be on an annual basis once patients are stabilized on their diet. This allows patients to be seen by a dietician as well as their physician and reinforces the need to comply with a strict diet. Compliance should also be checked by measuring antiendomysial antibody—it should be negative if the disease is in remission.

Complications

The two major complications of coeliac disease are an ulcerative jejunoileitis and a T-cell lymphoma, and some investigators consider the jejunoileitis to be a manifestation of a lymphoma. They usually occur in middle age and usually present with weight loss, anaemia, abdominal pain, and diarrhoea. Thus any coeliac presenting with these symptoms having been previously well on a gluten-free diet must be carefully screened for these complications. Biopsies should be snap-frozen in liquid nitrogen to allow immunohistochemical analysis of T-cell markers and the detection of T-cell receptor rearrangements. The prognosis of a lymphoma complicating coeliac disease is poor.

In addition, there is a slight increase in the frequency of small-bowel carcinoma, although this is still very rare. There is also an increased incidence of other gastrointestinal cancers, especially oesophageal tumours, although the reasons for this increase are obscure.

There is some evidence suggesting that the patients who develop malignant disease, especially lymphoma, are those who have been poor compliers with the diet. Although this association is not absolutely proven, it provides the basis for continuing to advise a strict diet and to monitor compliance on a regular outpatient review.

Osteoporosis

Bone density scans have shown that most patients with coeliac disease have reduced bone density at diagnosis, but that this improves after a year or so of a strict gluten-free diet. The recommended intake of calcium for individuals with coeliac disease is 1500 mg daily, which is high, and requires skilled dietetic advice. For those patients with frank osteoporosis, treatment with calcium and vitamin D is required. For those with osteopenia, a follow-up scan should be done following a year on a gluten-free diet and calcium supplementation.

Prognosis

Provided that patients adhere to a strict diet, the prognosis is excellent and there are no data which suggest that there is an excess mortality in this group. Children develop normally and proceed into adolescence without delay. However, as mentioned above, compliance with the diet is often poor in adolescents and some clinicians still believe that many of them can have a more liberal diet if they are asymptomatic. It is this group that often present some years later with anaemia, mouth ulcers, or more serious evidence of malabsorption.

Unresponsive disease

A rare group of patients who are found to have a flat small-intestinal biopsy fail to respond to a gluten-free diet despite meticulous attention to avoid even minute amounts of gluten over many months. By definition these patients do not have coeliac disease, although they are often referred to as 'non-responsive coeliacs', a phrase that is misleading and should be avoided. Treatment of this group is difficult. Corticosteroids with or without azathioprine may help some, and more recent case reports suggest oral cyclosporin may also be of benefit. Excluding other dietary items such as soya can be tried, or an elemental diet that removes all dietary antigens. Some of these patients have a variety of central and peripheral neurological signs that do not fit classic vitamin-deficiency syndromes. The aetiology and pathology of these neurological lesions is unknown and the initial suggestions that they represented vitamin E deficiency have not been substantiated. The prognosis for these patients is poor because the neurological damage is slowly progressive and patients gradually lose weight despite full nutritional support.

It is always worth reviewing the intestinal biopsies in patients who do not respond to gluten withdrawal. Small-intestinal lymphoma, loss of villous height with crypt hypoplasia, and collagenous sprue are alternative diagnoses that may not have been recognized during the initial assessment.

Further reading

Anderson RP, Jewell DP (2001). Coeliac disease. In: Hunt R, Irvine J, eds. *Evidence based gastroenterology*, pp.307–22. B. C. Decker Inc., Ontario.

Marsh MN (1992). Gluten, major histocompatibility complex, and the small intestine. *Gastroenterology* **102**, 330–54.

Sategna-Guidetti C, Grosso S (1994). Changing pattern in adult coeliac disease: a 24-year survey. *European Journal of Gastroenterology and Hepatology* **6**, 15–19.

van Berge-Henegouwen GP, Mulder CJJ (1993). Pioneer in the gluten-free diet: Willem-Karel Dicke 1905–1962, over 50 years of gluten free diet. *Gut* **34**, 1473–5.

Van De Wal Y *et al.* (2000). Coeliac disease: it takes three to tango! Gut **46**(5), 734–7.

14.9.4 Gastrointestinal lymphoma

P. G. Isaacson

Introduction

Gastrointestinal lymphomas, the most common extranodal lymphomas, are almost exclusively of non-Hodgkin's type, primary gastrointestinal Hodgkin's disease being extremely rare. A primary gastrointestinal lymphoma is defined as a lymphoma that has presented with the main bulk of disease in the gastrointestinal tract, with or without involvement of contiguous lymph nodes, necessitating direction of treatment to that site. The stomach is the commonest site of primary gastrointestinal lymphoma followed by the small intestine. Oesophageal and colorectal lymphomas are rare. The lymphomas that may arise in the gastrointestinal tract are listed in Table 1. Two of these, namely B-cell lymphoma of mucosa-associated

Table 1 Primary gastrointestinal non-Hodgkin's lymphoma

B cell
- Mucosa-associated lymphoid tissue (MALT) lymphoma (including immunoproliferative small intestinal disease (IPSID)) with or without evidence of high-grade transformation
- Mantle-cell lymphoma (lymphomatous polyposis)
- Burkitt lymphoma
- Other types corresponding to lymph node equivalents
  - follicular lymphoma
  - lymphocytic lymphoma
  - diffuse large B-cell lymphoma
- Immunodeficiency-related lymphomas
  - post-transplant
  - acquired (AIDS)
  - congenital

T cell
- Enteropathy-associated T-cell lymphoma (EATL)
- Other types not associated with enteropathy

Rare types (including conditions that may simulate lymphoma)

lymphoid tissue (**MALT**) and enteropathy-associated T-cell lymphoma (**EATL**), do not arise in peripheral lymph nodes and will be discussed in more detail in this section. Any of the lymphomas that normally arise in lymph nodes may present as a primary gastrointestinal tumour, the most frequent being diffuse large B-cell lymphoma and mantle-cell lymphoma, which usually manifests in the gut as lymphomatous polyposis. Burkitt's lymphoma, which is the commonest childhood gastrointestinal lymphoma, is an especially common primary small intestinal lymphoma in the Middle East. The increasingly important group of B-cell lymphoproliferative conditions associated with immunodeficiency commonly present in the gastrointestinal tract, but they are more properly considered in the context of immunodeficiency-related lymphoproliferative conditions as a whole.

MALT lymphomas

The term MALT-lymphoma is used to designate a group of low-grade B-cell lymphomas whose histology recapitulates the features of mucosa-associated lymphoid tissue (MALT) as exemplified by the Peyer's patch. Paradoxically, there is usually no lymphoid tissue in the sites where MALT lymphomas occur, but lymphoid tissue of MALT-type accumulates prior to the development of lymphoma. In the stomach this is usually the result of chronic inflammation in response to *Helicobacter pylori* infection and its associated autoimmune phenomena. Intestinal MALT lymphomas are less frequent but include the entity known as immunoproliferative small intestine disease (**IPSID**) that has interesting parallels with gastric MALT lymphoma.

Gastric MALT lymphoma

Clinical presentation

Gastric MALT lymphoma typically occurs in patients over 40 years of age but can occur at any age. The sex incidence is equal. The presenting symptoms are usually those of non-specific dyspepsia and more suggestive of gastritis or peptic ulcer than a neoplastic lesion. Likewise, endoscopy more often shows inflamed, sometimes eroded mucosa than a tumour mass.

Pathology

Most MALT lymphomas of the stomach arise in the antrum, and macroscopically are characterized by an ill-defined thickened inflamed and ulcerated mucosa. The histological features closely simulate those of MALT (Fig. 1). Reactive non-neoplastic follicles are surrounded by the lymphomatous infiltrate in the region corresponding to the Peyer's patch marginal

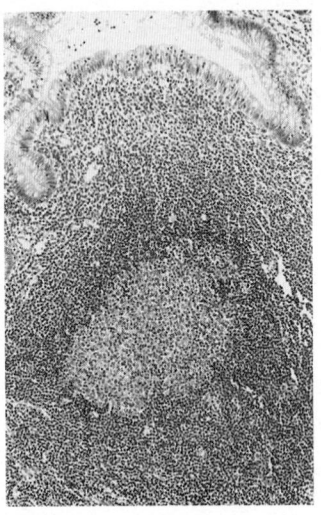 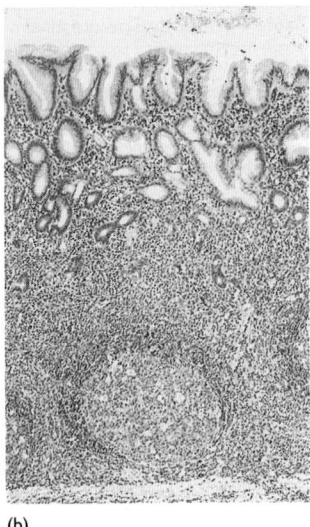

(a)   (b)

Fig. 1 (a) Peyer's patch comprising a B-cell follicle surrounded by a mantle zone external to which is the marginal zone. There are collections of small B lymphocytes within the dome epithelium. (b) Gastric MALT lymphoma. The tumour cells surround the reactive B-cell follicle in the marginal zone and invade gastric glands to form lymphoepithelial lesions. The overall structure is similar to the Peyer's patch.

zone. The infiltrate extends into the surrounding tissue and invades individual gastric glands to form characteristic lymphoepithelial lesions (Fig. 2). Although the term centrocyte-like is most commonly used to describe the cells of MALT lymphoma, their cytological characteristics are more variable and they may more closely resemble small lymphocytes or show the features of so-called monocytoid B-cells. Scattered transformed blasts are usually present and plasma-cell differentiation, characteristically maximal beneath the surface epithelium, is present in one-third of cases. The lymphoma cells may specifically colonize the reactive follicle centres in a way that may lead to an appearance closely resembling follicular lymphoma. Gastric MALT lymphoma is characteristically multifocal.

Biopsy appearances of gastric MALT lymphoma

There are many pitfalls in making the diagnosis of MALT lymphoma in small endoscopic biopsies. Amongst these are the retrieval of inadequate tissue, the presence of predominantly submucosal lymphoma, and the

presence of cryptic foci of high-grade lymphoma or an associated adenocarcinoma. The differential diagnosis between MALT lymphoma and florid *H. pylori*-associated chronic gastritis (follicular gastritis) can be especially difficult. Molecular evidence of B-cell monoclonality is also helpful, but a diagnosis of lymphoma should never be made unless the histological criteria are fulfilled.

Dissemination to lymph nodes and other sites

Most gastric MALT lymphomas are at clinical stage 1$_E$ at the time of diagnosis, but approximately 20 per cent have spread to the gastric lymph nodes or beyond. The more common distal sites include the small intestine, spleen, and bone marrow. In both lymph nodes and spleen the lymphomatous infiltrate tends to concentrate in the marginal zone.

The phenotype and genotype of gastric MALT lymphoma

The B-cells of MALT lymphoma express surface and, to a lesser extent, cytoplasmic immunoglobulin (usually IgM), which shows light-chain restriction. The cells express mature B-cell antigens including CD21 and CD35. They are CD5- and CD10-negative. This phenotype is homologous with that of marginal zone B cells, which are now acknowledged as the normal-cell counterpart. Various cytogenetic abnormalities have been described in MALT lymphomas, including trisomy 3, t(1;14) and t(11;18). The immunoglobulin (**Ig**) genes are mutated with ongoing mutations. Detection of monoclonal Ig gene rearrangement by Southern blotting or, more usually by the polymerase chain reaction (**PCR**), can assist in making the diagnosis of lymphoma in gastric biopsies, but caution is required since PCR evidence of monoclonality has been reported in biopsies from cases of florid *H. pylori*-associated gastritis.

High-grade transformation of gastric MALT lymphoma

Transformation of low- to high-grade MALT lymphoma is heralded by the emergence of increased numbers of transformed blast cells, which eventually form sheets or clusters (Fig. 3) and finally grow to confluence effacing any trace of the preceding low-grade tumour. This gives rise to difficulty both in grading some MALT lymphomas and in classifying large B-cell lymphomas of the stomach and other parts of the gastrointestinal tract. Those large-cell lymphomas in which no MALT component is evident are best classified as diffuse large B-cell lymphoma without reference to MALT.

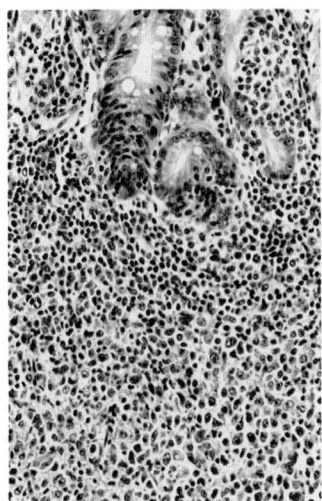

Fig. 2 Detail of the neoplastic infiltrate in a gastric MALT lymphoma showing 'centrocyte-like' cells invading gastric glands to form lymphoepithelial lesions (top left and bottom right).

Fig. 3 MALT lymphoma showing transformation from low-grade (small cell) histology (upper half of figure) to high-grade (large cell) lymphoma (bottom half of figure).

The clinical behaviour of gastric MALT lymphoma

In comparison with nodal low-grade B-cell lymphomas, such as follicular lymphoma, which, at the time of diagnosis are characteristically at an advanced stage, MALT lymphoma is usually at stage I_E or II_E when diagnosed and is slow to disseminate. Hence low-grade MALT lymphomas respond favourably to therapy and there is an excellent overall survival approximating 90 per cent at 10 years. The survival for cases in which there is evidence of high-grade transformation is significantly worse, 45 per cent at 10 years.

Helicobacter pylori and gastric MALT lymphoma

There are several lines of evidence that implicate *H. pylori* in the pathogenesis of gastric MALT lymphoma. These include the fact that normal gastric mucosa is devoid of organized lymphoid tissue which, however, accumulates as a consequence of *H. pylori* infection, and the observation that the organism can be detected in most cases. The epidemiological study of Parsonnet *et al.*, which showed that there was a significantly higher frequency of preceding *H. pylori* infection in patients with gastric lymphoma compared to matched controls with non-gastric lymphoma, added further support to this association. The evidence became even more compelling following *in vitro* studies, which showed that the cells of low-grade gastric MALT lymphoma respond to *H. pylori* antigens via a T-cell mediated mechanism. The clinical significance of these findings was first shown by Wotherspoon *et al.* who described the regression of gastric MALT lymphoma in patients following eradication of *H. pylori* using appropriate antibiotics. Subsequent studies have shown that eradication of *H. pylori* may result in striking regression of the lymphoma in approximately 75 per cent of cases. Deeply invasive lymphomas, those in which there are foci of high-grade transformation, and cases with t(11;18) are unlikely to respond.

Immunoproliferative small intestinal disease (IPSID)

This condition is a subtype of MALT lymphoma, which occurs most commonly in the Middle East, although small numbers of cases have been reported from elsewhere. It is a disease of young adults and usually presents with severe malabsorption. The histology of IPSID is similar to that of gastric MALT lymphoma, except that plasma-cell differentiation is much more prominent both in the intestine and mesenteric lymph nodes. These plasma cells synthesize large amounts of alpha heavy chain without light chain, which can be detected in the serum. Hence the term 'alpha chain disease' which was first used for this condition. IPSID remains localized to the small intestine for prolonged periods and patients usually die from the severe malabsorption. High-grade transformation may also occur.

In its early stages, IPSID may be responsive to broad-spectrum antibiotics, which presumably eradicate bacterial spp. from the intestinal lumen. Thus, there is a remarkable parallel with the relationship between *H. pylori* and gastric lymphoma, although no specific organism has yet been implicated in IPSID.

Enteropathy-associated T-cell lymphoma (EATL)

An association between malabsorption and intestinal lymphoma has long been recognized, and at first it was thought that the lymphoma was in some way responsible for the malabsorption. It subsequently became clear that the reverse is true, and that intestinal lymphoma, in common with a variety of other tumours, was a complication of the malabsorption, which was most likely due to coeliac disease (gluten-sensitive enteropathy). In 1978, Isaacson and Wright characterized the lymphoma associated with malabsorption as a single entity, namely a variant of malignant histiocytosis. Later, Isaacson *et al.* showed that both the phenotype and genotype of this lymphoma were those of T cells rather than histiocytes, hence the term 'enteropathy-associated T-cell lymphoma' (EATL) was coined to describe the disease.

Clinical features

EATL is characteristically a disease with an equal sex incidence that occurs in the sixth and seventh decades of life, although sporadic cases have been described in younger patients. The commonest presentation is the sudden onset of abdominal symptoms, usually with the reappearance of steatorrhoea, after a short (months to years) history of successfully treated adult coeliac disease. Some of the patients may have first presented with dermatitis herpetiformis. In a minority of cases there is a well-documented history of childhood coeliac disease. The lymphoma may also present as an abdominal emergency with no history of malabsorption, the features of coeliac disease are found in the uninvolved portion of the resected small intestine. Abdominal pain, weight loss, fever, finger clubbing, and an ichthyotic rash are all common presenting symptoms and signs. The lymphoma usually results in intestinal perforation or haemorrhage rather than obstruction.

Jejunal biopsy in patients with EATL usually shows villous atrophy with crypt hyperplasia, but it may show only minor changes that, in some cases, may be limited to an increase in intraepithelial lymphocytes. It is unusual to obtain lymphoma tissue in the biopsy, although evidence of active or healed ulcers is sometimes present.

Most patients with EATL are subjected to a laparotomy. The lymphoma may involve any segment of the small intestine but is more common in the jejunum where is occurs as multiple nodules, ulcers, and strictures or, less frequently, as a large mass. The small intestine may appear normal, although there is usually considerable enlargement of mesenteric lymph nodes.

The clinical course of EATL is very unfavourable, except in a minority of cases where resection of a localized tumour has been followed by long remission. In most cases the lymphoma involves multiple segments of intestine rendering resection impossible, or has already disseminated beyond the mesenteric lymph nodes and out of the abdomen.

Pathology

EALT may involve any part of the small intestine and, rarely, other parts of the gastrointestinal tract including the colon and stomach, but most cases arise in the jejunum. The tumour is usually, but not always, multifocal and forms ulcerating nodules or large masses that may be accompanied by benign-appearing ulcers and strictures. The mesentery is often infiltrated and mesenteric lymph nodes are commonly involved. There is sometimes remarkably little macroscopic evidence of disease in the intestine in contrast to mesenteric lymphadenopathy.

The histological features of EATL show great variation both between cases and within any single case. The tumour cells may be only slightly larger than normal small lymphocytes or resemble immunoblasts but, more usually, are strikingly pleomorphic (Fig. 4). Intraepithelial tumour cells may be prominent. Interpretation of the histology is further complicated by the heavy inflammatory component, often containing many eosinophils, and extensive necrosis, which, together, may mask the neoplastic infiltrate (Fig. 5). Granulomas may be present and cause confusion with Crohn's disease. Non-specific 'benign' ulcers are frequently present in EATL and microscopically these show only chronic inflammation (see below).

The histology of the small intestine remote from the site of the tumour is an important consideration in the diagnosis of EATL. In most cases the changes are identical with those of coeliac disease with villous atrophy with crypt hyperplasia, plasmacytosis of the lamina propria, and an increase in intraepithelial lymphocytes. The degree of intraepithelial lymphocytosis may be spectacular and so extreme as to virtually obscure the epithelial cells (Fig. 6). The lymphocytes are small, without neoplastic features, and in these extreme cases spill into the lamina propria where they may merge with the lymphomatous infiltrate.

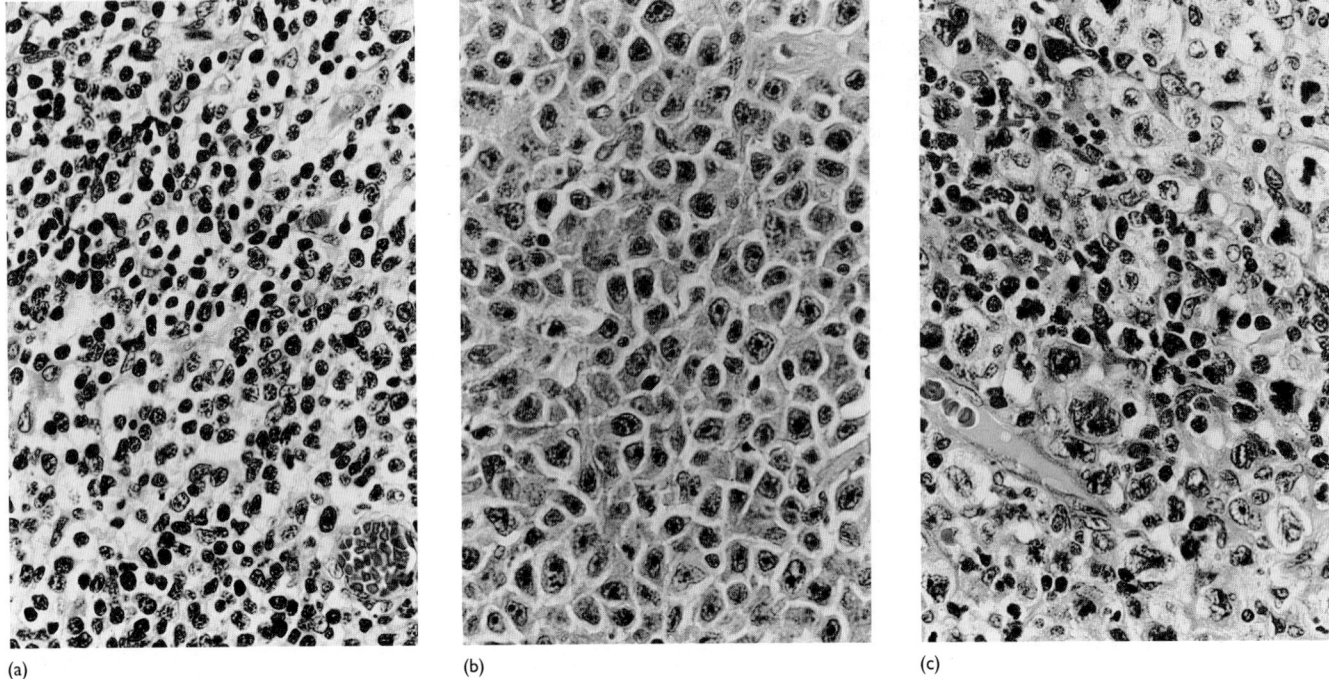

Fig. 4 Histological appearances of three different cases of EATL showing the cytological variability. In (a) the tumour is composed of small- to medium-sized lymphocytes; in (b) the tumour is composed of monomorphic, large immunoblasts; in (c) the tumour shows striking pleomorphism.

Episodes of ulceration followed by remission with healing may occur before the manifestation of EATL (so-called ulcerative jejunitis; see below). This can lead to a confusing appearance of the mucosa with scarring and distortion of mucosal architecture, and the appearance of cells of the ulcer-associated cell lineage.

Lymph node involvement

The mesenteric lymph nodes are commonly involved, and almost always show accompanying hyperplasia that may mask the malignant cells which may be present in remarkably small numbers. Selective necrosis of lymph nodes, often involving entire nodes, remote from the main lesion is a feature of some cases. The cause of this necrosis is obscure.

Immunophenotype and genotype

In most cases the cells are CD3+, CD7+, CD4−, CD8-, CD56-, CD103+ and contain cytotoxic granules. Although the cells are CD4/8-negative they do not express the γ/δ T-cell receptor. Occasionally the lymphoma cells fail to express CD3 and may be CD8+; more rarely they are CD56+. These properties suggest that EATL arises from intraepithelial T cells. No characteristic genotypic features have been described.

EATL and coeliac disease

There is strong evidence that the enteropathy in EATL is a consequence of coeliac disease. Its histology and distribution are those of coeliac disease,

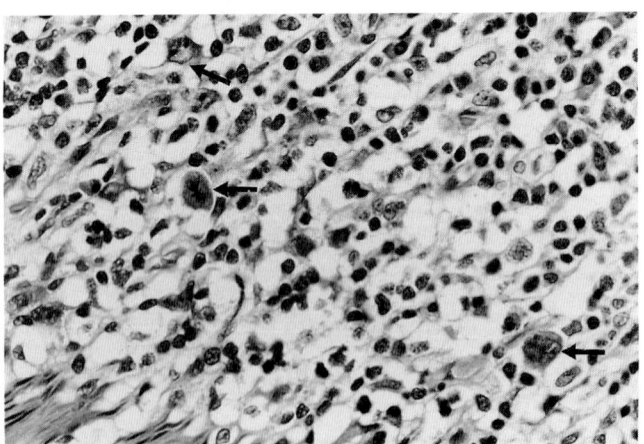

Fig. 5 A higher magnification of the ulcer base in which isolated malignant cells are evident (arrows).

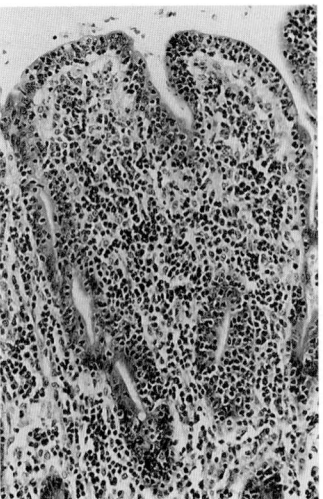

Fig. 6 Uninvolved mucosa from a case of EATL showing an extreme degree of intraepithelial lymphocytosis with spilling of lymphocytes into the lamina propria.

and the HLA type of patients with EATL and coeliac disease are identical. Moreover, gluten sensitivity has been demonstrated in numerous EATL patients and a gluten-free diet has been shown to protect against the development of lymphoma. There remains the dilemma posed by those cases with minimal or even absent enteropathy. These patients are thought to suffer from the so-called latent coeliac disease, which can be confirmed by the finding of a positive endomysial antibody test diagnostic of coeliac disease.

Refractory coeliac disease, chronic ulcerative jejunitis, and EATL

Patients with established coeliac disease who become resistant to a gluten-free diet are said to have developed refractory coeliac disease (refractory sprue). Patients with this disorder may present with gluten-resistant malabsorption *de novo*, and in these cases the diagnosis can be substantiated by the finding of endomysial antibodies. A subgroup of patients with refractory coeliac disease develops multiple intestinal ulcers, and this syndrome has been termed chronic ulcerative jejunitis. Patients with refractory coeliac disease, particularly those with ulcerative jejunitis, may progress to develop EATL. It has recently been shown that the intraepithelial lymphocytes in patients with refractory coeliac disease and ulcerative jejunitis comprise a monoclonal population with an abnormal immunophenotype (cCD3+, CD4–, CD8–) similar to that of EATL. Moreover, when these patients develop EATL there is clonal identity between the intraepithelial lymphocytes and the subsequent lymphoma. Interestingly, the intraepithelial lymphocytes in the 'non-lymphomatous' small intestinal mucosa of EATL likewise share the abnormal phenotype and clonal identity of the lymphoma. Thus, patients with refractory coeliac disease can be said to be suffering from a clonal T-cell disorder that is directly linked to EATL. The optimum treatment for this condition remains to be clarified.

Management

The treatment of EATL is most satisfactory in those cases with a localized tumour, when surgical excision may be followed by long remission or even cure. Most cases are multifocal or have already disseminated at diagnosis and require treatment appropriate for a high-grade, non-Hodgkin's lymphoma, which may include bone marrow autografting. This form of therapy is particularly hazardous in EATL because of the danger of intestinal perforation. Some cases of ulcerative jejunitis, even when small foci of lymphoma are present, may respond to steroids.

Further reading

MALT lymphoma

Akbulut H, *et al.* (1997). Five-year results of the treatment of 23 patients with immunoproliferative small intestinal disease: a Turkish experience. *Cancer* **80**, 8–14.

Isaacson PG, Norton AJ (1994). *Extranodal lymphomas.* Churchill Livingstone, Edinburgh.

Isaacson PG, Spencer J. (1987). Malignant lymphoma of mucosa associated lymphoid tissue. *Histopathology* **11**, 445–62.

Parsonnet J, *et al.* (1994). *Helicobacter pylori* infection and gastric lymphoma. *New England Journal of Medicine* **330**, 1267–71.

EATL

Bagdi E, *et al.* (1999). Mucosal intra-epithelial lymphocytes in enteropathy-associated T-cell lymphoma, ulcerative jejunitis, and refractory celiac disease constitute a neoplastic population. *Blood* **94**, 260–4.

Wright DH (1997). Enteropathy-associated T-cell lymphoma. In: Wotherspoon AC, ed. *Lymphoma, cancer surveys*, Vol. 30, pp. 249–61. Cold Spring Harbor Laboratory Press, Cold Spring Harbor.

14.9.5 Disaccharidase deficiency

T. M. Cox

Disaccharidases are specific glycosidases that are required for the complete assimilation of nearly all dietary carbohydrate apart from free glucose and fructose. The enzymes are found on the luminal surface of the small gut; their activity may be reduced by genetically determined deficiencies or acquired by generalized disease of the intestinal mucosa. Disaccharidase deficiency causes a characteristic syndrome of carbohydrate intolerance.

Physiology of carbohydrate digestion (Fig. 1)

Free disaccharides occur in the diet or are derived from the luminal hydrolysis of starch and glycogen by salivary and pancreatic α-amylase. Because amylase cannot hydrolyse the α-1,6 branching linkages and has little specificity for α-1,4 bonds adjacent to these points, the initial products of starch digestion are branched oligosaccharides containing at least one α-1,6 bond. Maltase-glucoamylase is a mucosal α-glucosidase that removes glucose moieties sequentially from the non-reducing terminus of linear oligosaccharides. α-Dextrinase (isomaltase) continues the hydrolysis of branched carbohydrate polymers by cleaving the α-1,6 glycosidic bonds of the limit dextrins that remain. α-Dextrinase is a component of the bifunctional enzyme complex, sucrase–isomaltase, the sucrase moiety of which hydrolyses sucrose into fructose and glucose. The disaccharides sucrose, lactose, and trehalose, like the α-dextrins, are poorly absorbed: to

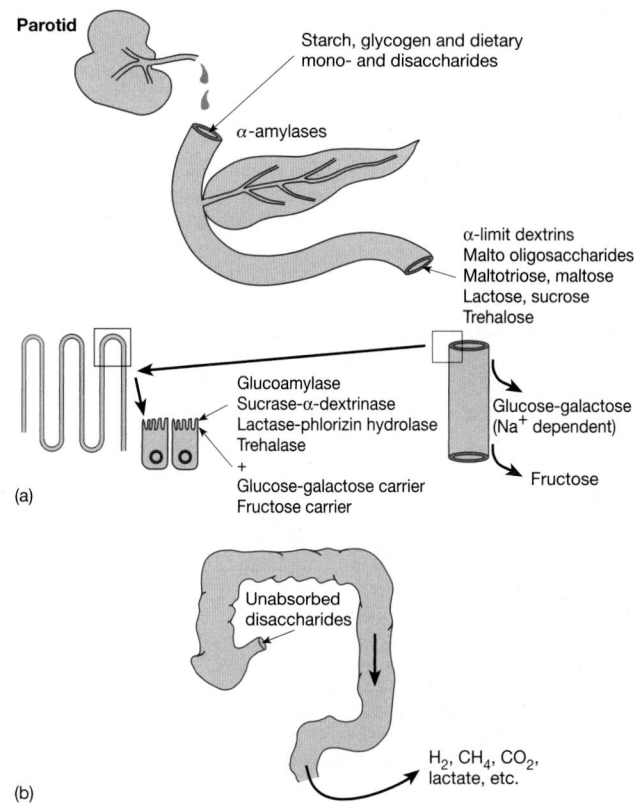

Fig. 1 Carbohydrate digestion and absorption.

be assimilated, they are also split into monosaccharides by glycosidases located on the brush-border membrane (sucrase, lactase, and trehalase). Mucosal disaccharidases are optimally active at pH 6.0 and are present principally in the duodenum and jejunum—activity also persists in the ileum but is absent in the colon.

Specific carriers in the microvilli for the transport of glucose and galactose, as well as fructose, mediate the uptake of monosaccharides released by the mucosal glycosidases—and absorption occurs rapidly. Active transport by the sodium-dependent glucose–galactose carrier is accompanied by the passive flux of water from the lumen. Maldigestion of osmotically active sugars thus leads to retention of fluid in the gut. For most carbohydrates, hydrolysis in the lumen and at the mucosal surface is sufficiently rapid to saturate the pathways for glucose and fructose transport. For lactose, however, the rate of hydrolysis, rather than glucose and galactose uptake by the mucosa, may become limiting. Hence the functional reserve of lactase in the human intestine is restricted and assimilation of lactose is often impaired in the early stages of mucosal disease.

Although the biosynthesis of surface disaccharidases continues throughout the life of the epithelium, the enzymes are only active in mature cells on the upper reaches of small-intestinal villi. Complete turnover of the enzyme molecules occurs several times during the lifespan of the mature enterocyte. Brush-border disaccharidases are complex glycoproteins that undergo proteolytic processing; extensive glycan modification in the Golgi apparatus occurs before insertion into the membrane. The mature enzymes are derived from large, single-chain polypeptides. The genetically determined mechanism by which lactase expression is normally reduced after infancy is not fully understood but in most individuals it appears to regulate transcriptional activity of the lactase gene. Unabsorbed carbohydrate resulting from the maldigestion of disaccharides is fermented by bacteria in the colon to short-chain organic acids, hydrogen, and methane. In these circumstances, ingestion of carbohydrate may cause pain by distension of the bowel with fluid and gas, accompanied by an irritant and watery diarrhoea.

Carbohydrate intolerance syndrome (Table 1)

Abdominal symptoms are usually noticed within an hour of the ingestion of foods containing the offending sugars. There is nausea, bloating, and distension of the abdomen accompanied by borborygmi and flatulence. Colicky pain precedes a watery diarrhoea, usually associated with flatus, and it may be explosive. Diarrhoea due to the maldigestion of carbohydrate can occur several hours after ingestion of the noxious food or drink. These symptoms may result from consumption of only a few grams of the offending sugar. Intestinal hurry aggravates fat malabsorption in disaccharidase deficiency and may obscure the underlying cause of the diarrhoea. Deficiency of particular disaccharidases is responsible for the dietary intolerance of specific foods and drinks: milk-containing products in the case of lactase deficiency; table sugar and starch in asucrasia; mushrooms (and

probably shellfish) in the rare trehalase deficiency. Identification of a cause-and-effect relationship between particular items and the intolerance syndrome is often impossible, given the ubiquity of sucrose and lactose in commercial foods.

Lactose intolerance

Most patients suffering from intolerance of lactose in the diet suffer either from lactase deficiency acquired as a result of intestinal disease, especially postinfective gastroenteritis in children, or as a result of genetically determined restriction of lactase expression.

Congenital lactase deficiency

A few infants have been reported in whom diarrhoea occurred after the first feed with breast milk and who responded completely to a lactose-free formula feed. This disorder is distinct from congenital glucose–galactose malabsorption, in which lactose exclusion alone is ineffective. Congenital lactose intolerance is associated with a severe inherited deficiency of mucosal lactase activity and, unlike the intolerance of lactose associated with prematurity or secondary to diffuse intestinal disease, remains lifelong. This syndrome leads to lactosuria due to the abnormal absorption of intact lactose, principally in the stomach; renal tubular acidosis and aminoaciduria have been recorded in this autosomal recessive disease that leads to vomiting, failure to thrive, and dehydration.

Lactase deficiency of prematurity

Unlike the other mucosal glycosidases, which appear early during fetal development, intestinal lactase activity is not fully expressed until after the 28th week of gestation and transient intolerance of milk feeds is common before this age. Abdominal distress due to gaseous distension and diarrhoea requires careful attention to the diet and fluid balance in premature infants.

Lactase restriction in children and adults

The capacity of the infant's intestine to digest lactose is retained into adult life by only a minority of individuals. Persistence of high intestinal lactase activity is an unusual state in adult mammals, and in humans is believed to have become prevalent in populations in which dairy culture was introduced about 10 000 years ago. Thus, tolerance of lactose in milk, dairy products, and many processed and ready-to-eat foods (Table 2) is found mainly in peoples of Northern European descent and those with a tradition of dairy farming. In about 5 per cent of Northern European adults, compared with more than 90 per cent in parts of Africa and Asia, there is a genetically determined and physiological decline in mucosal lactase activity after weaning. In most instances, reduction of mucosal lactose activity is associated with reduced synthesis of the precursor protein in the epithelial

---

Table 1 Carbohydrate intolerance syndromes due to deficiency of disaccharidases

Lactose intolerance
Congenital (inherited) lactase deficiency
Lactase restriction (genetically determined)
Lactase deficiency secondary to intestinal disease

Sucrose intolerance[*]
Congenital asucrasia (inherited)
Sucrase deficiency secondary to intestinal disease

Trehalose intolerance
Congenital atrehalasia

[*] Accompanied by reduced tolerance of starch.

Table 2 Foods containing lactose

Fresh, dried, skimmed, non-fat, and condensed milks
Cream
Yoghurt
Cheese
Processed meats and sausages
Sauces, stuffings, salad dressings
Custard powder
Canned and dried soups
Biscuits, cakes, cookies, pancakes, waffles, dried cereals
Confectionery
Frozen and canned fruits
Instant coffee
Lactose is also frequently used as a filler in powdered medicines and tablets

cells with apparently normal processing to the mature enzyme. The physiological decline in activity occurs between 3 and 5 years of age.

The element that determines lactase activity in adults acts in *cis* with the human lactase gene on chromosome 2q21. Recent studies of multiple polymorphic sites at this locus have identified a C/T polymorphism approximately 14 kb upstream of the gene that is tightly linked to the deficient/persistent lactase phenotype in several distinct populations. Homozygosity for the *C* allele at nucleotide −13910 is associated with adult lactase 'deficiency'—a finding consistent with the ancestral origin of lactase persistence. Although only low levels of lactase activity remain, this need be of no consequence when the consumption of dairy products is insignificant. Symptoms develop on exposure to excessive milk-and lactose-containing foods or medicines in late childhood or early adult life. The selective pressures that maintain this physiological reduction in mucosal lactase deficiency in childhood are unknown but the concept of 'lactase deficiency' in adults is difficult to justify, since lactase persistence is the least frequent variant. Nonetheless, with the increasing migration of peoples and their adoption of Western-style diets, this physiological loss of lactase activity is a prevalent cause of abdominal distress. A significant proportion of patients considered to have spastic colon, irritable bowel disease, or other 'functional' disturbances may prove to have lactase deficiency.

The speculative possibility arises that lactase-deficient subjects are at risk from osteoporosis in countries of the Northern hemisphere because of a dietary deficiency of calcium or vitamin D. A modest positive selection for the lactase persistence allele in Northern Europe would explain its present frequency if it arose at the time dairy farming was introduced. The relative lack of functional reserve of mucosal lactase activity also explains the frequency with which lactose malabsorption becomes manifest after partial gastrectomy and related procedures that enhance delivery of carbohydrate to the jejunum.

Diagnosis of lactose malabsorption

Intolerance of dietary carbohydrate caused by the maldigestion of lactose may be suspected from the dietary history of a patient typically complaining of abdominal pain, flatulence, and diarrhoea. Symptoms are often related to changes in social circumstances; they are frequently reported by Oriental immigrants to Western countries. The stool has an acidic pH (<6) and the osmolality of stool water is generally greater than 350 mosmol/kg due to the presence of lactate and other organic anions. Breath-hydrogen analysis is a useful confirmatory test. Hydrogen excretion determined by rebreathing 2 h after the ingestion of 50 g of lactose identifies patients with lactase deficiency diagnosed by enzymatic assay of jejunal mucosa. Other investigations, such as the lactose barium-meal examination and determination of blood glucose profile after oral challenge with lactose, are cumbersome and, because they give false-positive results, are now obsolete.

Secondary lactase deficiency

Lactase activity may be depressed by mucosal disease of the small intestine. This may occur transiently after infective gastroenteritis. It is particularly frequent in infants suffering from viral gastroenteritis, and continuing symptoms provoked by milk feeds can persist for days or some weeks. In infants, dehydration may develop rapidly, accompanied by prominent bloating; disacchariduria is found and acid, sour-smelling stools may be obvious. The symptoms resolve rapidly when dairy products are excluded from the diet. Decreased lactase activity also accompanies extensive and long-standing mucosal disease—the milk intolerance syndrome due to maldigestion may complicate coeliac disease, intestinal giardiasis, and Crohn's disease.

In secondary deficiencies of disaccharidases, because of the critical relationship between lactase activity and the rate of hydrolysis, intolerance of lactose predominates. However, the use of high-calorie supplements containing disaccharides other than lactose (especially maltose and sucrose) in patients with nutritional disturbances caused by intestinal disease may also cause the syndrome of carbohydrate maldigestion.

Sucrase–isomaltase (α-dextrinase) deficiency

This recessively inherited enzyme deficiency of the mucosal brush border is rare in all populations except the Inuit of Greenland, in whom the frequency of homozygotes is up to 10 per cent. Cetacean mammals also lack sucrase–isomaltase. Several defects of the human gene on chromosome 3q appear to be responsible; in some, there is aberrant glycosylation and the enzyme is inefficiently transported to the brush border. Substantial degradation of the abnormal polypeptide occurs within the epithelial cell.

Intolerance of sucrose is responsible for most of the symptoms, which develop as table sugar and sugar-containing foods are introduced during weaning. Intolerance of starch is less prominent because the osmotic contribution of the larger α-dextrin molecules that remain unsplit in the gut lumen is less. However, ingestion of large, starchy meals may induce cramping discomfort, flatulence, and diarrhoea. Whilst taking a normal diet, patients with deficiency of sucrase–isomaltase have persistent diarrhoea with the passage of acid and frothy stools containing increased concentrations of lactate.

The diagnosis may be suspected on the basis of the history of diarrhoea at weaning and on the character of the stools. Differentiation from coeliac disease, cow's milk allergy, infective or postinfective gastroenteritis, pancreatic failure, and disaccharide intolerance syndromes in relation to other inflammatory disease of the bowel is important, and biopsy of the jejunal mucosa for enzymatic assay and histological examination should be considered. In inherited sucrase–isomaltase deficiency, these activities are selectively reduced to less than 10 per cent of control values in histologically normal mucosa. Hydrogen breath tests after ingestion of sucrose and isomaltose may also prove to be useful in diagnosis, but experience is limited.

Trehalase deficiency

A few patients have been reported with mushroom intolerance due to the absence of mucosal trehalase. Trehalase is a brush-border α-glycosidase that cleaves the unusual 1α–1α bond of trehalase into its component glucose moieties. Trehalose is found in the haemolymph of arthropods and in fungi, so that intolerance of crustacean shellfish as well as mushrooms in the diet might be expected. Given that intolerance of edible fungi is not uncommon, trehalase deficiency may prove to be more frequent than previously supposed. Trehalase deficiency has also been reported to occur in 10 to 15 per cent of Greenland Inuit but the functional significance of this is unknown.

Treatment

Dietary exclusion of the offending sugar is the best method of preventing symptoms in individuals with primary or acquired disaccharidase deficiency. Symptoms recur as soon as excessive lactose or sucrose is reintroduced and advice from a professional dietitian may be needed to avoid indiscretions. In hypolactasia, complete elimination is not usually required, as lactase deficiency is rarely absolute; nevertheless, if symptoms persist there are many potential sources of lactose that warrant investigation (see Table 2).

An early, alternative method for preventing symptoms in lactose malabsorbers was the use of β-galactosidases obtained from yeast or other microorganisms. These enzymes were added to dairy products before consumption and often changed the taste. In the United States, β-galactosidase has been produced commercially from yeast ('LactAid') and has been shown to reduce symptoms as well as breath-hydrogen excretion in subjects with maldigestion of lactose. Similar studies have demonstrated the efficacy of β-galactosidase derived from *Aspergillus oryzae* ('Lactrase'), in children with late-onset intolerance of lactose. The enzymes are taken in tablet form immediately before challenge with lactose, but their cost, compared with dietary exclusion, may not be justified. In the future, microbial β-galactosidases might be used for food supplementation programmes in countries where lactose intolerance and nutritional deprivation in the adult population are widespread.

Complete absence of sucrase–isomaltase activity in most patients with sucrose intolerance together with the ubiquity of sucrose in modern diets complicates symptom management. Modest reduction of amylopectin-rich foods usually suffices to improve symptoms of starch intolerance but complete avoidance of sucrose-containing foods can be difficult especially in infants and young children. It has been reported that ingestion of dried brewer's yeast (containing invertase or sucrase but little lactase activity) after food is effective in patients with sucrase–isomaltase deficiency. However, dried yeast is rather unpalatable and not usually accepted by children. Recently, a high-potency liquid preparation of invertase used for the industrial manufacture of fructose from unrefined sugar cane juice ('Sacrosidase'; Universal Foods Corporation), which is approved by the Food and Drug Administration of the United States, has been used in a double-blind, randomized, controlled trial in patients with sucrase–isomaltase deficiency. The agent was found to be safe, acceptable, and effective for the treatment of all the associated symptoms and signs of this disease in patients receiving a low-starch diet.

Further reading

Anonymous (1992). Lactose intolerance. *Lancet* **338**, 663–4.

Clare H, Ruth M (1997). Phylogenetic analysis of the evolution of lactose digestion in adults. *Human Biology* **69**, 605–28.

Ennatah NS, *et al.* (2002). Identification of a variant associated with adult-type hypolactasia. *Nature Genetics* **30**, 233–7.

Gray GM (1975). Carbohydrate digestion and absorption. Rôle of the small intestine. *New England Journal of Medicine* **292**, 1225–30. [An informative and accessible review]

Hoskova A, *et al.* (1980). Severe lactose intolerance with lactosuria and vomiting. *Archives of Diseases in Childhood* **55**, 304–16.

King CE, Toskes PP (1983). The use of breath tests in the study of malabsorption. *Clinics in Gastroenterology* **12**, 591–610.

Madzarovova-Nohejlova J (1973). Trehalase deficiency in a family. *Gastroenterology* **65**, 130–3.

Medow MS, *et al.* (1990). β-Galactosidase tablets in the treatment of lactose intolerance in pediatrics. *American Journal of Diseases of Children* **144**, 1261–4. [Promising results with enzyme replacement therapy]

Simoons FJ (1978). The geographic hypothesis and lactose malabsorption. *American Journal of Digestive Diseases* **23**, 963–80.

Treem WR (1995). Congenital sucrase–isomaltase deficiency. *Journal of Pediatric Gastroenterology and Nutrition* **21**, 1–14.

Treem WR, *et al.* (1999). Sacrosidase therapy for congenital sucrase–isomaltase deficiency. *Journal of Pediatric Gastroenterology and Nutrition* **28**, 137–42.

Wang Y, *et al.* (1998). The genetically programmed down-regulation of lactase in children. *Gastroenterology* **114**, 1230–6.

14.9.6 Whipple's disease

H. J. F. Hodgson

Whipple's disease is an uncommon infection caused by the recently characterized actinomycete *Tropheryma whippelii*. The organism is widely distributed in tissues in affected individuals, and may cause disease in many systems. The condition is most commonly diagnosed when overt small intestinal disease occurs, leading to malabsorption, but systemic features such as arthralgia and fever may have been present for many years. The disease may also present with involvement of many other systems, including the brain and heart. Molecular techniques for identifying the organism

are increasing the frequency with which individuals with minimal or absent gastrointestinal disease are diagnosed, thus expanding the spectrum of manifestations of Whipple's disease. The condition responds well to antibiotics but may relapse. The organism is probably acquired as an enteric infection, because it has been identified in effluent samples from sewage plants.

Pathology and aetiology

Advanced or fatal cases of Whipple's disease predominantly show severe intestinal and intra-abdominal pathology. The presence of fatty deposits in the small intestine and mesenteric lymph nodes prompted Whipple to call the disease intestinal lipodystrophy. The small intestine is thick and oedematous, with stubby or absent villi and dilated lacteals (secondary lymphangiectasia reflecting obstructed lymph flow). The absorptive enterocyte layer is virtually normal, but the lamina propria is stuffed with macrophages containing foamy material which stains brilliant magenta with periodic acid-Schiff reagent (diastase resistant) (Fig. 1). There is little inflammation otherwise. There are fatty deposits, and occasionally granulomas, in the mesenteric nodes as well as the characteristic macrophages. Other organs are involved to a varying degree, with foamy macrophages in spleen, lymph nodes, central nervous system, liver, lung, heart, and joints. Valvular endocarditis and localized brain deposits account for two of the most severe forms of the disease.

Rod-shaped micro-organisms, the source of the periodic acid-Schiff-positive material, are identifiable at light and electron microscope level in affected tissues. After many decades of failure to identify these by conventional microbial culture methods, molecular characterization of the bacterial 16S ribosomal RNA gene in the tissues assigned the organism to a previously unrecognized class of actinomycetes. More recently human macrophages deactivated with anti-inflammatory cytokines and dexamethasone have allowed culture and passage of *Tropheryma whippelii*. The use of the polymerase chain reaction technique to identify sequences encoding the specific bacterial ribosomal RNA provides an invaluable diagnostic tool. The condition is an example of the value of molecular techniques in demonstrating that a disease process is infective in origin. The presence of the organism in sewage-exposed water suggests that infection occurs by invasion of the alimentary tract, and may explain the preponderance of

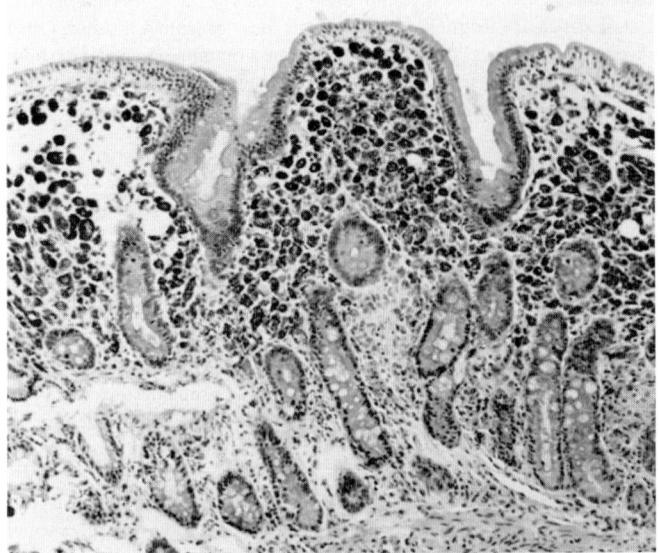

Fig. 1 Jejunal biopsy specimen from a 50-year-old man with Whipple's disease showing stunted villi and infiltration of the lamina propria with densely staining macrophages (periodic acid-Schiff stained, ×150).

small intestinal disease, with subsequent haematogenous or lymphatic dissemination. It remains unclear whether those who become infected have an underlying immunodeficiency, but host factors are probably relevant as there is evidence of diminished monocyte function persisting after successful treatment. A weak HLA B27 association has also been reported.

Demonstration of bacterial RNA-encoding sequences by means of the polymerase chain reaction now offers an alternative to the classical diagnostic techniques of biopsy and histology. However, some reports on saliva suggest the organism may reside as a commensal, emphasizing the need for clinical interpretation. Most patients continue to be diagnosed by the examination of the histology of the small intestine, reflecting the ease with which tissues can be obtained at routine upper gastrointestinal endoscopy. However, polymerase chain reaction positivity has been reported on peripheral blood, lymph nodes, synovial tissue, bone marrow, and even in faeces, and may yield positive results on small intestinal and other tissues in which characteristic histology cannot be identified. Application of diagnostic techniques based on the polymerase chain reaction to patients with arthritis, pyrexia of unknown origin, and other chronic undiagnosed conditions can identify cases in which small intestinal disease is not apparent, and this technique is likely to become widely used as it become available. The use of the polymerase chain reaction has suggested that intractable idiopathic thrombocytopenia, quadriparesis, isolated muscle weakness, and juvenile chronic arthritis may form part of the clinical spectrum of Whipple's disease.

Differential diagnosis

Histological appearances suggestive of Whipple's disease have been reported in AIDS patients affected with other organisms—atypical mycobacteria and rhodococci.

Clinical features and diagnosis

The condition is most frequently diagnosed in middle aged or elderly men but women and children may be affected. The typical patient is diagnosed with relatively advanced disease with malaise, weight loss, diarrhoea, and arthralgias, and on examination may show marked pigmentation, lymphadenopathy, anaemia, finger clubbing, hypotension, and oedema. Rarely gastrointestinal bleeding may also occur. In such cases, investigation of an obvious gastrointestinal complaint should quickly establish the diagnosis. Recognition is far more difficult if symptoms are limited to fever or arthritis, or another systemic manifestation, which may be present transiently or intermittently for many years before the disease is diagnosed. The arthritis is migratory, non-deforming, and seronegative, predominantly affecting peripheral joints and in some series affects up to 90 per cent of patients. Other early features include respiratory symptoms with pleurisy and pulmonary infiltrates, and pericarditis. Chylous or serous ascites, endocarditis, cardiac conduction defects, coronary arteritis, and neurological abnormalities may occur with progression of the condition. In a recent survey over 80 per cent of patients had gut disease at diagnosis but 15 per cent had no gastrointestinal disorder at any time. Joint symptoms were present at some time in 83 per cent of patients, 20 per cent had neurological disease, 17 per cent cardiovascular disease, and 15 per cent mucocutaneous manifestations (pigmentation or sarcoid-like plaques). The central nervous system manifestations are diverse and include depression, apathy, fits, and mycoclonus, and a variety of ocular manifestations including ophthalmoplegia, papilloedema, scotomata, pseudotumour, and uveitis. Meningitis and a hypothalamic syndrome with insomnia, hyperphagia, and polydipsia also occur. Oculomastatory myorhythmia is said to be diagnostic.

Supplementary investigations are of value in confirming the involvement of different organs, but are not diagnostic of the disease. Radiographs of the small intestine characteristically show dilatation. Ultrasonography and computed tomography of the abdomen may show lymphatic masses, and computed tomography or magnetic resonance imaging of the brain may show multiple lesions in the white matter and grey–white junction with characteristic appearances. The sedimentation rate is generally but not inevitably elevated and an anaemia due to folate or iron deficiency may be present. Eosinophilia and thrombocytosis may be apparent on blood films. Steatorrhoea, hypocalcaemia, vitamin deficiencies, and an elevated alkaline phosphatase occur with advanced gut disease, which may also give rise to hypoproteinaemia and a protein-losing enteropathy.

Treatment and prognosis

Whipple's disease progresses slowly, but unrecognized disease is eventually fatal. Antibiotic therapy is effective, although short-term corticosteroid therapy may occasionally be required in malnourished individuals to correct the metabolic and nutritional state. Administration of many different oral and parenteral antibiotics has been successful, including penicillin alone, penicillin plus streptomycin, tetracycline, and cotrimoxazole. A comparison of tetracycline versus cotrimoxazole (trimethoprine-sulphamethiazole) indicated superiority of the latter. Clinical improvement occurs within a few weeks, but prolonged treatment for at least a year is recommended. In particular it appears that the risk of a relapse with central nervous system manifestations is reduced if the initial regime involves drugs that pass the blood–brain barrier. The third-generation cephalosporin cefiximine has been reported to be effective in relapsing central nervous system Whipple's disease. A Herxheimer-like syndrome with fever and vasculitic manifestations has been reported at the start of treatment. The histological appearance of the gut mucosa returns to normal within a few months, although scattered periodic acid-Schiff-positive macrophages may persist for longer. Serial studies show that analysis of affected tissues by the polymerase chain reaction becomes negative in advance of histological improvement, and patients with clearance of tissues, documented by the polymerase chain reaction, appear to have a low risk of subsequent relapse. However, it is important to be aware of the possibility of relapse even after many years, especially when progressive central nervous system disease occurs in the absence of other systemic manifestations.

Further reading

Durand DV *et al.* (1997). Whipple disease. Clinical review of 52 cases. *Medicine Baltimore* **76**, 170–84.

Dutly F *et al.* (2000). *Tropheryma whippelii* DNA in saliva of patients without Whipple's disease. *Infection* **28**, 219–22.

Ectors NL *et al.* (1994). Whipple's disease: a histological, immunocytochemical, and electron microscopic study of the small intestinal epithelium. *Journal of Pathology* **172**, 73–9.

Gubler J *et al.* (1999). Whipple endocarditis without overt gastrointestinal disease *Annals of Internal Medicine* **131**, 112–16.

Louis ED *et al.* (1996). Diagnostic guidelines in central nervous system Whipple's disease *Annals of Neurology* **40**, 561–8.

Maizel H, Ruffin J, Dobbins W (1993). Whipple's disease: a review of 19 patients from one hospital and a review of the literature since 1950. *Medicine Baltimore* **72**, 343–55.

Marth T *et al.* (1997). Defects of monocyte interleukin 12 production and humoral immunity in Whipple's disease. *Gastroenterology* **113**, 442–8.

Misbah SA *et al.* (1997). Whipple's disease without malabsorption: new atypical features. *Quarterly Journal of Medicine* **90**, 765–72.

O'Duffy JD *et al.* (1999). Whipple's arthritis: direct detection of *Tropheryma whippelii* in synovial fluid and tissue. *Arthritis and Rheumatism* **42**, 812–17.

Playford RJ *et al.* (1992). Whipple's disease complicated by a retinal Jarisch–Herxheimer reaction. *Gut* **33**, 132–4.

Pron B *et al.* (1999). Diagnosis and follow-up of Whipple's disease by amplification of the 16S rRNA gene of *Tropheryma whippelii*. *European Journal of Clinical Microbiology and Infectious Diseases* **18**, 62–5.

Ramzan NN *et al.* (1997). Diagnosis and monitoring of Whipple disease by polymerase chain reaction. *Annals of Internals Medicine* **126**, 520–7.

Schoedon G *et al.* (1997). Deactivation of macrophages with IL4 is the key to the isolation of *Tropheryma whippelii*. *Journal of Infectious Diseases* **176**, 672–7.

Wilson K *et al.* (1991). Phylogeny of the Whipple's-disease-associated bacterium. *The Lancet* **338**, 474–5.

14.9.7 Effects of massive small bowel resection

R. J. Playford

Introduction

Large resections of the small bowel may cause multiple nutritional and other medical abnormalities, now commonly termed the 'short bowel syndrome'. More patients with this condition are surviving, due in part to improvements in anaesthetic and surgical techniques which have enabled patients previously considered to be inoperable to undergo radical procedures. The survivors present formidable medical problems, but scrupulous attention to their nutrition and general care, with the application of physiological principles, has improved their quality of life and independence.

Aetiology and prevention

The two main reasons why adults require massive intestinal resection are major vascular events involving the superior mesenteric artery, usually thrombosis or embolus, or multiple surgical resections of the small bowel in patients with Crohn's disease (regional ileitis). To reduce the number of those patients with Crohn's disease who will develop life-threatening consequences of recurrent disease in the residual intestine, it is imperative that the minimum amount of bowel is resected. Stricturoplasty, rather than resection, may be possible and multiple small segments of relatively normal intestine should be retained *in situ* and joined in series, rather than removed. Preservation of only a few additional centimetres of gut may be enough to allow the patient to be maintained on oral rather than parenteral nutrition.

The principal conditions requiring massive resection in children include segmental volvulus in the prenatal period and necrotizing enterocolitis postnatally. Rarer causes affecting all ages include trauma, retroperitoneal tumours, radiation enteritis, and strangulation, mainly resulting from adhesions.

Physiology

Although digestion and absorption of water, electrolytes, and nutrients occurs throughout the small intestine, there are regional differences. Regional functions of the jejunum include iron and folate absorption and disaccharide digestion and, in combination with the duodenum, the production of cholecystokinin and secretin.

The ileum is the principal site for absorption of vitamin B_{12} and bile salts and, in contrast to the jejunum, is capable of absorbing sodium against a steep gradient. It also plays a key role, in combination with the proximal colon, in mediating the 'ileal brake', in which intestinal transit and secretions are reduced when nutrients reach the terminal small bowel. Hormones, particularly peptide YY, probably mediate this phenomenon.

Factors, including adaptation, that influence the metabolic consequences of massive resection

The ability of the residual bowel to adapt after resection varies greatly between patients; it influences the development of symptoms and may determine the long-term requirement for parenteral nutrition. Four main factors influence the patient's ability to absorb nutrients:

(1) Extent and site resected. The length of the small intestine varies between individuals. As a general rule, patients who have an intact duodenum but less than 50 cm of additional small bowel if the colon is *in situ*, or less than 100 cm if the colon has been removed, will require long-term total parenteral nutrition. Conversely, a requirement for parenteral nutrition is unlikely if more than 25 per cent of the small bowel remains.

(2) Condition of the remaining intestine. The capacity of the residual bowel to adapt postoperatively is influenced by any underlying condition. Patients in which the residual bowel is damaged or abnormal due to conditions such as Crohn's disease or radiation enterocolitis are more likely to have metabolic disturbances.

(3) Presence of the ileocaecal valve. It is not unusual for part or all of the colon to be removed along with segments of small intestine. Removal of the ileocaecal valve has a major impact on subsequent clinical progress and troublesome watery diarrhoea that compounds malabsorption is frequent. Factors contributing to this include faster intestinal transit, possibly related to loss of the 'ileal brake' mechanism, and a much higher likelihood of bacterial overgrowth.

(4) Function of other digestive organs. Pancreatic hypofunction, resulting from malnutrition and reduced hormonal stimulation, may exacerbate fat malabsorption; this is sometimes compounded by gastric hypersecretion that inactivates pancreatic enzymes in the lumen.

Pathophysiology

Because regional differences in the function of the small intestine exist, the clinical sequelae of resection vary according to the site removed. Resection of most of the jejunum can usually be compensated for by the distal bowel, and the consequences of proximal resections are usually slight. Patients may experience iron and folic acid deficiency as well as lactose intolerance, resulting in abdominal bloating and watery diarrhoea.

Clinical problems are more likely to occur following large resections that include most of the ileum. Intractable (cholerheic) diarrhoea, often with steatorrhoea, and consequential metabolic abnormalities including vitamin B_{12} deficiency occur.

Diarrhoea

This is probably the most troubling symptom. Multiple factors are involved in its aetiology (Table 1):

- Transit time is decreased due to the reduced length of bowel and alteration in the control of its motility.

- Luminal osmolality is increased, partly due to reduced absorption of lactose and other carbohydrates, which are then metabolized by colonic bacteria. Severe metabolic (lactic) acidosis may develop—the increased 'anion gap' being due to the microbial generation of D-lactate.

- Disruption of the enterohepatic circulation of bile salts reduces the total body pool of bile salts. This is initially compensated for by a homeostatic upregulation of bile salt production by the liver. Increased

Table 1 Aetiology and therapy of diarrhoeal symptoms

Condition	Mechanism, effect	Potential therapy
Shortened bowel	Reduced time and surface for absorption	Antiperistaltic drugs
Lactose intolerance	Reduced mucosal surface area and lactase, increases luminal osmolality	Reduce dietary dairy products
Bile salt diarrhoea	Increased bile salts in colon stimulates fluid secretion	Bile salt sequestrants
Steatorrhoea	Bile salt deficiency, fatty acids stimulate colonic secretion and contractility, reducing transit time	Reduce fat intake, pancreatic supplements
Pancreatic hyposecretion	Malnutrition, exacerbates steatorrhea	Maintain nutritional support
Gastric hypersecretion	Increases gastric fluid secretion and inactivates pancreatic enzymes	Acid suppressants

delivery of bile salts into the colon, however, stimulates colonic adenylate cyclase activity, increasing colonic secretion of water and electrolytes, resulting in watery diarrhoea sometimes termed cholerheic diarrhoea.

- If most of the ileum has been removed, the compensatory upregulation of bile salt production may be insufficient to balance losses. This leads to decreased micelle formation in the lumen of the small bowel with a resultant reduction in absorption of water-insoluble fatty acids, causing the patient to have steatorrheic diarrhoea. Resection of the terminal 100 cm of ileum is typically associated with clinically significant malabsorption of bile salts. The presence of excess α-hydroxy fatty acids derived from bacterial metabolism in the colonic lumen stimulates adenylate cyclase, further increasing secretion of fluids and electrolytes.

- In massive intestinal resections, the reduced micellar solubilization of fat and consequential impairment of lipolysis is compounded by the loss of absorptive mucosa, thus aggravating the effects of maldigestion and fluid loss.

Stones

Gallstone formation is two to three times more common after ileal resection and may be of the cholesterol rich or pigment type. Reduced concentrations of bile salts within the bile due to depletion of the body pool of bile salts, in combination with gall bladder hypomotility, facilitate the formation of cholesterol crystals.

Renal stones (usually calcium oxalate) commonly result from increased absorption of oxalate and hyperoxaluria. The availability of free oxalate within the colon is increased by excessive complexation of calcium by fatty acids which normally promote formation of insoluble (non-absorbable) calcium oxalate. Although concentrations of bile salts in the small intestine may be reduced, the failure to reabsorb bile salts in the ileum increases luminal bile salts in the colon; this increases colonic permeability and further promotes oxalate absorption.

Gastric hypersecretion

This phenomenon occurs in some patients, although its severity tends to lessen over time. Hyperacidity may inactivate pancreatic enzymes by precipitating bile salts and lowering intraduodenal pH as in Zollinger–Ellison syndrome.

Nutritional status

Many patients undergoing resections will be malnourished preoperatively and energy consumption increases in the immediate postoperative period. If not appropriately managed, long-term protein-energy malnutrition, as well as life-threatening mineral and vitamin deficiencies develop.

Adaptation

Morphological and functional adaptive changes follow resection of the small intestine. The residual bowel undergoes mucosal hyperplasia and its capacity to absorb fluids and nutrients increases over a period of weeks or months. The molecular events that underly these changes are unclear but may include circulating trophic factors and growth factors present in pancreatic juice or secreted into the intestinal lumen. Early intervention is required to achieve maximal adaptation, and maintenance of a supply of luminal nutrients is a prerequisite for the adaptive changes. It is therefore important that luminal feeding is started as early as possible after surgery even if the patient also requires parenteral nutrition.

Management

Initial therapy

In the initial postoperative period, vigorous intravenous fluid and electrolyte replacement is required to prevent dehydration and to compensate for intestinal losses. Many patients will also require parenteral nutritional supplements while the residual bowel adapts. Ingestion of water may exacerbate diarrhoea and be counterproductive. The use of an oral iso-osmolar saline–glucose solution containing bicarbonate, similar to that used for the treatment of cholera, may often assist in reducing intravenous requirements without increasing intestinal fluid loss.

Nutrition

Oral nutrition, initially consisting of elemental or polymeric diets administered by nasogastric or enteral tube feeding, should ideally be started within the first few days of surgery. The introduction of luminal nutrition tends, however, to exacerbate the diarrhoea. Many high-calorie enteral supplements for use in malnourished patients who have little or no impairment of small intestinal function have a very high osmolality, thereby inducing catastrophic egress of luminal fluid and diarrhoea in patients with large resections. These preparations are to be used with great caution or avoided altogether in patients suffering the effects of massive bowel resections. Subsequently, small-volume, frequent, solid or semisolid meals with low fat and oxalate content should be introduced. Low-fat meals and supplements containing large quantities of medium-chain fatty acids tend to be unpalatable. Compliance of patients with dietary advice is therefore best if symptoms are used as a guide to the amount of fat that is included in the diet. Since much of the energy content of the ingested diet may well be lost in the stool, the daily intake of calories often has to be greater than expected. This is best provided in a complex form including glucose polymers and starch which have little osmotic effect in the lumen and are hydrolysed rapidly by brush-border hydrolases at the site of absorption. Lactose intolerance, seen particularly in patients following significant jejunal resections, may induce bloating and exacerbation of diarrhoea but usually responds to reduction in lactose-containing dairy products. Low-fibre diets are helpful in some patients although they may aggravate symptoms in others; treatment must be tailored to the individual. Patients should be encouraged to take multivitamin and mineral supplementation at levels two to five times the normal recommended daily requirements; vitamin B_{12} injections are required following terminal ileum resection. In all patients, regular long-term monitoring of fat-soluble vitamins (A, K, and D), vitamin B_{12}, folate, magnesium, zinc, and bone status is required.

In some patients, adequate fluid and nutritional balance cannot be maintained by the oral route alone and long-term total parenteral nutrition is needed. These patients should be encouraged to continue oral nutrition, for social and psychological reasons as well as to minimize the amount of parental nutrition required.

Drugs

Most patients will require antiperistaltic drugs to increase the time of contact between luminal contents and residual bowel. A step-wise approach should be used, starting with agents such as loperamide or codeine phosphate. Long-term administration of the more potent constipating, but potentially addictive, opiates should only be used in intractable cases. Since diarrhoea may be particularly troublesome in the initial postoperative period, liquid or occasionally intravenous formulations may be needed.

Administration of H₂-receptor antagonists or proton pump inhibitors may reduce diarrhoea and promote digestion, as well as prevent peptic ulceration, by decreasing gastric secretions and preventing inactivation of pancreatic enzymes. Cholerheic diarrhoeas may respond well to bile acid sequestrants such as cholestyramine but its use can worsen the fatty component of diarrhoea by exacerbating the deficiency of bile salts. Similarly, the use of long-acting somatostatin analogues can reduce gastrointestinal secretions and fluid loss but may exacerbate steatorrhea and formation of gallstones. In patients with marked steatorrhea who do not respond to restriction of fat intake, the addition of oral pancreatic enzyme supplements to food may assist lipolysis and improve digestion.

Bacterial overgrowth

Colonization of the small bowel by colonic or pathogenic bacteria results in exacerbation of diarrhoea, malabsorption, and nutritional deficiencies. Culture and analysis of small bowel aspirates is required for definitive diagnosis but is a moderately invasive procedure. Because results from many of the usual non-invasive tests, for example glucose or lactulose hydrogen breath tests, are abnormal in all patients after significant resection, empirical trials of antibiotics may be justified.

Surgical options

In patients with severe intractable diarrhoea further surgery should be considered, although it is usually of limited benefit. Although not in general clinical use, reversal of a small segment of small bowel can delay gut transit; however, if too long a segment is used, obstruction may occur. Longitudinal lengthening may also be of value, particularly in paediatric patients.

Small bowel transplantation is now available in a limited number of centres. Because of the high morbidity and mortality associated with transplantation, it is usually only offered to those patients who cannot be maintained on total parenteral nutrition. Patients who have undergone intestinal transplantation are particularly prone to infections and lymphoma. Problems with acute and chronic rejection are also common. Patients therefore require detailed counselling about the risks of any such procedure.

Future directions

Administration of gut trophic factors, such as glucagon-like peptide 2, hepatocyte growth factor, epidermal growth factor, and growth hormone (possibly in combination with glutamine supplements), during the early postoperative period may increase the rate and extent of mucosal adaptation that occurs in the intestine. In patients who prove not to adapt adequately, continuing advances in techniques for small bowel transplantation and in antirejection therapy offers future hope. In the longer term, advances in tissue engineering technology may allow intestinal mucosa to be obtained from humanized animal gut or to be reconstituted in culture from the patient's own residual bowel, thereby removing the problems of rejection and immunosuppression.

Further reading

Grand D (1999). Intestinal transplantation: 1997 report of the international registry. Intestinal Transplant Registry. *Transplantation* **67**, 1061–4. Review of the survival figures provided by 33 intestinal transplant programme centres.

Kim SS, Vacanti JP (1999). The current status of tissue engineering as potential therapy. *Seminars in Pediatric Surgery* **8**, 119–23.

Robinson MK, Ziegler TR, Wilmore DW (1999). Overview of intestinal adaptation and its stimulation. *European Journal of Pediatric Surgery* **9**, 200–6. Discusses the use of growth factors and dietary constituents to stimulate adaption.

14.9.8 Malabsorption syndromes in the tropics
V. I. Mathan

Introduction

Patients, in whom the 'digestive fire is weakened and food is expelled from the body without contributing to growth' were described in *Charaka-Samhita*, an ancient Indian treatise on medicine, compiled some time between the sixth and twelfth centuries BC. The clinical description in the section on '*Grahani Vyadhi*' or diseases of the organ of assimilation, clearly describes patients gradually wasting with chronic diarrhoea and loud borborygmi. Malabsorption of nutrients with its sequelae has therefore long been recognized as a clinical entity in some tropical regions.

Malabsorption is the result of the failure of intestinal function. It is multifactorial and may be due to failure in the luminal and mucosal phases of digestion and absorption, as well as of transport from the intestine. Detailed investigation of the individual patient is essential for diagnosing the causes of malabsorption.

In the context of the 'global village' of the third millennium, are there defined 'tropical' malabsorption syndromes? All the causes of nutrient malabsorption prevalent in temperate climates also occur in the tropics, but there are certain conditions: the majority being chronic enteric infections or infestations that are geographically limited to the tropics. Expatriates from other parts of the world to the tropics may have a higher susceptibility to some of these conditions.

Causes of malabsorption primarily prevalent in the tropics

The small intestinal and colonic mucosa of apparently healthy residents of many tropical countries, in comparison to residents of temperate-zone industrialized countries, show minor morphological and functional abnormalities. These changes, designated 'tropical enteropathy' and 'tropical colonopathy', are the normal background on which clinically significant malabsorption occurs.

Malabsorption in the tropics, as elsewhere, may have an identifiable underlying aetiology, when it is classified as secondary malabsorption. When no primary cause has yet been identified it is considered primary or idiopathic malabsorption (Table 1).

Table 1 Classification of tropical malabsorption syndromes

Secondary malabsorption	
Protozoal infections	*Giardia lamblia*
	Cryptosporidium parvum
	Isospora belli
	Enterocytozoon bieneusi
	Septata intestinalis
Helminthic infections	*Capillaria philippinensis*
	Strongyloides stercoralis
Bacterial infections	*Mycobacterium tuberculosis*
Viral infections	Human immunodeficiency virus
	Tropical (calcific) pancreatitis
	Immunoproliferative small intestinal disease (IPSID)
	Late-onset hypolactasia
Primary malabsorption	
Tropical sprue (idiopathic tropical malabsorption syndrome)	

The importance of a variety of protozoal infections, especially intracellular protozoans, was recognized in temperate-zone countries at the beginning of the AIDS epidemic, these organisms having been identified as opportunistic infections. In tropical countries these protozoa have been identified in symptomatic and asymptomatic immunocompetent subjects.

Capillaria philippinensis infestation has been reported in epidemics from The Philippines and as sporadic cases from other tropical countries including India. Hyperinfection with *Strongyloides stercoralis* can occur rarely. Both these helminths burrow into the mucosa and form tunnels.

Abdominal tuberculosis occurs much less frequently than pulmonary tuberculosis and is often secondary. Malabsorption in abdominal tuberculosis is the result of bacterial colonization of the small intestinal lumen secondary to strictures and extensive ulceration, or due to obstruction of the lymphatic outflow (*Tabes mesenterica*).

Progressive wasting in African people infected with the human immune deficiency virus (**HIV**) is known as 'slim disease', and is a consequence of malabsorption secondary to enteric opportunistic infections. There is some evidence to suggest that a primary HIV enteropathy can also contribute to malabsorption.

Calcific pancreatitis affecting young adults, particularly in economically disadvantaged sections of society, is another cause of malabsorption unique to the tropics.

Immunoproliferative small intestinal disease (**IPSID**) is due to the clonal expansion of immunocytes producing altered alpha heavy-chain immunoglobulin. This is also known as Mediterranean lymphoma and has been reported from several tropical countries. The characteristic histology in the premalignant stage is diagnostic and can be reversed by prolonged antibiotic therapy at this stage. Once malignant transformation has occurred the treatment is as for other lymphomas, but the prognosis is guarded.

In many tropical regions, particularly south and south-east Asia, the high lactase activity in the intestinal epithelium in the neonates declines rapidly after weaning. Since most adults in such countries do not regularly consume milk or lactose in their diets, this abnormality is of relatively small significance. The use of fermented milk and milk products (for example, yoghurt) can ensure that milk-based nutritional supplementation is still possible in such populations.

Malabsorption, or increased secretion, is an invariable part of all acute diarrhoeal infections. These episodes, most frequent in children, are of short duration, usually a few days. A small proportion of infants and young children have diarrhoea that persists for longer than 2 weeks following an acute episode. This persistent diarrhoea syndrome, seldom if ever seen in adolescents and adults, is also not considered as one of the malabsorption syndromes.

The concept of a 'postinfective malabsorption state' associated with the presence of a mixed bacterial flora in the small intestine has been postulated to explain, in particular, the persistent diarrhoea and malabsorption reported in many European travellers to the Indian subcontinent. By extension, it has been suggested that the syndrome of primary malabsorption in the tropics, tropical sprue, is only another form of postinfective malabsorption. Several factors contradict this assumption. Significant bacterial colonization of the small intestine has been found in apparently healthy asymptomatic adults resident in the tropics. Detailed investigation of many overland travellers from Europe to the Indian subcontinent identified several of the infections described earlier as the cause of persistent malabsorption, along with an altered luminal bacterial flora. The epidemiology of tropical sprue is distinctly different from that of acute infectious diarrhoea. Detailed clinical and laboratory investigations of adults and children in over 20 epidemics of acute diarrhoea, studied in south India, identified no single case of persistent malabsorption, other than the background prevalence of tropical enteropathy. There are also well-documented instances of expatriates from Europe who developed a primary malabsorption syndrome many years after their return to temperate climes. A careful analysis of the available literature therefore suggests that significant persistent and symptomatic malabsorption following acute enteric infectious diarrhoea is a rare event in the tropics.

When patients with conditions that can give rise to secondary malabsorption unique to the tropics or elsewhere are excluded, a group remain who have chronic diarrhoea, malabsorption, and its nutritional sequelae. Such patients are relatively rare in temperate climates, but they are frequently encountered in areas such as southern India and the Caribbean islands. This primary or idiopathic malabsorption syndrome has been called 'tropical sprue'. Tropical sprue occurs on the background of tropical enteropathy in the indigenous population of these regions.

Tropical enteropathy

The intestinal mucosal morphology of germfree and conventionally reared, litter-mate, rats is different; the latter having shorter villi, higher crypts, and increased mononuclear cells infiltrating the lamina propria and epithelium. These differences are attributed to the modulating effect of the microbial flora in the intestinal lumen of the conventionally reared litter-mates.

Similar morphological differences are found between the jejunal mucosa of apparently healthy asymptomatic individuals living in temperate-zone industrialized countries and those in tropical preindustrialized countries. The morphological features of this tropical enteropathy are characterized by the replacement of finger- and tongue-shaped villi by broader structures in the upper small intestine, reduction in the height of villi with an increase in crypt thickness, and an increased infiltration by mononuclear cells in the lamina propria and the epithelium. Similar mucosal morphological changes have also been shown to occur in the large intestine.

The morphology of fetal intestinal mucosa is identical in both geographical regions, the earliest differences appearing shortly after birth. The morphological changes are not apparent in biopsies from residents of Singapore—although this is a tropical country, it has standards of environmental hygiene and nutrition that equal those in temperate-zone industrialized countries. People expatriated from temperate countries to tropical countries develop these mucosal morphological changes over time. Even if expatriates from tropical countries living in a temperate zone continue to ingest a diet similar to that in their original home, they eventually revert to having a temperate-zone morphology. The evidence therefore suggests that the morphological alteration in the small intestine of residents of tropical countries is not a result of climatic differences, but is probably a reflection of an adaptation to environmental factors. *In vitro* organ culture studies have shown a slightly accelerated cell turnover in the jejunal mucosa of people living in the tropics, further supporting an adaptive response as the basis for the change.

Extensive bacterial colonization of the upper small intestinal lumen and mucosa, in apparently healthy adults, by aerobic and anaerobic bacteria, has been documented in studies from southern India. There is also circulation of enteric pathogens in asymptomatic individuals. It is also known that the first dose of oral immunization agents to enteric pathogens usually results in a secondary response, even in children as young as 2-years old living in the tropics. There is no evidence that the macronutrient deficiency widely prevalent in many tropical countries influences intestinal structure or function. No such information is available regarding micronutrient deficiencies. Conceptually, it may be useful to categorize 'specific pathogen-free' populations (temperate zone) and 'conventional' populations (tropical)!

Minor abnormalities in absorption can also be demonstrated in these healthy subjects, with xylose malabsorption in 40 per cent, mild steatorrhoea in 10 per cent, and vitamin B_{12} malabsorption in 3 per cent. The overall absorption of calories is reduced by about 5 per cent, while the colonic bacterial mass is increased. Colonic salvage of unabsorbed calories is thereby reduced. There is no evidence that these changes in the lining epithelium of the intestinal tract, a primary barrier between the internal and external environment of the body, significantly affects the health of these 'conventional' populations. However, the reduction in overall caloric absorption can raise the question as to whether the absence of tropical enteropathy can increase the effective availability of food without an increase in supply.

Tropical sprue

Definition

This primary (idiopathic) malabsorption syndrome affecting residents of, or visitors to, certain tropical regions, with characteristic enterocyte damage, is usually associated with chronic diarrhoea and the nutritional sequelae of persisting malabsorption. The aetiology(ies) underlying this syndrome is not yet understood. There are differences in the presentation, epidemiology, and clinical course in different geographical regions and between expatriates to endemic regions and indigenous residents affected by the syndrome.

History

William Hillary described a chronic wasting diarrhoea in European expatriates in Barbados in 1759, probably the first description of the syndrome in the English literature. The disease apparently attained epidemic proportions 3 years after he arrived in Barbados. The syndrome in expatriates was well recognized by British and Dutch physicians in south and south-east Asia with expanding colonization. However, no cases were described from tropical Africa. Tropical sprue assumed epidemic proportions during the Second World War and was a major factor for repatriation from the Assam and Burma theatres of war. Indian troops were also affected. It was only in the postcolonial era, with the work of Baker and colleagues in southern India and of Klipstein in Puerto Rico and Haiti, that the extent of the problem of tropical sprue was defined in indigenous populations.

Epidemiology

Endemic cases in indigenous and expatriate residents and epidemics in troops and indigenous populations have both been described. Endemic tropical sprue is apparently geographically restricted to south and south-east Asia and the Caribbean islands other than Jamaica, with a few case reports from Central and South America and Sub-Saharan Africa. In fact, much of the literature up to the 1960s is limited to expatriate populations. In India, only two large medical institutions, with well-developed laboratory facilities, have reported detailed studies, suggesting that in marginally nourished indigenous populations many cases may be missed due to the poor availability of diagnostic facilities.

Apart from the reports during the Second World War, large epidemics have only been described from southern India. The first such reported epidemic in 1960–61 affected approximately 100 000 patients, with a 40 per cent case fatality. This was reflected in the unusual death rates in the North and South Arcot Districts of Madras state in the 1961 census of India. The last epidemic was detected in 1978. In all the epidemics, patients initially developed an apparent episode of acute diarrhoea accompanied by vomiting in about 30 per cent and fever in 25 per cent of cases. Significant malabsorption of fat, carbohydrate, and vitamin B_{12} was present even during the first week of illness and 50 per cent of those affected had diarrhoea for longer than 1 month. The epidemics evolved over a period of months to years: adults had a significantly higher attack rate and were affected earlier during the course of the epidemic. The epidemiological data suggested an infective aetiology, but no causal viral, bacterial, or parasitic agent could be found.

Clinical features

The patient with tropical sprue is usually an adult with a history of loose or watery stools lasting for several weeks or months and with symptoms and signs of nutritional deficiency. There is usually anorexia, a feeling of abdominal distension, and loud abnormal borborygmi. The signs of nutritional deficiency include pallor due to anaemia, angular stomatitis, glossitis, oedema, and the skin and hair changes of severe hypoproteinaemia. The prevalence of nutritional deficiency, measured by clinical or laboratory parameters, is higher in those patients with a longer duration of symptoms. In the epidemic situation the prevalence of nutritional deficiency in patients during the first month of illness was no different from that in the unaffected people in the same village. However, in patients affected in the epidemics persistent malabsorption begins during the first few days of illness. The diarrhoea can be severe enough to produce life-threatening dehydration: in the epidemics the early deaths were mainly due to fluid and electrolyte imbalance. These could be prevented by maintenance of hydration. As the disease progresses the sequelae of severe malnutrition and consequential acute infections, especially of the respiratory tract, contribute to mortality. The natural history of the illness shows periods of remission, relapses, and spontaneous recovery, which make an evaluation of specific therapy difficult. Although patients have been followed for up to 25 years in southern India, intestinal neoplasms have not developed.

Investigation

Investigation of these patients should confirm the presence of intestinal malabsorption, exclude conditions that can give rise to secondary malabsorption, and evaluate the nutritional sequelae of malabsorption (Table 2).

A simple faecal smear stained with a fat stain such as Sudan 3 can often detect fat globules and fatty acid crystals associated with steatorrhoea. The extent of tests for confirming the presence of malabsorption is determined by the availability of facilities, which in many tropical areas is still limited. Tests of xylose absorption should be interpreted in the light of xylose malabsorption as a part of tropical enteropathy in the particular community.

The exclusion of conditions that can give rise to secondary malabsorption is of importance since many of these conditions are amenable to therapy. The diagnosis of the syndrome of primary malabsorption is one of exclusion.

Evaluation of the nutritional sequelae of malabsorption, especially the presence of megaloblastic anaemia, provides useful benchmarks for appropriate nutritional rehabilitation.

Pathology and pathogenesis

The wide availability of peroral mucosal biopsies confirmed the report, as early as 1924, that the primary lesion in tropical sprue was in the small intestinal mucosa. Electron microscopic examination of jejunal mucosal biopsies confirmed the presence of damage to enterocytes in the crypt

Table 2 Investigation of a patient with tropical malabsorption syndrome

1.	**Confirmation of the presence and extent of malabsorption**
	Steatorrhoea
	D-Xylose absorption
	Vitamin B_{12} absorption
	Breath hydrogen or CO_2 estimation with stable isotopes and other tests of absorption
	depending on availability
2.	**Exclusion of conditions leading to secondary malabsorption**
	Faecal examination for parasites
	Small intestinal luminal fluid cultures to exclude bacterial overgrowth
	Careful radiological examination of the small and large bowel including small bowel enema
	Duodenal or jejunal mucosal biopsy
	Serum protein electrophoresis for heavy-chain abnormality
3.	**Evaluation of the sequelae of malabsorption**
	Haemoglobin, haematocrit, reticulocyte count
	Bone marrow morphology, when indicated
	Serum protein and albumin
	Serum electrolytes
	Vitamin B_{12} and folate
	Estimation of other micronutrients based on availability

(regenerative) and villous (functional) compartments. This damage can be demonstrated in the first weeks of illness in patients affected during epidemics. Accelerated cell turnover in the regenerative compartment and increased loss of enterocytes from the functional compartment was demonstrated by *in vitro* culture of jejunal mucosal biopsies labelled with tritiated thymidine. In fact these changes in the enterocyte lifecycle explain the observed mucosal architecture, which has often been called partial villous atrophy. In contrast to the situation in coeliac disease, where the initial damage to enterocytes occurs in the functional compartment and the crypts are hypertrophied with normal enterocytes, in tropical sprue the primary lesion appears to affect the regenerative compartment. These findings have only been confirmed in patients studied in southern India.

The mucosal lesion in tropical sprue is not confined to the small intestine, since functional and structural abnormalities have also been demonstrated in the stomach and the colon. Significant water malabsorption in the colon may contribute to the severity of diarrhoea.

An appreciation of regional differences in the patient profile is essential for understanding the pathology and pathogenesis. All patients have malabsorption, but vitamin B_{12} malabsorption is only found in about 70 per cent of patients in southern Indian, while it is almost invariable in expatriates from the temperate zones and in the Caribbean. In Haiti and Puerto Rico the observed seasonal incidence is ascribed to small intestinal colonization by toxin-producing coliforms, probably secondary to the consumption of rancid pork fat. In southern India, the extent and severity of small bowel colonization by enterotoxin-producing coliforms is no higher than in matched controls. Identification of one or more 'agents' that can damage the mucosal epithelial cells will enable a clearer understanding of these differences.

Treatment

Provision of symptomatic relief from diarrhoea, correction of fluid and electrolyte abnormalities and nutritional deficiencies, and attempts at spe-

cific curative measures are the cornerstone of treatment. Diarrhoea and abdominal distension can be helped by the judicious use of loperamide and dimethyl polysiloxane. Increasing the nutrient intake and providing therapeutic supplements such as vitamin B_{12} and folic acid, as indicated, is beneficial. However, specific therapy to cure the condition awaits understanding of its aetiology.

Empirical evidence from patients in the Caribbean and European expatriate community, indicates that folic acid can alleviate symptoms in cases of less than 2 months' duration. In patients with a longer duration of symptoms, the addition of oral tetracycline for up to 6 months leads to the restoration of normal intestinal absorption. In southern India, the results of therapy with vitamin B_{12}, folic acid, and tetracyclines were not so clear-cut and a few patients were resistant to all therapy. Nevertheless, the recommended management includes the use of all three of these therapeutic agents for up to 6 months.

Areas needing further research

Malabsorption syndromes occur in tropical regions and there are conditions that are unique to this geographical region. While the advent of HIV infection has created an added dimension, it is important to continue the search for agents that can directly damage the endoderm-derived epithelial cells. The public health significance of tropical sprue is probably declining, with the last reported epidemic occurring over 20 years ago and the improving nutritional status of many tropical populations enhancing their ability to compensate for mild to moderate degrees of intestinal malabsorption.

Nevertheless, understanding tropical sprue, a primary or idiopathic malabsorption syndrome of the tropics, continues to be an intriguing challenge.

Further reading

Baker SJ (1973). Geographical variation in the morphology of the small intestinal mucosa in apparently healthy individuals. *Pathology and Microbiology* **294**, 222–37.

Baker SJ, Mathan VI (1972). Tropical enteropathy and tropical sprue. *American Journal of Clinical Nutrition* **25**, 1047–55.

Manson-Bahr PH (1924). The morbid anatomy and pathology of sprue and their bearing upon aetiology. *Lancet* **1**, 1148–51.

Mathan M, Mathan VI, Baker SJ (1975). An electron-microscopic study of jejunal mucosal morphology in control subjects and patients with tropical sprue in southern India. *Gastroenterology* **68**, 17–32.

Mathan M, Ponniah J, Mathan VI (1986). Epithelial cell renewal and turnover and its relationship to the morphological abnormalities in the jejunal mucosa in tropical sprue. *Digestive Diseases and Sciences* **31**, 586–93.

Mathan M, *et al.* (1990). Ultrastructure of the jejunal mucosa in human immuno deficiency virus infection. *Journal of Pathology* **16**, 119–27.

Mathan VI (1988). Tropical sprue in southern India. *Transactions of the Royal Society of Tropical Medicine and Hygiene* **82**, 10–14.

Ramakrishna BS, Mathan VI (1982). Water and electrolyte absorption by the colon in tropical sprue. *Gut* **23**, 843–6.

The Wellcome Trust (1971). *Tropical sprue and megaloblastic anaemia*. Churchill Livingstone, London.

14.10 Crohn's disease

D. P. Jewell

Crohn's disease is a chronic inflammatory disease of the gastrointestinal tract, the cause of which remains unknown. It is characterized by a granulomatous inflammation affecting any part of the tract, frequently in discontinuity, and by the tendency to form fistulas.

History

The first clear description of the disease affecting the terminal ileum (regional ileitis) was given by Crohn, Ginzburg, and Oppenheimer in 1932. However, the disease certainly existed long before then and many of the early descriptions of ulcerative colitis would now be regarded as Crohn's disease. Dalziel, in 1913, described an inflammatory process of the ileum and colon consisting of ulceration, submucosal oedema, fibrosis, and mesenteric lymphadenopathy. He reported the presence of granulomas on microscopy but could find no evidence of tuberculosis. Similar cases were described in the 1920s by Moschowitz and Willensky.

After the description by Crohn and his colleagues, it was clearly recognized that the colon could also be involved and, on occasions, it could be the sole site of the disease. The disease therefore became known as regional enteritis or, preferably, Crohn's disease. Colonic disease is often referred to as Crohn's disease of the colon, Crohn's colitis, or granulomatous colitis.

Epidemiology

Crohn's disease is well recognized in Europe, Scandinavia, North America, and Australia but is rarely seen in India, tropical Africa, and South America. This may be largely due to the difficulty of diagnosing Crohn's disease in areas where intestinal tuberculosis is common and to the problems of long-term follow-up. However, it is now being recognized in India in specialist gastrointestinal units. The disease is about 10 times less common in Japan than in the West, but its prevalence in Japan appears to be increasing.

There has been a striking increase in the incidence and prevalence of Crohn's disease in Europe and Scandinavia since 1950 (Table 1). This is also shown by examining the annual discharge rates in England and Wales. For Crohn's disease, the rate rose from 2.8 per 100 000 in 1958 to 7.2 per 100 000 of the population in 1971, whereas the rate for ulcerative colitis during the same period was unchanged at 10 to 12 per 100 000. Recent studies in Scotland and in Stockholm have suggested that the incidence has begun to decline in adults, but there is a widespread belief that Crohn's disease is increasing in children, supported by studies in Scotland.

The reasons for the changing patterns of incidence are not clear. Much of the increased incidence is due to an increased frequency of colonic disease and it might be argued that this represents diagnostic transfer from ulcerative colitis to Crohn's disease. The annual discharge rates for England and Wales, quoted above, make this explanation unlikely. Whether similar changes in frequency have occurred in North America is uncertain, although the data available suggest that the incidence has probably not altered. It is possible that the changing incidence may result from an infective or environmental factor.

Crohn's disease occurs in all age groups but it is rare in early childhood and most commonly affects young adults. There is no marked sex difference, and no association with social class or occupation. There may be an increased incidence amongst Ashkenazi Jews, especially in the United States.

Genetics

Evidence for a genetic susceptibility to developing Crohn's disease is suggested by a much higher concordance in monozygotic twins (approximately 45 per cent) compared with dizygotic twins (approximately 15 per cent), and by the finding that 10 to 15 per cent of patients will have at least one other family member affected. The highest risk is between siblings (λs 20 to 25—this is a measure of relative risk), but there is still an increased risk of affected offspring (λs 15) if a parent is affected. However, given the low incidence of Crohn's disease, the absolute risk to family members if one individual develops the disease is still low. Within a multiply-affected family, there is a remarkable concordance with respect to disease type (most will also have Crohn's disease, although Crohn's disease and ulcerative colitis can occur in the same family) and disease behaviour. However, there is no clear mode of inheritance and recent linkage studies utilizing microsatellite markers to link disease to areas of the genome have suggested that multiple genes are involved. It seems likely that there are a variety of genes which render individuals susceptible to 'inflammatory bowel disease' but that other genes determine the type and behaviour of disease. Crohn's disease has been linked to a pericentromeric region of chromosome 16 in many different populations, thus providing strong evidence that there is a

Table 1 Incidence of Crohn's disease per 100 000 population

Aberdeen	1955–61	1.7
	1964–66	3.3
	1967–69	4.5
	1970–72	4.3
	1973–75	2.6
Cardiff	1934–70	1.1
	1971–77	4.6
Malmö	1958–65	3.5
	1966–73	6.0
Uppsala	1956–61	1.7
	1962–67	3.1
	1968–73	5.0
Stockholm	1955–59	1.5
	1960–64	2.2
	1965–69	3.6
	1970–74	4.5
	1975–79	4.1

relevant gene in this region. In 2001 this gene was identified as *NOD2*, encoding a protein which is an intracellular receptor for bacterial lipopolysaccharide. A number of point mutations and a frameshift mutation are found in up to 40 per cent of patients with ileal disease but are not associated with colonic Crohn's disease. Linkages to chromosomes 6 and 14 have also been replicated.

Aetiology

The cause of Crohn's disease is unknown but clearly involves an interplay between genetic and environmental factors. The latter include smoking and intestinal luminal factors. There is a relative risk of 4 to 6 for Crohn's disease in smokers compared with non-smokers, which is in striking contrast to the reverse association seen in ulcerative colitis. Whether smoking predisposes to Crohn's disease by altering mucosal blood flow, synthesis of mucus, or by an effect on endothelial cells is unknown. The role of luminal factors is suggested by the tendency of Crohn's colitis to heal if the colon is rendered non-functional by an ileostomy and by the effectiveness of an elemental diet for the treatment of active disease. Other mechanisms may contribute to the pathogenesis and include diet, infective agents, ischaemia, and immune mechanisms. Recent claims that the measles virus or the **MMR** (measles, mumps, rubella) vaccine might predispose to Crohn's disease later in life have not been confirmed by subsequent data. Likewise there are no confirmatory data that *Mycobacterium paratuberculosis* is involved in disease pathogenesis.

Diet

Several investigators have reported that patients with Crohn's disease have a higher intake of refined sugar than a control population or a matched group of patients with ulcerative colitis. In addition, patients with Crohn's disease may also have a reduced intake of fibre, especially that derived from fruit and vegetables. However, the significance of these changes is unclear, especially as a controlled trial was unable to show that a low-sugar, high-fibre diet had any effect on the cause of the disease over a 2-year period. Claims have been made that many patients will benefit from dietary exclusion determined by a period on an elimination diet followed by challenge with individual foods. This might suggest a role for dietary factors, but the long-term benefit of dietary exclusion is by no means proven. Elemental diets consisting of glucose and amino acids have been shown to have equal efficacy to prednisolone for treating active Crohn's disease, but whether this effect is mediated by influencing bacterial populations, by removing dietary antigens, or by some other mechanism is unknown.

Infective agents

Viruses, cell-wall deficient bacteria, and atypical mycobacteria have been claimed to be the cause of Crohn's disease. Most of these claims have been discredited but there is current interest in the role of *M. paratuberculosis* and measles virus.

M. paratuberculosis is the organism that causes Johne's disease in cattle and other farm animals. This resembles Crohn's disease in so far as it is a granulomatous inflammatory disorder of the intestine. Over the last 20 years, an atypical mycobacterium has been isolated from intestinal tissue of a few patients with Crohn's disease and most of the isolated organisms have been shown to be identical to *M. paratuberculosis* using DNA analysis. The organism is very slow growing and it has taken 1 to 2 years of culture in order to demonstrate it. The possibility that such an organism might be involved in the aetiology of the disease was strengthened by the detection of *M. paratuberculosis* DNA in intestinal tissue in about two-thirds of patients using a specific probe and amplification by the polymerase chain reaction. However, specific DNA for the organism was also detected in 10 per cent of control tissue and other investigators have been unable to detect specific DNA in any patient with Crohn's disease. Antituberculous therapy has not proved effective so far. Thus, it is still very uncertain whether *M. para-*

tuberculosis is an aetiological agent, whether it is responsible for causing disease in all or just a subgroup of patients, whether some of the findings are laboratory artefacts, or whether it is a secondary invader of inflamed tissue.

The initial reports linking measles virus or the MMR vaccine to the risk of developing Crohn's disease later in life have not been substantiated by other investigators. At best, the case for measles virus remains unproven.

Ischaemia

Marked abnormalities of mucosal arterioles have been detected in resected specimens of intestine affected by Crohn's disease by making resin casts of the arterial tree. Many of the small vessels have been shown to be thrombosed, but in a rather patchy distribution, suggesting that much of the inflammation may arise from multifocal infarction. However, as many cytokines and inflammatory mediators released during an immunological or inflammatory response damage endothelium, it is not possible to be sure whether these vascular changes represent a primary abnormality or are merely secondary to the inflammation. It seems more likely that they occur as a consequence of the inflammation but, nevertheless, they may still contribute to the pathogenesis of chronic inflammation.

Immune mechanisms

Patients with Crohn's disease usually have normal serum concentrations of immunoglobulins and complement components, although raised concentrations may occur in association with active disease. Neutrophil and monocyte functions, *in vitro*, show no defect, although inhibitors of cell motility are often present in the serum of patients with active disease. The absolute number of peripheral blood T lymphocytes may be reduced but the proportion of phenotypic subsets (CD4, CD8) remains unchanged.

Within the inflamed tissue, there is a marked increase of plasma cells, lymphocytes, macrophages, and neutrophils. As with ulcerative colitis, the increased immunoglobulin production is predominantly of the IgG isotype, but in Crohn's disease, there is a greater proportional increase in the IgG2 subclass compared with the IgG1 or IgG3 subclasses. Antibodies to bacterial antigens and autoantibodies to epithelial and neutrophil antigens are much less common than they are in patients with ulcerative colitis, but antibodies to *Saccharomyces cerevisiae* (baker's yeast) have been frequently reported, especially with small intestinal Crohn's disease.

T cells and macrophages in the lamina propria are activated, as shown by the increased expression of activation markers and also, in the case of macrophages, by functional assays. The possibility that chronic inflammation results because of a defect in immunoregulation has been explored in a variety of assays but no consistent defect has been described. However, some evidence suggests that there may be an impaired facility to induce antigen-specific suppressor cells; if this is confirmed, it might explain some of the immunological overactivity that is characteristic of the disease. Cellular activation results in the release of cytokines and inflammatory mediators, which will influence the nature of the inflammatory response. Crohn's disease may reflect a predominant T_{H1} response. The possibility that the course of the disease, whether fibrosing or fistulating, may be determined by the cytokine profile is an attractive but unproven hypothesis.

Pathology

Crohn's disease may occur anywhere in the gastrointestinal tract, although the most common pattern is an ileocolitis. The disease is often discontinuous, giving rise to the so-called skip lesions. Isolated involvement of the mouth, oesophagus, stomach, and anus is recognized but such cases are extremely rare. Macroscopically the bowel is thickened and frequently stenosed. The serosal surface may be inflamed and the mesentery becomes oedematous. The regional mesenteric nodes are usually enlarged. The earliest macroscopic lesion on the mucosal surface is an aphthoid ulcer—a small, superficial lesion often surrounded by hyperaemia. In areas of more severe disease, deep, fissuring ulcers occur in the oedematous and inflamed mucosa, giving rise to a cobblestone pattern. Long, serpiginous ulcers are a further characteristic feature. Strictures occur as a result of submucosal fibrosis and, because of serosal inflammation, the affected intestine may become adherent to adjacent loops of intestine or other structures (such as the bladder or vaginal vault) with the subsequent formation of fistulas.

Histologically, the inflammation is transmural and consists principally of lymphocytes, histiocytes (tissue macrophages), and plasma cells. Granulomas are found in only 65 per cent of patients and they occur more commonly the more distal the disease; that is, they are present in most cases with rectal disease but are much less common in ileal disease. The granulomas appear to be in the walls of either blood vessels or lymphatics. The mucosal architecture is well preserved despite heavy inflammation and, in the colon, goblet cells are usually present even though the glands are being infiltrated with inflammatory cells. Fissures, penetrating into the submucosa and lined with histiocytic cells, are frequently present.

Quantitative histological and enzyme studies have suggested that the whole of the gastrointestinal tract is abnormal in patients with Crohn's disease even though only one segment may be overtly involved at any one time.

Immunofluorescent and immunoperoxidase studies have shown a large increase in IgG- and IgM-containing cells with a smaller rise in IgA-containing cells. Even in quiescent disease, the IgG- and IgM-containing cells appear to be increased compared with the normal intestine.

Clinical features

The manifestations of Crohn's disease are protean and are partly determined by the anatomical location of the disease. The majority of patients complain of diarrhoea (70 to 90 per cent), abdominal pain (45 to 66 per cent), and weight loss (65 to 75 per cent). Fever is also common (30 to 49 per cent). Obstructive symptoms (colic, vomiting) are much more commonly associated with ileal disease than colonic Crohn's disease. Colonic disease causes rectal bleeding more commonly than ileal disease, but even so, it is present in only about 50 per cent of patients with Crohn's colitis. Colonic disease is also associated with perianal disease (in about one-third of patients) and with extraintestinal manifestations, which are not commonly seen when the disease is confined to the ileum. Symptoms of anaemia are common and usually occur as a result of iron deficiency from intestinal blood loss or, less frequently, from vitamin B_{12} or folate deficiency. Other features of malabsorption are infrequent, but in patients with extensive small-bowel disease, symptoms and signs of osteomalacia may occur and there may be a bleeding tendency secondary to vitamin K malabsorption. Nutritional deficiencies may also be present, for example deficiencies of magnesium, zinc, selenium, ascorbic acid, and the B vitamins, but these are uncommon and are usually only seen in patients with diffuse small-intestinal disease.

A few patients present with the clinical features of acute appendicitis but at operation they are found to have an acute terminal ileitis. Only a minority of these prove to be due to Crohn's disease. Diagnostic difficulties may also occur when the disease presents without gastrointestinal symptoms. These include patients presenting with fever, weight loss, and anaemia without diarrhoea or abdominal pain, and those with ileocaecal disease presenting with urinary frequency and dysuria due to ureteric involvement.

Physical examination may be normal but many patients will show evidence of anaemia. Glossitis and aphthous ulcers in the mouth, beaking or frank clubbing of the nails, evidence of weight loss, and a tachycardia are common features. Abdominal examination usually reveals tenderness over the affected bowel, which can often be felt to be thickened. An abdominal mass is frequently palpable when small-intestinal disease is present. Anal examination often shows the presence of fleshy skin tags, which have a characteristic violaceous hue. Anal fissures, perianal fistulas, and abscesses are particularly associated with colonic disease.

The extraintestinal manifestations of Crohn's disease are similar to those of ulcerative colitis. Table 2 lists those that are most frequently seen.

Complications

Patients with Crohn's disease can develop an acute dilatation of the bowel (defined as a colonic diameter of 5.5 cm or more on a plain radiograph), perforation, or massive haemorrhage, especially when the disease involves the colon. However, these complications occur less frequently than they do in ulcerative colitis. The more usual complications are intestinal obstruction due to strictures in the small or large intestine and fistulas. The latter may occur between other parts of the gastrointestinal tract (such as gastrocolic, enterocolic) or between the affected loop of intestine and the bladder or vagina. Pneumaturia, the passage of faeces in the urine, or a faecal vaginal discharge are cardinal features of the latter forms of fistula formation. The gross malabsorption that occurs with a gastrocolic or ileocolic fistula is largely due to bacterial overgrowth of the small intestine. External

Table 2 Extraintestinal manifestations of Crohn's disease

	Frequency (%)	Comment
Related to disease activity		
Aphthous ulceration	20	
Erythema nodosum	5–10	
Pyoderma gangrenosum	0.5	
Acute arthropathy	6–12	Large joints affected; transient, non-destructive
Eye complications:	3–10	
Conjunctivitis		
Episcleritis		
Uveitis		
Unrelated to disease activity		
Sacroiliitis	15–18	Usually asymptomatic; may be present in up to 50 per cent using isotope scanning; unrelated to HLA B27
Ankylosing spondylitis	2–6	75 per cent of patients have the HLA B27 phenotype
Liver disease:	5–6	
Primary sclerosing cholangitis		Rare and poorly documented in Crohn's disease
Gallstones	Very common	Due to malabsorption of bile salts from ileum
Chronic active hepatitis	2–3	
Cirrhosis	2–3	
Fatty change	6	Very common in ill patients requiring surgery
Amyloid, granulomas	Rare	

fistulas to the skin also occur, but this is usually secondary to surgical intervention. Crohn's disease affecting the terminal ileum or the right side of the colon may involve the right ureter, giving rise to frequency with a sterile pyuria, a frank urinary tract infection, or a ureteric stricture with subsequent hydronephrosis. Left-sided disease may occasionally involve the left ureter, but this is very uncommon. Hyperoxaluria and oxalate stones may be complications of ileal disease associated with steatorrhoea. The mechanism is currently thought to be due to binding of calcium to unabsorbed fat, leaving the oxalate free to be absorbed from the colon.

Carcinoma of the colon may complicate Crohn's colitis. The incidence is about 3 to 5 per cent, a frequency similar to that of colonic carcinoma associated with ulcerative colitis. The risk factors are not yet established, however, although histological dysplasia has been noted in some cases of Crohn's disease. Small-bowel carcinomas have been reported in association with ileal Crohn's disease.

Amyloid is another complication of Crohn's disease; it may occur within the bowel or systemically, for example in liver, spleen, and kidney. It usually occurs in patients with poorly controlled Crohn's disease complicated by complex fistulas and abscesses. If renal function is deteriorating, the affected bowel should be resected as the amyloid may then regress with concomitant improvement in renal function.

Radiological appearances

A plain radiograph of the abdomen should always be obtained in patients with severe disease, together with decubitus films. These are often normal but may show evidence of intestinal obstruction or suggest an inflammatory mass in the right iliac fossa. In acute Crohn's colitis, evidence of mucosal oedema and ulceration may be clearly seen on the plain films. This appearance could obviate the need for barium studies, which should, if possible, be avoided in the presence of severe, active disease. The plain film can also provide evidence of sacroiliitis or ankylosing spondylitis.

Examination of the oesophagus, stomach, and duodenum is best done endoscopically because the radiological appearances are often non-specific and biopsies are required for histological confirmation. The small intestine may be examined with a standard barium meal and follow through, but more information is obtained with the barium infusion technique (small-bowel enema, enteroclysis). After colonic preparation, a tube is passed until the tip lies just beyond the ligament of Treitz and a dilute barium suspension is infused (800 to 1200 ml). The earliest lesions are thickening of valvulae conniventes and small, discrete aphthoid ulcers. In more severe disease, cobblestoning, fissure ulcers, and thickening of the wall occur (Fig. 1). Longitudinal ulcers may also occur but these are uncommon. Areas of stenosis and dilatation may be present, and sinus tracts and fistulas may be demonstrated. Asymmetry of the bowel is often present, although this may be an unreliable sign. The abnormal segment of the intestine is usually well demarcated from the normal bowel.

Radiological examination of the colon is made with a double-contrast barium enema after a thorough but gentle preparation. Characteristically there is rectal sparing but the appearances of Crohn's colitis are otherwise similar to those described for the small intestine (Fig. 2). Table 3 lists the main features that differentiate the radiological appearances of Crohn's colitis from ulcerative colitis. The barium enema is a good means of showing internal fistulas and fistulas to other organs.

If fistulas to the surface are present, sinograms should be taken to delineate the anatomy.

CT scans may be helpful in detecting intra-abdominal abscesses and also thickened loops of intestine. Magnetic resonance scans are particularly useful for visualizing peranal and perirectal fistulas, which often migrate between and through the sphincters and arbonize through the levator muscles.

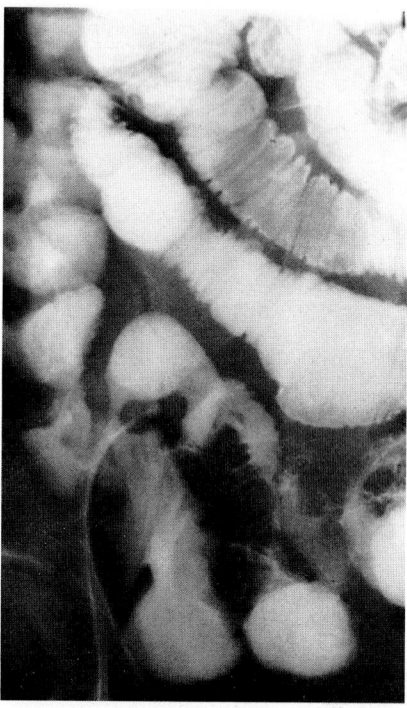

Fig. 1 Small-bowel enema demonstrating Crohn's disease of the terminal ileum with fissure ulcers, ileocaecal fistulas, and partial obstruction. (By courtesy of Dr D.J. Nolan.)

Endoscopy

Sigmoidoscopy and rectal biopsy should be done in all patients. The rectal mucosa is frequently normal but may show a granular proctitis and occasionally the typical appearances of Crohn's disease. Nevertheless, histological examination of a rectal biopsy specimen from a macroscopically normal rectum often shows an inflammatory infiltrate, which is often focal

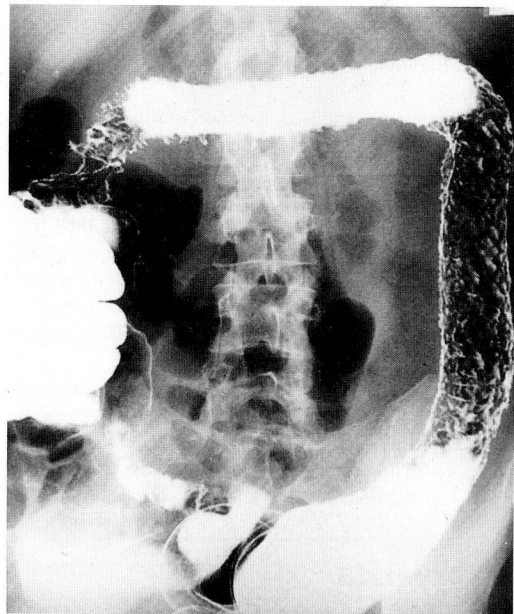

Fig. 2 Barium enema showing Crohn's disease of the colon and terminal ileum. Distal sigmoid, rectum, and a segment of ascending colon are normal. The diseased segments show loss of haustration, shortening, and fissure ulcers. (By courtesy of Dr D.J. Nolan.)

Table 3 Differential diagnosis of Crohn's disease and ulcerative colitis

	Crohn's disease	Ulcerative colitis
Clinical features		
Bloody diarrhoea	Less common	Common
Abdominal mass	Common	Rare
Perianal disease	Common	Less common
Malabsorption	Frequent (ileal disease)	Never
Radiological features		
Rectal involvement	Frequently spared	Invariable
Distribution	Segmental, discontinuous	Continuous
Mucosa	Cobblestones, fissure ulcers	Fine ulceration, 'double contour'
Strictures	Common	Rare
Fistulas	Frequent	Rare
Histological features		
Distribution	Transmural	Mucosal
Cellular infiltrate	Lymphocytes, plasma cells, macrophages	Lymphocytes, polymorphs, plasma cells, eosinophils
Glands	Gland preservation	Mucus depletion, gland destruction, crypt abscesses
Special features	Aphthoid ulcers, granulomas, histiocyte-lined fissures	None

and may contain granulomas. The indications for colonoscopy are: (i) to examine the colon and obtain biopsies in suspected cases where the barium enema is normal or equivocal; (ii) to obtain biopsies from strictures; (iii) to obtain biopsies when the differential diagnosis is in doubt; and (iv) to assess activity and extent of disease in symptomatic patients when there is little clinical evidence of activity. A further advantage of colonoscopy is that biopsies can often be obtained from the terminal ileum.

Endoscopically the earliest lesion of Crohn's disease is a small aphthoid ulcer surrounded by normal mucosa with a normal vascular pattern. This contrasts with the erythema and loss of vascular pattern seen in ulcerative colitis. In more severe disease the mucosa becomes oedematous and is penetrated by fissuring ulcers to give a cobblestone appearance. The ulcers are often linear and may eventually become confluent. A diffusely inflamed, granular, friable, and dark-red mucosa is more typical of ulcerative colitis, although discrete ulceration may occur in severe cases. Pseudopolyps and mucosal bridges occur in both diseases.

Multiple biopsies should be taken, even from apparently normal areas of mucosa, because granulomas may be present, which allows a precise diagnosis to be made.

Upper gastrointestinal endoscopy is not routinely required in these patients and is only indicated in the presence of appropriate symptoms or if abnormalities are noted on a barium meal. Although Crohn's disease of the stomach or duodenum may occur as an isolated phenomenon, most cases are associated with disease elsewhere in the gastrointestinal tract. Deep, longitudinal ulcers may occur in the stomach together with rugal hypertrophy and a cobblestone appearance. In the duodenum the major differential diagnosis is duodenal ulcer, but there is usually a 'cobblestone' mucosa surrounding the frank ulceration. Biopsies are usually helpful, although granulomas are found infrequently.

Examination of the small intestine is now possible using a push-type or sonde-type enteroscope (see Chapter 14.3.1). This is an expensive, lengthy procedure and, for these reasons, it is unlikely to become widely available. Nevertheless, it may be helpful for patients in whom the diagnosis is suspected but in whom the small-bowel enema is not diagnostic.

Laboratory data

Anaemia is common and is often due to mixed deficiencies. Iron deficiency from intestinal blood loss is the most common cause but serum folate and vitamin B_{12} concentrations may also be low. The blood film and mean corpuscular volume may therefore show microcytosis or macrocytosis. Serum ferritin is the best indicator of iron stores in those patients with chronic

disease. A neutrophil leucocytosis is usually, but not invariably, associated with active disease and there may also be a thrombocytosis. The total lymphocyte count and the absolute number of circulating T lymphocytes may be reduced.

Hypokalaemia is associated with severe diarrhoea and the plasma urea concentration is often low, reflecting a poor dietary intake of nitrogen. Serum albumin is reduced in the presence of active disease, largely due to down-regulation of albumin synthesis by cytokines such as interleukin 1 (**IL-1**), tumour necrosis factor, and IL-6, but studies using albumin labelled with chromium-51 often demonstrate a protein-losing enteropathy. Serum immunoglobulins are normal or mildly elevated and there may be a rise in the α_2-globulins. A low serum calcium, when corrected for albumin, is unusual unless there is extensive small-bowel disease, and a low urinary calcium is more likely to reflect a poor diet rather than osteomalacia. Liver function tests are frequently abnormal, usually consisting of mild elevations of the aspartate transaminase and alkaline phosphatase. Persistence of abnormal liver tests suggests associated liver disease and should be investigated by liver biopsy and visualization of the biliary tree. Patients with extensive ileal disease or with ileal stricture may have increased faecal fat excretion. This is usually secondary to bacterial overgrowth rather than loss of absorptive surface, and is compounded by the low circulating pool and increased excretion of bile salts, which is often present in patients with long-standing ileal disease. It is important not to miss magnesium, zinc, and selenium deficiencies, which are occasionally present.

Diagnosis

This may be delayed for several years. Intermittent abdominal symptoms and diarrhoea without systemic symptoms are often labelled as an irritable bowel syndrome. Weight loss, fever, and anaemia without gastrointestinal symptoms are another source of misdiagnosis. The diagnosis of Crohn's disease in children may be considerably delayed when it presents as failure to thrive or delayed puberty but without gastrointestinal symptoms.

Even when the clinical diagnosis seems sound, all patients must have: (i) stool examination to exclude pathogens; (ii) sigmoidoscopy and rectal biopsy—characteristic features (such as granuloma) may often be present in the biopsy specimen even when the mucosa is macroscopically normal; (iii) radiographs of the small and large intestine to confirm the diagnosis and establish the extent of the disease; and (iv) colonoscopy with multiple biopsies is indicated where the above investigations are equivocal or normal and there are strong clinical reasons for suspecting Crohn's disease.

Colonoscopy should also be done if the differential diagnosis is in doubt or if strictures are present.

Differential diagnosis

Few patients with an acute ileitis and a clinical picture of acute appendicitis subsequently develop Crohn's disease. Serological examination helps to diagnose those cases caused by yersinia; the aetiology of the remainder is unknown. The main differential diagnosis of ileal Crohn's disease is tuberculosis, especially when the disease occurs in patients from areas where intestinal tuberculosis is common. Laparoscopy may be helpful if serosal tubercles are present, as biopsies can be taken from them and cultured. Stool culture and circulating antibodies to mycobacteria are unhelpful. Colonoscopy with multiple biopsy specimens may be helpful. If genuine doubt exists, corticosteroid therapy for Crohn's disease must be covered with antituberculous therapy. Other differential diagnoses include abdominal lymphoma, α-chain disease, actinomycosis, amyloid, Behçet's disease, and carcinoma of the small bowel.

The major differential diagnosis of Crohn's colitis is ulcerative colitis (Table 3). Crohn's disease should also be considered in patients presenting with proctitis, as 30 per cent of patients with ileal Crohn's disease may have a proctitis and may present in this way. When a segmental colitis occurs, ischaemia, tuberculosis, and lymphoma have to be excluded. Young adults may present with an acute segmental colitis, which is self-limiting. The cause is unknown, although in women, oral contraceptives have been implicated. Crohn's disease can be overlooked on the barium enema when it occurs in association with severe diverticular disease.

As indicated above, Crohn's disease may have to be considered in the differential diagnosis of a fever with weight loss, malabsorption, and delayed development.

Assessment of activity

There is no satisfactory method of assessing activity of the disease and this poses a major clinical problem. Symptoms such as fever or continuing weight loss are obvious indicators, but severe disease can be present in the absence of any major symptom. Laboratory evidence of activity includes a reduced serum albumin, and a rise in acute-phase reactants (C-reactive protein, orosomucoid) and in the erythrocyte sedimentation rate. Recently, a number of activity indices have been developed in order to standardize assessment for the purpose of multicentre studies, two examples being the American Crohn's disease activity index and the Dutch activity index. However, they are mostly too complex for normal clinical use. Furthermore, they tend to measure different aspects of disease activity. At present it is worth remembering that disease activity can be assessed by the clinical picture (symptoms and signs), morphologically (for example by radiography or endoscopy), and by laboratory indices. Another technique for the assessment of activity is the use of indium-labelled neutrophils. The labelled cells preferentially migrate to inflamed mucosa and the increased uptake of isotope can be detected using a γ-camera (Fig. 3). Faecal excretion of the labelled cells can also be quantified and this has shown good correlation with the Crohn's disease activity index and albumin loss.

Labelling neutrophils with technetium-99 using hexamethyl propylene amine oxime (HMPAO) as a chelator is gradually replacing indium because it is easier, quicker, and less expensive. It appears to provide similar sensitivity and specificity but it cannot be used to assess faecal excretion of neutrophils.

Management

The management of Crohn's disease involves a team approach between physician and surgeon and includes nutritional support, medical therapy, and surgical treatment.

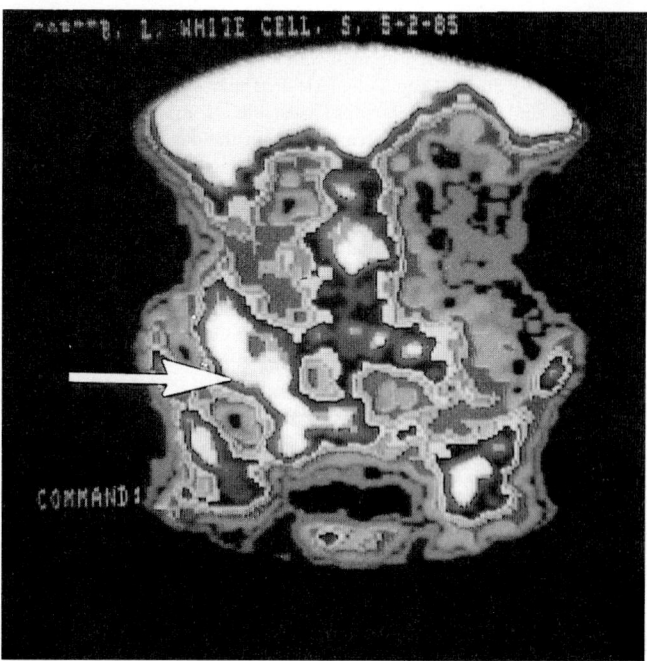

Fig. 3 A neutrophil scan labelled with indium-111 in a patient with active Crohn's disease. Active inflammation in distal ileal loops is well shown (arrow).

Nutritional support

For most patients, a well-balanced diet should be advised. A low-residue diet should be used for patients with strictures and a low-fat diet may be helpful for those with a steatorrhoea. Some centres claim good long-term results with elimination diets, but the value of this approach for all patients is far from proven. A lactose-free diet is obviously indicated for those with hypolactasia.

Iron and vitamin B_{12} deficiencies are common and need to be excluded. In patients with chronic active disease, the serum iron, binding capacity, and ferritin may all be low, making it difficult to know whether the anaemia is due to iron deficiency or to chronic inflammation. However, if the serum iron is less than 10 per cent of the iron-binding capacity it is reasonable to diagnose iron deficiency and treat accordingly. Many patients are intolerant of oral iron and for these a total-dose intravenous infusion is the best form of treatment. Patients with extensive small-intestinal disease may develop deficiencies of the fat-soluble vitamins (A, D, E, K). Deficiencies of folic acid and B vitamins may also occur because of poor dietary intake. Parenteral nutrition is often indicated for seriously ill patients who are being prepared for surgery or who have a short bowel syndrome.

Drug therapy

Active disease

In general, Crohn's disease is only treated if it is causing symptoms; there is no indication for treatment in asymptomatic patients. Active disease can usually be controlled with corticosteroids, the dose and route depending on the severity of the disease. Severe disease requires admission to hospital and treatment with intravenous prednisolone (60 to 80 mg daily) or hydrocortisone (400 mg daily), together with fluids and electrolytes. Most patients settle within 5 to 7 days and can then be given prednisolone orally (for example 40 mg daily). Patients with less severe disease can be treated with 20 to 40 mg of prednisolone daily. There is no defined duration of corticosteroid therapy but most patients will have made a good symptomatic response by 4 to 6 weeks; the dose can then be reduced over the next 3 to 6 weeks and finally stopped.

Active disease can also be treated with liquid diets. Elemental diets have been repeatedly shown to be as effective as prednisolone in controlling active Crohn's disease, but the major problem is one of compliance. Some patients intubate themselves at night with a fine-bore nasogastric tube and feed themselves during sleep. Polymeric diets may be as effective as elemental diets and are certainly more palatable. If an individual patient responds well and is willing to carry on with the diet, it should be continued until symptoms have settled and the laboratory indicators of inflammation have returned to normal. Experience then differs as to the course of the disease once normal food is introduced. Some data suggest that relapse occurs more rapidly than if remission has been achieved by the use of corticosteroids.

There is some evidence that antibiotics can be useful in treating active disease (for example metronidazole, ciprofloxacin, or clarithromycin), but the controlled trials are small and many are only published in abstract. However, they are often indicated to treat bacterial overgrowth, perianal sepsis, or abscesses associated with fistulas. Randomized controlled trials of antimycobacterial regimens have failed to confirm the optimism of anecdotal series.

The role of 5-aminosalicylic acid drugs for treating active disease is unclear. Using high doses of mesalazine (4 g daily), the initial trial showed benefit after 12 to 16 weeks but this has not been confirmed in subsequent trials. Meta-analysis of all trials shows no overall benefit compared with placebo.

Chronic active disease

There is good evidence from several trials, supported by meta-analysis, that azathoprine (2.0 to 2.5 mg/kg) or 6-mercaptopurine are effective treatment for steroid-dependent or steroid-resistant disease, although they act slowly and it may take up to 16 weeks before an effect is seen. Furthermore, both drugs are effective maintenance therapy in those patients who respond well. Retrospective studies suggest they maintain their effect over 4 to 5 years without inducing long-term side-effects. About 15 per cent of patients are unable to tolerate the drug (mostly because of gastrointestinal symptoms, myalgia, and occasionally hepatitis). Acute pancreatitis is rare. Bone marrow suppression is also rare and is confined to those who are homozygous for a deletion in the gene encoding the thiopurine methyl transferase enzyme (approximately 1 in 300 of the population). Interestingly, patients who develop nausea, diarrhoea, or myalgias on azathioprine are frequently able to tolerate 6-mercaptopurine. For patients failing to respond, or who are intolerant of these drugs, methotrexate may induce a response in two-thirds as shown by a clinical trial and by open series. In the trial, 25 mg of methotrexate by weekly intramuscular injection was used, but open series suggest a similar response when it is given orally. Recently, monoclonal antibodies to tumour necrosis factor have been developed. Infliximab is now licensed as a single infusion for chronic active disease unresponsive to steroids and immunosuppressants. It is an IgG1 chimeric antibody containing 75 per cent human immunoglobulin. A dose of 5 mg/kg by slow intravenous infusion over 2 h appears to give maximal response and this occurs in about 70 per cent of cases. Endoscopic healing can be shown but the response is usually temporary and, after a few months, patients begin to relapse. Side-effects are few (nausea, headaches, and rarely, infusion reactions can occur) but about 12 per cent of patients develop antibodies to double-stranded DNA, probably secondary to apoptosis induced by the antibody.

Maintenance of remission

There is no good maintenance therapy for Crohn's disease. The 5-aminosalicylic acid drugs have very little effect if remission has been induced by medical therapy, although high doses (3 g daily) can delay recurrence following surgical resection. However, eight such patients need to be treated to prevent one recurrence over a 5-year period. As described above, azathioprine and 6-mercaptopurine are effective long-term in steroid-dependent patients who make a good initial response to immunosuppression. Undoubtedly the best maintenance therapy is to stop patients smoking—that is associated with a more benign course and lower recurrence rates following surgical resection.

Osteoporosis

Many patients at the time of diagnosis have reduced bone density (chronic inflammation, poor nutrition) and this can be exacerbated subsequently if frequent courses of corticosteroids are required to control active disease. Dual energy X-ray absorptiometry (DEXA) scans should be obtained in patients with long-standing troublesome disease, and appropriate treatment begun (see Chapter 19.4).

Surgery

The majority of patients (70 to 80 per cent) will require at least one operation during the course of their disease. Indications for surgery include failure to respond to medical therapy, strictures causing mechanical obstruction, fistulas, and other complications such as abscess and perforation.

If surgery is required, the following principles apply. Resection should be limited to removing the most severely affected segment and an end-to-end anastomosis should be made, even if there is some inflammation in the tissue being anastomosed. Wide resections have not been shown to diminish the subsequent recurrence rate. Bypass procedures (such as ileotransverse colostomy) should not be done. If surgery is for internal fistulas, nutrition must be corrected, infection controlled, and active disease controlled with steroids before the operation. The anatomy of the fistulas must also be determined by sinograms or by CT scans or MRI. The fistula is excised together with the segment of affected intestine and the subsequent anastomosis is usually best protected with a temporary ileostomy. For colonic disease, the choice is a conservative operation of a split ileostomy or a proctocolectomy with terminal ileostomy. Colectomy with ileorectal anastomosis is associated with a high recurrence rate. Defunctioning the colonic disease with an ileostomy often allows the disease to settle and the patient's nutritional state to be restored. In Oxford, our practice is to reconnect after 12 to 18 months and the majority of patients then remain well. However, other clinicians claim a rapid relapse following restoration of continuity and will only use a split ileostomy as a means of getting patients fit for more radical surgery.

Perianal disease is common, both in ileal and colonic Crohn's disease. It may consist of simple fissures but, more frequently, consists of complex fistulas with abscess formation. Management has to include demonstration of the anatomy (e.g. a pelvic MRI scan), drainage of abscesses, control of infection and suppression of disease activity. The use of setons has been a major advance in allowing fistulas to heal by providing effective drainage and they can be kept in for months. Immunosuppression with thiopurines may allow some degree of healing but, recently, infliximab has been highly effective. In a randomized clinical trial, two-thirds of patients assigned to infliximab closed their fistulas, significantly more frequently than a placebo infusion. However, MRI scans have shown persistent fistula tracks even though the cutaneous orifice heals. Thus, it is not surprising that the apparent 'healing' is usually only temporary. Nevertheless, infliximab (usually an infusion of 5 mg/kg) at 0, 2, and 6 weeks) has been a major advance in the overall management of fistulas.

Some patients with small-intestinal disease present with multiple short strictures. Once active disease is controlled with corticosteroids, the strictures should be dealt with by stricturoplasty rather than by multiple resections. This gives good symptomatic relief and it is unusual for further stricturing to occur at sites of previous stricturoplasties. This conservative approach has greatly reduced the need for repeated resections and has therefore minimized the chances of a short bowel syndrome.

Management during pregnancy

Crohn's disease should be treated in the pregnant woman along the lines outlined above. Overall, the outcome of the pregnancy is not influenced by the disease except in very severe cases where there may be an increased risk of abortion. Corticosteroids and sulphasalazine are safe to use and have not been associated with fetal abnormalities. Likewise, azathioprine has not been clearly demonstrated to be teratogenic and can be used if there is sufficient clinical indication. Methotrexate is known to be teratogenic and is therefore completely contraindicated for women who are trying to conceive or who are pregnant.

Management in children

There is no essential difference in the principles of management from those described for adults, although dosages may need to be reduced. Alternate-day steroids should be employed, especially if long-term treatment seems likely. Excellent but uncontrolled results have been reported in adolescents using maintenance corticosteroids, as an alternate-day regimen, which allowed puberty and growth to develop normally. One of the major effects of the disease in children is growth retardation. Corticosteroid therapy often promotes a growth spurt but great emphasis should be paid to the child's nutrition. Dietary intake should be assessed and supplemented to provide a high-calorie, high-nitrogen intake. Many paediatric gastroenterologists use elemental or polymeric diets as first-line therapy for active disease, often administered via a percutaneous gastrostomy.

Course and prognosis

Patients are never cured of Crohn's disease and they are subject to relapses of their disease and to recurrence following surgical resection. Most patients (70 to 80 per cent) will receive surgical treatment at some point during the course of their illness. After a resection, the disease recurs in about 30 per cent of patients during the subsequent 5 years and in 50 per cent of patients during the subsequent 10 years; of these, half will require further surgery. Although there is still some controversy, the balance of evidence suggests that the risk of requiring second or third operations is no greater than the risk of requiring the initial operation. Patients with Crohn's colitis who have a proctocolectomy appear to have a lower risk of recurrence than those who have an ileal or ileocolic resection.

Recent endoscopic visualization of the neoterminal ileum has shown that the recurrence rates, when assessed by endoscopic appearance, are even higher than the rates quoted above, which are based on symptoms. For patients who have had an ileal or ileocolic resection, 70 to 80 per cent of them will show endoscopic lesions just proximal to the anastomosis within the first postoperative year. The more severe lesions, such as aphthoid ulcers, predict a high chance of symptomatic recurrence. Mesalazine has been shown to have no influence on the endoscopic recurrence rate and it remains to be seen whether steroid compounds with low systemic bioavailability (such as budesonide) will be effective in this context without inducing systemic side-effects.

The overall mortality of Crohn's disease varies from 10 to 15 per cent in different studies. Some of these reports have suggested a worse prognosis for women than for men, and for patients over the age of 50 years, although this was mainly associated with higher operative mortality. Overall, age and gender probably have little influence on the outcome of the disease. The Oxford experience has suggested that mortality is not appreciably increased during the first 15 years of the disease but then becomes progressively greater during subsequent follow-up. In contrast, however, data from Birmingham suggest that the highest mortality occurs in young people during the early stages of the disease.

In general, most patients with Crohn's disease will have a good prognosis with a mortality of only about twice that expected. Considerable morbidity can be expected but this will be intermittent and the overall quality of life should be good.

Further reading

Allan RN *et al.* (1997). *Inflammatory bowel diseases*, 3rd edn. Churchill Livingstone, Edinburgh.

Jewell DP, Warren BF, Mortensen NJ (2001). *Inflammatory bowel disease.*Blackwell Science, Oxford.

Kirsner JB (2000). *Inflammatory bowel disease*, 5th edn. WB Saunders Co., Philadelphia.

14.11 Ulcerative colitis

D. P. Jewell

Ulcerative colitis is a chronic inflammatory disease of the colon of unknown cause. It always affects the rectum and extends proximally to involve a variable extent of the colon. It is characterized by a relapsing and remitting course.

The disease was first described in 1859 by Samual Wilks, a physician at Guy's Hospital, who recognized that 'simple, idiopathic colitis' could be distinguished from other forms of colitis, mainly bacterial dysentery. It took many years for the concept to be accepted, but finally, in 1931, Sir Arthur Hurst was able to give a complete description of the disease including the sigmoidoscopic appearances. Nevertheless, he still considered the disease to be primarily infective, even though its chronic nature might be induced secondarily by other factors.

Epidemiology

Ulcerative colitis is a worldwide disease, although it may be difficult to diagnose in areas where infective colitis is prevalent. Accurate figures for incidence and prevalence are not universally available but the disease is now recognized in most countries. Table 1 lists data for the high-incidence areas and also shows that there have been no trends to suggest the disease is becoming more common, which is in contrast to Crohn's disease. The low-incidence areas include Eastern Europe, Asia, Japan, and South America where the incidence rates are at least tenfold less.

The age of onset peaks between 20 and 40 years but the disease may present at all ages from the first few months of life to the 80s. Some series show a secondary peak of onset in the 60- to 70-year-old age group, but this has not been a universal finding. Earlier series suggested a predominance of the disease in women, but more recently, there has been little difference between the sexes.

Table 1 Incidence of ulcerative colitis

	Period of study	Incidence (per 10^5)
USA		
Minnesota	1935–64	7.2
Baltimore	1960–63	4.6
UK		
Oxford	1951–60	6.5
Wales	1968–77	7.2
Aberdeen	1967–76	11.3
Denmark		
Copenhagen	1962–78	8.1
	1981–88	9.5
Holland		
Leiden	1979–83	6.8
Sweden		
Stockholm County	1975–79	4.3
Israel		
Tel-Aviv	1961–70	3.6

Both in the United States and Cape Town, Jews are more prone to ulcerative colitis than non-Jews by a factor of 3 or 4. Within Israel, Ashkenazi Jews have a higher incidence than Sephardim but it is still less than the incidence in Jews in the United States or, indeed, than the European incidence. This suggests that environmental factors may be involved in addition to genetic factors. However, the differences in incidence between urban as opposed to rural communities or between different socio-economic groups have been slight and inconstant.

Genetics

The familial incidence of ulcerative colitis has long been recognized, with 10 to 20 per cent of patients likely to have at least one other family member affected either with ulcerative colitis or with Crohn's disease. Most of the familial association is within first-degree relatives, but there is controversy about the precise relation, with a preponderance of parent–sibling combinations being found in the United States, whereas in the United Kingdom the disease is more commonly shared by siblings. Within a multiply-affected family there is a high degree of concordance for disease characteristics (for example extent, severity, presence of extraintestinal manifestations).

A study of twin pairs in Sweden showed that of 16 pairs of monozygotic twins in whom one member had ulcerative colitis, only one pair was concordant for the disease whereas all 20 dizygotic twins were discordant. This gave a proband concordance rate of 6.3 per cent, which is very much lower than 45 per cent for Crohn's disease.

This low concordance rate might suggest that familial clustering reflects environmental influence rather than inherited genetic susceptibility. However, the incidence of ulcerative colitis in spouses of probands is extremely low, although, of course, that does not exclude environmental factors operating early in life.

The mode of inheritance is unknown, but as with Crohn's disease, multiple genes are probably involved in determining disease susceptibility and its behaviour. Studies of multiply-affected families, using microsatellite technology, have demonstrated linkage to chromosome 12 and, less strongly, to chromosomes 3 and 7. These susceptibility loci are shared by patients with Crohn's disease although some evidence suggests that the locus on chromosome 12 contains two separate genes, one for ulcerative colitis and a second for Crohn's disease. In most studies, ulcerative colitis is more strongly linked to chromosome 6p (the HLA region) than Crohn's disease. Study of individual HLA alleles has shown that possession of HLA DR103 is likely to be associated with severe disease. In Japan and in the Jewish population of California, the disease is associated with HLA DR1502 (an allele of DR2 common in these populations but very uncommon in Europeans). The occurrence of extraintestinal manifestations also appears to be related to genetic make-up. For example, patients who develop a reactive, large joint arthropathy in association with active disease are likely to possess the HLA DR103 allele (35 per cent) compared with patients who do not (8 per cent) or healthy controls (3 per cent). In contrast, the small joint, seronegative arthropathy is associated with HLA B44 (77 per cent) and MICA-8 (98 per cent). Nevertheless, it is not possible to be sure on the basis of present knowledge whether these associations are biologically meaningful or whether they represent linkage disequilibrium with a nearby gene.

Aetiology

The cause of the disease remains unknown. The main hypotheses that have been proposed include infection, allergy to dietary components, immune responses to bacterial or self-antigens, an abnormality in epithelial cell integrity, and the psychosomatic theory. There are virtually no data to support a primary role for psychosomatic factors in the aetiology of the disease, although they may play a secondary role in determining the pattern of symptoms and must always be considered when managing individual patients.

Infection

No specific infective organism has been consistently isolated from patients with ulcerative colitis. However, the recognition that the strains of *Escherichia coli* in the normal colon are continually changing has led to the concept that patients may carry strains which, by releasing enzymes or other toxic products, might damage the mucosa. The demonstration that, even in remission, patients with ulcerative colitis are more likely to harbour *E. coli* expressing adhesins than control subjects is a particularly interesting observation, as these may allow the bacteria to adhere readily to the epithelium. The role of sulphate-reducing bacteria is also of interest as these organisms are found more commonly in those with colitis. They reduce sulphate to sulphide which, in turn, inhibits butyrate oxidation in epithelial cells. Several investigators have demonstrated reduced activity of butyrate dehydrogenase within colitic epithelium, even in remission, raising the possibility that luminal bacteria may have a deleterious effect on epithelial cell metabolism and, hence, integrity.

Food allergy

The early suggestions of allergic responses to milk proteins, eggs, and other dietary proteins have not been substantiated as an aetiological factor. Milk-free diets may be beneficial in a minority of patients but it is not clear whether this results from an associated hypolactasia, an immunological response, or some other mechanism. The failure of ulcerative colitis to respond either to intravenous nutrition avoiding oral food or to colonic isolation by means of a split ileostomy are further pointers that dietary factors play little part.

Environmental factors

As well as infection and diet, smoking and the use of oral contraceptives may influence disease. Many studies have now shown that ulcerative colitis is more common in non-smokers than smokers, with a relative risk of 2 to 6. Ex-smokers have a particularly high incidence and this is highest for former heavy compared with light smokers. Women taking oral contraceptives may have a slightly increased risk of the disease but this association is weak and loses significance when the data are corrected for smoking habits and social class.

Immunopathogenesis

The intense infiltration of the inflamed mucosa with plasma cells, B and T lymphocytes, and macrophages suggests immunological activity. Whether activation of both humoral and cellular immune mechanisms merely reflects increased antigenic absorption through an abnormal epithelium, a response to a specific aetiological agent, or an underlying defect in mucosal immunoregulation is unknown.

There is an increase in plasma cells synthesizing all three of the major immunoglobulin isotypes—IgA, IgG, and IgM. However, the largest pro-portional increase is in IgG-producing cells and this is predominantly of the IgG1 and IgG3 subclasses, which is in contrast to Crohn's disease where an IgG2 response is predominant. IgG1 and IgG3 are synthesized in response to protein antigen and are effective in fixing complement. Complement activation is known to occur in active colitis, probably as a result of the formation of antigen–antibody complexes, and is likely to be one of the principal effector mechanisms in establishing the inflammatory lesion. Some of the increased mucosal IgG synthesized is known to have antibody specificity for bacterial and epithelial antigens. As antibody to epithelial antigens, especially a 40-kDa protein, is a feature of ulcerative colitis, rather than Crohn's disease, it is possible that autoimmunity plays a part in ulcerative colitis. This concept is strengthened by the association with other auto-immune disorders and with circulating antibodies to neutrophils (pANCA), neither of which is associated with Crohn's disease. Nevertheless, whether anticolon antibodies or pANCA have a pathogenetic role is still very uncertain.

The main subsets of T cells (CD4+, CD8+) are present in increased numbers in the inflamed mucosa but their proportions do not change significantly. Several lines of evidence suggest that the T cells are activated and release a variety of cytokines. Whether there is a failure of T cells to either upregulate or downregulate the mucosal immune response has not been clearly shown. However, data suggest that there may indeed be a failure to induce suppression to specific antigens, which could lead to some of the immunological overactivity that is observed in this disease. Intraepithelial T lymphocytes isolated from colons resected for severe ulcerative colitis also fail to suppress T-cell proliferative responses to specific antigens, a property that is not due to the increased numbers of intraepithelial T lymphocytes using γδ T-cell receptors.

As well as T-cell activation, there is also a marked increase in the population of activated macrophages, which not only release inflammatory mediators (reactive oxygen metabolites, leukotrienes, platelet-activating factor) but serine proteases, metalloproteinases, and cytokines. The release of interleukin 1 (**IL-1**), IL-6, and tumour necrosis factor will not only lead to tissue damage but will initiate an acute-phase response, downregulate albumin synthesis, and induce fever. Release of interferon-γ from activated T cells induces HLA class II molecules on colonic epithelial cells, which, in turn, are able to present antigen to the adjacent CD4+ lymphocytes and to activate the CD8+ intraepithelial T lymphocytes. Changes in epithelial permeability induced by interferon-γ and inflammatory mediators, endothelial damage by a wide variety of cytokines and mediators leading to local ischaemia, and stimulation of collagen synthesis by transforming growth factor-β, IL-1, and IL-6 may all contribute to the inflammatory process.

Pathology
Macroscopic

Ulcerative colitis always involves the rectum but in about 40 per cent of patients the disease is limited to the rectum and sigmoid. In adults, only about 20 per cent will have the whole colon involved, although this proportion rises to about 50 per cent in children. In mild disease, the mucosa is hyperaemic and granular, but as the disease becomes more severe, small punctate ulcers appear, which may then enlarge and extend deeply into the lamina propria. The ulceration may be linear along the line of the taeniae coli. The mucosa can become intensely haemorrhagic. In patients with long-standing disease, inflammatory polyps (pseudopolyps) may develop. They are usually found in the colon and rarely in the rectum. Inflammatory polyps are of no significance and have no malignant potential. In occasional patients, they may regress.

When the disease goes into remission, the colonic appearances may return to normal, but, especially in patients who have had recurrent attacks, the mucosa becomes atrophic and featureless. There is often narrowing and shortening of the bowel. Fibrous strictures complicating long-standing chronic disease are extremely rare.

If an acute dilatation occurs in a patient with severe disease, the bowel becomes thin and congested. There is usually severe ulceration, with only small islands of mucosa remaining. An acute dilatation may be accompanied by a perforation.

Microscopic

The inflammation of ulcerative colitis is largely confined to the mucosa. The lamina propria becomes oedematous, with dilated and congested capillaries, and extravasation of red blood cells. There is a cellular infiltrate of acute and chronic inflammatory cells: neutrophils, lymphocytes, plasma cells, macrophages, mast cells, and eosinophils.

The neutrophils invade the epithelium, usually in the crypts, giving rise to a cryptitis and eventually to a crypt abscess. The triggers for this migration of neutrophils are unknown, but chemotactic peptides of colonic bacteria (for example formyl methionyl leucyl phenylalanine) as well as IL-8, leukotriene B4, platelet-activating factor, and activated complement are potential candidates. Damage to the crypts leads to increased epithelial cell turnover and a discharge of mucus from goblet cells. With increasing inflammation, the surface epithelial cells become flattened, irregular, and eventually ulcerate. Deep ulcers may extend into the lamina propria, leading to inflammatory changes in the submucosa—this may be accompanied by an acute dilatation or perforation.

Many of the acute changes of ulcerative colitis are non-specific and may also be seen in infective colitides. However, the diagnosis of ulcerative colitis can be made with some accuracy (more than 80 per cent probability) if features of a chronic inflammatory process are present. These include distorted crypt architecture, crypt atrophy, basal lymphoid aggregates, and a chronic inflammatory infiltrate.

Once the disease has gone into remission, the histological appearances may return to normal. However, there is frequent evidence of bifid or shortened crypts, hyperplasia of the muscularis mucosae, neuronal hypertrophy, and Paneth-cell metaplasia at the base of the crypts.

Clinical features

Patients usually present with a gradual onset of symptoms, often intermittent, but which become progressively more severe. Occasionally, ulcerative colitis can present much more rapidly and may mimic an infective colitis. Indeed, some patients begin with a documented infection (such as a campylobacter or salmonella colitis) but continue to have symptoms that ultimately lead to the correct diagnosis.

The principal symptoms include diarrhoea, rectal bleeding, the passage of mucus, and less frequently, abdominal pain. When the inflammation is confined to the rectum (proctitis), patients often pass fresh blood, which is usually mixed with the stool but can be streaked on the surface. These patients often complain of constipation rather than diarrhoea and, on clinical symptoms alone, may be mistakenly diagnosed as suffering from haemorrhoids. When the inflammation extends beyond the rectum, there is usually diarrhoea with the passage of partly altered blood. The diarrhoea is often accompanied by urgency and tenesmus, and patients can be incontinent. Nocturnal diarrhoea is a common symptom in the presence of severe inflammation. With a severe ulcerative colitis affecting most or all of the colon, patients are usually anorexic, nauseated, and have lost weight. They usually have severe diarrhoea (in excess of six motions daily) that becomes a slurry of faecal material, pus, and blood—it may resemble anchovy sauce and, indeed, some patients may fail to recognize that they are passing blood.

Patients may also complain of malaise, lassitude, and symptoms referable to chronic iron deficiency or to some of the extraintestinal manifestations, especially recurrent aphthous ulcers of the mouth.

On examination, patients with mild or moderate attacks usually look well and exhibit few abnormal physical signs. Weight should always be recorded and, for children and adolescents, both height and weight should be recorded on growth charts. Abdominal examination may reveal a tender colon but is often normal. Bowel sounds are normal and rectal examination is also normal apart from blood.

Patients with a severe attack may also look deceptively well and a tachycardia or a tender colon may be the only abnormal signs. However, many of these patients are obviously ill, with fever, salt and water depletion, anaemia, and evidence of weight loss. There may be oral candidiasis, aphthous ulceration, signs of iron deficiency, and finger clubbing. The skin changes of hypoalbuminaemia and dependent oedema may occur. The abdomen is often distended and tympanitic, with reduced bowel sounds and marked colonic tenderness.

Minor perianal disease, such as a fissure, may occur in patients with an active ulcerative colitis but it is never as severe as is seen in patients with Crohn's disease.

Assessment of disease severity

This can be done clinically, by grading the degree of inflammation seen endoscopically or histologically, and by using laboratory tests of inflammatory activity.

Clinical grading

1. Mild—there are less than four stools daily, with or without blood, with no systemic disturbance and a normal erythrocyte sedimentation rate.
2. Moderate—this is between mild and severe.
3. Severe—there are at least six stools daily, with bleeding, and evidence of systemic illness as shown by fever, tachycardia, a falling haemoglobin, hypoalbuminaemia, and raised erythrocyte sedimentation rate and C-reactive protein.

Laboratory markers of inflammation

Active disease is often accompanied by a neutrophil leucocytosis, thrombocytosis, and a rise in acute-phase proteins (C-reactive protein, orosomucoid) and in erythrocyte sedimentation rate. There may also be a fall in haemoglobin and albumin levels. These inflammatory markers are useful when measured serially during the course of treatment as an indicator of disease activity. However, if corticosteroids are used, the white cell count can no longer be used as a marker of disease activity because it will often rise in response to the steroids. Patients with a proctitis rarely have a rise in C-reactive protein unless the inflammation is particularly severe.

Diagnosis

The diagnosis is made on the basis of the history, the absence of faecal pathogens, and the endoscopic and histological appearances of the colon.

Stool cultures should be set up for all patients presenting for the first time and, ideally, for all those presenting with a relapse of established disease. Special culture conditions are required for campylobacter, yersinia, gonococci, and *Clostridium difficile*. The possibility of an infection with E. coli 0157 must also be considered, especially in patients in whom bleeding and abdominal pain are predominant symptoms. An infective colitis with opportunistic organisms in patients with immunodeficiency syndromes has become much more common and has to be remembered in differential diagnosis.

Sigmoidoscopy is safe, even in patients with a severe attack, and not only confirms rectal inflammation but also allows a biopsy specimen to be taken and an assessment of severity to be obtained. Although some centres use colonoscopy in severe attacks, this is rarely necessary for diagnosis, for assessment of severity, or for determining management. It is best avoided in the acute stage. The earliest signs of colitis on sigmoidoscopy are blurring of the vascular pattern associated with hyperaemia and oedema, leading to blunting of the valves of Houston. With increasing severity, the mucosa becomes granular and then friable. With severe inflammation, the mucosa shows spontaneous bleeding and ulceration. These changes begin in the rectum, they are diffuse, and extend proximally to affect a variable length of the colon. Pseudopolyps (inflammatory polyps) often occur in patients with long-standing disease but tend to be in the colon rather than the rectum.

Colonoscopy with multiple biopsies is useful for assessing the extent of disease and is mandatory for patients with a colonic stricture. It is also required for cancer surveillance (see later). Preparation of the colon should follow the normal methods and osmotic purgation is the most satisfactory. However, a more gentle approach is needed if colonoscopy is done in the presence of severe inflammation, but this is rarely indicated.

All patients with a severe attack must have a plain abdominal radiograph. Not only does this exclude a dilated colon but it may provide prognostic information (mucosal islands, distended small bowel loops) and demonstrate the extent of the disease. An abnormal haustral pattern, thickening of the bowel wall, and mucosal oedema can be detected on a plain film (Fig. 1). As an inflamed colon does not hold faecal material, the presence of faecal matter in the ascending or transverse colon will indicate that the inflammation is distal. In a severe attack, barium radiography is virtually never indicated, but if it is done, a single-contrast study in an unprepared colon with barium entering the colon at low pressure should be used. In less severe disease, a double-contrast barium enema can be safely given (Fig. 2), but the colon must not be overdistended and the procedure must be stopped if the patient complains of pain.

Biopsy specimens must be taken at sigmoidoscopy or colonoscopy, preferably with small, cupped forceps. Histological assessment contributes to grading severity as well as the differential diagnosis.

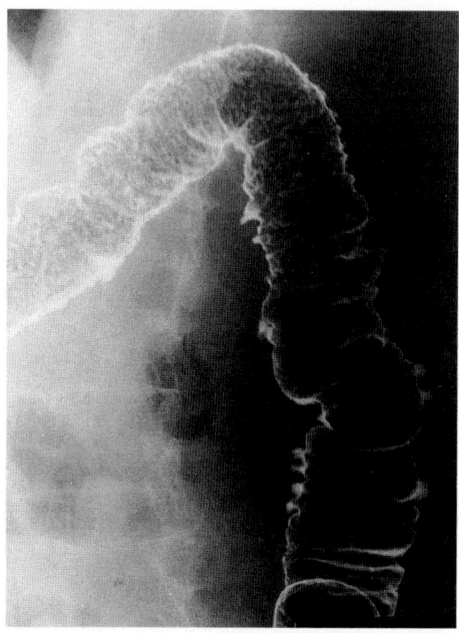

Fig. 2 A double-contrast barium enema in a patient with active ulcerative colitis. The figure is a close-up view of the splenic flexure to show extensive mucosal ulceration, loss of haustration, and narrowing of the colon. The patient also has diverticula in the descending colon.

Laboratory data

These are required for assessing severity, as discussed above, and to document haematological or biochemical complications.

Iron deficiency is common as a result of chronic iron loss; this can be exacerbated by a severe attack, in which 0.5 g of elemental iron can be lost. Thus, a hypochromic, microcytic anaemia is frequently present. A neutrophil leucocytosis, thrombocytosis, eosinophilia, or monocytosis may also be present and are indicators of active inflammation.

Biochemical abnormalities are rare in mild or moderate attacks, but hypokalaemia, hypoalbuminaemia, and a rise in α_2-globulin frequently accompany a severe attack. Minor elevations of the aspartate transaminase or alkaline phosphatase are also frequently seen in patients with a severe attack, but they return to normal when the disease goes into remission. They probably reflect a fatty liver, together with the effects of toxaemia or poor nutrition. Persistent elevation, especially of alkaline phosphatase, may indicate underlying chronic liver disease and needs further investigation (see below).

Serum immunoglobulins rarely exceed the upper limit of normal during a relapse, but usually fall as remission occurs.

Differential diagnosis

If the patient has a history of slow onset of symptoms, including blood and mucus, and has diffuse inflammation on sigmoidoscopy, the diagnosis of ulcerative colitis is highly probable. The major differential diagnosis is Crohn's disease (see Chapter 14.10). If clinical, radiological, endoscopic, and histological information is considered together, less than 10 per cent of patients fall into the category of indeterminate colitis. The recently recognized collagenous colitis usually has only a mild inflammation on colonoscopy and is diagnosed on the basis of a thickened subepithelial collagen band (wider than 15 µm) seen in a rectal biopsy specimen. Microscopic or lymphocytic colitis has a normal endoscopic appearance but shows a diffuse infiltration of the lamina propria with lymphocytes and eosinophils on histological examination. Although ischaemic colitis classically occurs around the splenic flexure, it may occur in the rectum, especially in the elderly, and can be diagnosed histologically. Radiation damage to the rectum may occur, especially in men who have had radiotherapy to the prostate.

Rarely, a drug-induced colitis may occur. The drugs that have been implicated include non-steroidal anti-inflammatory drugs, gold, penicillamine, and 5-aminosalicylic acid. The last drug may cause considerable diagnostic confusion in patients who already have ulcerative colitis. An

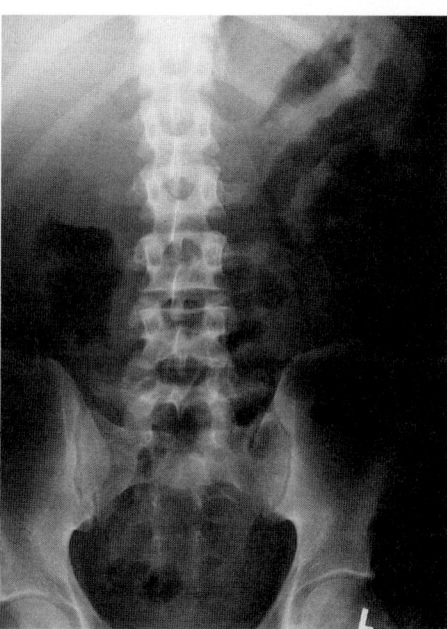

Fig. 1 Plain abdominal radiograph of a 24-year-old man with severe ulcerative colitis. The ascending and transverse colon are grossly oedematous and diseased with loss of the normal haustral pattern. In addition, there are multiple loops of distended small intestine.

antibiotic history must be taken but a pseudomembranous colitis secondary to *Cl. difficile* can occur in the absence of antibiotic usage, especially in the elderly.

For those patients presenting with a much more acute history, infective forms of colitis must be excluded by stool culture. A sudden onset of symptoms, the predominance of abdominal pain, the ingestion of potentially infected food (chicken, shellfish), and evidence of diarrhoeal disease in contacts are obvious pointers to an infection. Sigmoidoscopic appearances are usually very similar to ulcerative colitis but a rectal biopsy can be very useful in distinguishing an infective from a more chronic ulcerative colitis. The presence of a chronic inflammatory infiltrate, architectural disturbances of the glands, and basal lymphoid aggregates favour ulcerative colitis. The common organisms causing an infective colitis are salmonella, shigella, and campylobacter. Yersinial infections may also cause a colitis and can pursue a chronic course over many months before resolving. Special culture conditions may isolate the organism from stool, but a rising titre of serum antibody is often the more reliable method of identifying the infection. *E. coli* 0157 is a recognized cause of an acute colitis, especially in institutions, and massive bleeding is often a characteristic feature. Children may develop a haemolytic uraemic syndrome. Diagnosis is difficult because most laboratories are not equipped either to detect this strain of *E. coli* or to measure specific antibody. For patients who have travelled in endemic areas, amoebic and schistosomal colitis must be considered—stool examination and histological demonstration of amoebas or schistosomal ova in rectal biopsy specimens make the diagnosis.

Other causes of infective colitis can occur in immunosuppressed patients and include cytomegalovirus, herpes simplex, and *Mycobacterium avium intracellulare*. Although these organisms are usually associated with fairly characteristic sigmoidoscopic appearances, they can be associated with a more diffuse pattern of inflammation. Other sexually transmitted causes of proctitis (gonorrhoea, chlamydia, lymphogranuloma) do not usually cause diarrhoea and, especially with gonorrhoea, are associated with the passage of watery pus.

Ulcerative colitis also has to be differentiated from irritable bowel syndrome, colonic polyps or carcinoma, diverticular disease, solitary rectal ulcer syndrome, and factitious diarrhoea. Sigmoidoscopy usually clarifies the diagnosis, but if the ulceration of the solitary rectal ulcer syndrome becomes circumferential, this can be mistaken for ulcerative colitis. A biopsy specimen showing strands of smooth muscle radiating up into the lamina propria between the glands is characteristic of the solitary ulcer syndrome.

Extraintestinal manifestations

Table 2 lists the extraintestinal manifestations.

Table 2 Extraintestinal manifestations of ulcerative colitis

Related to activity of colitis
Aphthous ulceration of the mouth
Fatty liver
Erythema nodosum
Peripheral arthropathy
Episcleritis
Usually related to activity of colitis
Pyoderma gangrenosum
Anterior uveitis
Unrelated to colitis
Sacroiliitis
Ankylosing spondylitis
Primary sclerosing cholangitis
Cholangiocarcinoma

Skin

The most common skin rash seen in patients with ulcerative colitis is a hypersensitivity rash to sulphasalazine (related to the sulphapyridine moiety), which may be photosensitive. Erythema nodosum occurs in about 2 per cent of patients and is mostly associated with active disease. The lesions occur most commonly on the anterior aspect of the lower legs. Pyoderma gangrenosum is rare (1 to 2 per cent) and is usually seen in patients with active disease, but occasionally persists despite inactive colitis. The lesions usually begin as sterile pustules, usually on the limbs, which break down as they enlarge and finally coalesce. Ulceration leads to necrosis and the lesions become surrounded by black, necrotic tissue. Treatment of the colitis is usually followed by regression of the skin lesions.

Mouth

Crops of aphthous ulcers are common in patients with active disease. A sore tongue and angular stomatitis often accompany chronic iron deficiency.

Eyes

Episcleritis or an anterior uveitis occur in 5 to 8 per cent of patients. Local corticosteroids and treatment of active colitis usually lead to resolution.

Joints

An acute arthropathy occurs in 10 to 15 per cent of patients with active disease. It affects the larger joints (knees, hips, ankles, wrists, elbows) and is usually asymmetrical. It is a non-erosive condition and settles as the colitis goes into remission. A less common joint complication is a symmetrical small-joint polyarthropathy which is seronegative and is unrelated to the activity of the colitis.

Low back pain is a common symptom and is usually due to a sacroiliitis, which can be seen radiologically in 12 to 15 per cent of patients. It is unrelated to disease activity, is not strongly associated with HLA B27, and rarely progresses to ankylosing spondylitis. The latter disease occurs in only 1 to 2 per cent of patients and 60 per cent of these have the HLA B27 phenotype. There is a 2:1 ratio in favour of males with this complication. The spondylitis may present before the colitis becomes apparent or may follow the intestinal symptoms. Its natural history is independent to that of the colitis and should be treated with physiotherapy, hydrotherapy, and if necessary, non-steroidal anti-inflammatory drugs. However, these drugs can occasionally worsen the colitis and should therefore be used cautiously.

Liver disease

Patients with severe attacks of ulcerative colitis often have minor elevations of alkaline phosphatase or transaminases. The cause of these enzyme rises is probably multifactorial, including malnutrition, sepsis, and a fatty liver, which occurs in up to 60 per cent of patients coming to urgent colectomy. The liver enzymes return to normal activities when remission is achieved.

However, there may be persistent abnormalities in liver enzymes in about 3 per cent of patients, usually a rise in alkaline phosphatase. The overwhelming majority of these patients will have primary sclerosing cholangitis when the bile duct is visualized by endoscopic cholangiography. Histologically, liver biopsy specimens show evidence of chronic liver disease, but the spectrum of appearances ranges from those of an autoimmune hepatitis to the classic picture of concentric periductular fibrosis with obliteration of bile ducts.

Many patients with ulcerative colitis and sclerosing cholangitis remain well for many years. The colitis is often very mild, though frequently affecting the whole colon, but the liver disease is progressive and ultimately leads to portal hypertension and liver failure. Sclerosing cholangitis is a premalignant condition and explains the well-recognized association between ulcerative colitis and cholangiocarcinoma. Pathogenesis and treatment of the liver disease are discussed in Chapter 14.20.2.3.

Rare associations

Pericarditis with or without an effusion has been described in association with an acute attack of colitis but a true association is not yet proven. Autoimmune haemolytic anaemia has been reported in ulcerative colitis and may recur when the colonic disease becomes active. Amyloid rarely occurs in ulcerative colitis—it is much more likely to be associated with Crohn's disease. A rapidly progressing bronchiectasis has also been described in some patients with ulcerative colitis.

Medical management

The main principles of therapy for the treatment of ulcerative colitis are: to control active disease rapidly, to maintain remission, to select patients for whom surgery is appropriate, and to ensure as good a quality of life as possible.

Treatment of active disease

The most effective drugs for controlling active disease are the corticosteroids, which may be given systemically, topically, or in combination. Drugs containing 5-aminosalicylic acid (sulphasalazine, olsalazine, balsalaizide, mesalazine) are often used to treat a mild colitis but prednisolone has been shown to be more effective and to control symptoms more rapidly, which make it the drug of choice. The dosage and route of administration are largely governed by disease severity. Once active inflammation has been controlled and remission obtained, the corticosteroids should be tailed off because they are ineffective as maintenance therapy and prolonged use puts the patient at risk of long-term side-effects such as osteoporosis.

Proctitis

Proctitis refers to disease limited to the rectum—in practice, it refers to inflammation that does not extend beyond the limits of a rigid sigmoidoscope. It can be remarkably difficult to treat. Initial therapy is usually a 5-aminosalicylic acid drug by mouth in combination with topical therapy. The latter can be a corticosteroid or 5-aminosalicylic acid in the form of a suppository. For patients who do not respond, oral prednisolone may be given. Some have sufficiently severe proctitis to warrant intravenous steroids, and occasionally colectomy may be necessary. Many patients with a refractory proctitis develop a severe proximal constipation, which can cause considerable abdominal discomfort, bloating, and nausea. Relief of the constipation, usually by gentle osmotic purgation, will often give considerable symptomatic benefit but may also be associated with a marked improvement in the inflammation. Some patients appear to be refractory because foam or enema preparations are used: changing to a suppository allows a much higher concentration of drug in the rectum and is frequently associated with improvement in symptoms.

Mildly active disease

Patients who have no more than four motions daily on average, with inflammation extending beyond the limits of the rigid sigmoidoscope, should be given 20 mg of oral prednisolone daily, together with topical steroids or 5-aminosalicylic acid. Treatment should be given for at least 4 weeks before being tailed off over the subsequent 3 to 4 weeks. Clinical trials have shown that 5-aminosalicylic acid formulations are more effective than placebo in treating active disease, especially in high doses. However, corticosteroids achieve remission more quickly and in a higher proportion than 5-aminosalicylic acid drugs.

Moderately active disease

Patients who have, on average, more than four bowel motions daily but who are not systemically ill should be given 40 mg of prednisolone by mouth daily. Giving larger doses (such as 60 mg daily) provides only a marginally better effect but increases the frequency of side-effects quite considerably. The dose is reduced to 20 mg daily over 2 to 3 weeks and the regimen then follows that described for mild disease.

Severe disease

This is defined as an attack in which the patient has more than six bowel motions daily, with blood, and who is systemically ill as shown by tachycardia, fever, and anaemia. The colon is usually tender on palpation. These patients should be admitted to hospital and assessed by both physician and surgeon. Fluid and electrolyte losses are replaced intravenously; a blood transfusion should be given if the haemoglobin is less than 10 g/dl. Patients are given intravenous corticosteroids (such as 100 mg of hydrocortisone, 6-hourly) together with a twice daily rectal drip of hydrocortisone (100 mg in 100 ml water). Parenteral nutrition is indicated for patients who are malnourished, but for the majority, intravenous saline and dextrose–saline are sufficient, together with potassium supplements. Most patients with a severe attack prefer to have only clear fluids by mouth during the first 24 h. Thereafter, there is no evidence that a light diet has any adverse effect on the disease, but many clinicians will leave the patient on only clear fluids for the first few days.

Provided the patient is improving, treatment is continued for 5 to 7 days. At this time, a good response is one in which the patient feels well, there is no fever or tachycardia, the colon is not tender on abdominal palpation, and the diarrhoea has largely settled, usually to less than four motions daily. At this stage, the stools are rarely formed but macroscopic bleeding has stopped. These patients can then go on to oral prednisolone (for instance 40 mg daily), a retention enema, an oral 5-aminosalicylic acid drug, and a light diet. Patients who deteriorate during the first few days of intravenous treatment or those who have not made a substantial improvement by the end of the first week should be advised to have urgent surgery. The more difficult decision is when patients have made some improvement but are still not well—they may still be anorexic, have an intermittent low-grade fever, tachycardia, and continuing diarrhoea. Continuing intravenous therapy for more than 7 to 10 days is rarely beneficial and surgery is usually required. It is in this group of patients that the introduction of a light diet towards the end of the first week of treatment often provides a guide to future management. If the pulse rises or a fever develops in response to feeding, urgent colectomy is required. For the group of patients who do not make a rapid response to intravenous steroids, the addition of cyclosporin will induce remission in 60 to 80 per cent. The drug is usually given by continuous intravenous infusion (4 mg/kg), although the new oral formulation (Ne-oral) may be as effective. Intravenous cyclosporin should not be given in patients with a low cholesterol level (less than 3.00 mmol/l) as it can be complicated by fits. In these patients oral cyclosporin should be used as it is the cremaphor that is used to suspend the intravenous form that causes the fits. If cyclosporin is to be used, it should be added after 3 to 5 days of steroid therapy. Most patients respond very quickly (3 to 4 days) and thus, for those in whom surgery becomes necessary, a decision about colectomy can be made after a week or so of treatment. Those who do respond to drug therapy can be converted to oral treatment with decreasing doses of prednisolone. Practice varies between continuing oral cyclosporin for some months, changing to azathioprine, or using the two in combination. No controlled trial data are yet available to provide evidence-based guidelines.

So far, the use of cyclosporin has not been associated with major side-effects when used in the way described above, although prolonged use of high-dose steroids and cyclosporin can be associated with *Pneumocystis carinii* pneumonia. Minor, reversible side-effects are frequent with long-term use of oral cyclosporin.

Approximately 25 per cent of patients with a severe attack will require an urgent colectomy. These patients can often be identified early on using clinical and radiological features, which have been shown to have prognostic significance. These are the passage of more than nine stools daily, a pulse rate greater than 100/min, or a temperature greater than 38°C during the first 24 h of treatment. A serum albumin level of less than 30 g/l during the first few days or the failure of acute-phase proteins such as the serum C-reactive protein to fall are also poor prognostic signs. Seventy-five per cent of patients showing mucosal islands in the colon or having more than three loops of distended small bowel on a plain abdominal radiograph will come to urgent surgery. These findings, based on retrospective studies, have been confirmed by a prospective series which showed, in addition, that if, on day 3 of steroid therapy, patients were still having more than eight motions daily or four to six daily with a C-reactive protein greater than 45 mg/l there was an 85 per cent chance that urgent colectomy would be required. Thus, for patients falling into this category, cyclosporin should be added at this stage unless there are other reasons for proceeding directly to surgery.

Chronic active disease

Some patients repeatedly relapse when they come off corticosteroids or receive a daily dose of less than 10 to 15 mg of prednisolone. Immuno-suppression therapy with azathioprine or 6-mercaptopurine is often beneficial in this group. In the United Kingdom, azathioprine is the drug that is most used, in doses of 2.0 or 2.5 mg/kg, and may allow the prednisolone to be withdrawn. It usually takes 4 to 6 weeks before an effect is seen and the drug is then continued for several months. Although few long-term sequelae have been encountered, most clinicians do not usually continue therapy for more than 18 to 24 months. Oral cyclosporin (5 mg/kg) has also been used for chronic active disease but no formal clinical trials have been made. High-dose prednisolone (40 mg) given on alternate days is another approach that may be useful. However, if the patient's lifestyle is impaired by chronic disabling symptoms or by the side-effects of treatment, surgical management should be considered.

Maintenance of remission

Sulphasalazine and its active moiety, 5-aminosalicylic acid, are able to maintain the disease in remission when given over many years and reduce the relapse rate by about fourfold. Thus, provided they are well tolerated, they should be given indefinitely.

For sulphasalazine, the optimal dose to obtain good therapeutic efficacy with the least side-effects is 2 g daily. Common side-effects are nausea, anorexia, and headache, which are dose related and are caused by the sulphapyridine component. Other side-effects, which are also usually due to the sulphonamide but are not dose related, include hypersensitivity skin rashes, male infertility, agranulocytosis, and Heinz-body haemolytic anaemia. Overall, 10 to 15 per cent of patients are unable to take the drug, although the nausea and headache can often be overcome by starting at a low dose and gradually increasing it.

Sulphasalazine is an unusual drug in that it is poorly absorbed in the stomach and small intestine. When it reaches the colon, the azo-bond linking the 5-aminosalicylic acid and sulphapyridine moieties is split by bacterial azoreductases. The sulphapyridine is absorbed, metabolized in the liver, and excreted in the urine. The majority of the 5-aminosalicylic acid (about 70 per cent) is poorly absorbed and excreted in the faeces. As it is the 5-aminosalicylic acid that is the active compound, several drugs are now available that present 5-aminosalicylic acid to the colon without the sulphapyridine which causes the majority of the side-effects of sulphasalazine. The 5-aminosalicylic acid cannot simply be given by mouth as it is rapidly absorbed. Thus, it is either given as a delayed-release formulation (the mesalazine group) or as a prodrug (olsalazine, balsalazide). Table 3 lists these and details their characteristics.

Which drug containing 5-aminosalicylic acid should be prescribed as maintenance therapy for ulcerative colitis? Sulphasalazine is well tolerated by 85 per cent or so of patients, it is cheap, and serious side-effects (such as Stevens–Johnson syndrome, agranulocytosis, and pancreatitis) are very rare. The newer drugs are much more expensive than sulphasalazine but they have equal therapeutic efficacy. In general they are associated with fewer side-effects. However, occasional patients develop typical salicylate reactions (rhinitis, urticaria, and a colitis). About 10 to 12 per cent of patients will develop loose stools when given olsalazine. This gradually set-

Table 3 The salicylate drugs

	Characteristics
Mesalazine preparations	
Enteric coated:	
Asacol	Coated with Eudragit, S 5-ASA released at pH 7.0
Claversal, Salofalk	Coated with Eudragit, L 5-ASA released at pH 6.5
Controlled release:	
Pentasa	Tablets comprise 5-ASA granules coated with ethyl cellulose; released with time at pH greater than 6.5
Prodrugs	
Sulphasalazine (Salazopyrin)	5-ASA linked to sulphapyridine by an azo bond which is split by colonic bacteria
Olsalazine (Dipentum®)	Two molecules of 5-ASA linked with an azo bond
Balsalazide (Colazide)	5ASA linked to an amino acid by an azo bond
5-ASA	5-ASA linked to an amino bond by an azo bond

5-ASA, 5-aminosalicylic acid.

tles if treatment is continued, but about 5 per cent will develop a severe watery diarrhoea, which usually necessitates stopping the drug. The risk of diarrhoea can be minimized by taking the drug with food. There have been reports of renal failure, mainly due to an intestinal nephritis, and have been mostly associated with the delayed-release forms of mesalazine. It is a rare complication and the mechanism is unknown although 5-aminosalicylic acid has structural similarity to phenacetin. Both Asacol and, especially, Salofalk give higher plasma concentrations of 5-aminosalicylic acid than either Pentasa or the prodrugs (olsalazine, balsalazide, and sulphasalazine).

Diet

Patients with recurrent, severe disease have a slightly higher prevalence of hypolactasia and a lactose-free diet may be beneficial. Individual patients may be intolerant of dairy products, wheat, eggs, and other dietary constituents but the majority of patients should have a normal, well-balanced diet.

Local complications

Perianal lesions

Minor lesions such as fissures, perianal abscesses, or haemorrhoids may occur in patients with ulcerative colitis, but extensive lesions such as fistulas are exceptional and, if they occur, suggest Crohn's disease. Treatment of fissures involves treatment of active inflammation. Surgical treatment should be avoided wherever possible and, if necessary, should be conservative.

Massive haemorrhage

This occurs in association with severe attacks but is rarely seen. Intravenous corticosteroids and blood transfusion usually allow the bleeding to stop. However, if patients have already received six or more units of blood and are still bleeding, urgent colectomy must be considered.

Perforation

This is the most dangerous of the local complications and carries appreciable mortality. In patients receiving corticosteroids, the physical signs of peritonitis may not be obvious, and malaise, tachycardia, and reduced or absent bowel sounds may be the only clinical features. Plain abdominal films usually show free intra-abdominal gas. It may complicate an acute dilatation but can occur in its absence. Management consists of immediate intravenous fluid, electrolytes, antibiotics, and hydrocortisone. As soon as the patient's condition improves, urgent colectomy is performed immediately. The mortality of a perforation is as high as 16 per cent, even in specialist centres.

Acute dilatation

This is defined as a transverse colon with a diameter of greater than 5.0 to 6.0 cm with loss of haustration seen on a plain radiograph in a patient with a severe attack of ulcerative colitis. It occurs in about 5 per cent of patients with a severe attack and can be precipitated by hypokalaemia or the administration of opiates. Physical signs are often minimal but the patient is usually obtunded, the bowel sounds are reduced, and the abdomen may become distended. If the colon is already dilated on presentation of the severe attack, medical therapy with intravenous steroids should be given. Approximately 50 per cent of patients will settle on medical therapy alone, but urgent surgery is required for those who continue to deteriorate or do not improve within 24 h. If the colon dilates during the course of treating a severe attack, colectomy should be performed.

Strictures

These occur very rarely in patients with long-standing ulcerative colitis with a shortened, narrow colon. Colonoscopy with multiple biopsies must be carried out as there should be a high index of suspicion for carcinoma.

Pseudopolyps

These are common and may be filiform, sessile, or may form bridges. They can occur throughout the colon but often spare the rectum. They are not premalignant and may occasionally regress.

Colonic carcinoma

The risk of cancer is mainly in patients who have had extensive disease for more than 10 years, especially if they have had recurrent attacks. The most recent series studying primary cohorts suggest that the cumulative risk for patients with extensive disease is about 7 to 15 per cent at 20 years, with very little risk up to 15 years of disease.

Carcinoma is usually, but not always, preceded by dysplasia. This can be detected histologically and has led to the use of colonoscopic surveillance programmes for patients with long-standing ulcerative colitis affecting most or all of the colon. Provided no dysplasia is found, the examination is repeated every 1 to 3 years. If high-grade dysplasia is present, prophylactic colectomy is usually considered. For low-grade dysplasia, repeat colonoscopy within a few months is usually advised, but there are increasing reports of cancers occurring in association with low-grade dysplasia. Thus colectomy is increasingly being recommended whenever dysplasia is recognized regardless of grade. As large numbers of colonoscopies are involved in a surveillance programme the question of cost–benefit has been raised. However, two recent studies have shown that patients have a worse outcome with respect to cancer if they are not in a surveillance programme. The possibility of using flow cytometry to detect DNA aneuploidy in biopsy specimens as a means of increasing the sensitivity of surveillance has been explored, but is probably no better than a histological assessment given by an experienced intestinal pathologist.

Surgery

The indications for surgery have already been mentioned and are:

(1) severe inflammation unresponsive to medical therapy;

(2) acute complications—perforation, dilatation;

(3) for chronic active disease; and

(4) to prevent cancer.

The choice of operation is partly determined by the expertise available and the activity of the disease. When surgery is done for a severe attack, a

one-stage proctocolectomy with a Brooke ileostomy has been shown to be a safe and effective procedure. The major problems with the operation are poor healing of the perineal wound, adhesion obstruction, and ileostomy dysfunction. Sexual dysfunction in males rarely occurs if a perimuscular excision of the rectum is made. However, with the advent of restorative proctocolectomy with the formation of an ileoanal reservoir or pouch, many surgeons will do only a colectomy in the acute stage. The rectal stump is either oversewn (which is not recommended as it often leaks with abscess formation), or brought out as a mucous fistula either in the lower end of the wound or in the left iliac fossa. This allows histological examination of the whole colon to exclude Crohn's disease. The rectum is excised and the pouch formed some months later when nutrition has been restored and patients are not taking corticosteroids or immunosuppressive drugs.

Restorative proctocolectomy has become the procedure of choice for specialist centres provided the anal sphincter is intact. For this reason, this operation is not advised over the age of 65 years. Either the two-limb (J) or four-limb (W) pouch is now the favoured design and most surgeons preserve the anal transitional zone by anastomosing the pouch 1 to 2 cm above the dentate line. This allows for a stapled anastomosis which shortens the operation and is associated with better continence than a mucosectomy which inevitably requires anal dilatation by retractors. If the operation is being carried out for high-grade dysplasia or cancer, most surgeons will perform a mucosectomy and hand-sew the pouch to the dentate line.

The majority of patients who undergo a pouch operation have excellent function, with less than 10 per cent having any leakage, which is usually limited to night-time soiling. Nevertheless, all patients should be advised to wear a pad at first after a pouch procedure. The pouch usually requires emptying 6 to 12 times daily within the first few weeks of functioning and loperamide is usually needed. Adaptation occurs during the first few months, and by the end of a year the emptying frequency is around four to six times daily but without urgency. Complications of the pouch, once the immediate surgery is over, include anal stenosis, adhesion obstruction, and pouchitis. Pouchitis occurs in 10 to 20 per cent of patients and consists of diarrhoea with blood and evidence of inflammation on endoscopy. It usually responds to antibiotics such as metronidazole or ciprofloxacin but occasionally requires topical treatment with corticosteroids or 5-aminosalicylic acid.

The causes of pouchitis are heterogeneous and include ischaemia, infection with a recognized pathogen (such as campylobacter), and poor emptying, but most pouchitis attacks are unexplained.

Poor emptying can be recognized by isotopic scanning using a radiolabelled artificial stool and usually responds to regular catheterization of the pouch. The idiopathic pouchitis is particularly interesting in so far as it is only seen in patients who have previously had ulcerative colitis and is rarely, if ever, seen in patients who have a pouch for other reasons. After the formation of a pouch, for whatever indication, the ileal mucosa undergoes colonic metaplasia. The triggers for this are unknown but almost certainly involve luminal stasis. Thus, whatever factors first render an individual susceptible to developing ulcerative colitis also seem to render him/her susceptible to developing acute inflammation in ileal mucosa that has undergone colonic metaplasia.

Course and prognosis

Most patients with ulcerative colitis have intermittent attacks of the disease, but the duration of remission between attacks can vary from a few weeks to many years. About 10 to 15 per cent of patients will have a chronic continuous course and rarely achieve a full remission for any appreciable time. A few (5 to 10 per cent) will have a severe first attack requiring urgent surgery, but fewer, if any, have one attack only and never relapse.

Patients with extensive or total disease are much more likely to have a severe attack within 1 year of diagnosis than patients with distal disease and are therefore at greater risk of colectomy. However, a year from diagnosis the risk of colectomy is similar in all groups with a cumulative rate of about

1 per cent per year. Patients with disease limited to the rectum are a special group in so far as most of them continue to have very limited involvement. Only about 30 per cent will develop more extensive disease in the 20 years after diagnosis.

Despite having a chronic relapsing disease, 90 per cent or so of patients are able to work with very few days of sick leave each year. Nevertheless, quality of life can be impaired in many patients. During active inflammation, lassitude, discomfort, and urgency of defaecation are the major symptoms that limit everyday activities. Sexual and marital problems are not uncommon but may be no more frequent than that seen in other populations of patients with acute-on-chronic illnesses. Most of these problems disappear during remission, although fear of relapse and the need for continuing treatment and medical supervision can cause considerable anxiety. Many patients will alter their lifestyle with respect to daily activity, travel, and diet, but with prompt treatment of active disease and supportive medical care, most are able to have a normal life for most of the time. The development of patient self-help groups (such as The National Association for Colitis and Crohn's Disease in the United Kingdom) has been of tremendous value in providing education and an environment in which patients can regain their confidence and overcome the problem of isolation, an important and common factor in patients with an uncommon and socially unpleasant disease.

There has been a dramatic fall in the mortality rates for ulcerative colitis since the introduction of corticosteroids in the 1950s and the improvement in the management of severe attacks. The mortality rate for a severe attack, including urgent surgery, should now be less than 2 per cent. In the longer term, mortality differs hardly at all from that expected in a matched healthy population, a fact which the majority of life assurance companies fail to recognize.

Ulcerative colitis in pregnancy

Women with ulcerative colitis have normal fertility, are not at increased risk of having a spontaneous abortion, and there is no evidence that pregnancy is a risk factor for relapse. If they do become pregnant, the chance of having a normal baby is the same as for healthy women. Furthermore, there is no good evidence that corticosteroids, drugs containing 5-aminosalicylic acid, or even azathioprine are harmful. Therefore, maintenance treatment should be continued throughout the pregnancy and, if a relapse does occur, it should be treated aggressively with corticosteroids to obtain a rapid remission.

Ulcerative colitis in childhood

Ulcerative colitis is less common in children than in adults and, for the United Kingdom, the prevalence is about 6 to 7 per 100 000. Nevertheless it can present within the first few weeks of life, although the mean age of presentation is about 10 years. The symptoms are those of diarrhoea, rectal bleeding, abdominal pain, and failure to thrive. There may be evidence of delayed growth but this is more commonly a feature of childhood Crohn's disease. The proportion of children with a total colitis is about 50 per cent, which is higher than in adults, and probably accounts for the higher rate of colectomy reported in most series.

Treatment follows the same principles as for adults, although dosages are adjusted for the child's weight. In addition, great attention must be made to nutrition to allow for adequate growth. For children requiring repeated courses of corticosteroids, an alternate-day regimen usually controls the disease activity but prevents growth retardation. If colectomy becomes necessary, a restorative proctocolectomy should be done.

Further reading

Allan RN *et al.* (1997). *Inflammatory bowel diseases*, 3rd edn. Churchill Livingstone, Edinburgh.

Jewell DP, Warren BF, Mortensen NJ (2001). *Inflammatory bowel disease*.Blackwell Science, Oxford.

Kirsner JB (2000). *Inflammatory bowel disease*, 5th edn. WB Saunders Co., Philadelphia.

14.12 Functional bowel disorders and irritable bowel syndrome

D. G. Thompson

Introduction

Functional bowel disorders

Symptoms suggestive of disturbed lower gastrointestinal function without adequate explanation are very common in the adult population of the Western world. Surveys from the United Kingdom and United States indicate that up to 15 per cent of the adult population experience such symptoms at any one time, although most do not seek medical advice. The chief questions that remain largely unresolved are whether the symptoms of those individuals who do seek medical help have a different pathophysiological basis from those who do not, and whether the seeking of medical advice is an indication of a worried individual rather than of disturbed gut function.

Given these difficulties, it has to be accepted that most of the currently used terms are best viewed as an attempt by clinicians to provide some clinically useful categorization of such patients and their symptoms. Since knowledge of the physiology and the psychology of the problem remains incomplete, therapy remains largely empirical. Current observations about functional bowel disorders should therefore be regarded as the latest (but by no means the last) attempt at rationalizing a complex interrelationship between brain and gut function.

Definition of terms used

Over the last century many attempts were made to categorize functional bowel disorders. It is not surprising that most have failed to stand the test of time, as the symptoms suffered (whilst being genuine and troublesome to the patient) are often difficult to define, variable in their expression, and defy pathophysiological explanation. The latest and perhaps most comprehensive attempt has been made by a working group whose recommendations, known as the 'Rome criteria', are now accepted as useful research tools. Whether these criteria will stand the test of time as clinical diagnostic tools will, however, depend upon whether they turn out to provide a better understanding of the pathogenic mechanisms of the disease or to aid its therapy. The Rome Working Group has suggested the division of functional bowel disease into a number of symptom-based categories (Table 1). Because they do seem to have some practical value in guiding approaches to management, this chapter is based on some of the Rome categories, with emphasis on those previously encompassed by the term 'irritable bowel syndrome'. However, it must be recognized that the Rome criteria do not

Table 1 Categorization of functional bowel disease according to the 'Rome criteria'

Functional bowel disorders
Irritable bowel syndrome
Functional abdominal bloating
Functional constipation
Functional diarrhoea
Functional abdominal pain

necessarily include all symptoms presented by patients with abnormal bowel function. Failure to allocate a patient into one or other category should therefore not be taken to mean that the patient does not have a functional bowel disorder.

Irritable bowel syndrome

Definition

This syndrome is characterized by the presence of abdominal pain associated with defaecation, or a change in bowel habit, together with disordered defecation and the sensation of abdominal distension. For practical purposes, its recognition relies upon the presence of abdominal pain that is relieved by defaecation and of an associated change in frequency in defaecation and/or stool consistency, together with two or more of the following symptoms:

(1) altered stool frequency;

(2) altered stool consistency;

(3) altered ease of defaecation;

(4) passage of mucus;

(5) sensation of abdominal distension.

These criteria are themselves based on the studies of Manning and of Kruis, which identified that the above features were reported most frequently in patients with functional bowel problems but were very unusual in patients with structural disease of the colon.

Diagnosis

The diagnosis of irritable bowel syndrome is clinically based, and relies on a carefully taken history and examination, there being no specific endoscopic, radiological, or laboratory investigation that is yet capable of providing a positive diagnosis. Despite the absence of a specific pathological indicator, the identification of irritable bowel syndrome is usually not difficult, and in most cases it is unnecessary to investigate the patient extensively in an attempt to exclude other, more serious disease.

Clinical features

The history

In addition to the careful elicitation of the above specific symptoms, other features may be found that serve to increase clinical confidence. For example, many patients have upper-gut symptoms, for example food-related abdominal distension. Women may also complain of menstrual and bladder symptoms, and there is also an increased prevalence of psychosexual problems.

Examination

Clinical examination is important. Whilst there is no physical abnormality that is diagnostic of irritable bowel syndrome, a number of features occur commonly. Palpation over the site of the lower colon, particularly in the left iliac fossa, may produce discomfort, and a sigmoid colon containing faeces is often palpable. Similar tenderness may be present under the rib margins and in the right iliac fossa.

Rectal examination and sigmoidoscopy should be conducted as part of the initial clinical assessment. Characteristic findings are the presence of pellety stools in the rectum and a mucosa of normal appearance, evidence of mucosal inflammation is incompatible with the diagnosis. A further helpful pointer is the response to air insufflation during the sigmoidoscopy; abdominal discomfort is often reproduced and relieved by air expulsion. Evidence of a pigmented rectal mucosa (melanosis coli) may be found in patients who have been taking stimulant laxatives and is a useful indicator of the chronicity of the problem.

Further laboratory investigations remain at the discretion of the clinician, depending upon the confidence with which a clinical diagnosis is made. Routine haematological and biochemical screening is usually done on the assumption that they will be normal, and thus to provide reassurance both to the patient and the doctor. Radiological and endoscopic examination of the colon is not mandatory unless a clinical suspicion of a structural colonic disorder, particularly neoplasia, remains after the history and examination have been completed.

Features that raise the suspicion of organic disease and indicate a need for further investigation include the onset of symptoms in the middle-aged or elderly, weight loss, or blood in the stool. The development of new colonic symptoms in a patient with a long history of irritable bowel syndrome should also be taken seriously, as there is no evidence that the syndrome protects against the development of other disease and the incidence of colonic neoplasia increases with age.

Pathophysiology

Despite much interest and many painstaking clinical studies, our understanding of the pathophysiology of irritable bowel syndrome remains limited and the following hypotheses are discussed solely as a guide to current thinking.

Neuromuscular dysfunction

The most popular hypothesis is that these patients have a disorder of neuromuscular function of the gastrointestinal tract. However, whilst this seems eminently plausible, evidence is lacking. Manometric studies of the colon do show an increased contractile activity in patients with this syndrome, particularly after food, but the neurophysiological basis of this finding and its relationship to symptoms remains to be determined.

Visceral hypersensitivity

Another currently popular hypothesis is that visceral sensation from the gastrointestinal tract is somehow enhanced in these patients. This idea is based on the observation that distension of the rectum and colon produces greater discomfort than in people with normal bowel function. This increased sensory awareness appears to be viscerally specific, as cutaneous responsiveness is normal. However, it remains to be determined whether the mechanism for this hypersensitivity is peripheral (abnormal mechanoreceptor responsiveness in the gut) or central (abnormal sensory processing by the brain and spinal cord).

Psychiatric disease

There is convincing evidence that psychiatric disease and abnormal illness behaviour are more prevalent in patients with irritable bowel syndrome. The relationship between the psychological problem and any neuromuscular abnormality remains uncertain, although it is recognized that a heightened awareness of visceral sensation is a feature of affective disorders, particularly depression.

Diet

It is customary to regard diet as being a pathogenic factor and to attribute constipation symptoms to fibre deficiency, on the basis that irritable bowel syndrome is uncommon in those parts of the world where a high-fibre diet is consumed. While it is true that faecal bulk can be increased by ingesting more fibre and that constipation is improved, careful studies of fibre intake and symptom development do not show a clear causal relationship. Food 'allergy' or sensitivity is occasionally confused with irritable bowel syndrome because abdominal pain and diarrhoea can accompany both problems. Classic food allergy with measurable immunological alterations in response to a particular food (for example, eggs, shellfish) is readily distinguishable from irritable bowel syndrome by a clear relationship between ingestion of the implicated food and symptom development. More subtle forms of food intolerance (for example, lactose intolerance, fructose intolerance) that produce gut symptoms without an accompanying immune response are much more difficult to recognize because the nutrient in question is often present throughout the diet. Recognition requires a painstaking dietary history and the clear demonstration of a relationship between symptoms and food intake. In most patients such a relationship is not found.

Functional abdominal bloating
Definition

This is characterized by symptoms of abdominal fullness or distension, awareness of audible bowel sounds, and excessive flatus with no evidence of either maldigestion and malabsorption or excessive consumption of poorly absorbed fermentable carbohydrate.

Pathophysiology

Distension of the colon at sigmoidoscopy characteristically produces greater discomfort than normal, suggesting increased gut sensitivity. However, there is no evidence that intestinal gas production is increased. As in irritable bowel syndrome, the prevalence of psychological disorders is high.

Clinical features

The clinical assessment of such patients is identical to that for irritable bowel syndrome and features will be identical.

Functional constipation
Definition

This is arbitrarily defined as either persistently difficult, infrequent defaecation or the sensation of incomplete defaecation. Usually, two or more of the following are present: straining at defaecation; lumpy or hard stools; the sensation of incomplete evacuation; and two or fewer bowel movements per week.

Clinical evaluation

As with the other categories of functional bowel disorders, the diagnosis is based on a carefully conducted history and examination designed to exclude the possibility of more serious colonic disease, particularly cancer. When considering the diagnosis, it is important to enquire about immobility, concomitant drug therapy (particularly opiate analgesia), and a low roughage diet, which are well recognized as contributing to constipation, particularly in the infirm.

An abnormality of pelvic-floor function on attempted defaecation is an unusual cause of constipation that should be suspected in individuals who feel the need to defecate but cannot expel faeces despite severe straining.

Such a problem should be considered when symptoms develop following pelvic trauma or difficult childbirth. Clinical evidence of diabetes, hypothyroidism, and hypercalcaemia must also be sought, as these may also lead to altered colonic function and constipation.

Physical examination should include a rectal and vaginal examination. The absence of perineal descent on straining is a simple indicator of impaired pelvic-floor relaxation, while descent below the level of the ischial tuberosities indicates pelvic-floor weakness. Sigmoidoscopy is required to identify the presence of formed faeces, and to exclude faecal impaction and organic obstruction of the lower colon and rectum.

Laboratory examination

Extensive laboratory investigation is usually unnecessary in the absence of clinical indicators of systemic disease and in the presence of the above criteria. A plain abdominal radiograph is often helpful to confirm the presence of faecal material throughout the colon and to allow estimation of the diameter of the small intestine and colon, which helps to exclude the rare cases of intestinal pseudo-obstruction and megacolon caused by intestinal myopathies and neuropathies.

Transit studies using radio-opaque markers are commonly performed as part of the investigation of constipated patients to determine the severity of transit delay, and to distinguish those with a pancolonic abnormality from a more localized problem of pelvic relaxation. However, measurement of whole-gut transit should not be regarded as necessary for the diagnosis—documented infrequent defaecation is usually sufficient. The electrophysiological and radiological assessment of anorectal function is only indicated if there is evidence of abnormal perineal descent or rectal prolapse, as the accurate recognition of pelvic-floor dysfunction can influence the choice of therapy. Such investigations are indicated when Hirschsprung's disease is suspected.

Pathophysiology

The cause of functional constipation is uncertain. Factors likely to be of relevance are similar to those proposed for irritable bowel syndrome, in particular, enteric neural dysfunction.

In the mildest cases, dietary-fibre deficiency may be relevant; however, in the more severely affected patients, fibre supplementation does not abolish the problem and may even worsen symptoms, making, in such individuals, a causal role for fibre untenable. By contrast, a histological abnormality of the enteric nerves of the colon or muscle of the colon may be found in the most severe cases; for the great majority of constipated patients, however, no structural abnormality has been identified.

In a proportion of patients, almost invariably female, defecatory dysfunction appears to be the major factor. A failure of the pelvic-floor muscles to relax on attempted stool expulsion is identifiable in these patients; this appears to be a 'learned' phenomenon with a psychophysiological aetiology rather than peripheral nerve dysfunction. In other patients, low tone in the pelvic floor and rectal prolapse appear to be the result of damage to the pudendal nerve from straining at stool or parturition and thus may be a consequence of the constipation rather than its cause.

In some severely affected women, there is a relationship between symptom severity and the luteal phase of the menstrual cycle, which has led to the suggestion of a sex-hormonal aetiology. In support of this hypothesis is the fact that colonic muscle tone is reduced by progesterone and that constipation is a frequent accompaniment of normal pregnancies. Against the hypothesis, however, is the failure to demonstrate abnormal colonic sensitivity to progesterone in constipated women, leaving the possibility that the menstrual cycle-related events are merely the expression of a normal cyclical progesterone effect on a malfunctioning colon.

Functional diarrhoea

Definition

This is defined as the frequent passage of unformed stool without the presence of other features of irritable bowel syndrome. Neither abdominal pain nor the frequent passage of formed stools are included in the symptoms.

The diagnosis of functional diarrhoea depends on the presence of two or more of the following: unformed stool; three or more bowel movements per day; and increased stool weight, greater than 200 g/day.

Clinical features

This disorder is recognized only after excluding other, more medically serious conditions, in particular, inflammatory bowel disease and secretory diarrhoeas. The possibility of surreptitious laxative use should always be borne in mind. Some patients identify the time of onset of the problem to a specific life-event, particularly a bout of severe gastroenteritis. The possibility of a chronic intestinal infection needs to be considered carefully in such patients, although evidence of an infective agent will be lacking in most and the label 'postinfective diarrhoea' is usually applied.

Physical examination should determine the extent of nutritional deficiency, exclude metabolic disorders such as hyperthyroidism, and rule out intra-abdominal structural abnormalities. Careful examination of stool samples for pathogens and laxatives is required.

Laboratory investigations

Unlike the other functional diseases, it is important to make a careful search for a structural mucosal disease in such patients. Key diagnoses that must be excluded are: chronic malabsorption due to pancreatic insufficiency or gluten sensitivity, inflammatory bowel disease, infections, and infestations of the gastrointestinal tract.

Pathophysiology

In the absence of any definable structural abnormality, functional diarrhoea is generally assumed to be a disorder of neuroenteric control of intestinal epithelial transport.

In some patients, there is a clear relationship between psychological state and symptoms, with diarrhoea worsening whenever anxiety occurs. However, whether the relationship is truly causal is unknown.

Functional abdominal pain

Definition

While this symptom category is commonly included amongst the functional bowel disorders, the relationship between the abdominal pain and a disturbance of gastrointestinal-tract function is difficult to ascertain. Abdominal pain is frequent, recurrent, or continuous, and characteristically persists for many months. The relationship between pain and recognizable physiological events such as eating, defaecation, or menstruation is lacking, and evidence of organic disease in the abdomen is absent. Most of these patients show a major loss of daily functioning capacity and exhibit chronic illness behaviour.

Management of functional bowel diseases

The management of patients with functional bowel disorders remains empirical. Perhaps it should not be surprising that in an area of human suffering with such symptom diversity and in which the pathophysiological mechanisms remain obscure, no single pharmacological agent or group of agents have ever been found to be consistently effective.

A review of randomized, double-blind, placebo-controlled trials for the treatment of irritable bowel syndrome examined 43 trials and concluded that none offered convincing evidence that any therapy was effective, a conclusion which is perhaps as much an indictment of trial design as the efficacy of the drug therapy. Furthermore, in a condition in which the patient's mental state plays such an important part in defining symptom severity, it is not surprising that in most clinical trials placebo responses have been very high, usually up to 50 per cent. Also, short-term trials of therapeutic agents in diseases where symptoms are intermittent may be unable to distinguish a true drug effect from a placebo response.

So what can the clinician do to help patients with functional bowel disease? As in all chronic problems without a cure, a principal task is to give an explanation and reassurance. Therapy must be patient-centred and designed to provide a solution for the patient's personal needs and expectations. The clinician should give a full explanation of the likely nature of the problem and firm reassurance that organic disease is not likely to be present. Attention to the patient's psychological state is very important, as it is clear that mood is a powerful modulator of symptoms.

In more severe cases of irritable bowel syndrome, psychological treatment using a variety of techniques has been found to provide greater improvement in a patient's sense of well being than drug therapy alone. Good prognostic factors for improvement seem to be overt psychiatric symptoms, particularly anxiety or depression, together with intermittent pain exacerbated by stress. In contrast, patients in whom the abdominal pain is constant, and who exhibit evidence of chronic illness behaviour, do not seem to be helped by a psychotherapeutic approach but they may respond to antidepressants.

In mild cases, attention to the individual and his/her symptoms is usually the approach taken. In patients with predominant constipation, supplementary dietary fibre and poorly absorbed fermentable carbohydrates increase faecal bulk, soften the stool, and may ease defaecation. On occasion, however, this approach can exacerbate symptoms of abdominal distension, probably as a result of increased colonic gas produced by the fermentation of the unabsorbed carbohydrate. Wherever possible, long-term use of stimulant laxatives is best avoided because of the concern that such drugs may themselves damage the colonic enteric-neural function and eventually make the problem worse. Osmotic laxatives and enemas are the mainstay of therapy of the severely constipated patient with slow transit.

For the patient who appears unable to relax the pelvic floor musculature on attempted defaecation, a variety of biofeedback techniques are now available that help the individual to 'relearn' the process. Success is high in those able to engage closely with the therapist in the process.

For patients with diarrhoea-predominant symptoms, attention to diet is also often helpful, as the size of and timing of meals is likely to influence the frequency and social inconvenience of the diarrhoea. Fermentable carbohydrates are best taken in moderation because they can exacerbate symptoms. In the more persistent cases of diarrhoea, symptoms can be improved by simple antidiarrhoeal agents, the dose being adjusted according to the symptoms and administered before a meal.

In the management of patients with unexplained abdominal pain it is tempting to prescribe opiate-derivative analgesics. These are unlikely to be of benefit in the long term, however, and may even exacerbate symptoms because of their constipating effect. Antidepressants are often prescribed empirically in low doses, with evidence of benefit at least in mood elevation. Antispasmodics (for example, hyoscine butyl bromide) are frequently employed. Whilst there are undoubtedly a number of patients and doctors who are convinced of their value, a beneficial effect has yet to be proven beyond doubt by clinical trial.

Relaxation therapy, in particular hypnosis, seems to benefit those individuals who are prepared to participate. In the right conditions, programmes of self-delivered 'autohypnosis' may offer a satisfactory approach for some sufferers.

Surgical intervention for symptoms of functional bowel disorders is usually best avoided, as benefit is unlikely. On occasions, however, subtotal colectomy and ileorectal anastomosis will provide symptomatic benefit in carefully selected patients with severe constipation.

The management of patients with functional bowel disease therefore remains a major challenge that cannot be shirked by clinicians, with whom responsibility exists to provide a careful, individually oriented explanation, and support. The careful conduct of clinical trials of current and new therapies remains a priority for these disorders.

Further reading
Afzalpurkar RG, et al. (1992). The self-limited nature of chronic idiopathic diarrhoea. New England Journal of Medicine, 327, 1849–52.

Anuras S, ed. (1992). Motility disorders of the gastrointestinal tract. Raven Press, New York.

Christensen J (1992). Pathophysiology of the irritable bowel syndrome. Lancet, ii, 1444–7.

Creed FH, Craig T, Farmer RG (1988). Functional abdominal pain, psychiatric illness and life events. Gut, 29, 235–42.

Guthrie E, et al. (1991). A controlled trial of psychological treatment for the irritable bowel syndrome. Gastroenterology, 100, 450–7.

Klein KB (1988). Controlled treatment trials in the irritable bowel syndrome: a critique. Gastroenterology, 95, 232–41.

Kruis W, et al. (1984). A diagnostic score for the irritable bowel syndrome: its value in the exclusion of organic disease. Gastroenterology, 87, 1–7.

Manning AP, et al. (1978). Towards a positive diagnosis of the irritable bowel. British Medical Journal, 2, 653–4.

Read NW, Timms JM, Barfield LJ (1986). Impairment of defaecation in young women with severe constipation. Gastroenterology, 90, 53–61.

Wexner SD, et al. (1992). Prospective assessment of biofeedback for the treatment of paradoxical puborectalis contraction. Diseases of the Colon and Rectum, 35, 145–50.

Whorwell PJ, Prior A, Faragher EB (1984). Controlled trial of hypnotherapy in the treatment of severe refractory irritable bowel syndrome. Lancet, ii, 1232–4.

14.13 Colonic diverticular disease

N. J. McC. Mortensen and M. G. W. Kettlewell

Diverticula can be found throughout the gastrointestinal tract, but are seen most commonly in the sigmoid and descending colon.

Epidemiology

Asymptomatic diverticular disease is much more common than clinical diverticulitis. Autopsy studies in the United Kingdom and Australia have shown that the prevalence of colonic diverticula increases with age. It is rare in those under 30 years of age but occurs in more than 50 per cent of those over 70 years. On the other hand, colonic diverticulosis is very rare in African and Asian countries and right-sided disease predominates in Japan. This geographical distribution is not due to race, as West Indians and Asians living in Britain, American Blacks, and Japanese who have moved to Hawaii or the mainland United States are just as prone to the disease as Caucasians. Patients presenting with complicated diverticular disease have a low intake of dietary fibre, whilst vegetarians have a low incidence of the disease.

In Edinburgh, 23 per cent of all barium enemas demonstrated diverticula. The annual incidence increased from 0.17/1000 in those under 45 years to 5.7/1000 in those over 75 years of age. Women were affected more than men. In spite of the introduction of high-fibre diets, there is no evidence that the incidence of acute diverticulitis is declining.

Aetiology

Diverticular disease is said to be a disease of the twentieth century. It was rarely described in the nineteenth century literature, and in Britain there is a correlation between the rising incidence at the beginning of the twentieth century and an increased consumption of refined flour and sugar. Sugar consumption has trebled since 1860, and in the late 1870s the stone grinding of flour was replaced by roller milling, which removes more fibre. Modern white and some brown breads contain little fibre compared with the amount in wholemeal bread, which was previously a staple part of the diet.

The development of diverticula therefore can be ascribed to a lifelong diet deficient in dietary fibre. An unrefined, high-fibre diet produces swiftly passed, soft stools that subject the colon to little strain. Modern, fibre-deficient diets on the other hand give rise to stiff, viscous stools that need high intracolonic pressures to propel them. High luminal pressures cause a protrusion of the mucosa through vulnerable points in the sigmoid and descending colon. They usually occur at the site where colonic blood vessels penetrate the wall. This hypothesis is supported by the observation that, although basal intracolonic pressures are similar in health and diverticular disease, when the diseased colon is activated by emotion, eating, mechanical stimuli, or drugs such as morphine or prostigmine, high pressures are generated in those segments that have diverticula. This is due to hypersegmentation by the colonic smooth muscle, and the difference has been recorded in the earliest stage of disease and may explain its progressive nature. In symptomatic patients an increase in dietary fibre causes a relief of symptoms in many cases.

Changes in the colon wall also play a part. With age, and following episodes of diverticulitis, the colonic wall becomes stiff and less distensible, aggravating the effects of raised intracolonic pressure. An increase in elastin and changes in collagen have been reported. Diabetic patients are prone to diverticular disease at an earlier stage, suggesting a defect in glycolysation of colonic collagen with advancing age. In those with connective tissue disorders such as Ehlers–Danlos syndrome or Marfan's disease, diverticula are also seen at an unusually early age.

The distinction between symptomatic and asymptomatic diverticular disease is important, for whilst something is known about the formation of diverticula it is not known why some diverticula become symptomatic.

Pathology

A diverticulum consists of a herniation of mucosa through the colonic musculature, and as it enlarges its muscle covering atrophies, so that the fully developed diverticulum consists of mucosa, connective tissue, and peritoneum. The striking abnormality is in the thickening of the circular and longitudinal muscle, which both narrows the colonic lumen and shortens the sigmoid like a concertina to give a saw-tooth appearance on barium enema. The diverticula occur as slit-like apertures between the muscle clefts.

Inflammation in diverticular disease is the result of infection around diverticula, which spreads within the pericolic fat to form a dissecting abscess. Usually a single diverticulum is the cause of a pericolic abscess, perhaps initiated by the presence of a faecolith. Involvement of the peritoneum results in local peritonitis, which may become generalized in the event of a perforation. This may also give rise to intra-abdominal abscesses or fistulae to the bladder, small bowel, vagina, or uterus. Repeated episodes of diverticulitis lead to a contracted, narrowed sigmoid colon surrounded by fibrous tissue. Bleeding in diverticular disease can often be traced to an infected diverticulum. This may cause either the erosion of a vessel in its wall or the formation of granulation tissue inside the diverticulum, which then bleeds.

Clinical features

As diverticulosis is so common, most diverticula are asymptomatic. They are usually discovered incidentally and only some 10 per cent produce symptoms, and around 1 per cent require surgery. The symptoms usually result from disordered motility rather than secondary complications of the disease.

Uncomplicated diverticular disease

Pain can be felt along the course of the colon, particularly over the sigmoid, and is often accompanied by a change in bowel habit with the passage of broken, pellety stools after considerable straining. These symptoms may be indistinguishable from those of the irritable bowel syndrome. The passage

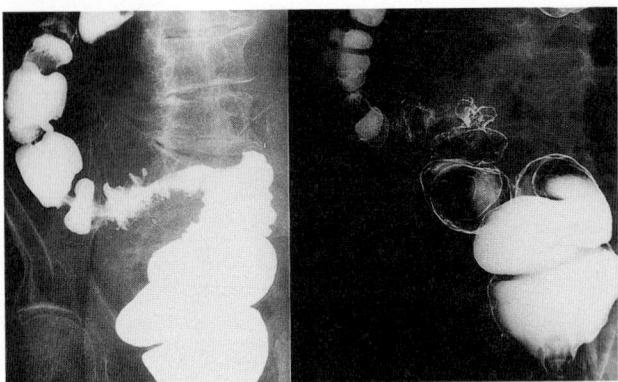

Fig. 1 Barium enema showing a narrowed sigmoid colon with a few diverticula. This appearance can be confused with those of a carcinoma and colonoscopy would be indicated to clarify the diagnosis.

of blood with an unformed stool is unusual and should alert one to the possibility of other pathology.

Management

All patients should have a rigid or flexible sigmoidoscopy in addition to a barium enema to exclude a rectal or sigmoid carcinoma (Fig. 1). They should be reassured that there is no serious underlying disease and a high-fibre diet should be recommended. This must include wholemeal bread, wholewheat breakfast cereals, rough porridge or muesli, and fresh fruit and vegetables daily. Fibre increases stool bulk in three ways—by holding water, by proliferation of bacteria, and from the byproducts of bacterial fermentation. The coarser the fibre the greater is the faecal bulk, and unpalatability, and although cooking bran improves its taste, it reduces its water-holding capacity. A good clinical response is usually achieved by including two tablespoons of bran with the morning cereal, but about half the patients will experience gaseous distension or cramps on starting the high-fibre diet. It is worth warning them that this is likely to happen and that it will resolve within a month or so if they persist with the diet.

In patients with pain, antispasmodics such as mebeverine may be useful, and in a minority with repeated severe attacks an elective resection is then indicated (Table 1). This is probably more effective than sigmoid myotomy, an operation popularized in the mid-1960s. In this procedure the circular muscle is divided with a longitudinal incision to widen the colonic lumen. The incision is made through the taenia so as to avoid opening diverticula, and is deepened until the mucosa is just seen. The operation lowers the sigmoid intraluminal pressures and improves symptoms but, after 3 years, pressures return to their former levels. The need for myotomy has declined but it may still be useful in some elderly or obese patients.

Table 1 Indications for surgery

Sepsis
    Recurrent diverticulitis
    Perforated diverticulitis
    Purulent peritonitis
    Faecal peritonitis
    Pelvic or paracolic abscess
Colonic obstruction
    Inflammatory stricture
    Fibrotic stricture
    Suspected malignancy
Fistulae
    Colovesical
    Colovaginal
    Ileocolic
Major haemorrhage

Complicated diverticular disease

It is important to distinguish the minority of patients who suffer from a febrile attack with left iliac-fossa peritonism, sometimes called left-sided appendicitis, from those with chronic pain and diarrhoea. The inflammation may settle with minimal symptoms or develop into a pericolic abscess or peritonitis.

Acute diverticulitis

Pain is felt over the left lower abdomen, and the patient may have pyrexia, malaise, anorexia, and nausea. The white blood count is raised.

Treatment is with rest, antibiotics, usually cefuroxime 750 mg and metronidazole 500 mg 8-hourly, and analgesia. Most cases settle and the diagnosis can be confirmed after 2 to 3 weeks by barium enema. A narrow segment can sometimes be difficult to distinguish from a carcinoma and any doubtful cases can be clarified by subsequent colonoscopy (Fig. 2).

If symptoms fail to resolve, or recur, resection of the sigmoid colon may be necessary. When it is necessary to resect an acutely inflamed and unprepared colon, a Hartmann's operation may be safer than a primary anastomosis.

For recurrent diverticulitis operated electively, a primary anastomosis would be ideal.

Diverticular abscess

Acute diverticulitis can lead to a local peritonitis with abscess formation, either in the paracolic or pelvic area. There may be a palpable mass and a swinging fever. When in doubt the diagnosis can be confirmed by ultrasound or computed tomography (**CT**) with rectal contrast (Fig. 3).

It is wise to let an abscess localize whilst treating the patient with rest, antibiotics, and analgesia. Some abscesses will be amenable to drainage by direct incision, over them or via the rectum or vagina. More complicated collections are best drained by CT-guided aspiration or drain placement. There is rarely any need to do a proximal transverse colostomy. If drainage persists, an elective sigmoid colectomy with primary anastomosis can be done at a later time. Even when an abscess is localized, however, the condition remains potentially dangerous as it may rupture into the peritoneal cavity giving rise to peritonitis.

Perforated diverticulitis

Acute diverticulitis can be complicated by generalized purulent peritonitis, either by direct spread from the inflamed colon or by rupture of a peridiverticular abscess. The clinical picture is of severe intraperitoneal sepsis

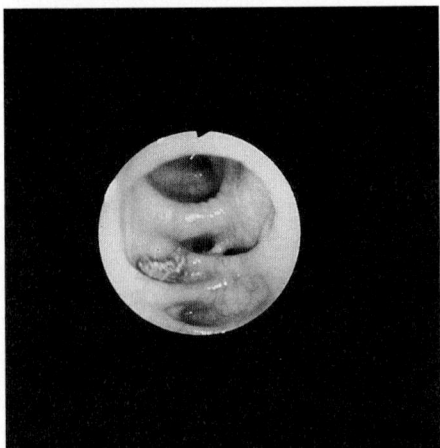

Fig. 2 The typical appearance of diverticula seen at colonoscopy. Note the muscular haustra and the mouths of diverticula—one with a faecolith. (Reproduced from the *Slide atlas of gastroenterology*, Gower Medical Publishing, London, with permission.)

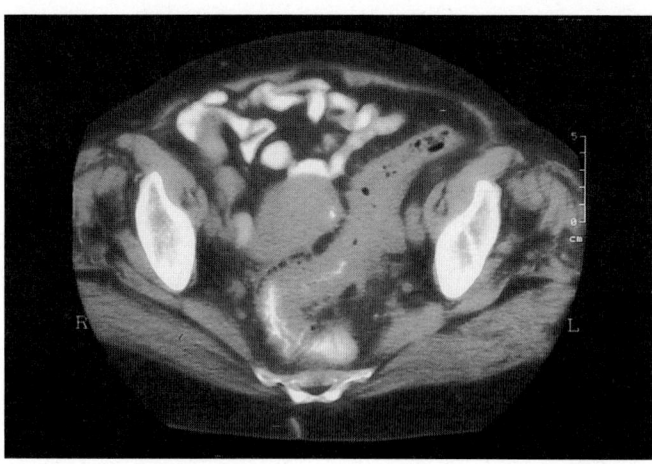

Fig. 3 Computed tomography of the pelvis in a patient with acute diverticulitis. The sigmoid colon is grossly thickened, the lumen narrowed, and pockets of air are seen in the diverticular disease.

with toxaemia, ileus, and abdominal pain, and septicaemia will often follow. Emergency laparotomy is almost always required, although time must be allowed for adequate rehydration, correction of electrolytes, and starting antibiotic therapy—again cefuroxime and metronidazole.

Other causes of the acute abdomen that may not require surgery should be excluded, including pelvic inflammatory disease, ureteric calculus, and even pulmonary embolus. In these circumstances a CT scan is invaluable.

There has been a shift away from the more conservative procedures in this situation. At one time, peritoneal toilet, pelvic drainage, and a defunctioning transverse colostomy was the favoured procedure, but this has the disadvantage that the 'septic colon' is left in place and that there is a column of faecal material below the stoma and above the perforation. There is the further problem of the unsuspected carcinoma within the inflammatory mass.

For these reasons more radical measures are favoured by experienced surgeons. A Hartmann's procedure—removing the diseased sigmoid, oversewing the distal rectum, and bringing out an end colostomy—is the most frequently used procedure (Fig. 4). In favourable cases it may be possible to do an on-table colonic lavage via the appendix stump and make an immediate anastomosis but this carries the risk of leakage.

Hartmann's procedure is safe and effective, although subsequent reconnection may involve a major operation in elderly patients. Purulent peritonitis carries a mortality of around 15 per cent.

Faecal peritonitis

This is a catastrophic complication with a mortality of around 50 per cent particularly in the elderly. A diverticulum ruptures, often with little or no inflammation, liberating quantities of faeces into the peritoneal cavity. Rapid and severe shock with septicaemia ensues. Energetic resuscitation is necessary, followed promptly by surgery and a Hartmann's operation. These patients often need to be stabilized in an intensive care unit postoperatively.

Intestinal obstruction

Recurrent inflammation with fibrosis and muscular hypertrophy can lead to progressive stenosis and colonic obstruction, which is usually chronic but may present acutely. Conservative treatment is worth trying at first, provided a carcinoma has been excluded. With the aid of a stool softener the symptoms may resolve and the stricture gradually dilate. If these measures fail, the bowel should be prepared for a resection, with care taken not to aggravate the obstruction.

Small-bowel obstruction is sometimes a complication of acute diverticulitis, as the bowel may adhere to the inflammatory mass. It usually resolves

as the inflammation subsides but on occasion a laparotomy and division of adhesions or even a small-bowel resection may be necessary.

Colonic fistulae

A colovesical fistula usually presents with recurrent urinary tract infections together with pneumaturia or faecuria. The fistula arises in the sigmoid, which has often folded over into the pouch of Douglas, and adheres to the apex of the bladder. This is the most frequent cause of colovesical fistula but carcinoma and Crohn's disease should be excluded.

Fistulae may also occur between the sigmoid and vagina, uterus, ureter, and ileum. They seldom heal spontaneously but do not always give rise to disabling symptoms and so represent a relative indication for surgery. Sigmoid colectomy as a one-stage procedure is the best option, and colostomy is rarely required. A fistula into the bladder is simply closed and urethral catheter drainage continued for a week.

Haemorrhage

Major haemorrhage is an uncommon but well-recognized complication. It is usually self-limiting, only requiring transfusion and supportive measures. The precise reason for the bleeding is not known but angiographic and colonoscopic studies suggest that many bleeds attributed to diverticula are caused by other lesions such as polyps and angiodysplasia.

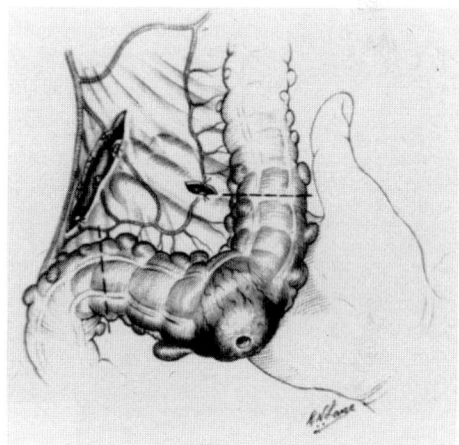

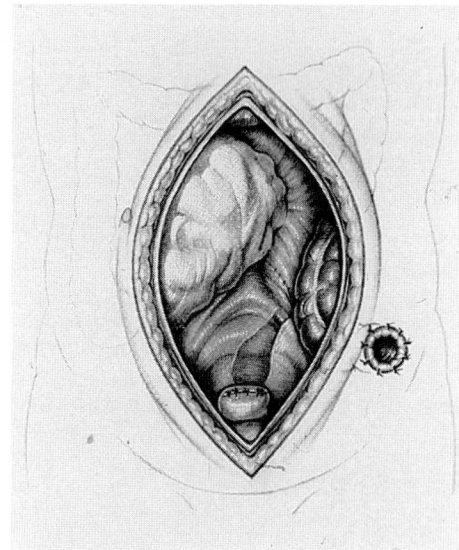

Fig. 4 (a) The area of sigmoid colon resected for perforated diverticular disease. (b) Hartmann's operation—the sigmoid colon has been resected, the rectum oversewn, and a left iliac fossa colostomy fashioned.

Repeated or minor haemorrhage is seldom caused by diverticula and is more likely to be due to carcinoma or polyps. It is therefore vital to exclude other sources of bleeding by barium enema or colonoscopy. The source of a persistent major bleed must be sought urgently, and selective angiography whilst the patient is bleeding is essential. As the haemorrhage can be from any part of the colon, good localization is an essential prelude to any operation. Blind colonic resections have a particularly poor record and if the site of bleeding has still not been located, on-table colonic lavage via the appendix stump and intraoperative colonoscopy will usually target the bleeding segment.

A recent study reported the results of urgent colonoscopy in bleeding diverticular disease. Instead of the tradititional conservative measures patients were given a bowel prep and colonoscoped within 12 h. Bleeding sites thus identified were treated by colonoscopic diathermy and the number of major bleeds, blood transfusions, and operations was reduced together with length of hospital stay. It remains to be seen whether this will result in a major shift of emphasis in management.

Further reading

Boulos BP et al. (1984). Is colonoscopy necessary in diverticular diverticula disease? The Lancet i, 95–6.

Eastwood MA et al. (1977). Variation in the incidence of diverticular disease within the city of Edinburgh. Gut 18, 571–4.

Eastwood MA et al. (1978). Comparison of bran, ispaghula and lactulose on colon function in diverticular disease. Gut 19, 1144–7.

Gear JSS et al. (1979). Symptomless diverticular disease and intake of dietary fibre. The Lancet i, 511–14.

Gianfranco JA, Abcarian H (1982). Pitfalls in the treatment of gastrointestinal bleeding with blind subtotal colectomy. Diseases of the Colon and Rectum 25, 441–5.

Grief JM, Fried DO, McSherry CK (1980). Surgical treatment of perforated diverticulitis of the sigmoid colon. Diseases of the Colon and Rectum 23, 483–7.

Heaton KW (1985). Diet and diverticulosis—new leads. Gut 26, 541–3.

Hughes LE (1969). Postmortem survey of diverticular disease of the colon. Gut 10, 336–51.

Hyland JMP, Taylor I (1980). Does a high fibre diet prevent the complications of diverticular disease? British Journal of Surgery 67, 77–9.

Jensen DM et al. (2000). Urgent colonoscopy for the diagnosis and treatment of severe diverticular haemorrhage. New England Journal of Medicine 342, 78–82.

Kettlewell MGW, Moloney GE (1977). Combined horizontal and longitudinal colomyotomy for diverticular disease: preliminary report. Diseases of the Colon and Rectum 20, 24–8.

Krukowski ZH, Mattheson NA (1985). Emergency surgery for diverticular disease complicated by generalised and faecal peritonitis: a review. British Journal of Surgery 71, 921–7.

Krukowski ZH, Koruth NM, Mattheson NA (1985). Evolving practice in acute diverticulitis. British Journal of Surgery 72, 684–6.

Painter NS (1975). Diverticular disease of the colon. Heinemann Medical, London.

Reilly M (1966). Sigmoid myotomy. British Journal of Surgery 53, 859–63.

Smith AN, Attisha RP, Balfour T (1969). Clinical and manometric results one year after sigmoid myotomy for diverticular disease. British Journal of Surgery 56, 895–9.

Whiteway J, Morson BC (1985). Elastosis in diverticular disease of the sigmoid colon. Gut 26, 258–66.

14.14 Congenital abnormalities of the gastrointestinal tract

V. M. Wright and J. A. Walker-Smith

Although present at birth, congenital abnormalities of the gastrointestinal tract usually manifest shortly after birth, but on occasion symptoms may be delayed for months or even years. For example duodenal atresia presents in the first few days of life whereas duodenal stenosis may not present until adult life.

The widespread use of ultrasound to assess the fetus allows many of these abnormalities to be recognized prenatally; in particular, abdominal wall defects, fluid-filled stomach in duodenal atresia, dilated bowel in the more distal atresias, and cystic masses. In addition, associated anomalies may indicate a major chromosome abnormality or cardiac lesion. This allows parental choice to continue with or terminate the pregnancy.

Embryology of the congenital abnormalities of the gastrointestinal tract

The primitive gut is initially a simple tube of endoderm, the muscle and connective tissue developing from the splanchnopleuric mesoderm. Cranially, the gut terminates at the buccopharyngeal membrane and caudally at the cloacal membrane. Both membranes disappear; failure of the cloacal membrane to do so results in one of the rarer forms of imperforate anus. The primitive foregut diverticulum gives rise to the respiratory system, oesophagus, stomach, duodenum to the level of the ampulla of Vater, liver, and pancreas. The primitive oesophagus lengthens rapidly, becomes narrow, and frequently the lumen is transiently obliterated. A longitudinal, ventral diverticulum of the foregut forms the trachea with ridges on either side that fuse, initially caudally with progression cranially, until the primitive respiratory system is separated from the oesophagus. Failure of this complex process results in the various forms of oesophageal atresia and tracheo-oesophageal fistula. Dilatation of the foregut distal to the oesophagus produces the stomach, initially slung from the dorsal body wall by the dorsal mesentery and from the septum transversum by the ventral mesentery. Rapid differential growth results in the stomach rotating through 90° on its long axis, the dorsal border becoming the greater curvature and the ventral border the lesser curvature. The dorsal mesentery forms the greater omentum. The ventral mesentery, into which the liver bud grows, forms the falciform ligament and coronary ligaments attaching the liver to the diaphragm, and the lesser omentum. Congenital abnormalities of the stomach are excessively rare. The liver arises as a shallow groove on the ventral aspect of the duodenum. The groove becomes tubular and invades the septum transversum and the ventral mesentery. Bile is secreted from the fifth month, and gives meconium its characteristic dark-green appearance. The mesoderm of the septum transversum forms the fibrous tissue of the liver.

The pancreas develops as two outgrowths of the duodenum. One comes from the dorsal aspect, the other from the ventral. The dorsal bud grows into the dorsal mesentery and the ventral bud is swept around dorsally into the mesentery when the duodenum rotates to the right. These two primordia fuse, the ducts fuse, and the main pancreatic duct joins the bile duct to enter the duodenum at the ampulla of Vater. If the ducts do not fuse, an accessory pancreatic duct persists. Annular pancreas is a congenital anomaly where the pancreas surrounds the duodenum, which may be atretic or intrinsically stenosed. Annular pancreas is not the primary cause of the duodenal obstruction in these cases.

The duodenum is derived partly from foregut and partly from the midgut. The loop of primitive duodenum is fixed at the pyloric end, and by the ligament of Treitz at the duodenojejunal flexure to the left of the first lumbar vertebra. By rotating to the right, the entire duodenum comes to lie retroperitoneally in a curve around the head of the pancreas. Failure of the duodenum to fix in this position is a fundamental reason for the gut failing to rotate correctly. During rapid growth the duodenal lumen is obliterated and partial or total failure of recanalization will result in the anomalies of duodenal atresia or stenosis. The small intestine and colon, suspended on the dorsal mesentery, rapidly lengthen and outgrow the primitive peritoneal cavity, and herniation occurs into the umbilical sac during the fifth week of development. Growth in length continues, the loop of bowel rotating through 90° anticlockwise, the cranial limb lengthening more than the caudal limb. About the tenth week the loops of bowel return to the peritoneal cavity, undergoing a further 180° anticlockwise rotation. The small intestine goes first, the large intestine subsequently. Thus the large intestine lies in front of the small. The caecum is initially subhepatic, the large liver occupying the right side of the abdomen, eventually retreating to the right upper quadrant and allowing growth in the length of the ascending colon. The caecum, ascending colon, and descending colon become fixed to the posterior abdominal wall; thus the small bowel is suspended from a mesentery that runs from the left side of the first lumbar vertebra to the right iliac fossa. Failure of the duodenum to rotate and fix, coupled with a failure of normal rotation of the bowel with consequent lack of normal fixation, gives rise to malrotation of the intestine. Abnormal bands run from the caecum, which lies to the left of the midline, to the region of the gallbladder and may compress the duodenum. The narrow mesentery of the small intestine predisposes to a volvulus of the entire midgut.

At the apex of the midgut loop, the primitive gut is in continuity with the extraembryonic yolk sac via the vitellointestinal duct, which runs in the umbilical cord. Obliteration and disappearance of this duct occurs, allowing the bowel to return from the umbilical sac to the enlarged peritoneal cavity. Failure of the duct to disappear may result in a Meckel's diverticulum, a band connecting the ileum to the umbilicus, a communication between the lumen of the ileum and the umbilicus, or failure of the gut to return completely to the peritoneal cavity, resulting in a small umbilical hernia.

Persistence of the umbilical sac will result in an exomphalos, with the sac containing a variable amount of gut and much of the liver. The embryology of gastroschisis is disputed. It may be due to early rupture of the umbilical sac allowing the primitive gut to extrude into the extraembryonic coelom, or failure of fusion of the lateral body folds producing a defect in the anterior abdominal wall adjacent to the umbilicus.

The midgut comprises the duodenum distal to the ampulla of Vater, jejunum, ileum, caecum, and colon as far as the left transverse colon. Atresia affecting the midgut may occur at single or multiple sites. The cause is probably intrauterine interference with the blood supply to that part of the gut which is affected, with consequent resorption of the ischaemic bowel.

The hindgut gives origin to the left third of the transverse colon, the descending colon, sigmoid, rectum, and upper part of the anal canal, and a considerable part of the urogenital system. The hindgut terminates in the primitive cloaca, which is separated from the proctodaeum (a shallow ectodermal depression) by the cloacal membrane. The primitive cloaca communicates with the hindgut and the allantois. Early in development the cloaca is joined by the pronephric ducts. A coronal septum (the urorectal septum) arises in the angle between the allantois and hindgut, grows caudally, fuses with the cloacal membrane, and divides the cloaca into a dorsal primitive rectum and a ventral primitive urogenital sinus. The cloacal membrane breaks down, establishing continuity between the endodermal hindgut and the ectodermal part of the anal canal. There are many varieties of imperforate anus. Absence of a variable length of rectum and anal canal, known as the 'high' anomaly, is frequently associated with the bowel terminating via a rectourethral or rectovaginal fistula. Ten per cent of babies with an imperforate anus will have oesophageal atresia, with or without a fistula, suggesting that the division of trachea and oesophagus and urogenital system and rectum must be occurring at a similar time in gestation, with possibly a similar mechanism producing the division. Anomalies of the urogenital system occur in a very high proportion of affected infants. Abnormalities of the ectodermal component of the anal canal result in 'low' imperforate anus.

The ganglion cells of the gut lie in the submucosa and intermyenteric plane. Ectodermal in origin, they migrate caudally along the length of the gut. Failure of migration down to the internal sphincter of the anal canal results in an aganglionic segment extending for a variable distance proximally, and is the underlying abnormality in Hirschsprung's disease.

Mucosal differentiation occurs in the early months. The inner circular muscle differentiates earlier than the outer longitudinal. Thus the fetal intestinal tract is prepared for digestion, absorption, and propulsion at a comparatively early stage in development.

Oesophageal atresia and tracheo-oesophageal fistula

The incidence of this condition is approximately 1 in 3500 live births.

The upper oesophagus ends in a blind pouch. In the majority of cases, the lower oesophagus communicates at its upper end with the trachea, that is there is a tracheo-oesophageal fistula. Although much less common, there are a number of well-recognized anatomical variations illustrated in Fig. 1.

Clinical features

Frequently the infant with oesophageal atresia is premature or small for gestational age. In 50 per cent there is a history of polyhydramnios. Shortly after birth, because swallowing is impossible, copious amounts of frothy

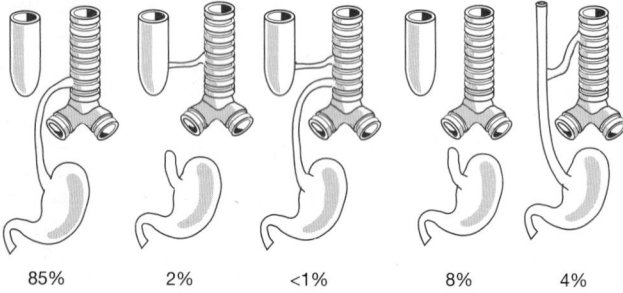

85%　　2%　　<1%　　8%　　4%

Fig. 1 Anatomical variations of oesophageal atresia and tracheo-oesophageal fistula, indicating the relative frequency.

saliva dribble from the mouth, associated with choking, dyspnoea, and cyanotic episodes. Frequent suction is required to keep the airway clear. The infant with a tracheo-oesophageal fistula without associated oesophageal atresia coughs, chokes, and becomes cyanosed during feeds. Because air escapes through the fistula into the oesophagus, gaseous distension of the abdomen is frequently present. Aspiration of feed into the airway results in pulmonary collapse/consolidation.

Over 50 per cent of infants with oesophageal atresia will have significant associated anomalies. Of particular importance are cardiac, anorectal, urogenital, and skeletal anomalies. The premature infant or the infant who is small for gestational age are more likely to have multiple anomalies than is the full-term infant.

Survival of infants with oesophageal atresia depends on birth weight and associated abnormalities. All infants with a birth weight greater than 1.8 kg and no associated abnormalities or pneumonia should survive; this is also true of the larger infant with a moderately severe associated abnormality or pneumonia. The mortality for the infant less than 1.5 kg, or one with multiple severe congenital abnormalities, remains in the region of 20 to 30 per cent.

Diagnosis

When oesophageal atresia is suspected a size 10 or 12 FG catheter is passed through the mouth and into the oesophagus. If the oesophagus is obstructed, the catheter meets a resistance 9 to 11 cm from the gum margin. A smaller catheter may curl up in the obstructed oesophagus. Contrast studies of the oesophagus are rarely necessary. A chest and abdominal radiograph will show the position of a radio-opaque tube in the upper oesophagus, and the presence of gas in the bowel if a tracheo-oesophageal fistula is present. Complete absence of gas in the abdomen is diagnostic of an oesophageal atresia without a distal tracheo-oesophageal fistula. The radiograph will also reveal any abnormalities of ribs or vertebrae, signs of pneumonia, and may provide evidence of an associated cardiac abnormality.

In isolated tracheo-oesophageal fistula, very careful contrast studies of the oesophagus are required to demonstrate the fistula. Endoscopic examination of trachea and oesophagus is usually diagnostic.

Management

Early division of the tracheo-oesophageal fistula and anastomosis of the oesophagus are possible in the majority of cases. Postoperatively, mechanical ventilation may be necessary, but usually the full-term infant with no preoperative complications only needs careful suction of the nasopharynx to maintain a clear airway. A gastrostomy or a transanastomotic nasogastric tube is usually used to enable the infant to be fed within 48 h of operation. A primary anastomosis may not be feasible in pure oesophageal atresia, extreme prematurity, or where the infant's general condition is poor. In such cases a tracheo-oesophageal fistula, if present, would be divided and a feeding gastrostomy established. Subsequently, an oesophageal anastomosis, after a delay of 4 to 6 weeks, having left the upper oesophageal pouch intact and kept empty of saliva by continuous suction, may be feasible. Alternatively, a cervical oesophagostomy is done with the intention, when the infant's condition permits, of establishing continuity between mouth and stomach, using a length of colon, a tube of stomach, or the whole stomach. The choice depends on the surgeon's preference.

Anterior abdominal wall defects

The incidence of exomphalos and gastroschisis is approximately 1 in 3000 births. An exomphalos occurs because the intra-abdominal contents herniate through the umbilical ring into the base of the umbilical cord and are covered by a translucent membrane composed of peritoneum and amnion. Exomphalos major indicates that the diameter of the defect is greater than 5 cm, exomphalos minor that the defect is less than 5 cm. The contents of the exomphalos almost always include liver and a variable amount of bowel. On occasion, a very small amount of bowel alone herniates into the base of the cord. The diagnosis is frequently made on a prenatal ultrasonographic scan and prompts a search for associated major abnormalities, particularly anencephaly, chromosomal trisomies, major cardiac anomalies, and the Beckwith–Wiedemann syndrome. Associated abnormalities occur in 40 per cent.

The Beckwith–Wiedemann syndrome also termed the exomphalos macroglossia gigantism (EMG) syndrome, usually presents as a large-for-dates infant with a small exomphalos. The tongue is strikingly large, there are frequently ridges in the ear lobes, and a prominent naevus flammeus on the forehead. Hypoglycaemia as a result of hyperinsulinism produced by islet-cell hyperplasia is a common early problem, which may require steroids, glucagon, and rarely subtotal pancreatectomy to effect control. In the long term, children with this syndrome have an increased incidence of solid tumours, particularly nephroblastoma and hepatoblastoma.

In gastroschisis there is a full-thickness defect in the anterior abdominal wall, usually to the right of the umbilical cord. The defect is small but most of the gastrointestinal tract may be extruded through it. In contrast to exomphalos, other intra-abdominal organs are rarely eviscerated and abnormalities outside the gastrointestinal are unusual. Again, prenatal diagnosis on ultrasonographic scan is common.

Exomphalos

Clinical features

The lesion will be obvious at birth. Occasionally the membrane will rupture during, or shortly after, delivery. Careful examination for associated defects is essential.

Management

A nasogastric tube is passed to decompress the bowel. The sac can be very satisfactorily covered and supported by wrapping clingfilm around the exomphalos and the baby's trunk. Plain radiographs of chest and abdomen are taken preoperatively in order to study the cardiac contour, the intestinal gas pattern, and to look for evidence of an associated diaphragmatic hernia. If the contents of the sac can be reduced into the peritoneal cavity, the abdominal wall can be closed in layers. If closure of all layers of the abdominal wall is impossible, skin closure alone may be used, or a synthetic material such as Silastic sheeting or Prolene mesh is used to enclose the sac after suturing it to the margins of the defect. Gradual reduction of the contents into the peritoneal cavity is then possible, with delayed closure of the abdominal wall. An alternative is to paint the sac with an antiseptic solution such as 70 per cent alcohol or one of the iodine-based preparations. This results in the formation of a dry eschar that separates after some weeks, leaving a granulating surface, which gradually epithelializes. Any method that does not achieve muscle closure will leave a ventral hernia, which requires surgery at a later date.

Postoperatively, ventilatory support may be necessary. Antibiotics commenced preoperatively are continued postoperatively, particularly if an artificial material is used. Parenteral nutrition will be necessary if oral feeds cannot be given. Survival is related to the size of the lesion and the severity of any associated abnormalities.

Gastroschisis

Clinical features

Babies with this abnormality are frequently small for gestational age. After delivery, heat loss from the exposed bowel rapidly causes hypothermia. Hypoproteinaemia is very common. The small size of the defect in the anterior abdominal wall and the often narrow pedicle from which the bowel is suspended may impair the blood supply and result in infarction of much of the extruded intestine. Atresia may have occurred because of intra-uterine impairment of the blood supply.

Management

A nasogastric tube is passed and the bowel decompressed. The bowel can be enclosed in clingfilm wrapped around the baby's trunk, or the baby can be placed in a large polythene bag taped around the chest. This keeps the bowel moist and prevents excessive heat loss. Antibiotics are commenced preoperatively and colloid is given to counteract the existing hypoproteinaemia and hypovolaemia. At operation the anterior abdominal wall is stretched and any meconium washed out *per rectum* to reduce bulk. Reduction of the extruded bowel is attempted and abdominal wall closure achieved where possible.

In about 10 per cent of cases, primary closure is not possible and a Silastic sheet or Prolene mesh is used to form an artificial sac to enclose the intestine. The material is sutured to the margins of the defect and the size of the sac gradually reduced over some days, squeezing the bowel back into the peritoneal cavity until closure of the abdominal wall becomes feasible—usually after 10 to 14 days. Ventilatory support postoperatively is often necessary. Parenteral nutrition is essential and may need to continue for many weeks until gastrointestinal motility and absorption are adequate. Sepsis is a considerable hazard. The mortality is now 5 to 10 per cent compared with 80 per cent 10 years ago. Improved postoperative management is largely responsible for this.

Congenital pyloric stenosis

Congenital hypertrophic pyloric stenosis is a disorder characterized by hypertrophy of the circular muscle of the pylorus and so obstruction to the gastric outlet. The incidence is 2 per 1000 live births. The aetiology is unknown. Theories include primary muscle hypertrophy, abnormalities of the maturation of ganglion cells, absence of a certain type of ganglion cell, or a response to abnormally high concentrations of circulating gastrin. Genetic and environmental factors play an important part. There is an increased incidence of pyloric stenosis in siblings of an affected child and in the offspring of a woman who has had the condition. Environmental factors include social class, type of feeding, and a seasonal variation with an increase in the winter months. In any large series the male:female ratio is 3 or 4:1 and half the cases will be first-born children.

Clinical features

The onset of symptoms is usually between 3 and 6 weeks of age, but may present shortly after birth. Vomiting of increasing severity is the cardinal symptom, eventually occurring after most feeds and becoming projectile. The vomitus is milk and mucus, and may contain altered blood suggesting an oesophagitis or gastritis; bile is never present. The baby stops gaining weight and becomes constipated. Characteristically the baby is alert, anxious, and hungry. If diagnosis is delayed, severe malnutrition may develop.

Examination reveals evidence of weight loss and in advanced cases signs of dehydration will be evident. When the stomach is full, waves of peristalsis travelling from left to right in the epigastrium will be seen (visible peristalsis). The thickened pylorus is felt as an olive-sized tumour lying deep to the edge of the right rectus and is often most easily felt when the stomach is empty. The diagnosis of pyloric stenosis is made on clinical grounds in the majority of cases. A plain radiograph of the abdomen may be very helpful in revealing a large stomach with a paucity of distal gas. A barium meal is diagnostic when the 'string' sign of the elongated pylorus is demonstrated. The barium study may also reveal gastro-oesophageal reflux, which is commonly associated with pyloric stenosis. Ultrasound is now widely used—pyloric length more than 1.2 cm and wall width more than 3 mm supporting the diagnosis.

Management

In the child presenting early, electrolyte disturbance and dehydration are minimal. In the later case, dehydration with hypochloraemic alkalosis and marked potassium depletion occurs. Preoperative correction of water and electrolyte deficits is essential. The operation of pyloromyotomy, described by Ramstedt in 1912, splits the hypertrophied muscle longitudinally allowing the mucosa to bulge through the defect, thus enlarging the pyloric canal. Postoperatively, various feeding regimens are advocated; all aim to have the baby on a normal feeds by 48 to 72 h postoperatively. The prognosis is excellent.

Atresia and stenosis of the small intestine

An intrinsic obstruction may produce either complete or partial obliteration of the bowel lumen. Complete obliteration may be due to a gap between the two ends of the small intestine, with or without a connecting band between these ends, or a complete mucosal diaphragm. Such complete obstruction is known as atresia. When obstruction is incomplete it may be due to a narrowing of the lumen—a stenosis—or a mucosal diaphragm with a hole. Small-intestinal atresia is a more common finding than is stenosis. The duodenum is most often affected, followed by jejunum, and least often ileum.

Associated abnormalities of the gastrointestinal tract, including malrotation, oesophageal atresia, imperforate anus, biliary atresia, and annular pancreas are a feature of duodenal atresia/stenosis. Localized volvulus and meconium ileus are associated with jejunoileal atresias.

Intrinsic obstruction of the small intestine of congenital origin presents most often in the neonatal period but when the obstruction is partial it may first present much later, in infancy and childhood.

Congenital intrinsic duodenal obstruction

When duodenal obstruction is complete, vomiting usually occurs within a few hours of birth and is bile stained unless the obstruction is proximal to the ampulla of Vater, when the vomiting is persistent and copious but not bile stained. Meconium may be passed normally and there may be obvious epigastric distension. In view of the association with other abnormalities, these should be sought carefully. In particular the infant should be examined for evidence of Down's syndrome. Duodenal lesions are an association of this syndrome and occur in 10 per cent of cases.

When obstruction is incomplete the symptoms may be intermittent and the diagnosis delayed.

Congenital intrinsic duodenal obstruction may be accompanied by an annular pancreas; this is a sign of failure of duodenal development rather than an obstructive lesion *per se*. In infants with duodenal atresia, at operation, it often looks as if there is an annular pancreas because there is interposition of the pancreas between the two ends of the duodenal atresia.

Congenital intrinsic duodenal obstruction is not, in general, associated with multiple atresias in the remainder of the small intestine, but there may be obstruction at two levels in the duodenum.

Jejunoileal obstruction

Symptoms, typically bile-stained vomiting and abdominal distension, usually occur within the first 2 days of life. Meconium may or may not be passed. When obstruction is incomplete the diagnosis may again be long delayed and the child may present with intermittent vomiting, abdominal distension, and even with features of malabsorption—a clinical picture that may resemble coeliac disease.

Diagnosis

Plain radiographs of the abdomen are usually diagnostic in infants who present with a complete obstruction. In duodenal atresia there is the characteristic 'double bubble' (Fig. 2). When duodenal obstruction is incomplete there may be small amounts of air in the lower bowel. A barium meal may be necessary to demonstrate the obstruction and may suggest an associated malrotation. When there is complete jejunoileal obstruction there are usually multiple dilated loops of intestine. A barium enema may reveal

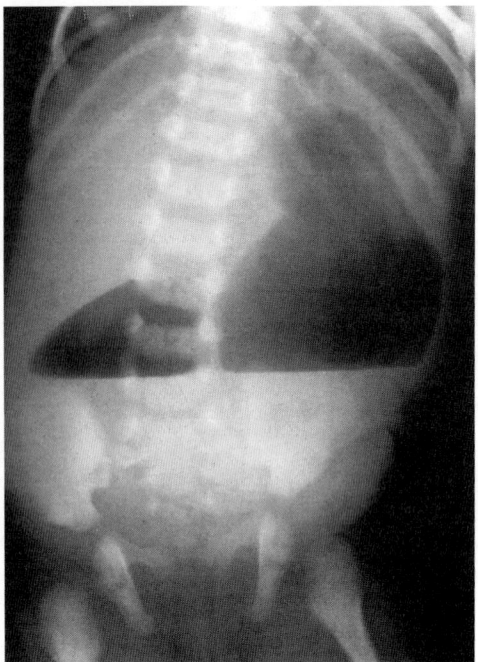

Fig. 2 Plain radiograph of the abdomen of an infant with duodenal atresia showing characteristic 'double bubble'.

an unused microcolon. When obstruction is incomplete a barium follow-through may be needed to establish the diagnosis. Rarely, laparotomy may be the final court of appeal.

Management

A nasogastric tube is passed to empty the stomach and allow accurate measurement of gastric losses. Correction of fluid and electrolyte disturbances, if present, should precede surgery, provided that gangrenous or ischaemic bowel is not suspected. At laparotomy, care should be taken to exclude any other gastrointestinal abnormality. In duodenal obstruction, the operation of choice is duodenoduodenostomy. In jejunoileal lesions, adequate resection of the proximal dilated gut reduces the great discrepancy in size between the two blind ends and so facilitates end-to-end anastomosis, although an oblique-to-end anastomosis is sometimes necessary. Leaving the dilated gut immediately proximal to the anastomosis results in ineffective peristalsis and delay in establishing enteral feeds.

Considerable loss of intestinal length may occur as a result of the intrauterine process producing the atresia; surgical correction, particularly of multiple atresias, will result in further loss. Every effort is made to preserve some ileum and the ileocaecal valve. Loss of considerable lengths of jejunum is well tolerated. Loss of ileum, particularly if the ileocaecal valve is also lost, presents management problems throughout childhood because malabsorption of a variety of important nutrients occurs. The enterohepatic circulation may be impaired. Early liver damage is a consequence of prolonged parenteral nutrition and episodes of sepsis.

Duplication of gastrointestinal tract

Definition

Duplications are cystic or tubular structures whose lumen is lined by a mucous membrane, usually supported by smooth muscle. They occur most often within the dorsal mesentery of the gut. They are also sometimes described as enteric cysts, neurenteric cysts, and reduplications. Duplications may occur anywhere along the alimentary tract but they are found most often in relation to the small intestine, particularly the ileum. They may not communicate with the lumen of the gastrointestinal tract. Duplications may be found in association with intestinal atresias. Sometimes those associated with the small intestine are lined by gastric mucosa and peptic ulceration of the adjacent small-intestinal mucosa, with bleeding, may occur. Those associated with the colon never contain ectopic gastric mucosa.

Clinical features

These are congenital malformations that present most often in early infancy. Later presentation, even into adult life, is well recognized. Duplications may present in infancy as a small-bowel obstruction, or a small cystic duplication may form the lead point of an intussusception. A palpable abdominal mass in infancy, as well as rectal bleeding and volvulus, may also be modes of presentation of this disorder. The clinical diagnosis is often difficult and the diagnosis may sometimes be made only at laparotomy. A technetium scan may be helpful by demonstrating ectopic gastric mucosa. Initial presentation may be a posterior mediastinal cystic mass, possibly associated with cervical or upper thoracic vertebral abnormalities. The mass is likely to communicate through the diaphragm with an intestinal duplication.

Management

Excision of a cystic duplication with or without the adjacent intestine is usually straightforward. Any associated thoracic cyst will also need excision. Short tubular duplications can be excised with the adjacent intestine; very extensive tubular duplications can be opened longitudinally and the mucosa stripped out, leaving the common muscle wall.

Small-intestinal malrotation with or without volvulus

Malrotation of the small intestine is due to disordered movement of the intestine around the superior mesenteric artery during the course of development of the embryo.

Two main abnormalities that produce symptoms may occur. First, there is a gross narrowing of the base of the mesentery, which may allow the midgut to twist around and cause a volvulus. This may occur acutely, causing complete obstruction, or it may occur intermittently, producing bouts of partial or complete obstruction that release themselves spontaneously. Secondly, there may be partial duodenal obstruction from extrinsic compression of the small intestine by peritoneal bands (Ladd's bands) that extend from the caecum to the subhepatic region.

Malrotation may be associated with duodenal atresia or stenosis. It is also found in association with diaphragmatic hernia, omphalocele, and gastroschisis. However, malrotation may be asymptomatic and is sometimes discovered only as an incidental finding on a barium study. The majority of children who develop symptoms related to malrotation do so within the neonatal period, presenting with features of intestinal obstruction, complete or incomplete. When there is a volvulus there may also be obstruction to the blood supply to the bowel, which if complete will lead to extensive gangrene of the small bowel. The passage of bloody stools may be an early sign of this complication.

Those children with malrotation who present later in childhood may do so with features of intermittent obstruction such as episodes of vomiting, often bile stained, and abdominal pain, but sometimes they may manifest with features of malabsorption and many clinical features suggestive of coeliac disease. This is due to intestinal stasis with bacterial overgrowth in the lumen of the small intestine. Steatorrhoea may be accompanied at times by protein-losing enteropathy from obstruction of the mesenteric lymphatics, and chylous ascites may also occur.

Diagnosis

The diagnosis needs to be considered in the differential diagnosis of small-intestinal obstruction in infancy.

Plain radiographs of the abdomen may be very useful, typically revealing an air-filled stomach with some gas scattered through the lower part of the abdomen. However, a malrotation may not be accompanied by any abnormality on the plain radiograph of the abdomen and a barium meal will then be necessary to reveal the presence of malrotation by outlining the failure of the duodenum to cross to the left of the vertebral bodies with the fourth part lying adjacent to the first lumbar vertebra. A barium enema may be useful if it demonstrates the abnormal position of the caecum, but a barium meal is more reliable.

Management

Surgical intervention is indicated when a firm diagnosis is established. Ladd's operation is usually the procedure of choice. This involves, in general, the placement of the colon on the left and the small intestine on the right, having divided any bands and adhesions between the duodenum and large bowel, and, by dissection, broadened the base of the mesentery as much as possible. After a volvulus, total bowel necrosis is untreatable, but severe bowel ischaemia can be reversible and a 'second look' laparotomy may be necessary.

Small-intestinal lymphangiectasia

Small-intestinal lymphangiectasia has been described as a primary, that is a congenital, abnormality or as a secondary manifestation of some other disease process such as constrictive pericarditis. The primary abnormality may be accompanied by generalized lymphatic abnormalities including lymphoedema, chylous ascites, and hypoplasia of the peripheral lymphatic system, but the lymphatic abnormality may be confined to the small bowel and its mesentery. It is usually, but not invariably, accompanied by hypoproteinaemic oedema. Radioisotope studies have demonstrated that the hypoproteinaemia is due to abnormal protein loss into the gut. The pathogenesis of the hypoproteinaemia has been attributed to the rupture of dilated lymphatic channels or to protein exudation from intestinal capillaries via an intact epithelium, where there is obstruction of lymphatic flow.

Clinical features

It is a rare condition, which may present throughout life but most often in the first 2 years with diarrhoea and failure to thrive and, later, generalized oedema with hypoproteinaemia. The clinical picture may resemble coeliac disease. There is lymphopenia in the presence of a normal bone marrow and reduction of serum albumin, serum IgG, and carrier proteins such as protein-bound iodine. The severe protein loss may be accompanied by enteric calcium loss, leading to hypocalcaemia. Steatorrhoea is often found in this disorder.

Diagnosis

Diagnosis is made by showing the characteristic lymphatic abnormality on small intestinal biopsy, that is dilated lacteals, but the lesion is patchy. One negative biopsy does not exclude the diagnosis. Radioisotope demonstration of abnormal enteric protein loss using a technique such as intravenous $CrCl_3$ is helpful in diagnosis but is not specific. Barium studies in most cases show coarse mucosal folds.

Pathology

Autopsy studies reveal a considerable variation in the distribution of the lymphatic abnormality along the length of the small intestine. Dilated lacteals may occur irregularly along the small bowel and there may be gross dilatation of lymphatics projecting into the lumen. Lymphatic proliferation and dilation may also occur within the mesentery, as well as the serosal, muscular, and submucosal layers of the small-intestinal wall, and extend into the lymph nodes and occupy part of the nodal tissue.

Treatment

This is usually dietetic, as the lymphangiectasia is rarely localized enough to allow surgical excision to effect a permanent cure. The amount of long-chain fat in the diet, which is normally absorbed via the intestinal lymphatics, should be limited. This leads to a reduction in the volume of intestinal lymph and in the pressure in the dilated lymphatics. It is best done by placing the child on a low-fat diet (5–10 g/day) and adding medium-chain triglycerides, instead of the usual long-chain dietary fats, in unrestricted amounts. A milk containing medium-chain triglyceride such as Pregestimil[R] may be used with medium-chain triglyceride oil for cooking. Some children may be resistant to this therapy when the abnormality is very extensive and, on occasion, death may result despite therapy. Albumin infusions are of little value in management as their benefit is so transitory. Steroids have been advocated but there is little evidence to justify their use. In a follow-up study of children, although there was a continuing chyle leak, as shown by persistent lymphopenia and hypoalbuminaemia, there was a rapid and sustained improvement in dependent oedema following the use of the diet recommended above, although asymmetrical oedema from peripheral lymphatic abnormalities was unaffected. Their growth rate improved on the diet. Clinical relapse occurred quickly when the diet was relaxed. Continued adherence to a strict diet, at least through puberty, is therefore recommended. Indeed it seems probable that this is a life-long disorder and that some dietetic management may usually need to be permanent.

Meckel's diverticulum

This diverticulum is the vestigial remnant of the vitellointestinal duct. Although most people who have such a diverticulum are asymptomatic, complications may arise, which may present in a variety of ways. In children, these complications chiefly arise in association with the presence of ectopic gastric mucosa in the diverticulum. Other ectopic tissue, for example pancreatic tissue and colonic mucosa, may be found in some cases.

The diverticulum is located in the distal ileum within 100 cm of the ileo-caecal valve. It is always antemesenteric.

Clinical features

Rectal bleeding is the main symptom. This is usually the passage of bright blood rather than tarry melaena stools. Typically the stool is at first dark in colour but later bright red. Bleeding may be acute, with shock requiring urgent blood transfusion, or it may be chronic. From a practical viewpoint any child who has a massive, painless, rectal bleed should be regarded as having a Meckel's diverticulum until proved otherwise. Most often bleeding from a Meckel's diverticulum is associated with ulceration of the small bowel adjacent to ectopic gastric or pancreatic mucosa but this is not always the case as bleeding may occur in the absence of ectopic mucosa.

Small-intestinal obstruction may also be a mode of presentation. This may be as a volvulus associated with a band, or an intussusception with the diverticulum as the lead point. Acute diverticulitis occurs and may produce a picture indistinguishable from acute appendicitis.

Diagnosis and management

This depends upon the mode of presentation. When rectal bleeding occurs, other causes need excluding. Investigation may include colonoscopy to exclude colonic causes and upper endoscopy to exclude peptic ulceration or oesophagitis.

Barium follow-through is usually an unrewarding investigation. a technetium scan is usually the most important investigation. The radionuclide technetium-99m concentrates in the gastric mucosa. When it is given intravenously, ectopic gastric mucosa appears as an abnormal localization on abdominal imaging with a gamma-camera. In this way a Meckel's diverticulum with ectopic gastric mucosa or indeed a duplication with such ectopic tissue may be diagnosed. A negative scan may prompt angiography. However, negative investigations in a child with severe bleeding should not deter a surgeon from proceeding with a diagnostic laparotomy, or laparoscopy if appropriately skilled. Indeed, when considering the other modes of presentation of Meckel's diverticulum it is often only at laparotomy that the role of a Meckel's diverticulum in the child's intestinal pathology is appreciated.

Meconium ileus

This is a manifestation of cystic fibrosis, the disorder sometimes known as fibrocystic disease of the pancreas. Meconium ileus is the earliest mode of presentation of this disorder during the neonatal period. A similar syndrome in older children and young adults who have cystic fibrosis may occur—the meconium ileus equivalent. The abnormally viscid consistency of the meconium produces an intraluminal obstruction. It may result from several factors including the lack of pancreatic enzymes during fetal life, which may account for the high protein content of the meconium. There is also evidence of reduced secretion of water and electrolytes in such infants, which may further render the meconium more viscid. The meconium, because of its high viscosity and tendency to adhere to the mucosa, cannot be propelled along the bowel and so small-intestinal obstruction results. This occurs most often in the distal ileum.

Clinical features

The neonate with this disorder usually develops signs of intestinal obstruction within the first 24 to 48 h of life, with the classical signs of bile-stained vomiting, progressive abdominal distension, and failure to pass meconium. In simple meconium ileus, the meconium is the sole source of the obstruction, but meconium ileus may be complicated by perforation of the gut and, when this occurs *in utero*, intraperitoneal calcification may be observed on a plain radiograph of the abdomen, providing evidence of meconium peritonitis. Perforation may also occur in the neonatal period. Volvulus and atresia may also complicate meconium ileus.

In simple meconium ileus, the plain radiograph of the abdomen may show dilated bowel but few fluid levels. Sometimes there is the appearance of bubbly meconium in the right lower quadrant. Bowel loops may be palpable. If a contrast enema is performed a microcolon, a consequence of disuse, will be demonstrated. Atresia associated with meconium ileus is frequently indistinguishable radiologically from an atresia of ischaemic origin.

Management

When meconium ileus is complicated by atresia or perforation, gangrene, peritonitis, or associated volvulus, surgical intervention is essential. Surgical options include the formation of a double-barrelled stoma with subsequent irrigation of the meconium from the distal bowel over a week or so, or intraoperative irrigation of the bowel with an immediate end-to-end anastomosis. In both options, an associated atresia or necrotic bowel are resected. The treatment of uncomplicated meconium ileus using enemas containing pancreatic enzymes, mucolytic agents such as acetylcysteine, and the detergent Tween 80 had been advocated for some time. Noblett in Melbourne, in 1969, used a Gastrografin enema to relieve intraluminal obstruction. Gastrografin is a radio-opaque, hyperosmolar solution that is effective because of its hypertonicity. This technique should not be used until a plain radiograph of the abdomen has excluded the possibility of complicated meconium ileus. An initial barium enema should exclude

Hirschsprung's disease and demonstrate a microcolon extending to the proximal colon. The retrograde passage of contrast medium through the ileocaecal valve should demonstrate intraluminal meconium with passage into proximal dilated ileum, thus excluding an ileal atresia. After a successful Gastrografin enema, large amounts of meconium will be passed.

Although there may be no signs clinically or radiologically of pulmonary complications in the neonatal period, physiotherapy should be started and any chest infections treated with antibiotics when they occur (as for older children with cystic fibrosis). A pancreatic enzyme preparation should also be started, at first in small dosage when milk feedings have begun. The diagnosis should be confirmed by sweat electrolyte estimations; concentrations of sweat sodium above 60 mmol/l are abnormal. In the majority of infants with cystic fibrosis, the finding of the abnormal gene $\delta F508$ or one of the other recognized mutations confirms the diagnosis. In a minority the abnormal gene is not identifiable.

Congenital short intestine

There is a syndrome of congenital short intestine in association with malrotation with clinical features similar to those that follow massive intestinal resection. There is also another syndrome of congenital short intestine in association with pyloric hypertrophy and malrotation. This latter syndrome is due to an absence or diminution of argyrophil ganglion cells in the small-intestinal wall. These cells normally organize peristalsis and ensure that the bolus moves forward at the correct speed. In the absence of such innervation, smooth muscle of the small-intestinal wall contracts spontaneously and rhythmically, but segmentation is not co-ordinated and the food bolus does not move forward, and there is work hypertrophy of smooth muscle. Both syndromes are rare and often only diagnosed at laparotomy.

Colonic atresia

Atresia of the large intestine is rare. In any series of cases of intestinal atresias, fewer than 10 per cent will have isolated colonic atresia.

Clinical features

The baby presents in the first 24 to 48 h with marked abdominal distension, vomiting, and failure to pass meconium.

Diagnosis

Abdominal radiographs reveal multiple dilated loops of bowel with fluid levels; the position of the loops may suggest a large bowel obstruction. Confirmation of the level of the atresia is obtained by barium enema.

Management

Nasogastric suction and intravenous fluids are commenced preoperatively. At laparotomy the lesion may be an isolated atresia or associated with multiple atresias of small and large bowel. If the atresia is solitary, it may be possible to perform an anastomosis after resection of the atresia and a length of the grossly dilated proximal bowel. Frequently a colostomy is fashioned to allow the dilated proximal bowel to contract before an end-to-end anastomosis some weeks later.

Hirschsprung's disease

In this condition, ganglion cells are absent in the bowel wall. The distal rectum is always aganglionic and the aganglionosis extends proximally for a variable distance. In 70 per cent the rectosigmoid is involved, in 20 per cent the aganglionosis extends proximal to the sigmoid for a variable distance up the colon, and in 10 per cent the aganglionosis extends into the small

intestine. The aganglionic bowel is incapable of co-ordinated peristalsis and passively constricts, resulting in a mechanical obstruction. The incidence is approximately 1 in 5000 births.

Clinical features

Hirschsprung's disease is not associated with a high incidence of prematurity, and most of the babies have a birth weight appropriate for gestational age. This contrasts sharply with most of the other congenital obstructions of the alimentary tract. Associated abnormalities are rare. The most important association is with Down's syndrome.

Symptoms of Hirschsprung's disease are present in the first few days of life in almost all cases. Exceptionally, a baby will have no symptoms during the early neonatal period. The major symptoms are failure to pass meconium within 36 h of birth, abdominal distension, vomiting, and poor feeding. These may occur singly or in combination. Frequently, a rectal examination will relieve the obstruction by passively dilating the aganglionic segment. Twenty to 50 per cent of patients with Hirschsprung's disease are not diagnosed in the early weeks of life. Later presentation is with constipation that dates back to the neonatal period. It is not accompanied by soiling and is frequently associated with failure to thrive. Presentation may be delayed for months or years.

Hirschsprung's enterocolitis may be the mode of presentation in the infant of a few weeks of age. This condition, the precise cause of which is unknown, presents with abdominal distension, profuse diarrhoea, and circulatory collapse. The infant is gravely ill and the mortality is 20 per cent. The child with this complication, successfully treated initially, may have absorptive problems for some time, suffer recurrent episodes of enterocolitis despite successful surgery, and the surgery is attended by a higher rate of complications. The incidence of enterocolitis can be greatly reduced if the diagnosis of Hirschsprung's disease is made in the first week of life.

Diagnosis

In the neonatal period a plain abdominal radiograph will reveal distension of small and large bowel. A barium enema may show the narrow aganglionic bowel with dilated proximal bowel (Fig. 3) but a normal barium enema does not exclude Hirschsprung's disease. A 24-h film showing retained barium in the colon is often more helpful than the actual enema in confirming the clinical suspicion of Hirschsprung's disease. The definitive diagnostic procedure is a rectal biopsy. Suction biopsy enables the pathologist to look for ganglion cells in the submucosal plexus; full-thickness biopsy provides the intermyenteric plexus as well but this is usually

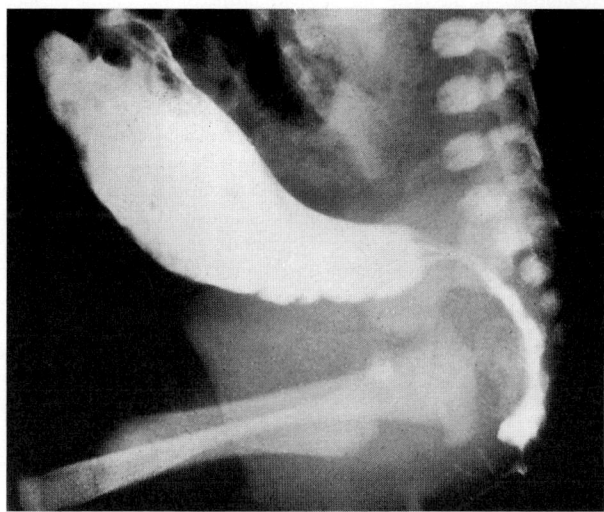

Fig. 3 Barium enema in Hirschsprung's disease illustrating a narrow aganglionic rectum with dilation proximally.

unnecessary. In Hirschsprung's disease, ganglion cells are absent, hypertrophic nerve trunks are present, and if a histochemical stain for acetylcholinesterase is used, this reveals excessive amounts of this enzyme in the bowel wall. Anorectal manometry in Hirschsprung's disease typically shows failure of relaxation of the internal sphincter in response to rectal distension but this reflex is frequently absent in normal term babies until after the second week of life. This method of diagnosis is therefore unreliable in the neonatal period, requires considerable expertise to obtain reliable results, and cannot be regarded as suitable for the routine diagnosis of Hirschsprung's disease.

Management

Following diagnosis, either definitive surgery is carried out or a colostomy is fashioned in ganglionic bowel and definitive surgery deferred for a period of time. Definitive surgery consists of excision of aganglionic bowel with a 'pull through' procedure, enabling an anastomosis to be made between the anus and ganglionic colon. The three operations most often performed are those described by Swenson, Duhamel, and Soave. Provided that the surgery is uncomplicated, the long-term complications, which include faecal and urinary incontinence, and impotence, should be minimal. Bowel control is likely to be imperfect for a number of years, with soiling as a major problem, but good bowel control will be achieved in the majority of patients treated by experienced surgeons.

Imperforate anus

The exact incidence of this abnormality is not known but the usual incidence quoted is 1 in 5000 births. The basic classification differentiates between the high anomalies, where the bowel terminates above the pelvic floor, the bowel narrowing down to communicate with the urethra in the male (a rectourethral fistula) and the vagina or vestibule in the female (a rectovaginal/vestibular fistula) in the majority of cases. In the low anomalies, the bowel passes through the pelvic floor and either opens on to the perineum in an ectopic position, or lies just beneath the skin-covered anus. The high anomaly is more likely to occur in boys, the low in girls. Overall, more boys than girls present with an imperforate anus. Associated anomalies of the urogenital tract, oesophagus, heart, and skeletal system are common.

Clinical features

Early examination of the perineum will establish the presence of an anorectal anomaly. In the male, the presence of meconium on the perineum usually indicates a low anomaly. In the female, careful inspection is necessary to differentiate meconium being passed *per vaginum*, indicating a high anomaly, from meconium emerging from a perineal site, suggesting a low anomaly. Careful probing of any opening will enable the direction in which the bowel is running to be established. In the female, doubt about the precise anatomy of the anomaly may be resolved by contrast studies. In the male, differentiating a completely covered anus from a high anomaly may be difficult in the early hours after birth. Examination of the urine microscopically may reveal the presence of squamous cells or debris, suggesting a fistula between bowel and urethra. Occasionally, meconium is passed *per urethra*.

A lateral film of the pelvis taken after the infant has lain 'bottom up' over a foam wedge for some minutes will often reveal the level at which the rectum terminates, but this film cannot be reliably interpreted in the first few hours after birth because air may not have reached the distal bowel. In boys, a micturating cystourethrogram will demonstrate a rectourethral fistula in a high proportion of cases, but is rarely necessary as an initial diagnostic procedure. Having defined the nature of the anorectal anomaly, evidence of any associated abnormality should be sought by careful clinical examination and radiographs of chest, abdomen, and the vertebral column.

Management

A low anomaly usually requires a perineal procedure to enlarge the opening. Dilatation alone may suffice, but in the majority of cases a simple anoplasty produces a more satisfactory result. In the long term, the functional results for the low anomalies should be very good. A high anomaly necessitates a defunctioning colostomy in the neonatal period. Definitive surgery involves division of any fistula and positioning the bowel accurately within the pelvic floor and sphincter muscles. Delay in achieving bowel control is common and a number of secondary operations designed to improve control have been advocated. However, if the initial surgery is meticulous, acceptable continence should be achieved in over 80 per cent of children within the first 10 years. A permanent colostomy should rarely be necessary. The high incidence of associated genitourinary abnormalities makes it mandatory to investigate carefully the urinary tract at an early stage. The mortality for anorectal anomalies is largely dictated by the presence of other serious abnormalities.

Further reading

Brown RL, Azizkhan RG (1999). Gastrointestinal bleeding in infants and children: Meckel's diverticulum and intestinal duplication. *Seminars in Pediatric Surgery* **34**, 202–9.

Dalla Vecchia LK, Grosfeld JL, Cono J, Khoury MJ, Weatherly MR, Moore CA (1998). Intestinal atresia and stenosis: a 25 year experience with 277 cases. *Archives of Surgery* **133**, 490–6.

De Backer AI, Parizel PM, De Schepper A, Vaneerdeweg W (1997). A patient with congenital short small bowel associated with malrotation. *Journal Belge Radiologie* **80**, 71–2.

Freeman NV, Burge DM, Griffiths DM, Malone PSJ, eds (1994). *Surgery of the newborn*. Churchill Livingstone, London.

Langer JC (1996). Gastroschisis and omphalocele. *Seminars in Pediatric Surgery* **5**, 124–8.

Larsen WJ (1997). *Human embryology*. Churchill Livingstone, New York.

Pierro A, Fasoli L, Kiely EM, Drake D, Spitz L (1997). Staged pull-through for rectosigmoid Hirschsprung's disease is not safer than primary pull-through. *Journal of Pediatric Surgery* **32**, 505–9.

Roberts HE, Cragan JD, Cono J, Khoury MJ, Weatherly MR, Moore CA (1998). Increased frequency of cystic fibrosis among infants with jejunoileal atresia. *American Journal of Medical Genetics* **78**, 446–9.

Shaul DB, Harrison EA (1997). Classification of anorectal malformations—initial approach, diagnostic tests, and colostomy. *Seminars in Pediatric Surgery* **6**, 187–95.

Swaniker F, Soldes O, Hirschl RB (1999). The utility of technetium 99m pertechnetate scintigraphy in the evaluation of patients Meckel's diverticulum. *Journal of Pediatric Surgery* **34**, 760–4.

Veereman-Wauters G (1996). Normal gut development and postnatal adaptation. *European Journal of Pediatrics* **155**, 627–32.

14.15 Tumours of the gastrointestinal tract

A. F. Markham, I. C. Talbot, and C. B. Williams

Introduction

Breakthroughs in our understanding of the basic molecular pathology of tumours of the gastrointestinal tract have provided a paradigm for explaining the development of malignancy. Insights into the mechanisms of carcinogenesis in specific tumours of the gut now inform aspects of their clinical management, but carcinomas of the digestive tract remain difficult to treat successfully. Indeed, only minor improvements in 5-year survival rates have been achieved over several decades. The realization that certain gene products are overexpressed early in the development of specific malignancies has led to the evaluation of known drugs in chemoprevention studies. The best example is the use of non-steroidal anti-inflammatory drugs (**NSAIDs**) to inhibit colorectal adenoma and cancer development in predisposed individuals. NSAIDs inhibit cyclooxygenase-2 (**COX-2**), which is upregulated in early colonic adenomas and may drive carcinogenesis. The ability to discriminate between genetic variants (phenocopies) of colorectal and other gastrointestinal cancers will allow more definitive clinical trials of specific treatments for particular forms of these conditions.

Screening strategies to detect surgically resectable gastrointestinal cancers at ever earlier stages are proving successful, particularly for gastric cancer in Japan and for colorectal malignancy in many countries. An appreciation of the natural history of colorectal cancer has informed the design of screening programmes, and also enables the diagnostic yields expected from faecal occult-blood testing, flexible sigmoidoscopy, or colonoscopic examination to be predicted. The complex health economic issues that such screening programmes raise are being subjected to examination.

As well as the gene encoding the adenomatous polyposis coli (**APC**) tumour suppressor protein, which is mutated in familial adenomatous polyposis (**FAP**) (OMIM175100; this refers to the number designation of the condition in McKusick's catalogue, *Online Mendelian inheritance in man*, available online at www.ncbi.nlm.nih.gov, which provides detailed clinical information on inherited conditions), seven different variants of hereditary non-polyposis colon cancer (OMIM114500) (**HNPCC** 1–7) are now recognized. Most of these involve mutation in one of the genes encoding components of the protein complex that repairs DNA mismatches introduced erroneously at replication. These Mendelian diseases are responsible for 5 per cent of colorectal cancers.

Genetic loci responsible for at least a proportion of the disease burden in juvenile intestinal polyposis (OMIM174900), mixed hereditary polyposis (OMIM601228), hyperplastic polyposis, and Peutz–Jeghers syndrome (OMIM175200) have been mapped and in some cases the mutant genes identified. Mutations in the E-cadherin gene have been shown to lead to familial gastric carcinoma (OMIM192090). The gene mutated in 'tylosis with oesophageal cancer' (OMIM148500) has been mapped to chromosome 17q24. Thus, there have been significant recent developments in all these disease areas.

Vogelstein and colleagues have added to their familiar model of the adenoma-to-carcinoma sequence of genetic alterations in colorectal cancer, with the concept of 'gate-keeper', 'caretaker', and 'landscaper' tumour suppressor genes in gastrointestinal cancer. *APC* is the classic example of a gate-keeper gene. The protein plays a key role in preventing carcinogenesis, and loss of such a tumour suppressor gene (**TSG**) leads inevitably to malignancy, with very high penetrance. The mismatch repair genes represent examples of genetic 'caretakers'. Mutations do not lead inevitably to cancer, but loss of their function leads to widespread genetic damage (characterized in the cell by 'microsatellite instability') including secondary mutation in gate-keeper genes, which can eventually generate a malignant phenotype. Thus, for example, colorectal cancer will develop in some 80 per cent of male carriers of an HNPCC mutation by the age of 85 years.

The concept of genetic 'landscaping' emerged from study of the paradox that colorectal cancers with microsatellite instability (**MSI**, sometimes referred to as 'replication error-positive' or **RER**+ tumours) did not contain the MLH1 mismatch repair protein, even though at least one allele of the gene encoding this protein appeared normal on DNA sequencing. This was the result of an epigenetic cause of tumorigenesis, which has proved to be a widespread factor in malignancy. DNA hypermethylation of CpG residues in the promoter regions of this or other genes starts a complex process involving histone deacetylation and permanent promoter silencing. This leads to the loss of function at a TSG allele, equivalent to that caused by a point mutation in the gene, or gene deletion.

In many cases, the roles of mutations in the genes discussed above in human cancers have been confirmed by introducing the corresponding mutations into transgenic mice. Although the phenotypes are by no means always identical, these animal models of human malignancy do act as model systems in which to develop the next generation of therapeutic agents.

The consensus emerging from these progressively more comprehensive, evidence-based surveys of the optimum approaches to the clinical management of gastrointestinal tumours has been incorporated herein. The reader is encouraged to consult these accessible sources directly.

Oesophageal tumours

Benign

Submucosal leiomyomas are the least rare of benign oesophageal lesions. Rarely, fibrovascular polyps, lipomas, haemangiomas, or other mesenchymal tumours are detected on barium-swallow examination. Endoscopic ultrasound can confirm the intramural localization of these lesions to exclude tracheal compression. Tumours large enough to cause dysphagia are removed by enucleation. Mucosal papillomas, foci of leucoplakia, or acanthosis nigricans also occur.

Malignant: oesophageal carcinomas

These constitute only 1 per cent of all malignancies and 6 per cent of gastrointestinal cancer, but cause some 10 per cent of all cancer deaths given their 5-year survival of less than 10 per cent. Historically, the majority of malignant tumours of the oesophagus were squamous carcinomas. However, there appears to be a current epidemic of adenocarcinoma in the lower third of the oesophagus, so that over 50 per cent of the disease in the Western world is now of this histological type.

Other malignant tumours are rare. They include metastases (primarily from the stomach), malignant melanoma, plasmacytoma, stromal tumours, and spindle-cell carcinoma. Some 50 per cent of patients dying with AIDS have gastrointestinal Kaposi's sarcoma. Although the incidence in the oesophagus is less than in the mouth or hypopharynx, oesophageal extension is associated with a poorer prognosis.

Epidemiology and aetiology

Squamous oesophageal carcinoma

Only half the 3000 cases of oesophageal cancer diagnosed annually in the United Kingdom are now squamous carcinoma. A threefold greater incidence in men may reflect an association with tobacco smoking and alcohol intake. The incidence is much higher in an area extending from the Caspian Sea to China. The high incidence in this 'oesophageal cancer belt' suggested that carcinogenic N-nitroso compounds in pickled foods in the diet might be responsible. The possibility that these may be population isolates with predisposing genotypes or even hereditary forms of the disease has only recently begun to be explored.

The incidence of squamous carcinoma is increased in patients with caustic oesophageal strictures due to the ingestion of corrosives, or after radiotherapy. Persistent achalasia predisposes to disease, possibly related to stasis above the narrowed segment. There is also an association with coeliac disease. The Patterson–Kelly (Plummer–Vinson) syndrome, characterized by iron deficiency anaemia, glossitis, postcricoid webs, and dysphagia, particularly in Scandinavian populations, has been associated with squamous carcinoma in up to 20 per cent of cases.

The autosomal dominant disease 'tylosis with oesophageal cancer' (OMIM148500) eventually causes carcinoma in 95 per cent of patients. Pedigrees segregating the characteristic hyperkeratosis of the palms and soles, have allowed the gene for this disease to be mapped to chromosome 17q24. Its identification can be anticipated. This may allow consideration of prophylactic oesophagectomy in carriers.

A number of loss-of-heterozygosity (LOH) studies have been performed with squamous carcinomas and several loci show consistent allelic losses compared with matched normal tissues, as would be expected at a tumoursuppressor gene locus. Pedigrees in northern China with consanguinity, and possibly segregating autosomal recessive forms of the disease, have recently been described.

Adenocarcinoma of the oesophagus

Barrett's oesophagus is attributed to chronic gastro-oesophageal reflux, resulting in replacement of the squamous epithelium by an abnormal columnar, metaplastic epithelium. This specialized intestinal metaplasia, with mucus-secreting goblet cells, is thought to increase the risk of developing adenocarcinoma 40-fold. Increasing epithelial atypia defines low to high grades of dysplasia. The frequent association of high-grade dysplasia with adenocarcinomas in surgical-resection specimens suggests that the former is a true precursor of the latter. The claimed annual incidence of adenocarcinoma in an established Barrett's oesophagus is approximately 1 per cent.

However, optimal surveillance of individuals with Barrett's oesophagus remains ill-defined. There is no correlation between the severity of symptoms and the extent of Barrett's metaplasia. The cancer risk in Barrett's oesophagus may have been overestimated because of publication bias towards reporting positive studies. The incidence of adenocarcinomas appears to be higher in long-segment than in short-segment metaplasia. Aggressive antireflux therapy or endoscopic ablation of the metaplastic epithelium have not been proved to decrease the risk of oesophageal cancer. There is no difference between proton-pump inhibitors and H_2-antagonists in preventing the progression of Barrett's oesophagus. Our lack of understanding of the pathophysiology of Barrett's metaplasia means it is not clear what endpoint in treating reflux disease (symptom relief, epithelial healing,

or elimination of reflux) is relevant in preventing progression to oesophageal cancer.

High-grade dysplasia may produce a much higher risk of disease progression. Given the cost implications of endoscopic surveillance programmes, which may not even measure progression effectively, there is an urgent need for reliable molecular markers of high risk. A few pedigrees have been described that apparently segregate an hereditary predisposition to Barrett's oesophagus and associated adenocarcinomas in an autosomal dominant, Mendelian fashion. These may provide the opportunity to identify predisposing mutant genes. Molecular markers associated with other malignancies in the gastrointestinal tract (TP53, RB1, E-cadherin, and cyclin D1) may be informative in that, for example, high levels of cyclin D1 expression in biopsy specimens appear to correlate with an increased risk of carcinoma.

Clinical features

Patients generally present with dysphagia, initially for solids but eventually also for liquids and even saliva. Unfortunately, dysphagia usually reflects circumferential disease. Impact pain from food, or pain in the front or back of the chest, are bad prognostic features. Loss of weight and appetite more often reflect the cachexia of advanced disease, rather than simply the difficulty in swallowing. Regional lymph node involvement is present in approximately 50 per cent of cases at diagnosis. Direct spread may involve the bronchi and aorta. Perforation may result in tracheo-oesophageal fistulas or mediastinitis. Hoarseness may be apparent on involvement of the recurrent laryngeal nerve. Obstruction with difficulty swallowing saliva may result in aspiration pneumonia. However, the physical signs may be limited to weight loss, anaemia, and/or cervical lymphadenopathy.

Diagnosis and staging

Barium swallow characteristically shows abrupt, irregular lumenal narrowing, in contrast to the smooth narrowing of a benign stricture. Endoscopy allows biopsy of the lesion, producing a diagnostic accuracy of over 95 per cent. Palliative dilatation or intubation may then be performed. **TNM** (primary tumour, regional nodes, and metastasis) staging is achieved using endoscopic ultrasound to image the tumour in the oesophageal wall and to assess regional lymph nodes. Computed tomography (**CT**) or magnetic resonance imaging (**MRI**) will highlight invasion of adjacent structures, more distal lymph node involvement, and metastatic disease.

Treatment

Patients with superficial carcinomas at stage T_1N0M0 may achieve 5-year survival rates of over 50 per cent. However, overall the results of treatment are dire, with a 5-year survival rate of less than 10 per cent. Unfortunately, perioperative mortality is rarely less than 10 per cent. Adjuvant chemo/radiotherapy has been advocated for otherwise inoperable disease that has spread beyond the oesophageal wall. Squamous-cell carcinomas are more sensitive to both these treatment modalities than adenocarcinomas. Chemotherapy and radiotherapy are the subjects of Cochrane Reviews, but there is no clear evidence of improved survival in patients with potentially resectable lesions. Palliative therapy is based on radiotherapy and therapeutic endoscopy for endoscopic dilatation or insertion of a stent to overcome dysphagia and bridge any fistulas which may have formed. Ablation of tumour growing into the lumen of the oesophagus may be attempted using laser photocoagulation or electrocautery. Ethanol injection induces tumour necrosis and is effective, particularly when combined with intubation.

Stomach tumours

Benign

Benign gastric tumours may be derived from the mesenchyme or epithelium. Gastrointestinal stromal tumours (GISTs) arising from the gastric wall are most frequent, though not common. These project into the gastric lumen and occasionally become superficially ulcerated leading to haemorrhage. When large, these tumours have low grade malignant potential (see section on small bowel tumours). Even rarer submucosal lesions include lipomas, haemangiomas, hamartomas, gastric carcinoids, and lymphoid hyperplasia. The latter may be difficult to discriminate from a mucosa-associated lymphoid tissue (**MALT**) lymphoma.

Gastric epithelial polyps are mainly hyperplastic or inflammatory and usually asymptomatic. The historical view that they are not susceptible to malignant change, may be questioned. Only 15 per cent of gastric polyps are adenomatous. Although the risk of gastric cancers in these adenomas is not as clear-cut as in the large bowel, their association with FAP in particular, the eventual development of gastric cancer in FAP, and their occurrence at the margins of gastric carcinomas indicate that they should be removed endoscopically. Villous adenomas and polyps larger than 2 cm have a particularly high malignant potential. Rarely, large pedunculated polyps may ulcerate and bleed, or obstruct the pyloric outflow. Gastric hamartomas occur in Peutz–Jeghers syndrome, Cronkhite–Canada syndrome, Cowden's disease, and juvenile intestinal polyposis and these polyps are associated with an increased incidence of malignancy, highest in Peutz–Jeghers syndrome. This is obscured by the higher risk of carcinomas elsewhere in the gastrointestinal tract in these conditions. Paradoxically the most numerous gastric polyps in FAP are cystic gland (mucus retention) polyps which have no malignant potential or clinical significance whatever.

Malignant: carcinoma of the stomach

Pathology

The antrum is the most frequent site of gastric adenocarcinoma. The incidence of proximal cancers (which are smoking-related) and gastro-oesophageal junction tumours is rising for reasons that are not fully understood. Pathological classification is not entirely clear-cut. The histological approach of Lauren defines two subtypes. The intestinal type (60 per cent) is glandular and polypoid, associated with metaplasia, chronic gastritis, and the presence of *Helicobacter pylori*. The diffuse type (30 per cent) consists of scattered clusters of cells and spreads submucosally to ultimately result in linitis plastica. It has a worse prognosis and occurs in younger individuals. Tumours of mixed type (10 per cent) are also recognized.

Morphological classifications have been attempted, including that of Borrmann for advanced gastric cancer: type 1, polypoid without ulceration; type 2, fungating with surface ulceration; type 3, ulcerated with a wall-like edge and surrounding infiltration; and type 4, diffusely infiltrative. This bears some resemblance to the Japanese classification of early gastric adenocarcinomas: type 1, protruded, polypoid; type 2, superficial (elevated, flat, or depressed); and type 3, excavated. An alternative histological classification defines early cancer as not penetrating the submucosa (T1 disease), with advanced disease involving extension through the submucosa to the muscularis propria or serosa (T2), breaching the peritoneum (T3), and into adjacent tissues (T4). The TNM classification defines lymph node status as N_1 when one to 6 nodes are involved, N_2 when 7 to 15 nodes are posistive and N3 when more than 15 nodes are involved. Differences in classification between Japanese and Western pathologists have resulted in attempts at International consensus statements: the Vienna and the Padova classifications—which, unfortunately, are not identical.

An autosomal dominant, familial form of gastric cancer of diffuse type occurs, with presentation at early ages (OMIM192090). This disease is caused by germline mutations in the E-cadherin gene. The finding is of significance because the intracellular domain of this protein interacts at the epithelial adherens junction with β-catenin, an important participant in colorectal carcinogenesis. Gastric cancers frequently demonstrate *P53* mutations and consistent LOH in a number of specific chromosome regions. HNPCC provides a fourfold increased risk of gastric cancer, presenting in 10 per cent of carriers. *APC* mutations also occur in early sporadic gastric cancers.

Epidemiology and aetiology

There are approximately 10 000 new cases in the United Kingdom annually, making gastric cancer the sixth commonest malignancy, and, like oesophageal cancer, accounting for about 10 per cent of cancer deaths. There has been a sustained slow decline in incidence in the United Kingdom, but an increase in the number of cases involving the cardia. There are marked geographic differences in incidence, the rate in Japan being eight times higher than amongst Whites in the United States. Gastric cancer rates in Japanese immigrants to the United States halve in one generation, suggesting an environmental factor in its aetiology. Mass radiographic screening for gastric cancer has been undertaken in Japan since 1960. Some 5 million barium studies conducted annually detect 6000 cases. Approximately half of these are early stage, offering the potential for curative resection. Screening in the United Kingdom cannot be justified given the lower incidence. The incidence in men still approaches twice that in women, worldwide.

H. pylori has emerged as a causative agent for distal gastric cancer and is now classified as a class 1 carcinogen. It causes gastritis, gastric and duodenal ulcers, and both adenocarcinoma and lymphoma in the stomach. Some 60 per cent of the world's population are infected. In the developing world most of the population is infected from early childhood. In contrast, the prevalence of infection is falling in the developed world. This probably reflects decreased childhood infection rates, rather than eradication of infection in adults. Bacterial isolates with the *Cag-A* genotype are particularly implicated in carcinoma of the middle and distal thirds of the stomach, of both intestinal and diffuse types.

The organism can be detected by urease breath-testing or immunologically by a serum enzyme-linked immunosorbent assay (**ELISA**). Initial infection induces pangastritis with achlorhydria. There is a brisk serum immune response and the appearance of IgA in gastric secretions. However, *H. pylori* is not eradicated and gastritis is maintained by a combination of *H. pylori*-induced cytokine release from gastric epithelium and a TH1-type T-cell response. A sustained period of antral gastritis ensues, associated with duodenal ulceration. Persistent reduction in acid secretion may lead to the reduced effectiveness of antioxidant mechanisms in the stomach. Eventually, multifocal atrophic gastritis develops with metaplasia, followed by dysplasia, leading on to malignancy. This pathway remains consistent with the model originally proposed by Correa in 1988 (Fig. 1).

The increased frequency of gastric carcinoma in lower socioeconomic groups may reflect their increased prevalence of *H. pylori* infection. A decreased incidence of *H. pylori* infection in childhood may explain the reduced rate of gastric carcinoma in Japanese immigrants to the United States. Eradication of the organism leads to resolution of the gastritis and normalization of basal acid secretion over several months. Reinfection rates

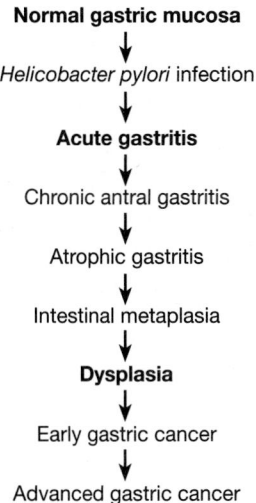

Normal gastric mucosa
↓
Helicobacter pylori infection
↓
Acute gastritis
↓
Chronic antral gastritis
↓
Atrophic gastritis
↓
Intestinal metaplasia
↓
Dysplasia
↓
Early gastric cancer
↓
Advanced gastric cancer

Fig. 1 Flow chart of the pathogenesis of gastric cancer.

in adults appear to be low in the developed world. This offers the possibility of achieving a long-term reduction in cancer incidence.

There is no convincing evidence that the prolonged use of H_2-blockers or proton-pump inhibitors is associated with an increased incidence of gastric cancer, secondary to prolonged suppression of acid secretion. Dietary factors such as nitrites or a lack of free-radical scavengers in the diet (for example, vitamin C, selenium) have long been suspected of causation in gastric carcinoma. Conversion of nitrates to nitrosamines by bacteria at neutral pH has been suggested to be carcinogenic. Smoking and increased alcohol use are associated with gastric cancer. Whether these dietary agents exert their effects indirectly through their influence on *H. pylori* infection rates remains to be established. An increased incidence in blood group-A individuals has been recognized since 1955. There is no direct connection between peptic ulcers and gastric cancers. Malignant ulcers may heal on initial treatment for dyspepsia, which can confuse the diagnosis. Furthermore, because they are both associated with *H. pylori* infection, the two conditions do tend to coincide.

Pernicious anaemia also leads to gastric atrophy in the body and fundus of the stomach and, presumably as a consequence, is associated with a threefold increase in the incidence of gastric cancer. The incidence may approach 10 per cent in patients followed up for 20 years. Intestinal metaplasia is recognized as a predisposing feature secondary to gastritis as it is found associated with carcinoma in resected specimens. However, this is again likely to be secondary to *H. pylori* infection in the main. Intestinal metaplasia and chronic active gastritis occur in gastric stumps postgastrectomy. These show an increased incidence of cancer, particularly after gastrojejunostomy. A prolonged bile reflux may be a cause of this gastritis. As in gastric atrophy, 10 per cent of patients may develop cancer during a 20-year follow-up for chronic gastritis. This is consistent with the need for multiple genetic hits to generate a malignant phenotype.

Clinical features

Although early gastric cancer may be asymptomatic, clinical suspicion of dyspepsia in older patients may lead to its early diagnosis, with the possibility of successful surgical intervention in early-stage disease. Common presenting symptoms include epigastric pain, which may be relieved or made worse by food. This pain can be constant and severe. The clinical features of anaemia, anorexia, early satiety, and weight loss suggest advanced disease at presentation. Large proximal tumours of the cardia may cause dysphagia. Tumours of the fundus are more likely to result in anaemia and nausea. Distal tumours of the antrum may cause outlet obstruction and result in vomiting.

Gross haematemesis from gastric cancers is unusual. Metastasis occurs to the peritoneum (with ascites and possibly ovarian involvement—Krukenberg's tumour), to the liver, and latterly to the lung and other sites. An epigastric mass may be palpable in 30 per cent of patients, and suggests advanced disease. Palpable lymphadenopathy (Virchow's node) in the left supraclavicular fossa (Troisier's sign) may be present. Carcinoma of the stomach is the malignancy most frequently associated with dermatomyositis or acanthosis nigricans.

Diagnosis

Although double-contrast plain imaging of the stomach can provide up to 90 per cent diagnostic accuracy, flexible endoscopy and biopsy has become the definitive diagnostic procedure (Fig. 2). Sensitivity increases with the number of biopsy samples taken from the base of an ulcer and its margins—10 biopsies of adequate depth will give a reliability approaching 100 per cent and eliminate false-negative results.

Staging of disease prior to attempted surgery relies on a number of imaging modalities. CT scanning defines the spread of the primary tumour and gross lymphatic and metastatic disease. CT is approximately 75 per cent accurate in detecting involved lymph nodes larger than 5 mm. However, it often fails to detect small involved lymph nodes and peritoneal deposits. Resolution may be improved with the use of intravenous contrast media. It is particularly important to detect distant involved lymph nodes because these would not normally be removed during surgery, and would therefore result in treatment failure. MRI scanning may help in this context.

Endoscopic ultrasound is useful in the local staging of gastric carcinoma. The normal stomach wall comprises five hyperechoic layers. Carcinomas present as hypoechoic lesions that disrupt the normal pattern. The depth of tumour invasion of the gastric wall can be assessed accurately, as can the presence of involved perigastric lymph nodes. T staging with 90 per cent accuracy and N staging with 70 per cent accuracy are achievable by correlation with pathological examination of specimen obtained during surgery. However, the technique is limited in its ability to detect distant enlarged lymph nodes. Classification of a tumour as stage T4 by endoscopic ultrasound renders surgical cure highly unlikely, so that palliative bypass or endoscopic techniques may be the preferred clinical option. Laparoscopy may be necessary to confirm the presence of peritoneal metastases. MRI or ultrasonography will identify hepatic metastases.

Treatment

Surgical resection of a tumour and involved lymph nodes is undertaken in the absence of metastases. The site of the tumour dictates the surgical approach. The goal is a tumour-free margin of 5 cm with lymphadenectomy to an uninvolved point along the arterial tree (defined as resection levels R1, R2, or R3, reflecting increasingly distal nodal involvement). This may require total gastrectomy, or some variant of a proximal or distal gastrectomy for tumours in these sites, ideally avoiding postoperative biliary reflux, which may itself predispose to disease recurrence. Endoscopic surgery for early gastric cancers may be possible, provided the tumours are small, confined to the mucosa, and non-ulcerated. This approach requires a

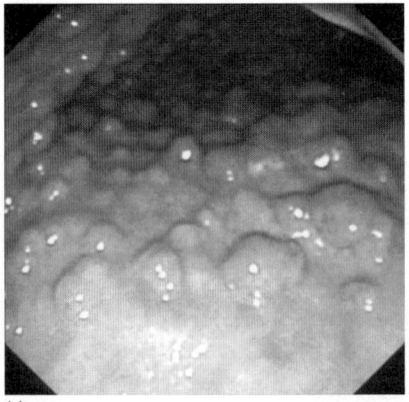
(a)

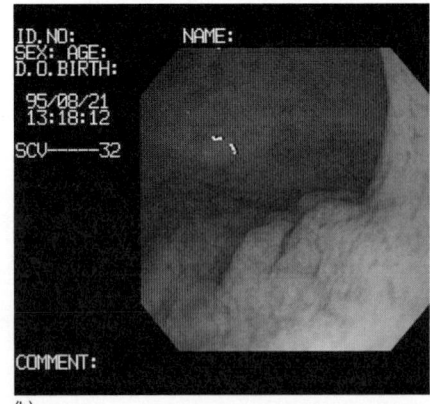
(b)

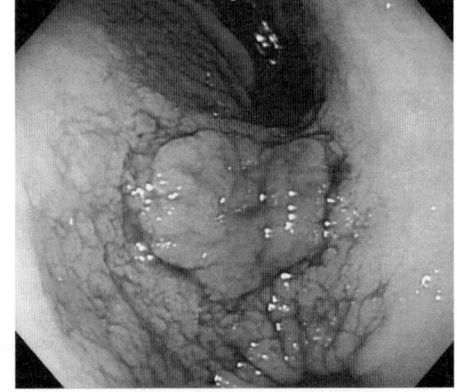

Fig. 2 Early gastric cancer – endoscopic appearance. (a) Initial view. Better view in retroversion (b) and (c) after dye-enhancement.

high degree of certainty that local lymph nodes are not involved. Endoscopic ultrasound-guided needle biopsy may be useful in this context.

Palliative procedures in symptomatic patients with disseminated disease may also include gastrectomy, which can double survival time, or less radical interventions including stenting, feeding gastrostomies, or laser photoablation. Adjuvant chemotherapy regimens including 5-fluorouracil (combined with various other agents) have produced small survival advantages in randomized clinical trials. Radiotherapy alone has not been shown to be beneficial.

Predicting the prognosis for an individual patient is complex. The stage of the cancer at operation is crucial and 5-year survival rates approaching 90 per cent have been reported for early gastric cancer detected by screening in Japan. However, apparently superior stage-specific survival rates in Japan may reflect a lower incidence of diffuse or proximal tumours. This dependence of 5-year survival rates on stage at presentation is mirrored in the United Kingdom, where new cases present with roughly a third each at stage 1/2, stage 3, and stage 4. Whilst patients in the first category may achieve a 30 to 50 per cent 5-year survival, this falls to less than 15 per cent in those with stage 3 disease. Those at stage 4 have less than a 3 per cent 5-year survival rate.

The 5-year survival rate is marginally lower for patients with proximal tumours than distal tumours, with those with tumours in the middle third showing a slightly better prognosis. Unfortunately, the latter category of tumours (20 per cent) is less common than the others (one-third of cases each), with disseminated diffuse cancer making up the remainder. Cancers with a diffuse histology appear to have a worse 5-year survival rate than those of intestinal type.

In summary, the combination of tumour stage, lymph node involvement, position in the stomach, and histological subtype all exert subtle influences on outcome in the absence of metastases. These factors and more sensitive detection of metastatic disease leading to less operations with intent to cure, make interpretation of possible improvements in 5-year survival rates after supposedly curative resections difficult to interpret. The need for *H. pylori* prophylaxis and for improved chemotherapy approaches are pressing. The requirement for vitamin B_{12} supplementation after gastrectomy should not be overlooked.

Malignant: gastric lymphoma

Mucosa-associated lymphoid tissue (MALT) lymphomas are B-cell, non-Hodgkin's lymphomas, associated with *H. pylori* infection in over 90 per cent of cases. These represent 5 per cent of all gastric malignancies. The disease arises as a low-grade MALT lymphoma in areas of chronic gastritis, characterized by large centroblast-like cells. High-grade lesions have immunoblastic features. The clinical presentations of these patients are not readily distinguishable from gastric carcinoma. *H. pylori* eradication can result in lymphoma regression or complete remission, especially for low-grade disease, with an overall response rate of over 60 per cent. Surgery to debulk the disease, chemotherapy (using CHOP (cyclophosphamide, hydroxydaunomycin, Oncovin, prednisone) regimens), and radiotherapy are effective in high-grade disease. The disease stage and histological grade determine prognosis. In the absence of distal lymph node involvement and bulky disease, the 5-year survival rate is over 70 per cent.

Cochrane Reviews have been published on the eradication of *H. pylori* (in the context of non-ulcer dyspepsia) and Protocols have appeared for Cochrane Reviews of extended-versus-limited lymph node dissection techniques for adenocarcinoma of the stomach.

Small-bowel tumours

Given the length of the small intestine, the incidence of neoplasia (5 per cent of all gastrointestinal tumours) is remarkably low. Some two-thirds of small-bowel tumours are malignant. Attempts to explain the rarity of these tumours on the basis of the reduced carcinogenic effects of small-bowel contents, their bacterial flora, or levels of protective secretory IgA are not convincing. There are, however, clear-cut associations between specific genetic traits, including FAP and Peutz–Jeghers syndrome, and small-bowel neoplasia.

The stem-cell compartment in the small bowel expresses low levels of the antiapoptotic protein, BCL-2, compared to the higher levels in the colonic crypt stem-cell compartment. It is possible that epithelial stem cells suffering genetic damage in the small intestine undergo apoptosis and are eliminated without the development of a neoplasm. In contrast, mutant colonic stem cells are resistant to apoptosis and persist to undergo further genetic hits, and a 50-fold increased rate of carcinoma compared to the small bowel. Paradoxically, the small bowel is the most common site in the gastrointestinal tract for metastatic melanoma.

Benign tumours

Adenomas and lipomas are the least rare, solitary benign tumours (with the exception of tumours arising in a variety of inherited forms of polyposis, discussed below). Adenomas predominate in the duodenum and are premalignant; haemangiomas and neurofibromas are more common in the jejunum; and fibromas and lipomas are more frequent in the ileum.

These tumours are frequently asymptomatic, incidental findings at operation. Symptoms where they do occur include obstruction, intussusception, pain or chronic haemorrhage with anaemia. Endoscopic examination and polypectomy in the duodenum, proximal jejunum and terminal ileum may be achievable. Barium follow-through is the appropriate diagnostic tool supplemented by angiography, for example where bleeding from an angioma or ectasia is suspected. Symptomatic benign small-bowel tumours are treated by surgical resection.

Gastrointestinal stromal tumours (GISTs) (formerly known as smooth muscle tumours) arise in the bowel wall, can grow to a large size and have low grade malignant potential, sometimes metastasizing to the liver many years after initial presentation and surgical resection. Evidence of malignancy is large size and more than 5 mitoses in 50 high power fields.

Malignant: carcinoma of the small bowel

Many adenocarcinomas of the small intestine occur in specific conditions. Management of FAP by total colectomy means that patients present with small-bowel adenomas, which have malignant potential. These occur commonly (50 per cent) in the duodenum (and rarely the stomach), particularly around the ampulla of Vater. Hamartomatous polyps are common in the jejunum in Peutz–Jeghers syndrome. These again undergo malignant change, imparting a 500-fold relative risk of small-bowel carcinoma. Coeliac disease is associated with an increased incidence of adenocarcinoma, as well as lymphoma, in the small bowel and an increased incidence of malignancies throughout the gastrointestinal tract (for example, the oesophagus) and elsewhere (for example, testes). Gluten-free diets do protect against the development of malignancy. Crohn's disease of prolonged duration slightly increases the incidence of small-bowel adenocarcinoma.

Clinical presentation usually involves abdominal pain, anorexia, cachexia, and/or anaemia. Patients may present with diarrhoea or, rarely, a palpable abdominal mass. Diagnosis involves radiological follow-through examination (Fig. 3) and CT or MRI scanning. Surgical treatment involves resection to uninvolved margins with any locally involved lymph nodes. The 5-year survival rates are dependent on tumour grade, lymph node involvement, and distant spread: with disease limited to the mucosa they approach 100 per cent, while the rate with lymph node involvement and distal metastases is essentially zero. The overall 5-year survival rate is around 25 per cent. There are very limited data on the value of adjuvant chemotherapy or radiotherapy. Combined preoperative radiotherapy and 5-fluorouracil have been claimed to be beneficial in duodenal adenocarcinoma. Where ampullary carcinomas are unresectable, palliation involves bile-duct stenting to avoid jaundice.

Carcinoid tumours are usually found in the ileum. Patients with these tumours have 5-year survival rates in excess of 75 per cent, in the absence of liver metastases. Multifocal small-bowel disease is present in approximately

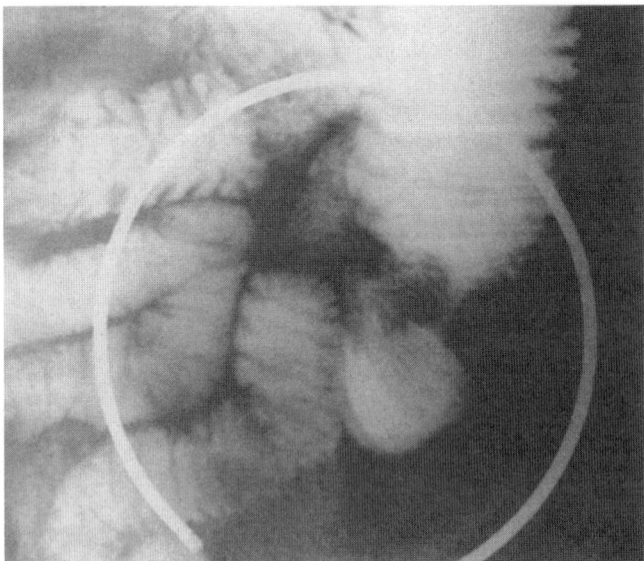

Fig. 3 Small bowel follow-through: compression view of mid-jejunum shows annular 'apple-core' appearance with pre-stenotic dilatation typical of an adenocarcinoma.

30 per cent of cases. Carcinoids that are more than 2 cm in diameter have frequently metastasized when detected. Carcinoid syndrome due to excessive amounts of serotonin occurs with liver metastases. Treatment involves resection of the primary tumour and hepatic metastases, with the use of somatostatin analogues (octreotide) to control the effects of hormone excess (see Chapter 14.8).

Malignant: lymphoma of the small bowel

Primary small-bowel lymphoma occurs not infrequently in the ileum (Fig. 4) and represents 5 per cent of all lymphomas. It is also a feature of disseminated lymphoma. Lymphomas constitute one-third of primary small-bowel malignancies: distinct groups of B- and T-cell lymphomas are recognized.

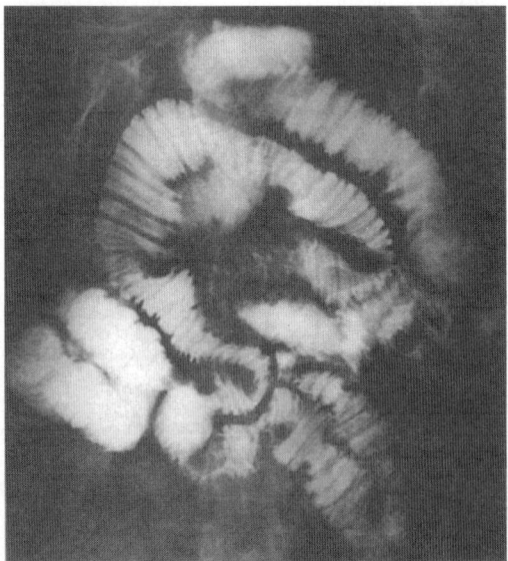

Fig. 4 Small bowel follow-through showing diffuse thickening of folds in ileum indicating submucosal infiltration (proved to be a lymphoma).

Immunoproliferative small-intestinal disease (IPSID)

These B-cell, non-Hodgkin's lymphomas occur mainly in the Middle East, Africa, and South America. This 'Mediterranean' lymphoma demonstrates an unusually strong association with low socioeconomic status. IPSID occurs in young adults as well as in the elderly. Initially the mucosa becomes infiltrated with plasma cells. It is sometimes associated with intestinal giardiasis, reminiscent of the association of gastric lymphoma with *H. pylori*. The clinical features resemble adenocarcinoma but with progressive diarrhoea, cachexia, and finger clubbing. Treatment of the infection, lymphoid infiltration, and secondary malabsorption is usually with tetracycline, or metronidazole and ampicillin. The progression to a large B-cell immunoblastic lymphoma histologically requires cytotoxic treatment with CHOP (cyclophosphamide, hydroxydaunomycin, Oncovin, prednisone) or one of its variants. IPSID frequently involves extensive areas of the small bowel so that surgical resection is often impossible. It tends to occur proximally and is associated with the production of monoclonal immunoglobulin heavy chains, which may be detectable in the serum.

Enteropathy-associated T-cell lymphoma (EATCL)

EATCL is less common than B-cell small-bowel lymphomas. The condition develops in patients with long-standing coeliac disease or dermatitis herpetiformis. Consequently, their relative risk of a T-cell lymphoma is 50-fold higher than the general population. Clinical suspicion should be raised in patients with coeliac disease who experience increased malabsorption despite maintaining their gluten-free diet. The disease is usually high-grade and consequently of poor prognosis. The lesions tend to ulcerate with a risk of intestinal perforation. They are notoriously unresponsive to standard lymphoma chemotherapy. Again surgical resection is precluded by the large areas usually involved, particularly in the jejunum.

Other small-bowel lymphomas

Non-IPSID, non-EATCL primary small-bowel lymphomas are usually distal, and unifocal, so that surgical resection to debulk them prior to chemotherapy with CHOP, may be appropriate. Small intestinal lymphoma is frequent in patients with the acquired immunodeficiency syndrome (**AIDS**), and a form of Burkitt's lymphoma has been described in the terminal ileum in susceptible populations.

Gastrointestinal polyps and the polyposis syndromes

A tumour projecting into the lumen of the gut is termed a polyp, from the Greek *polypous* for squid, which pedunculated polyps resemble. The nomenclature used to describe the wide range of gastrointestinal tumours encompassed by this general definition can be confusing (Fig. 5). However, recent advances in elucidating the genetic basis of several inherited polyposis syndromes have clarified some of these classification difficulties. These are autosomal dominant diseases in which multiple polyps (from five or more, to many thousands in particular conditions) of a given histological type occur. All these familial forms of polyposis predispose, to some extent, to the development of carcinoma in individual polyps.

Tubular adenoma   Tubulovillous adenoma   Villous adenoma

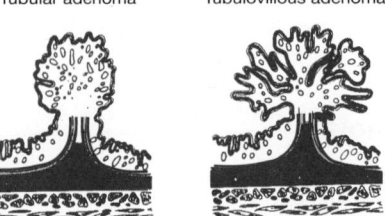
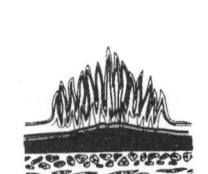

Fig. 5 Diagrammatic representation of the histology of adenomatous polyps.

In the subgroup of polyps which are adenomas, the progression from adenoma to carcinoma is well established. The molecular basis for this has been elucidated in the autosomal dominant disease familial adenomatous polyposis. The same mechanism has subsequently been shown to drive carcinogenesis in solitary adenomas occurring sporadically in individuals without the germline mutations present in the inherited condition.

Solitary hyperplastic (metaplastic), hamartomatous, or juvenile (retention) polyps have not been regarded as premalignant. However, the strong predisposition to malignancy in familial forms of polyposis of these histological types calls this into question. Identification of the different tumour-suppressor genes (TSGs) mutated in these familial diseases means that it is now possible to look for somatic mutations of the same TSGs in the corresponding histological types of sporadic polyps occurring in the general population. By analogy with adenomatous polyps, this may highlight other types of isolated polyp having a genotype suggestive of malignant potential.

Polyps can be classified simplistically on the basis of their gross shape and appearance as either sessile (villous), pedunculated, or flat. The latter type is of particular current interest as the significance of flat adenomas comes under greater scrutiny. However, these macroscopic descriptions offer little insight into the underlying histology. Polyps can range in size from almost invisible at less than 1 mm, to larger lesions several centimetres in diameter. They may occur singly or literally thousands of polyps may carpet the bowel in the polyposis syndromes. The system of classification of polyps as 'non-neoplastic' or 'neoplastic' requires revision. Many conditions historically included in the former category clearly predispose to the development of carcinoma. With this proviso, the traditional histological classification into non-neoplastic and neoplastic polyps is retained herein (Table 1). The majority of colorectal polyps are adenomas (neoplastic) in which a carcinoma may develop. Thus the detection and removal of these lesions are crucial. This can also be the case with many of the so-called non-neoplastic types of polyp.

Non-neoplastic polyps

Hyperplastic (metaplastic) polyps

These metaplastic lesions are a common finding on proctosigmoidoscopy, usually presenting as 2- to 4-mm pale shiny nodules. Metaplastic polyps are increasingly recognized to occur in association with so-called 'serrated adenomas' and mixed hyperplastic–adenomatous polyps, these latter demonstrating epithelial dysplasia. Large hyperplastic polyps are frequently found on the right side of the colon and are associated with the development of carcinoma. Multiple hyperplastic polyps (hyperplastic polyposis) are strongly associated with a family history of colorectal cancer. Hyper-

Table 1 Colonic polyps and polyposis: a classification

Pathogenesis	Polyps	Polyposis
Metaplastic	Hyperplastic	Hyperplastic polyposis
Inflammatory	Inflammatory	Inflammatory polyposis
Lymphatic	Benign lymphoid	Malignant lymphomatous polyposis
Traumatic	Mucosal prolapse syndrome	Inflammatory cap polyp polyposis
Neoplastic	Adenoma	Familial adenomatous polyposis, if >100
Hamartomatous	Juvenile	Juvenile polyposis
	Peutz-Jeghers	Peutz-Jeghers syndrome
		Cronkhite-Canada syndrome
Stromal origin		
Type/neoplastic	Leiomyomatous polyp Lipomatous polyp	Cowden's syndrome
Hamartomatous	Vascular hamartoma Neurofibroma Ganglioneuroma	

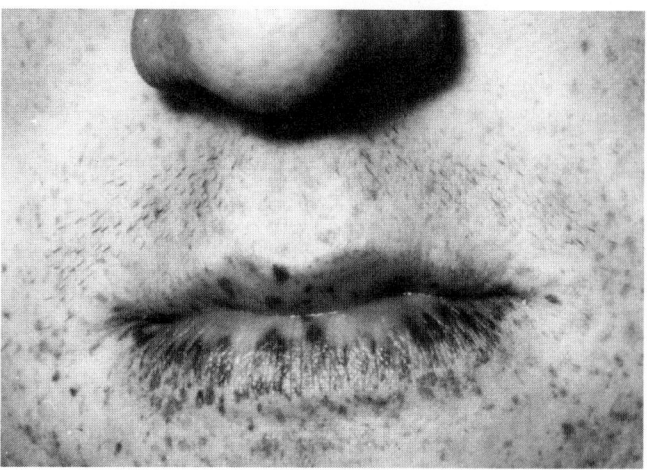

Fig. 6 Peutz-Jeghers patient showing characteristic lip pigmentation.

plastic polyposis appears to involve an early loss of chromosome 1p in about 25 per cent of patients. It seems increasingly likely that a metaplastic polyp–mixed hyperplastic/adenomatous polyp–carcinoma sequence occurs, reminiscent of the more familiar adenoma to carcinoma sequence.

Hamartomatous polyps

Polyps of this general histological type have usually been considered together as non-premalignant lesions. However, the natural history of familial diseases in which hamartomatous polyps are a feature casts doubt on this conclusion.

Peutz–Jeghers syndrome (OMIM175200) is an autosomal dominant disease characterized by hamartomatous polyps throughout the gastrointestinal tract, particularly in the jejunum, with mucocutaneous pigmentation of the buccal mucosa, perioral region (Fig. 6), and digits. Peutz–Jeghers hamartomatous polyps have a characteristic histopathological appearance distinct from other gastrointestinal polyps. They contain frond-like epithelium with cystic dilatation of glands overlying a network of characteristic fibromuscular bundles. Hypermucinous goblet cells are often prominent. Clinically there is a risk of intussusception or infarction of Peutz–Jeghers polyps that are more than 1 cm in diameter.

The disease has been mapped to chromosome 19p13.3 with possible genetic heterogeneity and a second locus on 19q. A putative tumour-suppressor gene, *STK11*, which encodes a serine/threonine kinase, harbours germline mutations in patients. Consistent with its function as a tumour suppressor, the normal allele of *STK11* is lost in hamartomas and in associated adenocarcinomas, suggesting that the former may be precursors of the latter.

Recent meta-analysis of the risk of a wide variety of malignancies in Peutz–Jeghers syndrome has confirmed the very high relative risks of developing cancer of the oesophagus (57 times higher than the general population), stomach (relative risk (**RR**) 213), small bowel (RR 520), colon (RR 84), and pancreas (RR 132), with increased risks also for lung, breast, uterine, and ovarian cancer. The cumulative risk for all cancer is over 90 per cent by the age of 65 years. Thus patients with the Peutz–Jeghers syndrome are at a very high relative and absolute risk for both gastrointestinal and non-gastrointestinal cancers. Endoscopic follow-up should be at 2-yearly intervals, barium follow-through series is needed at similar intervals. Periodic laparotomies may be needed to remove large (2 cm+) polyps and avoid the danger of intussusception and gangrene

Juvenile intestinal polyposis

Juvenile intestinal polyposis (OMIM174900) is another autosomal dominantly inherited hamartomatous polyposis syndrome that is genetically heterogeneous, with loci mapped to chromosomes 18q21.1 and 10q23.3. A further variant is the atypical juvenile polyposis syndrome called hereditary mixed polyposis syndrome (OMIM601228). These patients also have an increased incidence of inflammatory and metaplastic polyps. This autosomal dominant disease has been mapped to chromosome 6q, although identification of the actual gene involved has not yet been achieved.

Juvenile polyps are pedunculated hamartomas, prone to surface ulceration, which can cause bleeding and stalk torsion that can autoamputate the polyp with bleeding. The main distinction from Peutz–Jeghers syndrome is a lack of muscle fibres. Juvenile polyps are characteristically overlaid with a layer of normal epithelium in contrast to the dysplastic changes in adenomas. Single juvenile polyps are usually located in the distal colon and have a macroscopic cherry-red appearance. Up to 1 per cent of children may have a juvenile polyp, and in 70 per cent only a single polyp is present. Juvenile intestinal polyposis, defined by the presence of more than three to five polyps, is therefore relatively rare.

About one-quarter of juvenile intestinal polyposis pedigrees segregate mutations in the *SMAD4/DPC4* gene on chromosome 18q21.1. This gene was originally identified as a tumour suppressor deleted in pancreatic cancers. The protein functions in the signal transduction pathway of the inhibitory growth factor **TGF-β** (transforming growth factor-beta). Absence of this protein would be expected to lead to a loss of response to the growth inhibitory effects of TGF-β. Other pedigrees show genetic linkage to chromosome 10q23.3. The *PTEN* tumour-suppressor gene maps in this region. It encodes a phosphatase, which works through the PI3-kinase pathway to modulate the cell-cycle control protein p27. *PTEN* is mutated in pedigrees with the allelic conditions Cowden disease (OMIM158350) or Bannayan–Zonana syndrome (OMIM153480), in both of which hamartomas in multiple tissues and macrocephaly occur. Juvenile polyps are features of both these autosomal dominant diseases, but the number of polyps is not as high as in juvenile intestinal polyposis. The occurrence of *PTEN* mutations in juvenile intestinal polyposis remains unconfirmed and another gene at 10q23 may be involved.

Juvenile polyps also occur in patients with the Gorlin syndrome (OMIM 123456), an autosomal dominant disease primarily characterized by basal-cell carcinomas of the skin and odontogenic keratocysts in the mouth. The genes mutated in this condition encode the receptor for the sonic hedgehog (**SHH**) protein. Again, however, no mutations have been detected in pedigrees segregating juvenile intestinal polyposis. Interestingly, SHH signalling indirectly controls the expression of the *SMAD4/DPC4* gene, which is causative in some juvenile intestinal polyposis pedigrees. SHH signalling is also indirectly involved in wingless (**WNT**) expression. Loss of signalling control through the WNT pathway leads to FAP.

Juvenile intestinal polyposis predisposes to adenomatous transformation and an increased risk of colorectal cancer and cancers elsewhere in the gastrointestinal tract. The accepted view of solitary juvenile polyps has been that they do not predispose to malignancy in children, who do not therefore require follow-up. It will now be possible to confirm this if it can be shown that *DPC4* mutations (or mutations in the putative gene at 10q23) are not found in solitary retention hamartomas. The occurrence of mutations would suggest these tumours have malignant potential.

Cronkhite-Canada syndrome is a rare, non-Mendelian condition characterized by juvenile-type polyps throughout the gastrointestinal tract (with the exception of the oesophagus). Ectodermal abnormalities include nail dystrophy, alopecia, and brown hyperpigmentation of the skin. Patients present with severe diarrhoea, malabsorption, and weight loss. This condition is rapidly progressive with inflammation of the entire intestinal mucosa. In some cases the condition resolves spontaneously with corticosteroids, but up to one-third of patients die within months. Survivors have an increased incidence of adenomatous change and carcinoma warranting regular colonoscopic surveillance. Surgical resection is necessary for otherwise uncontrollable bleeding. The pathogenesis of this disease remains unknown.

Inflammatory polyps

These pseudopolyps arise during the healing phase after attacks of severe colitis (ulcerative colitis, Crohn's disease, and schistosomiasis).have led to extensive mucosal ulceration. Histologically the colonic epithelial-cell layer is often normal. Larger inflammatory polyps may be composed of granulation tissue in the healing mucosa. These polyps may be friable and bleed, and can be multiple (Cap polyposis). Biopsy may be necessary to distinguish between inflammatory polyps and adenocarcinoma but those over 1 cm diameter are usually removed endoscopically for surety.

Other types of non-neoplastic polyp

Lipomas are usually located in the right colon. With the exception of intussusception, they are asymptomatic and do not require removal. Other rare benign tumours arising from the colonic submucosa include leiomyomas, neurofibromas, and polypoid haemangiomas. Pneumocystic disease (also called pneumatosis cystoides or pneumatosis coli) leads to multiple submucosal cysts, which can be punctured and collapsed in patients when they cause abdominal pain. The cysts may resolve when treated with oxygen therapy.

Neoplastic (adenomatous) polyps and the adenoma to carcinoma progression

Adenomas are dysplastic epithelial growths with malignant potential. Most frequently they are tubular (Fig. 7), having glandular organization, with a peduncle of normal tissue. Adenomatous polyps with a tubulovillous mixed character occur as well as the less common villous adenomas, which are sessile lesions, frond-like histologically, often quite large, and with the highest tendency to malignant change. Our understanding of the molecular events during first adenoma then carcinoma development has mainly been gained from genetic studies of familial adenomatous polyposis.

Aetiology, epidemiology, and pathology (Table 2)

'Sporadic' colonic adenomas are extremely common and are usually asymptomatic. Adenomas are found in around 20 per cent of individuals in their sixth decade and the incidence increases steadily with age. The distribution of adenomas in the colon reflects the site-specific incidence of colorectal carcinomas, with only minor differences. The majority of adenomas are found on the left side of the colon and in the rectum, although more

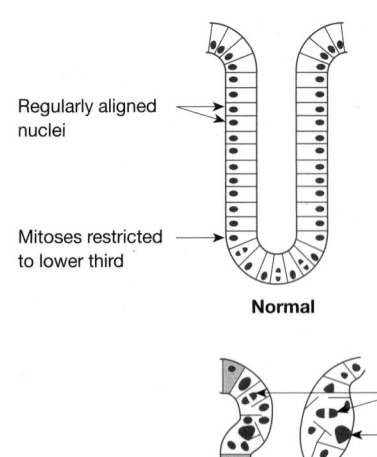

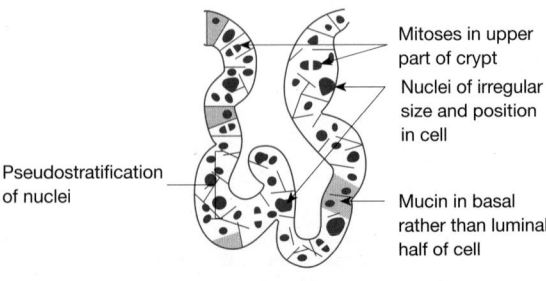

Fig. 7 Diagrammatic representation of the difference between the histology of a normal colonic crypt and the disorder of a neoplastic (dysplastic) crypt.

Table 2 Frequency of invasive carcinoma in different types of sizes of adenomas in an endoscopic series

	Type as percentage of all adenomas	Percentage with malignancy			
		<1.1 cm	1–2 cm	>2 cm	All sizes
Tubular	75	1	3.0	10	2
Tubulovillous	20		5.0	11	6
Villous	5		6.0	38	18
All adenomas		1	5.5	16	5 (overall)

From Gillespie PE *et al.* (1979). Colonic adenomas – a colonscopic survey. *Gut* **20**, 240–45.

right-sided lesions are found with increasing age. The role of environmental factors in adenoma development is suggested by their increased incidence in the developed countries. Furthermore, migrant communities such as the Japanese in the United States acquire an adenoma (and carcinoma) incidence comparable to the local population.

Around 60 per cent of adenomas can be accessed by flexible sigmoidoscopy. A distal adenoma is associated with the presence of a second more proximal adenoma in around 30 per cent of individuals. Like FAP adenomas, sporadic colorectal adenomas are thought to progress slowly over time. This means that only 5 per cent of 50-year-olds will eventually develop colorectal cancer, even though their incidence of adenomas is much higher than this. Because they are slow growing, only some 10 per cent of adenomas are greater than 1 cm in diameter when found. The incidence of malignant progression increases with tumour size.

Adenomas may arise in aberrant crypt foci, which are small areas of epithelium with irregular glandular organization, but without apparent dysplasia. These develop into single dysplastic crypts (unicryptal adenomas) so that the earliest recognizable adenomas have dysplastic epithelium. Dysplasia progresses through mild, moderate, to severe, which is reflected in the increasing malignant potential of the polyp. Adenomas may also be classified as early, intermediate, and late in histological appearance, and these histological changes have been correlated with the acquisition of a series of genetic alterations by Vogelstein and colleagues. Endoscopic excision is usually facilitated by the macroscopic difference in appearance between the normal mucosa and neoplastic epithelium, which appears hyperaemic and raised above the surrounding surface. In around 5 per cent of adenomas, carcinoma is detected (when neoplastic cells have breached the muscularis mucosae) (Fig. 8). Only at this stage is there access to the local lymphatics and blood vessels with the possibility of metastasis.

There is increasing recognition of the existence of flat adenomas. These polyps are only very slightly raised and indeed may appear as depressed lesions. Flat adenomas are difficult to see endoscopically, but pioneering studies by Japanese gastroenterologists using non-absorbable mucosal dyes to provide contrast has led to a more widespread recognition of these lesions. Their clinical significance is that they can be more severely dysplastic than polypoid adenomas of comparable size, and therefore may represent a much-increased risk of carcinoma. The difficulties of studying the natural history of flat adenomas and their progression to so-called 'flat carcinomas' is complicated by the fact that they are more common on the right side of the colon. Some individuals with germline *APC* mutations appear to develop a flat adenoma phenotype.

The location of colonic carcinoma within about 5 per cent of adenomas suggests that the adenoma is a precursor of carcinoma. The time for progression to carcinoma is slow, usually 10 years or more. Patients with large or villous adenomas have an increased risk of coexisting synchronous carcinomas, or for the subsequent development of another carcinoma and so merit colonoscopy and follow-up. Later stage cancers contain less adenomatous material, presumably because this is overgrown by the malignant cells. Epidemiological data also support the adenoma to carcinoma sequence.

Additional mutations accumulate as the adenoma moves through intermediate to late stages (Fig. 9). These include activating mutations in the K-*ras* proto-oncogene and loss of tumour-suppressor function at chromosome 18q21. It appears unlikely that this is the so-called 'deleted in colorectal cancer' (*DCC gene*) and is more likely to involve the *DPC4/SMAD4* pancreatic TSG. It is the accumulation of these different genetic changes rather than their stepwise occurrence that drives carcinogenesis. K-*ras* mutations occur in 50 per cent of sporadic colorectal tumours. Loss of function of the *P53* tumour-suppressor gene occurs in 70 per cent of sporadic colorectal cancers. The resulting lack of apoptosis correlates with a metastatic phenotype, in that the incidence of *P53* mutations in carcinomas is much higher than in associated adenomas. Additional mutations occur in distant metastases.

Clinical features, management, and surveillance

Colonic adenomas do not usually cause symptoms. Abdominal pain, altered bowel habit, or intermittent bleeding are unusual. Large villous adenomas of the rectum may rarely present with mucoid diarrhoea and hypokalaemia. Polyps are usually discovered accidentally on barium enema or scanning examination or during endoscopic screening. Histological discrimination from other types of polyp is mandatory. The detection of a distal adenoma by proctoscopy or flexible sigmoidoscopy justifies colonoscopy to exclude the presence of proximal adenomas. The health economic implications of this are considerable given the high incidence of adenomas in the adult population.

Polyps are removed by endoscopic snare polypectomy or electrocoagulation. This is painless except for polyps within 2-5 cm of the anal margin. Around 90 per cent of patients with polyps have only two lesions, the majority of which are under 1 cm, stalked, and easy to snare. The tendency to bleed after polypectomy is greater with larger tumours. Very large, sessile polyps may need to be removed in multiple portions, but few are so large as to need surgical resection. Endoscopic removal of an adenomatous polyp that subsequently proves to contain a focus of carcinoma is a satisfactory outcome not requiring subsequent operation if there are clear histological margins.

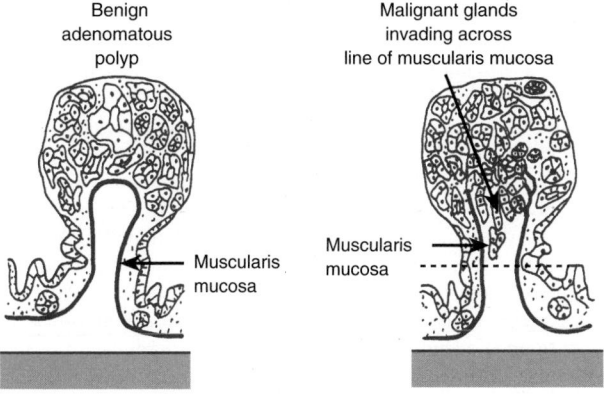

Fig. 8 Diagrammatic representation of the histology of a benign adenoma and a 'malignant polyp' showing adenoma and invasive adenocarcinoma (dotted line indicates transaction line to achieve complete removal).

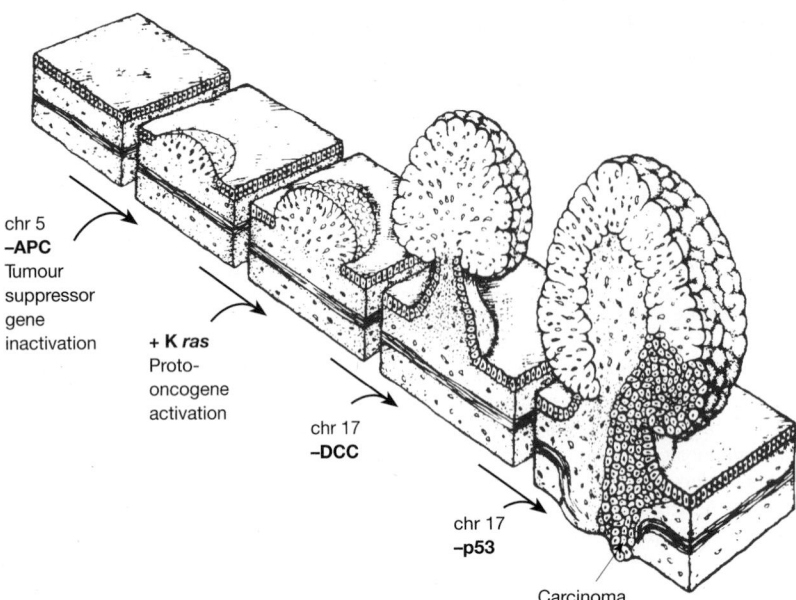

Fig. 9 The 'adenoma–carcinoma sequence' – a possible genetic model. Accumulated genetic changes to the stepwise progression from normal epithelium through increasing polyp size to eventual malignant change. Genetic alterations, which do not occur in a rigid sequence, include inactivation of tumour suppressor genes (adenomatous polyposis coli (APC), deleted in colorectal cancer (DCC) and p53, as well as the activation of proto-oncogenes such as K-ras. (Adapted from Fearon and Vogelstein (1990). *Cell* **61**, 759.)

Post-polypectomy surveillance is necessary in patients who have had an adenoma detected and removed. They are at higher risk of second adenomas, particularly when multiple (five or more) polyps are present at first examination. Villous adenomas are particularly liable to recur locally. Repeat colonoscopy is performed at 3 to 5 yearly intervals, depending on number and size of polyps found. The decision to cease surveillance at 75 years of age is justified after a negative examination because of the slow natural history of the disease, despite the increased incidence of both polyps and carcinoma with age.

Familial adenomatous polyposis (FAP)

The principal feature of FAP (OMIM175100) is the presence of hundreds to thousands of adenomatous polyps throughout the colon (Fig. 10). The condition is inherited as an autosomal dominant, although about one-quarter of cases arise without a family history, thus implying a high rate of new mutations. As well as the colonic polyps, adenomas are found in the

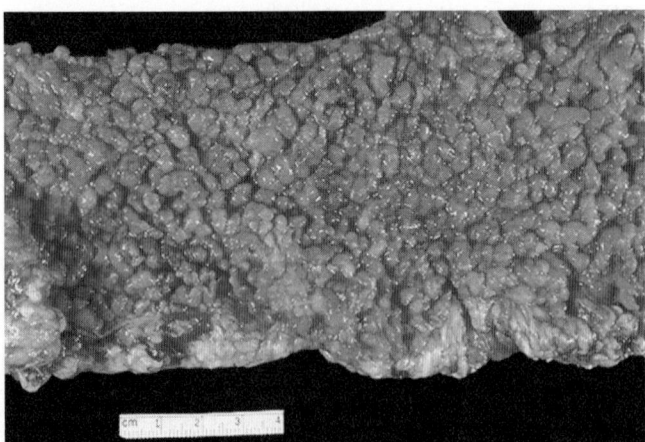

Fig. 10 Familial adenomatous polyposis (FAP) colectomy specimen, showing carpeting of the colon by hundreds of adenomas.

duodenum in the majority of patients, and also in the stomach and elsewhere in the small intestine. Adenomas usually begin to develop during the second decade so that screening is performed between 12 and 14 years of age. The risk of colorectal cancer developing in one of the adenomas is essentially 100 per cent by the age of 40 years, so that this condition is fully penetrant. Screening by flexible sigmoidoscopy with biopsy of polyps for histological diagnosis confirms the condition and allows surgery before the age of 20. Screening family members by flexible sigmoidoscopy confirms or eliminates the diagnosis in relatives. The creation of Polyposis registers makes FAP an example of practical colorectal cancer prevention.

There is a 10- to 20-year period between the appearance of an adenoma and its progression to colorectal carcinoma. Clinically, therefore, colectomy with ileorectal or ileoanal anastomosis is usually performed on FAP subjects in their late teens, as there is low risk of carcinoma before this age. Careful long-term follow up is required. There is a 10 per cent risk of carcinoma in any rectal stump over a 30-year period, although rectal polyps may undergo regression, suggesting that adenoma progression to carcinoma is not inevitable. Total proctocolectomy with ileostomy is also an option with large numbers of rectal polyps if the increased operative risks of ileoanal anastomosis with formation of a pelvic pouch are not regarded as acceptable.

Historically, FAP caused 1 per cent of all colorectal cancers. Surveillance programmes have reduced this incidence, but the prolonged survival of patients postcolectomy has highlighted the other features of FAP, which increasingly create clinical problems. Carcinomatous change occurs in adenomas in the duodenum, particularly around the ampulla of Vater and in the bile duct. It may also occur in the stomach. Follow-up is required to avoid these eventualities. Mesenchymal desmoid tumours, particularly those occurring in the retroperitoneum, can grow to an enormous size. Their position and tendency to re-growth makes them difficult to remove and they may cause devastating consequences due to pressure effects.

The wide range of additional features of FAP led to the description of Gardner's and Turcot's syndromes that have proved to be allelic with FAP. Additional features include osteomas of the mandible and skull, dental abnormalities, sebaceous cysts, and brain tumours. About one-half of patients with Turcot's syndrome have germline *APC* (adenomatous polyposis coli) mutations and develop cerebellar medulloblastomas. It is notable that the other 50 per cent have germline mutations in their DNA mismatch repair genes (that is, *HNPCC*). These individuals undergo somatic *APC* mutations but develop glioblastoma multiforme. This link between HNPCC and mutations in *APC* is intriguing.

FAP is caused by mutations in the *APC* gene on chromosome 5q21. This large 2843 amino-acid protein performs multiple functions in the cell, but in the context of colonic neoplasm development its key role is in the WNT pathway. In the absence of WNT signalling, APC forms a complex with two other proteins, axin and glycogen synthase kinase-3β (GSK-3β). This complex phosphorylates the β-catenin protein, which can then be tagged with ubiquitin and degraded by the proteasome system. In this manner, levels of cellular β-catenin are controlled. β-Catenin plays roles in intracellular signalling from E-cadherin in the epithelial adherens junction (which is also mutated in gastric cancer), but when present in the cell at high levels it can bind a second protein (TCF-4), enter the nucleus, and switch on the expression of a number of genes, including the c-*myc* oncogene and the cyclin D1 gene, and others. In the presence of a WNT signal, GSK-3β is inactivated and β-catenin levels rise to drive gene expression and cellular proliferation. With only mutant APC, the cell is also incapable of degrading β-catenin and again proliferation occurs.

APC expression increases as the colonocyte migrates up the crypt to the lumenal surface. This may reflect a role in controlling cell movement. In FAP, the vast majority of germline mutations are in the *N*-terminal half of the protein and are nonsense mutations leading to truncated proteins. The key region of APC for β-catenin binding lies between amino acids 1000 and 2000. Germline mutations occur almost exclusively before amino acid 1650. Some 85 per cent of sporadic colorectal adenomas and carcinomas also have mutations in the *APC* tumour-suppressor gene. The majority of these occur in the so-called 'mutation cluster region' between amino acids 1280 and 1500. Again, this creates truncated proteins that cannot properly degrade β-catenin. Consistent with Knudsen's hypothesis, the second normal *APC* allele is consistently lost in adenomas, so that the cell has no functional 'gate-keeper' tumour-suppressor protein.

Identical germline *APC* mutations can cause a variety of phenotypes, from polyposis alone to the full spectrum of Gardner's syndrome. This suggests that there are genetic modifier loci for FAP. Mutations at the extreme 5'-end of the gene may be associated with a milder 'attenuated' phenotype. Mutations towards the 3'-end of the gene (around amino acid 2600) cause the familial desmoid syndrome. Congenital hypertrophy of the retinal pigment epithelium (**CHRPE**) is another recognized clinical sign in FAP. Only germline mutations downstream of codon 422 cause CHRPE, for reasons that remain unclear. This means, however, that opthalmoscopic detection of CHRPE cannot be regarded as a reliable screening method.

Determination of the mutant sequence in FAP pedigrees now allows precise genetic counselling. However, the large size of this gene and protein make sequencing it difficult in individual patients. The protein truncation test (**PTT**) is used to detect *APC* mutations because so many generate truncated proteins. These are detected by electrophoresis after *in vitro* transcription and translation from patients' *APC* mRNA.

The critical role of APC in colorectal adenomas (and carcinomas) has been further emphasized by analysis of sporadic tumours that do not harbour *APC* mutations. These 15 per cent of colorectal neoplasms prove to have mutations in the β-catenin gene itself. Moreover, these mutations alter those amino acids which undergo phosphorylation by the APC–GSK-3β–axin complex. Thus, these mutant forms of β-catenin are constitutively active. This same mechanism seems to apply in melanoma. Mutations in the axin gene can also lead to colorectal neoplasia.

NSAIDs were serendipitously found to reduce the number and size of colorectal adenomas in FAP. The effect has been demonstrated with sulindac in particular. Aspirin also reduces the risk of colorectal cancer. Colorectal cancers overexpress cyclo-oxygenase-2 (COX-2). In *Apc* knockout mice, deletion of the murine *Cox-2* gene causes a significant reduction in the number of polyps formed. Aspirin or selective COX-2 inhibitors may delay the onset of FAP adenomas and hence their progression to carcinoma. The attraction of this possibility is the advantage of postponing elective colectomy into the third decade.

Polymorphic *APC* variants may exist in the population, which, although associated with an increased risk of adenoma development, are of such low penetrance that they do not seem Mendelian in character. This would be consistent with the marked familial clustering seen in colorectal cancer.

Colorectal cancer (Fig. 11)

The natural history of colorectal tumorigenesis now provides a rational basis for the introduction of screening programmes in an attempt to control this common malignancy, which is curable if detected early or at the precancerous (polyp) stage. Several screening modalities have been shown to decrease colorectal cancer (**CRC**) mortality, and screening guidelines have been published in several countries. The incidence of the disease is falling in the United Kingdom and United States as a result of increased detection and removal of adenomas.

Epidemiology and aetiology

Colorectal cancer is the most common malignancy in the United Kingdom after lung cancer: 19 000 deaths each year reflect a 5-year survival rate for CRC at all stages of approximately 50 per cent. The lifetime risk of colorectal cancer in the United States approaches 6 per cent. There is a higher incidence of rectal cancer in men. The estimate for the United States in 2000 was 130 200 new cases of colorectal cancer and 56 300 deaths, a lower population death rate than in the United Kingdom. The incidence of cancers of the colon and rectum increases with age, the mean age at diagnosis being 65 years. The 5-year survival rate is dependent upon the tumour stage at diagnosis: Dukes' stage A disease, over 90 per cent; Dukes' B disease, 65 per cent; stage C1 disease, 30 per cent; stage C2 disease, 20 per cent; and stage D disease, a 5-year survival of 2 per cent or less.

A small proportion of patients with Dukes' stage A colorectal cancer succumb to their disease. Although only 15 per cent of cases are diagnosed at this stage, it would be invaluable to identify the small proportion of them that might benefit from adjuvant therapies. This issue becomes more important in patients with Dukes' stage B carcinomas, which represent some 40 per cent of tumours diagnosed. It would be valuable to be able to discriminate those 35 per cent of patients at diagnosis who will go on to develop progressive disease and target adjuvant chemo/radiotherapy on them. Conversely, it would be desirable to avoid exposing patients who have had what proves to be curative surgery to the toxicity of adjuvant chemotherapy.

There are clearly environmental factors that influence the incidence of colorectal cancer. These are presumably mainly dietary. The incidence of colorectal cancer is higher in Northern Europe and North America than in the developing world. The risk of adenoma formation and colon cancer in Japanese peoples rises when they are exposed to a westernized diet. Although carcinogens or co-carcinogens may be produced by bacterial metabolism of bile salts, or from animal fat, or as a result of prolonged transit times of low-fibre diets, the evidence for this is not clear-cut.

It is increasingly recognized that genetic factors other than those causing Mendelian cancer syndromes are important in colorectal carcinoma with, for example, a threefold increased frequency of a family history of bowel cancer in individuals diagnosed as having an adenomatous polyp compared with normal controls. Thus the underlying aetiology of colorectal carcinogenesis is complex. Implantation of the ureters into the sigmoid colon (ureterosigmoidostomy) results in a high incidence of adenomas with subsequent carcinoma development 10 years and more after creation of the ureteric stoma. Long-term inflammation, as in extensive ulcerative colitis of over 20 years' duration (and probably also Crohn's colitis), provides a risk of ulcerative colitis-associated colorectal carcinoma (**UCACRC**). This may affect 5 per cent of these individuals, even where

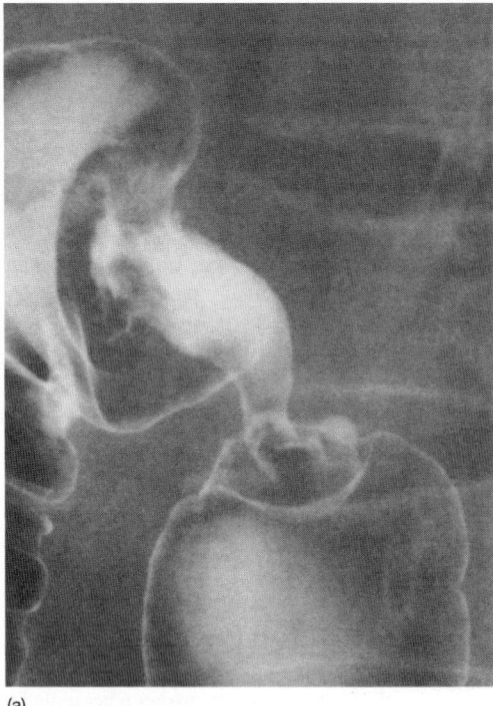

(a)

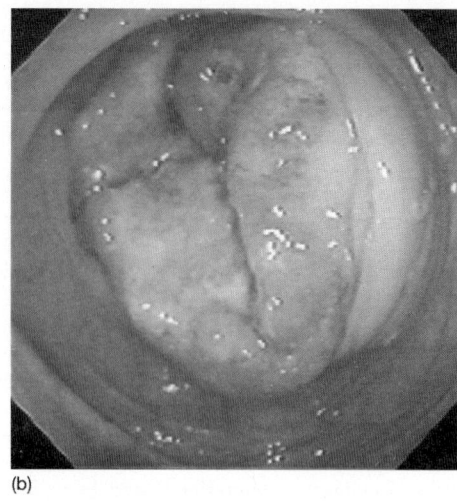

(b)

Fig. 11 Colonic carcinoma appearances. (a) Air-contrast barium study showing 'apple-core' stricture. (b) Colonoscopy appearance of encircling 'annular' tumour.

their disease is reasonably well controlled or healed. It may be multifocal. These cancers often have a mucinous appearance, with or without 'signet ring' cells. Ileorectal anastomosis to treat refractory inflammatory bowel disease (**IBD**) also leaves a risk of local malignant change in the rectum. Some protection is afforded by annual or biennial colonoscopy, with serial biopsies to detect any warning epithelial dysplasia.

Hereditary non-polyposis colon cancer

A second, autosomal dominant disease accounts for up to 5 per cent of cases of colorectal cancer. Hereditary non-polyposis colorectal cancer (HNPCC) was originally divided into Lynch syndromes type 1 and 2, with a range of other malignancies associated with the latter. A total of seven different mutant genes have now been characterized to define HNPCC types 1 to 7, superseding the Lynch definition. HNPCC kindreds were initially defined by the so-called 'Amsterdam' criteria, which are:

(1) at least three family members in two or more successive generations must have colorectal cancer;

(2) one of these must be a first-degree relative of the other two;

(3) cancer must be diagnosed before the age of 50 in at least one family member;

(4) FAP must be excluded.

HNPCC is associated with other malignancies in mutation carriers: endometrial cancer is the most common, ovarian cancer is frequent, and tumours in other organ systems are less common (breast, stomach, possibly prostate). The risk of uterine cancer may exceed that for colorectal cancer in females in pedigrees, emphasizing the necessity for uterine screening. HNPCC has an approximate penetrance of 74 per cent for colorectal cancer in men by the age of 70 compared with only 30 per cent in females. The risk of uterine cancer is 42 per cent in these women. Hysterectomy is usually accompanied by bilateral oophorectomy because of the risk of subsequent ovarian cancer.

The syndrome arises as a result of the germline transmission of mutations in one of six genes encoding components of the DNA mismatch repair enzyme system. Germline mutations in the TGF-β receptor II gene are now also classified as HNPCC. The encoded proteins repair DNA mismatches arising as a result of replication errors. These tumours were therefore described as RER+. Replication of DNA is particularly prone to error in those regions of DNA known as microsatellites where multiple short nucleotide repeat sequences occur. Loss of DNA repair function leads to the so-called 'microsatellite instability' of these regions. This means that the allele sizes of microsatellites are different in tumours than in normal cells from the same individual. PCR-based methods are readily able to detect this to establish that a given tumour has an RER+ phenotype. The extent of microsatellite instability varies between tumours and there is some disagreement as to how many loci need to be modified before a tumour can be classified as RER+.

In addition to patients with HNPCC, between 10 and 15 per cent of sporadic colorectal cancers are also RER+ to some extent. The inability to repair errors introduced during DNA synthesis renders the genome in HNPCC cells liable to mutation. Interestingly, the *APC* gene itself appears prone to mutation in mismatch repair deficiency, leading to a frame-shift mutation and premature termination of translation. Thus it is possible that colorectal adenomas arise in patients with HNPCC through a similar final common pathway to that in FAP.

The commonest mutations occur in the mismatch repair genes *MSH2* and *MLH1*. There is some evidence that HNPCC polyps and tumours occur predominantly on the right side of the colon. It has also been suggested that these have a better prognosis, although this may be confounded because right-sided lesions tend to be larger (given the reduced solidity of the stool in the ascending colon) at presentation and therefore likely to be at more advanced stages. It is clear that a variety of mutations can predispose to colorectal cancer, but intriguingly all of these seem to feed into a final pathway of tumorigenesis similar to that originally elucidated for FAP. Patients with HNPCC should be included in genetic counselling and surveillance programmes usually by colonoscopy performed at 2 to 3 yearly intervals.

Colorectal cancer screening and surveillance

A number of screening modalities have been evaluated. These include testing for faecal occult blood, flexible sigmoidoscopy, double-contrast barium enema examination, and colonoscopy. The health economic implications of implementing such screening programmes are considerable. However, there is clear benefit in screening and surveillance of high-risk individuals such as those with previously detected adenomas or with a strong family history. In these cases colonoscopic examination is justifiable, as in the follow-up of individuals who have had carcinomas resected.

In the average-risk population, there is increasing consensus that screening should begin at 50 years of age. A number of protocols are undergoing trial to establish their diagnostic yield in terms of cost per year of life saved. Despite its lack of sensitivity and specificity, annual faecal occult-blood testing (**FOBT**) can be considered. Others advocate flexible sigmoidoscopy every 5 years, with colonoscopy if any adenomas are detected. Whether repeat flexible sigmoidoscopy every 5 years in individuals in whom no polyps are found is worthwhile needs to be established, as its avoidance would generate considerable cost savings. Specific guidelines have been published in the United States and a Cochrane Review of FOBT screening has been published. Cochrane Reviews are in preparation on the benefits of colorectal adenoma surveillance programmes and on detecting colorectal cancer in patients with IBD. Population screening using flexible sigmoidoscopy is the subject of an ongoing, national multicentre study in the United Kingdom. There is the real possibility of achieving significant reductions in the incidence of this common, but avoidable, malignancy by screening. Colonoscopic surveillance of those with adenomas or significant genetic risk is at 2 to 5 year intervals thereafter.

Pathology

Most colorectal cancers occur distally, in the rectum and sigmoid colon. An approximate estimate is that one-third of cancers occur in the rectum, one-third in the sigmoid colon, and one-third more proximally. Carcinomas are typically polypoid masses with central ulceration, eroded edges that bleed easily, and which may result in strictures. Infiltrating scirrhous carcinomas are rare. Colorectal carcinoma initially spreads by local invasion, which accounts for its good prognosis when confined to the bowel wall. Invasion through the mucosal and muscle layers of the bowel may lead to involvement of adjacent organs including the bladder and prostate. Secondary complications may therefore include fistula formation. Venous and lymphatic spread results in the predominance of liver metastases. It is increasingly recognized that even multiple liver metastases may be amenable to surgical resection. Lymphatic spread is to local nodes (Dukes' stage C1 disease) then to more proximal nodes in the mesentery (Dukes' stage C2 disease).

The Dukes' classification of colorectal carcinomas (Fig. 12) remains the mainstay of tumour staging. Stage A disease is confined to the bowel wall with no extension to the serosal fat. Stage B disease involves the full thickness of the bowel wall with extension through to the serosa. Stages C1 and C2 involve the spread of tumour to draining lymph nodes. Stage D disease involves distant spread, primarily to the liver. These different stages very clearly correlate with 5-year survival. The alternative TNM staging system has the advantage over the Dukes' system in distinguishing early tumours involving only the submucosa (T1) and amenable to endoscopic resection, from slightly more advanced tumours (T2) which extend into the muscularis propria. T3 tumours extend into the serosal fat and T4 tumours are those which have perforated or involve the peritoneal surface or other viscera. The extent of histological differentiation is also an important prognostic indicator with poorly differentiated tumours particularly aggressive. As well as liver metastases, secondary deposits appear in the lung (50 per cent), peritoneum (15 per cent), and bones (15 per cent). Unfortunately, approximately 50 per cent of colorectal cancer is stage C or D at diagnosis because it remains asymptomatic, so that the overall 5-year survival rate is reduced. Skewing the stage of detection towards Dukes' A lesions would have a major impact on overall survival.

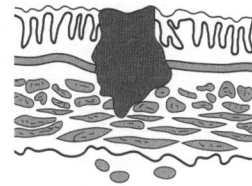

Dukes A
Tumour limited
to bowel wall

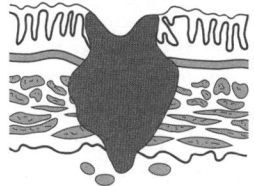

Dukes B
Tumour has penetrated
through the bowel wall
but lymph nodes are
not involved

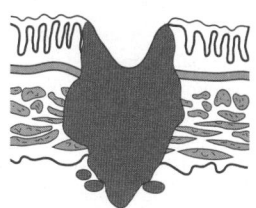

Dukes C
The lymph nodes
are now involved

Fig. 12 Dukes' classification of colorectal carcinoma.

Clinical features

The site of a colorectal cancer influences the resultant symptoms. Most colorectal neoplasms grow into the lumen of the bowel where they may cause obstruction or bleed because of their friable epithelial surfaces. Obstruction and bleeding are increasingly likely with more distal lesions as the stool becomes more solid. Blood is typically dark and mixed in with the stool, in contrast to the fresh or dripping bleeding observed from haemorrhoids. Alteration of bowel habit may involve frequency or increased constipation where solid stool flow is obstructed, particularly with left-sided lesions. Ascending colon tumours can grow large without affecting faecal flow. In these cases presentation is often with iron-deficiency anaemia as a consequence of long-standing but invisible blood loss. Diagnosis of right-sided lesions is further complicated by the difficulty of achieving complete evacuation, the challenge of barium enema or scanning studies in this region, and the difficulty of colonoscopic access. Pain in a patient with colorectal cancer suggests obstructive disease or invasion, and weight loss is a late symptom suggestive of advanced disease with poor prognosis. A palpable mass may reflect faecal retention, but the tumour itself may still be resectable. Thus the clinical picture in colorectal cancer is relatively nonspecific and must be differentiated from the anorectal bleeding of haemorrhoids or fissures, and the pain and altered bowel habit of irritable bowel disease.

The occurrence of so many tumours in the rectum makes digital rectal examination essential. Flexible sigmoidoscopy has become a routine procedure requiring a simple enema preparation and usually no sedation. It will detect 60 per cent of adenomas and carcinomas. Colonoscopic examination has the advantage that other synchronous polyps or tumours are detected. Other imaging modalities are becoming increasingly important, for example CT scanning as 'virtual colography' or to stage disease before operation in order to detect involvement of adjacent structures such as the ureters. MRI scanning is particularly useful to assess rectosigmoid disease. Transmural ultrasound is used in the rectum for assessing local invasion. Serological tests such as carcinoembryonic antigen levels are of some value in postoperative management and in the detection of tumour recurrence, but are secondary to accurate histological staging.

As a result of these investigations the differential diagnoses can usually be discounted. These include benign lesions such as areas of ischaemia, solitary rectal ulcer syndrome, masses of granulation tissue, endometriosis, or amoebomas, all of which may mimic carcinoma on radiography or endoscopy. An appendix abscess may mimic a caecal carcinoma, as may tuberculosis, actinomycosis, or Crohn's disease. Sigmoid diverticular disease with pericolic abscess formation may mimic distal carcinoma. Other malignancies of the colon, including lymphoma, sarcoma, and carcinoid tumours are rare. Kaposi's sarcoma presents as violaceous nodules in patients with AIDS. A variety of anal tumours occur that reflect the different structures and embryological derivation of this area. They include adenocarcinomas, condylomas, and squamous carcinomas (which are common in immunosuppressed patients due to papillomavirus infections), and malignant melanomas. Rarely, the anal margin may be the site of premalignant skin conditions such as leucoplakia, Paget's disease, or Bowen's disease.

Treatment

Surgical resection is the primary treatment and is potentially curative. The aim is to remove the neoplasm with an adequate uninvolved resection margin of normal tissue, as well as the entire draining lymphatic field. The need for careful mesorectal dissection to prevent local recurrence is established in rectal cancer surgery. In the presence of metastases, palliative resection of the primary tumour is usually desirable in order to prevent obstruction, so that 90 per cent of patients undergo surgery. The operative mortality for colorectal surgery is less than 1 per cent. Bowel preparation is essential, with oral purgatives and/or enemas, to avoid anastomotic complications. Prophylactic antibiotics minimize postoperative sepsis. Thorough preoperative preparation may be impossible in patients presenting in emergency with perforation or obstruction. Some 25 per cent of patients with colorectal cancer present in this manner, when the hazards of surgery are much increased.

The site of the tumour dictates the operation performed: caecal carcinomas are treated by right hemicolectomy; ascending and transverse colon tumours by extended right hemicolectomy; left hemicolectomy for descending colon cancer; and sigmoid colectomy for sigmoid tumours. All these operations involve resection back to the respective tributaries of the superior and inferior mesenteric arteries.

The operation performed for rectal cancer is also dependent on the tumour's position. An anterior resection is performed where it is possible to leave a disease-free margin above the anal canal. When the cancer is too low for this, an abdominoperineal resection is performed with resection of the distal sigmoid colon, rectum, and anus, and creation of a permanent sigmoid colostomy. Rectal surgery has been transformed by the availability of a variety of stapling instruments to reanastomose the bowel. Low anterior resections are now commonly performed with good results, so that anal excision is avoided. Abdominoperineal resection is unavoidable when the tumour involves the anal sphincter. A temporary colostomy is sometimes advisable, particularly acutely, when there is a high risk of postoperative anastomotic leakage.

There is increasing interest in the use of laparoscopic techniques to remove colorectal tumours. The great advantage of this approach is that surgery is less traumatic and postoperative recovery is accelerated. A variety of techniques have been developed to avoid the problem of disease recurrence at the sites of laparoscopic entry ports. Multicentre, randomized controlled trials are currently comparing outcomes, especially 5-year survival rates after laparoscopic versus open surgery for colorectal cancer. Given the different 5-year survival rates for tumours at different Dukes' stages, the outcomes of colorectal surgery essentially reflect the proportions of patients presenting at these different stages (Table 3).

Dukes' staging is also central to the appropriate use of chemotherapy and radiotherapy. 5-fluorouracil (with folinic acid) prolongs the survival of patients with stage D disease. Randomized trials have also shown that 5-fluorouracil (**5-FU**) improves survival in stage C disease when used as adjuvant therapy to surgery. It is not clear that portal vein infusion of 5-FU provides any additional advantage. The evidence of survival advantage from adjuvant chemotherapy in stage B disease is less clear-cut. The com-

Table 3 Modified Dukes' classification and life prognosis for potentially curative colorectal cancer

Dukes' classification	Cases resected (%)	5-year survival (%)[*]
A	15	95–100
B	40	65–75
C1 (local nodes)	35	30–40
C2 (apical nodes)	10	10–20

[*] Corrected for other causes of mortality.

plicating factor is that 60 per cent of these patients will survive for 5 years after surgery alone, and any additional survival advantage from chemotherapy must be balanced against the risk of life-threatening toxicity (stomatitis, leucopenia, etc.) in up to 5 per cent of patients. Intuitively, it has been assumed that agents beneficial in stage C disease should provide a therapeutic benefit in the 40 per cent of stage B patients (and 10 per cent of stage A patients) who do not survive for 5 years after surgery alone. Some newer drugs show promise in the treatment of colorectal cancer: these include other thymidylate synthase inhibitors and drugs that inhibit topoisomerase (the 'tecan' class). However, this begs the question of how patients with tumours with atypically poor prognosis can be identified.

Randomized clinical trials of preoperative radiotherapy versus surgery alone show a reduction in local recurrence rates and survival advantages, particularly in rectal cancer. However, this must be balanced against the disadvantages of radiotherapy: impaired bowel function in up to one-third of patients and minor increases in early postoperative morbidity. Based on the available evidence, preoperative radiotherapy is better than postoperative treatment because the incidence of surgical complications is lower. Thus, adjuvant chemotherapy combined with preoperative radiotherapy is established practice for Dukes' stage C colorectal cancer. Recurrent disease is incurable so complete tumour excision is vital, particularly total mesorectal excision of rectal carcinomas. Therefore, follow-up after potentially curative surgery is primarily aimed at detecting further adenomas or cancers in these patients, who are at increased risk. Colonoscopy at 5 years seems to be as effective as more intensive surveillance programmes.

Further reading

Cochrane Reviews have appeared on the clinical management of gastrointestinal tumours (available at www.update-software.com). Their topics include:
preoperative chemotherapy for resectable thoracic oesophageal cancer
preoperative radiotherapy for oesophageal carcinoma
palliative chemotherapy for advanced or metastatic colorectal cancer
screening for colorectal cancer using the faecal occult-blood test
Protocols have also been published for Cochrane Reviews on:
colorectal adenoma surveillance and colorectal cancer
surgery for obstructing left-sided colorectal cancer: primary or staged resection?
follow-up strategies for non-metastatic colorectal cancer
intravenous 5-FU-based regimes as adjuvant to surgery for colon cancer with local lymph node spread
local surgical treatment in early rectal cancer with or without adjuvant therapy
effect of preoperative radiotherapy and surgery for localized rectal carcinoma
strategies for detecting colon cancer or dysplasia in inflammatory bowel disease.

In addition, relevant material appears in publications from the NHS Centre for Reviews and Dissemination (e.g. Management of upper gastrointestinal cancers, *Reviews and Dissemination*, Vol. 6, 2000). Further authoritative reviews of United Kingdom best practice are published in *Clinical Evidence* (see Issue 4, December 2000). These include meta-analyses of randomized controlled trial evidence for or against:

treatment of gastro-oesophageal reflux disease in preventing progression of Barrett's oesophagus

adjuvant chemotherapy for stomach cancer

radical versus conservative surgical resection for stomach cancer

total mesorectal excision for rectal cancer

particular follow-up strategies after colorectal cancer

preoperative radiotherapy in colorectal cancer

adjuvant chemotherapy in colorectal cancer.

The consensus emerging from these progressively more comprehensive, evidence-based surveys of the optimum approaches to the clinical management of gastrointestinal tumours has been incorporated therein. The reader is encouraged to consult these accessible sources directly.

14.16 Vascular and collagen disorders

Graham Neale

Clinical disorders of the gastrointestinal tract caused by vascular and collagen disorders are rare in general medical practice. Vascular insufficiency (Table 1) may cause dramatic disease with infarction, perforation, bleeding, ulceration, or strictures, and in the very sick it may damage mucosal function and lead to ischaemia-reperfusion injury. In contrast, patients with collagen disorders often have abdominal symptoms due to disorder-related vasculitis, but such symptoms rarely dominate the clinical picture.

Causes of segmental mesenteric ischaemia

The blood supply to the gut may be impaired by compression, by intraluminal occlusion of vessels, or by intrinsic vascular pathology, including vasospasm.

Compression of mesenteric vessels

The mesenteric vessels may be compressed by torsion or strangulation of the mesentery, retroperitoneal haematomas, neoplastic infiltration, and rarely by proliferating fibrous tissue such as occurs in retroperitoneal fibrosis or occasionally around carcinoid or desmoid tumours. Venous occlusion with thrombosis is a rare complication of excessive gaseous pressure during laparoscopy.

Intraluminal occlusion of mesenteric vessels

Thrombosis

Thrombosis may occur in arteries or veins. In arteries thrombosis usually occurs on an ulcerated atheromatous plaque but it may occur spontaneously in polycythaemia, sickle cell disease, cryoglobulinaemia, and amyloidosis. Thromboangiitis obliterans (Buerger's disease) is a rare condition which does not usually affect mesenteric vessels but intestinal infarction has been described as a first manifestation of the disorder in women who

Table 1 Causes of ischaemia of the gut

Mechanical occlusion of vessels
  Torsion of the mesentery
  Strangulation of a loop of intestine
  Extraluminal compression
Intraluminal vascular occlusion
  Thrombosis—arterial or venous
  Emboli
  Diffuse microthrombosis
Intrinsic vascular pathology
  Atheromatous occlusion
  Inflammation of blood vessels
Non-occlusive mesenteric ischaemia which may cause
  Infarction
  Intestinal reperfusion injury

smoke. Mesenteric arterial thrombosis has also been described in cocaine addicts.

Mesenteric venous thrombosis is less common than arterial occlusion. An inherited thombophilia (such as deficiency of protein C, protein S, or antithrombin III) is the most likely cause. It may also occur in the primary antiphospholipid antibody syndrome and with dysfibrinogenaemia and has been described in women taking oral contraceptives (especially those who smoke) after splenectomy and in association with pancreatitis.

Arterial embolism

Emboli cause up to one-third of cases of mesenteric vascular occlusion. They arise from the heart, especially in patients with mitral stenosis and atrial fibrillation, with myocardial infarction and endomyocardial thrombosis, and with bacterial endocarditis. Paradoxical embolism through a patent foramen ovale and embolism from aortic mural thrombi are uncommon causes.

Diffuse microthrombosis

Diffuse thrombosis of small vessels may occur as a result of disseminated intravascular coagulation. The haemolytic–uraemic syndrome and thrombotic thrombocytopenic purpura are related conditions in which platelet aggregation occurs in small vessels (see Chapter 20.10.6 and Section 22). Renal failure usually dominates the clinical picture, but in most patients there is evidence of widespread involvement of the intestine and related organs. The haemostatic abnormalities and their relationship to microvascular injury are complex and give rise to diverse and often confusing clinical and laboratory findings. Infusions of platelets and fresh plasma are usually beneficial but therapy must be individualized depending on the nature of the underlying pathology and the site and severity of haemorrhage or thrombosis.

Intrinsic vascular pathology

Atheromatous occlusion

Atheroma is the most common cause of mesenteric vascular insufficiency, which often remains undiagnosed in life, probably because the slowness of the pathological process allows for the development of a compensatory collateral circulation. Intestinal infarction secondary to atheromatous occlusion of one major mesenteric vessel is uncommon. Indeed, all three vessels may be occluded without visceral damage.

Inflammation of blood vessels

Vasculitis is primarily a disorder of small vessels and affects many organs (Table 2). Involvement of the mesenteric circulation rarely causes infarction of long segments of the gut but may cause a wide spectrum of gastrointestinal disorders that are described later in this chapter.

Damage to the arterial wall in the splanchnic circulation sometimes occurs a few days after surgical correction of coarctation of the aorta. There is necrotizing arteritis with fibrinoid necrosis which is most marked at arterial bifurcations and appears to be related to the sudden sustained

Table 2 Vasculitides that may affect the gut

Involving vessels of all sizes
  Polyartertis nodosa
  (Churg–Strauss disease)
  Giant cell arteritis
  Takayasu's arteritis
  Transplant rejection
Involving predominantly medium and small vessels
  Wegener's granulomatosis
  Kawasaki disease
  Buerger's disease
Vasculitis of collagen–vascular disorders*
  Rheumatoid disease
  Systemic lupus erythematosus
  Progressive systemic sclerosis
  Dermatomyositis
Involving predominantly small vessels
  Hypersensitivity angiitis (microscopic polyarteritis)
  Henoch–Schönlein purpura
  Serum sickness
  Infective angiitis (e.g. typhoid, tuberculosis)

*The vasculitides of these disorders often involve only small vessels and the histological features may be indistinguishable from hypersensitivity angiitis. However, significant gastrointestinal pathology rarely occurs without the involvement of medium-sized vessels.

increase in blood pressure. It usually resolves spontaneously but may occasionally lead to intestinal infarction requiring operative intervention.

The walls of the mesenteric arteries may be involved in fibroelastic hyperplasia and in Takayasu's disease. In malignant hypertension, intimal hyperplasia and fibrinoid necrosis of arteriolar walls may lead to patchy ischaemia of the intestines. Irradiation of the abdomen leads to vascular necrosis and thrombosis, which in turn may cause ischaemic ulceration that on healing leaves a fibrosed intima and a poorly perfused segment of intestine.

Recently mesenteric veno-occlusive disease has been described as a discrete entity that may affect adults of any age. Previous cases were regarded as idiopathic venous thrombosis.

Non-occlusive mesenteric ischaemia (Table 3)

Sporadic and epidemic cases of necrotizing enteritis but without evidence of vascular occlusion have been described from many parts of the world and in all age groups. Neonatal necrotizing enterocolitis occurs in the first week of life of premature and low-birth-weight infants. Artificial hyperosmolar feeds may promote damage, whereas breast milk appears to be protective, possibly by providing passive enteric immunity. Lesions occur most frequently in the stomach, the distal ileum, and the colon; as mucosal integrity disintegrates bacterial invasion enhances the damage. The con-

Table 3 Intestinal infarction without acute vascular occlusion

Neonatal
  Necrotizing enterocolitis
Haemorrhagic enteritis or colitis
  Bacterial toxins (e.g. E. coli 0157:H7, Clostridium perfringens)
Focal ulceration
  Stress ulcers (especially stomach and duodenum)
  Drug-induced ulcers (e.g. potassium, NSAIDs*)
  Radiation enteritis
  Uraemic ulceration (especially in the colon)
After prolonged period of poor perfusion
  Low-output cardiac failure (?digitalis predisposed)
  Hyperviscosity syndromes
  Polycythaemia and haemoconcentration

*NSAIDs: non-steroidal anti-inflammatory drugs.

dition may also occur in infants of normal birth weight who have a hyperviscosity syndrome or who have been exposed to cocaine in utero.

In adults, infarction of the gastrointestinal tract without vascular occlusion is seen mainly in the elderly with severe low-output cardiac failure but it has been described in women in middle-life without obvious risk factors. In tropical and subtropical areas the condition is more common and may be related to environmental factors including diet, infection, and infestation.

Non-occlusive focal ischaemia appears to underlie the pathogenesis of uraemic colitis, radiation enteritis, potassium-induced ulcers, and multiple stress ulcers of the upper gastrointestinal tract. The verotoxin of *Escherichia coli* 0157:H7, which causes haemorrhagic colitis, is another aetiological agent. This is a particularly potent cause of disseminated intravascular coagulation, which may occur as a result of the absorption of bacterial endotoxin and thromboplastins from damaged tissues. It is associated with the development of the haemolytic–uraemic syndrome in children and more rarely with thrombotic thrombocytopenic purpura in adults (Table 2).

Intestinal ischaemia: the clinical syndromes

The clinical effects of mesenteric vascular insufficiency will be considered under four headings: acute mesenteric ischaemia, chronic mesenteric ischaemia, ischaemic colitis, and ischaemia-reperfusion injury. Focal ischaemia of the intestine will be considered in the section on collagen disorders.

Acute mesenteric ischaemia

Clinical features

Necrosis, incipient or complete, of that part of the gut supplied by the superior mesenteric artery is life-threatening. The onset is usually abrupt. Abdominal pain is the key symptom and at the onset it is usually colicky in nature. As the condition progresses the pain becomes constant and unremitting. Initially it is felt in the right iliac fossa and then spreads over the entire abdomen. Diarrhoea is usual and the motions may contain blood. Vomiting occurs in some cases but haematemesis is rare. There may be slight tenderness in the right iliac fossa and some exaggeration of bowel sounds. Over the course of hours (or at the most a day or two) the abdomen becomes distended and silent with increasing tenderness and a positive rebound sign. At this stage there are usually signs of peripheral circulatory failure. The patient is pale, anxious, sweating, and tachypnoeic. Later the blood pressure falls and the patient becomes cyanosed and anuric; by now damage to the intestine is irrecoverable.

Diagnosis is often delayed because there are no clinical signs apart from overwhelming patient distress which itself indicates the need for urgent specialist attention. Duplex Doppler ultrasonography and contrast-enhanced magnetic resonance imaging are probably the best means of confirmation but are rarely available. For practical purposes, the diagnosis still depends on the efficiency with which other causes of an apparent abdominal catastrophe can be excluded. Plain radiographs of the abdomen may show non-specific dilatation of loops of intestine with multiple fluid levels. The presence of gas bubbles in the portal vein is diagnostic of intestinal necrosis at a stage when the patient is beyond recovery. Needle aspiration of the peritoneal cavity may be a helpful procedure because intestinal infarction usually produces blood-stained fluid.

Management

Early laparotomy is essential. First the clinician has to combat the effects of loss of water, electrolytes, and protein leading to hypovolaemia and impaired tissue perfusion, bacterial invasion, and disseminated intravascular coagulation. The value of pharmacological agents (such as phenoxybenzamine, glucagon, or dopamine) for improving the mesenteric circulation remains uncertain.

As soon as the patient is sufficiently fit, the abdomen must be opened. If a large vessel is occluded, the surgeon may be able to undertake embolectomy or reconstruct an occluded artery. In both occlusive and non-occlusive vascular disease it is necessary to decide how much intestine to resect. If there is doubt about the viability of the residual intestine the abdomen should be closed and re-explored 24 h later. Infiltrating the coeliac and mesenteric plexuses with local anaesthetic may help relieve vascular spasm and should be used if there is no evidence of vascular occlusion. Treatment with anticoagulants may also be indicated.

Chronic intestinal ischaemia

Chronic intestinal ischaemia is usually due to atheroma. The coeliac axis and superior mesenteric artery are commonly affected and the inferior mesenteric artery to a much lesser extent. Stenotic lesions occur at the aortic origins of the vessels. Diffuse, severe atheroma throughout the intestinal arterial tree is uncommon and therefore arterial reconstruction may be very rewarding.

Clinical features

Patients with chronic ischaemia of the gut suffer poorly localized severe cramping abdominal pain. This occurs every day and is usually worse 20 to 60 min after eating. The pain may be relieved by simple analgesics or by vasodilator drugs. As the condition progresses the patient becomes afraid to eat and loses weight. There are no diagnostic physical signs and in particular it is not helpful to find a vascular bruit. Thus clinicians must request vascular imaging whenever there is reasonable suspicion and other tests (including computed tomographic scanning of the abdomen) have failed to give a diagnosis.

Magnetic resonance imaging is best able to provide functional information about the degree of arterial stenosis and quantitative information about blood flow and blood oxygenation. Unfortunately only a few specialized centres are likely to develop sufficient experience with this sophisticated technique.

Compression of the coeliac-axis

In occasional patients with chronic abdominal pain and an abdominal bruit (which may be exacerbated by inspiration), aortography shows apparent constriction of the coeliac axis by the median arcuate ligament. It has been claimed that the arteries in the territory of the coeliac axis 'steal' blood from that of the superior mesenteric artery, thereby causing an intestinal angina that may be relieved by dividing the median arcuate ligament and possibly by reconstructing the coeliac axis. The validity of this syndrome is uncertain.

Ischaemic colitis

The colon is more prone to ischaemic damage than the small intestine. The transverse and descending segments of the colon are supplied by marginal branches of the middle colic (superior mesenteric territory) and left colic (inferior mesenteric territory) arteries. An arterial and lymphatic watershed exists close to the splenic flexure, which is supported to a variable extent by an additional vascular arcade. This segment of the colon is at risk when the mesenteric circulation is compromised. In addition, distension of the colon may impair blood flow. Thus ischaemic colitis may occur in the segment of intestine immediately proximal to an obstructing lesion (stercoral ulceration) or with colonic pseudo-obstruction. Venous occlusion may also cause ischaemic colitis.

Clinical features

In the acute phase of ischaemic colitis the clinician has to differentiate between mild injury, which responds quickly and effectively to supportive measures and treatment with appropriate antibiotics, and severe injury, in which gangrene may develop. Typically the affected person complains of pain in the left iliac fossa, nausea, and vomiting followed by the passage of a loose motion containing dark blood.

Marked tenderness in the left iliac fossa is the most constant physical sign. At colonoscopy the mucosa may be blue and swollen without contact bleeding. The rectum is invariably spared. Plain radiographs of the abdomen may show an abnormal segment of large intestine outlined with gas.

Contrast enema examination of the colon is a most useful way of demonstrating ischaemic damage. In the early phase 'thumb printing' is the characteristic sign. This may persist for several days (Fig. 1). Subsequently the mucosal appearance may return to normal or progress to mucosal ulceration, giving an appearance that may be indistinguishable from segmental ulcerative colitis or Crohn's disease. These changes may resolve spontaneously or progress to tubular narrowing of the intestine with or without sacculation on the antimesenteric border.

Ischaemic colitis may be confused with dysenteric conditions, acute diverticular disease of the colon, acute inflammatory bowel disease, perforation of a hollow viscus, or left-sided peritonitis caused by pancreatitis. The most important distinguishing features are the association with degenerative cardiovascular disease and the distinctive, although not pathognomonic, radiographic and colonoscopic appearances.

Management

On establishing the diagnosis of ischaemic colitis the treatment is initially expectant. The patient should be given intravenous fluid as necessary, together with systemic broad-spectrum antibiotics. Well over 90 per cent of recognized cases resolve spontaneously. A stricture may develop in up to a third of patients but this is usually asymptomatic and only rarely needs to be resected. Surgery is indicated if there is evidence of peritonitis, persistent bleeding, or of an underlying colonic disorder (such as carcinoma).

Intestinal reperfusion injury

The gut mucosa may be transiently but seriously damaged after a period of ischaemia which is followed by apparently adequate reperfusion. The damage appears to be caused by the generation of reactive oxygen metabolites (including superoxide, hydrogen peroxide, and hydroxyl radicals). These alter the vascular permeability of endothelial cells and damage epithelial cells by peroxidation of cell membranes. The injured tissues are strongly

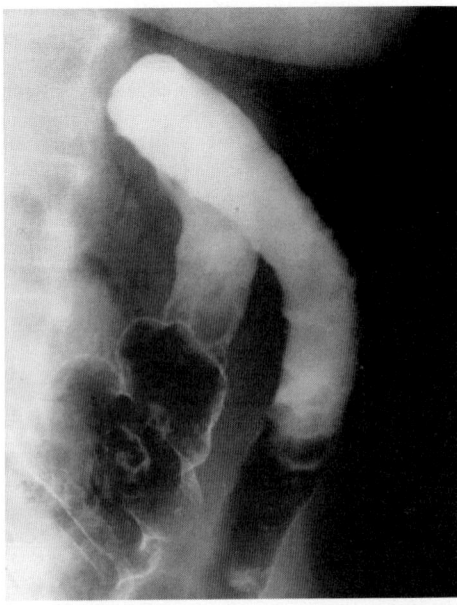

Fig. 1 Ischaemic colitis: barium enema showing thumb printing at the splenic flexure. (By courtesy of Dr A. Freeman, Addenbrooke's Hospital.)

chemotactic for neutrophils and this leads to an acute inflammatory response. Such damage diminishes the barrier function of the gut, increasing intestinal permeability and allowing the translocation of bacteria. Injury of the intestinal mucosa is now recognized as an important factor in the prognosis of critically ill patients in intensive care. Serial measurements of serum intestinal fatty acid protein (iFABP) have been shown to provide a sensitive marker of damage to intestinal mucosa.

Vasculitis and the collagen disorders: effects on the gut

The gut may be involved in any of the systemic collagen–vascular disorders. Vasculitis may cause focal ischaemic damage of the intestine (Table 2) but this is a feature of many conditions other than the collagen disorders, for example drug-induced ulceration (for example by potassium salts), the after-effects of blunt trauma to the abdomen, irradiation, and rarely infective disease (for example typhoid or leprosy) (Table 3).

In the collagen disorders the visceral muscle may be damaged and the resulting dysmotility may cause dysphagia, delayed gastric emptying, small intestinal stasis with bacterial overgrowth, or colonic inertia. Gas may infiltrate the tissues, giving rise to pneumatosis intestinalis.

The specific pathological diagnosis is usually based on the systemic features of the illness and the laboratory findings rather than on the mostly non-specific abdominal complications. But the inquisitive physician may also recognize curious associations in patients with multisystem disorders. Thus, intestinal malabsorption and protein-losing enteropathy have been described in association with systemic lupus erythematosus and rheumatoid arthritis, pancreatic insufficiency with systemic sclerosis, acute pancreatitis during the course of Behçet's disease, and apparently classical inflammatory bowel disease with systemic lupus erythematosus.

Systemic sclerosis

In primary systemic sclerosis (see Chapter 18.11.3), fibrous connective tissue proliferates. In the gastrointestinal tract it may replace smooth muscle, especially in the oesophagus (which is involved in 80 per cent of cases), to a lesser extent in the small intestine (although duodenal involvement is quite common), and rather rarely in the colon.

Overt vasculitis is a less common feature but occasionally causes intestinal infarction. Pneumatosis cystoides intestinalis is also described, especially in association with intestinal pseudo-obstruction or a pneumoperitoneum.

Clinical features

In systemic sclerosis progressive dysphagia is the most frequent gastrointestinal symptom. Initially there is a decrease in the incidence and amplitude of contractions of the lower oesophagus and incomplete relaxation of the lower oesophageal sphincter. In addition, the resting tone of the sphincter is reduced, allowing reflux of gastric juices, oesophagitis, shortening of the oesophagus, and occasionally stricture formation. Associated hiatal herniation is common.

More rarely the stomach is involved, causing delayed emptying that on occasion is exacerbated by associated stenosis of the pyloric canal. Changes lower down the gastrointestinal tract also occur. Characteristically the duodenum is dilated, the valvulae of the small intestine are thickened, and pseudodiverticula may form. These changes are associated with abdominal discomfort, distension, and borborygmi, especially after the taking of meals. The impaired motility of the small intestine leads to stasis of its contents and bacterial overgrowth causing malabsorption, especially of fat and vitamin B_{12} (see Chapter 14.9.2) (Fig. 2). Progressive constipation due to impaired colonic motility is uncommon.

Management

There is no specific treatment of primary systemic sclerosis. Lesions in the gastrointestinal tract need management on their merits. It is important to recognize early the patient with gastro-oesophageal reflux. A proton pump inhibitor should be given to prevent the ravages of acid-peptic digestion of the oesophageal mucosa. When strictures occur these should be dilated by bouginage. Surgical intervention is occasionally necessary.

A breath test (see Chapters 14.2.3 and 14.9.2) is a useful screening test for delayed passage of contents and bacterial proliferation in the small intestine. Patients with a positive breath test should be assessed for evidence of malabsorption, and if this is found intermittent therapy with antibiotics for an indefinite period may be of clinical value.

Systemic lupus erythematosus

Systemic lupus erythematosus (see Chapter 18.11.2) may cause abdominal symptoms arising from any part of the gastrointestinal tract. Anorexia, weight loss, nausea, vomiting, and diarrhoea are relatively common. Dysphagia, abdominal pain, distension due to ascites, and gastrointestinal bleeding are less frequent symptoms. Occasionally a patient with systemic lupus erythematosus develops an acute abdomen, which may be due to localized or widespread lupus vasculitis causing ischaemic damage to the gut or its related organs, including the gallbladder and pancreas. Arteriography may be helpful in diagnosis by revealing diffuse irregularities in the branches of mesenteric vessels.

Treatment with oral corticosteroids usually relieves minor abdominal symptoms and will lead to rapid resolution of simple ascites. In the acute stage of the disease, however, surgery may be necessary to deal with infarcted intestine, serious bleeding, or intestinal obstruction.

Other systemic disorders

In rheumatoid arthritis, vasculitis is associated with long-standing disease, seropositivity, and florid subcutaneous nodule formation (see Section 18.11). Occasionally, a severe diffuse and necrotizing angiitis causes infarction in the gallbladder, pancreas, or intestine. Symptoms vary from vague abdominal pain, with or without diarrhoea, to the development of an acute abdomen.

Dermatomyositis rarely causes damage to the viscera although thrombosis of small vessels occasionally causes gastrointestinal ulceration.

In Behçet's syndrome the triad of relapsing iritis, painful ulcers of the mouth, and genital ulceration is only part of the syndrome (see Chapter 18.11.5). Again, vasculitis appears to be the underlying histopathological lesion. In the gastrointestinal tract this may lead to ulceration of the colon, malabsorption (sometimes with lymphangiectasia), and pancreatitis.

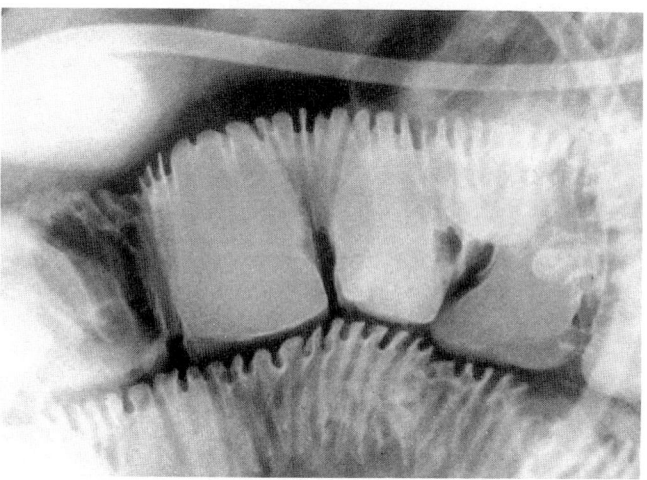

Fig. 2 Systemic sclerosis. Typical 'sacculation' appearance of the bowel.

Primary vasculitis

Henoch–Schönlein purpura (anaphylactic purpura)

This is a self-limiting disorder of unknown cause characterized by small-vessel vasculitis (see Section 18.11). Gastrointestinal disease occurs in at least two-thirds of cases and is manifest as abdominal pain and gastrointestinal bleeding. Intramural haematomas are common and rarely may be complicated by intussusception, perforation, or an infarcted segment of gut.

Polyarteritis nodosa

Abdominal pain and other gastrointestinal symptoms are common in patients with polyarteritis nodosa. The underlying cause is usually recognized by evidence of systemic disease such as skin lesions, renal involvement, hypertension, and eosinophilia. Mesenteric angiography is useful as a diagnostic tool because up to two-thirds of cases have recognizable aneurysms of mesenteric and renal vessels. A small proportion of patients with polyarteritis have acute abdominal episodes including ulceration, haemorrhage, perforation and segmental necrosis of intestine, cholecystitis, pancreatitis, and hepatic infarction. Kawasaki disease (infantile acute febrile mucocutaneous lymph node syndrome) (see Chapter 18.11.8) proceeds to a disorder indistinguishable histopathologically from infantile periarteritis nodosa. Cardiac involvement is most common, but the gastrointestinal tract is affected in up to a third of cases.

Antineutrophilic cytoplasmic antibody-positive vasculitides

Wegener's granulomatosis, Churg–Strauss syndrome, and microscopic polyarteritis are conditions frequently associated with the finding of antineutrophilic cytoplasmic antibodies. Gastrointestinal symptoms are common in these conditions, although the intra-abdominal pathology has not been well characterized except when angiitis has led to a life-threatening condition such as visceral perforation or infarction.

Giant cell arteritis

This characteristically affects the larger cranial arteries including the ciliary and central retinal arteries (see Chapter 18.11.4) and rarely limb arteries. Very occasionally a similar pathology affects mesenteric arteries and causes bowel infarction.

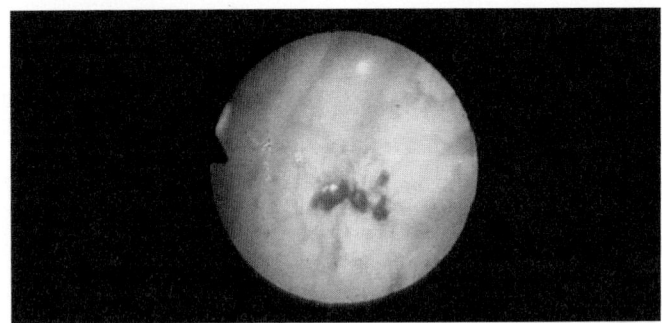

Fig. 3 Angiodysplastic lesion in the caecum, photographed through a colonoscope. (By courtesy of Dr R. Hunt, RN Hospital, Haslar.)

Localized arteritis

Arteritis has been described causing pathology solely in the appendix, the gallbladder, and the pancreas. The relationship of a localized arteritis to systemic polyarteritis is uncertain. Similarly, localized leucocytoclastic (hypersensitivity) vasculitis has been described in the abdominal cavities.

Other vascular disorders that may affect the gut

Aneurysms of the aorta and its major branches

Rarely, aneurysms fistulate into the stomach or duodenum. This usually causes catastrophic bleeding and rapid death. Even more rarely there is intermittent bleeding (for example from the splenic artery into the stomach), which may be difficult to diagnose.

Superior mesenteric artery syndrome

A syndrome of postprandial epigastric pain, distension, and vomiting may occur in asthenic young people, especially those who have lost weight or who are fixed in a position of hyperextension after spinal injury. Barium studies show a distended proximal duodenum with a sharp cut-off at the line where the superior mesenteric artery crosses the duodenum. Symptoms may be relieved if the patient adopts the prone position after meals

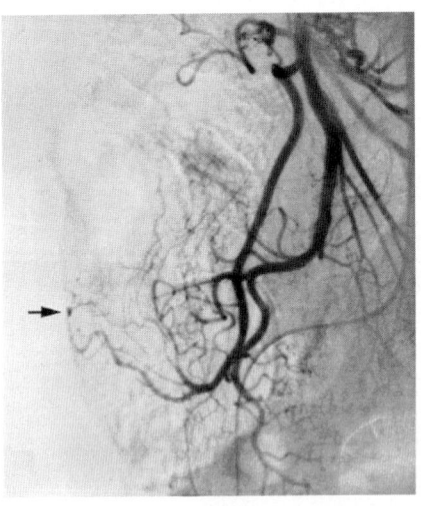

(a)

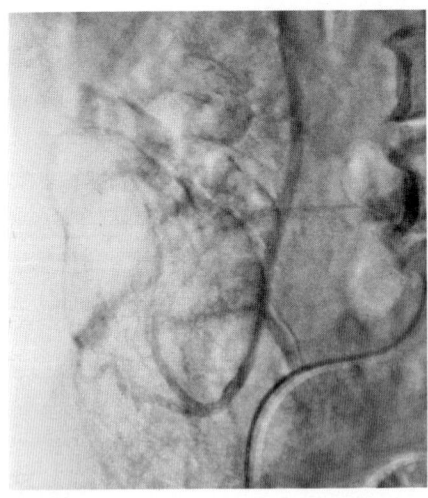

(b)

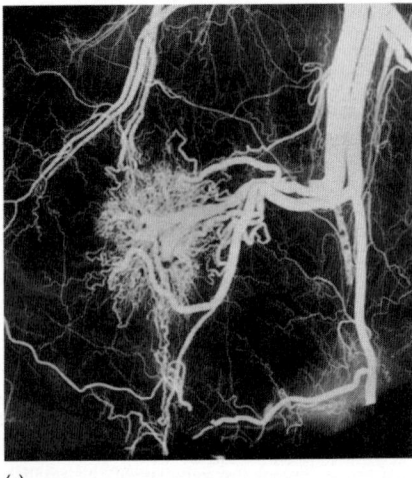

(c)

Fig. 4 (a) Angiodysplastic lesion in the caecum: superior mesenteric angiogram in a 53-year-old man with anaemia for 20 years (no lesion found at previous operations). Vascular lake in caecum (arrowed). (b) Angiodysplastic lesion in the caecum: superior mesenteric angiogram in a 53-year-old man with anaemia for 20 years (no lesion found at previous operations). Capillary phase, showing early filling vein arising from lesion. (c) Angiodysplastic lesion in the caecum: superior mesenteric angiogram in a 53-year-old man with anaemia for 20 years (no lesion found at previous operations). Injected specimen magnified ×30. (By courtesy of Dr D. J. Allison, Royal Postgraduate Medical School and previously published in *British Journal of Hospital Medicine*, 1980; **23**: 358.)

and usually disappear as the patient gains weight. Surgery is occasionally necessary. The condition must be distinguished from duodenal ileus caused by mesenteric bands, a condition that is associated with partial malrotation of the midgut.

Haemangioma

Haemangiomas are uncommon but they may cause painless bleeding especially in the jejunum.

Intestinal telangiectasia

These lesions occur most commonly with Osler–Weber–Rendu disease (see Section 22.04.04) and may lead to microscopic bleeding with anaemia, especially in adult life.

Vascular dysplasia

This is a more recently recognized and not uncommon disorder causing occult bleeding from the gut in older subjects. The lesions occur as small arteriovenous malformations or as foci of ectatic capillaries or veins with little supporting stroma. They are found predominantly in the caecum and ascending colon. There may be an association with aortic stenosis but none with cutaneous telangiectases and no familial aggregations have yet been described.

Patients give a history of recurrent anaemia or episodes of bleeding from the gut, have usually been investigated repeatedly without getting a firm diagnosis, and sometimes have had one or more operations (including resection of a segment of the gastrointestinal tract) without relief of symptoms. The diagnosis of vascular dysplasia should be considered in all cases of obscure gastrointestinal haemorrhage and may be made by direct visualization of the intestinal mucosa (Fig. 3) or by selective mesenteric arteriography (Fig. 4). The lesions may be multiple, in which case resection of the affected segment of gut may be necessary. Many patients, however, can be treated successfully by fulguration of the lesion through an endoscope. If the lesion(s) cannot be obliterated, in women a trial of treatment with an oestrogen–progesterone preparation is often effective.

Intramural bleeding

Bleeding into the wall of the bowel may occur as a result of treatment with anticoagulants or from the inflammation of small vessels (as occurs classically in Henoch–Schönlein purpura). The usual presentation is with colicky abdominal pain, with bleeding into the lumen of the gut. Appropriate barium examination may show the classical sign of 'thumb printing'. The condition usually resolves spontaneously providing that the underlying disorder can be treated. A blood transfusion may be needed.

Further reading

Bryant DS, Pellicane JV, Davies RS (1997). Non-occlusive intestinal ischemia: improved outcome with early diagnosis and therapy. *American Surgeon* **63**, 334–9. Good article on diagnosis and management of a poorly recognized condition.

Cappell MS (1998). Intestinal (mesenteric) vasculopathy (Parts I and II). *Gastro-enterological Clinics of North America* **27**, 783–860. Comprehensive review of the mesenteric vasculopathies.

Heiss SG, Li KC (1998) Magnetic resonance angiography of mesenteric arteries. A review. *Investigative Radiology* **33**, 670–81. Important non-invasive method of assessing mesenteric vessels and their blood flow.

Hunder GG, ed (1992). Vasculitic syndromes. *Current Opinion in Rheumatology* **44**, 1–55. Good review of vasculitic syndromes.

Jamieson CW (1986). Coeliac axis compression syndrome. *British Medical Journal* **293**, 159. Classical description of coeliac compression syndrome.

Lie JT (1997). Mesenteric inflammatory veno-occlusive disease (MIVOD): an emerging and unsuspected cause of digestive tract ischemia. *Vasa* **26**, 91–6. An newly described condition.

Marston A (1986). *Vascular disease of the gut.* Arnold, London. Classical book on vascular disease of the gut.

Pastores SM, Katz DP, Kvetan V (1996). Splanchnic ischemia and gut mucosal injury in sepsis and the multi-organ dysfunction syndrome. *American Journal of Gastroenterology* **91**, 1697–710. Description of the ischaemia-reperfusion syndrome.

14.17 Gastrointestinal infections

Davidson H. Hamer and Sherwood L. Gorbach

Introduction

Diarrhoea, the most common manifestation of intestinal tract infections, is a leading cause of death in most developing countries where its greatest impact is seen in infants and children. Infectious diarrhoea may be accompanied by numerous complications (Table 1). The financial burden associated with medical care and lost productivity due to infectious diarrhoea amounts to more than 20 billion dollars a year in the United States alone.

The aetiology and severity of gastrointestinal infections are determined by several epidemiological factors. Young children and the elderly are at greatest risk for more severe disease and complications. The presence of underlying medical conditions, especially those that compromise immunity, greatly enhances the risk of acquiring an infection and its ultimate severity. Poor sanitation, inadequate water supplies, and increasing globalization of food transport systems all predispose to the development of large epidemics of food- and water-borne outbreaks of gastrointestinal disease. Seasonal or cyclic weather variations also influence the epidemiology of diarrhoeal disease and food poisoning.

A wide array of bacterial, protozoal, and viral pathogens is responsible for gastrointestinal tract infections. The characteristics of specific organisms are described in detail in Section 7 of this book: here are presented the pathophysiology, common clinical syndromes, diagnosis, management, and prevention of gastrointestinal diseases.

Table 1 Complications of gastrointestinal infections

Complication	Causative pathogens
Dehydration	*Vibrio cholerae*, *Cryptosporidium parvum* (especially in immunocompromised hosts), enterotoxigenic *Escherichia coli* (ETEC), rotavirus
Severe vomiting	Staphylococcal food poisoning, Norwalk virus, rotavirus
Haemorrhagic colitis	*Campylobacter jejuni*, enterohaemorrhagic *E. coli* (EHEC), *Salmonella* and *Shigella* spp., *V. parahaemolyticus*
Toxic megacolon, intestinal perforation	EHEC, *Shigella* spp., *C. jejuni* (rare), *Clostridium difficile* (rare), *Salmonella* spp. (rare), *Yersinia* spp. (rare)
Haemolytic–uraemic syndrome (HUS), thrombotic thrombocytopenic purpura (TTP)	EHEC, *Shigella* spp., *C. jejuni* (rare)
Reactive arthritis	*C. jejuni*, *Shigella*, *Salmonella*, *Yersinia* spp.
Malabsorption/malnutrition	*Cyclospora cayetanensis*, *Giardia lamblia*, *C. parvum* (especially immunocompromised hosts)
Distant metastatic infection	*Salmonella*, *C. jejuni* (rare), *Yersinia* (rare)
Guillain-Barré syndrome	*C. jejuni* (rare)

Pathophysiology

Host factors

Normal intestinal flora

The proximal small bowel, including the stomach, duodenum, jejunum, and upper ileum, has a relatively sparse microflora, with most organisms being derived from the oropharynx. Colonization of the upper intestine by Gram-negative bacilli is an abnormal event, one that is characteristic of illness due to pathogens such as *Vibrio cholerae* and *Escherichia coli*. The large bowel has an abundant microflora, with total concentrations of 10^{11} bacteria per gram of content. Anaerobes including *Bacteroides* spp., *Clostridium* spp., and anaerobic streptococci outnumber aerobic bacteria, such as coliforms, by 1000-fold. During an episode of acute diarrhoea, regardless of the aetiology, the colonic flora becomes less anaerobic because of the rapid transit of intestinal contents. As a consequence, strictly anaerobic bacteria decrease in number while there is an increase in coliforms, which are often aberrant types such as *Enterobacter*, *Klebsiella*, and *Proteus* spp. The pathogen itself assumes a dominant position in the flora, so that the major faecal isolate may be *Salmonella* spp. or *V. cholerae*.

In addition to the longitudinal distribution of bacteria in the gastrointestinal tract, the bowel microflora is found both within the lumen and adherent to the mucous layer overlying epithelial cells. Invasive pathogens such as *Campylobacter*, *Shigella*, *Salmonella*, and *Yersinia* spp. can penetrate the mucosal surface and infect epithelial cells, or translocate into the mesenteric lymph nodes and bloodstream.

Control mechanisms

At the portal of entry, gastric acid suppresses most organisms that are ingested. In the setting of reduced or absent gastric acid, there is a higher incidence of bacterial colonization of the upper small intestine. Consequently, persons with hypochlorhydria, achlorhydria, or those using drugs such as proton-pump inhibitors that inhibit gastric acid secretion are susceptible to diarrhoeal diseases. A critical element in maintaining the sparse flora of the upper bowel is propulsive motility. The antibacterial properties of biliary fluid may control the intestinal flora. The glycocalyx and intestinal mucins secreted by epithelial cells provide a mechanical barrier to invasion by gut pathogens. Finally, antibacterial substances produced by the normal intestinal microflora help to maintain the stability of normal populations of organisms and to prevent the implantation of pathogens.

Intestinal immunity (see Chapter 14.4)

The intestinal immune system plays a major role in the host's response to enteric pathogens. The human gut contains a large amount of lymphoid tissue in the form of intraepithelial lymphocytes, lamina propria lymphoid cells, and Peyer's patches. The latter are lymphoid aggregates in the mucosa and submucosa of the distal small intestine which serve as sites for the presentation of antigens to B and T lymphocytes. After activation by antigens, bacteria, or viruses in the Peyer's patches, the lymphocytes migrate to the lamina propria and the intraepithelial portion of the intestinal lining where, along with macrophages and other types of white blood cells, they protect the host from specific pathogens. Plasma cells in the lamina propria produce secretory immunoglobulin A, which is released into the intestinal lumen. When the mechanical barrier of the gut fails, then the intraepithelial and lamina propria lymphocytes provide the next level of protection against pathogenic enteric organisms.

Microbial factors

The number of organisms that need to be ingested to establish a gastrointestinal tract infection varies from as few as 10 to 100 in the case of *Shigella* spp. to as many as 10^8 for *V. cholerae*. In the presence of reduced gastric acidity or underlying immunosuppression, the inoculum needed to establish infection is reduced.

Enteric pathogens can cause intestinal disease by means of enterotoxins, adherence to gut mucosa, or invasion of enterocytes.

Toxins

Bacterial enteric pathogens can elaborate enterotoxins that act directly on intestinal epithelial cells (for example, cholera toxin) or preformed toxins that are ingested in contaminated food (for example, *Bacillus cereus* toxin). While invasive bacteria penetrate the mucosal surface of the gut as the primary event, they may also secrete enterotoxins. Production of enterotoxin can be demonstrated in the laboratory by *in vivo* tests—such as the rabbit ileal loop model and the suckling mouse model, or by *in vitro* tests involving a tissue culture line, such as Y-1 adrenal cells or Chinese hamster ovary cells.

Many organisms elaborate enterotoxins that cause fluid and electrolyte secretion in the gut. Diarrhoeal toxins can be grouped into two categories: cytotonic, which produce fluid secretion by activation of intracellular enzymes such as adenylate cyclase, without causing any damage to the epithelial surface; and cytotoxic, which cause injury to the mucosal cell while also inducing fluid secretion, but not primarily by activation of cyclic nucleotides. *V. cholerae* and enterotoxigenic *Escherichia coli* (**ETEC**) are examples of pathogens that cause dehydrating diarrhoea by producing enterotoxins of the cytotonic type (see Chapter 7.11.7).

Intestinal fluid loss is the primary manifestation of cholera—this results from the action of enterotoxin on the small bowel epithelial cells. These organisms colonize the small intestine, adhering to epithelial cells and then elaborating enterotoxin. There is no invasion of the mucosal surface so there is no evidence of damage to the mucosal architecture and bacteraemia is not a complication. The faecal effluent is watery, often voluminous, and produces the clinical features of dehydration. The most sensitive areas are the upper bowel, particularly the duodenum and upper jejunum; the ileum is less affected, and the colon is usually in a state of absorption since it is relatively insensitive to the toxin. This is a form of 'overflow' diarrhoea, with a large volume of fluid produced in the upper intestine that overwhelms the capacity of the lower bowel to absorb.

ETEC produces two types of enterotoxins: a heat-labile (**LT**) and a heat-stable toxin (**ST**). LT is a protein that is destroyed by heat and acid; like cholera toxin, it activates adenylate cyclase, causing secretion of fluid and electrolytes into the lumen. In contrast, ST can withstand heating to 100 °C and acts by activating guanylate cyclase. Despite the differences between the two toxins, the ultimate effect of both enterotoxins is a non-inflammatory secretory diarrhoea.

Invasion

Whereas toxigenic organisms usually involve the upper intestine, invasive pathogens target the lower intestine, particularly the distal ileum and colon. Histological findings include evidence of mucosal ulceration with acute inflammation in the lamina propria. Principal pathogens in this group are *Salmonella* spp., *Shigella* spp., enterohaemorrhagic *E. coli* (**EHEC**), enteroinvasive *E. coli* (**EIEC**), *Campylobacter spp.*, and *Yersinia* spp. Although there are important differences among these organisms, they all have in common the property of mucosal invasion as the initiating event. To date, three theories have been invoked to explain the mechanism of fluid production in invasive diarrhoea. First, fluid production may result from an enterotoxin, at least in the initial phase of the illness. Most *Shigella* strains elaborate an enterotoxin that differs substantially from cholera toxin, but which does result in fluid and electrolyte secretion by the intestine. A similar toxin has been proposed for *Salmonella spp.*, and there is suggestive evidence that *Campylobacter* and *Yersinia* spp. elaborate enterotoxins. Second, invasive organisms lead to an increased local synthesis of prostaglandins at the site of the intense inflammatory reaction that may be responsible for fluid secretion and diarrhoea. Third, damage to the epithelial surface may prevent reabsorption of fluids from the lumen and thereby result in a net accumulation of fluid in the bowel lumen, resulting in diarrhoea.

A series of pathogenic factors, each controlled by plasmids or chromosomal loci, are used by pathogenic strains of *Salmonella*. Specific plasmids encode for bacterial spread from Peyer's patches to other sites in the body, for the ability of certain strains to survive within macrophages following phagocytosis, and for the ability of salmonellae to elicit transepithelial signalling to neutrophils (see Chapter 7.11.7). Invasion by *Shigella* spp. is also associated with diverse virulence factors related to various stages of invasion. The end result is the death of the intestinal epithelial cell, focal ulcers, and inflammation of the lamina propia. The shigella virulence factors are encoded by chromosomal and plasmid genes, all of which are needed for the full expression of virulence. Various genetic loci encode for an invasion plasmid antigen (*ipa*), which seems to determine recognition of the epithelial cell, *inv* invasion factors, and a series of *vir* loci that are involved in regulation within the infected cell. After penetrating the mucosal surface of the gut, *Shigella* spp. multiply within epithelial cells and extend the infected area by direct cell-to-cell migration of bacilli. *Shigella* species rarely penetrate beyond the intestinal mucosa and therefore do not usually invade the bloodstream.

Adherence

Specific fimbriae or adhesins mediate the attachment of pathogenic bacteria to gut mucosal cells. For example, the attachment of *V. cholerae* is mediated by a fimbrial colonization factor, known as the toxin-coregulated pilus. Some enteric pathogens such as enteropathogenic *E. coli* (**EPEC**) attach to the intestinal mucosa in a characteristic manner, producing ultrastructural changes known as attachment-effacement lesions; this leads to the elongation and destruction of microvilli. Protozoal parasites such as *Giardia lamblia* use a ventral adhesive disc to attach to the mucosal surface of the small intestine. Thus, enteropathogens have devised a number of different ways to adhere to the surface of the gut.

Clinical syndromes of gastrointestinal infections

Gastrointestinal infections usually result in three principal syndromes: non-inflammatory diarrhoea, inflammatory diarrhoea, and systemic disease. Non-inflammatory diarrhoea primarily involves the small intestine, whereas inflammatory diarrhoea predominantly affects the colon. The location of infection influences the clinical characteristics and certain diagnostic features of the diarrhoeal disease (Table 2). Thus, the organisms that target the small intestine tend to produce watery, potentially dehydrating diarrhoea, while those infecting the large intestine cause bloody mucoid diarrhoea associated with tenesmus.

Non-inflammatory diarrhoea
Bacteria

Cholera, the prototypic non-inflammatory diarrhoea, can cause dehydration and death within 3 to 4 h of onset. Like many other infectious diseases,

Table 2 Clinical features of diarrhoeal diseases

Feature	Site of infection	
	Small intestine	Large intestine
Pathogens	*Escherichia coli* (EPEC, ETEC)	*E. coli* (EIEC, EHEC)
	Cryptosporidium parvum	*Entamoeba histolytica*
	Giardia lamblia	*Shigella* spp.
	Norwalk virus	
	Rotavirus	
	Vibrio cholerae	
Location of pain	Mid-abdomen	Lower abdomen, rectum
Volume of stool	Large	Small
Blood in stool	Rare	Common
Faecal leucocytes	Rare	Common (except in amoebiasis)
Sigmoidoscopy	Normal	Mucosal ulcers, haemorrhagic foci, friable mucosa

there is a spectrum of clinical manifestations—from an asymptomatic carrier state to severe dehydration with shock. Initial symptoms of vomiting and abdominal distention are rapidly followed by diarrhoea, which accelerates over the next few hours to frequent purging of large volumes of 'rice-water' stools. The acutely ill patient has marked dehydration manifested by poor skin turgor, 'washerwoman's hands', feeble to absent pulses, reduced renal function, and hypovolaemic shock.

Non-01 cholera vibrios have also been associated with severe, dehydrating diarrhoea as well as wound infections and septicaemia. *V. vulnificus* is one of the most important non-cholera vibrios, based on the severity of illness that it causes, especially in patients with underlying liver disease and especially iron-storage disease. This infection can be acquired by direct consumption of seafood, usually raw oysters, or as a wound infection in people who have direct contact with salt water. Since this infection can be lethal in susceptible people, such persons should be warned about eating raw seafood, especially oysters.

ETEC infections are one of the most common causes of diarrhoea in travellers to less developed countries and children living in these regions. The incubation period of this infection is usually between 24 and 48 h, after which the disease often begins with upper intestinal distress, followed soon thereafter by watery diarrhoea. The infection can be extremely mild, with only a few loose movements, or it can be quite severe, mimicking cholera with profuse watery diarrhoea leading to severe dehydration. Other strains of *E. coli* such as enteroaggregative, diffusely adhering, and enteropathogenic *E. coli*, may also be associated with watery diarrhoea.

Viruses (see also Chapter 7.10.8)

Numerous viruses are responsible for as many as 30 to 40 per cent of self-limited episodes of non-inflammatory diarrhoea, especially in children. Rotavirus causes a range of clinical manifestations from asymptomatic carriage to severe, potentially fatal dehydration. The disease occurs primarily in children aged between 3 and 15 months; infections continue into the second year of life, but after this age are less common. Adults can develop mild infections with group A rotaviruses, especially if there is a sick child in the household. The disease process often begins with vomiting, followed shortly thereafter by watery diarrhoea. The incubation period is between 1 and 3 days, with an average duration of illness of 5 to 7 days, although some instances of chronic diarrhoea have been described.

Caliciviruses are single-stranded RNA viruses that are responsible for human and animal infections. Recent molecular studies have shown that the Norwalk and Norwalk-like viruses have a genetic composition that places them in the taxonomic family of Caliciviridae. This family of viruses typically causes disease mainly in infants and young children, especially in day-care centres. The illness is generally mild and indistinguishable from that due to rotavirus or even epidemic Norwalk disease. The Norwalk virus

causes explosive epidemics of diarrhoea that sweep through communities with a high attack rate. It shows no respect for age, as it can affect virtually all age groups except infants. Infections caused by the Norwalk agent tend to be relatively mild and short-lived, with common symptoms including diarrhoea, nausea, abdominal pain, vomiting, and myalgias. Generally, the clinical illness lasts no longer than 24 to 48 h.

Astroviruses are responsible for outbreaks of diarrhoea in day-care centres and in communities with infants. The disease is characterized by watery or mucoid stools, nausea, vomiting, and, occasionally, fever, but it tends to be milder than rotavirus diarrhoea as there is less dehydration. Adenovirus serotypes 40 and 41 are responsible for day-care centre and nosocomial outbreaks of gastroenteritis in children under two years of age. As opposed to rotavirus or Norwalk virus, infection with enteric adenovirus has a long incubation period lasting approximately 8 to 10 days, and the illness can be prolonged for as long as 2 weeks.

Other infestations (also see Section 7)

Giardia lamblia is responsible for clinical syndromes ranging from asymptomatic cyst passage, to self-limited diarrhoea, to chronic diarrhoea with malabsorption and weight loss. After an incubation period between 1 and 2 weeks, patients experience the onset of frequent, loose to watery bowel movements associated with abdominal cramps, bloating, belching, nausea, anorexia, and flatulence.

Patients with cryptosporidiosis present with watery diarrhoea associated with abdominal pain, nausea, vomiting, low-grade fever, malaise, and anorexia. Faecal output may be voluminous and dehydrating in immunocompromised patients, particularly those with underlying human immunodeficiency virus (**HIV**) infection. Symptoms usually resolve by 5 to 10 days. Infection with *Cyclospora cayetanensis* is manifested by anorexia, intermittent diarrhoea, and nausea. Diarrhoea is usually self-limiting, but it can last for several weeks in immunocompetent patients and result in significant weight loss. *Isospora belli* also causes a self-limited illness characterized by watery, non-bloody diarrhoea, abdominal cramping, anorexia, weight loss, and, less commonly, fever. Any of the parasitic infections is more severe and longer lasting in immunocompromised patients, such as those with HIV or organ transplants.

Food poisoning

Food poisoning is most commonly caused by the consumption of food contaminated with bacteria or bacterial toxins. Food poisoning can also be due to parasites (for example, trichinosis), viruses (e.g., hepatitis A), and other toxins (e.g., mushrooms see Section 8.3). The most well-recognized causes of bacterial food poisoning are the following: *Clostridium perfringens*, *Staphylococcus aureus*, *Vibrio* spp. (including *V. cholerae* and *V. parahaemolyticus*), *Bacillus cereus*, *Salmonella* spp., *C. botulinum*, *Shigella* spp., toxigenic *E. coli* (ETEC and EHEC), and certain species of *Campylobacter*, *Yersinia*, *Listeria*, and *Aeromonas*.

An enterotoxin elaborated by type A strains of *C. perfringens* is responsible for food-borne outbreaks with high attack rates but which are of short duration. *C. perfringens* food poisoning is characterized by severe, crampy abdominal pain and watery diarrhoea, usually without vomiting, beginning 8 to 24 h after the incriminating meal. Fever, chills, headache, or other signs of infection are usually absent. Strains of *C. perfringens* type C elaborate a similar enterotoxin that has been implicated in outbreaks of enteritis necroticans secondary to the consumption of rancid meat in Europe, also known as 'pigbel' in Papua New Guinea. This is a much more severe, necrotizing disease of the small intestine and carries a high mortality rate.

Staphylococcal food poisoning presents with severe vomiting, nausea, and abdominal cramps, often followed by diarrhoea. *B. cereus* is an aerobic, spore-forming, Gram-positive rod that has been associated with two clinical types of food poisoning—a diarrhoea syndrome and a vomiting syndrome. The latter has a short incubation period of about 2 h, after which nearly all affected persons experience vomiting and abdominal cramps. In contrast, the diarrhoea syndrome has a median incubation period of 9 h;

clinical illness is characterized by diarrhoea, abdominal cramps, and vomiting. *B. cereus* is particularly associated with the ingestion of contaminated rice that has been kept for a long time in a warm or partially cooked state in take-away food outlets. Fevers are uncommon with all three of these bacterial toxin-mediated syndromes. Episodes of staphylococcal and *B. cereus* food poisoning are short-lived, usually resolving within 24 h. Often the staphylococcus has been introduced by contamination from a small abscess, whitlow, or other discharging lesion present during preparation of food, which is allowed to remain warm and not fully cooked before serving.

Travellers' diarrhoea

People who travel from industrialized countries to less developed areas of the world are at risk of contracting traveller's diarrhoea, with as many as 25 to 50 per cent or more suffering from one or more episodes of diarrhoea. The greatest frequency of diarrhoea occurs in students or low-budget tourists. Business travellers are at intermediate risk, while travellers who are visiting relatives have the lowest risk. Young travellers—particularly those 20 to 29 years old—have the highest risk, whereas the lowest rates of travellers' diarrhoea are noted in those over 55 years of age. The disease does not begin immediately but generally starts 2 to 3 days after the traveller's arrival. While most people have three to five watery, loose stools daily, about 20 per cent can have as many as 6 to 15. A minority of patients, approximately 2 to 10 per cent, has fever, bloody stools, or both—these people are more likely to have shigellosis. Diarrhoea is frequently associated with gas, cramps, fatigue, nausea, abdominal pain, fever, and anorexia. The illness usually resolves without specific therapy within 3 to 5 days, although a few unfortunate travellers will have persistent diarrhoea.

Infectious micro-organisms in contaminated food and drink are the main source of travellers' diarrhoea. Especially risky foods include uncooked vegetables, meat, and seafood. Tap water, ice, unpasteurized milk and dairy products, salads, and unpeeled fruits are also associated with an increased risk. Although an array of pathogens has been found, the leading culprits are various forms of *E. coli*, particularly ETEC. *C. jejuni* is encountered in a significant proportion of cases, particularly during cooler seasons. Viruses, *Shigella*, *Salmonella*, *Giardia*, *Cryptosporidium*, and *Cyclospora* spp. are responsible for a minority of travellers' diarrhoea cases.

Prudent selection of beverages and foods can help reduce the risk of developing travellers' diarrhoea. Bottled carbonated beverages, hot coffee or tea, beer, and boiled water are generally safe choices for fluids. Avoiding salads, unpeeled fruit, ice, and undercooked or raw meat, poultry, and seafood can help lower the risk. Because the venue of food consumption determines the risk of contracting travellers' diarrhoea, travellers should be advised to avoid eating food from street vendors. While studies have shown high protection rates when prophylactic antimicrobial agents such as ciprofloxacin or cotrimoxazole are taken, this approach is generally not advised because of the risk of side-effects and emergence of antibiotic-resistant enteric flora.

Chronic non-inflammatory diarrhoea

Certain pathogens cause chronic diarrhoea of small intestinal origin. Some patients with giardiasis develop chronic diarrhoea associated with fatigue, steatorrhoea, weight loss, and intermittent constipation, along with malabsorption of fat, vitamins A and B$_{12}$, protein, and D-xylose. Acquired lactose intolerance is common, but a lactose-free diet should be recommended in such cases. Cryptosporidiosis can become a chronic, dehydrating diarrhoea in immunocompromised patients, especially in those with the acquired immunodeficiency syndrome (**AIDS**). Complications of chronic cryptosporidiosis include malabsorption, wasting, and biliary tract disease. Patients with AIDS are also at risk for chronic, non-inflammatory diarrhoea due to diffusely adherent *E. coli*, microsporidia, and *Isospora* and *Cyclospora* spp.

About 1 to 3 per cent of travellers returning from a developing country will have persistent diarrhoea that may last for 1 month or more. *Giardia*, *Cyclospora*, and, rarely, *Shigella*, *Salmonella* spp., or *C. jejuni* may be responsible for persistent diarrhoea in travellers. A causative agent is not identified in many travellers suffering from prolonged diarrhoea. Some of these unfortunate individuals will respond to empirical therapy with broad-spectrum antibiotics since they have 'tropical jejunitis' or a mild form of tropical sprue.

Bacterial overgrowth in the small intestine can result in chronic diarrhoea, steatorrhoea, bloating, abdominal pain, and wasting. Factors contributing to the development of this problem include achlorhydria, decreased motility (as may be seen in diabetes mellitus or scleroderma), and stasis due to diverticula or blind loops of bowel. Treatment with amoxicillin/clavulanic acid, erythromycin, or tetracycline in conjunction with a lactose-free diet will often lead to resolution of the diarrhoea.

Inflammatory diarrhoea

Acute inflammatory diarrhoea is the result of infection with bacterial enteropathogens such as *Shigella*, *Campylobacter*, *Salmonella* spp., EHEC, *V. parahaemolyticus*, and *C. difficile*. Among the parasites, *Entamoeba histolytica* is the most common cause of dysenteric illness although *Balantidium coli*, *Schistosoma mansoni*, *S. japonicum*, *Trichuris trichiura*, hookworms, and *Trichinella spiralis* can all cause bloody, mucoid diarrhoea (see Section 7).

Dysentery is an oft-used term that refers to a diarrhoeal stool that contains an inflammatory exudate composed of blood and polymorphonuclear leucocytes. Patients with bacillary dysentery classically present with crampy abdominal pain, rectal burning ('tenesmus'), and fever, associated with multiple small-volume, bloody mucoid, bowel movements. The most constant findings are lower abdominal pain and diarrhoea. Fever is present in less than half of patients and the typical dysentery stool, consisting of blood and mucus, in only one-third. Sigmoidoscopy reveals acute mucosal inflammation with ulcerations and focal haemorrhage.

Bacteria

The *Shiga* bacillus, *S. dysenteriae* type 1, produces the most severe form of dysentery, while *S. sonnei* produces the mild disease. *S. flexneri* is the most commonly encountered serogroup in tropical countries, whereas *S. sonnei* is the most common in industrialized nations. Many patients with shigellosis manifest a biphasic illness. The initial symptoms of fever, abdominal pain, and watery, non-bloody diarrhoea result from the action of enterotoxin. The second phase, starting 3 to 5 days after the onset of symptoms, is notable for tenesmus and small-volume bloody stools. This period corresponds to invasion of the colonic epithelium and acute colitis. Infection with *S. dysenteriae* type 1 and malnutrition, especially in young children, are factors associated with a more severe course. Complications of shigellosis include intestinal perforation, protein-losing enteropathy, hypoglycaemia, seizures, thrombocytopenia, and haemolytic–uraemic syndrome —the latter three being particularly common in children.

Campylobacter species, especially *C. jejuni*, have gained in prominence as invasive diarrhoeal pathogens. Clinically, disease manifestations range from frank dysentery, to watery diarrhoea, to asymptomatic excretion. Most patients have diarrhoea, fever, and abdominal pain—about 50 per cent will note bloody stools. Constitutional symptoms such as headache, myalgias, backache, malaise, anorexia, and vomiting are often present. The illness usually resolves in less than 1 week, although symptoms can persist for 2 weeks or more, and relapses occur in as many as one-quarter of patients. Rare complications include gastrointestinal haemorrhage, toxic megacolon, pancreatitis, cholecystitis, haemolytic uraemic syndrome, bacteraemia, meningitis, and reactive arthritis, and Guillain-Barré syndrome.

Recent years have seen an increasing frequency of outbreaks of *Salmonella enteritidis* associated with the consumption of uncooked or raw eggs. Salmonella gastroenteritis is characterized by initial symptoms of nausea and vomiting, followed by abdominal cramps and diarrhoea which is accompanied by fever in about 50 per cent of persons. The diarrhoea varies from a few loose stools, to dysentery with grossly bloody, purulent faeces, to a cholera-like syndrome.

Yersinia enterocolitica can cause illness ranging from acute non-bloody diarrhoea to invasive colitis and ileitis. Fever, abdominal cramps, and haem-positive diarrhoea that may persist for several weeks characterize yersinia enterocolitis. *V. parahaemolyticus* outbreaks have been associated with the consumption of raw fish or shellfish. Illness is generally characterized by explosive, watery diarrhoea, abdominal cramps, nausea, vomiting, and headaches. In some cases a bloody dysenteric syndrome is observed.

EIEC strains are capable of invading epithelial cells and producing a shiga-like toxin. Patients with EIEC present with diarrhoea, tenesmus, fever, and abdominal cramps. EHEC strains possess at least two virulence factors that produce intestinal damage: an adherence mechanism causing attachment-effacement lesions similar to those seen with EPEC; and the production of two shiga-like cytotoxins (SLT I and II). Some EHEC strains produce only SLT I or II, whereas others produce both toxins. After a mean incubation of 3 to 4 days, illness begins with watery, non-bloody diarrhoea associated with severe abdominal cramping, nausea, vomiting, chills, and low-grade fever. The diarrhoea then often progresses to visibly bloody stools. Leucocytosis with a shift to the left is usually present, but anaemia is uncommon unless infection is complicated by the development of the haemolytic–uraemic syndrome (**HUS**) or thrombotic thrombocytopenic purpura (**TTP**). The median duration of diarrhoea is 3 to 8 days—longer durations have been described in children and persons with bloody diarrhoea.

Parasites

While infection with a number of different intestinal nematodes and trematodes can be associated with an inflammatory diarrhoea, *E. histolytica* is by far the most common parasitic cause of dysenteric illness (see Chapter 7.13.1). Approximately 50 million cases of invasive colitis due to *E. histolytica* occur worldwide each year, primarily in developing countries. In industrialized countries, populations at high risk of infection include institutionalized persons, especially the mentally impaired, recent immigrants, returning travellers, and sexually active male homosexuals. Malnutrition, malignancy, glucocorticoid use, pregnancy, and young age are risk factors for greater severity of infection.

There are two distinct species of *Entamoeba* that can be differentiated on the basis of antigenic structure, isoenzyme analysis, host specificity, *in vitro* growth characteristics, *in vivo* virulence, and DNA characterization. The two species, *E. histolytica* and *E. dispar*, have the same lifecycle and are morphologically identical. However, *E. dispar* is associated with an asymptomatic carrier state, while *E. histolytica* is capable of invading tissue and causing symptomatic infection.

A spectrum of clinical illness occurs with *E. histolytica* infections including asymptomatic carriage, non-bloody diarrhoea, acute dysenteric colitis, fulminant colitis with perforation, chronic non-dysenteric colitis, and the formation of an amoeboma, an annular lesion of the colon that can be confused with colon cancer. Patients with acute amoebic dysentery usually present with a 1- to 3-week history of bloody diarrhoea, tenesmus, and abdominal pain. Fever and dehydration are present in a minority of patients. Complications of amoebic colitis include intestinal perforation and toxic megacolon. Although nearly all patients have blood in the stool, faecal leucocytes are usually absent, probably as a result of the lysis of inflammatory cells by trophozoites. Amoebic liver abscess can occur with or independent of acute colitis. The fulminant variant of amoebic colitis is characterized by the rapid onset of fever, bloody mucoid diarrhoea, diffuse abdominal pain with peritoneal signs, and leucocytosis. Chronic non-dysenteric amoebiasis is a syndrome usually lasting more than 1 year with intermittent diarrhoea, mucus, abdominal pain, flatulence, and weight loss.

Antibiotic-associated colitis

Although the mechanism has not been fully elucidated, it appears that the normal bowel flora inhibits overgrowth by *C. difficile* in the large intestine. Factors such as antibiotic use or chemotherapy disrupt the suppressive effects of the microflora and allow *C. difficile* to propagate and to secrete its toxins. This organism produces two cytotoxins, one of which, cytotoxin A, appears to be responsible for damaging the colonic mucosa, while the other, cytotoxin B, is used for diagnosis based on its cytotoxic effects in tissue culture.

Antibiotic-associated diarrhoea and colitis due to toxin-producing strains of *C. difficile* can be community-acquired or acquired in hospitals and chronic-care facilities. Recent treatment with antibiotics, especially cephalosporins and clindamycin, or chemotherapeutic agents such as methotrexate precedes the development of illness. Clinical findings range from asymptomatic carriage to fulminant colitis with perforation. Symptomatic patients have frequent, malodorous bowel movements that are not grossly bloody. Associated signs and symptoms include crampy abdominal pain, fever, and abdominal tenderness. Leucocytosis with an increase of immature neutrophil forms is often present. Complications of *C. difficile* colitis include toxic megacolon, perforation, electrolyte disturbances, and hypoalbuminaemia.

Invasive infections

There are many infections of the gastrointestinal tract that do not present with diarrhoea, but instead are manifested by a systemic illness in which constitutional symptoms and signs predominate. Enteric fever, particularly that caused by *S. typhi*, may be the most common invasive bacterial infection worldwide.

Typhoid fever

After ingestion in contaminated food or water, *S. typhi* penetrates the small bowel mucosa and makes its way rapidly to the lymphatics, the mesenteric nodes, and finally the bloodstream. Following an initial bacteraemia, the organism is sequestered in cells of the reticuloendothelial system where it multiplies and re-emerges several days later in recurrent waves of bacteraemia, an event that initiates the symptomatic phase of infection.

Typhoid fever is a febrile illness of prolonged duration, characterized by hectic fever, delirium, persistent bacteraemia, splenomegaly, abdominal pain, and a variety of systemic manifestations. Pulse–temperature dissociation is present in some patients. In approximately 50 per cent of patients, there is no change in bowel habits; in fact, constipation is more common than diarrhoea in children with typhoid fever. As a result of recurrent waves of bacteraemia, patients with typhoid fever can develop pneumonia, pyelonephritis, osteomyelitis, septic arthritis, and meningitis. Intestinal haemorrhage and perforation, the most common complications, often occur in the third week of infection or during convalescence.

While *S. typhi* is the main cause of typhoid fever, other serotypes of *Salmonella* occasionally produce a similar clinical picture, known as enteric or paratyphoid fever. These serotypes include *S. paratyphi*, *S. schottmülleri* (formerly *S. paratyphi B*), and *S. hirschfeldii* (formerly *S. paratyphi C*), as well as others such as *S. typhimurium*.

Parasitic infestations

Certain gastrointestinal parasites are associated with systemic signs and symptoms during the extraintestinal stages of their lifecycles. Gut infections with *Strongyloides stercoralis* manifest with vague symptoms such as abdominal pain, bloating, and diarrhoea, frequently associated with eosinophilia. During the migration of this parasite through the skin and lung, specific symptoms attributable to the local inflammatory response in these tissues may occur. Hyperinfection or disseminated strongyloidiasis develops in immunocompromised patients, especially those with HIV infection, haematological malignancies, or those treated with systemic steroids or other immunosuppressive agents. Individuals with the hyperinfection syndrome have heavy worm burdens that can lead to intestinal obstruction, meningitis, respiratory failure, or Gram-negative bacteraemia.

Other intestinal parasites such as hookworm, *T. trichiura*, and *Schistosoma* species can cause gradual blood loss from the intestine that, in prolonged infections, can lead to clubbing, severe malnutrition, pica, stunting of growth, and congestive heart failure secondary to severe anaemia. Chronic infections with all *Schistosoma* species with the exception of *S. haematobium* can cause significant morbidity and mortality as a result of granuloma formation in the intestine and liver. The resulting hepatic fibrosis leads to portal hypertension that can eventually be complicated by splenomegaly, oesophageal varices, haematemesis, and death.

Intestinal tuberculosis

Mycobacterium tuberculosis is responsible for most cases of intestinal tuberculosis. In some developing countries, however, cases caused by *M. bovis*, an organism found in unpasteurized dairy products, still occur. The most frequent sites of intestinal involvement are the distal ileum and caecum, although any region of the gastrointestinal tract can be involved. Most patients with intestinal tuberculosis are asymptomatic. The most common complaint is chronic, non-specific abdominal pain. Weight loss, fever, diarrhoea or constipation, and blood in the stool may be present. An abdominal mass, commonly located in the right lower quadrant of the abdomen, is appreciated in about two-thirds of patients. Complications include haemorrhage, obstruction, perforation, fistula formation, and malabsorption.

Peritoneal tuberculosis results from the haematogenous spread of *M. tuberculosis* to mesenteric lymph nodes. Ascites is the most common presenting feature and is often associated with fever, lethargy, and weight loss. The ascitic fluid is notable for an elevated white blood cell count with a lymphocytic predominance, and a high albumin concentration.

Diagnosis and management of gastrointestinal infections

Diagnosis

Although there is considerable overlap in presenting signs and symptoms, nevertheless a pathophysiological approach can be used to make a presumptive aetiological diagnosis in patients with infectious diarrhoea (Table 2). By separating micro-organisms that target the upper small intestine from those that attack the large bowel, the clinician can categorize the general type of pathogen based on the initial symptoms and the type of diarrhoea. In the case of the non-inflammatory bowel pathogens, microscopy of the stool reveals no leucocytes or erythrocytes, whereas these are often abundant in the faeces of patients with invasive diarrhoeal pathogens. Several organisms including *Salmonella*, *Yersinia* spp., *V. parahaemolyticus*, and *C. difficile* produce variable findings on microscopic examination of stools. Depending on the invasiveness of the strain and the extent of colonic involvement, there can be few to many red blood cells and/or polymorphonuclear leucocytes in the stool.

A diagnostic algorithm can be used to help decide which patients should be treated symptomatically and which require further diagnostic studies and treatment (Fig. 1). Approximately 90 per cent of cases of acute diarrhoea fall into the 'no studies–no treatment' category. Because of the significant morbidity and cost associated with infectious diarrhoea, making a specific laboratory diagnosis can be useful epidemiologically, diagnostically, and therapeutically. A definitive diagnosis is achieved mainly through study of faecal specimens, using bacteriological culture, viral culture, or

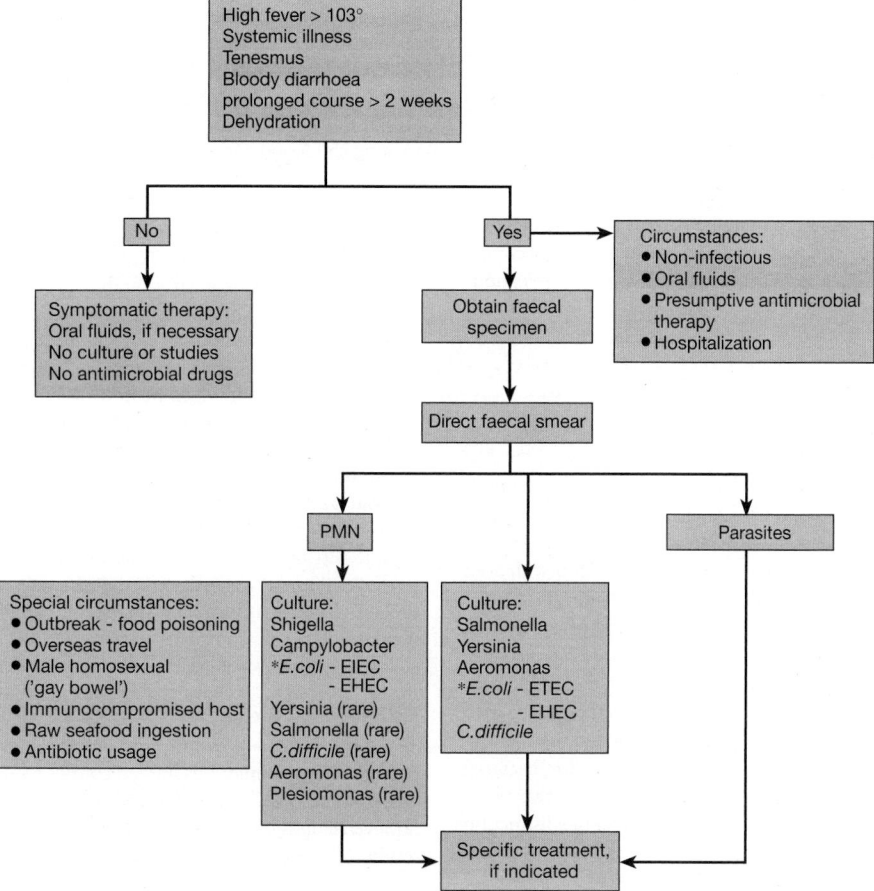

Fig. 1 Algorithm for the diagnosis and treatment of diarrhoea.

direct electron microscopy for viral particles, and identification of microbial antigens (viruses, bacteria, parasites, or toxins). DNA probes, polymerase chain reaction, and immunodiagnostic tests can now be used to identify several pathogens in stool specimens. Although some diseases can be diagnosed by elevations of serum antibody titres, this method is usually retrospective and often inaccurate.

Invasive procedures such as sigmoidoscopy or upper endoscopy generally play a limited role in the diagnosis of bacterial infections of the gastrointestinal tract. If performed, proctoscopy or sigmoidoscopy of patients with colitis due to *Shigella* spp., *Salmonella* spp., and other invasive pathogens will show a diffusely ulcerated, haemorrhagic, and friable colonic mucosa. Large bowel involvement with *C. difficile* manifests as an acute inflammatory colitis with or without pseudomembranes. While the demonstration of pseudomembranes by colonoscopy can provide a rapid diagnosis, this method is relatively insensitive. Sigmoidoscopy with biopsy of the rectal mucosa is often helpful in identifying parasitic infections such as *E. histolytica* or *S. mansoni*. Endoscopy with duodenal aspirates or biopsies may help to establish the diagnosis of giardiasis, cryptosporidiosis, microsporidiosis, or strongyloidiasis. These procedures should be carried out during the evaluation of patients with chronic diarrhoea if stool cultures and examinations for ova and parasites have failed to elucidate the aetiology.

Differential diagnosis

Non-inflammatory diarrhoea

A large number of non-infectious causes of food poisoning such as heavy metals (for example, arsenic or cadmium), mushrooms (for example, *Amanita phalloides*), and other chemical substances can result in acute diarrhoea, nausea, and vomiting. Various toxin-mediated forms of shellfish or seafood poisoning, including ciguatera, scombroid, and toxic encephalopathic shellfish poisoning, can all present with nausea, vomiting, and diarrhoea as part of a constellation of symptoms. A history of recent seafood consumption and the presence of other characteristic symptoms or signs should alert the clinician to the cause.

Endocrine disorders associated with diarrhoea include thyrotoxicosis and Addison's disease. Some secretory tumours such as carcinoid, medullary tumour of the thyroid, and vasoactive intestinal peptide-secreting adenomas have watery diarrhoea as a prominent symptom. Chronic, non-bloody diarrhoea is seen in patients with coeliac disease, laxative abuse, Whipple's disease, short-gut syndrome, and pancreatic insufficiency.

Inflammatory diarrhoea

Bloody diarrhoea due to invasive enteropathogens is difficult to distinguish from that caused by inflammatory bowel disease. Two features help to distinguish dysentery from an acute attack of idiopathic ulcerative colitis: a positive culture for a pathogen and a self-limited course without relapse. However, positive cultures are encountered in only 40 to 60 per cent of reported dysentery cases. Biopsy of colonic mucosa from patients with both bacterial dysentery and ulcerative colitis show oedema, neutrophils in the lamina propria, and superficial cryptitis with preservation of the normal crypt pattern. Yet, biopsy from idiopathic ulcerative colitis also reveals signs of chronicity such as crypt distortion and plasmacytosis in the lamina propria. In clinical practice, the main diagnostic quandary is the patient with severe, acute colitis who has failed to respond to antimicrobial therapy. Presumptive treatment should include a fluoroquinolone for bacterial pathogens and metronidazole for protozoa. The decision to use other treatments, such as corticosteroids and antimetabolites, rests on the distinction between these diseases, although it may be difficult to make this decision based on culture or histopathological findings. In addition to inflammatory bowel disease, often non-infectious causes such as ischaemic colitis, acute diverticulitis, and, rarely, colon cancer can present with bloody diarrhoea.

Enteric fever

Because the initial presentation of typhoid and paratyphoid fever is pyrexia, there is a large differential diagnosis during the early stages of enteric fever. Depending on epidemiological and clinical factors, a range of infectious (for example, malaria, Gram-positive sepsis, brucellosis, occult abscess) and non-infectious (for example, rheumatological diseases and malignancy) aetiologies need to be considered. Blood cultures are an essential part of the diagnostic evaluation for enteric fever.

Management

Rehydration

Since the most devastating consequences of acute infectious diarrhoea result from fluid losses, the major goal of treatment is the replacement of fluid and electrolytes. While the intravenous route of administration has been traditionally used, oral rehydration solutions (**ORS**) have been shown to be equally effective physiologically and logistically more practical and less costly to administer, especially in developing countries. ORS is the treatment of choice for mild-to-moderate diarrhoea in both children and adults, providing vomiting is not a major feature of the gastrointestinal infection. ORS can also be used in severely dehydrated patients after initial parenteral rehydration.

Although there is no doubt about the value of ORS in treating dehydrating diarrhoea, the optimal concentration of sodium that should be used remains in dispute, particularly in regard to the treatment of mild-to-moderate diarrhoea in well-nourished children in industrialized countries. The high concentration of sodium (90 mmol) in the standard World Health Organization ORS formulation may cause hypernatraemia and even seizures in children with non-cholera watery diarrhoea. Consequently, lower concentrations of sodium and a reduced osmolarity solution have been found to be effective for rehydration and not to be associated with any serious adverse clinical events. The substitution of starch derived from rice or cereals for glucose in ORS has been another approach. Rice-based salt solutions produce lower stool losses, a shorter duration of diarrhoea, and greater fluid and electrolyte absorption than do glucose-based solutions in treating childhood and adult diarrhoea.

Diet

The traditional approach to an acute diarrhoeal illness, dietary abstinence, restricts the intake of necessary calories, fluids, and electrolytes. During an acute attack, the patient often finds it more comfortable to avoid spicy, high-fat, and high-fibre foods, all of which can increase stool volume and intestinal motility. Although giving the bowel a rest provides symptomatic relief, continued oral intake of fluids and foods is critical for both rehydration and the prevention of malnutrition. In children, it is particularly important to restart feeding as soon as the child is willing to accept oral intake.

Because certain foods and fluids can increase intestinal motility, it is wise to avoid fluids such as coffee, tea, cocoa, and alcoholic beverages. Ingestion of milk and dairy products can potentiate fluid secretion and increase stool volume. Besides the oral rehydration therapy outlined above, acceptable beverages for mildly dehydrated adults include fruit juices and various bottled soft drinks. Carbonated drinks should be allowed to 'de-fizz' by letting them stand in a glass before ingestion. Soft, easily digestible foods are generally acceptable to the patient with acute diarrhoea.

Antimicrobial therapy

Since most patients with infectious diarrhoea, even those with a recognized pathogen, have a mild, self-limited course, neither a stool culture nor specific treatment is required for such cases (Fig. 1). For more severe cases, however, empirical antimicrobial therapy should be instituted, pending the results of stool and blood cultures. Gastrointestinal infections likely to respond to antibiotic treatment include cholera, giardiasis, cyclosporiasis, shigellosis, *E. coli* diarrhoea in infants, symptomatic travellers' diarrhoea, *C. difficile* diarrhoea, and typhoid fever. The choice of antimicrobial drug

Table 3 Non-specific treatments for diarrhoeal disease

Effective
Fluids
    Intravenous
    Oral rehydration therapy
Food
    Continue food intake
    Avoid caffeine, lactose, and methylxanthines
Antimotility drugs
    Diphenoxylate
    Loperamide
    Codeine, paregoric, tincture of opium
Bismuth subsalicylate
Antisecretory drugs (e.g., zaldaride maleate)
Lactobacillus GG (may be effective in rotavirus diarrhoea)

Not effective
Anticholinergics
Cholestyramine
Kaolin, pectin, charcoal
Lactobacilli
Hydroxyquinolones (may be harmful)

should be based on *in vitro* sensitivity patterns, which vary from region to region. A fluoroquinolone antibiotic is a good choice for empirical therapy, since these agents have broad-spectrum activity against virtually all bacterial pathogens responsible for acute infectious diarrhoea (except *C. difficile*) and resistance to this drug remains limited in most parts of the world. In patients with severe community-acquired diarrhoea—characterized by more than four stools per day lasting for at least 3 days or more with at least one associated symptom such as fever, abdominal pain, or vomiting—there is a high likelihood of isolating a bacterial pathogen. In this setting, a short course of a fluoroquinolone, namely 1 to 3 days' duration, will generally provide prompt relief with a low risk of adverse effects. Fluoroquinolones will not be effective for parasitic infections—specific antiparasitic drugs should be prescribed after identification of the offending pathogen in stool smears.

There are conflicting reports regarding the efficacy of antimicrobial drugs in several important infections, such as those caused by *Campylobacter* spp., and insufficient data for infections caused by *Yersinia and Aeromonas* spp., vibrios, and several forms of *E. coli*. In cases of EHEC, there is evidence that antibiotics are not helpful and may even be harmful.

The duration of antimicrobial therapy has not been clearly defined. While courses of anywhere from 3 to 10 days of treatment have been recommended, there are several studies that included severe forms of diarrhoea which suggested that a single dose is as effective as more prolonged therapy. For example, single-dose fluoroquinolone therapy is highly effective for infections due to *V. cholerae, V. parahaemolyticus,* and most *Shigella* species. On the other hand, short-course treatment of salmonella gastroenteritis with fleroxacin has not been found to be clinically beneficial. When treatment is indicated, a number of studies have shown that the combination of an antimicrobial drug and an antimotility drug provides the most rapid relief of diarrhoea.

Antidiarrhoeal agents (Table 3)
Antimotility drugs are particularly useful in controlling moderate-to-severe diarrhoea. These agents disrupt propulsive motility by decreasing jejunal motor activity. Opiates may decrease fluid secretion, enhance mucosal absorption, and increase rectal sphincter tone. The overall effect is to normalize fluid transport, slow transit time, reduce fluid losses, and ameliorate abdominal cramping.

Loperamide is the best agent because it does not carry a risk of habituation or depression of the respiratory centre. Treatment with loperamide produces rapid improvement, often within the first day of therapy. Although there has been a long-standing concern that antimotility agents might exacerbate cases of dysentery, this has largely been dispelled by clinical experience. Patients with shigellosis, even *S. dysenteriae* type 1, have been treated with loperamide alone and have had a normal resolution of symptoms without evidence of prolonging the illness or delaying excretion of the pathogen. However, as a general rule, antimotility drugs should not be used in patients with acute severe colitis, whether infectious or non-infectious in origin.

Bismuth subsalicylate (**BSS**), an insoluble complex of trivalent bismuth and salicylate, is effective in treating mild-to-moderate forms of diarrhoea. Bismuth possesses antimicrobial properties, while the salicylate moiety has antisecretory properties. In trials of diarrhoea among travellers in Mexico and West Africa, BSS reduced the frequency of diarrhoea significantly relative to placebo, but results were generally better when a high dose (for example, 4.2 g per day) was used. A number of studies have shown that the combination of an antimicrobial drug and an antimotility drug provides the most rapid relief of diarrhoea.

Prevention
Strict adherence to food and water precautions as outlined above will help travellers to less developed areas of the world to decrease their risk of acquiring gastrointestinal infections. Parasitic infections, such as strongyloidiasis and hookworms, can be avoided by the use of footwear. Avoiding contact with fresh water such as rivers and lakes in endemic areas serves to prevent schistosomiasis.

Immunization represents an ideal way to prevent certain bacterial and viral diseases, but has not yet proved successful for combating many gastrointestinal pathogens. The cholera vaccine that has been available for decades suffers from low efficacy, a moderate risk of side-effects, and a short duration of action. Newer oral cholera vaccines, including inactivated and live-attenuated forms, appear to be more promising. Immunization has been partially effective for the prevention of typhoid fever, especially in endemic areas. Although the efficacy of the currently available typhoid vaccines has not been determined in persons from industrialized regions, these vaccines are widely used for the prevention of typhoid fever in travellers to developing countries.

Further reading

Avery ME, Snyder JD (1990). Oral therapy for acute diarrhea: the underused simple solution. *New England Journal of Medicine* **323**, 891–4.

Acheson DWK, Keusch GT (1995). *Shigella* and enteroinvasive *Escherichia coli*. In: Blaser MJ, *et al.* eds. *Infections of the gastrointestinal tract*, pp 763–84. Raven Press, New York.

Blacklow NR, Greenberg HB (1991). Viral gastroenteritis. *New England Journal of Medicine* **325**, 252–64.

DuPont HL, Capsuto EG (1996). Persistent diarrhea in travellers. *Clinical Infectious Diseases* **22**, 124–8.

Echeverria P, Sethabutr O, Serichantalergs O (1993). Modern diagnosis (with molecular tests) of acute infectious diarrhea. *Gastroenterology Clinics of North America* **22**, 661–82.

Gerding DN, *et al.* (1995). *Clostridium difficile*-associated diarrhea and colitis. *Infection Control and Hospital Epidemiology* **16**, 459–77.

Gorbach SL (1997). Treating diarrhoea. *British Medical Journal* **314**, 1776–7.

Gorbach SL, Edelman R, eds. (1986). Travellers' diarrhea: National Institutes of Health Consensus Development Conference. *Reviews of Infectious Diseases* **8**(Suppl. 2), S109–S233.

Hamer DH, Cash RA (1999). Cholera and enterotoxigenic *Escherichia coli*. In: Armstrong D, Cohen J, eds. *Infectious diseases*, pp 22.1–22.4. Harcourt Brace, London.

Hamer DH, Gorbach SL (1998). Use of the quinolones for the treatment and prophylaxis of bacterial infections. In: Andriole VT, ed. *The quinolones*, 2nd edn, pp 267–85. Academic Press, San Diego.

Mishu Allos B, Blaser MJ (1995). *Campylobacter jejuni* and the expanding spectrum of related infections. *Clinical Infectious Diseases* **20**,1092–101.

Simon GL, Gorbach SL (1995). Normal alimentary tract microflora. In: Blaser MJ, *et al.* eds. *Infections of the gastrointestinal tract*, pp 53–69. Raven Press, New York.

Su C, Brandt LJ (1995). *Escherichia coli* 0157:H7 infection in humans. *Annals of Internal Medicine* **123**, 698–714.

14.18 Liver, pancreas, and biliary tree

14.18.1 The structure and function of the liver, biliary tract, and pancreas

A. E. S. Gimson

The liver and biliary tract

The liver weighs 1.2 to 1.5 kg and has a highly vascular architecture. The classic descriptions of liver anatomy demonstrating the complexity of different parenchymal and non-parenchymal elements have a long history, but only recently have they been united with an increasing understanding of the intricate functional organization and physiological compartmentalization of liver structure. This has had a profound effect on our understanding of the control of physiological processes and the development of liver surgery. A grasp of the hepatic anatomy is key to an appreciation of these complex functional arrangements.

Morphological anatomy

This describes the classic structure of the liver into two lobes, right and left, and the accompanying vascular structures, lymphatics, and biliary tract.

The liver, situated in the right upper quadrant of the abdomen, is covered by Glisson's capsule, a visceral continuation of the peritoneum. Three ligaments attach to surrounding structures—the falciform ligament anterior and superiorly, and the two posterior triangular ligaments which enclose the retrohepatic vena cava and the small bare area of the liver. Inferiorly Glisson's capsule attaches to the lesser curve of the stomach and at the hepatic hilus encases the hepatic pedicle consisting of hepatic artery, portal vein, and common hepatic bile duct.

Hepatic lobes

The two major lobes, right and left, and two accessory lobes, quadrate and caudate, are defined by points of surface anatomy (Fig. 1(a)). The larger right lobe comprises the dome of the liver under the diaphragm and is limited anteriorly and medially by the falciform ligament and posteriorly by the right border of the inferior vena cava. The quadrate lobe inferiorly abuts on to the antrum of the stomach and first part of the duodenum and is bordered by the posterior transverse hilar fissure, the gallbladder fossa laterally, and the umbilical fissure medially. The caudate lobe lies posterior and superior to the quadrate lobe limited by the vena cava and the ligamentum venosum. Finally, the left lobe has the umbilical fissure medially and the falciform ligament anteriorly.

Vascular anatomy

The portal vein, hepatic duct, and hepatic artery form the hepatic pedicle with the bile duct anterior in the free edge of the lesser omentum and the portal vein posteriorly (Fig. 1(b)). The latter is formed by the confluence of the superior mesenteric vein and the splenic veins running posteriorly in the pedicle, dividing into left and right branches to supply each lobe. The left gastric vein also drains into the portal vein and may, in the presence of portal hypertension, be a major feeding vessel for gastro-oesophageal varices.

The hepatic artery arises from the coeliac axis as the common hepatic artery before dividing into a gastroduodenal and the main hepatic artery. There are several common anatomical variants of the arterial supply of the liver, which are of no functional significance but which are of importance in liver transplantation and during surgical resection. The standard division into single left and right hepatic arteries is present in approximately 70 per cent of cases (Fig. 1(b)), but common variants include: a separate second right hepatic artery (10 per cent), a separate right and left hepatic arteries (8 per cent), and origin of the main hepatic artery off the superior mesenteric artery (2.5 per cent). Variants of the left hepatic arterial supply also occur with a separate left hepatic artery arising from the left gastric artery in 10 per cent of cases.

Venous drainage of the liver is through the three main hepatic veins, right, left, and middle, the latter two coalescing before joining the inferior vena cava. The caudate lobe drains separately through an array of small spigelian veins directly into the inferior vena cava. The functional anatomy of the liver (see below) describes the relationship between the main divisions of the portal vein and their draining hepatic veins running in the right, left, and main scissures (Fig. 2).

Biliary anatomy

Biliary canaliculi drain into left and right hepatic bile ducts forming the common hepatic duct until entry of the cystic duct after which it is designated the common bile duct and has a diameter of less than 8 mm. The left hepatic duct follows a nearly horizontal course, partially extrahepatic. Anatomical variants are again quite frequent, and are surgically important, the most common being drainage of the cystic duct directly into the right hepatic duct. The common bile duct passes behind the first part of the duodenum, through pancreatic tissue to the ampulla of Vater joining drainage of the pancreatic duct (Fig. 1(b)). The gallbladder lies in a shallow depression in the underside of the liver, may contain up to 50 ml of bile, and is connected to the cystic duct with a spiral valve.

Lymphatics

The liver has a high blood flow and a highly permeable microcirculation. The consequent production of interstitial fluid, intrahepatic lymph, is formed in the perisinusoidal space of Disse between the hepatocytes and sinusoidal lining endothelium. Lymphatic vessels drain via the portal tracts, closely applied to the hepatic arterial branches, to the hilum and thence to the thoracic duct. A smaller proportion drains with the hepatic veins and some interstitial fluid drains through Glisson's capsule into the peritoneum. Lymph flow acts to drain from the liver that interstitial fluid and protein that forms inevitably through microvascular filtration. The lymph flow rate in mammalian liver is approximately 0.5 ml/kg of liver per minute making up 25 to 50 per cent of thoracic duct lymph flow and may be increased either by elevated microvascular pressure (hydrostatic pressure) through increased hepatic venous pressure or increased inflow pressure, or by reduced transcapillary oncotic pressure.

Nervous system

Both sympathetic and parasympathetic efferent innervation of the liver are described, an anterior plexus around the hepatic artery and posterior around the portal vein. Sympathetic stimulation increases glucose release and glycogenolysis, and reduces oxygen consumption, ammonia uptake,

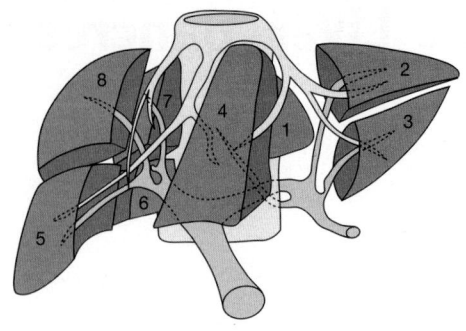

Fig. 2 Functional anatomy of the liver with Couinaud's segments.

and bile formation. Hepatic vascular resistance also rises as does portal pressure and there is rapid expulsion of blood out of the liver into the systemic circulation. An intrinsic nervous system with a wide variety of neurotransmitters including noradrenaline, prostanoids, neuropeptide Y, substance P, and vasoactive intestinal peptide is closely located to smooth muscle cells, fibroblasts, endothelial lining cells, and biliary epithelium within the liver and may be involved in chemoreception and osmoreception.

Extrinsic nervous regulation of hepatic physiological processes seems to be of minor importance as there is no apparent impairment of liver metabolism or bile formation following orthotopic liver transplantation. It may be more relevant during pathophysiological stress: the existence of a hepatorenal reflex is patients with cirrhosis has been postulated whereby an increase in sinusoidal pressure is associated with increased efferent renal sympathetic activity and reduced renal blood flow. In animal models of chronic liver disease, the metabolic consequences of sympathetic nerve stimulation are impaired but the haemodynamic responses exaggerated.

Functional anatomy

Following the initial descriptions by Cantlie in 1898, there has been an increasing appreciation of the importance of the functional anatomy of the liver, the culmination of which was the description by Couinaud of the present eight liver segments that underpins all modern hepatic surgery. Each segment is a complete functional unit with a single portal pedicle and a hepatic vein (Fig. 2). There are four portal pedicles, two for each lobe, each supplying a sector of the liver, divided from each other by the three hepatic veins lying in a right, middle, and left scissure. This separates the liver into a right and left liver, different from lobes, with independent vascular supply and biliary drainage. Within each sector of the liver there are further subdivisions into segments. The caudate lobe (segment 1) has its own venous drainage, manifest during the Budd–Chiari syndrome with thrombosis of hepatic veins when all venous drainage attempts to pass through this segment with consequent lobar hypertrophy.

The left liver consists of the left posterior sector of segment 2 alone, and a left anterior sector of segment 3 medially and segment 4 laterally separated by the umbilical fissure. The right liver comprises a posterior sector of segment 7 superiorly and segment 6 inferiorly and an anterior sector of segment 5 inferiorly and segment 8, being most of the dome of the liver, superiorly (Fig. 2).

Structural organization

Within the functional segments of the liver the structural unit is the hepatic lobule, a polyhedron (2 mm by 0.7 mm) surrounded by four to six portal tracts containing hepatic arterial and portal venous branches from which blood perfuses through sinusoids, surrounded by walls of hepatocytes that are a single cell thick and lined by specialized endothelial cells with 'windows' (fenestrae), to the centrilobular region and the central hepatic veins (Fig. 3).

The portal vein branches give off numerous terminal portal venules that run around the lobules in the interlobular septa accompanied by arterioles

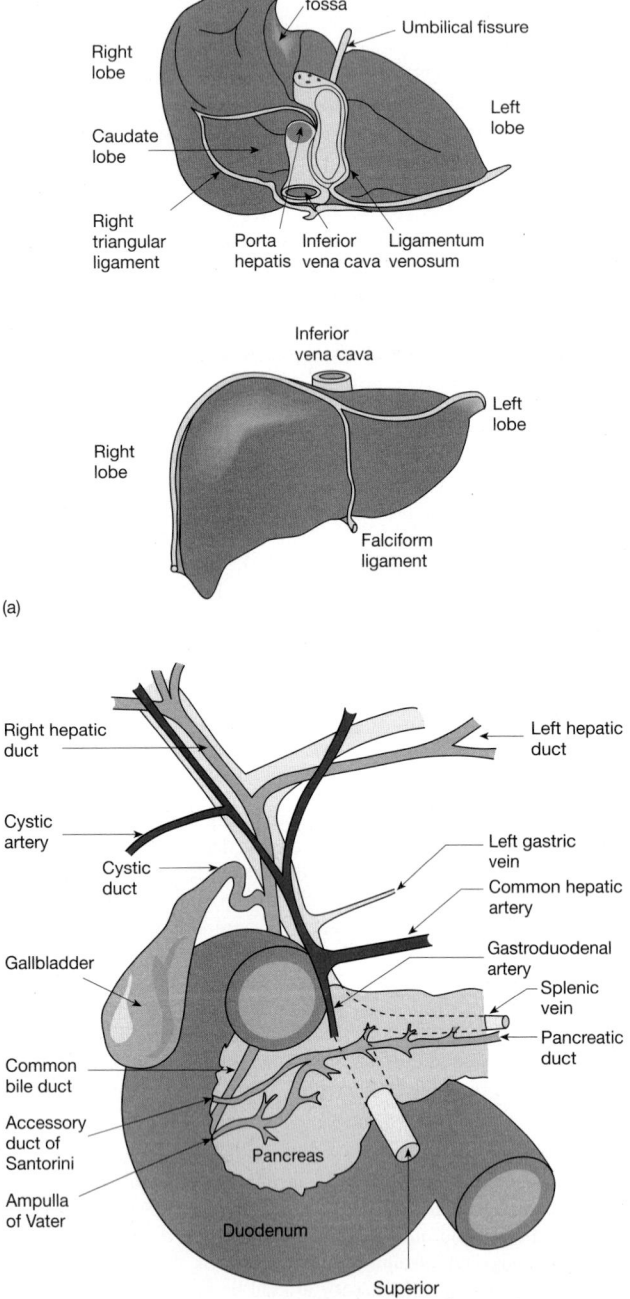

Fig. 1 (a) Lobar anatomy and relations. (b) Hilar, portal biliary tract, and pancreatic anatomy.

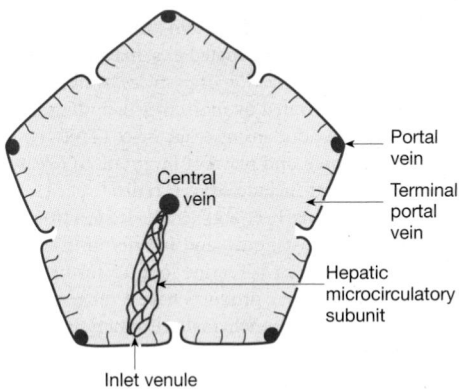

Fig. 3 Hexagonal lobule with portal venous branches and hepatic microcirculatory subunit—sinusoids.

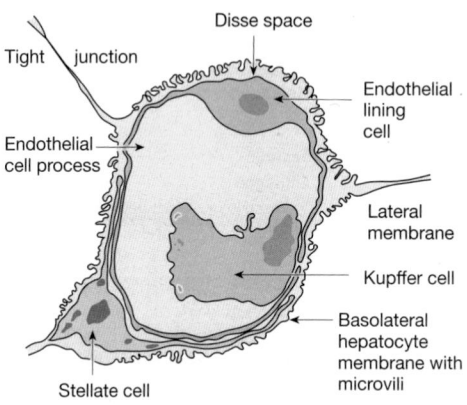

Fig. 4 Hepatic sinusoid, sinusoidal cells, and functional spaces.

and bile ductules, and subsequently branch into inlet venules which each supply a hepatic microcirculatory subunit consisting at the base of numerous interconnected sinusoids and, at the apex, the central vein (Fig. 3).

Sinusoids

Sinusoids are specialized capillaries without a basement membrane and lined with endothelial lining cells through which proteins of low molecular weight may percolate into the space of Disse. The sinusoidal membrane of the surrounding hepatocytes is covered by microvilli that increase the surface area sixfold (Fig. 4). Within the sinusoids, Kupffer cells and liver-associated lymphocytes may be found, and within the space of Disse, the hepatic stellate cells (also called Ito, fat storage, or perisinusoidal cells), which respectively make up 2, 0.2, and 1.4 per cent of the lobular parenchyma (Table 1).

Biliary canaliculi

Bile secreted through the canalicular membrane of the hepatocyte collects in biliary canaliculi, which pass around hepatocytes until draining through the short canal of Hering into the bile ductule. Cholangioles are lined by three or four cells that eventually become cuboidal epithelium.

The volume and flow rate of bile are low; secretion into the duodenum is controlled by gallbladder contraction and sphincter of Oddi tone. Agents that cause gallbladder contraction, including cholecystokinin, secretin, and motilin, also relax the sphincter of Oddi (Table 2). Factors modulating biliary motility have received increased attention recently with the realization that the syndrome of biliary dysmotility may be the cause of biliary-type pain in some cases. Changes in gallbladder motility may also be important in gallstone pathogenesis.

Table 1 Hepatic parenchymal cellular elements and physiological functions

Cell type	Percentage of parenchyma	Surface receptors	Cellular functions
Hepatocytes	94	Asialoglycoprotein receptors, IL-6, cytokine receptors, albumin, transferrin, mannose, annexin, MHC class 1, Fas ligand	Maintain glucose, amino acid, ammonia, and bicarbonate homeostasis. Bile acid synthesis and transport. Synthesis of most plasma proteins. Processing of absorbed nutrient fuels and xenobiotics. Lipoprotein metabolism. Processing of hormones and signal mediators
Endothelial lining cells	2.5	Scavenger receptor, Fc IgM, MHC class II (CD4), CD58, thrombospondin receptor	Acts as physical barrier lining to sinusoids allowing passage of molecules via fenestrations up to 100 nm or numerous pinocytotic vesicles. Receptor-mediated uptake of HDL, LDL by scavenger receptor. May express numerous adhesion molecules marginating leucocytes and lymphocytes to sites of inflammation
Kupffer cells	2	KP-1, (CD68), Fc and complement receptors, VCAM, ICAM-1	Phagocytosis of numerous particles including cellular debris, denatured albumin, bacteria, complement. After stimulation, release inflammatory mediators: oxygen radical species, nitric oxide, proteases, TNF-α, IL-1, -6, -10, TGF-β, prostanoids, interferons
Stellate, fat storage, or Ito cells	1.4	Retinoid, cytokine receptors, platelet-derived growth factor, TGF-β, endothelin receptor	Vitamin A storage. Under a wide range of stimuli, including TNF-α, TGF-β, acetaldehyde, CCL_4, prostanoids, cytokines, and oxygen species, transform into myofibroblasts. Secrete extracellular matrix proteins after activation (collagen, fibronectin, laminin, chondroitin sulphate, hyaluronic acid) resulting in fibrogenesis. Activated transformed stellate cells control sinusoidal blood flow
Pit cells	0.1	CD2, CD18	Natural killer cell activity that may be directed against tumour cells and virus-infected cells and occurs without prior activation

Table 2 Physiological effects of neurotransmitters and hormones on biliary function

Contraction	Relaxation
Gallbladder motility	
Acetylcholine	Secretin
Cholecystokinin	Glucagon
Motilin	Vasoactive intestinal peptide
β-Adrenergic agents	Pancreatic polypeptide
Endorphins	
Sphincter of Oddi	
Secretin	Cholecystokinin
Motilin	Vasoactive intestinal peptide
β-Adrenergic agents	Pancreatic polypeptide

Cellular elements

Hepatocytes are arranged in unicellular plates (Remak's plates) that branch and divide around sinusoids, and are covered by specific membranes at each surface: sinusoidal (70 per cent of surface area) for exchange of material between the Disse space and intracellular compartment (endo- and exocytosis); canalicular membrane (15 per cent) for exchange with the smallest of biliary canaliculi or hemicanals; and lateral membrane (15 per cent) separated from the former by tight junctions and involved in intercellular transport between hepatocytes. There is abundant smooth and rough endoplasmic reticulum, numerous mitochondria, and glycogen. There is an extensive cytoskeleton. Other cells making up 6 per cent of all parenchyma include sinusoidal-lining endothelial cells, Kupffer cells, hepatic stellate cells (Ito cells, fat-storing cells), and pit cells (intrahepatic lymphocytes) (Table 1). These cells each differ in morphology, patterns of function, reactions to stimuli and disease, and expression of surface molecules and receptors. Interplay between these cells is critical, with communication via tight junctions allowing complex modulation of hepatocyte growth and function by sinusoidal lining cells. Parenchymal cells may clear mediators, including cytokines, secreted by endothelial lining and Kupffer cells. Waves of cellular activity may pass down the length of sinusoids. Importantly some cells show heterogeneity of function relative to their zonal location. Periportal hepatocytes differ from perivenous cells in both the direction of carbohydrate metabolism and ammonia/glutamine synthesis. Ito cells show zonal differences in desmin and cytokeratin staining, vitamin A storage, and α-smooth muscle actin.

Endothelial lining cells

These cells are central to the processes that control entry and exit trafficking of molecules from the sinusoidal flow into the Disse space. Fenestrae with a diameter of 100 nm, occupying up to 8 per cent of the sinusoidal surface, act as a physical barrier to access of parenchymal cells by large molecules including lipids, cholesterol, vitamin A, and possibly some viruses. Endothelial cells also possess numerous specialized endocytotic mechanisms, some linked to specific receptors including mannose, transferrin, caeruloplasmin, modified high-density lipoprotein (**HDL**), low-density lipoprotein (**LDL**), glucosaminoglycans, and hyaluronic acid. Non-specific endocytosis of molecules and small particles up to 0.1 μm also occurs. Endothelial cells are also capable of expressing a range of surface adhesion molecules including E- and P-selectins, intercellular adhesion molecule 1 (**ICAM-1**), and lymphocyte function-associated antigen-4 (**LFA-4**) that enhance polymorphonuclear leucocyte and lymphocyte adherence, activation, and migration towards sites of inflammation.

Kupffer cells

These cells represent part of the mononuclear phagocyte system and are adherent to the sinusoidal surface of endothelial lining cells, predominantly in a periportal distribution. Covered with numerous microvilli and with a number of intracytoplasmic vesicles, their main function is to phagocytose a range of particulate material including cellular debris, senescent red blood cells, parasites, bacteria, endotoxin, and tumour cells. Phagocytosis is via a range of mechanisms including coated pits, macropinocytotic vesicles, and phagosomes aided by opsonization of particles by fibronectin or opsonin. Kupffer cells may be activated by molecules including *Escherichia coli* endotoxin, interferon-γ, tumour necrosis factor-α (**TNF-α**), and arachidonic acid as well as zymosan and phorbol myristate to release a range of inflammatory mediators that include oxygen radical species, nitric oxide, proteases, TNF-α, interleukins 1, 6, and 10 (**IL-1**, **-6**, **-10**), transforming growth factor-β (**TGF-β**), prostanoids, and interferon-α and -γ. Some of these may act in an autocrine or paracrine loop to further activate other Kupffer cells. These inflammatory products have a range of effects including significant modulation of parenchymal cell function (downregulation of albumin synthesis and upregulation of acute-phase protein gene expression), and induction of adherence of polymorphonuclear leucocytes and lymphocytes to endothelial lining cells due to enhanced expression of endothelial adhesion molecules.

Hepatic stellate cells

Stellate cells (Ito cells, fat-storing cells) have a similar morphology to fibroblasts with the addition of fat droplets, and are located within the Disse space. A fine branching array of cytoplasmic processes circle sinusoids under the endothelial cells. Stellate cells contain most of the body's stores of vitamin A. Retinoids are taken up from chylomicrons by specific receptors on hepatocytes and stellate cells and stored within the latter. These cells are central to the process of hepatic fibrogenesis, responding to mediators released by parenchymal and Kupffer cells, causing transformation into myofibroblasts. TGF-β initiates this process, stimulating production by the transformed stellate cell of extracellular matrix products (collagen type I, III, and IV, fibronectin, laminin, chondroitin sulphate, and hyaluronic acid) in addition to products for matrix degradation (collagenase, metalloproteinase, and its inhibitor TIMP-1). Activation of stellate cells is also an important mechanism for control of sinusoidal perfusion, through cytoskeletal actin within branching cellular processes beneath the endothelium.

Pit cells

Similar to large granular lymphocytes and located in clefts within endothelial lining cells, pit cells have natural killer cell properties with spontaneous activity against tumour cells in the absence of prior activation. They may also play a role in hepatic regeneration

Physiological processes

Hepatic blood flow

The liver receives approximately 25 per cent of cardiac output, one-third from the hepatic artery and two-thirds from the portal vein with a plasma flow at rest of 1600 ml/min in women and 1800 ml/min in men. Hepatic blood flow increases after feeding and with expiration and decreases with standing, inspiration, and sleep. In contrast to other organs, metabolic autoregulation of blood flow is not observed. Changes in hepatic oxygen consumption do not seem to control hepatic blood flow. Vascular autoregulation of hepatic arterial blood flow mediated by adenosine is present, but may not be of great physiological importance. Hepatic arterial resistance increases with increasing hepatic venous pressure due to a stepwise myogenic response in the hepatic artery to increased pressure. There is an important reciprocity between portal venous and hepatic arterial flow with a reduction in portal venous input being associated with significant compensatory decrease in hepatic arterial resistance and rise in arterial flow. The mechanism for this relationship is unproven but may be due to adenosine-mediated arterial vasodilatation.

The portal venous system is passive, without pressure-dependent autoregulation, and the major physiological factors controlling flow are those modulating supply to the intestines and spleen. The sites of portal venous resistance are not fully defined in humans but may be at sinusoidal or postsinusoidal levels. The significant capacitance of the hepatic circulation, with blood comprising up to 20 per cent of liver volume, is reflected in the important role of the liver and splanchnic circulation in acting as a blood reservoir. Sympathetic nerve stimulation may reduce hepatic blood volume by up to 50 per cent.

Sinusoidal perfusion

Blood pressure in sinusoids ranges from 4.8 to 1.7 mmHg, with flows of 270 to 410 ml/s. There is likely to be considerable heterogeneity of the uni-directional sinusoidal flow, control for which can be considered as either passive (haemodynamic) or active. Passive control mechanisms include: (i) the arterial input pressure and flow at the level of the arteriosinous twig at the origin of the sinusoid; and (ii) changes in right atrial pressure, central venous pressure, and hepatic venous pressure that are transmitted to the sinusoid from the centrilobular veins. Active control mechanisms include: (i) the presence of 'functional' sphincters at the inlet and outlet of the sinusoid due to indentations by the cell bodies of sinusoidal lining cells, which under different physiological stimuli may change dimension and alter sinusoidal perfusion; (ii) plugging by leucocytes, which are less compressible than erythrocytes and may under physiological stimuli adhere to endothelial lining cells; (iii) activation of Kupffer cells within sinusoids and release of other vasoactive mediators including nitric oxide, cytokines, and prostanoids; and (iv) transformation of hepatic stellate cells into activated contractile myofibroblasts that constrict the sinusoidal lumen. Sinusoidal flow will also affect the transendothelial traffic into and out of the Disse space by the processes of forced sieving and endothelial massage that may affect, respectively, the passage of lipoprotein particles and the appropriate mixing of the interstitial fluid. Therefore, sinusoidal flow is likely to have a profound effect on numerous hepatic metabolic functions and clearance of xenobiotics.

Bile formation

The formation of bile by hepatocytes and its modification by bile ductular epithelium serves many functions (Table 3). In humans the daily production of 600 ml of bile is made up of 75 per cent of canalicular origin and 25 per cent from ductules. Bile is formed by osmotic filtration, with the secretion of the two primary bile salt anions, taurine and glycine conjugates of cholic acid and chenodeoxycholic acid, across the canalicular membrane by an active transport mechanism against a concentration gradient of 5000:1 (Fig. 5). Negatively charged intercellular tight junctions prevent back diffusion of these anions, allowing the selective passage of cations, predominantly sodium, and to a smaller extent potassium, calcium, and magnesium, followed by the passive transit of water, transcellularly or between cells. The resulting bile salt-dependent bile flow makes up 50 per cent of canalicular bile flow, with the remaining bile salt-independent flow resulting from the active secretion of bicarbonate and glutathione.

Bile in biliary ductules is further modified by reabsorption of glucose, amino acids, and bile salts, as well as active secretion. Reabsorption of bile salts, the cholehepatic shunt pathway, occurs after their protonation in bile with the generation of further bicarbonate into bile stimulating bile flow.

Table 3 Physiological functions of bile

Digestion
Neutralization of duodenal pH
Bile salt activation of lipase, formation of micelles
Emulsification, lipolysis, and solubilization of fat
Absorption of fat-soluble substances
Excretion, including xenobiotics
Cholesterol
Bilirubin
Drugs
Environmental toxins
Heavy metals
Mucosal immunity
Secretory IgA

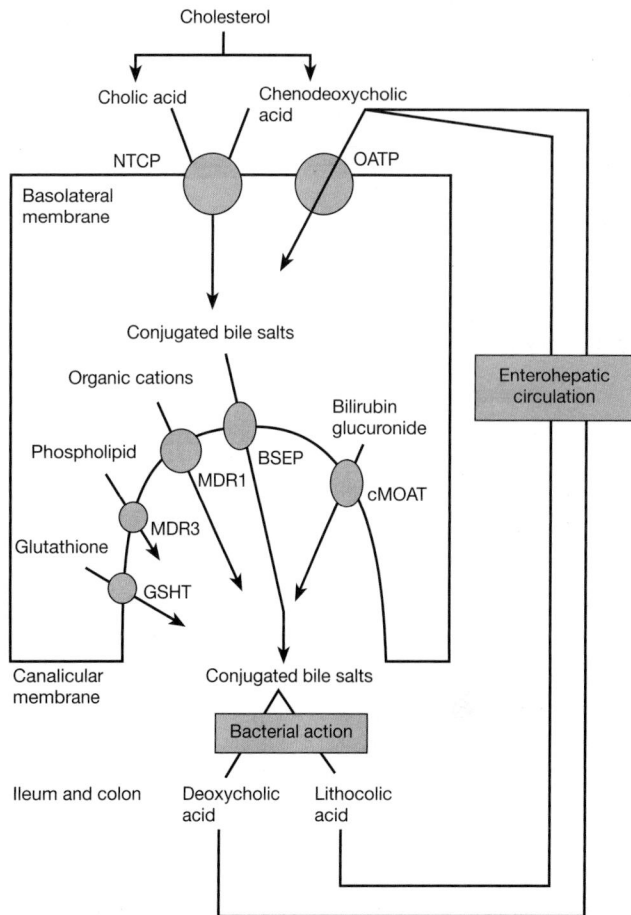

Fig. 5 Bile salt metabolism and enterohepatic pathway. NTCP, Na-taurocholate cotransporters; conjugated bile salt uptake from portal blood. OATP, organic anion transporter; bile salt, organic anion, and amphipathic solutes uptake. BSEP, bile salt export pump; ATP-dependent bile export—bile salt-dependent bile flow. MDR1, multidrug resistance-1 P glycoprotein; organic cation, xenobiotic export. MDR3, multidrug resistance-3 P glycoprotein; translocation of phosphatidylcholine. cMOAT, multispecific organic anion transporters; bilirubin glucuronide export; bile salt-independent bile flow. GSHT, glutathione transporter; gluthathione transport independent of bile flow.

Active secretion of bicarbonate and chloride within ductules is mediated by the secretin receptor and the cystic fibrosis transmembrane receptor. Gallbladder epithelium further modifies and concentrates bile by an active anion transport process.

Bile salt conjugates secreted from hepatocytes into bile are deconjugated in the jejunum and ileum with reabsorption and reuptake by the liver—this enterohepatic circulation conserves bile acids and maintains their high concentration within bile. The 5 per cent of bile acids passing through the ileocaecal valve are fully deconjugated by colonic bacteria and reabsorbed as the secondary bile acids deoxycholic acid and lithocolic acid, which are in turn secreted as taurine and glycine conjugates.

Metabolic processes

Hepatic metabolic processes have a central role in protein, carbohydrate, and lipid metabolism and fuel economy, orchestrating a diverse interplay between central splanchnic and peripheral organs. Interruption to these processes results in the major metabolic consequences of acute and chronic liver disease. Modulation of these metabolic processes can occur at a number of levels. Transport of molecules across membranes and through cells is an important control mechanism as are rate-limiting enzyme levels, controlled at a number of transcriptional and translational points. There is important zonal heterogeneity of hepatocyte function, with periportal zone 1 cells with a higher oxidative capacity and larger mitochondria involved in gluconeogenesis, β-oxidation of fatty acids, amino acid catabolism, ureagenesis, cholesterol synthesis, and bile secretion, whereas perivenular cells are more involved with glycolysis, lipogenesis, ammonia clearance with glutamine synthesis, detoxification, and biotransformation.

Bilirubin metabolism (Fig. 6) (see Chapter 14.19.3)

The first step in the production of bilirubin is the formation of biliverdin IXa by the action of haem oxidase on haem-containing proteins including catalases, cytochromes as well as haemoglobin in senescent red cells, with the release of carbon monoxide and Fe^{2+}. Biliverdin convertase within the cytosol reduces biliverdin to unconjugated bilirubin. Both biliverdin convertase and haem oxidase are predominantly found within reticuloendothelial cells.

Bilirubin is transported within plasma bound with high affinity to albumin. A few substances may displace bilirubin from albumin including sulphonamides and fatty acids. Unbound bilirubin, which is insoluble in water, is only present in nanogram quantities but may cause significant cellular toxicity in neonates and in the Crigler–Najjar syndrome.

Bilirubin uptake by hepatocytes occurs via an organic anion-binding protein receptor. Within the hepatocyte the unbound bilirubin is transported by organelles and a number of transport proteins including glutathione-S-transferase (ligandin) to the endoplasmic reticulum. This reduces back diffusion into sinusoids of the lipid-soluble unbound bilirubin. Glucuronidation to the mono- and diglucuronides renders bilirubin water soluble. Secretion across the canalicular membrane occurs at the canalicular multispecific membrane organic anion transporter.

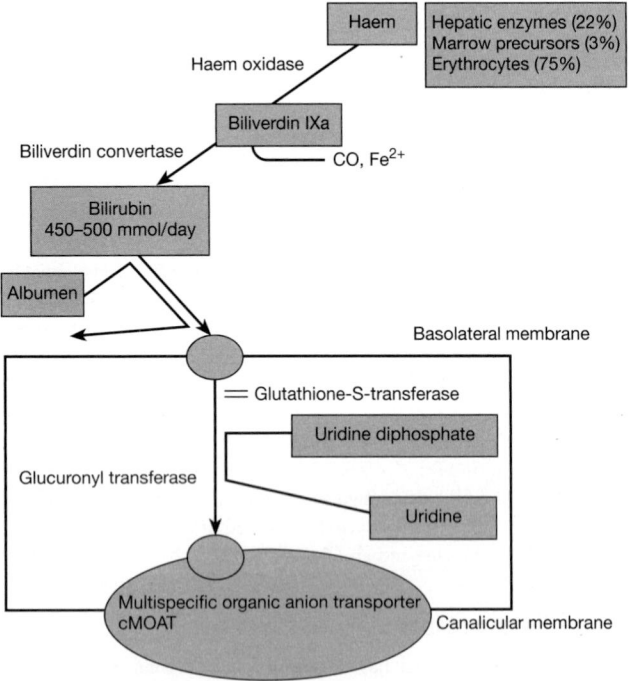

Fig. 6 Metabolism of haem and bilirubin with clearance through canalicular membrane to bile.

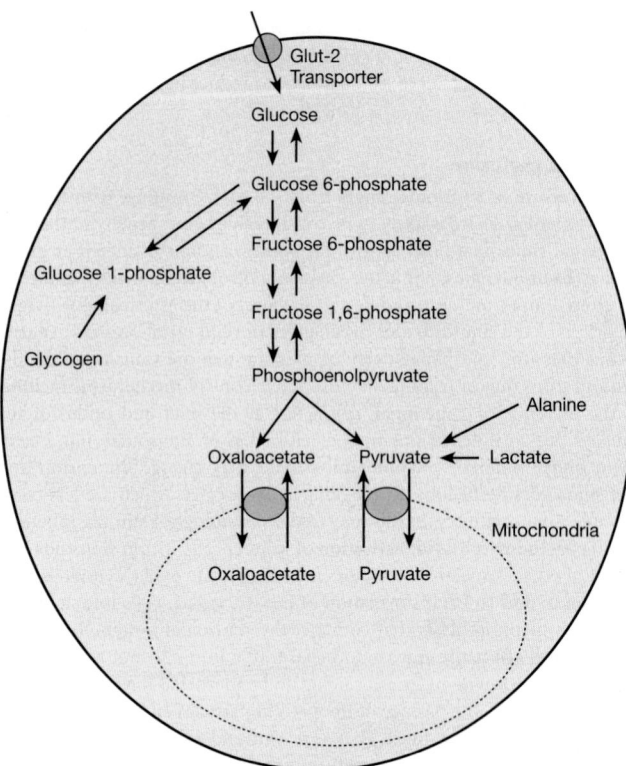

Fig. 7 Carbohydrate metabolism and pathways for glycolysis and glycogenesis.

Bile salt metabolism (Fig. 5)

In addition to their role in digestion, bile acids are the principal mechanism for clearance and metabolism of cholesterol, which acts as a substrate for their synthesis and in turn promotes biliary cholesterol secretion as lamellar vesicles. The first step in bile acid synthesis is rate limiting and involves cholesterol 7α-hydroxylase. Transcriptional control of the cholesterol 7α-hydroxylase gene has been demonstrated with thyroxine and glucocorticoids increasing, and glucagon decreasing, gene expression. Preformed (non-dietary) cholesterol and bile acids may also control this enzyme. The close association between bile acid and cholesterol metabolism is reflected in the often parallel activation of 7α-hydroxylase and HMG-CoA reductase, which is of critical importance in bile acid synthesis. The two major bile acids, cholic acid (60 per cent of bile acid pool) and chenodeoxycholic acid are secreted into bile as taurine and glycine conjugates.

Carbohydrate metabolism (Fig. 7)

The liver has a central role in maintaining blood glucose within a narrow margin. During fasting, hepatic glucose release is contributed to by both glycogenolysis (33 per cent) and gluconeogenesis (67 per cent) from lactate, pyruvate, glycerol, and the glucogenic amino acids alanine and glutamine. This process is regulated by at least four levels: (i) hormonal control, with glucagon accounting for up to two-thirds of basal fasted glucose output, and cortisol, growth hormone, and catecholamines also contributing; (ii) the supply of substrates, fatty acids, lactate, pyruvate, and amino acids for hepatic gluconeogenesis; (iii) metabolic regulation of hepatic enzyme activity; and (iv) the degree of hepatocellular hydration. The direction of gluconeogenesis or glycogenolysis is controlled at the level of three paired enzyme cycles—glucose/glucose-6-phosphate, fructose-6-phosphate/fructose-1,6-bisphosphate, and pyruvate/phosphoenolpyruvate. In contrast, after a glucose load, insulin suppresses hepatic glucose release and activates glucose synthetase, whilst autoregulation of hepatic glucose extraction by glucose itself within the portal venous circulation is an important factor in controlling the distribution of the load between liver and peripheral tissues.

Amino acid and ammonia metabolism

The liver is the most important organ in controlling the plasma concentration of amino acids. During prolonged starvation, hepatic proteolysis stimulated by glucagon increases splanchnic export of amino acids, whereas during the post-prandial absorptive state, amino acid uptake is significantly increased. The gluconeogenic amino acids are preferentially extracted and metabolized, whereas the branch-chain amino acids valine, leucine, and isoleucine are only cleared in the liver for protein synthesis and are catabolized in the muscle. During sepsis and under the influence of cytokines IL-1, IL-6, and TNF-α, the liver may significantly enhance gluconeogenesis and protein synthesis of acute-phase reactants (C-reactive protein, serum amyloid A).

The liver has a critical role in clearing portal venous ammonia generated within the gut lumen, by both formation of carbamoyl phosphate and entry into the urea cycle in periportal hepatocytes, and glutamine synthetase-driven glutamine synthesis in perivenous hepatocytes.

Protein synthesis

Most circulating plasma proteins with the exception of immunoglobulins and von Willebrand factor are produced by hepatocytes. The major controlling factors for this constitutive protein secretion are substrate delivery and the degree of hydration of hepatocytes. Acute-phase protein secretion is also specifically controlled by cytokines with a reciprocal relationship to albumin and other carrier protein synthesis.

Lipid and lipoprotein metabolism (Fig. 8) (see Chapter 11.6)

Plasma lipoproteins are particles with an outer layer of cholesterol, phospholipids, and apoproteins and an inner core of cholesterol esters and triglycerides. The various lipoproteins differ in the relative proportions of these elements. Dietary derived chylomicrons, consisting of more than 90 per cent triglyceride, are processed within muscle and adipose tissue by lipoprotein lipase, extracting free fatty acids and the remnant, enriched in

cholesterol, are extracted by the liver—an exogenous lipid pathway. During carbohydrate feeding, free fatty acids formed within the liver are exported as very-low-density lipoprotein (**VLDL**) and taken up by muscle and adipose tissue with extraction of free fatty acids, leaving intermediate-density lipoprotein and subsequently low-density lipoprotein (LDL). Specific LDL receptors on hepatocytes or scavenger receptors on Kupffer cells remove LDL where cholesterol may be utilized for bile salt metabolism or excreted into bile. Peripheral LDL receptors in extrahepatic tissues also extract cholesterol. Export of cholesterol from peripheral tissues in high-density lipoprotein is modified in plasma by lecithin; cholesterol acyltransferase (LCAT) and LDL is formed for further recirculation.

Pancreas structure and function

A retroperitoneal organ receiving arterial supply from splenic, superior mesenteric, and gastroduodenal arteries, the pancreas is composed of an exocrine portion centred on acini producing digestive enzymes draining through a ductal system into the duodenum, and the islets of Langerhans which make up 1 to 2 per cent of the whole volume and are predominantly located along arterioles.

Pancreas development and congenital anomalies

The pancreas develops from ventral and dorsal buds of the primitive duodenum. With rotation around the duodenum the two portions fuse together and the duct originating from the dorsal portion (duct of Santorini) forms the accessory duct whilst the main drainage of the gland is through the duct of Wirsung to the ampulla of Vater. Failure of ductal fusion, pancreas divisum, in which most of the gland drains through the duct of Santorini to the minor papilla, occurs in approximately 8 per cent of the population, and in a small proportion may lead to recurrent acute pancreatitis. Annular pancreas results from pancreatic tissue remaining wrapped around the duodenum during rotation of the ventral portion. Ectopic pancreatic tissue may occur in a submucosal location within the stomach and duodenum.

Exocrine pancreas

The pancreas secretes up to 2 litres of fluid per day although resting secretion rates are very low (0.3 ml/min). Acini are located in lobules draining into extralobular ducts. Cells lining the ducts secrete bicarbonate, the major anion within pancreatic juice. The acinar cells are pyramidal with the nucleus and endoplasmic reticulum towards the base and zymogen storage granules towards the apex and draining duct. Two classes of proteolytic enzymes are secreted—the serine proteases and the exopeptidases. Serine proteases all require activation either by intestinal endopeptidase in the case of trypsinogen or by trypsin itself in the case of chymotrypsin, elastase, and protease E. Serine protease act at various cleavage points whereas the carboxypeptidases A and B (exopeptidases) cleave C-terminal amino acids. The lipolytic enzymes include phospholipase A$_2$, lipase, and carboxylesterase. Other proteins found in pancreatic secretions include lysosomal proteins, ribonucleases, and amylase.

Control of the secretory process involves hormones as well as sympathetic and parasympathetic nerve fibres. Secretin is the main stimulus to ductal bicarbonate secretion, whereas cholecystokinin, acetylcholine, and to a lesser extent gastrin and neurotensin stimulate zymogen release of digestive enzymes at the apical membrane. Although often described as having cephalic, gastric, and intestinal phases to indicate the origin of the pancreatic stimulus, this distinction is physiologically artificial since the phases run concurrently. Somatostatin and glucagon inhibit pancreatic pro-enzyme secretion.

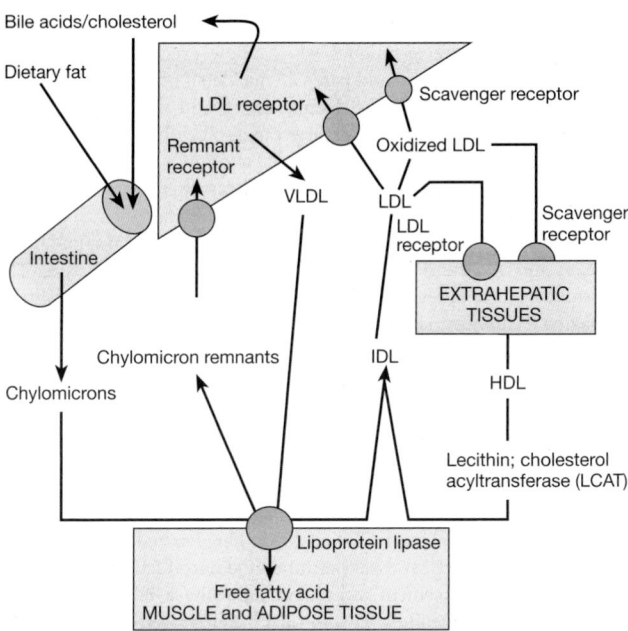

Fig. 8 Lipoprotein metabolism.

Table 4 Source and metabolic control of pancreatic endocrine function

	Source	Stimuli for release	Inhibitors of release	Physiological role
Insulin	B cells	Glucose, leucine, inosine, sulphonylureas Secondary stimuli: free fatty acids, arginine, alanine, acetylcholine, glucagon, GIP	Hypoglycaemia, adrenaline, noradrenaline, somatostatin, insulin-like growth factor	Increases rate of transport of glucose across cell membrane Enhances glycogen synthesis and inhibits gluconeogenesis; increases protein, triglyceride, and VLDL synthesis in hepatocytes Enhances protein and glycogen synthesis in muscle cells Enhances triglyceride deposition and inhibits lipolysis in adipocytes.
Glucagon	A cells	Glucose, catecholamines Secondary stimuli: glutamine, alanine, arginine, vasoactive intestinal peptide	Insulin, somatostatin	Stimulates glycogenolysis. Promotes gluconeogenesis from amino acids Increases lipolysis in adipose tissue
Somatostatin	D cells	Glucose, arginine, GIP, glucagon, sulphonylureas	Sympathetic nerve stimulation	Suppresses pancreatic exocrine release of insulin and glucagon Reduces gastric motility Inhibits growth hormone-releasing hormone
Pancreatic polypeptide	PP cells	Protein intake, sympathetic nerve stimulation	?	Probable inhibition of pancreatic acinar and ductal secretion

GIP, glucose-dependent insulinotropic polypeptide.

Endocrine pancreas

Islets of Langerhans represent an endocrine organ consisting of four cell types: A cells secreting glucagon, B cells secreting insulin, D cells secreting somatostatin, and PP cells secreting pancreatic polypeptide. B cells constitute 80 per cent of islet volume and form the central core around which the others cells form a mantle. The principal physiological function of these cells is to maintain stable glucose concentration irrespective of substrate delivery.

B cells act as a sensor of glucose concentration over a wide range, with rapid equilibration of glucose levels across the cell membrane by the GLUT-2 transporter. The molecular basis for this sensor is considered to be glucokinase, the activity of which closely follows glucose levels. Enhanced glucose metabolism increases adenosine triphosphate/adenosine diphosphate ratios, which in turn blocks potassium ion channels, and the subsequent change in membrane potential allows an influx of calcium that promotes exocytosis of insulin-containing granules. Many other hormones, neuropeptides, and neurotransmitters also modulate glucose-dependent insulin secretion (Table 4).

Further reading

Balabaud C *et al.* (1988). Light and transmission electron microscopy of sinusoids in human liver. In: Bioulac Sage P, Balabaud C, eds. *Sinusoids in human liver; health and disease*, pp 87–110. Kupffer Cell Foundation, Rijswik.

Erlinger S (1993). Intracellular events in bile acid transport by the liver. In: Tavoloni N, Berk PD, eds. *Hepatic transport and bile secretion. Physiology and pathophysiology*, pp 467–75. Raven Press, New York.

Gumucio JJ (1999). Functional organisation of the liver. In: Bircher J *et al. Oxford textbook of clinical hepatology*, pp 437–46. Oxford University Press.

Kang S, Davis RA (2000). Cholesterol and hepatic lipoprotein assembly and secretion. *Biochimica et Biophysica Acta* **1529**(1–3), 223–30.

Knook DI, Wisse E, eds (1982). *Sinusoidal liver cells*. Elsevier Biomedical Press, Amsterdam.

Tukey RH, Strassburg CP (2000). Human UDP-glucuronosyltransferases: metabolism, expression, and disease. *Annual Review of Pharmacology and Toxicology* **40**, 581–616.

14.18.2 Computed tomography and magnetic resonance imaging of the liver and pancreas

C. S. Ng, D. J. Lomas, and A. K. Dixon

Introduction

Computed tomography (**CT**) and magnetic resonance imaging (**MRI**) are cross-sectional imaging techniques which allow excellent, non-invasive evaluation of the anatomical and parenchymal detail of both these organs. Diffuse and focal lesions can be demonstrated, and information on the associated vascular and biliary structures can also be obtained.

Both imaging techniques rely on the detection of a variety of physical properties of tissues, in the case of CT, on X-ray attenuation (essentially physical density); and in the case of MRI, on multiple factors including the radiofrequency response, proton density, and T_1 (longitudinal spin–lattice) relaxation and T_2 (transverse spin–spin) relaxation times of tissues. The successful detection of focal lesions within tissues depends on the ability of the imaging technique to identify sufficient differences in the relevant physical properties between the lesions and background parenchyma of the organ in question.

Major technological advances have been made in recent years in the speed of image acquisition in both CT and MRI. The main contributions have been, in the case of CT, 'spiral' (or 'helical') and multidetector technology; and in the case of MRI, improvements in the speed at which magnetic field gradients can be switched. These advances now permit breath-hold imaging in both CT and MRI. This has reduced breathing-related imaging artefacts, and has permitted the introduction of multiphasic or dynamic enhancement techniques following a bolus intravenous injection of contrast medium. This in turn has improved lesion detection and characterization. Multiplanar or three-dimensional reformation of data can, on occasions, improve the spatial appreciation of the anatomy.

In general, body CT is more widely available than MRI. Combined with its relative flexibility in imaging more than one body region, CT can be regarded as the current optimal investigation for these organs, even though ultrasound is often used as a preliminary and sometimes definitive investigation. The lesion-detection sensitivities for CT and MRI are comparable. Unfortunately, some lesions can be overlooked by both, or one or other investigation. In general, MRI has an advantage over CT in characterizing lesions, and is often used as a problem-solving examination. Although lesions as small as 2 or 3 mm can be demonstrated, lesions smaller than 10 mm are very difficult to characterize. If necessary, and technically feasible, tissue specimens for cytopathology or histopathology can be obtained by imaging-guided, fine-needle aspiration (**FNA**) or histological core biopsy (Fig. 1). New developments such as CT fluoroscopy and open MRI machines are likely to improve the interventional scope of these techniques, which can include therapy (for example, radiofrequency or laser ablation of neoplastic lesions). However, such techniques are still under evaluation and only available in a very limited number of centres. Some of the relative merits of CT and MRI are presented in Table 1. In many instances, other imaging techniques, such as ultrasound, angiography, and nuclear medicine, provide complementary information.

CT and MRI of the liver

Modern spiral CT machines are able to obtain images of the liver in a single breath-hold (in the order of 15 to 25 s). Lesion detection is improved with the use of iodinated intravenous contrast media. In certain circumstances, the sensitivity and specificity of lesion detection is further improved by 'biphasic' imaging during the infusion of intravenous contrast media (that is, during arterial-dominant and portal-dominant phases). This is particularly true for hypervascular lesions, such as hepatoma, which may only be detected in the arterial-dominant phase of intravenous contrast medium infusion (Fig. 2). For the clinician, this means that the likely diagnosis(es) and clinical questions must be conveyed to the radiologists in order to adapt the CT protocol appropriately.

MR imaging of the liver centres on T_1-weighted and T_2-weighted images (the latter employing 'conventional' or 'fast' spin-echo sequences, often with 'fat suppression') (Fig. 3). As with CT, breath-hold imaging is now possible, and 'dynamic' images during infusion of intravenous contrast media (for example, gadolinium–diethylene-triamine-pentaacetic acid; **Gd-DTPA**) can add sensitivity and specificity. The addition of 'liver-specific' agents may also contribute to lesion detection (for example, paramagnetic iron particles which are taken up by Kupffer cells) or

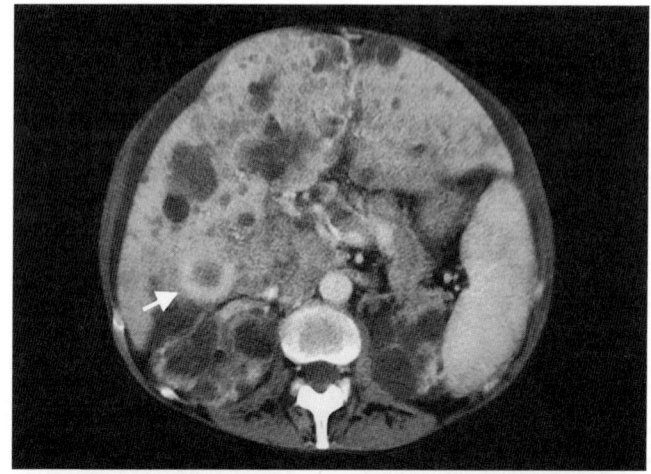

(a)

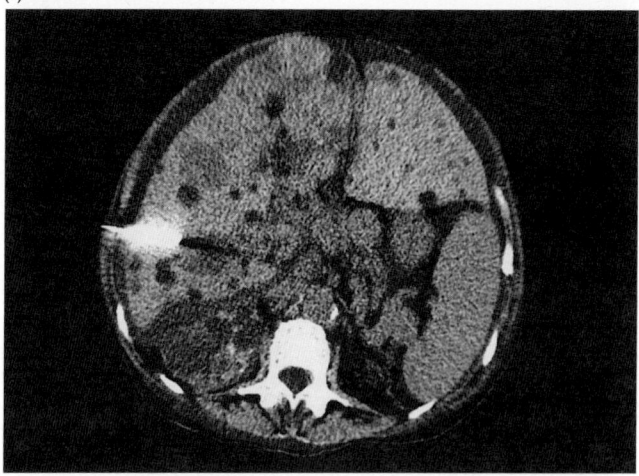

(b)

Fig. 1 (a) and (b). CT-guided biopsy of ring-enhancing liver lesion (arrow) in a complicated patient with polycystic liver and renal disease. This yielded adenocarcinoma. Note ascites.

Table 1 Relative merits of CT and MRI

	CT	MRI
Plane of section	Transaxial only (but improving resolution in reconstructed plane)	Multiplanar capability (typically, transaxial, coronal, sagittal)
Radiation source	Ionizing (X-rays)	Non-ionizing (radiofrequency)
Resolution	Better spatial resolution	Better tissue-contrast resolution
Contraindications		
– absolute	None	Ferromagnetic foreign bodies (e.g. cardiac pacemakers, intracranial aneurysm clips, intraocular metal
– relative	Pregnancy	Pregnancy, claustrophobia
Accessibility for 'ITU- type' patients	Generally straightforward	Generally difficult and requires 'compatible' equipment
Intravenous contrast media	Iodine-based	Gadolinium-based
– associated major reactions	More common; anaphylaxis, rashes, vomiting; renal impairment	Less common; anaphylaxis
Vascular occlusions	Inferior evaluation	Superior evaluation
Cost	Less expensive	More expensive
Duration of study	Approx. 15–30 min	Approx. 30–45 min
Body regions that can be evaluated	Wider coverage without significant additional time substantially, e.g. chest, abdomen, pelvis, brain	Evaluation of additional body regions generally increases imaging time
Imaging-guided procedures	Routine in most centres	Complex; requires special equipment

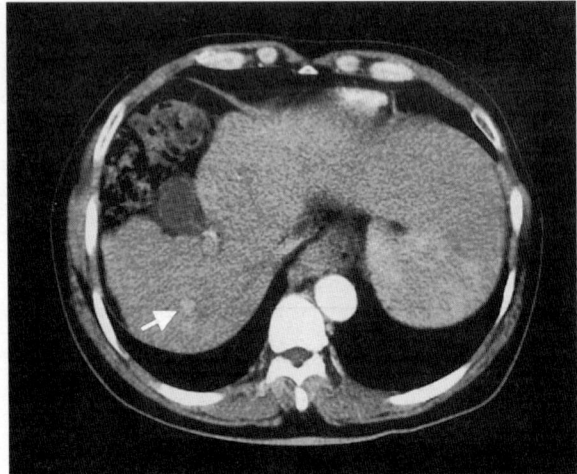

(a)

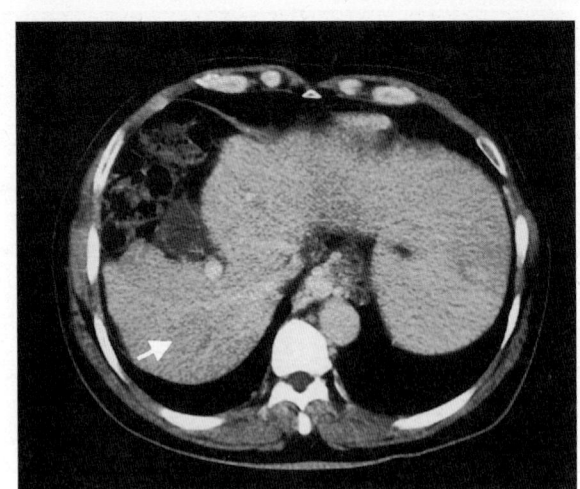

(b)

Fig. 2 CT showing hepatoma within a cirrhotic liver. Note the small shrunken right lobe. The small hepatoma (arrow) shows well in the arterial phase (a) due to the increased arterial supply. It is very much more difficult to see in the corresponding portal phase image (b), the conventional method of examining the liver.

manganese-based agents (which are taken up by hepatocytes). Flow-sensitive sequences can provide information on the patency or involvement of the major hepatic vessels.

CT arterioportography and CT following intra-arterial introduction of Lipiodol are further techniques that attempt to improve lesion detection; but these are invasive, requiring selective mesenteric intra-arterial catheterization. Both are subject to important artefacts, mainly due to minor anatomical vascular variants, which can cause false-positive results.

Focal liver lesions

The detection of focal liver lesions plays an important role in the management of patients with known or suspected malignancy. However, the differentiation between benign and malignant lesions can be extremely challenging. The former include cysts, focal nodular hyperplasia (Fig. 3), haemangiomas (Fig. 4), adenomas, focal fatty infiltration (and sparing), regenerating nodules in cirrhosis, and small abscesses/granulomas. Difficulties arise when lesions do not display their characteristic imaging appearances, and particularly when they are small (<1 cm). In addition, there is considerable overlap in the appearances of benign and malignant lesions. The overall accuracy of CT in the diagnosis of hepatic metastases is in the region of 60 to 80 per cent; high-quality MRI yields slightly better

results. Intraoperative ultrasound is generally considered to provide the best sensitivity. A key problem is the interpretation of a solitary small lesion in a patient with a known malignancy; such lesions are now commonly identified due to the advances in imaging technology; most will prove to be benign, even in patients with known malignancy.

Surgical resection for hepatic lesions, particularly metastases from colorectal carcinoma (Fig. 5), is a therapeutic option in many centres. CT and MRI can be used to determine the anatomical relationships of the tumour(s). For these purposes, the ability to delineate the functional divisions of the liver (Couinaud's nomenclature) is particularly useful from a surgical point of view (Fig. 6).

Diffuse liver lesions

Cirrhosis may be suggested in the presence of a distorted liver, an irregular liver surface, multiple hepatic nodules, or signs of portal hypertension (splenomegaly, ascites, or varices). However, in general, diffuse liver processes, which can include tumours and inflammatory conditions, are not reliably detected or characterized. Notable exceptions are the striking low CT attenuation caused by fatty infiltration (Fig. 7), and the abnormally high CT attenuation and low T_2-weighted MR signal intensity caused by heavy metal excess (usually iron; occasionally iodine following prolonged amiodarone therapy) (Table 2). In this regard, it is worth noting that the

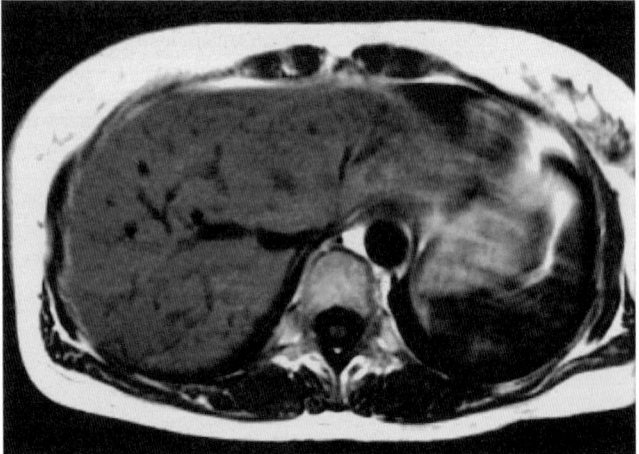

(a)

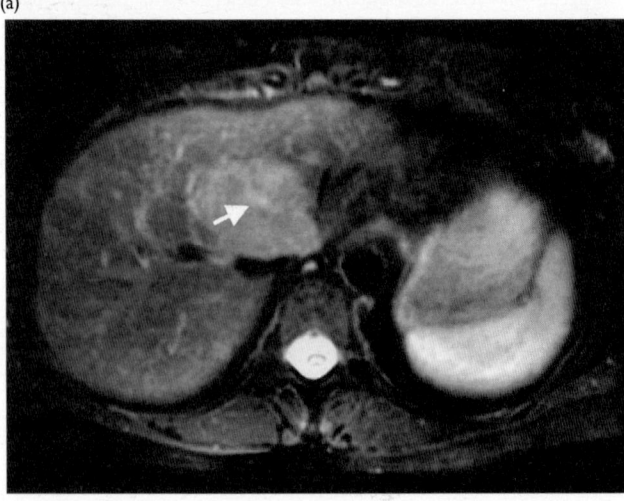

(b)

Fig. 3 Liver MRI. (a) T_1-weighted image. At first glance this appears normal. The intrahepatic veins are seen as signal voids because of the flowing blood. (b) T_2-weighted image. A large high-signal intensity lesion in segment IV is now apparent. This was focal nodular hyperplasia with a small central scar (arrow), which can just be identified on the T_1-weighted image in retrospect.

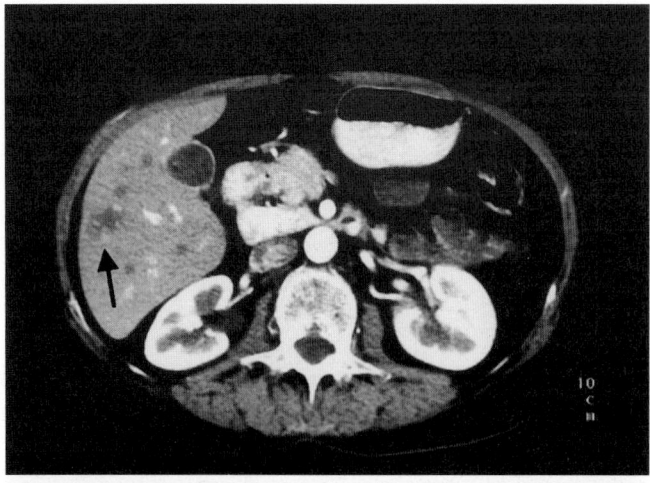

(a)

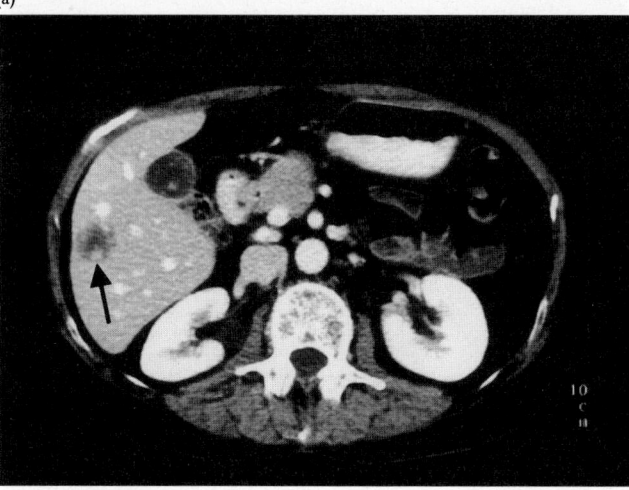

(b)

Fig. 4 CT showing liver haemangioma. On unenhanced images, the lesion had the same CT attenuation as blood in the aorta. It still shows as a low attenuation in the arterial phase (a). In the portal phase (b), it is filling in from venous lakes in the periphery (arrow).

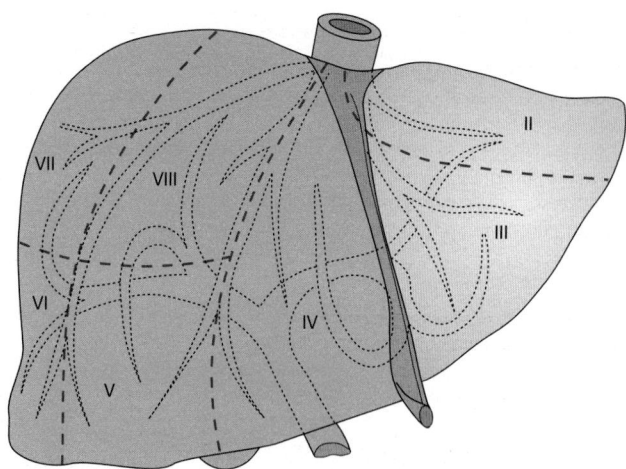

Fig. 6 Functional division of the liver and its segments according to Couinaud's nomenclature. (Reproduced from Merran S, Hureau J, Dixon AK, eds. (1989). *CT and MRI radiological anatomy*, with permission from Butterworth Heinemann.)

excess of copper found in Wilson's disease does not result in high CT attenuation; the excess is only in the microgram range; and the accompanying cirrhosis tends to reduce the attenuation.

Abnormalities involving the vascular tree can, on occasion, be detected, for example invasion or occlusion of the portal or hepatic veins by a tumour or thrombus. MRI, with its flow-sensitive capability, is superior to CT in this regard. Budd–Chiari syndrome produces a recognizable, but not entirely specific, parenchymal enhancement pattern. However, the key feature of an occlusion or thrombus within hepatic veins is not always reliably demonstrated by CT or MRI (nor indeed Doppler ultrasonography).

CT and MRI of the pancreas

The pancreas lies in a retroperitoneal location and its orientation in an oblique transverse plane is ideally suited to the axial planes of CT and MRI. Surrounding bowel and retroperitoneal fat are frequently helpful in delineating the pancreas in CT and MRI; conversely, these factors typically hinder ultrasound visualization of the organ. Although breath-hold, thin-section CT images of the pancreas are still anatomically superior to

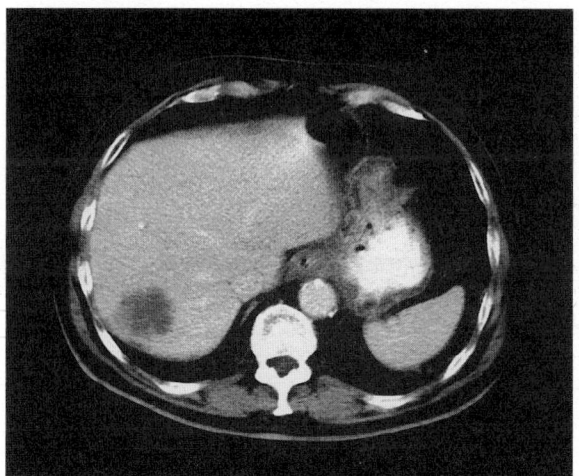

Fig. 5 CT showing liver metastasis from colorectal carcinoma.

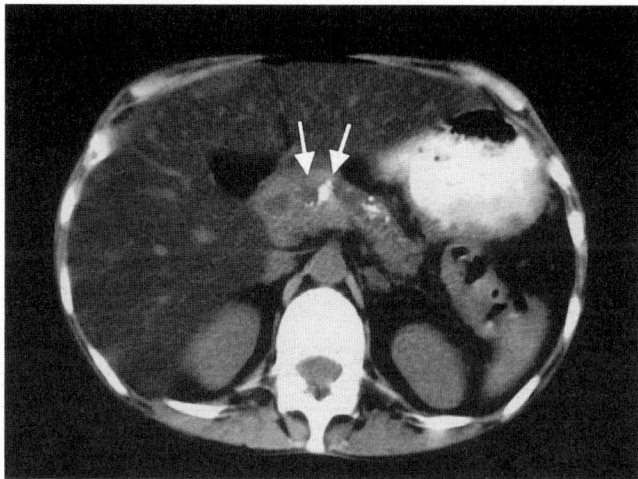

Fig. 7 CT showing a fatty liver and chronic pancreatitis. Dilated pancreatic duct (arrow), and calcification in pancreatic body (arrow). Note the markedly low attenuation of the liver (the normal density relationship of unenhanced hepatic vessels and liver is reversed), due to diffuse fatty infiltration (steatosis), which is turn is most commonly from alcoholic excess.

Table 2 Imaging patterns in diffuse liver disease

CT—diffuse low density (attenuation):
Fatty infiltration—excess alcohol ingestion, early cirrhosis, obesity, parenteral
    feeding, bypass surgery,
malnourishment, cystic fibrosis, steroids, Cushing's, late pregnancy, carbon
    tetrachloride exposure,
chemotherapy, high-dose tetracycline, glycogen storage disease
Malignant infiltration
Budd–Chiari
Amyloid infiltration

CT—diffuse high density (attenuation):
Haemochromatosis, haemosiderosis, iron overload
Glycogen storage disease
Amiodarone (iodine-containing), gold therapy (e.g. for rheumatoid arthritis)
Previous Thorotrast injection

MRI—diffuse low signal intensity:
Haemochromatosis, haemosiderosis (iron overload)

those obtained from MRI, the opportunities of magnetic resonance cholangiopancreatography (**MRCP**) images (heavily T_2-weighted, fluid-sensitive images) on modern MRI machines offer unique supplementary information about the biliary tree. The complementary role of endoscopic ultrasound, which continues to expand, should not be forgotten.

Acute pancreatitis

CT is generally considered the imaging investigation of choice, and can be valuable when the diagnosis is in doubt (Fig. 8(a)). On occasions, the causative distal common bile duct calculus can be identified (calculi in this location can be difficult to identify on ultrasound). Complications of acute pancreatitis may also be identified, these include necrotizing pancreatitis, abscess and/or pseudocyst formation, splenic vein thrombosis, and pseudoaneurysm formation. An assessment of the amount of viable pancreatic tissue can be made from the proportion of pancreas that enhances following administration of intravenous contrast media (Fig. 9). Differentiation between a simple pseudocyst and an infected collection can be difficult (Fig. 8(b)), but CT-guided diagnostic aspiration and/or drainage of collections can be undertaken.

Chronic pancreatitis

A diagnosis of chronic pancreatitis can be inferred on CT if there are the typical appearances of an atrophied gland with associated coarse parenchymal calcification and a dilated pancreatic duct (Fig. 7). However, the dilated and beaded pancreatic duct pattern that is the hallmark of early chronic pancreatitis on endoscopic retrograde cholangiography (**ERCP**) cannot be demonstrated by CT. At present, MRCP can only identify quite severe changes reliably; ERCP remains the 'gold standard' for subtle changes.

Focal pancreatic lesions

These include adenomas, adenocarcinomas (the most common), islet-cell tumours, cysts (which may be congenital, benign, or malignant), and focal pancreatitis. The role of imaging is in identifying the lesions, assessing treatment response, and evaluating surgical resectability.

Characterization of focal pancreatic lesions by CT or MRI is not well refined. Although, hypervascular lesions are typical of islet-cell tumours (Fig. 10), the majority of pancreatic lesions are hypovascular and there is considerable overlap in appearances. In particular, differentiation between pancreatic adenocarcinoma (Fig. 11) and focal pancreatitis can be difficult. So too may be the distinction between pancreatic pseudocyst, cystadenoma, and cystadenocarcinoma. In such circumstances, it may be necessary to perform to image-guided, fine-needle aspiration or biopsy. However, it should be emphasized that obtaining diagnostic material (for example, from pancreatic adenocarcinomas) is notoriously difficult, even for the surgeon who may have the pancreas exposed.

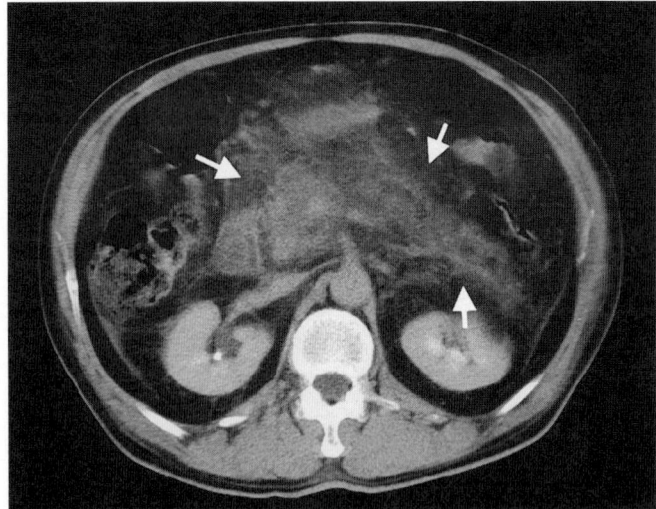

(a)

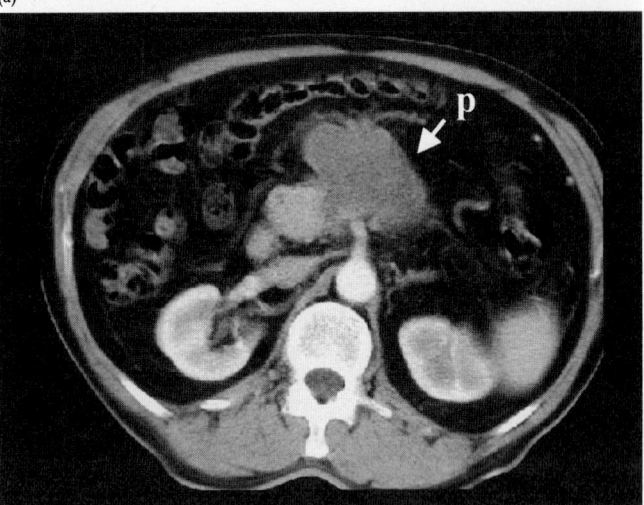

(b)

Fig. 8 CT showing acute pancreatitis progressing to pseudocyst formation. (a) In the acute phase note the poorly defined tissue planes (arrows), especially around the pancreatic head and Gerota's fascia. (b) One year later, the tissue planes around the pancreatic head are well defined, despite the distortion caused by the pseudocyst (p).

The accuracy of CT and MRI in assessing resectability in pancreatic adenocarcinoma is comparable.

Diffuse pancreatic changes

CT can show fatty changes within the pancreas. In type II diabetes, the outline of the pancreas can become irregular with increased fat within. In cystic fibrosis, the pancreas becomes fatty and will eventually atrophy. Similar appearances can be demonstrated by MRI.

Further reading

Bearcroft PW, Gimson A, Lomas DJ (1997). Non-invasive cholangio-pancreatography by breath-hold magnetic resonance imaging: preliminary results. *Clinical Radiology* **52**, 345–50.

Dixon AK, Walshe JM (1984). Computed tomography of the liver in Wilson disease. *Journal of Computed Assisted Tomography* **8**, 46–9.

Grainger RG, Allison DJ, eds. (1997). *Diagnostic radiology*, 3rd edn, pp 49–81, 1155–99, 1269–93. Churchill Livingstone, Edinburgh.

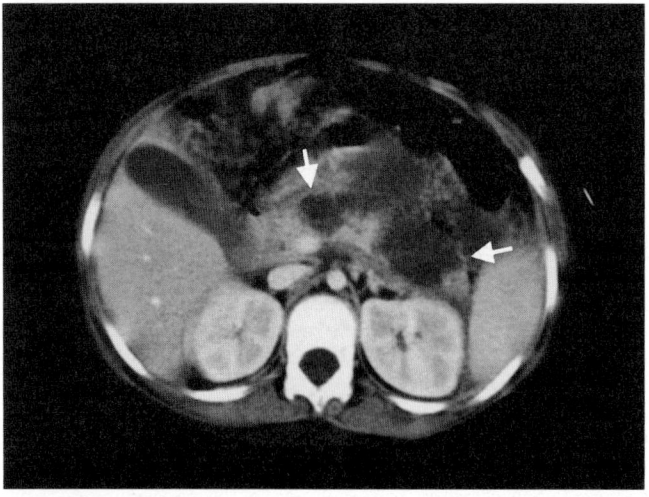

Fig. 9 CT of an acute necrotizing pancreatitis. Note ill-defined tissue planes due to retroperitoneal inflammation and non-enhancing foci following intravenous contrast medium (arrows), indicating areas of pancreatic necrosis.

Husband JES, Reznek RH, eds. (1998). *Imaging in oncology*, pp 129–90. ISIS Medical Media, Oxford.

Megibow AJ, *et al.* (1995). Pancreatic adenocarcinoma: CT versus MR imaging in the evaluation of resectability—report of the radiology diagnostic oncology group. *Radiology* **195**, 327–32.

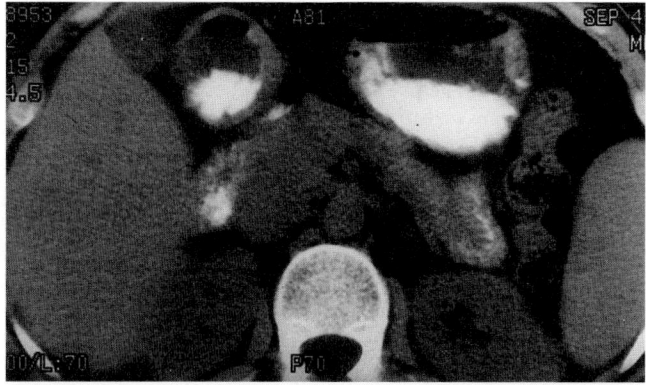

(a)

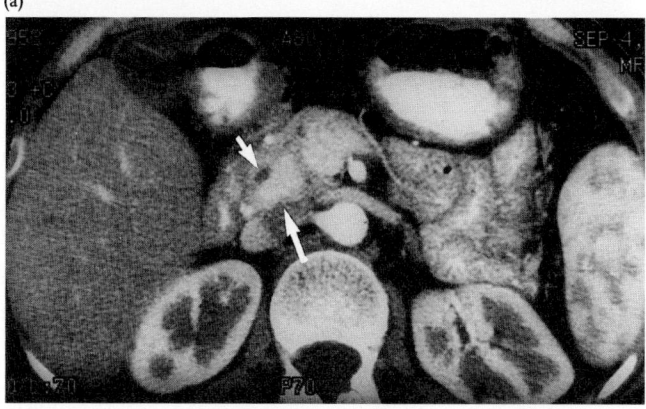

(b)

Fig. 10 (a) and (b). CT showing an islet-cell tumour of the pancreas. High-density lesion (arrow) adjacent to a normal common bile duct (small arrow) visualized on the arterial-dominant image (b) of intravenous contrast-medium enhancement (but not on the unenhanced image (a)).

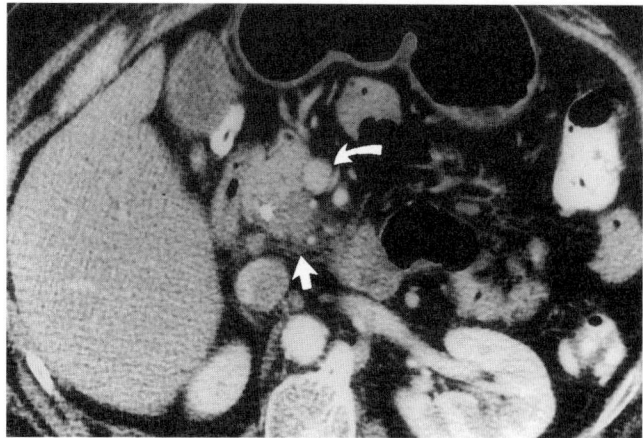

Fig. 11 CT showing a small pancreatic head carcinoma. A low-attenuation tumour (straight arrow), medial to a biliary stent, occupies the uncinate process and extends towards the normal pancreatic head. The superior mesenteric vein (curved arrow) and smaller accompanying artery are opacified well; they have normal adjacent fat planes.

Miller FH, *et al.* (1998). Using triphasic helical CT to detect focal hepatic lesions in patients with neoplasms. *American Journal of Roentgenology* **171**, 643–9.

Miller WJ, *et al.* (1994). Malignancies in patients with cirrhosis: CT sensitivity and specificity in 200 consecutive transplant patients. *Radiology* **193**, 645–50.

Ros PR, Payley MR. (1997). MR imaging of the liver – a practical approach. *Magnetic Resonance Imaging Clinics of North America* **5**, 415–29.

Ros PR, Taylor HM. (1998). Hepatic imaging: an overview. *Radiological Clinics of North America* **36**, 237–45.

Schwartz LH, *et al.* (1999). Prevalence and importance of small hepatic lesions found at CT in patients with cancer. *Radiology* **210**, 71–4.

14.18.3 Diseases of the pancreas

14.18.3.1 Acute pancreatitis

C. W. Imrie

Incidence and epidemiology

In different countries incidence figures vary from 40 to 500 new cases of acute pancreatitis per million of the population arise each year. Biliary disease and alcohol abuse are the main associated factors, gallstones accounting for 40 to 70 per cent of all cases. Older men and most women have biliary pancreatitis, while younger men develop pancreatitis due to alcohol abuse, as shown by studies of urban populations. This is typified by a study from Gothenburg, where, from the late 1950s to the mid 1970s, there was a change from a 68 per cent association with biliary disease to exactly same proportion with pancreatitis due to alcohol abuse.

In recent large population studies from Scotland and Finland the incidence of the disease has risen steadily to the current 400 patients per million population per year (higher figures from the United States are less reliable). From 1960 onwards, the mortality has reduced: it was 7.5 per cent overall in 1985 to 1994 with half the deaths occurring in the first week of illness. Death is usually due to multiple organ failure in which respiratory failure predominates.

Table 1 Aetiological factors in acute pancreatitis (according to frequency)

Major
    Biliary disease
    Alcohol abuse
Minor
    Post-ERCP
    Blunt trauma
    Coxsackie B virus
    Mumps virus
    Hyperlipoproteinaemia
    Ampullary tumour
    Hyperparathyroidism
    Worm infestation*
    Scorpion bites[†]
    Drugs
    Hereditary (trypsinogen gene defects)
    Sphincter of Oddi dysfunction

* Southeast Asia.
[†] Trinidad.
ECRP = endoscopic retrograde cholangiopancreatography.

Aetiological factors (Table 1)

Major factors

Biliary disease and alcohol abuse together account for over 80 per cent of patients in most prospective studies. With recent diagnostic advances, particularly the early use of endoscopic retrograde cholangiopancreatography (**ERCP**) and endoscopic ultrasound (**EUS**), it is clear that almost all the remaining patients have very small stones. Biliary sludge or bile crystals may also be indicative of a tendency to stone formation. Studies in the United Kingdom reveal that 40 to 65 per cent of patients have small gallstones. In Ohio in the United States a similar incidence has been detected, while in Argentina over 80 per cent of patients have been shown, by faecal sieving, to have small gallstones. The means by which the transient migration of small stones causes acute pancreatitis is not understood, but small stones which more easily exit the gall bladder to impact (usually transiently) in the ampullary area of the bile duct are a major factor.

Pancreatitis due to alcohol abuse occurs in over 80 per cent of patients from New York, and around 70 per cent in Helsinki. This association is usually found in young males who drink in excess of 80 g alcohol per day. Up to 10 per cent of patients have both biliary disease and abuse alcohol. Alcohol may provoke acute pancreatitis by acinar stimulation with simultaneous ampullary spasm.

Minor factors (Table 1)

Iatrogenic causes

Surgical or endoscopic procedures involving the ampulla of Vater can induce pancreatitis. The frequency of post-ERCP pancreatitis is increasing, even though the procedure only carries a risk for acute pancreatitis of about 1 per cent. Following a therapeutic endoscopic sphincterotomy the risk of acute pancreatitis is approximately 3 per cent. It is possible that failure to clear the duct of stones and inadequate sphincterotomies are the two most common predisposing features because they often allow stones to impact at the ampullary area. Manometric studies by patients themselves in a small group of patients with sphincter of Oddi dysfunction (SOD) are associated with acute pancreatitis in around 30 per cent of cases.

Viral infection

Viral infection, particularly mumps, coxsackie B, and viral hepatitis, can cause acute pancreatitis which is often missed. One clinical feature that may prove useful is prodromal diarrhoea, which is rare in all other types of acute pancreatitis.

Drug-induced acute pancreatitis

The drugs most commonly implicated in acute pancreatitis are valproic acid, azathioprine, L-asparaginase, and corticosteroids. However, unless viral titres have been determined, together with adequate biliary investigations, it is unwise to ascribe acute pancreatitis to a particular drug. Repeat exposure to the same drug again causing acute pancreatitis is the strongest evidence of a direct association.

Hyperparathyroidism

This is now recognized to be an uncommon accompaniment of acute pancreatitis. Indeed, many of the reported patients have also had gallstones. The association is calculated at 0.1 per cent. Removal of a parathyroid adenoma usually prevents further acute pancreatitis since persistent hypercalcaemia appears to be the provoking factor.

Hyperlipoproteinaemia

Patients with type I and V hyperlipoproteinaemia (see Chapter 11.6) may develop acute pancreatitis. The significance of this association can be difficult to validate. It has been found that acute pancreatitis associated with hyperlipoproteinaemia is rare in patients who do not, at the same time, have a high alcohol intake. Nevertheless, several experimental studies point to the importance of this association; patients with primary hyperlipoproteinaemia with chylomicronaemia and hypertriglyceridaemia are prone to attacks of acute pancreatitis in the absence of alcohol ingestion.

Hypothermia

This is a particularly important association in the elderly when pancreatitis may be associated with myxoedema coma. In younger patients, alcohol abuse may be linked, particularly if patients fall asleep out of doors or in a cold, unheated house.

Blunt trauma (Fig. 1)

This is a notable cause of acute pancreatitis, particularly in young children. Sports injuries from rugby, football, ice hockey, martial arts, and similar activities may result in acute pancreatitis, usually from a crush injury to the body of the pancreas against the vertebral column. Of greater importance numerically are victims of road traffic accidents when the diagonal section of seat belts is sometimes incriminated.

Periampullary adenoma or cancer

This is an important association, best diagnosed by ERCP. With the increase in this approach to diagnosis, tumours at or close to the ampulla have been shown to have a greater association with acute pancreatitis then hyperparathyroidism (0.4 per cent). Effective treatment of the tumour

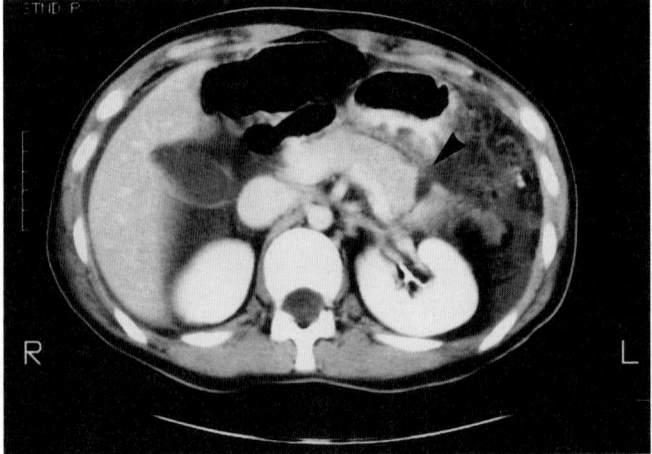

Fig. 1 Blunt trauma causing pancreatitis by transection at the arrowpoint on the CT scan.

Table 2 Rare associations with acute pancreatitis.

Hypothermia
Sclerosing cholangitis
α_1-Antitrypsin deficiency
Pancreatic cancer
Cancers metastatic to pancreas:
    Renal
    Stomach
    Breast
    Ovarian
    Lung
Virus infection:
    Hepatitis
    ECHO
Duodenal reduplication
Annular pancreas

abolishes recurrent attacks. This usually involves surgical resection, but in older less fit patients endoscopic laser therapy can be effective.

Hereditary

This form is increasingly being studied since the discovery of two genetic familial defects of trypsinogen (*N21I* and *RII7H*) have been identified with clinical acute pancreatitis usually presenting in children and young adults. Chronic pancreatitis follows from 20 to 50 years and an appreciable incidence of pancreatic carcinoma by 65 to 70 years. These cationic trypsinogen defects are autosomal dominant and shed light on the mechanism of acute pancreatitis.

Least common causes

The unusual causes of acute pancreatitis are listed in Table 2. The link with pancreatic cancer and metastases to the pancreas is well documented.

Microscopic pathology

All patients with acute pancreatitis have microscopic evidence of necrosis, while macroscopic changes, particularly black discoloration, are confined to the most severe cases. It is more frequent for this gross degree of necrosis to occur in the peripancreatic fatty tissue than in the pancreas itself. When present in the pancreas there is usually a panlobular necrosis and it is impossible to delineate where the disease initiated.

In a classical paper, Foulis claimed that the most common microscopic abnormality seen in humans, periductal necrosis, is typical of biliary and alcohol causation. Less commonly a perilobular necrosis is found, usually in patients with hypothermia or gross hypotension.

In experimental acute pancreatitis the initial lesion is now considered to be intracellular, featuring coalescence of lysozymes and zymogen granules. Acinar cell disruption is found with many of the hyperstimulation models such as caerulin-induced acute pancreatitis. It is now believed that this initial event may be associated with oxidative stress. Although this is very difficult to prove, it has formed the basis of some putative approaches to treatment.

Clinical presentation and laboratory abnormalities

Clinical features

Sudden onset of upper abdominal pain with vomiting is the most common manner of presentation.

The pain may focus in the epigastrium or right or left upper quadrant with penetration through to the back. Occasionally it encircles the upper abdomen. Patients who have experienced both a myocardial infarct and acute pancreatitis usually describe the latter pain as being much more severe. However, it tends to lessen in severity progressively over the first 72 h, and it is not usually a significant factor beyond this time. The pain on presentation is very similar to that of a perforated duodenal ulcer, but vomiting is less common in those with perforated ulcers.

Up to 90 per cent of patients with acute pancreatitis have troublesome vomiting in the first 12 h of illness, and this contributes to hypovolaemia and hypotension.

Patients with stones in the common bile duct may well be jaundiced and cholangitis can supervene in a minority. Much milder degrees of jaundice may occur from external compression of the lower bile duct in patients with alcohol-induced disease.

Hypotensive shock only occurs in very severe cases, but loss of circulating volume due to the extravasation of albumin, coupled with vomiting, leads to dehydration; the patient is thirsty, but fears drinking because of vomiting.

Bowel sounds are rarely present in the early phase of the disease and paralytic ileus may occasionally extend beyond 4 days. Despite these observations early nasojejunal feeding is possible even in clinically severe acute pancreatitis, and this is now a new therapeutic approach often begun within 48 h of the onset of disease.

The course of mild acute pancreatitis

Those patients who fail to meet objective criteria of severe acute pancreatitis tend to have a low mortality (maximum 2 per cent) and rarely need to be in hospital beyond 7 to 10 days. Simple therapeutic measures normally suffice through the first 24 to 48 h, at which time nasogastric suction and urinary catheterization can usually be discontinued. It is safer to assume that a patient may move into the more severe group and to provide early monitoring of the volume of nasogastric aspirate and hourly urinary output to maintain adequate fluid replacement. Even in this category of patients it may occasionally be necessary to provide 4 to 5 litres of intravenous fluid in the first 24 h of the illness. It is important to lower the risk of further attacks by clearing gallstones in the same admission.

The course of severe acute pancreatitis

Patients who meet objective criteria of severe acute pancreatitis may be pyrexial and are hypotensive, markedly tachypnoeic, and suffer from abdominal ascites, pleural effusions, and prolonged paralytic ileus. Body wall staining at the umbilical area (Cullen's sign) or in the flanks (Grey Turner's sign) can occur, usually appearing around the fourth day of illness.

Respiratory insufficiency or failure

Hypoxaemia is the hallmark of acute pancreatitis and reflects its severity. The basic mechanism of the hypoxaemia is unknown but high levels of various cytokines, as well as leucocyte elastase, are implicated, together with factors that contribute to localized intravascular coagulation. Shunting of blood occurs in the pulmonary vascular bed and accounts for up to 30 per cent of the cardiac output.

The initial clinical sign, which may easily be overlooked, is a fast respiratory rate; the patient may be cyanosed but there is no substitute for the measurement of arterial oxygen pressure. Almost all of the systems for objective monitoring of severity of disease include an arterial oxygen pressure of less than 60 mm Hg (8 kPa) as an index of severity. Hypoxaemia can usually be reversed by the provision of humidified oxygen, and in severe cases the pattern is similar to adult respiratory distress syndrome of other causes. Pleural effusions may be large enough to warrant aspiration, and when humidified oxygen is insufficient to reverse the hypoxaemia, assisted ventilation is necessary. Hyaline membrane formation has been found in severe cases, and even in milder cases complete reversal of the respiratory insufficiency takes many weeks.

Basal atelectasis and respiratory compromise are very common and must be expected. Urine output and arterial oxygen saturation must be monitored. Pulse oximetry is useful in monitoring, but arterial gas analysis may be needed three or four times in the first 24 h in order to make sensible decisions about humidified oxygen therapy and possible ventilator support. Single organ insufficiency or failure necessitates high-dependency care and often full intensive care management, as this may presage multiorgan failure.

The cardiovascular system

The initial hypovolaemia is of great importance in cardiac and renal function. Where cardiac output is more compromised and simple fluid replacement does not restore circulating volume, support drugs such as catecholamines may well be necessary. In the most severe acute pancreatitis the cardiovascular changes are very similar to those encountered in septic shock, with a high cardiac output and low peripheral vascular resistance. Stress on the heart may cause arrhythmias and ischaemic changes.

Renal impairment

Patients with acute pancreatitis are at risk from the development of acute renal failure which is related to hypovolaemic shock and the acute inflammatory changes associated with the illness.

The single most important corrective measure is to provide adequate fluid replacement. Low-dose dopamine may be a useful drug, and diuretics such as frusemide and mannitol may still have a place.

Additional measures are required in any patient failing to produce 30 ml of urine per hour. Most respond to increasing the rate of intravenous fluid replacement but more vigorous measures are necessary in the sickest patients, including haemoperfusion peritoneal dialysis or haemodialysis.

Biochemical abnormalities

A multitude of biochemical phenomena are found in acute pancreatitis—various pancreatic enzymes are released that are useful as diagnostic markers. With acinar cell disruption, high serum activities of amylase, lipase, trypsin, chymotrypsin, phospholipase, elastase, as well as breakdown products such as trypsinogen activation peptide and phospholipase activation peptide, are all found. The cheapest and most durable of these measurements as a diagnostic marker has been the total activity of serum amylase. Levels over four times the upper limit of normal in blood are usually taken as diagnostic of acute pancreatitis, provided the clinical course corresponds. The serum lipase activity is a more specific measure and is now almost as cheap to measure; levels of twice the upper limit of normal are significant. Other body fluids contain elevated activities of these enzymes.

Measurements of serum trypsin and chymotrypsin activity or antigens are expensive and the antiprotease defence mechanisms are efficient at releasing α_2-macroglobulin and α_1-antiprotease (also known as α_1-antitrypsin) which rapidly counteract free trypsin and chymotrypsin within body fluids. Thus measurement of both trypsin and chymotrypsin can be unrewarding while measurement of urinary trypsinogen activation peptide shows good potential. This small peptide molecule is excreted in urine very early in the disease course in patients with severe acute pancreatitis. It is therefore a good measure of the degree of disruption of acinar cells and a commercial assay is now available. This may be a valuable investigation for both diagnosis and for gauging severity of acute pancreatitis.

For many years it was believed that the antiprotease defence mechanisms required supplementation in patients with acute pancreatitis. Thus aprotinin (Trasylol), gabexate mesilate (FOY), and purified plasma derivatives have been administered intravenously in the hope of improving the clinical course. It is now clear, however, that the antiprotease defence system is intact and that there is no need to boost it—a conclusion that is supported by many clinical trials. Aprotinin was also given into the peritoneal cavity in the hope that it would improve survival and reduce complications, but was unsuccessful.

Very high concentrations of circulating cytokines are found in the blood at an early stage in the disease. The proinflammatory tumour necrosis factor-α, platelet activating factor, and interleukin 6 are present in greatest concentration in those with severe pancreatitis. The stimulus to the release of cytokines is thought to be endotoxin, probably from the gut, and there is great interest in the possibility of administering agents that inhibit endotoxin or the cytokines as a potential therapy. Alternatively exogenous interleukin 10 (an anti-inflammatory cytokine) may move from experimental to clinical use, but early clinical studies of post-ERCP pancreatitis have produced conflicting results.

Calcium-albumin

It has long been known that hypocalcaemia is a feature of acute pancreatitis; however, a significant proportion of patients have only a drop in protein-bound calcium and the primary pathology is the loss of albumin from the intravascular space rather than decreased ionized calcium. However, even after correction factors are applied there is an undoubted tendency for serum ionized calcium to fall; this is usually counteracted by a marked elevation in parathyroid hormone.

Haematological abnormalities

There is marked haemoconcentration associated with hypovolaemia so that initial haemoglobin levels of over 16 g/100 ml may be found. After rehydration, the haemoglobin level falls but it is unusual for blood transfusion to be required as the degree of haemorrhage in and around the pancreas is usually not of great moment. Later in the course of the disease, bleeding from gastric erosions, peptic ulcer, or haemorrhage into a pseudocyst may require blood products and endoscopic, angiographic, or surgical intervention.

In addition the acute-phase response results in high levels of liver-derived C-reactive protein, α_1-antiprotease, factor V, factor VIII, and fibrinogen. Platelet and α_2-macroglobulin levels fall in the first week, usually returning to normal by days 8 to 10. The common finding in patients with severe acute pancreatitis is hypercoagulation, and disseminated intravascular coagulation, while it does occur, is very uncommon; its management is considered in Section 22. The rapidity of mediator response makes leucocyte elastase, tumour necrosis factor-α, and interleukin 6 potentially excellent markers of severity; C-reactive protein levels in excess of 150 mg/litre, are another useful marker of severity.

Pyrexia

This reflects cell damage and necrosis as with any condition associated with tissue destruction. A low-grade fever is typical of the first 3 to 4 days of illness. Especially in those who have the clinical signs of obstructive jaundice, ascending cholangitis should be suspected and appropriate antimicrobials given. In the most severely ill patients, transudation of bacteria from the transverse colon into necrotic tissue around the pancreas, and occasionally in the gland itself, has been detected within 48 to 96 h of onset, although it is more typical to find such sepsis at a later stage.

Making an accurate diagnosis

The diagnosis is usually made from the clinical presentation, particularly the rapid onset of upper abdominal pain and vomiting. Gross elevations of amylase and lipase in blood usually support the diagnosis, while urinary amylase levels of greater than four times the upper limit of normal can be helpful in less typical cases.

Peritoneal aspiration (after catheterization of the urinary bladder and nasogastric intubation) can be used where diagnostic doubt still exists. The aspiration of more than 20 ml of free fluid without bacterial contamination (evident by smell and Gram stain) is indicative of a severe form of the disease. The darker the colour of the fluid, the more severe the disease. This

Table 3 Differential diagnosis of acute pancreatitis

Perforated duodenal ulcer
Acute cholangitis*
Acute cholecystitis*
Mesenteric ischaemia/infarction
Small bowel obstruction/perforation
Atypical myocardial infarction*
Ectopic pregnancy
Renal failure
Macroamylasaemia
Dissecting aortic aneurysm
Diabetic ketoacidosis

* Amylase is usually normal.

Table 4 Glasgow prognostic score—three or more prognostic factors indicates severe acute pancreatitis

WBC > 15 000/mm³
Glucose > 10 mmol/l (no diabetic history)
Urea > 16 mmol/l (despite intravenous infusion)
PO_2 < 8 kPA (60 mmHg)
Albumin < 32 g/l
Calcium < 2.0 mmol/l
LDH > 600 iu/l
AST/ALT > 200 units/l

Abbreviations: WBC, white blood count; LDH, lactate dehydrogenase; AST, serum aspartate aminotransferase; ALT, serum alanine aminotransferase; iu, international unit.

procedure is especially effective in patients with alcohol-induced acute pancreatitis. The presence of bacterial contamination indicates an alternative diagnosis and the need for an immediate laparotomy, as visceral perforation of the duodenum or small bowel is more likely.

Computed tomography (**CT**) will reveal pancreatic swelling, fluid collection, and change in density of the gland. Contrast enhanced CT scanning is mandatory to identify areas of pancreatic ischaemia and infarction. Magnetic resonance (**MR**) scanning may ultimately replace contrast enhanced CT scanning in this area. Either CT or MR can help in the difficult diagnosis.

Differential diagnosis (Table 3)

A dissecting aortic aneurysm usually presents with an initial history of chest pain in a known hypertensive; abdominal pain and loss of arterial pulses may occur later. A minor degree of pancreatitis due to ischaemia of the pancreas should not obscure the main diagnosis. Elevated amylase activities are frequently present in patients with renal failure, while a lifetime of high amylase occurs in those with macroamylasaemia; failure to filter the amylase complex results in very low urine levels.

High amylase activity in ectopic pregnancy derives from the fallopian tubes but the clinical presentation should not be mistaken for acute pancreatitis. Patients with diabetic ketoacidosis may occasionally have very high levels of amylase but this should not distract from the diagnosis.

Small bowel obstruction is associated with multiple gas–fluid interfaces on erect abdominal radiographs. The differentiation from an early perforated duodenal ulcer (less than 5 h) will rest on the combination of the finding of free gas under the diaphragm on radiographs and the lack of a significant rise in blood amylase to greater than twice the upper limits at the acute stage of illness. A more difficult diagnostic problem arises in the patient who has had a perforated duodenal ulcer for some hours because a marked elevation of serum amylase can occur. Similarly, mesenteric ischaemia or infarction can be associated with biochemical changes akin to those of acute pancreatitis, but in both these situations bacterial contamination of the peritoneal cavity will be detected by peritoneal aspiration.

Grading disease severity

The importance of objective grading of disease severity is that less experienced clinicians can direct the more serious cases to high-dependency or intensive care facilities at an early stage of their illness, or instigate contrast enhanced CT scanning and early ERCP for patients who will derive most benefit. Grading is also useful for trials of different forms of therapy.

The original Ranson grading system of 11 prognostic factors was developed for patients with acute pancreatitis due to alcohol abuse but later a system was introduced for those with gallstones. An alternative single system, validated for both the common causes, is the Glasgow scoring system of eight prognostic factors (Table 4). Validation came from a multi-

centre randomized British study that assessed the place of peritoneal lavage in the management of severe acute pancreatitis.

Atlanta criteria

In 1992 in Atlanta an international conference on disease nomenclature decided that severe acute pancreatitis was the presence of failure of one or more organs or the development of a major later complication—infected necrosis, abscess, or pseudocyst.

CT scanning

This can be very useful in confirming the diagnosis and also to grade severity of disease (Table 5). This is not a more accurate system of grading than the Glasgow score but it is very helpful in assessing an individual patient (Fig. 2). It is expensive and is not usually necessary in the initial few days of illness. The area of non-perfused pancreas corresponds to the extent of necrosis. Greater than 50 per cent necrosis (especially if the head of the pancreas is involved) is associated with the most severe disease.

The APACHE II system (Fig. 3)

This can be used to grade the severity of many diseases and has been shown to be useful in acute pancreatitis. It takes time for an individual clinician to learn to use the system, but it has the advantage that it can be applied throughout the first week of illness. The higher the score the worse the prognosis. Patients with the most severe acute pancreatitis have scores in excess of 10. A recent large (more than 1500 patients) clinical study assessing the potential role of a platelet activating factor antagonist in the management of higher-risk patients revealed major concerns about an entry criterion of an admission APACHE score of greater 6 or greater to select patients as the mortality rate in each of three groups of approximately 500 patients was less than 10 per cent.

Organ failure scoring

Clinical assessment by an expert is probably better than any of the other systems described at identifying the most ill patients. Quantification of the clinical assessment by scoring 0 to 4 points for each of several organ systems has revealed that 44 per cent of patients with an APACHE II score of 6 or more will show an organ failure score of 2 or more at admission. Most of these improve with supportive intravenous fluids and oxygen, but roughly a third continue with this degree of organ failure score or deteriorate.

It is this dynamic aspect of organ failure that is not recognized by the Atlanta criteria and probably caused most problems in previous grading

Table 5 Role of surgery in acute pancreatitis

To establish diagnosis without laparotomy
To remove gallstones within the same admission, if possible
To remove infected necrotic tissue in the most severe cases and possibly to remove non-infected necrotic tissue
To drain pseudocysts

systems. In the group who do not improve after admission with an organ failure score of 2 or more, and those who later develop this feature, we have found (in prospective data collected from 121 patients in Glasgow) a mortality in excess of 50 per cent. The application of such a scoring system for organ compromise and failure has the promise of greater accurary than Ranson, Glasgow, or APACHE II methods.

Obesity

Morbid obesity is usually described as a body mass index of over 40 kg/m^2. Acute pancreatitis carries a significantly higher mortality and morbidity in patients with a body mass index greater than 30 kg/m^2 (obesity) mainly because of increased risk of hypoxaemia but also from other associated factors.

C-reactive protein

Being an acute-phase reactant the main value of this marker is around 36 to 48 h of illness when the baseline levels of less than 10 mg/litre are far greater in those with severe acute pancreatitis. A cut-off at 150 mg/litre is a useful guide in groups of patients being assessed, but rogue results occur (Fig. 4). Of all the simple markers of severity, most experience has been gained with C-reactive protein. Values between 200 and 600 mg/litre are

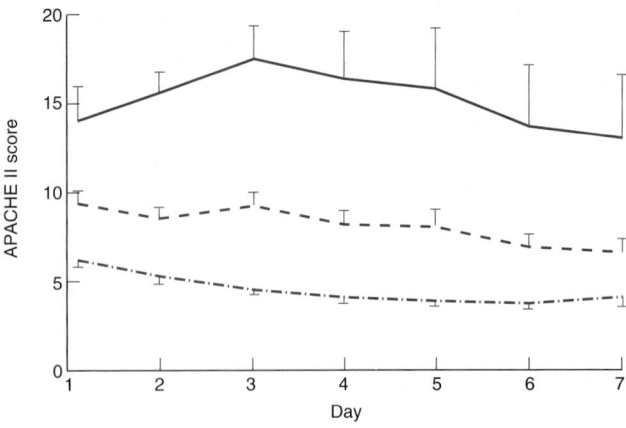

Fig. 3 Mean daily APACHE II scores by outcome in 119 patients with an uncomplicated course (–●–●–), 26 patients with a complicated course (– – – –), and 12 patients with a fatal outcome (—). The differences between fatal and uncomplicated and between complicated and uncomplicated were highly significant ($p < 0.001$) for each day (Mann–Whitney U test). (Published with permission from the *British Journal of Surgery*.)

found in the most severely ill patients. The test is cheap and easily performed.

Serum amyloid A

Prelimary studies measuring this substance hold considerable promise that it may be the most useful single marker of disease severity.

Trypsinogen activation peptide

The activation of trypsinogen releases trypsin and a small peptide (trypsinogen activation peptide) that passes unchanged in the urine, where its level can be used as a marker of severity. It has now been employed in two clinical studies with the promise of this being a valuable step forward in assessment of severity.

Clinical management

Pain is usually treated with intramuscular pethidine or buphrenorphine; intravenous benzodiazepines may also be required in severe cases. The effect of the combination of intravenous midazolam and pethidine can be particularly difficult to predict and the combination must be used with great care. Morphine has a strong spastic effect on the sphincter of Oddi and is contraindicated. Haloperidol is useful in managing the agitation of alcoholics with acute pancreatitis.

Correction of hypovolaemia requires the rapid infusion of high-volume electrolyte solutions. There is a tendency to underestimate fluid requirements in the initial 12 h of treatment and monitoring the central venous pressure is essential.

Catheterization of the bladder to monitor urine output should be done immediately and a minimum flow of 30 ml/h obtained. Nasogastric aspiration is beneficial and both this and urinary catheterization can be discontinued at an early stage if the disease proves to be mild. In such patients there is little justification for the routine use of antibiotics or H$_2$-receptor antagonists as nearly all of them improve within a few days. If gallstones have been identified by ultrasound scanning, laparoscopic or open cholecystectomy should be done in the same admission to minimize the risk of

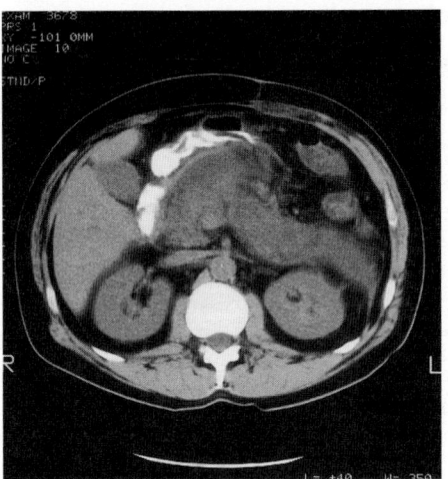

(a)

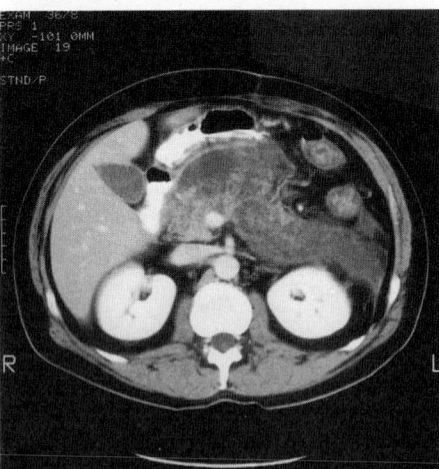

(b)

Fig. 2 (a) Severe acute pancreatitis with diffuse pancreatic swelling (CT scan). (b) Same scale level as in (a) with angiogram enhancement, revealing hypodense areas of poor perfusion.

recurrent attack. In older and infirm patients, ERCP sphincterotomy alone is considered a satisfactory alternative.

The severely ill patient

Those who are graded as having severe acute pancreatitis are usually particularly ill at the time of admission or within 24 h and warrant high-dependency or intensive care therapy. Monitoring for system failures and biochemical or haematological abnormalities is now routine. An algorithm for suggested steps in the management of severe acute pancreatitis (Fig. 5) is based on the United Kingdom National Guidelines published in 1998.

In addition to monitoring individual systems and providing support, early ultrasound scan and liver function test data may indicate consideration for diagnostic and therapeutic ERCP. Two controlled studies and a large body of clinical data indicate that endoscopic sphincterotomy in those with severe gallstone acute pancreatitis provides a significant therapeutic advantage. It has also been the author's experience that rapid improvement can occur in some of the most severely ill patients soon after early endoscopic duct clearance. The greatest advantage is in jaundiced patients with or without cholangitis. Intravenous antimicrobial therapy (as a single IV bolus) is recommended as a prophylactic measure during sphincterotomy

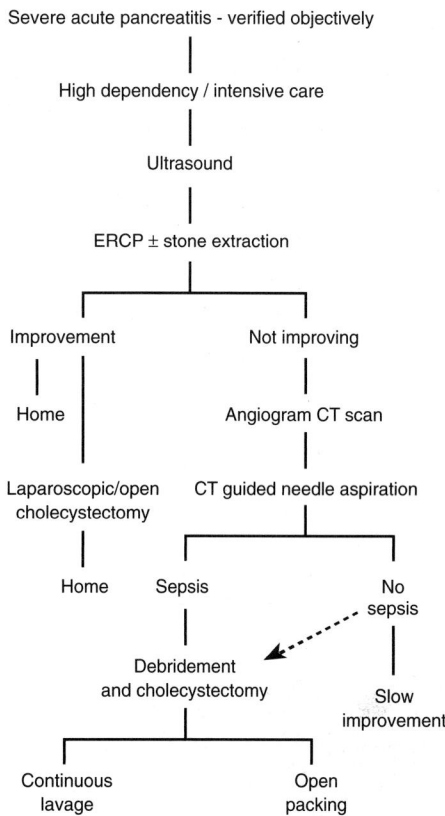

Fig. 5 Summary of management of acute pancreatitis.

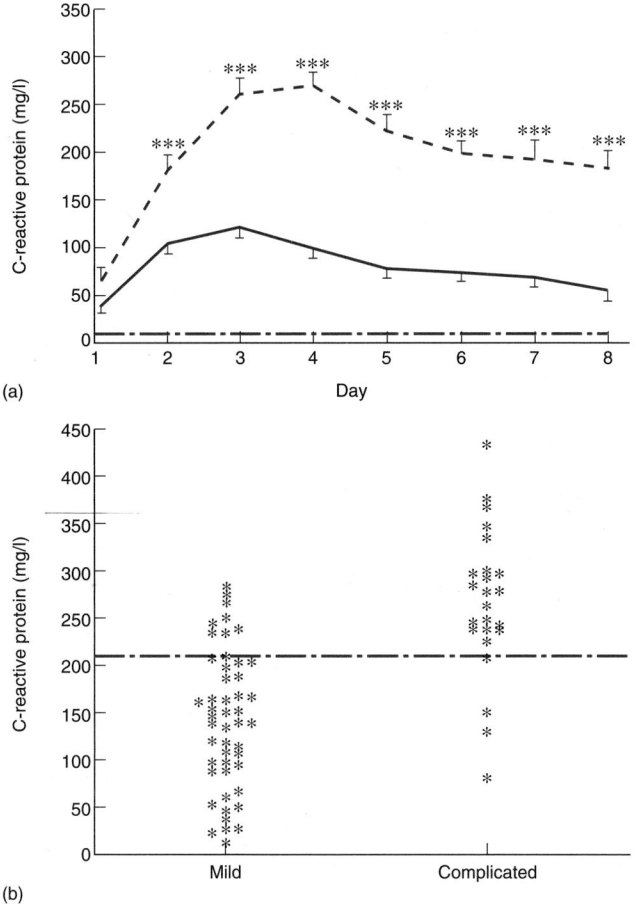

Fig. 4 (a) Sequential C-reactive protein concentrations in 47 patients with mild pancreatitis (—) and 25 with complicated attacks (– – –). Results are expressed as mean ± standard error of the mean: *$p < 0.05$; **$p < 0.01$; ***$p < 0.01$ (mild versus complicated); (— —), upper limit of normal for C-reactive protein. (b) Scattergram showing discrimination between mild and complicated attacks of pancreatitis based on the peak C-reactive protein concentration recorded on days 2 to 4 (— —). The peak concentration providing the best discrimination was greater than or equal to 210 mg/litre. (Published with permission from the *British Journal of Surgery*.)

and the drugs most widely used include the second-generation cephalosporins.

The prophylactic administration of parenteral imipenem to patients with objectively graded severe acute pancreatitis throughout the first 2 weeks of illness has been found to be of value in several studies, possibly because of its high tissue penetration. We advocate a more selective use of antibiotics depending on specific indications such as proven cholangitis, the use of ERCP, and evidence of infection by culture of organisms at percutaneous fine needle aspirate in patients with infected necrosis. Fungal infection can be a problem in long-term management of those with severe acute pancreatitis when broad-spectrum antibiotics are given for more than 10 days. The mortality of candida septicaemia was about 50 per cent in two recently published experiences.

Another approach has been to strive to reduce the concentration of intestinal organisms by selective gut decontamination combined with intravenous antimicrobial therapy, but this has only been done in one study of over 100 patients in The Netherlands; Gram-negative and fungal sepsis was reduced.

The reason for this attention to the lowering of the risk from sepsis is the belief that transudation of organisms from the transverse colon into the peripancreatic necrotic tissue is a life-threatening complication of this disease. While this is usually a late complication after the first week of illness, it has been claimed that it may occur much earlier. The majority expert view currently recommends parenteral use of broad spectrum antibiotics for the initial 10 to 14 days of illness in clinically severe disease but the randomized studies each contain fewer than 80 patients and the case has yet to be proved that parenteral antibiotics confer benefit other than lowering the incidence of pancreatic infection. Neither mortality nor morbidity have been significantly reduced.

Early nasoenteral feeding

The biggest single change in therapy of severe acute pancreatitis has been the revolutionary advocacy of early nasojejunal feeding previously considered impossible due to the supposed stimulatory effect on the inflamed pancreas. Clinical studies began with the experimental evidence (in acute pancreatitis) of very early loss of small bowel mucosal integrity and the possible protective effect of a peptide and carbohydrate feed. Encouragement was also provided by data from comparative studies of patients fed by intravenous and percutaneous jejunostomy in United States trauma units, which showed clinical advantage in terms of shorter intensive care and total hospital stay for enteral feeding.

A randomized study of 38 objectively graded patients with severe acute pancreatitis found that it was both safer and cheaper (fewer infective complications and £30 versus £100 per day) to immediately use nasojejunal feeding than parenteral feeding. Although there was no mortality difference, other trials demonstrated that early nasojejunal feeding was better than parenteral feeding in terms of enhanced antioxidant capacity, decreased levels of endotoxin antibodies, and a faster resolution of markers of systemic inflammatory response.

Clinical studies from Brussels and Glasgow involving almost 100 patients with severe acute pancreatitis have verified the practicality of early nasoenteral feeding within 48 h of onset, and this approach has now become standard practice in many hospitals. This is a rare instance of a clinical advance proving cheaper than its predecessor.

The role of surgery

Patients who develop infection in the necrotic tissue around the pancreas and in the pancreas itself require open surgical debridement of the necrotic tissue by a combination of gentle finger and forceps dissection; the necrotic material will not readily drain along percutaneously introduced tubes. After removal of the infected tissue there are two options. One is to establish a postoperative lavage system, which may necessitate up to three inflow and three outflow drains because of the tendency for retroperitoneal extension of the infected necrosis down the paracolic gutters and upwards towards the diaphragm. Alternatively, if venous ooze of blood is a particular problem, packing of the abdominal cavity with large cotton packs wrapped in non-adhesive paraffin gauze, together with limited or non-closure of the abdominal wall, has been advocated. Such patients are invariably in intensive care on ventilator therapy. The packs should be changed at intervals of 48 to 72 h, with removal of any extension of infection or necrosis. Abdominal wall closure and postoperative lavage may be established after the second or subsequent operations.

Debate continues as to whether only patients with infected necrosis warrant such surgical intervention Proof of infection depends on either the presence of retroperitoneal gas radiologically or the results of fine needle aspiration guided by ultrasound or CT scanning. Most experts advocate that uninfected necrosis can be managed successfully without surgical intervention, while others are concerned about the limitations of methods for detecting infection, and would therefore widen indications for surgical intervention. Irrespective of approach, the proportions of patients coming to this surgery vary between 4 and 15 per cent of those with objectively graded severe acute pancreatitis. Recently a method of minimally invasive decompression of pus and subsequent removal of necrotic tissue has been pioneered utilizing either a left flank retroperitoneal approach (80 per cent) or right anterior drainage (20 per cent); this is a promising development since it is less traumatic than open operation. A randomized comparison of the standard open approach with this minimally invasive one is now necessary to strive to identify which patients derive most benefit from each approach. Retroperitoneal pancreatic necrosectomy involves following the route of a radiologically placed guidewire at the time of fine needle aspiration (FNA). The track is dilated to 10 mm diameter using the Amplatz dilator system.

Gallstone eradication

Cholecystectomy and common duct clearance are indicated within the same admission in patients with stones or biliary sludge. The later complication of pancreatic pseudocyst has a higher morbidity and mortality in those with biliary than alcohol-abuse pancreatitis. This is largely attributable to postoperative complications of sepsis and haemorrhage, which are much more common in the gallstone group, particularly if they have not had the gallbladder removed at the primary operation. Thus all patients with severe acute pancreatitis coming to surgery should have a cholecystectomy, especially as it is often impossible to identify small stones/sand by either ultrasonography or palpation at operation.

Pancreatic pseudocyst

This condition is probably overdiagnosed. The 1992 Atlanta conference on nomenclature agreed that the fibrous wall around a pseudocyst took approximately 4 weeks to develop from the onset of acute pancreatitis. It recommended that the term 'acute fluid collection' be used at an earlier stage in the disease process because these frequently disappear spontaneously. Even established pseudocysts can spontaneously resolve in around 50 per cent of patients. For those not resolving, synthetic somatostatin therapy (octreotide) given subcutaneously three times a day may be helpful in speeding resolution although there is no evidence base for this view as no controlled study has yet been carried out.

Percutaneous aspiration alone invariably results in recollection of the fluid quite rapidly, while infection is potentially associated with long-term percutaneous drainage. In younger patients pseudocysts are best dealt with by internal surgical drainage to the stomach or a defunctioned Roux loop of jejunum. Cystogastrostomy has been done laparoscopically, an approach that can also be used combined with a cholecystectomy. Pancreatic pseudocyst most commonly occurs in the lesser sac and often represents a closed pancreatic fistula, as a breach in the main or major pancreatic duct can be demonstrated at ERCP. This investigation is potentially hazardous as it may lead to the introduction of infection and should not be done without an appropriate antimicrobial in the injection fluid or planned endoscopic or surgical drainage. In recent years endoscopic transgastric/duodenal decompression of pancreatic pseudocysts has been increasingly employed but the evidence that this is superior to surgery has yet to be provided. Likewise the alternative of the placement of a plastic stent along the main pancreatic duct across the breach in the duct has yet to be critically assessed against other approaches, but it can be very useful and is sometimes combined with transgastric/duodenal stent decompression. Endoscopic ultrasound increases safety by accurately identifying the optimum site of pseudocyst drainage.

Pancreatic ascites

This condition occurs either when a pancreatic pseudocyst spontaneously decompresses into the gut or peritoneal cavity or a major pancreatic duct disrupts after trauma (Fig. 1) or pancreatitis, with escape of pancreatic juice into the peritoneal cavity. Treatment comprises either a combination of intravenous nutrition and octreotide therapy or surgical excision of the disconnected segment of pancreas. Success has also been obtained with intrapancreatic main-duct stents placed endoscopically.

Rare complications

Rarer complications of severe acute pancreatitis include splenic vein thrombosis and subcutaneous fat necrosis. The latter condition can mimic erythema nodosum.

Further reading

Acosta JM, Ledesma CL (1974). Gallstone migration as a cause for acute pancreatitis. *New England Journal of Medicine* **290**, 480–7.

Balthazar EJ *et al.* (1990). Acute pancreatitis: value of CT in establishing diagnosis. *Radiology* **156**, 767–72.

Beger HG (1989). Surgical management of necrotising pancreatitis. *Surgical Clinics of North America* **69**, 529–69.

Bradley EL (1987). Management of infected pancreatic necrosis by open drainage. *Annals of Surgery* **206**, 542–50.

Bradley EL (1993). A clinically based classification system for AP: Atlanta International Symposium summary. *Archives of Surgery* **128**, 586–90.

Carter CR *et al.* (2000). Percutaneous necrosectomy and sinus tract endoscopy in the management of infected pancreatic necrosis: an initial experience. *Annals of Surgery* **232**, 175–80.

Corfield AP *et al.* (1985). Prediction of severity in acute pancreatitis: prospective comparison of three prognostic indices. *The Lancet* **ii**, 403–7.

Foulis AK (1982). Morphological study of the relation between accidental hypothermia and acute pancreatitis. *Journal of Clinical Pathology* **35**, 1244–8.

Gudgeon AM *et al.* (1990). Trypsinogen activation peptide assay in the early prediction of severe AP. *The Lancet* **i**, 4–8.

Heath DI *et al.* (1993). Role of interleukin-6 in mediating the acute phase protein response and potential as an early means of severity assessment in acute pancreatitis. *Gut* **34**, 41–5.

Imrie CW *et al.* (1977). Arterial hypoxia in acute pancreatitis. *British Journal of Surgery* **64**, 185–8.

Imrie CW *et al.* (1978). Parathyroid hormone and homeostasis in acute pancreatitis. *British Journal of Surgery* **65**, 717–20.

Imrie CW *et al.* (1978). A single centre double blind trial of Trasylol therapy in primary acute pancreatitis. *British Journal of Surgery* **65**, 337–41.

Kelly TR (1976). Gallstone pancreatitis: pathophysiology. *Surgery* **80**, 488–92.

Kivisaari L *et al.* (1984). A new method for diagnosis of acute haemorrhagic necrotising pancreatitis using contrast enhanced CT. *Gastrointestinal Radiology* **9**, 27–30.

Larvin M, McMahon MJ (1989). APACHE II score for assessment and monitoring of AP. *The Lancet* **ii**, 201–4.

Leese T *et al.* (1987). Multicentre clinical trial of low volume fresh frozen plasma therapy in acute pancreatitis. *British Journal of Surgery* **74**, 907–11.

London NJM *et al.* (1989). Contrast enhanced abdominal computed tomography scanning and prediction of severity of acute pancreatitis: a prospective study. *British Journal of Surgery* **76**, 268–72.

Lucarotti ME, Virjee J, Alderson D (1993). Patient selection and timing of dynamic computed tomography in acute pancreatitis. *British Journal of Surgery* **80**, 1393–5.

Luiten EJ (1995). Controlled clinical trial of selective decontamination for the treatment of severe acute pancreatitis. *Annals of Surgery* **222**, 57–65.

McKay CJ *et al.* (1999). High early mortality rate from acute pancreatitis in Scotland. 1984–1995. *British Journal of Surgery* **86**, 1302–6.

Murphy D, Pack A, Imrie CW (1980). The mechanisms of arterial hypoxia occurring in AP. *Quarterly Journal of Medicine* **49**, 151–63.

Neoptolemos JP *et al.* (1987). Acute cholangitis in association with acute pancreatitis: incidence, clinical features, outcome and the role of ERCP and endoscopic sphincterotomy. *British Journal of Surgery* **74**, 1103–6.

Pederzoli P *et al.* (1993). A randomised multicenter clinical trial of antibiotic prophylaxis of septic complications in acute necrotizing pancreatitis with imipenem. *Surgery, Gynaecology and Obstetrics* **176**, 480–5.

Pickford IR, Blackett RL, McMahon MJ (1977). Early assessment of severity of acute pancreatitis using peritoneal lavage. *British Medical Journal* **2**, 1377–9.

Poulakkainen P *et al.* (1987). C-reactive protein (CRP) and serum phospholipase A2 in the assessment of severity of AP. *Gut* **28**, 764–71.

Ranson JHC *et al.* (1974). Prognostic signs and the role of operative management in acute pancreatitis. *Surgery, Gynecology and Obstetrics* **139**, 69–81.

Viedma JA *et al.* (1992). Role of interleukin-6 in acute pancreatitis. Comparison with C-reactive protein and phospholipase A. *Gut* **33**, 1264–7.

Wilson C *et al.* (1989). C-reactive protein, antiproteases and complement factors as objective markers of severity of AP. *British Journal of Surgery* **76**, 177–81.

Wilson C *et al.* (1990). Prediction of outcome in acute pancreatitis: a comparative study of APACHE II, clinical assessment, and multiple scoring systems. *British Journal of Surgery* **77**, 1260–4.

Windsor AC *et al.* (1998). Compared with parenteral nutrition, enteral feeding attenuates the acute phase response and improves disease severity in acute pancreatitis. *Gut* **42**, 431–5.

14.18.3.2 Chronic pancreatitis

P. P. Toskes

Introduction

Patients with chronic pancreatitis usually come to medical attention with abdominal pain or maldigestion (diarrhoea, steatorrhoea, weight loss), but the frequency of chronic pancreatitis has been underestimated because of inadequate investigation of these symptoms. The realization that impaired pancreatic exocrine function can occur without obvious dilatation of the main duct, that is 'small-duct disease', has greatly influenced management. Symptomatic variability and the many causes of this disease have made its classification difficult.

There are three forms of chronic pancreatitis now recognized: (1) chronic calcifying, (2) chronic obstructive, and (3) chronic inflammatory. Alcohol abuse and/or malnutrition are the most common causes of the calcifying type. Obstruction of the main pancreatic duct with secondary fibrosis in that part of the pancreas proximal to the obstruction leads to the obstructive type. Chronic inflammatory pancreatitis is not well characterized and many patients with chronic pancreatitis of unknown cause fall into this group. Often irreversible changes occur in the gland, making a cure improbable. Nevertheless, the chief complaints of pain and/or maldigestion can be effectively treated.

Histologically, in advanced stages of chronic pancreatitis, the gland may be fibrotic and calcified and the main duct may be dilated. Inflammation and sclerosis with progressive damage to the acini and ducts are the histological hallmarks of chronic pancreatitis. Islet cells are usually lost more slowly than the exocrine part, so that diabetes is a late feature.

Aetiology

Table 1 classifies chronic pancreatitis into a number of different conditions associated with this disease. Chronic alcoholism and cystic fibrosis are the most frequent causes in adults and children, respectively. Gallstones rarely cause chronic pancreatitis because a cholecystectomy is almost always performed after the first or second attack of acute pancreatitis related to gallstones, after which the pancreas recovers. Hypertriglyceridaemia may cause chronic as well as acute pancreatitis. Some patients with chronic pancreatitis may have suffered autoimmune pancreatitis: they have had enlargement of the pancreas, strictures of the pancreatic duct, autoantibodies in the serum, elevated plasma immunoglobulins, and histology showing a dense lymphocytic infiltrate. A few have responded to steroid therapy. Tropical pancreatitis (Africa and Asia) is characterized by calcific disease, glucose intolerance, and infrequent pain. Pancreatic exocrine impairment occurs in patients with haemochromatosis and α_1-antitrypsin deficiency, but the pancreatic disease is usually asymptomatic. Secondary pancreatic exocrine insufficiency may occur after gastric surgery, leading to postcibal

Table 1 Conditions associated with chronic pancreatitis

Alcohol abuse
Cystic fibrosis
Malnutrition (tropical)
Pancreatic cancer
Gastrinoma
Trauma
Hereditary pancreatitis
Autoimmune pancreatitis
Hyperlipidaemic pancreatitis
Schwachmann's syndrome (pancreatic insufficiency and bone
    marrow dysfunction)
Trypsinogen deficiency
Enterokinase deficiency
Isolated deficiencies of amylase or lipase
Haemochromatosis
α_1-Antitrypsin deficiency
Postsurgery:
    pancreatic resection
    subtotal gastrectomy with Billroth I or II anastomosis
    truncal vagotomy and pyloroplasty
Idiopathic pancreatitis

(postprandial) asynchrony; usually the maldigestion is not very severe. Similarly, the acid hypersecretion associated with gastrinoma may irreversibly inactivate lipase, causing steatorrhoea. Hereditary pancreatitis and developmental anomalies leading to pancreatitis are discussed later.

Idiopathic chronic pancreatitis remains controversial and may account for up to 20 per cent of cases of chronic pancreatitis, depending on the population. Many patients with idiopathic pancreatitis present solely with unexplained abdominal pain and no evidence of maldigestion. These patients have small-duct disease, often without overt radiographic abnormalities. Direct intubation (hormone stimulation) tests are essential to identify this condition, although they are not universally carried out. Endoscopic retrograde cholangiopancreatography (**ERCP**), which is often used to diagnose chronic pancreatitis, may miss up to 30 per cent of patients with chronic pancreatitis who have abnormal hormone-stimulation tests. One questions how many patients with unexplained abdominal pain may indeed suffer from small-duct chronic pancreatitis! Some will be thought to have non-ulcer dyspepsia; others with idiopathic pancreatitis may present at an older age with painless diarrhoea, steatorrhoea, and secondary diabetes mellitus and often have pancreatic calcification.

Several investigators have documented mutations of the cystic-fibrosis, transmembrane-conductance regulator (**CFTR**) gene which functions as a cyclic AMP-regulated chloride channel in idiopathic chronic pancreatitis. More than 900 mutant alleles of the *CFTR* gene have been identified. Attempts to elucidate the relationship between the genotype and pancreatic manifestations have been hampered by the number of mutations. Two reports have shown *CF* (cystic fibrosis) gene mutations in 13 to 40 per cent of patients with idiopathic chronic pancreatitis (the observed frequency of a single *CFTR* mutation was 11 times greater than expected); moreover, the frequency of two mutant alleles was increased 80-fold. Most of these patients were adults with chronic pancreatitis, none of whom had any clinical evidence of pulmonary disease; the results of sweat chloride measurements were not diagnostic of cystic fibrosis. A further study examining all known *CFTR* mutations noted abnormalities in 55 per cent of 16 patients, 14 of whom had idiopathic chronic pancreatitis. Some of these patients with either one or two mutations had evidence of defective CFTR-mediated ion transport in nasal epithelium. It is not yet clear whether these CFTR abnormalities are primarily responsible for chronic pancreatitis or whether they are, at least in some cases, unrelated.

Pathophysiology

Although alcohol-induced chronic pancreatitis has been studied extensively, it remains uncertain as to whether the biochemical and histological lesions are caused by a reduced secretion of pancreatic-stone protein or alcohol toxicity. Ingestion of alcohol may decrease the stone protein secretion below a critical level, allowing calcium and other secretory components to precipitate and obstruct pancreatic ductules. On the other hand, alcohol may cause abnormalities in acinar cells, leading to an imbalance of proteases and their cognate inhibitors, resulting in the initiation of a necroinflammatory process. In tropical pancreatitis, a combination of protein deficiency and a dietary toxin that occurs in cassava or sorghum may be responsible. A primary defect in the permeability of the ductal epithelium to electrolytes in patients with cystic fibrosis reduces secretory fluxes, so that the hyperconcentrated proteinaceous fluid precipitates and obstructs the pancreatic ducts. The pathophysiology of the other causes of chronic pancreatitis is not understood.

Although it is widely believed that when a patient develops their first attack of acute alcoholic pancreatitis they have already sustained chronic damage to the pancreas, contemporary investigations indicate that some individuals who do not abuse alcohol regularly develop acute pancreatitis after ingesting uncommonly large quantities of alcohol (binge-drinking).

Incidence

The exact prevalence and incidence of chronic pancreatitis is unknown. Most opinions are based on clinical experiences, which vary greatly. The prevalence in autopsy studies varies from 0.04 to 5.0 per cent. The only prospective study (Copenhagen Pancreatic Study) found a prevalence of 26.4 cases per 100 000 population and an incidence of 8.2 new cases per 100 000 per year. However, this study mainly reflects alcohol-induced pancreatitis.

Clinical features

Abdominal pain is the cardinal symptom of chronic pancreatitis; its pattern, severity, and frequency vary considerably. Whereas the pain of acute pancreatitis is often located in the epigastrium and bores through to the back, the pain of chronic pancreatitis has no characteristic features and may be constant or intermittent. Eating often increases the severity of the pain, resulting in the avoidance of food and a subsequent weight loss. The pain may be mild, requiring no therapy, or severe, leading to the frequent use of analgesics and narcotic addiction.

Patients with abdominal pain may develop steatorrhoea and/or diarrhoea, or the abdominal pain may remain their primary symptom. Approximately 15 per cent of patients never suffer with abdominal pain but present with steatorrhoea, diarrhoea, and weight loss. In those who only have abdominal pain, there are few physical findings except for abdominal tenderness and mild pyrexia. There is a marked disparity between the severity of the abdominal pain and the physical findings.

Signs and symptoms of liver disease may be present in patients with maldigestion and weight loss due to alcohol-induced pancreatitis. Clinically apparent deficiencies of fat-soluble vitamins or vitamin B_{12} are uncommon.

Diagnosis

Computed tomographic (**CT**) scans may reveal diffuse enlargement of the pancreas and, occasionally, a pseudocyst (Fig. 1). Ultrasonography may reveal calcification and dilatation of the pancreatic duct (Fig. 2); calcification may also be seen on plain abdominal radiographs (Fig. 3). Blood tests rarely contribute to a diagnosis of chronic pancreatitis. The plasma

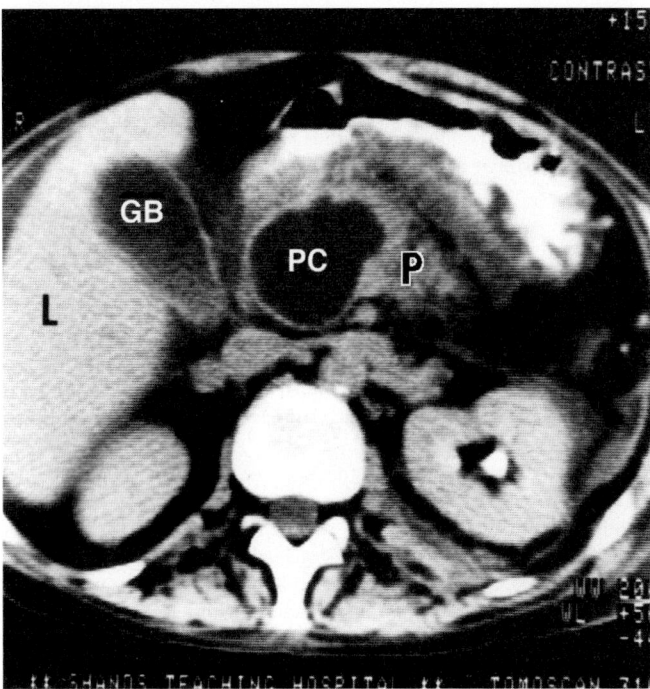

Fig. 1 CT scan demonstrating a pseudocyst (PC) in the head of the pancreas, diffuse enlargement of the pancreas (P), a normal liver (L), and normal gallbladder (GB).

activities of pancreatic enzymes (amylase, lipase, trypsin) are usually normal except in patients who have a pseudocyst of the pancreas. There may be evidence of cholestasis (elevated alkaline phosphatase, elevated bilirubin) caused by inflammatory reactions around the common bile duct. Some patients with severe disease may have raised fasting blood-glucose levels.

Table 2 lists selected tests of pancreatic function and structure, but abnormalities of function generally precede abnormalities in structure. The most sensitive tests are at the top of the table, the least sensitive at the bottom. Currently, the most accurate means of detecting chronic pancreatitis is a combination of a hormone-stimulation test and ERCP. As many as 30 per cent of patients with chronic pancreatitis may have a normal ERCP but an abnormal hormone-stimulation test. Occasionally the converse will

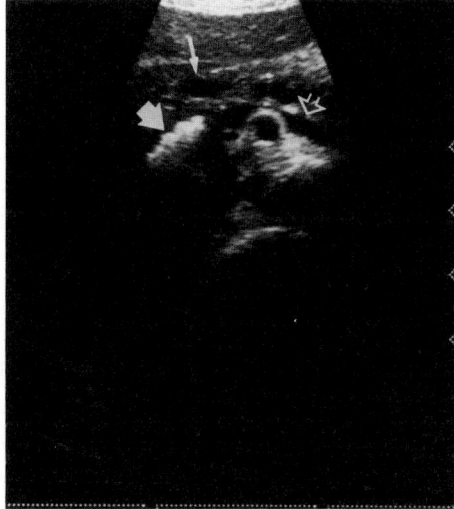

Fig. 2 Ultrasonogram of chronic pancreatitis. The large closed arrow points to pancreatic calcification; the small closed arrow shows a dilated pancreatic duct; and the open arrow identifies the splenic vein.

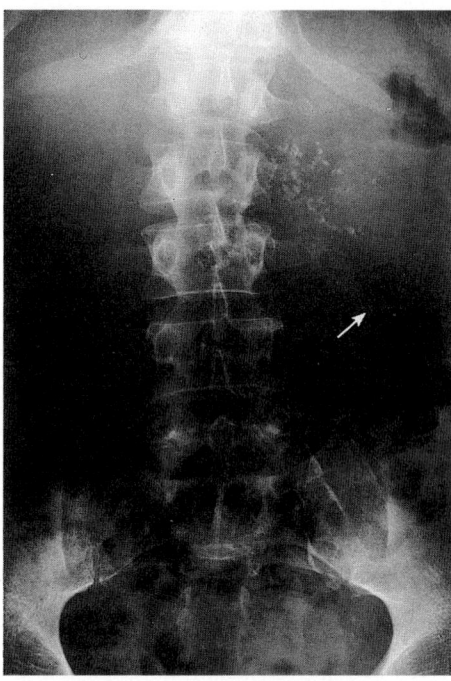

Fig. 3 Plain film of the abdomen showing diffuse pancreatic calcification; the arrow points to one of the calcified areas.

be true. The two significant causes of a false-positive (abnormal) ERCP are normal ageing and recent acute pancreatitis. Ageing does not appear to affect the hormone-stimulation test. Simple, non-invasive tests (bentiromide, pancreolauryl, trypsin) are not sensitive and are used to confirm the clinical impression. The same can be said for radiography other than ERCP.

Almost any test listed in Table 2 will identify patients with severe disease, but a hormone-stimulation test is often needed to diagnose those with abdominal pain only. Although it is generally accepted that a hormone-stimulation test is the most sensitive way to detect mild to moderate impairment of exocrine function, comparisons of the true 'gold standard' (histological examination of the pancreas) with any pancreatic test have been lacking until recently. The hormone-stimulation test correlates with the pancreatic histological findings obtained at surgery. A recent study found that the most discriminatory function was the maximum bicarbonate concentration, followed by volume and amylase output. A significant correlation was found between pancreatic function and histology. In 29 of the patients with histologically confirmed pancreatitis, the cholecystokinin–secretin test had a sensitivity of 79 per cent and ERCP 66 per cent. A simple, inexpensive test that has a sensitivity and specificity approaching that of hormone stimulation is needed. A cost-effective approach to the evaluation of patients suspected of having chronic pancreatitis would first be to use a simple non-invasive test like serum trypsin (or bentiromide) and to initiate pancreatic enzyme therapy if the result was abnormal. However, if this first-order test was normal, the next step would be to perform a hormone-stimulation test, and finally, if needed, an ERCP.

Relatively recent techniques for imaging the pancreas include magnetic resonance cholangiopancreatography (**MRCP**) and endoscopic ultrasonography (**EUS**). MRCP provides a satisfactory morphological assessment of the main pancreatic duct. However, this technique does not provide detailed imaging of the secondary ducts or even the main pancreatic duct if it is small. MRCP has been utilized successfully in elderly patients where the risk of pancreatitis from ERCP has influenced the clinician to not perform an ERCP. Endoscopic ultrasonography provides a detailed assessment of both the pancreatic duct and parenchyma. A total of nine abnormal features have been defined, and more than three criteria have been required in most studies for a diagnosis of chronic pancreatitis. EUS has replaced ERCP as a diagnostic modality in selected patients with suspected chronic pancreatitis. What is not yet clear is how sensitive and specific EUS is in defining abnormalities in patients considered to have early or mild chronic pancreatitis. In patients in whom only the hormone-stimulation test has been found to be abnormal will EUS be helpful in diagnosing chronic pancreatitis, but its sensitivity and specificity require further study.

Management

The cornerstone of the medical management of chronic pancreatitis is the use of pancreatic enzyme formulations. The principles of therapy are similar for treating pain or steatorrhoea. A potent enzyme formulation must be used to ensure that the relevant enzymes (protease for pain, lipase for steatorrhoea) escape destruction by gastric acid and reach the duodenum.

Abstinence from alcohol is recommended. The diet should be moderate in fat (30 per cent), high in protein (24 per cent), and low in carbohydrate (40 per cent). Non-narcotic analgesics are the pain-relieving medications of choice.

To date, three controlled trails have shown that pancreatic enzymes decrease abdominal pain in some patients with chronic pancreatitis. Pain relief was obtained in 75 per cent of the patients evaluated. Those most likely to respond have small-duct disease, that is to say a minimal to moderate impairment of exocrine function (abnormal hormone-stimulation test, minimal abnormalities on ERCP, normal fat absorption) (Fig. 4). Patients with severe (large-duct) disease (abnormal hormone-stimulation test, marked abnormalities on ERCP, steatorrhoea) (Fig. 5) do not respond well to enzyme therapy for pain. These clinical observations fit well with findings in experimental animals and humans, which demonstrate the negative-feedback regulation of pancreatic secretion controlled by the amount of proteases within the proximal small intestine. Treatment comprising eight tablets or capsules of a potent, non-enteric-coated enzyme preparation should be given at mealtimes and at bedtime, with appropriate adjuvant therapy (Table 3). Enteric-coated preparations are not the preparations of choice because they often release their proteases in the jejunum or ileum rather than the duodenum, thus failing to deliver to the feedback-sensitive segment of the intestine; these preparations may also cause acute colonic disease and rupture.

Figure 6 outlines an approach to patients with abdominal pain thought to be caused by chronic pancreatitis. After other causes of abdominal pain have been excluded, an ultrasonography should be obtained. If no pseudocyst or mass is found, a hormone-stimulation test should be performed; this will invariably be abnormal in patients with abdominal pain secondary to chronic pancreatitis. A 4-week trial of pancreatic enzymes (with adjuvant) is indicated, as described above. If pain is not relieved, ERCP is appropriate to characterize the pancreatitis as small- or large-duct disease, and possibly to define the surgical approach.

If there is large-duct disease (diameter of the main pancreatic duct greater than 7 mm), a lateral pancreaticojejunostomy (Peustow procedure) should be performed. Immediate pain relief occurs in 80 per cent of patients, with satisfactory pain relief sustained in about 50 per cent at 1 to 3 years' follow-up. If the ducts are not significantly dilated, most patients can eventually have their pain controlled by adjusting the enzyme and adjuvant therapy; for example, substitution of a proton-pump inhibitor for an H_2-receptor antagonist, total parenteral nutrition with no food orally for several weeks, or by performing a nerve block. It is now rare for a major pancreatic resection to be undertaken to control pain. In some preliminary controlled trials, octreotide in doses up to 200 µg three times daily given subcutaneously has been effective in reducing pain in patients with severe chronic pancreatitis. Whether ductal decompression or major resection are performed, enzyme therapy for enhancing digestion should be given.

Table 2 Selected pancreatic diagnostic tests

	Principle	Characteristics
Functional tests		
Hormone stimulation	Secretin stimulates HCO_3^- CCK stimulates enzyme output	Sensitive and specific, requires intubation
Pancreolauryl test	Fluorescein diaurate cleaved to release fluorescein which appears in urine	Will detect severe disease
Bentiromide test	Synthetic peptide cleaved to release PABA which is excreted	Similar to pancreolauryl
Faecal chymotrypsin Serum trypsinogen	Residual secretion Blood spillover	Insensitive, frequent false- positive/negative tests Highly specific; insensitive, inexpensive, and simple
Faecal elastase	Residual secretion	Unknown sensitivity, excellent specificity; inexpensive and simple
Quantitative faecal fat	Maldigestion of exogenous fat	'Gold standard'. Does not distinguish pancreatic from intestinal causes of fat maldigestion/malabsorption. Laborious; requires 3-day collection; expensive
Structural tests		
ERCP (see Figs 4 and 5)	Direct imaging of pancreatic ducts	Sensitivity 70%; specificity 90%. Differentiation of cancer may be difficult. Expensive, invasive—3% risk of acute pancreatitis
CT scan (see Fig. 1)	Detailed visualization of pancreas	Early detection of masses. Expensive; high-dose radiation; may not distinguish inflammation from cancer
Ultrasonography (see Fig. 2)		Simple, cheap, no radiation. Can provide information on cysts, phlegmon, calcification, abscesses
Plain abdominal radiographs (Fig. 3)	Diffuse calcification indicating severe damage; hallmark alcoholic pancreatitis	Simple, inexpensive; focal calcification seen in trauma, islet-cell tumours, hereditary pancreatitis, malnutrition, hypercalcaemia, idiopathic pancreatitis

CCK, cholecystinin; PABA, para-aminobenzoic acid; ERCP, endoscopic retrograde cholangiopancreatography; CT, computed tomography.

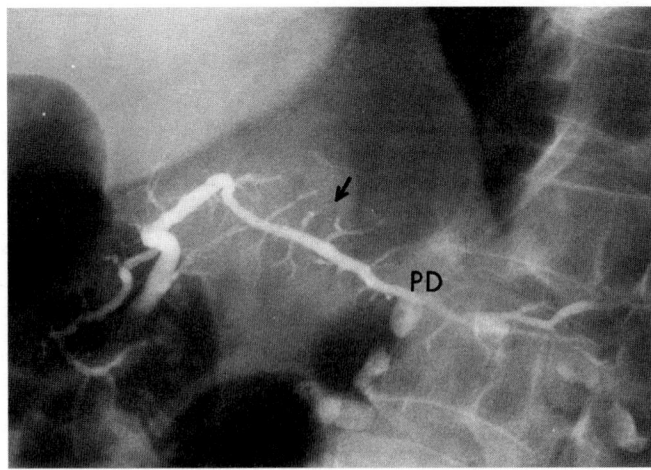

Fig. 4 Early ERCP changes of chronic pancreatitis. A non-dilated main pancreatic duct (PD) and accessory duct (AD) with mild dilatation and clubbing of the side branches (arrow) are shown.

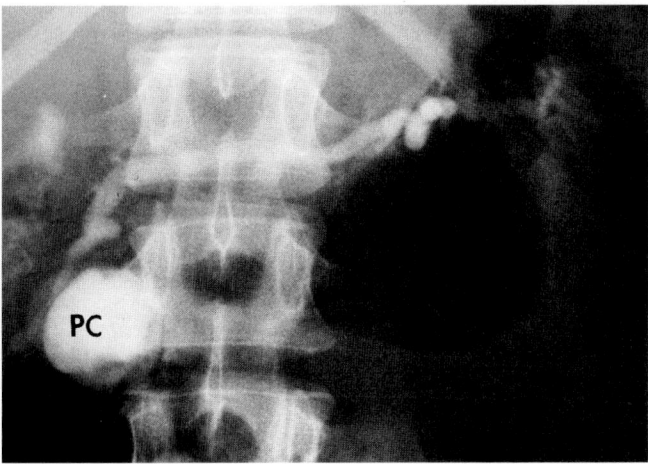

Fig. 5 ERCP showing a dilated main pancreatic duct with a communicating pseudocyst (PC).

Table 3 Frequently used pancreatic enzyme therapy

Pancrealipase
    Viokase 8 (C), 8 tablets each time
    Viokase 16 (C), 4 tablets each time

Pancreatin
    Creon (E), 3 capsules each time
    Pancrease MT (E), 3 capsules each time
    Ultrase (E), 3 capsules each time

Adjuvant
    H₂-receptor antagonist in usual acid-suppressive dose twice a day
    Proton-pump inhibitor in usual acid-suppressive dose once a day

The enzymes should be administered before meals; a bedtime dosage should be given if the enzymes are being used to treat pain.

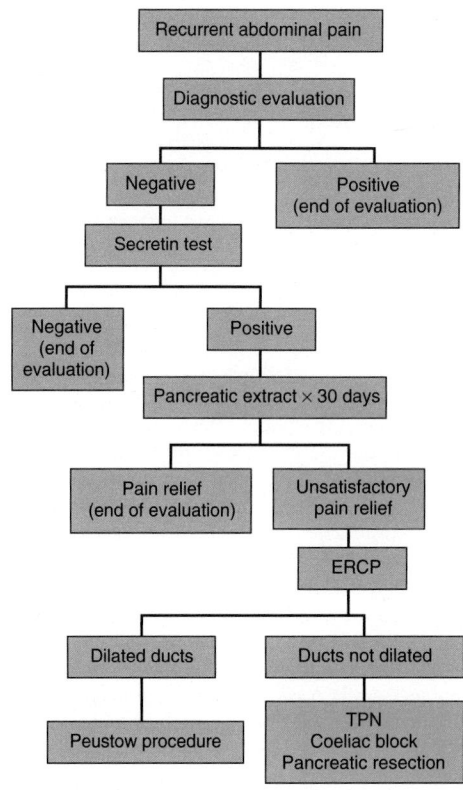

Fig. 6 Approach to the management of chronic pancreatitis and abdominal pain.

Endoscopic therapy for the pain of chronic pancreatitis has been disappointing. This therapy has included dilatation or stenting of duct strictures, removal of calculi, and treatment of biliary obstruction. With the exception of acute biliary decompression, none of these therapies has been shown to be effective. Complications such as bleeding, sepsis, pancreatitis, and perforation have occurred after stent placement; moreover, stents can induce progressive ductal changes similar to the abnormalities seen in chronic pancreatitis.

Steatorrhoea in chronic pancreatitis is a late finding and does not occur until lipase secretion is reduced by 90 per cent. With eight conventional or three enteric-coated enzyme tablets or capsules (Table 3), control of steatorrhoea and diarrhoea, and weight gain, can be readily achieved, even though some steatorrhoea persists. Formulations containing 25 000 units or more of lipase have recently been associated with the occurrence of colonic strictures in patients with cystic fibrosis who were taking large doses of these high-potency preparations. In the United States, all pancreatic enzyme preparations with more than 20 000 units of lipase per capsule have been taken out of clinical use.

Decreasing the amount of long-chain triglycerides in the diet and/or adding medium-chain triglycerides (which do not require pancreatic lipase for absorption) should decrease the steatorrhoea and enhance weight gain and energy.

Complications

Table 4 lists the structural and metabolic complications of chronic pancreatitis. Inflammatory masses are common. Ultrasonography and computed tomography greatly assist in discriminating phlegmon from a pseudocyst and from an abscess. The management of pseudocysts is currently being re-evaluated. Most clinicians have used drainage if the pseudocyst persists for longer than 7 weeks. However, the ability of pseudocysts to undergo late resolution may have been underestimated and the incidence of serious complications exaggerated. In patients with minimal symptoms who have

Table 4 Complications of chronic pancreatitis

Structural	Metabolic
Phlegmon	Narcotic addiction
Pseudocyst	Diabetes mellitus
Abscess	Cobalamin (vitamin B_{12}) malabsorption
	(deficiency rare)
Ascites	Subcutaneous fat necrosis
Common bile duct obstruction	Bone pain (osteomalacia)
Duodenal obstruction	Non-diabetic retinopathy
Splenic vein thrombosis	Pancreatic cancer
Gastrointestinal bleeding	

pseudocysts and do not actively abuse alcohol, a mature pseudocyst that has benign radiological appearances should be observed: nine out of ten such pseudocysts will resolve without complications.

Pancreatic ascites occurs when there is a rent in the pancreatic duct or a leaking pseudocyst. The amylase content in the ascitic fluid is extraordinarily high, averaging 20 000 IU/l. True pancreatic ascites should be distinguished from 'reactive ascites' in patients with pancreatitis. In reactive ascites the amylase content of the fluid while increased, is not nearly as high as in the pancreatic ascites. Pancreatic stimulation should be avoided in patients with pancreatic ascites, they should receive total parenteral nutrition and no food by mouth; proton-pump inhibitors or H_2-antagonists will reduce pancreatic stimulation resulting from gastric acid release into the duodenum. Surgery may be needed if the ascites persists after several weeks of conservative therapy. An ERCP may be needed to determine the site of duct leakage.

Although obstruction of the common bile duct is common, it may be temporary, due to the resolution of inflammation. Biliary obstruction due to fibrosis of the pancreas rarely leads to cholangitis. Conservative management is justified unless the alkaline phosphatase level remains very high or cholangitis develops. In a few patients, the obstruction may require surgical relief by anastomosing the dilated common bile duct to the duodenum or jejunum.

Gastrointestinal bleeding may arise from portal hypertension associated with splenic vein thrombosis caused by inflammation of the tail of the pancreas. Bleeding may also occur if a pseudocyst erodes into the duodenum or from a pseudoaneurysm within the wall of a pseudocyst. However, the most common cause of bleeding in chronic pancreatitis is a related duodenal ulcer or alcohol-induced gastritis.

Up to 30 per cent of patients with chronic pancreatitis have impaired glucose tolerance. Although pancreatic diabetes is usually manageable, destruction of glucagon-containing cells may render hypoglycaemia more likely. Diabetes retinopathy occurs as often in pancreatic diabetes as in other types of diabetes mellitus. Retinopathy due to a zinc or vitamin A deficiency may occur.

Cobalamin (vitamin B_{12}) malabsorption is common in chronic pancreatitis, but clinical vitamin B_{12} deficiency is rare. It is caused by the failure to release free cobalamin by proteolysis of transcobalamin complexes. The exogenous administration of pancreatic enzymes corrects the maldigestion.

Hereditary and familial diseases

Hereditary pancreatitis

Familial or hereditary pancreatitis is an autosomal dominant disorder with approximately 80 per cent penetrance. About 1 per cent of all cases of chronic pancreatitis is due to hereditary pancreatitis. Often these patients present in childhood with recurrent acute pancreatitis which causes chronic pancreatitis and often pancreatic insufficiency. The lifetime risk of developing pancreatic cancer is quite high. The genetic abnormality is a defect in the cationic trypsinogen gene that maps to chromosome 7, which appears to interfere with the inactivation of trypsin after it is cleaved. These

findings should prove to be revealing about the pathogenesis of idiopathic chronic pancreatitis.

Schwachmann's syndrome (pancreatic insufficiency and bone marrow disease)

This familial disorder affects the pancreas, bone marrow, and skeletal system. It is second only to cystic fibrosis as a cause of pancreatic insufficiency in infants. Unlike cystic fibrosis the sweat chloride test is normal. Neonates with this condition present with severe steatorrhoea. The associated neutropenia leads to frequent infections. The steatorrhoea is well treated by pancreatic enzymes, but severe skeletal defects result in dwarfism; there is a high lifetime risk of transformation into acute myeloid leukaemia for patients with Schwachmann's syndrome.

Isolated pancreatic enzyme deficiencies

Protease deficiencies result from a lack of enterokinase (proximal small-intestine mucosal enzyme) or trypsinogen. The addition of exogenous enterokinase to duodenal secretions will differentiate these two deficiencies; it will not activate duodenal secretions lacking trypsinogen. Both conditions respond to pancreatic enzyme therapy. Lipase and colipase deficiencies are also rare isolated deficiencies that cause steatorrhoea. Patients with these pancreatic lipase deficiencies retain a residual fat-absorbing capacity, presumably from the action of other lipases such as gastric lipase.

Developmental anomalies

Annular pancreas

A failure of the ventral and dorsal anlage of the pancreas to unite produces a ring of pancreatic tissue encircling the duodenum. This may lead to intestinal obstruction in the neonate or the adult. Non-specific symptoms of postprandial fullness, nausea, abdominal pain, and vomiting may be present for years before the diagnosis is made. The radiographs show fixed symmetrical dilatation of the proximal duodenum, with bulging of the recesses on either side of the annular band, effacement of the duodenal mucosa without obstruction of the mucosa, and accentuation of the findings in the right anterior oblique position. The differential diagnosis should include duodenal webs, tumours of the pancreas or duodenum, postbulbar peptic ulcer, Crohn's disease of the proximal intestine, and adhesions. Patients with an annular pancreas have an increased incidence of pancreatitis and peptic ulcer. Because of these and other intestinal complications, surgery may be necessary, even though the condition has been present for years. Retrocolic duodenojejunostomy is the procedure of choice, although some surgeons prefer a Billroth II gastrectomy with gastroenterostomy and vagotomy.

Pancreas divisum

Pancreas divisum is the most common, congenital, anatomical abnormality of the human pancreas. It occurs when the ventral and dorsal parts of the pancreas fail to fuse, so that pancreatic drainage is accomplished mainly through the accessory papilla. Current evidence indicates that this anomaly predisposes, albeit infrequently, to the development of pancreatitis. The combination of a pancreas divisum and a small accessory orifice could result in dorsal-duct obstruction. The challenge is to identify this subset of patients. Cannulation of the dorsal duct by ERCP is not as easy as cannulation of the ventral duct. Patients with pancreatitis and pancreas divisum demonstrated by ERCP should be treated conservatively, including pancreatic enzyme therapy. Many of them have idiopathic pancreatitis unrelated to the pancreas divisum and will respond well to pancreatic enzymes. Endoscopic or surgical intervention is indicated only when these methods fail. Surgical ductal decompression is indicated if marked dilatation of the dorsal duct can be demonstrated. However, the appropriate therapy for those patients without dilatation of the dorsal duct is not yet defined. It should be emphasized that the ERCP appearance of pancreas divisum (that is, a small-calibre ventral duct with an arborizing pattern) may be confused with an obstructed main pancreatic duct caused by a pancreatic tumour.

Further reading

Amann ST, Toskes PP (1998). Hyperlipidemia and pancreatitis. In: Berger HG, *et al.*, eds. *The pancreas*, pp 311–16. Blackwell Science, Oxford.

Forsmark CE (2000). The diagnosis of chronic pancreatitis. *Gastrointestinal Endoscopy* **52**, 293–8.

Josephson S, Toskes PP (1996). Chronic pancreatitis: medical management. *Practical Gastroenterology* **20**, 6–22.

Lowenfels AB, *et al.* (1994). Prognosis of chronic pancreatitis: an international multi-center study. International Pancreatitis Study Group. *American Journal of Gastroenterology* **89**, 1467–72.

Saforkas GH, *et al.* (2000). Long-term results after surgery for chronic pancreatitis. *International Journal of Pancreatology* **27**, 131–42.

Somogyi L, *et al.* (2000). Synthetic porcine secretin is highly accurate in pancreatic function testing in individuals with chronic pancreatitis. *Pancreas* **21**, 262–5.

Vitab GJ, Sarr MG (1992). Selected management of pancreatic pseudocysts: operative versus expectant management. *Surgery* **III**, 124–30.

Walsh TN, *et al.* (1992). Minimal change chronic pancreatitis. *Gut* **33**, 1566–71.

Whitcomb DC, *et al.* (1996). Hereditary pancreatitis is caused by a mutation in the cationic trypsinogen gene. *Nature Genetics* **14**, 141–5.

4.18.3.3 Tumours of the pancreas

Julian Britton

Every year an average of 10 individuals from a Western population of 100 000 people will develop a tumour of the pancreas. Nine of the 10 with ductal adenocarcinoma will be dead a year later. Very few will survive 5 years. Two-thirds of patients are over the age of 65 years and there are slightly more men than women. The incidence of pancreatic cancer is increasing and we have little understanding of the cause. Smoking is a definite risk factor and about one in seven patients either have or develop diabetes mellitus before the cancer becomes evident. Hereditary chronic pancreatitis, which is rare and for which the causative gene has recently been identified, is associated with an increased risk of developing pancreatic cancer. It is less certain that chronic pancreatitis due to other causes is a risk factor.

Pathology

Malignant tumours of the exocrine pancreas are the commonest histological type. Endocrine tumours and benign tumours are rare (Table 1). In clinical practice, two-thirds of ductal adenocarcinomas occur in the head and uncinate process of the gland. All the adenocarcinomas grow locally and then spread to the regional lymph nodes and the liver. Perineural and vascular invasion are common features on histology. Occasional patients develop secondaries in the lung. Cystic adenocarcinoma is a separate histo-

Table 1 Histological classification of pancreatic tumours

Type of tumour	Percentage of cases
Ductal adenocarcinoma	93
Mucinous cystadenocarcinoma	2
Serous cystadenoma	1
Acinar cell tumour	1
Cystic/papillary tumour	1
Endocrine tumours	2

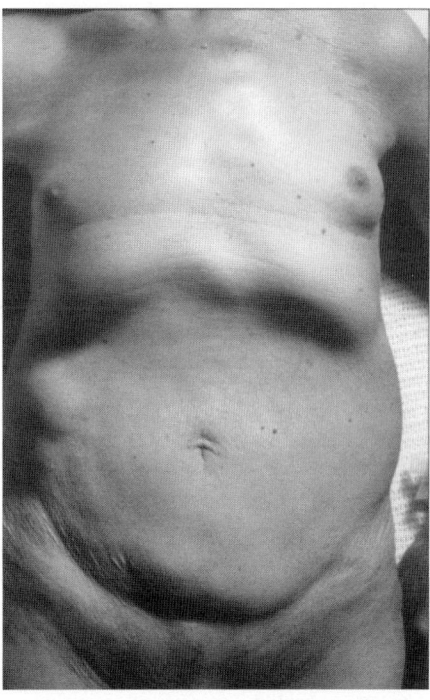

Fig. 1 This patient has cancer of the head of the pancreas and demonstrates Courvoisier's sign. The jaundice, the distended gall bladder, and the loss of weight are easy to see.

logical type with a better prognosis. Cystic/papillary tumours occur exclusively in young women. They grow to a large size and rarely metastasize. Adenocarcinomas of the ampulla, the bile duct, and the duodenum are separate and distinct tumours with a better prognosis.

Insulinomas are the most common endocrine tumour of the pancreas. Most are small, benign, and hard to find, but 10 per cent are multifocal or malignant. Gastrinomas have usually spread to the liver by the time they are discovered. About one in five islet cell tumours do not secrete sufficient hormones to produce clinical symptoms.

Breast cancer occasionally metastasizes to the pancreas and lymphoma can cause obstructive jaundice.

Diagnosis

A short history of epigastric abdominal pain which radiates through to the back, jaundice, and weight loss are the cardinal symptoms of a cancer in the head of the pancreas. About half the patients also complain of itching. Examination reveals a wasted and jaundiced patient with an enlarged palpable gall bladder (Courvoisier's sign) (Fig. 1).

Not all patients have a palpable gall bladder and not all tumours in the head and uncinate process of the gland cause jaundice. These tumours and tumours in the body and tail of the gland present with pain and disturbance of digestion. The symptoms are often initially diagnosed as gastritis or peptic ulceration. Occasional patients present with acute pancreatitis or thrombophlebitis migrans. Pancreatic tumours are rarely palpable, and they present late in the course of the disease.

Insulinomas release insulin and present with intermittent hypoglycaemia. Excess gastrin leads to severe peptic ulceration and steatorrhoea and vasoactive intestinal polypeptide causes diarrhoea. Often, however, the clinical picture is subtle and the key to diagnosis is appropriate biochemical analysis once the diagnosis is entertained. Non-functioning endocrine tumours behave like ductal adenocarcinoma and are discovered on investigation.

Investigation

Ultrasonography

Ultrasound examination of the bile ducts and the pancreas is the first investigation when a tumour in the pancreas is suspected. Dilatation of the bile ducts is easy to see. Experienced ultrasonographers may be able to identify the level of the obstruction or to see a mass in the pancreas. More commonly part or all of the pancreas is obscured by gas in the stomach, duodenum, or transverse colon. When ultrasound is unhelpful and there is a reasonable suspicion of pancreatic pathology then computed tomography is mandatory (Fig. 2). This is usually the only way to identify cancer of the body and tail of the gland. Magnetic resonance imaging is an alternative and has the advantage of imaging the pancreas and also obtaining a pancreatogram and a cholangiogram.

Endoscopic cholangio- and pancreatography, and percutaneous transhepatic cholangiography

Endoscopic cholangio- and pancreatography is the next preferred investigation. In cancer of the head of the gland, the bile duct and the pancreatic duct are usually narrow and irregular (the double-duct sign). In about three-quarters of these patients it is then possible to place a stent across the obstruction in the bile duct and so relieve the jaundice and pruritus. Percutaneous transhepatic cholangiography will also outline a biliary stricture but there is always a small risk of peritonitis because the needle, catheter and guide wire all cross the peritoneal cavity. However, it is slightly easier to place a biliary stent by this route (Fig. 3).

Biopsy

Biopsy of the duodenal wall is possible at endoscopic retrograde cholangio-pancreatography and biliary strictures can be brushed over a guide wire for

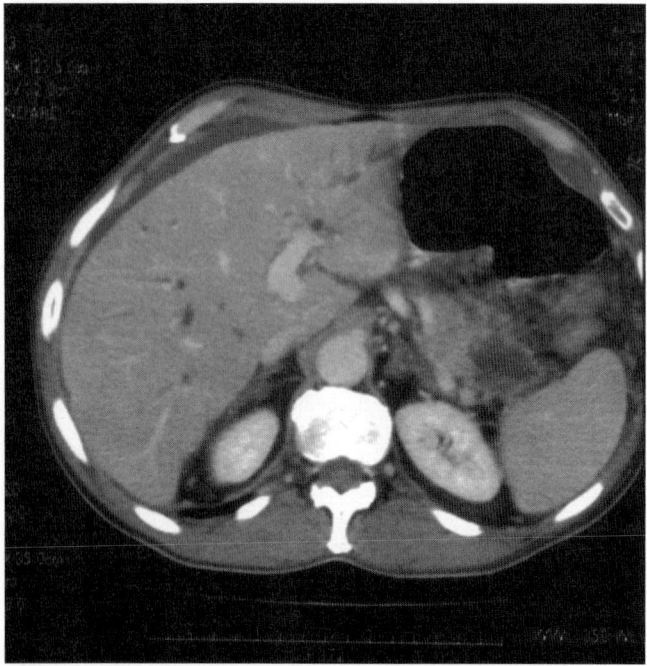

Fig. 2 The body and tail of the pancreas are swollen and enlarged and there is streaking in the peripancreatic fat. This patient had a biopsy proven carcinoma of the pancreas, but it can be very difficult to tell pancreatic cancer from chronic pancreatitis on radiological grounds.

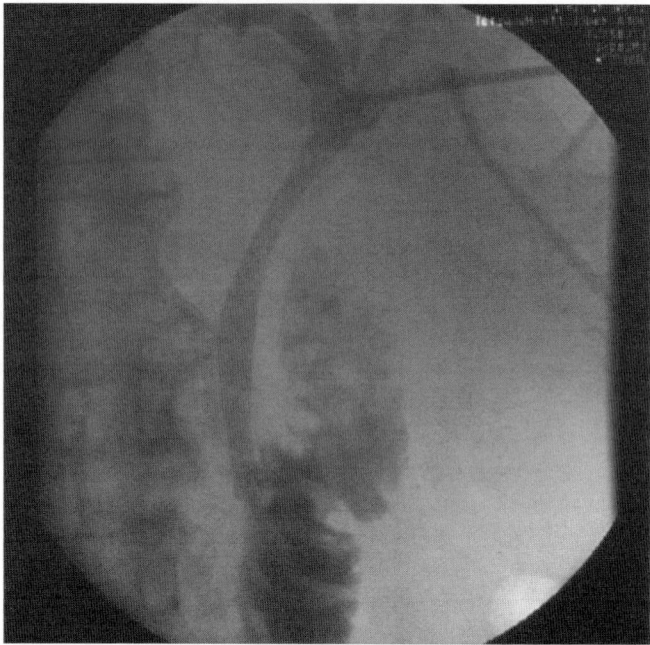

Fig. 3 Percutaneous transhepatic insertion of a biliary stent to relieve obstructive jaundice due to cancer of the pancreas. The catheter system to insert the self-expanding metal stent can be seen in the top left of the picture.

cytology. Alternatively a percutaneous biopsy can be obtained using computed tomography or ultrasonic guidance.

Computed tomography, magnetic resonance imaging, and angiography

Irregularity or narrowing of the arteries or veins around the pancreas on angiography indicate that a tumour is not resectable. Modern methods of imaging using three phase computed tomography or magnetic resonance imaging with suitable contrast agents can give the same information without a direct arterial injection. They are also more reliable at identifying liver metastases and a pancreatic resection is not justified if they are found.

Tumour markers

No serum marker has yet been found to be useful in the diagnosis of pancreatic cancer. During treatment an elevated CA 19-9 level will usually fall and this can be helpful in management.

Endocrine tumours

A high concentration of serum insulin in association with a low serum glucose is the key diagnostic feature of an insulinoma. Raised levels of other hormones will identify patients with other types of islet cell tumour. Although the tumours always develop in the pancreas or the duodenal wall most of them are less than a centimetre in size and they are hard to find. Ultrasound or computed tomography scanning and angiography are not worthwhile. Magnetic resonance imaging of the pancreas and endoscopic ultrasound are still developing and may be helpful. In most patients, once the diagnosis is established, a laparotomy by an experienced surgeon is the next best investigation. Most tumours can be seen or felt (Fig. 4), but when this is not the case intraoperative ultrasound with the probe applied directly to the pancreas will find the tumour. Transhepatic portal venous sampling, which will locate a tumour to a particular area within the pancreas, is best used after an initial unavailing laparotomy.

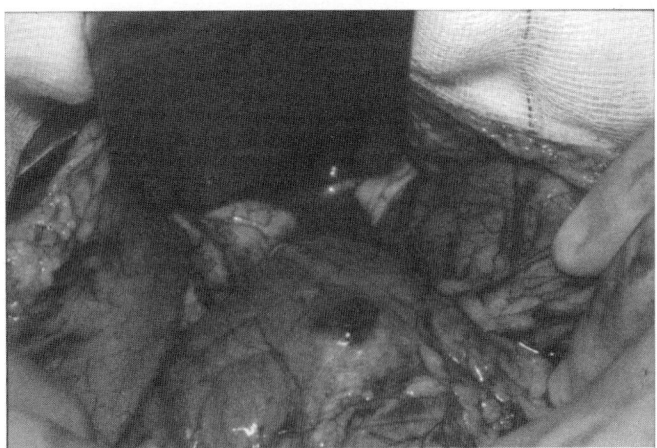

Fig. 4 The insulinoma is easily seen as a red swelling on the anterior surface of the body of the pancreas. It was a simple matter to enucleate the tumour. Leakage of pancreatic juice is rarely a problem afterwards.

Strategies for investigation

Cancer of the head of the pancreas commonly presents with jaundice. These patients need an urgent ultrasound examination which will confirm dilatation of the bile ducts. Either endoscopic retrograde cholangiopancreatography or percutaneous transhepatic cholangiography should be performed next and the choice depends on the available skills and local preference. In most patients, the jaundice can be relieved at the same time by inserting a stent across the biliary stricture. It is then necessary to identify those patients who would most likely benefit from surgery. Pancreatic resection is still a major procedure, despite a mortality rate now below 5 per cent. It is therefore preferable to offer radical surgery to patients under the age of 65 years, without significant other disease and whose tumour is less than 5 cm in diameter and apparently confined to the pancreas. Before surgery, this small group of patients should have portal venography carried out under computed tomography examination. In a few more patients this will show that the tumour is not resectable. The remaining patients should be offered an operation. Cancer of the body and tail of the pancreas is diagnosed on cross-sectional imaging and in most instances the computed tomography scan will also confirm that the tumour is not resectable.

Most patients with adenocarcinoma of the pancreas require palliative care. Biopsy of the pancreas or a liver metastasis is essential to confirm the diagnosis if chemotherapy is contemplated and is important for most other patients. Biopsy is not generally recommended in patients who are offered surgery because of the risk of seeding the tumour, despite the fact that a few are subsequently discovered to have a benign stricture.

Treatment

Palliation

Itching and intolerable pain are the two symptoms that require treatment. Itching rapidly improves once the bile duct is drained and the jaundice fades. Plastic stents last for an average of 4 months and can then be changed. Metal stents last rather longer. Most patients only survive a few months and never require a change of stent.

Pain from cancer of the pancreas is difficult to control. Early assistance should be sought from a specialist in palliative care. Regular opiate analgesia is usually required but a coeliac plexus block provides worthwhile pain relief in many cases. At operation 20 ml of absolute alcohol can be injected around the coeliac plexus to ablate sensory pathways. In other patients, the injection can be given by inserting the needle from the back alongside the lumbar spine and under the guidance of computed tomography.

A few patients will develop obstruction of the gastric outlet which will require a gastrojejunostomy. Surgical bypass of the biliary tract is now rarely required.

Radiotherapy has no part to play in palliation but many patients will wish to discuss chemotherapy with an oncologist. New drugs are being developed, and ideally most patients should be entered into a trial. About one in five patients will show some response to chemotherapy.

Surgery

Surgical resection of a localized pancreatic cancer is the only treatment that currently offers the possibility of long-term survival. Patients with apparently resectable tumours after investigation should therefore be offered an operation. A preliminary laparoscopy will identify patients with liver metastases which are too small to identify on scanning. Laparoscopic ultrasound in expert hands can identify involvement of the superior mesenteric or portal vein which also precludes resection. If the patient passes these tests the tumour should be assessed at a laparotomy. A trial dissection must show that the portal vein can be dissected off the tumour and that the superior mesenteric artery can be preserved. If this is the case then a pancreaticoduodenectomy (Whipple's operation) should be done (Fig. 5). The head and uncinate process of the pancreas along with the attached duodenum is removed. The antrum of the stomach is excised and the common bile duct is divided just above the duodenum. Some surgeons also remove the gall bladder. There are many techniques for restoring continuity. The pancreatic anastomosis is the most difficult and a pancreatic fistula is the cause of most postoperative complications. Occasionally a total pancreatectomy is required because the whole gland is diseased. In those rare cases in whom resection of a cancer in the body and tail of the gland is possible a splenectomy is always required as well. Even then tumour is often left around the origin of the splenic artery and postoperative radiotherapy to this area may be justified.

Insulinomas are well circumscribed and can be enucleated from the pancreas by careful blunt dissection. Multifocal tumours require a pancreatic

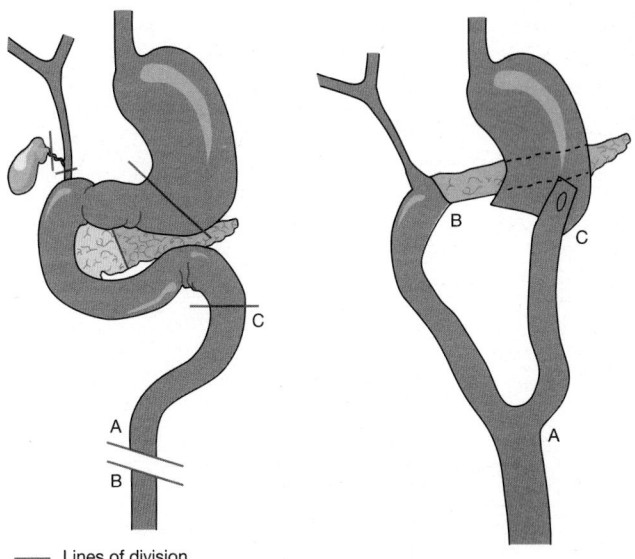

—— Lines of division

Fig. 5 The drawing on the left shows the structures that are removed in a classical pancreaticoduodenectomy (Whipple's operation). One method of restoring continuity is shown on the right.

resection or even total pancreatectomy. Metastases in the liver can be enucleated, although medical management is often more appropriate.

Prognosis

Most insulinomas are benign and patients are cured when the tumour is removed. Malignant endocrine tumours metastasize and kill patients either because of their mass effect or as a consequence of intractable hypoglycaemia, diarrhoea, and hypokalaemia or peptic ulceration unless the hormonal effects can be effectively blocked.

Overall the prognosis of adenocarcinoma of the pancreas is very poor. Ninety per cent of patients are dead within 12 months of diagnosis. In the small proportion who undergo successful surgery, about one in five will survive 5 years. This will include some patients with lymph node metastases at the time of the original surgery. A significant proportion of the long-term survivors of resection will develop both endocrine and exocrine pancreatic insufficiency. This will require replacement with insulin and enzyme supplements but surprisingly, digestion is often remarkably nor-

mal: the diabetes is not usually difficult to control and most survivors can lead a near normal life.

Overall most patients with pancreatic adenocarcinoma die rapidly once the diagnosis is made but a few will survive for a long time after successful surgery. Improving outcome in the future will depend on understanding the cause of this disease.

Further reading

Carter DC and Trede M (1993). Tumours of the exocrine pancreas and periampullary region. In : Trede M, Carter DC, eds. *Surgery of the pancreas*, pp 383–544. Churchill Livingstone, Edinburgh. [A comprehensive review of cancer of the pancreas from a European perspective.]

Yeo CJ, Cameron JL (2000). Pancreatic cancer. In: Morris PJ, Wood WC, eds. *Oxford textbook of surgery*, 2nd edn, pp. 1785–1808. Oxford University Press, Oxford. [A similar review from America.]

14.19 Disease of the gallblader and biliary tree

14.19.1 Congenital disorders of the liver, biliary tract, and pancreas

J. A. Summerfield

Pathogenesis of congenital disorders of the biliary tract

During the fourth week of gestation the liver arises as a bud of cells (the hepatic diverticulum) from the ventral wall of the foregut. At about the eighth week of gestation a layer of liver precursor cells around the portal vein branches differentiate to form a sleeve, termed the ductal plate. This sleeve duplicates to form a double layer of cells which by twelve weeks is remodelled by dilatation of segments of the double-layered ductal plate to form tubules that become the intrahepatic bile ducts. Non-tubular parts of the plate disappear and the bile ducts form part of the portal tracts.

Congenital disorders of the biliary tract are classified into two main groups: diseases characterized by inflammatory destruction of the bile ducts (the biliary atresias) and diseases marked by ectasia of the bile ducts with varying degrees of fibrosis (the fibropolycystic diseases). Both of these groups of disorders are related to the persistence or lack of remodelling of the embryonic ductal plate. They are termed 'ductal plate malformations'.

Ductal plate malformations can be seen on ultrasound or CT scans as a circular lumen containing a fibrovascular cord. Figure 1 shows ductal plate malformations in a CT scan of a patient with Caroli's disease (a fibropolycystic disease).

Biliary atresia

Classification

Biliary atresias are classified into extrahepatic biliary atresia and intrahepatic biliary atresia (paucity of intrahepatic bile ducts). Biliary atresia does not represent agenesis of the bile ducts but is the result of progressive bile duct destruction from an inflammatory disease of unknown cause. In extrahepatic biliary atresia the destructive cholangitis affects not only part or the whole of the extrahepatic bile duct but also intrahepatic bile ducts and leads to paucity of intrahepatic bile ducts. In intrahepatic biliary atresia the destructive cholangitis is restricted to the intrahepatic bile ducts. Intrahepatic biliary atresia can be classified further into a non-syndromatic or a syndromatic type (Alagille's syndrome or arteriohepatic dysplasia). About a quarter of patients with extrahepatic biliary atresia have evidence of ductal

plate malformation indicating that the destructive cholangitis started early in fetal life.

Symptoms and signs

Biliary atresia presents as cholestatic jaundice starting after the first two weeks of life. The infant develops jaundice with pale stools, dark urine, and hepatomegaly. Itching is often prominent. Bile pigments may stain the growing teeth greenish. The jaundice steadily deepens and xanthomas of the palm and knees, rickets, a bleeding tendency, and growth failure may develop. Biliary atresia may eventually causes biliary cirrhosis with pigmentation (due to melanin), portal hypertension, ascites, and liver failure.

The progress of biliary atresia depends on the type. Infants with extrahepatic biliary atresia (usually girls) have a steadily deepening jaundice and biliary cirrhosis soon develops. Untreated, these children usually die by six months of age. The fate of infants with intrahepatic biliary atresia depends on whether they have a syndromatic or non-syndromatic atresia. Children with non-syndromatic intrahepatic biliary atresia survive longer than those with extrahepatic biliary atresia, but biliary cirrhosis eventually develops in later childhood. In contrast, patients with syndromatic intrahepatic biliary atresia (Alagille's syndrome) tend to recover normal liver function as they become adolescent. Infants with Alagille's syndrome can be recognized by the associated features, which include a characteristic facies (a flattened and triangular-shaped face), pulmonary stenosis, vertebral abnormalities, and a change in the eyes (embryotoxon). Some patients have growth and mental retardation. Alagille's syndrome is associated with mutations in the Jagged 1 gene which encodes a Notch ligand.

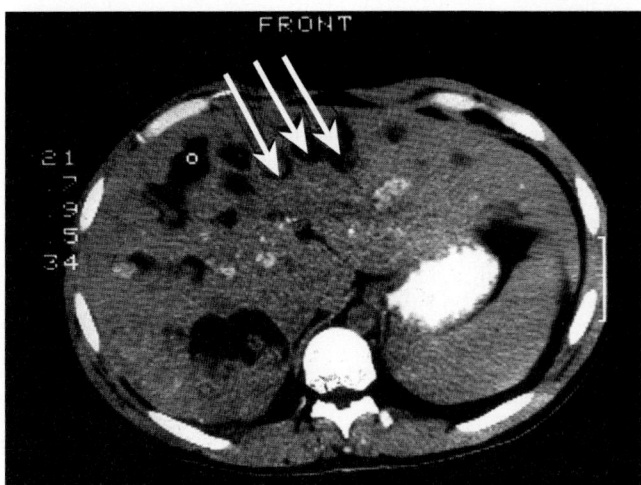

Fig. 1 Caroli's disease. Intravenous contrast enhanced CT scan of the liver shows dilated intrahepatic bile ducts containing filling defects which are portal vein branches (arrowed). This is an example of a ductal plate malformation. (From Sherlock S, Summerfield JA (1991), with permission.)

Differential diagnosis

Jaundice is common in early infancy. In the early neonatal period jaundice is usually due to haemolysis and impaired bilirubin conjugation. After two weeks, jaundice is usually cholestatic. There are many causes of cholestasis in infancy and childhood. The most common are extrahepatic and intrahepatic biliary atresias, neonatal hepatitis (such as hepatitis A, B, and C, rubella, and cytomegalovirus infection), metabolic causes (such as galactosaemia, α_1-antitrypsin deficiency, and tyrosinaemia), and the 'inspissated bile syndrome' (congenital spherocytosis).

Laboratory investigations

Liver function tests show a cholestatic (biliary obstructive) pattern. Serum bilirubin and alkaline phosphatase levels are markedly raised with only modest elevations of serum transaminases. Later, very high levels of serum cholesterol may develop.

Histological examination of the liver cannot distinguish between intrahepatic and extrahepatic biliary atresia. Liver biopsy shows severe centrizonal cholestasis and a prominent giant-cell reaction. In the portal tracts bile ducts are reduced. Later in the course of the disease the portal tracts are devoid of bile ducts and biliary cirrhosis is present.

Imaging

The initial step in the management of infants with cholestasis is to differentiate between intrahepatic and extrahepatic biliary atresia. Since the clinical and laboratory findings are similar, this distinction requires imaging techniques. In extrahepatic biliary atresia, scintiscanning with $^{99}Tc^m$ -labelled HIDA (dimethyl acetanilide iminodiacetic acid) shows accumulation of the label in the liver but none enters the biliary tree. Percutaneous and endoscopic cholangiography provide more precise anatomical detail.

Treatment and prognosis

General supportive measures include parenteral administration of fat-soluble vitamins A, D, K, and E. Medium-chain triglycerides as a source of fat, cholestyramine to relieve itching, and ursodeoxycholic acid as a choleretic help some patients.

Extrahepatic biliary atresia

Hepatic portoenterostomy (Kasai's operation) has been the treatment of choice for extrahepatic biliary atresia and is still widely performed. Approximately 25 to 35 per cent of patients who undergo a Kasai portoenterostomy will survive more than 10 years without liver transplantation. A third of the patients drain bile but develop complications of cirrhosis and require liver transplantation before the age of 10. For the remaining third of patients, bile flow is inadequate following portoenterostomy and the children develop progressive fibrosis and cirrhosis. The portoenterostomy should be done before there is irreversible sclerosis of the intrahepatic bile ducts. Consequently, a prompt evaluation for conjugated hyperbilirubinaemia is indicated for any infant older than 14 days with jaundice.

Intrahepatic biliary atresia

All infants should receive general supportive measures. Definitive treatment depends on the type of intrahepatic biliary atresia. Non-syndromatic intrahepatic biliary atresia eventually progresses to biliary cirrhosis and liver failure. Liver transplantation should be performed before the onset of liver failure. Syndromatic intrahepatic biliary atresia (Alagille's syndrome) has a good prognosis in most children and few develop biliary cirrhosis. General supportive measures are usually sufficient until the cholestasis disappears.

Fibropolycystic disease

Fibropolycystic disease encompasses a family of rare congenital hepatobiliary diseases that arise due to malformations of the embryonic ductal plate. These diseases include fibropolycystic disease (polycystic liver), congenital hepatic fibrosis, congenital intrahepatic biliary dilatation (Caroli's disease, Fig. 1), choledochal cysts, and microhamartomas (von Meyenberg complexes). Many patients will have more than one disease. The combination of congenital hepatic fibrosis and Caroli's disease is characteristic as these patients develop first variceal haemorrhage (due to congenital hepatic fibrosis) and later recurrent cholangitis (due to Caroli's disease). Associated kidney defects are common. Malignant change may complicate congenital hepatic fibrosis, Caroli's disease, choledochal cysts, and microhamartomas. These diseases are of widely differing severity and the prognosis in an individual patient is determined by the fibropolycystic diseases present.

Polycystic liver disease

The infantile type is inherited as an autosomal recessive disease and is usually rapidly fatal due to the associated renal disease. Adult polycystic liver disease is more common and has a dominant inheritance. The patient is usually a woman presenting in the fourth or fifth decade. The liver contains many thin-walled cysts filled with a clear or brownish liquid (due to altered blood). The cysts vary in size from a pinhead to about 10 cm in diameter. The remainder of the liver is normal. Patients present with right upper quadrant pain and increasing girth. Examination reveals an enlarged liver as the cause of the upper abdominal swelling. Liver function tests are normal. Provided no other fibropolycystic diseases are present, polycystic liver disease is benign. Some patients with polycystic liver disease also have polycystic kidneys or nephrocalcinosis. The associated renal disease may cause serious complications including renal failure. The diagnosis can be confirmed by ultrasound or CT scanning, which show numerous thin-walled cysts of low density (Fig. 2). The enlarged polycystic liver causes some patients considerable discomfort. It is best treated by percutaneous aspiration of the larger cysts using ultrasound guidance in order to reduce liver size. Percutaneous aspiration treatment can be performed repeatedly.

Congenital hepatic fibrosis

This is a rare autosomal recessive condition which is usually diagnosed before 10 years of age. The main complication is portal hypertension. Children present with a large, very hard liver and splenomegaly or bleeding from oesophageal varices. Congenital hepatic fibrosis may be misdiagnosed as cirrhosis. Liver function tests are normal or only slightly deranged. Ultrasound scans show the liver contains many bright areas due to the dense bands of fibrous tissue. The diagnosis is made by liver biopsy which

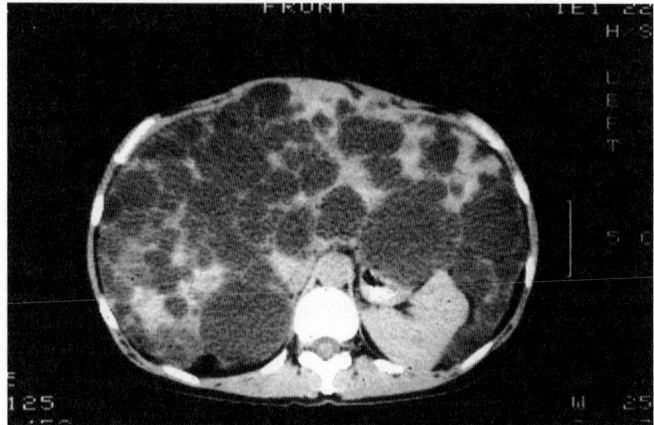

Fig. 2 Polycystic liver disease. CT scanning shows the liver contains many cysts of low density indicating that they are fluid filled. (From Sherlock S, Summerfield JA (1991), with permission.)

shows normal liver parenchyma surrounded by fibrous septa containing structures resembling bile ducts.

Patients with congenital hepatic fibrosis bleed repeatedly from oesophageal varices, but because liver function is well preserved they do not develop portosystemic encephalopathy. Portocaval shunts will stop the variceal bleeding and are well tolerated. Liver transplantation has also been used successfully.

The long-term prognosis in congenital hepatic fibrosis is usually determined by the associated renal disease. Renal lesions include renal dysplasia, medullary cystic disease, and infantile or adult-type polycystic kidneys. The kidneys are rarely normal and renal failure eventually develops in many patients. However, renal transplants have been successful.

Congenital intrahepatic biliary dilatation (Caroli's syndrome)

In Caroli's syndrome the common bile duct is normal but the intrahepatic ducts have bulbous dilatations with normal ducts between (Fig. 3). The mode of inheritance is unknown. While the cystic dilatations of the bile ducts remain uninfected the patient is symptom free. Eventually, ascending infection leads to cholangitis, which can be intractable with the formation of gallstones and liver abscesses. Caroli's syndrome usually presents in early adulthood as cholangitis. Most patients are male. Liver function tests show cholestasis with elevations of serum bilirubin and alkaline phosphatase and modest elevations of the transaminases. The diagnosis is made by endoscopic cholangiography. CT scans can also demonstrate the syndrome (Fig. 1). The natural history of Caroli's disease is of recurrent cholangitis which is very resistant to antibiotics. Biliary cirrhosis eventually develops. Bile duct cancer develops in about 10 per cent of cases. Treatment is difficult, antibiotics are usually only partially effective and liver transplantation is compromised by the extensive sepsis.

About half the patients with congenital hepatic fibrosis or Caroli's disease will also have the other disease. The clinical presentation in these patients is distinctive. As in Caroli's disease, males predominate. The first complication is variceal haemorrhage followed about 10 years later by recurrent cholangitis.

Choledochal cyst

Choledochal cyst is a congenital dilatation of part or the whole of the common bile duct (Fig. 4). It is more common in girls and usually presents in childhood but may appear in early adulthood. Choledochal cysts classically cause a triad of intermittent pain, jaundice, and a right hypochondrial mass. Choledochal cysts are particularly common in Japanese and Chinese

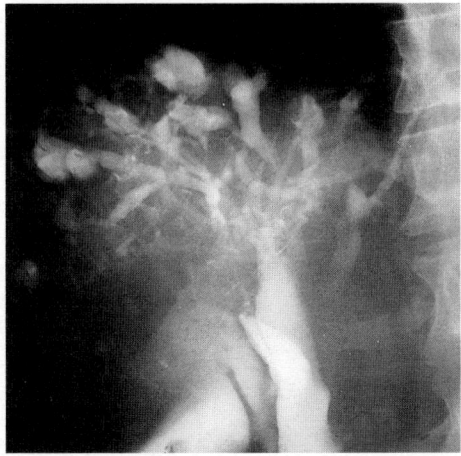

Fig. 3 . Caroli's disease. An endoscopic cholangiogram shows bulbous dilatations of the intrahepatic bile ducts. The rest of the biliary tree is normal. (From Sherlock S, Summerfield JA (1991), with permission.)

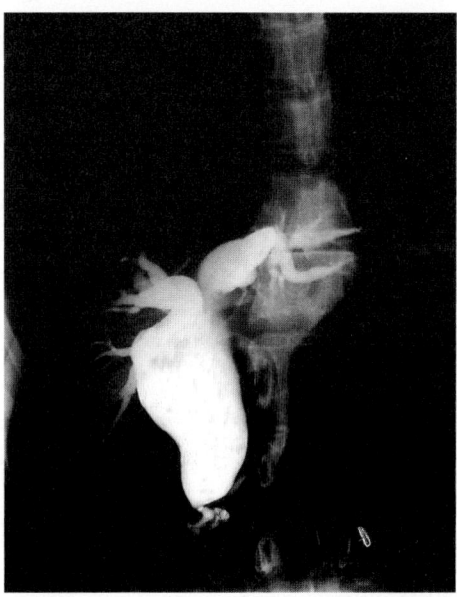

Fig. 4 Choledochal cyst in a 20-year-old woman. The endoscopic cholangiogram shows a massively dilated common bile duct. The gallbladder was normal but obscured by the dilated bile duct. (From Sherlock S, Summerfield JA (1991), with permission.)

individuals. Liver function tests show cholestasis, similar to Caroli's disease. Ultrasound and CT scans show cystic dilatation of the bile duct. The diagnosis is made by endoscopic or percutaneous cholangiography. Choledochal cysts should be treated by surgical excision because of the risk of bile duct malignancy. Caroli's disease is a common associated disease.

Microhamartomas (von Meyenberg complexes)

Microhamartomas are groups of rounded biliary channels embedded in a collagen stroma located around portal tracts. The appearances are of localized islands of congenital hepatic fibrosis. Microhamartomas are usually asymptomatic and discovered incidentally on liver biopsy. They may be associated with other fibropolycystic diseases and are a rare cause of portal hypertension. Bile duct and pancreatic cancers are commoner in these patients.

Congenital disorders of the pancreas

Agenesis of the pancreas

Pancreatic agenesis is rare and may occur as an isolated anomaly or be associated with other defects. These children usually die soon after birth. Agenesis of either the dorsal or ventral pancreas may occur, although agenesis usually involves the dorsal segment.

Annular pancreas

This is a rare condition where pancreatic tissue encircles the descending duodenum. It results from persistence of part of the ventral pancreas during embryonic development. Annular pancreas is the most common cause of duodenal obstruction in infancy and often involves growth of pancreatic tissue into the duodenal wall. However, the clinical presentation is variable and annular pancreas may first present as an incidental finding at surgery or autopsy.

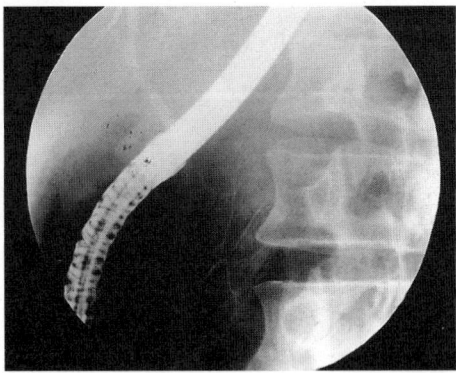

Fig. 5 Pancreas divisum. An endoscopic pancreatogram following injection of contrast medium into the ampulla of Vater shows only the ducts of the head of the pancreas, characterized by a trefoil pattern. The body and tail of the pancreas drain via the accessory ampulla.

Pancreas divisum

Pancreas divisum results from failure of fusion of the ducts of the dorsal and ventral portions of the pancreas. The body and tail of the pancreas drain through the narrow duct of Santorini into the accessory papilla. Only the head of the pancreas drains into the ampulla of Vater (Fig. 5). This is the commonest congenital abnormality of the pancreas occurring in about five per cent of patients. Pancreas divisum appears to be associated with an increased incidence of pancreatitis affecting the body and tail of the pancreas which drains into the accessory papilla. Endoscopic sphincterotomy of the accessory papilla is reported to lead to clinical improvement in this type of pancreatitis.

Hereditary pancreatitis

This rare form of pancreatitis is inherited as an autosomal dominant disorder. Recurrent attacks of abdominal pain start in childhood or the second decade. Hereditary pancreatitis tends to be troublesome rather than life-threatening and attacks become less severe as the patient gets older. They often disappear by middle age. Hereditary pancreatitis is associated with mutations in the cationic trypsinogen gene, which probably render the protease more resistant to autocatalytic trypsinogen breakdown.

Other rare abnormalities causing pancreatic disease

Congenital abnormalities adjacent to the pancreas are rare causes of pancreatitis. These include duodenal diverticulum, duplication of the duodenum, stenosis of the sphincter of Oddi, and choledochal cyst. These abnormalities seem to cause pancreatitis by obstructing the pancreatic duct.

Further reading

Chardot C *et al.* (1999). Prognosis of biliary atresia in the era of liver transplantation: French national study from 1986 to 1996. *Hepatology* **30**, 606–11.

Desmet VJ (1992) Congenital diseases of intrahepatic bile ducts: variations on the theme 'ductal plate malformation'. *Hepatology* **16**, 1069–83.

Sherlock S, Dooley JS (1997). *Diseases of the liver and biliary system*, 10th edn. Blackwell Scientific Publications, Oxford.

Sherlock S, Summerfield JA (1991). *A colour atlas of liver disease*, 2nd edn. Wolfe Medical Publications, London.

Summerfield JA *et al.* (1986). Hepatobiliary fibropolycystic diseases; a clinical and histological review of 51 patients. *Journal of Hepatology* **2**, 141–56.

14.19.2 Diseases of the gallbladder and biliary tree

J. A. Summerfield

Anatomy

The biliary system comprises the collection of ducts extending from the biliary canaliculus of each hepatocyte to the ampulla of Vater opening into the duodenum. The biliary canaliculi drain into interlobular and then septal bile ducts. These further ramify to form the intrahepatic bile ducts which are visible on cholangiography (Fig. 1). They eventually form the right and left hepatic ducts draining bile from the right and left lobes of the liver, respectively. The junction of the hepatic ducts at the porta hepatis forms the common hepatic duct. The cystic duct, linking the gallbladder to the bile duct, arises from the lower end of the common hepatic duct. The gallbladder rests in a fossa under the right lobe of the liver. Anatomical variations in the size and position of the gallbladder and the insertion of the cystic duct into the bile duct are of major surgical importance. The common hepatic duct becomes the common bile duct below the insertion of the cystic duct. The common bile duct passes through the head of the pancreas and the sphincter of Oddi to drain into the duodenum via the ampulla of Vater. The bile duct usually exits through a common channel

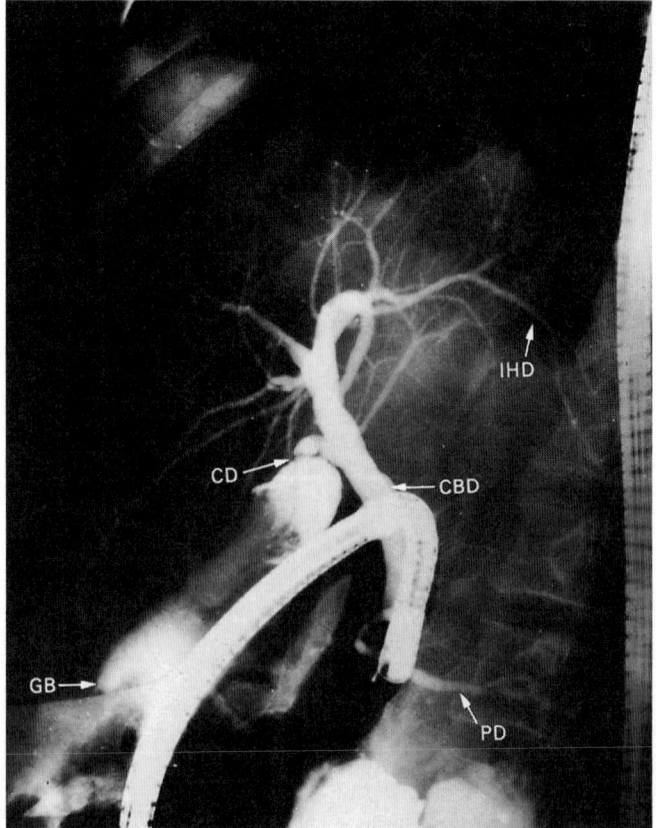

Fig. 1 The normal biliary tree. The intrahepatic bile ducts (IHD) taper smoothly and extend deep into the liver. The gallbladder (GB) drains via the cystic duct (CD) into the common bile duct (CBD). The pancreatic duct (PD) has also been opacified in this endoscopic retrograde cholangiogram.

with the pancreatic duct in the ampulla of Vater, although anatomical variations are frequent.

The investigation of biliary disease

Objectives

The clinical and laboratory features of biliary disease may also be caused by hepatic disorders. Consequently, the primary objective of investigations is to establish that the cause is due to biliary and not hepatic disease. The secondary objective is to define the anatomy of the lesion to permit a rational choice of the many surgical and non-surgical therapeutic options which are now available. To achieve these objectives requires not only a careful history and physical examination, but also the use of various imaging techniques and sometimes aspiration liver biopsy.

Symptoms and signs

Disorders of the biliary system usually give rise to the symptoms and signs of biliary obstruction (cholestasis). The repertoire is rather limited: pain, jaundice, itching, nausea and vomiting, fevers, and rigors. The pain can range from abdominal discomfort described as 'dyspepsia' to severe right hypochondrial colic caused by a sudden rise in biliary pressure. Jaundice, dark urine, and pale stools indicate obstruction of the bile duct. Itching is an important sign of biliary obstruction. Nausea and vomiting may be prominent in sudden obstruction of the bile duct, usually by a gallstone. The milder symptoms of flatulence and intolerance of fatty food are more common. Fever and rigors indicate bacterial infection of the biliary tract, which frequently accompanies partial obstruction. In jaundiced patients weight loss is usual and results from fat malabsorption due to the lack of bile acids reaching the gut; it may also indicate a malignant tumour. Prolonged biliary obstruction leads to skin changes: increased pigmentation (due to melanin) and cholesterol deposits (xanthelasma and xanthoma). Finally, biliary cirrhosis may develop causing the signs of portal venous hypertension and liver cell failure.

Laboratory investigations

In general, disorders of the biliary system give rise to the biochemical picture of biliary obstruction (cholestasis). A notable exception is gallstones in the gallbladder (cholelithiasis) where the liver function tests are usually normal. In cholestasis, the serum bilirubin concentration may be normal or raised and most of the bilirubin is esterified (conjugated). Bilirubinuria is present. The disappearance of urobilinogen from the urine indicates complete biliary obstruction. Elevation of the serum alkaline phosphatase is an important but not invariable sign of biliary obstruction; the rise is usually greater than three times normal. Other biliary canalicular enzymes accumulate in the blood, including γ-glutamyl transpeptidase. This enzyme is only found in the liver and is estimated if there is doubt as to whether the alkaline phosphatase is of bony or hepatic origin. This may be required in children and patients with malignancy. Serum transaminases, such as aspartate aminotransferase, show only modest elevation in contrast to the rises which occur in hepatitis. The serum cholesterol concentration rises and may cause abnormalities of red cell shape (target cells) (see Section 22). A raised concentration of serum bile acids is a sensitive index of biliary disease. A prolonged prothrombin time reflects intestinal malabsorption of fat-soluble vitamin K owing to a lack of bile acids. Vitamin A and D deficiency may also develop. The serum albumin and gammaglobulin levels are normal until biliary cirrhosis develops. A polymorphonuclear leucocytosis accompanies bacterial infections of the biliary system.

Imaging techniques

A plain radiograph of the abdomen may reveal an enlarged liver, calcified gallstones, or air in the biliary tree. Plain radiographs of the abdomen are now rarely performed. The preferred first investigation is ultrasonography

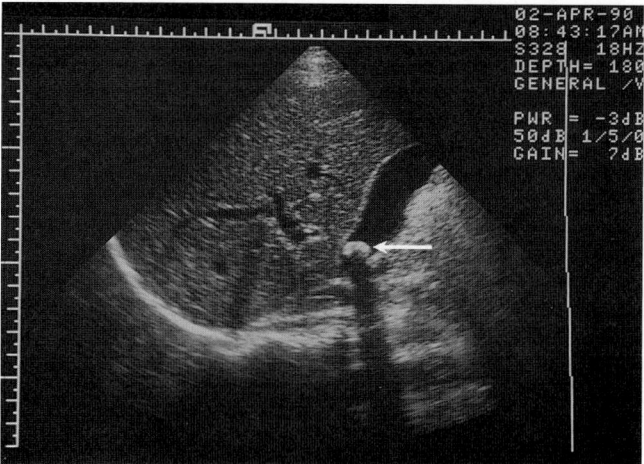

Fig. 2 Ultrasound scan of the gallbladder shows gallstones (arrowed) as bright round objects which cast acoustic shadows.

(Fig. 2). Computed tomography (**CT** scan) and magnetic resonance imaging (**MRI**) are used in complicated diagnostic problems. These tests reveal dilated bile ducts and may also indicate the position of the obstruction in the biliary tree and dense structures such as gallstones. Hepatic scintiscanning with ^{99}Tc^m -labelled HIDA (dimethyl acetanilide iminodiacetic acid) is an alternative and is of value in the diagnosis of acute cholecystitis. Oral cholecystograms are rarely performed nowadays but are useful to determine whether the gallbladder is functioning in patients with gallstones being assessed for oral bile acid dissolution therapy (see below). Intravenous cholangiography is obsolete. However, these non-invasive investigations usually provide insufficient anatomical detail for diagnosis or planning of treatment. An invasive cholangiographic technique such as percutaneous transhepatic cholangiography (**PTC**) or endoscopic retrograde cholangiopancreatography (**ERCP**) is necessary. ERCP is the preferred investigation in the first instance. PTC is reserved for patients in whom ERCP fails. Both these techniques carry small risks including haemorrhage, biliary peritonitis, and cholangitis (with PTC), and bowel perforation, cholangitis, and pancreatitis (with ERCP). Should cholangiography reveal a normal biliary system in a jaundiced patient, a liver biopsy is indicated.

This diagnostic approach is ideal but expensive both in terms of human and material resources. The apparatus required is costly and procedures such as ERCP require considerable expertise. Obviously local factors will determine the diagnostic pathway that is adopted. Nevertheless, these techniques have revolutionized the management of patients with biliary disease. It is now a routine matter to achieve a precise diagnosis rapidly. In addition, a series of non-operative therapeutic options ranging from the introduction of endoprostheses for the management of benign and malignant biliary structures to endoscopic sphincterotomy for the removal of the biliary calculi are direct consequences of these diagnostic approaches. Developments in MRI indicate that soon ERCP may be superseded by the non-invasive technique of magnetic resonance cholangiography (MRC).

Bile composition and gallstone formation

Bile composition

Bile is secreted by the hepatocytes and its water and electrolyte composition altered during its passage down the biliary system. Between meals much of the bile is diverted to the gallbladder where it is concentrated by the removal of sodium, chloride, bicarbonate, and water. In response to food, the gallbladder contracts, emptying bile into the duodenum. Apart from water (97 per cent) the major components of bile are bile acids, phospholipids, and cholesterol. Bile is also the major excretory route of other compounds including bilirubin and certain drugs and their metabolites. Cholesterol is insoluble in water but is held in solution by the detergent action of bile acids with the aid of phospholipids.

Cholesterol is synthesized primarily in the liver and small intestine. The rate-limiting enzyme for cholesterol production is hydroxymethylglutaryl-CoA reductase, which catalyses the first step, the conversion of acetate to mevalonate. Subsequently, non-esterified (free) cholesterol is secreted into bile. Dietary cholesterol also contributes to biliary cholesterol secretion. The control of cholesterol metabolism is complex. It is not yet clear what proportion of biliary cholesterol is derived from circulating lipoproteins and what proportion is newly synthesized by the liver.

The primary bile acids, cholic and chenodeoxycholic acid, are synthesized in the liver from cholesterol. The economy of the bile acid pool is preserved by efficient reabsorption, principally in the terminal ileum. About 95 per cent of the bile acids are reabsorbed and pass back to the liver in the portal venous system (enterohepatic circulation). The remainder enters the colon where bacteria form the secondary bile acids, deoxycholic and lithocholic acid, from cholic and chenodeoxycholic acid, respectively. Some of the secondary bile acids are absorbed from the colon but most are excreted in the faeces. The normal bile acid pool is about 3 to 5 g and circulates 6 to 10 times each day. Synthesis is controlled by the negative feedback of bile acids returning in the portal venous blood, which act on the rate-limiting hepatic enzyme, cholesterol-7α-hydroxylase. The principal phospholipid in bile is lecithin. It is produced in the liver and secreted into the bile. In the intestine lecithin is hydrolysed to lysolecithin by pancreatic phospholipase and is subsequently reabsorbed.

Above a certain level (the critical micellar concentration) bile acids coalesce to form micelles that have a hydrophilic external surface and hydrophobic internal surface. Cholesterol is incorporated into the hydrophobic interior. Phospholipids are inserted into the micellar wall so that the micelles are enlarged; these 'mixed micelles' are thus able to hold more cholesterol.

Consequently, the solubility of cholesterol in bile depends on the concentrations of bile acid and phospholipid. In the presence of a relative excess of bile acids and phospholipid (on a molar basis) the cholesterol-holding capacity of bile is increased and it is said to be unsaturated. However, if there are insufficient micelles of bile acid and phospholipid to hold the cholesterol, the solution is referred to as saturated and the excess cholesterol tends to precipitate. With a knowledge of the molar concentration of cholesterol, phospholipid, and bile acids, the cholesterol saturation of bile can be predicted using triangular co-ordinate diagrams.

Gallstone formation

Gallstone disease is common and afflicts between 10 and 20 per cent of the world's population. Gallstones are classified according to their composition into two main groups: cholesterol stones and bile pigment stones. Cholesterol stones are composed mainly of cholesterol (more than 70 per cent) and can be subdivided into pure cholesterol stones (usually solitary) and mixed stones which contain cholesterol in a matrix of calcium bilirubinate, calcium phosphate, and protein (Figs 3 and 4). Mixed stones are usually multiple and faceted. Bile pigment stones can also be divided into two main groups. Brown pigment stones are soft and friable and consist of calcium bilirubinate, cholesterol, and calcium soaps. Pure pigment stones ('black stones') are black, hard, and brittle and contain an insoluble black pigment, calcium bilirubinate, calcium carbonate and phosphate, calcium salts of fatty acids, and bile acids. All pigment stones contain a large amount of mucoprotein matrix (up to 70 per cent). Gallstones are rare before the age of 10 years. The incidence increases progressively with age. Cholesterol gallstones account for about 75 per cent of the gallstones in Europe and the United States.

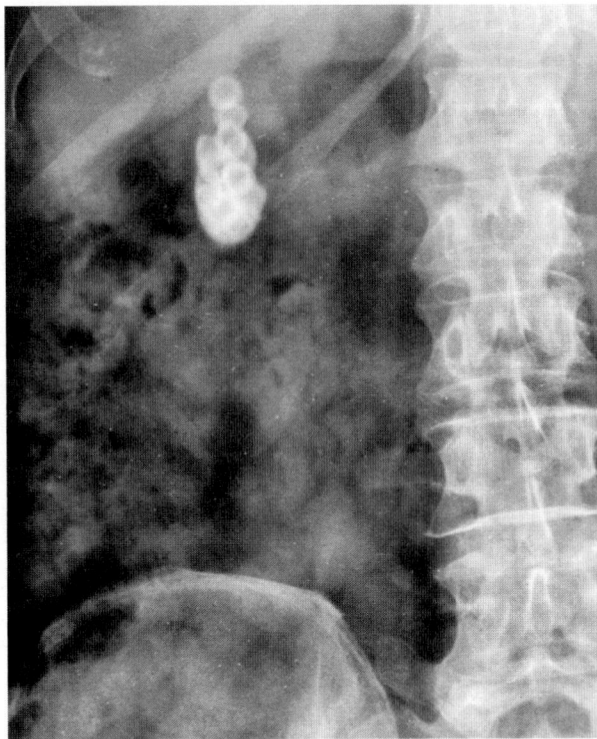

Fig. 3 Calcified gallstones. Gallstones contain sufficient calcium to be visible on a plain abdominal radiograph in about 10 per cent of patients. The gallbladder stones are surrounded by a ring of calcium slats. (Reproduced from Sherlock S, Summerfield JA, 1979, *A colour atlas of liver disease*, Wolfe Medical Publications, London, with permission.)

Cholesterol gallstones

Cholesterol gallstones result from the secretion of cholesterol-saturated bile by the liver. The cause of the saturation is unclear. Patients with gallstones usually have a smaller bile acid pool than controls and it circulates more

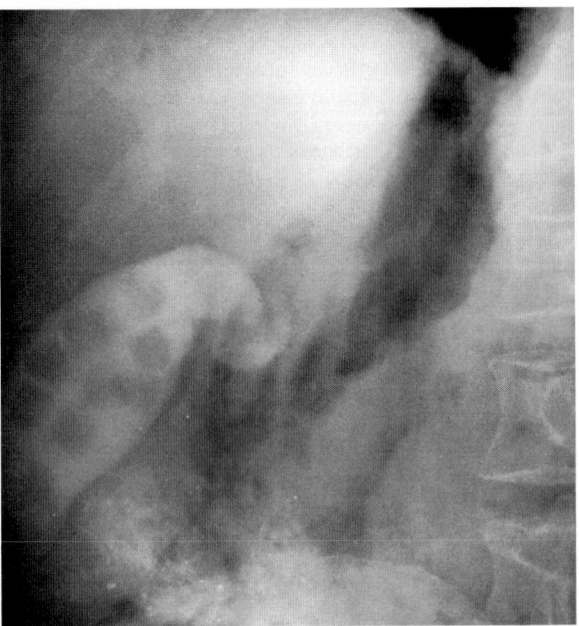

Fig. 4 Cholesterol gallstones. An intravenous cholangiogram has opacified the gallbladder showing multiple faceted radiolucent gallstones. These are typical features of cholesterol stones.

frequently. The rapid recycling of bile acids may be responsible for the smaller bile acid pool by excessive inhibition of the enzyme which controls bile acid synthesis, cholesterol-7α-hydroxylase. However, diminished bile acid synthesis is probably not the most important factor in the production of saturated bile. This appears to be an elevated biliary cholesterol secretion rate, due either to increased hepatic cholesterol synthesis or increased transfer of plasma lipoprotein cholesterol into bile. Nevertheless, saturated bile may be encountered in normal subjects, especially during fasting. It is therefore likely that other factors such as the condition of the gallbladder, the mechanism of seeding (nucleation) of gallstones, and the control of gallstone growth are important. Furthermore, racial differences, advancing age, female sex, obesity, diet, drugs (such as the contraceptive pill and clofibrate), and gastrointestinal disease (such as Crohn's disease) are known to have a significant influence on the development of gallstones.

Bile pigment gallstones

In contrast to cholesterol stones, little is known of the aetiology of bile pigment stones. The soft, friable brown-pigment stones are especially common in the Far East and are associated with *Escherichia coli*, bacteroides, and clostridium infection of the biliary tract. It is probable that these bacteria contribute to stone formation by producing β-glucuronidase that deconjugates bilirubin diglucuronide to form free unconjugated bilirubin. This combines with calcium to form sparingly soluble calcium bilirubinate that precipitates.

The black, hard, and brittle pure-pigment stones are the type commonly encountered in the West. The incidence of pure pigment stones increases with age and they are found in patients with cirrhosis, chronic bile duct obstruction (such as biliary strictures), chronic haemolytic anaemias including haemolysis induced by prosthetic heart valves, and malaria. Pure pigment stones affect both sexes equally. The mechanism of stones production is unclear, but does not appear to be due to cholesterol saturation of hepatic or gallbladder bile. About 50 per cent of all pigment stones are radio-opaque and they account for about 70 per cent of all opaque stones.

Natural history of gallstones

The majority of gallstones remain in the gallbladder (cholelithiasis) and may give rise to no symptoms ('silent' gallstones), being discovered incidentally during investigation or at autopsy. Impaction of a gallstone in the neck of the gallbladder results in gallbladder inflammation and the symptoms and signs of acute or chronic cholecystitis. Acute cholecystitis will subside if the stone spontaneously disempacts, or may progress to gangrene and perforation of the gallbladder or empyema of the gallbladder. Gallstones may pass through the cystic duct into the bile duct (choledocholithiasis) resulting in biliary obstruction and jaundice. Bacterial infection (cholangitis) commonly accompanies choledocholithiasis and can lead to a liver abscess. Gallstones may perforate through the inflamed gallbladder wall to form an internal fistula, usually to the small intestine or colon. A large gallstone passing into the small intestine may impact in the ileum resulting in intestinal obstruction (gallstone ileus). Finally, surgical treatment for gallstones, while usually curative, may result in a postcholecystectomy syndrome or a benign stricture of the bile duct.

Treatment

The usual treatment for gallstones remains cholecystectomy although medical treatments may be employed in selected patients (see below). The advent of laparoscopic cholecystectomy has swung the balance in favour of surgery since this technique carries so little morbidity and a very short hospital stay. Treatment is obviously indicated for symptomatic gallstones and for their complications. However, in patients in whom 'silent' gallstones are discovered incidentally and in patients with minimal symptoms it is by no means clear that treatment is always the best solution. The problem revolves around the probability of serious complications in the future.

It is appropriate to offer treatment to young patients (who, with many years ahead of them, will have a greater likelihood of developing the complications of gallstones) and to advise against treatment in the elderly with other major medical problems. However, in fit middle-aged patients with no or minimal symptoms it is reasonable to tell the patient of the finding and to withhold surgery until it is warranted by symptoms or complications.

Gallstone dissolution and disruption

Cholesterol gallstones can be removed from the gallbladder and bile ducts in a proportion of patients by medical treatments. These techniques avoid the discomfort, disability, and risks of general anaesthesia and surgical exploration of the abdomen and bile ducts. However, with the widespread availability of laparoscopic cholecystectomy these techniques are now used rarely. There are two types of medical method: chemical agents that dissolve gallstones, and physical methods such as endoscopic sphincterotomy and extracorporeal shock-wave lithotripsy (**ESWL**). Judicious combinations of chemical and physical methods yield the best results.

Chemical methods

Oral bile acid therapy

Oral treatment with chenodeoxycholic acid or ursodeoxycholic acid can dissolve cholesterol gallstones. These bile acids, normal constituents of bile, reduce the cholesterol saturation of bile and result in the leaching of cholesterol from gallstones. They act by reducing the hepatic synthesis and biliary excretion of cholesterol. Ursodeoxycholic acid has advantages over chenodeoxycholic acid in that it does not cause diarrhoea or elevations of serum transaminases. These bile acids differ in the way that they remove cholesterol from gallstones and have been shown to dissolve gallstones better in combination than singly. Combination therapy is the preferred treatment.

Contact dissolution of gallstones

Cholesterol stones in the gallbladder can be dissolved by the direct instillation of methyl tertbutyl ether (**MTBE**) into the gallbladder via a percutaneous catheter. MTBE is a foul-smelling, volatile, inflammable colourless liquid that remains liquid at body temperature. The gallbladder is catheterized by the transhepatic route, entering it through the area of attachment of the gallbladder to the liver and MTBE is continually infused and aspirated with vigour until the stones have disappeared (which typically takes 5 to 7 h).

Physical methods

Extracorporeal shock-wave lithotripsy

ESWL is a non-invasive and safe but expensive way of rapidly shattering gallstones into a coarse powder. The gallbladder must contain no more than three stones to allow accurate focusing of the shock waves.

Endoscopic sphincterotomy

Endoscopic sphincterotomy can remove gallstones from the bile duct. The bile duct is entered by a cannula passed via a duodenoscope and the bile duct is opened by diathermy cutting of the ampulla of Vater. Stones are removed by balloon or wire catheters.

Patient selection and results

Medical treatment with oral bile acid therapy, ESWL, or contact dissolution are suitable for patients with cholesterol gallstones in a functioning gallbladder (as judged by an oral cholecystogram). Calcified gallstones do not dissolve. Radiolucent gallstones are usually, but not always, composed of cholesterol. CT scans are useful for detecting low levels of gallstone calcification. These treatments should be reserved for patients with mild or no symptoms in whom the risk of cholecystectomy is high, including those with pre-existing disease, the elderly, and the very obese. They are also of value in patients who refuse surgery. Drugs which increase the cholesterol saturation of bile should be avoided; these include oestrogens, the oral contraceptive pill, and clofibrate.

Oral bile acid therapy is protracted but safe. It dissolves gallstones in about 25 per cent of patients fulfilling the selection criteria by 6 months. It should not be taken during pregnancy. The preferred treatment is combination therapy with chenodeoxycholic acid (7 mg/kg) and ursodeoxycholic acid (7 mg/kg). Proprietary combination tablets are available. Gallstone dissolution usually requires 6 to 24 months of therapy depending on stone size. Oral cholecystograms are performed every 6 months to assess progress. Combining oral bile acid therapy with ESWL speeds up the process greatly: gallstones will be cleared in more than 90 per cent of patients within 18 months. Furthermore, slightly calcified gallstones can be treated in this way. MTBE therapy is invasive and the ether is unpleasant to use, but dissolution is rapid. Endoscopic sphincterotomy removes gallstones from the common bile duct. Any type of stone can be removed up to about 20 mm in diameter.

Side-effects and toxicity

The most frequent side-effect of oral bile acid therapy is diarrhoea. It is dose related and usually mild and transient. It can be minimized by slowly increasing the dose to the required level. Transient elevations of serum transaminase activity are also common; liver function tests should be monitored. Ursodeoxycholic acid may cause calcification of gallstones. Gallstone recurrence remains a major problem with oral bile acid therapy. One year after gallstone dissolution about 30 per cent of patients will have had a recurrence. Unwanted effects of ESWL include biliary colic, skin petechias, and haematuria. The principal unwanted side-effects of MTBE are sedation, burning upper abdominal pain, nausea, and vomiting. Endoscopic sphincterotomy can cause gastrointestinal haemorrhage and acute pancreatitis.

Acute cholecystitis

Aetiology

Acute cholecystitis is associated with gallstones in over 90 per cent of patients. It follows the impaction of a gallstone in the cystic duct. Continued secretion by the gallbladder leads to a rise in pressure. Inflammation of the gallbladder wall results from the toxic effects of the retained bile and bacterial infection. The gallbladder bile is usually turbid but may become frank pus (empyema of the gallbladder). Intestinal organisms, especially anaerobes, are commonly cultured from the gallbladder. Ischaemia in the distended gallbladder wall may lead to infarction and perforation. Generalized peritonitis may follow, but the leak is usually localized to form a chronic abscess cavity. Some patients have repeated attacks of acute cholecystitis which are probably exacerbations of chronic cholecystitis. Acute cholecystitis in the absence of gallstones (acalculous cholecystitis) is usually very rare. However, acalculous cholecystitis is a particular problem in patients with the acquired immunodeficiency syndrome (**AIDS**). Cytomegalovirus and cryptosporidium are the most commonly associated organisms in acalculous cholecystitis in AIDS.

Symptoms and signs

The typical patient is an obese, middle-aged female, and the acute attack is often precipitated by a large or fatty meal. However, there are many exceptions to this pattern. The principal symptom is pain, of fairly sudden onset, which is severe, continuous or minimally fluctuating, and localized to the epigastrium or right hypochondrium. The pain often radiates to the back. The constancy of the pain is in contrast to the repeated short bouts of biliary colic. In uncomplicated cases the pain gradually subsides over 12 to 18 h. Flatulence and nausea are common but persistent vomiting suggests the presence of a stone in the common bile duct. Examination reveals an ill, sweating patient with shallow, jerky respiration. Fever indicates a complicating bacterial cholangitis. Jaundice may accompany acute cholecystitis but is usually a sign of a stone in the bile duct. The abdomen moves poorly with respiration. Right hypochondrial tenderness is present and is exacer-

bated by inspiration (Murphy's sign). Muscle guarding and rebound tenderness are common. The gallbladder is usually impalpable but occasionally a tender mass of omentum and gallbladder may be felt under the liver.

Laboratory investigations

The white cell count is usually moderately elevated (12 to $15 \times 10^9/l$) due to a polymorphonuclear leucocytosis. Serum bilirubin concentrations between 17 and 68 µmol/l (1 and 4 mg/dl) may be seen in uncomplicated acute cholecystitis, but should raise the suspicion of a stone in the bile duct. Modest rises in the serum alkaline phosphatase, aspartate transaminase, and amylase may also be seen. An abdominal radiograph will show gallstones in about 10 per cent of patients. Ultrasound scanning of the gallbladder is the preferred first investigation. Scintiscanning with $^{99}Tc^m$-labelled HIDA provides similar information. It is important to establish the correct diagnosis before surgery is performed.

Differential diagnosis

Acute cholecystitis may be confused with other abdominal emergencies including perforated peptic ulcer, acute pancreatitis, retrocaecal appendicitis, perforated carcinoma or diverticulum of the hepatic flexure of the colon, and liver abscess. Cardiac infarction and pneumonia with right-sided pleurisy should also be considered.

Complications

Gangrene of the gallbladder

Pain, tenderness, and fever progressively increasing or persisting for longer than 24 to 48 h are indications of gangrene of the gallbladder. The prognosis is poor if necrosis and perforation occur. In patients who are elderly and obese, perforation of the gallbladder can occur without definite signs. Perforation into an adjacent viscus may produce a cholecystenteric fistula and may lead to gallstone ileus.

Cholangitis

Intermittent high temperatures often accompanied by rigors indicate bacterial infection of the bile duct and usually follow the passage of a stone into the bile duct.

Treatment

In most patients acute cholecystitis subsides in a few days with conservative treatment. Cholecystectomy is performed either a few days after the symptoms have settled or 2 to 3 months later. In the latter event, if the symptoms recur during the interval, cholecystectomy is performed without delay. Immediate surgery is mandatory if signs of gangrene or perforation develop.

Conservative treatment

Oral feeding is stopped. Intravenous fluids, and analgesia with nalbuphine or pethidine (demerol) and atropine are administered. Antibiotics are given to all but the most mild cases; tetracycline, amoxicillin, or a cephalosporin are satisfactory for general use. The patient should be observed frequently with abdominal examination and sequential leucocyte counts to detect signs of gangrene of the gallbladder or cholangitis.

Surgical treatment

Cholecystectomy is the operation of choice. Laparoscopic cholecystectomy is the preferred approach. About 10 per cent of patients with acute cholecystitis will have stones in the common bile duct. The bile ducts should be assessed by ERCP and bile duct stones removed by endoscopic sphincterotomy. If an open cholecystectomy is performed, intraoperative cholangiography may be performed to determine whether bile duct stones are present. In high-risk patients and when technical difficulties are encountered a cholecystotomy may be performed.

Chronic cholecystitis

This is the most common form of gallbladder disease that results from gallstones. Pathologically it is characterized by chronic inflammation and thickening of the gallbladder wall. In addition to stones the gallbladder may contain a brown sediment ('biliary mud'). A proportion of these patients have cholesterolosis of the gallbladder ('strawberry gallbladder'). This describes the deposition of yellow specks of cholesterol in the pink gallbladder wall and is a consequence of cholesterol-saturated bile. Cholesterolosis of the gallbladder is asymptomatic but about half the patients develop gallstones. Chronic cholecystitis usually develops insidiously but may follow an attack of acute cholecystitis.

Symptoms and signs

Some patients complain of bouts of constant right hypochondrial or epigastric pain. If it is intermittent, that is, biliary colic, the height of the pain is separated by 15- to 60-min intervals. The pain may last several hours or be as brief as 15 to 20 min. It may radiate to the right shoulder or the back. More commonly the symptoms are vague and ill-defined and include abdominal discomfort and distension, nausea, flatulence, and intolerance of fatty foods. Unfortunately, many patients who do not have chronic cholecystitis complain of these symptoms. Examination of the abdomen may reveal tenderness over the gallbladder and a positive Murphy's sign. Laboratory investigations are usually unhelpful.

Imaging techniques

An ultrasound scan is used to detect gallstones. A plain radiograph of the abdomen may reveal calcified stones or opacification of the gallbladder caused by high concentrations of calcium carbonate ('limey bile') but is not often used now. If these investigations fail to show stones, but stones are still suspected on clinical grounds, an ERCP should be performed before surgery is undertaken.

Differential diagnosis

Dyspepsia and fat intolerance are common symptoms that may be caused by many conditions including peptic ulcers, hiatus hernia, irritable bowel syndrome, chronic relapsing pancreatitis, and tumours of the stomach, pancreas, colon, or gallbladder. Other functional disorders may also mimic chronic cholecystitis.

Complications

The complications of chronic cholecystitis include acute exacerbations (acute cholecystitis), passage of stones into the bile duct (choledocholithiasis or Mirizzi's syndrome), pancreatitis, cholecystenteric fistula formation and gallstone ileus, and rarely carcinoma of the gallbladder. Occasionally the accumulation of mucus and gallstones produces hydrops of the gallbladder, which is characterized by a tender mass without the symptoms of acute cholecystitis.

Treatment

In established cases of chronic cholecystitis the treatment of choice is cholecystectomy. When the diagnosis is in doubt, especially when vague symptoms are associated with a well-functioning gallbladder containing stones, a conservative approach is worth trying. This includes weight reduction and a low-fat diet, especially if fatty food is associated with the symptoms. Oral bile acid therapy may also be considered (see above).

Prognosis

Chronic cholecystitis carries a good prognosis. Cholecystectomy is curative and should have a mortality below 1 per cent. However, if cholecystectomy is performed indiscriminately on patients with 'dyspeptic' symptoms who happen to have incidental gallstones, the results will be unpredictable and often unsatisfactory.

Choledocholithiasis

Most stones in the common bile duct originate in the gallbladder. About 15 per cent of patients with cholelithiasis have common duct stones. This proportion rises with age so that in the elderly nearly 50 per cent of patients with cholelithiasis may have common duct stones. Stones may develop in the bile duct in diseases causing chronic biliary obstruction such as benign bile duct strictures and sclerosing cholangitis.

Clinical features

The classic triad of symptoms is right upper abdominal pain, jaundice, and fever. The abdominal pain is typically colicky, severe, and persists for hours. It is often associated with vomiting. Fever and rigors indicate cholangitis, which commonly accompanies bile duct stones. Jaundice is variable; it may be mild or deep and is often intermittent. The urine is dark due to conjugated bilirubin and the faeces are pale. Frequently, the amount of pigment in the faeces varies. Itching may be prominent. However, common bile duct stones may also be silent, especially in the elderly. Alternatively, only one of the triad of symptoms may be present; the patient presenting with jaundice, abdominal pain, or cholangitis. The liver is moderately enlarged and there may be tenderness in the right upper quadrant. Prolonged biliary obstruction lasting months or years eventually leads to biliary cirrhosis with portal venous hypertension and liver cell failure.

Laboratory investigations

Liver function tests show a cholestatic (biliary obstructive) pattern. The prothrombin time may be prolonged due to inadequate absorption of vitamin K. A polymorphonuclear leucocytosis is common and indicates biliary infection. Blood cultures should be performed repeatedly during the fevers to isolate the organism and determine sensitivities.

Imaging techniques

A plain radiograph of the abdomen will show calcified gallstones in 10 per cent of patients, but is rarely performed now. Ultrasonography is useful for demonstrating the dilated biliary tree that results from obstruction and may reveal biliary gallstones. Unfortunately, ultrasound frequently fails to detect common duct stones obstructing the lower end of the bile duct. Cholangiography by ERCP is required in these patients (Fig. 5). Common bile duct stones should be removed by endoscopic sphincterotomy before the patient is submitted to cholecystectomy.

Differential diagnosis

Common duct stones are the most common cause of cholestatic (biliary obstructive) jaundice. Next in frequency are carcinomas of the head of the pancreas, bile duct, and ampulla of Vater (Table 1). Intrahepatic diseases may also cause a cholestatic jaundice; the causes include viral and alcoholic hepatitis, drugs, and pregnancy.

Treatment

Common bile duct stones must be removed. The optimal treatment is endoscopic sphincterotomy to remove bile duct stones followed by laparoscopic cholecystectomy. This approach avoids the hazards of open exploration of the common bile duct. Endoscopic removal of common duct

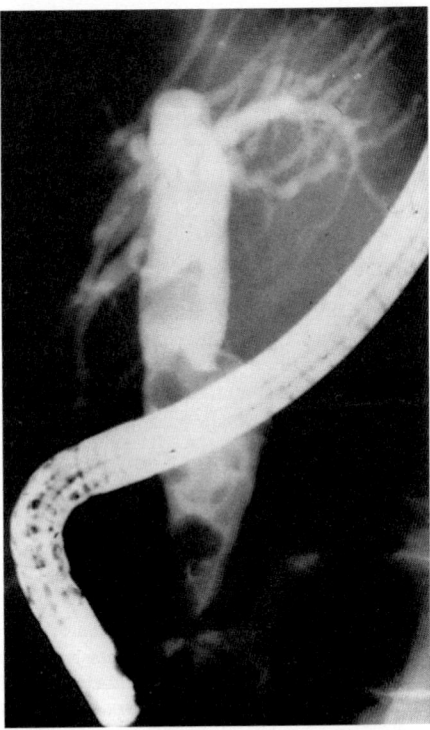

Fig. 5 Choledocholithiasis. An endoscopic retrograde cholangiogram shows multiple faceted radiolucent stones in a dilated bile duct. The gallbladder has not been opacified.

gallstones without cholecystectomy is appropriate in patients unfit for surgery. Few patients will have further problems from the gallbladder that remains. Stones overlooked at surgery (residual calculi) are best treated by endoscopic sphincterotomy or, if a T-tube is in place, removed by a steerable basket-catheter manipulated down the T-tube track. Open exploration of the common bile duct is required if gallstones are too large to be removed endoscopically (more than 2 cm). Preoperative preparation includes appropriate antibiotics for cholangitis, the correction of fluid and electrolyte balance, nutrition, and anaemia, and if the prothrombin time is prolonged, parenteral vitamin K.

Table 1 Causes of bile duct obstruction

Intrinsic causes
Common bile duct gallstones
Cholangitis
Carcinoma of the bile duct
Carcinoma of the gallbladder
Benign post-traumatic stricture
Sclerosing cholangitis (primary and secondary)
Haemobilia
Extrinsic causes
Carcinoma of the pancreas
Carcinoma of the ampulla of Vater
Metastatic carcinoma
Lymphoma
Pancreatitis (acute and chronic)
Pancreatic cysts
Congenital causes
Biliary atresia
Choledochal cyst
Congenital intrahepatic biliary dilatation (Caroli's disease)

Postcholecystectomy syndromes

After cholecystectomy a proportion of patients continue to complain of symptoms such as right upper quadrant pain, flatulence, and fatty food intolerance. However, the vast majority of patients with gallstones are improved by surgery. The persistence of symptoms in many is probably a consequence of the wrong diagnosis being made before surgery and other diseases such as oesophagitis, pancreatitis, or functional bowel disease should be sought. In others, technical problems during surgery may have resulted in a benign post-traumatic biliary stricture or residual calculi. However, there remains a group of patients where the cause appears to be due to less common biliary disorders such as long, dilated cystic duct remnants, amputation neuromas of the cystic duct, and spasm or stenosis of the sphincter of Oddi. The biliary tract must be carefully investigated in these patients, especially if colicky pain, fever, jaundice, or cholestatic liver function tests persist. Biliary tract manometry is of value when spasm or stenosis of the sphincter of Oddi is suspected.

Biliary infections

Bacterial cholangitis (suppurative cholangitis)

This is usually associated with common bile duct calculi and benign biliary structures. Malignant structures produce complete obstruction and the bile remains sterile. Other conditions associated with cholangitis are biliary enteric fistulas—both spontaneous and surgical—sclerosing cholangitis, and congenital intrahepatic biliary dilation (Caroli's disease). Organisms of the gut flora are usually cultured in these infections, including aerobes such as *E. coli*, *Streptococcus faecalis*, *Proteus vulgaris* and staphylococci, and anaerobes such as bacteroides, aerobacter, and anaerobic steptrococci.

Clinical features and treatment

The onset of malaise, fever, and rigors is followed by pain, vomiting, jaundice, and itching. The urine turns dark and the faeces pale. The biliary obstructive features are probably due to oedema of the bile duct wall. Recurrent attacks are common. Hepatic abscesses may result. Repeated blood cultures are performed during the fever to isolate the organisms. Culture of a liver biopsy fragment may also yield the organism. The main element of treatment is drainage of the biliary tract, which is best achieved by emergency endoscopic sphincterotomy. Additionally, appropriate antibiotics such as cefuroxime and metronidazole are given. For recurrent attacks of cholangitis, tetracycline, amoxicillin, or cephalexin are usually effective.

Infestations

Infestations (see Section 7) with the roundworm *Ascaris lumbricoides* and the liver fluke *Clonorchis sinensis* are particular problems of the Far East. Both lead to cholangitis. *C. sinensis* infestation predisposes to bile duct carcinoma and primary liver cancer. The common sheep fluke *Fasciola hepatica* may be encountered as a cause of cholangitis in Europe during wet summers.

Benign biliary strictures

In about 95 per cent of patients these are a consequence of biliary tract surgery. The remainder are caused by gallstones eroding the bile duct and, rarely, blunt injury to the abdomen. Signs of biliary stricture may be detected in the immediate postoperative period but are often delayed. Disasters such as ligation or section of the bile duct present early with jaundice and drainage of bile from the wound drains. With lesser damage to the duct the patient presents after an interval with cholangitis and jaundice. Liver function tests reveal a cholestatic pattern and blood cultures may yield an organism. The precise delineation of the stricture requires ERCP or PTC.

Biliary stricture is not a benign condition; untreated it will usually progress to biliary cirrhosis with portal venous hypertension and liver failure. Treatment is surgical and should be performed by a surgeon skilled in this difficult repair.

Malignant biliary stricture

This is most commonly due to adenocarcinoma of the head of the pancreas but may also be caused by adenocarcinomas of the bile ducts, of the ampulla of Vater, and rarely of the gallbladder. Occasionally the cause is lymph node enlargement at the porta hepatis due to malignant metastases or lymphoma.

Symptoms and signs

Cancers of the pancreas and biliary tree (Figs 6 and 7) usually affect middle-aged and elderly individuals. The onset is insidious with deepening jaundice, itching, and weight loss. A dull nagging upper abdominal pain which radiates to the back is common. In contrast to choledocholithiasis and benign strictures, cholangitis is unusual. Examination reveals a deeply jaundiced patient often excoriated from scratching. The liver is enlarged but not tender. If the malignant obstruction is below the level of the cystic duct, the gallbladder is distended and may be palpable (Courvoisier's law). The urine is dark and the stools pale. In cancer of the ampulla of Vater, a film of blood on the pale stool may give it a silvery colour ('silver stools').

Laboratory investigation

Liver function tests reveal a cholestatic pattern. The serum bilirubin may be very high (600 μmol/l; 35 mg/dl). A microcytic hypochromic anaemia indicates blood loss from the tumour.

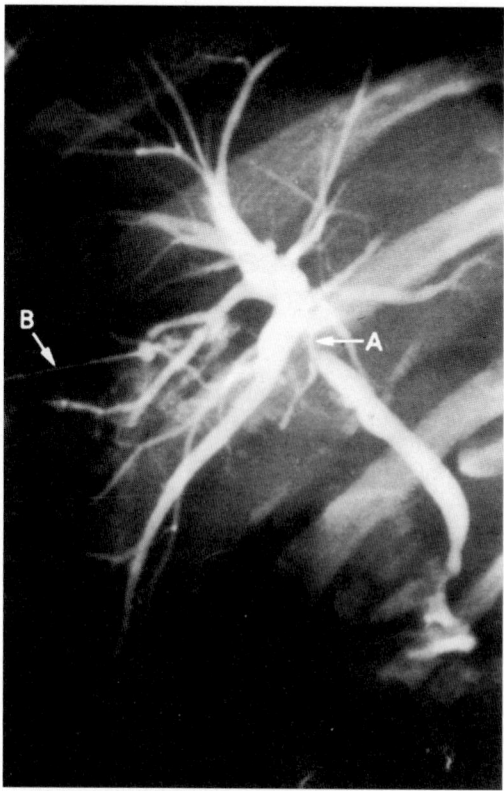

Fig. 6 Carcinoma of the bile duct. A percutaneous transhepatic cholangiogram (PTC) shows a stricture (a) high in the bile duct at the porta hepatis intrahepatic bile ducts are moderately dilated. The transhepatic track of the 'skinny' needle used for the PTC is also visible (b).

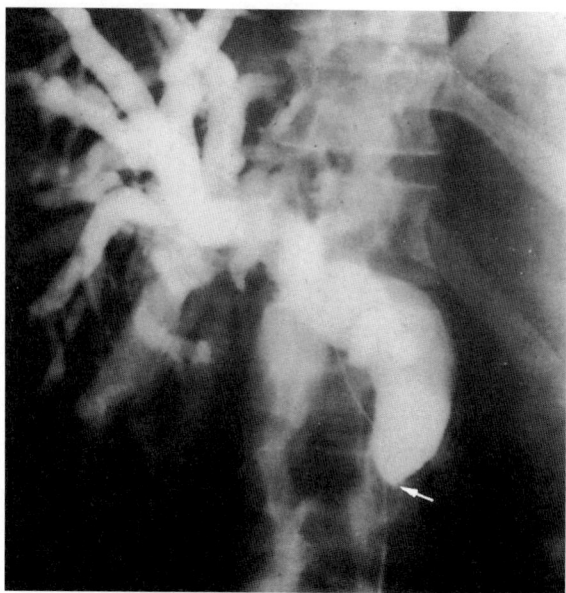

Fig. 7 Carcinoma of the pancreas. The percutaneous transhepatic cholangiogram shows a very dilated biliary tree which terminates in a blunt 'nipple-like' obstruction (arrow) at the lower end of the common bile duct. This is the usual finding in the cancers of the head of the pancreas which obstruct the bilary system.

Imaging techniques

An ultrasound or CT scan examination will reveal dilatation of the biliary tree and may demonstrate the level of the obstruction. Ultrasound-guided percutaneous needle biopsy may be employed to provide a histological diagnosis. Bile duct carcinoma frequently causes obstruction at the porta hepatis and, consequently, at laparotomy the extrahepatic biliary tract appears non-dilated. Even if operative cholangiography is performed, the constrast medium frequently fails to pass the obstruction and fill the dilated intrahepatic biliary tree. Therefore it is important to establish the diagnosis precisely before surgery is contemplated by performing an ERCP or PTC. This is particularly important because most of these patients are best treated by endoscopic or percutaneous biliary stents rather than surgery (see below).

Treatment

Occasionally small tumours confined to the head of the pancreas and ampulla of Vater may be treated curatively by a Whipple's operation. Unfortunately the great majority of pancreatic and bile duct cancers can only be treated palliatively with a bypass procedure such as a cholecystojejunostomy. The prognosis for these patients is poor. An alternative treatment is endoscopic or percutaneous transhepatic introduction of prostheses (stents) through the biliary stricture. Patients with endoscopic prostheses have the same median survival as those with surgical bypass procedures, but the operative mortality and morbidity rate is much lower for endoscopic prostheses. Endoscopic prostheses are the preferred treatment for unresectable biliary and pancreatic cancers. The prostheses may block after about 3 months and need to be replaced.

Other causes of bile duct obstruction

Pancreatitis may obstruct the common bile duct during its passage through the head of the pancreas. Transient jaundice is common in acute pancreatitis due to compression by pancreatic oedema. In chronic pancreatitis, especially alcoholic, persistent jaundice can develop requiring a surgical bypass procedure such as a cholecystojejunostomy. This biliary obstruction is probably a consequence of pancreatic fibrosis. Pancreatic cysts may rarely cause extrinsic compression of the bile duct. Haemobilia or haemorrhage into the biliary tract is uncommon but may follow trauma, liver biopsy, biliary tumours, and gallstones. In addition to jaundice, the blood clots cause biliary pain. Massive gastrointestinal haemorrhage may occur. The diagnosis of these conditions relies on accurate cholangiography (usually ERCP).

Sclerosing cholangitis

Sclerosing cholangitis is the description applied to multiple strictures and bead-like dilatations of the intrahepatic and extrahepatic biliary tree.

Primary sclerosing cholangitis (Fig. 8)

This should only be diagnosed if the following criteria are satisfied: (i) absence of gallstones; (ii) absence of previous biliary surgery; and (iii) sufficiently long follow-up to exclude carcinoma of the bile duct. Primary sclerosing cholangitis affects males more than females (2:1) and about 70 per cent of patients have ulcerative colitis. The usual clinical presentation is cholestatic jaundice and cholangitis. However, a significant proportion of patients are asymptomatic or present with cirrhosis and portal venous hypertension. There is associated retroperitoneal fibrosis or Riedel's thyroiditis in some cases. Serum biochemistry shows cholestatic liver function tests. A raised serum alkaline phosphatase is almost invariable. Consequently the diagnosis should be considered in patients with cirrhosis whose liver function tests show cholestatic features. The IgM concentration is commonly elevated. Liver biopsy may be helpful and usually indicates large bile duct obstruction. The diagnosis is established by cholangiography with ERCP or PTC. Laparotomy should not be performed. Lone tight strictures and stones can be treated by endoscopic techniques. Primary sclerosing cholangitis is being recognized more frequently as a result of the widespread use of ERCP and PTC. It may be confused with primary biliary cirrhosis, but the serum mitochondrial antibody is always negative in primary sclerosing cholangitis. Treatment is unsatisfactory, neither corticosteriods nor azathioprine are of proven value. Ursodeoxycholic acid improves liver function tests but has not been shown to prolong survival.

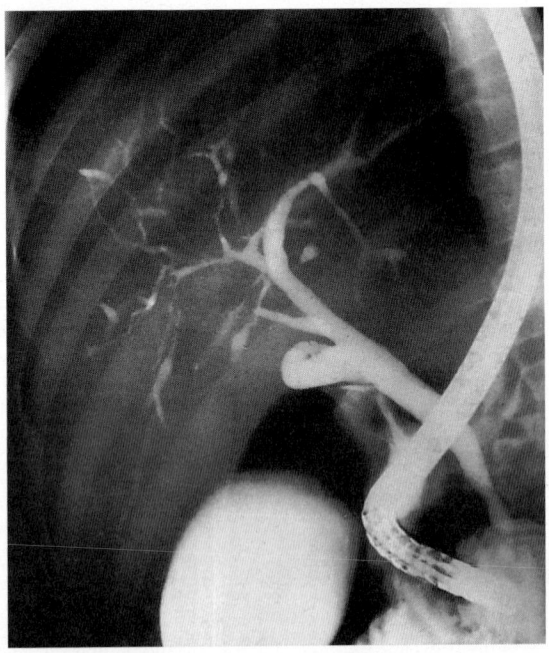

Fig. 8 Primary sclerosing cholangitis. The intrahepatic bile ducts show alternate strictures and dilatations ('beading'). The common bile duct, cystic duct, and gallbladder appear normal in this study but may also be involved.

Pruritus may be helped by cholestyramine. The prognosis is variable but most patients eventually develop cirrhosis and liver failure. Liver transplantation yields excellent results in these patients. Bile duct adenocarcinoma is a late complication.

Secondary sclerosing cholangitis

Several causes of secondary sclerosing cholangitis are now recognized. These include recurrent bacterial cholangitis due to gallstones or benign biliary strictures. Children with primary immunodeficiency syndromes and patients with AIDS also develop sclerosing cholangitis. Cytomegalovirus and cryptosporidium are the organisms most commonly associated with AIDS-related sclerosing cholangitis. Sclerosing cholangitis may also develop in patients treated by hepatic arterial infusion of cytotoxic drugs and after the introduction of caustics into hydatid cysts.

Congenital disorders of the gallbladder and biliary tract

This subject is discussed in Chapter 14.19.1.

Further reading

Angulo P, Lindor KD (1999). Primary sclerosing cholangitis. *Hepatology* **30**, 325–32.

Donovan JM (1999). Physical and metabolic factors in gallstone pathogenesis. *Gastroenterology Clinics of North America* **28**, 75–97.

Ko CW, Lee SP (1999). Gallstone formation. Local factors. *Gastroenterology Clinics of North America* **28**, 99–115.

Schiff L, Schiff ER (1993). *Diseases of the liver*, 7th edn. Lippincott, Philadelphia.

Sherlock S, Summerfield JA (1991). *A colour atlas of liver disease*, 2nd edn. Wolfe Medical Publications, London.

Sherlock S, Dooley JS (1997). *Diseases of the liver and biliary system*, 10th edn. Blackwell Scientific Publications, Oxford.

14.19.3 Jaundice

R. P. H. Thompson

Jaundice is the clinical sign of hyperbilirubinaemia, and hence usually indicates disease of the liver or biliary tree. The pigment in the tissues in best seen as yellowing of the sclera; eventually the skin and soft palate become tinted, but not saliva or sputum. The urine usually becomes dark. Rarely, carotenaemia, from eating excessive carrots or vitamin A, can mimic jaundice, but its colour is more prominent in the palms than the sclera.

Physiology of bilirubin (Fig. 1)

All haem molecules in haemoglobin or cytochrome enzymes are stoichiometrically (1:1) degraded to bilirubin, especially in the spleen and liver, but also in macrophages in other tissues, including skin, and in renal tubular cells. Haem oxygenase enzymes break open the asymmetric tetrapyrrole haem molecule specifically at the α-methene bridge, releasing carbon monoxide and iron. One principal isomer of biliverdin, namely IXα, is formed, although small amounts of the other three possible isomers (β, γ, and δ) can be detected in bile. The excretion of carbon monoxide in breath can be used quantitatively to determine the breakdown of haem to bilirubin, of which 200 to 350 mg (340 to 600 μmol) is produced daily. About 85 per

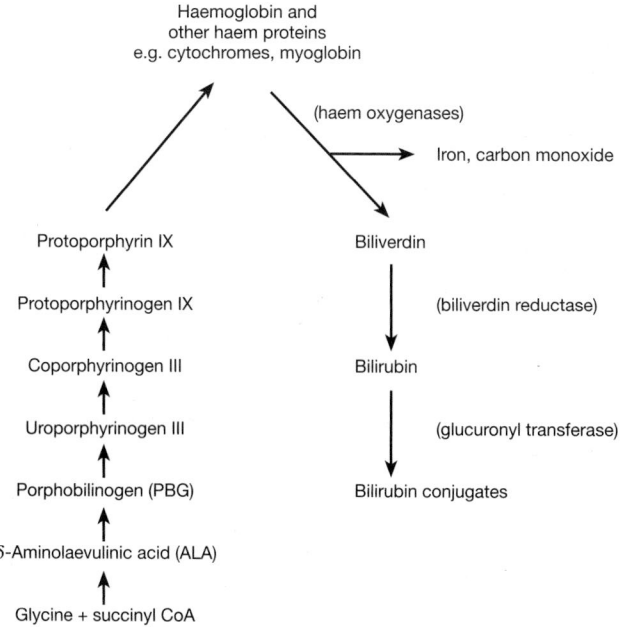

Fig. 1 The porphyrin–bilirubin pathway.

The diagram shows: HAEM at the top, with:
- Haemoglobin and other haem proteins e.g. cytochromes, myoglobin
- (haem oxygenases)
- Iron, carbon monoxide

Left branch (upward):
- Protoporphyrin IX
- Protoporphyrinogen IX
- Coporphyrinogen III
- Uroporphyrinogen III
- Porphobilinogen (PBG)
- δ-Aminolaevulinic acid (ALA)
- Glycine + succinyl CoA

Right branch (downward):
- Biliverdin
- (biliverdin reductase)
- Bilirubin
- (glucuronyl transferase)
- Bilirubin conjugates

cent of biliverdin and bilirubin is derived from the delayed breakdown of the haemoglobin in effete red blood cells, while the remainder is either from the breakdown of haem proteins, chiefly in the liver, or from ineffective erythropoiesis in the bone marrow; these constitute the so-called 'early labelled' bilirubin, defined by isotopic studies *in vivo*.

Biliverdin is green and is directly excreted in bile by birds, amphibians, and reptiles but not by mammals. Biliverdin is reduced by the cytosolic enzyme biliverdin reductase in liver and spleen to the yellow bilirubin IXα, which has then to be excreted. The reason for this difference was obscure, for bilirubin is lipid soluble, and potentially toxic, and has to be conjugated before it is excreted in bile, while biliverdin is water soluble and can be readily excreted in urine and bile by mammals. However, bilirubin is an antioxidant or free radical scavenger in plasma and bile, particularly when bound to copper, and this may be especially important in the neonate, especially when levels of the antioxidant ascorbate are low. Hence bilirubin probably has a function and is not just a waste product. Bilirubin is surprisingly lipid soluble, this being due to internal hydrogen bonding in the molecule so that it forms a tight, non-polar, non-linear, three-dimensional structure. After its release from macrophages, it is firmly bound to plasma albumin, so that none enters the urine. At high concentrations in the blood it slowly diffuses into tissues, where it can be toxic, particularly in the neonatal brain (kernicterus) or kidney. Jaundice is usually less obvious in unconjugated hyperbilirubinaemia since its diffusion into the tissues is more limited.

The circulating pool of bilirubin in the plasma (about 100 μmol) is almost all unconjugated. Routine measurements still rely on the Van den Bergh diazo reaction, which yields either an indirect (unconjugated bilirubin) or direct reaction (conjugated) and, although this overestimates the true level of conjugated bilirubin, the results indicate whether or not circulating bilirubin is wholly unconjugated. The direct and indirect reactions depend on the slow reaction of the unconjugated bilirubin with the reagent, which is accelerated when solvents such as methanol, which break the internal hydrogen bonding, are added. The normal range of plasma bilirubin is wide (about 5 to 19 μmol/l), reflecting wide variation in the rate of conjugation in the liver, and is higher than in most other mammals in whom clearance and excretion are more efficient. The distribution of values

is Gaussian, so that the true upper limit of normal is arbitrary (see Gilbert's syndrome). Hepatic enzyme-inducing drugs reduce the plasma level by increasing conjugation and hence clearance.

Bilirubin is selectively removed by hepatocytes from sinusoidal blood, although its plasma clearance (about 50 ml/min) is low compared, for instance, with that of bile acids, and hence its extraction (1.5 per cent of plasma pool/min) is dependent more upon hepatocyte distribution and function than on blood flow. It is initially surprising that bilirubin can be displaced from its plasma binding sites and enter hepatocytes, and specific hepatic cytoplasmic binding proteins have been described. Nevertheless, binding to the active site of the microsomal conjugating enzyme uridyl diphosphate (**UDP**)-glucuronyl transferase should be sufficient to maintain a low level of free bilirubin in the cytoplasm, which, without the need for specific transfer proteins, should alone produce a gradient sufficient to allow bilirubin slowly to enter the hepatocyte. Uptake of bilirubin is facilitated by the direct contact of plasma with the hepatocyte in the interstitial space of Disse through fenestrations in the endothelium of hepatic blood capillaries. Although uptake into the cell predominates, dynamic studies show that there is considerable reflux of bilirubin back out of the cell to the plasma.

Within the hepatocyte bilirubin is principally conjugated by one of the two specific isoforms of the microsomal enzyme UDP-glucuronyl (glucuronate-glucuronosyl) transferase, chiefly with two glucuronic acid moieties. Conjugated bilirubin is excreted out of the endoplasm reticulum and then across the microvillous intercellular canalicular membrane by the anionic conjugate transporter protein (**mrp2**; or cMOAT). Hepatocytes have a separate canalicular bile salt export pump protein (bsep). mrp2 also transports other multivalent anions, such as conjugated bromsulphthalein. Minor quantities of bilirubin are conjugated with one glucuronic acid molecule (monoglucuronide) or with combinations of related sugars (xylose, glucose); a small amount of unconjugated bilirubin also appears in bile. The chemical properties of the conjugated molecules are quite different from those of unconjugated bilirubin, for there is no internal hydrogen bonding of bilirubin—they now become more linear, fully water-soluble molecules and are efficiently excreted in bile. In many liver diseases conjugated bilirubin readily refluxes back into blood and, since it is water soluble and less firmly bound to albumin than unconjugated bilirubin, about 1 per cent is filtered across the glomerular membrane and enters the urine (choluria). Excretion of conjugated bilirubin is increased by the bile acids that also accumulate in cholestasis. If renal function is normal, renal excretion of bilirubin matches production when conjugated bilirubin levels in the plasma reach about 600 μmol/l. With renal failure, or haemolysis, plasma levels rise higher. Little bilirubin, even conjugated bilirubin, diffuses through renal dialysis membranes.

Recently it has been shown that deconjugated bilirubin can undergo a substantial enterohepatic circulation; it is absorbed from the colon, particularly when there is bile acid malabsorption and hence the concentration of bile acids is increased in the colon, for example as a result of ileal disease or resection. This reabsorption increases the concentration of bilirubin re-excreted in bile, and may in part explain the increased incidence of pigment gallstones in patients with ileal disease. Similarly, fasting increases unconjugated bilirubin levels in the plasma by increasing the reabsorption of bilirubin.

In the distal intestine, conjugated bilirubin is deconjugated and reduced to a series of sterco- and urobilinogens that give the normal colour to faeces. Some colourless urobilinogen is normally absorbed from the colon and undergoes an enterohepatic circulation, with a small amount being excreted in urine. If this circulation and biliary excretion is impaired in liver disease, or increased in haemolysis, then excess urobilinogen is excreted in urine, where it can oxidize on standing to brown urobilins. Urobilinogen is easily detected by routine clinical 'stix'. Ehrlich's aldehyde reagent was at one time used, and when added to urine containing excess urobilinogen it turns it red; the urobilinogen pigment can then be extracted into an organic solvent such as chloroform, unlike the pigment formed from the

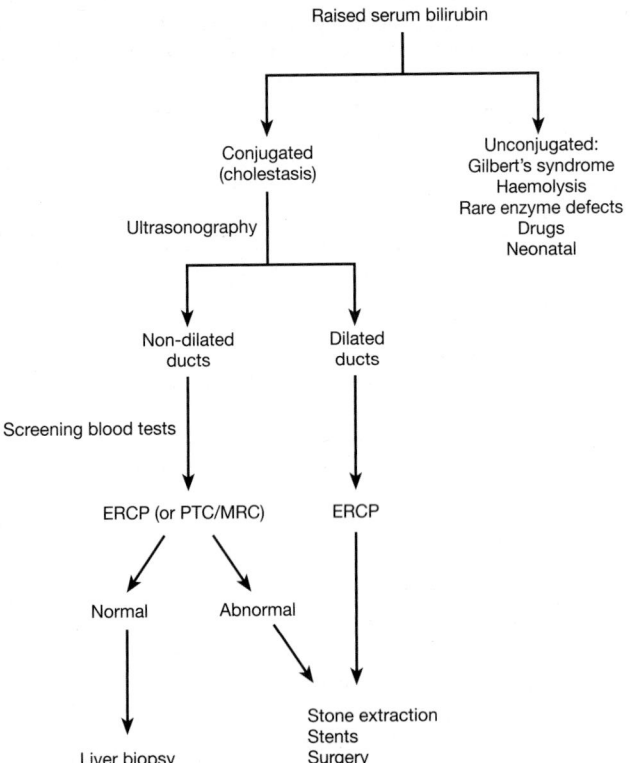

Fig. 2 Investigation of jaundice.

more polar porphobilinogen adduct in acute porphyria, which remains in the aqueous phase.

Management of jaundice

Complex algorithms of management of the patient with hyperbilirubinaemia or jaundice have been published, but a simple pragmatic approach is proposed here (Fig. 2).

Raised plasma bilirubin levels, and eventually frank jaundice, are due primarily to excessive unconjugated or conjugated bilirubin in blood, depending on whether the abnormality in bilirubin metabolism is in its production and/or conjugation, or in the subsequent hepatic excretion of conjugated bilirubin, respectively. Impaired excretion is almost always combined with impaired bile flow and is best termed cholestasis. When other liver-related blood tests are abnormal, especially the biliary enzymes alkaline phosphatase and γ-glutamyl transpeptidase, serum bile acids are also raised, there is often itching, and the microvilli lining the biliary canaliculi are injured. Examination of a liver biopsy specimen taken from a patient with cholestasis under light microscopy may show bile plugs. This finding is, however, often termed 'obstructive jaundice', an unfortunate term, since this implies extrahepatic obstruction of the biliary tree. The molecular events underlying some forms of cholestasis are now being unravelled (see below).

History

Dark urine and, less commonly, pale stools indicate cholestasis. Many drugs, including alcohol, can be a cause of unconjugated and conjugated hyperbilirubinaemia and should be rigorously enquired about. Fever (hepatitis, cholangitis, abscesses), travel (hepatitis, amoebiasis), sexual history (hepatitis A, B, or C), surgery and anaesthesia (postoperative jaundice, see below; biliary tract disease), herbal medicines (e.g. West Indian teas,

Chinese herbs), and transfusions and blood products (hepatitis B or C) can be important clues.

Clinical examination

Stigmata of chronic liver disease (e.g. spider naevi, facial telangietases, parotid enlargement, Dupuytren's contractures, muscle wasting, hepatosplenomegaly, and ascites) are important, but do not define the cause of jaundice.

Testing for unconjugated hyperbilirubinaemia

If serum bilirubin alone is abnormal among the liver-related blood tests, unconjugated hyperbilirubinaemia should first be excluded by testing whether the bilirubin in blood is predominantly conjugated or unconjugated. A normal reticulocyte count will usually exclude haemolysis severe enough to cause raised bilirubin levels and blood film examination may be additionally informative. Suspected haemolysis is investigated as described elsewhere. If no cause of unconjugated hyperbilirubinaemia is identified, then benign constitutional unconjugated hyperbilirubinaemia (Gilbert's syndrome) is diagnosed (see below).

Conjugated hyperbilirubinaemia

The familial syndromes without cholestasis (Dubin–Johnson and Rotor) are rare (see below).

Routine liver-related blood tests cannot differentiate between intra- or extrahepatic causes of jaundice, unless the transferases are very high (e.g. more than 1000 IU/l), in which case hepatitis (e.g. viral, alcoholic) is certain. A greatly raised alkaline phosphatase level does not necessarily imply an extrahepatic lesion; intrahepatic causes are common (Table 1). Research methods for assessing liver function (e.g. galactose tolerance test, aminopyrine breath test) are of no value in the management of the patient with jaundice.

Cholestasis should be investigated first with abdominal ultrasonography, which should accurately detect a dilated intra- and/or extrahepatic biliary tree and often also reveal its cause (e.g. gallstones, tumour). Cholecystography or intravenous cholangiography will fail in the presence of jaundice. If biliary disease is thus suspected, then an endoscopic retrograde cholangiogram (ECRP) or, failing that, a fine-needle, percutaneous, transhepatic cholangiogram (PTC), will define the anatomy more accurately and often provide definitive therapy (removal of biliary stones, stenting), thus often avoiding surgery. Magnetic resonance cholangiography (MRC) is

Table 1 Intrahepatic cholestasis

Infection	Viral hepatitis A, B, or C
	Bacterial: sepsis, miliary tuberculosis, leptospirosis
	Neonatal hepatitis syndrome
Toxins	Alcohol.
	Drugs: hepatotoxic, idiosyncratic
	Oestrogens: pregnancy, contraceptive pill
	α_1-Antitrypsin deficiency
Infiltration	Carcinoma: metastases
	Lymphoma
	Adenocarcinoma of kidney (non-metastatic)
	Sarcoidosis
Familial	Benign recurrent
	Neonatal cholestatic syndromes
Reduced blood flow	Perioperative hypoperfusion/shock
	Sickle-cell anaemia
Intrahepatic ducts	Biliary atresia
	Primary biliary cirrhosis
	Sclerosing cholangitis
	Malignant infiltration of ducts
Autoimmune	Chronic active hepatitis

increasing in sensitivity and availability and can now produce high-quality non-invasive images of the biliary tree and pancreas; it is useful even for intrahepatic biliary disease. It cannot, of course, be therapeutic. Endoscopic ultrasonography (EUS) can show accurately the presence of stones, biliary or pancreatic tumours, and sclerosing cholangitis, while γ-camera scans with technetium-labelled **HIDA** (hepato-iminodiacetic acid) can be used to indicate biliary obstruction, particularly in the neonate, if ultrasonography is normal.

If intrahepatic cholestasis is suspected because of a non-dilated biliary tree on ultrasound, the following tests should be considered: hepatitis A, B, or C serology, autoantibodies (antimitochondrial for primary biliary cirrhosis, smooth muscle and liver–kidney microsomal for autoimmune chronic hepatitis), serum caeruloplasmin and copper for Wilson's disease if less than 40 years of age, or plasma α_1-antitrypsin concentrations for homozygous deficiency. Intrahepatic masses on ultrasound will prompt measurement of α-fetoprotein for primary hepatoma and other tumour markers. A percutaneous needle liver biopsy (or aspiration of an abscess) may then be indicated, provided that blood coagulation parameters and the platelet count are normal. Guidelines for liver biopsy have recently been published. A transjugular venous approach for the biopsy is appropriate if the risks of bleeding are increased.

Unconjugated hyperbilirubinaemia

Plasma bilirubin levels are exponentially and positively related to the half-life of circulating red blood cells (i.e. bilirubin load), and negatively to the hepatic clearance rate of bilirubin. This relationship is analogous to that of muscle breakdown, plasma creatinine, and glomerular filtration rate. Hence, as the rate of haemolysis rises or clearance falls, bilirubin levels may rise rapidly in response to small changes of the input load or removal rate from plasma, or both.

Haemolytic jaundice is most commonly encountered in the haemoglobinopathies of sickle-cell anaemia (homozygous SS or heterozygous SC disease) or homozygous thalassaemia major, although dark skin may render it difficult to detect. The 'acholuric jaundice' of hereditary spherocytosis is rare. Mildly elevated bilirubin levels are described in ineffective erythropoiesis of the bone marrow, in vitamin B_{12} deficiency (pernicious anaemia), or in thalassaemia minor.

Drugs may cause haemolysis (e.g. methyl DOPA, sulphasalazine), or impair hepatic bilirubin clearance (e.g. rifampicin). Infections (e.g. malaria) or mismatched blood transfusions can produce massive haemolysis, but this overshadows the raised bilirubin levels. Autoimmune haemolytic anaemia, glucose-6-phosphate dehydrogenase deficiency, and haemolysis due to leaking prosthetic cardiac valves may cause obvious clinical jaundice that may escape diagnosis before the true nature of the hyperbilirubinaemia is recognized.

Familial unconjugated hyperbilirubinaemia

A series of defects of the hepatic conjugating enzyme UDP-glucuronyl transferase produce various degrees of unconjugated hyperbilirubinaemia due to impaired bilirubin clearance; they have long fascinated physiologists and more recently molecular biologists.

At least 3 per cent of the normal adult population have mildly raised unconjugated bilirubin levels in blood that rise excessively on fasting. This 'phenomenon' is commonly termed Gilbert's syndrome, although it is unclear whether the eponym is justified. The raised concentrations of bilirubin develop in early adult life and are often associated with mild degrees of haemolysis. Various associated defects of hepatic drug metabolism have also been described and these are probably linked genetic abnormalities. Any combination of an increased bilirubin load from the haemolysis and a mildly impaired clearance will increase plasma bilirubin concentrations more than would either alone, and hence together they bring the condition to notice. It is probably not a discrete entity but rather different defects of conjugation that elevate bilirubin levels above an arbitrary upper limit of normal. Determination of the bilirubin-conjugating capacity of liver biopsy tissue has shown that the activity of glucuronyl tranferase is reduced by 60 to 70 per cent, and this impairs bilirubin clearance.

Gilbert's syndrome is recognized by a fluctuating, raised serum bilirubin concentration with other routine liver-related blood tests being normal, and a normal reticulocyte count to exclude overt haemolysis. It can be confirmed by measuring the unconjugated fraction of the bilirubin, which should be greater than 90 per cent. Measuring the pronounced increase of plasma bilirubin that occurs after a 48-h fast on 400 kcal/day or provocation with intravenous nicotinic acid are now generally considered to be research procedures of little clinical value. A liver biopsy is rarely needed. Reassurance that the results do not indicate liver disease and will not affect life insurance is important. Plasma bilirubin concentrations rise in patients with Gilbert's syndrome during intercurrent illness when frank jaundice may be observed.

It is said that Gilbert's syndrome can follow an attack of viral hepatitis, although this may be simply due to ascertainment bias in a population with a high underlying prevalence of the biochemical anomaly.

Crigler–Najjar syndromes

Two syndromes of more severe unconjugated hyperbilirubinaemia have been described, namely the rare type I (100 cases reported), which often causes neonatal death, and the more common, and benign type II. Both are due to severe deficiency in the UDP-glucuronyl transferase enzymes.

In type I, first reported in 1952, with an autosomal recessive inheritance, neonates rapidly become progressively jaundiced in the first days of life (bilirubin levels reach 350 to 950 μmol/l) and, if untreated, develop kernicterus or brain damage. Death usually occurs within a year but delayed kernicterus has been reported. There is no conjugated bilirubin in bile, but small quantities of unconjugated bilirubin can be found in bile and cross the intestinal wall.

The inheritance of type II is complex, and is reported both to be dominant with incomplete penetrance or autosomal recessive. Bilirubin levels are lower (less than 350 μmol/l), and persistent mild jaundice is only noticed in childhood. Brain damage does not occur, and the only problem is cosmetic. One-third of the conjugated bilirubin in bile is present as the monogluronide (normally less than 10 per cent).

In the Gunn strain of rat, severe unconjugated hyperbilirubinaemia occurs and glucuronyl transferase activity is absent in the liver, as it is in Crigler–Najjar type I. In type II, enzyme activity is less than 10 per cent of normal, but measurable.

It has long been known that there is a spectrum of bilirubin levels in type II Crigler–Najjar and Gilbert's syndromes and indeed both conditions have been observed within families, suggesting different degrees of enzyme activity. Phenobarbitone or other hepatic microsomal enzyme-inducing agents markedly reduce bilirubin levels in Gilbert's and Crigler–Najjar type II syndromes, although unfortunately not in Crigler–Najjar type I, and increase the activity of glucuronyl transferase. Such treatment, however, is not needed, except possibly for cosmetic purposes.

Molecular analysis of the genes encoding human UDP-glucuronyl transferases has clarified the genetic basis and inheritance of these disorders. The two complementary DNAs for the two human bilirubin UDP-glucuronyl transferase isoforms have been sequenced; they differ from those that encode the other glucuronyl transferases that conjugate, for instance, steroids. The UDP-glucuronyl transferases map to human chromosome 2, where at least seven exons encode the specific mRNAs of the isozymes, together with a common region for the glucuronyl transferases. Analysis of DNA from five patients with type I Crigler–Najjar syndrome has identified homozygous or heterozygous defects in the common structural exons encoding the two bilirubin glucuronyl transferase isoforms—similar defects occur in the Gunn rat.

In Crigler–Najjar type II syndrome, initial studies have found mutations in the upstream regulating region of the gene encoding the active bilirubin glucuronyl transferase isoform. Phenobarbitone induces the expression of the abnormal enzyme, explaining its efficacy in this condition. Probably a heterozygous combination of an abnormality of the promoter region (Gilbert's defect; see below) and this Crigler–Najjar defect is responsible for the phenotype of type II Crigler–Najjar syndrome. This explains the presence of patients with Gilbert's syndrome within families with type II Crigler–Najjar.

The genetic basis of Gilbert's syndrome remains controversial but it appears that it is an autosomal recessive condition in which there is a homozygous abnormality in the promoter region affecting expression of the specific glucuronyl transferase gene. Heterozygotes have normal bilirubin levels. There must be another factor responsible for the increased bilirubin concentrations as the heterozygote abnormality occurs in 40 per cent of healthy individuals without hyperbilirubinaemia. Moreover, some individuals who are homozygous for the defect have normal plasma concentrations of conjugated bilirubin. The bilirubin load from red cell breakdown will influence plasma concentrations.

Crigler–Najjar type I syndrome can now be successfully treated by whole-body blue-light phototherapy for 16 h daily (see below), or by plasmapheresis until orthotopic liver transplantation can be carried out as a definitive cure. Severe kernicterus is a contraindication to transplantation as it is not reversible. About 20 patients have so far received transplants, with two deaths. Hepatocyte transplantation, in which donor hepatocytes are infused into the portal vein, has been partially successful, and clearly has potential for development. Drugs that displace unconjugated bilirubin from albumin (sulphonamides, salicylates, penicillin) will increase brain damage in Crigler–Najjar syndrome and must be avoided.

Neonatal jaundice

Unconjugated hyperbilirubinaemia, often with mild clinical jaundice, occurs in all full-term newborn infants. Bilirubin concentrations are maximal at 2 to 5 days after birth but the plasma bilirubin rarely exceeds 90 µmol/l; neonatal jaundice is more severe in premature infants. It is attributed to a combination of immaturity of hepatic glucuronyl transferase and the added load of bilirubin from rapid haemolysis of surplus fetal red blood cells in the neonatal period. Before birth, fetal bilirubin is excreted by the mother, and meconium as well as stools are pale because of the reduced excretion of bilirubin.

If haemolysis is increased, as in rhesus or other fetomaternal incompatibility of red cell antigens, causing haemolysis of fetal red blood cells by maternal antibodies, then severe jaundice and kernicterus can occur. Acidosis and some drugs (sulphonamides, salicylates, penicillin) may increase kernicterus by displacing unconjugated bilirubin from albumin. Glucose-6-phosphate deficiency can also cause jaundice and anaemia in the neonatal period and is usually observed in infants of Mediterranean, African, or Chinese ancestry.

Treatment with phenobarbitone induces hepatic glucuronyl transferase but its effect is slow unless given to the mother before birth. Exchange transfusion or plasmapheresis are more effective. Phototherapy, namely exposure of the near-naked infant to blue light in an incubator, is also very effective. Being yellow, bilirubin absorbs light at approximately 450 nm and is sensitive to light, which oxidizes it to water-soluble, non-toxic products. Hence, exposure of the bilirubin in skin capillaries to light reduces plasma concentrations; the breakdown products are excreted safely in urine and bile. Reabsorption of bilirubin from the intestine can also be reduced by giving agar by mouth, thus interrupting the enterohepatic circulation.

Breast feeding slightly increases bilirubin levels and about 1 in 40 breast-fed infants develop jaundice, which remits on transfer to cow's milk for 24 h; this jaundice does not always recur when breast milk is reintroduced. Breast feeding increases the enterohepatic cycling of bilirubin from the intestine, since stool weights and frequency are less than with formula feeds. A further effect of steroid molecules that inhibit glucuronyl transferase activity in the neonatal liver and that are present in breast milk has also been postulated.

Hypothyroidism increases jaundice and should be sought in patients with unexplained hyperbilirubinaemia since it may not be associated with obvious neonatal cretinism. The rare Crigler–Najjar type I syndrome presents with florid jaundice in the first few days of life.

Sickle-cell anaemia and β-thalassaemia

Jaundice is common in homozygous sickle-cell anaemia due to the unconjugated hyperbilirubinaemia from persistent haemolysis. During crises jaundice often deepens in association with increasing anaemia, suggesting accelerated haemolysis although transient bone marrow failure may also occur. Occasionally, conjugated hyperbilirubinaemia with dark urine occurs during these episodes, and hepatic histology may show areas of necrosis due to thrombosis and bile thrombi. Patients with sickle-cell anaemia are also prone to pigment gallstones, due to the excessive bilirubin excreted, and these can cause extrahepatic biliary obstruction. Unconjugated and conjugated hyperbilirubinaemia both occur in homozygous thalassaemia as a result of increased red cell destruction and intramedullary haemolysis associated with ineffective erythropoiesis.

Cholestasis

There are many causes of intrahepatic cholestasis (Table 1).

Neonatal cholestasis

Conjugated hyperbilirubinaemia or cholestasis in the neonate, with dark urine and pale stools, is always pathological and if it continues beyond 2 weeks of age requires urgent investigation. There are many causes.

In many instances the cause is never established and although once called neonatal hepatitis, it is better termed the hepatitis syndrome; hepatic histology shows hepatitis, sometimes with giant cells. Some babies recover, while perhaps half progress to hypoplasia of the intrahepatic bile ducts, which then overlaps with extra- and intrahepatic biliary atresia.

Infections, particularly urinary, can cause transient cholestasis. Syphilis is now rare, as is toxoplasmosis. Various viral infections (rubella, cytomegalovirus) can cause neonatal jaundice. The hepatotrophic hepatitus B virus contracted from an HBe antigen-positive mother rarely causes jaundice. Metabolic diseases that may be causes of neonatal jaundice include galactosaemia, hereditary fructose intolerance (fructosaemia), and tyrosinosis—all of which need to be diagnosed quickly so as to start dietary treatment early—as well as homozygous α_1-antitrypsin deficiency, and intravenous feeding per se. Other genetic diseases include trisomy 13 and trisomy 18 (one-quarter of babies developing the hepatitis syndrome) and cystic fibrosis.

Several familial syndromes presenting with neonatal cholestasis have been described, some with other congenital abnormalities, such as arteriohepatic dysplasia (Alagille's syndrome), and others solely with progressive familial cholestasis, with persistent jaundice, raised serum bile acids, hepatosplenomegaly, steatorrhoea, and failure to thrive, such as Byler's syndrome in Amish families. Bile duct hypoplasia, cirrhosis, and liver failure often follow, unless liver transplantation is carried out. There are several different mutations in the various syndromes of progressive familial cholestasis that affect the function of the FIC-1 gene, so that canalicular biliary bile acid and conjugated bilirubin excretion are severely impaired, and hence cholestasis develops.

Extrahepatic cholestasis in the neonate is most commonly due to biliary atresia, but choledochal cyst or bile duct perforation can also cause jaundice at this age. Biliary atresia appears to represent a form of sclerosing cholangitis with progressive loss of intra- and extrahepatic ducts. HIDA scans, percutaneous liver biopsy, and retrograde cholangiography can establish the diagnosis without laparotomy.

Benign recurrent intrahepatic cholestasis

In this rare syndrome, recurrent reversible episodes of cholestasis start in childhood or adult life. Each attack is characterized by jaundice, anorexia, and itching for several months, which then subsides with no residual effects. Hepatic histology only shows cholestasis. Phenobarbitone or ursodeoxycholic acid may shorten and attenuate attacks. A locus for benign recurrent intrahepatic cholestasis has been mapped to chromosome 18, and the abnormality is similar to some cases of progressive familial cholestasis.

Postoperative jaundice

Jaundice due to halothane hepatitis, post-transfusion viral hepatitis, incompatible blood transfusion, drugs, and bile duct damage is described elsewhere.

Prolonged intrahepatic cholestasis used to be common after cardiac surgery, and for no clear reason is much less commonly seen in intensive care units. It is related to the length of surgery and intraoperative cardiac function, and may be due to reduced hepatic blood flow during surgery. Improvement in intra- and postoperative care seems to have improved hepatic function and rendered the syndrome uncommon. Transfused red blood cells are prone to rapid haemolysis and this increases the bilirubin load, while impaired renal function reduces the urinary excretion of conjugated bilirubin. Drug-induced liver injury should be considered.

Cholestasis of pregnancy

Slight impairment of the hepatic excretion of bilirubin can be demonstrated during normal pregnancy or after the administration of oestrogens, but rarely bilirubin and alkaline phosphatase levels rise during the third trimester and intolerable itching and frank jaundice develop, all of which rapidly remit after delivery. The severity of the syndrome increases in successive pregnancies. The fetus is probably not affected, but premature induction of labour may be needed for the mother's sake. The contraceptive pill frequently causes a milder syndrome in the same susceptible women. Ursodeoxycholic acid is reported to ameliorate the condition and is safe, at least during late pregnancy. Phenobarbitone may help the itching, although there may be a small risk of impairing neonatal respiration. Cholestyramine has also been used.

Other causes of jaundice in late pregnancy should be remembered, including acute fatty liver, extrahepatic biliary obstruction, such as from gallstones, and toxaemia.

Pregnancy, by affecting bilirubin excretion, may bring the jaundice of primary biliary cirrhosis or the Dubin–Johnson/Rotor syndromes to notice.

Sepsis

Abnormal liver-related blood tests, and occasionally cholestatic jaundice, often develop during bacterial/viral infections, unrelated to the administration of drugs. In animals this has been shown to be due to endotoxins and cytokines that rapidly down-regulate and translocate the canalicular transport protein mrp2, which excretes conjugated bilirubin into the canaliculus. At the same time other pump proteins are up-regulated, a complex rearrangement that may protect the hepatocyte against oxidative damage. The degradation and impaired synthesis of mrp2 may explain the strange, slow time courses of some of the remitting cholestatic syndromes. Jaundice is especially common in patients with glucose-6-phosphatase deficiency when they develop sepsis, such as pneumonia, since the haemolysis exacerbates the jaundice. The combination of high bilirubin levels and sepsis is particularly damaging to the kidney.

Dubin–Johnson and Rotor syndromes

There are two rare, familial forms of non-haemolytic, conjugated hyperbilirubinaemia without cholestasis.

The Dubin–Johnson syndrome, first described in 1954, is a chronic, relapsing jaundice, without itching or raised serum bile acids. Other liver-related blood tests are normal, but there are associated defects in the excretion of other anions, such as bromsulphthalein, radiographic dyes, and urobilinogen. Hence cholecystography fails, there is excess urobilinogen in the urine, and a delayed rise of the plasma levels of bromsulphthalein after an injection of the dye due to reflux of the conjugated anion from hepatocytes. Jaundice increases during pregnancy or when taking the contraceptive pill because oestrogens impair bilirubin excretion further. A black pigment accumulates in the liver so that at laparoscopy the liver appears strikingly black, as do needle biopsy specimens. Urinary coproporphyrin excretion is abnormal. The inheritance seems to differ between families, and a similar condition occurs in a mutant strain of Corriedale sheep, although in this instance photosensitivity also occurs. Other families have been described in which there are similar findings but no hepatic pigment, the so-called Rotor syndrome. No treatment of either syndrome is required apart from reassurance, and support when seeking life assurance.

Further reading

Chowdury JR, Chowdury NR (1993). Unveiling the mysteries of inherited disorders of bilirubin glucuronidation. *Gastroenterology* **105**, 288–92.

Elferink RPJO, van Berge Henegouwen GP (1998). Cracking the genetic code for benign recurrent and progressive familial intrahepatic cholestasis. *Journal of Hepatology* **29**, 317–20.

Grant A, Neuberger J (1999). Guidelines on the use of liver biopsy in clinical practice. *Gut* **45**(Suppl IV), 1–11.

Jansen PLM (1996). Genetic diseases of bilirubin metabolism: the inherited unconjugated hyperbilirubinemias. *Journal of Hepatology* **25**, 398–404.

Jansen PLM, Müller M (1998). Early events in sepsis-associated cholestasis. *Gastroenterology* **116**, 486–8.

Soloway RD (1996). The increasingly complex molecular life cycle of bilirubin. *Gastroenterology* **110**, 2013–14.

14.20 Hepatitis and autoimmune liver disease

14.20.1 Viral hepatitis—clinical aspects

H. J. F. Hodgson

Many viruses can infect the liver (Table 1). In some patients, hepatic involvement is merely one facet of a systemic infection, and the liver involvement is generally trivial, although occasionally it can be dominant. The liver bears the brunt of infection with the major hepatitis viruses. Thus far, five such viruses have been clearly delineated—A, B, C, D, and E. Other hepatitis viruses are being described and their clinical relevance is under investigation. Viral hepatitis is a major clinical problem worldwide, particularly in developing countries, but no society is exempt.

The clinical effects of infection with a hepatitis virus depend on the severity of the inflammation induced in the liver, and on whether the virus is rapidly cleared from the liver or persists long-term. These in turn reflect the characteristics both of the virus and of the host's immune response. The clinical picture of viral hepatitis is very variable, including fatal fulminant acute hepatitis, acute hepatitis with complete recovery, or chronic infection leading to cirrhosis and predisposing to hepatocellular carcinoma. This chapter will describe the clinical and pathological consequences of viral hepatitis in general, identify virus-specific clinical patterns, and discuss the investigation, management, and prophylaxis of viral hepatitis.

Clinical outcome of hepatitis virus infection

The commonest clinically recognized manifestation of viral hepatitis is an episode of acute icteric hepatitis, generally a self-limited condition with a low mortality and complete recovery. In a typical attack, after an initial prodrome lasting from several days to a couple of weeks—comprising malaise, anorexia, mild fever, and upper abdominal discomfort—jaundice appears. The icteric period typically lasts for a few days to a few weeks, after which the jaundice slowly subsides. Pruritis may occur, generally after the onset of jaundice. Development of ascites or oedema is uncommon but

Table 1 Viruses affecting the liver

Major hepatotrophic viruses	A, B, C, D, E
Minor hepatotrophic viruses	G, transfusion-transmitted virus (**TTV**)
Systemic viruses capable of causing hepatitis*	Herpesviruses, Epstein–Barr virus (**EBV**), cytomegalovirus (**CMV**), varicella virus, adenovirus
Tropical viruses	Yellow fever, dengue, haemorrhagic viruses

* More frequently in immunosuppressed patients.

may occur in more severe cases. Return to normality after an attack of hepatitis may take several weeks to a few months and residual fatigue is common.

There are a number of variations on the clinical course of acute hepatitis. Often jaundice does not occur (anicteric hepatitis), and the episode is asymptomatic or dismissed as 'flu-like'. This may occur more frequently than clinically recognized attacks. In cholestatic hepatitis, jaundice with pruritus, pale stools, and dark urine persists for up to 2 or 3 months. Before recovery eventually occurs, a small number of patients have relapsing hepatitis with a transient worsening of jaundice after an initial improvement. Acute hepatitis is only rarely fatal. If it is, patients usually rapidly develop hepatic encephalopathy, and the timing of onset of this has been used to define a variety of syndromes of fulminant hepatitis. One definition is that in 'fulminant hepatitis' encephalopathy develops within 2 weeks of jaundice. Encephalopathy occurs later than this in patients with 'subfulminant hepatitis'. Hepatitis A, B, C, and E can all initiate an acute self-limited hepatitis, although hepatitis C is particularly unlikely to give rise to the fulminant form. Only hepatitis B and C have the propensity to cause chronic viral hepatitis: generally an indolent disease, in which viral carriage in the liver persists over years or decades, with inflammation that varies in intensity. Hepatitis D, which coinfects patients infected with hepatitis B, can contribute to either acute or chronic inflammation. *

Features of acute hepatitis caused by different viruses

Hepatitis A virus (HAV)

This causes acute self-limited hepatitis, but not chronic viral carriage or chronic liver disease. The RNA virus is acquired orally. The incubation period is between 2 and 6 weeks. Transmission generally follows the ingestion of food or water contaminated with faeces from an HAV-infected individual. Viral shedding in the faeces ceases at approximately the onset of clinical symptoms. Transmission may occur in epidemics, following floods, or after sewage contamination of shellfish beds. The disease is also endemic in all parts of the world. In developing countries, infection is frequent; there is serological evidence of past infection in up to 100 per cent of 10-year-olds in some countries. In Western countries, evidence of prior infection varies, typically ranging from 5 to 40 per cent dependent on age, social class, and other factors. Promiscuous homosexual males have a high incidence of infection. Very rarely, pooled blood products have transmitted the disease parenterally. Clinically the disease is often anicteric or mild, particularly in young children. About 10 per cent of patients have a relapse before recovery. The mortality rate is low, about 0.3 per cent. Deaths occur predominantly in the elderly amongst whom mortality rates may exceed 2 per cent, and pre-existing chronic viral hepatitis B or C may predispose to a fatal outcome. A rare sequel is aplastic anaemia some months after recovery from hepatitis.

Hepatitis B virus (HBV)

Hepatitis B viral infection was recognized by its parenteral transmission route, classically as serum- and then transfusion-associated hepatitis. The incubation period of this DNA virus varies from 4 to 24 weeks. In between 90 and 95 per cent of adult cases the infection is self-limited and the HBV is cleared. In infants, clearance rates are as low as 5 to 10 per cent. The incidence of acute hepatitis B varies widely, and is very high in the Far East and Africa. Transmission may be vertical—that is, infection of a newborn or infant child usually by a chronically infected mother, either at the time of birth or during close family contact. Horizontal transmission routes include blood transfusion and blood products, the use of contaminated needles medically or by drug addicts, exposure in dialysis units, tattooing, and sexual contact. Promiscuous homosexuals and heterosexuals are at risk.

Anicteric attacks of acute HBV are common. If the acute infection is recognized clinically, in addition to the typical clinical features of any acute hepatitis, the preicteric prodrome may include prominent arthritis, fever, and an urticarial rash, due to immune complex deposition. Hepatitis B is fulminant in about 0.3 per cent of cases, and both the strain of HBV and a very active host immune response may contribute. In the great majority of cases, in which HBV is cleared after acute infection, **HBsAg** (hepatitis B surface antigen) disappears from the blood within weeks to a few months. Failure to clear within 6 months defines 'chronic carriage'.

Hepatitis C virus (HCV)

This was recognized as a cause of transfusion-associated hepatitis. The incubation period ranges from 2 to 26 weeks, but usually between 5 and 12. Apart from blood transfusion and blood product administration, drug addiction and renal dialysis are strong epidemiological associations. Sexual transmission and horizontal transmission are uncommon, but not unknown. Fulminant hepatitis due to HCV is rare. Indeed, the initial acute episode is most often subclinical, but after acquiring the infection 85 per cent of individuals fail to clear the virus. HCV infection is therefore usually not recognized until the chronic phase.

Hepatitis D virus (HDV)

The unique position of hepatitis D virus, an RNA virus 'parasitic' on HBV, has been discussed (Chapter 7.10.19). If HBV and HDV coinfect simultaneously, either unremarkable acute hepatitis, or on occasion fulminant disease, result. If HBV is cleared, HDV must be so also. Acute HDV infection can superinfect a chronic HBV carrier, and result in worsening of liver function, particularly if the hepatitis B virus has previously caused significant liver disease. In such a carrier, the superinfection with HDV may be transient, or chronic hepatitis D carriage may persist. Both coinfection and superinfection are recognized initiators of fulminant hepatitis. In the West, intravenous drug abuse is a prominent epidemiological association, but all parenteral modes demonstrated by HBV occur, including sexual transmission. The southern Mediterranean, the Far East, and South America are areas of high or moderate incidence.

Hepatitis E virus (HEV)

This enterally acquired RNA virus, as is HAV, causes acute hepatitis without chronic carriage. Most major epidemics of acute hepatitis in the Indian subcontinent and the Far East are due to the HEV. Such epidemics affect adults as well as children, indicating that immunity in those areas is not regularly acquired in childhood. Flooding and sewage contamination often precede epidemics. The incubation period is about 6 weeks, and faecal excretion of the virus may persist for nearly 2 months after the onset of hepatitis. A striking feature of HEV infection, and the main clinical difference from HAV, is the propensity to induce fulminant hepatitis if acquired during mid-trimester pregnancy, and mortality rates of 10 to 40 per cent are recorded amongst pregnant women.

Other hepatotrophic viruses

Other hepatotrophic viruses remain to be described, in particular to explain non-A/B/C/D/E fulminant and transfusion hepatitis. Although the hepatitis G virus and transfusion-transmitted virus (**TTV**) have been well characterized, they do not appear to give rise to significant disease.

Clinical examination

Jaundice and right upper-quadrant abdominal tenderness characterize acute hepatitis. Skin manifestations include spider naevi (which often disappear after recovery), scratch marks in the pruritic phase, and rarely a vasculitic or urticarial rash. Mild hepatomegaly is common, but a rapid shrinkage in hepatic size may occur in severe or fulminant hepatitis. Splenomegaly is uncommon, and suggests alternative viral causes such as Epstein–Barr virus or cytomegalovirus, or pre-existing liver disease. Marked nausea and persistent vomiting indicate a severe hepatitis and increase the chance of developing hypoglycaemia. Stools become pale and urine darkens as jaundice is established. Ascites and peripheral oedema may occur in prolonged or severe episodes. The most significant clinical indicator of deterioration is the development of hepatic encephalopathy, indicating the onset of hepatic failure.

Laboratory investigations

Virological investigations depend on serological testing as outlined in Table 2. Figures 1 and 2 indicate the typical serological evolution of self-limited episodes of A and B viral hepatitis.

Typically, hepatocellular enzyme levels in blood (AST, aspartate aminotransferase; ALT alanine aminotransferase) are prominently raised at the time of the onset of symptoms, often more than 10-fold above normal, whilst the serum alkaline phosphatase level is only slightly increased, less than 2.5-fold (Fig. 3). As an episode evolves, transaminase levels fall and alkaline phosphatase may rise, notably if there is prolonged intrahepatic cholestasis. Urinary analysis shows excess urobilinogen in early and late phases of an episode, with excess bilirubin at the height of jaundice. The severity of the attack is best reflected in the synthetic parameters of albumin and clotting factors: in particular, progressive prolongation of the prothrombin time mirrors the onset of liver failure. A low factor V (below about 30 per cent of normal) level has been used as an indicator of irreversible failure.

Hepatic imaging techniques such as ultrasound contribute to diagnosis primarily by excluding other causes. Patients with uncomplicated hepatitis do not require a liver biopsy, but hepatic histology is very helpful if there is diagnostic uncertainty or an unusual course in severity or duration (Fig. 4 and Plate 1). In such cases, biopsy may require correction of clotting factors and use of the transjugular route or 'plugged' biopsy techniques.

Differential diagnosis

Drug-induced jaundice is the most common differential diagnosis, and its course may be very similar. Drug history and drug screening should particularly enquire about the use of acetaminophen and non-steroidal anti-inflammatory drugs. Other potential drugs and toxins include halothane, antituberculous drugs, carbon tetrachloride, and mushroom poisoning. Alcoholic hepatitis often presents with less marked elevations of serum transaminases and a high circulating leucocyte count. About one-third of patients with autoimmune hepatitis present with a clinical picture of acute hepatitis. Autoantibody testing is generally helpful: the majority of patients with autoimmune disease having high levels of circulating autoantibodies.

Table 2 Serological tests used in the assessment of acute hepatitis

Test	Interpretation	Timing in relation to jaundice
HAVAg	Not tested in routine practice	Disappears at time of onset
HAVAb-IgM	Acute or recent infection	From onset for approximately 4 months
HAVAb-IgG	Acute, recent, or past infection	Persists till old age
HBsAg	Viral protein in blood	Cleared by 6 months in >90% of cases; persistence beyond 6 months confirms chronicity
HBsAb	Viral clearance occurring	Few weeks after jaundice—persists lifelong
HBsAg	Infectious phase, high-titre HBV-DNA	Cleared by 1 month in >90% of cases
HbeAb	Immune response to infectious virus indicates that the virus will be cleared	Appears as HbeAg cleared
HBcAb-IgM	Acute infection	Present at onset, persists for approximately 4 months
HBcAb-IgG	Acute, recent, or past infection	Persists for 2–5 years if virus cleared
HBV-DNA	Infectious virus in blood	Cleared in 2 months in >90% of cases
HCV-RNA	Active viral replication	Present at onset
HCVAb	Acute, recent, or past infection	May not appear until a few weeks after onset
HDVAg	Presence of viral protein in blood	Present at onset
HDVAb-IgM	Acute or chronic infection	Present at onset, persists in chronic carriage
HEVAb-IgM	Acute or recent infection	From onset for 4–6 months
HEVAb-IgG	Acute, recent, or past infection	From onset for several years

HBs, hepatitis B surface; HBc, hepatitis B core; Ag, antigen; Ab, antibody.

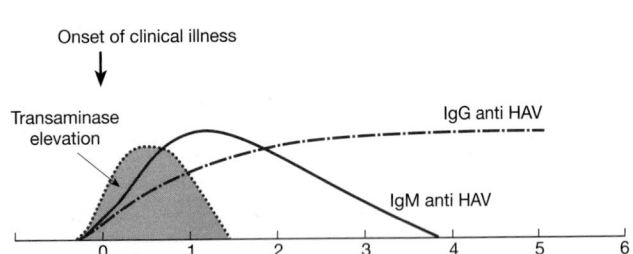

Fig. 1 Typical serology of hepatitis A infection.

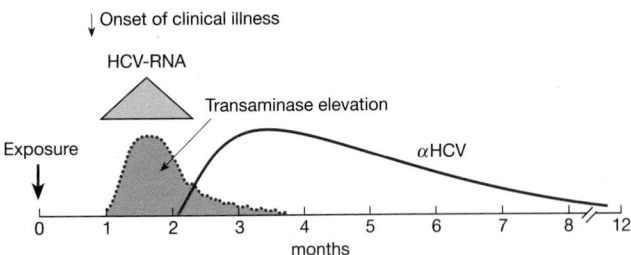

Fig. 3 Serological changes during acute hepatitis C with viral clearance.

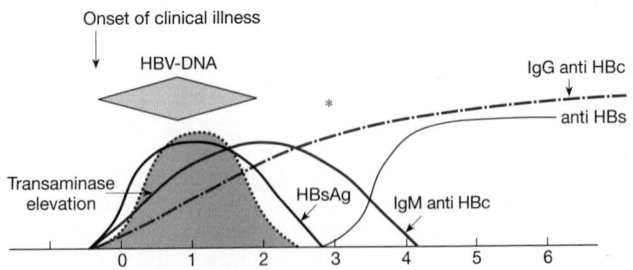

Fig. 2 Serological changes during acute hepatitis B with viral clearance. *, 'Window phase' after elimination of HBsAg and before the emergence of anti-HBs, during which anti-HBc may be the sole indicator of infection.

However, there are often low- or moderate-titre antinuclear and anti-smooth muscle antibodies in uncomplicated viral hepatitis. Similarly, there may be some increase of immunoglobulin levels in acute hepatitis, though not the doubling characteristic of autoimmune hepatitis. Although uncommon, acute Wilson's disease is an important diagnosis to make, because of the high incidence of acute liver failure and the rapid necessity for transplantation. 'Surgical' obstructive jaundice tends not to raise transaminase levels markedly, but serum alkaline phosphatase levels are high. Obstruction is generally confirmed by imaging techniques, notably ultrasound. Individual causes may be suspected from features in the history such as nausea and biliary colic in cholelithiasis, and painless jaundice without systemic upset in an elderly patient with pancreatic cancer. Pregnancy-associated syndromes—acute fatty liver and **HELLP** (haemolysis, elevated liver function tests, low platelets)—are in fact less common in pregnancy than acute hepatitis. Occasionally ischaemia, generally after profound hypotension over many hours, and rapidly progressive malignant infiltration may mimic acute viral hepatitis.

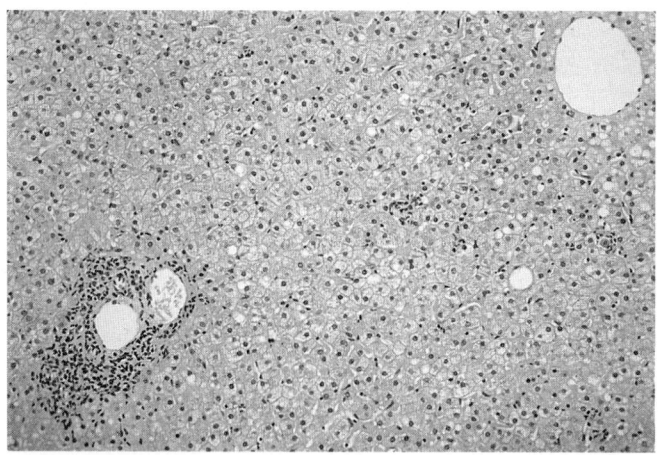

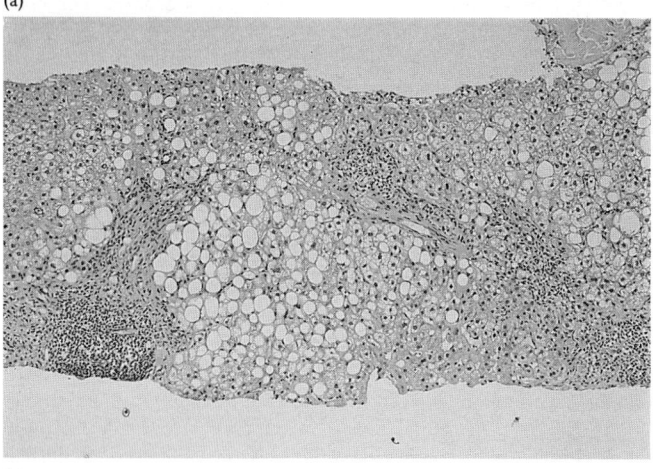

Fig. 4 Haematoxylin and eosin staining of liver biopsies from (a) mild hepatitis with inflammation restricted to the portal tracts and minimal fibrosis, and (b) severely active but still precirrhotic liver with bridging necrosis (by courtesy of Professor P. Dhillon). (See also Plate 1.)

Management

Uncomplicated cases of hepatitis recover spontaneously. Classical studies in military personnel demonstrated no benefit from bed rest, though whether the same applies to the elderly is unknown. In any case malaise and nausea often enforce rest. Clinicians must be alert to signs of impending liver failure and ensure that hypoglycaemia is avoided, if necessary by parenteral administration of glucose. No diets are of established benefit, but dietary fat is often poorly tolerated. There is no rationale for protein restriction unless evidence of hepatic encephalopathy has emerged. Alcohol and potentially hepatotoxic drugs should be withdrawn. Troublesome pruritus can be treated with colestyramine, which is preferable to antihistamines because of potential hepatotoxicity. There is no proven therapy to enhance recovery. Corticosteroids do not speed recovery or improve survival, although they do lower serum bilirubin levels. In hepatitis B, and particularly hepatitis C, the use of interferon has been advocated to enhance the chance of elimination of the virus. There is little evidence of its efficacy with HBV, but some reports in HCV infection are very encouraging.

In fulminant hepatic failure, which in the setting of viral hepatitis carries a mortality risk of 80 per cent, patients should, if possible, undergo orthotopic liver transplantation. Criteria for listing differ in different centres, but include a marked abnormality of clotting parameters (e.g. prolongation of the prothrombin time to >50 s or a factor V level <20–30 per cent) and the development of significant encephalopathy. Patients awaiting transplant-

ation require glucose supplementation, full intensive-care monitoring, and prophylaxis of infection. Some patients require renal support, such as haemofiltration, and ventilation. Some units invasively monitor intracerebral pressure, which may rise dangerously, so that cerebral oedema may be treated with intravenous mannitol.

Prevention of viral hepatitis

Sanitation and hygiene reduce the frequency of the enteric-borne infections HAV and HEV. Passive protection against hepatitis A (to close family contacts) and hepatitis B (after exposure to risk factors such as sexual contact with an individual incubating acute hepatitis B, or a needlestick injury) are available using gammaglobulin preparations (standard preparations for protection against HAV, specific high-titre preparations for HBV). Active immunization to HAV, using formalin-inactivated viral preparations, provides a high level of protective immunity within a few days—suitable, for example, for use prior to travel from the West to highly endemic areas, and also advisable in patients with established chronic liver disease, particularly chronic viral hepatitis. Active immunization to HBV is discussed below, which also protects against HDV. Vaccines are not yet available for HCV or HEV.

Chronic viral hepatitis—hepatitis B

Up to 10 per cent of adults and more than 90 per cent of infants become chronic B carriers after infection, defined by the persistence of HBsAg in the blood for more than 6 months. Subsequently, a low proportion of patients will clear the virus spontaneously each year, but most are infected long-term. Failure to clear the virus is more common in neonates or those infected as infants, in males, and those with natural or iatrogenic immunosuppression. Carriage rates in the population vary widely geographically, and are notably high in the Far East and Southern Africa (10–20 per cent), and low in Northern Europe and North America (<1 per cent).

The consequences of long-term carriage are varied, reflecting the strength of the immune response mounted by the host, the duration of infection, and alteration in the mechanisms of viral replication with time (Fig. 5). Viral mutation may also contribute to modulation of the host response and viral replication. During the early years, the 'replicative' phase, HBeAg (hepatitis B e antigen)-expressing virus replicates independently of the host chromosomes, resulting in the production of fully infectious viral particles in the blood with high levels of HBV-DNA (Table 3). The early replicative phase is associated with a state of relative immune tolerance by the host, and may be very prolonged if infection is acquired as an infant. In the later replicative phase there is expression of immune responses associated with inflammation. Thereafter, HBeAg expression is often lost, HBV-DNA in the blood may be at low or undetectable levels, and HBsAg production may be driven by viral sequences integrated into the genome (integrative phase).

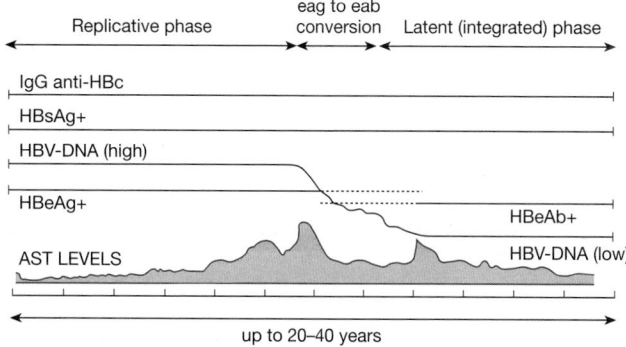

Fig. 5 Serological markers during chronic hepatitis B. Note that HBV mutants not expressing HBeAg may emerge and that HBV-DNA quantitation is required to assess their replicative phase.

Table 3 Serological tests in chronic HBV carriage

First few months	
HBsAg+	HBsAb−
HBeAg+	HBeAb−
HBcAb IgM+*	
HBcAb IgG+	
HBV-DNA+	

Replicative phase (several years but variable)	
HBsAg+	HBsAb−
HBeAg+	HBeAb−
HBcAb IgM−*	
HBcAb IgG+	
HBV DNA+	

Late phase (variable duration)	
HBsAg+	HBsAb−
HBeAg−	HBeAb+
HBcAb IgM−*	
HBcAb IgG+	
HBV-DNA−, or minimal	

+, Positive; −, negative; see Table 2 for other abbreviations.

* HbcAb-IgM tests are set to only be positive at high titre and thus detect acute infections. Lower titres of IgM antibody persist long-term and the test may again become positive during flares.

Infection with the pre-core mutant of HBV does not lead to HbeAg expression but is associated with HBV-DNA in blood and with active disease. Patients with this mutant form are often HbeAb+.

Chronic hepatitis B infection is associated with a spectrum of histological damage and clinical manifestations. The inflammatory response to the virus may sometimes be so slight that the histological appearances of the liver are virtually normal, with the exception of evidence of virally infected hepatocytes seen as 'ground-glass' cells on routine eosin staining or by histochemistry. More commonly, the immune response is adequate to inflame the liver but inadequate to clear the virus. The resulting chronic inflammation may be confined to the portal tracts, with a chronic lymphocytic infiltration, associated to varying extent with periportal and/or lobular inflammation, a tendency to develop fibrosis spreading from the portal tracts, and in some cases eventually cirrhosis. These appearances can be categorized in terms of inflammatory activity and fibrosis (Table 4). In general, the replicative phase of HBV infection with HBeAg-positivity, particularly in its later phase, is associated with more marked inflammation than the subsequent HBeAb-positive stage.

Table 4 Grading of chronic hepatitis

Activity

I	Minimal inflammation in portal tracts; scanty piecemeal necrosis; no lobular necrosis
II	Mild portal inflammation; piecemeal necrosis; scanty lobular necrosis
III	Moderate portal inflammation; piecemeal necrosis; lobular necrosis
IV	Marked portal inflammation; prominent piecemeal necrosis; lobular necrosis including confluent bridging necrosis between portal tracts

Staging

I	Mild fibrous expansion of portal tracts
II	Periportal fibrosis, only fine strands of fibrosis into parenchyma
III	Bridging of fibrosis with confluent portal tracts or portocentral vein bridging
IV	Cirrhosis—bridging fibrosis and nodular regeneration

Chronic hepatitis B infection may be clinically silent for years, or give rise only to non-specific symptoms of fatigue. The condition may be recognized on screening (for example, during pregnancy) or the investigation of coincidentally detected abnormal liver function tests. Some patients present with non-specific indications of chronic liver disease (malaise or hepatomegaly), or at a late stage with a complication of established cirrhosis. Episodes of enhanced inflammation ('flares') may give rise to transient worsening of liver function tests, particularly transaminase elevations and jaundice at any stage of the disease; precipitating events may include a reduction of prior immunosuppression, or the time of conversion from HBeAg- to HBeAb-positivity. Usually the progression to cirrhosis takes many years, but the rate varies. The incidence of hepatocellular cancer in chronic hepatitis B is high, probably increased 100-fold over non-infected controls. Most, but not all, patients with hepatocellular cancer will have cirrhosis.

Chronic HBV infection may also give rise to a number of extrahepatic manifestations. These include membranous glomerulonephritis, polyarteritis nodosa, and cryoglobulinaemia.

After establishing the diagnosis of chronic HBV infection, it is necessary to define the virological status of the patient with respect to infectivity and viral replication (see Table 3), and the hepatic status with respect to the presence of inflammation and liver damage. Interpretation of viral status may be complicated by the emergence of viral mutants, particularly the 'pre-core' mutant that results in absent HBeAg expression, but which, none the less, is associated with active inflammation and circulating HBV-DNA levels.

Treatment

The general measures relevant to chronic liver disease of any aetiology are discussed elsewhere.

With respect to HBV infection, the prospects for inducing viral clearance in an individual patient are relatively low, but the viral load, infectivity, and intensity of hepatic inflammation can often be reduced. The two current approaches are the use of α-interferons, which have both immunomodulatory and antiviral properties, and the use of inhibitors of viral replication, currently nucleoside analogues.

Patient selection is important. Those with active inflammation, viral replication independent of host DNA, but low levels of HBV-DNA have the greatest potential to benefit. Most patients treated will have circulating HBeAg present. In the absence of elevated transaminases the response to treatment is very poor. Whilst some patients will clear HBsAg from the blood in response to treatment, loss of HbeAg is a more common event.

α-Interferons (**IFN-α**) act predominantly by enhancing T-cell-mediated viral clearance, by processes including the enhancement of hepatocyte class I-HLA expression. Treatment involves parenteral IFN-α (5 MU daily or 10 MU three times weekly, for 4 months). If viral clearance or HBeAg to HBeAb conversion occurs, there is generally an inflammatory flare during the second or third month. Side-effects include malaise, fever (particularly in the first weeks of treatment), anaemia, alopecia, and depression. HBeAg to HBeAb conversion or loss of HBV-DNA occurs in 30 to 40 per cent of cases, HBsAg clearance in about 10 per cent. Women, those with a shorter duration of carriage, occidentals, and those without an additional immunosuppressed background (for example, human immunodeficiency virus (**HIV**) infection) respond more favourably. Relapse after the clearance or sustained loss of HBV replication is rare (5–10 per cent). Successful treatment slows histological progression and reduces liver-related mortality (including hepatocellular cancer).

Nucleoside analogues can inhibit viral reverse transcriptase and inhibit replication. Drugs such as lamivudine are orally bioavailable and now licensed for use. Lamivudine for 12 months markedly reduces HBV-DNA for the duration of treatment, leads to HBeAg to HBeAb conversion in one-third of patients, and reduces inflammatory activity on histological and liver-function test criteria in 50 per cent of cases. However, the loss of

HBsAg is infrequent. One difficulty with this drug is that cessation of therapy can occasionally be followed by a disease flare. Moreover, in a significant proportion of cases lamivudine-resistant strains emerge due to mutations in DNA polymerase (*YMDD* mutants). The inflammatory response to this mutant form of the virus may however be diminished. The role of lamivudine and other nucleoside analogues such as famciclovir is under intensive investigation.

Prevention of hepatitis B

Active immunization for the prevention of HBV infection initially involved the use of a vaccine derived from viral proteins in infected blood, but it now uses recombinant HBsAg proteins. Vaccination strategies range from universal vaccination in infancy to the vaccination of only high-risk individuals. In areas of high carriage in the Far East, universal vaccine programmes have already reduced the national incidence of infection, carriage, and hepatocellular cancer. Conventional three-dose immunization in adults leads to protective immunity, as judged by anti-HBsAg, in 90 per cent of individuals.

Passive immunization with anti-HBsAg hyperimmune globulin provides rapid protection after exposure (e.g. after needlestick injury). A combination of passive and active immunization is recommended for children born to infected mothers. In some infants, chronic infection with a mutant 'escape' virus has subsequently occurred.

Chronic hepatitis C

Around 85 per cent of patients who become infected with HCV fail to clear the virus and become chronic carriers. In the majority of cases the initial presentation will have been asymptomatic, and HCV infection is generally recognized in the chronic phase. Following the availability of tests to diagnose HCV infection, it is clear that an asymptomatic indolent necroinflammatory response to the virus in the liver may persist long term, and often, but not inevitably, lead to cirrhosis after 15 to 25 years and predispose to hepatocellular cancer thereafter.

Mechanisms of transmission and prevalence rates vary geographically. In the West, blood transfusion and treatment of clotting disorders with plasma concentrates prior to the early 1990s, and intravenous drug abuse constitute the main routes of transmission. Medical use of unsterilized needles, including in vaccination programmes, tattooing, dentistry, and communal shaving practices, may all contribute worldwide. Vertical transmission is rare. Sexual transmission is low (<5 per cent in stable heterosexual relationships).

As with HBV, the severity of liver damage reflects host–virus responses. Severe inflammation is less common if the virus is acquired in childhood and progression to cirrhosis less frequent and probably slower. HBV coinfection and alcoholism worsen disease and increase the likelihood and rate of developing cirrhosis. The histological response of the liver shows a similar variety of response to that seen in HBV infection, from minimal to severe portal inflammation, periportal hepatocyte necrosis, and progressive fibrosis leading to cirrhosis. The presence of lymphoid follicles in portal tracts and parenchymal steatosis are characteristic of the response to HCV.

Patients may be diagnosed coincidentally during the investigation of fatigue or abnormal liver function tests, or with manifestations of chronic liver disease. In addition, there are a variety of extrahepatic manifestations thought to reflect either antigen–antibody complex formation or the induction of crossreacting autoimmunity. These include a vasculitic rash associated with cryoglobulinaemia (type 2, polyclonal immunoglobulin plus rheumatoid factor), glomerulonephritis, abnormal thyroid function, thrombocytopenia, and porphyria cutanea tarda. As in HBV, assessment of a patient with HCV involves both the virological and the hepatic status.

The initial screening test for HCV is detection of circulating anti-HCV antibody. If present, confirmation is required either by more specific antibody testing using immunoblots, or more often by using **PCR** (polymerase

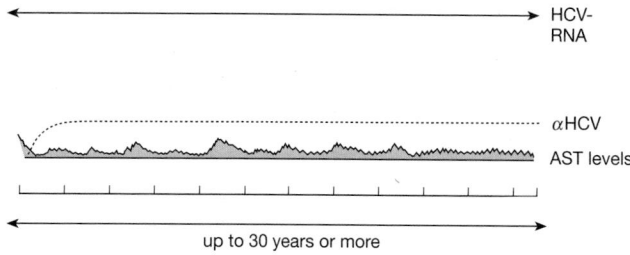

Fig. 6 Serological changes during chronic hepatitis C.

chain reaction) for viral RNA (Fig. 6). Quantitative PCR and viral genotyping (types 1–4) are becoming more relevant as treatment strategies evolve (see below). Changing sensitivities of antibody tests, and varying techniques for PCR testing, render specialist interpretation mandatory.

The severity of inflammation in the liver is poorly judged from routine liver function tests such as aminotransferase level measurements. Histological assessment may reveal both significant inflammation and progressive fibrosis despite normal serum enzyme levels, and are necessary if treatment is to be considered. There is consensus that moderate or severe precirrhotic disease as judged by activity grading and well-compensated cirrhosis should be considered for treatment. The position in minimal or mild disease is uncertain, in part because patients with mild disease histologically, and normal aminotransferase levels, do not respond well to current treatment.

Treatment of chronic HCV

The main aim of treatment in chronic HCV infection is to clear the virus, which has been established to be associated with a reduction in necroinflammation and slowing in the rate of accumulation of fibrosis in the liver.

Initial studies using IFN-α monotherapy demonstrated that between 25 and 50 per cent of patients responded temporarily, with normalization of aminotransferase levels and loss of PCR-positivity for viral RNA recorded at the end of 6 months' therapy. However when assessed 6 to 12 months later this response was sustained in far fewer patients—overall sustained virological response rates were only between 10 and 12 per cent. Rates were higher with more prolonged treatment, but did not exceed 20 per cent. Clearance rates were lower with genotype 1 infection and when initial aminotransferase levels were normal.

Subsequently, the combination of interferon with ribavirin has been shown strikingly to enhance sustained response rates, with an approximate doubling of clearance rates after both 24 and 48 weeks. For genotypes 2 and 3 however, 6 months' treatment appears adequate. Currently, for these genotypes, the combination of 3 MU of IFN-alpha three times weekly plus ribavirin 1000 to 1200 mg orally is recommended. For genotype 1, treatment for 12 months is recommended. With this regime, in addition to the side-effects of IFN-α listed discussed above for HBV treatment, ribavirin induces cough, rash dyspnoea, and insomnia in about 25 per cent of patients, and there is predictably a dose-dependent haemolytic anaemia. Both pregnancy and fathering children need to be avoided whilst taking ribavirin. Strategies for the early identification of non-responders, by assessing whether there is a reduction in viral load in the blood, are evolving. The full role of therapy in established cirrhosis, and the long-term benefits of reducing inflammation with these therapies in patients in whom viral clearance has not been achieved, are currently under investigation. Improved interferon formulations (such as interferon conjugated to polyethylene glycol, PEG) and other antiviral drugs are being introduced.

Prevention of hepatitis C

There is no vaccine available for HCV. Passive immunization with HCV-antibody-containing gammaglobulin in not protective.

Hepatitis D

Chronic HDV generally follows superinfection of a chronic HBV carrier in whom ample HbsAg to permit HDV encapsulation is already present. The spectrum of chronic liver disease associated with the double chronic infection is as variable as with HBV alone. Overall, however, the liver tends to be more severely affected, and in 10 to 15 per cent of chronic carriers there may be a rapid (1 to 2 year) evolution to cirrhosis. HDV acts to suppress HBV infection, so that markers of HBV activity, such as HBV-DNA, in the serum may become suppressed. Many patients with HDV may therefore be HBeAb positive.

The treatment of HDV mirrors that for HBV. Prolonged courses of IFN-α (6 or more months) may transiently clear HDV in some patients in whom HbsAg persists. In general, HbsAg clearance is required to cause sustained HDV clearance.

Liver transplantation

Liver transplantation is indicated both in fulminant hepatic failure due to acute hepatitis and in advanced chronic hepatitis with cirrhosis. Recurrence of viral hepatitis after transplantation is a major concern. The use of hyperimmune globulin, interferon, and nucleoside analogues allows control in most cases of HBV. Severe recurrence remains a significant problem after transplantation for HCV.

Further reading

Alter MJ (1997). Epidemiology of hepatitis C. *Hepatology* 26(Suppl 1), 62S–65S.

Bell BP, et al. (1998). The diverse patterns of hepatitis A epidemiology in the United States—implications for vaccination strategies. *Journal of Infectious Diseases* 178, 1579–84.

Chang MH, et al. (1997). Shau Universal hepatitis B vaccination in Taiwan and the incidence of hepatocellular carcinoma in children. *New England Journal of Medicine* 336, 1855–9.

Farci P, et al. (1994). Treatment of chronic hepatitis D with interferon alfa-2a. *New England Journal of Medicine* 330, 88–94.

Feitelson MA (1994). Biology of hepatitis B virus variants. *Laboratory Investigation* 71, 324–49.

Guillevin L, et al. (1995). Polyarteritis nodosa related to hepatitis B virus. A prospective study with long-term observation of 41 patients. *Medicine* 74, 238–53.

Hoofnagle JH (1997). Hepatitis C: the clinical spectrum of disease. *Hepatology* 26(Suppl 1), 15S–20S.

Irshad M (1997). Hepatitis E virus: a global view of its seroepidemiology and transmission pattern. *Tropical Gastroenterology* 18, 45–9.

Lai CL, et al. (1998). A one-year trial of lamivudine for chronic hepatitis B. *New England Journal of Medicine* 339, 61–8.

Lee WM (1997). Medical progress: hepatitis B virus infection. *New England Journal of Medicine* 337, 1733–45.

Lemon SM, Thomas DL (1997). Vaccines to prevent viral hepatitis. *New England Journal of Medicine* 336, 196–204.

Poynard T, et al. (1998). Randomised trial of interferon alpha2b plus ribavirin for 48 weeks or for 24 weeks versus interferon alpha2b plus placebo for 48 weeks for treatment of chronic infection with hepatitis C virus. *Lancet* 352, 1426–32.

Scheuer PJ, Davies SE, Dhillon AP (1996). Histopathological aspects of viral hepatitis. *Journal of Viral hepatitis* 3, 277–83.

Sjogren MH (1996). Serologic diagnosis of viral hepatitis. *Medical Clinics of North America* 80, 929–56.

Thursz MR, Thomas HC (1997). Host factors in chronic viral hepatitis. *Seminars in Liver Disease* 17, 345–50.

Vento S, et al. (1998). Fulminant hepatitis associated with hepatitis A virus superinfection in patients with chronic hepatitis C. *New England Journal of Medicine* 338, 286–90.

14.20.2 Autoimmune liver disease

14.20.2.1 Autoimmune hepatitis

H. J. F. Hodgson

Autoimmune hepatitis describes chronic inflammation in the liver attributed to immune responses against self-antigens in the liver. Patients generally have circulating autoantibodies, and 60 per cent have other autoimmune diseases in addition. In severe cases autoimmune hepatitis can lead to acute liver failure, and untreated there is often progression to cirrhosis. There is generally a good response to corticosteroid therapy.

The term 'autoimmune hepatitis' should be reserved for patients with clinically significant liver disease, and not used to describe the very mild chronic inflammation often seen in the livers of patients with systemic autoimmune conditions. Previous terms for autoimmune hepatitis include 'autoimmune chronic active hepatitis' and 'lupoid hepatitis'.

Aetiology

Autoimmune hepatitis is often familial, and a constellation of autoimmune diseases (for example, thyroiditis, type-1 diabetes) may occur in affected families. Some of the predisposing genetic factors have been characterized. There are strong HLA associations. In the United Kingdom and United States the strongest association is with HLA DR haplotype B1*030 (50 per cent of patients compared with 20 per cent of controls), and a secondary association with *0401, but in other geographical areas there are different associations. The DR4 association is strongest in Japan. Deficiency of the C4 component of complement also predisposes to the disease. In the West, DR3 is associated with more severe disease and a younger onset, and DR4 with an older onset and better treatment response. In most cases there is no clear initiating event for the development of autoimmune hepatitis, but occasionally drugs (α-methyldopa, oxyphenisatine, nitrofurantoin, isoniazid, minocycline, pemoline, dihydralazine, tienilic acid) can precipitate the condition. As discussed below, in some patients with chronic hepatitis C, autoimmune manifestations develop and may contribute to the inflammatory processes in that chronic viral condition.

Histological appearances and immunopathogenesis

The histological appearances used to be referred to as 'chronic active hepatitis', but pathologists now grade chronic hepatitis in respect of aetiology, disease activity (grading), and progression (staging). There is a marked portal tract infiltrate containing both plasma cells and T cells. Cytotoxic T cells spread out across the limiting plate of the portal tract, associated with piecemeal necrosis of periportal hepatocytes, and lymphocytes are often present diffusely within the parenchyma (Fig. 1). Compared with the inflammation seen in chronic hepatitis B and C, the plasma-cell component of the portal tract infiltrate is more prominent, as is regenerative 'rosette' formation by the hepatocytes. The portal tract lymphoid aggregates and steatosis common in hepatitis C are less frequent in autoimmune hepatitis. With progression, periportal fibrosis, bridging necrosis linking portal tracts to central veins, and hyperplasia of regenerating hepatocytes all occur leading to cirrhosis.

Antibody and T-cell reactivity to a panel of hepatic antigens, both intracellular and on the cell surface, are described. Some of these may be the primary mechanism of liver damage, and others a secondary response to

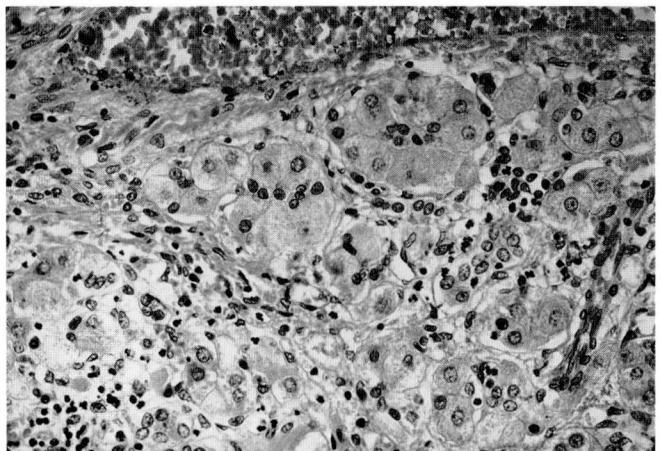

Fig. 1 Haematoxylin and eosin stained liver histology showing 'rosettes' of regenerated hepatocytes, surrounded by lymphocytes that have spread into the hepatic parenchyma.

tissue injury. Cell-surface targets such as the hepatocyte-specific asialoglycoprotein receptor may be particularly relevant to the development of tissue damage.

Epidemiology

Most reported cases are of European ancestry, although cases occur worldwide. Most patients are female—with female:male ratios of up to 8:1 reported in some series. Northern European prevalence figures are about 100 to 200 per 100 000, similar to those for primary biliary cirrhosis and primary sclerosing cholangitis. The age of onset varies widely, but young adults and children are most commonly affected. Perhaps 20 per cent of cases occur after the age of 65.

Clinical manifestations

In about 30 per cent of cases the onset is indistinguishable clinically from acute viral hepatitis, with anorexia, nausea, hepatic discomfort, and the development of jaundice. Other patients present just with malaise, or with extrahepatic manifestations such as arthralgia, arthritis, or fever, and subsequent investigation demonstrates high circulating transaminase levels. Despite an acute onset, many patients have cirrhosis at the time of presentation.

Clinical signs may therefore vary greatly. Cutaneous manifestations of palmar erythema and prominent spider naevi, a maculopapular or acneiform rash, and occasionally abdominal striae (without corticosteroid therapy) may be found both in acute and insidious presentations. In an acute presentation, jaundice and tender hepatomegaly may be prominent, with severe cases demonstrating ascites and most sinisterly the development of encephalopathy. Acute severe autoimmune hepatitis may progress to fulminant hepatic failure. Splenomegaly, which is often marked, indicates that cirrhosis has already developed. There may also be evidence of other autoimmune conditions (Table 1).

Investigations

High transaminase levels, marked hyperglobulinaemia (particularly IgG), and circulating autoantibodies characterize the condition. Transaminase levels are often five or ten times the upper normal limit. Hyperglobulinaemia may include IgG levels of more than 30 g/l when the condition is active. The major serological diagnostic markers are the presence of autoantibodies demonstrated by tissue immunofluorescence, prominently antinuclear

antibodies (**ANA**), titre 1:40 or greater, and an anti-smooth muscle (**SMA**) titre 1:80 or greater. In addition, other autoantibodies may be present, in particular to liver–kidney microsomes (liver and proximal renal tubule, LKM-1). However, the antibody profiles in the disease are variable and may alter over time: some cases identified on clinical and histological grounds may lack circulating antibodies on routine testing. Other autoimmune associations of the disease may be manifest with antithyroid, parietal cell, and intrinsic factor antibodies, or antibodies leading to immune thrombocytopenia or haemolysis. Other positive immune tests include a moderate frequency of antibodies to double-stranded and single-stranded DNA. The positive lupus erythematosus cells described in early reports of the condition led to the designation of 'lupoid hepatitis'.

Diagnostic criteria

There are no critical signs, symptoms, or liver test abnormalities that are sufficiently specific to provide diagnostic criteria. The diagnosis is therefore made on a constellation of features, each of which may also occur in other conditions. Diagnosis during the active phase of the disease generally reflects the presence of elevated serum transaminase levels without marked elevation of alkaline phosphatase, elevated globulins, positive antibodies to ANA, SMA, or LKM-1, seronegativity for hepatitis viruses (although the overlap with hepatitis C is discussed below), and characteristic or compatible liver histology. A 'scoring system' to identify definite or probable autoimmune hepatitis from a combination of clinical and histological features has been proposed.

Differential diagnosis

The differential diagnosis during investigation includes not only viral and drug-induced hepatitis, but the metabolic conditions of Wilson's disease and α1-antitrypsin deficiency. Some alcoholic patients may manifest histological appearances overlapping with autoimmune hepatitis. The immune biliary diseases primary biliary cirrhosis (**PBC**) and primary sclerosing cholangitis (**PSC**) are generally easy to differentiate by the predominant elevation of serum alkaline phosphatase and the antimitochondrial antibody in PBC, and antineutrophil cytoplasmic antibodies (**ANCA**) and cholangiography in PSC. However, as already mentioned, each of the suggestive indicators for autoimmune hepatitis may be absent in particular cases, and in some series up to 20 per cent of cases lack any ANA, SMA, and anti-LKM-1 antibodies. Furthermore, there is overlap in the autoimmune profiles of various immunological liver diseases, with, for example, low titres of ANCA often found in autoimmune hepatitis, and SMA in both

Table 1 Associated conditions

Arthropathy****	Skin rashes****
Keratoconjunctivitis sicca****	
Autoimmune thyroiditis***	Diabetes***
Renal tubular acidosis***	
Peripheral neuropathy**	
Fibrosing alveolitis*	Ulcerative colitis*
Coeliac disease*	Immune thrombocytopenia*
Rheumatoid arthritis*	Glomerulonephritis*
Autoimmune haemolytic anaemia*	

Approximate relative frequency of finding in patients with autoimmune hepatitis: ****20–40 per cent; ***10–20 per cent; **5–10 per cent; *1–5 per cent.

In the rare autoimmune polyendocrine syndrome -Type 1 (adrenal insufficiency, mucocutaneous candidiasis, hypoparathyroidism) about 20 per cent of patients have hepatic involvement.

PBS and PSC. Autoimmune hepatitis is not part of the spectrum of systemic lupus erythematosus.

Autoimmune hepatitis subtypes

A subclassification of autoimmune hepatitis into four groups according to a combination of autoantibody profiles and clinical features has also been suggested (Table 2):

Type I—Classical autoimmune hepatitis with high-titre ANA and SMA. Typically, patients are young adult females. The SMA antibody has anti-F-actin specificity, as can be demonstrated using cell lines as immunofluorescent substrates.

Type II—Anti-LKM-1 antibodies are present, with specificity for a cytochrome P-450 antigen, CYP4502D. The disease may be particularly severe, and tends to affect children. However anti-LKM-1 may also be found in sera from patients with chronic hepatitis C infection, which can itself also predispose to a variety of autoimmune manifestations. It has therefore been suggested that Type-II autoimmune hepatitis should be further subdivided to separate those with a primary autoimmune condition (IIa) from those in whom hepatitis C has triggered an autoimmune response (IIb). This, however, introduces further confusion as some patients with hepatitis C have ANA and SMA but not anti-LKM.

Type III—Antibodies to a soluble liver antigen (**SLA**), often without ANA, SMA, or LKM antibodies.

Type IV—No antibodies detectable.

The value of this classification has been questioned, and the issue is complex. Many other autoantibodies are being described in these patients, to both intracellular and surface antigens of liver cells (for example: antibodies to the hepatocyte-specific asialoglycoprotein receptor, to other hepatic membrane antigens, and to cytosolic enzymes; and to a 'liver–pancreas' antigen). Furthermore, antibodies identified by immunofluorescence are often relatively non-specific, and reactions to different epitopes may give similar staining patterns. Many of the newly described antibodies are found in more than one type of autoimmune hepatitis and in other immune conditions affecting the liver. Also, as described below, there are well-described 'overlap' cases, with patients with autoimmune hepatitis also showing manifestations of another immune liver disease. Subtyping on autoantibody criteria alone is therefore unlikely to be definitive. The delineation of Type IV, with no detectable autoantibodies, serves to emphasize that if other clinical and laboratory features are present, a trial of corticosteroids may be worthwhile even if autoantibodies have not been identified.

Associated liver diseases and overlap conditions

Up to 10 per cent of cases may show mixed autoimmune hepatitis and immune biliary disease, generally PBC and less frequently PSC. The disease may also coexist with autoimmune cholangitis (which resembles PBC but is antimitochondrial antibody-negative).

Natural history

Untreated, autoimmune hepatitis may occasionally spontaneously remit, but there is a marked tendency for progression with the development of hepatic fibrosis and cirrhosis, and subsequently the complications thereof. Childhood-onset and Type-II autoimmune hepatitis have a bad prognosis. Over half of the patients with severe disease die within 5 years if untreated. Epidemiological features suggest that inapparent autoimmune hepatitis is the cause of a significant number of cases of cryptogenic cirrhosis. Cirrhosis arising as a consequence of autoimmune hepatitis only rarely leads to hepatocellular carcinoma.

Treatment regimes

Specific therapy for autoimmune hepatitis is aimed at reducing or abolishing inflammation. Patients, particularly those with cirrhosis, may require treatment for the complications of portal hypertension and liver failure discussed in Chapter 14.21.2.

There is consensus that severe cases of autoimmune hepatitis should be treated with an immunosuppressive regime for 1 to 2 years. Evidence of benefit is firm in patients with transaminase levels more than five times normal, and those with histological evidence of bridging necrosis on biopsy. Whether patients with mild disease (minor elevations of transaminase, minor inflammation on biopsy without developing fibrosis) benefit from immunosuppressive therapy is unclear, and in such patients a period of observation followed by repeat biopsy to gauge progression may be helpful. The finding of established cirrhosis should not be taken as a reason to prevent treatment, provided there is active inflammation.

Corticosteroid treatment of patients with severe disease reduces inflammation in 80 to 90 per cent of cases, reduces the chance of progression to cirrhosis if it has not already occurred, and prolongs survival. In assessing the short-term effects of corticosteroid or other therapy, responses are characterized as 'complete' if transaminase levels normalize and remain so for a year or more, or if repeat histology shows only minimal activity. A 'partial response' describes improvement but the persistence of transaminase abnormalities at more than twice the upper limit of normal, or persistent histological activity despite the normalization of transaminase levels. In the most successful cases, complete responses with regression of fibrosis and normalization of architecture have been reported.

Table 2 Subtypes of autoimmune hepatitis based on autoantibody profiles

Disease	Antibody profile	Descriptive features	Treatment
Autoimmune hepatitis			
Type I	ANA++, SMA++	Classical AIH 70–80% of cases	Corticosteroids
Type II	LKM-1++	Often childhood or adolescent 5% of cases Overlap with hepatitis C	Corticosteroids(except hepatitis C)
Type III	Anti-SLA++; ANA+/–; SMA+/–	Rare—mimics Type I	Corticosteroids
Type IV	ANA–; SMA–; LKM–	15% of cases	Corticosteroids
Drug-induced	Variable—includes LM+		Drug withdrawal and corticosteroids
Hepatitis C	ANA+/–; SMA+/–; LKM-1 +/–	About 30% hepatitis C Less female preponderance	IFN-α/ribavirin Corticosteroids contentious

AIH, autoimmune hepatitis; ANA, antinuclear antibody; SMA, anti-smooth muscle (F-actin specificity); SLA, anti-soluble liver antigen (specificity contentious—includes glutathione-S-transferase); LKM, liver–kidney microsomal antibody: LKM-1, anti-CYP450II; LM, liver microsomal antibodies; IFN-α, interferon-alpha. ++ = highly positive; + = positive; +/- = variable; - = negative.

A variety of corticosteroid-based regimes are in use. Comparative studies demonstrate equivalent anti-inflammatory efficacy of a solely corticosteroid regime of prednisolone 20 mg daily, and a steroid-sparing combination of 75 mg azathioprine plus 10 mg prednisolone, but a lesser incidence of side-effects over 2 years with the latter. Many physicians use higher doses of prednisolone initially, 30 to 45 mg, until there is a definite improvement in liver function tests. Amongst those who respond, corticosteroid treatment will significantly reduce or normalize transaminase levels within a few weeks to a few months. Symptoms tend to resolve over a similar period, but corticosteroids may not abolish inflammation, as judged histologically, for a year or more. Therefore, if a complete clinical and biochemical remission is established, generally within a few months, most physicians advocate treatment for between 1 and 2 years and a repeat liver biopsy after that to see if there is still histological evidence of inflammation. A biopsy at this interval may also demonstrate that cirrhosis has supervened, despite clinical and biochemical control of the disease. If there is no active inflammation, or only mild inflammation, on the follow-up biopsy, cautious withdrawal of corticosteroids—for example, reducing the dose at a rate of 1 mg per month—may allow their discontinuation. However, the chances of relapse are high (perhaps 70 per cent) either during withdrawal or later, in which case immunosuppressive therapy will again be required and should then be continued long-term. When this is required, azathioprine alone may be all that is required. For patients who have only partially responded to corticosteroids—judged by the failure to reduce transaminase levels significantly or by persisting inflammation on follow-up biopsy—long-term immunosuppression is advocated, and increased corticosteroid or azathioprine dosage may be required to achieve remission.

Minimizing the incidence and severity of corticosteroid side-effects is very important. Glucose intolerance and hypertension should be screened for, and the enhanced risk of infection warrants increased vigilance. Strategies to reduce bone loss include oral supplementation with calcium and vitamin D, or the use of bisphosphonates to restore lost bone mass. The orally administered halogenated corticosteroid budesonide is rapidly metabolized by the liver, and reports indicate that it may be effective in treating autoimmune liver disease with less effect on the pituitary–adrenal axis than prednisolone. Theoretically, lesser effects on bone would also be anticipated.

For patients who fail to respond to corticosteroid-based immunosuppression there is anecdotal evidence of a reasonable response rate to ciclosporin. A number of alternative immunosuppressive agents—methotrexate, mycophenylate, and tacrolimus—have also been anecdotally reported to be useful. Failure to respond should also prompt reconsideration of the diagnosis, in particular exclusion of previously unrecognized Wilson's disease.

In the overlap syndrome of primary biliary cirrhosis-autoimmune hepatitis, the periportal inflammatory element of the condition and the serum transaminase elevations generally respond to corticosteroid therapy, but the biliary component is not improved. Conversely, bile acid therapy with ursodeoxycholic acid can improve the biliary manifestations whilst leaving the transaminase levels and periportal inflammation unaffected. Combination of the two therapeutic approaches may be necessary to restore normal biochemical markers of liver disease. Patients with the autoimmune hepatitis-PSC overlap syndrome respond poorly to treatment.

Prognosis after treatment

Amongst patients presenting without cirrhosis, long-term survival is excellent (over 95 per cent at 10 years), whilst the 10-year survival rate is about 65 per cent if cirrhosis is present initially. Corticosteroid therapy increases the survival of both cirrhotic and non-cirrhotic patients.

Transplantation

Endstage cirrhosis due to autoimmune hepatitis, and acute non-responsive autoimmune hepatitis leading to acute or subacute liver failure, provide firm indications for orthotopic liver transplantation. Failure to achieve an early response in acute disease, with a shrinking liver volume, should prompt consideration of transplantation. Overall, the prognosis after transplantation is good, with 5-year survival rates in excess of 80 per cent, and a similar incidence of acute rejection episodes (50–60 per cent) to that seen in other immunological liver diseases. Autoantibodies persist after transplantation, though at lower titre. There is a tendency for the disease to recur in the transplanted liver, with a frequency of about 20 per cent at 5 years, sometimes necessitating retransplantation. Whether more aggressive immunosuppressive antirejection regimes will prevent this remains to be established.

Further reading

Alvarez F et al. (1999). International Autoimmune Hepatitis Group Report: review of criteria for diagnosis of autoimmune hepatitis. Journal of Hepatology 31, 929–38.

Bansi D, Chapman R, Fleming K (1996). Antineutrophil cytoplasmic antibodies in chronic liver disease: prevalence, titre, specificity and IgG subclass. Journal of Hepatology 24, 581–6.

Cassani F, et al. (1997). Serum autoantibodies in chronic hepatitis C: comparison with autoimmune hepatitis and impact on the disease profile. Hepatology 26, 561–6.

Chazouilleres O, et al. (1998). Primary biliary cirrhosis-autoimmune hepatitis overlap syndrome: clinical features and response to therapy. Hepatology 28, 296–301.

Czaja AJ (1998). Frequency and nature of the variant syndromes of autoimmune liver disease. Hepatology 28, 360–5.

Czaja AJ, Carpenter HA (1993). Sensitivity, specificity, and predictability of biopsy interpretations in chronic hepatitis. Gastroenterology 105, 1824–32.

Dufour JF, DeLellis R, Kaplan MM (1997). Reversibility of hepatic fibrosis in autoimmune hepatitis. Annals of Internal Medicine 127, 981–5.

Fernandes NF, et al. (1999). Cyclosporine therapy in patients with steroid resistant autoimmune hepatitis. American Journal of Gastroenterology 94, 241–8.

Johnson PJ, McFarlane IG, Williams R (1995). Azathioprine for long term maintenance of remission in autoimmune hepatitis. New England Journal of Medicine 333, 958–63.

Meyer zum Buschenfelde KH, Dienes HP (1996). Autoimmune hepatitis. Virchows Archiv 429, 1–12.

Newton JL, et al. (1997). Autoimmune hepatitis in older patients. Age and Ageing 26, 441–4.

Ratziu V, et al. (1999). Long term follow up after liver transplantation for autoimmune hepatitis, evidence of recurrence of primary disease. Journal of Hepatology 30, 131–41.

Strettell MD, et al. (1997). Allelic basic for HLA encoded susceptibility to type 1 autoimmune hepatitis. Gastroenterology 112, 2028–35.

14.20.2.2 Primary biliary cirrhosis

M. F. Bassendine

Primary biliary cirrhosis is a chronic, cholestatic liver disease in which the biliary epithelial cells lining the small intrahepatic bile ducts are the target for immune-mediated damage leading to progressive ductopenia. The cause is unknown but evidence points to an autoimmune aetiology, in particular the strong association with disease-specific autoantibodies. It affects women in over 90 per cent of cases and usually has an insidious onset in middle age. Patients with early disease are often recognized following the incidental discovery of antimitochondrial antibodies or elevated levels of serum alkaline phosphatase. Progression may be slow but eventually many patients develop cirrhosis and, ultimately, death may occur from liver failure or complications of cirrhosis such as bleeding oesophageal varices. It is a common indication for liver transplantation.

Epidemiology

There is a marked geographical variation in the prevalence of the disease; it is commonest in Northern Europe but rare in the Indian subcontinent and Africa. It was rare and accounted for fewer than 5 per cent of patients dying of cirrhosis in Western communities, but its incidence appears to be increasing. In the North-East of England the prevalence rose from 202 per million adults and 541 per million women over 40 in 1987 to 335 per million adults and 940 per million women over 40 in 1994. It remains unclear whether this increase represents better diagnosis or a true increase in prevalence. Death rates from all causes are nearly three times greater in patients with biliary cirrhosis compared with the general population after adjusting for age and sex.

Aetiology and pathogenesis

In common with most autoimmune disorders, genetic factors partially determine susceptibility to primary biliary cirrhosis, but the pattern of inheritance is very complex. Familial clustering is well documented, and the sibling relative risk is 10.5, similar to values seen in other autoimmune disorders where it is thought that genetic factors may contribute up to 50 per cent of the total risk. There is no association of the disorder with major histocompatibility complex (**MHC**) class I antigens but several associations with class II antigens have been reported, in particular HLA DR8 with a two- to sixfold increase in patients compared with controls. Information on MHC class III associations is conflicting. The genetic predisposition conferred by HLA is however neither sufficient nor necessary for disease development and other genes are likely to be involved. The gene encoding cytotoxic T lymphocyte-associated antigen-4 has recently been examined as a candidate gene and this locus is important for conferring susceptibility not only to primary biliary cirrhosis but also to autoimmunity in general.

Over 95 per cent of patients have antibodies to mitochondria, with the dominant autoantibody response being directed against two components (dihydrolipoamide acetyltransferase (E2) and E3-binding protein) of pyruvate dehydrogenase complex (**PDC**) (Table 1). The loss of tolerance to these autoantigens is an early event in this progressive disease with antimitochondrial antibodies (**AMA**) being detectable in serum before abnormalities in liver function and long before the onset of symptoms. One

hypothesis is that the development of these AMA marks the exposure of a genetically susceptible individual to an initiating environmental factor. Autoreactive T cells play a central role in the development of various autoimmune diseases and an immunodominant T-cell epitope within pyruvate dehydrogenase complex E2 (peptide 163 to 176) has been identified in patients with primary biliary cirrhosis. T-cell clones reactive to this peptide can also be activated by mimicry peptides derived from several microbial proteins, supporting the hypothesis that autoreactive T cells present in the peripheral blood can be activated and clonally expanded by antigenic stimulation by mimicry peptides derived from environmental non-self antigen.

Aberrant expression of pyruvate dehydrogenase complex occurs on the apical surface of biliary and salivary epithelial cells in patients with primary biliary cirrhosis and secretory IgA autoantibodies have been found in bile and saliva. IgA autoantibodies to pyruvate dehydrogenase complex may thus interact with components of pyruvate dehydrogenase complex within the epithelial cells leading to metabolic consequences and subsequent cell damage.

Antinuclear antibodies occur in a minority of patients with primary biliary cirrhosis (Table 1) and display unique immunofluorescence patterns such as nuclear dots or a nuclear ring-like pattern. Disease-specific nuclear antigens include a 210-kDa glycoprotein of the nuclear pore membrane (gp 210), nucleoporin p62, and Sp100, an interferon-inducible nucleoprotein with a molecular mass of 100 kDa.

Despite progress in characterizing the reactivity of the disease-specific autoantibodies, little is understood of the way in which the autoimmune response is induced or the effector mechanisms that cause tissue damage. The concept of the T_{H1}/T_{H2} paradigm has gained importance in autoimmune reactions; in primary biliary cirrhosis there is dominance of T_{H1} cells. Interferon-γ is the main cytokine in the liver and CD8+ cytotoxic T cells infiltrate the portal tract as part of the chronic inflammation that characterizes primary biliary cirrhosis. The cytotoxic lymphocyte must interact closely with its putative target in order to recognize peptide in association with MHC class 1 and this is facilitated by adhesion to intercellular adhesion molecule 1 (ICAM-1) and CD58, both of which are increased on inflamed biliary cells. Biliary epithelial cells undergo apoptosis but the mechanisms involved and the role of the other effector systems are less clear.

Table 1 Disease-specific autoantibodies and their reactivity in primary biliary cirrhosis

Antigen	MW ($\times 10^3$)	Occurrence of autoantibodies (%)
Mitochondrial antigens		
Pyruvate dehydrogenase complex (PDC):		
E2 acetyltransferase	74	95
PDC E3-binding protein	52	95
PDC E1α decarboxylase	41	40–66
PDC E1β decarboxylase	36	2–10
2-oxoglutarate dehydrogenase complex:		
E2 succinyl transferase	48	39–88
Branched-chain 2-oxo-acid dehydrogenase complex:		
E2 acyltransferase	50	53–89
Nuclear antigens		
Glycoprotein of the nuclear-pore membrane	210	10–47
Nucleoporin p62	62	32
Sp100	100	20

MW, molecular weight.

Clinical features

Patients with early disease may complain only of fatigue or symptoms of coexisting autoimmune disease. Those with more advanced disease have evidence of cholestasis, with jaundice, pruritus, light stools, easy bruising, and weight loss. The pruritus may first be noticed during pregnancy or when the patient is on the contraceptive pill. Occasionally, patients present with gastrointestinal bleeding from oesophageal varices or associated peptic ulcer.

Findings on examination vary widely. At one extreme, there may be no abnormality, whereas at the other the patient is jaundiced, with scratch marks and signs of long-standing cholestasis. The planus form of xanthoma occurs characteristically as xanthelasmas around the eyes and in the palmar creases. Tuberous lesions develop late on the extensor surfaces around the knees, elbows, wrists, ankle, and on pressure points such as buttocks. Occasionally they affect tendon sheaths and nerves, producing xanthomatous peripheral neuropathy.

The liver is often enlarged and firm, and splenomegaly may be present, with or without portal hypertension. Spider naevi and palmar erythema are less frequent than in patients with alcoholic cirrhosis. Fluid retention with ascites and oedema is usually a late complication, as is bleeding from oesophageal varices. Steatorrhoea occurs primarily in patients who have advanced cholestasis, leading to malabsorption of fat-soluble vitamins, especially vitamin D. Bone pain due to osteomalacia, with tenderness and fractures involving vertebrae, can occur, as can liver failure with encephalopathy. Such late manifestations of disease are now rarely seen in Western countries as liver transplant is performed in most patients before their development. Osteoporosis is also well recognized but may largely reflect the gender and age of patients with primary biliary cirrhosis. Deficiency of vitamin K sometimes results in easy bruising or other haemorrhagic phenomena. Clubbing of the fingers and leuconychia are rare findings. There is an increased incidence of gallstones and peptic ulceration, and features of these conditions may form part of the clinical picture.

Primary biliary cirrhosis is associated with past smoking and a number of other autoimmune diseases. These include Sjögren's syndrome, seropositive and seronegative arthropathy, thyroiditis, scleroderma, and renal tubular acidosis. The CREST syndrome (calcinosis, Raynaud's phenomenon, sclerodactyly, and telangiectasia), pulmonary fibrosis, psoriasis, and coeliac disease have also been reported.

Pathology

The characteristic early lesion of primary biliary cirrhosis is inflammatory duct destruction. Later there is fibrosis, often patchy, and eventually a frank cirrhotic picture. Histologically this disease appears to evolve from a florid duct lesion to cirrhosis. This has led to a morphological classification into four stages. It must be recognized, however, that overlap between stages is common in different parts of the liver. In stage 1, the duct lesion is florid (Fig. 1) with the epithelium irregular, hyperplastic, or ulcerated. There is a heavy infiltrate of lymphocytes, plasma cells, and neutrophils, with occasional eosinophils. Aggregates of histiocytes with granulomas ranging from foci of epithelioid cells to rounded lesions with multinucleated giant cells are present. In stage 2 there is established duct destruction and the bile ducts may be replaced by lymphoid aggregates with fibrosis. In stage 3 there is relatively little inflammation, though lymphoid aggregates may be present and fibrous septa extend from the portal tract. In stage 4 there is an established cirrhosis, paucity of bile ducts, and lymphoid infiltration (Fig. 2). Mallory bodies similar to those seen in alcoholic liver disease may be present adjacent to the areas of inflammation and there is excess stainable copper-binding protein, a reflection of the cholestasis.

Malignancy

There is a dramatically increased risk for the development of hepatobiliary malignancies in patients with primary biliary cirrhosis with a reported relative risk of 46 for women and 55 for men. Hepatocellular carcinoma is a

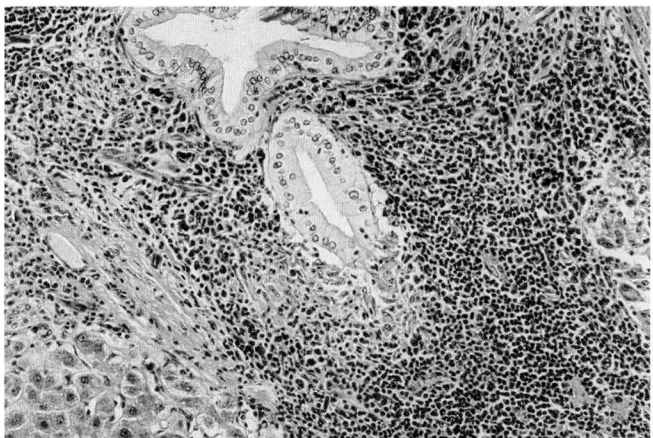

Fig. 1 Bile duct lesion in primary biliary cirrhosis. There is granulomatous destruction of a medium-sized bile-duct radicle in which the epithelium appears hyperplastic. Epithelioid macrophages are surrounded by a chronic inflammatory cell infiltrate. Haematoxylin and eosin stain. (By courtesy of A.D. Burt.)

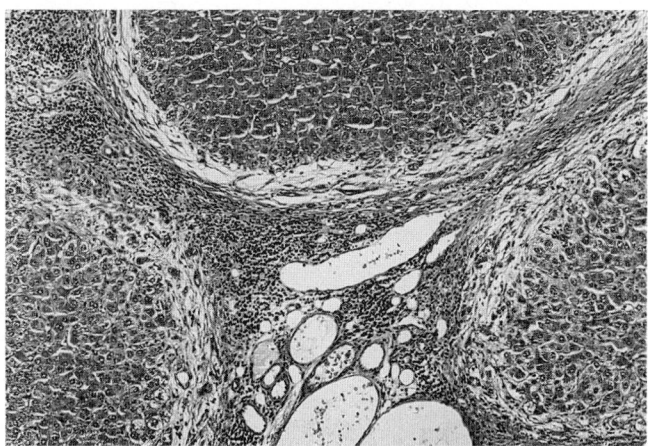

Fig. 2 Stage 4 primary biliary cirrhosis: an established micronodular cirrhosis; the halo effect seen around the nodules is a characteristic feature of biliary cirrhosis. Haematoxylin and eosin stain. (By courtesy of A.D. Burt.)

recognized complication of cirrhosis from any cause. Men are afflicted at least twice as often as women, and primary biliary cirrhosis is no exception to this rule. Hepatocellular carcinoma is a relatively common cause of death in male patients with concomitant primary biliary cirrhosis and liver cirrhosis and screening with regular liver ultrasound is recommended.

Diagnosis

The diagnosis is based on the serological and biochemical changes, together with the clinical findings and liver histology. A positive AMA may antedate all other abnormalities. Liver function tests reflect cholestasis, with increases in serum alkaline phosphatase and γ-glutamyl transferase, but only modest changes in transaminases. At presentation, total serum bilirubin is usually normal or only modestly increased. The serum globulins are usually raised, particularly the IgM, but the serum albumin is usually maintained until late in the disease. Other tests such as erythrocyte sedimentation rate, cholesterol, and autoantibodies other than AMA are less specific. In a patient with a strongly positive AMA and the typical symptoms and biochemical abnormalities, a liver biopsy may not be essential, but is helpful. The features are very specific, and although several different histological stages may be found in one biopsy, the presence of fibrosis or cirrhosis indicates a worse prognosis.

The main differential diagnosis is from other causes of cholestasis. Good ultrasound examination of the liver and biliary tree is mandatory to exclude extrahepatic biliary obstruction or gallstones. Computed tomography, magnetic resonance cholangiopancreatography (**MRCP**), or endoscopic retrograde cholangiopancreatography (**ERCP**) may be necessary for patients without detectable AMA, many of whom have a positive antinuclear antibody and may be thought to have 'autoimmune cholangitis'. There is an overlap with autoimmune hepatitis, which can be diagnosed on liver histology, whilst primary sclerosing cholangitis will be evident on MRCP or ERCP.

Treatment

This consists of therapy aimed at modifying the disease process and progression to cirrhosis, and treatment of symptoms and late complications.

Numerous trials of specific therapy have been undertaken in the last 30 years; the agents that have been assessed are shown in Table 2. Over recent years the naturally occurring bile acid, ursodeoxycholic acid, has become an established treatment for primary biliary cirrhosis. Many randomized controlled trials comparing ursodeoxycholic acid with placebo have been published. All the trials reported an improvement in standard

Table 2 Drugs evaluated as monotherapy in primary biliary cirrhosis

Agent	Dosage	Comment
Cyclosporin	2.5 to 4 mg/kg.day	Improved hepatic function but renal toxicity and hypertension
Methotrexate	15 mg/week	Under evaluation; some benefit, but toxicity possible
Prednisolone	30 reducing to 10 mg/day	Improved hepatic function in one small study
Azathioprine	1 to 2 mg/kg.day	Minor benefits; ? improved survival
Chlorambucil	0.5 to 4 mg/day	Potentially toxic; benefits unclear
Colchicine	0.6 to 1.2 mg/day	Minor benefits
Malotilate	1.5 mg/day	Minor benefits
D-Penicillamine	250–1000 mg/day	No convincing benefit; excessive toxicity
Ursodeoxycholic acid	10 to 15 mg/kg.day	Improvement in biochemistry; may delay progression to cirrhosis; well tolerated

liver enzyme tests and serum bilirubin levels. Results from three large studies have been included in a combined analysis, which indicated that treatment with ursodeoxycholic acid was associated with a significant delay in the time to death or transplantation. However, this was not confirmed in a long-term study (median follow-up of 3.4 years), nor in a meta-analysis of published randomized controlled trials. Data suggest that ursodeoxycholic acid does not prevent ongoing bile-duct destruction but that it exerts its beneficial effect by protecting against the consequences of bile duct destruction. Ursodeoxycholic acid therapy does not benefit the symptom of fatigue and has a variable effect on pruritus. At best ursodeoxycholic acid, in a dose of 12 to 15 mg/kg per day, may retard progression to cirrhosis (histological stage 4), but it does not halt the disease and cannot be seen as a cure. However, it is safe and well tolerated.

Trials of combination therapy using ursodeoxycholic acid with methotrexate, colchicine, prednisolone, oral budesonide, and mycophenolate mofetil have been reported; most are too small to evaluate the efficacy adequately, but one pilot study suggests ursodeoxycholic acid plus budesonide is superior in patients with early disease.

Itching can be an intolerable symptom in primary biliary cirrhosis and the first line of treatment is with cholestyramine. Improvement in itching has also been reported with rifampicin and opioid antagonists (nalmifene and naloxone). There is no indication for a fat-free diet unless the patient has symptoms related to steatorrhoea or xanthelasma with high serum cholesterol levels. Supplementation with medium-chain triglycerides may be necessary if adequate weight or nutrition cannot be sustained. A prolonged prothrombin time is treated with intramuscular vitamin K at a dose of 10 mg monthly. Injections of vitamin A (100 000 iu) and vitamin D (100 000 iu) are usually given every 2 months in jaundiced patients and vitamin E supplements may also be required. Osteomalacia is now rare, given such treatment. The principles developed for monitoring and treating postmenopausal osteoporosis can be followed for patients with primary biliary cirrhosis. The complications of portal hypertension and of liver failure are treated appropriately.

Liver transplantation is now the accepted treatment for endstage primary biliary cirrhosis. Referral to a transplant centre should be considered as the bilirubin approaches 100 μmol/l, although patients with disabling symptoms such as intractable itching may need to be considered individually. Recurrence of primary biliary cirrhosis occurs in about 10 per cent of patients in the first few years after liver transplantation; the cumulative risk increases with time and may be affected by the immunosuppression used.

Prognosis

The progression of primary biliary cirrhosis is extremely variable. Asymptomatic patients have a reduced survival compared with an age-and gender-matched general population and about 40 per cent develop symptoms within 5 to 7 years. The most reliable determinant of prognosis is the serum bilirubin concentration; other factors associated with poor prognosis include weight loss, hepatomegaly, splenomegaly, histological stage, patient age, and impaired liver synthetic function. Several prognostic models have been validated in clinical studies; the most widely used is the Mayo risk score.

Quality of life aspects

Fatigue is present in more than 80 per cent of patients and is one of the worst symptoms. It is not related to disease severity and may be associated with depression. The Fisk Fatigue Severity Score is a reproducible measure of fatigue severity and can be used in the clinical assessment of patients and in therapeutic trials.

Further reading

Adams DH, Shields PL (2000). Lymphocyte recruitment and activation in primary biliary cirrhosis. *Immunological Reviews* 174, 15–26.

Agarwal K, Jones DEJ, Bassendine MF (1999). Genetic predisposition to primary biliary cirrhosis. *European Journal of Gastroenterology and Hepatology* 11, 603–6. [Part of 'Review in depth' of primary biliary cirrhosis.]

Gershwin ME *et al.* (2000). Primary biliary cirrhosis: an orchestrated immune response against epithelial cells. *Immunological Reviews* 174, 210–25.

Goulis J, Leandro G, Burroughs AK (1999). Randomised controlled trials of ursodeoxycholic-acid therapy for primary biliary cirrhosis: a meta-analysis. *Lancet* 354, 1053–60.

Heathcote JE (1999). Evidence based therapy for primary biliary cirrhosis. *European Journal of Gastroenterology and Hepatology* 11, 607–15. [Part of 'Review in depth' of primary biliary cirrhosis.]

Heathcote EJ (2000). Management of primary biliary cirrhosis. *Hepatology* 31, 1005–13. [Guidelines developed under the auspices of, and approved by, the Practice Guidelines Committee of the American Association for the Study of Liver Diseases.]

James OFW *et al.* (1999). Primary biliary cirrhosis once rare, now common in the United Kingdom? *Hepatology* 30, 390–4.

Jones DEJ, James OFW, Bassendine MF (1998). Primary biliary cirrhosis: clinical and associated autoimmune features and natural history. In: Lindor KD, Dickson ER, eds. *Clinics in liver disease: primary biliary cirrhosis, primary sclerosing cholangitis, and adult cholangiopathies*, Vol 2, pp 265–82. WB Saunders, Philadelphia. [Part of an in depth review of adult cholangiopathies, including primary biliary cirrhosis.]

Jones EA, Bergasa NV (1999). The pathogenesis and treatment of pruritus and fatigue in patients with PBC. *European Journal of Gastroenterology and Hepatology* 11, 623–31. [Part of 'Review in depth' of primary biliary cirrhosis.]

Kim WR, Dickson ER (1998). Predictive models of natural history in primary biliary cirrhosis. In: Lindor KD, Dickson ER, eds. *Clinics in liver disease: primary biliary cirrhosis, primary sclerosing cholangitis, and adult cholangiopathies*, Vol 2, pp 313–31. WB Saunders, Philadelphia. [Part of an in depth review of adult cholangiopathies, including primary biliary cirrhosis.]

Metcalf JV, James OFW (1997). The geoepidemiology of primary biliary cirrhosis. *Seminars in Liver Disease* 17, 13–22.

Neuberger J (1997). Primary biliary cirrhosis. *Lancet* 350, 875–9.

Nijhawan PK *et al.* (1999). Incidence of cancer in primary biliary cirrhosis: The Mayo experience. *Hepatology* 29, 1396–8.

Shimoda S *et al.* (2000). Mimicry peptides of human PDC-E2 163–176 peptide, the immunodominant T-cell epitope of primary biliary cirrhosis. *Hepatology* **31**, 1212–16.

Yeaman SJ, Kirby JA, Jones DEJ (2000). Autoreactive responses to pyruvate dehydrogenase complex in the pathogenesis of primary biliary cirrhosis. *Immunological Reviews* **174**, 238–49.

Table 1 Causes of secondary sclerosing cholangitis

Previous bile-duct surgery with stricturing and cholangitis
Bile-duct stones causing cholangitis
Intrahepatic infusion of 5-fluorodeoxyuridine
Formalin insertion into hepatic hydatid cysts
Alcohol insertion into hepatic tumours
AIDS—probably infective (cytomegalovirus or cryptosporidium)

14.20.2.3 Primary sclerosing cholangitis

R. W. Chapman

Primary sclerosing cholangitis is a chronic cholestatic liver disease characterized by an obliterative inflammatory fibrosis of the biliary tract. It may lead to bile-duct obstruction, biliary cirrhosis, hepatic failure, and in some patients, cholangiocarcinoma. Primary sclerosing cholangitis was initially considered to be a rare disease; however, the advent of endoscopic retrograde cholangiopancreatography (**ERCP**) in the early 1970s established the diagnosis in a progressively larger number of patients. This led to the realization that primary sclerosing cholangitis has a much wider clinical and pathological spectrum than was previously recognized.

The generally accepted diagnostic criteria of primary sclerosing cholangitis are: (i) generalized bleeding and stenosis of the biliary system on cholangiography (Fig. 1); (ii) absence of choledocholithiasis or a history of bile-duct surgery; and (iii) exclusion of bile-duct cancer, usually by prolonged follow-up.

The term secondary sclerosing cholangitis is used to describe the typical bile-duct changes when a clear predisposing factor to duct fibrosis, such as previous bile-duct surgery, can be identified. The causes of secondary sclerosing cholangitis are shown in Table 1.

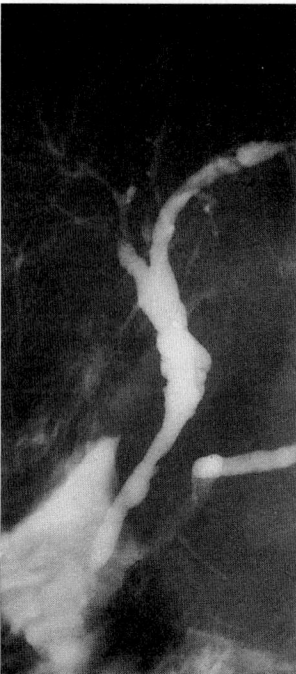

Fig. 1 Endoscopic retrograde cholangiogram showing the typical features of primary sclerosing cholangitis with stricturing and dilatation of the intra- and extrahepatic biliary tree.

Aetiology

The cause of primary sclerosing cholangitis remains unknown. There is a very close association, however, between primary sclerosing cholangitis and inflammatory bowel disease, particularly ulcerative colitis. Approximately two-thirds of Northern European patients with primary sclerosing cholangitis have coexisting ulcerative colitis, and primary sclerosing cholangitis is the most common form of chronic liver disease found in ulcerative colitis. In Southern Europeans about one-half of patients with primary sclerosing cholangitis will have ulcerative colitis. This difference in populations may be real or may represent differences in case finding as not all the patients studied had had colonoscopy and colonic biopsies performed. Three to 10 per cent of patients with ulcerative colitis will develop primary sclerosing cholangitis, and the prevalence is greater in patients with substantial or total colitis than in those with distal colitis only. In a Swedish study, the prevalence of ulcerative colitis was 171 per 100 000 population and primary sclerosing cholangitis 6.3 per 100 000 population. It is clear that any proposed factors in the aetiopathogenesis of primary sclerosing cholangitis must explain this close association with inflammatory bowel disease. Current studies have suggested that genetic and immunological factors are important in the pathogenesis of primary sclerosing cholangitis.

Immunogenetic factors

Case reports of families in whom members developed ulcerative colitis and primary sclerosing cholangitis led to the search for an HLA association. A close link with the *HLA A1-B8-DR3* haplotype has been found, in common with other organ-specific autoimmune diseases such as autoimmune chronic active hepatitis. *HLA DRw52a*, which is in linkage disequilibrium with *DR3*, is also closely linked to the development of primary sclerosing cholangitis. In British patients who are *DR3* and *Drw52a* negative, an increased prevalence of *HLA DR2* is found. *HLA A1-B8-DR3* and *DR2* are equally distributed in patients with primary sclerosing cholangitis, with or without ulcerative colitis. An independent association with *HLA DR6* has also been documented. It has been suggested that *DRw52a*, *DR6*, and *DR2* encode for amino acids in the HLA β-chain that may enhance antigen presentation by the HLA molecule to the T-cell receptor. Further evidence of an autoimmune basis for this condition has been provided by many studies that have shown humoral and cellular immune abnormalities.

Humoral immune abnormalities

Like primary biliary cirrhosis, a disease with which it shares many features (see Chapter 14.27.2), symptomatic primary sclerosing cholangitis is characterized by hypergammaglobulinaemia, often with a disproportionate elevation of serum IgM concentrations in adult patients. In contrast, high concentrations of serum IgG are found in all children with primary sclerosing cholangitis. Smooth-muscle antibody and antinuclear factor are also found in approximately one-third of patients with primary sclerosing cholangitis, usually in low titres.

Recently, a cytoplasmic antineutrophil antibody was found in the serum of 80 per cent of patients with primary sclerosing cholangitis and approximately 30 per cent of patients with ulcerative colitis. However, it is not specific for primary sclerosing cholangitis and is found in 50 per cent of patients with autoimmune chronic active hepatitis (type 1). It is not found in primary biliary cirrhosis. The antigens in primary sclerosing cholangitis are distinct from those found in Wegener's granulomatosis, which have been shown to be proteinase 3 and myeloperoxidase. Current evidence suggests that the antigen may be a nuclear envelope protein. The pathogenetic significance of the circulating antibody is not clear, but it may prove to be useful in a diagnostic test. Titres of the antibody do not change after hepatic transplantation.

Cellular immune abnormalities

Elevated circulating immune complexes associated with activation of complement via the classic pathway have been found in the serum and bile of patients with primary sclerosing cholangitis. In common with other autoimmune diseases, there are reduced levels of T-suppressor cells circulating in the serum of these patients, leading to an increased ratio of T-helper to T-suppressor cells. Infiltration of portal tracts by increased numbers of mononuclear cells is seen in liver biopsies from patients with primary sclerosing cholangitis. The majority of these cells are activated T lymphocytes.

Current evidence suggests that primary sclerosing cholangitis is an immunologically mediated disease, perhaps triggered in genetically susceptible subjects by acquired toxic or infectious agents, which are presented through antigen-presenting cells to activated T lymphocytes. Unlike normal biliary cells, the biliary epithelial cells in primary sclerosing cholangitis express HLA class II molecules and also intercellular adhesion molecules (**ICAM**) such as ICAM-I. It has not yet been confirmed, however, that bile-duct cells can act as antigen-presenting cells, as expression of other costimulatory molecules such as B7, which are needed for antigen presentation, are not consistently found on biliary epithelial cells (cholangiocytes).

Alternative hypothesis—exposure to bacterial components

An alternative hypothesis has been proposed in which the initial event is the reaction of an immunologically susceptible host to bacterial cell wall products. This reaction would result in hepatic macrophages producing tumour necrosis factor-α and endotoxin. The exposure to bacterial components and increased gut permeability would be increased by the presence of inflammatory bowel disease, but could also, in theory, occur during episodes of gut infection. The resulting increase in peribiliary cytokine and chemokine secretion would attract activated neutrophils, monocyte/macrophages, T cells, and fibroblasts. The deposition of concentric fibrosis could result in atrophy of the biliary epithelial cells secondary to ischaemia. The resulting bile duct loss would lead to progressive cholestasis, fibrosis, and secondary biliary cirrhosis. This hypothesis does not explain the relative scarcity of patients with Crohn's colitis and does not take into account the strong circumstantial evidence of immune mediation and autoimmunity, previously described.

Clinical features

There is a clear male predominance, with a male:female ratio of 2:1. The majority of patients present between the ages of 25 and 40 years, although primary sclerosing cholangitis may be diagnosed at any age. Indeed, it has become recognized recently as an important cause of chronic liver disease in children.

The clinical presentation is variable: some patients may present with fatigue, intermittent jaundice, weight loss, right upper quadrant pain, and pruritus. Attacks of acute cholangitis are surprisingly rare and usually follow instrumental biliary intervention, such as ERCP. Physical examination is abnormal in approximately half of symptomatic patients; the most common findings are jaundice and hepatosplenomegaly. Many patients with primary sclerosing cholangitis are asymptomatic at diagnosis, which is made incidentally when a persistently raised serum alkaline phosphatase is discovered, usually in the setting of ulcerative colitis.

Serum biochemical tests usually indicate cholestasis, but primary sclerosing cholangitis may cause no abnormalities of serum biochemistry. The

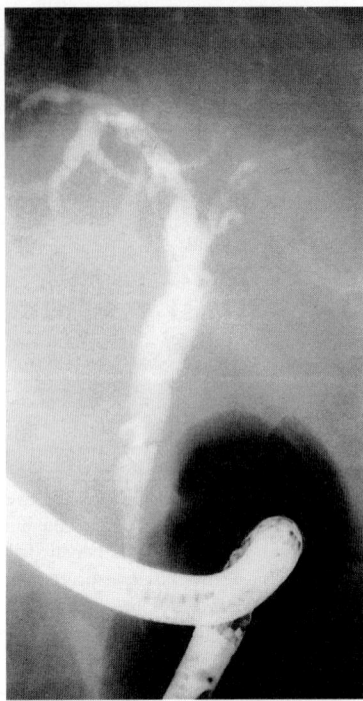

Fig. 2 Endoscopic retrograde cholangiogram from a patient with primary sclerosing cholangitis showing a diverticular appearance of the common bile duct.

serum alkaline phosphatase is often raised to greater than three times normal, and mild elevations in liver transaminases are seen in the majority of patients. Serum bilirubin is not usually elevated until later stages of the disease. Levels of bilirubin and alkaline phosphatase may fluctuate widely in an individual patient during the course of the disease. Hypoalbuminaemia is unusual until the disease becomes advanced. As mentioned above, increased serum IgM concentrations are seen in about half of the symptomatic adult patients, but high concentrations of IgG are always found in children with primary sclerosing cholangitis.

In addition to the serum antineutrophil antibodies, low levels of antinuclear antibody and smooth-muscle antibody may be found in approximately one-third of patients, but serum mitochondrial antibodies are absent.

Diagnosis

Radiological features

The cholangiographic appearances on ERCP are usually diagnostic and consist of multiple, irregular stricturing and dilatation (beading of the intrahepatic and extrahepatic biliary ducts) (Fig. 1). Occasionally, involvement is localized to the intrahepatic system, and even more rarely, only the extrahepatic bile ducts may be involved. Small diverticula are found along the common bile duct in about 20 per cent of patients and are pathognomonic (Fig. 2). Magnetic resonance cholangiopancreatography provides a non-invasive method of imaging the biliary tree, and will become the standard technique for the diagnosis of primary sclerosing cholangitis. (Fig. 3) Approximately 20 per cent of patients have stricturing of the main pancreatic duct, although exocrine pancreatic insufficiency is rare.

Pathological features

The histological appearances of liver are not usually diagnostic for primary sclerosing cholangitis, although some form of biliary disease can usually be identified. The characteristic early features of primary sclerosing cholangitis are periductal 'onion skin' fibrosis and inflammation, portal oedema,

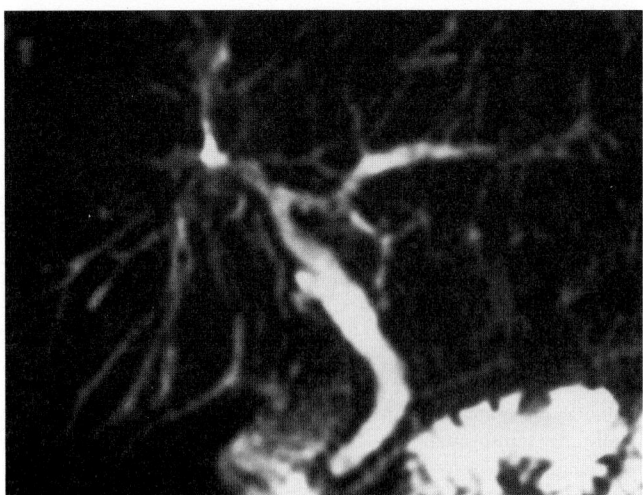

Fig. 3 Magnetic resonance cholangiogram demonstrating hilar stricture and intrahepatic involvement of the biliary tree.

and bile ductular proliferation resulting in the expansion of the portal tracts (Fig. 4). Later, fibrosis spreads into the liver parenchyma to form fibrous septa, leading inevitably to biliary cirrhosis. As in primary biliary cirrhosis, with disease progression an obliterative cholangitis occurs, leading to complete replacement of the intralobular bile ducts by connective tissue—the so-called vanishing bile-duct syndrome. In addition, piecemeal necrosis, copper-binding protein, cholestasis, and occasional portal phlebitis may be present.

Association with other diseases

A large number of diseases have been associated with primary sclerosing cholangitis (Table 2). The most important association, as discussed above, is with inflammatory bowel disease, particularly ulcerative colitis. The extent of the colitis is usually total but symptomatically, and paradoxically, mild, often with no rectal bleeding and characterized by prolonged remission. Rectal sparing is found in 20 per cent of patients with ulcerative colitis and primary sclerosing cholangitis compared with 5 per cent of patients with ulcerative colitis alone. Although the symptoms of ulcerative colitis usually develop before those of primary sclerosing cholangitis, the onset of the latter may precede the symptoms of colitis by some years. The outcome of primary sclerosing cholangitis is completely unrelated to the activity, severity, or clinical course of the colitis, and colectomy has no effect on the

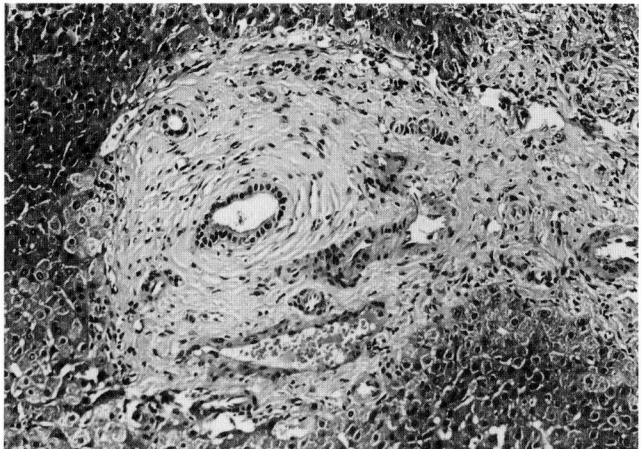

Fig. 4 The hepatic histological changes of early primary sclerosing cholangitis showing a concentric (onion skin) fibrosis around the bile ducts.

Table 2 Diseases associated with primary sclerosing cholangitis

Ulcerative colitis
Crohn's colitis
Chronic pancreatitis
Retroperitoneal fibrosis
Riedel's struma
Retro-orbital tumours
Immunodeficiency states
Sjögren's syndrome
Angioimmunoblastic lymphadenopathy
Histiocytosis X
Autoimmune haemolytic anaemia

progression of the cholangitis. Primary sclerosing cholangitis is less common in Crohn's disease, occurring in less than 1 per cent of patients and only in those with Crohn's colitis. Patients with primary sclerosing cholangitis and ulcerative colitis are at greater risk of developing colorectal dysplasia and colonic cancer than those with ulcerative colitis alone. In a Swedish study, the absolute accumulative risk of developing colorectal dysplasia/cancer in the primary sclerosing cholangitis/ulcerative colitis group was 9, 31, and 50 per cent, respectively, after 10, 20, and 25 years of disease duration. In the group with ulcerative colitis alone, the corresponding risk was 2, 5, and 10 per cent, respectively.

Natural history and prognosis

The course of primary sclerosing cholangitis is highly variable. The median survival from presentation to death or liver transplantation in symptomatic patients is approximately 10 to 12 years, whilst approximately 75 per cent of asymptomatic patients survive 15 years or more. The majority of patients die in hepatic failure following deepening cholestatic jaundice. However, approximately 10 to 30 per cent of patients with long-standing primary sclerosing cholangitis die from the development of bile duct carcinoma, which often follows a very aggressive course. The mean survival after the diagnosis of cholangiocarcinoma is only 9 months. Unfortunately, there are no factors that will predict which patients will develop this cancer. Tumour markers such as CEA and CA 19–9 have been investigated as potential serum markers of the development of bile duct cancer in primary sclerosing cholangitis. Although some centres have found elevations in serum CA 19–9 a useful predictor, these results have not been confirmed in other units. Attempts to model factors that will predict the risk of progression to liver failure and death have yielded conflicting data from different centres. It is probable that the majority of asymptomatic patients will progress insidiously to symptomatic liver disease, liver failure, and death.

Treatment

Symptomatic measures

There is no curative treatment for primary sclerosing cholangitis. This is indicated by the plethora of medical, endoscopic, and surgical approaches that has been advocated.

Management of cholestasis

Symptomatic patients are frequently troubled by pruritus. This is best managed initially by cholestyramine and the dose should be increased until relief is obtained. Second line treatments include rifampicin and the opioid antagonist naltrexone. In addition, replacement of fat-soluble vitamins is necessary when patients become jaundiced. Metabolic bone disease (usually osteoporosis) is a common complication of advanced primary sclerosing cholangitis. Calcium supplementation with vitamin D_3 should be given prophylactically in jaundiced patients and bisphosphonates considered in patients with osteoporosis.

Management of complications

Broad-spectrum antibiotics such as ciprofloxacin should be given for acute attacks of cholangitis, but they have no proven prophylactic value and should not be used in the long term routinely. If cholangiography shows a well-defined obstruction to the main extrahepatic bile ducts, then mechanical relief must be considered. In many patients the best approach is to introduce a prosthesis (stent) through the obstruction. This may be placed non-operatively by the percutaneous transhepatic route or at ERCP. Balloon dilatation of the strictures before stenting may prove useful in a minority of patients with well-defined localized strictures and can lead to a striking improvement in symptoms and serum biochemistry.

Another common complication is the development of small biliary stones (brown pigment) and biliary sludge, which can lead to a rapid clinical or biochemical deterioration. In these patients, endoscopic sphincterotomy with extraction of the biliary debris can be beneficial.

Small duct disease

A few patients with ulcerative colitis will have persistently abnormal cholestatic liver function tests with typical histological appearances such as concentric fibrosis but with normal bile ducts at cholangiography. The term 'small-duct primary sclerosing cholangitis' has been proposed to replace the term 'pericholangitis' in this group of patients as the evidence suggests that these conditions are all part of the same disease spectrum. Only a minority of patients with 'small-duct disease' will progress to develop extrahepatic biliary involvement and they are not predisposed to develop cholangiocarcinoma.

Specific treatment

Medical

The medical treatment of primary sclerosing cholangitis has included trials of corticosteroids, immunosuppressive drugs, cholecystogogues, and antibiotics, either alone or in combination. The results have been universally disappointing, although assessment of treatment of this uncommon disease is difficult because the clinical course fluctuates, survival is variable, and some patients may remain asymptomatic for long periods of time. The role of corticosteroid therapy is unclear. There have been no large controlled trials, but corticosteroids have been used topically and systemically in small and generally uncontrolled studies. However, there is evidence that, even in male patients, metabolic bone disease may be accelerated by corticosteroids and in general they should not be used in this condition.

Ursodeoxycholic acid is a non-hepatotoxic hydrophilic bile acid which has been used widely for the treatment of cholestasis—it reduces levels of cholestatic liver enzymes. Controlled trials in concentrated doses (10 to 15 mg/kg body weight) have shown no effect on symptoms, histology, or survival. Recent trials suggest that larger doses are needed to produce a beneficial effect, with improvement in histology at 2 years.

A number of immunosuppressant agents have been tried, either alone or in combination, including azathioprine, methotrexate, and cyclosporin. Overall, the results have been disappointing.

Surgical

The role of hepatobiliary surgery in the treatment of primary sclerosing cholangitis remains controversial. Good results have been claimed for the resection of the extrahepatic biliary tree followed by biliary reconstruction with silastic transhepatic stents. However, controlled trials are needed to confirm the efficacy of these and other surgical techniques, as previous biliary surgery will increase perioperative mortality from hepatic transplantation.

Transplantation

Orthotopic liver transplantation is the only option available in young patients with primary sclerosing cholangitis and advanced liver disease. Primary sclerosing cholangitis is now the second most common indication for liver transplantation in the United Kingdom. Recent results have been very encouraging, with 5-year survival rates of 80 to 90 per cent being obtained in most centres. These rates compare favourably with those for other forms of chronic liver disease. It has become clear that primary sclerosing cholangitis recurs in the transplanted liver in 20 per cent of patients at 1 year post-transplant, but only rarely has recurrence led to problems with liver decompensation requiring retransplantation. Proven cholangiocarcinoma is a contradiction to transplantation because the tumour recurs rapidly after transplantation with immunosuppression. As patients suffering from primary sclerosing cholangitis in combination with ulcerative colitis have an increased risk for the development of colon cancer after transplantation, yearly colonoscopy has been recommended in this group. Several centres have noted a worsening in the symptoms of ulcerative colitis after transplantation; the explanation for this phenomenon remains unclear.

Further reading

Broome U *et al.* (1995). Primary sclerosing cholangitis and ulcerative colitis: evidence for increased neoplastic potential. *Hepatology* **22**, 1404–8.

Broome U, Olsson RK, Loof L (1996). Natural history and prognostic factors in 305 Swedish patients with primary sclerosing cholangitis. *Gut* **38**, 610–15.

Chalasami N *et al.* (2000). Cholangiocarcinoma in patients with primary sclerosing cholangitis: a multicentre case–control study. *Hepatology* **31**, 7–11.

Chapman RW *et al.* (1980). Primary sclerosing cholangitis—a review of its clinical features, cholangiography and hepatic histology. *Gut* **21**, 870–7.

Donaldson PT *et al.* (1991). Dual association of HLA DR2 and DR3 with primary sclerosing cholangitis. *Hepatology* **13**, 129–33.

Graziadei IW *et al.* (1999). Long term results of patients undergoing liver transplantation for primary sclerosing cholangitis. *Hepatology* **30**, 1121–7.

Graziadei IW *et al.* (1999). Recurrence of primary sclerosing cholangitis following liver transplantation. *Hepatology* **29**, 1050–6.

Johnson GK *et al.* (1991). Endoscopic treatment of biliary tract strictures in sclerosing cholangitis: a large series and recommendations of treatment. *Gastrointestinal Endoscopy* **37**, 38–43.

Lindor KD (1997). Ursodiol for primary sclerosing cholangitis. Mayo Primary Sclerosing Cholangitis–ursodeoxycholic Audit Study Group. *New England Journal of Medicine* **336**, 691–5.

Lo SK, Fleming KA, Chapman RW (1992). Prevalence of antineutrophil antibody in primary sclerosing cholangitis and ulcerative colitis using an alkaline phosphatase method. *Gut* **33**, 1370–5.

Ludwig J *et al.* (1981). Morphological features of chronic hepatitis associated with primary sclerosing cholangitis and ulcerative colitis. *Hepatology* **1**, 632–40.

Manns MP *et al.* (1998). *Primary sclerosing cholangitis.* Kluwer Academic Publishers, London.

Mitchell SA *et al.* (2001). A preliminary trial of high dose ursodeoxycholic acid in primary sclerosing cholangitis. *Gastroenterology* **122**, 900–7.

Terjung B *et al.* (1998). Atypical antinuclear cytoplasmic antibodies with perinuclear fluorescence in chronic inflammatory bowel diseases and hepatobiliary disorders colocalise with nuclear lamina proteins. *Hepatology* **28**, 332–40.

14.21 Other disorders of the liver

14.21.1 Alcoholic liver disease and non-alcoholic steatosis hepatitis

O. F. W. James

Alcoholic liver disease

Only 10 to 30 per cent of heavy, persistent, alcohol drinkers develop cirrhosis, although well over 50 per cent have fatty livers. Individual susceptibility depends on many factors. The contribution of nutrition remains controversial, but is seems possible that both undernutrition and obesity act synergistically with direct alcohol toxicity to increase the likelihood of liver damage. High alcohol consumption in patients infected with hepatitis C virus also increases the possibility of severe liver disease.

In a large group of males with alcoholic cirrhosis, average alcohol consumption was 160 g/day (equivalent to over two bottles of wine, 4.5 litres of normal strength lager or two-thirds of a bottle of spirits) over 8 years. In females the corresponding figure was 110 g/day. It seems likely that almost no risk of significant alcohol-related liver damage exists below about 40 g/day equivalent to 30 units per week in men, rather less in women, assuming no other associated risk factors. Current 'sensible' limits recommended in the United Kingdom are 21 units (200 g) for men and 14 units (130 g) for women, but these figures are arbitrary.

Susceptibility to alcoholism and to alcoholic liver damage each have genetic components; probably one in three alcoholics will have at least one parent who is alcoholic. Analysis of twin studies suggests hereditability of excess drinking of alcohol in the range of 0.3–0.6 (where 0 = no hereditability, 1.0 = complete hereditability).

Pathology

Fatty liver is the first histological lesion; it occurs in most heavy drinkers at one time or another, but is completely reversible on alcohol withdrawal. More serious is alcoholic hepatitis, which may occur in up to 40 per cent chronic ethanol abusers. The most severe changes are seen in the perivenular area; including ballooning and necrosis of liver cells, in some of which Mallory bodies may be seen; pericellular fibrosis around hepatic venules ('chicken wire' fibrosis); and a patchy inflammatory-cell infiltrate, mainly polymorphs, often only seen around a few hepatocytes. Ultimately, fibrous septa link hepatic veins to portal veins and regeneration occurs, disturbing normal liver architecture with the formation of nodules and cirrhosis.

Clinical features

Symptoms and signs of alcoholic liver disease (Table 1) correlate only very broadly with underlying histology or abnormal tests of liver function.

Patients with fatty liver may have no symptoms or complain only of nausea and malaise. Liver function tests may be mildly deranged but in severe cases, there may be cholestasis or even, very rarely, liver failure and portal hypertension.

Mild alcoholic hepatitis is often indistinguishable clinically from fatty liver, with which it usually coexists, but in more severe cases anorexia, nausea, abdominal pain, and weight loss may develop. Severe alcoholic hepatitis, with or without cirrhosis, is a medical emergency; patients are at risk of ascites, bleeding, and encephalopathy. They may also become infected—urinary tract infection, pneumonia, spontaneous bacterial peritonitis, or septicaemia. Detection of such infection is complicated by the fever and leucocytosis caused by the liver disease itself. Those most severely affected may develop profound cholestasis and hypoglycaemia.

The picture in established cirrhosis is variable. In some who have stopped drinking there may be no symptoms and liver function tests may

Table 1 Clinical signs of alcoholism

Undernutrition
Thin arms and legs (reduced muscle mass), frequently with swollen abdomen
Red tongue
Dry, scaly, cracked skin (zinc and/or essential fatty-acid deficiency)

Endocrine
Gynaecomastia
Testicular atrophy
Loss of body hair
Signs of pseudo-Cushing's (red face, hump, striae)

Face/skin
Parotid enlargement
Spider naevi
Paper-money skin
Easy bruising
Dupuytren's contracture

Neuromuscular
Tremor
Proximal myopathy
Painful peripheral neuropathy
Specific neurological syndromes
Memory loss and cognitive impairment

Cardiovascular
Hypertension
Signs of heart failure (cardiomyopathy)
Hyperdynamic circulation (in advanced liver disease)

Bone
Unexplained rib fractures on chest radiographs
Spinal osteoporosis (often in men)

General
Signs of personal neglect
Smells of drink

be near normal. More often, patients suffer malaise and will have lost weight and show classical physical signs (Table 1), may be jaundiced, and may bleed from varices. Zieve's syndrome of marked jaundice from a combination of cholestasis and haemolysis with hyperlipidaemia is rare.

History and investigation

Many patients are reluctant to admit their alcoholism, even when liver disease is gross (see Chapter 26.7.2). Liver function tests are often unhelpful in establishing severity, except at the late stage. Early abnormalities may include raised serum γ-glutamyl transferase and macrocytosis. Measurement of blood or urinary ethanol is helpful if high levels are found. There may be a disproportionate elevation of serum aspartate transaminase compared to alanine transaminase. Serum ferritin may be very elevated in active heavy drinkers. Alcoholism is a common cause of combined hyperlipidaemia, indeed serum may be very hyperlipaemic. Liver biopsy allows confirmation of histological severity and exclusion of other pathologies. White-out on colloid liver scan implies severe alcoholic hepatitis.

Prognosis

Prognosis is above all related to whether the patient continues to drink or stops. In patients with fatty change alone the outlook is excellent, provided patients stop or substantially cut down drinking, although some may progress to more advanced liver disease. Mild alcoholic hepatitis has a similar prognosis to fatty change. In severe, acute alcoholic hepatitis, whether or not superimposed upon cirrhosis, there is a 12 to 50 per cent mortality within 6 months of presentation. Particularly adverse features are raised bilirubin level and abnormal blood clotting. This had led to the use of a discriminant function to help assess prognosis and decide upon treatment (Table 2). In alcoholic cirrhosis overall survival at 5 years is about 50 per cent, among abstainers 70 per cent, and in those who continue to drink 35 per cent. A second important prognostic feature is age at presentation. In a recent United Kingdom study, 3-year survival was 77 per cent in patients under the age of 60, and 46 per cent in those presenting over that age. Nutrition (possibly reflecting socio-economic status) also influences survival. Unfortunately, hepatocellular cancer can arise in patients with long-standing, often inactive, alcoholic cirrhosis, particularly men.

Treatment (see also Section 26.7)

The best treatment remains total withdrawal of alcohol and subsequent long-term abstinence in all patients with liver disease worse than moderate fatty change alone, in which case, very moderate drinking after a period of abstinence may be an option. Good prognostic features include recognition of the problem by the patient, a supportive family, steady employment, and willingness to accept treatment. No other treatment is required for patients with fatty liver or mild alcoholic hepatitis.

Severe alcoholic hepatitis

Meta-analysis of more than 10 trials of high-dose corticosteroid treatment added to conventional therapy has led to the following recommendations. In patients with discriminant function over 32 (Table 2) but who have no overt sepsis or active bleeding, 40 mg prednisolone for 21 days probably provides a 20 per cent improvement in mortality. Insulin and glucagon, anabolic steroids, colchicine, enteral and parenteral nutrition, and a variety of other so-called 'hepato-protective drugs' have all been used in trials but without real evidence of benefit with respect to mortality.

Table 2 Alcoholic liver disease discriminant function

Discriminant function (number) = [4.6 × (prothrombin time – control PT) + serum bilirubin (mg%)

Over 32 = poor prognosis

Cirrhosis

Treatment is directed against its complications, particularly portal hypertension, ascites, spontaneous bacterial peritonitis, and encephalopathy.

Transplantation

The indications for transplantation in alcoholic cirrhosis are similar to those for other endstage liver diseases (see later), with the caveat that even in advanced alcoholic cirrhosis, abstention can lead to enormous clinical improvement and long-term survival. Many transplant units consider patients only after a 6-month period of abstention, both to detect patients in whom transplantation is no longer necessary and to exclude individuals who continue to drink heavily. Estimated 5-year survival following transplantation is now over 70 per cent.

Non-alcoholic steatosis hepatitis

This is increasingly recognized as an important distinct clinical entity. Originally described in, usually very, obese females and in diabetics, or patients with hyperlipidaemia, also in patients following jejunoilial bypass surgery for obesity. This condition is now recognized in individuals of both sexes who are only marginally obese but who may have changed weight recently. Patients often present because of detection of abnormal liver function tests. It is important to make this diagnosis both for prognostic reasons and to clearly state the non-alcoholic nature of this disease in an individual for purposes of employment and insurance.

Pathology

This is identical to alcoholic liver disease, most patients having simple steatosis, others develop an alcoholic hepatitis-like appearance with or without fibrosis, a small proportion (perhaps 5–10 per cent) develop cirrhosis.

Clinical features

Most are asymptomatic but are 'accused' of having alcoholic liver disease. Up to 40 per cent have persistent right upper abdominal pain and may complain of lethargy and malaise. About 5 to 10 per cent, usually very obese and diabetic, develop cirrhosis with its complications.

Investigations

Patients must have a history of high alcohol consumption exhaustively excluded as a cause for their liver disease. Liver function tests show raised serum transaminases, unlike alcoholic liver disease serum alanine transaminase is raised compared with aspartate transaminase. Serum γ-glutamyl transferase is also raised. Liver ultrasound shows a fatty appearance but cannot reliably distinguish the extent of fibrosis.

Prognosis

This is excellent except in the small proportion of those who develop cirrhosis where complications and clinical course are as for other causes of cirrhosis.

Treatment

No treatment has yet been proven to be effective. Probably slow weight reduction, a reduced fat diet, and a period of abstinence from any alcohol consumption are most effective.

Further reading

Day CP, Bassendine MF (1992). Genetic predisposition to alcoholic liver disease. *Gut* **33**, 1344–7.

Hislop WS, *et al.* (1983). Alcoholic liver disease in Scotland and north-eastern England; presenting features in 510 patients. *Quarterly Journal of Medicine* **206**, 232–3.

Sherlock S, Dooley J (2001). *Diseases of the liver and biliary system*, 2nd edn. Blackwell Science, Oxford.

14.21.2 Cirrhosis, portal hypertension, and ascites

Kevin Moore

Introduction

Ascites is the accumulation of fluid in the peritoneal cavity. It has fascinated doctors for many years, and studies on its pathogenesis were initiated as long ago as the seventeenth century. Richard Lower (1631–1691), a physician based in Oxford, demonstrated that ascites developed in dogs following ligation of the inferior vena cava. Ernest Henry Starling (1866–1927), a physiologist based at University College London, made the greatest contribution to the study of oedema formation, with the demonstration that both hydrostatic forces and oncotic forces were involved. He also showed that the increase in thoracic lymph flow following obstruction of the inferior vena cava is mainly derived from the liver.

Aetiology

Ascites is a common complication of cirrhosis and indicates the presence of portal hypertension and hepatic decompensation. It occurs in at least 50 per cent of patients within 10 years of the diagnosis of cirrhosis, which accounts for over 75 per cent of cases presenting with ascites. Ascites may be due to malignancy, pancreatitis, tuberculosis, cardiac failure, myxoedema, or other rarer causes, each of which may also occur in patients with cirrhosis (Table 1). Ascites does not occur in patients with portal vein thrombosis or other forms of non-cirrhotic portal hypertension such as congenital hepatic fibrosis, except as a transient finding following a gastrointestinal haemorrhage. It frequently occurs in patients with the Budd–Chiari syndrome or late-onset hepatic failure (subfulminant hepatic failure), and, to a lesser extent, where small amounts of peritoneal fluid accumulate in cases of acute liver failure.

Other (rare) causes of ascites include constrictive pericarditis, malnutrition, stromal tumours and Meigs' syndrome, hypothyroidism, Budd–Chiari syndrome, veno-occlusive disease, or lymphatic leak (chylous ascites). Rare infections include candidiasis and filariasis. Granulomatous liver disease such as sarcoidosis may cause severe portal hypertension, and occasional ascites. Although ascites commonly occurs in patients with cardiac failure, it is not usually a presenting feature. Ascites may also occur in the ovarian hyperstimulation syndrome in women undergoing fertility treatment.

Table 1 Underlying causes of patients presenting with ascites in the United States

Cause	% Total
Cirrhosis (ALD)	65
Cirrhosis (viral)	10
Cirrhosis (other)	6
Malignancy	10
Heart failure	3
Tuberculosis	2
Pancreatic disease	1
Other causes	3

ALD, alcoholic liver disease

Epidemiology

Cirrhosis is the eleventh leading cause of death in the United States. It heralds the beginning of a usually rapid decline of liver function so that about half the patients die within 2 years of the onset of ascites.

Pathogenesis of ascites due to cirrhosis

The presence of portal hypertension is essential for the development of ascites: fluid accumulation does not occur at a portal pressure below 8 mmHg. However, factors other than portal pressure are important, since ascites does not develop spontaneously in patients with portal vein thrombosis. Ascites develops as a consequence of sodium and water retention, which in the presence of portal hypertension causes transudation of fluid into the peritoneal cavity, and together with an increased production of hepatic lymph may cause a massive accumulation of fluid—a moderate to marked ascites will comprise about 5 to 25 litres of fluid. Portal hypertension is an essential prerequisite for the development of ascites, since it does not develop when salt and water retention is due to mineralocorticoid excess (for example, Conn's syndrome or a secreting adrenal carcinoma), in which the cardinal manifestation is hypertension. Whilst it is well recognized that abnormal sodium handling occurs in patients with advanced cirrhosis, it less well known that sodium handling is abnormal even in the preascitic stage. Experiments by Dudley and colleagues have shown that the proximal tubular reabsorption of sodium is enhanced in early cirrhosis, and that some patients exhibit glomerular hyperfiltration. Sodium retention does not occur as a result of hyperaldosteronism, for approximately 60 per cent of patients with ascites have normal aldosterone levels at initial presentation. There is no doubt, however, that aldosterone plays a role in sodium balance, as it increases sodium retention in the distal tubules. The administration of high doses of spironolactone increases natriuresis in patients with cirrhosis and ascites, despite apparently normal plasma aldosterone levels. This has given rise to the concept that renal sensitivity to aldosterone may be enhanced in cirrhosis. Other factors known to be involved in sodium homeostasis include the sympathetic nervous system, which is activated in decompensated liver disease and which enhances sodium reabsorption along the proximal tubules. A third important factor is the rate of sodium delivery to the tubules. Renal blood flow is decreased in cirrhosis, and decreases further with decompensation. During decreased sodium delivery, sodium reabsorption is enhanced. Other factors such as atrial natriuretic peptide, endothelin-1, or urodilatin may be involved, but their role is as yet undefined.

The underlying cause of the activation of sodium-retaining pathways is still disputed, but data are available to support both the underfill and overfill hypotheses. There is no doubt that at different stages of disease development the same patient may exhibit signs of both an expanded and a contracted central blood volume. A unifying hypothesis, known as the 'vasodilatation hypothesis', was put forward to explain the observations regarding the development of salt-retaining states (Fig. 1). In this, the central stimulus for activation of neurohumoral pathways is a decrease in the central blood volume, which differs in severity depending on the intensity of liver disease. Whilst superficially attractive, this hypothesis fails to explain why many patients develop salt retention in the presence of normal aldosterone concentrations, and why systemic vasodilatation is only observed in the supine state.

Clinical features

Ascites is graded 1 to 3 depending on its severity. Grade 1 ascites is mild, and only detectable by ultrasound examination. Grade 2 ascites is moderate, and is manifest by moderate symmetrical distension of the abdomen; whereas grade 3 ascites is large or gross, with marked abdominal distension. A grade 2 ascites is most easily detected by a shifting dullness. Grade 3 ascites is usually tense and easily detected by the presence of a fluid thrill on

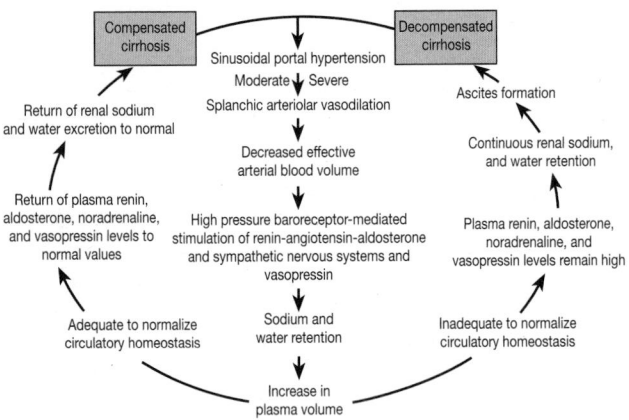

Fig. 1 Outline of peripheral vasodilation hypothesis (Schrier *et al.* (1988). Peripheral arterial vasodilation hypothesis: a proposal for the initiation of renal sodium and water retention in cirrhosis. *Hepatology* **8**, 1151–7).

palpation. There is often divarification of the rectus abdomini muscles, and prominent veins may be evident on the abdominal wall (see Fig. 2). Paraumbilical hernias develop in about 20 per cent of patients with ascites, an incidence that increases to up to 70 per cent in those with long-standing recurrent tense ascites. The main risks are rupture and strangulation. Pleural effusions (hepatic hydrothorax) develop in about 5 per cent of patients with cirrhosis. Hepatic hydrothorax may develop in patients with no discernible ascites. The pleural effusions are right-sided in 85 per cent of cases, left-sided in 13 per cent and bilateral in 2 per cent of cases.

Laboratory diagnosis

The cause of ascites or its precipitation is often self-evident. Where there are no obvious clues to its aetiology, tests must be directed at diagnosing both the presumed cause of liver disease and/or at excluding other causes of ascites such as malignancy or tuberculosis, etc. Other causes of abdominal distension such as huge masses, Meigs' syndrome, or pregnancy should be considered. The essential investigations on admission of a patient to hospital include:

* *Serum urea and electrolyte concentrations*—patients with ascites due to cirrhosis are prone to hyponatraemia or renal impairment, either spontaneously or following diuretic therapy.

* *Ascitic aspiration* with microscopy, determination of albumin or protein content, culture, cytology, and amylase measurement should be performed to confirm or exclude spontaneous bacterial peritonitis,

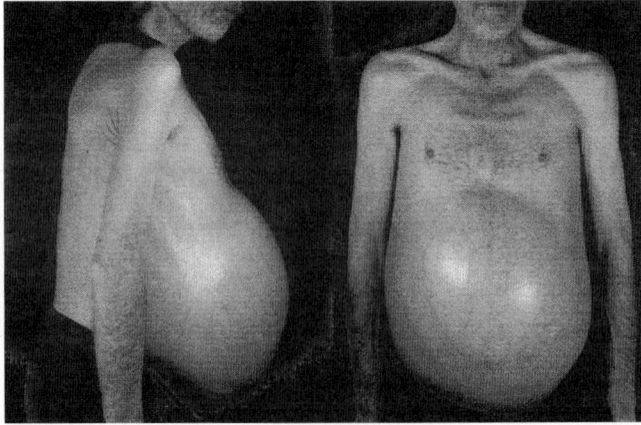

Fig. 2 Alcoholic cirrhosis with ascites is often associated with marked anorexia.

tuberculosis, malignancy, or pancreatic disease. A Gram stain is usually uninformative.

* *Ultrasound scans* are needed to evaluate liver appearance (nodular and cirrhotic) or congested (for example, congestive cardiac failure (CCF)), as well as blood flow in the portal vein (to exclude the portal vein thrombosis that occurs in 8 per cent of patients with cirrhosis, and which may precipitate hepatic decompensation), a semi-quantitation of the amount of ascites, and the presence of tumour in the liver or other masses.

Paracentesis

An ascitic tap is used for either diagnostic purposes or for the therapeutic removal of large volumes of ascites. The most common site for aspirating ascites is about 15 cm lateral to the umbilicus, with care being taken to avoid an enlarged liver or spleen. The epigastric arteries run just lateral to the umbilicus towards the mid-inguinal point and should also be avoided.

For diagnostic purposes, between 20 and 50 ml of ascitic fluid should be withdrawn, and 3 to 5 ml placed under aseptic conditions (i.e. the needle changed) into each of two blood culture bottles (tuberculin cultures have to be requested specifically). Fluid for culture should **not** be sent in plastic containers for culture—when a sample of infected ascites is placed into such containers the culture positivity is only 40 per cent, whereas it is more than 90 per cent positive when inoculated into blood culture bottles. A 5-ml aliquot of fluid should be sent in a plastic container to the microbiology department for a polymorphonuclear neutrophil (PMN) or lymphocyte count. The microbiologist should report a neutrophil count (e.g. < 250 PMNs/mm³) together with a limited differential (i.e. PMN or lymphocytes). Ascitic fluid occasionally clots, in which case a sample should be placed in a tube containing EDTA (ethylenediaminetetraacetic acid). Coulter-counter estimations of ascitic neutrophil numbers are probably unreliable at the lower end of a pathologically increased white blood cell count. A 5-ml aliquot should be sent for measurement of ascitic protein content or, ideally, ascitic albumin. Ascitic cytology should involve liaison with the cytopathologist. Cytology requires 20 to 50 ml of ascitic fluid. There is little diagnostic value in an analysis of ascitic fluid pH or of lactate or glucose concentrations.

Ascitic fluid investigations

Ascitic protein
The use of ascitic protein in the differential diagnosis of the causes of ascites is much over-rated, and misinterpreted. Conventionally, the type of ascites is divided into exudates and transudates: ascitic protein concentration over 25 g/l or under 25 g/l, respectively. The purpose of this subdivision is to narrow the differential diagnosis of the causes of ascites. However, many physicians assume that cardiac ascites will have a low level of ascitic protein, when this is rarely the case, and that patients with tuberculous peritonitis have a high ascitic protein content, when in fact it is low in 30 per cent of patients. Moreover, about 15 per cent of cases of cirrhotic ascites have an ascitic protein level of more than 25 g/l, while 20 per cent of patients with a malignancy have a low ascitic protein level. The causes of transudative and exudative ascites are given in Table 2. For those patients with cirrhosis, a very low ascitic protein level (< 10 g/l) is associated with an increased risk of spontaneous bacterial peritonitis (**SBP**) at the time of hospital admission. SBP is present in about 15 per cent of all patients admitted with cirrhotic ascites. The use of ascitic protein estimations to subdivide patients into exudative or transudative causes of ascites is considerably enhanced by measuring the difference between ascitic and serum albumin levels (see below).

Serum-ascites albumin gradient
Several studies have compared the value of ascitic protein with serum-ascitic albumin gradient measurements in patients with ascites resulting from cirrhosis and other causes. In one study comprising 44 patients, it was

Table 2 Subdivision into exudative and transudative ascites

Exudative ascites (protein >25 g/l)	Transudative ascites (protein <25 g/l)
Malignancy (80%)	Cirrhosis (85%)
Tuberculosis (70%)	Malignancy (20%)
Congestive cardiac failure	Protein-losing enteropathy
Cirrhosis (15% of cases)	Tuberculosis (30%)
Pancreatitis	
Budd–Chiari syndrome	
Myxoedema	
Constrictive pericarditis	
Nephrotic syndrome	

reported that 5/29 (17 per cent) patients with cirrhotic ascites had an ascitic protein level above 25 g/l, whereas 3/15 (20 per cent) with malignant ascites had an ascitic protein level below 25 g/l. In contrast, the overlap in each group was reduced to 1/29 and 1/15 respectively when a serum-ascitic albumin gradient above 11 g/l was used. Based on the many inaccurate predictions of aetiology based on the measurement of ascitic protein, it is clearly preferable to measure the serum-ascitic albumin gradient in patients presenting with ascites. This method, which involves subtraction of the ascitic albumin concentration from that observed in ascites, very accurately divides patients into two groups: those with a high gradient (>11 g/l) and those with a low gradient (< 11 g/l). The overall accuracy of this method is 97 per cent. (Table 3)

Ascitic amylase

The ascitic fluid amylase level should always be measured in patients with an exudative or unexplained ascites. A very high value is obtained when ascitic fluid results from a pancreatic pseudocyst or mass.

Ascitic fluid microscopy

An ascitic neutrophil count of more than 250 PMNs/mm³ is diagnostic of spontaneous bacterial peritonitis. An elevated lymphocyte count should raise the possibility of tuberculous peritonitis. Excess red blood cells are most commonly due to a traumatic tap, but should raise the possibility of malignancy.

Ascitic fluid culture

Classically, aspirated fluid is placed in a sterile container and sent to the microbiology department for microscopy and culture. For infected fluid handled in this way, a positive culture will be obtained in only about 40 per cent of samples. However, if ascitic fluid is treated in the same way as blood cultures, and fluid inoculated directly into blood culture bottles at the bedside, the positive culture rate increases to 92 per cent (see above). A single study has evaluated the effectiveness of cytospin with cell lysis to improve the efficacy of culturing ascitic fluid, and again found that direct inoculation of ascitic fluid into blood culture bottles was far superior (79 per cent positivity) compared with the cell-lysis method (46 per cent culture-positive).

Table 3 Subdivision of patients into high and low ascitic albumin gradient

Serum-ascites albumin gradient <11 g/l (Low gradient)	Serum-ascites albumin gradient >11 g/l (High gradient)
Malignancy	Cirrhosis
Tuberculosis	Cardiac failure
Pancreatic	Budd–Chiari syndrome
Biliary	Myxoedema
Nephrotic syndrome	
Connective tissue disease	

Ascitic fluid cytology

Ascitic cytology should involve liaison with the cytopathologist so that the index of suspicion and type of potential tumour are discussed. A 20- to 50-ml sample of ascitic fluid is required to produce a cell concentrate for cytology—obtained by centrifuging the ascites fluid, removing supernatant, and resuspending the cells. A sample of the concentrate then undergoes a cytospin to deposit cells on to microscope slides, following which the cells are stained. Typical stains include the Papanicolaou and May-Grunwald–Giemsa stain.

Ascitic volume

Ascitic volume is not usually determined in clinical practice. It can, however, be quantified radiologically or by indicator-dilution. As a rough guide, patients with barely detectable ascites usually harbour between 1 and 4 litres, those with moderate ascites 4 to 8 litres, and those with marked ascites more than 8 litres of fluid. Ultrasonographic determination of ascitic volume involves measurement of the abdominal circumference and the deepest vertical depth of the fluid, and modelled as a segment of a sphere. Isotopic determination of ascitic volume involves the injection of radiolabelled ⁹⁹Tc- macroalbumin.

Treatment

Patients with ascites can be divided into those that are easy to treat and those that are difficult. In general, patients with their first presentation of ascites and normal renal function, who have a spot urine sodium concentration of more than 20 mmol/l, or an identifiable source of dietary sodium excess, respond well to simple measures. Likewise, when ascites has developed as a consequence of bleeding or infection, it usually resolves more readily. The treatment of ascites is summarized in Table 4.

Bed rest

Bed rest is probably of no benefit in patients with a preserved renal function, as indicated by a serum creatinine concentration of less than 125 μmol/l and a good initial response to diuretics. However, there is data to suggest that it may be beneficial in those with a poor response to diuretics, but further studies are required.

Dietary salt restriction

There is a general consensus that dietary salt restriction is important in the management of patients with cirrhosis and ascites. However, it is important to maintain an adequate level of nutrition in patients with cirrhosis. Therefore it is generally agreed that sodium intake should be restricted to less than 90 mmol/day, which in effect amounts to a 'no added salt' diet with avoidance of preprepared meals. It is also generally agreed that salt restriction should be an adjunct to diuretic therapy, and that it is rarely effective alone.

Table 4 Summary of treatment of ascites

- Bed rest is of little value
- Sodium restriction to 90 mmol/day
- Water restriction should only be used in severely hyponatraemic patients with caution
- Diuretic therapy should employ spironolactone as the first-line drug
- Total paracentesis should initially be carried out on patients with moderate or marked ascites
- Shunts may be used in those with refractory ascites in whom recurrent paracentesis is too frequent or poorly tolerated, or in those with a hepatic hydrothorax

Role of water restriction

There are no studies evaluating the role of water restriction on the resolution of ascites. In many studies from the United States and Europe, it has been customary to restrict water intake to between 1 and 1.5 litres/day, a recommendation that has appeared in many major texts for the last 20 to 30 years. It would appear that this treatment has simply crept into current dogma, with no clinical or scientific basis to support this treatment. It is well known that water follows salt, and thus fluid loss will occur with salt restriction or adequate diuresis. In a study of 55 patients with ascites, none of whom had taken any diuretics for 2 weeks, 21 had spontaneous hyponatraemia and 34 were normonatraemic. In all patients with normonatraemia, the free-water clearance was normal. Of those with hyponatraemia, 13 had a marked reduction in free-water clearance and glomerular filtration rate. The remaining 8 hyponatraemic patients had a relatively normal free-water clearance. The patients with hyponatraemia and poor renal function did not respond to diuretic therapy, and had a poor prognosis: 60 per cent inpatient mortality compared with 15 per cent in the remaining patients. Hyponatraemia is caused by excessive water retention, primarily as a result of increased circulating vasopressin levels. Since the hyponatraemia is due to water excess, patients with significant hyponatraemia are usually subject to a water restriction of less than 500 ml/day. The response, however, is slow, and many regard this approach as being relatively ineffective. It is sometimes more prudent to try and improve renal function with volume expansion, in the first instance with colloid.

Thus, patients with ascites who are normonatraemic or mild/moderately hyponatraemic (serum sodium concentration above 125 mmol/l) should not be water-restricted. Water restriction should be reserved for those with severe hyponatraemia in whom the free-water clearance is decreased, after ensuring that their intravascular volume is adequate.

Diuretics

Since they first became available, diuretics have been the mainstay of the treatment of ascites. Diuretic dosage should be increased stepwise if there is an insufficient diuretic response, as defined by a weight loss of less than 1 kg in the first 7 days and/or 2 kg every 7 days thereafter, until the ascites is adequately controlled. The safe upper limit of the rate of weight loss is contentious. However, most experts agree that, in clinical practice, the diuretic dose should be adjusted to achieve a rate of weight loss below an average of 500 g per day in patients without peripheral oedema or 1 kg per day in those with peripheral oedema. Best practice is to add a loop diuretic (furosemide (frusemide) 40 mg/day) once a patient fails to respond to the equivalent of 200 mg spironolactone per day. Many diuretic agents have been evaluated over the years, but in the United Kingdom and Europe this has been mainly confined to spironolactone, amiloride, furosemide (frusemide), and bumetanide.

Diuretic agents

Spironolactone

Spironolactone is an aldosterone antagonist, acting mainly on the distal tubules to increase natriuresis and conserve potassium. In a controlled study comparing the efficacy of spironolactone in 40 non-azotaemic patients with ascites who were excreting less than 12 mmol of sodium/day, 18 of 19 patients responded to spironolactone alone, whereas only 11 of 21 patients responded to furosemide (frusemide) alone. Most patients responding to spironolactone required 150 mg/day, and a few required 300 mg/day. In all cases diuresis occurred by the third day. For those given furosemide, most responders required 80 mg/day, but a few required 160 mg/day. Furosemide was associated with a decrease in the serum potassium concentration, which necessitated potassium supplementation. In those given spironolactone, serum potassium concentrations increased appreciably. The side-effects of spironolactone include gynaecomastia, hyponatraemia, hyperkalaemia, impotence, menstrual disturbance (although most ascitic patients are amenorrhoeic), and osteomalacia.

Amiloride

Amiloride was first used in 1968, and, combined with either furosemide (frusemide) or ethacrynic acid, resulted in a satisfactory diuresis in most cirrhotic subjects with ascites. In a larger study, Yamada and Reynolds evaluated the efficacy of amiloride in patients with cirrhosis and ascites resistant to bed rest and a very low salt diet (<20 mmol Na/day). When used alone it induced a satisfactory response in 80 per cent of patients at doses of 15 to 30 mg/day.

Furosemide (frusemide)

Furosemide is a loop diuretic that causes a marked natriuresis and diuresis in normal subjects. Its efficacy compared with spironolactone is discussed above. In normal subjects it has a half-life of about 75 min, increasing to about 130 min in patients with cirrhosis. It is generally used as an adjunct to spironolactone treatment and has poor efficacy when used alone in cirrhosis. This is probably because there is salt retention in the distal tubules in the subset of patients with high plasma aldosterone concentrations. Furosemide should be used in a dose not exceeding 160 mg/day; its use is associated with severe electrolyte disturbance, and therefore should be prescribed cautiously.

Complications and benefits of diuretic therapy

Diuretic therapy generally improves morbidity and well being, since it causes resolution of ascites, allows a more liberal diet, decreases portal pressure, and increases the opsonic activity of ascitic fluid thereby decreasing the risk of spontaneous bacterial peritonitis. However, diuretic use is associated with complications in between 10 and 70 per cent of patients. The high incidence of side-effects from diuretics seen earlier is now becoming less common. The main complications of diuretic therapy are shown in Table 5.

Therapeutic paracentesis

Paracentesis has been in use for at least 2000 years, and was widely used in the earlier part of the last century. When diuretics first became available in the 1940s the practice declined but it was still used as an adjunct to therapy until the early 1960s. It gradually fell into disrepute with the recognition that repeated paracentesis resulted in salt depletion and oliguria, and became virtually banned as a treatment. The use of paracentesis re-emerged in the mid-1980s when several controlled clinical studies demonstrated that paracentesis with colloid replacement was safe and associated with fewer complications than diuretic therapy. In a large controlled study, patients with tense ascites were randomized to receive either paracentesis with intravenous albumin (40 g after each paracentesis) or diuretics (spironolactone 200–400 mg/day plus furosemide (frusemide) (40–240 mg/day). Patients with significant renal impairment (serum creatinine concentration > 250 μmol/l) were excluded. Paracentesis (4–6 litres/day) was effective in all patients, and no significant change in electrolytes or renal function was observed. Diuretics were effective in 28 out of 34 patients. There was, however, a significant increase and decrease in serum creatinine and sodium levels, respectively, in the diuretic-treated group, and the duration of inpatient treatment was considerably longer. Total paracentesis does, however, ensure a decrease in blood pressure (Fig. 3) by 7 to 10 mmHg. This research was followed by many other studies evaluating the speed of paracentesis, the haemodynamic changes following paracentesis, and the need for colloid replacement therapy.

Table 5 Complications of diuretics in the management of ascites

- Hyponatraemia (50%)
- Hyperkalaemia (spironolactone) or hypokalaemia (loop diuretics)
- Hepatic encephalopathy (secondary to electrolyte disturbance)
- Hyperuricaemia (30%)
- Renal impairment
- Gynaecomastia, osteomalacia, and mild metabolic acidosis with spironolactone

Practical aspects of therapeutic paracentesis

The most important feature of a paracentesis cannula is that it should have multiple side perforations to avoid obstruction by omentum. All ascitic fluid should be drained in a single session as rapidly as possible over 1 to 4 h. If 25 litres of ascites can be drained within 2 to 4 h it is quite safe to do so. The old dogma that rapid paracentesis causes marked hypotension is false, and the haemodynamic changes that occur do so after the removal of as little as 1 litre of ascites. There is a rapid increase in cardiac output, and a corresponding decrease in systemic vascular resistance that peaks at 3 h. There is an immediate fall in right atrial pressure (within 30 min), due to a decrease in intra-abdominal pressure and a decrease in compression of the right atrium. Pulmonary capillary wedge pressure remains constant for 6 h (in the absence of colloid), and decreases after this interval in the absence of colloid replacement. Mean arterial pressure decreases by about 8 mmHg. These changes are shown in Fig. 3. The drainage system should never be left in place overnight since this carries a risk of infection.

Colloid replacement

It is very important that colloid replacement is given following paracentesis to prevent circulatory disturbances. After total paracentesis, synthetic plasma substitutes may be used if the volume of ascites removed is less than 5 litres. However, albumin should be used when more than 5 litres is removed. All or most trials have used albumin at a dose of 8 g/l of ascites removed. There are no data on whether smaller or larger amounts of albumin have differing degrees of efficacy. Based on studies of the haemodynamic changes that follow paracentesis, it is clear that colloid should be given after paracentesis has been completed.

Contraindications to paracentesis

It is generally agreed that there are no contraindications to paracentesis, although studies to date have excluded several subsets of patients, primarily because of inadequate data. In practice, some clinicians have concerns about carrying out paracentesis in patients who have a severe coagulopathy or marked thrombocytopenia in case localized bleeding complications arise, but there are no data to support this view.

Benefits of paracentesis

Paracentesis provides immediate relief from ascites and a tense abdomen. There is a suspicion that paracentesis makes patients more responsive to diuretic therapy. Whilst there is no direct evidence to support this, the observation that plasma arginine vasopressin (AVP) levels are proportional to intra-abdominal pressure lends credibility to this idea. Despite the assumption that during paracentesis the observed exacerbation of vasodilatation involves the splanchnic bed, studies have shown that paracentesis causes a significant reduction of portal pressure. A further benefit includes the relief on respiratory muscles. Tense ascites clearly restricts breathing, and increases both the workload of respiration and energy expenditure. Paracentesis provides immediate relief. Likewise, patients who present with fluid overload and ascites can be rapidly relieved by paracentesis. Ascites increases the resting energy expenditure, and this may be improved following paracentesis. One potential beneficial effect of paracentesis may be to enhance salt and water excretion, due to the acute reductions of renal venous pressure and the increase in renal perfusion that follow. A second and unexpected benefit may relate to water metabolism. Studies by Solis-Herruzo have shown that paracentesis is followed by an acute fall in plasma arginine vasopressin levels—this hormone is implicated in water homeostasis, since it directly affects the water permeability of the collecting tubules and ducts. This acute decrease in plasma concentrations is directly related to intrathoracic or intra-abdominal pressure, since inflation of the abdomen with air to form a pneumoperitoneum, which increases intrathoracic and intra-abdominal pressure, had a similar effect.

Role of albumin infusion

There is a persistent belief that the infusion of albumin is beneficial to patients with cirrhosis. The role of albumin infusion has already been mentioned in the section relating to paracentesis, and it also has a role in the treatment of SBP. The identification of new hepatitis viruses, HIV, and the advent of new-variant Creutzfeldt–Jakob disease should make all clinicians cautious in the administration of human products. During the 1940s, several studies evaluated the effect of fractionated human albumin solution in patients with cirrhosis. These studies demonstrated that the infusion of albumin could correct the low plasma levels observed and result in a modest diuresis in some patients, but overall the results were disappointing.

Role of angiotensin-converting enzyme (ACE) inhibitors

The therapeutic effect of ACE inhibitors is attractive since they directly target the system involved most intimately with salt and water retention. However, the acute administration of either captopril or enalapril may cause an acute fall in blood pressure. Some studies have suggested that in patients with ascites, the chronic administration of enalapril suppressed plasma aldosterone levels and increased urinary sodium excretion and glomerular filtration rate (GFR), as well as increasing urinary prostaglandin (PG) E_2 and 6-oxo-PGF$_{1\alpha}$. More studies on the efficacy of these drugs and of angiotensin antagonists on portal pressure and the treatment of ascites are expected. Recent studies have suggested that low doses of ACE inhibitors may enhance salt excretion, but they should be used very carefully.

Treatment of patients with severe liver dysfunction and ascites

Patients with endstage liver disease often have subclinical renal impairment, with a typical GFR of around 60 ml/min. For patients with alcoholic liver disease with or without alcoholic hepatitis, the presence of ascites does not generally affect the clinical outcome, unless the ascites becomes a focus for infection. Up to 90 per cent of patients dying from alcoholic hepatitis develop renal failure. For those with alcoholic hepatitis that resolves spontaneously or with treatment, the ascites usually improves as salt and water excretion increase with improvement of the liver disease. Most patients

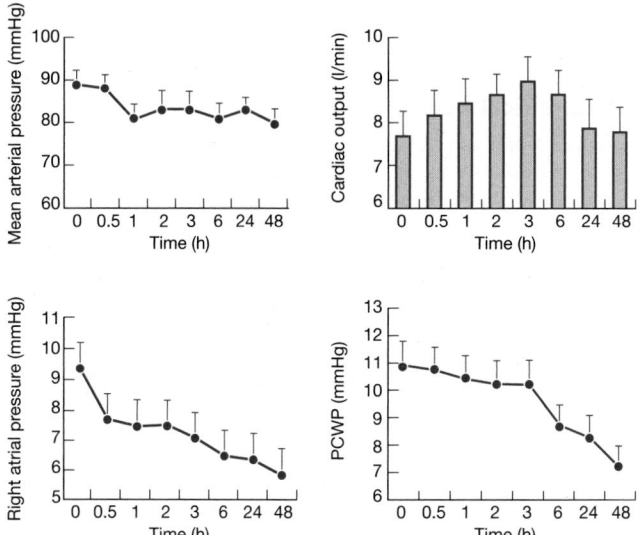

Fig. 3 Haemodynamic changes following acute total paracentesis of approximately 10 litres of ascites over 1 h. Paracentesis was commenced at time 0 h and sequential changes were monitored by a Swan–Ganz catheter, without albumin replacement (modified from Panos *et al.* 1990).

with severe liver failure have been excluded from clinical studies assessing the efficacy of diuretics or paracentesis. It is recommended that extreme caution is exerted when trying to diurese patients with endstage liver disease. It is probably safer to paracentese such patients rather than give potentially nephrotoxic drugs, although few studies have been conducted in such patients.

Treatment of refractory ascites

Diuretics may be ineffective for a variety of reasons. Approximately 5 to 10 per cent of patients do not respond adequately to diuretics. This may be because the diuretics induce an electrolyte disturbance or encephalopathy, necessitating a temporary and recurrent withdrawal of medication. Alternatively, the patient may be genuinely resistant to the diuretics given. In both these groups, there is invariably significant renal dysfunction when assessed by creatinine clearance or other techniques measuring GFR. Because of confusion over the random use of the term 'refractory ascites' in the literature, in 1994 the International Ascites Club agreed the following definition: 'refractory ascites is defined as ascites that cannot be mobilized or the early recurrence of which cannot be satisfactorily prevented by medical therapy'. It is subdivided into diuretic-resistant ascites and diuretic-intractable ascites (see below); however, it should be noted that the amount of sodium restriction used in the following definitions is now below the recommended sodium restriction:

- *Diuretic-resistant ascites* is defined as an ascites that cannot be mobilized or prevented postparacentesis because of the lack of a response to dietary sodium restriction (<50 mmol/day) and maximal diuretic therapy. Maximal diuretic therapy is defined as spironolactone 400 mg/day together with furosemide (frusemide) 160 mg/day.
- *Diuretic-intractable ascites* is defined as an ascites that cannot be mobilized or prevented postparacentesis because of the development of diuretic-induced complications that preclude the use of an effective or maximal dose of diuretics.

The mainstay of treatment for these patients is repeated paracentesis.

Shunts

Transjugular intrahepatic portosystemic shunts (TIPS) for refractory ascites

Several studies have suggested that TIPS may improve natriuresis in patients with diuretic-resistant ascites. In one study, 50 patients with refractory ascites were treated by TIPS, sufficient to decrease the portal pressure gradient by over 60 per cent. Some 75 per cent of all patients showed complete resolution of their ascites by 3 months, and 20 per cent achieved a partial response. A new onset of hepatic encephalopathy occurred in a further 10 per cent of patients. Other studies, however, have reported a 45 per cent incidence of hepatic encephalopathy post-TIPS, which was severe and disabling in 15 per cent of all treated patients, and this has been confirmed. TIPS was also associated with a decrease in the mean serum creatinine concentration from 133 μmol/l to 80 μmol/l at 6 months. The mean 1-year survival post-TIPS is less than 50 per cent. The effect of TIPS on sodium excretion and renal function is, for some reason, delayed, not being apparent until about 1-month postinsertion. Insertion of a TIPS is associated with a deterioration of liver function, and some patients develop severe haemolysis.

Peritoneovenous shunts (Le Veen shunts or Denver shunts)

Peritoneovenous shunting became very popular in the 1970s, with numerous publications on its benefits to renal function and resolution of ascites. However, it soon became apparent that many shunts became blocked or infected and caused scarring of the peritoneum, which can make liver transplantation difficult. There have been three clinical trials evaluating the efficacy of the peritoneovenous shunt. This technique offers no survival advantage over medical therapy or repeated paracenteses. With respect to

Table 6 Complications of ascites

- Pleural effusion
- Paraumbilical hernia
- Hepatorenal syndrome
- Respiratory difficulties
- Hypercatabolic state
- Spontaneous bacterial peritonitis

its effects on renal function, it has been shown that shunting had no overall effect on mortality in patients with the hepatorenal syndrome.

Prognosis

The occurrence of ascites in patients with cirrhosis is associated with a poor prognosis. Survival rates vary between 50 per cent at 1 to 2 years, but a somewhat better survival in alcoholic patients with ascites who stop drinking. The development of bacterial peritonitis in patients with ascites is associated with a mortality of 75 per cent at 1 year. Thus, the development of this complication is associated with an overall poor prognosis, and, unless contraindicated, all patients should be considered for orthotopic liver transplantation.

Important complications

The complications of ascites are shown in Table 6 and discussed below.

Pleural effusion

Pleural effusions (hepatic hydrothorax) develop in about 5 per cent of patients with cirrhosis. Fluid tracks up into the pleural cavity via defects in the diaphragm (for example, holes or blebs), which occasionally close spontaneously. Hepatic hydrothorax may develop in patients with no discernible ascites. The pleural effusions are right-sided in 85 per cent of cases and bilateral in 2 per cent of cases. To confirm the diagnosis, if doubt exists, a radiotracer should be injected under aseptic conditions into the abdomen and its appearance followed in the pleural fluid. A pleural effusion should be managed as for conventional ascites unless it is unresponsive and causing severe dyspnoea, in which case a TIPS (transjugular intrahepatic portosystemic shunt) should be inserted. TIPS is a highly effective treatment for hepatic hydrothorax.

Paraumbilical hernia

Paraumbilical hernias develop in about 20 per cent of patients with ascites, an incidence that increases up to 70 per cent in those with long-standing recurrent tense ascites. The main risks are rupture and strangulation.

Hepatorenal syndrome

Hepatorenal syndrome is the development of renal failure in patients with advanced liver disease (acute or chronic) in the absence of any pathological cause of renal failure. It is due to a reduction of renal blood flow, an increased renal sympathetic drive, and increased circulating or increased renal production of various vasoactive mediators such as endothelin-1, cysteinyl-leukotrienes, thromboxane A_2, or F(2)-isoprostanes. This syndrome is discussed in detail elsewhere.

Hypercatabolic state

Many patients with ascites present in a hypercatabolic state. This may be secondary to the low-grade endotoxaemia present in many patients, together with their general state of malnutrition. This can be reversed, particularly in alcoholic patients who stop drinking and improve their nutritional lifestyle. However, successful TIPS can also improve the nutritional status of these patients, although this may of course be secondary to their cessation of alcohol intake.

Respiratory difficulties

Increasing abdominal distension due to the accumulation of peritoneal fluid increases the effort required for breathing. Occasionally, this may precipitate extreme difficulty in breathing and should be treated by rapid paracentesis.

Spontaneous bacterial peritonitis (SBP)

The spectrum of bacterial peritonitis includes spontaneous bacterial peritonitis, monomicrobial bacterascites, culture-negative neutroascites, and secondary bacterial peritonitis. Spontaneous bacterial peritonitis is now defined as the combination of a positive ascitic fluid culture, an ascitic fluid neutrophil count of more than 250 cells/mm³, and no evident intra-abdominal source of infection. Secondary bacterial peritonitis is identical, except that an intra-abdominal source is apparent and the organisms are frequently polymicrobial.

The risk of SBP has been evaluated. Of patients presenting with ascites, about 11 per cent will develop SBP within 1 year and 15 per cent within 3 years. For those with an ascitic protein level below 10 g/l the risk is 24 per cent within 3 years. For patients admitted to hospital with ascites with or without other complications (for example, bleeding) the incidence of SBP on admission, based on a review of several reports, is about 10 per cent.

The symptoms of SBP are shown in Table 7.

The pathogenesis of bacterial peritonitis is shown below in Fig. 4. It is apparent that a source for bacteraemia gives rise to organisms in the hepatic lymph and thence the ascitic fluid. Before an inflammatory reaction occurs, an ascitic tap will yield a positive culture, but a low neutrophil count. This is termed 'monomicrobial bacterascites'. If there is a polymicrobial growth with a low ascitic neutrophil count, then the tap is likely to have been traumatic. This occurs in 0.6 per cent of all ascitic taps. In the absence of any intervention it is estimated that two-thirds of these cases will resolve as a consequence of complement-mediated bacterial lysis: that is to say, it will not develop into SBP but will be resolved by the normal antimicrobial defences of the body. If the organisms multiply and neutrophils are mobilized, the ascitic neutrophil count increases. An ascitic tap at this stage yields a positive culture and an elevated white blood cell count. If the infection resolves at this stage (that is, the organisms are lysed) and an ascitic tap is then performed, the ascitic neutrophil count will be increased but the ascitic fluid will be sterile. This is termed 'culture-negative neutrocytic ascites' (**CNNA**). The most common cause is, however, a poor culture technique. As shown, the opsonic activity is important in determining whether the monomicrobial bacterascites resolves or develops into SBP. The organisms isolated are shown in Table 8, and the risk factors for the development of SBP are summarized in Table 9 and discussed below.

Risk factors

Decreased opsonic activity

The protein concentration of ascitic fluid does not change with the advent of SBP. Patients with a low protein content have an increased risk of developing SBP, compared to those with a high ascitic protein content. Patients with cirrhotic and nephrotic ascites are prone to infection, whereas those with malignant ascites or cardiac ascites are not. The risk of SBP is

Table 7 Symptoms of spontaneous bacterial peritonitis

• Asymptomatic	25%
• Abdominal pain	60%
• Abdominal tenderness	10%
• Fever	50%
• Encephalopathy	10%
• Shock	<5%

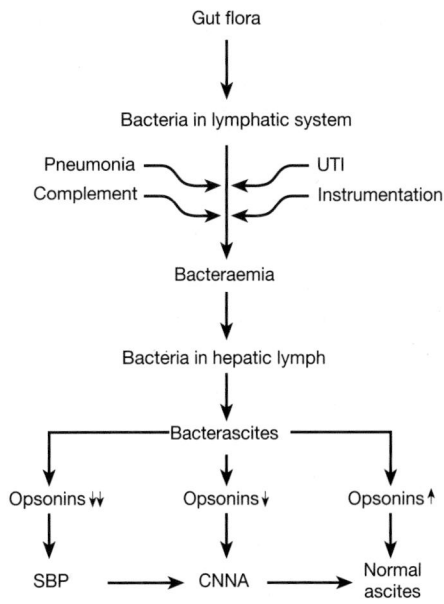

Fig. 4 Pathogenesis of spontaneous bacterial peritonitis. Bacteria can enter ascites through the lymphatic system. In many cases this is resolved through complement mediated bacterial lysis. When opsonins are decreased (e.g. low ascitic protein) or host defence is poor, bacteria multiply and cause spontaneous bacterial peritonitis (SBP). CNNA = culture negative neutrocytic ascites.

Table 8 Organisms causing spontaneous bacterial peritonitis

The gut and urine are the most frequent source of organisms
Enteric organisms (75%)
    Enterobacteria (mainly *E. coli* (60%))
    Other Gram-negative bacilli, e.g. *Klebsiella* spp. (8%)
    Enterococcus faecalis (6%)
    Anaerobes (1–5%)

Non-enteric organisms (25%)
    Gram-positive cocci
        Streptococcus pneumoniae (12%)
        Other *Streptococcus* spp. (7%)
        Staphylococcus spp. (4%)
        Others (2%)

Table 9 Risk factors for spontaneous bacterial peritonitis (SBP)

- Instrumentation procedures (endoscopy, sigmoidoscopy, balloon tamponade)
- Gastrointestinal haemorrhage
- Bacterial infections (e.g. chest, urinary tract infections, bacteraemia)
- Previous episodes of SBP
- Decreased opsonic activity
    Low ascitic protein (<10 g/l)
    Low ascitic C3 concentration
    Complement deficiency

increased sixfold for those with an ascitic protein of less than 10 g/l. When bacteria enter ascitic fluid they may be lysed by the activity of complement if they are serum-sensitive, or they may be coated with opsonins such as IgG or the third component of the complement pathway (C3). Complement deficiency also predisposes to infection. The opsonic activity of ascitic fluid correlates with the total protein, as well as that of CH100 (total haemolytic complement), C3, and C4 concentration. These concentrations may be increased by diuresis, thus decreasing the risk of SBP. Paradoxically, diuretics may also increase the neutrophil count in ascitic fluid.

Recent instrumentation

Recent instrumentation such as endoscopy or sigmoidoscopy increases the risk of SBP. However, the risk of developing SBP is not increased by paracentesis. A study compared the risk of SBP in two groups of patients and found that it was slightly less, if anything, in those treated with paracentesis than in those treated with diuretics.

Gastrointestinal haemorrhage

There is a 21 per cent incidence of SBP in patients admitted to hospital with a gastrointestinal haemorrhage. Whilst it is assumed that bleeding predisposes to infection, there is data to suggest that infection may predispose to bleeding. Since the incidence of SBP immediately following a gastrointestinal bleed is high, many clinicians now advocate the prophylactic use of broad-spectrum antibiotics in such situations.

Previous spontaneous bacterial peritonitis

SBP is a recurrent condition. The recurrence rate for SBP is 47 per cent at 6 months and 69 per cent at 1 year.

Treatment of SBP

The mortality associated with SBP is approximately 30 per cent in most series. Therefore, SBP must be treated as soon as a presumptive diagnosis is made following microscopy of ascitic fluid. For patients with bacterascites but no rise in the neutrophil count, the ascitic tap should be repeated, while those with an increased neutrophil count should be treated. The following therapeutic regimen is used in the United Kingdom, which is based on the types of organism most frequently encountered during SBP: treatment is continued until complete resolution of all signs of infection and the ascitic neutrophil count decreases to within the normal range. This is generally achieved within 1 week of treatment. Appropriate antibiotics include cefotaxime, ciprofloxacin with amoxicillin, and piperacillin with tazlocillin (PIP/TAZ). Recent studies from Barcelona have also shown that the administration of albumin at a dose of 1.5 g/kg at the time of diagnosis and 1 g/kg at 48 h decreases the incidence of renal dysfunction, and improves survival. The treatment of SBP is summarized in Table 10.

Prevention and control

The prevention and control of ascites have already been covered under the treatment of ascites. Currently there is an ongoing National Institutes of Health (**NIH**)-funded multicentre study evaluating the efficacy of β-blockade on the development of portal hypertension, but the results of this are not yet available. However, there have been many studies investigating prophylaxis against SBP.

Table 10 Treatment of spontaneous bacterial peritonitis (SBP)

1.	Diagnosis of SBP on ascitic microscopy (>250 PMNs/mm³)
2.	Commence third-generation cephalosporin or ciprofloxacin with amoxicillin
3.	Infuse albumin at 1.5 g/kg at diagnosis and 1g/kg at 48 h
4.	Treat until resolution (~1 week, mortality up to 30%)
5.	Commence prophylaxis against future SBP
6.	Consider liver transplantation as 1-year mortality is 75%

Prophylaxis against SBP

Many clinicians in the United Kingdom now use ciprofloxacin. A French study has evaluated the efficacy of this antibiotic in patients with cirrhosis who have an ascitic protein level below 15 g/l. This study observed that the administration of 750 mg ciprofloxacin given in a single dose per week decreased the incidence of SBP from 22 per cent to 4 per cent at 6 months, with a corresponding decrease in hospital admission over this period (18 days to 9 days). These authors concluded that prophylaxis with ciprofloxacin was effective, and cost-analysis studies have shown such antimicrobial prophylaxis to be cost-effective.

Special problems in pregnant women

Women with cirrhosis and ascites rarely, if ever, become pregnant, since ovulation has usually ceased before the onset of ascites.

Occupational, quality of life, and psychological aspects

Ascites is significant because it indicates the development of hepatic decompensation, and a corresponding poor prognosis. It also carries a significant morbidity—increasing the workload on the patient, causing backache, etc.—and may be associated with the development of electrolyte disturbance and hepatic encephalopathy. It has enormous cost implications to the National Health Service in terms of repeated hospital admissions, long-term treatment of salt and water retention, and iatrogenic complications. It may also be complicated by the development of spontaneous bacterial peritonitis, which is itself associated with gastrointestinal haemorrhage, and a high mortality.

Areas of controversy

Current areas of controversy include the use of albumin or plasma substitutes following paracentesis. Although albumin has been shown to be superior to plasma substitutes in preventing the activation of hormonal systems that indicate hypovolaemia, there is no hard data to show that albumin is more effective than colloid substitutes in terms of overall patient survival or duration of hospital stay. There is also controversy over the issue of central blood volume, with two groups reporting diametrically opposite findings. This is a crucial argument since the current peripheral vasodilatation hypothesis is based on the premise of a decreased central blood volume. Studies by Mauro Bernardi's group have shown that vasodilatation disappears during upright posture, and it appears that patients may exhibit features of both underfill and overfill depending on their posture and severity of liver disease.

Areas needing further research

Ideally, longitudinal studies conducted over many years need to be performed in newly diagnosed patients with cirrhosis, including baseline clinical, hormonal, and sodium-balance studies, as well as long-term (10 years or more) investigations of systemic haemodynamics and portal pressure. Why do patients develop vasodilatation? Although current ideas favour a role for nitric oxide, the evidence to support this is unclear. Why do patients develop ascites after liver transplantation? This complication is unusual but can be very striking and disruptive to management. Finally, controlled studies are needed to determine whether it is beneficial to para-centese patients with spontaneous bacterial peritonitis.

Further reading

Arroyo V, Ginés P (1992). Arteriolar vasodilatation and the pathogenesis of the hyperdynamic circulation and renal sodium and water retention in cirrhosis. *Gastroenterology* **102**, 1077–8. [This paper reviews the vasodilatation hypothesis of cirrhosis.]

Arroyo V, *et al.* (1976). Prognostic value in spontaneous hyponatremia in cirrhosis with ascites. *Digestive Diseases* **21**, 249–56. [This paper highlights the incidence and prognostic value of serum sodium or free-water clearance in cirrhosis with ascites.]

Bernard B, *et al.* (1995). Prognostic significance of bacterial infection in bleeding cirrhotic patients a prospective study. *Gastroenterology* **108**, 1828–34. [Many patients with variceal haemorrhage have an underlying bacterial infection.]

Bernardi M, *et al.* (1995). Hyperdynamic circulation of advanced cirrhosis: a re-appraisal based on posture-induced changes in haemodynamics. *Journal of Hepatology* **22**, 309–18. [Several papers from Bernardi's group have shown that the vasodilatation is only evident in patients when they are supine, and this affects the renal handling of sodium and glomerular filtration.]

Campra JL, Reynolds TB (1978). Effectiveness of high-dose spironolactone therapy in patients with chronic liver disease and relatively refractory ascites. *Digestive Diseases* **23**, 1025–30. [This paper highlights the use of spironolactone in the management of ascites.]

Dolz C, *et al.* (1991). Ascites increases the resting energy expenditure in liver cirrhosis. *Gastroenterology* **100**, 738–44. [This study demonstrates that patients with ascites have an increased energy expenditure rate which decreases with treatment of ascites.]

Henriksen JH, *et al.* (1989). Reduced central blood volume in cirrhosis. *Gastroenterology* **97**, 1506–13. [This paper demonstrates the reduction of central blood volume in cirrhosis.]

Inadomi J, Sonnenberg A (1997). Cost-analysis of prophylactic antibiotics in spontaneous bacterial peritonitis. *Gastroenterology* **113**, 1289–94. [It is cost-effective to give prophylactic antibiotics to prevent SBP in at-risk individuals.]

Luca A, *et al.* (1994). Favorable effects of total paracentesis on splanchnic haemodynamics in cirrhotic patients with tense ascites. *Hepatology* **20** (Part 1), 30–3. [This study shows that paracentesis is followed by a reduction of portal pressure.]

Nevens F, *et al.* (1996). The effect of long-term treatment with spironolactone on variceal pressure in patients with portal hypertension without ascites. *Hepatology* **23**, 1047–52. [This paper shows that treatment with spironolactone also lowers the portal pressure.]

Panos MZ, *et al.* (1990). Single, total paracentesis for tense ascites: sequential haemodynamic changes and right atrial size. *Hepatology* **11**, 662–7. [This study demonstrated the haemodynamic changes over 48 h following a single, total, large-volume paracentesis.]

Pare P, Talbot J, Hoefs JC (1983). Serum-ascites albumin concentration gradient: a physiologic approach to the differential diagnosis of ascites. *Gastroenterology* **85**, 245–53. [Several papers have shown that measurement of serum-ascites albumin gradient is far superior to measurement of ascitic protein in helping with the differential diagnosis of causes of ascites.]

Perez-Ayuso RM, *et al.* (1983). Randomized comparative study of efficacy of furosemide versus spironolactone in non-azotemic cirrhosis with ascites. *Gastroenterology* **84**, 961–8. [One of the few controlled trials on the use of diuretics in the management of ascites.]

Rolachon A, *et al.* (1995). Ciprofloxacin and long-term prevention of spontaneous bacterial peritonitis: results of a prospective controlled trial. *Hepatology* **22**, 1171–4. [One of several studies of antibiotic prophylaxis for SBP.]

Runyon BA (1986). Low-protein-concentration ascitic fluid is predisposed to spontaneous bacterial peritonitis. *Gastroenterology* **91**, 1343–6. [Low ascitic protein concentration is a risk factor for the development of SBP.]

Runyon BA (1997). Treatment of patients with cirrhosis and ascites. *Seminars in Liver Disease* **17**, 249–60. [This provides a view from the US on the management of ascites, and extensively reviews the historical and recent literature.]

Runyon BA, Hoefs JC (1984). Culture-negative neutrocytic ascites a variant of spontaneous bacterial peritonitis. *Hepatology* **4**, 1209–11. [This was one of several landmark papers by Runyon that helped us to understand the pathogenesis of SBP.]

Runyon BA, *et al.* (1990). Bedside inoculation of blood culture bottles with ascitic fluid is superior to delayed inoculation in the detection of spontaneous bacterial peritonitis. *Journal of Clinical Microbiology* **28**, 2811–12. [Inoculation of blood culture tubes with ascitic fluid is far superior to conventional methods.]

Salerno F, *et al.* (1991). Randomized comparative study of hemaccel vs. albumin infusion after total paracentesis in cirrhotic patients with refractory ascites. *Hepatology* **13**, 707–13. [This study suggests that plasma expanders are equally effective in the prevention of postparacentesis complications.]

Simón M-A, Díez J, Prieto J (1991). Abnormal sympathetic and renal response to sodium restriction in compensated cirrhosis. *Gastroenterology* **101**, 1354–60. [This study suggests that sodium restriction causes activation of the sympathetic nervous system in non-ascitic patients with cirrhosis.]

Solà R, *et al.* (1995). Spontaneous bacterial peritonitis in cirrhotic patients treated using paracentesis or diuretics results of a randomized study. *Hepatology* **21**, 340–4.

Solis-Herruzo J, *et al.* (1991). Effect of intra-thoracic pressure on plasma arginine vasopressin levels. *Gastroenterology* **101**, 607–17. [This shows that plasma AVP levels decrease following paracentesis.]

Stanley MM, Ochi S, Lee KK, and the Veterans Administration Co-operative Study on Treatment of Alcoholic Cirrhosis with Ascites (1989). Peritoneovenous shunting as compared with medical treatment in patients with alcoholic cirrhosis and massive ascites. *New England Journal of Medicine* **321**, 1632–8. [A controlled trial comparing two therapies.]

Strauss RM, Boyer TD (1997). Hepatic hydrothorax. *Seminars in Liver Disease* **17**, 227–32. [This is a good review of the subject.]

Tító L, *et al.* (1988). Recurrence of spontaneous bacterial peritonitis in cirrhosis frequency and predictive factors. *Hepatology* **8**, 27–31. [SBP is a recurrent disease.]

14.21.3 Hepatocellular failure

E. Anthony Jones

Introduction

Hepatocellular failure is the syndrome that occurs when loss of hepatocytes and/or hypofunction of hepatocytes exceeds the capacity of hepatocytes to regenerate and/or repair hepatocellular injury. Its clinical manifestations include hepatic encephalopathy, a haemorrhagic diathesis, ascites, and hepatocellular jaundice. The syndrome may complicate any disease in which the pathophysiology includes hepatocellular necrosis or apoptosis, or hypofunction of hepatocellular organelles. The duration of evidence of hepatic dysfunction before the onset of hepatocellular failure is variable, ranging from a few days to many years. The term hepatocellular failure does not necessarily imply impaired function of hepatic cells other than hepatocytes. Although many biochemical lesions induced by specific chemical, immunological, or cytopathic hepatotoxic factors have been documented, with the notable exception of hypoxia, the precise mechanisms by which such factors induce hepatocellular failure are poorly understood. Factors that may contribute to hepatocellular injury include immunological damage mediated by cytotoxic T lymphocytes, macrophage activation, direct cytopathic effects of viruses, cytokine-induced activation of cellular interactions, and oxidative stress. An influx of calcium ions into hepatocytes appears to be a late phenomenon in the sequence of biochemical events culminating in hepatocellular necrosis.

Definitions

Acute hepatocellular failure

The syndrome of hepatocellular jaundice, hypertransaminasaemia, and prolongation of the prothrombin time associated with an acute liver disease.

Fulminant hepatic failure

Classically defined as the syndrome of acute hepatocellular failure complicated by hepatic encephalopathy occurring within 8 weeks of the onset of clinical evidence of liver disease. The King's College Hospital (London) group have introduced the terms hyperacute liver failure for the occurrence of encephalopathy within 7 days of the onset of jaundice and late-onset liver failure for the syndrome in which hepatic encephalopathy occurs 8 to 24 weeks after the onset of clinical evidence of liver disease. In addition, the Beaujon Hospital (Paris) group has proposed that the term fulminant hepatic failure be applied to acute liver failure with a plasma factor V level less than 50 per cent of normal and hepatic encephalopathy occurring less than 2 weeks after the onset of jaundice, and that the term subfulminant hepatic failure be used for acute liver failure with a plasma factor V level less than 50 per cent of normal and hepatic encephalopathy occurring 2 weeks to 3 months after the onset of jaundice.

Chronic hepatocellular failure

This is the syndrome of decompensated chronic liver disease, which is chronic hepatocellular disease complicated by hepatic encephalopathy, coagulopathy, ascites, and/or hepatocellular jaundice.

Hepatic encephalopathy (portosystemic encephalopathy)

This is the complex neuropsychiatric syndrome attributable to impaired hepatocellular function and increased portosystemic shunting. The terms hepatic encephalopathy and portosystemic encephalopathy are usually used interchangeably. However, whereas the term portosystemic encephalopathy may be appropriate for encephalopathy complicating increased portosystemic shunting in the absence of overt hepatocellular failure, it may be inappropriate to use the term hepatic encephalopathy in this context.

Aetiology

Acute hepatocellular failure

The most common causes of fulminant hepatic failure are acute viral hepatitis and drugs. About one-third of cases appear to be due to non-A, non-B, non-C hepatitis of undetermined aetiology. Markers of acute infection with specific hepatitis viruses (such as IgM anti-HAV, IgM anti-HBc, IgM anti-HDV) may be useful in suggesting the aetiology. A syndrome similar to acute liver failure with encephalopathy associated with infection by other viruses (such as herpes, varicella) may occur, particularly in immunocompromised patients. Only drugs that can cause acute hepatocellular injury (rather than cholestasis) have the potential of inducing fulminant hepatic failure. Examples are paracetamol, halothane, and antiretroviral drugs. Fulminant hepatic failure caused by poisoning may be due to *Amanita* mushrooms or industrial solvents, particularly chlorinated hydrocarbons. Hypoxic hepatocellular injury may be attributable to reduced hepatic perfusion, but rarely leads to fulminant hepatic failure (for example following cardiac arrest). Important vascular causes of fulminant hepatic failure include the Budd–Chiari syndrome and veno-occlusive disease. The latter

may be induced by pyrrolizidine alkaloids, chemotherapy, or irradiation. A rare cause of fulminant hepatic failure is heat stroke. Intravascular haemolysis suggests Wilson's disease. Autoimmune chronic active hepatitis may present with a syndrome similar to subfulminant hepatic failure with type 1 antibodies to liver and kidney microsomes. Fulminant hepatic failure may be precipitated by partial hepatectomy (removal of more than 80 per cent of a normal liver). Fulminant hepatic failure soon after orthotopic liver transplantation may be due to hyperacute allograft rejection or hepatic arterial thrombosis. In carriers of the hepatitis B or C viruses, fulminant hepatic failure may be precipitated by modulation of the host's immune response to the virus as a consequence of immunosuppressive chemotherapy or its withdrawal. In Reye's syndrome a fulminant hepatic failure-like syndrome may occur, but there are, in addition, mitochondrial changes in the brain which are not specific for liver failure.

Chronic hepatocellular failure

Chronic hepatocellular failure may complicate any progressive chronic hepatocellular disease or any lesion causing chronic hepatic central venous congestion.

Manifestations

Cardinal features

Hepatic encephalopathy

Impaired mental function in liver failure may lead to a wide spectrum of psychiatric and neurological changes. Impaired psychometric test results and/or abnormal brain electrophysiological function in a patient with chronic liver disease, in whom a routine neurological examination is normal, may imply subclinical hepatic encephalopathy. The earliest clinical signs are psychiatric and behavioural changes. These changes are primarily due to subtle impairment of intellectual function that reflects predominantly bilateral forebrain dysfunction. Conventionally, four clinical stages of hepatic encephalopathy are recognized (Table 1). Increased muscle tone with cogwheel and neck rigidity, and myoclonic twitching may occur. Asterixis ('liver flap') can often be elicited (Table 1, Fig. 1). The mouth may be difficult to open. With progression, deep tendon reflexes may be increased and subsequently decreased. One or both plantar responses may be extensor. With progression, the frequency of the electroencephalogram decreases and its amplitude increases. With further progression, the amplitude decreases and triphasic waves may occur. Both the clinical and electrophysiological manifestations of hepatic encephalopathy are non-specific. Hepatic encephalopathy complicating chronic liver disease may be acute or chronic. When acute it is usually associated with one or more recognized precipitating factors (Table 2). With the notable exception of sedative hypnotic drugs, the mechanisms by which common precipitating factors exacerbate encephalopathy are poorly understood. Failure to identify a precipitating factor may imply deterioration of hepatocellular function. The term chronic portosystemic encephalopathy is often preferred when hepatic encephalopathy complicating chronic liver disease is persistent or episodic.

Hepatic encephalopathy is considered to be a reversible metabolic encephalopathy with a multifactorial pathogenesis. Traditionally, gut factors have been considered to play important roles (Tables 2 and 3). In liver failure there is decreased hepatic extraction and metabolism of constituents of portal venous plasma and decreased exposure of hepatocytes to these constituents as a consequence of their passage through intrahepatic and extrahepatic portosystemic venous collateral channels. Consequently, constituents of portal venous plasma tend to accumulate in the systemic circulation. If some of these compounds are neuroactive and can cross the blood–brain barrier, modulation of brain function may occur. The blood–brain barrier is normally highly permeable to non-polar substances, such as non-ionic ammonia and benzodiazepines, but has a low permeability to polar compounds. However, in liver failure the permeability of the barrier

Table 1 Clinical stages of hepatic encephalopathy

Stage	Mental status	Asterixis	Electroencephalographic changes
I (prodrome, often diagnosed in retrospect)	Mild confusion, euphoria or depression, decreased attention, slowing of ability to perform mental tasks, untidiness, slurred speech, irritability, reversal of sleep rhythm	Usually absent	Often lacking
II (impending coma)	Drowsiness, lethargy, gross deficits in ability to perform mental tasks, obvious personality changes, inappropriate behaviour, intermittent disorientation (usually for time), lack of sphincter control	Present (with or without incoordination)	Generalized slowing
III	Somnolent but rousable, unable to perform mental tasks, persistent disorientation with respect to time and/or place, amnesia, occasional fits of rage, speech present but incoherent, pronounced confusion	Usually present (if patient can co-operate)	Always present
IV	Coma; with (IV-A) or without (IV-B) response to painful stimuli	Usually absent	Always present

to polar compounds, such as the inhibitory neurotransmitter GABA, may increase. Most of the manifestations of hepatic encephalopathy appear to be attributable to a global suppression of central nervous system function, due predominantly to a net increase in inhibitory neurotransmission, as a consequence of increased neurotransmission mediated by inhibitory neurotransmitters (such as GABA) and/or decreased neurotransmission mediated by excitatory neurotransmitters (such as glutamate). Currently, the two factors considered to be most important in pathogenesis are raised brain concentrations of ammonia and increased GABA-mediated neurotransmission.

Increased GABAergic neurotransmission is associated with impaired motor function and decreased consciousness, two of the cardinal manifestations of hepatic encephalopathy. Potential mechanisms for increased GABAergic tone in hepatic encephalopathy include: (i) increased availability of GABA at GABA_A receptors in synaptic clefts; (ii) increased astrocytic synthesis and release of neurosteroids that are agonists of the GABA_A receptor; and (iii) increased brain concentrations of natural benzodiazepine receptor agonist ligands.

Ammonia was originally implicated in pathogenesis because it was recognized to be neurotoxic, plasma concentrations tend to be raised in liver failure, and plasma ammonia readily enters the brain. Plasma ammonia

Table 2 Factors that may precipitate encephalopathy in a patient with cirrhosis

Precipitating factor	Comments
Constipation Oral protein load Upper gastrointestinal bleed	Gut factors contribute to hepatic encephalopathy
Diuretic therapy Paracentesis Diarrhoea and vomiting	Dehydration, electrolyte and acid–base imbalance
Hypoglycaemia Hypoxia Hypotension Anaemia	Factors with adverse effects on both liver and brain function
Sedative/hypnotic drugs[1]	Benzodiazepines and barbiturates enhance the action of GABA
Azotaemia[2] Infection[3] Induction of a portosystemic shunt[4] General surgery	

[1] Includes drugs acting on the GABA_A/benzodiazepine receptor complex.
[2] Blood urea is a source of intestinal ammonia.
[3] May cause dehydration and increased release of nitrogenous substances.
[4] For example, a transjugular intrahepatic portosystemic stent (TIPSS).

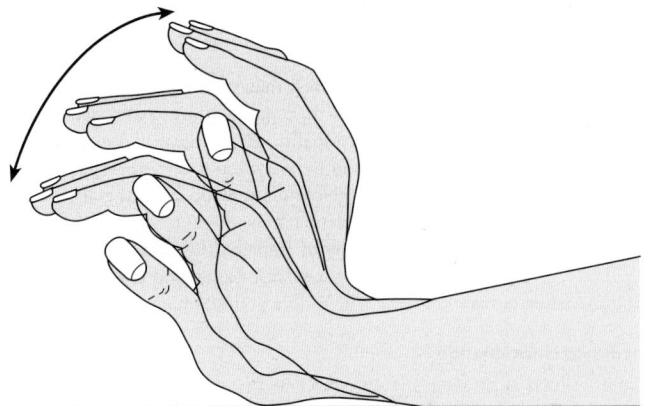

Fig. 1 The 'liver flap' is a slow, flapping tremor (one flap every 1 to 2 s), which can be elicited by asking the patient to dorsiflex the hands with the arms outstretched and the fingers extended and parted. It is due to neuromuscular incoordination between flexor and extensor muscles (negative myoclonus). The hands tend to fall forward, but this involuntary movement is rapidly corrected by readoption of the dorsiflexed position, thereby creating a 'flap'. The same phenomenon may be elicited by asking the patient to squeeze the physician's extended finger. Neuromuscular incoordination is indicated by repeated intensification and relaxation of the intensity of the squeeze ('milkmaid's grip').

Table 3 Treatment of hepatic encephalopathy

Treatment	Comments
1. Correction or removal of precipitating factors	Mandatory
2. Institution of manoeuvres to minimize absorption of nitrogenous substances: Dietary protein restriction Evacuation of the bowel Non-hydrolysed disaccharide (lactulose or lactitol) and/or oral poorly absorbed broad-spectrum antibiotic (such as neomycin)	Routine
3. Reduction of portosystemic shunting	Rarely practical
4. Drugs that directly reverse brain pathophysiology, such as flumazenil	Experimental

concentrations higher than those usually found in liver failure (more than 1 mmol/l) are associated with increased neuronal excitation and seizures. In contrast, plasma ammonia concentrations typically found in patients with precoma stages of hepatic encephalopathy (stages I to III) (100 to 400 μmol/l) may enhance neuronal inhibition by: (i) directly facilitating GABA-gated chloride conductance; (ii) selectively increasing the binding of agonist ligands to the GABA$_A$/benzodiazepine receptor complex; and (iii) stimulating astrocytic synthesis and release of neurosteroids that are potent GABA$_A$ receptor agonists.

Possible roles for neurotransmitter systems, other than the GABA system, have been postulated. Some of the symptomatology of hepatic encephalopathy can be explained by disturbances in functional loops of basal ganglia, which could arise as a consequence of an imbalance between glutamatergic and GABAergic neurotransmission.

Haemorrhagic diathesis

The basis of the haemorrhagic diathesis is multifactorial. Of major importance is impaired synthesis of hepatocyte-derived blood clotting factors; this leads to prolongation of the prothrombin time (see Chapter 22.5.1), which is not corrected by parenteral vitamin K. Thrombocytopenia is often present; it may be secondary to the hypersplenism of portal hypertension (see Chapter 14.21.2). However, in fulminant hepatic failure, platelet structure and function are abnormal and the capillary bleeding time is greater than that predicted from the platelet count. Mild disseminated intravascular coagulation is often detectable, but is rarely of clinical significance. Upper gastrointestinal haemorrhage (for example from gastritis, gastro-oesophageal varices, or ulcers) frequently occurs. A common clinical manifestation of the bleeding tendency is bruising around venepuncture sites.

Ascites

Ascites due to hepatocellular failure complicates lesions that cause sinusoidal portal hypertension (such as cirrhosis) or impaired hepatic venous drainage. However, hepatocellular failure is not invariable when ascites is associated with hepatic venous congestion (see Chapter 14.21.2).

Hepatocellular jaundice

The jaundice of hepatocellular failure has an orange tint and is attributable to conjugated hyperbilirubinaemia due to impaired secretion of conjugated bilirubin into the bile canaliculus; the transport maximum for conjugated bilirubin across the bile canaliculus is reduced relative to bilirubin production and conjugation (see Chapter 14.19.3). In acute hepatitis the degree of conjugated hyperbilirubinaemia reflects the extent of hepatocellular necrosis, but even when jaundice is deep, other features of hepatocellular failure (such as a prolonged prothrombin time) are often absent, reflecting the large normal hepatic reserve. In contrast, in chronic noncholestatic liver disease, hepatocellular jaundice usually reflects severe hepatocellular failure.

Other features

Increased susceptibility to infection

About 80 per cent of infections are bacterial, but about one-third are complicated by tissue invasion by fungi (such as aspergillosis, candidiasis). There may be no fever or leucocytosis. The mortality is high. Fungal infection is suggested by antibiotic-resistant fever. The increased frequency of infections may be related to reduced levels of complement components and opsonins, reduced phagocytic and bactericidal properties of polymorphonuclear leucocytes, and reduced clearance function of Kupffer cells. Spontaneous bacterial peritonitis is a common complication of ascites (see Chapter 14.21.2).

Fetor hepaticus

Fetor hepaticus is the term applied to a particular smell of the breath that commonly occurs in patients with cirrhosis and extensive portosystemic shunts or fulminant hepatic failure. Descriptions vary and include a sweet-ish, slightly pungent, or faecal smell, similar to that of a rotten apple, mice, or a freshly opened corpse. Being subjective there is considerable variation in its recognition. It has been attributed to gut-derived, sulphur-containing products of methionine metabolism.

Acid–base and electrolyte changes

A wide range of abnormalities occur, particularly in fulminant hepatic failure, and may contribute to altered neurological and cardiac function. Hyponatraemia may be due to impaired free-water clearance, failure of the sodium pump, or diuretics. Hypernatraemia is usually iatrogenic. Respiratory alkalosis, secondary to hyperventilation of central origin, is common in fulminant hepatic failure. Loop diuretics often precipitate a hypokalaemic metabolic alkalosis. Metabolic acidosis may be associated with extensive tissue damage, hypoxia, and lactic acidaemia. Respiratory acidosis may be associated with hypercapnia and respiratory infection.

Cerebral oedema and raised intracranial pressure

Cerebral oedema and raised intracranial pressure frequently complicate fulminant hepatic failure, occurring in about 80 per cent of patients with stage IV encephalopathy, but are uncommon in patients with chronic hepatocellular failure. These complications may be classified separately from hepatic encephalopathy. Herniation of the cingulate, uncus, or cerebellar tonsil secondary to raised intracranial pressure is a frequent cause of death in fulminant hepatic failure. Antemortem diagnosis of cerebral oedema and raised intracranial pressure is suggested by sudden deterioration of consciousness, increased muscle tone, unequal pupils, abnormally reacting pupils, myoclonus, focal seizures, decerebrate posturing, fixed pupils with spontaneous respiration, and/or absent ciliospinal reflexes. Sudden changes in pulse and blood pressure unrelated to haemorrhage, rapid deterioration of the electroencephalogram, sweating, tachycardia, arrhythmias, intermittent systemic hypertension, sudden severe hypotension, bursts of hyperventilation, and fever may all be manifestations of raised intracranial pressure. Papilloedema is rare. Signs of raised intracranial pressure become apparent when intracranial pressure exceeds 30 mmHg. A failure of cellular osmoregulation, with intracellular accumulation of osmolytes, such as glutamine, appears to be a pathogenic mechanism (cytotoxic). Compensatory loss of other intracellular osmolytes, such as inositol, may be more effective in chronic liver disease than in fulminant hepatic failure. Increased blood-to-brain transfer of fluid across the blood–brain barrier (vasogenic), and expansion of the extravascular space (interstitial or hydrocephalic) may also contribute to pathogenesis.

Hypoglycaemia

Severe hypoglycaemia (blood glucose less than 40 mg/dl) occurs in about 40 per cent of patients with fulminant hepatic failure (particularly children) and may exacerbate encephalopathy. The clinical and electroencephalographic features of hepatic and hypoglycaemic encephalopathies are similar. In acute liver failure, hypoglycaemia may occur in the absence of hepatic encephalopathy. Hypoglycaemia may develop rapidly and may recur with sepsis. It is due primarily to impaired hepatic glucose release secondary to glycogen depletion. In contrast to hepatic encephalopathy, hypoglycaemic coma may cause irreversible brain damage.

Cardiovascular changes

Hepatocellular failure is associated with systemic vasodilation and a hyperdynamic circulation. Cardiac output is increased, peripheral vascular resistance decreased, blood pressure reduced, and splanchnic and capillary flow increased, but perfusion of the renal cortex is decreased. Features of a hyperdynamic circulation include a bounding pulse, capillary pulsation, vasodilated extremities, a precordial heave, and an ejection systolic murmur. The increased cardiac output has been attributed to an increased vascular capacitance and hence relative hypovolaemia with low jugular venous pressure.

Recently, endogenous cannabinoids acting at vascular CB_1 receptors have been implicated in this state of vasodilation. Arrhythmias, other than sinus tachycardia, frequently occur with hypoxia and stage IV encephalopathy due to fulminant hepatic failure. Cardiac arrest (unrelated to respiratory arrest) may occur.

Hepatorenal syndrome

Renal failure is common and may be rapidly progressive. In only a minority of cases is it attributable to hypovolaemia or a lesion of the urinary tract. It is typically functional and characterized by reduced glomerular filtration rate and oliguria. Acute tubular necrosis may supervene. Absorption of large quantities of nitrogenous substances from the gut after a gastrointestinal haemorrhage may contribute to azotaemia. Plasma urea and creatinine are not reliable indices of renal function in fulminant hepatic failure; hepatic synthesis of urea is reduced and tubular secretion of creatinine is increased. Functional renal failure is associated with intense renal arterial vasoconstriction. The kidneys in this syndrome function normally when transplanted into subjects without liver disease. Several humoral systems have been implicated in pathogenesis (see Chapter 14.20.2).

Hepatopulmonary syndrome

This syndrome is defined as the triad of liver disease, intrapulmonary peripheral vascular dilatation with decreased pulmonary vascular resistance (right to left shunt), and an increased alveolar–arterial oxygen gradient. Hypoxaemia (Pao_2 less than 70 mmHg) is common and may be associated with cyanosis. The hypoxaemia is usually reversed by 100 per cent oxygen and is attributable to abnormal ventilation–perfusion ratios and impaired diffusion capacity, but uncommonly in cirrhosis hypoxaemia, not reversible by 100 per cent oxygen, may be due to large pulmonary arteriovenous shunts. Portopulmonary shunting and pulmonary hypertension may develop. Chest radiographs may show a high diaphragm, basal pulmonary infiltrates, or pulmonary oedema. Pulmonary oedema, not attributable to left ventricular failure, occurs in fulminant hepatic failure. Respiratory arrest of central origin may occur. The mechanism of the pulmonary vasodilation is unknown. Oxygen does not diffuse readily into the centre of dilated vessels and increased cardiac output limits the time for gas exchange.

Skin changes

Recognition of certain skin changes in a patient with chronic liver disease alerts the clinician to the possibility of incipient or overt chronic hepatocellular failure. However, no skin changes are specific for hepatocellular failure. Spider naevi are often present in patients with cirrhosis. They consist of a central protuberant arteriole from which small vessels radiate in a manner that has been likened to the appearance of a spider's legs (Fig. 2 and Plate 1). Their diameter is usually less than 0.5 cm. They occur in the area of drainage of the superior vena cava and should be distinguished from telangiectasia, corkscrew scleral vessels, and purpura. Development of new

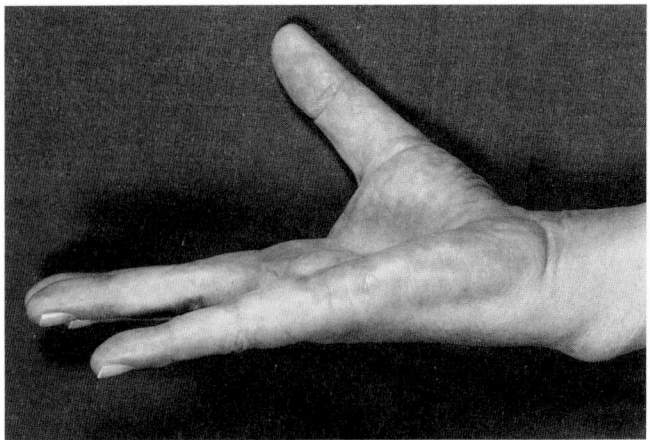

Fig. 3 Palmer erythema in a patient with cirrhosis. (See also Plate 2.)

'spiders' suggests progressive hepatocellular disease. Palmar erythema occurs less frequently than spider naevi. It is characterized by an exaggeration of the normal mottling of palmar surfaces of the hands, resulting in well-demarcated redness of the thenar and hypothenar eminences, and of the pulps of the fingers (Fig. 3 and Plate 2). Dilated, thread-like blood vessels in the skin, having an apparently random distribution, may occur, and may resemble a United States dollar note ('paper money' skin). White nails with loss of demarcation of the lunulae (leuconychia, Terry's nails) (Fig. 4 and Plate 3) and finger clubbing (Lovibond's angle greater than 180°) (Fig. 5 and Plate 4) may also occur.

Endocrine changes

Chronic liver disease may be associated with reduced concentrations of testosterone. Some male patients with cirrhosis develop hypogonadism and feminization. The former is characterized by testicular atrophy, decreased potency and libido, and a reduced need to shave; the latter is characterized by gynaecomastia and female hair distribution and body habitus. Some female patients with cirrhosis develop infertility, scanty irregular menstruation, and an asexual appearance due to loss of female characteristics. Unilateral or bilateral (tender) gynaecomastia may be a complication of cirrhosis (Fig. 6) or spironolactone therapy.

Fatigue

Severe disabling fatigue that seems to be out of proportion to a patient's general condition may occur in chronic liver disease, before the onset of overt hepatocellular failure.

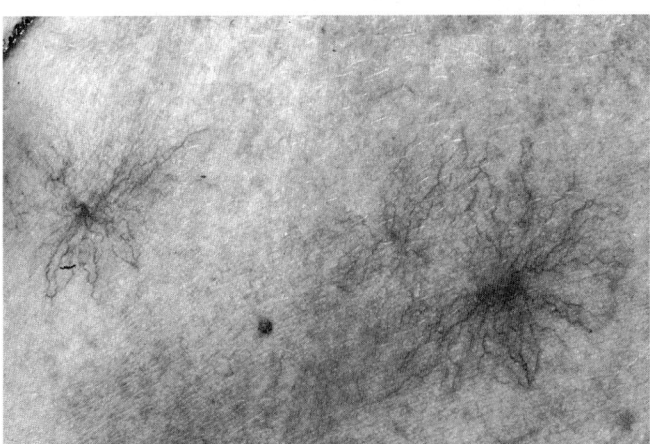

Fig. 2 Spider naevi in a patient with cirrhosis. (See also Plate 1.)

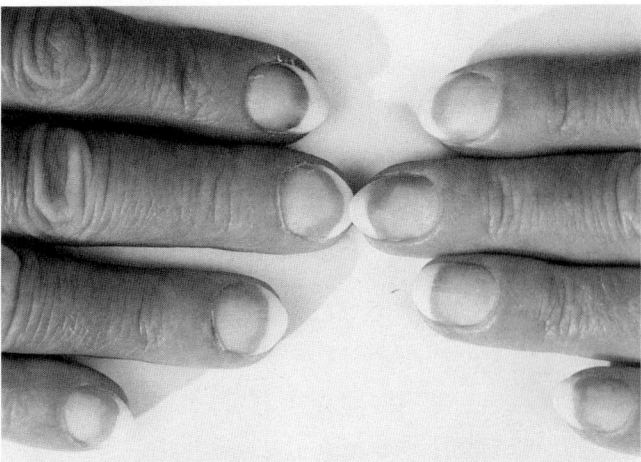

Fig. 4 White nails in a patient with cirrhosis. (See also Plate 3.)

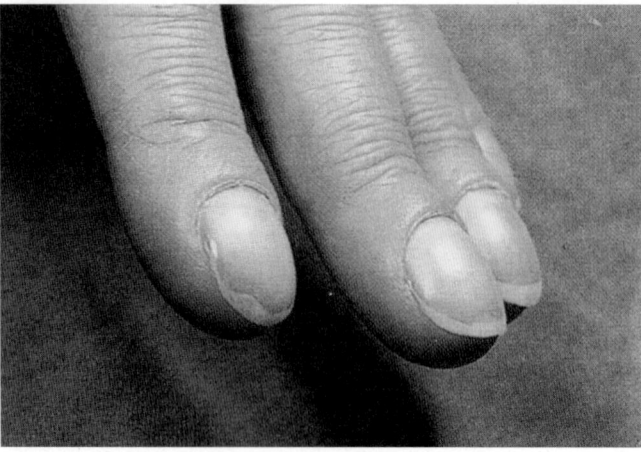

Fig. 5 Finger clubbing in a patient with cirrhosis. (See also Plate 4.)

Abnormal protein metabolism

In cirrhosis the degree of hypoalbuminaemia reflects both decreased hepatic synthesis and an increase in plasma volume. Because of albumin's long plasma half-life, hypoalbuminaemia may not be present early in the course of fulminant hepatic failure. Chronic hepatocellular failure is associated with increased protein catabolism and a loss of skeletal muscle mass.

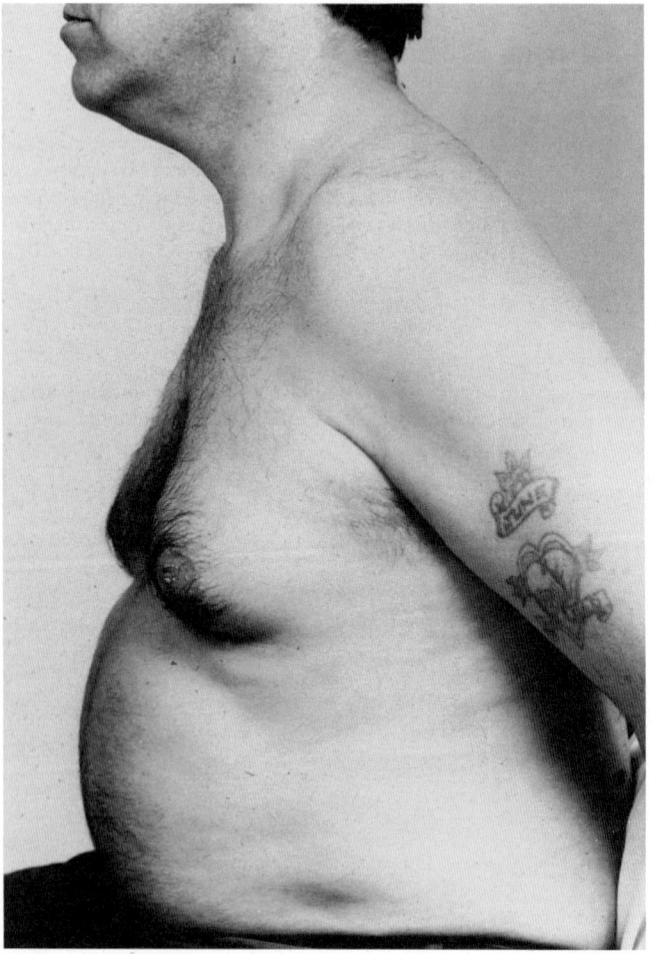

Fig. 6 Gynaecomastia in a male patient with cirrhosis.

Fever

A low-grade fever may occur with severe active hepatocellular disease (such as acute alcoholic hepatitis) in the absence of infection.

Anaemia

A normochromic normocytic anaemia is a feature of chronic hepatocellular failure.

Osteopenia

Osteopenia is common in patients with decompensated cirrhosis.

Diagnosis

The syndrome of hepatocellular failure constitutes a clinical spectrum from acute liver failure at one extreme to decompensated chronic hepatocellular disease at the other. A patient dying of hepatocellular failure usually exhibits all four of the cardinal manifestations with or without complicating sepsis.

Hepatic encephalopathy

This is a clinical diagnosis that is usually made by recognizing the presence of encephalopathy and excluding non-hepatic causes. No individual clinical or laboratory abnormality is specific for hepatic encephalopathy. Special attention is paid to changes in personality, hypersomnia, and deterioration of performance at work or school. Asterixis (liver flap) is not pathognomonic. Signs of portal hypertension, non-specific cutaneous stigmata of liver disease, and/or fetor hepaticus may be present. It is necessary to recognize disorders with neurological manifestations that may mimic hepatic encephalopathy, such as Wernicke's encephalopathy, alcohol intoxication, or subdural haematoma. More than one type of encephalopathy may coexist. Psychometric tests are useful in detecting and monitoring subtle mental dysfunction in patients with subclinical or prestupor stages of hepatic encephalopathy. The quantitiative number connection test is frequently applied, but allowance must be made for the effects of learning and age on test scores. Electroencephalographic abnormalities are non-specific. There is usualy a fairly good correlation between the clinical stage of encephalopathy and the degree of abnormality of the electroencephalogram. The electroencephalogram is of value in differential diagnosis; it can reveal focal lesions in the brain, seizure activity, and other findings that might suggest an alternative diagnosis. Visual event-related potentials that depend on cognitive function, such as P300 potentials, are sensitive in the detection of electrophysiological changes in the brain in patients with cirrhosis who do not have overt encephalopathy. Routine laboratory tests aid in the differential diagnosis of encephalopathies, and in the detection of factors that may precipitate hepatic encephalopathy (Table 2). Plasma ammonia concentrations are modestly increased in the majority of patients with hepatic encephalopathy, but correlate poorly with the clinical stage and are not useful in management. An elevated plasma ammonia may be helpful in suggesting a hepatic origin for an undiagnosed encephalopathy.

Haemorrhagic diathesis

The most important readily obtainable laboratory markers of this diathesis are the prothrombin time and the platelet count. Plasma activities of individual clotting factors that are synthesized in the liver are reduced (see Chapter 22.5.1).

Ascites

When the presence of ascites on physical examination is in doubt, the issue may be resolved by ultrasonography of the abdomen, which can detect as little as 100 to 200 ml of intraperitoneal fluid. Careful examination of the jugular veins is necessary in the exclusion of cardiac causes. On ultrasonography diffuse inhomogeneity of the liver suggests cirrhosis, and difficulty in visualizing major hepatic veins suggests the Budd–Chiari syndrome. A small diagnostic ascitic fluid tap is done routinely; analysis of the fluid includes determination of concentrations of leucocytes and protein, examination for malignant cells, and culture.

Hepatocellular jaundice

The conjugated hyperbilirubinaemia of hepatocellular failure has to be distinguished from acquired intrahepatic cholestatic disease, cholestasis due to large duct biliary obstruction, and rare congenital hyperbilirubinaemias in which other routine serum biochemical liver tests are normal. Recognition that conjugated hyperbilirubinaemia is attributable to hepatocellular failure is usually possible from clinical and routine haematological and serum biochemical data and an ultrasound showing no evidence of dilated bile ducts. Unconjugated hyperbilirubinaemia is not a feature of hepatocellular failure.

Acute hepatocellular failure

Acute hepatocellular disease associated with a conjugated hyperbilirubinaemia may be classified as acute liver failure when prolongation of the prothrombin time occurs. If acute liver failure is due to hypoxia, a cause is usually obvious, such as a hypotensive episode during surgery.

The diagnosis of fulminant hepatic failure requires the presence of encephalopathy, elevated serum alanine aminotransferase levels early in the course, and marked prolongation of the prothrombin time. Serum alanine aminotransferase concentrations exceeding 50 times the upper limit of normal are common in massive hepatocellular necrosis, but may be less than three times the upper limit of normal with minimal hyperbilirubinaemia when fulminant hepatic failure is associated with microvesicular hepatic steatosis (see Pathology). Abdominal pain may occur with poisoning. Rarely, hepatic encephalopathy precedes jaundice and abnormal behaviour may have to be distinguished from non-hepatogenous acute psychiatric disease. However, patients with fulminant hepatic failure due to massive hepatocellular necrosis, who survive more than a few days, develop deep jaundice. Lumbar puncture should usually be avoided, because of the coagulopathy and possible raised intracranial pressure. However, a baseline CT scan of the brain may be useful. Evidence for the presence of other types of encephalopathy is routinely sought. The syndrome of fulminant hepatic failure may occasionally be mimicked by severe sepsis or falciparum malaria. In subfulminant hepatic failure, ultrasonography may reveal inhomogeneity of the liver due to nodular transformation.

Chronic hepatocellular failure

The diagnosis of chronic hepatocellular failure requires the demonstration of an appropriate chronic liver disease and evidence of hepatocellular failure. Mild conjugated hyperbilirubinaemia and a modest prolongation of the prothrombin time tend to occur before the development of overt hepatic encephalopathy or ascites. In contrast to diseases that lead to sinusoidal portal hypertension (such as cirrhosis), those that cause presinusoidal portal hypertension (such as schistosomiasis) do not usually progress to hepatocellular failure.

Pathology

There is no single hepatic histological change that is pathognomonic of hepatocellular failure. Fulminant hepatic failure is usually associated with massive or confluent hepatocellular necrosis. However, occasionally, when due, for example, to acute fatty liver of pregnancy, or hepatotoxicity caused by intravenous tetracycline, valproic acid, or antiretroviral drugs, liver histology reveals microvesicular hepatocellular steatosis, in which the nucleus retains its central location within hepatocytes. In an appreciable proportion of autopsies on patients who succumb to fulminant hepatic failure, there is evidence of cerebral oedema and raised intracranial pressure, such as increased brain weight, tense dura, flattened cortical gyri, dilated ventricles,

and cingulate, uncal, or cerebellar herniation. The histological appearances of the brain in fulminant hepatic failure are essentially normal. In contrast, histology of the brain of patients who died from chronic liver failure typically shows an increase in the number and size of Alzheimer type 2 astrocytes. Functional renal failure is associated with no gross pathological changes in the kidney.

Course and prognosis

Acute hepatocellular failure

In patients with acute liver failure, who do not develop encephalopathy, such as the typical case of acute icteric viral hepatitis, complete recovery is the rule.

The course of fulminant hepatic failure is variable. There are no reliable criteria that enable prediction of whether an individual patient will die or regain consciousness and ultimately survive. Overall survival appears to have improved with advances in intensive supportive care, and may currently be about 40 per cent without liver transplantation. Mortality tends to be greater when the encephalopathy is severe and prolonged, and when coagulopathy is profound (prothrombin time greater than 100 s). Mortality also tends to be greater if the patient's age is below 5 or over 40 years, or if encephalopathy occurs more than 8 days after the onset of jaundice. The mortality is particularly high (more than 80 per cent) in cases caused by halothane, or drugs other than paracetamol, but is about 50 per cent when paracetamol is implicated. Major complications increase mortality. Small or decreasing liver size, convulsions, cardiac arrhythmias (other than sinus tachycardia), and marked fetor hepaticus are ominous signs. Serum concentrations of aminotransferases may decrease abruptly, but have no prognostic value. The course of fulminant hepatic failure can be divided into five phases.

Pre-encephalopathy

In acute liver failure a progressive increase in prothrombin time is ominous and often precedes the onset of hepatic encephalopathy. After paracetamol overdosage the onset of encephalopathy may be predicted from plasma concentrations of the drug.

Encephalopathy

About one-third of patients die within 2 days of the onset of stage IV encephalopathy. In about 20 per cent of cases, death appears to be due to acute liver failure with progressive encephalopathy. In other cases, death can be attributed to one or more complications of the syndrome, such as upper gastrointestinal haemorrhage, cerebral oedema and raised intracranial pressure, sepsis, and renal failure. In subfulminant hepatic failure, death due to raised intracranial pressure and/or sepsis is more common than in fulminant hepatic failure.

Hepatic regeneration

The key factor in determining the outcome of fulminant hepatic failure, in the absence of liver transplantation, is the ability of the liver to regenerate. Nodules of hyperplastic regenerating liver tissue may be found at autopsy in patients who survive more than 10 days after the onset of encephalopathy. In general, such patients have usually died of a complication of fulminant hepatic failure at a time when indices of hepatocellular function were improving. Serum concentrations of α-fetoprotein, which are regarded as an index of hepatic regeneration, do not usually become elevated until at least 10 days after the onset of encephalopathy. The concentrations tend to correlate fairly well with the amount of hepatic regeneration found at autopsy. Recovery is usually heralded by clinical improvement in encephalopathy, which may be preceded by a decreasing prothrombin time. The electroencephalogram may remain abnormal for several days after consciousness is regained.

Cholestasis

A phase of profound cholestasis often develops 2 to 3 weeks after patients regain consciousness. When death has occurred during this phase, large regenerative nodules and intense cholestasis in hepatocytes have been found at autopsy.

Long-term sequelae

Complete restoration of normal hepatic function and structure usually occurs in survivors of fulminant hepatic failure, even after cerebral oedema, decerebrate rigidity, and episodes of flattening of the electroencephalogram. Serum biochemical liver tests and hepatic histology typically return to normal 45 to 75 days after the onset of hepatic encephalopathy. Permanent neurological sequelae have been reported when recovery has occurred after respiratory arrest.

Chronic hepatocellular failure

In patients with chronic hepatocellular disease, hepatic encephalopathy is often reversible, particularly if a precipitating factor is identified. An MRI of the brain typically reveals symmetric pallidal hyperintensities, possibly due to increased deposition of manganese in the basal ganglia. These hyperintensities appear to correlate with the degree of impairment of hepatocellular function, but not with hepatic encephalopathy. Elevated serum conjugated bilirubin in cirrhosis or precirrhotic alcoholic liver disease is associated with a poor prognosis. An increasing serum conjugated bilirubin in a patient with a chronic cholestatic liver disease may reflect progression of the disease and/or the development of hepatocellular failure. The serum bilirubin is regarded as a good index of prognosis in primary biliary cirrhosis. When ascites first develops in a patient with cirrhosis, 1-year survival is about 50 per cent and 5-year survival about 20 per cent. Survival after the onset of the hepatorenal syndrome is usually only a few weeks or months.

Management

The first issue is whether there is any effective therapy for the underlying liver disease. A treatment that suppresses the pathological process responsible for impairing hepatocellular function may decrease or reverse manifestations of hepatocellular failure. For acute liver failure, corticosteroids are ineffective and may be harmful, except in uncommon patients in whom the underlying lesion is an autoimmune hepatitis, and in carriers of the hepatitis B or C virus in whom acute liver failure has been precipitated by the withdrawal of immunosuppressive chemotherapy. Antiviral therapy has not been shown to be efficacious for acute viral hepatitis. Acetylcysteine has been shown to improve survival in patients who have taken an overdose of paracetamol, and this may apply even when the antidote is given after hepatic encephalopathy has developed. When viral infections, other than viral hepatitis, are diagnosed, antiviral treatment is instituted. Interruption of pregnancy has been advocated to improve survival in patients with fulminant hepatic failure due to acute fatty liver of pregnancy. It is useful to consider management of acute and chronic hepatocellular failure separately. The chronic syndrome accounts for the great majority of cases of hepatocellular failure, whereas the acute syndrome, when severe, is one of the most challenging in clinical medicine, presenting the physician with a unique constellation of difficult problems. In addition to discontinuing drugs that might have contributed to the clinical condition, especially neuroactive, hepatotoxic, and nephrotoxic drugs, it is necessary to take into account hepatocellular disease-associated alterations in drug pharmacokinetics and pharmacodynamics when prescribing for the patient in hepatocellular failure. Drugs may modify the clinical manifestations of hepatocellular failure. For example, patients with cirrhosis exibit increased sensitivity to the central neuroinhibitory and muscle relaxant effects of benzodiazepines. Whether liver transplantation is an appropriate therapeutic option must be considered in all patients with hepatocellular failure (see Chapter 14.21.4).

Chronic hepatocellular failure

As the patient has irreversible architectural changes in the liver, there is no potential for complete recovery with medical treatment. In such cases, management consists of trying to reduce the manifestations of hepatocellular failure that are amenable to treatment, especially encephalopathy and ascites; optimizing nutritional status with a high protein diet, if tolerated; treating complicating infections; and assessing suitability for liver transplantation. Non-specific clinical deterioration raises the possibility of bacteraemia, spontaneous bacterial peritonitis, or hepatocellular carcinoma.

Hepatic encephalopathy

The following general principles are relevant in the management of hepatic encephalopathy: (i) removal or correction of any precipitating factor (Table 2); (ii) reduction of absorption of nitrogenous substances from the gut; (iii) reduction of increased portosystemic shunting; and (iv) reversal of contributing neuropathophysiological mechanisms with drugs that act directly on the brain (Table 3).

Acute hepatic encephalopathy

All drugs that might contribute to encephalopathy, including diuretics, are stopped, and consideration is given to administering an appropriate antidote, such an naloxone or flumazenil. Meticulous attention is paid to maintaining fluid and electrolyte balance, and an adequate urine flow. Dietary protein intake is restricted, and enemas, such as magnesium sulphate or phosphate, are given. Lactulose, or another disaccharide with similar properties, such as lactitol, is given routinely. There is no disaccharidase on the microvillus membrane of enterocytes that hydrolyses lactulose. Its metabolism by colonic bacteria leads to production of lactic acid and other organic acids, a fall in colonic pH, and increased ionization of nitrogenous compounds. These changes may lead to a decrease in the absorption of nitrogenous compounds, including ammonia. Lactulose is a cathartic and is widely believed to be efficacious in the management of hepatic encephalopathy. It may induce hypernatraemia due to increased faecal fluid loss. In addition, an enterically administered, broad-spectrum, poorly absorbed antibiotic may be given to reduce the enteric bacterial flora. Neomycin (up to 6 g daily) has been most extensively used; potent alternatives include kanamycin and paramomycin. Metronidazole, which is effective against anaerobes, may also be given. If improvement in consciousness occurs, dietary protein is increased incrementally.

Chronic portosystemic encephalopathy

In the absence of protein intolerance a nutritious diet that includes a high protein content (80 to 100 g/day) is encouraged to maintain a positive nitrogen balance and optimize liver function. Vitamins are given empirically and thiamine replacement may be indicated in malnourished patients who are alcoholic. Vegetable protein diets seem to be well tolerated and tend to be cathartic due to their fibre content. Oral branched-chain amino acids may decrease protein catabolism and facilitate maintenance of a positive nitrogen balance. When protein intolerance develops, management consists of reducing dietary protein intake to as low as 40 g/day. Lactulose or lactitol is given in doses sufficient to produce two or three semiformed bowel actions daily, and precipitating factors are carefully avoided. If disaccharide intolerance develops, a broad-spectrum antibiotic may be tried. However, long-term neomycin should be avoided because of the risk of ototoxicity and nephrotoxicity. Metronidazole may induce a peripheral neuropathy.

If intractable chronic portosystemic encephalopathy occurs in a patient with a large spontaneous or surgically-induced portosystemic shunt, the invasive technique of balloon occlusion, coupled with embolization of a collateral vein, may reverse portal blood flow from hepatofugal to hepatopetal, improve hepatocellular function, and ameliorate the encephalopathy. Similarly, in a patient with chronic portosystemic encephalopathy and a patent transjugular intrahepatic portosystemic stent (TIPSS) the shunt can be narrowed or closed.

A new approach

A new therapeutic approach is to give a drug that acts on the target organ of hepatic encephalopathy, the brain, by reversing contributory neuropatho-physiological mechanisms. The benzodiazepine antagonist, flumazenil, is the first promising drug of this type. It competes with high specificity with other benzodiazepine receptor ligands for binding to central benzodiazep-ine receptors, and rapidly and completely reverses the sedative and other neurological effects of benzodiazepine agonists, such as diazepam. When given as a bolus intravenously, flumazenil induces transient, incomplete clinical and electrophysiological ameliorations of overt encephalopathy in an appreciable proportion of patients with encephalopathy complicating acute liver failure or cirrhosis.

Ascites

Treatment is discussed in Chapter 14.21.2.

Acute hepatocellular failure

Prevention

The incidence of fulminant hepatitis B should be substantially reduced by widespread vaccination. Fulminant hepatic failure can be prevented by avoiding re-exposure to an agent that has induced an idiosyncratic acute hepatitis (such as halothane), and may be prevented by giving *N*-acetylcysteine after paracetamol overdose.

Acute liver failure

Treatment of acute liver failure in the absence of encephalopathy is expect-ant, but frequent monitoring is necessary when the prothrombin time is prolonged and prompt admission to hospital is indicated at the first sign of encephalopathy. Referral to a specialized liver unit has been recommended before encephalopathy develops if levels of clotting factors fall to less than 50 per cent of normal.

Fulminant and subfulminant hepatic failure

Routine management for acute hepatic encephalopathy is instituted (by extrapolation from the management of hepatic encephalopathy complicat-ing chronic liver disease). With the onset of stage II hepatic encephalopathy, intensive supportive care should be instituted and transfer of the patient to a unit with the potential of undertaking orthotopic liver transplantation is recommended. All patients are considered to have potentially reversible disease. Treatment is designed to buy time for hepatic regeneration to take place and to avoid iatrogenic deterioration. No factor reported to stimulate hepatic regeneration experimentally is of proven clinical benefit. Conven-tional intensive care for the unconscious patient is instituted. A fluid intake of 1 to 2 litres daily is usually adequate. A nasogastric tube is used to decompress the stomach and detect upper gastrointestinal haemorrhage. Despite the coagulopathy, an arterial catheter is useful for continuous blood-pressure monitoring, frequent blood sampling, and measurement of blood gases. Caloric intake is maintained by infusing hypertonic dextrose (10 to 50 per cent), usually 200 to 300 g/day into a central vein. Intravenous lipids and amino acids may also be given. Vitamins may be given empiric-ally. Unless the aetiology is known to be non-infectious, blood and all secretions are considered to be infectious. In this circumstance, attending personnel should wear gowns, gloves, and masks. Enteric isolation pro-cedures are enforced and all specimens from the patient are labelled as infectious.

Blood is withdrawn at the outset for serological markers (such as for hepatitis viruses, cytomegalovirus), screening for common drugs, and esti-mation of serum copper. Blood glucose is monitored as frequently as every 1 to 2 h. The following investigations are carried out every 12 h: haemo-globin, total and differential leucocyte count, platelet count, urea, creati-nine, potassium, sodium, chloride, and bicarbonate. Daily investigations include prothrombin time, total and direct bilirubin, alkaline phosphatase, alanine and aspartate aminotransferases, albumin, amylase, calcium, phos-phate, magnesium, fibrinogen, and fibrinogen split products. Chest radio-graphs are obtained daily. Serial ultrasonic determinations of liver size may be useful in following the course. Needle biopsy of the liver is contraindi-cated. Frequent semiquantitative assessment of neurological status (such as the Glasgow coma score) and continuous monitoring of the electrocardio-gram and electoencephalogram should be instituted. Patients should be monitored frequently for complications, which must be treated promptly and vigorously. A major goal is the prevention of brain damage. If agitation, piercing cries, delirium, or seizures occur, the patient should be restrained in a dark quiet room and the temptation to administer sedatives should be resisted.

Specific problems

Susceptibility to infections

Intensive microbiological monitoring is necessary. In fulminant hepatic failure, daily cultures of blood, urine, sputum, and swabs of intravenous cannulas are recommended. For patients admitted to a liver failure unit, prophylactic antimicrobial therapy has been advocated, such as intraven-ous, broad-spectrum antibiotics, oral or nasogastric amphotericin B sus-pension, and in females, vaginal clotrimazole cream. Nephrotoxic aminoglycosides are avoided. Antibiotics are recommended to cover inva-sive procedures. Potential sources of infection, such as intrauterine devices, are removed.

Acid–base and electrolyte disturbances

Alkalosis does not require treatment. Acidosis should be managed by spe-cific treatment of the cause; intravenous sodium bicarbonate increases body sodium. Hypokalaemia (potassium less than 3.5 mmol/l) is corrected by adding potassium chloride to intravenous fluids. The serum potassium is not increased above 4.0 mmol/l if liver transplantation is an option, as graft reperfusion may precipitate hyperkalaemia. Addition of sodium chloride to intravenous fluids is not indicated in the presence of hypona-traemia unless there is clear evidence of excessive loss of sodium. Sudden changes in sodium concentration should be avoided; they have been caus-ally related to central pontine myelinolysis.

Cerebral oedema and raised intracranial pressure

Hepatic encephalopathy in fulminant hepatic failure may be compounded by cerebral oedema and raised intracranial pressure, hypoglycaemia, hyp-oxia, renal failure, and acid–base/electrolyte changes. Cerebral oedema pre-cedes raised intracranial pressure and is not always demonstrable on CT scan; it may be indicated by a loss of demarcation between grey and white matter. To avoid precipitating an increase in intracranial pressure, patients are nursed in a quiet room with the trunk and head elevated 40°; jugular venous compression is avoided. To measure intracranial pressure, direct monitoring is necessary. A parietal or temporal bur hole is required to place an extradural or subdural pressure transducer. This procedure is controversial—it is potentially hazardous due to the coagulopathy and should be undertaken by a neurosurgeon in an operating theatre. Epidural monitoring is safer, but less accurate, than subdural monitoring. The cere-bral perfusion pressure (mean arterial pressure minus intracranial pres-sure) should be maintained at a minimum of 60 mmHg. The best time to introduce a transducer is uncertain, but may be when progression to stage III encephalopathy occurs or when the patient becomes a candidate for liver transplantation. Although monitoring intracranial pressure has not been associated with increased survival, it may facilitate optimal manage-ment before liver transplantation. Mannitol has been shown to reduce ele-vated pressures that are not greater than 60 mmHg. It is given as an intravenous bolus of a 20 per cent solution (1 g/kg), which can be repeated every 4 h (0.5 g/kg) if the previous infusion induced a diuresis, plasma osmolarity does not exceed 315 mosmol/l, and azotaemia is not present. Mannitol has variable and potentially deleterious effects on intracranial pressure when the initial pressure is over 60 mmHg, and should probably not be given without prior measurement of intracranial pressure. Thio-pentone (185 to 500 mg intravenously over 15 min), indomethacin, or induced hypothermia may reduce intracranial pressure if mannitol is ineffective. Corticosteroids and controlled hyperventilation do not appear to be effective treatments.

Haemorrhagic diathesis

The haemorrhagic diathesis requires no treatment in the absence of overt bleeding. Vitamin K (10 mg) is usually given intravenously, in spite of the low risk of inducing anaphylaxis. Fresh frozen plasma is not given routinely, so that plasma levels of clotting factors can be used as indices of prognosis. Skin puncture sites may require protracted pressure to achieve haemostasis. Administration of an H_2-antagonist to maintain gastric pH above 5.0 decreases transfusion requirements in fulminant hepatic failure; dose reduction may be necessary in the presence of renal failure. Infusion of platelets and fresh frozen plasma may be indicated to cover invasive procedures. Clotting factor concentrates, which exacerbate disseminated intravascular coagulation, are contraindicated. Heparin is not indicated for mild disseminated intravascular coagulation. Standard regimens of endoscopic diagnosis and therapy are instituted when haemorrhage occurs from the gastrointestinal tract. A haematocrit of at least 30 to 35 per cent should be maintained. A substantial increase in intracranial pressure may be due to an intracranial haemorrhage and is an indication for a CT scan of the head.

Hypoglycaemia

Hypoglycaemia must be prevented. Dextrose is administered intravenously to maintain a plasma glucose of 60 to 200 mg/dl. Occasionally, massive amounts of dextrose are required (for example more than 2 kg).

Cardiovascular changes

Maintenance of a normal blood pressure may reduce the risk of cerebral oedema or lessen its severity. Ionotropes may increase tissue hypoxia and have not been shown to be beneficial. However, if sepsis is suspected as a cause of hypotension, an ionotrope infusion may be warranted. If hypertension occurs, hypotensive or vasodilator drugs, which might adversely affect intracranial pressure, are not given. Arrhythmias may subside with correction of hypoxia, or acid–base or electrolyte disturbances.

Hepatorenal syndrome

Optimization of blood volume by infusing 20 per cent albumin may transiently improve renal function by correcting haemodynamic disturbances. Care is taken not to overload the circulation to avoid an adverse effect on intracranial pressure. Any therapeutic agents that may contribute to impaired renal function, including diuretics, are avoided. Severe acid–base/electrolyte disturbances or fluid overload, and rarely azotaemia, may be an indication for ultrafiltration or renal dialysis. Such procedures, which must be undertaken carefully because of cardiovascular instability and coagulopathy, may be necessary to optimize a patient's condition before liver transplantation, but would not be expected to alter the course of the hepatic or renal dysfunction. In the presence of raised intracranial pressure, ultrafiltration is preferred. Continuous venous access may be obtained using a double-lumen tube. The left femoral vein may not be used to facilitate venovenous bypass during liver transplantation. Use of vasopressin analogues is experimental.

Hepatopulmonary syndrome

No attempt should be made to correct hyperventilation. Hypoxaemia is an indication for 100 per cent oxygen by face mask. Endotracheal intubation is recommended at the onset of stage III encephalopathy. A tube large enough to permit bronchoscopy should be used. The procedure may be facilitated by curarization. Assisted mechanical ventilation is indicated for patients with stage IV encephalopathy, respiratory failure (increasing P_{CO_2}), or pulmonary oedema. Positive end-expiratory pressure, which may reduce hepatic blood flow and increase intracranial pressure, should be avoided.

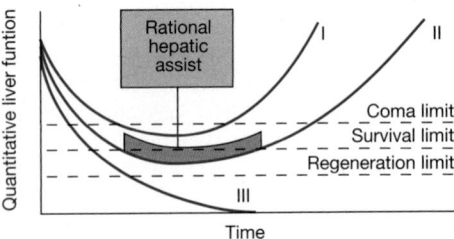

Fig. 7 Three hypothetical courses of fulminant hepatic failure (as envisaged by N. Tygstrup). In group I patients, liver function deteriorates below the coma limit, but does not fall below the survival limit; these patients should survive with intensive conventional medical supportive care alone. In group II patients, liver function deteriorates below the survival limit, but, if it can be maintained above this limit for a sufficient time by providing effective temporary hepatic support (rational hepatic assist), liver function would not fall below the regeneration limit and these patients should also survive. In group III patients, liver function deteriorates below the survival and regeneration limits irrespective of whether temporary hepatic support is provided. Liver transplantation offers the only hope of survival for group III patients. To facilitate optimal selection of patients for temporary hepatic support and liver transplantation, it is necessary to develop reliable criteria that indicate which course an individual patient will follow.

Convalescence

Abstinence from alcohol for a period of 6 months is recommended after recovery from an episode of acute liver failure not precipitated by alcohol. If alcohol was implicated in such an episode, lifelong abstinence is advocated. Other identified precipitants, such as halothane, must be rigorously avoided.

Temporary hepatic support

The original rationale for providing temporary hepatic support was based on the assumption that the hepatic lesion in fulminant hepatic failure is potentially reversible, provided that the patient can be kept alive sufficiently long for hepatic regeneration to take place. Theoretically, the patient selected for treatment with temporary hepatic support would die if treated by conventional intensive supportive care alone and would survive if the functions of the liver could be provided artificially over a finite period (Fig. 7). Temporary hepatic support should not only maintain the general condition of the patient, but also prevent life-threatening complications of fulminant hepatic failure. As there is a lack of detailed understanding of the biochemical disturbances that need to be corrected in fulminant hepatic failure, the design of artificial liver support systems has been largely empirical. Attempts have been made to (i) remove substances that have accumulated in the body using non-biological systems, such as charcoal haemoperfusion; (ii) provide deficient factors normally synthesized by the liver as well as clear accumulated substances using biological systems, for example haemoperfusion using devices containing hepatocyte preparations; and (iii) combine both approaches (hybrid systems). It has not yet been established that the risk/benefit ratio associated with application of any liver support device favours the patient. The provision of temporary hepatic support in the management of chronic irreversible liver disease (such as cirrhosis) may be limited to preparing a patient for liver transplantation. When a patient with fulminant hepatic failure or cirrhosis is a candidate for liver transplantation, effective temporary hepatic support may not only reduce operative or perioperative mortality but may also beneficially increase the waiting time for a donor liver.

Further reading

Basile AS, Jones EA, Skolnick P (1991). The pathogenesis and treatment of hepatic encephalopathy: evidence for the involvement of benzodiazepine receptor ligands. *Pharmacological Reviews* **43**, 27–71.

Batkai S, *et al.* (2001). Endocannabinoids acting at vascular CB$_1$ recptors mediate the vasodilated state in advanced liver cirrhosis. *Nature Medicine* 7, 827–32.

Blei AT, Butterworth RF, eds (1997). Hepatic encephalopathy. *Seminars in Liver Disease* 16, 233–338.

Chang S-W, Ohara N, eds (1996). The lung in liver disease. *Clinics in Chest Medicine* 17, 1–169.

Gines P, Arroyo V, Rodes J (1998). Ascites and hepatorenal syndrome: pathogenesis and treatment strategies. *Advances in Internal Medicine* 43, 99–142.

Jones EA, Weissenborn K (1997). Neurology and the liver. *Journal of Neurology, Neurosurgery and Psychiatry* 63, 279–93.

Pappas SC, Jones EA (1983). Methods for assessing hepatic encephalopathy. *Seminars in Liver Disease* 3, 298–307.

Williams R, ed. (1996). Fulminant hepatic failure. *Seminars in Liver Disease* 16, 341–444.

14.21.4 Liver transplantation

Graeme J. M. Alexander and M. Allison

Introduction

Pioneer work in the dog in the 1950s laid the basis for human liver transplantation, which was first undertaken in 1968 but liver transplantation was only established as a treatment for human therapy for liver failure in the mid 1980s. The number of centres and countries providing liver transplant services and the number of recipients continue to rise, accompanied by a combination of increased surgical and anaesthetic competence, more effective immune suppression, and improved organ preservation.

Liver transplantation services are now part of a sophisticated, multidisciplinary specialty. One-year survival of over 90 per cent should be achieved for low-risk elective cases. Successful liver transplantation enables most patients with severe liver disease to return to normal life.

The donor organ

Size match between donor and recipient is critical. Transplantation can be performed across the ABO barrier in exceptional circumstances but at the expense of long-term graft function. Matching for blood group is routine. Donor organ quality has a major impact on the immediate postoperative outcome and is influenced by many factors including experience of the surgical retrieving team, ensuring adequate, healthy artery, vein, and bile duct for the anastomoses. The introduction of cold University of Wisconsin solution *in situ* to the donor organ has prolonged the acceptable cold ischaemia time and transplantation can now be undertaken during working hours.

Fatty changes in the donor liver (the most common cause of primary graft non-function and the most frequent reason that a retrieval team refuse a liver) is important since such livers are less tolerant of cold and warm ischaemia. Relative donor shortage, increasing waiting lists, and prolonged waiting time compel the use of donors of marginal viability. Early postoperative graft function is likely to become more prevalent. Learning to use donor livers of impaired quality is a critical area for future research.

Surgical aspects

After recipient hepatectomy, the donor liver is implanted into the abdomen and anastomoses of the upper inferior vena cava, portal vein, lower inferior vena cava, and the hepatic artery are carried out. Surgeons may have to improvise the hepatic artery anastomosis, since about 20 per cent of donor hepatic arteries have anomalous anatomy. Venovenous bypass with extracorporeal circulation of blood via the portal vein back into the systemic circulation is associated with improved outcome in difficult cases and reduced rates of renal failure and sepsis.

Biliary anastomosis is carried out end-to-end, duct-to-duct unless there are doubts about the vascular supply to the biliary tree, with a second or subsequent transplant, or with biliary tract disease when a Roux loop is used. Whether this is appropriate in primary sclerosing cholangitis is contentious, since residual biliary tissue may retain a risk of future cholangiocarcinoma. In the past, the gall bladder was used as a conduit between recipient and donor ducts and was associated with a high rate of biliary strictures and gallstones.

Living-related donation has the advantages of a planned procedure, avoidance of cold ischaemia, minimal warm ischaemia time, and donor/recipient relatedness. However, the risk to such donors is not negligible. Auxiliary transplantation is one option for metabolic disease and acute liver failure but is not established because of difficulties in establishing an additional supply of blood. In an era of donor shortage, split livers are attractive, whereby the liver is divided and offered to two recipients, is an attractive option. Multiple organ transplantation is associated with reduced rates of rejection of organs transplanted with the liver, at the expense of prolonged delay waiting for a suitable donor.

Complication rates are higher in paediatric recipients because of size, the increased likelihood of in congenital anomalies and the use of 'cut-down' livers. Previous surgery is associated with an increased risk of haemorrhage. Established portal vein thrombosis is also a relative contraindication to transplantation.

Indications

There are no fixed rules for liver transplantation, which should be considered for patients with progressive disease where death is a likely end point (Table 1). It should be considered for patients with poor quality of life (a subjective assessment) who are able to withstand the procedure. For certain disorders guidelines are available to aid decisions.

Table 1 Indications for liver transplantation

Acute liver failure
Paracetamol overdose
Viral hepatitis
hepatitis A
hepatitis B
non-A, non-B hepatitis
Drugs
Subacute liver failure
Viral hepatitis
Autoimmune hepatitis
Budd–Chiari syndrome
Chronic liver disease
Chronic viral hepatitis
hepatitis C
hepatitis B
Alcoholic liver disease
Primary biliary cirrhosis
Primary sclerosing cholangitis
Autoimmune hepatitis
Haemochromatosis
Wilson's disease
Tumours
Metabolic disease

Complications of liver disease

Liver transplantation may be used to treat the complications of liver disease: hepatic encephalopathy, ascites, subacute bacterial peritonitis, variceal haemorrhage (particularly gastric varices), jaundice, malnutrition, hepatic osteodystrophy, hepatopulmonary syndrome, hepatorenal syndrome, reversed portal vein flow, and superimposed hepatocellular carcinoma.

Early referral

Early referral allows time for the introduction of the patient to the concept of liver transplantation and improves outcome. Patients with a small body habitus and blood group O have a prolonged wait and should be assessed early. Increasing age, renal dysfunction, poor nutritional status, high Child–Pugh score, and jaundice are associated with a poor outcome.

Assessment

As well as assessing the severity of their underlying liver disease, patients should be assessed for fitness for surgery. The presence of hepatopulmonary syndrome and pulmonary hypertension might complicate anaesthesia, but are not absolute contraindications. Some patients require psychiatric evaluation for alcohol or drug addiction. Early nutritional assessment is advised, to address weight loss in advance.

Accepted contraindications

Patients with AIDS and those with viraemia would not be considered without introduction of antiviral therapy. Extrahepatic malignancy is considered a contraindication, with the exceptions of neuroendocrine tumours and some cases of haemangioendothelioma. Metastatic disease involving liver is a contraindication.

Relative contraindications

The presence of HIV antibody may be regarded as a contraindication, despite an adequate CD4 count and absence of viraemia. Age alone is not a contraindication. Severe psychiatric disease requires psychiatric assessment. Continued alcohol or substance abuse, or a history of recidivism, are relative contraindications. Portal vein thrombosis in the absence of an adequate alternative vessel is a surgical contraindication. The likelihood of non-compliance with hospital attendances and immunosuppressive medication is difficult to assess but those deemed incapable of complying with these demands should not be considered.

Waiting list

Whilst waiting for transplantation, patients may develop new complications of their liver disease. Sepsis is common and requires suspension from the waiting list for treatment. Hyponatraemia (<125 mmol/l) is a risk factor and should be corrected in advance to avoid the risk of central pontine myelinolysis. Non-specific deterioration should prompt imaging of the portal vein and liver for new thrombosis or tumour respectively, and a search for sepsis. A proportion of patients develop the hepatorenal syndrome whilst under surveillance.

Specific disorders

Acute liver failure

Compared with chronic liver disease, the outcome for acute liver failure is less favourable (Table 2). However, the patients are often younger and may be cured by transplantation. For patients with paracetamol (acetoaminophen) poisoning, the decision to proceed to transplantation is made on the basis of prothrombin time, bilirubin, hepatic encephalopathy, renal failure, and acidosis; late rises in prothrombin time denote a grave prognosis and often indicate the presence of sepsis. Such patients require psychiatric

Table 2 Patient survival (data from European Liver Transplant Registry, January 1988 to December 1996)

	Number	Patient survival at 1 year (%)
All patients	19381	76
Acute liver failure		
Fulminant hepatic failure	1311	61
Subacute liver failure	101	69
Hepatic malignancy		
Hepatocellular carcinoma	1344	67
Cholangiocarcinoma	124	58
Cirrhosis		
Virus-related cirrhosis	4631	77
Alcoholic liver disease	2954	80
Primary biliary cirrhosis	1939	81
Primary sclerosing cholangitis	881	81
Autoimmune cirrhosis	436	78
Budd–Chiari syndrome	209	73
Wilson's disease	182	86
Secondary biliary cirrhosis	126	82

assessment at the earliest opportunity to identify treatable conditions and to assess future compliance with medication and follow-up.

For patients with acute liver failure of other cause (drugs, hepatitis A, hepatitis B) the decision to proceed to transplantation is based on considerations of age, aetiology, jaundice to encephalopathy time, bilirubin, and prothrombin time.

Subacute hepatic failure

The prolonged period between onset of jaundice and encephalopathy allows patients with subacute hepatic failure to be identified. These are likely to survive long enough to be offered a liver and have an excellent outcome. Without transplantation, most patients with subacute hepatic failure die.

Chronic liver disease

Primary biliary cirrhosis

Several models have justified the introduction of transplantation for patients with primary biliary cirrhosis based on knowledge about life expectancy without liver transplantation. Such analyses are useful in decision making since definitive, controlled trials have never been done. A bilirubin in excess of 100 µmol/l predicts high mortality without transplantation. Some patients require transplantation because of extreme fatigue and pruritus prior to the onset of significant jaundice.

Primary sclerosing cholangitis

Patients suffering from primary sclerosing cholangitis are amongst the hardest to assess for liver transplantation. The presence of frequent episodes of jaundice, increasing jaundice, or cholangitis should prompt consideration of liver transplantation. There is a significant lifetime risk of cholangiocarcinoma (which would be a contraindication) and an ever-present concern that it may have evolved. Patients with primary sclerosing cholangitis should be considered for a transplant early in the course of their illness rather than late. Measurement of serum CA19.9 identifies patients with an evolving cholangiocarcinoma, but this value can rise very significantly in the presence of severe biliary disease and sepsis and should not be relied upon alone. Inflammatory bowel disease should be sought and treated before transplantation, even when asymptomatic.

Autoimmune hepatitis

Transplantation is indicated for complications of autoimmune hepatitis, poor control despite adequate therapy, or those patients who are slow to achieve control or escape control with immunosuppressant drugs.

Chronic viral hepatitis

Patients with chronic hepatitis B virus infection (HBV), chronic hepatitis C virus infection (HCV), and chronic hepatitis D virus infection (HDV) should be considered on merit according to the presence or absence of the complications of chronic liver disease and symptoms.

Alcohol

Patients with alcoholic liver disease undoubtedly constitute the most contentious group: liver transplantation is restricted largely to those with progressive disease despite abstinence. Most centres insist on complete abstinence from alcohol, first because the liver disease improves with prolonged abstinence and second because it is thought that patients who are able to maintain abstinence for six months have a lower risk of recidivism after transplantation. Assessment of abstinence is difficult and the ethics of random testing for alcohol abuse without consent are complex. It is important that details of any contract between patient and doctor are recorded accurately. In practice, those patients able to maintain a stable home life, job, and partner are more likely to be offered a liver transplant than those who are homeless, jobless, and isolated.

Tumours

For the treatment of hepatocellular carcinoma evolving on a background of cirrhosis, there are two options—resection and liver transplantation. Resection is unrealistic for most with cirrhosis and restricted to those with accessible tumours and Child–Pugh class A. Transplantation is indicated for those with a low risk of tumour recurrence. Accurate assessment of the extent of disease is therefore critical. Patients with tumours greater than 5 cm, or more than three nodules, or evidence of extrahepatic disease are likely to have recurrent disease after the transplant procedure. Radiological assessment of the extent of disease usually includes multiple modalities (hepatic angiogram, CT, MR, and ultrasound scans). Despite this, capsular or vascular invasion is often discovered at the time of transplantation.

The fibrolammellar variant of hepatocellular carcinoma usually occurs in young patients without cirrhosis and is probably more slow growing. However, resection is more appropriate for this group but although the 5-year survival figures for fibrolammellar disease are good, a significant risk of tumour recurrence remains.

Cholangiocarcinoma

The risk of postoperative recurrence is so high that this condition is regarded as a contraindication to hepatic transplantation.

Neuroendocrine tumour

Where disease is limited to the liver with a long lead-time, transplant offers reasonable 5-year survival. Recurrence after transplantation is frequent, although recurrent disease may be amenable to other strategies—chemotherapy, hormone modulation, radiotherapy, and direct tumour ablation.

Haemangioendothelioma

The reported prognosis after transplantation varies from early recurrence to none. A firm recommendation is impossible and the decision to go ahead with the procedure is often based on factors other than histology.

Budd–Chiari syndrome

Patients with acute liver failure in relation to the Budd-Chiari Syndrome should be managed as any other patient with acute liver failure. For chronic disease, there are alternative approaches, including surgical shunts and transplantation. One expressed view is that liver transplantation is the most reliable and effective shunt procedure. Most patients with Budd–Chiari syndrome have an underlying disorder predisposing to thrombosis, which should be thoroughly investigated and treated before the transplantation procedure is carried out.

Metabolic/genetic disease

Transplantation is successful in a number of metabolic/genetic disorders associated with liver disease, including Wilson's disease, α-1-antitrypsin deficiency (with maintained respiratory function), Gaucher's disease, glycogen storage disease, Crigler–Najar syndrome, and Bylers syndrome. Patients with haemochromatosis have increased morbidity, perhaps as a consequence of associated disorders (diabetes and cardiomyopathy), as well as an increased incidence of sepsis in the early postoperative stages that may be related to systemic iron overload.

Polycystic liver disease rarely requires liver transplantation but where associated with renal polycystic disease, combined liver/kidney transplantation is considered. The Rendu–Osler–Weber syndrome may be associated with hepatic haemangiomas causing portal hypertension or shunting that result in biliary ischaemia, and thus is best treated by liver transplantation.

Patients with cystic fibrosis represent a difficult group, presenting with portal hypertension and cardiorespiratory disease requiring heart/lung transplantation. Waiting for a triple organ donation for a recipient with a small body habitus may be futile, while proceeding with single organ transplantation in a patient with several diseased organs that will ultimately require transplantation procedures in their own right, may also be mistaken.

Metabolic disorder with a structurally normal liver

Patients with a structurally normal liver have undergone liver transplantation for hypercholesterolaemia and hyperoxaluria. In the former, it is essential to address the cardiovascular complications before transplantation. For the latter, it is important to recognize that the kidneys transplanted simultaneously remain at risk of oxalate-induced damage for several years after otherwise successful hepatic transplantation has been carried out.

Complications

Immediate

The most immediate, usual complication of transplantation is perioperative haemorrhage.

The presence of one or more of: coma following withdrawal of sedation, a rapidly rising prothrombin time, acidosis, high insulin requirement, thrombocytopenia, and hyperkalaemia, prompts consideration of three diagnoses—primary non-function of the graft, non-thrombotic graft infarction, or vascular thrombosis. Imaging of the hepatic artery and portal vein with ultrasound and angiography may greatly aid distinction between these possibilities. The patient may need a further hepatic graft as an emergency and delay in this situation can be catastrophic for survival.

Hyperacute rejection of the liver is rare (in contrast to the kidney) and liver transplantation can be undertaken successfully in the presence of a positive cross-match.

Early

Hepatic artery thrombosis may be identified by worsening liver function tests (confirmed by ultrasound and/or angiography), by ischaemia seen on liver biopsy, or biliary leak due to ischaemia of the bile duct. Portal vein thrombosis may present with either an ischaemic graft (less acute than that seen in the immediate postoperative phase) or the presence of ascites. Caval stricture might present with rapid accumulation of ascites and peripheral oedema. With an abdominal drain *in situ*, many litres of ascites might need to be removed daily. Cholangitis can be recognized by fever, neutrophilia, pain, and jaundice. A stricture should be sought by ultrasound.

Acute rejection

Acute rejection of the grafted organ may present with pain, fever and jaundice. Most often however, acute rejection is identified by noting a deterioration in liver biochemistry (particularly bilirubin) associated with peripheral blood eosinophilia. A liver biopsy is essential to determine severity and may confirm the presence of tissue eosinophils in association with lymphoblasts. The target tissues are bile duct and endothelial cells (hepatic artery, portal vein, and, less frequently, central vein). Not all acute rejection requires therapy but patients with acute rejection are prescribed supplemental high-dose corticosteroids. Severe rejection, steroid resistant rejection, and multiple episodes of acute rejection carry a poor long-term prognosis for the graft.

Graft-versus-host disease

Graft-versus-host disease is characterized by a skin eruption, gastrointestinal disturbance, and malnutrition. Often, patients with graft-versus-host disease are malnourished, have alcohol-related liver disease, are lymphopenic, and do not develop acute rejection. The diagnosis is confirmed by identification of host and recipient lymphocytes in the circulation. The best form of therapy is likely to be monoclonal antibody directed against activated T cells. Overall, the prognosis is poor.

Hepatic artery and portal vein strictures

These are identified usually as a consequence of abnormal liver biochemistry or a slow recovery following transplantation; occasionally, however, liver biochemistry may be normal. Ultrasound is unreliable for identification of vascular strictures and CT perfusion scanning or angiography are recommended.

Biliary strictures

Persistent elevation of the alkaline phosphatase and an ultrasound revealing intrahepatic duct dilatation reveal strictures of two types. The most common is anastomotic and usually amenable to dilatation at ERCP. With recurrence, reconstruction should be considered. A hilar stricture should prompt a search for ischaemia. In these circumstances reconstruction and/or retransplantation are considered.

Bacterial infection

Bacterial sepsis is common in chest, urine, blood, abdomen, and intravascular cannulae. There is no universal recommendation for antibiotics although most physicians recommend the use of antimicrobial prophylaxis for up to 48 h. Thereafter, antimicrobial therapy is based on careful observation, clinical assessment, culture, and local knowledge of likely pathogens.

Viral infections

Herpes simplex virus infections are often clinically apparent and can be managed with topical acyclovir, unless there is a suspicion of systemic disease, requiring parenteral acyclovir. It seems probable that genital herpes will also be reactivated.

In the past, cytomegalovirus (CMV) infection has been the principal viral cause of infection in this period but there have been significant advances in the past decade. Prophylaxis with oral ganciclovir to prevent clinical expression of disease has proved effective but it may occur with reduced severity once ganciclovir is withdrawn at 3 months. For patients who have completed prophylaxis and recipients with antibody at transplantation, recrudescence or infection with a donor strain can be investigated by means of PCR for CMV DNA in serum. CMV viraemia is associated closely with clinical disease, affecting the gastrointestinal tract, central nervous system, respiratory system, the bone marrow, retina, and liver. Patients who become CMV PCR positive should receive systemic ganciclovir. Newer, quantitative assays might guide therapy more accurately. Ganciclovir resistance has been reported. Shingles is a common complication of the early postoperative period and should be treated with systemic antiviral therapy with acyclovir. Amitriptyline and carbamazepine reduce the risk of postneuralgic syndrome.

Fungal infections

Candidal species are isolated commonly and prophylaxis is in routine use. Fluconazole is effective, but drug interactions, particularly with immunosuppressive agents, may render its use problematic. Oral therapy with nystatin or amphotericin is recommended at a later stage, up to 3 months. Systemic candidal or *Aspergillus* infections are more likely in those with severe liver disease, ischaemic grafts, a poor postoperative course, and renal impairment.

Protozoal infections

Co-trimazole prophylaxis for lymphopenia has almost eradicated *Pneumocystis carinii* infection in many centres. Toxoplasmosis is rare since the introduction of prophylaxis with pyrimethamine or co-trimazole for 6 weeks for patients with prior serological evidence of infection.

Late

Multiple biliary strictures may present with recurrent cholangitis and may be a late expression of ischaemia. A proportion comes ultimately to retransplantation, usually after a period of years.

Lymphoproliferative disease

This affects 2 to 4 per cent of patients and is less common with liver than with other solid organ grafts. Usually the disorder is a B-cell lymphoma and most are Epstein–Barr virus related. The most frequent location for lymphoma is the liver. Management is by reducing immunosuppression to a minimum and chemotherapy according to conventional guidelines.

Carcinoma

There is a substantial increase in the incidence of almost all carcinomas, including squamous and other skin cancers.

Osteodystrophy

A large proportion of patients has severe bone disease at presentation, which then worsens so that there is an increased fracture rate in the postoperative period. The severity of bone disease has improved considerably over the past decade because of the reduced dose of corticosteroids used. Bone mass improves significantly over the first 2 to 3 years after transplantation but it is wise to use bisphosphonates (and sex hormones) for patients who show clear evidence of reduced bone density.

Chronic rejection

This is a devastating consequence of liver transplantation and is rarely reversible. It can be predicted on the basis of severe acute rejection, steroid-resistant acute rejection, or multiple episodes of acute rejection. It leads to graft loss and the requirement for a further transplant. It is uncertain what the main target for the process is and the precise immunological nature of the process remains to be determined. However, the main branches of the hepatic artery become obliterated with foamy macrophages and the histological pattern resembles chronic rejection of other solid organs. Bile ducts are lost (the vanishing bile duct syndrome), probably as a consequence of chronic ischaemia.

Cardiovascular disease

Patients who have undergone liver transplantation have a significant increase in their cardiovascular risk profile in the early postoperative phase, which extends long term. It is probable that this represents a consequence of immunosuppression, since hyperlipidaemia, hypertension, renal impairment, and weight gain are common features.

Recurrent disease

It is recognized that immunosuppressive regimes should be modified according to the primary indication for transplant, especially for prevention or treatment of recurrent graft disease.

Hepatitis B virus

Serum HBV DNA at the time of transplantation or the presence of HBcAg in host liver predicts accurately the likelihood that the graft will become infected with HBV. Graft infection without treatment is associated with a significant morbidity and mortality such that in the 1990s many patients with HBV were not considered.

The situation has been revolutionized. Hepatitis B immunoglobulin, although expensive, reduces the rate of graft infection, particularly in those HBV DNA negative in serum at the time of transplantation. Lamivudine prevents graft infection if given prior to transplantation and is effective therapy for graft infection. Regrettably, lamivudine resistance evolves rapidly and mutated virus can cause liver damage. Adefovir for patients with lamivudine resistant virus post-transplantation has been useful and resistance to the combination has not yet been reported. The role of adefovir in preventing graft infection has not been assessed. Corticosteroids should be withdrawn by week 6 and maintenance on single therapy with tacrolimus rather than cyclosporin is recommended.

Hepatitis C virus

HCV infects the graft inevitably, and is associated with a rapidly progressive fibrosis which is not usual in HCV-positive patients not treated by hepatic transplantation. A significant proportion of patients have cirrhosis by 5 to 10 years and a small proportion of patients lose the graft to HCV infection within 1 to 2 years of transplantation. Trials of interferon-α and ribavirin in the transplant setting are underway but there is no evidence yet that this combination is able to prevent graft infection or to prevent liver damage once graft infection occurs. Most established transplant units recommend minimal immunosuppression for this group of patients.

Autoimmune hepatitis

Undoubtedly this can affect the graft and cause graft loss. It may be predicted in advance of significant deterioration by monitoring immunoglobulins. A small proportion of patients develops 'autoimmune hepatitis' de novo. Triple therapy with long-term azathioprine and long-term low dose prednisolone, tacrolimus, or cyclosporin is advised.

Primary sclerosing cholangitis

This may affect the graft and is associated with an increased incidence of biliary complications. Immunosuppression does not appear to prevent recurrence in the graft, which may be lost.

Primary biliary cirrhosis

This can affect the graft and cause graft loss. It appears that immunosuppression does not prevent recurrence. Indeed, cirrhosis with portal hypertension has occurred within 2 years of grafting for this indication.

Alcohol

Recidivism for alcoholism and the development of alcohol-related liver disease after transplantation for alcohol-related disease are well recognized but uncommon. Liver damage can lead to graft loss within a period of 12 months if the consumption of alcohol is resumed.

Immune regulation

Tolerance

Tolerance is probably rare and there are no adequate tests to identify tolerance in human grafts when it does occur. Studies of liver tissue in well patients with normal liver biochemistry have invariably shown many with abnormal liver histology; only a small minority are normal (and probably tolerant). It is recognized that calcineurin inhibitors prevent the development of tolerance, which is an active process. Nevertheless, these drugs are currently the best available for transplantation. Murine and other animal models indicate that a range of antibodies to T-cell markers can induce tolerance experimentally (including CD4, CD2, CD3, CTLA-4, CD45RB and CD40L).

Immunosuppression

Over the past decade the introduction of additional immunosuppressive agents has been a major therapeutic advance: individual disorders and individual patients can receive tailored therapy (Table 3). Maintenance in the early stages is based on triple therapy—cyclosporin or tacrolimus, which are prescribed indefinitely, azathioprine for 1 year, and prednisolone for a variable period. Our current practice is to stop prednisolone at 3months, adrenal function permitting. The daily dose of prednisolone used nowadays rarely exceeds 20 mg and the daily dose of azathioprine rarely exceeds 1 mg/kg. Large, parenteral doses of prednisolone are given for acute rejection.

Table 3 Immunosuppressive agents

Agent	Mechanism of action	Side-effects
Prednisolone	Acts at a number of levels including inhibition of cytokine gene transcription	Weight gain Hyperglycaemia Osteoporosis
Azathioprine	Metabolized to purine analogue and hence impairs proliferation	Marrow suppression Pancreatitis
Cyclosporin A	Inhibition of signalling downstream of the T-cell receptor	Renal dysfunction Hypertension Hyperlipidaemia Neuropsychiatric
FK506	Inhibition of signalling downstream of the T-cell receptor	Renal dysfunction Hypertension Hyperlipidaemia Neuropsychiatric
Mycophenylate mofetil	Inhibition of de novo purine synthesis, thereby more lymphocyte-specific than azathioprine	Diarrhoea
Rapamycin	Inhibition of interleukin-2 receptor signalling	Poor wound healing Bone pain Peripheral neuropathy
Antilymphocyte globulin (ALG)	Lymphocyte depletion	Profound immunosuppression
Antithymocyte globulin (ATG)	Lymphocyte depletion	Profound immunosuppression
OKT3	T-lymphocyte depletion	Profound immunosuppression

Cyclosporin causes significant cardiovascular morbidity with hypertension, hyperlipidaemia, and weight gain. Neuropsychiatric illness is also reported. Peculiar to cyclosporin is the development of hirsutism and gum hypertrophy, making this particularly unsuitable for females. Renal impairment is a common problem which is probably under-reported and under-recognized. Renal grafting has been required for cyclosporin-induced renal failure.

Tacrolimus

Tacrolimus shares most of the side effect profile of cyclosporin, in particular the cardiovascular complications (hypertension, hyperlipidaemia, and weight gain) as well as neuropsychiatric disease and renal toxicity. The question of whether diabetes mellitus is induced by tacrolimus remains contentious.

Other immunosuppressive agents

Other agents used are unproven and at present lack clear clinical indications. These include rapamycin, which is associated with poor wound healing, bone pain, gastrointestinal upset, bone marrow suppression, and hypertriglyceridaemia. The absence of hypertension, weight gain, or renal toxicity may prove invaluable for those complications arising with calcineurin inhibitors. Mycophenolate mofetil is another unproven agent for liver transplant patients. It reduces cell proliferation in similar fashion to azathioprine but appears to be more lymphocyte-specific—gastrointestinal disturbances are common with this agent.

Antilymphocyte globulin and antithymocyte globulin are T-cell antibodies utilized in the treatment of steroid-resistant acute rejection. Some utilize one or other in the initial induction regime. They carry an increased risk of infection, long-term lymphopenia, and lymphoproliferative disease; the use of these compounds in routine immunosuppression is in decline.

A number of newer, monoclonal antibodies are in development or subject to evaluation in clinical trials. These are directed largely at activated T cells or adhesion molecules. Their clinical role remains to be defined.

Future

Three main areas can be identified for the future development of hepatic transplantation. First, increasing the number and quality of donor livers; at the same time research to improve rescue of damaged donor organs is critically important. Second, donor-specific tolerance remains a goal—in this respect, considerable encouragement has been gained by the successful induction of tolerance in experimental animals as a result of continued world-wide investment in basic transplantation research by immunologists. Finally, improved management of the long-term complications of transplantation, in particular cardiovascular and malignant disease, would greatly extend the duration and quality of life of the many patients who have received donor livers for otherwise fatal hepatic diseases.

Further reading

Balen V, Marsh JW, Rekele J (1999). Liver transplantation. In: Bircher J, Benhamou J-P, McIntyre N, Rizzetto M, Rodes J, eds. *Oxford textbook of clinical hepatology*, 2nd edn, pp. 2039–63. Oxford University Press, Oxford.

Carrithers RL Jr (2000). Liver transplantation: American Association of the Study of Liver Diseases practice guidelines. *Liver Transplantation* **6**, 122–35.

Devlin J, O'Grady J (1999). Indications for referral and assessment in adult liver transplantation: a clinical guideline. *Gut* **45** (Suppl. 6).

Morris RE (1996). Mechanism of action of new immunosuppressive drugs. *Kidney International* (Suppl.), S26–S38.

14.21.5 Primary and secondary liver tumours

Iain M. Murray-Lyon

Benign and malignant tumours may arise in the liver from the hepatocytes, bile-duct epithelium, or supporting mesenchymal tissue. With the exception of hepatocellular carcinoma all the primary malignant tumours are rare, but the liver is frequently the site of secondary (metastatic) deposits of malignant tumours elsewhere in the body.

Hepatocellular carcinoma

This occurs either as a single mass or as scattered nodules of tumour, and in around 80 per cent of patients there is pre-existing cirrhosis. The tumour tends to invade the portal and hepatic veins, and spreads to the abdominal lymph nodes and bone. Histologically the tumour is typically composed of cells resembling hepatocytes, which are arranged in cords. A number of other distinct histological subtypes are now recognized, including the fibrolamellar variant in which clumps of eosinophilic carcinoma cells are surrounded by a characteristic fibrous stroma. This tumour occurs in young adults in a non-cirrhotic liver.

Epidemiology

Although this is a comparatively rare tumour in Western Europe and North America where the annual incidence is around 1 to 2 per 100 000 of the population, there is recent evidence that it is becoming more common, and in Africa and South-East Asia the incidence is 20 to 30 times higher. In patients with underlying cirrhosis, males greatly outnumber females but in non-cirrhotic cases this sex difference is less striking. In areas of high incidence the peak age is in the third and fourth decades of life but in Europe and North America most cases occur in the fifth and sixth decades.

Aetiology

In all countries in the world, cirrhosis, particularly the macronodular form, is present in about 80 per cent of cases. In Western Europe and the United States this is usually due to chronic alcoholism or chronic hepatitis B or C, and at least 10 per cent to 15 per cent of such patients will develop a hepatocellular carcinoma. In Africa and Asia, chronic liver disease is usually associated with hepatitis B or C virus infection. Rare cases may complicate cirrhosis due to other causes, and may follow prolonged use of the oral contraceptive pill or prior investigations using the radioactive contrast agent Thorotrast.

In parts of Africa and the Far East there is increasing evidence implicating aflatoxin. This is a potent carcinogen derived from the mould *Aspergillus flavus*, which often contaminates food.

The hepatitis B virus (**HBV**) is now recognized to have an important role in the development of hepatocellular carcinoma, particularly in areas of high incidence. Long-term, follow-up studies of large numbers of HBV carriers have confirmed that the risk of developing hepatocellular carcinoma is at least 100 times higher than in matched uninfected controls. The HBV can be identified in the tumour as well as the surrounding liver, and integration of viral DNA in the genome of hepatocellular carcinoma has been shown. This HBV DNA integration may result in major structural rearrangements in adjacent cellular DNA, and a range of deletions, duplications, and translocations between chromosomes has been reported. In geographical areas of high endemicity of HBV as well as exposure to aflatoxins, one of a variety of mutations of the *p53* gene on chromosome 17 is a frequent finding. How these molecular events are initiated and progress is still unclear.

The hepatitis C virus (**HCV**) is also closely linked with the development of hepatocellular carcinoma, especially in geographical areas such as North America, Western Europe, and Japan where HBV is not hyperendemic. Almost all cases are associated with cirrhosis. Prospective studies of patients with chronic post-transfusion HCV infection indicate the latent period before tumour development may be as long as 25 to 30 years.

Hepatocellular carcinoma is a largely preventable disease, and the extensive use of hepatitis B vaccination has already led to a reduction in the incidence of this tumour in Taiwan. Until such time as a vaccine against HCV is available, introduction of all possible measures to reduce transmission of this virus is important. Furthermore, there are indications that the successful treatment of chronic hepatitis B and C will reduce the cancer risk.

Clinical features

In Africa and other high-incidence areas, patients usually present with a short history of right upper abdominal pain, often associated with fever and weight loss. There may be considerable abdominal swelling due to liver enlargement, with or without ascites. Catastrophic intraperitoneal bleeding sometimes occurs due to tumour rupture. In low-incidence areas the disease is often more insidious and presents as a general deterioration in the health of a patient already known to have cirrhosis. There is usually hepatomegaly and a bruit may be heard over the liver. A number of non-metastatic systemic manifestations may also rarely occur, such as hypoglycaemia, hypercalcaemia, and porphyria cutanea tarda.

Because of the use of screening in high-risk groups, more small (less than 3-cm diameter), asymptomatic tumours are now being detected.

Investigations

Haematological and biochemical indices

The haematological and biochemical changes, apart from alpha-fetoprotein, are non-specific and reflect the space-occupying lesion as well as the underlying cirrhosis present in about 80 per cent of cases.

Alpha-fetoprotein is a glycoprotein synthesized by the fetal liver and its plasma concentrations reach their maximum at the end of the first trimester (3 to 4 mg/ml) and then decline. After birth, concentrations fall rapidly to adult levels (1 to 10 ng/ml). Raised levels are found in about 80 per cent of patients with hepatocellular carcinoma and tend to be higher in African and Far-Eastern populations than in those in low-incidence areas and in those patients with small tumours. Concentrations above 500 ng/ml in a patient with liver disease are highly suggestive of hepatocellular carcinoma. However, in interpreting alpha-fetoprotein levels it should be remembered that high plasma levels are found in some patients with germinal-cell tumours of the testis and ovary as well as occasional patients with carcinoma of the stomach or pancreas, usually with hepatic metastases. Below 500 ng/ml there is a diagnostic 'grey zone', for such levels may be found in patients with severe viral hepatitis and active cirrhosis. But subsequent readings tend to fall towards normal in patients with these conditions, whereas in patients with hepatocellular carcinoma the levels rise progressively. Sequential readings are therefore of great diagnostic value, and the measurement of hepatoma specific isoforms may improve diagnostic specificity and sensitivity.

Other tumour markers for hepatocellular carcinoma have been described in the serum, including an abnormal vitamin B_{12} binding protein which is usually present with the fibrolamellar histological variant.

Liver imaging

Real-time ultrasound

This is a sensitive and specific test and picks up hepatocellular carcinoma in 85 to 90 per cent of cases. False-negative results usually occur in patients with tumours of less than 2 cm in diameter.

Abdominal computed tomographic (**CT**) scanning

This technique is probably no more accurate in detecting hepatocellular carcinoma than ultrasound and should be reserved for cases in which doubt persists. Sensitivity can be increased by contrast enhancement. Dynamic spiral contrast-enhanced CT scanning is even more sensitive.

Magnetic resonance imaging (MRI)

This technique, particularly with the addition of a contrast agent, is proving useful in identifying and characterizing focal liver masses. Manganese dipyridoxyl diphosphate (**Mn-DPDP**) targets hepatocytes and super-paramagnetic iron oxide (**SPIO**) targets reticuloendothelial cells, resulting in increased prominence of the lesion with respect to normal liver tissue (Fig. 1). Lesions that do not contain reticuloendothelial cells or hepatocytes (haemangiomas and metastases) do not have their signal intensities altered.

Hepatic arteriography

Excellent visualization of the hepatic artery can usually be obtained by selective catheterization using the Seldinger technique. As the major vascular supply to a hepatocellular carcinoma is usually arterial, diagnostic changes are seen in a high proportion of cases. Information gained on the

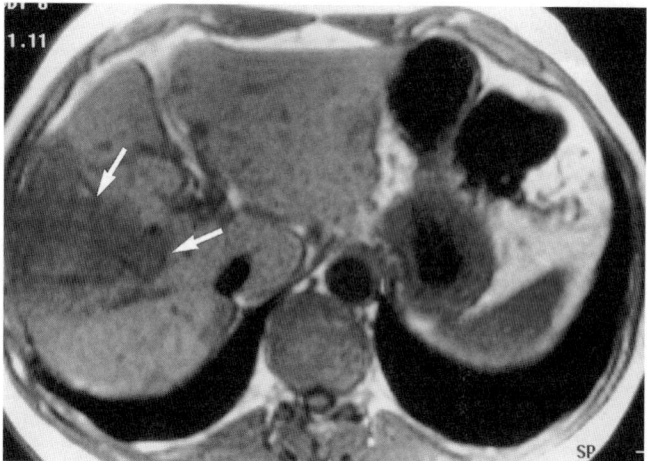

(a)

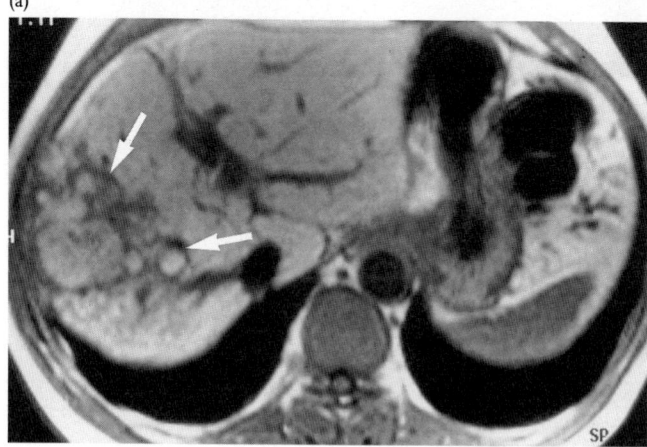

(b)

Fig. 1 (a) Axial T_1-weighted image through the liver in a patient with hepatitis C. An ill-defined area of reduced signal in the right lobe of the liver at the junction of segments 7 and 8 is suspicious for a liver tumour (arrowed). (b) Axial T_1-weighted image through the liver in the same patient following an infusion of Mn-DPDP, a hepatocyte specific contrast agent. There is a general increased signal in the normal liver and a heterogeneous increased signal in the liver tumour, characteristic of uptake by a hepatocellular carcinoma (arrowed).

anatomical distribution of the tumour and the vascular anatomy is essential if surgical resection or transplantation is being contemplated, and consideration can also be given at the time of arteriography to intra-arterial chemotherapy and hepatic artery embolization. The sensitivity of arteriography can be increased by combining it with dynamic spiral CT scanning together with late films to show the portal venous system, as well as injection of the iodine-containing contrast medium Lipiodol. CT scanning 10 to 14 days later can visualize Lipiodol selectively retained in tumours as small as 2 to 3 mm in diameter.

Liver biopsy

For definitive diagnosis, liver biopsy is essential, although this is not always possible because of the prolongation of the prothrombin time. The diagnosis can be considered highly likely without liver biopsy proof if the alpha-fetoprotein level is greater that 500 ng/ml and the hepatic arteriogram shows a tumour circulation. Biopsy may be conveniently done at the time of laparoscopy or ultrasonography and suspicious areas can be sampled under direct vision. Because of the risk of tumour spread, biopsy is often avoided if curative resection or transplantation is planned.

Screening

Patients with an increased risk of developing hepatocellular carcinoma, such as those with cirrhosis or chronic HBV or HCV infection, should be considered for regular screening by alpha-fetoprotein assay and abdominal ultrasonography. While such a strategy has been shown to pick up early tumours, and there is evidence of improved survival figures for these patients in the Far East, the benefits of screening have so far proved disappointing in Europe.

Prognosis

This is a highly malignant tumour and the mean survival in most series is around 4 to 6 months. In Africa the disease tends to run a more malignant course. Patients with cirrhosis have a poorer prognosis than those without. Encapsulated tumours and the fibrolamellar histological variant, as well as small tumours picked-up at screening, have a better prognosis.

Treatment

Curative

Only complete resection or orthotopic transplantation hold out any chance of cure and these procedures should be considered in every case.

Resection

Resection is only possible in about 10 per cent of cases because of underlying cirrhosis or tumour in both lobes. Often a major resection is needed and the anatomical possibilities are illustrated in Fig. 2. In the presence of cirrhosis only a limited resection is possible as liver regeneration is defective, but this procedure may be curative if the tumour is small. In China, screening programmes to detect early hepatocellular carcinoma have led to higher rates of tumour resection in cirrhotic patients and improved long-term survival figures.

The best results are achieved in patients with well-compensated cirrhosis and small tumours (less than 3 cm), but 5-year survival rates of only 20 to 30 per cent are usually quoted due to progression of the underlying liver disease, tumour recurrence, and the development of new tumours.

Transplantation

This is an attractive option for patients with cirrhosis and a hepatocellular carcinoma and the procedure can cure both the tumour and the underlying cirrhosis. Long-term results are best with tumours less than 5 cm in diameter when survival figures up to 70 per cent at 5 years are recorded. The best results are obtained when a hepatocellular carcinoma is discovered incidentally in the resected liver when transplantation is performed for liver failure, and with the fibrolamellar histological variant.

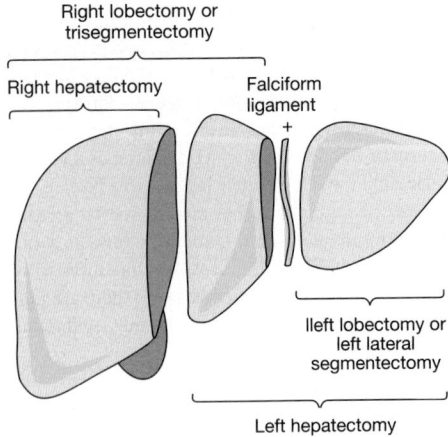

Fig. 2 Diagram to illustrate the main types of hepatic resection.

Palliation

Radiotherapy

External-beam X-irradiation does not produce consistent improvement. Intra-arterial injection of Lipiodol mixed with iodine-131 has given some encouraging preliminary results.

Cytotoxic drugs

Doxorubicin (Adriamycin) is one of the few drugs that may produce worthwhile regression, but only 20 to 30 per cent of cases respond and no survival benefit has been established. Mitoxantrone (mitozantrone), which is structurally similar to doxorubicin, gives a similar response rate and has fewer toxic side-effects.

The presence of hormone receptors in hepatocytes has prompted attempts to modify tumour growth. Results are poor with tamoxifen but octreotide has been reported to be of value.

Targeted therapies

A wide variety of local targeted therapies have been developed and assessed in recent years. Very few, however, have yet been submitted to a prospective, randomized controlled trial.

Percutaneous ethanol injection

Sterile alcohol is injected directly into the tumour under ultrasound guidance causing tumour necrosis. Repeated injections may be given into more than one tumour mass. The best results are obtained with tumours less than 3 cm in diameter and the survival figures are comparable with those of limited surgical resection.

Lipiodol-targeted chemotherapy

Cytotoxic drugs may be emulsified with Lipiodol (see above) and delivered directly into the liver at selective hepatic arteriography. There are some data to show that the duration of action of the drugs is prolonged because of the retention of Lipiodol in the tumour. There is, however, no convincing evidence of benefit.

Transcatheter arterial embolization (**TAE**)

Embolization with foreign materials, such as gel foam, can be achieved at the time of hepatic arteriography and may result in substantial tumour necrosis, particularly in highly vascular tumours, which derive the bulk of their blood supply from the hepatic artery. In patients with decompensated cirrhosis and those with portal vein occlusion the procedure is contraindicated. Broad-spectrum antibiotics are given for some days because of the risk of anaerobic infection in the ischaemic liver. As tumour necrosis is never complete, embolization of the tumour should be combined with targeted chemotherapy (chemoembolization). The gel foam particles may be soaked in doxorubicin or cisplatin or the TAE may be immediately preceded by Lipiodol targeted chemotherapy. While such treatment may result in tumour necrosis, shrinkage, and symptomatic improvement, three controlled trials have not established survival benefit.

Cryoablation and thermal ablation

These techniques are intended to destroy tumour cells by physical means. No controlled trials have been reported. Cryotherapy probes are inserted into the tumour either at laparotomy or laparoscopy and liquid nitrogen is circulated through them. Thermal energy can be applied via probes placed percutaneously in the tumour using either laser, radiofrequency, or microwaves. All three techniques have proved safe, have few side-effects and can be repeated. Current data are insufficient to allow comparison of the efficacy of these ablative techniques.

Cholangiocarcinoma

Carcinoma may arise in any part of the biliary tree from the small intrahepatic bile ducts down to the lower end of the common bile duct. Two clinical varieties occur in the liver—a peripheral form, which consists of one single or multiple nodules; and the much commoner hilar form usually situated at the confluence of the right and left hepatic duct. This invades locally and causes obstruction of the biliary tree. The histological appearances are identical whatever the site of origin. It is an adenocarcinoma with a simple ductular arrangement of columnar or cuboidal cells, usually with a prominent fibrous stroma.

Epidemiology

This tumour is much less common than hepatocellular carcinoma and accounts for about 7 to 10 per cent of primary malignant tumours, except in the Far East where it makes up about 20 per cent. The peak age is in the sixth and seventh decades and the sex incidence shows only a slight male predominance.

Aetiology

Thorium dioxide (Thorotrast) is a well-recognized but rare cause of the intrahepatic variety of the tumour. In the Far East, infestation of one of a variety of distomes (*Clonorchis sinensis*, *Opisthorchis viverrini*) is probably commonly related.

Patients with long-standing ulcerative colitis occasionally develop carcinoma in the biliary tree, and the risk is about 10 times greater than for the general population. Primary sclerosing cholangitis— whether or not associated with inflammatory bowel disease and various types of cystic disease of the biliary tree such an congenital hepatic fibrosis, polycystic disease of the liver, and Caroli's disease—may all be complicated by the development of malignant change. Unlike hepatocellular carcinoma neither long-standing HBV or HCV infection nor cirrhosis seem to predispose to cholangiocarcinoma.

Signs and symptoms

In the peripheral intrahepatic type, patients present with upper abdominal pain, anorexia, malaise, and weight loss. With hilar tumours, jaundice is an early feature. Hepatomegaly is usual and splenomegaly may be found if secondary biliary cirrhosis develops owing to prolonged biliary obstruction.

Diagnosis

The liver function tests show cholestatic features with elevation of bilirubin and alkaline phosphatase levels. Alpha-fetoprotein concentrations are usually normal or only slightly raised. Levels of Ca 19.9 and carcinoembryonic antigen (**CEA**) may also be raised, although sensitivity and specificity do not approach 100 per cent as raised levels are found in obstructive jaundice due to other causes.

Ultrasonography and CT scanning may demonstrate the tumour mass and with hilar tumours show dilatation of the intrahepatic biliary tree. On hepatic angiography the tumour tends to be avascular but encasement and occlusion of vessels occurs. Biliary tree obstruction in the hilum may be demonstrated on MRI cholangiography or by endoscopic retrograde cholangiography (**ERCP**) prior to insertion of a stent (see below).

Prognosis

Most patients deteriorate progressively, with an average survival from diagnosis around 12 to 18 months. If biliary drainage can be achieved in patients with hilar tumours, the prognosis may be better, for these tumours are often slow growing.

Treatment

For the peripheral tumours the principles of treatment are the same as for hepatocellular carcinoma (see above). The response to therapy is disappointing and no controlled trials have been reported. Hilar tumours may sometimes be suitable for curative resection with anastomosis of a Roux loop of jejunum to the biliary tree in the hilum. More usually curative excision is not possible, and the aim must be to establish biliary drainage. A stent can be placed through the growth at laparotomy, or at ERCP, or via the percutaneous transhepatic route thus avoiding surgery. The use of self-expanding metal stents is a recent advance.

Conventional radiotherapy and high-dose local irradiation within the biliary tree by means of iridium-192 wire may sometimes produce useful symptomatic relief. If biliary drainage can be achieved by these procedures, survival for 1 to 2 years is not unusual. Because of the high risk of tumour recurrence, liver transplantation is seldom indicated.

Angiosarcoma (Kupffer-cell sarcoma)

This is a rare tumour consisting of spindle-shaped malignant endothelial cells. It is often multifocal and may arise in a cirrhotic liver.

Considerable progress has been made in identifying aetiological agents. Like hepatocellular carcinoma and cholangiocarcinoma, it occurs in patients who were exposed to Thorotrast 15 to 25 years earlier, and chronic exposure to arsenic has also been implicated. More recently the tumour has been found in workers in the vinyl chloride industry, particularly those exposed to high concentrations of vinyl chloride monomer while cleaning the autoclaves. Since this discovery strict safety regulations have been introduced but because of the long latent period new cases continue to present. A few cases have occurred in long-term androgen takers, but no aetiological factor has yet been identified in the majority of cases. As with other liver tumours, patients present with abdominal pain and hepatic enlargement and blood-stained ascites is common.

This is a highly malignant tumour and curative resection is rarely possible. No form of palliative treatment has so far proved effective.

Epithelioid haemangioendothelioma

This is a rare malignant tumour of vascular endothelial origin with a characteristic histological appearance. It is usually multifocal. It occurs in younger patients than angiosarcoma and does not have the same aetiological associations. The tumour is usually slow growing and prolonged survival has been reported after resection and liver transplantation.

Other primary malignant tumours

These are extremely rare and include fibrosarcoma, leiomyosarcoma, and lymphoma. Children develop both hepatoblastoma and hepatocellular carcinoma.

Hepatic metastases

The liver is a favoured site for metastatic spread and about 50 per cent of malignant tumours in the portal venous drainage area eventually gives rise to hepatic metastases.

Diagnosis

The diagnosis is easy when physical examination reveals a large nodular liver but detection of small or solitary deposits is difficult. Liver function tests may be normal, but the alkaline phosphatase usually rises as the tumour mass enlarges. Ultrasound scanning should pick up tumours greater than 1 cm in diameter but accuracy is greatest when the metastases are large or numerous. The diagnosis can be confirmed by targeted liver biopsy at the time of laparoscopy or ultrasonography.

Prognosis

The prognosis is obviously worse when there is extensive liver replacement by tumour with severe disturbance in liver function tests or ascites. The site of the primary growth is also relevant and deposits from colorectal cancer have a better prognosis (untreated mean survival 9 to 12 months) than most other tumours.

Treatment

The range of possible treatments is the same as has been discussed for hepatocellular carcinoma. Partial hepatectomy to remove deposits may occasionally lead to prolonged survival or cure and, as mentioned above, the results are best in patients with colorectal cancer. A special situation exists with respect to hepatic metastases from the carcinoid tumour. This is often a slow-growing neoplasm and the main problem is the distress caused by flushing and diarrhoea. Resection of tumour bulk with no attempt at total removal often gives symptomatic relief for some years, as does embolization. Transplantation should be considered for slow-growing tumours.

The choice of chemotherapy will be determined by the origin of the primary tumour and this will not be discussed here. As with hepatocellular carcinoma the poor results with systemic chemotherapy led to trials with intra-arterial perfusion. Such treatment has been simplified by the development of implantable pumps, but while objective tumour regression may occur with improved quality of life, as yet there is little convincing evidence that survival is prolonged.

Benign tumours

Haemangioma

This is the most common benign tumour and is usually asymptomatic, being found incidentally either during ultrasonography or CT scanning. Occasionally when large it may cause abdominal pain or shock due to rupture leading to surgical excision.

Although the appearances with ultrasonography are usually diagnostic, it may be necessary to proceed to CT scanning with contrast, angiography, or MRI for diagnostic certainty.

Hepatic adenoma

The incidence of this tumour seems to have increased markedly since the introduction of the oral contraceptive pill, with most reported cases having occurred in females who have been on the pill for 5 years or more. It should be emphasized, however, that the risks for the individual woman is infinitesimal. Patients are often asymptomatic and a mass is discovered on physical examination or incidentally on ultrasound examination. Some patients complain of upper abdominal pain and others present acutely with shock due to intraperitoneal bleeding. The tumour is usually solitary but may be multiple. It consists of cords or acini of hepatocytes without bile ducts or

portal tracts, and fibrous tissue septa are sparse. It may be encapsulated. There is little or no disturbance in liver function and alpha-fetoprotein concentrations are normal.

Ultrasonography shows a focal lesion of variable echogenicity, CT scanning shows marked arterial enhancement and sometimes areas of haemorrhage within the tumour which can be confirmed on MRI scanning.

In some cases the tumour has regressed after withdrawal of the contraceptive pill, but surgical resection is usually recommended because of the risk of intraperitoneal bleeding and the occasional development of malignant change.

Focal nodular hyperplasia

This is a benign condition of uncertain pathogenesis that is frequently confused with hepatic adenoma. The lesion is composed mainly of hepatocytes and Kupffer cells. Typically it has a central stellate scar with radiating septa containing arterial and venous channels and bile ductules. It is much more frequent in women than men, but no relationship to the oral contraceptive pill has been established. The mass is usually solitary and asymptomatic but rupture with intraperitoneal bleeding occasionally occurs. The findings on imaging are often different from those of hepatic adenoma and may allow definitive diagnosis. In particular Doppler ultrasound may show an arterial signal within the tumour, CT scanning or MRI scanning may demonstrate the central stellate scar and biliary scintiscanning may show a late hotspot in the tumour.

The prognosis is excellent and malignant change is not recorded. If the imaging techniques do not provide a definite diagnosis, however, surgical excision is often recommended.

Other benign tumours

These are very much rarer and include fibroma, lipoma, leiomyoma, and cystadenoma.

Further reading

Cherqui D, *et al.* (1995). Management of focal nodular hyperplasia and hepatocellular adenoma in young women: a series of 41 patients with clinical, radiological, and pathological correlations. *Hepatology* **22**, 1674–81.

Clavien P-A, ed. (1999). *Malignant liver tumours. Current and emerging therapies.* Blackwell Science, Malden, MA.

De Groen PC, *et al.* (1999). Biliary tract cancers. *New England Journal of Medicine* **341**, 1368–78.

Mathurin P, *et al.* (1998). Review article: overview of medical treatments in unresectable hepatocellular carcinoma—an impossible meta-analysis? *Alimentary Pharmacology and Therapeutics* **12**, 111–26.

Schafer DF, Sorrell MF (1999). Hepatocellular carcinoma. *Lancet* **353**, 1253–7.

Vauthey J-N, *et al.* (1996). Arterial therapy of hepatic colorectal metastases. *British Journal of Surgery* **83**, 447–55.

Williams R, Rizzi P (1996). Treating small hepatocellular carcinomas. *New England Journal of Medicine* **334**, 728–9.

14.21.6 Hepatic granulomas

C. W. N. Spearman, P. de la Motte Hall, and S. J. Saunders

Introduction

Granulomas are localized collections of modified macrophages, known as 'epithelioid' cells, that have become transformed from a predominantly phagocytic cell to a more secretory cell in response to ingested antigens. The epithelioid cells, which are derived from blood monocytes, have abundant amounts of eosinophilic cytoplasm. Langhans' or foreign body-type giant cells, which form by fusion of the epithelioid cells, are often seen in granulomas. Granulomas are usually surrounded by a rim of mononuclear cells, predominantly lymphocytes. Granulomas may be progressively replaced by collagen.

The aetiology of hepatic granulomas varies with the patient population and geographical origin. In the developed world, sarcoidosis, primary biliary cirrhosis, and drug-induced hepatic granulomas probably account for most, whilst infectious causes such as mycobacterial infections, schistosomiasis, and AIDS-related infections predominate in the developing world.

The diagnosis of granulomatous hepatitis is usually made during the investigation of a systemic illness, frequently presenting as a pyrexia of unknown origin (**PUO**). However, granulomas are found in 10 to 15 per cent of all liver biopsies and may be an unexpected finding. The histomorphology of the granuloma, their distribution in the liver, and special stains, for example Ziehl–Neelsen for mycobacteria and a methenamine silver for fungi, may yield a definite diagnosis.

Pathogenesis

Granuloma formation represents a specialized cellular immune-mediated response involving the presentation of antigen, either endogenous or exogenous, by activated macrophages to CD4 lymphocytes, which are in turn activated by the secretion of macrophage-derived interleukin-1 (IL-2). The activated CD4 lymphocytes secrete interferon, resulting in the upregulation of MHC class II molecules on the surface of the activated macrophages. Upregulation of the HLA DR-positive macrophage and the resulting increased interaction with stimulated CD4 lymphocytes, is accompanied by the consequent increase in IL-2 receptor expression and IL-2 secretion. This results in a clonal increase in the CD4 lymphocytes, leading to the recruitment of B cells which are activated and produce immunoglobulins, antibodies, and autoantibodies. Persistent antigenaemia or poorly degradable antigens, such as chemicals or toxins, provide an ongoing stimulus for the cytokine cascade which results in the focal accumulation of activated lymphocytes and macrophages, with the macrophages undergoing epithelioid transformation.

In infections, the micro-organisms, together with their by-products, are the sensitizing exogenous antigens, whereas in malignancy, or immune complex disease, sensitizing endogenous antigens may trigger an interaction between the activated macrophages and lymphocytes.

Depending on the cause, differences are seen in the above-described structural/functional arrangement of the granuloma. The well-studied sarcoid granuloma has a central core of HLA DR-positive macrophages, epithelioid cells, and giant cells with a peripheral rim of CD4 lymphocytes. The macrophages surrounding the central core are distinguishable from those in the centre by their reactivity with the macrophage monoclonal antibody RFD-1 as opposed to RFD-2. CD8 suppresser cells, and some CD4 cells, may be found at the periphery but not in the centre of the granuloma. The epithelioid cells in sarcoid granuloma secrete a number of compounds, including angiotensin-converting enzyme, lysozyme, glucuronidase, collagenase, elastase, and calcitriol. In AIDS patients with *Mycobacterium avium intracellulare* (**MAI**) infection, there is a paucity of CD4 lymphocytes in the granulomas. While in granulomas infected with *Schistosoma mansoni*, the CD4 cells show increased Th2 co-operation. The granulomas in tuberculoid leprosy contain very few bacilli, while bacilli are profuse in lepromatous leprosy.

Aetiology

The many causes of hepatic granulomas are shown in Table 1. Granulomas are frequently non-specific in appearance and a clinicopathological correl-

ation is essential for diagnosis. In 10 to 30 per cent of hepatic granulomas, the aetiology remains unknown. However, caseating granulomas (Fig. 1 and Plate 1) are characteristic of mycobacterium tuberculosis; the presence of ova and non-caseating granulomas permit the diagnosis of schistosomiasis; fat droplets are seen in the granuloma (lipogranuloma) that accompanies mineral oil ingestion; and fibrin-ring granulomas are highly suggestive of Q fever.

Clinical presentation

Fever (PUO) is the most common presenting symptom. The diverse clinical features, which include weight loss, anorexia, fatigue, hepatosplenomegaly, and abdominal pain, depend on the underlying aetiologies. Serum transaminase activities are frequently normal, but alkaline phosphatase activity may be elevated. Jaundice is uncommon unless there is bile-duct injury, for example primary biliary cirrhosis and sarcoidosis.

Infectious causes

Mycobacterium tuberculosis infection

Tuberculosis is a common cause of hepatic granuloma in the developing world. There may be evidence of pulmonary tuberculosis or of tuberculosis elsewhere, or the patient may present with a pyrexia of unknown origin. Hepatic granulomas are common in miliary tuberculosis. Caseation occurs in about one-third of cases but, while characteristic of tuberculosis, is not unique to it, occurring also in candidiasis, histoplasmosis, and cryptococcosis. Acid-fast bacilli are seen in 10 to 15 per cent of cases, and in 31 per cent of autopsy specimens, and therefore the biopsy must always be cultured. More recently, use of the polymerase chain reaction (**PCR**), based on amplification of IS6110 insertion sequences, was shown to have a sensitivity of 58 per cent in the diagnosis of hepatic granulomas of definitive tuberculosis origin and a specificity of 96 per cent, and is a useful test as it can be performed on paraffin-embedded tissue. BCG vaccination may also cause hepatic granulomas.

HIV/AIDS

Currently more than 30 million people worldwide test positive for the human immunodeficiency virus (**HIV**). Opportunistic infections, especially *Mycobacterium avium intracellulare* (**MAI**), are an important cause of hepatic granulomas in patients with AIDS. The MAI granulomas are composed of epitheliod cells with striated bluish cytoplasm, due to the presence of large numbers of micro-organisms (Fig. 2 and Plate 2).

Histoplasmosis, cryptococcosis, toxoplasmosis, and cytomegalovirus may also cause granulomas in AIDS patients. However, an infectious cause is not always found, presumably there are as yet unidentifiable infections.

Drugs, Hodgkin's disease, and non-Hodgkin's lymphoma may also cause hepatic granulomas in AIDS patients.

Leprosy

Millions of people living in the Indian subcontinent have leprosy and this disease is also common in Africa. Hepatic granulomas are more common in lepromatous leprosy. The diagnosis is usually made from the characteristic skin and peripheral nerve lesions, and only occasionally, the physician is alerted to the diagnosis by the finding of an otherwise unexplained hepatic granuloma.

Histoplasmosis

Histoplasmosis is an important cause of hepatic granuloma in the United States. The fungus may be seen in the granulomas and may be cultured from liver biopsies, blood, or bone marrow. The chest radiograph is usually abnormal and the diagnosis is confirmed serologically.

Q fever

The patients usually present with a PUO or an illness resembling viral hepatitis. The typical granuloma contains inflammatory cells and fat droplets and has a fibrin ring within or at its margin. However, fibrin-ring granulomas may be seen in patients with cytomegalovirus infection, Hodgkin's disease, and leishmaniasis, and in drug reactions to, for example, allopurinol.

Schistosomiasis

Schistosoma japonicum and *Schistosoma mansoni* infestation occurs commonly in Africa, South America, and in the Far East. Ova are usually deposited in the portal tracts within the portal vein radicles where a granulomatous reaction occurs around the ova. Presinusoidal portal hypertension may occur with a 'pipe-stem' cirrhosis. Common presenting features are hepatomegaly and portal hypertension. Eosinophilia also occurs.

Hepatitis C virus (HCV)

Sparse non-caseating hepatic granulomas have been described in patients with chronic hepatitis C infection and in liver-transplanted patients who have subsequent recurrent HCV infections. There is controversy as to whether the presence of hepatic granulomas is predictive of a favourable response to interferon therapy.

Non-infective causes

Sarcoidosis

This is the most common non-infectious cause of hepatic granuloma formation. Although thought to be immunologically mediated, the triggering factor remains unknown. Hepatic granulomas are found in 60 per cent of liver biopsies performed on patients with sarcoidosis.

Well-formed, non-caseating granulomas occur in clusters in the parenchyma and the portal tracts. There may be associated portal fibrosis, which in some patients, progresses though bridging fibrosis to cirrhosis. Other features that are sometimes seen include bile duct damage and loss, which needs to be differentiated from primary biliary cirrhosis, other causes of ductopenia, and acute cholangitis associated with bile-duct obstruction. A lobular hepatitis, portal inflammation with interface hepatitis may also occur. The development of nodular regenerative hyperplasia as well as fibrosis and cirrhosis may be associated with granulomatous phlebitis of the portal and hepatic veins.

Hepatic sarcoidosis is frequently asymptomatic. While significant hepatomegaly is uncommon, splenomegaly is often present. The liver enzymes may be normal or there may be elevated levels of alkaline phosphatase and aminotransaminases. Portal hypertension and cholestasis are rare complications occurring in only 1 in 300 European patients, but appear to be more common in the United States, and particularly in Black males. Patients may present with intrahepatic cholestasis and later cirrhosis. Differentiation from primary biliary cirrhosis is often difficult. The portal hypertension is presinusoidal and is thought to be due to granulomatous involvement of the portal venous radicals. These patients may present with variceal bleeds in the absence of cirrhosis.

Treatment with steroids often results in the reduction of the size of the hepatosplenomegaly and in improvement in liver enzymes. Steroids have little effect on portal hypertension but may benefit patients with intrahepatic cholestasis.

Primary biliary cirrhosis

Hepatic granulomas are found in approximately 25 per cent of patients with primary biliary cirrhosis (**PBC**). The granulomas are found in portal

Table 1 Causes of hepatic granulomas

1.	**Infections**	2.	**Chemicals**
	Mycobacteria		Beryllium
	Tuberculosis		Copper
	Leprosy		Talc
	Atypical		Silicone
	Bacteria	3.	**Immunological or systemic disease**
	Brucella spp.		Sarcoidosis
	Francisella tularense		Inflammatory bowel disease
	Yersinia pseuodomallei (melioidosis)		Primary biliary cirrhosis
			Immune complexes
	Spirochaetes		Hepatic granulomatous disease
	Treponema spp.		AIDS
	Fungi	4.	**Enzyme defect**
	Blastomyces spp.		Chronic granulomatous disease
	Coccidioides spp.		of children
	Histoplasma spp.	5.	**Neoplasia**
	Cryptococcus spp.		Lymphoma—Hodgkin's disease
	Protozoa spp.		Carcinoma
	Leishmania spp.		Melanoma
	Toxoplasma spp.	6.	**Miscellaneous**
	Metazoa		BCG vaccine
	Schistosoma spp.		Cholestasis
	Toxocara spp.		Polymyalgia rheumatica
	Rickettsia	7.	**Drugs** (see Table 2)
	Q fever		
	Boutonneuse fever		
	Viruses		
	EBV		
	CMV		
	HCV		
	Helminths		

EBV, Epstein–Bar virus; CMV, cytomegalovirus; HCV, hepatitis C virus.

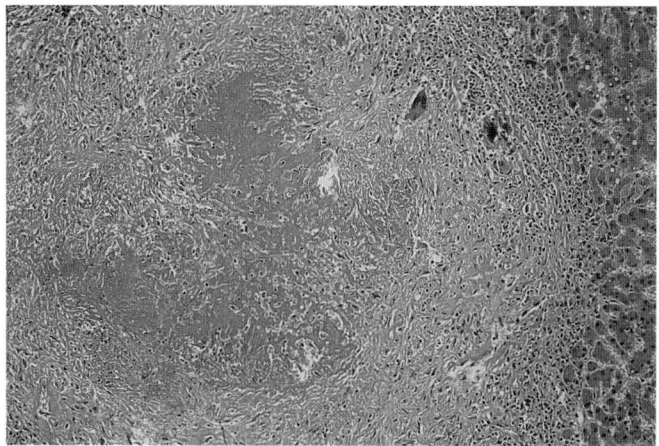

Fig. 1 Liver showing a portion of a large caseating granuloma from a patient with miliary mycobacterium tuberculosis. Several Langhans' giant cells are also seen. (Haematoxylin and eosin, total magnification 25.) (See also Plate 1.)

tracts and tend to surround damaged bile ducts. Occasionally, granulomas are seen in the parenchyma. The granulomas are seen in the early stages of PBC. PBC has a female to male ratio of 8:1, tends to present in the fifth decade of life, and usually has no extrahepatic systemic manifestations. Pruritis tends to be marked, clubbing and hepatomegaly is frequent. These clinical features help to differentiate PBC from sarcoidosis. The latter has an equal female to male ratio, occurs in the third and fourth decades of life, and frequently has extrahepatic manifestations such as erythema nodosa, uveitis, pulmonary involvement, hilar adenopathy, and abnormalities of calcium metabolism with hypercalcaemia and hypercalciurea. Antimitochondrial antibodies are positive in over 95 per cent of patients with PBC. The serum angiotensin-converting enzyme activity test may be elevated in both conditions.

Neoplasia

Non-caseating hepatic granulomas occur with a variety of neoplasms, including lymphoma and carcinoma. These granulomas may occur in the absence of tumour deposits and may represent an immune response to tumour antigens.

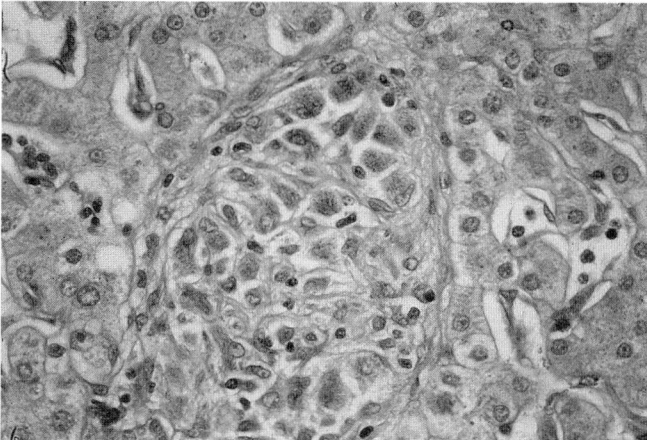

Fig. 2 Liver from an HIV/AIDS patient infected with *Mycobacterium avium intercellulare*, showing a granuloma composed of epithelioid cells which contain large numbers of micro-organisms. (Diastase/periodic acid–Schiff stain, total magnification 100.) (See also Plate 2.)

Lymphoma

Hepatic granulomas may occur in both Hodgkin's and non-Hodgkin's lymphoma. Granulomas may mask the infiltrates of malignant lymphoma and in Hodgkin's disease. Immunohistochemistry may demonstrate a clonal lymphocytic population in or around the granulomas associated with lymphoma.

Chronic granulomatous disease of childhood

This is a classical X-linked disorder, usually presenting at about 5 years of age with hepatosplenomegaly, generalized lymphadenopathy, granulomatous skin lesions, and diffuse miliary lung infiltration. The neutrophils of children with chronic granulomatous disease are unable to kill ingested bacteria, as they are deficient in those enzymes required for the superoxide respiratory burst. The diagnostic test for this condition is the inability of neutrophils to reduce nitroblue tetrazolium from colourless to blue-black formazan granules in their cytoplasm in the presence of a bacterial infection.

Crohn's disease

Non-caseating granulomas are found in the intestine, perineum, lip, and, occasionally, in the liver. The clinical manifestations are typical of Crohn's disease and diagnosis is not usually problematic.

Hepatic granulomatous disease

Hepatic granulomatous disease is a diagnosis of exclusion. The granulomas are seen in the portal tracts and lobules but there is no evidence of hepatitis. There appear to be two variants: one an acute febrile illness characterized by respiratory symptoms, a high white-cell count, and splenomegaly; and the other a more chronic condition presenting more frequently in middle-aged men with recurrent fevers, rigor, sweating, general malaise, and loss of weight. Neuralgia and arthralgia are common, there may be mild, tender hepatomegaly, and liver enzyme abnormalities are non-specific, including bilirubinaemia, mild elevation of transaminases, as well as elevated alkaline phosphatase levels. There is usually a good response to steroid therapy, with pyrexia resolving and liver enzymes improving. The cause is unknown.

Drugs and chemicals

Many drugs cause granulomatous hepatitis (Table 2). Drug-induced liver injury is frequently due to a hypersensitivity reaction. Although drug reactions may result in eosinophil-rich granulomas, in most cases the granulomas are non-specific.

Table 2 Drugs causing hepatic granulomas

Allopurinol	Flucloxacillin	Perhexiline
Amiodarone	Glibenclamide	Phenylbutazone
Amoxicillin	Gold	Phenytoin
Ampicillin	Halothane	Penicillin
Aspirin	Hydralazine	Procainamide
Berylium	Isoniazid	Procarbazine
Carbamazepine	Methyldopa	Quinidine
Carbutamide	Metolazone	Ranitidine
Cephalexin	Mineral oil	Salicylazo-sulphapyridine
Chlorpromazine	Nitrofurantoin	Silica
Chlorpropamide	Nomifensine	Sulphonamides
Copper salts	Oral contraceptive	Tetrahydro-aminoacridine
Dapsone	Steroids	Tocainide
Diazepam	Oxacillin	Tolbutamide
Diltiazem	Papaverine	Trichlor-methiazide
Fenfluramine		

Drug-induced hepatic granulomas may be completely asymptomatic or present with features suggestive of a drug allergy with a swinging fever, skin rash, eosinophilia, and abnormal liver enzymes. Although the diagnosis of drug-induced granulomatous hepatitis is one of exclusion, drugs should always be considered when granulomas are found in the liver.

Exposure to various chemicals such as beryllium, silicone, starch, talc, and suture material has also been associated with the development of hepatic granulomas.

Investigation and management of hepatic granulomas

To obtain the correct diagnosis and determine the appropriate therapy, it is important always to consider the epidemiological background of the patient. In the Western world, the common causes of granulomas in the liver are sarcoidosis, PBC, drugs, and neoplasms, whilst in patients in developing countries infectious causes must be considered first and excluded before considering others. However, the global problem of HIV/AIDS may well place mycobacterial and other infections as the most frequent causes of granulomatous hepatitis.

Further reading

Barceno R, *et al.* (1998). Post-transplant liver granulomatosis associated with hepatitis C. *Transplantation* **65**, 1494–5.

Denk H, *et al.* (1994). Guidelines for the diagnosis and interpretation of hepatic granulomas. *Histopathology* **25**, 209–18.

Devaney K, *et al.* (1993). Hepatic sarcoidosis. Clinicopathologic features in 100 patients. *American Journal of Surgical Pathology* **17**, 1272–80.

Diaz ML, *et al.* (1996). Polymerase chain reaction for the detection of *Mycobacterium tuberculosis* DNA in tissue and assessment of its utility in the diagnosis of hepatic granulomas. *Journal of Laboratory and Clinical Medicine* **127**(4), 359–63.

Emile JF, *et al.* (1993). The presence of epithelioid granulomas in hepatitis C virus-related cirrhosis. *Human Pathology* **24**, 1095–7.

Farrell GC (1995). Drug-induced granulomatous hepatitis. *Drug-induced liver disease*, pp 301–17. Churchill Livingstone, Edinburgh.

Goldin RD, *et al.* (1996). Granulomas and hepatitis C. *Histopathology* **28**, 265–7.

Ishak KG (1998). Sarcoidosis of the liver and bile ducts. *Mayo Clinic Proceedings* **73**, 467–72.

Lee RG, *et al.* (1981). Granulomas in primary biliary cirrhosis: a prognostic feature. *Gastroenterology* **81**, 983–6.

Lefkowitch JH (1999). Hepatic granulomas. *Journal of Hepatology* **30**, 40–5.

O'Connell MJ, *et al.* (1975). Epithelioid granulomas in Hodgkin's disease: a favourable prognostic sign. *Journal of the American Medical Association* **233**, 886–9.

Simon HB, Wolff SM (1973). Granulomatous hepatitis and prolonged fever of unknown origin: a study of 13 patients. *Medicine* (Baltimore) **52**, 1–20.

14.21.7 Drugs and liver damage

J. Neuberger

Introduction

Drug-induced liver injury is relatively uncommon, but unless it is recognized early and the drug discontinued it may cause death. Adverse drug reactions are responsible for between 0.1 and 3 per cent of all hospital admissions. Reliable data are difficult to come by: a relatively recent study has shown that in 1986 to 1987 about 1600 cases per year of adverse drug reactions were reported in England. Hepatic reactions accounted for 3.5 per cent of which 7 per cent were fatal. Similar figures were found by Pillans in New Zealand. A total of 205 drugs were associated with 943 reports of adverse liver injury between 1974 and 1994: 20 drugs accounted for nearly 60 per cent of reports. Most reactions are of jaundice and hepatitis; the more common are due to antibiotics and non-steroidal anti-inflammatory drugs. Halothane, perhexiline, and erythromycin were common causes of death and diclofenac, augmentin, and flucloxacillin were the most important causes of liver damage. In Denmark, Dossing and colleagues estimated that drug-induced liver injury accounts for between 1 in 600 and 1 in 3500 hospital admissions, amounting to 2 to 3 per cent of all hospital admissions due to adverse reactions and about 3 per cent of all jaundiced patients. In general practice, the spectrum of liver damage is slightly different: drugs associated with a high incidence of acute liver injury (greater than 100 per 100 000 users) were chlorpromazine and isoniazid; drugs with intermediate incidence of acute liver damage (more than 10 per 100 000 users) were amoxicillin/clavulanic acid and cimetidine.

Drug-induced liver damage may be caused by agents not considered as conventional drugs, such as herbal remedies, and by 'recreational drugs' such as ecstasy (methylenedioxymethampfetamine) and cocaine (see Box 1). The wide regional and individual variation in reporting rates and failure to report reactions after deliberate overdose combine to underestimate the frequency and severity of adverse drug reactions. Most adverse drug reactions are not fatal and withdrawal of the drug will usually lead to resolution of the liver damage. A study reporting the outcome of 110 cases of presumed drug-induced liver damage found a significant proportion of continuing liver damage, sometimes associated with continuing use of the hepatotoxic drug.

Almost all patterns of liver disease can be induced by drugs (Table 1) and some drugs may be associated with more than one type reaction. For example, oral contraceptives are associated not only with the development of cholestasis but also with adenoma, hepatocellular carcinoma, peliosis hepatis, and Budd–Chiari syndrome. It is important therefore to consider the possible contribution of drugs in a patient with any type of hepatic abnormality.

The diagnosis of drug-induced liver damage is largely circumstantial and by exclusion of other causes of liver disease. It must be remembered that the reporting of an associated drug reaction does not prove causality. The temporal association between the onset of damage and timing of drug exposure, and the response to drug withdrawal (Table 2) and the known patterns

Box 1 The 'rules' of drug-induced liver disease

- Assume that all drugs may cause liver damage
- All patterns of liver damage have been associated with drug toxicity
- Some drugs may cause more than one pattern of liver damage
- Always take a full drug history
- Ask about other drugs—including herbal remedies, recreational drugs, vitamins
- The diagnosis of an adverse drug reaction is one of exclusion and temporal relationship
- Drug withdrawal is not always associated with improvement in liver function
- Reports of drug-associated liver damage do not necessarily mean causality
- Clinical challenge is rarely justified, may be fatal, and may be misleading

of drug reaction all help in establishing a drug as the cause of liver damage. Rarely, the presence of specific serological markers may help confirm the association between the drug and liver damage. For example, an antibody to tifluoroaceylated proteins is found in halothane-associated hepatitis, and antiliver–kidney microsomal antibodies occur in tienilic acid-associated hepatitis. Use of a clinical challenge is rarely justified, may be rnisleading, and may prove fatal.

Acute hepatitis

The severity of liver cell necrosis associated with drugs varies from a mild elevation of serum transaminases without symptoms to fulminant hepatic failure. Many drugs have been associated with acute liver failure (Table 3). Clinically, the picture may be indistinguishable from that of viral hepatitis. Occasionally, right upper quadrant pain may he so severe as to lead to the mistaken diagnosis of acute cholecystitis. The serological changes are those of acute hepatitis with initial elevations of serum aminotransferases. Prolongation of the prothrombin time and jaundice may occur in more severe cases. Histologically, the appearances vary from a mild focal necrosis to massive liver cell damage. In some cases, paracetamol for example, the damage is predominantly centrilobular, whereas in others, such as α-methyldopa, the whole lobule is affected. Steatosis, granulomas, and eosinophilia are variable features. The most common causes of drug-asso-

ciated fulminant hepatic failure are paracetamol overdose and halothane hepatitis. Liver failure may also be associated with 'recreational' drugs.

The development of abnormalities of liver tests during prolonged drug use poses particular problems, as for example with antituberculous therapy. Derangement of serum aminotransferases occurs in approximately 10 per cent of patients and, if the noxious drug is continued, up to l0 per cent of these develop severe hepatic necrosis. Identification of those patients who will develop severe hepatic failure is difficult and the clinician has to decide whether the risks of continuing therapy outweigh the potential benefits. Drugs such as heparin are commonly associated with abnormal liver enzymes but very rarely with liver disease. The reason is not known but it may be due to loss of a few sensitive hepatocytes or to adaptation.

Conventionally, hepatic drug reactions are classified into predictable and idiosyncratic (Table 4). Predictable reactions are dose dependent; that is, the greater the amount of drug ingested, the greater the probability of developing liver damage. Because animal models can usually be developed, screening will detect many of these drug reactions and the drug withdrawn before reaching the market. Hence this type of drug reaction is relatively uncommon, except in overdose. The classic example is paracetamol toxicity, which is described in detail elsewhere.(Irene: cross reference?) None the less, between individuals there may exist great variability in the probability of developing predictable drug reactions.

With very few exceptions, drugs require metabolism before cytotoxicity develops. Variations in susceptibility may, therefore, be a consequence of genetic variations in drug metabolism. Well-recognized genetic polymorphisms include variations in the cytochrome P450 isoenzymes, drug oxidation, acetylation, and hydroxylation. Age, too, is associated with differences in susceptibility to toxicity. In general, younger children metabolize drugs differently from adults. Those taking enzyme inducers such as alcohol, rifampicin, or phenobarbital are at a greater risk of increased metabolism of the drug and hence of forming toxic metabolites. Those with reduced glutathione stores, due to fasting, malnutrition, or associated disease for example, may be at greater risk of developing paracetamol toxicity because detoxification mechanisms are impaired. Other factors determining susceptibility include smoking and coexisting diseases, so that, for example, methotrexate toxicity is more common in those with diabetes. Finally, liver disease itself may alter susceptibilities to drug toxicity. However, because of potential alterations in absorption, volume of distribution, protein binding, detoxification, and excretion it is difficult to predict the effect of disease on susceptibility to drug toxicity. Many drugs induce hepatitis by apoptosis which may be accompanied by simultaneous or secondary necrosis.

In contrast, idiosyncratic drug reactions are dose independent and may be due either to metabolic idiosyncrasy or the involvement of immune mechanisms. Immune involvement rather than metabolic idiosyncrasy is suggested by a rapid onset after subsequent exposure and the appearance of markers such as peripheral and intrahepatic eosinophilia, granulomas, circulating immune complexes, autoantibodies, and other autoimmune phenomena, for example haemolytic anaemia. Two drugs in particular have been well studied with respect to immune-mediated hepatitis—halothane

Table 1 Patterns of adverse hepatic drug reactions

Adverse reaction	Drug
Hepatitis	
Fulminant	Paracetamol, halothane
Acute	
Subacute	
Chronic	Methyldopa, nitrofurantoin
Cholestatic	Phenothiazines
Granulomatous	Phenytoin
Cirrhosis	
Cholestasis	
Bland	Anabolic steroids, oestrogens
Vanishing bile duct syndrome	Chlorpromazine, penicillins
Sclerosing cholangitis	Floxuridine
Granulomas	sulphonamides
Steatosis	
Macrovesicular	Amiodarone
Microvesicular	Valproic acid
Tumours	
Adenoma	Oestrogens
Carcinoma	Oestrogens
Angiosarcoma	Arsenicals, thorium dioxide
Cholangiocarcinoma	Thorium dioxide
Vascular lesions	
Peliosis	Oestrogens
Budd–Chiari syndrome	Oestrogens
Veno-occlusive disease	Azathioprine
Fibrosis	Vitamin A, arsenicals

Table 2 Criteria for defining adverse drug reactions. (From Danan O (1990). Consensus meeting. Criteria of drug induced liver disorders. *Journal of Hepatotogy* **11**, 272–6)

Drug reaction	Suggestive compatible		Incompatible		
	From onset	From onset	From cessation	From onset	From cessation
Hepatitis					
Initial exposure	5–90 days	< 5 or > 90 days	< 15 days	Drug started after onset	> 15 days
Subsequent exposure	1–15 days	> 15 days	< 15 days	Drug started after onset	> 15 days
Cholestasis					
Initial exposure	5–90 days	> 5 days	< 1 month	Drug started after onset	> 1 month
Subsequent exposure	1–90 days	> 90 days	< 1 month	Drug started after onset	

Table 3 Drugs associated with hepatocellular necrosis

Area of drug use	Drug
Anaesthesia	Chloroform
	Cyclopropane
	Enflurane
	Ethyl ether
	Fluroxene
	Halothane
	Isoflurane
	Methoxyflurane
	Trichloroethylene
	Vinyl ether
Antineoplastic disorders	Carmustine
	Chlorozotocin
	Cyclophosphamide
	Cytarabine
	Dacarbazine
	Hydroxycarbamide
	Flutamide
	Mithramycin
	Procarbazine
	Streptozotocin
	Vincristine
Cardiovascular disease	Captopril
	Coumarins
	Enalapril
	Frusemide
	HMG Co-A reductase
	Hydralazine
	Lisinopril
	Metoprolol
	Methyldopa
	Nicotinic acid
	Nifedepine
	Papavarine
	Quinidine
	Tienilic acid
	Verapamil
Gastroenterological disorders	Chenodeoxycholic acid
	Omeprazole
	Salazopyrine
	Ebrotidine
Endocrine disorders	Acetohexamide
	Carbutamide
	Flutamide
	Metahexamide
	Propylthiouracil
	Troglitazone
Infectious disorders	p-Aminosalicylic acid
	Amiodaquine
	Carbenicillin
	Ciprofloxacillin
	Clindamycin
	Cotrimoxazole
	Dapsone
	Dideoxyinosine
	Erythromycin
	Fluconazole
	Fusidic acid
	Hycanthone
	Isoniazid
	Ketoconazole
	Levamisole
	Mebendazole
	Mepacrine
	Minocycline
	Oxacillin

Table 3 continued

Area of drug use	Drug
	Piperazine
	Sulphonamides
	Zidovudine
Neuropsychiatric disorders	Amitriptyline
	Bromocryptine
	Carbamazepine
	Dantrolene
	Desipramine
	Disulphiram
	Ferpexide
	Feltamate
	Imipramine
	Iproniazid
	Isaxonine
	Lergotrile
	Levodopa
	Loxapine
	Methylphenidate
	Nomifensine
	Oxapozin
	Pemoline
	Pergomide
	Phenacetamide
	Phenelzine
	Pheniprazine
	Phenoxyproperazine
	Phenytoin
	Phethenylate
	Valproate
	Viloxazine
Nutritional and metabolic diseases	Clofibrate
	Fenofibrate
	Gemfibrozil
	Nicotinamide
Radiological examinations	Iodapamide
	Iopanoic acid
Rheumatic and musculoskeletal disorders	Allopurinol
	Aspirin
	Baclofen
	Benorylate
	Benoxaprofen
	Clomacetin
	Dantrolene
	Glafenine
	Nimesulide
	Paracetamol
	Piroxicates
	Salicylates
Skin diseases	Elretinate
	Methoxsalen
	Povidone-iodine
	Tannic acid
Herbal remedies	Germander
	Chinese herbal tea
	Mistletoe
	Pennyroyal oil
Others	Ampfetamine
	Cocaine
	Ecstasy[*]

[*] Methylenedioxymethampfetamine.

and tienilic acid. Halothane hepatitis occurs rarely and after multiple exposures. Risk factors include female sex, obesity, and repeated or subsequent exposure within 3 months. Immune involvement is suggested by an increased incidence of organ non-specific autoantibodies, peripheral

Table 4 Patterns of acute hepatitis associated with drugs

Type	Onset	Reaction on re-exposure	Dose dependent	Reproducible in animals	Hyper-sensitivity features
Predictable Idiosyncratic	Rapid	Rapid	++	+	−
Metabolic	Variable	Delayed	+/−	−	−
Immune mediated	Variable	Rapid	−	−	+

eosinophilia, and circulating immune complexes, and the presence of antibodies reacting with a variety of halothane-associated liver cell macromolecules. In other examples. antibodies to drug-metabolizing enzymes are present in serum. Tienilic acid-associated hepatitis is associated with a circulating liver–kidney microsomal antibody that reacts with the cytochrome P450, CYP 2C9, associated with metabolism of the drug; antibodies to CYP 1A2 are associated with hydralazine and disulfiram hepatitis; alcohol and halothane hepatitis are associated with antibodies to CYP 2E1. Iproniazid hepatitis is associated with antibodies to MAO-B. Whether these antibodies are involved in the pathogenesis of the disease remains uncertain.

Cross-reaction between two drugs may occur. Thus, halothane sensitization may predispose to toxicity from other halogenated hydrocarbon anaesthetic agents such as isoflurane. This may be due to the two drugs inducing similar antigenic determinants, leading to cross-sensitization, or to a different mechanism of toxicity, as suggested for captopril and enalapril hepatotoxicity, where a similar metabolic pathway of toxicity has been postulated.

Acute cholestatic hepatitis

Acute cholestatic hepatitis is characterized by jaundice, pruritus, pale stools, and dark urine. There are usually few clinical findings, although the liver may be enlarged. Serologically, in the early stages there is elevation of the serum alkaline phosphatase and γ-glutamyl transpeptidase; as the disease progresses, hepatocellular enzymes start to rise. Histologically, the liver shows dilated sinusoids with cholestasis often predominating in the centrilobular region. There may be an associated portal inflammation and liver cell necrosis. In the majority of cases there is rapid resolution following withdrawal of the drug, although with chlorpromazine and other phenothiazines the cholestasis may take up to 1 to 2 years to resolve. Many drugs cause a mixed hepatitis, where there are features both of cholestasis and liver cell damage (Table 5).

Bland cholestasis

Bland cholestasis is characterized by cholestasis in the absence of hepatitis and is due to specific interference with bile secretion. The two main groups of drugs associated with this condition are oral contraceptives and oestrogens and anabolic steroids. Cholestasis occurs in women taking oral contraceptives and in pregnancy. Prevalence varies, being low in southern Europe and North America (1 in 10 000) and high (1 in 4000) in parts of Chile and Scandinavia. Cholestasis associated with anabolic and contraceptive steroids is well recognized and may occur in association with virtually all the anabolic steroids with a C17 group; these drugs include norethandrolone, oxymethalone, danazol, stanozalol, and methyltestosterone. Other drugs are listed in Table 6. In some cases, drug induced cholestasis leads to a progressive, vanishing bile duct syndrome. Treatment is symptomatic: the itching may be intense and sometimes responds to cholestyramine or colestipol; other therapies include antihistamines, ursodeoxycholic acid, rifampicin, androgenic anabolic steroids, and opiate receptor antagonists.

Steatosis

Steatosis may be micro- or macrovesicular. Differentiation is important because the clinical features and outcomes are different. (Table 7).

Microvesicular steatosis

In microvesicular steatosis, the fat is distributed in small lipid droplets and the hepatocellular nucleus is not displaced. There may be an associated hepatitis. Extensive microvesicular steatosis, even in the absence of liver cell necrosis, may lead to a serious clinical syndrome with haemorrhage, syncope, hypotension, lethargy, coma, and hypoglycaemia. In some cases, renal failure and pancreatic inflammation may occur. Biochemically, serum aminotransferases and bilirubin are not greatly increased, although the prothrombin time may be greatly prolonged. Microvesicular steatosis is thought to be related to drug inhibition of mitochondrial oxidation of fatty acids.

Macrovesicular steatosis

In contrast, macrovesicular steatosis is usually far less serious. The hepatocyte contains a large droplet of fat, which displaces the nucleus to the periphery. Liver tests are usually only minimally deranged. Damage is thought to be related to impaired release of lipids from liver cells.

Granulomatous hepatitis

The spectrum of granulomatous hepatitis varies from an asymptomatic finding to a systemic illness characterized by generalized aches and pains, pruritus, jaundice, and hepatomegaly. Serologically. the main abnormality is an increase in serum alkaline phosphatase. Histologically the liver is infiltrated by granulomas—small, rounded foci of epithelioid cells with multinucleated giant cells. Drugs associated with granulomatous hepatitis are listed in Table 8.

Phospholipidosis

Phospholipidosis is characterized by the accumulation of phospholipids in liver cell lysosomes. The major drugs associated with this form of liver damage, perhexiline and amiodarone, are cationic, amphiphilic compounds that accumulate within the liver cell lysosomes where they form complexes with phospholipids. Accumulation can be detected by immunohistochemistry or electron microscopy. The compounds are stored in these complexes and may be released very slowly, even after ingestion has stopped. The extent to which these complexes accumulate in patients without toxicity remains uncertain.

Non-alcohol steatotic hepatitis

Long-term treatment with perhexiline and amiodarone may be associated with a syndrome that is clinically and histologically identical to alcoholic hepatitis. The disease develops insidiously and is characterized by hepatomegaly, jaundice, ascites, and encephalopathy. Other drugs implicated in this syndrome include diltiazem and nifedipine.

Table 5 Drugs associated with cholestatic hepatitis

Area of drug use	Drug
Cancer	Aminoglutethimide
	Arabinoside
	Azathioprine
	Chlorambucil
	Chlorotozotocin
	Cisplatin
	Cytosin
	Mitomycin
	Streptozotocin
Cardiovascular disease	Ajmaline
	Captopril
	Diltiazem
	Disopyramide
	Flecanide
	Hydrallazine
	Methyldopa
	Mexilitine
	Nifedepine
	Phenindione
	Prajmaline
	Procaineamide
	Propafenone
	Quinine
	Spironolactone
	Ticlopidine
	Verapamil
	Warfarin
Gastroenterological disorders	Cimetidine
	Ranitidine
Endocrine disease	Acetohexamide
	Carbimazole
	Chlorpropamide
	Glibenclamide
	Metahexamide
	Methimazole
	Propylthiouracil
	Tamoxifen
	Thiouracil
	Tolbutamide
Infectious and parasitic disease	p-Aminosalacylic acid
	Arsphenamine
	Cefalexin
	Chloramphenicol
	Claxacillin
	Cotrimoxazole
	Erythromycin
	Griseofulvin
	Nalidixic acid
	Nitrofurantoin
	Quinine
	Rifampicin
	Sulphadiazine
	Sulphonamides
	Tiabendazole
	Troleandomycin
	Tryparsamide
Neuropsychiatric disease	Amitryptaline
	Bromocriptine
	Carbamazepine
	Chlordiazepoxide
	Chlorpromazine
	Desipramine
	Diazepam
	Fluphenazine

Table 5 continued

	Flurazepam
	Haloperidol
	Imipramine
	Iprindole
	Mianserin
	Phenobarbital
	Phenytoin
	Prochlorperazine
	Promazine
	Thioridizine
	Triazolam
	Trifluoperazine
	Zimeldine
Rheumatic and musculoskeletal diseases	Allopurinol
	Baclofen
	Colchicine
	Diclofenac
	Diflunisal
	Fenbrufen
	Feprazon
	Flurbiprofen
	Gold salts
	Ibfenac
	Ibuprofen
	Indomethacin
	Kebuzone
	Naproxen
	Oxyphenbutazone
	Penicillamine
	Phenopyrazone
	Phenylbutazone
	Piroxicam
	Probenacid
	Propoxyphene
	Proquazone
	Sulindac
	Zoxazolamine
Skin disease	Isoretanoin

Fibrotic and vascular disease (Table 9)

Perisinusoidal fibrosis

Perisinusoidal fibrosis is characterized by accumulation of collagen within the space of Disse. This may be asymptomatic or lead to hepatomegaly and portal hypertension. The most common causes of perisinusoidal fibrosis due to drugs are large doses of vitamin A given for prolonged periods, or methotrexate. Liver damage may be associated with alopecia. Characteristically the liver shows hyperplasia of the Ito cell as a consequence of vitamin A accumulation. Serum concentrations of vitamin A may he normal, even in the presence of marked liver damage. Patients with a high intake of alcohol are at greater risk of fibrosis.

Peliosis hepatis

Peliosis hepatis is a histological diagnosis and is characterized by blood-filled cavities, bordered by hepatocytes, which may be distributed throughout the liver. Originally described in association with tuberculosis, it is now appreciated that peliosis hepatis may be drug induced and is often asymptomatic. The major drugs involved are the anabolic steroids, androgenic steroids, azathioprine, vinyl chloride, and pyrizolide derivatives.

Hepatic venous damage

Obstruction of the large hepatic veins results in the Budd–Chiari syndrome, characterized by the onset of abdominal pain and ascites, often with

Table 6 Drugs associated with acute cholestasis

Class of drug/area of drug use	Drug
Antimicrobials	Amoxicillin/clavulinic acid
	Cephalosporins
	Cotrimoxazole
	Erythromycin
	Flucloxacillin
	Griseofulvin
	Nitrofurantoin
	Ketoconazole
	Penicillins
	Rifampicin
	Sulphones
	Thiobendazole
	Trimethoprim
Antithyroid drugs	Thiouracil
	Carbimazole
	Methimazole
Hypoglycaemic agents	Chlorpropamide
	Glibenclamide
	Tolbutamide
Anticancer drugs	Azathioprine
	Busulfan
	Chlorambucil
	Cytarabine
Steroids	Aminoglutethemide
	Anabolic steroids (C17)
	Danazol
	Stanozolol
	Tamoxifen
Cytokines	Interleukin-2
	Tumour necrosis factor
Anti-inflammatory and analgesic agents	Benoxaprofen
	Dextropropoxyphene
	Diflunisal
	Gold
	Naproxen
	Nimesulide
	Penicillamine
	Phenylbutazone
	Piroxicam
Anticonvulsants	Carbamazepine
	Phenobarbitone
	Phenytoin
Psychiatric disease	Amitryptiline
	Chlordiazepoxide
	Chlorpromazine
	Flurazepam
	Haloperidol
	Imipramine
	Nomifensine
	Thioridizine
	Prochlorperazine
	Zemeldene
Cardiovascular drugs	Ajmaline
	Captopril
	Chlorthalidone
	Disopyramide
	Hydralazine
	Nifedepine
	Thiazides
	Verapamil
Other	Cyclosporin A
	Warfarin

Table 7 Drugs associated with steatosis

Type of steatosis	Drug
Microvesicular	Amineptine
	Aureomycin
	Bleomycin
	Cisplatin
	Mitomycin C
	Pirprofen
	Tetracycline
	Valproate
Macrovesicular	Asparaginase
	Glucocorticosteroids
	Methotrexate
	6-Mercaptopurine

diarrhoea. In the acute form the patient may develop liver failure. Most cases of Budd–Chiari syndrome are due to myeloproliferative disorders, either clinically apparent or latent, but it may be associated with the use of oral contraceptives and some antineoplastic drugs such as dacarbazine, doxorubicin, and cyclophosphamide.

Obstruction of the small veins leads to hepatic veno-occlusive disease, characterized by non-thrombotic, concentric narrowing of the small centrilobular veins. Clinical presentation is often chronic but rarely may be acute. Veno-occlusive disease was initially described in association with ingestion of the pyrrolizidine alkaloids present in senecin plants but may be seen in patients treated with immunosuppressives, especially with organ transplantation.

Table 8 Drugs associated with hepatic granulomas

Area of drug use	Drug
Antineoplastic	Procarbazine
Cardiovascular	Amiodarone
	Diltiazem
	Hydralazine
	Methyldopa
	Procaineamide
	Quinidine
	Quinine
	Tocainade
Endocrine	Chlorpropamide
	Glibenclamide
	Tolbutamide
Gastroenterological	Ranitine
	Sulphasalazine
Infectious disease	Amoxicillin/clavulinic acid
	Cephalexin
	Dapsone
	Isoniazid
	Nitrofurantoin
	Oxacillin
	Penicillin
	Sulphonamides
Neuropsychiatric disease	Carbamazepine
	Chlorpromazine
	Diazepam
	Nomifensine
Rheumatological	Allopurinol
	Aspirin
	Gold
	Oxyphenbutazone
	Phenylbutazone

Table 9 Drug-related vascular diseases of the liver

Vascular disorder	Drug
Veno-occlusive disease	Actinomycin D
	Azathioprine
	Busulfan
	Cyclophosphamide
	Mercaptopurine
	Mitomycin
	Pyrrolizidine alkaloids
	Thioguanine
	Vincristine
	Herbal remedies—comfrey, ilex plants, Chinese medicinal teas*
Budd–Chiari syndrome	Actinomycin
	Dacarbazine
	Oral contraceptives
Perisinusoidal fibrosis	Arsenicals
	Azathioprine
	Mercaptopurine
	Methotrexate
	Vitamin A excess
Nodular regenerative hyperplasia	Azathioprine
	Busulfan

* May be due to pyrrolizidine alkaloids.

Hepatic tumours

Hepatic tumours may be benign or malignant (Table 10). Hepatocellular adenoma has been associated with the use of oral contraceptives and anabolic steroids. These tumours have a potential for malignant transformation. Usually withdrawal of the steroid results in a reduction in the size of the tumour.

In contrast, hepatocellular carcinoma is also associated with the anabolic and androgenic steroids, oral contraceptives, and thorium dioxide. Although the risk of malignancy increases with the prolonged use of oral contraceptives, up to eightfold after 8 years, it must be emphasized that the overall risk of developing hepatocellular carcinoma with oral contraceptives is extremely small, and must be balanced against their beneficial, therapeutic effects. Angiosarcomas and cholangiosarcomas may also be related to drugs, although the association is less clear-cut.

Chronic disease

Cirrhosis and chronic hepatitis

Some drugs are associated with chronic liver disease. It may be that the initial lesions develop subclinically and that only prolonged use of the drug will result in cirrhosis. Rarely, a short-term exposure to a drug results in chronic liver disease. In some instances, there is a syndrome resembling autoimmune hepatitis: although corticosteroids may be given, withdrawal of the drug usually leads to resolution of the hepatic inflammation. Some of the drugs associated with the development of cirrhosis and chronic hepatitis are listed in Table 11.

Table 10 Malignant liver tumours associated with drugs

Type of tumour	Drug
Hepatocellular carcinoma	Anabolic/androgenic steroids
	Oral contraceptives
	Thorium dioxide
Cholangiocarcinoma	Thorium dioxide
Angiosarcoma	Anabolic/androgenic steroids
	Arsenicals
	Thorium dioxide

Intrahepatic chronic cholestasis

In some instances of drug-related cholestasis, jaundice or cholestatic liver tests persist for 6 months or more (Table 12). In these cases it is important to exclude other causes of cholestatic disease, such as primary biliary cirrhosis or primary sclerosing cholangitis, which may have been brought to light by drug-induced disorders. However, some drugs may be associated with a chronic vanishing bile duct syndrome, which may be indistinguishable from primary biliary cirrhosis. A syndrome virtually identical to primary sclerosing cholangitis can be induced by infusion into the hepatic artery of floxuridine for the treatment of intrahepatic malignancy. Sclerosing cholangitis may develop several months after starting chemotherapy. The outcome is variable. A vanishing bile duct syndrome has been associated with carbamazepine, thiobendazole, flucloxacillin, haloperidol, ajmaline, cyproheptidine, and chlorpromazine. There has been a suggestion that primary biliary cirrhosis is associated with the use of benoxaprofen. The cause of the chronic cholestasis is uncertain; both immune mechanisms and the recirculation of toxic metabolites have been implicated.

Table 11 Commoner drugs associated with subacute and chronic hepatitis and cirrhosis

Acetohexamide
Amiodarone
Amodiaquine
Aspirin
Benzarone
Busulfan
Chlorambucil
Cimetidine
Clometacin*
Dantrolene
Doxorubicin*
Diclofenac*
Etridonate*
Iproniazid
Isoniazid*
Methotrexate
Methyldopa*
Minocycline*
Nicotinic acid
Nitrofurantoin*
Oxyphenisatin*
Perhexiline
Propylthiouracil
Sulphonamides*
Tienilic acid*
Urethane
Valproate
Vitamin A (excess)

* May also be associated with autoimmune hepatitis.

Table 12 Drugs associated with chronic cholestasis

Phenothiazines
Tricyclic antidepressants
Sex steroids
Sulphonylureas
Penicillins
Others—arsenicals, cyproheptidine, haloperidol, thiobendazole, troleandomycin, piroxicam

the anterior abdominal wall. The condition usually resolves without treatment, although the use of penicillin promotes more rapid resolution. Abnormalities of liver function may occur in gonococcal bacteraemia, peritonitis, and endocarditis. Perihepatitis is also reported in association with syphilis and chlamydial infections. Chlamydial infection is today the most frequent cause of chronic perihepatic adhesions.

In childhood, some infections with *Escherichia coli* may be associated with hepatitis and jaundice. Jaundice is rare in older patients, although pregnant women seem more susceptible. Abnormalities of liver function occur in systemic streptococcal and staphylococcal infection and in enteric fevers, paratyphoid, and typhoid. Hepatomegaly is common in typhoid infection and jaundice occurs in about 10 per cent of patients, although up to a third have abnormal liver function tests with increased levels of aminotransferase and normal values for alkaline phosphatase. The hepatomegaly rapidly responds with treatment. In gas gangrene, deep jaundice may occur may occur in up to a fifth of patients. The liver may be infected and a plain radiograph of the abdomen may show gas within the liver. Liver damage and jaundice are associated with *Listeria monocytogenes* and *Legionella pneumophila* infections

Brucellosis may also be associated with jaundice and abnormal liver function tests. All three species of *Brucella* have been associated with abnormal liver function. Characteristically, the liver biopsy shows a marked inflammatory infiltrate and fibrosis with multiple large or small granulomas scattered throughout the parenchyma. Some reports have suggested that granulomatous hepatitis due to *Brucella* may cause cirrhosis, but this is questionable. The common causes of liver granulomas, including infections, are listed in Table 4. The liver damage asociated with leptospirosis (Weil's disease) is described elsewhere (Section 7).

Actinomyces spp. are commensal organisms that rarely cause disease. Actinomycotic infection of the liver may occur, the patient presenting with abdominal pain, anorexia, and fever. In one case report the liver was found to have small, multilocular abscesses.

Tuberculosis may present with granulomatous hepatitis, biliary tuberculosis, a solitary tuberculoma, or tuberculosis of the biliary tract. The liver is involved in up to 85 per cent of patients with tuberculosis, especially in those with miliary disease. The presence of multiple granulomas in the liver should raise the possibility of tuberculosis, although the differential diagnosis of granulomatous hepatitis is long (see Table 4). With the increasing incidence of atypical mycobacterial infections, lesions similar to tuberculosis can be found. In those infected with *Mycobacterium avium intracellulare* there are numerous acid-fast bacilli, often in the absence of granulomas.

Leptospirosis

Leptospiral infections are described in Section 7. Acute leptospirosis is frequently accompanied by jaundice, although frank liver failure is uncommon. The jaundice is mainly cholestatic, although there may be liver cell injury.

Rickettsial infection

Liver injury in Q fever (*Coxiella burnetti*) is recognized, although symptoms of liver disease are uncommon. Hepatomegaly is frequent and liver function tests may show an elevation of serum alkaline phosphatase and, rarely, a picture resembling viral hepatitis. Histologically, the liver has areas of focal necrosis, Kupffer cell proliferation, lipogranuloma formation, and mononuclear cell infiltration in the portal tracts. The characteristic histological feature of Q fever is eosinophiliic fibrinoid necrosis but this is not specific. Treatment is with chloramphenicol or tetracycline. Liver disease is much more frequent in Rocky Mountain spotted fever (*Rickettsia rickettsia*).

Fungal infections

The liver may be involved in fungal infection, often in patients with immunodeficiency such as with AIDS, following chemotherapy, and after organ transplantation. Histoplasmosis, cryptococcosis, aspergillosis, blastomycosis, and candidiasis are all causes of liver damage. The liver is usually involved in disseminated fungal infections. Cryptococcal infection has also been associated with a primary biliary cirrhosis-like condition.

Protozoal infections

Protozoal infections are described in detail in Section 7.13 many of them involve the liver. In toxoplasmosis, while most patients are asymptomatic and liver involvement is mild, hepatitis may occur and *Toxoplasma gondii* may be found in liver biopsy samples. In malaria, due to either *Plasmodium falcipartun* or *P. vivax*, abnormalities of liver tests may be observed. Hepatomegaly is common and is often associated with jaundice. The jaundice is in part due to haemolysis but liver tests may provide a picture suggestive of viral hepatitis. Histological examination may show characteristic features of Kupffer cell proliferation with black malarial pigment and mononuclear cell infiltrate. Frank hepatic failure is extremely rare.

Schistosomiasis is one of the most common causes of liver disease worldwide. A heavy infection of fertile schistosomes in the portal system results in deposition of eggs that induce an immune response, leading to portal fibrosis and granuloma formation, portal hypertension with consequent splenomegaly, ascites, and variceal haemorrhage. Hepatocyte function is well preserved. There is a complex interaction between schistosomal eggs and the immune system; the degree of fibrosis is directly related to the number of eggs and the duration of infection. The diagnosis is made on stool examination or finding schistosomes in the liver. Serological tests are unreliable at present. Treatment is described in Chapter 7.16.1. Successful treatment is associated with a significant but variable improvement in the degree of portal hypertension. Treatment of the portal hypertension is dependent on the medical facilities available. As parenchymal function is well preserved, these patients usually tolerate a portosystemic shunt.

Coinfection of patients with schistosomiasis and hepatitis B or C virus is associated with an aggressive progression.

Table 4 Common causes of hepatic granulomas

Infective	Bacterial
	Mycobacteria
	Brucellosis
	Rickettsial
	Spirochaetal
	Parasitic
	Amoebiasis
	Ascariasis
	Giardiasis
	Schistosomiasis
	Toxocara
	Viral
	Cytomegalovirus
	Epstein–Barr virus
	Fungal
Drugs	Allopurinol
	Sulphonamides
	Phenylbutazone
Parenchymal disease	Primary biliary cirrhosis
	Primary sclerosing cholangitis
Malignancy	Hodgkin's disease
Other	Sarcoid
	Systemic lupus erythematosus
	Whipple's disease
	Collagen disease
	Erythema nodosum
	Crohn's disease
	Toxins: beryllium and silicon

Table 5 Sources of a pyogenic abscess

Source	Percentage of cases
Obstructive biliary tree	30–40
Intra-abdominal infection	15–25
Systemic infection	15–20

Viral infections

Hepatitis may be a significant feature of viral infection other than with the classical hepatitis viruses. Thus, infection with cytomegalovirus, Epstein–Barr virus, herpesviruses, measles, rubella, coxsackievirus, adenoviruses, and echoviruses may all cause a significant hepatitis. Such viral infections (especially cytomegalovirus) are more common in immunosuppressed patients. The diagnosis is made serologically, but in some cases, such as with cytomegalovirus, herpes, and adenoviral infections, the liver histology may show characteristic features.

Pyogenic liver abscess

Pyogenic liver abscesses may occur as part of a systemic illness, or as a consequence of portal phlebitis. Abscesses are often associated with bowel sepsis, biliary tract disease, direct trauma, septicaemia, and in association with carcinoma of the colon or bacterial endocarditis. They most commonly arise out of portal phlebitis, with the primary focus being the appendix, colon, diverticular disease, or in the pelvis (Table 5). Although abscesses may occur in patients with inflammatory bowel disease, this is relatively rare. The patient presents with abdominal pain, pyrexia, nausea, and weight loss. However, fever is less common in children. Hepatomegaly may be present and the liver is sometimes tender. The serum albumin is often reduced and alkaline phosphatase elevated. There is usually marked neutrophil leucocytosis, but this is not invariable. The diagnosis is made on imaging of the liver. A chest radiograph may show elevation of the right hemidiaphragm with an associated pleural effusion or even lung consolidation. Ultrasound, computed tomography, and magnetic resonance imaging may define a hepatic abscess. With the increasing sensitivity of these techniques, radio-isotope scanning is now less important.

Treatment of a solitary abscess is by percutaneous drainage in the first instance. Under the guidance of ultrasound or computed tomography, a percutaneous drain should be established for single abscesses, and even in some cases of multiple abscesses. The abscesses should be drained to dryness, and antibiotics should be given according to the sensitivities of the organisms isolated. Pathogens are usually anaerobic or aerobic gut coliforms, especially *Streptococcus milleri*, but in children *Staphylococcus aureus* is common. The success rate of treatment with drainage and systemic antibiotics is 80 to 90 per cent. Fatality is high in children and the elderly, in those with coexisting disease such as diabetes mellitus, and in those with delayed diagnosis. Once the abscess has been drained, the primary source of infection must be sought and appropriate management instituted. Surgery may be required for patients with multiple abscesses or for those with abscesses that do not respond to simple drainage and antibiotic therapy. Liver abscess due to hydatid and amoebal infection is discussed elsewhere.

AIDS and liver disease

Liver disease in patients with human immunodeficiency virus (HIV) infection may be due to pre-existing hepatitis virus, opportunistic infections, or neoplasms. In some cases the abnormality of liver function may be due to virus itself. Such patients have non-tender hepatomegaly with anorexia, weight loss, and low-grade fever. Liver function tests show slight derangement with cholestasis. The liver biopsy shows non-specific features including Kupffer-cell hyperplasia, fat infiltration, non-caseating granulomas, and portal-tract inflammation; Mallory hyaline bodies may occasionally be present.

Other causes of hepatobiliary abnormality in patients with HIV include primary hepatic infection due to viral hepatitis.

Other causes of liver damage in AIDS

Many patients with AIDS are also at risk from hepatitis B, C, and D. As discussed elsewhere, these patients respond less well to interferon than do those who are HIV negative. Other infections that are more common in HIV-positive patients include cytomegalovirus, herpesvirus, cryptosporidiosis, and mycobacterial infections including tuberculosis and *Mycobacterium avium intracellurare*. Drug-induced liver damage must always be considered in HIV patients with abnormal liver tests, and it has been suggested that such patients are more susceptible to drug hepatotoxicity. Thus, many of the anticonvulsants, analgesics, and antimicrobials are associated with hepatocellular damage, and antibiotics may also be associated with cholestasis. Other abnormalities that may be of less significance clinically include peliosis hepatis and fatty infiltration.

The biliary tree may also be affected in HIV infection inducing a syndrome superficially resembling primary sclerosing cholangitis. This is characterized by a rapid elevation of the serum alkaline phosphatase, which may be associated with pain in the right upper quadrant and, later, jaundice. Ultrasonography may be unhelpful, although dilated and thickened walls of the bile duct may be seen. Otherwise, endoscopic retrograde cholepancreatography will show the characteristic changes of sclerosing cholangitis with bleeding, dilatation, and stricture. Both cryptosporidial and cytomegaloviral infections have been associated with this form of sclerosing cholangitis.

The liver may be affected by HIV in other ways. There is an association between AIDS and lymphomas, be they Burkitt's, large cell, or immunoblastic lymphomas. The liver and/or spleen may be the site of these tumours and hepatic infiltration may be present in up to a third of those with gastrointestinal lymphomas. Tumours may be microscopic or macroscopic. The hepatic masses are often asymptomatic but if large they may cause pain in the right upper quadrant, fever, jaundice, and abnormalities of serum liver tests, especially of the serum alkaline phosphatase. Kaposi's sarcoma may affect the liver and biliary tree but is often asymptomatic.

Liver and rheumatological disease

Liver abnormalities occur in patients with rheumatological disorders, although they rarely prove to be clinically significant. Hepatic disease may either be a consequence of treatment or occur in association with other autoimmune diseases. For example, those diseases assumed to have an autoimmune basis, such as autoimmune hepatitis or primary biliary cirrhosis, may be associated with extrahepatic rheumatological diseases such as the sicca syndrome.

Rheumatoid arthritis

Abnormalities of liver structure and function are uncommon in patients with rheumatoid arthritis, although minor abnormalities of liver function tests occur in 20 to 50 per cent of cases. Nodular regenerative hyperplasia may cause complications of portal hypertension.

Felty's syndrome

Felty's syndrome is characterized by the triad of splenomegaly, hypersplenism, and seropositive rheumatoid arthritis. Liver function tests tend to be more commonly deranged than in uncomplicated rheumatoid arthritis. Anti-inflammatory therapy may contribute to the abnormal liver tests. Histological examination of the liver shows lymphocytic infiltration and, rarely, an established cirrhosis. Nodular regenerative hyperplasia occurs in patients with Felty's syndrome, as with rheumatoid arthritis. Although portal hypertension and variceal haemorrhage may occur, jaundice is unusual.

Hepatic arterial occlusion

This is a rare condition. It usually follows surgical trauma but has been found in association with arteritis and bacterial endocarditis.

The condition is characterized by an acute onset of pain in the upper abdomen, tenderness over the liver, and progressive shock and liver failure. Most cases have a fatal outcome.

Hepatic arterial aneurysm

This condition is recognized by the triad of upper abdominal pain, jaundice, and haematemesis following rupture of the aneurysm into the stomach or duodenum. The diagnosis is made by hepatic angiography. Treatment is by surgical resection.

Septic venous thrombosis of the portal system

This condition results from infection anywhere in the abdominal cavity leading to pylephlebitis of the portal venous system. It may occasionally result from a systemic septicaemia or from inflammatory disorders of the bowel, such as ulcerative colitis.

The acute phase of the disorder is usually characterized by features related to the underlying abdominal sepsis. This is followed by an episode of high fever, worsening abdominal pain, and rigors. There may be obvious evidence of septic embolization to the liver. This may lead to abdominal pain and hepatic tenderness with mild jaundice. All the systemic features of a severe infection develop and there is usually a polymorphonuclear leucocytosis and abnormal liver tests. Occasionally, multiple large intrahepatic abscesses may develop.

The condition should be suspected in any patient with abdominal sepsis who develops an acute systemic illness with abdominal pain and deranged liver tests. Management consists of intensive antibiotic treatment directed particularly towards Gram-negative organisms and micro-aerophilic streptococci. In some patients the clinical picture associated with portal venous thrombosis may develop after the acute phase has settled.

Protein-losing enteropathy

Rarely, hypoproteinaemia may result from excessive loss of plasma proteins into the gastrointestinal tract. All plasma proteins are affected; those showing the greatest reduction in concentration are the ones with the longest half-lives, including albumin. The resulting oedema is largely due to the low level of albumin, this being the main molecule responsible for the plasma colloid osmotic pressure. Although uncommon, this is an important condition to recognize because the resulting oedema or ascites may overshadow the intestinal symptoms and hence the underlying condition is easily missed.

This condition has been found in association with a wide variety of inflammatory or neoplastic disorders of the small bowel and abdominal lymphatic system. It is an almost inevitable consequence of intestinal lymphangiectasia, an inherited or congenital disorder caused by maldevelopment of the lymphatic system. It is also associated with allergic disorders involving the small bowel. In most of these conditions protein loss is mild and incidental. Severe protein loss occurs mainly in lymphatic disorders and in Ménétrier's disease, a curious condition characterized by the presence of giant gastric rugae.

Clinical features

When severe, the condition is characterized by peripheral oedema and occasionally by ascites and pleural effusions. There is marked hypoalbuminaemia in the absence of liver or renal disease. There may be associated steatorrhoea, particularly if the condition occurs in association with lymphoma of the bowel.

Diagnosis

The diagnosis is made by determining the rate of loss of protein into the intestine using a radioactive label, usually chromium(III) chloride ($^{51}CrCl_3$), which attaches to all plasma proteins, or as chromium-51 albumin, which redistributes the label, to some extent, to other proteins. $^{67}Copper$-labelled caeruloplasmin is theoretically a better marker but has a short half-life. The proportion of radioactivity in the stool is measured during the succeeding 4 days; 0.7 per cent is taken as the upper limit of normal. In comparison with plasma radioactivity, more sophisticated measures of plasma clearance can be derived to give quantitative data. Alternatively, measurement of α_1-antitrypsin in the stool has been shown to be a useful marker of protein-losing enteropathy, without necessitating radioactive labelling.

The further diagnosis of the condition is directed towards determining the underlying cause.

Treatment

Treatment is directed towards raising the plasma albumin and correction of the underlying disorder. For example, cases associated with neoplasm of the stomach or colon require surgical resection. Those secondary to coeliac disease, sprue, Whipple's disease, or allergic gastroenteropathies should be treated appropriately.

Jejunoileal bypass

Most patients with massive obesity have fatty infiltration of the liver. After jejunoileal bypass, 55 per cent of them show further fatty change, although this is usually asymptomatic. The increase in fat is due entirely to an accumulation of triglyceride. There is frequently a mild elevation of liver enzymes in serum but this returns to normal once weight reduction has been achieved. The mechanism for the increased fatty change is unknown but it may be a result of protein–calorie malnutrition. An alternative possibility is that the steatosis may be secondary to bacterial overgrowth in the excluded loop of small intestine, as steatosis may diminish with metronidazole therapy.

Acute liver failure may develop in a few patients and is associated with considerable mortality. It is thought to be due to bacterial colonization of the included and excluded small intestine with the production of 'hepatotoxins', which are then absorbed. Treatment consists of intravenous amino acids and broad-spectrum antibiotics. If the condition recurs, further treatment should be given and the ileal bypass reversed.

A micronodular cirrhosis may develop 1 to 6 years after a bypass operation. Histologically, the liver often shows appearances similar to those induced by alcohol. If liver function deteriorates, small-bowel continuity should be restored. Patients may still progress to liver failure and death, but there are reports of the cirrhosis arresting or even reversing with complete recovery of the histology.

Parenteral nutrition and the liver

Abnormalities of serum liver enzymes and bilirubin are commonly seen in patients receiving total parenteral nutrition. Thirty to 60 per cent of patients will show a rise in at least one liver test of greater than 50 per cent of baseline, a rise in alkaline phosphatase being the most frequent abnormality. The changes occur towards the end of the first week and peak between 9 and 12 days. Patients receiving intravenous lipid are particularly at risk, but biochemical cholestasis can occur when no fat is given. Liver histology shows steatosis, mild portal inflammation and fibrosis, bile-duct proliferation, and bile plugs. The changes in serum liver tests and in liver histology are reversible once parenteral nutrition is discontinued, although persistent histological changes have been reported. The abnormal concentrations of liver enzymes may also return to normal if the calorie–nitrogen ratio is lowered by reducing the amount of dextrose given, or may even settle spontaneously if parenteral nutrition is continued without change.

The cause of the intrahepatic cholestasis is unknown. Direct toxicity of the intravenous solutions (especially those containing tryptophan), calorie excess, or a deficiency of essential fatty acids have been proposed as possible mechanisms. A more likely explanation is the possibility of an overgrowth of anaerobic bacteria in the intestine with subsequent production of endotoxin and lithocholic acid, both of which induce liver damage in animals with similar histological features to those seen in humans receiving total parenteral nutrition. Patients who develop a rise in serum transaminases and alkaline phosphatase have a high concentration of lithocholic acid in the bile compared with patients being parenterally fed who do not have abnormal liver tests. Furthermore, metronidazole has been shown to prevent cholestasis developing in these patients. Hence, the situation may be analogous to the cholestasis associated with a jejunoileal bypass (see above).

Peliosis hepatitis

This consists of venous lakes within the liver, which probably occur as a result of sinusoidal ectasia. It may be seen in association with oral contraceptive usage, terminal cachexia from carcinoma, and with androgenic steroid therapy. Clinically there are usually few symptoms, although hepatomegaly may be present. Mild to moderate increases in transaminases may occur. Diagnosis is usually made coincidentally on liver biopsy and the prognosis is that of the underlying condition.

Further reading

Adibi BA, Stanko RT (1984). Perspective on gastrointestinal surgery for the treatment of morbid obesity: the lesson learned. *Gastroenterology* **87**, 1381.

Baddeley RM (1980). Surgical management of severe obesity. In: Truelove SV, Kennedy HJ, eds. *Topics in gastroenterology*, Vol 8. Blackwell Scientific, Oxford.

Bolt RJ (1976). Disease of the hepatic blood vessels. In: Backus HL, ed. *Gastroenterology*, 3rd edn, p 471. Saunders, Philadelphia.

Chatel A et al. (1979). L'arteriographie dans la periartérite noueuse. *Journal of Radiology* **60**, 113–20.

Dockerty MB (1972). Primary malakoplakia of the colon. *Mayo Clinic Proceedings* **47**, 114.

Drenick EJ, Fisler J, Johnson D (1982). Hepatic steatosis after intestinal bypass—prevention and reversal by metronidazole, irrespective of protein–calorie malnutrition. *Gastroenterology* **82**, 535.

Lambert JR, Thomas SM (1985). Metronidazole prevention of serum liver enzyme abnormalities during total parenteral nutrition. *Journal of Parenteral Nutrition* **9**, 501.

Lazenby AJ et al. (1989). Lymphocytic ('microscopic') colitis: a comparative histopathologic study with particular reference to collagenous colitis. *Human Pathology* **20**, 18–28.

Long R, James O (1974). Polymyalgia rheumatica and liver disease. *Lancet* **i**, 77.

Ranney B (1975). The prevention, inhibition, palliation and treatment of endometriosis. *American Journal of Obstetrics and Gynecology* **123**, 778.

Runyon BA, La Brecque DR, Anuras S (1980). The spectrum of liver disease in systemic lupus erythematosus. *American Journal of Medicine* **69**, 187.

Sheldon GF, Peterson SR, Sanders R (1978). Hepatic dysfunction during hyperalimentation. *Archives of Surgery* **113**, 504.

Sherlock S (1981). *Diseases of the liver and biliary system*, 6th edn. Blackwell Scientific, Oxford.

Sleisenger MH, Fordtran JS (1993). *Gastrointestinal disease*, 4th edn. Saunders, Philadelphia.

Steer HD, Colin-Jones DG (1975). Melanosis coli. Studies of toxic effects of irritant purgatives. *Journal of Pathology* **115**, 119.

Whaley K, Webb J (1977). Liver and kidney disease in rheumatoid arthritis. *Clinics in Rheumatic Diseases* **3**, 527.

15

Cardiovascular medicine

15.1 Cardiovascular biology, atherosclerosis, and thrombosis

15.1.1 The blood vessels

15.1.1.1 Introduction

Peter L. Weissberg

The scale of the problem

All organs require an adequate blood supply to survive and function normally, yet in the Western world we are in the midst of an epidemic of disease caused by atherosclerosis in which lipids are deposited in the subendothelial space of major arteries initiating a process that results in narrowing and occlusion of vessels and consequent ischaemia and necrosis of organs and limbs. Although atherosclerosis is manifested most dramatically as acute myocardial and cerebral infarction (heart attack and stroke), it also has a substantial impact on limb, gut, and renal function. Indeed, there is no other single disease that has such a potent and diverse impact on health. Coronary, cerebrovascular, and peripheral vascular disease together account for approximately 40 per cent of male and 30 per cent of female deaths in the United Kingdom in those under 75 years of age. In recent years there has been a gratifying fall in the incidence of deaths from cardiovascular causes in middle-aged adults in the so-called developed world. However, since most heart attacks and strokes occur in the elderly and life expectancy is increasing, the prevalence of cardiovascular disease is bound to increase. Also, there is clear evidence that the epidemic of cardiovascular disease is spreading rapidly, particularly in former Eastern Block countries and, alarmingly, in the Third World. It therefore follows that if atherosclerosis could be understood and overcome, the impact on world health would be substantial.

The atherosclerotic plaque

An atherosclerotic plaque comprises a subendothelial accumulation of oxidized lipid at its core with an inflammatory cell infiltrate covered by a fibrous cap consisting of modified vascular smooth muscle cells and their extracellular matrix. Plaques begin in early life as asymptomatic fatty streaks. Symptoms arise later on, either because a plaque has grown large enough to limit flow, or because a plaque erodes or ruptures causing platelet aggregation and evolution of an occlusive thrombosis within the vessel lumen.

Large plaques eventually declare themselves through the emergence of inducible ischaemia, manifested as angina pectoris (coronary disease, Fig. 1) or intermittent claudication (peripheral vascular disease), which resolves when oxygen demand is reduced, either by stopping the triggering activity or by drug therapy. Plaque erosion or rupture is sudden and usually precipitates an acute ischaemic event such as unstable angina (Fig. 1), myocardial infarction, transient cerebral ischaemia, or stroke depending on the vascular bed involved. Tissue viability then depends on whether or not flow

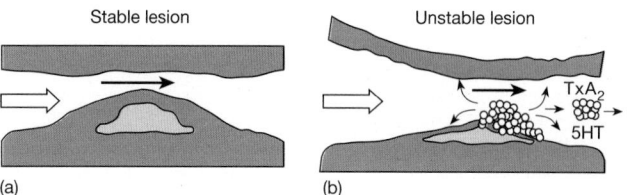

Fig. 1 Mechanisms by which atherosclerotic plaques induce symptoms. (a) Large stable atherosclerotic plaque limits blood flow in response to increased demand causing stable angina. (b) Platelet aggregation and thrombus formation on an unstable atherosclerotic plaque limit blood flow and cause vasoconstriction and embolization at rest, leading to unstable angina (TxA_2 thromboxane A_2, 5HT, 5-hydroxytryptamine). (Redrawn from Weinberg PL (1999). In: *Angina in clinical practice* (ed. P. Schofield). Martin Dunitz Ltd.)

can be restored and how quickly. In the coronary circulation removal of the offending thrombus is achieved either with drug therapy or by angioplasty. Pharmacological and mechanical strategies for restoring cerebral blood flow after ischaemic stroke are less well established.

The inflammatory basis of atherosclerosis

It is now recognized that atherosclerosis is a destructive inflammatory process, probably initiated and maintained by modified (oxidized) lipids, involving endothelial dysfunction, and mediated by activated macrophages, T cells, and possibly also mast cells. The inflammatory process is isolated from the circulation by a protective fibrous cap synthesized by intimal vascular smooth muscle cells. If the inflammatory process predominates, then plaque rupture and thrombosis results (Fig. 2). The inflammatory basis of

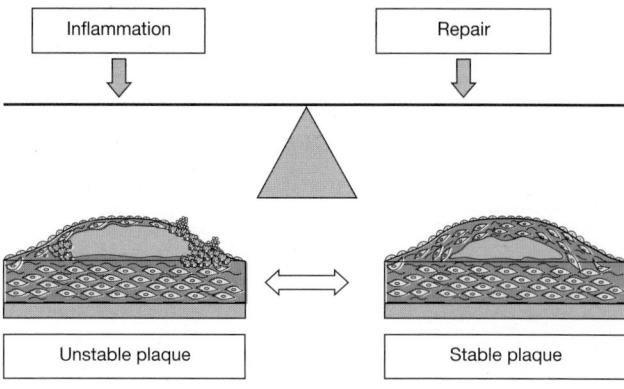

Fig. 2 The balance of atherosclerosis. The stability of atherosclerotic plaque is determined by the net effect of the destructive inflammatory process tending to plaque rupture and thrombosis balanced by the stabilizing influence of the fibrous cap synthesized by intimal smooth muscle cells. (Redrawn from Weinberg PL (1999). *Atherosclerosis*, **147** (suppl. 1), S3–S10.)

atherosclerosis is reflected in a close correlation between circulating markers of inflammation, for example fibrinogen, C-reactive protein, serum amyloid A, and serum albumen (inverse) and clinical outcome in patients with known disease.

The changing treatment of atherosclerosis

Atherosclerosis has traditionally been regarded as a collection of end-stage organ-based diseases such as myocardial infarction, stroke, and limb ischaemia, treated by specialists from a variety of disciplines concerned more with its consequences than its cause. Therapy has therefore relied largely on mechanical procedures such as bypass surgery, endarterectomy, and balloon angioplasty to relieve obstruction and improve blood flow. However, whilst these procedures have been very successful at relieving symptoms, they have had little impact on survival, except in a few specific patient groups. The main impact on survival has come from advances in drug therapy.

Since thrombosis is the commonest terminal event in atherosclerosis it is not surprising that fibrinolytic, antithrombotic, and antiplatelet drugs are all effective in acute events caused by plaque rupture, such as myocardial infarction, unstable angina, and transient ischaemic attacks. However, the most important recent therapeutic development has been the introduction of inhibitors of HMG Co-A reductase (the statins), which reduce low-density lipoprotein cholesterol and triglycerides, increase high-density lipoprotein cholesterol, and improve endothelial function. Treatment with statins reduces the risk of a vascular event (both heart attack and stroke) by about 30 per cent in patients with and without symptoms of atherosclerosis (secondary and primary prevention) and with high or 'normal' cholesterol levels, yet they produce little, if any, haemodynamically meaningful plaque regression. The optimistic message from these observations is that statins have a greater effect on plaque stability than on plaque size and that atherosclerosis is therefore a dynamic process that can be modified, even in advanced disease.

In the twenty-first century atherosclerosis is best viewed as a single dynamic disease in which complex interactions between endothelial cells, smooth muscle cells, inflammatory cells, and platelets dictate its course. The development of effective medical therapies for atherosclerosis argues for a common approach to its management regardless of its presentation. Thus all patients with established atherosclerotic disease should have the opportunity to benefit from treatment with lipid-lowering and antiplatelet therapies. Since it is now possible to prevent clinical events in asymptomatic patients with occult vascular disease, the challenge is to target expensive therapies to those at highest risk. In the future this is likely to include assessment of 'classical' risk factors (family history, smoking, diabetes, cholesterol levels) but also possibly indices of inflammation and measures of genetic variations (polymorphisms) in molecules known to play a central role in plaque progression and stability.

Further reading

LIPID Study Group (1998). Prevention of cardiovascular events and death with pravastatin in patients with coronary heart disease and a broad range of initial cholesterol levels. *New England Journal of Medicine* 339, 1349–57.

Ridker P *et al.* (1997). Inflammation, aspirin, and the risk of cardiovascular disease in apparently healthy men. *New England Journal of Medicine* 336, 973–9.

Ridker P *et al.* (1998). Inflammation, pravastatin, and the risk of coronary events after myocardial infarction in patients with average cholesterol levels. Cholesterol and Recurrent Events (CARE) Investigators. *Circulation* 98, 839–44.

Ross R (1986). The pathogenesis of atherosclerosis–an update. *New England Journal of Medicine* 314, 488–500.

Ross R (1993). The pathogenesis of atherosclerosis: a perspective for the 1990s. *Nature* 362, 801–9.

Ross R (1999). Atherosclerosis—an inflammatory disease. *New England Journal of Medicine* 340, 115–26.

Ross R, Glomset J (1976). The pathogenesis of atherosclerosis. Part 1. *New England Journal of Medicine* 295, 369–77.

Ross R, Glomset J (1976). The pathogenesis of atherosclerosis. Part 2. *New England Journal of Medicine* 295, 420–8.

Sacks FM *et al.* (1996). The effect of pravastatin on coronary events after myocardial infarction in patients with average cholesterol levels. Cholesterol and Recurrent Events Trial investigators. *New England Journal of Medicine* 335, 1001–9.

Scandinavian Simvastatin Survival Group (1994). Randomised trial of cholesterol lowering in 4444 patients with coronaryheart disease: the Scandinavian Simvastatin survival study (4S). *Lancet* 344, 1383–9.

Shepherd J *et al.* (1995). Prevention of coronary heart disease with pravastatin in men with hypercholesterolemia. *New England Journal of Medicine* 333, 1301–7.

Treasure CB *et al.* (1995). Beneficial effects of cholesterol-lowering therapy on the coronary endothelium in patients with coronary artery disease. *New England Journal of Medicine* 332, 481–7.

15.1.1.2 Vascular endothelium: its physiology and pathophysiology

P. Vallance

A monolayer of endothelial cells lines the intimal surface of the entire vascular tree (Fig. 1) to form the largest endocrine/paracrine organ in the body. These cells are metabolically very active and exert a profound influence on vascular reactivity, thrombogenesis, and the behaviour of circulating cells. Abnormalities of endothelial function have been implicated in a wide variety of diseases ranging from atheroma and hypertension to acute inflammation and septic shock (Table 1). Recent advances in endothelial research have led to the development of new therapies and re-evaluation of those that exist. This section provides an introduction to the biology of the vascular endothelium and describes how endothelial dysfunction may contribute to cardiovascular disease.

Development of endothelium

During early development the endothelium forms the first layer of the circulatory system and extends to produce a network of interconnecting tubes; this ability of endothelial cells to form tube-like structures is retained even when they are grown *in vitro* (Fig. 1). *In vivo*, the endothelial tubes differentiate into arteries, arterioles, capillaries, veins, and lymph vessels, and regional differences in function and structure evolve such that the properties of endothelial cells vary between arterial and venous beds, between micro- and macrovasculature, between organs, and between different parts of individual organs—perhaps the most striking example being the specialized layer of endothelial cells that forms the blood–brain barrier. Heterogeneity of endothelial cell function undoubtedly has implications for physiology, pathophysiology, and therapeutics. However, endothelial cells from different vessels also have many features in common and a number of pathologies, including those causing premature vascular disease, are associated with widespread changes in the behaviour of endothelial cells.

Anatomy of endothelium

Each endothelial cell is between 25 and 50 μm long, 10 and 15 μm wide, and up to 5 μm deep, and lies with its long axis aligned in the direction of the blood flow (Fig. 1). The underlying smooth muscle cells lie radially, are about 5 to 10 μm wide, and taper at either end so that a single endothelial cell can communicate with many smooth muscle cells, and vice versa. The endothelium also comes into intimate contact with circulating cells, and the total area of the luminal surface of endothelium is in excess of 500 m². This thin layer of cells is particularly susceptible to injury, and changes in endothelial cell morphology and turnover occur in experimental hypertension, diabetes, and atheroma. Antibodies directed against endothelium can be found in a number of inflammatory and immune conditions.

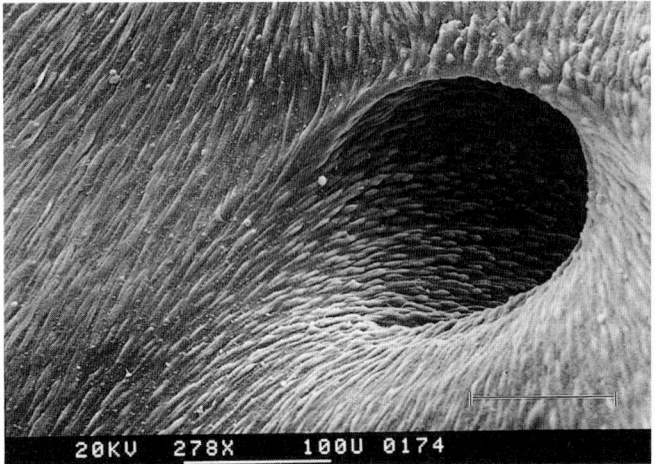

(a)

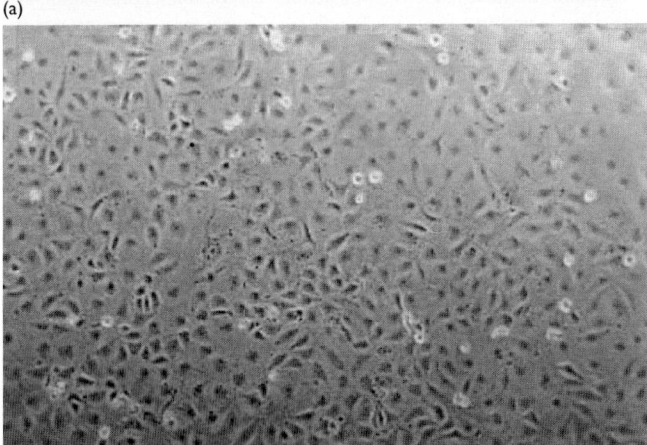

(b)

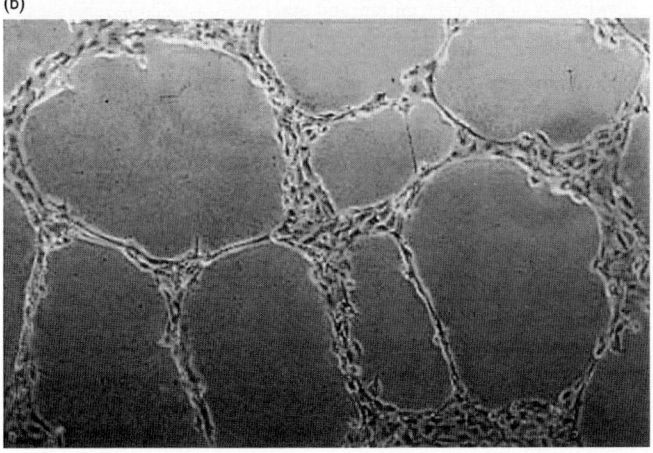

(c)

Fig. 1 Panel (a) shows a scanning electron micrograph of the endothelium of a human coronary vessel at a branch area (supplied by P. M. Rowles). Panel (b) shows endothelial cells grown in culture in the absence of angiogenic factors. With stimulation by the correct angiogenic factors, endothelial cells form a tube-like structure (Panel (c)).

Table 1 Diseases associated with endothelial dysfunction

Atherosclerosis	
Atherosclerotic risk factors	Hypertension
	Diabetes
	Hypercholesterolaemia
	Smoking
	Elevated homocysteine
Pulmonary hypertension	
Connective tissue disorders	Raynaud's disease
	Systemic sclerosis
Vascular inflammation	Kawasaki's disease
	Haemolytic uraemic syndrome
	Transplant rejection
	Systemic infection
Drug induced	Cyclosporin toxicity
Malignant haemangioendothelioma	

Signal detection by endothelial cells

The endothelial cell membrane expresses a large number of receptors for circulating hormones, local mediators, and vasoactive factors released from blood cells. It can also sense local changes in pressure and flow; stretch of the cell membrane leads directly to opening of a cation channel permeable to calcium, and flow across the cell surface leads to opening of a potassium channel, which hyperpolarizes the cell. The precise mechanisms linking the various stimuli received to the response of the endothelial cell have yet to be determined, but calcium is undoubtedly important. Receptor occupation, stretch, or shear stress all lead to changes in the concentration of intracellular free calcium, and the profile of change influences which endothelial functions are activated and therefore which message is produced by the cell. In addition, it is clear that the endothelial cell can adjust both the expression and localization of certain key enzymes in response to physical or chemical stimuli. Translocation of enzymes from cytosol to cell surface or to specialized invaginations in the cell surface (caveolae) in response to stimuli can greatly alter the metabolic activity of the endothelial cell. The endothelium acts as a signal transducer and exerts a profound influence on the cardiovascular system by virtue of the way in which it alters its phenotype in response to signals.

Control of vascular tone

Endothelium extracts and inactivates circulating hormones, converts inactive precursors into active products, and synthesizes and releases a variety of vasoactive mediators (Fig. 2). Vasoconstrictor and vasodilator mediators are produced and allow the vessel to respond to changes in the local milieu, but the predominant background influence of the endothelium is dilator, with removal of the endothelium leading to vasoconstriction. Basal endothelium-dependent dilator tone seems to provide a physiological counterbalance to the continuous constrictor tone of the sympathetic nervous system.

Vasodilators

The endothelium produces at least three vasodilator mediators (Fig. 2): nitric oxide, prostanoids, and hyperpolarizing factor.

Nitric oxide

Physiology

The production of nitric oxide is responsible for basal endothelium-dependent dilator tone. This simple gas is a potent vasodilator: its synthesis and main actions through the second messenger cyclic GMP are described in Fig. 3. In addition, nitric oxide inhibits cytochrome c oxidase, initially in

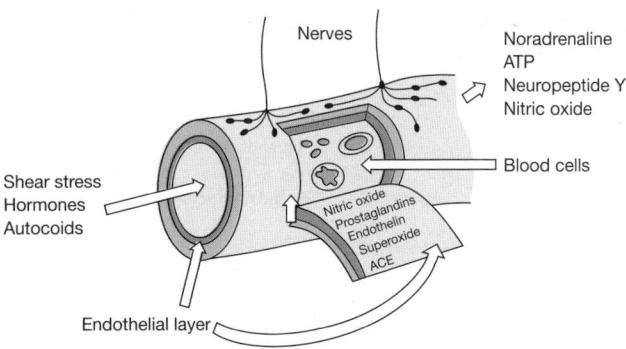

Fig. 2 Vascular endothelial cells lie at the interface between blood and the smooth muscle cells. They detect chemical and physical signals in the lumen of the blood vessel and adjust their output of biologically active mediators accordingly. This provides a mechanism of local regulation of vascular function. Rapid adjustment of vascular tone is probably achieved through a balance of endothelium-derived nitric oxide and neuronally derived noradrenaline. Endothelin provides a slowly modulating constrictor tone and angiotensin II has the capacity to fine-tune neuronal, endothelial, and smooth muscle function. Abbreviations: ACE (angiotensin converting enzyme), ATP (adenosine triphosphate).

a reversible manner, but irreversibly under certain conditions. Inhibition of this enzyme decreases oxygen utilization, and the release of nitric oxide by endothelial cells appears to be an important determinant of oxygen consumption in the vasculature. It is possible that there are additional important targets for nitric oxide, including ion channels and other enzymes, but the physiological significance of these effects is not yet clear. Nitric oxide modifies the adhesiveness of the endothelial cell for circulating white cells, but rapid inactivation by haemoglobin prevents any significant downstream effect.

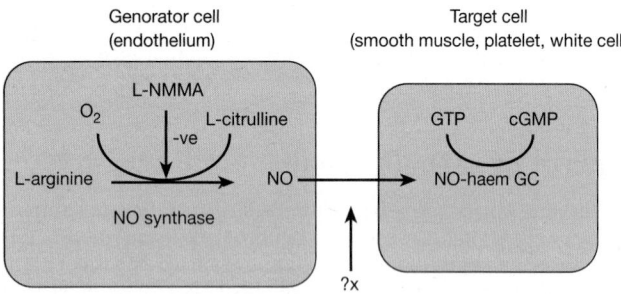

Fig. 3 Nitric oxide (NO) is synthesized from L-arginine by the action of nitric oxide synthase. Citrulline is the byproduct of the reaction. Nitric oxide, which has a half-life of only a few seconds, diffuses from the endothelial cell to reach a target cell—this may be vascular smooth muscle, a platelet, or a white cell. In the process of diffusion nitric oxide may interact with other molecules (X) which may stabilize or destroy the mediator. A major physiological target for nitric oxide is guanylyl cyclase (GC). Nitric oxide binds to the haem moiety of this enzyme and this leads to enzyme activation and generation of cyclic guanosine monophosphate (cGMP). Elevation of cGMP relaxes smooth muscle and inhibits platelet aggregation and adhesion. The platelet-derived mediators adenosine diphosphate (ADP) and 5-hydroxytryptamine (5-HT; serotonin) stimulate endothelial cells to synthesize nitric oxide and this provides a negative-feedback system to prevent activated platelets from causing vasospasm and further platelet adhesion and aggregation. The synthesis of nitric oxide can be inhibited by certain guanidino-substituted analogues of L-arginine such as N^G-monomethyl-L-arginine (L-NMMA) and this substance as well as asymmetric dimethylarginine (ADMA) occurs naturally and may contribute to nitric oxide deficiency in disease states. Nitric oxide synthase activity can be stimulated by calcium, provision of co-factors, phosphorylation of the enzyme, and by altered intracellular localization

Nitric oxide is a free radical (it has an unpaired electron in its outer orbit) and as such reacts readily with other free radicals and reactive oxygen species. The reaction between nitric oxide and superoxide anion (O_2^-) is extremely fast and can result in the formation of either the toxic product peroxynitrite ($ONOO^-$) or the inactive breakdown product nitrate (NO_3^-). Such interactions between radicals can greatly influence the overall behaviour of the wall of the blood vessel and can lead to an apparent defect in endothelial function even when the output of endothelial mediators is normal.

The arterial circulation of animals and humans is vasodilated continuously and actively by endothelium-derived nitric oxide, and inhibition of the synthesis of nitric oxide with certain guanidino-substituted analogues of L-arginine, including N^G-monomethyl-L-arginine, leads to vasoconstriction, hypertension, and sodium retention. Shear stress—the force caused by the viscous drag of flowing blood—is probably an important physiological stimulus for the continuous production of nitric oxide. As shear stress increases more nitric oxide is produced and the blood vessel relaxes, reducing the stress. This process of flow-mediated dilatation appears to be a homeostatic mechanism to prevent shear stress from increasing to levels that might initiate activation of platelets or other cells and may also help co-ordinate tissue perfusion. Flow-mediated dilatation is an autoregulatory property of blood vessels that tends to oppose classical myogenic autoregulation—the process by which a blood vessel constricts in response to an increase in intraluminal pressure.

Synthesis of nitric oxide is stimulated by acetylcholine, bradykinin, and substance P, and in many vessels release of nitric oxide accounts for the vasodilator actions of these mediators, which are known as 'endothelium-dependent vasodilators'. Circulating hormones, including insulin and oestrogens, may also act on receptors on or within the endothelial cell to stimulate the release of nitric oxide acutely or to alter the expression of endothelial nitric oxide synthase chronically.

Veins differ from arteries and arterioles, and do not seem to be actively dilated by continuous release of nitric oxide. Venous endothelium releases nitric oxide when stimulated by acetylcholine or bradykinin, but not under basal conditions. Furthermore, human veins do not release much nitric oxide in response to platelet-derived mediators. Indeed, aggregating platelets constrict veins, due to the unopposed action of the platelet-derived mediators on vascular smooth muscle. The reasons for the arteriovenous difference in nitric oxide production are not fully understood, but one consequence is that the guanylyl cyclase in venous smooth muscle is relatively upregulated and veins respond to smaller amounts of nitric oxide than do arteries or arterioles. This is of therapeutic relevance; nitric oxide is the active moiety of glyceryl trinitrate and other nitrovasodilators, and the low basal synthesis of endogenous nitric oxide by venous endothelium accounts, in part, for the venoselective action of these drugs.

Pathophysiology

Loss of nitric oxide leads to arterial vasoconstriction, has the potential to enhance platelet and white cell adhesion, and in experimental models may enhance atherogenesis. Several clinical conditions, including atherosclerosis, hypertension, hypercholesterolaemia, and diabetes, are associated with a functional loss of nitric oxide-mediated effects.

In the coronary vasculature, loss of nitric oxide predisposes to vasospasm and may contribute to the onset of anginal symptoms. Atherosclerotic coronary arteries constrict in response to the platelet-derived mediator serotonin (5-hydroxytryptamine), whereas healthy vessels are stimulated to produce more nitric oxide and dilate (Fig. 3). Flow-dependent dilatation is also lost in such vessels, and the response to sympathetic stimulation is converted from dilatation to unopposed constriction. Endothelial dysfunction precedes the development of overt atheroma and there is a relationship between risk factors for ischaemic heart disease and impaired responsiveness of coronary arteries to endothelium-dependent vasodilators. Furthermore, hypercholesterolaemia, even in the absence of angiographic evidence of atheroma in large vessels, is associated with abnormal endothelium-dependent vasodilatation in coronary and peripheral arterioles. Modified low-density lipoproteins appear to inhibit nitric oxide synthesis or speed its destruction, possibly by enhancing production of superoxide anion.

Basal endothelium-dependent dilatation is also impaired in patients with essential hypertension and the degree of impairment increases with increasing blood pressure. It is not known whether the defect is a consequence or a cause of the raised pressure, but the fact that endothelial function appears to be restored by antihypertensive therapy argues in favour of dysfunction being a response to raised pressure. Patients with diabetes show diminished endothelium-dependent dilatation, and this defect does not reverse with treatment. Thus patients with uncontrolled hypertension, diabetes, and hypercholesterolaemia all display defects of nitric-oxide-mediated vasodilatation and this could provide a common mechanism of vascular dysfunction in these diseases. Impaired endothelium-dependent dilatation associated with hypercholesterolaemia is partially reversed by supplementation with L-arginine (see below).

In addition to the effects of disease states on nitric oxide, genetic variation in endothelial nitric oxide synthase may predispose to cardiovascular disease. Common variations occur in promoter and coding regions of the gene encoding endothelial nitric oxide synthase and certain variants appear to be associated with excess cardiovascular risk, but the data are not yet conclusive. Nor is it clear how the genetic variations alter nitric oxide synthesis or endothelial cell function.

Overproduction of nitric oxide may also contribute to disease. Bacterial endotoxin, and certain cytokines, including interleukin 1 and interferon-γ, induce expression of a second nitric oxide synthesizing enzyme which appears in the endothelium, vascular smooth muscle, and inflammatory cells invading the vessel wall. Unlike the constitutive enzyme present in healthy endothelium (endothelial nitric oxide synthase), this inducible isoform of nitric oxide synthase is not regulated by calcium and produces large amounts of nitric oxide. In these quantities nitric oxide, either alone or in combination with superoxide, may contribute to tissue damage in addition to causing profound vasodilatation and hypotension. Excess production of nitric oxide from endothelial nitric oxide synthase due to stimulation of certain essential cofactors including tetrahydrobiopterin may also contribute to these effects. The therapeutic potential of specific inhibitors of nitric oxide synthase as anti-inflammatory agents has not yet been established. In contrast to the general increase in nitric oxide seen in response to inflammation, certain proinflammatory cytokines (particularly tumour necrosis factor-α) may impair normal endothelium-dependent relaxation and nitric oxide synthesis. This might be an important mechanism linking infection or inflammation to increased risk of cardiovascular events including arterial or venous thrombosis.

Prostanoids

Nitric oxide appears to be the dominant vasoactive factor released from endothelial cells under basal conditions, but it is by no means the only mediator produced. The endothelium is a rich source of prostanoids, including the vasodilators prostacyclin and the prostaglandins E_2 and D_2. However, whereas inhibition of nitric oxide leads to profound and widespread changes in vascular tone, inhibition of prostanoid synthesis with aspirin, or other non-steroidal anti-inflammatory drugs, does not. Renal vasculature is an exception, and dilator prostanoids do appear to be important in the regulation of basal renal blood flow; aspirin and other non-steroidal anti-inflammatory drugs lead to vasoconstriction in the kidney, indicating tonic release of vasodilator prostanoids in this vascular bed. Furthermore, in the fetus and newborn, indomethacin leads to closure of the ductus arteriosus and a fall in cerebral blood flow suggesting a significant contribution of endothelium-derived prostanoids to tonic vasodilatation in these beds, at least during development. Cerebral blood flow in adults also falls in response to indomethacin, but not to aspirin and other cyclo-oxygenase inhibitors, and so the role of prostanoids is unclear. Vasodilator prostanoids are important in the vascular changes of inflammation, although whether the prostanoids derive exclusively from the endothelium is not known. A cytokine-inducible isoform of cyclo-oxygenase (cyclo-oxy-

genase II) has been identified and this probably contributes to the increased synthesis of vascular prostaglandins in inflammation.

Hyperpolarizing factor

An endothelium-derived hyperpolarizing factor has been identified in certain animal and human blood vessels. Hyperpolarization of vascular smooth muscle cells leads to a fall in calcium entry and vascular relaxation. Increasing evidence suggests that endothelium-dependent hyperpolarization may be particularly important in small arteries and arterioles. The chemical identity of endothelium-derived hyperpolarizing factor has not been clearly established, but products of activity of cytochrome P450, the cannabinoid anandamide, and the potassium ion have all been suggested as possible candidates. Only when a clear identify for endothelium-derived hyperpolarizing factor has been established, or a specific inhibitor produced, will it be possible to determine the precise role of this mediator in vascular physiology and pathophysiology.

Vasoconstrictors

Although the predominant background influence of the endothelium is dilator, important vasoconstrictor factors are also synthesized and released.

Endothelin

The endothelins are a family of potent vasoconstrictor peptides containing 21 amino acids that are closely related to the snake venom toxin of the Israeli burrowing asp. Three types of endothelin have been described, endothelin 1, 2, and 3, and there are at least two endothelin receptors in human blood vessels: endothelin A receptor and endothelin B receptor. Endothelins vasoconstrict and can promote the growth of vascular smooth muscle cells. Effects are mediated in part through stimulation of increases in calcium and in part through calcium-independent mechanisms including activation of protein kinases.

Endothelin 1 is synthesized from 'big endothelin' within human endothelial cells (Fig. 4). It is a potent and long-lasting constrictor of human blood vessels, and causes widespread vasoconstriction, hypertension, and sodium retention when infused into healthy volunteers. Antagonists of the

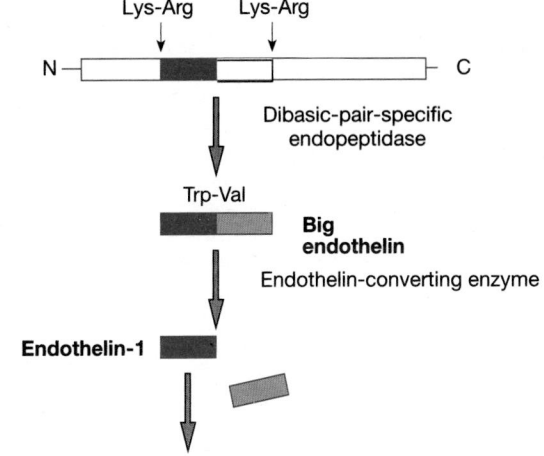

Fig. 4 Biosynthesis of the vasoconstrictor peptide endothelin 1. Endothelin 1 produces profound vasoconstriction, through activation of endothelin A receptors. Activation of endothelin B receptors on smooth muscle also causes vasoconstriction, but stimulation of endothelin B receptors on the endothelium stimulates nitric oxide and prostacyclin production.

endothelin A receptor cause vasodilatation when infused locally, and mixed endothelin A/B antagonists lower blood pressure in normotensive and hypertensive individuals. These findings indicate that there is a tonic synthesis and release of endothelin. A number of studies suggest that there may be important interactions between the sympathetic nervous system, the renin–angiotensin system, and the endothelin system and that these may act in concert to control constrictor tone, with the endothelin system providing a slowly modulating background constrictor tone.

Paradoxically, endothelin can also produce transient vasodilatation. This seems to be mediated by activation of endothelin B receptors. Although activation of endothelin B receptors on vascular smooth muscle causes constriction, activation of endothelial endothelin B receptors leads to the generation of vasodilator prostanoids and/or nitric oxide. Binding of endothelin to endothelin B receptors also seems to be important to clear the peptide from the circulation. Stimuli for endothelin production include thrombin, insulin, cyclosporine, adrenaline, angiotensin II, cortisol, various proinflammatory cytokines, hypoxia, and shear stress.

The concentrations of endothelins circulating in plasma are low and may not reflect local concentrations achieved within the vessel wall. It is difficult to interpret the elevated values reported in many conditons. A role for endothelin in the pathogenesis of vasospasm associated with subarachnoid haemorrhage and some types of renal ischaemia is suggested by results from experiments in animals, and endothelin A/B antagonists produce short-term changes in haemodynamics in patients with heart failure that suggest a possible beneficial therapeutic effect. It seems likely that the precise role of endothelin in these diseases, and other vasospastic conditions, will become apparent as inhibitors of endothelin synthesis, and specific endothelin receptor blockers become more widely used in clinical trials.

Increased production of endothelin has been clearly implicated in the pathogenesis of a very rare form of secondary hypertension caused by malignant haemangioendothelioma, a vascular tumour characterized by intravascular proliferation of atypical endothelial cells. In this condition the degree of hypertension correlates with plasma levels of endothelin and when the tumour is removed blood pressure and plasma endothelin levels fall.

Angiotensin converting enzyme

Angiotensin converting enzyme is located primarily on the luminal surface of the endothelium. This enzyme converts angiotensin I to angiotensin II and also metabolizes bradykinin to inactive products (see Fig. 2). The pulmonary vasculature provides the largest area of endothelium, and is important in the regulation of circulating levels of angiotensin II, but activity of endothelial angiotensin converting enzyme in systemic vessels may be more important in determining the final concentrations of angiotensin II and bradykinin reaching the blood vessel wall. Furthermore, endothelial cells also have the ability to synthesize renin and its substrate. It therefore seems as though the enzymatic machinery for a complete renin–angiotensin system is present within the vessel wall.

The activity of the renin–angiotensin system is clearly important in cardiovascular diseases including hypertension and heart failure, but the relative importance of local compared with systemic regulation of angiotensin II production is not yet clear. Furthermore, the full clinical significance of bradykinin metabolism by endothelial angiotensin converting enzyme (see Fig. 2) has yet to be determined. It has been demonstrated that at least part of the vasodilator action of angiotensin converting enzyme inhibitors in certain isolated blood vessels is due to accumulation of bradykinin which stimulates nitric oxide synthesis.

Prostanoids

The endothelium synthesizes thromboxane and the unstable prostaglandin endoperoxides prostaglandin G_2 and prostaglandin H_2. Overproduction of constrictor prostanoids by the endothelium has been implicated in animal models of diabetes and hypertension, but the significance of these findings for human disease remains uncertain.

Superoxide

The superoxide anion (O_2^-) is synthesized within endothelial cells. There are several possible enzymatic sources including co-factor deplete nitric oxide synthase and cyclo-oxygenase. In neutrophils, NADH/NADPH oxidase is the major source of superoxide. Components of this system have been detected in endothelial cells and they are now assumed to be the major site of superoxide generation. Superoxide is usually destroyed by superoxide dismutase, but under certain conditions it seems as though it may act as an endothelium-derived contracting factor or interact with nitric oxide as described above.

Regulation of platelet function and haemostasis

The endothelium synthesizes and releases prothrombotic and antithrombotic factors. However, healthy endothelium presents a thromboresistant surface, indicating that the antithrombotic factors predominate under basal conditions.

Platelets

Endothelial cells inhibit the aggregation and adhesion of platelets, and disaggregate aggregating platelets. Two mediators are of particular importance: nitric oxide and prostacyclin (or prostaglandin E_2 in microvascular endothelium). They act synergistically through different second messenger systems: cyclic guanosine monophosphate for nitric oxide and cyclic adenosine monophosphate for prostacyclin.

Thiols and sulphydryl-containing molecules react with nitric oxide to produce more stable adducts, including nitrosocysteine, nitrosoglutathione, nitrosoalbumin, and even nitrosohaemoglobin. Some of these compounds are formed *in vivo* and may enhance the antiplatelet effects of endothelium-derived nitric oxide. Furthermore, interaction between nitric oxide and tissue plasminogen activator leads to the formation of nitrosotissue plasminogen activator, a molecule with fibrinolytic, antiplatelet, and vasorelaxant properties. It is not yet clear how important these nitric oxide adducts are in human physiology or pathophysiology.

Deficient production of nitric oxide has been implicated in a wide variety of cardiovascular diseases (see above) and abnormalities of prostanoid synthesis occur in experimental models of atherosclerosis and diabetes. In the presence of a quiescent healthy endothelium, loss of basal nitric oxide alone does not lead to significant systemic platelet activation. However, loss of nitric oxide and prostacyclin at sites of endothelial damage, dysfunction, or activation promotes the formation of platelet aggregates and may contribute to thrombosis and vessel occlusion. In animals, stenosed endothelium-denuded vessels lead to cyclical variations in flow as platelets stick to the vessel wall and release vasoactive and proaggregant mediators. If this also occurs in human vessels *in vivo*, it might be an important mechanism of vasospasm and thrombosis.

Under basal conditions the endothelium inhibits platelet activation, but in response to certain stimuli, proaggregant, proadhesive mediators may be synthesized and released. Unstable prostaglandin endoperoxides activate platelets, platelet activating factor may be produced, and von Willebrand factor, which is synthesized and stored within endothelial cells, increases platelet adhesion. These changes occur in response to inflammatory mediators and may also result from repeated endothelial 'injury'.

Coagulation

Heparan sulphate is a glycosaminoglycan closely related to heparin, but less potent, which is found on the surface of endothelial cells. Antithrombin III is also expressed on the endothelial cell surface and together with heparan sulphate provides a mechanism for binding and inactivating thrombin. In addition, endothelial cells participate in the activation of the anticoagulant protein C; protein S is secreted and thrombomodulin is found on the cell surface.

In the quiescent state, expression of anticoagulant factors predominates, but when activated the endothelium may promote coagulation. Receptors for clotting factors appear on the endothelial surface, von Willebrand factor is secreted, and tissue factor—the principal cellular initiator of coagulation—is expressed. Bacterial endotoxin, inflammatory cytokines, and glycosylated proteins activate the endothelium and shift the balance in favour of coagulation. This may occur in response to infection, inflammation, or endothelial injury. Circulating levels of von Willebrand factor are increased in certain patients with diabetes or hypertension.

Fibrinolysis

The endothelial cell surface has a fibrinolytic pathway. Urokinase and tissue plasminogen activator are secreted and there are specific binding sites for plasminogen activators and plasminogen. Thrombin, adrenaline, vasopressin, and stasis of blood may be physiological stimuli for the release of tissue plasminogen activator from human endothelium.

Plasminogen activator inhibitor 1 is also synthesized and bound by endothelium, providing a pathway for local inhibition of the fibrinolytic system. Under basal conditions fibrinolysis is dominant, but the balance may be altered by a variety of local and circulating factors, including inflammatory cytokines and the atherogenic particle lipoprotein (a), which inhibits plasminogen binding and hence plasmin generation. In the presence of atherosclerosis the fibrinolytic properties of endothelium are diminished.

Cellular adhesion

The resting endothelium prevents cells from adhering fully to the vessel wall but allows leucocytes to roll along its surface. The regulation of 'rolling', adhesion, and migration is governed largely by specialized glycoproteins known as cell adhesion molecules, which are expressed in varying amounts on the endothelial cell surface and interact with complementary adhesion molecules on circulating cells. Endothelial-leukocyte adhesion molecule 1 (also known as E-selectin), vascular adhesion molecule 1, intercellular adhesion molecule 1, and P-selectin (also known as GMP 140) are all expressed on cytokine-activated endothelium. The degree of expression and the type of adhesion molecules expressed determines the 'stickiness' of the endothelium for different cell types.

Expression of adhesion molecules is an important mechanism of cellular adhesion during inflammation and is also important in recruitment of T cells and monocytes in atherosclerosis. Increased expression of endothelial-leukocyte adhesion molecule 1 is seen in the coronary arteries of transplanted hearts and has been implicated in the rapid development of atherosclerosis in these vessels. Nitric oxide and prostacyclin inhibit the adhesion of white cells to endothelium and this effect may be mediated by changes in the expression or configuration of adhesion molecules. Certain endothelial cell adhesion molecules are shed into the plasma: changes in their concentration have been detected in a variety of cardiovascular diseases, but the significance of this is uncertain.

Proinflammatory cytokines

Cytokines are released from activated leucocytes in response to infection and immunological stimulation and are also produced by the vessel wall itself; interleukins 1, 6, and 8, and colony stimulating factors are synthesized by endotoxin-stimulated endothelial cells, and tumour necrosis factor by human smooth muscle cells. A large number of cytokines alter endothelial functions, upsetting the balance of vasoactive mediators, altering thrombotic activity and the expression of adhesion molecules, or initiating apoptosis (programmed cell death). Interleukin 1 and certain other proinflammatory cytokines alter the synthesis of nitric oxide (see above) and a

variety of prostaglandins, enhance the generation of thrombin, platelet activating factor, von Willebrand factor, and plasminogen activator inhibitor, alter endothelial permeability, increase expression of intercellular adhesion molecule 1 and vascular adhesion molecule 1, and may also cause endothelial cell damage and death. These findings are of direct relevance to the vascular changes occurring in inflammation and sepsis, but might also provide a link between acute or chronic immunological stimulation (for example infection) and the development of cardiovascular disease including atherosclerosis or acute cardiovascular events.

Cell growth and angiogenesis

The endothelium of healthy differentiated vessels inhibits proliferation of the underlying smooth muscle. Endothelium-derived vasodilator, antiplatelet, and antithrombotic mediators (nitric oxide, prostacyclin) tend to inhibit the growth of vascular smooth muscle cells whereas vasoconstrictor and prothrombotic mediators (endothelin, angiotensin) tend to promote it. Thus the basal state of the endothelium, in which dilatation and thromboresistance predominates, also prevents the growth of smooth muscle. The heparin-like molecules prevent cell growth and molecules similar or identical to platelet-derived growth factor and fibroblast growth factor are endothelium-derived growth promoters. Others such as transforming growth factor-β produced by endothelial cells may either inhibit or promote cell growth, and the precise role of this molecule *in vivo* is unclear. The basal antiproliferative effects of the endothelium may retard the development of atherosclerosis and intimal proliferation.

In addition to affecting the growth of underlying smooth muscle, endothelial cells are essential for the formation of new blood vessels. The ability of endothelial cells to initiate the formation of new vessels (angiogenesis and vasculogenesis) is retained in adults, but the only place this occurs physiologically is in the female reproductive tract. However, angiogenesis occurs in a wide range of disease states including atherosclerosis, rheumatoid arthritis, and tumour growth and during wound healing or in response to ischaemia. Positive and negative regulators of angiogenesis have been identified and a wide variety of cytokines, growth factors, and local autacoids can act alone or in concert to promote endothelial cell growth, migration, and tube formation. Of particular interest is vascular endothelial growth factor, a growth factor produced by smooth muscle cells in response to hypoxia, inflammatory cytokines, and certain other growth factors. There is good evidence that vascular endothelial growth factor can promote angiogenesis in a variety of animal models and in humans. Intriguingly, it appears as though vascular endothelial growth factor can increase the production of nitric oxide by endothelial cells and this may be one of the effector molecules mediating some of the actions of this growth factor. In order to form tubes through tissues, endothelial cells must degrade matrix and they are capable of synthesizing and releasing a variety of matrix metalloproteinases. Some of these matrix metalloproteinases may in turn affect endothelial function by regulating cell attachment, proliferation, and migration. Failure of endothelial cells to initiate appropriate angiogenesis in response to ischaemia may lead to tissue hypoxia, whilst excessive or inappropriate angiogenesis may contribute to a sustained inflammatory response in the vessel wall, disrupt vessel wall architecture, or lead to haemorrhage into atherosclerotic plaques.

Transport and metabolism

The endothelium presents a permeability barrier for molecules in the bloodstream. Transfer of molecules from the bloodstream into the vessel wall across the endothelium can occur by transport through the endothelial cells or between them. The junctions between endothelial cells are maintained by specialized molecules, including cadherins, and are actively regulated. Transport between cells occurs when endothelial cells contract to leave intercellular gaps. This is an important mechanism for formation of localized oedema. Transport through cells occurs by transcytosis and is an important mechanism for the passage of certain macromolecules, including insulin. In addition, specialized channels for transport of water have been identified—the aquaporins.

The endothelium is intimately involved in lipid metabolism. Lipoprotein lipase is located on the endothelial cell surface and receptors for low-density lipoproteins are present in varying amounts. In quiescent endothelium lipoprotein lipase is active but there are few low-density lipoprotein receptors, indicating that healthy endothelium provides a barrier for entry of low-density lipoprotein into the vessel wall. However, under conditions in which low-density lipoprotein is taken into the endothelium, modification by oxidation occurs and this step may stimulate atherogenesis.

Therapeutic implications

The balance of mediators produced by quiescent healthy endothelium promotes vasodilatation, inhibits activation of platelets and white cells, prevents thrombosis, prevents the growth of smooth muscle cells, and does not support angiogenesis. However, the endothelium also has the capacity to constrict blood vessels, promote cellular adhesion, initiate thrombosis, stimulate the growth of smooth muscle cells, and initiate the formation of new vessels. Whilst all of these properties of the endothelium may be considered as appropriate in the correct physiological context, the term 'endothelial dysfunction' is usually taken to mean impairment of the usual vasodilator and thromboresistant properties of the endothelium and this seems to be a marker of enhanced atherogenesis and increased cardiovascular risk. Therapeutic implications of endothelial dysfunction are now emerging.

Certain therapeutic interventions cause endothelial damage. Antibodies directed against the endothelium are found after heart transplantation and endothelial dysfunction may contribute to the rapid development of coronary artery disease seen in transplant recipients. Balloon angioplasty leads directly to severe disruption of the endothelium and this has been implicated in the development of postangioplasty vasospasm, thrombosis, and restenosis due to the growth of smooth muscle. Venous coronary artery bypass grafts are more prone to occlusion than arterial grafts, and this may reflect differences between arterial and venous endothelium including reduced basal release of nitric oxide by venous endothelium or differential production of growth factors. Acute disruption of endothelial function may promote vasospasm, thrombosis and occlusion, while chronic changes enhance atherogenesis.

Drugs also affect endothelial function. Nitrovasodilators mimic endogenous nitric oxide: glyceryl trinitrate is metabolized to nitric oxide within the vessel wall while sodium nitroprusside liberates nitric oxide spontaneously. Like the endogenous mediator, certain nitrovasodilators inhibit platelet activation and this may provide an additional mechanism to explain the beneficial effects of these drugs in coronary artery disease. Other drugs of benefit in acute coronary artery disease may also replace endothelial mediators, or restore a healthy balance of mediators released by endothelium and blood-borne cells; heparin mimics heparan sulphate proteoglycans on the cell surface, plasminogen activators replace the endogenous molecule, and low-dose intermittent aspirin preferentially inhibits thromboxane synthesis in platelets while sparing endothelial prostanoid production. Furthermore, angiotensin converting enzyme inhibitors block the breakdown of bradykinin and this mediator stimulates the release of nitric oxide from endothelial cells. Recently it has been demonstrated that oestrogens modify endothelial function and enhance endothelium-dependent vasodilatation. Antioxidants may restore a redox balance within the vessel wall which reduces superoxide levels and protects and stabilizes nitric oxide. In experimental systems fish oils may enhance the generation of antiplatelet prostanoids and increase the generation of nitric oxide. Thus all of these interventions appear to work in part by affecting endothelial function and restoring the usual vasculoprotective balance.

There has been considerable interest in the possibility that the amino acid arginine might have therapeutic utility. Theoretically giving extra arginine should have no effect on the synthesis of nitric oxide since the intracellular concentrations of arginine are far in excess of the amounts needed for nitric oxide synthesis. However, in practice several studies have shown that arginine supplementation restores endothelium-dependent relaxation towards normal in patients with certain conditions including hypercholesterolaemia and some types of renal failure. The discrepancy between biochemical theory and experimental observation is known as the 'arginine paradox'. Improvement of endothelium-dependent relaxation is a surrogate end-point of uncertain significance and clinical trials of the effects of arginine on clinically relevant end-points are currently under way.

A greater understanding of the normal protective functions of vascular endothelium and how these are altered by disease is bound to lead to therapies designed to modify endothelial function. New drugs based on nitric oxide, endothelin, adhesion molecules, and growth factors are in development and likely to enter clinical practice, and seeding of genetically altered endothelial cells on to blood vessels or genetic manipulation of the expression of enzymes that generate key endothelial mediators is a possibility. Indeed gene transfer experiments with endothelial nitric oxide synthase and vascular endothelial growth factor have already shown promise in studies in animals and appear to be technically feasible in humans.

Further reading

Feletou M, Vanhoutte PM (1999). The alternative: EDHF. *Journal of Molecular and Cellular Cardiology* **31**, 15–22.

Furchgott RF, Zawadzki JV (1980). The obligatory role of endothelial cells in the relaxation of arterial smooth muscle. *Nature* **288**, 373–6.

Gerlach H, Esposito C, Stern DM (1990). Modulation of endothelial hemostatic properties: an active role in the host response. *Annual Review of Medicine.* **41**, 15–24.

Hayden MR, Reidy M (1995). Many roads lead to atheroma. *Nature Medicine* **1**, 22–3.

Haynes WG, Webb DJ (1998). Endothelin as a regulator of cardiovascular function in health and disease. *Journal of Hypertension* **16**, 1081–98.

Isner JM, Asahara T (1999) Angiogenesis and vasculogenesis as therapeutic strategies for postnatal neovascularization. *Journal of Clinical Investigation* **103**, 1232–6.

Kinlay S, Libby P, Ganz P (2001). Endothelial function and coronary artery disease. *Current Opinion in Lipidology*, **12**, 383–9.

Krishnaswamy G *et al.* (1999). Human endothelium as a source of multifunctional cytokines: molecular regulation and possible role in humans disease. *Journal of Inteferon and Cytokine Research* **19**, 91–104.

Lüscher TF *et al.* (1992). Endothelium-derived contracting factors. *Hypertension* **19**, 117–30.

Mason JC, Haskard DO (1994). The clinical importance of leucocyte and endothelial cell adhesion molecules in inflammation. *Vascular Medicine Review* **5**, 249–75.

Maxwell AJ, Tsao PS, Cooke JP (1998). Modulation of nitric oxide synthase pathway in atherosclerosis. *Experimental Physiology* **83**, 573–84.

Noll G, Luscher TF (1998). The endothelium in acute coronary syndromes. *European Heart Journal*, **19** (Suppl. C), C30–C38.

Panes J, Perry M, Granger DN (1999). Leukocyte-endothelial cell adhesion: avenues for therapeutic intervention. *British Journal of Pharmacology* **126**, 537–50.

Papapetropoulos A, Rudic RD, Sessa WC (1999). Molecular control of nitric oxide synthases in the cardiovascular system. *Cardiovascular Research* **43**, 509–20.

Ross R (1999). Atherosclerosis—an inflammatory disease. *New England Journal of Medicine* **340**, 115–26.

Vallance P (1998). Nitric oxide in the human cardiovascular system. *British Journal of Clinical Pharmacology* **45**, 433–9.

Vallance P, Collier J, Bhagat K (1997). Infection, inflammation and infarction: does acute endothelial dysfunction provide a link? *The Lancet* **349**, 1391–2.

Vane JR, Bakhle YS, Botting RM (1998). Cyclooxygenases 1 and 2. *Annual Review of Pharmacology and Toxicology* **38**, 97–120.

15.1.1.3 Vascular smooth muscle cells

Peter L. Weissberg

Introduction

Normal human arteries comprise an intima made up of a single layer of endothelial cells and a few underlying vascular smooth muscle cells, separated from the tunica media by an internal elastic lamina. The media comprises only vascular smooth muscle cells and elastic lamellae arranged circumferentially. The number of layers of vascular smooth muscle cells varies, being fewest in small arterioles and greatest in large arteries like the aorta. On the outer boundary of the media is the external elastic lamina that separates the medial vascular smooth muscle cells from the adventitia containing connective tissue, small blood vessels (the vasa vasora), nerves, and adventitial myofibroblasts. The main function of the medial vascular smooth muscle cells is to contract and relax in response to exogenous stimuli, thereby altering the calibre of the arterial lumen and regulating vascular tone. However, unlike cardiac and skeletal myocytes, which are terminally differentiated and can only perform a contractile role, mature vascular smooth muscle cells are highly reactive and can respond to changes in their extracellular environment by dramatic alterations in gene expression, a process often referred to as phenotypic modulation. Thus vascular smooth muscle cells have the ability to migrate and proliferate and to change from a contractile cell to one that produces large quantities of extracellular matrix and other proteins (Fig. 1). This phenotypic plasticity means that vascular smooth muscle cells can play multiple roles in the pathogenesis and progression of vascular disease.

Vascular development

The versatility of the vascular smooth muscle cell is best exemplified during vascular development. Most of what is understood about this process comes from observations in developing rodents, in particular rats and mice, where the vascular smooth muscle cell is the main cell responsible for vessel growth and development. Blood vessels begin to develop in very early fetal life as endothelial tubes that recruit cells from the surrounding tissues to form the vascular smooth muscle cells of the vessel media. Vascular smooth muscle cells in some vessels are derived from mesoderm and in others from neural crest tissue or both under the influence of local morphogens. It still remains to be determined whether the heterogeneous origin of vascular smooth muscle cells in different arteries has any influence upon development of disease, and in particular the propensity of some, particularly the coronary arteries, to develop atherosclerosis.

Expression of smooth muscle specific genes is first detectable in early fetal development, implying an early commitment to muscle development, but expression of contractile proteins remains low until well after birth. During late fetal and very early neonatal development vascular smooth muscle cells proliferate in the media as the vessels grow. However, shortly after birth, the proliferation of vascular smooth muscle cells decreases rapidly and thereafter vessel growth is achieved by a combination of vascular smooth muscle cell hypertrophy (enlargement) and, particularly, accumulation of extracellular matrix. As blood pressure increases after birth there is an increase in expression of the contractile proteins required to regulate vascular tone, such as smooth muscle myosin heavy chain and actin, and a corresponding decrease in production of matrix and basement membrane proteins. Thus, mature vascular smooth muscle cells in the adult vascular wall undergo little if any proliferation, contain abundant myofilaments, and produce only small amounts of extracellular matrix proteins. This 'contractile' phenotype is maintained thereafter by the combined influences of mechanical forces and extracellular matrix components, particularly sulphated proteoglycans and basement membrane proteins, which signal into the cell and dictate gene expression via receptors on the vascular smooth muscle cell surface.

Vascular smooth muscle cell phenotype

When adult vascular smooth muscle cells are removed from their extracellular environment and placed in cell culture, they immediately reduce production of contractile proteins and increase production of matrix proteins, in particular collagen and elastin. This change from a contractile phenotype to what has been called a 'synthetic' phenotype is characterized ultrastructurally by loss of contractile myofilaments and a dramatic increase in synthetic organelles. The cells also become more responsive to growth factors and gain the ability to take up lipids and to elaborate matrix-degrading enzymes (Fig. 1). This phenotypic change does not occur if the cells are maintained in a medium containing proteoglycans and basement membrane proteins that mimic their natural extracellular environment in the vessel wall, indicating that vascular smooth muscle cells posses an inherent tendency to 'default' to a phenotype resembling that of the developing vessel if not actively stimulated to do otherwise.

Electron microscopic studies have shown that intimal vascular smooth muscle cells in atherosclerosis contain a higher proportion of synthetic organelles and fewer myofilaments than medial vascular smooth muscle cells and therefore resemble the synthetic phenotype observed in cell culture. These observations contributed to the emergence of the 'response to injury' hypothesis of atherosclerosis, initially proposed in the 1960s and still widely quoted today. This hypothesis proposed that the initiating event in atherosclerosis was endothelial cell loss or injury leading to local platelet aggregation and recruitment of vascular smooth muscle cells into the intima where a switch to the synthetic phenotype facilitated proliferation and accumulation of lipids to form the atherosclerotic lesion. This paradigm therefore portrayed the vascular smooth muscle cell as being central to the initiation and maintenance of the atherogenic process, a view reinforced by the contemporaneous suggestion that restenosis after angioplasty was due to excessive proliferation of intimal vascular smooth muscle cells. However, over the past 20 years this view of the role of vascular smooth muscle cells has changed completely, such that vascular smooth muscle cells are now considered to be the main cell type in the plaque protecting against the thrombotic complications of atherosclerosis.

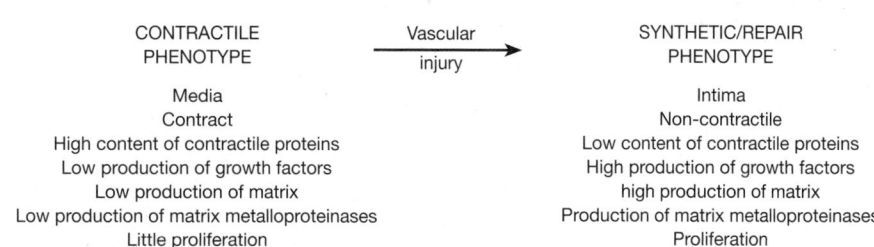

Fig. 1 Characteristics of vascular smooth muscle cell phenotypes.

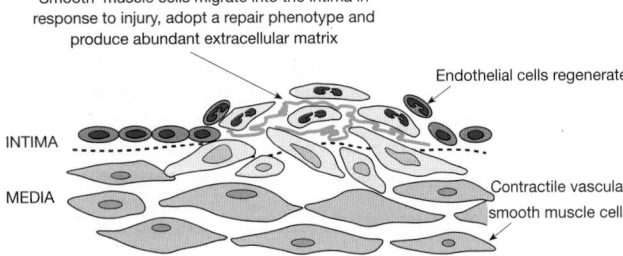

Fig. 2 The response of vascular smooth muscle cells to mechanical intimal damage.

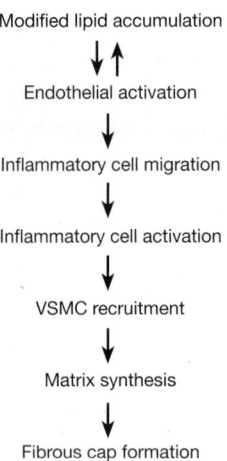

Fig. 3 Events leading to formation of the protective fibrous cap in atherosclerosis.

The response of the vascular smooth muscle cell to injury

When the intima of an artery is damaged, for example by a balloon catheter, there is a wave of DNA synthesis in medial vascular smooth muscle cells which is quickly followed by migration of vascular smooth muscle cells into the intima where they change phenotype to form a neo-intima comprising vascular smooth muscle cells and their extracellular matrix (Fig. 2). It remains unclear whether the neo-intimal population of vascular smooth muscle cells is derived directly from contractile medial vascular smooth muscle cells or arises from a clonal expansion of a small subpopulation of vascular smooth muscle cells with inherently different properties from normal adult medial cells. It is also possible that adventitial myofibroblasts may also migrate into the intima to contribute to neo-intima formation. The resulting endothelialized neo-intima 'heals' the damage and may be sufficiently large to narrow the vessel lumen, as occurs in restenosis following therapeutic balloon angioplasty.

Vascular smooth muscle cells in atherosclerosis

The recent recognition that atherosclerosis is an inflammatory process driven by the interaction between oxidized lipids and reactive inflammatory cells has brought about a complete re-evaluation of the role of vascular smooth muscle cells in its pathogenesis. Intimal vascular smooth muscle cells protect against plaque rupture and therefore the thrombotic consequences of atherosclerosis by migrating into the intima and changing phenotype to elaborate the matrix components of the all-important fibrous cap. Indeed, vascular smooth muscle cells are the only cells capable of making the fibrous cap, such that loss of vascular smooth muscle cells from the cap is one of the major determinants of plaque rupture. By reverting to a phenotype very similar to that of vascular smooth muscle cells in the neonatal blood vessel, they are adopting a beneficial 'repair' phenotype, in which the genes they express facilitate their reparative role. When reacting to either mechanical injury or the chemotactic influence of inflammatory cells they synthesize plasminogen activators and matrix metalloproteinases. These interact to digest the basement membrane of the vascular smooth muscle cells and thereby allow the vascular smooth muscle cells to migrate into the intima to form the fibrous cap by a combination of proliferation and matrix production, the latter being predominant (Fig. 3).

A paucity of vascular smooth muscle cells in the fibrous cap predisposes the lesion to plaque rupture. Vascular smooth muscle cells can be destroyed by inflammatory cells within the lesion, as discussed later in this chapter. Also, intimal vascular smooth muscle cells lose their capacity to regenerate and become highly susceptible to spontaneous 'suicide' by apoptosis (programmed cell death). Unless senescent vascular smooth muscle cells are replaced by those that are active, the capacity to repair and maintain the

fibrous cap is lost, thereby tipping the balance in favour of plaque rupture. Indeed, senescence could be a feature of all vascular smooth muscle cells as they get older, possibly explaining why plaque rupture, leading to heart attacks and strokes, occurs increasingly frequently with age.

Atherosclerosis does, therefore, involve the response of vascular smooth muscle cells to injury, but it is not an initiating event, rather it is secondary to, and protective against, the destructive lipid-driven inflammatory process that leads to plaque instability, thrombosis, and patient death. However, vascular smooth muscle cells do contribute to some extent to plaque progression in as much as the formation of a new fibrous cap over a subclinical erosion or rupture necessarily increases the size of the lesion.

The role of vascular smooth muscle cells in restenosis

In approximately 30 to 40 per cent of patients undergoing successful balloon angioplasty for symptomatic coronary disease, symptoms will return because of restenosis at the site of the procedure. Initially this was thought simply to be due to excessive proliferation of intimal vascular smooth muscle cells in response to the injury. However, it has now become apparent that several factors in addition to the proliferation of vascular smooth muscle cells contribute to restenosis in man. Firstly, there is the early elastic recoil of the vessel wall that occurs soon after the balloon has been removed. Secondly, there is less vascular smooth muscle cell proliferation than anticipated from animal models and the bulk of the neo-intima comprises relatively few vascular smooth muscle cells scattered throughout an abundant extracellular matrix. Thus the production of vascular smooth muscle cell matrix is probably more important than the proliferation of vascular smooth muscle cells in determining neo-intimal bulk. Thirdly, eventual lumen diameter is determined by the capacity of the vessel to remodel. Angioplasty induces a vigorous adventitial response characterized by proliferation of adventitial myofibroblasts: these also express smooth muscle cell genes and synthesize a dense extracellular matrix that splints the vessel and prevents outward remodelling. As mentioned above, these cells may also migrate through the damaged media and contribute to the formation of neo-intima. Most of these consequences of balloon angioplasty can be abrogated by the deployment of an intravascular stent that prevents elastic recoil and negative remodelling. Although proliferation of intimal vascular smooth muscle cells and matrix synthesis still occur in stented vessels, their impact on the final diameter of the lumen is offset by the

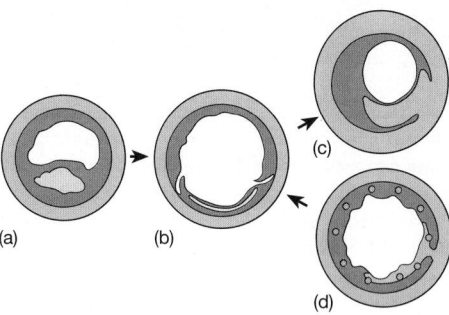

Fig. 4 Restenosis after balloon angioplasty. (a) Stenotic atherosclerotic lesion before angioplasty. (b) Lesion immediately after angioplasty showing expansion of the whole artery with fissuring through the media into the adventitia. (c) Restenosis occurs because of formation of neo-intima in response to balloon injury. The neo-intima arises in part through medial smooth muscle cell proliferation and matrix synthesis and invasion of adventitial myofibroblasts. Note also that the adventitia has thickened and in effect 'splints' the vessel, preventing outward remodelling to compensate for the formation of neo-intima. The net result is lumen narrowing and restenosis. (d) Stent deployment after balloon dilatation prevents elastic recoil and negative remodelling induced by the adventitial response. Although there is still neo-intima formation it is insufficient to induce significant lumen narrowing.

initial gain in diameter achieved by balloon dilatation and maintained by the stent (Fig. 4).

Summary

The vascular smooth muscle cell is highly adaptable and can serve multiple roles. In the normal vessel wall it acts principally as a contractile cell. However, in response to any form of vascular insult it rapidly assumes a wound-healing role and expresses the repertoire of genes necessary to repair the vessel wall. In the context of the chronic inflammatory stimulus of atherosclerosis, this response creates the protective fibrous cap responsible for conferring stability to the plaque and preventing plaque rupture. Following balloon angioplasty the reactive vascular smooth muscle cells act primarily to 'heal' the damage caused by the balloon. In so doing, they create a neo-intima that stabilizes the lesion but which may also cause restenosis if adequate compensatory remodelling does not occur.

Further reading

Bennett MR *et al.* (1997). Increased sensitivity of human vascular smooth muscle cells from atherosclerotic plaque to p53-mediated apoptosis. *Circulation Research* **81**, 591–9.

Bennett MR *et al.* (1998). Co-operative interactions between RB and p53 regulate cell proliferation, cell senescence and apoptosis in human vascular smooth muscle cells from atherosclerotic plaques *Circulation Research* **82**, 704–12.

Campbell GR *et al.* (1988). Arterial smooth muscle. A multifunctional mesenchymal cell. *Archives of Pathology and Laboratory Medicine* **112**, 977–86.

Clowes AW, Reidy MA, Clowes MM (1983). Mechanisms of stenosis after arterial injury. *Laboratory Investigation* **49**, 208–15.

Glagov S *et al.* (1987). Compensatory enlargement of human atherosclerotic coronary arteries. *New England Journal of Medicine* **316**, 371–5.

Shanahan C, Weissberg P (1998). Smooth muscle cell heterogeneity—patterns of gene expression in vascular smooth muscle cells *in vitro* and *in vivo*. *Arteriosclerosis Thrombosis and Vascular Biology* **18**, 333–8.

Weissberg P, Clesham G, Bennett M (1996). Is vascular smooth muscle cell proliferation beneficial? *The Lancet* **347**, 305–7.

15.1.2 Atherosclerosis and thrombosis

15.1.2.1 The pathogenesis of atherosclerosis

R. P. Naoumova and J. Scott

Introduction

Atherosclerosis, the underlying cause of heart attacks, strokes, and peripheral vascular disease, is one of the major killers in the world. The disease develops slowly over many years in the innermost layer of large and medium-sized arteries. It does not usually manifest before the fourth or fifth decade of life, but may strike with devastating suddenness. At least 30 per cent of individuals die from their first heart attack. In England and Wales coronary heart disease accounts for 31 per cent of all deaths in men and 23 per cent of all deaths in women, and morbidity from the disease is significant, with a profound impact on health-care services and on the industrial economy.

Epidemiology

The demonstration of coronary heart disease in an individual is taken as a reliable index of the presence of more general atherosclerosis. The highest death rates from coronary heart disease are found in Britain, northern Europe, the United States, Australia, and New Zealand. Deaths from coronary disease rose dramatically after the First World War, peaked in the late 1960s in the United States, and have since declined. In western Europe this peak and decline lagged behind the United States by some 10 years. Changes in diet, exercise, smoking, and affluence account for much of this decline. Better medical and surgical interventions have also been important. By contrast, the countries of eastern Europe and the former Soviet Union are showing a marked increase in the prevalence of coronary heart disease. This can be attributed to the influence of the risk factors that operate in the industrialized West (Table 1). Substantially lower death rates are found in southern Europe, Latin America, Japan, and China. For further discussion see Chapter 15.4.1.2.

Table 1 Risk factors for atherosclerosis

Risk factor	Modifiable
Male gender	No
Race	No
*Diet high in saturated fat and cholesterol, low in fruit, grain, and vegetables	Yes
Family history of premature coronary heart disease in first degree relative (men < 55 years; women < 65 years)	No
*Hypercholesterolaemia (total cholesterol > 5.0 mmol/litre (190 mg/dl))	Yes
*Cigarette smoking	Yes
*Hypertension	Yes
Low high-density cholesterol (<1 mmol/litre (40 mg/dl))	Yes
*Diabetes mellitus	Possibly
Obesity	Yes
High lipoprotein (a)	Possibly
High fibrinogen	Possibly
High homocysteine	Yes
Physical inactivity	Yes

*Major modifiable risk factors.

The lesions of atherosclerosis

Autopsy studies show that in humans atherosclerosis begins in early life and develops slowly over many years (Fig. 1) before becoming symptomatic. Atherosclerosis is a focal intimal disease of arteries ranging in size from the aorta down to those of approximately 3 mm external diameter. The arteries most commonly involved with atherosclerosis include the aorta, coronaries, carotid, cerebral, and femoral. Branch points and curvatures, the sites of blood turbulence, favour the development of atherosclerotic lesions.

The earliest lesions of atherosclerosis are fatty streaks. These consist of an accumulation of lipid-engorged macrophages (foam cells), and T lymphocytes in the arterial intima. The fatty streaks progress to intermediate lesions (or transitional plaque), composed mainly of macrophage foam cells and smooth muscle cells which migrate into the intima from the media. With time these develop into raised fibrous (advanced) plaques, characterized by a dense fibrous cap of connective tissue and smooth muscle cells overlying a core containing necrotic material and lipid, mainly cholesteryl esters, which may form cholesterol crystals on histological section. The necrotic core is a result of apoptosis and necrosis, increased proteolytic activity and lipid accumulation. Fibrous plaques also contain a large number of macrophage foam cells, T cells, and smooth muscle cells. This collection of cells, surrounding the necrotic core, promotes plaque growth. The plaque undergoes vascularization and microvessels develop in connection with the artery's vasa vasorum. The new vessels provide a channel for the access of inflammatory cells and may also lead to intraplaque haemorrhage and thus weaken the plaque. Advanced atherosclerotic plaques frequently accumulate calcium, due to the presence of proteins specialized in binding calcium (osteocalcin, osteopontin, bone morphogenic proteins).

The advanced plaque is the substrate from which the complicated plaque develops, leading almost inevitably to clinical symptoms. The complicated plaque has a thin cap, especially at the shoulders or margins of the lesion, and may contain ulcerations, fissures, erosions, or cracks. These provide sites of platelet adherence, aggregation, and thrombosis. The thin fibrous cap may break or tear leading to haemorrhage into the necrotic core and thrombosis.

Arterial remodelling and clinical syndromes associated with atherosclerosis

Arterial remodelling is a clinically important feature in the evolution of the atherosclerotic lesion. It delays the development of significant luminal narrowing and is a compensatory process in human atherogenesis. During early phases of plaque formation the lesion grows away from the lumen, so affected vessels increase in diameter (compensatory enlargement) and the plaque will not cause flow-limiting stenosis. Most plaques of this type will not be visible angiographically.

When the plaque covers more than 40 per cent of the elastic lamina, the artery cannot compensate by dilatation and the lesion begins to intrude into the arterial lumen, becoming angiographically detectable. It may impede the blood flow to an organ, giving rise to ischaemia, the symptoms of stable angina, and intermittent claudication. If the atherosclerotic lesion undergoes superficial erosion of the endothelium with limited thrombosis, this may result in unstable angina or myocardial infarction, even when the lesion is not flow limiting. Deep fissuring or frank rupture of the plaque with complete sudden occlusion of coronary arteries may cause myocardial infarction or sudden death. In the cerebral circulation, the same process causes transient ischaemic attacks and completed stroke. In arteries weakened by the ageing process and complicated by atherosclerosis, aneurysmal dilatation and rupture may occur.

Plaque stability and plaque rupture

Rupture of atherosclerotic lesions can trigger the thrombosis that precipitates clinical events. However, plaques have different propensities to rupture. Plaques with dense extracellular matrix, relatively thick fibrous caps, and limited lipid cores are generally unlikely to initiate thrombosis followed by an acute vascular event.

Culprit lesions, causing myocardial infarction or unstable angina, characteristically have thin fibrous caps, large cores of extracellular lipids, and an abundance of macrophages and T lymphocytes at the site of plaque rupture. Plaques usually contain limited numbers of smooth muscle cells, leading to decreased synthesis of extracellular matrix and weakening of the plaque's fibrous cap. The integrity of the fibrous cap is also attacked by cytokines derived from activated macrophages, which can promote the expression of proteinases that can degrade the extracellular matrix. Plaque rupture usually occurs at the 'shoulders' of the plaque. Angiography cannot accurately predict the stability of a lesion.

The pathogenesis of atherosclerotic lesions

Atherosclerosis develops as a healing response of the intima to repeated vascular wall injury, where risk factors (Table 1) operate by promoting chronic cycles of damage and repair. In the broadest terms, atherosclerosis is now recognized to be a chronic inflammatory process.

Endothelial dysfunction is the first step in the development of atherosclerosis. Modified low-density lipoprotein, toxins in tobacco smoke, the shear stress of hypertension, elevated plasma homocysteine concentrations,

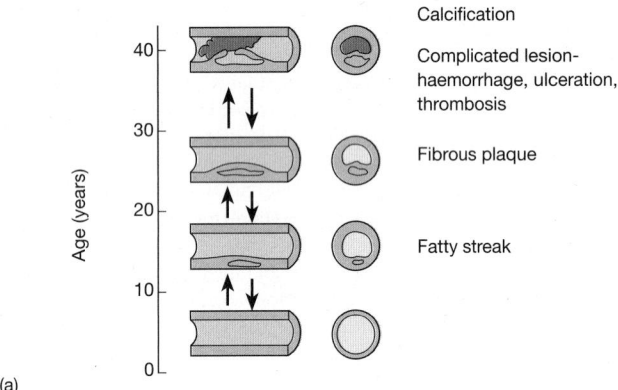

(a)

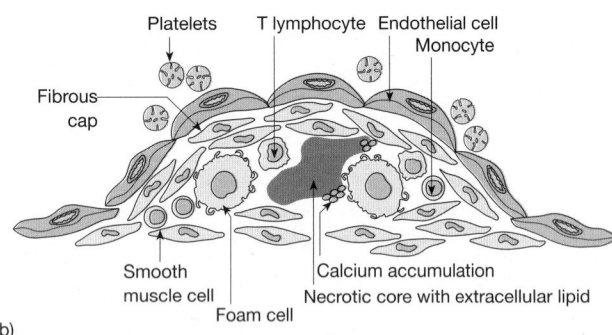

(b)

Fig. 1 (a) Natural history of atherosclerosis. (Reprinted with permission from McGill HC Jr, *et al.* In: Sandler S and Bourne N, eds. *Atherosclerosis and its origin*, Academic Press, New York, 1963). (b) Schematic diagram of an advanced atherosclerotic lesion. As fatty streaks progress to advanced lesions, they form a fibrous cap due to migration and proliferation of smooth muscle cells. This represents a type of healing response to injury. The cap covers a mixture of foam cells, T lymphocytes, lipids, and debris, forming a necrotic core—the result of apoptosis and necrosis.

diabetes mellitus, and infectious micro-organisms can all cause dysfunction of endothelial cells. The dysfunctional endothelium undergoes a protective response that alters normal homeostatic properties due to expression of adhesion molecules, growth-promoting substances, and activation of the blood coagulation cascade. Monocytes and T lymphocytes adhere to the activated endothelium, become activated, and produce growth factors, cytokines, and chemoattractants. Adherent white blood cells migrate into the arterial intima and smooth muscle cells are recruited from the media into the intima. With repeated rounds of injury and repair, palisades of smooth muscle cells, matrix proteins, lipid-laden macrophages, and T lymphocytes accumulate to form atherosclerotic plaques (Fig. 1).

Low-density lipoprotein has a central role in the pathogenesis of atherosclerosis. It may enter the intima through the damaged endothelium or, more commonly, by transcytosis across the intact endothelium, becoming 'trapped' in the subendothelial space. There, low-density lipoprotein undergoes low-grade modification by oxidative free radicals, secreted by cells of the artery wall, forming minimally modified low-density lipoprotein (Fig. 2). Although still recognized by the low-density lipoprotein receptor, minimally modified low-density lipoprotein can stimulate the release of macrophage colony-stimulating factor and monocyte chemoattractant protein 1 from endothelial cells: these facilitate monocyte recruitment and their differentiation into tissue macrophages. Minimally modified low-density lipoprotein adheres to matrix proteins of the arterial wall, where it undergoes more extensive oxidation. Free radicals are produced from macrophages and from nitric oxide derived from endothelial cells. This is compounded by the products of tobacco smoke and by homocysteine. Highly oxidized/modified low-density lipoprotein is characterized by changes not only of the lipid but also of the protein portion of low-density lipoprotein, leading to loss of recognition by the low-density lipoprotein receptor. Thus oxidized low-density lipoprotein becomes the major ligand for the scavenger receptor family (scavenger receptor A, scavenger receptor B, and others), expressed in the macrophages accumulating at the site of the injury to the vessel wall. This shift in receptor recognition leads to uptake of oxidized low-density lipoprotein by receptors, not regulated by the cholesterol content of the cell. The result is massive accumulation of cholesteryl esters in the macrophages, giving the cytoplasm its characteristic foamy appearance and transforming the macrophage into a foam cell.

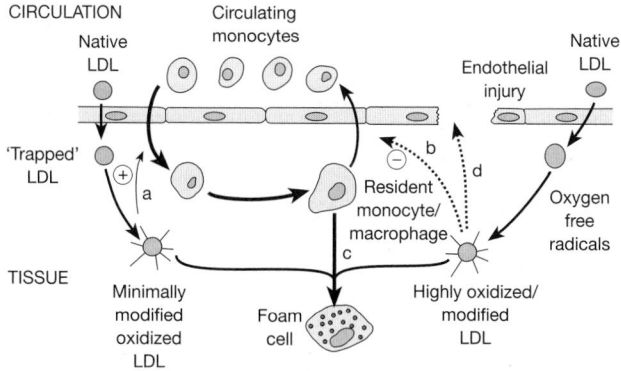

Fig. 2 Oxidation of low-density lipoprotein. The figure shows the mechanisms by which oxidized low-density lipoprotein contributes to atherosclerosis. (a) Oxidized low-density lipoprotein is chemotactic for circulating monocytes. (b) Oxidized low-density lipoprotein inhibits the movement of resident macrophages out of the arterial intima. (c) Resident macrophages generate free radicals and contribute to production of oxidized low-density lipoprotein, leading to the generation of foam cells. (d) Oxidized low-density lipoprotein is cytotoxic and this leads to endothelial cell damage and loss of integrity. (Reproduced from Quinn MT *et al.* (1987). Oxidatively modified low density lipoproteins: a potential role in recruitment and retention of monocyte/macrophages during atherogenesis. *Proceedings of the National Academy of Sciences of the United States of America* **84**, 2995–8, with permission.)

Hypertension accelerates atherogenesis by activating genes in response to increased sheer stress, the products of which perturb vascular tone and promote the accumulation of smooth muscle cells. Hypertension also increases the formation of hydrogen peroxide and free radicals that worsen oxidative damage, reduces the formation of nitric oxide by the endothelium, and increases leucocyte adhesion. In diabetes mellitus hyperglycaemia may promote non-enzymatic glycation of low-density lipoprotein, which may initiate atherosclerosis in the same way as oxidatively modified low-density lipoprotein. A high plasma homocysteine concentration is toxic to endothelium, decreases the availability of nitric oxide, and has prothrombotic activity.

The cells of the atherosclerotic plaque

Endothelial cells

In the earliest stages of atherogenesis, damaged endothelial cells become dysfunctional. Sloughing of the endothelium occurs at a later stage, when plaques become complicated and split or fissure. Dysfunctional endothelial cells produce growth factors, cytokines, chemoattractants, clotting factors, and adhesion molecules. The result is recruitment and transformation of monocytes into macrophages, and recruitment and proliferation of smooth muscle cells and T cells. Thrombotic processes are activated. There is chronic alteration of vascular tone as a result of disordered nitric oxide production and signalling.

Monocyte/macrophages

The lipid-laden macrophage is the hallmark of atherosclerosis and is instrumental in its development. Monocyte conversion from a quiescent cell to a phagocytically active macrophage is associated with expression of scavenger receptors and oxidized low-density lipoprotein receptors which avidly take up highly oxidized low-density lipoprotein, the latter no longer being recognized by the low-density lipoprotein receptor. The cholesteryl ester released from low-density lipoprotein is broken down in lysosomes and re-esterified in the cytoplasm.

Activated macrophages secrete a wide variety of growth-modulating substances and chemoattractants. Phagocytic macrophages produce free radicals and are induced to produce nitric oxide, which generates free radicals, promoting further oxidative damage to low-density lipoproteins (Fig. 2). Macrophages also secrete proteolytic enzymes (collagenase, elastase, stromelysin, and gelatinases): these contribute to the necrosis and liquefaction of the core of advanced fatty plaques and also render the plaque prone to rupture by thinning the fibrous cap.

Vascular smooth muscle cells

Smooth muscle cells in the walls of normal arteries mainly contain contractile proteins, such as actin and myosin, and are said to display a contractile phenotype. They respond to vasoregulatory substances—catecholamines, angiotensin II, prostaglandins, leukotrienes, endothelin, nitric oxide, and other regulatory compounds. However, under the influence of proinflammatory cytokines and growth factors, smooth muscle cells in the atherosclerotic plaque switch from a contractile to a secretory phenotype and produce extracellular matrix. In the media of normal arteries, the matrix consists of types I and III collagen, whereas in the atherosclerotic lesion it comprises largely proteoglycans, intermixed with loosely scattered collagen fibrils. The local release of growth factors, cytokines, and chemoattractants leads to autocrine and paracrine effects on growth and cell recruitment. Smooth muscle cells also express scavenger receptors and they, too, become lipid-loaded.

T lymphocytes

T cells (both CD4 and CD8) are present in the atherosclerotic lesion in all stages of the process. These are activated when they bind antigen processed and presented by macrophages, resulting in the secretion of proinflammatory cytokines, including interleukin 1, interferon-γ, and tumour necrosis factor α and β, which amplify the inflammatory response and compound the atherosclerotic process by attracting further macrophages and T lymphocytes and perpetuating endothelial cell activation. T cells in the plaque become sensitized to new antigens in the lesion, such as modified low-density lipoprotein.

Platelets

Platelets undergo activation in response to agonists such as thrombin, ADP, adrenaline, and platelet activating factor. When activated, platelets release their granules, containing cytokines and growth factors. The activation is also triggered when peripheral blood is exposed to thrombogenic agents at the site of blood vessel damage. Here agonists such as collagen present in the extracellular matrix, exposed in the subendothelium along with von Willebrand factor and fibrinogen produced at the wound site, initiate the cascade of events that leads to platelet aggregation and the formation of a platelet plug. In this process platelet-specific integrins act as receptor tyrosine kinases (glycoprotein, GP IIb/IIIa), initiating the intracellular changes that mediate platelet activation and aggregation, and later the binding to fibrin and clot retraction.

Molecular and cell interactions

The formation of the atherosclerotic plaque is brought about by a complex series of cellular and molecular interactions. Substances expressed at the cell surface and secreted in response to cellular activation bring about these events. Intracellular co-ordinating mechanisms, such as the NF_B system, operate at the site of the lesion. NFκB is a ubiquitous transcription factor that can be activated by diverse proatherogenic stimuli and provides a potential common link to co-ordinate the expression of series of genes involved in atherogenesis.

Growth factors

Molecules controlling the proliferation of smooth muscle cells include platelet-derived growth factor, fibroblast growth factor, heparin-binding epidermal growth factor, insulin-like growth factor I, interleukin 1, tumour necrosis factor-α, transforming growth factors α and β, thrombin, and angiotensin II.

Platelets contain platelet-derived growth factor and other growth regulatory substances, such as epidermal growth factor, transforming growth factors α and β, insulin-like growth factor I, and thromboxane, which are released during platelet aggregation and activation. Platelet-derived growth factor is also produced from activated endothelial cells and secretory smooth muscle cells in response to the macrophage cytokines interleukin 1, tumour necrosis factor-α, and transforming growth factor-β. Fibroblast growth factor, the other potent mitogen for vascular smooth muscle cells, also has mitogenic activity for endothelial cells. Heparin-binding epidermal growth factor is a potent growth factor and chemoattractant for smooth muscle cells only. Transforming growth factor-β is a multifunctional cytokine, expressed with its receptor system on smooth muscle cells. It is a potent inhibitor of mitosis of smooth muscle cells and also stimulates elaboration of matrix proteins such as fibronectin and vascular collagen.

Vascular endothelial cell growth factor is a potent and specific mitogen for endothelial cells and also promotes permeability of small veins and venules. It is produced by endothelial cells and macrophages in response to ischaemia and acts as a potent chemoattractant for macrophages, also inducing endothelial cells to produce collagenase as well as urokinase-type plasminogen activator, tissue plasminogen activator, and their inhibitor plasminogen activator inhibitor 1.

Cytokines

Cytokines are multipotent mediators of inflammation and immunity with generalized action in host defence and pathology. They can affect key functions of vascular wall cells and may participate as autocrine and paracrine mediators in atherogenesis.

The cytokines interleukin 1, interleukin 2, tumour necrosis factor-α, γ-interferon, and granulocyte–macrophage and macrophage colony stimulating factors are secreted from macrophages, T lymphocytes, activated endothelial cells, and secretory smooth muscle cells. Interleukin 1, tumour necrosis factor-α, and transforming growth factor-β induce endothelial cell activation, with the release of mitogens and chemoattractants for smooth muscle cells, and activate the coagulation cascade. Colony stimulating factors attract further inflammatory cells. Cytokines can also inhibit the proliferation of smooth muscle cells, and thus may either promote or retard atherogenesis.

Chemokines (chemoattractants)

Chemokines are members of a superfamily of small polypeptides that share the ability to induce migration, growth, and activation of subsets of leucocytes and other cells present in atherosclerotic lesions. They are also involved in regulating angiogenesis at inflammatory sites of the atherosclerotic plaque. More than 30 human chemokines have been identified. Interleukin 8 acts predominantly on neutrophils; monocyte chemoattractic protein 1 acts on lymphocytes, monocytes, mast cells, and eosinophils; whereas lymphotactin acts solely on lymphocytes. Chemokines mediate their actions via specific cell surface receptors, members of the seven transmembrane-spanning G-protein-linked molecules.

Adhesion molecules

Dysfunctional endothelial cells undergo activation, with the production of cell surface proteins that mediate the adherence of inflammatory cells. This inductive process is mediated by cytokines. The adhesion molecules induced include E-selectin, which is a membrane glycoprotein specific to endothelial cells that mediates the adhesion of neutrophils. It is a member of the selectin gene family, which also includes L-selectin and P-selectin. These molecules are implicated in the initial 'rolling step' of leucocyte extravasation.

Vascular cell adhesion molecule 1 is induced on endothelial cells by interleukin 1, tumour necrosis factor-α, lipopolysaccharide, and oxidized low-density lipoprotein. Vascular cell adhesion molecule 1 binds cells expressing integrins α4β1 (VLA4), such as monocytes and lymphocytes, but not neutrophils. Another adhesion molecule is intercellular adhesion molecule 1, a receptor for integrins, which binds all leucocytes. Thus vascular cell adhesion molecule 1 and intercellular adhesion molecule 1 serve to anchor activated leucocytes after the initial 'rolling step'.

Platelet endothelial cell adhesion molecule exists at the tight junctions of endothelial cells and is required for the transmigration of neutrophils and monocytes and for platelet adhesion.

Matrix proteins

Smooth muscle cells that have taken on a secretory phenotype are the primary source of extracellular matrix. Matrix proteins comprise collagens, elastin, proteoglycans, and microfibrillar protein. Their production is controlled by interleukin 1, tumour necrosis factor-α, and transforming growth factor-β, which mediate the switch between proliferative and secretory smooth muscle cell phenotypes, whereas γ-interferon suppresses collagen expression.

In the normal artery both synthesis and degradation of matrix are very slow, whereas atherosclerosis and injury lead to increased synthesis of many matrix proteins. The degree of ongoing matrix degradation is a highly controlled and essential component of the homeostasis of the normal artery. Increased matrix degradation, due to high activity of proteases in the plaque, is common in unstable atherosclerotic lesions. Ageing is associated with a reduction of elastin in the extracellular matrix, leading to hardening of the arteries.

Cellular death

Advanced fibrous caps that have ruptured have twice as many macrophages, but only half as many smooth muscle cells, as unruptured fibrous caps. The relative decrease in the number of smooth muscle cells may result from growth inhibition due to γ-interferon or cellular death from lytic injury and necrosis. Recent studies show that smooth muscle cells of the atheromatous plaque undergo programmed cell death, apoptosis.

Coagulation factors

The activation of endothelial cells initiates cell-surface assembly of the prothrombinase complex and subsequent deposition of fibrin and platelet activation. The process is initiated by plasma membrane expression of tissue factor, which activates factor VIIa and, in turn, factors IX and X. Thrombin is generated in the presence of endothelial cell factor V. Thrombin contributes to the inflammatory response by induction of the adhesion molecule P-selectin and platelet activating factor. Platelet arachidonic acid is released by activity of phospholipase C and phospholipase A2. The enzyme cyclo-oxygenase generates platelet endoperoxides, and the enzyme thromboxane synthase generates thromboxane, which in turn increases phospholipase C activity, stimulating platelet activation and degranulation. Together these substances promote neutrophil and platelet adhesion. Thrombin also induces plasminogen activator inhibitor 1, and increases tissue factor synthesis and expression of platelet-derived growth factor. E-selectin is induced and serves as a site for leucocyte attachment. Thus the control of coagulation by cytokines closely mimics that of the inflammatory response, indicating the interdependence of the two processes.

Restenosis

Surgical treatment of arteries narrowed by atherosclerosis is by arterial or venous bypass grafting or endarterectomy. Medical treatment is by percutaneous transluminal balloon angioplasty. Immediate complications of this procedure are thrombosis and arterial wall dissection. There is also a high failure rate due to restenosis of the arterial lumen (30–40 per cent within 3–6 months).

Restenosis is a complex reparative process involving the following sequence of events after angioplasty: recoil, remodelling, mural thrombus formation with subsequent organization by connective tissue, followed by smooth muscle cell activation, migration, proliferation, and increased synthesis of extracellular matrix. Growth factors originating from the thrombus, vessel wall, and circulating cells contribute to these events. After 2 to 6 months the stenotic region becomes organized and consists of a maturing scar, but little thrombus or lipid. The NFκB pathway plays a central role in triggering the transcription of genes encoding leucocyte adhesion molecules, chemokines, and enzymes that can influence extracellular martix metabolism, leading to restenosis. Satisfactory regimens for the prevention of restenosis have yet to be established.

Transplant atherosclerosis

Cardiovascular disease is emerging as the major cause of late morbidity and mortality in transplant patients, accounting for 45 per cent of deaths in renal transplant recipients and being the major factor limiting survival of cardiac allografts.

Recipients of organ transplant often have multiple classical risk factors before transplantation and contributing to accelerated atherosclerosis

afterwards (Table 1). Immunosuppressive agents such as prednisolone and cyclosporine have adverse effects on lipid metabolism, whereas tacrolimus (FK506) affects lipid metabolism to a lesser extent. Cytomegalovirus infection and abnormal platelet aggregation also contribute to accelerated atherogenesis.

Specific immunological factors contribute to the development and progression of transplant atherosclerosis, especially in the accelerated form of coronary arteriopathy that plagues heart transplant recipients.

Future perspectives

Despite changes in lifestyle and the use of potent lipid-lowering agents, cardiovascular disease continues to be the major cause of death in western Europe and North America. Furthermore, end-point clinical trials using statins show at best a 30 per cent decrease in total mortality, with a 42 per cent decrease in coronary deaths. Clearly new therapeutic targets need to be pursued.

Serum levels of high-density lipoprotein cholesterol are inversely related to coronary heart disease. Reduced levels of high-density lipoprotein are found in half of the patients with coronary heart disease. The discovery of the pivotal role of the *ABC1* transporter gene, encoding the cholesterol-efflux regulatory protein, in the generation of high-density lipoprotein provides opportunities for new drug targets.

Better understanding of the pathogenesis of the initiation, progression, and complications of atherosclerotic lesions will provide new potential therapeutic approaches, different from plasma lipids. An understanding of the central role of oxidized low-density lipoproteins and of the macrophage in the pathogenesis of atherosclerotic lesions points to a new direction for prevention and treatment—antioxidants.

Since atherosclerosis is a multigenic disease, understanding the patterns of gene expression will shed light on differences in susceptibility to agents causing disease, on genetic variability in prediction of risk and response to therapy, and may provide clues for designing new therapeutic approaches.

Further reading

Davies MJ, Woolf N (1993). Atherosclerosis—what is it and why does it occur? *British Heart Journal* **69** (Suppl.), S3–S11.

Kiechl S, Willeit J for the Bruneck Study Group (1999). The natural course of atherosclerosis. Part II: vascular remodelling. *Arteriosclerosis, Thrombosis and Vascular Biology* **19**, 1491–8.

Krieger M (1997). The other side of scavenger receptors: pattern recognition for host defence. *Current Opinion in Lipidology* **8**, 275–80.

Libby P *et al.* (1998). Current concepts in cardiovascular pathology: the role of LDL cholesterol in plaque rupture and stabilization. *American Journal of Medicine* **104** (Suppl. 2A), 14S–18S.

McGill HC Jr, Geer JC, Strong JP (1963). The natural history of human atherosclerotic lesions. In: Sandler M, Bourne G, eds. *Atherosclerosis and its origins*, pp 396–405. Academic Press, New York.

Quinn MT *et al.* (1987). Oxidatively modified low density lipoproteins: A potential role in recruitment and retention of monocyte/macrophages during atherogenesis. *Proceedings of the National Academy of Sciences of the United States of America* **84**, 2995–8.

Ross R (1993). The pathogenesis of atherosclerosis: a perspective for the 1990s. *Nature* **362**, 801–9.

Ross R. (1999). Atherosclerosis—an inflammatory disease. *New England Journal of Medicine* **340**, 115–25.

Scott J (1999). Good cholesterol news. *Nature* **400**, 816–19.

Seinberg D (1997). Oxidative modification of LDL and Atherogenesis. Lewis A. Conner Memorial Lecture. *Circulation* **95**, 1062–71.

15.1.2.2 The haemostatic system in arterial disease

T. W. Meade, P. K. MacCallum, and G. J. Miller

Introduction

General recognition of the thrombotic component in arterial disease, particularly coronary heart disease, is comparatively recent. The term 'coronary thrombosis' appears to have first been used by Herrick very early in the 1900s and it continued to be used until coronary heart disease became the preferred terminology after the Second World War, when the condition had reached epidemic proportions.

Epidemiological studies which started in the late 1940s—the work in the community of Framingham being the best known—began to establish the characteristics of those at particular risk of heart attacks. The main emphasis, however, was on the part played by lipid infiltration, which has tended to dominate thinking in North America ever since in comparison with a readier acceptance in Europe of a thrombotic component (as well as of atherogenesis). There was good reason for supposing that lipids play a major part: it was easy to demonstrate lipid-rich material, including cholesterol crystals, in the coronary arteries and it seemed logical to suggest that high-fat diets and blood cholesterol levels might contribute to atheroma. In the 1950s, however, J. N. Morris and his colleagues at the (now Royal) London Hospital showed very clearly that while advanced atheroma obviously contributed, it could not explain the whole of the coronary heart disease epidemic, although the implication that there must be another process involved—almost certainly thrombosis—was not fully recognized for another 20 years.

Interest in a thrombotic component to coronary heart disease started to re-emerge in the 1970s but was initially characterized by a rather sterile debate as to whether thrombosis causes or is a consequence of myocardial infarction. Evidence for the role of thrombosis in myocardial infarction was provided in convincing form when angiographic monitoring of the early use of thrombolytic therapy showed the development of occlusive thrombi preceding full manifestation of the clinical event. As for sudden coronary death, one reason for doubting the involvement of thrombosis had been the failure to demonstrate thrombi at autopsy in many cases. Apart from limitations in methods for detecting thrombi, the very striking increase in fibrinolytic activity associated with the agonal process of dying from a heart attack is likely to result in the dissolution of some thrombi that were nevertheless responsible for the event. In 1984, a particularly careful study comparing the prevalence of thrombosis in sudden death from coronary heart disease with sudden death from other causes gave the results summarized in Table 1, indicating that a degree of thrombosis is demonstrable in nearly all sudden coronary deaths. Other studies have generally confirmed this. It is now also recognized that the pathology of unstable angina pectoris is similar to that of myocardial infarction and of sudden coronary death in consisting of a significant thrombotic component and in responding to antithrombotic treatment (see Chapter 15.4.2.1).

Table 1 The presence of thrombus in 100 sudden coronary and 78 sudden non-coronary deaths

Thrombus type	Coronary (%)	Non-coronary (%)
Intraluminal	74	0
Intraluminal with plaque fissure	19	3.8
Intraintimal only	2	6
None	5	89.8

(From Davies MJ and Thomas A (1984). Thrombosis and acute coronary-artery lesions in sudden cardiac ischemic death. *New England Journal of Medicine* **310**, 1137–40.)

Further evidence for the role of thrombosis in coronary heart disease came with recognition of the effects of aspirin in modifying the aggregation of platelets and with the results of observational studies and early trials showing the reduction in coronary heart disease attributable to aspirin. Morphological observations and striking cine film pictures of platelet aggregation at sites of vascular injury have put the role of platelets in the thrombotic process beyond any doubt for many years now. However, no tests of platelet behaviour have convincingly been shown to be associated with the subsequent risk of first events of coronary heart disease, although spontaneous platelet aggregation and increased platelet volume may help predict those at risk of recurrent episodes.

Until fairly recently, the contribution of the coagulation system to arterial thrombosis through fibrin formation was not considered to be of clinical significance. This was partly because platelet aggregation in response to vascular injury is very rapid, and hence possibly more relevant than the allegedly slower-acting coagulation system, and also because of the value of aspirin in reducing coronary heart disease. However, epidemiological studies of the coagulation system in thrombosis and coronary heart disease have now demonstrated its involvement and implications for the management and prevention of coronary heart disease. This section summarizes, first, the mainly epidemiological evidence regarding coagulability and coronary heart disease (also arterial disease at other sites), and secondly, implications for long-term management and prevention (the treatment of acute events being described in Chapter 15.4.2.3).

Epidemiological evidence

Population-based studies started from the general proposition that high levels of procoagulatory clotting factors and low levels of anticoagulatory factors would predispose to coronary heart disease. Sceptics argued that (other than in obvious deficiency conditions such as haemophilia) clotting factors circulate well in excess of concentrations required for haemostasis under normal conditions and that no associations with coronary heart disease would therefore be demonstrable. However, requirements for haemostasis may not be a reliable guide to the influence of different levels of clotting factors on thrombosis, where a high level of a procoagulatory factor might facilitate thrombosis and a major coronary heart disease event. By analogy with blood pressure, a certain level of pressure is necessary to maintain normal circulatory function while raised levels predispose to the pathological processes involved in coronary heart disease and stroke.

Studies that demonstrate associations between different characteristics and the risk of coronary heart disease have two main purposes. One is to contribute to our understanding of the pathogenesis of the condition. The other is to identify characteristics with reasonably clear implications either for screening purposes and/or for treatment and prevention.

Figure 1 shows the main features of the coagulation system. Here and in the text the letter 'a' signifies the activated form of the clotting factor. The coagulation process, resulting in the generation of thrombin, can be initiated either through the extrinsic system, so called because it depends on the availability of tissue factor which has not generally been considered a component of the circulating blood, or through the contact system which is not dependent on biochemical properties outside the circulating blood. Tissue factor becomes available when atheromatous lesions leak or rupture, and other evidence strengthens the conclusion that the extrinsic system predominates in coronary heart disease, though not to the exclusion of an influence of factors XII and VIIIa on the intrinsic system (see below). As well as its well-known function in converting soluble fibrinogen into insoluble fibrin, thrombin has numerous other properties, of which the principal ones are shown in Table 2. It is a potent platelet-aggregating agent and may exert this action at least as soon as (if not before) its action on fibrinogen, so that the coagulation system has a strong influence on platelet behaviour as well as on the deposition of fibrin. Other actions of thrombin include the activation of protein C, which together with protein S inhibits the coagulation process; it also has both activating and inhibiting effects on the fibrinolytic system (see Fig. 1 and Table 2).

There have now been numerous cohort (prospective) and case-control or case-comparison studies of associations between different components of the coagulation system and the risk of coronary heart disease.

Fibrinogen

A recent overview of 18 cohort studies based on 4018 cases of coronary heart disease demonstrated that those in the top third of the fibrinogen distribution are at 1.8 times the risk of coronary heart disease compared with those in the bottom third, the findings being similar in the 12 studies concerned with first events and the other six with individuals known to have had previous episodes and followed for recurrences. The association of fibrinogen with the incidence of coronary heart disease is independent of other risk factors, is of a similar magnitude to the risk due to raised cholesterol, and is probably the same in women as in men. Besides first and recur-

rent events of coronary heart disease, high fibrinogen levels are also associated with the onset, recurrence, and progression of cerebrovascular and lower extremity arterial disease, with the incidence of graft occlusion following bypass surgery, and possibly with an increased risk of restenosis following coronary or lower limb angioplasty.

Factor VII

The possible involvement of factor VII activity in coronary heart disease is of theoretical as well as practical interest: when tissue factor is exposed it binds with factor VII, such that high levels of the latter might affect the amount of thrombin produced. However, the evidence is equivocal. Two cohort studies suggest that high levels increase risk, whilst others do not. Case-control and cross-sectional studies have also given conflicting results. Several assay techniques have been used and it has been established that these may vary in their sensitivity to factor VII activity, which might partly account for the differing results.

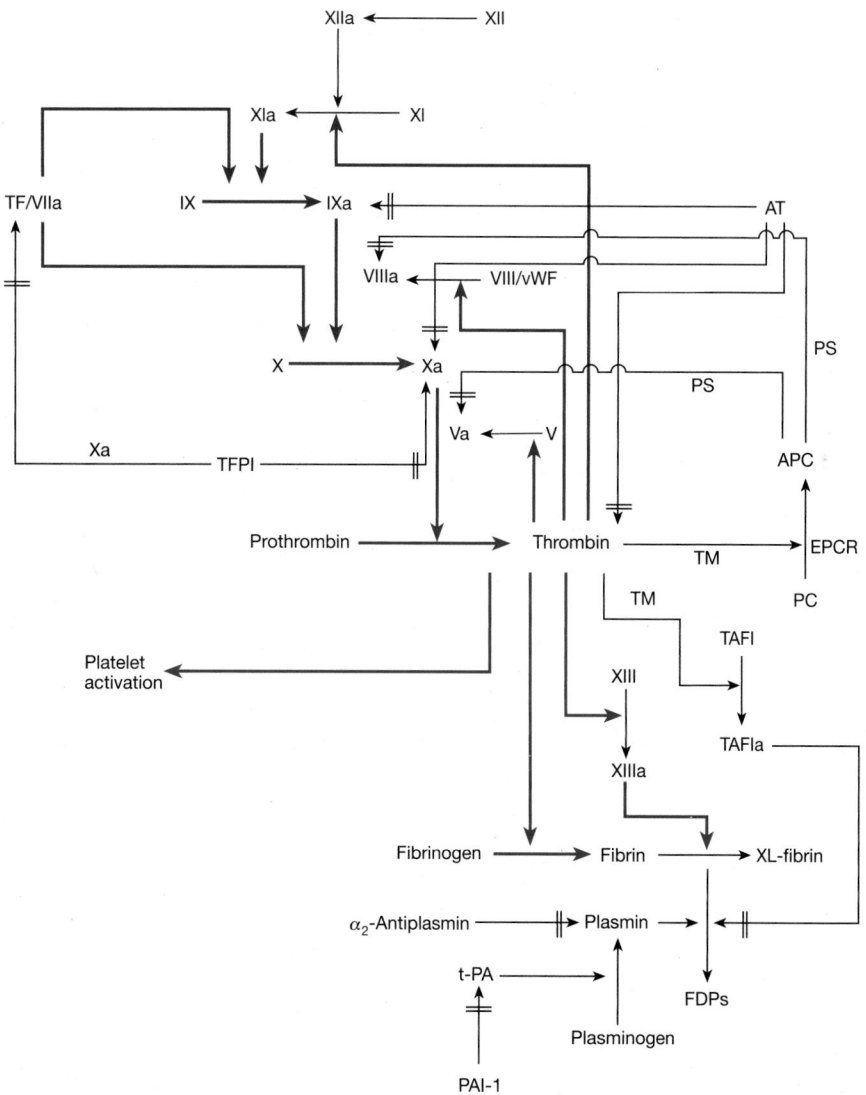

Fig. 1 Outline of the coagulation system and its regulation. The bold arrows represent the main pathways of generation of thrombin and thrombin's key role in fibrin formation and platelet activation: – reflects inhibitory activities; TF = tissue factor; TFPI = tissue factor pathway inhibitor; AT = antithrombin; PC = protein C; APC = activated protein C; PS = protein S; TAFI = thrombin activatable fibrinolysis inhibitor; XL-fibrin = cross-linked fibrin; FDPs = fibrin degradation products; t-PA = tissue-type plasminogen activator; PAI-1 = plasminogen activator inhibitor type 1; vWF = von Willebrand factor; EPCr = endothelial protein C receptor.

Table 2 Described effects of thrombin on the haemostatic and cardiovascular systems

Conversion of fibrinogen to fibrin
Activation of platelets
Activation of clotting factors V, VIII, XI, and XIII
Activation of protein C
Inactivation of protein S
Activation of thrombin activatable fibrinolysis inhibitor (TAFI)
Increased plasma levels of tissue-type plasminogen activator, urokinase-type plasminogen activator, and plasminogen activator inhibitor type 1
Increased synthesis of interleukin-1 and interleukin-8
Increased transforming growth factor-β
Increased endothelin 1
Promotion of neutrophil activation
Chemotactic for monocytes, neutrophils and fibroblasts
Mitogenic for vascular smooth muscle cells and fibroblasts
Activation of nuclear factor κB
Activation of endothelial cells with release of contents of Weibel–Palade bodies
Endothelial expression of cellular adhesion molecules

Factor VIII and von Willebrand factor

Factor VIII circulates in a complex with von Willebrand factor. The two proteins serve different haemostatic functions and have different sites of production, but they are closely correlated in a statistical sense so that independent contributions of the two proteins cannot easily be demonstrated, if at all. Four cohort studies have shown high levels of factor VIII to confer an increased risk of coronary heart disease. Haemophiliac patients appear to have a lower than expected incidence of coronary heart disease (though a considerable excess of cerebrovascular disease because of bleeding) and carriers of haemophilia have a reduced standardized mortality rate from coronary heart disease. Autopsy data show that haemophilia does not prevent the development of atheroma, suggesting that the decreased risk of coronary heart disease in patients with haemophilia is due to the effect of low levels of factor VIII on fibrin formation and thrombogenic potential. Case-control data show that elevated levels of factor VIII are associated with an increased relative risk of venous thrombosis, which also supports a prothrombotic role for factor VIII since vessel wall disease is not a consideration on the venous side. The association of factor VIII with coronary heart disease therefore appears to be due to a direct contribution of the level of factor VIII in circulating blood and not to a chronic phase response to atheromatous vessel wall changes.

Fibrinolytic activity

Several cohort studies, whether concerned with first events or in patients with previous episodes of coronary heart disease, have led to the conclusion that impaired fibrinolytic activity is an independent risk factor for coronary heart disease or its recurrence. Different studies have used different methods. These have included global tests of fibrinolytic activity such as the dilute clot lysis time, which takes account of both activators and inhibitors, and assays of specific components of the fibrinolytic system, principally plasminogen activator inhibitor type 1 and of D-dimer, the main degradation product of fibrinolysis. The principal determinants of the dilute clot lysis time are plasminogen activator inhibitor type 1 and, in men, activity of tissue-type plasminogen activator. Several studies have shown that fibrinogen does not make an independent contribution to measures of fibrinolytic activity so that the latter is not simply a reflection of the fibrinogen level. Fairly consistently, high levels of tissue-type plasminogen activator antigen have been associated with both coronary heart disease and stroke, which seems counterintuitive since high levels of tissue-type plasminogen activator would be expected to confer protection. The explanation may be that tissue-type plasminogen activator antigen, which is what the studies in question have measured, complexes with plasminogen activator inhibitor type 1 that is present in higher concentration and for which tissue-type

plasminogen activator antigen is a surrogate marker. Raised levels of D-dimer, indicating increased fibrin turnover, have been found to be predictive of future cardiovascular events—again, independent of fibrinogen. The association of activity of plasminogen activator inhibitor type 1 with coronary heart disease is not seen after adjustment for the features of insulin resistance (body mass index, triglyceride, high-density lipoprotein cholesterol, blood pressure, and diabetes) so that the prognostic value of plasminogen activator inhibitor type 1 may be related chiefly to this syndrome.

Other factors

Whereas inherited deficiencies of the naturally occurring inhibitors of coagulation such as antithrombin, protein C, and protein S clearly increase the risk of venous thromboembolism, the contribution that alterations in the levels of these proteins makes to arterial thrombosis is unclear. Anecdotally, case reports and case series have described deficiencies of these inhibitors in patients who have sustained arterial events. More formal studies have given conflicting and inconclusive results. What evidence there is suggests that low antithrombin levels may predispose to coronary heart disease.

Controversy surrounds the role in arterial disease of two recently recognized clotting factor polymorphisms, the factor V Leiden mutation and the prothrombin G20210A mutation (a polymorphism in the 3' untranslated region of the gene associated with higher prothrombin levels), in contrast to their generally accepted role in venous thromboembolism (see Chapter 15.15.3.1). Resistance to activated protein C, the laboratory phenotypic abnormality which led to discovery of the factor V Leiden mutation at one of the activated protein C cleavage sites on factor Va, has been described in patients with arterial disease. The roles in coronary heart disease of particular polymorphisms of platelet surface glycoprotein receptors and circulating levels of thrombomodulin, an endothelial receptor that binds thrombin, thereby leading to activation of protein C (anticoagulant effect) and thrombin-activatable fibrinolysis inhibitor (antifibrinolytic effect), are also uncertain. The antiphospholipid syndrome, which is characterized by both venous and arterial thrombosis together with laboratory evidence of anticardiolipin antibodies and/or the lupus anticoagulant, is discussed in Chapters 13.14 and 18.10.2.

The contact system consists of factor XII, factor XI, prekallikrein, and high molecular weight kininogen. Regulation of the system is provided in part by the multifunctional inhibitor, C1 inhibitor. The step which initiates activity is the conversion of factor XII to its derivative enzyme, factor XIIa, in response to exposure to biological substances with a negatively charged surface, for example lipopolysaccharide and phosphotidylinositol. The generation of factor XIIa triggers several activating reactions along pathways concerned with the response to injury, including activation of factor XI (which activates factor IX in the intrinsic pathway of coagulation), the production of kallikrein (which cleaves high molecular weight kininogen to bradykinin), the production of plasmin and renin, degranulation of neutrophils, activation of collagenase, and activation of the first component of complement. This range of activities raises the possibility that the contact system plays a co-ordinating role in the response to injury. A high level of factor XIIa is associated with raised levels of a number of familiar risk factors for coronary heart disease, including plasma triglyceride and systolic blood pressure, and it is an independent predictor of coronary heart disease.

Overall, the evidence shows that predisposition to thrombosis and coronary heart disease is associated with changes in several components of the coagulation system, as well as with platelet behaviour, and the question arises as to whether they represent causality. If so, what are the pathways involved and what are the implications for management and prevention through measures affecting the haemostatic system? There are three main ways in which these questions can be approached: first, detailed laboratory studies; secondly, the extent to which the associations of clotting factor with coronary heart disease are consistent with the effects of known risk factors such as smoking; and thirdly, the ability of agents used in randomized controlled trials (for whatever reason and with whatever clinical outcome) to affect particular pathways.

Laboratory studies

The effects of fibrinogen have been extensively studied and are summarized in Fig. 2. High fibrinogen levels make a substantial contribution to the viscosity of whole blood and plasma and to the amount of fibrin deposited when coagulation is initiated, they increase platelet aggregability, enhance the binding of leucocytes to platelets and endothelial cells, decrease clot deformability, and contribute to the atheromatous process—all of which have been shown to, or are likely to, increase the risk of thrombosis and thus of clinical events. The fibrinogen level itself is influenced by a range of characteristics, including smoking (increase), moderate alcohol consumption (decrease), and genetic characteristics. As an acute and chronic phase protein, fibrinogen levels also rise in response to inflammatory stimuli, of which underlying vessel wall pathology may be an example. This has sometimes led to the view that fibrinogen is no more than a marker of the risk of coronary heart disease, whereas the likelihood seems to be that, whatever the original explanations for raised fibrinogen levels may be, these will increase risk. If so, fibrinogen may be considered to be both a marker and a causal feature.

A number of metabolic studies have shown associations of factor VII with dietary fat intake and with serum triglyceride concentrations. Factor VIIa is also associated with plasma levels of the activation peptide fragment 1 + 2, an indicator of thrombin generation that is released from prothrombin upon its conversion to thrombin. Dietary and other studies have shown a pivotal role for factor IXa on the level of blood coagulability. Binding of factor VIIa to tissue factor may also lead to intracellular signalling, the consequences of which may include augmented macrophage activation. Factor VIII has been shown to increase the rate of activation of factor X by factor IXa in a dose-dependent manner.

Consistency with known risk factors

Very generally, associations of haemostatic variables with coronary heart disease are similar to the effects of more familiar risk factors. This is best illustrated for fibrinogen in Fig. 2 in which many of the personal or lifestyle characteristics apparently influencing fibrinogen levels are known to be associated with the risk of coronary heart disease itself—for example the increased risk due to smoking and the protective effect of a moderate intake of alcohol. Indeed, the associations of smoking and alcohol with fibrinogen are likely to explain, at least in part, how these aspects of lifestyle affect coronary heart disease itself.

One feature absent from Fig. 2 is dietary intake, particularly of saturated fat, but diet undoubtedly exerts a major effect on factor VII activity. Obesity and the other features of the insulin resistance syndrome impair fibrinolytic activity, as does smoking. The general conclusion, therefore, is that the personal and lifestyle influences on the risk of coronary heart disease operate through effects on the haemostatic system and thrombotic tendency as well as through more familiar lipid pathways. The implications for pharmacological intervention are considerable (see below).

Other effects of haemostatic variables in arterial disease

Response to injury

It is becoming increasingly clear that besides coagulability the haemostatic system plays a major role in the response to injury (although in evolutionary terms these two functions serve the same common purpose of repair of injury). Fibrinogen, for example, serves as a cell–cell adhesion protein for binding between platelets, monocytes, neutrophils, and endothelial cells. Fibrin forms a temporary matrix at sites of vessel wall injury, providing a framework for infiltration of smooth muscle cells and fibroblasts. Factor Xa stimulates proliferation of smooth muscle cells, and by limited proteolysis of protease-activated receptors, thrombin induces many cellular inflammatory responses including the expression of cytokines and adhesion molecules. Factor XIIa and kallikrein activate neutrophils and trigger the degranulation reaction. Inflammatory products have actions on components of the haemostatic system. For example, leucocytosis with neutrophil activation is a feature of atherosclerotic disease. Neutrophil elastase and cathepsin-G have diverse actions (at least *in vitro*) on the haemostatic pathway including limited proteolytic cleavage of factor IX, factor VII, factor

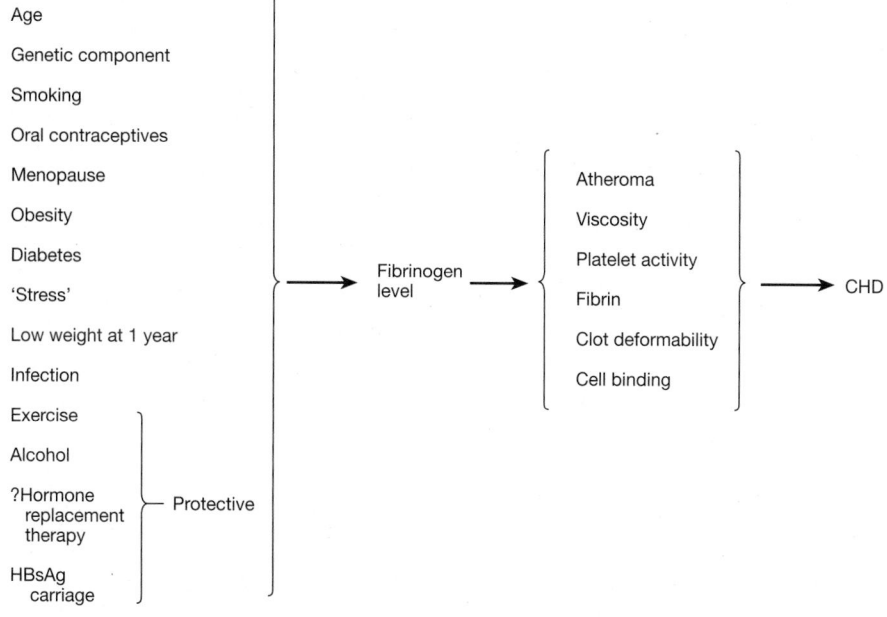

Fig. 2 Summary of determinants and thrombogenic pathways of fibrinogen in the pathogenesis of coronary heart disease.

VIII, factor V, and of platelets, and degradation of fibrinogen, fibrin, antithrombin, and tissue factor pathway inhibitor. The significance of interactions such as these between the haemostatic system and the inflammatory/immune mechanism is poorly understood, but they are likely to be pivotal in ensuring an integrated response to injury and tissue defence and repair. In summary, the original hypothesis that the haemostatic system contributes to coronary heart disease simply by a direct effect on thrombogenic potential, and thus through 'hypercoagulability', probably now requires modification. Account must also be taken of other processes involved in the pathogenesis of coronary heart disease to which changes in the coagulation system may be a secondary response, although some of these changes may then contribute to thrombotic potential.

Inflammatory markers and arterial disease

Recent years have seen the widespread recognition that atherosclerosis is an inflammatory process and the emegence of evidence that circulating markers of inflammation might be used to predict the risk of coronary events.The most consistently observed association has been that of the acute-phase reactant, C-reactive protein (CRP), with coronary risk. In healthy, asymptomatic adults, a single CRP measurement (using a sensitive assay) in the high normal range is associated with an increased risk of angina, acute myocardial infarction and death. The association is independent of lipids and its strength is similar to that observed with other risk factors including cholesterol and fibrinogen. CRP is also associated with the risk of recurrent events in those with established coronary heart disease.

CRP is synthesized in the liver and, stimulated by cytokines (particularly interleukin 6), its level rises more than 100-fold in response to severe infection. In this setting, it binds to phosphocholine on the surface of invading microbes and assists their killing by complement and phagocytes. It also diminishes adherence of leucocytes to the vascular endothelium, releasing marginated neutrophils to infected sites while preventing the accumulation of leucocytes in uninflamed tissues. By these and other mechanisms, CRP (together with other inflammatory markers) provides an important survival function.

By contrast with this beneficial effect, repeated or prolonged low-grade stimulation of the acute phase response might have harmful consequences (see below). In the context of arterial disease, debate continues as to whether CRP is merely a marker of the inflammation that characterizes atheroma or is directly involved in the pathogenesis of atherothrombosis. In support of the latter view, CRP is deposited in human atherosclerotic lesions and is capable of binding to both enzymatically-degraded, non-oxidized low-density lipoprotein and to the terminal complement complex, C5b-9, thereby promoting inflammation. It is chemotactic for monocytes and may play a role in the recruitment of monocytes during atherogenesis. It may contribute to the expression on the endothelium of adhesion molecules such as intercellular adhesion molecule I (ICAM-I), vascular-cell adhesion molecule I (VCAM-I), and E-selectin, further enhancing the local inflammatory response within atheromatous plaques. CRP may also promote thrombosis by enhancing tissue factor expression by monocytes. Therefore, like fibrinogen, CRP may be both a marker of the underlying pathological process and a direct contributor to the development of atherothrombosis.

It is uncertain whether the acute phase stimulus for increased CRP levels comes from the atheromatous plaques themselves, from arterial infection, or from chronic extravascular stimuli. Causes of the latter may include smoking, chronic mucosal infections such as bronchitis, gastritis and periodontitis, and obesity, with strong associations having been made between the levels of body fat and inflammatory markers with adipose tissue increasingly recognized as a source of cytokines including interlukin 6. Indeed different mechanisms might operate within one individual. As yet little is know about the genetic determinants of CRP.

Statin therapy, administered to lower cholesterol levels in those at risk of coronary events, also lowers levels of CRP, an effect which appears to be independent of their effect on lipid levels. The possibility has therefore been raised that CRP might be added to an individual's risk factor profile when deciding whether or not to use a statin for the primary prevention of coronary heart disease but this requires confirmation in prospective trials.

Associations between many other inflammatory markers and coronary heart disease risk have been reported. Inflammatory markers are synthesized in a number of different sites including the liver (CRP, serum amyloid A), macrophages (lipoprotein-associated phospholipase A_2, soluble phospholipase A_2), the vessel wall (ICAM-I, VCAM-I, E-selectin), and adipocytes (cytokines including interleukin-1β, interleukin 6, tumour necrosis factor α). It is possible that each makes a contribution to the chronic process of atherosclerosis, although in prospective studies they have generally been less clearly associated independently with coronary heart disease than has CRP. However, this may be for assay-related rather than biological reasons and independent associations of soluble ICAM, interleukin 6, and lipoprotein-associated phospholipase A_2 with coronary disease have been reported.

Homocysteine

Although not itself a component of the haemostatic system, the sulphur-containing amino acid homocysteine has emerged in recent years as a potentially important risk factor for arterial disease (and also for venous thromboembolism), with postulated mechanisms of effect that may be mediated in part through components of the haemostatic system.

It was first recognized in the 1960s that premature atherothrombosis was often seen in individuals with the rare inherited metabolic disorder homocystinuria, in which the plasma level of homocyteine is very high. Within the past decade evidence has emerged from observational studies showing an association between homocysteine levels and the risk of vascular disease within the general population, although the causal nature of this association remains to be established.

Homocysteine is a byproduct derived from the metabolic demethylation of dietary methionine. Study of the metabolic pathway of homocysteine metabolism (Fig. 3) shows that it can be metabolized either by trans-sulphuration, with vitamin B_6 (pyridoxine) as a cofactor, or by remethylation to methionine, with vitamin B_{12} as a cofactor and N^5-methyltetrahydrofolate (derived from dietary folate) as the methyl donor. In the liver, betaine can act as an alternative methyl donor.

Homocysteine is present in plasma in several forms: 70 to 80 per cent is disulphide-bound to plasma proteins, 20 to30 per cent combines either with itself to form the disulphide homocystine or with other thiols such as cysteine to form mixed disulphides, and about 1 per cent circulates as the free thiol. Homocysteine (usually as the combined total of the different forms) can be measured either in the fasting state or post- methionine-loading with a standard amount of methionine. The latter estimate may be particularly sensitive to disturbances in the trans-sulphuration pathway, thereby enabling additional cases of hyperhomocysteinaemia to be detected, but it is inconvenient for patients. Blood samples should ideally be centrifuged immediately because homocysteine is progressively released from blood cells with the passage of time. If this is not possible, samples should be placed on ice following collection and centrifuged as soon as possible. The fasting reference range in Western populations is approximately 5 to 15 μmol/1, reflecting levels 2 standard deviations above and below the mean, and higher levels are arbitrarily categorized as moderate (16–30 μmol/l), intermediate (31–100 μmo/l), and severe (>100 μmol/l) hyperhomocysteinaemia. However, although such a range can be defined statistically, there is no clear threshold effect in studies that have reported positive associations between homocysteine levels and atherothrombotic disease, an analogous situation to that observed with other CHD risk factors such as cholesterol and blood pressure where risk rises even within the 'normal range'.

Plasma homocysteine levels are influenced by a number of factors, both genetic and environmental. Nutritional deficiency of folate is the most common cause of hyperhomocysteinaemia and deficiencies of vitamin B_{12} and vitamin B_6 also contribute. Other acquired causes of hyperhomocysteinaemia include renal impairment, hypothyroidism, malignancy, severe psoriasis and drugs that interfere with folate or B6 metabolism. Levels rise with age and are higher in males than females and in smokers compared to non-smokers. The combined oral contraceptive pill and hormone replacement therapy appear to lower the concentration. Homocysteine should probably not be measured immediately after an occlusive vascular event as levels may be transiently depressed.

The most common genetic cause of moderate hyperhomocysteinaemia is a point mutation (C-to-T substitution at nucleotide 677) in the coding region of the gene for N^5, N^{10}-methylenetetrahydrofolate reductase (MTHFR) that results in a thermolabile variant of the enzyme with about half normal activity. The homozygous MTHFR polymorphism is present in 10 to 15 per cent of Caucasians and is associated with an increase in homocysteine levels particularly if folate status is suboptimal. Rarer inherited causes are covered in Chapter 11.1

The data linking homocysteine and atherothrombotic disease are somewhat inconsistent, perhaps inevitable given that the relationship has been examined in over 12 000 patients in more than 100 observational studies. Data from case-control studies have mostly reported a positive association between homocysteine and arterial disease. Data from prospective cohort studies have been less consistent, although the association has been in a positive direction, even if not significantly so, in the majority. Moreover, the association appears to be independent of traditional CHD risk factors such as age, sex, smoking, blood pressure, and cholesterol. Critics of the association of homocysteine and atherothrombosis point to the lack of consistent findings in the prospective studies, the lack (so far) of an associ-

ation between the common genetic marker of raised homocysteine (the thermolabile MTHFR genotype), and vascular disease despite the association of genotype with homocysteine level, and the possibility that homocysteine may be simply a marker of another causal risk factor. Overall, it seems probable that homocysteine is an independent risk factor and the results of further genetic analyses and intervention trials will hopefully resolve this uncertainty.

The mechanism(s) by which homocysteine might promote atherothrombosis remains speculative. A number of possible explanations have been put forward but have often been based on *in vitro* studies that have used higher levels of homocysteine than those typically found clinically and therefore should be interpreted with caution. They include effects on platelet adhesiveness or activation, activation of clotting factors V and X, and inhibition of fibrinolysis through enhanced binding of lipoprotein(a) to fibrin. Possible effects on the endothelium may result from oxidative damage and include increased tissue factor and decreased thrombomodulin expression, and inhibition of nitric oxide. Proliferation of smooth muscle may be enhanced.

Folic acid (pteroylmonoglutamic acid) is the single most effective treatment for hyperhomocysteinaemia. It is the synthetic version of dietary folate with twice the bioavailability and it lowers homocysteine levels even in those who are not folate deficient. For most people the maximum reduction of about 25 per cent is seen with a dose of 0.8 mg daily although patients with renal impairment need much higher doses. Vitamin B_{12} produces a smaller 7 per cent decrease in homocysteine. Dietary sources of folate include green vegetables and fortified breakfast cereals. In the United States flour has been fortified with folic acid since 1998 in order to reduce the risk of neural tube defect by ensuring improved folate status in women of child-bearing age. The level of fortification is likely to produce an extra 0.1 mg at least of folic acid per day in the diet and therefore lead to a partial lowering of homocysteine in the general population. Discussions are ongoing as to whether similar measures should be adopted in the United Kingdom. Concerns have been expressed about increasing the risk of subacute combined degeneration of the cord in patients with undiagnosed B_{12} deficiency through correction of the haematological manifestations by administration of folic acid potentially masking development of the neurological condition. The extent of this theoretical risk is uncertain and is probably extremely small but no consensus has yet been reached on whether B_{12} deficiency should be excluded before starting higher doses of folic acid or whether vitamin B_{12} should be administered in conjunction with folic acid.

A number of clinical trials with therapy that lowers homocysteine (with folic acid alone or in combination with vitamin B_6 or B_{12}) are under way in an effort to prevent coronary and cerebrovascular disease and venous thromboembolism and the results should become available within the next few years.

Implications for clinical practice

Screening and diagnosis

Recent work on the haemostatic system has certainly led to improved understanding of the pathogenesis of coronary heart disease, but only some of the information gained so far has implications for clinical practice—in particular, attempting to identify those at increased risk of first or recurrent events. Measuring fibrinogen and assessing fibrinolytic activity are the two investigations that may be helpful. A high fibrinogen level is sometimes the only identifiable risk factor in a patient referred for investigation because of a strong family history of coronary heart disease, for example, or in some patients who have recovered from myocardial infarction and in whom there are no other obvious risk factors. It may also, of course, be an additional finding in those with other risk factors. Although there is only limited evidence on the value of lowering fibrinogen levels (see below), information about these may be useful in deciding whether, for example, to recommend low-dose aspirin for primary prevention—a measure that should almost

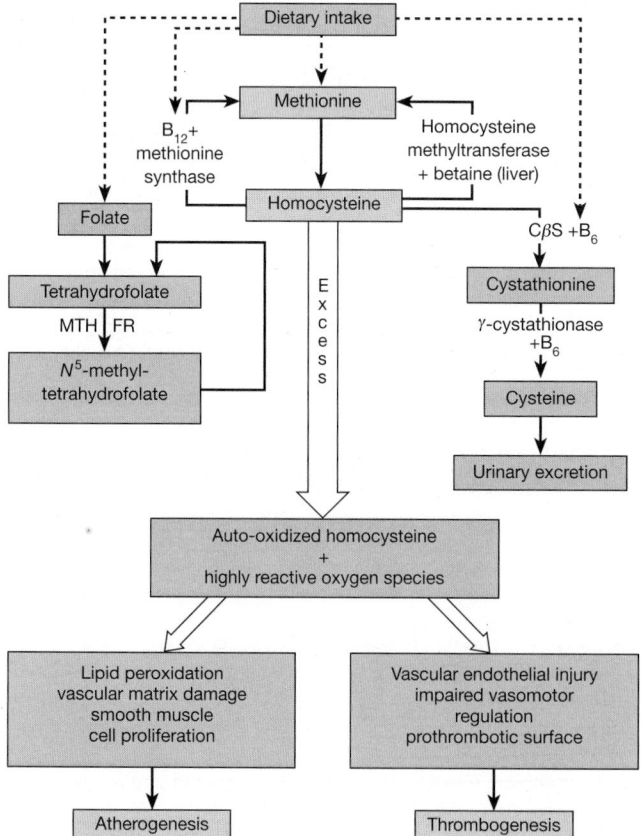

Fig. 3 Homocysteine metabolism. MTHFR, methylenetetrahydrofolate reductase; CβS, cystathionine β synthase

certainly be taken only after much more careful consideration than is often the case—even though aspirin does not lower fibrinogen. Measuring the euglobulin lysis time and the activity of plasminogen activator inhibitor type 1 can also be helpful, though they are often to be explained by obesity and other features of the insulin resistance syndrome.

Fibrinogen and fibrinolytic activity should only be measured some time after an acute episode of coronary heart disease and in the absence of recent infection. As for other risk factors such as cholesterol and blood pressure, they should be measured several times before an individual's habitual level can be established with any certainty. There is now a World Health Organization standard for fibrinogen, which means that ranges and values can be much more confidently compared between different centres than previously. Assays of factor VII activity are difficult to perform and the interpretation of results is uncertain. There are no established interventions for lowering levels of activity of factor VIII. While there is some evidence that low levels of antithrombin increase the risk of coronary heart disease, there are no specific agents for raising them.

Prevention

Primary prevention

In contrast to the value of aspirin in reducing recurrent major vascular events and mortality after a first attack (secondary prevention, see below), its value in primary prevention seems on present evidence to be confined mainly to reducing non-fatal myocardial infarction. There is no evidence for a reduction in fatal episodes of coronary heart disease and it is possible that the risk of cerebral haemorrhage is actually increased. It is also possible that the reduction in non-fatal events is mainly confined to those who are normotensive. Thus, those with raised blood pressure may not only experience more cerebral haemorrhage but also be exposed to the risk of gastrointestinal haemorrhage while deriving no protection against coronary heart disease. These conclusions need to be strengthened or refuted by results from further studies, but they do justify considerably more thought than is commonly given to the use of aspirin in primary prevention: many middle-aged men take aspirin indiscriminately and not necessarily beneficially and safely.

One trial has evaluated low-dose aspirin (75 mg daily) and low-intensity oral anticoagulation with warfarin (aiming at an international normalized ratio of 1.5) either singly or in combination in men at increased risk of coronary heart disease. Both agents reduced the incidence of major coronary heart disease by about 20 per cent. However, in common with other evidence in primary prevention, aspirin achieved this as a result of reducing non-fatal events by just over 30 per cent (and, if anything, slightly increasing the risk of fatal episodes). Warfarin reduced fatal episodes by 39 per cent but had little effect on non-fatal events. The combination of both agents reduced events, whether fatal or non-fatal, by 34 per cent. Warfarin may also have reduced the onset of angina pectoris slightly. There was no demonstrable difference in serious bleeding between the three active treatment groups (warfarin and aspirin together, warfarin alone, and aspirin alone) or between them and the placebo group (although minor bleeding was clearly more frequent in those on active treatment regimens). The assumption that warfarin is intrinsically more dangerous than aspirin was therefore not supported. The disadvantage of the need for international normalized ratio and dose monitoring when using warfarin is balanced by the possibility of a substantial reduction in fatal events which needs to be considered alongside the inability to predict which first major events of coronary heart disease will be fatal and the high proportion of those experiencing their first major event who die.

There is still only limited agreement about the optimal dose of aspirin: the evidence mostly points to the need for no more than 75 mg and certainly no more than 300 mg daily, both for antithrombotic effect and safety.

Secondary prevention

Antithrombotic treatment in the early stages of myocardial infarction, in which a combination of aspirin and thrombolytic treatment is used, merges into the longer-term secondary prevention of further episodes. Aspirin in the early stages reduces further major vascular events (myocardial infarction, stroke, or vascular death) by some 25 per cent, the reduction in non-fatal episodes of coronary heart disease being somewhat more than for fatal outcomes. The proportional benefits of aspirin are similar in older and younger patients, in men and women, in normotensive and hypertensive patients (which contrasts with the possible difference in primary prevention), and in non-diabetic and diabetic patients. Absolute reductions, however, are greater in the higher-risk groups (for example older, hypertensive, or diabetic patients) because of their higher event rates. There is little or no formal evidence on how long aspirin should be taken after an initial event, but since those who have already experienced episodes of arterial disease are likely to remain at high risk indefinitely, antithrombotic treatment should probably also be continued long term.

Despite the clear value of aspirin in secondary prevention, the benefits of oral anticoagulation should not be overlooked. First, it is possible that anticoagulation confers slightly greater protection against recurrence than aspirin, perhaps because of the effect of thrombin, which is reduced by warfarin, on platelets as well as fibrinogen. Despite the disadvantages of anticoagulation, this extra benefit (if real) may still be worthwhile for a common condition with a high risk of recurrence. Secondly, the value of oral anticoagulants in modifying fibrin production may add to the value of aspirin in reducing platelet aggregability. The value of combined antithrombotic regimens has been well illustrated through the concurrent use of aspirin and thrombolytic therapy in early myocardial infarction and in the postoperative treatment with aspirin and warfarin of patients undergoing heart valve surgery. Aspirin with heparin followed by warfarin is also beneficial in the setting of acute coronary syndromes. Other trials have cast doubt on the possible benefit of combined antithrombotic therapy for recurrent coronary heart disease, but they used fixed or capped low-dose warfarin, whereas it is almost certainly necessary to give warfarin in a dose-adjusted manner, i.e. to achieve a target international normalized ratio. Combined regimens of agents modifying different aspects of platelet function such as aspirin and dipyridamole in the secondary prevention of stroke further illustrate the potential value of modifying more than one pathway at a time, provided the risk of serious bleeding is not unacceptably increased. An obvious question not so far tested in randomized trials is the potential value of the simultaneous use of antithrombotic and lipid-modifying agents. While intravenous antagonists of the platelet glycoprotein IIb/IIIa receptor are effective in the early postacute management of acute coronary syndromes, oral therapy does not appear to confer benefit.

Further reading

Antiplatelet Trialists' Collaboration (1994). Overview of randomised trials of antiplatelet therapy—I: Prevention of death, myocardial infarction, and stroke by prolonged antiplatelet therapy in various categories of patients. III: Reduction in venous thrombosis and pulmonary embolism by antiplatelet prophylaxis among surgical and medical patients. *British Medical Journal* **308**, 81–106, 235–46.

Banerjee AK et al. (1992). A six year prospective study of fibrinogen and other risk factors associated with mortality in stable claudicants. *Thrombosis and Haemostasis* **68**, 261–3.

Cairns JA et al. (2001). Antithrombotic agents in coronary heart disease. *Chest* **119 (suppl)**, 228S–252S.

Danesh J, Collins R, Peto R (1997). Chronic infections and coronary heart disease: is there a link? *Lancet* **350**, 430–6.

Danesh J et al. (1998). Association of fibrinogen, C-reactive protein, albumin, or leukocyte count with coronary heart disease. Meta-analyses of prospective studies. *Journal of the American Medical Association* **279**, 1477–82.

Davies MJ, Thomas A (1984). Thrombosis and acute coronary-artery lesions in sudden cardiac ischemic death. *New England Journal of Medicine* **310**, 1137–40.

Ernst E *et al.*, eds (1992). *Fibrinogen: a 'New' Cardiovascular Risk Factor.* Blackwell-MZV, Vienna.

Gillis S, Furie BC, Furie B (1997). Interactions of neutrophils and coagulation proteins. *Seminars in Hematology* **34**, 336–41.

Hankey GJ, Eikelboom JW (1999). Homocysteine and vascular disease. *Lancet* **354**, 407–13.

MacCallum PK, Meade TW, eds (1999). *Thrombophilia*, 2nd edn. *Baillière's Clinical Haematology* **12**, London.

Medical Research Council's General Practice Research Framework (1998). Thrombosis prevention trial: randomised trial or low-intensity oral anticoagulation with warfarin and low-dose aspirin in the primary prevention of ischaemic heart disease in men at increased risk. *The Lancet* **351**, 233–41.

Mennen LI *et al.* (1996). Coagulation factor VII, dietary fat and blood lipids. *Thrombosis and Haemostasis* **76**, 492–9.

Miller GJ *et al.* (1996). Activation of factor VII during alimentary lipemia occurs in healthy adults and patients with congenital factor XII and factor XI deficiency, but not in patients with factor IX deficiency. *Blood* **87**, 4187–96.

Morris JN (1951). Recent history of coronary disease. *Lancet* **1**, 1–7, 69–73.

Munford RS (2001). Statins and the acute-phase response. *New England Journal of Medicine* **344**, 2016–8.

Pulmonary Embolism Prevention (PEP) Trial Collaborative Group (2000). Prevention of pulmonary embolism and deep vein thrombosis with low dose aspirin: Pulmonary Embolism Prevention (PEP). *Lancet* **355**, 1295–302.

Rader DJ (2000). Inflammatory markers of coronary risk. *New England Journal of Medicine* **343**, 1179–82.

Ridker PM *et al.* (1997). Inflammation, aspirin, and the risk of cardiovascular disease in apparently healthy men. *New England Journal of Medicine* **336**, 973–9.

Ridker PM *et al.* (2000). C-reactive protein and other markers of inflammation in the prediction of cardiovascular disease in women. *New England Journal of Medicine* **342**, 836–43.

Ross R (1999). Atherosclerosis – an inflammatory disease. *New England Journal of Medicine* **340**, 115–26.

Samis JA *et al.* (1998). Neutrophil elastase cleavage of human factor IX generates an activated factor IX-like product devoid of coagulant function. *Blood* **92**, 1287–96.

15.1.3 The heart

15.1.3.1 Biochemistry and cellular physiology of heart muscle

P. H. Sugden, N. J. Severs, K. T. MacLeod, and P. A. Poole-Wilson

Introduction

The heart of a normal human weighs 250 to 300 g, contracts at a rate of 70 to 75 beats/min at rest, and pumps approximately 5 litres of blood/min. The cardiac content of the energy transducing molecule ATP is only sufficient to support contraction for a few beats (about five to ten) and the supply of endogenous fuels (for example glycogen, endogenous triglyceride) is limited given the amount of work the heart has to perform. In order to maintain fuel oxidation, ATP regeneration, and cardiac contraction, a highly developed coronary circulation and a maintained coronary blood flow are necessary to ensure adequate delivery of O_2 and fuels, and to remove the major product of fuel oxidation (CO_2). Thus, about 5 per cent of the cardiac output is used to perfuse the heart itself (about 1 ml/min/g of myocardium). On maximal exercise both heart rate and cardiac output can increase substantially—to 200 beats/min and 20 litres/min respectively—and these changes are accompanied by an almost immediate increase of coronary blood flow to about four times its normal amount. The magnitude of the potential increase is known as the coronary reserve.

The heart is made up of many different cell types. Cardiac myocytes (the contractile cells of the heart) constitute about 75 per cent of the ventricular mass but, as they are large cells, they account for only about 25 per cent of the cell number. Other types of myocytes are specialized for the initiation of the cardiac action potential (sinoatrial nodal cells) and its transmission in a regular and co-ordinated manner to the working ventricular myocardium (conduction myocytes of the atrioventricular node, the bundle of His, and the Purkinje fibres). In addition, the heart is innervated by neurones of the autonomic nervous system. Cardiac fibroblasts synthesize and maintain the extracellular matrix. The extensive vasculature contains smooth muscle cells and pericytes, and is lined by a monolayer of endothelial cells. The endothelium is more than simply a barrier lining the blood vessels and heart chambers. Release of signalling molecules such as endothelin and nitric oxide from the endothelial cells regulates vascular smooth muscle tone and the biological properties of the myocytes themselves (see Chapter 15.1.1.2).

Interrelationships between structure and function in the ventricular myocyte and myocardium

The adult ventricular myocyte is a large cell, approximately 100 to 120 μm long and 20 to 35 μm wide (Fig. 1). Each is physically joined to approximately 10 adjacent myocytes and lies close to an extensive capillary network. The ventricular myocyte contains a highly developed contractile apparatus and a large complement of mitochondria. These fit it for its major role *in vivo*, namely the rhythmic contraction that provides the force

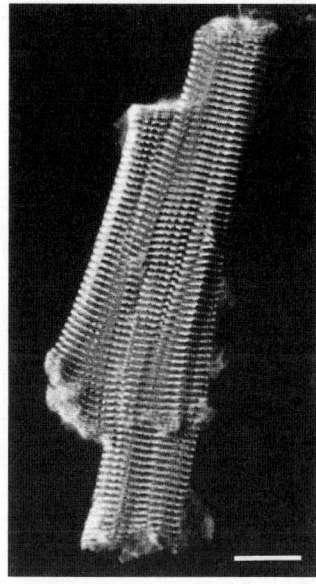

Fig. 1 Ventricular myocyte viewed by confocal microscopy. The image was prepared by combining a stack of serial optical sections through the cell. The striated myofibrils are visualized by the immunostaining of α-actinin, a component of the Z bands. The bar is 10 μm. (From Severs NJ (2000) *BioEssays* **22**, 188–99, with permission.)

needed for the ejection of blood from the ventricles. Atrial myocytes have a less well developed myofibrillar apparatus than ventricular myocytes, in accordance with the lesser contractile demand on the atria compared with the ventricles.

Intercommunication between the myocytes and extracellular matrix

The myocardial cell is surrounded by the sarcolemma which comprises the plasma membrane (about 10 nm thick) and an outer layer (70 nm thick) called the surface coat or glycocalyx (Fig. 2). As with all biological membranes, the plasma membrane consists of a phospholipid bilayer with numerous intercalated and associated proteins. Transmembrane proteins include the channels, transporters, and pumps that allow passage of ions through the membrane, and receptor sites for hormones, pharmacologically active substances, and components of the extracellular matrix. The glycocalyx lies outside the plasma membrane (but is attached to it) and is made up of polysaccharides conjugated to protein or lipid.

At the ends of its long axis and at branches along its length, each myocyte makes contact with neighbouring myocytes through a characteristic area of plasma membrane called the intercalated disc. The intercalated disc contains three types of cell junction: the fascia adherens, the desmosome, and the gap junction. The fasciae adherentes link adjacent myocytes mechanic-

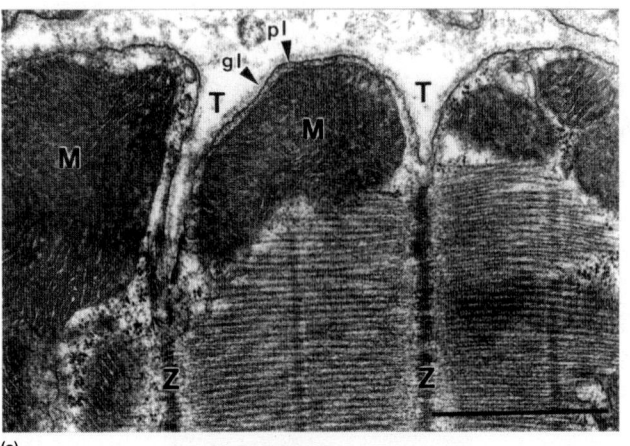

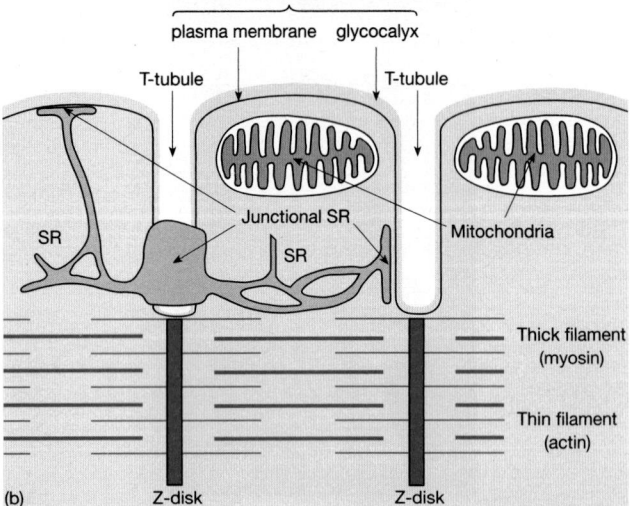

Fig. 2 Electron micrograph (a) and explanatory diagram (b) illustrating the organization of T tubules and sarcoplasmic reticulum. Labels on the micrograph as follows: T, T tubule; Z, Z disc of myofibril; M, mitochondrion; pl, plasma membrane; gl, glycocalyx. The bar is 1 μm.

ally so that force can be transmitted between them. The contractile apparatus is anchored to the fascia adherens by a series of linking proteins such as α-actinin, filamin, and vinculin; these bind to adhesive proteins (cadherins) which are transmembrane proteins that bond across the extracellular space. The desmosomes form sites at which the intermediate filaments of the cytoskeleton attach to the plasma membrane, the cytoskeleton being important in the establishment and maintenance of myocyte shape as it provides an intracellular supporting lattice structure. As with the fasciae adherentes, bonding at the desmosome is mediated by proteins of the cadherin superfamily. The gap junctions are the sites in the intercalated disc where the membranes of adjacent myocytes come into intimate contact. Here, clusters of channels, each made of dodecamers of the protein connexin surrounding a central pore, permit myocyte-to-myocyte communication. The permeability of these pores to ions allows electrical impulses to pass easily between myocytes. The gap junctions also allow the passage of other small molecules (< 1 kDa) between the cytoplasmic compartments of adjacent cells.

The lateral (non-intercalated disc) plasma membrane is strengthened on its cytoplasmic aspect by a net-like skeleton composed of the structural proteins dystrophin and spectrin. As well as being responsible for the skeletal muscle abnormalities of Duchenne and Becker muscular dystrophy, mutations in dystrophin are responsible for the cardiomyopathy associated with these syndromes. The skeletal structure of the membrane is further reinforced by rib-like transverse bands of vinculin, termed costameres, which contain transmembrane proteins (for example integrins) that bind to components of the extracellular matrix, thereby allowing lateral transmission of the mechanical force of contraction from the cell to the matrix.

The extracellular matrix is important for the overall morphology of the heart and provides an anchoring structure against which the myocytes contract. It is made principally of collagen and fibronectin. Fibronectin fills the spaces between the cells and possesses binding sites for the integrins of the plasma membrane and for collagen. Collagen types I and III form a fibrous network that weaves around the myocytes, maintaining their alignment, preventing overstretching, and transmitting force. This network preserves the overall shape and architecture of the heart, and acts as a spring to store energy during systole. The normal heart contains about 5 per cent collagen but, in pathological conditions, this can increase to 25 per cent. This increases myocardial 'stiffness' and can impede contraction.

Contraction

The contractile apparatus is highly ordered, consisting of bundles of striated myofibrils (approximately 1 μm in diameter with around 150 per cell) running the length of the cell (Fig. 3). As in skeletal muscle, myofibrils (which are responsible for contraction) are made up of a repeating sarcomeric unit that is about 2 μm in length in the relaxed state. Each sarcomere consists of thick filaments that interdigitate with thin filaments (Fig. 4). The thick filament is a polymer of the protein myosin, a hexamer of two myosin heavy chains and four myosin light chains. The myosin heavy chain has an elongated rod-like domain and a globular head, to each of which two light chains are bound (Fig. 5). The rod-like regions of two myosin heavy chains intertwine to form the hexamer. The thin filaments consist of a double-beaded strand of the globular protein actin with which the rod-like protein tropomyosin and members of the troponin family (troponin I, troponin C, and troponin T) are associated (Fig. 5). The thin filaments within adjacent sarcomeres are linked at the Z line. The alignment and the overlapping of thick and thin filaments gives the myofibril its striated appearance in micrographs (Figs. 3 and 4).

Myofibrillar contraction in the heart is essentially similar to that in skeletal muscle. The globular heads of myosin interact with actin, and the myofibrillar actomyosin adenosine triphosphatase (**ATPase**) transduces the chemical energy released by ATP hydrolysis into external mechanical work (Fig. 5). In the absence of Ca^{2+}, troponin I maintains the actomyosin ATPase in an inactive state. Binding of cytoplasmic Ca^{2+} ions to troponin C

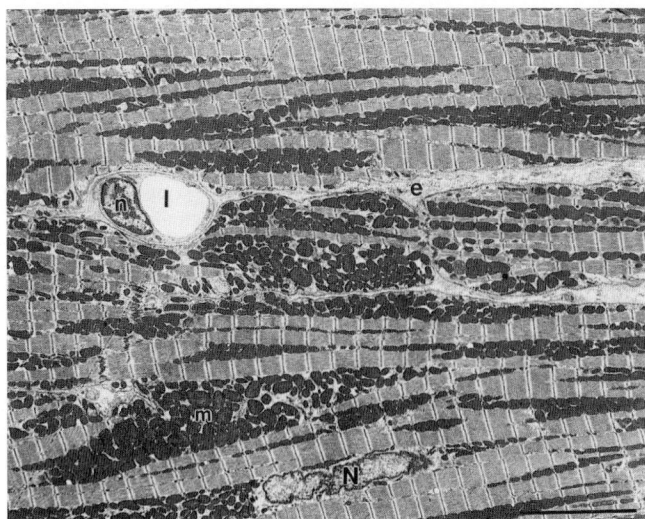

Fig. 3 Structure of ventricular myocardium by thin-section electron microscopy. The major components of the myocytes, the striated myofibrils and the mitochondria (m, seen as abundant dark-stained rounded objects), dominate the view. N, nucleus of myocyte; n, nucleus of endothelial cell; l, lumen of capillary; e, extracellular matrix. The bar is 10 μm.

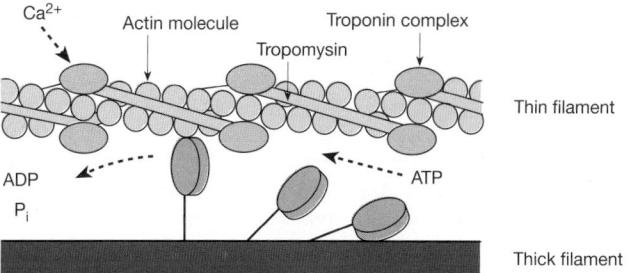

Fig. 5 Diagrammatic representation of myofilament structure and contraction. The thick filament is a polymer of myosin, the double beaded helix of the thin filament is a polymer of actin. Increases in intracellular Ca^{2+} ion concentrations are detected by troponin C of the troponin complex and this relieves the inhibition of the actomyosin ATPase by troponin I. The hydrolysis of ATP by the ATPase provides the energy for contraction. The globular myosin heads, which form crossbridges with the thin filaments, move as shown causing shortening of the sarcomere.

removes this restraint and contraction occurs by the movement of the myosin heads in the thick filaments along the actin beads in the thin filaments, with concomitant hydrolysis of ATP. Mutation of specific amino acid residues in the myosin heavy chain in particular (but also in other myofibrillar proteins) can give rise to an inheritable disease generically known as hypertrophic cardiomyopathy (see Chapter 15.8.2).

Since Ca^{2+} is intimately involved in the regulation of contractile activity, a well-developed apparatus controls the intracellular (subscript 'i') concentration of Ca^{2+} ions. The ventricular myocyte possesses an array of T tubules and an extensive sarcoplasmic reticulum, a specialized form of endoplasmic reticulum. The T tubules are finger-like invaginations from

the cell surface with openings of up to 200 nm in diameter, spaced so that a T tubule lies alongside each Z disc of most (or even all) of the myofibrils (Fig. 2). Both the T tubule and the sarcoplasmic reticulum are involved in regulation of the movement of Ca^{2+}. The T tubules regulate the entry of extracellular (subscript 'o') Ca^{2+} into the myocyte, and the sarcoplasmic reticulum 'stores' Ca^{2+}_i during diastole. The regulation of movement of Ca^{2+} in the myocyte is described in more detail below.

Although much of the intracellular volume of the ventricular myocyte is occupied by myofibrils, about 30 per cent is taken up by mitochondria (Fig. 3). As in other oxidative tissues, these subcellular organelles oxidize metabolic fuels and convert the energy released by this oxidation to drive regeneration of ATP (from ADP and inorganic phosphate). In the myocyte, the majority of the energy released by ATP hydrolysis is used to power myofibrillar contraction, but there are also other essential processes that require energy (for example macromolecule synthesis and other biosynthetic pathways, ion transport, etc.).

The nucleus and the cell cycle

The mammalian ventricular myocyte is believed to lose its ability to divide during the perinatal period, hence most maturational growth occurs through cellular enlargement. However, complicating factors are that the myocyte may be multinucleate, and its nucleus may possess more that two chromosome pairs (polyploidy). Thus the arrest in the cell cycle appears to reside at the stage of cell division (cytokinesis) rather than nuclear division (karyokinesis). The reasons for the withdrawal of the myocyte from the cell cycle are not understood, and although some molecules which regulate the cell cycle are present in the ventricular myocyte, it has not yet been experimentally possible to drive the cell into division. This means that the myocardium cannot regenerate, and the loss of myocytes following, for example, an ischaemic insult is potentially disastrous. An ability to restore entry of ventricular myocytes into the cell cycle in a controlled manner might well have considerable clinical significance as it would be one step towards allowing the damaged heart to regenerate its contractile capacity. As it is, the myocyte can only increase its contractile capacity by cell enlargement (hypertrophy), and this leads to the clinical entity of cardiac hypertrophy.

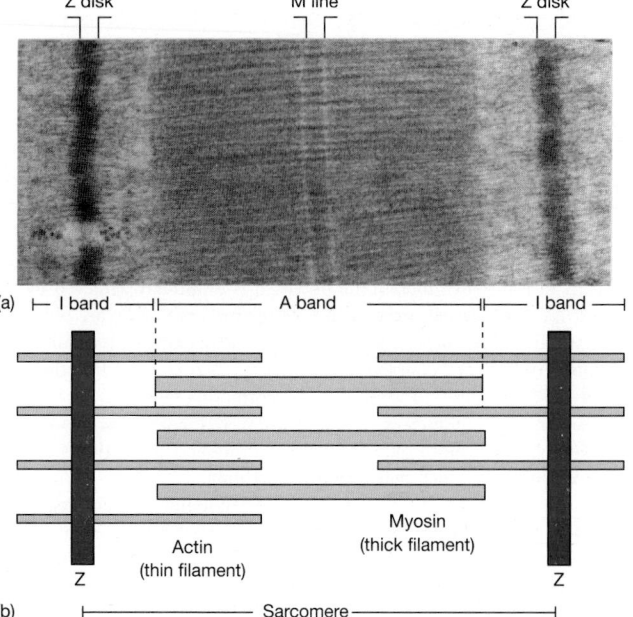

Fig. 4 High-power electron micrograph of a single sarcomere (a), the basic contractile unit of heart muscle, with explanatory diagram (b) of the organization of the thick and thin filaments, Z discs, and bands.

Cardiac electrophysiology

Each heartbeat is initiated by a spontaneous electrical discharge in the sinoatrial node. The electrical signal passes across the atrium to the atrioventricular node, through the bundle of His, and down the Purkinje fibres to the ventricular myocardium. This incremental excitation of the heart provides a means of co-ordinating the contractile activities of the four chambers and is the basis for the electrocardiogram (see Chapter 15.3.2).

Electrical excitation of each myocyte involves the movement of ions through ion channels. These are 'excitable' macromolecules embedded in the plasma membrane which contain pores that open or close in response to a stimulus. This stimulus could be a change in membrane potential, a neurotransmitter or hormone, an intracellular second messenger or ion, or mechanical stretch of the membrane. When a channel opens, it becomes selectively permeable to a restricted series of ions, selectivity being determined by the interaction of the various ions with the channel pore. There are a large number of different types of channel, often named after the most important permeant ion they pass, for example the Na$^+$, Ca^{2+}, and K$^+$ channels. The groups of channels are functionally distinct and can be further divided into subgroups on the basis of amino acid sequence and tertiary structure. Ions move down their electrochemical gradients through the channels at high rates ($> 10^6$ ions/s), which distinguishes them from other ion transport proteins (for example, the Na$^+$,K$^+$-ATPase or pump, and the Na$^+$,Ca^{2+} exchanger, see below) which move ions across plasma membranes several orders of magnitude more slowly.

When a ventricular myocyte is at rest (diastole), there is a potential difference of -80 mV across the plasma membrane, the inside of the cell being negative with respect to the outside. This is due to K$^+$ channels being open, making the plasma membrane more permeable to K$^+$ than any other ion. The concentration of K$^+$ is about 4 mmol/litre outside the cell and about 140 mmol/litre inside, so K$^+$ tends to leave the cell by diffusing down its concentration gradient, which results in the inside becoming negatively charged since there is no movement of anions to balance the K$^+$ loss. An equilibrium is established where the electronegative force retaining K$^+$ inside the cell balances its tendency to diffuse out of the cell down its concentration gradient. This is termed the equilibrium potential (E), and can be calculated from the Nernst equation. The calculated equilibrium potentials for important ions are shown in Table 1.

The actual transmembrane potential difference at rest and the calculated equilibrium potential for K$^+$ are rarely the same owing to a small leakage of other ions (mainly Na$^+$) into the cell. To counteract this leak of Na$^+$ down its concentration gradient and to maintain the concentration gradients of Na$^+$ and K$^+$ upon which the generation of the membrane potential depends, the sarcolemmal Na$^+$,K$^+$-ATPase uses energy derived from the hydrolysis of ATP to pump these ions against their concentration gradients. This process is electrogenic (three Na$^+$ are extruded for two K$^+$ entering) and generates 3 to 10 mV of the membrane potential.

Table 1 Intracellular and extracellular concentrations of pertinent ions in the quiescent myocyte, and their calculated equilibrium potentials (*E*). *E* is calculated from the Nernst equation:

$$E = \frac{RT}{zF} \ln (a_o/a_i)$$

where *E* is in volts, *T* is the absolute temperature, *R* is the gas constant, *F* is the Faraday constant, *z* is the valency, and a_o and a_i are the extracellular and intracellular activities of the ion in question, respectively.

Ion	Intracellular concentration (mmol/litre)	Plasma concentration (mmol/litre)	Calculated *E* (mV)
Na$^+$	10	140	+ 70
K$^+$	140	4.5	− 91
Ca^{2+}	0.0001	2.3	+ 131
Cl$^-$	20	110	+ 45

When a myocyte is electrically excited, Na$^+$ channels open and allow Na$^+$ ions to enter the cell. Positive charge is taken into the cell, the membrane potential increases towards the equilibrium potential for Na$^+$ (Table 1), and the cell depolarizes (Fig. 6). This causes the rapid upstroke (phase 0) of the action potential. The rate of change of the potential is related to the propagation velocity of the action potential across the heart. The current (*I*) generated by the inward movement of Na$^+$ (I_{Na}), like the same current in nerve tissue, is inhibited by tetrodotoxin, lidocaine, and quinidine. Na$^+$ channels close very rapidly and so I_{Na} almost entirely inactivates within the first 4 ms of the action potential. A small proportion of Na$^+$ channels do not inactivate as rapidly and allow a small inward current to persist for up to 100 ms, i.e. during the plateau phase of the action potential (phase 2).

The characteristic notch observed in phase 1 of the action potential in ventricular myocytes (Fig. 6) (the notch is also particularly apparent in the Purkinje cell action potential; see Fig. 7) is caused by a transient outward current (I_{TO}), mainly carried by K$^+$ ions, that partially repolarizes the membrane. A number of different currents flow during phase 2 (the action potential plateau): the most important, from the point of view of the generation of contraction, is I_{Ca}. Ca^{2+} channels, which take longer to activate and inactivate than Na$^+$ channels, open within 3 ms of the start of the upstroke. The inward flow of Ca^{2+}, mainly through the L-type Ca^{2+} channel, maintains depolarization (Tables 1 and 2) and can be inhibited by 'Ca^{2+} antagonists' such as verapamil and the dihydropyridines. The influx of Ca^{2+} initiate Ca^{2+}-induced Ca^{2+} release from the sarcoplasmic reticulum through the sarcoplasmic reticulum Ca^{2+}-release channels, and the increase in cytoplasmic Ca^{2+} concentration causes the myocyte to contract (see below).

The plateau phase (phase 2) of the action potential (Fig. 6) is prolonged in ventricular myocytes because of the properties of several types of K$^+$ channel. The repolarizing current I_K flows through a channel that opens at positive membrane potentials and closes at negative potentials, akin to its counterpart in nerve. However, the kinetics of this channel are much slower than in nerve so that a much longer time is taken for it to start to repolarize, this being one of the reasons that a cardiac action potential is so much longer than a nerve action potential. In addition, ventricular myocytes possess another K$^+$ channel with peculiar characteristics. The current I_{K1} flows through a channel that first increases its conductance but then decreases it as the cell depolarizes away from E_K (anomalous rectification). The combined effect of these K$^+$ currents is that, despite the membrane potential approaching 0 mV during the plateau phase, a large outward K$^+$ current does not occur and the action potential is prolonged.

Repolarization (phase 3) starts to occur because of an increase in K$^+$ conductance via I_K and the termination of I_{Ca} (Fig. 6). As repolarization proceeds, the Na$^+$,Ca^{2+} exchanger responds to the increase in cytoplasmic Ca^{2+} concentration and produces an inward current ($I_{Na,Ca}$) through the exchange of three Na$^+$ entering the cell for one Ca^{2+} expelled. By producing an inward current, the Na$^+$,Ca^{2+} exchanger helps to prolong the plateau and slows repolarization. In ventricular myocytes, complete repolarization and a return to a negative membrane potential is eventually achieved by the current I_{K1}. The clinical consequences of the presence of I_{K1} are profound and result from this channel being acutely sensitive to the extracellular concentration of K$^+$. For example, shortly after myocardial infarction there is a loss of K$^+$ from cells and local K^+_o concentrations increase. Because K^+_o increases channel conductance and outward movement of K^+_i, I_{K1} increases accordingly. Thus, more outward current flows and the action potential duration shortens, which may lead to arrhythmia.

The configuration of the cardiac action potential differs regionally (Fig. 7) because of the presence or absence of different ionic currents. In the sinoatrial node (the pacemaker), I_{Na} is very small and the main current responsible for the depolarizing upstroke is I_{Ca}. The only repolarizing current is I_K. I_{K1} is absent and this partially explains why sinoatrial node cells have a more depolarized diastolic potential than ventricular myocytes. Sinoatrial node cells also depolarize spontaneously (phase 4), probably owing to the absence of I_{K1} and the presence of a current activated on hyperpolarization called I_f. Phase 4 is often termed the 'pre- or pacemaker potential' and is caused by the gradual decrease in I_K and increase in I_f (Figs. 6 and 7). Once the cell has depolarized to the point where Ca^{2+} channels open (the threshold), a more rapid depolarization takes place forming

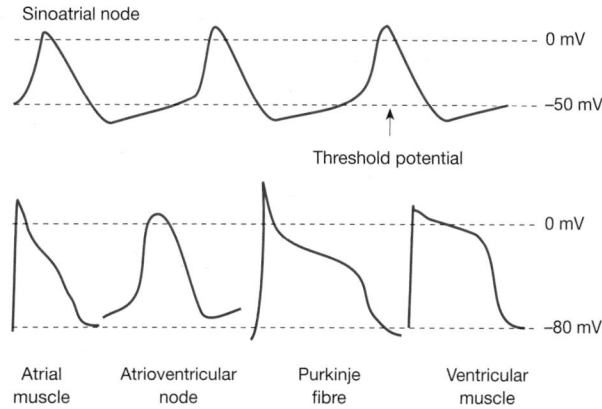

Fig. 7 Regional configuration of the action potential. In the sinoatrial and atrioventricular nodes, the cells spontaneously depolarize during diastole (phase 4 depolarization). When the membrane potential reaches a threshold value, the complete action potential is initiated. Because the sinoatrial nodal cells have the fastest phase 4 depolarization, they act as the cardiac pacemaker.

the upstroke of the sinoatrial node action potential. Atrial and ventricular myocytes do not have pacemaker potentials and spontaneously discharge only when injured or when there is abnormal intracellular Ca^{2+} balance. The longest action potential is in Purkinje fibres; this acts as a gate preventing retrograde activation by depolarization of adjacent ventricular myocytes. The action potential is longer in the epicardium than in the endocardium, and in the apex than in the base of the heart: the reason for this is not clear, but the discrepancy is the probable explanation for the upright T wave on the electrocardiogram.

When the cholinergic drive from autonomic neurones to the nodal cells is increased, the slope of the pacemaker potential is decreased (Fig. 8). Acetylcholine (**ACh**) opens another group of K^+ channels and activates $I_{K, ACh}$, which counters the decline in I_K and slows the rate of depolarization. I_f and I_{Ca} are also reduced and the overall effect is a reduction in the rate of production of action potentials. Conversely, upon stimulation of the sympathetic cardiac nerves, noradrenaline activates I_f and facilitates the opening of L-type Ca^{2+} channels, so increasing I_{Ca}. The net effect is to depolarize the membrane to the threshold level more quickly and increase the rate of production of action potentials. A summary of the ionic currents flowing during the cardiac action potential is given in Table 2.

Intracellular calcium ions—regulators of contraction

The electrical events throughout the heart initiate and regulate contraction (Fig. 9). The coupling of the electrical excitation of the heart to the production of contraction (called EC coupling) by Ca^{2+} ions involves the interaction of a number of cellular proteins involved in Ca^{2+} homeostasis. The T tubules allow the wave of depolarization of the action potential to reach deeply into the cell. The sarcoplasmic reticulum is an intracellular membranous lace-like structure surrounding the myofibrils, with swellings called junctional sarcoplasmic reticulum where the membrane of the sarcoplasmic reticulum comes close to the T tubules, (Figs. 2 and 10). During diastole, when cytoplasmic Ca^{2+} concentrations are low (around 0.1 μmol/litre), Ca^{2+} is sequestered by the Ca^{2+} buffering protein calsequestrin within the junctional sarcoplasmic reticulum. When opened, the L-type Ca^{2+} channels (also known as dihydropyridine receptors because of their sensitivity to the dihydropyridine Ca^{2+} channel antagonists) allow influx of Ca^{2+} across the sarcolemma (Fig. 10). This influx increases the local Ca^{2+} concentration around clusters of Ca^{2+} release channels in the sarcoplasmic reticulum (the ryanodine receptors, so-called because of their sensitivity to interference by the plant alkaloid ryanodine) sufficiently to open them, the

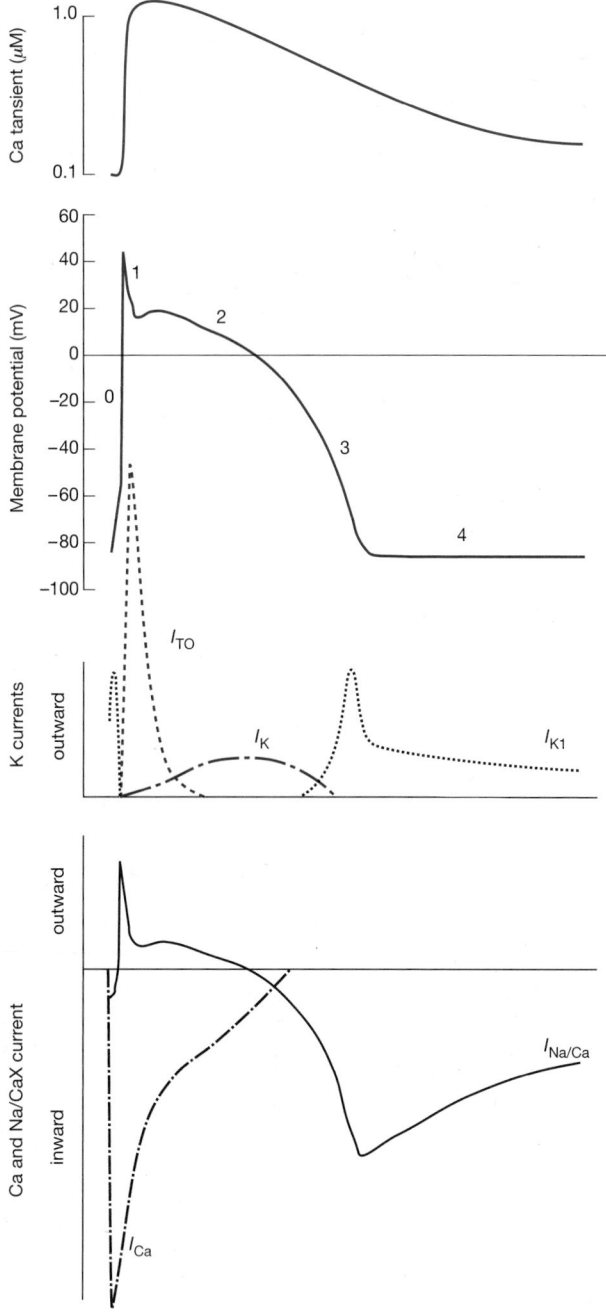

Fig. 6 Major ionic currents flowing during a ventricular myocyte action potential. Top trace: changes in cytoplasmic Ca^{2+} concentration during the action potential (Ca^{2+} transient). Second trace: the action potential recorded from a ventricular myocyte. Third and fourth traces: time courses and relative sizes of current flows during one beat. All K^+ currents (I_{TO}, I_K, and I_{K1}, seen in the third trace) repolarize the cell because of outward K^+ movement. Because of the inward movement of Ca^{2+}, Ca^{2+} current (I_{Ca}, seen in the fourth trace) is depolarizing. The Na^+,Ca^{2+} exchanger (Na/CaX, fourth trace) produces both outward and inward current ($I_{Na,Ca}$). Note that the inward Na^+ current that produces the rapid upstroke of the action potential is not shown: it is roughly eight to ten times the size of the Ca^{2+} current and has largely inactivated by the time the peak of the Ca^{2+} current is reached.

number of channels activated in this way being mainly, though not exclusively, determined by the size of the Ca^{2+} current. This allows Ca^{2+} stored by the sarcoplasmic reticulum to be released into the cytoplasm (Ca^{2+}-induced Ca^{2+} release). The fluxes of Ca^{2+} combine to raise the cytoplasmic concentration of Ca^{2+} to between 5 and 10 µmol/litre, when contraction is initiated by the binding of Ca^{2+} to troponin C, relieving the inhibition of the actomyosin ATPase by troponin I.

Contraction is terminated by two principal mechanisms:

- By the activation of an ATP-requiring Ca^{2+} pump present in the sarcoplasmic reticulum membrane (the sarcoplasmic (endoplasmic) reticulum ATPase type 2 (**SERCA2**)), which catalyses ATP-dependent reuptake of Ca^{2+} into the sarcoplasmic reticulum.

- By the response of the sarcolemmal Na^+,Ca^{2+} exchanger to the increase in cytoplasmic Ca^{2+} (Fig. 10).

On a beat-to-beat basis, these are the main systems involved in removing Ca^{2+} from the cytoplasm and so inducing relaxation. Ca^{2+} is pumped back into the sarcoplasmic reticulum by SERCA2, which is regulated by the extent of phosphorylation of the SERCA2-associated protein, phospholamban. Hypophosphorylated phospholamban tonically inhibits SERCA2; as more phospholamban is phosphorylated (see below) the inhibition is removed and more Ca^{2+} is pumped into the sarcoplasmic reticulum. This, along with increased troponin I phosphorylation (see below), accounts for

the more rapid relaxation of myocytes when the intracellular concentration of cyclic adenosine 3_,5_-monophosphate (**cAMP**) and the activity of cAMP-dependent protein kinase (see below) are increased by, for example, heightened sympathoadrenal tone.

Ca^{2+} is extruded from the cell by the sarcolemmal Na^+,Ca^{2+} exchanger that utilizes the energy associated with the concentration and electrical gradients for Na^+ to expel Ca^{2+} from the cell. It couples the transport of three Na^+ into the cell with the expulsion of one Ca^{2+}. It is thus electrogenic, and for every Ca^{2+} removed from the cell, one positive charge enters. It can be predicted thermodynamically that the direction of ion movement mediated by the exchange can vary according to the membrane potential and the intracellular and extracellular concentrations of Na^+ and Ca^{2+}. The exchange is sensitive to the intracellular Na^+ concentration (normally about 7 to 10 mmol/litre in ventricular myocytes). When membrane potential is near diastolic levels and intracellular Na^+ concentration at normal physiological levels, the Na^+,Ca^{2+} exchanger will eject Ca^{2+} from the cell. However, if the intracellular Na^+ concentration increases by a few mmol/litre and the membrane potential becomes depolarized, the exchanger can reverse and mediate Ca^{2+} entry. Although ventricular myocytes possess other systems to decrease cytoplasmic Ca^{2+} concentrations (namely the sarcolemmal Ca^{2+} ATPase and mitochondrial Ca^{2+} uptake), these contribute less than 5 per cent towards relaxation of a normal twitch. SERCA2 and Na^+,Ca^{2+} exchange contribute about 70 and 25 per cent respectively

Table 2 Sarcolemmal currents in the myocyte

Symbol	Name	Activated by	Blocked by	Function
Inward currents				
I_{Na}	(Fast) Na^+ current	Depolarization	Tetrodotoxin, local anaesthetics	Rapid upstroke of action potential
$I_{Ca,L}$	L-type Ca^{2+} current	Depolarization	Verapamil, Cd^{2+}, dihydropyridines	Ca^{2+} influx that activates calcium-induced calcium release, provides some Ca^{2+} for contraction
$I_{Ca,T}$	T-type Ca^{2+} current	Activates on depolarization but at more negative potentials than L-type current	Ni^{2+}	Channel density high in pacemaker and conducting tissue and may contribute to pacemaker activity. Role in ventricular cells unclear
I_f	Pacemaker current	Hyperpolarization, noradrenaline, cAMP	Cs^+	Present in SA node and Purkinje fibres, brings membrane potential slowly to threshold
Inward and outward current				
$I_{Na,Ca}$	NaCaX current	Ca^{2+}_i	Ni^{2+}	Expels Ca^{2+} from the cell, maintains inward current flow near end of action potential; at positive potentials may reverse and mediate Ca^{2+} influx
Outward currents				
I_{TO}	Transient outward current (mainly K^+)	Depolarization	4-aminopyridine	Early repolarization (notch)
I_{Cl}	Chloride current	cAMP		Early repolarization
$I_{Cl,Ca}$	Ca^{2+}-activated chloride current	Ca^{2+}		Early repolarization
I_K	Delayed rectifier, (consists of three components, ultra-rapid (I_{Kur}), rapid (I_{Kr}) and slow (I_{Ks})	Depolarization	Tetraethylammonium ions, Cs^+, Ba^{2+}	Repolarization of cell
I_{K1}	Inward (anomalous) rectifier	Depolarization from E_K. Conductance of channel increases then decreases to zero close to 0 mV	K^+_o	Prolongs action potential duration, background K^+ conductance
I_p	Na^+/K^+ pump current	Na^+_i, K^+_o	Cardiac glycosides (digoxin)	Maintains low $[Na^+]_i$
$I_{K,ACh}$	Acetylcholine-activated K^+ current (inward rectifier)	Acetylcholine		Muscarinic receptor-coupled. Activates additional K^+ channels so slowing pacemaker potential
$I_{K,ATP}$	ATP-sensitive K+ current	A decrease in intracellular ATP, hypoxia, lemakalim	Intracellular ATP, glibenclamide	Responsible for shortening the action potential during hypoxia and ischaemia

Abbreviations: I, current; E_K, equilibrium potential for K^+; NaCaX, Na^+,Ca^{2+} exchanger; SA, sinoatrial; cAMP, cyclic adenosine 3′,5′-monophosphate; ATP, adenosine 5′-triphosphate. Non-sarcolemmal (intracellular) currents are not shown.

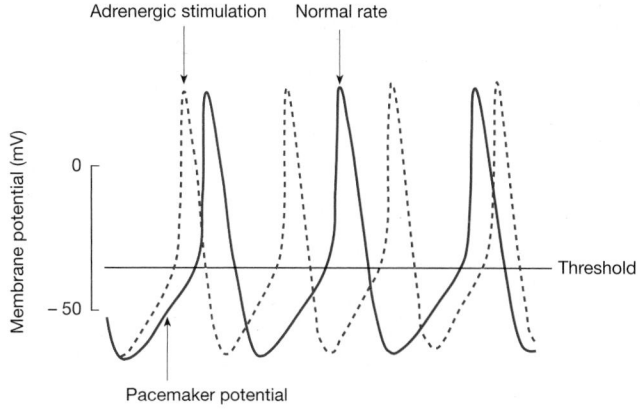

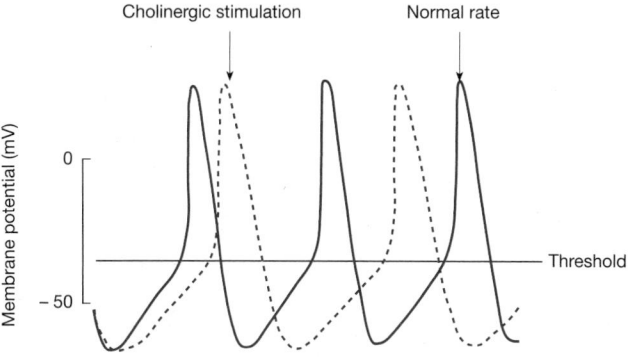

Fig. 8 Change in heart rate produced by altering the phase-4 slope of the pacemaker potential. Adrenergic stimulation increases and cholinergic stimulation decreases the slope, affecting the time taken to reach threshold.

towards relaxation, though these figures vary greatly between animal species. In steady-state conditions, the amount of Ca^{2+} leaving the cell via the Na^+,Ca^{2+} exchanger is the same as the amount entering (via I_{Ca}) to evoke Ca^{2+}-induced Ca^{2+} release, hence precise Ca^{2+} homeostasis is achieved.

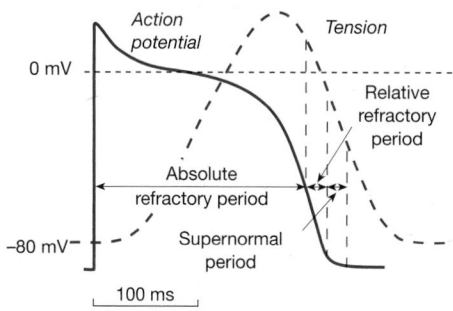

Fig. 9 The relationship between the action potential and the generation of force. The peak of force production is not achieved until near the end of the plateau phase of the action potential. This reflects the time required for Ca^{2+}-induced Ca^{2+} release. For a period between phase 0 and about halfway through phase 3, cardiac muscle cannot be excited with another stimulus no matter how strong. The muscle is in its absolute refractory period. Thus, tetanic contraction of the type seen in skeletal muscle cannot occur. When cardiac muscle is in its relative refractory period, an abnormally strong stimulus can initiate an action potential. In the supernormal period that follows, a slightly weaker stimulus that would normally fail to reach threshold can also initiate an action potential. The states of refractoriness are related to the ability of ion channels to recover from a stimulus. This recovery is both voltage- and time-dependent.

Cardiac mechanics

Four key factors determine the contraction of isolated cardiac muscle preparations; these are also applicable to the intact heart. The first factor is the relationship between the initial fibre length and the force it produces: initial 'preload' stretches the sarcomeres, increasing the sensitivity of the myofilaments to Ca^{2+} and allowing them to produce force that is directly proportional to the preload (i.e. resting length). The second factor determining contraction is termed the 'afterload': if a mass is attached to a muscle just before it contracts isotonically, it represents a constant force (afterload) against which the muscle must work during contraction, and the amount and speed of contraction are inversely proportional to this. If preload and afterload are held constant, the maximum force and speed of contraction can be altered by changing the inotropic state of the muscle, which is generally brought about by chemical or hormonal influences (for example, increasing concentrations of catecholamines). In the whole heart, these three factors (preload, afterload, and inotropic state) influence the stroke volume (the volume of blood ejected by the ventricle during each systole), which, along with heart rate (the fourth factor), determines the cardiac output. These issues are discussed in Chapter 15.1.3.2.

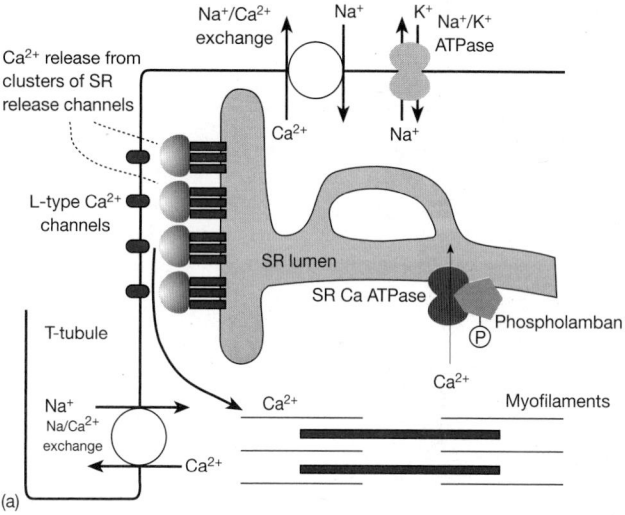

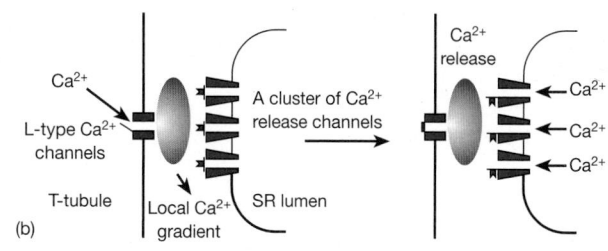

Fig. 10 EC coupling in the heart. Panel A: L-type Ca^{2+} channels allow Ca^{2+} influx across the sarcolemma and this creates I_{Ca}. This influx increases the local Ca^{2+} concentration around a cluster of Ca^{2+} release channels in the sarcoplasmic reticulum (SR) in sufficient amounts to open them (Ca^{2+}-induced Ca^{2+} release). Panel B: The opening of clusters of Ca^{2+} release channels in the sarcoplasmic reticulum allows Ca^{2+} stored by the sarcoplasmic reticulum to be released into the cytoplasm. The fluxes of Ca^{2+} combine to initiate contraction. The process is terminated by the sarcoplasmic reticulum Ca^{2+} ATPase (regulated by phospholamban) which removes Ca^{2+} from the cytoplasm and pumps it into the sarcoplasmic reticulum, and by the sarcolemmal Na^+,Ca^{2+} exchanger which expels Ca^{2+} from the cell. In steady-state conditions, the amount of Ca^{2+} leaving the cell (via the Na^+,Ca^{2+} exchanger) balances the amount entering (via the L-type Ca^{2+} channel).

Energy for contraction

As mentioned earlier, the heart is principally reliant on aerobic metabolism for its energy supply. In normal humans at rest, the heart extracts 60 to 65 per cent of O_2 passing through it. This corresponds to a rate of O_2 utilization of about 4.5 µmol/min/g wet weight (0.1 ml/min/g wet weight), which may increase by three- to fourfold during exercise. The comparable rates (in µmol/min/g wet weight) in other organs are: brain, 1.7; kidney, 7.1; liver 1.6; skeletal muscle at rest, 0.08; and skeletal muscle during exercise, 6.4. Thus, the maximal physiological O_2 uptake of the heart is higher than that of any other tissue.

In terms of metabolic fuels, the heart utilizes any fuel presented to it, within the constraints of metabolic regulation. Furthermore, because the heart is contracting continuously, an uninterrupted exogenous provision of fuels through the coronary circulation is essential. The major substrates for oxidation in man are lipid-derived fuels (long-chain fatty acids, principally palmitate, triglycerides, and ketone bodies (acetoacetate and 3-hydroxybutyrate)) and the carbohydrate-derived fuels (glucose, lactate, and pyruvate) (Fig. 11). Although the heart can oxidize amino acids, these probably represent a relatively minor fuel. The relative contribution of each substrate to cardiac fuel supply depends principally on the individual concentrations of substrates in the plasma (which are largely hormonally regulated).

Carbohydrate metabolism

Glucose crosses the myocardial plasma membrane by two carrier-mediated mechanisms (the type 1 and the type 4 glucose transporters). The activity of the type 1 glucose transporter is largely independent of insulin but is controlled by the intra- and extracellular concentrations of glucose. Insulin can increase glucose uptake by recruiting intracellular type 4 glucose trans-

porter to the plasma membrane. The principal use of intracellular glucose is to provide energy for contraction. In addition, the heart has a limited capacity to store carbohydrate as the polysaccharide glycogen. Whilst glycogen breakdown may not be quantitatively significant under normal conditions, it represents a fuel that can be used for a limited period in pathological conditions (e.g. during myocardial infarction, when the supply of fuels and O_2 is disrupted).

Each molecule of glucose is degraded through the exclusively cytoplasmic glycolytic pathway to pyruvate, the chemical energy released allowing the regeneration of two molecules of ATP (from ADP) per glucose molecule utilized and the concomitant reduction of the electron carrier nicotinamide adenine dinucleotide (**NAD+**) to NADH (Fig. 11). This pathway occurs anaerobically but is inefficient in terms of the quantity of ATP regenerated per glucose utilized. Under the aerobic conditions that normally exist in the heart, pyruvate is transported into the mitochondria and the glycolytically derived reducing equivalents enter on a shuttle mechanism (the malate/aspartate shuttle) regenerating cytoplasmic NAD^+. The remaining steps of carbohydrate metabolism take place in the mitochondria: pyruvate is oxidized to acetyl CoA and NADH (NAD^+ accepting the reducing equivalents) by the pyruvate dehydrogenase multienzyme complex, and acetyl-CoA then enters the tricarboxylic acid cycle, with the net result being the complete oxidation of the glucose molecule (glucose + $6O_2$ → $6CO_2$ + $6H_2O$). The bulk of the mitochondrially generated ATP is then exchanged with cytoplasmic ADP, making it available for myofibrillar contraction and other processes.

In some pathological circumstances (for example in coronary artery disease), the heart may become intermittently hypoxic. When this happens, glucose is increasingly metabolized anaerobically (glucose → 2 lactate + $2H^+$), and lactate and protons are released into the circulation. By contrast, under aerobic conditions exogenous lactate or pyruvate can also be utilized by the heart, entering oxidative metabolism in the same way as glycolytically derived pyruvate and NADH.

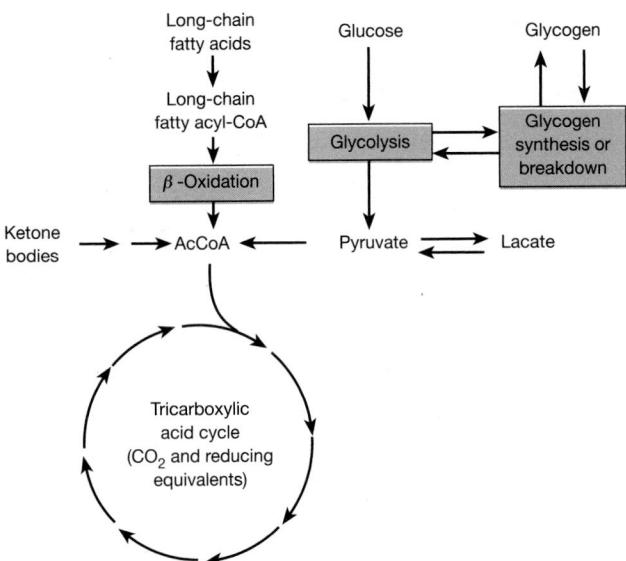

Fig. 11 Fuel utilization. Multistep processes are shown in boxes. In aerobic metabolism, the key intermediate acetyl CoA (AcCoA) is oxidized to CO_2 and water. Reducing equivalents produced mainly in the mitochondria by the tricarboxylic acid cycle and β-oxidation are passed between a series of carriers (the electron transport chain), the chemical energy released at each transfer step being used to drive regeneration of ATP from ADP and inorganic phosphate (oxidative phosphorylation). The ultimate electron acceptor for the reducing equivalents is O_2, which is reduced to water.

Metabolism of fatty fuels

Long-chain fatty acids, triglycerides, and ketone bodies are all capable of providing energy for the heart. Long-chain fatty acids (principally palmitate) are present in the plasma either non-covalently bound to albumin or covalently bound as triglycerides, which are in turn complexed with apolipoproteins. The albumin-bound long-chain fatty acids enter the ventricular myocyte by a carrier-mediated process that is still relatively ill-defined. Triglycerides are hydrolysed by the ectoenzyme lipoprotein lipase on the capillary wall to form long-chain fatty acids (and glycerol). Ketone bodies are synthesized hepatically from long-chain fatty acids and are (compared with long-chain fatty acids) a relatively soluble, readily diffusible, non-toxic fuel.

Long-chain fatty acids and ketone bodies can only be metabolized aerobically, and their catabolism takes place exclusively in the mitochondria (Fig. 11). Two-carbon fragments are successively removed from long-chain fatty acids (as long-chain fatty acid CoA) in a series of reactions known generically as β-oxidation to form acetyl CoA. Each turn of β-oxidation generates sufficient reducing equivalents to regenerate five ATP molecules. Acetyl CoA is then oxidized through the tricarboxylic acid cycle to regenerate more ATP, hence the energy yield from long-chain fatty acid oxidation is considerable. Lipid-derived fuels are preferentially used by the heart and their utilization diminishes the use of carbohydrate, thereby conserving glucose for tissues that are obligatorily dependent on carbohydrate as an energy source. This is achieved by the inhibitory phosphorylation of pyruvate dehydrogenase multienzyme complex, which is stimulated by increased acetyl CoA and NADH concentrations, and by inhibition of the glycolytic pathway by intermediates of the tricarboxylic acid cycle, such as citrate.

Transmembrane and intracellular signalling pathways in the heart

Systemic stimuli in the form of neuroendocrine factors (for example catecholamines and insulin) impinge on the extracellular face of the sarcolemma of the myocyte. These molecules bind to transmembrane receptors that transfer information carried by the stimuli into the inside of the cell. Intracellular signalling pathways then transmit information from one part of the cell to another. Many of these pathways involve reversible protein phosphorylation (catalysed by protein kinases) and dephosphorylation (catalysed by protein phosphatases). Some hormones (for example thyroid hormone and oestrogen) interact directly with intracellular receptors. This group is mainly concerned with signalling at the level of transcription, which is achieved by the formation/presence of the signal–receptor complex in the nucleus.

Extraneous signals that utilize transmembrane receptors mediate their intracellular responses through signalling pathways that, although limited in number compared with the variety of receptors, produce diverse intracellular responses in different cellular contexts. End responses are cell specific because of the variety of proteins expressed in a given cell and the wide range of cell structures.

Intracellular signalling processes are discussed elsewhere. Those relevant to the heart are shown in Fig. 12.

G protein-coupled receptors

The ventricular myocyte is heavily dependent on signalling through transmembrane G protein-coupled receptors. The intracellular domains of these receptors interact with one or more of the large family of heterotrimeric ($\alpha\beta\gamma$) guanine nucleotide-binding proteins (G proteins). In their inactive state, guanosine diphosphate (GDP) is bound to the G protein α subunit (α.GDP). The binding of agonists to the extracellular domain of their individual receptors and the receptor-G protein interaction that follows stimulates exchange of GDP for guanosine triphosphate (GTP) on the α subunit and dissociation of $\alpha\beta\gamma$ into α.GTP and $\beta\gamma$. This dissociation is reversed by the innate GTPase activity of the α subunit and α(GDP). $\beta\gamma$ is reformed. α.GTP (and possibly $\beta\gamma$) are effectors of membrane-bound enzymes that produce so-called 'second messengers'.

The archetypal second messenger is cAMP, which is formed from ATP by the membrane enzyme adenylyl cyclase following β-adrenergic receptor activation (Fig. 12). The interaction of the β-adrenergic receptor with the G_s protein causes formation of α_s.GTP which stimulates adenylyl cyclase and the cAMP formed activates cAMP-dependent protein kinase. The activation of this protein kinase is terminated by hydrolysis of cAMP to AMP by a group of phosphodiesterases. The β-adrenoceptor also activates G_i proteins ($\alpha_i.\beta\gamma$) which counteract the effects of α_s on adenylyl cyclase and act as a negative feed-back mechanism. In the heart, β-adrenergic agonists are positively inotropic, positively lusitropic (i.e. they increase the rate of relaxation), and positively chronotropic. The positive inotropism is the result of a cAMP-dependent protein kinase-catalysed phosphorylation of the L-type Ca^{2+} channel which enhances Ca^{2+} entry into the cell, and the direct activation of the L-type Ca^{2+} channel by α_s.GTP. The positive lusitropism involves increased phosphorylation of the sarcoplasmic protein phospholamban and the myofibrillar protein troponin-I. In its hypophosphorylated state, phospholamban is an inhibitor of SERCA2. Phosphorylation removes this inhibition and thus activates SERCA2, stimulating re-uptake of Ca^{2+} ions into the sarcoplasmic reticulum and increasing the rate of myofibrillar relaxation. Phosphorylation of troponin I stimulates dissociation of Ca^{2+} from troponin C, again increasing the rate of relaxation. The positive chronotropic effect of catecholamines is probably exerted at the level of the pacemaker and presumably also involves cAMP. The loss of β-adrenoceptor responsiveness in heart failure is due to increased inhibition of adenylyl cyclase by G_i and loss of cell surface

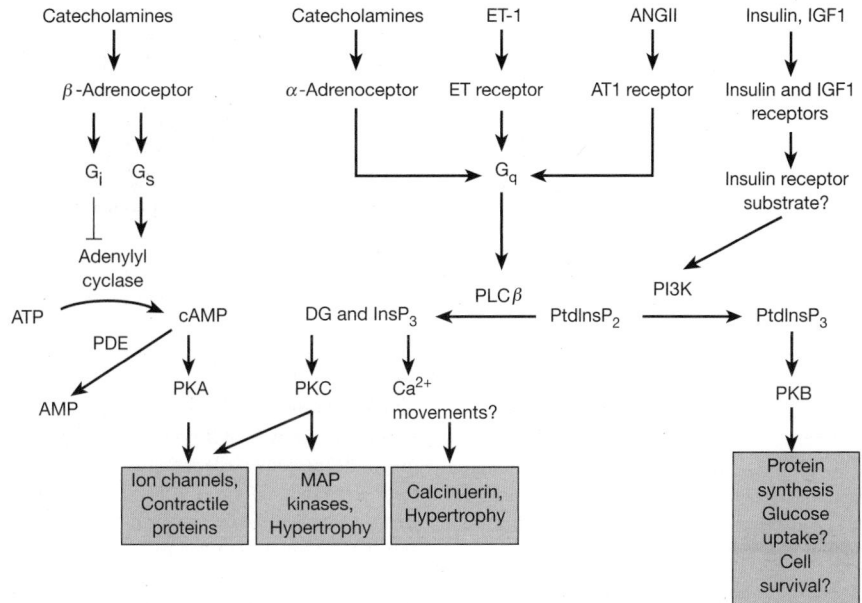

Fig. 12 Intracellular signalling pathways. Neurohumoral agonists bind to their transmembrane receptors and stimulate the formation of a variety of small molecule second messengers (cAMP, diacylglycerol (DG), inositol 1,4,5-trisphosphate (InsP₃), phosphatidylinositol 3,4,5,-trisphosphate (PtdInsP₃)). These then often activate enzymes, many of which catalyse reversible protein phosphorylation (protein kinases) or dephosphorylation (protein phosphatases) and alter the phosphorylation states of proteins which regulate biological processes, thereby modulating the rates of those processes. With the exception of the effect of the G_i protein on adenylyl cyclase, all stages shown are stimulatory. Other abbreviations: ANGII, angiotensin II; ET-1, endothelin-1; G_i, G_q, and G_s, heterotrimeric G_i, G_q, and G_s proteins; IGF 1, insulin-like growth factor 1; MAP kinases, mitogen-activated protein kinases; PDE, cyclic nucleotide phosphodiesterase; PI3K, phosphatidylinositol 3-kinase; PKA, PKB, and PKC, protein kinase A, B, and C, respectively.

β-adrenoceptors by an internalization pathway involving heightened activity of a β-adrenoceptor kinase and arrestin.

Receptor protein tyrosine kinases

Receptor protein tyrosine kinases (which include the insulin and the insulin-like growth factor 1 receptors) are a second group of transmembrane receptors. These possess an intracellular domain with a protein tyrosine kinase activity essential for signalling. The ventricular myocyte possesses receptors for both insulin and insulin-like growth factor 1 which mediate the stimulatory effects of these hormones on glucose uptake, protein synthesis and cell survival (Fig. 12). Activation of the insulin or insulin-like growth factor 1 receptor stimulates formation of another signalling molecule, phosphatidylinositol 3,4,5,-trisphosphate (**PtdInsP3**), which is formed in the membrane by phosphorylation of PtdInsP$_2$ by phosphatidylinositol 3-kinase (Fig. 12). This leads to the activation of the recently-identified protein kinase B (or Akt),which is intimately concerned with regulation of cell growth, protein synthesis, and cell survival (although its role in the ventricular myocyte has not yet been extensively investigated). However, activation of protein kinase B may account for the observed amelioration of heart failure by insulin-like growth factor 1.

Other signalling pathways

In addition to endothelin, the endothelial cells that line the coronary circulation and the endocardium produce nitric oxide, which induces the relaxation of smooth muscle (thus causing vasodilatation and increasing coronary blood flow) and is negatively inotropic. There is immense current interest in nitric oxide: see Chapter 15.1.1.2 for further information.

Positive and negative inotropes

The action of drugs on the myocardium can be due to an effect on the Ca^{2+} transient (upstream regulation) or on the sensitivity of the contractile proteins to Ca^{2+} (downstream regulation). No inotrope in general use in clinical practice increases the force of contraction by a direct effect on the myofibrils.

Upstream Ca^{2+} regulation—positive effects

The importance of increases in cytoplasmic Ca^{2+} concentrations and of β-adrenoceptor-mediated increases in cAMP concentrations in regulating myocardial contractility were described earlier. These two processes are the points of action of many useful drugs. Catecholamines (adrenaline and the pharmacological β-agonist isoprenaline) raise cAMP and protein kinase activity and are powerful positive inotropic drugs. Cyclic nucleotide phosphodiesterase inhibitors (for example caffeine, amrinone, and milrinone) raise cAMP concentrations by inhibiting its breakdown and thereby also activate protein kinase. Increased concentrations of cAMP and increased protein kinase activity increase Ca^{2+} entry through L-type Ca^{2+} channels; relaxation is also augmented by phosphorylation of phospholamban and the ensuing activation of SERCA2, as described previously. The positive chronotropicity of these agents probably results from cAMP facilitating the opening of L-type Ca^{2+} channels and augmenting I_f in the conduction tissue.

Cardiac glycosides (for example digoxin) inhibit the Na$^+$,K$^+$-ATPase, preventing the extrusion of Na$^+$$_i$. This in turn inhibits Ca^{2+}$_i$ extrusion through the Na$^+$,Ca^{2+} exchanger and may, when the cell is depolarized, augment Ca^{2+} entry by reversing the direction of the exchanger. Ca^{2+} may also be taken up in increased amounts by the sarcoplasmic reticulum, thereby increasing the cardiac Ca^{2+} pool and facilitating Ca^{2+}-induced Ca^{2+} release. The net effect is to increase the cytoplasmic concentration and availability of Ca^{2+} resulting in an increased force of contraction.

Upstream Ca^{2+} regulation—negative effects

In some circumstances, a decrease in myocardial contractility is desirable. This can be achieved with β-blockers that compete with catecholamines for occupancy of β-adrenoceptors. These lower cAMP and can exert an anti-ischaemic effect by lowering heart rate, increasing diastolic blood flow, and reducing myocardial contractility, thereby diminishing O$_2$ demand and improving O$_2$ delivery.

The 'calcium antagonists' (verapamil, nifedipine, diltiazem) inhibit Ca^{2+} entry through the L-type Ca^{2+} channel in both cardiac myocytes and vascular smooth muscle cells. They reduce myocardial contractility, relax smooth muscle, and reduce conduction in the sinoatrial and atrioventricular nodes. Therapeutically, their major effects are through their vasodilator activity (which increases blood flow and O$_2$ delivery to the myocardium).

Downstream Ca^{2+} regulation—positive effects

A group of drugs known as Ca^{2+}-sensitizing agents was initially believed to provide a fresh approach to the treatment of chronic/congestive heart failure. This heterogeneous group of positive inotropic agents mediate their effects by increasing the sensitivity of the contractile elements to Ca^{2+}, either by increasing the affinity of troponin C for Ca^{2+} or by direct effects on the actin–myosin complex. They were envisaged as being able to enhance myocardial contractility without changing the cytosolic Ca^{2+} concentration. Pimobendan, levosimendan, MCI-154, EMD-53998, and CGP-48506 have been studied as possible therapies for chronic/congestive heart failure: all have positive inotropic effects on isolated cardiac tissue, but their clinical usefulness has not yet been established.

Myocardial ischaemia

The three important consequences of myocardial ischaemia are failure of contraction, increased frequency of arrhythmias, and cell death. The general pathophysiology of this condition is discussed in Chapter 15.1.1.3 and the clinical aspects in Chapters 15.4.2.2 and 15.4.2.3: the following discussion is limited to the biochemical consequences of ischaemia for heart muscle.

Regulation of cardiac fuel and adenine nucleotide metabolism during hypoxia

In myocardial ischaemia the coronary blood flow to the affected area is insufficient to meet the demands for O$_2$ and fuels and to remove the products of metabolism. Maintenance of ATP regeneration is impossible, given the lack of O$_2$ supply and the fact that, given its high work output, the heart contains relatively little of the endogenous fuel polysaccharide glycogen. Anaerobic carbohydrate metabolism would have to increase about tenfold (not possible given the activity of the glycolytic pathway) and lactate would have to be removed (not possible in ischaemia). ATP concentrations eventually fall and contractile activity decreases. Two mechanisms operate in the short term to maintain ATP. First, ATP is buffered by the operation of the creatine phosphokinase equilibrium (phosphocreatine + ADP + H$^+$ ⇌ creatine+ATP) which is driven to the right by proton production from glycolytic lactate. Second, the small amount of glycogen present is broken down (glycogenolysis) and glycolysis is increased.

In partial ischaemia, changes similar to those described above are also observed. Additionally, these hearts show increased accumulation of endogenous triglyceride droplets. These probably arise because, during ischaemia, the intermediates of fatty acid metabolism accumulate (for example long-chain fatty acid CoA and long-chain fatty acid carnitine, the long-chain fatty acid derivative which actually traverses the inner mitochondrial membrane). Combined with accumulation of glycerol-

3-phosphate (formed from the reduction of the glycolytic intermediate 3-phosphoglyceraldehyde by accumulating NADH), this leads to synthesis of triglycerides. Long-chain fatty acid CoA and long-chain fatty acid carnitine are also powerful detergents. Their accumulation may therefore lead to disruption of membrane systems within the myocyte, to the detriment of cellular integrity.

Metabolic and mechanical consequences of ischaemia

Total ischaemia results in cessation of contraction within 60 s. Two important causes of the decline in contractility are the rapid development of intracellular acidosis through production of lactate and protons (see above), and an increase in intracellular concentrations of inorganic phosphate. The latter is caused by an inability to regenerate ATP from ADP and inorganic phosphate by fuel utilization. ATP concentrations are maintained in the short term (~ 60 s) because they are 'buffered' by creatine phosphate (see above). Thus, the inability to regenerate ATP by fuel utilization is reflected in a rapid decline in concentration of creatine phosphate. Both the fall in pH and the rise in inorganic phosphate decrease the maximum force that the myofilaments can produce, by shifting the Ca^{2+} sensitivity of the myofilaments to the right. The result is that higher concentrations of Ca^{2+} are required to produce the equivalent amount of force (Fig. 13). During ischaemia there is also a gradual increase in the resting (diastolic) level of cytoplasmic Ca^{2+}, probably because of a progressive failure of Ca^{2+} seques-

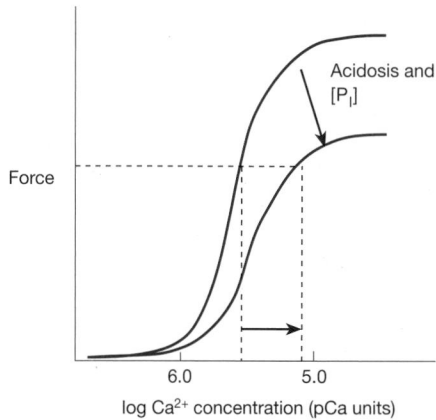

Fig. 13 Intracellular pH, inorganic phosphate, and myofilament Ca^{2+} sensitivity. The normal sigmoidal force/Ca^{2+} concentration relationship is shown by the line on the left. Acidosis or an increase in increased intracellular inorganic phosphate (P_i) decrease the sensitivity of myofilaments to Ca^{2+} and shift the relationship downwards and to the right. The maximum force produced is reduced.

tration and efflux mechanisms. The effects of inorganic phosphate and acidosis would be larger if it were not for this increase in Ca^{2+} concentration. If ischaemia is prolonged, the sequestration and efflux mechanisms fail completely and this accounts for the cessation of the Ca^{2+} transient.

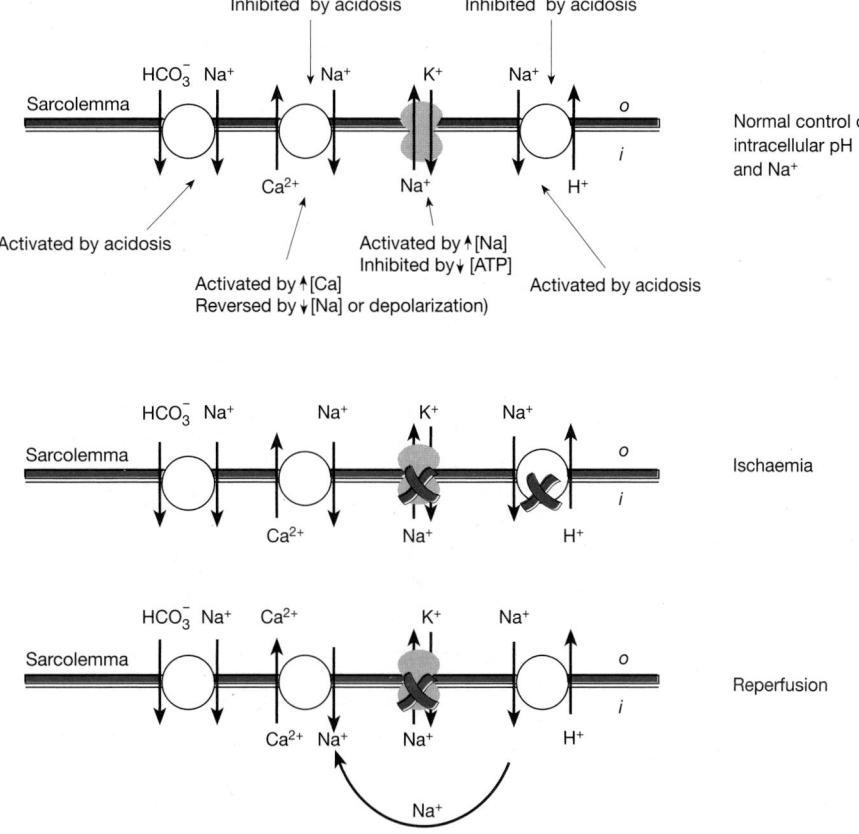

Fig. 14 Control of intracellular pH and Na^+ concentration. The membrane Na^+,H^+ exchanger and the Na^+,HCO_3^- symport counteract a fall in pH_i. Intracellular Na^+ concentration is controlled by the Na^+,K^+-ATPase and influences the direction of Ca^{2+} transport by the Na^+,Ca^{2+} exchanger. If ischaemia is prolonged, the decrease in extracellular pH inhibits the Na^+,H^+ exchanger and a decrease in intracellular ATP inhibits the Na^+,K^+-ATPase. On reperfusion, rapid normalization of extracellular pH reactivates the Na^+,H^+ exchanger and results in a large influx of Na^+ which cannot be expelled quickly owing to inhibition of the Na^+,K^+-ATPase. The increase in intracellular Na^+ concentration coupled with a depolarized membrane potential reverses the normal direction of the Na^+,Ca^{2+} exchange and mediates Ca^{2+} entry. Abbreviations: o, extracellular; i, intracellular.

In addition to intracellular buffering, there are other mechanisms to protect myocytes against acidosis. Two systems in the sarcolemma (the Na^+,H^+ exchanger and the Na^+,HCO_3^- symport) are activated by intracellular acidosis (Fig. 14). The Na^+,H^+ exchanger expels intracellular protons in exchange for extracellular Na^+ and is inhibited by the amiloride group of compounds. The Na^+,HCO_3^- symport transports HCO_3^- and Na^+ into the cell to buffer H^+.

Under normal resting conditions, the myocardium will recover almost completely after 10 to 15 min of ischaemia if adequate flow is restored. More prolonged periods of ischaemia cause the plasma membrane to become permeable to cations and recovery is reduced. If limited blood flow is present from collateral coronary arteries or from 'stuttering ischaemia' (periodic opening and closing of the native coronary artery), the onset of necrosis is delayed. After 60 to 90 min of ischaemia, the plasma membrane is destroyed. This may be attributable to low ATP concentrations, acidosis, activation of phospholipases, and lysosomal activity.

Reperfusion of ischaemic heart muscle results in further damage (reperfusion injury). This is characterized by an immediate swelling of the cell, release of intracellular enzymes (creatine phosphokinase, lactate dehydrogenase) and a large influx of Ca^{2+}. Ca^{2+} is taken up by the mitochondria and can be detected by electron microscopy as deposits of insoluble calcium phosphate. A large gain of Ca^{2+} is indicative of cell damage since it prevents the normal functioning of mitochondria and the regeneration of ATP. Many theories exist to explain the sudden influx of Ca^{2+}. A popular hypothesis is that the reintroduction of O_2 causes increased generation of reactive oxygen species, normal 'byproducts' of electron transport, which damage the plasma membrane through lipid peroxidation and render it permeable to Ca^{2+} in particular. The normal mechanisms within the cell for the removal of reactive oxygen species may be insufficient to protect against the sudden increased production of reactive oxygen species. Another hypothesis involves the Na^+,H^+ exchanger. If ischaemia is prolonged, there is a fall in extracellular pH that can often exceed the intracellular decline. Na^+,H^+ exchange is activated by intracellular acidosis, but is inhibited by extracellular acidosis. Thus, in prolonged ischaemia, the initial stimulation of the exchange will be followed by inhibition. On postischaemic reperfusion, there will be a rapid washout of extracellular protons that will reactivate the exchanger and result in a large influx of Na^+. The preceding ischaemia will have caused a decline in intracellular ATP so the Na^+,K^+ pump will be inhibited and thus the influx of Na^+ will lead to an increase in intracellular Na^+ concentration. As described earlier, the increase in intracellular Na^+ concentration coupled with a depolarized membrane potential reverses the normal direction of the Na^+,Ca^{2+} exchange and mediates excessive Ca^{2+} entry (Fig. 14).

Recovery from a period of ischaemia is slow. This is partly because the myocyte loses nucleotides. ATP is hydrolysed to ADP and operation of the adenylate kinase equilibrium ($2ADP \rightleftharpoons ATP + AMP$) leads to AMP production. AMP is hydrolysed to adenosine (a vasodilator in its own right), but adenosine is rapidly broken down to inosine, thence oxidized to hypoxanthine and xanthine by xanthine oxidase, producing reactive oxygen species. Regeneration of nucleotides is slow and is the probable reason why, even if a cell does not die, total recovery is prolonged.

At present, treatments which are used in an attempt to reduce the size of a myocardial infarction act either by reducing ATP consumption (cardioplegic solutions, hypothermia, afterload reduction, negative inotropic agents) or by increasing coronary flow (afterload reduction, coronary vasodilators) through collaterals or the native coronary. The use of thrombolytic therapy in many patients with myocardial infarction reduces infarct size if the occlusion is due to thrombus, if the thrombus can be dissolved, and if the occlusion has not been present for more than 6 to 12 h. The only treatments that may benefit the ischaemic myocyte by mechanisms that act directly on the cell metabolism or cell structure are insulin, glucose and K^+ therapy, corticosteroids, and hyaluronidase.

Further reading

Bers DM (2001). *Excitation-contraction coupling and cardiac contractile force*, 2nd edn. Kluwer, Dordrecht.

Bolli R and Marban, E. (1999) Molecular and cellular mechanisms of myocardial stunning. *Physiological Reviews* **79**, 609–34.

Chien KR (1999). *Molecular basis of cardiovascular disease*. WB Saunders, Philadelphia.

Fozzard HA *et al.* (1991). *The heart and cardiovascular system. Scientific foundations*. Raven Press, New York.

Jennings RB, Steenbergen C Jr, Reimer KA (1995). Myocardial ischemia and reperfusion. *Monographs in Pathology* **37**, 47–80.

Kastor JA (1994). *Arrhythmias*. WB Saunders, Philadelphia.

Katz AM (1992). *Physiology of the heart*. Raven Press, New York.

Milnor WR (1990). *Cardiovascular physiology*. Oxford University Press, Oxford.

Nelson DL, Cox MM (2000). *Lehninger principles of biochemistry*. Worth, New York.

Newsholme EA, Leech AR (1983). *Biochemistry for the medical sciences*. Wiley, Chichester.

Opie LH (1995). *Drugs for the heart*. WB Saunders, Philadelphia.

Opie LH (1998). *The heart. Physiology, from cell to circulation*, 3rd edn. Lippincott Raven, Philadelphia.

Severs NJ (2000). The cardiac muscle cell. *BioEssays* **22**, 188–99.

Sheridan DJ (1998). *Left ventricular hypertrophy*. Churchill-Livingstone, London.

15.1.3.2 Clinical physiology of the normal heart

D. E. L. Wilcken

Introduction

The function of the heart is to pump sufficient oxygenated blood containing nutrients, metabolites, and hormones to meet moment to moment metabolic needs and preserve a constant internal environment. The heart has two essential characteristics, contractility and rhythmicity. The nervous system and neurohumoral agents modulate relationships between the venous return to the heart, the outflow resistance against which it contracts, the frequency of contraction, and its inotropic state; there are also intrinsic cardiac autoregulatory mechanisms. This section describes normal cardiac function and discusses the principal mechanisms contributing to its regulation.

The cardiac cycle

Electrical events initiate the cardiac cycle with depolarization of the sinoatrial node in the upper right atrium near the orifice of the superior vena cava (Fig. 1). Cardiac muscle acts as a functional syncytium. Cell to cell conduction is possible because the intercalated discs offer a low electrical resistance. The action potential in an active cell causes current flow, which depolarizes the adjacent cells. The generated action potential spreads from the sinoatrial node across the functional syncytium at a speed of 1.0 to 1.2 m/s. The first mechanical response is atrial systole.

The valvular attachments and connective tissue in the atrioventricular groove normally prevent cell to cell conduction of the electrical impulse from atrium to ventricle. This conduction occurs only through the specialized cells of the atrioventricular node (Fig. 1). The atrioventricular node is a region of slow conductance, from 0.02 to 0.1 m/s. This delays activation of the cells of the bundle of His and allows time for completion of ventricular filling. The conduction velocity in the bundle of His is from 1.2 to 2.0 m/s. The impulse passes via the right bundle branch and the two

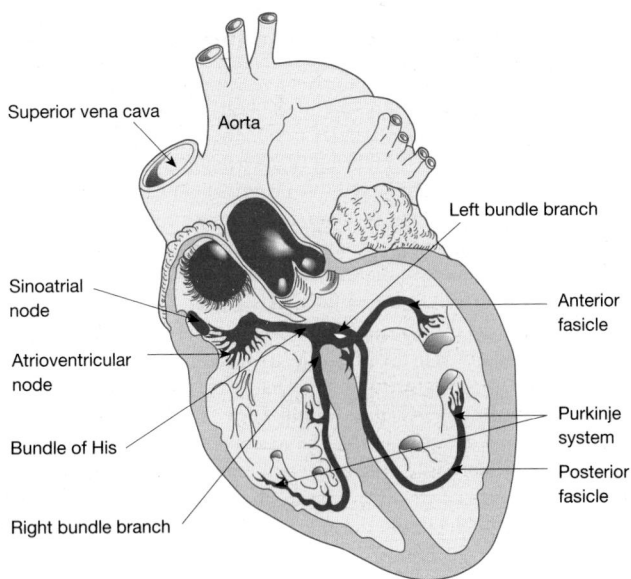

Fig. 1 Diagram of the heart showing the impulse-generating and impulse-conducting system. (Reproduced with permission from Junqueira LC, Carneiro J, Kelley RO (1998). *Basic histology*, 7th edn. Appleton and Lange, Norwalk, CT.)

branches of the left bundle, and spreads rapidly (2.0 to 4.0 m/s) through the Purkinje fibres and each muscle cell to produce an orderly sequence of ventricular contraction (Fig. 1). Atrial and ventricular depolarization (P wave and a QRS complex) and repolarization (T wave) can be recorded on the electrocardiogram as the summation of the spread of the electrical potentials over all the cells of the heart (Fig. 2). Electrocardiography is considered in Chapter 15.3.2.

The specialized cells of pacemaker tissue have an inherent rhythmicity which is shared by the sinoatrial node, the atrioventricular node, and Purkinje tissue. Unlike other myocardial cells these cells do not maintain a diastolic intracellular potential of about –90 mV but tend to depolarize spontaneously. Because the sinoatrial node has the fastest inherent discharge (depolarization) rate, and because there is a brief period after

depolarization of the whole heart during which a further stimulus is ineffective—the absolute refractory period—the sinoatrial node is normally the pacesetter for the heart. However, if this does not occur, pacemaker tissue in the atrioventricular node, the bundle of His, or the Purkinje system, will assume this role. The heart rate is then considerably slower.

Mechanical events

The mechanical events following depolarization of the atrial and ventricular muscle and their timing in relation to the electrocardiogram, to pressure and flow changes, and to heart sounds are shown in five phases in Fig. 3. After the P wave, and coinciding with atrial systole, 'a' waves appear in left atrial and right atrial pressure tracings due to atrial contraction, and an 'a'

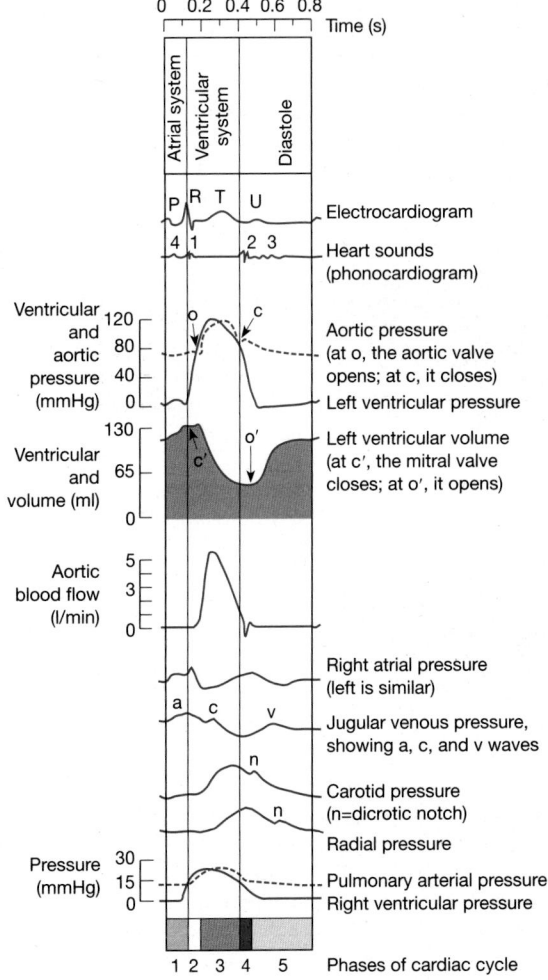

Fig. 3 Events of the cardiac cycle at a heart rate of 75 beats/min. The phases of the cardiac cycle identified by the numbers at the bottom are: (1) atrial systole; (2) isovolumetric ventricular contraction; (3) ventricular ejection; (4) isovolumetric ventricular relaxation; and (5) ventricular filling. Note that late in systole, aortic pressure actually exceeds left ventricular pressure. However, the momentum of the blood keeps it flowing out of the ventricle for a short time. The pressure relationships in the right ventricle and pulmonary artery are similar. The jugular venous pulse is similar in form to that seen in the right atrial pressure tracing. The 'c' wave interrupts the 'x' descent of the 'a' wave. The decline in pressure from the peak of the 'v' is the 'y' descent; the rate of decline reflects speed of ventricular filling. Atr. syst, atrial systole; ventric. syst, ventricular systole. (Modified with permission from Ganong WF (2001). *Review of medical physiology*, 20th edn. Appleton and Lange, Norwalk, CT.)

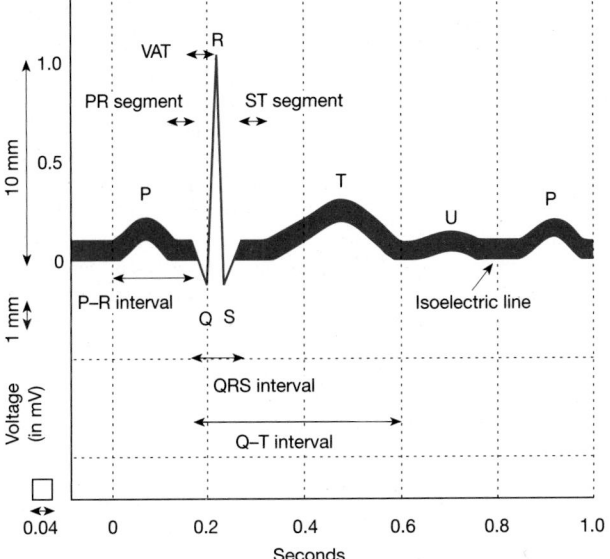

Fig. 2 Diagram of electrocardiographic complexes, intervals, and segments. VAT, ventricular activation time. (Reproduced with permission from Goldman MJ (1986). *Principles of clinical electrocardiography*, 12th edn. Lange, Los Altos, CA.)

wave can be seen in the jugular venous pulse. Atrial contraction increases ventricular filling by about 10 per cent (phase 1).

The onset of ventricular contraction coincides with the peak of the R wave of the electrocardiogram and there is a rapid rise in intraventricular pressure, which closes the mitral and tricuspid valves. The first heart sound is heard at the time of maximum displacement of these valves as they reach their closing positions. During this short isovolumetric period (phase 2 of Fig. 3) the pressure rises rapidly in the ventricle. When ventricular pressures exceed those in the pulmonary artery and aorta, the outflow valves open and ventricular ejection follows, with the highest flow rate occurring in early systole, and pressures in the aorta and pulmonary artery rise. Normally between 50 and 70 per cent of the ventricular volume is ejected during systole, and this can be seen in the volume curve included in Fig. 3 (phase 3).

The jugular venous pulse during ventricular contraction has a positive deflection in early systole, the 'c' wave, due to right ventricular contraction and bulging of the tricuspid valve into the right atrium. Descent of the tricuspid ring caused by ventricular contraction then produces a negative 'x' descent, but as atrial inflow continues the pressure rises in the atria and great veins, producing the 'v' wave. This reaches its peak just before the opening of the tricuspid valve, declining during early ventricular filling as the negative 'y' descent. The changes in the pulmonary veins and left atrium are similar.

As the strength of ventricular contraction declines, and coinciding with the end of the T wave of the electrocardiogram, the aortic and pulmonary valves close, producing the dicrotic notch seen on both aortic and pulmonary artery pressure tracings in Fig. 3. Aortic closure slightly precedes pulmonary closure, and together these are responsible for the two components of the second heart sound. A short period of further rapid decline in ventricular pressure ensues without change in the ventricular volume (the period of isovolumetric ventricular relaxation, phase 4) and at the end of this the mitral and tricuspid valves open. There is a pressure gradient from atrium to ventricle so that a period of rapid ventricular filling follows, which coincides with the timing of the third heart sound. The rapid ventricular filling is reflected in the shape of the ventricular volume curve, and is followed by a period of slower filling (phase 5) with a final sudden small increment from the next atrial contraction as diastole ends (phase 1).

Third heart sounds are audible with the stethoscope in normal children and young adults, but over the age of about 40 years this usually indicates elevation of ventricular end-diastolic pressure (most frequently in the left ventricle). This is probably because the myocardium and valvular structures become stiffer with ageing, and large increases in ventricular end-diastolic pressure are then required to tense valvular structures and generate audible vibrations. The hearing of a fourth heart sound almost always indicates abnormal ventricular function. The end-diastolic pressure in the affected ventricle (usually the left) is increased, and the already stretched inflow valve responds to atrial systole and further filling with oscillations, producing a low-pitched sound that is often palpable as well as audible at the cardiac apex. A fourth heart sound precedes the Q wave of the electrocardiogram and must be distinguished from a normal splitting of the two components of the first heart sound. The latter occurs after the Q wave (Figs 2 and 3).

Normal volumes, pressures, and flows

The blood volume in normal adults is about 5 litres (haematocrit 45 per cent), and of this about 1.5 litres are in the heart and lungs—the central blood volume. The pulmonary arteries, capillaries, and veins contain about 0.9 litres, with only about 75 ml being in the pulmonary capillaries at any one instant. The volume of blood in the heart is about 0.6 litres. Left ventricular end-diastolic volume is about 140 ml, the stroke volume about 90 ml, so that the end-systolic volume is around 50 ml, and the ejection fraction (stroke volume/end-diastolic volume) is between 50 and 70 per cent. The right ventricular ejection fraction is similar.

Of the 3.5 litres in the systemic circulation most, at least 60 per cent of the total blood volume is in the veins. The term 'mean circulatory pressure' introduced by Guyton is useful and refers to the equilibrium pressure measured in the entire circulation within a few seconds of stopping the heart; in dogs this is about 7 mmHg. The systemic veins containing most of the blood volume are easily distensible, and input of blood into the contracting heart is associated with only small changes in venous pressure. By contrast, ejection of blood into the much less distensible arterial tree produces large pressure changes.

The normal values for pressures generated in the heart and great vessels during the cardiac cycle are shown in Table 1. Pressures are measured with reference to a zero pressure arbitrarily set at 5 cm below the sternal angle with the patient recumbent. 'Normal' arterial blood pressure is considered later (see below).

Cardiac output is the product of stroke volume and heart rate. It is related to body size and is best expressed as litre/min/m^2 of body surface area: the 'cardiac index'. The mean cardiac index under resting and relaxed conditions is 3.5 litre/min/m^2, and values below 2 and above 5 are abnormal. The cardiac index declines with age. In persons of average size, resting oxygen consumption is about 240 ml/min, and the difference in oxygen content between arterial and mixed venous blood is about 40 ml/litre (arteriovenous oxygen difference), giving a basal cardiac output of 6 litre/min from the direct Fick equation. In normal subjects the arteriovenous difference in oxygen content at rest is maintained within narrow limits, from 35 to 45 ml/litre; values of 55 ml/litre and above are always abnormal.

Pulmonary or systemic vascular resistance is estimated by dividing the difference between mean inflow pressure (pulmonary artery or aortic) and mean outflow pressure (left atrial or right atrial) in mmHg by the flow in litre/min through the respective circulations. In normal subjects and patients without intracardiac shunts this flow is the cardiac output. Normal pulmonary vascular resistance is less than 2 mmHg/litre/min (160 dyn/s/cm^5). Arterial blood pressure is the product of cardiac output and total peripheral resistance.

Stroke work is the integral of instantaneous ventricular pressure with respect to stroke volume, but is usually estimated as the product of stroke volume and mean ejection pressure. The orderly sequence of contraction in the normal cardiac cycle co-ordinates changes in instantaneous pressure and flow, so maximizing the transfer of energy to the circulation. Normal left ventricular work output at rest is about 6 kg/m^2/min.

Table 1 Normal resting values for pressures in the heart and great vessels

Site	Systolic pressure (mmHg)	Diastolic pressure (mmHg)	Mean pressure (mmHg)
Right atrium	'a' up to 7, 'v' up to 5	'y' up to 3, 'x' up to 3	Less than 5
Right ventricle	Up to 25	End pressure before 'a' up to 3; end pressure on 'a' up to 7	Not applicable
Pulmonary artery	Up to 25	Up to 15	Up to 18
Left atrium (direct or indirect pulmonary capillary wedge)	'a' up to 12, 'v' up to 10	'x' up to 7, 'y' up to 7	Up to 10
Left ventricle	120	End pressure before 'a' up to 7; end pressure on 'a' up to 12	Not applicable

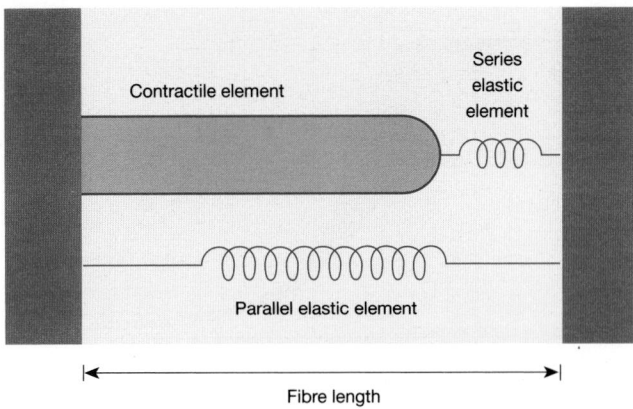

Fig. 4 A representation of the model used by A. V. Hill to illustrate the three mechanical components of functioning muscle.

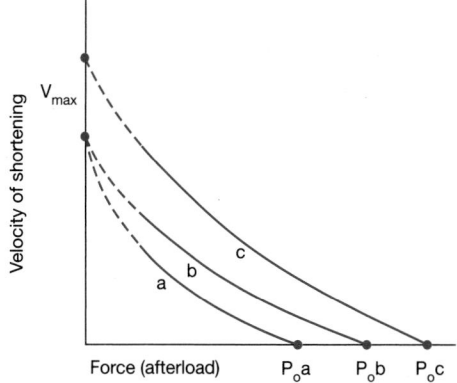

Fig. 5 Idealized relationships between velocity of fibre shortening and afterload or force developed during contraction of a strip of cardiac muscle under three different conditions. Curves a and b were obtained with the muscle in the same inotropic state but with a longer initial fibre length (greater preload) for curve b. Curves b and c were obtained with initial fibre length the same but with contractility increased in c by the addition of a drug producing a positive inotropic effect. The terms V_{max} and P_0 were used by Hill to describe, respectively, a hypothetical maximum shortening velocity in the absence of any load (hence the broken lines), and the force developed in an isometric contraction. An increase in initial fibre length increases P_0 but not V_{max}; a positive inotropic change increases both P_0 and V_{max}.

Myocardial mechanics

A more rational approach to the understanding of cardiac muscle contraction and altered performance in disease states has come from renewed interest in the results of classic experiments in skeletal muscle physiology. The three-component model for muscular contraction proposed by Hill in 1938 (Fig. 4) comprises, first, a contractile element which, when activated, develops force and shortens; second, a series elastic element that is stretched passively during shortening and produces a dampening effect; and, third, a parallel elastic element which supports resting tension. The latter, together with the series elastic element, is responsible for the extensibility or compliance of relaxed muscle. It is not known which precise structures are responsible for the series elastic and parallel elastic components, but there is no doubt about their functional significance.

When a muscle is activated to contract, it develops a potential for doing work. In isolated skeletal and heart muscle preparations the stretching force applied to the muscle, and therefore the length of the muscle, can be varied before contraction; this is the preload. The activated muscle will begin to shorten when it has generated a force sufficient to overcome that exerted by the attached weight or load against which it contracts. When the force exerted by the load is so arranged that it is not applied to the relaxed muscle and is applied only after the muscle has begun to develop tension it is termed the afterload. If this load is so large that the activated muscle is unable to overcome it, and so cannot shorten, the contraction produces tension only, and the contraction is isometric. When shortening does occur, external work is done. If the load is constant during the shortening, the contraction is said to be isotonic; if it changes it is auxotonic.

The tension produced by both skeletal and cardiac muscle during contraction depends on initial fibre length; during afterloaded isotonic contractions from a particular length, the amount and the speed of fibre shortening and the tension developed all depend upon the afterload. Over a range of loads the initial velocity of muscle shortening is most rapid and the most extensive shortening occurs when the load is smallest.

The inverse relationship between initial velocity of fibre shortening and load in an isotonic contraction is a fundamental one for both skeletal and cardiac muscle (Fig. 5). There is, however, a major difference between the two types of muscle in that the relationship at any one length is constant in a skeletal muscle, whereas in cardiac muscle there are variations in inotropic state that are accompanied by considerable changes in the relationship between force and velocity. A positive inotropic effect produces a more extensive contraction from the same initial length and afterload, and a faster maximum velocity of shortening (V_{max}). An increase in initial fibre length with no increase in inotropic state increases the force of contraction but does not, however, change the maximum velocity of shortening. This is illustrated in Fig. 5.

The contraction of the intact heart can be visualized as being similar mechanically to the afterloaded contraction of an isolated muscle strip. For the left ventricle, the preload is the distending force which stretches the muscle fibres in end-diastole, and the initial afterload is the force the ventricle must generate in order to open the aortic valve and eject blood. At the end of ejection, the ventricular muscle is isolated from the peripheral circulation, with the afterload then supported by the competent aortic valve, and the muscle relaxes against a comparatively small force. Relaxation of the heart is an active process due to withdrawal of calcium ions from the cytoplasm surrounding the myofibrils. 'Active' relaxation is still proceeding in the ventricular wall when the atrioventricular valves open, and, if it is delayed, as in the hypoxic heart, the slower relaxation increases the stiffness of the ventricular wall and reduces filling. Wall thickness is also a determinant of relaxation rate and compliance. For this reason filling pressures are higher for the thicker and stiffer left ventricle than for the thinner and more distensible right ventricle (Table 1). When the left ventricle is hypertrophied due to chronic pressure overload, as in systemic hypertension or aortic stenosis, it becomes stiffer and filling pressures may then be abnormally high.

Regulation of cardiac function

Four essential factors determine the performance of the heart:

(1) venous return;

(2) outflow resistance (afterload);

(3) inotropic state or contractility;

(4) heart rate.

Changes in cardiac performance are accomplished by mechanisms that alter these four determinants.

Venous return, preload, and the Frank–Starling relationship

The relationship described independently by Frank and Starling between end-diastolic fibre length and force of contraction is shown in Fig. 6. When the right or left ventricle ejects against a constant pressure, variations in venous return alter the degree of stretch of the muscle fibres in diastole, and

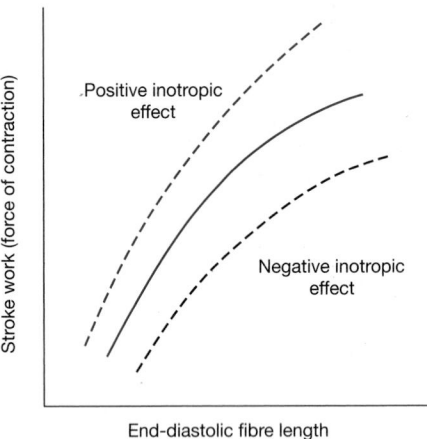

Fig. 6 The relation between left ventricular end diastolic fibre length and left ventricular stroke work showing displacement upward and to the left with an increase in contractility and downward and to the right with a reduction in contractility. Similar but not identical curves are obtained by plotting left ventricular stroke work as one measure of the force of contraction against ventricular end-diastolic pressure or volume (see text). Similar function curves may be obtained from both ventricles and both atria.

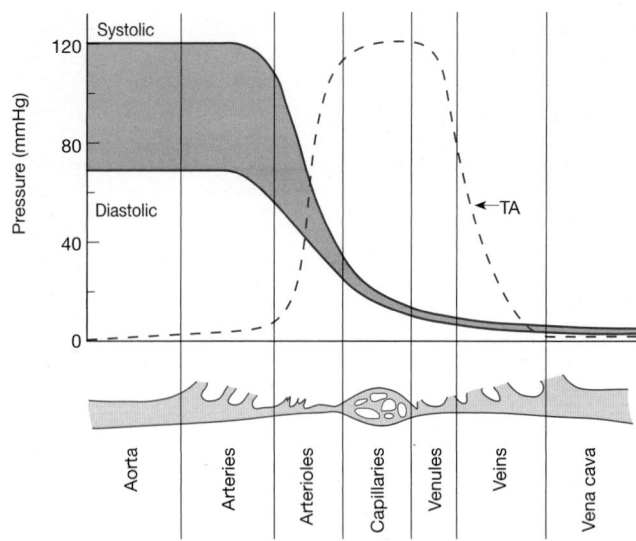

Fig. 7 Diagram of the changes in pressure as blood flows through the systemic circulation. TA, total cross-sectional area of the vessels. This increases from 4.5 cm² to 4500 cm² in the capillaries. The major resistance to flow is at the arteriolar level. (Modified and reproduced with permission from Ganong WF (2001). *Review of medical physiology*, 20th edn. Appleton and Lange, Norwalk, CT.)

this determines contraction strength and work output. The number of active force-generating sites in each fibre increases as it lengthens so that, within limits, the force of contraction and stroke work are positively related to end-diastolic fibre length. The relationship is curvilinear when stroke work is plotted against end-diastolic pressure as an index of preload, reflecting the exponential relationship between end-diastolic pressure and end-diastolic volume. When stroke work is plotted against end-diastolic volume the relationship between stroke work and preload is linear.

The response of the heart at any particular time depends upon:

1. The intrinsic state of the muscle, i.e. the nature of its own biochemistry and contractile machinery.

2. The prevailing neurohumoral state, i.e. increased sympathetic outflow produces a more forceful contraction at any end-diastolic fibre length and shifts the curve upward and to the left.

3. Extrinsic inotropic influences; drugs which have a positive inotropic effect also shift the curve upward and to the left, whereas myocardial depressants have a negative inotropic effect and shift the curve downward and to the right.

End-diastolic fibre length is determined by the force distending the ventricle at end-diastole, and end-diastolic pressure provides a reasonable indication of this force when the ventricle has normal distensibility or compliance; this is the preload. The systemic venous return and the elastic properties of the myocardium produce the end-diastolic distending pressure for the right ventricle, and the pulmonary venous return and myocardial elasticity that for the left ventricle. For clinical purposes it is convenient to equate venous return with preload because, as it changes from beat to beat, it adjusts the strength of the subsequent ventricular (and atrial) contraction by varying the force stretching the relaxed cardiac muscle and changing end-diastolic fibre length.

Outflow resistance or afterload

The pressure which the ventricle must develop to exceed that in the pulmonary artery and the aorta and open the pulmonary and aortic valves is determined largely by the pulmonary and systemic vascular resistances, as shown for the latter in Fig. 7. These resistances, together with an inertial component dependent upon the mass of blood within the vessels, the compliance (stiffness) of the vessels, and the physical characteristics of each vascular tree combined with the pulsatile nature of the flow, constitute the impedance to ventricular outflow. This is the load against which the ven-

tricle must contract and shorten. As this load is not applied in diastole to the relaxed muscle, it then being supported by competent aortic and pulmonary valves, it is usefully described clinically as the afterload; it becomes applied to the muscle only after the ventricle has begun to develop tension.

Regulation of systemic arterial blood pressure

The regulation of the systemic circulation is well adapted to the vital function of maintaining constant, adequate cerebral perfusion. There is a need to maintain a relatively constant arterial blood pressure when there are changes in posture and circulating blood volume. The baroreceptors mediate rapid responses to alterations in aortic pressure, whilst a variety of hormonal and physical factors regulate the circulating blood volume.

Baroreceptors

The baroreceptor regulatory system comprises two groups of stretch receptors: one group in the carotid sinuses near the bifurcations of the common carotid arteries in the neck and a second group in the arch of the aorta. These respond to an increase in central arterial pressure by the firing of impulses, which pass by the glossopharyngeal and vagus nerves to the solitary tract nucleus in the medulla and inhibit sympathetic outflow. Efferent impulses from these central connections pass via the right vagus nerve mainly to the sinoatrial node, and via the left vagus mainly to the atrioventricular node. The effect is to decrease the heart rate and the force of atrial contraction. There is also attenuation of sympathetic discharge via the thororacolumbar sympathetic outflow to arteriolar smooth muscle in the limbs and visceral circulation, resulting in a release of peripheral arteriolar constriction and therefore peripheral vasodilatation. Thus the immediate response to a rise in arterial pressure is slowing of the heart rate, reduced force of atrial contraction, and reduced vascular resistance. The net effect of this negative feedback system is to offset the elevation in blood pressure. Conversely a lowering of blood pressure diminishes stimulation of the stretch receptors and reduces afferent traffic to the solitary tract nucleus resulting in reduced inhibition of sympathetic outflow. As a consequence there is a quickening of the heart rate and peripheral vasoconstriction so that the blood pressure increases. The changes in heart rate take place within 1 to 2 s and changes in vasomotor control within 5 or 6 s.

Baroreceptor mechanisms effectively modulate the responses of blood pressure to postural change. Additionally they adapt to maintain the normal circadian variation in blood pressure (see below). They also maintain elevated arterial blood pressure in systemic hypertension. Sensory input to the reflex is reduced in disorders of the autonomic nervous system, and in the prolonged weightlessness of space flight.

Blood volume

The circulating blood volume is relatively small and a large proportion is contained in the veins (Fig. 7) so that any change in blood volume will affect venous return and therefore cardiac output and blood pressure. When blood volume is large and the veins full there is little reduction in venous return on standing and cardiac output is maintained. However, when effective blood volume is reduced and the veins are relatively empty, on standing there is pooling of blood in the veins of the legs and a reduction in venous return and cardiac output so that arterial blood pressure falls. Baroreceptor responses become evident within a couple of beats, the heart rate increases, and cardiac output and blood pressure are restored. Circulating blood volume is kept relatively constant by a combination of mechanisms which involve the actions of natriuretic peptides, the renin–angiotensin–aldosterone system, vasopressin, and osmolality.

The natriuretic peptides The discovery of secretory granules in the atria of the heart and the demonstration in 1981 that they produce a natriuretic factor that inhibits the reabsorption of sodium in the distal tubule of the kidney enhanced understanding of the regulation of blood volume and cardiac performance. Three natriuretic peptides have subsequently been identified.

Atrial natriuretic peptide is present in the circulation and concentrations increase during volume expansion. The right atrium contains about two to four times as much activity as the left, and release of the hormone is mediated largely by atrial distension. The effect is to produce a diuresis and to reduce cardiac and circulating blood volume. Atrial natriuretic peptide also has a vasodilator action and opposes the vasoconstricting effects of noradrenaline and angiotension II.

The second natriuretic peptide was identified in brain tissue, and is referred to as brain natriuretic peptide. Large amounts were later shown to be in the ventricles of the heart and circulating levels are increased in ventricular hypertrophy and cardiac failure. Brain and atrial natriuretic peptides have similar actions. The third to be identified was C-type natriuretic peptide. It is distributed widely in tissues, circulating concentrations are low, and it appears also to have actions similar to the other two peptides, but with a greater vasodilator effect on veins.

Thus these three peptides contribute to the regulation of cardiac and circulating blood volume and of blood pressure. The therapeutic potential of manipulating the effects of these peptides is currently being assessed.

The renin–angiotensin system This system, which is both local and systemic, is of major importance in the regulation of circulating blood volume and the maintenance of normal blood pressure. Enhanced activity of systemic renin and angiotensin increases the production of aldosterone, which promotes reabsorption of sodium by the kidney and expansion of circulating blood volume. All components of the renin–angiotensin system are distributed widely throughout tissues, including the brain and the heart, and increased activation of the system increases the risk of cardiovascular events. Angiotensin II is a potent vasoconstrictor that also enhances the proliferation of smooth muscle cells. The angiotensin converting enzyme inhibitors in clinical use diminish angiotension II production locally and in the circulating blood. Both local and general effects appear important in mediating the benefits that accrue from the use of these drugs in the management of hypertension and congestive cardiac failure, and in the reduction in rates of recurrence of coronary events in ischaemic heart disease. The mechanisms mediating this latter effect in particular await clarifica-

tion. It is yet to be determined whether the use of the more recently developed angiotensin II receptor blocking drugs will result in similar outcomes.

Ventricular volume and afterload

Ventricular volume also has a major effect on afterload, as pressure is equal to force per unit area. The force acting radially on the inner surface of the whole ventricle at any time during systole is the product of the intraventricular pressure and ventricular surface area at that time. If the left ventricle is assumed to be a sphere (surface area = πd^2), the force opposing ejection at any time during contraction is the product of the intracavity pressure and πd^2 at that time. Thus, a change in left ventricular diameter from a normal value of 5 cm to one of 10 cm would result in a fourfold increase in the force opposing ejection for the same intracavity systolic pressure; the ventricle would need to develop greatly increased wall tension to overcome that force. Because wall tension developed during systole is the major determinant of myocardial oxygen consumption, the contraction will clearly be much less efficient in the larger heart for the same stroke volume and ejection pressure (stroke work).

During a normal heartbeat the afterload is greatest at the beginning of ejection (rapid rise in pressure and maximum volume; Fig. 3), but thereafter decreases as the pressure reaches a plateau and then declines as the ventricle becomes smaller. There is therefore a matching of the afterload to the declining intensity of the contraction as it proceeds to completion, and fibres shorten at a relatively constant rate. This is less obvious in a large heart where the volume change during ejection is a smaller proportion of the total ventricular volume.

The end-diastolic volume is influenced by preload, afterload, circulating blood volume, the inotropic state of the ventricle, heart rate, and neurohumoral influences. For example, it is smaller in the erect than in the horizontal position because of reduced venous return, and it decreases with a moderate increase in heart rate because of an associated positive inotropic effect. The proportion of end-diastolic volume ejected during systole, the ejection fraction (normal 50 to 70 per cent), is a useful index of overall left ventricular function and is easily measured non-invasively by gated blood pool scanning and two-dimensional echocardiographic techniques. The ejection fraction increases with exercise and with positive inotropic interventions. Values for right ventricular ejection fraction are of the same order as those for the left side of the heart.

Myocardial contractility and inotropic state

Myocardial function is greatly altered by changes in inotropic state or contractility. Positive inotropic effects are thought to be mediated by activation of excitation–contraction coupling mechanisms and are associated with an increased influx of calcium ions into myocardial cells and a more powerful contraction. Changes in the intensity of excitation–contraction coupling are independent of the Frank–Starling mechanism. Increases in the intensity shift the curve upwards and to the left and decreases shift it downwards and to the right (Fig. 6). With a positive inotropic effect, the force of contraction, however measured, is increased for a given end-diastolic fibre length and, if the afterload is the same, the initial velocity of fibre shortening is also increased (Fig. 5); in the intact heart, there is more complete emptying during systole. Increased sympathetic stimulation, some drugs, and an increase in heart rate itself (the staircase or Bowditch phenomenon; postectopic potentiation, see below) have positive inotropic effects. Myocardial depressants, such as hypoxia and most anaesthetic drugs, have negative inotropic effects. Increased parasympathetic stimulation produces acetylcholine-mediated negative inotropic effects that are confined almost entirely to the atria because of the anatomical distribution of vagal endings in the myocardium.

It is difficult to measure inotropic changes accurately in the human heart because changes in the intensity of excitation–contraction coupling and changes in the Frank–Starling relationship, though separate, are nevertheless closely linked. Whilst Hill's classic model (Fig. 4) has been important conceptually, attempts to define contractility as predicted by the model—by deriving an extrapolated maximum velocity of fibre shortening which would obtain with the muscle contracting against zero load—have not been rewarding. The peak rate of change of intraventricular pressure (peak dp/dt) is a useful index of change in contractility provided that preload, afterload, and heart rate remain constant.

An approach that appears relatively insensitive to changes in both preload and afterload is that of Suga and Sagawa, using the ventricular pressure–volume loop diagram. There is an approximately linear relationship between end-systolic pressure (or wall stress) and end-systolic volume when measured over a narrow physiological range in the human left ventricle. Increased contractility shifts the relationship upward and to the left, as illustrated in Fig. 8, allowing the separation of enhanced from reduced contractility in the same heart, and poorly contracting from normally contracting ventricles. Stroke volume is shown on the abscissa as the difference between end-diastolic and end-systolic volumes. The efficacy of reduction in afterload in assisting reduced ventricular function is also easily explained from the diagram. With a reduced afterload, the aortic valve opens at a lower pressure and a greater stroke volume is ejected; a new end-systolic pressure–volume point is reached, which is shifted downwards on the same linear relationship. There has been no change in contractile state.

Heart rate

Frequency of contraction is the fourth essential determinant of cardiac performance. Heart rate during rest and exertion may vary from 45 to 200 beats/min in the healthy young adult. As changes can occur within seconds, an increase in heart rate is the usual and most effective way of producing a rapid increase in cardiac output. It plays the major role in the response to exercise, during which stroke volume does increase (more so in athletes and when in the erect rather than the supine position) but the changes are less marked than those of rate. In addition, an increase in contraction frequency itself produces a positive inotropic effect, whereby the force of contraction increases and reaches a new steady state within a few beats. This is termed the 'positive staircase', Treppe, or Bowditch effect. It may be a consequence of an augmented movement of calcium ions into myocardial cells with increased frequency of action potentials, combined with diminished time for outward movement of calcium between beats. More forceful contractions also follow premature beats—the phenomenon of postextrasystolic potentiation—and the mechanism is probably the same. The

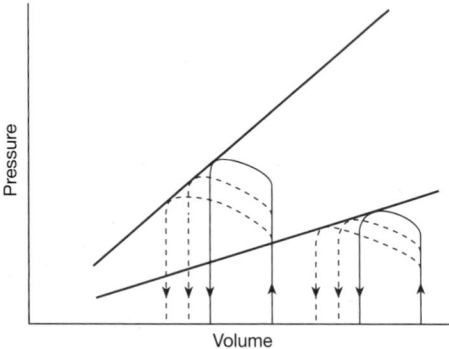

Fig. 8 Diagrammatic representation of intraventricular pressure and volume relationships during the cardiac cycle at two levels of myocardial contractility; three separate beats with the same end-diastolic volume are shown for each. The loops on the left of the diagram were obtained when contractility is increased and those on the right when it is reduced. There is a linear end-systolic pressure–volume relationship with different afterloads (pressures) for each level of contractility. The slope of the end-systolic pressure–volume relationship for any inotropic state is relatively insensitive (see text) to changes within physiological ranges in afterload and preload, although changes in preload are not shown in this diagram. The volume change seen on the horizontal axis for each beat is the stroke volume. This increases with reduction in pressure (afterload).

extrasystole occurring prematurely is a weak contraction because of decreased filling time and an unco-ordinated activation of the ventricle when the ectopic focus is within the ventricle. The next beat is delayed because of the refractory period of the extrasystolic beat, but is a more powerful contraction because of increased filling time and ventricular volume, and increased contractility. Calcium-dependent changes similar to those of the Bowditch effect are probably responsible for the latter.

Coronary blood flow

Coronary blood flow accounts for about 4 per cent of the cardiac output. The heart extracts most (70 per cent) of the oxygen carried in the coronary circulation; the arteriovenous difference for oxygen across the heart being about 110 ml/litre, whilst that for the whole body is only about 40 ml/litre under resting conditions. Therefore, large increases in myocardial oxygen requirements must be met largely by increases in coronary blood flow, and this may increase five- or sixfold during strenuous exercise. The greater part of this flow is to the left ventricle, of which at least two-thirds occurs during diastole because of the throttling effect systole has on myocardial perfusion. The main coronary arteries are on the superficial surface of the heart, and because of this, and the hindrance to coronary flow during systole, the subendocardial region of the left ventricle is more vulnerable to perfusion deficits in relation to oxygen need than the outer two-thirds of the muscle wall. Despite these mechanical problems, flow is normally evenly distributed throughout the myocardium so that, when regional coronary blood flow is measured using injected radioactive microspheres (in dogs), the ratio of endocardial to epicardial flow is approximately unity. In fact the inner layers of the heart probably receive slightly more blood (up to 10 per cent) than the outer layers. This is consistent with the subendocardium developing more tension than the subepicardium, and is evidence for a greater rate of myocardial oxygen consumption in the inner layers.

Myocardial oxygen requirements and coronary blood flow are finely adjusted. The regulation of coronary blood flow is described elsewhere.

The nervous system and the heart

The heart is richly supplied with adrenergic nerves. Terminals reach atrial and ventricular muscle fibres and impinge upon all pacemaker tissue including the sinoatrial and atrioventricular nodes and Purkinje fibres. Sympathetic stimulation leads to an increase in myocardial contractility and heart rate, and in the rate of spread of the activation wave through the atrioventricular node and the Purkinje system. This is mediated by local noradrenaline release, which interacts with β-adrenergic receptors. The key elements in these regulatory mechanisms are calcium ions and cyclic AMP. The activated β-receptor increases adenylcyclase activity and the conversion of ATP to cyclic AMP. Peptide cotransmitters released with noradrenaline and acetylcholine have recently been isolated and also influence autonomic function. Neuropeptide Y is a peptide of 36 amino acids that is collocated with noradrenaline in most sympathetic nerves and is released with sympathetic stimulation. It is a powerful pressor agent with direct arteriolar vasoconstrictor action and also potentiates the pressor action of noradrenaline.

The distribution of parasympathetic fibres is much more limited, being confined to the sinoatrial and atrioventricular nodes and the atria, with few if any fibres reaching the ventricles in humans, except perhaps in relation to coronary arteries and Purkinje tissue. The effects of parasympathetic nerve stimulation are mediated by local acetylcholine release, which slows the heart rate and speed of conduction through the atrioventricular node and Purkinje tissue, and depresses atrial contractility. The negative inotropic effects are associated with a lowering of the concentration of intracellular cyclic AMP.

The effect of the nervous system on the heart at any one time is the sum of the activities of these two opposing control systems. They usually vary reciprocally. Under resting conditions, vagal inhibitory effects predominate, maintaining a slow heart rate, there being virtually no sympathetic outflow. With exercise, there is withdrawal of vagal activity and an increase in sympathetic outflow. Afferents from stretch receptors in the carotid sinus and aortic arch—the baroreceptors—also have a considerable effect on cardiac performance, this effect being mediated via the adrenergic nervous system and vagal withdrawal. A fall in blood pressure reduces stretching in the carotid sinus and inhibitory afferent traffic so that the sympathetic outflow increases. As a consequence of this combined vagal and adrenergic effect there is a quickening of the heart rate within one or two beats, a positive inotropic effect, and also a constriction of veins and arterioles that increases preload and afterload. Elevation of pressure in the carotid sinus has the reverse effects. In cardiac failure there is a reduced variability in heart rate due to these autonomic mechanisms as there is then a predominance of adrenergic activity.

There are also mechanoreceptors in all four chambers of the heart (in dogs) and in the coronary vessels, which give rise to depressor reflexes. Their clinical relevance is uncertain, but they may contribute, for example, to the bradycardia and hypotension occurring in some patients with acute myocardial infarction and to the syncope that patients with critical aortic stenosis may experience with the onset of exercise when there is sudden left ventricular distension. Vagal afferents from reflexogenic areas in the infarcting left ventricle may be responsible for the bradycardia, gastric distension, nausea, and vomiting which frequently occur with the onset of inferior or posterior myocardial infarction, but not usually of anterior infarction, which is generally associated with a marked increase in sympathetic activity. The cardiac receptors connected to afferent fibres running in cardiac sympathetic nerves, however, are very important because they are responsible for the perception of cardiac pain. Receptors have also been identified (in animals) at the junction of pulmonary veins with the atrial wall. These respond to mechanical distension with increased sympathetic outflow to the sinus node and inhibition of secretion of antidiuretic hormone from the posterior lobe of the pituitary gland. The result is a quickening of the heart rate and diuresis, effects that could contribute to the regulation of cardiac volume.

Autonomic efferent activity

The autonomic outflow to the heart is controlled by multiple integrative sites within the central nervous system, with complex interactions between afferent and central inputs. Autonomic responses are mediated through the suprapontine and bulbospinal pathways, both those arising 'reflexly' and those arising from various types of volitional or central 'command'. Nevertheless, intrinsic mechanisms are sufficient for adequate cardiac function in the absence of autonomic control, as prolonged survival after cardiac transplantation has shown. But in the denervated heart there is blunting of the normally rapid physiological adjustments mediated by the autonomic nervous system.

Diurnal variation in autonomic function

Variations in vascular tone and control of blood pressure and of hormone secretion and platelet function occur in a predictable way throughout the 24-h cycle. In normal subjects there is a circadian rhythm of blood pressure changes that is not seen in patients after cardiac transplantation who have denervated hearts. There is a decline in blood pressure at night and an increase soon after wakening. This is due to a normal adrenergic surge in the early morning, which results in increased vascular tone and blood pressure. Increased forearm vascular resistance in the morning with a reduction in the afternoon and evening can be clearly identified in humans by assessing responses to α-adrenergic blockade. It is presumed that this occurs in coronary vessels as well. Measurable early morning increases in circulating catecholamines and in the propensity for platelets to aggregate can also be documented.

The circadian rhythm of autonomic function is correlated with a significant tendency for myocardial infarction and sudden cardiac death to occur more frequently in the morning soon after wakening. There is also an increase in the occurrence of angina pectoris in the early morning, independent of the level of physical activity.

Exercise and the heart: cardiac reserve

The heart responds to exercise with an increase in cardiac output, and values of 30 litre/min may be achieved in a trained athlete. Exercising muscles extract more oxygen from the blood perfusing them, but the response of the cardiac output is the ultimate determinant of delivery of oxygen to tissues and is the limiting factor for aerobic exercise.

The cardiac response to exercise involves all the mechanisms already discussed. Interaction within the central nervous system between higher and autonomic centres augments sympathetic discharge and there is a withdrawal of parasympathetic outflow. The heart rate increases immediately, and redistribution of peripheral flow increases venous return and preload. There is venoconstriction, particularly in the large-volume splanchnic circulation, and vasoconstriction and increased oxygen extraction in non-active parts. In active parts there is vasodilation. This is most evident in the vascular beds of the exercising skeletal muscles and of the heart. The overall effect is a marked lowering of total peripheral vascular resistance, which reduces afterload and encourages greater systolic emptying of the left ventricle. Stroke volume increases during exercise in the upright position. During light to moderate exercise (running or cycling), up to about 80 per cent of maximum exercise capacity, there is an almost linear relationship between work intensity and heart rate response, cardiac output, and oxygen uptake. With further exercise the heart rate and cardiac output responses level off whilst additional increases in oxygen consumption (about 500 ml) occur by increased oxygen extraction and a greater widening of the arteriovenous difference for oxygen.

The venous return increases in relation to the elevated cardiac output. Vasodilation in the working muscles that receive the bulk of the redirected blood permits high flow rates into the capacitance vessels. Because of adrenergically mediated venoconstriction the capacity of this system is reduced, so that blood moves rapidly into the right atrium. Venous return is also enhanced by the pumping action of the rhythmically contracting working muscles, by a decrease in intrathoracic pressure with forced inspiration, and by an increase in intra-abdominal pressure. The augmented pulmonary blood flow results in only slight increases in pulmonary artery pressure because of the distensibility of the large pulmonary arteries, an increased area of the pulmonary capillary bed due to the recruitment of more capillaries, and the low resistance offered by the normal pulmonary circulation (see Table 1).

The elevated cardiac output and larger stroke volume result in increased systolic blood pressure and pulse pressure even though the afterload itself is reduced. Enhanced neurohumoral activity from adrenergic stimulation of the heart and the suprarenal glands (increased circulating adrenaline and noradrenaline) effect positive inotropic changes, to which tachycardia also contributes because of the Bowditch effect. There is a shift in the Frank–Starling relationship to the left, increased speed and force of cardiac contraction, and elevated ejection fraction and stroke volume. Peak dp/dt is increased and there is a rapid rise in coronary blood flow to meet myocardial oxygen requirements that increase linearly with the product of systolic blood pressure and heart rate. During moderate exercise these changes together result in a decreased or unaltered end-diastolic volume and decreased end-systolic volume. With severe exercise, end-diastolic dimensions and end-diastolic fibre length are slightly increased and the Frank–Starling mechanism then operates and further augments the force of contraction.

The haemodynamic and ventilatory responses evoked by an increase to a new steady workload take about 2 to 3 min to equilibrate and adjust oxygen supply to the greater demand. Protocols for exercise testing are therefore usually based on work increments at 3-min intervals to allow time for a new 'steady state' to occur as, for example, in the standard Bruce Exercise

Protocol. A steady state becomes progressively more difficult to maintain as maximal exercise capacity is approached. Glycogen is used by the working skeletal muscles as a source of stored energy and the anaerobic metabolism which ensues produces lactic acidosis and thereby further increases ventilation. As all cardiopulmonary transport mechanisms reach maximum levels, shortness of breath, fatigue, and muscle pain become limiting symptoms; motivation is then the final determinant of the duration of exercise. Ageing reduces the efficacy of cardiopulmonary transport mechanisms and, of course, exercise capacity. The heart rate response at peak exercise reflects this. In healthy individuals aged 20 years it is about 200 beats/min and at 65 years about 170 beats/min.

When exercise stops, the cardiopulmonary and metabolic changes return rapidly to resting levels, the rate following an exponential pattern in the first few minutes; the excretion and metabolism of lactate and other substances, and the dissipation of heat generated take longer (time constant of about 15 min or more). Reduced circulatory function slows the recovery rate.

Training effects

Regular exercise to about 60 per cent of maximal heart rate for 20 to 30 min three times a week is the minimum requirement for improved effort tolerance due to a training effect. The resting heart rate becomes slower whilst the cardiac output is maintained by an increased end-diastolic volume and ejection fraction, and therefore stroke volume. In a 'trained' exercising individual there is a reduced heart rate response to a standard submaximal work load, and systemic blood flow is more effectively distributed away from visceral and skin circulations to working muscles. Adaptive changes occur in muscle mitrochondria, permitting improved extraction of oxygen from perfusing blood so that maximum oxygen consumption increases. There is suggestive evidence that prolonged endurance training increases the calibre of coronary arteries and enlarges the capillary surface area relative to cardiac muscle mass (in animals). Myocardial protein synthesis increases. Adrenergic mechanisms appear to be involved in mediating this response. It should be noted that rhythmic exercise (such as running) and isometric exercise (such as weightlifting) have different physiological effects. The blood pressure rises disproportionately during the latter. The mechanisms are partly reflex and partly mechanical from the contracting muscles. Isometric exercise training is not recommended for cardiac patients because of the increased afterload it imposes on the heart.

Regular exercise may also partly prevent the now well documented endothelial dysfunction associated with ageing. The age-related reduction in availability of nitric oxide resulting from reduced activity of the L-arginine–nitric oxide pathway in the endothelium has now been established and is thought to be a consequence of oxidative stress. Regular exercise improves the availability of nitric oxide. Vascular effects related to nitric oxide are considered elsewhere.

There is now good evidence for exercise-induced mood changes resulting in feelings of well-being. Increased concentrations of circulating β-endorphin occur during exercise, and studies using the opiate receptor antagonist naloxone to block the effects of opioid peptides suggest that β-endorphin release may reduce exercise-induced adrenaline and noradrenaline responses. Regular exercise lowers blood pressure in normotensive and mildly hypertensive subjects, and modulation of catecholamine release by changes in endogenous opioid peptide secretion may be a possible contributing mechanism. There are other diverse exercise-induced hormonal changes, but one of particular clinical relevance is reduced glucose-stimulated insulin secretion. This is beneficial for type II diabetics, whose basal hyperinsulinaemia is the result of both hypersecretion and hypocatabolism of insulin, and for patients with insulin resistance and hyperinsulinaemia, obesity, hypertension, and dyslipidaemia—so-called syndrome X.

To summarize, changes in the four essential determinants of cardiac function—preload, afterload, heart rate, and contractility—combine to augment cardiac output and oxygen delivery during exercise. Measurement of the cardiovascular response to exercise is essential for the objective assessment of cardiac function.

Further reading

Braunwald E, Zipes DP, Libby P (2001). *Heart disease: a textbook of cardiovascular medicine*, 6th edn. WB Saunders, Philadelphia.

Ganong WF (2001). *Review of medical physiology*, 20th edn. McGraw Hill, New York.

Hill AV (1970). *First and last experiments in muscle mechanics*. Cambridge University Press, Cambridge.

Jones NL, Killian KJ (2000). Exercise limitation in health and disease. *New England Journal of Medicine* **243**, 632–41.

Suzuki T, Yamazaki T, Yazaki Y (2001). The role of natriuretic peptides in the cardiovascular system. *Cardiovascular Research* **51**, 489–94.

15.2 Clinical presentation of heart disease

15.2.1 Chest pain

J. R. Hampton

Introduction

Chest pain is one of the commonest causes of emergency admission to hospital (Table 1). In the hospital context the commonest cause of chest pain is myocardial ischaemia, but in primary care other causes predominate. The majority of those admitted with chest pain will have evidence of pre-existing coronary disease (a previous myocardial infarction or known previous angina) and their pain is likely to be a manifestation of this. Perhaps 20 per cent of this group will have a definite myocardial infarction. A misdiagnosis of chest pain can have serious consequences for both patient and doctor, but the number of patients seen in accident and emergency departments with chest pain is so large that it is impracticable for all to be admitted to hospital for investigations to be completed. Similarly, it is neither necessary nor sensible for every patient with chest pain seen in primary care to be referred to hospital.

The initial management of patients with chest pain depends on an accurate history, the physical examination and simple investigations being of lesser importance.

Table 1 The diagnoses of the patients admitted to an admissions ward of a district general hospital over a period of 18 months

Diagnosis	Number of admissions	Percentage of total admissions
Chest pain	4865	29
Asthma	1171	7
Overdose	1153	7
Stroke	935	6
Heart failure	886	5
Collapse	783	5
Infection (not chest)	755	4
Chest infection	740	4
Gastrointestinal bleed	731	4
Falls/social admission	657	4
Arrhythmia	581	3
Deep vein thrombosis	496	3
Diabetes	462	3
Abdominal pain/ diarrhoea and vomiting	444	3
Headache	369	3
Fits	292	2
Other	1482	9

The patient's history

Myocardial ischaemia

Coronary artery insufficiency, usually the result of atheroma but occasionally the result of arterial spasm, leads to a spectrum of conditions which can be grouped together as 'myocardial ischaemia'. The common end result is chest pain.

Stable angina

Angina was first recognized by William Heberden in 1768, and his description of the pain of myocardial ischaemia can hardly be bettered. He wrote:

> The seat of it, and the sense of strangling and anxiety with which it is attended may make it not improperly called angina pectoris.

> They who are afflicted with it, are seized while they are walking (more especially if it be uphill, and soon after eating) with a painful and most disagreeable sensation in the breast, which seems as if it were to extinguish life, if it were to increase or continue; but the moment they stand still, this uneasiness vanishes....The pain is sometimes situated in the upper part, sometimes in the middle, sometimes at the bottom of the os sterni, and often more inclined to the left than to the right side. It likewise very frequently extends from the breast to the middle of the left arm.

Whether myocardial ischaemia is due to stable angina, myocardial infarction, or the acute coronary syndromes, the distribution of the pain is much as Heberden described it. It is central, or sometimes left sided; rarely it is felt only in the back. The most classical—but not the most common—radiation is to the front of the neck, and the lower jaw or the teeth. The most common radiation is to the left arm, though the pain of other chest problems may also radiate here. Radiation from the front of the chest to the back is not uncommon.

The nature of the pain is usually described as 'tight', 'crushing', 'squeezing', or 'heavy'. Many patients describe a 'sensation', or an 'ache' rather than a pain. The pain of myocardial ischaemia is seldom described as 'sharp'.

The duration of the pain in stable angina depends on whether or not the patient rests: typically the pain will disappear within a minute or two when exercise ceases. Sometimes the pain will disappear if exercise continues; this has been called 'walk through' angina.

Stable angina, as opposed to the other manifestations of myocardial ischaemia, can be recognized by factors that precipitate or relieve it. Stable angina is, above all, predictable. It occurs after a constant amount of exercise—often on a particular hill, after so many metres walking, on climbing so many stairs, or on hurrying. Pain that is unpredictable is unlikely to be stable angina, though it may be due to an acute coronary syndrome. The pain of stable angina is worse on exercise in cold or windy weather, and on exercise after a meal. It is often induced by sexual intercourse, or by any emotional stress. Any chest pain, whatever its distribution, that occurs with emotional stress is likely to be angina.

Table 2 Checklist for angina

Is the pain characteristic?	Predictable
	Related to exercise
	Worse in cold or windy weather
	Worse on exercise after food
	Induced by sexual intercourse
	Induced by emotional stress
	Relieved by nitrate
Is the distribution characteristic?	Central
	Radiating to jaws and teeth
	Radiating to arm or back
Is the nature of the pain characteristic?	Dull
	Crushing
	A dull sensation, rather than a pain
Are there factors unlike angina?	Pain lasts hours
	Occurs at the end of a busy day
	'Relieved' by nitrates but only after 30 min
	Pain that is sharp or stabbing
	Pain that comes on or goes away suddenly (in an instant)

Stable angina is relieved rapidly by rest, and very rapidly by a tablet or sublingual spray of a short-acting nitrate. If the problem is not relieved within 3 or 4 min by a nitrate either it is not stable angina (it could be a myocardial infarction) or the nitrate has exceeded its shelf-life and has become inactive.

Chest pain, even with the characteristic distribution of angina, that occurs at the end of a busy day rather than during exercise, that lasts for hours, and which is not helped by nitrate is most unlikely to be angina.

Angina may be associated with breathlessness, and sometimes breathlessness on exertion is the dominant symptom. Table 2 gives a check list of the features that are characteristic of angina.

Myocardial infarction

The distribution of pain due to myocardial infarction is similar to that of stable angina. It is usually in the centre of the chest, and may radiate to the jaw, teeth, arms, or back. The nature of the pain is also similar—typically squeezing or crushing—but it is usually much more severe and can be one of the worse of all pains. It is often associated with a cold sweat, and with vomiting. The pain is frightening, and many will volunteer that they thought that they were going to die. The pain typically lasts a few hours. It may occasionally be associated with heavy exertion (particularly any activity that causes a sudden rise in heart rate and blood pressure) but usually there is no obvious precipitating cause. Nothing other than a strong analgesic such as diamorphine will relieve the pain, and nitrates are completely ineffective. Some patients need a second injection of diamorphine, but few need three, and if chest pain lasts more than 24 h a diagnosis other than myocardial infarction should be considered.

Myocardial infarction can be 'silent', meaning that it occurs without much in the way of pain. Population surveys of older people suggest that some 15 per cent of previous myocardial infarctions demonstrated on ECG are unrecognized. 'Silent' infarction is more likely to happen in diabetics.

The symptoms of myocardial infarction are, of course, modified by complications such as heart failure, arrhythmias, heart block, and pericarditis.

Unstable angina

The chest pain of unstable angina is difficult to describe because unstable angina is difficult to define. The term has been used to describe the first attack of what later proves to be stable angina, stable angina of increasing frequency and severity (sometimes called 'crescendo' angina), and angina at rest. The development of new markers of myocardial infarction such as the troponins has widened the possible definition of myocardial infarction, and unstable angina with a positive troponin test merges into 'non-Q-wave' infarction.

The distribution and intensity of the pain of unstable angina resembles that of stable angina, though patients with non-Q-wave infarction can have severe chest pain indistinguishable from that of Q-wave infarction.

Typically the chest pain of unstable angina will occur at rest. Many patients with unstable angina will gain relief from nitrates, but those with non-Q-wave infarction will not.

The pain of unstable angina is seldom associated with symptoms due to immediate complications such as heart failure, though unstable angina is associated with a relatively high risk of myocardial infarction and death in the next 3 months.

Prinzmetal's variant angina and syndrome X

There are two further varieties of angina that cause ischaemic chest pain, but both are somewhat nebulous concepts and are probably overdiagnosed. In Prinzmetal's 'variant' angina, chest pain characteristic of angina occurs either on exercise or at rest. The pain is believed to result from spasm of the coronary arteries. The diagnosis is only made if an ECG shows ST segment elevation, rather than the usual depression, during an attack of pain. The ST segment returns to normal as the pain disappears, which differentiates the ECG change from that of acute myocardial infarction.

'Syndrome X' is a term used to describe the occurrence of exercise-induced stable angina with a positive exercise test but a normal coronary angiogram. The problem is assumed to be in vessels too small to be demonstrated angiographically, and the term 'microvascular angina' is sometimes used. While the syndrome undoubtedly exists, the diagnosis should only be accepted after very careful investigation.

Dissection of the aorta

Perhaps one patient in a thousand of those who are admitted to hospital with chest pain has a dissection of the aorta. It can be very difficult to diagnose aortic dissection unless the possibility is considered in all of these patients. This is important: the treatments for myocardial infarction and aortic dissection are very different.

The typical patient has a pain similar to that of myocardial infarction, but the pain is more usually sudden in onset. Like infarction, it is in the centre of the chest. It is usually very severe and it often radiates to the back. It is often described by the patient as 'tearing', and it lasts much longer than the pain of myocardial infarction. The onset of pain is often associated with a 'collapse' or with sudden neurological deficit suggesting a stroke. The position of the pain gives a rough guide to the site of dissection; anterior chest pain correlates to some extent with proximal dissection, while pain in the back correlates with distal dissection. The pain may move from the front to the back of the chest as the dissection spreads distally.

If the dissection affects the ostium of a coronary artery, myocardial infarction with its own pain may result.

Unfortunately not all patients with aortic dissection give a typical story. Since the physical examination is not always helpful and the ECG may be normal, patients are not infrequently discharged from the accident and emergency department, or from the ward, with some such diagnostic label as 'myocardial infarction excluded'. Since patients with dissection who survive the first few hours have a reasonable chance of successful surgical repair, it is essential that the diagnosis should at least be considered (if only to be rapidly excluded) before any patient presenting with acute chest pain is discharged.

Pericarditis

The most common cause of pericarditis is myocardial infarction, and the pain of infarction is sometimes replaced by that of pericarditis. Viral infection is a common cause, and pericarditis should be suspected in anyone presenting with chest pain in the context of a 'flu-like illness, particularly if they are likely to be at low risk of coronary artery disease (young men or premenopausal women with few risk factors).

Pericardial pain has some features in common with those of myocardial ischaemia and aortic dissection. It is central, and may have the same radiation. It differs, however, in being (usually) less severe and lasting longer.

The most typical feature of pericardial pain is the effect of posture. The pain is worst when the patient lies on his or her back: the pericardial fluid drains to the back of the pericardial sac, leaving the inflamed anterior visceral and parietal pericardial surfaces to come into contact and so cause pain. Sitting up and leaning forward, which allows the fluid to drain to the front, separates the pericardial layers and relieves the pain.

Pericardial pain often has a pleuritic element, being worse on deep breathing.

Pleuritic pain

Pain from the pleura—the old term was 'pleurisy'—is usually on one side of the chest only. Whatever the cause (and the main causes are infection, pulmonary embolism, and pneumothorax) it is identified because it is worse on inspiration. As a result the patient will need to take shallow and therefore rapid breaths. Unlike the pain of myocardial ischaemia it is usually described as sharp or knife-like. It can be severe, though seldom as severe as myocardial infarction or aortic dissection. Its onset can be sudden (especially when due to pneumothorax or pulmonary embolism) or slow (infection). Pleuritic pain can often be identified because it is associated with symptoms of lung disease such as breathlessness, cough, sputum production, or haemoptysis.

Oesophageal pain

Pain originating in the oesophagus can be difficult to differentiate from the pain of myocardial ischaemia. Both are common, so patients not infrequently suffer from both, and cannot always tell one from the other.

Typical oesophageal pain is central and anterior, and is often described as 'burning'. It usually has some relation to eating. It is commonly due to oesophagitis caused by acid reflux from the stomach because of a hiatus hernia. The pain is often induced by bending, when the patient can be aware of an acid and bitter taste in the mouth. Oesophagitis can cause spasm which is itself painful, and the spasm may be relieved by nitrate, sometimes leading to confusion with angina. More commonly, oesophageal pain is relieved by an antacid.

Rupture of the oesophagus causes severe central chest pain very similar to that of a myocardial infarction. It always follows vomiting, as opposed to the vomiting which can accompany myocardial infarction, which occurs after the pain has become intense.

Musculoskeletal chest pain

Pain can arise in any of the structures of the chest wall, and can mimic all other causes of pain. Pain that is induced or relieved by postural change is likely to be musculoskeletal in origin, as is highly localized pain reproduced by pressure at the affected site. Nerve root compression due, for example, to vertebral disease (collapse, metastasis, abscess) can cause pain to radiate round the ribs. If the pain results from bony collapse it can be of sudden onset, but musculoskeletal pain seldom has the time course of ischaemic pain.

Pain to the left of the sternum, with tenderness over the costochondral junctions, is common in middle-aged men. Sometimes thought to have an inflammatory basis, it is not associated with arthritis elsewhere or with a rise in inflammatory markers. It is sometimes called Tietze's syndrome.

Under the same heading comes the pain of herpes zoster. Patients, especially the elderly, may be admitted to a coronary care unit with a severe left-sided chest pain with tenderness, and the cause becomes obvious the following day as the characteristic rash appears.

Chest pain ? cause

After all the possible causes of chest pain have been excluded there remains a group of patients, usually middle-aged men, in whom no firm diagnosis can be made. It is entirely proper to label these as 'chest pain ? cause'. Making a diagnosis of 'musculoskeletal pain' in such patients is not only incorrect, but it may prevent the diagnosis being properly reassessed on a later occasion.

'Chest pain ? cause' is the discharge diagnosis in about 10 per cent of patients admitted to hospital with suspected myocardial infarction. The pain can be similar to that of acute ischaemia, though it is seldom very severe, and while it may radiate to the left arm it never spreads to the jaw or teeth. By definition, detailed investigation fails to explain the pain, which is not infrequently recurrent. Long term follow-up of such patients shows that their prognosis is essentially that of the healthy population.

'Chest pain ? cause' is also a proper diagnosis in patients with recurrent chest pain in whom the alternative is stable angina. Here the pain is nearly always left-sided, is not predictable, is not clearly related to exercise or emotional stress, and is never brought on by sexual intercourse. This sort of pain merges into Da Costa's syndrome, which was first identified in the American Civil War. Soldiers complained of sharp, lancinating or burning pain, often on a background of a duller pain with a feeling of 'uneasiness' around the heart. The patients described by Da Costa were also troubled by palpitation and hyperventilation. The same thing was observed in the First World War, and this type of pain is considered functional: older terms used to describe it were 'soldiers' heart' and 'cardiac neurosis'. However, nonspecific 'chest pain ? cause' also occurs in people who are not apparently under stress.

Physical signs in patients with chest pain

In patients with severe pain the findings on examination may be dominated by those due to pain itself: pallor, cold and clammy extremeties, and a sinus tachycardia. The blood pressure may be high due to intense peripheral vasoconstriction, or low if there has been severe myocardial damage. After pain relief, or in between episodes of pain, there may be few physical abnormalities.

When the pain sounds like chronic stable angina it is important to look for possible causes other than coronary disease, including aortic stenosis, anaemia, and brady- or tachyarrhythmias. There may be evidence of peripheral vascular disease: absent peripheral pulses, or bruits over the carotid or femoral arteries, suggesting that coronary disease is likely. There may be signs of risk factors such as those associated with hypercholesterolaemia, and hypertension may be present.

All these physical signs should be sought in patients with persistent chest pain. In addition there may be evidence of myocardial dysfunction, including heart failure (raised jugular venous pressure, a gallop rhythm, pulmonary crackles), mitral valve regurgitation due to papillary muscle dysfunction or rupture, and ventricular septal defect.

Although there are classical signs of aortic dissection, these are by no means uinversal. About one-third of the patients will have high blood pressure; a third will have a murmur of aortic regurgitation due to distortion of the aortic root; and perhaps half will have a pulse missing or a different blood pressure in each arm. A pericardial friction rub or pericardial tamponade due to blood tracking backwards into the pericardium is uncommon, but when associated with aortic regurgitation the diagnosis of aortic dissection becomes almost certain.

Pericarditis is diagnosed from the presence of a pericardial friction rub, which is best heard with the patient lying flat. It may be associated with signs of tamponade which include a rise in the jugular venous pressure and fall in the arterial pressure on inspiration. Similarly, pleuritic pain can be identified from the pleural rub if one can be heard. Otherwise there may be sounds of pulmonary consolidation or pleural effusion that make associated pleurisy likely.

Patients with viral pericarditis are likely to have a fever. In those with pleurisy, a high fever (over 38.5 °C) makes pneumonia a more likely diagnosis than pulmonary embolism. Myocardial infarction causes a low-grade fever, but this not often seen until a day or two after the event.

There are few physical signs in patients with oesophageal pain, though there may be tenderness in the epigastrium. Musculoskeletal pain is suspected when there is bony tenderness (fractures, metastases) or when the pain is reproduced by local pressure or movement. 'Chest pain ? cause', virtually by definition, has no physical signs other, perhaps, than those of anxiety.

The immediate management of patients with chest pain

Patients seen in the accident and emergency department with chest pain need urgent assessment and treatment. Those with a possible acute coronary syndrome need rapid sorting into those who need immediate reperfusion of a blocked coronary artery (identified by raised ST segments on the ECG) and those with non-Q-wave infarction or unstable angina, who have less need for immediate treatment but who will need more detailed investigation and treatment over the next few days. All these patients should be admitted to hospital, ideally to a coronary care unit, though it is frequently impracticable to admit all patients seen in an accident and emergency department with chest pain.

If the initial ECG is normal but the patient has significant pain, the ECG should be recorded again after 1 and 2 h. Patients with persistent pain at that point will have to be admitted. Early plasma markers of myocardial necrosis—the creatine kinase and creatine kinase myocardial band enzymes, and the troponins—are helpful if positive, but will often not be elevated until about 6 h after the onset of pain. Although one possible treatment strategy is to hold patients in the accident and emegency department until 6 h have elapsed and the enzymes and troponins have been shown to be normal, this is not foolproof because the troponins may not become elevated for as long as 18 h.

Chest radiographs are seldom helpful in patients with chest pain, and if anteroposterior films are taken they can be positively misleading. Obtaining a posteroanterior film may mean transferring the patient to an X-ray department where close monitoring cannot easily be maintained, but using portable X-ray equipment in the accident and emergency department will almost inevitably produce a distorted cardiac and mediastinal shadow. It is under these circumstances that widening of the mediastinum, which may be the first indication of an aortic dissection, will be missed. Portable X-ray equipment is only reliable for assessing the lung fields, and to some extent for detecting heart failure. If aortic dissection seems at all possible, then a departmental posteroanterior chest radiograph is essential.

Patient management inevitably depends to some extent on the patient's perception of what has happened and whether, for example, the pain that has led to his or her hospital attendance is like or unlike previous angina. In general, however, if the patient becomes pain free and there are no important physical abnormalities, if an ECG repeated after 2 h shows no change from the initial recording, and if a departmental chest radiograph and plasma troponin or creatine kinase are normal, then it is not unreasonable to allow the patient to go home (with notification for their general practitioner and arrangements for further investigation, for example cardiac treadmill testing, as appropriate). Total safety of diagnosis and management requires hospital admission and observation for perhaps 18 h, but in the real world this is often impracticable.

The diagnosis depends on the synthesis of the patient's history, the physical examination, and simple investigations. A carefully taken history, coupled with a high index of suspicion for important problems such as an acute coronary syndrome or aortic dissection, is the key to a successful patient management.

Further reading

Bakker AJ *et al.* (1993). Failure of new biochemical markers to exclude acute myocardial infarction at admission. *The Lancet* **343**, 1220–2.

Bayliss RIS (1985). The silent coronary. *British Medical Journal* **290**, 1093–4.

Cannon RO (1993). Chest pain with normal coronary angiogram. *New England Journal of Medicine* **328**, 1706–8.

DeSanctis RW *et al.* (1987). Aortic dissection. *New England Journal of Medicine* **317**, 1060–7.

Hampton JR, Gray A (1998). The future of general medicine: lessons from an admissions ward. *Journal of the Royal College of Physicians of London* **32**, 39–42.

Ohman EM *et al.* (1996). Cardiac troponin T levels for risk stratification in acute myocardial ischaemia. *New England Journal of Medicine* **335**, 1333–41.

Ryan J *et al.* (1996). ACC/AHA Guidelines for the Management of patients with acute myocardial infarction. *Journal of the American College of Cardiology* **28**, 1328–1428.

Slater EE, DeSanctis RW (1976). The clinical recognition of dissecting aortic aneurysm. *American Journal of Medicine* **60**, 625–33.

Spittell PC *et al.* (1993). Clinical features and differential diagnosis of acute dissection: experience with 236 cases (1980 through 1990). *Mayo Foundation for Medical Education and Research* **68**, 642–51.

Thadani U *et al.* (1971). Pericarditis after acute myocardial infarction. *British Medical Journal* **2**, 135–7.

15.2.2　The syndrome of heart failure

Andrew J. S. Coats

Introduction

Heart failure is a common condition, carrying a high burden of disability and mortality. Many treatments have now been established that ameliorate, at least partially, its debilitating effects, but despite this it is increasing in both prevalence and cost in the developed and developing worlds as the population ages. Much disability remains, and there are many shortfalls between treatment possibilities and that which is achieved in everyday practice around the world. Major advances seem possible with the advent of greater understanding about the causes of cardiovascular disorders, including molecular mechanisms, and the development of newer, effective treatments, including surgical advances and gene therapies.

Definitions

'Heart failure' is an unfortunate term. It has negative connotations for the patient and describes imprecisely several different clinical situations. Left and right heart failure are quite distinct clinical syndromes, although they frequently coexist (biventricular failure). Historically heart failure has been further subdivided on the basis of presumed pathophysiological mechanisms into: (1)'forward' or 'backward' heart failure, depending on whether congestion or organ underperfusion was the predominant clinical feature; (2)'congestive' or 'non-congestive', depending on the presence or absence of oedema; and (3)'high-output' or 'low-output'. These subdivisions have not proved to be particularly useful. A more recent and more useful classification is dependent on the predominant pattern of left ventricular dysfunction, be it systolic, diastolic or mixed. Whatever the complexities of the ventricular pathophysiology that initiates events, a well-recognized clinical pattern is identifiable as 'heart failure' and has proved a useful description of a complex clinical syndrome for many years.

The important features of any definition of heart failure (of which there have been several) are that the clinical picture is:

(1) initiated by a reduction in effective cardiovascular (usually ventricular) functional reserve;

(2) associated with symptoms either at rest or at an unexpectedly low level of exertion; and

(3) associated with characteristic pathophysiological changes in many disparate organ systems.

These latter can include biochemical, hormonal, metabolic, or functional alterations. In simple terms heart failure is a syndrome in which a reduction in left ventricular function causes pathophysiology that produces symptoms and exercise limitation.

A clinical picture similar to that of heart failure can develop when ventricular function itself is normal, but where there is an extreme volume or pressure overload on the ventricle. These include volume overload conditions such as endotoxic high-output shock, severe anaemia, arteriovenous fistulas or shunts, and pressure overload conditions such as acute hypertensive crisis or prosthetic heart valve occlusion. It is appropriate both clinically and for research purposes to separate these from cases where the initiating cause is a reduction in ventricular function.

Acute and chronic heart failure

It is conventional, because of differences in assessment and management, to separate acute from chronic heart failure. Both are different stages of a single disease process, and in the clinical course of a patient with chronic heart failure acute exacerbations may be common, often described as 'acute decompensation' or 'acute on chronic' heart failure. Acute heart failure is typically a dramatic clinical presentation with an acutely dyspnoeic patient demonstrating visible signs of cardiovascular insufficiency such as tachycardia, pulmonary or peripheral oedema, and underperfusion of systemic organs. Chronic heart failure, by contrast, can be a subtle disorder, which if gradual in onset can be missed by both patient and physician. The salient features are the initiation and persistence of left ventricular dysfunction, and the pathophysiological changes in other organs that produce symptoms and which limit exercise. A persistent state of circulatory insufficiency can exist in severe chronic heart failure, with pulmonary and peripheral oedema and symptoms and signs of distress even at rest.

Epidemiology, aetiology, and pathogenesis

Epidemiology

Heart failure is a common condition with an estimated incidence of 20 to 30 per thousand of the adult population per year and an overall prevalence of about 1 per cent. The prevalence increases in frequency with increasing age, reaching 30 per cent in those aged over 80 years, and in developed countries the average age of patients with heart failure is now in excess of 75 years. It is one of the most expensive medical conditions, and is an increasing major healthcare cost. Because of its many debilitating symptoms, heart failure is a frequent cause for both acute hospital and long-stay residential care admissions, indeed it is the most common discharge diagnosis from hospitals in the developed world in people over the age of 65, and the second most common overall. Heart failure is a feature of the clinical condition of approximately 5 per cent of patients in hospital at any time, and also the one with the greatest rate of hospital re-admission.

Paradoxically, improvements in the management of acute myocardial infarction and chronic coronary heart disease have led to more instances of heart failure rather than less, as more people survive to develop heart failure later in life. However, preventive therapies do work: multiple trials of antihypertensive treatment and the 4S trial of cholesterol reduction have shown a significant reduction in the incidence of new cases of heart failure in high-risk populations. Smoking reduction also reduces the number of new cases of heart failure, as does the selective use of angiotensin-converting enzyme inhibitors in high-risk patients after a myocardial infarction or for those with asymptomatic left ventricular systolic dysfunction. Appro-

priate use of thrombolytic therapy at the time of myocardial infarction will also reduce the incidence of new cases of heart failure.

Whilst there is reasonable consensus as to the prevalence of heart failure in younger and middle-aged populations, where most cases demonstrate significant deterioration in systolic function of an enlarged heart, in the elderly an increasing proportion of cases of clinically suspected cases of heart failure have small ventricular cavities and preserved systolic function. In these cases diastolic dysfunction can be frequently demonstrated, and many experts feel that the majority of cases in an older population will be due primarily to diastolic dysfunction. However, methods of assessing diastolic function are less developed than those for systolic function, and interventional trials have historically concentrated on systolic dysfunction as a cause of heart failure. As a result we know much less about how best to diagnose diastolic heart failure and how best to teat it once diagnosed. This remains a major challenge to the cardiological community in the twenty-first century.

Aetiology

Heart failure is a clinical syndrome, not a single diagnosis, and it can have many different aetiologies. In Western industrialized societies the most common underlying causes are ischaemic heart disease, hypertension, and idiopathic dilated cardiomyopathy (see Chapter 15.8.2). The Framingham study suggested that hypertension, especially when complicated by left ventricular hypertrophy, was by far the most common antecedent of heart failure. Recent intervention trials in heart failure have usually included a preponderance of patients whose heart failure was secondary to ischaemic heart disease. In recent cross-sectional studies of heart failure in the community, hypertension is cited to be a relatively minor cause of heart failure. This change has been attributed to better detection and treatment of hypertension, but it may also reflect re-labelling, with coronary artery disease more likely to be blamed for heart failure than hypertension in the many patients who have evidence of both. Some cases of hypertension may proceed to a dilated poorly functioning heart with an eventual normalization in arterial pressure. These cases may be labelled as idiopathic dilated cardiomyopathy, with the only clue to the correct underlying diagnosis being a greater than expected degree of left ventricular hypertrophy.

In industrialized societies previously common causes of heart failure such as nutritional deficiency disorders or chronic complications of rheumatic valvular disease are now rare. In less developed societies infective causes still underlie the majority of cases. Some disorders may be common in particular societies and these should always be borne in mind when assessing an individual patient: examples would include Chagas' disease in Central and Southern America, iron overload in certain tribes in southern Africa, and nutritional deficiency states in the world's poorest countries.

Classification of cause

More than one underlying cause of heart failure can coexist, such as hypertension and ischaemic heart disease. Table 1 lists the major causes of heart failure, subdivided according to the mechanisms by which ventricular disease leads to the clinical syndrome. Such a differentiation is important because of specific strategies available for certain diagnoses, such as nutritional support, cardiac valve or bypass surgery, endocrine therapy, and avoidance of a toxic agent.

Pathogenesis

There is no unique pathological finding in the heart or elsewhere that defines the presence of heart failure. Heart failure can be the result of a wide variety of cardiovascular disorders: anything that puts an excessive demand on the heart for a prolonged period can lead to myocardial failure. Alternatively, loss of myocytes or an abnormal myocardial interstitium can lead to loss of effective heart function and cause the clinical syndrome of heart failure.

Although the more severe the loss of myocyte number or reduction in cardiac pumping capacity, the more likely is clinical heart failure, there is no strict relationship between measures of global cardiac function and the presence or severity of the features of the heart failure syndrome. The severity of heart failure is measured by the severity of symptomatic limitation, and by the extent of pathophysiological abnormalities, which closely correlate with the reduction in survival. Important amongst these changes of heart failure are the body's responses such as neurohormonal overactivity, autonomic dysfunction, and immunological and metabolic derangements.

Oxygen and energy supply

Myocardial dysfunction can result from a deficient oxygen supply to the myocardium, whether caused by occlusive coronary artery disease or by a reduced blood-carrying capacity such as in anaemia or certain toxic states. In addition, endothelial dysfunction, raised ventricular myocardial tissue pressures, and reduced diastolic blood pressure and diastolic time intervals all contribute to a reduction in the net effective coronary flow. Energy metabolism is frequently abnormal within the myocardium in cases of chronic heart failure. This can be a primary defect in familial cardiomyopathies or an acquired defect, such as in the insulin resistance that complicates chronic heart failure.

Defects in myocardial contractile performance

There remains considerable controversy as to whether individual myocytes are functionally deficient in most cases of human chronic heart failure.

Table 1 Causes of heart failure

1. **Loss of myocytes**
   Ischaemic heart disease
   Idiopathic dilated cardiomyopathy
   Familial cardiomyopathies
   Infective cardiomyopathies, e.g. Chagas' disease, AIDS cardiomyopathy
   Toxic cardiomyopathies including alcoholic cardiomyopathy
   Infiltrative conditions: sarcoid, amyloid, iron overload
   Cardiac neoplasms
   Senile cardiomyopathy (apoptosis)

2. **Myocyte dysfunction**
   Nutritional deficiencies
   ? Chronic ischaemia ('hibernating myocardium')
   Hypertrophic cardiomyopathy
   Restrictive cardiomyopathy
   Secondary to chronic tachyarrhythmia
   Endocrine disorders, e.g. thyrotoxic, hypocalcaemic, acromegalic

3. **Alterations in myocardial interstitium**
   Senile myocardial fibrosis
   Endomyocardial fibrosis

4. **Valvular disorders**
   Rheumatic heart disease
   Congenital valve disease
   Senile valve calcification
   Mitral valve prolapse
   Paravalvar dysfunction: e.g. paraprosthetic leak, dissection of aortic valve
   Infective endocarditis
   Non-infective endocarditis, e.g. secondary to connective tissue diseases

5. **Pericardial disorders**
   Constrictive pericarditis
   Cardiac tamponade

6. **Extracardiac causes**
   Volume overload, e.g. anaemia, arteriovenous shunt
   Pressure overload, e.g. coarctation, severe hypertension

There are isolated cardiomyopathies where such defects are likely, but in most cases the major defect is a loss of myocyte number with compensatory myocyte hypertrophy. This leads to dysfunction of myocyte relaxation, due in part to an intracellular accumulation of calcium, rather than deficient contraction. Isolated single gene defects can be the cause of rare familial cardiomyopathies and in these, and presumably in more cases in the future as we understand more of the genetic processes underlying the control of myocardial contraction, specific abnormalities of myocyte contraction can be implicated in the cardiac dysfunction evident at the organ level.

Defects in the control of myocardial function

Although in theory an abnormal control of contraction could lead to cardiac dysfunction sufficient to cause heart failure, examples of clinical syndromes demonstrating this pathophysiological mechanism are rare. Myocyte necrosis can occur in cases of persistent sympathetic overactivity such as phaeochromocytoma, and more commonly excessive blockade of sympathetic nerve endings can acutely remove this support to myocardial contractility leading to acute heart failure.

Changes in the interstitium of the heart

Excessive myocardial fibrosis, such as that seen in senile changes in the heart and as a complication of sustained hypertension and aortic stenosis, can reduce the effective myocardial performance despite individual myocyte hypertrophy. Similarly, rare cases such as endomyocardial fibrosis can cause a syndrome of cardiac failure despite individual myocytes being functionally normal if studied in isolation. The importance of the intracellular milieu has only recently been fully recognized, and this may be a target for future interventions to modify the processes of ageing of the myocardium and progression in the syndrome of chronic heart failure.

Pathophysiology

Cardiac

Structural changes

Structural changes in the heart are common, both at macroscopic and microscopic levels. The clinical picture usually includes enlargement of the left ventricular cavity (with the exception of diastolic dysfunction and restrictive or constrictive cardiomyopathies). The shape of the ventricle also changes, becoming more spherical. This can occur rapidly after a myocardial infarction via a passive process of stretching of the infarcted territory (infarct expansion), or more slowly over a period of weeks to months in a process termed 'remodelling' (see Chapter 15.4.2). A similar change in shape is seen in dilated cardiomyopathies, but not in the restrictive cardiomyopathies. The more spherical shape of the 'remodelled' and enlarged ventricle increases the stress of the myocardial wall and may thereby worsen myocardial ischaemia. The shape change may also disrupt the complex conformational change that normally occurs during the isovolumic contraction phase, in which the apex of the ventricle constricts in a twisting motion and pushes the blood into the ventricular base. Where the ventricle is already spherical at rest, this intraventricular redistribution of blood during isovolumic contraction is not possible and the net effect is a reduction in the efficiency with which the blood is ejected.

Cardiac enlargement has long been known to be an adverse prognostic sign, even when estimated crudely as the cardiothoracic diameter on chest radiographs. More precise measurements of the internal dimensions of the left ventricle by echocardiography have confirmed the prognostic value of cardiac enlargement in patients recovering from myocardial infarction, even when accounting for the size of the myocardial infarct. Prevention of the late remodelling process was the theory behind the use of angiotensin-converting enzyme (**ACE**) inhibitors after myocardial infarction. These agents have been shown to reduce ventricular size and to reduce late mortality if given early after infarction, but whether this beneficial effect is directly related to any reduction in ventricular remodelling is not known.

Changes at the microscopic level

The failing heart also shows alterations in cardiac structure at microscopic and ultrastructural levels. There is an increase in the collagen content of the extracellular matrix, a process thought to be partly related to increased wall stress and partly due to neurohormonal activation, particularly aldosterone. This change reduces ventricular wall distensibility and may affect the efficiency with which active restorative forces can assist the diastolic filling process. Hence this microscopic structural change may help to explain the frequent coexistence of systolic and diastolic functional deterioration in an enlarging ventricle in chronic heart failure.

The enlargement of the ventricle is associated with thinning of the ventricular wall and, as there is believed to be no increase in the total myocyte population, there must be a realignment of the intercellular attachments between individual myocytes. This process, whereby there is a continual breaking and reforming of cell-to-cell junctions to allow remodelling, has been termed 'cell slippage', although exactly how this occurs has not been established. There are changes in the microscopic structure of the failing ventricle, with a reduced number of tight junctions between myocytes, and this may be involved in this process.

Overall circulatory function

The description of an objective measurement of systolic function in intact humans has proved difficult. In simplest terms, the left ventricle is a pump that generates both pressure and flow. It has a theoretical operating range from a pure pressure generator to a pure flow generator, although it always functions as a mixed pump. The function of this pump can be described in terms of the kinetic and potential energy it imparts to the blood ejected each beat, or in terms of the average power output of the circulation (flow multiplied by the mean pressure drop), assuming the left ventricle is the only significant power source in the circulation. Thus, overall ventricular function can be described as cardiac output multiplied by the pressure drop across the systemic circulation, a quantity described as cardiac power output. Cardiac power output is well preserved at rest even in severe heart failure, but the maximal reserve of cardiac power output is reduced progressively as heart failure progresses, and a significant reduction in maximal power output during inotropic stimulation is a poor prognostic sign.

The measurement of cardiac power output tells us little, however, of the mechanisms underlying any reduction in ventricular performance. This may be due to reduced ventricular filling, or emptying, or to wasted myocardial power such as in aortic stenosis. Hence, attempts have been made to define the components of ventricular function to explain the nature of a reduced overall circulatory function and to assist in monitoring a patient's clinical course and response to treatment.

Systolic dysfunction

Systole can be defined either clinically as the ejection phase between mitral valve closure and aortic valve closure, or in terms of ventricular dynamics as the phase of contraction of the myocytes within the ventricle. These two definitions do not coincide, for there is a period of isovolumic contraction at the onset of ventricular systole in which myocyte contraction generates a pressure increase within the ventricle and a conformational change in its shape, but during which no blood is ejected. Similarly during the latter phase of ventricular ejection, the blood is flowing out of the left ventricle passively and the myocardial elements may be already relaxing.

In clinical practice, systolic dysfunction is most easily recognized by direct haemodynamic measurements showing a reduced peak rate of pressure rise within the ventricle (positive dP/dt max), an increased filling pressure (left ventricular end-diastolic pressure, **LVEDP**), or by indirect measurement of ventricular volumes (see Chapter 15.3.6). If there is a reduction in myocardial contractile function an enlargement of the ventricle will develop, in which a greater preload will enhance ventricular emptying via the Frank–Starling mechanism. As a result the ventricle will operate at an increased end-diastolic and end-systolic volume. This can be measured by pressure and volume estimations, such as by ventriculography (either radiographic or radionuclear) or echocardiography. Although not a direct measure of ventricular performance, ejection fraction, being the fractional emptying of the ventricle with each beat, carries information about ventricular volumes and global ventricular function. This is only a poor predictor of the severity of symptomatic limitation, but it has been shown to be an important predictor of longevity in heart failure, independent of other measures of severity, and it has the advantage of simplicity. At the most simple level, therefore, systolic heart failure can be recognized by signs of cardiac insufficiency in the presence of an enlarged ventricle, and clinically is most conveniently estimated by the left ventricular ejection fraction.

Diastolic dysfunction

Diastole is the opposite of systole, the period of filling of the ventricle or the period of relaxation of the myocytes. Objective measurements of diastolic function are, however, more problematic than for systolic function. Whereas systole occurs rapidly and in one action, diastole is complex, with an initial rapid and active ventricular recoil producing filling of the ventricle, then a period of relative stasis as atrial and ventricular pressures equilibrate, followed by a second period of ventricular filling due to atrial contraction. These processes are affected by many factors including heart rate, atrioventricular delay, atrial contractility, active myocardial recoil, passive ventricular wall stiffness, the efficacy of ventricular systole, and the residual end-diastolic volume and pressure within the ventricle. As a result of all these interacting factors, it is not surprising that no simple measure of 'diastolic function' has been developed, and those measures that have been used clinically are profoundly affected by systolic function and heart rate. However, diastolic functional disturbance is important: there are cases of definite clinical heart failure in which the patient has a small heart, with normal or even increased left ventricular ejection fraction, and in whom the only demonstrable abnormalities of ventricular mechanics are those related to diastolic filling. These may include increased filling pressures, delayed pressure fall within the ventricle, and a greater than normal dependence on the effects of atrial contraction for ventricular filling. Such cases form the minority of cases of heart failure (estimates vary from a few per cent to about one-fifth of cases), but are seen with increasing frequency in older patients in whom senile myocardial fibrosis occurs more frequently as the major pathology underlying the heart failure. Other rarer causes include hypertrophic cardiomyopathy, infiltrative conditions such as amyloid heart disease, and the acute effects of ischaemia or the chronic effects of advanced hypertrophy in response to hypertension.

Diastolic dysfunction can be quantified by a variety of measurements: haemodynamic; echocardiographic; radionuclear; or ventriculographic. Those most commonly employed are the rate constant of isovolumic relaxation of the ventricle during early diastole (tau), the early to late peak filling velocity ratio (*E/A*) across the mitral valve on Doppler echocardiography, and the peak rate of ventricular filling on radionuclear gated acquisition (MUGA) scans in end-diastolic volumes per second. None of these parameters are independent of the loading conditions of the ventricle, nor of atrioventricular delay and heart rate, nor of the effect of systolic dysfunction.

Pure diastolic dysfunction is rare, as indeed is pure systolic dysfunction, as the two are almost inseparably interdependent. One can speak, however, of cases where the heart failure is predominantly due to systolic or diastolic impairment of the ventricle, and the simplest separation is via the size of the end-diastolic volume; if large, systolic dysfunction is likely to be the major abnormality; if small, diastolic. As will be discussed, this differentiation is important because of differing effects of treatment, in particular vasodilators, which may be less useful in diastolic dysfunction because of the requirement for high ventricular filling pressures in this condition.

Non-cardiac

General syndrome

Although initiated by ventricular dysfunction, in its chronic form heart failure is a multisystem disorder: the syndrome of chronic heart failure. The causes of many of the disparate organ pathologies that develop are poorly understood, as are the mechanisms by which these are (slowly) corrected by effective therapy, including transplantation of the heart. Much remains uncertain about this non-cardiac pathology and pathophysiology, including its genesis, symptomatic effects, and correct management. Evidence suggests, however, that non-cardiac factors become responsible both for the symptoms and the objective limitation of exercise capacity in chronic heart failure.

Specific organ systems

The microvasculature

Changes occur in the microvasculature in many organ systems and these may contribute to the organ underperfusion seen in this syndrome. There have been few reports of definite structural changes in the microvasculature, but functionally the endothelial-dependent vasomotor control systems are disordered. The endothelial-dependent vasodilator system is impaired both in the myocardial vessels and in the periphery. Tumour necrosis factor-alpha, which is elevated in some cases of chronic heart failure, has been implicated in impaired endothelial vasodilator function in addition to the enhanced activity of the endothelin vasoconstrictor system. This generalized endothelial dysfunction may contribute to some of the organ dysfunction described below, including renal, hepatic, and pulmonary vascular impairment. Specific treatments for endothelial abnormalities have not been established for heart failure, although promising results have been seen with improved endothelial function after localized exercise training or administration of the nitric oxide precursor L-arginine.

Large arterial function

In heart failure there is a reduction in large arterial compliance, which in turns leads to an increase in the impedance to ventricular outflow. Thus the efficiency of ventriculoaortic coupling is reduced, the impaired ventricular reserve is further stressed, and there is an increase in myocardial wall stress. The cause of the changes in large arteries probably relate to sympathetic and possibly local renin–angiotensin activation. In acute heart failure counterpulsation by intra-aortic balloon pumping probably helps forward aortic blood flow, at least partially by a mechanism involving improved ventriculoaortic coupling, in addition to the beneficial effects of enhanced diastolic coronary perfusion pressures.

The respiratory system

The lungs

Despite the frequency of dyspnoea as a central complaint of a patient with heart failure, relatively little is known of the role of the lung in chronic heart failure. In acute heart failure, changes within the lung are profound and easily explain much of the acute respiratory distress of the syndrome. With an acute reduction in left ventricular performance a rapid increase in left ventricular filling pressures, and hence pulmonary venous pressures, will lead to fluid accumulation in the lung parenchyma. Initially this will decrease the compliance of the lung, thereby reducing vital capacity and increasing the work of breathing. It may also, via oedematous swelling of the bronchial mucosa, cause a non-asthmatic bronchial constriction that can mimic asthma and further increase respiratory muscle work. With more severe pulmonary venous hypertension the alveolar membrane becomes thickened and oedematous and this may impair gas exchange, leading to an increase in the alveolar–arterial oxygen gradient and eventually arterial hypoxaemia. Eventually frank pulmonary oedema can form, further exacerbating the processes described above and leading to the clinical picture of gross dyspnoea, hypoxaemia, lung crepitations, and the production of copious quantities of pink frothy sputum (the alveolar oedema fluid itself).

In chronic heart failure, the patient is dyspnoeic but the changes in the lungs are far less marked. Pulmonary venous pressures may be normal if diuretic treatment is effective, and in well-diuresed and non-oedematous patients very few changes can be detected in lung histology. The changes of pulmonary siderosis seen with chronic untreated mitral stenosis are not seen in well-treated chronic heart failure cases. There have been reports of subtle changes in lung function in chronic heart failure, including a reduction in gas diffusing capacity, intermittent non-asthmatic bronchial constriction, and a purported increase in dead-space ventilation, but these are largely functional changes without an established anatomical cause. One pathophysiological change that can lead to respiratory distress is an alteration in the volume, structure, strength, and fatiguability of the respiratory musculature. The effects of these changes on the sensation of dyspnoea, or most appropriate therapy, are unknown. Similar changes are seen in skeletal muscle (see below).

Pulmonary oedema is not synonymous with heart failure. In addition to the acute respiratory distress syndrome (see Chapter 16.5.1) there are other causes of pulmonary oedema that need to be considered as differential diagnoses for heart failure: these are discussed in Section 15.15.

Respiratory control

The mechanisms of normal control of ventilation during exercise are not fully understood. It is not surprising, therefore, that the mechanisms underlying the abnormal respiratory response seen in chronic heart failure are also unclear. Patients with heart failure, even in the absence of pulmonary oedema, have an increased ventilatory response to exercise, whilst maintaining normal arterial blood gas tensions. They show reduced maximal oxygen consumption, an early dependence on anaerobic metabolism, and an increased ventilatory equivalent for carbon dioxide even at low work levels. This latter feature can be best appreciated by the plot of ventilation against the rate of carbon dioxide production (the $Vus.\dot{V}CO_2$ slope) during progressive exercise: this is significantly steeper (up to threefold) throughout both aerobic and anaerobic levels of exercise, and its steepness correlates closely with the reduction of maximal oxygen consumption. Although it is clear that this increased ventilation relative to the external work rate must indicate wasted ventilation, exactly why this occurs in non-oedematous patients is not certain. It has been assumed that there is a primary increase in dead-space ventilation due to a reduction in the ability of the right ventricle to perfuse adequately all lung regions, or the development of significant ventilation/perfusion mismatching within the lung, but these hypotheses have not been proven. An alternative hypothesis is that something other than the rate of carbon dioxide production causes the increased exertional ventilation in patients with heart failure, which is supported by the finding that, rather than being abnormal, arterial carbon dioxide during exercise is often lower than in normals, suggesting relative hyperventilation and the action of a non-carbon dioxide ventilatory stimulus. There are several candidate stimuli including an increased release of, or sensitivity to, known ventilatory stimuli such as lactate, arterial potassium, or adenosine. Skeletal muscle is abnormal in heart failure cases (see below) and releases metabolites earlier in exercise than age-matched normal controls.

There is also a neural pathway (the ergoreflex or metaboreflux) in the control of ventilation, utilizing group III and IV afferents from skeletal muscle. These are sensitive to the metabolic state of exercising muscle and transmit signals via the lateral spinothalamic tract to mediate reflex increases in ventilation as well as peripheral vasoconstriction and sympathoexcitation. Both this reflex control system and the arterial chemoreflexes that control ventilatory effort are abnormally active and oversensitive in chronic heart failure, possibly contributing to the excessive ventilation during exercise and playing a role in causing the subjective dyspnoea during low-level exercise seen in cases of chronic heart failure.

Airflow

Expiratory airflow can be restricted in patients with heart failure, even when all smokers and patients with a history of intermittent bronchospasm have been excluded. These patients can exhibit considerable dips in their peak expiratory flow rate on occasion, especially at night, which may lead to episodes of respiratory distress as well as adding to the work of breathing, and through that to the perception of dyspnoea. The mechanisms of this 'bronchoconstriction' are not known but they may involve oedema of the bronchial mucosa. Thus, a variety of lung factors can add together to contribute to dyspnoea in chronic heart failure, even in the absence of frank pulmonary oedema. Recently methoxamine in an opening of airways has been reported to improve peak flow rates and lead to an increase in exercise tolerance in these patients.

Gas exchange

Although arterial oxygen desaturation and carbon dioxide retention are rare in well-diuresed patients with heart failure, a more mild alteration in the gas exchange function of the lung can occur. These factors could reduce the rate of delivery of oxygen to the metabolizing tissues and act as a stimulus to increased ventilation. They may also explain the compensatory increase in arterial oxygen content seen in chronic heart failure if mild but intermittent hypoxia develops in this condition. This could also explain the beneficial effects of oxygen supplementation, even acutely, on exercise tolerance in patients with chronic heart failure.

It is not certain, however, that in chronic heart failure a reduction in diffusing capacity is either quantitatively important, or that oxygen supplementation works via increasing net oxygen delivery to the tissues. Alternative explanations are that the effect of a high inspired concentration of oxygen is non-specific in reducing peripheral chemoreflex drive and thereby relieving the sensation of dyspnoea, in a way akin to that produced by narcotic analgesics. Similarly, reduced gas exchange, especially for oxygen, may have more to do with inadequate expansion of the pulmonary capillary network and an inadequate time for gas transfer rather than to any alteration in the alveolar blood–gas barrier itself. The very low mixed venous oxygen saturations seen in chronic heart failure may mean that even a normal capillary transit time is inadequate for full oxygen exchange.

The sleep-apnoea syndrome

Nocturnal oxygen saturation monitoring of patients with chronic heart failure has demonstrated the presence of episodes of desaturation, often to below 80 to 85 per cent. These episodes coincide with and are caused by episodes of apnoea; they are also followed by semi-arousal from sleep and hyperventilation that may awaken and frighten the sleeping partner. In addition to obstructive sleep apnoea, which is common in patients with heart disease due to similar antecedent risk factors, the pattern is reminiscent of the Cheyne–Stokes respiratory patterns that are well recognized in patients with severe heart failure.

The mechanisms of both abnormalities of respiratory rhythm are incompletely understood. In some cases of nocturnal desaturations there is an obstructive element with obesity and pharyngeal occlusion by the tongue flopping back. In other cases there appears to be an alteration in the central sensitivity to carbon dioxide so that oscillating levels of respiratory drive, and hence of arterial oxygen saturation, develop. This second mechanism may be partly the cause for Cheyne–Stokes breathing as well. Another finding that may be related is that patients with chronic heart failure exhibit reduced total and high-frequency heart rate variability, but relatively enhanced variability of heart rate at very low frequencies (less than 0.01 Hz, or 1 cycle every 100 s). Although rhythmic variations in heart rate at higher frequencies are related to homeostatic mechanisms controlling blood pressure, in particular the vagal and sympathetic limbs of the arterial baroreflex, the genesis of this very low-frequency rhythm is not known. It does, however, have several features to suggest that chemoreflex activity may play a role in its genesis. First, this rhythm is particularly prominent in heart failure, where the circulation time is long; second, it is of similar frequency to the more obvious rhythm of Cheyne–Stokes breathing; and third, the chemoreflex loop has sufficient delay characteristics and possesses sufficient interactions with the baroreflexes and control of heart rate for a harmonic of oscillatory arterial gas concentrations to set up a similar

harmonic oscillation in respiration, which would then entrain heart rate via an effect of the baroreflex. Finally, similar rhythms are particularly prominent in heart failure in pulmonary arterial pressure tracings, hence it may be that periodic sleep-apnoea (at least that which is not obviously obstructive), very low-frequency rhythms of heart rate variability, and Cheyne–Stokes respiration may all be reflections of harmonic oscillation of chemoreflex–baroreflex interactions. If this is the case then they may respond to therapies that alter chemoreflex gain or drive, and in this regard the promising reports of nocturnal oxygen supplementation and of nasal positive-pressure ventilation may be supportive for this theory. It is in any case surprising, and perhaps chastening, to note that in a condition so associated with dyspnoea that the state of the chemoreflex drive at rest, during sleep, or exercise is not known.

Musculoskeletal

Structure

Skeletal muscle biopsies in patients with moderate to severe chronic heart failure have shown a variety of pathological changes. These include individual fibre atrophy, a shift in the distribution frequency of types IIa and IIb fibres, and changes at an ultrastructural level, including a reduction in mitochondrial density, volume, and the number of cristae. It has proved impossible to define a specific pathological change characteristic of heart failure, partly because of the enormous variation in a control population, but also because muscle becomes abnormal in a limited number of ways in a variety of diseases associated with skeletal myopathy. It is also important to be sure of studying a specific heart failure-related change and not some subclinical skeletal myopathy as part of an inherited cardioskeletal myopathy. That such changes are seen with equal frequency and severity in ischaemic heart failure makes this unlikely to be the only explanation of the findings.

One of the most marked structural changes in peripheral muscle is the substantial reduction in total skeletal muscle bulk. Although it has long been recognized that in some cases of end-stage heart failure a catabolic wasting syndrome can develop (cardiac cachexia), it has only recently been stressed that more subtle evidence of muscle wasting may be both common and functionally important in chronic heart failure. If less muscle is available to do the work of the limb then each fibre will be more easily fatigued, be able to accept a lower total blood flow, and will appear metabolically more stressed and require anaerobic metabolism at an earlier point in exercise. These findings have all been taken as indicators of a deficiency in blood and oxygen delivery, rather than the alternative explanation that there simply is too little muscle for exercise to be performed efficiently.

Function

In chronic heart failure there is a reduction in the peak strength of both small and large muscle groups. In the case of the small muscles of the hand this clearly cannot be due solely to a reduced cardiac pumping capacity because of their tiny blood flow requirement. This suggests that there may be inherent defects in the quality of the muscle itself, but given the difficulty of exactly matching for active muscle bulk the difference may, however, be partly a reflection of muscle wasting.

In addition to reduced peak strength, there is an early fatiguability of muscle in heart failure. As a result, patients frequently complain that muscle fatigue is the major limitation to the performance of their daily tasks, and weakness and fatigue may both contribute to reduced physical activity that may induce physical deconditioning and further muscle wasting and dysfunction.

Metabolism

Skeletal muscle metabolism during exercise has been investigated by magnetic resonance spectroscopy. This technique allows an exploration of the rate of utilization of high-energy phosphate bonds associated with phosphocreatine and of intracellular pH, and through these the efficiency of aerobic and anaerobic metabolism within the muscle. These experiments have shown that there is an early depletion of phosphocreatine, an early acidification and accumulation of inorganic phosphate, a reduction in the rate of resynthesis of phosphocreatine, and in the removal of adenosine diphosphate (**ADP**). These changes cannot be explained by the acute effect of impaired blood flow, because the difference between normal controls and heart failure patients is seen even when both groups perform exercise in ischaemic conditions produced by regional circulatory occlusion. The metabolic abnormalities described by magnetic resonance spectroscopy probably reflect alterations in the oxidative enzymatic content of skeletal muscle described in biopsy studies. The causes of these metabolic changes are not understood, but it has been estimated that muscle wasting alone cannot explain them, because the half-time of ADP removal is independent of both the workload per unit muscle mass and the blood flow.

The only treatment that has been definitely shown to correct these metabolic abnormalities is physical exercise conditioning of the muscle, either localized or general. The time course of the possible correction of the muscle changes after cardiac transplantation has not been determined, nor has any definite effect of ACE-inhibitor treatment been described.

Autonomic and neuroendocrine systems

Much has been written about the importance of neuroendocrine activation in chronic heart failure, partly because of the established benefits of blocking two aspects of this with the ACE inhibitors and β-blockers. There is an undoubted activation of neuroendocrine systems involved in the 'fight or flight' reaction. These probably evolved, in a teleological sense, as a way of compensating for blood or fluid loss or sodium depletion, but in heart failure, although initially helping to support the circulation, continuous activation may be harmful. The neuroendocrine systems involved include the renin–angiotensin–aldosterone system, the sympathetic nervous system, and the vasopressin system, as well as that of the counteracting cardiac natriuretic peptides. Simultaneously with neuroendocrine activation there is a reduction in vasodilator influences and in vagal tone which, when maintained chronically, may be harmful. Adverse consequences have been described such as organ hypoperfusion, myocardial toxicity, an increased susceptibility to ventricular arrhythmias, and a possible progression of the underlying disease process, whether it be myocardial ischaemia or cardiomyopathy.

The renin–angiotensin–aldosterone system

In untreated heart failure there is mild activation of the renin system, which is dramatically augmented by the first use of diuretics in the treatment of the heart failure. After that there is a reasonable relationship between the severity of the heart failure and further increases in circulating renin and angiotensin II levels. In addition, all the components of the circulating renin–angiotensin system also exist in tissue sites and there is probably activation of these local tissue systems in the heart, kidney, brain, and blood vessel walls. The role and effects of these in health and in the progression of heart failure are unknown, but some of the beneficial effects of ACE inhibition described in other sections stress how important these systems may be in the syndrome of chronic heart failure.

At an organ level, the effects of elevated local and circulating angiotensin II can be very profound. In the kidney it can cause either a preservation of glomerular filtration rate (**GFR**) in the presence of low arterial pressure, or a reduced renal blood flow and GFR if the kidney is already dependent on angiotensin II-mediated efferent arteriolar constriction to maintain an adequate filtration pressure in the glomerulus. Such dependence can be seen in renal artery stenosis. In the heart, local increases in angiotensin II can cause coronary vasoconstriction and toxic effects on the myocytes, and in the periphery local angiotensin activation can elevate systemic vascular resistance and thereby increase the afterload to the failing heart.

The clinical effects of inhibition of the renin–angiotensin–aldosterone system are dealt with more fully in other chapters, but it is important to note that we still do not know how they mediate their beneficial effects, whether by reduced circulating or tissue-based angiotensin II, or by augmentation of bradykinin or other kinin systems.

The autonomic nervous system

Early in the progression of heart failure from mild asymptomatic left ventricular dysfunction to the full clinical picture of chronic heart failure there is an activation of the sympathetic nervous system and a concomitant reduction in resting vagal tone. These changes are further enhanced by the administration of diuretics. There is no clear mechanism for either the activation of the sympathetic system in mild heart failure, or to explain why the activation should persist and progress in the chronic syndrome. In severe heart failure there may be a reduction in blood pressure, but this is often the result of aggressive therapy. By contrast, in asymptomatic left ventricular dysfunction, or mild heart failure, sympathetic activation commences at a stage when there is no perceptible change in blood pressure. It has been said that the activation is secondary to the withdrawal of the chronic sympathoinhibitory effects of the arterial baroreflexes, but there are flaws in this explanation. Even complete denervation of the baroreceptors does not lead to such persistent sympathoexcitation as seen in chronic heart failure, and in heart failure it also begs the question as to what caused the baroreceptor inhibition in the first place. If it is thought to be sympathetic activation, as seems likely, then we are left with a circular argument. No significant sympathoexcitatory influence has been demonstrated to underlie the very high levels of sympathetic tone in established heart failure. Two candidate mechanisms that have received little attention are the skeletal muscle ergoreceptor system and an interaction between the arterial chemoreflex and the baroreflex and cardiovascular autonomic centres. Both the ergoreflex and the chemoreflex cause sympathetic activation and may be abnormal throughout the progression of chronic heart failure.

The investigation of sympathovagal balance is limited by the lack of precise and quantifiable methods. Apart from a measurement of plasma norepinephrine (noradrenaline) levels there is no easily available clinical test for the activity of the sympathetic limb, and for the vagal limb the problem is even more difficult. Analysis of variations of heart rate variability has identified characteristic frequency harmonic oscillations in cardiovascular parameters, the relative oscillatory power of which show promise in the estimation of sympathovagal balance. The pattern in heart failure is very abnormal, with a dramatic reduction in total heart rate variability and a selective loss of the higher frequency (predominantly vagally mediated) rhythm characteristic of respiratory sinus arrhythmia, and a relative preservation of low- and very low-frequency rhythms which have their genesis more in the action of the sympathetic (low frequency) and renin–angiotensin or chemoreflex systems (very low frequency). Analysis of total heart rate variability, and in particular of individual frequency components, has shown that the pattern seen in heart failure is one associated with a high risk for the development of unstable ventricular arrhythmias and cardiac sudden death, although why this should be the case is not certain.

Beta-receptor function

With chronic sympathetic activation there is depletion of myocardial catecholamine stores and a downregulation of β1-receptors on the myocardium. There is also a decoupling of receptors from the postreceptor response, all of which lead to a loss of myocardial response to increased sympathetic drive. Clinically this manifests as chronotropic incompetence, loss of response to sympathomimetic stimulation, and a further impairment of exercise tolerance. Specific treatments are few, but there has been some improvement after β-blockade, ACE inhibition, and even very shortduration intermittent sympathomimetic stimulation.

The natriuretic peptide systems

The atria and ventricles contain granulated cells that release peptides, atrial natriuretic peptide (**ANP** or **ANF**) and brain natriuretic peptide (**BNP**), in response to stretch. In addition, the vasculature of the heart and other organs is the site of production of a closely related peptide, C-type natriuretic peptide (**CNP**), the physiological role and normal modulation of which is less clearly understood. These peptides are natriuretic agents that also relax peripheral vasculature and thereby oppose the actions of the sympathetic and renin–angiotensin systems. There is an increased release of these peptides in chronic heart failure associated with cardiac enlargement, but the significance of the increased plasma levels is uncertain. The use of exogenous ANP or neutral endopeptidase inhibitors, to increase endogenous levels by inhibiting the breakdown of these peptides, have produced only minor natriuretic and haemodynamic effects in heart failure, although the effects may be greater if administered on the background of inhibition of the opposing renin–angiotensin–aldosterone system. BNP has been shown to be quite accurate in determining the degree of systolic dysfunction of the heart in selected hospital series, and there is such a close relationship between myocardial stretch and BNP release that estimation of BNP has been shown to quite accurately predict in population surveys which patients are likely to be diagnosed as suffering from heart failure.

The vasopressin system

Elevated plasma concentrations of vasopressin, also known as antidiuretic hormone (**ADH**), are found in chronic heart failure, but the importance of vasopressin in the pathophysiology of the condition is not certain. Its actions are a combination of haemodynamic, with profound arteriolar vasoconstriction increasing peripheral resistance, and renal, with an action on the collecting duct to increase reduce free water reabsorption and thereby cause antidiuresis.

Other hormonal systems

Abnormalities have been described in several other hormonal systems in chronic heart failure, but the significance of these changes is uncertain. Thyroid hormone metabolism is deranged, with an increase in reverse T3 similar to that seen in the so-called 'sick cell syndrome'. Plasma insulin levels are increased in heart failure, whether of ischaemic, valvular, or idiopathic aetiology, and this is associated with a decreased sensitivity to the glucose transport effects of insulin. Alterations in sex hormones and growth factors are likely in advanced cardiac cachexia, but to what extent these are specific to the syndrome of chronic heart failure is uncertain.

The kidney

Control of fluid and electrolyte balance is impaired in heart failure. This is due to the reduced renal perfusion pressure in advanced disease, to the effects on intrarenal haemodynamics of the neuroendocrine activation described above, and to the effects and side-effects of commonly prescribed medications.

Fluid overload and hence oedema is common in heart failure, and electrolyte disturbances are both common and important. In mild heart failure fluid retention is due to the effects of aldosterone, vasopressin and catecholaminergic renal vasoconstriction. The kidney itself is partly a passive organ, responding to neuroendocrine activation outside its control, but it is also an active endocrine and autocrine organ responding to reduced renal perfusion pressure in heart failure.

The renin–angiotensin–aldosterone system

The juxtaglomerular apparatus, adjacent to the distal convoluted tubule, senses a reduction in the rate of delivery of sodium to the distal tubule and releases renin in response, thereby playing an important part in the activation of the circulating renin–angiotensin system described above. Activation leads, via aldosterone, to an increased reabsorption of sodium in the distal renal tubules, and an additional effect of angiotensin on thirst and possibly salt hunger completes the response, all encouraging the retention of sodium and water in the body.

All the components of the renin–angiotensin system also exist within the kidney and there can be local autocrine activation with important effects on intrarenal haemodynamics. These may either increase or decrease GFR, depending on the level of renal perfusion pressure and other factors operating on the kidney, such as the renal sympathetic nerves and circulating vasoactive factors.

The kallikrein–kinin system

This second autocrine system of the kidney is less well studied because of the short half-life of some of its active components and the difficulty in isolating them. In simple terms the kinin system appears complementary to the renin–angiotensin system, causing vasodilatation where the latter causes vasoconstriction. It is also thought to be involved in the control of renal tubular function, but its precise role in heart failure and the effects of ACE inhibitors (which also block the enzyme that breaks down bradykinin) are unknown.

The cardiorenal syndrome

Some of the causes of heart failure, most notably atherosclerotic arterial disease and hypertension, can have direct effects on the kidney. This is one reason for an increased coexistence of cardiac and renal failure. Other less common conditions that can cause both organs to fail include amyloid, sarcoid, and certain vasculitidies. A more common finding is that an apparently reasonably well-functioning kidney can progressively fail in the presence of severe heart failure. This is partly the effect of hypovolaemia and low blood pressure (prerenal azotaemia), but is also due to the circulating and intrarenal neurohormonal systems described above, and the renal effects of drugs used in treatment. The net effect is that renal failure is an extremely common and clinically important complication of severe heart failure. Aggressive diuretic therapy can precipitate a significant worsening of renal function that then blunts their effectiveness. The ACE inhibitors usually lead to a small increase in serum creatinine concentrations, but in a few patients they can precipitate clinically important renal failure.

Electrolyte disturbances

Electrolyte disturbances are not common in untreated heart failure, except when this is severe. There is an initial retention of sodium and a loss of potassium due to the effects of increased levels of aldosterone. Later, and especially after diuretics have been administered, there is a further depletion of potassium and also of magnesium. Both these disturbances may be important in generating cardiac arrhythmias, especially in digoxin toxicity. A dilutional hyponatraemia can develop in patients with severe heart failure: this can be both difficult to manage and is a poor prognostic sign.

The careful management of fluid and electrolyte balance in patients with heart failure can lessen renal complications and improve both symptoms and prognosis. There is no simple therapeutic regime that will ensure this, just careful repeated clinical examination and monitoring, judicious use of drugs, with knowledge of their potential side-effects.

Haematological system

Haemoglobin

Increased haemoglobin content has been described as an adaptive response in heart failure. This may be secondary to chronic tissue hypoxia, perhaps most importantly in the kidney in which it may stimulate an increase in erythropoietin production. It is doubtful if the increase in haemoglobin is very effective in increasing oxygen delivery to the tissues, for if the haematocrit increases too much then the resulting increased whole blood viscosity will reduce net tissue perfusion by increasing the resistance to blood flow. In more severe chronic heart failure anaemia becomes more common. It is similar to the anaemia seen in other chronic illnesses.

Other haematological changes

Impaired clotting factor production can result from hepatic dysfunction (see below) and resulting abnormalities in haemostatic function are not uncommon. The white blood cell count may be mildly elevated in heart failure as part of a more generalized, but poorly understood, immune activation.

Other organ systems

The liver

In heart failure the liver can be affected by an increased venous back-pressure, by an impaired arterial supply, and by the metabolic complications of the syndrome. The underlying process that leads to heart failure, for example alcohol excess or haemachromatosis, can also affect it.

The most common hepatic abnormality in chronic heart failure is congestion due to the effects of right heart failure on venous pressures. This leads to increased venous engorgement of the liver and can result in a noticeable increase in hepatic size, local tenderness, and minor derangements in liver function, causing modest increases in transaminase levels in its mildest form. In more severe cases, nausea and right hypochondrial discomfort develop, and in severe cases jaundice, impaired albumin and clotting factor production, and malabsorption of fats may result. These changes can have clinically important effects on clotting, especially as warfarin is commonly prescribed, and also on the hepatic metabolism of certain drugs. The nausea and malabsorption can worsen the catabolic state of the patient and can contribute to the wasting seen in cardiac cachexia. There is no specific treatment for this complication of chronic heart failure, other than the correct dosage of diuretics and the maximization of cardiac function with vasodilators.

Gastrointestinal tract

This is mainly affected by the increased venous pressure of right heart failure. Intestinal mucosal oedema can contribute to malabsorption and possibly nausea. Cardiac conditions are also associated with a higher rate of intestinal angiodysplasia: this can lead to recurrent blood loss, which can be a considerable management problem in the patient who requires anticoagulation.

Central nervous system

Certain conditions that cause heart failure can also produce neurological effects: these include alcoholism, amyloid, and heavy metal poisoning. Apart from the abnormalities of autonomic and neuroendocrine function described earlier, specific neural complications of heart failure are not common.

Immune function

Immune abnormalities in heart failure include both an excess of proinflammatory cytokines and a deficiency of inhibitory and immunomodulatory cytokines. Some cytokines are released in excessive amounts in both acute heart failure and in cases of relapsing or severe heart failure. Important amongst these is tumour necrosis factor-alpha (**TNF-α**), important because it has been shown to produce harmful effects that are common in chronic heart failure. These include endothelial dysfunction, myocyte depression, necrosis and apoptosis (programmed cell death), and loss of skeletal muscle mass. This cytokine has been implicated in the generation of severe wasting, both in cancer-related cachexia and in the syndrome of cardiac cachexia. Although the exact pathogenic mechanisms for the high cytokine levels in chronic heart failure are unknown, several theories have been proposed. These include the possibility that the failing heart itself is a site of production, or that recurrent bacterial loads due to bowel-wall oedema and bacterial-product translocation to the circulation cause an endotoxaemia that is known to be able to stimulate cytotoxic cytokine release. TNF-α has the properties to be harmful in heart failure and studies are underway to evaluate whether antitumour necrosis-factor strategies, such as the use of monoclonal antibodies or subantibody fusion-protein fragments, which neutralize tumour necrosis factor, would benefit the clinical course of patients with advanced chronic heart failure.

Cause of non-cardiac pathophysiology in heart failure

The changes described in different organ systems as part of the syndrome of chronic heart failure remain largely unexplained. We have proposed a 'muscle hypothesis' in which we explain the generation of many of these abnormalities via the combined effect of physical deconditioning and metabolic dysfunction, combining a release of catabolic factors with a loss of normal anabolic function. Figure 1 describes the general pathway by which these changes could lead to skeletal and respiratory muscle abnormalities, and via these to fatigue, dyspnoea, exercise limitation, and sympathoexcitation.

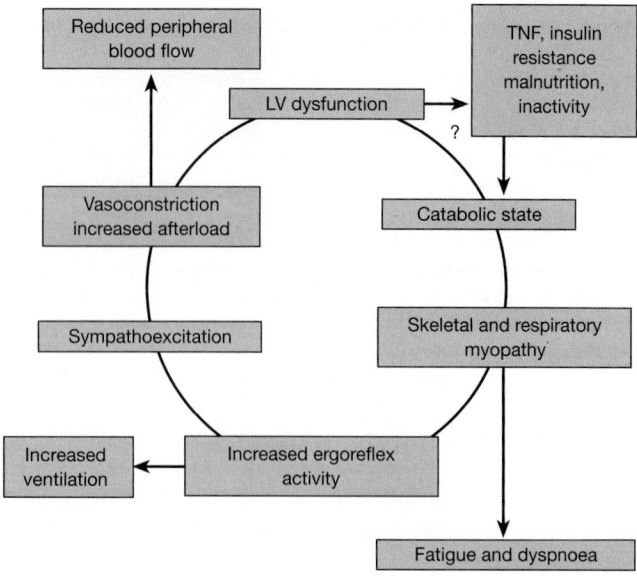

Fig. 1 The Muscle hypothesis in chronic heart failure. A proposal to explain the genesis and effects of several components of the non-cardiac pathophysiology of heart failure. As proposed by Coats *et al.* 1996. TNF, tumour necrosis factor.

Clinical assessment

The assessment of a patient with heart failure requires a careful history and examination, both at initial presentation and when assessing progress and response to treatment. Confirmation of heart failure can be aided by chest radiography, echocardiography, and, in selected cases, by cardiac catheterization, radionuclide ventriculography, and other imaging modalities. Invasive haemodynamic monitoring has a role in the assessment of acute severe heart failure. The use of a biochemical test (such as estimation of brain natriuretic peptide, BNP) to detect heart failure shows promise, but is not yet recommended in routine clinical practice.

Cardiopulmonary exercise testing with respiratory gas analysis can help to establish the cause of symptoms in patients with coexisting heart and lung disease, and to determine whether heart failure is causing the symptoms limiting the patient. When the respiratory exchange ratio (CO_2 produced per unit of oxygen consumed) exceeds 1.0, muscle metabolism has become anaerobic, indicating that a point of limiting cardiac reserve has been approached. If it does not exceed 1.0 at peak exercise then the true cardiac limitation cannot be assessed. Significant hypoxaemia and/or hypercapnia on exercise are rare in non-oedematous chronic heart failure, and when present suggests the limiting factor is pulmonary or (less commonly) a right to left shunt.

Regular assessment of the severity of heart failure is usually made by a history of symptomatic limitation and by clinical examination. The occasional use of chest radiography, echocardiography, and cardiopulmonary exercise testing can also help. Repeated haemodynamic monitoring has little role in chronic heart failure. Whether monitoring levels of plasma norepinephrine (noradrenaline) or atrial natriuretic peptides would materially assist in clinical management is uncertain: regular assessment of clinical biochemistry is certainly essential.

Symptoms

Heart failure is defined as symptomatic left ventricular dysfunction. As a result classical symptoms must be present to make the diagnosis. These most commonly are dyspnoea or fatigue, but initial presentation can be collapse, syncope, oedema, chest pain, or palpitations (Table 2).

Table 2 Symptoms of heart failure

Major symptoms
Fatigue, dyspnoea, and ankle oedema

Minor symptoms
Nocturia, urinary frequency, chest discomfort, or picked up at screening

Clinical examination

The physical examination of any patient with suspected heart failure is important. It can be a way of detecting the cause of the heart failure, such as the detection of aortic stenosis, leading to a definitive treatment option. Most cases of treated heart failure do not demonstrate florid signs such as seen in acute or decompensated heart failure, hence skilled clinical examination is necessary to obtain all the available clues as to cause, severity, and complicating factors (Table 3).

Investigations

Investigations may be necessary to confirm the diagnosis of heart failure, to establish the cause, and to stratify for the risk of complications or deterioration. A chest radiograph, an electrocardiogram, and an assessment of full blood count, urea, and electrolytes are essential in all cases of suspected heart failure. The electrocardiogram may give specific evidence of ischaemia/infarction, left ventricular hypertrophy, arrhythmia, and other causes of pathological Q-waves, and can combined with stress testing to detect reversible myocardial ischaemia.

Many studies have demonstrated the inaccuracy of diagnosis and assessment of the cause of heart failure in primary-care settings without the use of more specialized investigations, with up to one-third of cases being misclassified. As a result it is now a recommendation that all suspected cases of heart failure should have, if at all possible with local resources, an echocardiogram to assess the nature and extent of ventricular dysfunction and to detect those causes of heart failure identifiable by echocardiography. It can be used to detect and grade valvular disease, for the differentiation of a globally impaired left ventricle (for example, dilated cardiomyopathy) from segmental dysfunction (for example, ischaemic heart disease), and may also reveal ventricular hypertrophy, aneurysms, amyloid and other infiltrates, and specific forms of cardiomyopathy.

Specific blood tests can be used to check for certain rare causes of cardiac failure: hypocalcaemic cardiomyopathy; thyroid heart disease (hyper- or hypothyroidism); iron storage diseases; anaemia; heavy metal poisons; amyloid (serum electrophoresis); and sarcoid (serum ACE). Occasionally coronary angiography, and rarely ventricular biopsy, may be indicated in cases where the presentation is at a young age or specific features suggest a high likelihood of a treatable condition.

Certain investigations may be useful in assessing the severity of ventricular dysfunction in addition to or as alternatives to echocardiography, for

Table 3 Signs of heart failure

Acute heart failure

Signs of fluid retention:	oedema, raised JVP, lung crepitations
Signs of impaired perfusion:	cold clammy skin, low blood pressure
Signs of ventricular dysfunction:	displaced apex, right ventricular heave, third and/or fourth heart sound, functional mitral or tricuspid regurgitation, tachycardia

Chronic heart failure
Can be free of objective signs, but also can include all the signs of acute heart failure with, in addition, skeletal muscle wasting and cachexia

Signs of underlying disorder
Valvular disease, atherosclerotic vascular disease, severe hypertension, severe anaemia or volume overload, e.g. AV shunt, pathological arrhythmia, evidence of generalized myopathy or poisoning

JVP, jugular venous pressure; AV, arteriovenous.

Box 1 Treatment of chronic heart failure

General	No added salt	Treat hypertension
	Maintain optimal weight	Detect alcohol abuse
	Stop smoking	Prevent coronary disease
	Encourage exercise	
Mild	Thiazide/loop diuretic	β-blocker
	ACE inhibitor	
	Digoxin if atrial fibrillation	
Moderate	Loop diuretic	β-blocker
	ACE inhibitor	
	Combine diuretics	
Severe	Increase loop diuretic	Spironolactone
	Combine diuretics	? β-blocker
	Metolazone	? digoxin
	ACE inhibitor	Transplant

example rest or exercise radionuclide ventriculography. Monitoring by 24-h Holter electrocardiography to detect ventricular arrhythmias and blood tests for associated renal or liver dysfunction or electrolyte disturbances can be used to give a rough guide to prognosis, although this is rarely reliable on an individual patient basis.

Other specialized investigations such as cardiopulmonary exercise testing, CT or MR scanning, cardiac catheterization, and myocardial biopsies are covered in other chapters to which the reader is referred for more detailed explanation.

Treatment

The major elements of treatment of heart failure are listed in Boxes 1 and 2. This has undergone a revolution in the last two decades, with substantial treatment efficacy established first for the ACE inhibitors and more latterly for β-blockers (a group previously considered absolutely contraindicated in heart failure) and the aldosterone antagonist spironolactone.

Diuretics

Diuretics remain the mainstay of the management of oedema in heart failure and are often the first agents to be used in new cases. This is not because their role for this indication has been proven, but rather they are used to treat what is frequently the first manifestation of heart failure, peripheral or pulmonary oedema. In acute heart failure intravenous loop diuretics lead

Box 2 Options in the treatment of severe chronic heart failure

1.	Drugs	Diuretics	Loop, thiazide, and potassium-sparing combination
		ACE inhibitors	
		Vasodilators	Nitrates, hydralazine
		Positive inotropes	Digoxin, IV intermittent inotrope
		Anticoagulants	
		β-blockers, calcium antagonists, or anti-arrhythmics	
2.	Implantable cardiac defibrillator—ICD		
3.	Haemofiltration		
4.	Peritoneal dialysis or haemodialysis		
5.	Aortic balloon pump or ventricular assist device		
6.	Transplantation or cardiomyoplasty		

ACE, angiotensin-converting enzyme; IV, intravenous.

to a dramatic and rapid improvement in condition, and in almost all patients with moderate or severe heart failure diuretics will be essential for adequate symptom control. Concern has been expressed about the potential adverse effects of diuretic agents, including activation of the sympathetic and renin–angiotensin systems, but until an alternative mechanism for the control of oedema fluid is achieved there remains no viable alternative.

In the modern era of evidence-based therapies diuretic use remains an example of the art of medicine surviving despite a marked lack of proof. No single placebo-controlled trial of a loop diuretic has proven a convincing improvement in either mortality or morbidity rates: the treatment was introduced and popularized before the modern era of randomized controlled trials. The only significant treatment trial of diuretics was with a low dose of the weak diuretic spironolactone 25–50 mg per day, which showed a significant reduction in total mortality in severe heart failure in the RALES study published in 1999. This effect was probably due to the inhibition of the harmful effects of the neurohormonal factor aldosterone than to the diuretic effect of spironolactone.

Initially the thiazide diuretics may be sufficient in patients with mild heart failure, but in more severe cases of heart failure one of the loop diuretics—furosemide (frusemide), bumetanide, or torasemide—will be necessary. These are very familiar agents, particularly furosemide, but there remains some confusion about the best mode of treatment. Furosemide and bumetanide both give an acute and relatively short-acting diuresis that some patients find disabling. Others actually prefer this, as they can time their outings to avoid periods of diuresis. The newer torasemide has a much more prolonged action over 24 h and the increase in urine flow is said to be much less obvious to the patient.

Initially 40 mg of furosemide or its equivalent (about 1 mg of bumetanide) may be sufficient to control oedema, but some patients will need much higher doses (e.g. furosemide 80 or 120 mg twice daily) for oedema control. A better alternative to increasing the dose of loop diuretic is to use combination diuretics by adding agents with different modes of action, such as amiloride, thiazides, or spironolactone, or all three together. This is often far more effective than even extremely high-dose intravenous loop diuretics. The potassium-sparing drugs have the added advantage of ameliorating the loss of potassium produced by the other agents, although this is now less of a problem because the majority of patients with heart failure will be taking an ACE inhibitor, which has potassium-sparing effects.

In an acute exacerbation, switching to intravenous administration can boost response, as can a short period of bed rest, or the use of a short period of positive inotropic therapy with dopamine or dobutamine, especially as these have some renal vasodilator action.

It should also never be forgotten that diuretic therapy should go hand in hand with sodium and fluid restriction. The 'Chinese take-away syndrome', due to the effects of an acute sodium load and water retention, describes an episode of acute pulmonary oedema occurring several hours after a high sodium meal in a previously stable patient with chronic heart failure. This should remind us of the effects of excessive sodium intake.

In patients with severe heart failure fluid restriction may be necessary, but care should be taken not to produce dehydration and further deterioration in renal function. In the long term, fluid restriction should not be to less than 1500 ml per day.

Metolazone is a thiazide-like diuretic with a profound diuretic action when given on the background of loop-diuretic therapy. This combination therapy can be very powerful, often considerably stronger than the intravenous administration of furosemide alone, even in high doses. As little as 2.5 or 5 mg of metolazone given in this way can lead to several litres of extra urine output; this should never be started for the first time in an outpatient, but should be reserved for specialist hospital use, except under special instruction. Profound electrolyte disturbance can accompany this diuresis. A small number of outpatients with severe oedematous heart failure require chronic administration of metolazone, but often only 2.5 mg on alternate days or once or twice a week may be needed. Care should be taken

to monitor electrolytes, urea, and creatinine very carefully in patients so treated.

Digoxin

Digoxin is the oldest drug therapy available for heart failure, and it still retains a place as the only safe chronically administered positive inotropic agent. Its use in patients with sinus rhythm remains controversial, for although it is considered as first-line standard therapy in the United States and many European countries, cardiologists in the United Kingdom point to the lack of any data demonstrating its long-term benefits in a large prospective placebo-controlled trial. The only definitive large-scale trial of digoxin against placebo, the DIG trial, showed no significant effect on mortality, despite a significant reduction in the number of hospital admissions. With its narrow therapeutic window the routine use of digoxin in patients with sinus rhythm remains a matter of debate. In severe heart failure, where the patient remains very symptomatic, it may be worth trying: some respond with an improvement in symptomatic status. (See Chapter 15.5.1 for further information.)

Direct-acting vasodilators

The major agents in this class in regular use for heart failure are the combination of hydralazine and isosorbide dinitrate. Although an advance at the time, their use has been largely supplanted by the more effective ACE inhibitors. Other agents such a prazosin have proved less effective, and the calcium-antagonist vasodilators, particularly the short-acting dihydropyridine group, such as nifedipine, are significantly negatively inotropic and can worsen heart failure. Longer acting agents that cause less reflex tachycardia appear to be preferable, with amlodipine in particular seeming to be at least safe in chronic heart failure if its use is needed for its antianginal profile. The routine use of vasodilators in chronic heart failure cannot be supported by clinical trial data. (See Chapter 15.5.1 for further discussion.)

Angiotensin-converting enzyme (ACE) inhibitors

In heart failure

The introduction of ACE inhibitors has had a profound effect on the treatment of heart failure. Their benefits are not restricted to patients with end-stage heart failure, but extend also to patients with mild to moderate heart failure, and even to modifying the progression of the disease in patients with asymptomatic left ventricular dysfunction or extensive left ventricular dysfunction after myocardial infarction. The ACE inhibitor enalapril was the first agent to be shown to dramatically reduce mortality in severe heart failure: 253 patients in the CONSENSUS I study were randomly allocated to enalapril or control and, with an overall 6-month mortality in the placebo group of 44 per cent, there was a significant 40 per cent reduction in mortality in those randomized to enalapril. These patients were in end-stage heart failure, symptomatic at rest or on minimal effort, and this treatment was a clear therapeutic breakthrough, so much so that almost immediately ACE inhibitors became standard therapy in this situation.

Within a few years of the CONSENSUS I study similar evidence of benefit was shown for ACE inhibitors in the treatment of mild to moderate heart failure (New York Heart Association, NYHA class II and III), patients in whom moderate exertion led to symptoms, but in whom the 1-year mortality rate was 10 to 20 per cent rather than the 50 per cent or more of the CONSENSUS I study patients. Despite the lower overall mortality rate in these patients, the ACE inhibitor enalapril produced further significant reductions in mortality. The SOLVD treatment study looked at 2569 patients with mild to moderate heart failure randomized to enalapril or control and showed a statistically significant 16 per cent reduction in mortality. The V.HefT II study looked at 804 patients randomized between enalapril and the vasodilator combination of hydralazine and isosorbide dinitrate and found a significantly lower mortality with enalapril.

The prevention limb of the SOLVD trial, despite not showing any significant reduction in overall mortality, did show a reduction in the rate of progression of disease, with less new diagnoses of clinical heart failure, and a reduction in the rate of hospital admissions for heart failure. This suggests there may be both clinical and economic gains from the use of ACE inhibitors in this clinical situation.

See Chapter 15.5.1 for further discussion of the use of ACE inhibitors in heart failure.

After myocardial infarction

After a myocardial infarction the area of infarcted myocardium does not form a stable scar immediately, but rather undergoes a complex series of changes over weeks to months and even years (see Chapter 15.4.2). Some of these changes are beneficial and some are not, and this process may hold some of the clues to why patients after a myocardial infarction can develop heart failure months or even years later, without any evidence of further infarction.

In the first few days after the infarction there is an increased load on the residual myocardium, which undergoes compensatory hypertrophy, partly stimulated by activation of some of the neurohormonal pathways described earlier. The infarcted area is not protected from these influences, and as it is under increased mechanical stress as well, the overstimulation of the adjacent myocardium by the sympathetic and renin–angiotensin systems can lead to an even greater mechanical stress on the freshly infarcted region. These processes can lead to infarct expansion, a process whereby the infarcted wall is stretched and thinned by the mechanical stress exerted upon it, and to an apparent increase in the extent of infarcted myocardium expressed in absolute size or as a percentage of the total left ventricular wall. This should be distinguished from infarct extension, where previously living myocardium at the fringes of the infarcted area itself infarcts, leading to an increased size of wall motion abnormality.

Over a period of weeks to months and possibly years, a second process develops where the wall of the whole myocardium becomes thinned and enlarged. This affects the residual myocardium and involves realignment between myocytes, a process called 'cell slippage', leading to a progressive alteration in the shape of the ventricle, not requiring any further episodes of infarction. The shape of the ventricle becomes more globular and enlarges and the ventricle is said to have 'remodelled'. Very good animal experimental data and observational data on patients have shown that this remodelling process precedes and predicts the development of heart failure, and that the administration of an ACE inhibitor could delay or prevent left ventricular remodelling and reduce mortality in this setting.

The first large trial reported orally was the CONSENSUS II study. This indicated a non-significant trend towards an adverse effect on mortality when enalapril was given to relatively high-risk patients recovering from infarction. Therapy was commenced with intravenous enalaprilat within 24 h of the infarct, and included subjects with quite low blood pressure at entry. The trial was terminated early with no definite effect on mortality. This trial was rapidly followed by the SAVE trial, which studied captopril in a target dose of 50 mg thrice daily in patients recovering from a myocardial infarction. Unlike the CONSENSUS II study the patients were recruited after the initial infarct-healing phase had been completed, after most infarct expansion and scar formation had begun, but before the later remodelling process had become established. The patients were all thoroughly investigated, including documentation of significantly impaired left ventricular function by a radionuclide ventriculogram ejection fraction of 40 per cent or less, and all had undergone correction of clinically important residual myocardial ischaemia by either angioplasty or bypass surgery prior to entry to the trial. A total of 2231 patients were randomized between 3 and 16 days after infarction to receive captopril or placebo and followed for 42 months. After the first 6 months of follow-up the survival curves for the two groups separated and at the end of the trial there was a significant 19 per cent reduction in total mortality; there was also a 22 per cent decrease in the rate of hospital admission for heart failure.

Following the SAVE trial there was rapid confirmation of its results. The AIRE study, co-ordinated from Leeds, recruited 2006 patients who had clinical evidence of transient heart failure after a myocardial infarction, including radiological evidence of pulmonary oedema or chest crepitations, or the presence of a third heart sound on auscultation. Patients were randomized to ramipril (5 mg twice daily) or placebo between 3 and 10 days postinfarction: there was a significant 27 per cent reduction in mortality at 15 months of follow-up. The survival benefit appeared to commence within the first few weeks of follow-up.

These beneficial effects have been confirmed with a number of ACE inhibitors in different trial settings. The overwhelming conclusion from these studies is that ACE inhibitors beneficially affect the recovery process after a myocardial infarction, and in the longer term reduce mortality by preventing the progression to heart failure. Based on available evidence, the vast majority of patients either with heart failure or at high risk of developing heart failure, should be on long-term ACE inhibitor therapy. These large trials have shown benefits postinfarction and in heart failure, with a variety of ACE inhibitors, including enalapril, captopril, ramipril, lisinopril, and trandolapril. It would seem a reasonable conclusion that the benefit of the ACE inhibitors is largely a class effect.

β-Blockers

This is an interesting therapeutic area because everything from total β-receptor antagonists (for example, metoprolol), through partial agonists (xamoterol), to totally positive agonists has been tried or suggested for the treatment of heart failure. Until recently β-blockers were routinely prohibited for patients with heart failure. However, the last few years have seen a sequence of well-designed randomized controlled trials that have demonstrated a profound reduction in mortality, improvement in left ventricular function, and a reduction in the need for hospital admission in patients with mild, moderate, and severe heart failure. This has been shown for metoprolol in a slow-release preparation, bisoprolol, and the combined β- and α-receptor antagonist carvedilol, but it is too early to say if the beneficial effects are a class effect.

The difficulty of using β-blockers in significant heart failure should not, however, be underestimated. Patients were carefully selected in the major trials, almost always stable outpatients at the time of treatment initiation, and with recent episodes of oedema or decompensation. β-Blockade was commenced at very low initial starting doses and increased slowly under careful observation. In addition, treatment was commenced and monitored by physicians expert in the care of patients with heart failure. Those with stable heart failure should not be denied the benefits of β-blockade, but only specialists in the care of patients with heart failure should start this therapy, which can sometimes be difficult. (See Chapter 15.5.1 for specific guidance.)

Antiarrhythmic agents

Ventricular arrhythmias are extremely common in those with heart failure. As sudden death is a common mode of demise for these patients it is tempting to think that antiarrhythmic therapy, which can suppress the ventricular arrhythmias, may reduce the incidence of sudden death. Unfortunately this approach has not proved to be effective, and many agents that have been tried appear to induce more sudden deaths than they prevent. The most promising drug is amiodarone, despite its formidable list of side-effects. The GESICA trial in South America, which included a high proportion of patients with Chagas' cardiomyopathy, even suggested a net reduction in mortality in heart failure patients regardless of the presence of ventricular arrhythmias, but subsequent trials in ischaemic left ventricular dysfunction failed to confirm this promise. By and large, unless symptomatic, non-sustained episodes of ventricular tachycardia are best left alone. The implantable defibrillator is more effective at reducing mortality in patients resuscitated from sudden death or those with frequent potential fatal ventricular tachycardia, but costs are high and they are not uniformly available to all patients who might benefit from their use. (See Chapter 15.6 for further discussion.)

Oral, positive inotropic agents

This group of drugs, including the phosphodiesterase inhibitors and calcium sensitizers, were heralded as a major advance when introduced into practice, but trial after trial comparing them against placebo have not only shown a loss of effect with time, but have suggested an increased mortality. With the exception of digoxin there is no safe, chronically administered, positively inotropic agent.

Anticoagulants and antiplatelet agents

There is clear evidence for the benefits of aspirin or other antiplatelet agents in patients recovering from a myocardial infarction. As most people with heart failure in the developed world appear to have extensive ischaemic heart disease, it is likely the majority will be treated with aspirin to reduce the chance of coronary arterial occlusion. Another indication for aspirin is in the prevention of cerebral embolism in chronic atrial fibrillation in patients with significantly impaired left ventricular function. Several studies have shown a positive effect of aspirin in this situation, although it is probably less effective than full anticoagulation with warfarin, although there are some patients in whom it would be preferable. This indication for aspirin would incorporate patients with dilated cardiomyopathy as well as those with extensive ischaemic heart disease. However, some as yet unconfirmed fears have arisen that aspirin may interfere with some of the beneficial effects of ACE inhibitors in heart failure, so it is not considered routine to use aspirin in all patients with this condition. Full anticoagulation is usually reserved for those with heart failure who also have chronic or regularly recurrent atrial fibrillation, who have suffered a prior thrombotic or embolic stroke, or who suffer from transient ischaemic attacks. (See Chapter 15.5.2 for further discussion.)

Angiotensin-II receptor antagonists

Following the great success of the angiotensin-converting enzyme inhibitors in heart failure, much was expected of a group of agents that specifically blocked the harmful effects of angiotensin-II at its main site of action, the AT-1 receptor. However, the trials published to date have failed to prove that these agents are superior to ACE inhibitors in terms of reducing mortality, nor can it yet be said with confidence whether they are as good as the older agents. They do appear to be better tolerated, with less likelihood of producing cough as a side-effect, but their role, if any, in the management of patients with heart failure remains unclear. The largest trial to date, ELITE-II, of approximately 2000 elderly patients with chronic heart failure, compared captopril 50 mg three times a day with losartan 50 mg once a day. There was no significant difference in mortality between the two treatments. The trial was not large enough to prove that the angiotensin-II receptor antagonist was equivalent or an alternative to the ACE inhibitors. (See Chapter 15.5.1 for further information.)

Non-pharmacological treatments

Patient education

Patients and their families are often confused and bewildered by the term 'heart failure'. Alternatives such as 'weak heart', 'congestion', or 'large heart' may be better at giving the correct impression as to the nature of the condition. In can be extremely useful for long-term adherence to treatment recommendations to spend some time explaining to the patient and partner some simple physiology of left ventricular dysfunction, the body's compensatory mechanisms, and why these lead to symptoms and signs that the patient may have already noted. The patient will then be much more aware of the need for diuretics and vasodilators, and the effects of alterations in fluid and salt intake, intercurrent illness, etc. This could improve oedema control and lessen the frequency with which a patient needs to attend the outpatient department or be admitted to hospital for stabilization. Simple measures such as information on low-salt diets, fluid restrictions, and monitoring daily weight at home can significantly improve long-term heart failure management.

Specialist heart failure clinics and outreach nursing services

Recent trials have suggested that there can be a reduction in the need for emergency hospital admissions if patients are enrolled into specialist services to help them, their relatives, and their general practitioners manage their heart failure after discharge from hospital. Important amongst these services is adequate education about the correct way to take their heart failure medication. Specialized nursing services with home visits and improved liaison between the primary care and secondary care of patients with heart failure appears to be particularly helpful in improving the quality of care.

Rest and exercise

There is very good evidence in acute heart failure, or in an acute decompensation in chronic heart failure, that bed rest can improve renal blood flow and the response to diuretics. This is presumably via a reduction in the level of stimulation of the sympathetic and renin–angiotensin systems. Admission to hospital for a few days' rest is thus a common treatment for heart failure, and one with a very long history. Initial enthusiasm for the benefits of longer periods of bed rest (weeks to months) as a management strategy for chronic heart failure and cardiomyopathy have not been borne out; in fact this practice is accompanied by the considerable and well-known complications of prolonged bed rest. On the contrary, benefits have been shown after exercise training in carefully selected patients with chronic heart failure. Improvements are seen in exercise tolerance, skeletal muscle and respiratory function, and in autonomic balance. This raises the possibility that profound physical deconditioning may be contributing to some of the pathophysiological changes described in the sections above. In a patient with stable chronic heart failure, with no evidence of exercise-induced ventricular arrhythmias, regular exercise should be encouraged rather than prohibited. The reader is referred to Chapter 15.5.3 for a discussion of the benefits that can be obtained from a careful and selected use of exercise training programmes in patients with stable chronic heart failure.

Other treatments

Cardiac transplantation and mechanical assist device therapies are described in Chapter 15.5.4.

Prognosis

In severe heart failure, where patients are symptomatic at rest (NYHA class IV), the prognosis is dire, with survival expected to be 1 year or less. The prognosis remains poor even in mild heart failure (class II–III), being comparable to that of many solid tissue malignancies with a mortality rate of between 20 and 30 per cent per year. Although major treatment advances have been achieved in mild, moderate, and even severe heart failure, these have led to only a very partial correction of the excess mortality associated with this condition.

Prognostic factors and markers

Many different parameters have been described as having prognostic value in patients with heart failure. It is important to differentiate between prognostic factors, which have a direct functional link to increased mortality,

Plates for Section 11
Chapter 11.5 The porphyrias

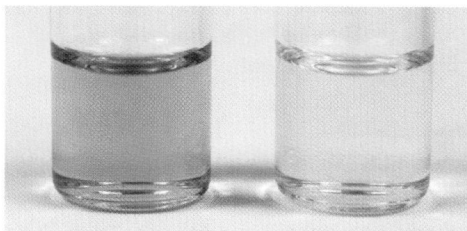

Plate 1 Urine from a patient with acute intermittent porphyria around the time of an acute attack (left); control urine (right). A positive reaction with Ehrlich's diazo reagent is shown in the patient following the addition of 50 μl of urine to 1 ml of 2 per cent acidic dimethyl benzaldehyde. Subsequent tests showed that the pink diazo adduct was insoluble in chloroform and other organic solvents indicating the presence of excess porphobilinogen. (Urobilinogen in excess may give a positive reaction with the diazo reagent but the product is readily extracted into organic solvents.)

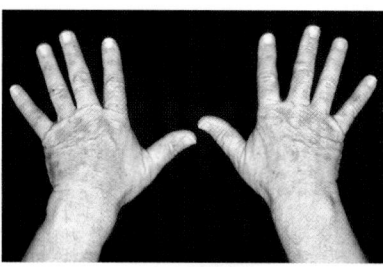

Plate 2 Porphyria cutanea tarda in a 60-year-old heterozygote for the *HFE* C282Y mutation. This man, a taxi driver, had noticed irritation after exposure of his hands to light transmitted through the windscreen. He had noticed fragility and blistering combined with pigmentary changes typical of this disorder. After treatment by controlled phlebotomy his skin complaint has regressed.

Plate 3 Fluorescent microscopy of an unstained blood film from a patient with erythropoietic protoporphyria. Note the red fluorescence of increased free protoporphyrin within individual young erythrocytes and reticulocytes.

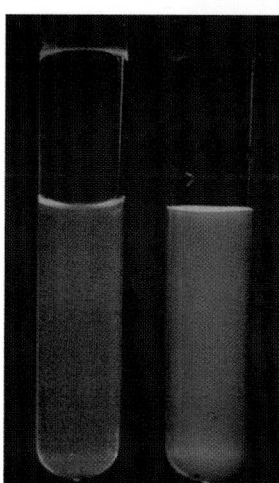

Plate 4 Examination of human plasma under long-wave ultraviolet light. Plasma on the right was obtained from a patient with protoporphyrin hepatopathy and greatly increased photosensitivity and is compared with plasma obtained from a healthy subject on the left. Note the bright red fluorescence due to the presence of high concentrations of free protoporphyrin. Maximum fluorescence was obtained by exposure to visible light in the violet and green–yellow spectral regions corresponding to the absorbance bands of porphyrins.

Chapter 11.6 Lipid and lipoprotein disorders

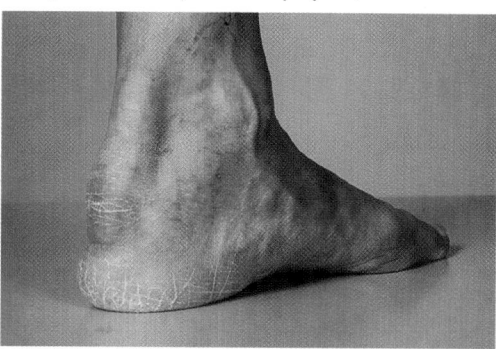

Plate 1 Achilles tendon xanthoma (heterozygous familial hypercholesterolaemia).

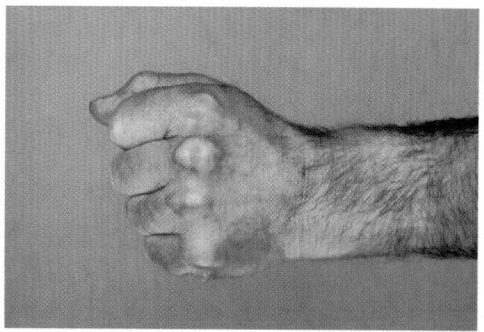

Plate 2 Tendon xanthomata on the dorsum of a hand (heterozygous familial hypercholesterolaemia).

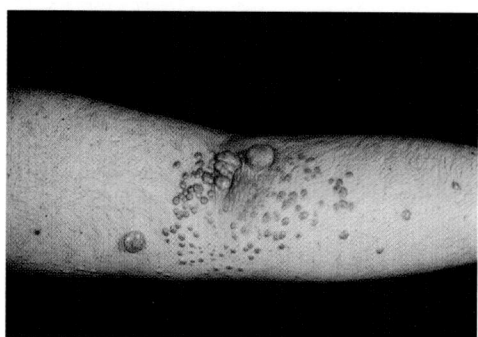

Plate 3 Eruptive and tuberous xanthomata on an arm (type III hyperlipoproteinaemia with marked hypertriglyceridaemia).

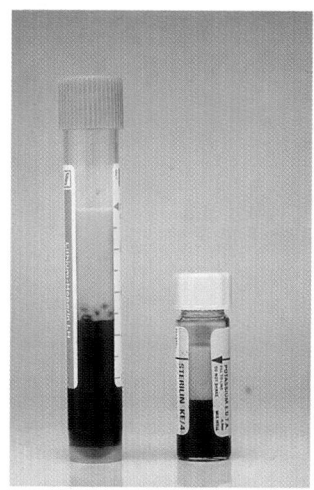

Plate 4 Milky plasma indicating marked hypertriglyceridaemia (blood samples from a patient with acute abdominal pain).

Chapter 11.7.1 Hereditary haemochromatosis

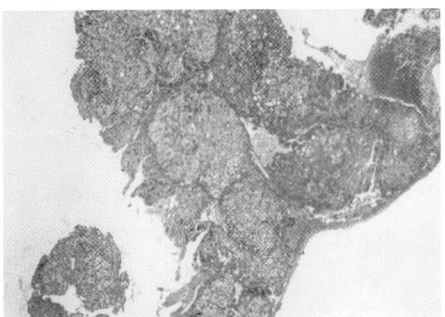

Plate 1 Low-power, needle-biopsy appearance of liver specimen stained with haematoxylin and eosin from a 67-year-old man with adult haemochromatosis due to homozygosity for the *C282Y* mutation. Note the large hyperplastic nodules and fibrosis.

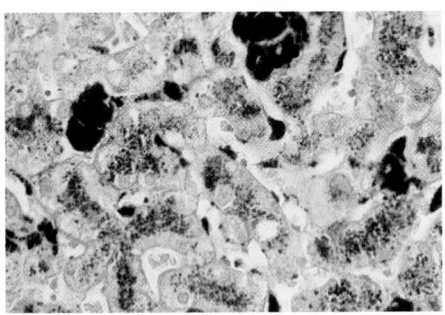

Plate 2 High-power micrograph of the liver biopsy specimen shown in Plate 1 stained with Perls' reagent. Note extensive deposits of ferric iron in all cell types including Kupffer cells, cells lining small biliary radicles, and in a punctate distribution within parenchymal hepatocytes. Liver cells are hyperplastic.

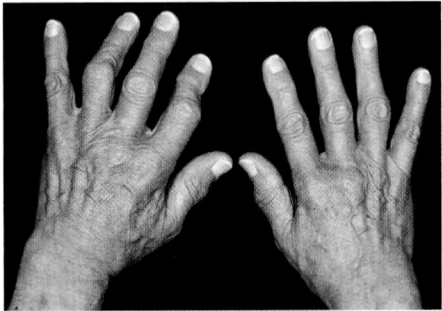

Plate 3 Arthropathy in a man with adult haemochromatosis forced to stop manual work because of painful arthritis especially in the second and third metacarpophalangeal joints; note increased skin pigmentation.

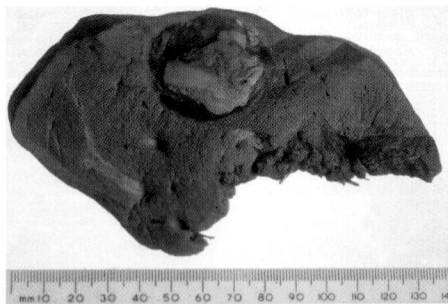

Plate 4 Adult haemochromatosis. Section of liver lobe after surgical resection to remove a primary hepatocellular carcinoma arising in an iron-loaded but, unusually, non-cirrhotic liver in this disorder. The patient, aged 62 years, had been partially treated by venesection but recently noticed increasing lethargy: a raised serum α-fetoprotein concentration led to the diagnosis; moderate histochemical evidence of iron storage was found in the non-malignant tissue excised at surgery.

Chapter 11.7.2 Wilson's disease, Menke's disease: inherited disorders of copper metabolism

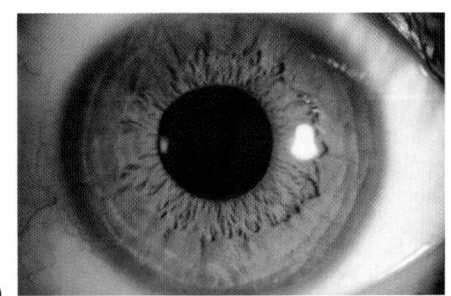

(a)

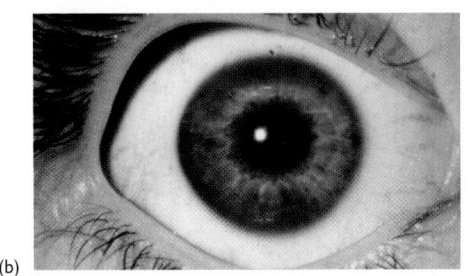

(b)

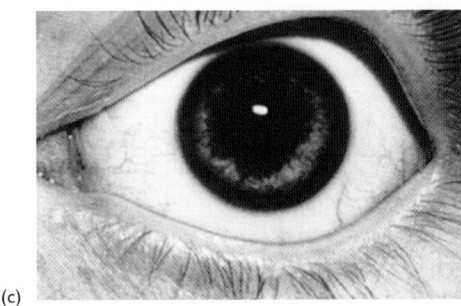

(c)

Plate 1 (a–c) Kayser–Fleischer ring in Wilson's disease.

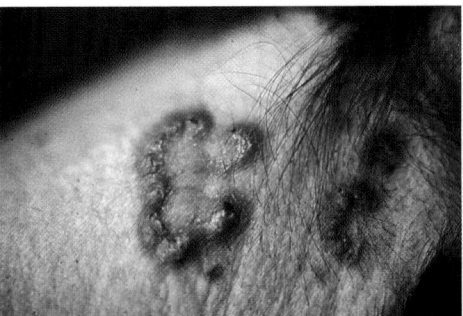

Plate 2 Penicillamine dermatopathy—elastosis perfringens serpiginosa.

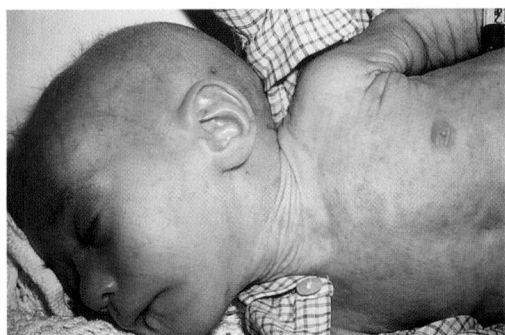

Plate 3 Appearance in Menkes' disease.

Chapter 11.8 Lysosomal storage diseases

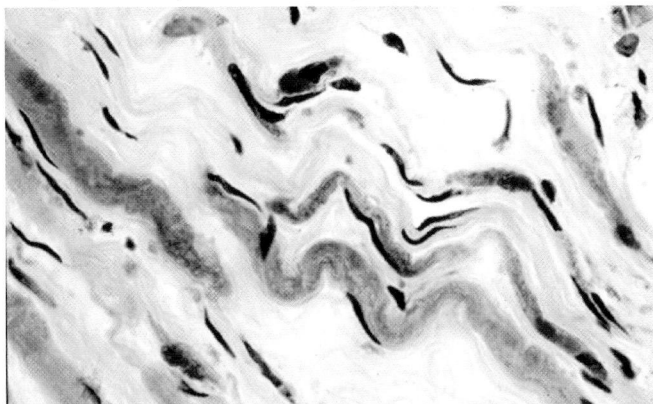

Plate 1 Sural nerve biopsy stained with toluidine blue from the patient shown in Plate 2 with metachromatic leucodystrophy. Note the brown-staining granular material within Schwann and perineurial macrophages typical of this disorder due to the deposition of the glycolipid sulphatide. (By courtesy of Dr J. Xuereb, Addenbrooke's Hospital).

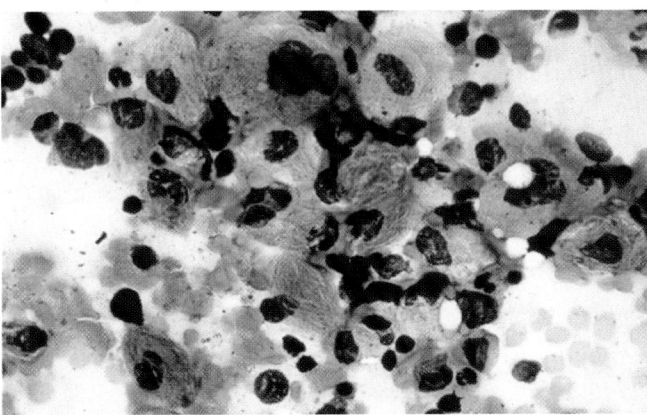

Plate 2 Light micrograph of a Leishmann-stained bone marrow biopsy obtained from a 23-year-old man with type 1 Gaucher's disease. Note that the large, pale-blue staining Gaucher's cells with striated cytoplasm replace the Kupffer cells of the liver, alveolar macrophages of the lung, and of the bone marrow.

Chapter 11.13 α₁-Antitrypsin deficiency and the serpinopathies

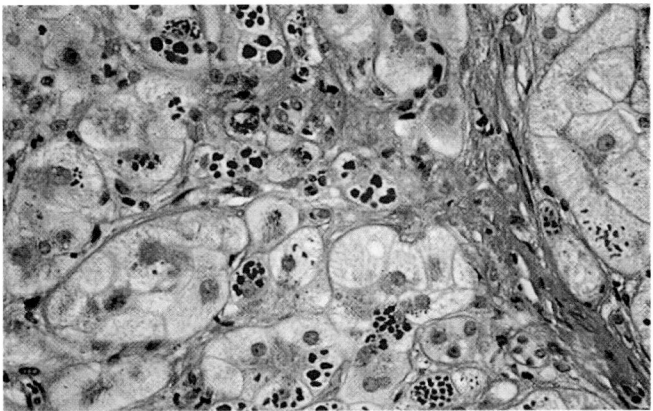

Plate 1 A chain of loop-sheet polymers isolated from a patient with α_1-antitrypsin deficiency. These polymers can form filaments or circlets that tangle within the endoplasmic reticulum of the hepatocyte to form the inclusions which are the hallmark of the disease. These intrahepatic inclusions are characteristically periodic acid–Schiff (**PAS**)-positive and diastase-resistant and stain positive for α_1-antitrypsin on immunohistochemistry.

Plates for Section 12
Chapter 12.4 The thyroid gland and disorders of thyroid function

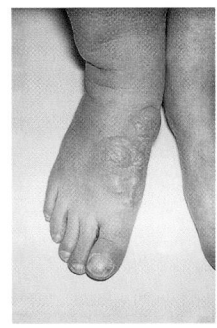

Plate 1 Thyroid dermopathy (pretibial myxoedema) affecting the lateral aspect of the shin and the dorsum of the foot; the patient also had thyroid acropachy.

Chapter 12.7.1 Diseases of the adrenal cortex

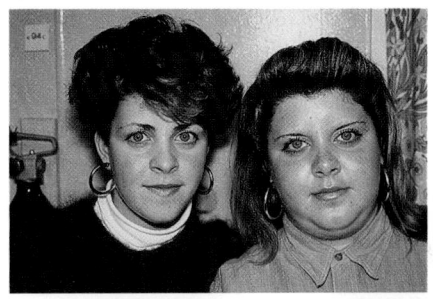

(a)

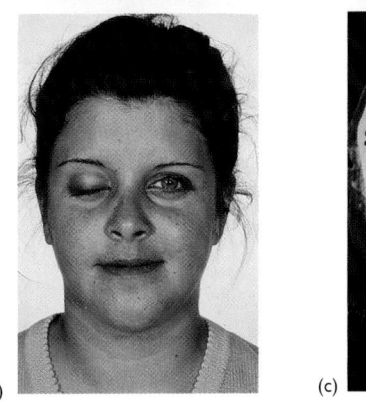

(b)

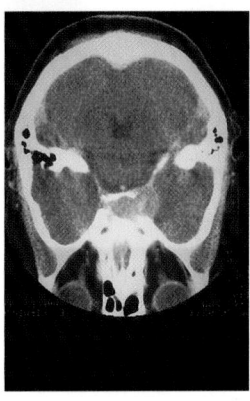

(c)

Plate 1 A young woman with Cushing's disease, photographed initially alongside her identical twin sister (a). In this case treatment with bilateral adrenalectomy was undertaken and several years later the patient re-presents with Nelson's syndrome and a right III cranial nerve palsy due to cavernous sinus infiltration from a locally invasive corticotrophinoma.

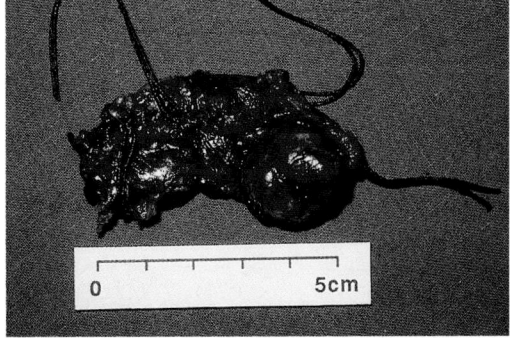

Plate 2 A solitary adrenal adenoma. The characteristic yellow appearance of the cut surface of the excised tumour reflects the high cholesterol content.

Chapter 12.8.1 Approach to the patient with ovarian disorders

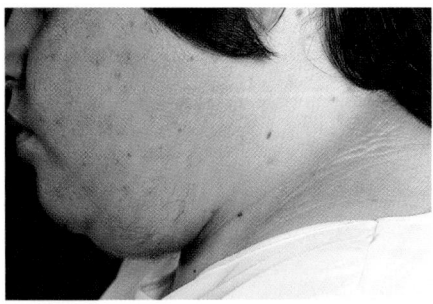

Plate 1 Acanthosis nigricans in a young woman with polycystic ovary syndrome.

Chapter 12.10 Non-diabetic pancreatic endocrine disorders and multiple endocrine neoplasia

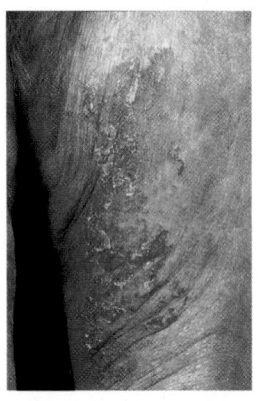
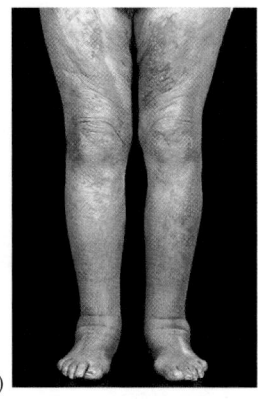

Plate 1 (a) Necrolytic migratory erythema in a patient with the glucagonoma syndrome. (b) Pigmentation in healed areas.

Chapter 12.11.1 Diabetes mellitus

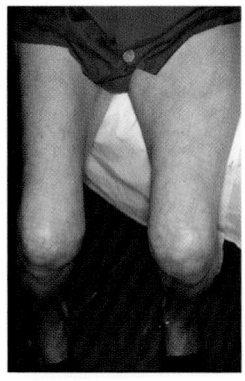

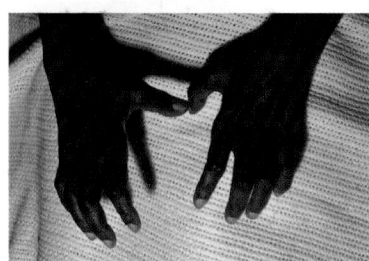

Plate 1 (a) Diabetic amyotrophy: quadriceps right wasting due to femoral neuropathy (with thanks to Dr Geoff Gill, University Hospital, Aintree, Liverpool). (b) Wasting of small muscles of the hands due to both ulnar and median nerve lesions.

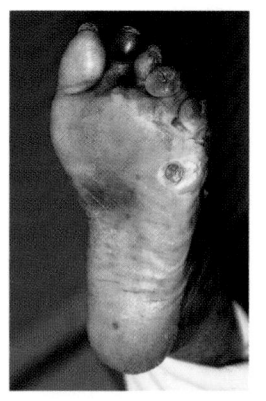
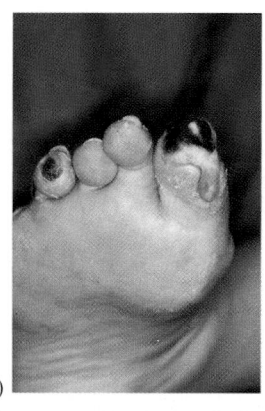

Plate 2 The diabetic foot. (a) Typical punched-out neuropathic ulcer on the lateral aspect of the sole in an ischaemic foot with gangrene of the second, fourth, and fifth toes. (b) Ulceration and digital gangrene, caused by wearing tight shoes on a severely ischaemic foot.

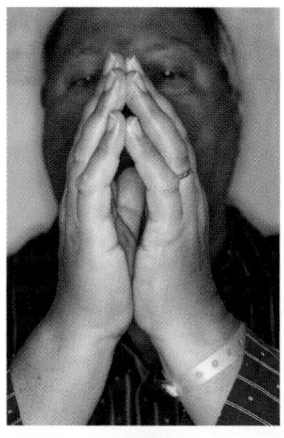

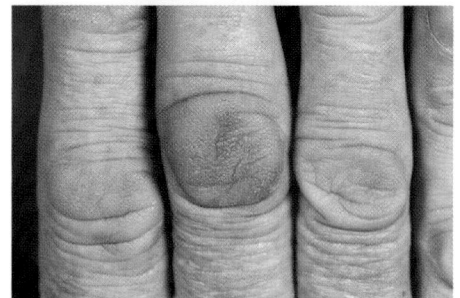

Plate 3 The hands in long-standing diabetes. (a) Limited joint mobility (cheiroarthropathy), showing the 'prayer sign'. (b) Thickening of the skin over the knuckles and proximal interphalangeal joints (Garrod's pads).

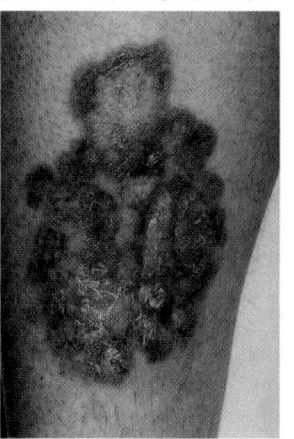

Plate 4 Necrobiosis lipoidica diabeticorum (with thanks to Dr Geoff Gill, University Hospital, Aintree, Liverpool.

Plates for Section 13
Chapter 13.13 The skin in pregnancy

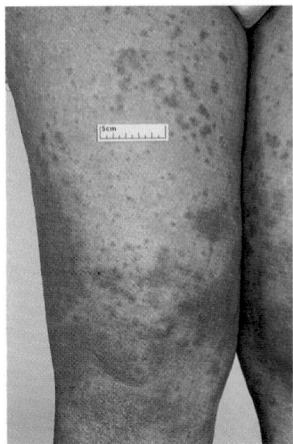

Plate 1 Polymorphic eruption of pregnancy: urticated papules and plaques on the thigh.

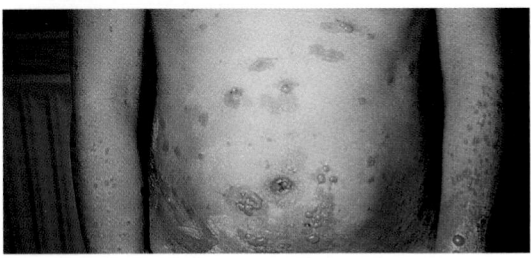

Plate 2 Pemphigoid gestationis: urticated papules and plaques and blisters (reproduced with permission from Charles-Holmes R, Black MM (1990). Herpes gestationis. In: Wojnarowska F, Briggaman RA, eds. *Management of blistering disease*, pp. 93–104. Chapman and Hall, London).

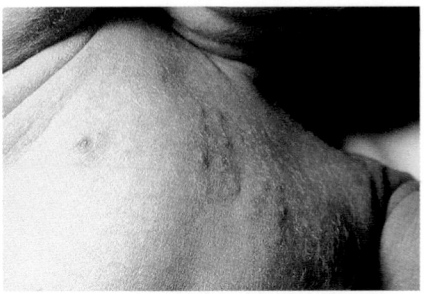

Plate 3 Pemphigoid gestationis: urticated papules in the neonate (reproduced with permission from Charles-Holmes R, Black MM (1990). Herpes gestationis. In: Wojnarowska F, Briggaman RA, eds. *Management of blistering disease*, pp. 93–104. Chapman and Hall, London).

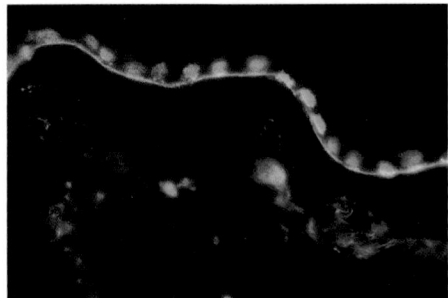

Plate 4 Pemphigoid gestationis: linear deposition of C3 at the amnion basement membrane zone as demonstrated by immunofluorescence. The nuclei are counterstained with propidium iodide. (Provided by B.S. Bhogal and M.M. Black, St John's Institute of Dermatology, St Thomas's Hospital, London.)

Plates for Section 14
Chapter 14.4 Immune disorders of the gastrointestinal tract

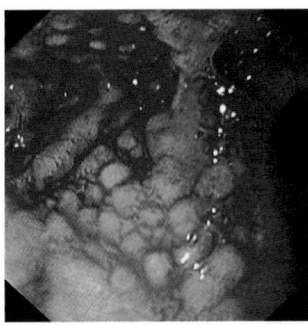

Plate 1 The appearance of nodular lymphoid hyperplasia on upper gastrointestinal endosocpy.

Chapter 14.20.1 Viral hepatitis – clinical aspects

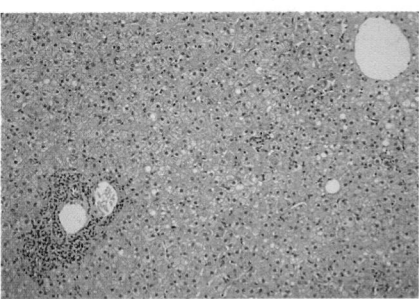

Plate 1 Serological changes during chronic hepatitis C.

Chapter 14.20.2.1 Autoimmune hepatitis

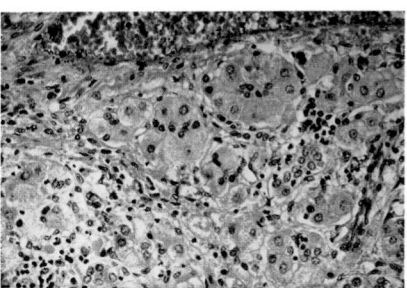

Plate 1 Haematoxylin and eosin stained liver histology showing "rosettes" of regenerated hepatocytes, surrounded by lymphocytes that have spread into the hepatic parenchyma.

Chapter 14.21.3 Hepatocellular failure

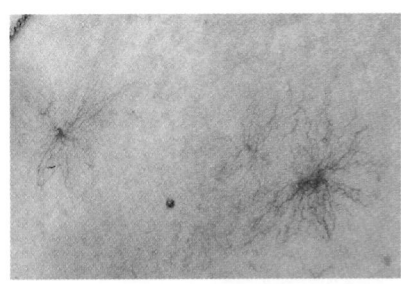

Plate 1 Spider naevi in a patient with cirrhosis.

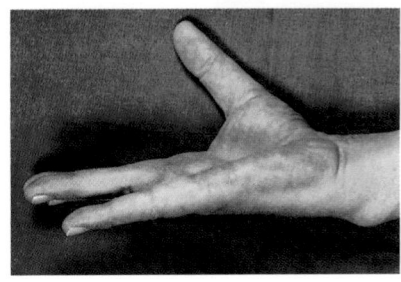

Plate 2 Palmer erythema in a patient with cirrhosis.

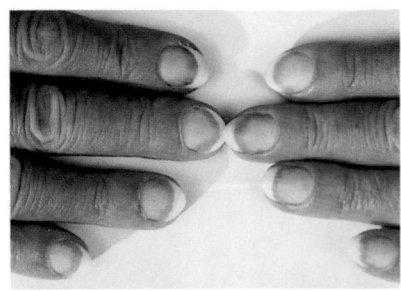

Plate 3 White nails in a patient with cirrhosis.

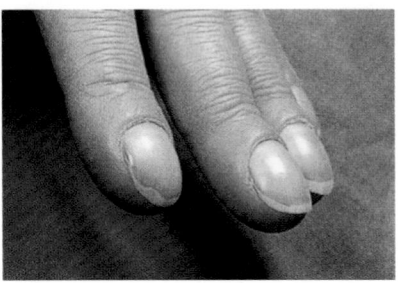

Plate 4 Finger clubbing in a patient with cirrhosis.

Chapter 14.21.6 Hepatic granulomas

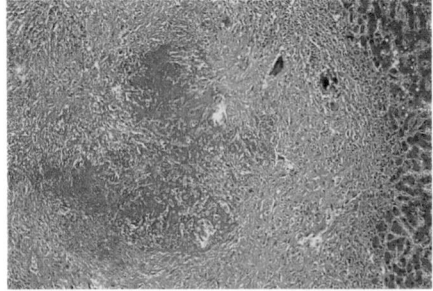

Plate 1 Liver showing a portion of a large caseating granuloma from a patient with miliary mycobacterium tuberculosis. Several Langhans' giant cells are also seen. (Haematoxylin and eosin, total magnification 25.)

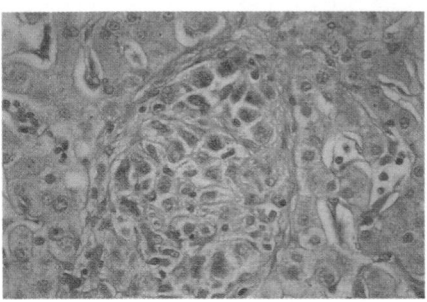

Plate 2 Liver from an HIV/AIDS patient infected with *Mycobacterium avium intracellulare*, showing a granuloma composed of epithelioid cells which contain large numbers of micro-organisms. (Diastase/periodic acid–Schiff stain, total magnification 100.)

Plates for Section 15
Chapter 15.3.3 Echocardiography

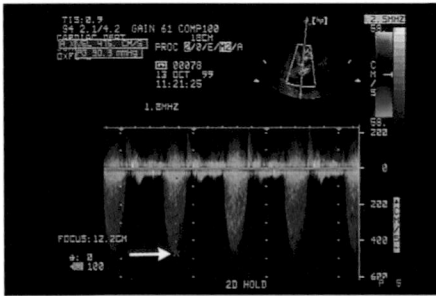

Plate 1 Apical continuous wave Doppler across the aortic valve in a patient with severe aortic stenosis. The peak velocity is greater than 4.5 m/s consistent with a peak instantaneous gradient across the aortic valve of 90 mmHg.

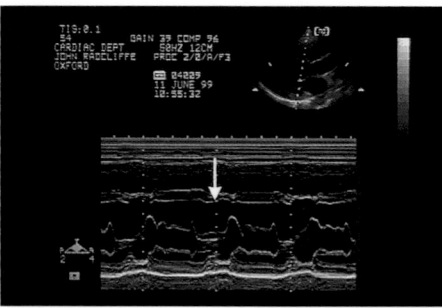

Plate 2 M-mode echocardiogram through the mitral valve in a normal patient. Opening of the leaflets during ventricular diastole and closing during systole (arrow) can be observed.

Chapter 15.8.2 The cardiomyopathies: hypertrophic, dilated, restrictive, and right ventricular

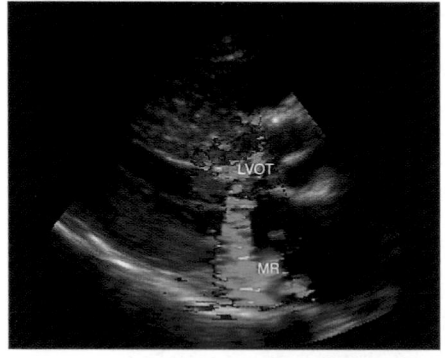

Plate 1 Colour flow Doppler image (parasternal long axis view) of the same patient as shown in Fig. 3 of Chapter 15.8.2, demonstrating left ventricular outflow tract (LVOT) turbulence (shown in red) and mitral regurgitation (MR) with a posteriorly directed jet (shown in blue/green).

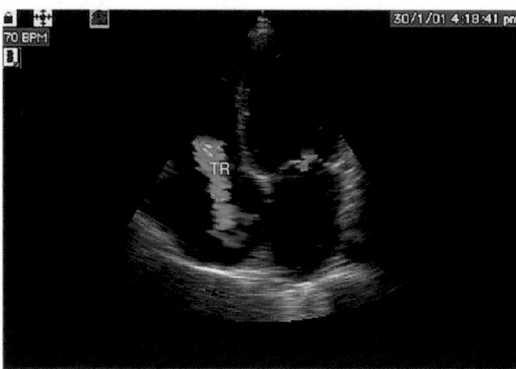

Plate 2 Colour flow Doppler image of the same patient as shown in Fig. 5 of Chapter 15.8.2 showing a regurgitant tricuspid jet (TR, shown in blue).

Chapter 15.10.2 Infective endocarditis

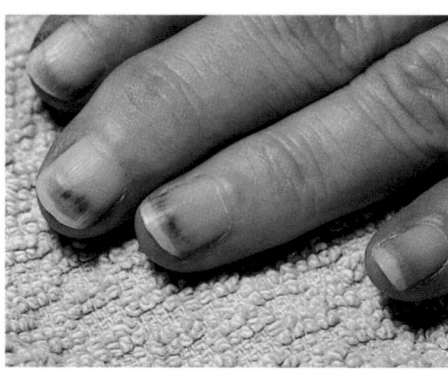

Plate 1 Splinter haemorrhages in a case of infective endocarditis.

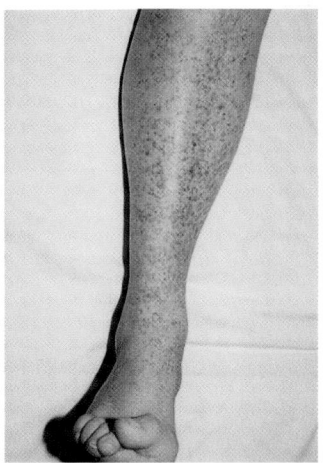

Plate 2 Vasculitic rash on lower limb of a patient with infective endocarditis.

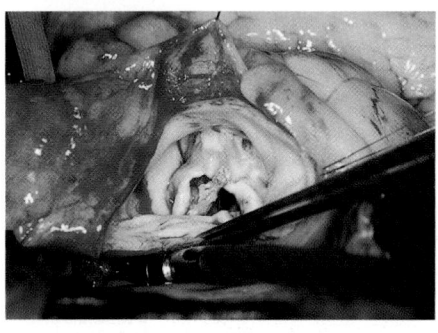

Plate 3 A large vegetation on the aortic valve of a patient with infective endocarditis as seen at the time of surgery.

Chapter 15.14.1 Thoracic aortic dissection

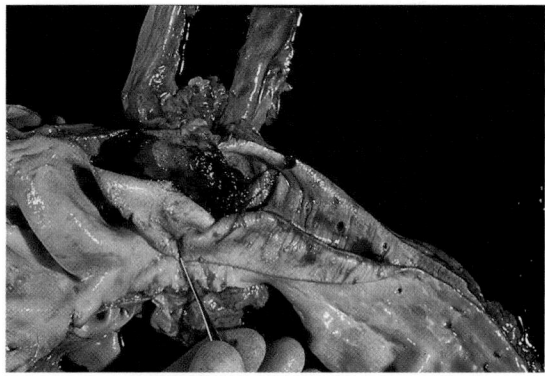

Plate 1 Post-mortem specimen of aortic dissection. The intimal/medial flap is pulled back with a retractor to show the false lumen parallel to the true lumen.

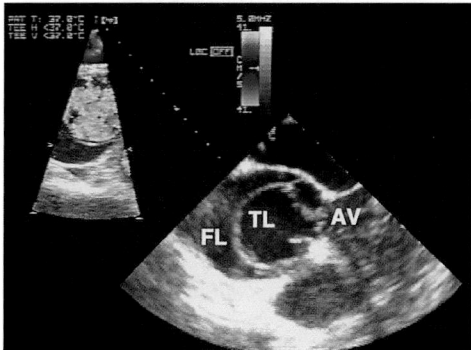

Plate 2 Transoesphageal transverse two-dimensional and colour Doppler echo images of the ascending aorta showing a dissection membrane partitioning the true (TL) and false lumen (FL). Upper left panel shows systolic flow in the true but not the false lumen.

Chapter 15.14.2 Peripheral arterial disease

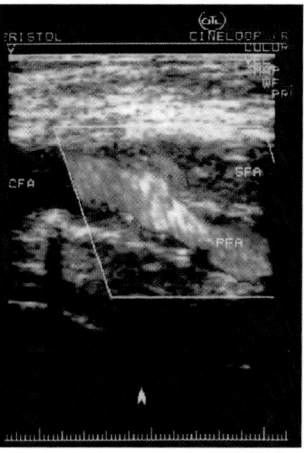

Plate 1 Occlusion of the superficial femoral artery demonstrated by colour-coded duplex ultrasonography. On the left, the common femoral artery (CFA) lies outside the colour box. In the colour box antegrade flow through the profuma femoris artery (PFA) is shown in blue. The red flash represents rebound flow against the occluded origin of the superficial femoral artery (SFA).

Chapter 15.14.3 Cholesterol embolism

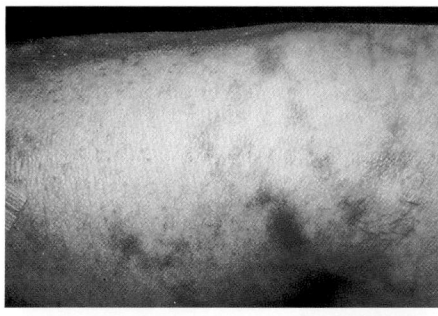

Plate 1 Livedo reticularis and vasculitic-like erythematous nodules on the leg of a patient in whom cholesterol-crystal embolization occurred after coronary angiography.

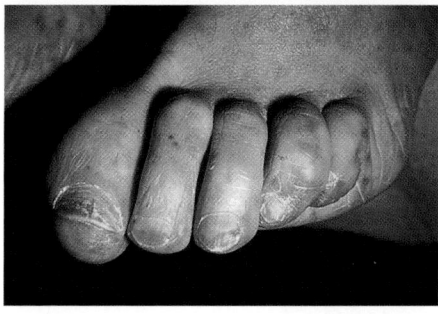

Plate 2 Purpuric spots and acral cyanosis of the toes from cholesterol embolism after aortic aneurysm repair.

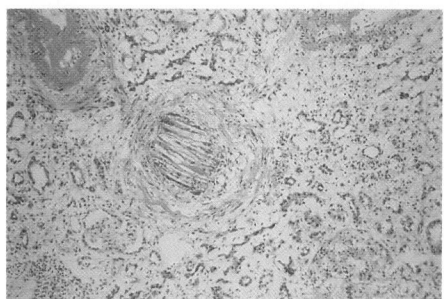

Plate 3 Renal biopsy demonstrating the characteristic needle-shaped cholesterol clefts occluding a medium-sized renal arteriole with surrounding inflammatory cell infiltration, intimal proliferation, thickening, and concentric fibrosis. There is extensive autolysis (postmortem sample).

Chapter 15.14.4 Takayasu arteritis

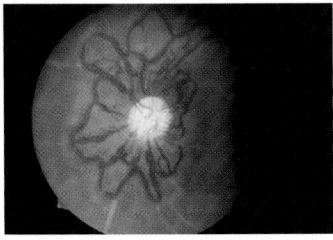

Plate 1 Typical coronary anastomosis of retinal vessels in Takayasu arteritis.

Chapter 15.15.2.1 Primary pulmonary hypertension

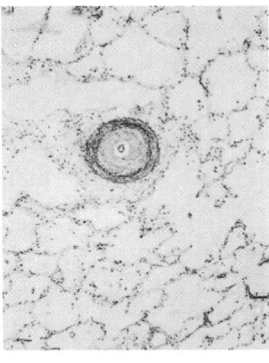

Plate 1 Intimal thickening of a pulmonary artery in pulmonary hypertension (Chazova I *et al.*, 1995. Pulmonary artery adventitial changes and venous involvement in primary pulmonary hypertension. *American Journal of Pathology* **146**, 389–97).

Chapter 15.16.3 Hypertensive emergencies and urgencies

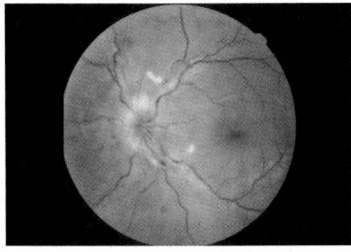

Plate 1 Ocular fundus in hypertension, showing papilloedema, exudates, and a few haemorrhages.

Plates for Section 17
Chapter 17.3.4 Diagnostic bronchoscopy, thoracoscopy, and tissue biopsy

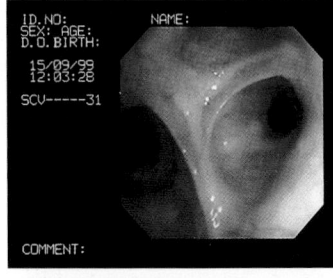

(a)

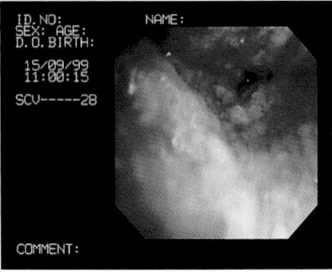

(b)

Plate 1 Appearances at bronchoscopy. The normal thin mucosa and sharp interlobar carinae of the normal left side (a) are in contrast to the irregular exophytic appearance of an advanced non-small cell tumour of the right main bronchus (b) in the same 73-year-old patient.

Chapter 17.11.2 Cryptogenic fibrosing alveolitis

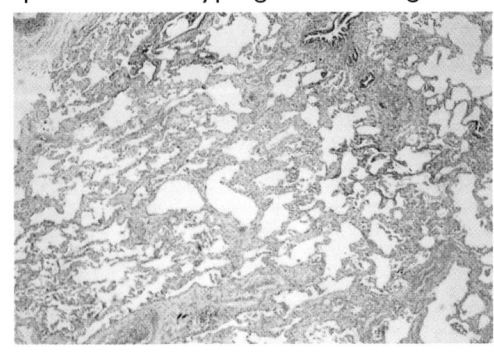

(a)

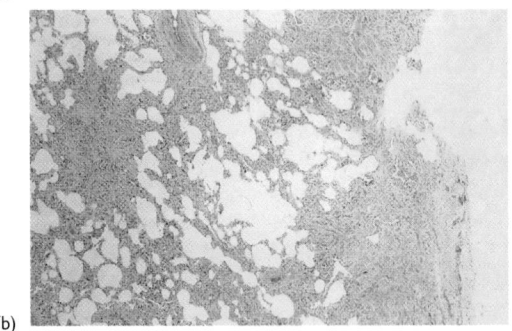

(b)

Plate 1 Histopathological appearance of cryptogenic fibrosing alveolitis and the non-specific interstitial pneumonia 'mimic'. (a) Usual interstitial pneumonia, the histopathological pattern seen in cryptogenic fibrosing alveolitis. Note the pale, fibroblast foci that are the hallmark of usual interstitial pneumonia. (b) The non-specific interstitial pneumonia 'mimic' of cryptogenic fibrosing alveolitis. This is much less common than usual interstitial pneumonia. Note the uniformity of the pathology throughout the section.

Chapter 17.11.3 Bronchiolitis obliterans and organizing pneumonia

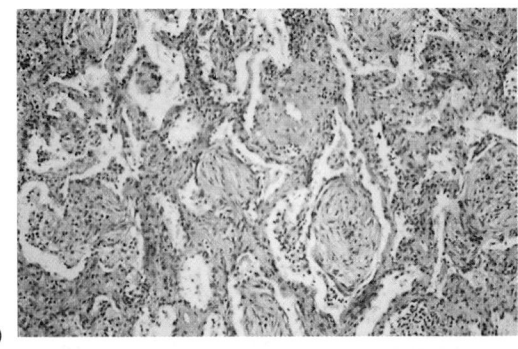

(a)

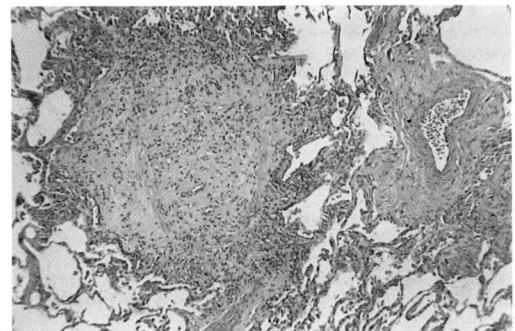

(b)

Plate 1 Histopathology. (a) Proliferative bronchiolitis. (b) Constrictive bronchiolitis. Note the loosely packed granulation tissue in (a) in contrast to the more established scarring in (b).

and prognostic markers which merely reflect a worse prognosis, without themselves being involved in the mechanism. It can be dangerous to base treatments on the supposition that improving an adverse prognostic feature will improve outlook: treatment may improve a marker but have either a neutral, or even a detrimental effect on survival.

The presence of non-sustained ventricular tachycardia on Holter monitoring is a sign of an increased mortality risk for sudden death. Class I antiarrhythmic agents can reduce the frequency of ventricular tachycardia, and as a result they were suggested for this purpose in heart failure. However, the Cardiac Arrhythmia Suppression Trial (**CAST**), a randomized controlled trial of three such agents in left ventricular dysfunction, showed that despite reducing the frequency of ventricular arrhythmias there was an increased rate of sudden death, presumably due to some proarrhythmic effect. Similarly, a low ejection fraction is an adverse prognostic sign in heart failure, and it was expected that agents that improve ejection fraction should increase survival. However, in controlled studies, positively inotropic agents such as milrinone (a phosphodiesterase inhibitor) increase ejection fraction but reduce survival. Hence, improving a risk marker should never be used as the justification for treatment, unless we have proof that in so doing we improve survival. The only justifications for treatment are to slow the progression of the underlying disease, to relieve symptoms that trouble the patient, or to use agents proven to improve survival.

Specific prognostic indicators

These can be divided into several relatively independent groups. The most important factors are:

(1) the extent of the left ventricular dysfunction;

(2) the degree of functional limitation;

(3) electrolyte disturbances;

(4) the degree of neurohormonal or autonomic dysfunction; and

(5) certain electrophysiological or electrocardiographic indicators of ventricular arrhythmogenesis.

There are also general factors such as age or the presence of comorbidities. It has not been established whether estimation of these predictive variables materially improves patient management. An improved scheme for accurate risk stratification can be used to prioritize patients for more careful and regular medical follow-up, or to select patients for expensive or limited treatment options such as transplantation. Table 4 lists some of the established risk markers for poor survival in patients with chronic heart failure.

Further reading

Anon. (2000). Heart failure drugs: what's new? *Drug and Therapeutics Bulletin* **38**, 25–7.

Coats AJ (1996). The 'muscle hypothesis' of chronic heart failure. *Journal of Molecular and Cellular Cardiology* **28**(11), 2255–62.

Flather MD, *et al.* (2000). Long-term ACE-inhibitor therapy in patients with heart failure or left-ventricular dysfunction: a systematic overview of data from individual patients. ACE-Inhibitor Myocardial Infarction Collaborative Group. *Lancet* **355**,1575–81.

Kannel WB, Belanger AJ (1991). Epidemiology of heart failure. *American Heart Journal* **121**, 951–7.

McMurray JJ, Stewart S (2000). Epidemiology, aetiology, and prognosis of heart failure. *Heart* **83**(5), 596–602.

Westaby S (2000). Non-transplant surgery for heart failure. *Heart* **83**, 603–10.

(See Chapter 15.5.1 for more complete referencing of the medical treatment of heart failure.)

Table 4 Adverse prognostic markers in heart failure

1. **Left ventricular dysfunction**
   Low ejection fraction
   Increased cardiothoracic ratio
   Increased left ventricular end-diastolic diameter
   Reduced peak cardiac power output

2. **The degree of functional limitation**
   Reduced exercise time
   Reduced peak oxygen consumption
   Advanced New York Functional Class

3. **Electrolyte disturbances**
   Hyponatraemia
   Hypomagnasaemia

4. **Neurohormonal or autonomic dysfunction**
   Increased plasma norepinephrine (noradrenaline)
   Increased cardiac natriuretic peptide levels
   Reduced heart rate variability
   Impaired baroreflex sensitivity

5. **Markers of ventricular arrhythmogenesis**
   Non-sustained ventricular tachycardia on Holter monitoring
   Late potentials

6. **Other markers**
   Cytokines such as tumour necrosis factor–alpha or its receptors
   Erythrocyte sedimentation rate
   Uric acid
   Creatinine
   Abnormal liver function tests

15.2.3 Syncope and palpitation

A. C. Rankin and S. M. Cobbe

Syncope and palpitation are symptoms that are commonly of cardiovascular origin, which may be related to abnormalities of cardiac rhythm. However, there are a number of aetiologies for both, and the prognosis for either can range from benign to life-threatening, hence a major priority in assessment is the identification of patients who may be at risk of dying. Treatment options may also range from reassurance with no therapy, to curative or lifesaving treatments for cardiac arrhythmia. The investigation, diagnosis, and management of cardiac arrhythmias are described in more detail in Section 15.6.

Syncope

Syncope is defined as a transient loss of consciousness with the loss of postural tone, and is most commonly due to cardiovascular mechanisms resulting in reduced cerebral perfusion. It is a common presentation, resulting in 1 to 2 per cent of emergency department visits and up to 6 per cent of hospital admissions. The cause is often initially uncertain and assessment must first differentiate syncope from other causes of loss of consciousness, in particular epileptic seizures. The next priority is to identify high-risk patients.

Syncope can be considered in three categories, namely (1) neurally-mediated, (2) cardiac, and (3) neurological or psychiatric (Table 1). The commonest cause is reflex-mediated or vasovagal syncope, which has a benign prognosis, whereas cardiac causes of syncope have been reported to have 1-year mortality rates as high as 18 to 33 per cent. Patients without underlying heart disease in whom no aetiology of syncope is established have a good prognosis, but they may have recurrent syncope.

Where a cause is eventually identified, the diagnosis is indicated by the initial clinical assessment—including history, physical examination, and an electrocardiogram (**ECG**)—in up to 50 per cent of cases. The history is most important and may strongly suggest a vasovagal origin or an epileptic seizure. However, the diagnosis may be complicated by an overlap in features, such as convulsive movements during a vasovagal episode due to anoxic convulsive seizures. It is increasingly recognized that many patients who attend clinics for epilepsy have been misdiagnosed and are suffering from recurrent syncope. Some of these patients have potentially lethal ventricular arrhythmias and should be receiving treatment.

Aetiology

Neurally mediated syncope

There are many disorders of autonomic control that can cause orthostatic intolerance and thereby syncope. To simplify, these can be considered as causing either reflex syncope, due to an increased sensitivity of normal reflex responses, or autonomic dysfunction, where abnormal neurovascular control results in orthostatic hypotension.

Vasovagal syncope

Vasovagal or neurocardiogenic syncope is the most common cause of syncope. It can affect all age groups and varies from infrequent episodes associated with obvious triggering factors to frequent unprovoked collapses, which may be debilitating. The pathophysiology most commonly involves the upright posture with venous pooling of blood and reduced venous return to the heart. Reduced cardiac output and blood pressure stimulate arterial baroreceptors with resultant increased sympathetic activity and cat-

Table 1 Causes of syncope

1.	**Neurally mediated**	
	(a)	*Reflex-mediated*
		Vasovagal or neurocardiogenic syncope
		Carotid sinus hypersensitivity
		Situational (micturition, defaecation, cough, swallow)
	(b)	*Autonomic dysfunction*
		Pure autonomic failure
		Multiple system atrophy (parkinsonian, cerebellar)
		Postural orthostatic tachycardia syndrome
		Secondary autonomic failure
2.	**Cardiac syncope**	
	(a)	*Bradycardia*
		Atrioventricular block
		Sinoatrial disease
	(b)	*Tachycardia*
		Ventricular arrhythmia
		previous myocardial infarction
		cardiomyopathy
		Long-QT syndrome
		Supraventricular arrhythmia
	(c)	*Structural cardiovascular disease*
		Aortic stenosis
		Hypertrophic cardiomyopathy
		Atrial myxoma or thrombus
		Pulmonary embolism
3.	**Neurological or psychiatric**	
	(a)	*Neurological*
		Migraine
		Subclavian steal
		Vertebrobasilar disease
	(b)	*Psychiatric*
		Anxiety, depression
		Hyperventilation

echolamine levels. The vigorous contraction of relatively empty ventricles results in the activation of mechanoreceptors that would normally respond to stretch in the left ventricular wall. Afferent nerve fibres conduct to the cerebral medulla and activate the reflex withdrawal of peripheral sympathetic tone and activation of vagal parasympathetic activity. The resultant vasodilatation and bradycardia cause reduced cerebral perfusion and loss of consciousness. However, there is debate about these mechanisms and other factors may be involved in the aetiology of syncope, as illustrated by the documentation of neurocardiogenic syncope, despite cardiac denervation, in orthotopic heart transplant recipients. Certainly, it is well recognized that vasovagal syncope can result from other stimuli, such as pain, emotional shock, or the sight of blood. In these instances, the reflex activation is central in origin.

The development of tilt-testing has allowed the study of the pathophysiology of neurocardiogenic syncope. The patient is strapped to a tilt-table and is tilted, head upright, usually at 70 degrees for up to 45 min. Protocols that use additional provocation with isoprenaline or nitrates are also commonly used. Blood pressure and cardiac rhythm are monitored throughout the tilt-test. In neurocardiogenic syncope, the patient classically maintains normal blood pressure initially, until the sudden onset of syncope is associated with severe hypotension and bradycardia, often preceded by tachycardia. These features resolve with return to the supine posture. Some patients have a mainly vasodepressor response, with hypotension and little change in heart rate, while others have a marked cardioinhibitory response, with severe bradycardia or asystole of several seconds' duration (Fig. 1). However, most patients exhibit a mixed response, and those patients with marked cardioinhibition also have a preceding vasodepressor response. This is an important observation when treatment is considered since permanent pacing to maintain cardiac rhythm may not cure all symptoms, because falls in blood pressure may still occur even when bradycardia is prevented.

Carotid sinus hypersensitivity

This is an abnormal sensitivity of a normal reflex that is responsible for syncope. Activation of the carotid sinus baroreceptors (for example by physical pressure, such as carotid sinus massage) results in sympathetic withdrawal and parasympathetic activation. Bradycardia is usually a prominent feature.

Situational reflex-mediated syncope

In susceptible individuals, similar abnormal reflex sensitivity can result in syncope in response to afferent activity from other mechanoreceptor activation. Syncopal responses to cough, micturition, defaecation, or swallowing have been reported.

Autonomic dysfunction

Hypotension may occur in patients in whom there are abnormalities in the autonomic control of cardiovascular function. Abnormalities of afferent or efferent pathways, or of peripheral vascular control, can result in low blood

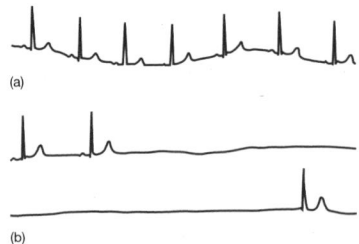

(a)

(b)

Fig. 1 Cardioinhibitory response to tilt-testing. (a) After 6 min of head-up tilting at 70° the patient complained of presyncope. Heart rate was 60 per min but blood pressure was 70 mmHg. (b) By 7 min the patient had lost consciousness, associated with an asystolic pause of 10 s duration and an unrecordable blood pressure. Recovery was rapid following the patient's return to the supine position.

pressure in the upright posture, that is to say orthostatic hypotension. This may be diagnosed by a fall in systolic pressure of more than 20 mmHg, or to less than 90 mmHg, within 3 min of standing. During tilt-testing there may be an immediate drop in blood pressure with head-upright tilting, or a progressive fall may be observed in some patients, in contrast to those with reflex-mediated syncope in whom blood pressure is maintained until the sudden onset of symptoms. Orthostatic hypotension is more common in elderly patients, where it may be multifactorial, often exacerbated by drugs (Table 2). Nocturnal symptoms may occur, with a fall in blood pressure exacerbated by sudden rising from a warm bed.

Autonomic failure is an uncommon cause of syncope and patients may present with other features, including disturbances of bowel, bladder, or sexual function. Pure autonomic failure can be acute or chronic, primary (of unknown origin) or secondary to systemic disease. Multiple system atrophy is characterized by autonomic dysfunction, parkinsonism, and ataxia. Orthostatic hypotension may be a marked feature (the Shy–Drager syndrome), with additional parkinsonian features or cerebellar symptoms. Secondary autonomic failure can result from the central or peripheral involvement of certain diseases, including multiple sclerosis, a cerebral tumour, diabetes, and amyloidosis. A recently reported milder form of autonomic dysfunction, the postural orthostatic tachycardia syndrome (**POTS**), causes symptoms because of inappropriate tachycardia on standing, and occasionally syncope secondary to hypotension.

Cardiac syncope

Loss of consciousness of cardiac origin may result from abnormalities of heart rhythm, due to extremes of rate, either fast or slow, or from some major disturbance of cardiovascular function, with resultant reduced cerebral perfusion. The importance in establishing the diagnosis of cardiac syncope is the associated adverse prognosis, which may be improved with appropriate treatment. The probability of cardiac syncope is increased in the presence of structural cardiovascular disease identified from the history, clinical examination, or investigation.

Bradycardia

A sudden decrease in heart rate, onset of ventricular standstill, or asystole may be a cause of syncope. When due to sinoatrial dysfunction (Sick-sinus syndrome) this is not associated with a poor prognosis, but syncope due to intermittent complete atrioventricular (**AV**) block is. Syncope in a patient with a permanent pacemaker may indicate pacemaker malfunction.

Tachycardia

Syncope may be caused by tachycardia, most commonly ventricular, but supraventricular tachycardia can also be associated with loss of consciousness if it is very fast or in patients with structural heart disease (Fig. 2). Syncope, rather than cardiac arrest, may result from self-terminating ventricular tachycardia or from sustained tachycardia with hypotension at the onset, but with a subsequent recovery of blood pressure. Whether or not a tachycardia causes syncope is related to its rate, underlying left ventricular

Table 2 Drugs that may cause postural hypotension

Diuretics
α-Adrenergic receptor blockers
β-Adrenergic receptor blockers
ACE inhibitors
AII receptor antagonists
Calcium-channel blockers
Nitrates
Opiates
Ethanol
Tricyclic antidepressants
Bromocriptine
Phenothiazines
Levodopa

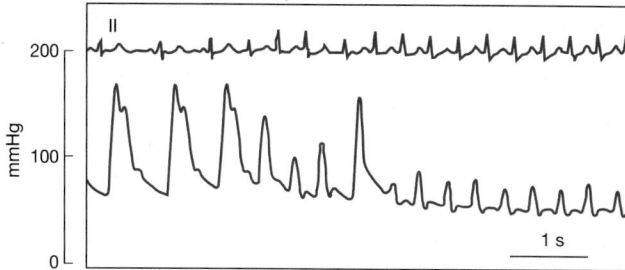

Fig. 2 Hypotension with the onset of supraventricular tachycardia. Surface ECG lead II and intra-aortic pressure are shown.

function, and to the patient's baroreceptor sensitivity. Structural heart disease, for example prior myocardial infarction, is the commonest substrate for ventricular tachycardia, but this may also occur in patients with structurally normal hearts. *Torsade de pointes* in a patient with the Long-QT syndrome is an important diagnosis to consider in young people with a history of loss of consciousness and possible epilepsy, in whom the episodes of collapse may be due to syncope caused by ventricular arrhythmia.

Structural cardiovascular disease

Aortic stenosis may be associated with syncope, particularly during sudden exertion when the demand for increased cardiac output cannot be met because of the mechanical obstruction. Hypertrophic cardiomyopathy may also be associated with syncope, either because of outflow obstruction or ventricular arrhythmia. Obstruction of blood flow through the mitral valve by an atrial myxoma or thrombus is an extremely uncommon cause of syncope, and a number of other cardiac diseases may be associated with loss of consciousness by a variety of mechanisms (arrhythmia, reflex-mediated or haemodynamic), including myocardial infarction, pulmonary embolism, congenital heart disease, or cardiac tamponade. Vascular diseases may also be involved, such as aortic dissection and extracranial vascular disease.

Neurological or psychiatric causes of syncope

When epilepsy is excluded, neurological aetiologies are rare causes of loss of consciousness, but possible causes include migraine, transient ischaemic attacks, vertebrobasilar vascular disease, and subclavian steal syndrome. A psychiatric origin of syncope implies the absence of neurally mediated, neurological or cardiac abnormalities, and may occur in association with anxiety, depression, and conversion disorders. For instance, apparent syncope may occur during tilt-testing but with normal pulse and blood pressure. Hyperventilation may be an associated mechanistic factor in psychogenic syncope.

History

The importance of the clinical history in assessing a patient with syncope cannot be overemphasized. If possible an eyewitness description of the patient during the syncopal event should always be obtained.

Provocative factors

Vasovagal syncope is classically associated with upright posture, often with aggravating circumstances such as prolonged standing, a hot environment, or hunger. However, episodes may also occur when seated, including when driving. Specific stimuli may be responsible for neurocardiogenic syncope in susceptible individuals. Ventricular arrhythmia, in particular *torsade de pointes* in the Long-QT syndrome, may be provoked by sudden stimuli such as a noise, for example an alarm clock. Exertional syncope is a feature of aortic stenosis or hypertrophic cardiomyopathy.

Preceding symptoms

Sweating and feeling hot or nauseated may precede vasovagal syncope. Cardiac arrhythmia may be associated with palpitation, chest pain, or breathlessness. Bradycardia, such as intermittent complete heart block, may produce no preceding symptoms and may cause loss of consciousness without warning. Sinoatrial dysfunction is a cause of symptoms of dizziness and light-headedness in addition to syncope. A psychiatric origin may be suggested by multiple associated symptoms including hyperventilation, paraesthesiae in fingers and lips, palpitation and chest pain, which may precede syncope. Epilepsy may be preceded by a characteristic aura, which would strongly point away from syncope as the diagnosis.

The syncopal episode

The duration of loss of consciousness is usually short in syncope, with recovery after a few minutes. A longer duration of loss of consciousness would suggest an alternative diagnosis. An exception to this is when the patient has remained upright during the attack, possibly aided by well-meaning but misguided helpers. Incontinence is a feature of epileptic seizure but may also occur (uncommonly) with syncope. Description of the patient during the episode is of great value. The classic description of an episode of syncope due to cardiac arrhythmia, in particular sudden-onset severe bradycardia, is of a sudden loss of colour, becoming deathly pale, with flushing on recovery (Stokes–Adams attack). Cyanosis may be a feature of an arrhythmic origin of syncope. Convulsive movements during the episode would raise the possibility of epilepsy, but they also occur with syncope.

The recovery period

By contrast to the postictal phase following epilepsy, there is commonly a rapid recovery of cerebral function following syncope. Vasovagal syncope may be followed by persisting nausea or vomiting.

Family history

There are a few specific causes of syncope in which a family history of syncope or sudden death may have prognostic significance. Long-QT syndrome is hereditary and may be associated with sudden death. A family history of syncope is of adverse prognostic significance in hypertrophic cardiomyopathy.

Associated injury

In addition to concern about prognosis in cardiac syncope, there is the possibility of injury occurring with any cause of syncope. The exception to this is syncope of psychiatric origin when injuries are absent despite frequently recurring symptoms.

Investigation

The investigation of cardiac disease and arrhythmia are dealt with in the appropriate chapters, but the approach to the patient with syncope will be described briefly.

Electrocardiogram

An ECG should be performed on all patients with syncope. This may provide evidence of either aetiology of syncope, such as the Long-QT syndrome, or of structural heart disease, such as prior myocardial infarction or left ventricular hypertrophy. An arrhythmia may be documented if it is sustained. There may be evidence of arrhythmia, or sinoatrial disease or conduction system disease, such as trifasicular block, bundle-branch block, or first- or second-degree block. In the absence of carotid bruits, carotid sinus massage, with digital pressure to the carotid artery for up to 5 s, may cause marked bradycardia, with pauses of more than 3-s duration, in carotid sinus hypersensitivity.

Ambulatory monitoring

Documentation of cardiac rhythm during syncope is desirable but is difficult to obtain because of the intermittent and usually infrequent nature of the symptom. Holter monitoring is unlikely to record the rhythm during an episode but may provide evidence of lesser degrees of abnormality, which may support a diagnosis such as sinoatrial dysfunction. Real-time event-recorders are also of limited value in the investigation of syncope because they require a conscious patient to make the recording. Patient-activated loop-recorders, which can store the rhythm prior, during, and following an episode, may be of more value. Implantable loop-recorders are of value in difficult cases.

Tilt-testing

When the history is suggestive of vasovagal syncope, the tilt-test is of value in confirming the diagnosis, allowing reassurance of the patient and clarification of treatment options. However, if cardiac syncope is likely then tilt-testing may be deferred until cardiac investigations are completed. A negative tilt-test does not exclude neurocardiogenic syncope and repeating the test with provocation (isoprenaline or nitrate) may increase its sensitivity.

Electrophysiological testing

Abnormal sinus node function or evidence of atrioventricular conduction disease may be elicited by electrophysiological testing, but demonstrating bradycardia during ambulatory monitoring more reliably makes both these diagnoses. In patients with structural heart disease in whom arrhythmia is suspected, programmed electrical stimulation of the ventricles can induce sustained monomorphic ventricular tachycardia. This is a relatively specific response and shows that the patient is at risk of recurrent ventricular arrhythmia, and makes an arrhythmic origin of syncope likely. The diagnostic yield of electrophysiological testing is low in patients with a structurally normal heart.

Other investigations

Assessment for structural heart disease is important. Physical examination will detect most significant valve disease, but other diagnoses, for example hypertrophic cardiomyopathy or atrial myxoma, may produce little in the way of clinical signs. An echocardiogram is therefore worthwhile. A strong suspicion of diagnoses other than syncope should lead to other investigations, including EEG and brain imaging, but these have a low diagnostic yield in patients with syncope and should not be routine.

Treatment

Neurocardiogenic syncope may require no treatment other than reassurance and avoidance of provocative factors. Treatments of vasovagal syncope, bradycardia, and cardiac arrhythmia are discussed in Chapters 24.13.5 and 15.6. In up to one-third of patients the aetiology of syncope may not be found: these patients have a good outcome unless they have underlying heart disease.

Palpitation

The symptom of palpitation is defined as an awareness of one's heart beating. This may be due to an awareness of an abnormal heart rhythm but it may also be due to an abnormal awareness of normal rhythm. A careful and detailed history can provide a likely diagnosis. The most important aim in investigation is to correlate symptoms with cardiac rhythm.

History

A description of the symptom should include an estimate of heart rate, duration of symptom, regularity of rhythm, suddenness of onset and offset. It may be helpful to ask the patient to tap with their finger on a desk to describe their palpitation. Trigger factors, including exercise, and aggravating factors such as alcohol and caffeine should be detailed. The length of history may be of interest.

Sinus tachycardia

An awareness of a rapid heart rate of gradual onset and offset is often associated with feelings of alarm and panic in patients with anxiety.

Premature beats

Atrial and ventricular beats commonly occur in normal individuals and may be associated with symptoms. The patient may describe 'missed beats' or forceful beats. These symptoms relate to the pause that follows a premature beat. The premature beat produces a short diastolic filling interval and the low ventricular volume results in reduced ventricular contraction with a small stroke volume. However, the subsequent pause provides a long diastolic filling period and the resultant stretching of the ventricular walls is associated with an increased and forceful systolic contraction. The combination of the diminished premature beat and the enhanced postextrasystolic beat is responsible for the symptoms.

Atrial fibrillation

This common arrhythmia may produce a variety of symptoms depending on ventricular rate, irregularity, and persistence. Paroxysmal atrial fibrillation is typically associated with self-terminating episodes of atrial fibrillation when there is a rapid and irregular ventricular response. The patient is aware of an increased heart rate and often describes the irregular nature of the symptom. The variations in diastolic interval produce symptoms by similar mechanisms to that described above for premature beats, with 'missed' and 'forceful' beats. Patients with sinoatrial dysfunction may be most symptomatic on termination of the atrial fibrillation, which can be followed by sinus bradycardia or prolonged sinus pauses. Atrial fibrillation may be persistent or permanent, and the severity of symptoms will be related to the ventricular rate and irregularity.

Paroxysmal junctional re-entry tachycardia

A history of sudden onset, rapid, regular palpitation in a healthy patient with no underlying structural heart disease is suggestive of paroxysmal junctional re-entry tachycardia. It may stop spontaneously or with vagotonic manoeuvres, or the patient may have had to attend hospital for intravenous therapy. In addition to palpitation, patients commonly report fatigue, malaise, light-headedness, or dyspnoea, but because they have normal hearts such episodes of tachycardia are usually well tolerated. Polyuria is a common associated symptom, which results from the release of atrial natriuretic peptide secondary to atrial stretch.

Ventricular tachycardia

Ventricular arrhythmias can present with the symptom of palpitation, but more severe symptoms such as syncope or cardiac arrest also occur. Characteristically the symptom of palpitation would be of sudden onset and offset of a rapid regular heart rhythm. A history of structural heart disease should be sought.

Investigation

Electrocardiogram

The first aim is to document cardiac rhythm during symptoms. This may be possible with a standard ECG if the arrhythmia is sustained or persistent. Atrial or ventricular premature beats, or evidence of structural heart disease, for example myocardial infarction, may be documented. The presence of pre-excitation indicates the diagnosis of Wolff–Parkinson–White syndrome and suggests symptoms due to episodes of junctional re-entry tachycardia.

Ambulatory monitoring

The success of ambulatory monitoring in documenting the rhythm during symptoms will be dependent on the frequency of symptoms. If they occur daily then a 24- or 48-h Holter recording should suffice. However, palpitation is often infrequent and other patient-activated devices can be of more value. These include handheld, patient-activated event recorders that allow the transtelephonic transmission of recordings. These devices do not allow retrospective recording and require symptoms of sufficient duration to allow their use. Shorter episodes may be captured using loop-recorders.

Electrophysiological studies

Invasive studies are of most value in determining the mechanism of a previously documented tachyarrhythmia, particularly with a view to treatments such as radiofrequency catheter ablation.

Management

Documentation of the cardiac rhythm during palpitation allows appropriate management, with reassurance as the only treatment in those with sinus tachycardia or premature beats. The treatment of other cardiac arrhythmias is discussed in Chapter 15.6.

Further reading

Benditt DG, *et al.* (1999). Pharmacotherapy of neurally mediated syncope. *Circulation* **100**, 1242–8.

Fitzpatrick AP, *et al.* (1993). Vasovagal syncope may occur after orthotopic heart transplantation. *Journal of the American College of Cardiology* **21**, 1132–7.

Grubb BP (1999). Pathophysiology and differential diagnosis of neurocardiogenic syncope. *American Journal of Cardiology* **84**, 3Q–9Q.

Kapoor WN, *et al.* (1983). A prospective evaluation and follow-up of patients with syncope. *New England Journal of Medicine* **309**, 197–203.

Kenny RA, *et al.* (1986). Head-up tilt: a useful test for investigating unexplained syncope. *Lancet* **2**, 1352–4.

Linzer M, *et al.* (1997). Diagnosing syncope. Part 1: Value of history, physical examination and electrocardiography. *Annals of Internal Medicine* **126**, 989–6.

Linzer M, *et al.* (1997). Diagnosing syncope. Part 2: Unexplained syncope. *Annals of Internal Medicine* **127**, 76–86.

Muller T, *et al.* (1991). Electrophysiologic evaluation and outcome of patient with syncope of unknown origin. *European Heart Journal* **12**, 139–43.

Schatz IJ, Low P, Polinsky RJ. (1997). Disorders of the autonomic nervous system. *New England Journal of Medicine* **337**, 278–80.

Zaidi A, *et al.* (2000). Misdiagnosis of epilepsy: many seizure-like attacks have a cardiovascular cause. *Journal of the American College of Cardiology* **36**, 181–4.

15.2.4 Physical examination of the cardiovascular system

J. R. Hampton

Introduction

The cardiovascular system is perhaps more accessible to physical examination than any other. Examination is most helpful if it is approached logically: there is a group of general abnormalities that can be detected in cardiovascular disease, there is a group of signs associated with the arterial side of the circulation, a group associated with the venous side, and a group associated with the heart itself.

General examination

Pain due to cardiovascular disease (as in myocardial infarction or aortic dissection) may cause pallor, cold and clammy extremities, and a sinus tachycardia.

Breathlessness and an inability to lie flat (orthopnoea) may result from pulmonary congestion due to left heart failure. Pulmonary oedema will cause extreme breathlessness with the coughing up of frothy and sometimes bloodstained sputum, and peripheral vasoconstriction will cause cold and clammy extremities.

Central cyanosis (affecting the lips and tongue as well as the hands and feet) may indicate heart failure or pulmonary disease but may be due to polycythaemia. Central cyanosis, especially when associated with finger clubbing, is characteristic of a right to left shunt. Peripheral cyanosis indicates a high tissue oxygen extraction, and will be seen when the hands or feet are cold, or when there is peripheral arterial occlusion.

Infection of the heart valves (infective endocarditis) will cause fever, anaemia, weight loss, finger clubbing, 'splinter haemorrhages' under the finger and toenails, a large spleen, loss of arterial pulses and/or neurological abnormalities due to embolization of infected material, and skin lesions such as petechiae and nodules in the fingertips (Osler's nodes).

Physical signs in the arterial circulation

Peripheral pulses

A pulse can be felt whenever an artery is near the surface of the body. In fat or muscular people some pulses may be difficult to feel, but asymmetry of pulses is usually abnormal. Pulses may be lost through atheromatous disease, embolization, or injury. Pulses that are unusually easy to feel—for example in the abdomen, or the popliteal pulses—may be due to aneurysmal dilatation.

The pulses that should be checked are the superficial temporals, carotids, brachials, radials, the aorta, femorals, popliteals, dorsalis pedis, and posterior tibials. Tenderness over the superficial temporal pulses may indicate temporal arteritis. Auscultation over the carotid and femoral pulses, and over the aorta, should be routine as bruits will indicate narrowing, usually atheromatous.

Blood pressure

The blood pressure should be measured in the brachial artery using a cuff around the upper arm. It is essential to use a large cuff in fat people, because a small cuff will result in the blood pressure being overestimated. The diastolic pressure is taken as the point where the sound disappears (Karotkov V). For further discussion see elsewhere in Section 15.

In patients with chest pain, or if ever the radial pulses appear asymmetric, the pressure should be measured in both arms because a difference between the two may indicate aortic dissection.

Heart rate and rhythm

Although the heart rate is usually—and most conveniently—counted in the radial artery, this can be unreliable. In uncontrolled atrial fibrillation there may be a 'pulse deficit', with the true rate being faster than is apparent at the radial artery. The 'apex rate', counted by listening to or feeling the cardiac apex, is more reliable. Similarly, it is easier to distinguish irregularities of the heart rhythm by auscultation than by feeling a peripheral pulse.

Arterial waveform

Descriptions like 'strong' and 'weak' should not be used: these essentially reflect systolic pressure and are best indicated by the blood pressure itself.

The true 'waveform' in an artery can only be obtained by recording the intra-arterial pressure, and the 'pulse character', which describes the rate of rise and fall of pressure, is a crude reflection of this and an unreliable phys-

ical sign. It is best felt in large arteries such as the carotid or brachial. In aortic stenosis the rise is slow and the waveform feels flat—the 'plateau' pulse. In aortic regurgitation the arterial pressure falls rapidly, as it does in the left ventricle, causing a 'collapsing' or 'water hammer' pulse. These abnormalities are not easy to detect and are an unreliable guide to the severity of disease. Severe aortic regurgitation, classical of syphilitic aortitis, can cause the head to jerk with each pulse (de Musset's sign).

Abnormalities of the venous circulation

Peripheral veins

Venous thrombosis can occur in the arms, but is much more common in the legs. Thrombosis of an arm vein probably indicates local obstruction (perhaps by a tumour) or a thrombotic tendency. In the legs, superficial phlebitis causes local inflammation in the line of a vein, and the vein is usually palpable and tender. There may be associated swelling. Detecting deep venous thrombosis is much more difficult, but it must be suspected in any painful leg and particularly when there is unilateral swelling. The 'classical' signs of deep vein thrombosis—calf or thigh tenderness, warmth, and Homan's sign (pain in the calf on dorsiflexion of the foot)—are all unreliable.

The jugular venous pulse

The abbreviation 'JVP' may be used for jugular venous pulse or jugular venous pressure. The importance of the jugular venous pressure is that it directly reflects the pressure in the right atrium and is the best clinical indication of heart failure.

A pulse can be detected in either the external or internal jugular vein. The external vein (running diagonally from the midpoint of the clavicle to the midpoint of the mandible) is usually easy to see. Unfortunately it is a less reliable guide to venous pressure than the internal jugular vein, because flow can be obstructed in the external vein as it passes through the fascia in the neck. The internal jugular vein runs with the carotid artery from the sternoclavicular joint to the lateral end of the mandible, crossing under the sternocleidomastoid muscle and the external jugular vein. The pulsation in the internal jugular is usually seen as a flickering movement under the skin, rather than as an obvious venous pulsation.

The jugular venous pressure is taken as the highest point at which a pulsation can be seen, measured vertically above the manubriosternal angle. The position of the patient does not affect this measurement, because the height of the manubriosternal angle above the right atrium varies little as position changes. The patient should therefore be placed at whatever angle allows the pulsation to be seen most clearly. A patient with a high jugular venous pressure might need to sit upright, whilst a patient with a low pressure might need to lie flat. The key to successful observation of the jugular venous pulse is careful positioning of the patient, and arranging a tangential light, which will make movement under the skin of the neck more obvious.

A jugular venous pulsation has characteristics that allow it to be differentiated from an arterial pulse:

- The position of the pulsation in the neck varies with the patient's posture, reflecting its constant vertical height above the manubriosternal angle.

- A venous pulsation has a complex waveform compared with the single peak of an arterial pulse. In the venous pulse there is the 'a' wave due to atrial contraction, which is followed quickly by the 'c' wave. This has been variously attributed to tricuspid valve closure or to transmission from the carotid artery, and while it can be detected with an external pressure transducer, it is seldom possible to see it. There is then the 'x' descent due to the downward movement of the tricuspid valve as the right ventricle contracts. This is followed by a rise called the 'v' wave, which corresponds with the late stage of atrial filling during ventricular systole, followed by the 'y' trough as the atrium drains into the right ventricle.

- A venous pulse cannot be felt (except sometimes in triscupid regurgitation).
- A venous pulse can be obliterated by light pressure at the root of the neck.
- The height of the pulsation is affected by respiration, becoming less as intrathoracic pressure falls during inspiration.
- Pressure on the abdomen increases venous return and raises the jugular venous pressure (hepatojugular reflux).
- A prominent external jugular vein, which does not pulsate or move with respiration, may indicate superior mediastinal obstruction by a tumour.

The jugular venous pulse is abnormal in a number of disease states:

- The 'a' wave is lost in atrial fibrillation.
- The 'a' wave becomes more prominent (sometimes described as 'flicking') when the right atrial pressure is high, as in pulmonary hypertension.
- When the atrium contracts against a closed tricuspid valve, as occurs intermittently in complete heart block, large 'a' waves called 'cannon' waves are seen.
- If the tricuspid valve is incompetent the right ventricle expels part of its stroke volume through the right atrium and up the jugular veins, causing a 'cv' or 'systolic' wave. This is followed by a sudden and deep 'y' descent.
- If there is pericardial constriction the jugular venous pressure will rise rather than fall on inspiration.

The liver

If the right atrial pressure is high the liver will be distended and be palpable below the costal margin. It will be smooth and tender. With tricuspid regurgitation the liver will pulsate, and pulsation may also be seen in varicose veins in the legs. With marked and longstanding right heart failure there may also be splenic enlargement. Heart failure causes liver malfunction and—especially when tricuspid regurgitation is present—there may be jaundice.

Oedema

A combination of a high right heart pressure and hormonal changes cause fluid retention, with oedema fluid collecting in dependent areas. There will be symmetrical ankle and leg swelling, and if the patient is in bed for a prolonged period there will be oedema over the sacrum. Fluid can collect in all serous cavities causing pleural and pericardial effusions and ascites.

It is logical to think of the lungs at the same time as the veins: a rise in left atrial pressure will cause pulmonary congestion and eventually pulmonary oedema. These can be recognized by a soft wheeze ('cardiac asthma') and crackles at the lung bases.

Examination of the heart

Palpation

The apex beat is the furthest point outward from the midline, and downwards, where a cardiac impulse can be felt. It is important to accept this definition, and not to confuse the apex beat with the 'point of maximum impulse', because it provides the best guide to the size of the heart. The normal position of the apex beat is in the fifth rib interspace in the midclavicular line. The apex beat may be displaced by:

- left ventricular hypertrophy or dilatation
- right ventricular hypertrophy

- mediastinal shift.

Right ventricular hypertrophy is detected from a diffuse 'heaving' movement just to the left of the sternum; remember that the right ventricle forms the anterior surface of most of the heart. Mediastinal shift is identified if the trachea is moved to one side of the suprasternal notch. If the apex beat is displaced laterally and downwards but the trachea is central and there is no parasternal heave, then the left ventricle must be enlarged. A diffuse and abnormal movement medial to the apex may indicate a left ventricular aneurysm.

The precordium should be felt with the flat of the hand over the cardiac apex and the upper right sternal edge where thrills may be present. A thrill is simply a palpable murmur. A loud first sound may be felt as a tapping apex beat.

Heart sounds

There are four possible heart sounds and various extra sounds called clicks or snaps. These discrete noises arise from sudden movements in the circulating blood; they are not the result of valve cusps coming into contact with each other. Their pitch varies, and it is necessary to listen with the bell of the stethoscope for low-pitched sounds, and with the diaphragm for high-pitched sounds. Auscultation should be performed at the cardiac apex, to the left side of the top and bottom of the sternum and at the top of the right sternal edge. These positions are sometimes called the mitral, tricuspid, pulmonary, and aortic areas, but these descriptions are inappropriate because murmurs from these valves are not localized in these areas. The terms should be abandoned.

The first sound is associated with closure of the mitral and tricuspid valves at the beginning of systole. It is sometimes possible to hear separation, or splitting, of these two components but this is not a useful sign.

The second sound, best heard at the upper left sternal edge, is associated with closure of the aortic and pulmonary valves. The aortic valve closes first, and in inspiration, when pulmonary closure becomes delayed due to the increased blood flow through the right heart, the two components separate more widely. Variable splitting of the second heart sound is heard almost invariably in the young, but becomes less marked with age. Fixed splitting of the second sound is associated with right bundle branch block on the electrocardiogram, and may indicate an atrial septal defect. Reverse splitting is associated with left bundle branch block on the electrocardiogram. Aortic valve closure is delayed in left bundle branch block, so pulmonary closure is heard first. On inspiration pulmonary closure becomes delayed, so the pulmonary sound moves back to join the sound of aortic closure and the second sound becomes single.

The third and fourth sounds are due to rapid ventricular filling. The third sound is in early diastole soon after the second sound, and the fourth sound is associated with atrial contraction and therefore comes just before the first sound. Both are low pitched and are best heard at the apex with the patient rolled slightly onto the left side. A third sound is normal in children and young adults, but after middle age it is a sign of heart failure. A fourth sound (which can be difficult to differentiate from a split first sound) is nearly always abnormal and is said to indicate reduced ventricular distensibility. Right ventricular third and fourth sounds can sometimes be heard at the lower left sternal edge; they are louder on inspiration.

An ejection click, occurring just after the first sound, indicates a deformed but mobile aortic or pulmonary valve. The click may be associated with 'doming' of the valve before it opens. Late systolic clicks are heard with mitral valve prolapse.

An opening snap is a diastolic sound, just after the second sound, and is associated with the opening of a stenosed but mobile mitral or tricuspid valve. Unlike a third sound it is high pitched, and an opening snap can often be heard towards the left sternal edge while a third sound is always localized to the apex.

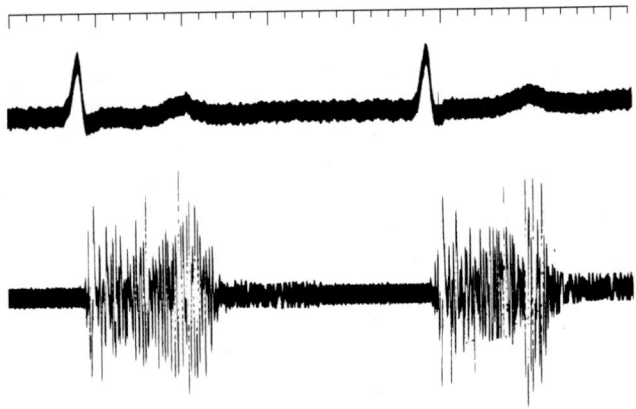

Fig. 1 Phonocardiographic recording of a patient with mitral regurgitation. The ECG recording (top line) determines that the murmur is systolic.

Heart murmurs

Heart murmurs are the result of turbulent blood flow associated with stenosed, leaking, or incompetent valves (when the murmur is said to be 'regurgitant') and with abnormal connections between the pulmonary and systemic circulation. A loud murmur can sometimes cause a palpable thrill. Murmurs can be systolic or diastolic (referring to the ventricles). A systolic murmur occurs when the mitral and tricuspid valves are shut, and the aortic and pulmonary valves are open. Conversely, diastolic murmurs are heard when the aortic and pulmonary valves are shut and the mitral and tricuspid valves are open.

Most murmurs originate in the left heart. Right heart murmurs are usually quiet but may become louder on inspiration. It should be remembered that the loudness of a murmur is only an extremely crude guide to its haemodynamic significance.

Murmurs originating in the mitral valve are best heard at the cardiac apex with the patient rolled a little to the left side. Mitral regurgitation (or incompetence) causes a medium pitch 'pansystolic' murmur, which begins immediately after the mitral valve closes and persists throughout systole. Murmurs can be recorded and displayed pictorially by the old technique of phonocardiography: Figure 1 shows a murmur of mitral regurgitation.

Murmurs spread, or radiate, in the direction of flowing blood and the murmur of mitral regurgitation radiates round the axilla and through to the back, as turbulent blood flows into the left atrium which forms the posterior part of the heart. When mitral regurgitation is due to mitral valve prolapse the murmur is still systolic, but it comes late in systole and is not pansystolic.

In mitral stenosis the opening snap is followed by a murmur, which rises to a peak and then falls, making a 'diamond' shape on a phonocardiogram (Fig. 2). This sort of murmur is called 'ejection'.

Tricuspid regurgitation causes a systolic murmur similar to that of mitral regurgitation, but it is loudest at the low left sternal edge, on inspiration. However, many patients with tricuspid regurgitation also have mitral regurgitation, and it can be difficult to differentiate the two. Tricuspid

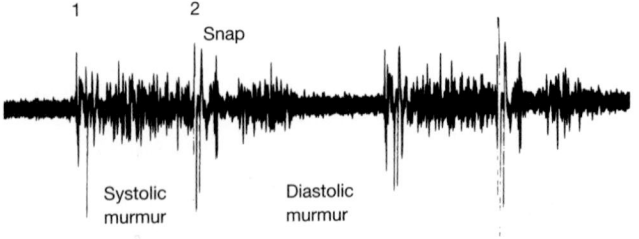

Fig. 2 Phonocardiographic recording of a patient with mixed mitral valve disease.

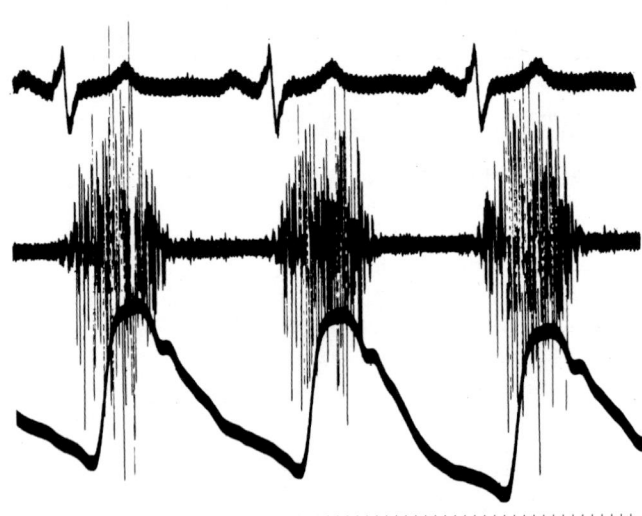

Fig. 3 Phonocardiographic recording of a patient with aortic stenosis. The ECG recording (top line) determines that the murmur is systolic. The bottom line records intra-arterial pressure.

regurgitation is diagnosed from the large 'cv' wave with a steep 'y' descent in the jugular venous pulse, and from an enlarged and pulsating liver. Tricuspid stenosis can occur with congenital or rheumatic heart disease and causes a similar ejection diastolic murmur to mitral stenosis, but the murmur of tricuspid stenosis occurs at the lower left sternal edge and is loudest on inspiration. Such a murmur is also heard as a 'flow' murmur in patients with an atrial septal defect, because increased flow through the right heart causes turbulence even through a normal valve.

Aortic stenosis causes the classic ejection systolic murmur (Fig. 3) heard at the upper right sternal edge. It radiates up the carotids, and this radiation has to be differentiated from a bruit due to narrowing of the carotid arteries. Carotid artery bruits are usually asymmetrical. An aortic ejection systolic murmur may also be heard when the valve is abnormal (for example, when it is bicuspid) but does not impede blood flow, or where there is an increased flow through a normal valve as in anaemia or pregnancy.

Aortic regurgitation causes a high-pitched murmur that begins immediately after aortic valve closure and dies away, usually by mid-diastole. It is described as an 'early diastolic' murmur, and is best heard at the mid left sternal edge—hence the fallacy of calling the upper right sternal edge the aortic area. The murmur of aortic regurgitation is best heard with the patient leaning forward and breathing out. The regurgitant jet of aortic regurgitation may impinge on the anterior cusp of the mitral valve causing it to flutter. This can cause a murmur (the Austin Flint murmur) that is very similar to that of mitral stenosis, but there is no associated opening snap.

Pulmonary systolic and diastolic murmurs share many of the characteristics of aortic stenosis and regurgitation and are also heard at the left sternal edge. They are quieter and are heard best on inspiration. Pulmonary regurgitation, characteristic of pulmonary hypertension, is sometimes called the Graham Steell murmur.

Murmurs associated with congenital heart disease may be systolic, diastolic, or continuous. The systolic and diastolic murmurs depend on obstruction to flow or regurgitant flow. Continuous murmurs occur in both systole and diastole, with their greatest intensity at the time of the second heart sound. The most typical is the murmur of a patent ductus arteriosus, heard under the left clavicle, but similar sounds are made by artificial shunts such as a Blalock operation.

A ventricular septal defect causes a murmur at the low left sternal edge: it is typically pansystolic, but a small defect can cause a very loud ejection murmur that radiates up the left sternal edge. An atrial septal defect does not cause a murmur itself, but increased right heart blood flow can cause a pulmonary systolic and a tricuspid diastolic murmur.

The importance of the physical examination

An accurate diagnosis of cardiovascular disease depends on the history and on the identification of a group of physical signs. It is always more efficient to look for things rather than at things. In a patient with chest pain look for signs of risk factors (smoking, hypertension, hypercholesterolaemia), evidence of vascular disease elsewhere (absent pulses, arterial bruits), and cardiac damage (signs of heart failure, mitral regurgitation due to papillary muscle dysfunction, postinfarct ventricular septal defect). In patients with palpitations check the rhythm and look for evidence of cardiac disease (especially rheumatic disease) or of other diseases such as thyrotoxicosis. In patients with breathlessness look for signs of heart failure (a rapid heart rate, raised jugular venous pressure, distended liver, ankle swelling, a gallop sound at the cardiac apex).

Individually, almost all physical signs are fallible. Finger clubbing, the identification of which varies between individuals, can be a congenital abnormality totally unrelated to cardiac disease. Splinter haemorrhages may be due to trauma. Cyanosis may be due to polycythaemia rubra vera. A raised jugular venous pressure may due to a 'high output' state such as pregnancy. The loudness of a murmur gives little information about its importance—and so on. But grouped together (for example a mitral regur-

gitant murmur with a displaced apex beat due to left ventricular hypertrophy) and used intelligently they become much more reliable.

It is true that there is considerable variability in the identification of physical abnormalities, particularly between non-specialists. But to abandon physical signs in favour of the ECG, the echocardiogram, and the chest radiograph is impracticable and expensive. In appropriate patients all these and other investigations may be essential. But for the initial assessment of patients, and for monitoring progress of disease, physical examination is both essential and adequate. It maintains a holistic approach to patient care, and can be an extremely satisfying art.

Further reading

Butman SM et al. (1993). Bedside cardiovascular examination in patients with severe chronic heart failure: importance of rest or inducible jugular venous distension. *Journal of the American College of Cardiologists* 22, 968–74.

Fletcher RH, Fletcher RW (1992). Has medicine outgrown physical diagnosis? *Annals of Internal Medicine* 117, 786–7.

Ishmail AA et al. (1987). Interobserver agreement by auscultation in the presence of a third heart sound in patients with congestive heart failure. *Chest* 91, 870–3.

Spiteri MA, Cook DG, Clarke SW (1988). Reliability of eliciting physical signs in examination of the chest. *The Lancet* 1, 873–5.

Stevenson LW, Perloff JK (1989). The limited reliability of physical signs for estimating hemodynamics in chronic heart failure. *Journal of the American Medical Association* 261, 884–8.

15.3 Clinical investigation

15.3.1 Chest radiography in heart disease

M. B. Rubens

Introduction

The chest radiograph is often abnormal in patients with congenital heart disease, but in most patients with acquired heart disease it is normal and rarely provides a precise diagnosis. Nonetheless, a chest radiograph remains part of the routine work-up of virtually all patients with known or suspected heart disease because it is relatively inexpensive and non-invasive and it provides a record of cardiac size and shape, sometimes also suggesting specific chamber enlargement. Abnormal cardiac calcification may be visible, and analysis of the pulmonary vessels may indicate particular physiological disturbances. Analysis of the skeleton may provide evidence of associated systemic disease or previous surgery, and abnormalities of situs may be apparent. Occasionally, unsuspected non-cardiac abnormalities are discovered.

A routine examination always includes a frontal view and sometimes a lateral view. Ideally, the frontal view is posteroanterior, with the patient upright and at end-inspiration. Patients who are too ill to be taken to the X-ray department may be examined with mobile equipment when an anteroposterior film is taken. In this projection the heart appears magnified because it is further from the film. A lateral film may give additional information on heart size and shape, and cardiac calcification is often best demonstrated in this view. Frontal and lateral films combined with a barium swallow may provide data on left atrial size and the presence of aberrant branches of the great vessels.

As in all areas of clinical examination, the chest radiograph should be analysed in a careful, systematic manner. It must be remembered that poor radiographic technique may produce spurious appearances. Moreover, the cardiovascular silhouette is such an obvious focus of attention that the bones, soft tissues, and upper abdomen may be overlooked. The cardiac shadow provides information about anatomy, but the lungs provide information about haemodynamics. A recommended order of analysis is as follows: technical factors, the bones, the upper abdomen, the lungs, and, finally, the cardiovascular silhouette. Discussion in this chapter will focus on the appearance of the heart and vessels and other changes on the chest radiograph produced by cardiovascular disease.

The normal chest radiograph

The cardiovascular silhouette

The right border of the cardiovascular silhouette (Fig. 1) comprises, from above downwards, the superior vena cava, the body of right atrium, and the

inferior vena cava. The normal superior vena cava produces a low-density vertical shadow, just lateral to the spine. The azygos vein may be visible as a convex density above the origin of the right main bronchus and superimposed on the superior vena cava. The lower part of the right cardiovascular silhouette is convex and produced by the body of the right atrium. Occasionally, the inferior vena cava is visible as a short vertical shadow in the right cardiophrenic angle.

The left border of the cardiovascular silhouette comprises, from above downwards, the aortic knuckle, the pulmonary trunk, the left atrial appendage, and the left ventricle. The aortic knuckle is produced by the posterior part of the aortic arch. The proximal descending aorta may be visible as a vertical shadow, continuous with the knuckle and eventually merging with the left paraspinal shadow. The pulmonary trunk is situated below the aortic knuckle, and below this is a short segment of left atrial appendage. The bulk of the left heart border is formed by the body of the

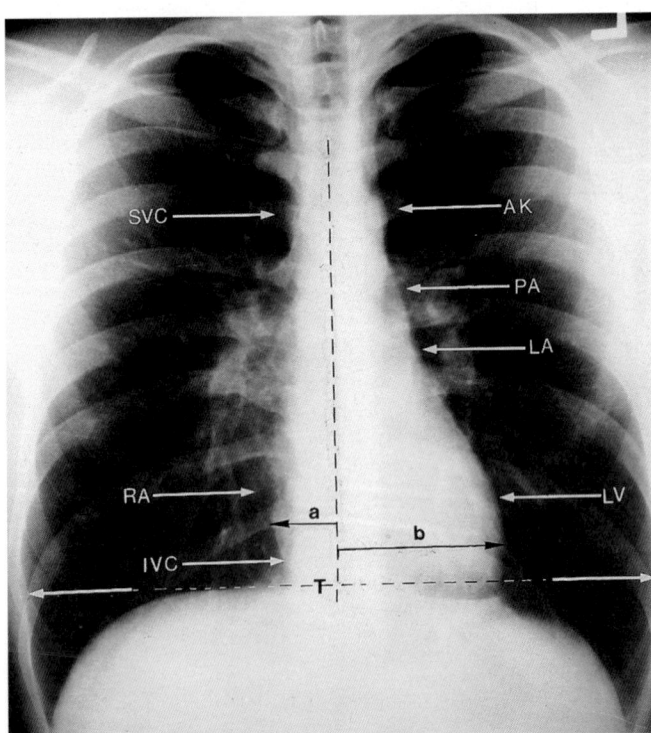

Fig. 1 Normal chest radiograph. The right border of the cardiovascular silhouette comprises superior vena cava (SVC), right atrium (RA), and inferior vena cava (IVC), and the left border comprises aortic knuckle (AK), pulmonary trunk (PA), left atrial appendage (LA), and left ventricle (LV). Transverse cardiac diameter=a+b. Cardiothoracic ratio=(a+b)/T.

left ventricle. The left cardiophrenic angle may be occupied by a low-density shadow representing an apical pericardial fat pad. Less often, a fat pad is visible in the right cardiophrenic angle.

On the lateral film (Fig. 2) the heart is seen immediately posterior to the inferior half of the sternum. The anterior border of the cardiac shadow is formed almost entirely by the right ventricle, although in atrial diastole the right atrial appendage may come in contact with the sternum. The right ventricular outflow tract is continuous with the main pulmonary artery that arches posteriorly and continues into the left pulmonary artery. The branches of the right pulmonary artery cast an ovoid shadow anterior to the right bronchus. Part of the ascending aorta may be visible above the pulmonary trunk, and the aortic arch is seen passing posteriorly and then descending for a variable distance. The aortic arch is separated from the left pulmonary artery by the subaortic fossa. The upper part of the posterior aspect of the cardiac silhouette is formed by the body of left atrium and the pulmonary veins, and the lower part by the left ventricle. The inferior vena cava may be visible as a short, straight vertical shadow extending from the diaphragm and overlapping the posterior heart border.

The normal cardiovascular silhouette changes with age. In infancy, the thymus occupies much of the anterior mediastinum and may obscure the aorta, the pulmonary trunk, and the right ventricular outflow tract. By early adolescence, the thymus is no longer visible on the chest radiograph, and the normal pulmonary trunk is often prominent. In adulthood, the pulmonary trunk is less prominent, and with advancing years the left ventricular contour becomes more convex. In old age, the ascending aorta may become tortuous and project lateral to the superior vena cava, and the aortic knuckle and descending aorta may be increasingly prominent.

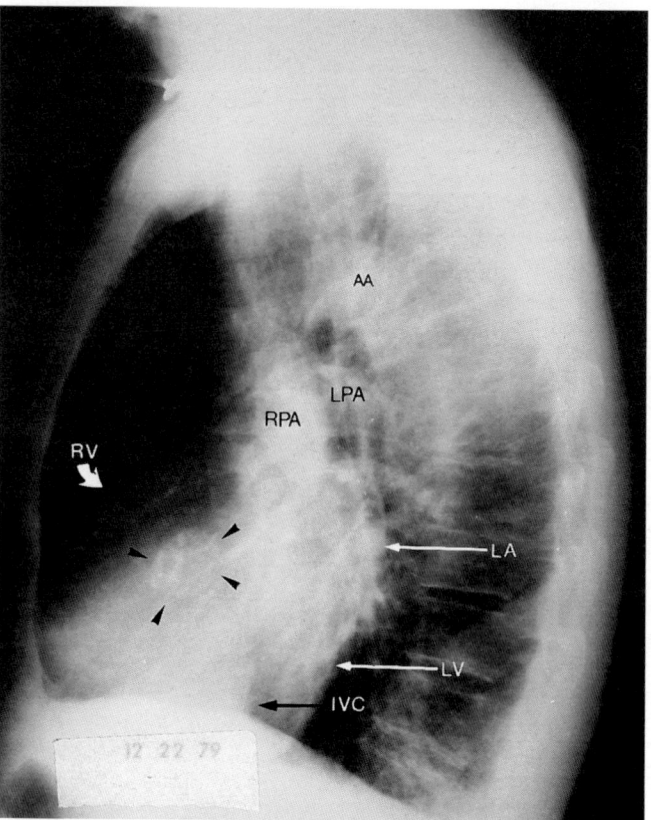

Fig. 2 Lateral chest radiograph. Patient with calcific aortic stenosis. The aortic valve is heavily calcified (arrowheads). AA=aortic arch; IVC=inferior vena cava; LA=left atrium; LPA=left pulmonary artery; LV=left ventricle; RPA=right pulmonary artery; RV=right ventricle.

Heart size

The commonest methods of assessment of cardiac size using the chest radiograph are the measurement of the transverse cardiac diameter and the measurement of cardiothoracic ratio (Fig. 1).

The transverse cardiac diameter is measured on a posteroanterior film by adding the maximum distance of the right heart border from the mid-line to the maximum distance of the left heart border from the mid-line. The upper limit of normal is 16 cm for men and 15 cm for women. A change of 1.5 cm in cardiac diameter should be regarded as significant. Apparent increase in heart size may be due to a poor inspiration; on anteroposterior films geometric magnification of the heart shadow occurs.

The cardiothoracic ratio is the ratio of transverse cardiac diameter to maximum internal diameter of the thorax. There are racial differences in the normal ratio, which should not exceed 50 per cent in white subjects or 55 per cent in black subjects.

The pulmonary vasculature

The pulmonary trunk normally forms a short segment of the left cardiovascular silhouette. The pulmonary arteries are not visible on the chest radiograph until they emerge from the pericardium and are surrounded by aerated lung. The right pulmonary artery lies anterior to the right main bronchus and usually divides into upper lobe and descending arteries just before emerging from the pericardium. The descending branch is usually clearly seen lateral to the right heart border, where it forms the bulk of the right hilum. Its diameter should not exceed 15 mm in women and 16 mm in men. The left pulmonary artery arches posteriorly over the left main bronchus, and the left hilum is therefore higher than the right. The branching pattern of the pulmonary arteries is similar to that of the bronchi. As the pulmonary arteries pass peripherally, they taper smoothly and are not normally visible in the outer third of the lung.

The anatomy of the pulmonary veins is variable. The upper lobe veins run lateral to the corresponding pulmonary arteries and can often be identified crossing the pulmonary arteries at the hilum prior to the left atrium. The lower lobe veins run more horizontally and medially than the accompanying arteries.

On the frontal chest radiograph of a normal, erect subject the pulmonary vessels should be clearly visible and are larger in the lower zones than in the upper zones. The upper zone veins in the first anterior intercostal space should not exceed 3 mm in diameter. On a supine film, the upper zone and lower zone vessels appear similar in size.

The abnormal chest radiograph

Technical considerations

On an over-exposed chest radiograph the lungs appear blacker than usual and may mimic pulmonary oligaemia. Conversely, an under-exposed film may accentuate the pulmonary vascular pattern, or even suggest diffuse lung disease. A chest radiograph taken on expiration may show increased basal shadowing and suggest pulmonary oedema or other some other interstitial pulmonary abnormality, and the heart may appear enlarged. A rotated film may make some structures appear unusually prominent and others unusually small.

The bones

Deformity of the thoracic skeleton may alter the appearance of the heart. Sternal depression (pectus excavatum) usually displaces and rotates the heart to the left producing a characteristic straight left heart border). In the 'straight back syndrome', the anteroposterior diameter of the thorax is decreased and the heart may be compressed between sternum and spine producing a spurious appearance of cardiomegaly on the frontal chest radiograph. Severe scoliosis may not only alter the shape of the mediastinum but may actually cause cardiopulmonary disease.

Congenital deformity of the thoracic skeleton may be associated with cardiac disease. Both sternal depression and 'straight back' are associated with mitral valve prolapse. Many systemic diseases and congenital syndromes which involve the cardiovascular system may also have skeletal manifestations, for example in Down's syndrome there may be an atrioventricular septal defect and only 11 pairs of ribs.

Rib notching is usually associated with coarctation of the aorta, but may also be seen in pulmonary atresia and vena caval obstruction or following creation of a Blalock–Taussig shunt. Evidence of previous surgery, such as rib deformity, sternal sutures, and prosthetic valves, may be seen on the chest radiograph.

The upper abdomen

Rarely, patients presenting with chest pain have a hiatus hernia or gallstones that may be visible on the chest radiograph. In those with congenital heart disease, information about situs may be visible on the chest radiograph and it is worth noting if the stomach and liver are normally situated, also the visibility and location of the spleen. The best indication of atrial situs, however, is given by the tracheobronchial anatomy.

The lungs

The normal radiographic appearance of the lung is produced by pulmonary vessels outlined by aerated lung. Any opacity that is not a vessel should be carefully considered. Since smoking is an important aetiological factor in both cardiovascular and pulmonary disease, it is not surprising that the routine chest radiograph in a cardiac patient may uncover previously unsuspected lung disease.

The pulmonary vascular pattern may be normal, increased, decreased, or uneven. Normal pulmonary vascularity does not exclude significant myocardial disease, mild valvular disease, or a small intracardiac shunt.

Increased pulmonary vascularity

There are four distinct patterns of increased pulmonary vascularity:

(1) pulmonary venous hypertension;

(2) pulmonary arterial hypertension;

(3) pulmonary over-circulation;

(4) systemic supply to the lungs.

Any of these patterns may coexist.

Pulmonary venous hypertension

Pulmonary venous hypertension is most commonly caused by left ventricular failure, mitral valve disease, or aortic valve disease. Rarely, it is due to pulmonary venous obstruction. When pulmonary venous pressure rises, the upper lobe veins distend, becoming similar in size to the lower lobe veins and eventually larger. This phenomenon may be described as 'upper lobe blood diversion' (Fig. 3). When the pulmonary venous pressure exceeds the plasma osmotic pressure, fluid accumulates in the interstitial spaces of the lung. This appears radiographically as interstitial pulmonary oedema: the lower zone and hilar vessels may become indistinct (perihilar haze) and interstitial lines may appear. Kerley B lines are caused by fluid-filled interlobular septa and appear as fine, non-branching horizontal lines in the periphery of the lower zones (Fig. 4). Kerley A lines are less common and are longer, fine-line shadows that radiate from the hila into the mid and upper zones. They also represent distended interlobular septa. Excess interstitial fluid around bronchi may appear as peribronchial cuffing. A further rise in pulmonary venous pressure leads to accumulation of fluid in the alveolar spaces (Fig. 5). Classically, alveolar oedema is perihilar, but it may be patchy and asymmetric, or even nodular, and it may be indistinguishable from other forms of pulmonary consolidation. Pleural effusions are common in pulmonary venous hypertension.

In the untreated patient there is a fairly close correlation between the pulmonary capillary wedge pressure and the radiographic signs of pulmonary venous hypertension. A normal vascular pattern corresponds to a

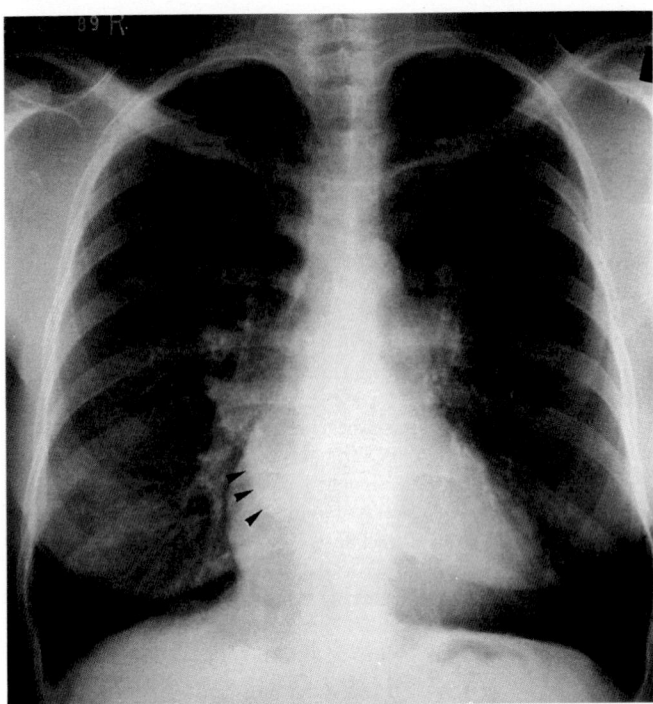

Fig. 3 Upper lobe blood diversion. Patient with mitral valve disease. The extra density over the right heart border (arrowheads) is due to left atrial enlargement.

wedge pressure of less than 12 mmHg, redistribution of blood flow corresponds to 12 to 18 mmHg, interstitial oedema corresponds to 18 to 22 mmHg, and above 22 mmHg there is usually overt alveolar oedema. If a patient has received diuretic therapy, this correlation is less reliable.

In patients with long-standing pulmonary venous hypertension, radiographic signs of pulmonary arterial hypertension may also be present.

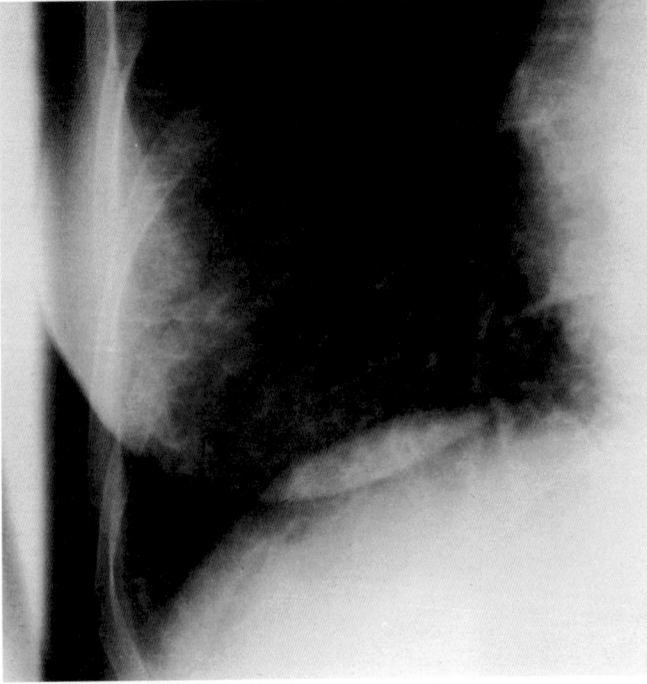

Fig. 4 Kerley B lines. Patient with interstitial pulmonary oedema due to mitral stenosis.

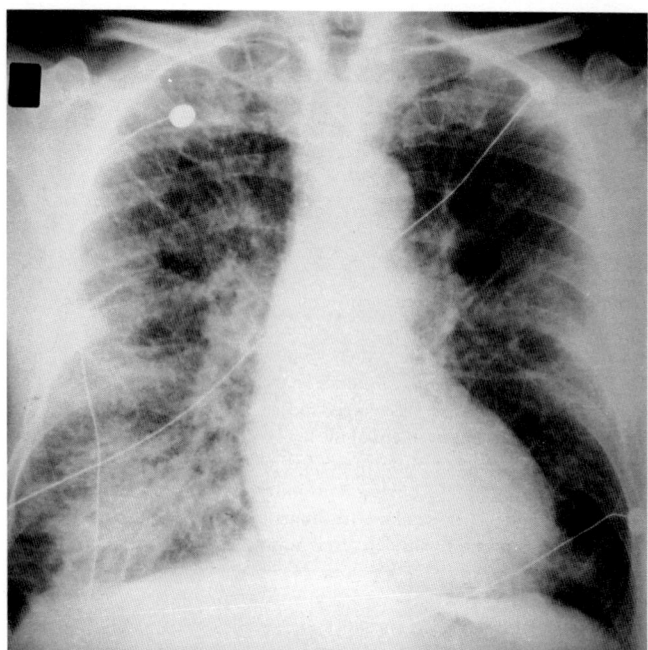

Fig. 5 Severe pulmonary venous hypertension. Patient with acute myocardial infarction. In addition to upper lobe blood diversion, perihilar haze and basal septal lines indicate interstitial oedema, and right lower zone consolidation indicates alveolar oedema.

Chronic pulmonary venous hypertension may also be associated with pulmonary haemosiderosis or pulmonary ossicles. The former appears as a fine nodular pattern throughout both lungs, and the latter as calcified basal nodules of up to 1 cm in diameter.

Although redistribution of blood flow and septal lines are most often a manifestation of pulmonary venous hypertension, there are other causes that should be considered. Redistribution of blood flow may occur in patients who have basal emphysema and no evidence of pulmonary venous hypertension. Septal lines may be seen in non-cardiogenic pulmonary oedema, lymphangitis carcinomatosa, sarcoidosis, and silicosis.

Pulmonary arterial hypertension

Pulmonary arterial hypertension may be defined as a pulmonary artery systolic pressure exceeding 30 mmHg. The commonest causes of this condition are chronic lung disease, pulmonary emboli, pulmonary venous hypertension, and intracardiac shunts. It may also be idiopathic. The typical radiographic appearances are enlargement of the central pulmonary arteries and attenuation of the peripheral arteries. In severe, long-standing pulmonary arterial hypertension, calcification may be seen in the central pulmonary arteries.

An indication of the underlying cause may be present on the chest radiograph; for example there may be signs of chronic obstructive airways disease or pulmonary embolism. Bilateral hilar lymph node enlargement may mimic enlarged central pulmonary arteries, but usually lymphadenopathy is lobulated, whereas enlarged arteries have a smooth outline.

Pulmonary over-circulation

Pulmonary over-circulation or plethora implies increased blood-flow through the lungs. It is usually due to a left-to-right shunt, less commonly due to bidirectional shunting and rarely due to increased cardiac output. Small shunts may not be perceptible on the chest radiograph, but shunts with a pulmonary-to-systemic flow ratio of 2:1 or greater should be apparent unless there is coexisting heart failure. The central pulmonary arteries are larger than normal and peripheral pulmonary vessels are visible in the outer third of the lung (Fig. 6). Pulmonary plethora in a non-cyanosed

patient indicates a left-to-right shunt, whereas in the presence of cyanosis it indicates bidirectional shunting.

Systemic supply to the lungs

Systemic arterial supply to the lungs, which is sometimes referred to as 'bronchial circulation', develops in patients with severe right ventricular outflow obstruction. The pulmonary trunk is either small or absent, and the peripheral vessels are disorganized and may produce a reticular or nodular pattern that mimics diffuse lung disease.

Decreased pulmonary vascularity

Pulmonary oligaemia

Pulmonary oligaemia implies decreased blood flow through the lungs. It is usually due to right ventricular outflow obstruction in association with a right-to-left shunt, for example tetralogy of Fallot. The lungs appear to have fewer and smaller vessels than usual, and the pulmonary trunk may be small or inapparent. Pulmonary oligaemia due to restricted filling of the right heart, such as occurs in cardiac tamponade, is rarely perceptible on the chest radiograph.

Uneven vascularity

Uneven pulmonary vascularity is most commonly due to pulmonary disease. A previous lung resection will obviously alter the vascular pattern. Apart from pulmonary thromboembolism, cardiovascular causes of uneven vascularity are rare but include previous shunt operations for congenital heart disease, pulmonary artery stenoses, and pulmonary arteriovenous fistulae.

Abnormalities of the heart and great vessels

The systemic veins

Enlargement of the superior vena cava may be caused by either increased flow or increased pressure. Increased flow occurs in supracardiac anomalous pulmonary venous return. Increased pressure occurs in right heart failure, tricuspid valve disease, cardiac tamponade, and constrictive pericarditis. The superior vena cava may also dilate secondary to obstruction caused by mediastinitis or mediastinal tumour. The superior vena cava may be displaced laterally by a tortuous or dilated ascending aorta or a right-sided aortic arch.

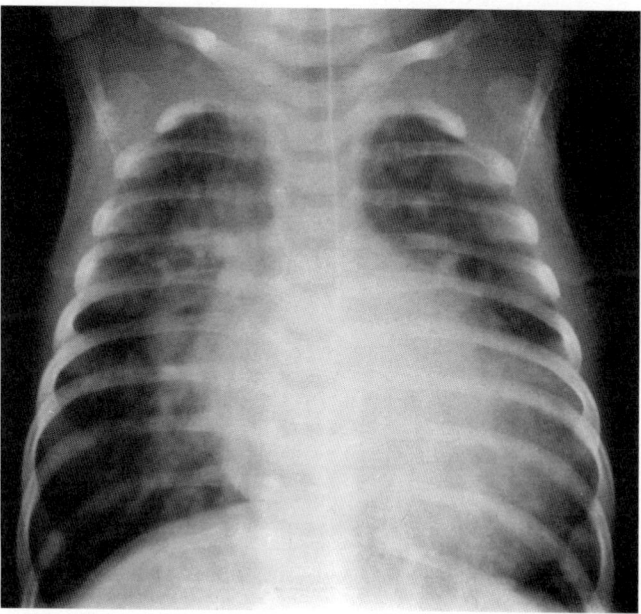

Fig. 6 Pulmonary plethora. Infant with transposition of the great arteries. The pulmonary vascular pattern is accentuated; there is also cardiomegaly.

The azygos vein may enlarge for the same reasons as enlargement of the superior vena cava. An enlarged azygos vein is also seen in superior vena caval obstruction, portal vein obstruction, and absence of the hepatic portion of the inferior vena cava in polysplenia.

The inferior vena cava may enlarge in secondary to tricuspid valve disease and right heart failure.

The right atrium

Right atrial enlargement rarely occurs in isolation, and is usually associated with right ventricular enlargement. Classically, right atrial enlargement produces increased prominence of the lower half of the right side of the cardiac shadow. It occurs in right heart failure, tricuspid valve disease, and in atrial septal defect and other shunts that enter the right atrium.

The right ventricle

The normal right ventricle is not a border-forming structure on the frontal chest radiograph. An enlarging right ventricle tends to displace the left ventricle laterally so that the cardiac apex becomes elevated. In gross right ventricular enlargement, the right ventricle may actually form the left heart border, and dilatation of its outflow tract may produce a bump just below the pulmonary trunk. On the lateral view, right ventricular enlargement may manifest as increased contact of the heart with the sternum. Right ventricular enlargement occurs in pulmonary arterial hypertension, tricuspid valve disease, pulmonary valve disease, left-to-right shunts, and tetralogy of Fallot.

The pulmonary trunk

Enlargement of the pulmonary trunk is due to increased pressure, increased flow, poststenotic dilatation, or idiopathic dilatation (Fig. 7). In pulmonary arterial hypertension, it may be associated with enlargement of the central pulmonary arteries and peripheral pruning. In situations of

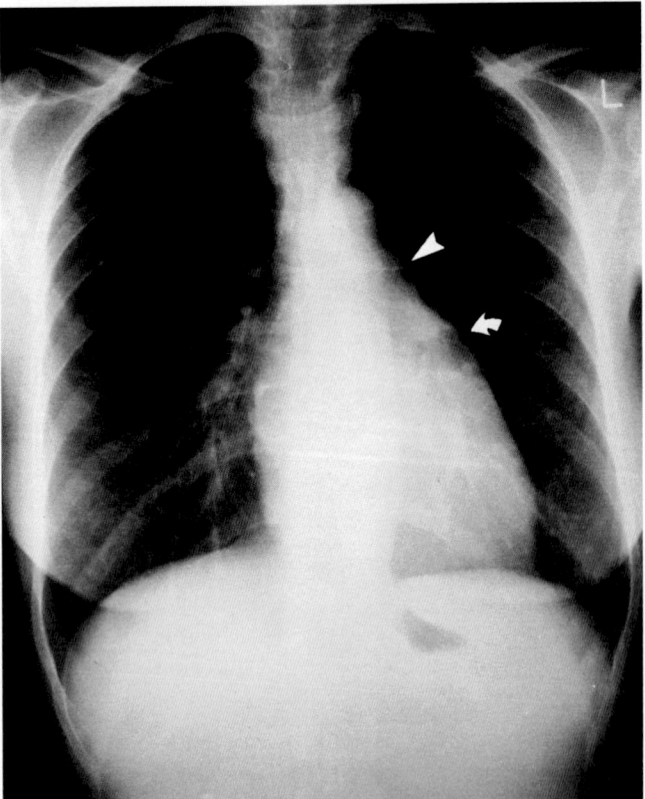

Fig. 7 Patient with mitral stenosis. The transverse cardiac diameter size is normal, but the left atrial appendage is enlarged (curved arrow), and there is also prominence of the pulmonary trunk (arrowhead).

increased flow, it is associated with pulmonary plethora. In cases of poststenotic and idiopathic dilatation, it is usually associated with enlargement of the left pulmonary artery and normal peripheral vascularity.

In corrected transposition of the great arteries, the pulmonary trunk is not visible on the chest radiograph. In tetralogy of Fallot and pulmonary atresia, the pulmonary trunk is small, producing an obvious pulmonary bay.

The left atrium

The body of the left atrium is situated beneath the carina and in front of the oesophagus. Enlargement superiorly may increase the angle between the left and right bronchi by elevating the left bronchus and displacing it posteriorly. Posterior enlargement may displace the oesophagus posteriorly. Enlargement to the right may produce an extra density over the right heart border (Fig. 3), and if grossly enlarged the left atrium may actually form the right heart border. Enlargement of the left atrial appendage causes straightening or convex bulging of the upper left heart border (Fig. 7). Left atrial enlargement occurs most obviously in mitral valve disease, but is seen in other forms of left heart failure, in shunts at ventricular and great vessel level, and in association with left atrial tumours.

The left ventricle

Left ventricular hypertrophy produces increased convexity of the left heart border, but not cardiac enlargement unless heart failure develops. Left ventricular dilatation causes displacement of the cardiac apex downward and to the left, and on the lateral view the heart shadow extends more posteriorly than usual. Left ventricular hypertrophy results from systolic overload, and dilatation from diastolic overload. In left ventricular aneurysm, a discrete bulge may develop on the left heart border.

The aorta

Selective enlargement of the ascending aorta is seen in poststenotic dilatation due to aortic valvar stenosis and in association with aneurysms. The aortic knuckle may be prominent due to aneurysm, patent ductus arteriosus, tetralogy of Fallot, and pulmonary atresia. In coarctation of the aorta, the knuckle always appears abnormal—it may be prominent, flat, high, low, or have an abnormal contour. In non-obstructing coarctation or pseudocoarctation, the arch appears elongated and kinked. Selective enlargement of the descending aorta may be due to aneurysm. Generalized prominence of the thoracic aorta may be part of the ageing process but is also seen in systemic hypertension and aortic regurgitation.

The aortic arch is usually left-sided, arching posteriorly over the left main bronchus. However, it can be right-sided, when it arches over the right bronchus and indents the right side of the trachea, the usual shadow of the left arch is absent, and the superior vena cava may be displaced laterally. A right arch with an aberrant left subclavian artery is not usually associated with heart disease, but if its branches are the mirror image of normal there is a high incidence of congenital heart disease. Tetralogy of Fallot, pulmonary atresia, truncus arteriosus, and ventricular septal defect may be associated with a right arch. An aberrant subclavian artery can be identified on a barium swallow.

The pericardium

Pericardial effusion may produce non-specific globular enlargement of the heart shadow and rapid increase in heart size on serial films is suggestive of this condition. Pulmonary vascularity is usually normal. A pericardial cyst may appear as a well-circumscribed, rounded opacity adjacent to the heart. Partial pericardial defects may allow herniation of the left atrial appendage causing a prominent bulge on the left heart border. In congenital absence of the pericardium there is usually displacement of the entire heart to the left.

Cardiac calcification

Calcification may occur in any cardiovascular structure, and is usually the result of inflammatory disease or infarction. Although cardiac calcification may be visible on the chest radiograph it is better demonstrated by fluoroscopy when movement of an abnormally calcified structure aids its detection, in contrast to the chest radiograph where movement causes blurring.

Myocardial and endocardial calcification most commonly occur in the left ventricle secondary to coronary artery disease. Curvilinear calcification may occur in the wall of left ventricular aneurysms, in thrombi, and in infarcts. Left atrial wall calcification may be due to rheumatic myocarditis, and left atrial thrombi may calcify.

Aortic valve calcification usually lies over the spine on the frontal chest radiograph and may, therefore, be obscured. It is best seen on the lateral view (Fig. 2), and tends to lie mostly above a line drawn from the carina to the anterior costophrenic angle. Mitral valve calcification usually lies to the left of the spine, and on a lateral view lies below the line drawn from carina to the anterior costophrenic angle. Calcification is rarely seen in the tricuspid and pulmonary valves, but commonly occurs in right ventricular outflow tract homografts.

Calcification is frequently seen in the aortic arch of older patients as part of the normal ageing process. Extensive aortic calcification is most likely to be due to atheroma, but it may be the result of an arteritis or syphilitic aortitis, which characteristically involves the ascending aorta. Calcification in a healed dissecting aneurysm may be seen in any part of the aorta. Chronic traumatic aneurysms in the region of the aortic isthmus may calcify. Coronary artery calcification indicates atheroma, but does not necessarily correspond to significant coronary artery narrowing. A patent ductus arteriosus may calcify, and calcification may develop in the central pulmonary arteries in long-standing, severe pulmonary arterial hypertension.

Pericardial calcification may be a sequel to pericarditis and haemopericardium, and it may be associated with pericardial constriction. Rare causes of cardiac calcification include tumours, hydatid disease, and coronary artery fistulae.

Further reading

Elliott LP (1991). *Cardiac imaging in infants, children and adults.* Lippincot, Phildelphia.

Elliott LP, Schiebler GL (1979). *X-ray diagnosis of congenital cardiac disease,* 2nd edn. Charles C. Thomas, Springfield.

Jefferson K, Rees S (1980). *Clinical cardiac radiology,* 2nd edn. Butterworth, London.

15.3.2 Electrocardiography

D. J. Rowlands

The resting 12-lead ECG

Historical introduction

The first electrocardiographic recording of the human heart was made in 1887 by A. D. Waller, who expressed the view that it was unlikely that such recordings would be of much use in clinical practice. This view was not shared by Einthoven, who noted the differences between recordings taken from healthy and from sick persons and was, in consequence, convinced that the technique would prove to be of great clinical value. Einthoven suggested the P, QRS, T, U terminology which is in universal use today, and recognized that a better recording device than the capillary electrometer (used by Waller) would be necessary. He modified and developed the string galvanometer for this purpose. The resulting instrument was unwieldy, weighing over a quarter of a ton (254 kg) and requiring five people for its operation, but it produced electrocardiograms of remarkable quality. The

first commercially available machine for recording the electrocardiogram (ECG) was made in England in 1911 by the Cambridge Scientific Instrument Company and was delivered to Sir Thomas Lewis at University College Hospital in London. In the early 1900s Einthoven and Lewis were undoubtedly the pioneers who did most to advance the clinical study of electrocardiography. In the early 1930s the most productive research worker in this field was Frank N. Wilson of Ann Arbor, Michigan, who had been stationed in England during World War I in a rehabilitation hospital under the command of Sir Thomas Lewis. Wilson's early research work was, therefore, undertaken in England and, whereas Lewis had concentrated on the cardiac rhythm, Wilson's work was centred on the QRS complexes and T waves. It was Wilson who developed the unipolar recording system, by developing an 'indifferent' electrode that gave a stable reference potential with respect to which the potential at a single exploring electrode could be measured. This reference potential was obtained from a central terminal connected to the left arm, the right arm, and the left leg through equal resistors.

The development of electrocardiographic recording techniques continues (witness the rapidly expanding use of electrophysiological studies of the heart), but the standard 12-lead ECG still forms an essential part of any full clinical cardiological assessment more than 100 years after the first human ECG recording was made. It is estimated that in excess of 100 million 12-lead ECGs are recorded annually worldwide, a fact that would surely have astonished Waller. Electrocardiography developed empirically and its basic diagnostic criteria remain empirical. The criteria given in this chapter represent a reasonable compromise between sensitivity and specificity.

Normal ECG appearances

The basic ECG waveform

The basic ECG waveform consists of three recognizable deflections termed 'P wave', 'QRS complex', and 'T wave', by Einthoven (Fig. 1). The P wave is the surface electrocardiographic manifestation of atrial myocardial depolarization. Depolarization of the sinoatrial node is not recognizable on the surface ECG and can only be inferred from the shape and direction of the P wave. The QRS complex is the surface electrocardiographic manifestation of ventricular myocardial depolarization. The S–T segment and T wave represent ventricular myocardial repolarization. Atrial myocardial repolarization is indicated by the Ta wave, which is a small, asymmetrical negative wave following the P wave, usually obscured by the QRS complex which occurs at the same time. The Ta wave usually becomes easily recognizable during sinus tachycardia (especially during exercise), since it then increases in size and becomes a rounded negative wave beginning before the QRS complex and extending into the S–T segment. A prominent atrial repolarization wave occurring during an exercise stress test is frequently wrongly interpreted as S–T-segment depression. The key to avoiding this error is to recognize that the negativity begins before the QRS complex. The P wave and T wave have relatively simple shapes which exhibit few variations. The QRS complexes exhibit more readily recognizable differences in pattern in different leads within the same ECG.

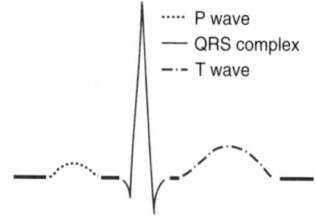

..... P wave
— QRS complex
–·– T wave

Fig. 1 The basic ECG waveform.

QRS waveform nomenclature

The QRS complexes usually have the largest voltages and virtually always the highest frequency components of the various ECG deflections, and typically consist of 'sharp', pointed deflections. The presence and relative size of the several possible components of the QRS complex may be indicated by a convention using combinations of the letters q, r, s, Q, R, S (Fig. 2). If a given component is considered to be large, an UPPER CASE letter is used, if it is considered to be small a lower case letter is used.

The 12 conventional ECG leads

Unipolar, bipolar, and augmented leads

Leads I, II, and III are the bipolar limb leads, introduced originally by Einthoven. The remaining three limb leads and the six precordial leads are unipolar (they involve the use of the central reference terminal of Wilson) and are termed V leads (the 'V' originally stood for 'voltage', to reflect the fact that these unipolar leads effectively measure the voltage at the location of the recording electrode). All currently available ECG machines use augmented (a) limb leads (that is to say they record aVR, aVL, and aVF as opposed to VR, VL, and VF; VR (right arm), VL (left arm), VF (left leg)) as a result of the use of a standard, but no longer necessary, modification of

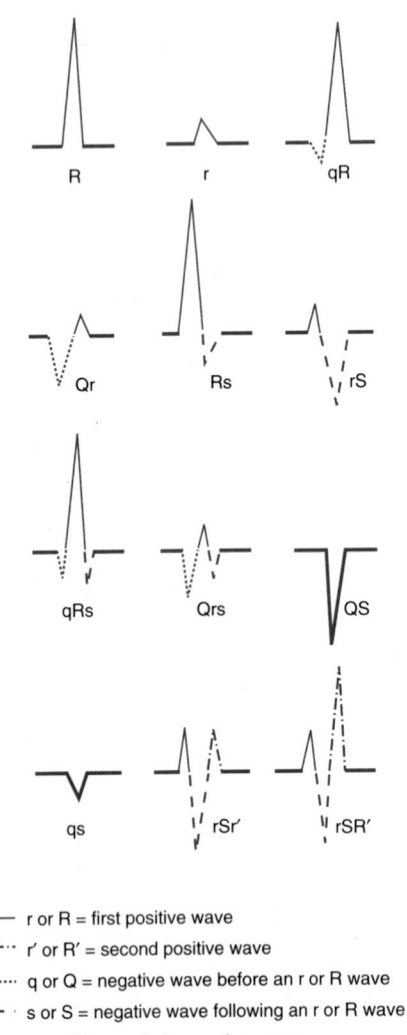

Fig. 2 QRS waveform nomenclature.

— r or R = first positive wave

–·–·– r' or R' = second positive wave

·········· q or Q = negative wave before an r or R wave

– – – s or S = negative wave following an r or R wave

—— qs or QS = entirely negative wave

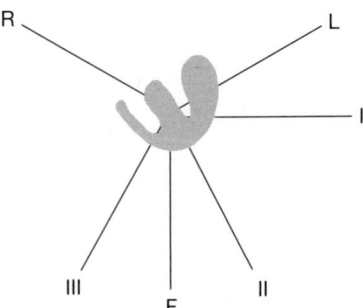

Fig. 3 The arrangement of the frontal plane leads. Note that leads II, III, and F are inferior to the heart, I and L are anterolateral to the heart, and R looks into the cavity of the heart.

the original Wilson central terminal, designed to produce a 1.5-fold amplification in the recorded voltage.

The six limb leads (frontal plane leads)

The limb leads are remote from the heart and give (spatially) general rather than localized (spatially specific) information. In this respect they differ markedly from the precordial leads. The limb leads consist of the three bipolar leads (leads I, II, and III) and the three augmented, unipolar leads aVR, aVL, and aVF. The orientation around the heart of the six limb leads is illustrated in Fig. 3. The orientation of leads aVR, aVL, and aVF with respect to the heart is intuitively obvious since the limbs act as linear conductors (like wires). The left arm connection is therefore effectively 'looking at the heart' from the left shoulder (i.e. the left arm is acting as part of the wire connecting the ECG machine to the patient's left shoulder). Similarly, the right arm connection 'looks at the heart' from the right shoulder and the foot lead connection from the pelvic area. One practical consequence of the fact that the limbs act as linear conductors is that it does not matter whereabouts on any given limb the electrode is attached. The orientation of the bipolar leads with respect to the heart is not intuitively obvious (simply because they are bipolar leads), but may be worked out from the known polarities of the conventional connections used in the bipolar leads. Thus, for example, since lead I is recorded with the left arm connected to the positive and the right arm to the negative terminal of the recorder, the position of lead I is effectively that obtained by subtracting the right arm vector from the left arm vector. To subtract vector R from vector L one reverses the direction of vector R and adds it to vector L. Inspection of Fig. 3 reveals that if this is done the resulting 'direction' of lead I is effectively horizontally to the left of the heart. In a similar manner it can be shown that the effective orientations of leads II and III with respect to the heart are as shown in Fig. 3.

The six precordial leads (chest leads)

For each precordial lead, the positive (recording) terminal is connected to an electrode at an agreed site on the chest wall. Since the connection to the negative terminal of the recorder is the 'indifferent' one formed by joining together leads R, L, and F, the chest leads are 'V' leads and are designated V_1, V_2, V_3, V_4, V_5, and V_6. Because the torso, unlike the limbs, acts as a volume conductor, the waveform obtained depends critically on the siting of the recording electrode. A standard anatomical siting of the precordial electrodes was agreed between the British Cardiac Society and the American Heart Association and is shown in Fig. 4. The important relationships of the precordial leads to the cardiac chambers are shown in Fig. 5.

The 12 conventional ECG leads

Figure 6 shows the relationship of the 12 conventional electrocardiographic leads to one another and to the heart.

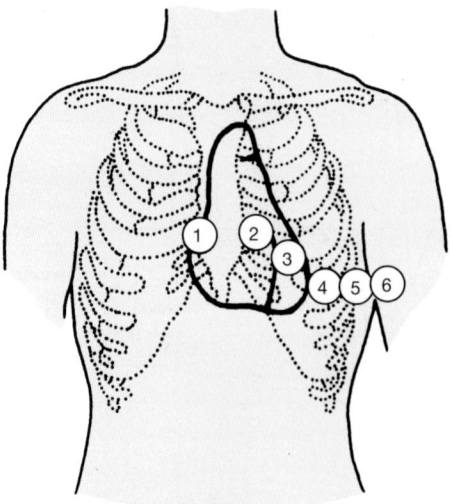

Fig. 4 The positions of the precordial leads. V1 is located at the right sternal margin in the fourth intercostal space, V₂ at the left sternal margin at the fourth intercostal space, V₄ at the intersection of the left midclavicular line and left fifth intercostal space, V₃ midway between V₂ and V₄, V₅ at the intersection of the left anterior axillary line with a horizontal line through V₄, and V₆ at the intersection of the left midaxillary line with a horizontal line through V₄ and V₅.

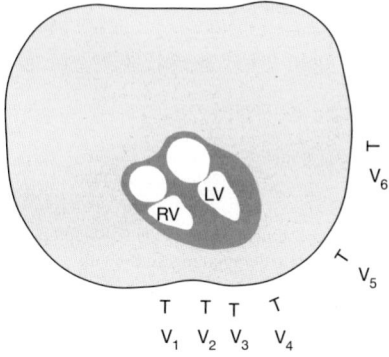

Fig. 5 The precordial leads and their important anatomical relationship to the main cardiac chambers.

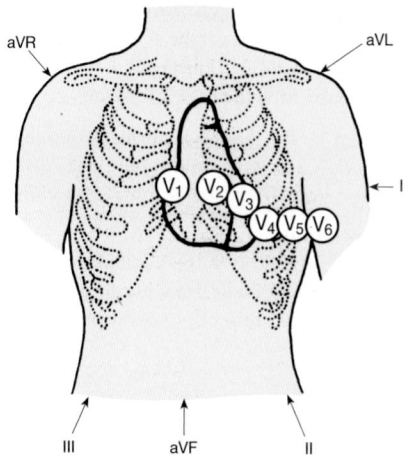

Fig. 6 The conventional 12 ECG leads and their relationships to the heart.

Recognizing the normal electrocardiogram

This is the most difficult and the most important aspect of understanding the electrocardiogram, which is recognized as being within or beyond normal limits by the normality or otherwise of the shape and dimensions of its various substituent deflections, and by the frequency of the deflections and their relationship in time to the deflections preceding and succeeding them. This introduction to the subject considers only morphological normality or abnormality. The presence of sinus rhythm will therefore be assumed. The criteria for normality of the P waves obtain in any rhythm where atrial depolarization is of sinus origin (sinus tachycardia, sinus bradycardia, sinus arrhythmia, first-, second-, or third-degree heart block). Those for the QRS complexes, S–T segments, and T waves obtain in any rhythm of supraventricular origin, provided the rate is not so rapid as to induce functional bundle-branch block. A supraventricular rhythm is one initiated at a site above the bifurcation of the His bundle.

All the criteria described below are dependent upon a normal (standard) calibration and a normal paper recording speed.

Precordial leads

Normal precordial P waves

The P waves are usually upright from V₄ to V₆. Upright or biphasic P waves may occur in V₁ and V₂. If the P waves are biphasic, the negative (terminal) component of the P wave should have an area no greater than the positive (initial) component.

Normal QRS appearances in the precordial leads

QRS morphology The QRS complex in V₁ typically shows a small initial positive wave followed by a larger negative wave, and in V₆ a small initial negative wave followed by a large positive wave. In general, the size of the initial positive wave (r or R wave) increases progressively from V₁ to V₆ (Fig. 7(a)) The direction of the initial part of the QRS is generally upward (i.e. positive) in V₁ to V₃, and downward (i.e. negative) in V₄ to V₆. That is, V₁ to V₃ show initial r waves and V₄ to V₆ initial q waves. Leads showing an rS complex are being primarily influenced by right ventricular myocardium, and leads showing a qR complex by left ventricular myocardium. The transition zone between right and left ventricular epicardial leads is seen (Fig. 7(b)) to be between V2 and V4. When the transition zone falls outside this region the heart is said to be rotated. If the transition zone occurs further to the left in the precordial series (for example, between V₅ and V₆) then the heart is said to be clockwise rotated. Conversely if the transition zone is moved to the right in the precordial series, the heart is said to be counter-clockwise rotated. Clockwise and counter-clockwise rotation refer to a normal state of variability between one subject and another and are not in themselves indicative of abnormality. More extensive works should be consulted for a detailed understanding of clockwise and counter-clockwise rotation. Although, as stated above, V₁ usually shows an rS complex and V₆ a qR complex, it is also possible for V₁ to show a QS complex and for V₆ to show a monophasic R wave, a QRS complex, or an Rs complex (Fig. 7(c)).

QRS dimensions The dimensions of the individual waves making up each part of the precordial QRS complexes are of crucial importance in determining normality or otherwise. Figure 8 shows how measurements within the QRS complexes are obtained. The criteria for normality of these individual waves are:

(1) *minimum voltage*: at least one R wave in the precordial leads must exceed 8 mm in height;

(2) *maximum voltage*: (a) the tallest R wave in the left precordial leads must not exceed 27 mm, (b) the deepest S wave in the right precordial leads must not exceed 30 mm, (c) the sum of the tallest R wave in the left precordial leads and the deepest S wave in the right precordial leads must not exceed 40 mm;

(3) *maximum duration*: the total QRS duration in any one precordial lead must not exceed 0.10 s (2.5 small squares);

(4) *q-wave criteria*: (a) no precordial q wave should equal or exceed 0.04 s (1 small square), (b) precordial q waves must not have a depth greater than a quarter of the height of the R wave in the same lead; and

(5) *the ventricular activation time*, also known as 'intrinsic deflection time', in leads facing the left ventricle (i.e. showing qR complexes) must not exceed 0.04 s (one small square).

Normal precordial S–T segments

There is a single rule for normality of the S–T segment. It must not deviate by more than 1 mm above or below the isoelectric line in any precordial lead. The isoelectric line is that vertical position of the ECG recording when no part of the heart is being depolarized or repolarized (i.e. the interval between the end of one T wave and the beginning of the next P wave—the T–P interval).

Normal precordial T waves

The criteria given below for normality of the T waves are applicable to adults only.

T waves in lead V_1 In this lead 80 per cent of normal adults have upright T waves and 20 per cent have flat or inverted T waves. Therefore, the finding

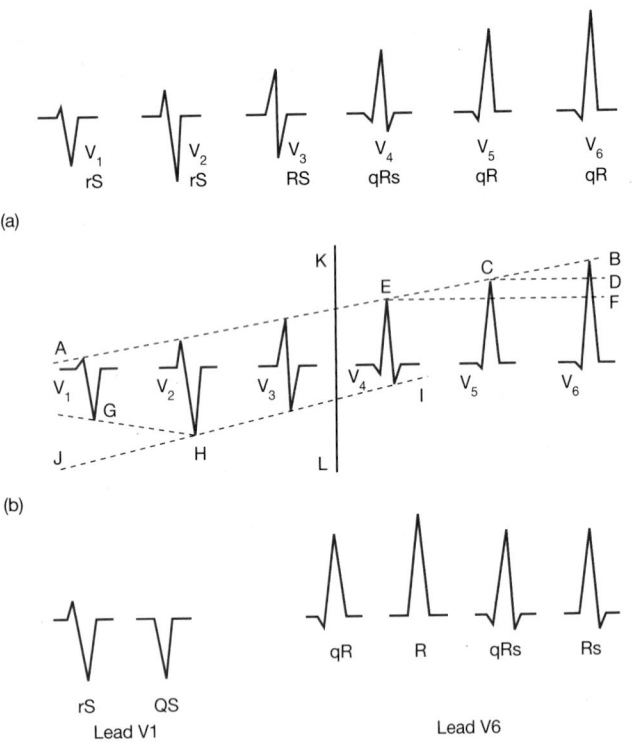

Fig. 7 Morphology of the precordial QRS complexes. (a) Typical normal QRS morphology of the precordial leads. (b) Normal variations of R-wave amplitude and S-wave depth in the precordial leads. The R wave in each precordial lead is usually larger than in the preceding lead in the series from V_1 to V_6 (line AB). However, it is quite normal for the R wave in V_6 to be smaller than that in V_5 (line CD) or for the R wave in V_5 to be smaller than that in V4, provided that the R wave in V_6 is also smaller than that in V_5 (line EF). The size of the S wave diminishes progressively across the precordial leads (line JI), although the S wave in V_2 is often greater than that in V_1 (line GHI). Leads before line KL have an initial deflection which is positive, while those after line KL have an initial deflection which is negative. This line marks the transition zone between right and left ventricular QRS configurations (i.e. between rS and qR configurations, respectively). (c) Possible normal QRS configurations in leads V1 and V6. Typically, V_1 has an rS configuration, but a QS configuration is also normal in this lead. Typically, V_6 has a qR configuration, but it is also normal for V_6 to show an R wave, a qRs complex, or an Rs complex.

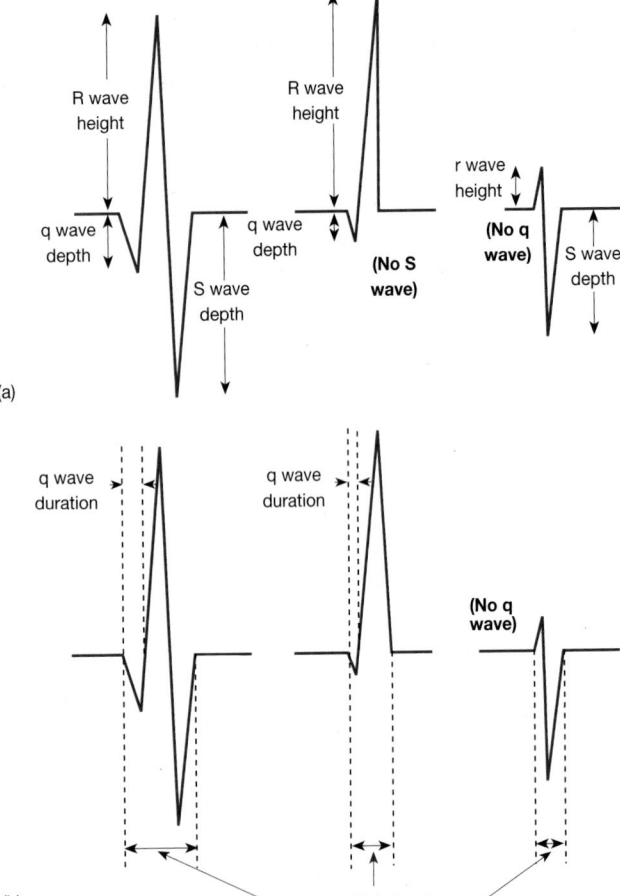

Fig. 8 The dimensions of constituent waves within QRS complexes. (a) Wave voltage measurements. (b) Wave duration measurements.

of an inverted T wave in Vl cannot be considered an abnormality (unless it was upright in a previous ECG).

T waves in lead V_2 About 95 per cent of normal adults show upright T waves and 5 per cent have flat or inverted T waves in V_2. Therefore there is a 1 in 20 possibility of inverted T waves in V_2 occurring by chance and not indicating an abnormality. However, if the T wave in V_2 is inverted when it was formerly upright, it is abnormal. Further, if there is T-wave inversion in V_2 with an upright T wave in V_1 then the T wave in V_2 is abnormal.

T waves in leads V_3 to V_6 The T wave is normally upright in these leads. T-wave inversion in V_4, V_5, or V_6 is always abnormal. T-wave inversion in V_3, as well as in V_1 and V_2, may (rarely) be found in healthy young adults.

T-wave size There are no strict criteria for T-wave size. In general, the tallest precordial T wave is found in V_3 or V_4, and the smallest in V_1 and V_2, and, as a general rule, the T wave should not be less than one-eighth and not more than two-thirds of the height of the preceding R wave in each of the leads V_3 to V_6.

Limb leads

Normal limb lead P waves

The limb lead that normally best shows the P wave is lead II. In this lead the normal P-wave duration does not exceed 0.12 s and its height does not exceed 2.5 mm

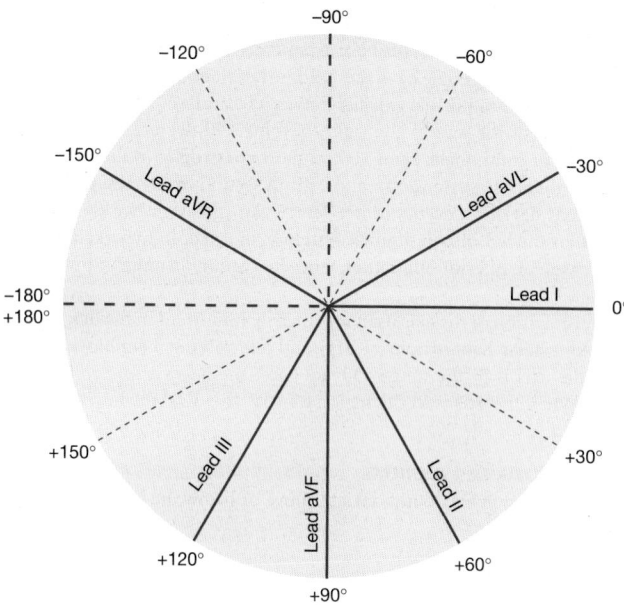

Fig. 9 The hexaxial reference system. The hexaxial reference system is constructed by taking each of the six frontal plane limb leads (continuous lines) and extrapolating them through the origin to create six additional lines (discontinuous), thereby producing 12 lines each at 30° to its neighbour on either side thus dividing the 360° of the frontal plane into equal (30°) sections.

Normal limb lead QRS complexes

Only three criteria need to be applied to the limb leads to determine the normality or otherwise of the QRS complexes:

(1) *the size of any q waves in aVL, I, II, or aVF;*

(2) *the size of the R waves in aVL and aVF;* and

(3) *the electrical axis of the heart.*

Q waves Any q wave present in lead I, II, or aVF must not exceed one-quarter the height of the ensuing R wave and must not equal or exceed 0.04 s in duration. Any q wave present in aVR or lead III should be ignored, irrespective of its size. Q waves present in aVL should fulfil the same criteria as those in leads I, II, or aVF unless the frontal plane QRS axis is more positive than +60°, in which case large q waves in aVL are acceptable, since aVL is then a cavity lead (and may therefore have a QS complex as aVR, which is virtually always a cavity lead, usually has).

R-wave size The R wave in aVL must not exceed 13 mm, while that in aVF must not exceed 20 mm.

The frontal plane axis The value of the axis is determined using the hexaxial reference system (Fig. 9) in which lead I is arbitrarily assigned the value 0°, with the convention that rotation clockwise from this point is denoted positive ('+') and rotation anticlockwise is denoted negative ('−'). The mean frontal plane QRS axis in the adult lies within the range from −30° to +90° (travelling clockwise). The frontal plane axis represents the dominant direction of ventricular myocardial depolarization on the frontal plane. The axis is closest to that frontal plane lead with the tallest QRS complex, but because of the uneven distribution of the limb leads the axis cannot reliably be determined by simple inspection of the limb lead QRS complexes.

The general direction of ventricular depolarization in the frontal plane in a normal record is typically towards lead II (60°), but can lie anywhere between aVL (−30°) and aVF (+90°). When the axis lies within the range −30° to +30° the heart is said to be horizontal and the tallest QRS complexes will be found in aVL and I. When the axis lies within the range +60° to +120° the heart is said to be vertical and the tallest QRS complexes will be found in aVF and II. With a typical normal axis of +60° there are up-

right QRS complexes in lead II, and to a lesser extent in aVF, and smaller QRS complexes in III and aVL. Lead aVR 'looks into' the cavity of the heart. Since depolarization of the ventricles is from endocardium (where the Purkinje tissue is) to epicardium, the cavity leads record depolarization travelling away from them and therefore have negative QRS deflections.

A knowledge of the axis is helpful in understanding the variation in appearances in the limb leads between different subjects with similar (normal or abnormal) precordial ECG appearances. Thus, for example, in a patient with left ventricular hypertrophy, if the heart is horizontal (axis lies in the region of −30° to +30°) appearances similar to those in V₅ and V₆ will be seen in aVL and I (Fig. 10), whereas if the heart is vertical (axis +60° to +120°) appearances similar to those in V₅ and V₆ will be seen in II and aVL.

Determination of the mean frontal plane QRS axis

To determine the mean frontal axis to the nearest 30° requires two steps, which can be illustrated using Fig. 10 as follows:

(1) Inspect the six frontal plane (limb) leads to find the lead in which the algebraic sum of the deflections in the QRS complexes approximates to zero (i.e. the lead in which the sum of all the positive deflections minus all the negative deflections gives a result closest to zero). In doing this one is looking for the smallest mean QRS deflection. The axis will always be approximately at right angles to the lead with the smallest QRS. Let the lead showing the smallest net QRS size be called lead 'x'. (In the example of Fig. 10 this is lead II.)

(2) Using the hexaxial reference diagram (Fig. 9), decide which other lead (y) is at right angles to lead 'x'. (In Fig. 10 this is aVL.) There will always be one such lead. The axis must either be: (a) in the same direction as or very close to lead y (in this example, aVL, i.e. −30°) or (b) directly opposite to y or very close to that position (in this example, +150°), both of which possible positions are approximately at right angles to x. To determine which of these two possibilities indicates the correct orientation of the axis look again at the given ECG and inspect the QRS in lead y (in this case aVL). It must either have a large dominant positive wave, or a large dominant negative wave. If the former, the axis of the heart is along lead y (i.e. approximately −30°), if the latter the axis is directly away from lead y (i.e. approximately +150°). To the nearest 30°, therefore, the axis in the ECG of Fig. 10 is −30°.

To assess the axis to the nearest 15° it is necessary to take one further step

(3) Look again at the QRS in that lead where the algebraic sum of QRS deflections is close to zero (II in Fig. 10). Assess whether that sum is (a) indistinguishable from zero, (b) close to zero but clearly slightly positive, or (c) close to zero but clearly slightly negative. If (a), then the current estimate of the axis is now correct to the nearest 15°; if (b), then the axis estimate must be 'bent' from the 30° accuracy estimate, 15° towards the lead where the QRS algebraic sum is close to zero; if (c), then the axis estimate must be 'bent' from the 30° accurate estimate, 15° away from the lead where the QRS algebraic sum is close to zero. In this case the QRS in II is clearly slightly positive and the 30° accuracy estimate (−30°) must be 'bent' 15° towards lead II, giving an axis of −15 (to a 15° accuracy). (Had the algebraic sum of QRS deflections in lead II, Fig. 10, been negative it would have been necessary to 'bend' the estimated axis 15° away from lead II, giving −45°).

Significance of the mean frontal plane QRS axis

The normal range for the frontal plane axis in adults is from −30° to +90° (travelling clockwise). Axes that are more negative than −30° are described as left-axis deviation (LAD). Axes more positive than +90° are described as right-axis deviation (RAD). These terms (LAD and RAD) are descriptive, in the same manner as the term 'hypertensive' is descriptive. Axes of −60° and −90° are both examples of left-axis deviation, but the difference is significant. It is therefore preferable to describe the axis in an individual case in degrees, just as it is preferable to give their measured blood pressure in mmHg. The other reason for preferring to describe the axis in degrees is that axes in the quadrant from −180° to −90°, which are uncommon, could be described either as extreme left- or as extreme right-axis shift.

The axis in the newborn tends to be around +120°. As the child grows the axis swings towards the left. In adult life the normal axis lies within the range −30° to +90°. In older age groups the axis typically lies between −30° and +30°. Tall, thin people have axes nearer the right end of the normal range and short fat people have axes nearer the left end of the normal range. The most common normal axis lies between 0° and +60°.

Deviation of the axis to the right, beyond +90 degrees (that is, RAD) occurs in cor pulmonale, right ventricular hypertrophy (pulmonary stenosis, pulmonary hypertension), and ostium secundum atrial septal defect.

Left-axis deviation occurs in left ventricular disease, when the superior division of the left bundle-branch system is blocked, in hyperkalaemia, in some cases of inferior infarction, and in ostium primum atrial septal defect.

Determination of the axis itself is primarily important in the diagnosis of right ventricular hypertrophy (RVH) and left anterior hemiblock (LAH). When the axis is in the range −30° to +30°, the heart is said to be 'horizontal'. When the axis is in the region of +60° to +120° the heart is said to be 'vertical'.

Normal limb lead S–T segments

Normal S–T segments do not deviate above or below the isoelectric line by more than 1 mm.

Normal limb lead T waves

In general, the T waves and QRS complexes in the limb leads are concordant: that is to say, when the QRS complexes are upright, the T waves are upright, and when the QRS complexes are negative, the T waves are negative. A normal T wave will always be negative in aVR and positive in I and II. T waves can be positive or negative in aVL, aVF, and II without necessarily indicating abnormality. A rough guide to assess normality of the T waves in the limb leads is:

(1) in any lead in which the QRS is predominantly upright, the T wave must be clearly upright;

(2) in any lead in which the QRS is predominantly negative, the T wave should be clearly negative;

(3) in any lead in which the algebraic sum of QRS deflections is close to zero, the T wave may be positive or negative (though small in either case) or isoelectric (flat); and

(4) the normal T wave is always upright in leads I and II.

Myocardial hypertrophy

Appreciable hypertrophy of the right or left ventricle produces characteristic changes in the electrocardiogram. Lesser degrees of hypertrophy may be present without electrocardiographic changes or with only minor, non-specific changes. This is more often true of right than of left ventricular hypertrophy.

Left ventricular hypertrophy

Left ventricular hypertrophy is not an all-or-none phenomenon, and the same is true of its recognition on the ECG. Several scoring systems have been devised. The most sensitive (and least specific) criteria consider the precordial lead voltages. The increased bulk of the left ventricle increases the voltage that is induced during left ventricular depolarization. This results in taller R waves in the left precordial leads and deeper S waves in the right precordial leads. The increased ventricular wall thickness also results in prolongation of the time taken for the depolarization wave to travel from endocardium to epicardium, that is to say it increases the ventricular activation time. In addition, secondary changes in depolarization occur, altering the S–T segments and T waves. The electrocardiographic criteria for left ventricular hypertrophy are:

(1) at least one R wave in the left precordial leads exceeds 27 mm;

(2) at least one S wave in the right precordial leads exceeds 30 mm:

(3) the sum of the tallest R wave and the deepest S wave in the precordial leads exceeds 40 mm;

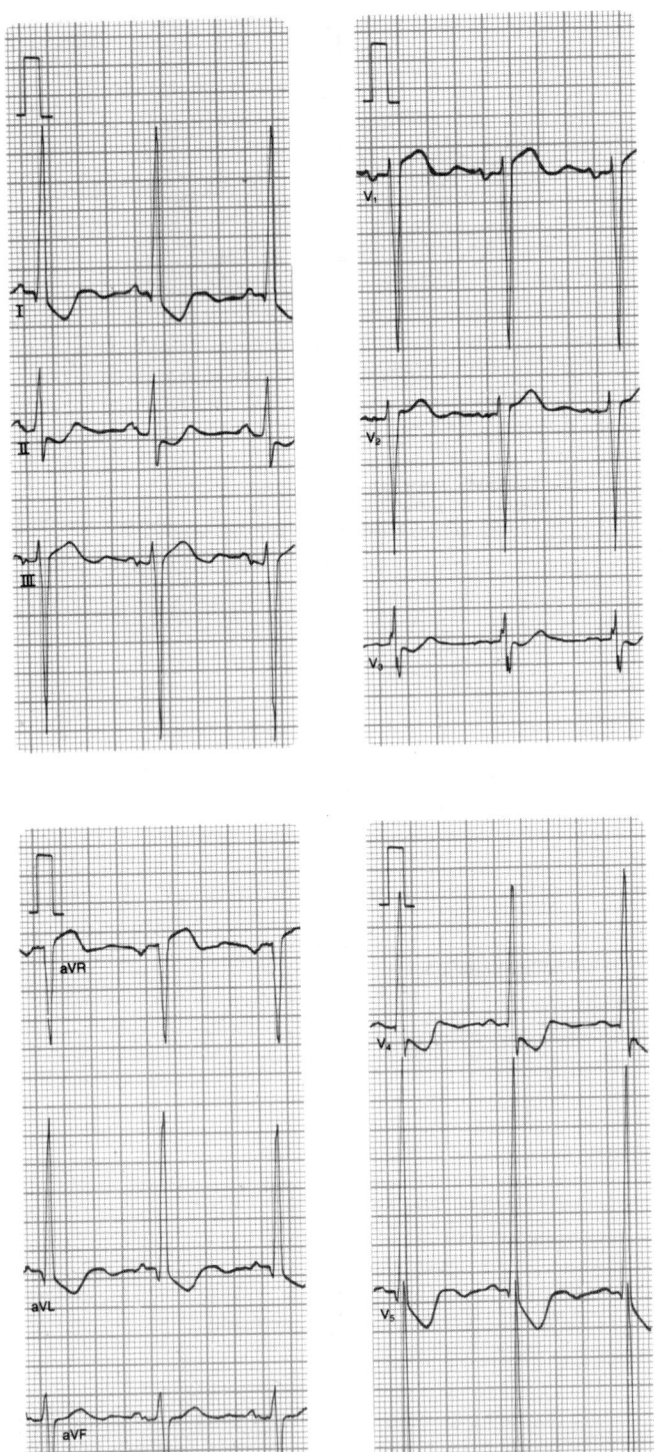

Fig. 10 Left ventricular hypertrophy. There is also evidence of left atrial hypertrophy.

(4) the largest positive or negative deflection in the limb leads exceeds 20 mm;

(5) the intrinsic deflection time (ventricular activation time) exceeds 0.04 s;

(6) S–T-segment depression and T-wave inversion may occur in the left precordial leads and in those limb leads that face the left ventricle.

The presence of one or more of the above abnormalities suggests the presence of left ventricular hypertrophy, only provided that the total QRS duration does not exceed 0.10 s. The greater the number of criteria fulfilled, the more confident one can be of the diagnosis. The voltage criteria have the greatest sensitivity, and the intrinsic deflection time the greatest specificity. However, one must exercise caution in diagnosing left ventricular hypertrophy on the basis of voltage criteria alone, especially if the patient is slim—and also note that the sensitivity for the diagnosis of left ventricular hypertrophy is very low in those who are obese. An example of clear-cut electrocardiographic changes of left ventricular hypertrophy is shown in Fig. 10.

Right ventricular hypertrophy

Increased bulk of the right ventricle gives rise to higher voltages during right ventricular depolarization, increasing the size of the positive deflection in the right precordial leads. In addition, it shifts the electrical axis towards the right and changes the S–T segments and T waves in leads facing the right ventricle, because of secondary changes in the repolarization process. The electrocardiographic criteria for right ventricular hypertrophy are:

(1) a positive deflection equal to or greater than the negative deflection in V_1 (RS, Rs, qR, rR') in the presence of a normal total QRS duration;

(2) a mean frontal plane QRS axis more positive than +90°; and

(3) S–T-segment depression and T-wave inversion in right precordial leads.

The more features present, the more convincing is the electrocardiographic evidence for right ventricular hypertrophy, but, in general, the combination of a dominant positive deflection of the QRS in V_1 and an abnormal degree of right-axis deviation (axis more positive than +90°) establishes the diagnosis. Examples are shown in Figs 11(a) and (b). In both examples there is abnormal right-axis deviation and a dominant R wave in V_1. Figure 11(a) shows an Rs complex in V_1 and Fig. 11(b) shows a qR complex. The more common finding is of an Rs in V_1. An initial q wave (qR complex) can appear in V_1 in right ventricular hypertophy, which results from hypertrophy of the right side of the upper part of the interventricular septum with resultant redirection of initial septal depolarization relatively posteriorly and therefore away from (and negative with respect to) V_1. Figure 11(b) also shows pronounced clockwise cardiac rotation, which often accompanies right ventricular hypertrophy.

Atrial hypertrophy

The electrocardiographic changes produced by left atrial hypertrophy are those produced by an increase in the voltage and duration of the left atrial depolarization wave. Since the terminal part of the normal P wave is produced by left atrial depolarization, it follows that the total P-wave duration is prolonged in left atrial hypertrophy. In addition, the P wave tends to be bifid in lead II and biphasic in V_1. In V_1 the area of the (terminal) negative component exceeds the area of the (initial) positive component (Figs 10 and 12). Left atrial hypertrophy is most commonly seen in association with left ventricular hypertrophy and (in countries where rheumatic heart disease is rare) is most commonly due to systemic hypertension. The finding of left atrial hypertrophy in the absence of evidence of left ventricular hypertrophy suggests mitral valve obstruction (mitral stenosis or, very rarely, left atrial myxoma).

The electrocardiographic change produced by right atrial hypertophy is an increase in the peak voltage of the P wave. This is usually best seen in

lead II. In lead II the P-wave voltage is abnormal when it exceeds 3 mm (see Fig. 11(b)). Right atrial hypertrophy is most commonly seen in the presence of right ventricular hypertrophy. The finding of right atrial hypertrophy in the absence of right ventricular hypertrophy suggests tricuspid valve obstruction.

Bundle-branch block

Total failure of conduction in the right or left branches of the bundle of His (bundle-branch block) can only be diagnosed with confidence from the appearances in the precordial leads, although necessarily there are also changes in the appearances in the limb leads.

Right bundle-branch block

In right bundle-branch block, the primary change induced is a delay in depolarization in the right ventricular free wall. This results in the development of a second positive wave in the right ventricular leads (and a second negative wave in left ventricular leads), and prolongs the total QRS duration. The essential electrocardiographic features of right bundle-branch block are:

(1) a total QRS duration of 0.12 s or more; and

(2) the presence of a secondary positive wave in V_1 (rsR', rR').

In addition, secondary changes occur, but these are not in themselves essential for the definitive diagnosis. They include:

(3) deep and slurred S waves in lead I, aVL, and V_4–V_6; and

(4) secondary S–T, T changes in leads V_1–V_3.

An example of the appearances in right bundle-branch block is shown in Fig. 13.

Left bundle-branch block

Left bundle-branch block induces changes in the ECG which are more extensive than those produced by right bundle-branch block. In left bundle-branch block not only is depolarization of the free wall of the left ventricle delayed (a precise corollary of the changes in right bundle-branch block), but also the direction of depolarization of the interventricular septum is from right to left instead of from left to right as in the normal electrocardiogram. This reversal of the direction of septal depolarization gives rise to widespread and major alterations in the QRS complexes in every lead of the electrocardiogram. The diagnostic criteria for left bundle-branch block are:

(1) a total QRS duration equal to or in excess of 0.12 s; and

(2) absence of the normal (septal) q waves in lead I, aVL, and V_4–V_6; and

(3) absence of a secondary r wave in V_1.

This latter criterion is necessary to prevent confusion in cases of right bundle-branch block occurring in the presence of pronounced clockwise cardiac rotation, which gives a loss of q waves in left ventricular leads. (The finding of a secondary r wave in V_1 in the presence of an abnormally wide QRS complex indicates the presence of right bundle-branch block.) Secondary changes also inevitably occur, but these are not part of the diagnostic process. These include:

(4) secondary S–T depression and T-wave inversion in leads I, aVL, and V_4–V_6;

(5) broad QS waves in V_1–V_3;

(6) notching of the R waves giving rise to rsR' or 'M-shaped' QRS complexes, and

(7) broad, R waves in leads I, aVL, and V_4–V_6.

An example of the ECG appearances in left bundle-branch block is shown in Fig. 14. The changes in left bundle-branch block so disturb the normal pattern of the ECG that none of the usual criteria can be applied for determining any other abnormality of the QRS complexes, S–T segments,

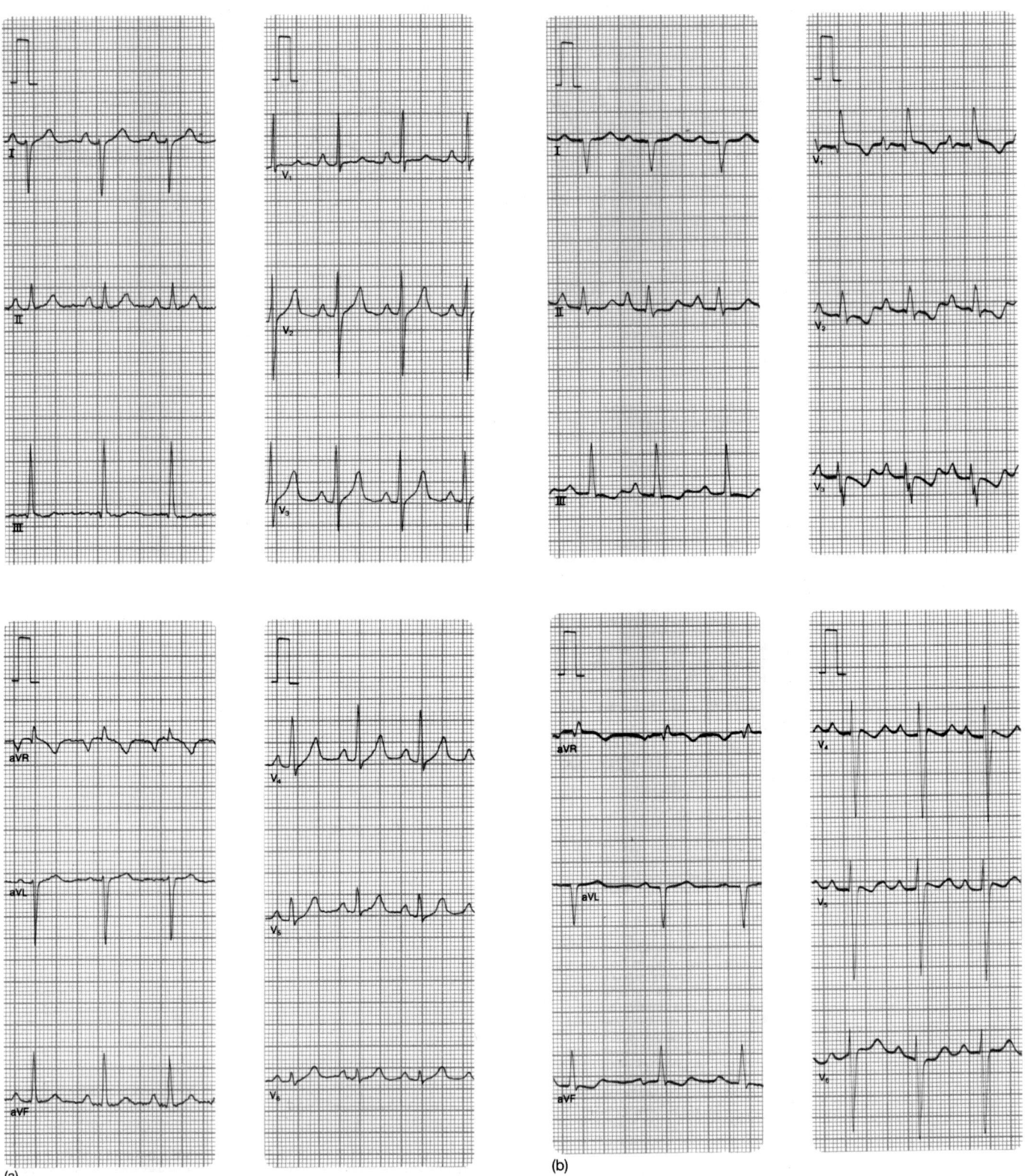

Fig. 11 Two examples of right ventricular hypertrophy. There is also right atrial hypertrophy. Fig. 11(a) shows an Rs complex in V₁; (b) shows a qR complex.

or P waves. When left bundle-branch block is present, a diagnosis of right or left ventricular hypertrophy, myocardial ischaemia or infarction, or of non-specific changes in the S–T segments and T waves cannot easily or reliably be made.

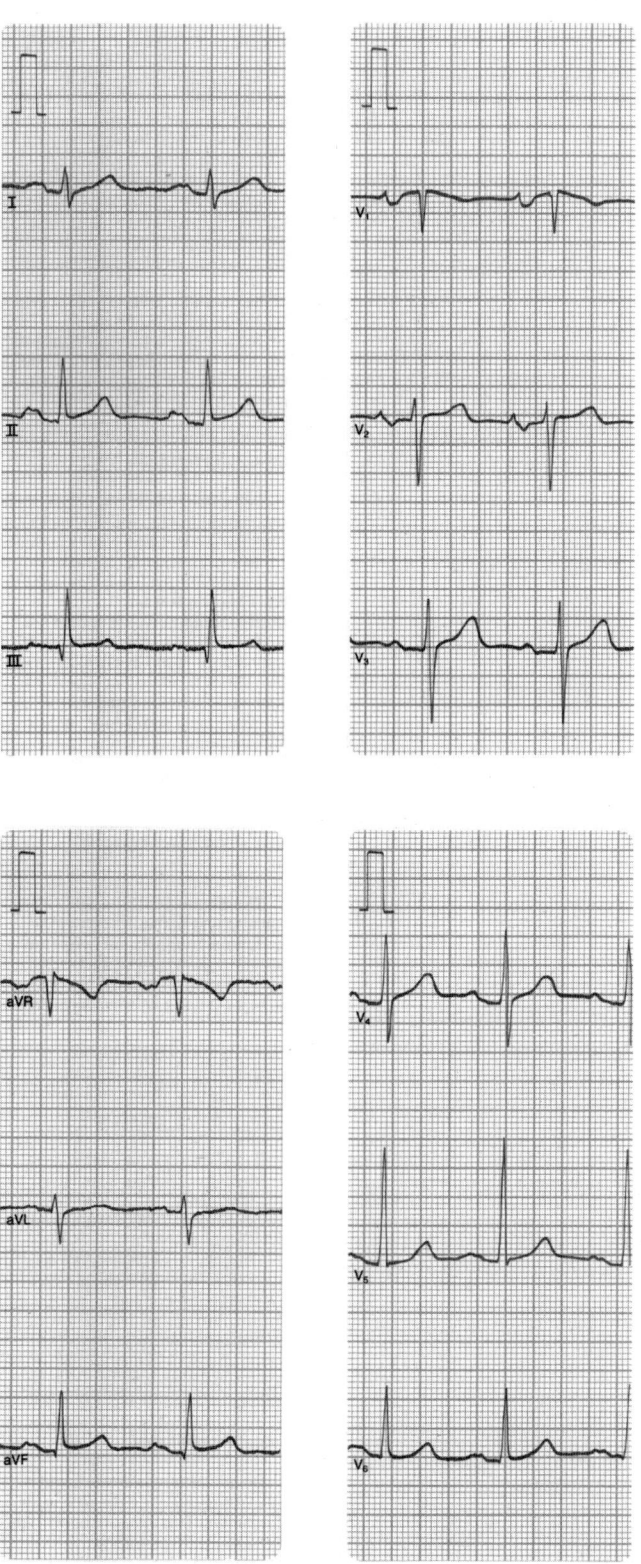

Fig. 12 Left atrial hypertrophy. Broad, bifid P waves in lead II. Biphasic P waves in V1, with dominant negative component. Since there is no evidence of left ventricular hypertrophy, the most likely cause of the left atrial hypertrophy is mitral valve obstruction. The patient had mitral valve stenosis.

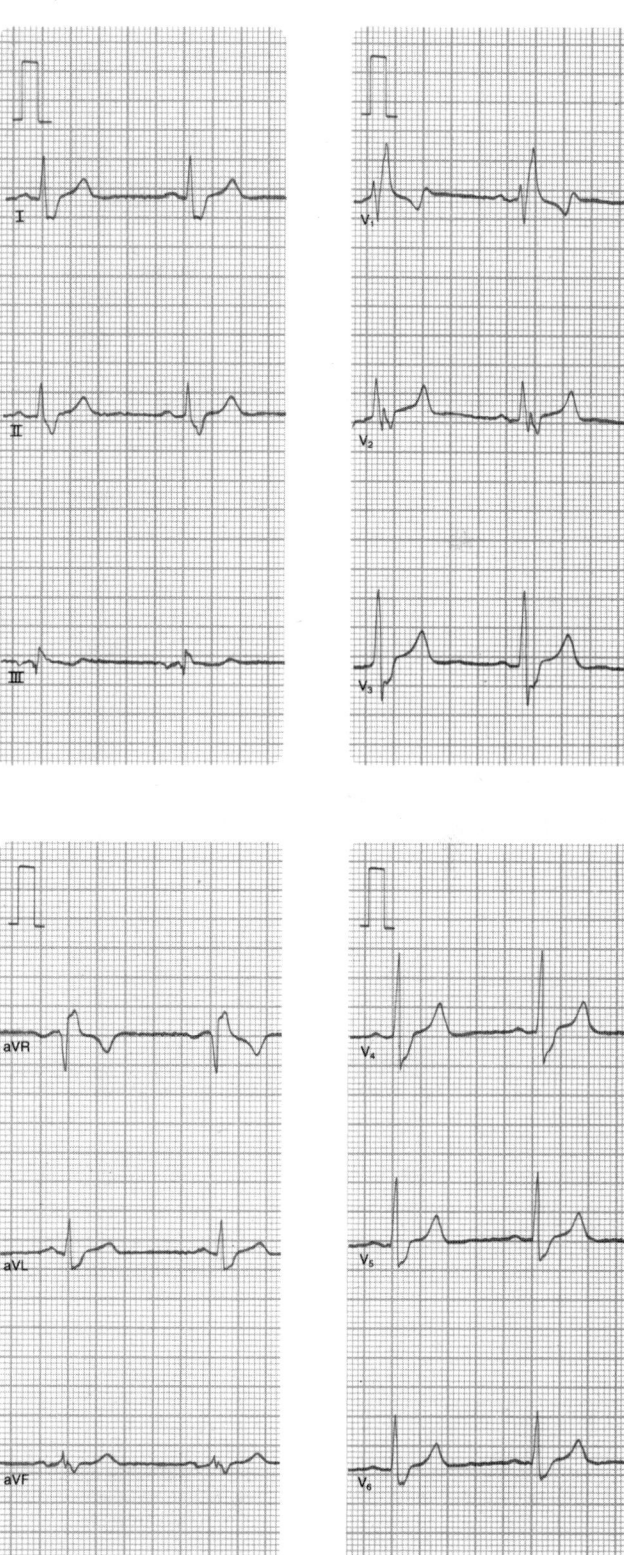

Fig. 13 Right bundle-branch block. The total QRS duration is prolonged. There is an rsR' in V₁ and there are broad, slurred S waves in V₃–V₆.

The hemiblocks

During normal intraventricular conduction the anterosuperior and the posteroinferior divisions of the left bundle-branch system conduct more or

less simultaneously. This has the result that the dominant direction of depolarization of left ventricular myocardium lies midway between these two divisions and is therefore downwards and to the left, giving an axis in the range −30° to +90° and most typically in the region of +60°.

Left anterior hemiblock

When there is failure of conduction in the anterosuperior division of the left bundle branch ('left anterior hemiblock') the direction of the initial part of the QRS vector moves marginally to the right as a result of the loss of the opposing initial leftward voltage. However, the bulk of the QRS vector is slightly delayed and moves strongly to the left. This is because depolarization of the superior and left part of the left ventricular myocardium is dependent upon spread from the initially depolarized rightward and inferior aspects of the ventricle. The resulting changes in the ECG are therefore (1) a trivial increase in the QRS duration (but the QRS duration is not prolonged beyond normal limits) and (2) a shift of the axis to the left (more negative than −30°). The other common cause of abnormal left-axis deviation is inferior myocardial infarction. The ECG criterion for left anterior hemiblock is a mean frontal plane QRS axis more negative than −30° in the absence of abnormal q waves in aVF (which would indicate inferior infarction).

Left posterior hemiblock

Left posterior hemiblock, as would be expected from the above, gives rise to abnormal right-axis deviation (axis more positive than +90°). Unfortunately, there are numerous causes of abnormal right-axis deviation. It is therefore not possible, from the 12-lead ECG, to diagnose left posterior hemiblock. One can only raise the possibility of this in those situations in which there is an abnormal degree of right-axis deviation without any clear electrocardiographic or clinical explanation.

Ischaemic heart disease

ECG changes in ischaemic heart disease are very variable, depending on the site and severity of ischaemic damage. However, certain patterns are commonly produced.

Acute coronary syndromes (Q-wave infarction, non-Q-wave infarction, and unstable angina)

The terms 'transmural infarction' and 'Q-wave infarction' are often used interchangeably, as are the terms 'subendocardial infarction' and 'non-Q-wave infarction'. These two types of myocardial infarction are not separable on clinical grounds alone, and the distinction between the two depends entirely on the presence or absence of abnormal Q waves on the ECG. It is generally agreed that the terms 'Q-wave infarction' and 'non-Q-wave infarction' are preferable to 'transmural infarction' and 'subendocardial infarction', because autopsy data indicate that the ECG does not have sufficient sensitivity and specificity to guarantee reliable distinction between transmural and subendocardial infarction. However, the distinction between Q-wave and non-Q-wave infarction should not be used to determine management. The full spectrum of Q-wave infarction and unstable angina is now designated under the overall label of 'Acute coronary syndromes'.

Patients presenting clinically with an acute coronary syndrome may or may not have initial S-T elevation. Most (75 per cent) of those with S-T elevation subsequently develop abnormal Q waves and most of the remaining 25 per cent develop reduction in R wave height. Occasionally the ECG may return entirely to normal after initial S-T elevation. Those who present without initial S-T elevation do not usually develop abnormal Q waves. In such cases there may be (non-specific) S-T segment depression (flat, down sloping or up sloping), flattening or inversion of the T waves or a combination of non specific S-T and T changes and the final diagnosis can then be either non-Q-wave infarction or unstable angina. The distinction between

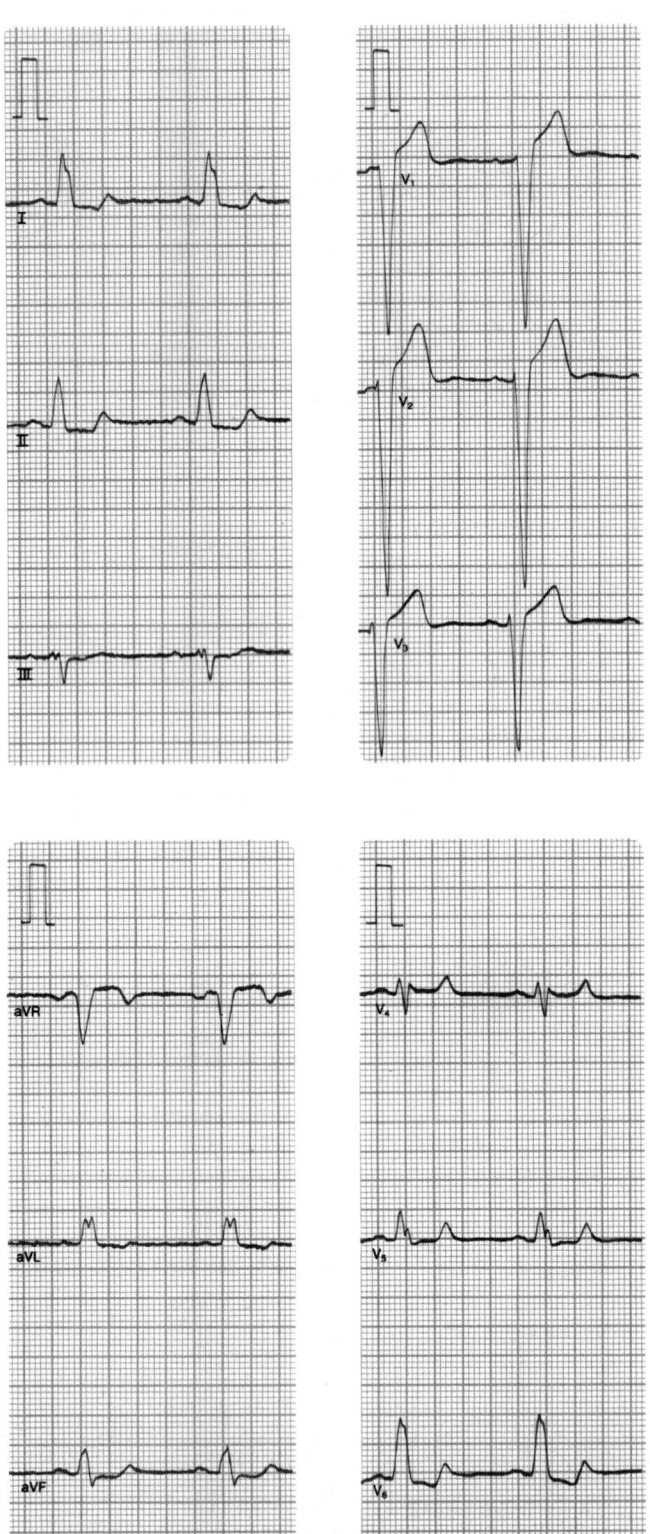

Fig. 14 Left bundle-branch block. The total QRS duration is prolonged and no q wave is seen in I, avL, and V₄–V₆. In addition there is no secondary R wave in V₁.

these two depends entirely on whether or not serum markers of infarction are present.

In contrast to the typical, striking evolutionary changes of acute Q-wave infarction, the ECG findings in non-Q-wave infarction are less dramatic and less predictable. The electrocardiographic evidence consists of primary S–T-segment depression ('primary' implies in the absence of any detectable S–T elevation) or of deep, symmetrical T-wave inversion without any change in the QRS complexes. Each of these changes can be produced by myocardial ischaemia without infarction, and the diagnosis of non-Q-wave infarction cannot be made on a single electrocardiogram alone. Either (1) a single such record accompanied by clinical or enzyme evidence of infarction, or (2) serial records that persistently show primary S–T depression or that show deep symmetrical T-wave inversion, is required. The persistence of non-specific S–T and/or T changes that were not formerly present, and which accompany clinical and enzymatic evidence of acute infarction, are the hallmark of non-Q-wave infarction. When the primary change is S–T depression it will often be visible in all or most leads, with the exception of the cavity leads (aVR is always a cavity lead, aVL is a cavity lead if the heart is vertical (axis +60° or more positive) and lead III is a cavity lead if the heart is (axis +30° or further to the left)). The cavity leads may also show reciprocal S–T elevation. The only exception to the rule 'that when S–T elevation and S–T depression are both present in the same recording, it is the elevation which is the primary change' occurs when, as in this case, the reciprocal S–T elevation occurs in cavity leads (which, by definition, all show QS complexes).

QRS changes of myocardial infarction

Two QRS changes are indicative of myocardial infarction. These are:

(1) inappropriately low R-wave voltage in a local area; and

(2) abnormal q waves.

These two changes represent parts of the same process. The development of increased negativity (abnormal q waves) and the reduction in the normal positivity (loss of R-wave height) of QRS complexes in the precordial leads each results from a loss of underlying viable muscle, with a consequent reduction in the normally generated positive voltage. When there is full-thickness (transmural) myocardial infarction in an area of myocardium underlying the precordial leads there is total loss of the positive deflection. In this situation a totally negative wave (QS complex) occurs. This totally negative wave occurs as a result of depolarization of the posterior wall of the ventricle travelling (posteriorly) from endocardium to epicardium in the normal way, which is no longer swamped by the usual simultaneous and dominant depolarization towards the exploring electrode of the anterior wall of the ventricle.

The normal precordial QRS complexes show a progressive increase in the R-wave height from V₁ to V₆ (Fig. 15). The positive (upgoing) part of the deflection in each precordial lead is predominantly the result of depolarization from underlying endocardium to epicardium. In the presence of infarction of part of the left ventricle, the positive waves overlying the necrotic area will be reduced in size (Fig. 16). Loss in R-wave height can only be used as a criterion for myocardial infarction if either: (1) larger, normal R waves are visible on both sides of the infarcted zone, or (2) previous ECGs are available demonstrating the normal R-wave height for that particular lead in that particular subject. If a major part of the thickness of

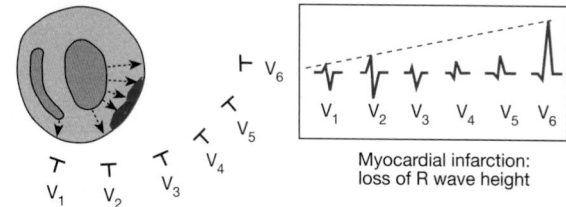

Fig. 16 Loss of R-wave height in myocardial infarction. The R-wave height is reduced in leads V3 to V5.

the myocardial wall is infarcted, the positive wave generated by any remaining viable left ventricular myocardium underlying the electrode is insufficient to overcome the negative deflection induced by the normal depolarization of the interventricular septum, from left to right, and of the free wall of the right ventricle (or the posterior wall of the left ventricle) from endocardium to epicardium. In this situation an abnormal q wave will develop. In the precordial leads, a q wave is abnormal if its duration is equal to or in excess of 0.04 s or if its depth is equal to or greater than a quarter the height of the ensuing R wave in that lead. In Fig. 16, the q wave in V₄ satisfies this criterion. If the infarction involves the full thickness of the ventricular wall (transmural infarction), no R wave is generated at all and an entirely negative (QS) wave develops (Fig. 17). Figure 18 shows (in diagrammatic form) the appearances produced in the precordial leads when infarcts of varying thickness occur under each of three precordial electrodes. The QRS complex in V₃ is of QS type and indicates transmural infarction at this site. The appearances in V₄ indicate a substantial loss of myocardium underlying that electrode. The q wave is abnormal in duration and depth. The appearances in V₅ indicate a thinner zone of infarction. The q wave is not, in itself, abnormal, but the R-wave height is less than would be predicted from the height of the R waves present in V₂ and V₆.

The diagnosis of myocardial infarction from the limb leads depends entirely on the presence of abnormal q waves. Q waves of any size may be seen in the normal ECG in aVR and in lead III. In leads I, II, and aVF, q waves which are equal to or greater than 0.04 s in duration or which have a depth in excess of a quarter the height of the ensuing R wave are abnormal and, unless a defect of intraventricular conduction is known to be present, indicate myocardial infarction. The same is also true of abnormal q waves in aVL, except when the mean frontal plane QRS axis is equal to or more positive than +60°, for in this situation aVL becomes a cavity lead like aVR.

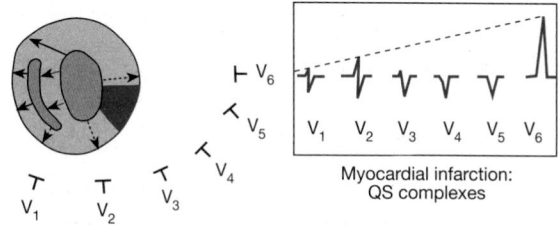

Fig. 17 Transmural myocardial infarction. QS complexes are seen from V₃ to V₅.

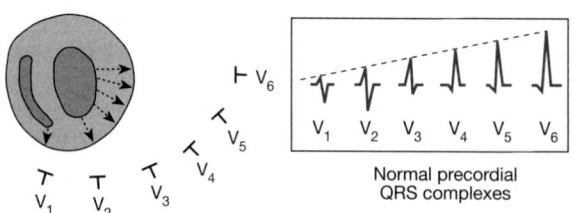

Fig. 15 Normal R-wave progression in the precordial series.

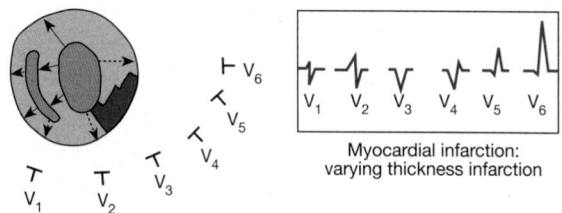

Fig. 18 Varying thickness infarction.

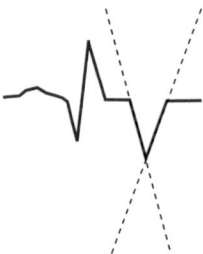

Fig. 19 Deep, symmetrical T-wave inversion. This is not truly specific but is typically found in association with myocardial ischaemia or infarction.

S–T-segment changes of infarction

Only changes in the QRS complexes provide definitive electrocardiographic evidence of infarction, but an S–T-segment shift occurs in the acute stages of Q-wave infarction. Strictly speaking, this shift is evidence of injury to, rather than infarction of, the myocardium. Thus, although in the vast majority of cases the development of typical S–T-segment elevation is followed by the development of definitive QRS changes, occasionally the ECG with S–T-segment elevation of myocardial injury will revert to normal within hours. This does not happen if definitive QRS changes of infarction are also present. It is marginally more likely to occur following the use of thrombolytic therapy but is still relatively uncommon. The essential change of myocardial injury is deviation of the S–T segment above the isoelectric line. The S–T-segment shift must be in excess of 1 mm to be significant. Minor degrees of S–T-segment elevation in the right precordial leads are very common in normal ECGs, and S–T-segment elevation of up to 2 mm may be accepted as being within normal limits in V_1 and V_2. Significant S–T-segment elevation occurs in transmural and subepicardial infarction in leads facing the infarct. S–T-segment depression occurs in leads facing the infarct when it is subendocardial. Secondary S–T-segment depression also occurs as a reciprocal change (see below) in leads opposite to those showing the primary changes of acute infarction.

T-wave changes of infarction

A variety of T-wave changes occur in association with myocardial infarction. These include flattened, biphasic, and inverted (negative) T waves. None of these changes is specific. Whilst they are always abnormal in leads V_4 to V_6 and in those limb leads showing clearly upright QRS complexes, they may be caused by factors other than infarction or ischaemia, including electrolyte changes, digitalis effect, pericarditis, myocarditis, changes in body position, and changes in oesophageal temperature. T-wave changes are never, in themselves, reliable indicators of infarction, although characteristic T-wave changes do occur in relation to the latter. The most typical T-wave change associated with infarction is the development of deep, symmetrically inverted T waves (Fig. 19).

The sequence of ECG changes in Q-wave infarction

Any combination of the QRS, S–T-segment, and T-wave changes described above may occur in relation to acute infarction of the myocardium, but commonly a typical sequence of changes can be recognized in relation to Q-wave infarction (Fig. 20). Typically, S–T-segment elevation (which is convex upwards) appears within hours of the onset of symptoms. At this stage no change in the QRS complex can be recognized. Within 1 to 3 days,

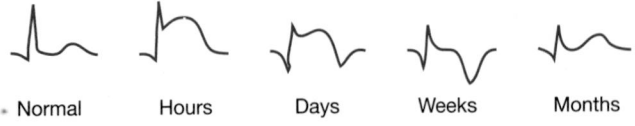

Normal   Hours   Days   Weeks   Months

Fig. 20 Sequential changes in acute myocardial infarction.

Table 1 Electrocardiographic location of changes occurring in Q-wave infarction

Location of infarction	Leads showing primary changes
	Typical changes
Anteroseptal	V_1, V_2, V_3
Anterior	V_2, V_3, V_4
Anterolateral	V_4, V_5, V_6, I, aVL
Extensive anterior	$V_1, V_2, V_3, V_4, V_5, V_6$, I, aVL
High lateral	aVL (plus high precordial leads)
Inferior	II, III, aVF
Inferolateral (apical)	II, III, aVF, V_5, V_6, I, aVL
Inferoseptal	II, III, aVF, V_1, V_2, V_3
	Other changes
Posterior	V_1, V_2
Subendocardial	Any lead (usually multiple leads)

reduction in the R-wave height occurs, abnormally deep and broad q waves develop, some reduction in the extent of S–T-segment elevation occurs, and there is development of T-wave inversion. After the first few days the S–T-segment elevation disappears completely. The deep, symmetrical T-wave inversion typically persists for weeks before reverting to normal. The changes in the QRS complex are usually permanent. The QRS changes may occasionally disappear altogether if the infarct is small and the myocardial scar subsequently shrinks.

Location of ECG changes in myocardial infarction

Primary ECG changes of the type described above occur in leads facing the infarct. It follows that the leads in which such primary changes occur indicate the location of the infarct (Table 1).

Reciprocal changes

In addition to the primary changes, 'reciprocal' changes occur in leads opposite those facing the infarct. Reciprocal changes are the inverse of primary changes (e.g. S–T-segment depression instead of S–T-segment elevation and tall, pointed T waves instead of symmetrical T-wave inversion). The inferior limb leads (II, III, and aVF) are reciprocal to the anterior leads (the precordial leads, lead I, and aVL) and vice versa. Examples of ECGs showing recent and old anterior and inferior infarctions are shown in Figs 21, 22, 23, 24, and 25.

Pitfalls in the diagnosis of myocardial infarction

Left bundle-branch block

Left bundle-branch block so distorts the normal ECG that the usual criteria for the diagnosis of myocardial infarction are no longer applicable. It is sometimes possible to diagnose myocardial infarction in the presence of left bundle-branch block, but commonly the presence of left bundle-branch block obscures all other possible ECG diagnoses involving the QRS complexes, S–T segments, or T waves. The reason for this is that the two most important determinants of ventricular myocardial depolarization (and therefore also of repolarization) are radically altered in left bundle-branch block. These two determinants are (1) the direction of depolarization of the interventricular septum (which is reversed in left bundle-branch block), and (2) depolarization of the free wall of the left ventricle (which is appreciably delayed in left bundle-branch block). However, the changes of acute myocardial infarction can sometimes be recognized against a background of pre-existing left bundle-branch block, in which situation three independent criteria have been shown to have value in the diagnosis of acute infarction. These are: (1) S–T-segment elevation concordant with (i.e. in the same direction as) the QRS complex in a given lead; (2) S–T-segment depression of 1 mm or more in leads V_1, V_2, or V_3; and (3) S–T-segment elevation of 5 mm or more discordant with the QRS complex.

Figure 26 shows an example of acute anterior infarction with pre-existing left bundle-branch block. There is in excess of 5 mm of S–T elevation con-

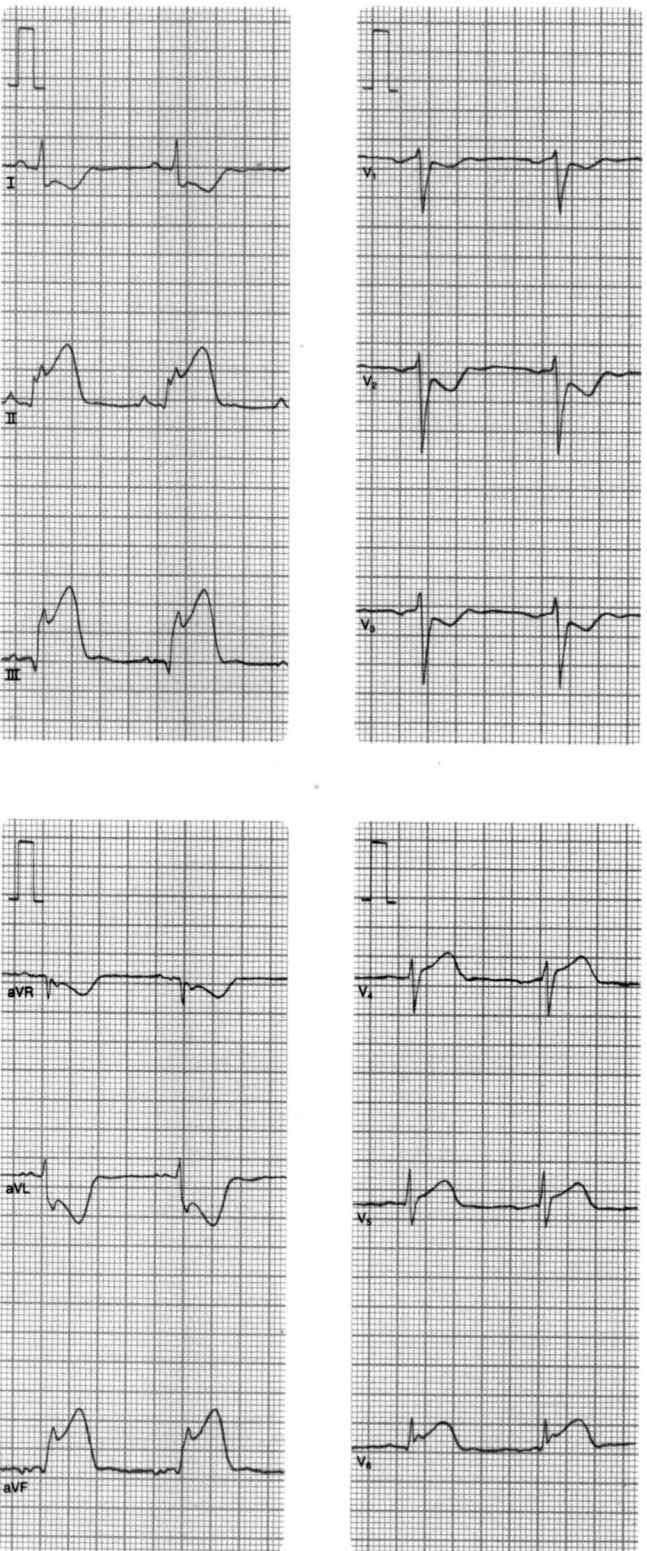

Fig. 21 Acute inferior myocardial ischaemic damage. Primary S–T elevation is visible in leads II, III, and aVF. S–T elevation is also visible in V4–V6, indicating that the damage extends to the lateral wall of the ventricle. There is reciprocal S–T-segment depression in I, aVL, aVR, and from V1 to V3.

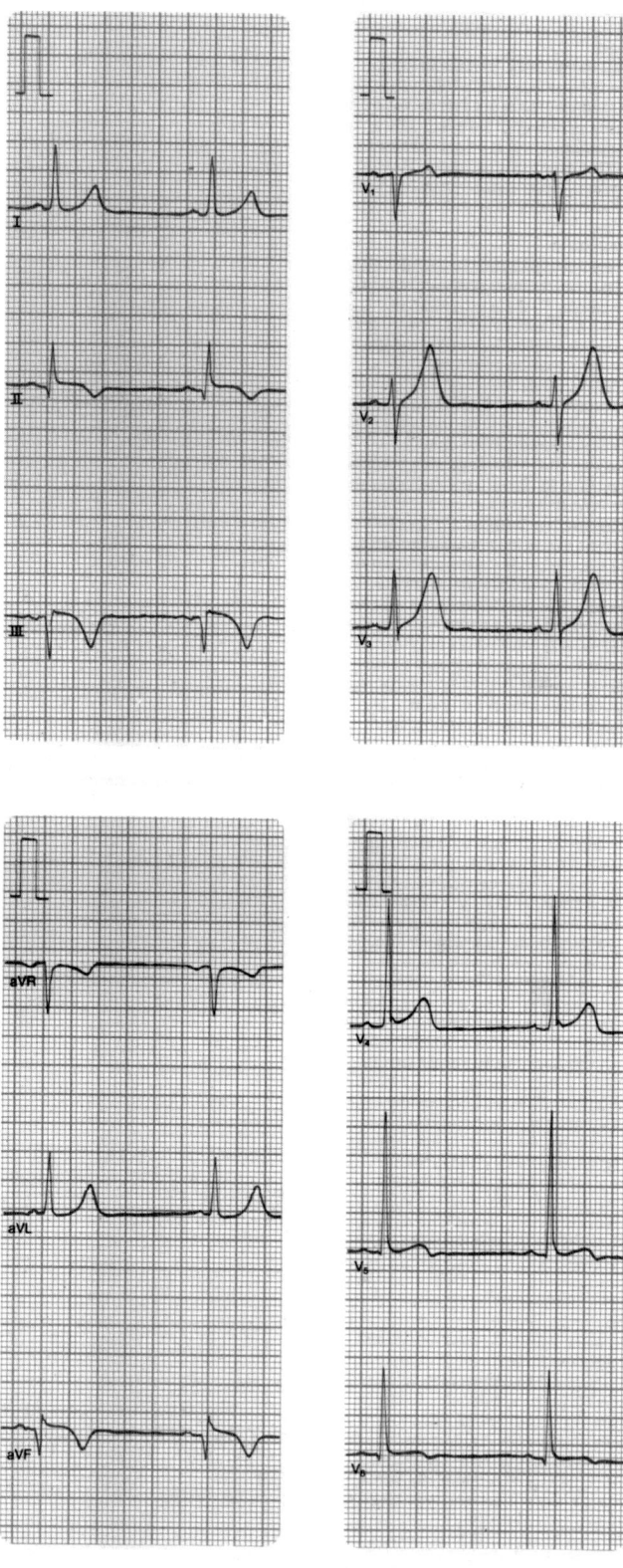

Fig. 22 Inferior myocardial infarction of intermediate age. The Q waves are abnormal in aVF (and also in III) and the q waves in II are borderline abnormal. There is T inversion in II, III, and aVF. The S–T segments are still minimally elevated in these leads. There is inversion of the terminal part of the T wave in V5 and V6, suggesting that the ischaemic area extends to the lateral wall of the ventricle. The T waves are strikingly tall in V2 and V3. This is not necessarily abnormal but could indicate true posterior ischaemia.

cordant with the QRS in leads V_2 to V_4 and there is concordant S–T elevation in V_4 and V_5.

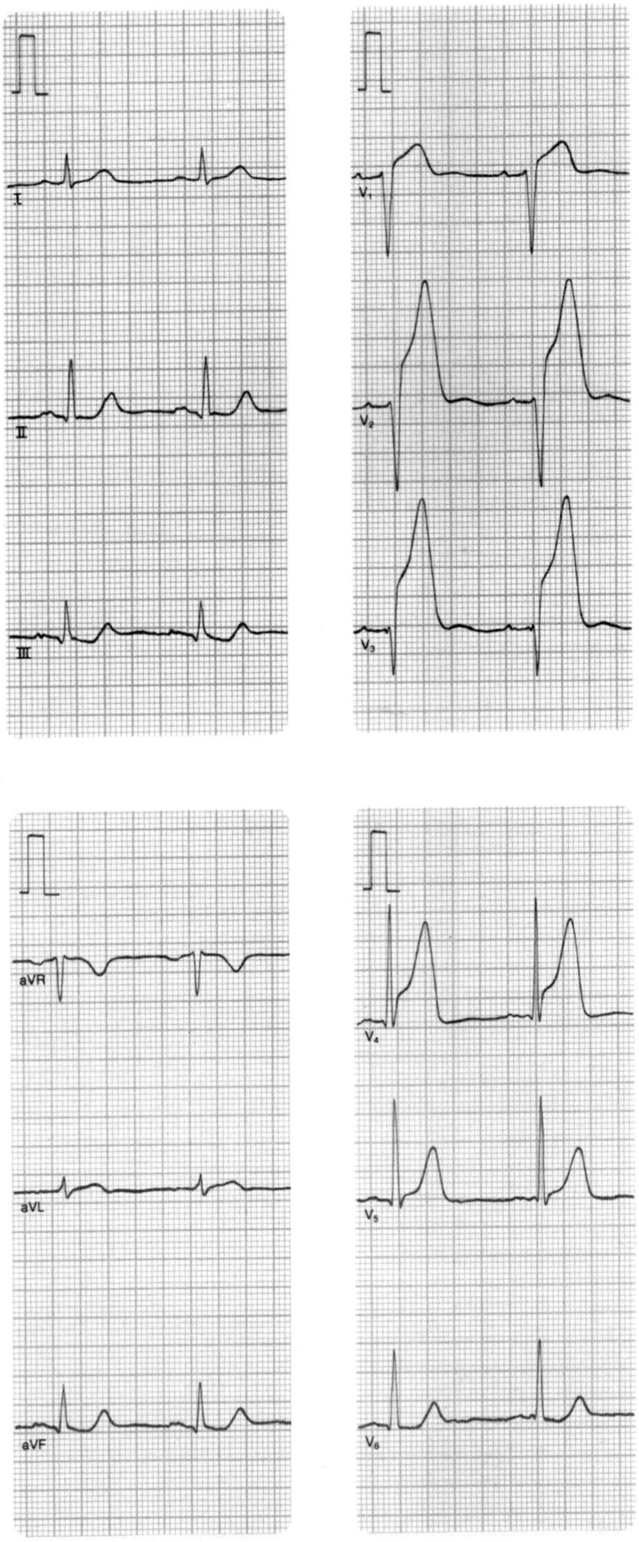

Right bundle-branch block

Right bundle-branch block does not interfere with the diagnosis of acute or of old myocardial infarction. (Fig. 27)

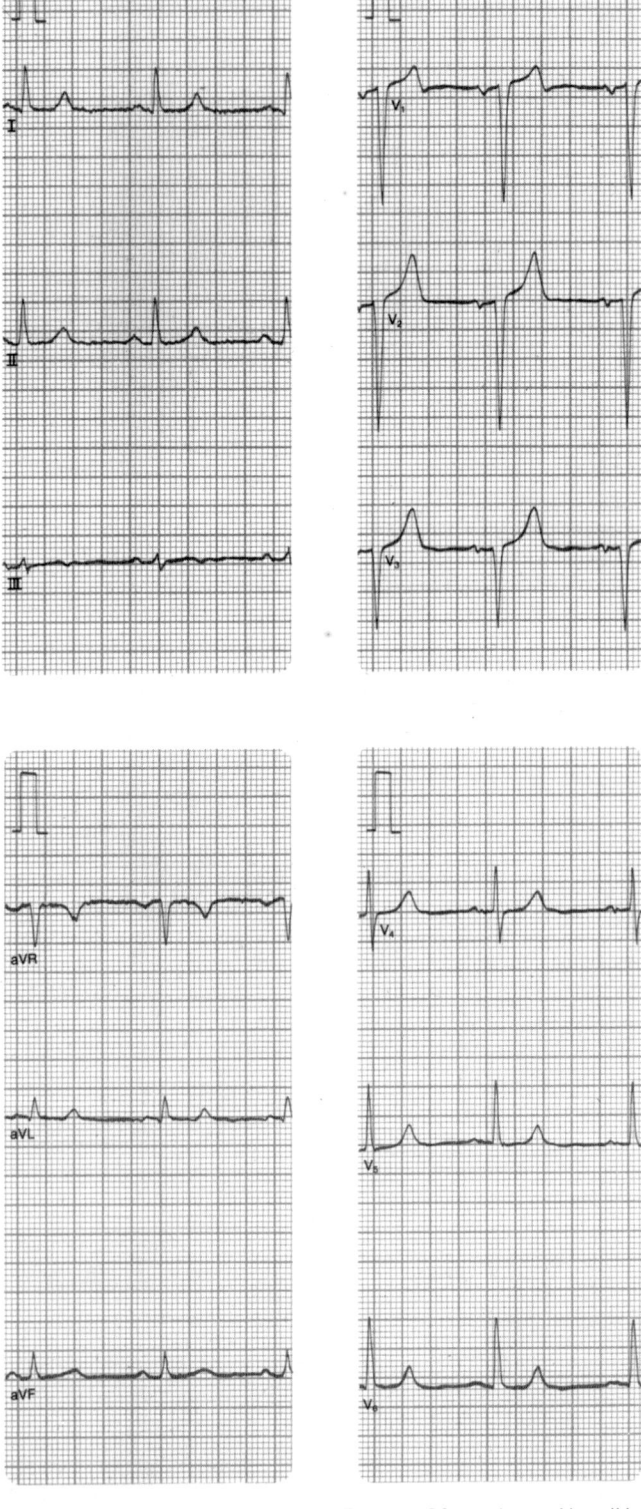

Fig. 23 Acute anteroseptal infarction. There is obvious S–T elevation in V_1–V_4 with minimal reciprocal S–T depression in III and aVF. There is obvious loss of initial R-wave height in V_2 and V_3.

Fig. 24 Old anterior myocardial infarction. There are QS complexes in V_2 and V_3.

Ventricular pre-excitation

When present, ventricular pre-excitation effectively precludes the diagnosis of left bundle-branch block and of myocardial infarction (see below). Very

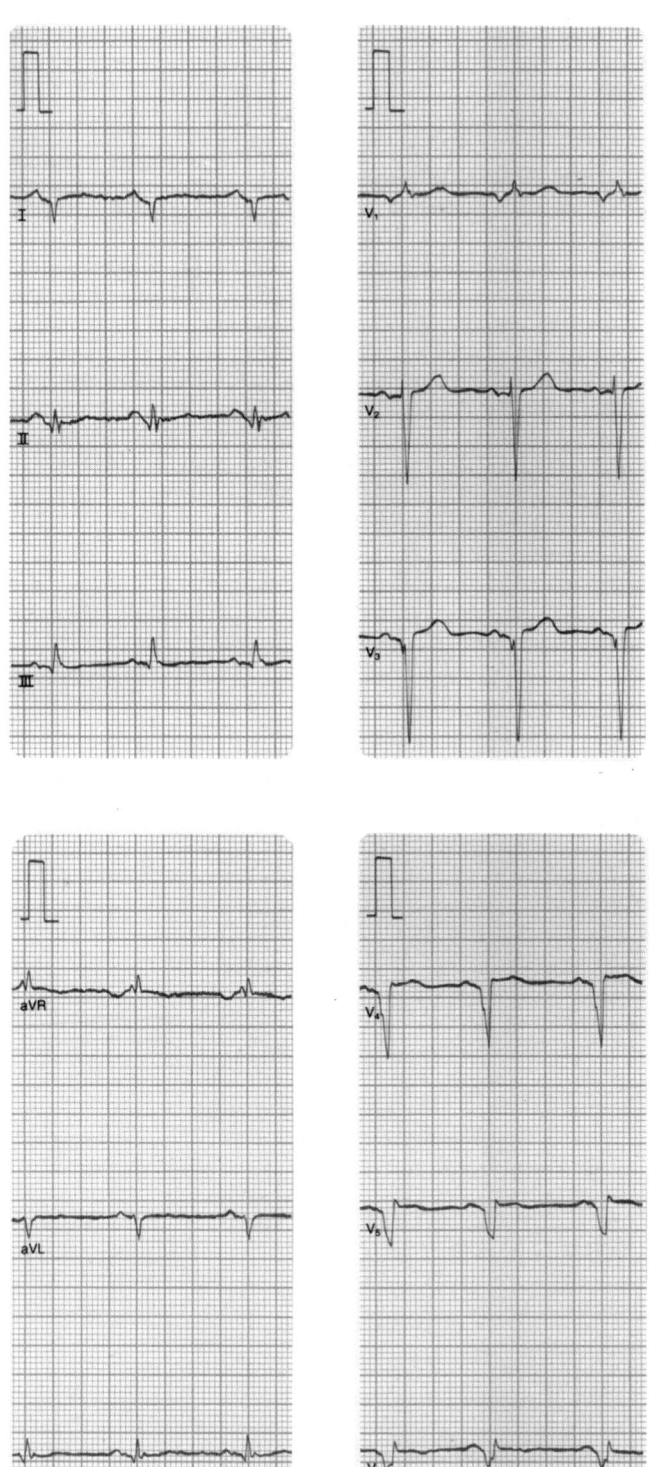

Fig. 25 Extensive anterior infarction. There are abnormally wide, abnormally deep Q waves from V₃ –V₆ and in I. The T waves are of low voltage in most leads. This latter abnormality is non-specific.

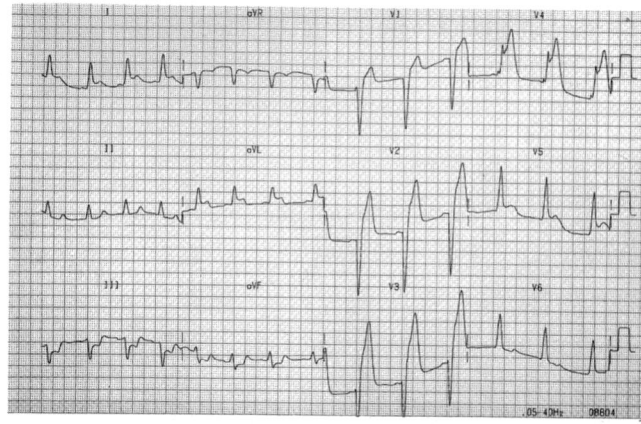

Fig. 26 Acute myocardial infarction with pre-existing left bundle-branch block. There is in excess of 5 mm of S–T elevation in leads V₂–V₄ and concordant S–T elevation in V₄ and V₅.

occasionally, substantial S–T elevation may provide an important clue to the diagnosis of acute infarction even when pre-excitation is seen.

Miscellaneous abnormalities

Abnormalities associated with the effects of drugs (including digitalis), hypokalaemia, hyperkalaemia, pericarditis, and hypothyroidism are discussed in other parts of this textbook. It is appropriate here, however, to mention ventricular pre-excitation, even though this is also dealt with in more detail elsewhere. The reason for this is that an incorrect diagnosis of bundle-branch block (right or left), ventricular hypertrophy (right or left), or myocardial infarction may easily be made if ventricular pre-excitation is present but not recognized.

Ventricular pre-excitation

Ventricular pre-excitation is found in approximately 0.1 per cent of the general population and failure to recognize it may lead to serious misdiagnosis. The term 'ventricular pre-excitation' implies that some part of the ventricular myocardium is depolarized (during normal sinus rhythm or any supraventricular rhythm) earlier than would be anticipated. This occurs as a result of the presence of one or more accessory (anomalous) pathways linking atrial and ventricular myocardium in such a way as to permit the depolarization wave descending through the atria from the sinoatrial node to bypass the atrioventricular node, partially or completely, intermittently or consistently. A variety of pathways exist which may, for example, pass (1) from atrial myocardium to ventricular myocardium, (2)

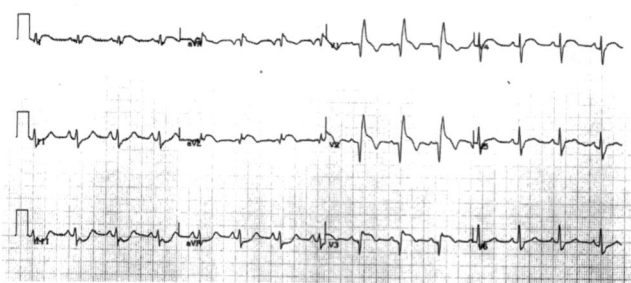

Fig. 27 Anteroseptal myocardial infarction with right bundle-branch block. Right bundle-branch block is diagnosed by the combination of (a) a total QRS duration of 0.12 s or more, plus (b) a secondary R wave in V₁. Anterior myocardial infarction is indicated by the presence of abnormally deep, abnormally wide Q waves in V₁–V₃. The presence of S–T elevation from V₂ to V₅ suggests that the infarct is recent.

from atrial myocardium to the distal part of the atrioventricular node, or (3) from the atrioventricular node to the ventricular myocardium. The commonest are those that link atrial and ventricular myocardium directly, and such pathways can exist at any point around the atrioventricular junction since, embryologically, the atrial and ventricular muscle masses were in continuity around the whole atrioventricular junction. These muscular remnants bear no resemblance to the junctional structures described by Kent; the use of the term 'Kent bundle' to describe the anomalous atrioventricular muscular connections that form the anatomical substrate for ventricular pre-excitation, though in widespread usage, is anatomically unjustifiable.

The presence of dual atrioventricular (AV) conduction routes (an accessory atrioventricular conduction pathway and the AV node) provides a substrate that facilitates the development of circus movement tachycardia. Patients with such pathways are at risk of developing paroxysmal tachycardia, but only a proportion do so: 10 per cent in the 20 to 39 age group and 36 per cent in the over-60s. In the presence of such a pathway, an appropriately timed atrial or ventricular premature beat may initiate atrioventricular node re-entrant tachycardia (AVNRT).

Recognition of the presence and of the location of such pathways has assumed greater practical importance with the advent of the technique of radiofrequency ablation. This makes it possible to destroy, or at least to render non-functional, the accessory conduction pathway, thereby removing the anatomical substrate upon which the occurrence of AVNRT is dependent.

ECG appearances in the presence of anomalous AV pathways

Space constraints prevent a detailed discussion of this important topic, but the typical ECG appearances have the following features:

(1) an abnormally short PR interval (0.11 s or less); and

(2) an abnormally wide QRS complex (0.11 s or more), and

(3) slurring of the initial 0.03 s of the QRS complex (a delta wave).

An example is shown in Fig. 28. This figure also illustrates the point that the presence of an accessory pathway does not guarantee that atrioventricular conduction will always occur via this route. Atrioventricular conduction can occur:

(1) always via the accessory pathway;

(2) always via the AV node;

(3) sometimes via the pathway and sometimes via the AV node;

(4) simultaneously via the pathway and the AV node (giving 'fusion beats in respect of the QRS complexes.

When, in a given patient, conduction never occurs via the pathway, the 12-lead ECG never shows any evidence of ventricular pre-excitation and the pathway is said to be 'concealed'. Such pathways can sustain AVNRT in just the same way as revealed pathways: ventriculoatrial conduction in the re-entrant arrhythmia being via the pathway (which can therefore conduct backwards), and atrioventricular conduction occurring via the AV node.

When ventricular pre-excitation is seen on the 12-lead ECG no further interpretation of the electrocardiogram should be attempted in respect of the QRS complexes, S–T segments, or T waves, except in respect of assessment of the QRS complexes to try to determine the location of the accessory pathway. Ventricular pre-excitation may mimic left bundle-branch block, right bundle-branch block., left ventricular hypertrophy, right ventricular hypertrophy, and myocardial infarction.

Location of the accessory pathways

Accessory pathways may remain at any site around the atrioventricular junction, but the sites can be broadly categorized as:

(1) left free wall (lateral) (55 per cent),

(2) posteroseptal (25 per cent),

(3) right free wall (15 per cent), and

(4) anteroseptal (5 per cent).

The 12 lead ECG provides some information concerning the approximate location of any manifest accessory pathway (i.e. any pathway along which conduction is occurring at the time of the recording). Anterograde conduction along the pathway initiates early ventricular depolarization at the site of insertion of the pathway into the ventricular myocardium. Thus the initial part of the QRS complex (the delta wave in the case of a pre-excited beat) is determined by the ventricular location of the pathway and will be positive in V) in left sided accessory pathways (just as it is in right bundle branch block and in the case of left ventricular premature beats — two other situations in which left ventricular depolarization is initiated earlier than right ventricular depolarization). Similarly the initial part of the QRS in V, will be negative in right-sided accessory pathways (just as it is in left bundle branch block and in the case of right ventricular premature beats—two other cases which right ventricular depolarization is initiated earlier than left ventricular depolarization).

Numerous algorithms have been proposed to predict the location of accessory pathways from the QRS configuration. However, the majority of each QRS complex (i.e. excluding the delta wave) is determined by the relative contribution of (a) conduction along the accessory pathway and (b) conduction via the normal AV nodal route. This relative distribution varies greatly between subjects and can vary very significantly within subjects (being influenced, for example, by autonomic effects on AV nodal function). Furthermore the physical orientation of the heart within the chest,

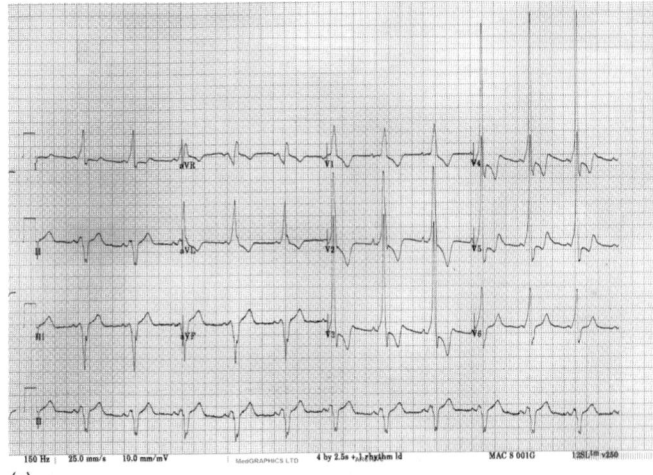

(a)

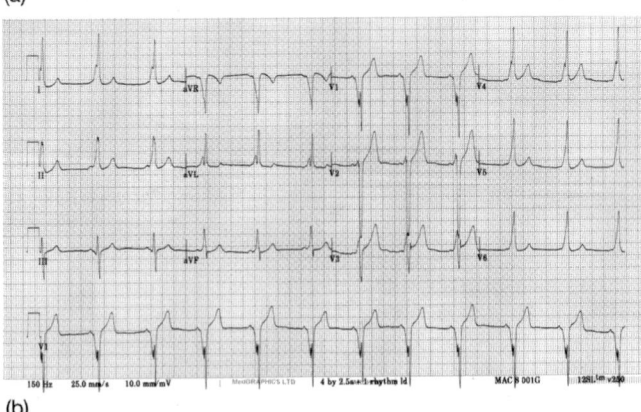

(b)

Fig. 28 Ventricular pre-excitation. (a) and (b) both show the essential features of ventricular pre-excitation. The PR interval is short in both and delta waves are seen in leads I, II, aVR, aVL, and V₂–V₆ in (a), and in leads I, II, III, aVR, aVL, aVF and V₂–V₆ in (b). In (a) the dominant R wave in V₁ and the 'pseudo RBBB' pattern indicates a left-sided AP. In (b) the small r waves in V₁ and the 'pseudo LBBB' pattern indicates a right sided AP.

the presence of QRS abnormalities unrelated to pre-excitation, and the possibility of multiple accessory pathways are all potential confounding factors. It follows that the value of the surface ECG in determining the location of accessory pathways is limited.

As a general guide to the approximate location of an accessory pathway (AP), the following features are helpful. A left sided AP will typically give rise to a positive QRS in V_1 (i.e. a dominant R wave or an equiphasic RS complex) with a 'pseudo RBBB' pattern (Fig. 28(a)). A right sided AP will typically give rise to a small r wave in V_1 and V_2. There may be delta waves in V_6 with a 'pseudo LBBB' pattern (Fig. 28(b)). The smaller the r waves in the right precordial leads and the later in the precordial leads the RS transition (from dominant S in the right precordial leads to dominant R in the left precordial leads), the further to the right of the septum is the accessory pathway. The more posterior the location of the pathway, the more likely it is that there will be negative delta waves in the inferior leads and that there will be a superior QRS axis. The more anterior the pathway location the more likely it is that the QRS axis will be inferior.

The exercise ECG

Historical background

The present-day use of the exercise stress electrocardiogram in the diagnosis of coronary heart disease (in the form of the graded-exercise stress test—GXT) has evolved as a result of numerous observations and developments.

In 1908, Einthoven observed S–T depression after exercise but did not comment on it. In 1918, Blousfield recorded S–T-segment depression in leads I, II, and III during spontaneous angina. Feil and Siegel, in 1928, exercised patients known to have angina and observed S–T-segment and T-wave changes. Master and Oppenheimer, in 1929, developed an exercise test to assess 'circulatory efficiency' (using pulse and blood pressure) but did not use the ECG. In 1931, Wood and Wolferth described S–T changes associated with exercise, but felt that the test was too dangerous to use in patients with coronary disease. In 1932, Goldhammer and Scherf reported S–T depression in 75 per cent of patients with angina—a figure indicating a remarkably similar false-negative rate to that of current-day studies. In 1941, Master and Jaffe suggested that the ECG recorded before and after exercise could be used to detect 'coronary insufficiency'. Paul Wood and colleagues, in 1950, at the National Heart Hospital in London, described their experience of a test in which the patients had to run up 84 steps adjacent to the laboratory. They showed an 88 per cent reliability (compared with 39 per cent in the Master's test) and emphasized that the amount of work required should be adjusted to the patient's physical capacity.

The era of modern, stress testing began in 1956 when Bruce reported his findings and established guidelines for a standardized GXT procedure. Subsequently, the application of Bayesian techniques of analysis; the addition of nuclear techniques (myocardial scintigraphy and cardiac blood pool analysis) and echocardiographic stress testing; and the use on non-exercise stress techniques (using dipyridamole, dobutamine, and adenosine) have all brought greater sophistication and applicability to cardiac stress testing.

This section will be confined to the use of the exercise stress ECG in the assessment of the heart and circulation and, in particular, to the role of the GXT in the detection and assessment of ischaemic heart disease.

Current usage

Although the exercise ECG may be used for several purposes, its commonest uses are in the diagnosis and assessment of ischaemic heart disease (IHD). In this respect, however, it is extremely important at the outset to recognize that the test has a significant false-negative rate, even in populations with an appreciable prevalence of IHD, and that the false-negative rate may be unacceptably high in populations with a low prevalence. The test is therefore of very limited value in screening low-risk, asymptomatic subjects. Most subjects who have undergone exercise stress testing as a screening procedure and who subsequently experience sudden cardiac death are found in retrospect to have had a normal exercise test result. A meta-analysis of 147 consecutive studies involving a total of 24 074 patients who had undergone both exercise stress testing and coronary angiography revealed sensitivities ranging from 23 to 100 per cent (mean 68) and specificities ranging from 17 to 100 per cent (mean 77). In patients with multi-vessel coronary disease the sensitivities ranged from 40 to 100 per cent (mean 81) and the specificities from 17 to 100 per cent (mean 66). For patients with single-vessel disease a positive GXT is most likely for lesions in the left anterior descending artery. Patients with lesions in the circumflex artery are least likely to give a positive result, while those with lesions in the right coronary artery occupy an intermediate position.

Exercise electrocardiography is also used in the estimation of prognosis in patients with known IHD, for risk stratification following myocardial infarction, for screening of professionals in high-risk situations (e.g. pilots and professional athletes), and in the assessment of some cardiovascular symptoms (e.g. palpitations, tachyarrhythmias, and syncope) when these are exercise related. The database for the evaluation of the usefulness of the technique in these situations is less well established than is the case in relation to its use in the assessment of IHD.

Exercise testing in females

The specificity of exercise testing is less in women than in men. It seems likely that this is, in part at least, related to their lower prevalence of IHD. However, biological differences might be relevant. It has been suggested that oestrogens (with certain chemical structural similarities to digitalis) contribute to S–T-segment depression, but it has also been pointed out that women secrete more catecholamines during exercise than men. Both of these postulated mechanisms have been thought possibly to act via coronary vasoconstriction.

Risks

High-level exercise carries a cardiovascular mortality risk, and a maximal-exercise stress ECG is, basically, supervised high-level exercise. Inevitably, therefore, a GXT carries a risk, but multiple studies have shown the risk to be remarkably low. In 1971 a survey of 73 medical centres summarized the risks in relation to approximately 170 000 stress tests. A total of 16 deaths were reported (mortality rate 0.01 per cent), and 0.04 per cent required admission within 24 h because of arrhythmia or prolonged chest pain. The risks are greater when the test is conducted soon after an ischaemic event. Even in this situation, however, the test is still remarkably safe. A survey of 151 941 tests undertaken within 4 weeks of acute myocardial infarction revealed a mortality rate of 0.03 per cent and a 0.09 per cent rate of non-fatal reinfarction or (successfully resuscitated) cardiac arrest.

Contraindications

Exercise stress testing is contraindicated to some extent whenever the pre-existing clinical state indicates a significantly increased risk of mortality or morbidity. In some situations the additional risk is so great as to constitute an absolute contraindication. In other situations the presenting clinical state indicates the need for more vigilant supervision than usual. Exercise, whilst not 'contraindicated', is of limited or negligible value in situations where abnormalities of the resting ECG make interpretation of the exercising record difficult or impossible.

Absolute contraindications

These include:

- acute ischaemic syndromes:

  unstable angina,

  suspected acute myocardial infarction,

  known acute myocardial infarction within 5 days;

- known left main-stem stenosis;

- acute myocarditis;
- acute pericarditis;
- severe aortic stenosis;
- severe congestive cardiac failure;
- recent acute pulmonary oedema;
- current acute systemic illness;
- absence of trained supervisory staff or of resuscitation equipment;
- failure of the patient to understand the procedure or to give informed consent

Situations requiring intensive supervision

These include:

- known severe coronary disease;
- known moderate or mild aortic stenosis;
- severe or moderate systemic hypertension;
- severe or moderate pulmonary hypertension;
- severe impairment of ventricular function;
- known history of ventricular tachycardia;
- known history of supraventricular tachycardia;
- existing second- or third-degree atrioventricular block;
- hypertrophic cardiomyopathy;
- severe congestive cardiomyopathy;
- known hypokalaemia.

Situations where interpretation of the exercising record is difficult or impossible

Abnormalities of the resting ECG that preclude effective interpretation of the exercising record include:

- left bundle-branch block;
- ventricular pre-excitation;
- currently paced ventricular rhythm;
- widespread S–T,T changes;
- widespread QS complexes (especially across the precordial leads).

Procedures

Lead positioning

During exercise it is not possible to maintain adequate physical and electrical stability in relation to limb lead connections at their usual (for the standard 12-lead ECG) location. Instead, the 'limb' lead electrodes are positioned on the torso: with the right and left arm connections situated at the most lateral aspects of the respective infraclavicular fossa, and the right and left leg electrodes positioned halfway between the respective anterior iliac crest and the rib margin. This Mason–Likar modification of the standard 12-lead ECG results in a rightward shift of the axis, which is more marked in the standing than in the recumbent position. This rightward shift (typically giving an axis of +90° to +120°) sometimes results in the appearance of new q waves in aVL (but it should be noted that, whenever the mean frontal plane QRS axis is +90° or more positive, aVL becomes a 'cavity' lead and the finding of a q wave in a cavity lead is not abnormal).

Exercise protocols

Various exercise modalities can be used, including static or dynamic exercise, arm or leg exercise, and bicycle ergometry or treadmill procedures, but the commonest procedure by far is dynamic treadmill exercise. The most popular protocol is the Bruce protocol. This has a starting walking speed of 1.7 mph (1 km/h) at a 10 per cent slope, giving an oxygen consumption of about four metabolic equivalents, which in general use has proved very

satisfactory. One major advantage of the Bruce protocol is that large diagnostic and prognostic databases exist for this test.

Exercise endpoints

Exercise is continued until one of the following endpoints is reached:

- subject wishes to stop (chest pain, dyspnoea, fatigue, leg weakness, light headedness, exhaustion, claudication);
- target endpoint is reached (target heart rate or exercise level);
- operator terminates the procedure:

   early or severe (>2 mm) S–T depression,

   S–T elevation,

   ventricular tachycardia,

   second- or third-degree heart block,

   fall in heart rate (20 beats/min or more),

   fall in blood pressure (20 mmHg or more),

   perceived patient distress,

   failure of monitoring equipment.

Assessment of the exercise electrocardiogram

As the heart rate increases with exercise, the PR, QRS, and QT intervals all reduce in normal subjects. The P-wave amplitude increases and the atrial repolarization wave (the Ta wave) increases in amplitude.

Atrial repolarization wave

Sinus tachycardia is associated with an increase in the depth and duration of the Ta wave. This gives a curved upsloping segment between the QRS complex and the T wave, often misconstrued as S–T-segment depression, and a common cause of an incorrect conclusion that an exercise test is positive. A Ta wave can be recognized when it is noted that back-extrapolation of a depressed S–T segment shows it to be continuous with downsloping depression in front of the QRS complex (Fig. 29).

Standard criteria for a positive test

By definition, a positive test occurs when 1 mm (0.1 mV) of horizontal or downsloping S–T depression occurs during exercise (usually at peak exercise) or in the early recovery period. Upsloping S–T depression is less reliably predictive of the presence of coronary disease than flat or downsloping S–T depression. Greater (than 1 mm) degrees of S–T depression are more reliably predictive of coronary disease, as are S–T depression occurring

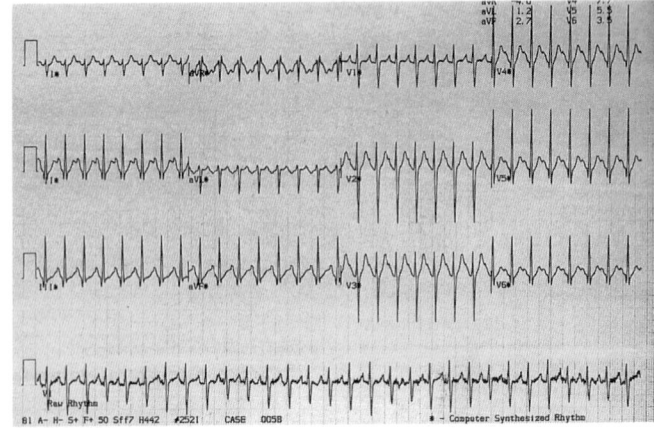

Fig. 29 Negative exercise ECG. This ECG is the record taken at peak exercise in a maximal stress test. The heart rate is 180 beats/min. There is no S–T depression. A prominent atrial depolarization wave (Ta wave) is clearly seen in II, III, aVF, and V₄–V₆ (best in II). As would be expected aVR shows an 'upside down' Ta wave (since it is a cavity lead).

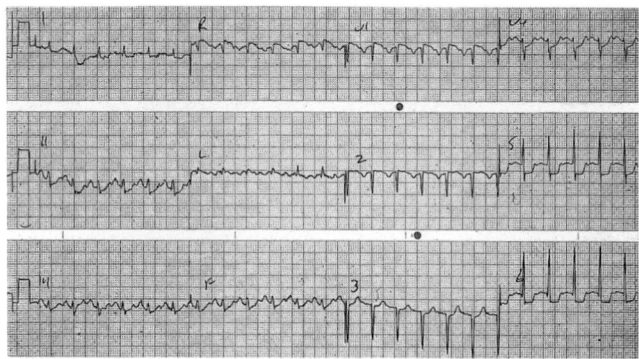

Fig. 30 Positive exercise ECG. This ECG is the record taken at peak exercise in a maximal stress test. The heart rate is only 136 beats/min. The test was stopped before the 'target' heart rate was reached because the patient had chest pain and the test was already clearly giving a positive result. There is 2 mm of S–T depression in the left precordial leads.

earlier in the exercise period, more prolonged S–T depression, and a more widespread (within the ECG recording leads) S–T change. Figure 30 shows an example of significant (2 mm) S–T depression in the left precordial leads.

Sometimes the S–T depression is most marked or only occurs during the recovery period (Fig. 31).

An example of a negative stress test is shown in Fig. 29.

Interpretation of the test result

Positive or negative. Pre- and post-test probability. Bayesian analysis

The criterion for positivity of an exercise ECG is widely accepted as being 1 mm of flat or downsloping S–T segment depression during or early after exercise. The interpretation of a positive result is more problematical. Usually the question being asked is whether or not the test result indicates a high probability that the patient has coronary heart disease. Bayesian analysis of this problem indicates the enormous impact of the prevalence of coronary disease in the population group from which the subject is drawn (the prior probability of the condition) in answering this question. In essence, Bayes's theorem states the self-evident truth that interpretation of the future (probability of disease in the given subject) is helped by a knowledge of past experience (prevalence of the disease in the population from which the subject comes) as well as present observations (the test result).

Bayesian analysis expresses the probability that a subject with a positive exercise test result does actually have coronary heart disease, in terms of the sensitivity and specificity of the test and the prevalence of the disease, as follows:

$$\text{Probability} = [\text{prevalence} \times \text{sensitivity}]/[\text{prevalence} \times \text{sensitivity} + (1 - \text{prevalence}) (1 - \text{specificity})].$$

If one inserts reasonable (on the basis of published results of exercise testing) values for the sensitivity (say 0.8, i.e. 80 per cent) and specificity (say 0.9, i.e. 90 per cent) into this equation and then looks at the impact of variations in prevalence on the predictive value of a positive test, then the values shown in Table 2 are obtained. Clearly the false-positive rate is very high in low-prevalence populations (the healthy population) and this limits the value of exercise testing as a screening procedure in asymptomatic, presumptively healthy groups.

The likelihood that a subject with a positive stress-test result has coronary artery disease (the 'post-test or posterior probability') is therefore dependent on the prevalence of the disease in the population from which the subject is derived (the 'pretest or prior probability'). Equally, of course, the likelihood that a subject with a negative stress-test result does not have coronary artery disease (the 'post-test probability') is also dependent on the prevalence of the disease in the population from which the subject is

derived (the 'pretest probability'). This concept is shown graphically in Fig. 32.

Degree of abnormality of the test result

The degree of abnormality of the stress-test result also has a powerful bearing on the predictive value of the result. Greater or lesser degrees of abnormality may be shown by:

(1) the depth of the S–T depression;

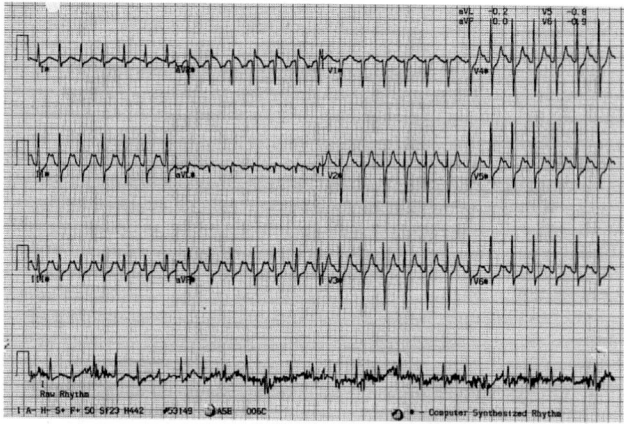

(a)

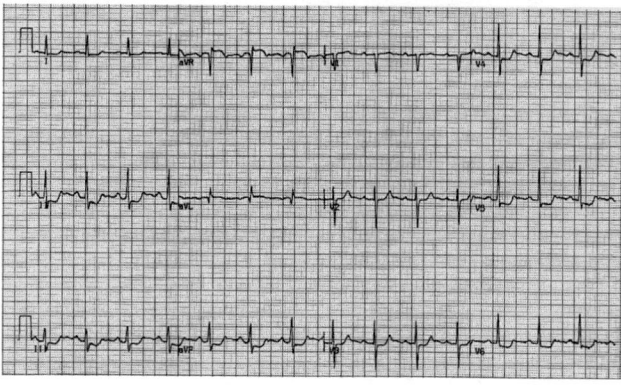

(b)

Fig. 31 Positive exercise ECG. Record (a) was taken at peak exercise. It is not abnormal. It shows a prominent atrial repolarization wave. Record (b) was taken 6 min into the recovery period (after 9 min of exercise). Although no S–T depression occurred during exercise (a) there is clearly abnormal S–T depression during recovery. Coronary angiography confirmed the presence of significant disease in the anterior descending and diagonal branches of the left coronary artery.

Table 2 Impact of prevalence of coronary disease in the study population (prior probability) on the value of a positive exercise test in predicting the presence of coronary disease (posterior probability) and therefore on the false positive rate of the test

Prevalence	Probability of disease	False-positive rate (%)
1.0	1.0	0
0.9	0.99	1
0.5	0.89	11
0.03	0.2	80
0.01	0.04	96

(2) the time of onset of the S–T depression;

(3) the duration of the S–T depression;

(4) the number of ECG leads showing significant S–T depression.

Only in respect of the depth of S–T depression, however, is there currently a large database of information. The effect of varying degrees of S–T depression on the predictive value of a positive test is shown in Fig. 33.

Confounding ECGs

Interpretation of the exercise ECG is dependent upon the assessment of the timing, duration, degree, and distribution of S–T depression occurring during exercise. When the pre-exercise ECG shows significant S–T-segment abnormalities (left bundle-branch block, ventricular pre-excitation, ven-

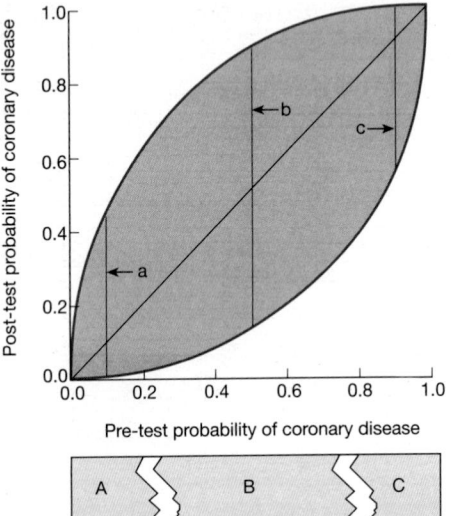

Fig. 32 Predictive value of positive and of negative exercise stress tests. The pretest probability of the condition (prevalence) is shown on the abscissa and the post-test probability (likelihood of the condition in the light of the test result and in the population from which the subject exercised was drawn) on the ordinate. The 45° line shows the impact of a completely non-predictive test result (for example, tossing a coin), the post-test probability being unchanged by the test result. Curves for clearly positive (= 2 mm flat or downsloping S–T depression) and clearly negative (no S–T depression at peak exercise with target heart rate achieved) test results are shown. The upper curve is for positive and the lower curve for negative results. The vertical distance between the curves shows the relative diagnostic 'benefit' (additional diagnostic probability) from the test result. This is greatest (b) where the pretest probability is intermediate (B). In a low-prevalence population (A), such as young, asymptomatic persons being screened, the pretest probability of the condition is (by definition) very low, and even the contribution of a strongly positive test result (upper curve) only results in a post-test probability of 40 per cent, i.e. the false-positive rate in this low-prevalence population is 60 per cent. In such a low-prevalence population a clearly negative result (lower curve), i.e. one concordant with the initial statistical probability, would be powerfully effective in confirming the initial likelihood. In this case a pretest probability of about 10 per cent would give way to a very low post-test probability of about 1 per cent. In a high-prevalence population (C) the pretest probability in this case is about 89 per cent and the post-test probability of a positive result would give about a 99 per cent probability of coronary artery disease. In such a population a clearly negative result would give about a 55 per cent probability of coronary disease, i.e. there would be a very significant false-negative rate. In general, therefore, a positive exercise stress-test result in a high-prevalence population is likely to be a true-positive and a negative result in a low-prevalence population is likely to be a true-negative. Conversely, a positive result in a low-prevalence population and a negative result in a high-prevalence population are both significantly likely to be false results. The stress test will make its greatest diagnostic contribution (b) where the prevalence is intermediate (B), i.e. where the initial diagnostic position is unclear.

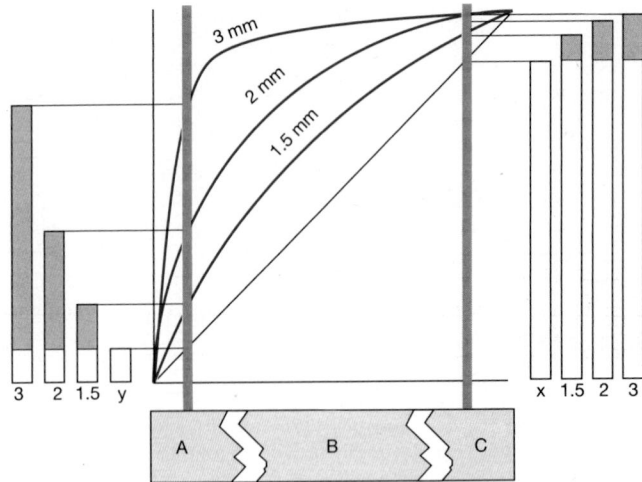

Fig. 33 Predictive value of different degrees of positivity of exercise stress tests. In a high-prevalence population (C) the pretest probability of coronary disease is high (×) and positive test results of increasing degree (1.5, 2, and even 3 mm S–T depression) only minimally increase the probability of the condition. In a low-prevalence population (A) a 1.5-mm and a 2-mm S–T depression result still leave less than a 50 per cent probability that the subject has significant ischaemic heart disease. In such a population only a really strikingly positive result (3-mm depression) would result in a significant (75 per cent) probability of the condition.

tricular paced rhythm, non-specific S–T-segment depression, etc.), interpretation of changes in the S–T segments occurring during exercise is virtually impossible. In these situations the exercise stress ECG makes no useful contribution to the diagnosis of or to the exclusion of significant coronary artery disease.

Further reading

Bruce RA, *et al.* (1963). Exercise testing in adult normal subjects and cardiac patients. *Pediatrics* **32** (Suppl.) 742–56.

Casale PN, *et al.* (1987). Improved sex-specific criteria of left ventricular hypertrophy for clinical and computer interpretation of electrocardiograms: validation with autopsy findings. *Circulation* **75**, 565–72. [The Cornell gender-specific voltage criteria give the best correlation with left ventricular mass]

Chaitman BR (1997). Exercise stress testing. In: Braunwald E, ed. *Heart disease: a textbook of cardiovascular medicine*, pp 153–76. WB Saunders, Philadelphia. [The standard textbook of cardiovascular medicine]

Ellestad MH, *et al.* (1996). History of stress testing. In: Ellestad MH, ed. *Stress testing: principles and practice*, pp 1–9. FA Davies, Philadelphia. [An excellent reference textbook of exercise stress testing]

Fletcher GF, *et al.* (1995). Exercise standards. A statement for healthcare professionals from the American Heart Association. *Circulation* **91**, 580–615. [Standard protocols and procedures]

Gianrossi R, *et al.* (1989). Exercise-induced ST segment depression in the diagnosis of coronary artery disease: a meta-analysis. *Circulation* **80**, 87–98. [Comprehensive, authoritative meta-analysis]

Hamm LF, *et al.* (1989). Safety and characteristics of exercise testing early after acute myocardial infarction. *American Journal of Cardiology* **63**, 1193–7. [The largest report of the risks of exercise stress testing early after acute myocardial infarction]

Macfarlane PW, Lawrie TDV, eds (1989). *Comprehensive electrocardiography. Theory and practice in health and disease.* Pergamon Press, Oxford. [A three-volume encyclopaedia of electrocardiography.]

Rochmis P, Blackburn H (1971). Exercise test: a survey of procedures, safety and litigation experience in approximately 170,000 tests. *Journal of the American Medical Association* **217**, 1061–1066. [The first large survey of the risks of exercise stress testing]

Romhilt DW, *et al.* (1969). A critical appraisal of the electrocardiographic criteria for the diagnosis of left ventricular hypertrophy. *Circulation* **40**, 185–95.

Rowlands DJ (1978). The electrical axis. *British Journal of Hospital Medicine* **19**, 472–81. [A detailed description of the technique for estimating the clinical significance of the measurement]

Rowlands DJ (1991). *Clinical electrocardiography.* Gower, London. [A detailed explanation (extensively illustrated) of the basis of electrocardiography]

Schamroth L (1976). *An introduction to electrocardiography.* Blackwell Scientific, Oxford. [A simple, basic introduction to the ECG]

Sgarbossa EB, *et al.* (1996). Electrocardiographic diagnosis of evolving acute myocardial infarction in the presence of left bundle-branch block. *New England Journal of Medicine* **334**, 481–7.

Sokolow M, Lyon TP (1949). The ventricular complex in left ventricular hypertrophy as obtained by unipolar precordial and limb leads. *American Heart Journal* **37**, 161–86.

Weinstein MC, Fineberg HV (1980). *Clinical decision analysis.* WB Saunders, Philadelphia.

15.3.3 Echocardiography

A. P. Banning

Introduction

Modern transthoracic echocardiography combines real-time two-dimensional imaging of the myocardium and valves with information about velocity and direction of blood flow obtained by Doppler and colour flow mapping. It is non-invasive and a complete examination can be performed in most patients in less than 30 min.

Doppler echocardiography has revolutionized the diagnosis and follow-up of patients with valvular heart disease. Serial cardiac catheterization to assess severity and progress of valvar stenosis has been almost completely superseded by echocardiography, and the role of invasive investigation is increasingly limited to assessment of the coronary arteries prior to corrective surgery.

Transoesophageal echocardiography is available in larger cardiac centres. Under sedation, an ultrasound probe is passed into the oesophagus to a position behind the heart producing excellent resolution of cardiac structures. It is used diagnostically in many emergency situations, including aortic dissection and suspected prosthetic mechanical valve dysfunction, and as an additional method of monitoring cardiac performance during cardiac and non-cardiac surgery.

The dramatic expansion in the availability of echocardiography has been accompanied by continuing technological development. Stress echocardiography can be used to detect occult coronary disease and predict cardiac risk, whilst the administration of contrast agents may allow visualization of myocardial perfusion. Although three-dimensional reconstruction is currently a research tool, real-time three-dimensional imaging is an increasingly realistic goal. In the future, these and other developments seem likely to ensure that echocardiography will maintain its central role in the diagnosis and management of most cardiac and many non-cardiac patients.

Principals of echocardiography

The transducer used for most echocardiographic examinations contains piezo-electric crystals that emit ultrasound frequencies of 2.5 to 5 MHz. Most of the sound energy is scattered or absorbed, but reflection occurs at interfaces between tissues of different acoustic impedance (e.g. between blood and muscle). The transducer collects these reflections and the time delay between emission and reception is calculated. This allows the depth of the reflection to be derived and its position to be displayed on a screen as a dot (pixel). The brightness of the dot is related to the magnitude of the reflected signal. In general, higher frequency transducers allow better discrimination between structures but more ready attenuation leads to reduced penetration.

There are three main echocardiographic techniques: cross sectional (two-dimensional), M-mode, and Doppler.

Cross sectional echocardiography (two-dimensional echo)

Cross sectional (two-dimensional) images are constructed as the ultrasound beam sweeps across the heart. Between 50 and 100 cross sections are presented each second and this gives the impression of a moving picture. These images are readily interpretable by an observer with a knowledge of cardiac anatomy and this technique is the cornerstone of modern echocardiography.

M-mode echocardiography

M-mode echocardiography preceded modern two-dimensional imaging. Unlike two-dimensional imaging, which uses a series of sweeps across the heart, M-mode uses a single static beam of very frequent ultrasound pulses. The narrow beam is analogous to a vertical mineshaft passing through various layers of rock. Displayed in real time this results in reflections from cardiac structures being displayed as horizontal lines with superficial structures at the top of the screen and the deeper structures at the bottom. These data are interpretable when one knows which structure each line represents and the technique has excellent spatial resolution. With the advent of two-dimensional and Doppler, M-mode is now principally used for measurement of cardiac chamber dimensions and observation of the relative movement of cardiac structures to each other, for example the relationship of the anterior leaflet of the mitral valve to the septum in hypertrophic cardiomyopathy.

Doppler echocardiography

The Doppler principal allows the velocity and direction of movement of an object (or moving blood in the case of cardiac ultrasound), to be calculated from the shift in the frequency of a reflected waveform relative to the observer. Cardiac imaging employs pulsed wave, continuous wave, and colour Doppler techniques.

Pulsed wave Doppler allows information about flow to be obtained from a particular point within the heart. The range of detectable velocities is limited, and it is used for sampling normal and low velocities, for example mitral valve flow.

Continuous wave Doppler measures the peak velocity encountered along the ultrasound beam and is particularly valuable for measuring high velocity jets, for example aortic stenosis. It is important to remember that failure to align the transducer exactly parallel to flow results in measurement of artefactualy low velocities and an underestimation of the valvular stenosis.

Colour Doppler allows a dynamic representation of the direction and velocity of flow to be superimposed onto a two-dimensional image of the heart. Velocities towards the transducer are coded in red and velocities away are coded in blue. Turbulent flow produces variable velocities and results in a mosaic pattern that is ideal for characterization of regurgitant lesions. This technique is now so sensitive that it can detect trivial regurgitation during the closure of many normal heart valves.

Imaging

Imaging is usually performed with the patient lying on their left hip in the left lateral position, with their left arm behind their head (Fig. 1). Ultrasound cannot travel through bone and thus cardiac imaging is performed

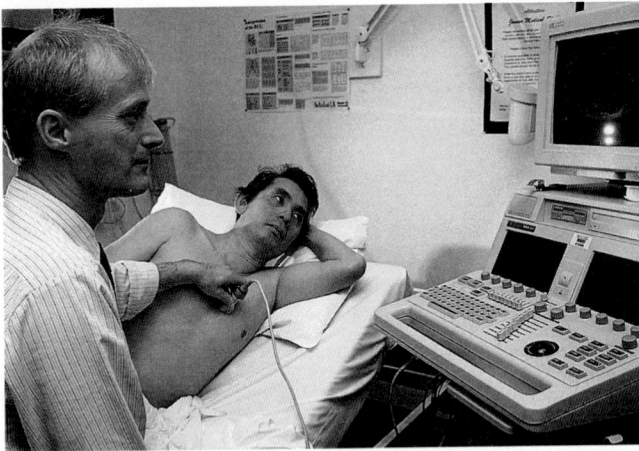

Fig. 1 Patient in the standard position undergoing transthoracic echocardiography.

in intercostal spaces to the left of the sternum and at the apex of the heart in the axillary line. These 'echo windows' provide standard views described as the parasternal short and long axis and apical two, four, and five chamber. Useful additional views can be obtained from the subxiphoid and suprasternal approach in some patients.

A standard echo examination involves two-dimensional imaging from the parasternal approach followed by M-mode measurements and colour Doppler. Apical two-dimensional views are followed by colour and continuous and pulsed Doppler interrogation.

Applications of echocardiography

Valvular heart disease

Transthoracic Doppler echocardiography is the investigation of choice for patients with suspected valvular heart disease. All four cardiac valves can be visualized and interrogated by Doppler. Concomitant abnormalities in ventricular performance can be assessed simultaneously.

Aortic stenosis

Two-dimensional echocardiography can usually image the aortic valve cusps and if they are thin and freely mobile it is unlikely that there is significant aortic stenosis. However, if the valve cusps are thickened and calcified, interrogation by continuous wave Doppler is mandatory. The severity of aortic stenosis is expressed as the peak pressure difference (or gradient) across the valve, and is calculated from the maximum flow velocity (V) using the modified Bernoulli equation (pressure gradient=$4V^2$). The gradient measured by continuous wave Doppler is not directly comparable with a gradient measured at cardiac catheterization, which can lead to confusion. Doppler measures the peak instantaneous gradient and is higher than peak-to-peak gradient measured by catheterization (Fig. 2). In patients with normal left ventricular systolic function a peak-to-peak catheter gradient of 50 mmHg suggests significant aortic stenosis (Fig. 3 and Plate 1): this corresponds to a peak instantaneous gradient measured by Doppler of about 70 to 80 mmHg.

When chronic critical outflow obstruction results in declining left ventricular function and reduced cardiac output, the gradient produced by any degree of valve obstruction also falls. Doubt about the severity of the stenosis can usually be resolved by calculating the valve area using the continuity equation which uses data from Doppler and two-dimensional echo. In experienced hands this provides valuable additional information, but accurate measurement of the left ventricular outflow tract diameter can be difficult and if the findings are not consistent with other data, the investigation should be either be repeated or the patient should be referred for cardiac catheterization.

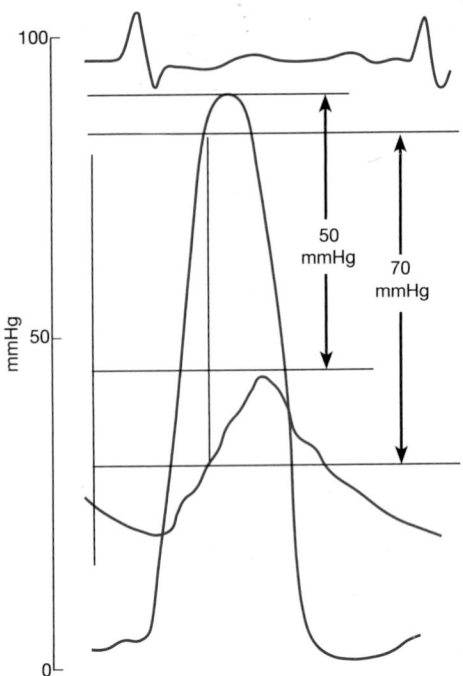

Fig. 2 Representative pressure traces of left ventricular pressure (lower line) and aortic pressure (upper line). The measured gradient at cardiac catheterization is the difference between the two peak pressures (peak-to-peak) and in this case it is 50 mmHg. Continuous wave Doppler measures the maximum difference between the pressures or the peak instantaneous gradient which in this case is 70 mmHg.

Aortic regurgitation

Assessment of the mechanism and severity of aortic regurgitation requires a combination of all three echo modalities. M-mode may demonstrate fluttering of the anterior leaflet of the mitral valve and in the setting of acute severe aortic regurgitation, premature closure of the mitral valve. Two-dimensional will occasionally demonstrate prolapse of one more of the aortic cusps, but even severe aortic regurgitation can occur through an aortic valve that appears to be structurally normal.

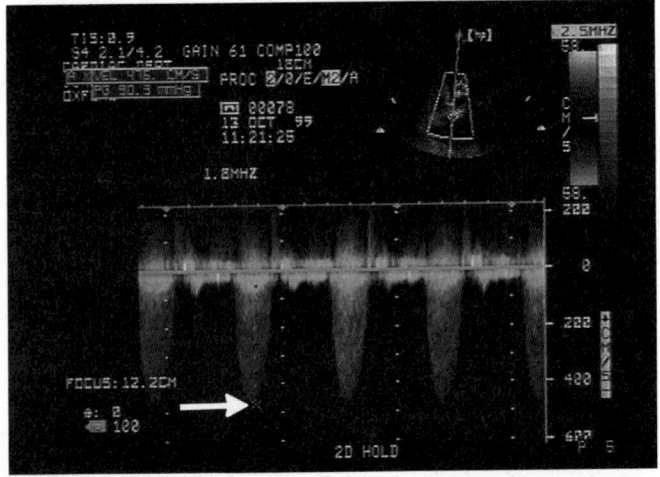

Fig. 3 Apical continuous wave Doppler across the aortic valve in a patient with severe aortic stenosis. The peak velocity (arrow) is greater than 4.5 m/s consistent with a peak instantaneous gradiant across the aortic valve of 90 mmHg. (See also Plate 1.)

The severity of aortic regurgitation can be estimated using continuous wave and colour Doppler, although assessment can be difficult as it is influenced by left ventricular function. Doppler-derived pressure half-time and measurement of regurgitant fraction and/or flow convergence zone are valuable when there is uncertainty over lesion severity. M-mode and colour Doppler can be combined and when the regurgitant jet fills more than 50 per cent of the left ventricular outflow tract the regurgitation is classified as severe.

In patients with severe asymptomatic aortic regurgitation, a serial increase in left ventricular dimensions or a progressive fall in ejection fraction are indications for surgery. However, any increase in ventricular dimension should be at least 0.5 cm before it is regarded as significant given the limited reproducibility of echocardiographic parameters.

Mitral stenosis

Mitral valve stenosis is well visualized using either M-mode or cross-sectional echocardiography. Its severity can be determined by estimating the area of the valve orifice either by direct planimetry of the two-dimensional short axis image or from the Doppler pressure half-time ($MVA = 220/Pt_{1/2}$). A valve area of less than 1.0 cm² indicates severe mitral stenosis. Transthoracic echocardiography is also used to assess the suitability of the mitral valve for balloon dilation, although transoesophageal imaging is necessary to exclude left atrial thrombus.

Mitral regurgitation

Transthoracic echocardiography will usually demonstrate the mechanism and severity of mitral regurgitation. Two-dimensional imaging identifies abnormalities of the valve leaflets and colour flow shows jet direction and area. Severe mitral regurgitation is suggested by increased left ventricular end-diastolic dimension and hyperdynamic wall motion due to volume overload. Precise quantification of the amount of regurgitation is demanding as it is influenced by left ventricular function, the direction of the jet, and left atrial size. Various algorithms have been devised to improve quantitation of mitral regurgitation, including measurement of the flow convergence zone and the PISA method, but most centres simply classify the extent of regurgitation as mild, moderate, or severe.

Pulmonary and tricuspid valve disease

In adults, two-dimensional imaging of the pulmonary valve may be difficult, particularly if there is lung disease. Despite this, accurate Doppler information is usually obtainable. Tricuspid stenosis is very uncommon but some degree of tricuspid regurgitation is detectable even in healthy individuals. Measurement of the peak velocity of tricuspid regurgitation (V) is valuable as in the absence of pulmonary valve disease it can be used to estimate pulmonary artery systolic pressure:

$$\text{PA systolic pressure (mmHg)} = 4V^2 + \text{right atrial pressure (usually assumed to be 5–10 mmHg)}$$

Prosthetic valves

Transthoracic echo is commonly performed as part of the routine follow-up of prosthetic valves. It is usually able to assess biological valves accurately, but for mechanical mitral valve prostheses in particular, attenuation artefact produced by the metal may be problematic. Transoesophageal imaging is recommended when transthoracic imaging is suboptimal or if improved resolution is required, for example suspected prosthetic valve endocarditis.

Abnormal left ventricular function

In most patients a full transthoracic echo study will confirm or refute a clinical suspicion of left ventricular dysfunction and identify the likely aetiology of any abnormality. Systolic and diastolic left ventricular function can be assessed and a variety of methods can be used to derive an estimate of left ventricular ejection fraction. In patients with ischaemic heart disease, assessment of regional wall motion is valuable and may occasionally dem-

onstrate evidence of aneurysm formation. Left ventricular hypertrophy is detected by echocardiography and a measurement of left ventricular mass can be derived.

Echocardiography is a pivotal investigation in suspected heart failure, particularly as an ejection fraction of less than 40 per cent has been used as an inclusion criteria for most therapeutic trials in this condition. Community studies have demonstrated that many patients treated with diuretics for mild heart failure (usually ankle swelling) do not have left ventricular systolic impairment, and screening with echocardiography was initially recommended before initiation of treatment with angiotensin-converting enzyme inhibitors. However, subsequent studies have shown that impaired systolic function is very unlikely when the ECG and clinical examination are normal, and conversely that angiotensin-converting enzyme inhibitors can be initiated without waiting for echocardiography in patients with evidence of ischaemic heart disease and radiographic evidence of pulmonary oedema, as the ejection fraction is almost invariably less than 40 per cent under these circumstances.

Transthoracic echo may detect mural thrombus, particularly in patients with impaired systolic ventricular function. However, differentiation between thrombus and myocardium can be problematic at the left ventricular apex and tissue harmonic imaging and/or contrast agents may be necessary.

Minor concentric left ventricular hypertrophy is common in patients with hypertension. In hypertrophic cardiomyopathy, two-dimensional imaging may demonstrate asymmetrical septal hypertrophy with disproportionate thickening of the interventricular septum compared with the left ventricular free wall, or dramatic concentric hypertrophy with left ventricular cavity obliteration. Other characteristic features of hypertrophic cardiomyopathy include systolic anterior motion of the mitral valve (Figs 4 and 5 and Plate 2) and partial mid-systolic closure of the aortic valve, which usually correlates with the presence of outflow tract obstruction. In the absence of conditions that may induce ventricular hypertrophy, for example aortic stenosis, these findings are diagnostic of hypertrophic cardiomyopathy. Colour Doppler can demonstrate turbulence in the outflow tract and continuous wave Doppler may detect characteristic 'dynamic' gradients that increase in severity as systole progresses. Other associated echocardiographic abnormalities in hypertrophic cardiomyopathy include mitral regurgitation and severe diastolic dysfunction.

Atrial fibrillation

Echocardiography readily excludes a structural cause for atrial fibrillation (e.g. mitral stenosis) and facilitates thromboembolic risk stratification. It

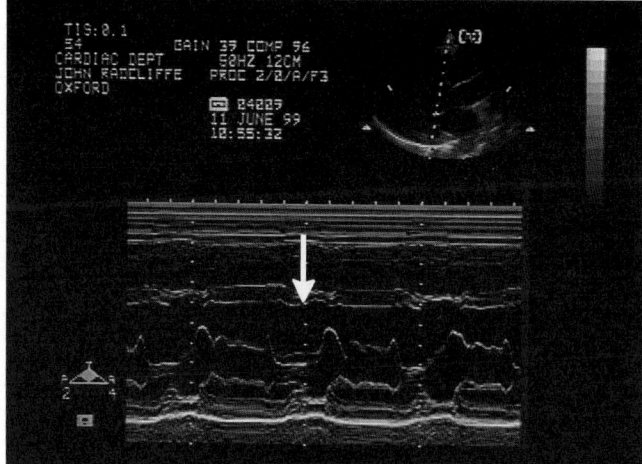

Fig. 4 M-mode echocardiogram through the mitral valve in a normal patient. Opening of the leaflets during ventricular diastole and closing during systole (arrow) can be observed. Contrast the behaviour of the mitral valve with that in Fig. 5. (See also Plate 2.)

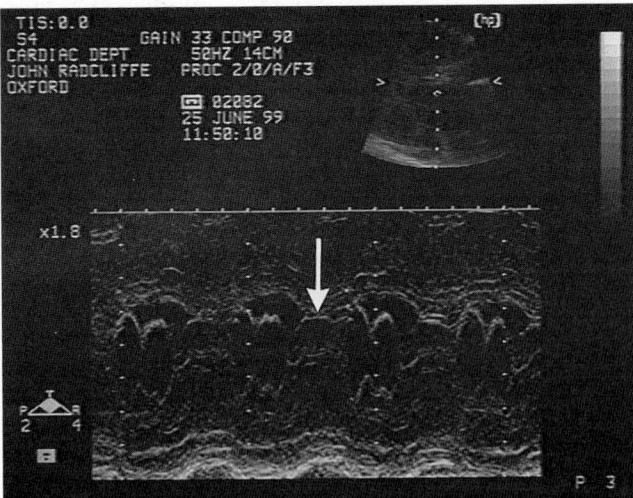

Fig. 5 M-mode echocardiogram through the mitral valve in a patient with obstructive hypertrophic cardiomyopathy. Closure of the valve during systole is accompanied by marked movement of the valve apparatus towards the left ventricular septum (arrow)—this is referred to as systolic anterior motion (SAM) of the mitral valve.

also allows measurement of left atrial dimension, which is valuable as cardioversion is less likely to be successful when this is large.

Following an embolic event/stroke

Echocardiography is the investigation of choice when a cardiac source of an embolus is suspected. It is mandatory in all patients presenting with embolic occlusion of a peripheral artery, or thromboembolic episodes in more than one vascular territory. Echocardiography should not, however, be performed in circumstances when the result is unlikely to influence patient management, but in patients with ischaemic stroke and a low likelihood of atheromatous arterial disease an echo can be considered as occasionally it will detect occult abnormalities such as atrial myxoma or cardiac thrombus.

Pericardial disease

Echocardiography readily diagnoses the presence of pericardial fluid and is useful when percutaneous drainage is attempted. Echocardiographic signs of pericardial tamponade include exaggerated respiratory variation in the mitral valve Doppler, presystolic closure of the aortic valve, and (particularly) right atrial and right ventricular diastolic collapse. Constrictive pericarditis is a difficult diagnosis to make using standard echocardiographic techniques and patients complaining of episodic breathlessness/fluid retention with characteristic abnormalities of the venous pressure require particularly careful interrogation by Doppler.

Pulmonary embolism

Echo can be useful in patients with pulmonary embolism as it can demonstrate right ventricular dilation and/or impaired right ventricular systolic function. Tricuspid regurgitant velocity can be used to estimate pulmonary artery systolic pressure, although it is unusual for this to be more than 70 mmHg acutely. Exceptionally, two-dimensional imaging may show thrombus within the right heart and/or the proximal pulmonary arteries. Although echocardiography is useful diagnostically when it demonstrates features consistent with pulmonary embolism, it cannot exclude the diagnosis.

Infective endocarditis

Echocardiography cannot be used to exclude endocarditis but is valuable when endocarditis is suspected clinically but there is insufficient data to make a formal diagnosis. Under these circumstances a typical vegetation detected by an experienced observer is regarded as a major criterion in the Duke diagnostic classification, and this may facilitate appropriate management. Transoesophageal echo should be performed when there is a suspicion of aortic root abscess, if prosthetic endocarditis is suspected, or occasionally in cases where there is persistent diagnostic doubt and the additional sensitivity and spatial resolution might be valuable.

Congenital heart disease

Echocardiography is the diagnostic modality of choice for patents with suspected congenital heart disease. Detailed transthoracic cardiac imaging is possible in co-operative babies and children but occasionally sedation or a short anaesthetic may be required. Rates of cardiac catheterization have been reduced by miniaturization of transoesophageal probes that facilitate diagnosis and follow-up of complex congenital heart disease. Fetal echocardiography is performed when surveillance obstetric ultrasound is abnormal or in cases where previous history suggests a possible cardiac problem.

Transoesophageal echocardiography

Transoesophageal echocardiography is available in cardiac centres and some smaller hospitals. The ultrasound probe is similar to the endoscope used for upper gastrointestinal investigation, except that there are no optical fibres. With the patient under sedation, the probe is manipulated into the oesophagus where its position behind the heart produces excellent resolution, particularly of posterior cardiac structures.

Transoesophageal echocardiography is an invasive procedure and the patient's written consent is required. After fasting for a minimum of 4 h, local anaesthetic spray (10 per cent lidocaine) is applied to the upper pharynx and the patient is usually sedated with a short acting benzodiazopine (e.g. midazolam). Blood pressure and oxygen saturation are monitored throughout and both resuscitation equipment and the benzodiazepine antagonist flumazanil should be readily available (Fig. 6).

Even though transoesophageal echo is commonly performed in high-risk haemodynamically unstable patients, the rate of serious complications (aspiration and oesophageal rupture/tears) is less than 1 per cent. Absolute contraindications to transoesophageal echo include oesophageal tumours, strictures, varices, and diverticulae.

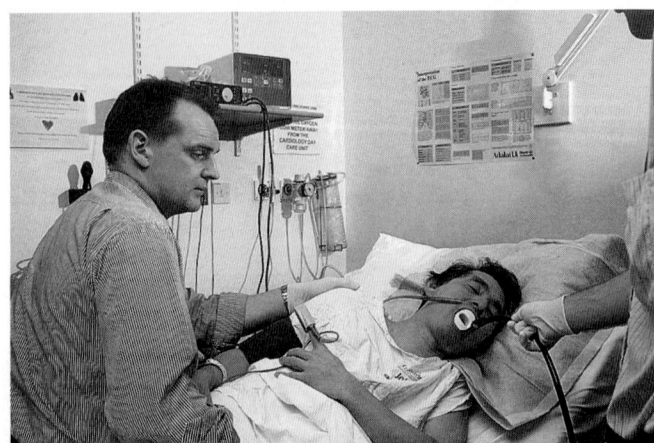

Fig. 6 Patient in the standard position undergoing a transoesophageal echocardiogram. Non-invasive monitoring of pulse rate, oxygen saturation, and blood pressure is mandatory when intravenous sedation is being administered.

Who should have a transoesophageal echocardiogram?

The principal indications for transoesophageal echocardiography are listed in Table 1. Its principal advantages over transthoracic imaging are improved spatial resolution and the ability to image posterior structures such as the left atrium and descending aorta. It is valuable in a number of emergency situations including suspected aortic dissection, prosthetic mechanical valve failure, and possible endocarditis. It may be used to image patients in whom data from transthoracic imaging is unsatisfactory because of obesity, lung disease, or chest deformity. Other indications include screening for left atrial thrombus before cardioversion of atrial fibrillation and monitoring cardiac performance during cardiac and some non-cardiac surgery.

Valve disease

Patients with mitral stenosis are at particular risk of thromboembolism and transthoracic echo has limited sensitivity for the detection of left atrial thrombus (Fig. 7). Transoesophageal echocardiography is recommended in those with mitral stenosis if embolic events occur despite therapeutic anticoagulation and may demonstrate spontaneous echo contrast (smoke-like echoes produced by the interaction of erythrocytes and plasma proteins under conditions of stasis). This is an independent predictor of left atrial thrombus and/or cardiac thromboembolic events. Transoesophageal echo is also used to assess anatomy and exclude left atrial thrombus before balloon valvuloplasty in patients with mitral stenosis and to assess anatomy, severity, and suitability for surgical repair in patients with mitral regurgitation. In patients with mitral prostheses, reverberation artefact overlying the left atrium limits the ability of transthoracic imaging to detect paraprosthetic regurgitation. Transoesophageal imaging provides excellent visualization of the left atrium and is particularly recommended under these circumstances.

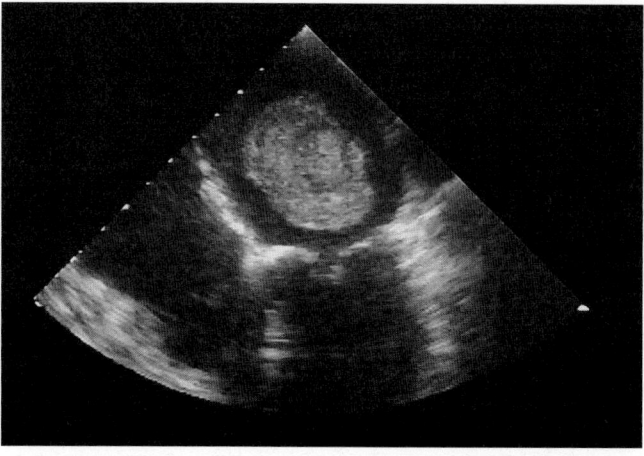

Fig. 7 Two-dimensional transoesophageal echocardiogram of the left atrium demonstrating a large mobile thrombus in a patient with mitral stenosis.

Endocarditis

Characteristic vegetations or evidence of abscess formation identified by echocardiography are increasingly used as diagnostic criteria in patients with possible endocarditis. The excellent spatial resolution (less than 1 mm) of transoesophageal echo makes it superior to transthoracic imaging for the detection of vegetations and its sensitivity may exceed 90 per cent. Transoesophageal echo should be considered when there is a high clinical suspicion of endocarditis but blood cultures are sterile and transthoracic imaging is not diagnostic, or under circumstances when the sensitivity of transthoracic imaging is particularly poor, for example prosthetic valves or calcific valvular disease. Transoesophageal echo is also recommended if there is a possibility of aortic root abscess formation as this complication is not easily identified using transthoracic imaging and surgery is usually necessary.

Aortic disease

Transthoracic imaging of the aorta is limited to the proximal aortic root and the arch in most patients. Using transoesophageal imaging most of the ascending and all of the descending thoracic aorta can be visualized and image quality is improved. This is particularly useful in patients with suspected acute aortic dissection and in many cases it is the only imaging necessary before emergency surgery. Large, mobile or pedunculated aortic atheroma in the descending aorta may be detected by transoesophageal echocardiography and several studies have suggested an association with ischaemic stroke. Transoesophageal imaging of the aorta has also been recommended in suspected cases of cholesterol embolization and to assess thromboembolic risk prior to cardiac intervention or surgery.

Thromboembolism

In patients with thromboembolism, there has been extensive debate over the value of imaging with transoesophageal echocardiography. Clinical examination, electrocardiography, and transthoracic echocardiography provide sufficient information to determine optimal management in the majority. However, transoesophageal echocardiography is indicated when embolic events occur in anticoagulated patients with native or prosthetic valvular heart disease, especially if endocarditis is suspected, or when transthoracic images are inconclusive.

In patients with unexplained or cryptogenic ischaemic stroke, wider use of transoesophageal echo has been advocated. Transthoracic echo and exclusion of alternative pathologies such as thrombophilia and carotid stenoses should precede the transoesophageal examination as under these circumstances minor cardiac structural abnormalities are more likely to be clinically relevant.

The transoesophageal approach is superior to transthoracic echocardiography for imaging the interatrial septum for atrial septal aneurysm (a

---

Table 1 Principal indications for transoesophageal echocardiography

Valve disease

(1) Mitral stenosis—to assess anatomy and exclude left atrial thrombus before balloon valvuloplasty

(2) Mitral regurgitation—to assess anatomy, severity, and suitability for surgical repair

(3) Prosthetic valves—particularly to assess prosthetic mitral regurgitation

Infective endocarditis

(1) Possible aortic root abscess

(2) Failure to respond to antibiotics or recurrent fever in a patient with endocarditis

(3) Clinical suspicion of endocarditis but no diagnostic abnormality on transthoracic imaging

(4) Possible prosthetic valve endocarditis

Aortic disease

(1) Possible acute aortic dissection

(2) Follow up of patients with known aortic pathology

(3) Imaging aortic atheroma before surgery or patients with possible cholesterol embolization

Potential cardiac source of embolism

(1) Before elective cardioversion of atrial fibrillation

(2) Patients with valvular heart disease and a definite embolic episode despite anticoagulation

(3) Patients with a definite embolic episode and a 'normal heart'

Incomplete or impractical transthoracic imaging

(1) Chest deformity or pulmonary disease

(2) Patients undergoing mechanical ventilation

(3) Congenital heart disease

Perioperative imaging of cardiac performance

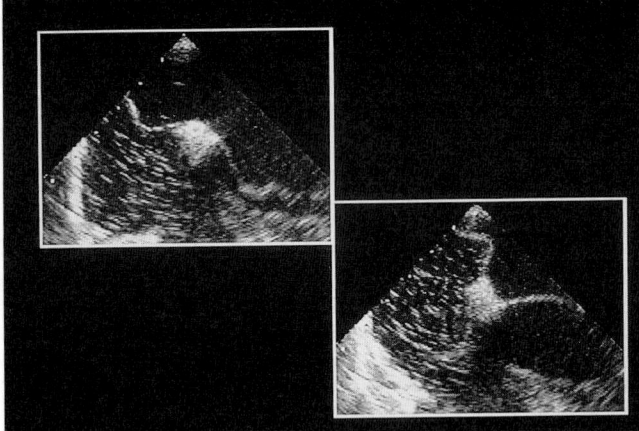

Fig. 8 Two-dimensional transoesophageal echocardiogram of the atria. In the upper panel contrast is principally contained within the right atrium although two bubbles can be seen in the left atrium. There is marked excursion of the atrial septum towards the left atrium during expiration (lower panal). These appearances are consistent a diagnosis of an atrial septal aneurysm with patent foramen ovale.

redundant bulge in the area of fossa ovale, with respiratory movement greater than 10 mm) and assessing patency of the foramen ovale (Fig. 8). The clinical relevance of these atrial septal abnormalities can be questionable as the relationship to the thromboembolic event is commonly speculative. Currently, anticoagulation is the usual management following a otherwise unexplained single embolic event, but occasionally percutaneous or surgical correction of the defect is recommended.

Stress echocardiography

Diagnosis of reversible ischaemic myocardial dysfunction is now possible using echocardiography. Imaging can be performed either during or immediately after exercise, but more commonly an intravenous infusion of dobutamine is used to mimic the cardiac response to exercise. Development of reversible systolic regional wall motion abnormalities suggests coronary artery disease and stress echo is used increasingly as a diagnostic test in patients with chest pain. Stress echo also has an increasing role in risk stratification prior to general surgical procedures and in assessing myocardial viability prior to revascularization.

Further reading

Cheitlin MD *et al.* (1997). ACC/AHA guidelines for the clinical application of echocardiography: executive summary. *Journal of the American College of Cardiology* **29**, 862–79.

Flachskampf FA, Decoodt P, FraserAG, Daniel WG, Roelendt JRTC (2001). Recommendations for performing transesophageal echocardiography. *European Journal of Echocardiography* **2**, 8–21.

Kerut EK, McIlwain EF, Plotnick GD. *Handbook of echo-Doppler interpretation.* Futura, New York. [A good integration of clinical and more technical echocardiography.]

Oh JK, Seward JB, Tajik AJ (1999). *The echo manual*, 2nd edn. Lipincott-Raven. [A well presented practical guide.]

Rimington H, Chambers J (1998). *Echocardiography: a practical guide for reporting.* Parthenon, London. [A short guide to reporting echocardiograms including normal ranges and how to interpret data.]

15.3.4 Nuclear techniques

H. J. Testa and D. J. Rowlands

Nuclear imaging of the heart plays an important role in the investigation of patients with heart disease, giving valuable information for the practical management of patients and contributing to the understanding of the physiology of myocardial perfusion. The techniques may be used to:

(1) localize areas of ischaemia induced by exercise or by drugs;

(2) demonstrate the extent and distribution of viable myocardium;

(3) provide an assessment of global and of regional left ventricular function; and

(4) demonstrate recent myocardial cell damage.

The investigations are scarcely invasive and of little discomfort or inconvenience to the patient.

In recent years, the use of nuclear imaging tests has increased dramatically. This increase is largely due to two factors: (i) development of new radiopharmaceuticals labelled with technetium to aid in the imaging process, and (ii) recognition of the value of pharmaceuticals for the induction of cardiovascular stress, permitting stress studies to be undertaken without exercise, which is particularly useful when exercise is difficult or contraindicated. There has also been considerable improvement in the quality of the images obtained thanks to substantial improvement in gamma-camera technology and to the widespread use of single photon emission computer tomography (SPECT). Recent estimates suggest that, in the United States, the annual number of procedures undertaken has doubled from 2.9 million in 1990 to 5.8 million in 1997. In our department, the number of cardiac studies has increased from 300 per year in 1995 to more than 1000 in 1999; the main area of increase being in the use of myocardial perfusion studies to investigate myocardial ischaemia.

Myocardial perfusion imaging in the recognition and assessment of myocardial ischaemia

Myocardial perfusion imaging is undertaken using an injection of a radiopharmaceutical that is taken up by the myocardium in proportion to the myocardial blood flow at the time of the injection and which remains in the myocardial cells during the period of the imaging. Studies are performed both at rest and under stress, in order to evaluate differing regional perfusion in these two states. The three compounds mainly used in current clinical practice are thallium[201], technetium-99m-Cardiolite (sestamibi-MIBI), and technetium-99m-Myoview (tetrofosmin).

Thallium[201] is an analogue of the potassium ion. It is taken up only by myocardial cells that are both viable and adequately perfused. A dose of 75 MBq, (approximately 2 mCi) is injected intravenously (i) at maximal chosen or achievable exercise, or (ii) after pharmacological stress, or (iii) in association with a combination of these procedures (exercise plus pharmacological stress). Pharmacological stress can be induced with powerful vasodilators (dipyridamole or adenosine) or with inotropic and chronotropic stimulators (dobutamine). The initial myocardial distribution of thallium[201] reflects regional blood flow. Redistribution of the isotope to all viable myocardial cells occurs approximately 3 to 4 h later. Images are taken immediately after exercise (to reflect blood flow) and 3 to 4 h later to reflect viable myocardium.

The patient is positioned supine on the SPECT couch with the left arm placed over the head to avoid attenuation artefacts. The gamma camera rotates around the patient through 180° from the right anterior oblique 30° to the left posterior oblique 30°, at 6° increments of 30 s duration. The orbit of rotation may be circular or non-circular; the latter is preferred. The acquired data is computer analysed and slice images are constructed using the techniques of filtering back projection at approximately 1-cm intervals. Short axis (SA), vertical long axis (VLA), and horizontal long axis (HLA) slices are reconstructed for clinical evaluation. An example of images obtained in this way is shown in Fig. 1.

Any localized defects occurring in association with stress are indicative of non-viability (infarction) or of underperfusion (ischaemia). Defects of thallium uptake occurring at rest or after redistribution during a period of rest following stress (exercise or pharmacological) correlate well with areas of infarction. A defect in tracer uptake immediately post-exercise or stress that shows redistribution after rest is indicative of myocardial ischaemia. It is now known that redistribution can be very slow in hypoperfused but viable myocardium, and a further injection of thallium may help to improve the differentiation between reversible and fixed perfusion defects. Furthermore, the comparison of images taken immediately after injection at rest with those taken at rest 3 to 4 h later (rest-redistribution protocol) can be used in viability assessment and investigation of hibernating myocardium.

The drawback of thallium is its long physical half-life of 72 h (which limits the dose that can be used so as to minimize radiation exposure to the patient) and the low photon energy (60–90 keV) which cause significant attenuation and degradation of the images.

As a consequence of the physical limitations of thallium[201], technetium-labelled radiopharmaceuticals have been developed. Technetium[99m] has a higher photon energy (140 keV) than thallium[201] and a shorter physical half life of 6 h. Two compounds are used in routine practice—technetium-99m-MIBI and technetium-99m-Myoview. Both are lipophilic and, like thallium, are taken up by the myocardium in proportion to myocardial blood flow. The maximum dose injected to the patient for the study (stress/rest) is of 1000 MBq (approximately 25 mCi).

Technetium-99m-MIBI is an isonitrile complex which after intravenous injection diffuses from the blood into cardiac myocytes and it is retained by the mitochondria within the cell. Its clearance from the blood is rapid, but only 40 to 60 per cent is extracted on the first pass through the myocardium. However, at about 20 min the percentage uptake by the myocardium is similar to thallium. This compound does not have a significant clinical redistribution (less than 15 per cent from its initial uptake) and the concentration in the myocardium remains constant over a period of 4 or 5 h. Images can be taken several hours after injection, when they still represent the distribution of coronary blood flow in the myocardium at the time of injection. Because of this lack of redistribution it is necessary to inject the patient twice, at maximum stress/exercise and at rest.

Technetium-99m-Myoview is also a lipophilic compound which, after intravenous injection, is rapidly cleared from the blood, taken into myocytes and retained in the mitochondria. Myocardial uptake is of the order of 1.2 per cent of the injected dose and reaches this level at about 5 min. It shows little redistribution and, as with technetium-99m-MIBI, two injections are necessary for a comparison of rest and stress/exercise uptake. Its

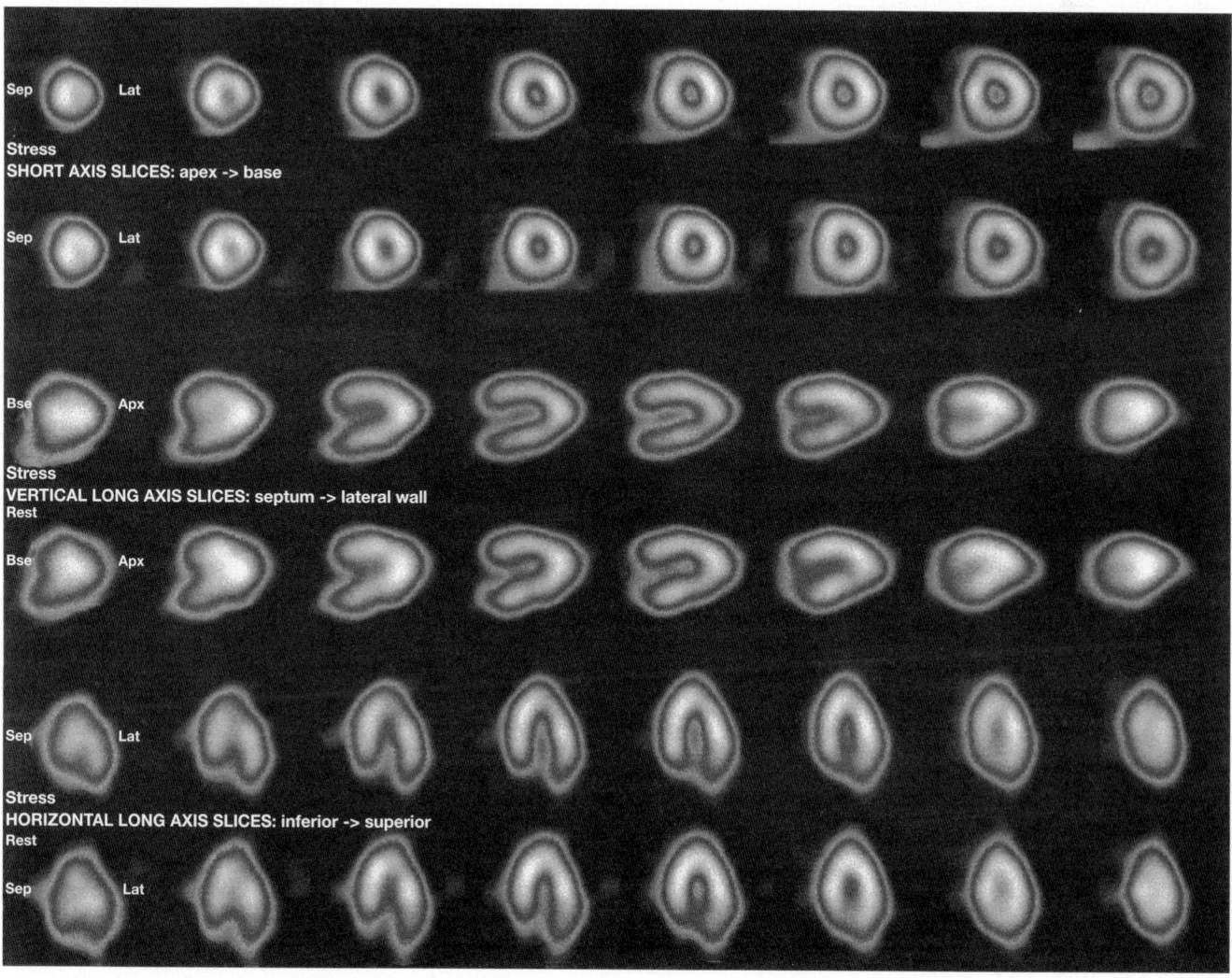

Fig. 1 Normal stress and rest study with thallium-201.

advantage is that it has less liver uptake than technetium-99m-MIBI with resulting improvement in the interpretation of images in the inferior wall.

Several imaging protocols have been developed for the technetium compounds including rest and stress injections either on 1 or 2 days. Ideally the two studies should be carried out on separate days, but if they are performed on the same day at least a three times larger dose is given with the second injection in order to swamp activity from the first. It is also possible to use thallium[201] to obtain resting images and technetium compounds for stress studies. This later protocol permits stress and rest studies to be completed in about 2 h.

Interpretation of the images is, in practical terms, similar to that of thallium: any localized defects occurring in association with stress or exercise indicate either infarction or ischaemia. Defects of uptake occurring on the rest study are indicative of areas of infarction. A defect in tracer uptake immediately postexercise or stress that improves during the rest study is indicative of myocardial ischaemia. Figure 2 shows an example of a patient with myocardial ischaemia mainly affecting the apex.

The main clinical indications for myocardial perfusion scintigraphy, in patients without a clear diagnosis of coronary artery disease, include:

(1) the assessment of patients with acute chest pain and non-diagnostic electrocardiograms;

(2) use as a screening test in patients with

    (a) familial hyperlipidaemia,

    (b) a family history of coronary artery disease, and

    (c) a perceived cardiac ischaemic risk in relation to proposed non-cardiac surgery.

In patients with known coronary artery disease the main indications include:

(1) evaluating the functional significance of coronary stenoses detected by angiography;

(2) assessment of the most significant functional stenoses in patients with multiple coronary lesions;

(3) evaluation of postinfarction patients to establish the size of the infarct and the presence or absence of ischaemia in other areas of the myocardium.

It is also of value in the investigation of restenosis after revascularization with angioplasty or coronary artery bypass grafting.

The procedure is useful in relation to exercise stress testing (both for patients with known coronary disease and in those with no definite evidence of ischaemic disease) where the ECG in not able to yield useful information on stress-induced ischaemia (pre-existing left bundle branch block, ventricular pre-excitation, functioning ventricular pacemaker, or initial widespread abnormality).

SPECT perfusion studies for the diagnosis of coronary artery disease have a higher sensitivity and specificity than electrocardiography, particularly when state of the art systems are used (average sensitivity of about 90 per cent and specificity 80 per cent). They also provide better localization with respect to the vascular beds of the three coronary arteries. Sensitivity is higher for lesions occurring in the left anterior descending artery and lower for the right coronary artery. Sensitivity and specificity appear to be lower for female than for male populations. Stress tests or exercise tests have similar diagnostic performances, but exercise testing in patients who do not reach the target heart rate (220–age) has decreased sensitivity.

It is important to recognize that patients with left bundle branch block may have perfusion abnormalities in the septum that are not due to coronary artery disease; in these patients pharmacological stress studies improve the sensitivity of the test. Reversible perfusion defects have also been reported in patients with hypertrophic cardiomyopathy, aortic stenosis, and left ventricular hypertrophy.

Scintigraphic determination of ventricular function

The assessment of left ventricular function is one of the most important aspects of the evaluation of the cardiac status. Scintigraphy can provide the following information:

(1) estimates of ventricular ejection fraction (the proportion of the ventricular end-diastolic volume ejected per beat, i.e. the stoke volume expressed as a percentage of the end diastolic volume), which is an overall measure of left ventricular performance;

(2) estimates of regional ventricular performance by observation of the movements of the margins of the ventricle.

Two approaches can be taken: the 'first pass technique' and the 'gated equilibrium' method. Both involve the intravenous injection of technetium[99m], which for first pass studies may be used in its ionic form as technetium-99m-pertechnetate, and for gated equilibrium studies by labelling the patient's own red blood cells. Both techniques (first pass and gated equilibrium) can be performed with a single injection of radioactive tracer.

In the first pass technique the first circulation of the radioactive bolus through the heart is studied and sequential images show the passage of the tracer through the right and left ventricles, separated in time. The single most useful view is probably the right anterior oblique (the projection of choice in single plane contrast radiography of the left ventricle). Images are taken at 1-s intervals and stored in the computer. A region of interest for the left ventricle is outlined and a high frequency activity–time curve for that region is plotted. Each point on the curve represents accumulated counts for a period of 0.04 s. The amount of radioactivity in the heart is proportional to the volume of blood in the cardiac cavities. Thus the change in the precordial count rates reflects the cyclical volume changes in the heart. A second region of interest is taken (usually as a horse-shoe-shaped region surrounded the left ventricular region of interest) to sample

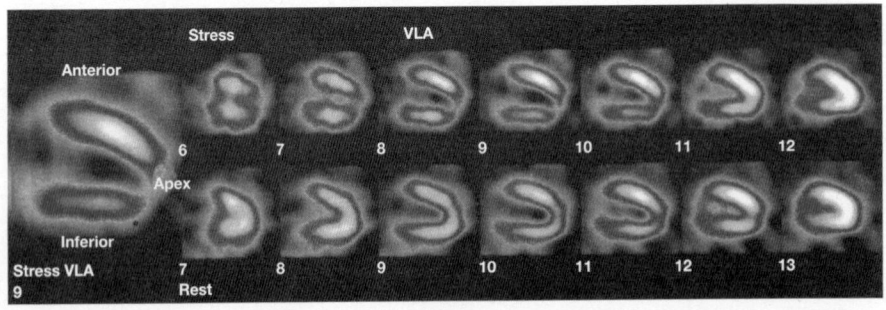

Fig. 2 Myocardial study carried out with Myoview showing, in the vertical long axis (VLA) view, an area of decreased tracer uptake at the apex on the images obtained after exercise (stress—row of seven images at the top of the figure) and improvement in this area at rest (row of seven images at the bottom of the figure). Views in other axes would be obtained simultaneously but are not shown.

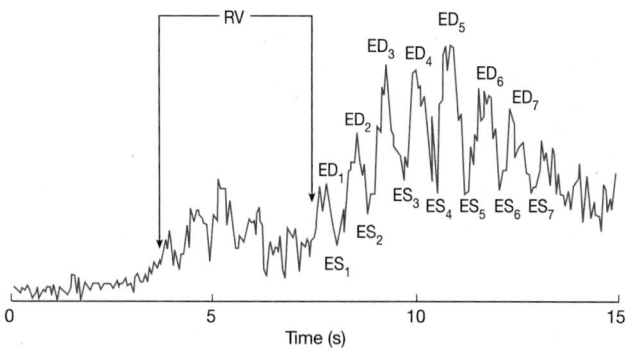

Fig. 3 High frequency activity—time curve recorded from the region of the left ventricle during the first passage of radioactive tracer through the central circulation. The time, in seconds, after the injection is shown on the abscissa. The ordinate displays the scintillation counting rate on a linear scale, after background correction. The early hump shows increased activity during the passage of the tracer through the right ventricle (RV). The later, larger hump shows the count rate during the passage through the left ventricle. Peaks and troughs are visible in relation to each cardiac cycle. Estimates of ejection fraction can be made for each cardiac cycle: $(ED_1-ES_1/ED_1, ED_2-ES_2/ED_2$, etc).

background activity variation with time. The background curve is 'normalized' to the left ventricular curve and then subtracted point-for-point from the high frequency left ventricular activity–time curve to give the corrected high frequency left ventricular activity–time curve (Fig. 3). It is usual to take two to six cycles around the peak of the left ventricular curve and then average the calculated ejection fraction for these cycles.

The gated equilibrium technique, referred to as gated cardiac blood pool imaging or as multigated acquisition (MUGA) imaging, depends upon complete mixing of the marker throughout the circulating blood volume

and it therefore requires a marker that remains intravascular. The marker of choice is technetium-99m-labelled red blood cells. The cells do not have to be removed from the patient to be labelled: the 'in vivo labelling' technique may be used, which involves predisposing the patient's red cells to accept the technetium label by the administration, 30 min prior to technetium, of non-active stannous pyrophosphate. Subsequently, 600 to 800 MBq (approximately 15 to 20 mCi) of technetium-99m-pertechnetate are injected intravenously and imaging is begun after 10 min or so. As there is complete mixing of the marker throughout the blood volume, all four cardiac chambers are seen simultaneously and various degrees of superimposition of the chambers inevitable. Proper alignment of the gamma camera is therefore crucial for the optimal separation of the cardiac chambers. In general, maximal separation of the right and left ventricles is achieved in the left anterior oblique view, to which a caudal tilt of 15° may be added.

For the determination of ejection fraction, a region of interest over the left ventricle and a second region of interest for background correction are assigned in the same manner as for the first pass technique. A background-corrected activity–time curve of the left ventricular area is obtained: Fig. 4 (normal), Fig. 5 (abnormal). With the equilibrium technique this is usually displayed as a single cycle representative activity–time curve being produced as a composite of many (typically hundreds) consecutive cycles, synchronization of the cycles being achieved by means of the R wave of the electrocardiogram.

Regional wall motion studies can also be carried out with this technique. Left ventricular images are collected for each of many short time intervals (typically 0.03 s, giving 25 images per cardiac cycle at a heart rate of 80/min) and images for corresponding parts of numerous cardiac cycles (typically several hundred) are summed to produce a composite. In this way 25 'frames' of a 'representative cine cycle' are produced. Figures 4 and 5 show examples of end-diastolic and end-systolic 'frames' of such a representative cine-cycle. Comparison of the end-diastolic and end systolic ventricular boundaries permits the assessment of regional wall motion. In

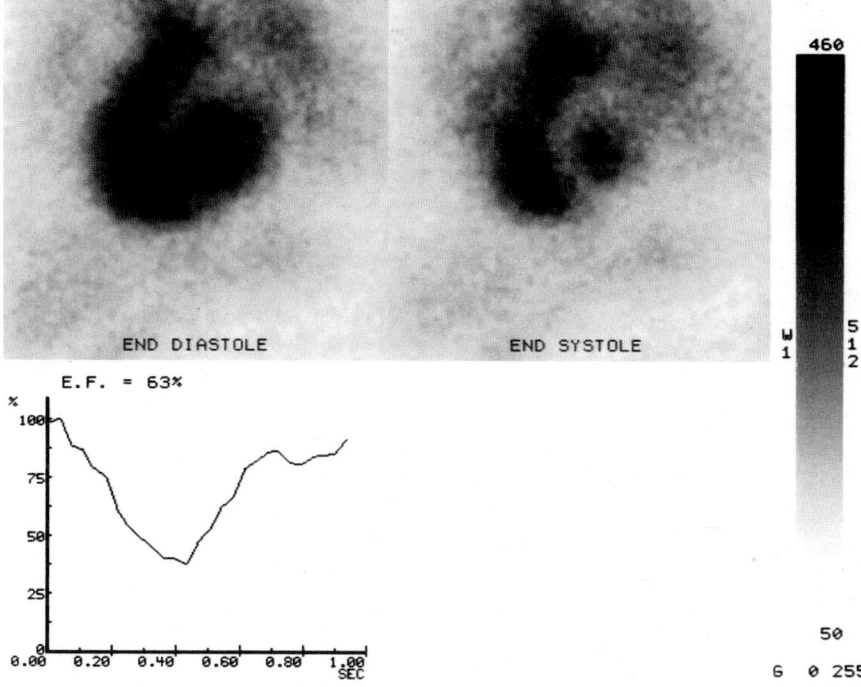

Fig. 4 Normal, resting multigated acquisition scan in the left anterior oblique 45° view. *Top view*, end-diastolic frame. The circular outline of the left ventribular cavity and the crescentic outline of the right ventricular cavity are seen. The curved zone of decreased activity between the two represents the interventricular septum. *Top right*, end-systolic frame. The left ventricular end systolic volume is clearly much smaller than in the end-diastolic frame and all regions of the left ventricule have contracted well. *Bottom left*, background corrected activity–time curve showing the overall count rate from the region of the left ventricle with the end-diastolic count rate normalized to 100 per cent. The ejection fraction is normal at 63 per cent.

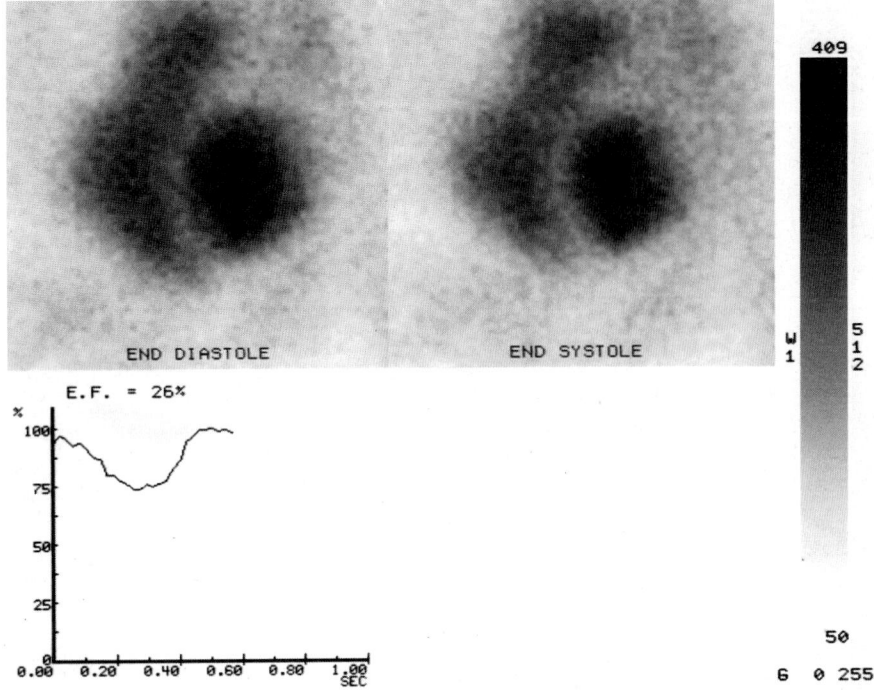

Fig. 5 Abnormal, resting multigated acquisition scan in the left anterior oblique 45° view. The format and layout are as in Fig. 4

Fig. 4 this reveals normal contraction of those parts of the ventricular wall that are displayed in the view shown. In Fig. 5, from a patient with congestive cardiomyopathy, there is uniformly reduced myocardial contraction.

Currently available non-scintigraphic techniques for the assessment of ventricular function (echocardiography, angiography, etc.) are, in general, less satisfactory when applied to the right than to the left ventricle. The differences are less marked in respect of nuclear techniques, such that scintigraphic procedures currently offer one of the best approaches to the assessment of right ventricular function. The basic techniques involved are the same as for the left ventricle. First pass radionuclide angiography provides adequate temporal anatomical separation of activity within right-sided and left-sided cardiac structures and provides a valuable method for the assessment of right ventricular ejection fraction. The gated equilibrium technique is less useful in the assessment of right ventricular function because of the overlap between the two ventricles, but it is possible to obtain useful information concerning right ventricular size and regional wall motion (usually visually assessed) from this technique. The best approach is to combine the two techniques to obtain a gated first pass study.

Radionuclide imaging in the diagnosis of myocardial infarction

Two general approaches have been used for the detection of myocardial infarction:

1. Recent myocardial damage may be demonstrated using radiopharmaceuticals that concentrate selectively in acutely injured cells. This 'positive imaging', 'infarct-avid imaging', or 'hot spot scanning' can clearly only be applied when infarction has occurred recently (within several days).

2. Non-viable myocardium (i.e recent or long-standing infarction) may be demonstrated by the absence of uptake of several tracers such as thallium[201], technetium-99m-MIBI, or technetium-99m-tetrofosmin as previously described (see above). This is called 'negative imaging' or 'cold-spot scanning'.

Infarct-avid imaging

Three main radiopharmaceuticals have been used for infarct avid imaging: technetium-99m-stannous pyrophosphate, indium-111-antimyosin and, more recently and still in process of investigation, technetium-99m-glucaric acid.

Technetium-99m-stannous pyrophosphate is the compound most extensively used to date. The observation that calcium is deposited in irreversibly damage myocardial cells led to the idea of using this tracer, a bone scanning agent, as a mean of demonstrating myocardial necrosis. The cellular death of myocardial infarction is accompanied by an influx of calcium ions, which are deposited in crystalline and subscrystalline form within the mitochondria, and it has been suggested that calcium accumulation in this way is an index of irreversible cell damage. However, it has also been suggested that the tracer is associated with cytoplasmic denatured macromolecules rather than with mitochondrial hydroxyapatite. Irrespective of the mechanism of tracer uptake, research and clinical work confirm that this radiopharmaceutical localizes in infarcted and severely injured myocardium. For a scan to be positive there must be both (i) significant myocardial necrosis (to give rise to myocardial uptake) and also (ii) persistent residual collateral coronary blood flow into the area of myocardial damage (to permit delivery of the tracer to the infarcted myocardium).

The time interval between the clinical onset of the infarction and scanning is critical. Scans are unlikely to be positive within the first 12 h and the optimum scanning time is 24 to 96 h, but scans can occasionally be positive 2 weeks after an isolated episode of infarction. Between 200 and 600 MBq (approximately 5 to 15 mCi) of technetium-99m-stannous pyrophosphate are given intravenously, with scanning undertaken 60 to 90 min later. Figure 6 shows a normal study and Fig. 7 one of a patient with myocardial infarction.

False negative and false positive results occur. In 14 different series involving 562 patients with acute myocardial infarction, the false negative rate was 6 per cent. A further group of 15 different series involving 1083 patients with no evidence of acute infarction showed a false positive rate of 17 per cent. The 'efficiency' of the procedure (i.e. its overall ability correctly to classify patients as to whether or not they have acute infarction) is 86 per cent. False positive results have been described in patients with unstable

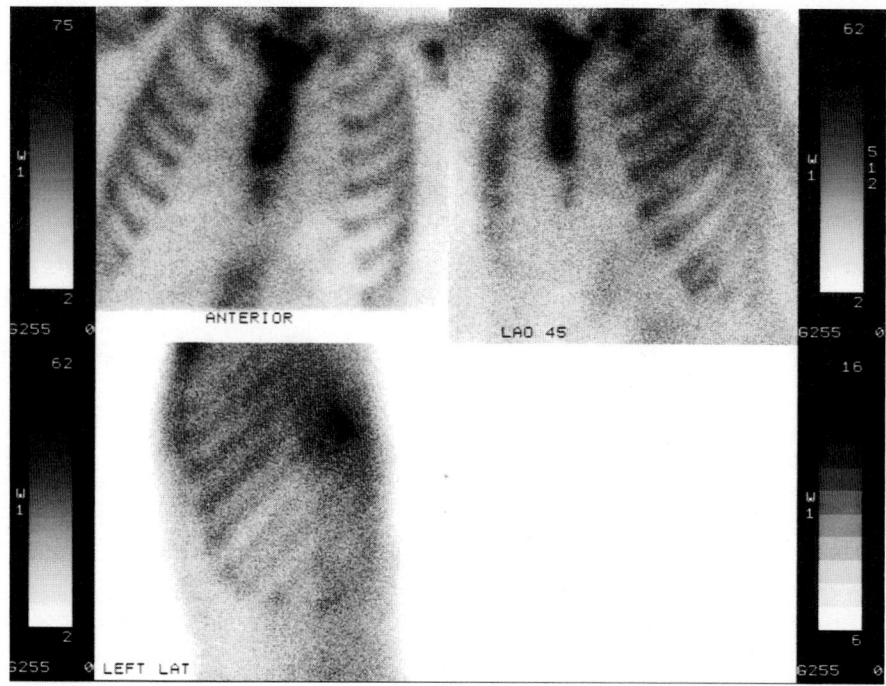

Fig. 6 Normal technetium-99m-stannous pyrophosphate scan, seen in the anterior 45°, and left lateral views. Normal uptake is seen in the sternum and ribs. There is no recognizable activity in the region of the myocardium.

angina, left ventricular aneurysms, cardiomyopathy, valvular calcification, myocardial contusion, persistent blood pool activity, rib fractures, breast tumours, calcified costal cartilages, skeletal muscle damage, and recent cardio-version (the latter giving either skeletal muscle or cardiac damage).

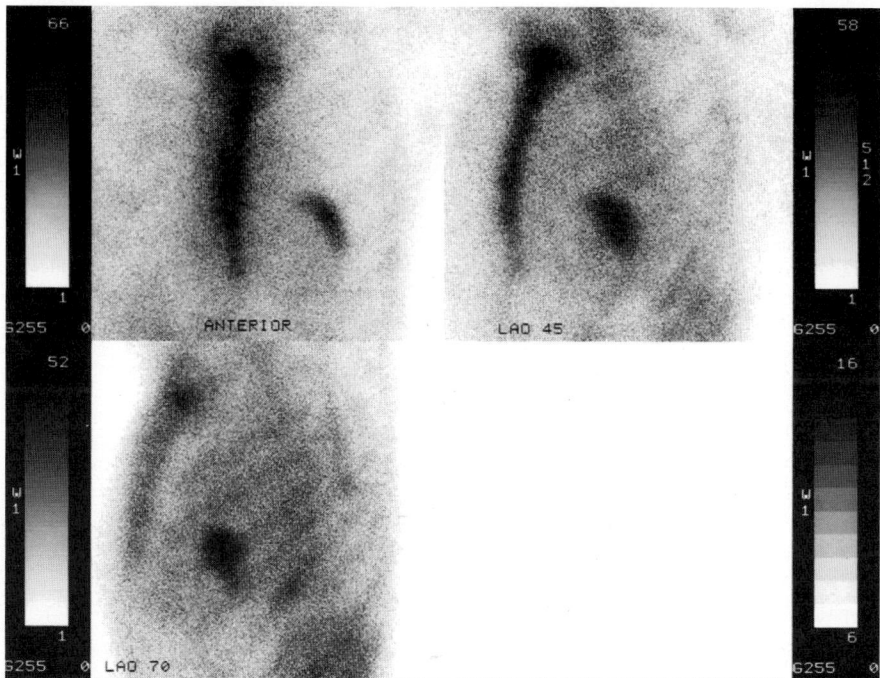

Fig. 7 Abnormal technetium-99m-stannous pyrophosphate scan, seen in the anterior, left anterior oblique 45°, and left lateral views. In addition to the normal uptake in the sternum (well seen) and ribs (less well seen), there is clearly a large area of localized uptake lateral and posterior to the sternum, in the region of the left ventricle. The patient had had an acute myocardial infarction.

The drawback of this technique is the delay of 1 day before reliable diagnosis of infarction in the non-reperfused myocardial infarction can be made. It is clearly of no value in identifying patients who will benefit from thrombolytic therapy and this is one reason why the technique has not been commonly used in clinical practice.

Indium-111-labelled monoclonal antimyosin, which binds selectively to irreversibly damaged myocytes, has also been used for the investigation of acute myocardial infarction. Clinical studies have shown a sensitivity between 87 and 98 per cent and a specificity of 93 per cent. Because of the high sensitivity and specificity, the technique has been used in the investigation of equivocal myocardial infarction, and in the investigation of right ventricle myocardial infarction. The main drawback is again delay: 12 to 24 h between the administration of tracer and imaging, due to very slow clearance from blood.

More recently, some experience has been gained with the use of technetium-99m-glucaric acid, developed with the hope of achieving an early diagnosis of myocardial infarction. This is a natural dicarboxylic acid sugar which clears from the blood with a very short half-life, allowing images to be carried out within a few hours after injection. Uptake is due to its affinity for the histone of the necrotic myocytes. The clinical usefulness of this compound remains to be determined.

Functional images

Functional images of the heart can be obtained by applying the mathematical technique of Fourier analysis to the left ventricular volume–time curve. The time activity curve is fitted with the first Fourier harmonic, a cosine function with a period equal to the period of the cardiac cycle. The amplitude and phase of this function are adjusted to match the left ventricular curve optimally. The amplitude image reflects the change in ventricular volume through the cycle. It is similar to the stroke volume but may give a more reliable index of the change in chamber volume. The phase image represents the time at which the maximum contraction occurs, and gives information on the mechanical contractility of the heart. Phase data are also presented as histograms in which the number of pixels in an image with a particular phase is plotted against the phase.

Positron emission topography (PET)

This technique uses positron emitting radionuclides and emission computed axial tomography to produce tomographic images of coronary flow and cardiac metabolism. The instrumentation consists of detector systems working in coincidence to register the paired annihilation photons emitted from the radiopharmaceuticals.

PET devices record multiple slices (usually between three and 18) of the heart simultaneously. Perfusion studies can be carried out after injecting radiopharmaceuticals such as ammonia-13, $H_2^{15}O$, or rubidium-82. Because of the short half life of this radiopharmaceutical, it is necessary to inject the patient twice, at rest and during maximum exercise. Metabolic studies of the heart have been carried out using carbon-11-palmitate or glucose analogues such as fluorine-18-deoxyglucose. Although these procedures are now more commonly used, they are only performed in routine clinical practice in selected centres. The main drawback of these techniques is cost: they require expensive detectors and a cyclotron on site for the production of radionuclides.

Further reading

Rigo P (1998). Other cardiac applications. In: Maisey MN, Britton KE, Collier BD, eds. *Clinical nuclear medicine*, 3rd edn. Chapman and Hall, London.

Rigo P, Benoit T (1998). Myocardial ischaemia. In: Maisey MN, Britton KE, Collier BD, eds. *Clinical nuclear medicine*, 3rd edn. Chapman and Hall, London.

The heart (1995). In: Wagner HN, Szabo Z, Buchanan JW, eds. *Principles of nuclear medicine*. WB Saunders, USA.

Travin M, Wexler JP (1999). Cardiovascular nuclear medicine (Part 1). *Seminars in Nuclear Medicine* **24**.

Wexler JP, Travin M (1999). Cardiovascular nuclear medicine (Part 2). *Seminars in Nuclear Medicine* **24**.

15.3.5 Cardiovascular magnetic resonance and computed X-ray tomography

S. Richard Underwood, Raad H. Mohiaddin, and M. B. Rubens

Magnetic resonance

Cardiovascular magnetic resonance imaging (**MRI**) has an established clinical role, particularly for the assessment of congenital heart disease and diseases of the aorta and pericardium. However, its clinical impact is currently more limited than that of echocardiography, nuclear cardiology, and invasive investigation. As MRI technology evolves, rapid imaging techniques allow acquisition within a breath-hold and even in real-time. Such techniques promise to extend the capabilities of cardiovascular magnetic resonance to imaging of the coronary arteries and assessment of myocardial perfusion, when it may then play a more important clinical role. For information on the technical aspects of magnetic resonance imaging and spectroscopy, the reader is referred to other texts (see bibliography).

Congenital heart disease

Spin echo images in multiple contiguous slices and in several planes provide excellent anatomical information (Fig. 1). Magnetic resonance compares favourably with echocardiography and cardiac catheterization in providing a complete anatomical diagnosis in 90 per cent of cases, although congenital anomalies of the valves and small defects of the interatrial and interventricular septum are often difficult to visualize on spin echo images alone. Cine gradient echo images provide additional information such as ventricular function, particularly on the right. They also show turbulent blood flow in a manner similar to colour-coded Doppler, and this improves the detection of small ventricular and atrial shunts. The combination of cine imaging with velocity mapping provides further information, improving the detection of shunts and allowing flow to be measured in conduits, great vessels, and within the heart. Shunts can be measured either from the difference in stroke volumes of left and right ventricles or, more flexibly, by measuring flow directly in the aorta and pulmonary artery.

Pulmonary arteries

Several studies have shown the ability of MRI to identify the central pulmonary arteries in patients with pulmonary atresia, which is particularly helpful for determining the feasibility of creating a shunt surgically and for monitoring the growth of the pulmonary artery after shunting. In these patients, magnetic resonance is also able to assess shunt patency accurately, although complete evaluation of systemic collateral arteries, particularly their distal connections, may require selective angiography. Peripheral pulmonary artery stenoses can be missed by MRI.

Pulmonary and systemic veins

Normal pulmonary veins can be identified in most patients and 95 per cent of pulmonary venous abnormalities can be diagnosed. This is superior to

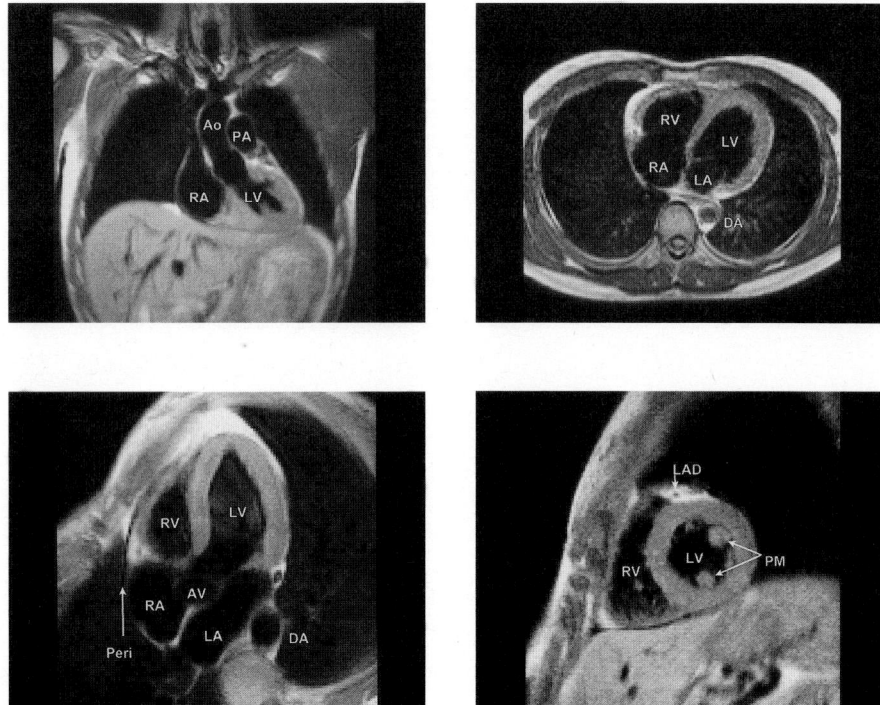

Fig. 1 Spin echo images showing normal anatomy. Top left, coronal; top right, transverse; bottom left, horizontal long axis; bottom right, short axis. LV, left ventricle; RV, right ventricle; LA, left atrium; RA, right atrium; Ao, aorta; DA, descending aorta; PA, pulmonary artery; AV, aortic valve; LAD, left anterior descending coronary artery; peri, pericardium; PM, papillary muscles.

cardiac catheterization and to transthoracic echocardiography. Abnormalities of the systemic veins such as a left-sided superior vena cava and its drainage are clearly seen.

Transposition of the great arteries

Postoperative follow-up with MRI is a valuable addition to transthoracic echocardiography for the detection of superior vena caval obstruction in patients with a transposition that has been surgically repaired. Cine gradient echo imaging can improve the assessment by demonstrating abnormal flow patterns associated with residual ventricular septal defects, subpulmonary stenosis, obstruction of the pulmonary venous atrium, and baffle leaks. Because the right ventricle supports the systemic circulation in these patients, outcome is partly determined by right ventricular function and competence of the tricuspid valve. Magnetic resonance can be used to monitor both of these accurately and reproducibly. In a minority of patients, artefacts caused by sternal wires may preclude complete assessment of the right ventricle.

Surgical conduits

Obstruction of conduits between the right ventricle and the pulmonary circulation, such as in tricuspid atresia after the Fontan operation (Fig. 2), may be difficult to detect clinically because patients may be asymptomatic despite having significant obstruction. Magnetic resonance imaging can demonstrate the anatomy of the proximal and distal anastomoses, and of obstruction within the conduit caused by intimal proliferation or 'peel'. A pressure gradient can be determined by velocity mapping and invasive investigation avoided in many cases. By contrast, echocardiography often fails to visualize the conduit because of its position behind the sternum. Palliative systemic to pulmonary shunts are also difficult to assess by echocardiography, but MRI is able to provide anatomical and functional information in most patients.

Complex disease

Another group of patients in whom MRI has advantages over other techniques are those with complex congenital disease such as single or common ventricles. These anomalies are frequently associated with abnormal thoracic or abdominal situs, and abnormal venous and ventriculoarterial connections. Spin echo imaging is as effective as angiography in demonstrating ventricular morphology and size, the orientation of the septum relative to the atrioventricular valves, and the origins and relationships of the great vessels. Magnetic resonance imaging is superior to other imaging techniques for assessing thoracic and abdominal situs and systemic and pulmonary venoatrial connections.

The aorta

The advantages of magnetic resonance in imaging aortic dissection are its ability to image in oblique planes and the fact that it does not require contrast injection, but it is undoubtedly more difficult to image sick patients in the current generation of scanners than to use other techniques that might be applied in this clinical context (computed tomography (**CT**) or transoesophageal echocardiography). Dissection is readily detected and its extent can be seen, including the involvement of the arch and other vessels (Fig. 3). The ability to demonstrate aortic regurgitation and rupture into the pericardial space are important additional features when assessing these patients. Because the intimal flap is thin it may not always be revealed in spin echo images unless static blood in the false lumen leads to natural contrast with the true lumen. If there is any doubt, then the flap will be more easily seen using a gradient echo sequence, and velocity mapping will confirm the diagnosis by demonstrating the differential flow velocities in each lumen.

Comparisons of MRI with other imaging techniques have concluded that magnetic resonance should be the primary investigation in stable patients and transoesophageal echocardiography the primary investigation in patients who are too ill to be imaged by magnetic resonance. In most

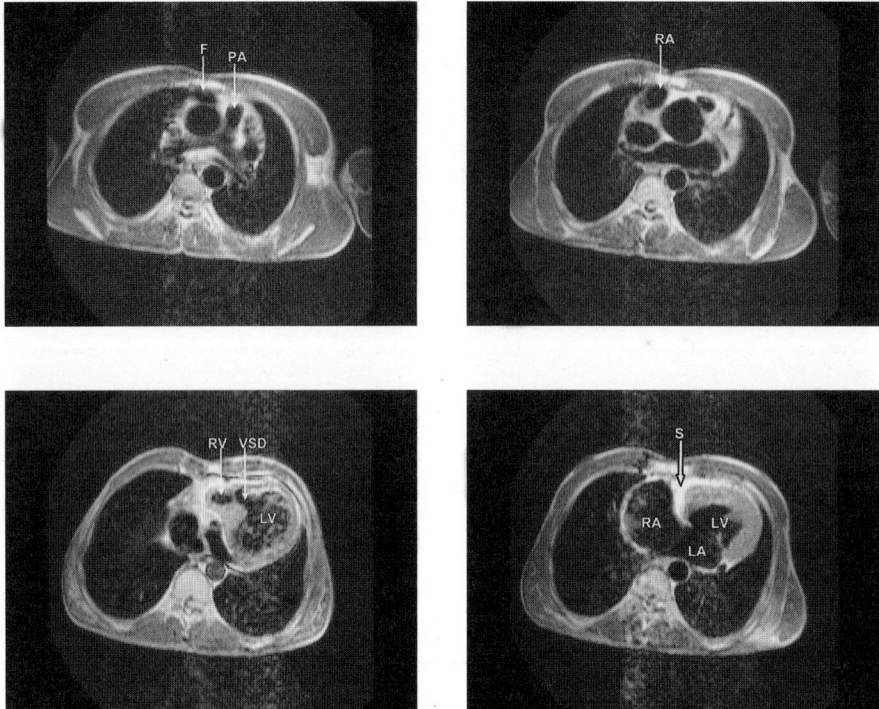

Fig. 2 Transverse spin echo images from superior (top left) to inferior (bottom right) in a patient with tricuspid atresia (S) and a Fontan conduit (F) connecting the right atrial appendage (RA) to the pulmonary artery (>PA). The right ventricle (RV) is hypoplastic and has a ventricular septal defect (VSD) connecting it to the left ventricle (LV). There is also an atrial septal defect connecting the right atrium and left atrium (LA).

cases the investigation performed will depend upon practical issues such as local expertise and availability of equipment.

Other aortic abnormalities that can be seen by magnetic resonance are aneurysms and coarctation. The combination of anatomical imaging and velocity mapping to assess the gradient across the coarctation means that surgical decisions can be taken without invasive investigation in many cases. It is an ideal method for the long-term follow-up of patients following coarctation repair and those with Marfan's syndrome. A further application is in suspected myocardial or mediastinal abscess in postoperative patients with infection that is difficult to control. Echocardiography is often equivocal in such patients and magnetic resonance will usually produce a definitive answer.

Tumours

Magnetic resonance imaging can provide additional information in many patients with masses previously identified by echocardiography. Although it is not possible to identify the nature of a mass from its signal with certainty, the high signal of lipomas and the appearance of angiomas are often characteristic. Gadolinium–diethylene-triamine-pentaacetic acid (**Gd-DTPA**) may be helpful for demonstrating vascularity and for distin-

guishing a myxoma from a thrombus. However, even in the absence of a typical signal, a diagnosis can often be made from the site and size of the tumour and from its involvement of neighbouring tissues.

Metastatic tumours are much more frequent than primary cardiac tumours. These can also be imaged successfully, whether as direct invasion of the heart, for example in carcinoma of the bronchus, or distant metastases as in melanoma. Involvement of the myocardium or pericardium can be identified, with the large field of view having a considerable advantage over echocardiography for determining the extent of a tumour.

Thrombus

Atrial or ventricular thrombus is easily identified by MRI, although trans-oesophageal echocardiography is also reliable in the left atrium, and the transthoracic approach often provides clear images in the ventricles. It is important to combine spin echo MRI with cine gradient echo imaging because it may be difficult to distinguish signal from thrombus and from slowly moving blood in spin echo images. Although the contrast is not as great in cine gradient echo images, it is more consistent, and the presence of a fixed filling defect is characteristic of a thrombus.

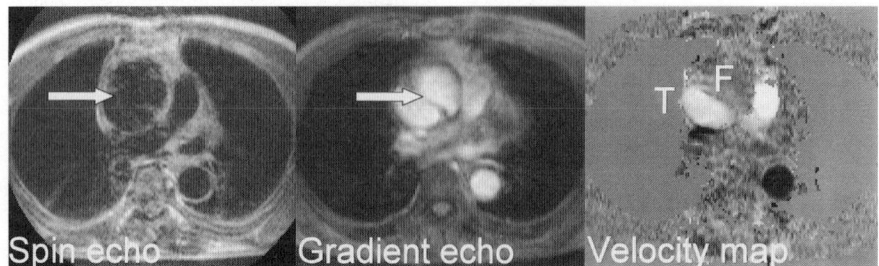

Fig. 3 Three images in the same plane in a patient with aortic dissection. The ascending aorta is dilated and there is an intimal flap (arrow), better seen in the gradient echo image. The velocity map shows rapid systolic flow in the true lumen (T—in white), and absent flow in the false lumen (F—in grey).

Pericardium

Pericardial thickening is readily demonstrated by magnetic resonance and by computed X-ray tomography: both techniques are more accurate than echocardiography. The commonest clinical question is to distinguish between pericardial constriction and myocardial restriction. Visualizing a thickened pericardium with the haemodynamic features of constriction makes the distinction reliably. Cine imaging shows immobility of the pericardium; additional features that indicate constriction are dilated atria and caval veins, small ventricles with retained systolic function, and a reduced diastolic caval flow peak, suggesting impaired right ventricular filling. Magnetic resonance cannot detect calcification reliably and this may be a drawback if pericardectomy is planned.

Pericardial effusion is clearly seen on spin echo images but its appearance is variable (Fig. 4). Moving fluid gives no signal but static fluid gives a high signal, particularly if haemorrhagic. It can also appear with varying signal in cine gradient echo imaging because rapid through plane refreshment of fluid reduces magnetic saturation. Cine imaging is therefore particularly helpful to distinguish thickened pericardium from a pericardial effusion.

Myocardium

Hypertrophy

The measurement of myocardial volume and mass has been extensively validated in animal experiments and in humans and, because of its accuracy, magnetic resonance should now be the standard against which other techniques are judged. Increased muscle volume (and hence mass) can be observed in athletes and patients with left ventricular hypertrophy, and the regression of hypertrophy following treatment of hypertension can be monitored.

Hypertrophic cardiomyopathy

The location and severity of hypertrophic cardiomyopathy is readily assessed (Fig. 5). Many patients do not have the classical form of asymmetrical septal hypertrophy, and apical hypertrophy in particular is better shown by MRI than by echocardiography. Metabolic abnormalities have also been observed using phosphorus-31 spectroscopy, with a reduced ratio of phosphocreatine to adenosine triphosphate compared with control subjects and patients with dilated cardiomyopathy, and a lower myocardial pH. It is not yet clear whether these changes are specific and whether they will be helpful in distinguishing hypertrophic cardiomyopathy from other forms of hypertrophy.

Dilated cardiomyopathy

Chamber dilatation and impaired myocardial thickening are clearly demonstrated. Because of the reproducibility of MRI measurements even modest changes of systolic and diastolic function can be monitored serially. Metabolic abnormalities have been demonstrated by magnetic resonance spectroscopy, with a reduced ratio of phosphocreatine to ATP in patients with heart failure and an improvement with therapy.

Other myocardial disease

Non-coronary myocardial disease can manifest itself by abnormalities of global and regional left ventricular function or by abnormalities of relaxation times that lead to differential contrast within the myocardium. Myocardial sarcoidosis is an example of a condition where magnetic resonance may have a useful role because there is a high incidence of subclinical involvement: conventional methods of detection include electrocardiography, echocardiography, and thallium-201 or gallium-67 scintigraphy, but the sensitivity of all these techniques is limited; magnetic resonance can show active involvement either by an increased myocardial signal, indicating active inflammation, or by regional wall motion abnormalities.

Generalized thickening of the myocardium and valves is seen in advanced cardiac amyloidosis. Early involvement may not be apparent, although abnormal diastolic function may be suggestive. Other myocardial diseases in which abnormalities have been demonstrated include myocarditis, systemic lupus erythematosus, Pompe's disease, and Fabry's disease.

Endocardium

Magnetic resonance is not as good as echocardiography at demonstrating small moving structures such as thickened valves and vegetations, but it is able to detect complications of infective endocarditis such as aneurysms and abscesses. The interpretation of spin echo images is only minimally compromised by the presence of a prosthetic valve and, because infection of these valves is a frequent cause of perivalvular abscess, MRI should be used if there is any doubt after echocardiography.

Valve disease

Regurgitation

If only a single valve is regurgitant, comparison of the left and right ventricular stroke volumes allows the regurgitant fraction to be calculated. If single valves on both sides of the heart are regurgitant, the method can be extended by comparing ventricular stroke volumes with flow in the great vessels, the latter measured by magnetic resonance velocity mapping. The regurgitant fraction then compares well with the regurgitant grade assessed by Doppler echocardiography. The method still fails if both valves on one side of the heart are regurgitant, but flow studies in the proximal aorta (or

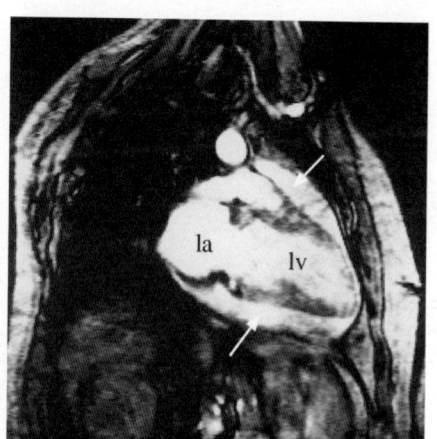

Fig. 4 End diastolic frames from a gradient echo cine acquisition in the horizontal (left) and vertical (right) long axis planes in a patient 3 weeks after heart transplantation. There is a large pericardial effusion (arrows). la, Left atrium; ra, right atrium; rv, right ventricle.

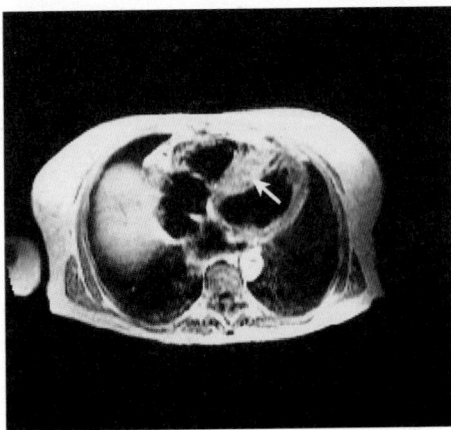

Fig. 5 Transverse spin echo image acquired at mid-ventricular level in a patient with hypertrophic cardiomyopathy. The interventricular septum is asymmetrically thickened (arrow).

pulmonary artery) can be used to measure aortic (or pulmonary) regurgitation alone from the amount of retrograde diastolic flow in the artery, and it is then possible to assess even the most complex cases.

Regurgitation can also be detected using cine gradient echo imaging when a turbulent jet of regurgitation is seen as an area of signal loss (Fig. 6). The size of the jet can be used as a semiquantitative measure of regurgitation, although factors other than the size of jet can affect the area of signal loss.

Stenosis

As with regurgitant jets proximal to a valve, a turbulent distal jet can be used to detect potential stenosis, although abnormal valves that are not stenosed can also generate turbulence. The best method of assessing stenosis is therefore to use cine velocity mapping to measure the peak velocity within the jet. The modified Bernoulli equation, commonly used in Doppler echocardiography, can then be used to estimate the pressure gradient across the stenosis. A disadvantage of magnetic resonance is that it is not yet

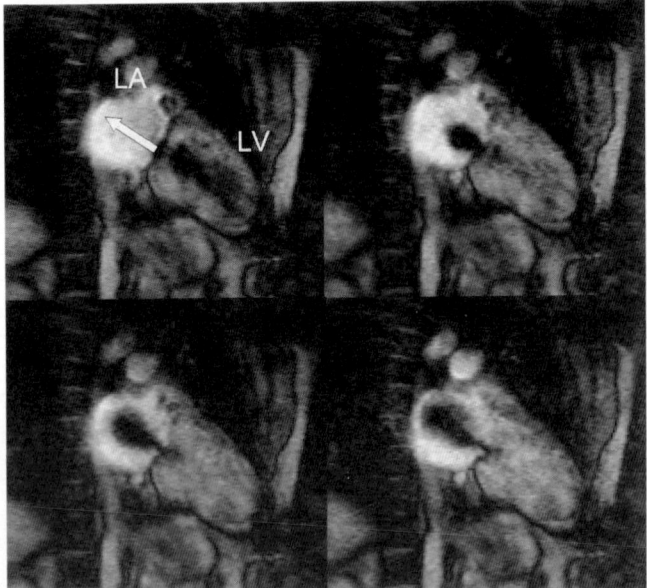

Fig. 6 Four systolic frames from a cine gradient echo acquisition in the vertical long axis plane in a patient with rheumatic mitral stenosis and regurgitation. The regurgitant jet from the left ventricle (LV) to the left atrium (LA) is seen by virtue of signal loss (black) from the turbulence. The size of the jet indicates that regurgitation is moderate.

real-time and so careful alignment of the imaging plane is required in order to obtain an accurate measurement.

Ischaemic heart disease

Myocardial infarction

Magnetic resonance imaging can be used in a number of ways to detect and measure the extent of acute myocardial necrosis. The simplest methods are to use spin echo or cine gradient echo imaging to image the associated wall motion abnormality: the findings agree well with X-ray left ventriculography. Alterations in the myocardial signal can also be observed, an increase of signal in T2-weighted spin echo images occurring only a few hours after occlusion of a coronary artery. The changes are most likely related to oedema and the abnormal area may include viable as well as necrotic myocardium.

Abnormal signal can also be observed in T1-weighted images, but these changes follow a different time course to the changes of T2 and are maximal at 6 weeks, possibly corresponding to cellular infiltration and repair rather than to oedema. Intravenous contrast agents can highlight the abnormalities and have helped to distinguish reperfused from continuing ischaemia in animal models. The same has not been possible in humans.

Reversible ischaemia

Dynamic exercise is impractical within a scanner, but pharmacological intervention using dipyridamole or dobutamine is a suitable alternative. Regional function is assessed using cine gradient echo imaging and global function can also be measured from cine velocity mapping of aortic flow. New wall motion abnormalities imply myocardial ischaemia, and there is a close correspondence between these abnormalities and regional perfusion assessed by radionuclide perfusion imaging. The sensitivity of this approach for detecting coronary artery disease depends upon whether a vasodilator or a β-agonist is used. Because the heterogeneities of myocardial perfusion provoked by dipyridamole do not always cause myocardial ischaemia, sensitivity is not as high (60 per cent) as with dobutamine (91 per cent). The latter is therefore the preferred agent for provoking abnormalities when using a wall motion technique.

An alternative method of assessing reversible perfusion abnormalities is to study the transit of a bolus of magnetic resonance contrast medium through the myocardium. This is not possible using conventional triggered images, but with ultra-fast gradient echo (or echo planar) techniques, images can be acquired in more than 100 ms (or more than 50 ms). Images in each cardiac cycle show the arrival and transit of a bolus of contrast (Gd-DTPA) injected into a central vein. Territories supplied by diseased arteries have a delayed arrival of contrast and a reduced signal increase, and abnormalities can be provoked by dipyridamole vasodilatation. Such bolus-tracking studies of perfusion cannot yet replace radionuclide techniques, but they do have the advantage of higher resolution and the potential to provide measurements of myocardial perfusion in absolute terms.

Coronary vessels

Bypass grafts

Coronary artery bypass grafts can be imaged relatively easily using conventional spin echo or gradient echo techniques. In spin echo images, the appearance of a low intraluminal signal, contrasting with the high signal of the surrounding fat or other soft tissue, implies that the graft contains moving blood and is patent, particularly if it can be followed distally to its insertion. If a graft cannot be identified, or if its origin is seen but it cannot be followed distally, then it is likely to be occluded. Using these criteria, sensitivity and specificity for the detection of patent grafts in the region of 90 per cent can be achieved. Internal mammary artery grafts are more difficult to visualize than saphenous vein grafts, partly because of their smaller size and partly because they can be tortuous and therefore more difficult to follow through multiple slices.

Cine gradient echo imaging has been used with similar results and the cine technique is helpful for identifying a graft if there is doubt from the

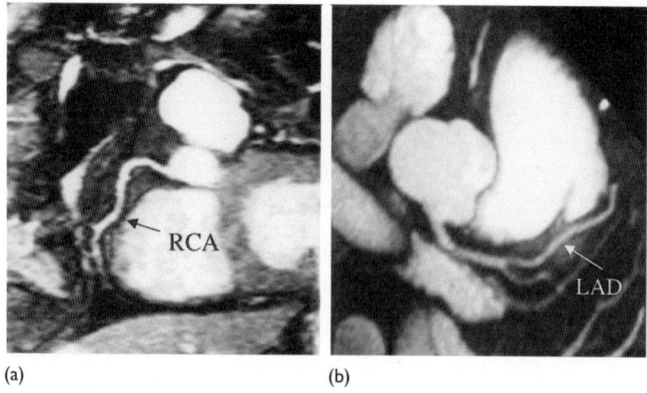

Fig. 7 Breath-hold, contrast-enhanced magnetic resonance angiogram of the right (a) and left (b) coronary arteries in a healthy volunteer. RCA, right coronary artery; LAD, left anterior descending artery.

spin echo images alone. Metallic clips and sternal sutures produce larger artefacts in gradient echo than in spin echo images. They are not ferromagnetic and imaging is perfectly safe, but the artefacts can complicate image interpretation. More recently, contrast-enhanced magnetic resonance angiography has proved useful for demonstrating the anatomy of the tortuous bypass coronary graft.

Native arteries

The coronary arteries are small, tortuous, and rapidly moving: three properties that conspire against successful imaging. Despite this, the proximal vessels can nearly always be identified in conventional spin echo images and their appearance with a low intraluminal signal implies that they contain moving blood and are patent. Unfortunately, resolution is not sufficient to identify stenoses reliably. Rapid gradient echo techniques and acquisition within a single breath-hold provide much better images; moreover, the resolution is adequate for detecting atheromatous disease (Fig. 7). Spiral and echo planar imaging have also been used, all of which can be combined with velocity mapping. Rapid, magnetic resonance flow measurement techniques allow quantification of coronary blood flow reserve, but there is a need to improve the resolution and the reliability of coronary artery imaging and flow measurements non-invasively by magnetic resonance.

Computed X-ray tomography

Computed X-ray tomography (CT) is widely available and has an established clinical role in imaging the heart, particularly the pericardium and great vessels (Table 1). Resolution was degraded on earlier generation scanners by cardiac and respiratory motion. State-of-the-art spiral scanners can image the entire heart volume within a single breath-hold, but even the

Table 1 Applications of conventional (CT) and electron-beam (EBCT) computed X-ray tomography

Mechanical CT	Electron-beam CT
Clinical	
Pericardium and pericardial fluid	Pericardium and pericardial fluid
Aortic dissection	Aortic dissection
Cardiac tumours	Cardiac tumours
	Coronary calcification
Specialist	
Bypass graft patency	Bypass graft patency
	Intracardiac masses
	Cardiac structure and function
Research	
	Myocardial perfusion

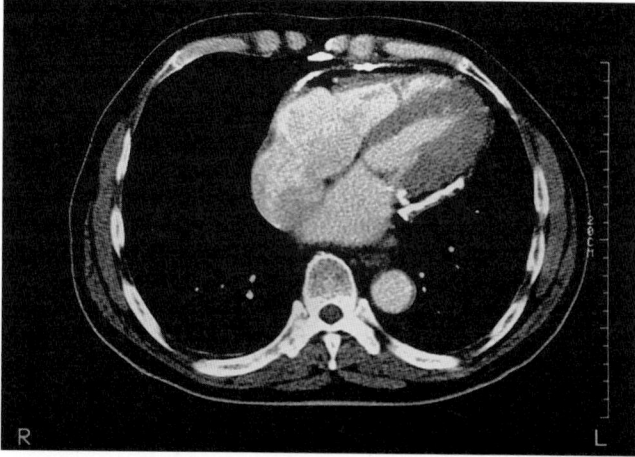

Fig. 8 Constrictive pericarditis. Electron-beam CT scan with contrast showing thickened and calcified pericardium, dilated atria, and normal-sized ventricles.

fastest conventional scanner requires 300 ms to acquire a single slice. The best temporal resolution is achieved with electrocardiographic gating and an electron-beam CT scanner (**EBCT**). This uses an electron beam that is focused and deflected on to a stationary target to generate a fan of X-rays that pass through the patient (Fig. 8). In its fastest mode this scanner can acquire two contiguous 8-mm thick slices in 50 ms with a repetition rate of 34 images a second.

Pericardium

The normal pericardium is seen in 95 per cent of patients by conventional CT, particularly over the anterior surface of the heart. The posterior pericardium is most frequently seen at its caudal insertion into the central tendon of the diaphragm, where it may be 3 to 4 mm thick. It is less easily seen laterally and posteriorly because of the absence of epicardial fat. Pericardial cysts, thickening, calcification, and effusion can be readily identified. The presence of thickening can differentiate pericardial restriction from restrictive cardiomyopathy, although thickening is also seen in a variety of conditions without necessarily implying constriction (Fig. 8).

Aortic dissection

CT is sensitive (83 to 100 per cent) and highly specific (90 to 100 per cent) for the identification of thoracic aortic dissection. This is similar to MRI and transoesophageal echocardiography, but CT is more widely available. The true and false lumens are commonly seen separated by an intimal flap (Fig. 9). Other features that indicate dissection include differential opacification of the true and false lumens, compression of the true lumen by a thrombosed false lumen, inward displacement of intimal calcification, and intramural haemorrhage. Although CT is particularly successful in identifying the distal extent of dissection and the presence of a haemopericardium, it has limitations. Artefacts may create difficulties, and the intimal tear or flap may not be identified in all cases. Therefore, if findings are negative despite strong clinical suspicion of dissection, further investigation is necessary.

Intracardiac masses

The presence, location, and extent of a thrombus and tumour in the cardiac chambers can be defined with both CT and EBCT. In patients with right heart lesions appropriate windowing of the images will allow assessment of the lungs for pulmonary embolism, and in patients with malignant tumours for metastatic disease.

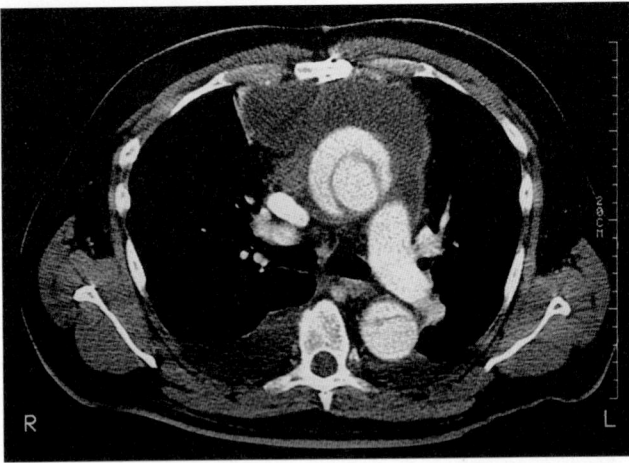

Fig. 9 Aortic dissection. Electron-beam CT scan with contrast showing a dilated ascending aorta with almost circumferential dissection. The descending aorta is also involved.

Cardiac structure and function

Using electrocardiographic gating and intravenous contrast medium, EBCT provides cine images at multiple contiguous levels in approximately eight cardiac cycles. This allows a qualitative assessment of ventricular function and morphology. Planimetry can then provide cavity, muscle area, and hence volume at any part of the cardiac cycle. Regional and segmental left ventricular wall motion can be assessed at rest and during pharmacological stimulation, and changes induced by exercise in patients with ischaemic heart disease can be measured.

Coronary calcification

Coronary artery calcification occurs only in the intima, and microcalcification detected by EBCT indicates the presence of atheroma (Fig. 10), arising when lipid pools first collect within the plaque and not necessarily a sign of advanced disease. A reliable and reproducible scoring system for quantifying calcium has been developed, and a significant relationship between the calcium score and the extent and severity of coronary artery disease as

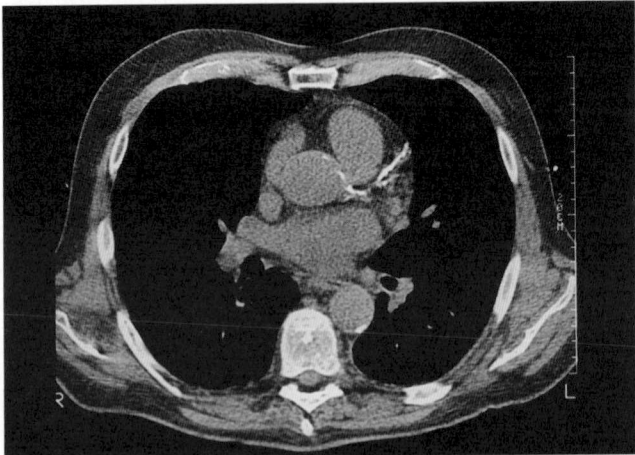

Fig. 10 Coronary calcification. Electron-beam CT scan without contrast. There is high-intensity calcification in the aortic root, the left main stem, left anterior descending, and diagonal coronary arteries.

assessed by coronary angiography has been established. However, there is only a weak relationship between the presence of calcium and the severity of luminal stenosis at the same site. The absence of calcification on EBCT does not exclude the presence of coronary atheroma, but it does make significant stenosis unlikely.

EBCT offers the possibility of a non-invasive screening test for coronary artery disease, but this use is controversial because the implications of a positive scan are uncertain. It is likely that the incidence of future coronary events is related to the degree of calcification, but the evidence is conflicting. If a relationship between calcium and coronary risk were firmly established, then the technique could play an important role in detecting individuals at risk of coronary events, in selecting people who may benefit most from primary prevention such as lipid-lowering therapy, and in monitoring the progression of disease.

Although EBCT technology is expensive and not widely available, it is possible that modern mechanical CT scanners may also be used to detect coronary calcification, even if in a less sensitive and reproducible fashion.

Coronary angiography

When combined with intravenous X-ray contrast media, EBCT can be used to image the lumen of the coronary arteries and bypass grafts, and three-dimensional images of the coronary tree can be reconstructed from multiple contiguous tomograms. The patency of the arteries and grafts can be determined accurately, but individual stenoses are detected with lesser accuracy and so the technique does not currently provide an alternative to invasive angiography. It is roughly equivalent in terms of accuracy and capability to magnetic resonance coronary angiography. Disadvantages include incomplete visualization of the distal coronary arteries and their branches, and the lack of opportunity to proceed to an intervention if a suitable lesion is demonstrated.

Further reading

Axel L (1998). Physics and technology of cardiovascular MRI. *Cardiology Clinics* **2**, 125–33.

Higgins CB, Hricak H, Helms CA (1992). *Magnetic resonance imaging of the body*, 2nd edn. Raven Press, New York. [Covers the whole field of magnetic resonance in the body, but excludes neurological applications.]

Marcus ML, *et al.*, eds. (1991). *Cardiac imaging: a companion to Braunwald's heart disease*. WB Saunders, Philadelphia. [Reviews of all non-invasive imaging techniques in cardiology, including several chapters on magnetic resonance and computed X-ray tomography.]

Mohiaddin RH, Pennell DJ (1998). MR blood flow measurement. Clinical application in the heart and circulation. *Cardiology Clinics* **16**, 161–87.

Neubauer S, *et al.* (1998). The clinical role of magnetic resonance in cardiovascular disease. *European Heart Journal* **19**, 19–39. [Extensive literature review with recommended indications for MRI in clinical practice.]

Nienaber CA, *et al.* (1993). The diagnosis of thoracic aortic dissection by noninvasive imaging procedures. *New England Journal of Medicine* **328**, 1–9.

Shellock FC, Morisoli S, Kanal E (1993). MR procedures and biomedical implants, materials, and devices: 1993 update. *Radiology* **189**, 587–99. [An ideal entry to the literature on the safety of magnetic resonance imaging.]

Underwood SR, Firmin DN (1991). *Magnetic resonance of the cardiovascular system*. Blackwell Scientific, Oxford. [Textbook covering all aspects of cardiovascular magnetic resonance.]

Wexler L, *et al.* (1997). Coronary artery calcification: pathophysiology, epidemiology, imaging methods, and clinical implications. A statement for health professionals from the American Heart Association. *Circulation* **94**, 1175–92.

15.3.6 Cardiac catheterization and angiography

Edward D. Folland

Introduction

Invasive cardiac diagnosis by means of catheterization and angiography developed hand-in-hand with cardiac surgery throughout the twentieth century. It answered the need for precise information about cardiac physiology and anatomy, which arose in the 1940s when surgical techniques for the treatment of congenital and rheumatic heart disease first became available. A few years earlier, in 1929, Werner Forsman of Germany successfully and safely passed a filiform urinary catheter from a median basilic vein into the right atrium of his own heart and documented it on X-ray film. Although this feat cost him his own job, it enabled Andre Cournand and Dickenson Richards a decade later to use catheters for sampling blood, measuring pressure and flow, and injecting radio-opaque contrast medium (angiography) into the intact, beating human heart, ushering in the era of invasive cardiac diagnosis. Cournand and Richards later won the Nobel Prize for their important work. This chapter will review the diagnostic applications of cardiac catheterization and angiography.

Indications for cardiac catheterization and angiography

Because catheterization is expensive and entails some degree of risk and discomfort, patients should be carefully selected. In broadest terms, it is indicated for detailed evaluation of patients having coronary, valvular, and congenital heart disease once they have been identified as candidates for surgery or other forms of intervention. It may also be indicated for patients whose diagnosis is uncertain from non-invasive evaluation.

Coronary artery disease

The vast majority of patients presenting for cardiac catheterization have coronary artery disease. Angiography of the coronary arteries performed during cardiac catheterization is essential for patients in whom revascularization is indicated. In spite of the limitations discussed later in this chapter, no other imaging modality, including magnetic resonance imaging and computed tomography, can provide the detailed anatomy of the entire coronary circulation that is needed for planning revascularization procedures such as coronary artery bypass surgery and percutaneous intervention.

Coronary angiography is indicated for patients having chronic stable angina, which persists in spite of reasonable efforts at pharmacological therapy. It is also indicated for patients whose survival would be improved, regardless of symptoms. Such patients are those with severe stenosis of the main left coronary artery and those with severe two- and three-vessel coronary artery disease in combination with impaired left ventricular function. These patients may be identified by the following features of stress testing: ischaemia at low workload (especially in stage 1 of the Bruce Protocol), marked depression of the electrocardiographic ST segment (greater than 2 mm), failure to augment systolic blood pressure during exercise, and large exercise-induced defects or increased lung uptake during radionuclide perfusion imaging. In addition, patients having high-risk clinical presentations such as unstable angina and postmyocardial infarction ischaemia are candidates for angiography. Depending upon the availability of emergency revascularization, patients having acute myocardial infarction may be best served by immediate catheterization. The indications for emergency catheterization and percutaneous revascularization instead of thrombolytic therapy will be covered in more detail in Chapter 15.4.5. Finally, catheterization is sometimes indicated for obtaining a definitive diagnosis when non-invasive testing has yielded equivocal or inconsistent results.

Valvular disease

Catheterization was once considered essential prior to the surgical treatment of valvular heart disease. This is no longer the case because of advances in non-invasive testing using ultrasound and Doppler techniques. Nevertheless, catheterization is a frequently helpful technique for gathering the information needed to properly select patients for surgical therapy and to guide the surgeon in providing optimum treatment. The most common reason for catheterization in these patients is to assess the need for coronary artery revascularization, particularly amongst those with aortic stenosis since coronary artery disease is often present in the age group in which this disease commonly occurs. Haemodynamic study may also be necessary in cases where non-invasive diagnostic data are limited or equivocal. By contrast, it is often possible to avoid catheterization in young patients in whom non-invasive studies yield unequivocal conclusions and there is no evidence of coronary artery disease.

Congenital disease

Most patients with congenital heart defects can be definitively diagnosed by transthoracic or transoesophageal ultrasound. As in valvular disease, catheterization is most useful in cases where the abnormality is unusually complex, the non-invasive data incomplete, or the patient is suspected of having coronary artery disease. Catheterization is particularly useful in quantifying shunt flow and pulmonary vascular resistance, both of which are important considerations in the treatment of intracardiac defects. The physical passage of a systemic venous catheter across the atrial septum into a pulmonary vein or the left ventricle is diagnostic of an atrial septal defect.

Pericardial disease

Pericardial tamponade and constriction lend themselves particularly well to diagnosis by catheterization. Although ultrasound has superseded catheterization as a rapidly available method of confirming the clinical diagnosis of tamponade, it is usually inconclusive for patients with pericardial constriction. At catheterization, patients with both conditions usually demonstrate equalization of all intracardiac diastolic pressures. In addition, unique pressure waveforms are exhibited in the right atrium and right ventricle, which usually distinguish the two diagnoses (Fig. 1).

Congestive heart failure

The aetiology and pathophysiology of congestive heart failure are readily elucidated by catheterization. States of pressure and volume overload as well as systolic and diastolic dysfunction of the ventricles can be easily identified, as explained in detail later in this chapter. Furthermore, catheterization is uniquely suited for identifying transient or reversible causes of left ventricular dysfunction caused by ischaemia or myocardial hibernation due to underlying coronary artery disease. Sometimes exercise or other interventions are performed during a catheter study to elicit transient abnormal haemodynamic function. Myocardial biopsy performed during catheterization can often identify the aetiology of primary myocardial dysfunction.

Pulmonary vascular disease

Patients with primary pulmonary hypertension (see Chapter 15.15.2.1) should undergo catheterization to measure pulmonary vascular pressure and resistance. Certain vasodilating drugs may or may not benefit the

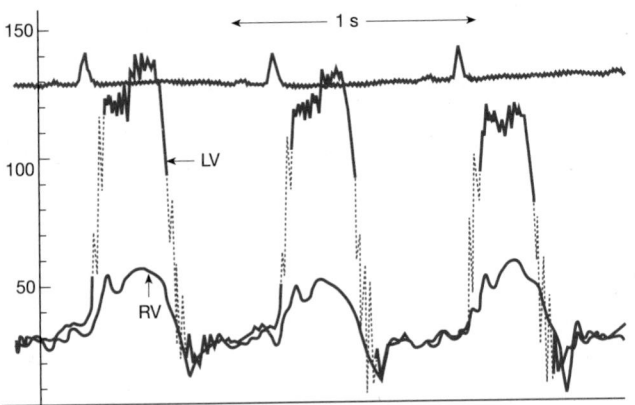

Fig. 1 Pericardial constriction. This is a tracing of simultaneous left ventricular (LV) and right ventricular (RV) pressure in a patient with pericardial constriction. Generally, the diastolic pressure of the left ventricle is higher than that of the right ventricle. For patients with a constriction, the pericardium determines the diastolic compliance of both chambers, causing the diastolic pressures to be equal. Note also the typical 'dip-plateau' pattern or 'square-root sign' of both chambers in diastole. Although diastolic ventricular pressures are also equal for patients having tamponade, the dip-plateau pattern is usually absent.

patient, depending upon their effect on pressure and resistance during acute administration. Pulmonary angiography performed during right heart catheterization is still regarded as the most definitive test for pulmonary embolism, in spite of advances in radioisotope lung scanning and spiral computed tomography.

Preparing the patient for catheterization

Precatheterization evaluation should consist of a careful history and examination particularly aimed at eliciting details of prior cardiac procedures, reactions to contrast medium, renal function, peripheral vascular status, and haemostatic function. The patient should be carefully advised of the indications, alternatives, risks, discomforts, and expected benefits of the procedure. The skilled clinician does this while building the patient's confidence and avoids creating undue alarm. Following an uncomplicated diagnostic catheterization the patient should usually expect to go home the same day and to resume customary physical activities within a day or two.

Approaches to cardiac catheterization and angiography

Vascular access

The traditional approach to vascular access is via a cut-down near the antecubital fossa. Isolating and mobilizing the brachial or antecubital vein and the brachial artery for right and left heart catheterization may thereby achieve arterial and venous access. Following the procedure the arterial entry site is repaired by suture and the vein is usually tied off. This approach has the advantages of enabling earlier postprocedure ambulation and the security of direct arterial closure in anticoagulated patients. It has the disadvantage of being more time-consuming for most physicians and less cosmetic for the patient.

Percutaneous vascular access is achieved by direct puncture with a needle through which a flexible spring guidewire is passed into the vessel. Catheters may then be passed into the vessel over the guidewire. (The

guidewire is placed in the catheter to maintain access during catheter exchanges.) Following the procedure haemostasis is achieved by applying pressure over the puncture site until bleeding stops. Percutaneous access is most frequently employed at the femoral site, although it may also be used at brachial, axillary, internal jugular, and radial locations. It has the advantage of speed, simplicity, and, when performed from the femoral vessels, frees the upper body and arms during angiographic filming. However, percutaneous access has the disadvantage of requiring several hours' immobilization of the catheterization site following the procedure, which is particularly troublesome after femoral puncture since 6 h of postprocedure bedrest is frequently required. Nevertheless, the percutaneous femoral approach has become the preferred choice in 90 per cent of cases, with the recent use of smaller catheters (4 and 5 French) and closure devices for the arterial puncture site enabling earlier ambulation. The percutaneous radial approach is becoming increasingly popular for outpatients.

Right heart catheterization

Right heart catheterization can be performed from any of the approaches described above. Although traditionally performed with a stiff, woven Dacron, end-hole catheter, it is often done with a flexible, balloon-tip, flow-directed catheter (Swan–Ganz) because this is safer and enables the measurement of cardiac output by thermodilution.

Catheterization of the right heart is indicated by itself for the study of pulmonary vascular disease and haemodynamic response to exercise or drug administration. It is indicated in combination with left heart catheterization for patients requiring haemodynamic study of valvular, congenital, or myocardial disease, and for patients being studied primarily for coronary artery disease who also have heart failure, valvular, or pulmonary disease.

Left atrial pressure can be measured indirectly via right heart catheterization by wedging the tip of the catheter in a pulmonary arteriole, or by occluding a pulmonary artery branch with the inflated balloon at the tip of a Swan–Ganz catheter. In either case, this creates a static column of blood from the tip of the catheter, through the pulmonary capillary bed, to the left atrium. This static column of blood has the effect of extending the tip of the catheter to the left atrium for pressure-measuring purposes. The resulting pressure is identical to the directly measured left atrial pressure, except that it is delayed temporally by approximately 80 milliseconds. This pressure, commonly known as the pulmonary (artery) capillary wedge (**PCW**) pressure, is very useful in the management of left heart failure and shock, and for estimating the diastolic gradient across the mitral valve in patients with mitral stenosis.

Left heart catheterization

Left heart catheterization is generally performed in conjunction with coronary angiography, but is specifically required for the assessment of left ventricular function and assessment of stenosis or regurgitation of the left-sided valves (mitral and aortic). It is most often accomplished by femoral or brachial arterial access, and by retrograde crossing of the aortic valve to enter the left ventricle. Left heart catheterization may also be achieved by controlled puncture of the interatrial septum with a catheter originating from the right femoral vein (trans-septal left heart catheterization): this can then be used to measure left atrial pressure directly, and be passed antegradely through the mitral valve to measure pressure and perform angiography of the left ventricle. Retrograde access of the left atrium from the left ventricle is technically difficult and seldom done. The left ventricle may also be entered via transthoracic needle puncture. This approach, known as direct left ventricular puncture, is occasionally necessary for studying patients who have mechanical prosthetic valves at both mitral and aortic positions. The passage of the needle into the left ventricle from the cardial apex is facilitated by echocardiographic guidance.

Information obtained from cardiac catheterization and angiography

Intracardiac pressures

Methodology

Pressure at the tip of the catheter is transmitted through the fluid inside the catheter (usually saline) to a device called a transducer, which converts the pressure signal to an electrical signal that can then be amplified and displayed on a television screen or on a strip-chart paper recording. Once calibrated, the pressure at the tip of the catheter can be read graphically from the recording screen or paper. The fidelity of recording depends upon the physical characteristics of the fluid-filled catheter, stopcocks, connecting tubing, and the pressure transducer itself. A fluid-filled system is usually capable of responding to transient pressure changes up to 20 or occasionally 30 Hz. This is sufficient fidelity to reproduce diagnostically useful pressure waveforms from the heart. However, it is not responsive enough to accurately reproduce the rate of rise of left ventricular pressure during the isovolumic phase of systole (dP/dt). This requires responsiveness to transient pressure changes of at least 60 Hz, of which fluid-filled catheter systems are not capable. For such applications catheter-tip manometers are available (Millar catheters) in which the transducer is placed at the tip of catheter, eliminating the need for an intervening column of fluid. These devices are expensive and are used only when such fidelity is required, usually in research applications.

Normal intracardiac pressures

The upper limits of all normal intracardiac pressures measurable from a right heart catheter are approximate multiples of six, hence they are easily remembered by 'The Rule of Sixes' (Table 1). For example, the mean right atrial pressure is 6 mmHg or less, mean left atrial pressure is 12 mmHg or less. A further aid to remembering normal pressures is the 'Corollary of Continuity', which means that contiguous chambers have a common pressure when the intervening valve is open. For example, the right ventricle and right atrium are essentially a common chamber when the tricuspid valve is open in diastole, therefore the upper limit of right ventricular end-diastolic pressure is the same as the upper limit of the normal right atrial pressure, or 6 mmHg. This assumes there is no significant stenosis or regurgitation across the tricuspid valve, and that the right ventricle has normal compliance. The same condition applies to the mitral valve in diastole and the pulmonic and aortic valves in systole. Another practical rule is that the pulmonary artery diastolic and pulmonary artery capillary pressures approximate each other in the absence of severe pulmonary vascular dis-

Table 1 Normal intracardiac pressures[*]

Location	Phasic pressure (mmHg)	Mean pressure (mmHg)
Right atrium		3 ± 2
Right ventricle		
Systole	24 ± 4	
Diastole	5 ± 3	
Pulmonary artery		13 ± 5
Systole	24 ± 6	
Diastole	13 ± 5	
Pulmonary capillary wedge		9 ± 3
Left atrium		9 ± 3
Left ventricle		
Systole	120 ± 18	
Diastole	10 ± 5	

[*] These values are derived from 100 consecutive catheterization studies of patients proven to have no evidence of heart disease at the West Roxbury Veterans Administration Hospital from 1955 to 1980. An easy way to remember the upper limits of normal values (≤2 standard deviations above mean) is that they are generally multiples of the number six.

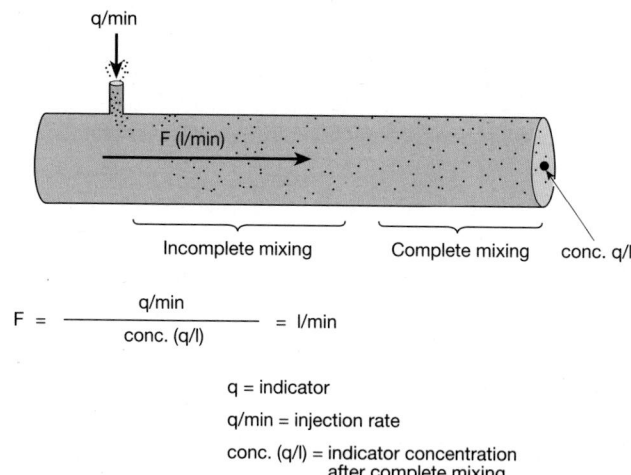

$$F = \frac{q/min}{conc.\ (q/l)} = l/min$$

q = indicator

q/min = injection rate

conc. (q/l) = indicator concentration after complete mixing

Fig. 2 The Fick principle. The flow rate (F) through a vessel (cardiac output, in this case) can be measured if an indicator is added to the flowing liquid at a known rate (q/min) and the concentration (q/L) of the indicator is measured after complete mixing has occurred.

ease. Once this has been established for any given patient, the pulmonary artery diastolic pressure can be followed as a surrogate for pulmonary capillary wedge pressure in situations where a pulmonary artery catheter is used for intensive-care monitoring.

All intracardiac pressures rise and fall phasically with breathing due to transmission of shifting intrapleural pressure during respiratory effort. Usually this variation is no more than a few mmHg from inspiration to expiration, but it can be quite marked in patients with obstructive lung disease. Standards of normal pressure are based upon measurements taken during resting respiration, averaging several respiratory cycles. Pressures in the catheterization laboratory should be similarly measured: asking a patient to hold his or her breath may generate misleading data.

Waveforms

The shape of intracardiac pressure waveforms carries useful diagnostic information. Atria and ventricles have characteristic waveforms, the left-sided chambers normally demonstrating similar patterns at relatively higher pressures than right-sided chambers. The state of volume loading and the relative compliance or 'stiffness' of the respective ventricles during diastolic filling determines pressures in the right and left atria. The left ventricle is generally thicker, stiffer, and less compliant to the stretch of increasing volume than the right ventricle; hence the left atrial and left ventricular diastolic pressures are higher than the respective pressures in the right heart. Conditions such as pericardial constriction and tamponade alter this normal relationship (Fig. 1).

Cardiac flow and output

Measurement of cardiac output was one of the earliest applications of catheterization. Most methods entail application of the indicator dilution theory (the 'Fick' principle), summarized graphically in Fig. 2. Stated simply: the rate of flow can be measured if an indicator substance is added to the moving vehicle (for example, blood) at a known rate, and the concentration of the indicator is also known proximal and distal to the point where the indicator is added. The indicator can be any readily measured substance such as oxygen, indocyanine green dye, or saline, the temperature of which is known and different from that of the bloodstream.

Cardiac output by oximetry

In this method, commonly called the 'Fick method', the indicator is oxygen which is carried physiologically by the blood. The method requires that the subject be in a metabolic steady state where the use of oxygen is constant.

Such a steady state exists at rest and also during exercise, provided that the workload is constant for at least 3 min. As seen in Fig. 3, the pulmonary blood flow can be calculated when the oxygen consumption rate is known and the oxygen contents of blood in systemic and pulmonary arteries are known. In the absence of intracardiac shunts the pulmonary blood flow equals the systemic blood flow, or cardiac output.

Dye dilution

This method entails the rapid injection of a known quantity of indocyanine dye into the pulmonary artery. Blood is then sampled by withdrawal at a constant rate from a systemic artery. The sampled blood passes through a spectrophotometer, which is calibrated to measure the concentration of dye. A concentration curve is inscribed when the injected bolus of dye passes the sampling point (Fig. 4). Dividing the quantity of dye injected by the area of the time–concentration curve (corrected for recirculation) yields the cardiac output.

Thermodilution

Measurement of cardiac output by thermodilution uses the same principle as dye dilution, with the indicator being 'negative calories' (the difference in caloric content of the injected bolus of cool saline compared to the caloric content of the same quantity of the subject's blood). The downstream 'concentration' of injected negative calories is measured as a transient drop in temperature by a thermistor at the tip of the injection catheter several centimetres from the point of injection. Dividing the negative calories injected by the area of the distal time–temperature curve yields cardiac output. The advantages of speed, automaticity, and repeatability of this method make it particularly suitable for serial measurements during different haemodynamic states.

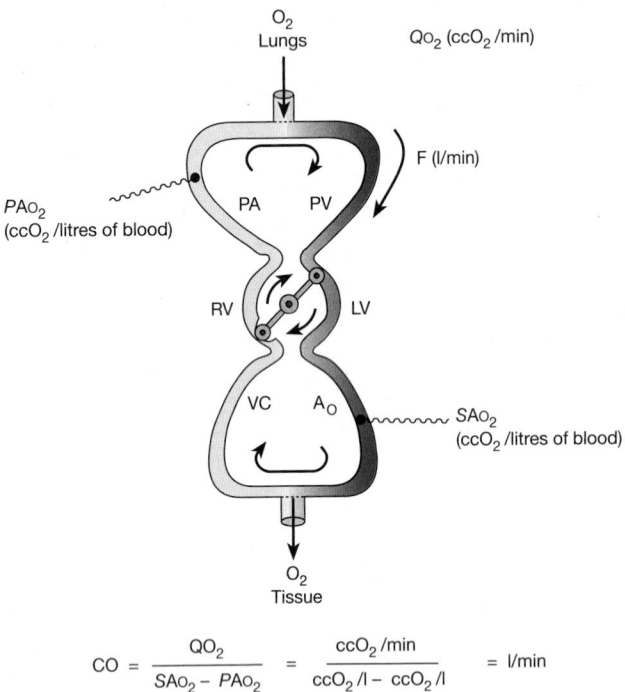

$$CO = \frac{QO_2}{SAO_2 - PAO_2} = \frac{ccO_2/min}{ccO_2/l - ccO_2/l} = l/min$$

Fig. 3 Cardiac output measured by oximetry. This is an application of the Fick principle in which oxygen is the indicator carried by flowing blood. The patient's metabolism must be at steady state, a condition where oxygen consumption and utilization are matched. It requires three measurements: oxygen consumption rate (QO_2), systemic arterial oxygen content (SAO_2), and pulmonary arterial oxygen content (PAO_2). Other abbreviations: Ao, aorta; CO, cardiac output; LV, left ventricle; PV, pulmonary vein; RV, right ventricle; VC, vena cava; cc, cm³.

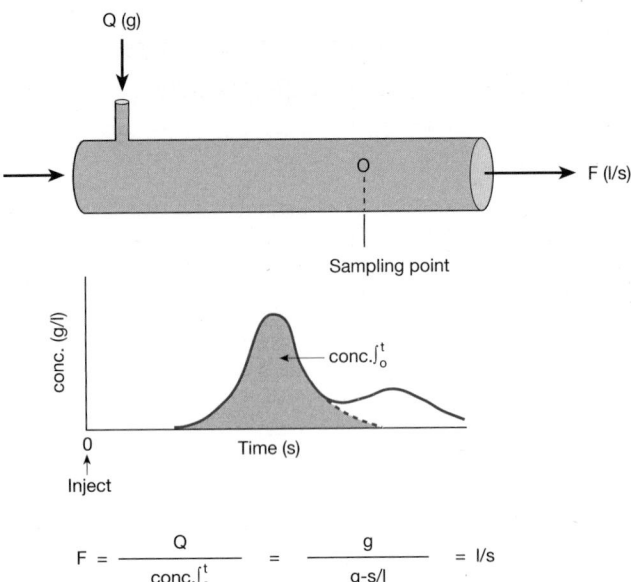

$$F = \frac{Q}{conc.\int_o^t} = \frac{g}{g\text{-}s/l} = l/s$$

Fig. 4 Cardiac output measured by dye curve. The concentration curve of indocyanine green dye generated by sampling distal to an injection point can be analysed to yield cardiac output. See text for more details. Thermodilution cardiac output employs the same principle, except that temperature is the measured indicator. F, flow or cardiac output; Q, quantity of indicator injected.

Angiographic output

This is the only commonly used method that does not employ the indicator dilution or Fick principle. The left ventricular stroke volume calculated from quantitative angiography is multiplied by the heart rate to yield the left ventricular output. In the absence of valvular regurgitation this is the same as cardiac output. As explained in greater detail later in the chapter, this method is particularly useful in assessing mitral and aortic valvular regurgitation.

Quantitative angiography

Quantitative left ventricular angiography enables the measurement of left ventricular volume at instants throughout the cardiac cycle. Radiographic contrast medium is rapidly injected into the left ventricle and the shadow image of the opacified ventricle captured on film or electronically at a particular frame rate in any chosen projection. The most common projection is 30 degrees right anterior oblique at a filming rate of 30 frames per second. In this view the image of the left ventricle is parallel to its long axis, resembling an ellipse, or an American football/rugby ball. Arvidsson and Greene first suggested that the volume of the left ventricle could be calculated from the volume formula for an ellipsoid, the three-dimensional structure created by rotating an ellipse on its long axis. Dodge and Sandler improved upon this concept by deriving the minor hemi-axes from an idealized ellipse of the same length and area as the projected image of the ventricle. This method is still commonly used and is often referred to as the area–length method. Images captured at end-diastole and end-systole are analysed and corrected for magnification to yield end-diastolic and end-systolic volumes, the difference between these volumes being the stroke volume and the product of the stroke volume and heart rate, the angiographic left ventricular output. These indices are useful in the assessment of left ventricular function and valvular regurgitation as discussed later in this chapter.

Intracardiac shunts

The same methods of oximetry and indicator dilution utilized in measuring cardiac output can be employed for the detection and quantitation of intracardiac shunts. Under normal resting conditions, blood is approximately 75 per cent saturated as it returns from the body to the right heart and pulmonary artery. As it leaves the lungs in the pulmonary veins blood is 99 per cent saturated. Intracardiac shunts can be detected, localized, and quantified by measuring the oxygen saturation in various locations. Left to right shunts will cause a step-up in the saturation of the blood at the location of the shunt; for example, in a patient with an atrial septal defect the saturation will rise in the right atrium, whereas with a ventricular septal defect the saturation will rise in the right ventricle. A patient with Eisenmenger's syndrome (pulmonary hypertension and right to left shunting) will exhibit a drop in saturation at the location of the shunt, namely at the left atrium or ventricle in the case of atrial and ventricular septal defects, respectively. The degree of the change in saturation is proportional to the size of the shunt, and enables calculation of the shunt flow in either direction in litres per min. Figure 5 presents a scheme and formulas for calculating shunt volume.

Vascular resistance

Methodology

Blood flow through the pulmonary and systemic circulations can be compared to the flow of an electric current through a circuit. Pressure is the driving force analogous to voltage, flow rate is analogous to current, and the impediment to flow through the vascular bed is resistance. Pressure, flow, and resistance relate to each other in a fashion analogous to Ohm's law:

$$\text{Resistance} = \text{pressure}/\text{flow}.$$

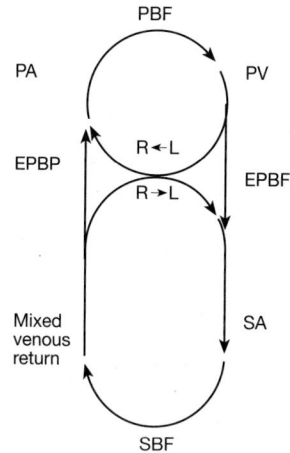

$$SBF \text{ (l/min)} = \frac{O_2 \text{ consumption (ml/min)}}{(SA_{O_2} - \text{mixed } V_{O_2}) \times 10}$$

$$PBF \text{ (l/min)} = \frac{O_2 \text{ consumption (ml/min)}}{(PV_{O_2} - \text{mixed } PA_{O_2}) \times 10}$$

$$EPBF \text{ (l/min)} = \frac{O_2 \text{ consumption (ml/min)}}{(PV_{O_2} - \text{mixed } V_{O_2}) \times 10}$$

Shunt flow (l/min):
$$L \to R = PBF - EPBF$$
$$R \to L = SBF - EPBF$$

Fig. 5 Quantitation of intracardiac shunts. Shunts between the left and right sides of the heart due to septal defects can be quantified by oximetry using this scheme. PBF, pulmonary blood flow; SBF, systemic blood flow; EPBF, effective pulmonary blood flow, which is that part of the systemic venous return that actually passes through the lungs and is oxygenated; PA_{O_2}, pulmonary artery oxygen content; PV_{O_2}, pulmonary vein oxygen content; SA_{O_2}, systemic artery oxtygen content; mixed V_{O_2}, mixed systemic venous oxygen content.

Table 2 Normal vascular resistance*

Location	Resistance (dynes s^{-5})
Total systemic resistance	1276 ± 371
Total pulmonary resistance	185 ± 57
Pulmonary vascular resistance	55 ± 18

* The values are derived from 100 consecutive catheterization studies of patients proven to have no evidence of cardiac disease at the West Roxbury Veterans Administration Hospital during the years 1955–1980.

In the above formula 'pressure' is the difference in mean pressure across the systemic vascular bed (systemic arterial pressure—right atrial pressure) or the pulmonary vascular bed (pulmonary artery pressure—left atrial pressure). In the absence of intracardiac shunts 'flow' is the same for both circulations and is measured as cardiac output by methods already described. In cases of intracardiac shunting the systemic and pulmonary flows will differ according to the degree of shunting, and can be calculated as described under the section on cardiac shunts. Normal values for pulmonary vascular and systemic vascular resistance are expressed either in dyne s cm^{-5} or Wood units and are displayed in Table 2. Total pulmonary resistance is a useful concept for expressing the total resistance against which the right ventricle must work, and includes not only the pulmonary vascular resistance, but also the resistance engendered by the static pressure in the left atrium. Hence, pulmonary vascular disease, left heart failure, or both, can increase the total pulmonary resistance.

Clinical application

Measurement of resistance is useful for assessing the state of the pulmonary circulation in congenital heart disease with intracardiac shunting: high pulmonary vascular resistance may preclude the safe correction of an intracardiac shunt, particularly if the shunt is from right to left. It is also useful in diagnosing the relative contribution of left heart failure and pulmonary vascular disease in patients with pulmonary hypertension, and is the best indicator of the effectiveness of vasodilating drugs for patients with pulmonary hypertension.

Valvular stenosis

Valvular stenosis is assessed by measuring the transvalvular pressure gradient and by calculating the valvular orifice area using a formula introduced in the late 1940s by cardiologist Richard Gorlin and his father, an engineer. The Gorlin formula for valve area was initially developed for patients with rheumatic mitral stenosis. It is based upon a study which utilized data from right heart catheterization alone, validated by relatively crude intraoperative estimates of valve area using the index finger of surgeon Dwight Harken during closed mitral commissurotomy operations at the Peter Bent Brigham Hospital in Boston, Massachusetts. In spite of this, the formula has stood the test of time and remains the standard for the haemodynamic assessment of valvular stenosis. In its generalized form it is expressed as follows:

$$\text{Valve area} = \text{transvalvular flow rate}/K \sqrt{\text{gradient}}.$$

In the above formula K is a constant unique to mitral or aortic valve analysis (38 and 44.5, respectively). The transvalvular flow rate (**TFR**) is cardiac output normalized for the time that the valve is actually open. In aortic valve applications TFR is the cardiac output divided by the product of heart rate and systolic ejection period. In mitral valve applications it is the cardiac output divided by the product of heart rate and diastolic filling period. Cardiac output is the effective systemic blood flow as determined by Fick, thermodilution, or dye dilution methods unless there is associated valvular regurgitation, in which case it is the total left ventricular output as determined by quantitative left ventricular angiography. Gradient is the mean pressure gradient in mmHg during the time when the valve is open.

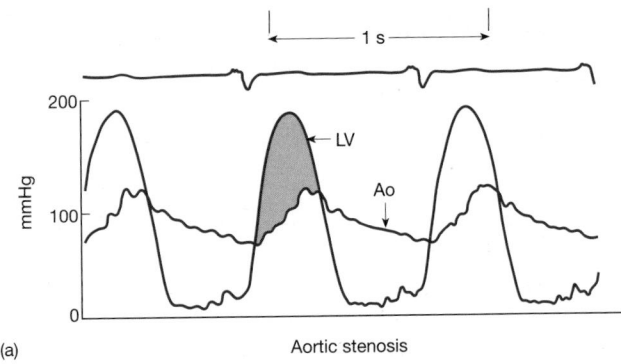

(a)   Aortic stenosis

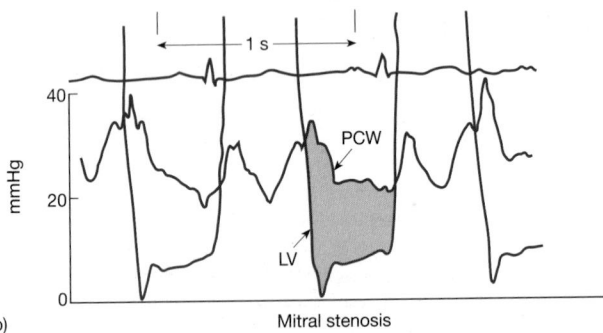

(b)   Mitral stenosis

Fig. 6 Pressure gradients associated with valvular stenosis. The upper panel shows simultaneous tracings of left ventricular (LV) and ascending aortic (Ao) pressure in a patient with severe aortic stenosis. The mean systolic gradient across the aortic valve is 60 mmHg. The lower panel shows simultaneous tracings of left ventricular (LV) and pulmonary capillary wedge (PCW) pressure in a patient with severe mitral stenosis. The mean diastolic pressure gradient across the valve is 16 mmHg. The respective valvular gradients are cross-hatched.

Figure 6 shows tracings that demonstrate typical gradients from patients with aortic and mitral stenosis. The ranges of calculated valve area associated with various levels of stenosis for both aortic and mitral valves are displayed in Table 3. In general, procedures performed for the relief of anatomical stenosis are expected to be beneficial in symptomatic patients with severe valvular obstruction. However, many factors enter into such a decision and individual clinical judgement is required. Although patients with large transvalvular gradients generally experience the best result from intervention, the gradient by itself can be misleading due to its exponential relationship to cardiac output.

Valvular regurgitation

Qualitative assessment

Regurgitation of all four cardiac valves can be qualitatively assessed by angiography. The downstream side of the valve in question is opacified by a rapid injection of radiographic contrast medium. Regurgitation is visualized as upstream leakage of contrast across the closed valve. In the case of

Table 3 Calculated valve areas associated with various degrees of mitral and aortic stenosis

| | Valve area (square cm) | |
Severity	Aortic	Mitral
Mild	>1.2	>2.0
Moderate	0.8–1.2	1.1–2.0
Severe*	<0.8	≤1.0

* 'Severe' stenosis is generally considered to be sufficient to warrant surgical correction.

mitral regurgitation systolic opacification of the left atrium occurs during injection of the left ventricle. In aortic regurgitation diastolic opacification of the left ventricle occurs during supravalvular injection of the aorta. The degree of regurgitation is graded on an arbitrary scale from mild (1+) to severe (4+).

Quantitative assessment

Aortic and mitral regurgitation can be quantified in terms of regurgitant flow in litres per min or regurgitant fraction as a percentage of left ventricular output. The method requires measurement of the total left ventricular output by the angiographic method and subtraction from that of the effective forward output measured by the Fick or indicator dilution methods (both described earlier). It is the best method for measuring the severity of regurgitation, provided that the left ventricular angiogram, which itself changes cardiac output, is performed soon after the Fick measurement. Furthermore, both measurements must be made with considerable care to ensure accuracy. Regurgitation is considered clinically severe when 50 per cent or more of the total left ventricular output is simply shuttling or regurgitating across the defective valve. The ability to quantify regurgitation across either valve is lost when both mitral and aortic valves are leaky.

Left ventricular function

Global function

Global function of the left ventricle is broadly described by its ability to generate pressure and flow under particular conditions of preload and afterload. Plotting the pressure and volume of the left ventricle at instants in time for a single cardiac cycle generates a pressure–volume loop displayed in Fig. 7. Most of the commonly used indices of left ventricular function can be derived from such a loop, including end-diastolic volume, end-systolic volume, stroke volume, ejection fraction, end-diastolic pressure, and dP/dt. Of these, the ejection fraction is most useful because it correlates with prognosis in a variety of cardiac diseases.

Grading angiographic wall motion in various segments of the left ventricle as normal, hypokinetic, akinetic, or dyskinetic assesses the regional

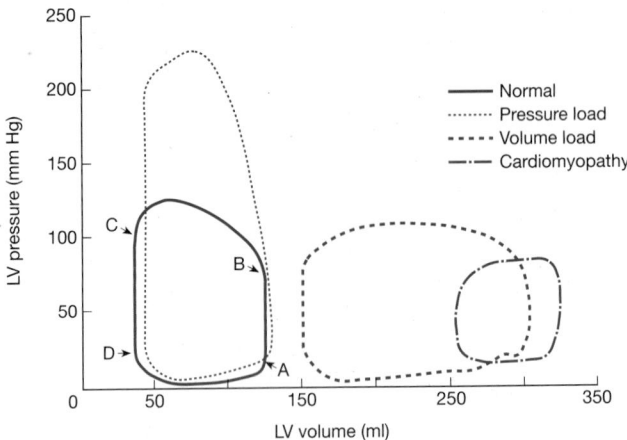

Fig. 7 Pressure–volume loops. Simultaneously plotting the instantaneous pressure and volume of the left ventricle throughout a single cardiac cycle produces these loops. The loop is a synthesis of most information relevant to left ventricular function. In this figure a loop from a normal patient is contrasted with those from patients with pressure load (hypertension or aortic stenosis), volume load (aortic or mitral regurgitation), and cardiomyopathy. Point A represents mitral valve closure; segment A–B, isovolumic contraction; point B, aortic valve opening; segment B–C, systolic ejection; point C, aortic valve closure; segment C–D, isovolumic relaxation; point D, mitral valve opening; and segment D–A, diastolic filling.

function of the left ventricle. Regions of abnormal function generally correspond to locations of infarcted myocardium.

Contractility

This parameter is difficult to assess in the intact heart, because all pressure and volume indices are dependent upon preload and afterload. Although ejection fraction is clinically useful it can be misleading in situations of high afterload (for example, severe aortic stenosis) and low afterload (for example, severe mitral regurgitation). The concept of 'elastance' has gained favour as a useful index of intrinsic contractility, because it is relatively independent of loading conditions. Elastance is the slope of the line generated by plotting the end-systolic left ventricular pressure from a series of pressure–volume loops generated at differing afterloads created by the infusion of pressor or vasodilator drugs. The method is laborious and generally reserved for research applications.

Diastolic function

Diastolic function of the left ventricle is best appreciated from the slope of the pressure–volume loop during the period from mitral valve opening to its closure at the onset of systole. The curve becomes steeper as the left

ventricle becomes less compliant due to the effects of hypertrophy, ischaemia, or infiltrative disease. In general, left ventricular end-diastolic pressure (**LVEDP**) rises as diastolic compliance falls, accounting for the high left atrial pressure and heart failure seen in diastolic left ventricular dysfunction.

Assessment of coronary arterial anatomy and function

Disease of the coronary arteries may be characterized at catheterization by both anatomical and functional assessment. Coronary angiography images the lumen of the vessel, which has been rendered radio-opaque by injection of radiographic contrast medium. It is a shadowing technique, which displays the impact of the lesion on the arterial lumen, but does not image the plaque *per se*. Intracoronary ultrasound provides a tomographic image of the vessel wall and is capable of demonstrating the thickness and sonic density of the vessel wall and any associated plaque. Angiography and intravascular ultrasound are complementary methods of assessing vascular anatomy. To learn the haemodynamic importance of a coronary lesion it may be necessary to analyse its effect on function by measuring pressure

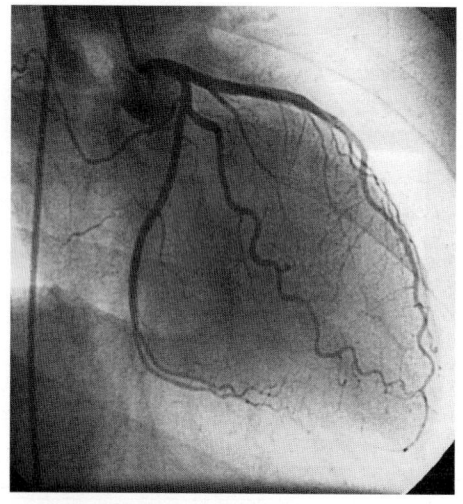
(a)

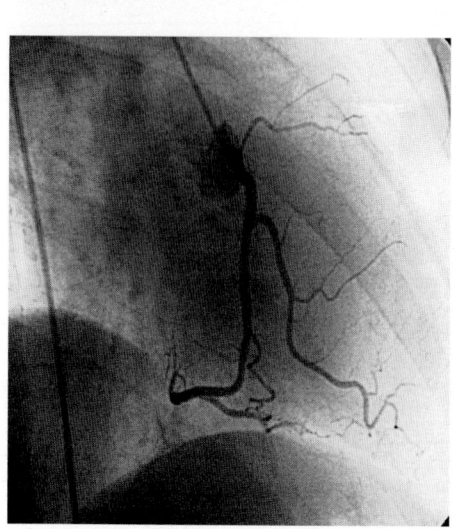
(c)

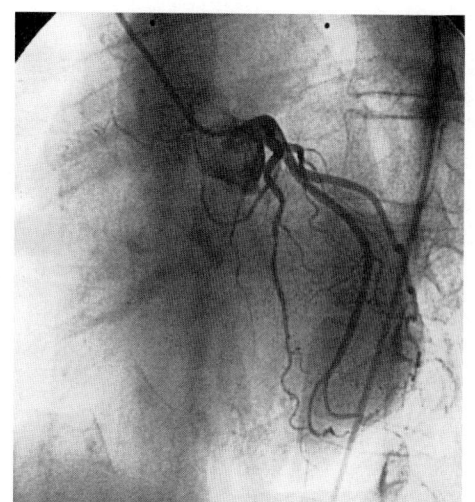
(b)

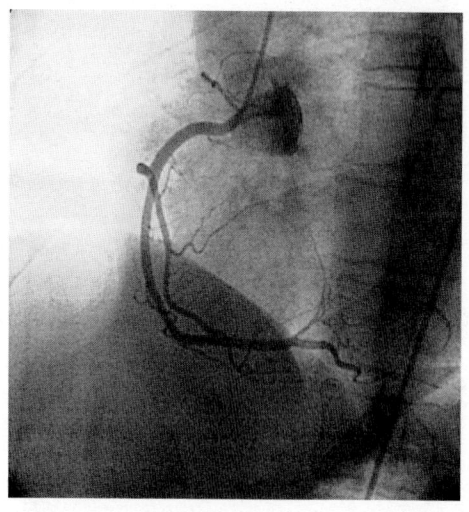
(d)

Fig. 8 Normal coronary anatomy. Left coronary angiogram showing main stem, left anterior descending, and left circumflex arteries from right anterior oblique (RAO) view (a) and left anterior oblique (LAO) view (b). Right coronary angiogram showing right coronary and posterior descending arteries from RAO view (c) and LAO view (d).

and flow in the affected vessel. All these anatomical and functional modalities may be accomplished by catheterization.

Coronary arteriography or angiography

Coronary arteriography or angiography is presently the single most essential application of cardiac catheterization. The anatomy of coronary arteries in living, conscious humans was first demonstrated by non-selective injection of the aortic root. In the early 1960s David Littmann developed a loop catheter that enabled the injection of contrast medium preferentially in the outer circumference of the aortic root, opacifying the left and right coronary arteries simultaneously. At the time it was commonly believed that selective injection of contrast material into a coronary artery would have fatal consequences. This changed when Mason Sones accidentally performed the first selective coronary angiogram without harm. He was intending to inject the left ventricle, but the catheter recoiled across the aortic valve and into the right coronary artery. Sones, a cardiologist by training, went on to develop a safe method of selective coronary angiography from the brachial artery cut-down approach using the flexible-tip catheter bearing his name. At the same time Melvin Judkins, a radiologist by training, was perfecting his own method of selective coronary angiography, using preshaped catheters, from a percutaneous femoral artery approach. Both methods have continued to be practised, although the percutaneous femoral, or Judkins' approach, has become most popular because of its speed and simplicity. In recent years there has been a return to the brachial and even radial artery approach using percutaneous methods, which enable more rapid patient ambulation.

Normal coronary anatomy is demonstrated in Fig. 8. A patient's anatomy is considered to be right- or left-dominant, depending upon whether the posterior descending artery arises from the right or left coronary artery, respectively. Approximately 80 per cent of humans are right-dominant.

Atherosclerotic disease is manifest by lesions that encroach upon the opacified lumen of the coronary artery (Fig. 9). Various approaches are used to grade the severity of these lesions. Most commonly a visual estimate of the percentage of the diameter of stenosis is given to each lesion. Lesion severity may be quantified by comparing the minimal lumen diameter within a lesion to the diameter of the nearest normal segment of artery. This can be done manually using callipers or automatically using computer-based systems for edge detection and contrast densitometry. Quantitative coronary angiography is a complex subject because it requires attention to many variables, such as selection of view and frame, and choice made from among several analytical techniques.

Early work by Lance Gould determined that a lesion must impair coronary blood flow to be clinically important. Although flow at rest is usually not reduced until the diameter of the stenosis exceeds 90 per cent, flow under stress may be reduced when the diameter of the stenosis is 70 per cent. The clinical impact of a stenosis of any given severity is also dependent upon the degree of collateral flow into the vascular bed distal to the stenosis.

Flow and pressure may be directly measured in the coronary artery by means of special guidewires that have pressure transducers or Doppler flow transducers mounted near their tips. As mentioned above, the flow at rest may be normal across a particular coronary artery stenosis. Coronary flow normally increases after maximal vasodilatation induced by local vasodilators. The quotient of the vasodilated flow divided by the resting flow is called the coronary flow reserve, which is normally greater than two. If not, the lesion in question is considered to be haemodynamically important. Pressure can be measured in the coronary artery at a location distal to a lesion using a guidewire with a transducer at its tip. The quotient of pressure distal to a lesion compared to the proximal pressure during maximal vasodilatation is called the fractional flow reserve. A quotient less than 0.75 is considered to be clinically important.

Intravascular ultrasound

Intravascular ultrasound (**IVUS**) is accomplished by advancing a catheter over a guidewire previously placed into a coronary artery. The catheter has a miniature ultrasound transducer near its tip, which enables rotational Doppler imaging of the vessel wall in a plane perpendicular to its axis. IVUS is particularly useful for assessing the nature of angiographically questionable lesions, determining the true size of the vessel prior to stent deployment, and assessing the completeness of stent deployment. It is also probably the best method for serial studies of coronary anatomy during drug treatment trials, because it is able to image the plaque itself and is therefore a more sensitive method than angiography.

Table 4 Complications of cardiac catheterization from a prospective study of 1559 procedures performed on 1483 United States Veterans having valvular heart disease during the years 1977–1982[*]

Type of complication	Frequency (%)
Death within 24 h	0.1
Death between 24 h and 30 days	0.1
Stroke	0.3
Transient cerebral ischaemia	0.1
Myocardial infarction	0.2
Peripheral arterial embolism	0.1
Occlusion of arterial access site	1.5
Brachial artery	2.9
Femoral artery	0.4
Bleeding	0.2
Cardiac tamponade	0.3
Ventricular fibrillation	0.5
Arrhythmia other than ventricular fibrillation	1.5
Primary hypotension	0.5
Reaction to contrast medium (allergic and renal)	1.8
Arterial perforation or dissection	0.3
Miscellaneous complications	1.4
Patients having one or more of the above complications	6.9

[*] Although this is a high-risk group of patients undergoing extensive study, the rates are very comparable to what should be expected today. In fact, some complications, especially bleeding, are now more frequent due to aggressive anticoagulation and antiplatelet treatments given to many patients prior to and during catheterization.

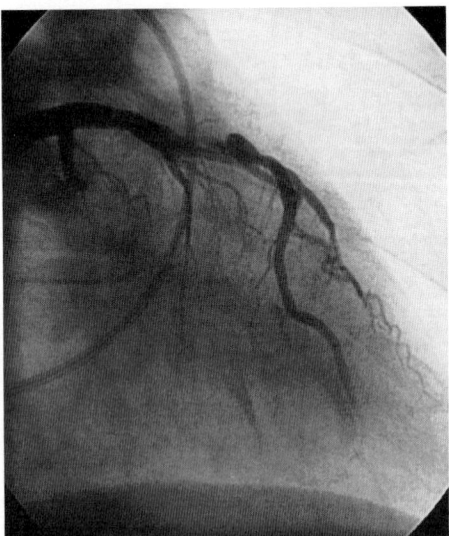

Fig. 9 Atherosclerotic coronary artery disease. The constrictions and blunt terminations seen in this patient's coronary angiogram represent atherosclerotic lesions.

Complications

Although cardiac catheterization is a relatively safe procedure, it is nevertheless important for both the patient and the referring physician to recognize the nature and likelihood of potential complications. Table 4 lists the complications of bilateral heart catheterization including coronary, left ventricular, and aortic angiography in a prospective study of valvular heart disease from the United States Veterans Administration. Even though these data were collected over 20 years ago from a particularly high-risk group of patients, the frequency of complication is a realistic estimate of what should currently be expected. The rate of each particular complication will vary with the age and general health of the patient. For example, the risk of vascular complication is considerably increased by the presence of vascular disease, and the risk of renal failure due to contrast medium is particularly high in diabetic patients with pre-existing renal dysfunction. Therefore, in counselling the patient regarding the likelihood of untoward events it is important to give individualized advice based upon the patient's particular circumstances. Finally, the decision to recommend catheterization must be based upon the anticipation that its benefits justify its cost and risk.

Further reading

Baim DS, Grossman W, eds (2000). *Cardiac catheterization, angiography, and intervention*, 6th edn. Williams and Wilkins, Baltimore. [This is a standard textbook for the field of invasive cardiology. It covers all the subjects presented in this chapter in greater detail and gives detailed references to primary sources.]

15.4 Ischaemic heart disease

15.4.1 Epidemiology

15.4.1.1 Influences acting *in utero* and early childhood

D. J. P. Barker

The fetal origins hypothesis

Over the past 10 years epidemiological studies have shown that people who had low birthweight, or who were thin or short at birth, are at increased risk of developing ischaemic heart disease and the related disorders stroke, hypertension, and non-insulin dependent diabetes (NIDDM). Associations between small size at birth and later disease, first recorded in Britain, have now been extensively replicated in studies in Europe and the United States. The associations extend across the whole range of birthweight and depend on lower birthweights in relation to the duration of gestation rather than the effects of premature birth. They are not the result of confounding variables acting in later life, such as low socio-economic status and smoking.

These observations have given rise to the 'fetal origins hypothesis', which proposes that cardiovascular disease originates through adaptations which are made by a fetus when it is under-nourished. Unlike adaptations made in adult life, those made during early development tend to have permanent effects on the body's structure and function—a phenomenon sometimes referred to as programming.

Fetal nutrition

In common with other living creatures, human beings are 'plastic' in their early life, and are shaped by their environment. Although the growth of a fetus is influenced by its genes, studies in humans and animals suggest that it is limited by the environment, in particular by the nutrients and oxygen the fetus receives from the mother. The fetus responds to undernutrition in a number of ways. It can redistribute its cardiac output to protect key organs, the brain in particular; it can alter its metabolism, for example by switching from glucose to amino acid oxidation; and it can change the production of, or tissue sensitivity to, hormones regulating growth, in which insulin has a central role. Slowing of growth is also adaptive because it reduces the requirement for substrate. Experiments show that even minor modifications to the diets of pregnant animals may be followed by life-long changes in the offspring in ways that can be related to human disease, for example raised blood pressure and altered glucose–insulin metabolism.

Birthweight serves as a marker of fetal nutrition and growth, but it is an imperfect one. The fetus can adapt to undernutrition and continue to grow at the same rate, but with permanently altered physiology and metabolism. Furthermore, the same birthweight may be the outcome of many different paths of growth. Where more detailed measurements of body size at birth are available they can give insights into adaptations that the fetus has made. For example babies that are thin, though within the normal range of birthweight, tend to be insulin resistant as children and adults and are therefore liable to develop NIDDM. It seems that the thin baby responds to undernutrition through endocrine changes.

Ischaemic heart disease

An important clue suggesting that ischaemic heart disease might originate during fetal development came from studies of death rates among babies in Britain during the early 1900s. The usual certified cause of death in newborn babies at that time was low birthweight. Death rates in the new-born differed considerably between one part of the country and another, being highest in some of the northern industrial towns and the poorer rural areas in the north and west. This geographical pattern in death rates was shown to closely resemble today's large variations in death rates from ischaemic heart disease, variations that form one aspect of the continuing inequalities in health in Britain. One possible conclusion suggested by this observation is that low rates of growth before birth are in some way linked to the development of ischaemic heart disease in adult life.

The subsequent studies that confirmed the association between ischaemic heart disease and small size at birth were based on the simple strategy of examining men and women in middle and late life whose body measurements at birth were recorded. In the first study of this kind, 16 000 men and women born in Hertfordshire, United Kingdom, during 1911 to 1930 were traced from birth to the present day. Death rates from ischaemic heart disease fell two-fold between those at the lower and upper ends of the birthweight distribution (Fig. 1). A study in Sheffield, United Kingdom, showed that it was people who were small at birth because they failed to grow, rather than because they were born early, who were at increased risk of the disease. The association between low birthweight and ischaemic heart disease has been confirmed in studies of men in Uppsala (Sweden), Helsinki (Finland), and Caerphilly (Wales), and among women in Helsinki and the United States. Among 80 000 women in the American Nurses Study there was a two-fold fall in the relative risk of non-fatal ischaemic heart disease across the range of birthweight. An association between low birthweight and prevalent ischaemic heart disease has recently been shown in a small study in South India. Among Indian men and women aged 45 years and over the prevalence of the disease fell from 18 per cent in those who weighed 5.5 lb (2.5 kg) at birth to 4 per cent in those who weighed 7 lb (3.2 kg) or more.

Some of these epidemiological studies included birth length, and other measurements of size at birth, in addition to weight. In Sheffield and in India, rates of ischaemic heart disease were higher in men who had short body length at birth. Thinness at birth, as measured by a low ponderal index (birthweight/length^3), has also been found to be associated with ischaemic heart disease. Among men born in Helsinki, Finland, while low

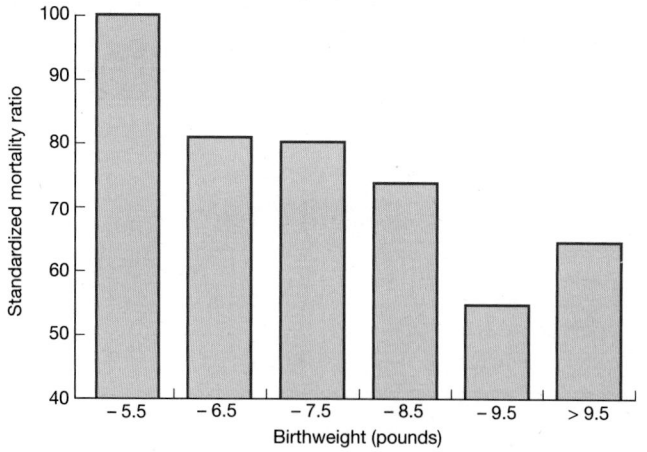

Fig. 1 Death rates from ischaemic heart disease in 15 726 men and women born in Hertfordshire according to their birthweights.

birthweight was associated with raised death rates for ischaemic heart disease, there was a stronger association with thinness at birth, especially in men born at term (Fig. 2). Among women in the same cohort, those who developed ischaemic heart disease also had low birthweight but were short at birth rather than thin. Since the men and women were born to the same group of mothers this difference may reflect intrinsic differences between the sexes in their paths of fetal growth. In the whole cohort, body proportions at birth differed in the sexes: the girls tended to be short while the boys tended to be thin. This may reflect differences in rates of fetal growth at similar levels of maternal nutrition. Female fetuses grow more slowly from an early stage of gestation and are therefore less vulnerable to undernutrition. The lower rates of ischaemic heart disease among women could be related to their slower rates of growth *in utero*.

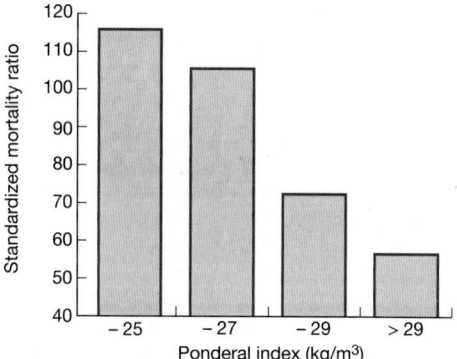

Fig. 2 Death rates from ischaemic heart disease in 3302 Finnish men born at term according to their ponderal indices at birth (birthweight/length³).

Stroke

The pattern of body proportions at birth which predicts stroke is different to that which predicts ischaemic heart disease. Whereas stroke is similarly associated with low birthweight it is not associated with thinness or shortness. Instead, the studies in Sheffield and Helsinki found increased rates among men who had a low ratio of birthweight to head circumference. One interpretation of this is that normal head growth was sustained at the cost of interrupted growth of the body in late gestation. 'Brain-sparing' patterns of growth can result from diversion of cardiac output to the brain at the expense of the abdominal viscera, importantly the liver. Preliminary evidence suggests that this has lasting effects on liver function including altered regulation of low density lipoprotein cholesterol and raised plasma fibrinogen concentrations, a known risk factor for stroke.

Hypertension

Studies of the mechanisms linking low birthweight with ischaemic heart disease have shown that the progressive fall in disease rates across the range of birthweight (Fig. 1) is paralleled by progressive falls in two of its major biological risk factors—hypertension and NIDDM. Associations between low birthweight and raised systolic and diastolic pressure in childhood and adult life have been extensively documented around the world. Averaged across 69 studies, the difference in systolic pressure associated with a 1-kg difference in birthweight is around 3.5 mmHg. In clinical practice this would be small, but it is a large difference between the mean values of populations. Available data suggest that lowering the mean systolic pressure in a population by 10 mmHg would correspond to a 30 per cent reduction in total attributable mortality. Although in these studies alcohol consumption and higher body mass were also associated with raised blood pressure, the associations between birthweight and blood pressure were independent of them. Nevertheless, body mass remains an important influence on blood pressure and, in humans and animals, the highest blood pressures are found in those who were small at birth but become overweight as adults.

Table 1 shows the systolic pressures of a group of 50-year-old men and women who were born at term in Preston, United Kingdom. The subjects are grouped according to their birthweights and placental weights. Consistent with findings in other studies, systolic pressure fell between subjects with low and high birthweight. In addition, however, there was an increase in blood pressure with increasing placental weight. Subjects with a mean systolic pressure of 150 mmHg or more, a level sometimes used to define hypertension in clinical practice, comprised a group who as babies were small in relation to the size of their placentas. A rise in blood pressure with increasing placental weight has also been found in children in Salisbury, United Kingdom, and Adelaide, Australia, but in studies of children and adults the association between placental enlargement and raised blood pressure or ischaemic heart disease has been inconsistent.

As yet, we know little about the mechanisms which underlie the association between low rates of fetal growth and raised blood pressure. One suggestion is that retarded fetal growth leads to a reduced number of nephrons which in turn leads to increased pressure in the glomerular capillaries and the development of glomerular sclerosis. Another hypothesis

Table 1 Mean systolic blood pressure (mmHg) of men and women aged 50, born after 38 completed weeks of gestation, according to placental weight and birthweight

Birthweight lb (kg)	Placental weight lb (g)				
	−1.0 (454)	−1.25 (568)	−1.5 (681)	>1.5 (681)	All
− 6.5 (2.9)	149 (24)	152 (46)	151 (18)	167 (6)	152 (94)
− 7.5 (3.4)	139 (16)	148 (63)	146 (35)	159 (23)	148 (137)
> 7.5 (3.4)	131 (3)	143 (23)	148 (30)	153 (40)	149 (96)
All	144 (43)	148 (132)	148 (83)	156 (69)	149[a] (327)

[a] s.d. = 20.4

Figures in parentheses are number of subjects.

which is being actively investigated is that fetal undernutrition leads to life-long changes in the fetus' hypothalamic–pituitary–adrenal axis and these in turn reset homeostatic mechanisms controlling blood pressure. Excessive cortisone production, as occurs in Cushing's syndrome, is associated with raised blood pressure and people who were small at birth have elevated plasma cortisol concentrations within the normal range. A third hypothesis derives from the observation that men and women in Sheffield who were small at birth had reduced elasticity in the large arteries of the trunk and legs, and raised blood pressure. The elasticity of larger arteries depends on elastin, which is laid down *in utero* and during infancy and thereafter turns over slowly: its half-life is 40 years. The amount of elastin laid down *in utero* increases with blood flow. 'Brain-sparing' diversion of blood to the brain could therefore lead to permanent loss of elasticity in the large arteries of the trunk.

Non-insulin dependent diabetes

Both insulin resistance and deficiency in insulin production are thought to be important in the pathogenesis of NIDDM. There is evidence that both may originate during fetal life. Men and women with low birthweight and a low ponderal index have a high prevalence of the 'insulin resistance syndrome', in which impaired glucose tolerance, hypertension, and raised serum triglyceride concentrations occur in the same patient. The patients are insulin resistant and hyperinsulinaemic. A number of studies have shown that people who had low birthweight are already insulin resistant in childhood. A study of men and women who were *in utero* during the war-time famine in Holland provides direct evidence that maternal undernutrition can programme insulin resistance and NIDDM in the offspring. The 'Dutch famine' began abruptly in November 1944 and ended with the liberation of Holland in 1945. The official rations varied between 400 and 800 calories per day. Men and women exposed to the famine *in utero* had higher 2-h plasma glucose concentrations after a standard oral glucose challenge than those born before or conceived after it. They also had higher fasting plasma proinsulin and 2-h plasma insulin concentrations, suggesting insulin resistance.

Figure 3 brings together some of the ideas and findings about the mechanisms through which ischaemic heart disease may be programmed *in utero*. It is a working hypothesis and will need to be re-evaluated as more information becomes available.

Ischaemic heart disease and childhood growth

As already described, babies that have low birthweight and are thin or short are at increased risk of ischaemic heart disease in adult life. We are beginning to learn how childhood growth modifies this risk. In the Helsinki study, ischaemic heart disease was commonest among men who were thin at birth, but who 'caught-up' in weight before the age of 7 years and had above average body mass index thereafter. Among women in the same cohort, those who developed ischaemic heart disease were short at birth but had accelerated growth in height in childhood. Table 2 shows that among men with the lowest ponderal indices at birth, but the highest body mass indices in childhood, the risk of ischaemic heart disease was five times that of men with the highest ponderal indices but lowest body mass indices in childhood. It is not known why accelerated postnatal growth is detrimental. One speculation is based on the observation that restricted fetal growth leads to permanently reduced cell numbers in tissues such as the kidney, in which there is no further cell replication after birth. Accelerated postnatal growth could be deleterious either because overgrowth of a limited cell mass disrupts cell function or because large body size imposes an excessive metabolic demand on a limited cell mass.

Whatever underlies the association between death from ischaemic heart disease and accelerated growth in height and weight in early childhood,

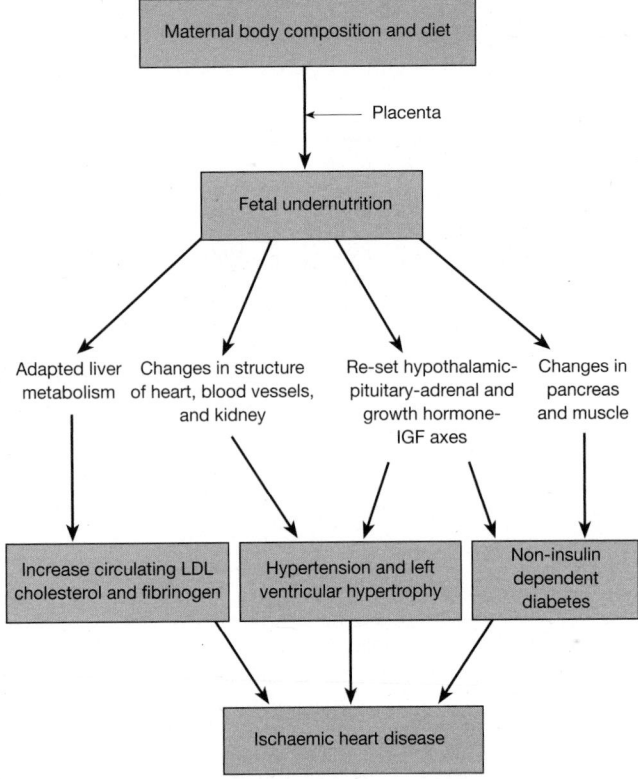

Fig. 3 Framework of possible mechanisms linking fetal undernutrition and ischaemic heart disease.

imbalances between prenatal and postnatal growth seem to be important in the genesis of adult disease. The effects of adult obesity are a further illustration of this. The highest prevalence of NIDDM is found in people who had low birthweight but become obese as adults. The Dutch famine had its greatest effect on the glucose tolerance of men and women who were overweight as adults.

Maternal nutrition

The nutrition of the fetus depends on the nutrition of the mother. In recent years 'maternal nutrition' has been equated with the diets of pregnant women. This is too limited a definition. Mellanby wrote in 1933 that 'it is certain that the significance of correct nutrition in child-bearing does not begin in pregnancy itself or even in the adult female before pregnancy. It looms large as soon as a female child is born and indeed in its intrauterine life'. Maternal nutrition defined in this way encompasses the nutritional experience of the mother from her own conception, through fetal life, childhood, and into adolescence and adult life. The Helsinki study shows

Table 2 Hazard ratios for death from ischaemic heart disease according to ponderal index at birth and body mass index at age 11 years, adjusted for length of gestation

Ponderal index (kg/m³) at birth	Body mass index (kg/m²) at age 11 years			
	– 15.5	– 16.5	– 17.5	> 17.5
≤ 25	2.7 (21)	3.3 (26)	3.7 (19)	5.3 (14)
– 27	1.5 (14)	3.2 (40)	4.0 (35)	2.7 (14)
– 29	2.2 (17)	1.6 (18)	1.8 (19)	3.2 (21)
> 29	1.0 (4)	1.7 (11)	1.5 (12)	1.9 (12)

Figures in parentheses are number of deaths.

BMI cutpoints are approximately quartiles.

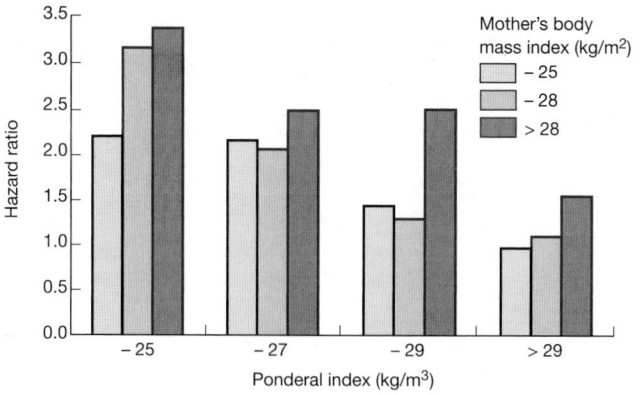

Fig. 4 Hazard ratios for ischaemic heart disease in Finnish men according to their ponderal indices at birth (birthweight/length^3) and their mother's body mass indices (weight/height^2).

that the mother's body composition before and during pregnancy is an important influence in programming the fetus. Figure 4 shows mortality from ischaemic heart disease according to the men's ponderal indices and their mothers' body mass indices (weight/height^2) in late pregnancy. At any ponderal index, death rates were higher in men whose mothers had a high body mass, so that the highest rates were in men who were thin at birth but whose mothers had a high body mass. The effect of body mass was confined, however, to the offspring of mothers of below average stature (below 1.58 m). The processes by which high body mass in short mothers compounds the increased risk of ischaemic heart disease that is associated with thinness at birth are currently under investigation. The findings already described suggest that raised plasma glucose concentrations in overweight women, which necessarily lead to higher glucose intakes by the fetus, may be one influence.

There is now a body of evidence suggesting that mothers who are thin also afford an unfavourable environment to their fetuses, leading to insulin resistance and raised blood pressure in the offspring. In the Dutch famine, for example, it was people born to mothers with the lowest weights in pregnancy who had the highest 2-h plasma glucose concentrations. Maternal thinness may have different consequences for the fetus depending on whether it is reflected in a low body mass index, low weight gain in pregnancy, or low skinfold thickness. Mothers' diet in pregnancy has been directly related to cardiovascular risk factors in the offspring during adult life in studies in Aberdeen, Scotland. The blood pressures of men and women were related to the balance of animal protein and carbohydrate in their mothers' diets in late pregnancy, while high intakes of fat and protein were associated with insulin deficiency. The findings of this small study are currently being examined in a larger study in Scotland.

Conclusion

Studies of programming in fetal life and infancy are now established in the agenda for medical research. They have refocused attention on maternal nutrition and fetal growth. The search for the environmental causes of ischaemic heart disease has hitherto been guided by a 'destructive' model. The causes to be identified act in adult life and accelerate destruction processes: the formation of atheroma, rise in blood pressure, and loss of glucose tolerance. There is now a 'developmental' model for the disease. The causes to be identified act on the baby. In responding to them the baby ensures its continued survival and growth at the expense of premature death from ischaemic heart disease.

Further reading

Barker DJP (1998). *Mothers, babies and health in later life*, 2nd edn. Churchill Livingstone, Edinburgh.

Bateson P, Martin P (1999). *Design for a life*. Jonathan Cape, London.

O'Brien PMS, Wheeler T, Barker DJP (1999). *Fetal programming: influence on development and disease in later life*. RCOG Press, London.

15.4.1.2 The epidemiology of ischaemic heart disease

A. R. Ness and G. Davey Smith

Introduction

Ischaemic heart disease (IHD) is defined by a joint International Society and Federation of Cardiology and World Health Organization task force as 'myocardial impairment due to an imbalance between coronary blood flow and myocardial requirements caused by changes in the coronary circulation.' In this chapter we will focus on the epidemiology of the clinical manifestations of IHD. These include angina pectoris, myocardial infarction, and coronary death.

Atherosclerosis is clearly an important underlying pathological process in IHD. Other non-coronary manifestations of atherosclerotic disease include stroke, peripheral vascular disease, and aortic aneurysm. These different conditions share some epidemiological features but show distinct patterns in other respects. For example there is little correlation between IHD and stroke mortality across countries, and within Britain aortic aneurysm mortality correlates negatively with both stroke and IHD mortality. It therefore makes more sense to consider the epidemiology of these conditions separately rather than together.

The process of atheroma deposition and arterial narrowing in the coronary vasculature cannot be observed directly in life without the use of invasive clinical procedures such as coronary angiography. The thickness of carotid arteries measured ultrasonically is currently under evaluation and may prove to be a useful marker of atheroma. Even so, the study of symptomatic disease rather than the underlying process of atheroma deposition may actually be more appropriate. The clinical disease is, after all, what is experienced and may represent the culmination of a number of pathological processes. Indeed, the fact that changes in atherosclerosis at post mortem over time do not mirror changes in clinical IHD rates suggest that it would be unwise to concentrate on the epidemiology of a single pathological process.

IHD is a—or the—leading cause of death in most developed countries. The rates of such deaths in men and women from the populations participating in the World Health Organization MONICA (monitoring trends and determinants in cardiovascular disease) study, which established arrangements to monitor the mortality and incidence of coronary disease (using comparable coding criteria) over a 10-year period in 37 defined populations (in 21 countries), are shown in Fig. 1. Large differences in disease rates between countries, evidence that risk of disease changes on migration, large differences within countries according to socioeconomic position and area of residence, and relatively rapid changes (both increases and decreases in rates of IHD mortality and incidence over time) suggest that the disease is preventable. In this chapter as we describe the epidemiology of IHD we will attempt to relate these findings to the potential for IHD prevention, considering medical therapy only to the extent that it informs our understanding of disease aetiology and prevention.

The burden of ischaemic heart disease

Around one-quarter of all deaths amongst men and one-fifth of all deaths of women in Britain are due to IHD. Among women the proportion is relatively stable throughout the adult years, whilst in men it peaks among 55 to 64-year-olds, for whom IHD accounts for a third of all deaths. Around 6 per cent of 55 to 64-year-old men and 3 per cent of 55 to 64-year-old women report experiencing angina; this increases to 13 per cent and 9 per cent respectively for those aged 75 and over. The National Health Service in England deals with around 200 000 inpatient episodes due to IHD for men and 100 000 for women each year, representing around 5 per cent of all hospital inpatient episodes for men and 3 per cent for women. In addition, there are around 30 million work days lost due to certified incapacity for IHD amongst men and over 4 million amongst women each year in Britain.

A historical perspective

Ischaemic heart disease was until recently viewed largely as a twentieth-century epidemic. In retrospect it seems clear that IHD and IHD deaths occurred before the formal medical description of myocardial infarction in the early years of the twentieth century. William Heberden described the typical symptoms of angina pectoris and the fact that sudden death occurred as a complication in 1768. Later in the eighteenth century, Dr Samuel Black of Newry, County Down, described many cases of angina pectoris and produced a list of factors associated with increased and decreased susceptibility to angina (Table 1). While angina pectoris was

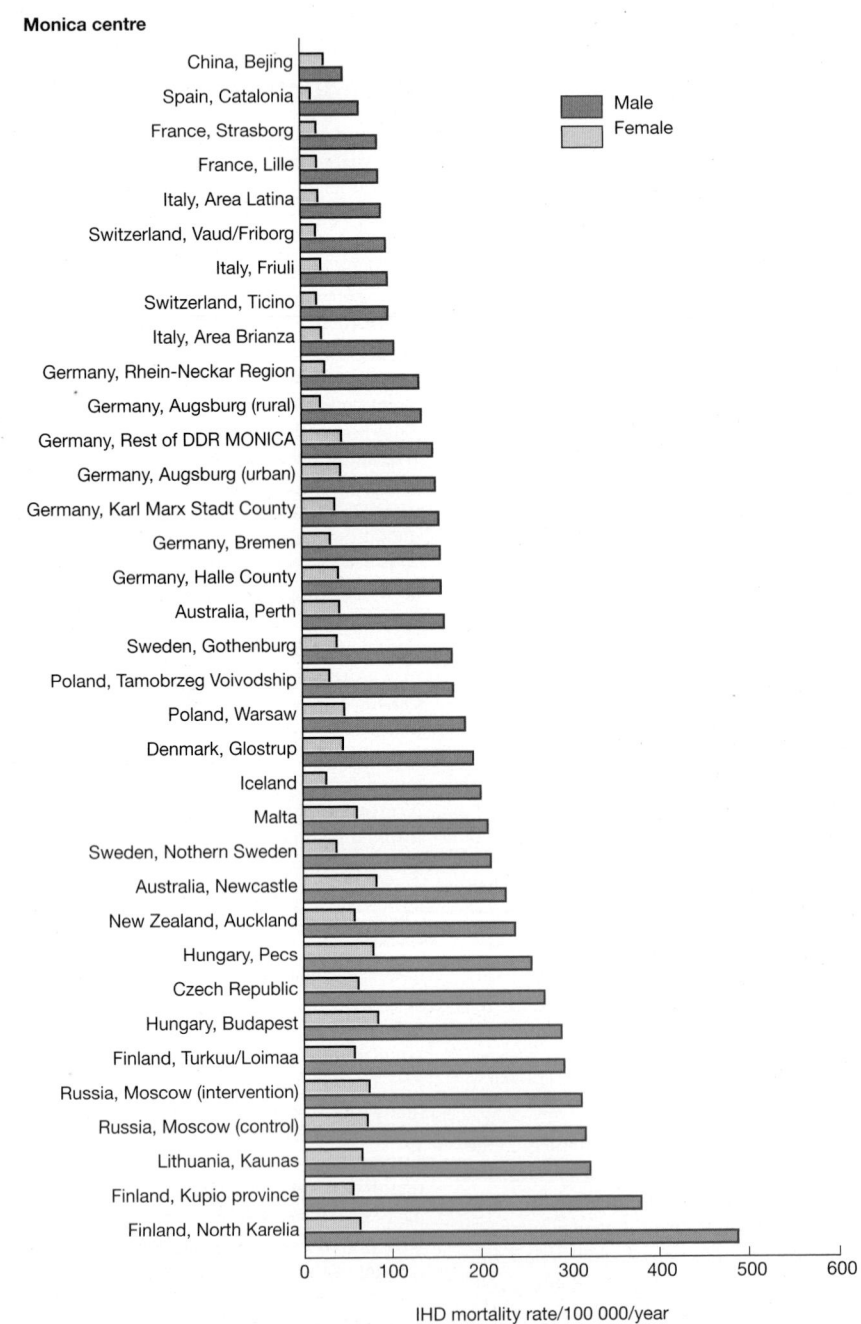

Fig. 1 Male and female IHD mortality rates in men and women aged 35 to 64 in 35 MONICA populations in the 1980s. Source: Lawlor DA, Ebrahim S, Davey Smith G (2001). *British Medical Journal*, **323**, 541–5.

Table 1 Dr Samuel Black's categorization of factors related to liability and exemption from angina pectoris

Liable
The male sex
The better ranks of society
The psychologically stressed
Those with an ossific diathesis
Those with an accumulation of fat around the heart
Those with full and plethoric habits who live luxuriously
Those with insufficient exercise
The obese
Exempt
The female sex
The poor
The laborious
Those who use strong exercise
The foot-soldier
The French

Source: Evans A (1995). Dr Black's favourite disease. *British Heart Journal* **74**, 676–7.

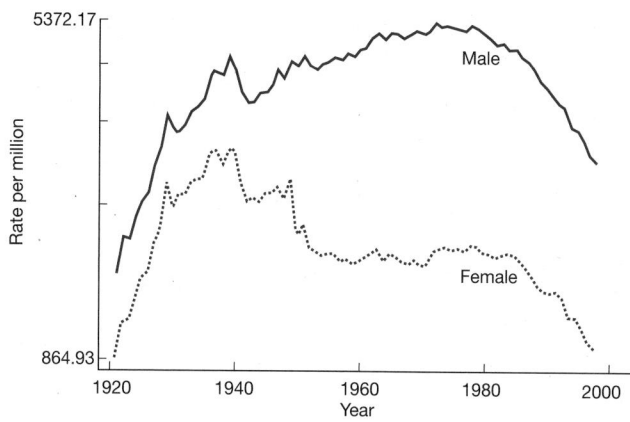

Fig. 2 Mortality from IHD, 1921 to 1998, ages 35 to 74, for England and Wales. Deaths per million population, age standardized to European population. Source: Lawlor DA, et al. (2001). *British Medicial Journal* **323**, 541–5.

occasionally recorded as a cause of death, less than 2 per cent of all deaths attributed to heart disease in Britain fell into this category even by the early part of the twentieth century.

In the middle of the nineteenth century, Richard Quain described a condition he called 'fatty disease of the heart'. A retrospective review of his case series suggests that 52 out of 83 cases probably suffered from IHD. The pathologist Carl Weigert and clinician Carl Huber in Leipzig described the myocardial lesions induced by acute ischaemia and speculated that myocardial infarction and angina both reflected underlying coronary artery disease. Before the turn of the century myocardial infarction and coronary thrombosis were thought of as terminal events. The first diagnosis of acute coronary thrombosis in the living patient is generally attributed to two Russian doctors, Obrastzow and Straschesko, in 1910. By 1918 Herrick was able to link clinical information with electrocardiogram patterns shown to reflect myocardial infarction in experimental canine studies, making the antemortem diagnosis of myocardial infarction easier.

Atherosclerosis has retrospectively been demonstrated in Egyptian mummies, but the first contemporary descriptions occurred in the sixteenth century. As IHD is generally associated with advanced coronary atherosclerosis the dramatic increase in IHD mortality in the first half of this century would be expected to be accompanied by increasing evidence of severe atheroma. However, studies of post-mortem records of the London Hospital suggested that there was no such increase between 1908 and 1949; in fact the degree of coronary atheroma declined. This was interpreted as indicating that an increase in the risk of thrombosis was responsible for the increase in IHD incidence and mortality. Later data comparing the coronary arteries at post mortem of United States soldiers who died in the Korean and Vietnam War show a higher prevalence of atheroma in young men in the early 1950s (77 per cent with atherosclerosis, 15 per cent with clinically significant narrowing of vessels) than the 1960s (45 per cent and 5 per cent, respectively), while IHD mortality in the United States was high and stable over this period. A study in the United States covering the period 1980 to 89—when IHD mortality was declining rapidly—found no reduction in the prevalence of atherosclerosis. Hence the relative contribution of atherosclerosis and thrombotic tendency to trends over time and differences between countries in IHD mortality remain difficult to elucidate.

Trends in ischaemic heart disease in Britain

Despite problems of changing definition, IHD rates in Britain clearly increased from the beginning of the century until the 1980s for men, the pattern of change in women being somewhat different (Fig. 2, and see 'Gender', below). Since the late 1970s, IHD mortality has declined steadily in both men and women.

In men, total circulatory disease mortality increased in the early decades of the century until the 1970s, although not as dramatically as IHD mortality. In women, total circulatory disease has tended to decrease over the century and the rise of IHD has been less consistent (with some decreases in the decades before the mid-century), and much less marked in women than men. Between the 1920s and 1960s the male to female ratio of IHD death rates increased from around 1.5 to around 6 for those under 55; males showed excess mortality at older ages but to a less extreme degree, with the ratio being around 2.5 for 65 to 74 year olds. Sex ratios have remained stable since the 1960s. The rapid rise and fall in rate of death attributed to IHD suggests that these differences were environmental rather than genetic and point to the scope for prevention.

International trends in ischaemic heart disease

Non-socialist, developed countries other than Britain have shown a similar pattern of rise and then fall in IHD mortality. Some, such as the United States and Australia, have experienced an earlier and more rapid fall in mortality than that seen in the United Kingdom. The United Kingdom (and in particular Scotland and Northern Ireland) has one of the highest death rates in the world from IHD, while rates in Japan and the Mediterranean countries of Europe, such as Greece, are low. These international time trends for men are illustrated in Fig. 3.

More detailed data on recent trends in IHD incidence is available from the WHO MONICA study, which has shown that large differences between rates of death attributed to IHD do exist (Fig. 1), also that the recent trends in mortality are in part attributable to changes in event rates and in part to changes in case fatality. Other studies suggest that the recent falls in mortality attributed to IHD observed in the United States are largely due to reductions in case fatality rather than incidence. This suggests that interventions after myocardial infarction—such as aspirin, thrombolytics, β-blockers, and statin cholesterol lowering drugs—are reducing future mortality in groups with existing IHD.

Migrant studies

Studies of groups that migrate from a low-risk population to a high-risk population can provide valuable insights into the heritability of disease and the key stage of life at which risk is determined. Studies of Japanese migrants to Hawaii and mainland America suggest that as those of Japanese ancestry adopt Western lifestyles their risk of IHD increases. Thus the difference in risk between populations is at least in part environmental, rather than genetic. More puzzling is the fact that migrants to Australia from Greek islands, despite adopting many of the detrimental habits of their host country, are at lower risk of IHD. The acculturation process is clearly complex and it may be that Greek Australians adopt healthier lifestyles in other respects that counterbalance their increased fat consumption and smoking prevalence. Nevertheless, the experience of Greek migrants to Australia further emphasizes the ability of groups of individuals to modify their risk of subsequent IHD.

Overview of risk factors for IHD

There are a number of personal attributes, often described as risk factors, associated with the development of IHD. Some of these—such as age, sex, and family history—are fixed. Others, such as smoking and diet, are modifiable environmental exposures. Some, such as serum cholesterol and blood pressure, though modifiable, are really intermediate processes in the development of IHD and are a product of the interplay between an individual's genetic make-up and environmental exposures. A list of attributes associated with subsequent IHD, by no means exhaustive, is set out in Table 2. This list is not dissimilar to that proposed by Samuel Black over a 100 years earlier (Table 1).

Stamler suggests that the established major risk factors amenable to change are smoking, high blood pressure, high serum cholesterol, and diet. In a large study of middle-aged men in the United States, smokers in the

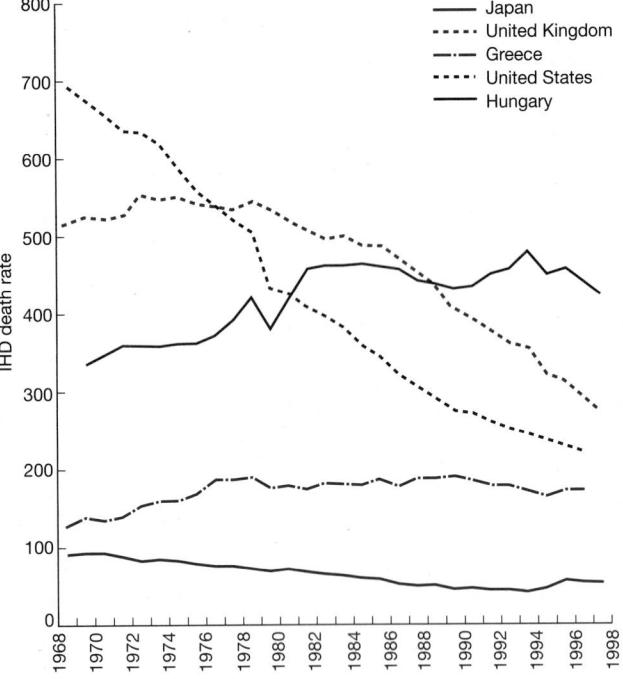

Fig. 3 Age-standardized death rates attributed to ischaemic heart disease from 1968 to 1997 in men aged 35 to 74 in selected countries. Source: Peterson S, Mockford C, Rayner M. *Coronary heart disease statistics 1999 edition.* British Heart Foundation, London, 1999.

Table 2 Personal attributes associated with ischaemic heart disease

Fixed factors	Exposure	Composite markers of risk
Age	Smoking	Serum lipids
Sex	Physical inactivity	Blood pressure
Family history	Diet	Lung function
Race of origin	Psychosocial stress	Haemostatic factors
Genotype	*In utero* experience	Obesity
	Infections	Insulin resistance
	Climatic factors	Hormonal status
		Homocysteine

highest quintiles for serum total cholesterol and systolic blood pressure were around 20 times as likely to die from IHD over the next 11.6 years as non-smokers in the lowest quintiles of serum cholesterol and blood pressure (Table 3). However, although these factors are powerful predictors of risk within a population, they only account for 23 per cent of the variance in IHD incidence in men and 14 per cent of the variance in women observed between 25 populations in the WHO MONICA study. Since these established major risk factors were described, many more risk factors have been suggested.

In the following sections we will discuss attributes associated with IHD, starting with fixed and relatively fixed risk markers, then covering the social environment and behavioural factors, finally considering physiological mediating processes.

Age

Age is the strongest risk indicator for IHD incidence and mortality. Compared to men aged 40, 50 year-old-men have five times the risk, 60 year-old-men have 15 times the risk, and 70-year-old men have over 40 times the risk of dying from IHD. A similar steep gradient with age is seen for women. Risk continues to increase into older age groups and recent evidence that the elderly benefit from risk factor control, blood pressure lowering, cholesterol lowering, and probably smoking cessation, combined with their much higher absolute level of risk than younger people, indicates that this is a group for whom sizeable absolute reductions in IHD risk can be achieved and therefore for whom therapies may be particularly cost effective.

Gender

Rates of death attributed to IHD in men are consistently three to four times higher than those in women across countries with differing background levels of disease. The rates of death attributed to IHD in women correlate closely with those in men, suggesting that environmental factors common to both sexes explain the international differences in ischaemic disease rates.

The temporal pattern of mortality attributed to IHD over the last 100 years in Britain has been different in women to that observed in men (Fig. 2). In men, mortality increased from the 1920s until the 1980s, when it began to decline. In women, the mortality rates have always been considerably lower than those observed in men. As with men, mortality in women increased in the early years of this century, but peaked around 1940. Mortality then declined until the 1960s, increased again until the mid-1970s, and has declined since then.

Despite the fact that women have been under represented in epidemiological studies of IHD, it nevertheless appears that classical risk factors such as serum total cholesterol, blood pressure, and smoking (shown to predict coronary disease in men) perform similarly in women. But as the disease is commoner in men the differences in absolute risk are much greater for men than for women.

Men are more likely to smoke than women are, but differences in smoking and other established coronary risk factor levels do not appear to fully explain the observed excess of IHD seen in men. The lower risk of coronary heart disease among women has understandably led to studies of sex hormones as potential protective or risk factors for IHD. There is, however, little empirical evidence to support an important role for sex hormones. It has often been stated that women are only protected against ischaemic heart disease premenopausally, and that their risk progressively increases towards that of men after the menopause. This supposition, which has recently been challenged, provided support for the notion that hormone replacement therapy taken after natural or artificial menopause would reduce the risk of IHD among women. Many observational studies (of women who had elected to take hormone replacement therapy) appeared to support this contention, but the preliminary findings of randomized, controlled trials (where women were allocated at random to hormone

Table 3 Baseline cigarette smoking, quintiles of serum cholesterol, systolic blood pressure, and age-adjusted IHD mortality per 10 000 person years in 361 662 men enrolled in the Multiple Risk Factor Intervention Trial (MRFIT) after 11.6 years

Serum total cholesterol (mg/l)	Systolic blood pressure (mmHg)					
	<118	118–124	125–131	132–141	142+	Q5/Q1[a]
Non- smokers						
<182[b]	3.09	3.72	5.13	5.35	13.66	4.42
182–202	4.39	5.79	8.35	7.66	15.80	3.60
203–220	5.20	6.08	8.56	10.72	17.75	3.41
221–244	6.34	9.37	8.66	12.21	22.69	3.58
245+	12.36	12.68	16.31	20.68	33.40	2.70
Q5/1[a]	4.00	3.41	3.18	3.87	2.45	–
Smokers						
<182[b]	10.37	10.69	13.21	13.99	27.04	2.61
182–202	10.03	11.76	19.05	20.67	33.69	3.36
203–220	14.90	16.09	21.07	28.87	42.91	2.88
221–244	19.83	22.69	23.61	31.98	55.50	2.80
245+	25.24	30.50	35.26	41.47	62.11	2.46
Q5/1[a]	2.43	2.85	2.67	2.96	2.30	–

[a] Q5 is the highest quintile and Q1 is the lowest quintile.

[b] <182 mg/dl ≈ <4.68 mmol/l,

182–202 mg/dl ≈ 4.68–5.19 mmol/l,

203–220 mg/dl ≈ 5.22–5.66 mmol/l

221–244 mg/dl ≈ 5.68–6.27 mmol/l

> 245 mg/dl ≈ >6.30 mmol/l.

Source: Stamler J (1992). Established major coronary risk factors. In: Marmot M, Elliott P, eds. *Coronary heart disease epidemiology: from aetiology to public health*. Oxford University Press.

replacement therapy or placebo) suggest no such protection is given by hormone replacement therapy.

Further studies should allow more detailed study of the determinants of IHD in women. If these can also shed light on the reasons for the consistent sex difference in coronary disease they may, through uncovering important determinants of IHD risk, benefit both men and women.

Family history and genetic factors

A family history of IHD in first-degree relatives is associated with an increased risk of IHD over and above that produced by a shared environment. Currently identified, major, single gene conditions—for example familial hypercholesterolaemia—are of low prevalence, so that while they are associated with a large increase in relative risk for an individual, they contribute little to the overall population prevalence of IHD. Other polymorphisms with lower relative risks but greater prevalence are under investigation. The marked secular trends in IHD risk, change in risk on migration, and large differences between countries indicate that at the population level genetic factors must act in concert with environmental influences to produce population IHD rates, and that there is thus large scope for prevention. At the individual level, however, a strong family history of premature IHD means that an individual may have more to gain from intensive risk factor control than other members of the population.

Early-life influences

Until relatively recently the majority of epidemiological research on IHD focused on behavioural, physiological, socioeconomic, and psychological risk factors acting in adulthood. However, more recently it was noted that risk factors acting during adulthood could not account for all of the geographical and socioeconomic variation in IHD mortality, leading some to postulate that early-life influences could have a long lasting impact on IHD risk independent of adulthood risk factors. A series of studies have demonstrated that birth weight is inversely related to risk of IHD, suggesting that suboptimal intrauterine environments result in offspring who, many years later, are more likely to succumb to IHD. Furthermore, several conventional IHD risk factors have been shown to be related to birth weight—blood pressure, glucose tolerance, respiratory capacity, and (less consistently) haemostatic factors demonstrate associations with birthweight which would generate the observed inverse birthweight–IHD relationships. However, taking these risk factors into consideration does not appear to fully account for the influence of fetal development on IHD risk, which seems to involve other, as yet unspecified, pathways. It is possible that the birthweight–IHD associations, while they exist, are not causal and therefore not of public health significance. Genetic factors could underlie both low birthweight and increased disease risk in adulthood, and there is evidence that some polymorphisms could indeed act in this way. Whether modifying fetal development will modify later IHD risk is a matter that requires further investigation. These issues are discussed in detail in Chapter 15.4.1.1.

In addition to intrauterine influences, exposures acting in infancy, childhood, and adolescence may be of importance. A frequently replicated and long-standing observation is that taller individuals are at reduced risk of IHD. Growth occurs during infancy and childhood, being influenced by nutrition and infections, as well as genetic factors. Recently it has been shown that stature in childhood is inversely related to later IHD risk, indicating that the association between height and IHD mortality is not due to differential shrinkage occurring in adulthood amongst individuals most prone to IHD. Of the components of stature, leg length—rather than trunk length—is the one of importance, and this is particularly responsive to changes in nutrition and other environmental exposures acting during early childhood. Of the infections acquired in childhood *Helicobacter pylori* infection has been most widely investigated, but the overall evidence does not strongly point in the direction of a direct causal association between this infection and IHD risk. The role of nutrition and other infections acting in childhood requires more study if the intriguing associations between stature and IHD risk are to be understood.

Socio-economic position

In most industrialized countries, IHD risk is higher amongst people living in worse social circumstances. Whether the apparent gradients in the opposite direction seen during the early stages of the IHD epidemic in industrialized countries, and in newly industrialized countries currently, are genuine or due to differential classification of disease remains uncertain. Studies that have taken population samples and standardized measures of IHD prevalence or incidence—rather than simply using certified causes of death—have consistently shown a gradient of increasing risk with decreasing affluence. Social disadvantage can influence IHD risk in a wide variety of ways, and act across an individual's entire lifetime. People born into worse social circumstances are likely to have lower birthweight, which appears to influence later IHD risk. Socio-economic deprivation in childhood is associated with poor nutrition and growth, and possibly higher incidence of childhood infections, which may increase later IHD risk. Behavioural patterns—in particular with relation to diet, physical activity, alcohol consumption, and smoking—are developed in childhood in a socially-patterned manner and track into adulthood. In most industrialized countries, smoking and dietary patterns associated with increased IHD risk are more common amongst poorer adults. Unemployment and job insecurity in adulthood may also increase IHD risk.

Given the wide array of exposures associated with socio-economic deprivation that could increase the risk IHD, it is not surprising that studies which have taken into account a limited number of these (generally smoking, blood cholesterol, body mass index, alcohol consumption, leisure time physical activity, and blood pressure) find they fail to account fully for the socio-economic distribution of IHD. The large (and in many countries increasing) socio-economic differentials in IHD risk provide both a model for testing aetiological hypotheses and also evidence of an important potential for public health interventions. Figure 4 shows the three-fold difference in IHD mortality between men in unskilled manual occupations in Britain compared to those in managerial and professional occupations, and the graded difference in risk between these occupational extremes. Clearly, reducing IHD risk amongst the less socio-economically advantaged to the same level as that of the most advantaged would have a dramatic influence on overall diseases rates in the population. A further implication is that since socio-economically disadvantaged people have a considerably increased risk of IHD, which is not purely dependent upon conventional risk factors, they have the most to gain from interventions, such as the statin cholesterol-lowering drugs that produce a consistent proportional risk reduction amongst different groups of people treated. A 30 per cent reduction in risk for an unskilled manual labourer in Britain is, in absolute terms, a considerably greater risk reduction than a 30 per cent risk reduction in a manager.

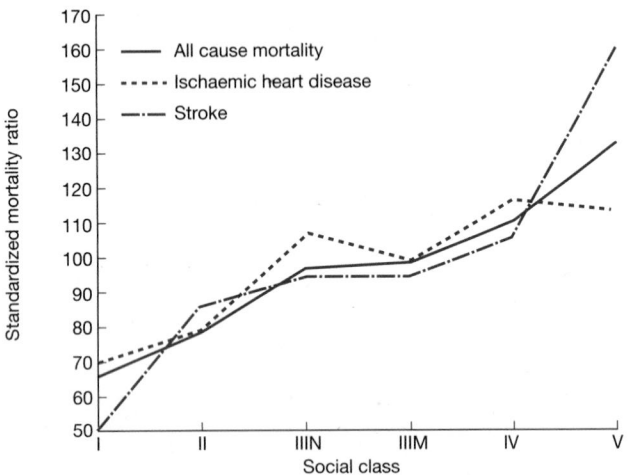

Fig. 4 Social class differences in mortality of men 15 to 64 between 1976 and 1989 from various causes of death. Source: Harding S. Social class differences in mortality of men: recent evidence from the OPCS Longitudinal Study. *Population Trends* 1995; **80**: 31–7.

Table 4 Diet and ischaemic heart disease[a]

Food pattern	Foods	Constituents
Vegetarian	Fruits	Energy intake
Mediterranean	Vegetables	Saturated fat (adverse)
Pacific	Fish	Monounsaturated fat
	Alcoholic drinks (in moderation)	Trans fat (adverse)
	Garlic	Antioxidant vitamins
	Coffee (adverse)	Antioxidant minerals
	Tea	Other antioxidants
	Nuts	Fibre
	Olive oil	Complex carbohydrates
		Phyto-oestrogens
		Sodium (adverse)
		B$_6$ and folate

[a]The dietary patterns, foods, or constituents are believed to be protective unless marked as adverse.

Diet

The association of diet and IHD can be thought of on three levels: the overall dietary patterns, the foods eaten, and the constituents of the diet. The dietary features thought to be associated with IHD are summarized in Table 4.

Overall dietary patterns

Certain regional dietary patterns are associated with low risk of IHD, for example the Mediterranean diet, which contains more fish, fresh fruit, fresh vegetables, and olive oil than the English diet. One small, randomized trial allocated people with a recent myocardial infarction to receive either advice to eat a Mediterranean diet (more bread, more vegetables, more fruit, more fish, and less meat) and to replace butter and cream with rapeseed margarine, or to usual dietary advice. After 27 months the trial was stopped early because there was a marked reduction in the relative risk of death in those given advice to eat a Mediterranean diet. Of particular interest is the observation that these dietary changes did not alter blood cholesterol levels, implying that the protective effect was not mediated through an effect on cholesterol. The results of this study require confirmation in further trials, and while it is unlikely that the very substantial reduction in IHD risk seen in this trial will be seen in future studies, it is clear that such dietary advice could produce a worthwhile influence on IHD rates.

The dietary patterns in East Asia (the pacific diet) are probably one reason for the low IHD rates there. The broad characteristics of the United States, Japanese, and Mediterranean diets are summarized in Table 5. These so-called traditional diets have changed considerably over recent years so that, for example, the Japanese diet now contains more meat and dairy products and less salted foods. Such changes make it difficult to interpret comparisons of dietary differences and time trends in IHD between countries. Within countries, vegetarians have a lower risk of IHD, but are different in a number of other ways that could influence IHD risk from non-vegetarians.

Foods eaten

Various foods have been linked to risk of IHD. These include alcoholic beverages, fish, fruits, and vegetables. Moderate consumption of alcoholic drinks appears to protect against IHD, with higher rates of IHD in teetotallers and heavy drinkers. Ecological comparisons suggest that wine may exert additional protection, but cohort studies appear to show that the type of beverage is unimportant. Recent studies have looked at the pattern of alcohol consumption as well as the average weekly consumption. People who indulge in sporadic- or binge-drinking appear to be at increased (rather than reduced) risk of IHD.

The low reported rates of IHD among the Inuit (formally known as Eskimos) led to work on the effect of eating fish on IHD risk. Some studies have

Table 5 Diet and rate of ischaemic heart disease in middle age in Greece, Japan, and the United States in the 1960s

		USA	Greece	Japan
Standardized IHD rates				
Age 0–64 (per 100 000 people)	Male	189	33	34
	Female	54	14	21
Diet in the 1960s				
Fat (% energy)		39	37	11
Saturated fat (% energy)		18	8	3
Vegetables (g/day)		171	191	198
Fruit (g/day)		233	463	34
Legumes (g/day)		1	30	91
Bread and cereals (g/day)		123	453	481
Meat (g/day)		273	35	8
Fish (g/day)		3	39	150
Alcohol (g/day)		6	23	22

Source: Willett WC (1994). Diet and health: what should we eat? *Science* **264**, 532–7.

shown that regular consumers of fish are at reduced IHD risk, while others have not. Two large trials of advice to eat more fish or fish oil capsules in people following a myocardial infarction suggest that intake of dietary fish or fish oil reduces total mortality by around 20 per cent.

The regular consumption of fresh fruit and vegetables is widely believed to be protective against IHD, but the exact size and nature of any beneficial effect is unclear. It is even possible that the observed protective associations represent residual confounding by other lifestyle factors, since people who eat more fruit and vegetables differ in many ways from those who eat less.

Dietary constituents

A number of dietary constituents have been associated with risk of IHD. These include energy intake, intake of various fats, antioxidants, and cereal fibre. The more energy consumed per day the lower the risk of IHD. Though obese people under-report food consumption, reported energy intake also reflects energy expenditure—that is level of physical activity. Hence this finding may reflect higher participation in exercise protecting against IHD.

The Seven Countries Study compared the diets of individuals from populations with different rates of IHD. It showed a strong association between IHD mortality and both total dietary fat and saturated fat consumption. The results of this study are shown in Fig. 5. Studies comparing individuals within cohorts have mostly failed to confirm this relationship, perhaps because of the problem of measuring diet accurately. The relationship between fats and IHD may also be more complex than first thought, with different fatty acids increasing, decreasing or having no effect on disease risk. There is some evidence that high intake of trans fatty acids, produced when oils are solidified by hydrogenation to form margarine, increases risk of IHD.

There is laboratory evidence that suggests that oxidation of cholesterol is an important step in atherosclerosis. This laboratory work has generated interest in the association between the intake of dietary antioxidants and rates of IHD. These include minerals such as copper, zinc, manganese, and selenium, vitamins (and provitamins) such as β-carotene, vitamin C, vitamin E, and other chemicals such as flavonoids. Though cohort studies have observed protective associations, the results of randomized trials—where they have been carried out—have not confirmed these observations.

Prospective observational studies of β-carotene intake showed a significantly lower pooled risk of cardiovascular death among those consuming more β-carotene. The results from the randomized trials, however, indicated a moderate adverse effect of β-carotene supplementation (Fig. 6). Various explanations have been put forward to account for these results, including the use of the wrong isomer of β-carotene, the wrong dose, and a

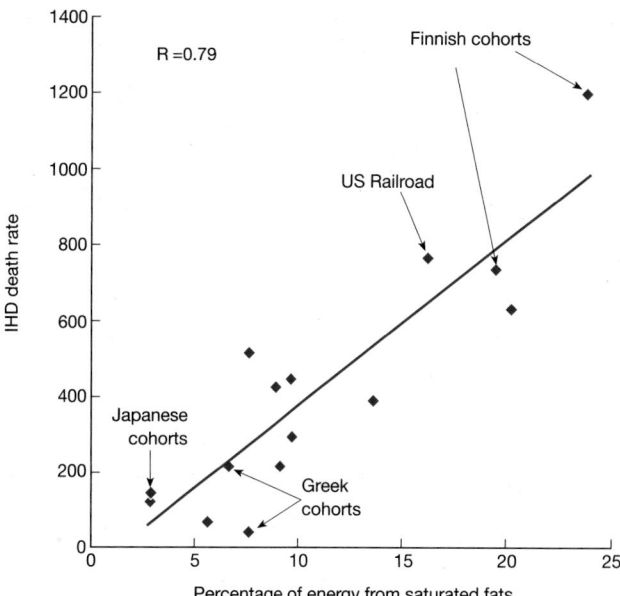

Fig. 5 Ecological comparison between percentage of calories from saturated fat consumed at baseline and IHD mortality over 15 years in 15 cohorts from seven countries recruited between 1958 and 1962. Source: Keys A, Menotti A, Karvonen MJ *et al*. The diet and 15-year death rate in the seven countries study. *American Journal of Epidemiology* 1986; **124**: 903–15

detrimental effect of supplementation on levels of other carotenoids. It is more likely that the apparent protective association in observational studies represents confounding, as people who eat diets rich in β-carotene or who take supplements are more socio-economically advantaged and adopt a number of protective health-related behaviours.

Similarly, most observational studies of vitamin E intake and IHD have reported a protective association, but cardiovascular mortality in trials is essentially unchanged in those receiving vitamin E (Fig. 7). In the case of β-carotene it was suggested that inappropriate supplements were used and that the trials were too short. These arguments are difficult to sustain for vitamin E, as the protective observational association was observed in

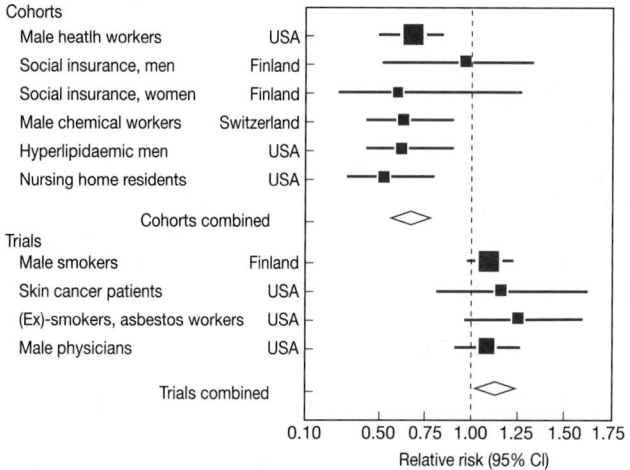

Fig. 6 Meta-analysis of the association between β-carotene intake and cardiovascular mortality: Results from observational studies indicate considerable benefit whereas the findings from randomized, controlled trials show an increase in the risk of death. Source: Egger M, Schneider M, Davey Smith G. Spurious precision? Meta-analysis of observational studies. *British Medical Journal* 1998; **316**: 140–144.

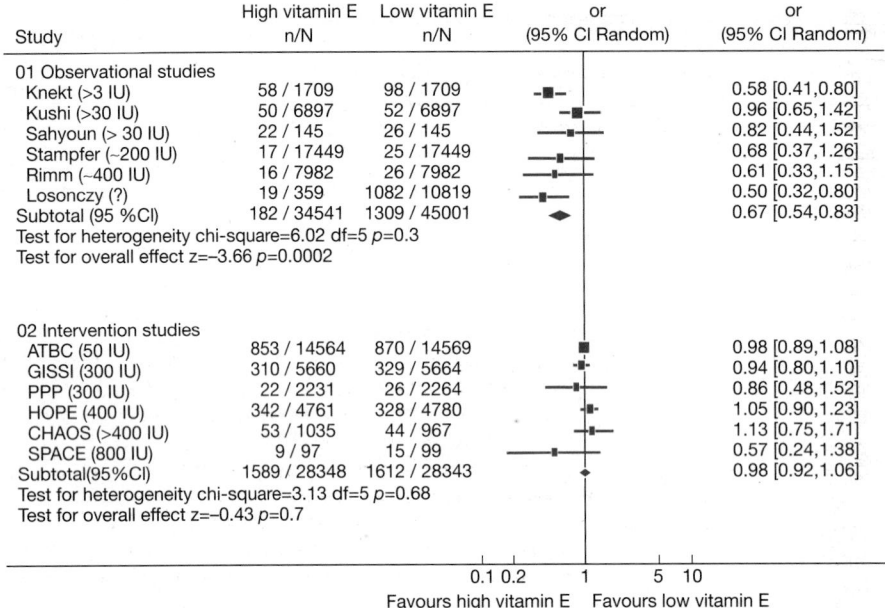

Study	High vitamin E n/N	Low vitamin E n/N	or (95% CI Random)	or (95% CI Random)
01 Observational studies				
Knekt (>3 IU)	58 / 1709	98 / 1709		0.58 [0.41,0.80]
Kushi (>30 IU)	50 / 6897	52 / 6897		0.96 [0.65,1.42]
Sahyoun (> 30 IU)	22 / 145	26 / 145		0.82 [0.44,1.52]
Stampfer (~200 IU)	17 / 17449	25 / 17449		0.68 [0.37,1.26]
Rimm (~400 IU)	16 / 7982	26 / 7982		0.61 [0.33,1.15]
Losonczy (?)	19 / 359	1082 / 10819		0.50 [0.32,0.80]
Subtotal (95 %CI)	182 / 34541	1309 / 45001		0.67 [0.54,0.83]

Test for heterogeneity chi-square=6.02 df=5 p=0.3
Test for overall effect z=−3.66 p=0.0002

	High vitamin E n/N	Low vitamin E n/N		
02 Intervention studies				
ATBC (50 IU)	853 / 14564	870 / 14569		0.98 [0.89,1.08]
GISSI (300 IU)	310 / 5660	329 / 5664		0.94 [0.80,1.10]
PPP (300 IU)	22 / 2231	26 / 2264		0.86 [0.48,1.52]
HOPE (400 IU)	342 / 4761	328 / 4780		1.05 [0.90,1.23]
CHAOS (>400 IU)	53 / 1035	44 / 967		1.13 [0.75,1.71]
SPACE (800 IU)	9 / 97	15 / 99		0.57 [0.24,1.38]
Subtotal(95%CI)	1589 / 28348	1612 / 28343		0.98 [0.92,1.06]

Test for heterogeneity chi-square=3.13 df=5 p=0.68
Test for overall effect z=−0.43 p=0.7

0.1 0.2   1   5   10
Favours high vitamin E   Favours low vitamin E

Fig. 7 Meta-analysis of the effect of high versus low vitamin E intake on cardiovascular mortality for observational and intervention studies. Source: Hooper L, Ness AR, Davey-Smith G (2001). *Lancet*, **357**, 1705. *n* = number of deaths; *N* = number at risk.

people taking supplements and in people who had only taken supplements for a few years. As with β-carotene, it is more likely that the protective association in observational studies represents confounding, but with vitamin E there is little evidence that supplements are harmful.

Cohort studies consistently report a protective association between increased intake of dietary fibre from cereals and reduced rates of IHD. One large trial randomized men with a recent history of myocardial infarction to receive advice to increase their dietary fibre intake (without making other changes to their diets) or no fibre advice. After 2 years there was no survival benefit in those randomized to receive fibre advice, indeed mortality was increased by about 20 per cent, though this increase was not statistically significant.

Summary of effect of diet on ischaemic heart disease

Dietary differences between populations and over time probably explain a considerable proportion of the temporal and geographical variation in IHD. The broad dietary patterns associated with reduced risk of IHD are not in dispute, but the relative importance of specific dietary features is less clear.

Smoking

Smoking was convincingly identified as a cause of lung cancer by German researchers in the 1930s and 1940s and suggestions about a detrimental effect on IHD were also made at this time, although backed by less elegant epidemiological evidence. Since the results of prospective epidemiological studies in the 1950s it has been clear that heavy cigarette smokers have an approximately two-fold elevation in risk of IHD incidence and death, which is reduced by giving up the use of cigarettes, the risk returning to close to that of non-smokers after about 10 years. Cigar smokers who have not previously smoked cigarettes do not have an increased risk of IHD, although amongst those who were previously cigarette smokers an increased risk is seen, presumably because cigarette smokers who switch to cigars continue to inhale some of the smoke.

The mechanism linking cigarette smoking and IHD remains unclear. Initially it was thought that nicotine was the important component of tobacco smoke, but the lack of elevated risk among primary cigar and pipe smokers who absorb nicotine through their buccal membranes suggests

this is not the case. In Sweden (among other countries), raw or porous-bagged tobacco ('snuss') is widely used, applied to the buccal membrane this leads to high nicotine absorption but no increased risk of IHD.

Smoking accounts for some of the international variation in IHD rates, but it is noticeable that some countries with a high prevalence of smoking, such as Japan, have low IHD rates. This is borne out by data from the MONICA study that found that smoking alone (when included in models that adjust for cholesterol and blood pressure) accounts for only 5 per cent of the variance in rates of death attributed to IHD across countries. At a cross-national level a relatively high level of saturated fat intake and circulating cholesterol level may be required for smoking to translate into high population rates of IHD. Similarly some populations—for example women of Indian subcontinent family origin living in Britain—have high rates of IHD despite having low rates of smoking.

Obesity

For nearly 100 years insurance data have demonstrated that very obese individuals have an increased risk of death, including death from heart disease. However, studying the association between degree of overweight and IHD risk has produced conflicting findings. In most studies, body mass index (BMI) (weight (in kilograms) divided by height (in metres) squared) is used as the index of adiposity. A U-shaped association between BMI and all-cause mortality has been seen in many studies, with a similar pattern observed for IHD mortality. The reasons for this have been hotly debated, but it seems likely that the high mortality among thin individuals reflects a subset of people who have low BMI because they are ill, or because behavioural patterns—heavy smoking or heavy alcohol consumption—are associated with thinness. The greater the degree to which studies have been able to take this into account, the less evident is the elevated mortality amongst the thin.

Obesity is at least partially related to higher IHD risk because it is in turn associated with higher blood pressure and an unfavourable blood lipid profile (higher low-density lipoprotein (LDL) cholesterol and lower high-density lipoprotein (HDL) cholesterol). Reducing weight is accompanied by reductions in blood pressure and an improvement in blood lipid profile, therefore the risk factor profile associated with obesity should be considered to contribute to the mechanism linking overweight to IHD, rather than being seen as confounding factors. In some early epidemiological studies this issue was confused and investigators statistically adjusted the association between degree of overweight and IHD risk for these physiological measures, which is clearly inappropriate given that they are themselves influenced by the degree of overweight.

Obesity is associated with insulin resistance (which is covered in the next section) and this may also contribute to the elevated IHD risk amongst the obese. However, compared to a simple relative weight measure, such as BMI, the distribution of body fat is more strongly associated with insulin resistance. In epidemiological studies, the ratio of a waist measurement to a hip measurement (waist–hip ratio) has been used as an indicator of central adiposity. People with higher waist–hip ratios are at increased risk of IHD above and beyond the fact that people with high BMI tend to have higher waist–hip ratios; they also demonstrate adverse profiles of factors associated with insulin resistance. Prospective studies are currently examining other measures of adiposity such as impedance (which estimates percentage of body fat) and abdominal height (which estimates the amount of abdominal fat) to see if they are better predictors of IHD risk than BMI and waist–hip ratio.

Conventional hereditability models applied to studies of twins, adoptees, and siblings suggest that obesity is, to a remarkable degree, a genetic characteristic of individuals, with only a small proportion of the population variance being accounted for by environmental factors. This finding probably reflects the limitations of the methods available to study genetic contributions to population levels of risk factors. The substantial changes in the prevalence of obesity that have occurred within populations such as the United States or the United Kingdom over a relatively short period of time—during which there is essentially no genetic change of the population—indicate that environmental factors are of great importance. Low levels of physical activity and a high calorie intake to physical activity ratio are particularly implicated in the rising prevalence of obesity. Though mapping of the human genome may identify those at risk of obesity earlier and more precisely (and offers the possibility in the future of targeted treatments or genetic manipulation), tackling the current obesity epidemic requires measures to reduce population levels of physical inactivity and to encourage energy intake appropriate to activity levels.

Insulin resistance and diabetes

A spectrum of metabolic disorder running from frank diabetes to minor levels of glucose intolerance is of relevance when considering IHD risk. Examining fasting glucose levels or glucose levels after standardized intakes (e.g. in glucose tolerance tests) demonstrates this, with somewhat arbitrary cut-offs being used for 'impaired glucose tolerance (IGT)' and non-insulin dependant diabetes mellitus (NIDDM). This is not the case with insulin-dependant diabetes mellitus (IDDM), where in most instances people either have the disease or do not, but this is a considerably rarer condition that contributes substantially less to the population levels of IHD than NIDDM and IGT.

A cluster of physiological risk factors for IHD have been grouped into the insulin resistance syndrome (also known as the metabolic syndrome or syndrome X). These involve resistance to insulin-stimulated glucose uptake, high circulating levels of insulin, high triglyceride levels, low HDL cholesterol levels, and elevated blood pressure. The degree to which this truly constitutes a syndrome remains disputed, but it is clear that these risk indicators are correlated within populations and contribute to IHD risk.

The epidemiology of diabetes is discussed in detail elsewhere (see Chapter 12.11.1). By far the most important environmental factor influencing diabetes risk and level of glucose intolerance is obesity, in particular central obesity. Physical activity also appears to protect against NIDDM and IGT, while findings have been mixed with respect to alcohol intake and smoking, which have been both positively and negatively associated with disease risk.

Unlike risk factors such as circulating blood cholesterol or blood pressure, fasting glucose does not show a continuous association with IHD risk

in prospective epidemiological studies. Only the top 5 or 10 per cent of the population levels of fasting glucose levels are associated with increased risk in studies in the United States and United Kingdom. Thus, the use of fasting glucose as a means of predicting risk in individuals is limited. The clear increased risk of IHD amongst people with frank NIDDM, which seems above and beyond their level of conventional IHD risk factors, indicates that these people have much to benefit from cholesterol and blood pressure lowering if they are eligible for these therapies.

Physical inactivity

In the early days of the coronary heart disease epidemic in industrialized countries it was thought that exercise may predispose to ischaemic heart disease through cardiac strain. However, research starting in the mid-twentieth century suggested that occupational physical activity was associated with reduced risk of IHD. With the increasingly sedentary nature of many occupations this has become a less important risk indicator for IHD and attention has shifted to physical activity in leisure time.

Clearly, health-related selection is a serious problem in studying the relationship between leisure time physical activity and ischaemic heart disease, since those with early signs of the disease will be less physically active. There is also considerable confounding as engagement in leisure time physical activity is associated with other important risk factors for IHD, such as smoking and socioeconomic position. However, the general picture suggests that increased physical activity does protect against IHD, although there is uncertainty about the type, intensity, and frequency of exercise that is required to confer such protection.

The key question has been whether the physical activity needs to be vigorous or not, with some studies suggesting that only vigorous exercise is protective, while others indicate that any form of increased physical activity is effective. This may reflect difficulties in measuring usual physical activity accurately, particularly at low levels. Differences in the findings between studies may also reflect the fact that the type of exercise that is vigorous for one group may not be vigorous for another. For example the elderly or unfit will find relatively low intensity physical activity results in increased cardiorespiratory fitness, while lower intensity activity will have no such training effect in fit young adults. A formulation that is consistent with the current data is that physical activity which is at a sufficient level to produce cardiorespiratory training reduces the risk of IHD, while the value of lower intensity physical activity is unclear.

Stress

Stress is widely considered by the general public to be an important cause of IHD. Indeed, several surveys of lay beliefs have shown that it is one of the most widely recognized risk factors for the disease. Stress is, however, difficult to define or measure. Epidemiological studies have examined a wide range of potential exposures that fall under the general heading of 'stress'. These include measures which are essentially of personality traits—such as the well-known Type A behaviour pattern—through to records of stressful life events or global measures of perceived stressfulness of daily activities. A broader conceptual category of 'psychosocial factors' is now widely used in the epidemiological literature. This includes aspects of social life such as the strength of social support networks or the level of control that people have over their work.

The type A behaviour pattern was investigated from the 1950s, particularly in the United States, as a potential cause of IHD. Type A individuals—those who are involved in an incessant struggle to achieve more and more in less and less time—were found to have higher risk of IHD in several early prospective studies, and type A personality was included in official publications (produced by august bodies such as the American Heart Association) as a cause of IHD, along with smoking, high blood pressure, and high saturated fat diet. More recent studies have failed to find any association between type A behaviour and IHD. It may be that this association no longer exists because IHD is not now considered a disease of the wealthy, stressed, business man, who in the past was more likely to be diagnosed with the condition. Research on behavioural traits now focuses on those elements of the original type-A classification that are related to adverse social background, for example hostility: these may predict IHD risk because of this, rather than because of any causal link with the disease.

Measures of self-reported global stress and other self-reported indicators, such as low control at work or poor social networks, tend to be related to self-reported IHD symptoms (usually angina or severe chest pain indicative of a myocardial infarction). They less consistently relate to objective measures of IHD, such as ECG changes or IHD mortality. This may reflect an underlying reporting tendency, such that people who report higher levels of adversity in their lives also report higher levels of symptoms. Given the history of the association between type A behaviour and IHD it is also important to consider whether associations between stress and IHD are generated by confounding. People with low control over their work (e.g. shift workers in a factory) are, almost by definition, in less favourable social locations than those with higher control over their work (e.g. managers or senior academics). It is not surprising that the former have higher rates of IHD, given the strong social patterning of the disease. Whether these adverse psychosocial factors are one of the causes of the high IHD mortality in the less advantaged or merely another consequence of material inequalities is not clear.

More methodologically robust studies employing objective measures of both stress and IHD outcomes are required. In particular, it is remarkable that the supposed biological mediators between stress and disease (disturbed functioning of the hypothalamo–pituitary–adrenal axis and possible immune system outcomes of this) have not themselves been related to IHD risk in prospective observational studies, some 70 years after the basic concept was advanced by Hans Selye. The current controversy—with enthusiastic proponents of stress as a cause of IHD on one side (feeding into a popular propensity for accepting this view) lined up against the majority of academic and research cardiologists and epidemiologists who dismiss the association as spurious—will only be resolved when studies employing better methods report their findings.

Cholesterol

Circulating blood cholesterol is strongly and positively associated with ischaemic heart disease risk in men and women, both young and old. A series of large-scale, randomized, controlled trials of blood cholesterol reduction demonstrate that this process is reversible and risk reductions of the magnitude predicted from the observational data can be produced through lowering blood cholesterol.

One issue not directly relevant to ischaemic heart disease that led to controversy regarding cholesterol reduction was the suspicion that low circulating blood cholesterol caused an increased risk of morbidity and mortality from non-coronary causes, including cancer, psychiatric disease, and gastrointestinal and respiratory disease. Observational studies tended to report inverse associations between blood cholesterol and these conditions, though it was clear that these associations could be generated through early stages of ill-health or adverse health-related behaviours leading to lower circulating cholesterol levels. Findings from randomized, controlled trials of cholesterol reduction were initially ambiguous, in that there was evidence of elevation of non-coronary morbidity and mortality in some studies. This now appears to reflect specific adverse effects of certain cholesterol lowering drugs, in particular the fibrates. More recent studies in which circulating cholesterol levels were reduced more profoundly than in earlier studies, through the use of statins, suggest there are no detrimental effects of cholesterol lowering itself.

Early epidemiological studies only measured total circulating cholesterol, but it is evident that subfractions of cholesterol have differential effects on ischaemic heart disease risk. The adverse effects are restricted to the low-density lipoprotein cholesterol fraction, with high-density lipoprotein cholesterol (HDL) levels being inversely associated with ischaemic heart disease risk. Alcohol consumption increases HDL cholesterol and increased HDL levels are a potential mediator of the apparent protective effect of low to moderate alcohol consumption on IHD. Trials of raising HDL cholesterol are difficult to interpret as the agents employed also decrease trygliceride levels and, to an extent, LDL cholesterol. Current evidence suggests that there may be a protective effect of raising HDL cholesterol, but this requires confirmation.

Blood pressure

There is a strong, consistent dose–response relationship between increased casual blood pressure measured in middle age and increased risk of IHD. In observational studies a 10 mmHg increase in diastolic blood pressure is associated with a 37 per cent increase in the risk of coronary disease. Large, randomized trials of pharmacological blood pressure reduction in middle age have confirmed that blood pressure reduction reduces subsequent risk of coronary disease. Several observational studies have also shown that increased blood pressure in early adult life is associated with increased coronary mortality in later life, suggesting that risk trajectory may be set early.

Blood pressure is continuously distributed in populations and increases in blood pressure across the range of blood pressure measures are associated with increased risk of IHD. There is therefore no natural dichotomy between normotensives and hypertensives. Hypertension has to be defined by weighing up the risks of disease at a given level of blood pressure against the risks of treatment to lower blood pressure.

Blood pressure is determined both by environmental factors, such as increased sodium intake (increases blood pressure), increased alcohol intake (increases blood pressure), increased fruit and vegetable intake (lowers blood pressure), and genetic factors. While individual blood pressure response to environmental factors may be influenced by genetic factors, migrant studies illustrate the substantial and relatively rapidly acting effects of environmental factors. In one study of migrants from a rural community in western Kenya to urban Nairobi, mean diastolic blood increased by around 6 mmHg from that measured 10 months previously.

Not all environmental factors that increase blood pressure increase risk of coronary disease. For example increased alcohol intake results in increased blood pressure and people who drink heavily are at increased risk of coronary disease, but those that consume alcohol in moderation have lower risks of coronary disease than teetotallers. Though there are a number of explanations for this particular protective association, this example illustrates the more general point that effects on risk factors may not necessarily translate into changes in risk of IHD.

Haemostatic factors

Studies of changes in prevalence of atherosclerosis (discussed earlier) provide indirect evidence that another pathological process, such as thrombosis, influenced trends in symptomatic disease over the last century. Over the last 20 years a number of cohort studies have examined the association between haemostatic factors and coronary disease. There is a consistent, independent association between increased fibrinogen levels and increased risk of coronary disease. The subsequent risk of IHD comparing those in the highest third with those in the lowest third of the fibrinogen distribution at baseline is increased by around 80 per cent. Some prospective studies have reported increased coronary risk with factors VII and VIII but the data are less extensive and less consistent. Other studies have reported associations with tissue-type plasminogen activator (t-PA) and with plasminogen activator inhibitor-1 (PAI-1), while platelet function tests do not appear to predict subsequent coronary risk. These associations need to be confirmed. Smokers have higher fibrinogen levels than non-smokers and this may in part explain their excess coronary risk. Fibrinogen levels are also associated with higher levels of other acute phase reactants suggesting that chronic inflammatory or infective processes may increase fibrinogen levels and thus risk of symptomatic coronary disease. Alternatively, fibrinogen may merely be a marker for these underlying processes. These issues are discussed elsewhere.

The prevention of ischaemic heart disease

As we have seen, there are marked differences in the rate of death attributed to IHD over time, between countries, between regions, within countries, and between groups of individuals within countries. These differences point to the potential scope for prevention.

Attempts at prevention can be roughly classified as primary, secondary, or tertiary. Tertiary prevention is the treatment and rehabilitation of people with symptomatic disease: it clearly offers important opportunities for preventing further symptomatic episodes since many who experience an acute myocardial infarction will have known coronary disease. The recent results from the WHO MONICA study would seem to confirm that the widespread use of effective treatments can reduce the number of symptomatic episodes and deaths attributed to IHD. Secondary prevention is the identification and treatment of early, often asymptomatic, disease: this is not currently (and may never be) a discrete option, because most people in Western populations have at least some atherosclerotic disease in their coronary arteries and there are no proven non-invasive tests that are able to detect reliably those with early disease before they develop symptoms. Primary prevention is the prevention of the onset of disease. In IHD the distinction between primary, secondary, and tertiary prevention is blurred: people identified as being at high risk of disease on the basis of risk factor profiles will comprise those with symptomatic disease, those with asymptomatic disease, and those without manifest disease.

There are two differing but complementary approaches to primary prevention: the high-risk approach and the population approach. The high-risk approach seeks to identify those at highest risk of developing disease with time to intervene to prevent disease. This approach has the advantage that it may be easier to encourage people at high risk to alter their lifestyles and to take tablets as these individuals have a considerable amount to gain personally from accepting change. Such an approach, however, requires that those at high risk be identified and ignores the many people who develop symptomatic disease who are at moderate rather than high risk. For example, in the Whitehall study, 42 per cent of the coronary deaths (and 36 per cent of all deaths) occurring over a 15-year follow-up occurred in the 20 per cent at highest risk (on the basis of smoking status, blood pressure, and plasma cholesterol). The majority of coronary deaths (58 per cent), however, occurred in those who were not at high risk (Table 6). Thus, even a universally effective package of interventions for people at high risk could only hope to prevent around 40 per cent of coronary deaths, and a (more plausible) package of interventions that halved coronary mortality in those at high risk could only hope to prevent around 20 per cent of coronary deaths. The alternative approach is the population approach, which seeks to alter risk-factor levels or behaviour across the whole population, its advantage being that for fairly modest changes in mean population risk-factor levels it is likely to produce larger overall improvements in the health of the population as a whole than the high-risk approach. The disadvantage is that the absolute benefit for each individual who makes a lifestyle change is likely to be small. This mismatch between the likely size of the benefits to the individual and population has been called the 'prevention paradox'.

In terms of IHD prevention, smoking cessation strategies are potentially of high impact. It has been shown that brief advice from physicians leads to small, but (in population terms) worthwhile reductions in smoking rates among their clients. Nicotine replacement gum can also aid smoking cessation. More problematic are attempts to reduce the initiation of smoking in adolescents. School-based antismoking programmes have shown disappointing results, which is perhaps not surprising given the nature of experimental behaviour among this age group. While smoking is an option it is likely that a high percentage of the population will experiment with the behaviour and strategies for early cessation—which also occurs amongst a high proportion of those who try the behaviour—should be built upon.

The detection and treatment of high blood pressure reduces the risk of IHD in the primary prevention setting and has the added benefit of also substantially reducing the risk of stroke. Similarly, lowering cholesterol levels with the statin drugs reduces IHD risk in primary prevention, although the absolute benefit is small for those who are not at increased risk of IHD for other reasons.

A series of multiple risk factor intervention trials have been carried out at both the community and individual participant level in which encouragement to modify diet, reduce smoking, increase physical activity, and (in some studies) increase medical treatment of elevated risk factors have been explored. Beyond the evident benefits of pharmacological reduction of blood pressure, the findings have been disappointing.

These results emphasize the degree to which health-related behaviours—such as dietary consumption, smoking, heavy drinking, and physical activity patterns—are strongly influenced by societal legislative and fiscal forces and are less to do with individual levels of knowledge and degree of willpower. This is clearly the pattern for smoking, where smoking levels in a country, smoking initiation rates, and the social distribution of smoking are all responsive to the profit-making incentives offered to tobacco companies. The diversification of tobacco companies to other products (within the 'home' advanced capitalist markets) and shifts to export to newly industrializing countries reflects the unfavourable economic environment that has been created for the companies in some countries. The prevention of smoking—one of the most important modifiable health risks globally—can only be ultimately successful if the world community accepts the need to restrict the profitability of growing and selling tobacco.

The differences between countries and over time in both behaviour and IHD disease rates clearly illustrate the capacity for populations to alter their behaviour and to adopt healthier lifestyles. While simple invocations to change have modest effects on behaviour and IHD risk, social change can result in profound improvements in health. Conversely, where cultures fail to adapt or social structures demise (as happened in Russia with the collapse of the Soviet Union) disease rates can increase. Effecting societal change is complex, but the potential public health benefits of even modest population change are profound. The concentration of IHD (and many other diseases) in those in society who are least advantaged suggest that policies will be more effective if they seek to improve the lot of the poor by improving their income, opportunities, and self-esteem. More inclusive and extensive programmes that seek to reduce inequalities in health and improve health for all offer real opportunities to reduce IHD incidence and mortality.

Table 6 Distribution of 15-year ischaemic and all cause mortality by quintile of risk (based on smoking status, systolic blood pressure, and plasma cholesterol) in the Whitehall study

Quintile of risk	Percentage of deaths	
	IHD	All causes
1	7	10
2	11	13
3	17	17
4	24	24
5	42	36

Source: Rose G (1992). Strategies of prevention: the individual and the population. In: Marmot M, Elliott P, eds. *Coronary heart disease epidemiology: from aetiology to public health.* Oxford University Press.

Summary

IHD is a globally important cause of morbidity and mortality. Epidemiological studies provide evidence that IHD is preventable and give some estimate of how much IHD might indeed be prevented. Current favourable trends in mortality in developed countries may not be maintained in the face of the current epidemic of obesity. Equally, the reductions in IHD case fatality (leading to reductions in mortality) achieved through use of effective treatments may not be viable solutions in less wealthy countries. While there are genuine areas of uncertainty that require further research, much is known about the aetiology and prevention of IHD. Invocations to individuals to adopt healthier lifestyles have produced disappointing results. At the population level, however, the will and capacity to modify behaviour exists. If coronary care units are to meet the same fate as sanatoriums, major societal and structural changes will be required to improve the material conditions of the least advantaged throughout their lives and to shape the diets, activity levels, alcohol consumption patterns, and smoking behaviour of us all.

Further reading

Anonymous. NIH Consensus development panel on physical activity and cardiovascular health (1996). *Journal of the American Medical Association* **276**, 241–6.

Barker DJP (1998). *Mothers, babies, and health in later life.* Churchill Livingstone, Edinburgh.

Burr ML, Fehily AM, Gilbert JF, *et al* (1989). Effects of changes in fat, fish, and fibre intakes on death and myocardial reinfarction: diet and reinfarction trial (DART). *Lancet* **ii**, 757–61.

Charlton J, Murphy ME, Khaw KT, Ebrahim SB, Davey Smith G (1997). Cardiovascular diseases. In: Charlton J, Murphy ME, eds. *The health of adult britain 1841–1994*, Vol. 2, pp. 60–75. Stationery Office, London.

Collins R, Peto R, Macmahon S, *et al* (1990). Blood pressure, stroke, and coronary heart disease. Part 2, short term-reductions in blood pressure: overview of randomised drug trials in their epidemiological context. *Lancet* **335**, 827–38.

Davey Smith G (1997). Down at heart: the meaning and implications of social inequalities in cardiovascular disease. *Journal of the Royal College of Physicians* **31**, 414–24.

de Lorgeril M, Renaud S, Mamelle N, *et al* (1994). Mediterranean alpha-linolenic acid-rich diet in secondary prevention of coronary heart disease. *Lancet* **343**, 1454–9.

Ebrahim S, Davey Smith G (1998). Health promotion for coronary heart disease: past, present and future. *European Heart Journal* **19**, 1751–7.

Ebrahim S, Davey Smith G, McCabe C, *et al* (1999). What role for statins? *Health Technology Assessment* **3**, 1–91.

Hart CL, Davey Smith G, Hole D, Hawthorne VM (1999). Alcohol consumption and mortality from all causes, coronary heart disease, and stroke: results from a prospective cohort study of Scottish men with 21 years of follow up. *British Medical Journal* **318**, 1725–9.

Hulley S, Grady D, Bush T, *et al* (1998). Randomized trial of estrogen plus progestin for secondary prevention of coronary heart disease in postmenopausal women. *Journal of the American Medical Association* **280**, 605–13.

Isles CG, Hole DJ, Hawthorne VM, Lever AF (1992). Relation between coronary risk and coronary mortality in women of the Renfrew and Paisley survey: comparison with men. *Lancet* **339**, 702–6.

Jarrett RJ (1996). The cardiovascular risk associated with impaired glucose tolerance. *Diabetic Medicine* **13**, S15–S19.

Kuh D, Ben Shlomo Y (1997). *A lifecourse approach to chronic disease epidemiology.* Oxford University Press, Oxford.

Kuulasmaa K, Tunstall-Pedoe H, Dobson A, *et al* (2000). Estimation of contribution of changes in classic risk factors to trends in coronary-event rates across the WHO MONICA project populations. *Lancet* **355**, 675–87.

Labarthe DR (1998). *Epidemiology and prevention of cardiovascular disease: a global perspective.* Aspen, Gaithersburg, Maryland.

Macmahon S, Peto R, Cutler J, *et al* (1990). Blood pressure, stroke, and coronary heart disease. Part 1, prolonged differences in blood pressure: prospective observational studies corrected for the regression dilution bias. *Lancet* **335**, 765–74.

McKeigue PM, Marmot MG, Adelstein AM, *et al* (1985). Diet and risk factors for coronary heart disease in Asians in Northwest London. *Lancet* **ii**, 1086–90.

Meade TW, Mellows S, Brozovic M, *et al* (1986). Haemostatic function and ischaemic heart disease: principal results of the Northwick Park Heart Study. *Lancet* **ii**, 533–7.

Ness AR, Powles JW (1997). Fruit and vegetables and cardiovascular disease: a review. *International Journal of Epidemiology* **26**, 1–13.

Powles JW (1994). Greek migrants in Australia: Surviving well and helping their hosts. In: Marks L, Worboys M, eds. *Migrants, minorities and medicine: historical and contemporary perspectives.* Routledge, London.

Rimm EB, Klatsky A, Grobbee D, Stampfer MJ (1996). Review of moderate alcohol consumption and reduced risk of coronary heart disease: is the effect due to beer, wine, or spirits? *British Medical Journal* **312**, 731–6.

Rose G (1992). *The strategy of preventive medicine.* Oxford University Press, Oxford.

Steinberg D, Parthasarathy S, Carew TE, Khoo JC, Witztum JL (1989). Beyond cholesterol. Modifications of low-density lipoprotein that increase its atherogenicity. *New England Journal of Medicine* **320**, 915–24.

Tunstall-Pedoe H, Kuulasmaa K, Mähönen M, *et al* (1999). Contribution of trends in survival and coronary-event rates to changes in coronary heart disease mortality: 10-year results from 37 WHO MONICA project populations. *Lancet* **353**, 1547–57.

Tunstall-Pedoe H, Vanuzzo D, Hobbs M, *et al* (2000). Estimation of contribution of changes in coronary care to improving survival, event rates, and coronary heart disease mortality across the WHO MONICA project populations. *Lancet* **355**, 688–700.

Ulbricht TLV and Southgate DAT (1991). Coronary heart disease: seven dietary factors. *Lancet* **338**, 985–93.

Willett WC (1994). Diet and health: What should we eat ? *Science* **264**, 532–7.

World Health Organization MONICA Project (1994). Ecological analysis of the association between mortality and major risk factors of cardiovascular disease. *International Journal of Epidemiology* **23**, 505–16.

15.4.2 Pathophysiology and clinical features

15.4.2.1 The pathophysiology of acute coronary syndromes

Peter L. Weissberg

Introduction

An acute coronary syndrome arises when there is sudden total or partial occlusion of a coronary artery leading to myocardial ischaemia and its consequences. The syndrome therefore encompasses the clinical entities of unstable angina, acute myocardial infarction, and many cases of sudden cardiac death. In the vast majority of instances, an acute coronary syndrome is due to the thrombotic consequences of rupture or erosion of an atherosclerotic plaque. To understand the pathophysiology of acute coronary syndromes it is therefore important to understand the cellular and molecular events leading to the development and progression of an atherosclerotic plaque.

Atherosclerosis: stable and unstable plaques

Atherosclerosis

Endothelial function is crucially important in the development of atherosclerosis. Normal endothelial cells form a physical barrier between the thrombogenic matrix of the underlying vessel wall and the circulation. However, by producing a variety of antithrombotic and anti-inflammatory molecules the endothelium also protects against the development of atherosclerosis. In particular nitric oxide, which is constitutively produced from arginine by the action of endothelial nitric oxide synthase in normal endothelial cells, prevents accumulation of inflammatory cells and, along with prostacyclin, prevents activation and adhesion of platelets. Patients with established atherosclerosis have abnormal endothelial function, particularly if they smoke, as do apparently healthy individuals with high cholesterol levels.

Endothelial dysfunction is manifest in the coronary and peripheral circulations as reduced vasodilation in response to infused acetylcholine, a pharmacological stimulator of nitric oxide production, and in the brachial artery as reduced flow-mediated vasodilation in response to hyperaemic forearm blood flow. However, it remains unclear how these abnormalities of endothelial function relate to the development of atherosclerosis. Indeed, whilst it is accepted that the endothelium is abnormal in atherosclerosis, it is still unclear whether a primary endothelial abnormality predisposes to lipid accumulation and therefore the development of atherosclerosis, or whether endothelial dysfunction is secondary to hyperlipidaemia and/or the presence of subclinical atherosclerosis in apparently healthy subjects. The fact that the endothelium can respond to changes in shear stress by increasing or decreasing production of a number of molecules known to be involved in the atherogenic process suggests that subtle perturbations in endothelial function induced by local haemodynamic factors may contribute to the tendency of atherosclerosis to develop only at particular sites within the arterial tree.

The pathogenesis of the atherosclerotic plaque is discussed in detail in Chapter 15.1.2.1, but in brief, in the earliest atherosclerotic lesion, the fatty streak, there is subendothelial accumulation of oxidized lipid. This is associated with activation of the overlying endothelium and recruitment of inflammatory cells, predominantly monocytes and some T cells, into the subendothelial space. Once in the subendothelial space, the monocytes mature into macrophages and express a variety of surface molecules, in particular the scavenger receptors that allow them to bind and ingest lipid to become macrophage foam cells, the most abundant cell in the core of the atherosclerotic plaque. There is good evidence that oxidation of lipids is an essential step in the formation of foam cells and a mature atherosclerotic lesion. T cells are also activated and there is expression of major histocompatibility complex (MHC) molecules in surrounding vascular smooth muscle cells, some of which may also take up lipids to become foam cells. The activated inflammatory cells within the plaque produce a variety of cytokines that serve to recruit further inflammatory cells into the lesion. A crucial aspect is that some of these molecules also induce migration of vascular smooth muscle cells from the vessel media into the intima where they become incorporated into the atherosclerotic lesion. During the process of migration the vascular smooth muscle cells change from a contractile to a repair phenotype, as discussed in Chapter 15.1.1.3, which allows them to proliferate and elaborate the matrix proteins required to form a fibrous cap over the lipid core. Vascular smooth muscle cells are the only cells capable of synthesizing the fibrous cap, and their participation is therefore essential for plaque stability. Stable atherosclerotic plaques characteristically contain few inflammatory cells, large numbers of vascular smooth muscle cells, and have a thick fibrous cap that is resistant to rupture. They only cause symptoms if they are large enough to compromise flow through the artery, in which case they cause reversible ischaemia in the form of stable angina.

Plaque instability

Atherosclerotic plaques give rise to acute coronary syndromes when there is a sudden reduction in coronary blood flow. In most cases this is due to aggregation of platelets, with or without subsequent thrombosis. Spontaneous haemorrhage, presumably from immature microvessels within the plaque, causes rapid expansion of the plaque and a sufficient reduction in coronary blood flow to precipitate either myocardial infarction or unstable angina in a few cases. Most thrombotic events are due to rupture or fissuring of the fibrous cap with consequent exposure of the thrombogenic lipid core, but in some cases, variably reported to be between 25 and 44 per cent of thrombotic coronary events, thrombosis occurs because of accumulation of platelets at the site of endothelial erosion without obvious disruption of the fibrous cap or exposure of the lipid core.

Thrombosis due to endothelial erosion appears to be particularly common in female smokers dying suddenly with coronary disease, which may reflect a greater tendency to thrombosis in women than men rather than a difference in underlying plaque pathology. The mechanism of plaque erosion still remains to be determined, but it is possible that plaque inflammatory cells may produce cytokines that are toxic to the overlying endothelium, thereby inducing endothelial cell death and exposure of the underlying collagenous matrix of the atherosclerotic lesion. Alternatively, there may be a detrimental interaction between endothelial cells and underlying smooth muscle cells. Further studies are required to resolve the mechanism of endothelial erosion before therapies aimed at its prevention can be developed.

Plaque rupture, with the development of a thrombus that occludes the lumen and extends into the core of the lesion, is the commonest substrate for an acute coronary syndrome. In contrast to endothelial erosion, the pathophysiological mechanisms underlying plaque rupture are now beginning to be resolved. Modelling of the structural characteristics of atherosclerotic plaques has predicted that plaques with a large lipid core and a thin fibrous cap are subject to increased circumferential tensile stress, increasing the chance of rupture, whereas a thick fibrous cap confers structural stability by reducing tensile stress. The interaction between the physical properties of the plaque and local haemodynamic forces are therefore likely to play a part in determining stability and resistance to rupture, particularly in circumstances where the clinical event is related to physical activity, there being a well-recognized association between activities such as shovelling snow and the development of an acute coronary syndrome.

However, the most important determinant of plaque instability is the balance between the activity of inflammatory cells and the healing, fibrotic reaction of the smooth muscle cells in the fibrous cap. Plaque rupture occurs in lesions containing few vascular smooth muscle cells and abundant inflammatory cells, suggesting that inflammatory cells are responsible for the breakdown of the plaque: there are a number of ways in which they might weaken the fibrous cap. Firstly, they produce proinflammatory cytokines that inhibit vascular smooth muscle cell proliferation and matrix production. Secondly, inflammatory cytokines such as interleukin 1β, tumour necrosis factor-α, and interferon-γ act synergistically to induce vascular smooth muscle cell death. Thirdly, activated macrophages can induce vascular smooth muscle cell death by direct cell to cell contact. Fourthly, and probably most importantly, inflammatory cells, particularly macrophages, produce and activate a number of matrix metalloproteinases that digest the matrix of the fibrous cap. Thus inflammatory cells exert a potent negative influence on the turnover of matrix protein within the lesion. Furthermore, as discussed in Chapter 15.1.1.3, vascular smooth muscle cells in the fibrous cap become senescent and develop an inherent tendency to undergo apoptosis (programmed cell death). The overall effect is that inflammatory cell activity destroys the fabric of the fibrous cap and at the same time reduces the number and synthetic activity of intimal vascular smooth muscle cells, leading inevitably to weakening of the cap and eventual rupture under the stress of local haemodynamic forces (Fig. 1). The clinical importance of individual inflammatory cytokines and matrix metalloproteinases in the progression and rupture of plaque has yet to be established. However, evidence is beginning to emerge that subtle, genetically determined differences in production and activity of inflammatory mediators and matrix metalloproteinases, measured as polymorphisms in the genes coding for their

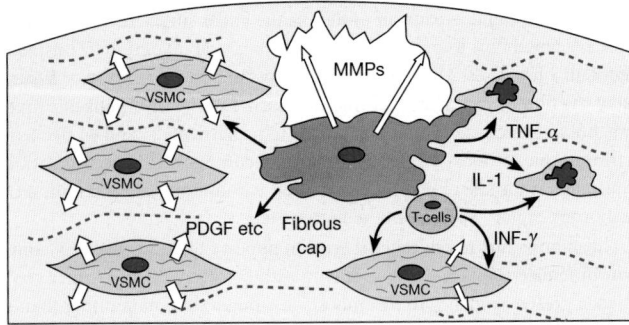

Fig. 1 Cellular interactions within the fibrous cap of an established atherosclerotic lesion leading to plaque rupture and an acute coronary syndrome. In early lesions cytokines produced by macrophages recruit vascular smooth muscle cells that produce the matrix proteins of the fibrous cap. In advanced lesions the cytokines produced by inflammatory cells inhibit vascular smooth muscle cell protein production and are cytotoxic. The vascular smooth muscle cells become senescent and die and macrophages produce matrix metalloproteinases that destroy the fibrous cap, leading to plaque rupture.

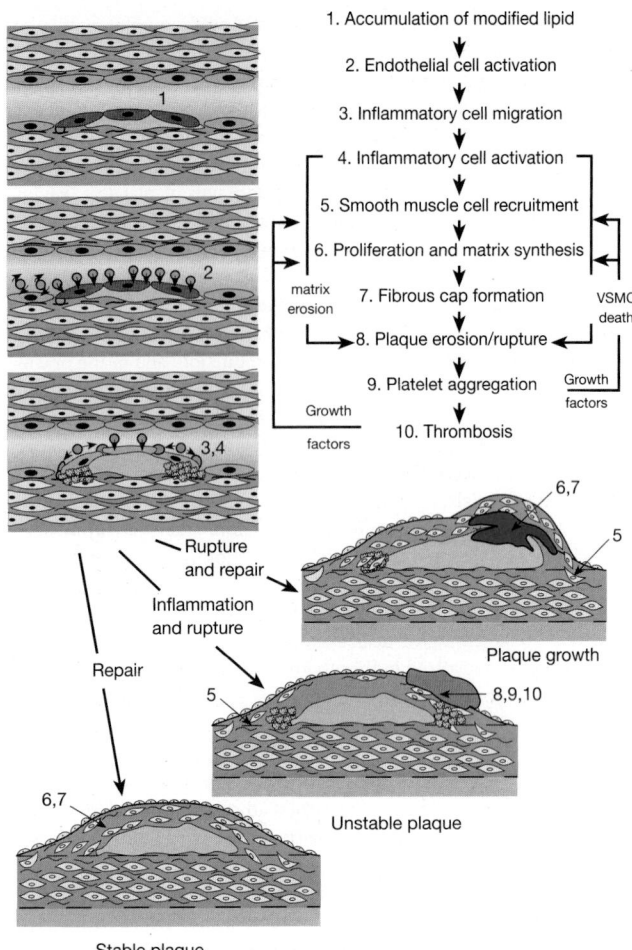

Fig. 2 Cellular interactions leading to the development and progression of atherosclerosis. (Reproduced from Weissberg PL (2000). *Heart* **83**, 247–52, with permission.)

production, may influence the rate of progression and outcome of atherosclerosis in different individuals.

Modification of plaque stability

For many years symptomatic atherosclerosis was thought to represent the end stage of a slowly progressive, irreversible disease process that had developed over decades and which was therefore unlikely to be influenced favourably by medical therapy. Consequently, therapy for ischaemic heart disease focused either on abrogating the consequences of atherosclerosis, for example with antianginal, antiplatelet, and thrombolytic drugs, or relieving stenoses by interventions such as angioplasty or bypass surgery. However, as described above, it is now recognized that atherosclerosis is a dynamic inflammatory condition involving constant or cyclical recruitment and activation of inflammatory cells, with repeated subclinical episodes of plaque rupture and repair leading to episodic growth of individual plaques (Fig. 2). Encouragingly, results of several recently published large-scale trials of lipid-lowering agents, in particular the HMG CoA reductase inhibitors or 'statins', have shown that medical therapy can modify the pathophysiology of atherosclerosis.

Aggressive, sustained lipid lowering, by whatever means, reduces the risk of myocardial infarction. However, it is only since the introduction of statins that doctors have had access to powerful lipid-lowering drugs that are well tolerated and relatively free of toxicity. Angiographic studies in patients with angina have shown that statins reduce the rate of appearance of new lesions and reduce the incidence of spontaneous, clinically silent, vessel occlusions (occurring when there is plaque rupture and thrombosis in the context of a good collateral circulation that maintains viability of the tissue downstream of the occlusion). However, statin therapy has only a marginal and probably haemodynamically insignificant effect on the size of established stenotic atherosclerotic lesions. Despite this disappointing effect on plaque size, treatment with statins reduces mortality and the risk of a coronary event (unstable angina, myocardial infarction, or the need for surgical intervention) by about 30 to 40 per cent, both in asymptomatic individuals at high risk of a coronary event (primary prevention) and in patients who have already experienced a coronary event (secondary prevention). Results of theses studies suggest strongly that statins are stabilizing atherosclerotic plaques.

The inflammatory basis of atherosclerosis

The cellular and molecular interactions described above all point to an important role for inflammation in the development and progression of atherosclerosis. Evidence in support of this contention comes from recent

clinical studies in which circulating levels of acute-phase proteins such as C-reactive protein, fibrinogen, and serum amyloid A have been shown to correlate closely with the risk of an acute coronary syndrome, or indeed stroke. This applies both in apparently healthy subjects without overt coronary disease and in those who have already survived a myocardial infarction. Recognition of this association led to the speculation that atherosclerosis or its consequences may be precipitated by infection, and several early studies demonstrated an association between serological evidence of recent infection with *Helicobacter pylori*, *Chlamydia pheumoniae*, and cytomegalovirus and coronary events. The case for *Chlamydia pheumoniae* was particularly plausible since these organisms can be found in vascular smooth muscle cells and macrophages within atherosclerotic lesions. However, recent more rigorous studies have suggested that these associations may be spurious, due to inadequate control for confounders, particularly for *Helicobacter pylori* infection, and do not indicate a strong association between infection and the development of coronary artery disease. The outcome of several ongoing studies on the effects of antibiotic therapy on coronary events should help resolve this important question. Evidence that elevated levels of C-reactive protein reflect inflammatory activity within atherosclerosis rather than infection comes from studies of inhibition of hepatic HMG CoA reductase with pravastatin. Compared with patients treated with placebo, whose C-reactive protein levels rose, patients treated with pravastatin, which lowers low-density lipoprotein cholesterol but has no known effect on bacteria, experienced a substantially reduced risk of a coronary event with an associated fall in level of circulating C-reactive protein.

The causes of acute coronary syndromes

Unstable angina versus myocardial infarction

The pathogenesis of unstable angina and myocardial infarction is similar in that both occur because of plaque erosion or rupture and subsequent aggregation of platelets. Lesions causing unstable angina are characteristically eccentric and ulcerated with associated non-occlusive thrombus, whereas angiographic studies have shown that myocardial infarction is usually due to complete thrombotic occlusion of the relevant vessel. Treatment of myocardial infarction therefore includes aspirin to prevent further platelet aggregation and a fibrinolytic drug to lyse the occluding thrombus. In unstable angina the accumulation and activation of platelets causes local release of a number of peptides, such as thromboxane A2, 5-hydroxytryptamine, and platelet derived growth factor, all of which are potent vasoconstrictors. Thus, vasoconstriction superimposed on partial occlusion of the lumen is often responsible for myocardial ischaemia (Fig. 1). Although the thrombus in unstable angina may be non-occlusive, it provides the substrate from which embolization of platelet aggregates downstream can produce microinfarcts that are not apparent electrocardiographically, but which may be detectable through release of sensitive markers of myocyte necrosis, such as troponins I or T. Patients with unstable angina and an associated increase in circulating troponin levels are at particularly high risk of subsequent coronary events if not treated aggressively.

The logical result of this analysis is that the management of unstable angina includes inhibition of platelet aggregation with aspirin, heparin to prevent progression to a fibrin clot, and nitrates to offload the myocardium and relieve any local coronary artery spasm. Although aspirin continues to be the first-line antiplatelet drug, newer drugs such as ADP and glycoprotein IIb/IIIa antagonists are rapidly establishing their role in the management of unstable angina and other acute vascular syndromes such as transient cerebral ischaemic attack.

Plaque instability often occurs in small, haemodynamically insignificant atherosclerotic plaques that are clinically silent (not causing stable angina) and which may not be apparent at angiography. Approximately 70 per cent of coronary lesions that break down to cause thrombosis and subsequent myocardial infarction cause less than a 50 per cent stenosis of the relevant coronary artery. This is probably because arteries can remodel to accommodate large atherosclerotic lesions without reducing lumen diameter, but it explains why so many patients (about 50 per cent) suffer myocardial infarction without experiencing any prior symptoms of coronary disease. It also serves to emphasize the relatively greater importance of plaque composition than plaque size in determining the outcome of coronary disease.

Other causes of acute coronary syndromes

Not all acute coronary syndromes arise as a result of rupture of atherosclerotic plaque. Rarely, acute myocardial infarction can occur in the absence of significant coronary artery disease. Acute coronary artery dissection is a rare event that occurs more commonly in women than men and which can cause myocardial infarction and even sudden death. The underlying aetiology is unknown. Coronary artery spasm may also precipitate an acute coronary syndrome and even myocardial infarction, but the reasons for coronary spasm in the absence of atherosclerosis are poorly understood, although they almost certainly arise from endothelial dysfunction. Angina due to spasm, so-called Prinzmetal's variant angina, is characterized by marked ST segment elevation on the ECG, by contrast with ischaemia due to atherosclerotic plaque rupture or erosion that are characterized by ST segment depression. It usually responds to treatment with calcium channel blockers, particularly nifedipine. Finally, acute coronary syndromes can be precipitated by legitimate and illegitimate drug therapy. For example, symptoms of myocardial ischaemia can be provoked in some patients by the use of HT1 agonists to treat migraine or sildenafil for impotence, particularly when combined with nitrates. Recreational drug abuse, particularly cocaine derivatives, may also precipitate an acute coronary syndrome and should be considered when clinically appropriate.

Consequences of acute coronary syndromes

Sudden reduction in blood flow through a coronary artery inevitably leads to myocardial ischaemia unless the myocardium is supplied by an adequate collateral blood supply from another coronary artery. The three main clinical consequences of such ischaemia are arrhythmias, reduced contractile function, and, less commonly, myocardial rupture: these are discussed in Chapter 15.4.2.3. However, it is becoming clear that ischaemia has complex effects on the myocardium, and considerations of myocardial stunning and hybernation and of ischaemic preconditioning are likely to be increasingly important in the development of new therapies.

Myocardial stunning and hibernation

Contractile dysfunction after infarction does not always imply irreversible necrosis of myocytes. The myocardium may be either stunned or hibernating. Viable myocardium is said to be stunned when it fails to contract appropriately after the obstruction to coronary blood flow has been removed or bypassed. This may be due to what is called the 'no reflow' phenomenon in which there is a failure of flow through the previously ischaemic tissue, despite there being a patent feeding artery. The underlying mechanism for this phenomenon is unknown, but probably relates to local endothelial dysfunction. Stunned myocardium usually recovers normal or near normal function with time.

The term hibernating myocardium is used to describe viable myocardium that fails to contract properly because it has an inadequate blood supply. The importance of this concept lies in the fact that restoration of an adequate blood flow, by angioplasty or bypass surgery, usually results in recovery of contractile function. Identification of hibernating myocardium is crucial in determining which patients will experience an improvement in myocardial function if subjected to a revascularization procedure: revascularization of dead myocardium clearly confers no benefit. Techniques based on the echocardiographic measurement of left ventricular wall motion under pharmacological stress or which compare myocardial metabolism and blood flow with positron emission tomography (see above) can identify those with myocardial dysfunction due to hibernation.

Ischaemic preconditioning

Over recent years it has become clear that episodes of myocardial ischaemia may protect the myocardium from the consequences of a further ischaemic event. Thus it has been found that a transient interruption of myocardial blood flow delays the onset of infarction if blood flow is subsequently permanently interrupted. The biochemistry of this phenomenon is complex and incompletely understood and its clinical importance is currently unclear. However, its recognition heralds the possibility of future development of drugs that will protect the myocardium from the consequences of ischaemia.

Further reading

Arbustini E *et al.* (1999). Plaque erosion is a major substrate for coronary thrombosis in acute myocardial infarction. *Heart* **82**, 269–72.

Davies MJ (1995). Stability and instability—2 faces of coronary atherosclerosis—the Paul-Dudley-White-Lecture. *Circulation* **94**, 2013–20.

Fuster V, Fayad Z, Badimon J (1999). Acute coronary syndromes: biology. *Lancet* **353**, 5–9.

Libby P (1995). Molecular bases of the acute coronary syndromes. *Circulation* **91**, 2844–50.

Redwood SR, Ferrari R, Marber MS (1998). Myocardial hibernation and stunning: from physiological principles to clinical practice. *Heart* **80**, 218–22.

Yellon D *et al.* (1998) Ischaemic preconditioning: present position and future directions. *Cardiovascular Research* **37**, 21–33.

15.4.2.2 Management of stable angina

L. M. Shapiro

Introduction

Coronary artery disease is the predominant cause of death in the developed world, causing 300 000 deaths per year in the United Kingdom, and is increasing in importance in developing countries and the previous Communist bloc. Coronary artery disease is also a major cause of hospital admission and clinic consultation.

The syndrome of stable angina pectoris is clinically defined as consistent exertional- or stress-related cardiac symptoms, usually of chest pain and, less frequently, shortness of breath. In the last decade there have been major advances in the management of patients with stable symptoms and coronary artery disease: particularly in the areas of lifestyle modification, medical treatment, and revascularization. The management of patients with stable angina is the subject of this chapter.

General patient management

The diagnosis of angina pectoris in a patient should be accompanied by a detailed explanation of the disorder. In particular, that angina pectoris has an unpredictable nature, with the possibility of deterioration as well as stabilization or an improvement with treatment. The treatments available include lifestyle modification, pharmacological intervention, and revascularization. These need to be individualized and usually ameliorate symptoms, and in most circumstances improve prognosis.

In the initial management of patients with chronic angina pectoris, a search should be made for treatable conditions which increase myocardial oxygen demand or reduce oxygen delivery—for example, marked obesity, thyrotoxicosis, fever, anaemia, tachycardia, or aortic stenosis.

The medical management of stable angina pectoris then depends upon consideration of the following options to improve symptoms and/or prognosis:

(1) control of risk factors and lifestyle modification;

(2) pharmacological management;

(3) revascularization.

Risk-factor management and lifestyle modification

Lifestyle modification, if sufficiently rigorous, has the advantage of providing a modest degree of symptom relief and a reduction in the rate of further development of coronary artery disease.

Hypertension

The relationship between the development of coronary artery disease and hypertension is well established. Hypertension increases myocardial oxygen demand and leads to ischaemia in patients with obstructive coronary artery disease. Elevation of left ventricular mass is a strong predictor of mortality due to coronary artery disease. Treatment of hypertension, especially in the elderly, has been shown to reduce the mortality from cardiovascular causes by nearly one-third.

Cigarette smoking

Not only is smoking a powerful risk factor for the development of coronary artery disease, it also leads to more severe and premature atherosclerotic plaques. Cigarette smokers with documented coronary artery disease have an increased 5-year mortality risk, and cessation of smoking lessens the risk of adverse cardiovascular events. Smoking may also lead to exacerbation of angina pectoris by increasing myocardial oxygen demand and reducing coronary blood flow by a direct effect on coronary artery tone. Passive smoking may also be important.

Hyperlipidaemia

Reduction of cholesterol by diet, and more especially by drugs therapy, has been shown in primary prevention trials to reduce the risk of the development of coronary disease. Treatment with the statin group of drugs in patients with established coronary artery disease (secondary prevention) has only a modest effect on angiographically documented, coronary artery obstruction, but significantly reduces the number of new cardiovascular events. The Scandinavian Simvastatin Survival Study treated patients with a cholesterol level in excess of 5.5 mmol/l, but a value of 4.8 mmol/l or less is currently seen as a treatment threshold.

Recent evidence from the AVERT study (atorvastatin versus revascularization treatment) suggests that, in patients with mild and stable angina pectoris, aggressive cholesterol lowering with atorvastatin had a similar effect in reducing ischaemic events as treatment with percutaneous transluminal coronary angioplasty, although the latter group had better symptom control.

Antioxidants

Oxidized low-density lipoproteins (**LDL**) may play an important role in the pathogenesis of atherosclerosis. Agents that prevent lipid peroxidation of LDL particles might therefore influence the development of atherosclerosis and its clinical consequences. Epidemiological data suggests that high vitamin E levels are protective of coronary artery disease. Giving β-carotene does not appear to confer an advantage, whereas vitamin E may show some benefits in secondary prevention in doses of 400 or 800 IU per day.

Aspirin

Activated, aggregating platelets play an important role in the development of acute coronary events. A meta-analysis of 300 studies—including 140 000 patients with chronic coronary heart disease, stroke, or previous bypass surgery—has shown aspirin to have a prophylactic benefit. Aspirin is therefore widely used in the dose range of 75 to 150 mg per day in patients with chronic angina pectoris.

Physical inactivity

Regular aerobic exercise allows a greater workload to be performed for any level of oxygen consumption, allowing patients with coronary heart disease to increase their exercise tolerance. The physiological benefits of exercise training have largely been described from postmyocardial infarction rehabilitation. However, smaller studies have confirmed significant benefits in improved quality of life, effort tolerance, and possibly morphology of coronary artery lesions, from a graded supervised physical exercise programme in those with chronic stable angina.

Obesity

The presence of obesity most probably acts via increased blood pressure and serum cholesterol as coronary artery disease risk factors. However, it may lead to symptom development in chronic angina and weight loss may have a profound influence on symptoms.

Diabetes mellitus

This is a powerful and independent risk factor for the development of coronary artery disease. Control of blood glucose levels is vital in the management of patients with stable angina pectoris.

Pharmacological management

Basic treatment includes the use of aspirin, sublingual glycerol trinitrate (**GTN**), and β-blockade. Other antianginal agents may also be helpful, including calcium antagonists, long-acting nitrates, and potassium-channel openers.

Nitrates

In 1867, Brunton first described the clinical benefit of organic nitrates. These are prodrugs and are biotransformed by denitration, thereby liberating nitric oxide. This endothelium-derived relaxing factor (**EDRF**) exerts a vasodilatory effect, even in the absence of the endothelium, and also reduces platelet aggregation and adhesion. The antianginal and haemodynamic effects are mediated predominantly by vasodilatation of the venous system, leading to a fall in left ventricular preload and cardiac work, but also by vasodilatation of arteries, including the coronary arteries.

GTN remains the most commonly used preparation. Single doses of tablets or spray rapidly relieve angina pectoris and may be repeated every 5 min if symptoms persist. GTN is particularly effective when used prophylactically 2 to 5 min before activity. Many patients need no other antianginal medication if their angina is predictable and not particularly severe. Adverse effects of GTN are common and include flushing, headache, and hypotension. GTN is best used in the sitting or lying position to avoid hypotensive syncope, particularly for the first few doses.

Various nitrate preparations are widely used in the chronic treatment of angina pectoris, but are all limited by the development of nitrate tolerance. The mechanism leading to a reduction in clinical efficiency is not well understood, but its clinical effects can be overcome by intermittent nitrate dosing.

Nitrates can be given transdermally. Dermal absorption from ointment and patches has been shown to improve exercise duration. The ointment is applied in strips, often to the chest, and is particularly useful in those with nocturnal angina, or in immobile patients with severe symptoms. Transdermal application is also subject to nitrate tolerance.

Isosorbide dinitrate has a low bioavailability and marked variations in plasma concentration occur. Isosorbide-5-mononitrate is the active metabolite of the dinitrate and has excellent bioavailability, with a standard preparation yielding clinical effects for 4 to 8 h. Long-acting preparations, given at doses of 20 to 60 mg, are beneficial for up to 12 h. Single daily dosing does not induce tolerance, but such dosing regimes can lead to rebound myocardial ischaemia during the nitrate-free period. However, this is uncommon in clinical practice, particularly if the timing of the dose covers the period when the patient is physically active.

β-Blocking agents

These are the cornerstone of the pharmacological management of chronic angina pectoris. β-Blocking agents are well tolerated and reduce the frequency and duration of anginal episodes and improve exercise tolerance. They are also effective antihypertensive agents and prevent some arrhythmias. They act by competitively inhibiting catecholamine effects on the β-adrenergic receptor. This reduces heart rate and improves coronary perfusion (by prolonging diastole), thereby reducing an exercise-induced rise in blood pressure and contractility.

There are increasing numbers of β-blocking agents available. Factors that influence their usage include selectivity, elimination half-life, intrinsic sympathomimetic activity, and vasodilatory properties. However, for the standard treatment of patients with chronic angina pectoris, most agents will have a similar beneficial effect.

The β-receptor has two major subtypes: β1 and β2. The former predominates in the heart and the latter in the lungs. Non-selective β-blocking agents (propanolol, nadolol, pindolol, sotalol, and timolol) block both receptors, whereas selective agents (atenolol, bisoprolol, metoprolol) predominantly influence β1 receptors. These effects are relative and as doses rise selectivity becomes less prominent, so that bronchoconstriction may occur at effective antianginal doses.

Acebutolol, celiprolol, and pindolol have intrinsic sympathomimetic activity, inducing low-grade stimulation when sympathetic activity is low. The clinical significance of this is uncertain. Lipid-soluble agents such as propranolol and metoprolol are readily absorbed and have shorter half-lives.

Most agents are started in relatively small doses which are titrated against symptoms and markers of β-blockade such as heart rate, particularly on exercise. They are generally well tolerated, but bradycardia, atrioventricular block, heart failure, central nervous system effects (fatigue, depression, and nightmares) are often seen. Cold hands and feet, sexual dysfunction, and lethargy are also common. If β-blockers are to be stopped, this should be done gradually. Abrupt cessation can lead to worsening of angina pectoris with reflex tachycardia and anxiety.

The most appropriate recipient of β-blockade is an individual with exercise-induced angina, possibly with coexisting hypertension or arrhythmias. These patients should commence treatment with, for example, atenolol 50 to 100 mg once daily, metoprolol 50 to 100 mg twice daily, or propanolol 80 mg twice or three times per day. There is additional benefit after myocardial infarction. However, such agents are best avoided in the presence of reversible airways obstruction, diabetes, and impaired left ventricular function. Depression is often worsened, as is peripheral vascular disease.

Calcium antagonists

Calcium antagonists constitute a heterogeneous group of compounds with various degrees of effect on heart muscle, atrioventricular conduction, and peripheral and coronary vessels. They act by inhibiting calcium ion movement through slow channels in cardiac and smooth muscle membranes by non-competitive blockade of voltage-sensitive calcium channels. The effect of calcium antagonists in angina pectoris is related to a reduction in myocardial oxygen demand with some increase in oxygen supply. The latter is particularly important in patients with a vasoconstrictor component to their disease. While calcium antagonists may be effective on their own, some can be particularly useful when taken in combination with β-blocking agents. There are three main first-generation, calcium-channel blocking agents (verapamil, diltiazem, and nifedipine), which have quite diverse physiological actions and clinical effects.

Verapamil

This acts by slowing the heart rate and reducing myocardial contractility as well as dilating systemic and coronary vessels. It is markedly negatively inotropic, but this rarely causes clinical effects. Verapamil is started orally in the range of 40 to 80 mg three times daily. Adverse effects are hypotension, facial flushing, and constipation.

Diltiazem

The cardiac depressant effect of diltiazem is rather less than that of verapamil, but rather more than that of nifedipine. It is well tolerated. Although it causes little vasodilatation of coronary arteries, it does block exercise-induced coronary vasoconstriction and reduces afterload. It is usually started at a dose of 60 mg three times daily, but a number of long-acting preparations are now available (200–300 mg once daily).

Nifedipine

Nifedipine is a dihydropyridine derivative and there are a number of second-generation agents of a similar type (nicardipine, isradipine, and amlodipine). It is a more potent vasodilator than verapamil or diltiazem. Its beneficial effect in angina is due to its capacity to reduce myocardial oxygen requirement by afterload reduction and increase oxygen delivery through coronary vasodilatation. Nifedipine is usually started as 10 mg three times daily, but there are number of long-acting preparations that deliver 30 to 90 mg per day. Adverse effects are quite prominent and relate to vasodilatation, including headache, dizziness, palpitations, flushing, hypertension, and leg oedema. The adverse effects of nifedipine are reduced by the use of sustained-release preparations and short-acting formulations should probably not now be used. Nifedipine may increase in mortality. Second-generation dihydropyridine derivatives may have some advantages in side-effect profiles.

Other pharmacological agents

The potassium-channel opener nicorandil has been show to have effective antianginal properties. It is currently prescribed to patients with persisting symptoms despite 'maximal' medical therapy. Whether patients would benefit from an earlier introduction of nicorandil is yet to be determined.

Revascularization

Coronary angiography, with a view to revascularization, is recommended in patients who remain symptomatic or have documented ischaemia, despite maximal medical therapy. Other indications include the results of non-invasive testing suggesting poor prognosis despite milder symptoms (exertional hypotension, arrhythmias, and marked ischaemia), or for occupational reasons. While in younger, more active, patients, revascularization may be considered earlier in the disease course, age itself is not a restriction. However, whilst percutaneous transluminal coronary angioplasty can be performed safely in the elderly, the mortality from bypass surgery will rise unacceptably in very old patients with coexisting disease (see later). Coronary angiography is underutilized but clinically very useful in patients with diagnostic doubt as to the cause of chest pain, as normal findings considerably simplify management.

Exercise electrocardiography (or similar tests of ischaemia) give positive results in only 60 to 80 per cent of patients with coronary artery disease. The remainder are false-negative tests. Also, some normal individuals have an ischaemic response—these are false-positives. Such lack of sensitivity and specificity makes these tests too unreliable for screening normal individuals for coronary artery disease (for a fuller discussion of these important issues see Chapter 15.3.2).

Summary of the medical management of patients with chronic stable angina

1. Confirm the diagnosis by demonstrating myocardial ischaemia.
2. Control risk factors and modify lifestyle: in particular, weight loss may improve symptoms.
3. Treat with aspirin and GTN for both symptom relief and prophylaxis.
4. Add a β-blocking agent.
5. If angina is not controlled, add a long-acting nitrate or calcium-channel blocker.
6. If angina persists, and there are no contraindications, consider coronary revascularization.

Further reading

Diaz MN, et al. (1997). Antioxidants and atherosclerosis heart disease. *New England Journal of Medicine* 337, 408–11. [Overview of the importance of antioxidants.]

O'Connor GT, et al. (1989). An overview of randomised trials of rehabilitation with exercise after myocardial infarction. *Circulation* 80, 234–44. [Overview of the importance of exercise in coronary artery disease.]

Parker JD, Parker JO (1998). Nitrate therapy for stable angina pectoris. *New England Journal of Medicine* 338, 520–6. [Important review of nitrate therapy and tolerance.]

Pitt B, et al. (1999). Aggressive lipid-lower therapy compared with angioplasty in stable coronary artery disease. *New England Journal of Medicine* 341, 70–6. [First study to compare lipid-lowering therapy with PTCA]

Shuler G, Hambrecht R, Schlierf G et al. (1992). Myocardial perfusion and regression of coronary artery disease in patients with a regime of intensive physical exercise and low fat diet. *Journal of the American College of Cardiology* 19, 34–8. [Effect of lifestyle modifications on symptoms.]

15.4.2.3 Management of acute coronary syndromes: unstable angina and myocardial infarction

Keith A. A. Fox

Introduction

Acute coronary syndromes comprise a clinical spectrum of conditions that extend from new-onset angina through unstable angina and minimal myocardial injury (enzyme release without diagnostic changes of infarction) to myocardial infarction based upon ECG and enzyme criteria. These different clinical presentations share important pathophysiological features. They occur in patients with underlying symptomatic or occult coronary artery disease and flow-limiting or non-flow-limiting atheromatous plaques in the coronary arterial wall.

The acute coronary syndrome is precipitated in an abrupt change in an atheromatous plaque, resulting in increased obstruction to perfusion and ischaemia or infarction in the territory supplied by the affected vessel. For discussion of the mechanisms involved, see Chapter 15.4.2.1. The clinical manifestations are dependent not only upon the degree of obstruction to perfusion, but also on the presence or absence of collateral perfusion, the extent and distribution of fragmented microthrombi, and myocardial oxygen demand in the perfused territory. Thus, the clinical consequences of plaque rupture can range from an entirely silent episode through to a development of abrupt occlusion with profound ischaemia and infarction or sudden death.

Rational management, including pharmacological treatment and percutaneous or surgical revascularization strategies, are critically dependent on the underlying pathophysiological mechanisms and on the extent and severity of myocardial ischaemia. Despite sharing key pathophysiological mechanisms with ST-segment elevation, acute myocardial infarction (**MI**), unstable angina, and non-ST elevation MI demand special attention. Whereas acute reperfusion strategies (thrombolysis or primary percutaneous coronary intervention, **PCI**) are of proven benefit in ST-segment elevation infarction (or that associated with new bundle-branch block), there is no evidence that thrombolytic treatment improves outcome in the remainder of the syndrome. For this reason a pragmatic division is made between acute coronary syndromes with ST-segment elevation, and those without.

Unstable angina/non-ST elevation MI

Outcome based upon trial data and large-scale observational registry studies

Imprecision in the definition and characterization of unstable angina or non-ST elevation MI has previously resulted in underestimation of the risk of this syndrome. The inclusion of patients with chest pain, but without diagnostic features of acute ischaemia, masked the true hazards of the syndrome.

Table 1 Clinical presentation of unstable angina

I	New-onset angina	Onset within 8 weeks, at least CCS grade III
II	Crescendo angina	Previously stable angina becomes more frequent, more easily induced, severe, or prolonged, or less responsive to nitroglycerin(at least CCS grade III)
III	Rest angina	Angina occurring at rest and lasting longer than 15–20 min

- New Q waves or the elevation of cardiac enzymes to more than twice normal (or >99th centile of normals: new ACC/ESC definition of MI) defines the occurrence of MI
- Within this spectrum of symptomatic manifestations of ischaemic heart disease are variant or Prinzmetal's angina and angina in the early post-MI period (>24 h). Non-Q wave MI cannot be differentiated from unstable angina on initial clinical presentation and the initial management is not different. ST- and T-wave abnormalities are common. (See Fig. 1.)

CCS grade III: Canadian Cardiovascular Society angina grade III, which is angina on minor exertion or emotion.

Patients with acute coronary syndrome (without persistent ST elevation) are at substantial risk of subsequent cardiac events despite current therapy. Based on data from randomized trials and prospective registry studies, about 9 to 11 per cent suffer death or myocardial infarction at 6 months, with almost half of this risk within the first 7 days (GUSTO IIb, OASIS Registry, GRACE Registry). Between one-quarter and a third of patients suffer death, myocardial infarction, or readmission for unstable angina within 6 months (GRACE Registry, PRAIS Registry).

Clinical presentation and definition of the syndrome

Unstable angina may present *de novo* (new-onset angina) with episodes of typical ischaemic discomfort at rest (rest angina) or on minimal exertion. Alternatively, a previously stable pattern of angina may deteriorate abruptly or progressively, resulting in episodes of typical rest angina or angina provoked by minor exertion (crescendo angina). Although new-onset exertional angina is not generally recognized as part of the acute coronary syndrome, the outcomes are similar (7 per cent develop non-fatal MI and 4 per cent die, and a further 19 per cent require revascularization within 15 months) (Table 1).

As a clinical syndrome, unstable angina is conventionally diagnosed by the presence of new-onset angina or angina of worsening severity in terms of frequency or duration. The syndrome must be distinguished from noncardiac pain, stable angina, and infarction. To improve the specificity of the diagnosis, and for the purposes of clinical trials, a more restricted definition has been employed which requires at least 15 to 20 min of typical, ischaemic discomfort, or two 5-min episodes at rest. The specificity is further improved when the definition requires objective evidence of ischaemia or evidence of underlying coronary artery disease. ST-segment depression on the electrocardiogram, especially in association with typical pain, is highly predictive, whereas the less specific ECG abnormalities including T-wave inversion are less strong predictors. Markers of myocardial damage (troponins or cardiac enzymes) are powerfully predictive. The ECG changes and the markers also indicate an adverse prognostic outcome. In the absence of such markers, documented evidence of underlying coronary artery disease (prior infarction or angiographically demonstrated coronary disease) helps to confirm the diagnosis.

Minimal myocardial damage—infarction without ST elevation or Q-wave development ('including non-Q-wave MI')—lies between unstable angina and Q-wave myocardial infarction in its prognostic significance (Fig. 1). It is best considered as part of the continuous spectrum of acute coronary syndromes rather than as a separate entity (Fig. 2). Management strategies are the same as for other higher risk patients with unstable angina. Minimal myocardial injury arises as a result of episodes of transient occlusion and/or embolization of thrombus into the distal circulation of the affected coronary vessel. Injury to myocytes results in the release of enzymes from the contractile apparatus (troponins) and cardiac enzymes, indicating irreversible injury (creatine kinase (CK) or CK-MB (**CK-MB**)). Thus, although the management of ST-*segment-elevation MI* differs, the remainder of the acute coronary syndrome should be managed as a continuous spectrum, but influenced by risk stratification.

Variant angina

A condition characterized by recurrent episodes of angina at rest, often accompanied by ST-segment elevation, was originally described by Prinzmetal. Such patients may have relatively a well-preserved exercise capacity and specific diurnal periodicity to the symptoms, with occasional clustering of symptomatic episodes and symptom-free periods. Coronary vasospasm has been implicated in the syndrome, and in some instances the coronary arteries appear angiographically normal, or with only minor occlusive disease. However, the vast majority of patients with symptomatic ischaemia and ST-segment elevation or depression have occlusive coronary artery disease with superimposed thrombosis, and they should be managed as such. Indeed, vasospasm very frequently accompanies plaque rupture and thrombosis. With the use of modern cardiac enzyme studies and coronary angiographic techniques, variant angina is a rare diagnosis that

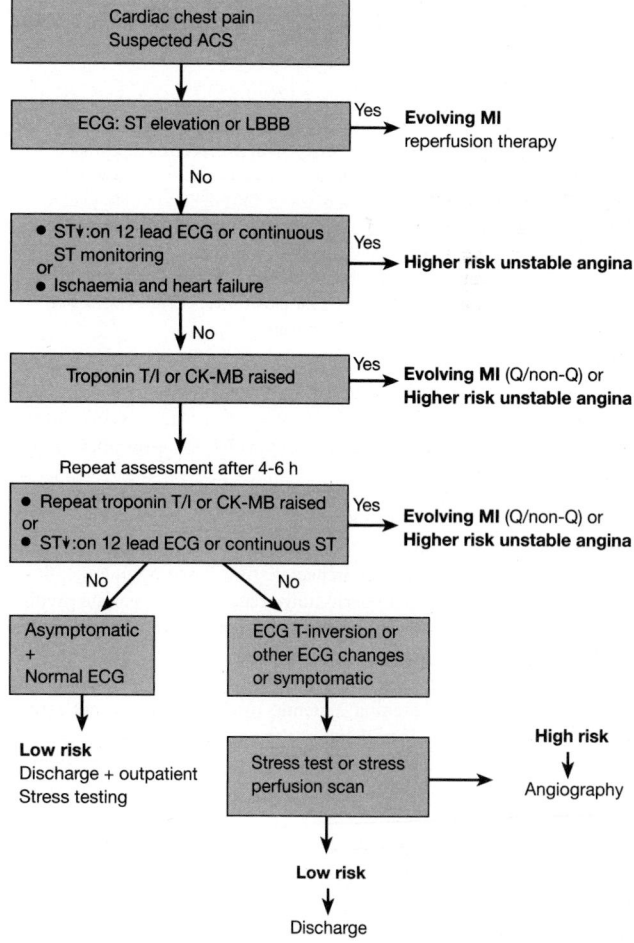

Fig. 1 Diagnostic triage for suspected acute coronary syndromes. Flow chart to illustrate the key diagnostic features for evolving myocardial infarction, for higher risk unstable angina and for low-risk patients.

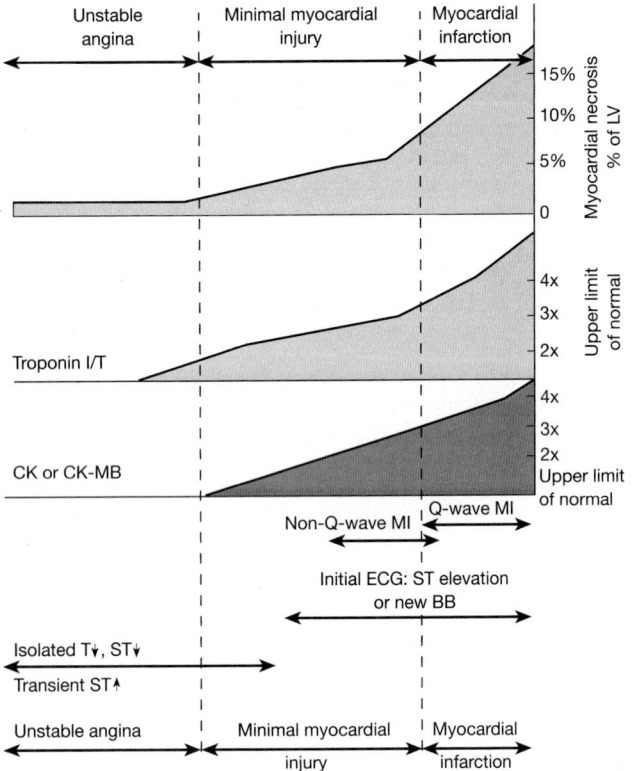

Fig. 2 Schematic of the spectrum of acute coronary syndromes. The relationship between the extent of myocardial necrosis (upper panel) and the release of cardiac enzymes (troponin I or T, or CK or CK-MB) and electrocardiographic changes. The schematic illustrates that unstable angina is associated with minor myocardial necrosis without the release of CK or CK-MB but with the release of troponin in approximately one-third of cases. With minimal myocardial injury, more extensive myocardial necrosis is associated with the release of cardiac enzymes and ECG changes (non-ST elevation-wave MI). With Q-wave MI the most extensive myocardial necrosis and release of cardiac enzymes occurs in association with the electrocardiographic changes.

should only be considered if atherosclerotic acute coronary syndromes have been excluded. It is possible that erosion of a minor plaque, superimposed thrombosis and embolization may be responsible for a number of such clinical cases.

Risk characterization and outcome

In patients with acute coronary syndromes, risk can be separated into two components: prior risk and acute ischaemic risk. Based upon large observational studies it is possible to derive univariate and multivariate predictors of outcome. Prior risk is determined by patient characteristics (age and gender), prior ischaemic heart disease (myocardial infarction, heart failure, prior angina), and systemic factors that influence risk (hypertension, diabetes, and other life-threatening systemic disorders). These are largely unchangeable and can be considered as the background level of risk that the patient brings with them to the point of presentation. The extent of underlying coronary artery disease and prior heart failure require assessment and management.

The second component of risk, 'acute ischaemic risk' is determined by the severity of ischaemia induced by plaque rupture and thrombosis and the extent of the territory affected. Collateral perfusion and myocardial oxygen demand both influence the extent of ischaemia. Patients may experience transient complete occlusion, or severe subtotal occlusion complicated by distal embolization of fragments of a platelet-rich thrombus, also by changes in vascular tone in the distal territory. Clinical markers of acute ischaemic risk include electrocardiographic changes, enzyme release

into the systemic circulation, and mechanical and arrhythmic complications of the ischaemic episode.

The first priority in the management of patients with acute coronary syndromes is to deal with acute ischaemic risk. Assessment of the extent of underlying coronary artery disease (for example with stress testing and/or angiography) and assessment of left ventricular function can take place later in the management of these patients. Simplistically, 'prior risk' can be regarded as the 'baggage' that the patient carries with them, and 'acute ischaemic risk' as an 'acquired hazard' arising from the new ischaemic event. The distinction is important because management strategies for prior risk aim to treat heart failure, underlying coronary and systemic disease, and risk factors. The management of acute ischaemic risk aims to reverse the impact of acute coronary obstruction and thrombosis.

The clinical syndrome and outcome

The Braunwald classification categorizes unstable angina according to the mode of onset and time course (Table 2). It was empirically based but has been validated by prospective studies. Patients with unstable angina at rest (Braunwald Class 3) have the highest risk of an adverse cardiac event (approximately 11 per cent in hospital event rate). Similarly, those with unstable angina following acute myocardial infarction are at an increased risk. Although useful, many of the patients that present with acute coronary syndromes are in Braunwald Class 3B and additional methods of risk characterization are required to optimize management.

A diagnostic triage system can be developed for patients with suspected acute coronary syndromes (Fig. 1). This is based upon electrocardiographic changes, enzyme release, and stress or perfusion testing. As a result, those with evolving infarction are identified and those with higher risk unstable angina are separated from those with lower risk. These categories of patients require different management strategies.

The electrocardiogram and outcome

The 12-lead electrocardiogram (performed on admission) provides direct prognostic information (Table 3).

The greatest risk of death and subsequent MI is seen in patients with simultaneous ST elevation and depression. The next highest risk is seen in those with transient ST-segment elevation or ST-segment depression. Isolated T-wave inversion carries a lower risk (Table 3). The number of leads demonstrating ST deviation also yields prognostic information: among those with ST deviation in the anterior leads a rate of death or myocardial infarction of 12.4 per cent was seen at 1 year, higher than seen with similar changes in other locations (TIMI III trial). Patients with a left main and three-vessel coronary artery disease may show a combination of ST-segment elevation and depression.

Holter ST-segment recording can identify patients with unstable angina and either silent or symptomatic myocardial ischaemia with an increased risk for major subsequent cardiac events. However, they provide off-line analysis and are not suitable for the prediction of imminent events. Computer-assisted, continuous, multi-lead, ECG monitoring techniques have become available for real-time ECG and ST-segment monitoring. The occurrence and extent of ischaemic territory identified by such continuous recordings can provide additional prognostic information over and above the admission ECG. They can be combined with serial enzyme markers; recent studies have indicated that together they provide additional prognostic information (FRISC study).

Biochemical markers and outcome

Enzymes are gradually released into the systemic circulation following complete or transient occlusion of the coronary artery, or fragmentation of a thrombus and embolization. Following total occlusion of the vessel, creatine kinase (or more specifically CK-MB) will be released and detectable at clearly abnormal levels about 6 to 8 h after the event, unless there is extensive collateral perfusion. By convention, CK values greater than twice the upper limit of normal are associated with infarction, and this is categorized

Table 2 Classification of unstable angina (Braunwald)

Class		A Secondary unstable angina	B Primary unstable angina	C Postinfarction (<2 weeks) unstable angina
I	New-onset, severe or accelerated angina	IA	IB	IC
II	Subacute rest angina (<48 h ago)	IIA	IIB	IIC
III	Acute rest angina (within 48 h)	IIIA	IIIB	IIIC

An empirical classification of unstable angina based upon the mode and time course of presentation (Taken with permission from Braunwald E. *Circulation* 1989, **80**, 410–14).

into those with Q-wave development and those without. However, a continuous spectrum of injury exists from unstable angina through non-Q-wave myocardial infarction to Q-wave infarction. The evolution of Q waves on the ECG (or none) provides prognostic information by the time of hospital discharge, but cannot be used to guide early treatment.

The measurement of myocardial isoforms of troponins in the blood are more sensitive markers of injury. The cardiac isoforms of troponin I and troponin T are exclusively expressed in cardiac myocytes and provide specific evidence of myocardial damage. Only a few patients with renal dysfunction will have falsely elevated troponin measurements. Following marked ischaemia or infarction, troponins are released from the cytosolic pool and first appear in the circulation in detectable concentrations between 3 and 4 h after the ischaemic event and reach diagnostic concentrations at 6 to 8 h. Troponin release may be regarded as evidence of myocardial injury and it carries a prognostic significance worse than that of patients without troponin release but less severe than those with acute infarction diagnosed by by a rise of more than twofold in CK-MB (Fig. 3) unless the concentrations in the blood are markedly elevated. The greater the troponin release the greater the risk of subsequent myocardial infarction and death.

When should the cardiac enzymes be measured? The time course of the release of enzymes from myocardium is such that diagnostic concentrations may not be achieved until between 6 and 8 h after an ischaemic event. Thus, normal values for a patient on arrival do not exclude infarction or unstable angina. However, elevated values on arrival are highly predictive of subsequent infarction (for CK, or CK-MB, or troponins). The CK and CK-MB measurements should be repeated between 8 and 12 h later and also after any suspected ischaemic event. Troponins should be measured on arrival and at approximately 8 h: these provide the highest predictive accuracy.

Among those with persistently negative troponins and without significant ECG changes there is a very low risk of subsequent infarction and death (provided that severe underlying coronary artery disease is excluded). Ideally such patients should undergo predischarge stress testing; the most accurate test being that accompanied by myocardial perfusion scanning or stress echocardiography. Treadmill electrocardiograms on exercise are less accurate but more widely available (see Chapter 15.3.2).

Among patients in whom myocardial infarction is excluded by standard criteria, about one-quarter will have elevated troponin levels (minor myo-

cardial damage) and these patients have the same frequency of cardiac events during follow-up as seen for conventionally diagnosed infarction.

Markers of inflammation

Inflammatory changes in the vessel wall promote plaque fissuring or erosion, and inflammatory changes also follow episodes of minor myocardial damage. In unstable angina there is evidence that inflammatory markers (C-reactive protein (**CRP**), interleukin-6, and interleukin-1) are independent predictors of adverse outcome. Only 50 to 70 per cent of patients with Braunwald class IIIB unstable angina have elevated CRP levels. After the acute phase, continuing inflammation—with, for example, elevated CRP—occurs in half of those whose levels are acutely elevated and identifies a category of patients at increased risk. Although inflammatory mechanisms are implicated in plaque growth and plaque destabilization, specific anti-inflammatory therapy of surface integrins (including the inhibition of surface integrins or inhibition of polymorph infiltration with anti-CD11/CD18 antibodies) has not yet been demonstrated to improve outcome.

Treatment

Antiplatelet therapy

Aspirin

Exposure of the contents of atheromatous plaque to circulating blood triggers platelet activation by several different pathways. Aspirin is a potent and irreversible inhibitor of platelet cyclo-oxygenase, blocking the formation of thromboxane A_2 and inhibiting platelet aggregation. Although the effects of aspirin can be overcome in the presence of potent thrombogenic stimuli, nevertheless the benefits of aspirin treatment in unstable angina are clearly defined and substantial. The Antiplatelet Trialists Collaboration demonstrated a reduction of 36 per cent in death or MI with antiplatelet treatment (predominantly aspirin) versus placebo in unstable angina trials. Aspirin treatment significantly reduces subsequent myocardial infarction, stroke, and vascular death, with the largest reductions seen amongst patients at highest risk. In patients with unstable angina, four key studies have demonstrated that aspirin significantly reduces the risk of cardiac death or non-fatal MI by approximately 50 per cent.

The efficacy of lower dose aspirin (75 mg day) therapy has been demonstrated in several studies, including those of Wallentin and colleagues where long-term effects were evaluated in men under 70 years of age with unstable

Table 3 Prognostic value of admission ECG for early risk stratification in 12 142 patients with an acute coronary syndrome

	ST elevation + ST depression (%)	ST elevation (%)	ST depression (%)	T wave inversion (%)	*p*
Patients	15	28	35	23	
Acute infarction on admission	87	81	47	31	<0.0001
Death	6.8	5.0	5.0	1.8	<0.001
(Re)infarction	6.9	5.1	6.7	4.3	<0.001

Death and reinfarction at 30 days' follow-up. Data from the GUSTO IIb trial.

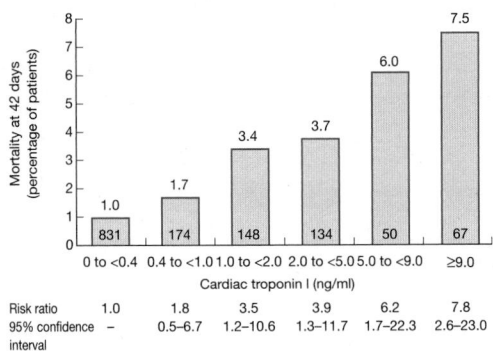

Fig. 3 Cardiac troponin I and subsequent risk of death among patients with unstable angina or non-ST-elevation MI. Mortality rates at 42 days (without adjustment for baseline characteristics) are shown for ranges of cardiac troponin I levels measured at baseline. The numbers at the bottom of each bar are the numbers of patients with cardiac troponin I levels in each range, and the numbers above the bars are percentages. $p < 0.001$ for the increase in the mortality rate (and the risk ratio for mortality) with increasing levels of cardiac troponin I at enrolment. (Reproduced with permission from Antman *et al*. *New England Journal of Medicine* 1996, **335**, 1342–9.)

coronary artery disease. After 6 and 12 months of aspirin treatment the risk of myocardial infarction or death was reduced by 54 per cent and 48 per cent, respectively (risk ratio 0.52 with 95 per cent confidence intervals 0.37–0.72). The strength of evidence and magnitude of benefit demonstrated with aspirin treatment in unstable angina or non-ST-*segment-elevation MI* is such that aspirin forms the reference standard against which alternative or adjunctive antiplatelet therapies are judged.

- Aspirin treatment is indicated in all patients with acute coronary syndromes unless there is good evidence of aspirin allergy.

Nevertheless, patients with acute coronary syndromes are at significant risk despite aspirin therapy. In prospective registry studies of unstable angina/non-ST-*segment-elevation MI*, and in spite of aspirin treatment in more than 80 per cent of patients, the risk of death or myocardial infarction is approximately 10 per cent at 6 months and the risk of death/myocardial infarction or refractory angina is approximately 22 to 33 per cent over the same period (OASIS Registry, PRAIS Registry).

ADP antagonists (thienopyridines)

Ticlopidine and clopidogrel reduce thrombotic events following angioplasty and stenting. Clopidogrel has now replaced ticlopidine as it lacks the side-effect of thrombocytopenia.

Clopidogrel has now been tested in a large-scale trial of patients with unstable angina/non-ST-elevation MI (*N*=12 562 CURE trial). The agent was used on top of existing therapy and in addition to aspirin. It reduced death, non-fatal MI and stroke from 11.4 per cent to 9.3 per cent (95 per cent CI 0.72-0.90 *P* = <0.001). For every 1000 patients treated there were 28 fewer major cardiovascular complications but six more transfusions. Importantly, benefits were seen across risk groups (diabetics, hypertensives, CK or troponin elevation or not, revascularization or not). In a sub-study (PCI-CURE) clopidogrel also reduced death and myocardial infarction in those undergoing percutaneous revascularization (2.9 per cent clopidogrel versus 4.4 per cent for placebo). Thus, with the combination of clopidogrel and aspirin there is evidence of early and sustained reductions in the risks of death and myocardial infarction in patients that present with acute coronary syndromes, irrespective of their risk group and irrespective of baseline conditions. New guidelines are likely to incorporate this treatment in the management of the syndrome.

Glycoprotein IIb/IIIa inhibitors

Platelet adhesion is the initial step in haemostasis after disruption of an atheromatous plaque. It is triggered by damage to the vessel wall and exposure of the subendothelium, and is followed by platelet activation and aggregation. Regardless of the agonist, the final common pathway leading to the formation of a platelet aggregate is mediated by the glycoprotein (**GP**) IIb/IIIa receptor (up to 80 000 per platelet). GPIIb/IIIa receptor antagonists inhibit platelet aggregation irrespective of the agonist, and they prevent binding of fibrinogen to its receptor on the platelet surface.

To date, three GPIIb/IIIa inhibitors have been tested in large-scale randomized clinical trials. Abciximab is a chimeric human–murine monoclonal antibody that binds with high affinity to the receptor: it has a long biological half-life of 6 to 12 h, and low levels of receptor occupancy are detected even 2 weeks after treatment. Eptifibatide is a synthetic cyclic heptapeptide with high affinity for the arginine–glycine–aspartic acid ligand adhesion site of the IIb/IIIa receptor. It inhibits platelet aggregation in a dose-dependent manner and is readily reversible due to competitive binding and a short half-life of approximately 2.5 h. Tirofiban is a non-peptide tyrosine derivative which also binds to the arginine–glycine–aspartic acid site with high specificity. It inhibits platelet aggregation in a dose- and concentration-dependent manner and is rapidly reversible, with platelet function approaching normal levels in 90 per cent of patients within 4 to 8 h.

Although it is convenient to group glycoprotein IIb/IIIa receptor antagonists together, and undoubtedly there is evidence of a class effect, there are nevertheless biological and pharmacological differences between the agents.

Trials of GPIIb/IIIa inhibitors

More than 32 000 patients have been randomized in clinical trials involving GPIIb/IIIa inhibitors (16 trials). A highly significant ($p < 0.001$) benefit is observed for the combined endpoint of death or MI at 48 to 96 h, 30 days, and 6 months. At 30 days the odds ratio is 0.76, or 20 fewer events per 1000 patients treated. Similarly, a highly significant benefit is observed for the combined endpoint of death/MI or revascularization at all time points. By contrast, mortality benefits are seen only at 48 to 96 h with no significant benefit at 30 days or 6 months. However, a pooled analysis of abciximab trials has revealed a net mortality benefit.

The effects of GPIIb/IIIa inhibitors may be greater in higher risk groups: trials involving percutaneous intervention (angioplasty with or without stent) have demonstrated significantly greater reductions in events with GPIIb/IIIa inhibitors in comparison with trials where angiography or intervention were not a prerequisite. In the interventional trials, death or MI was reduced by 27 fewer events per 1000 patients treated (odds ratio 0.64; confidence interval (95 per cent CI 0.51–0.80). In trials of GPIIb/IIIa inhibitors in acute coronary syndromes without mandatory intervention, there were 13 fewer events per 1000 patients treated (with an odds ratio of 0.88; 95 per cent CI, 0.81–0.97).

Subsequent analyses have been performed for those patients with elevated troponin levels and data from the CAPTURE study, the PRISM PLUS, and the PRISM study indicate that almost all the benefit is seen amongst those higher risk patients demonstrating troponin release.

Indications for treatment with GPIIb/IIIa inhibitors

Because of the variability in trial design, it is not yet feasible to assess differences, if any, in clinical benefit among the GPIIb/IIIa inhibitors. Head-to-head trials in acute coronary syndromes would be needed to resolve this issue. Nevertheless, robust evidence supports the following conclusions:

- Treatment with glycoprotein IIb/IIIa inhibitors results in improved outcome in unstable angina or non-Q-wave MI patients treated with aspirin and heparin. Most benefit is seen in high-risk patients (ST depression and/or troponin-elevation).

- Glycoprotein IIb/IIIa inhibitors result in improved outcome in patients requiring urgent percutaneous intervention for unstable angina or non-ST-*segment-elevation MI*.

Antithrombins

Unfractionated heparin

Unfractionated heparin has been adopted as standard antithrombin therapy in guidelines for the treatment of unstable angina/non-ST-elevation MI. However, the evidence upon which this is based is less robust than for other widely adopted treatment strategies. In practice, unfractionated heparin is difficult to control due to its unpredictable levels of binding to plasma proteins, and this may be amplified by the acute-phase response. In addition, heparin has reduced effectiveness against platelet-rich and clot-bound thrombin. In the absence of aspirin, heparin treatment is associated with a lower frequency of refractory angina/myocardial infarction and death (as a combined endpoint) compared to placebo.

Oler and colleagues have conducted a meta-analysis of the influence of adding heparin to aspirin in the treatment of patients with unstable angina. Only six randomized trials were available: there were 55 deaths or myocardial infarctions out of 698 in the aspirin plus heparin arm and 68 out of 655 in the aspirin-alone arm, giving a risk reduction of 0.67 and a 95 per cent confidence interval of 0.44 to 1.02. Thus, these results do not produce conclusive evidence of benefit from adding heparin to aspirin, but it must be stressed that appropriately powered, larger scale trials have not been conducted. Nevertheless, clinical guidelines have adopted unfractionated heparin treatment with aspirin as a pragmatic extrapolation of the available evidence.

Low-molecular-weight heparins versus placebo

The 1996 FRISC trial tested dalteparin against placebo in aspirin-treated patients with unstable angina/non-ST-elevation MI. Some 1506 patients were randomized to receive dalteparin (twice daily for the first 6 days and then once daily at a lower dose for approximately 6 weeks), and the trial showed a highly significant reduction in the frequency of death or new myocardial infarction at 6 days (1.8 per cent versus 4.8 per cent, with a risk ratio of 0.37). The effects were sustained to 42 days but were attenuated at 6 months, the differences no longer maintaining significance. Nevertheless, this trial clearly showed the benefit of low-molecular-weight heparin over placebo, in the presence of aspirin, and the feasibility of administering such treatment over a prolonged time.

Low-molecular-weight heparins possess enhanced anti-Xa activity in relation to anti-IIa (antithrombin) activity compared with unfractionated heparin. They also exhibit decreased sensitivity to platelet Factor 4, have more predictable anticoagulant effect, and lower rates of thrombocytopenia. In view of their enhanced bioavailability they offer the substantial practical advantage of subcutaneous administration, based on a dose per kilogram of body weight, and without the need for laboratory monitoring.

Low-molecular-weight heparin versus unfractionated heparin

Acute-phase treatment (approximately 2 to 8 days) In the FRIC trial dalteparin was tested against unfractionated heparin in 1400 patients with unstable angina: it had limited power to show a difference, and no significant difference was seen between unfractionated heparin and dalteparin.

The ESSENCE trial was double-blinded and placebo-controlled and tested enoxaparin against unfractionated heparin. The treatments were given for 2 to 8 days (median 2.6 days) and the primary endpoints were death, myocardial infarction, or recurrent angina. Enoxaparin reduced the primary endpoint from 19.6 per cent to 16.6 per cent at 14 days (odds ratio 0.80 and confidence intervals 0.67–0.98). A similar and significant odds ratio was maintained at 30 days and 1 year. At 1 year there were 3.7 fewer events/100 patients ($p = 0.022$). The study was not powered for death/myocardial infarction alone but demonstrated corresponding trends for these endpoints.

The TIMI 11b trial was also double-blinded and tested enoxaparin *versus* unfractionated heparin, but additionally it examined 72 h of treatment *versus* 43 days of treatment. The results up to 14 days mirrored those seen in the ESSENCE trial: at 14 days the primary outcome occurred was 16.6 per cent (heparin) *versus* 14.2 per cent (enoxaparin), risk ratio 0.85 ($p = 0.03$).

A combined analysis of ESSENCE and TIMI 11b in 1999 indicated an absolute reduction of 3.1 per 100 for death/MI/refractory angina, and showed a similar risk ratio of 0.79 (CI 0.65–0.96) for death and myocardial infarction. Taken together, these findings indicate that short-term treatment with enoxaparin results in about 3 per 100 fewer major cardiac endpoints compared to unfractionated heparin treatment, and this is achieved without additional major bleeding.

Prolonged outpatient treatment The FRAXIS trial reported in 1999 tested fraxaparin, for 6 or 14 days, against unfractionated heparin. A total of 3468 patients were randomized within 48 h of symptom onset; no difference was seen at 6 days, 14 days, or 43 days, but there was a significant excess of major bleeds with longer term outpatient treatment. In TIMI 11b the curves remained separated over the succeeding treatment interval: at 43 days there were 19.6 per cent events (heparin) *versus* 17.3 per cent (enoxaparin) ($p = 0.049$), with no evidence of a further separation of the curves. However, only about 60 per cent of the patients entered the chronic-treatment phase of the study and it must be recognized that the study does not exclude a moderate treatment for more prolonged treatment. There was 1.4 per cent absolute excess in major bleeds over the chronic phase.

One component of the FRISC II trial compared long-term *versus* short-term low-molecular-weight heparin (dalteparin) treatment. After 5 days of open-phase treatment with dalteparin, patients were randomized to placebo or weight-adjusted dalteparin for a period of 3 months. The primary endpoint of death/MI occurred in 6.7 per cent of patients at 90 days in the dalteparin arm and 8 per cent in the placebo arm (a non-significant difference). The risk ratio was 0.82 but confidence intervals were between 0.6 and 1.11. The secondary analysis at earlier time points indicated a difference in favour of the low-molecular-weight heparin but this diminished by 3 months.

Conclusions from the low-molecular-weight heparin studies There is convincing evidence in aspirin-treated patients that low-molecular-weight heparin is better than placebo (FRISC trial). The two trials using enoxaparin have provided consistent data in favour of low-molecular-weight heparin over unfractionated heparin when administered as an acute regimen. The other trials have produced a similar outcome for the acute phase of treatment and it can be concluded that acute treatment is at least as effective as unfractionated heparin. To date, the evidence to support longer term treatment with low-molecular-weight heparin is less convincing. Low-molecular-weight heparins offer significant practical advantages with simplicity of administration, more consistent antithrombin effects, lack of the need for monitoring, and a safety profile similar to that of unfractionated heparin. Evidence supports the following conclusions:

- Low-molecular-weight heparin is superior to placebo in aspirin-treated patients.
- Low-molecular-weight heparin is at least as effective as unfractionated heparin.
- Low-molecular-weight heparin can be used in place of unfractionated heparin and has practical advantages over unfractionated heparin.

Hirudin

Hirudin is a more potent and specific antithrombin than heparin, and large-scale trials have been conducted against unfractionated heparin. A combined analysis of the OASIS-1, OASIS-2, TIMI 9b, and GUSTO IIb trials indicates a 22 per cent relative-risk reduction in cardiovascular death or MI at 72 h, 17 per cent at 7 days, and 10 per cent at 35 days. This combined analysis is significant at 72 h and 7 days and the *p* value at 35 days is 0.057. Hirudin has specific indications for patients with heparin-induced thrombocytopenia. None of the hirudins are currently licensed in the United Kingdom for the treatment of acute coronary syndromes.

Anti-ischaemic therapy

Specific antithrombotic treatment will have an impact on limiting the progression of occlusion and improving perfusion, hence such treatment has an anti-ischaemic impact. In addition, other pharmacological treatments reduce myocardial oxygen demand and may induce coronary vasodilatation, thus reducing ischaemia. Mechanical revascularization (percutaneous intervention and coronary bypass surgery) also aims to relieve obstruction and reduce a patient's susceptibility to ischaemia and these interventions will be considered separately (see below).

Nitrates

Nitrates act by venodilatation, and in higher dose arteriolar dilatation, and hence reduce preload and afterload, thereby decreasing oxygen demand (see Chapter 15.4.2.2). In addition, nitrates can also induce coronary vasodilatation. They are effective in relieving symptoms of ischaemia. In the acute phase of the syndrome, where dose titration is required, they are most conveniently administered intravenously. Once dose titration is no longer required, buccal, oral, or topical administration is feasible.

The main limitation of continuous administration is the development of tolerance. Increased doses of nitrates may be required, with the dose adjusted on the basis of heart rate, blood pressure response, and relief of symptoms.

Large outcome trials have been conducted with nitrates in acute myocardial infarction but not in the remainder of acute coronary syndromes. However, patients without ST-segment elevation or bundle-branch block were randomized within the ISIS-4 trial. Their mortality was 5.3 per cent for nitrate treatment and 5.5 per cent for placebo treatment, a non-significant difference.

Following acute-phase treatment, patients may be switched to an outpatient oral administration of nitrates. However, if tolerance has been induced in the acute phase, such treatment may have reduced efficacy. Nevertheless, on the basis of current evidence:

- nitrates are effective in reducing ischaemia in the inhospital management of unstable angina/non-ST-elevation MI.

β-Blockers

β-Adrenoceptor antagonists reduce heart rate and blood pressure and myocardial contractility. They are primarily employed to reduce ischaemia in acute coronary syndromes. Large-scale trials have not been conducted in patients with unstable angina or non-Q-wave myocardial infarction. However, in the context of acute myocardial infarction β-blockers reduce mortality by approximately 10 to 15 per cent. They may act be reducing ventricular arrhythmias, reinfarction, and myocardial rupture. A meta-analysis of five trials involving 4700 patients with threatened MI (treated with intravenous β-blockers followed by oral therapy for approximately 1 week) resulted in a 13 per cent reduction in the risk of MI.

β-Blockers may exacerbate acute heart failure. By contrast, recent trials have produced strong evidence of a benefit for the gradual introduction of β-blockers in ambulant patients with heart failure (see Chapter 15.2.2).

On the basis of current evidence:

- Patients with suspected acute coronary syndromes should be initiated on β-blocker therapy unless contraindicated in the individual case.

Calcium-entry blockers

These agents inhibit the slow inward current induced by the entry of extracellular calcium through the cell membrane, especially in cardiac and arteriolar smooth muscle. They act by lowering myocardial oxygen demand, reducing arterial pressure, and reducing contractility. Some agents induce a reflex tachycardia (nifedipine, nicardipine, amlodipine) and are best administered in combination with a β-adrenoceptor antagonist. By contrast, diltiazem and verapamil are suitable for patients who cannot tolerate a β-blocker because they inhibit conduction through the atrioventricular (AV) node and tend to cause bradycardia. All calcium antagonists reduce myocardial contractility and may aggravate heart failure. Calcium-entry blockers have been demonstrated to reduce the frequency of angina in patients with variant angina.

A meta-analysis of calcium-entry blockers in acute coronary syndromes indicates a non-significant trend towards a higher mortality in treated *versus* control patients (5.9 per cent *versus* 5.2 per cent, in 7551 patients). In

individual trials, diltiazem has been compared with propranolol and both agents produced a similar reduction in anginal episodes. Subgroup analysis suggests that diltiazem is efficacious in the group with rest angina, but the clinician should always be cautious in extrapolating from subgroup analyses.

- Dihydropyridine calcium-entry blockers should be employed with β-blockers in acute coronary syndromes to avoid reflex tachycardia. In patients unable to tolerate β-blockers, a heart rate-slowing calcium antagonist may be appropriate. Short-acting dihydropyridines should not be used in isolation in acute coronary syndromes.

Potassium-channel activators

These agents (for example, nicorandil) have arterial and venous dilating properties but do not exhibit the tolerance seen with nitrates. They have been shown to be better than placebo in relieving the symptoms of angina, but little convincing evidence exists in comparison with other antianginal agents. Nicorandil possesses both potassium channel and nitrate properties and may be considered as an alternative to nitrate administration.

Conclusions: anti-ischaemic therapy

The following strategy is based upon available clinical and trial evidence:

- Patients with suspected acute coronary syndromes should be initiated on nitrate and β-blocker therapy unless there are contraindications to the use of β-blockers.

- In patients with contraindications to β-blockers, heart rate-slowing calcium antagonists should be employed.

- The combination of a calcium antagonist and β-blocker is superior to either agent alone.

- Angiography and revascularization should be considered in patients with recurrent ischaemia (with ECG abnormalities) or patients with troponin elevation (including non-ST elevation MI).

Revascularization

In chronic, stable angina strong evidence supports the use of surgical revascularization for the relief of symptoms and also for improved prognosis in patients with left main or three-vessel coronary artery disease (especially with left ventricular impairment). Percutaneous revascularization (percutaneous intervention, PCI) is primarily employed for the relief of symptoms in chronic stable angina and in patients with one- or two-vessel coronary artery disease. By contrast, until 1999 evidence to support revascularization in the acute coronary syndrome was inconclusive. The feasibility of PCI or coronary artery bypass grafting (CABG) had been established, but they were associated with an increased risk of complications in comparison with equivalent procedures performed in patients with chronic stable angina.

Observational studies

Large-scale observational studies have demonstrated wide variations between countries in the use of cardiac catheterization and revascularization for patients with acute ischaemic syndromes (OASIS Registry 1998, GRACE Registry 2001). Unsurprisingly, a direct correlation was demonstrated between the availability of revascularization facilities and the frequency with which such procedures were performed. Thus, highest revascularization rates were demonstrated in the United States, with lower rates in Poland and Hungary. By contrast, no significant differences in the rates of death or myocardial infarction were seen, despite rates of invasive procedures of 59 per cent in high revascularization countries *versus* 21 per cent in low revascularization countries. Furthermore, the higher rates of revascularization were associated with an increased frequency of procedural complications, including stroke and major bleeding. These observational data highlighted the importance of performing randomized trials to resolve the role and timing of revascularization in patients with acute coronary syndromes, and to test the impact of adjunctive antithrombotic therapy.

Randomized trial data

Early comparisons of CABG and medical therapy for patients admitted with unstable angina were performed in two studies in the 1970s and 1980s, but these produced inconclusive results. The TIMI IIIB trial was conducted in the early 1990s: 1473 patients were randomized to an early invasive strategy or an early conservative strategy. Unfortunately, the trial was rather underpowered in size and was further underpowered by the high crossover rate from the conservative to invasive strategy (61 per cent revascularization in the invasive arm *versus* 49 per cent in the conservative arm). Mortality or myocardial infarction occurred in 7.2 per cent of patients randomized to the invasive strategy *versus* 7.8 per cent in those randomized to conservative strategy (at 6 weeks), and the corresponding rates at 1 year were 10.8 per cent *versus* 12.2 per cent. These differences were not significant, but the revascularization strategy was supported by a low frequency of hospital readmission. On the basis of this trial, guidelines have suggested that either strategy is acceptable.

The **VANQWISH** study (Veterans Affairs Non-Q Wave Infarction Strategies in Hospital) randomized 916 patients with evolving non-*ST-segment* elevation myocardial infarction. These patients had a high prevalence of comorbidity; moreover, the rate of death or reinfarction at 1 year was 24 per cent in the surgical group *versus* 19 per cent in the medical group (risk ratio of 1.29, $p = 0.05$). There was a high 30-day mortality in those undergoing surgical revascularization, but most of the deaths occurred amongst those randomized to revascularization but in whom the procedure was not performed. Furthermore, the study had a significant crossover rate, with 29 per cent crossing from the conservative to the revascularization arms within 30 days.

The FRISC-II trial compared an invasive strategy with a conservative strategy in patients who were initially stabilized with approximately 6 days of treatment with low-molecular-weight heparin. Coronary angiography was performed within the first 7 days and revascularization performed in 71 per cent of those in the invasive arm and 9 per cent of those in the non-invasive arm within 10 days. This was therefore the first trial to achieve substantial separations in strategy and to include an appropriately powered population. After 6 months, death or myocardial infarction occurred in 9.4 per cent of the invasive group compared with 12.1 per cent of the non-invasive group (a risk ratio of 0.78, $p = 0.031$) and the results remained significant at 1 year. Greatest benefits were demonstrated in higher risk patients.

Can the apparently discordant findings be resolved?

Early trials of revascularization predated modern techniques, and stenting was not performed in the TIMI IIIB study. The VANQWISH trial had no deaths among those undergoing percutaneous revascularization; however, it did demonstrate a high postoperative surgical mortality and a substantial death rate in those assigned revascularization but in whom the procedure was not performed. In addition, the strategy in the 'conservative arm' was more aggressive than in many other studies, in that it aimed to detect ischaemia with nuclear perfusion scanning and undertake revascularization where such tests revealed significant ischaemia. The FRISC-II trial demonstrated the feasibility of a revascularization strategy and a low surgical complication rate. It must be interpreted in the context of an initial stabilization of several days' infusion with low-molecular-weight heparin. Up until 30 days the invasive arm had an excess rate of death or myocardial infarction due to periprocedure complications. Such complications may be reduced with the use of glycoprotein IIb/IIIa receptor antagonists (used in only 10 per cent of cases in FRISC-II). This strategy was tested in the TACTICS trial where all patients received a GPIIb/IIIa inhibitor (tirofiban) and no early excess hazard was observed in the intervention arm of the trial. The results support the findings of FRISC-II. As discussed above, GPIIb/IIIa antagonists reduce the frequency of peri and postprocedure myocardial infarction in patients with acute coronary syndromes and therefore their use is indicated, especially in those high-risk patients with positive troponins or marked *ST-segment* depression.

In conclusion, an invasive strategy of revascularization can result in a lower frequency of major cardiac complications when performed in patients who are initially stabilized with low-molecular-weight heparin treatment. The FRISC-II trial should not be interpreted as supporting very early revascularization in the absence of an initial stabilization period. The results of FRISC-II are supported by TACTICS indicating that an early invasive strategy is preferable to a conservative strategy in treating higher risk patients with acute coronary syndromes. Although very unstable patients have not been randomized in these trials (for example, those with profound ischaemia or haemodynamic complications) and emergency revascularization may provide their best therapeutic option. It is also important to note that the vast majority of patients in FRISC-II had evidence of ischaemia on the electrocardiogram and most had a positive troponin test: the results should not be extrapolated to low-risk patients, including those without clear-cut ischaemia or without troponin release.

An integrated approach to the patient with unstable angina/non-ST-elevation MI

The at-risk patient

Among patients presenting with an acute coronary syndrome approximately 40 per cent have evidence of prior coronary artery disease (**CAD**) (myocardial infarction, angiographically demonstrated CAD, documented angina with a positive stress test). Appropriate lifestyle, dietary, and non-smoking measures should be introduced for all such patients in addition to the prescription of long-term aspirin (75 mg per day). Implementation of secondary prevention drug treatment will also reduce the risk of subsequent acute coronary syndrome events and deaths, for example lipid-lowering therapy and angiotensin-converting enzyme inhibitors (**ACE** inhibitors).

Access to hospital care

Patients with acute coronary syndromes may present to primary care physicians or directly to emergency hospital services. In addition, 15 to 20 per cent of those presenting directly to chest-pain clinics may have acute coronary syndromes. Patients with previously documented coronary artery disease need specific advice about seeking emergency medical care for episodes of typical anginal pain that persist beyond 20 min at rest, especially if unrelieved by glyceryl trinitrate, or if symptoms are consistent with crescendo angina.

Emergency department triage

For the patient with chest pain, two issues must be resolved urgently:

- Is the chest pain/discomfort thought to be of cardiac origin? This is a clinical judgement and requires prompt and skilled assessment.

- In those with suspected cardiac pain, is there evidence of evolving infarction?

Patients with evolving infarction (*ST-segment* elevation or bundle-branch block and clinical features of infarction) require 'fast-track' reperfusion with thrombolysis or primary angioplasty (see Fig. 1 and below). The remaining patients can be triaged into low- or high-risk categories:

- Patients with typical clinical features of ischaemia and ST-segment depression or transient ST-segment elevation or with cardiac enzyme or troponinelevation are high-risk acute coronary syndrome. Those with elevated levels of cardiac enzymes (troponins or CK, CK-MB) are termed minimal myocardial injury or non-ST-elevation MI.

- Patients with clinical features of acute coronary syndrome and non-specific ECG changes (T-wave inversion, T-wave flattening, minor conduction abnormalities) have intermediate or low-risk acute coronary syndrome (unless enzymes/markers are elevated).

- Patients with a normal electrocardiogram and normal cardiac examination have a potentially low-risk acute coronary syndrome or alternative diagnosis.

Evaluation of patients at intermediate or low risk

Patients who initially seem to be at intermediate or low risk require further assessment to determine their risk status and management. They should be admitted to a cardiac or medical acute assessment area, where further clinical, electrocardiographic, and enzyme assessments will resolve them into relatively high- and low-risk groups.

- Patients with an indeterminate risk and those with a suspected evolving infarction require repeat 12-lead electrocardiography or continuous ST-segment analysis, ideally in a cardiac-care or intensive-care unit setting. Such patients require baseline and repeat troponin estimations to identify those at higher risk (see Fig. 1).

- Clinically stable patients with minor or non-specific ECG abnormalities can be separated into those at very low risk on the basis of negative troponins and the absence of diagnostic ECG changes on repeat evaluation. Such patients may nevertheless have significant underlying coronary artery disease. They require stress testing or perfusion scanning, ideally prior to discharge.

Patients with an indeterminate or low risk on clinical grounds can therefore be resolved into those that require further investigation and treatment for acute coronary syndromes (ECG evidence of ischaemia, positive troponins, or positive stress test) and those without (Fig. 4). Follow-up studies have demonstrated that those without significant ECG abnormality, without troponin elevation (at 12 h after the acute event), and with a low-risk stress test have a very low risk of subsequent cardiac events and prompt hospital discharge should be appropriate. In studies from Hamm and colleagues only one such patient out of 850 went on to have a cardiac event.

Management of patients at high risk

High-risk patients with acute ischaemia at initial presentation, and especially those with haemodynamic compromise, require emergency assessment for possible revascularization. Such patients should also benefit from glycoprotein IIb/IIIa inhibition (Fig. 5). Trial evidence also supports an improved outcome with glycoprotein IIb/IIIa inhibition amongst the remainder of patients with troponin positivity or *ST-segment* depression. Those proceeding to emergency revascularization should receive aspirin, unfractionated heparin, and glycoprotein IIb/IIIa inhibition. Large-scale safety studies have not yet been completed for the combination of low-molecular-weight heparin with glycoprotein IIb/IIIa inhibition, especially in the context of acute revascularization.

Coronary artery bypass surgery

As demonstrated by the FRISC II study, those with three-vessel or left main coronary artery disease and an acute coronary syndrome can be stabilized in the acute phase on low-molecular-weight heparin and aspirin, and can proceed to coronary artery bypass surgery (median 17 days) which carries a low perioperative and postoperative morbidity and mortality in experienced centres (2 per cent, 30-day mortality). A substantial part of the benefits seen in the FRISC II study were amongst those patients undergoing surgical revascularization.

Secondary prevention and rehabilitation

These issues are the same in those patients with unstable angina/non-ST-elevation MI as they are in those with ST-elevation MI (see below for details).

ST-segment-elevation MI

Introduction

In *ST-segment*-elevation myocardial infarction (MI), outcome is critically determined by the extent and severity of myocardial ischaemia. In addition,

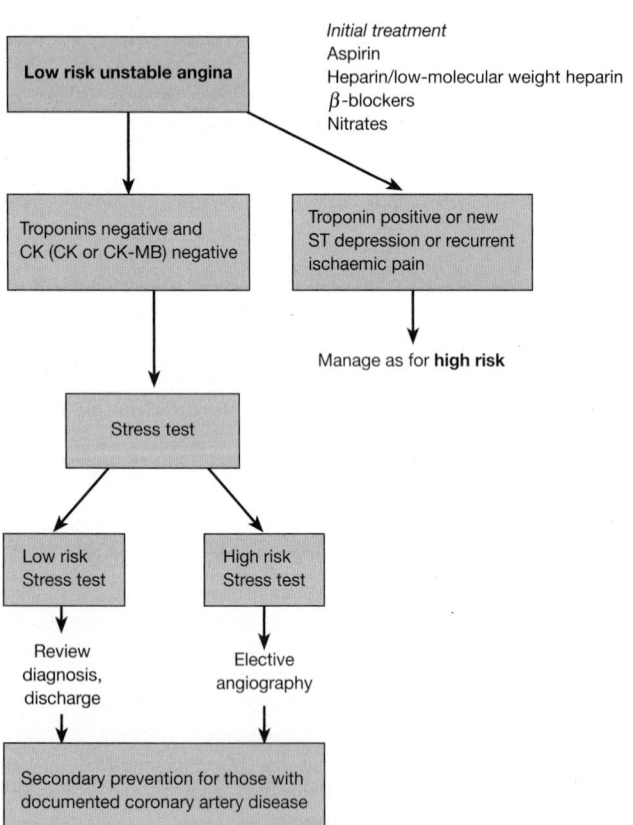

Fig. 4 Uncertain and low-risk unstable angina: initial treatment and diagnostic triage.

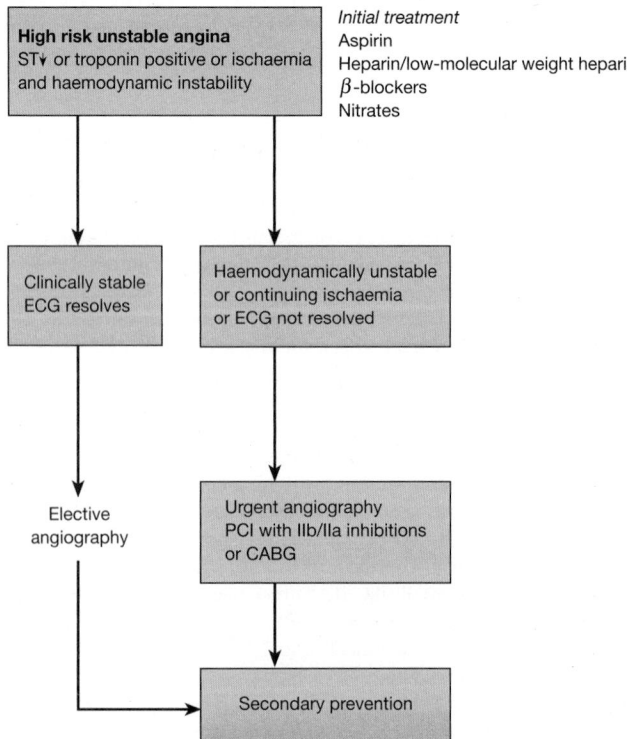

Fig. 5 High-risk unstable angina: initial treatment and diagnostic triage.

the eventual extent of irreversibly injured myocardium is influenced by residual myocardial perfusion, the duration of myocardial ischaemia, and cytoprotective mechanisms including preconditioning (see Chapter 15.4.2.1). As a result, the clinical consequences of abrupt coronary occlusion can range from an entirely silent episode, to profound ischaemia with major cardiac rhythm disturbances (ventricular fibrillation or asystole), to acute mechanical decompensation with heart failure. The outcome and management are influenced by the presence or absence of such complications, especially arrhythmias and acute heart failure.

The priorities in the management of *ST-segment*-elevation MI are to relieve acute distress and to limit the extent of infarction, mainly by reperfusion, and to treat complications. Beyond the acute phase, attention focuses on secondary prevention and rehabilitation.

Outcome in ST-segment-elevation MI

Community-based studies in various populations have demonstrated that the case fatality from acute MI is approximately 50 per cent by 1 month after the onset (MONICA studies). Approximately half of the deaths occur within the first 2 h. However, the risks of death, prior to hospitalization, vary with age: 80 per cent of those above 85 years die reaching hospital but only 40 per cent below 55 years. Prior to the introduction of cardiac care units in the 1960s, inpatient mortality was in the range of 25 to 30 per cent and in the 1980s, prior to the introduction of thrombolysis, inpatient mortality averaged approximately 18 per cent. More recently, the MONICA study from five cities has indicated that the 28-day mortality for patients admitted to hospital with a myocardial infarction ranged from 13 to 27 per cent, and other studies have provided figures of 10 to 20 per cent.

A marked discrepancy exists between mortality figures from randomized clinical trials and those from observational studies. Recent thrombolytic clinical trial data have consistently found that the 30-day mortality ranges from 6 to 8 per cent for those randomized within the trials. Some trials have analysed the outcome for individuals ineligible for inclusion and have demonstrated substantially higher death rates. Thus, although clinical trial data are accurate for the populations studied, they do not provide a comprehensive picture of outcome. This is the result of the exclusion of higher risk and complicated patients, including the elderly. In addition, the standards of care achieved in trial centres are not necessarily achieved in routine clinical practice. Although there is relatively little possibility of improving outcome amongst those eligible for randomization in clinical trials, substantial scope does exist in the remainder. Special attention needs to be drawn to the provision of acute resuscitation and defibrillation in the community.

Prehospital care

The priorities in prehospital care are to establish a prompt diagnosis of suspected acute infarction, to treat ventricular fibrillation, and to arrange emergency hospital admission for reperfusion therapy. In rural and other communities with more than a 30-min transfer time to hospital appropriate equipment and training facilities need to be established to allow prehospital thrombolysis to be administered safely and effectively.

The diagnosis of suspected infarction

A working diagnosis of suspected infarction is based upon typical severe chest discomfort of more than 15-min duration and which is unresponsive to glyceryl trinitrate. Characteristically, the pain may radiate to the neck, lower jaw, and arms and is often accompanied by autonomic features including sweating and pallor. Unless complications are present, physical examination may reveal no significant abnormalities, other than those associated with autonomic disturbance, but signs can include tachycardia or bradycardia, the presence of a third or fourth heart sound, and features of heart failure.

The initial electrocardiogram is seldom normal but may not show the classical features of *ST-segment* elevation or the development of Q-waves. Within minutes of the onset of ischaemia hyperacute T-wave changes can be present, and this may be followed by the evolution of characteristic

ST-segment elevation, but minor or non-specific ECG abnormalities in conjunction with a characteristic history may signal the early stages of infarction. The working diagnosis relies heavily on the clinical history, and when this suggests myocardial infarction repeat electrocardiography within 30 to 60 min will frequently reveal the evolution of recognizable electrocardiographic changes.

In the prehospital setting a primary care physician may have to rely on the clinical findings to establish the working diagnosis and to initiate immediate treatment. Prompt relief of pain is important, not only for humanitarian reasons, but because pain is associated with sympathetic activation, vasoconstriction, and increased myocardial work. Effective analgesia is achieved by the titration of intravenous opioids, but paramedic crews only have access to non-opioid analgesia. Side-effects of analgesia include nausea and vomiting, hypotension, and respiratory depression. Antiemetics can be administered concurrently; hypotension and bradycardia will usually respond to atropine and respiratory depression to naloxone. Oxygen should be administered, especially to those who are breathless or those with any features of heart failure or shock (see Chapter 16.3 for information on basic and advanced life support in the management of cardiac arrest or ventricular fibrillation).

The logistics of providing acute care for patients with myocardial infarction depend upon the locally available facilities. Guidelines recommend integrated planning involving the emergency care system (ambulance and paramedic personnel), primary care physicians (general practitioners), and hospital-based specialists, including cardiologists and emergency care physicians. Within an urban setting, with relatively short transfer times, the shortest delays and the most prompt initiation of reperfusion occurs when the patient seeks an emergency medical ambulance and direct access to the hospital emergency department.

Prehospital versus inhospital thrombolysis

If patients initially call their primary care physician, this inevitably produces additional delays prior to reperfusion therapy. However, a general practitioner can administer intravenous opioids for the relief of pain. In the ideal scenario, the primary care physician and paramedic ambulance crew arrive together, analgesia is administered, acute complications managed, and the patient transferred rapidly to hospital. Telemetry of the electrocardiogram is possible, with physician-guided thrombolysis administered by paramedic and ambulance crews: the feasibility and safety of this approach has been established in The Netherlands. If a doctor is available in the ambulance, then after assessment and electrocardiography, thrombolysis can be initiated prior to transfer to hospital. In remote settings the feasibility and efficacy of prehospital thrombolysis administered by the general practitioner has been established (GREAT study).

To date, eight trials have been conducted comparing prehospital with inhospital administration of thrombolytic therapy. Depending upon the clinical setting, between 30 and 130 min are saved by prehospital thrombolysis (fibrinolytic drug plus aspirin). Overall, for the complete study population of 6607 patients, the 30-day mortality was 10.7 per cent for those receiving inhospital administration of thrombolysis and 9.1 per cent for those where it was administered prior to hospital admission. This amounts to a 17 per cent relative reduction in early mortality with a p value of 0.02 (1.6 per cent absolute reduction). Complication rates were similar for community-treated and hospital-initiated thrombolysis, although ventricular fibrillation occurred more frequently with community administration and necessitated well-trained staff and the availability of defibrillators. The greatest benefit is seen where prehospital treatment is applied in remote settings where transport delays are more than 1 h. Several studies have indicated that about 20 patients with chest pain require evaluation for each patient found to be eligible for thrombolytic therapy in the community. Nevertheless, with appropriate training and facilities prehospital care can provide a gain of approximately 20 lives per 1000 treated, amongst eligible patients.

Prehospital cardiac arrest

The management of prehospital cardiac arrest requires special attention. At least as many lives can be saved by prompt resuscitation and defibrillation as by prompt thrombolysis. For these reasons, emergency assessment of the patient with suspected infarction necessitates that the clinician or paramedic has access to a defibrillator and the skills to manage cardiac arrest promptly and effectively. The provision of basic or advanced life support training to paramedic ambulance crews, together with semiautomatic defibrillators, has resulted in a substantial increase in the number of patients surviving out-of-hospital cardiac arrest. Prior to the institution of such programmes successful resuscitations were opportunistic and often relied on the availability of a medical- or nursing-trained bystander. Nationwide figures indicate that resuscitation now achieves survival in 7 to 10 per cent of those patients found with cardiac arrest and in whom the initial rhythm is thought to be ventricular fibrillation. With effective integrated programmes higher success rates have been achieved. In the southeastern region of Scotland about 14 per cent survive to reach hospital alive, and in Seattle, with a well-established community training and resuscitation programme, the figure exceeds 20 per cent. Of those reaching hospital alive, approximately half survive to be discharged home.

Emergency inhospital management and patient triage

The priority immediately after arrival at the hospital is to identify those patients with ST-elevation infarction for prompt reperfusion therapy (Fig. 6). The triage is usually performed in a casualty or similar emergency receiving department, but in some institutions patients with a high probability of infarction gain direct access to a cardiac-care assessment area. An integrated strategy involving the paramedic or ambulance system, the emergency physicians, and the cardiologists is required. 'Fast track' systems have been developed to minimize inhospital delay to thrombolysis: these are facilitated by specifically trained medical and nursing staff, with the aim of ensuring clinical assessment and electrocardiography within 15 min of arrival and the institution of thrombolytic therapy within 30 min. Audit programmes and continuous training are necessary for centres to achieve this 30-min median 'door to needle time'. Prior to the advent of 'fast track' systems, door to needle times of between 60 and 90 min were frequently recorded in clinical trials and in observational studies.

Definite versus suspected infarction

Rapid triage systems allow the identification of patients with clearly defined clinical and electrocardiographic features of infarction (characteristic symptoms of infarction which persist at rest and are not relieved by glyceryl trinitrate, in the presence of at least 1-mm ST-segment elevation in two or more contiguous leads, or the development of bundle-branch block). Clinical trials have employed ECG criteria of a 1-mm ST elevation for limb leads and 2 mm for chest leads. Although this definition improves specificity it is associated with reduced sensitivity.

Amongst those without diagnostic ECG changes a working diagnosis of suspected myocardial infarction or possible unstable angina can be established. Such patients require repeat clinical and electrocardiographic assessments to detect those with evolving infarction and to separate them from the remainder of patients with unstable angina or non-ST-elevation infarction (see Figs 1 and 6). Patients with unstable angina or non-ST-segment elevation infarction do not benefit from thrombolytic treatment, and large-scale clinical trials and meta-analyses have demonstrated that they experience the hazards of bleeding complications from thrombolytic treatment with no evidence of improved survival.

The rationale for minimizing delays to thrombolysis

Experimental and clinical data demonstrate that the duration of ischaemia, prior to reperfusion, is a critical determinant of the eventual extent of myocardial damage. These data are supported by the improved outcome seen with prehospital *versus* inhospital thrombolysis and observational data from large clinical trials in which survival gain diminishes with each additional hour of ischaemia. The Fibrinolytic Trials Overview (Fig. 7) suggests about 1.6 additional deaths per hour of delay per 1000 treated.

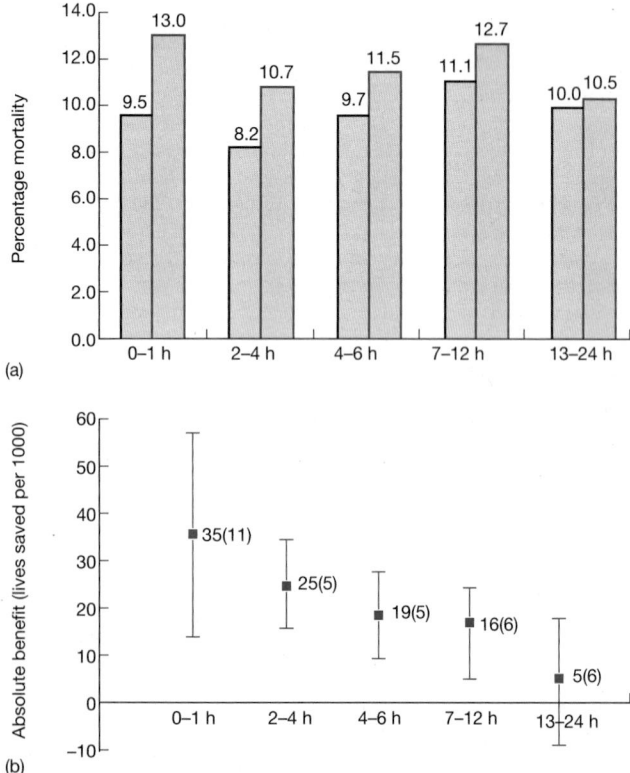

Fig. 7 Effects of thrombolytic therapy on mortality in subsets of patients with suspected MI, according to the time from the onset of symptoms. (a) Mortality rates in the fibrinolytic group (grey bars) versus control groups (pink bars); (b) absolute benefit (lives saved per 1000 treated, standard deviation in parentheses) by time to presentation. (Based on data from the FTT Collaborative Group and reproduced with permission.)

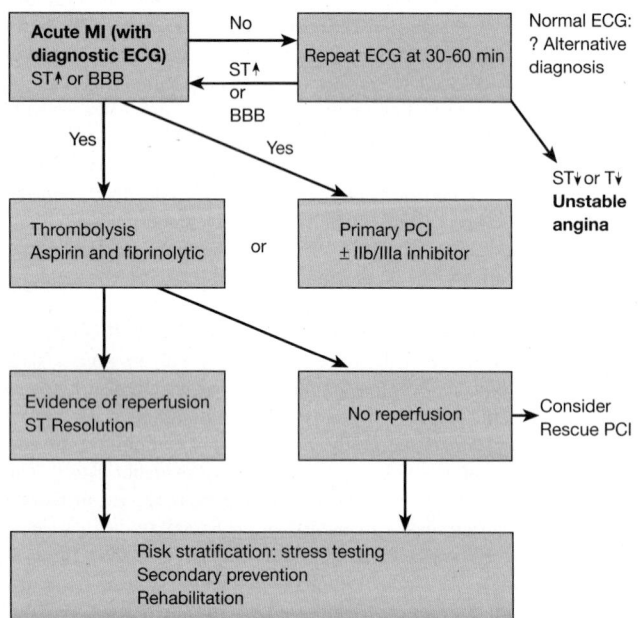

Fig. 6 Management of acute MI.

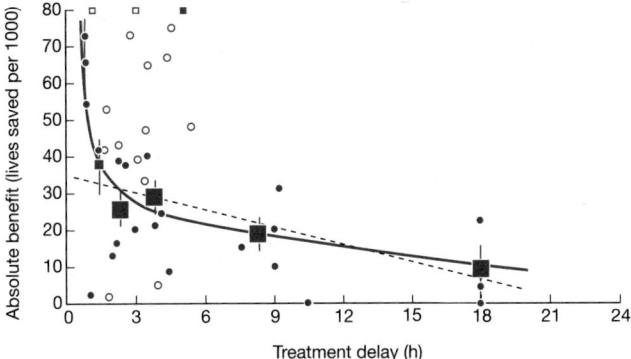

Fig. 8 Absolute benefit in lives saved per 1000 patients treated versus treatment delay. The relationship is non-linear, with most benefit occurring within the first 1 h of symptom onset. Small closed circles, information from trials included in the FTT analysis; open circles, information from additional trials; small squares, data beyond the scale of x/y cross. The linear (34.7 − 1.6x) and non-linear (19.4 − 0.6x +29.3x⁻¹) closed regression lines are fitted within these data, weighted by the inverse of the variance of the absolute benefit at each data point. The pink squares denote the average effects in six time-to-treatment groups (areas of the squares are inversely proportional to the variance of the absolute benefits described). (From Boersma E, Maas ACP, Deckers JW, et al. Early thrombolytic treatment in acute myocardial infarction: reappraisal of the golden hour. Lancet 1996, **348**, 771–5 and reproduced with permission.)

The relationship between the duration of ischaemia and the extent of infarction is non-linear: the greatest potential for salvage occurs when reperfusion is initiated within 60 min of the onset of infarction (Fig. 8). Under such circumstances, a proportion of patients (5 to 7 per cent) will have the infarction aborted and will not develop Q-waves or significant enzyme elevation despite characteristic ST elevation on the initial electrocardiogram. Minimizing the time delay is therefore critical in salvaging myocardium. Based on data from individual trials, and from the Fibrinolytic Trials Overview, most benefit occurs within the first 3 h of the onset of infarction, and highly significant benefits still occur at up to 6 h (Fig. 7). Statistically significant gains are still present at 12 h, but beyond 12 h the benefits are marginal. However, some patients present with a stuttering pattern and in the presence of persistent or intermittent ST-segment elevation and continuing symptoms of ischaemia, reperfusion beyond 12 h may salvage a significant proportion of ischaemic myocardium.

Differential diagnosis

It is important to remember that thrombolytic therapy or angiography for anticipated primary angioplasty will be of no benefit to those who do not have myocardial infarction. Such patients suffer the dual hazards of thrombolysis or angiography in the acute phase of their illness and the delay in initiating appropriate treatment. Furthermore, those treated inappropriately with thrombolysis will experience the bleeding hazards of the drug (a net increase in intracerebral haemorrhage of approximately 0.5 per cent) and the disrupted coagulation system will render other emergency surgery (for example, for perforated peptic ulceration) more hazardous. Alternative cardiac diagnoses include unstable angina and non-ST-*segment-elevation MI*, myocarditis, pericarditis, and aortic dissection. Non-cardiac diagnoses include gastrointestinal pain of oesophageal, peptic, or biliary origin; pancreatitis; respiratory and musculoskeletal abnormalities.

Aortic dissection presents a particular problem when it extends proximally to the origin of the right coronary artery and produces inferior infarction. Computed tomography, magnetic resonance imaging, or transoesophageal echocardiography may be required to establish the diagnosis (see Chapter 15.14.1).

Transthoracic echocardiography can be valuable when infarction is suspected but characteristic electrocardiographic features are absent. Normal left ventricular function excludes significant infarction. Conversely, a regional contraction abnormality helps to confirm the diagnosis of ischaemia or possible infarction. However, in those with prior myocardial damage the differentiation of new from old mechanical dysfunction is complex and requires specialist assistance.

Cardiac enzymes are helpful when abnormal, but most patients present within 3 h of the onset of symptoms and insufficient time has elapsed to produce a diagnostic release of creatine kinase (CK) or CK-MB, or troponins. Patients with suspected infarction, but normal electrocardiograms, require further clinical electrocardiographic and enzyme estimations 4 to 6 h after the suspected event.

Among elderly and very elderly patients (over 90 years of age) the presentation of infarction is often atypical. They may not experience a typical pattern of symptoms and concomitant multisystem disorders may obscure the diagnosis. Myocardial infarction must be considered in the differential diagnosis of abrupt collapse, haemodynamic disturbance of sudden onset, or severe non-specific symptoms in elderly patients.

Treatment

Thrombolytic treatment

Thrombolytic treatment refers to the combination of antiplatelet therapy (usually aspirin) with fibrinolytic treatment. The fibrinolytic agent directly or indirectly converts plasminogen to plasmin and plasmin lyses fibrin in the clot. Crosslinked fibrin is more resistant to fibrinolytic drugs than a newly formed fibrin clot.

The combination of aspirin and a fibrinolytic agent has undergone extensive clinical testing in trials involving more than 100 000 patients. Additional trials have been conducted comparing one fibrinolytic agent with another. For patients presenting within 6 h of symptom onset, and with ST elevation or bundle-branch block, approximately 30 deaths are prevented per 1000 patients treated. For those presenting between 7 and 12 h, approximately 20 deaths are prevented per 1000 patients treated, and beyond 12 h the benefits are inconclusive.

The ISIS-2 trial demonstrated that the benefits of aspirin treatment were additional to those of fibrinolytic treatment, each achieving about 25 lives saved per 1000 patients treated (for the whole of the study population). Thus, in combination, about 50 lives are saved per 1000 patients treated, but the benefits are larger than this among those presenting within 3 h of infarction with ST-segment elevation or bundle-branch block. Overall, the largest *absolute* benefit is seen in patients at highest risk, although the proportional benefit may be similar for all. High-risk patients include those over 65 years of age, those with a systolic blood pressure below 100 mmHg, and those with anterior infarction or more extensive ischaemia (see primary angioplasty below). The absolute benefit in lives saved per 1000 treated is 11 ± 3 for those under 55 years of age; 18 ± 4 for those between 55 and 64; 27 ± 5 for those 65 to 74; and 10 ± 13 for those over 75 (Fibrinolytic Trials Overview). Similarly, for those patients with more extensive infarction or hypotension, the absolute benefit for the following systolic blood pressures is: 62 ± 18 for less than 100 mmHg; 18 ± 3 for 100 to 149 mmHg; 15 ± 4 for between 150 and 174 mmHg; and 11 ± 8 for those more than 174 mmHg (Fibrinolytic Trials Overview). For patients with bundle-branch block and acute MI, the absolute benefit in lives saved per 1000 treated is 49. For those with anterior ST elevation it is 37, and for inferior ST elevation it is 8. However, for ST depression there is a net hazard of 14 lives lost per 1000 treated, and for those with a normal ECG 7 lives lost per 1000 treated (Fibrinolytic Trials Overview). Thus, evidence supports thrombolysis treatment only for those patients with ST elevation or bundle-branch block.

Hazards of thrombolysis

Thrombolytic therapy is associated with a significant excess of haemorrhagic complications, including cerebral haemorrhage. Overall, about two non-fatal strokes occur per 1000 patients treated, and of these half are moderately or severely disabling. An additional two strokes per 1000 patients are fatal, and the net impact on mortality includes such patients. The risk of stroke increases with age, especially for those over 75 years of age, and for those with systolic hypertension. The excess of non-cerebral bleeds is about 7 per 1000 treated, including those that require blood transfusion, or are life-threatening, or result in a longer hospital stay. Bleeding occurs at arterial and venous puncture sites, hence blood sampling or cannulation of vessels should be limited to sites where external compression can achieve haemostasis.

Streptokinase and other streptokinase-containing agents (anistreplase) can produce hypotension and, rarely, allergic reactions. Routine administration of hydrocortisone is not indicated. When hypotension occurs it can be managed by interrupting the streptokinase infusion, lying the patient flat or head down and by the administration of atropine, or intravascular volume expansion.

Comparison of thrombolytic agents

The most widely used thrombolytic agents are streptokinase and alteplase (tissue plasminogen activator, **tPA**). The GISSI International Trial and ISIS-3 international trial both failed to find a difference in outcome between streptokinase and tissue plasminogen activator. However, the **GUSTO** trial (Global Utilization of Streptokinase and Tissue plasminogen active for Occluded coronary arteries) employed an accelerated administration of alteplase over 90 min, and intravenous heparin adjusted using the activated partial thromboplastin time (Table 4). The GUSTO trial resulted in 10 fewer deaths per 1000 patients treated with alteplase compared with the streptokinase group. However, this was partially offset by 1 per 1000 additional non-fatal strokes (with residual neurological deficit).

Newer fibrinolytic agents

Novel agents have been developed with the aim of improved clot lysis and simpler administration. Such agents include mutants of native tPA (reteplase, lanoteplase, tenecteplase (TNK-tPA)), and a derivative of streptokinase with increased fibrin specificity and reduced antigenicity, staphylokinase.

Only reteplase, lanoteplase, and tenecteplase have been tested in large-scale comparative trials. Reteplase is administered as two 10-IU boluses given 30 min apart, and the mortality outcome is very similar to that of alteplase (0.23 per cent in favour of alteplase with confidence intervals of −1.11 per cent to +0.66 per cent). The impact on death or disabling stroke is also similar, with stroke occurring in 1.64 per cent of those treated with reteplase and 1.79 per cent of those treated with alteplase (results that are not significant). Lanoteplase or n-PA is a deletion mutant of alteplase that is administered as a single bolus. In the large In-TIME-2 trial 15 078 patients were randomized to lanoteplase versus alteplase, and the results were broadly similar with respect to mortality (6.77 per cent versus 6.60 per cent, respectively), but lanoteplase treatment was associated with slightly more bleeding events. Tenecteplase (TNK-tPA), administered as a single bolus, has been tested against the reference standard of accelerated tPA in a large-scale ASSENT-2 trial involving 17 000 patients. The 30-day mortality figures were virtually identical to those of alteplase (6.18 per cent versus 6.15 per cent, respectively); bleeding events were also similar (intracerebral

haemorrhage 0.93 per cent versus 0.94 per cent and blood transfusions 4.25 per cent versus 5.49 per cent, respectively).

Neither staphylokinase nor prourokinase (saruplase) have been tested in large-scale trials, but patency studies have produced encouraging data for both agents.

Conclusion: comparison of thrombolytic agents

The current reference standard for the comparison of fibrinolytic agents is the accelerated infusion regimen of alteplase (tPA). However, streptokinase remains the most widely used fibrinolytic agent internationally. This is largely because the cost of alteplase is substantially higher than that of streptokinase. Newer agents are more convenient to administer than the rather complex infusion regimen of alteplase and have a lower frequency of hypotension and bradycardia than streptokinase. However, there is no evidence that any 'third generation' fibrinolytic agent has improved clinical outcome nor substantially different bleeding complications compared with alteplase. Their main advantage lies in ease of administration. Indeed, recent trials have been associated with a modest but progressive increase in intracerebral bleeding, which may be associated with more aggressive heparin anticoagulation.

In summary:

- The limit appears to have been reached in achieving reperfusion with fibrinolytic agents, and alternative strategies involving adjunctive glycoprotein IIb/IIIa inhibitor therapy have not demonstrated improved outcome or substantially improved safety profile.

- The limit in treating all potentially eligible patients with reperfusion therapy has not been reached. Between 45 per cent (Europe, ENACT study) and 60 per cent (United States, NRMI Registry) of all myocardial infarctions receive neither thrombolysis nor primary angioplasty (percutaneous coronary intervention, **PCI**).

- Thrombolysis is a very cost-effective treatment for acute MI. A sustained benefit on survival has been demonstrated 14 years after thrombolysis.

Combination of fibrinolytic agents with glycoprotein IIb/IIIa inhibitors

The importance of combining antiplatelet agents with fibrinolytic agents was demonstrated in the original ISIS-2 trial, where the benefits of aspirin treatment were additive to those of fibrinolysis. More potent and specific platelet inhibition with glycoprotein IIb/IIIa inhibitors offered the potential for enhanced thrombolysis, and dose-ranging studies were encouraging (TIMI-14).

The large scale randomized trials (ASSENT-S and GUSTO V) have not fulfilled the promise of the earlier studies. In GUSTO V patients were randomized to thrombolytic (reteplase) or the combination of half dose reteplase and abciximab. The combination was not superior to the thrombolytic alone. Nevertheless, there were reductions in secondary points including reinfarction. In ASSENT-S there were significantly fewer endpoints for the combination of abciximab plus thrombolytic (11.1 per

Table 4 Clinical endpoints in comparative thrombolytic trials

Endpoints (%)	GISSI-2/international		ISIS-3			GUSTO-1		
	SK (n = 10 396)	**tPA** (10 372)	**SK** (13 607)	**tPA** (13 569)	**APSAC** (13 599)	**SK** (20 173)	**tPAa** (10 344)	**SK+tPA** (10 328)
Death	8.5	8.9	10.6	10.3	10.5	7.3	6.3*	7.0
Reinfarction	3.0	2.6	3.5	2.9*	3.6	3.7	4.0	4.0
Any stroke	0.9	1.3*	1.0	1.4*	1.3	1.3	1.6	1.7
Haemorrhagic stroke	0.3	0.4	0.2	0.7*	0.6	0.5	0.7*	0.9
Non-CNS bleeds	0.9	0.6*	4.5	5.2*	5.4	6.0	5.4*	6.1

*p <0.05; statistical comparisons are only listed for SK vs tPA.

aAccelerated dose tPA

SK, streptokinase; tPA, alteplase (tissue plasminogen activator); APSAC, anistreplase (anisoylated plasminogen streptokinase activator complex).

cent versus 15.4 per cent) compared with thrombolytic and unfractionated heparin, but a similar benefit was achieved with low- molecular-weight heparin (enoxaparin) and thrombolytic: 11.4 per cent endpoints. There were fewer bleeding events with enoxaparin than with abciximab (major bleeds 3 per cent versus 4.4 per cent). Thus the glycoprotein Hb/IDas do not appear to offer any advantage over the combination of low-molecular-weight heparin and thrombolytic (TNKtPA). A combination ofTNKtPA and enoxaparin appears to provide the best combination of efficacy and safety based on the ASSENT-3 trial.

If the results of ASSENT-3 are confirmed in a separate study, the new standard of care for fibrinolysis will be aspirin plus a fibrinolytic agent plus antithrombin therapy with low-molecular-weight heparin (enoxaparin).

Primary angioplasty

In an attempt to overcome the limitations of fibrinolysis (bleeding hazards and delayed or incomplete reperfusion) studies of primary angioplasty have been undertaken. Primary angioplasty is defined as percutaneous coronary intervention (PCI) without concomitant fibrinolytic therapy. It requires a highly skilled interventional cardiology team with substantial experience of the procedure.

Patients are transferred as an emergency to the cardiac catheterization laboratory and angiography undertaken to establish coronary anatomy and the nature of the vessel occlusion. A flexible guidewire is then passed across the occluded lesion and balloon angioplasty (usually accompanied by stent implantation) performed, thereby restoring patency. Several moderate-sized comparative trials have demonstrated the feasibility of this approach, and in highly skilled centres the data suggest an improved outcome for primary angioplasty compared to conventional thrombolysis. The American College of Cardiology (ACC) and the American Heart Association (AHA) guidelines for the management of MI recommend primary PCI as an alternative to thrombolysis, provided it can be performed within 60 to 90 min of admission, and by individuals skilled in the procedure (those performing more than 75 cases per annum) and in a high-volume centre (more than 200 cases per annum). However, larger scale studies have been performed (GUSTO 2) and these reveal that the quality of the results achieved, in broad clinical practice, are not as high as those of very experienced interventional centres. In consequence, the differences in outcome between primary angioplasty and thrombolysis are less apparent in such large international comparisons. Nevertheless, primary angioplasty is effective in securing and maintaining coronary patency and avoids the intracerebral bleeding complications of thrombolysis. Randomized trials indicate that, in experienced centres, it is more effective in restoring patency and achieves better ventricular function, with trends towards improved clinical outcome (compared to thrombolysis). Particular gains are seen in haemodynamically compromised patients and those with cardiogenic shock. Thus:

- Primary percutaneous transluminal coronary angioplasty (PCI) is specifically indicated in individuals with a contraindication to thrombolytic therapy and in haemodynamically compromised patients.

- In highly experienced interventional centres primary PCI may provide an effective alternative to thrombolysis.

The choice of reperfusion strategy will clearly continue to depend upon available resources and the expertise of each centre. Unless primary angioplasty can be performed within approximately 1 h of hospital admission, the potential gains do not appear to outweigh the hazards when compared with thrombolysis.

Angioplasty combined with thrombolysis

The combination of angioplasty and thrombolytic therapy has proved disappointing in a number of trials, with a tendency to an increased risk of complications. Although many of these trials predate current instrumentation and drug therapy, the routine combination of angioplasty and thrombolysis is not recommended.

Rescue angioplasty

Patients in whom thrombolysis fails to achieve reperfusion may benefit from 'rescue' angioplasty. Such patients can be identified by the failure to resolve ST-segment elevation, in combination with persistent clinical features of ischaemia, with or without haemodynamic compromise. Limited experience from relatively small randomized trials suggests a trend towards an improved benefit from rescue angioplasty.

Coronary artery bypass surgery

In the acute phase of myocardial infarction the role of coronary artery bypass grafting (CABG) is limited to those patients with acute mechanical complications, such as ventricular septal defect or mitral regurgitation due to papillary muscle rupture. Unless such mechanical complications are present the hazards of acute bypass surgery are significantly increased compared to delayed revascularization in a stabilized patient. The Danish DANAMI study investigated the role of revascularization in those with ischaemia during the recovery phase of myocardial infarction. It suggested that, following infarction, individuals with symptomatic or electrocardiographic ischaemia on stress testing experience significant long-term benefit from surgical revascularization.

Later inhospital management

The main aims of later inhospital management are the:

- identification and treatment of acute complications of infarction;

- identification of patients at increased risk for subsequent cardiac events; and

- initiation of secondary prevention and rehabilitation.

The distinction between early treatment and later phase treatment is clearly arbitrary. Major complications may be apparent at the time of presentation and haemodynamic, arrhythmic, or ischaemic complications may be evident shortly thereafter. Nevertheless, in the period beyond the first 12 to 24 h it is appropriate to focus attention on the points listed above.

Identification and treatment of complications of infarction

Failure of reperfusion

Electrocardiographic markers of failed reperfusion are the persistence of ST-segment elevation together with clinical and haemodynamic features of continuing ischaemia. Continuous computed ST analysis allows the most accurate definition of ECG changes, but an approximation can be obtained with repeated 12-lead ECGs and measurement of ST-segment elevation.

- In those with successful reperfusion, ST segments decrease to less than 50 per cent of peak elevation within 60 min.

In addition, some patients exhibit reperfusion arrhythmias (ventricular tachycardia, idioventricular rhythm, and, rarely, ventricular fibrillation). Such arrhythmias are more common in the presence of marked ischaemia and prompt reperfusion within 60 to 90 min of occlusion.

The most effective treatment for failed reperfusion has not yet been validated in large-scale clinical trials. However in those without successful reperfusion:

- rescue angioplasty is feasible, consisting of mechanical recanalization of the occluded vessel with percutaneous intervention, often accompanied by stent implantation.

This strategy achieves an 'open artery' and may be associated with improved mechanical function and improved longer term prognosis.

Repeat thrombolysis A thrombolytic agent may fail to achieve recanalization as a result of an extensive organized thrombus (crosslinked fibrin), platelet-rich thrombi, and mechanical obstruction to flow due to intraplaque haemorrhage. In addition, among patients treated with streptokinase, previous exposure to a streptococcus or to streptokinase can induce an antibody response that can block at least half of the 1.5 million unit standard dose of streptokinase. Thus, previous exposure to streptokinase or known antistreptococcal antibodies are indications to use an alternative thrombolytic in the first instance. Feasibility studies have been undertaken of partial- or full-dose alteplase following (unsuccessful) streptokinase, but large-scale outcome trials are needed to establish the safety and efficacy of this strategy.

Cardiogenic shock, left ventricular dysfunction, and heart failure

Cardiogenic shock In cardiogenic shock mechanical contractile abnormalities of the left ventricle or acute haemodynamic complications (papillary muscle rupture or ventricular septal defect) lead to reduced blood pressure and impaired tissue perfusion. Clinically, the condition is recognized by a systolic blood pressure of less 90 mmHg together with impaired tissue flow, as reflected by oliguria, impaired cerebral function, and peripheral vasoconstriction. Between 5 and 20 per cent of those patients admitted to hospital with acute MI demonstrate cardiogenic shock. There is evidence that its frequency has been reduced by thrombolytic therapy and primary PCI. The mortality rate when cardiogenic shock complicates an acute coronary event is in excess of 70 per cent if acute revascularization is not possible.

Time delay is critically important in the management of cardiogenic shock: mortality rises progressively if more than 2 h have elapsed since its onset. Treatment aims to improve the recovery of acutely ischaemic myocardium (mechanical and surgical revascularization) and to support the circulation with a combination of inotropes, vasodilators, and loop diuretics. Evidence suggests that the most important treatment may be to reopen the infarct-related artery with either thrombolysis or primary angioplasty. Once cardiogenic shock has developed observational studies of primary angioplasty have demonstrated improved outcome (PAMI trial). In addition, the SHOCK trial has demonstrated that aggressive treatment with intra-aortic balloon pumping (**IABP**) followed by surgical revascularization may also significantly reduce mortality.

Aside from attempts to induce reperfusion, management of the patient with cardiogenic shock after myocardial infarction traditionally includes inotropes. Dopamine is commonly used, initially at a low 'renal dose' (1–5 µg/kg per min) that activates dopaminergic receptors (but also has an effect on the circulation), but if necessary at higher doses of 5 to 20 µg/kg per min that have positive inotropic and chronotropic effects. In doses above 20 µg/kg per min there is activation of α-adrenoceptors with undesirable peripheral vasoconstriction and a decline in renal perfusion. Dobutamine acts mainly as a β1-adrenoceptor agonist and is used in the range of 2 to 40 µg/kg per min. Phosphodiesterase inhibitors have both inotropic and vasodilator effects and, although they have produced favourable haemodynamic responses, the studies conducted have not shown an improvement in outcome.

The management of pulmonary oedema consists of opiates (to relieve distress and to reduce vascular resistance), oxygen, vasodilators, and diuretics. Vasodilators (including nitrates, salbutamol, and sodium nitroprusside) reduce venous and pulmonary arterial pressure, but tachycardia may be a limiting feature and their use is limited in those who are profoundly hypotensive. Loop diuretics are employed in bolus intravenous doses or by infusion.

Left ventricular dysfunction and heart failure Large-scale trials of angiotensin-converting enzyme (ACE) inhibitors have been conducted in patients with left ventricular dysfunction and those with clinical and radiological features of heart failure (see Chapter 15.5.3). Clear evidence demonstrates the improved short- and long-term outcome with ACE inhibitors in patients with heart failure and those with asymptomatic left ventricular dysfunction.

• In patients with left ventricular dysfunction or heart failure, ACE inhibitors improve the short- and long-term prognosis.

Caution must be exercised with the introduction of ACE inhibitors in patients with intravascular volume depletion: they can cause hypotension. ACE inhibition should commence with very small doses (for example,

6.25 mg of captopril) with dosages increased progressively in conjunction with clinical monitoring. They can provoke deterioration in renal function in patients with renal artery stenosis, which is not uncommon in those with atheromatous coronary disease. Hence, it is important to check serum electrolytes and creatinine during follow-up. Angiotensin receptor blockers appear to provide similar benefits to those seen with ACE inhibitors (ELITE 2 study), but most evidence exists for ACE inhibition.

Arrhythmias

A wide variety of arrhythmias can be seen in the context of acute myocardial infarction and its treatment. In the early days of coronary-care units, great emphasis was placed on the treatment of even minor rhythm disturbance. This is now thought to have been misplaced: antiarrhythmic agents are almost invariably negatively inotropic and they may also be proarrhythmic in the context of acute coronary ischaemia. An overview of randomized trials into the use of prophylactic lidocaine (lignocaine) showed that it increased mortality. Ventricular fibrillation should be treated with DC cardioversion, and treatment with lidocaine or other antiarrhythmics (for example, amiodarone) reserved for those who have had ventricular fibrillation or another symptomatic arrhythmia (see Chapter 15.6 for details of the diagnosis and treatment of arrhythmias).

Heart block Heart block of any degree can occur after acute myocardial infarction. It is more common with inferior than anterior infarction because the right coronary artery supplies the atrioventricular node, and also because vagal reflexes are more likely from this area. It is often transient, and does not necessarily imply a large infarct, except when it occurs with anterior infarction, in which case the prognosis is grave. Temporary pacing is justified when bradycardia compromises the circulation, but not advocated 'prophylactically' for a first- or second-degree block.

Ventricular septal defect, papillary muscle rupture, and myocardial rupture

Rupture of the interventricular septum occurs in up to 3 per cent of acute infarctions and is responsible for about 5 per cent of deaths due to myocardial infarction. Rupture in the apical area may complicate anterior infarction and in the basal inferior area may complicate inferior infarction. Clinically, the condition is associated with the development of a new pansystolic murmur and clinical features of a left to right shunt with increased pulmonary congestion. Surgery should be undertaken as soon as possible: the outlook for those who are not operated upon is very bleak, few survive. However, a very few patients with small shunts survive the acute phase, but they may suffer the later consequences of the shunt.

Papillary muscle rupture occurs as a result of acute ischaemic damage due to obstruction of either the left anterior descending or circumflex coronary arteries. It causes the abrupt onset of severe mitral regurgitation and accounts for 5 per cent of deaths after acute MI. The complication generally occurs within the first week after infarction and may be recognized as the abrupt onset of acute pulmonary oedema. It is often accompanied by a new systolic murmur, but when the left atrial pressure rises acutely the murmur may be insignificant. The management is acute surgical repair with or without revascularization (for further discussion of acute mitral regurgitation, see Chapter 15.7).

In the patient who deteriorates haemodynamically after myocardial infarction—with hypotension, pulmonary oedema, or both—it is important to consider the possibility of a ventricular septal defect or acute mitral regurgitation. However, it can be impossible to distinguish between the two on clinical grounds. Both classically produce a new pansystolic murmur, and although differences between the murmurs have been described, these are not robust enough to discriminate with certainty in the individual case. Acute mitral regurgitation is best diagnosed by echocardiography, but transthoracic echocardiography may be unable to detect a ventricular septal defect in a reliable manner. Transoesophageal echocardiography is better, as is the use of a contrast-enhanced technique. If unavailable, an alternative approach is to pass a flow-directed pulmonary catheter and take blood samples from the pulmonary artery, right ventricle, and right atrium. A step up in oxygen tension between the right atrium and the pulmonary artery indicates the presence of a left to right shunt and confirms the diagnosis of a ventricular septal defect.

Myocardial rupture may follow acute infarction, usually involving the free wall of the left ventricle. It is responsible for approximately 10 per cent of all deaths in acute MI. Half of the ruptures occur within the first week, and 90 per cent within 2 weeks. The location of rupture is usually within the infarcted area, but may be at the junction with adjacent normal myocardium. In most cases death is immediate and due to electromechanical dissociation. The patient is unresponsive to resuscitation measures but, rarely, with subacute rupture, patients can be supported until surgical repair is performed. The diagnosis is made on clinical and echocardiographic criteria with assessment for possible cardiac tamponade (see Chapter 15.9). In some patients, partial rupture of the free wall can result in the late development of a false aneurysm.

Left ventricular thrombus

A left ventricular thrombus can be detected using echocardiography in up to 40 per cent of patients with acute anterior MI. The thrombus is usually located at the apex in association with a dyskinetic or aneurysmal section of myocardium with impaired contractile function. The thrombus may be large and is associated with risks of embolization (in 15 to 20 per cent of cases). Anticoagulation with heparin followed by warfarin is advised in patients with extensive infarction and those in whom apical aneurysms or mural thrombi are detected. Both thrombolysis and surgical repair have been successfully conducted. However, there is no clear evidence that either strategy is superior (provided there is no evidence of embolization).

Pericarditis

Pericarditis is a frequent complication of transmural myocardial infarction and may be manifest clinically as a pericardial friction rub accompanied by pleuritic chest pain. A small pericardial effusion may be detected using echocardiography. Dressler's syndrome is associated with pericarditis between 2 weeks and 3 months after acute infarction and has an autoimmune basis, often accompanied by pleural and pericardial effusions. It is managed with salicylates or non-steroidal anti-inflammatory agents. The frequency of both pericarditis and Dressler's syndrome is reduced with acute reperfusion (see Chapter 15.9 for further discussion).

Shoulder hand syndrome

This is a syndrome of rheumatic pain in the left shoulder, with restricted movement, which can occur in the weeks after myocardial infarction. The pathogenesis is unknown. It is treated symptomatically and usually resolves spontaneously.

An integrated approach to the management of ST-segment-elevation MI

Management of the at-risk patient

Secondary prevention measures in patients with documented coronary artery disease reduce the frequency of subsequent infarction (aspirin, lipid lowering, ACE inhibitors, cessation of smoking, treatment of hypertension). Preventive strategies in those at risk of subsequent infarction can reduce the frequency of both MI and sudden cardiac death.

Prehospital management

In a patient with suspected acute infarction prehospital management aims to treat acute arrhythmic complications, including ventricular fibrillation and other forms of cardiac arrest, to provide analgesia and oxygen, and to minimize delays to reperfusion. Prehospital thrombolysis may be given where transfer times to hospital exceed 30 min, and appropriate facilities exist with trained paramedic crews.

Table 5 Benefits of single or short-term treatments for acute myocardial infarction

Treatment	Duration of initial follow-up	Problems prevented per 1000 patients treated
Aspirin	5 weeks	24 deaths
Streptokinase	5 weeks	27 deaths
Streptokinase and aspirin	5 weeks	52 deaths
ACE inhibitors—all patients	5–6 weeks	5–8 deaths

Adapted with permission from Sivers F (1999). *Evidence-based strategies for secondary prevention of coronary heart disease*, 2nd edn, 1999. A&M Publishing, Guildford, Surrey.

Early inhospital management

Initial assessment involves the identification of those with clear-cut evidence of infarction (based on clinical and diagnostic ECG criteria). Such patients require immediate triage to reperfusion therapy (thrombolysis with a fibrinolytic agent plus an antiplatelet agent or primary PCI (Table 5). The remaining patients in whom the diagnosis of MI is suspected but the ECG criteria are not diagnostic should be managed in an intensive-care setting (in the Emergency Department or CCU) with repeat ECG evaluation at 30-min intervals (or ST-segment analysis). Cardiac enzymes may be elevated when the index episode of pain occurs more than 6 h prior to the obtained blood sample. Such patients may be resolved into those with evidence of non-ST elevation infarction (ECG and enzyme or troponin elevation) and those with unstable angina (T-wave inversion, ST-segment depression, or transient ST-segment elevation, without elevated cardiac troponins). Among those with minor or non-specific ECG changes and no enzyme elevation, re-evaluation should take place for alternative diagnoses, and stress testing performed subsequently to detect underlying coronary artery disease (Figs 1 and 3).

Management of the later inhospital phase

During this phase the management of complications, initiation of secondary prevention, and early cardiac rehabilitation should take place. In high-risk patients (those with recurrent acute ischaemia or those with failure of ST-segment resolution and continuing pain) emergency angiography and possible revascularization can be performed in appropriately equipped centres (Fig. 6).

Regular clinical and electrocardiographic assessments are required during the recovery phase to detect acute mechanical and arrhythmic complications, and to identify impaired contractile function in patients who will benefit from ACE inhibitor treatment. ACE inhibitor treatment is indicated in those with overt heart failure in the acute phase. Based on the HOPE trial, patients with documented vascular disease benefit substantially from ACE inhibition (ramipril 10 mg). Cardiovascular deaths are reduced from 8.1 per cent to 6.1 per cent and myocardial infarction from 12.3 per cent to 9.9 per cent (relative risk reductions 0.73 and 0.80 respectively, $p < 0.001$ in both instances). Treating 1000 patients with ramipiril for 4 years prevents approximately 150 cardiovascular events in 70 patients. Thus, ACE inhibition is indicated for those with vascular disease irrespective of whether there is evidence of overt heart failure or impaired LV function in acute phase. Prior to discharge, patients also require assessment for lipid-lowering therapy (current evidence suggests that all patients with MI will benefit unless their total cholesterol concentration is below 4.8 mmol/l or their low-density lipoprotein (LDL) concentration is below 3.0 mmol/l). There is evidence to support management of diabetes with glucose and insulin during the in-hospital and early post-hospital phase (see Chapter 12.12.1).

All patients will benefit from smoking cessation and the management of hypertension (systolic pressure to less than 140 mmHg). Dietary advice is required for those with a basal metabolic index (**BMI**) above 25 kg/m².

Summary of secondary prevention measures in those with unstable angina and myocardial infarction

Following an acute coronary syndrome, patients require dietary and life-style advice including the support necessary to discontinue smoking (including nicotine replacement therapy). Lipids should be measured within the first 24 h of admission and evidence supports the use of lipid-lowering therapy with statins in almost all patients, excepting those with very low LDL or total cholesterol levels. Based on data from the HOPE study, individuals with documented coronary artery disease have reduced long-term risks of death and myocardial infarction if maintained on ACE inhibition. In addition, such patients may require antianginal therapy and all should receive long-term, low-dose aspirin.

Non-pharmacological interventions

Evidence supports the following non-pharmacological interventions in secondary prevention:

- cessation of smoking (including the avoidance of passive smoking);
- dietary modification;
- exercise;
- rehabilitation; and
- management of obesity.

Modification of high-risk conditions

Trial evidence supports therapeutic interventions to modify the following conditions:

- hyperlipidaemia;
- left ventricular dysfunction and heart failure;
- diabetes mellitus;
- hypertension.

Pharmacological interventions

Evidence (summarized in Tables 6 and 7) supports the following therapies to reduce the risk of subsequent cardiovascular events:

Table 6 Estimated benefits of long-term secondary prophylactic treatment/intervention after myocardial infarction

Treatment/intervention	Problems prevented per 1000 patient-years of treatment	
All post-MI patients (unless specific contraindications exist)		
Aspirin (meta-analysis)	7	vascular deaths
	9	non-fatal reinfarctions
	3	non-fatal strokes
Oral β-blocker	21	deaths
	21	reinfarctions
Statin (hyperlipidaemia, post-MI)	7	deaths
	11	revascularizations
	12	non-fatal MIs
	3	strokes
	4	congestive heart failure
	13	angina
Statin (average cholesterol, post-MI, CARE)	2	deaths
	9	revascularizations
	4	non-fatal MIs
	2	strokes
	4	unstable angina
Smoking cessation (observational studies)	15	deaths
	46	reinfarctions
Post-MI patients with LVD or heart failure (additional treatment unless specific contraindications exist)		
ACE inhibitor (left ventricular ejection fraction ≤ 40%)	12	deaths
	9	MIs
	10	congestive heart failure (requiring hospital admission)
ACE inhibitor (heart failure)	45	deaths
	26	congestive heart failure (severe)

LVD, left ventricular dysfunction.

Adapted with permission from Sivers F (1999) *Evidence-based strategies for secondary prevention of coronary heart disease*, 2nd edn. A&M Publishing, Guildford, Surrey.

Table 7 Comparison of the treatment benefits from interventions to prevent cardiovascular events

Problems/therapy	Events prevented	NNT*
Severe hypertension (DBP 115–129 mmHg)	Death or stroke or MI	3
Coronary artery bypass surgery for left main stem stenosis	Death	6
Aspirin for transient ischaemic attack	Death or stroke	6
Statin for hyperlipidaemia, post-MI/angina (4S)	Death or non-fatal MI or CABG/PTCA or cerebrovascular event	6
Warfarin for atrial fibrillation	Stroke	7
ACE inhibitor for LV dysfunction post-MI	CV death or hospitalization for CHF	10
Statin for average cholesterol post-MI (CARE trial) or stroke	Death or non-fatal MI or CABG/PTCA	11
Aspirin post-MI	CV death or stroke or MI	12
Statin for average/elevated cholesterol, post-MI/unstable angina (LIPID trial)	Death or non-fatal MI or CABG/PTCA or stroke	15
Beta-blocker post-MI	Death	20
ACE inhibitor for LV dysfunction	CV death or hospitalisation for CHF	21
ACE inhibitor for vascular disease (HOPE)	Deaths	50
	MI	42
	Stroke	67
Statin for hypercholesterolaemia in primary prevention	Death or non-fatal MI or CABG/PTCA or stroke	26
Mild hypertension (DBP 90–109 mmHg)	Death or stroke or MI	141

*NNT, estimated number of patients that need to be treated for 5 years to prevent one event.

DBP, diastolic blood pressure; MI, myocardial infarction; CABG, coronary artery bypass grafting; PTCA, percutaneous transluminal coronary angioplasty; ACE, angiotensin-converting enzyme; LV, left ventricle; CV, cardiovascular; CHF, congestive heart failure; CARE, Cholesterol and Recurrent Events Trial; LIPID, Long-term Intervention with Pravastatin in Ischaemic Disease Trial; HOPE, Heart Outcomes Prevention Evaluation Trial.

Adapted with permission from Sivers F (1999) *Evidence-based strategies for secondary prevention of coronary heart disease*, 2nd edn. A&M Publishing, Guildford, Surrey.

- antiplatelet therapy (usually aspirin in a dose of 75 mg/day);
- β-blockers in those without contraindications;
- lipid lowering with 3-hydroxy-3-methylglutaryl coenzyme A (**HMG CoA**) reductase inhibitors (statins);
- ACE inhibitors in those with left ventricular dysfunction and heart failure, and based on the results of the HOPE study, in other patients with vascular disease (Table 6).

Anticoagulants

These are indicated in those with high risks of embolism due to left ventricular or atrial thrombus. There is evidence to support the use of anticoagulants in post-MI patients but no definitive evidence that such treatment is superior to aspirin therapy.

Hormone replacement therapy (HRT)

HRT is associated with a reduced risk of coronary heart disease in observational studies, but in the only randomized study (HERS) it resulted in no overall reduction in the risk of non-fatal MI or CHD death.

Calcium-channel blockers

An overview of data from 19 000 patients based on all randomized trials of acute infarction and unstable angina suggests that the available calcium-channel blockers are unlikely to reduce the rate of subsequent infarct development, infarct size, or subsequent infarction. They may, however, have indications for the relief of angina (especially heart-rate lowering calcium antagonists).

Antiarrhythmic agents

A review of the effects of antiarrhythmic agents (with the exception of β-blockers) does not demonstrate a beneficial impact on mortality.

Further reading

Antman EM, *et al.* (1996). Cardiac-specific troponin I levels to predict the risk of mortality in patients with acute coronary syndromes. *New England Journal of Medicine* **335**(18), 1342–9. [Troponin levels are key determinants of mortality risk in acute coronary syndromes.]

Antman EM, *et al.* (1999). Assessment of the treatment effect of enoxaparin for unstable angina/non-Q-wave myocardial infarction. TIMI IIB–ESSENCE meta-analysis. *Circulation* **100**, 1602–8. [Combined analysis of TIMI IIB and ESSENCE (enoxaparin) indicating 20 per 1000 fewer death/MIs compared with unfractionated heparin.]

ASSENT-2 Investigators (1999). Single-bolus tenecteplase compared with front-loaded alteplase in acute myocardial infarction: the ASSENT-2 double-blind randomised trial. *Lancet* **354**, 716–22. [Tenecteplase and alteplase have almost identical outcomes in acute MI.]

ASSENT-3 Investigators (2001). Efficacy and safety of tenecteplase in combination with enoxaparin, abciximab, or unfractionated heparin: the ASSENT-3 randomised trial in acute myocardial infarction. *Lancet* **358**, 605–13.

Bode C, *et al.* (1999). Randomised comparison of coronary thrombolysis achieved with double-bolus reteplase (recombinant plasminogen activator) and front-loaded, accelerated alteplase (recombinant tissue plasminogen activator) in patients with acute myocardial infarction. *Circulation* **94**, 891–8. [Reteplase and alteplase have an almost identical outcome in acute MI.]

Braunwald E. (1989). Unstable angina: a classification. *Circulation* **80**, 410–14. [Classification of unstable angina based upon mode of presentation and time course (excludes ECG changes and predates troponins).]

Cannon CP, *et al.* (2001). Comparison of early invasive and conservative strategies in patients with unstable coronary syndromes treated with the glycoprotein IIb/IIIa inhibitor tirofiban. The TACTICS-Thrombolysis in Myocardial Infarction 18 Investigators. *New England Journal of Medicine* **344**, 1879–87.

CAPTURE Investigators (1997). Randomised placebo-controlled trial of abciximab before and during coronary intervention in refractory unstable angina: the CAPTURE study. *Lancet* **349**, 1429–35. [Reduced cardiac events with abciximab before and following PCI (mostly MI).]

Cox J, Naylor CD (1992). The Canadian Cardiovascular Society grading scale for angina pectoris: is it time for refinements? *Annals of Internal Medicine* **117**, 677–83. [A scoring system for the severity of angina pectoris.]

CURE (Clopidogrel in Unstable Angina to Prevent Recurrent Events Trial) Investigators (2001). *New England Journal of Medicine* **345**, 494–502. [Key study demonstrating impact of clopidogrel, with aspirin, in reducing deaths, MI, and stroke.]

DANAMI—Madsen JK, *et al.* (1997). Danish multicentre randomised study of invasive versus conservative treatment in patients with inducible ischaemia after thrombolysis in acute myocardial infarction (DANAMI). *Circulation* **96**, 748–55. [Improved outcome with revascularization for spontaneous or exercise-induced ischaemia.]

ELITE II—Pitt B, *et al.* (1999). Effects of losartan versus captopril on mortality in patients with symptomatic heart failure: rationale, design, and baseline characteristics of patients in the Losartan Heart Failure Survival Study—ELITE II. *Journal of Cardiac Failure* **5**, 146–54. [Equivalent effects of angiotensin receptor blocker (losartan) versus ACE inhibitor (captopril).]

ESSENCE—Cohen MD, *et al.* (for the Efficacy and Safety of Subcutaneous Enoxaparin in Non-Q-Wave Coronary Events Study Group: ESSENCE) (1997). A comparison of low-molecular-weight heparin with unfractionated heparin for unstable coronary artery disease. *New England Journal of Medicine* **337**, 447–52. [First study to demonstrate the superiority of low-molecular-weight heparin (enoxaparin) over unfractionated heparin in unstable coronary artery disease.]

Fibrinolytic Therapy Trialists' (FTT) Collaborative group (1994). Indications for fibrinolytic therapy in suspected acute myocardial infarction: collaborative overview of early mortality and major morbidity results from all randomised trials of more than 1000 patients. *Lancet* **343**, 311–22. [Definitive combined analysis of fibrinolytic trials with more than 1000 patients and outcome.]

Fox KAA (1999). Comparing trials of glycoprotein IIb/IIIa receptor antagonists. *European Heart Journal Supplements* **1**(Suppl R), R10–R17. [Analysis of trials of glycoprotein IIb/IIIa antagonists in acute coronary syndromes.]

FRAX.I.S. Study Group (1999). Comparison of two treatment durations (6 days and 14 days) of a low molecular weight heparin with a 6-day treatment of unfractionated heparin in the initial management of unstable angina or non-Q wave myocardial infarction: FRAX.I.S. (FRAxiparine in Ischaemic Syndrome). *European Heart Journal* **20**, 1553–62. [Fraxiparine and unfractionated heparin have similar outcomes in unstable angina or non-Q-wave MI.]

FRISC Study Group—Lindhal B, Venge P, Wallentin L (1996). Relation between troponin T and the risk of subsequent cardiac events in unstable coronary artery disease. *Circulation* **93**, 1651–7. [Increased risks with troponin elevation in unstable coronary artery disease.]

FRISC II. FRagmin and Fast Revascularisation during inStability in Coronary artery disease (FRISC II) Investigators (1999). Invasive compared with non-invasive treatment in unstable coronary artery disease: FRISC II prospective randomised multicentre study. *Lancet* **354**, 708–15. [Revascularization after initial stabilization with low-molecular-weight heparin results in improved outcome compared with conservative management.]

Gandhi MM, Lampe FC, Wood DA (1995). Incidence, clinical characteristics, and short-term prognosis of angina pectoris. *British Heart Journal* **73**, 193–8. [Community-based study on the incidence and characteristics of new-onset angina pectoris.]

GISSI (Gruppo Italiano per lo Studio Della Streptochinasi Nell'Infart Miocardico) (1988). Effectiveness of intravenous thrombolytic treatment in acute myocardial infarction. *The Lancet* **i**, 397–402. [The first large-scale study of thrombolysis in acute MI: marked survival advantage with streptokinase treatment.]

GRACE—Foxkaa *et al.* (2001). Management of acute coronary syndromes. Variations in practice and outcomes: findings of the Global Registry of Acute Coronary Events (GRACE). *European Heart Journal* (in press).

GREAT—Rawles J, *et al.* (1994). Halving of mortality at 1 year by domiciliary thrombolysis in the Grampian Region Early Anistreplase Trial (GREAT). *Journal of the American College of Cardiology* **23**, 1–5. [Reduced mortality following domiciliary thrombolysis compared to delayed hospital thrombolysis (3 h time separation).]

GUSTO Investigators (1993). An international randomised trial comparing four thrombolytic strategies for acute myocardial infarction. *New England Journal of Medicine* **329**, 673–82. [Key large-scale international comparison of streptokinase and alteplase in acute MI: approximately 10 per 1000 survival advantage for alteplase; small excess of haemorrhage.]

GUSTO-IIb Investigators—Savonitto S, *et al.* (1997). Prognostic value of the admission electrocardiogram in acute coronary syndromes. Results from the GUSTO-IIb trial. *European Heart Journal* **18**(Suppl.), **335**, 5–82. [The importance of the admission electrocardiogram in determining prognosis in acute coronary syndromes.]

GUSTO-IIb—Armstrong PW, *et al.* (1998). Acute coronary syndromes in the GUSTO-IIb trial: prognostic insights and impact of recurrent ischemia. The GUSTO-IIb Investigators. *Circulation* **98**, 1860–8. [Prognostic factors based upon the GUSTO-IIb trial.]

GUSTO-V Investigators (2001). Reperfusion therapy for acute myocardial infarction with fibrinolytic therapy or combination reduced fibrinolytic therapy and platelet IIb/IIIa inhibition: the GUSTO V trial. *Lancet* **357**, 1905–14.

Hamm CW, *et al.* (1992). The prognostic value of serum troponin T in unstable angina. *New England Journal of Medicine* **327**, 146–50. [The important prognostic value of troponin in acute coronary syndromes.]

Held PH, Yusuf S, Furberg CD (1989). Calcium channel blockers in acute myocardial infarction and unstable angina: an overview of randomized trials. *British Medical Journal* **299**, 1187–92. [Combined analysis of calcium channel blockers.]

HERS–NHANES—Herrington DM (1999). *Erratum*, Comparison of the Heart and Estrogen/Progestin Replacement Study (HERS) cohort with women with coronary disease from the National Health and Nutrition Examination Survey III (NHANES). *American Heart Journal* **138**, 800. [First published in *American Heart Journal* 1998, **136**, 115–24]. [No advantage for HRT in this first randomized trial of women with coronary disease.]

HOPE Study Investigators (The Heart Outcomes Prevention Evaluation) (2000). Effects of an angiotensin-converting-enzyme inhibitor, ramipril, on death from cardiovascular causes, myocardial infarction, and stroke in high-risk patients. *New England Journal of Medicine*, **342**, 145–53. [Marked and sustained impact of ACE inhibitor (ramipril) on survival and cardiac and cardiovascular events among patients with vascular disease. No benefits from vitamin E.]

ISIS-2 (Second International Study of Infarct Survival) Collaborative Group (1988). Randomised trial of intravenous streptokinase, oral aspirin, both, or neither among 17,187 cases of suspected acute myocardial infarction. *Lancet* **ii**, 349–60. [Landmark thrombolysis trial of streptokinase and aspirin demonstrating a survival advantage with either but an additive benefit with both.]

ISIS-3 (Third International Study of Infarct Survival) Collaborative Group (1992). A randomised comparison of streptokinase *vs* tissue plasminogen activator *vs* anistreplase and of aspirin plus heparin *vs* aspirin alone among 41 299 cases of suspected acute myocardial infarction. *Lancet* **339**, 153–70. [Comparison of streptokinase versus tPA versus anistreplase in acute MI, similar outcome (tPA regimen differed from that of GUSTO, duteplase versus alteplase and slower administration).]

ISIS-4 (Fourth International Study of Infarct Survival Collaborative Group) (1995). A randomised factorial trial assessing early oral captopril, oral mononitrate, and intravenous magnesium sulphate in 58,050 patients with suspected acute myocardial infarction. *Lancet* **345**, 669–85. [Impact of ACE inhibitor in acute MI (modest benefit in 5 per 1000 treated). No benefit demonstrated with mononitrate nor with magnesium.]

Kong DF, *et al.* (1998). Clinical outcomes of therapeutic agents that block the platelet glycoprotein IIb/IIIa integrin in ischemic heart disease. *Circulation* **98**, 2829–35. [Pooled analysis of glycoprotein IIb/IIIa inhibitors in acute coronary syndromes, including those undergoing percutaneous intervention.]

Lewis WR, Amsterdam EA (1994). Utility and safety of immediate exercise testing of low-risk patients admitted to the hospital for suspected acute myocardial infarction. *American Journal of Cardiology* **74**, 987–90. [Benefits and safety of early exercise testing in low-risk patients with suspected MI.]

Maas ACP, *et al.* (1999). Sustained benefit at 10–14 years follow-up after thrombolytic therapy in myocardial infarction. *European Heart Journal* **20**, 819–26. [Sustained survival benefit following thrombolytic therapy.]

MONICA—Tunstall-Pedoe H, *et al.* (1996). Sex differences in Myocardial Infarction and Coronary Deaths in the Scottish MONICA Population of Glasgow 1985–1991. *Circulation* **93**, 1981–92. [Prospective study of myocardial infarction in death in a community-based population.]

OASIS—Yusuf S, *et al.* for the Organisation to Assess Strategies for Ischaemic Syndromes Registry Investigators (1998). Variations between countries in invasive cardiac procedures and outcomes in patients with suspected unstable angina or myocardial infarction without initial ST elevation. *Lancet* **352**, 507–14. [Outcome and clinical characteristics in a prospective registry of acute coronary syndromes.]

Oler A, *et al.* (1996). Adding heparin to aspirin reduces the incidence of myocardial infarction and death in patients with unstable angina. A meta-analysis. *Journal of the American Medical Association* **276**, 811–15. [Pooled analysis suggests benefit of adding heparin to aspirin in unstable angina, individual trial data not significant and overall result marginally significant.]

PAMI-I—Nunn CM, *et al.* (1999). Long-term outcome after primary angioplasty, Report from the primary angioplasty in myocardial infarction (PAMI-I) trial. *Journal of the American College of Cardiology* **33**, 640–6. [Long-term outcome of primary angioplasty.]

PCI-CURE Study—Mehta *et al.* (2001). (Clopidogrel in unstable angina to prevent recurrent events trial Investigators). *Lancet* **358**, 528–33.

Pocock SJ, *et al.* (1995). Meta-analysis of randomised trials comparing coronary angioplasty with bypass surgery. *Lancet* **346**, 1184–9. [Combined analysis of all the randomized trials (up to 1995) comparing coronary angioplasty and bypass surgery.]

PRAIS-UK Investigators—Collinson J, *et al.* (2000). Clinical outcomes, risk stratification and practice patterns of unstable angina and myocardial infarction without ST elevation: Prospective Registry of Acute Ischaemic Syndromes in the UK (PRAIS-UK). *European Heart Journal* **21**, 1450–7. [12 per cent rate of death/MI and 30 per cent rate of death/MI, refractory angina at 6 months in those presenting with unstable angina or non-ST elevation MI.]

PRISM. The Platelet Receptor Inhibition in Ischemic Syndrome Study Investigators (1998). A comparison of aspirin plus tirofiban with aspirin plus heparin for unstable angina. *New England Journal of Medicine* **338**, 1498–505. [Tirofiban versus heparin in unstable angina.]

PRISM-PLUS. The Platelet Receptor Inhibition in Ischemic Syndrome Management in Patients Limited by Unstable Signs and Symptoms Study Investigators (1998). Inhibition of the platelet glycoprotein IIb/IIIa receptor with tirofiban in unstable angina and non-Q-wave myocardial infarction. *New England Journal of Medicine* **338**, 1488–97. [Improved outcome with tirofiban in unstable angina (high-risk population).]

Ravkilde J, *et al.* (1995). Independent prognostic value of serum creatine kinase isoenzyme MB mass, cardiac troponin T and myosin light chain levels in suspected acute myocardial infarction. Analysis of 28 months of follow-up in 196 patients. *Journal of the American College of Cardiology* **25**, 574–81. [Prognostic value of cardiac enzymes in suspected acute MI.]

Ryan TJ (1999). Early revascularisation in cardiogenic shock—a positive view of a negative trial. *New England Journal of Medicine* **341**, 687–8. [Beneficial trends for early revascularization in cardiogenic shock.]

Sivers F (1999). Evidence-based strategies for secondary prevention of coronary heart disease, 2nd edn. A&M Publishing, Guildford, Surrey. [Systematic and comprehensive analysis of evidence based strategies for secondary prevention in CHD.]

TIMI III—Braunwald E, *et al.* (1994). Effects of tissue plasminogen activator and a comparison of early invasive and conservative strategies in unstable angina and non-Q-wave myocardial infarction, results of the TIMI III trial. *Circulation* **89**, 1545–56. [No significant difference in death/MI for early invasive versus conservative strategy in unstable angina (but fewer hospital readmissions).]

TIMI-III—Cannon CP, *et al.* (1995). Prospective validation of the Braunwald classification of unstable angina: results from the Thrombolysis in Myocardial Ischemia (TIMI) III Registry. *Circulation* **92**, 1-19. [Outcome in relation to the Braunwald classification.]

TIMI-14—Antman EM, *et al.* (1999). Abciximab facilitates the rate and extent of thrombolysis: results of the thrombolysis in myocardial infarction (TIMI) 14 trial. *Circulation* **99**(21), 2720–32. [Abciximab plus half-dose tPA results in angiographic opening rates similar to primary angioplasty (approximately 70 per cent at 60 min).]

TRIM Study group—Luescher MS, *et al.* (1997). Applicability of cardiac troponin T and I for early risk stratification in unstable coronary disease. *Circulation* **96**, 2578–85. [Similar data for troponin T and troponin I in risk stratification.]

VANQWISH—Boden WE, *et al.* (1998). Outcomes in patients with acute non-Q-wave myocardial infarction randomly assigned to an invasive as compared with a conservative management strategy. Veterans Affairs Non-Q-Wave Infarction Strategies in Hospital (VANQWISH) Trial Investigators. *New England Journal of Medicine* **38**(25), 1785–92. [Increased mortality with an invasive strategy compared to a conservative strategy.]

White HD, Van de Werf FJ (1998). Thrombolysis for acute myocardial infarction. *Circulation* **97**, 1632–46. [Review of thrombolysis for acute myocardial infarction.]

Yusuf S, *et al.* (1985). B-blockade during and after myocardial infarction: an overview of the randomized trials. *Progress in Cardiovascular Disease* **27**, 335–71. [Combined analysis demonstrating the benefits of β-blockers during and after acute MI.]

15.4.2.4 Percutaneous interventional cardiac procedures

Edward D. Folland

Introduction

The birth of interventional vascular medicine is generally credited to Charles Dotter, a radiologist from Portland, Oregon, who in 1964 first dared to relieve atherosclerotic stenosis of a patient's femoral artery by passage of a percutaneously introduced dilator. Although Dr Dotter had a few notable successes, which were widely publicized in the lay press, the scientific community scorned him. His radical concept lay dormant until a decade later when Andreas Gruentzig, a young German radiologist studying in Zurich, revived it. Dr Gruentzig was convinced that percutaneous dilatation of atherosclerotic stenosis was a sound concept and proposed that Dotter's solid dilator be replaced by a catheter with an inflatable cylindrical balloon at its tip. Using catheters he created in his own kitchen, he proceeded carefully and logically in applying his technique first to animal models, then to human peripheral vessels, and finally in 1977 to his ultimate goal, the human coronary artery. News of Gruentzig's percutaneous transluminal coronary angioplasty (**PTCA**) was quickly embraced by the medical community, and the era of percutaneous coronary intervention (**PCI**) was born. This chapter will deal with percutaneous approaches to treating coronary, valvular, and congenital heart disease.

Percutaneous coronary intervention

Percutaneous coronary intervention or PCI is the current general term applied to a variety of percutaneous, catheter-based procedures that accomplish revascularization either by angioplasty (enlargement of a vessel lumen by modification of plaque structure), stenting (deployment of an internal armature or stent), atherectomy (removal or ablation of plaque), or thrombectomy (removal of thrombus). Several different devices have been developed to perform these procedures. The interventional cardiologist chooses among these approaches to best suit the particular requirements of each individual patient.

Indications

The indications for percutaneous revascularization have expanded dramatically during the past 25 years. In the early days of PTCA it was indicated for subtotal, proximal occlusions of single vessels in patients with chronic, stable angina pectoris who had failed medical therapy. As experience grew and equipment improved, patients with unstable angina, total occlusions, bypass grafts, multivessel disease, and acute myocardial infarction were added to the list. Currently, the most common single indication for PCI is acute coronary syndrome (unstable angina or acute myocardial infarction).

PCI has traditionally been performed only in hospitals having cardiac surgical backup. However, as the procedure has become safer and the need for emergency bypass surgery less common (currently under 1 per cent of all cases), it has become more common, particularly in Europe, for these procedures to be performed in facilities where surgical backup is not on-site. Likewise, all patients undergoing PCI were once required to be potential candidates for bypass surgery in case of failure of the percutaneous procedure. Now some patients who are poor surgical candidates may undergo salvage intervention as their best or only avenue for revascularization. The choice of initial treatment (pharmacological, interventional, or surgical) for patients with each of the above coronary syndromes has been guided by evidence from a number of randomized clinical trials and will be treated in more detail in the later section headed 'Outcomes'.

Devices

Balloon angioplasty

Balloon angioplasty is the traditional, basic technique of coronary intervention, although it is now uncommonly employed as a stand-alone treatment. Nevertheless, it is fundamental to the deployment of coronary stents, which are currently the most widely utilized of the interventional devices. The equipment for angioplasty is displayed in Fig. 1 and consists of a

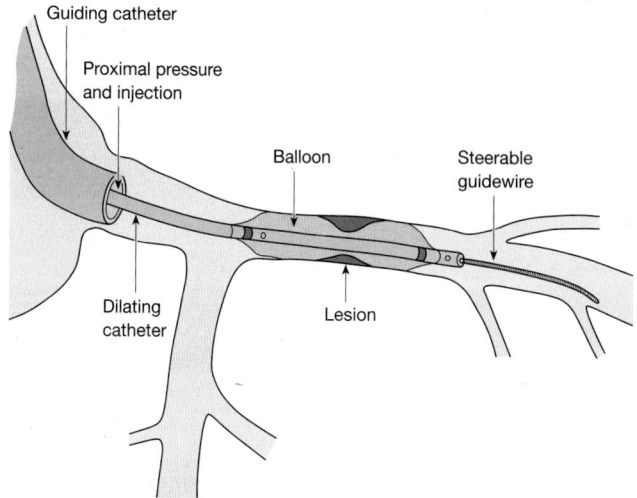

Fig. 1 Balloon angioplasty. The guiding catheter gives access to the coronary artery and provides a platform against which the dilating apparatus can be advanced. The steerable guidewire is passed down the vessel being treated and provides a rail over which the balloon catheter can be advanced. Once centred on the atherosclerotic lesion, the balloon is inflated under pressure to dilate the narrowed segment of artery.

coaxial array of guiding catheter, balloon catheter, and steerable guidewire. The procedure is accomplished by first engaging the left or right coronary orifice with the tip of the guiding catheter to access the vessel containing the target lesion and to provide backup support during advancement of the guidewire and balloon across the lesion (Fig. 2(a)). Next, the guidewire is advanced through the guide catheter into the appropriate vessel and across the lesion to be treated. Typical guidewires are 14-thousandths of an inch in diameter (about 0.36 mm) and have a flexible spiral coil tip that can be directed by rotating its proximal end outside the body. The balloon catheter is then advanced over the guidewire until the deflated balloon lies across the target lesion. Finally, the balloon is inflated with a solution of dilute contrast medium to a pressure sufficient to expand the cylindrical balloon to its nominal manufactured diameter (Fig. 2(b)). The balloon size is selected to match the estimated diameter of the nearest segment of normal vessel and the length of the target lesion. Sometimes intravascular ultrasound is used to assist in this choice. The balloon is then withdrawn and the result assessed by angiography and, occasionally, by ultrasound (Fig. 2(c)).

Traditional angioplasty now finds its chief application in deployment of balloon expandable stents. However, angioplasty may serve as a stand-alone interventional technique for the treatment of lesions of small vessels (less than 2.5 mm in diameter) and lesions located far distally or beyond tortuous segments where more rigid devices such as stents cannot reach. In experienced hands, with appropriate case selection, the initial success rate of balloon angioplasty should exceed 95 per cent. Abrupt closure of the vessel might be expected in about 3 per cent of cases (usually due to dissection), but the majority of these can be corrected by deployment of a stent, resulting in a need for emergency bypass surgery in less than 1 per cent of cases. The clinical consequence of vessel closure is often insufficient to justify surgery in vessels too small or distal for stenting.

The technology of guide, balloon, and guidewire systems has advanced to the point where few locations in the coronary anatomy are inaccessible. Totally occluded vessels can usually be successfully crossed with appropriate manipulation of the right guidewire, enabling successful angioplasty. The success rate for angioplasty of totally occluded vessels depends upon the age, length, and composition (thrombus versus plaque) of the occlusion; it is well over 90 per cent in cases of acute thrombotic occlusion, and over 50 per cent in cases of chronic occlusion (longer than 3 months).

The chief disadvantage of balloon angioplasty is the phenomenon of restenosis, which will be discussed in more detail later in this chapter, and which spurred the development of newer devices in the hope of circumventing restenosis.

Stenting

Stenting has become the intervention of choice in approximately 90 per cent of cases undergoing PCI. The term 'stent' is believed to originally derive from the name of an eighteenth-century British dentist who devised a compound for creating impressions of human teeth. A modern-day vascular stent is actually an armature, or internal skeleton, for restoring and maintaining the cylindrical structure of a diseased vessel. Most stents are made from a thin-walled, stainless-steel tube in which slots have been carved. The slotted tube is then mounted securely on a deflated angioplasty balloon and deployed at the target lesion of the coronary artery by inflating the balloon at high pressure with dilute contrast medium. When the balloon is deflated the stent remains expanded against the vessel wall, its slots stretched into diamond-shaped apertures (Fig. 3). Approximately 20 per cent of the vessel wall is covered by metal, the remainder being an intrastrut aperture. This accounts for the surprisingly high patency of side branches following stent deployment, and the ability to access these side branches when necessary for further intervention. A variation of the slotted-tube stent is a balloon-deployed coiled wire. Many recent stent designs are hybrids, which incorporate desirable properties of both the slotted-tube and coiled-wire designs.

A somewhat different approach to stenting is the self-deploying, coiled-wire stent called the Wallstent. A coiled wire made from nitinol or another alloy with shape-retaining characteristics is compressed into a tubular delivery sheath, which is advanced over a guidewire across the target lesion. Once in its proper position the sheath is drawn back, allowing the stent to expand to its original size and shape (Fig. 4). As with slotted-tube stents, pre- or postdeployment dilation with a balloon may be necessary depending upon the nature of the lesion treated and the device used. Although it is one of the original stent designs, the self-expanding stent is used less commonly for coronary artery applications, but still finds use in many peripheral vascular cases.

Stents have gained remarkable popularity mainly for three reasons. First, immediate complications are reduced because abrupt closure of the vessel due to dissection is less likely, emphasized by the fact that a stent is the best treatment for a balloon-induced dissection. Second, the immediate result is better in terms of the diameter and smoothness of the lumen, which turns out to be of more than cosmetic value because the early gain in lumen size relates directly to the late outcome. Finally, stents have been demonstrated in randomized clinical trials to be effective in reducing the likelihood of late restenosis.

However, stents do have some disadvantages, which include their propensity to subacute thrombosis, the persistence of some degree of restenosis (depending upon the size of the vessel and length of the lesion), and the fact

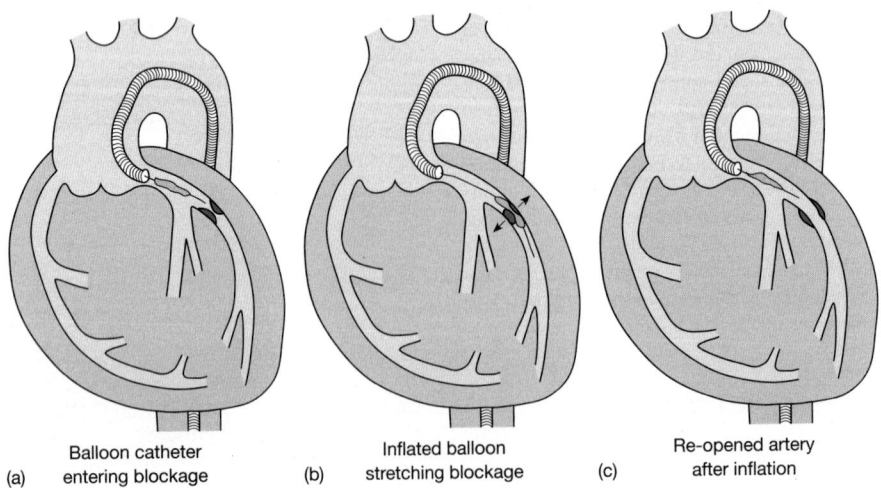

(a)	(b)	(c)
Balloon catheter entering blockage	Inflated balloon stretching blockage	Re-opened artery after inflation

Fig. 2 A typical lesion before (a), during (b), and after (c) balloon angioplasty.

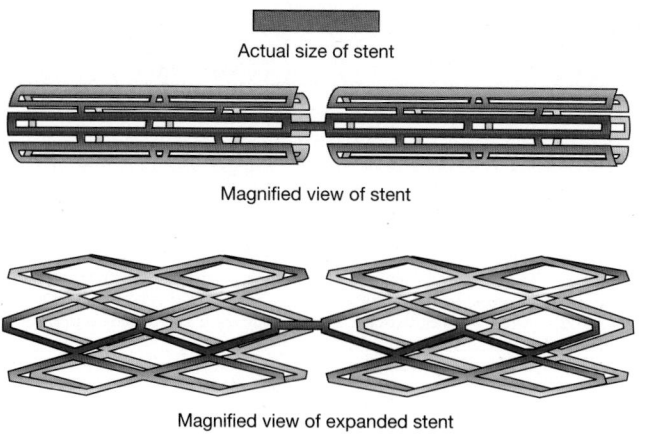

Fig. 3 A balloon-deployed coronary artery stent before (a) and after (b) deployment.

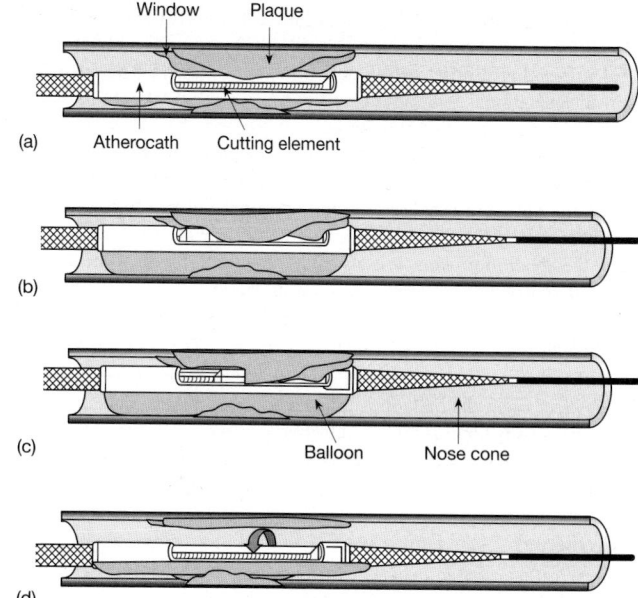

Fig. 5 Directional coronary atherectomy. The rotating cylindrical blade is advanced across the window of the housing and cuts away plaque, packing it into the nose cone.

that they cannot be deployed under some circumstances. Subacute thrombosis, a complication unique to stents, usually occurs within 10 days after stent deployment. By contrast to restenosis, which is a gradual phenomenon, stent thrombosis is usually sudden, presenting as acute myocardial infarction and requiring emergency revascularization, usually by balloon angioplasty. The likelihood of subacute thrombosis has been reduced to less than 3 per cent by antiplatelet therapy with a combination of aspirin and clopidogrel or ticlopidine.

Directional coronary atherectomy

Directional coronary atherectomy (**DCA**) is achieved with a device illustrated in Fig. 5, which utilizes a rotating cylindrical blade that is advanced across an open aperture near the tip of a cone-shaped, guidewire-directed catheter. Opposite the aperture is an eccentric balloon, which when inflated compresses plaque of the opposite vessel wall into the aperture, where it is cut away by the rotating blade and pushed into the nose cone. The direction of the aperture can be rotated so that slices of plaque are removed in a radial fashion by multiple cuts taken at different locations around the circumference of the vessel. The catheter can then be withdrawn and the excised plaque removed from the nose cone. The catheter may be reintroduced, if necessary, for more atherectomy.

Although DCA was originally devised with the hope of reducing the incidence of restenosis, it has failed to outperform balloon angioplasty in most circumstances. It has therefore assumed the role of a 'niche' technology, which is useful in particular situations such as very eccentric proximal lesions, and lesions involving the ostia of major side branches. Removal of plaque at branch points seems to reduce the likelihood of plaque shifting from one branch to another as the respective lesions are

dilated with balloons or stents. DCA has the disadvantage of requiring a rather large, stiff device, limiting its application to proximal lesions of large vessels. Furthermore, the removal of plaque seems to have surprisingly little effect on restenosis. DCA is currently employed in less than 5 per cent of interventional cases.

Rotational ablation (Rotablator)

Rotational ablation (Rotablator) is a method of pulverizing plaque into particles smaller than the size of a capillary, which wash away with the circulating blood. This process is accomplished by means of a diamond-studded burr, which rotates at approximately 150 000 revolutions per min (Fig. 6) and is advanced along a guidewire into the plaque. The diamond studs on the forward face of the olive-shaped burr selectively cut into hard substances such as plaque and calcium, sparing the soft surface of normal tissue. During rotational atherectomy a vasodilating solution is infused into the artery proximal to the burr to prevent spasm and to maintain maximal coronary flow, which carries away particulate debris. Burrs are manufactured in sizes ranging from 1.5 mm to 2.5 mm in diameter. Atherectomy often requires the use of two or three burrs of progressively larger size until an adequate lumen size is achieved. Although occasionally used as a stand-alone procedure, rotational ablation is usually employed to 'debulk' lesions prior to final dilatation with a balloon or stent.

Like directional atherectomy, rotational ablation was originally conceived as a potential solution to the problem of postintervention restenosis. Unfortunately, it too has failed to outperform balloon angioplasty in this regard and has also assumed the role of a 'niche' device for special situations. It is most commonly used to treat restenosis within previously

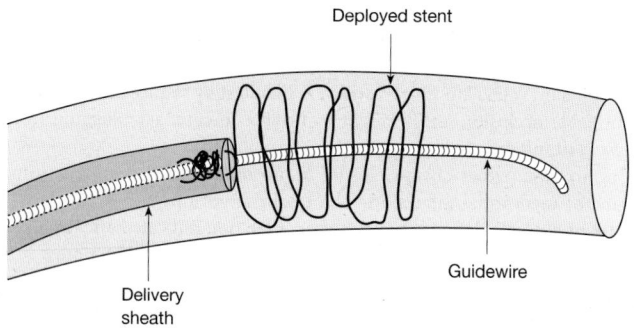

Fig. 4 A self-deploying coil stent. The stent unfurls as its delivery (containment) sheath is pulled back.

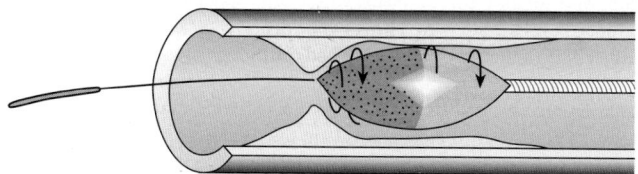

Fig. 6 Rotational atherectomy. The rotating burr pulverizes plaque as it is advanced over the guidewire into the lesion.

deployed stents, but it also finds application in the treatment of heavily calcified lesions that do not respond well to balloons and stents. It is also useful in treating diffuse, osteal, and bifurcating lesions. The frequency with which rotational ablation is employed varies by operator, but averages 5 to 10 per cent of most centres' cases.

Rotational ablation has the disadvantage of being a relatively expensive addition to other interventional modalities. It is unable to adequately increase the lumen of large vessels, and is contraindicated in lesions containing thrombus. Due to its tendency to transiently decrease contractility during the ablation process, it is also relatively contraindicated in patients whose left ventricular function is severely impaired.

Cutting balloon

The cutting balloon has several tiny longitudinally mounted blades which become erect when the balloon is inflated and create linear cuts along the vessel wall. This balloon is preferred by many cardiologists for initial treatment of stent restenosis. Its use is often followed by brachytherapy in order to reduce further the likelihood of another episode of stent restenosis.

Brachytherapy

The local, catheter based delivery of beta or gamma radiation is currently considered the best method for prevention of recurrent episodes of stent restenosis. Radiation is delivered with the assistance of a radiation therapist after initial treatment of stent restenosis with a cutting balloon, Rotablator, or conventional balloon. The benefit of brachytherapy appears to be limited to treatment of stent restenosis. It is not recommended following initial deployment of a stent. Brachytherapy also prolongs the period of risk for subacute thrombosis, making it necessary to treat patients with both aspirin and clopidogrel for at least 6 months following treatment.

Drug eluting stents

Polymer coated stents can be used locally to deliver drugs which inhibit the vessel's proliferative response to injury and therefore reduce the likelihood of stent restenosis. Drugs which have shown promise in preliminary trials include sirolimus (Rapamycin), taxol (and its derivative paclitaxel), and actinomycin.

Other devices

Distal protection devices are methods of capturing and collecting thrombus and other debris that may embolize distally from the target lesion during the use of many of the interventional tools mentioned above. They may be particularly beneficial during the treatment of old, degenerated vein grafts in which distal embolization is especially common.

Excimer laser coronary atherectomy (**ELCA**) employs a guidewire-directed fibreoptic catheter to deliver bursts of excimer laser energy to the plaque. Disintegrated plaque washes away in the circulation. However, ELCA has also failed to solve the restenosis problem, is used uncommonly at most centres, but remains the sole surviving member of a number of laser applications that have been tried and failed over the past 25 years. It finds its most frequent application in treatment of osteal lesions, stent restenosis, and diffuse calcified disease. Due to limitations of fibre size it is usually followed by balloon or stent treatment.

The transcutaneous excision catheter (**TEC**) device was developed at approximately the same time as directional coronary atherectomy and employs a rotating conical blade, which cuts away plaque and clot as it is advanced over a guidewire. The resulting debris is sucked back through the catheter into a reservoir outside the body. Although originally developed as an atherectomy device, it has found its chief application in treating clot-laden lesions. Nevertheless, it has not gained wide usage. More recently devised approaches to clot removal are the AngioJet and Excisor devices. The AngioJet uses the Venturi effect from a high-velocity jet of water, which draws thrombus into a window near the tip of a guidewire-directed catheter and propels it into a reservoir. The Excisor employs a helical screw at the end of a catheter, which breaks up the clot so that it can be withdrawn

Table 1 Complications of percutaneous coronary intervention*

Complication	Frequency (%)
Death	0.5–2
Acute myocardial infarction	2–5
Emergency bypass surgery	0.5–3
Abrupt closure	1–2
Subacute stent thrombosis	1–3
Peripheral arterial complications	5
Restenosis (clinical)	10–30

*These rates are approximate and vary widely with the clinical setting and patient characteristics. These are in addition to the usual complications of cardiac catheterization presented in Chapter 15.3.6.

through the catheter. Both these devices currently find their chief application in the treatment of degenerated and clot-laden vein-graft lesions.

Complications

Percutaneous coronary intervention exposes the patient to all the potential complications of cardiac catheterization presented in Chapter 15.3.6. In addition, it carries the risk of other complications unique to interventional procedures. Most of these complications stem from four general processes, which account for most of the adverse outcomes from coronary artery intervention: abrupt closure, distal embolization, subacute stent thrombosis, and restenosis. When considering PCI for a patient, it is important to weigh the likelihood of these adverse outcomes against the expected chance of adverse events without intervention. The approximate frequencies of various specific complications from percutaneous coronary intervention are listed in Table 1. As in diagnostic catheterization, the likelihood of these complications is also dependent upon patient characteristics and operator skill.

Abrupt closure and distal embolization

Abrupt closure and distal embolization account for most of the immediate complications of PCI, especially acute myocardial infarction and emergency coronary artery bypass surgery. Dissection, spasm, and thrombosis are the leading causes of abrupt closure. The availability of stents has reduced the need for emergency bypass surgery to less than 1 per cent, because these are an effective treatment for acute dissection in most cases. Nevertheless, dissection sometimes extends with the addition of each stent, and occasionally the stent itself can be the cause of dissection at one of its edges. Acute thrombosis may occur in spite of routine prophylactic treatment with heparin and aspirin: glycoprotein IIb and IIIa inhibitors may stop this process and are often given prophylactically, especially in high-risk cases. Incomplete stent deployment seems to be a leading cause of thrombotic occlusion.

Distal embolization is surprisingly uncommon, except when patients have acute coronary syndromes or visible thrombus. It is especially troublesome for patients with degenerated or thrombus-laden vein grafts. Embolization may result in discrete occlusion of branch vessels or the phenomenon called 'no reflow', which is manifest by reduced flow without identifiable occlusion and thought to be due to capillary plugging from showers of microemboli.

In any case, either abrupt closure or no reflow often results in some degree of myocardial infarction. The frequency of this complication is a matter of how it is defined. Non-Q-wave infarction indicated only by a rise of creatine kinase enzyme is more common than Q-wave infarction.

Subacute thrombosis

Subacute thrombosis is a complication unique to stents, which occurs between 2 and 10 days following intervention and is manifest by acute myocardial infarction. It is a medical emergency that should be managed in a fashion similar to spontaneous acute infarction. Emergency reperfusion by balloon angioplasty is usually preferred, unless a catheterization laboratory is unavailable, in which case thrombolytic therapy is recommended. In the early days of stenting this complication occurred in over 3 per cent of cases in spite of vigorous anticoagulation including intravenous heparin and warfarin. This treatment required several days of hospital stay for the initiation of warfarin therapy and delayed the widespread acceptance of stenting. However, once the current treatment consisting of oral antiplatelet agents was proven to be superior, the length of hospital stay and local bleeding complications were reduced, and the use of stents grew rapidly. Subacute thrombosis now occurs in approximately 1 to 3 per cent of cases.

Restenosis

Restenosis remains the 'Achilles heel' of coronary intervention. In patients undergoing balloon angioplasty the likelihood of restenosis at 6 months following intervention is between 30 and 50 per cent if defined by angiographic stenosis of 50 per cent or greater, and approximately 25 per cent if defined by the clinical recurrence of symptoms. The use of stents has reduced the angiographic rate of restenosis to approximately 25 per cent and the clinical rate to as little as 10 per cent. The risk of restenosis varies depending upon the individual circumstances of each case: factors associated with restenosis include long lesions, small vessels, and suboptimal initial results.

Restenosis typically presents clinically as exertional angina at 1 to 6 months following intervention: if it is not present at 6 months, it is unlikely to occur. It is a gradual phenomenon, caused by the proliferation and migration of smooth muscle cells into the lumen of the treated vessel. Stents have been effective in reducing restenosis because they eliminate elastic recoil and generally result in a large lumen. However, smooth muscle cell migration is triggered by any form of vascular injury and takes place after stenting as well as other interventions. Attempts at reducing restenosis by pharmacological and mechanical means other than stenting have been largely unsuccessful. Brachytherapy, described above, is successful in reducing smooth muscle cell proliferation following repeat intervention. Other promising approaches under investigation include local gene therapy and local drug therapy delivered by coated stents or 'leaky' balloons.

Outcomes

Chronic stable angina

Randomized clinical trials have shown that patients with single- and double-vessel disease experience a more rapid and complete resolution of symptoms, and a greater improvement in treadmill exercise performance, when treated by balloon angioplasty rather than by pharmacological therapy for chronic stable angina pectoris. However, this comes at the price of a greater likelihood of repeat intervention or bypass surgery at 6 months, largely due to the need to treat restenosis. Nevertheless, the rate of bypass surgery becomes equal in both groups by 3 years.

When compared to coronary bypass surgery, angioplasty provides similar relief of symptoms and similar rates of mortality and myocardial infarction at 5 years' follow-up, with the exception of diabetic patients who have somewhat better 5-year survival rates when treated surgically. Otherwise, the main difference between patient groups randomly assigned to surgery or angioplasty is that repeat catheterization or revascularization is less frequent for those having surgery. Again, this difference is largely due to the effect of restenosis in the angioplasty group. Few of the interventionally treated patients in these trials received stents, so the likelihood of repeat procedures might be expected to be less using current devices.

Unstable angina

The choice between initial aggressive treatment (catheterization and revascularization) and initial conservative treatment (medical therapy with catheterization and revascularization only for those who have continued evidence of ischaemia) for patients with unstable angina has been controversial. However, one of the most recent studies favours an aggressive approach to these patients.

Acute myocardial infarction

Percutaneous intervention has been shown to be an effective treatment for acute myocardial infarction, both as a salvage procedure after failed thrombolytic therapy and as a direct, initial approach to reperfusion. Randomized trials have shown that direct intervention is superior to initial thrombolytic therapy when performed in centres with expert interventionists and catheterization facilities that are available around the clock. In the general community setting this advantage has not yet been proven. In any case, direct PCI is the treatment of choice for patients in whom thrombolytic therapy is contraindicated and for patients who are haemodynamically unstable.

Economic considerations

The cost of equipment and supplies for percutaneous coronary procedures may become a limiting factor, particularly in developing countries and in healthcare systems with stringent budgets. Most catheters, guidewires, and other supplies are intended for one-time use. Expendable supplies alone cost approximately £500 ($US 800) for a simple balloon angioplasty procedure. That cost may be multiplied severalfold as multiple stents and Rotablator burrs are added to the list. Nevertheless, the cost of a single percutaneous revascularization procedure usually remains less than that of a comparable coronary bypass operation. However, when the added cost of repeat percutaneous revascularizations necessitated by restenosis is considered, the price difference between the two therapeutic approaches narrows.

Percutaneous balloon valvuloplasty

Allain Cribier of France developed the treatment of valvular stenosis by means of balloon catheters in the 1980s. The clinical utility of the procedure depends upon the valve treated and the age of the patient.

Mitral stenosis

Balloon valvuloplasty of the mitral valve has become the treatment of choice for selected patients with rheumatic mitral stenosis. The concept is similar to the aortic valvuloplasty illustrated in Fig. 7. The most common

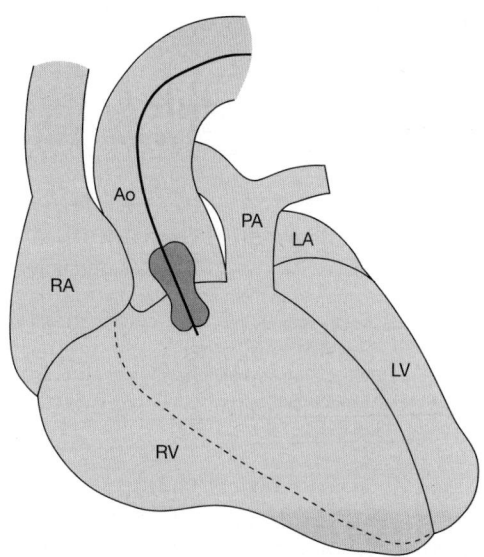

Fig. 7 Percutaneous balloon aortic valvuloplasty. The balloon is centred on the stenotic valve and inflated to tear open the fused commissures.

approach to the mitral valve is via trans-septal puncture of the left atrium from percutaneous access of the right femoral vein. After passing a stiff guidewire with a curved soft tip across the mitral valve, an appropriately sized balloon is centred on the valve and inflated with dilute contrast medium, tearing open the fused commissures and allowing the valve to open more normally. A dumbbell-shaped balloon, named after Dr Inoue, is often utilized, preventing the balloon from slipping off the valve during inflation. Clinical improvement, complications, and durability of the outcome from balloon mitral valvuloplasty have been shown to be comparable to surgical commissurotomy in appropriately selected patients. To be a candidate for balloon mitral valvuloplasty a patient must have no evidence of thrombus in the left atrium. Other features which auger poorly include immobility of the valve leaflets, severe calcification, thickening of the chordae tendineae, and more than mild regurgitation.

Aortic stenosis

Experience with balloon valvuloplasty for patients with aortic stenosis has been disappointing, largely due to an almost universal tendency for the stenosis to recur within 1 year. Consequently, the procedure is now performed only under unusual circumstances. It is occasionally used as a bridge to later surgery for patients who are initially too ill to safely undergo valve replacement. It is also sometimes performed for the temporary palliation of patients who are not candidates for valve replacement. In addition, it has a role for children with congenital aortic stenosis, where temporary treatment by valvuloplasty may allow the child to complete growth before requiring surgical valve replacement.

Pulmonic stenosis

Balloon valvuloplasty is the treatment of choice for patients with pulmonary stenosis. The majority are children whose valves respond well to this treatment. The advantage of avoiding surgery outweighs the moderate tendency for restenosis of these valves.

Percutaneous closure of cardiac defects

Atrial septal defects and patent ductus arteriosus can be closed percutaneously with catheter-delivered devices. One such device called a clamshell has been used for this purpose for a number of years, but has not yet gained wide acceptance.

Further reading

General reading

Topol EJ, ed (1999). *Textbook of interventional cardiology*, 3rd edn. WB Saunders, Philadelphia. [This is a standard textbook of interventional cardiology. It covers the topics discussed in this chapter in greater detail and gives complete references.]

Interventional versus medical therapy

Hartigan P, *et al.* (1998). Two to three year follow-up of patients with single vessel coronary artery disease randomized to percutaneous transluminal angioplasty or medical therapy (results of a VA Cooperative Study). *American Journal of Cardiology* 82, 1445–50.

RITA-2 Investigators (1997). Coronary angioplasty versus medical therapy for angina: the second Randomised Intervention Treatment of Angina (RITA-2) trial. *Lancet* 350, 461–8.

Interventional versus surgical therapy

Henderson R, *et al.* (1998). Long term results of RITA-1 trial: clinical and cost comparisons of coronary angioplasty and coronary-artery bypass grafting. *Lancet* 352, 1419–5.

The BARI Investigators (2000). Seven-year outcome in the Bypass Angioplasty Revascularization Investigation (BARI) by treatment and diabetic status.

Journal of the Anmerican College of Cardiology 35, 1122–9. [These are two of several randomized trials yielding similar conclusions regarding the relative benefits of interventional versus surgical therapy.]

Unstable angina

FRISC II Investigators (1999). Invasive compared with non-invasive treatment in unstable coronary-artery disease: FRISC II prospective randomised multicentre study. *Lancet* 354, 708–15. [The latest of several studies on this subject, and the first to show a clear advantage for invasive treatment.]

Acute myocardial infarction

Grines CL, *et al.* (1993). A comparison of primary angioplasty with thrombolytic therapy for acute myocardial infarction. *New England Journal of Medicine* 328, 673–9.

Gibbons RJ, *et al.* (1993). Immediate angioplasty compared with the administration of a thrombolytic agent followed by conservative treatment for myocardial infarction. *New England Journal of Medicine* 328, 685–91.

Zijlstra F, *et al.* (1993). A comparison of immediate coronary angioplasty with intravenous streptokinase in acute myocardial infarction. *New England Journal of Medicine* 328, 680–4.

[These three studies all appeared in the same journal issue and presented similar data supporting immediate intervention over thrombolytic therapy. Such an advantage is yet to be proven in the community setting.]

15.4.2.5 Coronary artery bypass grafting

A. J. Ritchie and L. M. Shapiro

Introduction

Coronary artery bypass grafting (CABG) is one of the most effective therapeutic surgical interventions that can be undertaken. It can reliably be performed with a mortality of 1 to 3 per cent in complex groups of high risk patients, providing sustained and proven relief from the symptoms of angina, and high quality, event-free survival in up to 80 per cent of patients 10 years later. It is a unique procedure that has to be immediately effective if the patient is to survive: there is no room for recovery and rest of the organ as in almost all other forms of surgery. The role of CABG in the treatment if ischaemic heart disease is constantly evolving. Over the past decade, advances in all fields of cardiovascular medicine and surgery have taken place at an astonishing pace. This continues, such that discerning the role of the changing therapeutic options requires continuous reassessment. The purpose of this chapter is to define the role of CABG as it currently stands, discuss issues of particular relevance to physicians, to outline work currently under study, and to delineate likely future developments.

Historical perspectives of CABG

Cardiac surgery is the youngest surgical specialty. The earliest attempts by surgeons to treat ischaemic heart disease were aimed at avoiding operating on the heart altogether, for example endeavours to control the symptoms of angina by denervation with alcohol and phenol injections. Subsequently, it was claimed that 80 per cent of patients could have their angina abolished if the thyroid gland was removed, but the price was obvious—profound hypothyroidism.

In the early part of the twentieth century efforts were made to address the root cause, occlusive coronary artery disease, by indirect attempts at revascularization. These took the forms of attaching omentum to the heart, or inducing a pericarditis and inflammatory response. More directly, arterialization of the coronary sinus was achieved by connecting a vein graft from the aorta. In 1946, Vineberg implanted the bleeding end of the left internal mammary artery into the left ventricular wall.

Seminal to the development of modern cardiac surgery were technological advances that gave surgeons the time and opportunity to construct direct aortocoronary artery bypass grafts with the expectation of a successful outcome. These came in the form of cardiopulmonary bypass circuits and angiography, which allowed the identification and targeting of the epicardial arteries. Saphenous vein bypass conduits attached directly to coronary arteries by Johnson and Favaloro made direct coronary revascularization possible and this became achievable in routine operations, associated with low mortality and morbidity, and which were applicable to the vast majority of patients. They offered substantial benefits over previous therapeutic modalities for intractable angina pectoris. CABG passed from being possible to achievable.

Questions then arose about the applicability and affordability of CABG when compared to medical treatment, which was also evolving at the same time. The most important clinical trials that had a bearing on this were conducted in the 1970s and 1980s. The Veterans Administration Coronary Artery Surgery Study and the European Coronary Surgery Study were multicentre studies examining the efficacy of CABG versus medical management in different clinical situations. These landmark studies each had problems controlling variables and could not compensate for important improvements in treatment within each group and cross over from medical to surgical groups. In addition, different types of patient were enrolled in the various studies, making comparison between them difficult. However, in essence, they showed that surgery provided better relief of symptoms, improved functional capacity, and reduced the incidence of fatal myocardial infarction. They demonstrated that patients with left main stem and/or significant flow obstructing lesions in all three major coronary arteries (triple vessel disease) enjoyed a significant prognostic benefit compared with medical treatment. Those with impaired ventricular function benefited likewise from surgery. Hence, these flawed but crucial studies led to the development of broad clinical indications for CABG. These indications, together with others that are widely accepted in clinical practice, are summarized in Table 1.

The objectives of CABG

Rapid revascularization of ischaemic myocardium, no matter how achieved, dramatically improves outcome and survival. Complete reversibility of the changes that occur due to ischaemia can be achieved when perfusion is restored, providing the rational basis for thrombolytic therapy and mechanical revascularization, whether achieved by balloon angioplasty or CABG. The simplistic aim is to rematch oxygen supply with demand. However, recent studies indicate that where there is disease at the microvascular level, then epicardial revascularization alone is likely to be only of partial benefit. Advances in medical therapy that reduce mortality in ischaemic heart disease, such as aspirin, β blockade, aggressive treatment of hyperlipidaemia by HMG CoA reductase inhibition, and angiotensin-converting enzyme (ACE) inhibition were not available at the time of the early CABG versus medical trials outlined previously. These are likely to affect the microvasculature in addition to effects on disease of the main epicardial (coronary) arteries. We are therefore moving into an era where the control of risk factors may lead not only to a slowing of the progression of coronary disease, but even to its regression. This has major implications for defining the modern role of CABG, but the core objectives of mechanical revascularization remain the same:

(1) revascularization of ischaemic areas of myocardium;

(2) relief of anginal symptoms;

(3) prolongation of patient survival;

(4) prevention of myocardial infarction;

(5) preservation of cardiac function;

(6) improvement of quality of life, for example exercise tolerance.

The broad indications for CABG are to control symptoms where medication has failed and the patient remains unacceptably incapacitated by pain, and to improve prognosis when this is possible. Increased survival after coronary artery bypass surgery is seen in the following groups: left main stem stenosis, triple vessel disease, double vessel disease with left ventricular impairment, and left ventricular aneurysm.

The standard CABG operation

This involves the use of the left internal mammary artery and saphenous vein obtained from the leg as bypass conduits via a median sternotomy incision. The patient is then fully heparinized and cardiopulmonary bypass instituted, usually by cannulation of the ascending aorta and right atrium. When it is difficult to access these vessels safely, then femoral artery and vein cannulation provide a satisfactory alternative. The cardiopulmonary bypass machine provides continuous or pulsatile flow, oxygenates and removes carbon dioxide, and regulates the temperature of the blood. This leaves the heart isolated, allowing the operation to proceed. A range of techniques is then employed to reduce or stop heart movement and allow the construction of anastomoses. Inevitably these compromise the circulation to the heart and create myocardial ischaemia, creating a time limit within which the surgery must be completed. As directed by the angiogram, and in the knowledge that incomplete revascularization is a risk factor for premature death or recurrent angina, all technically suitable coronary arteries are bypassed distal to occlusive lesions. Where diffuse disease exists, or there is no lumen, an endarterectomy can be performed. As many bypass grafts as necessary can be constructed from available conduits using 'jump' grafts, but the usual number is three or four in patients with triple vessel

---

Table 1 Clinical indications for CABG and factors related to outcome

Definite indications

Angina unresponsive to medical treatment (NYHA Class III)[1]

Unstable angina/acute coronary syndrome unresponsive to medical treatment

Left main coronary artery stenosis

Triple vessel disease (left circumflex and anterior descending and right coronary artery involvement)

Failed PTCA with acute ischaemia

Relative indications

Stable but limiting angina pectoris unresponsive to medical therapy (NYHA Class II)[1]

Two vessel disease with significant obstruction of left anterior descending artery

Coronary artery disease associated with ventricular arrhythmias

Coronary artery disease in severely depressed LV function with reversible ischaemia

Factors related to outcome of CABG[2]

Left ventricular dysfunction

Extent of coronary disease both proximal and distal (around and distal to site of anastomosis)

Arrhythmias

Advanced age

Diabetes

Hypertension

Hyperlipidaemia

Peripheral and carotid vascular disease

Left ventricular hypertrophy

---

[1]NYHA Class I—asymptomatic; Class II—slight limitation, mild shortness of breath on ordinary activity; Class III—marked limitation, shortness of breath on minimal exercise; Class IV—inability to carry out any activity, shortness of breath at rest.

[2]The presence of any of the factors listed is associated with increased risk and poorer outcome.

PTCA = percutaneous transluminal coronary angioplasty.

Table 2 Patients at increased risk from cardiopulmonary bypass

Previous stroke
Chronic obstructive pulmonary disease
Renal disease
Haematological disorder
> 75 years of age
Steroid therapy
Calcific aortic disease

disease. At the end of the procedure the patient is weaned from cardiopulmonary bypass and returned to the intensive care unit.

Perioperative morbidity

Following a standard CABG procedure the patient must recover from the effects of cardioplegia and cardiopulmonary bypass as much as from the operation per se. The use of cardioplegia rarely causes perioperative myocardial infarction or more diffuse global myocardial ischaemia, thought to be due to reperfusion injury and resulting in myocardial stunning. This can result in a low cardiac output state, seen particularly in patients with impaired ventricular function or evolving infarction. Although this occurs in less than 2 per cent of cases, the changing case mix of the population undergoing cardiac surgery is resulting in operations on older, sicker, and higher risk patients (Table 2), such that these problems are likely to become more common. Several strategies are under investigation to improve cardioprotection, but in general the risk of complications rises with prolonged ischaemia and cardiopulmonary bypass times and in older patients; they are rare in routine elective cases.

The use of cardiopulmonary bypass results in local and systemic complications as outlined in Table 3. The most common form of arrhthymia after CABG is atrial fibrillation, occurring in up to 30 per cent of cases. This often delays patient discharge and carries extra risks for the patient, despite its usually transient nature. Ventricular arrhymias are much less frequently seen, but potentially much more serious, and usually indicate ongoing ischaemia.

Transient but diffuse cerebral injury resulting in short term memory and concentration loss are detectable by neurobehavioural comparison pre- and postsurgery in most patients undergoing CABG. By contrast, stroke is very rare, affecting less than 1 per cent of cases. Damage to other organs, in particular the development of acute renal failure, can follow cardiopulmonary bypass and the occurrence of a low output state.

Medical treatment and longer-term complications of patients who have undergone CABG

Routine medication in the immediate and long term almost always includes lifelong aspirin or other antiplatelet agent. There is little place for the use of warfarin, except in those patients who have undergone endarterectomy. Medications to control hypercholesterolaemia (statins) and hypertension (β blockers and ACE inhibitors) are increasingly being associated with improved survival and are usually lifelong treatments.

Table 3 Complications associated with cardiopulmonary bypass

Local	Systemic
Thrombosis	Neurological
Embolus	Pulmonary
Dissection	Renal
Haemorrhage	Haematological

The patient has to recover from the operation before CABG can achieve its long-term goals. In the vast majority of cases there are no complications, when ambulation and return to exercise occurs within days. Initial stiffness and muscular aches can be expected, but there is no reason to advise against exercise or resumption of sexual activities for any specified period of time. By far the most frequent complaint that patients make is in relation to the saphenous vein harvest site. The ankle has a tendency to swell and the wound may be inflamed. This usually subsides quickly with rest and elevation. The increasing use of radial artery for conduits is associated with quickly healing, trouble-free wounds. A dull ache or burning pain in the chest can be associated with mammary artery harvest but usually recedes after 2 to 3 months.

Driving, riding bicycles, or other activities that put similar tensions on the chest should not be undertaken until the sternal base has a solid union, usually 6 to 8 weeks postoperatively. It is normally expected that patients who are working up until the time of their operation will be fit to resume work at 2 months postoperatively, although those employed in hard physical labour should be advised to recommence this carefully.

Other complications that can develop in the medium and long term are very rare. Postcardiotomy syndrome (Dressler's syndrome) presents as pain in the chest, which may be similar to angina but is associated with a pericardial friction rub and relieved by non-steroidal anti-inflammatory agents. Return of angina is the most sinister symptom, requiring further investigation and usually due to incomplete revascularization or occlusion of a bypass conduit. In diabetics this may be due to microvascular disease, the operation being conducted to confer prognostic benefit rather than relief of angina as its main aim.

Mortality

CABG is currently performed in over 1000 per million population in the United States and 300 to 700 per million population in Europe and Australia. It is the most documented and assessed operation ever performed. In the United Kingdom, mortality for first time CABG that includes elective and emergency cases has remained constant at 2 to 3 per cent over the last decade, with comparable figures in the United States. These data do not yet take account of risk stratification, the different nature, increased complexity, and age of patients currently referred, but there is clearly a range of outcomes, from less than 1 per cent mortality for a routine elective case to up to 10 per cent for rescue from acute percutaneous transluminal coronary angioplasty (PTCA) dissection.

Non-standard CABG procedures

Prior to the introduction of percutaneous transluminal coronary angioplasty (PTCA), CABG resulted in longer survival and better quality of life for patients with multivessel disease compared to medical treatment alone. Technological advances in PTCA and stenting now offer strategies in this group. The Bypass and Angioplasty Investigation (BARI) trial, a 5-year prospective comparison of CABG and PTCA in patients with multivessel disease, found no statistically significant difference in survival between the two groups (except for diabetic patients). However, the rate of reintervention or revascularization was 42 per cent in the PTCA group, compared with only 3 per cent in the CABG group, with 31 per cent of patients initially undergoing PTCA ultimately receiving CABG.

Standard CABG still has a major role to play in patients with multivessel disease, yet the invasive, expensive, and time-consuming nature of the operation are unattractive to physician and patient alike. While much has been done to limit the deleterious effects of cardiopulmonary bypass, reports in the last decade have continued to highlight the morbidity and mortality associated with its use. The introduction of PTCA has been seen as a way of avoiding these problems altogether and resulted in a dramatic shift of treatment paradigms, as well as driving new technical developments in surgery.

Total arterial revascularization

Cardiac surgeons no longer dispute the use of the left internal mammary artery as the choice for revascularizing the left anterior descending artery, pioneered in 1968. Critics doubted its ability to deliver enough flow and worried about morbidity associated with its harvest, particularly in diabetic patients. However, the use of single as well as double internal mammary artery grafts instead of saphenous vein has been convincingly demonstrated to improve survival and reduce recurrent angina and infarction without adding to morbidity or mortality. The outcome for the patient is longer survival and higher quality of life where revascularization is maintained by continued patency.

In the past, the issue of conduit patency was not accorded primary importance because progression of disease distal to the original site of anastamosis was thought to be the major determinant of outcome. However, this view has changed with appreciation of the time-related failure of saphenous veins due to accelerated atherosclerosis and the advent of a new era of medical interventions (aggressive lipid lowering strategies etc.). These may prevent progression of disease and stabilize acute plaque fissure, or even lead to disease regression, meaning that the long-term patency of the conduit becomes the major determinant of success or failure of CABG. The current trend in CABG is therefore to utilize a range of arterial conduits with similar biological properties, for example radial artery, gastroepiploic artery. Increased use of total arterial revascularization in combination with control of risk factors is likely to reduce significantly the requirement for redo CABG, with its attendant risk for the patient and cost to society.

Off pump coronary artery bypass

The initial work in coronary artery bypass grafting was done in an era before cardiopulmonary bypass was established. In 1967, Kolessov performed grafts to left anterior descending and circumflex through a left thoracotomy without bypass, and various reports over the following 7 years demonstrated the safety of off pump CABG in large, single centre cohorts of patients. However, the introduction and refinement of cardiopulmonary bypass made an extraordinary difference to our ability to provide definitive surgical management. Additionally, dramatic improvements in survival at and beyond surgery came with advances in cardioplegia, allowing a dry operative field and a protected myocardium. Such was the rapid advance in these technologies that the original method of CABG was abandoned, but off pump techniques are now being used again.

Minimal access CABG procedures, conducted through minimally invasive incisions, are capable of producing effective and long lasting anastomosis off pump in single vessel disease. The main shortcomings of this approach are the limited number of vessels that can be bypassed, that is primarily the left internal mammary to left anterior descending arteries, and morbidity from minithoracotomy wounds. It is likely to be applicable to less than 10 per cent of the overall patient population, but because of the significant reintervention rate following PTCA and the associated problem of in-stent stenosis, the off bypass and minimal access CABG procedure has immense potential and may revolutionize coronary revascularization in a large group of patients.

Minimally invasive procedures in cardiology and surgery can have significant advantages for both patients and institutions: reduced recovery time, reduced requirement for intensive care, and shorter hospital stay. Costs can potentially be reduced in the short and long term, with quicker return to normal life. These procedures are patient and industry driven: audit data is disseminated on the internet, and many patients in the United States and Europe now actively seek off pump CABG procedures. Well-designed, randomized, prospective, controlled trials are needed in this area.

The future for CABG

The last decade has seen marked and rapid advances across all aspects of medical and surgical management of ischaemic heart disease, making it difficult to discern the optimal treatment strategy. Innovation in CABG surgery is likely to utilize total arterial conduits in short operations, possibly done without the use of cardiopulmonary bypass. It remains to be seen in whom these advances are best applicable, and how affordable they are in competition with percutaneous interventional techniques. However, single episode, short duration operations with unrivalled long-term patency provided by arterial conduits and backed up by preventative cariological medications are likely to be cheaper and more efficacious than currently available interventional alternatives.

Further reading

Bergsma TM *et al.* (1998). Low recurrence of angina pectoris after coronary artery bypass graft surgery with bilateral internal thoracic and right gastroepiploic arteries. *Circulation* 97, 2402-5.

Buffalo E *et al.* (1996). Coronary artery bypass grafting without cardiopulmonary bypass. *Annals of Thoracic Surgery* 61, 63–6.

Cooley DA (1998). Coronary bypass grafting with bilateral internal thoracic arteries and right gastroepiploic artery. *Circulation* 97, 2384–5.

Loop FD *et al.* (1986). Influence of internal mammary artery graft on 10 year survival and other cardiac events. *New England Journal of Medicine* 314, 1–6.

Pepine CJ, Deedwania PC (1998). How do we best treat patients with ischaemic heart disease? *Circulation* 98, 1985–6.

Society of Cardiothoracic Surgeons of Great Britain and Ireland (1998). National adult cardiac surgical database report.

15.4.2.6 The impact of coronary heart disease on life and work
M. C. Petch

Introduction

Coronary heart disease is common and lethal (Tables 1 and 2). In developed countries, heart attacks account for about a quarter of all deaths. Death is usually sudden. These facts are well known and have a profound influence on attitudes towards the victims of heart disease. Employers are reluctant to take back people who have lost time off work as a result of a heart attack. Spouses become overprotective. The survivors are acutely aware that they have received an intimation of their mortality; some fail to cope. The first manifestation of coronary heart disease, which is usually chest pain, prompts re-evaluation of the remainder of life and work. The spectre of cardiac pain and death hangs over many a middle-aged man, including employers, politicians, public health physicians, journalists, and others in positions of influence. In most developed countries there is therefore public pressure to prevent the development of coronary disease (primary prevention), to prevent a recurrence (secondary prevention), and to put in place measures which will reduce the risk of harm to the individual and others in the event of sudden incapacity/death of a worker in a 'safety-critical' job.

Women are not of course immune, but coronary heart disease does tend to strike later, often after usual retirement age. Nevertheless the impact of coronary heart disease can be as devastating: older women are often the most important carers in a family. Whilst there are minor differences between the sexes in the presentation and management of coronary heart disease, the comments in this chapter should be taken to apply to both sexes.

Table 1 Deaths by cause, sex, and age in 1997 in the United Kingdom

		All ages	Under 35	35–44	45–54	55–64	65–74	75 and over
All causes	Men	300 739	10 887	6610	15 656	33 710	77 883	156 047
	Women	330 210	5 670	4 286	10 389	21 024	55 801	233 088
	Total	630 949	16 557	10 896	26 045	54 734	133 684	389 135
All diseases of	Men	124 768	604	1 548	5 699	14 127	34 195	68 595
the circulatory	Women	136 547	338	658	1 905	5 820	21 336	106 491
system	Total	261 315	942	2 206	7 604	19 947	55 531	175 086
(390–459)								
Coronary heart	Men	76 490	143	955	4088	10 300	22 619	38 385
disease	Women	64 069	38	207	828	3 238	11 779	47 979
(410–414)	Total	140 559	181	1 162	4 916	13 538	34 398	86 364
Stroke	Men	24 898	148	246	713	1 741	5 567	16 483
(430–438)	Women	41 502	118	244	598	1 318	4 971	34 253
	Total	66 400	266	490	1 311	3 059	10 538	50 736

ICD codes in parentheses.

Sources:

Office for National Statistics (1998) Deaths registered in England 1997 by cause, and area of residence, personal communication.

Office for National Statistics (1998) Deaths registered in Wales in 1997 by cause, and area of residence, personal communication:

General Register Office (1998) Annual Report 1997, General Register Offices, Edinburgh

General Register Office (1998) Annual Report 1997, Statistics and Research Agency, Northern Ireland.

Life before coronary heart disease

Most people do not think about their health until it goes wrong. With advancing years people become aware that their contemporaries are suffering from mortal diseases. They then belatedly begin to look at their own lifestyle. Many believe the results of the latest research quoted in the press and attempt to adapt their habits by increasing their intake of vitamin E, or fish oil, or red wine, or by reducing the amount of coffee and animal fat that they consume, or by undergoing stress counselling, or by purchasing an exercise machine which they never use. Then along comes a new report which sets another fashion.

There are a few public health issues on which the medical profession can speak with authority. Cigarette smoking is the prime example. Doctors, nurses, and other health-care professionals have a duty to discourage this habit by example and by persuasion. No other habit enjoys such powerful evidence that mandates a lifestyle change. Regular exercise is to be commended. A prudent diet is capable of different interpretations, but the old adage 'a little of what you fancy does you good' dates back many generations to a time when coronary heart disease was much less common. Food can be one of life's great pleasures. The current political ambition to change national lifestyles is not heeded by those most at risk and has never been clearly shown to have lasting benefit.

A sensible compromise for most societies is to prevent smoking, encourage exercise, promote the sale of fruit, vegetables, and so on, and to reduce the availability of 'junk' foods in shops and workplace canteens, but not to go to such lengths that people feel guilt when faced with a delicious steak. The fact that this Epicurean attitude is shared by most doctors makes it all the more persuasive. The use of drugs such as aspirin and statins to reduce

Table 2 Inpatient cases by main diagnosis, sex, and age in National Health Service hospitals in 1994/95, England

		All ages	Under 15	15–44	45–64	65–74	74–84	85 and over
All diagnoses	Men	4 016 453	699 261	968 550	983 621	719 263	498 436	145 737
	Women	5 384 009	508 456	2 363 687	966 038	624 692	605 761	313 395
	Total	9 400 462	1207 717	3 332 237	1 949 659	1 343 955	1 104 197	459 132
All diseases of	Men	503 202	2 561	43 699	183 314	148 004	98 258	27 196
the circulatory	Women	419 648	1 975	44 480	96 426	102 960	113 551	60 050
system	Total	922 850	4 536	88 179	279 740	250 964	211 809	87 246
(390–459)								
Coronary heart	Men	195 679	38	10 410	92 725	58 355	28 333	5 773
disease	Women	106 140	14	2 301	28 795	33 684	29 296	12 009
(410–414)	Total	301 819	52	12 711	121 520	92 039	57 629	17 782
Acute myocardial	Men	63 160	3	3 111	25 047	20 595	13 346	3 034
infarction	Women	38 737	3	494	6 938	11 896	13 351	6 028
(410)	Total	103 897	6	3 605	31 985	32 491	26 697	9 062
Stroke	Men	66 836	275	2 698	15 213	21 152	20 691	6 774
(430–438)	Women	72 963	157	2 614	9 760	16 328	26 852	17 213
	Total	139 799	432	5 312	24 973	37 480	47 543	23 987

ICD codes in parentheses; ordinary admissions and day cases combined.

Source: Department of Health (1996) Hospital Episode Statistics, Vol. 1, England, 1994/95. DII, Blackpool.

the risk of a coronary event can likewise only be justified in those individuals whose risk is especially high, as judged by their family history and other risk factors.

Health screening is another controversial topic. In (over)developed societies screening services have become very popular and assessment of cardiovascular risk in businessmen is a useful source of income for some clinics. Certainly the measurement of blood pressure can be supported and, in some circumstances, the estimation of serum lipids. Beyond that the advice that may be offered boils down to common sense—don't smoke, take more exercise, eat less.

Occasionally health screening can create extreme anxiety, for example when an electrocardiogram or exercise test suggests silent coronary disease. These investigations can only be justified when the individual is aware of the possible outcomes of screening and/or is in a safety-critical job.

Life and work with coronary heart disease

The risk of sudden disability and death through ventricular fibrillation is the major factor affecting work capacity amongst victims of coronary heart disease. The risk is greatest in the early days following the development of symptoms and in those with most myocardial damage.

Common sense and experience (i.e. clinical judgement) remain the best tools for assessing an individual's fitness to resume his life and work following the development of coronary heart disease. The onset of cardiac pain, or change in the nature of pain in someone with known ischaemic heart disease, should prompt rapid evaluation. Stable angina pectoris, preferably confirmed by exercise testing, usually requires no change in lifestyle: modern drug therapy is very effective and often comprises just aspirin, glyceryl trinitrate, and a statin. Unstable angina or myocardial infarction is a different matter and necessitates hospital admission, with further investigation. Even then clinical judgement remains the basis for advice about lifestyle changes, supplemented by 'non-invasive' tests.

The presence of myocardial failure and/or significant areas of ischaemia are the principal determinants of prognosis. The former may be identified by history, clinical examination, chest radiography, and echocardiography; the latter by the development of angina and electrocardiographic ST-segment shift on exercise testing. An exercise test may also reveal cardiovascular incapacity in other ways, for instance exhaustion, inappropriate heart rate and blood pressure responses, and arrhythmia.

Following myocardial infarction or unstable angina, assessment of prognosis along the lines outlined above is recommended: those with no complications and good exercise tolerance may return to work in about 4 weeks. This applies particularly to younger individuals whose employers need have little hesitation in taking them back to their former job, perhaps part-time initially. A few will take longer to recover, and some will need a change of job.

Limitation of working capacity and the risk of sudden incapacity can both be well judged in populations by specialist opinion, aided by the results of 'non-invasive' tests. However, the progression of coronary disease can be unpredictable, and individuals judged to be at low risk from further cardiovascular events can suffer recurrences. This difference between the individual and the population is not well understood by employers and employees and can be a source of misunderstanding and confusion. Nevertheless, individual exceptions do not invalidate the principles on which recommendations for individuals are made.

Coronary angioplasty/stenting

Patients with persistent angina, or those with a very abnormal exercise response, should undergo coronary arteriography with a view to myocardial revascularization. Coronary angioplasty is nowadays straightforward, safe, and effective in relieving angina. Resumption of normal activities, including work, is normally possible a few days afterwards. Recurrent angina is much less common with the more widespread use of stents, but it remains a problem in 10 to 20 per cent of patients and hence regulatory

authorities remain cautious about those individuals whose performance might be compromised by a return of cardiac pain.

Coronary artery bypass grafting

Coronary artery bypass grafting is also remarkably safe, with most centres reporting mortality rates of less than 1 per cent for elective operations. Recovery is rapid and most patients resume work within 2 to 3 months of surgery. Most are relieved of their angina. Patients who were able to work before surgery should generally be able to do so afterwards, and restrictions that may have been appropriate previously should no longer be relevant. However, since surgery is a dramatic event, it may prompt overprotective attitudes amongst family members, friends, employers, or even medical advisers. Many individuals who could and should return to work fail to do so for this reason, rather than because of continuing incapacity. No special restrictions are usually necessary after return to work. Coronary graft stenosis and occlusion leads to recurrence of angina at a rate of about 4 per cent per annum. This is generally less severe than previously but will affect long-term occupational planning. Unfortunately, waiting times for coronary arteriography and bypass surgery in some countries (such as the United Kingdom) are very long, so that many patients do not return to work.

Rehabilitation programmes

Rehabilitation programmes are now well established in many hospitals and communities. These enable patients to make a full physical and psychological recovery following a cardiac event such as myocardial infarction or coronary artery bypass grafting. An acceptable exercise response is a prerequisite for enrolment into a rehabilitation programme. The participants are thus the fittest survivors, selected for physical retraining on the strength of their satisfactory performance on the treadmill. Definite measures of benefit, such as reduction in recurrent myocardial infarction or death, are lacking.

However, the fashion for cardiac rehabilitation is undeniable and seems to owe much to the enthusiasm of the participants—patients and staff alike. This may be a comment on modern cardiology with its mechanistic approach, haste, and failure to recognize the psychological effects of heart attacks, with concomitant need for lifestyle advice. Sex, for example, is rarely discussed except in rehabilitation classes, yet for many patients it is a burning issue. The mechanistic view is that the physical effort required is equivalent to two flights of stairs or stage 3 of the Bruce protocol. The psychological aspects are probably better dealt with in a rehabilitation class (or perhaps the bar afterwards). With health-care budgets always under pressure, it is reasonable to suggest that the demand for rehabilitation might perhaps best be satisfied on a voluntary basis, and that scarce resources may be better directed elsewhere, for example towards the drug budget, where outcome benefits are measurable.

Risk evaluation: the 1 per cent rule

Workers whose sudden incapacity would place themselves and others at risk are described as being in 'safety-critical' jobs. The traditional approach to this dilemma was to exclude anyone with heart disease from working in such an environment. This may still be appropriate in certain occupations where any increased risk of incapacity is unacceptable: drivers of mainline passenger trains and captains of ocean-going vessels are two current examples. This blanket exclusion is patently unfair to some, and may waste the skills and experience of a valued employee. Also, no individual is totally free of risk of an incapacitating event, so a few accidents as a result of sudden illness are inevitable in apparently normal people. A better approach is therefore to define what level of risk is acceptable, and then decide whether the medical condition places that individual within the predetermined limits of acceptability. This has the great merit of objectivity and is a well-tried engineering practice.

The Civil Aviation Authority was the first to adopt this approach with what is now known as the '1 per cent rule'. Aircraft engineers have always recognized that a disaster may occur as a result of component failure, and have recommended design and safety features so that the risk of failure is 'extremely improbable' (1/10^{-9} flying hours). This approximates to a risk of an incapacitating event in a pilot of 1 per cent per annum if a number of assumptions are made. A pilot with a medical condition may therefore be regarded as a component of aircraft safety and hold a licence if his risk of a cardiovascular event is comparable, that is, his risk is no greater than his peers or other parts of the aircraft.

There are a number of difficulties in applying the approach described above in other situations and in other industries. First, who decides an acceptable level? Second, the epidemiological data in cardiovascular medicine generally describe events such as death or heart attack, which may not be the relevant parameter. Heart attacks are a rare cause of road traffic accidents; more commonly the driver is found in his vehicle on the verge, 'slumped over the wheel with the engine still running'. Death may have been sudden in epidemiological terms, but it was not instantaneous; the victim had sufficient warning to pull over to the side of the road. Third, some incapacitating events, neurocardiogenic syncope for example, are clearly relevant to many safety-critical jobs, and yet there are scant data on which to base an objective decision. Fourth, cardiovascular event rates have fallen since the 1 per cent rule was formulated.

Risk evaluation: exercise testing

The data on exercise testing in coronary heart disease are the best established for evaluating the risk of incapacity in employees in safety-critical jobs, for example vocational driving. The guidelines relating to vocational drivers were developed in the United Kingdom and adapted by a Task Force of the European Society of Cardiology. They are now being applied more widely to other groups of workers whose occupation may involve an element of risk to themselves or others should that individual suffer cardiovascular collapse.

The protocol for which most information is available is that described by Bruce. He and Fisher examined strategies for risk evaluation of sudden cardiac incapacitation in men in occupations affecting public safety: 2373 men with clinically manifest coronary artery disease who had undergone exercise evaluation were followed up for a mean of 61 months; 300 sudden cardiac incapacitations (cardiac arrest or sudden cardiac death) occurred. Exercise testing in all age groups defined low- and high-risk populations with annual incapacitation rates of 1 and 3 per cent, respectively. The former were those who could reach stage 3 of the Bruce protocol with no chest pain, attain 85 per cent of age-predicted maximal heart rate, and manifest less than 1 mm of ischaemic ST-segment depression. A similar message came from the study of 4083 medically treated patients in the Coronary Artery Surgical Study registry. The 32 per cent of patients who could exercise into stage 3 of the Bruce protocol with less than 1 mm ST-segment depression on ECG (10 METS) had an annual mortality of 1 per cent or less. By contrast, the annual mortality rate of the 730 patients with 2 mm or greater ST depression was 3.6 per cent, ranging from 5.6 per cent for those patients achieving stage 1 or less of exercise to 2.0 per cent for those patients achieving stage 3. The study also confirmed the overriding prognostic importance of left ventricular function and the poor survival of patients with heart failure. An ability to exceed stage 3 of the Bruce protocol with less than 2 mm of ST-segment depression is the best criterion for identifying a population with an annual risk of death of less than 2 per cent.

Driving

Since decisions concerning fitness to drive should be objective and evidence-based whenever possible, a similar approach to that described for pilots is being adopted. An attempt is also being made to be consistent, so that all forms of illness that might cause sudden incapacity should be considered in comparable manner. One condition for which good data are available is epilepsy. Currently the agreed, annual, acceptable levels of risk in the United Kingdom are 2 per cent for vocational drivers and 20 per cent for ordinary drivers: a driver's licence entitlement can be determined by

reference to well-validated tables of risk, for example following a head injury. Risks for drivers with cardiovascular disorders are less easy to quantify because of the poor relationship between the presence of the disease process and the risk of incapacity. However, some drivers with heart disease can be identified as being at an increased risk of an incapacitating event, and attempts are being made in the transport industry and elsewhere to provide objective criteria, which will be applicable across a range of disease processes.

The '2 per cent rule' may prove to be the correct criterion for vocational drivers and other workers in similar occupations who suffer from cardiovascular disorders. Society already accepts drivers with vocational licences up to the age of 80 years, by which time their annual risk of a cardiovascular event is 4 per cent. If the assumption is made that half of the events are incapacitating then the acceptable risk accords with the epilepsy criteria, so those drivers whose annual risk of a cardiovascular event is 4 per cent (or death 2 per cent) or greater should not be entitled to hold a vocational licence.

For ordinary drivers a 20 per cent annual risk also seems reasonable for cardiovascular disorders; such level of risk is in accord with existing guidelines, for instance shortly after a heart attack. Ordinary driving may be resumed 1 month after a cardiac event provided that the driver does not suffer from angina which may be provoked at the wheel. Vocational driving may be permitted at 6 weeks, subject to a satisfactory outcome from non-invasive testing. In the United Kingdom, ordinary driving licence holders do not need to notify the Driver and Vehicle Licensing Agency (**DVLA**), Swansea if they have made a good recovery and have no continuing disability, but vocational drivers must notify the DVLA. Insurance companies vary in their requirements, but most policies are temporarily invalidated by illness.

Special circumstances

Toxic substances

Work involving exposure to certain hazardous substances may aggravate pre-existing coronary heart disease and careful consideration should be given to patients who are returning to jobs involving exposure to chemical vapours and fumes. Methylene chloride, a main ingredient of many commonly used paint removers, is rapidly metabolized to carbon monoxide in the body and, in poorly ventilated work areas, blood levels of carboxyhaemoglobin can become elevated enough to precipitate angina or even myocardial infarction. A blood carboxyhaemoglobin level of 2 to 4 per cent has been shown to be associated with impairment of cardiovascular function in patients with angina pectoris. The World Health Organization recommends a maximum carboxyhaemoglobin level of 5 per cent for healthy industrial workers and a maximum of 2.5 per cent for susceptible persons in the general population exposed to ambient air pollution: this level may also be applied to workers whose jobs entail specific exposure to carbon monoxide, such as car park attendants and furnace workers. To ensure that the 2.5 per cent carboxyhaemoglobin level is not exceeded, the ambient carbon monoxide concentration should not be higher than 10 ppm over an 8-h working day: equivalent to exposure to the current occupational exposure standard (50 ppm) for no more than 30 min. Occupational exposure to carbon disulphide in the viscose rayon manufacturing industry is a recognized causal factor of coronary heart disease but the mechanism remains unclear.

Reports of sudden death from angina are well recognized in dynamite workers, particularly after a period of 36 to 72 h away from work and following re-exposure, an effect almost certainly related to direct action of nitroglycerine on the blood vessels of the heart or peripheral circulation. Persons with clinical evidence of coronary heart disease should avoid occupational exposure to these substances.

Solvents, such as trichloroethylene or 1,1,1-trichloroethane, may cause sudden death in workers receiving heavy exposure in poorly ventilated workplaces. The chlorofluorocarbon CFC-113 has been implicated in sudden cardiac deaths and CFC-22 has been reported to cause arrhythmias.

Some industrial workers will need proper assessment of their workplace by an occupational physician and occupational hygienist so that they can be advised on their suitability for work handling chlorinated hydrocarbon solvents or involving exposure to gases.

There are no formal medical requirements for workers who have to enter confined spaces where there may be hazards of oxygen deficiency or a build up of toxic gases. Those with heart disease or severe hypertension may need to be excluded. Certain occupations may require the use of special breathing apparatus either routinely (e.g. asbestos-removal workers), or in emergencies (e.g. water workers handling chlorine cylinders). The additional cardiorespiratory effort required whilst wearing a respirator, combined with the general physical exertion that may be required, usually means that people with a previous history of coronary heart disease are excluded from such work.

Hot conditions

Working in hot conditions may prove difficult for some patients with heart disease. High ambient temperatures or significant heat radiation from hot surfaces or liquid metal, added to the physical strain of heavy work, will produce quite profound vasodilatation of muscle and skin vessels. Compensatory vascular and cardiac reactions to maintain central blood pressure may be inadequate and lead to reduced cerebral or coronary artery blood flow. The resulting weakness or giddiness could prove dangerous. Since many cardioactive drugs have vasodilating and negative inotropic actions, some reduction in dosage may be necessary.

Cold conditions

Cold is a notorious trigger of myocardial ischaemia and caution must therefore be exercised for individuals who suffer from coronary heart disease. Impaired circulation to the limbs will result in an increased risk of claudication, risk of damage to skin (frostbite), and poor recovery from accidental injury to skin and deeper structures.

Stress

The idea that psychological stress has a role in the aetiology of coronary heart disease is a persistent one, owing much to the work of Friedman and his colleagues who suggested that hectic work patterns marked by long hours, competitiveness, time urgency, and aggression (so-called type A behaviour) may predispose to the development of coronary heart disease. The results of other epidemiological and clinical studies have been conflicting, much of the difficulty arising from the criteria for identifying a type A personality. The idea that a stressful incident may trigger a heart attack is also well embedded in Western culture. Some studies have shown a relationship, for example after earthquakes. But generally psychological stress is not regarded as sufficient provocation to form the basis of a legal settlement. Such stress may, however, on occasion provoke angina in susceptible individuals. Patients and their relatives can almost invariably point to a stressful incident prior to a heart attack and may fail to appreciate that life is a series of stressful incidents, heart attacks are extremely common, and coincidences are inevitable. The only trigger of a heart attack that has withstood critical scrutiny (and legal cross-examination) so far is sudden unaccustomed vigorous effort within 2 h of the attack.

Travel

Following a cardiac event such as myocardial infarction, individuals should convalesce at home and not travel far for 4 to 6 weeks. Those with no evidence of continuing myocardial ischaemia or heart failure can then travel freely within their own country for pleasure, for example a holiday. Business and overseas travel is more problematical because the physical and psychological demands are greater. Additional difficulties for the overseas traveller include the uncertain provision of coronary care facilities in some countries and the justifiable reluctance of insurance companies to provide health cover. Such travel is best deferred until 3 months have elapsed and any necessary further investigations and treatment have been carried out to ensure cardiovascular fitness.

Overseas travel for those with continuing cardiovascular unfitness need not be ruled out. Utilizing the airport services for disabled travellers can ease a passenger through customs, passport control, and so on, at major airports. Modern aircraft can be very comfortable. The cabins are kept at a pressure equivalent to 2000 m so that those with angina are not likely to experience an attack. Businessmen with continuing cardiac disorders may therefore fly to Europe, North America, and other countries with good coronary care services with very little risk. But flights in unpressurized aircraft, work in undeveloped countries or in remote areas of the world, and work in a hostile environment (both climatic and political) are best avoided.

Aircrew are subject to guidelines drawn up by the Joint Aviation Authorities. In the United Kingdom the regulatory agency is the Civil Aviation Authority, whose advice should always be sought.

Cardiac deaths are uncommon in trekkers or workers at high altitude (2440 to 4570 m.). The increase in cardiac output at altitude will exacerbate symptoms in those who already experience symptoms at sea level, but asymptomatic individuals with coronary heart disease are unlikely to be at special risk.

Implanted devices

Cardiac pacemakers are generally implanted into older patients who have idiopathic degeneration of their conduction system. However, both heart block and sinoatrial disorder are well-recognized complications of coronary heart disease. Single- and dual-chamber (VVI and DDD in most) pacemakers are rarely subject to electromagnetic interference and no modification of lifestyle is necessary, with the exception that the device can trigger alarms at airports and elsewhere.

The implantable cardioverter defibrillator (**ICD**) has the capacity to detect and treat ventricular tachycardia and fibrillation, either by antitachycardia pacing or by a shock, in patients in whom a further cardiac arrest is anticipated. Both shock and arrhythmia are potentially incapacitating. In North America and Europe, patients with ICDs have restrictions placed upon them, for example driving. They commonly have severe underlying heart disease and may well not be able to work, but if they can do so, then this should be in an environment that is free from electromagnetic interference. There has been one report of ICD malfunction in the vicinity of an electronic antitheft surveillance system.

There has been considerable interest in the possibility that mobile telephones might interfere with pacemakers and ICDs. Studies have shown that this is a theoretical possibility and that reprogramming of a pacemaker can be achieved under exceptional circumstances if the telephone is held close (less than 20 cm) to the pacemaker. In practice no clinically significant interference has yet been reported, but individuals are advised to use the hand and ear furthest from the pacemaker and not to 'dial' with the telephone near to the pacemaker.

Seafarers

The Merchant Shipping (Medical Examination) Regulations in the United Kingdom currently state that any manifestation of ischaemic heart disease renders the individual permanently unfit to return to sea. This regulation has been in force since 1983 and applies to all those seafarers who serve in vessels registered in the United Kingdom above a certain size (a small coaster upwards). This does not necessarily apply to vessels registered in other countries. These regulations will almost certainly change, the likely outcome of current discussions being that acceptable levels of risk will be defined, both for the individual and for the job.

Retirement and end of life

Despite modern treatments some patients will experience multiple coronary events which eventually lead to extensive ventricular damage and persisting symptoms of fatigue and dyspnoea, with signs of heart failure. Such individuals should be warned of their limited prognosis. Some should be advised to retire, which is never an easy decision.

There is often a discrepancy between the symptoms and the objective cardiac data. Some patients—typically the overweight, smoking, manual worker in his forties, who has always enjoyed robust good health—appear to be very symptomatic despite good ventricular function and no evidence of myocardial ischaemia. A heart attack proves devastating. One explanation for this is the profound psychological disturbance that sometimes follows the development of cardiovascular disease. At the other extreme some patients seem well and active despite appalling ventricular function. As always, common sense has to override the results of investigations, but the latter group are still liable to experience sudden cardiac death, when apparently 'so well'.

Patients (with their partners if appropriate) should be given the opportunity of a frank discussion about their prognosis, but some would rather not know and that attitude should be respected. However, most need to put their affairs in order: what to say exactly is one of the most difficult problems in cardiology. The victim's quality of life may be excellent. There is no point in advising a restricted lifestyle or retirement. The only lifestyle trigger of a heart attack, namely sudden unexpected vigorous exercise, should be avoided. Otherwise, normal activities should continue, with the knowledge that the chance of successful resuscitation following a coronary event are greater in developed countries, in fact better in most of Europe and North America than the United Kingdom.

Early retirement on grounds of ill health following a heart attack is sometimes seen as an attractive option. However, most permanent sickness policies contain a clause which states that benefit will only be payable if the subscriber is 'totally unable to follow his former occupation', which is often not the case after a heart attack or coronary artery bypass grafting. Advice about retirement should only be given after due consideration and a review of the job description.

Further reading

Baxter PJ, Petch MC (2000). Cardiovascular disorders. In: Cox RAF, Edwards FC, Palmer K, eds. *Fitness for work*, 3rd edn, pp. 349–70. Oxford Medical Publications.

Joy MD, ed. (1999). Second European Workshop in Aviation Cardiology. *European Heart Journal* Suppl D.

Petch MC (1998). Task Force Report: driving and heart disease. *European Heart Journal* **19**, 1165–77.

Taylor J (1995). In: *Medical aspects of fitness to drive*. Medical Commission on Accident Prevention, London.

15.5 Treatment of heart failure

15.5.1 Pharmacological management of heart failure

J. K. Aronson

There are three aims in treating heart failure: if possible, to remove causative factors and so reverse the condition; otherwise, to relieve symptoms and to improve survival. Examples of reversible causes include valvular disease, hypertension, anaemia, and hyperthyroidism. Symptomatic relief can be produced by the use of diuretics to relieve fluid retention, vasodilators to reduce the workload of the heart, and digitalis to increase cardiac contractility. Positive inotropic drugs other than digitalis (for example, inhibitors of phosphodiesterase type III) are not currently used in the long-term treatment of congestive heart failure, because they are associated with increased mortality. By contrast, reduction in mortality during long-term treatment of heart failure can be achieved with angiotensin-converting enzyme (**ACE**) inhibitors, spironolactone, beta-blockers, and the combination of hydralazine with a nitrate.

Mechanisms of action of drugs used to treat heart failure

The ways in which drugs affect the major pathophysiological abnormalities of heart failure are shown in Fig. 1, and a list of the drugs used is given in Table 1.

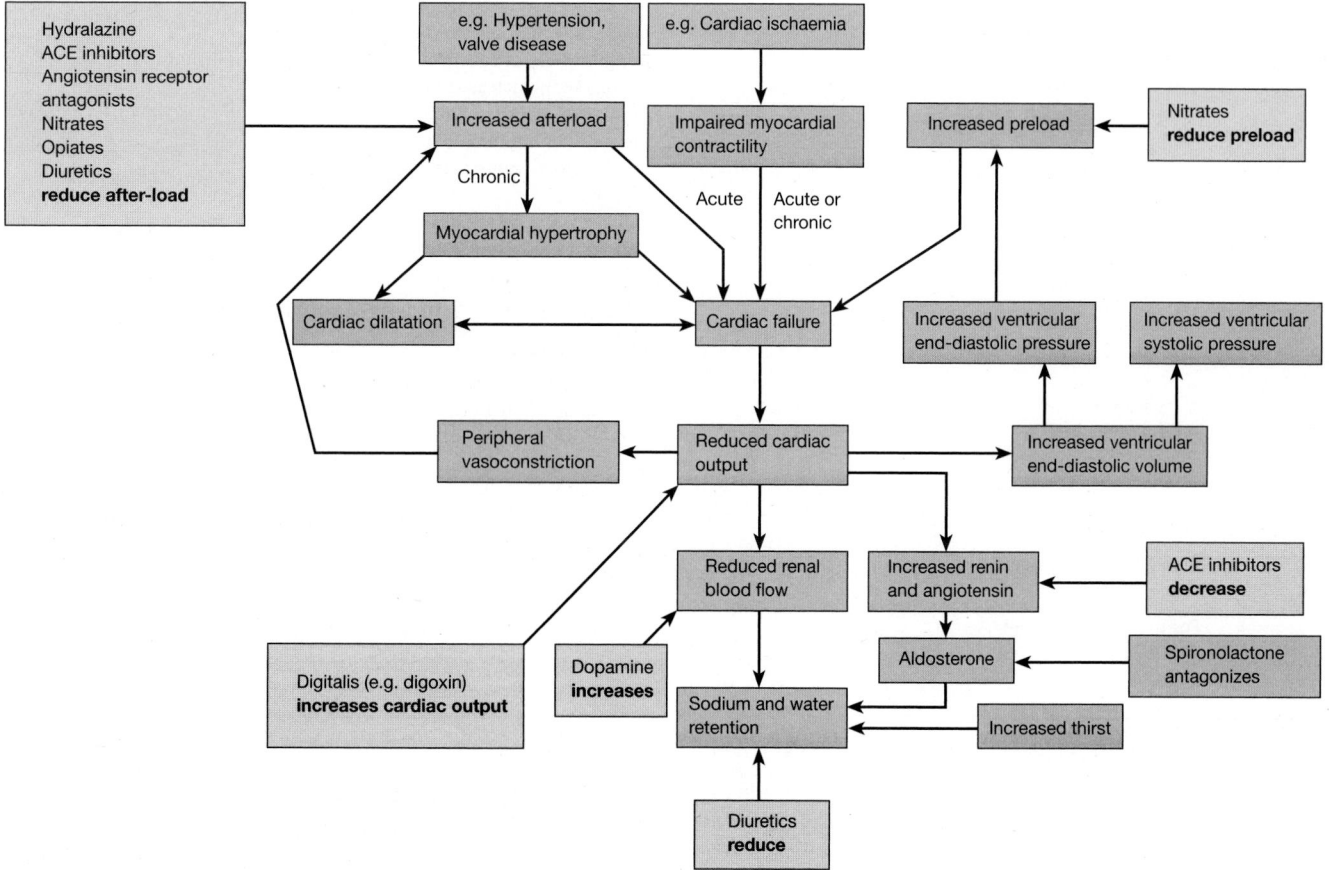

Fig. 1 The pathophysiology of cardiac failure and the sites and mechanisms of action of drugs used in its treatment. (Taken with permission from Grahame-Smith DG, Aronson JK (2001). *The Oxford textbook of clinical pharmacology and drug therapy*, 3rd edn. Oxford University Press, Oxford.)

The effects of heart failure and of some of the drugs used to treat it on the relation between cardiac output and ventricular end-diastolic pressure (the Frank–Starling curve) are shown in Fig. 2. In established heart failure the curve is displaced downwards. It may be possible to increase cardiac output (for example, by increased endogenous sympathetic drive), but that can only happen at the expense of an increased ventricular end-diastolic pressure, and eventually signs and symptoms of congestion occur. If cardiac output cannot be increased, the signs are of low output (for example in cardiogenic shock).

Diuretics

Sodium and water retention occur in heart failure through a combination of mechanisms, including reduced renal blood flow, increased ADH secretion, and increased renin secretion, leading to increased secretion of angiotensin and aldosterone. Diuretics reduce the body sodium and water content. Their sites of action in the renal tubule are shown in Fig. 3.

The loop diuretics furosemide and bumetanide inhibit sodium and chloride reabsorption in the ascending limb of the loop of Henle, with a resulting increase in sodium excretion and a reduction in free-water clearance. They do this by inhibiting Na/K/2Cl cotransport. In addition potassium secretion in the distal convoluted tubule is increased, because of the exchange of potassium for sodium under the influence of aldosterone and an increased intraluminal sodium concentration. Note, however, that the effects of furosemide and bumetanide in the treatment of acute left ventricular failure occur more quickly than would be expected from the rate of onset of their diuretic actions; vasodilator effects may be involved in their acute actions.

The thiazide diuretics act by inhibiting sodium and chloride reabsorption in the distal convoluted tubule of the nephron, resulting in increased sodium and free-water clearance. The molecular mechanism of this effect is through the inhibition of a Na/Cl cotransport system. A secondary effect is the loss of potassium by increased secretion in the distal tubule in response to the increased intraluminal sodium concentration.

Spironolactone and its active metabolite canrenone are aldosterone receptor antagonists; they counteract the effects of hyperaldosteronism that can occur from heart failure itself, and as a secondary response to the natriuresis produced by other diuretics. In a low dosage (25 mg/day) spironolactone reduces mortality in congestive heart failure, presumably by inhibiting the effects of aldosterone, circulating concentrations of which are markedly increased in heart failure. Other potassium-sparing diuretics (amiloride and triamterene) do not interfere with the action of aldosterone; instead they inhibit sodium channels in the distal tubule. They are used only as potassium-sparing diuretics and have not been shown to affect mortality.

The effect of diuretics on the Frank–Starling curve is to lower the ventricular end-diastolic pressure.

ACE inhibitors and angiotensin receptor antagonists

ACE inhibitors, which reduce mortality in chronic heart failure, reduce the production of angiotensin II and prevent the breakdown of bradykinin, both of which are mediated by the angiotensin-converting enzyme (ACE). They are mixed arteriolar/venular vasodilators, mostly by their action on angiotensin production. Because angiotensin causes aldosterone release, the ACE inhibitors also reduce aldosterone production, which reduces sodium retention, leading to reduced blood volume and a fall in cardiac preload.

The ACE inhibitors do not completely prevent the effects of angiotensin on the myocardium, because some angiotensin II is produced by the action of a convertase that is not inhibited by ACE inhibitors. Angiotensin II receptor antagonists, which are selective for angiotensin II type 1 receptors, act beyond this point and prevent the effects of angiotensin II at its site of action. They do not affect the production of bradykinin.

β-Adrenoceptor antagonists

In chronic heart failure, particularly in patients with milder disease, the risk of sudden death is increased; β-blockers reduce that risk through an antiarrhythmic action. They also mitigate the effects of catecholamines, which are produced in excess due to increased sympathetic nervous system activity in heart failure. In some patients there is poor ventricular relaxation

Table 1 Drugs used in the treatment of acute or chronic heart failure

1. **Diuretics**
   Thiazide diuretics
   - Bendroflumethiazide
   - Cyclopenthiazide
   - Hydrochlorothiazide
   - Hydroflumethiazide
   - Polythiazide

   Thiazide-like diuretics
   - Chlortalidone
   - Clopamide
   - Clorexolone
   - Indapamide
   - Mefruside
   - Metolazone
   - Quinethazone
   - Xipamide

   Loop diuretics
   - Furosemide
   - Bumetanide

   Potassium-sparing diuretics
   - Amiloride
   - Triamterene
   - Spironolactone

2. **Drugs affecting the renin–angiotensin system**
   ACE inhibitors
   - Captopril
   - Cilazapril
   - Enalapril
   - Fosinopril
   - Imidapril
   - Lisinopril
   - Moexipril
   - Perindopril
   - Quinapril
   - Ramipril
   - Trandolapril

   Angiotensin receptor antagonists
   - Candesartan
   - Irbesartan
   - Losartan
   - Telmisartan
   - Valsartan

3. **Positive inotropic drugs**
   Cardiac glycosides
   - Digoxin
   - Digitoxin

   Adrenoceptor agonists
   Phosphodiesterase type-III inhibitors
   - Enoximone
   - Milrinone

4. **β-Blockers**
   - Bisoprolol
   - Carvedilol
   - Metoprolol

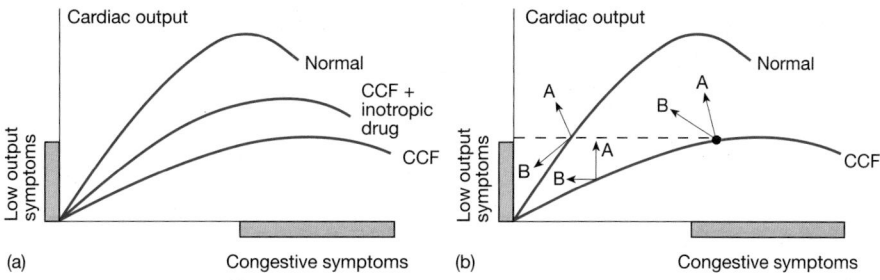

Fig. 2 The Frank–Starling curve, shown here as the relation between ventricular end-diastolic pressure and cardiac output. (a) The effect of positive inotropic drugs: inotropic drugs increase the cardiac output for any given value of end-diastolic pressure. (b) The effects of vasodilators: the effects of vasodilators depend on whether they are predominantly arterial vasodilators (A: for example hydralazine) or mixed vasodilators (B: for example ACE inhibitors). ((a) Adapted with permission from Mason DT (1973). *American Journal of Cardiology* **32**, 437–48. (b) Adapted with permission from Braunwald E (1980). *Heart disease*, p. 548. WB Saunders, Philadelphia.)

during diastole, which can be obviated by β-blockers. However, great care must be taken, because their negative inotropic effect can lead to worsening of heart failure. In addition to being a β-blocker, carvedilol is an α₁-adrenoceptor antagonist and therefore also a vasodilator.

Positive inotropic drugs

Positive inotropic drugs increase cardiac output at any given value of ventricular end-diastolic pressure, thus shifting the Frank–Starling curve upwards. Of drugs with positive inotropic effects only the cardiac glycosides are currently used in the long-term treatment of congestive heart failure. They act by inhibiting sodium transport out of cells, through inhibition of the Na+/K+ pump enzyme Na+/K+-ATPase. The resultant increase in the intracellular sodium concentration leads to altered calcium flux via the Na+/Ca2+ exchange mechanism, and thus to an increased intracellular calcium concentration. This leads to increased contractility through excitation–contraction coupling. The long-term use of other positive inotropic drugs increases mortality in heart failure; digoxin does not.

Other vasodilators

Vasodilators reduce the workload of the heart by dilating arterioles or venules, or both. Dilatation of arterioles results in a reduction in cardiac afterload; dilatation of venules results in a reduction in cardiac preload. A pure reduction in afterload increases the cardiac output at a given ventricular end-diastolic pressure, while a pure reduction in preload reduces the ventricular end-diastolic pressure and hence the cardiac output along the Frank–Starling curve. In practice, vasodilators cause both these effects. This is because a reduction in arterial resistance (reduction in afterload) increases ventricular emptying (which in turn reduces preload), and venous dilatation (reduction in preload) reduces ventricular volume (which in turn reduces afterload). In both cases cardiac output increases and ventricular end-diastolic pressure falls. However, the extent to which these two effects occur depends on whether the vasodilator acts predominantly on arterioles or venules. For example, nitrates are mixed vasodilators, but the venous element predominates, reducing filling pressure. The effects of different vasodilators on arterioles and venules are shown in Table 2.

Clinical pharmacology of drugs used to treat heart failure

Diuretics

All the thiazide diuretics are well absorbed and excreted unchanged by the kidney. They have a slow onset and long duration of action, with half-lives of about 8 to 12 h, and are given once a day. Hypokalaemia, hyponatraemia, and dehydration are their most important adverse effects, and hypomagnesaemia can also occur. Hypokalaemia due to thiazide diuretics potentiates the effects of cardiac glycosides and can cause ventricular arrhythmias, such as *torsade de pointes*, in patients taking antiarrhythmic drugs that prolong the QT interval. Hypercalcaemia can occur in susceptible patients, due to reduced urinary calcium excretion. Hyperglycaemia occurs but is usually not of clinical importance, although occasionally diabetes mellitus may be

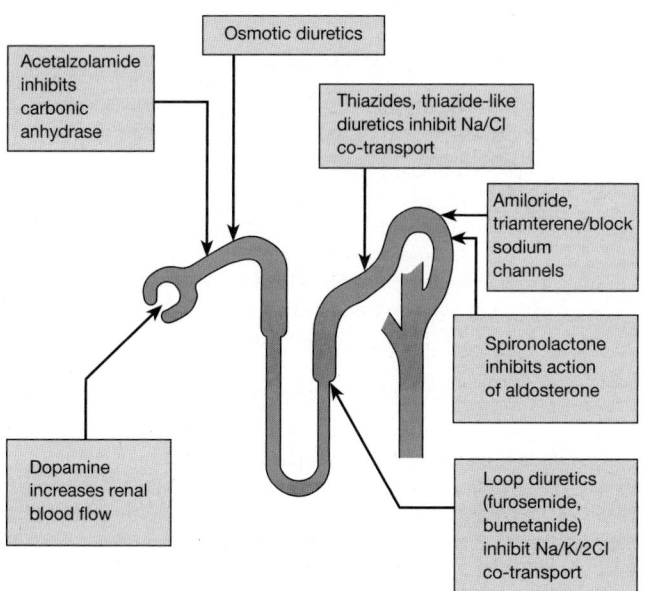

Fig. 3 The sites of action of diuretics in the nephron (Taken with permission from Grahame-Smith DG, Aronson JK (2001). *The Oxford textbook of clinical pharmacology and drug therapy*, 3rd edn. Oxford University Press, Oxford.)

Table 2 Effects of different vasodilators on arterioles and venules

Drug	Arterial dilatation	Venous dilatation
Hydralazine	++	–
Calcium channel blockers	++	+
ACE inhibitors	++	++
Prazosin	++	++
Salbutamol	++	++
Nitroprusside	++	++
Nitrates	+	++
Opiates	+	++

precipitated in a susceptible patient; increased doses of oral hypoglycaemic drugs may be required in diabetics. Hyperuricaemia occurs, but acute gout is uncommon. Erectile impotence can occur in men. Thiazide diuretics reduce the clearance of lithium by the kidney; lithium dosages should be halved initially and adjusted with careful serum concentration monitoring.

In contrast to the thiazide diuretics, furosemide and bumetanide have a rapid onset and short duration of action (about 6 to 8 h), with half-lives of between 1 and 2 h. Bumetanide is well absorbed after oral administration, but furosemide is not, and its absorption may be slowed in patients with congestive heart failure. For this reason patients who do not respond to oral furosemide should be given intravenous furosemide or oral bumetanide instead. Despite their short duration of action these drugs are usually given only once a day, partly to avoid night-time diuresis and partly because, at least in the case of furosemide, the kidney is refractory to further diuresis for about 8 h after an effective dose. If furosemide is given intravenously in doses of 80 mg or more it should be infused at a rate of 4 mg/min, partly to avoid ototoxicity and partly because it is more effective when infused slowly, for reasons that are not understood. The adverse effects and interactions of the loop diuretics are similar to those of the thiazides, except that the loop diuretics are calciuric. Acute urinary retention can be precipitated by too rapid a diuresis in patients with prostatic hyperplasia. Encephalopathy can be precipitated in patients with hepatic insufficiency, particularly if hypokalaemia occurs. Rapid intravenous injection of high doses of furosemide can cause cochlear damage, which is usually reversible. Bumetanide can occasionally cause muscle cramps, independent of hypokalaemia.

Spironolactone is well absorbed. It has a short half-life (about 10 min) but is metabolized to the active compound canrenone (half-life 16 h), which is excreted by the kidney. Partly because of the long half-life of its metabolite, spironolactone has a long duration of action and its maximum effects develop over several days. Nausea and vomiting are common, but not with the low doses currently used to treat heart failure. Hyperkalaemia can occur and is dose-related. Gynaecomastia is common, even with low dosages, and is often painful. Other less frequent effects include menstrual disturbances, impotence, testicular atrophy, and peptic ulceration.

Amiloride is very poorly absorbed. It is almost completely excreted unchanged in the urine and has a half-life of 6 h. Triamterene is incompletely but fairly rapidly absorbed from the gastrointestinal tract. It is extensively metabolized before urinary excretion and its half-life is 2 h. It has variable biliary excretion. Both amiloride and triamterene commonly cause hyperkalaemia, dehydration, and hyponatraemia. The incidence of hyperkalaemia (about 5 per cent) is unaffected by the concurrent administration of potassium-depleting diuretics. Nausea and vomiting occur occasionally. Triamterene can cause crystalluria and rarely causes interstitial nephritis, particularly when it is used in combination with thiazide diuretics; renal prostaglandins may protect the kidney against this damage and this protection may be lost if patients also take non-steroidal anti-inflammatory drugs.

Angiotensin-converting enzyme inhibitors

The ACE inhibitors are variably absorbed: captopril and enalapril are well absorbed, ramipril is moderately well absorbed, and lisinopril is slowly and poorly absorbed (25 per cent or less); the absorption of captopril and enalapril is reduced to 50 per cent by food. Lisinopril is eliminated unchanged in the urine; captopril is 50 per cent excreted unchanged and 50 per cent metabolized to inactive compounds; and the other ACE inhibitors are pro-drugs that are metabolized to active forms. The half-lives of the ACE inhibitors are long, because they bind to ACE in the plasma.

Hypotension can occur with ACE inhibitor overtreatment—particularly if the intravascular volume is depleted by concurrent diuretic therapy—and is most common after the first dose, which should therefore be low and taken whilst the patient is lying down. Cyclo-oxygenase inhibitors, such as indometacin, can reduce the hypotensive effects of the ACE inhibitors.

The ACE inhibitors can cause renal function impairment, particularly in those with renovascular disease and especially unilateral renal artery stenosis; this is because the perfusion pressure in the ischaemic kidney depends on the action of locally produced angiotensin. Proteinuria and the nephrotic syndrome are uncommon adverse effects; the latter is due to a membranous glomerulonephritis. ACE inhibitors inhibit the excretion of lithium.

The ACE inhibitors cause potassium retention by inhibiting aldosterone secretion, and potentiate the effects of other drugs that cause hyperkalaemia, for example, potassium-sparing diuretics or potassium chloride supplements.

Rashes are common (up to 10 per cent) and may be accompanied by fever and eosinophilia. Taste disturbance, which is usually transient, occurs in up to 5 per cent of patients. Cough is the commonest adverse effect requiring drug withdrawal. Angio-oedema occurs rarely. Although neutropenia is rare, it may progress to agranulocytosis.

β-Adrenoceptor antagonists (β-blockers)

Some properties of some commonly used β-blockers are shown in Table 3. Most are well absorbed; atenolol, nadolol, and sotalol, being relatively polar, are exceptions, at 50 per cent or less. During their first passage through the liver carvedilol, metoprolol, and propranolol are extensively metabolized to active compounds, which are excreted in the urine. Bisoprolol is 50 per cent metabolized, but without first-pass elimination. Atenolol and sotalol are mostly eliminated unchanged in the urine. Those β-blockers that are used to treat patients in heart failure (bisoprolol, carvedilol, and metoprolol) have durations of action that roughly correlate with their half-lives.

Blockade of β_2-adrenoceptors in the lungs in susceptible subjects can cause bronchoconstriction, which can lead to life-threatening acute severe asthma. Hence, non-selective β-blockers should not be given to asthmatics, and even relatively selective β-blockers should be used with caution, if at all, since none is completely devoid of some β_2-adrenoceptor antagonist activity.

β-Blockers have negative inotropic effects: careful dosage titration and monitoring of therapy is therefore important in patients in whom they are being used to treat heart failure. In patients with poor left ventricular function after myocardial infarction D-sotalol increased mortality from 3 to 5 per cent (the SWORD trial), probably because of cardiac arrhythmias secondary to prolongation of the QT interval.

Central nervous system effects (depression, hallucinations, sleep disturbances) are more common with lipophilic drugs, which enter the brain well (see Table 3). Peripheral vasoconstriction, resulting in Raynaud's phenomenon, which is particularly troublesome in cold weather, is a common complaint, the precise mechanism of which is still not understood.

If a β-blocker is to be withdrawn, this should be done slowly, since abrupt withdrawal can cause a rebound increase in anginal symptoms or frank myocardial infarction, possibly related to adaptive β-adrenoceptor supersensitivity in response to chronic blockade.

Carvedilol can cause postural hypotension because of its α-blocking action.

Drug interactions with β-blockers occur through a variety of mechanisms:

- The effects of insulin and oral hypoglycaemic drugs are potentiated by β-blockers, and hypoglycaemia can result. There is some evidence that this effect is more pronounced with non-cardioselective β-blockers. This interaction is distinct from the effect of β-blockers in blocking the peripheral clinical response to hypoglycaemia, except for sweating, which is a sympathetic nervous function not served by catecholamines.

- Cimetidine inhibits the first-pass metabolism of propranolol and metoprolol and the metabolism of bisoprolol.

Table 3 Some properties of some β-adrenoceptor antagonists. (Adapted with permission from Dukes MNG, Aronson JK, eds (2000). *Meyler's side effects of drugs*, 14th edn, p. 580. Elsevier, Amsterdam.)

Drug	Lipid solubility[a]	Cardio-select-ivity	Partial agonist activity	Membrane-stabilizing activity	Mean half-life (h)
Acebutolol	0.7	±	+	+	7
Atenolol	< 0.02	+	–		7
Betaxolol		+	–	±	18
Bisoprolol		++	–	–	12
Carvedilol	++	–	–		6
Labetalol	+	–	–		3
Metoprolol	0.2	+	–	±	4
Nadolol	0.03	–	–	–	20
Oxprenolol	0.7	–	+	+	2
Pindolol	0.2	–	++	±	4
Propranolol	4.3	–	–	++	4
Sotalol[b]	0.02	–	–	–	12
Timolol	0.03	–	±	±	4

[a]Octanol:water partition coefficient.

[b]As well as being a non-selective β-blocker, sotalol, through its isomer D-sotalol, has class III antiarrhythmic activity.

- When β-blockers and verapamil are used concurrently there is an increased incidence of bradyarrhythmias and an increased risk of heart failure. There have also been reports of asystole attributed to the use of the combination.

- Sotalol should not be used in combination with other antiarrhythmic drugs that prolong the QT interval (for example, amiodarone, disopyramide, procainamide, quinidine), nor with the antimalarial drug halofantrine, which does the same.

- Monitoring the plasma digoxin concentration during carvedilol therapy is recommended, since carvedilol has been reported to increase plasma digoxin concentrations.

Cardiac glycosides

Digoxin is moderately well absorbed from tablets (about 67 per cent) and better from elixir (80 per cent) and encapsulated elixir (more than 90 per cent). It is mostly eliminated unchanged by the kidneys, with a half-life of about 40 h when renal function is normal, increasing to about 5 days in complete anuria. Dosages must therefore be reduced in renal insufficiency (see below). It has a fast onset of action after oral administration so that intravenous administration is rarely justified; intramuscular injection is painful and causes muscle necrosis and should be avoided.

Digitoxin, in contrast, is almost completely absorbed after oral administration, has a long half-life (about 5 days), and is eliminated by hepatic metabolism. This makes its effects less predictable than those of digoxin, because hepatic metabolism is more variable than renal excretion. However, some prefer it to digoxin, particularly when there is severe renal insufficiency. There are no advantages to using other cardiac glycosides (such as ouabain, acylated forms of digoxin, gitoformate, gitoxin, k-strophanthin, pengitoxin, and proscillaridin).

The adverse effects of the cardiac glycosides are dose-related. Common non-cardiac effects include: anorexia, nausea, vomiting, and diarrhoea; confusion and acute psychiatric disturbances, particularly in old people; and visual disturbances (photophobia, blurring of vision, disturbances of colour vision). Virtually any cardiac arrhythmia can occur, the commonest being ventricular and supraventricular ectopic arrhythmias. Atrioventricular nodal conduction can be impaired, leading to heart block. The combination of an ectopic arrhythmia and heart block (for example, paroxysmal supraventricular tachycardia with block) is particularly suggestive of glycoside toxicity. Bradycardia occurs occasionally, but is often simply an effect of parasympathetic stimulation in a resting patient without glycoside intoxication.

The adverse effects of cardiac glycosides are enhanced by electrolyte disturbances, especially: hypokalaemia, hypercalcaemia, and hypomagnesaemia; hypoxia and acidosis; hypothyroidism; and old age (due to increased tissue sensitivity).

Drug interactions are common with digoxin. Hypokalaemia due to other drugs (for example diuretics) markedly enhances its effects and should be avoided. Drugs that inhibit P-glycoprotein, which mediates the renal tubular secretion of digoxin, increase plasma digoxin concentrations and the risk of toxicity; these include amiodarone, ciclosporin, quinidine, spironolactone, and many of the calcium channel blockers, notably verapamil. Quinidine also alters the tissue distribution of digoxin and reduces its non-renal clearance; this combination is better avoided. The antibiotics erythromycin, clarithromycin, and tetracycline increase the oral systemic availability of digoxin by inhibiting its breakdown by intestinal bacteria, mainly *Eubacterium glenum*. The metabolism of digitoxin is increased via enzyme induction by drugs such as rifampicin and barbiturates.

Cardiac glycoside plasma concentrations should be carefully monitored. This can be of value in individualizing therapy, in monitoring compliance, and in diagnosing digitalis toxicity. It is worth measuring the plasma (or serum) concentration during the initial stages of therapy to ensure that a reasonable target concentration has been achieved (1.0 to 2.0 nmol/l for digoxin, 10 to 20 nmol/l for digitoxin). A cautious increase in dosage is justifiable if there is still a poor response to treatment, but the risk of toxicity starts to rise markedly at plasma concentrations above 2.0 and 20 nmol/l respectively. If there are subsequent changes in the patient's condition, for example renal insufficiency in a patient taking digoxin, measurement of the plasma concentration may help in readjusting dosages. Toxicity is highly likely at plasma concentrations above 3.0 nmol/l (digoxin) or 30 nmol/l (digitoxin); at concentrations below 1.5 or 15 nmol/l respectively, toxicity is unlikely. However, toxicity can occur even with low concentrations and should particularly be suspected if there is hypokalaemia. Certain factors besides potassium depletion increase the risk of digitalis toxicity at a given plasma concentration (see above); these alter the interpretation of the plasma concentration and lower the threshold of suspicion of toxicity.

Other vasodilators

Hydralazine

Hydralazine is well absorbed and extensively metabolized, principally by acetylation. This has a bimodal distribution in the general population, but the half-life of hydralazine (about 4 h) does not differ much between people who are slow and fast acetylators. This is because acetylation occurs mainly during the first passage through the liver, hence the subsequent rate of clearance is not appreciably related to the rate of acetylation; however, patients who are slow acetylators are exposed to more of the parent compound.

Palpitation and tachycardia, nausea, vomiting, diarrhoea, and postural hypotension are all common adverse effects. An arthropathy resembling rheumatoid arthritis or a syndrome similar to that of systemic lupus erythematosus (so-called lupus-like syndrome) can occur with dosages over 200 mg/day, especially in those who are slow acetylators. Hydralazine-induced lupus is more common in patients with the HLA phenotype DR4.

Nitrates

In contrast to glyceryl trinitrate, which is completely metabolized in the liver after oral administration and cannot therefore be given orally, isosorbide dinitrate is absorbed from the gut and extensively metabolized to its active metabolites: especially isosorbide mononitrate, which is itself metabolized. Isosorbide dinitrate and isosorbide mononitrate are therefore active after oral administration, the half-life of isosorbide dinitrate being 1 h and that of isosorbide mononitrate being 4 h, which rate-limits the kinetics of isosorbide dinitrate.

Vasodilatation can cause throbbing headache, sinus tachycardia, and hypotension. Tolerance to the actions of the nitrates occurs with prolonged administration, for example if transdermal patches are left on the skin continuously, or if modified-release formulations are taken without a long enough gap between doses. This can be minimized or avoided by removing the patch for a few hours each day (for example, overnight) or by leaving at least 14 h between the night-time dose of a modified-release formulation and the next morning's dose. The mechanism of this tolerance is not known, but hypotheses include depletion of tissue sulphydryl groups (causing reduced transformation of organic nitrates to nitric oxide), desensitization of guanylyl cyclase, increased vascular production of superoxide anions, changes in plasma volume, and increased production of vasopressin. An attractive theory is that chronic vasodilatation in response to nitric oxide causes a compensatory increased production of the vasoconstrictor endothelin via activation of the renin–angiotensin system.

Patients who take sildenafil concurrently with a nitrate may experience profound hypotension; this combination should be avoided.

Angiotensin receptor antagonists

Candesartan esters are rapidly and completely de-esterified during absorption to candesartan, the systemic availability of which is low, and which is partly metabolized and partly excreted in the bile. Irbesartan is rapidly and completely absorbed and subject to only slight presystemic metabolism; it is metabolized by glucuronidation and oxidation by CYP2C9. Losartan is well absorbed but is subject to extensive presystemic metabolism by CYP2C9 and CYP3A4—one metabolite is active, and is inactivated by further metabolism. The metabolites are excreted in the bile and systemic availability is doubled in patients with liver disease. Valsartan has a systemic availability of about 0.25, which is reduced to about 0.15 by food. It is mostly excreted in the bile. The half-lives of these drugs or their active metabolites range from 6 to 12 h.

As with the ACE inhibitors, hypotension can occur with overtreatment, particularly if the intravascular volume is depleted by concurrent diuretic therapy. Similarly, the angiotensin receptor antagonists should be used with caution in patients with renal insufficiency, since they can cause impairment of renal function, particularly in those with renovascular disease. Hyperkalaemia can occur, but is uncommon. Angio-oedema is rare. Because they do not affect kinins the angiotensin receptor antagonists do not cause cough.

Practical management of heart failure

Acute left ventricular failure

Acute left ventricular failure producing pulmonary oedema is a medical emergency, requiring treatment with oxygen, morphine or diamorphine, a loop diuretic, and vasodilators if required.

Oxygen should be given in a high concentration by face-mask or nasal cannulae. Furosemide 40 mg, or bumetanide 1 mg, is given intravenously (**IV**), followed by 10 mg of morphine IV, via the same needle. If there is a poor response to this regimen, the dose of morphine is repeated and a higher dose of diuretic given. Intravenous vasodilators should be used in patients with severe left ventricular failure, for example glyceryl trinitrate or isosorbide dinitrate, but glyceryl trinitrate can be given sublingually (0.5 mg) or by transdermal patch (5 mg) as a stop-gap. Such treatment should ideally be monitored with the measurement of pulmonary artery wedge pressure using a Swan–Ganz catheter, but this may not be practicable, in which case careful monitoring of the systemic blood pressure is necessary to avoid a systolic pressure below 95 mmHg. Glyceryl trinitrate is given as an IV infusion through a syringe pump in a dosage of 10 to 200 μg/min—starting with no more than 10 μg/min, increasing as necessary, and monitoring the response. The dose of isosorbide dinitrate by IV infusion is between 2 and 10 mg/h.

Cardiac glycosides can also be used in the treatment of acute left ventricular failure, particularly when this is associated with fast atrial fibrillation. However, they increase the risk of cardiac arrhythmias after myocardial infarction.

In the rare circumstance of acute left ventricular failure due to acute severe hypertension, the blood pressure should be lowered rapidly (see Chapter 15.16.3).

Acute left ventricular failure due to iatrogenic fluid overload can be prevented by the use of a loop diuretic. For example, during blood transfusion in a patient with chronic anaemia and therefore a normal intravascular volume, furosemide 20 mg IV should be given immediately before each unit of blood, which should be infused as slowly as possible.

Chronic heart failure

Diagnosis on the basis of symptoms and signs, assisted where possible by echocardiography, should be made as soon as possible, because of the improvement in prognosis promised by ACE inhibitors and spironolactone; such therapy should be begun as early as possible. Information on left ventricular function is immensely helpful in assessing severity, appropriate treatment, response, and prognosis. Appropriate action is indicated if a primary cause is selectively correctable, unsuspected aortic valve disease in the elderly being a common example.

A drug history is essential. Non-steroidal anti-inflammatory drugs cause sodium retention and can tip patients into heart failure. Many calcium channel blockers are negatively inotropic, and short-acting calcium blockers increase the risk of heart failure and should be avoided. Some antiarrhythmic agents are negatively inotropic. Most β-blockers (outside of their careful use, as described below) can be deleterious. Tricyclic antidepressants are best avoided.

Salt intake should be moderated. Hypertension must be treated, and ACE inhibitors can relieve both heart failure and hypertension. It is important that plasma electrolytes, urea, and creatinine be measured, so that renal function can be monitored during treatment.

Assuming that drug therapy is indicated and there is left ventricular dysfunction, then, although diuretics may bring symptomatic relief, an ACE inhibitor should also be used. These two drug categories are now the mainstay of therapy and can be supplemented by spironolactone, which also reduces mortality. In severe cases or when ACE inhibitors are contraindicated or poorly tolerated, there is a case for further vasodilator therapy with hydralazine plus isosorbide dinitrate or mononitrate. Cardiac glycosides as positive inotropic agents still have a place.

It is not yet known whether different types of heart failure require different types of pharmacological management. Currently there is not enough evidence to guide the selection of therapy in different patients, and choices among different types of drugs are generally made on the basis of contraindications and adverse effects rather than positive indications.

Diuretics

The choice of diuretic depends on the severity of heart failure. In mild heart failure a thiazide or thiazide-like diuretic is sufficient (see Table 1). The most commonly used of these diuretics in the United Kingdom are bendroflumethiazide (5 to 10 mg once daily, orally) and cyclopenthiazide (0.5 to 1.0 mg once daily, orally), but there is no particular advantage in using one thiazide rather than another.

Oral loop diuretics are used in cases of more severe heart failure; for example, furosemide 40 to 160 mg once daily or bumetanide 1 to 5 mg once daily. If there is a poor response to either a thiazide or a loop diuretic, the two types can be combined.

In the Randomized Aldactone Evaluation Study (RALES), 822 patients were randomly assigned to receive spironolactone 25 mg/day and 841 to receive placebo. There were significantly fewer deaths in the spironolactone group (284 versus 386), with fewer deaths from progressive heart failure and fewer sudden deaths from cardiac causes. There was also a reduced frequency of hospital admission for worsening heart failure and a significant improvement in the symptoms of heart failure. Most of the patients were taking an ACE inhibitor. Spironolactone 25 mg/day should be given routinely to all patients with congestive heart failure.

In using potassium-wasting diuretics care should be taken to avoid hypokalaemia, especially in old people and in patients taking cardiac glycosides. In patients who are also taking an ACE inhibitor and even a low dose of spironolactone, extra measures to conserve potassium are generally unnecessary. It is not known whether higher doses of spironolactone than 25 mg/day are also associated with a beneficial effect on mortality. If extra potassium-sparing is required it is probably wise to use potassium chloride supplements (to repair depletion) or another potassium-sparing diuretic (amiloride or triamterene) (to prevent further depletion).

ACE inhibitors

ACE inhibitors are now widely considered to be the first-line treatment for chronic heart failure, in combination with a diuretic. Several large studies have shown they improve symptoms and reduce morbidity and mortality in patients with left ventricular dysfunction. A systematic review of 32 randomized, controlled clinical trials in symptomatic heart failure showed that ACE inhibitors reduced mortality by 28 per cent, independent of the ACE inhibitor used. Treatment with an ACE inhibitor also reduced the number and duration of hospital admissions. There was a reduction in mortality of about 8 per cent in patients with asymptomatic heart failure (but see the results of the HOPE study mentioned below).

When starting treatment with an ACE inhibitor in a patient who is already taking a diuretic, particularly a high-efficacy (so-called 'high ceiling') loop diuretic, care must be taken not to cause serious hypotension. If a patient is in severe heart failure and taking a large dosage of a loop diuretic, or is hypovolaemic, or has hyponatraemia (plasma sodium concentration of 130 mmol/l or less), has renal impairment, is taking other vasodilator therapy, or is frail and elderly, it is wise to admit them to hospital for initiation of therapy. Diuretics should be stopped for 24 h, a low dose of a short-acting ACE inhibitor (preferably captopril) should be given, blood pressure should be monitored both when the patient is lying and standing, and the dosage of the ACE inhibitor should only be increased when one is satisfied that serious hypotension has not occurred. If the systolic blood pressure is less than 100 mmHg, if there is clinical heart failure, and if diuretic therapy has already been given, it is unlikely that ACE inhibitor therapy will be tolerated, but each case must be taken on its merits.

Despite all these cautions, it is possible to start some patients on an ACE inhibitor in the community. Diuretics should be stopped for at least 24 h; the first low dose should preferably be given in an environment in which blood pressure monitoring is possible; and the dosage should be increased very gradually.

The effects of ACE inhibitors in the treatment of heart failure are dose-related. The recommended maximal doses are those that have been shown to be efficacious and set as limits beyond which toxicity, namely hypotension, becomes a frequent and unacceptable problem. Thus, the maximal dose for captopril is 50 mg three times a day, for enalapril 20 mg/day, and for lisinopril 20 mg/day. Of these, the author prefers enalapril, which has a longer duration of action than captopril and is better absorbed than lisinopril. However, since the publication of the results of the Heart Outcomes Prevention Evaluation (HOPE) study, ramipril has become more widely used. In this study 9297 high-risk patients (aged 55 or over), with vascular disease or diabetes plus one other cardiovascular risk factor and who were not known to have a low ejection fraction or heart failure, were randomly assigned to receive ramipril (10 mg/day) or placebo. Ramipril reduced the death rates from cardiovascular causes (relative risk 0.74), myocardial infarction (0.80), stroke (0.68), death from any cause (0.84), revascularization procedures (0.85), cardiac arrest (0.63), heart failure (0.77), and complications related to diabetes (0.84).

β-Adrenoceptor antagonists (β-blockers)

Despite much evidence that β-blockers are beneficial in patients with chronic heart failure, particularly in preventing sudden death in patients with mild or moderate disease, there is understandable reluctance to use them, because of the risk of worsening heart failure through impaired myocardial contractility. Certainly they should not be used in patients with severe heart failure (New York Heart Association class IV); indeed, in patients with severe heart failure the β-blocker xamoterol increases mortality. However, if β-blockers are used in patients with milder forms of heart failure, and in very low initial doses with very gradual dosage increases, the evidence is that they are relatively safe and reduce all-cause mortality (risk ratio about 0.7) and cardiac deaths (risk ratio about 0.6). As yet, however, there is no evidence about their efficacy in direct comparison with ACE inhibitors and spironolactone, nor information about whether the combination of a β-blocker with such drugs produces further increases in benefit. Current trials are comparing different β-blockers with each other and β-blockers with ACE inhibitors. It is not known whether digoxin can mitigate the negative inotropic effect of β-blockers in patients with chronic heart failure (although one would expect it to do so), nor how such a combination would affect mortality.

In my view, β-blocker therapy should currently be initiated only by a specialist in hospital. It should be limited to patients with moderate heart failure at worst, despite optimal doses of diuretics, an ACE inhibitor, spironolactone, and digoxin, if indicated. For carvedilol the initial dose should be 3.125 mg and the patient should be observed for a few hours after the first dose. If there is no evidence of worsening heart function 3.125 mg can be given twice daily for 2 weeks, after which a further dosage increase to 6.25 mg twice daily can be attempted. The dosage can be further increased, no more often than every 2 weeks, to a maximum of 50 mg twice daily, and at each stage the patient should be carefully monitored for a few hours after the first dose for evidence of worsening cardiac function. Daily monitoring of body weight is also important, and if a patient's weight increases by 2 kg or more they should report to their doctor; an increase in the dosage of diuretic may help in such cases. The corresponding initial and maximum doses of other β-blockers of proven efficacy in heart failure are: bisoprolol 1.25 mg/day and 10 mg/day; metoprolol 12.5 mg/day and 200 mg/day. The class III antiarrhythmic drug D-sotalol increases mortality after myocardial infarction, suggesting that the racemic form DL-sotalol, which also has β-blocking activity, should be avoided in such patients.

Cardiac glycosides

The positive inotropic effects of cardiac glycosides can be useful in reducing symptoms (mainly breathlessness) in patients already taking diuretics and ACE inhibitors. However, the beneficial effect is small and digoxin does not reduce mortality during long-term therapy. However, it does have a small effect in reducing hospital admission rates; there is also evidence that heart function deteriorates in about 25 per cent of patients after withdrawal, so there may still be a role for digoxin in a few patients who need extra symptomatic relief. It is also the drug of choice for treating atrial fibrillation in patients with congestive heart failure. Set against this is the difficulty in using it properly and the high risk of toxicity, particularly in older people, who have poor renal function and are prone to hypokalaemia, particularly if they are also taking diuretics.

Cardiac glycosides should not be used, or are ineffective, in the following conditions:

- left ventricular outflow obstruction (for example, aortic stenosis, hypertrophic obstructive cardiomyopathy), since they increase the force of contraction against a fixed obstruction;

- constrictive pericarditis, for an analogous reason;

- chronic cor pulmonale, because of reduced efficacy and an increased risk of toxicity, perhaps secondary to hypoxia and acidosis;

- hyperthyroidism, because of reduced efficacy and an increased risk of toxicity, although they may be useful in addition to a β-adrenoceptor antagonist in patients with atrial fibrillation and to some extent protect the heart against the negative inotropic effects of β-blockers;

- arrhythmias associated with accessory conduction pathways (for example Wolff–Parkinson–White syndrome), since they impair conduction through the normal conducting pathways without affecting the accessory pathways.

Digoxin is given orally in an initial loading dose of 15 μg/kg, preferably in three divided doses at 6-hour intervals, monitoring for evidence of toxicity (for example, cardiac arrhythmias or symptoms of nausea and vomiting) before the second and third doses. In severe renal insufficiency the initial loading dose should be reduced to 12 μg/kg and increased only in the face of a plasma concentration below the target range (see above). The subsequent maintenance dose should be based on renal function, as shown in Table 4. In patients with atrial fibrillation, in whom the response to digoxin can be easily measured by counting the ventricular rate, an extra dose of 5 μg/kg (in other words, a total loading dose of 20 μg/kg) can be given if necessary; in that case the daily maintenance dose should be increased proportionately. There is no advantage in giving digoxin intravenously; moreover, intramuscular injection is painful and causes muscle necrosis. If digoxin has to be given parenterally in a patient who cannot swallow, it should be infused intravenously over no less than 30 min to avoid the acute hypertension that can occur during rapid intravenous administration. Monitoring therapy by plasma concentration measurement is discussed above.

Other vasodilators

The combination of hydralazine (300 mg/day) with a nitrate (isosorbide dinitrate 160 mg/day) has beneficial haemodynamic effects, improves symptoms, and also reduces mortality, although not as markedly as ACE inhibitors. This combination is also less well tolerated than ACE inhibitors. It should be reserved for patients in whom renovascular disease militates against the use of ACE inhibitors and angiotensin receptor antagonists. It has been suggested that the addition of hydralazine and a nitrate to ACE

Table 4 Maintenance dosages of digoxin according to renal function

Creatinine clearance (ml/min)	Daily elimination rate (fraction of total body load)	Usual maintenance dose (μg/kg per day)*
100	1/3	5.00
50	1/4	3.75
25	1/5	3.00
10	1/6	2.50
0	1/7	2.14

*Based on a loading dose of 15 μg/kg; alter proportionately for different loading doses.

inhibitor therapy should improve mortality even further, but this hypothesis has not yet been tested in a large clinical trial.

Short-acting calcium channel blockers increase cardiovascular mortality in patients with coronary heart disease and should be avoided in long-term treatment. Modified-release formulations of short-acting calcium blockers and long-acting drugs (such as amlodipine) seem to be safe in this regard, but there is as yet no evidence that they reduce mortality in patients with chronic heart failure. Amlodipine may delay the time to and reduce the number of admissions to hospital in connection with ventricular arrhythmias. However, there is currently no place for the use of calcium blockers in patients with congestive heart failure, except in the treatment of associated conditions such as hypertension or angina pectoris.

Alpha-blockers, such as prazosin, neither improve symptoms nor reduce mortality in chronic heart failure; they should not be used.

Angiotensin receptor antagonists

In patients who cannot tolerate ACE inhibitors because of adverse effects, such as cough or renal insufficiency, angiotensin receptor antagonists seem a logical alternative, and they are certainly better tolerated than ACE inhibitors. However, although there is some evidence that angiotensin receptor antagonists improve symptoms in congestive heart failure, there is currently no evidence that they are better than ACE inhibitors at reducing mortality. There is some early evidence that a combination of an ACE inhibitor with an angiotensin receptor antagonist may be more efficacious than either alone, but this hypothesis awaits proper testing. Until further information becomes available, angiotensin receptor antagonists should be reserved for patients who cannot tolerate ACE inhibitors. Typical once-daily doses are: candesartan 4 to 16 mg; irbesartan 75 to 300 mg; losartan 25 to 100 mg; and valsartan 40 to 160 mg.

Other positive inotropic drugs

Other positive inotropic drugs, including the phosphodiesterase inhibitors (such as amrinone, milrinone, and vesnarinone), ibopamine, and intermittent intravenous dobutamine, all increase mortality during long-term treatment of congestive heart failure and should not be used. However, there is evidence that short-term intravenous milrinone for a few weeks can help achieve haemodynamic stability and tide suitable patients over to heart transplantation. Milrinone has also been used to help wean patients off cardiopulmonary bypass.

Other antiarrhythmic drugs

If sudden death in chronic heart failure is due to cardiac arrhythmias, one would expect other antiarrhythmic drugs to be beneficial. However, the results of the few available studies of the class III antiarrhythmic drug amiodarone are not impressive. In one trial amiodarone 300 mg/day produced a small reduction in mortality, but this has not been confirmed. Some of the data suggest that amiodarone may be more beneficial in patients with non-ischaemic heart failure, but it should currently be reserved for patients with identified ventricular arrhythmias. Class I antiarrhythmic drugs increase mortality after myocardial infarction and should be avoided.

Anticoagulants

There is an increased risk of venous thrombosis in immobile patients who have severe heart failure and have swollen legs due to oedema. Prophylactic anticoagulation is therefore advisable, using either an oral anticoagulant (for example, warfarin) or low-dose subcutaneous heparin. Other patients with cardiomyopathy, severe left ventricular dilatation, or demonstrable intracardiac thrombus on echocardiography should be given anticoagulants to prevent systemic emboli. These issues are discussed in Chapter 15.5.2.

Monitoring therapy in heart failure

Drug therapy in heart failure should be monitored for evidence of therapeutic efficacy and drug toxicity.

Fluid and electrolyte balance and the response to diuretics should be monitored by body weight and serum electrolyte measurements. Potassium depletion can occur, even in patients taking potassium-sparing drugs (ACE inhibitors, angiotensin receptor antagonists, and spironolactone), in which case potassium chloride should be given to replace any deficit and additional amiloride or triamterene to prevent further potassium loss.

Renal function should be monitored before giving an ACE inhibitor or angiotensin receptor antagonist during the first few days or weeks of therapy, and whenever the dosage is increased. Worsening renal function will dictate dosage reduction or drug withdrawal.

Blood pressure should be measured at each visit. It will often fall after the first dose of an ACE inhibitor but will usually improve thereafter.

Serum or plasma digoxin concentration measurement is discussed above.

During anticoagulant therapy with warfarin the target International Normalized Ratio (**INR**) is 2.0 to 2.5 for the prevention of deep vein thrombosis, 2.5 to 3.0 for patients with atrial fibrillation, dilated cardiomyopathy, or mural thrombosis, and 3.5 for recurrent deep vein thrombosis or pulmonary embolism and in patients with prosthetic heart valves.

Further reading

Acute Infarction Ramipril Efficacy (AIRE) Study Investigators (1993). Effect of ramipril on mortality and morbidity of survivors of acute myocardial infarction with clinical evidence of heart failure. *Lancet* **342**, 821–8.

Australia/New Zealand Heart Failure Research Collaborative Group (1997). Randomised, placebo-controlled trial of carvedilol in patients with congestive heart failure due to ischaemic heart disease. *Lancet* **349**, 375–80.

Bart BA, *et al.* (1999). Contemporary management of patients with left ventricular systolic dysfunction. Results from the Study of Patients Intolerant of Converting Enzyme Inhibitors (SPICE) Registry. *European Heart Journal* **20**, 1182–90.

CIBIS-II Investigators and Committees (1999). The Cardiac Insufficiency Bisoprolol Study II (CIBIS-II): a randomised trial. *Lancet* **353**, 9–13.

Cohn JN, *et al.* (1986). Effect of vasodilator therapy on mortality in chronic congestive heart failure. Results of a Veterans Administration Cooperative Study. *New England Journal of Medicine* **314**, 1547–52.

Cohn JN, *et al.* (1991). A comparison of enalapril with hydralazine–isosorbide dinitrate in the treatment of chronic congestive heart failure. *New England Journal of Medicine* **325**, 303–10.

CONSENSUS Trial Study Group (1987). Effects of enalapril on mortality in severe congestive heart failure. Results of the Cooperative North Scandinavian Enalapril Survival Study (CONSENSUS). *New England Journal of Medicine* **316**, 1429–35.

Cruickshank JM (1993). The xamoterol experience in the treatment of heart failure. *American Journal of Cardiology*, **71**, 61C–64C.

De Vries RJ, Van Veldhuisen DJ, Dunselman PH (2000). Efficacy and safety of calcium channel blockers in heart failure: focus on recent trials with second-generation dihydropyridines. *American Heart Journal* **139**, 185–94.

Dickstein K, Kjekshus J (1999). Comparison of the effects of losartan and captopril on mortality in patients after acute myocardial infarction: the OPTIMAAL trial design. Optimal Therapy in Myocardial Infarction with the Angiotensin II Antagonist Losartan. *American Journal of Cardiology* **83**, 477–81.

Digitalis Investigation Group (1997). The effect of digoxin on mortality and morbidity in patients with heart failure. *New England Journal of Medicine* **336**, 525–33.

Doughty RN, *et al.* (1997). Effects of β-blocker therapy on mortality in patients with heart failure. A systematic overview of randomized controlled trials. *European Heart Journal* **18**, 560–5.

Doval HC, *et al.* (1994). Randomised trial of low-dose amiodarone in severe congestive heart failure. Grupo de Estudio de la Sobrevida en la Insuficiencia Cardiaca en Argentina (GESICA). *Lancet* **344**, 493–8.

Eichhorn EJ, Bristow MR (1997). Practical guidelines for initiation of β-adrenergic blockade in patients with chronic heart failure. *American Journal of Cardiology* **79**, 794–8.

Furberg CD, Psaty BM, Meyer JV (1995). Nifedipine. Dose-related increase in mortality in patients with coronary heart disease. *Circulation* **92**, 1326–31.

Garg R, Yusuf S (1995). Overview of randomized trials of angiotensin-converting enzyme inhibitors on mortality and morbidity in patients with heart failure. Collaborative Group on ACE Inhibitor Trials. *Journal of the American Medical Association* **273**, 1450–6.

Havranek EP, *et al.* (1999). Dose-related beneficial long-term hemodynamic and clinical efficacy of irbesartan in heart failure. *Journal of the American College of Cardiology* **33**, 1174–81.

Heart Outcomes Prevention Evaluation Study Investigators (2000). Effects of ramipril on cardiovascular and microvascular outcomes in people with diabetes mellitus: results of the HOPE study and MICRO-HOPE substudy. *Lancet* **355**, 253–9.

Heart Outcomes Prevention Evaluation Study Investigators (2000). Effects of an angiotensin-converting-enzyme inhibitor, ramipril, on cardiovascular events in high-risk patients. *New England Journal of Medicine* **342**, 145–53.

Kober L, *et al.* (1995). A clinical trial of the angiotensin-converting-enzyme inhibitor trandolapril in patients with left ventricular dysfunction after myocardial infarction. Trandolapril Cardiac Evaluation (TRACE) Study Group. *New England Journal of Medicine* **333**, 1670–6.

Krum H (1999) Beta-blockers in heart failure. The 'new wave' of clinical trials. *Drugs* **58**, 203–10.

Massie BM, *et al.* (1996). Effect of amiodarone on clinical status and left ventricular function in patients with congestive heart failure. CHF-STAT Investigators. *Circulation* **93**, 2128–34.

Mehra MR, *et al.* (1997). Safety and clinical utility of long-term intravenous milrinone in advanced heart failure. *American Journal of Cardiology* **80**, 61–4.

MERIT-HF Study Group (1999). Effect of metoprolol CR/XL in chronic heart failure: Metoprolol CR/XL Randomised Intervention Trial in Congestive Heart Failure (MERIT-HF). *Lancet* **353**, 2001–7.

Packer M, *et al.* (1993). Withdrawal of digoxin from patients with chronic heart failure treated with angiotensin-converting-enzyme inhibitors. RADIANCE Study. *New England Journal of Medicine* **329**, 1–7.

Packer M, *et al.* (1996). The effect of carvedilol on morbidity and mortality in patients with chronic heart failure. US Carvedilol Heart Failure Study Group. *New England Journal of Medicine* **334**, 1349–55.

Packer M, *et al.* (1999). Comparative effects of low and high doses of the angiotensin-converting enzyme inhibitor, lisinopril, on morbidity and mortality in chronic heart failure. ATLAS Study Group. *Circulation* **100**, 2312–18.

Pennell DJ, *et al.* (2000). The Carvedilol Hibernation Reversible Ischaemia Trial, Marker Of Success (CHRISTMAS) study. Methodology of a randomised, placebo controlled, multicentre study of carvedilol in hibernation and heart failure. *International Journal of Cardiology* **72**, 265–74.

Pfeffer MA, *et al.* (1992). Effect of captopril on mortality and morbidity in patients with left ventricular dysfunction after myocardial infarction. Results of the survival and ventricular enlargement trial. The SAVE Investigators. *New England Journal of Medicine* **327**, 669–77.

Pitt B, *et al.* (1997). Randomised trial of losartan versus captopril in patients over 65 with heart failure (Evaluation of Losartan in the Elderly Study, ELITE). *Lancet* **349**, 747–52.

Pitt B, *et al.* (1999). Effects of losartan versus captopril on mortality in patients with symptomatic heart failure: rationale, design, and baseline characteristics of patients in the Losartan Heart Failure Survival Study—ELITE II. *Journal of Cardiac Failure* **5**, 146–54.

Pitt B, *et al.* (1999). The effect of spironolactone on morbidity and mortality in patients with severe heart failure. Randomized Aldactone Evaluation Study Investigators. *New England Journal of Medicine* **341**, 709–17.

SOLVD Investigators (1991). Effect of enalapril on survival in patients with reduced left ventricular ejection fractions and congestive heart failure. *New England Journal of Medicine* **325**, 293–302.

Swedberg K, *et al.* (1999). Candesartan in heart failure—assessment of reduction in mortality and morbidity (CHARM): rationale and design. Charm–Programme Investigators. *Journal of Cardiac Failure* **5**, 276–82.

Uretsky BF, *et al.* (1993). Randomized study assessing the effect of digoxin withdrawal in patients with mild to moderate chronic congestive heart failure: results of the PROVED trial. PROVED Investigative Group. *Journal of the American College of Cardiology* **22**, 955–62.

Xamoterol in Severe Heart Failure Study Group (1990). Xamoterol in severe heart failure. *Lancet* **336**, 1–6.

15.5.2 Therapeutic anticoagulation in atrial fibrillation and heart failure

David Keeling

Atrial fibrillation

Atrial fibrillation is present in 5 per cent of the population over 65 years of age and in 10 per cent of those over 70 years. It increases the risk of stroke fivefold and is present in 15 per cent of all stroke patients. The overall risk of ischaemic stroke in atrial fibrillation without rheumatic heart disease is about 5 per cent per year, but this can be modified by other risk factors. The risk increases with age: those over 75 years old are at high risk; by contrast, those less than 65 years old with no other risk factors have a risk of stroke of 1 per cent per year. Other factors that increase the risk of stoke in atrial fibrillation have been well characterized (Table 1). It is not clear for how long one must successfully treat patients with hypertension before their risk of stroke decreases, and pending further studies treated hypertension should still be regarded as a major risk factor.

Warfarin decreases the risk of ischaemic stroke in atrial fibrillation by 68 per cent, compared with a reduction of approximately 21 per cent with aspirin. The risk of ischaemic stroke has to be balanced against the risk of intracranial haemorrhage on anticoagulant therapy. The risk of intracranial haemorrhage on warfarin is approximately 0.5 per cent per year, and although this increases with age, so does the risk of ischaemic stroke.

Long-term oral anticoagulation should be considered for those patients with atrial fibrillation who are at high risk of stroke. They should receive warfarin if they are over 75 years old or have one or more of the major risk factors in Table 1 and no contraindication. Oral anticoagulation is recommended instead of aspirin because of the large absolute risk reduction: when the risk of stroke is 7.5 per cent per annum only 20 patients need to be treated for 1 year to prevent a stroke. Patients between 65 and 75 years are at greater risk than those less than 65 years: if they have additional minor risk factors such as diabetes or coronary artery disease, they too should be offered warfarin. Patients between 65 and 75 years of age with no other risk factors and those less than 65 years old with only minor risk factors are at intermediate risk and the choice of oral anticoagulation or aspirin will be significantly affected by patient preference. Those less than 65 years old with no risk factors should receive aspirin (Table 2).

For warfarin the target INR should be 2.5 (range 2.0 to 3.0): lower intensity anticoagulation is not effective and higher intensity increases the risk of bleeding. For those on aspirin it is unnecessary to give more than 75 mg /day.

Anticoagulation after an acute ischaemic stroke should be delayed until most of the deficit has resolved, or for 2 weeks in the case of severe strokes.

Oral anticoagulation should be given for 3 weeks before elective cardioversion of patients who have been in atrial fibrillation for more than 48 h and continued until sinus rhythm has been maintained for 4 weeks. It is not needed if atrial fibrillation has lasted for less than 48 h.

Heart failure

The trials of oral anticoagulation (with high target INRs) after myocardial infarction showed reductions in recurrent myocardial infarction, ischaemic stroke, and all-cause mortality similar to those observed with aspirin. However, aspirin is recommended for long-term therapy in preference to warfarin because of its safety. Warfarin is given to survivors of myocardial infarction at high risk of systemic embolization because of severe left ventricular dysfunction, congestive heart failure, mobile mural thrombus, or atrial fibrillation. In these cases the target INR is 2.5 (target range 2.0 to 3.0). Although it is not clear if this lower intensity protects as effectively against vascular disease, aspirin is not given concurrently because of the increased risk of bleeding. Warfarin should also be considered in congestive heart failure due to causes other than myocardial infarction to reduce the high risk of thromboembolism.

Further reading

Laupacis A *et al.* (1998). Antithrombotic therapy in atrial fibrillation. *Chest* **114**, 579S–589S.

Table 1 Factors increasing the risk of stroke in atrial fibrillation.

Major
Previous stroke or TIA
Hypertension
Poor left ventricular function*
Rheumatic mitral valve disease
Prosthetic heart valve†
Minor
Diabetes
Coronary artery disease

*Either clinically or on echocardiography.
†Mechanical or tissue.

Table 2 Warfarin or aspirin for atrial fibrillation?

Warfarin
Major risk factor
Age >75 years
Age 65–75 years with minor risk factor
Warfarin or aspirin
Age 65–75 with no risk factor
Age < 65 years with minor risk factor
Aspirin
Age <65 years with no risk factor

Risk factors are as in Table 1.

15.5.3 Cardiac rehabilitation

Andrew J. S. Coats

Introduction

Cardiac rehabilitation constitutes the use of pharmacological and non-pharmacological treatment modalities to restore a patient to premorbid health, outlook, and activity. It is more than treating a disease: it is the systematic attempt to correct all factors limiting a subject from full participation in the healthy aspects of their predisease lifestyle.

The conventional four phases of rehabilitation constitute: the early interventions during hospital stay (phase 1); followed by the first 6 weeks after discharge (phase 2); then full participation in sport, work, and family life over the next 6 to 12 months (phase 3); and, last, the maintenance of the new healthier condition and lifestyle (phase 4). Secondary prevention of cardiovascular disease by the full use of available techniques is an important part of rehabilitation. The components of a successful cardiac rehabilitation programme, which needs to be well monitored and adequately staffed with a multidisciplinary team, are listed in Table 1.

It has been established that cardiac rehabilitation can increase quality of life, exercise capacity, and the chance of return to work in patients recovering from a myocardial infarction. Meta-analyses of published randomized controlled trials of cardiac rehabilitation programmes which include a structured exercise training component have shown that these are able to produce an approximately 25 per cent reduction in mortality. Rehabilitation programmes also give an opportunity for the effective implementation of secondary preventive measures to reduce the risk of subsequent cardiovascular events.

Rehabilitation in special populations

The benefits and risks of taking part in a cardiac rehabilitation programme after a myocardial infarction depend on the prior morbidity and prognosis of the individual. The lower the cardiovascular risk, and the better the exercise tolerance and state of health of the patient at the start, the lower the chance of any adverse events occurring during rehabilitation. However, such low-risk patients may have relatively little to gain from the programme if their degree of fitness and motivation are already high. By contrast, patients at a higher risk of reinfarction, or with a lower level of motivation and exercise tolerance, may achieve more substantial benefit. However, there is a tendency for rehabilitation to be offered to the lower risk younger patient rather than the higher risk older patient with more medical problems. But given the benefits that can be achieved in those at high risk, special procedures should be instituted to make sure these patients receive rehabilitation services.

Table 1 Components of a successful cardiac rehabilitation programme

1. **Administrative**
   Committed medical leadership
   Adequate funding and staffing
   Proper resuscitation and exercise facilities in an accessible location
   Documentation, audit, and development strategies
   Up-to-date standard operating procedure manuals

2. **Professional input**
   Multidisciplinary team:
   - medical
   - nursing
   - physiotherapy
   - exercise physiology
   - dietetics
   - pharmacy
   - clinical psychology
   - occupational therapy

3. **Patient selection**
   Inclusive
   Not ageist
   Able to cater for minority cultures and languages
   Special facilities for high-risk patients:
   - elderly
   - heart failure
   - chronic angina

The elderly

There is often an effective age restriction for entry to many cardiac rehabilitation programmes, but, physiologically and medically, there is no reason for age *per se* to be a contraindication to rehabilitation. The risk factors for cardiovascular disease may differ in the elderly, with dys- and hyperlipidaemias being quantitatively less important and systolic blood pressure being more important, but it can still be advantageous to identify and reduce these risk factors. Exercise tolerance is more markedly impaired at the outset, but it can be increased by training even in the very elderly. Other diseases frequently coexist in the elderly, and they are more likely to be taking multiple medications, to have a poorer memory, and to have less adequate social support networks for their greater needs. These and many other factors make rehabilitation programmes with an exercise component more problematic and associated with a higher rate of complications. This does not mean, however, that elderly patients should not be encouraged to participate.

The elderly are likely to need a longer and gentler introduction to rehabilitation, more frequent and prolonged contact throughout the programme, and closer attention from medical staff. They will often present with other non-cardiac problems, requiring assistance from various medical specialties and paramedical staff and social workers. It is wise to involve all relevant parties in the rehabilitation visits of the elderly patient, so that no conflict of advice ensues about, for example, activities and lifestyle. However, the benefits of recruiting elderly patients can be very great, enabling them to achieve a greater degree of independence and avoiding the need for long-term residential care.

Rehabilitation in those with specific cardiac conditions

Angina

Continuing angina frequently prevents a patient from participating in a formal rehabilitation programme. In some, participation can be delayed until completion of further investigation and revascularization procedures, but there remain many patients with persistent angina in whom revascularization procedures are either impossible or incompletely successful. These patients may gain benefit in terms of secondary prevention and in improving exercise tolerance by participating in a rehabilitation programme. There is good evidence for a modest antianginal effect of physical training, and risk factor reduction is of considerable importance for angina sufferers. Training in the presence of exercise-induced angina may also promote the development of new collateral vessels to the myocardium.

Heart failure

In the past, heart failure was frequently listed as an absolute contraindication to participation in cardiac rehabilitation. Whilst active myocarditis or acute heart failure with congestion remain contraindications to exercise training, research over the last decade has shown that carefully selected patients with stable chronic heart failure can achieve significant and worthwhile benefits from exercise training. This is now an important area in cardiac rehabilitation research.

Like the situation for the elderly, those with heart failure are significantly limited and in need of considerable medical care. They are also likely to benefit substantially from even modest improvements in their ability to perform exercise, as many daily tasks will stress them to close to their cardiopulmonary exercise reserve. These patients are frequently well motivated and co-operate fully with the rehabilitation programme. Several practical difficulties arise, however, including the need for closer supervision, more detailed preparticipation assessment, and a greater likelihood of complications including serious ventricular arrhythmia. Perhaps most importantly from a practical point of view, these patients may need a lifelong attachment to the programme for continuing benefit.

Research in specialist units has shown possible training benefits for patients with moderate and severe heart failure, provided their condition is stable. Improvements of between 20 and 25 per cent have been seen in exercise capacity, associated with reduced sympathetic tone, reduced breathlessness and exercise ventilation, and improved exercise haemodynamics. However, in each case the training exercise needs to be tailored specifically to the patient's reduced capacity. The level of exercise prescription may start at a very low level, such as 70 per cent of their existing maximal capacity for as little as 5 to 10 min a session. This is then gradually increased in duration and absolute intensity as the patient's maximal capacity increases.

It is recommended that patients with heart failure undergo cardiopulmonary exercise assessment in a specialist unit to establish accurately their exercise capacity prior to entry into a rehabilitation programme. Detailed evaluation is needed, such as the detection of ventricular arrhythmias either by 24-h ECG monitoring or on exercise testing. The presence of ventricular tachycardia is common in patients with moderate and severe heart failure, and may increase the risk during exercise. Whether these arrhythmias negate possible benefits of rehabilitation because of the risk of precipitating arrhythmias remains unknown.

No patient with heart failure should take part in an exercise programme in the presence of acute decompensation, such as with pulmonary or peripheral oedema, active myocarditis, or febrile illnesses. Although there is no lower limit on ejection fraction for the participation of those with heart failure, the patient must be comfortable at rest and be able to exercise for 5 min at an exercise level of 2 **METS** (metabolic equivalents (of oxygen consumption)) or greater. A left ventricular ejection fraction of 20 per cent or less is still compatible with participation, and patients can still usefully participate when they are stable on a cardiac transplantation waiting list.

Further reading

Coats AJS, *et al.* (1992). Controlled trial of physical training in chronic heart failure: exercise performance, hemodynamics, ventilation and autonomic function. *Circulation* **85**, 2119–31.

Coats AJS. (1993). Exercise rehabilitation in chronic heart failure. *Journal of the American College of Cardiology* **22**(Suppl. A), 172A–177A.

Oldridge NB, *et al.* (1988). Cardiac rehabilitation after myocardial infarction. Combined experience of randomized clinical trials. *Journal of the American Medical Association* **260**, 945–50.

Todd IC, Ballantyne D (1990). Antianginal efficacy of exercise training: a comparison with beta blockade. *British Heart Journal* **64**, 14–19.

15.5.4 Cardiac transplantation and mechanical circulatory support

John H. Dark

Introduction

The basic surgical technique and the first clinical attempts at heart transplantation were described over 30 years ago, but poor results lead to a quiescent phase during the 1970s. This hiatus stimulated the development of a range of pumps intended to replace the function of the heart.

Effective immunosuppression, particularly with the introduction of ciclosporin A in 1981, enormously improved transplant results and there

was a rapid expansion of activity over the next decade. This reached a plateau during the 1990s, with 3000 to 4000 heart transplants worldwide and up to 300 in the United Kingdom, although the total is now declining.

The size of the problem

The incidence of heart failure is increasing, not only because of an ageing population but also because of the longer survival of existing patients, benefiting from greatly improved medical management. In the United States, a conservative estimate is that 35 000 patients per year would benefit from cardiac replacement therapy, and enthusiasts put this figure above one million. By extrapolation, a figure of 5000 patients per year can be derived for the United Kingdom.

Transplantation brings with it unavoidable morbidity, both from immunosuppression and progressive graft failure, and long-term survival is limited. The limited number of donors means that it is only an option for a tiny proportion of those with congestive cardiac failure, and furthermore, transplantation is not always available when required, as demonstrated by a mortality rate of 15 to 40 per cent amongst those accepted on to transplant waiting lists. There is thus a huge need for an alternative to transplantation for patients with heart failure that is readily available, will provide an adequate cardiac output, and will have better long-term performance.

Mechanical circulatory support

Mechanical means of assisting or replacing the heart have evolved through short-term (days) postoperative support and medium-term (weeks to months) devices for 'bridge to transplant', to those on the verge of being accepted for long-term permanent implantation (Fig. 1).

Devices

Intra-aortic balloon pump

Counterpulsation with an intra-aortic balloon pump (**IABP**), usually placed via the femoral artery into the proximal descending aorta, was introduced in the late 1960s and is now used primarily for the short-term support of patients with postoperative low cardiac output or unresolved ischaemia. It is sometimes used as an adjunct to intravenous inotropes in potential transplant recipients who are deteriorating, but has no proven role except perhaps in those with ischaemic cardiomyopathy. The balloon pump has not found a role in the management of cardiogenic shock after myocardial infarction, unless there is a surgically remediable problem such as an acquired ventricular septal defect or papillary muscle rupture.

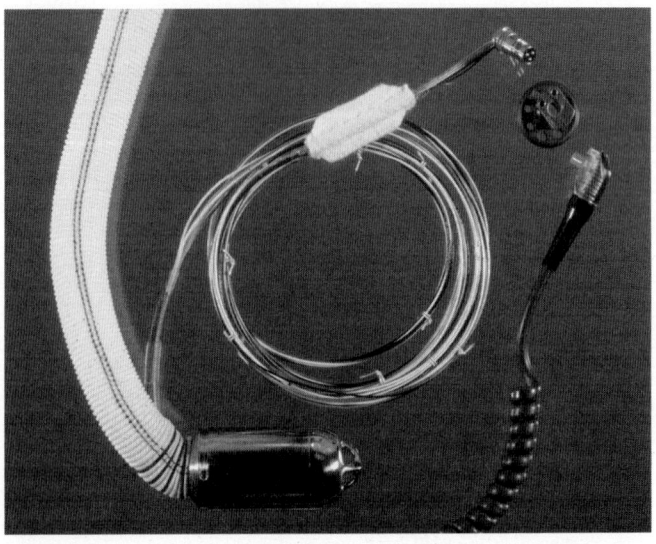

Fig. 1 The Jarvik pump (by courtesy of Mr Steve Westaby).

Centrifugal pumps

There are a number of paracorporeal pumps, developed as alternatives to roller pumps for cardiopulmonary bypass, that can be used for short-term circulatory support. Their use is limited to about 96 h, and there are significant problems with bleeding because of the need for partial heparinization. However, they are very inexpensive and have a role in support after cardiac surgery, or for assistance of the right ventricle.

Paracorporeal, pulsatile, ventricular assist devices

A variety of relatively simple, external, pneumatically powered pumps, connected to the heart with pipes traversing the skin, are available. The best known is the 'Thoratec' system, but others include the 'ABIOMED' pump, and in Europe, various forms of the 'Berlin' Heart. They can be used for either univentricular or biventricular support, for days or even weeks. The principal application is in 'bridging to transplant'. Morbidity and mortality is high, and complications include bleeding, thromboembolic events, and infection.

'Pusher-plate' implantable devices

This category includes the two most successful left ventricular assist devices, the 'Novacor' and the broadly similar 'HeartMate', which have the electrically powered pump lying deep to the abdominal wall. Connections are to the apex of the left ventricle and ascending aorta, with inflow and outflow valves. Power is supplied via a percutaneous cable and there is also a pipe to vent the air displaced with each beat. Transcutaneous transmission of electrical power is possible using induction loops, but a reliable implantable expansion chamber to deal with the displaced air has yet to be perfected. Portable batteries and control systems have been developed for both devices to allow discharge of the patient from hospital. Some patients fitted with such a device have survived for several years.

The principal difference between these two pumps lies in their blood interface. In the Novacor there is a seamless polyurethane sac, which is rhythmically compressed by the pusher plate. Anticoagulation with both warfarin and antiplatelet agents is required. By contrast, the blood-contacting surfaces of the HeartMate are textured to encourage deposition of circulating cells. The resulting autologous tissue lining is resistant to thrombus formation and only aspirin is required.

Both these pumps are large and expensive—typically £50 000 for the implantable components, batteries, and controllers. They cannot be used in small adults and children, and there are risks of infection and thromboembolism. Typically, 40 per cent of patients fitted with the HeartMate will experience driveline infections, although these can be contained in the 'bridge to transplant' setting and do not preclude successful transplant. The Novacor may be more prone to thromboembolic complications: in one study, 17 per cent of 36 patients who had the device for more than a year had major emboli; in another group 24 strokes occurred in 36 patients treated for a mean of 200 days.

Implantable impeller pumps

The next stage in the evolution of mechanical support is represented by a variety of axial-flow pumps. These are electrically driven, but with much lower power requirements than their predecessors, and consist of a turbine, usually in a tube connecting the left ventricular apex with the aorta. There are no valves, and the whole of the moving parts are bathed in blood. The earliest reports are only just appearing, but these pumps, if laboratory reliability can be repeated in clinical practice, have considerable potential.

Aims of mechanical support

Apart from postoperative support, which will not be discussed further, there are three uses for mechanical pumps. The commonest is 'bridge to transplant', with the intention of stabilizing or improving a deteriorating patient until a transplant can be performed. In a small minority of patients, myocardial function improves to the extent that the device can be removed. This is termed 'bridge to recovery'. The longer term aim of all these devices, and particularly for the impeller pumps, is permanent implantation.

Bridge to transplant

Patients with heart failure who deteriorate rapidly may die before they can be transplanted, or they develop progressive end-organ failure that significantly worsens the outcome after transplantation. Mechanical pumps, principally the Thoratec device and the two implantable pusher-plate pumps, have been used in thousands of patients for periods of up to several years, before they eventually receive a transplant. Only 60 to 70 per cent of such patients will receive a transplant. Most of the remainder do not survive, either developing irreversible failure of other organs despite a good cardiac output, or succumbing to problems such as stroke, haemorrhage, or infection whilst on the pump.

The 1-year survival rate after transplantation for bridged patients is between 80 and 90 per cent, at least as good as for routine patients, and probably better than that for very sick patients who do not receive a pump but survive to transplant in a precarious state.

Many patients develop anti-HLA and other antibodies whilst on a pump, either as a result of multiple transfusions, or due to the inflammatory response that occurs secondary to prolonged exposure of the blood to foreign surfaces. This delays transplantation, sometimes for years, and makes the implantable systems and discharge home economically attractive despite the high initial cost.

Bridging does not result in more transplants, but biases the transplant population towards younger, sicker recipients, and away from older, more stable candidates. The costs are huge: sums of $300 000 to 400 000 per subsequent transplant have been quoted from centres in the United States. A cynical view is that it is a very expensive way of selecting a slightly different group of patients for transplantation, and it has not yet been adopted in the United Kingdom to any significant extent.

Bridge to recovery

The reduction in afterload when the left ventricle is completely decompressed by a mechanical pump results in shrinkage of the heart and an improved ejection fraction. In some patients this improvement is real (in other words, it is not just load-dependent), sustained, and the pump can eventually be removed. Such myocardial recovery occurs particularly after postpartum cardiomyopathy and in those supported for an acute myocarditis. However, recovery in idiopathic dilated cardiomyopathy can also result: an improvement in histological appearance is seen, with a more regular arrangement of myocytes accompanied by a reduction in their diameter to normal. Other markers of heart failure, such as levels of tumour necrosis factor-α (**TNF-α**) and anti-β-receptor antibodies, which may be involved in the aetiology of the cardiomyopathy, also improve.

Only a few patients recover to the point where transplantation is not needed, and such recovery is not always sustained. In the Berlin series, one of the largest, 7 out of 19 patients who had pumps removed had either died or had been transplanted within 12 months. The remaining 12 were alive 1 year after the device was removed. However, in the future, mechanical support combined with manoeuvres to reverse some of the causes of cardiomyopathy – control of inflammatory elements, reconstitution of β receptors – may be applicable to significant numbers of patients, avoiding the need for transplantation.

Permanent implantation

A number of patients have been sustained for years with various implantable, left-ventricular assist devices, and indeed such pumps were designed as an alternative to transplant. It is not known whether the current devices can be used in the very long term. A clinical trial of left-ventricular assist devices against medical treatment in patients deemed unsuitable for heart transplant (the REMATCH trial) reportED its results in November 2001. For these critically ill patients, there was a survival advantage in receiving an assist device but even for such patients the mortality at 2 years was

Table 1 Presenting diagnoses in patients accepted for cardiac transplantation

Common indications
Idiopathic dilated cardiomyopathy
Ischaemic cardiomyopathy

Less common indications
Congenital heart disease
Valvular heart disease
Infiltrative conditions:
　　sarcoid
　　amyloid
Anthracycline toxicity
Associated with skeletal myopathies

Table 2 Components of a scoring system to estimate the prognosis of ambulatory patients with heart failure

Characteristic	Implication for prognosis
Presence of ischaemic heart disease	Bad if present
Left ventricular ejection fraction	Bad if low
Resting heart rate	Bad if high
Intraventricular conduction delay (QRS duration >0.12 s)	Bad if present
Mean resting blood pressure	Bad if low
Peak oxygen consumption (peak V_{O_2})	Bad if low: a value of <14 ml/kg per min often being used to define low
Serum sodium concentration	Bad if low

Adapted with permission from Aaronson et al.

77 per cent. The implication is that the pusher plate type of pump used in this trial is not yet suitable for long-term implantation.

Cardiac transplantation

For a minority of patients with endstage cardiac failure, transplantation remains an excellent form of treatment. Crucial to a successful outcome are patient selection and donor management. Post-transplant, the avoidance of acute rejection, minimization of the side-effects of chronic immunosuppression, and steps to reduce late graft failure are important issues.

Patient selection

Almost all adults presenting for transplant will have either a dilated idiopathic or ischaemic cardiomyopathy. The latter predominates in older patients: other diagnoses in patients accepted for transplantation are shown in Table 1. Amongst children, dilated cardiomyopathy now exceeds congenital heart disease as a reason for transplantation. Young adults who underwent successful palliative procedures (such as Mustard or Senning operations for transposition of the great vessels) 20 or more years ago now need a transplant.

Regardless of the aetiology of the disease, referral for consideration for cardiac transplantation should only be made when conventional treatment, both medical and surgical, has been exhausted. Thus most patients with heart failure will have had the benefit of state-of-the-art medical therapy—angiotensin-converting enzyme inhibitors, β-blockade, diuretics including spironolactone, and often digoxin and amiodarone. Reversible ischaemia should be sought when there is coronary disease.

The outlook for patients with severe and deteriorating cardiac failure is clearly poor, indeed a proportion of these patients will either need urgent transplantation or a mechanical assist device. Consideration of the ambulant patient with controlled heart failure is more difficult: improvements in medical management have rendered obsolete many of the accepted markers of poor prognosis, and it has been suggested that transplantation only improves the 1-year survival rate of patients with the most severe heart failure.

Exercise testing with measurement of maximum oxygen uptake has been a useful objective test, with values below 14 ml/kg per min suggesting a 1-year survival rate of only 30 per cent. Its combination with other markers (Table 2) into a scoring system for likely survival has allowed the stratification of this group of patients, a system that has been validated both in North America and Europe.

Contraindications to transplantation

Careful screening of individuals with irreversible failure of other organs is essential and a list of standard exclusions is shown in Table 3. The absolute contraindications mainly relate to other life-threatening conditions that would not be reversed by the presence of a new heart. Active infection clearly has to be avoided in any patient who is about to be aggressively immunosuppressed. The relative contraindications are more difficult to judge, a good example being elevation of pulmonary vascular resistance. All patients with left-heart failure have some degree of pulmonary vasoconstriction and the chance of failure of the unprepared right ventricle of the donor heart, the risk of early death being correlated in a continuous fashion with the pulmonary vascular resistance or transpulmonary gradient. Higher values contribute the greatest risk but, of course, are more likely to be found in the sickest patients. An individual assessment has to be made in each case, considering not only the patient's need but also the best use of a limited number of donor organs.

Perioperative management

The cardiac donor

Although the heart continues to beat after brainstem death occurs, there is a progressive loss of homeostatic control. This includes hypotension with loss of vascular tone, compounded by a polyuria and hypothermia. Appropriate corrections include the administration of ADH analogues (usually intranasal **DDAVP**, 1-deamino-8-D-arginine vasopressin; desmopressin), intravenous fluids, and often peripheral vasoconstrictors as well.

The initial damage to the brain is usually intracerebral or subarachnoid haemorrhage, or head trauma. Positive serology for the human immunodeficiency virus (**HIV**) and hepatitis B, previous cardiac surgery, or a known history of ischaemic heart disease are contraindications to cardiac

Table 3 Contraindications to cardiac transplantation

Absolute
Solid-organ malignancy during the last 5 years
Another life-threatening medical condition
Continued abuse of alcohol or drugs
Psychiatric history likely to result in non-compliance with postoperative treatment regimen
Positive serology for HIV or hepatitis B
Active extracardiac infection
Severe peripheral or cerebrovascular disease
Active peptic ulcer disease

Relative
Age >65 years
Pulmonary vascular resistance >6 Wood units, or transpulmonary gradient >15 mmHg
Renal impairment with GFR <40 ml/min unless a candidate for simultaneous renal transplant
Obesity (BMI >30)
Recent pulmonary infarction
Diabetes with significant end-organ damage
Giant-cell myocarditis
COPD with FEV_1 <40% predicted
Osteoporosis

GFR, glomerular filtration rate; BMI, body-mass index; COPD, chronic obstructive pulmonary disease; FEV1, forced expiratory volume in 1 s.

donation, as are prolonged periods of hypotension. Intravenous drug abuse (because of its association with HIV infection) is a contraindication, as is more than the occasional use of cocaine. Brainstem death following tricyclic antidepressant overdose or carbon monoxide poisoning is associated with specific damage to the heart and such donors would not usually be acceptable.

Older donors, into their fifties or even sixties, are acceptable if they have normal coronary arteries, but the use of such hearts is associated with a poorer long-term outcome since they are much less tolerant of longer ischaemic times. However, with falling mortality rates from trauma and an increasing demand for transplantation, donors are now more likely to be older and to die as a result of intracerebral haemorrhage, often being hypertensive with left ventricular hypertrophy and premature coronary artery disease.

Matching of recipient and donor

The donor should be blood-group compatible (but not necessarily identical) with the recipient, and size discrepancies of more than 20 to 30 per cent should be avoided. Although HLA matching, particularly for the DR antigens, may reduce rejection rates, time constraints make this impossible.

Some 5 to 10 per cent of recipients are presensitized to HLA antigens by blood transfusion, pregnancy, or a previous transplant. Moreover, preformed antibodies can cause immediate rejection, which is often fatal. Before a transplant is performed from a particular donor, recipient serum is tested against donor cells to exclude a positive or cytotoxic crossmatch in this group of patients.

The operation

After removal of the native heart, the standard implantation was, in the past, with anastomoses to the pulmonary artery, aorta, and cuffs of the left and right atrium. Whilst technically straightforward, this was somewhat clumsy and sometimes resulted in distortion of the interatrial septum. The standard approach now is to perform separate caval anastomoses, thus keeping the donor right atrium intact. Better right ventricular filling, fewer arrhythmias, and almost complete elimination of the need for permanent pacing has followed this modification.

Postoperative management is as for any other cardiac surgical procedure, with transfer from an intensive care unit to the recovery ward within a few days, and discharge from hospital after approximately 2 weeks.

Immunosuppression and rejection

A host's immune response is most vigorous early after the transplant and gradually diminishes with time. Immunosuppression is based principally on one of the calcineurin-inhibitor group of drugs, ciclosporin A or tacrolimus (FK506), in conjunction with corticosteroids and usually one other agent. There are few clinically important differences between the two calcineurin inhibitors: both are nephrotoxic and both have neurological side-effects, both require monitoring by measurement of trough drug levels. Tacrolimus does not cause the hirsuitism or gum hypertrophy seen with ciclosporin A and is therefore preferable in adolescents and females: it is, however, associated with a much higher rate of glucose intolerance.

Steroid treatment is initially with large intravenous doses of methylprednisolone, which is then converted to oral prednisolone, with dosage titrated down from 1 mg/kg to between 0.1 and 0.2 mg/kg over 2 to 4 weeks. Approximately 50 per cent of patients can be weaned off steroids entirely. However, in practice, continuation of a small dose (5–10 mg per day) allows lower doses of the other drugs with different toxicities to be tolerated.

The other component of so-called 'standard triple-drug regimens' is azathioprine in a dose of 1.5 to 2.5 mg/kg, adjusted against the white blood cell count. The principal side-effects are marrow toxicity and cholestatic jaundice, but azathioprine is effective, inexpensive, and easy to control. An alternative with broadly similar actions is mycophenolate mofetil (**MMF**).

In comparative studies, patients treated with MMF have slightly lower rejection rates and there may be some reduction in the rate of progression of allograft vasculopathy (see below), but these advantages have not been translated into a demonstrable improvement in survival. Mycophenolate is much more expensive than azathioprine and its role in cardiac transplant patients has yet to be determined.

Monitoring rejection episodes

Acute rejection, a loss of the control of the immune response caused by drug therapy, leads to an infiltration of inflammatory cells and myocardial oedema. This causes diastolic rather than systolic dysfunction. Clinical signs may be sparse; a third sound, elevated filling pressures or atrial flutter, together with pyrexia and sometimes influenza-like symptoms can occur. The 'gold standard' for detecting rejection is transvenous endomyocardial biopsy, performed under local anaesthetic and radiological control. Non-invasive methods are not as sensitive or specific, although echocardiography may have a role in children. Biopsy is done weekly for the first month, then at decreasing intervals over the first year. Dense infiltrates with myocyte necrosis require augmented treatment, usually with intravenous steroids. Between 20 and 40 per cent of patients will have at least one such episode of acute rejection. Regular biopsies allow the titration of treatment against the histological picture, effectively tailoring therapy to the individual.

Infection after transplantation

The need for high levels of immunosuppression creates a substantial risk of infection, particularly during the first few months. Within the first few weeks this is typically bacterial (chest, urinary tract, intravenous catheters) and with commonplace rather than opportunistic organisms. Patients who receive augmented immunosuppression are at risk of fungal infections, of which aspergillosis is the most significant.

Cytomegalovirus (**CMV**) is the most important viral infection, occurring between 1 and 2 months' post-transplantation. This may be either a reactivation of a previous exposure (50 per cent of recipients are seropositive at the time of transplant), or acquired with the heart from a donor who was seropositive. For those at greatest risk, prophylaxis with oral ganciclovir has become routine. If an infection occurs with pyrexia, leucopenia, and organ involvement (for example, pneumonitis or gastritis), it can be life-threatening and requires treatment with intravenous ganciclovir.

Patients with fever should be investigated aggressively to make a specific diagnosis, often with invasive means such as bronchoscopy. Except for life-threatening sepsis, empirical antibiotics should be avoided. Unusual, opportunistic organisms (for example, *Aspergillus* spp., *Pneumocystis carinii*, and *Legionella* spp.) should all be considered.

For further discussion of infective complications after solid-organ transplantation, see Chapter 20.6.3 and chapters dedicated to particular pathogens.

Long-term complications

Despite excellent survival and functional rehabilitation, drug side-effects, the risks of continuous immunosuppression, and graft vasculopathy can lead to morbidity. The combination of these factors results in an attrition rate of 4 per cent per year after the first 12 months.

Side-effects of immunosuppressants

All the drugs used have relatively poor therapeutic profiles, and a degree of drug toxicity is almost invariable. For the calcineurin inhibitors (ciclosporin, tacrolimus) the most troublesome are hypertension and nephrotoxicity. Some 80 per cent of patients require an antihypertensive agent, with ACE inhibitors as the first choice, followed by nifedipine. Many other calcium-channel blockers interact with ciclosporin metabolism. Both ACE inhibitors and calcium-channel blockers may benefit graft vasculopathy.

Renal impairment is due to a combination of drug toxicity and pre-existing renal disease: by 10 years' post-transplant, between 5 and 10 per cent of patients need renal replacement therapy, but their prognosis is very poor.

Effects of chronic immunosuppression

The transplant patient remains at risk, diminishing with time, of opportunistic infections. Malignant change in the skin exposed to sunlight is very common, and appropriate precautions should be taken from the beginning.

Post-transplant lymphoproliferative disease (**PTLD**)

All immunosuppressants inhibit suppressor T cells, which usually exert immunological control over Epstein–Barr virus (**EBV**)-infected lymphocytes. Reduction of this control after transplantation may result in the proliferation of lymphocytes with a histological picture of B-cell 'lymphoma'. The clinical picture ranges from something akin to primary EBV infection (infectious mononucleosis) to a highly malignant, multifocal lymphoma. In most cases, reduction of immunosuppression results in restoration of control, and the 'lymphoma' is seen to shrink. Sometimes this is inadequate (or rejection of the heart occurs) and chemotherapy is required, when the outlook for the patient is much poorer.

PTLD affects about 2 per cent of transplant patient in the first year, and 1 per cent per year thereafter. It is much commoner (up to 40 per cent) if acquired as a primary infection from the donor organ. Use of polymerase chain reaction (**PCR**) technology to monitor viral load may have a role in predicting those at risk, and for allowing a pre-emptive reduction in immunosuppression.

Graft vasculopathy

There is continued immunological damage to the endothelium of the coronary arteries of the transplanted heart. (A similar process is seen in other solid-organ grafts.) Endothelial abnormalities can be detected as early as 6 weeks' post-transplant, and intravascular ultrasound (**IVUS**) can detect thickening of the subintimal layer over the first year. This process is accelerated in individuals with repeated rejection episodes and is worsened by hyperlipidaemia and hypertension. It is commoner in older donor hearts, even when free of disease at transplant. By 5 years, between 40 and 70 per cent of patients will have angiographically visible disease, and this is the commonest cause of death after the first year.

Control of risk factors, particularly hyperlipidaemia, is very important. The statin group of drugs are of proven benefit, and all adult patients with heart transplants should be given these agents (if tolerated).

Because the heart is denervated, clinical presentation is subtle. There is a spectrum of disease from exercise dyspnoea, through silent myocardial infarction, to sudden death. Detection is by surveillance angiography: non-invasive alternatives (for example, thallium scintigraphy and stress dobutamine echocardiography) have yet to prove themselves useful.

Treatment of established disease is unsatisfactory. Localized lesions may respond to angioplasty or coronary stenting, but graft vasculopathy is a diffuse process and restrictions to flow from small-vessel narrowing remain. The very occasional patient may require coronary grafting for a

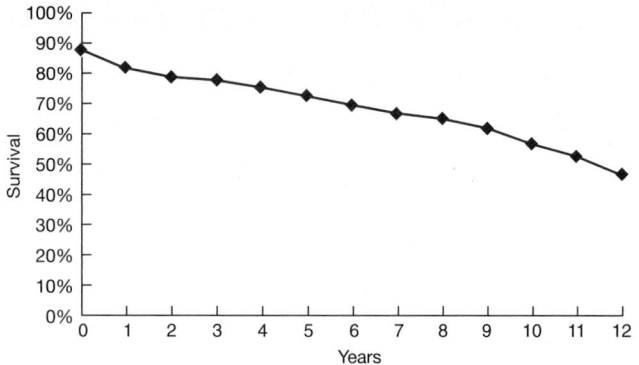

Fig. 2 Actuarial survival curve after cardiac transplantation.

collection of proximal, focal lesions, but the only definitive treatment is retransplantation, which gives satisfactory results for carefully selected patients.

Results

Voluntary registries and publications from single institutions report a 1-year survival rate between 80 and 85 per cent, falling to 70 per cent at 5 years, and perhaps 50 per cent at 10 years (Fig. 2). Figures for a typical transplant programme may be a little worse. Rehabilitation is excellent, with 90 to 95 per cent of patients in **NYHA** (New York Heart Association) class I or II, although a disappointing proportion, perhaps only 20 per cent, return to work.

Further reading

Aaronson KD, *et al.* (1997). Development and prospective validation of a clinical index to predict survival in ambulatory patients referred for cardiac transplant evaluation. *Circulation* **95**, 2660–7.

Hunt SA (1998). Current status of cardiac transplantation *Journal of the American Medical Association* **280**, 1692–8.

Hunt SA, Frazier OH (1998). Mechanical circulatory support and cardiac transplantation. *Circulation* **97**, 2079–90.

Kobshigawa JA, *et al.* (1995). Effect of pravastatin on outcomes after cardiac transplantation *New England Journal of Medicine* **333**, 621–7.

Perreas KG, *et al.* (2000). Donor management tactics for cardiothoracic transplantation. *Transplantation Reviews* **14**, 127–30.

Society of Thoracic Surgeons (2001). Fifth International Conference on Circulatory Support Devices for Severe Cardiac Failure. *Annals of Thoracic Surgery* **71**(Suppl.), S55–S222.

Westaby S, *et al.* (2000). First permanent implant of the Jarvik 2000 Heart. *Lancet* **356**, 900–3.

Young JB (2000). Perspectives on cardiac allograft vasculopathy *Current Atherosclerosis Reports* **2**, 259–71.

15.6 Cardiac arrhythmias

S. M. Cobbe and A. C. Rankin

General principles

Definition

The term cardiac arrhythmia (or dysrhythmia) is used to describe an abnormality of cardiac rhythm of any type. The spectrum of cardiac arrhythmias ranges from innocent extrasystoles to immediately life-threatening conditions such as asystole or ventricular fibrillation. Arrhythmias may occur in the absence of cardiac disease, but are more commonly associated with structural heart disease or external provocative factors.

Normal cardiac electrophysiology is discussed in Chapter 15.3.2. Abnormalities in cardiac impulse formation or propagation may give rise either to an abnormally slow heart rate (bradycardia) or fast heart rates (tachycardia).

Symptoms of cardiac arrhythmias

The symptoms produced by bradyarrhythmias depend on the extent of cardiac slowing. They may include sudden death, syncope (Stokes–Adams attacks), or dizziness (presyncope). Continuous bradycardia without asystolic pauses may produce symptoms of fatigue, lethargy, dyspnoea, or mental impairment.

The symptoms caused by tachyarrhythmias depend on a variety of factors including the heart rate, the difference between the rate during the arrhythmia and the preceding heart rate, the degree of irregularity of the rhythm, and the presence or absence of underlying cardiac disease. Symptoms of tachycardia include a feeling of rapid palpitation, angina or dyspnoea, syncope or sudden death. The differential diagnosis of palpitation and syncope is discussed in Chapter 15.2.3.

Investigation of arrhythmias

History taking must include a detailed description of the symptoms associated with the arrhythmia. Evidence should be sought for factors that may precipitate the arrhythmia (for instance, exercise, alcohol) and for the presence of underlying cardiac disease, in particular valvular heart disease, myocardial ischaemia/infarction, or congestive heart failure. Examination of the pulse will be unremarkable if the arrhythmia is intermittent. Physical examination for evidence of structural heart disease is essential. Further investigations to establish the presence of structural heart disease and to determine ventricular function may include 12-lead electrocardiography, chest radiography, echocardiography, exercise stress testing, and coronary arteriography.

Electrocardiography

The key to the successful diagnosis of cardiac arrhythmias is the systematic analysis of an electrocardiogram (**ECG**) of optimal quality obtained during the arrhythmia (Table 1). Ideally, this should comprise all 12 leads recorded on a multichannel recorder, which can allow the identification of P-waves in one lead while they may be absent or equivocal in another.

Ambulatory electrocardiography

Continuous monitoring is necessary for identification where arrhythmias are intermittent. This may involve monitoring in the cardiac care unit, particularly in the acute stages of myocardial infarction, or ambulatory (Holter) monitoring. Ambulatory electrocardiography is normally performed for periods of between 24 and 48 h using a portable recorder, which records every heartbeat on to magnetic tape or into solid-state memory. High-speed or automatic replay facilities enable the identification of intermittent arrhythmias, as well as the quantification of extrasystoles and assessment of parameters of heart rate variability.

Interpretation of recordings requires knowledge of possible artefacts, such as variations in tape speed in magnetic tape-based recorders, or movement artefact. It is important to allow for physiological variability in the sinus rate, also to appreciate that minor abnormalities such as extrasystoles or brief (3 to 4 beat) runs of supraventricular arrhythmias are usually of no significance. Ambulatory electrocardiographic recordings are of most value when they provide correlation between the patient's symptoms and the cardiac rhythm at that moment. Patients should therefore be issued with a diary card to report any symptoms suggestive of arrhythmia during the recording.

Conventional 24- to 48-h ambulatory electrocardiography is unlikely to yield useful results if the frequency of arrhythmic symptoms is less than every day or two. Alternative strategies include the use of a patient-activated recorder, which is applied and activated during symptoms, or an external or implanted 'loop' recorder. Loop recorders continually record the electrocardiographic signal, but only have sufficient buffer memory to retain a few minutes' data. In the event of symptoms, the patient activates the device, thus 'fixing' the previous few minutes' recording for analysis. Loop recorders are particularly useful in the diagnosis of infrequent brief, but disabling, symptoms, where the use of a patient-activated recorder is not feasible.

Table 1 Principles of ECG diagnosis of arrhythmias

• **Obtain 12-lead or multichannel recordings if possible**	
• **Atrial activity**	P-waves visible?
	Normal P-wave morphology and axis?
	Flutter/fibrillation waves?
	Atrial rate?
• **Ventricular activity**	Ventricular rate?
	Regular or irregular?
	Normal QRS morphology and duration?
	Bundle-branch block or bizarre QRS morphology?
	Variation in QRS morphology/axis?
• **Atrioventricular relationship**	PR interval—fixed or varied?
	Retrograde P-waves?
	Atrial versus ventricular rate?

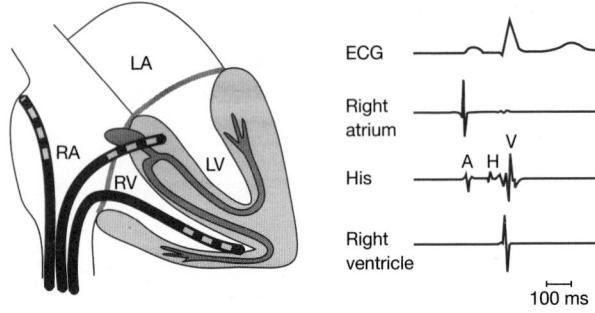

Fig. 1 Electrophysiological study. Illustration of lead placement (left). Quadripolar leads have been inserted from the femoral vein and the tips are shown positioned to allow recording and pacing from the high right atrium, the His bundle, and the right ventricular apex. Intracardiac electrograms (right) show recordings from atrium (A), His bundle (H), and right ventricle (V).

Cardiac electrophysiological study

More detailed investigation of cardiac arrhythmias is undertaken by invasive cardiac electrophysiological testing. Multipolar electrodes are inserted to record electrograms from the atrium, ventricle, His bundle, and commonly from the coronary sinus (Fig. 1). The site of conduction delays within the heart may be identified, or accessory pathways localized. Sustained arrhythmias may be initiated and terminated by extrastimuli (Fig. 2), and their pattern of activation in the heart studied in detail. Electrophysiological mapping is an essential part of radiofrequency ablation (see below).

Bradycardias

Aetiology and mechanisms

Bradycardia is defined as a ventricular rate of less than 60 per min, and results from a reduction in the rate of normal sinus pacemaker activity, or from disturbances of atrioventricular (**AV**) conduction. Sinus bradycardia may be physiological—for example, during sleep, in athletes, and in young people. Pathological bradyarrhythmias can result from intrinsic degenerative disease of the sinus or atrioventricular node, or the conducting system. Changes may also be due to extraneous factors such as sympathetic withdrawal, vagal stimulation, drug effects, myocardial ischaemia/infarction, infiltration, or surgical trauma, also miscellaneous conditions such as hypothyroidism, hypothermia, jaundice, or raised intracranial pressure.

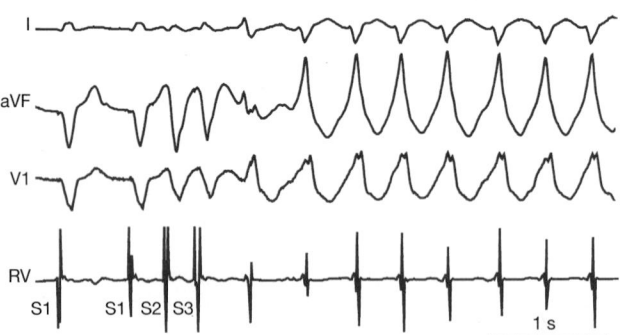

Fig. 2 Induction of ventricular tachycardia by programmed stimulation. Ventricular pacing stimuli (S1) at 100 beats per min are followed by two extra stimuli (S2, S3). Sustained monomorphic ventricular tachycardia is induced. Surface leads I, aVF, V₁, and the intracardiac electrogram from right ventricular apex (RV) are shown.

Specific disorders

Sinoatrial disease

Sinoatrial disease, often referred to as 'sick sinus syndrome', results in inappropriate sinus bradycardia, sinus pauses, or junctional rhythm (Fig. 3) in the absence of extrinsic factors. The condition is most commonly caused by idiopathic degeneration of the sinus nodal cells, particularly in the elderly, and is associated in about 20 per cent of cases with idiopathic bundle-branch fibrosis (see below). Occasionally, sinoatrial disease is caused by ischaemia due to obstruction of the right coronary artery. Conduction block may occur between the sinus node and the atrium (sinoatrial block), resulting in 'dropped' P-waves (Fig. 4). More prolonged suppression of sinus node activity results in periods of sinus arrest, which are terminated by an escape beat from the sinus node, atrioventricular junction, or ventricle (Fig. 5(a)). Where the sinus rate is permanently slower than the junctional rate, continuous AV junctional rhythm will be present. Patients with sinoatrial disease have an increased predisposition to atrial tachyarrhythmias (bradycardia/tachycardia syndrome), and prolonged pauses may follow termination of tachycardia (Fig. 5(b)).

Sinoatrial disease can cause symptomatic bradycardia, dizziness, or syncope, but may be asymptomatic. The diagnosis is normally made from 12-lead or ambulatory ECG recording. Investigation should focus on excluding extrinsic causes of bradycardia, and on demonstrating the correlation between bradycardia or pauses and symptoms.

Neurocardiogenic syncope

Conditions where patients suffer reflex-induced attacks of bradycardia or hypotension are described in Chapter 15.2.3.

Atrioventricular conduction disorders

Impairment of atrioventricular conduction may occur either within the atrioventricular node (intranodal) or within the His–Purkinje system (infranodal). Intranodal block is not associated with QRS abnormalities, while distal (infranodal) block is commonly associated with bundle-branch block.

First-degree atrioventricular block

The normal upper limit of the PR interval is 0.20 s, and if the value exceeds this then first-degree atrioventricular block is present (Fig. 6). A prolonged PR interval may be associated with bifascicular block (for example, right bundle-branch block plus left anterior hemiblock). This condition, termed trifascicular block, implies the presence of slowed conduction through the remaining fascicle.

Second-degree atrioventricular block

In second-degree atrioventricular block, there is intermittent failure of conduction from atrium to ventricle. In type I (Wenckebach) second-degree block, a characteristic pattern of increasing PR interval duration followed by a non-conducted P-wave is seen (Fig. 7). The QRS morphology is commonly normal. In type II second-degree AV block there is a sudden failure of conduction, without a preceding increase in the PR interval (Fig. 8). Regular non-conducted P-waves may result in high-degree block, with 2:1 or 3:1 conduction.

Third-degree atrioventricular block

The characteristic feature of third-degree (complete) atrioventricular block is complete dissociation between atrial and ventricular activity (Fig. 9). The ventricular rate is regular and slower than the atrial rate. An escape rhythm arising above the bifurcation of the bundle of His will produce a narrow QRS morphology, commonly with a relatively rapid escape rhythm (50 to 60 per min). A more distal escape rhythm results in widened, bundle branch block morphology complexes with a slower escape rate (20 to 30 per min). When complete AV block coexists with atrial fibrillation, it is recognized by the presence of a slow, regular ventricular response.

High-degree AV block can be intermittent, and the resting ECG may be normal or only show evidence of mild conducting system disturbance such

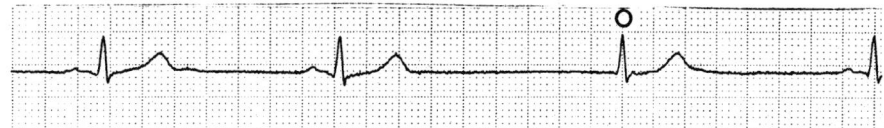

Fig. 3 Sinus bradycardia. The heart rate is less than 40 beats/min, and the sinus rate is so slow that an escape junctional beat is seen (open circle), preceding the P-wave.

as first-degree AV block or bundle-branch block. If there is clinical suspicion, ambulatory ECG recording, for prolonged periods if necessary, is required to obtain evidence of higher degrees of AV block.

Aetiology of atrioventricular block

The causes of atrioventricular block are shown in Table 2: the commonest is idiopathic fibrosis of the His–Purkinje system, which occurs with increasing frequency from the seventh decade of life onwards, is associated with sinoatrial disease in up to 25 per cent of cases, and results in progressive impairment of atrioventricular conduction.

Atrioventricular block may occur acutely in myocardial infarction (Fig. 10). Inferior myocardial infarction predominantly affects atrioventricular nodal conduction by vagal overactivity, and possibly adenosine release from ischaemic myocardium. First-degree, type I (Wenckebach) second-degree block or third-degree atrioventricular block may occur, but these are commonly transient. Spontaneous recovery of normal conduction generally occurs within 7 to 10 days. By contrast, atrioventricular block secondary to anterior myocardial infarction is normally due to extensive infarction of the interventricular septum involving the left and right bundle branches after the division of the bundle of His. This may result in type II second-degree block or complete atrioventricular block, with a lower probability of recovery of normal conduction.

Any drug slowing atrioventricular conduction may potentially produce atrioventricular block. The risk is greater when such drugs are used in combination, the combination of intravenous verapamil in patients already receiving β-adrenoceptor blockers being particularly hazardous. Vagally mediated conduction disturbances occur as a physiological finding in highly trained athletes, or in neurocardiogenic syncope. Atrioventricular conduction disturbances arise in structural congenital heart disease such as endocardial cushion defects, but also as an isolated congenital abnormality, commonly in association with maternal systemic lupus erythematosus.

Management of bradycardias

The principal indications for active intervention in bradycardia are symptomatic (disturbances of consciousness, fatigue, lethargy, dyspnoea, or bradycardia-induced tachyarrhythmias) or prognostic (prevention of sudden cardiac death). Drugs interfering with sinoatrial or atrioventricular nodal function should be withdrawn if possible, although under certain circumstances (for example, tachybradycardia syndrome) it may be necessary to combine pacemaker implantation with continued drug therapy. Transient increases in sinus rate or the ventricular escape rate in complete atrioventricular block may be obtained with atropine or isoproterenol (isoprenaline). However, drug treatment is only of temporary value, and pacing is indicated for persistent bradycardia.

Management of specific disorders

Sinoatrial disease

Pacemaker implantation is indicated for the relief of symptoms (see below). Prognosis is not improved by pacemaker implantation in sinus nodal disease and thus pacemaker implantation in asymptomatic patients is not indicated.

Neurocardiogenic syncope

Patients with carotid sinus hypersensitivity and symptoms of presyncope or syncope should undergo permanent pacemaker implantation (see below). In vasovagal syndrome, the optimal treatment is uncertain: medical therapy with agents as diverse as α-agonists, β-blockers, vagolytic agents (disopyramide, hyoscine), ephedrine, or antidepressants is often tried, but the evidence base for the efficacy of drug therapy is weak, and spontaneous

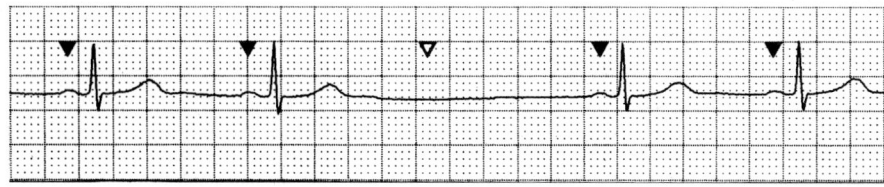

Fig. 4 Sinoatrial block. A pause occurred because of the absence of a P-wave (open arrow). The timing of the sinus beats, however, is not interrupted, indicating that the sinus node discharged but the impulse failed to excite the atria.

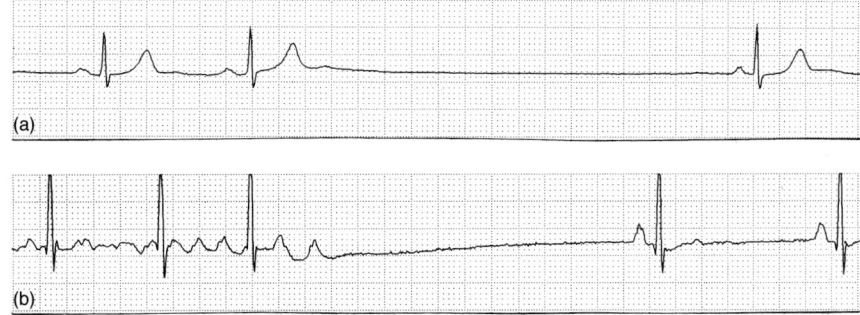

Fig. 5 Sinus arrest. (a) Pause of 4 s results from failure of the sinus node to discharge. (b) Termination of atrial fibrillation is followed by a sinus pause of 2.5 s due to sinus arrest in a patient with bradycardia/tachycardia syndrome.

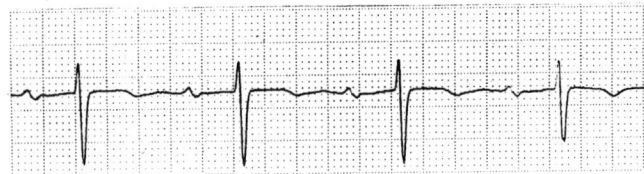

Fig. 6 First-degree heart block. The PR interval is prolonged (0.32 s).

resolution of symptoms occurs in many patients. Those whose symptoms persist despite drug therapy, particularly if bradycardia is a major component of the response to tilt-testing, are candidates for pacemaker implantation.

Atrioventricular conduction disturbances

First-degree AV block produces no symptoms and does not require treatment. The risk of progression from chronic bifascicular block to complete heart block is low, and patients with asymptomatic bifascicular block do not require prophylactic pacemaker implantation. The presence of trifascicular block implies advanced conducting system disease, and permanent pacing should be considered if there are symptoms or evidence of intermittent complete heart block.

Type I (Wenckebach) second-degree AV block is normally associated with a reliable subsidiary pacemaker and a low risk of progression to complete heart block. In the majority of instances active treatment is not necessary unless recurrent presyncope or syncope suggest the occurrence of an intermittent higher degree block, requiring consideration of pacemaker implantation. Type II second-degree AV block is generally indicative of extensive infranodal conduction abnormality, with a high risk of progression to complete AV block. Most authorities therefore recommend permanent pacemaker implantation even in the absence of symptoms. The presence of complete atrioventricular block, except in the context of an acutely reversible condition, should be regarded as an indication for permanent pacemaker implantation. This is urgent in cases where Stokes–

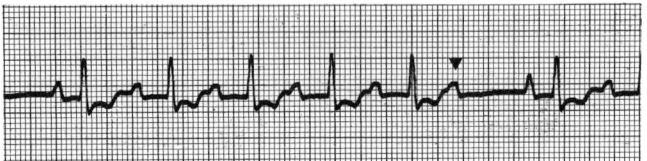

Fig. 7 Second-degree heart block, type I (Wenckebach). The PR interval progressively prolongs until there is a failure of conduction following a P-wave (arrow).

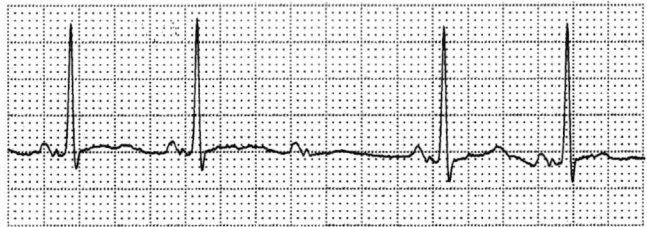

Fig. 8 Second-degree heart block type II. A non-conducted P-wave occurs without preceding prolongation of the PR interval.

Adams attacks are occurring, but even in asymptomatic patients the prognosis appears to be improved by permanent pacing. One exception to this general rule is congenital complete heart block, where the escape rhythm is often relatively fast (50 to 60 per min) with a narrow QRS morphology. Many patients remain asymptomatic well into adult life, although there is a small risk of syncope or sudden death. Pacemaker implantation should be considered if there are symptoms, or if the ventricular rate on ambulatory recording remains persistently below 50 beats/min, or in patients over 40 years of age.

Temporary pacemaker implantation is indicated where frequent Stokes–Adams attacks are occurring, or where the conduction disturbance is likely to be transient such as in cases of drug intoxication or inferior myocardial infarction. In the latter case, even the presence of complete heart block may be associated with an adequate ventricular rate and pacing need only be undertaken if there is haemodynamic compromise. Temporary pacing can only be used for a few days, owing to the risk of introducing infection along the electrode track.

Prognosis The prognosis of patients with complete atrioventricular block having Stokes–Adams attacks is poor without pacemaker implantation, and is improved markedly by permanent pacing. Following pacing, the prognosis will depend on the nature and extent of underlying cardiac disease.

Asystole

The term asystole is used when the electrocardiogram shows a complete cessation of both atrial and ventricular activity: this appearance may be mimicked by disconnected ECG cables or other artefacts, but since asystole causes cardiac arrest the distinction is usually obvious. The management of asystole is discussed in Chapter 16.3.

Pacemaker therapy

Basic principles

The basis of pacemaker therapy is the local depolarization of the myocardium by an electric current passed through an electrode in contact with the heart (atrium or ventricle). Activation of the remainder of the atria or ventricles occurs by direct cell-to-cell conduction. The minimum current necessary to stimulate the heart during diastole is known as the pacing *threshold*. Pacemaker systems normally comprise one or more intracardiac catheter *electrodes*, introduced into the heart via the venous system, and a *pulse generator*, which contains the circuitry for generating and timing the pacing stimulus, as well as for sensing spontaneous cardiac depolarizations. The pacing stimulus is delivered between the active pole at the tip of the electrode catheter and an indifferent electrode. This is sited either on the same electrode catheter 1 to 2 cm proximal to the tip (bipolar pacing), or utilizes the can of the implanted pulse generator (unipolar pacing). An essential prerequisite for satisfactory pacing is that the electrode maintains a stable electrical contact with the myocardium. This is most likely to occur when the endocardial surface is trabeculated rather than smooth, and for this reason the standard sites for endocardial atrial and ventricular pacing are the right atrial appendage and the right ventricular apex, respectively (Fig. 11).

The pulse generator is sited externally for temporary pacing. For permanent pacing, it is usually implanted deep to the subcutaneous fat layer in the prepectoral region (Fig. 11). The generator contains a timer set to deliver pacing stimuli at a preset *pulse interval* (for example, 1000 ms). The amplitude and duration of the pacing stimulus (*pulse width*) are usually set at nominal values (for example, 5 volts, 1 ms), but are adjustable and can be

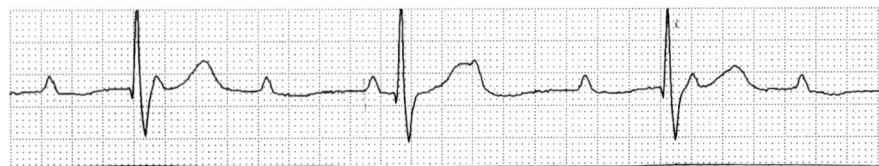

Fig. 9 Third-degree (complete) heart block. Atrial activity does not conduct to the ventricles, and there is a regular escape rhythm of 35 beats per min.

Table 2 Causes of atrioventricular block

- Idiopathic conducting-system fibrosis
- Acute myocardial ischaemia/infarction
- Infiltration—calcific aortic stenosis, sarcoid, scleroderma, syphilis tumour
- Infection—diphtheria, rheumatic fever, endocarditis, Lyme disease
- Drugs—digoxin, verapamil, β-blockers, class I antiarrhythmics
- Surgical trauma, radiofrequency ablation
- Congenital heart block, congenital heart disease
- Vagal—athletic heart, carotid sinus, and vasovagal syndrome
- Dystrophia myotonica

reduced to prolong the life of the battery, providing there is a sufficient safety margin between the pulse generator output and the pacing threshold. Most pulse generators are powered by lithium batteries and have a life of approximately 5 to 7 years, after which the generator is replaced. Pacemakers normally operate in the *demand* mode, whereby if spontaneous activation of the cardiac chamber is sensed via the electrode, the delivery of a pacing stimulus is *inhibited,* and the timer circuit of the generator is reset. Pacing in the *fixed rate* mode results in the delivery of stimuli regardless of the spontaneous activity of the chamber being paced.

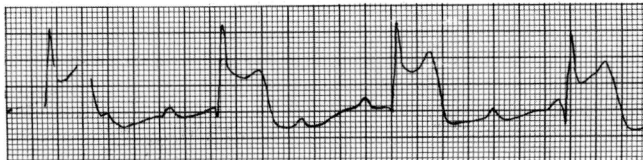

Fig. 10 Complete heart block in a patient with acute myocardial infarction. There is a narrow QRS-complex escape rhythm with ST segment elevation, ventricular rate 45 beats/min.

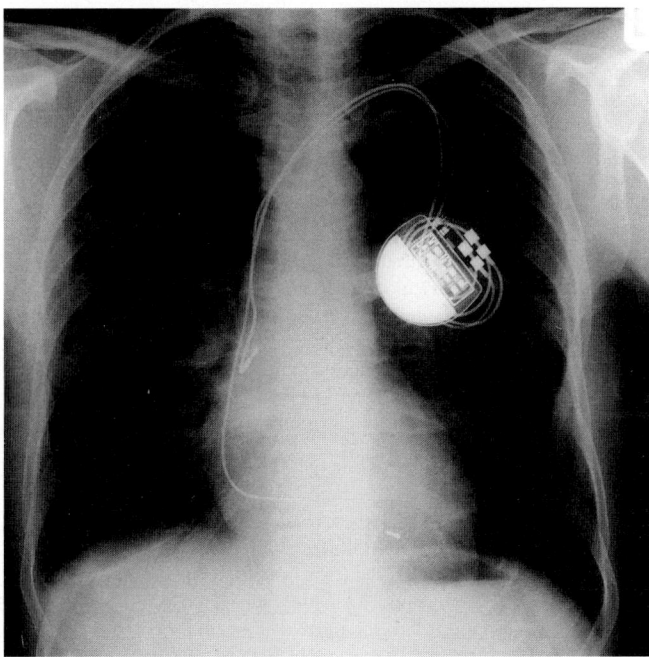

Fig. 11 Dual-chamber permanent pacemaker. Chest radiograph showing the pacemaker generator (in a subcutaneous pocket in the pectoral region) which is connected to electrodes that pass via the left subclavian vein and superior vena cava to the heart. The tips of the electrodes are in the right atrial appendage and the right ventricular apex.

Temporary ventricular pacing

Facilities for radiographic screening, continuous electrocardiographic monitoring, and defibrillation are necessary for the performance of temporary ventricular pacing. The temporary pacing electrode is introduced under aseptic conditions via an intravascular sheath inserted into the subclavian, internal jugular, or femoral vein and passed under radiographic control to the right atrium. The electrode tip is advanced across the tricuspid valve and impacted as distally as possible at the right ventricular apex. Non-sustained ventricular tachycardia, or occasionally ventricular fibrillation, may occur during catheter manipulation. Once the electrode is in an acceptable site, pacing is initiated, and the minimum output necessary to achieve stable ventricular capture is determined. The pacing threshold should normally be less than 1 volt, at a pulse width of between 0.5 and 2 ms. If the pacing threshold is unsatisfactory, the electrode is repositioned until an acceptable site is found. Care should be taken to determine that the electrode is stable by asking the patient to take deep breaths or to cough while pacing at threshold. The electrode is then secured at the site of insertion and the pulse generator set to an output of at least 3 volts above the pacing threshold.

Permanent pacemaker implantation

The technique of permanent pacemaker implantation is essentially similar to that of temporary pacing, except that the electrodes are much more flexible to minimize the risk of late myocardial perforation, and they are stiffened by a stylet during manipulation. Insertion is normally via the left subclavian or cephalic vein. Once the electrode is in a satisfactory position, it is secured and connected to the implanted pulse generator. The rate, output voltage, pulse width, and other pacemaker functions can be modified non-invasively by means of telemetry via a transmitter/receiver placed on the skin over the pulse generator.

Pacing mode selection The nomenclature used to describe pacing mode is given in Table 3, and electrocardiographic examples of the principal pacing modes are given in Fig. 12. Atrial demand (AAI) pacing is used for sinoatrial disease in the absence of atrioventricular block. Ventricular pacing (VVI) is the simplest and technically easiest mode of pacing, and is required for atrioventricular conduction disturbances. However, VVI pacing does not permit atrioventricular synchrony or an increase in pacing rate in response to an increase in sinus (atrial) rate. Dual-chamber (DDD) pacemakers have electrodes in both the right atrium and ventricle. If the sinus cycle length is greater than the pulse interval, atrial demand pacing occurs. Following the atrial stimulus, a programmable atrioventricular delay commences. If no spontaneous ventricular depolarization is sensed before the end of this interval, a pacing stimulus is delivered via the ventricular electrode. If the sinus cycle length is shorter than the pulse interval, no atrial stimulus is given, but the atrioventricular delay is *triggered*, followed by spontaneous or paced ventricular activation. By this means, the ventricular rate tracks the atrial rate up to a programmable maximum, allowing the heart to increase its rate in a physiological manner in response to metabolic demand. An alternative, and simpler, approach to achieve a rate response is the use of an activity sensor such as an accelerometer in the pulse generator. Such devices detect bodily movement and increase the pacing rate according to a programmable algorithm. Rate response can be

Table 3 Pacemaker-mode nomenclature

Chamber-paced	Chamber-sensed	Mode	Additional features
A—atrium	A—atrium	I—inhibited	R—rate responsive
V—ventricle	V—ventricle	T—triggered	
D—dual	D—dual (A and V)	D—dual (I and T)	
(A and V)	O—neither	O—fixed rate	

See text for examples.

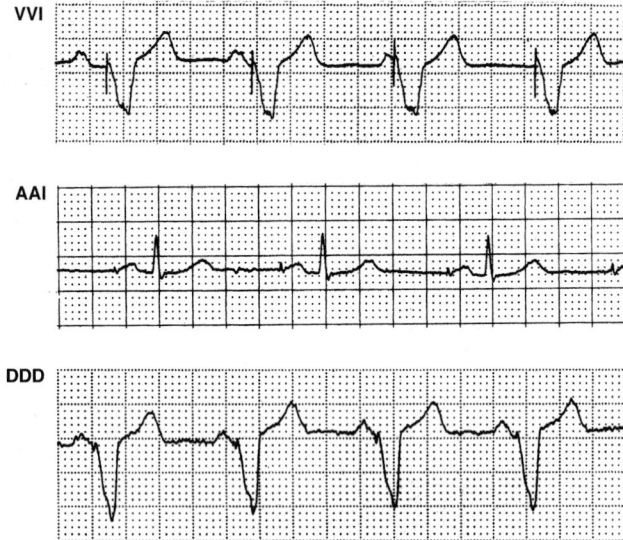

Fig. 12 Permanent pacemaker modes. Ventricular demand pacing, VVI (upper) with broad-complex ventricular complexes following the stimulus. Dissociated atrial activity can be seen. Atrial demand pacing, AAI (middle) with low amplitude bipolar pacing spike preceding the P-waves. Dual-chamber pacemaker, DDD (lower) with paced ventricular complexes following each P-wave (atrial tracking).

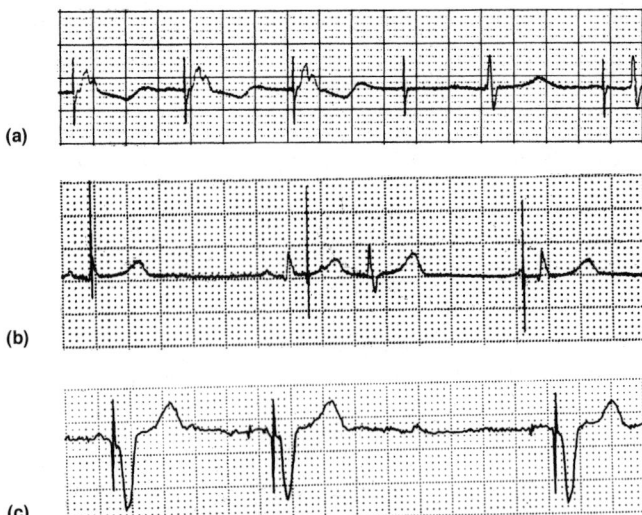

Fig. 13 Pacemaker malfunction. (a) Failure to capture. The fourth stimulus fails to capture the ventricle. (b) Undersensing. The atrial pacemaker has failed to sense the preceding atrial activity and therefore delivered the second stimulus. This has captured the atrium, with the P-wave in the ST segment, and subsequent conduction to the ventricle. (c) Oversensing. This dual-chamber pacemaker has sensed an electrical artefact through the ventricular lead and as a result has suppressed ventricular pacing, with the absence of ventricular activation following the third P-wave.

utilized in either single- or dual-chamber pacemakers, and is designated by the suffix 'R' (e.g. AAIR, VVIR, DDDR).

The advantage of dual-chamber (DDD) pacing over VVI pacing lies in the maintenance of atrioventricular synchrony and rate responsiveness, but this is achieved at the expense of increased complexity, complications, and cost. Observational studies have suggested that dual-chamber pacing reduces the risk of atrial fibrillation by virtue of pacing the atrium and avoiding retrograde atrial activation via the atrioventricular node. Additional suggested benefits include a lower incidence of the pacemaker syndrome (see below) and reduction in the risks of stroke, heart failure, and death. However, two recent large-scale randomized trials comparing DDD with VVI(R) pacing have failed to substantiate important prognostic or symptomatic benefits from DDD pacing, at least during follow-up periods of up to 3 years.

Complications Complications of temporary or permanent pacemaker implantation include those of central venous cannulation (for instance, pneumothorax), perforation of the heart by the electrode tip leading to pericardial effusion and cardiac tamponade, and macroscopic or microscopic displacement of the electrode resulting in an increase in the pacing threshold or failure to capture. A chest radiograph should always be taken after pacemaker insertion to exclude pneumothorax and to confirm that the electrode position is satisfactory.

Permanent pacing may be complicated by the development of infection around the pulse generator, or by mechanical erosion of the generator through the skin. Once infection is established, or the skin is breached, it is almost never possible to eradicate infection with antibiotics: removal and replacement of the pacing system is required. Following electrode implantation, oedema and inflammation around the electrode tip result in a steady rise in the pacing threshold over the first few weeks. This may occasionally result in an increase of the pacing threshold such that capture is lost (Fig. 13(a)), although the process is normally mild and self-limiting. Demand pacemakers require an adequate intracardiac signal to recognize activation of the chamber in question, in order to inhibit output. If the intracardiac signal is of insufficient amplitude the pacing stimulus will not be suppressed (*undersensing*), resulting in inappropriate pacemaker firing (Fig. 13(b)). This phenomenon is commoner in atrial pacing, owing to the lower amplitude of atrial compared with ventricular electrograms. Alternatively, detection of extraneous electrical activity (for example, skeletal

muscle activity) via the pacing electrode can result in inappropriate inhibition of the pacemaker output (*oversensing*) (Fig. 13(c)). Oversensing is commoner with unipolar than bipolar pacing modes because of the inclusion of the pulse generator can in the electrical circuit, and its proximity to the pectoral muscles. For the same reason, unipolar pacemaker systems are more prone to the problem of local skeletal muscle stimulation. Damage to the conductor or insulation of the pacing electrode may occur due to trauma at the site of ligation or to compression between the clavicle and first rib. This may result in oversensing, skeletal muscle stimulation, or to short-circuiting leading to premature battery depletion.

Patients receiving atrial demand (AAI) pacemakers may subsequently develop atrioventricular block, resulting in a recurrence of syncope and requiring upgrade of the pacing system to a dual-chamber (DDD) unit. A proportion of patients with ventricular demand (VVI) pacemakers, particularly those with sinoatrial rather than atrioventricular disease, will manifest retrograde ventriculoatrial conduction during ventricular pacing. This sometimes causes symptoms of fatigue, dizziness, or hypotension ('pacemaker syndrome'), which are associated with the presence of atrial cannon waves occurring as a result of simultaneous atrial and ventricular contraction. Upgrade of the system to a dual-chamber unit is necessary if symptoms are troublesome.

Follow-up Patients with permanent pacemakers require follow-up by a pacemaker clinic. As well as detection of the complications described above, the function of such a clinic is to assess the status of the pulse generator battery, and to maximize its life by programming the pulse generator output to the minimum consistent with a satisfactory safety margin. The design of pulse generators and the battery characteristics normally allow prediction of the expected replacement date several months if not years ahead. However, premature battery depletion or pacemaker failure does occur, and patients should therefore be assessed at least annually by the clinic. It must be borne in mind that many patients who have long-standing heart block treated by permanent pacing have no underlying cardiac rhythm, and that failure of the pacing system for whatever reason may be fatal.

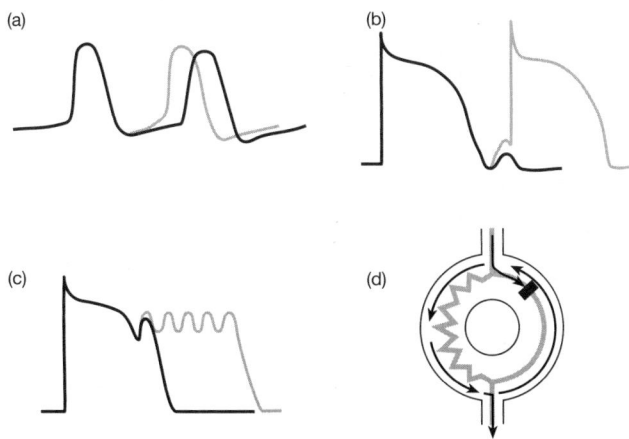

Fig. 14 Mechanisms of arrhythmia. (a) Increased automaticity. (b) Triggered activity due to early after-depolarizations. (c) Triggered activity due to delayed after-depolarizations. (d) Re-entry circuit. See text for details.

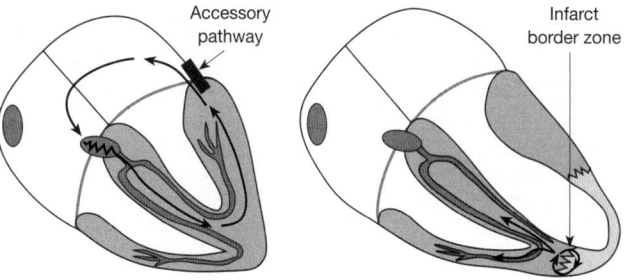

Fig. 15 Clinical examples of re-entry tachycardias. (a) Macro re-entry circuit involving an accessory pathway, which results in atrioventricular re-entry tachycardia. (b) Micro re-entry circuit at the border zone of a myocardial infarction.

Tachycardias

Mechanisms of arrhythmogenesis

The exact electrophysiological mechanism responsible for tachyarrhythmias is not known in all cases. There is a complex interaction between an underlying substrate such as previous myocardial infarction, a triggering event such as an extrasystole, and modulating influences, of which sympathetic stimulation and myocardial ischaemia are the most important. The principal mechanisms responsible for tachyarrhythmias are those of abnormal automaticity, triggered activity, and re-entry (Fig. 14).

Automaticity

Abnormal automaticity is defined as an inappropriate increase in the rate of discharge of a tissue that has physiological pacemaker properties (namely, sinus node, atrioventricular node, or Purkinje fibres) (Fig. 14(a)). Such abnormalities are most commonly seen in the presence of ischaemia, sympathetic stimulation, or drug toxicity, especially digoxin. Automatic tachycardias are characterized by an absence of initiation by extrasystoles, either spontaneously or during electrophysiological testing.

Triggered activity

The term 'triggered activity' is used to define the appearance of automaticity immediately associated with a preceding action potential, and can be induced *in vitro* in tissues that do not demonstrate physiological automaticity. Two characteristic forms of depolarization may cause triggered activity:

1. *Early after-depolarizations* occur during the plateau phase of the action potential, prior to repolarization (Fig. 14(b)), and are more evident at slow heart rates, particularly in the presence of hypokalaemia and hypomagnesaemia. Mutations in cardiac Na^+ or K^+ channels, or drugs that prolong myocardial repolarization by inhibiting one or more components of the outward potassium current I_k (for example, class IA and class III antiarrhythmics, tricyclic antidepressants, antihistamines, organophosphorous insecticides, and many others) predispose to the appearance of early after-depolarizations *in vitro*. These changes are associated with the congenital and acquired long QT syndromes and the arrhythmia *torsade de pointes* (see below).

2. *Delayed after-depolarizations* are small subthreshold depolarizations occurring after full repolarization of the action potential (Fig. 14(c)). Their amplitude is increased by tachycardia or intracellular calcium overload, and may reach a level at which a spontaneous action potential is generated, potentially initiating a sustained tachycardia. Delayed after-depolarizations can be induced experimentally by digitalis overload, and are the likely mechanism of digitoxic arrhythmias.

Re-entry

The majority of the clinically important sustained tachycardias, whether of atrial, junctional, or ventricular origin, appear to arise on the basis of re-entry. The establishment of a re-entry tachycardia requires the presence of a potential circuit comprising two limbs with different refractoriness and conduction properties (Fig. 14(d)). A premature beat can be conducted in one limb of the circuit, but the other limb may still be refractory, resulting in unidirectional conduction block. If conduction is sufficiently slow, the tissue distal to the site of block in the refractory limb will have regained excitability before the arrival of the depolarizing wavefront, and can conduct the activity retrogradely. This results in reactivation of the initial conducting pathway and thus a circus movement tachycardia is established. Macro re-entry is defined as the occurrence of a re-entry circuit over a large area of the heart, such as in the presence of an accessory pathway (Fig. 15(a)). Micro re-entry occurs in a relatively small area of the heart, for example at the border zone of an old myocardial infarction, where effective conduction velocity is markedly slowed (Fig. 15(b)). The characteristic feature of a re-entrant tachycardia is that an appropriately timed extrastimulus can induce unidirectional block and initiate the arrhythmia. The tachycardia may be terminated by extrastimuli that depolarize the tissue ahead of the circulating wave front and thus interrupt the circus movement.

Management of tachyarrhythmias

Differential diagnosis of tachycardias

The first and most important step in the diagnosis and management of tachycardias is to determine whether the arrhythmia arises within the atria and/or atrioventricular junction, or from the ventricles. An essential element in the differential diagnosis is to distinguish between tachycardias with normal QRS-complex morphology and duration ('narrow-complex tachycardias'), and those where the QRS complexes are abnormal in morphology and increased in duration ('wide-complex tachycardias').

Narrow-complex tachycardias

Narrow-complex tachycardias arise through mechanisms that result in ventricular activation via the atrioventricular node and His–Purkinje system and therefore show normal QRS morphology and duration (≤0.12 s) during tachycardia. The principal narrow-complex tachycardias and their characteristic ECG features are listed in Table 4. Careful study of all leads of the electrocardiogram is necessary to identify the presence of retrograde P-waves. Atrial flutter waves are most commonly evident in the inferior limb leads or in lead V1. Transient interruption of atrioventricular nodal conduction by vagal stimulation or intravenous adenosine is of particular value in revealing the tachycardia mechanism. Atrial tachyarrhythmias will not normally be terminated by adenosine, but an increase in AV block

Table 4 Diagnosis of narrow QRS tachycardias

Arrhythmia	P waves Rate	Morphology/axis	P–R relationship	Comment
Sinus tachycardia	100–150	Normal	1:1 normal PR	Rarely >150 except exercise
Sinus node re-entry	100–140	Normal	1:1 normal PR	Abrupt ↑ heart rate at onset
Atrial tachycardia	150–200	Abnormal	1:1 with prolonged PR or 2:1	
Atrial flutter	300	Flutter waves -ve in II, III, aVF (commonly)	Variable 1:1 to 4:1 or Wenckebach	Ventricular response regular or irregular
Atrial fibrillation	450–600	'f' waves or isolectric	–	Irregular ventricular response
AVNRT	140–220	Retrograde	Usually simultaneous	Normal resting ECG
AVNRT fast/slow	120–150	Retrograde	RP' > P'R	Frequent/incessant
AVRT	150–220	Retrograde	RP' < P'R Inverted P' in ST segment	WPW or concealed accessory pathway

AVNRT, atrioventricular nodal re-entry tachycardia; AVRT, atrioventricular (orthodromic) re-entry tachycardia; P', retrograde P wave; RP', interval between onset QRS and P'; P'R, interval between P' and following QRS onset.

reveals the underlying atrial tachyarrhythmia. By contrast, tachycardias utilizing the atrioventricular junction as part of the re-entry circuit will be terminated by transient AV block.

Wide-complex tachycardias

Few areas in cardiology cause more difficulty, or result in more mismanagement, than the diagnosis of wide-complex tachycardias. Whilst it is safe to assume that virtually all narrow-complex tachycardias have a supraventricular origin, wide-complex tachycardias (QRS duration ≥0.12 s) may arise either from the ventricle or from supraventricular mechanisms, the latter occurring if there is pre-existing bundle-branch block in sinus rhythm or if functional bundle-branch block (aberration) occurs as a result of the tachycardia. An additional cause is activation of the ventricles via an accessory pathway. The electrocardiographic features of wide-complex tachycardias are described in Table 5.

Difficulties in diagnosis and management most commonly arise when ventricular tachycardia is not recognized and is misdiagnosed as 'SVT with aberration'. This usually happens as a result of a number of failings and misconceptions, the commonest being that the clinical context is not considered:

Table 5 Diagnosis of wide-complex tachycardias

	Atrial rhythm	AV relationship	ECG morphology	
			Tachycardia	Sinus rhythm
Irregular ventricular response				
AF/AFl with previous BBB	'f' or flutter waves	Irregular	Typical BBB	Typical BBB
AF/AFl with functional BBB	'f' or flutter waves	Irregular	Typical BBB	Normal
Pre-excited AF	Obscured	Irregular	Varying normal/pre-excited	Pre-excitation (WPW)
Polymorphic VT	Obscured	–	Varying QRS axis and morphology	
Torsades de pointes	Obscured	–	Varying QRS axis and morphology	Long QT
Regular ventricular response				
Ventricular tachycardia	Sinus or retrograde VA conduction	AV dissociation or 1:1/2:1 VA conduction	Abnormal wide complexes QRS >0.14 s Extreme axis deviation Fusion/capture beats Concordance RBBB tachycardia with Rsr' in V1 or qS in V6	Commonly old MI
AFl with BBB	Flutter waves	Variable 1:1 to 4:1	Typical BBB	Typical BBB
AVRT with functional BBB	Retrograde atrial activation	1:1	Typical BBB	WPW or normal
AVNRT with functional BBB	Synchronous with QRS	1:1	Typical BBB	Normal
Antidromic tachycardia	Obscured in QRS	1:1	Pre-excited	WPW

AF/Fl, atrial fibrillation/flutter; BBB, bundle-branch block; WPW, Wolff–Parkinson–White syndrome; VT, ventricular tachycardia; AV, atrioventricular; VA, ventriculoatrial; MI, myocardial infarction; AVRT, atrioventricular (orthodromic) re-entry tachycardia; AVNRT, atrioventricular nodal re-entry tachycardia.

Table 6 Diagnostic use of intravenous adenosine

Arrhythmia	Response
Atrial tachycardia Atrial flutter Atrial fibrillation	Transient AV block reveals atrial arrhythmia. Rarely terminated
AVNRT AVRT	Terminates tachycardia by anterograde (AV) block
Ventricular tachycardia	Not terminated 1:1 VA conduction may be blocked, revealing AV dissociation

For abbreviations, please see Table 5.

1. *The age of the patient*: middle-aged or elderly individuals presenting with a recent history of wide-complex tachycardia, and who give a history of myocardial infarction or congestive heart failure, are more likely to have ventricular than supraventricular tachycardia. Ventricular tachycardia can also arise in young patients.

2. *The haemodynamic status of the patient*: it is often assumed that ventricular tachycardia should cause haemodynamic collapse, whereas patients may in fact be haemodynamically stable if the rate is not excessively fast or if underlying cardiac function is good. Conversely, supraventricular tachycardias may cause syncope, hypotension, or shock if sufficiently rapid.

3. *The nature of the episodes of palpitation*: it is often not appreciated that ventricular tachycardia can present with a typical history of paroxysmal self-terminating episodes, just as in the case of supraventricular tachycardia.

In addition to attention to the history and 12-lead ECG, which must be analysed carefully during tachycardia, the response to transient AV nodal blockade with adenosine will assist considerably in diagnosis in many patients (Table 6). The importance of making a correct diagnosis in wide-complex tachycardia is twofold. First, inappropriate acute therapy of the tachyarrhythmia can be avoided. In particular, the use of verapamil in ventricular tachycardia misdiagnosed as supraventricular tachycardia is associated with a high risk of haemodynamic collapse as a result of the negative inotropic effect of verapamil, coupled with its lack of efficacy in terminating ventricular tachycardia. Adenosine is a safer diagnostic aid. Second, the correct diagnosis has prognostic implications. Although any wide-complex tachycardia can be terminated effectively by cardioversion, if the original arrhythmia has been misdiagnosed then the adverse prognostic significance of ventricular tachycardia will be overlooked. Appropriate investigation and long-term management may not be instituted.

Objectives of therapy

Many cardiac arrhythmias are benign and require no intervention. The main indications for treatment are the relief of symptoms, prevention of complications such as myocardial ischaemia, cardiac failure, or embolism, or an attempt to prevent arrhythmic sudden death. Precipitating factors such as myocardial ischaemia/infarction, infection, thyrotoxicosis, alcohol, electrolyte disorders, or drug toxicity must be sought and treated if possible. The type of therapy used will commonly be influenced by the presence of underlying structural heart disease such as myocardial ischaemia/infarction or left ventricular impairment.

Antiarrhythmic drug therapy

All antiarrhythmic drugs have potentially serious side-effects. They may worsen existing arrhythmias or produce new, possibly life-threatening ones (proarrhythmia), and the possibility of a proarrhythmic response should be borne in mind as part of the risk–benefit assessment whenever such drugs are prescribed. No classification exists that provides an accurate predication of the efficacy of a given drug for a given arrhythmia, thus therapy is initiated partly on the basis of trial and error, supported if neces-

sary by more detailed investigation such as ambulatory ECG monitoring or cardiac electrophysiological testing.

The Vaughan Williams classification is based on the effects of antiarrhythmic drugs in isolated tissue. The effects of the major classes of antiarrhythmic drug activity at the tissue level, and the associated electrocardiographic changes, are listed in Table 7. Individual drugs are described in Table 8.

Class I activity

Class I antiarrhythmic drugs act by inhibiting the rapid inward sodium current and have local anaesthetic activity. Class Ia agents (for example, quinidine, procainamide, and disopyramide) increase the action potential duration and have intermediate effects on the onset and recovery kinetics of the sodium channel and hence on intracardiac conduction. Class Ib agents (for example, lidocaine and mexiletine) shorten the cardiac action potential duration and have very rapid offset kinetics that result in minimal slowing of normal intracardiac conduction. Class Ic drugs (for example, flecainide and propafenone) have no major effect on action potential duration, but produce the most long-lasting effect on cardiac sodium channel kinetics and the most marked slowing of intracardiac conduction.

Class II activity

Class II activity is defined as antagonism of the arrhythmogenic effects of catecholamines. The commonest agents in this class are the competitive β-adrenoceptor blockers. Other agents such as propafenone have a weak β-receptor blocking activity, while amiodarone (see below) exhibits a noncompetitive sympatholytic effect.

Class III activity

The class III mode of antiarrhythmic activity comprises lengthening of the cardiac action potential duration and hence of the effective refractory period. Drugs in this class possess a broad spectrum of activity against atrial, supraventricular, and ventricular arrhythmias. Currently available class III agents act by inhibiting the rapid component of the outward potassium current I_{kr}. Dofetilide and ibutilide are examples of drugs with 'pure' class III antiarrhythmic actions. Sotalol is a non-selective β-adrenoceptor antagonist that also possesses class III activity. Amiodarone possesses antiarrhythmic activity in all four Vaughan Williams classes.

Class IV activity

Class IV drugs (for example, verapamil and diltiazem) reduce the inward calcium current I_{Ca} in sinoatrial and atrioventricular nodal tissues. They are used to prevent or interrupt re-entry arrhythmias involving the atrioventricular node (for example, atrioventricular nodal re-entry tachycardia), or to slow the ventricular response in atrial fibrillation or flutter. The dihydropyridine calcium antagonists such as nifedipine have no antiarrhythmic action.

Digoxin

The antiarrhythmic activity of digoxin is not explained within the Vaughan Williams classification. Although its inotropic actions are based on inhibition of cardiac $Na^+K^+ATPase$, the antiarrhythmic activity appears to be mediated predominantly through vagal stimulation. Digoxin is used to slow ventricular rate in atrial fibrillation.

Adenosine

Adenosine, a naturally occurring purine nucleoside, is used pharmacologically to produce transient slowing or block of the sinus node or atrioventricular node, and is effective for the termination of re-entry arrhythmias involving the atrioventricular node. Adenosine is of particular value in view of its extremely short plasma half-life (about 2 s), which confers safety. It must be administered by rapid intravenous bolus injection, using incremental doses from 3 to 12 mg, to achieve the desired therapeutic effect.

Table 7 Classification of antiarrhythmic drug activity

		ECG effect				Tissue effect			
		HR	PR	QRS	QT	SA node	Atrium	AV node	Ventricle
Class	Ia	0	0/–	+	++	0	++	–	++/–
	Ib	0	0	0	0/–	0	0	0	++/–
	Ic	0	+	++	+	0	++	0/+	++/–
Class	II	–	+	0	0	++	++	++	+/0
Class	III	0/–	0/+	0	++	0/+	++	0/+	++/–
Class	IV	0/–	+	0	0	0/+	+/–	++	0
Digoxin		0/–	+	0	0	0/+	0/–	++	0/-
Adenosine		–	+	0	0	++	0/–	++	0

ECG effect: +, increases; –, decreases; 0, no effect; HR, heart rate.

Tissue effect: +, antiarrhythmic activity; –, potential adverse or proarrhythmic effect; 0 no effect

Non-pharmacological therapy

Physical manoeuvres

Tachycardias involving the atrioventricular node may be terminated by manoeuvres that produce transient vagal stimulation, and patients with recurrent supraventricular tachycardias should be taught to perform these techniques in order to abort attacks and avoid the need for hospital treatment. The Valsalva manoeuvre, performed in the supine position, is the most effective technique.

Antitachycardia pacing

Re-entry tachycardias may be terminated by the delivery of appropriately timed extrastimuli that depolarize part of the re-entry circuit prior to the arrival of the wave front and interrupt the arrhythmia. Simple overdrive pacing can be effective in the termination of atrial flutter, AV nodal re-entry, AV (orthodromic) re-entry tachycardia, or sustained ventricular tachycardia (Fig. 16). The cardiac chamber in question is paced for brief periods at a rate just above that of the tachycardia, for example 6 to 12 beats, with repeated attempts sometimes necessary at gradually increasing rates. Overdrive atrial or ventricular pacing may result in degeneration into atrial and ventricular fibrillation, respectively, hence facilities for defibrillation must be available. Implantable antitachycardia pacing facilities are incorporated into implantable cardioverter-defibrillators (see below).

External cardioversion/defibrillation

R-wave synchronized, direct current cardioversion under general anaesthesia or deep sedation is the most effective and immediate means of terminating sustained tachycardias, and is commonly used in the termination of atrial flutter, atrial fibrillation, or sustained ventricular tachycardia (Fig. 17). Although atrial flutter may respond to low-energy cardioversion (50 to 100 joules), the other arrhythmias normally require energies of 100 to 360 joules for termination. The use of non-synchronized DC shock in the termination of ventricular fibrillation is discussed in Chapter 16.3.

Internal cardioversion

Failure of external cardioversion of atrial fibrillation occurs in a significant proportion of patients as a result of various factors, including increased transthoracic impedance due to obesity, prolonged atrial fibrillation, left ventricular dysfunction, and left atrial dilatation. Internal cardioversion can still be achieved in a proportion of these patients. The procedure involves the introduction of specialized electrode catheters that permit DC-shock delivery between electrodes in the right atrium and the pulmonary artery or coronary sinus, providing a current field that achieves depolarization of both atria.

Implantable cardiovertor-defibrillators

Patients identified as being at high risk of sudden cardiac death, owing to a history of spontaneous or inducible sustained ventricular arrhythmias or out-of-hospital cardiac arrest, may be treated with an implantable cardio-verter-defibrillator (**ICD**). However, these devices are expensive, complex, and require regular specialist follow-up. A transvenous rate-sensing/-shocking electrode is introduced via the subclavian vein to the right ventricular apex, with the generator implanted in the pectoral region (Fig. 18). The shock is delivered between the intracardiac shocking electrode and the generator can. Some devices also include a right atrial electrode to sense atrial activation. This improves the distinction between sinus or atrial tachyarrhythmias and ventricular tachycardia, and reduces the risk of an inappropriate shock being delivered. ICDs can be programmed to deliver initial antitachycardia ventricular pacing for slower tachycardias, with shock delivery available for faster rates or if pace-termination fails.

Implantable atrial defibrillators have been developed for use in those patients with frequent paroxysmal atrial fibrillation, but the value of these has not been fully evaluated.

Radiofrequency ablation

Selective ablation of part of a re-entry circuit, an arrhythmic focus, or of the atrioventricular node is used increasingly in the management of troublesome arrhythmias, and offers the opportunity of curative treatment. Radiofrequency energy is delivered between the tip of an intracardiac electrode positioned at the appropriate site and an indifferent surface electrode placed over the scapula. The energy produces a localized necrotic lesion 2 to 3 mm in diameter, which results in local conduction block. The success of the procedure depends on the accuracy of the placement of the lesion in relation to the re-entry circuit or arrhythmic focus. Current indications for radiofrequency ablation are listed in Table 9, and specific issues are discussed below in relation to individual arrhythmias.

Arrhythmia surgery

The 'Maze' procedure for atrial fibrillation involves creating a series of linear incisions in the left and right atria, which are then sutured, creating lines of conduction block. This prevents the development of atrial re-entry circuits while permitting atrioventricular conduction. Surgical management of recurrent ventricular tachycardia by mapping and resection of the re-entry circuit is occasionally performed, but is being superceded by ablation or ICD therapy.

Individual arrhythmias

Extrasystoles

The term extrasystole is used to describe a premature beat arising from a focus other than the sinus node. Extrasystoles are also described as premature beats, premature contractions, premature depolarizations, or ectopic beats.

Atrial extrasystoles

Atrial extrasystoles are recognized by a premature P-wave of different morphology from the sinus P-wave (Fig. 19(a)), which can be hidden within the ST segment or T wave of the preceding sinus beat. Premature atrial extrasystoles that occur before full recovery of the atrioventricular node will be followed by prolongation of the PR interval, or, if sufficiently premature, complete failure of conduction (Fig. 19(b)). Non-conducted atrial extrasystoles must be distinguished from sinus arrest or second-degree atrioventricular block.

Atrial extrasystoles are a common finding in healthy people, particularly with increasing age, but are more frequent in the presence of increased atrial pressure or stretch such as in cardiac failure or chronic mitral valve disease. Patients should be reassured that the arrhythmia is benign and that drug treatment is rarely necessary. If treatment is required on symptomatic grounds, β-adrenergic blockers may be used, but class I antiarrhythmic drugs should be avoided in view of their proarrhythmic risk.

Junctional extrasystoles

Junctional extrasystoles are identified by the appearance of a premature, normal QRS complex in the absence of a preceding atrial extrasystole. The atria as well as the ventricles may be activated, resulting in an inverted P-wave simultaneous with the QRS complex, or inscribed within the ST segment. The significance and management of junctional extrasystoles are similar to those of atrial extrasystoles.

Ventricular extrasystoles

Ventricular extrasystoles are identified by the appearance of a bizarre, wide QRS complex not preceded by a P-wave (Fig. 20). There is commonly ST segment depression and T wave inversion. Ventricular extrasystoles may be intermittent, or occur with a fixed association to the preceding normal

Table 8 Commonly used antiarrhythmic drugs

Class Ia	Principal indication	Dose		Adverse effects
		IV	oral	
Quinidine	AF cardioversion	–	1–2 g/day	Hypersensitivity, GI symptoms, QT prolongation, hypotension
Disopyramide	AF prophylaxis VT termination	2 mg/kg	300–600 mg/day	Negative inotropy, QT prolongation, Parasympathetic blockade(accelerated AV conduction, urinary retention, dry mouth, blurred vision)
Procaineamide	AF cardioversion VT termination	100 mg/5 min up to 1000 mg 1–6 mg/min	2–6 g/day	Hypotension, QT prolongation GI upset, lupus syndrome
Class Ib				
Lidocaine (lignocaine)	VT termination VT/VF prophylaxis	100 mg bolus 1–4 mg/min	Ineffective	CNS—confusion, dysarthria, fits
Class Ic				
Flecainide	AF cardioversion AF prophylaxis WPW prophylaxis	2 mg/kg	100–300 mg/day	Proarrhythmia, negative inotropy, CNS disturbance
Propafenone	AF cardioversion AF prophylaxis WPW prophylaxis	–	450–900 mg/day	Proarrhythmia, negative inotropy, CNS disturbance
Class II				
Various, e.g. atenolol	AF prophylaxis AF rate control SVT prophylaxis Sudden death prophylaxis	–	50–100 mg/day	Bradycardia, -ve inotropy, cold extremities, bronchoconstriction, lethargy
Class III				
Sotalol	AF termination AF prophylaxis WPW prophylaxis VT prophylaxis	2 mg/kg	160–480 mg/day	Bradycardia, negative inotropy, cold extremities, bronchoconstriction, lethargy, QT prolongation
Amiodarone	AF termination AF prophylaxis WPW prophylaxis VT prophylaxis	300 mg in 30 min then 1200 mg/24 h	0.6–1.2 g/day loading first 2 weeks, then 100–400 mg/day	Bradycardia, photosensitivity, skin pigmentation, hypo- or hyperthyroidism, alveolitis, hepatitis, peripheral neuropathy, epidydimitis
Class IV				
Verapamil	SVT termination SVT prophylaxis AF rate control	5–10 mg IV	240–480 mg/day	Negative inotropy, AV block flushing, constipation
Other				
Digoxin	AF rate control		0.125–0.5 mg/day	Anorexia, nausea, vomiting, AV block, atrial and ventricular arrhythmias
Adenosine	SVT termination	3–12 mg by incremental bolus	ineffective	Flushing, chest pain, bronchospasm, transient AV block

AF, atrial fibrillation; SVT, supraventricular tachycardia (atrioventricular nodal and atrioventricular re-entrant tachycardia); VT, ventricular tachycardia; WPW, Wolff–Parkinson–White syndrome.

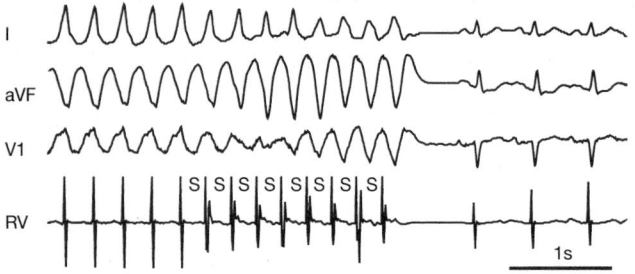

Fig. 16 Termination of ventricular tachycardia by overdrive ventricular pacing. During ventricular tachycardia a burst of eight stimuli (S) results in termination of the tachycardia and resumption of normal sinus rhythm. Surface leads I, aVF, V₁, and intracardiac electrograms from the right ventricular apex (RV) are shown.

beats, that is 1:2, 1:3 (bigeminy or trigeminy). Where extrasystoles are of differing morphologies, the terms 'multifocal' or 'multiform' are used.

Ventricular extrasystoles occur in otherwise normal hearts, but are found particularly in the presence of structural heart disease. They occur commonly in the acute phase of myocardial infarction, but are also seen in the postinfarction phase, and in the presence of severe left ventricular hypertrophy or dysfunction of whatever cause. Extrasystoles may produce symptoms that require treatment in a minority of cases. The safest option is β-blockade.

Atrial arrhythmias

Atrial fibrillation

Atrial fibrillation is the commonest sustained tachycardia. The underlying mechanism is thought to be re-entry in most instances, with multiple wavelets (probably a minimum of six) circulating through the atria. Studies of patients with frequent paroxysmal 'lone' atrial fibrillation suggest that the arrhythmia may be triggered by one or more rapidly discharging foci, which are commonly situated in the pulmonary veins. Such patients often have frequent premature 'P-on-T' atrial extrasystoles on ambulatory ECG monitoring. Recent experimental and clinical studies have helped to explain the long-standing clinical observation that the longer the duration of atrial fibrillation, the more difficult it is to restore and maintain sinus rhythm ('atrial fibrillation begets atrial fibrillation'). Rapid atrial activation induces a process of electrical remodelling, resulting in shortening of the atrial refractory period and loss of the normal lengthening of the atrial refractory period at slower heart rates. The initial mechanism is thought to be intracellular Ca²⁺ overload, although more prolonged atrial tachyarrhythmias result in downregulation of Ca²⁺ entry and de-differentiation of atrial myocytes towards a fetal phenotype. Preliminary clinical data suggest that atrial electrical remodelling is reversible following cardioversion. The possibility exists that short-term treatment after cardioversion, during the period of regression of atrial electrical remodelling, could have long-term benefits in the prevention of relapse.

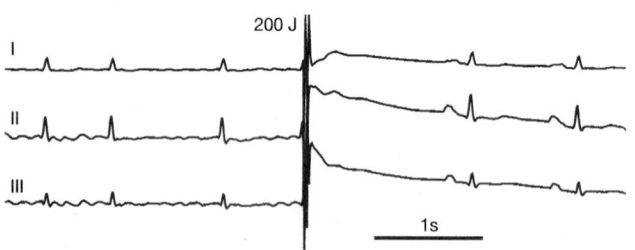

Fig. 17 Synchronized DC cardioversion of atrial fibrillation. A direct current shock, 200 joules, is delivered during atrial fibrillation to coincide with the R-wave of the QRS complex. This shock terminates the arrhythmia with restoration of normal sinus rhythm.

The characteristic ECG findings in atrial fibrillation of recent onset are of rapid, irregular 'f' waves at a rate of 350 to 600/min. These are associated with an irregular ventricular response because of variable conduction through the AV node (Fig. 21). With increasing duration of chronic atrial fibrillation, the amplitude of the 'f' waves diminishes until they are no longer visible. Under these circumstances, atrial fibrillation is diagnosed by the absence of P-waves and the irregular ventricular response (Fig. 21(b)).

Clinical features of atrial fibrillation The prevalence of atrial fibrillation increases with advancing age and may be as high as 5 per cent in the elderly. There are numerous causes of the arrhythmia (Table 10), but in many instances no obvious aetiological factor can be identified, and the individual is described as having 'lone' atrial fibrillation. Atrial fibrillation carries adverse prognostic significance, due in part to its association with organic heart disease. In addition, atrial fibrillation is an important risk factor for the development of stroke and systemic embolism as a result of stasis and thrombus formation in the left atrium. The risk of stroke is particularly high in patients with mitral stenosis or mitral valve replacement and chronic atrial fibrillation. The thromboembolic risk in non-rheumatic

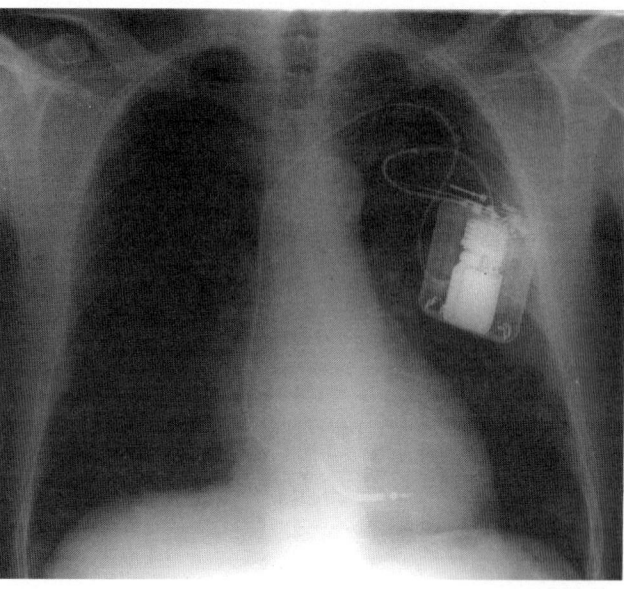

(a)

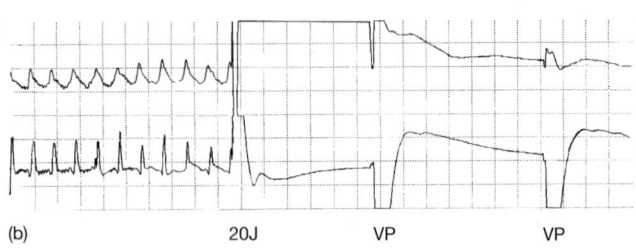

(b)   20J   VP   VP

Fig. 18 Implantable cardioverter-defibrillator (ICD). (a) Chest radiograph showing the ICD generator in the left pectoral region, connected to a lead which passes via the left subclavian vein and superior vena cava to the heart. The tip of the lead is in the right ventricular apex. Cardiac rhythm is sensed from the electrodes at the tip of the lead, and shocks can be delivered between the metal casing of the generator and the right ventricular coil (thickened portion of lead). (b) Discharge from an ICD. A rapid polymorphic ventricular tachycardia is terminated by a 20-joule shock from the device. Electrograms shown are retrieved from the memory of the device, upper tracings from the shocking circuit (generator can to ventricular coil) and lower tracings from the sensing circuit (bipolar electrodes at the tip of the catheter in the right ventricle. The shock is followed by ventricular pacing (**VP**).

Table 9 Indications for radiofrequency ablation

Diagnosis	Ablation target	Success	Comments
AVRT	Accessory pathway	+++	
Pre-excited AF	Accessory pathway	+++	
AVNRT	Slow pathway	+++	1–2 % risk of CHB
Atrial flutter	TVA–SVC isthmus	++	
Focal atrial tachycardia	Tachycardia focus	++	
Paroxysmal AF	Pulmonary vein focus	+	High recurrence rate
Uncontrolled AF	AV node	+++	Requires permanent pacing
Scar-related ventricular tachycardia	Re-entry circuit	+	High recurrence rate
RVOT ventricular tachycardia	Site of origin	++	

AVRT, atrioventricular (orthodromic) re-entry tachycardia; AF, atrial fibrillation; AVNRT, atrioventricular nodal re-entry tachycardia; CHB, complete heart block; TVA, tricuspid valve annulus; SVC, superior vena cava; RVOT, right ventricular outflow tract.

atrial fibrillation is related to age, previous left ventricular dysfunction, hypertension, and diabetes mellitus (Table 11).

Atrial fibrillation results in loss of the atrial contribution to left ventricular filling, which results in a modest reduction in cardiac output. In the presence of impaired ventricular function this can result in a worsening of heart failure. More commonly, symptoms and impairment of left ventricular function ('tachycardiomyopathy') arise as a result of a rapid uncontrolled ventricular rate. In addition, uncontrolled atrial fibrillation can cause further impairment of ventricular filling in mitral stenosis and conditions associated with left ventricular diastolic dysfunction, or the development of angina in patients with coexisting coronary artery disease.

Atrial fibrillation is classified into three patterns: paroxysmal, persistent, or permanent. In paroxysmal atrial fibrillation, spontaneously terminating attacks of palpitation last anything from a few seconds to a few days. The

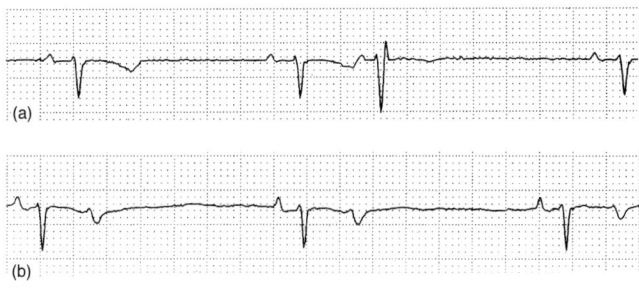

Fig. 19 Atrial extrasystoles. (a) An atrial extrasystole, with an abnormal P-wave at the end of the preceding T wave, occurs following a sinus beat. (b) Blocked atrial extrasystoles. In the same patient, atrial extrasystoles occur following each sinus beat. They are earlier than those in (a), and the AV node is refractory because of the proximity of the atrial extrasystoles to the preceding beat, and conduction is blocked.

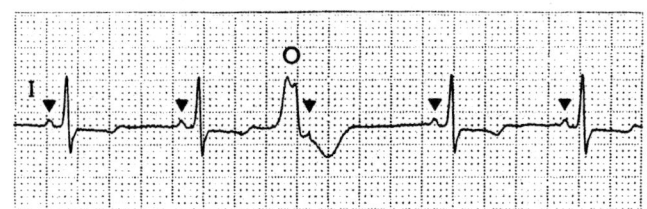

Fig. 20 Ventricular extrasystole (open circle). No retrograde atrial activation occurs, and the P-wave sequence is undisturbed (arrowed).

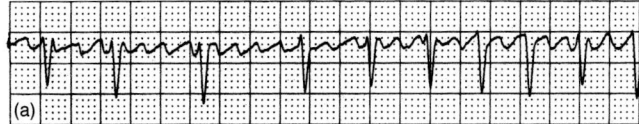

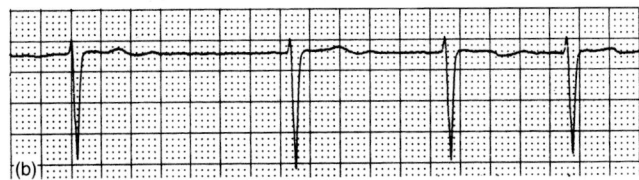

Fig. 21 Atrial fibrillation. (a) Coarse atrial fibrillation of recent onset. (b) Fine atrial fibrillation in a patient with long-standing valvular disease. Surface V₁ leads are shown.

Table 10 Aetiology of atrial fibrillation

- Increased atrial pressure—mitral valve disease, congestive heart failure, left ventricular hypertrophy, restrictive cardiomyopathy, pulmonary embolism
- Atrial volume overload—atrial septal defect
- Myocardial ischaemia/infarction
- Thyrotoxicosis
- Alcohol
- Sinoatrial disease
- Infiltration—constrictive pericarditis, tumour
- Infection—myo/pericarditis, pneumonia
- Retrograde activation—WPW syndrome, ventricular pacing
- Cardiac or thoracic surgery
- Idiopathic—'lone' atrial fibrillation

Table 11 Thromboembolic risk and anticoagulation in atrial fibrillation

High risk (annual risk of CVA 8–12 per cent)
- Previous transient ischaemic attack or stroke
- Patients ≥ 75 years with diabetes and/or hypertension
- Patients with clinical evidence of valvular heart disease, heart failure, thyroid disease, and/or impaired left ventricular function on echocardiography

Moderate risk (annual risk of CVA ≈ 4 per cent)
- Patients under 65 years with clinical risk factors: diabetes mellitus, hypertension, peripheral arterial disease, ischaemic heart disease
- Patients over 65 years of age not in high-risk group

Low risk (annual risk of CVA ≈ 1 per cent)
- All other patients under 65 with no history of embolism, hypertension, diabetes, or other clinical risk factors

Treatment
- High risk: Warfarin (target INR 2.0–3.0) if no contraindications and if practicable
- Moderate risk: Either warfarin or aspirin. In view of insufficient evidence, treatment may be determined on an individual basis. Echocardiography may be helpful.
- Low risk: Aspirin 75–300mg daily

Reproduced with permission from Lip G (1999). *Lancet*, **353**, 4–6.

ventricular rate is often rapid and the patient may be severely symptomatic. The term 'persistent atrial fibrillation' is used to describe instances where the arrhythmia is not self-terminating, but where sinus rhythm can be restored by electrical or pharmacological cardioversion. In paroxysmal and persistent atrial fibrillation, the objectives of therapy are the restoration and maintenance of sinus rhythm. Permanent atrial fibrillation describes the situation where restoration of sinus rhythm is no longer possible, and the principal objective of therapy is control of the ventricular rate. At this stage, the ventricular rate is often slower and the patient may be unaware of the irregular pulse or of palpitations.

Management of atrial fibrillation The management of a patient in atrial fibrillation depends upon the duration of the episode, the presence of organic heart disease, and any precipitating factors. Atrial fibrillation of recent onset (for example, less than 12 h) may terminate spontaneously. If fibrillation is persistent, an attempt to restore sinus rhythm should be made unless the arrhythmia is obviously long-standing or is associated with advanced organic heart disease. Underlying precipitating factors such as thyrotoxicosis should be corrected before attempting cardioversion. Chemical cardioversion may be achieved with class Ia, Ic, or III agents. Class Ia agents accelerate the ventricular rate by virtue of their anticholinergic action on the AV node and must be used in combination with digoxin. Traditionally, the commonest agent used was quinidine (1–2 g/day), but use of this drug has declined with the increasing recognition of adverse effects, in particular the risk of *torsade de pointes*. For patients without significant underlying heart disease, the current drugs of choice are the class 1c agents (for example, flecainide 2 mg/kg intravenously over 30 min). Class III drugs are somewhat less effective but are safer in the presence of left ventricular dysfunction or ischaemic heart disease. Options include sotalol (1.5 mg/kg intravenously over 30 min) or amiodarone (300 mg intravenously over 30 min followed by 1200 mg per 24 h until cardioversion). The pure class III agent ibutilide is approved for this indication in the United States. Normally, only one drug should be tried in any individual patient. If drug therapy fails, direct current cardioversion is commonly effective.

Following successful cardioversion, or in the presence of paroxysmal atrial fibrillation, prophylactic therapy should be considered, particularly if multiple episodes have occurred. No drug is entirely satisfactory. Quinidine, the traditional mainstay of prophylaxis, increases mortality and is best avoided. Class 1c agents (flecainide or propafenone) are effective and safe in the absence of underlying ischaemia or left ventricular dysfunction. Sotalol (80 to 160 mg twice daily) is also effective and well tolerated. A randomized clinical trial comparing amiodarone, sotalol, and propafenone in the prophylaxis of atrial fibrillation showed amiodarone to be clearly superior to the other two drugs in the prevention of recurrent fibrillation following DC cardioversion. However, the side-effect profile is such that it is rarely indicated for long-term use unless the arrhythmia is troublesome and fails to respond to other drugs.

In permanent atrial fibrillation, restoration of sinus rhythm is not feasible or is unsuccessful and chronic management involves control of ventricular rate. The mainstay of treatment is digoxin, at a dose titrated to achieve adequate slowing in the ventricular rate at rest, with therapeutic plasma concentrations. Despite adequate rate control at rest, patients with atrial fibrillation commonly have an uncontrolled heart rate on exercise. Control of rate response with additional atrioventricular nodal blocking drugs such as verapamil or β-blockers does not improve exercise tolerance in the short term, but improved rate control reduces the risk of development of tachycardiomyopathy and chronic heart failure. Rate control is especially important if the duration of diastole is critical, as in mitral stenosis or ischaemic heart disease.

If drug therapy fails to control paroxysmal atrial fibrillation, particularly in the absence of underlying heart disease, consideration should be given to the possibility of a focal mechanism, which may be amenable to radiofrequency ablation. Atrioventricular nodal ablation and implantation of a permanent pacemaker may be indicated if such treatment fails, or in the case of permanent atrial fibrillation with uncontrolled ventricular rate. Ablation and pacing may improve symptoms and function, but it is wise to defer therapy if possible in view of the irreversible nature of the procedure and the need for lifelong permanent pacing. Furthermore, many patients with paroxysmal atrial fibrillation revert into permanent atrial fibrillation with a marked improvement in symptoms.

Prophylaxis against thromboembolism should be considered in all patients in atrial fibrillation. Cardioversion may be associated with embolism, hence patients who are scheduled to have elective chemical or electrical cardioversion should ideally be treated with warfarin for up to 4 weeks before admission. If the arrhythmia is known to have started within the previous 24 h, intravenous heparin for 24 to 48 h is acceptable. Once warfarin has been started, it should be continued for a minimum of 4 weeks after cardioversion since atrial mechanical function recovers slowly and there is a high risk of recurrent fibrillation.

Chronic anticoagulation with warfarin is indicated in patients in atrial fibrillation with mitral stenosis or regurgitation. Recent studies have shown that patients with non-rheumatic atrial fibrillation will also benefit from prophylaxis against thromboembolism. Meta-analysis of these trials shows that warfarin anticoagulation with a target range for the International normalized ratio (**INR**) of between 2.0 and 3.0 reduces the risk of thromboembolic events by about 60 per cent. Aspirin is a significantly less-effective alternative, achieving a risk reduction of around 20 per cent. The choice of antithrombotic prophylaxis depends on balancing the risk of thromboembolism (Table 11) against the risk of haemorrhagic complications, as well as the local facilities for anticoagulant control.

Atrial flutter

Atrial flutter is caused by a macro re-entrant circuit in the right atrium (Fig. 22), which produces a typical electrocardiographic 'saw tooth' pattern of atrial activity with a rate close to 300/min (Fig. 23). In the common form of the arrhythmia, flutter waves are negative in leads II, III, and aVF and positive in lead V1. Atrial flutter may be associated with either a regular or irregular ventricular response. Flutter with 2:1 atrioventricular conduction produces a regular tachycardia of 150/min and should always be considered in the differential diagnosis of a regular, narrow-QRS tachycardia of this rate. Occasionally, flutter occurs with 1:1 atrioventricular conduction producing a ventricular rate approaching 300/min. The flutter waves may not be seen easily with faster ventricular rates, and transient slowing of AV conduction may be necessary to make the diagnosis (Fig. 23).

The underlying causes of atrial flutter are the same as those of atrial fibrillation (Table 10). Although atrial flutter may last for many months or occasionally years, it usually degenerates into chronic atrial fibrillation unless cardioversion is undertaken. Atrial flutter also carries a risk of

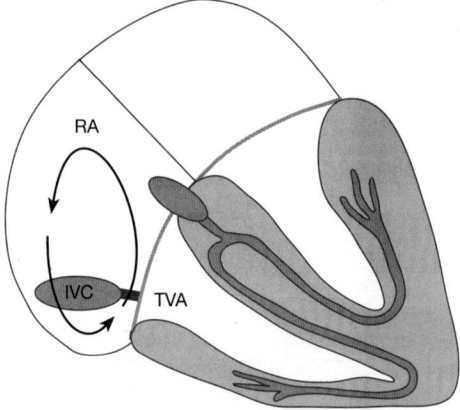

Fig. 22 Mechanism of atrial flutter. Typical atrial flutter results from a counter-clockwise re-entry circuit in the right atrium. The isthmus between the tricuspid valve annulus (**TVA**) and inferior vena cava (**IVC**) forms a critical part of this circuit, and linear ablation to create block can prevent recurrent atrial flutter.

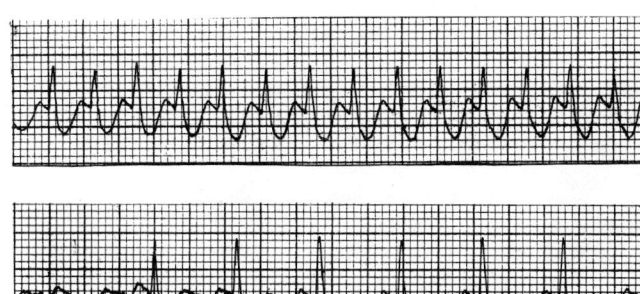

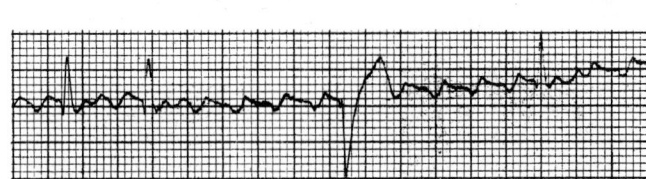

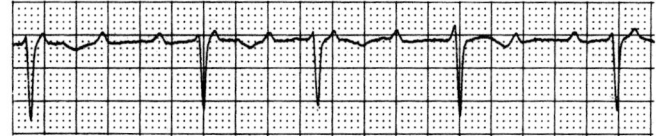

Fig. 23 Atrial flutter with 1:1 AV conduction (above), 2:1 conduction (middle), and following adenosine administration (below) (6 mg intravenous injection 10 s previously).

thromboembolism, and anticoagulation is indicated before and after cardioversion as for atrial fibrillation.

It is important to attempt to terminate atrial flutter since the ventricular rate is often poorly controlled by atrioventricular nodal blocking drugs. Termination may be achieved by chemical or electrical cardioversion as described above for atrial fibrillation. Bursts of atrial overdrive pacing at a rate approximately 10 per cent above the atrial flutter rate are also used: this may restore sinus rhythm or precipitate atrial fibrillation. Prophylaxis against atrial flutter is undertaken using the same agents as in paroxysmal atrial fibrillation, indeed the conditions often coexist and patients may manifest either flutter or fibrillation at different times.

Curative treatment of atrial flutter by radiofrequency ablation can be achieved by creating a line of conduction block between the tricuspid valve annulus and the inferior vena cava. This interrupts the isthmus through which the re-entry circuit must pass (Fig. 22).

Atrial tachycardia

Atrial tachycardia usually results in an atrial rate between 120 and 250/min. As in atrial flutter, there may be a degree of AV block, although 1:1 AV conduction may occur. The ECG shows regular P-waves which do not show the same 'saw tooth' appearance as in atrial flutter (Fig. 24). Atrial tachycardia may occur as a result of sinus node re-entry, when sudden paroxysms of tachycardia with a normal P-wave morphology will arise. Automatic atrial tachycardia manifests an abnormal P-wave morphology, commonly with a longer PR interval. The rate characteristically accelerates or 'warms up' before reaching a rate of 125 to 200/min. This arrhythmia is not started or terminated by atrial extrasystoles. Atrial tachycardia with atrioventricular conduction block is a manifestation of digitalis toxicity. Multifocal atrial tachycardia, in which rapid, irregular P-waves of three or four different morphologies are seen, may occur in severely ill elderly patients or in association with acute exacerbation of pulmonary disease.

The approach to management is identical to that of atrial fibrillation. Focal atrial tachycardia can be treated by radiofrequency ablation.

Fig. 24 Atrial tachycardia, with variable AV conduction. Lead V₁.

Junctional re-entry tachycardias

The majority of regular narrow-complex tachycardias are junctional re-entry tachycardias, which involve the atrioventricular node in the re-entry circuit. Correct recognition of these arrhythmias has achieved additional importance with the development of effective curative measures.

Atrioventricular nodal re-entry tachycardia

This is the commonest cause of paroxysmal re-entry tachycardia manifesting regular, normal QRS complexes. The basis of the arrhythmia is the presence of two functionally distinct pathways in the region of the atrioventricular node (Fig. 25). The 'fast' pathway conducts more rapidly, but has a longer refractory period. The 'slow' pathway has slower conduction properties but a shorter refractory period. During sinus rhythm, atrioventricular nodal conduction occurs via the fast pathway with a normal PR interval (Fig. 25(a)). If a sufficiently premature atrial extrasystole arises, conduction in the fast pathway is blocked, but slow pathway conduction may continue, resulting in an abrupt increase in the AH interval as recorded in the His–bundle electrogram and corresponding to an increased PR interval on the surface ECG. Conduction down the slow pathway may be sufficiently tardy to allow the fast pathway to recover excitability before activation reaches the distal end of the pathways, allowing retrograde activation to occur via the fast pathway (Fig. 25(b)). The stage is then set for a re-entry circuit with anterograde conduction via the slow pathway and retrograde conduction via the fast pathway ('slow/fast atrioventricular nodal re-entry') (Fig. 25(c)). The arrhythmia circuit is functionally distinct from the atria and ventricles, which may be perturbed by extrastimuli without interruption of the tachycardia. Characteristically, anterograde activation of the ventricles and retrograde activation of the atria occur virtually simultaneously, resulting in the P-wave being 'buried' within the QRS complex, or producing a very small distortion of the terminal QRS, which requires careful comparison with the ECG during sinus rhythm (Fig. 26). The tachycardia is readily initiated by atrial premature stimulation, and terminated by appropriately timed extrastimuli or by overdrive pacing.

A less common variant of atrioventricular nodal tachycardia may arise where anterograde conduction during tachycardia is via the fast pathway with retrograde conduction via the slow pathway ('fast/slow atrioventricular nodal re-entry'). Under these circumstances, the atrium is activated well after the QRS complex, characteristically producing an inverted P' wave with the RP' interval greater than the P'R interval during tachycardia (Fig. 27). Occasionally, slow/fast and fast/slow tachycardias may coexist in the same patient.

Atrioventricular nodal re-entry tachycardia commonly presents for the first time in childhood or adolescence, although it may appear at any age. The natural history is of episodic paroxysmal tachycardia. Attacks occur at random intervals, although clustering of attacks may occur interposed with periods of relative freedom from symptoms. Atrioventricular nodal re-entry tachycardia has no specific association with other organic heart disease. Palpitations are normally well tolerated unless the tachycardia is particularly rapid, prolonged, or if the patient has other heart disease.

Management Termination of an attack of atrioventricular nodal re-entry tachycardia is achieved by producing a transient AV nodal block. This may be achieved by vagotonic manoeuvres, by intravenous verapamil (5 to 10 mg), or by intravenous adenosine (3 to 12 mg) (Fig. 26). Drug prophylaxis of AV nodal re-entry tachycardia is undertaken with β-blockers, a combined β-blocker/class III agent such as sotalol, or with atrioventricular nodal blocking drugs such as verapamil or digoxin. Curative treatment of AV nodal re-entry tachycardia is readily achieved by ablation and is indicated if patients are refractory to drugs, intolerant of side-effects, or unwilling to take long-term medication. Radiofrequency energy is delivered to the 'slow' pathway, which lies between the compact atrioventricular node and the tricuspid annulus. Ablation at this site is normally curative but carries a small risk (1 to 2 per cent) of inducing complete heart block.

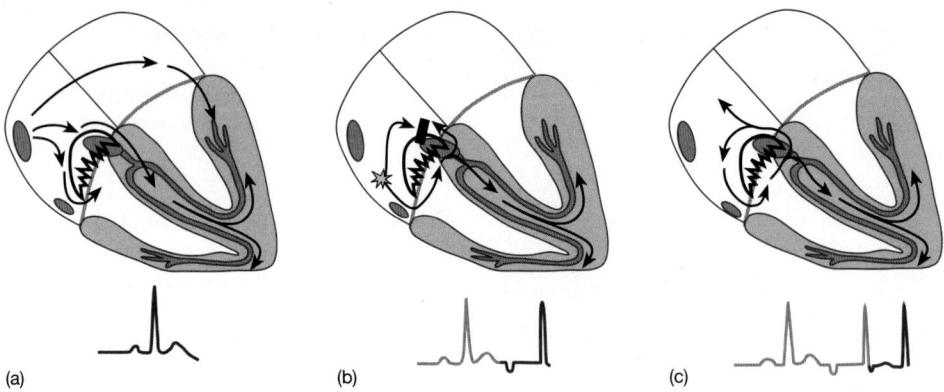

Fig. 25 Atrioventricular nodal re-entry tachycardia. Mechanism of initiation by atrial extrasystole. See text for details.

Pre-excitation syndromes (Wolff–Parkinson–White syndrome)

The term 'pre-excitation' refers to the premature activation of the ventricle via one or more accessory pathways that bypass the normal atrioventricular node and His–Purkinje system. The commonest of the pre-excitation syndromes is the Wolff–Parkinson–White syndrome, in which accessory pathways with electrophysiological properties of normal myocardium may lie at any point in the atrioventricular ring, the commonest sites being in the left free wall and the posteroseptal region. The characteristic electrocardio-graphic appearance is of early activation of the myocardium adjacent to the ventricular insertion of the accessory pathway (Fig. 28(a)). There is no atrioventricular delay, hence the PR interval is shortened, but slow intraventricular conduction results in slurred initiation of the QRS complex (the delta wave) (Fig. 29), although the remainder of the ventricle is excited via the normal His–Purkinje system. The ECG appearances of a delta wave occur in approximately 1.5 per 1000 of the population, but many individuals never experience paroxysmal tachycardias. The degree of pre-excitation during sinus rhythm is variable: it may be *intermittent* if the refractory period of the accessory pathway is close to the sinus cycle length (Fig. 29), or *inapparent* if the delta wave is obscured due to rapid AV nodal conduction. In such instances, transient slowing of AV nodal conduction (for example, by adenosine) will enhance the proportion of the ventricle excited by the accessory pathway and reveal pre-excitation.

In many instances, accessory pathways conduct only in the retrograde (ventriculoatrial) direction, and do not cause ventricular pre-excitation. Such pathways are termed *concealed*, since there is no clue to their presence

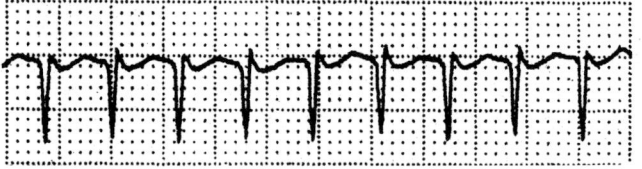

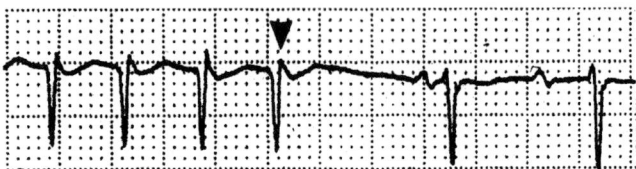

Fig. 26 Atrioventricular nodal re-entrant tachycardia. Rapid narrow-complex tachycardia with no apparent P-waves (upper) responding to 6 mg adenosine with restoration of sinus rhythm (lower). Close inspection reveals a positive deflection of the terminal QRS during tachycardia (arrow) which is absent during sinus rhythm. This is due to retrograde atrial activity coincident with ventricular activation. Lead V₁.

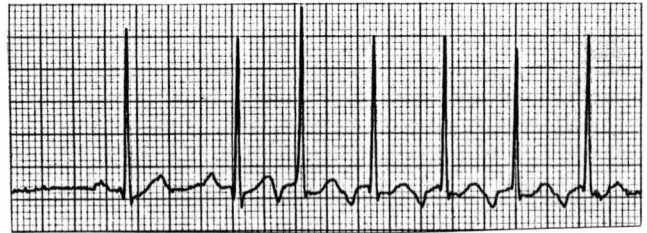

Fig. 27 Atypical atrioventricular nodal re-entry tachycardia (long RP'). Inverted P-waves precede the QRS complex during tachycardia (compare with preceding sinus beats).

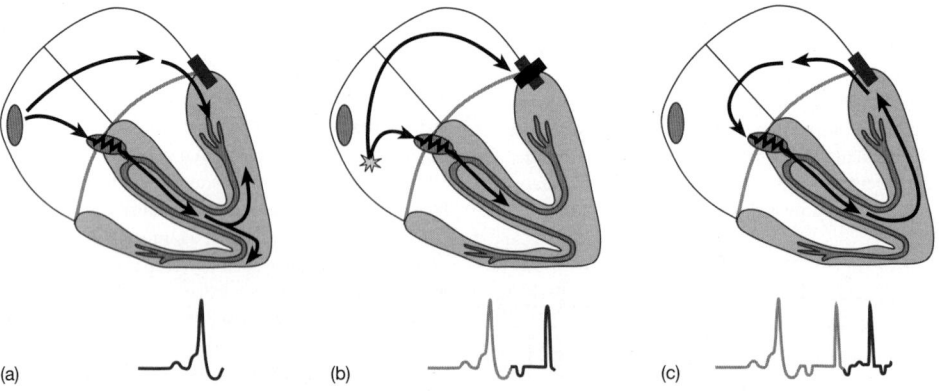

Fig. 28 Atrioventricular re-entry tachycardia. Mechanism of initiation by atrial extrasystole. See text for details.

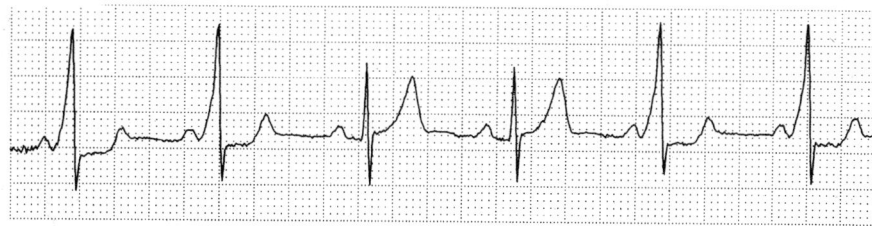

Fig. 29 Intermittent pre-excitation in Wolff–Parkinson–White syndrome. The first two beats show the characteristic short PR interval and delta wave. The middle two beats, however, show that the pre-excitation was intermittent. The pathway has become refractory, with normal PR interval and QRS morphology. Pathway conduction returns to cause pre-excitation in the final two beats.

on the resting ECG. These patients are not at risk of pre-excited atrial fibrillation (see below), but either overt or concealed accessory pathways can lead to episodes of atrioventricular re-entry tachycardia.

Atrioventricular re-entry tachycardia

The mechanism of orthodromic tachycardia, the common form of atrioventricular re-entry tachycardia, is illustrated in Fig. 28. A premature atrial extrasystole may find the accessory pathway refractory, but be conducted through the atrioventricular node to the ventricles (Fig. 28(b)). If sufficient delay has occurred by the time the ventricular insertion of the accessory pathway is depolarized, the pathway will have recovered excitability and allow retrograde activation from the ventricle to atrium, with the establishment of a re-entry circuit (Fig. 28(c)). Since the circuit involves activation of the ventricles via the His–Purkinje system, the QRS morphology during re-entry tachycardia is normal, unless a rate-related, bundle-branch block develops. Retrograde atrial activation can be identified by the presence of a characteristic inverted P' wave early in the ST segment, an important diagnostic feature of atrioventricular tachycardia (Table 7, Fig. 30).

Antidromic tachycardia

A rarer form of atrioventricular tachycardia has anterograde conduction via the accessory pathway and retrograde conduction via the atrioventricular node (antidromic tachycardia). The QRS morphology of this tachycardia is grossly abnormal with appearances dependent upon the site of insertion of the accessory pathway.

Other forms of pre-excitation include the Mahaim pathway, a direct atrioventricular or atriofasicular connection with slow conduction properties typical of AV nodal tissue. Evidence for direct atrionodal pathways associated with a short PR interval but no delta wave (Lown–Ganong–Levine syndrome) remains controversial and has not been established histologically.

Pre-excited atrial fibrillation

The major prognostic concern in Wolff–Parkinson–White syndrome is pre-excited atrial fibrillation. Conduction via an accessory pathway with a short refractory period, bypassing the normal AV nodal slowing, results in very rapid ventricular conduction that may degenerate into ventricular fibrillation (Fig. 31). The degree of pre-excitation during atrial fibrillation varies, giving a characteristic pattern of an irregular ventricular response with QRS morphology ranging from normal to fully pre-excited.

Patients with symptomatic Wolff–Parkinson–White syndrome should be evaluated carefully for the risk of pre-excited atrial fibrillation. If pre-exci-

tation is intermittent, this is commonly associated with a long accessory-pathway refractory period and a low risk of life-threatening tachycardias. Disappearance of the delta wave in response to administration of a class Ia or Ic antiarrhythmic drug also suggests a low risk. The risk of sudden death due to rapid pre-excited atrial fibrillation is very low among patients who have not had any symptomatic tachycardias, but is higher in symptomatic patients, particularly if episodes of pre-excited atrial fibrillation have been documented. Risk can be assessed by analysis of the shortest pre-excited RR intervals during spontaneous or induced episodes of pre-excited atrial fibrillation, a value of less than 250 ms identifying a higher risk group. Patients who have experienced atrial fibrillation with relatively slow ventricular rates are unlikely to develop faster ventricular responses subsequently. The general tendency is for accessory pathway conduction to become slower with increasing age, and spontaneous disappearance of conduction is well documented.

Management of patients with accessory pathways

Orthodromic re-entry tachycardia may be terminated by AV nodal blocking manoeuvres such as vagal stimulation, verapamil, or adenosine. Pre-excited atrial fibrillation requires particular care, since digoxin or verapamil may paradoxically accelerate the ventricular rate and are contraindicated. Electrical cardioversion is indicated in the presence of severe haemodynamic disturbance. Where patients are stable, agents such as intravenous flecainide, sotalol, or amiodarone, which both slow anterograde conduction through the accessory pathway and also restore sinus rhythm, are used. Drug prophylaxis is used to minimize the risk of recurrent orthodromic re-entry tachycardia or atrial fibrillation. Drugs acting only on the AV node, such as verapamil, are less effective than agents having additional action on the accessory pathway such as flecainide and sotalol. Although amiodarone is effective, its use is not desirable in otherwise fit young people who may require long-term drug therapy.

Patients with symptomatic Wolff–Parkinson–White syndrome are increasingly offered radiofrequency ablation as first-line therapy. This approach abolishes the risk of pre-excited atrial fibrillation as well as preventing further attacks of atrioventricular re-entry tachycardia. Careful electrode mapping of the atrioventricular annulus is necessary to identify the accessory pathway, the site at which the interval between the atrial and ventricular electrograms is at a minimum, ideally with a discrete accessory pathway potential between the signals. Passage of the radiofrequency current results in the disappearance of accessory pathway conduction within a few seconds (Fig. 32). The success rate of ablation varies according to the

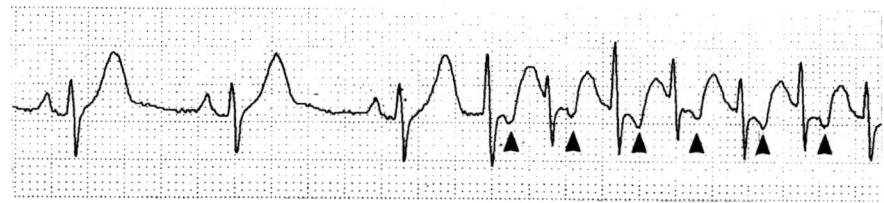

Fig. 30 Initiation of atrioventricular re-entry tachycardia. The third sinus beat is followed by the onset of narrow-complex tachycardia, initiated by an atrial extrasystole (obscured by T-wave). Retrograde atrial activation, with inverted P-waves in the ST segment (arrows), are seen during tachycardia.

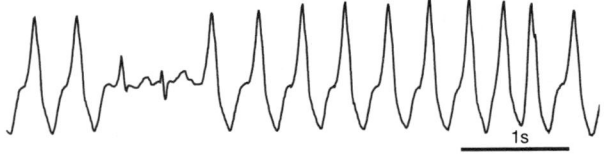

Fig. 31 Pre-excited atrial fibrillation. Conduction via an accessory pathway results in an irregular wide-complex tachycardia. The third and fourth beats show less pre-excitation, with activation mainly through the normal conducting system, with more normal QRS-complex morphology. Lead V₁.

location of the pathway, but is usually over 90 per cent in experienced hands.

Radiofrequency ablation is indicated in patients with tachycardias due to concealed accessory pathways if they are not well controlled on drugs, intolerant of side-effects, or unwilling to take long-term medication. Localization of the accessory pathway is performed as described above, except that mapping is performed during ventricular pacing or during stable atrioventricular tachycardia, and the earliest site of retrograde atrial activation at the atrioventricular annulus is the site of ablation.

Ventricular tachyarrhythmias

Definitions

Ventricular tachycardia is defined as the presence of three or more consecutive ventricular beats at a rate of 120 per min or greater. Ventricular tachycardia is considered *sustained* if an individual salvo lasts for 30 s or more, and *non-sustained* if the duration is between 3 beats and 30 s. *Monomorphic* ventricular tachycardia demonstrates a consistent QRS morphology during each paroxysm, although patients may have paroxysms of monomorphic ventricular tachycardia of different morphologies at different times. *Polymorphic* ventricular tachycardia demonstrates a constantly changing QRS morphology, often without discrete QRS complexes. Polymorphic ventricular tachycardia may degenerate into ventricular fibrillation and the electrocardiographic distinction between the two is difficult. *Torsade de pointes* is a characteristic type of polymorphic ventricular tachycardia with a typical undulating variation in QRS morphology as a result of variation

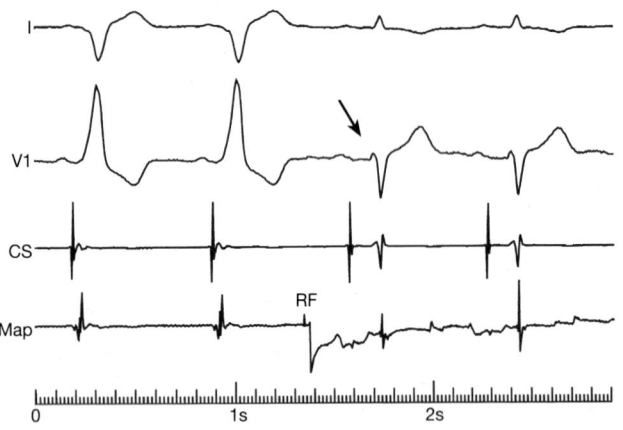

Fig. 32 Radiofrequency ablation of an accessory pathway. The patient had Wolff–Parkinson–White syndrome with evidence of ventricular pre-excitation on the surface electrogram during sinus rhythm (short PR interval, delta wave). One beat after switching on the radiofrequency (**RF**) current the QRS becomes normal, indicating successful ablation of the accessory pathway. This was a left-sided accessory pathway, as shown by the short interval between left atrial and left ventricular activation recorded from the coronary sinus (**CS**). This interval is prolonged following ablation of the pathway. Surface leads I, V₁, and intracardiac electrograms from CS and mapping catheter (**Map**) are shown.

in axis. The term is reserved for the arrhythmias arising in association with QT interval prolongation.

Sustained monomorphic ventricular tachycardia

Aetiology Sustained monomorphic ventricular tachycardia commonly occurs in the presence of structural heart disease, but also arises in structurally normal hearts. It rarely occurs in the acute phase of myocardial infarction, but may be seen in the subacute phase (>48 h), or may arise many years after the index infarction, particularly in association with left ventricular dilatation and aneurysm formation. The arrhythmia also occurs in other conditions associated with ventricular dilatation or fibrosis such as dilated cardiomyopathy, hypertrophic cardiomyopathy, or previous ventriculotomy (for example, following repair of Fallot's tetralogy). Sustained monomorphic tachycardia can occur as a proarrhythmic response to antiarrhythmic drugs, particularly class I agents.

Although ventricular tachycardia normally occurs in individuals with overt heart disease, it is also seen in young, apparently healthy, subjects. Arrhythmogenic right ventricular cardiomyopathy (dysplasia) is an autosomal dominant condition associated with replacement of the right ventricular free wall with fat and fibrous tissue. These patients may have no symptoms or signs of cardiac disease, but typical ECG changes (T wave inversion in the right precordial leads) are associated with variable degrees of dilatation of the right ventricle demonstrated on echocardiography or magnetic resonance imaging. There remains a minority of patients with documented ventricular tachycardia in whom no structural heart disease is evident on clinical, ECG, or echocardiographic examination. The tachycardia may arise from the outflow tract of the right or, rarely, left ventricle, or from one of the fascicles of the left bundle branch.

ECG characteristics The presence of atrioventricular dissociation is a particularly important feature to seek in a wide-complex tachycardia as it makes the diagnosis of ventricular tachycardia virtually certain (Table 8, Fig. 33(a)). A careful search for P-waves perturbing the QRS complex or T-waves is necessary, ideally using multichannel recordings. Occasionally, a fortuitously timed P-wave allows the development of a capture beat of normal QRS morphology without interrupting the tachycardia. A fusion beat occurs when activation of the ventricle is partly via the normal His–Purkinje system and partly from the tachycardia focus (Fig. 33(b)). Fusion and capture beats are diagnostic of ventricular tachycardia, but are commonly present only if the ventricular rate is relatively slow. Where dissociated P-wave activity cannot be recognized with certainty on the surface ECG, direct recording of atrial activity by an oesophageal or right atrial electrogram may aid the diagnosis. Although atrioventricular dissociation

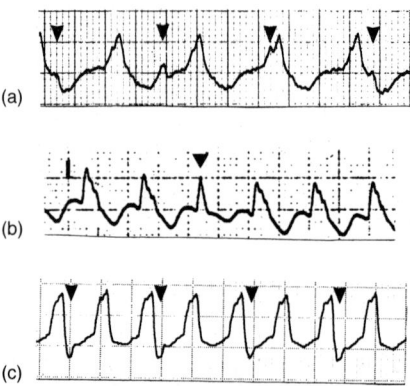

Fig. 33 Sustained monomorphic ventricular tachycardia. (a) Ventricular tachycardia with atrioventricular dissociation. P-waves (arrowed) are seen to have no relationship to the ventricular activation. Lead V₁. (b) Ventricular tachycardia with fusion beat (arrow). Lead V₁. (c) Ventricular tachycardia with 2:1 ventriculoatrial conduction. Lead III. Inverted P-waves (arrows) follow every second ventricular complex.

is diagnostic of ventricular tachycardia, it is not invariable. Retrograde ventriculoatrial conduction may occur, giving either 1:1 conduction or higher degrees of block (Fig. 33(c)).

The QRS duration in ventricular tachycardia is commonly greater than 0.12 s, and values greater than 0.14 s are particularly suggestive of ventricular tachycardia. Although the QRS morphology may superficially resemble left or right bundle-branch block, the morphology is commonly atypical (Table 8). Ventricular tachycardia arising from the right ventricular free wall has a left bundle-branch block-like pattern, whilst left ventricular free wall tachycardias show right bundle-branch block morphology. The presence of concordant positive or negative QRS complexes across the chest leads is suggestive of ventricular tachycardia, as is the existence of extreme axis deviation.

Acute management of ventricular tachycardia Rapid ventricular tachycardia may present with cardiac arrest, syncope, shock, anginal chest pain, or left ventricular failure, but slower tachycardias in patients with good cardiac function may be well tolerated.

Sustained ventricular tachycardia is a medical emergency. If the patient is pulseless or unconscious, immediate DC cardioversion is necessary. If the patient is conscious but hypotensive, urgent DC cardioversion under general anaesthesia or deep sedation is used. Haemodynamically tolerated tachycardias may be terminated by drug therapy. The commonest agent used is intravenous lidocaine (lignocaine) 100 mg, repeated if necessary after 5 min. Sotalol 1.5 mg/kg intravenously is more effective, but its use is restricted by its negative inotropic action. Second-line drugs for the termination of ventricular tachycardia include procainamide, disopyramide and amiodarone. Amiodarone normally has a slow onset of action but may be effective if the tachycardia is well tolerated. Flecainide is contraindicated in view of the risk of developing incessant tachycardia. All antiarrhythmic drugs have significant negative inotropic actions that may further impair the haemodynamic status of the patient if sinus rhythm is not restored. For this reason, no more than one antiarrhythmic drug should normally be given before recourse to alternative therapy, usually DC cardioversion. Overdrive termination of ventricular tachycardia following insertion of a temporary pacing lead may be effective (Fig. 16), particularly if the tachycardia is relatively slow. Facilities for cardioversion must be available in view of the risk of acceleration or degeneration into ventricular fibrillation.

Prophylaxis of ventricular tachycardia Ventricular tachycardia is a potentially life-threatening condition. Unless the acute episode was clearly precipitated by some transient or reversible factor, there is a high probability of recurrent attacks, which may result in sudden death rather than a sustained tachycardia. The 3-year cardiac survival rate varies from 80 per cent in patients in whom arrhythmia induction is suppressed by antiarrhythmic drug therapy, to 40 per cent in those in whom no effect of suppression is achieved and/or empirical therapy is used.

Clinical evaluation of the patient after restoration of sinus rhythm should be supported by electrocardiography, echocardiography, and/or radionuclide ventriculography. In those with ischaemic heart disease, exercise testing should be undertaken to identify the presence of reversible ischaemia, which may act as a trigger to ventricular tachycardia, and coronary arteriography to determine the extent of arterial disease. Particular attention should be paid to the possibility of right ventricular dysplasia in young patients.

Unless there is a clear precipitating factor such as drug toxicity, electrolyte abnormality, or acute ischaemia, patients who have had documented ventricular tachycardia require antiarrhythmic prophylaxis. The most reliable form of prophylaxis against arrhythmic sudden death or recurrent sustained ventricular tachycardia is provided by the implantable cardioverter-defibrillator (Fig. 18). The Antiarrhythmics versus Implantable Defibrillators Trial (**AVID**) showed defibrillators to be superior in preventing death from any cause, in comparison to drug therapy with amiodarone or sotalol in patients resuscitated from ventricular fibrillation or ventricular tachycardia causing haemodynamic compromise (Fig. 34).

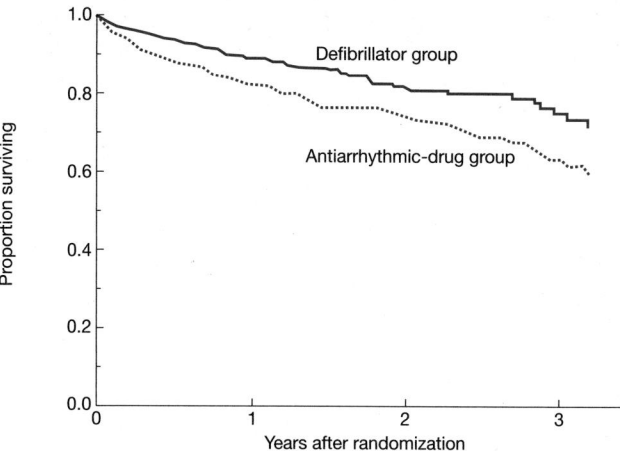

Fig. 34 Improved survival with the implantable cardioverter defibrillator compared to antiarrhythmic drugs in patients resuscitated from near-fatal ventricular arrhythmia. (Taken with permission from the AVID investigators (1997). *New England Journal of Medicine* **337**, 1576. Copyright 1997, Massachusetts Medical Society. All rights reserved).

Those with non-sustained ventricular tachycardia (see below) and left ventricular dysfunction, in whom sustained tachycardia can be induced at electrophysiological testing, also have a better survival with defibrillator implantation compared with drug therapy. Indeed, the indications for such treatment are expanding to include a wide range of patients with sustained or non-sustained ventricular tachyarrhythmias who are at risk of sudden death.

In view of the cost and complexity of implantable defibrillator therapy, it is not affordable in all countries, and not appropriate for patients with advanced congestive heart failure or other conditions with a severely limited prognosis. Medical therapy is necessary for many patients, but is limited by a relative lack of randomized, controlled-trial evidence. Beta-adrenoceptor blockers have been shown to reduce the risk of sudden death in unselected survivors of myocardial infarction, and to be comparable to conventional antiarrhythmic agents in the prevention of recurrent ventricular tachyarrhythmias. Since β-adrenoceptor blockers are now shown to be of prognostic benefit even in the presence of severe left ventricular dysfunction, they should be used routinely in the prophylaxis of ventricular tachycardia if tolerated. Of the conventional antiarrhythmic agents, there is evidence that the class III drugs sotalol and amiodarone are superior to class I antiarrhythmic agents, which should no longer be used for this indication. However, sotalol and amiodarone have not been tested against placebo or conventional β-adrenoceptor blockers in randomized trials, although observational studies suggest they are of benefit in the prevention of arrhythmic death.

The efficacy of any given antiarrhythmic drug cannot be predicted, thus it is necessary to demonstrate antiarrhythmic drug efficacy and to exclude proarrhythmic responses in each patient. If episodes of ventricular tachycardia, sustained or non-sustained, are occurring frequently, it is sufficient to administer antiarrhythmic drugs under continuous electrocardiographic monitoring, and to demonstrate that salvoes of tachycardia have been completely suppressed. If episodes of ventricular tachycardia are infrequent, cardiac electrophysiological testing is indicated. The initial objective of such testing is to initiate a tachycardia of similar rate and QRS morphology to the spontaneous arrhythmia (Fig. 2): drug therapy is then administered and a repeat study is undertaken once stable plasma levels of the drug have been achieved. Suppression of inducibility of the tachycardia is associated with a reduced risk of arrhythmia recurrence and an improved prognosis in comparison with patients whose arrhythmia is not suppressed. Even if ventricular tachycardia is still inducible, the presence of marked slowing (increase in cycle length greater than 100 ms) associated with good haemodynamic tolerance appears to indicate a good long-term prognosis.

Radiofrequency ablation is used in the management of ventricular tachycardia, particularly in right ventricular outflow tract or fascicular tachycardia. Location and ablation of critical areas of slow conduction in ventricular tachycardias due to previous myocardial infarction are feasible but technically difficult, with lower rates of success than for other types of ablation.

Direct surgical management of recurrent ventricular tachycardia involves aneurysmectomy, endocardial mapping, and resection of the subendocardial area containing the micro re-entry circuit. The indications for surgery have been reduced considerably since the advent of the implantable cardioverter-defibrillator, since the surgical mortality is up to 10 to 15 per cent, compared with 0.5 per cent for defibrillator implantation. Where medically intractable ventricular tachyarrhythmias are associated with very poor left ventricular function, the only possible therapeutic option is cardiac transplantation.

Non-sustained ventricular tachycardia

Clinical features The mechanism and causes of non-sustained ventricular tachycardia (Fig. 35) are similar to those of sustained ventricular tachycardia. There is often slight variation in the RR interval, particularly if the salvo involves only a few beats. Short salvoes of non-sustained ventricular tachycardia are often asymptomatic; more prolonged episodes may result in dizziness or presyncope, and occasionally in syncope. Apart from the instances where non-sustained ventricular tachycardia produces troublesome symptoms, the major clinical significance of the arrhythmia is as a risk marker for sustained ventricular tachycardia or sudden cardiac death. However, long-term follow-up of patients with non-sustained ventricular tachycardia in the absence of structural heart disease has indicated a good prognosis with no excess risk, although non-sustained ventricular tachycardia recorded by ambulatory ECG monitoring in the convalescent phase or after remote myocardial infarction is an independent risk factor for subsequent sudden cardiac death, especially if it is associated with impaired left ventricular function. The risk of arrhythmic death is particularly high if sustained ventricular tachycardia can be initiated in these patients by electrophysiological testing. Non-sustained ventricular tachycardia is also an adverse prognostic feature in patients with hypertrophic cardiomyopathy. Asymptomatic non-sustained ventricular tachycardia is commonly recorded in patients with advanced congestive heart failure: it is associated with an increased risk of cardiac death, but not selectively of sudden death.

Management The management of non-sustained ventricular tachycardia involves the identification of underlying organic heart disease, as described in the section on sustained monomorphic ventricular tachycardia. Patients should be evaluated non-invasively by echocardiography or radionuclide ventriculography. If no significant organic heart disease is present, and the patient is asymptomatic, no treatment is indicated. Treatment of symptoms in the absence of significant heart disease should be with β-blockers in the first instance to minimize the risk of proarrhythmic reactions. Calcium-channel blockers are effective occasionally and may be tried. Failing these, sotalol or a class I agent may be necessary.

Patients with structural heart disease but well-preserved ventricular function and a normal signal-averaged electrocardiogram are at low risk of sustained ventricular tachycardia and may be treated empirically with β-blockers. If non-sustained ventricular tachycardia is associated with impaired ventricular function, there is likely to be a substrate for sustained ventricular tachyarrhythmias. Patients in whom sustained ventricular tachycardia or fibrillation is inducible have an improved survival following defibrillator implantation compared with patients treated medically.

Low-dose amiodarone therapy has been recommended in the management of patients with hypertrophic cardiomyopathy and non-sustained ventricular tachycardia, although the evidence for its efficacy is based on comparison with historical controls rather than on a randomized prospective study.

Accelerated idioventricular rhythm

The term 'accelerated idioventricular rhythm' is used to describe a continuous ventricular rhythm with a rate less than 120/min. Idioventricular rhythm commonly occurs in the setting of acute myocardial infarction and appears to be a marker of successful thrombolytic therapy. No active treatment is necessary.

Polymorphic ventricular tachycardia

Polymorphic ventricular tachycardia is an unstable rhythm with varying QRS morphology. It is most commonly seen in the acute phase of myocardial infarction and is due to unstable re-entry circuits. As such, it commonly undergoes spontaneous termination, although it may degenerate into ventricular fibrillation. If episodes of polymorphic ventricular tachycardia are frequent in the early hours of myocardial infarction, they can be suppressed by intravenous lidocaine (lignocaine). However, short, infrequent episodes are commonly left untreated.

The Brugada syndrome is an autosomal dominant condition due to a mutation of one of the genes encoding the rapid sodium channel (SCN5a), causing partial inactivation. There is an unusual pattern of variable ST-segment elevation and partial right bundle-branch block in the right precordial leads, associated with a risk of polymorphic ventricular tachycardia and sudden death.

Torsade de pointes and the long QT syndromes

ECG characteristics *Torsade de pointes* is an atypical ventricular tachycardia characterized by a continuously varying QRS axis ('twisting of points') (Fig. 36). Episodes of *torsade de pointes* are commonly repetitive and normally self-terminating, although they may degenerate into ventricular fibrillation. Paroxysms of *torsade de pointes* are associated in the preceding beats with evidence of marked QT prolongation, and frequently with morphological abnormalities of the T-waves such as T–U fusion, gross increases in T-wave amplitude, or T-wave alternans. Paroxysms of *torsade de pointes* in the congenital syndromes are often associated with increases in sinus rate, while in the acquired syndromes a slowing of the heart rate, and in particular a postextrasystolic pause, is often associated with initiation of the arrhythmia. This produces a characteristic 'short–long–short' sequence of initiation (Fig. 36). The combination of QT interval prolongation during sinus rhythm with intermittent *torsade de pointes* is described as the long QT syndrome.

Congenital long QT syndromes The underlying arrhythmic mechanisms in the congenital syndromes involve mutations in genes encoding proteins in the ion channels conducting either the inward sodium current I_{Na}, or the rapid or slowly inactivating components of the outward potassium current (I_{kr} and I_{ks}, respectively). Multiple mutations have been described and the long QT syndromes are subclassified according to the underlying gene

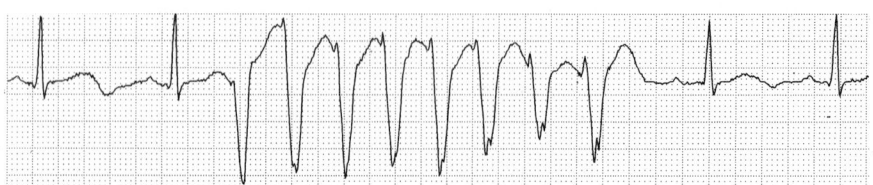

Fig. 35 Non-sustained ventricular tachycardia.

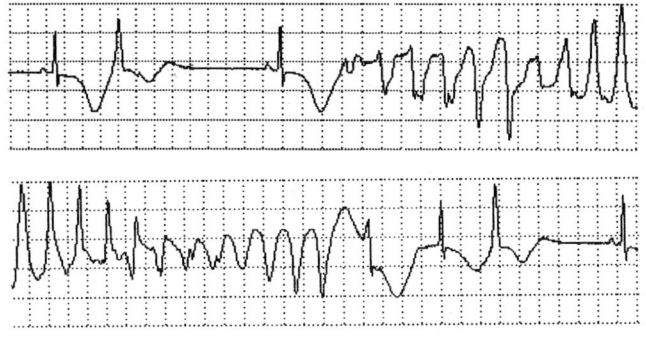

Fig. 36 *Torsade de pointes*. Note the marked QT interval prolongation in the sinus beats. Ambulatory monitoring recording is shown (continuous tracing).

defect (Table 12). All the currently recognized subgroups show an autosomal dominant mode of inheritance. Lengthening of ventricular repolarization, and hence of the QT interval, occurs as a result either of increased duration of current flow via I_{Na}, or inhibition of outward current flow via I_{kr} or I_{ks}. The arrhythmias have characteristics consistent with triggered activity. A variety of congenital long QT syndrome phenotypes have been identified. In the Jervell–Lange–Nielsen syndrome, the long QT gene disorder is inherited as an autosomal dominant, but neural deafness as an autosomal recessive. The other long QT syndromes are not associated with deafness. Sporadic cases of idiopathic, presumed congenital long QT syndrome have been reported.

Attacks of *torsade de pointes* in the congenital syndromes are commonly associated with sympathetic stimulation such as exercise, waking, or fright. Paroxysms may produce syncope, which if prolonged may be complicated by convulsion, leading to misdiagnosis as epilepsy. A family history of recurrent syncope or sudden death may be obtained. Sinus bradycardia is commonly seen in these syndromes.

Acquired long QT syndromes Many drugs and other factors predispose to the development of the acquired long QT syndrome (Table 13). Although class Ia and III antiarrhythmic drugs are best known for this complication, it is important to recognize that a very large number of non-cardiac drugs inhibit the outward potassium current I_{kr}, and may cause significant lengthening of the QT interval singly or in combination. Episodes of *torsade de pointes* often occur as a result of a combination of factors, including prolongation of the QT interval in association with bradycardia or pauses, hypokalaemia, and hypomagnesaemia. All of these predispose to early after-depolarizations *in vitro* and this mechanism appears to be the likely cause of *torsade de pointes* in the acquired syndromes. It is increasingly recognized that there is a genetic predisposition to the development of acquired long QT syndrome in the face of predisposing factors, leading to the concept that patients developing acquired long QT syndrome have reduced 'repolarization reserve' as a result of a *forme fruste* of the congenital syndrome.

Acute management of *torsade de pointes* The common clinical presentation is of recurrent dizziness or syncope, and the condition may easily be misdiagnosed as self-terminating polymorphic ventricular tachycardia or ventricular fibrillation unless the characteristic morphology of *torsade de pointes* and the associated QT interval prolongation is recognized. It is essential to discontinue predisposing drugs or other agents and to avoid empirical antiarrhythmic drug therapy, which may worsen the arrhythmia. Individual paroxysms of *torsade de pointes* are normally self-limiting, but if they are persistent, cardiac arrest will occur and emergency defibrillation is necessary. Intravenous magnesium sulphate (8 mmol over 10–15 min, repeated if necessary) is a safe and effective emergency measure for the prevention of recurrent paroxysms of tachycardia. If *torsade de pointes* is associated with bradycardia and pauses, the heart rate should be increased to between 90 and 100/min by atrial or ventricular pacing or isoproterenol (isoprenaline) infusion. Hypokalaemia should be sought and corrected if necessary.

Long-term management of long QT syndromes The prognosis of untreated congenital long QT syndrome is poor, with a high incidence of sudden death in childhood. Patients with the congenital long QT syndrome presenting with attacks of syncope are initially treated with high-dose β-blockade for example, propranolol. If this is unsuccessful, selective high left stellate ganglionectomy has been employed successfully. Permanent pacing at rates of 70 to 80/min, in combination with β-blockers, may also be effective in reducing symptoms. Defibrillator implantation is necessary for resistant cases, and is commonly used as first-line therapy if episodes of *torsade de pointes* have resulted in cardiac arrest. Retrospective data from the International Registry have indicated that the 15-year survival in patients following their first episode of *torsade de pointes* has been improved from 50 per cent in untreated cases to 90 per cent following treatment with β-blockade and/or left stellate ganglionectomy. The prognosis of the acquired long QT syndromes are excellent, provided the underlying predisposing factors are identified and avoided.

Ventricular fibrillation

Ventricular fibrillation is defined as a chaotic, disorganized arrhythmia with no identifiable QRS complexes (Fig. 37). The mechanism is of multiple, unstable re-entry circuits. The electrocardiographic pattern depends on the duration of fibrillation: recent-onset fibrillation is described as 'coarse', with a peak-to-peak amplitude of around 1 mV (1 cm); with increasing duration of cardiac arrest, the amplitude of ventricular fibrillation diminishes and 'fine' ventricular fibrillation is less likely to be amenable to successful electrical defibrillation.

Ventricular fibrillation may represent the endpoint of cardiac disease of many aetiologies. Fibrillation may occur during acute myocardial ischaemia, and is the principal cause of death in the first 2 hours following acute myocardial infarction (Fig. 37). Ventricular fibrillation during myocardial infarction is subdivided into primary, occurring without warning in an otherwise stable patient, and secondary, where fibrillation occurs in the

Table 12 Congenital Long-QT syndromes

Genotype	Relative frequency*	Chromosome/gene affected		Phenotype
LQT1	+++	11	*KvLQT1*	$\downarrow I_{ks}$
LQT2	++	7	*HERG*	$\downarrow I_{kr}$
LQT3	+	3	*SCN5a*	$\uparrow I_{Na}$
LQT4	–	Not known		Not known
LQT5	+/–	21	*KCNE1*	$\downarrow I_{ks}$
LQT6	–	21	*KCNE2*	$\downarrow I_{kr}$

*Relative frequencies among genotyped families in the International long QT Registry (+++, most frequent;– least frequent). The products of *HERG* and *KCNE1* and those of *KvLQT1* and *KCNE1* form the subunits of the channels carrying the rapid (I_{kr}) and slow (I_{ks}) components, respectively, of the outward potassium current. Modified with permission from Viskin S (1999). *Lancet*, **354**, 1625–33.

Table 13 Acquired Long-QT syndromes

Drug induced

Antiarrhythmic drugs	Classes Ia, III
Macrolide antibiotics	Erythromycin
Antifungals	Ketoconazole
Vasodilators	Prenylamine, ketanserin, lidoflazine
Psychotropics	Tricyclic/tetracyclic antidepressants, antipsychotics
Antihistamines	Terfenadine, astemizole
Cholinergic antagonists	Cisapride

Electrolyte disturbances

Hypokalaemia, hypomagnesaemia, hypocalcaemia

Metabolic

Hypothyroidism, starvation, anorexia nervosa, liquid protein diet

Bradycardia

Sinoatrial disease, AV block

Toxins

Organophosphorous insecticides, heavy metal poisoning

context of left ventricular failure and cardiogenic shock. In acute myocardial infarction, ventricular fibrillation is often initiated by an R on T extrasystole. Ventricular fibrillation occurring in chronic heart disease is most commonly a result of degeneration of rapid ventricular tachycardia, whose causes have been described above. Rarer causes of fibrillation are listed in Table 14.

Ventricular fibrillation is rarely self-terminating, and normally causes cardiac arrest with the rapid onset of pulselessness, unconsciousness, and apnoea. The management of cardiac arrest due to ventricular fibrillation is discussed in Chapter 16.3.

Management of survivors of ventricular fibrillation Patients who survive an episode of ventricular fibrillation should be assessed carefully to determine the risk of recurrence. If ventricular fibrillation has occurred in the first few hours of a typical Q-wave myocardial infarction, the risk of recurrent cardiac arrest is low, and no specific prophylactic therapy other than conventional postinfarction β-blockade is indicated. In many instances ventricular fibrillation arises as a result of acute ischaemia in patients with known, extensive heart disease who have not sustained an acute infarction. These patients remain at high risk of recurrent ventricular fibrillation, and should be evaluated fully by exercise testing and coronary arteriography

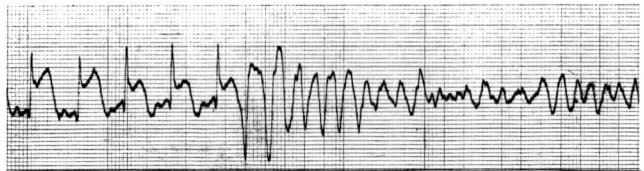

Fig. 37 Ventricular fibrillation complicating acute myocardial infarction. The arrhythmia is initiated by an 'R on T' ventricular extrasystole.

Table 14 Causes of ventricular fibrillation

- Acute myocardial ischaemia
- Acute myocardial infarction—primary or secondary
- Advanced organic heart disease with poor LV or RV function
- Severe LV hypertrophy
- Ventricular tachycardia/torsade de pointes
- Electrical—electrocution, lightning, unsynchronized DC shock, competitive ventricular pacing
- Pre-excited atrial fibrillation
- Profound bradycardia
- Hypoxia, acidosis

with a view to revascularization. Patients may sustain a cardiac arrest without any preceding chest pain, but in the presence of a known risk factor for ventricular tachycardia such as previous myocardial infarction. In these individuals, it is likely that ventricular fibrillation arose as a result of degeneration of rapid ventricular tachycardia. These patients are at risk of further cardiac arrest, and are managed with an implantable cardioverter-defibrillator or antiarrhythmic therapy as discussed in the section on ventricular tachycardia.

Further reading

Andersen HR, *et al.* (1997). Long-term follow-up of patients from a randomized trial of atrial versus ventricular pacing for sick sinus syndrome. *Lancet* **350**, 1210–16.

Atiga WL, Rowe P, Calkins H (1999). Management of vasovagal syncope. *Journal of Cardiovascular Electrophysiology* **10**, 874–86.

Atrial Fibrillation Investigators (1994). Risk factors for stroke and efficacy of anti-thrombotic therapy in atrial fibrillation: analysis of pooled data from five randomised controlled trials. *Archives of Internal Medicine* **154**, 1449–57.

Brugada J, Brugada R, Brugada P (1998). Right bundle-branch block and ST-segment elevation in leads V1 through V3: a marker for sudden death in patients without demonstrable structural heart disease. *Circulation* **97**, 457–60.

Connolly SJ (1999). Evidence-based analysis of amiodarone efficacy and safety. *Circulation* **100**, 2025–34.

Connolly SJ, *et al.* (2000). Effects of physiological pacing versus ventricular pacing on the risk of stroke and death due to cardiovascular cause. *New England Journal of Medicine* **342**, 1385–91.

Domanski MJ, Zipes DP, Schron E (1997). Treatment of sudden cardiac death. Current understandings from randomized trials and future research directions. *Circulation* **95**, 2694–9.

Drew BJ, Scheinman MM (1995). ECG criteria to distinguish between aberrantly conducted supraventricular tachycardia and ventricular tachycardia: practical aspect for the immediate care setting. *Pacing and Cardiac Electrophysiology* **18**, 2194–208.

Echt DS, *et al.* (1991). Mortality and morbidity in patients receiving encainide, flecainide, or placebo. *New England Journal of Medicine*, **324**, 781–8.

Fitzpatrick A, Sutton R (1992). A guide to temporary pacing. *British Medical Journal* **304**, 365–9.

Ginks W, Leatham A, Siddons H (1979). Prognosis of patients paced for chronic atrioventricular block. *British Heart Journal* **41**, 633–6.

Gregoratus G, *et al.* (1998). ACC/AHA guidelines for implantation of cardiac pacemakers and arrhythmia devices. A report of the American College of Cardiology/American Heart Association Task Force on Practice Guidelines (Committee on Pacemaker Implantation). *Journal of the American College of Cardiology* **31**, 1175–209.

Haïssaguerre M, *et al.* (1998). Spontaneous initiation of atrial fibrillation by ectopic beats originating in the pulmonary veins. *New England Journal of Medicine* **339**, 659–66.

Kay GN, Plumb VJ (1996). The present role of radiofrequency catheter ablation in the management of cardiac arrhythmias. *American Journal of Medicine* **100**, 344–56.

Lamas GA, *et al.* (1998). Quality of life and clinical outcome in elderly patients treated with ventricular pacing as compared with dual-chamber pacing. *New England Journal of Medicine* **338**, 1097–104.

Lévy S, *et al.* (1998). Atrial fibrillation: current knowledge and recommendations for management. Working Group on Arrhythmias of the European Society of Cardiology. *European Heart Journal* **19**, 294–320.

Lip GYH (1999). Thromboprophylaxis for atrial fibrillation. *Lancet* **353**, 4–6.

Mehta D, *et al.* (1988). Relative efficacy of physical manoeuvers in the termination of junctional tachycardia. *Lancet* **i**, 1181–5.

Morady F (1999). Radio-frequency ablation as treatment for cardiac arrhythmia. *New England Journal of Medicine* **340**, 534–44.

Morley-Davies A, Cobbe SM (1997). Cardiac pacing. *Lancet* **349**, 41–6.

Moss AJ, *et al.* (1996). Improved survival with an implanted defibrillator in patients with coronary disease at high risk for ventricular arrhythmia. *New England Journal of Medicine* **335**, 1933–40.

Priori SG, *et al.* (1999). Genetic and molecular basis of cardiac arrhythmia; impact on clinical management. Study group on molecular basis of arrhythmias of the working group on arrhythmias of the European Society of Cardiology. *European Heart Journal* **20**, 174–95 (also published in *Circulation* **99**, 518–28, 674–81.)

Priori SG, *et al.* (2001). Task Force on Sudden Cardiac Death of the European Society of Cardiology. *European Heart Journal* **22**, 1374-450.

Rankin AC, Rae AP, Cobbe SM (1987). Misuse of intravenous verapamil in patients with ventricular tachycardia. *Lancet* **ii**, 472–4.

Rankin AC, *et al.* (1989). Value and limitations of adenosine in the diagnosis and treatment of narrow and broad complex tachycardias. *British Heart Journal* **62**, 195–203.

Roden DM (2000). Antiarrhythmic drugs: from mechanisms to clinical practice. *Heart* **84**, 339–46.

Roy D, *et al.* (2000). Amiodarone to prevent recurrence of atrial fibrillation. *New England Journal of Medicine* **342**, 913–20.

Task Force of the Working Group on Arrhythmias of the European Society of Cardiology (1991). The 'Sicilian Gambit'. A new approach to the classification of antiarrhythmic drugs based on their actions and arrhythmogenic mechanisms. *Circulation* **84**, 1831–51.

The Antiarrhythmic Versus Implantable Defibrillators (AVID) Investigators (1997). A comparison of antiarrhythmic-drug therapy with implantable defibrillators in patients resuscitated from near-fatal ventricular arrhythmias. *New England Journal of Medicine* **337**, 1576–83.

Shaw DB, Holman RR, Gowers JI (1980). Survival in sinoatrial disorder (sick sinus syndrome). *British Medical Journal* **280**, 139–41.

Viskin S (1999). Long QT syndromes and *torsade de pointes*. *Lancet* **354**, 1625–33.

Wijffels MCEF, *et al.* (1995). Atrial fibrillation begets atrial fibrillation: a study in awake chronically instrumented goats. *Circulation* **92**, 1954–68.

Zipes DP, Wellens HJJ (1998) Sudden cardiac death. *Circulation* **98**, 2334–51.

15.7 Valve disease

D. G. Gibson

Mitral stenosis

Aetiology

Chronic rheumatic heart disease is much the commonest cause of mitral stenosis, though there are a number of other well defined conditions in which blood flow across the mitral valve is limited to a variable extent.

1. Congenital mitral stenosis is a rare condition with thick, rolled leaflets and short chordae, with the spaces between them obliterated. The papillary muscles may be abnormally inserted, either directly from the free wall of the ventricle or from the septum. In parachute mitral valve, there is only one papillary muscle. Congenital mitral stenosis may be associated with left ventricular outflow obstruction, hypoplasia of the left ventricular cavity and the aorta, or endocardial fibroelastosis.

2. A calcified mitral valve ring may rarely cause mild mitral stenosis.

3. In infective endocarditis, bulky vegetations may occasionally interfere with transmitral flow.

4. Nodular rheumatoid arthritis may be associated with thickening of the valve cusps, but true mitral stenosis does not occur.

5. In systemic lupus erythematosus, treatment of Libman–Sachs endocarditis with steroids has led to fibrosis of the cusps with commissural fusion.

6. The combination of ostium secundum atrial septal defect and rheumatic mitral stenosis, Lutembacher syndrome, is probably fortuitous.

Rheumatic mitral stenosis

Incidence

The incidence of rheumatic mitral stenosis parallels that of acute rheumatic fever (see Chapter 15.10.1). It is thus much commoner, and presents earlier, in the Middle East, the Indian sub-continent, and the Far East than in the West.

Pathology

Rheumatic mitral stenosis is due to distortion of the normal mitral valve anatomy with fusion of the commissures. The cusps themselves become vascularized, thickened, and frequently develop thrombus on their atrial surfaces. The chordae become thickened and fused, and the papillary muscles scarred. Finally, the cusps may become calcified. The left ventricle is usually normal or small in pure mitral stenosis, but occasionally dilates. The left atrium is characteristically enlarged with scarring and disruption of muscle fibres. Mural thrombosis is common, particularly on the free wall just above the posterior mitral valve cusp (McCallum's patch). In long-standing cases, calcification of the left atrial wall may develop in plaques on its endocardial surface. In the lungs, the changes of pulmonary venous congestion, pulmonary hypertension, and haemosiderosis develop. These lead to dilatation and hypertrophy of the right ventricle with functional tricuspid regurgitation.

Pathophysiology

The main disturbance in mitral stenosis is due to left ventricular filling. When mitral valve area falls to around 2.5 cm², peak early diastolic ventricular filling rate falls and diastasis is lost. This does not matter at rest when the heart rate is slow and filling period relatively long, but during exercise as the heart rate increases, flow is maintained only by a pressure drop between atrium and ventricle. With a smaller valve area, a pressure drop is present at rest, and mean left atrial pressure rises. Patients with symptomatic mitral stenosis have a valve area of 0.75 to 1.25 cm², and a pressure drop as high as 20 to 30 mmHg across the valve during diastole. Cardiac output falls and pulmonary vascular resistance usually increases.

The subvalvular apparatus may interfere with left ventricular filling by restricting wall movement, so reducing stroke volume and increasing left atrial pressure in the absence of any diastolic pressure drop across the valve itself. Left ventricular cavity size, usually normal in young patients, may increase in the middle aged or elderly, and end-diastolic pressure may rise. A number of factors contribute to such left ventricular disease, including restriction of filling, coronary emboli, and distortion of the septum by right ventricular hypertrophy and overload. In addition, disturbed filling interferes in some way with systolic function, since after successful surgery cavity size usually falls, particularly at end-systole, as stroke volume increases.

Chronic left atrial hypertension causes a corresponding rise in pulmonary capillary pressure; clinical evidence of pulmonary congestion appears when it reaches around 25 mmHg. Further lung disease may be caused by active pulmonary hypertension, repeated pulmonary emboli or chest infections, haemosiderosis, or even bone formation.

Clinical features

Symptoms

The symptoms of mitral stenosis usually appear insidiously, and may have been present for several years before the patient seeks medical attention. They may be apparent within 3 or 4 years of the attack of acute rheumatic fever, or be delayed by up to 50 years. Less frequently, their onset is abrupt with an attack of acute pulmonary oedema, systemic embolism, or the onset of atrial fibrillation.

The commonest manifestation of mitral stenosis is a reduction in exercise tolerance by breathlessness, or less frequently, by fatigue or palpitation in patients in atrial fibrillation. Later in the disease, nocturnal dyspnoea occurs, though florid acute pulmonary oedema has become uncommon. Recurrent chest infections or winter bronchitis are very characteristic; the resulting infected pulmonary oedema responds poorly to antibiotics, and often leads to fluid retention and haemoptysis. Occasionally, massive or recurrent haemoptysis may be the presenting or only symptom of mitral stenosis. Systemic embolism from the left atrium is common in untreated mitral stenosis, particularly when atrial fibrillation is present. Any organ may be affected, but the commonest sites are cerebral, coronary, splenic, renal, mesenteric, or the arteries of the limbs. Salt and water retention is common in untreated mitral stenosis, and leads to peripheral oedema, ascites, pulmonary oedema, and pleural effusion.

Physical examination

Prolonged low cardiac output leads to weight loss and a malar flush.

The character of the pulse is normal, although its amplitude may be decreased and the rhythm irregular due to atrial fibrillation. The arterial pulses should always be checked in view of the possibility of previous arterial emboli.

The venous pressure is usually normal unless tricuspid regurgitation is present. An 'a' wave in the venous pulse of a patient with what appears to be pure mitral stenosis should always raise the possibility of additional tricuspid stenosis or severe pulmonary hypertension.

Palpation of the precordium at the apex may reveal a palpable first sound, previously called a 'tapping apex', and less frequently, a palpable opening snap. It may also be possible to feel pulmonary valve closure at the base of the heart if severe pulmonary hypertension is present. A left parasternal heave is usually due to right ventricular hypertrophy caused by pulmonary hypertension, but may also be due to tricuspid regurgitation, or increased prominence of a normal right ventricle secondary to an enlarged left atrium. In pure mitral stenosis, a sustained apex beat is unusual, but may be seen when the right ventricle is very considerably enlarged or more commonly, because of coexistent left ventricular disease.

On auscultation at the apex, the classic findings are a loud first sound, preceded by a presystolic murmur if the patient is in sinus rhythm, an opening snap, and a mid-diastolic murmur. A loud first sound is less specific for rheumatic mitral stenosis than a palpable one, since it also occurs in high cardiac output states, such as hyperthyroidism. A soft or absent first sound in mitral stenosis strongly suggests that the anterior cusp of the mitral valve is calcified or immobile. An opening snap is a very characteristic physical sign. It is usually loudest at the lower left sternal edge, less commonly the apex or the base. It is a sign of a pliable anterior cusp, and is absent if the valve structure is severely disorganized. The mid-diastolic murmur starts after the opening snap; it is low pitched and persists for a variable period throughout diastole. If the mitral stenosis is mild, the murmur is short, but if the murmur lasts throughout diastole at a normal ventricular rate, then the degree of stenosis is likely to be at least moderately severe. When the rate is rapid due to atrial fibrillation, the murmur may no longer be audible, although in these circumstances, the diagnosis can be suspected from the palpable first sound. However, there are some patients in whom no mid-diastolic murmur is audible even when the heart rate is controlled: so-called 'silent' mitral stenosis. These patients frequently either have severe pulmonary hypertension or a very disorganized and immobile mitral valve.

Investigations

Chest radiography (Fig. 1)

Heart size may be normal or increased. Selective enlargement of the left atrium is the commonest radiographic abnormality, 'selective' implying that the degree of enlargement is proportionately greater than that of the heart shadow as a whole. It appears on the penetrated posteroanterior film as a double outline on the right side of the heart shadow, with elevation of the left main bronchus, and enlargement of the left atrial appendix which forms that part of the left heart border just below the main pulmonary artery. Mitral valve calcification may be visible on the posteroanterior film just to the left of the spine.

In the lung fields, the upper lobe veins may be dilated with the patient in the erect position, indicating that left atrial pressure is raised. The size of the main pulmonary artery can be increased due to pulmonary hypertension. Upper lobe blood diversion occurs when pulmonary vascular resistance is greatly increased: this can be recognized from decreased

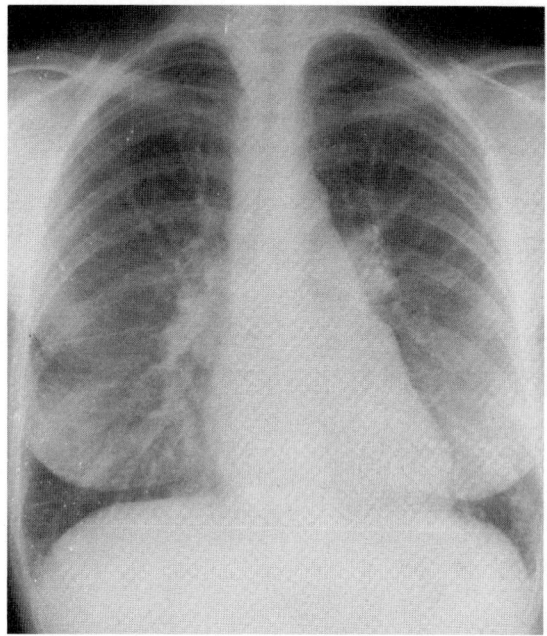

Fig. 1 Chest radiograph from a patient with pure mitral stenosis. Heart size is normal, but the left atrial appendage is enlarged. The upper lobe vessels are dilated and there are Kerley lines at both bases.

prominence of the vessels to the lower zones, while those to the upper zones are normal or increased. Pulmonary oedema occurs when the left atrial pressure reaches approximately 25 to 30 mmHg. It gives rise to lymphatic (Kerley B) lines in the lower zones, basal pleural effusions, generalized hazy shadowing, and finally, obvious interstitial oedema. Pulmonary haemosiderosis is due to long-standing pulmonary congestion. Bone formation, appearing as dense nodules of a few millimetres in diameter, is rarely seen.

ECG

The ECG is not very informative in mitral stenosis. Atrial fibrillation can be confirmed. If the patient is in sinus rhythm, then left atrial hypertrophy causes a bifid P wave in lead II and a dominant negative deflection in V1. ECG evidence of right atrial hypertrophy suggests tricuspid stenosis in addition to mitral stenosis. The electrical axis is usually vertical: right ventricular hypertrophy, if severe, is shown by a dominant R wave in V1.

Echocardiography

On M-mode echocardiography (Fig. 2) the mid-diastolic closure rate of the anterior cusp of the mitral valve is less than 50 mm/s in mild mitral stenosis and 0 to 20 mm/s in severe disease. Cusp fusion causes forward rather than backward movement of the posterior cusp during diastole.

On cross-sectional echocardiography the mobility of the anterior cusp is reduced, particularly near its tip (Fig. 3(a)). Valve area can be estimated semiquantitatively from the parasternal minor axis view (Fig. 3(b)), provided that the cusps are not calcified. The degree of subvalve involvement can be assessed and occasionally atrial thrombus can be detected (Fig. 4).

The diastolic pressure drop across the valve can be estimated by cross-continuous-wave Doppler. Peak right ventricular pressure is derived from the systolic velocity of tricuspid regurgitation. The aortic and tricuspid valves can also be checked.

Transoesophageal echocardiography is particularly useful for demonstrating thrombus in the body of the left atrium or in the left atrial appendix. Spontaneous contrast within the left atrial cavity is probably due to stasis resulting from a combination of atrial fibrillation, low forward flow, and increased cavity size. It indicates an increased risk of thrombus formation. Finally, the degree of thickening and calcification of the cusps and

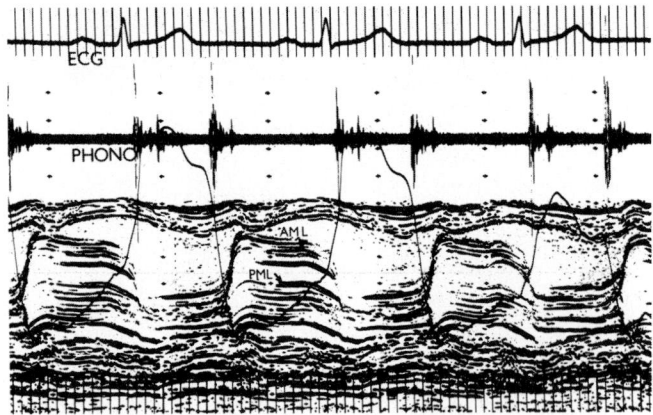

Fig. 2 M-mode echocardiogram from a patient with mitral stenosis. The anterior cusp (AML) is thickened, and its diastolic closure rate is reduced. The posterior leaflet (PML) moves forward during diastole. There is an opening snap on the phonocardiogram, coinciding with maximum forward motion of the anterior cusp.

the extent to which the subvalve apparatus is involved can be assessed particularly well by this approach.

Cardiac catheterization

This is rarely necessary, either to make the diagnosis or to assess severity. It is performed only to determine the state of the coronary arteries in older patients and as a prelude to balloon valvuloplasty, or very occasionally in patients in whom diagnostic echocardiograms cannot be obtained.

Diagnosis

The diagnosis of mitral stenosis is usually straightforward on the basis of history, physical signs, and chest radiography, and can rapidly be confirmed by echocardiography. When the ventricular rate is rapid, the diastolic murmur may be inaudible, but becomes apparent when the ventricular rate is controlled by digoxin. Silent mitral stenosis may mimic primary pulmonary hypertension, but the correct diagnosis is easily made by echocardiography. Mild mitral stenosis should be suspected as a source of systemic emboli and as a cause of unexplained atrial fibrillation, particularly in the elderly.

Differential diagnosis

(1) Left atrial myxoma (see Chapter 15.11.1);

(2) cor triatriatum (see Chapter 15.13);

(3) pulmonary veno-occlusive disease (see Section 15.15.2); or

(4) Austin–Flint murmur (see Aortic regurgitation section, below).

Treatment

Medical

In patients under 30 years of age, longer in some cases, penicillin prophylaxis against further attacks of acute rheumatic fever should be given (see Chapter 15.10.1 for further discussion).

Atrial fibrillation should be treated with a digitalis preparation to control ventricular rate. Anticoagulant therapy must be given to reduce the risk of systemic embolism to all patients with atrial fibrillation, unless there are very strong contraindications. It is also advisable to give anticoagulants to patients in sinus rhythm with mitral stenosis, particularly the middle aged and elderly: the incidence of embolism is significant, especially if they go into atrial fibrillation. The risk of embolism is particularly high when a patient with atrial fibrillation not receiving anticoagulants is admitted to hospital with a rapid heart rate and pulmonary oedema. In this situation intravenous heparin should be given until therapeutic anticoagulation with an oral agent is established.

Fluid retention associated with mitral stenosis responds well to treatment with diuretics. Chest infections should be treated promptly with appropriate antibiotics, and patients should be given a supply of antibiotic to take prophylactically at the start of a head cold. A diuretic is also useful because chest infections often precipitate, or may be precipitated by, fluid retention.

In all patients with valvular heart disease, prophylactic antibiotics should be given for all dental manipulations and other potentially septic hazards (see Chapter 15.10.2).

Mitral valvuloplasty

Rheumatic mitral stenosis results from fusion of the commissures between the two mitral cusps, which is susceptible to rupture by inflating a catheter-mounted balloon across the valve orifice (Fig. 5). Mitral valvuloplasty has the great advantage over surgery of avoiding thoracotomy. A catheter is introduced through the inferior vena cava to the right atrium. The atrial septum is crossed, and the catheter stabilized across the mitral valve, usually by a guidewire passed out through the aortic valve. The balloon itself

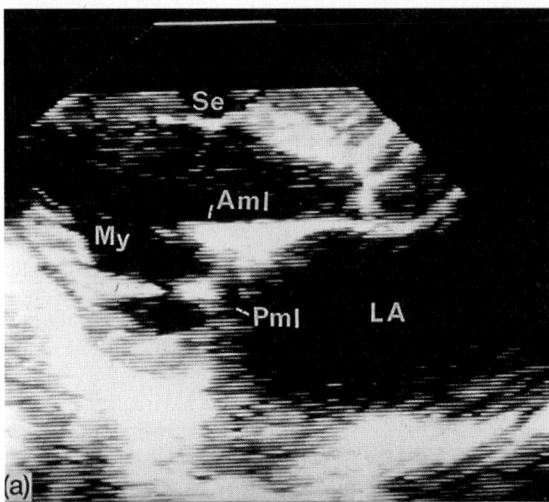

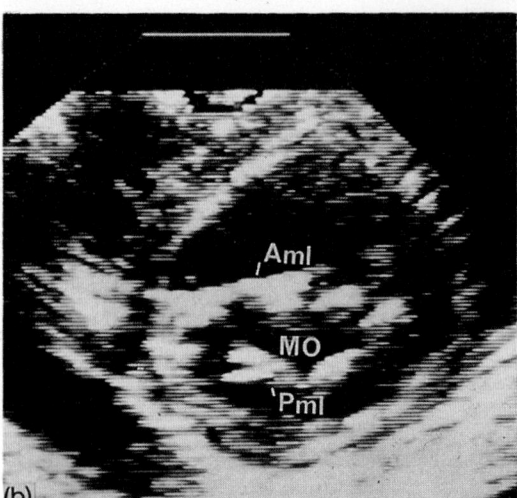

Fig. 3 (a) Two-dimensional echocardiogram from a patient with mitral valve disease; parasternal long-axis view taken in mid-diastole. The anterior cusp (Aml) of the mitral valve is thickened, and fails to open normally. LA, left atrium; Se, septum; My, myocardial echoes; whose intensity is increased due to scarring of the subvalve apparatus; Pml, posterior mitral leaflet. (b) Two-dimensional echocardiogram. Rheumatic mitral valve disease, parasternal minor-axis view during mid-diastole, at the level of the mitral valve orifice (MO), anterior cusp of the mitral valve (AML), and posterior mitral leaflet (Pml).

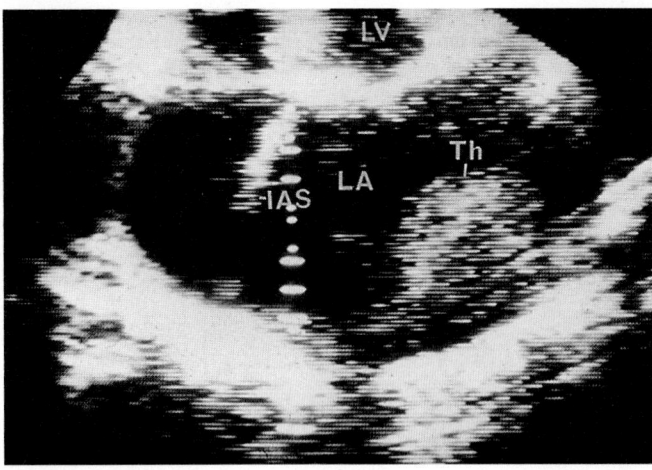

Fig. 4 Left atrial thrombus (Th) in a patient with mitral valve disease. LA, left atrium; LV, left ventricle; IAS, interatrial septum. The left atrium is considerably enlarged.

may be single, often with a waist; less commonly, two balloons are placed simultaneously across the orifice. The balloon is inflated to a predetermined size for 20 s.

Not all patients are suitable for valvuloplasty. It is unsatisfactory in those with calcified and immobile valve cusps, who constitute the majority with mitral stenosis in the developed world. There should be no more than minimal regurgitation. Ideally, the cusps should be thin and mobile, without calcification in the commissures, shortening of the chordae, or scarring of the papillary muscles. Clot in the left atrial appendix must have been excluded by transoesophageal echocardiography. In appropriately selected patients, valvuloplasty gives a satisfactory fall in transmitral pressure drop, maintained in the short and medium term. Mitral regurgitation may be provoked, sometimes severe enough to require valve replacement on an elective or even an emergency basis. The majority of patients are left with a small ASD at the site of passage of the catheter, but this is not of any haemodynamic significance.

Mitral surgery

Surgical procedures available include mitral valvotomy, open or closed, and mitral valve replacement. The choice of operation depends on the anatomy of the mitral valve determined on the basis of the physical signs and the echocardiogram, the age of the patient, and the surgical resources available.

Closed mitral valvotomy is a relatively simple procedure in terms of the resources that are required, although a satisfactory result presupposes con-

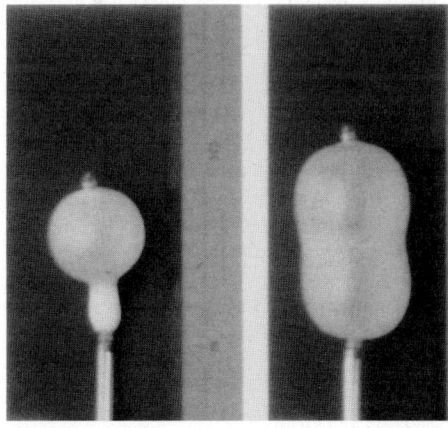

Fig. 5 The Inoue balloon catheter, as used for mitral valvuloplasty, partially (left) and completely (right) inflated.

siderable experience with the operation, experience that is now becoming rare in the developed world. It is particularly suitable in a Third World country, where the major radiographic and expensive disposables necessary for balloon valvuloplasty are not available. It is most effective in a young patient, in sinus rhythm, with evidence of a mobile anterior cusp. It can be regarded as a form of beating heart surgery, and when performed with intraoperative transoesophageal echocardiographic monitoring is particularly effective. Symptom-free follow-up of 40 years or more regularly occurs after this procedure.

Open valvotomy requires cardiopulmonary bypass but allows a more complete procedure to be undertaken, and in particular the subvalvular apparatus can be inspected and adherent chordae divided. If the results of valvotomy are found to be unsatisfactory, it is possible to proceed to valve replacement at the same operation. In general, significant mitral regurgitation is a contraindication to a conservative procedure; although the early results of repair may be excellent, replacement is usually necessary within 5 years.

Valve replacement is necessary when the valve cusps are greatly thickened or calcified. This operation should not be considered in patents in whom the haemodynamic disturbance caused by the valve disease is mild, since the prosthesis causes a resting diastolic pressure drop across it, as well as interfering with systolic and diastolic left ventricular function.

Indications for interventional procedures

It is difficult to lay down hard and fast indications for intervention in patients with mitral stenosis. If the clinical and echocardiographic evidence suggests that valvuloplasty is feasible, then the presence of definite limitation of exercise tolerance is an adequate indication, particularly in a young person. It may also be used in patients with asymptomatic but well developed mitral stenosis before pregnancy. Open valvotomy should be considered if there is any significant contraindication to valvuloplasty. Closed valvotomy is unfortunately no longer available in most developed countries, but it remains a most attractive possibility where medical and surgical resources are limited. In avoiding the use of either radiographic screening or cardiopulmonary bypass, it may be an attractive option for the patient who develops acute pulmonary oedema during pregnancy, provided that local surgical expertise is available.

If valve replacement is likely to be required, then limitation of exercise tolerance should be more severe. In individual patients the decision is not usually difficult when there has been definite progression of symptoms. It is not often necessary to advise operation in a patient with normal exercise tolerance. Unless it is due to coronary artery disease, the presence of left ventricular dilatation is not a contraindication to operation, however severe it may appear to be in terms of increased cavity size or reduced amplitude of wall motion. The same applies to pulmonary hypertension, which is not a contraindication, since it increases the benefits of operation to a greater extent than the risks.

Prognosis

In the absence of surgical treatment, mitral stenosis is usually a progressive disease, although the rate is unpredictable. Unfavourable features include a gradual increase in the severity of the valve disease with disorganization of its structure and superimposed calcification, an increase in pulmonary resistance, and the development of functional tricuspid valve disease, with chronic elevation of the venous pressure leading to cardiac cirrhosis and impaired liver function.

Surgical treatment has considerably improved the prognosis, although conservative mitral surgery does not prevent progression of the rheumatic process, nor does it reduce the risk of infective endocarditis. It has also become clear that the life of biological mitral valve substitutes, particularly the porcine xenograft, is limited to no more than 10 years in the majority of patients above the age of 21, and considerably less than this in children. These valves should thus be confined to the very elderly, and to young women who wish to undertake pregnancy, knowing that repeat surgery will be needed. There are minor differences in haemodynamics between the different types of mechanical valve substitutes, but in individual cases, these are of little consequence.

Mixed mitral valve disease

Mixed mitral valve disease is nearly always rheumatic in origin. The mitral regurgitation is not usually severe in terms of the volume load that it imposes on the left ventricle, though the increased stroke volume increases the diastolic pressure drop across the valve. In general, it occurs in older patients than pure mitral stenosis, and the valve is more disorganized. It is more likely to be calcified with limited cusp mobility and scarred subvalve apparatus. The symptoms are similar. On examination, a pansystolic murmur is evident along with the mid-diastolic murmur. The first sound is not palpable or accentuated. The pansystolic murmur is usually loudest towards the axilla, reflecting the frequent scarring and retraction of the posterior cusp. Chest radiography (Fig. 6) may show more advanced changes than in pure mitral stenosis, and in particular, the left atrium may be very large indeed. ECG is unhelpful. Echocardiogram is likely to show thickened cusps whose motion is reduced as well as mitral regurgitation. Valvuloplasty or conservative surgery are both unsatisfactory, and when symptoms merit, mitral replacement is usually required.

Mitral regurgitation

Aetiology

There are many causes of mitral regurgitation. Any of the components of the mitral valve apparatus may be involved (Table 1).

Degenerative mitral valve disease is the commonest condition to affect the cusps. It has been described under a number of other names, based either on its pathology or on its clinical features: degenerative mitral valve disease, mucinous or myxomatous degeneration, or floppy or ballooning mitral valve. It is a non-inflammatory process partially or completely

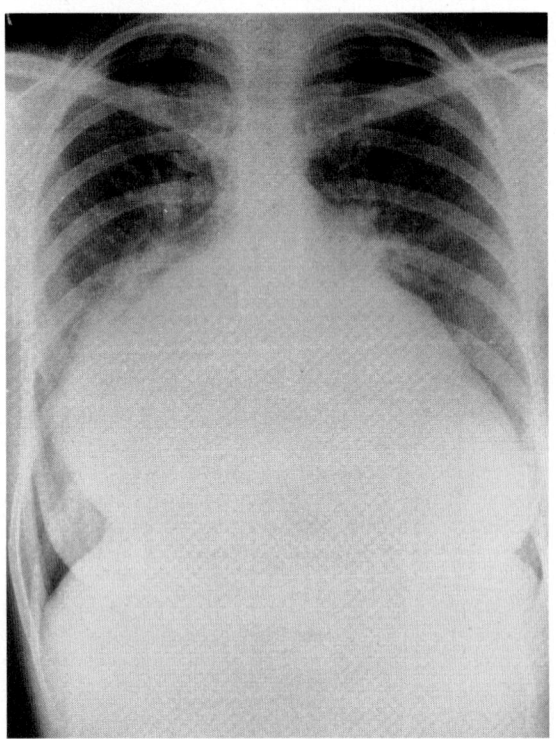

Fig. 6 Chest radiograph from a patient with mixed mitral valve disease, showing gross cardiac enlargement, due mainly to dilation of the left atrium.

Table 1 Common causes of pure mitral regurgitation

Structure affected	Anatomical fault	Pathogenesis
Valve cusps	Congenital cleft	Primary atrial septal defect Isolated
	Redundant cusps	Floppy valve Marfan's syndrome
	Perforation	Infective endocarditis
	Scarring	Rheumatic
	Iatrogenic	
Chordae	Redundant	Floppy valve Marfan's syndrome Other CT diseases
	Rupture	Floppy valve Marfan's syndrome Other CT diseases Infective endocarditis Rheumatic
	Shortening	Rheumatic EMF
Papillary muscle	Dysfunction	Ischaemic heart disease
Cardiomyopathy	Prolapsing cusp	Various
	Rupture	Acute myocardial infarction
Valve ring	Dilatation	Severe LV disease
	Calcification	Various

CT, connective tissue; EMF, endomyocardial fibrosis, LV, left ventricular.

affecting either cusp. Cusp area is increased, causing folding and upward doming into the left atrium during systole. The chordae may become elongated, tortuous, and thinned, predisposing to chordal rupture. Ulceration of the cusps may predispose to thrombosis on their surface and infective endocarditis. Ring circumference may increase. The papillary muscles are normal. Histologically, the centre of the cusp—the fibrosa—is abnormal, with large areas in which collagen bundles are fragmented or absent altogether, and a dense layer of laminated collagen forms on the atrial surface. There is no evidence of vascularization or of inflammatory cells in the absence of secondary infective endocarditis.

The cause of sporadic cases of floppy mitral valve is unknown. However, similar appearances may complicate Marfan's syndrome, pseudoxanthoma elasticum, Ehlers–Danos syndrome, and osteogenesis imperfecta. The incidence of the sporadic condition tends to rise with age, and individual case histories suggest that it can be a very benign and chronic process.

Infective endocarditis is a major cause of symptomatic mitral regurgitation (see Chapter 15.10.2).

Systemic lupus erythematosus can affect both mitral and aortic valves, causing thickening of the cusps and the appearance of sterile vegetations (Libman–Sachs endocarditis). Their appearance and severity fluctuates in individual patients, and does not correlate with other markers of activity of the underlying disease. They rarely give rise to significant haemodynamic disturbance, but may predispose to emboli and to infective endocarditis.

Pathophysiology

Pure mitral regurgitation increases left ventricular output. Since the pressure in the left atrium is lower than that in the aorta, the net force opposing left ventricular ejection is reduced, and stroke volume may be up to three times normal. Ejection begins almost immediately after the start of left ventricular contraction, and by the time the aortic valve opens, up to one-quarter of the stroke volume may already have entered the left atrium. Left atrial pressures are therefore increased, with the V or systolic wave sometimes reaching 50 to 60 mmHg. These high pressures shorten the phase of isovolumic relaxation and greatly increase the velocity of early diastolic left ventricular filling, thus causing the third heart sound. When mitral regurgitation is very severe indeed, left ventricular and left atrial pressure may equalize at mid-ejection. Left ventricular end-diastolic cavity size is not greatly increased, particularly when the history is short, but end-systolic size is considerably smaller than normal due to the low force opposing ejection. Resting left ventricular output is maintained by a sinus tachycardia that is nearly always present when mitral regurgitation is severe.

Clinical features

The clinical picture of pure mitral regurgitation depends on the underlying pathology, the severity of regurgitation, and whether or not the left ventricle is diseased. Different clinical patterns will be described separately, recognizing that they overlap and that the relation between the clinical picture and the underlying aetiology is not fixed.

Ruptured chordae tendineae

Ruptured chorda is a complication of degenerative mitral valve disease and often causes severe mitral regurgitation. It usually occurs spontaneously but may be caused by infective endocarditis. A murmur may have been heard in the past, often many years previously, and described at the time as 'innocent' or 'benign'. The onset of symptoms is usually gradual, but in a minority may be so sudden that patients are able to describe exactly what they were doing at the time. In such cases the symptoms are most severe at their onset, improving over the next few weeks as the ventricle adapts to the volume load. However, even in this more compensated phase, exercise tolerance may be severely limited by breathlessness or fatigue. When the regurgitation is only moderately severe, it can be tolerated remarkably well for many years with minimal symptoms. However, the most severe cases can present in intractable pulmonary oedema, requiring immediate intermittent positive-pressure ventilation.

Physical examination

Patients are usually in sinus rhythm until late in the course of the disease when mitral regurgitation is non-rheumatic. Sinus tachycardia is frequent, and the pulse 'jerky', implying that its amplitude is normal although the upstroke is rapid. The venous pressure is normal unless severe pulmonary hypertension or associated tricuspid regurgitation is present.

The precordial impulse at the apex is prominent and sustained, and may be double due to a palpable third sound. A systolic thrill may also be present. A left parasternal heave reflects systolic expansion of the left atrium rather than right ventricular hypertrophy.

On auscultation, the first sound is normal or reduced in intensity. The most prominent findings are a loud pansystolic murmur and a third heart sound. The third sound may be rather more high-pitched than that associated with left ventricular disease, reflecting the high early diastolic inflow velocity, and may be confused with the second sound. The murmur may thus be mistimed. This mistake can be avoided by starting auscultation at the base of the heart, where the true second sound can be appreciated, and 'inching' the stethoscope towards the apex, when the second heart sound can be heard to bury itself in the murmur as the third sound appears. If the mitral regurgitation is so severe as to cause left atrial and left ventricular pressures to equalize before the end of systole, the murmur stops early. In the most severe cases, presenting with acute pulmonary oedema and shock, the mitral valve is effectively absent and there may be no murmur at all. Unlike rheumatic mitral regurgitation, the position at which the amplitude of the murmur appears maximal is variable: it may be at the apex, down the left sternal edge, at the back, to the left of the spine, or even the top of the head.

Investigations

Chest radiography

The radiographic picture reflects the haemodynamic disturbance (Fig. 7). Overall heart size is normal or only moderately enlarged, with selective enlargement of the left atrium, though not to the same extent as in rheumatic mitral valve disease. The pulmonary vasculature reflects the increase in

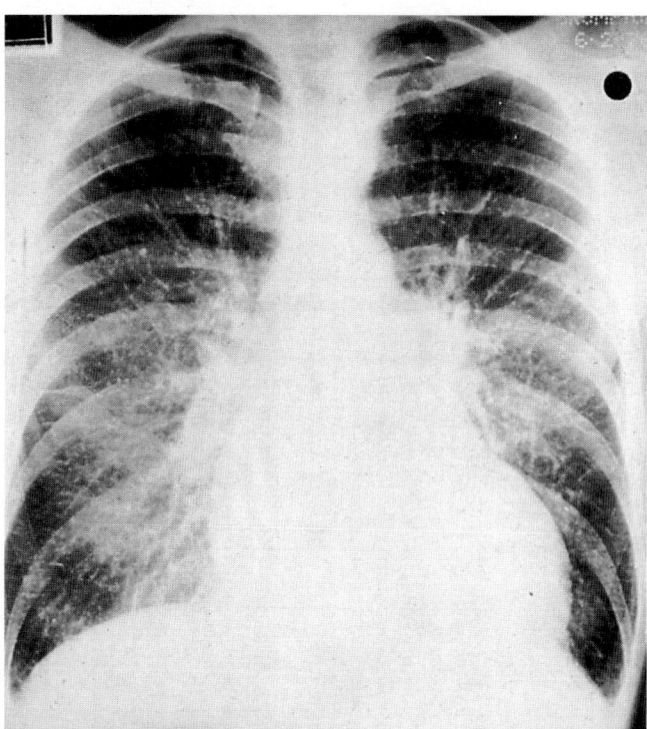

Fig. 7 Chest radiograph showing acute pulmonary oedema due to acute mitral regurgitation resulting from ruptured chordae tendineae.

mean left atrial pressure. A chest radiograph taken soon after the onset of severe mitral regurgitation may show pulmonary oedema with a normal-sized heart. If the condition is severe and long-standing, considerable cardiac enlargement develops due to secondary left ventricular disease.

ECG

The ECG usually shows sinus rhythm with only moderate left ventricular hypertrophy. There may, in addition, be evidence of left atrial hypertrophy. Frequent ventricular ectopic beats are characteristic of mild or moderate mitral regurgitation.

Echocardiography

M-mode echocardiography may show cusp prolapse, with cusp remnants visible in the left atrium during systole. The amplitude of left ventricular wall motion is increased. Initially the end-systolic cavity dimension is small, but it gets larger as the left ventricle adapts, increasing progressively when irreversible left ventricular disease supervenes.

Cross-sectional echocardiography confirms the presence of very active left ventricular wall motion. It allows a clearer view of the extent of systolic cusp prolapse into the left atrium, and the affected cusp is identified more reliably.

Continuous wave Doppler confirms the presence and timing of regurgitation, (Fig. 8) and the jet can be mapped within the left atrium by colour flow. Apparent jet area, whether or not normalized to left atrial cavity size, has proved a disappointing measure of the severity of the regurgitation.

Transoesophageal echo may give more information about valve anatomy, allowing ruptured chordae and small vegetations to be seen in detail. Severe regurgitation causes retrograde flow in the pulmonary veins.

Cardiac catheterization

This is not usually necessary to make the diagnosis when the clinical features and echocardiography are typical, though many surgeons require views of the coronary arteries in older patients when planning operation.

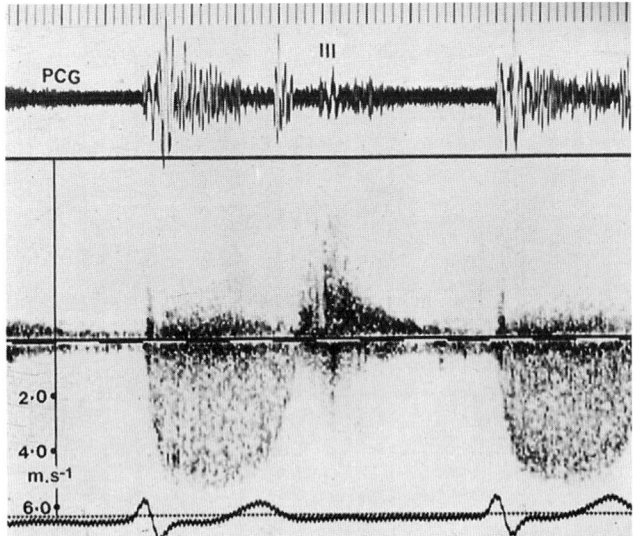

Fig. 8 Doppler cardiogram from a patient with pure mitral regurgitation, showing regurgitant flow as a downward deflection during systole. Diastolic flow velocity pattern is normal, with peak velocity coinciding with the third heart sound (III) on the phonocardiogram (PCG).

Functional mitral regurgitation

Normal mitral closure depends on the integrity of the myocardium as well as that of the valve apparatus itself. In part, the position of the cusps during systole is maintained by contraction of the papillary muscles as the left ventricular cavity gets smaller. This mechanism can be disturbed in a number of ways. The papillary muscles themselves may be affected by ischaemic or other left ventricular disease, so that their ability to contract is impaired. If left ventricular cavity size is greatly increased, the relation between wall movement and papillary muscle shortening becomes abnormal. In hypertrophic cardiomyopathy (see Chapter 15.8.2), the greatly hypertrophied papillary muscles and abnormal cavity shape may contribute to the characteristic forward movement of the whole mitral valve apparatus during systole. Loss of support for the mitral ring itself may occur due to impairment of the function of circumferentially arranged myocardium at the base of the heart.

The term functional mitral regurgitation thus represents the combination of the regurgitation itself, a structurally intact valve apparatus, and left ventricular disease, usually cavity dilatation. It may also be referred to as papillary muscle dysfunction, although this mechanism has not been confirmed directly in humans.

The mitral regurgitation itself is usually mild, though in a minority it may be as severe as that due to ruptured chorda. However, even when mild it may last more than 500 ms, particularly when left bundle branch block is present, so that it limits the time available for ventricular filling when the heart rate is rapid. The clinical picture is therefore usually dominated by impaired left ventricular function. The presence of mitral regurgitation is demonstrated by either a late or a pansystolic murmur, which often varies in its intensity and timing from day to day, and which becomes softer with successful treatment as cavity size and left ventricular diastolic pressures fall.

Echocardiography shows a large cavity with poor wall movement, quite different from the picture seen in severe organic mitral regurgitation. The mitral regurgitation itself can be detected by continuous wave and colour flow Doppler. Cardiac catheterization confirms the presence of a raised left atrial pressure, secondary to a corresponding elevation of the left ventricular end-diastolic pressure. Left ventricular angiography shows a dilated and poorly functioning left ventricle with reflux of contrast into the left atrium, where it tends to accumulate due to poor forward flow. Coronary artery disease as the underlying cause can only be confirmed or excluded by coronary arteriography.

Ruptured papillary muscle

This is a rare and catastrophic complication of acute myocardial infarction, and is quite different from chordal rupture. Papillary muscle rupture is usually complete, though less commonly a single head may be involved. Rupture usually occurs 2 to 5 days after the infarct, and is rarely associated with survival for more than 24 h without very prompt surgical intervention. Whether partial or complete, papillary muscle rupture causes very severe mitral regurgitation, occurring on top of left ventricular impairment caused by the infarct itself. A pansystolic murmur may sometimes be audible at the apex. Death is due to cardiogenic shock and pulmonary oedema.

Partial rupture occurs rather later after the infarct than complete rupture, but similarly causes a striking deterioration in clinical state, along with the development of a pansystolic murmur. The posteromedial papillary muscle is involved more frequently than the anterolateral, both by partial and complete rupture. Since patients are likely to be ventilated, papillary muscle rupture is best diagnosed by transoesophageal echo (Fig. 9), which shows a very active left ventricle and an abnormally mobile mitral valve. The condition requires emergency mitral valve replacement, but even when this can be achieved the prognosis is much worse than that after chordal rupture due to associated left ventricular disease.

Mitral prolapse

Mitral prolapse consists of systolic displacement of one or both mitral valve cusps into the left atrial cavity by 2 mm or more from the line joining the hinge points of the cusps as shown by cross-sectional echocardiography. There may or may not be associated thickening of the cusps themselves. The mid-systolic click occurs as the valve cusps move abruptly backwards into the left atrium during systole (Fig. 10).

The incidence of mitral prolapse, diagnosed on these strict criteria, is less than 2 to 3 per cent in a normal population. In the past, when the diagnosis was made on M-mode alone, or other less specific criteria, a much higher incidence was claimed, approaching 25 per cent in some populations. The majority of well documented cases occur on the basis of mild degenerative mitral valve disease.

From the point of view of clinical manifestations, the main determining factor is the extent to which the margins of the cusps remain apposed during systole, that is, on the extent of secondary mitral regurgitation. It is

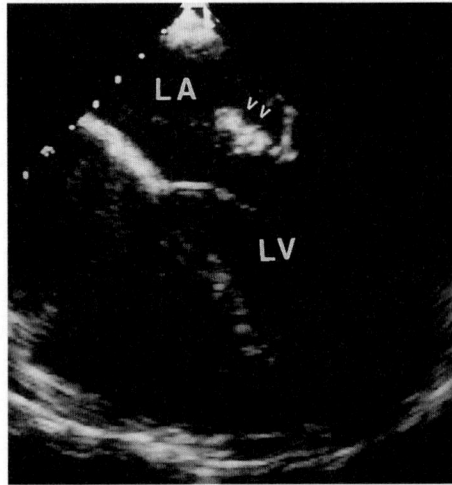

Fig. 9 Transoesophageal cross-section echocardiogram from a patient presenting with ruptured papillary muscle 48 h after acute myocardial infarction. Note the abnormal mobility of the papillary muscle head (indicated by arrows) attached to the anterior mitral valve cusp. LA, left atrium; LV, left ventricle.

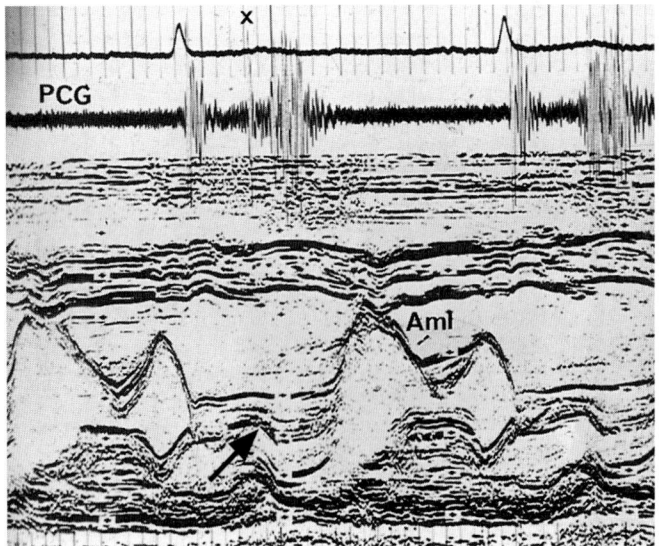

Fig. 10 Mitral valve prolapse, M-mode echocardiogram. Mid-systolic prolapse occurs, marked by the arrow. This is associated with a mid-systolic click (x) and late systolic murmur on the phonocardiogram (PCG).

usually insignificant and unrecognized until a mid-systolic click or late systolic murmur are heard at routine examination. Indeed, in the absence of both the diagnosis may be questioned.

In the past, it was thought that the condition was associated with non-specific chest pain, potentially life-threatening arrhythmias, and cerebral embolism. There is no good evidence for any of these clinical associations. However, mitral prolapse does predispose to infective endocarditis, so that antibiotic prophylaxis is essential. In addition, over the long term, simple mitral prolapse may gradually progress to more severe mitral regurgitation, either by chordal stretching or rupture, particularly when there is evidence of cusp thickening. This type of mitral valve disease is common in Marfan's syndrome and other connective tissue diseases.

Endomyocardial fibrosis

Endomyocardial fibrosis causes fibrosis of the endocardium and underlying myocardium of either or both ventricles. It also involves the papillary muscles, and thus causes secondary mitral regurgitation. It is common in Uganda and surrounding countries in East Africa, where it accounts for approximately 10 per cent of hospital admissions with heart disease, and also in Nigeria in West Africa. It occurs less commonly in south India and Sri Lanka. Occasionally, it is seen in European individuals who have lived in affected areas and very rarely in those who have never been to the tropics.

When the right ventricle is involved, fibrosis starts at the apex and spreads upwards towards the tricuspid valve, involving the papillary muscles and chordae, but sparing the outflow tract. In the left ventricle, the inflow tract, apex, and lower part of the outflow tract are usually involved, and also the posterior mitral valve cusp and its papillary muscle. In both ventricles there is involvement of the underlying myocardium and mural thrombosis. The result is atrioventricular valve regurgitation, an abnormally stiff ventricle, and very high atrial pressures.

The aetiology is unknown, but it does not appear to be related to rheumatic fever or any vector-borne virus, although the incidence increases with malnutrition.

The clinical picture is of progressive mitral or tricuspid insufficiency of insidious onset, together with restriction of ventricular filling by subendocardial scarring. When the tricuspid valve is mainly involved, there is gross fluid retention, whereas mitral or combined involvement leads to pulmonary oedema. Emboli from the right or left ventricle are common.

Medical treatment consists of high doses of diuretic and vasodilators, preferably an ACE inhibitor, if valvular regurgitation is severe. Decortica-

tion of the ventricular cavities may be possible surgically, along with replacement of mitral or tricuspid valve.

Mitral ring calcification

Heavy calcification of the mitral valve ring is a disease of the elderly, and is particularly common in women. Although it appears to be a degenerative condition, it occurs more frequently with left ventricular hypertrophy. It does not usually cause symptoms, and is detected incidentally by calcification in the mitral ring on chest radiography or on echocardiography. The central fibrous body may also be involved, with calcium spreading down the anterior cusp. However, the condition is not totally benign. The valve is a potential source of platelet emboli, and a focus for infective endocarditis. Approximately half the patients have abnormalities of conduction, including high-grade atrioventricular block, sinus node disease, or bundle branch block. Mild mitral regurgitation is common, but rarely is it severe enough to need valve replacement. Very occasionally the condition has been reported as causing mitral stenosis, with a diastolic pressure drop of up to 20 mmHg.

In the absence of complications, no treatment is required other than low-dose aspirin and prophylaxis against infective endocarditis. Complications are treated on their own merits.

Diagnosis of mitral regurgitation

The diagnosis of mitral regurgitation is usually straightforward on the basis of the physical signs, with a pansystolic murmur and third heart sound when it is haemodynamically significant, and a late systolic murmur when it is due to mitral prolapse and mild. Cardiac enlargement and pulmonary congestion on chest radiography reflect the extent both of the regurgitation itself and of associated left ventricular disease. Echocardiography is invaluable in assessing such cases. Abnormalities of mitral valve anatomy can be detected and associated abnormalities of left ventricular function quantified, whether due to volume overload or associated ventricular disease.

Difficulties in diagnosis may arise when mitral regurgitation is of acute origin and very severe. Patients may present with pulmonary oedema of sudden and unexplained onset with a chest radiograph showing a normal-sized heart shadow. Echocardiography demonstrates very active left ventricular wall movement, showing that the poor peripheral blood flow is due to valvular regurgitation rather than left ventricular disease, and in addition, one or both mitral valve cusps may be abnormally mobile, usually as the result of chordal or papillary muscle rupture. However, the Doppler echocardiogram may be atypical, showing an abbreviated regurgitant flow signal of low velocity reflecting near equalization of ventricular and atrial pressures. Such low blood velocities make colour flow Doppler particularly misleading.

In patients who present with more typical signs, the main diagnostic problem is to decide the relative contributions of valvular regurgitation and left ventricular disease to the overall clinical state. In such cases, intrinsic disease of the mitral valve apparatus suggests that ventricular disease is secondary to long-standing regurgitation, while normal mitral valve anatomy suggests the reverse.

Differential diagnosis

1. Ventricular septal defect (see Chapter 15.13).

2. Aortic valve disease—The ejection systolic murmur of aortic valve disease is frequently audible at the apex, where it may be louder than at the base, and have a slightly different quality. However, this is not an adequate basis for diagnosing additional mitral regurgitation and it is essential to establish that the timing of the murmur is pansystolic, either from its relation to the second heart sound, or in aortic regurgitation, from its relation to the start of the early diastolic murmur.

3. Tricuspid regurgitation—The pansystolic murmur of tricuspid regurgitation may be mistaken for that of mitral regurgitation, particularly when the right ventricle is greatly enlarged. The presence of tricuspid

regurgitation can be suspected from an elevated venous pressure with systolic waves, and confirmed by Doppler echocardiography. In severe mitral regurgitation, however, additional tricuspid regurgitation may be present.

Treatment of mitral regurgitation

Mild or moderately severe mitral regurgitation is well tolerated and does not require treatment apart from prophylactic antibiotic for all dental manipulations and potentially septic hazards. If left ventricular size is increased either on chest radiograph or echocardiogram an ACE inhibitor should be added. Such patients should be followed up at annual intervals, since mitral regurgitation may be progressive, particularly when due to degenerative disease.

When mitral regurgitation is functional and mild, treatment is again medical and that of the underlying left ventricular disease. However, in a minority of patients with severe ischaemic ventricular disease, a more aggressive surgical approach may be warranted. Mitral regurgitation due to hypertrophic cardiomyopathy does not require specific treatment.

Severe mitral regurgitation, which causes significant symptoms in spite of medical treatment, is best managed by mitral valve surgery. This will involve either mitral valve replacement, or in suitable cases, mitral valve repair. The long-term prognosis following mitral repair is better than that after replacement, both with respect to survival and functional result. The exact reasons for the difference are not clear, but are probably because replacement involves insertion of a rigid mitral ring and section of the papillary muscles with very abnormal flow patterns into the ventricle. Mitral repair is thus to be preferred whenever possible, and in suitable cases can be recommended earlier in the course of the disease. It is particularly satisfactory with non-rheumatic regurgitation due to posterior cusp prolapse, and in an increasing number of patients with anterior cusp prolapse as surgical techniques develop.

The timing of operation is critical. After acute chordal rupture, it is often possible to treat the patients medically with rest, diuretics, and vasodilators for 1 to 2 weeks, while the left ventricle enlarges to compensate for the increased volume load. Clinical improvement may be striking, so that surgery becomes a less hazardous procedure than an emergency operation in the acute stage would have been. By contrast, those with a ruptured papillary muscle should undergo surgery at the earliest opportunity. Until this is possible, their pulmonary oedema is best treated by intermittent positive-pressure ventilation. Any benefit of pharmacological treatment or balloon counterpulsation is marginal at best, and probably only distracts attention from the main aim, which should be to get the patient to surgery as soon as possible.

The treatment of papillary muscle dysfunction is that of the underlying ventricular disease, with the particular aim of reducing the left ventricular diastolic pressures. In a minority of cases, hibernating myocardium will respond to vein grafting. Mitral valve replacement should be avoided whenever possible, since the deterioration in ventricular function caused by the valve replacement itself usually outweighs any benefit from correction of the regurgitation. A more promising approach is to insert an undersized mitral ring, leaving the mitral apparatus otherwise intact. This not only corrects the regurgitation but also may reduce basal left ventricular cavity size and thus systolic wall stress.

Aortic stenosis

Aortic stenosis represents a fixed obstruction to left ventricular ejection into the aorta. The obstruction is most commonly at the level of the valve itself, aortic valvar stenosis, but may also be immediately above the sinuses, supravalvar stenosis, or within the left ventricle, subvalvar stenosis.

Table 2 Types of aortic stenosis

Valvular
Congenital
Fused commissure 'bicuspid'
Rheumatic
'Senile' (calcified tricuspid valve)
Infective endocarditis (rare)
Hyperlipidaemia (rare)
Fixed subaortic
Membrane
Tunnel
Supravalvular

Aetiology

Types of valvar aortic stenosis are summarized in Table 2. Valvar aortic stenosis is an important cause of cardiac disability, and though it is commonest in the elderly, it may present at any time of life. Congenital aortic stenosis, due to a valve with only a single commissure, is most frequent in infancy or childhood. Congenital bicuspid valve, consisting of fusion of one of the three commissures, is a much commoner abnormality. It may be detected as an incidental finding early in life, but does not usually give rise to significant haemodynamic abnormality unless it becomes calcified or involved by infective endocarditis. Rheumatic aortic stenosis develops as the result of commissural fusion in a tricuspid valve and may subsequently become calcified. Senile or degenerative aortic stenosis results from deposition of calcium in a tricuspid valve, initially on the aortic surface by a process similar to atherosclerosis. Calcification of a tricuspid valve is becoming an increasingly important cause of disability in the elderly. Very rarely, vegetations in infective endocarditis or lipid deposits in hyperlipidaemia may be bulky enough to cause significant left ventricular outflow tract obstruction.

Pathophysiology

Blood flow across a stenotic aortic valve causes a pressure drop between the left ventricular cavity and the aorta, which in symptomatic cases, may be greater than 60 mmHg at rest, and reach over 200 mmHg on exertion. Stroke work is therefore increased and left ventricular hypertrophy develops. Wall thickness increases although cavity size remains normal or even falls. A corresponding increase in the coronary vascular bed does not occur, predisposing to myocardial ischaemia, particularly in the subendocardial region. Hypertrophy, ischaemia, and associated fibrosis cause the diastolic stiffness of the myocardium to increase so that the end-diastolic pressure may rise causing pulmonary congestion. Increased left ventricular wall thickness also predisposes to ventricular arrhythmias. Late in the disease, when left ventricular involvement is severe, the cavity dilates and becomes more spherical. Calcification may spread from the aortic valve to the anterior cusp of the mitral valve or into the septum where it can involve the conducting system which runs nearby.

Aortic stenosis is most common in patients with a high incidence of ischaemic heart disease, so that obstructive coronary artery disease may contribute coincidentally to symptoms or impairment of left ventricular function.

Clinical features

Symptoms

The three characteristic clinical features of aortic stenosis are breathlessness, chest pain, and syncope.

Breathlessness in aortic stenosis is frequently associated with an elevated left ventricular end-diastolic pressure and occurs at first on exercise, but later at rest. Paroxysmal nocturnal dyspnoea and episodic pulmonary oedema—breathlessness persisting for 5 min or more after exercise—are both common in late stages of the disease and indicate the need for urgent treatment. The length of the history of breathlessness from its onset until it becomes severe is usually only of the order of 1 to 2 years, and thus considerably shorter than that in mitral stenosis.

Angina occurring in aortic stenosis is clinically indistinguishable from that due to coronary artery disease, which in many cases is the main cause. However, typical anginal pain can occur in patients in whom the large and medium-sized coronary arteries are normal. The mechanism for this is uncertain, but disproportion between muscle mass and coronary vascular bed, and the direct effects of abnormal myocardial relaxation in left ventricular hypertrophy are both likely to contribute.

There are several causes of syncope in aortic stenosis. In some patients it is clearly related to exertion and appears to be due to hypotension resulting from the combination of exercise-induced vasodilation and a fixed cardiac output. In other cases it results from transient complete atrioventricular block due to involvement of the atrioventricular node by calcification, carotid sinus hypersensitivity, or even from short periods of ventricular tachycardia or fibrillation.

Physical examination

The physical signs of well developed aortic stenosis are very characteristic.

1. The carotid pulse is slow rising with a reduced amplitude and an early notch on the upstroke, followed by a thrill.

2. The venous pressure is usually normal until late in the disease, but a small 'a' wave is frequently present. This cannot be taken as evidence of pulmonary hypertension, but appears to be related in some way to the presence of left ventricular hypertrophy (Bernheim 'a' wave).

3. The apex beat is sustained and is often double, due to an additional left atrial impulse.

4. On auscultation, the first sound is normal or soft, and may be preceded by a fourth heart sound. The second sound is single when the valve is calcified, due to lack of the aortic component. In younger patients with mobile valve cusps, aortic valve closure may be audible, but delayed, so that splitting of the second sound is reversed. When left ventricular disease is severe, pulmonary valve closure is accentuated. The characteristic ejection systolic murmur is maximal at the base of the heart, and is also audible over the right common carotid artery. It may seem longer than the ejection systolic murmur of, for example, anaemia or thyrotoxicosis because in aortic stenosis, ventricular systole is prolonged and aortic valve closure delayed. A soft early diastolic murmur is nearly always present, although this does not imply haemodynamically significant aortic regurgitation.

As ventricular disease progresses and stroke volume falls, these physical signs are modified. Pulse volume drops and loses its slow rising quality. The aortic murmur becomes shorter and softer, and a third heart sound and functional mitral regurgitation appear.

Investigations

Chest radiography

Heart size is normal in uncomplicated aortic stenosis. If it is increased, the underlying cause is likely to be unsuspected aortic regurgitation, left ventricular cavity dilatation, or very severe left ventricular hypertrophy, when the cavity may be normal in size, but the myocardium up to 50 mm thick. Increased left ventricular filling pressure may cause left atrial hypertension and thus dilatation of the upper lobe vessels as well as selective enlargement of the left atrium in the absence of organic mitral valve disease. The aortic root is nearly always dilated and the aortic valve calcified in older patients: this is best seen on the lateral chest radiograph or with screening.

ECG

The ECG characteristically shows changes of left ventricular hypertrophy, although it may be entirely normal, even in the presence of severe aortic stenosis. Left atrial hypertrophy is shown by a bifid P wave in lead II or a dominant negative deflection in V1. Conduction disturbances include left

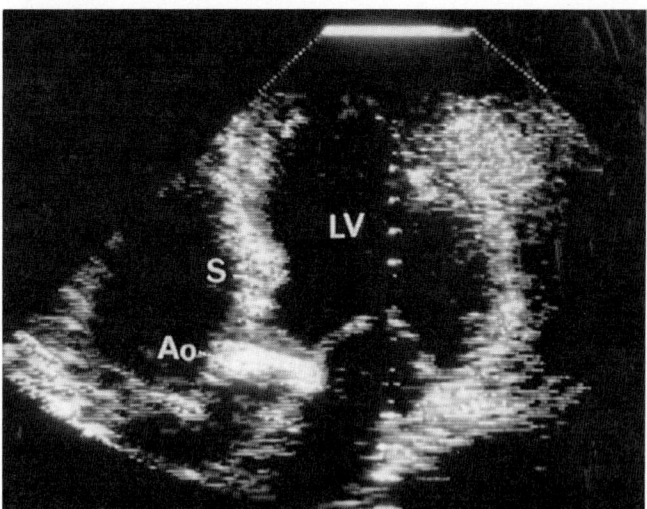

Fig. 11 Aortic stenosis, two-dimensional echocardiogram from apical four-chamber view, showing left ventricle (LV) and heavily calcified aortic valve (Ao). S, septum.

axis deviation, left bundle branch block, prolonged P–R interval, or complete heart block. Poor progression of R waves across the chest leads is common, and suggests septal hypertrophy rather than anterior myocardial infarction.

Echocardiography

Cross-sectional echocardiography demonstrates thickening and reduced mobility of the valve cusps. In young patients with a bicuspid valve, doming of the cusps during systole can be seen, while in older patients, a calcified aortic valve appears as an immobile mass (Fig. 11).

The pressure drop across the outflow tract can be reliably measured by continuous wave Doppler. Additional aortic regurgitation can also be detected. Left ventricular anatomy and function, both in terms of the extent of hypertrophy and cavity size and ejection fraction can be studied.

Transverse dimension and myocardial thickness can be measured by M-mode. Late in disease, the left ventricle becomes enlarged and its ejection fraction falls to values commonly seen in dilated cardiomyopathy.

Cardiac catheterization

The abnormal haemodynamics of aortic stenosis and associated left ventricular disease can usually be comprehensively demonstrated by echocardiography. The role of cardiac catheterization is thus to confirm the pressure drop across the valve in the minority of patients in whom this is not possible for technical reasons using continuous wave Doppler, and to display coronary artery anatomy.

Diagnosis

A complete diagnosis of aortic stenosis depends not only on establishing the anatomical abnormality, but also its severity and the degree of associated left ventricular disease. When cardiac output is normal, a peak pressure drop across the valve of greater than 60 mmHg indicates significant stenosis, and corresponds to a valve area of 0.9 cm^2 or less. The corresponding peak velocity, as measured by continuous wave Doppler is 4.0 m/s.

Mild aortic stenosis is associated with a normal carotid pulse and a short systolic murmur which stops well before the second sound, since a pressure difference between the left ventricular cavity and the aorta is present only during the first part of systole. In addition, both components of the second heart sound are audible and splitting is normal. An uncalcified bicuspid aortic valve causes mild stenosis, with an ejection click and systolic murmur, often followed by a short early diastolic murmur.

Left ventricular hypertrophy can be inferred from a sustained apical impulse with a palpable left atrial contraction. A raised left ventricular end-diastolic pressure can be deduced from accentuation of pulmonary valve closure, which forms the only component of the second sound and, in the late stages of the disease, a third heart sound. In such patients the stroke volume is low, the pressure drop across the valve falls, and significant stenosis may be associated with values of 30 to 40 mmHg. To allow for this, it is necessary to measure valve area.

Differential diagnosis

1. Hypertrophic cardiomyopathy—This can present with a history very similar to that of aortic stenosis. By contrast, the carotid pulse is normal or jerky rather than slow rising. The diagnosis is confirmed by echocardiography, which reveals a normal aortic valve and shows characteristic ventricular features (see Chapter 15.8.2).

2. Congestive cardiomyopathy—Patients with long-standing untreated aortic stenosis can present with severe breathlessness, a large heart on radiography, a small volume pulse with a normal upstroke, a third heart sound, and pansystolic murmur due to papillary muscle dysfunction. These features can all be found in congestive cardiomyopathy (see Chapter 15.8.2). In endstage aortic stenosis, the echocardiogram shows a calcified valve with a significant (more than 35 mmHg) pressure drop across it: in congestive cardiomyopathy it shows a dilated and poorly contractile ventricle, but the aortic valve is normal.

3. Fixed subaortic stenosis—This is usually discovered in asymptomatic children and young adults in whom a systolic murmur is detected on routine examination. An ejection click is absent, and a short early diastolic murmur usually heard. There is clinical and ECG evidence of left ventricular disease, which may be severe. The two-dimensional echocardiogram usually demonstrates the site and type of obstruction (see also Chapter 15.13).

Prognosis

The prognosis of symptomatic aortic stenosis is poor with a 50 per cent survival of only 1 to 2 years. Approximately half the deaths are due to relentless haemodynamic deterioration, and the remainder are 'sudden' and unexpected. The prognosis of asymptomatic but haemodynamically severe aortic stenosis is somewhat better. However, older patients with a peak velocity of 4 m/s or more across the aortic valve are likely to become symptomatic in a period of 2 years or less.

Exercise testing is as safe in aortic stenosis as it is in coronary artery disease, and using it a significant number of 'asymptomatic' patients can be shown to have reduced exercise tolerance. The truly asymptomatic patient, often below the age of 30 years, with normal ECG and without left ventricular hypertrophy or cavity dilatation on echocardiogram, can safely be watched. Regular follow-up of such patients is essential, and surgery should be considered with any evidence of deterioration.

Treatment

Medical treatment has little to offer in aortic stenosis: in mild cases it is unnecessary and in severe cases ineffective. However, it is essential that all patients with aortic stenosis, of whatever severity, have prophylactic antibiotic for any potentially septic hazard. Patients with severe left ventricular disease and fluid retention will benefit from a period of bed rest and treatment with a diuretic before operation is contemplated. ACE inhibitors are contraindicated.

Severe aortic stenosis requires intervention. Unfortunately, aortic balloon valvuloplasty, though satisfactory in infants and children, is either ineffective or harmful in adults in whom the cusps are calcified, and the procedure has been largely abandoned, even as a temporizing manoeuvre in very ill patients. Aortic valve replacement for aortic stenosis is amongst the most effective of all surgical operations. In uncomplicated cases, it can be carried out with low mortality and morbidity, and should therefore be considered in all patients in whom the disease causes significant symptoms. It is likely to relieve breathlessness, angina, and syncope, whether due to ischaemic heart disease or to the aortic stenosis itself. Associated coronary artery disease is usually treated with bypass grafting at the same operation. Aortic valve replacement is also effective when significant aortic stenosis is complicated by severe left ventricular enlargement. Although the risks of surgery are greater, so are the benefits, and the remarkable improvement in symptoms and prognosis that may follow surgery for this combination of valve and ventricular disease is amongst the most gratifying in cardiology.

Mixed aortic valve disease

Mild to moderate aortic regurgitation often accompanies aortic stenosis, but does little to alter the overall clinical picture. The combination may result from a bicuspid aortic valve, chronic rheumatic heart disease, or be the result of conservative surgery or endocarditis on a stenotic valve. The main haemodynamic disturbance remains increased resistance to ejection rather than a volume load. In addition, superimposition of even a moderately increased stroke volume due to regurgitation on the small, stiff left ventricular cavity of pure aortic stenosis may lead to high filling pressures, left atrial enlargement, and even pulmonary hypertension. Breathlessness and chest pain thus remain the most prominent symptoms. The arterial pulse is bisferiens, with a notch half way up the upstroke, rather than slow rising. Atrial fibrillation usually points to a rheumatic basis; less commonly to high filling pressures in an incompliant cavity. The early diastolic murmur is audible down the left sternal edge. The extent of the volume load, the aortic pressure drop, and the presence or absence of rheumatic mitral involvement can all be determined by echocardiography. Treatment of symptomatic patients is likely to require valve replacement.

Aortic regurgitation

Aortic regurgitation increases stroke volume and when severe and uncorrected causes irreversible left ventricular disease. Its causes are summarized in Table 3.

Pathology

Chronic rheumatic involvement leads to a tricuspid valve whose cusps are thickened, with rolled edges and fused commissures. There may be superimposed calcification or thrombosis. Infective endocarditis may lead to cusp destruction or perforation and may spread to involve the sinus of Valsalva, the atrioventricular node and the interventricular septum, where abscess formation may occur. Organisms may also be carried to the anterior cusp of the mitral valve, where they cause 'jet lesions', localized aneurysms, or perforations. Dilatation of the aortic ring may cause aortic

Table 3 Causes of aortic regurgitation

Cusp	
Distortion	
Rheumatic	
Rheumatoid	
Perforation	
Infective endocarditis	
Traumatic	
Ring	
Dilatation	
Dissecting aneurysm	
Marfan's syndrome	
Syphilis	
Ankylosing spondylitis	
Reiter's syndrome, ulcerative colitis	
Loss of support	
Subaortic ventricular septal defect	

regurgitation with normal cusps. This can result from a 'flask-shaped' aneurysm of the ascending aorta, complicating Marfan's syndrome, or isolated medionecrosis. Syphilitic aortitis causes dilatation of the valve ring, with aneurysm formation of the ascending aorta and involvement of the coronary ostia. Dilatation of the ring may occur on its own or with connective tissue disease such as ankylosing spondylitis, rheumatoid arthritis, Reiter's syndrome, or relapsing polychondritis. Dissecting aneurysm involving the aortic root may separate the cusps from the valve ring; and the presence of a high ventricular septal defect or Fallot tetralogy may leave the cusps unsupported from below.

Pathophysiology

Aortic regurgitation is associated with an increase in left ventricular stroke volume and cavity size. Ventricular mass is therefore increased, but wall thickness is usually within normal limits. In moderately severe aortic regurgitation, the stroke volume is twice normal, and in severe cases, up to three or even four times normal. The characteristics of ejection are altered in that the end-diastolic pressure in the aorta is low, so that the resistance to ejection of blood by the left ventricle is reduced and ventricular systole is prolonged. These factors together with the large stroke volume, explain the characteristic rapid upstroke and large volume pulse. Peripheral vasodilatation also contributes to the large forward stroke volume. In long-standing cases, left ventricular cavity size increases out of proportion to the stroke volume, with loss of the normal myocardial architecture, so that the cavity becomes more spherical in shape; the walls become stiffer and the end-diastolic pressure increases.

Clinical features

Symptoms

Patients with aortic regurgitation remain asymptomatic for many years. When symptoms develop, they are those of left ventricular disease, with limitation of exercise tolerance by breathlessness or chest pain the most prominent one. Less commonly, the presenting symptom may be nocturnal dyspnoea, or an attack of acute pulmonary oedema. Retrosternal pain, aggravated by exertion, may develop in patients with aneurysms of the ascending aorta in whom the coronary arteries are normal. This seems to originate from the aortic root itself. Aortic dissection (see Chapter 15.14.1) may also cause severe central chest pain.

Physical signs

The physical signs of aortic regurgitation are characteristic.

1. The carotid pulse has a large amplitude and a rapid upstroke. Visible arterial pulsation in the neck (Corrigan's sign) excludes significant aortic stenosis. Other physical signs which depend on a large pulse volume and peripheral vasodilation include capillary pulsation, visible in the nail beds, and the de Musset sign, nodding of the head in time with the heart beat. The Durosiez sign, which is of greater clinical value, is elicited by compression of the femoral artery and listening proximally with the stethoscope for a diastolic murmur. It may be positive even when an aortic diastolic murmur is inaudible, and implies retrograde flow in the femoral artery due to aortic regurgitation that is at least moderately severe. The peripheral pulses should always be checked to exclude the presence of coarctation of the aorta.

2. The venous pressure is normal until late in the course of the disease, although the venous pulse may show a dominant 'a' wave (a Bernheim 'a').

3. The left ventricular impulse is sustained, indicating hypertrophy. A palpable 'a' wave is much less common than in aortic stenosis, and when present usually denotes additional left ventricular disease.

4. On auscultation, the characteristic finding is an early diastolic murmur, maximal down the left sternal edge. Less commonly it is loudest at the apex or even in the left axilla (the Cole–Cecil murmur). An ejection

systolic murmur is nearly always present, due to the increased stroke volume, and not necessarily to additional stenosis. Aortic valve closure is usually inaudible, but P2 may be accentuated due to passive pulmonary hypertension. At the apex, a mid-diastolic murmur may be heard, indistinguishable from that of mitral stenosis (Austin–Flint murmur). This may continue throughout diastole, with presystolic accentuation and even a loud first heart sound, though the last is never palpable. With the development of ventricular disease, a soft mitral pansystolic murmur or a third sound may appear.

These classic signs of aortic regurgitation may be modified in a number of circumstances. If infective endocarditis has caused cusp perforation, then the early diastolic murmur may have a high-pitched musical quality, a 'seagull murmur'. In the presence of severe left ventricular disease, or less commonly, of rheumatic mitral stenosis or severe pulmonary hypertension, the collapsing pulse, and other evidence of aortic regurgitation may be lost, although the aortic diastolic murmur persists. It is worth noting, however, that Durosiez' sign frequently remains positive in these circumstances if the regurgitation is moderate or severe. In severe aortic regurgitation of rapid onset, usually due to infective endocarditis affecting the aortic valve, the patient presents with a low cardiac output state, normal or reduced pulse volume, and sinus tachycardia. On auscultation the main abnormality is a loud third sound, due to a very short period of forward flow across the mitral valve. A short early diastolic murmur may be audible. Durosiez' sign is usually positive.

Investigations

Chest radiography

Significant aortic regurgitation nearly always causes cardiac enlargement on chest radiography (Fig. 12). The aortic root is often dilated, but the aortic valve not necessarily calcified. The pulmonary vessels remain normal until severe left ventricular disease develops.

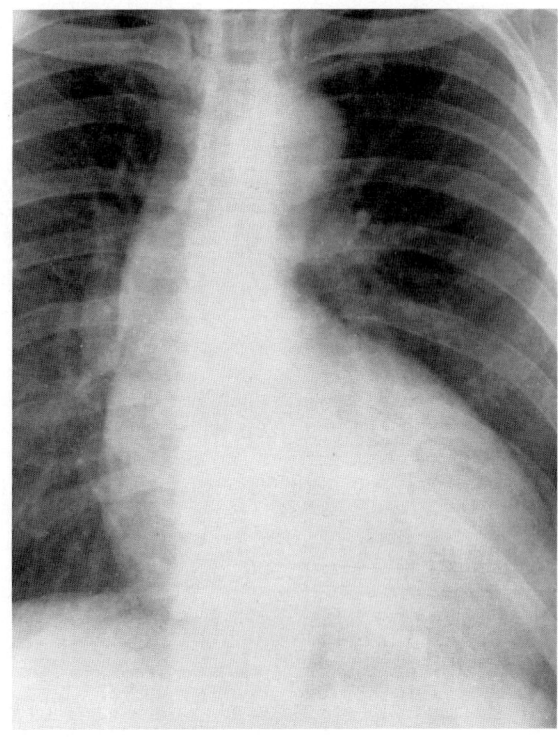

Fig. 12 Chest radiograph from a patient with chronic aortic regurgitation showing cardiac enlargement and dilation of the ascending aorta.

ECG

This usually shows left ventricular hypertrophy on voltage and T-wave criteria, with left atrial enlargement. The duration of the QRS complex increases and left bundle branch block may develop, indicating the presence of intrinsic left ventricular disease. A long P–R interval in association with aortic regurgitation is very suggestive of disease of the aortic root.

Echocardiography

The anatomy of the aortic valve and root can be determined. Dissection and aortic root abscesses can sometimes be detected; vegetations on the aortic valve are well. When infective endocarditis is suspected, transoesophageal echo may give further useful information, particularly if the P–R interval is prolonged. It is also the means of choice for demonstrating aortic root aneurysms. Colour flow Doppler allows the presence of regurgitation to be confirmed and a semiquantitative estimate made of its severity. Left ventricular cavity size is determined from the M-mode record (Fig. 13).

In acute aortic regurgitation, the mitral valve closes prematurely. This is the result of severe regurgitation into a relatively non-compliant left ventricle causing the cavity pressure to rise, closing the mitral valve in mid-diastole (Fig. 14). As ventricular diastolic pressure rises, the pressure drop from the aorta to the ventricle in diastole may fall to 20 mmHg or less, which is reflected in the continuous wave Doppler record across the valve in diastole. This is pathophysiologically significant, since the pressure difference between aorta and left ventricle during diastole supports coronary flow. Hence, as aortic regurgitation becomes more severe, coronary flow to a volume-loaded ventricle becomes progressively compromised.

Cardiac catheterization

It is not usually necessary to resort to cardiac catheterization to make the diagnosis of aortic regurgitation. Although an aortogram may give useful information, it should be avoided in seriously ill patients because radiographic contrast medium expands the plasma volume and depresses ventricular function. The anatomy of the aortic root is best demonstrated by

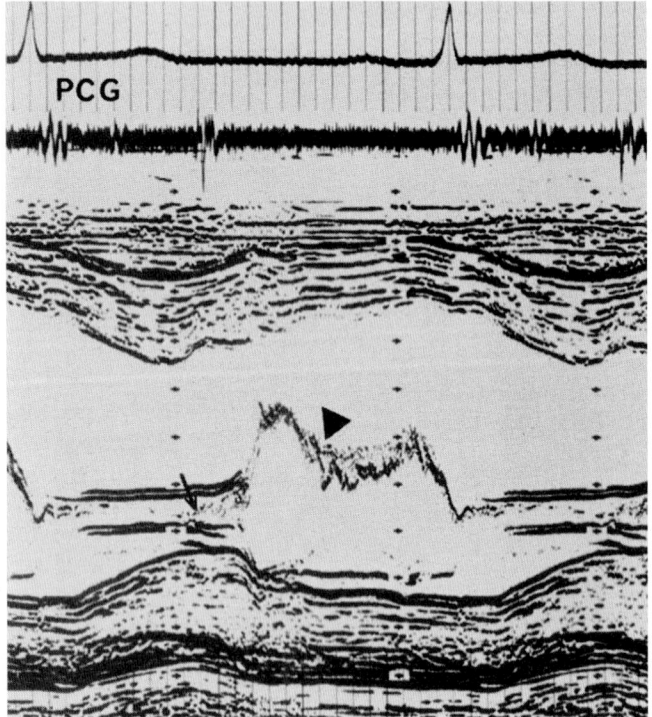

Fig. 13 Chronic aortic regurgitation. M-mode echocardiogram, showing dilatation of the left ventricular cavity; also 'flutter' on the anterior cusp of the mitral valve, marked by arrow, caused by the regurgitant aortic jet striking the cusp. PCG, phonocardiogram.

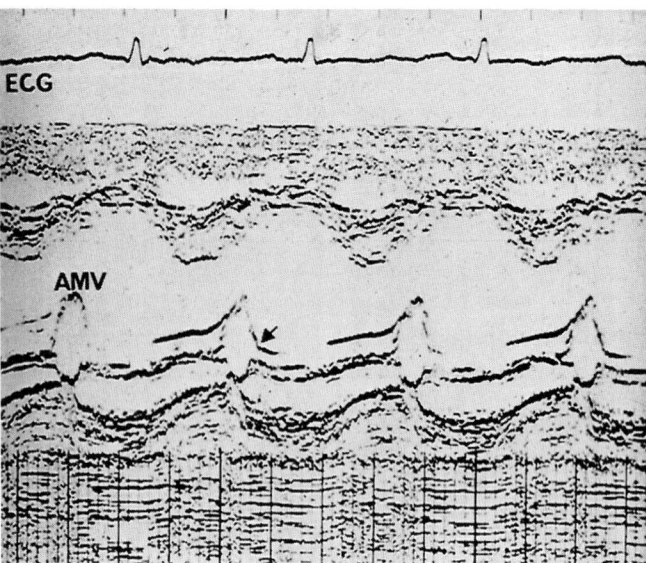

Fig. 14 M-mode echocardiogram showing premature mitral valve closure (arrow) in a patient with acute aortic regurgitation due to infective endocarditis.

MRI. Coronary arteriography is usually performed in older patients as a prelude to surgery, even in the absence of clinical evidence of significant coronary artery disease.

Diagnosis

As with aortic stenosis, it is not enough merely to establish the presence of aortic regurgitation; its severity must be estimated, and also the state of the left ventricle. In uncomplicated cases, the severity can be judged indirectly from the carotid pulse and from the heart size on chest radiography, but direct measurement of left ventricular cavity size and stroke volume by echocardiography, MRI, or angiography is more satisfactory. Left ventricular disease can be suspected clinically from accentuated pulmonary valve closure, and from chest radiography by the presence of pulmonary vascular congestion and inappropriate cardiac enlargement. However, left ventricular function is most satisfactorily assessed by direct measurement, the characteristic feature being enlargement of end-diastolic, and in particular, end-systolic cavity size out of proportion to stroke volume such that ejection fraction falls.

Acute aortic regurgitation may present difficulties in diagnosis when the classic physical signs are modified due to a low forward output. Echocardiography is particularly useful in making a definite diagnosis non-invasively, demonstrating aortic vegetations, a large left ventricular stroke volume, and premature mitral valve closure. It is also important to confirm or exclude other types of valve disease.

Coexistent aortic stenosis is often diagnosed on the basis of an ejection systolic murmur, but this does not constitute adequate evidence, and in order to confirm its presence clinically, a bisferiens pulse should be present. Additional rheumatic mitral stenosis is best confirmed or excluded by echocardiography, although the presence of atrial fibrillation, a palpable first sound, or an opening snap makes its presence very likely on clinical grounds. Mitral regurgitation leads to an additional pansystolic murmur at the apex, which may sound continuous with the early diastolic murmur across the second sound. It is usually caused by a dilated valve ring in the absence of organic mitral valve disease, and thus indicates considerable left ventricular enlargement.

It is usually not necessary to establish the exact aetiology of aortic regurgitation, although it is important to exclude infection and look for the presence of disease of the aortic root and ascending aorta. This should be suspected if there is a history of chest pain that is not clearly anginal in nature, and also from excessive dilatation of the ascending aorta on chest radiography or a long P–R interval on ECG. Proximal aortic root diameter can be measured by echocardiography, and the anatomy of the whole aortic arch demonstrated by MRI.

Differential diagnosis

In the presence of severe pulmonary hypertension, the pulmonary artery may dilate, causing functional pulmonary regurgitation and a soft early diastolic murmur (Graham–Steell murmur). The carotid pulse is normal. Difficulty in diagnosis usually arises when the patient has mitral valve disease, pulmonary hypertension, and an early diastolic murmur. In these circumstances, aortic regurgitation may not necessarily cause an abnormal carotid pulse. In many cases, the differential diagnosis can only be made by Doppler echocardiography, but on clinical grounds, pulmonary incompetence is more likely when there is other evidence of severe pulmonary hypertension, and in particular, when chest radiography shows the main pulmonary artery to be appreciably dilated.

Aortic regurgitation should also be distinguished from other causes of aortic run-off (see Chapter 15.13):

(1) persistent ductus arteriosus;

(2) ruptured sinus of Valsalva aneurysm; and

(3) coronary arteriovenous fistula.

These all cause an increase in pulse pressure, but a continuous rather than an early diastolic murmur down the left sternal edge.

Additional abnormalities that may give rise to confusion are the combination of aortic regurgitation and either mitral regurgitation or a ventricular septal defect. Here the combination of pansystolic and early diastolic murmurs may lead to a continuous quality.

Treatment

Chronic aortic regurgitation

Mild or moderately severe aortic regurgitation is well tolerated and requires no treatment other than prophylactic antibiotic to prevent infective endocarditis.

Severe aortic regurgitation in a symptomatic patient should be treated by aortic valve replacement.

In an asymptomatic patient with severe regurgitation, the decision is more difficult. Without treatment, the outlook is very favourable, with the clinical state remaining stable over many years. Premature operation should be avoided. The most reliable basis for recommending surgery is evidence of progression of disease, such as an increase in heart size on chest radiography, deterioration in the ECG, or an enlarging left ventricular cavity or aortic root on echocardiography. A policy of depending on the results of any single investigation or 'parameter', convenient as it may seem, is inflexible in practice and subject to the limited reproducibility of all cardiological measurements.

Prophylactic administration of nifedipine or ACE inhibitor has been shown to delay the necessity for operation by 2 to 3 years in asymptomatic patients with aortic regurgitation. Severe ventricular disease may become apparent over a period as short as 1 to 2 years, so patients being treated conservatively must be kept under regular review.

Acute aortic regurgitation

Acute aortic regurgitation is a surgical emergency. With a native valve, it is nearly always due to infective endocarditis, and blood cultures should be taken so that the organism can be isolated retrospectively, whilst antibiotics are started preoperatively.

One of the most useful criteria for emergency aortic valve replacement is premature mitral valve closure on the M-mode echocardiogram (Fig. 14). The aim should always be to transfer the patient as soon as possible to a centre capable of performing open heart surgery. As with mitral regurgitation, pharmacological treatment is usually a distraction, but intermittent positive-pressure ventilation is effective treatment for pulmonary oedema.

An increasing P–R interval is a sign of a septal abscess, and requires urgent pacemaker insertion, preferably before transfer, since bradycardia due to complete atrioventricular block can be fatal in severe aortic regurgitation. A prolonged preoperative course of antibiotics is contraindicated in such patients, since the valve is rarely sterilized, and the delay causes further deterioration in left ventricular function with a correspondingly poor outcome. The appearance of aortic regurgitation of any severity with acute dissection of the ascending aorta is also a very strong indication for surgery.

Acquired tricuspid valve disease

Tricuspid stenosis

Although functional tricuspid stenosis may occur with a large flow through the right heart such as occurs in an atrial septal defect, organic tricuspid stenosis is nearly always the result of chronic rheumatic heart disease. Rheumatic tricuspid stenosis virtually always coexists with rheumatic mitral valve disease, although its incidence is about one-tenth. The two conditions are similar both with respect to their pathology and to the functional disturbance that they cause. The valve cusps become thickened, and the commissures fused, so that the cross-sectional area of the orifice is reduced. The tricuspid subvalvar apparatus, though, is not usually involved, nor does calcification occur. The primary functional abnormality is obstruction to right ventricular filling associated with a diastolic pressure drop across the valve. In clinically severe tricuspid stenosis, however, this drop is smaller than it would be with clinically severe mitral stenosis, and is usually within the range of 3 to 10 mmHg. This causes a corresponding increase in right atrial pressure, which leads to ascites and peripheral oedema.

True acquired cusp fusion with severe tricuspid stenosis has recently been described in association with pacemaker catheters, when it presumably represents the effect of chronic trauma. Why it occurs so infrequently with simple pacing catheters, and whether its incidence will increase with the stiffer and more massive catheters needed for automatic implanted cardioverter devices is still not clear.

Clinical features

In patients with chronic rheumatic heart disease, the clinical problem is to recognize the presence of additional tricuspid stenosis in a patient known to have mitral and perhaps also aortic valve disease. This is not always possible on clinical grounds, but a number of indications may be sought. There are no specific findings in the history.

If the patient is in sinus rhythm, tricuspid stenosis is often associated with an 'a' wave in the venous pulse and with evidence of right atrial hypertrophy on ECG. These findings are unusual in the presence of pulmonary hypertension and mitral stenosis alone. The venous pulse is usually otherwise unremarkable.

On auscultation, a separate tricuspid mid-diastolic murmur may be audible. This is similar in timing to a mitral one, but it is higher in pitch, resembling an aortic diastolic murmur in this respect. It is maximal down the left sternal edge or in the epigastrium. A tricuspid opening snap may also be present; it is later than a mitral one and its timing with respect to pulmonary valve closure varies with respiration.

Investigations

Chest radiography may be suggestive, since right atrial enlargement causes the heart shadow to enlarge to the right of the midline. These appearances, however, are non-specific, and may be present with functional tricuspid regurgitation, or even a giant left atrium.

Echocardiography gives the diagnosis. Cross-sectional echocardiography shows doming of the tricuspid valve into the right ventricle during systole (Fig. 15) in the apical four-chamber view. The diastolic pressure drop can be estimated by continuous wave Doppler.

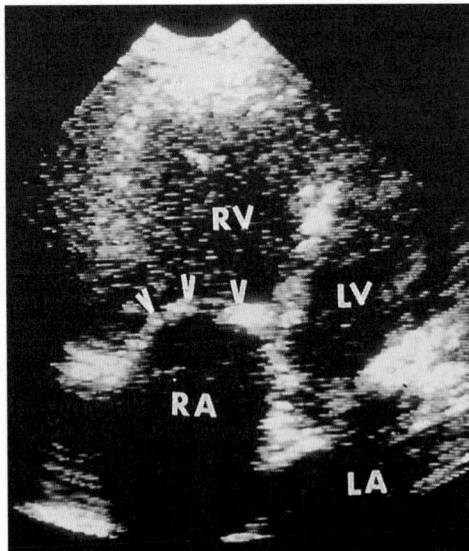

Fig. 15 Rheumatic tricuspid stenosis, apical four-chamber view showing doming and thickening of the tricuspid valve during diastole (arrows). LA, left atrium; LV, left ventricle; RA, right atrium; RV, right ventricle.

Cardiac catheterization is now rarely performed to diagnose tricuspid stenosis, but it may show a small diastolic pressure drop across the valve.

Cases of organic tricuspid stenosis may still reach operation for mitral or aortic valve disease without the diagnosis having been made. When they do so, the previously undiagnosed tricuspid stenosis may be unmasked by successful left-sided surgery, which allows cardiac output to increase. This causes a corresponding increase in the tricuspid diastolic pressure drop, which leads to salt and water retention, so that a patient thought to have had a satisfactory operation develops striking ascites or peripheral oedema afterwards.

Treatment

Medical treatment is not very satisfactory but consists of diuretic administration to control fluid retention. Prolonged administration of inappropriately large doses leads to potassium depletion. Definitive treatment is surgical, consisting of either valvotomy or repair at the time that the other valve lesions are dealt with. Isolated tricuspid stenosis, developing after mitral valve surgery, has been dealt with by balloon valvuloplasty. Tricuspid valve replacement is avoided whenever possible in view of the physiological significance on the right side of the heart of the diastolic pressure drop across all normally functioning prostheses. An additional procedure on the tricuspid valve increases the operative risk of mitral valve surgery, with greater postoperative incidence of jaundice and arrhythmias.

Tricuspid regurgitation

As with mitral regurgitation, a number of different pathological processes can cause tricuspid regurgitation (Table 4).

Table 4 Causes of tricuspid regurgitation

Organic
  Rheumatic
  Infective endocarditis
  Ebstein's anomaly
  Atrioventricular defect
  Carcinoid syndrome
  Cirrhosis of the liver
  Endomyocardial fibrosis
  Prolapsing cusp
Functional

The tricuspid valve is much more liable to develop functional regurgitation than the mitral valve, and tricuspid regurgitation is often functional, occurring in association with dilatation of the right ventricular cavity. It is particularly common in patients with pulmonary hypertensive mitral valve disease, but may also occur with primary pulmonary hypertension, or in the terminal stages of many types of congenital heart disease, particularly those with a significant left to right shunt.

Severe, non-rheumatic tricuspid regurgitation is being increasingly recognized as occurring late after mitral valve replacement, in the absence of significant left-sided disease or pulmonary hypertension. Its cause is not clear, but there is no evidence of disease of the valve cusps or subvalve apparatus.

Organic tricuspid regurgitation may be congenital, as an isolated abnormality, or associated with the Ebstein anomaly. A cleft right-sided atrioventricular valve may also occur in ostium primum atrial septal defect. Acquired, organic tricuspid regurgitation may be rheumatic in origin, or result from infective endocarditis of a previously normal valve, which occurs particularly commonly in intravenous drug users. Right-sided endomyocardial fibrosis causes progressive obliteration of the right ventricular cavity with scarring and distortion of the tricuspid subvalvular apparatus.

Mid-systolic prolapse of the tricuspid valve can occur in exactly the same way as that of the mitral valve, and is common in Marfan's syndrome. Organic tricuspid regurgitation has been described as a long-term consequence of radiotherapy to the thorax, when it may be associated with features of pericardial constriction or restrictive myocardial disease, making its diagnosis difficult.

Clinical features

The clinical features of tricuspid regurgitation are those of severe and chronic elevation of the venous pressure, often in association with disease on the left side of the heart.

The symptoms are non-specific, although when tricuspid regurgitation supervenes in a patient with mitral stenosis, it is often associated with an increase in the prominence of fatigue as a factor limiting exercise tolerance instead of breathlessness. Symptoms may also be related to the development of oedema or ascites: hepatic enlargement may be associated with nausea and upper abdominal or epigastric pain aggravated by exercise.

The main physical sign of tricuspid regurgitation is a raised venous pressure with a prominent systolic wave, which is almost a *sine qua non* for the diagnosis. The mean venous pressure may be very high, greater than 15 cmHg, with pulsations visible in the retinal vessels or palpable in the femoral veins. The high venous pressure is also responsible for the protein-losing enteropathy that sometimes occurs in the same way as with constrictive pericarditis (see Chapter 15.9). In approximately two-thirds of patients, there is associated systolic expansile pulsation of the liver, which may be considerably enlarged and tender. In long-standing cases, hepatic fibrosis develops so that this physical sign disappears. The hepatic dysfunction may also cause mild jaundice, which with increased skin pigmentation can give these patients a very characteristic appearance.

In approximately one-third of cases, a tricuspid pansystolic murmur is present, audible down the left sternal edge. An increase in intensity during inspiration is difficult to demonstrate, so that the murmur is usually indistinguishable from that of functional mitral regurgitation.

Investigations

Chest radiographic findings depend mainly on other cardiac disease present, but, as with tricuspid stenosis, there may be enlargement of the heart shadow towards the right.

The ECG may show right atrial hypertrophy in isolated tricuspid regurgitation if the patient is in sinus rhythm, but otherwise is dominated by other cardiac disease present.

Echocardiography is the best way of making the diagnosis. Cusp disease, either rheumatic or 5-hydroxytryptamine (carcinoid, see later) induced, and right ventricular function are assessed by the cross-sectional technique, while the extent of the regurgitation can be measured by continuous wave and colour flow Doppler. The nature and extent of left-sided disease and pulmonary hypertension can also be documented. Cardiac catheterization is rarely necessary either to make the diagnosis or assess its severity.

Treatment

Medical treatment with diuretics deals with associated fluid retention, and may even allow right ventricular cavity size to decrease, restoring competence to the tricuspid valve. Isolated tricuspid incompetence, unless very severe or accompanied by right ventricular disease, is reasonably well tolerated. Surgical treatment is avoided if possible. However, if regurgitation is very severe and fluid retention requires doses of diuretics large enough to cause significant metabolic consequences, then intervention may be considered. Unfortunately, repair and replacement of the tricuspid valve are unsatisfactory operations: the former does not usually control regurgitation and the latter leads to a very significant diastolic pressure drop between right atrium and right ventricle. In addition, the risks of surgery are high in these patients, and postoperative jaundice and renal failure are common.

When tricuspid regurgitation occurs in association with rheumatic heart disease involving the left side of the heart, it may subside spontaneously after the latter has been dealt with surgically, although there is a case for routine tricuspid valve plication or repair to prevent tricuspid regurgitation developing postoperatively.

Serotonin-induced heart disease

Increased levels of 5-hydroxytryptamine (**5HT**, serotonin) associated with metastatic carcinoid disease cause severe tricuspid and pulmonary regurgitation, and similar findings are associated with anorectic agents. Fenfluramine also causes 5HT release and thus has similar effects on the right-sided valves.

5HT is normally cleared by the lungs, so that in the absence of a right to left shunt, the left side of the heart is not usually affected in carcinoid disease. However, fenfluramine has been used in combination with phentermine, which blocks pulmonary uptake of 5HT, so that together these drugs can lead to involvement of the mitral and aortic valves as well.

The valves are thickened, with a glistening appearance, due to the deposition of plaques of fibrosis. Vascularization and cusp fusion do not occur. However, the cusps themselves become retracted, so that the dominant lesion is regurgitation through a central jet. Subendocardial thickening may also occur, so that the effects of reduced cavity compliance are superimposed on those of volume overload. On the left side of the heart, the regurgitation may be severe enough to require valve replacement.

Not all patients with carcinoid disease develop cardiac manifestations, but when they are present they may progress, even after removal of the tumour. In slowly progressive cases, tricuspid valve replacement has been successfully undertaken.

Pulmonary valve disease

Acquired pulmonary valve disease is unusual. The commonest form is that associated with severe pulmonary hypertension and dilatation of the pulmonary valve ring, causing mild regurgitation. This commonly occurs in association with pulmonary hypertensive mitral valve disease, causing a soft early diastolic murmur (the Graham–Steell murmur), but an identical picture may be present with severe pulmonary hypertension from any cause. Although the murmur itself is early diastolic in timing, there is no associated abnormality of the carotid pulse as would be expected in aortic regurgitation. Nevertheless, the differential diagnosis on clinical grounds can be difficult when mitral valve disease is severe. Mild pulmonary regurgitation is effectively a normal finding on colour flow Doppler; a more extensive jet in a patient with pulmonary hypertension being required to confirm the diagnosis. Aortic regurgitation can be confirmed or excluded by Doppler. Rheumatic pulmonary regurgitation is extremely rare, although it has been reported in populations living at high altitudes. How-

ever, even when present it contributes little to overall disability. Pulmonary regurgitation may also form part of the carcinoid syndrome, but its effect on the clinical picture is less than that of the tricuspid or left-sided valves. It may also be iatrogenic, following pulmonary valvotomy for pulmonary stenosis, when it contributes to the elevated venous pressure that can persist for a variable period after this operation. It is of no clinical consequence and requires no specific treatment.

Valve disease and pregnancy

For information of the effect of pregnancy on patients with valve disease, see Chapter 13.6.

Management of patients with valve prostheses

Many patients have received heart valve replacements over the past 40 years, with very significant improvement in their quality of life. However, although the haemodynamic performance of these prostheses is greatly superior to the diseased valves that they replaced, it is not normal, and survival with any valvular prosthesis is significantly less than that for age-matched normal individuals. Having a valve replacement should now be regarded as the commonest form of valve disease in Western society.

Valve prostheses can be mechanical or biological. Mechanical prostheses include the Starr–Edwards ball and cage prosthesis, which has the advantage of a 30-year follow-up and remarkable reliability; single tilting disc valves (Bjork–Shiley); but those inserted over the last 10 years are likely to be bileaflet (St Jude). The more modern types have a larger effective orifice area than the Starr–Edwards in relation to the size of their ring.

Biological prostheses usually consist of a plastic stent on which cusps made from some biological material are mounted. The cusps may be derived from porcine aortic valve or pericardium. More recently, unstented xenografts (e.g. the Toronto) have been used, where the aortic homograft is mounted on a ring of native aortic root. In the Ross operation, the patient's own pulmonary valve is inserted into the aortic position (pulmonary autograft) and replaced by an aortic homograft in the right ventricular outflow tract.

There are minor differences in performance between the various valve substitutes, but these are not of great clinical significance. Apart from the pulmonary autograft, all fall short of their natural counterpart *in vivo*. Under normal working conditions, pressure differences are present across mitral prostheses, which range from 4 to 5 mmHg for the Starr–Edwards to 2 to 4 mmHg for the others. In addition, all mitral valve substitutes have a rigid mitral ring which interferes with ventricular function. Apart from the autograft, and to a lesser extent the homograft, whose performance approximates to that of the native valve, systolic gradients across aortic prostheses are in the range 10 to 25 mmHg at rest, increasing on exercise.

The main factors guiding choice of valve prosthesis are durability and the likely incidence of thrombotic complications. Present operative mortality is in the region of 3 to 5 per cent for single valve replacement and approximately 10 per cent for double valve replacement. These values are higher if simultaneous coronary artery grafting is necessary. Long-term survival studies have shown that 10-year survival after single valve replacement is approximately 70 to 75 per cent, and after double valve replacement 50 to 65 per cent. For reoperation, mortality is higher, the exact figure depending on the circumstances in which surgery is performed.

Late complications of valve replacement

Thromboembolism

This is a major complication associated with all mechanical prostheses. Long-term anticoagulant therapy with a drug of the warfarin type is essential in all patients in whom these prostheses have been inserted, and even with satisfactory control (international normalized ratio, **INR**, between 3 and 4.5), an incidence of significant events including transient weakness, dysphasia, or visual disturbances of 1 to 2 per cent per annum can be expected. At the same time, anticoagulant therapy itself causes bleeding complications severe enough to require admission to hospital with an incidence of approximately 1 per cent per annum.

In a small minority of patients, emboli are frequent in spite of good anticoagulant control. Initially, such patients should be given an antiplatelet agent such a dipyridamole, and the anticoagulant dose adjusted accordingly. The possibility of some other cause for the neurological manifestations, such as cerebrovascular disease, must always be considered. However, frequent embolization may be associated with thrombosis of the prosthesis, and if this is proven beyond all question and cannot be suppressed medically, reoperation and replacement with a biological prosthesis may be necessary.

The incidence of thromboembolic complications is much lower with biological prostheses, so that long-term anticoagulant therapy can be dispensed with in patients in sinus rhythm after aortic or mitral valve replacement. However, many surgeons recommend a short course of 2 to 3 months in such patients whilst suture lines become endothelialized. Patients with atrial fibrillation require standard long-term anticoagulant therapy.

In developing countries, mitral replacement may have to be performed in children under the age of 15 years, in whom biological valves are unsuitable. The use of a mechanical prosthesis might seem appropriate, but facilities for regular anticoagulant monitoring are not available, while uncontrolled administration of standard doses of warfarin is associated with unacceptable risk of haemorrhage. This therapeutic dilemma is, at present, unsolved.

Limited prosthetic function

In a minority of patients, valve replacement may give rise to severe haemodynamic disturbances, such that in extreme cases the condition of the patient may be worse after the operation than before. This usually arises when the valve ring or the ventricular cavity is very small, and a correspondingly small prosthesis was inserted. In the mitral position, resting diastolic pressure differences as high as 20 mmHg may be present, or of 50 mmHg across the aortic valve on this basis. A related problem is the insertion of a prosthesis that is too large, particularly of the ball and cage type. In the mitral position, the cage may impinge on the septum, and obstruct the left ventricular outflow tract, causing subaortic stenosis; whilst in the aortic position, obstruction may develop between the ball and the aorta. These complications are now avoided by the use of low-profile prostheses, such as the St Jude bileaflet prosthesis.

Infection

Patients with prostheses, mechanical or biological, are at greatly increased risk of infective endocarditis. The infecting organism may have been introduced at the time of operation, when it usually manifests within 2 months of surgery. Later infections are bloodborne. It is therefore essential that all patients receive full antibiotic prophylaxis immediately after surgery and subsequently for dental manipulations and other potentially septic hazards, rather than the single dose of single agent currently recommended for routine dental prophylaxis in those at lower risk (see Chapter 15.10.2).

Infective endocarditis is a very serious complication, and rarely responds to antibiotic therapy alone. A second valve replacement is nearly always required, often in a seriously ill patient in whom the valve ring may be infected and friable. The clinical features of endocarditis on a mechanical prosthesis differ very significantly from those on a native valve. Vegetations are uncommon. The infection is often confined to the tissue around the prosthesis, including the sewing ring, and may rot the sutures, so that the first manifestation is sudden death due to displacement of the valve to the aortic bifurcation. Partial dehiscence leads to severe regurgitation with a rocking prosthesis, demonstrable by simple screening or cross-sectional echocardiography. The main disturbance may be stenosis, due to ingrowth

of infected clot. Abscess formation around the prostheses is particularly common in the aortic position, which may cause complete heart block or perforation to the right side of the heart. These difficulties are compounded by the acoustic properties of the mechanical valves themselves which limit the value of echocardiography. Para-aortic abscesses are well demonstrated by transoesophageal echo.

Prosthetic dysfunction

This is an important cause of morbidity in patients who have undergone valve replacement. There may be structural damage to the prosthesis itself, which is uncommon in mechanical valves, though occasional batches may undergo strut fracture due to metal fatigue, a well known example being the concavo-convex Bjork–Shiley valves inserted in the late 1970s.

Malfunction is much commoner with biological prostheses, when cusps may become calcified, perforated, or detached. Calcification of porcine bioprostheses regularly occurs within 1 to 2 years of insertion in children under the age of 15 years. This complication takes much longer to develop in the aortic homograft, usually 10 to 15 years. Once cusp degeneration has occurred, the valve should be regarded as unstable, since sudden cusp detachment or perforation can occur, and it is therefore inadvisable to adhere to haemodynamic guidelines appropriate to native valves when deciding on the timing of further surgery. It is an advantage of the homograft valve that sudden deterioration in haemodynamic function is much less common.

Mechanical prostheses are subject to thrombosis. This may take two forms. Deterioration in function may be insidious over a period of several months or years due to ingrowth of organized clot (pannus), usually from the atrial side (Fig. 16). This may be associated with an increased incidence of emboli in spite of adequate anticoagulant therapy. Alternatively, the prosthesis may clot acutely: this is particularly likely to occur with the Bjork–Shiley in the mitral position, and represents a surgical emergency. It can often be recognized clinically, the patient presenting with pulmonary oedema or in a low cardiac output state, and the closing click of the prosthesis no longer audible. Operation is required as soon as possible, since deterioration may occur within hours. If the condition of the patient is so poor as to preclude anaesthesia, then thrombolysis should be used, in spite of the risk of systemic embolism. Improvement may be expected within a few hours, when the thrombolysis can be neutralized and surgery undertaken.

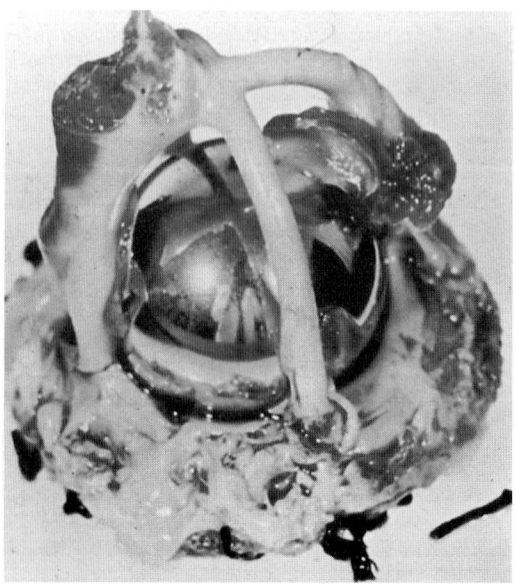

Fig. 16 Thrombosed Star–Edwards prosthesis, removed at emergency operation.

Finally, paraprosthetic regurgitation may develop. In the aortic position, this may have been present since the original operation, because heavy calcification of the original valve extended into the valve ring. Paraprosthetic regurgitation that appears suddenly always raises the possibility that the prosthesis might have become infected. Mitral paraprosthetic regurgitation usually results from part of the valve sewing ring tearing away. Again, infection should always be considered, but regurgitation is well documented in its absence.

Recognizing prosthetic dysfunction

Stenosis or regurgitation associated with a prosthesis does not have the same physical signs as the corresponding lesion of the native valve. In general, it presents as deterioration in cardiac state, whose progress may be acute or chronic. The clinical picture is of 'heart failure'. On examination, the venous pressure is raised, the liver enlarged, and chest radiography shows that the heart has enlarged and pulmonary congestion appeared. When a mitral prosthesis is involved, there are characteristically no murmurs, other than those of tricuspid regurgitation; an aortic systolic murmur may be present, but its intensity and timing differs little from that of a normally functioning prosthesis. It is essential, therefore, that the possibility of a prosthesis-related complication is considered in all such patients in whom a diagnosis of 'heart failure' is entertained. The differential diagnosis is exacting, and requires echocardiography, Doppler, and possibly cardiac catheterization by an experienced operator. All patients presenting in this way should therefore be referred to a unit where these investigations can be performed reliably, and emergency surgery can be undertaken if necessary.

Haemolysis

All mechanical prostheses are associated with increased intravascular haemolysis. This rarely gives rise to clinical problems when the prosthesis is functioning normally, and anaemia does not occur. The extent of haemolysis can be estimated from a peripheral blood film, which shows fragmented forms, from depression or absence of serum haptoglobin, and from an increase in lactate dehydrogenase levels.

Haemolysis may become significant with a normally functioning prosthesis when the patient has a compensated haemolytic state of some different aetiology, such as congenital spherocytosis or thalassaemia minor. In these circumstances, there is a risk of haemolysis becoming severe.

Mild paraprosthetic regurgitation whose severity is insufficient to give rise to any haemodynamic complications can cause clinically significant haemolysis. In such cases, it may be undesirable to expose the patient to the risk of reoperation, particularly if the original valve leak was due to some predictable cause such as heavy calcification of the valve bed, and so likely to recur. Provided that haemolysis is not severe, such patients can usually be treated medically on maintenance therapy with iron and folic acid. A requirement for transfusion, however, is a strong indication for reoperation.

Left ventricular disease

This is a major cause of morbidity and mortality after valve replacement. There is no single cause. In many patients, severe left ventricular disease was present preoperatively, and though some improvement frequently occurs with correction of the valve disease, function never returns to normal. Operation itself causes additional damage. Methods of myocardial preservation during the period of cardiopulmonary bypass have improved very considerably over the last 20 years with the general introduction of cold blood cardioplegia, but before then ischaemic arrest appears to have been associated with myocardial damage that may take several years to become manifest. A rigid prosthetic mitral ring invariably leads to abnormal function, and there is increasing evidence that section of the papillary muscles may have the same effect. Coronary emboli may arise from the prosthesis. Many patients are of an age to have additional coronary artery disease.

Whatever the cause, left ventricular disease after valve replacement presents its usual clinical features. There is progressive limitation of exercise tolerance and breathlessness due to reduction in cardiac output and pulmonary congestion. Venous pressure becomes raised, and the earliest clinical evidence may relate to right rather than left ventricular disease, with elevated venous pressure, fluid retention, and hepatic congestion. Auscultatory signs may be modified, and in particular third and fourth heart sounds are not audible in patients with mechanical mitral prostheses. Chest radiography shows an increase in heart size and pulmonary congestion. ECG may show Q waves, but their absence is of no significance.

The differential diagnosis of ventricular disease after valve replacement is prosthetic dysfunction, and it is essential that a correct diagnosis is established in any patient who fails to progress, or whose improvement after operation is not maintained. Echocardiography, transthoracic and transoesophageal, has proved of great value in such patients, since it allows the very active left ventricular wall motion that accompanies a paraprosthetic leak to be distinguished from the dilated cavity and poor shortening fraction of left ventricular disease. Continuous wave Doppler can be used to detect significant gradients across biological valves. However, unless the diagnosis is clear from non-invasive investigation, cardiac catheterization is required to settle the diagnosis beyond doubt.

The prognosis once clinically apparent left ventricular disease has developed is poor, usually being of the order of 1 to 2 years, so it is essential that no remediable cause is overlooked.

Follow-up of patients after valve replacement

Patients must be followed up after valve replacement for life. This must at least be at annual intervals, with regular chest radiography and ECG in an experienced clinic. Echocardiography should be performed early, not only to detect immediate postoperative complications such as a pericardial fluid collection, which can be potentially fatal if delayed tamponade occurs, but also to establish a baseline from which to detect future change. Deterioration must be detected early, and investigated in detail so that life-threatening complications are not missed. Dental prophylaxis is essential.

Valve disease and pregnancy

The circulatory changes associated with pregnancy modify the physiology of valve disease and thus its management. These changes are hormonally mediated, and result in an increase in cardiac output by 40 to 45 per cent above control values and a corresponding fall in peripheral resistance, maximal in the middle trimester. This elevation in cardiac output is mediated in approximately equal parts by increases in stroke volume and heart rate. The raised stroke volume, in particular, can lead to the development of a soft ejection systolic murmur, whose benign origin can normally be clarified by echocardiography, chest radiography being avoided where possible.

The effects of the circulatory changes of pregnancy on those of pre-existing valve disease are very predictable. Since the increase in cardiac output is brought about mainly by a fall in peripheral resistance, patients with valvular regurgitation do well. The main problems are with stenotic lesions. In mitral stenosis, the increased stroke volume and tachycardia combine to increase the diastolic pressure drop across the valve, thus predisposing to pulmonary oedema. Pulmonary oedema in a pregnant patient is a medical emergency, and prompt transfer to a surgical centre should be arranged if the symptoms are more than mild. Medical treatment with digoxin and β-blocking agents, aimed at slowing the heart rate, may be satisfactory, but surgery is often necessary. Mitral valve anatomy in young women is usually compatible with a conservative operation. Closed mitral valvotomy has a long and proven record, and is available if the surgical expertise is still available. In its absence balloon valvuloplasty, with appropriate screening to minimize radiation, is also satisfactory.

The combination of aortic stenosis and pregnancy is also difficult to manage, since an increase in the pressure drop across the valve combined with a fall in peripheral resistance is particularly liable to cause syncope as well as aggravating left ventricular disease, and leading to pulmonary oedema and death. Cardiopulmonary bypass for valve replacement during pregnancy is associated with a 20 to 30 per cent fetal loss, but there may be no alternative. In young female patients with mitral and particularly with aortic stenosis, therefore, there is a strong case for dealing with the valve lesion before pregnancy.

Prosthetic valves and pregnancy

Pregnancy

Clinical problems in pregnancy arise from the anticoagulant therapy needed for mechanical prostheses. Pregnancy is accompanied by an increase in coaguability and a decrease in fibrinolysis. Coumarin anticoagulants lead to an incidence of spontaneous abortion of approximately 30 per cent, particularly during the sixth to ninth weeks, while in the third trimester, they are associated with fetal haemorrhage and post-partum bleeding, even when the INR is well controlled. In the absence of large-scale trials, a commonly used regime is to give heparin for the first trimester, followed by warfarin until just before delivery, when heparin is substituted. Heparin does not cross the placenta, and can readily be discontinued or neutralized with protamine. There is recent evidence to suggest that the incidence of fetal abnormality is low if the warfarin dose can be maintained below 5 mg/day.

Further reading

Benjamin EJ *et al.* (1992). Mitral annular calcification and the risk of stroke in an elderly cohort. *New England Journal of Medicine* **327**, 374–9.

Blackstone EH, Kirklin JW (1992). Recommendations for prophylactic removal of heart valve prostheses. *Journal of Heart Valve Disease* **1**, 3–14.

Bulkley BH, Roberts WC (1976). The heart in systemic lupus erythematosis, and change induced in it by corticosteroid therapy. *American Journal of Medicine* **58**, 243–64.

Cohen DJ *et al.* (1992). Predictors of long-term outcome after percutaneous balloon mitral valvuloplasty. *New England Journal of Medicine* **327**, 1329–35.

Connolly HM *et al.* (1997). Valvular heart disease with flenfuramine-phentermine. *New England Journal of Medicine* **337**, 581–8.

Fowler N, van der Bel-Kahn JM (1979). Indications for surgical replacement of the mitral valve with particular reference to common and uncommon causes of mitral regurgitation. *American Journal of Cardiology* **44**, 157.

Freed LA *et al.* (1999). Prevalence and clinical outcome of mitral prolapse. *New England Journal of Medicine* **341**, 1–7.

Groves PH, Hall RJC (1992). Late tricuspid regurgitation following mitral valve surgery. *Journal of Heart Valve Disease* **1**, 80–6.

Hehoe JA, Carpenter DF, Golden A (1968). Cardiac valvular lesions in rheumatoid arthritis. *Archives of Internal Medicine* **122**, 141–6.

Leatham A, Brigden W (1980). Mild mitral regurgitation and the mitral prolapse fiasco. *American Heart Journal* **99**, 659–64.

Ling LH *et al.* (1996). Clinical outcome of mitral regurgitation due to flail leaflet. *New England Journal of Medicine* **335**, 1417–23.

Oakley CM, Burkhardt D (1993). Optimal timing of surgery for chronic mitral or aortic regurgitation. *Journal of Heart Valve Disease* **2**, 223–9.

Rahimtoola SH (1983). Valvular heart disease; a perspective. *Journal of the American College of Cardiology* **1**, 199–215.

Roberts WC *et al.* (1981). Congenital bicuspid aortic valve causing severe, pure aortic regurgitation without superimposed infective endocarditis. *American Journal of Cardiology* **47**, 206–9.

Ruttley MST (1992). The chest radiograph in adult heart valve disease. *Journal of Heart Valve Disease* **2**, 205–17.

Selzer A (1987). Changing aspects of the natural history of aortic stenosis. *New England Journal of Medicine* **317**, 91–8.

Smith HJ *et al.* (1976). The natural history of rheumatic aortic regurgitation and the indications for surgery. *British Heart Journal* **38**, 147–54.

Smith N, McAnulty JH, Rahimtoola SH (1978). Severe aortic stenosis with impaired left ventricular function and clinical heart failure: results of valve replacement. *Circulation* **58**, 255–64.

Vijayaraghavan G *et al.* (1977). Rheumatic aortic stenosis in young patients presenting as combined aortic and mitral stenosis. *British Heart Journal* **39**, 294–8.

Wood P (1954). An appreciation of mitral stenosis. Part 1. Clinical features. *British Medical Journal* **i**, 1051–63.

Wood P (1954). An appreciation of mitral stenosis. Part II. Investigations and results. *British Medical Journal* **I**, 1113–24.

15.8 Diseases of heart muscle

15.8.1 Myocarditis

Jay W. Mason

Introduction

Myocarditis is a disease that has captured the interest of clinicians and scientists. This interest is generated by its varied aetiology, its diagnostic and therapeutic challenges, the possibility that myocarditis may be the primary cause of dilated cardiomyopathy, and the availability of numerous, easily manipulated animal models of the disease.

Clinical features

Myocarditis affects young people. The average age of patients in the United States Myocarditis Treatment Trial was 42 years. There was a slight male predominance (62 per cent) in that trial, but other series have not demonstrated a sex predilection. The true incidence of myocarditis is unknown. Autopsy studies have reported up to a 3 per cent incidence, but varying histological criteria were used, and myocarditis may occur as an incidental complication of other fatal illnesses. About 10 per cent of patients with influenza infections have electrocardiographic abnormalities, but it is not know if these are the result of myocarditis. The incidence of fatal myocarditis was estimated in a retrospective review of United States Air Force recruits undergoing boot camp training. There were eight such deaths over 1 606 167 person days, which yields an estimate of 4/100 000 per year in people aged 17 to 28 years. This incidence is probably greater than would be expected in the general population in the United States, who would not be exposed to similar levels of intense exercise or high probability of transmission of viral illnesses.

In Europe and North America most cases of myocarditis present with congestive heart failure of unknown cause. In many cases there is a history of recent upper respiratory tract infection or of a 'flu-like' illness. This is followed by symptoms of cardiac decompensation, usually fatigue, breathlessness, and cough. Chest pain occurs in a substantial minority of patients. A small proportion of patients with myocarditis present with ventricular tachyarrhythmias and minimal or no cardiac dilatation. Typically, the duration of symptoms due to infection is brief, less than 1 month in approximately 50 per cent of patients and nearly always less than 1 year. Myocarditis should always be suspected when a patient presents with unexplained congestive heart failure with a rapid onset, especially if there is a viral prodrome.

Clinical examination typically reveals signs of cardiac failure. The ECG may show conduction abnormalities and ST/T-wave changes, or arrhythmias (atrial or ventricular). The chest radiograph shows cardiomegaly and pulmonary oedema. The echocardiogram reveals four-chamber dilatation and reduced contractility, and is notable for the fact that valvular disease is absent or minimal. Should coronary angiography be performed, the vessels are normal or show only minor abnormalities. The role of myocardial biopsy will be discussed later. CPK-MB elevation is common.

Although viruses are thought to be the most common cause of myocarditis, viral titres are rarely useful in diagnosis and treatment. Although the cardiotrophic enteroviruses, including echoviruses and coxsackieviruses, are the predominant aetiological agents, dozens of viruses have been implicated and many more, undoubtedly, cause myocarditis in humans. Thus, it is impractical to exclude all. In addition, patients usually present a substantial period of time after the viral infection has cleared, making it difficult or impossible to document an acute rise in titre. Knowledge of a specific virus, or any virus, as the cause in a given case of myocarditis has little, if any, therapeutic relevance. Even if virocidal therapy (which is not yet a proven treatment; see below) is being considered, negative titres for the common viral agents do not exclude a viral aetiology.

A small number of patients, perhaps about 10 per cent, present with a secondary form of myocarditis. These special presentations are discussed below.

Aetiology and pathogenesis (Table 1)

The most common form of myocarditis in Europe and North America is known as lymphocytic myocarditis or non-specific lymphocytic myocarditis. Other frequently applied terms are viral or post-viral myocarditis, because an antecedent viral infection is common. Indeed, some experts believe that nearly all lymphocytic myocarditides are the result of viral infections, presumed to be subclinical in those patients with no awareness of a viral prodrome.

In animal models enteroviruses, such as coxsackie B3, can cause two phases of myocarditis. The first is the result of direct injury of myocytes by replicating virus and the resulting acute immune response. A delayed immune response brings about the second phase, and it is this which is thought to be the more common cause of overt congestive heart failure. The underlying mechanisms are complex and incompletely understood, but most hypotheses suggest that autoimmune phenomena play a major role. In some instances molecular mimicry may be involved, in which the similarity of a viral antigen to a myocardial protein triggers an autoimmune reaction. In others an autoimmune response to cellular proteins released during the viral replication phase may occur, and myosin has been implicated in this regard. Cytokines arising from immune activation and cellular necrosis probably play a role in some cases, bringing about further cellular damage. Although all of these mechanisms have been well delineated in murine models, they have not been proven to account for myocarditis in humans.

Myocarditis may result from a hypersensitivity reaction to a drug or other agent (see Table 1). In these cases eosinophils accompany the inflammatory lymphocytic infiltrate. A number of other specific causes of myocarditis, each with differing pathogenises and presentations, are discussed below.

Relationship to idiopathic dilated cardiomyopathy

Classic lymphocytic myocarditis usually resolves, with resultant improvement in cardiac function over weeks or months. In the United States Myocarditis Treatment Trial, the mean left ventricular ejection fraction improved during the year after initial presentation by more than 10 EF units (from 24 to 36 per cent; normal more than 55 per cent). However, residual cardiac dilatation and dysfunction were common, and mortality was high, reaching 55 per cent at 5 years. In those patients who do not recover fully, the ensuing clinical picture cannot be distinguished from that of idiopathic dilated cardiomyopathy. The possibility that myocarditis may occur without an obvious viral prodrome therefore raises the interesting possibility that viral myocarditis may be a common covert cause of idiopathic dilated cardiomyopathy. In the United States trial, only 10 per cent of patients with suspected myocarditis had positive biopsies. Hence, the fact that endomyocardial biopsy does not reveal myocarditis in patients with idiopathic dilated cardiomyopathy may be the result of timing of the biopsy. The lymphocytic infiltrate usually resolves spontaneously, and it may be that earlier biopsy might have detected myocarditis in a portion of the 90 per cent with negative biopsies. The presence of viral genomic material in a minority of these negative biopsies lends support to the viral aetiology hypothesis. Absence of viral genome in the rest of them does not eliminate post-viral autoimmune processes, proceeding despite complete viral clearing, as a possible aetiology.

Treatment of post-viral and non-specific lymphocytic myocarditis

As stated above, non-specific lymphocytic myocarditis is believed by most to have a viral aetiology, even in the absence of a clinically apparent viral prodrome. In the acute phase of viral myocarditis, the direct cytolytic effect of viral myocyte infection may lead to congestive heart failure, although this is uncommon. In this early phase, the immune response is likely, on balance, to be beneficial. Thus, antiviral therapy might be expected to be helpful, on theoretical grounds, but immunosuppressive therapy would not. However, no antiviral therapies have been adequately tested in humans. Although hyperimmune globulin is thought to be effective on the basis of retrospective studies, its efficacy has not been proved in a prospective trial. In the second stage, thought to result from an adverse immune response to previous infection, immunosuppressive therapy has appeared to be beneficial in uncontrolled trials. However, no benefit was demonstrated in the United States Myocarditis Treatment Trial, the only prospective, randomized trial performed in patients with myocarditis defined histologically. In that trial the 'Dallas' criteria defined myocarditis histologically as a lymphocytic infiltrate with associated myocyte necrosis (Fig. 1). Treatment with prednisone combined with either cyclosporin or with azathioprine did not improve outcome, as defined by change in left ventricular ejection fraction.

Table 1 Aetiologies of myocarditis

INFECTION	INFECTION (cont.)
Viruses	**Protozoa**
Adenovirus	*Entamoeba histolytica*
Arbovirus	*Leishmania* spp.
Arenavirus	*Toxoplasma gondii*
Coronavirus	*Trypanosoma cruzi* (Chagas'
Coxsackievirus (A, B)	disease)
Cytomegalovirus	**Helminths**
Echovirus	*Echinococcus* spp.
Encephalomyocarditis	*Schistosoma* spp.
Epstein–Barr	*Toxocara* spp.
Hepatitis B	*Trichinella* spp.
Hepatitis C	**Fungal**
Herpes simplex	*Actinomyces* spp.
Human immunodeficiency	*Aspergillus* spp.
Influenza (A, B)	*Blastomyces dermatitides*
Junin	*Candida* spp.
Mumps	*Coccidioides immitis*
Polio	*Cryptococcus neoformans*
Rabies	*Histoplasma capsulatum*
Respiratory syncytial	Mucormycosis-related
Rubella (German measles)	organisms
Rubeola (measles)	*Nocardia* spp.
Vaccinia	*Sporothrix schenckii*
Varicella-zoster virus	**DRUGS AND CHEMICALS**
Bacteria, spirochaetes, and	**Toxicity**
bacteria-like organisms	α_2-Interferon
β-Haemolytic streptococci	Anthracyclines
Borrelia burgdorferi (Lyme	Catecholamines
disease)	Cocaine
Brucella spp.	5-Fluorouracil
Campylobacter jejuni	Interleukin 2
Chlamydia psittaci (psittacosis)	**Hypersensitivity**
Chlamydia trachomatis	Aminophylline
(trachoma)	Ampicillin
Clostridia spp.	Benzodiazepines
Corynebacterium diphtheriae	Digoxin
Francisella tularensis	Ephedrine
(tularaemia)	Frusemide
Haemophilus influenzae	Hydrochlorthiazide
Legionella pneumophila	Methyldopa
Leptospira spp.	Penicillin
Listeria monocytogenes	Phenytoin
Mycobacterium spp.	Tetracycline
Mycoplasma pneumoniae	Tricyclic antidepressants
Neisseria gonorrhoeae	**AUTOIMMUNITY**
Neisseria meningitidis	**Antigenic mimicry**
Salmonella typhi	**Autoimmune disease associated**
Streptococcus pneumoniae	**Cardiac myosin**
Staphylococcus spp.	**Cytokines**
Treponema pallidum (syphilis)	**Dressler's syndrome**
Rickettsia	**Post-cardiotomy syndrome**
Coxiella burnetii (Q fever)	**Postinfectious**
Orientia tsutsugamushi (scrub	**Post-radiation**
typhus)	
Rickettsia rickettsii (Rocky Mountain	
spotted fever)	
Rickettsia prowazekii (typhus)	

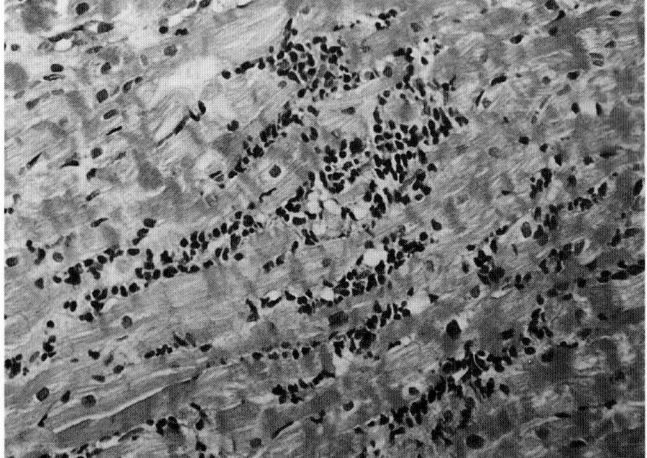

Fig. 1 An example of acute myocarditis, with lymphocytic infiltration adjacent to frayed myocytes.

An algorithm for the diagnosis and treatment of suspected myocarditis is shown in Fig. 2. Spontaneous improvement in left ventricular function can be anticipated in many patients with myocarditis. In most cases it is reasonable to use standard therapy for congestive heart failure, without performing a biopsy or administering steroids, and to observe the patient, using echocardiography to monitor left ventricular function. However, in patients who deteriorate, or who present in cardiogenic shock, an endomyocardial biopsy should be performed. If myocarditis is present, many would regard it as appropriate to administer immunosuppressive therapy,

typically beginning with prednisone at 1.25 mg/kg per day, tapering to 0.15 mg/kg per day over 1 month. It must be admitted, however, that the efficacy of such treatment has not been proved.

Ventricular tachyarrhythmias

Lymphocytic myocarditis, with or without a viral prodrome, may present with ventricular tachyarrhythmias and little or no cardiac dilatation and

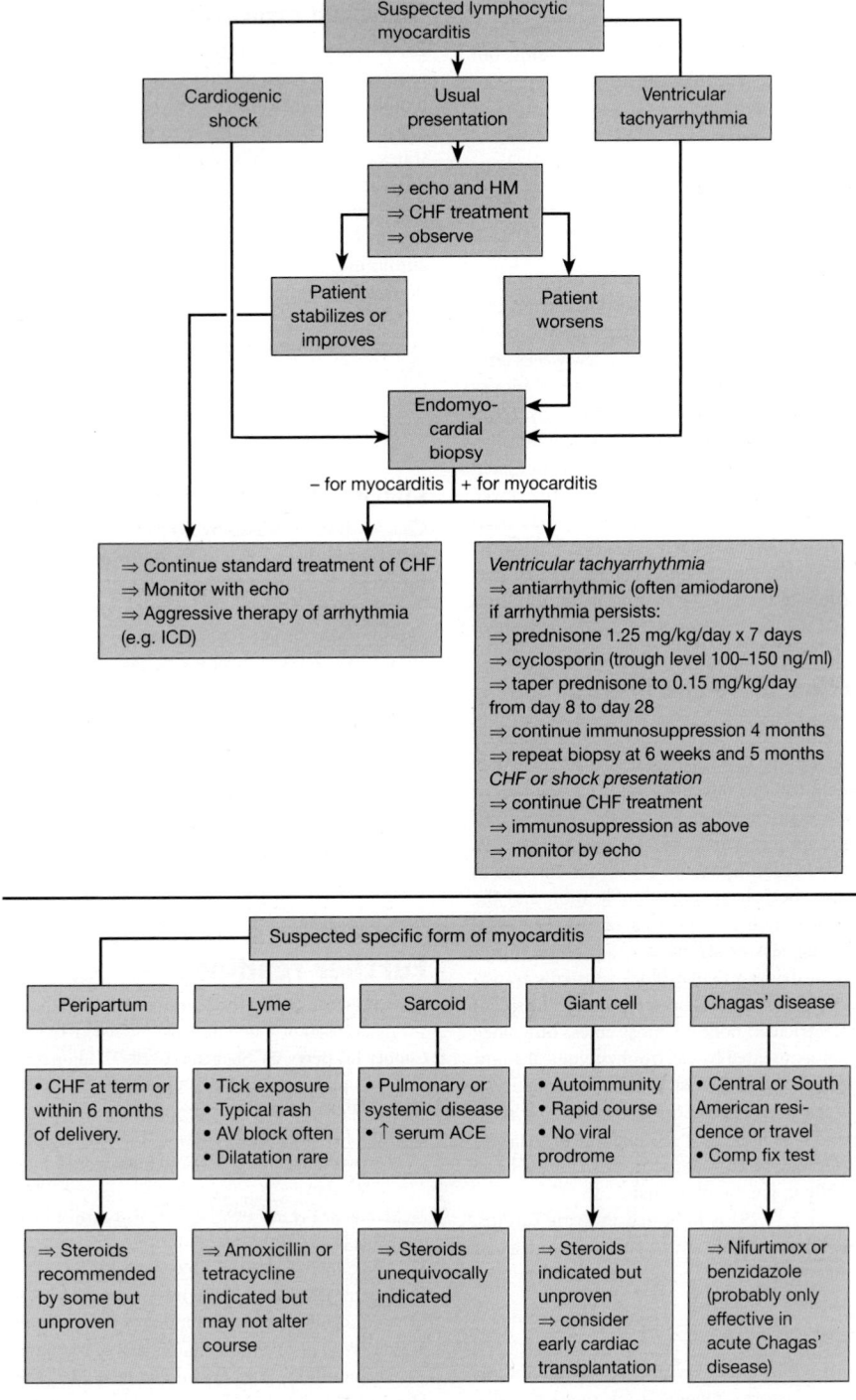

Fig. 2 Algorithm for diagnosis and treatment of suspected myocarditis. Abbreviations: CHF, congestive heart failure; ICD, implantable cardioverter device; ACE, angiotensin-converting enzyme; echo, echocardiogram; HM, Holter monitor.

dysfunction. An endomyocardial biopsy should be considered in all cases of ventricular tachycardia of recent onset if no aetiology is apparent, because the presence of myocarditis can substantially change treatment strategy. Since myocarditis is often a self-limiting disorder, the patient's risk of recurrent ventricular tachyarrhythmias may resolve, and it may be unnecessary to subject the patient to electrophysiological study and/or cardioverter-defibrillator implantation. If arrhythmia does not improve spontaneously, a trial of immunosuppressive therapy should be considered. In such cases it is difficult to know how long to continue with anti-arrhythmic drugs. The risks of ventricular arrhythmia should not be underestimated, but nor should those of long-term treatment with agents such as amiodarone. If 24-h ECG monitoring at 6 months shows no sinister abnormalities, then many would withdraw anti-arrhythmic treatment at that point, but others advocate repeat endomyocardial biopsy to document complete resolution of myocarditis before taking this step.

Specific forms of myocarditis

Peripartum myocarditis

Dilated cardiomyopathy developing during the last trimester of pregnancy or within 6 months of delivery is known as peripartum or postpartum cardiomyopathy (see also Chapter 13.6). In some series the dominant cause is myocarditis. When heart failure develops rapidly in the first few weeks after delivery, myocarditis is more likely to be found on endomyocardial biopsy than when the onset is insidious and delayed, and those with early, rapid onset are more likely to recover quickly and completely. While steroid therapy has been used and is recommended by some, its efficacy has not been proved, and spontaneous resolution of peripartum cardiomyopathy is well documented. The usual prohibition against future pregnancy has been debated; it is very clear that some women risk recurrent heart failure, while others do not. In those women in whom severe heart failure persists, cardiac transplantation is an appropriate therapy. After transplantation, successful pregnancies have occurred without recurrence of cardiomyopathy.

Lyme carditis (see Section 15.10 and Chapter 7.11.29)

Borrelia burgdorferi, a spirochaete, infects humans following *Ixodes* tick bites. Lyme disease, which results from this infection, has been reported in 48 of the 50 United States as well as in Europe and Asia. It is characterized by an erythema migrans rash and flu-like symptoms, followed by arthritis, carditis, and neurological disorders in some patients. Carditis is detected in approximately 8 per cent of cases. Both lymphocytic infiltration and the bacterium itself can be demonstrated by endomyocardial biopsy. The usual cardiac manifestation is varying degrees of atrioventricular block. Infrequently, cardiac dilatation occurs. Atrioventricular block is usually transient, though permanent complete heart block has been reported. The site of block appears to be the atrioventricular node in most cases, but block within the His bundle has been documented by electrophysiological study, and the common occurrence of intraventricular conduction delays suggests that bilateral bundle branch block may also occur. Temporary pacing is usually sufficient, though recovery of antegrade conduction may take a week or longer. Lyme carditis should be considered in any case of heart block of unknown cause, especially in young individuals.

Antibiotic therapy (see Chapter 7.11.29) is indicated in Lyme carditis, but it is not known if this alters the course of carditis and atrioventricular block.

Cardiac sarcoidosis

Less than 10 per cent of patients with pulmonary or systemic sarcoidosis have clinically manifest cardiac involvement, ranging from conduction disturbances and arrhythmias to cardiac dilatation. Endomyocardial biopsy reveals typical sarcoid granulomas. The most serious complications of cardiac sarcoidosis are complete heart block, ventricular tachyarrhythmias, and dilated cardiomyopathy. The relatively high incidence of sudden death in patients with sarcoidosis is thought to result from sudden complete heart block or ventricular fibrillation. Patients with sarcoidosis who develop significant conduction disease, arrhythmias, or congestive heart failure should receive steroids. Occasionally, cardiac involvement will occur without detectable systemic manifestations of sarcoidosis. Thus, cardiac sarcoidosis is in the differential diagnosis of any undiagnosed ventricular arrhythmia, dilated cardiomyopathy, or atrioventricular block.

Giant cell myocarditis

Early recognition of this rapidly progressive form of myocarditis is required, as it has a prognosis considerably worse than that of non-specific lymphocytic myocarditis. The endomyocardial biopsy is distinguished by the presence of multinucleated giant cells and scattered lymphocytic infiltrates with eosinophils. The aetiology of giant cell myocarditis is unknown, but thought to be autoimmune, given its association with myasthenia gravis and other immune disorders, thymoma, and Crohn's disease. It should be suspected in patients, particularly those with a history of an autoimmune condition, who present with disease which progresses unusually rapidly, without viral prodrome, and who do not respond to standard therapy of congestive heart failure. Endomyocardial biopsy should be performed if giant cell myocarditis is suspected, because immunosuppressive therapy appears to be helpful, though not yet proved. Patients with giant cell myocarditis should be considered for early cardiac transplantation if they do not respond to therapy.

Chagas' disease (see Chapter 7.13.11)

Chagas' disease, caused by *Trypanosoma cruzi*, is the leading cause of myocarditis and dilated cardiomyopathy in some Central and South American countries, but uncommon in the United States. Overt acute myocarditis with congestive heart failure, arrhythmias, and conduction disease may develop, but cardiac involvement in early Chagas' disease is usually subclinical. Years later, chronic Chagas' disease may develop and may involve the heart. In the chronic phase, right bundle branch block and biventricular failure are present, and right heart failure predominates. Myocarditis occurs in both the acute and chronic phases, when immune mediation of myocyte injury is well documented. Antiprotozoal treatment with nifurtimox or benznidazole is beneficial in the acute phase. These agents are also indicated in the chronic phase, but, while they do reduce or eliminate serological immune markers of disease, it is not known if they improve outcome.

Further reading

Aretz HT *et al.* (1987). Myocarditis. A histopathologic definition and classification. *Cardiovascular Pathology* **1**, 3–14.

Cooper LT, Berry GJ, Shabetai R (1997). Idiopathic giant-cell myocarditis—natural history and treatment. *New England Journal of Medicine* **336**, 1860–6.

Gauntt CJ *et al.* (1995). Molecular mimicry, antcoxsackievirus B3 neutralizing monoclonal antibodies, and myocarditis. *Journal of Immunology* **154**, 2983–95.

McManus BM *et al.* (1993). Direct myocardial injury by enterovirus: a central role in the evolution of murine myocarditis. *Clinical Immunology and Immunopathology* **68**, 159–69.

McNamara DM *et al.* (1997). Intravenous immune globulin in the therapy of myocarditis and acute cardiomyopathy. *Circulation* **95**, 2476–8.

Mason JW *et al.* (1995). A clinical trial of immunosuppressive therapy for myocarditis. *New England Journal of Medicine* **333**, 269–75.

Matsumori A (1997). Molecular and immune mechanisms in the pathogenesis of cardiomyopathy. Role of viruses, cytokines and nitric oxide. *Japanese Circulation Journal* **61**, 275–91.

Midei MG *et al.* (1990). Peripartum myocarditis and cardiomyopathy. *Circulation* **81**, 922–8.

Rose NR, Hill SL (1996). The pathogenesis of postinfectious myocarditis. *Clinical Immunology and Immunopathology* **80**, S92–S99.

15.8.2 The cardiomyopathies: hypertrophic, dilated, restrictive, and right ventricular

William J. McKenna

Introduction

Heart muscle disease has traditionally been classified as idiopathic or specific. The former, termed the cardiomyopathies, are classified as hypertrophic, dilated, right ventricular, and restrictive. This descriptive classification is useful in relation to natural history, treatment, and prognosis, but recent discoveries of disease-causing mutations in genes encoding sarcomeric contractile proteins in hypertrophic, cytoskeletal proteins in dilated, and a desmosomal protein in right ventricular cardiomyopathy, all indicate that developing knowledge of aetiology/pathogenesis will ultimately require a new classification of the 'idiopathic cardiomyopathies'. The term specific heart muscle disease incorporates myocardial involvement as part of a systemic disease (such as sarcoidosis, systemic hypertension) or when the mechanism of myocardial damage is recognized (such as ischaemia).

Hypertrophic cardiomyopathy

Definition

Hypertrophic cardiomyopathy is defined clinically as an idiopathic heart muscle disorder that is characterized by a hypertrophied and non-dilated left ventricle in the absence of a cardiac or systemic cause. Such a diagnosis of exclusion often presents problems. Does the patient with moderate systemic hypertension and 1.5-cm left ventricular hypertrophy have one or two diseases? Is 1.5-cm hypertrophy a physiological response in a highly trained athlete? Diagnostic uncertainty in the presence of other causes of left ventricular hypertrophy highlights a major limitation of the current definition of hypertrophic cardiomyopathy.

Genetics

Hypertrophic cardiomyopathy is usually familial with autosomal dominant transmission. Clinical presentation with left ventricular hypertrophy under the age of 3 years is usually caused by metabolic or mitochondrial disorders (Table 1) and is unusual in autosomal dominant hypertrophic cardiomyopathy, where morphological and clinical features typically present during or following periods of childhood or adolescent growth. Clinical history reveals familial disease in 40 to 50 per cent, but when cardiovascular evaluation of first-degree relatives includes ECG and echocardiography, 90 per cent of patients have familial disease. Variable expression of the disease is common, even within families bearing the same gene defect.

Mutations in the DNA encoding cardiac β-myosin heavy chain, essential and regulatory myosin light chain, α-tropomyosin, cardiac troponin T and I, cardiac myosin binding protein C, and cardiac actin have been identified in families with hypertrophic cardiomyopathy. Mutations in these genes are found in 60 to 70 per cent of pedigrees evaluated, with those in the β-myosin heavy chain accounting for 20 to 30 per cent, defining hypertrophic cardiomyopathy as a disease of sarcomeric contractile proteins. Most mutations involve a single base-pair change, resulting in amino acid substitutions in exons encoding highly conserved regions. *De novo* mutations occur, but appear to account for 10 per cent of cases or less.

There is allelic heterogeneity with respect to penetrance, morphology, and prognosis. β-Myosin heavy chain mutations that are fully penetrant are associated with worse prognosis (such as Arg403Glu, Arg453Cys), while disease complications are uncommon in patients with mutations that cause mild or no clinical expression (such as Leu908Val). This contrasts with troponin T disease, which may cause premature sudden death in asymptomatic patients who have only minor ECG and/or echocardiographic abnormalities. Troponin T mutations cause 5 to 15 per cent of disease and are associated with incomplete penetrance, disease expression in adolescence, severe myocyte disarray despite mild hypertrophy, and sudden death in adolescents and young adults. Diagnostic difficulties in relatives of sudden death victims who had myocyte disarray with normal or near normal heart weights underscores the importance of implementing a DNA diagnostic test for troponin T. Mutations in myosin binding protein C cause 20 to 30 per cent of disease; most are major deletions rather than single base-pair changes. Myosin binding protein C disease differs in that disease expression occurs later in life, often associated with the recent onset of mild hypertension. However, once disease expression occurs (abnormal ECG and/or echocardiogram) patients may develop symptoms and are at risk from arrhythmia, emboli, and sudden death. Disease caused by the other five recognized gene abnormalities appears to account for less than 10 per cent of all cases of hypertrophic cardiomyopathy. Recently mutations have been identified in the γ subunit of AMP dependent protein kinase in families with hypertrophic cardiomyopathy, premature conduction disease, and pre-excitation cosegregating to a locus on chromosome 7.

Pathology

Hypertrophic cardiomyopathy may involve the left or both ventricles. Hypertrophy in the left ventricle is usually asymmetric, involving the anterior and posterior septum and the free wall to a greater extent than the posterior wall. Right ventricular hypertrophy, which is usually symmetric, is seen in over 30 per cent of patients; isolated right ventricular hypertrophy

Table 1 Causes of left ventricular hypertrophy at age 3 years or less

Metabolic*
Pompe disease (GSD II)
Forbes disease (GSD III)
Total lipodystrophy
Hurler's syndrome
Fabry's disease
Infant of a diabetic mother
Hypertrophic cardiomyopathy with associated syndromes
Noonan syndrome
LEOPARD syndrome
Friedreich's ataxia
Beckwith–Wiedemann syndrome
Mitochondrial myopathy
MELAS
MERFF
NADH—coenzyme Q reductase deficiency
Cytochrome b deficiency
Miscellaneous causes
Hypertension
In utero ritodrine HCl exposure
Swyer's syndrome (46, XY pure gonadal dysgenesis)

*The main metabolic causes of left ventricular hypertrophy.

GSD, glycogen storage disorder; MELAS, myopathy, encephalopathy, lactic acidosis, stroke-like episodes; MERFF, myoclonic epilepsy and ragged red fibres has not been reported. Over 60 per cent of patients have structural abnormalities of the mitral valve, including increased leaflet area, elongation of the leaflets, and malposition or anomalous insertion of the papillary muscles. Another common macroscopic finding is a patch of endocardial thickening just below the aortic valve, which results from contact of the septum with the anterior mitral leaflet in patients with mitral leaflet abnormalities and/or left ventricular outflow tract obstruction.

The histological findings in hypertrophic cardiomyopathy are distinctive and provide the basis for the pathological diagnosis (Fig. 1). Affected myocardium shows interstitial fibrosis with gross disorganization of the muscle bundles resulting in a characteristic whorled pattern. The cell-to-cell orientation of muscle cells is lost (disarray) and there is disorganization of the myofibrillar architecture within cells. Myocardial cells are wide, short, and often bizarre in shape. Foci of disorganized cells are often interspersed among areas of hypertrophied muscle cells that are otherwise normal in appearance. Such changes are not completely specific: small amounts of fibre disarray may be seen in congenitally abnormal hearts and in secondary left ventricular hypertrophy, and something similar is found at the junction of the septum with the anterior and posterior walls of the left ventricle in normal subjects. However, the extent of myocyte disarray in normal subjects rarely exceeds 5 per cent, whilst in hypertrophic cardiomyopathy up to 40 per cent of the myocardium may be involved. Extensive myocyte disarray is occasionally found in the macroscopically normal heart of a patient who experienced typical clinical features: this highlights the broader phenotype and suggests that hypertrophy may be a secondary rather than a primary abnormality.

Pathophysiology

Disarray

Myocardial disarray and hypertrophy, hyperdynamic systolic function, and impaired diastolic function account for many of the clinical features of hypertrophic cardiomyopathy. The extent and distribution of myocardial disarray can only be determined at autopsy. It is probable that the disorganized architecture with abnormal myofibre and myofibrillar alignment provides a substrate for electrical instability and contributes to diastolic abnormalities, but the precise relationship between myocardial disarray and spontaneous arrhythmia, in particular the threshold for ventricular fibrillation, has not been established.

Diastole

Diastolic abnormalities are common but variable. Typically, left ventricular end-diastolic pressure and atrial pressures are elevated as consequences of abnormal left ventricular diastolic filling and reduced compliance. The isovolumic relaxation time is prolonged, filling is slow, and the proportion of filling volume that results from atrial systolic contraction (while still preserved) may be increased. Occasionally, there is rapid early filling with

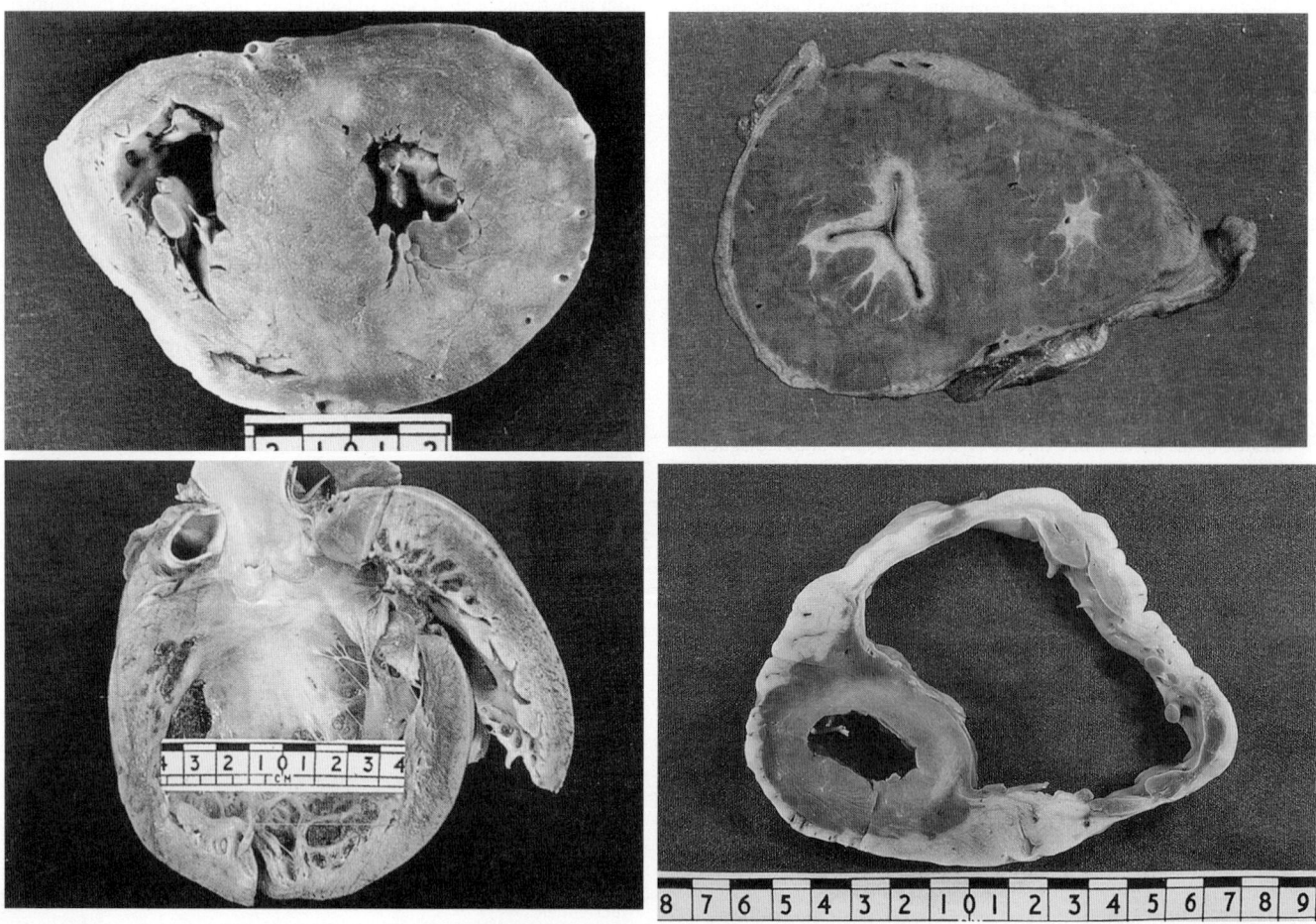

Fig. 1 Transverse short axis section through the ventricles from patients with cardiomyopathy. Upper left shows symmetrical left ventricular hypertrophy in hypertrophic cardiomyopathy. Upper right shows dense white fibrous tissue obliterating the apex of both ventricles in endomyocardial fibrosis. Lower left shows a globular, dilated left ventricle in a child with dilated cardiomyopathy. Lower right shows a grossly dilated right ventricle with adipose infiltration of the right ventricular free wall in arrhythmogenic right ventricular dysplasia. (Reproduced with permission from Davies MJ, 1986, *Colour atlas of cardiovascular pathology*, Oxford University Press.)

restrictive physiology that resembles the situation in patients with constrictive pericarditis or endocardial fibrosis (see Chapter 15.9). Altered diastolic function may be caused by myocardial hypertrophy, ischaemia, and architectural abnormalities including myocyte disarray and fibrosis. In an individual patient it is often difficult to identify the major determinant of diastolic disease.

Systole

Most young and some old patients have evidence of hyperdynamic systolic function with rapid, early, and near complete ventricular emptying. Approximately 30 per cent of patients with hyperdynamic systolic function have recordable gradients between the body and outflow tract of the left ventricle at rest; an additional 20 to 25 per cent develop such a gradient following manoeuvres that increase myocardial contractility or result in a decrease in ventricular volume with reduced afterload or venous return. The presence and magnitude of a gradient is determined not only by systolic contractile performance, but also by left ventricular outflow tract size and geometry, which are determined by the extent of upper septal hypertrophy, mitral leaflet morphology, and papillary muscle size and position. The conventionally accepted mechanism of the gradient is that Venturi forces from increased ejection velocity in the narrowed outflow tract draw the anterior and posterior mitral leaflets (which are often large and redundant) toward the septum. However, the significance of such gradients has been controversial. Many workers have claimed that the development of a left ventricular gradient in close temporal association with the development of systolic anterior motion (**SAM**) of the mitral valve and a fall in peak aortic velocity represents impediment or obstruction to left ventricular emptying, but another interpretation of these findings is that they are generated by a dynamic left ventricle that has almost completely emptied. Assessment of the significance of a left ventricular gradient in an individual patient is aided by knowledge of the relative volume ejected by the onset of the gradient. In most patients with resting left ventricular gradients (i.e. 30 to 70 mmHg), at least 70 per cent of stroke volume has already been ejected by the onset of the gradient. By contrast, patients with larger gradients usually have a significant residual volume in the left ventricle at the onset of SAM-septal contact and can be considered to have obstruction.

Ischaemia

Myocardial ischaemia despite normal epicardial coronary arteries is common and caused by several features that relate to myocardial hypertrophy (Table 2). Evidence of ischaemia, however, is not limited to those with severe hypertrophy, and abnormalities of the intramural arteries and of coronary vasomotor behaviour may also be important.

Diagnosis

Hypertrophic cardiomyopathy has been described in Western, African, and Asian populations. The prevalence in adults is estimated to be 1:500 of the population. The diagnosis of hypertrophic cardiomyopathy is based upon the demonstration of unexplained myocardial hypertrophy, which is best done using two-dimensional echocardiography. The diagnosis requires that measurements of wall thickness exceed two standard deviations for gender-, age-, and size-matched populations. In practice, in an adult of normal size, the presence of a left ventricular myocardial segment of 1.5 cm or greater in thickness, in the absence of a recognized cause, is usually considered to be diagnostic. Less stringent criteria should be applied to first-

Table 2 Potential causes of ischaemia in hypertrophic cardiomyopathy

Increased muscle mass
Elevated diastolic filling pressures
Enhanced myocardial oxygen demand (increased wall stress)
Systolic compression of arteries
Inadequate capillary density
Impaired vasodilatory reserve

degree relatives of an affected individual, where the probability of carrying the disease gene drops from 1:500 to 1:2. Unexplained symptoms or minor ECG or echocardiographic abnormalities have a high probability of representing disease expression when there is a 50 per cent chance of carrying the gene defect. Modified diagnostic criteria are applied in the context of proven familial disease (Table 3).

In children and adolescents the diagnostic features, particularly the ECG and echocardiographic manifestations of myocardial hypertrophy, often develop during or following growth spurts. The finding of a normal ECG and echo in a child or adolescent reduces the probability of their developing hypertrophic cardiomyopathy, but re-evaluation—ideally annually during adolescence—is warranted because disease expression may not occur until adolescent growth has been completed. In adults, however, the *de novo* development of unexplained left ventricular hypertrophy has so far only been seen with myosin binding protein C disease. Hence an asymptomatic adult with familial disease of onset before age 30 years who has a completely normal ECG and two-dimensional echocardiogram is at very low risk of developing hypertrophic cardiomyopathy and in practical terms does not need re-evaluation in this regard. By contrast, when there is a family history of disease presentation in later life, the possibility of late-onset disease caused by a myosin binding protein C mutation warrants re-evaluation every 3 to 5 years, or sooner if symptoms or ECG changes develop. This represents a clinical situation where a diagnostic DNA test could be cost-effective and aid clinical management.

Problems in diagnosis often arise in highly trained athletes and in patients with mild hypertension in whom the hypertrophic response appears greater than expected from the apparent stimulus. Competitive athletes normally have an increase in myocardial mass, with maximum increase of 2 to 3 mm in left ventricular wall thickness. The determinants of the hypertrophic response in a patient with hypertension are unknown, but at least in part racially determined; the Afro-Caribbean response appears to be greater than the Caucasian one. In athletes and hypertensive subjects, the diagnosis or exclusion of hypertrophic cardiomyopathy is dependent on the whole clinical picture. An athlete who has 1.5-cm left ventricular hypertrophy with either a small left ventricular cavity or a family history of hypertrophic cardiomyopathy probably does have the condition, whereas an athlete who has negative family history and normal or increased left ventricular cavity dimensions probably does not.

There is the potential for molecular genetic evaluation to provide a 'gold standard' when the clinical diagnosis is equivocal, or when preclinical diagnosis would be of value, for instance in families where there have been multiple sudden deaths in children and adolescents (namely troponin T disease). The finding of a mutation in one of the identified contractile protein genes would confirm disease, but absence of mutation would not exclude the possibility. Identification of the remaining gene(s) for hypertrophic cardiomyopathy would increase the potential value of DNA diagnostic testing.

Though less common than in young children (under 3 years), hypertrophic cardiomyopathy in adults may also be caused by metabolic and mitochondrial diseases. Fabry's disease may account for up to 2 per cent of adult hypertrophic cardiomyopathy: the distinguishing cardiovascular features of this autosomal recessive disorder remain to be fully elucidated, but reduced α-galactacidase enzyme activity is diagnostic. Enzyme replacement therapy is feasible and potentially may improve symptoms and decrease cardiac hypertrophy. Occasionally fatigue or extreme limitation of exercise that is out of proportion to the morphological and haemodynamic severity of the cardiomyopathy are the predominant symptoms. These are characteristics of mitochondrial myopathies and in the absence of severe cardiac failure, sleep apnoea, chronotrophic incompetence, and/or excessive β-blockade should lead to appropriate investigations. In Friedreich's ataxia the cardiac manifestations may precede neurological features by years, necessitating mutation analysis of the frataxin gene for diagnosis. Reduced peak oxygen consumption and early acidification during maximal

Table 3 Major and minor criteria for the diagnosis of hypertrophic cardiomyopathy in adult members of affected families

Major criteria	Minor criteria
Echocardiography	
Left ventricular wall thickness ≥ 13 mm in the anterior septum or posterior wall or ≥ 15 mm in the posterior septum or free wall	Left ventricular wall thickness of 12 mm in the anterior septum or posterior wall or of 14 mm in the posterior septum or free wall
Severe SAM (septal-leaflet contact)	Moderate SAM (no septal-leaflet contact)
	Redundant mitral valve leaflets
Electrocardiography	
Left ventricular hypertrophy + repolarization changes (Romhilt and Estes)	Complete bundle branch block or (minor) interventricular conduction defect (in LV leads)
T-wave inversion in leads I and aVL (≥ 3 mm) (with QRS–T-wave axis difference ≥ 30°), V3–V6 (≥ 3 mm) or II and III and aVF (≥ 5 mm)	Minor repolarization changes in LV leads
Abnormal Q (> 40 ms or > 25 per cent R wave) in at least two leads from II, III, aVF (in absence of left anterior hemiblock), V1–V4; or I, aVl, V5–V6.	Deep S V2 (> 25 mm)
Clinical	Unexplained chest pain, dyspnoea, or syncope

LV, left ventricular; SAM, systolic anterior motion of the mitral valve. (McKenna WJ *et al.* 1997, *Heart* **77**, 130–2. Reproduced with permission.)

Criteria fulfilled if: (1) one major or (2) two minor echocardiographic or (3) one minor echocardiographic plus two minor electrocardiographic abnormalities seen.

exercise testing with metabolic gas exchange measurements suggest a coexistent skeletal myopathy. The coexistence with the hypertrophic cardiomyopathy of other somatic features including conduction disease, accessory pathways, eye abnormalities, and diabetes are also suggestive of mitochondrial disease. However, routine neurological examination often fails to elicit abnormalities and muscle biopsy with enzyme analysis is often required for diagnosis.

Clinical features

History

Symptomatic presentation may be at any age with breathlessness on exertion, chest pain, sustained palpitation, syncope, or sudden death. Hypertrophic cardiomyopathy is occasionally found at autopsy in a stillborn baby or presents during infancy with cardiac failure, which is usually fatal. In children and adolescents the diagnosis is most often made during screening of siblings and offspring of affected family members. Paroxysmal symptoms or mild impairment of exercise tolerance are often present, but in the absence of a murmur may not elicit a diagnostic cardiac evaluation. Approximately 50 per cent of adults present with symptoms; in the remainder the diagnosis is made during family screening or following the detection of an unsuspected abnormality on physical, electrocardiographic, or echocardiographic examination.

In adults dyspnoea is common (over 50 per cent) and thought to be a consequence of elevated left atrial and pulmonary capillary wedge pressures resulting from impaired left ventricular relaxation and filling. Approximately 50 per cent of patients complain of chest pain, which is exertional, atypical, or both in similar proportions of patients. Atypical pain may have no obvious precipitant; more commonly it follows exercise or anxiety-related tachycardia, when it persists for up to several hours after the stress has been removed without enzymatic evidence of myocardial damage. Approximately 15 to 25 per cent of patients have experienced syncopal episodes, but in only a minority are there findings suggestive of an arrhythmia or evidence of overt conduction disease: in most patients the mechanism cannot be determined. Patients rarely present with symptoms attributable to left or right heart failure, for example recurrent paroxysmal nocturnal dyspnoea, ascites, or peripheral oedema. Thus, there is a wide spectrum of clinical presentation in hypertrophic cardiomyopathy, from severe cardiac failure in infancy to an incidental finding at any age.

Physical examination

In most patients with hypertrophic cardiomyopathy the physical examination is unremarkable and the detection of abnormalities is dependent on the elucidation of subtle physical signs. There is usually a rapid upstroke arterial pulse, best felt in the carotid area, which reflects dynamic left ventricular emptying. Most patients also have a forceful left ventricular cardiac impulse, best appreciated on full-held expiration in the left lateral position. In about one-third of patients the jugular venous pulse may demonstrate a prominent 'a' wave, reflecting diminished right ventricular compliance secondary to right ventricular hypertrophy. The first and second heart sounds are usually normal, and—unless patients are in atrial fibrillation—there is either a loud fourth heart sound, reflecting increased atrial systolic flow into a non-compliant ventricle, or a palpable atrial beat reflecting forceful atrial systolic contraction that may or may not be associated with significant forward flow of blood.

The most obvious physical sign in hypertrophic cardiomyopathy is an ejection systolic murmur present in those patients (20 to 30 per cent) who have a resting left ventricular outflow tract gradient. This murmur starts well after the first heart sound and ends well before the second. It is best heard at the left sternal border, radiating towards the aortic and mitral areas but not into the neck or the axilla. The intensity varies with changes in ventricular volume; it can be increased by physiological and pharmacological manoeuvres that decrease afterload or venous return (amyl nitrate, standing, Valsalva), and decreased by manoeuvres that increase afterload and venous return (squatting, phenylephrine). Occasionally, ejection systolic murmurs are associated at their onset with an ejection sound.

Most patients with a left ventricular gradient also have mitral regurgitation, which may be difficult to distinguish by auscultation. Doppler examination reveals that mitral regurgitation usually begins just before (30 to 40 ms) the onset of the gradient and continues for the duration of systole. Radiation of the systolic murmur to the axilla is often the best auscultatory clue to the presence of coexistent mitral regurgitation, which may be moderate to severe, either alone or in association with a left ventricular outflow tract gradient. A mid-diastolic rumble may sometimes result from increased transmitral flow in patients with severe mitral regurgitation; more commonly it occurs in isolation, presumably reflecting inflow tract turbulence.

Early diastolic murmurs of aortic incompetence may develop following surgical myotomy/myectomy or infective endocarditis involving the aortic valve. Although such murmurs are rare in the absence of such complications, they appear to occur more commonly than would be expected by chance and may reflect traction on the non-coronary cusp of the aortic valve by the septum. An ejection systolic murmur in the pulmonary area, reflecting right ventricular outflow tract obstruction, is also rare; when present it is usually associated with severe biventricular hypertrophy in the young or in those with coexistent Noonan's syndrome and a dysplastic pulmonary valve (see Chapter 15.12).

Prognosis

Patients with hypertrophic cardiomyopathy experience slow progression of symptoms, gradual deterioration of left ventricular function, and a significant incidence of sudden death, which occurs at all ages. Referral centre data from the 1970s and 1980s reveal an annual mortality from sudden death of 2 to 3 per cent in adults and 4 to 6 per cent in children and adolescents. It is even greater in young patients with recurrent syncope or a family history of 'malignant' hypertrophic cardiomyopathy. Although the mortality figures from non-referral hospitals are lower, the risk of sudden death is still present. More recent data in managed patients reveal annual mortality rates related to sudden death and disease of 1 and 2 per cent, respectively.

Symptomatic deterioration is usually slow. However, severe symptoms may develop in association with progressive myocardial wall thinning, presumably reflecting myocyte necrosis or fibrosis and severe reduction in left ventricular systolic performance and/or diastolic filling. Patients who experience such deterioration occasionally present with a clinical picture resembling restrictive cardiomyopathy with grossly enlarged atria, signs of right heart failure, and relative preservation of left ventricular systolic performance.

Atrial dilatation and the development of atrial fibrillation/flutter are important features in the clinical course, representing a risk of embolic stroke as well as of acute and/or chronic deterioration. Earlier onset of atrial fibrillation was considered to be an ominous development but is part of the evolution of patients with diastolic dysfunction and with appropriate management need not represent a major cause of morbidity or mortality. The largest study of patients with atrial fibrillation revealed that their 5-year survival was similar to that of age- and sex-matched patients who remained in sinus rhythm and, if the ventricular response was controlled, symptomatic status remained stable.

Left ventricular hypertrophy develops during childhood and adolescence but is not progressive in adults. The trigger and other determinants of disease expression in late-onset myosin binding protein C disease are uncertain, but (as with the other disease-causing genes) left ventricular hypertrophy does not appear to be progressive beyond the limited phase of disease expression.

Investigations

Cardiological evaluation of patients with hypertrophic cardiomyopathy is performed to confirm or make the diagnosis, to characterize the functional and morphological features to guide symptomatic therapy, and to assess the risk of complications, particularly that of sudden death.

Electrocardiography

The 12-lead electrocardiogram is the most sensitive diagnostic test, although occasionally normal (around 5 per cent), particularly in the young. Five to ten per cent are in atrial fibrillation at the time of diagnosis. Many patients have an intraventricular conduction delay, 20 per cent have left axis deviation, while complete right bundle or left bundle branch block are uncommon (less than 5 per cent). The latter may develop following surgery and is occasionally seen in the elderly. ST-segment depression and T-wave changes are the most common abnormalities and are usually associated with voltage changes of left ventricular hypertrophy and/or deep S waves in the anterior chest leads V1–V3. Isolated repolarization changes or giant negative T waves are occasionally seen. Voltage criteria for left ventricular hypertrophy are rare in the absence of repolarization changes. Approximately 20 per cent of patients have abnormal Q waves, either inferiorly (II, III, and aVF), or less commonly in leads V1–V3. P-wave abnormalities of left and/or right atrial overload are common. The distribution of the P–R interval is similar to that in the normal population, but occasionally a short P–R interval may be associated with a slurred upstroke to the QRS complex, similar to that seen in the Wolff–Parkinson–White syn-

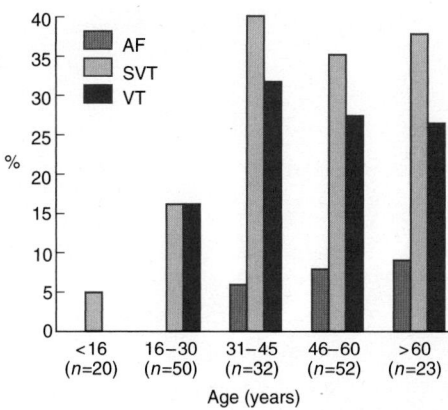

Fig. 2 The relation of arrhythmias and age in hypertrophic cardiomyopathy. SVT, supraventricular tachycardia; VT, ventricular tachycardia; AF, atrial fibrillation.

drome. At electrophysiological study such changes are not usually associated with evidence of pre-excitation, although patients with hypertrophic cardiomyopathy and accessory pathways have been described. Despite the many electrocardiographic abnormalities, there is no electrocardiogram that is typical of hypertrophic cardiomyopathy; a useful rule is to consider the diagnosis whenever the electrocardiogram is bizarre, particularly in younger patients.

The incidence of arrhythmias during 48-hour ambulatory electrocardiographic monitoring increases with age (Fig. 2). Non-sustained ventricular tachycardia is detected in 20 to 25 per cent of adults and, although usually asymptomatic, is associated with an increased risk of sudden death. Supraventricular arrhythmias are also common in adults: these are poorly tolerated if sustained (more than 30 s)—unless the ventricular response is controlled—and they carry an increased risk of embolism. By contrast, most children and adolescents are in sinus rhythm and arrhythmias during ambulatory electrocardiographic monitoring are uncommon (Fig. 2). The increased incidence of supraventricular arrhythmias with age is not surprising: their development is related to increased echocardiographic left atrial dimensions and increased left ventricular diastolic pressure, both of which increase with age. The aetiology of ventricular arrhythmias is not known, but may relate to myocyte loss and myocardial fibrosis, which appear to be related to age. Documented sustained ventricular tachycardia is uncommon, but a recognized complication in patients with an apical outpouching or aneurysm, which may develop as a consequence of midventricular obstruction.

Imaging

Chest radiography

The chest radiograph may be normal or show evidence of left and/or right atrial or left ventricular enlargement; if left atrial pressure has been chronically elevated, there may be evidence of redistribution of blood flow to upper lung zones. Mitral valve annular calcification is seen, particularly in the elderly.

Echocardiography

The extent and severity of myocardial hypertrophy is best evaluated with two-dimensional echocardiography/Doppler (Fig. 3). Left ventricular hypertrophy may be symmetric or asymmetric and localized to the septum or the free wall, but most commonly to both the septum and free wall with relative sparing of the posterior wall. 'Apical' hypertrophic cardiomyopathy appears to be common in Japan, but is rare in the West, although approximately 10 per cent of patients have left ventricular hypertrophy that is maximal in the distal ventricle from the level of the papillary muscles down to the apex. Approximately one-third of patients also have hypertrophy of the right ventricular free wall, the presence and severity of which is strongly

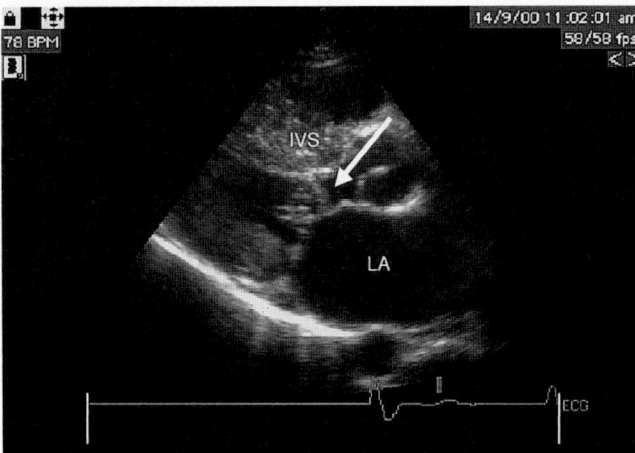

Fig. 3 An echocardiogram (parasternal long axis view) of a patient with hypertrophic obstructive cardiomyopathy demonstrating hypertrophy of the interventricular septum (IVS), enlargement of the left atrium (LA), and systolic anterior motion of the mitral valve, bringing it into contact with the septum (arrow).

related to the severity of left ventricular hypertrophy. Typically, left ventricular end-systolic and end-diastolic dimensions are reduced, and the left atrial dimension is increased. Indices of systolic function such as ejection fraction may be increased, but systolic function is often impaired, which may be best appreciated by measurement of long axis rather than short axis function.

Colour Doppler provides a sensitive method of detecting left ventricular outflow tract turbulence (Fig. 4 and Plate 1), and when combined with continuous wave Doppler the peak velocity (Vmax) of left ventricular blood flow can be measured and left ventricular outflow tract gradients calculated. Doppler-calculated gradients (pressure gradient (mmHg) = $4V$max^2) are seen in 20 to 30 per cent of patients and correlate well with those measured invasively. Systolic anterior motion of the mitral valve is usually present when the calculated outflow tract gradient is more than 30 mmHg. Early closure or fluttering of the aortic valve leaflets and Doppler evidence of mitral regurgitation are often seen in association with systolic anterior motion of the mitral valve. A posteriorly directed mitral

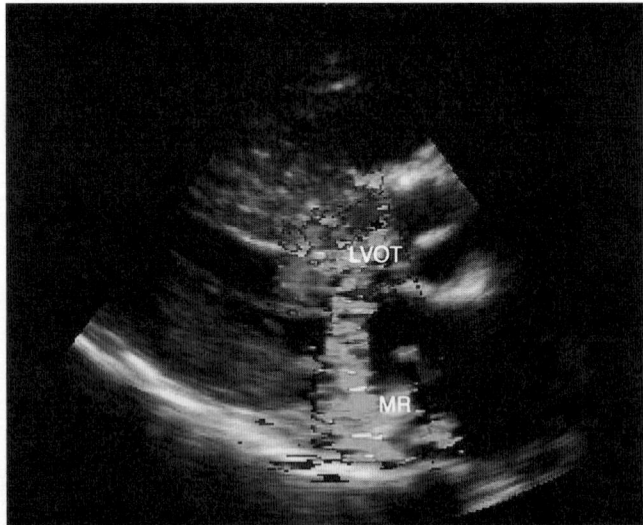

Fig. 4 Colour flow Doppler image (parasternal long axis view) of the same patient as shown in Fig. 3, demonstrating left ventricular outflow tract (LVOT) turbulence and mitral regurgitation (MR) with a posteriorly directed jet. (See also Plate 1.)

regurgitant jet is seen in association with and related to the magnitude of the outflow tract gradient (Fig. 4). An anterior regurgitant jet or mitral regurgitation in the absence of obstruction suggest the coexistence of structural mitral valve abnormalities.

Other imaging techniques
There is no role for routine magnetic resonance or computed tomographic imaging, but these modalities may be helpful when echocardiography fails to visualize cardiac structures adequately, particularly the left ventricular apex.

Cardiac catheterization
Two-dimensional echo/Doppler evaluation has replaced invasive haemodynamic measurements and angiography as the method of assessing left ventricular structure and function in hypertrophic cardiomyopathy. Cardiac catheterization is not necessary for diagnosis and is rarely indicated unless symptoms are refractory and direct measurement of cardiac pressures is potentially informative, particularly in assessing the severity of mitral regurgitation. Coronary arteriography may be necessary to exclude coexistent coronary artery disease in older patients who have significant angina or ST-segment changes during exercise. The left coronary arteries are usually large in calibre. The left anterior descending and septal perforator arteries may demonstrate phasic narrowing during systole in the absence of fixed obstructive lesions, but such changes do not appear to relate to symptoms.

Left ventricular angiography is rarely indicated, but recognition of the abnormally shaped ventricle, which typically ejects at least 75 per cent of its contents in association with mild mitral regurgitation, may provide a valuable diagnostic clue when hypertrophic cardiomyopathy was not suspected before catheterization.

Exercise testing
Maximal exercise testing in association with respiratory gas analysis provides useful functional and prognostic information, which can be monitored serially. Peak oxygen ventilatory capacity (peak V_{O_2}) is often moderately and occasionally severely reduced, even in patients who claim their exercise tolerance is not limited. Continuous measurement of the blood pressure during upright treadmill or bicycle exercise reveals that approximately one-third of younger patients (less than 40 years) have an abnormal blood-pressure response, with either drops of more than 20 mmHg from peak recordings or a failure to rise by 20 mmHg or more despite an appropriate increase in cardiac output. Such changes are usually asymptomatic but are associated with an increased risk of sudden death. The mechanism of the hypotensive response during exercise in hypertrophic cardiomyopathy is uncertain, but may relate to myocardial mechanoreceptor activation and altered baroreflex control causing inappropriate drops in systemic vasculature resistance despite maintenance of an appropriate cardiac output. ST-segment depression of 2 mm from baseline is documented in 25 per cent of patients. The relation of such changes to metabolic markers of ischaemia requires further evaluation and their prognostic significance has yet to be determined.

Electrophysiological studies
Electrophysiological studies may occasionally be necessary in patients with sustained, rapid palpitation to identify associated accessory pathways or aid management of sustained monomorphic ventricular tachycardia. Conventional programmed ventricular stimulation does not aid the identification of high-risk patients (see below).

Management

Pharmacological
The goal of therapy is to improve symptoms and prevent complications, in particular sudden death. β-Adrenoceptor blockers, particularly propranolol, and calcium antagonists, especially verapamil, are the mainstay of

symptomatic pharmacological therapy. Both drugs have several potentially beneficial actions, including a decrease in the determinants of myocardial oxygen consumption and blunting of the heart-rate response during exercise, providing increased time for filling at equivalent workloads in those with poor relaxation and slow filling. Both agents exert a negative inotropic effect, thereby reducing hyperdynamic systolic function and left ventricular gradients; it is also claimed they improve diastolic filling, verapamil by improving relaxation and propranolol by increasing compliance. The side-effects of propranolol are rarely serious, but the suppressant effect of verapamil on atrioventricular nodal conduction may cause problems in patients with unsuspected pre-existing conduction disease, and its vasodilatory and negative inotropic effects have resulted in acute pulmonary oedema and death. In practice, both drugs are effective but it is safer to use propranolol. If this is ineffective, verapamil can then be tried, but it should be started in hospital in patients with conduction abnormalities, resting or provocable gradients, or impaired systolic function.

Surgical

Surgery is a therapeutic option in patients with obstruction and/or mitral valve abnormalities. The conventional indication for surgery has been a resting left ventricular outflow tract gradient of more than 50 mmHg in patients refractory to medical therapy, and the commonest operation has been to remove a segment of the upper anterior septum (myotomy/myectomy) via a transaortic approach. Transventricular approaches have been used, but these are associated with a higher incidence of late complications, particularly of cardiac failure. Mitral valve 'repair' and papillary muscle repositioning or remodelling may be required, and mitral valve replacement has also been advocated; excellent results have been achieved, particularly in elderly patients with severe mitral regurgitation. Specialist hypertrophic cardiomyopathy centres report perioperative mortality of 2 per cent or less, with 80 per cent success in abolishing gradients and improving symptoms. It is unlikely, however, that such excellent results are obtained in centres with more limited experience of the medical and surgical aspects of the condition. Obstruction is a function of several features including septal hypertrophy, outflow tract dimensions, ventricular geometry and flow patterns, mitral valve/papillary muscle anatomy and position, and left ventricular contractile performance. The approach to gradient reduction needs to be individualized to a greater extent than has been recognized, perhaps contributing to mortality rates of 5 to 10 per cent in early operative series.

Pacing

The pacing option was promoted following recognition that alteration of the ventricular activation sequence, with optimization of filling characteristics by DDD pacing, may result in reduction of gradients and filling pressures and improved symptoms in selected patients. The role of DDD pacing in symptomatic management of obstruction was evaluated in three randomized multicentre trials, demonstrating symptomatic improvement and gradient reduction (50 per cent), but no change in exercise capacity. However, the placebo effect of the procedure was considerable: 40 per cent reported significant symptomatic improvement with the pacemaker programmed to a standby mode. Overall, the initial enthusiasm for DDD pacing has not been substantiated by greater experience and trials. Nevertheless, pacing offers a therapeutic option in patients with obstruction that is refractory to drug treatment, and in whom surgery is either not acceptable or inappropriate. It appears that elderly patients with localized septal hypertrophy and without significant free wall involvement or mitral regurgitation may do particularly well.

Other techniques

Injection of alcohol into the septal artery that supplies the 'obstructing' septal muscle has been developed as a percutaneous, non-pharmacological approach to gradient reduction. Most experienced centres have reported excellent results. As for surgery and DDD pacing, patient selection—in particular regarding the mechanism of the gradient—and technical consider-

ations are important determinants of outcome. The major complication has been the need for a pacemaker in 5 to 10 per cent, and concerns remain about long-term left ventricular function and arrhythmia risk from the 'controlled myocardial infarction'. At present alcohol septal ablation offers a therapeutic option in older patients with suitable anatomy who are refractory to drugs.

Particular symptoms

Dyspnoea

Dyspnoea most often occurs in patients who also experience chest pain or discomfort. Treatment depends on the predominant mechanism. In patients with dyspnoea who have slow filling that continues throughout diastole, β-blockers and verapamil are appropriate. Conversely, those with rapid early filling may benefit from a relative tachycardia and do better without negative chronotrophic agents. When dyspnoea is associated with significant obstruction, that is, at least 50 per cent of stroke volume in the left ventricle at the onset of the gradient, β-blockers, disopyramide, and—failing this—myotomy/myectomy or the other non-pharmacological options may be beneficial. Disopyramide should be used in the maximum tolerated dose (anticholinergic side-effects may limit higher doses) in conjunction with a conventional β-blocker. Occasionally, dyspnoea is associated with severe mitral regurgitation and responds well to mitral valve replacement. Endocarditis is a rare complication of hypertrophic cardiomyopathy; it occurs in patients with left ventricular outflow tract turbulence and/or mitral regurgitation, may involve the mitral and/or aortic valve, and is usually associated with increased dyspnoea. Antibiotic prophylaxis is important in appropriate patients, such as those with intracardiac transvalvular turbulence.

Chest pain

When chest pain is severe, associated with significant ST-segment changes during exercise, or refractory to therapy, the performance of coronary arteriography is warranted to exclude coexistent coronary artery disease. The results of coronary artery bypass grafting in hypertrophic cardiomyopathy are good, even when additional procedures such as myectomy/mitral valve replacement are performed. Exertional chest pain usually responds to therapy with propranolol or verapamil, and when refractory has responded to very high doses of these agents (propranolol at 480 mg daily, verapamil at 720 mg daily). Short-acting nitrates, diuretics, and high-dose verapamil may be useful in selected patients, perhaps by reducing filling pressures and improving coronary flow to subendocardial layers. Atypical chest pain may persist long after the initial stimulus has been removed.

Arrhythmia

Arrhythmias are a common complication of hypertrophic cardiomyopathy. Treatment with anticoagulants and digoxin, with or without verapamil or β-blockers, is appropriate once atrial fibrillation is established. The aim of therapy is to control the ventricular response and prevent emboli. Most patients who develop atrial fibrillation during electrocardiographic monitoring are unaware of changes from sinus rhythm to atrial fibrillation as long as the ventricular response is well controlled. However, in a few cases the loss of atrial systolic contribution to filling volume is important, when electrical cardioversion can be facilitated by prior therapy (4 to 6 weeks) with amiodarone (300 mg daily) if pharmacological cardioversion does not occur first.

Sustained (more than 30 s) episodes of paroxysmal atrial fibrillation or supraventricular tachycardia occur, representing a risk of haemodynamic collapse and emboli. Low-dose amiodarone (1000 to 1400 mg weekly) is effective in suppressing such episodes and also provides control of the ventricular response should breakthrough occur. If episodes persist, the threshold for anticoagulation should be low as embolic complications are common, even when atrial dimensions are only moderately increased.

Non-sustained episodes of supraventricular arrhythmia are common. Though often asymptomatic they are a marker (albeit of low positive predictive accuracy) for the subsequent development of established atrial fibrillation. If they occur in the presence of atrial enlargement, the threshold to introduce amiodarone with or without anticoagulation should be low. Episodes of non-sustained ventricular tachycardia are common but are rarely symptomatic: therapy is warranted only if it can be shown to improve prognosis (see below).

Prevention of sudden death

Sudden death is probably a consequence of multiple interacting mechanisms. The histological abnormalities, particularly myocyte disarray, small vessel disease, and replacement scarring, contribute to the underlying substrate. Events may be triggered by haemodynamic alterations, myocardial ischaemia, and arrhythmias, including ventricular tachycardia, atrial fibrillation, atrioventricular block, and rapid conduction of a supraventricular arrhythmia via an accessory pathway. Intense physical exertion may also contribute to the above triggers. The interaction of triggers and substrate may be modified by inappropriate peripheral vascular responses and the development of ischaemia.

Risk factor stratification

Prevention of sudden death relies on risk factor stratification to identify the high-risk cohort. Several adverse features, which can be elicited from the clinical history and non-invasive evaluation, have been identified (Table 4). Their relative importance varies with age; for example, the finding of non-sustained ventricular tachycardia on 24-h electrocardiographic monitoring in children and adolescents is uncommon (less than 5 per cent), but is associated with an eightfold increased risk of sudden death, whereas in adults this arrhythmia is common (20 to 25 per cent), but in isolation confers only a twofold increased risk.

In the young (less than 25 years) the finding of non-sustained ventricular tachycardia, severe and diffuse left ventricular hypertrophy, unexplained syncope (particularly if recurrent or exertional), or a family history where a high proportion of affected individuals experienced premature (less than 40 years) sudden death warrants prophylactic treatment. Such patients usually also exhibit abnormal exercise blood-pressure responses, indeed the finding of a normal exercise blood-pressure response appears to identify the low-risk younger (less than 40 years) patient (negative predictive accuracy 97 per cent), allowing appropriate reassurance that is also clinically important. In adults aged 25 to 60 years the positive predictive accuracy for each of the risk factors is lower (15 to 20 per cent): in general prophylactic treatment is reserved for those with two or more risk factors who will have a predicted risk of sudden death of at least 2 per cent per year.

It is important to consider risk in all patients, even those who are asymptomatic or who have mild echocardiographic features of hypertrophic cardiomyopathy. Though children and adolescents with severe congestive symptoms may be at greater risk, the data reveals that the severity of chest pain, dyspnoea, and exercise limitation are not reliable predictors of the risk of sudden death in adults. In addition it is recognized that most patients who die suddenly have mild (1.5 to 2.0 cm) or moderate (2.0 to 2.5 cm) left ventricular hypertrophy, while some genetic defects (for instance cardiac troponin T) may cause sudden death in the absence of symptoms or hypertrophy. The presence of a left ventricular outflow tract gradient is not associated with sudden death, although data on patients

Table 4 Risk factors for sudden death

Family history of sudden death (≥ 2 premature [< 40 years] sudden deaths)
Unexplained syncope within previous year
Abnormal exercise blood pressure
Non-sustained ventricular tachycardia (≥ 3 beats at ≥ 120 beats/min)
Severe left ventricular hypertrophy (> 3 cm)
Cardiac arrest (or sustained ventricular tachycardia)

with large gradients (more than 100 mmHg) are limited. Diastolic impairment with abnormal Doppler filling patterns and atrial enlargement is associated with symptomatic limitation and poor prognosis, but not with premature sudden death.

Some investigators have suggested that the induction of sustained ventricular arrhythmias during programmed electrophysiological stimulation is associated with a higher risk of sudden death. However, the predictive accuracy is low, and as most high-risk patients can be identified using non-invasive clinical markers, the inherent risks and inconvenience associated with programmed stimulation dictate that it should not be used routinely to assess risk in hypertrophic cardiomyopathy.

Dilated cardiomyopathy

Definition

Dilated cardiomyopathy is characterized by unexplained dilatation and impaired contractile performance of the left ventricle. Potential causes of ventricular dysfunction, particularly coronary artery disease and systemic hypertension, must be excluded for the diagnosis to be made. Typical angina pectoris, fluctuating ST and T-wave changes, and regional abnormalities on two-dimensional echocardiography or thallium scintigraphy, which reflect damage to a specific vascular territory, suggest ischaemic heart disease. Renal and ocular hypertensive changes may provide a useful marker of previous systemic hypertension, but are often unremarkable in the decompensated phase in the normotensive patient. Calcific aortic stenosis may be overlooked as a cause of heart failure, particularly when the murmur is soft or absent.

Specific heart muscle disorders should also be considered in differential diagnosis (see Chapter 15.8.3). A primary cardiac presentation of diabetes mellitus, connective tissue disorders, and neuromuscular disease is rare, but arrhythmias or progressive conduction disturbance with mild left ventricular dysfunction may provide the earliest evidence of cardiac sarcoidosis.

Since the definition of dilated cardiomyopathy is a diagnosis of exclusion, it is likely that structural and functional abnormalities result from heterogeneous pathogenic processes. In North America and Europe symptomatic dilated cardiomyopathy has an incidence and prevalence of 20 and 38 per 100 000, respectively, and is the commonest indication for cardiac transplantation.

Genetics

Pedigree analysis reveals familial disease in at least 25 per cent of cases and an additional cohort (10 to 20 per cent) with mild abnormalities of left ventricular performance who possibly have early presymptomatic dilated cardiomyopathy. Inheritance is usually autosomal dominant with incomplete penetrance, although families with X-linked transmission have been reported. Different patterns of disease expression are recognized. Disease progression appears to be slow (over decades) in most cases, and conduction disturbance is a late complication related to disease severity. However, in some families (less than 20 per cent) the early stages are characterized by progressive conduction disease, and left ventricular dilatation and impairment are later manifestations, which typically occur in the 4th to 6th decade. Families are also recognized in whom dilated cardiomyopathy develops in later decades in individuals who have had sensorineural hearing loss since childhood, or in association with skeletal myopathy.

Penetrance is age dependent and has been estimated to be 10 per cent in those aged less than 20 years, 34 per cent in young adults aged 20 to 30 years, 60 per cent in adults aged 30 to 40 years, and 90 per cent in those over 40 years. Familial evaluation is recommended: guidelines have been proposed, based on the identification of major and minor criteria for the diagnosis (Table 5). It has been proposed that the diagnosis of familial dilated cardiomyopathy is fulfilled in a first-degree relative of a proband in

Table 5 Major and minor criteria for the diagnosis of familial dilated cardiomyopathy in adult members of affected families (see text for details)

Major criteria	Minor criteria
• A reduced ejection fraction of the left ventricle (< 45%) and/or fractional shortening (< 25%) as assessed by echocardiography, radionuclide scanning, or angiography • An increased left ventricular end-diastolic diameter corresponding to > 117% of the predicted value corrected for age and body surface area (Manolio *et al.* 1992)	• Unexplained supraventricular or ventricular arrhythmia • Mitral dilatation (> 112% of the predicted value) • An intermediate impairment of left ventricular dysfunction • Conduction defects • Segmental wall motion abnormalities in the absence of intraventricular conduction defect or ischaemic heart disease • Unexplained sudden death of a first-degree relative or stroke before 50 years of age

the presence of one major criterion, or left ventricular dilatation plus one minor criterion, or three minor criteria.

Disease-causing genes have been reported in dystrophin (X-linked), taffazin (X-linked Barth syndrome), metavinculin (X-linked), cardiac actin (two small autosomal dominant families), lamin A/C (families with premature conduction disease), and desmin (1 of 44 probands with gene-positive affected family members). Lamin A/C mutations may also cause Emery–Dreifuss and limb girdle muscular dystrophy and familial partial lipodystrophy, desmin may cause conduction disease, and dystrophin mutations cause childhood (Duchenne) and adult (Becker) forms of muscular dystrophy. Mutations in these genes appear to account for less than 5 per cent of cases of dilated cardiomyopathy, but they provide potentially valuable clues in relation to aetiology and pathogenesis. The function of taffazin is unknown, but the other genes all encode cytoskeletal proteins that are involved in force transmissions between cells. The recent identification of mutations in genes which encode for sarcomere proteins (TropT, βMHC) involved in force generation may change this paradigm.

Pathogenesis

Based on the molecular genetic findings described above, dilated cardiomyopathy is hypothesized to be a disease of the cardiac cytoskeleton, but pathogenesis is poorly defined. Macroscopic examination of hearts with dilated cardiomyopathy taken at autopsy or explanted reveals dilated cardiac chambers (Fig. 1), mural thrombi, and platelet aggregates with normal extra- and intramural coronary arteries. Histology shows features consistent with healed myocarditis—patchy perimyocyte and interstitial fibrosis, various stages of myocyte death, as well as myocyte hypertrophy and rare isolated inflammatory cells (see Chapter 15.8.1). These postinflammatory findings are non-specific and do not suggest a particular pathogenesis.

The myocardial depressant effects of alcohol in normal and diseased myocardium are established. Alcohol, like pregnancy, may precipitate cardiac failure in predisposed individuals, but an additional specific aetiological or pathogenetic role remains uncertain. Viral involvement is supported by viral myocarditis progressing to dilated cardiomyopathy in specific genetic strains of a murine model, as well as in isolated rare patients, also by an association with abnormal coxsackievirus serology and hybridization studies that show non-replicating enteroviral genome in a variable proportion (0 to 30 per cent) of dilated cardiomyopathy hearts. The potential for immune pathogenesis is supported by development of autoimmune murine myocarditis and by the findings of a cardiac- and disease-specific autoantibody in over 30 per cent of patients with dilated cardiomyopathy and their first-degree relatives, inappropriate MHC class II expression on endothelial cells from cardiac tissue, and a weak HLA DR4 association.

In summary, pathogenesis of dilated cardiomyopathy remains controversial, with resolution hampered by clinical presentation at 'endstage' when pathogenesis may be largely completed. A reasonable working hypothesis proposes an immune pathogenesis, with or without a viral trigger, in genetically predisposed individuals who carry a cytoskeletal or sarcomere gene mutation.

Clinical features

Dilated cardiomyopathy has been described in Western, African, and Asian populations, affecting both genders and all ages. Initial presentation is usually with symptoms of cardiac failure (fatigue, breathlessness, decreased exercise tolerance), but an arrhythmia (atrial fibrillation, ventricular tachycardia, atrioventricular block), a systemic embolus, or the finding of an electrocardiographic or radiographic abnormality during routine screening may prompt earlier diagnosis. Symptoms, physical signs, and chest radiographic changes are those of cardiac failure (see Chapter 15.2.2) and depend on the stage of the disease.

Physical examination may be entirely normal or may reveal evidence of myocardial dysfunction with cardiac enlargement and signs of congestive heart failure. Systolic blood pressure is usually low with a narrow pulse pressure and a low volume arterial pulse. In patients with severe left ventricular failure, pulsus alternans may be present and the jugular veins may be distended, with a prominent V wave reflecting tricuspid regurgitation. In such patients the liver is often engorged and pulsatile, and there is usually peripheral oedema and ascites. The precordium often reveals a diffuse and dyskinetic left and occasionally a right ventricular impulse. The apical impulse is usually displaced laterally, reflecting ventricular dilatation. The second heart sound is usually normally split, but paradoxical splitting may be present when there is left bundle branch block, which occurs is approximately 15 per cent of patients. With severe disease and the development of pulmonary hypertension, the pulmonary component of the second heart sound may be accentuated. Characteristically, a presystolic gallop or fourth heart sound is present before the development of overt cardiac failure. However, once cardiac decompensation has occurred, ventricular gallop or third heart sound is often present. When there is significant ventricular dilatation, systolic murmurs are common, reflecting mitral and (less commonly) tricuspid regurgitation.

The development of unexplained cardiac failure during pregnancy or within the 3 months following parturition is often labelled as peripartum cardiomyopathy. Unrecognized pre-eclamptic heart disease may also present with cardiac failure and should be excluded by careful examination of the antenatal records; this has a different prognosis and recurs with increasing severity during subsequent pregnancies unless treated. Antecedent cardiac evaluation is often absent in those with peripartum cardiomyopathy, and there is usually uncertainty whether the cardiac failure is acute (for instance potentially myocarditic) or chronic and exacerbated by the haemodynamic stress of pregnancy and labour (for instance dilated cardiomyopathy). When the heart failure is acute and there is persistence of left ventricular chamber dilatation or impaired systolic performance, the diagnosis of peripartum cardiomyopathy can legitimately be made. The mechanism and true natural history is uncertain, though it is probable that the adverse prognostic effect of subsequent pregnancies is less important than the literature would suggest, particularly in those with only mild residual abnormalities of left ventricular structure and function. For further discussion of cardiac disease in pregnancy, see Chapter 13.6.

Arrhythmia

Atrial arrhythmias and particularly atrial fibrillation are common and are associated with the severity of symptoms, left ventricular dysfunction, and poor prognosis. Atrial fibrillation is a marker of disease severity, but not an independent predictor of disease progression or sudden death. Occasionally, however, focal atrial tachycardia or atrial fibrillation may cause a tachycardia that results in gradual deterioration in left ventricular function, resembling dilated cardiomyopathy. Systolic function usually returns to normal with control of the arrhythmia.

Ventricular arrhythmias are also common and like supraventricular arrhythmias are markers of disease severity. Non-sustained ventricular tachycardia during ECG monitoring is seen in approximately 20 per cent of asymptomatic or mildly symptomatic patients and in up to 70 per cent of those who are severely symptomatic. The prognostic significance of this arrhythmia is controversial: its presence early in the course of disease, when left ventricular function is relatively preserved, is probably an independent marker of sudden death risk, whereas in general, markers of haemodynamic severity (such as ejection fraction, left ventricular end-diastolic dimension, filling pressures) are more predictive of disease-related mortality and sudden death. Sudden death risk in patients with severe disease (NYHA Class III, IV) increases approximately threefold when syncope is present.

Prognosis

The prognosis of dilated cardiomyopathy is uncertain because the diagnosis is usually not made until clinical features, which are late manifestations of the disease, become obvious. However, recent follow-up of a large cohort of asymptomatic first-degree relatives suggests that disease progression is insidious over decades. An upper respiratory tract infection or a salt or fluid load (pregnancy) often precipitates clinical presentation. Symptoms develop when filling pressures rise or stroke volume diminishes sufficiently to cause salt and water retention and oedema. Once clinical symptoms of impaired ventricular performance are apparent, prognosis is poor and related to the degree of left ventricular dilatation and impaired contractile performance. Data from adult and paediatric referral centres in the 1970s and 1980s indicate 50 per cent mortality from progressive heart failure or its complications in the 2 years following referral diagnosis. Survival will undoubtedly be improved by recognition of asymptomatic family members as well as of others with early/mild disease, and by modern management including the early introduction of ACE inhibitors, β-blockade, aggressive treatment of arrhythmias, and the availability of cardiac transplantation. Treatment will usually stabilize or improve the patient's condition once symptoms develop, with a reduction in cardiac dimensions and improvement in myocardial performance. However, conventional evaluation of cardiovascular structure and function does not permit accurate prediction of outcome and there is an annual mortality of up to 4 per cent, predominantly from sudden death, even in those who improve or stabilize.

The recent recognition of the familial nature of dilated cardiomyopathy indicates that a correct diagnosis is of practical importance for family members as there is now the potential to identify individuals with dilated cardiomyopathy at an early or preclinical stage.

Investigation

Cardiological evaluation of patients with dilated cardiomyopathy is performed to confirm the diagnosis, to determine objective measurements of functional capacity as a guide to symptomatic treatment, and to assess risk of complications, particularly progressive deterioration, arrhythmias, and sudden death.

By the time of diagnosis in a referral centre, a normal ECG is rare (less than 5 per cent) and most patients show features consistent with diffuse myocardial abnormalities. Twenty per cent are in established atrial fibrillation and paroxysmal supraventricular and ventricular arrhythmias during 24-h ECG monitoring are common.

Patient perception of functional limitation relates to many factors, including the time course of the illness, and is very variable. Maximal exercise testing, ideally with respiratory gas analysis, provides a simple reproducible measure of functional capacity and is also useful to exclude ischaemia and assess risk of arrhythmia. Similarly two-dimensional echocardiography is important in providing an easily repeated measure of cardiac cavity dimensions and systolic performance, assessment of regional wall motion as well as mural and intracavitary thrombi (Figs 5 and 6 and Plate 2). In the young patient the origins of the right and left main coronary arteries can often be visualized to exclude mainstem coronary anomalies as the cause of myocardial dysfunction. Symptoms, exercise testing, and two-

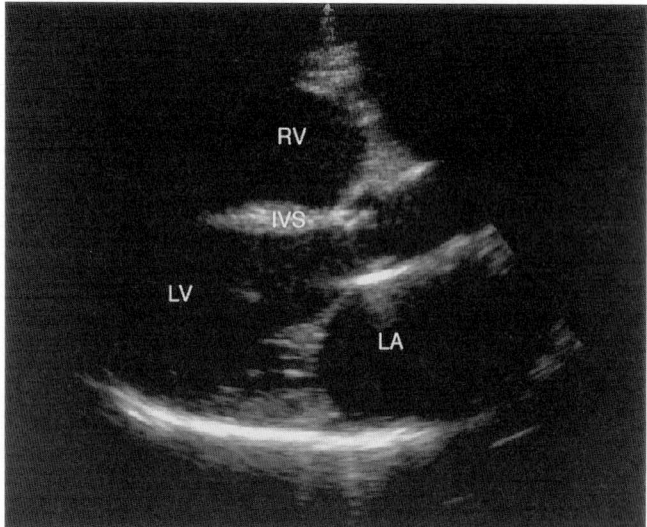

(a)

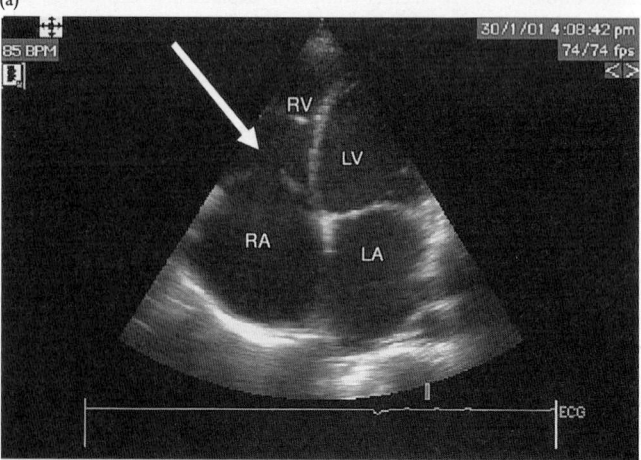

(b)

Fig. 5 Echocardiographic appearances of a young patient with familial dilated cardiomyopathy. Panel A: parasternal long-axis view showing significant left atrial (LA) and biventricular dilatation with a thin intraventricular septum (IVS). Panel B: apical four-chamber view demonstrating dilatation of all four chambers. There is failure of the tricuspid leaflets to coapt in systole (arrow). LV, left ventricle; RA, right atrium; RV, right ventricle.

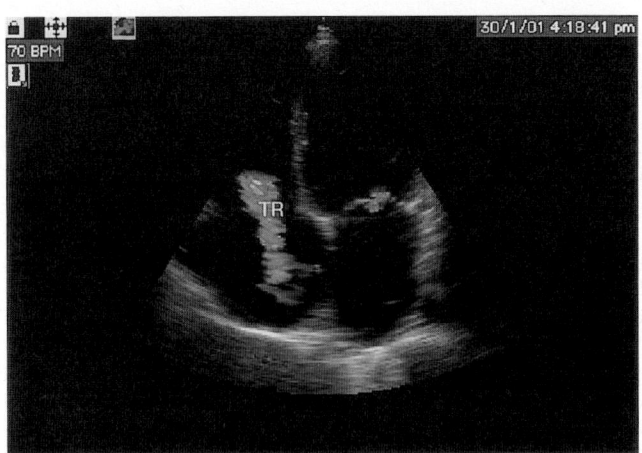

Fig. 6 Colour flow Doppler image of the same patient as shown in Fig. 5 showing a regurgitant tricuspid jet (TR). (See also Plate 2.)

dimensional echocardiography provide the basis for assessment of treatment and monitoring of disease progression.

Many of the systemic diseases that are associated with heart muscle disorders have typical clinical, immunological, and biochemical features (see Chapter 15.8.3), and in the absence of evidence to suggest a systemic disease an exhaustive 'routine screen' is probably not cost-effective. There are, however, several potential reversible secondary causes of heart muscle disorder that may simulate dilated cardiomyopathy, and basic screening tests should include serum phosphorus (hypophosphataemia), serum calcium (hypocalcaemia), serum creatinine and urea (uraemia), thyroid function tests (hypothyroidism), and serum iron/ferritin (haemochromatosis).

Electrophysiological testing

Programmed electrical stimulation is of limited clinical value in the identification of high-risk patients. Polymorphic ventricular tachycardia is inducible in up to 30 per cent of cases, but this is a non-specific endpoint. Approximately 10 per cent of patients have inducible sustained monomorphic ventricular tachycardia; about one-third of these die suddenly, but most (75 per cent) who die in this way do not have inducible ventricular tachycardia during programmed stimulation.

Inducible ventricular tachycardia usually arises from diseased myocardium. However, bundle branch re-entry ventricular tachycardia may occur, and in one selected series was seen in up to 40 per cent of patients. This tachycardia is typically rapid (mean cycle length 280 ms) and uses a macrore-entrant circuit that involves the His Purkinje system, usually with right bundle branch anterograde conduction and left bundle branch retrograde conduction. Differentiation from myocardial ventricular tachycardia is confirmed by the presence of a His or right bundle branch potential preceding each QRS: diagnosis is important since catheter ablation of either the left or right bundle branch usually is curative.

Cardiac catheterization/biopsy

Coronary arteriography should be performed if doubt remains regarding potential ischaemic aetiology of left ventricular dysfunction. Cardiac catheterization is also warranted for measurement of pulmonary vascular resistance in those with very severe or rapidly progressive disease in whom cardiac transplantation may be required. However, if coronary artery disease can be confidently excluded and transplantation is not an imminent consideration, then cardiac catheterization is not required for a diagnosis or symptomatic management. Useful prognostic information regarding cardiac enlargement and systolic performance can be more readily provided from echocardiographic or radionuclide studies.

The role of endomyocardial biopsy is controversial. It is warranted to exclude myocarditis and specific heart muscle disorders and to characterize patients for the presence of viral genome and markers of immune acti-

vation, but these evaluations require specialist expertise in cardiac pathology that may not be readily available and the therapeutic implications of findings are uncertain.

Management

Management in dilated cardiomyopathy is aimed at improving symptoms, attenuating disease progression, and preventing arrhythmia, stroke, and sudden death. Such non-specific therapy is unsatisfactory and will remain so until the aetiology and pathogenesis of dilated cardiomyopathy are better delineated.

Pharmacological

Symptomatic therapy is the treatment of heart failure with reliance on ACE inhibitors, β-blockers, and diuretics (see Chapters 15.2.2 and 15.5.1). Evidence-based therapy of cardiac failure has, with few exceptions, not specifically been evaluated in dilated cardiomyopathy in a randomized fashion, but is likely to be as effective as in others with this condition. Vigorous exercise and significant alcohol intake are proscribed. Moderate- to high-dose ACE inhibition is probably the goal, although in advanced disease this may be limited by hypotension and take time to achieve. The use of low-dose β-blockade with gradual dosage augmentation as tolerated over months is increasingly supported by trial evidence, with metoprolol (6.25 to 50 mg twice daily), bisoprolol (1.25 to 10 mg once daily), and carvedilol (3.125 to 50 mg twice daily) proven to be beneficial. Note, however, that rapid increase in dosage of β-blockers or their sudden withdrawal after chronic administration may precipitate deterioration and dosage changes should be made gradually. Diuretics should be reserved for patients with congestive symptoms as their inappropriate use will limit the ability to achieve optimal dose of ACE inhibitor and β-blocker.

If sustained or symptomatic arrhythmias are documented during 24-h ECG monitoring or exercise testing, conventional treatment is warranted (see Chapter 15.6). Amiodarone (100 to 400 mg daily) has no negative inotropic effect and is effective in suppressing both supraventricular and ventricular arrhythmias. Most class I antiarrhythmics will depress left ventricular function and are likely to be poorly tolerated. The use of low-dose amiodarone (200 mg od) with low to moderate dose of a β-blocker is often effective, but the combination of sotalol and amiodarone represents a proarrhythmic risk because of their additive effects on repolarization. If drug treatment is unsuccessful, the threshold for implantation a cardioverter defibrillator should be low, although concomitant antiarrhythmic therapy may still be required.

Non-pharmacological

Non-pharmalogical alternatives for the treatment of heart failure are increasingly available. Permanent pacing can correct two important intracardiac conduction abnormalities. First, a small subset of patients who have marked P–R interval prolongation (more than 220 ms), usually secondary to atrioventricular nodal disease, experience deleterious effects on left ventricular haemodynamics with reduction in diastolic ventricular filling time and the development of end-diastolic tricuspid and mitral regurgitation. Correction of P–R interval prolongation with short atrioventricular delay dual-chamber pacing may increase stroke volume and blood pressure, and decrease mitral regurgitation with dramatic clinical improvement. Second, patients with marked intraventricular conduction delay (for example left bundle branch block greater than 150 ms) experience asynchronous contraction of the left ventricular free wall and interventricular septum (which may decrease ejection fraction) and late activation of the anterolateral papillary muscle (which may increase functional mitral regurgitation). Biventricular or left ventricular pacing with specialized leads via the coronary sinus can correct both problems and early anecdotal reports of dramatic amelioration of symptoms have been confirmed in randomized trials with subjective and objective evidence of clinical improvement. In addition, the resultant increase in blood pressure and pacemaker maintenance of the desired minimum heart rate permits use of higher doses of β-blockade and ACE inhibition with potential secondary benefit.

Surgical removal of non-viable (Dor procedure) and/or viable myocardium (Batista procedure) to improve haemodynamics by reducing left ventricular volume has been advocated. Though mitral valve repair may occasionally be helpful, these and other surgical volume reduction procedures (partial left ventriculotomy) probably have no role in dilated cardiomyopathy.

Cardiac transplantation has provided a lifeline in those with progressive deterioration. However, the improvements in the pharmacological and non-pharmacological treatments of heart failure in dilated cardiomyopathy appear to be attenuating the progression to endstage disease requiring transplantation. In addition, improvements in left ventricular assist devices and artificial heart technology provide alternatives that are now reasonably seen as viable future treatment options. These issues are discussed in Chapter 15.5.4.

Prevention of disease progression, thromboembolism, and sudden death

With awareness of the importance of familial disease, patients with asymptomatic mild left ventricular dysfunction are increasingly being recognized. Though there is no proof that early treatment will attenuate or prevent disease progression, the recognition that dilated cardiomyopathy is characterized by insidious progression during the asymptomatic phase, and that analogous patients who were in the treatment limb of the Studies of Left Ventricular Dysfunction (SOLVD) prevention trial had improved survival, suggests a role for the introduction of ACE inhibitors at a presymptomatic stage.

Systemic and pulmonary emboli are common. In the retrospective series from the Mayo Clinic, 25 per cent of patients experienced a documented embolic event during 5 years of follow-up. Precise guidelines for anticoagulation are not established. However, patients with mural or intracavitary thrombi and those with established or paroxysmal atrial fibrillation should be fully anticoagulated. Those with severe left ventricular dysfunction (ejection fraction less than 20 per cent) or atrial dilatation (more than 40 mm) should also be anticoagulated, with the INR (international normalized ratio) maintained at the lower end of the therapeutic range (1.5 to 2.5).

The other major complication is sudden death, which may occur in those who are stable or improving as well as in those who are deteriorating. The mechanism is probably ventricular arrhythmia, although bradyarrhythmias may be more likely in those who are severely ill, such as those awaiting cardiac transplantation. Myocyte loss and replacement by fibrous tissue is common in dilated cardiomyopathy, creating a milieu for anisotropic conduction and re-entrant arrhythmias. At autopsy, extensive subendocardial scarring in the left ventricle is seen in approximately one-third of patients, with multiple patchy areas of replacement fibrosis in the majority. Catecholamine excess in such patients may result in several maladaptive responses, including down-regulation of β-adrenergic receptors, inappropriate sinus tachycardia, increased transmural dispersion of refractoriness, and enhanced automaticity of both atrial and ventricular ectopic foci, all of which may increase the risk of both atrial and ventricular arrhythmias.

Recent large, prospective, randomized trials have redefined the role of β-blockade in the treatment of patients with dilated cardiomyopathy and congestive heart failure, demonstrating a substantial reduction not just in sudden death rates but in total mortality, heart failure mortality, and rates of admission to hospital for heart failure. These studies underscore the importance of β-blockers as first-line therapy for symptoms and prognosis in patients with dilated cardiomyopathy.

Though ACE inhibition and angiotensin II (AT$_1$) receptor antagonism also improve prognosis, the effects in reducing sudden death are less consistent. ACE inhibition usually results in only a transient decrease in aldosterone concentrations. The recent Randomised Aldactone Evaluation (RALES) study, which enrolled approximately 800 patients with severe dilated cardiomyopathy (ejection fraction less than 35 per cent and NYHA class IV symptoms), showed that the addition of low-dose spironolactone (25 mg) to conventional heart failure treatment reduced sudden death as well as progressive heart failure deaths.

Primary prevention of sudden death has been limited by the absence of an accurate risk factor stratification algorithm to identify the appropriate high-risk patients and by the complications of antiarrhythmia therapy. Earlier trials of class I antiarrhythmics were associated with increased mortality from sudden death, presumably due to ventricular proarrhythmia and possibly also related to drug-related worsening of ventricular performance. Recent survival trials (involving only small numbers of patients with dilated cardiomyopathy) provide reassurance that amiodarone is safe and possibly effective and, though unproven, it is reasonable to treat those with frequent episodes of asymptomatic, non-sustained ventricular tachycardia during ECG monitoring, as well as those with symptomatic or documented ventricular arrhythmia, with low-dose amiodarone (200 to 300 mg/day). Ongoing prospective trials are examining the role of implantable cardioverter defibrillators in the primary prevention of sudden death. They will probably be shown to be effective: the challenge, however, is to identify those patients whose disease-related life expectancy is adequate and whose arrhythmia risk is sufficient to warrant an implantable cardioverter defibrillator.

Restrictive cardiomyopathy

Definition

Restrictive cardiomyopathy, the least common of the cardiomyopathies, is characterized by restrictive filling of one or both ventricles. This is usually caused by endomyocardial fibrosis. Two variants with similar pathology are recognized. Tropical endomyocardial fibrosis is more common and accounts for 10 to 20 per cent of deaths from heart disease is Africa. Endomyocardial fibrosis in temperate countries is rare and typically associated with hypereosinophilia. The pathology is similar in advanced cases with or without hypereosinophilia, and both variants are considered to be different manifestations of the same disease process. Idiopathic myocardial restrictive cardiomyopathy occurs with and without myocardial fibrosis, but is rare. Myocardial infiltrative diseases (amyloid, sarcoid, Gaucher's), storage diseases (haemochromatosis, glycogen, and Fabry's), and endomyocardial disease associated with malignancies (metastases, carcinoid, radiation, anthracycline toxicity) may also have restrictive physiology and mimic restrictive cardiomyopathy.

Pathology

In endomyocardial fibrosis the cardiac pathology is distinctive, with endocardial fibrosis and overlying thrombosis involving the inflow tracts and the apices, but sparing the outflow tracts of one or both ventricles. Necrotic, thrombotic, and fibrotic stages have been defined in patients with endomyocardial fibrosis and hypereosinophilia. In the necrotic stage there is an acute inflammatory reaction characterized by eosinophilic abscesses in the myocardium, with associated necrosis and arteritis. The endocardium is often thickened and mural thrombi may develop. The thrombotic stage is characterized by endocardial thrombus formation that may be severe, with massive intracavitary thrombosis causing restriction to ventricular filling and a low-output state with high filling pressures. There is a risk of systemic emboli. During the necrotic and thrombotic stages the disease may mimic a hyperacute rheumatic carditis (see Chapter 15.10.1). If the patient survives, healing by fibrosis with hyaline fibrous tissue occurs. There is no further evidence of inflammation and the impact of the disease is caused by the effect of the dense fibrous tissue on ventricular filling volume and atrioventricular valve function.

Clinical features and investigation

Disease onset is usually insidious. Clinical presentation relates to endomyocardial fibrosis: left-sided disease may present with symptoms of pulmonary congestion and/or mitral regurgitation, right-sided disease with raised jugular venous pressure, hepatomegaly, ascites, and tricuspid regurgitation. Radiographic and electrocardiographic appearances are non-specific, showing evidence of raised left and/or right atrial pressure and cardiomegaly with left ventricular hypertrophy. Pulmonary infiltrates, non-specific repolarization changes, and fascicular blocks may occasionally develop.

Two-dimensional echocardiography provides the best non-invasive means of confirming the diagnosis, allowing visualization of the structural abnormalities involving the endocardium and atrioventricular valves as well as demonstration of the abnormal physiology with restriction to filling. There may be intracavitary thrombus with apical cavity obliteration, or bright echoes from the endocardium of the right or left ventricle with tethering of the chordae and reduced excursion of the posterior mitral valve leaflet. Typically, ventricular dimensions and wall thickness are normal, whereas the atria are grossly enlarged. Left ventricular filling terminates early and is followed by a plateau phase coincident with the third heart sound.

The principal haemodynamic consequence of endomyocardial scarring is a restriction to normal filling. Early diastolic pressures are normal, but there is a rapid mid-diastolic rise (square root sign), which plateaus and is not associated with impairment of systolic performance. A similar functional haemodynamic abnormality is seen in pericardial constriction (see Chapter 15.9), but in the latter condition end-diastolic pressures are usually closely similar within the two ventricles, whereas in endomyocardial fibrosis there is usually inequality of the end-diastolic pressures. Mitral and tricuspid regurgitation may be severe and both ventricles appear abnormal in shape on angiography due to obliteration of the apices. This may be particularly marked in the right ventricle in which the infundibulum is hypertrophied and hypocontractile. In addition, the fibrotic process results in smoothing of the internal architecture of the ventricle with loss of the normal trabeculas. The presence of intracavitary thrombi in the left ventricle may give rise to the erroneous diagnosis of a cardiac tumour.

The structural and physiological abnormalities that can be demonstrated with two-dimensional echocardiography or during cardiac catheterization result from the thrombotic and fibrotic stages of the disease. During the early acute phase the appearances of the left and right ventricle are far less abnormal and the diagnosis can best be confirmed at this stage by endomyocardial biopsy. In later stages, diagnosis should be apparent and the risk of biopsy is excessive.

Management

Medical treatment of advanced disease is not particularly effective and the prognosis is poor, with 35 to 50 per cent 2-year mortality. Congestive symptoms from raised right atrial pressure can be improved with diuretics, though too great a reduction in ventricular filling pressure will lead to a reduction in cardiac output. Arrhythmias are common, but their prognostic significance is uncertain and they should therefore not be treated unless they are sustained or associated with symptoms. Antiarrhythmic drugs that significantly slow the heart rate may be deleterious because of the small stroke volume. Digoxin may be helpful to control the ventricular response in atrial fibrillation, but cannot be expected to improve congestive symptoms as systolic function is usually well preserved. Anticoagulants may help to prevent venous thrombosis and systemic emboli; both warfarin and antiplatelet drugs are advised.

Surgery with either mitral and/or tricuspid valve replacement, with or without decortication of the endocardium, has been carried out in some patients. Good long-term symptomatic results have been obtained, but there is significant perioperative mortality (15 to 20 per cent).

Arrhythmogenic right ventricular cardiomyopathy

Definition

Arrhythmogenic right ventricular dysplasia or cardiomyopathy has only recently been recognized. It is characterized pathologically by fibrofatty replacement of the right ventricular myocardium and by clinical presentation with arrhythmia and sudden death. The prevalence is unknown, but estimated to be between 1:1000 and 1:5000. It occurs worldwide, but the high incidence of disease recognized in the Veneto region of Northern Italy raises the possibility of a founder effect. In young athletes (under 25 years) who die suddenly a cardiovascular cause is identified in over 80 per cent, most commonly hypertrophic cardiomyopathy and arrhythmogenic right ventricular cardiomyopathy.

Genetics

The disease is often familial (at least 30 per cent) with autosomal dominant inheritance and incomplete penetrance. Six loci have been reported in autosomal dominant families. The identification of gene abnormalities has been slow, perhaps because of problems in diagnostic ascertainment caused by age-related penetrance, which is seen even in the later decades. Mutations in the ryanidine receptor gene have been found in families with adrenergically mediated ventricular tachycardia which may overlap with the disease phenotype. In an autosomal recessive family from the Greek island of Naxos, in whom palmoplantar keratoderma and woolly hair cosegregated with arrhythmogenic right ventricular cardiomyopathy, a disease-causing mutation has been identified in the plakoglobin gene. Plakoglobin has signalling and intracellular adhesion properties and is an important constituent of the cell-to-cell junction.

Aetiology/pathogenesis

The identification of the plakoglobin gene abnormality in an autosomal recessive form of arrhythmogenic right ventricular cardiomyopathy provides a candidate gene pathway for evaluation. Whether the paradigm that arrhythmogenic right ventricular cardiomyopathy is a disease of the cell-to-cell junction is correct, analogous to hypertrophic cardiomyopathy as a disease of the sarcomere, remains to be determined. Segmental disease is usual in arrhythmogenic right ventricular cardiomyopathy, with involvement of the diaphragmatic, apical, and infundibular regions of the right ventricular free wall. Evolution to more diffuse right ventricular involvement and left ventricular abnormalities with heart failure are more common than the earlier literature suggested. The fibrofatty replacement of the myocardium may be focal or widespread, usually involves the subepicardial layer of the right ventricular free wall, and when severe may appear transmural. Two morphological patterns are recognized: lipomatous replacement of the myocardium without fibrosis is usually seen with preservation of normal right ventricular free wall thickness in the absence of an inflammatory infiltrate, whilst the fibrolipomatous pattern is characterized by replacement myocardial fibrosis with thinning and discrete bulges of the right ventricular free wall, often in association with lymphocytic infiltrates surrounding degenerating or necrotic myocytes. Animal and *in vitro* studies support the hypothesis that mutations in plakoglobin or analogous genes involved in cell adhesion may cause myocytes under mechanical stress to detach and die, with subsequent fibrofatty replacement.

Clinical presentation and management

Clinical manifestations of the disease include structural and functional abnormalities of the right ventricle, electrocardiographic depolarization/repolarization changes, and presentation with sudden death or arrhythmias of right ventricular origin. Structural and functional evaluation of the right ventricle is problematic. There is no ideal method: reliance on invasive

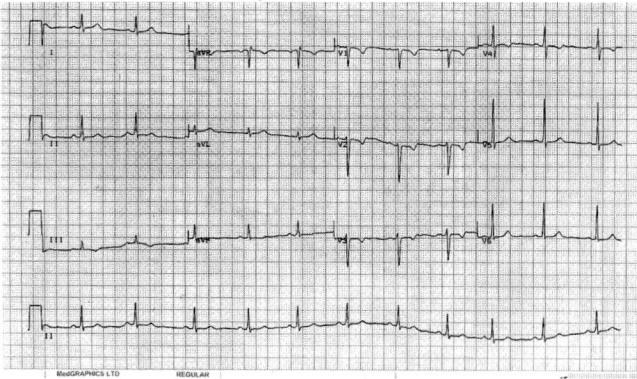

Fig. 7 A 12-lead ECG from a young woman showing the most common electrocardiographic abnormality found in arrhythmogenic right ventricular cardiomyopathy, T-wave inversion in the precordial leads V1–V4.

angiography, two-dimensional echocardiography, radionuclide angiography, computed tomography, and/or magnetic resonance imaging will depend on local expertise and facilities. Quality imaging usually reveals segmental dilatation or localized aneurysm(s) of the right ventricular free wall with minimal but occasionally severe left ventricular impairment. The typical ECG presents inverted T waves in right ventricular precordial leads (V1–V3(4)) (Fig. 7) and ventricular postexcitation 'epsilon waves'. These waves are the surface ECG manifestation of late potentials that are found on the time domain signal-averaged electrocardiogram in 40 to 50 per cent of patients who present with arrhythmia. They occur as a consequence of the inhomogenous and delayed right ventricular depolarization.

Symptomatic presentation is usually with palpitation and/or syncope from sustained ventricular arrhythmia. Ventricular tachycardia is of left bundle branch block morphology suggesting a right ventricular origin. Sudden death related to exercise may be the initial manifestation, especially in the young.

The diagnosis of right ventricular dysplasia is based on histological demonstration of fibrofatty replacement of right ventricular myocardium at either autopsy or surgery. Diagnosis based on biopsy specimens from the right ventricular endomyocardium is inherently difficult because the segmental nature of the disease causes false negatives (Fig. 8), and because the amount of tissue usually obtained is insufficient to differentiate fibrofatty replacement from islands of adipose tissue that are not infrequently seen

between myocytes in the right ventricle of normal subjects. Nevertheless, the positive finding of fibrofatty replacement of myocytes on biopsy can be a valuable diagnostic clue.

Diagnostic criteria are based on evidence of familial disease and on the clinical demonstration of structural, functional, and electrophysiological abnormalities that are caused by or reflect the underlying histological changes (Table 6). The presence of two major or one major and two minor or four minor features provides specific though possibly insensitive diagnostic criteria.

The natural history of arrhythmogenic right ventricular dysplasia is uncertain because patients at autopsy and/or those presenting with sustained ventricular arrhythmias bias published series. In the absence of sustained ventricular arrhythmia most patients will be asymptomatic. Progression from localized (with no or minor symptoms) to more diffuse right ventricular involvement with features of right ventricular failure has been reported. The left ventricle may be involved in long-standing disease, making differentiation from dilated cardiomyopathy with biventricular involvement difficult.

Table 6 Criteria for the diagnosis of arrhythmogenic right ventricular cardiomyopathy (ARVC)

Major	Minor
1. Family history	
Familial disease confirmed at autopsy or surgery	Family history of premature sudden death (< 35 years) caused by ARVC
	Family history (clinical diagnosis based on present criteria)
2. ECG depolarization/conduction abnormalities	
Epsilon waves or localized prolongation (> 110 ms) of the QRS complex in the right precordial leads (V1–V3)	Late potentials seen on signal-averaged ECG
3. Repolarization abnormalities	
	Inverted T waves in right precordial leads (V2 and V3) in people over 12 years and in the absence of right bundle branch block
4. Tissue characterization of walls	
Fibrofatty replacement of myocardium on endomyocardial biopsy	
5. Global and/or regional dysfunction and structural alterations*	
Severe dilatation and reduction of right ventricular ejection fraction with no (or only mild) left ventricular impairment	Mild global right ventricular dilatation and/or ejection fraction reduction with normal left ventricle
Localized right ventricular aneurysms (akinetic or dyskinetic areas with diastolic bulging)	Mild segmental dilatation of the right ventricle
Severe segmental dilatation of the right ventricle	Regional right ventricular hypokinesia
6. Arrhythmias	
	Left bundle branch block type ventricular tachycardia (sustained or non-sustained) documented on ECG, Holter monitoring or during exercise testing
	Frequent ventricular extrasystoles (more than 1000/24 h) on Holter monitoring

Diagnosis of ARVC = 2 major criteria or 1 major +2 minor criteria or 4 minor criteria.
*Detected by echocardiography, angiography, magnetic resonance imaging, or radionuclide scintigraphy (McKenna *et al.* 1994).

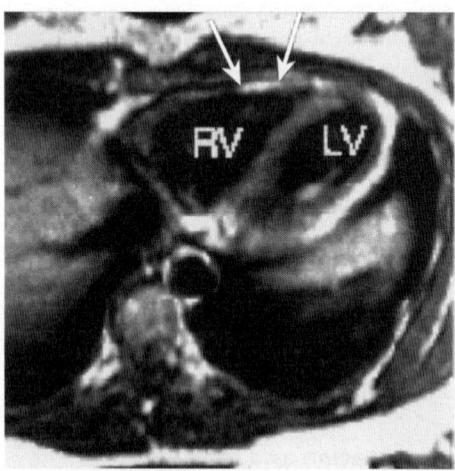

Fig. 8 A transverse plane spin-echo MRI in a young woman with arrhythmogenic right ventricular cardiomyopathy demonstrating a circumscribed area of enhanced MR signal intensity in the right ventricular (RV) free wall (arrows) due to fatty infiltration. (By courtesy of Dr Dudley Pennell, Cardiovascular Magnetic Resonance Unit, Royal Brompton Hospital, London.)

Management aims to identify those at risk of sustained ventricular arrhythmia and to prevent sudden death. Assessment of asymptomatic patients should include exercise testing and Holter monitoring for detection of occult arrhythmia. Antiarrhythmic treatment guided by electrophysiological studies is warranted in patients with palpitation, syncope, or documented sustained ventricular arrhythmia, and should also be considered in those with a markedly abnormal signal-averaged electrocardiogram who are at increased risk. The morphology of ventricular arrhythmia may vary, suggesting multiple sites of origin. Arrhythmias are usually progressive and therapy—whether pharmacological, ablation, or surgical—is not usually definitive. Implantable cardioverter defibrillators are the treatment of choice in patients resuscitated from haemodynamically compromising ventricular tachycardia or ventricular fibrillation.

Further reading

Hypertrophic cardiomyopathy

Braunwald et al. (1964). Idiopathic hypertrophic subaortic stenosis. I. A description of the disease based upon an analysis of 64 patients. Circulation 30(Suppl IV), 3–119.

Elliott PM et al. (2001). Relation between the severity of left ventricular hypertrophy and prognosis in patients with hypertrophic cardiomyopathy. Lancet 357, 420–4.

Maron BJ et al. (2000). Efficacy of the implantable cardioverter-defibrillator for the prevention of sudden death in hypertrophic cardiomyopathy. New England Journal of Medicine 342, 365–73.

McKenna WJ et al. (1985). Improved survival with amiodarone in patients with hypertrophic cardiomyopathy and ventricular tachycardia. British Heart Journal 53, 412–16.

Spirito P et al. (1997). The management of hypertrophic cardiomyopathy. [Review.] New England Journal of Medicine 336, 775–85.

Teare D (1958). Asymmetrical hypertrophy of the heart in young adults. British Heart Journal 20, 1–8.

Thierfelder L et al. (1994). α-Tropomyosin and cardiac troponin T mutations cause familial hypertrophic cardiomyopathy: a disease of the sarcomere. Cell 77, 1–20.

Vosberg H-P, McKenna WJ (2002). Cardiomyopathies. In: Rimoin DL, Connor JM, Pyeritz RE, eds. Emery and Rimoin's principles and practice of medical genetics, 4th edn. Churchill Livingstone, New York, in press.

Watkins H et al. (1992). Sporadic hypertrophic cardiomyopathy due to de novo myosin mutations. Journal of Clinical Investigation 90, 1666–71.

Wigle ED et al. (1985). Hypertrophic cardiomyopathy. The importance of the site and the extent of hypertrophy. A review. Progress in Cardiovascular Diseases 28, 1–83.

Dilated cardiomyopathy

Baboonian C, Treasure T (1997). Meta-analysis of the association of enteroviruses with heart disease. Heart 78, 539–43.

Caforio ALP et al. (1994). Autoimmunity in dilated cardiomyopathy: evidence from family studies. Lancet 344, 773–7.

Mestroni L et al. (1999). Collaborative research group of the European human and capital mobility project on familial dilated cardiomyopathy. Guidelines for the study of familial dilated cardiomyopathy. European Heart Journal 20, 93–102.

Michels VV et al. (1992). The frequency of familial dilated cardiomyopathy in a series of patients with idiopathic dilated cardiomyopathy. New England Journal of Medicine 326, 77–82.

Noutsias M et al. (1999). Expression of cell adhesion molecules in dilated cardiomyopathy: evidence for endothelial activation in inflammatory cardiomyopathy. Circulation 99, 2124–31.

Pauschinger M et al. (1999). Dilated cardiomyopathy is associated with significant changes in collagen type I/III ratio. Circulation 99, 2750–6.

Tracy S et al. (1990). Molecular approaches to enteroviral diagnosis in idiopathic cardiomyopathy and myocarditis. Journal of the American College of Cardiology 15, 1688–94.

Vosberg H-P, McKenna WJ (2002). Cardiomyopathies. In: Rimoin DL, Connor JM, Pyeritz RE, eds. Emery and Rimoin's principles and practice of medical genetics, 4th edn. Churchill Livingstone, New York, in press.

Restrictive cardiomyopathy

See Chapter 15.8.3.

Arrhythmogenic right ventricular dysplasia

Corrado D et al. (1997). Spectrum of clinicopathologic manifestations of arrhythmogenic right ventricular cardiomyopathy/dysplasia: a multicenter study. Journal of the American College of Cardiology 30, 1512–20.

Marcus FI et al. (1982). Right ventricular dysplasia: a report of 24 adult cases. Circulation 65, 384–98.

McKenna WJ et al. (1994). Diagnosis of arrhythmogenic right ventricular dysplasia/cardiomyopathy. British Heart Journal 71, 215–18.

McKoy G et al. (2000). Identification of a deletion in plakoglobin in arrhythmogenic right ventricular cardiomyopathy with palmoplantar keratoderma and woolly hair (Naxos disease). Lancet 355, 2119–24.

15.8.3 Specific heart muscle disorders

William J. McKenna

Cardiac manifestations of musculoskeletal and connective tissue diseases

The cardiac manifestations of musculoskeletal and connective tissue diseases often go undetected. Every anatomical structure in the heart may be involved, there usually being no correlation between the extent of systemic disease and cardiac involvement. For details of the cardiac manifestations of musculoskeletal and connective tissue diseases, see Tables 1 and 2.

Systemic lupus erythematosus

Systemic lupus erythematosus is a multisystem immune disorder characterized by the formation of autoantibodies to numerous organ systems. The prevalence of cardiovascular involvement is reported to be greater than 50 per cent. The pericardium is most commonly affected, with as many as 30 per cent of patients with lupus having clinical pericarditis at some stage, and up to 66 per cent affected at autopsy. Progression to constrictive pericarditis or tamponade remains extremely rare.

Myocardial involvement occurs less frequently, although reported in up to 30 per cent of patients at autopsy: signs and symptoms are uncommon, but patients may occasionally present with heart failure or arrhythmias.

As many as one-third of patients have systolic murmurs, but these usually represent hyperdynamic flow states due to other causes. The classic verrucous vegetations adherent to the endocardium described by Libman and Sachs in 1924 can be identified in up to 30 per cent of patients at autopsy. These lesions most commonly affect the mitral valve but rarely become clinically significant, although thromboembolism, valvular incompetence, and infective endocarditis are all described.

Conduction abnormalities are common: various degrees of heart block and bundle branch block can be seen, but complete heart block is rare. Arrhythmias such as atrial fibrillation and flutter may also occur, particularly in association with pericarditis. Myocardial infarction is very rarely reported in patients with systemic lupus erythematosus, atherosclerosis usually being implicated in the pathogenesis, although arteritis and steroid use may also play a role.

Table 1 Cardiac manifestations of musculoskeletal and connective tissue diseases

Disease	Cardiac manifestation
Systemic lupus erythematosus	Accelerated atherosclerosis
	Non-infective endocarditis (Libman–Sach's)
	Myocarditis
	Pericarditis
Systemic sclerosis	Myocarditis
	Pericarditis
	Arrhythmias
Polyarteritis nodosa	Hypertension
	Congestive heart failure
	Partial or complete coronary artery occlusion
	Pericarditis
	Arrhythmias
Churg–Strauss syndrome	Congestive cardiac failure
	Pericarditis
	Coronary arteritis/myocardial infarction
	Arrhythmias
Wegener's granulomatosis	Constrictive pericarditis
	Atrioventricular block
Rheumatoid arthritis	Coronary arteritis
	Aortic and mitral regurgitation
Takayasu's syndrome	Pericarditis
	Aortic arch vasculitis
	Heart failure
Seronegative arthropathies :	
Ankylosing spondylitis	
Reiter's syndrome	Pancarditis
Psoriatic arthritis	Proximal aortitis
Ulcerative colitis	Conduction disease
Crohn's disease	

Death from the cardiac complications of lupus is rare. Mild pericardial disease may respond to non-steroidal anti-inflammatory drugs, heart failure is treated conventionally, and conduction defects may require pacing. Corticosteroids are thought to be useful in patients with coronary vasculitis and myocarditis, but there is no evidence for the use of other immunosuppressants.

Antiphospholipid syndrome

The antiphospholipid syndrome is recognized both in patients without (primary) and with systemic lupus erythematosus. It is a thrombophilic disorder characterized by arterial and venous occlusions, recurrent fetal loss, thrombocytopenia, and increased maternal complications of pregnancy. It is associated with persistently raised titres of anticardiolipin antibodies or the Lupus anticoagulant. Involvement of the mitral and aortic valves is particularly common and dramatic response to prednisolone has been described (see Chapter 13.14 for further information).

Systemic sclerosis

Heine in 1926 and Weiss *et al.* in 1943 first described cases of myocardial involvement: it has now been shown that up to 60 per cent of patients have cardiac involvement at autopsy. Gradual obliteration of the microvasculature leads to a 'Raynaud's' type of phenomenon in the heart, which is thought to be responsible for ischaemia that may then progress to patchy myocardial fibrosis. This pathological process most commonly affects the left ventricle. Right ventricular dysfunction is usually secondary to pulmonary vascular disease or pulmonary hypertension, but an associated right ventricular cardiomyopathy may coexist.

Dyspnoea is the most common symptom and usually attributable to pulmonary involvement, though it may be secondary to left ventricular systolic and/or diastolic dysfunction. Atypical chest pain may be secondary to pulmonary hypertension or fibrosis, pericarditis, or oesophageal reflux.

Diffuse narrowing of intramural coronary arteries may be associated with myocardial infarction or angina. Clinical pericarditis is reported in

Table 2 Cardiac involvement in the more common connective tissue disorders

	Pericardial involvement	Myocardial involvement	Valvular involvement	Coronary/arteritis	Conduction system involvement
Rheumatoid arthritis (RA)	16–40% at autopsy; 10–15% clinical pericarditis	4–20% at autopsy; symptomatic in under 5%	> 50% valvulitis at autopsy; symptoms rare	11–20% involvement of coronary vessels at autopsy; vasculitis affecting the aorta rare	Any part of conduction system involved; varying degrees of heart block in 0.1%
Systemic lupus erythematosus (SLE)	45–66% at autopsy; 20–30% clinical pericarditis	30% at autopsy; symptomatic in < 10%	Libman–Sach's lesions in 30% at autopsy	Coronary vessels involved in < 10%; vasculitis affecting the aorta rare	Any part of conduction system involved; varying degrees of heart block in < 1%
Systemic sclerosis and variants	70% at autopsy; 7–15% clinical pericarditis	Up to 60% at autopsy; symptoms rare	Rare, AR and MVP described	Reversible perfusion defects in up to 40%; symptoms in < 10%	Any part of conduction system involved; abnormal ECG in 50%
Polymyositis/ dermatomyositis (PM/DM)	Clinical involvement rare (usually in children with DM)	Up to 25% at autopsy; symptoms in 13–26%	MVP common, other lesions rare	Vasculitis demonstrated rarely	Any part of conduction system involved (symptoms extremely rare)
Seronegative spondyloarthro-pathies (ankylosing spondylitis, AS, and Reiter's syndrome)	< 1% incidence of pericarditis in AS and Reiter's	Myocardial involvement/ dysfunction common on ECHO in AS; symptoms rare	Aortic incompetence most common: 1–10% in AS, 1–15% in Reiter's; MR very rare	Aortitis: 1–10% in AS, 1–15% in Reiter's	Heart block: 8% in AS, 8% in Reiter's; rare in other forms of spondyloarthropathy

MR, mitral regurgitation; MVP, mitral valve prolapse; AR, aortic regurgitation

15 per cent of patients and up to 70 per cent demonstrate pericardial involvement at autopsy.

ECG abnormalities are reported in 75 per cent of patients with scleroderma. Conduction abnormalities are seen in as many as 50 per cent of those with cardiac disease and may present with palpitations, syncope, or sudden death. The presence of left bundle branch block or bifascicular block suggests significant myocardial involvement: a septal infarct pattern or interventricular conduction abnormalities may also be seen. Ambulatory electrocardiograms frequently reveal a high prevalence of atrial and ventricular premature beats: supraventricular tachycardias are seen in 30 per cent of patients and ventricular tachycardia (which may predict future sudden death) in up to 15 per cent. The echocardiogram typically shows features of dilated or restrictive cardiomyopathy. Resting thallium perfusion abnormalities are seen in the majority of affected individuals, whilst arteriography usually reveals normal coronary arteries. Endomyocardial biopsy is rarely performed.

Treatment for pulmonary involvement may involves prostacyclin, long-term oxygen therapy, and anticoagulation. Treatment for heart failure is along conventional lines; calcium channel antagonists, nitrates, and vasodilators may improve resting myocardial perfusion.

The major cause of death in scleroderma is pulmonary hypertension, with a 5-year mortality rate of 60 per cent. Although nothing has been shown to alter the cardiac manifestations, D-penicillamine and isoretinoin have been used with some success. Symptomatic cardiac involvement predicts a poor prognosis, with a 2-year mortality of approximately 60 per cent.

Rheumatoid arthritis

Cardiac involvement is found in up to 60 per cent of patients on echocardiography, but only in 10 to 15 per cent clinically. The presence of cardiac disease tends to correlate with the severity of joint disease and the presence of rheumatoid nodules. Histological changes consist of a non-specific inflammatory infiltrate, myocyte necrosis, and fibrosis affecting any part of the heart. Rheumatoid nodules may accompany this, and the heart may also be affected by secondary amyloidosis. Myocarditis is reported in up to 20 per cent at autopsy, but symptoms are uncommon. Pericarditis occurs more frequently, and up to 40 per cent of patients have an effusion on echocardiography, but progression to constrictive pericarditis or tamponade is rare. Acute vasculitis involving the larger epicardial arteries has been reported but is uncommon. Non-specific valvitis may affect the mitral and particularly the aortic valve: this may eventually lead to scarred, hyalinized, and even incompetent valves. Rheumatoid nodules may occasionally deform the mitral valve and lead to valvular incompetence. Conduction disturbances may be secondary to infiltration by rheumatoid nodules: the commonest ECG abnormality is first-degree heart block, but left bundle branch block and complete heart block are also described. Although pericarditis is usually responsive to steroids, it is unclear whether steroids or disease-modifying drugs alter the other cardiac manifestations.

Polymyositis and dermatomyositis

Cardiac involvement in polymyositis or dermatomyositis is present in up to 15 per cent of patients clinically and as many as 55 per cent on echocardiography. Histological changes consist of non-specific inflammatory cell infiltrate, myocyte necrosis, and fibrosis, involving particularly the cardiac conducting tissue and leading to various degrees of conduction block and arrhythmias.

There is echocardiographic evidence of pericardial disease in up to 25 per cent of patients, but this usually remains asymptomatic. Myocarditis may be present in 25 per cent of patients at autopsy, although the development of clinically apparent heart failure is uncommon. The ECG is often abnormal, particularly in children. Abnormalities consist mostly of non-specific 'ST' and 'T' wave changes and conduction delays. Treatment is based on symptomatology.

Seronegative arthropathies

This group of disorders is characterized by the absence of rheumatoid factor and includes ankylosing spondylitis, Reiter's syndrome, and psoriatic and gastrointestinal arthropathies. These may all be associated with cardiac involvement, in particular pancarditis, proximal aortitis, aortic incompetence, and varying degrees of conduction abnormalities. They may also result in amyloid deposition. On occasion cardiac disease may present before joint disease. Treatment is empirical and based on symptomatology.

Neuromuscular diseases

The muscular dystrophies are a group of disorders characterized by progressive skeletal and cardiac muscle involvement (Table 3). Dystrophic effects on skeletal muscle result in fibre necrosis, followed by fibrosis and fatty replacement. The heart is commonly affected and cardiac disease tends to be progressive. The structural and functional changes, which occur in the ventricles, can lead to the development of cardiomyopathy, in particular dilated cardiomyopathy and heart failure. The effect on the specialized conducting tissue may lead to bradyarrhythmias, conduction defects, malignant arrhythmias, and sudden death.

Duchenne and Becker muscular dystrophy are progressive disorders arising from abnormalities (deletion, duplication, or point mutation) in the genes involved in the manufacture of the extra-sarcomeric cytoskeletal protein dystrophin. In addition to defects in dystrophin, other defects that might be responsible for muscular dystrophy and dilated cardiomyopathy include those affecting the genes for the intracellular proteins, emerin and laminin. Emerin is a transmembrane protein that is embedded in the inner nuclear cell membrane. Laminin A–C are filament-like proteins that form a proteinaceous mesh underlying and attached to the inner nuclear membrane. The exact mechanism by which alterations in these proteins may lead to cardiomyopathy remains unclear.

In general, treatment of the cardiomyopathy of neuromuscular disorders is empirical and based on symptomatology and evidence of arrhythmia or conduction block. Should advances in the treatment of neuromuscular disorders by gene therapy or other means result in prolonged survival, then cardiac failure may become the limiting factor.

Amyloid

Amyloidosis describes a group of diverse protein-deposition diseases. The biochemical nature of the proteinaceous deposits and the aetiology of the underlying associated diseases differ (Table 4).

As many as 50 per cent of patients with systemic AL (primary) amyloidosis have cardiac involvement and this will manifest clinically in up to half of these. Systemic AA (secondary) amyloidosis is almost never associated with clinical cardiac amyloidosis. The heart is frequently involved in familial amyloid polyneuropathy, which is the most common type of hereditary amyloidosis and caused by more than 70 mutations in the transthyretin gene. Senile amyloidosis is extremely common, indeed almost all individuals over the age of 80 years will have scattered deposits of amyloid, particularly affecting the aorta. Clinical involvement is variable, depending on the extent of deposition, but tends to be unimportant in senile amyloidosis.

The extracellular deposition of amyloid results in a firm, thickened, non-compliant myocardium. Deposition occurs throughout the atrial and ventricular muscle. Conducting as well as nodal tissue may be affected: fibrosis of these structures may occur. Valvular function is rarely affected, although deposition in and thickening of cardiac valves is common. Intramural coronary arteries and veins frequently contain deposits, which can occasionally compromise the lumina of these vessels.

Amyloid heart disease most frequently mimics hypertrophic cardiomyopathy with restrictive physiology. The reduced compliance of the myocardium produces the characteristic diastolic dip and plateau (square root

Table 3 Cardiovascular abnormalities in neuromuscular disorders

Condition	Inheritance	Cardiac disease	Non-cardiac manifestations	Genetic defects
Duchenne	X-linked 1:3500 male births	Begins in first decade, 62% have ECG changes by age 10 years: short PQ, prolonged QT, tall R in V1. Conduction system anomalies/HCM and DCM reported. Symptoms uncommon	Severe muscle weakness, proximal-girdle distribution at 2–5 years in males. Calf pseudohypertrophy, mild cognitive impairment, high CPK. Wheelchair dependency by age 12. Death in adolescence	Xp21; dystrophin gene mutations
Becker	X-linked 1:15 000 male births	High incidence of clinical cardiac involvement, heart failure is the most common cause of death. DCM seen. ECG usually abnormal: reduced R wave or prominent Q in 1, AVL and V6	Mild to moderate muscle weakness, proximal girdle distribution from childhood, and ambulation preserved at least until late teens. Calf pseudohypertrophy, high CPK	Xp21; dystrophin gene mutations
		Arrhythmias and heart block in less than 10%	Lifespan usually dependent on severity of cardiac involvement	
X-linked dilated cardio-myopathy	X-linked (rare)	Second or third decade onset CM and heart failure, rapid cardiac progression. Milder variants possible. Heart block not reported, arrhythmias in less than 10%	No muscular weakness. Muscle cramps, myalgias. CPK usually elevated	Xp21; altered or selective loss of cardiac dystrophin
Limb girdle 1B (allelic to AD-EDMD)	AD	Variable degrees of AV block, AF, with high degree block, bradycardia, palpitations, and syncope	Mild to moderate muscle weakness, proximal limb girdle distribution. CPK elevated	Lamin A–C gene, 1q11–21. This disorder is allelic to AD-EDMD and isolated cardiomyopathy with conduction system disease mapped to 1q
		DCM in 5%		
Limb girdle 2A	AR	Cardiac involvement rare	Muscle weakness, proximal-girdle distribution. CPK elevated	15q15 Calpain-3 (calcium activated neutral protease)
Limb girdle with sarcoglycan deficiency	AR	DCM reported. Arrhythmias uncommon	Proximal-girdle distribution of muscle weakness. Calf pseudohypertrophy. CPK elevated. Severity varies from Duchenne to Becker like	α-Sarcoglycan, 17q12 β-Sarcoglycan, 4q12 γ-Sarcoglycan, 13q12 δ-Sarcoglycan, 5q3
Congenital	AR	Cardiac involvement usually insignificant. Cardiomyopathy has been reported	Severe hypotonia and muscle weakness from birth, elevated CPK. Maximal ability: sitting without support	16q22–23; α-2 laminin chain mutations (Merosin)
Myotonic 1:8000	AD	Conduction defects and arrhythmias common yet most remain asymptomatic. ECG changes in 23–80%: prolonged PR and QRS intervals. Left and right bundle branch block, AF, aflutter and bradycardias. MVP common. DCM and HCM detected rarely	Muscle weakness, may be associated with frontal balding, cataracts, hypogonadism, and myotonia	19q13.3; myotonin-protein kinase gene mutations (unstable CTG trinucleotide repeats)
Emery–Dreifuss	X-linked	AV block is the most common feature, high incidence of sudden death (pacemaker advised). Sinus node disease as well as tachyarrhythmias are common. DCM is rare	Childhood onset of contractures, mild muscle weakness in humeroperoneal distribution. Lower extremities affected first. CPK elevated moderately. No calf pseudohypertrophy	Xq28 defect of nuclear transmembane protein emerin
	AD (it is actually more common than X-linked)	DCM associated with conduction system disease commonly seen. Ventricular fibrillation reported despite pacing	Same as X-linked form. May be little evidence of skeletal myopathy	1.q11–21 Laminin A–C mutation (this disorder is allelic to LGMD1B)

AD, autosomal dominant; AR, autosomal recessive; AF, atrial fibrillation; CPK, creatinine phosphokinase; DCM, dilated cardiomyopathy; HCM, hypertrophic cardiomyopathy; AV, atrioventricular; EDMD, Emery-Dreifuss muscular dystrophy; MVP, mitral valve prolapse.

Table adapted from Gerald et al.(1997). Dystrophies and heart disease. *Current Opinion in Cardiology* **12**, 329–42.

Table 4 Classification of amyloidosis

Type	Fibril precursor protein	Associated conditions	Clinical syndrome
AL 'Primary amyloidosis'	Monoclonal Light chains	Monoclonal gammopathy; myeloma	Systemic amyloidosis with frequent cardiac involvement
AA 'Secondary amyloidosis'	Serum amyloid light chains	Chronic inflammatory diseases; rheumatoid arthritis; familial Mediterranean fever	Systemic amyloidosis with predominant renal disease
ATTR	1. Wild-type transthyretin	1. Senile systemic amyloidosis	1. Cardiac amyloidosis in the very elderly
	2. Genetically variant forms of transthyretin	2. Familial amyloid polyneuropathy	2. Cardiac amyloid frequent, and may predominate
Other hereditary forms	Genetically variant forms of ApoAI, lysozyme, and fibrinogen		Hereditary renal amyloidosis

ATTR, amyloid associated with transthyretin.

sign) in the ventricular pressure waveform that may simulate constrictive pericarditis. An impaired rate of early diastolic filling is characteristic and systolic dysfunction may also occur, leading to congestive heart failure.

Progressive infiltration of the autonomic nervous system results in orthostatic hypotension in 10 per cent of cases. Arrhythmias are common, in particular ventricular premature beats and atrial fibrillation. Complex ventricular arrhythmias may be harbingers of sudden death.

The chest radiograph may show cardiomegaly in patients with systolic dysfunction but is often normal in those with restrictive cardiomyopathy, although pulmonary congestion may be prominent. The ECG shows diminished voltages in approximately 50 per cent of patients, and loss of 'R' waves in precordial leads; the presence of 'Q' waves in the inferior leads may simulate myocardial infarction. Echocardiography reveals an increased thickness of the ventricular walls with small ventricular chambers, dilated atria, intra-atrial septal thickening, left ventricular dysfunction, and a characteristic 'sparkling' appearance to the myocardium. Asymmetrical septal hypertrophy has also been recognized. Scintigraphy with technetium-99-pyrophosphate may be strongly positive. CT and MRI may also be helpful, as may endomyocardial biopsy.

Symptomatic heart disease typically presents late in the course of amyloidosis and the presence of clinical signs is an ominous feature with mortality approaching 100 per cent at 2 years. Treatment is supportive in combination with measures to suppress the underlying amyloidogenic condition. This ranges from myeloma-type chemotherapy in AL amyloidosis to liver transplantation in familial amyloid polyneuropathy. Digoxin and calcium channel antagonists should be used with caution as they selectively bind to amyloidal fibrils, enhancing their effect. Patients with symptomatic conduction system disease require a pacemaker. Diuretics and vasodilators should be used cautiously as they may aggravate hypotension. Transplantation is feasible in selected cases but is a palliative procedure without treatment of the underlying process.

Inherited infiltrative disorders causing cardiomyopathy

Various disorders may lead to infiltration of the myocardium by an abnormal metabolic product, resulting in abnormal systolic and/or diastolic function of the heart. The disorders include glycogenoses, the mucopolysaccharidoses, Fabry's disease, and Gaucher's disease.

Fabry's disease (angiokeratoma corporis diffusum universale)

An X-linked disorder present in 1 in 40 000 live-born babies in which an inherited deficiency of the enzyme α-galactosidase results in the intracellular accumulation of a glycolipid substrate in numerous organs, including the myocardium. Most patients eventually develop symptomatic cardiovascular manifestations including hypertension, mitral valve prolapse, and

congestive heart failure. The electrocardiogram often shows left ventricular hypertrophy, 'P' wave abnormalities, conduction defects, and arrhythmias. Echocardiography usually demonstrates increased thickness of the left ventricle, which may simulate hypertrophic cardiomyopathy. Differentiation from other hypertrophic or restrictive processes may require MRI or endomyocardial biopsy. A low leucocyte α-galactosidase activity is diagnostic.

Gaucher's disease

A deficiency of the enzyme β-glucosidase results in the accumulation of cerebrosides in the spleen, liver, bone marrow, lymph nodes, brain, and myocardium. Diffuse interstitial infiltration of the left ventricle leads to a reduction in left ventricular compliance and cardiac output. Clinical evidence of cardiac involvement is uncommon, but when present is characterized by left ventricular dysfunction, haemorrhagic pericardial effusion, thickened left ventricle, and calcification of left-sided valves.

Sarcoid

Sarcoid is a multisysytem granulomatous disorder of unknown aetiology. Myocardial involvement is seen in 20 to 30 per cent of patients at autopsy but is clinically apparent in less than 10 per cent of cases. Primary cardiac involvement is extremely rare.

Non-caseating granulomas may involve any region of the heart, although the left ventricular free wall and interventricular septum are the most commonly affected sites. The granulomas can be localized or widespread, and healing may result in the formation of scars. The ventricular muscle eventually becomes increasingly non-compliant; this can lead to defects in contractile function as well as wall motion. Replacement of large portions of the ventricle by sarcoid tissue may lead to aneurysm formation. Granulomas and fibrosis may also extend to involve nodal or conducting tissue. Isolated pericardial involvement is rare, although pericardial effusions are commonly seen on echo. Valvular dysfunction occurs in fewer than 5 per cent of patients and may be the result of infiltration of papillary muscles or direct valvular involvement, which is less common.

Clinical manifestations of myocardial sarcoidosis are shown in Table 5. Chest pain has been described in up to 28 per cent of patients, and since about half of these will have abnormal thallium perfusion scans despite arteriographically normal coronary arteries, this is thought to be secondary to microvascular spasm.

Sudden death is one of the most common and feared manifestations of myocardial sarcoidosis, occurring in about 65 per cent of affected patients. It is thought to be predominantly secondary to arrhythmias, including ventricular tachycardia and fibrillation. The presence of a ventricular aneurysm may be associated with resistant ventricular arrhythmias and necessitate its resection. Conduction disturbances such as complete heart block are a frequent occurrence and may also predict sudden death. The electrocardiogram is frequently abnormal with 'T' wave abnormalities and varying degrees of interventricular or atrioventricular block. Pathological

Table 5 Clinical manifestations in myocardial sarcoidosis

Abnormality	Reported percentage of patients affected
Atrioventricular block	41–52
Ventricular ectopics	31–47
Congestive heart failure	12–19
Sudden death	21–38
Bundle branch block	26–34
Supraventricular tachycardia	11–25
Ventricular tachycardia	12–23
Simulating myocardial infarction on ECG	14–18
Pericarditis/pulmonary embolism	4–8

'Q' waves may simulate myocardial infarction when myocardial involvement becomes extensive. Echocardiography most commonly shows features of restrictive or occasionally dilated cardiomyopathy. Systolic and/or diastolic dysfunction as well as regional wall motion abnormalities may also be seen. Gallium or technetium pyrophosphate scanning and MRI have all been used to detect affected areas of myocardium. Endomyocardial biopsy can be diagnostic but is rarely done due to the patchy nature of the disease.

Steroids have been shown to lead to improvements in symptoms as well as electrocardiographic and echocardiographic features and myocardial perfusion defects, although there is a theoretical risk of increased aneurysm formation. Amiodarone may be of benefit in resistant arrhythmia and the insertion of an implantable defibrillator may protect against sudden death in susceptible patients. Transplantation may improve prognosis and quality of life in patients who remain symptomatic despite these measures, although recurrence has been documented. The average survival from the onset of symptomatic cardiac involvement has been reported as 1 to 2 years.

Haemochromatosis

Hereditary haemochromatosis is the most common single-gene disorder in people of northern European origin, where approximately 3 to 5 persons per 1000 are homozygous for the disease. It results in excessive and inappropriate mucosal absorption of iron, which is then deposited predominantly in the heart, liver, gonads, and pancreas. Deposition in the heart results in thickening of the ventricular walls together with dilatation of the ventricular chambers and heart failure. Histopathologically, myocardial degeneration and fibrosis occur over time and may extend to involve the conducting system of the heart.

The ECG most commonly reveals 'ST' and 'T' wave changes. Supraventricular arrhythmias are also characteristic, with atrioventricular conduction defects and ventricular arrhythmias being less common. Echocardiography typically shows a mixed dilated and restrictive cardiomyopathy with thickened ventricular walls, ventricular chamber enlargement, systolic and/or diastolic dysfunction. Endomyocardial biopsy may be useful to confirm the diagnosis but cannot rule it out. Treatment involves repeated phlebotomy and/or desferrioxamine.

There is evidence that the type of the inherited mutation may determine the development of cardiomyopathy. Two new mutations have recently been described which may predispose to the development of hereditary haemochromatosis and dilated cardiomyopathy. These affect the haemochromatosis gene on chromosome 6p (termed the HPE gene) and probably act as disease-modifying genes in dilated cardiomyopathy, although having little effect on iron status. The pathogenesis of cardiomyopathy here may be unrelated to excessive iron.

Diabetes

A man with diabetes has a relative risk of developing heart failure that is 2.4 times higher than that of a man without diabetes, and the equivalent relative risk for a woman is 5:1. The risk has been shown to be independent of age, systolic blood pressure, serum cholesterol, and weight. People with diabetes have been shown to have elevated end-diastolic pressures, reduced ejection fractions, left ventricular dilatation, and hypertrophy, even in the absence of coronary artery disease. Diastolic dysfunction as well as a diffuse hypokinesis of the myocardium has also been demonstrated. Implicated mechanisms include small vessel disease and autonomic neuropathy.

The most prominent histopathological finding is that of myocardial fibrosis. Occasionally a picture resembling restrictive heart disease is seen, with a small left ventricular chamber and reduced compliance of the left ventricle.

The treatment of heart failure is the same as in patients without diabetes, although β-blockers with intrinsic sympathomimetic activity are preferred. Preload and after-load reducing agents should be used cautiously because of autonomic dysfunction. It is unclear whether tight glucose control affects the progression of diabetic 'cardiomyopathy', but it is clearly prudent for other reasons to optimize control as well as to reduce obesity and control hypertension.

Hyperthyroidism

In general, excess thyroid hormone results in a high output state with tachycardia, increased cardiac contractility, and peripheral vasodilatation. In the long term this can result in ventricular hypertrophy and an increase in ejection fraction. However, some patients may develop a low output state with symptoms of heart failure and echocardiographic demonstration of dilated cardiomyopathy and systolic dysfunction. These changes may be a result of long-standing tachycardia and increased cardiac work, but thyroxine itself may directly alter the expression of certain cardiac proteins involved in cardiac function, and there is also some evidence that direct autoimmune attack on the myocardium may occur in Graves' disease.

Typical symptoms of hyperthyroidism include angina-like chest pain, fatigue, palpitations, and exertional dyspnoea. Cardiac findings include sinus tachycardia and atrial flutter or fibrillation in 17 to 20 per cent. These may be complicated by thromboembolism in up to 40 per cent; also by congestive heart failure. Mitral valve prolapse has been reported in patients with Graves' disease.

Control of the ventricular rate in atrial fibrillation may be obtained with digoxin, β-adrenergic antagonists, or calcium channel antagonists. The increased metabolic clearance of digoxin may necessitate a higher maintenance dose. Cardioversion should generally be deferred until euthyroid. β-Adrenergic antagonists offer prompt control of sympathomimetic manifestations. The presence of an already dilated vascular bed means that diuretics should be used with caution and vasodilators are generally contraindicated. Treatment of hyperthyroidism *per se* is discussed elsewhere.

Hypothyroidism

Patients suffering from hypothyroidism, whether in its mild form or full-blown myxoedema, present a wide variety of symptoms. Complaints of fatigue, lethargy, mental slowness, and cold intolerance usually dominate. Less frequently, symptoms suggestive of cardiac dysfunction such as dyspnoea on exertion, syncope, or angina-like chest pain may be prominent. The most common cardiac abnormality is pericardial effusion, which is usually asymptomatic but reported in at least 30 per cent of untreated patients. Heart failure generally represents exacerbation of pre-existing cardiac disease by the superimposed haemodynamic consequences of thyroid deficiency—bradycardia, diminished myocardial contractility, and increased peripheral vascular resistance. Rarely, hypothyroidism alone can closely resemble cardiomyopathy severe enough to cause heart failure.

Echocardiographic evidence of asymmetric thickening of the interventricular septum as well as reduced left ventricular outflow tract dimensions has been reported. The characteristic ECG findings are sinus bradycardia, prolongation of the QT interval, and a reduction in voltages if there is an associated pericardial effusion.

The management of heart failure involves the identification of any primary cardiac disease that may coexist; both ischaemic heart disease and aortic stenosis may be exacerbated by thyroid replacement. L-Thyroxine (T_4) significantly enhances myocardial performance within 1 week. It is generally used as first-line treatment of hypothyroidism, but in those with known or suspected coronary artery disease it should be initiated at a lower dose than usual, typically 25 µg/day, and increased slowly at 4- to 6-week intervals until the thyroid-stimulating hormone is within the normal range. Tri-iodothyronine (T_3) may be preferable in severe cases as clinical improvement occurs sooner. β-Blockade can be used prophylactically or added if treatment with L-thyroxine exacerbates ischaemic heart disease.

Further reading

Benson MD (1997). Aging, amyloid, cardiomyopathy. *New England Journal of Medicine* **336**, 502–4.

Braunwald E, ed. (1998). *Heart disease: a textbook of cardiovascular medicine*, 5th edn, pp 1427–35. WB Saunders, Philadelphia.

Cox GF, Kunkel LM (1997). Dystrophies and heart disease. *Current Opinion in Cardiology* **12**, 329–42.

Landerson PW (1990). Recognition and management of cardiovascular disease related to thyroid dysfunction. *American Journal of Medicine* **88**, 638–41.

Shabina H, Isenberg DA (1999). Autoimmune rheumatic diseases and the heart. *Hospital Medicine* **60**, 95–9.

Shammas RL (1993). Sarcoidosis of the heart. *Clinical Cardiology* **16**, 462–72.

Topol EJ (1998). *Comprehensive cardiovascular medicine*, volume 1, chapter 27, pp. 690–726.

15.9 Pericardial disease

D. G. Gibson

Anatomy of the pericardium

The normal pericardium consists of serous and fibrous components. The fibrous pericardium is thick and unyielding, separating the heart from surrounding organs. It fuses with the central tendon of the diaphragm below and with the great vessels above, 1 to 2 cm beyond their origins. Inside the fibrous pericardium is the serous pericardium, in which the heart is invaginated. It has two layers, a parietal layer which lines the inner aspect of the fibrous pericardium and a visceral layer, sometimes called the epicardium, which covers the surfaces of the heart and the origins of the great vessels. The pericardial cavity is the potential space between the visceral and parietal layers of the serous pericardium. It normally contains only a few millilitres of fluid, but it has a considerable capacity where fluid may accumulate.

Physiology of the pericardium

The normal pericardium is not essential to life: the pericardial space is often obliterated after open heart surgery, and both layers may be removed in patients with constrictive pericarditis without apparent ill effect. Whether restraint by the normal pericardium is of any pathophysiological importance as a mechanism limiting stroke volume in disease remains uncertain.

Congenital abnormalities of the pericardium

Congenital abnormalities of the pericardium are uncommon with an incidence of 1 to 2 per 10 000 autopsies. Congenital absence of the pericardium may be partial or complete. A partial defect, involving the left side of the pericardium is about four times as common as the complete form. Either type may be associated with additional congenital anomalies in about one-third of cases, including Fallot tetralogy, atrial septal defect, or sequestered pulmonary segments. Clinical features include non-specific chest pain and sinus bradycardia, with an ECG showing right axis deviation. A chest radiograph is characteristic, with a shift of the heart to the left and prominence of the main pulmonary artery. Heart size is increased and the lower border of the cardiac shadow ill-defined. Echocardiography shows increased right ventricular size and reversed septal motion, as occurs in atrial septal defect. If the defect is partial, the left atrial appendix may herniate through it, and even strangulate leading to a clinical picture suggesting acute pericarditis. If the defect is larger, the left ventricle may herniate and undergo torsion. Alternatively, lung may become trapped in the pericardial space. These complications are treated surgically by enlarging the defect.

Pericardial cysts

These are rare, have a variety of embryological origins, and may be continuous with the pericardium or separate from it. They do not usually cause symptoms, but can be discovered on chest radiographs taken for any reason. Their nature becomes obvious with CT scanning or MRI, but the exact diagnosis is often established only when they are removed surgically.

Mulibrey nanism

Mulibrey (**mu**scle, **li**ver, **br**ain, **ey**e) nanism is an autosomal recessive condition characterized by growth failure, a triangular face, often with a hydrocephaloid skull, hypotonia, a peculiar voice, large liver, and yellowish dots and pigment dispersion in the optic fundi. The majority of cases have pericardial constriction due to congenital thickening of the pericardium, and this may be responsible for some of the clinical features. Histologically, the pericardium shows simple fibrosis. Considerable improvement follows pericardiectomy.

Acquired pericardial disease

Diseases of the pericardium may be considered from two points of view. The first is aetiological, the second is in terms of the physiological and clinical disturbances that result. There is no fixed relation between the two, so that an account will be given of the different diseases affecting the pericardium and then of the three main syndromes: acute pericarditis, pericardial tamponade, and pericardial constriction.

Aetiology

Diseases affecting the pericardium are given in Table 1.

Acute idiopathic pericarditis

Acute idiopathic pericarditis is a disease occurring in young adults, usually sporadically. Prospective studies have suggested a viral basis for around half. Coxsackie B is most commonly involved, but others including ECHO type 8, rubella, hepatitis B, mumps, and influenza have also been identified. Epidemics can occur, with approximately equal numbers of patients developing pericarditis and myocarditis.

The commonest clinical feature is chest pain, but 'flu-like' symptoms, palpitations, orchitis, encephalitis, and radiographic appearances of pneumonitis or pleural effusion have all been reported. The condition is usually self-limiting, but a minority of cases follow a relapsing course over the succeeding 6 to 12 months. A virus may be identified from paired blood samples taken 2 weeks apart, or recovered from throat or rectal swabs, but in many cases no clear cause is identified and positive virology is not necessary for the diagnosis.

HIV infection

Pericardial effusion can occur in AIDS, usually as a late manifestation with poor prognosis. For further information see Chapter 15.10.4.

Pyogenic infection

Pyogenic infection of the pericardium is uncommon. It is usually due to bloodborne infection of a previously sterile pericardial effusion, or the

Table 1 Diseases affecting the pericardium

Acute idiopathic pericarditis
Infections:
  viral
  bacterial (including tuberculosis)
  toxoplasmosis
  amoebiasis
  histoplasmosis
  actinomycosis
  nocardiosis
  echinococcal
Other inflammatory:
  postcardiotomy
  Dressler's syndrome
In association with systemic disease:
  connective tissue disorders (rheumatoid arthritis, systemic lupus
    erythematosus, systemic sclerosis, rheumatic fever, polyarteritis
    nodosa, Churg–Strauss syndrome, giant cell arteritis)
  uraemia
  hypothyroidism
Neoplastic:
  primary or secondary
Physical agents:
  radiotherapy
  blunt trauma
Haemorrhage:
  trauma
  aortic dissection
Drug-induced chylopericardium

result of direct spread from the lungs or pleural space. The organisms most commonly involved are staphylococci, pneumococci, or streptococci. Bacterial infection of the pericardium is not usually an isolated event and occurs more frequently in an immunologically compromised patient.

Tuberculous infection

Tuberculous infection is an important cause of pericardial disease, particularly in the Third World. It may take the form of acute pericarditis, pericardial effusion, or constriction. Acute pericarditis appears to be a 'primary' response, and can be regarded as an exudative lesion whose main basis is allergic. Chronic pericardial effusion and constriction both reflect granulomatous disease, often with fibrosis and calcification in the late stages. Both parietal and visceral layers of the pericardium may be involved, and spread of the disease to the myocardium follows. In the first instance, treatment is with antituberculous drugs. In both effusion and constriction in HIV-negative patients, adding steroids for the first 11 weeks reduces the need for pericardiectomy, increases the speed with which heart rate and venous pressure fall to normal, and expedites return to work. In the absence of specific contraindication, therefore, steroids should be added to standard antituberculous chemotherapy.

In Sub-Saharan Africa, patients with tuberculous pericarditis now have a more than 80 per cent chance of being HIV positive. Pericardial constriction severe enough to require surgery is rare, possibly reflecting depressed ability to form dense fibrosis in HIV infection. Treatment is with standard antituberculous drugs which, apart from thiacetazone, are well tolerated and effective. It is uncertain whether there is an adjuvant role for additional steroid in such patients. Long-term survival is shorter than in HIV-negative patients, due to other opportunistic infections rather than recurrence of tuberculosis.

Fungal infection

Fungal pericarditis is uncommon, but infection with actinomycosis, coccidioidomycosis, and histoplasmosis have all been recorded, the last leading to constriction and calcification. Pericardial calcification by hydatid disease

is increasingly recognized in areas where the disease is endemic and may require surgical treatment if cardiac compression occurs.

Myocardial infarction

Evidence of acute pericarditis can be found in up to 15 per cent of patients in the first 24 to 72 h after acute myocardial infarction. This may take the form of a friction rub when infarction was transmural. It seldom gives rise to symptoms other than dull retrosternal pain, which differs from that due to the infarction itself by varying with posture and respiration. Patients with pericarditis have more extensive ST segment changes and a slightly higher risk of supraventricular arrhythmia. There is no evidence to suggest increased risk of complication with thrombolysis. Echocardiography may demonstrate a small pericardial effusion, but this is unlikely to require treatment.

Post-cardiotomy syndrome

Pericardial involvement is an important component of the post-cardiotomy syndrome. This is an acute febrile illness occurring up to 1 year after cardiac surgery. The onset is usually sudden, with pleural or precordial pain and pyrexia of up to 40°C. Chest radiography may show an enlarged heart or a pleural effusion. ECG is unaffected. The condition is usually self-limiting, but can recur. Diagnosis is by excluding, in particular, infective endocarditis or cytomegalovirus infection from blood transfusion. Treatment is with aspirin or indomethacin. Rarely a large pericardial effusion may develop, requiring surgical drainage.

Dressler's syndrome

Dressler's syndrome is similar to post-cardiotomy syndrome. It follows 2 to 4 weeks after acute myocardial infarction, in 3 to 4 per cent of cases. It is a self-limiting febrile illness, accompanied by pericardial or pleural pain, and by pneumonitis in more severe cases. Like the post-cardiotomy syndrome, it responds to aspirin, indomethacin, and (if necessary) steroids.

Rheumatic fever

A small pericardial effusion accompanies virtually all cases of acute rheumatic fever, where it is associated with epicardial inflammation and sometimes acute pericarditis. Less commonly, the effusion may be large enough to cause cardiac enlargement on chest radiography and so suggest myocardial disease. Healing is virtually complete, although rheumatic pericarditis may be responsible for adhesions found at the time of subsequent valve replacement, and it has also been invoked as a cause of subsequent constriction. The diagnosis is made echocardiographically, and the condition must be distinguished from myocarditis or severe valve disease.

Autoimmune rheumatic disorders

Pericardial involvement can be a serious manifestation of rheumatoid disease, particularly in male patients with positive serology. Transient pericardial pain, symptomatic pericardial effusion, and particularly pericardial constriction may all occur. Pericardial involvement is also common in systemic lupus erythematosus, whether spontaneous or precipitated by procainamide or hydralazine. Pericardial pain, asymptomatic effusion, and chronic constriction have all been reported. Pericardial effusion can also be seen in association with scleroderma, polyarteritis nodosa, and the Churg–Strauss syndrome, when it may accompany myocardial involvement and functional mitral regurgitation.

Renal failure

Pericarditis, commonly fibrinous and associated with a bloody effusion, is often seen in untreated or inadequately treated chronic renal failure. The usual presentation is with pericardial pain and a rub, both of which subside if an effusion develops. Tamponade is common in untreated cases. Collagenous thickening of the epicardium is less common, but may give rise to myocardial constriction. Either of these complications may need surgical relief.

Hypothyroidism

Clinically silent pericardial effusion is common in untreated hypothyroidism. The effusion itself has a high cholesterol content which may produce an unusual secondary pericarditis with cholesterol deposits of 'gold paint' appearance. The pericardial effusion very rarely needs to be treated in its own right, and subsides when thyroid replacement therapy is given.

Malignancy

Malignant involvement of the pericardium may be due to a primary tumour, or much more commonly to secondary involvement. The least rare primary tumours are mesothelioma or myosarcoma. Clinical manifestations of malignant involvement include supraventricular arrhythmias or atrial fibrillation as well as pericardial tamponade or constriction. Malignant effusion is a very common cause of tamponade, and likely to need drainage. Positive diagnosis is best made by a limited surgical approach, allowing open biopsy and the fashioning of a window into the pleural cavity to prevent recurrence.

Irradiation

Pericarditis can be caused by irradiation. This is usually asymptomatic and a rub is unusual, but transient cardiac enlargement and minor ECG changes occur. It may occur at the time of the irradiation or at any time thereafter, and can be large enough to require drainage. The clinical picture needs to be distinguished from recurrence of malignancy. At operation, the pericardium is found to be thickened with fibrosis and dense adhesions. In a small minority of patients, pericardial constriction can develop up to 40 years after irradiation.

Haemorrhage

Haemorrhage into the pericardium is an important cause of tamponade. It may occur with aortic dissection involving the ascending aorta. If the leak is large it causes pericardial tamponade and death, but a small volume of blood is not uncommon with dissection. It can be detected by echocardiography, and may be responsible for ST segment changes on the ECG.

Pericardial haemorrhage may be the result of stab wounds or blunt injury, or may occur after cardiac surgery. It may also be induced by excessive anticoagulant therapy, or follow invasive procedures such as myocardial biopsy or pacemaker insertion.

Symptoms can occur at the time of bleeding, or may be delayed by 2 to 3 weeks, possibly because autolysis of clotted blood increases the volume of fluid within the pericardial space. Delayed tamponade causes a characteristic syndrome of elevated venous pressure, fluid retention, and low cardiac output that resembles myocardial disease. Haemorrhage into the pericardial space may also be the basis of delayed pericardial constriction occurring up to 10 years after open heart surgery.

Clinical syndromes associated with pericardial disease

Acute pericarditis

Clinical findings

There are three main components to the clinical syndrome of acute pericarditis: chest pain, pericardial rub, and ECG changes. The pain is usually retrosternal, continuous, and sharp or 'raw' in character. It is frequently aggravated by sudden movements or deep inspiration, and is relieved by sitting up. Less commonly it may resemble angina pectoris, or may be mild and 'atypical'. Painful breathing causes dyspnoea. The onset of the pain is usually sudden, but in idiopathic pericarditis, it may have been preceded by several days' malaise or other non-specific symptoms.

On examination, the main abnormality is a pericardial rub, audible in any position over the precordium. In patients in sinus rhythm it has two components, corresponding to atrial and ventricular systole. Rubs are frequently evanescent, and may vary with posture. They are often louder in inspiration. An irregular pulse due to supraventricular ectopic beats is common, particularly in patients with renal failure or after cardiac surgery. Atrial fibrillation or flutter are also seen.

The third clinical feature of the syndrome of acute pericarditis is an abnormal ECG. Symmetrical elevation of the ST segments by 1 mm or more in all leads other than aVr is seen in over 90 per cent of patients in whom the diagnosis is confirmed. Early in the illness, the T waves are upright, but over the next 2 to 3 weeks, they become flattened and inverted as the ST-segment changes regress. These T-wave changes are variable in incidence, direction, and extent. They usually resolve completely, but a minority of patients may be left with minor T-wave inversion, only to be detected many years later at a routine ECG.

Chest radiography is usually uninformative. It may show cardiac enlargement, but it is not possible to tell whether this is due to pericardial fluid, an increase in wall thickness, or enlargement of one or more cardiac chambers.

Echocardiography is the method of choice for detecting pericardial effusion (see section xxx). Cross-sectional echo may also detect pericardial adhesions that are responsible for the rub. However, acute pericarditis can occur without demonstrable pericardial effusion.

Diagnosis

The is usually straightforward, although it is possible that either the late systolic murmur of mitral prolapse or the systolic 'scratch' of Ebstein's anomaly may be mistaken for a pericardial rub. An underlying cause for acute pericarditis should always be sought, though it may not be found, and a final diagnosis of idiopathic pericarditis is probably the commonest outcome. The possibility of additional myocarditis should always be considered.

Treatment

Idiopathic acute pericarditis is usually self-limiting, requiring simple analgesics only. Since additional myocarditis is possible, the patient should rest until pain has subsided. Pericarditis due to Dressler's or the post-cardiotomy syndrome responds well to aspirin, or if more severe, to a non-steroidal anti-inflammatory drug. When symptoms are severe, repeated, or prolonged, steroids may be given empirically. Associated pericardial effusion is treated on its own merits: only rarely does it need to be drained. Supraventricular arrhythmias are treated in the standard way. When pericarditis is part of a generalized disease, this should obviously be treated appropriately.

Pericardial tamponade

Pathophysiology and clinical features

Pericardial tamponade occurs when the pressure of fluid within the pericardial cavity becomes high enough to interfere with ventricular filling. The volume of fluid needed to cause tamponade varies considerably between patients. If the fluid has collected slowly, 1 to 2 litres may be present, but if it has collected rapidly, or the pericardium is rigid, a much smaller volume will cause tamponade.

When pericardial pressure increases, right and left atrial pressures must necessarily rise to allow cardiac filling. The presence of fluid in the pericardium also reduces the volume of blood that can be accommodated in the cardiac chambers, such that stroke volume becomes small and fixed. Patients with cardiac tamponade therefore present with a high jugular venous pulse and clinical evidence of low cardiac output: the skin is cold, the pulse rate rapid but the volume small, and urine flow reduced, though systolic arterial pressure may be above 100 mmHg.

An important and characteristic physical sign in cardiac tamponade is arterial 'pulsus paradoxus'. Arterial pressure normally falls on inspiration by up to 10 mmHg. This fall is more obvious in patients with obstructive lung disease. Arterial paradox is unfortunately named: it is an accentuation of the normal response and not paradoxical. What is abnormal is the extent to which the arterial pressure falls. In severe tamponade the reduction in pulse pressure can readily be palpated at the radial artery, and with critical circulatory embarrassment the pulse may disappear altogether on inspiration. In milder cases, arterial paradox is sought using the sphygmomanometer.

The mechanism of pulsus paradoxus is still uncertain. Direct measurement of the pericardial pressure shows it to rise during inspiration, probably because the cavity is distorted by downward motion of the diaphragm. This increase is accompanied by a corresponding rise in right atrial and central venous pressure so that filling of the right side of the heart is maintained. By contrast, on the left side of the heart there is no corresponding increase in pulmonary venous pressure, which can fall to a low level compared with that in the pericardium and compromise left ventricular filling. During inspiration the interventricular septum then shifts from right to left, right ventricular stroke volume is maintained only by almost complete obliteration of the left ventricular cavity, left ventricular stroke volume drops dramatically, and profound inspiratory hypotension results. Finally, as pericardial pressure rises higher, there is diastolic collapse of right atrium and right ventricle.

Abnormal right ventricular filling is reflected in the venous pulse. The pressure is always raised: if it is not, the diagnosis of tamponade must be questioned. Usually it is very high, and it may be difficult to see the top. If a central venous line is in place, a further increase occurs with inspiration (Kussmaul's sign). This is a much less specific finding that arterial paradox and merely reflects the inability of the right heart to deal with an increase in stroke volume. It is seen in a variety of conditions including right ventricular disease and pulmonary hypertension. Although X and Y descents are visible, their amplitude is small, since the main disturbance is an increase in mean venous pressure. Unlike pericardial constriction, therefore, abnormalities in the form of the venous pulse are not particularly helpful in making the diagnosis.

Investigations

Chest radiography shows a large globular heart (Fig. 1), similar to that seen in dilated cardiomyopathy. More useful in making the diagnosis, therefore, is the absence of any evidence of pulmmonary congestion, which would be expected if myocardial disease were the main abnormality. Pulmonary oedema is most unusual in pure tamponade: if it is present, it suggests additional myocardial disease.

ECG shows tachycardia, often with low-voltage QRS complexes, but without Q waves or conduction disturbances. If the effusion is large, electrical alternans is present, when alternate QRS complexes show differing morphology (Fig. 2), because the heart swings to and fro in a large (therefore usually malignant) effusion.

Echocardiography is a most important investigation since it allows rapid and unequivocal diagnosis of pericardial effusion, which is usually large with tamponade (Fig. 3). Evidence for circulatory embarrassment is diastolic collapse of the right ventricle or right atrium (Fig. 4), and a striking increase in the amplitude of septal motion with respiration. If electrical alternans is present, motion of the heart within the pericardium can be confirmed.

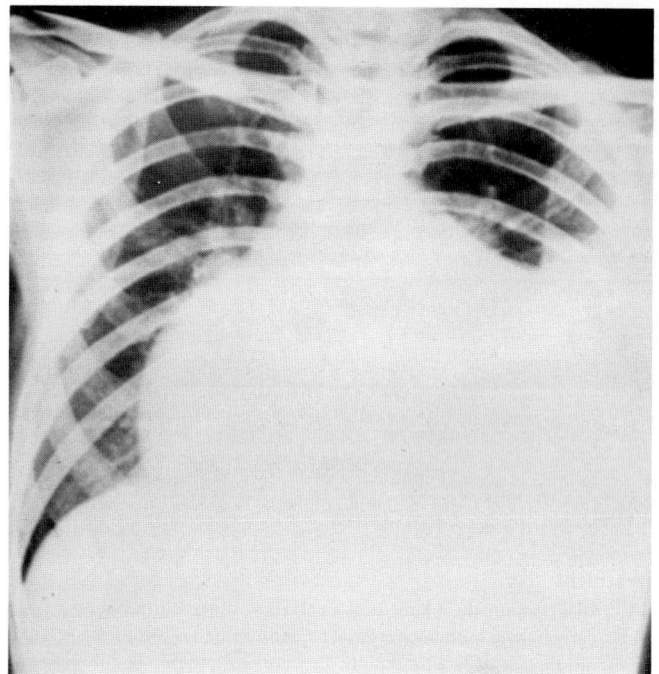

Fig. 1 Posteroanterior chest radiograph of a patient with a large pericardial effusion. The heart shadow is greatly enlarged and globular in configuration. The lung fields are normal.

Arterial pulsus paradox can be confirmed or excluded from a simultaneous trace of respiration and peripheral arterial Doppler (Fig. 5).

The circulatory embarrassment occurring with pericardial effusion varies in its exact nature between cases. 'Tamponade' does not therefore represent a uniform diagnosis. In the small minority of patients in whom an echocardiographic diagnosis of pericardial effusion cannot be made for technical reasons, some other imaging method such as CT or MRI may have to be used. Cardiac catheterization is no longer necessary.

Differential diagnosis

The main step in making the diagnosis of pericardial tamponade is to think of it in a patient presenting with clinical evidence of a low cardiac output. The condition must be distinguished from severe ventricular disease, massive pulmonary embolism, hypovolaemia, or overwhelming sepsis. Hypovolaemia is ruled out by the high venous pressure, whilst the absence of added heart sounds and pulmonary congestion makes severe ventricular disease unlikely. Massive pulmonary embolism is accompanied by a right ventricular third sound and characteristic ECG abnormalities.

An echocardiogram should be obtained early in all patients with low cardiac output for which the cause is not apparent, and if there is a large pericardial effusion the diagnosis of tamponade becomes very likely. It is essential for the occasional echocardiographer to distinguish pericardial effusion from pleural effusion. This is done by locating the high-intensity echo from the fibrous pericardium posterior to the left ventricle on the left parasternal view. A pericardial effusion is inside this structure, and a pleural effusion outside. Rarely, a large pleural effusion may compress the heart and cause a clinical picture very similar to tamponade in the absence of any pericardial fluid. This seems to occur when the pleural effusion is

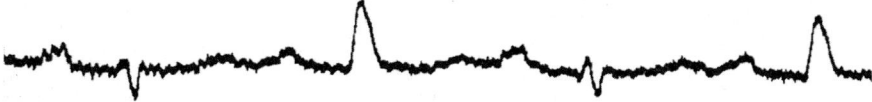

Fig. 2 Electrocardiogram from a patient with massive malignant pericardial effusion showing electrical alternans. Note that all are sinus beats with the same PR interval, but that the QRS axis alternates.

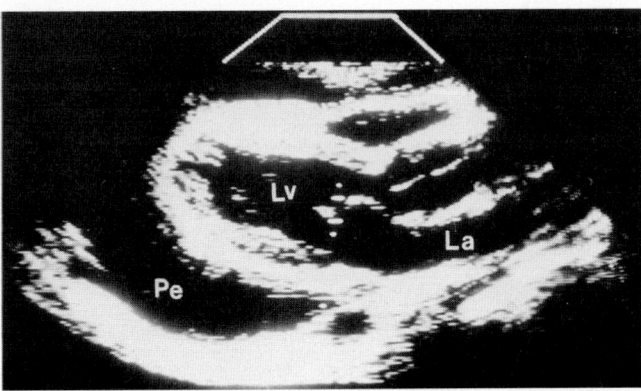

Fig. 3 Two-dimensional echocardiogram, parasternal long-axis view, showing a large pericardial effusion (Pe) posterior to the left ventricle (Lv). La, left atrium.

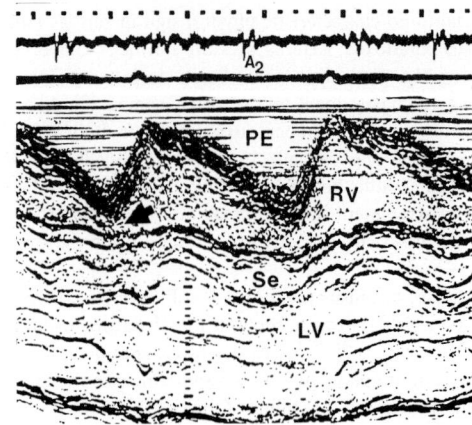

Fig. 4 M-mode echocardiogram showing diastolic collapse of the right ventricle (marked by arrow) in a patient with a large pericardial effusion. Note the minimum dimension of the right ventricle occurs at the end of the diastole. PE, pericardial effusion; RV, right ventricle; Se, interventricular septum; A2, aortic valve closure on phonocardiogram; LV, left ventricle (time marker = 200 ms)

under pressure, and haemodynamics rapidly return to normal with pleural drainage.

Treatment

Pericardial tamponade is a medical emergency. It needs urgent treatment, particularly if there is obvious arterial paradox, or if the effusion is of recent onset and fluid is collecting rapidly. Pericardial aspiration should be performed in an area where resuscitation facilities are available. Echocardiography is used to determine where to insert the needle, and to get some idea of the direction and depth. Subcostal or apical routes are possible, but the former is preferable if the heart is accessible in this way, since damage to the anterior descending coronary artery is possible from the apex. The depth of the pericardial fluid can usually be confirmed when the local anaesthetic is inserted. A larger needle or polythene cannula is then introduced into the effusion and a pig-tail catheter inserted over a guide wire. A maximum of 500 ml of fluid is removed initially and relieves any haemodynamic problem: rapid withdrawal of larger volumes can provoke cardiovascular collapse. Continuous drainage is then instituted and the remainder of the effusion drained over 12 to 24 h.

Many pericardial effusions, particularly malignant ones, are heavily bloodstained. They can be distinguished from blood associated with puncture of a chamber by their colour, since they are very desaturated, and by

their failure to clot, since they are defibrinated. If necessary, the haematocrit of the fluid can be compared with that of blood taken simultaneously.

Aspiration of a pericardial effusion is necessary when there is any suspicion of tamponade. It should also be considered when the volume is large, even in the absence of specific evidence of resting circulatory embarrassment, since exercise tolerance is commonly limited before overt tamponade develops. In addition, such patients are unstable and tamponade can develop quickly with the accumulation of a relatively small additional volume of fluid.

Aspiration is not necessarily the best way of definitively managing pericardial effusion. It does not prevent recurrence, and it is not usually possible to make a diagnosis from the pericardial fluid alone. The most satisfactory line of treatment, therefore, is to undertake limited thoracotomy, either through the fifth interspace, or subcostally, the latter operation being possible with local anaesthetic. This allows an adequate specimen of pericardium to be removed under direct vision for histology, and drainage of the pericardial space can be assured by making a window to the pleura. It

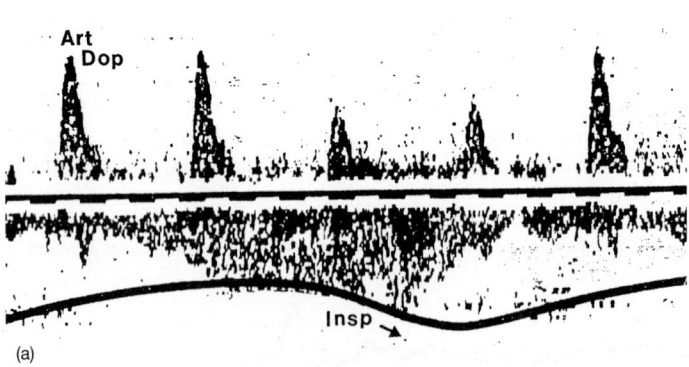

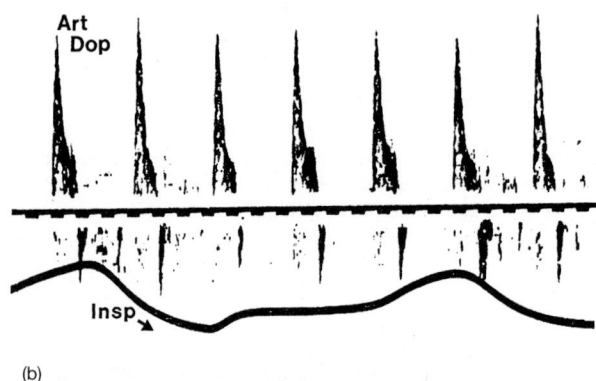

Fig. 5 (a) Arterial Doppler variation with respiration recorded from a patient with a large pericardial effusion. Note that peak arterial velocities drop to approximately half their peak values with inspiration. Art Dop, arterial Doppler; insp, inspiration. (b) The same patient after aspiration of the pericardial effusion. Note that the arterial pulse no longer varies with respiration (time marker = 100 ms).

is also possible to deal with a loculated effusion and to remove blood clots whose presence can give rise to delayed tamponade.

Pericardial constriction

Pericardial constriction is the haemodynamic disturbance caused when ventricular filling is limited by the pericardium. The pericardium itself is usually, but not always, thickened. The myocardium may also be involved, particularly in its subepicardial layers, by atrophy and fibrosis. Constriction usually affects both ventricles symmetrically, but in rare cases it may be localized. The majority of cases, particularly in the developed world, show no evidence of inflammation, acute or chronic, so 'pericardial constriction' is a better name than 'constrictive pericarditis'.

Pathophysiology and clinical features

Pericardial constriction prevents cardiac filling in late diastole. Since the two sides of the heart are usually affected symmetrically, right and left atrial filling are equally compromised. Early diastolic ventricular pressure is normal, but since the pericardium is effectively indistensible, a normal or reduced stroke volume causes a striking increase in filling pressure. End-diastolic pressures are equal to within 1 to 2 mmHg in all four cardiac chambers. This persists with respiration or even with fluid loading, and is the main criterion on which the invasive diagnosis of constriction is based. The ventricular pressure trace during filling is also characteristic. It rises rapidly in early diastole, and then stops rising abruptly, often with a slight rebound, and remains constant for the remainder of diastole. This pattern is often referred to as the 'square root sign' from a fancied resemblance to the mirror image of the mathematical symbol for a square root. Abnormal early diastolic filling is also reflected in the transmitral Doppler trace, which shows a rapid early diastolic deceleration, and reduced or absent flow across the valve during atrial systole.

The jugular venous pulse is also characteristic. Overall pressure is raised, with the dominant descent during systole, the X descent (Fig. 6). This descent is independent of right atrial systole, occurring later in the cardiac cycle than the A wave and persisting with atrial fibrillation. Flow towards the heart in the superior cava is also systolic, meaning that right atrial volume must also be increasing at this time. The unexpected combination of an increase in right atrial volume with a simultaneous fall in right atrial pressure is caused as follows. In pericardial constriction, an increase in the transverse dimension of the ventricle is limited by the pericardium, but increase in the longitudinal axis is not. Long-axis changes are brought about mainly by motion of the atrioventricular ring, and during ventricular ejection both atrioventricular rings move towards the cardiac apex. This enlarges the capacity of the atria, draws blood in from the vena cavae, and manifests as a dramatic X descent in the jugular venous pulse.

The clinical picture of pericardial constriction is dominated by obstruction to right ventricular filling. The jugular venous pressure is always raised, in well developed cases by 15 cm or more, showing abrupt systolic, and to a lesser extent, early diastolic descents whether or not the patient is in atrial fibrillation. Tachycardia and atrial fibrillation are common. The precordial impulse is not usually palpable, and on auscultation the heart sounds are soft. There may be an early diastolic sound, whose timing corresponds to the end of rapid filling, and which should therefore be classified as a third sound, though it is sometimes referred to as a ventricular 'knock'. It is often earlier than the classic third heart sound, but only because rapid filling ends earlier in constriction than in uncomplicated ventricular disease. The liver is enlarged, and in patients with long-standing disease, there may be wasting and jaundice. Ascites is often more prominent than peripheral oedema, particularly when the patient is stabilized on large doses of diuretic.

Investigations

The chest radiograph is usually normal, but the heart may be enlarged and it is important to look for pericardial calcification. This appears as multiple plaques or, more frequently, as a rim covering the diaphragmatic and anterior surfaces of the heart.

The ECG often shows atrial fibrillation, low-voltage QRS complexes and non-specific T-wave abnormalities. There are no diagnostic features.

CT scanning or MRI can demonstrate the extent and distribution of pericardial thickening. While this does not make the diagnosis of constriction, it is often very useful to know that the pericardium is actually abnormal in a patient in whom this diagnosis is suspected on clinical grounds. M-mode and cross-sectional echocardiography are unhelpful in making the diagnosis of constriction. Doppler may be useful in demonstrating abnormalities of ventricular filling.

Unless the diagnosis is very obvious, cardiac catheterization is still usually performed. To establish the diagnosis, three features should be present:

(1) a difference of less than 5 mmHg between the equal end-diastolic pressures in the two ventricles, persisting with respiration;

(2) a peak right ventricular pressure of less than 50 mmHg; and

(3) a ratio of end-diastolic to peak right ventricular pressure of more than 0.33.

It is still uncertain whether the normal pericardium can ever cause constriction in humans. The pericardium can stretch and accommodate a gradual increase in heart size. If constriction were to occur, it would probably be in the setting of rapid increase in ventricular size, for example in myocarditis or valvular regurgitation of acute onset. In these circumstances it would be difficult to dissociate from the primary manifestations of ventricular disease.

Alternative clinical presentations

A number of less common clinical presentations have been described.

1. Localized constriction may compress the outflow tract of the right ventricle or may mimic mitral or tricuspid stenosis.

2. A greatly raised venous pressure may lead to the clinical features of a protein-losing enteropathy or classic nephrotic syndrome.

3. The possibility that occult pericardial constriction might exist has been raised. In these patients, the resting venous pressure is normal and the symptoms are non-specific, including mild limitation of exercise tolerance or fatigue. There may be a history of previous acute pericarditis. The diagnostic haemodynamics of constriction can be unmasked by rapid volume infusion.

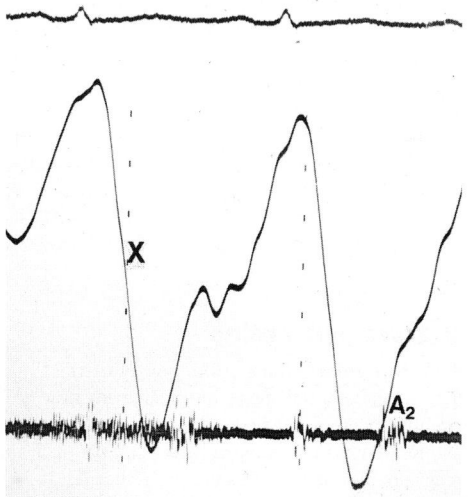

Fig. 6 Jugular venous pulse recording showing a dominant X descent in a patient with pericardial constriction. A2, aortic valve closure; (time marker = 500 ms).

Differential diagnosis

The main differential diagnosis of pericardial constriction is restrictive myocardial disease, where the passive properties of the myocardium itself are abnormal, usually as the result of fibrosis or infiltration. The haemodynamics are very similar in the two conditions: ventricular early diastolic pressure is normal, but that at end-diastole is greatly increased. The differential diagnosis is important: both are debilitating and life-threatening conditions, but whereas constriction can frequently be treated effectively by surgery, restrictive myocardial disease cannot (other than by transplantation). Approaches used to distinguish between the two conditions include the following.

Anatomical

If the pericardium is thickened or calcified, a diagnosis of constriction is very likely. Similarly, if echocardiography shows the characteristic appearances of amyloid then it is very likely that restrictive myocardial disease is present. The same applies when only one ventricle is greatly dilated with a reduced ejection fraction. In typical restrictive disease, however, left ventricular end-systolic cavity size is normal, although stroke volume may be reduced. Tricuspid regurgitation severe enough to lead to a clinical picture resembling either condition can readily be diagnosed by echocardiography.

Haemodynamics

Raised ventricular filling pressures, with a square root sign on the pressure pulse, increased early diastolic filling velocities, and shortened early filling periods do not distinguish between the two. All three catheter criteria mentioned above should be present before a definitive diagnosis of constriction is made. A dominant systolic X rather than Y descent on the jugular venous pulse is also very characteristic of constriction, probably because longitudinal as well as circumferential filling is impaired in restrictive myocardial disease.

Clinical progress

With diuretic treatment, the venous pressure usually drops in patients with restrictive myocardial disease, albeit at the cost of causing fatigue and hypovolaemia. It is very rare to be able to bring the venous pressure down to normal in a patient with well developed constriction.

This discussion is based on the assumption that constriction and restriction are independent conditions, and that a patient has either one or the other. However, this is not always the case. When the visceral pericardium (epicardium) is involved, fibrosis can spread to involve the myocardium and such cases may show features of both constriction and restriction. This state of affairs is analogous to that seen with subendocardial thickening as occurs in eosinophilic heart disease, which is usually classified as a form of restrictive cardiomyopathy. For this reason, in particular, the differential diagnosis between constriction and restriction may not be clear even after extensive investigation, and in a minority of cases it is not possible to avoid an exploratory thoracotomy. This enables the diagnosis of constriction to be made and treated accordingly, or to be definitively excluded, so that the patient can be reconciled to medical treatment, unsatisfactory as it may be.

Pericardial constriction must also be distinguished from other causes of raised venous pressure. Superior caval obstruction is excluded by the presence of venous pulsation. Right ventricular inflow may be obstructed by tricuspid stenosis or, very rarely, by a right ventricular tumour. Elevation of the venous pressure is also a feature of selective right atrial compression by blood clot occurring in the postoperative period (see later). Severe tricuspid regurgitation may occur on its own, or because of right ventricular disease. It seems to be becoming increasingly common as a long-term complication following mitral valve replacement. These possibilities can all be excluded by echocardiography.

Treatment

Mild pericardial constriction can usually be managed by diuretics. Although the venous pressure does not fall to normal, fluid retention can often be controlled. However, if fluid retention persists, or if an excessive dose of diuretic is needed, as shown by an increase in blood urea or impaired exercise tolerance due to fatigue, then surgery should be considered. The thickened pericardium must be removed from the anterior and inferior surfaces of the heart, and from the atrioventricular sulci. Cardiopulmonary bypass is usually needed to expose and decompress the heart satisfactorily. The operation is often a long and difficult one, particularly when the pericardium is calcified or when there is fibrosis of the myocardium. In many patients, the venous pressure is as high after the operation as it was before, though the X descent is lost and the Y descent becomes dominant. However, with digitalis and diuretic treatment, the pressure gradually falls over the succeeding weeks, as the condition of the patient improves.

Other manifestations of pericardial disease

Postoperative pericardial disease

A modified type of pericardial tamponade occurs after open heart surgery due to blood clots within the pericardium, particularly behind the left atrioventricular sulcus. Clinically this presents as a fall in urine flow and cardiac output, a reduction in skin temperature and finally hypotension. The atrial pressures may be normal or raised, and the classic arterial and venous pulse abnormalities are absent. Chest radiography and ECG show no specific abnormality. The transthoracic echocardiographic window is often poor immediately after surgery, but transoesophageal echo may show clot alongside the heart, compressing one or more chambers. The condition should be suspected in a patient who may have bled rather heavily after operation, particularly when the blood flow from the chest drains suddenly falls, and is most satisfactorily diagnosed by reopening the chest and removing the blood clots.

Clot may also compress the right atrium. This characteristically occurs towards the end of the first postoperative week, after the chest drains have been removed and when the patient is being mobilized. The main clinical features are fluid retention and elevation of the venous pressure. The diagnosis can usually be made by transthoracic echocardiography, which demonstrates distortion of the right atrial cavity by blood clot and sometimes increased right atrial filling velocities. If the precordial window is poor, transoesophageal echocardiography is required. Treatment is by drainage.

Pericardial constriction is increasingly being recognized as a long-term complication of cardiac surgery. It has a major effect on the clinical course of 1 to 2 per cent of patients; minor degrees are probably rather more common. It presents as chronic elevation of the venous pressure, and is often diagnosed as postoperative 'heart failure'. The diagnosis is suspected from the absence of any intracardiac cause of the syndrome of heart failure, such as ventricular disease, valvular regurgitation, or pulmonary hypertension, and from pericardial thickening demonstrated by CT or MRI. It can usually be controlled by a small dose of diuretic, but in a minority of cases, pericardial surgery may be needed.

Recurrent acute pericarditis

Recurrent acute pericarditis is an uncommon but clinically demanding form of pericardial disease to manage. It occurs at any time up to 10 years after an apparently uncomplicated episode of acute pericarditis of any aetiology. The commonest manifestation is chest pain, although rarely it may present as recurrent pericardial effusion. ECG changes and echocardiographic evidence of effusion occur in about half of cases. As with the original attack, immunological studies are likely to be indecisive. The clinical problem is that repeated episodes can become debilitating to the patient, particularly as they occur after what was represented as a self-limiting disease. Constriction and myocardial disease are significant complications. Management consists of maintaining a positive outlook and controlling the manifestations of acute pericarditis. Simple analgesia with aspirin is the most satisfactory means, but this may not always be adequate. Non-steroidal anti-inflammatory agents or corticosteroids may be required, the latter sometimes in large enough doses to lead to Cushingoid manifestations. There is no evidence to suggest that immunosuppressive agents have a therapeutic role. Pericardiectomy may be necessary, but is not necessarily effective, presumably because all pericardium cannot be removed. The overall prognosis of the condition is good.

Tuberculous pericardial constriction in the Third World

This runs a very different course from that seen in developed countries. In the absence of HIV infection, it occurs early in the disease and may be the presenting feature. Alternatively, it may supervene after an effusion has been drained. Patients present with sinus tachycardia rather than atrial fibrillation, a very high venous pressure, ascites, and weight loss. The venous pressure often does not show the characteristic pattern of systolic dip, and a third heart sound is present in about 50 per cent of cases. Chest radiography shows a normal-sized heart, but characteristically a 'shaggy' left heart border. There is no pericardial calcification. ECG shows sinus tachycardia and non-specific T-wave abnormalities. Cross-sectional echocardiography is very helpful, showing the two layers of pericardium separated by amorphous echoes often enclosing small loculated pockets of fluid (Fig. 7). This pattern is sometimes referred to as 'effusive-constrictive' pericarditis. The amplitude of ventricular wall motion is reduced, and the pericardial

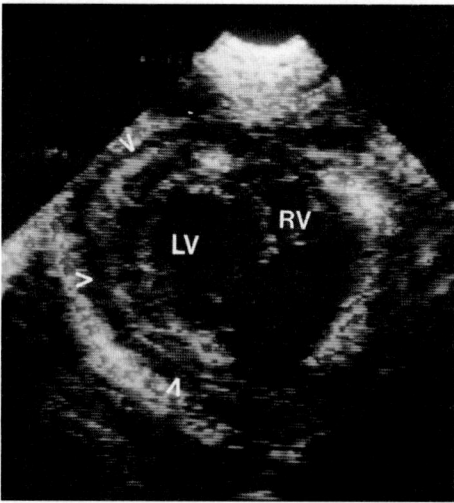

Fig. 7 Cross-sectional echocardiogram showing effusive-constrictive pattern of pericardial involvement (marked with arrow) in a patient with tuberculous pericarditis.

surface shows a very characteristic 'frozen' appearance. Treatment is with antituberculous chemotherapy. Added steroids help, with heart rate and venous pressure returning more rapidly to normal. They also reduce the risk of death and the requirement for operation. When possible, fluid retention should be controlled by diuretics. During the early subacute phase, surgery is demanding and unsatisfactory. It may be needed, however, in a minority of seriously ill patients who cannot be held on medical treatment. In the absence of AIDS, ultimate prognosis is excellent, being indistinguishable from that of the population at large whether treatment is medical or surgical.

Further reading

Baldwin JJ, Edwards JE (1976). Uremic pericarditis as a cause of tamponade. *Circulation* **53**, 896–901.

Caird R, Conway N, McMillan IKR (1973). Purulent pericarditis followed by early constriction in young children. *British Heart Journal* **35**, 201–3.

Carty JE, Deverall PB, Losowsky MS (1975). Retrosternal pain, widespread T wave inversion and collapse of left lower lobe with effusion, strangulated atrial appendix. *British Heart Journal* **37**, 98–100.

Dresler W (1959). The post-myocardial infarction syndrome. A report of 44 cases. *Archives of Internal Medicine* **103**, 28–20.

Fowler NO, Harbin III AD (1986). Recurrent acute pericarditis: follow-up study of 31 patients. *Journal of the American College of Cardiology* **7**, 300–5.

Hatle LK, Appleton CP, Popp RL (1989). Differentiation of constrictive pericarditis and restrictive cardiomyopathy by Doppler echocardiography. *Circulation* **79**, 357–70.

Heidenreich PA *et al.* (1995). Pericardial effusion in AIDS. *Circulation* **92**, 3229–34.

Kahn AH (1975). Pericarditis of myocardial infarction. *American Heart Journal* **90**, 788–94.

Martin RG *et al.* (1975). Radiation induced pericarditis. *American Journal of Cardiology* **35**, 217–20.

Perheentupa J *et al.* (1973). Mulibrey nanism, an autosomal recessive syndrome with pericardial constriction. *Lancet* **ii**, 351–5.

Spodick DH (1974). ECG in acute pericarditis. *American Journal of Cardiology* **40**, 470–4.

Strang JIG (1984). Tuberculous pericarditis in Transkei. *Clinical Cardiology* **7**, 667–70.

Tubbs OS, Yacoub MH (1968). Congenital pericardial defects. *Thorax* **23**, 598–607.

Vaitkus PT, Kussmaul WG (1991). Constrictive pericarditis versus restrictive cardiomyopathy: a reappraisal and update of diagnostic criteria. *American Heart Journal* **122**, 1431–41.

Watters DAK (1997). Surgery for tuberculosis before and after human immunodeficiency virus infection: a tropical perspective. *British Journal of Surgery* **84**, 8–14.

Wood P (1961). Chronic constrictive pericarditis. *American Journal of Cardiology* **7**, 48–55.

15.10 Cardiac involvement in infectious disease

15.10.1 Acute rheumatic fever

Jonathan R. Carapetis

Introduction

Acute rheumatic fever is an immunologically mediated, multisystem disease induced by recent infection with group A streptococcus. Most medical practitioners in industrialized countries will rarely, if ever, see a case. However, the dramatic decline in incidence of acute rheumatic fever in industrialized countries during the second half of the twentieth century is not replicated in many developing countries, or among some indigenous and other populations living in poverty in industrialized countries. Moreover, acute rheumatic fever has recently returned as an important public health problem in some middle-class regions of the United States. Rheumatic heart disease remains the most common acquired heart disease of childhood in the world.

Epidemiology

The highest reported annual incidence of acute rheumatic fever, more than 500/100 000, occurs in the Aboriginal population of the Northern Territory of Australia. Populations in developing countries commonly have incidence rates between 50 and 200/100 000 per year. There have been dramatic declines in recent decades in many Latin American and Asian countries with improving economic and living conditions. In most populations with high incidence rates, the predisposing conditions are those that promote endemicity and high levels of transmission of group A streptococci: these include overcrowded housing, poor personal and community hygiene, poor access to medical services and, in some circumstances, widespread skin infection and scabies infestation.

Outbreaks of acute rheumatic fever occurred in middle-class areas of the United States during the 1980s and 1990s. These outbreaks arose because of the emergence of virulent strains of group A streptococci, particularly belonging to M serotypes 1, 3, and 18. By contrast, outbreaks of acute rheumatic fever have rarely, if ever, been described from developing countries; most cases appear to arise from the ongoing circulation of pathogenic group A streptococcal strains in the population.

Recurrent episodes are almost as common as primary episodes in many populations with high incidence rates of acute rheumatic fever, and account for approximately 40 per cent of all episodes among the Aboriginal population of northern Australia. Recurrences may lead to accumulated cardiac valvular damage and are therefore responsible for many cases of rheumatic heart disease, yet they are almost entirely preventable using secondary prophylaxis (see later).

In many developing countries females are affected more than males, usually in the ratio between 1.3 and 2 to 1. In affluent countries males and females appear to be affected equally. The gender association is stronger for rheumatic heart disease (especially mitral stenosis) than acute rheumatic fever; this may reflect a greater tendency to recurrences among females. Any female preponderance may relate to inherited characteristics, to greater exposure to group A streptococci because of the increased involvement of girls and young women in child-rearing in most cultures, or to reduced access by females to primary and secondary prophylaxis.

The maximum incidence of acute rheumatic fever is between the ages of 5 and 15 years in all populations. Approximately 5 per cent of cases occur in children younger than 5 years, but very rarely are children younger than 3 years affected. This age distribution parallels that of group A streptococcal pharyngitis, and supports the hypothesis that all cases of acute rheumatic fever follow this condition. However, it may be that cases do not occur in infants or very young children because of the need for maturity of the immune system (particularly of cellular immunity), or sensitization of the immune response by prior streptococcal infections. New cases occur occasionally up to age 30, but rarely beyond. Hypotheses to explain the reduced incidence in adulthood include development of non-type-specific immunity to primary group A streptococcal infections, further maturation of immune responses, or reduced sensitization by recurrent streptococcal infections.

Pathogenesis

Despite a century of research, the pathogenesis of acute rheumatic fever remains incompletely understood. The presumed pathogenetic pathway is summarized in Fig. 1.

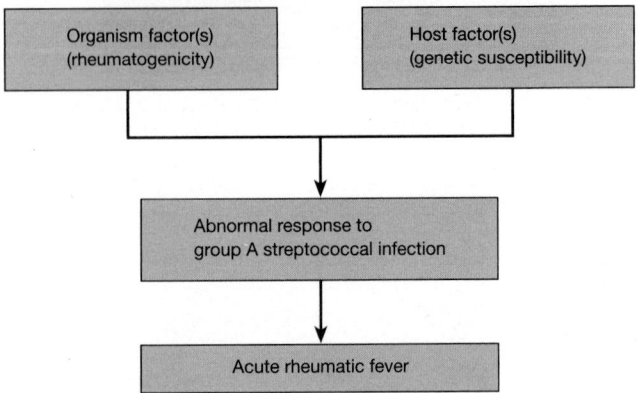

Fig. 1 Simplified approach to understanding the pathogenesis of acute rheumatic fever. (Adapted with permission from Carapetis JR, Currie BJ, Good M (1996). Editorial review: Towards understanding the pathogenesis of rheumatic fever. *Scandinavian Journal of Rheumatology* **25**, 127–31.)

Host factors

Epidemiological evidence suggests that less than 5 or 6 per cent of people have the potential to develop acute rheumatic fever after relevant streptococcal exposure, and that this proportion does not vary substantially between populations. Attack rates of acute rheumatic fever after untreated group A streptococcal pharyngitis vary from less than 1 to 3 per cent. Genetic susceptibility to acute rheumatic fever was first suggested by its familial aggregation and by a greater concordance in monozygotic than in dizygotic twins. The mode of inheritance is uncertain; autosomal recessive or autosomal dominant with partial penetrance have been suggested.

The basis for genetic susceptibility is not known. Recent work suggests an association of rheumatic heart disease with certain HLA class II alleles. A B-cell alloantigen (D8/17) is expressed in a high percentage of B cells from patients with acute rheumatic fever and their family members in many populations. However, D8/17 may not predict susceptibility in all populations; recent studies in India suggest that different B-cell alloantigens may identify patients with acute rheumatic fever there. It is not yet clear whether these putative markers are genetic or induced by streptococcal infection as part of the pathogenesis of acute rheumatic fever.

Organism factors

The observation that outbreaks of pharyngitis due to certain serotypes of group A streptococcus resulted in high attack rates of acute rheumatic fever, whereas no cases occurred after infection with other serotypes, led to the concept of 'rheumatogenicity'—that only some strains of group A streptococcus have the potential to cause acute rheumatic fever. M serotypes 1, 3, 5, 6, 14, 18, 19, 24, 27, and 29 have been most frequently implicated. However, there may be substantial genetic diversity among strains belonging to a particular M serotype, and not all strains of 'rheumatogenic serotypes' appear to cause acute rheumatic fever. Therefore, rheumatogenicity may be strain specific rather than serotype specific; that is, any group A streptococcus may acquire the potential to cause acute rheumatic fever.

The pathogenic factor(s) are not known. Parts of the organism have immunological cross-reactivity with human tissue; there is close homology between regions of the M protein and human myosin, tropomyosin, and keratin. Other components of group A streptococci, including the hyaluronic acid capsule, the cell-wall associated group-specific carbohydrate, and the cell membrane, cross-react with a variety of human tissues damaged in acute rheumatic fever, including components of heart muscle and valves, joints, and brain. Acute rheumatic fever-associated strains of group A streptococcus also tend to be heavily encapsulated with hyaluronic acid, and not to express opacity factor. Group A streptococci possess components which act as superantigens, selectively stimulating subsets of T cells without the need for antigen presentation. Their role in acute rheumatic fever pathogenesis is not yet clear.

Site of infection

Although it is widely accepted that acute rheumatic fever may result from group A streptococcal infection of the upper respiratory tract, but not of the skin, there is some evidence that this may not always be the case. Upper respiratory tract infection certainly accounts for most, if not all, episodes of acute rheumatic fever in countries with a temperate climate. However, in tropical countries where streptococcal impetigo is highly endemic but group A streptococcal pharyngitis less common, it may be that skin infection accounts for many cases of acute rheumatic fever, either *de novo* or after subsequent throat infection. Determining whether group A streptococcal skin infection may have a role in pathogenesis of acute rheumatic fever would have enormous public health implications, as it may redirect present approaches to primary prevention (see later).

The immune response

The finding of immunological cross-reactivity led to initial enthusiasm for the role of humoral immunity in the pathogenesis of acute rheumatic fever.

This was supported by the finding of anti-group A streptococcal antibodies cross-reactive with heart, joint, and brain in the sera of patients with acute rheumatic fever. Immunoglobulin and complement deposits have also been demonstrated in damaged heart tissue.

More recently, patients with acute rheumatic fever were found to have elevated levels of most markers of cellular immune activation, including circulating CD4 lymphocytes, interleukins (**IL**)-1 and -2, IL-2 receptor-positive T cells, neopterin, tumour necrosis factor-α receptors, natural killer cell cytotoxicity, T-cell responsiveness to group A streptococcal antigens, and others. T-cell and histiocytic-cell infiltrates are also present in valvular and myocardial tissue during acute rheumatic fever. This has led to theories that the primary damage in acute rheumatic fever may be due to cell-mediated immune responses and that the humoral response may be secondary to antigens released from already damaged tissues. Cross-reacting antigens of group A streptococci may be presented to the immune system abnormally, or they may be abnormally recognized by helper T cells, resulting in uncontrolled activation of cellular immunity. The resulting damage targets those tissues for which the inducing strain has sequence mimicry.

Clinical manifestations

There is always a latent period between group A streptococcal infection and the development of acute rheumatic fever. This varies from 1 to 5 weeks in most cases (usually about 3 weeks), but may be shorter in recurrences. Chorea may occur up to 6 months after the precipitating streptococcal infection. The preceding infection is asymptomatic in about two-thirds of cases.

The tissues most commonly affected are the heart, joints, and brain. Although the symptoms due to each can be disabling in the short term, only cardiac damage may be permanent and progressive. Therefore, the focus in controlling or treating acute rheumatic fever is always to prevent the development of rheumatic heart disease.

The frequency with which the various clinical manifestations have occurred in recent descriptions of acute rheumatic fever is listed in Table 1.

Carditis

Although inflammation in acute rheumatic fever may affect the pericardium (causing pericardial rubs and occasionally pleuritic chest pain) or the myocardium (sometimes causing cardiac failure, and evident on biopsy with pathognomonic Aschoff bodies), endocardial inflammation is the most important cause of cardiac damage. If acute cardiac failure or chronic cardiac disease occur, they are almost always due to damage to the cardiac valves.

A murmur is the most common evidence of acute valvular disease, usually the apical pan-systolic murmur of mitral regurgitation, with or without a low-pitched mid-diastolic (Carey–Coombs) murmur. Occasionally an

Table 1 Frequency of clinical manifestations in acute rheumatic fever

Manifestation	Proportion of patients with manifestation (%)	
	Chorea absent*	Chorea present*
Carditis	40–60	20–30
Polyarthritis	50–75	<10
Erythema marginatum	1–10	0–1
Subcutaneous nodules	1–10	0–1
Fever > 37.5°C	> 90	10–25
Arthralgia	< 10–20	< 5
Elevated acute-phase reactants	> 90	10–25
Prolonged P–R interval	30–50	5–10

*Chorea is present in less than 10 per cent to over 30 per cent of patients with acute rheumatic fever, depending on the population.

aortic regurgitant murmur may be heard, mainly in older adolescents or young adults. Murmurs of tricuspid or pulmonary regurgitation are rare and are usually secondary to increased pulmonary venous pressures resulting from mitral regurgitation or stenosis. Sinus tachycardia or gallop rhythms may also be present in acute carditis.

Valves affected by rheumatic carditis may have a characteristic appearance or pattern of regurgitation on Doppler echocardiography (when interpreted by experienced technicians), which may be found even in the absence of a cardiac murmur. This may be useful for diagnosis when other clinical manifestations are not definitive. However, echocardiographic criteria have not yet been standardized, and it is difficult to distinguish acute carditis from previous rheumatic valve damage.

Mitral or aortic stenosis may develop as later complications of severe and/or recurrent acute carditis due to scarring and contraction following the acute inflammatory process. Rarely, mitral stenosis may occur in young children with acute rheumatic fever—so-called 'juvenile mitral stenosis'—the reasons for the development of this condition are not clear.

Damage to the electrical conduction pathways may result in prolongation of the P–R interval on electrocardiography. Although a subset of healthy people may have this finding, the presence of a prolonged P–R interval that resolves over the ensuing few days to weeks may be a useful diagnostic feature in cases where the clinical manifestations are not clear. Occasionally, in the acute phase, second- or third-degree heart block or a nodal rhythm may be present (Fig. 2).

Arthritis

The characteristic joint manifestation of acute rheumatic fever is severe, large-joint, migratory polyarthritis. The knees, ankles, wrists, and elbows are most commonly involved; only rarely, and usually only when the

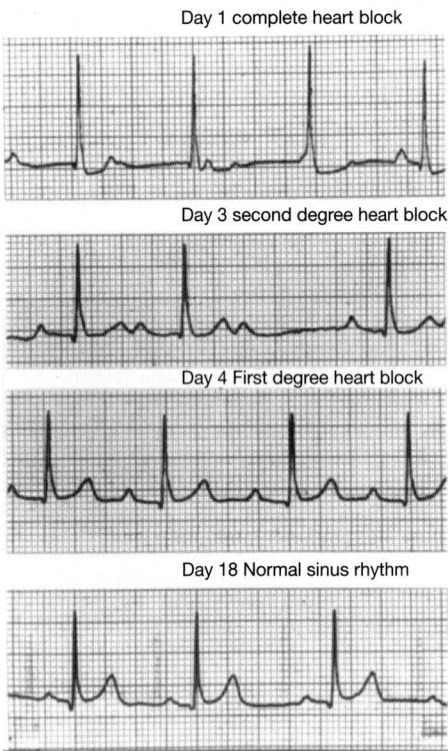

Day 1 complete heart block

Day 3 second degree heart block

Day 4 First degree heart block

Day 18 Normal sinus rhythm

Fig. 2 Electrocardiographic changes in a young adult with acute rheumatic fever, showing evolution over 18 days from complete heart block, to second-degree (Wenckebach) block, to first-degree block, and then to normal sinus rhythm. (Reproduced with permission from Bishop W *et al.* (1996). A subtle presentation of acute rheumatic fever in remote northern Australia. *Australian and New Zealand Journal of Medicine* **26**, 241–2.)

patient is untreated for several days, are the hips or small joints of the hands or feet inflamed. One joint characteristically becomes exquisitely painful and inflamed as another is waning. Most patients have only one or two joints affected at any one time, and each joint may be involved for just a few hours or up to 1 or 2 days. The arthritis is so responsive to non-steroidal anti-inflammatory medication that its persistence more than 1 or 2 days after commencing high-dose aspirin should lead one to consider alternative diagnoses.

Arthritis of a single large joint may occur in acute rheumatic fever, although other causes (including septic arthritis) should first be excluded. Arthralgia (joint pain without objective evidence of inflammation) is usually migratory and affects large joints, and like the arthritis of acute rheumatic fever is very responsive to anti-inflammatory medication.

Sydenham's chorea

In 1686 the English physician Thomas Sydenham described rheumatic chorea, initially naming it 'St Vitus' dance'. It is the most intriguing manifestation of acute rheumatic fever, particularly as it commonly occurs in the absence of other manifestations, usually follows a prolonged latent period (up to 6 months) after the precipitating group A streptococcal infection, and occurs most commonly in females (and almost never in post-pubertal males). The rapid, jerky, involuntary movements affect predominantly the upper limbs and face, may be asymmetrical, and may be sufficiently severe to render the patient unable to eat, drink, walk, or perform other activities of daily living. Mild chorea can sometimes be detected by having the patient join palms above the head to reveal occasional twitches of the arms or the head. Typical signs include the 'milk-maid's grip' (rhythmic squeezing when the patient grasps the examiner's fingers), spooning of extended hands (caused by flexion of the wrists and extension of the fingers), darting of the protruded tongue, and the 'pronator sign' (the arms and palms turn outwards when held above the head). As with other forms of chorea, the disorder usually becomes more evident with anxiety or purposeful movements (such as drinking or writing). Movements may appear semi-purposeful, and symptoms subside during sleep. Sydenham's chorea often is associated with excessive emotional lability or personality changes: these may precede the abnormal movements.

Most patients can be reassured that Sydenham's chorea will resolve completely and leave no long-lasting effects, usually within 6 weeks and almost always within 6 months, but rarely lasting up to 3 years.

Subcutaneous nodules and erythema marginatum

Both of these manifestations are found in less than 2 per cent of patients with acute rheumatic fever, although they were described in up to 10 to 20 per cent of patients in earlier studies from the United States and the United Kingdom. Subcutaneous nodules are firm, painless lumps, usually between 0.5 and 2 cm in diameter, commonly found in crops of three or more, and usually appear 2 to 3 weeks after the onset of acute rheumatic fever. They occur mainly over extensor surfaces or bony protuberances, particularly the hands, feet, occiput, and back. The nodules are similar, though often smaller, to those found in rheumatoid arthritis, and are most likely to be associated with severe carditis. Nodules usually last from a few days to 2 or 3 weeks.

The characteristic rash, erythema marginatum, appears as a light pink macule that spreads outwards with a serpiginous, well-demarcated edge, while the central portion clears. It appears, disappears, or moves before the observer's eyes. Multiple areas are often involved, usually over the trunk, occasionally over the proximal portions of the limbs, but rarely, if ever, the face. It usually appears together with the other initial symptoms of acute rheumatic fever, but may recur intermittently for weeks or even months. This does not indicate ongoing rheumatic inflammation, and patients can be reassured that the rash will eventually disappear without complications.

Fever

With the exception of those with pure chorea, 90 per cent of patients will have a temperature at presentation higher than 37.5°C. Although it has been reported that the temperature usually exceeds 39°C, others have found only 25 per cent of confirmed cases with fever to that level. Any temperature above 37.5°C should be considered a minor manifestation. As with arthritis, fever is very sensitive to anti-inflammatory medication, usually resolving completely within 1 or 2 days of commencing high-dose salicylates.

Elevated acute-phase reactants

Almost all patients, except those with pure chorea, have a dramatically elevated erythrocyte sedimentation rate or serum C-reactive protein. There appears little difference between these measurements in their diagnostic usefulness. The C-reactive protein may return to normal more rapidly than the sedimentation rate when rheumatic activity subsides. Mild to moderate peripheral leucocytosis is common, although this is a less sensitive marker of rheumatic inflammation.

Other features

Severe, central abdominal pain is found at presentation in a small proportion of patients. It may be associated with other features of acute rheumatic fever; if not, these features usually appear within 1 or 2 days. The pain responds quickly to anti-inflammatory medication. Epistaxis was reported frequently in historical accounts of acute rheumatic fever, but does not feature prominently in recent descriptions. Pulmonary infiltrates may be found in patients with acute carditis; this has been labelled 'rheumatic pneumonia' although it is not clear whether the infiltrates represent rheumatic inflammation or another process. There may be microscopic haematuria, pyuria, or proteinuria; also mild elevations of liver transaminases: these are non-specific and not usually severe.

Associated post-streptococcal syndromes

Post-streptococcal reactive arthritis has been differentiated from rheumatic fever by some authors because it has a shorter incubation period after streptococcal infection, sometimes follows non-group A β-haemolytic streptococcal infection, may have a different pattern of arthritis (including small joint involvement), and is less responsive to anti-inflammatory medication. Because of the lack of cardiac involvement, these patients are said not to require secondary prophylaxis. However, a few patients who have subsequently developed carditis have led other authors to question the distinction between post-streptococcal reactive arthritis and rheumatic fever. If post-streptococcal reactive arthritis is diagnosed, secondary prophylaxis should be prescribed for at least 1 year and discontinued if there is no evidence of carditis. In populations with high incidence rates of acute rheumatic fever, it may be prudent to treat all cases of possible post-streptococcal reactive arthritis as acute rheumatic fever.

The frequent finding of emotional lability, motor hyperactivity, and occasional obsessive–compulsive symptoms in patients with Sydenham's chorea led to the observation that group A streptococcal infections may precipitate or exacerbate other disorders of the basal ganglia. These include tic disorders, Tourette syndrome, and obsessive–compulsive disorder, and the term **PANDAS** (paediatric autoimmune neuropsychiatric disorders associated with streptococcal infections) has been coined. Patients with PANDAS appear not to be at risk of developing carditis. There is evidence that these patients, and some children with autism, have high proportions of circulating B cells expressing D8/17 antigen, which is a proposed marker of rheumatic fever susceptibility. It is not yet clear whether these syndromes are linked with acute rheumatic fever.

Table 2 The Jones criteria for guidance in the diagnosis of the initial attack of acute rheumatic fever, updated in 1992

Major manifestations	Minor manifestations
Carditis	Fever
Polyarthritis	Arthralgia
Chorea	Elevated acute-phase reactants
Subcutaneous nodules	Prolonged P–R interval
Erythema marginatum	
Plus	
Supporting evidence of a recent group A streptococcal infection:	
Positive throat culture or rapid antigen test	
Elevated or increasing streptococcal antibody titre	

The presence of two major or one major and two minor manifestations, plus evidence of a preceding group A streptococcal infection, indicates a high likelihood of acute rheumatic fever. Reprinted with permission from Special Writing Group of the Committee on Rheumatic Fever, Endocarditis and Kawasaki Disease, American Heart Association (1992). Guidelines for the diagnosis of rheumatic fever: Jones criteria, 1992 update. *Journal of the American Medical Association* **15**, 2069–73.

Diagnosis

Because of the diversity of symptoms and signs, and the non-specific nature of most of them, Dr T. Duckett Jones developed a set of criteria to aid in the diagnosis of acute rheumatic fever in 1944. The Jones criteria have subsequently been revised and updated a number of times to improve their positive and negative predictive values. The most recent version, the 1992 update, is shown in Table 2. The manifestations are divided into: major, those which are most predictive of acute rheumatic fever, and minor, those which are commonly found in acute rheumatic fever but are less specific.

The diagnosis requires the presence of either two major, or one major and two minor criteria, plus the demonstration of a current or recent group A streptococcal infection. Evidence of group A streptococcal infection is not required for chorea, where the onset may be delayed up to 6 months after streptococcal infection, and late-onset carditis, when low-grade inflammation may persist for prolonged periods after the precipitating infection.

The 1992 updated Jones criteria are to be used only for the diagnosis of the initial episode of acute rheumatic fever. Patients with a previous history of acute rheumatic fever or rheumatic heart disease need have only one major or two minor manifestations, have evidence of recent group A streptococcal infection, and have no other plausible explanation for their symptoms. The Jones criteria are a guideline, but cases not fulfilling the criteria should only be diagnosed as acute rheumatic fever once all other possible diagnoses have been excluded.

Proof of a recent group A streptococcal infection can include demonstrating the organism in the upper respiratory tract, either by culture or rapid antigen techniques. However, most children with acute rheumatic fever no longer have a group A streptococcus detectable by these methods, and up to 15 to 25 per cent of normal children in temperate climate countries may carry the organism in their throats. Therefore, serological techniques are most commonly used, particularly the anti-streptolysin O, anti-DNase B, or anti-hyaluronidase titres. One of any two of these tests will be positive in well over 90 per cent of recent streptococcal infections. Their usefulness is increased by performing more than one serological test, or by demonstrating rising titres in paired sera. Serology is of limited value in regions with high prevalence rates of streptococcal impetigo, where children may have positive anti-streptococcal titres most of the time. The diagnosis of acute rheumatic fever in these circumstances can be very difficult. There is therefore a need for a better diagnostic test of recent streptococcal infection, or an objective diagnostic test for acute rheumatic fever itself.

The most common clinical presentation, that of a child with fever and polyarthritis, raises multiple differential diagnoses that will vary by region. Table 3 lists some alternative diagnostic possibilities for the three most common major manifestations.

Table 3 Some differential diagnoses for the three most common major manifestations of acute rheumatic fever

Manifestation		
Polyarthritis	**Carditis**	**Chorea**
Connective tissue disease	Innocent murmur	Systemic lupus
Immune complex disease	Mitral valve prolapse	erythematosus
Septic arthritis (including	Congenital heart disease	Drug reaction
gonococcal)	Infective endocarditis	Wilson's disease
Viral arthropathy	Hypertrophic cardio-	Tic disorder
Reactive arthropathy	myopathy	Choreoathetoid cerebral
Lyme disease	Myocarditis:	palsy
Sickle cell anaemia	viral or idiopathic	Encephalitis
Infective endocarditis	Pericarditis:	Huntington's chorea
Leukaemia or lymphoma	viral or idiopathic	Intracranial tumour

Treatment

If untreated, acute rheumatic fever lasts on average for 3 months. Except in the case of life-threatening acute carditis, there is no evidence that presently available treatments alter the outcome. Most treatments are designed to provide symptomatic relief or are based on theoretical (but unproven) approaches to attenuating the long-term damage.

All patients with acute rheumatic fever should be admitted to hospital (if practical) to confirm the diagnosis, to perform baseline investigations to ascertain the status of the heart, to provide adequate treatment for the acute phase, to commence secondary prophylaxis, to allow communication of details to personnel responsible for long-term follow-up of the patient, and to begin education of the patient and family. The mainstays of treatment are bed rest, penicillin, and salicylates.

Bed rest

Previous recommendations that children with acute rheumatic fever be rested in bed until all signs of active inflammation abated were probably more extreme than is necessary. Once symptoms of arthritis have subsided and any cardiac failure is controlled, the child may begin gentle mobilization, which may be increased as tolerated. There is no evidence that bed rest beyond the period where mobilization leads to exacerbation of pain or cardiac failure has any long-term benefit.

Penicillin

All patients with acute rheumatic fever should be given penicillin to eradicate the group A streptococcus that precipitated the attack. This is based on an early finding that, in some cases, prolonged group A streptococcal infection led to more severe acute rheumatic fever. Although in most cases the precipitating organism cannot be cultured, a treatment course of penicillin is prudent in case the strain remains present in low numbers, and to prevent its transmission to other contacts. As the aim is eradication of group A streptococcal infection, penicillin may be administered either as a single intramuscular injection of benzathine penicillin G at a dose of 1.2 million units (600 000 U for patients less than 30 kg) into the gluteal or quadriceps muscles, or as a 10-day course of oral phenoxymethyl penicillin (V) at a dose of 500 mg (adolescents and adults) or 250 mg (children) given either two or three times daily. In the case of penicillin allergy, the present recommendation is to use oral erythromycin at 20 to 40 mg/kg per day given two to four times daily for 10 days, although in some regions levels of erythromycin-resistance among group A streptococci are increasing.

Salicylates

Children with arthritis or severe arthralgia should be treated with non-steroidal anti-inflammatory medication; salicylates have been most widely used. Aspirin at a dose of 80 to 100 mg/kg per day (4 to 8 g/day in adults) usually results in defervescence and resolution of arthritis and arthralgia within 1 to 2 days. Sometimes these doses lead to nausea or vomiting; this can be minimized by increasing from lower starting doses. When the diagnosis is uncertain, salicylates should be withheld for a day or two to observe for the development of characteristic migratory polyarthritis. In such cases, codeine can be used to control pain until the diagnosis is confirmed.

There is no evidence that salicylates reduce the severity of acute carditis or the risk of chronic cardiac valve damage. Nevertheless, many clinicians administer salicylates until acute-phase reactants have returned towards normal in the belief that this may reduce the risk of long-term cardiac damage. After 2 weeks, the dose is often reduced to 60 to 70 mg/kg per day for the remaining 2 to 4 weeks. Arthritis or arthralgia may return up to 2 to 3 weeks after discontinuation of therapy; this is usually a brief and mild recrudescence, often associated with increased erythrocyte sedimentation rate or C-reactive protein, and can be managed either with rest and reassurance or a short course of lower-dose anti-inflammatory medication.

Corticosteroids

For many years, corticosteroids have been used in acute rheumatic fever, particularly for patients with severe carditis. As with salicylates, the evidence that they reduce either the severity of acute carditis or the risk of long-term valve damage is conflicting. Many clinicians continue to use them, commonly oral prednisone or prednisolone at a dose of 40 to 60 mg/day, tapering after 2 or 3 weeks.

Treatment of cardiac failure

Although the use of corticosteroids is controversial, there is no doubting the need to treat cardiac failure. Diuretics, angiotensin-converting enzyme inhibitors (especially in aortic regurgitation), and fluid restriction are most commonly employed. Digoxin is usually restricted to cases where atrial fibrillation coexists with cardiac failure, often found in older patients with established mitral stenosis.

If medical therapy fails, cardiac surgery should be considered, even during the acute phase. In populations where fulminant acute carditis is relatively common (e.g. South Africa), mitral valve repair or replacement can be life saving and surgeons have developed techniques for undertaking these procedures despite friable, acutely inflamed valvular and perivalvular tissues. In recent years, there has been a greater tendency to undertake valve repair rather than replacement, or to use homografts or xenografts rather than mechanical prostheses. This is to avoid high rates of thromboembolic complications associated with mechanical prostheses, particularly in populations where compliance with anticoagulation chemotherapy is suboptimal and there are difficulties in monitoring coagulation indices.

Treatment of chorea

Sydenham's chorea always resolves, and if mild there may be no need for specific treatment. However, medications may reduce abnormal movements in moderate or severe chorea. Haloperidol is commonly used as a first-line treatment. Other medications employed include sodium valproate, pimozide, chlorpromazine, or benzodiazepines. Occasionally, low doses of minor tranquillizers are necessary for associated anxiety and emotional lability. All of these medications should be used sparingly and only for defined periods. Salicylates and steroids have no role in treatment of chorea. Psychotherapeutic interventions have little role in the short to medium term, and may increase the stigma of this self-limited organic disease. However, if longer-term behavioural abnormalities persist (e.g. emotional lability, obsessive–compulsive traits), behavioural therapy should be considered.

Newer therapies

Because of the autoimmune nature of acute rheumatic fever, immunomodulatory therapies have been tried. Intravenous immune globulin (IVIG) has been given in some small trials. One study showed no apparent benefit on rate of improvement of clinical, laboratory, or echocardiographic parameters of acute carditis, but another suggested that it may accelerate recovery from chorea. Other therapies have yet to be formally assessed.

Prognosis and follow-up

The most important prognostic factors are the severity of the acute carditis and the number of recurrences. Overall, approximately 30 to 50 per cent of patients with a first episode of acute rheumatic fever will develop chronic rheumatic heart disease. This increases to more than 70 per cent in patients with severe carditis at the first episode, or in those who have had at least one recurrence.

Any patient with acute rheumatic fever requires long-term follow-up. Follow-up assessments should focus on cardiac status, adherence to secondary prophylaxis, early treatment of group A streptococcal pharyngitis, and prevention of streptococcal pyoderma (including hygiene and treatment or prevention of scabies infestation). Patients with evidence of cardiac valve damage should be assessed regularly by specialist physicians and considered for cardiac surgery before substantial left ventricular dysfunction occurs. Vasoactive drugs, particularly angiotensin-converting enzyme inhibitors, may delay the need for operation in asymptomatic patients with chronic aortic regurgitation. Regular echocardiography may be useful to follow the progress of rheumatic heart disease, especially in populations where follow-up may be irregular or in whom communication or cultural differences make clinical assessment difficult.

Recurrences

Approximately 75 per cent of all recurrences occur within 2 years of an episode of acute rheumatic fever. The reasons for this are not known, but are thought to relate to a time-dependent sensitization of the immune response. The clinical features of recurrences tend to mimic those present at the initial episode, particularly in the case of chorea. However, this rule is not absolute, and the risk of developing other manifestations increases with each recurrence. For example, in the Australian Aboriginal population 40 per cent of patients without carditis at the initial episode of acute rheumatic fever developed it at the first recurrence, and 70 per cent developed carditis at either of the first two recurrences. The practical implication of this is that the absence of carditis at the first episode does not help to identify patients who may not need secondary prophylaxis.

Prevention of acute rheumatic fever

Secondary prophylaxis

Every patient with acute rheumatic fever should immediately commence secondary prophylaxis: long-term, regular antibiotics to prevent primary group A streptococcal infections. This strategy is proven to reduce the incidence of recurrences and the risk of developing chronic rheumatic heart disease.

The optimal regimen is 1.2 million units of intramuscular benzathine penicillin G every 3 weeks, and this is commonly given in populations with high incidences of acute rheumatic fever and programmes in place to support the regimen. Higher doses (1.8 or 2.4 million units) given every 4 weeks may have similar effect, but further evidence is needed before such regimens can be recommended routinely. An alternative strategy is to use oral penicillin V at a dose of 250 mg twice daily; this is almost as effective as using benzathine penicillin G, but adherence is usually less reliable.

The most effective strategy for patients proven to be allergic to penicillin is to attempt desensitization using an approved protocol. If this is unsuccessful, the present recommendation is to use oral erythromycin at a dose of 250 mg twice daily. Recent trials have shown newer oral cephalosporins to be effective at eliminating upper respiratory tract carriage of group A streptococci. However, none of these antibiotics have been evaluated for their ability to prevent acute rheumatic fever.

The duration of secondary prophylaxis is dictated by the reducing risk of recurrence with increasing age, with time since the last episode, and the possible consequences of recurrences. Secondary prophylaxis should continue for at least 5 years following the most recent episode or until age 21 years, whichever comes last. However, in patients with substantial valvular disease (e.g. moderate or severe mitral or aortic regurgitation, or any mitral or aortic stenosis), secondary prophylaxis should be continued longer—to age 30 or 35 years in most populations. If the damage is severe, or in patients who have had valve surgery, the possibility that recurrence might be catastrophic mandates that secondary prophylaxis be continued for life.

Primary prophylaxis

A full course of penicillin treatment commencing within 9 days of the onset of symptomatic group A streptococcal pharyngitis will prevent the subsequent development of acute rheumatic fever in most cases. After the diagnosis has been confirmed by a throat culture or rapid antigen diagnostic test, the treatment of choice is penicillin, administered either as a single intramuscular injection of benzathine penicillin G (600 000 U for children who weigh less than 30 kg, or 1.2 million U for larger children and adults) or as a full 10 days of oral (phenoxymethyl) penicillin V (250 mg for children or 500 mg for adults given two to three times daily). The importance of completion of the 10-day course, even if symptoms abate quickly, should be stressed to patients and parents. Shorter courses of oral penicillin treatment are associated with higher risks of acute rheumatic fever. There has never been a clinical isolate of group A streptococcus that is resistant to penicillin; therefore, the use of other antibiotics for primary prophylaxis should be restricted to patients who are allergic to penicillin.

In the case of penicillin allergy, a 10-day course of an oral macrolide such as erythromycin is recommended. First-generation oral cephalosporins also may be considered. However, these agents have not been evaluated in populations with high incidences of acute rheumatic fever. Shorter courses (e.g. 5 days) of some later-generation oral cephalosporins appear to be effective in eradicating carriage, but because of their expense and broader spectrum of antimicrobial activity they should be considered as second-line agents.

It is not possible to predict which episodes of group A streptococcal pharyngitis will precipitate acute rheumatic fever, so this treatment must be offered in all cases to be effective. Unlike prevention of recurrent episodes, which is virtually complete using secondary prophylaxis, penicillin treatment of streptococcal pharyngitis will prevent only the one-third or so of cases of acute rheumatic fever that follow a sore throat. However, this important intervention may arrest the spread of pathogenic group A streptococci in the community. Penicillin treatment of group A streptococcal pharyngitis should begin as early as possible in patients with a history of acute rheumatic fever, should they not be taking secondary prophylaxis, but even then may not prevent a recurrence, hence the need for secondary prophylaxis.

In recent years the use of primary prophylaxis has been questioned in some industrialized countries where acute rheumatic fever is now rare. It is argued that the strategy prevents few cases of acute rheumatic fever but contributes to overuse of antibiotics. Similar arguments were raised in the United States during the 1970s, but faded somewhat with the resurgence of acute rheumatic fever in that country during the 1980s. Any country considering abandoning primary prophylaxis should first have in place effective surveillance to detect changes in the epidemiology of primary group A streptococcal infections and the appearance of cases of acute rheumatic fever.

Primary prophylaxis is unsuccessful in many developing countries. It requires trained health workers, microbiology laboratories, transportation and communication infrastructure, the availability of penicillin, and a population likely to seek and adhere to treatment for sore throats. In some high-risk populations, all patients with sore throats receive intramuscular benzathine penicillin G without further attempts at diagnosis; the cost-effectiveness of this strategy has not been fully determined. Clinical algorithms to identify patients with group A streptococcal pharyngitis without resorting to laboratory tests have not been validated sufficiently for them to be recommended universally. Even if primary prophylaxis were to be instituted effectively in developing countries, acute rheumatic fever would not disappear, as most cases do not follow a sore throat.

Other methods of primary prevention are clearly needed in developing countries. Improved living standards and access to primary health care appear years or decades away in many places. Although streptococcal skin infections may be linked to acute rheumatic fever pathogenesis, there are no trials of impetigo control programmes to prevent acute rheumatic fever. There is a current focus on attempts to develop a group A streptococcal vaccine. Clinical trials of prospective vaccines are imminent, but the process will take many years, and recent experience suggests that new vaccines are often beyond the financial reach of most developing countries. For the foreseeable future at least, acute rheumatic fever prevention in many developing countries will depend on improving adherence to secondary prophylaxis and developing new strategies for primary prophylaxis.

Further reading

Anonymous (1995). Strategy for controlling rheumatic fever/rheumatic heart disease, with emphasis on primary prevention: memorandum from a joint WHO/ISFC meeting. *Bulletin of the World Health Organization* **73**, 583–7. [Recommendations for prevention in developing countries.]

Bach JF *et al.* (1996). Ten-year educational programme aimed at rheumatic fever in two French Caribbean islands. *Lancet* **347**, 644–8. [Demonstrates dramatic impact of comprehensive public health approach in developing countries.]

Bisno AL (1991). Group A streptococcal infections and acute rheumatic fever. *New England Journal of Medicine* **325**, 783–93. [Concise summary, including pathogenesis.]

Carapetis JR, Currie BJ, Kaplan EL (1998). The epidemiology and prevention of group A streptococcal infections: acute respiratory tract infections, skin infections and their sequelae at the close of the twentieth century. *Clinical Infectious Diseases* **28**, 205–10. [Comparison of epidemiology and public health approaches in industrialized and developing countries.]

Committee on Rheumatic Fever, Endocarditis, and Kawasaki Disease of the Council on Cardiovascular Disease in the Young, the American Heart Association (1995). Treatment of acute streptococcal pharyngitis and prevention of rheumatic fever: a statement for health professionals. *Pediatrics* **96**, 758–64. [Updated recommendations for prophylaxis.]

Kaplan EL (1993). Global assessment of rheumatic fever and rheumatic heart disease at the close of the century. Influences and dynamics of populations and pathogens: a failure to realize prevention? *Circulation* **88**, 1964–72. [Summary of epidemiological aspects, and their contribution to understanding pathogenesis.]

Martin DR *et al.* (1994). Acute rheumatic fever in Auckland, New Zealand: spectrum of associated group A streptococci different from expected. *Pediatric Infectious Diseases Journal* **13**, 264–9. [Important study suggesting a link between skin streptococci and rheumatic fever.]

Quinn RW (1989). Comprehensive review of morbidity and mortality trends for rheumatic fever, streptococcal disease, and scarlet fever: the decline of rheumatic fever. *Reviews of Infectious Diseases* **11**, 928–53. [Exactly as the title suggests.]

Stollerman GH (1975). *Rheumatic fever and streptococcal infection*. Grune & Stratton, New York. [Landmark review of all aspects of rheumatic fever, with comprehensive clinical information.]

Stollerman GH (1997). Rheumatic fever. *Lancet* **349**, 935–42. [Excellent summary of recent advances in rheumatic fever research.]

15.10.2 Infective endocarditis

W. Littler and S. J. Eykyn

Historical background

Lazerous Riverius recorded the first case of what is now known as infective endocarditis in 1723. He described a French magistrate with an irregular pulse, oedema, and congestion, who at autopsy had fleshy masses 'the size of hazelnuts' obstructing the aortic ostia. Fifty years later Morgani (1769) made the link between infection (fulminating gonorrhoea) and 'whitish polypus concretions on the upper part of the aortic valve near its borders'.

The clinical picture of endocarditis was first described by Jean Baptiste Bouillard in 1835: 'fever, an irregular pulse, cardiomegaly (by percussion) and a bellows murmur in the heart'. He gave the disease the name 'endocarditis' or an inflammation of the inner membrane of the heart and fibrous tissues of the valve and was the first to use the term 'vegetations' for the valvular lesions.

Winge used the term 'mycoses endocardi' for the groups of micro-organisms that he saw when he examined vegetations under the microscope in 1870. In 1886 Wyssecokowitch cultured *Staphylococcus aureus* from an endocardial vegetation. Lenthartz in 1901 was the first to use blood cultures in the diagnosis of endocarditis. 'Infective endocarditis' was the term used by Thomas Horder in 1901 to describe the syndrome consisting of (i) the presence of valvular disease, (ii) the occurrence of systemic embolism, and (iii) the discovery of micro-organisms in the bloodstream.

Epidemiology

Infective endocarditis was universally fatal before the advent of antibiotic therapy. Since 1944 deaths from endocarditis have fallen by 80 per cent: about 200 deaths are recorded each year in the United Kingdom, which is probably an underestimate. The true incidence of the condition is unknown, but it is at least 25 cases per 1 000 000 of population. The incidence is greater in men, in those over 65 years of age, and in those with prosthetic heart valves. About 20 per cent of patients with infective endocarditis die and they account for about 0.1 per cent of the total deaths from diseases of the circulatory system (ICD codes 390–429).

Endocarditis does occur in children but is rare, especially in the first decade of life. In the older literature tetralogy of Fallot was the commonest cardiac problem associated with infective endocarditis, but nowadays cardiac surgery is the most likely predisposing cause.

Pathogenesis

Normal vascular endothelium is resistant to microbial infection and very few patients potentially at risk actually develop infective endocarditis. Since low-grade bacteraemia occurs frequently in everyone, a defence mechanism must exist that can eradicate microbes adherent to vegetations. Platelets play a pivotal role in the antimicrobial host defence mechanism and human platelets have been found to contain at least 10 different bactericidal proteins or 'thrombocidins'.

Damage to the endothelial surface of the heart or blood vessels induces platelet and fibrin deposition, producing a sterile thrombotic vegetation; infective endocarditis is initiated by the binding of microbes, discharged into the general circulation from a peripheral site, to these vegetations. These microbes become encased in further depositions of platelets and fibrin and multiply.

The pathogenesis of infective endocarditis involves complex interactions between microbes and the host defence mechanisms, both circulating and at the site of endothelial damage. An essential step is the activation of the clotting system and the formation of a fibrin clot on the endothelial surface. Experimental evidence suggests that the main pathogens in infective endocarditis (streptococci and staphylococci) can bind to endothelial cells and induce functional changes within these cells, causing monocyte adhesion. The combination of damaged endothelial cells, bacteria, and endothelial-bound monocytes results in the induction of tissue factor-dependent procoagulant activity which initiates clot formation. Polymorphonuclear leucocytes that are recruited to the infected endothelial site subsequently may be involved in the disease progression: probably the contents of lysosomes released by the activated leucocytes cause softening and separation of valve tissue leading to its destruction.

In endocarditis the vegetations are found predominately on the left side of the heart (95 per cent). In a large autopsy series of more than 1000 cases reported over 50 years ago the mitral valve was involved in 86 per cent, the aortic in 55 per cent, the tricuspid in 20 per cent, and the pulmonary valve in only 1 per cent. The predominance of left-sided lesions led to the belief that the higher pressures and velocities encountered in the left side of the heart and the proximal aorta must impose a greater mechanical stress on the valves and endocardium, which in turn leads to local damage.

Endocarditis is classically associated with 'jet lesions', where blood flowing from a high pressure area through an orifice to an area of lower pressure produces a high velocity jet. Vegetations are usually found in the lower pressure area, for example on the atrial surface of the mitral valve in mitral regurgitation, or the ventricular surface of the aortic valve in aortic regurgitation. This particular deposition of vegetations has been explained on the basis of the Venturi effect.

Once a vegetation is established it determines the subsequent clinical picture by four basic processes: bacteraemia, local tissue destruction, embolization, and the formation of circulating immune complexes.

Clinical features

Early reports of infective endocarditis described a low-grade febrile illness caused by viridans streptococci from the patient's mouth in those with chronic rheumatic heart disease. Night sweats, anorexia, and weight loss were followed by the development of splinter haemorrhages and Osler nodes, finger clubbing, and splenomegaly. The infection progressed relentlessly with increasing cachexia and the patient died from cardiac failure or a major embolic episode. The term 'subacute bacterial endocarditis' was used to describe this illness. 'Acute or malignant endocarditis' described an aggressive form of the disease usually caused by *S. aureus*, or other virulent bacteria.

During the past 50 years there has been a striking change in the pattern of endocarditis. The dramatic decrease in rheumatic fever in developed countries, the use of antibiotics, and the emergence of antibiotic-resistant organisms, together with surgical advances have all contributed to many clinical variants and modes of presentation.

The proportion of patients in developed countries with endocarditis with no known pre-existing cardiac lesion has risen to over 50 per cent. This change is related to both the decline in rheumatic heart disease and to

the increase in extracardiac predisposing factors including intravenous narcotic abuse, haemodialysis, and the use of intravascular devices. Prosthetic heart valves are an important predisposing factor and cardiac surgery for complex congenital lesions has increased the lifespan of patients who would previously have died prematurely. The longevity of the populations in developed countries has resulted in an increasing age of patients with infective endocarditis. The mean age has risen from under 40 years before 1940 to between 60 and 70 years today.

Features of a bacteraemic illness

Discharge of the infecting agent into the circulation produces constant bacteraemia, which may present as pyrexia, rigors, malaise, anorexia, headache, confusion, arthralgia, and anaemia. However, some cases of endocarditis may present without fever, particularly in the elderly.

Features of tissue destruction

Endocarditis initially affects valve cusps, leaflets, or chordae tendineae. Tissue destruction results in valvular incompetence, cusp perforation, or rupture of the chordae producing an appropriate cardiac murmur that may change in character during the course of the illness. Large vegetations rarely obstruct a native valve, but mechanical obstruction of prosthetic valves is more common and clinically more difficult to detect. As the infective process progresses it may extend beyond the valve into the paravalvular structures. This is more common in native aortic valve endocarditis than in mitral valve infection. Aortic root abscess is a serious complication and a destructive lesion. When the abscess extends through the aortic wall into other tissues or cavities a fistula may be formed or pseudo-aneurysms produced. Involvement of the conducting tissue leads to heart block. Infection of a mechanical valve involves the sewing ring and may lead to valve dehiscence. Endocarditis involving an aortic mechanical valve is often localized to the junction between the sewing ring of the aortic valve and the aortic annulus: a large false aneurysm may develop in this area.

Features of systemic or pulmonary emboli

Fragments of an infected vegetation may be dislodged into the general or pulmonary circulation, depending on the site of the vegetation, producing the emboli that are reported in 20 to 40 per cent of cases; a higher incidence (50 per cent) has been reported in autopsy series. Emboli may lodge in any part of the circulation and present as a cerebrovascular accident, arterial occlusion of a limb, myocardial infarction, sudden unilateral blindness, or infarction of the spleen or a kidney. In right-heart endocarditis, recurrent septic pulmonary emboli may be misinterpreted as 'pneumonia'. Mycotic aneurysms arise from embolism of the vasa vasorum weakening the arterial wall: they have been reported in almost 3 per cent of clinical cases, but are found in up to 15 per cent of cases at autopsy. In the cerebral circulation such aneurysms may produce subarachnoid haemorrhage. The popliteal artery is a common site for mycotic aneurysms.

Emboli are characteristic of *S. aureus* infections and large emboli are a feature in HACEK (see below) and fungal endocarditis. Emboli usually occur before or within the first few days after starting antimicrobial therapy. The risk of emboli decreases with time during appropriate antimicrobial treatment. There is no significant difference between mitral valve and aortic valve vegetations with respect to embolization. Vegetation size does not predict systemic embolization, but large vegetations (greater than 10 mm) are associated with a poor outcome overall.

Features of circulating immune complexes

The infected vegetation contains antigens that trigger an immune response. The length of the illness seems to determine the extent of this response; chronic antigenaemia stimulates generalized hypergammaglobulinaemia, so that after several weeks of infection a variety of autoantibodies can be detected. Immune complex deposition may cause many of the extracardiac

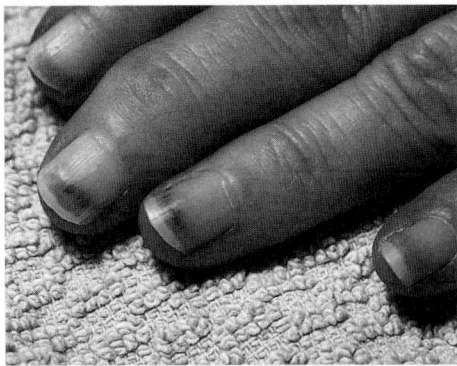

Fig. 1 Splinter haemorrhages in a case of infective endocarditis. (See also Plate 1.)

manifestations of infective endocarditis, but these classic signs are relatively uncommon and are often absent in individual patients.

Splinter haemorrhages

These are found in the nail bed of the fingers, less commonly the toes, and are linear in form (Fig. 1 and Plate 1).

Osler nodes

These transient painful erythematous nodules are found at the ends of fingers and toes and the thenar and hypothenar eminences. An alternative explanation is that Osler nodes are due to minute infected emboli.

Janeway lesions

These irregular painless erythematous macules are found in roughly the same distribution as Osler nodes. They tend to blanche with pressure.

Vasculitic rash

Immunoglobulin and complement deposits are found in the walls of skin capillaries (Fig. 2 and Plate 2). Vasculitis may account for some of the neurological findings in infective endocarditis.

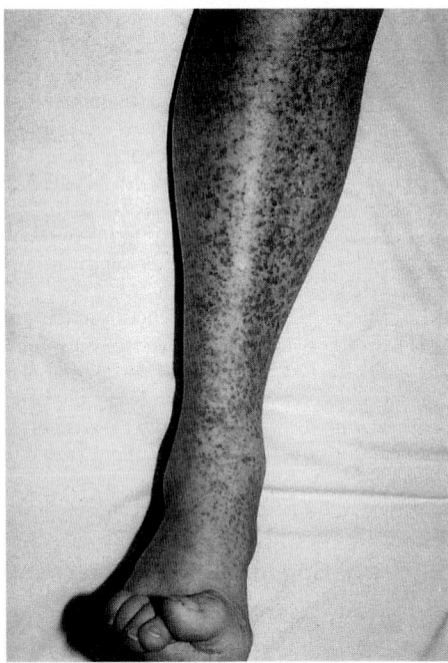

Fig. 2 Vasculitic rash on lower limb of a patient with infective endocarditis. (See also Plate 2.)

Roth spots

Boat-shaped haemorrhages in the retina are often called Roth spots, but true Roth spots are white retinal exudates that may be surrounded by haemorrhage. They consist of perivascular collections of lymphocytes.

Splenomegaly

Clinical splenomegaly is now less common than reported in the earlier literature. CT scanning of the abdomen shows the spleen to be enlarged in at least 50 per cent of cases and often demonstrates splenic infarcts.

Nephritis

Immune complexes can cause glomerulonephritis, with immunofluorescence demonstrating deposition of immunoglobulins and complement in irregular granular deposits in the glomerular basement membrane and mesangium. Proteinuria, haematuria, and cellular urinary casts may be present.

Arthralgia

The joint manifestations of infective endocarditis may result from immune complex deposition in the synovial membrane.

Other features

Up to 30 per cent of patients with endocarditis present with neurological symptoms; these are most common in staphylococcal infection, in which one-third present with the clinical features of meningitis. Headaches, confusion, and toxic psychosis can be present as well as encephalomyelitis. Cerebral embolism, which may produce a stroke as a result of cerebral infarction, is more characteristic of viridans streptococcal and enterococcal endocarditis. Mycotic aneurysms may rupture causing subarachnoid or intracerebral bleeding. Septic embolism may result in the formation of a cerebral abscess. It is not certain whether some of these neurological manifestations arise from repeated small emboli or from a vasculitic process within the cerebral circulation resulting from immune complex deposition. The cerebrospinal fluid can show an increase in white cells, but is usually sterile on culture, although very occasionally positive in staphylococcal infection.

Immune-mediated glomerulonephritis has been regarded as the typical lesion of infective endocarditis, but this assumption was based on small series pre-dating modern treatment regimens. More recent work indicates that the commonest renal histological finding is infarction, usually septic. Glomerulonephritis is usually vasculitic. Acute postinfective glomerulonephritis and membranoproliferative glomerulonephritis are less common. Circulatory compromise can cause severe renal impairment as a result of acute tubular necrosis or (very rarely) renal cortical necrosis.

Finger clubbing is one of the classic features of infective endocarditis, usually seen after 1 or 2 months of the illness. It is seldom seen now, but remains a useful sign since it rarely occurs in conditions with which infective endocarditis is confused.

Specific types of endocarditis

Prosthetic valve endocarditis

Patients with prosthetic heart valves have a small but constant risk of infective endocarditis, estimated at 0.2 to 1.4 events per 100 patient years. The incidence of prosthetic valve endocarditis is about 3 per cent in the first postoperative year, with the highest risk during the first 3 months. Prosthetic valve endocarditis is five times more common with aortic than mitral prostheses, and may involve mechanical, xenograft, and homograft valves.

Prosthetic valve endocarditis has been classified as early or late according to its temporal relationship to the time of surgery. Early prosthetic valve endocarditis accounts for 30 per cent of cases and usually occurs within 60 days of open heart surgery. It is caused either by contamination of the prosthetic valve at implantation or by perioperative bacteraemia. The commonest organisms are usually coagulase-negative staphylococci.

Late prosthetic valve endocarditis accounts for 70 per cent of cases and usually occurs 60 days or more after surgery. The pathogens are usually those seen in native valve endocarditis with a preponderance of viridans streptococci and staphylococci, but with a higher incidence of other organisms. Some patients with late prosthetic valve endocarditis will have acquired the infection at the time of surgery, but a bacteraemia is usually the principal cause.

Bacteraemia in a patient with a prosthetic valve must always be taken seriously, but it may not always be the result of endocarditis. The clinical picture of prosthetic valve endocarditis is usually fever, malaise, and weakness, but the more classic signs are usually absent. The condition is often insidious and difficult to diagnose clinically. A new murmur may appear and heart failure and embolic phenomena result in a high mortality (20 to 50 per cent). Infection in a mechanical valve is located in the sewing ring; the infection can spread into the host tissues producing annular abscesses, paravalvular leak, and prosthetic dehiscence. Myocardial abscesses can develop as a consequence of an annular abscess with xenograft or homograft valves. Infection usually involves the valve leaflets, resulting in destruction or perforation and consequent valvular incompetence. The infection involves the valve annulus less commonly than with a mechanical prosthesis. Vegetations may cause obstruction with all forms of prosthetic valve.

The diagnosis of prosthetic valve endocarditis requires a high index of clinical suspicion, blood cultures, and transoesophageal echocardiography. This technique is far superior to the transthoracic approach for finding vegetations and identifying periprosthetic spread of the infection. Vegetations are more difficult to identify in patients with mechanical valves than those with bioprostheses.

Right-sided endocarditis

Right-sided infective endocarditis accounts for only 5 per cent of cases overall, but centres that treat large numbers of intravenous drug users will have a higher incidence. The clinical picture differs significantly from left-sided disease. It is usually associated with intravenous drug addiction or indwelling intravascular devices, and in the former is found particularly in a younger population. *S. aureus* is the commonest pathogen and the tricuspid valve is more commonly affected that the pulmonary. Fever is almost always present and a cardiac murmur is found in 80 per cent of cases. Right-sided endocarditis is associated with septic pulmonary emboli, and the resultant pulmonary infarcts may cavitate. Symptoms include cough, haemoptysis, and pleuritic chest pain, while a chest radiograph shows pulmonary infiltrates often misdiagnosed as 'patches of pneumonia' (Fig. 3). Renal involvement has been described in over half the cases; most commonly abscess formation or diffuse pyelonephritis. Myocarditis is more common in right-sided involvement than left. Peripheral stigmas of infective endocarditis, splenomegaly, and central nervous system involvement are rare, being described in 5 per cent or less of cases. Death is most commonly due to sepsis, rarely to heart failure.

Endocarditis in intravenous drug users

Endocarditis is a serious complication of intravenous drug abuse. The right side of the heart is affected most commonly, but the left may also be involved in a substantial number of patients (37 per cent), and both right and left side in a minority (7 per cent). On the right side the tricuspid valve is affected in 80 per cent of cases, while the mitral and aortic valves are equally infected in left-sided disease. A history of previous heart disease is only found in some 25 per cent of cases. *S. aureus* is responsible for 40 per cent of all cases. Gram-negative bacilli are the next most frequent, with *Pseudomonas aeruginosa* and *Serratia marcescens* accounting for the majority of these. Candida can cause endocarditis in intravenous drug users and polymicrobial endocarditis accounts for 5 per cent of cases.

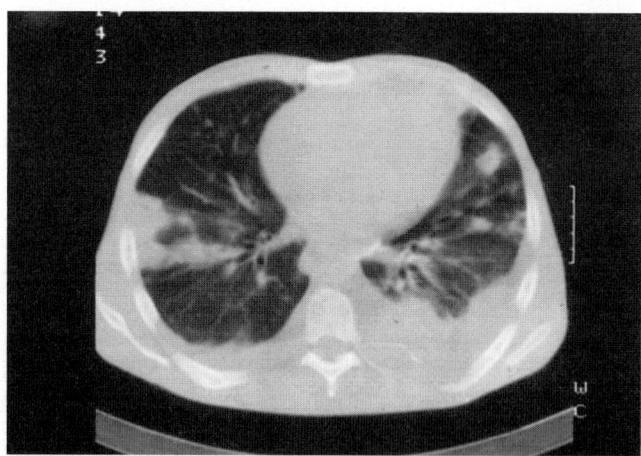

Fig. 3 CT scan of the chest showing multiple pulmonary infarcts in a case of right-sided endocarditis of the tricuspid valve in an intravenous drug user.

The skin is the commonest site from which pathogens enter the bloodstream via needles. Gram-negative bacilli are rarely recovered from needles or the drug itself and it has been suggested that these organisms come from tap water, sinks, or lavatory pans.

The clinical picture of drug-associated endocarditis depends on which side of the heart is affected. Right-sided disease is associated with fever, a murmur of tricuspid incompetence, and pulmonary infiltrates on the chest radiography. Left-sided disease behaves like that seen in cases not associated with intravenous drugs, with a high incidence of heart failure, arterial embolism, central nervous system involvement, and peripheral stigmas.

The overall mortality depends on when the patient presents: it is high if they present late and reflects, among other things, the difficulty in dealing with addicts because of their poor compliance and reluctance to discontinue their drug habit. The principles of management are similar to those for patients who do not abuse drugs. The duration of intravenous antibiotics should be at least 4 weeks, but it is usually impossible to do this in practice; while in right-sided endocarditis simple removal of the valve without replacement appears to be the best strategy.

The diagnosis of infective endocarditis

Laboratory diagnosis

Blood culture

This is the most important laboratory investigation in the diagnosis of endocarditis. Isolation of the pathogen enables an effective antibiotic treatment regimen to be devised. Blood cultures should be taken before antibiotics are given; if they have already been given, cultures should still be done, and if possible the giving of further antibiotics delayed for a few days. However, previous antibiotics may render the blood sterile for some time and the chances of recovering the pathogen, particularly when it is a viridans streptococcus, are very low. Much mystique has been attached to the number and timing of blood cultures in cases of suspected endocarditis. What is known is that the bacteraemia is usually constant and that whenever the blood is obtained for culture, and however many sets are taken, in most cases all bottles will grow the pathogen. There are of course rare exceptions when only a small proportion of bottles cultured are positive, and this is one reason why it is conventional to take two or three sets. Another reason for several cultures is to assess the relevance of the common skin contaminants, particularly the coagulase-negative staphylococci but also *Corynebacterium* spp., which can cause endocarditis.

In most laboratories blood culture systems are automated, with continuous monitoring which flags up growth for further investigation. Most cultures become positive within 48 h and after this the chances of isolating the pathogen recede, with the exception of fastidious organisms of the HACEK group (see below) that may take much longer to recover from the blood. In most laboratories blood cultures are incubated for 5 to 7 days, but this may not be long enough for the rare fastidious slow grower. The onus is on the clinical microbiologist or clinician to request prolonged incubation of blood cultures from patients in whom endocarditis is strongly suspected on clinical grounds and echocardiography who have not had previous antibiotics and whose blood cultures are sterile after a week's incubation.

Blood tests

In infective endocarditis an elevated erythrocyte sedimentation rate and C-reactive protein are almost invariable and these inflammatory markers are used most commonly to monitor the activity of the disease. A normochromic normocytic anaemia is often present and a polymorphonuclear leucocytosis is found in the majority of cases. Hypergammaglobulinaemia and a low serum complement may be present, together with a false-positive rheumatoid factor. Circulating immune complexes may be detected.

Dipstick testing of the urine may reveal the presence of proteinuria or haematuria, indicating renal involvement. When haematuria is present the pellet of a centrifuged specimen of urine should be resuspended and examined microscopically for the presence of red cell casts, which clinch the diagnosis of glomerulonephritis in this context.

Serology

Serum antibodies are used to diagnose *Coxiella burnetii* (Q fever), bartonella, and chlamydia endocarditis and should be done in any patient with convincing evidence of endocarditis and negative blood cultures. Candida antibodies are of no diagnostic value.

Echocardiography

In suspected cases of endocarditis echocardiography should be performed as soon as possible and interpreted by an experienced cardiologist. Its principal role is to detect vegetations. Echocardiography is not sufficiently sensitive to allow the clinician to exclude the diagnosis confidently on the basis of a negative result. The sensitivity depends on the size of the vegetations and the time course of the disease. Echocardiography can resolve vegetations as small as 1 to 2 mm, but it is more difficult with prosthetic than native valves, and more difficult with mechanical than biological prostheses.

Vegetations appear as thick, ragged, non-uniform echoes oscillating on or around a cardiac valve or in the path of a regurgitant jet. They do not usually restrict leaflet mobility and exhibit valve-dependent motion. On native valves vegetations are usually attached to the ventricular side of the aortic valve and the atrial side of the mitral and tricuspid valves.

Two-dimensional echocardiography should be employed initially in all cases of suspected endocarditis (Fig. 4). Transoesophageal echocardiography has improved the rate of diagnosis of infective endocarditis over that of transthoracic echocardiography, particularly in the presence of a prosthetic valve. Transoesophageal echocardiography has made it easier to recognize many complications of prosthetic valve endocarditis, such as abscesses, fistulas, and paravalvular leak (Fig. 5). In addition to vegetations, echocardiography may demonstrate indirect signs of valvular integrity, such as excessive systolic expansion of the left atrium in mitral incompetence or fluttering of the anterior leaflet of the mitral valve in aortic incompetence. Ventricular size and contractility are both easily assessed. The diagnosis of right-sided endocarditis has been greatly facilitated by echocardiography, particularly transoesophageal echocardiography. Vegetations, which in general tend to be larger on the right side, can be demonstrated in 80 to 100 per cent of cases.

Vegetations need to be differentiated from other conditions that produce echo density on cardiac valves, including calcification, myxomatous degeneration, and atrial myxoma. Echocardiography does not provide direct information on blood flow, but Doppler echocardiography complements the technique and adds significantly to the diagnosis of valvular function. It is able to diagnose valvular regurgitation with great accuracy.

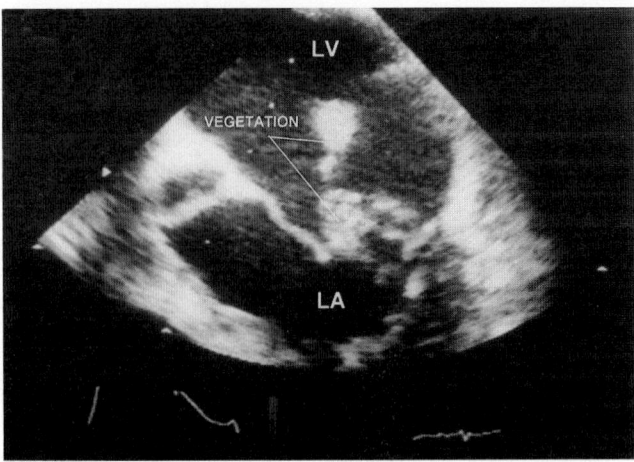

Fig. 4 Two-dimensional echocardiogram showing a large vegetation involving the posterior leaflet of the mitral valve and prolapsing into the left ventricle. LA, left atrium; LV, left ventricle.

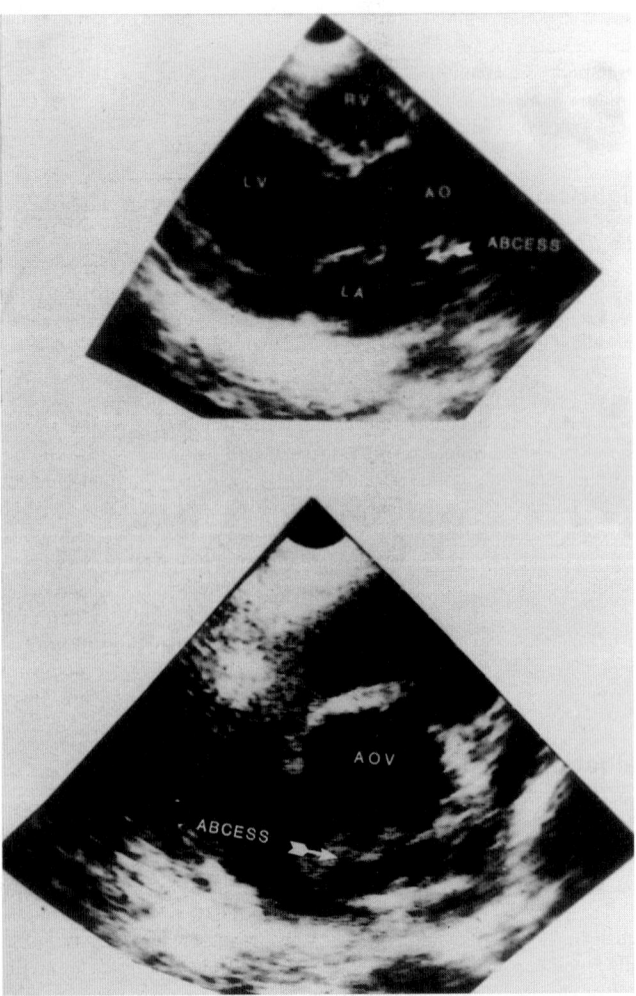

Fig. 5 Transoesophageal echocardiogram showing a large abscess communicating with aortic root. RV, right ventricle; LV, left ventricle; LA, left atrium; AO, aorta; AOV, aortic valve.

Criteria for the diagnosis of infective endocarditis

In 1994 Durack and his colleagues introduced criteria for the diagnosis of infective endocarditis that have been accepted as 'the Duke Criteria' (Table 1). These include two major criteria (typical blood culture and positive echocardiogram) and six minor criteria (predisposition, fever, vascular phenomena, immunological phenomena, suggestive echocardiogram, and suggestive microbiological findings). Application of these criteria is used to define three diagnostic categories: definite, possible, or rejected cases of infective endocarditis.

Modifications of the Duke Criteria to increase their sensitivity have been suggested by others. These include the following additional minor criteria: the presence of newly diagnosed clubbing, splenomegaly, splinter haemorrhages and petechias, a high erythrocyte sedimentation rate or a high C-reactive protein, and the presence of central non-feeding lines, peripheral lines, and microscopic haematuria.

Microbiology

While almost any micro-organism can cause infective endocarditis, particularly when this involves a prosthetic valve, certain species do so much more commonly than others and the predominant species involved in the infection have not changed significantly in their incidence in the past three decades. Overall, viridans streptococci and staphylococci account for about two-thirds of all cases. However, endocarditis cannot be considered as a microbiologically homogeneous entity as the incidence of any specific organism depends: (i) on the patient—whether an intravenous drug user or not; (ii) on the valve—whether native or prosthetic; if native whether previously abnormal or not, and if prosthetic whether mechanical or a bioprosthesis, and whether the infection was acquired early or late; and (iii) where (and how) the infection was acquired—whether in the community or (and increasingly these days) in hospital, usually via an infected intravascular device. The more common species encountered will be considered individually.

Streptococci

The genus *Streptococcus* includes species of differing virulence and pathogenicity as well as differing normal habitat in man. It has undergone numerous taxonomic revisions over the past decade or more and the previous dependence on haemolytic activity on blood agar and serological reactions has been superseded in many cases by molecular and chemotaxonomic approaches. Examples of such taxonomic change include the assignment of the faecal streptococci to the genus *Enterococcus*, of *Streptococcus morbillorum* to *Gemella morbillorum*, and of the nutritionally dependent streptococci previously known as *Streptococcus adjacens* and *Streptococcus defectivus* to the genus *Abiotrophia*. There are many other examples, but taxonomic change is of limited interest to clinicians and has no bearing on the management of infection.

Viridans streptococci

For many years it has been conventional to refer to a group of streptococci that produce greening (α-haemolysis) on blood agar as viridans streptococci, indeed many still refer (inaccurately) to a microbe 'Streptococcus viridans'. While most of these streptococci are virtually specific to the normal oropharyngeal flora and are rarely encountered at other sites, some are not found in the oropharynx at all, for example *S. bovis*, and others are found at many sites including the oropharynx, for example the milleri group of streptococci. The viridans streptococci are the commonest cause of community-acquired native valve endocarditis and community-acquired late-onset prosthetic endocarditis. The commonest species of the viridans streptococci that are specific to the oropharynx are *S. sanguis*, *S. oralis*, and *S. mutans*, but there are others. Dextran formation may be a virulence factor in these streptococci. Contrary to popular belief they do not require a dental extraction to enter the bloodstream and cause frequent bacteraemias after chewing, tooth brushing, and so on. They are organisms of low virulence and thus usually only infect previously abnormal heart valves. Whereas *S. oralis* and *S. sanguis* are occasionally isolated from blood cultures of patients who do not have endocarditis, the isolation of *S. mutans* from the blood is virtually synonymous with endocarditis.

Table 1 Definitions of terms used in the Duke criteria for the diagnosis of infective endocarditis

Major criteria	Minor criteria
1. Positive blood culture for infective carditis A. Typical micro-organism consistent with infective carditis from two separate blood cultures as noted below: (i) viridans streptococci[a], *Streptococcus bovis*, HACEK group or (ii) community-acquired *Staphylococcus aureus* or enterococci, in the absence of a primary focus or B. Micro-organisms consistent with infective carditis from persistently positive blood cultures defined as: (i) at least two positive cultures of blood samples drawn > 12 h apart or (ii) all three of these or a majority of four or more separate cultures of blood (with first and last sample drawn at least 1 h apart). 2. Evidence of endocardial involvement A. Positive echocardiogram for infective carditis as defined as: (i) oscillating intracardiac mass on valve or supporting structures, in the path of regurgitant jets, or on implanted material in the absence of an alternative anatomical explanation or (ii) abscess or, (iii) new partial dehiscence of prosthetic valve. B. New valvular regurgitation (worsening or changing of pre-existing murmur not sufficient)	1. Predisposition: predisposing heart condition or intravenous drug use 2. Fever: temperature > 38°C 3. Vascular phenomena: major arterial emboli, septic pulmonary infarcts, mycotic aneurysm, intracranial haemorrhages, and Janeway's lesions 4. Immunological phenomena: glomerulonephritis, Osler's nodes, Roth spots, and rheumatoid factor 5. Microbiological evidence: positive blood culture but does not meet a major criterion as noted in column one[b] or serological evidence of active infection with organism consistent with infective carditis 6. Echocardiographic findings: consistent with infective carditis but do not meet a major criterion as noted in column one

HACEK, *Haemophilus* spp., *Actinobacillus actinomycetemcomitans*, *Cardiobacterium hominis*, *Eikenella corrodens*, and *Kingella kingae*.

[a] Includes nutritionally variant strains.

[b] Excludes single positive cultures for coagulase-negative staphylococci and organisms that do not cause endocarditis.

Streptococcus bovis

This streptococcus, which may appear 'viridans' on blood agar, is part of the normal intestinal flora but may initially be mistaken for an oral streptococcus. In common with the enterococci it bears the Lancefield group D antigen and thus can also be mistaken for *Enterococcus faecalis*, though it is sensitive to penicillin whereas the latter is resistant. There is a significant association between *S. bovis* bacteraemia (and hence endocarditis) and colonic pathology, and any patient with *S. bovis* endocarditis thus warrants appropriate investigation for this. *S. bovis* endocarditis is much less common than that caused by oral streptococci.

Pyogenic streptococci

These organisms, often referred to as β-haemolytic streptococci, cause endocarditis less frequently than the viridans streptococci, but are more aggressive microbes and are likely to affect (and often rapidly destroy) a previously normal valve. The commonest pyogenic streptococcus to cause endocarditis is the Lancefield group B β-haemolytic streptococcus (**GBS**) sometimes referred to as *S. agalactiae*. This organism is found as normal flora in the genital and gastrointestinal tracts. As with *S. aureus,* any patient with community-acquired GBS bacteraemia should be assumed to have infection in bone, joint, or on a heart valve until proved otherwise. Groups C and G β-haemolytic streptococci occasionally cause endocarditis and group A even more rarely. The milleri group of streptococci are best regarded as pyogenic streptococci. These streptococci form part of the normal flora of all mucous membranes and occasionally cause endocarditis, though much more often abscesses at many different sites. The milleri group consists of three species, *S. constellatus, S. intermedius,* and *S. anginosus*. Interestingly these streptococci can bear the Lancefield antigens A, C, G, or F (or none); all group F streptococci are milleri but not all milleri are group F.

Streptococcus pneumoniae (pneumococcus)

Pneumococcal endocarditis accounted for about 10 per cent of cases of endocarditis in the preantibiotic era, but is now rarely seen, although it is sometimes diagnosed at autopsy of patients with fatal pneumococcal infection. The pneumococcus is a virulent pathogen and attacks normal heart valves. Patients with endocarditis generally have pneumonia and sometimes meningitis, the organism originating in the upper respiratory tract.

Enterococci

Enterococci form part of the normal gastrointestinal flora. They are more virulent than viridans streptococci and more resistant to antibiotics. The past decade has seen an increase in enterococcal endocarditis, particularly in the elderly, but this infection is still much less common than that caused by viridans streptococci. While there are many species of enterococci, those causing endocarditis are usually *E. faecalis* and occasionally *E. faecium*. Most cases are community acquired but the infection can be acquired in hospital, sometimes as a result of urological instrumentation. Any patient admitted from the community with *E. faecalis* in the blood should be investigated for endocarditis.

Staphylococci

Staphylococci now account for about a third of cases of community-acquired endocarditis and are the commonest cause of hospital-acquired endocarditis. Most of these staphylococci are *S. aureus*, but an increasing proportion is now due to coagulase-negative staphylococci. All staphylococci are skin organisms and patients become infected from their own skin flora, or in the case of methicillin-resistant *S. aureus* (**MRSA**) from that of others by cross-infection.

Staphylococcus aureus

S. aureus is an important and aggressive pathogen in community-acquired native valve endocarditis. Sometimes a trivial skin lesion can be identified as the source of the organism, but there is often no obvious lesion. *S. aureus*, and increasingly now MRSA, is the commonest cause of hospital-acquired endocarditis. Prosthetic valves can become infected with *S. aureus* both early as result of sternal wound sepsis and late as with native valves. *S. aureus* is the commonest pathogen causing endocarditis in intravenous drug users.

Coagulase-negative staphylococci

Although still regarded by many as pathogens of prosthetic rather than native valves, coagulase-negative staphylococci also cause native valve infection and this has become more common, or certainly more commonly recognized, in the last two decades. The infecting species is most often *S. epidermidis* (*sensu stricto*) but in many reports the designation *S. epidermidis* tends to be used for any unspeciated coagulase-negative staphylococcus. Many other species have been reported in native valve endocarditis including *S. lugdunensis, S. simulans, S. warneri, S. capitis, S. caprae,* and *S. sciuri*. Coagulase-negative staphylococci are normal skin flora and different species vary in their distribution throughout the body. As in community-acquired *S. aureus* endocarditis, there is sometimes a presumptive predisposing skin lesion. Most patients have a pre-existing cardiac abnormality. Many of these staphylococci can be as virulent as *S .aureus* and actually share some of the same virulence factors.

Other organisms

A wide variety of organisms account for the small percentage of cases of endocarditis that are not caused by streptococci, staphylococci, or enterococci. Only a few warrant a specific mention here.

HACEK group

These are fastidious slow-growing species that are oropharyngeal commensals and have a predilection for heart valves, such that their presence in blood cultures is virtually synonymous with this infection. The group consists of *Haemophilus aphrophilus/paraphrophilus, Actinobacillus actinomycetemcomitans, Cardiobacterium hominis, Eikenella corrodens,* and *Kingella kingae*. *A. actinomycetmcomitans* in particular seems more likely to infect prosthetic than native valves. The large vegetations thought to be characteristic of HACEK organisms in native valve infection may be the result of diagnostic delay and prolonged illness rather than any inherent property of the microbes *per se*.

Organisms that cannot be cultured by routine techniques

Endocarditis is a rare (and late) sequel of acute *Coxiella burnetii* (Q fever) infection. Most infections occur in middle-aged men with pre-existing valve disease. The reservoir of the organism is usually sheep or cattle, but the source and mode of transmission in many human cases is unknown. The diagnosis is usually made serologically, although *C. burnetii* can be recovered from the blood and excised valves by special techniques. The disease is almost certainly underdiagnosed and some cases are labelled 'culture negative' endocarditis.

Bartonella quintana endocarditis was first recognized in 1995 in homeless alcoholic patients; *Bartonella henselae* infection may be associated with cat or cat flea contact and other species of bartonella have also been described causing endocarditis. Bartonella infection is usually diagnosed by serology, although these bacteria can also be recovered from the blood and excised valves by special culture techniques and their presence detected by polymerase chain reaction (PCR). False-positive serology for *Chlamydia* spp. has been reported with bartonella infections, but *Chlamydia* spp.— and particularly *C. psittaci*—can also cause endocarditis (very rarely); it is possible that some cases attributed to chlamydia in the past on the basis of serology may have been caused by bartonella.

Fungi

Fungal endocarditis is very rare and more likely to occur on prosthetic than native valves, except in intravenous drug users. Most infections are acquired in hospital, when infection at intravascular access sites and broad-spectrum antibiotics predispose to candida infections. *Candida* spp., usually *C. albicans*, are the commonest fungi, but *Aspergillus* spp. and more exotic genera have also been reported. Blood cultures are only likely to be positive with *Candida* spp., and then often only intermittently; for other fungi the diagnosis must be made by serology and culture of the fungus from the excised valve or detection on valve histology.

Blood culture negative endocarditis

The possibility that the illness is not endocarditis should always be entertained when blood cultures are repeatedly negative. However, in 5 to 10 per cent of definite cases of endocarditis the blood cultures will be negative. The commonest explanation for this is previous antibiotics. In a few cases the pathogen will be recovered from another site, including the excised valve, excised emboli, or specifically in right-sided endocarditis, respiratory specimens. Other causes of negative blood cultures are infection with organisms that cannot be grown by conventional blood culture methods and infections that are diagnosed by serology such as *C. burnetii*, *Bartonella* spp., and *Chlamydia* spp.

Treatment

Initial therapy

In those patients who have been chronically unwell for many weeks, antibiotic treatment can be deferred until the blood cultures are positive and the pathogen known. In patients who are acutely ill, antibiotic treatment should be started after taking blood cultures, using a broad-spectrum combination that can be adjusted when the pathogen is known. However, in many who are acutely ill with native valve infection, endocarditis is often not suspected initially—there may be no obvious signs of this—and the antibiotics are started for 'septicaemia'. There are many possible combinations for acutely ill patients, but intravenous vancomycin and gentamicin will encompass most possible pathogens. When methicillin-resistant staphylococci (whether *S. aureus* or coagulase-negative staphylococci) are likely pathogens, vancomycin or teicoplanin are an essential component of any combination.

Definitive therapy

There are various national guidelines for the treatment of specific organisms. It is important to realize that very few are based on clinical trials that show efficacy of any particular regimen. It is possible to conduct such trials in endocarditis caused by viridans streptococci, but well nigh impossible in cases caused by virulent organisms such as staphylococci as the patients are seldom comparable, with many needing surgery after varying periods of antibiotic treatment. It is conventional to estimate the minimum inhibitory concentration (**MIC**) of the antibiotic for the pathogen, though in practice routine disc sensitivity tests are quite satisfactory in many cases. Although it is widely believed that prosthetic endocarditis requires a longer duration of antibiotic treatment than native valve infection, there are few data to support this. Recommendations for the commonest causative organisms will be given.

Penicillin-sensitive streptococci (MIC < 0.1 mg/l)

It was shown 30 years ago that native valve endocarditis caused by sensitive streptococci could be treated effectively with 2 weeks of intravenous penicillin and an aminoglycoside (originally streptomycin but now gentamicin). The purpose of the aminoglycoside is to achieve synergy, so a full therapeutic dose is not given. This regimen is seldom used in practice in the United Kingdom. Patients allergic to penicillins should be given vancomycin or teicoplanin and gentamicin.

Table 2 Treatment regimens for adults not allergic to the penicillins

Viridans streptococci and streptococcus bovis
(A) Fully sensitive to penicillin (MIC < 0.1 mg/l)
Benzylpenicillin, 7.2 g daily in six divided doses by intravenous bolus injection for 2 weeks plus intravenous gentamicin, 80 mg twice daily for 2 weeks*
(B) Reduced sensitivity to penicillin (MIC > 0.1 mg/l)
Benzylpenicillin, 7.2 g daily in six divided doses by intravenous bolus injection for 4 weeks plus intravenous gentamicin, 80 mg twice daily for 4 weeks*

Enterococci
(A) Gentamicin sensitive or low level resistance (MIC < 100 mg/l)
Ampicillin or amoxycillin, 12 g daily in six divided doses by intravenous bolus injection for 4 weeks plus intravenous gentamicin, 80 mg twice daily for 4 weeks.*
(B) Gentamicin highly resistant (MIC > 2000 mg/l)
Ampicillin or amoxycillin, 12 g daily in six divided doses by intravenous bolus injection for a minimum of 6 weeks. Streptomycin can be given if strain is sensitive

Staphylococci
(A) Penicillin sensitive
Benzylpenicillin, 7.2 g daily in six divided doses by intravenous bolus injection for 4 weeks plus intravenous gentamicin, 80–120 mg three times daily for 1 week*
(B) Penicillin resistant, methicillin sensitive
Flucloxacillin, 12 g daily in six divided doses by intravenous bolus injection for 4 weeks plus intravenous gentamicin, 80–120 mg three times daily for 1 week*
(C) Penicillin and methicillin resistant
Vancomycin, initially 1 g by intravenous infusion given over at least 100 min twice daily. Determine blood concentration and adjust dose to achieve 1-h postinfusion concentrations of about 30 mg/l and trough levels of 5–10 mg/l. Give for 4 weeks plus intravenous gentamicin, 80–120 mg three times daily for 1 week*

* Gentamicin levels must be monitored.

Streptococci with reduced sensitivity to penicillin (MIC > 0.1 mg/l)

The regimens given above should be continued for 4 weeks

Enterococci

Enterococci are rather more sensitive to amoxicillin and ampicillin than penicillin and thus these agents are recommended rather than penicillin. Many enterococci are still relatively sensitive to gentamicin and this drug is given with amoxicillin (for synergy, not a full therapeutic dose) for 4 weeks. Patients allergic to penicillin should be given vancomycin and gentamicin. Some enterococci are now resistant to high levels of gentamicin and for such strains gentamicin should not be given. Some gentamicin-resistant strains are sensitive to streptomycin and, if so, this can be used instead of gentamicin. If not, high-dose amoxicillin should be given for 4 to 6 weeks. Unfortunately some enterococci (usually *E. faecium*) are resistant to amoxicillin, gentamicin, and vancomycin and for them expert help should be obtained.

Staphylococci

The same antibiotic regimens should be used whether the staphylococcus is *S. aureus* or a coagulase-negative strain—it is the antibiotic sensitivity that matters not the infecting species. Strains that are sensitive to penicillin should be treated with this, those that are penicillin resistant but methicillin sensitive should be treated with flucloxacillin, and methicillin-resistant strains with vancomycin. There is no evidence that the addition of gentamicin (for gentamicin-sensitive strains) to the β-lactam antibiotic improves cure rates, but it may result in more rapid defervescence and clearance of bacteraemia.

Practical treatment recommendations are shown in Tables 2 and 3.

Table 3 Treatment regimens for adults allergic to the penicillins

Viridans streptococci, streptococcus bovis, and enterococci

Initially, **either** vancomycin, 1 g by intravenous infusion given over at least 100 min twice daily. Determine blood concentrations and adjust dose to achieve 1-h postinfusion concentrations of about 30 mg/l and trough concentrations of 5–10 mg/l

or teicoplanin, 400 mg by intravenous bolus injection 12-houly for three doses and then a maintenance intravenous dose of 400 mg daily.

Give vancomycin or teicoplanin for 4 weeks **plus** intravenous gentamicin, 80 mg twice daily. Viridans streptococcal and *Strep bovis* endocarditis should be treated with gentamicin for 2 weeks and enterococcal endocarditis for 4 weeks*

Staphylococci

Vancomycin, initially 1 g by intravenous infusion given over at least 100 min twice daily. Blood concentrations should be monitored as above. Give for 4 weeks plus intravenous gentamicin, 80–120 mg three times daily for 1 week*

* Gentamicin blood levels must be monitored.

Monitoring of treatment

Serum bactericidal titres against the infecting organism are no longer recommended. There was always great variation in the monitoring methods used for these tests and in the interpretation of their results. At best they could only predict bacteriological not clinical cure and bacteriological failure is very rare. The most useful laboratory test for monitoring the response to treatment (which is usually obvious clinically) is serial C-reactive protein estimation. This is of much more use than the erythrocyte sedimentation rate, which is much slower to fall.

Prevention and prophylaxis

While antibiotic prophylaxis in 'at-risk patients' is accepted as reasonable, there are many uncertainties about its value and data confirming its effectiveness are lacking. The rationale for antibiotic prophylaxis depends on indirect data from *in vitro* studies, experimental animal models, and clinical bacteraemia studies. Despite this uncertainty, all authorities continue to recommend antibiotic prophylaxis to cover certain procedures associated with a predictable and significant bacteraemia in patients known to be at risk, but accept that prophylaxis may fail, even with the recommended regimens, and that adverse reactions to the antibiotics are important even if relatively uncommon.

An international consensus group has recently undertaken a comparative analysis of the published national guidelines, which in the main are quite similar, though the antibiotic regimen for a given procedure may vary according to the perceived cardiac risk. Controversial areas include fibreoptic bronchoscopy, colonoscopy, vaginal hysterectomy, and vaginal delivery. Based on their analysis the consensus group have proposed universal guidelines for cardiac (Tables 4 and 5) and procedural (Table 6) risks. Prophylactic regimen are shown in Table 7.

Table 4 Cardiac conditions at risk for infective endocarditis requiring antibiotic prophylaxis—international consensus

Cardiac diseases with the highest risk

Prosthetic valves (5 to 10 times higher risk than native valves)

Congenital heart disease causing cyanosis

Previous infective carditis

Other cardiac diseases at risk

Valvular heart disease. Aortic regurgitation, mitral regurgitation, aortic stenosis, mitral stenosis including mitral valve prolapse with mitral regurgitation and bicuspid aortic valve

Congenital heart disease that does not cause cyanosis, except interatrial communication

Hypertrophic obstructive cardiomyopathy

Tables 4, 5, and 6 produced from Catherine Leport and the Endocarditis Working Group of International Society of Chemotherapy (1998). Antibiotic prophylaxis for infective endocarditis. *Clinical Microbiology and Infection* **4**, 3S56–3S61, with permission.

Table 5 Cardiac disease not at risk for infective carditis—international consensus

Interatrial communications

Mitral valve prolapse without mitral regurgitation, functional mitral insufficiency, or mitral ring calcifications

Coronary artery bypass grafting

Cardiac pacemakers

Implantable defibrillators

Corrected left-to-right shunts

Surgical treatment of infective endocarditis

Surgery will be required in about 30 per cent of cases during the acute phase (first 4 months) of endocarditis and 20 to 40 per cent of cases thereafter (Fig. 6 and Plate 3). Since surgery may be required at any time during an episode of endocarditis, it is essential to involve a cardiac surgeon in the overall management from the outset: in practical terms this means transferring the patient to a centre with cardiac surgery wherever possible. Even so, surgery for endocarditis carries a risk of 10 to 25 per cent mortality, and up to 25 per cent of patients develop a paravalvular leak requiring a further operation. The main predictive factors for mortality associated with surgery are prosthetic valve endocarditis, infections due to staphylococci or candida, perioperative shock, or late referral. The timing of surgery is all important and demands experience and clinical judgement, which is best achieved by a team approach with cardiologists, cardiac surgeons, and microbiologists.

The main indications for surgery are haemodynamic instability and persistent infection. In such cases surgery should never be delayed, even if only hours or days of antibiotic treatment have been given. The primary goals of the surgeon are to remove all infected material and to reconstruct the heart and/or restore valvular function at the lowest operative risk. An understanding of the surgical anatomy of infective endocarditis is a precondition for surgical success, which means the involvement of an experienced surgical team. Wherever possible surgeons now strive to preserve the native valve, either by removal of the vegetation(s) or valve repair. In prosthetic valve endocarditis removal of all foreign material is mandatory.

There are two unresolved issues with regard to the surgical treatment of endocarditis. The first concerns the timing of surgery in patients who have had a cerebrovascular accident either as a result of an embolic stroke or from haemorrhage due to a ruptured mycotic aneurysm. As a general rule,

Table 6 Procedures at risk for infective endocarditis requiring antibiotic prophylaxis—international consensus

Dental	All procedures
Upper respiratory tract	Tonsillectomy, adenoidectomy
Gastrointestinal	Oesophageal dilatation or surgery
	Endoesophageal laser procedures
	Sclerosing procedures of oesophageal varices
	Abdominal surgery
Urological	Instrumental procedures involving the ureter or the kidney
	Biopsy or surgery of prostate or urinary tract

Procedures for which the risk of infective endocarditis is controversial

Upper respiratory tract	Fibreoptic bronchoscopy
	Endotracheal tube insertion
Gastrointestinal	Colonoscopy with or without biopsy
Genital	Vaginal hysterectomy, vaginal delivery*

* Antibiotic treatment is required in cases of concomitant infection.

if haemorrhage is detected by CT scanning, delay of at least 1 week is suggested; if there is no haemorrhage, surgery can be undertaken within 72 h.

The second issue concerns the duration of antibiotic treatment postoperatively. If the excised valve is sterile it is doubtful whether further antibiotics are of any benefit. If the pathogen is isolated from the excised valve,

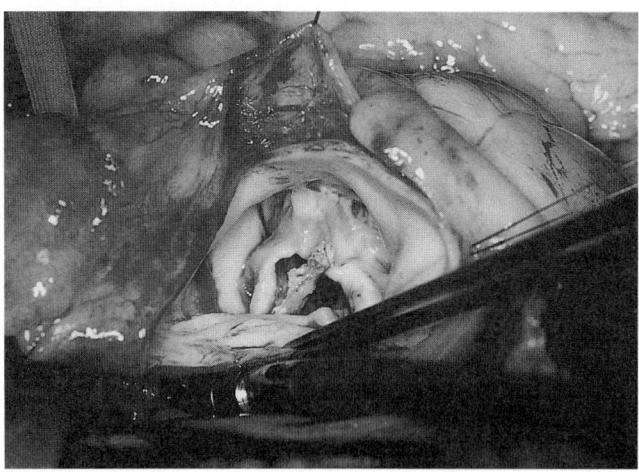

Fig. 6 A large vegetation on the aortic valve of a patient with infective endocarditis as seen at the time of surgery. (See also Plate 3.)

antibiotics should be given for a further 2 weeks. If debridement is incomplete, whatever antibiotics are given may fail.

Table 7 Prevention of endocarditis in patients with known cardiac risk[a]

Dental procedures[b] (under local or no anaesthesia)

Patients who have not received more than a single dose of a penicillin[3] in the previous month, including those with a prosthetic valve (but not those who have had endocarditis), oral amoxycillin 3 g 1 h before the procedure; **child** under 5 years, quarter of adult dose; 5–10 years, half adult dose

Patients who are penicillin-allergic shall receive oral clindamycin 600 mg 1 h before procedure; **child** under 5 years, quarter adult dose; 5–10 years, half adult dose

Patients who have had previous endocarditis, amoxycillin + gentamicin, as under general anaesthesia

Dental procedures[b] (under general anaesthetic)

No special risk (including patients who have not received more than a single dose of penicillin in the previous month)

Either intravenous amoxicillin 1 g at induction, then oral amoxicillin 500 mg 6 h later; **child** under 5 years, quarter of adult dose

Or oral amoxicillin 3 g 4 h before induction, then oral amoxicillin 3 g as soon as possible after the procedure; **child** under 5 years, quarter adult dose; 5–10 years, half adult dose

Or oral amoxicillin 3 g + oral probenecid 1 g 4 h before procedure

Special risk (patients with a prosthetic valve or who have had endocarditis), intravenous amoxicillin 1 g + intravenous gentamicin 120 mg at induction, then oral amoxicillin 500 mg 6 h later; **child** under 5 years, amoxicillin quarter adult dose, gentamicin 2 mg/kg; 5–10 years, amoxicillin half adult dose, gentamicin 2 mg/kg

Patients who are penicillin-allergic or who have received more than a single dose of penicillin in the previous month,

Either intravenous vancomycin 1 g over at least 100 min then intravenous gentamicin 120 mg at induction or 15 min before procedure; **child** under 10 years, vancomycin 20 mg/kg, gentamicin 2 mg/kg

Or intravenous teicoplanin 400 mg + gentamicin 120 mg at induction or 15 min before procedure; **child** under 14 years, teicoplanin 6 mg/kg, gentamicin 2 mg/kg.

Or intravenous clindamycin 300 mg over at least 10 min at induction or 15 min before procedure, then oral or intravenous clindamycin 150 mg 6 h later; **child** under 5 years, quarter adult dose; 5–10 years, half adult dose

Upper respiratory-tract procedures

As for dental procedures; postoperative dose may be given parenterally if swallowing is painful

Genitourinary procedures

As for special-risk patients undergoing dental procedures under general anaesthesia except that clindamycin is not given, see above; if urine infected, prophylaxis should also cover infective organism

Obstetric, gynaecological, and gastrointestinal procedures

Prophylaxis required for patients with prosthetic valves or those who have had endocarditis only, as for genitourinary procedures

Multistage procedures

For multistage procedures alternating oral doses of amoxycillin 3 g + clindamycin 600 mg 1 h before procedure are recommended

[a] Advice on the prevention of endocarditis reflects the recommendations of a Working Party of the British Society for Antimicrobial Chemotherapy, *Lancet* 1982, **ii**, 1323–6; *idem* 1986, **i**, 1267; *idem* 1990, **335**, 89; *idem* 1992, **339**, 1292–3; *idem* 1997, **350**, 1100; also *Journal of Antimicrobial Chemotherapy* 1993, **31**, 437–8.

[b] Antibiotic prophylaxis for dental procedures may be supplemented by with chlorhexidine gluconate gel 1 per cent or chlorhexidine gluconate mouthwash 0.2 per cent used 5 min before procedure.

Further reading

Amoury RA, Bowman EO, Malm JR (1966). Endocarditis associated with intracardiac prostheses. Diagnostic management and prophylaxis. *Journal of Thoracic and Cardiovascular Surgery* **51**, 36–48. [One of the earliest papers setting out the problems of endocarditis associated with prosthetic heart valves.]

Baine RJI *et al.* (1988). Impact of a policy of collaborative management on mortality and morbidity from infective endocarditis. *International Journal of Cardiology* **19**, 47–54. [This paper demonstrates the benefit of a 'team approach' to the management of infective endocarditis.]

Birmingham GD, Rahko PS, Ballantyne R (1992). Improved detection in infective endocarditis with transoesophageal echocardiogram. *American Heart Journal* **123**, 774–821. [This paper describes the benefits of using the transoesophageal approach to echocardiography in the diagnosis of infective vegetations.]

Cohen PS, Maguire JH, Weinstein L (1980). Infective endocarditis caused by Gram-negative bacteria: a review of the literature 1945–1977. *Progress in Cardiovascular Diseases* **22**, 205–41. [Even after 20 years this is still one of the best reviews of this particular aspect of endocarditis.]

Durak DT, Lukes AS, Bright DK (1994). New criteria for diagnosis of infective endocarditis: utilisation of specific echocardiographic findings. *American Journal of Medicine* **96**, 200–9. [This paper describes the application of criteria to increase the number of definite diagnoses of infective endocarditis.]

Durak DT (1995). Prevention of infective endocarditis. *New England Journal of Medicine* **332**, 38–44. [An excellent review of prophylaxis against endocarditis.]

Gutschik E and The Endocarditis Working Group of the International Society of Chemotherapy (1998). Microbiological recommendations for the diagnosis and follow-up of infective endocarditis. *Clinical Microbiology and Infection* **4**, 3S10–3S16. [A comprehensive review of investigations currently available for the diagnosis of infective endocarditis.]

Hoen B *et al.* (1995). Infective endocarditis in patients with negative blood cultures: analysis of 88 cases from a one year nationwide survey in France. *Clinical Infectious Diseases* **20**, 501–6. [An excellent review of the problems involved in culture-negative endocarditis. How the problem might be tackled.]

Report of a Working Party of the British Society of Antimicrobial Chemotherapy (1998). Antibiotic treatment of streptococcal, enterococcal and staphylococcal endocarditis. *Heart* **79**, 207–10. [Recommendations for the treatment of the common causes of infective endocarditis in the United Kingdom.]

15.10.3 Cardiovascular syphilis

B. Gribbin and I. Byren

Introduction

Cardiovascular syphilis is a feature of tertiary syphilis and no longer a prominent cause of heart disease: even in specialized cardiac units it is now a rarity. Left untreated, about 12 per cent of patients with syphilis will eventually develop cardiovascular complications. Although gummas can occur in the pericardium, myocardium, and endocardium, and have been the cause of Stokes–Adams attacks when present in the atrioventricular node or the bundle of His, the characteristic lesion is an aortitis. This follows spirochaetal infection of the aortic wall, leading to an endarteritis and periarteritis of the aortic vasa vasorum, initially in the adventitia and subsequently in the media. Lymphocytes and plasma cells surround these small feeding vessels and obliterative changes result in the loss of medial smooth muscle and elastic fibres, occasionally with frank necrosis and eventually with fibrous tissue replacement. This causes scarring of the aortic wall and weakening of its structure. Macroscopically the intima becomes thickened in a gelatinous patchy fashion and fibrosis produces an irregular linear thickening that has been termed the tree-bark appearance. Intimal scarring may involve the ostia of the coronary arteries, which are susceptible to further narrowing by accelerated and superimposed atheroma.

The ascending aorta is involved in about half of all cases, the arch is next in frequency, and the descending aorta in only 10 per cent, with changes virtually limited to that part of the vessel lying above the renal arteries. As the aortic wall structure weakens, so dilatation occurs, resulting in aneurysm formation, which in turn leads to further dilatation and the risk of rupture. The major branches of the aorta may also be affected, especially the innominate artery.

Enlargement of the aortic root and separation of the cusp commissures causes aortic reflux, and although thickening and retraction of the leading edges of the cusps also occurs, this is thought to be a secondary change due to abnormal turbulence rather than a consequence of direct syphilitic involvement of cusp tissues.

Clinical features

Because cardiovascular syphilis can take up to 40 years after primary infection to become apparent, most patients are middle aged or elderly, although tertiary syphilis has been known to occur within a year or two of primary infection. Men are more often affected. Patients with aortitis can present in four main ways: asymptomatic aortitis (most common), aneurysm formation (10 per cent), aortic reflux (25 per cent), and lastly as the result of coronary artery ostial stenosis (25 per cent). The last three are not mutually exclusive and aortic reflux plus ostial stenosis may coexist with aneurysm formation. Gummatous disease of the myocardium is extremely rare.

Aortitis in asymptomatic patients is usually diagnosed as the result of radiographic findings of a dilated ascending aorta with calcification in the wall (Fig. 1). Although aortic calcification is common, particularly in the elderly and hypertensive population, it is then virtually limited to the aortic knuckle and descending aorta. More generalized thoracic aortic calcification is sometimes seen in patients with widespread atheromatous disease, but when visible in the ascending aorta, particularly in a linear fashion, syphilitic aortitis should come to mind and supporting evidence, such as mild aortic reflux, be sought. Serology is likely to be positive.

Syphilitic aortic aneurysms tend to be saccular rather than fusiform and occur most commonly in the ascending aorta, also in the arch, and with increasing rarity down the descending aorta. This is in contrast to athero-

sclerotic aneurysms, which tend to involve the distal aorta below the renal arteries. The clinical features vary depending on the site of the aneurysm, its size, and whether or not compression and even erosion of adjacent structures occurs. A large aneurysm may cause no symptoms, but pain can be a prominent feature, often sustained and boring in nature, influenced by position, and exacerbated by impending rupture. Pain due to ascending aortic aneurysms is felt in the upper chest wall to the right of the sternum, and with large aneurysms a bulge may appear at this site and erosion of ribs and even sternum may be apparent on radiographs. Aneurysms of the arch

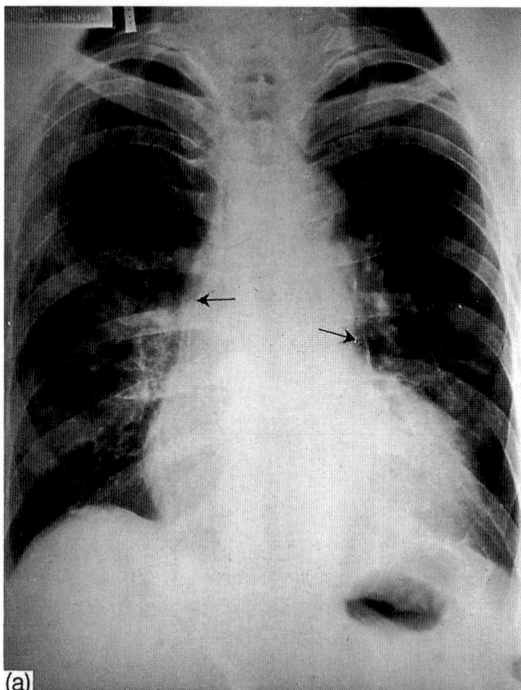

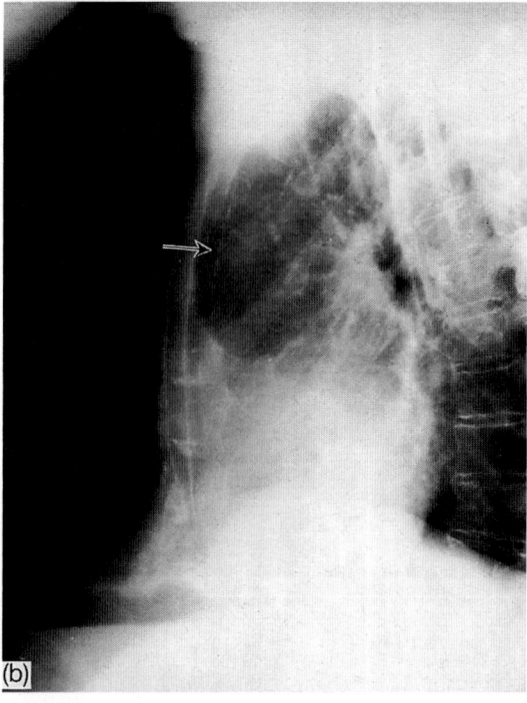

Fig. 1 Posteroanterior and lateral radiographs showing evidence of syphilitic aortitis. A line of calcification (arrowed) is visible in the wall of the dilated ascending aorta.

produce pain over the upper sternum and occasionally in the throat and there may be visible arterial pulsation in the root of the neck with tracheal deviation. Pressure on upper mediastinal structures can produce superior vena caval obstruction, dysphagia, stridor, and a tracheal tug in time with the pulse. Involvement of the upper descending aorta causes pain between the scapulae or to the left of the spine, and there is a risk of hoarseness from pressure on the left recurrent laryngeal nerve and complications arising from compression of the left main bronchus. Rupture can occur into the bronchus, into the left pulmonary artery, or the left pleural space, and erosion of vertebrae may result in chronic and debilitating pain.

Syphilitic aortic reflux may have a number of features to help distinguish it from the more usual varieties (see Chapter 15.7). Radiographic or clinical evidence of aneurysmal dilatation of the ascending aorta is one, and explains the fact that the early diastolic murmur may be heard better at the right, rather than the more usual left, sternal edge position. Furthermore, an ejection click may be audible, probably as a result of sudden distention of the dilated aortic root by the large stroke volume. However, these auscultatory signs are not entirely specific and may be found in patients with annuloaortic ectasia, now a more common condition, and characterized by a flask-like dilatation of the proximal ascending aorta. Even severe aortic reflux may be tolerated well for years, but eventually the volume overload of the left ventricle leads to cardiac failure: this carries a poor prognosis without, and sometimes despite, surgical intervention.

Coronary ostial stenosis is not restricted to cases of syphilitic aortitis and may occur as a variant of the more usual atheromatous coronary artery disease. It presents as angina, the true cause of which may be missed unless a thin line of calcification is noted in the ascending aorta, or there is other evidence of syphilitic disease in the cardiovascular system or elsewhere. Myocardial infarction may occur as a complication.

Diagnosis

The diagnosis of cardiovascular syphilis is usually made by detecting a positive serum antibody test in a patient who may give a history of past syphilitic infection, and who has evidence of aortitis or one of its complications. It is important to note that 10 to 25 per cent of patients with cardiovascular syphilis also have central nervous system involvement.

Non-specific antibody tests such as the Venereal Diseases Research Laboratory (**VDRL**) or rapid plasma reagin (**RPR**) may be negative in cardiovascular syphilis. If positive in high titre, they may indicate active untreated disease and can be used to gauge response to treatment. However, they have drawbacks: false positive results are not uncommon, and they are invariably positive in patients with endemic non-venereal treponematosis. Specific tests such as the fluorescent treponemal antibody absorption test (FTA-ABS) and *Treponema pallidum* haemagglutination test (TPHA) are almost always positive. They remain positive despite treatment and therefore cannot be used to assess response to treatment. Sexual and vertical transmission does not occur with cardiovascular syphilis, but nevertheless it is prudent to consider testing of known sexual partners and the children of women with cardiovascular syphilis. For more detailed information see Chapter 7.11.33.

Treatment

It is generally accepted that antibiotic treatment is indicated for patients with cardiovascular syphilis who have not received effective antibiotic treatment in the past. There is, however, no evidence that this reduces the severity of aortitis or improves prognosis. All patients with active cardiovascular syphilis should be examined for neurosyphilis and treated accordingly (see Chapter 24.14.4). If absent, treatment consists of 2.4 million IU of benzathine penicillin intramuscularly at weekly intervals for a total of three doses, alternatively 600 000 IU of procaine penicillin daily by intramuscular injection for 21 days. For patients known to be allergic to penicillin some practitioners desensitize and then use penicillin and others use doxycycline (200 mg orally, twice a day, for 28 days). There are insufficient data to unequivocally recommend the use of other drugs such as ceftriaxone and azithromycin.

Following treatment patients should be reviewed and those with positive non-treponemal tests (VDRL/RPR) should be checked serologically at 6-monthly intervals, with a declining titre used to confirm the adequacy of treatment.

There has been a concern that provocation of a Jarisch–Herxheimer reaction might lead to inflammatory swelling of the aortic wall with the risk of rupture or further critical narrowing of ostial stenoses. However, large numbers of patients with cardiovascular syphilis have been given penicillin without untoward effects, and whereas the Jarisch–Herxheimer reaction can occur rarely, it has never been shown to cause life-threatening changes in the aortic wall.

Surgery may be required to deal with the complications of aortitis. Symptoms of ischaemic heart disease caused by severe ostial stenosis have been relieved successfully by endarterectomy of the coronary orifices, although coronary bypass grafting is the usual treatment of choice. Theoretically, coronary stenting may offer another therapeutic option, although the degenerative changes apparent in the surrounding aortic wall make this seem even less attractive than when atheromatous disease is the cause. Aortic valve replacement has been carried out successfully for severe aortic reflux. Saccular and the less common fusiform aneurysms have been excised and scarred aortic tissue replaced by grafts. Indications for the latter form of surgery are based on: the need to relieve pain; to prevent rupture, the risk of which is considerable when the aneurysm reaches 6 to 7 cm in diameter; and the need to decompress adjacent organs such as the left main bronchus, pulmonary artery, or oesophagus.

Further reading

Augenbraun MH, Rolfs R (1999). Treatment of syphilis, 1998: nonpregnant adults. *Clinical Infectious Diseases* **28** (Suppl 1), S21–8. [Evidence-based recommendations for treatment of syphilis.]

Frank MW *et al.* (1999). Syphilitic aortitis. *Circulation* **100**, 1582–3. [Contemporary imaging of syphilitic aortitis with histology.]

Heggtveit HA (1964). Syphilitic aortitis. A clinicopathologic autopsy study of 100 cases, 1950 to 1960. *Circulation* **29**, 346–55.

Jackman JD, Radolf JD (1989). Cardiovascular syphilis. *American Journal of Medicine* **87**, 425–33. [A case report of a patient with syphilitic aortitis and a literature review of the condition.]

Vlahakes GJ, Hanna GJ, Mark EJ (1998). Case records of the Massachusetts General Hospital. *New England Journal of Medicine* **338**, 897–903. [Syphilitic aortitis with coronary ostial stenosis.]

15.10.4 Cardiac disease in HIV infection

N. Boon

Some form of heart disease is demonstrable at autopsy in approximately 40 per cent of patients with AIDS, and by echocardiography in approximately 25 per cent. However, many of these lesions are mild and heart disease probably causes symptoms in less than 10 per cent and death in only 1 to 2 per cent of all patients infected with HIV.

The common cardiac manifestations of HIV infection are listed in Table 1. Although, tuberculous pericarditis is a major problem in Africa (see section 15.09), heart muscle disease is the most important cardiac complication of AIDS in the Western world.

Table 1 Cardiac manifestations of HIV infection

Pericardial effusion
Idiopathic
Infectious:
    viral
    bacterial (especially tuberculosis)
    fungal
Neoplastic:
    Kaposi's sarcoma
    non-Hodgkin's lymphoma
Heart muscle disease
Myocarditis:
    idiopathic lymphocytic (autoimmune)
    specific infections
    toxic (e.g. penicillin)
Dilated cardiomyopathy
Endocarditis
Marantic (non-bacterial thrombotic endocarditis)
Infective
Pulmonary hypertension
Primary or idiopathic
Secondary:
    repeated chest infections
    thromboembolism
Sudden death
Autonomic dysfunction
Proarrhythmic drug effects

Pericardial effusion

HIV-related pericardial effusions are usually exudates and tend to occur in patients with advanced disease. The annual incidence of pericardial effusion in AIDS is approximately 10 per cent and the prevalence in all forms of HIV infection is approximately 20 per cent. The development of an HIV-related pericardial effusion is an independent risk factor for early death and when this complication occurs in AIDS the median survival is less than 6 months.

Less than 5 per cent of HIV-related pericardial effusions are associated with pericardial pain or friction rubs. Breathlessness, however, is common and approximately 10 per cent of effusions are associated with the symptoms and signs of tamponade.

Small subclinical effusions do not usually have an identifiable cause and often resolve spontaneously; they can therefore be managed conservatively. By contrast, moderate and large effusions are often symptomatic and are frequently due to specific opportunist infections or malignancy: aspiration is usually advisable. A wide variety of viral, bacterial, and fungal pericardial infections have been reported and conventional antimicrobial therapy combined with drainage procedures can produce good results in those with early disease.

Pericardial tuberculosis is a frequent complication of HIV infection and has become the commonest cause of pericardial effusion in many parts of the world, particularly sub-Saharan Africa. The clinical features vary widely but most patients present with prolonged fever, breathlessness, and pleuropericardial pain. Antituberculous chemotherapy is usually effective but it is not clear whether the benefits of corticosteroids seen in HIV-negative tuberculous pericarditis extend to patients who are HIV positive (see Chapter 15.9).

Malignant effusions are usually due to non-Hodgkin's lymphoma.

Malignant cardiac tumours

Kaposi's sarcoma, which is associated with human herpesvirus-8, is the most common cardiac tumour in HIV disease. The heart is involved in approximately 25 per cent of patients with disseminated Kaposi's sarcoma

and there have been a few reports of primary cardiac disease. The tumour shows a predilection for subepicardial adipose tissue and seldom infiltrates the myocardium. Pericardial effusion is a surprisingly rare complication and the diagnosis is usually made at autopsy.

Non-Hodgkin's lymphoma can also involve the heart and is more likely to cause cardiac symptoms and signs. These tumours are usually derived from B cells and may be associated with Epstein–Barr virus or human herpesvirus-8. They are usually metastatic, although primary cardiac tumours do occur, and tend to invade the epicardium. In contrast to Kaposi's sarcoma, this tumour often causes symptomatic pericardial effusion and can also infiltrate the myocardium, provoking fatal arrhythmias including ventricular fibrillation and all forms of heart block.

Heart muscle disease

HIV-related heart muscle disease tends to occur in the late stages of HIV infection and usually presents with heart failure or otherwise unexplained cardiomegaly. Left ventricular systolic dysfunction (dilated cardiomyopathy) is present in approximately 15 per cent of patients with AIDS and overt heart failure will develop in approximately 25 per cent of these patients.

The symptoms and signs of heart muscle disease include breathlessness, fatigue, tachycardia, a high jugular venous pressure, a gallop rhythm, and crepitations at the lung bases; they can be subtle and are sometimes mistakenly attributed to anaemia or chest infection. The ECG is usually abnormal, but changes are non-specific and seldom aid diagnosis; increased ventricular ectopic activity, a variety of repolarization changes, and features of left atrial hypertrophy, left ventricular hypertrophy, and left bundle branch block have all been documented. Although chest radiographs may reveal cardiomegaly and pulmonary venous congestion, the diagnosis usually depends on echocardiography, which typically shows global left ventricular dysfunction with enlargement of all the cardiac chambers.

HIV-related dilated cardiomyopathy carries an exceptionally poor prognosis with a median survival of approximately 100 days compared with 500 days for patients with similar disease and normal hearts (Fig. 1); death is often due to progressive heart failure or arrhythmia. Conventional therapy for heart failure is given, but many patients tolerate vasodilators poorly, possibly because peripheral vascular resistance tends to be low due to recurrent sepsis.

The aetiology of HIV-related heart muscle disease has not been established beyond doubt and is almost certainly complex and multifactorial. However, it seems likely that an autoimmune lymphocytic myocarditis is the usual substrate for HIV-related dilated cardiomyopathy. There are intriguing parallels between HIV-related heart muscle disease and idiopathic dilated cardiomyopathy (see Chapters 15.8.1 and 15.8.2), and the pathogenesis of the two conditions may be very similar. Autopsy and endomyocardial biopsy studies have shown that some form of myocarditis is present

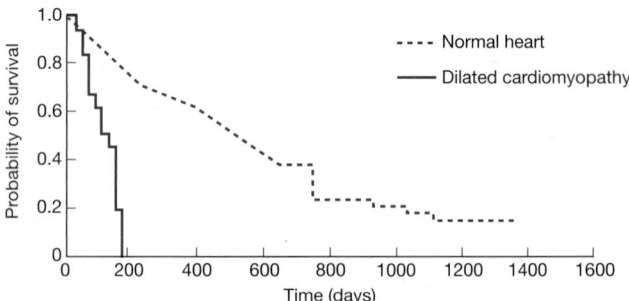

Fig. 1 Kaplan Meir survival curves for patients with HIV-related dilated cardiomyopathy and patients with structurally normal hearts and otherwise similar HIV disease (CD4 count < 20 × 10⁶ cells per litre). (Modified from Currie *et al.* (1994). *British Medical Journal* **309**, 1605–7, with permission.)

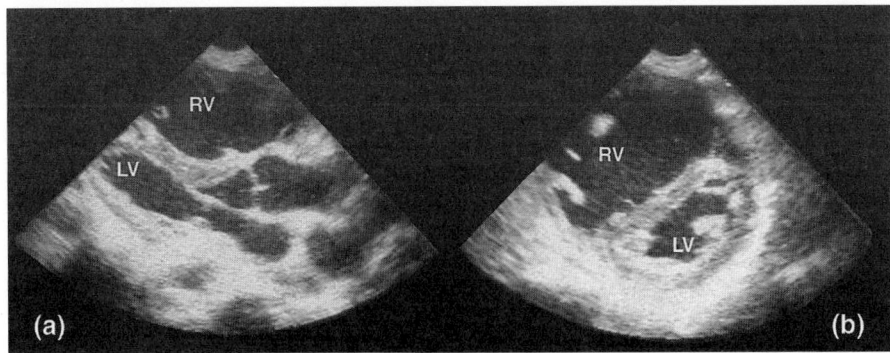

Fig. 2 (a) Long-axis and (b) short-axis parasternal view of a two-dimensional echocardiogram from an HIV-positive intravenous drug user with idiopathic pulmonary hypertension illustrating dilatation of the right ventricle and flattening of the interventricular septum.

in approximately 40 per cent of patients with AIDS and up to 80 per cent of patients with HIV-related heart muscle disease. The Dallas criteria for the diagnosis of myocarditis are seldom satisfied but it can be argued that these are not appropriate in the presence of marked immunodeficiency. Specific forms of myocarditis (e.g. *Toxoplasma gondii* and penicillin hypersensitivity) have been described but these are rare and a non-specific focal lymphocytic myocarditis appears to be the underlying problem in the majority of patients with HIV-related heart muscle disease. The inflammatory infiltrates are composed mainly of CD8+ lymphocytes with increased MHC (major histocompatibility complex) class I antigen expression. In some cases there are excess circulating cardiac autoantibodies.

A variety of molecular techniques have demonstrated that a few transcripts of HIV-1 are present in the myocardium of many patients with heart muscle disease. Myocardial damage is unlikely to be due to direct HIV toxicity because the viral load is low and there is no CD4 receptor on the myocyte; nevertheless, it is possible that the presence of the virus could trigger an autoimmune reaction. Other factors that might contribute to or amplify cardiac damage include increased oxidative stress due to micronutrient (particularly selenium) deficiency, coinfection with cardiotropic viruses (e.g. cytomegalovirus), and direct cytokine-mediated injury.

The antiretroviral drug zidovudine can cause a specific dose-related reversible skeletal myopathy by inhibiting mitochondrial γ-DNA polymerase; it can also damage cardiac muscle in rats and may be implicated in some cases of HIV-related heart muscle disease.

Infective endocarditis

Non-bacterial thrombotic (marantic) endocarditis is a disease of unknown aetiology, in which friable clumps of platelets and red blood cells adhere to the cardiac valves. The condition is sometimes complicated by systemic embolism and is associated with a variety of debilitating illnesses. It is a recognized complication of AIDS, but is infrequent and seldom causes clinical problems.

HIV infection is not associated with an increased incidence of infective endocarditis. However, intravenous drug use is an important risk factor for infective endocarditis in this patient group. *Staphylococcus aureus* is the most common pathogen in this setting and the clinical features of the condition appear to be identical in HIV-positive and HIV-negative drug users; the tricuspid valve is usually involved and infected pulmonary emboli may occur. Survival rates are around 80 per cent.

There have been surprisingly few reports of infective endocarditis in HIV-positive individuals who do not use intravenous drugs. Nevertheless, infections with a wide variety of unusual organisms (e.g. *Aspergillus fumigatus* and *Pseudoalleschira boydii*) have been described and it has been suggested that severe immunodeficiency may modify the presentation and course of disease. Salmonella endocarditis, which is usually associated with devastating cardiac complications in HIV-negative patients, appears to carry a surprisingly good prognosis in HIV-positive patients and it is conceivable that, in some situations, even minor changes in the inflammatory reaction may impair vegetation formation and limit valvular damage. On the other hand, there is evidence that other forms of infective endocarditis run a more fulminant course when they occur in the late stages of HIV infection.

Pulmonary hypertension

Significant pulmonary hypertension occurs in approximately 5 per cent of patients with advanced HIV infection. This usually presents with increasing breathlessness and right heart failure. The ECG typically shows right ventricular hypertrophy and the diagnosis is often established by echocardiography which shows characteristic dilatation of the right ventricle with flattening of the interventricular septum (Fig. 2).

The common causes of HIV-related pulmonary hypertension are recurrent chest infections, thromboembolism, and idiopathic or primary pulmonary vascular disease. Patients with left heart failure do not usually live long enough to develop pulmonary hypertension.

The symptoms and signs of right heart failure in patients with cor pulmonale due to recurrent chest infections often improve with appropriate antibiotic therapy and oxygen supplementation . Pulmonary thromboembolism is particularly common in active intravenous drug users, who can sometimes obliterate their pulmonary vascular bed by inadvertently injecting themselves with particulate material.

Approximately 2 per cent of patients with advanced HIV infection develop idiopathic pulmonary vascular disease. The clinical and histological features of this condition are indistinguishable from those of primary pulmonary hypertension (see Chapter 15.15.2.1) and it has been suggested that both conditions may have an autoimmune basis. Treatment is usually ineffective and the outlook is extremely poor.

Sudden death

Sudden death due to ventricular arrhythmias or heart block is a rare but recognized complication of HIV infection. It is usually attributed to a combination of factors including autonomic dysfunction, heart muscle disease, and drug effects. Autonomic dysfunction is a common and disabling complication of AIDS and may cause syncope, presyncope, symptomatic hypotension, and a broad range of arrhythmias, including ventricular tachycardia and ventricular fibrillation. Many potentially proarrhythmic drugs are used in the treatment of HIV infection; these include pentamidine and ganciclovir, which prolong the QT interval and can cause the form of ventricular tachycardia known as Torsades des Pointes (see Chapter 15.6).

Further reading

Barbaro G *et al.* (1998). Incidence of dilated cardiomyopathy and detection of HIV in myocardial cells of HIV-positive patients. *New England Journal of Medicine* **339**, 1093–9.

Chen Y *et al.* (1999). Human immunodeficiency virus-associated pericardial effusion: report of 40 cases and review of the literature. *American Heart Journal* **137**, 516–21.

Currie PF *et al.* (1994). Heart muscle disease related to HIV infection: prognostic implications. *British Medical Journal* **309**, 1605–7.

Heidenreich PA *et al.* (1995). Pericardial effusion in AIDS: incidence and survival. *Circulation* **92**, 3229–34.

Lipshultz SE, ed. (1998). *Cardiology in AIDS.* Chapman & Hall, New York.

Nahass RG *et al.* (1990). Infective endocarditis in intravenous drug users: a comparison of human immunodeficiency virus type 1-negative and -positive patients. *Journal of Infectious Diseases* **162**, 967–70.

Pisani B, Taylor DO, Mason JW (1997). Inflammatory myocardial diseases and cardiomyopathies. *American Journal of Medicine* **102**, 459–69.

Petitpretz P *et al.* (1994). Pulmonary hypertension in patients with human immunodeficiency virus infection: comparison with primary pulmonary hypertension. *Circulation* **89**, 2722–7.

15.11 Tumours of the heart

15.11.1 Cardiac myxoma

Thomas A. Traill

Introduction

Cardiac myxomas are benign, typically golfball-sized tumours that grow in the lumen of the atria, usually the left, attached by a stalk to the atrial septum. They are not common, but are important because they can present in a number of ways to general physicians, and because most can easily and permanently be removed by heart surgery. They are easily demonstrated by conventional transthoracic echocardiography, and it is usually the echocardiographer who makes the diagnosis; seldom has the patient been referred with this possibility in mind. Estimates of the prevalence of such a rare condition are necessarily approximate and range from 1 to 5 per 10 000 in autopsy series, or 2 per 100 000 in the general population, with a sex ratio of 2:1 in favour of women. As a cause of left atrial obstruction, myxomas are 200 to 400 times less common than mitral stenosis. The majority of patients are between 30 and 60 years, but there are reports of tumours occurring in infants and in the elderly.

Most myxomas are sporadic, unassociated with other diseases, but there is at least one mendelian syndrome involving myxoma, best named the Carney complex. This is characterized by lentiginosis, multiple myxomas (most of them cardiac), skin fibromas, and various kinds of endocrine overactivity, which has included Cushing's syndrome caused by pigmented adrenocortical hyperplasia, acromegaly, and Sertoli cell tumour. Unlike the usual kind of atrial myxoma, myxomas in Carney's syndrome may arise anywhere in the heart, are commonly multiple, and frequently recur. Inheritance of this rare disease is autosomal dominant, with centrofacial freckling as the most obvious outward marker of the phenotype. This freckling often involves unusual areas, for instance the lips, conjunctiva, and vulva.

Pathology

Cardiac myxomas are benign. Local invasion is unknown and metastatic growth is exceptional, despite the lesions' situation in the bloodstream. They take the form of polypoid masses arising from a stalk, ranging in size from 3 cm to as much as 10 cm or more, with a smooth or lobulated surface and gelatinous consistency. They are frequently covered with more or less adherent thrombus. More than 75 per cent occur within the left atrium, with the base of the pedicle arising from the fossa ovalis or its rim. Occasionally they arise from the base of the mitral valve leaflets, from the posterior part of the left atrium, or from within the right atrium. Sometimes they grow in both atria, in the form of a dumb-bell. Ventricular myxomas are exceptional and seen almost exclusively as part of Carney's syndrome. Because they are in the systemic circulation, left atrial myxomas usually draw attention to themselves at a size smaller than those on the right side.

The histology is that of a loosely woven, sparsely cellular, connective tissue tumour with very infrequent mitotic figures. Several cell types are identifiable, including undifferentiated stellate and polygonal cells, as well as smaller numbers of fibroblasts, smooth muscle cells, and endothelial cells. Among these are found macrophages and plasma cells, and rarely other mesodermal tissues, including bone. Cytogenetic studies fit with the general presumption that these indolent masses are indeed neoplastic, but immunohistochemical studies of differentiation markers do not clearly define the cell type of origin. It is suggested that the source is a primitive multipotential mesenchymal cell and that the predilection of these tumours for the atrial septum reflects the abundance of such cells in this region.

Clinical features

Presentation

Although the wide availability of echocardiography has made the diagnosis of atrial myxoma straightforward, it remains true that the prerequisite for recognizing this rare lesion is to include it in the differential diagnosis of patients presenting with symptoms and signs of much more common conditions. Left atrial myxomas may mimic mitral stenosis and cause left atrial obstruction. They may be the source of emboli to the systemic circulation, and occasionally they may present as an obscure constitutional illness with fever. Right atrial myxomas seldom cause symptoms until they are very large, when they cause right atrial obstruction with elevated systemic venous pressure, splanchnic congestion, and oedema.

Left atrial obstruction

The most common symptoms and signs mimic those of mitral stenosis, with left ventricular inflow obstruction as the chief pathophysiological change. The presenting symptoms are progressive breathlessness, orthopnoea, paroxysmal nocturnal dyspnoea, fluid retention, and atrial arrhythmias. Examination suggests rheumatic heart disease, and before the routine use of ultrasound a few such patients were referred for mitral valve surgery and the lesion was first diagnosed at operation. Some patients may develop pulmonary hypertension before the diagnosis becomes apparent.

Systemic embolism

Systemic emboli occur in about 40 per cent of patients and are frequently the first manifestation of disease. By contrast to mitral stenosis, such emboli often occur while patients are in sinus rhythm. Emboli may be sizeable, large enough even to occlude the aortic bifurcation, and besides thrombus they frequently contain tumour material, so that histological examination may be diagnostic. Thus, when systemic emboli are removed from patients they should always be sent for histological analysis. Typically, patients with systemic embolism are referred for echocardiography, and the diagnosis is then easily made.

Constitutional effects

Constitutional effects of the neoplasm predominate in a few patients. These include fever, weight loss (which is more conspicuous than in mitral stenosis and often occurs without severe left atrial obstruction), Raynaud's phenomenon (rare), finger clubbing (rare), a raised erythrocyte sedimentation rate (present in about 60 per cent of patients), and abnormal serum proteins with elevated immunoglobulin levels. These changes are usually attributed to abnormal proteins secreted by the tumour, although the nature of these has not been determined. Other haematological abnormalities include anaemia, which may be due to mechanical haemolysis, polycythaemia, associated particularly with right atrial tumours, leucocytosis, and thrombocytopenia. Such constitutional changes may prompt an initial diagnosis of infective endocarditis in patients who have heart murmurs, or lead to the suspicion of collagen vascular disease or occult cancer.

Physical signs

In many patients specific cardiovascular signs of myxoma are inconspicuous or absent. In others they vary from a prominent first heart sound to obvious changes similar to those of mitral valve disease. These include apical systolic murmurs, somewhat more common than diastolic rumbles, and signs of pulmonary hypertension with accentuated pulmonary closure and tricuspid regurgitation in some patients. Some may have an audible 'tumour plop' in early diastole, analogous to a mitral opening snap, but this is often heard best only after echocardiographic diagnosis. On combined echocardiographic and phonocardiographic recordings the plop is seen to coincide with the end of the tumour's downward movement into the ventricle, usually a short time after mitral valve opening. A rare but specific feature of the condition is variation of the auscultatory findings with change in posture; this may be particularly obvious in right atrial tumours.

Investigations

Chest radiography and electrocardiography do not help to distinguish myxoma from mitral valve disease. Left atrial enlargement is common but seldom marked and signs of pulmonary venous hypertension are infrequent. Calcification within the tumour is rarely demonstrable.

Echocardiography

While the first account of left atrial myxoma diagnosed during life was not until 1951, it is now exceptional for the diagnosis to be made first at autopsy. This is chiefly attributable to the wide availability of echocardiography, which has proved itself both reliable and specific for recognizing these tumours. The characteristic pattern of left atrial myoma is easily recognized, and it is no accident that the echocardiographic appearance of these lesions was among the first clinical reports by ultrasonographers, in 1959. Figure 1 illustrates a typical two-dimensional echocardiogram from a patient with left atrial myxoma. This 'four-chamber view' shows the characteristic dense mass of echoes from the tumour lying just above the mitral valve orifice. A video recording would demonstrate the mobility of the mass as it flops to and fro within the atrium, restrained only by its peduncle. Trans-oesophageal echocardiography affords the opportunity to examine the tumour and its attachment with great precision; generally this extra clarity is unnecessary, but on occasion the trans-oesophageal technique is helpful if there is difficulty in differentiating tumour from an atrial thrombus.

The differential diagnosis of left atrial myxoma is seldom difficult. Large masses may occasionally be difficult to distinguish from left atrial ball thrombus, a lesion that is even rarer than myxoma. Smaller left atrial masses may be papillary fibroelastomas or infective vegetations caused by endocarditis. These can usually be distinguished by their clinical context. Masses in the right atrium may also represent thrombus, sometimes propagated from the inferior vena cava, or occasionally venous extension of

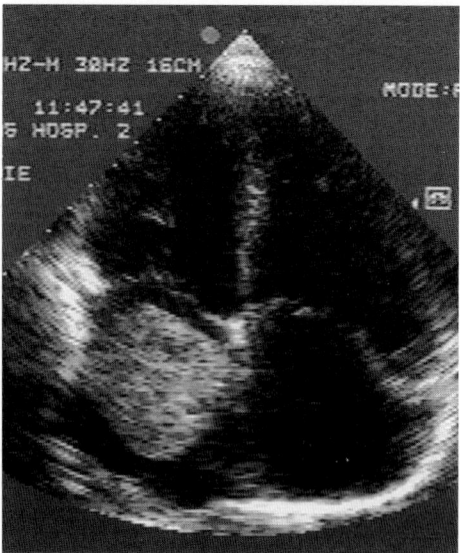

Fig. 1 Echocardiogram in the four-chamber view showing a myxoma occupying much of the left atrium.

abdominal cancers, particularly renal cell cancer. In a few patients abundant strands of the Chiari network of right atrial trabeculation may give rise to similar echocardiographic appearances.

Cardiac catheterization

The echocardiographic appearance is so characteristic that angiography no longer has a role in diagnosis of myxoma. The only time to undertake it is in an older patient in whom there is fear of occult coronary artery disease.

Treatment and prognosis

Atrial myxoma is treated by urgent surgical removal. The risk is low, comparable with that of surgery for mitral valve disease. It is important to ensure complete removal of the base by excising a full-thickness button of the atrial septum. The resulting defect is repaired with a small patch.

Functional results of surgery are good. Some patients are left with mitral regurgitation, but this is seldom severe. Recurrence is uncommon, provided excision has been complete, except in Carney's syndrome. In these patients regular echocardiographic follow-up is required, at intervals of 6 months. The rare occurrence after excision of the usual kind of myxoma generally occurs within the first 2 years; thereafter follow-up can safely be infrequent.

Further reading

Casey M *et al.* (2000). Mutations in the protein kinase A r1alpha regulatory subunit cause familial cardiac myxomas and Carney complex. *Journal of Clinical Investigation* **106**, R31–8.

Greenwood WF (1968). Profile of atrial myxoma. *American Journal of Cardiology* **21**, 367–75.

Krikler DM *et al.* (1992). Atrial myxoma: a tumour in search of its origins. *British Heart Journal* **67**, 89–91.

Murphy MC *et al.* (1990). Surgical treatment of cardiac tumors: a 25-year experience. *Annals of Thoracic Surgery* **49**, 612–18.

Schaff HV, Mullany CJ (2000). Surgery for cardiac myxomas. *Seminars in Thoracic and Cardiovascular Surgery* **12**, 77–88.

15.11.2 Other tumours of the heart

Thomas A. Traill

While each individually is rare, taken together the other tumours of the heart have an incidence that roughly equals that of myxoma. They include benign lesions, seen especially in children, sarcomas, and secondary involvement by metastasis or direct tumour extension. They are generally first recognized or suspected during echocardiography. Magnetic resonance imaging, or occasionally echo-directed transvenous biopsy, usually yield the diagnosis.

Benign cardiac tumours

Papillary fibroelastoma

The most common tumour seen in adult patients is the papillary fibroelastoma, a small pedunculated mass that hangs off one of the left-sided valve leaflets, usually the mitral valve. Its echocardiographic appearance is very characteristic. The size of the mass and presence of a peduncle distinguish this small tumour from the usual kind of Lambl's excrescence, but histologically they are identical and, like Lambl's excrescences, papillary fibroelastomas probably arise through organization of fibrinous material that collects at the trailing edges of the valve leaflets. Their importance lies in the fact that they have been labelled as a potential source of systemic embolism, and that some authors have recommended that they should be removed as a matter of routine. The evidence to support this view is thin, and this author's recommendation is to remove them only if they have been discovered in the search for a source of otherwise unexplained embolism. If they are an incidental echocardiographic finding then it is safe to leave them alone; aspirin treatment may be recommended.

Fibroma, rhabdomyoma, hamartoma, haemangioma

These are tumours of childhood, rhabdomyoma being the characteristic cardiac tumour in patients with tuberous sclerosis. By contrast to myxomas and fibroelastomas they grow within the myocardium, not into the lumen of the heart. Rhabdomyomas are usually asymptomatic, and when they are they should be left alone, since most regress spontaneously. Fibromas and hamartomas are both very rare, and may present with arrhythmias (particularly ventricular hamartomas, or Purkinje cell tumours) or with hae-

modynamic abnormalities caused by their mass effect. They require surgical excision, and when this is feasible the long-term results of treatment are very good. Haemangiomas, also very rare, tend to grow, and to develop multiple feeding vessels, so that surgical excision is usually recommended.

Cardiac sarcoma

Primary cardiac sarcomas can have one of several cell types. They are found more often in the right heart than in the left. Haemangiosarcoma is the most common, and typically develops in the right atrium. Rhabdomyosarcoma may develop in the ventricular septum or in the right ventricular outflow tract, as may the still rarer osteosarcoma, or tumours that are undifferentiated. Since these tumours often present with mechanical effects, typically obstruction at the atrial or outflow tract level, surgical resection is often attempted. However, recurrence and metastasis are common, and long-term results are very poor.

Cardiac involvement by other malignancies

Microscopic secondary deposits within the myocardium can often be found in patients who die of metastatic cancer, but intramyocardial secondaries of a size large enough to be of clinical importance are very rare. By contrast, pericardial involvement by lymphoma, or by cancers of the lung, breast, pancreas, and other tumours is not uncommon, and may sometimes be the first presentation of the tumour (see Chapter 15.9). Treatment is analogous to that of malignant pleural effusions, with drainage, creation of a window, or intrapericardial chemotherapy depending on the rest of the clinical situation.

Intraluminal spread of cancer, by direct extension up the inferior vena cava, is a particular feature of renal cell cancers. Diagnosis by echocardiography is generally obvious as the tumour has a very characteristic appearance as it waves, like seaweed in the right atrium and even dangles through the rest of the right heart. It may prove possible to resect the cava, along with the kidney and the tumour mass, under circulatory arrest.

Further reading

Case Records of the Massachussetts General Hospital (1999). *New England Journal of Medicine* **341**, 1217–24.

Olinger GN, ed (2000). Cardiac neoplasms. *Seminars in Thoracic and Cardiovascular Surgery* **12**, 76–129.

15.12 Cardiac involvement in genetic disease

Thomas A. Traill

Introduction

Singling out a few of the more prominent mendelian disorders seen by cardiologists may seem a somewhat arbitrary basis for a chapter, especially in an age when we are exploring the molecular genetic basis for so many more of the common heart diseases. However, this is a grouping that works in practice. Many clinicians find themselves faced from time to time with a patient who has a family history of a known disorder, such as Marfan's syndrome, or who has non-cardiac features that suggest a syndrome, perhaps Noonan's. They may wonder how to make the diagnosis, what else to look for, and how to screen family members.

Two important familial heart diseases are covered elsewhere in this book, namely familial hypertrophic cardiomyopathy (see Chapter 15.8.2), and the long QT syndromes (see Chapter 15.6). Both are genetically heterogeneous: familial hypertrophic cardiomyopathy is caused by mutations in any of a number of the sarcomere proteins responsible for contraction, and the long QT syndromes are caused by mutations of ion channels that affect the cardiac action potential.

The first part of this section deals with syndromes that include congenital cardiac structural defects and is restricted to a few relatively common disorders seen in adult patients. The second part describes the two common connective tissue disorders—Marfan's and Ehlers–Danlos syndromes. A number of other heritable diseases that affect the heart are listed in a table, without discussion in the text. Haemochromatosis (Chapter 11.3) and Friedreich's ataxia (Chapter 24.13.12) are discussed elsewhere in this book; the others, though important to other organ systems, offer little opportunity to the cardiologist for diagnosis or management.

Syndromic congenital heart disease

Aneuploidy disorders

The two commonest chromosomal disorders in adult patients are Down's and Turner's syndromes, and each includes characteristic cardiac abnormalities. A third, Klinefelter's syndrome, does not. Twenty-five to fifty per cent of patients with Down's syndrome have congenital heart disease. The characteristic lesion, present in about half of the affected hearts, is atrioventricular canal defect. This ranges from the relatively simple primum atrial septal defect to the complete type, in which the defect involves both the atrial and ventricular septa, between which there lies a single atrioventricular valve ring. In other patients, ventricular septal defect, tetralogy of Fallot, and persistent ductus arteriosus are seen in roughly equal numbers. Some suspect that patients with Down's syndrome are especially prone to develop pulmonary vascular disease, and hence Eisenmenger reaction, but growing experience with surgical repair for affected children seems to show that this suspicion is ill-founded. Patients with Down's syndrome undergo surgery most easily when they are infants, and the tendency has shifted away from a nihilistic approach to operating on patients with serious cardiac malformations early in life.

Turner's syndrome causes abnormalities of the aorta. The two principal lesions are coarctation and congenital abnormalities of the aortic valve, usually a bicuspid valve. Most patients with coarctation have a bicuspid aortic valve as well, and patients with a bicuspid valve frequently have some degree of anuloaortic ectasia. In some patients with Turner's syndrome the whole aorta is abnormal, either hypoplastic or weakened by the presence of cystic medial necrosis. Aortic dissection may occur, and aortic surgery, to repair coarctation for example, can sometimes be very difficult. Other congenital heart abnormalities are not common in Turner's syndrome, except for anomalies of pulmonary venous return.

Mendelian 'single-gene' disorders causing congenital heart disease

Noonan's syndrome

Noonan's syndrome is the most common heritable syndrome that characteristically causes congenital heart disease. The syndrome shares a number of features with the Turner phenotype, and the two were confused between 1930 and Noonan's studies in the 1960s, which coincided with the advent of karyotyping. In 1963 Noonan described a small series of patients with pulmonary stenosis who shared a characteristic facial appearance. Since then the phenotype has been well described, associated with a normal karyotype and autosomal dominant inheritance. Cardiac involvement has been recognized to include not only pulmonary stenosis, but a wide variety of other lesions, much wider than in Turner's syndrome. A locus has been mapped to chromosome 12.

Patients with Noonan's syndrome are of short stature, with a facies that is variously described as elfin or triangular. There is ocular hypertelorism, and the palpebral fissure may slope downwards (the antimongoloid slant), which may be emphasized by ptosis or an epicanthal fold. The ears are set low and rotated forwards so that the lobes are prominent, and there is characteristic webbing of the neck, the most obvious of the features that may lead to confusion with Turner's syndrome. Pectus deformities are common, as are other miscellaneous skeletal abnormalities, including cubitus valgus. Patients with Noonan's syndrome are prone to develop keloid scars. Cryptorchidism is common, as is delayed sexual maturation, but not infantilism as in Turner's syndrome. Unlike Turner's syndrome, a proportion of patients with Noonan's syndrome have a degree of mental retardation, but this is quite variable. Among this author's patients with Noonan's syndrome are a physician, an architect, a certified accountant, and a high-school mathematics teacher.

The frequency of cardiac involvement in Noonan's syndrome is unknown, since the diagnosis is so easily missed in the absence of congenital heart disease. The most characteristic lesion is pulmonary stenosis, but in contrast to the almost stereotypical cardiovascular findings in Turner's syndrome, the range of congenital heart abnormalities in Noonan's syndrome is broad. In many patients the stenotic pulmonary valve leaflets are not simply fused, as in non-syndromic pulmonary stenosis, but may be dysplastic, thickened, and immobile, unsuitable for simple balloon or surgical valvotomy. Other congenital lesions found in Noonan's syndrome are ventricular and atrial septal defects, tricuspid atresia, single ventricle, and abnormalities of the left ventricle including congenital mitral stenosis, subaortic stenosis, and a combination of these two lesions. The electrocardiogram often shows a superior axis (left axis deviation), even when there is pulmonary stenosis and right ventricular hypertrophy.

The most ominous complication of Noonan's syndrome is cardiomyopathy, taking the form of myocardial hypertrophy complicated by progressive fibrosis. This leads over the course of 5 to 15 years to low cardiac output with very high ventricular diastolic pressures—the pathophysiology of restrictive cardiomyopathy. Since the valvular abnormalities are for the most part correctable, this hypertrophic restrictive cardiomyopathy is the main factor limiting life-expectancy.

Williams' syndrome and familial supravalve aortic stenosis

Williams' syndrome is a contiguous gene phenomenon, caused by a macro-deletion that includes the elastin gene on chromosome 7. A loss-of-function mutation or hemizygosity of the elastin gene alone causes familial supravalve aortic stenosis, inherited as a dominant trait, in which a tight constriction develops in the aorta just above the sinuses of Valsalva. The aortic lesion is generally accompanied by a similar abnormality of the left and right pulmonary arteries, leading to peripheral pulmonary artery stenosis. In Williams' syndrome more far-reaching effects caused by deletion of contiguous genes accompany these cardiac abnormalities. The full syndrome comprises a characteristic facial appearance, with round blue eyes, a distinctive stellate pattern of the irises, depression of the nasal bridge, outwards tilting of the nostrils, abnormal dentition, and big lips, together with small stature, mental retardation, and a history of infantile hypercalcaemia. Mental retardation in Williams' syndrome takes on very individual forms, the patients often being articulate and socially adept: several purported idiots savants have had Williams' syndrome. Supravalve aortic stenosis in either of these syndromes can lead to severe left ventricular outflow obstruction, with left ventricular failure or even sudden death: surgical treatment may be required.

DiGeorge and velocardiofacial syndromes (chromosome 22 deletion syndrome)

DiGeorge syndrome, described in 1965, comprises abnormalities of the parathyroid glands, absence or hypoplasia of the thymus, and conotruncal abnormalities of the heart such as pulmonary atresia and severe forms of tetralogy of Fallot. A number of affected patients have learning disabilities or schizophrenia. It was recognized soon after the original description that the syndrome is generally caused by deletions in a region of chromosome 22.

Velocardiofacial syndrome, or Shprintzen's syndrome, described in 1981, comprises similar cardiac abnormalities along with cleft palate, a characteristic facies, and learning difficulty. It has since proved to be caused by deletions in the same region of chromosome 22, now often referred to as the DGCR (DiGeorge critical region). A third syndrome, known as 'conotruncal anomalies face', also linked to this site has been described.

With a broad spectrum of phenotypic variation, and deletions that are often quite large, it was suspected for some time that these syndromes are related manifestations of a contiguous gene phenomenon, just as in Williams' syndrome. However, it has emerged that the size of the deletion does not predict the extent of the phenotype, and that within a family the same (presumably stable) deletion can be the cause of a wide range of phenotypes. Mutations that may well account for the entire range of phenotypes have been recently been discovered in a single gene (*Ufd1*) within the region, in which case renaming as a single gene syndrome will become appropriate.

Heart–hand syndromes

The two commonly recognized heart–hand syndromes are Holt–Oram syndrome and Ellis–van Creveld syndrome.

Holt–Oram syndrome

Holt–Oram syndrome, inherited as an autosomal dominant trait, was described in 1960, comprising a secundum atrial septal defect and skeletal abnormalities, principally affecting the upper limbs and shoulder girdle, never the legs, and more pronounced in the left arm. Within a family, affected individuals may have skeletal abnormalities, congenital heart disease, or both. The limb abnormalities cover a wide spectrum from just a triphalangeal thumb to phocomelia. Abnormalities of the hand and forearm always involve the radial side and thumb (in contrast with Ellis–van Creveld syndrome). The characteristic cardiac abnormality is fossa ovalis (secundum) atrial septal defect, but affected patients may have other relatively simple lesions, for example ventricular septal defect or pulmonary stenosis.

Holt–Oram syndrome has been mapped and cloned. The mutation is in a transcription factor known now as TBX5, a close homologue of a transcription factor seen as phylogenetically far back as the fruit fly. Mutations of the homologous gene in the fruit fly produce abnormalities of the wing.

Ellis–van Creveld syndrome

Ellis–van Creveld syndrome is inherited as a recessive trait, hence the more complete clinical descriptions have come from studies in genetically circumscribed communities, notably the Old Order Amish of Pennsylvania where thanks to a founder effect the gene is common and homozygotes abound. The syndrome, described in 1940, includes dwarfism, caused mainly by shortening of the forearms and lower legs, and symmetrical polydactyly affecting the ulnar side with accessory sixth and even seventh digits attached to or beyond the little finger. Cardiac involvement is very common, present probably in three-quarters of homozygotes. The characteristic lesion is common atrium—a lesion that has the appearance on echocardiography and to the surgeon of a very large primum atrial septal defect. A few patients have more complete forms of atrioventricular canal defect, and, at least among the Amish, there is a high perinatal mortality rate among affected infants, suggesting the possibility of still more extensive cardiac involvement. The gene has been mapped to chromosome 4 and sequenced, but the protein's function is unknown.

Connective tissue disorders

Marfan's syndrome

Thanks principally to the work of McKusick and his collaborators, beginning in 1955, Marfan's syndrome has become the paradigm for the clinical and genetic investigation of the heritable disorders of connective tissue. The importance of the syndrome is heightened by the fact that its recognition and treatment have had a dramatic impact on survival among those affected. In 1896 Marfan described a patient with what he termed arachnodactyly. In the century since, it has been appreciated that the syndrome is mendelian and pleiotropic, involving several apparently unrelated organs whose common feature proves to be the importance of elastic tissue to their structural integrity. Ocular involvement, with the lens subluxed because of failure of its suspensory ligament, was recognized early in the twentieth century. Cardiovascular involvement was noted incidentally in the 1940s, and studied systematically from the 1950s onwards. Skeletal involvement includes—besides long limbs and arachnodactyly—scoliosis and other abnormalities of the thoracic cage. The sternum may be pushed outwards or inwards by the abnormally long ribs, hence pectus carinatum and/or excavatum, often asymmetrical. Skin involvement is identified by light-coloured striae, which should be looked for over the deltopectoral groove and the flanks. Less common findings are dural ectasia, which can sometimes be so marked as to cause radicular symptoms, and spontaneous pneumothorax or apical blebs.

The characteristic cardiovascular findings in Marfan's syndrome are aneurysmal dilatation of the aorta, and occasionally other large arteries, and floppy mitral valve. The former was recognized in the 1920s but not really addressed until McKusick showed that it was the principal cause of early death in the disease. Shortly afterwards, echocardiography became available to identify and follow these abnormalities, and surgical techniques were developed by Bentall and Gott to repair the aneurysms. Until then, median life expectancy for men with Marfan's syndrome had been 45 years, for women a year or two longer.

Fibrillin gene mutations

The syndrome is caused in almost all patients by mutations of the fibrillin gene on chromosome 15. Fibrillin is a pleated protein laid down in sheets, and a mutation functions as a dominant negative by coding for a misshapen protein that interferes with this polymerization. This is a common mechanism among the connective tissue disorders, seen in Ehlers–Danlos syndrome and in osteogenesis imperfecta. It appears from animal models that in Marfan's syndrome the stage is set for abnormal arterial wall development early in fetal life.

The fibrillin molecule is large and most of the disease-causing mutations have yet to be described, hence genetic diagnosis by screening for known mutations is seldom possible and diagnosis usually depends on applying clinical criteria. There are a number of polymorphisms within the gene, so in some kindreds it is possible by tracking particular alleles to determine which is associated with the disease, and therefore contains the pathogenetic mutation. This has allowed diagnosis of the syndrome in individual family members in whom the clinical findings were uncertain, and has been used for prenatal diagnosis. Furthermore, the technique makes it possible to infer the existence of a fibrillin mutation in kindreds where the phenotype has not met clinical criteria for Marfan's syndrome; if aortic ectasia segregates with a particular copy of the fibrillin gene, then the chances are high that a fibrillin mutation somewhere in that copy is the pathogenetic mechanism.

Diagnostic criteria

The clinical diagnosis of Marfan's syndrome rests on major and minor criteria. In an index case, involvement of three organ systems is required, with major criteria in two. Major criteria can be aortic aneurysm, lens subluxation, characteristic skeletal abnormalities, or dural ectasia. Minor criteria can be striae, mitral valve prolapse, joint laxity, the facies, or moderate pectus excavatum. Characteristic skeletal abnormalities can be: arachnodactyly (encircling the wrist with the thumb and little finger, the 'wrist sign', and making a fist with a protruding thumb, the 'thumb sign'), marked pectus deformity, increased wing-span to 5 per cent more than the height, and scoliosis. In the relative of an index case, the positive family history becomes another major criterion.

In clinical practice, determining whether a patient satisfies these criteria may be fairly subjective and requires experience with the syndrome. Often it is enough to know whether or not there is cardiovascular involvement, and there are numerous families with aortic aneurysms or ectasia whose full phenotype does not satisfy clinical criteria for Marfan's syndrome, yet whose long-term management is identical. Equally, a lanky patient who has a normal aorta needs only infrequent follow-up, even though there may be a suspicion that he has a mild case of the syndrome.

Clinical management

Patients with Marfan's syndrome should be followed up with annual or 6-monthly echocardiograms to examine the aortic root. If there is reason to suspect that the aorta may be dilated above the echo plane then CT scanning or MRI is required at least once to validate the echo measurement. When the maximum measurement across the aorta reaches 5 cm, we generally recommend surgical replacement of the aortic root, to prevent aortic dissection (see Chapter 15.14.1), which becomes a real risk once the dimension reaches 6 cm. The traditional and very successful approach is with the composite graft: a mechanical aortic valve prosthesis to which is indissolubly attached a tubular vascular prosthesis is used to replace the entire aortic root and annulus. The coronary artery ostia are excised from the native aorta and reattached to the prosthetic root. Recently, to avoid anticoagula-

tion in certain patients, there has been interest in a valve-sparing technique of root replacement in which a vascular prosthesis is fitted snugly over the aortic valve commissures, with the native leaflets suspended in their normal anatomical arrangement. Long-term success with this approach will depend on the degree to which the valve leaflets themselves degenerate because of the connective tissue abnormality. The Ross (pulmonary autograft) procedure is not appropriate in Marfan's syndrome. After surgery, and especially in patients whose surgery was done as an emergency for dissection, follow-up is with periodic imaging by CT or MRI to keep the remaining aorta under surveillance. Management of mitral prolapse and regurgitation in Marfan's syndrome is the same as in other patients. Surgery is required for severe or symptomatic regurgitation; mitral valve repair has proved surprisingly successful.

It is usual to treat patients who have aortic involvement with β-blockers, to slow the progression to aneurysm. We generally advise against excessively demanding sports, particularly competitive basketball, but in all affected children it is important to balance the risks of aortic disease against the importance of normal psychological development. Pregnancy is not contraindicated in all women with Marfan's syndrome, but genetic counselling should be offered, and it is advised that people not become pregnant if the aorta is enlarged to over 4 cm.

Ehlers–Danlos syndromes

In the early part of the twentieth century Ehlers and Danlos described an association between hyperextensibility of the skin, atrophic scarring, and hypermobility of the large joints. Several different mendelian Ehlers–Danlos syndromes are now defined, caused by mutations of different collagen molecules (and some others besides collagen). Since phenotypes may be highly variable, even within a single family, the details of classifying these diseases according to their pathogenesis are still not completely worked out.

Three principal cardiovascular manifestations of the Ehlers–Danlos syndromes are recognized, namely vascular fragility and rupture, mitral valve prolapse, and aortic root ectasia. The first of these is the potentially fatal feature of the vascular type of Ehlers–Danlos (formerly type IV), inherited as a dominant trait and caused by mutations in the type III procollagen molecule. Patients with this form are prone to spontaneous rupture of large and medium-sized arteries. The aorta does not dilate as in Marfan's syndrome and dissection is less common than simple through and through tearing. Less common, but also potentially fatal complications of the vascular type, are spontaneous perforations of the bowel: with severe vascular fragility, treatment of this or other surgical emergencies can be difficult or impossible.

The classic form of Ehlers–Danlos syndrome (formerly types I and II), inherited as a dominant trait, is characterized by marked skin extensibility, joint laxity, and characteristic wide, atrophic ('cigarette paper') scars at the sites of previous injury or surgery. Patients frequently have mitral valve prolapse, as do many people with joint laxity who do not have diagnosable Ehlers–Danlos syndrome, but only a few progress to develop severe mitral reflux or to the point of requiring surgery. Enlargement of the aortic sinuses of Valsalva may occur, but this is seldom severe or progressive. Surgical replacement of the aortic root, as is performed in Marfan's syndrome, is exceptional in Ehler–Danlos syndrome.

Other heart-related connective tissue and metabolic disorders

Osteogenesis imperfecta causes aortic and mitral regurgitation, as do several of the mucopolysaccharidoses (Table 1). It is striking, particularly in the case of osteogenesis imperfecta, how healing is almost non-existent where there is foreign material. If the opportunity arises, even years later, to inspect the operative result in a patient who has undergone valve replacement, the sutures look as though they had only just been placed, with minimal endothelial reaction and scar tissue formation.

Inherited disorders of heart muscle

All three principal groupings of cardiomyopathy—dilated, hypertrophic, and restrictive—include mendelian forms, but familial hypertrophic cardiomyopathy is by far the best studied (see Chapter 15.8.2). Mutations in the actin molecule have been implicated in some families with dilated cardiomyopathy, as have inborn errors of metabolism affecting high-energy phosphate production, for example carnitine deficiency. Other types of familial dilated cardiomyopathy are seen in several striated myopathies, notably Becker's muscular dystrophy, and in mitochondrial dystrophies. The severity of cardiac involvement in muscular dystrophy is quite variable, and the converse, so that some cases involving both kinds of myopathy may be missed. For example, muscle wasting caused by limb-girdle dystrophy may be ascribed to cardiac cachexia in a case of severe cardiomyopathy, and cardiomegaly in a patient with endstage muscular dystrophy may be wrongly attributed to cor pulmonale.

Arrhythmogenic right ventricular dysplasia is a familial disease, inherited as a dominant trait, that affects almost exclusively the right ventricle. The pathology consists of replacement of islands of right ventricular myocardium with fatty and fibrous connective tissue. Generally these islands are small and the disease seldom leads to any detectable mechanical deficit. However, the areas of fibrous replacement create the substrate for ventricular arrhythmias and the clinical presentation is with palpitations, syncope, and even sudden death. Exercising may unmask the tendency to arrhythmias, so the disease is particularly recognized among athletes. Echocardiography or MRI usually establishes the diagnosis. Treatment is by management of the arrhythmia; severely affected patients may require implantation of an automatic defibrillator.

Further reading

Dietz HC *et al.* (1991). Marfan syndrome caused by a recurrent *de novo* missense mutation in the fibrillin gene. *Nature* **352**, 337–9.

Gott VL *et al.* (1999). Replacement of the aortic root in patients with Marfan's syndrome. *New England Journal of Medicine* **340**, 1307–13.

Lowery MC *et al.* (1995). Strong correlation of elastin deletions, detected by FISH, with Williams syndrome: evaluation of 235 patients. *American Journal of Human Genetics* **57**, 49–53.

McKusick VA (2000). Ellis–van Creveld syndrome and the Amish. *Nature Genetics* **24**, 203–4.

Noonan JA (1999). Noonan syndrome revisited. *Journal of Pediatrics* **135**, 667–8.

Pepin M *et al.* (2000). Clinical and genetic features of Ehlers–Danlos syndrome type IV, the vascular type. *New England Journal of Medicine* **342**, 673–80.

Pyeritz RE (1983). Cardiovascular manifestations of heritable disorders of connective tissue. *Progress in Medical Genetics* **5**, 191–302.

Yamagishi H *et al.* (1999). A molecular pathway revealing a genetic basis for human cardiac and craniofacial defects. *Science* **283**, 1158–61.

Table 1 Rare Mendelian disorders affecting the cardiovascular system

	Biochemical abnormality	Non-cardiac features	Cardiovascular features
Osteogenesis imperfecta	Heterogeneous, abnormalities of type 1 procollagen	Bony fractures and deformity, blue scleras (four types described)	Mitral valve prolapse and regurgitation. Aortic root enlargement and aortic regurgitation
Pseudoxanthoma elasticum		Areas of thickened skin and pseudoxanthomas Vascular fragility and haemorrhage. Fundus: angioid streaks	Extensive vascular narrowing and calcification with angina, claudication, and limb ischaemia
Hunter's syndrome (MPS II)	Iduronate sulphate sulphatase	X-linked usually severe with dwarfing, mental retardation, gargoylism	Cardiomyopathy, coronary narrowing, valve lesions
Scheie's syndrome (MPS I S)	α-Iduronidase (as in the much more severe, allelic, Hurler's syndrome, MPS I H)	Arthropathy, hepatosplenomegaly, corneal clouding	Aortic regurgitation. Abnormal valve leaflets
Morquio's syndrome (MPS IV)	Galactosamine-6-sulphate sulphatase or α-galactosidase	Dwarfism, deafness, spinal cord compression and injury	Aortic regurgitation and stenosis
Homocystinuria	Cystathionine-α-synthase	Osteoporosis, sternal deformity, lens subluxation, mental retardation	Vascular thrombosis, precocious coronary atherosclerosis
Fabry's disease	α-Galactosidase A	Painful neuropathy, CNS disease, renal failure, corneal opacity	Coronary artery disease, myocardial infarction, mitral valve dysfunction
Friedreich's ataxia	Unknown	Spinocerebellar degeneration	Cardiomyopathy with increased wall thickness and restrictive physiology. Ventricular arrhythmias
Duchenne's muscular dystrophy	Dystrophin	X-linked muscular dystrophy with rapid progression during childhood and adolescence	Dilated cardiomyopathy, characteristic ECG
Becker's muscular dystrophy	Dystrophin	X-linked muscular dystrophy, less severe than Duchenne's	Dilated cardiomyopathy, variable severity
Dystrophia myotonica	Myotonin protein kinase	Weakness and myotonia, ptosis, cataracts, frontal balding, intellectual slowing	Bundle branch block, bradyarrhythmias, less frequently VT
Haemochromatosis	HFE protein	Diabetes, liver disease, pigmentation, arthritis, pituitary dysfunction	Dilated or restrictive cardiomyopathy
Arrhythmogenic right ventricular dysplasia	Unknown	None	Palpitations, syncope, sudden death

CNS, central nervous system; MPS, mucopolysaccharidosis.

15.13 Congenital heart disease in adolescents and adults

S. A. Thorne and P. J. Oldershaw*

Introduction

Doctors in all areas of medicine and surgery will encounter the growing number of patients with congenital heart disease who survive beyond childhood. It is therefore important that all doctors have an understanding of the principles of congenital heart disease and enough knowledge to know when to refer such patients to a specialist centre.

The future size of the population of long-term survivors will be influenced by a number of factors. In the era before paediatric and neonatal cardiac surgery, 70 per cent of the approximately 4 per 1000 live-born babies diagnosed as having congenital heart disease died before their 10th birthday. However, with advances in medical and surgical care during childhood the majority can now expect to survive into adulthood, increasing the numbers of patients with operatively modified disease. The advent of echocardiography has allowed less severe lesions that previously presented later in life to be diagnosed in infancy, so that the true incidence of congenital heart disease is around 10 per 1000 live-born babies. In societies where termination of pregnancy is available, prenatal diagnosis by fetal echocardiography may result in a reduced incidence of live-born infants with severe congenital heart disease, but its full impact on the population of long-term survivors remains to be determined.

Many of those who survive to adulthood do so with surgically modified lesions, and the continuing evolution of new surgical techniques creates a population with different residual lesions, long-term complications, and survival than earlier generations with the same initial diagnosis. Careful follow-up is therefore crucial, not only to provide high standards of clinical care, but also to provide feedback about late results in order to inform initial management in infancy. For example, as a result of such long-term follow-up information, the operation of choice for transposition of the great arteries is now the arterial switch, because of the late problems encountered in patients who had undergone interatrial repair with the Senning or Mustard operations.

The concepts of congenital and acquired heart disease are arbitrary, lesions may change and develop during a patient's lifetime either as part of the natural history, or in response to surgical intervention. For example, aortic regurgitation may be acquired in the presence of a subaortic ventricular septal defect because the aortic valve which forms the roof of the defect is unsupported and becomes incompetent as a result of the Venturi effect 'sucking' one of the valve leaflets into the defect. In double-inlet left ventricle with ventriculoarterial discordance, the aorta arises from the rudimentary right ventricle via a ventricular septal defect that is usually non-restrictive and hence does not limit aortic flow. However, age-related or surgically induced ventricular hypertrophy and interventions that reduce the volume load on the ventricle may reduce the size of the ventricular septal defect, causing subaortic stenosis. Changing lesions can also be observed *in utero*, further challenging the division between congenital

and acquired disease. In some cases of pulmonary atresia with intact interventricular septum, serial fetal examinations may show pulmonary stenosis evolving into pulmonary atresia, with concomitant failure of development of an initially normal-looking right ventricle.

Molecular genetics in congenital heart disease

Advances in molecular genetics are changing our understanding of congenital heart disease, not only in terms of recurrence risks, but also in embryogenesis and in genetic–environmental interactions. Recently, single gene abnormalities have been identified in Holt–Oram syndrome (skeletal and cardiac anomalies, especially atrial septal defect) and in non-Down's atrioventricular septal defect. New technologies have begun to explain the overlapping phenotypes of di George syndrome and velocardiofacial syndrome which comprise a variety of defects of neural crest-derived tissues, and are also known by the acronym, CATCH 22. In both syndromes there is deletion or microdeletion of a region of chromosome 22q11, the phenotypic spectrum being dependent on the degree and position of the deletion. This discovery has implications for genetic counselling: if a patient has tetralogy of Fallot with 22q11 microdeletion, the chances of their offspring inheriting the microdeletion and a phenotypic abnormality are higher than if there is no microdeletion.

Some cardiac defects have a clear environmental cause, such as patent arterial duct and peripheral pulmonary arterial stenosis in maternal rubella and ventricular and atrial septal defects in maternal alcohol abuse. However, in up to 80 per cent of congenital heart defects, no clear single genetic or environmental factor is implicated, that is, the cause is multifactorial and due to interactions between gene(s) and the environment. Candidate genes for specific stages in embryogenesis are beginning to be identified. For example, septation of the ventricular outflow tract appears to be dependent on the HIRA gene regulating migration of neural crest cells; attenuated expression of this gene may play a role in di George and velocardiofacial syndromes.

Cyanotic congenital heart disease

Cyanosis and pulmonary vascular disease are common problems in congenital heart disease and are discussed in general terms below.

Eisenmenger syndrome: defects with secondary pulmonary vascular disease

The Eisenmenger reaction describes the pathophysiology of patients who have pulmonary hypertension at systemic level as a result of high pulmonary vascular resistance with a reversed or bidirectional shunt. The shunt is usually a non-restrictive communication between the systemic and pulmonary circulations and may occur at atrial, ventricular, or arterial levels. Pulmonary vascular disease is established early in life when the shunt is at

---

* We acknowledge the pioneering work of Jane Somerville in the field of adult congenital heart disease.

ventricular or arterial level. A continuing large left to right shunt at systemic pressure causes the pulmonary vascular resistance to rise progressively until it exceeds systemic vascular resistance and the shunt reverses, establishing Eisenmenger physiology. By comparison, the pulmonary hypertension associated with non-restrictive shunts at atrial level usually occurs later in life.

Clinical findings

Whatever the underlying defect, some examination findings are shared. Patients have cyanosis and clubbing and may be plethoric. There is a right ventricular heave and the pulmonary component of the second heart sound is palpable and loud. A pulmonary ejection click may be audible, also a soft early diastolic murmur of pulmonary regurgitation (Graham–Steell murmur). A soft systolic flow murmur may be heard from the dilated pulmonary artery. No systolic murmur can be heard from the lesion responsible for the pulmonary vascular disease since the chambers on both sides of it are at equal pressures. Thus the presence of a loud systolic murmur brings in to doubt a diagnosis of Eisenmenger syndrome, although the murmur of associated tricuspid regurgitation may occasionally be loud.

It is frequently possible to distinguish between the common lesions associated with the Eisenmenger syndrome on clinical grounds (Table 1). The patient with an Eisenmenger duct has differential cyanosis and clubbing since fully saturated blood from the left ventricle supplies the aortic arch and its branches before mixing occurs with desaturated pulmonary arterial blood via the patent duct. The right hand may therefore be pink with no clubbing, the left may be slightly more cyanosed because of the origin of the left subclavian artery opposite the duct, and the toes are more deeply cyanosed and clubbed (see Taussig–Bing anomaly for reversed differential cyanosis). The second heart sound may be closely or normally split. By contrast, cyanosis and clubbing is uniform when the right to left shunt occurs at atrial, ventricular, or ascending aortic (as in truncus arteriosus) levels. The second sound is single in ventricular septal defect, atrioventricular septal defect, and truncus but may be split in an atrial septal defect.

Natural history and complications

Survival into adulthood with the Eisenmenger syndrome is common. Symptoms of breathlessness relate to the degree of hypoxia; many patients feel worse in hot weather or after a hot bath because the resulting systemic vasodilation is not accompanied by a reduction in pulmonary vascular resistance, so the right to left shunt is enhanced and the patient becomes more hypoxic.

The patient with Eisenmenger syndrome is prone to all the complications of cyanotic heart disease discussed below. In addition, exercise-induced syncope may occur and is exacerbated by hot weather and dehydration. Haemoptysis is common and may be fatal. It is usually due to rupture of small hypertensive intrapulmonary vessels, or more rarely to thrombosis *in situ* and pulmonary infarction. All patients with haemoptysis should be admitted and the systemic pressure kept low by bed rest and β-blockade; the pulmonary artery pressure is the same as that measured in the brachial artery. Any non-steroidal anti-inflammatory agents should be stopped and vasodilators should not be used. If the haemoptysis is massive, diamorphine should be administered and consideration given to selectively intubating the non-bleeding lung. Fresh frozen plasma or cryoprecipitate may be given. Bronchoscopy has no role and may worsen the haemorrhage. Spiral CT differentiates pulmonary artery thrombosis from intrapulmo-

nary haemorrhage. Few data exist to direct management of patients with pulmonary arterial thrombus. Warfarin may increase the risk of bleeding whilst failing to reduce the thrombus, and aspirin should be avoided as it may exacerbate haemorrhage associated with thrombocytopenia.

Right ventricular failure may be precipitated by atrial arrhythmia and usually occurs after the age of 30 years. Decline may be heralded by the onset of right ventricular failure, supraventricular arrhythmia, and haemoptysis. Death is sudden in about 30 per cent of patients and results from arrhythmia or massive haemoptysis. In some patients death appears to follow progressive hypoxia, terminating in bradycardia and asystole from which resuscitation is impossible.

Pregnancy (see below) and non-cardiac surgery pose major risks. The latter is particularly dangerous when carried out without the benefit of expert cardiological anaesthetic and perioperative care. A sound understanding of the pathophysiology and the importance of avoiding vasodilators, dehydration, hypotension, and air emboli are vital.

Investigations

The chest radiograph shows a dilated pulmonary trunk because of high pulmonary blood flow in earlier life, but the lung fields are oligaemic (Figs 1 and 2). Unless cardiac failure intervenes, the cardiac silhouette is usually normal, the effects of volume overload having regressed as pulmonary vascular resistance increased and the left to right shunt diminished and disappeared. The electrocardiogram shows p pulmonale and biventricular hypertrophy. The echocardiogram should establish the site of the shunt and allow an estimation of pulmonary arterial pressure and ventricular function.

Cardiac catheterization is unnecessary and potentially dangerous for patients with established pulmonary vascular disease. The only indication is for those patients whose pulmonary vascular disease is suspected to be reversible and who would be considered for surgical repair if reversibility can be confirmed. This situation is rarely encountered in the adult population. Histologically, pulmonary vascular disease progresses from medial hypertrophy through intimal proliferation with migration of smooth muscle cells, to progressive fibrosis and obliteration, dilatation, the development of angiomas, and finally fibrinoid necrosis. Those who have developed fibrotic and obliterative changes are likely to have irreversible pulmonary vascular disease. Routine lung biopsy is not recommended; it carries a high risk in the adult with pulmonary hypertension and is unlikely to show reversible pathology. In addition, thoracotomy scars are a relative contraindication to heart–lung transplantation.

Treatment options in the Eisenmenger syndrome

Avoiding unnecessary intervention is the mainstay of management. Heart failure and arrhythmia should be treated with care to avoid overdiuresis and vasodilation. The limited role of phlebotomy for symptomatic hyperviscosity is discussed below.

Heart–lung transplantion, or lung transplantion with repair of the cardiac defect, are often seen as the ultimate options. However, current donor shortages and the high risk of transplanting patients with long-standing cyanosis who are prone to excessive haemorrhage, renal failure, and technical surgical difficulties due to previous thoracotomy, mean that many patients never receive a transplant. Whether chronic therapy with oxygen or with pulmonary vasodilators, such as prostaglandin or nitric oxide, has a role in improving morbidity or mortality in adults remains to be seen.

Table 1 Clinical differentiation between lesions associated with the Eisenmenger syndrome

	Ventricular septal defect or truncus arteriosus	Atrial septal defect	Persistent ductus arteriosus
Cyanosis and clubbing	Uniform	Uniform	Differential (toes more than fingers)
Second heart sound	Single	Usually closely split, becomes widely split as right ventricle fails	Closely or normally split, more widely split as right ventricle fails

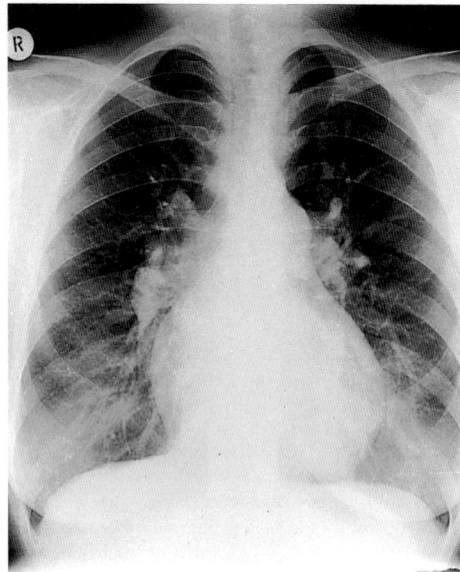

Fig. 1 Chest radiograph of a 35-year-old woman with Eisenmenger secundum atrial septal defect. The aortic knuckle is small and the central pulmonary arteries enlarged, indicating pulmonary arterial hypertension; the lung fields are clear. The cardiac silhouette is not enlarged.

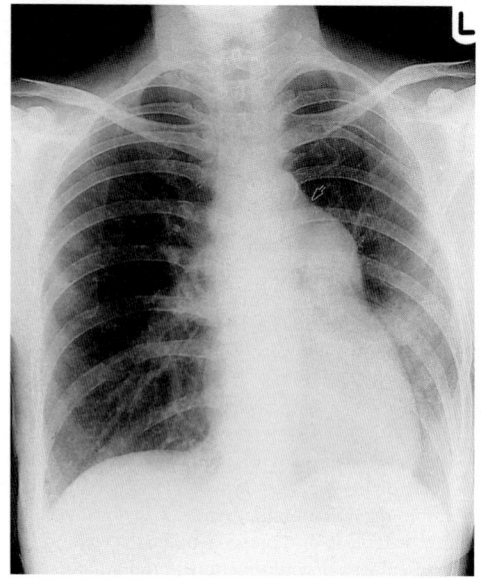

Fig. 2 Chest radiograph of a 45-year-old woman with Eisenmenger arterial duct which is calcified and fills the indentation between the aortic knuckle and main pulmonary artery (arrow). There has been an exploratory left thoracotomy.

Given the shortage of organ donors, it may not be realistic to consider such approaches as a temporary bridge to transplantation.

Cyanotic heart disease: a multisystem disorder

Cyanotic heart disease is a multisystem disorder; its manifestations are listed in Table 2.

Secondary erythrocytosis

Chronic hypoxia is the stimulus to the increased red blood cell mass and high haematocrit found in cyanotic heart disease. This physiological response increases the oxygen carrying capacity of the blood and may improve tissue oxygenation sufficiently to reach a new equilibrium at a higher haematocrit. However, adaptive failure occurs if the increase in blood viscosity brought about by the high haematocrit impairs oxygen delivery and negates the beneficial effects of erythrocytosis.

The secondary erythrocytosis of cyanotic heart disease is a physiological response, often associated with thrombocytopenia. It is fundamentally different to the generalized increase in all haemopoietic stem cell lines found in the malignant disease, polycythaemia rubra vera. Failure to differentiate

Table 2 Complications of cyanotic congenital heart disease

Haematological	Secondary erythrocytosis	→ Hyperviscosity
	Iron deficiency (over venesection, menorrhagia)	→ Hyperviscosity ↑ Risk of CVA
	Thrombocytopenia	
	Haemorrhage	
	Coagulopathy	
Neurological	CVA	Secondary to paradoxical embolism
	Cerebral abscess	
Hyperuricaemia	Impaired renal clearance	→ Gout
	Increased production?	
Renal abnormalities	↓ Uric acid clearance	
	Glomerular proteinuria	
	Mesangial matrix thickening	
	Capillary and hilar arteriole dilatation	
Bilirubin kinetics	↑ Haem breakdown	→ Pigment gallstones
Digits and long bones	Clubbing	
	Hypertrophic osteoarthropathy	
Dental	Gingival hypertrophy	→ ↑ Risk of endocarditis
Infection	Endocarditis	
	Cerebral abscess	
Skin	Acne	

Table 3 Symptoms of hyperviscosity

Headache
Faint, dizzy, light headed
Depressed mentation, sense of distance
Blurred vision, amaurosis fugax
Paraesthesiae
Tinnitus
Fatigue, lethargy
Myalgia, muscle weakness
Chest and abdominal pain

between these two phenomena has contributed to the persistent misman-agement of erythrocytosis in cyanotic heart disease. Three misconceptions lead to inappropriate venesection in cyanotic heart disease:

Misconception 1—volume replacement is not necessary. If venesection is performed without simultaneous volume replacement, the sudden fall in systemic blood flow, oxygen delivery, and cerebral perfusion may result in cardiovascular collapse. Simultaneous infusion of an equal volume of 0.9 per cent saline or colloid should be given.

Misconception 2—venesection is performed to reduce the risk of stroke. The risk of stroke in adults with cyanotic heart disease does not relate to the haematocrit, but rather to microcytosis and iron deficiency brought on by injudicious venesection.

Misconception 3—venesection should be done routinely to keep the haem-atocrit less than 65 per cent. The only indication for venesection is for the temporary relief of symptoms of hyperviscosity in hydrated, iron-replete individuals with a haematocrit greater than 60 to 65 per cent (Tables 3 and 4). If the patient does not gain symptomatic improvement then further venesection is unlikely to be beneficial. Any dehydration should be cor-rected before assessing the need for venesection. Some patients reach a stable equilibrium with a haematocrit greater than 70 per cent; venesection is not indicated if there are no symptoms of hyperviscosity. The only excep-tion is the preoperative patient with thrombocytopenia and a high haem-atocrit, when venesection may cause a temporary rise in platelet count and a reduction in perioperative bleeding.

Microcytic iron-deficient erythrocytes have a reduced oxygen carrying capacity and are less deformable than biconcave iron-replete cells and so increase blood viscosity, negating any beneficial effect of venesection in reducing the haematocrit. Iron deficiency also causes muscle weakness and myalgia independent of its effect on blood viscosity. If standard doses of iron supplements are given, uncontrolled erythropoiesis occurs and the haematocrit rises rapidly, resulting in a cycle of excessive venesection and iron deficiency, leaving the patient symptoms of hyperviscosity induced by both the haematocrit level and iron deficiency. Low-dose iron replacement (ferrous sulphate, 200 mg daily) combined with close monitoring of the blood count so that iron therapy is withdrawn as soon as the haematocrit rises (often within a week) should allow the gradual recovery of iron stores and the avoidance of counterproductive venesection and further iron defi-ciency. Hydroxyurea is an antitumour agent that may have a role in sup-pressing the erythrocytotic response to iron therapy in patients with a high haematocrit. It also causes thrombocytopenia and neutropenia, so should be used with caution.

Disorders of coagulation

Why patients with cyanotic disease are at increased risk of haemorrhage and thrombosis is poorly understood. There is often a mild thrombocyto-penia that may be partly due to shortened platelet survival time, and the large multimeric forms of von Willebrand factor and other clotting factors may be depleted. Bleeding may be minor and mucocutaneous, but major haemorrhage can occur during surgery, or from pulmonary haemorrhage (see above). Coagulation testing may yield spurious results in patients with a haematocrit greater than 55 per cent unless the amount of citrate anti-coagulant is reduced, according to the following equation:

$$\text{Volume of anticoagulant per ml blood} = \frac{100 - \text{haematocrit}}{595 - \text{haematocrit}}$$

Other complications of cyanotic heart disease

Right to left shunting creates a risk of paradoxical embolism causing stroke and cerebral abscess as well as air emboli from venous lines not fitted with filters. Patients who require transvenous pacing should be formally anti-coagulated with warfarin to prevent paradoxical thromboembolism from pacing leads.

Despite the high incidence of hyperuricaemia, attacks of acute gout are uncommon and asymptomatic hyperuricaemia does not require treatment. Acute attacks should be treated with colchicine, avoiding non-steroidal anti-inflammatory agents because of their detrimental effects on haemo-stasis and renal function. As in primary hyperuricaemia, allopurinol is use-ful in preventing recurrence. The renal abnormalities outlined in Table 2 are rarely associated with abnormal baseline renal function. However, renal failure may be precipitated by hypotension and dehydration, especially in combination with radiographic contrast media or non-steroidal anti-inflammatory agents. Acne is a common complaint in adolescents and adults with cyanotic disease and may be widespread and psychologically debilitating. When severe it may also increase the risk of bacteraemia and endocarditis.

Digital clubbing is almost universal in cyanotic heart disease, and some degree of hypertrophic osteoarthropathy of the long bones may occur in up to one-third of patients. Symptoms include aching and tenderness of the long bones of the forearms and legs. There is oedema and cellular infil-tration, causing lifting of the periosteum that is visible radiographically, and new bone formation and resorption. Localized activation of endothe-lial cells by an abnormal platelet population, with the ensuing release of fibroblast growth factors, may play a central role in the pathogenesis of both phenomena.

Table 4 Guidelines for venesection in adults with cyanotic heart disease

Symptoms of hyperviscosity	Haematocrit	Action
No	Any	Venesection not indicated
Yes	> 60–65%, iron replete, no dehydration	Isovolumic venesection (400–500 ml)
Yes	< 65%, iron deficient	Seek underlying cause of iron deficiency
		Low-dose iron therapy, closely monitoring haematocrit
Yes	> 65%, iron deficient	Seek underlying cause of iron deficiency
		Avoid venesection if possible
		Consider cautious low-dose iron

Cyanotic patients become more hypoxic during air travel as the partial pressure of oxygen in a pressurized aircraft is lower than that at sea level. However, such travel seems to be well tolerated and supplemental oxygen should not normally be necessary. Travellers should be warned to avoid dehydration and to plan their journeys to avoid having to carry baggage long distances within large airports.

Classification of congenital heart disease

A classification according to pathophysiological groups allows discussion of the basic physiological principles of congenital heart disease (Tables 5 and 6). A full morphological classification and discussion of segmental sequential analysis is beyond the scope of this chapter.

Specific lesions

Anomalies of pulmonary venous drainage

Total anomalous pulmonary venous drainage

Total anomalous pulmonary venous drainage occurs in 1 per 17 000 live-born babies. All four pulmonary veins drain into the right atrium either directly, or via a common vein into a systemic vein. The anomalous veins may follow:

(i) a supracardiac course draining to the superior vena cava, azygos, or brachiocephalic veins;

(ii) a cardiac course, draining to the right atrium directly or to the coronary sinus directly or via a persistent left superior vena cava connection; or

(iii) an infradiaphragmatic course, draining to the portal vein or inferior vena cava.

The presence of pulmonary venous obstruction is the most important predictor of a poor outcome. Associated anomalies include an obligatory right to left shunt, nearly always at atrial level.

The condition presents in infancy and 98 per cent of patients reaching the adolescent or adult clinic will have survived corrective surgery in early life. Unless there is residual pulmonary hypertension most such adults

should be asymptomatic, have a normal cardiovascular examination, and an excellent prognosis. In the long term, atrial arrhythmias may develop, probably with a similar incidence to that following repair of secundum atrial septal defect. Patients who are still growing may develop obstruction of the redirected pulmonary venous pathway and present with dyspnoea, signs of pulmonary oedema, evidence of pulmonary venous congestion on the chest radiograph, and an obstructive Doppler flow signal at the site of the stenosis.

The rare patient who reaches adulthood without an operation is likely to have survived because of a large atrial septal defect and unobstructed pulmonary venous drainage. They will be cyanosed, have developed pulmonary vascular disease, and be at risk of atrial tachyarrhythmias and right heart failure. The chest radiograph has the appearance of a large atrial septal defect with a small aortic knuckle, cardiomegaly, and a dilated main pulmonary artery. In addition the anomalous veins may cause an abnormal vascular shadow.

Partial anomalous pulmonary venous drainage

There is anomalous drainage of some of the pulmonary veins to the right atrium. In 90 per cent of cases the anomalous pulmonary venous connection is between the right upper or middle pulmonary vein to the superior vena cava or right atrium, usually in association with an atrial septal defect. Ten to fifteen per cent of all atrial septal defects and 80 to 90 per cent of superior vena cava-type sinus venosus atrial septal defects are associated with partial anomalous pulmonary venous connection.

Partial anomalous pulmonary venous drainage may present in adult life with signs of a left to right shunt at atrial level, and the pathophysiological consequences are the same as for an atrial septal defect with an equivalent shunt. When in coexistence with an atrial septal defect, the clinical findings of the two lesions are inseparable. If the atrial septum is intact, physiological splitting of the second heart sound enables anomalous venous drainage to be distinguished from atrial septal defect.

The chest radiograph may reveal the abnormally draining pulmonary vein. Transthoracic echocardiography may be indicative of a shunt at atrial level, but in adults it may not be possible to image the pulmonary veins and a transoesophageal approach is likely to be necessary. The identification of all the pulmonary veins is crucial in assessing the suitability of a secundum

Table 5 Acyanotic congenital cardiac lesions

No shunt			Left to right shunt	
	Site	Specific lesion	Level of shunt	Specific lesion
Left sided	LA inflow obstruction	Pulmonary vein stenosis	Atrial	ASD Partial anomalous pulmonary venous drainage (Lutembacher)
	LV inflow obstruction	Cor triatatrium, mitral stenosis		
	Left atrioventricular valve regurgitation	AVSD, cTGA, parachute mitral valve	Ventricular	VSD, AVSD
	LVOTO Aortic regurgitation	Subvalvar, valvar, supravalvar	Arterial	Coronary arteriovenous fistula, ruptured sinus of Valsalvar aneurysm, coronary artery from pulmonary artery
	Coarctation of the aorta			
Right sided	RV inflow obstruction	Tricuspid stenosis	Aortopulmonary	Aortopulmonary window, PDA
	Tricuspid regurgitation	Ebstein with intact interatrial septum		
	RVOTO	Infundibular, valvar, supravalvar	Multiple	AVSD, ASD and VSD, VSD and PDA
	Pulmonary regurgitation			

Key: see Table 6

Table 6 Cyanotic congenital cardiac lesions

Normal/↓ pulmonary blood flow		↑ Pulmonary blood flow		Potential for shunt reversal due to development of pulmonary vascular disease	
Level of shunt	Specific lesion	Level of shunt	Specific lesion	Level of shunt	Specific lesion
Atrial	Ebstein with PFO, Severe PS with PFO, SVC to LA, Unroofed coronary sinus	Atrial	Unoperated TAPVD, Common atrium	Atrial	ASD (rare)
Ventricular, with obstruction to pulmonary blood flow	Tetralogy of Fallot, DORV with PS	Ventricular, no obstruction to pulmonary blood flow	DORV (Taussig–Bing)	Ventricular	Any non-restrictive VSD and no PS including: AVSD, univentricular heart, TGA with VSD
Complete mixing with obstruction to pulmonary blood flow	Fallot with pulmonary atresia, TGA with PS, Univentricular heart with PS	Complete mixing, no obstruction to pulmonary blood flow	Fallot with pulmonary atresia and large collaterals, TGA no PS, Univentricular heart with no PS, HPLHS, Truncus arteriosus	Arterial	Truncus arteriosus PDA Aortopulmonary window Fallot with pulmonary atresia and large aortopulmonary collaterals
Pulmonary AVM	HHT Cirrhosis, Late complication of Glenn anastomosis				

Key to Tables 5 and 6: ASD, atrial septal defect; AVM, arteriovenous malformation; AVSD, atrioventricular septal defect; CTGA, congenitally corrected transposition; DORV, double-outlet right ventricle; HHT, hereditary haemorrhagic telangectasia; HPLHS, hypoplastic left heart syndrome; LA, left atrium; LV, left ventricle; LVOTO, left ventricular outflow tract obstruction; PAPVD ?; PFO, patent foramen ovale; PDA, persistent ductus arteriosus; PS, pulmonary stenosis; RV, right ventricle; RVOTO, right ventricular outflow tract obstruction; SVC, superior vena cava; TAPVD, total anomalous pulmonary venous drainage; TGA, transposition of the great arteries; VSD, ventricular septal defect.

atrial septal defect for transcatheter device closure, this technique being contraindicated in the presence of anomalous pulmonary veins (see later).

The indications for surgical repair are the same as those for repair of an atrial septal defect. In the most common variant of right pulmonary venous connection to the superior vena cava in association with a sinus venosus defect, the patch closing the atrial septal defect is placed to direct the anomalous vein into the left atrium.

Scimitar syndrome (Fig. 3)

Partial anomalous pulmonary venous drainage also occurs as part of the rare familial 'scimitar syndrome' in which part or all of the right pulmonary venous drainage is to the inferior vena cava below the diaphragm. The affected lung lobes are usually hypoplastic and are supplied with arterial blood from the descending aorta. Recurrent infection and bronchiectasis may develop in the hypoplastic lung. Magnetic resonance imaging demonstrates the abnormal arterial supply and venous drainage of the affected lung segment, and may obviate the need for diagnostic cardiac catheterization. Surgical repair may be complicated by difficulty in maintaining perfusion to the affected lung, and lobectomy may by required. In view of this it should be remembered that patients presenting with scimitar syndrome for the first time in adult life have a good prognosis without an operation, similar to that of a small atrial septal defect.

Anomalies of systemic venous drainage

These anomalies frequently form part of a more complex lesion, particularly atrial isomerism.

Superior caval vein anomalies (Fig. 4)

A persistent left-sided superior vena cava occurs in 0.3 per cent of the general population, around 3 per cent of patients with congenital heart disease, and 15 per cent of those with tetralogy of Fallot. The left superior vena cava

may be visible on the chest radiograph; it drains to the right atrium via the coronary sinus which is seen to be dilated on two-dimensional echocardiography. A right-sided superior vena cava is usually also present and the two cavae do not usually communicate via the brachiocephalic vein. This common anomaly should be sought routinely at cardiac catheterization; although it does not have any haemodynamic significance, it may cause technical difficulties during transvenous pacemaker insertion and cardiac surgery (Fig. 5).

Other superior vena cava anomalies are the following.

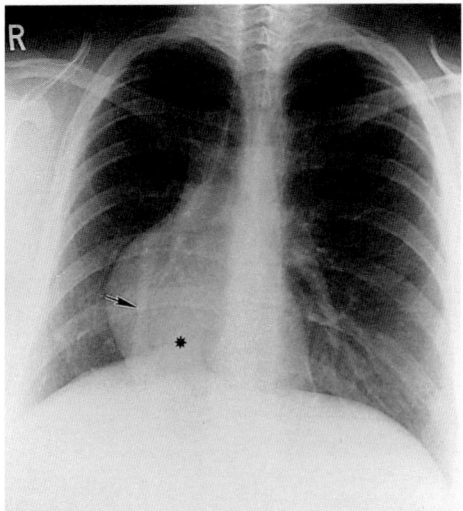

Fig. 3 Chest radiograph of a 25-year-old woman with scimitar syndrome. The heart is shifted into the right hemithorax because the right lung is small. The 'scimitar' shadow (arrow) is produced by the anomalous descending venous channel which drains into the dilated inferior vena cava(*).

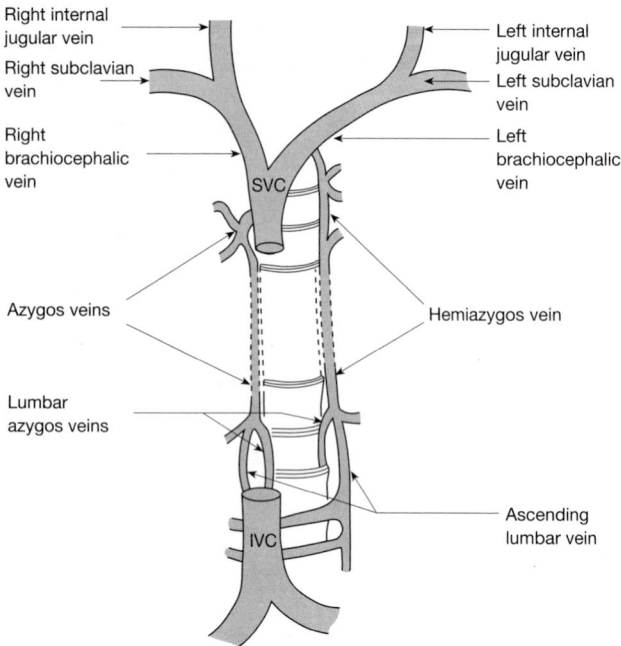

Right internal jugular vein
Right subclavian vein
Right brachiocephalic vein
SVC
Left internal jugular vein
Left subclavian vein
Left brachiocephalic vein
Azygos veins
Hemiazygos vein
Lumbar azygos veins
IVC
Ascending lumbar vein

Fig. 4 Schematic diagram of normal systemic venous drainage.

1. An absent right superior vena cava is associated with arrhythmias including atrioventricular block, sinus node dysfunction, and atrial fibrillation.

2. The left, or rarely the right superior vena cava may connect directly to the left atrium, causing an obligatory right to left shunt and cyanosis. It is associated with isomerism of the atrial appendages.

Inferior caval vein anomalies

Azygos continuation of the inferior vena cava occurs in 0.6 per cent of patients with congenital heart disease. The infrahepatic portion of the inferior vena cava is absent and continues to the superior vena cava via an azygos vein; the hepatic veins drain directly into the right atrium. It is often associated with complex lesions, particularly left atrial isomerism. The chest radiograph reveals an absence of the inferior vena cava at the junction of the diaphragm with the right heart border and a dilated azygos vein

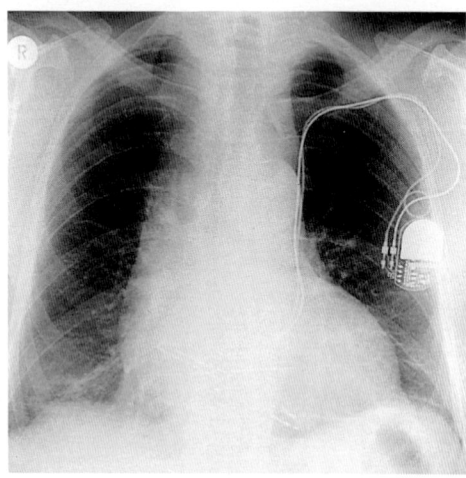

Fig. 5 Chest radiograph of a 56-year-old man with bicuspid aortic valve, aortic regurgitation, and coarctation. A left superior vena cava draining via the coronary sinus to the right atrium is marked by the path taken by the transvenous pacing leads, inserted for complete heart block.

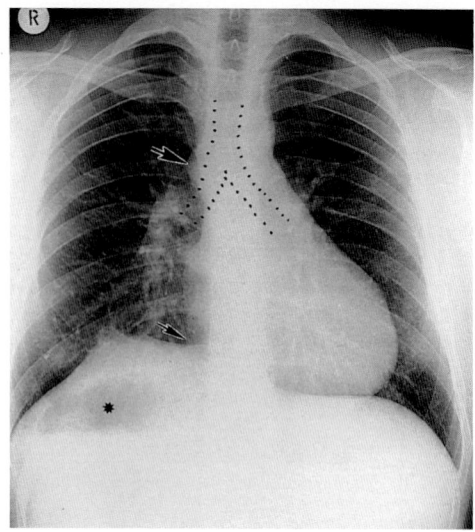

Fig. 6 Chest radiograph of a 50-year-old man with abdominal situs inversus (*) and laevocardia. Left atrial isomerism is inferred from the symmetrical long bronchi. The inferior vena cava is absent at the level of the diaphragm (small arrow), and the azygos vein receiving inferior caval venous blood is prominent (large arrow).

(Fig. 6). Direct connection of the inferior vena cava to the left atrium is rare; the patient is cyanosed, as in the superior vena cava to left atrium connection.

Atrial arrangement and isomerism of the atrial appendages

Atrial situs solitus is the term used to describe normal atrial arrangement, that is, a right atrium with right-sided morphology and a left atrium with left-sided morphology. Atrial situs inversus is a mirror image arrangement: the right-sided atrium has left morphology and that on the left is a morphological right atrium. The term isomerism refers to abnormal symmetry of paired structures which are normally asymmetrical and have laterality. In right isomerism, both atrial appendages are of right morphology; both are of left morphology in left isomerism. A full description is beyond the scope of this book, but the major features of different atrial arrangements are outlined in Table 7 and illustrated in Figs 6 and 7.

The key for the physician is to be alerted by the presence of isomerism to the coexistence of complex associated lesions, including a variety of abnormalities of venous connections which may cause technical difficulties at cardiac catheterization and permanent pacemaker insertion. Right isomerism is commoner in males and left in females. Survival to adulthood with right isomerism is uncommon because of associated asplenia and severe cyanotic heart disease, including obstructed anomalous pulmonary venous drainage (the pulmonary venous confluence is a left atrial structure), complete transposition of the great arteries, atrial septal defect, atrioventricular septal defect, absent coronary sinus (a left atrial structure), severe pulmonary stenosis or atresia, and univentricular heart. The lesions associated with left isomerism tend to produce left to right shunts and little if any cyanosis. They include atrioventricular block, atrioventricular septal defect, common atrium, and left ventricular outflow tract obstruction.

Atrial septal defects

Atrial septal defects account for approximately 10 per cent of congenital heart disease. The exact figure depends on the definition of atrial septal defect, since small or probe-patent foramen ovale occurs in around 10 per cent of the population. The sites of the various types of atrial septal defect are shown in Fig. 8.

Ostium secundum atrial septal defect

Secundum atrial septal defect accounts for 40 per cent of left to rights shunts in adults over 40 years of age. It is commoner in females, with a sex ratio of 2:1, and may be familial. Atrial septal defect may be an incidental finding in a geriatric patient at autopsy and diagnosis in life may be delayed well into adulthood because of the absence of symptoms and subtlety of clinical signs. However, the natural history of this lesion is not benign, only 50 per cent of those with non-restrictive atrial septal defects surviving without operation to the age of 40 years, and 10 per cent beyond 60 years of age.

Presentation in adulthood may be with symptoms or as a result of incidental clinical or radiographic findings. Patients over the age of 30 years with unrepaired atrial septal defect commonly develop paroxysmal and eventually chronic atrial arrhythmia, but also flutter and ectopic atrial tachycardia. Most patients over the age of 60 years are symptomatic with exertional dyspnoea and palpitation. A left to right shunt at atrial level predisposes to paradoxical embolus since simple manoeuvres such as the Valsalva are sufficient to increase right atrial pressure and reverse the shunt. Patients with unoperated atrial septal defect are therefore at risk of embolic stroke, and should not dive because of the risk of paradoxical gas embolism. An age-related reduction in left ventricular compliance augments the left to right shunt and is one of the causes for the progression of symptoms with age. In addition, modest pulmonary arterial hypertension increases with age so the right ventricle is exposed to pressure as well as volume overload and may eventually fail.

Clinical signs

If the defect is non-restrictive, the a and v waves of the jugular venous pulse tend to be equal. In older patients with reduced left ventricular compliance, the left and therefore right atrial pressure is raised, reflected in an elevated jugular venous pressure. A right ventricular heave may be felt at the left sternal border and the dilated pulmonary artery may be palpable in the left second intercostal space. The first sound is loud due to increased diastolic flow across the tricuspid valve. The second heart sound is widely split and fixed, and there is loss of normal sinus arrhythmia if the left to right shunt is equal to 2:1 or greater. There may be a pulmonary flow murmur at the upper left sternal edge. Only if the atrial septal defect has a high gradient across it will it generate a murmur itself, usually a soft continuous murmur. This is the case if the defect is small and restrictive and the left atrial pressure high, for example if there is associated mitral stenosis. If the patient has pulmonary vascular disease, the signs will be the same as for pulmonary hypertension with right to left shunt (see above).

Associations

Acquired disease may coexist and interact with congenital heart disease, especially in the ageing patient. Left ventricular dysfunction due to coronary artery disease and systemic hypertension may increase the left to right interatrial shunt, resulting in a more rapid clinical deterioration than would be expected. Similarly, mitral regurgitation increases the effective interatrial shunt and mitral valve abnormalities may be acquired secondary to the effects of a secundum atrial septal defect. There may be distortion of the anterior mitral valve leaflet with fibrotic shortened chordae due to the abnormal position of the interventricular septum as a result of chronic right ventricular overload. Concomitant pulmonary stenosis may be overestimated in the presence of an atrial septal defect, since Doppler velocities are increased in the presence of a left to right shunt.

Lutembacher's syndrome is the association of mitral stenosis with secundum atrial septal defect. The presence of mitral stenosis increases the left to right shunt at atrial level, causing an overestimation of the significance of the atrial septal defect and an underestimation of the severity of mitral

Table 7 Diagnosis of atrial arrangement

	Atrial situs solitus	Atrial situs inversus	Right isomerism	Left isomerism
Atrial morphology	Normal: R-sided morphological RA, L-sided morphological LA	Mirror image: R-sided morphological LA, L-sided morphological RA	Bilateral morphological RA, extensive pectinate muscles	Bilateral morphological LA, pectinate muscles confined to appendages
Atrial appendages*	Normal: Broad-based RA appendage, long narrow LA appendage	Mirror image	Bilateral broad-based RA appendages	Bilateral long narrow LA appendages
Sinus node	Single, R-sided	Single, L-sided	Bilateral	Absent
Pulmonary morphology	R lung trilobed L lung bilobed	R lung bilobed L lung trilobed	Bilateral trilobed lungs	Bilateral bilobed lungs
Bronchial morphology**	R-sided main bronchus: short, morphological R L-sided main bronchus: long, morphological L	Mirror image	Bilateral short morphological R bronchi	Bilateral long morphological L bronchi
Abdominal arrangement***				
Aorta IVC	To L of spine To R of spine	Normal or mirror image	Aorta and IVC on same side; IVC anterior to aorta	Aorta and azygos on same side; azygos posterior to aorta
Stomach Liver Spleen	L-sided R-sided R-sided	Normal or mirror image	Usually L-sided Midline Usually absent	Usually R-sided Midline Often polysplenia

IVC, inferior vena cava; L, left; LA, left atrium; R right; RA, right atrium; SVC, superior vena cava

*Readily identified on transoesophageal echocardiography.

**Since bronchopulmonary situs nearly always follows atrial situs, atrial situs can be inferred from the chest radiograph.

***Echocardiography shows the intra-abdominal relations of the great vessels. In left isomerism, there is usually interruption of the IVC, and the abdominal venous return connects to the heart via a (right-sided) azygos or (left-sided) hemiazygos vein. The hepatic veins can be identified draining separately into the atria.

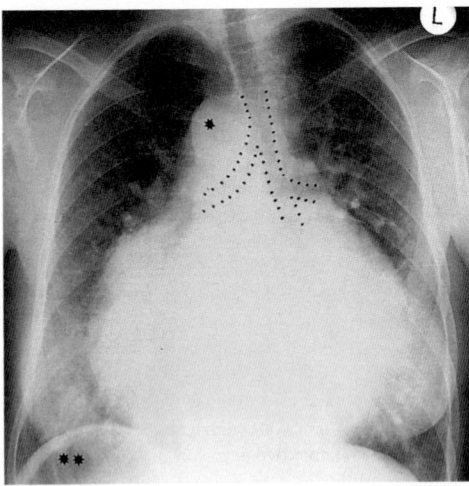

Fig. 7 Chest radiograph of a 21-year-old woman with abdominal situs inversus (**), bronchial and inferred atrial situs inversus, mesocardia, and right aortic arch (*). She has tetralogy of Fallot with pulmonary atresia, palliated with an aortopulmonary shunt via a left thoracotomy.

stenosis. Repair of the atrial septal defect alone may unmask severe mitral stenosis.

Pulmonary vascular disease and atrial septal defect

Only around 10 per cent of atrial septal defects develop a right to left shunt secondary to pulmonary vascular disease, and a causal relationship between atrial septal defect and the Eisenmenger reaction remains controversial. In atrial septal defect, unlike other lesions which may cause the Eisenmenger reaction such as large ventricular septal defect, the pulmonary vasculature is not exposed to increased flow at systemic pressure.

Atrial septal defect with a right to left shunt due to pulmonary vascular disease and pulmonary hypertension occurs most commonly in young women and in some cases may be due to primary pulmonary hypertension with an incidental atrial septal defect. In this combination, the prognosis may be better than for primary pulmonary hypertension with intact atrial septum, the septal defect protecting the right heart from pressure overload by allowing right to left shunting. Persistence of the fetal pulmonary vascular pattern may be implicated in the development of pulmonary hypertension in some young patients with atrial septal defect. Patients living or born at high altitude have a higher incidence of pulmonary vascular disease. In older patients with atrial septal defect there may be a relationship with *in situ* pulmonary arterial thrombosis and the development of pulmonary hypertension.

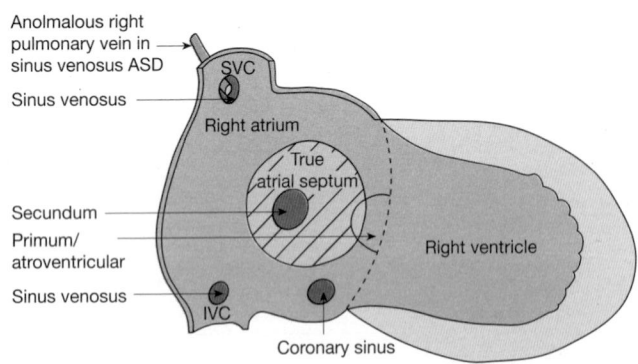

Fig. 8 Sites of atrial septal defects. The shaded area delineates the true atrial septum. Sinus venosus and coronary sinus defects are therefore not strictly atrial septal defects although they permit shunting at atrial level.

Investigations

The electrocardiogram may show sinus node dysfunction and, less commonly, prolongation of the P–R interval. The QRS axis is usually vertical. The QRS complex may be prolonged with rSr' in lead V1: this does not represent incomplete right bundle branch block, but occurs because the last part of the myocardium to depolarize is the right ventricular outflow tract, which is enlarged and thickened due to volume overload. The sinus node may be damaged when the superior vena cava is cannulated during surgery: occasionally perioperative sinus bradycardia and sinus pauses persist and a permanent pacemaker is required. The P–R interval may return to normal as right atrial size decreases. Macro-reentry circuits at the site of atrial surgery may result in postoperative ectopic atrial tachycardias.

The typical chest radiograph shows dilated proximal pulmonary arteries with a small aortic knuckle, plethoric lung fields, and cardiomegaly secondary to dilatation of the right atrium and ventricle.

Transthoracic echocardiography demonstrates the volume overloaded right atrium and ventricle. The size of the shunt can be estimated and colour flow Doppler facilitates the detection of the site of the shunt. If transcatheter device closure is considered, a transoesophageal approach is necessary to define the site and size of the atrial septal defect precisely and to identify the pulmonary veins.

Cardiac catheterization is only indicated to calculate pulmonary vascular resistance if there is a suspicion of pulmonary hypertension, or to exclude coexisting congenital or acquired cardiac pathology such as coronary artery disease.

Indications for closure of atrial septal defect

Surgical repair carries low mortality and morbidity. However, vigilance is required to detect postoperative pericardial effusions, which appear to be more common than following other operations. Closure of an atrial septal defect is indicated if there is exertional dyspnoea, if the left to right shunt is greater than 1.5:1, if there is right heart volume overload, or in order to prevent recurrent paradoxical embolism. Repair of an isolated secundum atrial septal defect by the third decade results in a normal life expectancy, between the ages of 25 and 41 years it results in a good but shorter than normal life expectancy, and beyond the age of 41 years, morbidity and mortality remain significantly higher than normal. None the less, functional status and longevity are improved following repair over the age of 40 years, 5- and 10-year survival being estimated as 98 and 95 per cent, respectively, for patients who underwent repair, and 93 and 84 per cent for those treated medically. Surgical repair in older patients does not reduce the risk of late atrial arrhythmia, particularly if there is right ventricular dysfunction, elevated pulmonary artery pressure, or pre-existing atrial arrhythmia. Whether the incorporation of a modified maze procedure or cryoablation into the surgical repair of atrial septal defect will reduce the long-term incidence of existing or *de novo* atrial arrhythmia remains to be determined.

Secundum atrial septal defects up to 3 cm in stretched diameter may be closed by transcatheter devices as long as the surrounding rim of atrial septal tissue is sufficient. Criteria for device closure of secundum atrial septal defect are: size less than 3 cm; a situation away from the atrioventricular valves, pulmonary and caval veins; and normal pulmonary venous drainage. Following closure, antiplatelet or anticoagulant therapy is recommended for 3 months. Device closure is the procedure of choice for patent foramen ovale complicated by paradoxical embolism.

Sinus venosus defect

Sinus venosus defects account for 2 to 3 per cent of atrial septal defects and have an equal sex incidence.

They are not truly defects of the atrial septum, but since they allow shunting at atrial level, they are included in the classification of atrial septal defects. The inferior border of the more common superior vena cava type of sinus venosus defect is made by the superior limbus of the fossa ovalis, and the upper border comprises the junction of the superior vena cava with the atrial mass. The superior caval vein overrides the atrial septum, connecting to both atria, and the right upper pulmonary vein usually drains anomalously into the superior vena cava. There may be an ectopic atrial pacemaker because the defect is located in the area of the sinoatrial node. This may be reflected by a leftwards p-wave axis and an inverted p wave in lead III.

Coronary sinus defect

The rarest form of atrial septal defect, this defect is at the site of entry of the coronary sinus to the right atrium. The unroofed coronary sinus is a variation of coronary sinus defect in which the partition between the coronary sinus and the left atrium is absent as the coronary sinus runs posteriorly along the floor of the left atrium. In this condition, a left superior vena cava commonly connects directly to the left atrium, producing a right to left shunt and cyanosis.

Atrioventricular septal defect

The sites of ostium primum and atrioventricular septal defects are shown in Fig. 8, and the leaflet patterns in atrioventricular septal defects in Fig. 9.

Ostium primum defect describes the atrial component of the atrioventricular septal defect, previously termed endocardial cushion defect or atrioventricular canal. The atrioventricular septum is absent and the atrioventricular valves share a common junction and fibrous ring, with a five leaflet atrioventricular valve. Since they share common leaflets, the valves are not correctly called mitral and tricuspid valves, but left and right atrioventricular valves. As a consequence the normal offsetting of the right atrioventricular valve towards the right ventricular apex is absent. In addition, the aorta is 'unwedged' from its normal position between the left and right atrioventricular valves, with loss of the normal fibrous continuity between the 'mitral' and aortic valves. The left ventricular outflow tract is therefore elongated ('gooseneck') and has the propensity to develop obstruction. 'Cleft mitral valve' refers to the commissure between the anterior and posterior bridging leaflets which renders the left atrioventricular valve potentially regurgitant. The left ventricular papillary muscles are abnormally placed anteriorly and posteriorly instead of in the normal anterolateral and posteromedial positions. A partial atrioventricular septal defect has a common atrioventricular junction, but the right and left atrioventricular valves have separate orifices and the ventricular component of the defect is usually small or absent. There are both a common atrioventricular junction and a common valve orifice in a complete atrioventricular septal defect, and the ventricular component of the defect is usually large.

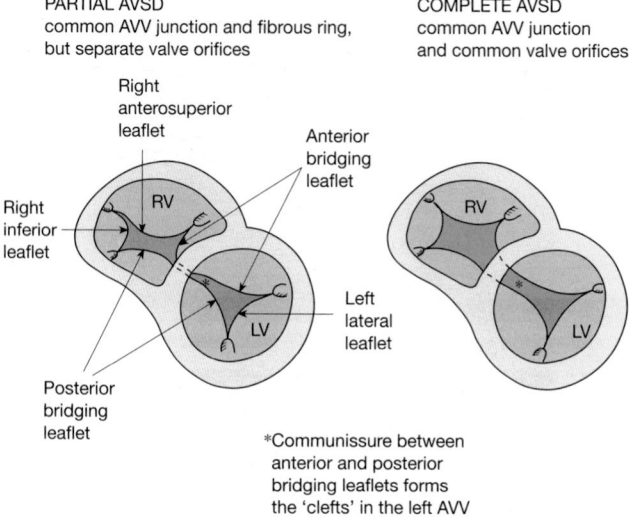

PARTIAL AVSD
common AVV junction and fibrous ring, but separate valve orifices

COMPLETE AVSD
common AVV junction and common valve orifices

Right anterosuperior leaflet

Anterior bridging leaflet

Right inferior leaflet

RV

RV

Left lateral leaflet

LV

LV

Posterior bridging leaflet

*Communissure between anterior and posterior bridging leaflets forms the 'clefts' in the left AVV

Fig. 9 Leaflet patterns in atrioventricular septal defect. Diagrams are in short axis, as imaged by two-dimensional echocardiography. (Modified from Anderson RH et al., 1983, *Morphology of congenital heart disease*. University Park Press, Baltimore.)

Atrioventricular septal defect occurs with equal sex incidence. The complete form of the defect is most commonly associated with Down's syndrome. A single gene defect may be responsible for atrioventricular septal defect with normal chromosomes; the recurrence risk is high: around 10 per cent if the mother has an atrioventricular septal defect, less if the father is affected.

The physiological consequences of an atrioventricular septal defect are the same as for other conditions with left to right shunting at atrial or ventricular level, but may be complicated by left atrioventricular valve regurgitation or left ventricular outflow tract obstruction. If the ventricular septal defect is large and non-restrictive, pulmonary vascular disease may develop. Patients with Down's syndrome are at particular risk of this complication; coexisting upper airway obstruction and sleep apnoea, and abnormal pulmonary parenchyma may be contributory factors.

Investigations

The electrocardiogram is distinctive, with a left and superior QRS axis and notching of S waves in the inferior leads. The chest radiograph appearances depend on the degree of interatrial shunting and left atrioventricular valve regurgitation; the former producing cardiomegaly due to left heart dilatation and the latter, left atrial enlargement. There may be increased pulmonary vascularity, particularly in young patients with complete atrioventricular septal defect and high pulmonary blood flow. Transthoracic echocardiography reveals the detailed anatomy of the defect and establishes the site and degree of shunting, the presence of left ventricular outflow tract obstruction, and the function and anatomy of the atrioventricular valves, including the classic 'fish mouth' deformity of the left atrioventricular valve during diastole. The indications for cardiac catheterization are the same as for secundum atrial septal defect, namely to exclude inoperable pulmonary vascular disease. In addition, useful information may be obtained regarding the severity of left atrioventricular valve regurgitation and left ventricular outflow tract obstruction.

Clinical course

First presentation may occur in adulthood if the left to right shunt is small and the left atrioventricular valve is competent. Physical signs are the same as in other atrial septal defects: there may also be an apical pansystolic murmur. Paradoxical embolism is less common than in secundum atrial septal defect, since the position of the primum defect low in the interatrial septum avoids the streaming of inferior vena cava blood which is most likely to carry emboli and is directed towards the mid-portion of the septum.

Most adult patients have undergone surgery to repair the defect and left atrioventricular valve. Others have survived without an operation and may have developed pulmonary vascular disease.

Whether or not it has previously been repaired, the abnormal left atrioventricular valve may become regurgitant in later life, particularly in response to changes in the left ventricle due to ageing, ischaemia, or systemic hypertension. The risk of endocarditis relates largely to the abnormal left atrioventricular valve. Atrial arrhythmias occur in the same way as in secundum atrial septal defect, however there is a higher incidence of postoperative atrioventricular block in atrioventricular septal defect because of the proximity of the atrioventricular node to the site of repair.

Lesions affecting ventricular inflow

Cor triatriatum

This is a very rare defect in which one of the atria (nearly always the left) is partitioned by a fibromuscular membrane into an upper chamber that receives the pulmonary veins, and a lower chamber connecting with the atrial appendage and mitral valve. The membrane usually inserts into the atrial septum at the fossa ovalis, where an atrial septal defect coexists in around 50 per cent of cases, allowing communication between the right and left atria. The membrane may be intact, or pierced by one or more holes that are usually restrictive, causing supramitral stenosis. First presentation in adulthood is unusual unless the membrane is non-restrictive or coexists with a large atrial septal defect. Patients may have signs of an atrial septal defect or mitral stenosis. The diagnosis is made by echocardiography. The chest radiograph is also characteristic, showing signs of pulmonary venous congestion, but not the left atrial appendage enlargement that accompanies valvar mitral stenosis, since the appendage lies in the low pressure atrial chamber. The lateral chest radiograph may show enlargement of the pulmonary venous compartment of the left atrium. Treatment is surgical resection and the postoperative prognosis is good.

Congenital mitral valve anomalies

These anomalies are rare and frequently coexist with other lesions. A supramitral ring often coexists with congenital mitral stenosis. It differs from cor triatatrium in that the ring is sited inferiorly to the os of the appendage and lies immediately above the mitral valve.

Shone syndrome comprises four levels of left heart obstruction: supramitral ring, parachute mitral valve, subaortic stenosis, and coarctation of the aorta. Parachute mitral valve exists when the two papillary muscles are fused or there is hypoplasia or absence of one papillary muscle; the valve and its apparatus are often additionally dysplastic. Obstruction occurs at the level of the abnormal papillary muscles. The parachute mitral valve may also be regurgitant if the chordae are elongated and not significantly fused.

Isolated cleft mitral valve differs from the 'cleft' seen in an atrioventricular septal defect in being in the anterior (aortic) leaflet, directed towards the aortic outflow tract, rather than being in the space between the bridging leaflets and pointing towards the septum. The isolated cleft can be readily repaired to resemble a competent normal mitral valve.

Ebstein's anomaly of the tricuspid valve

This rare condition occurs in 1 per 20 000 live-born babies and affects both sexes equally. The risk may be increased by maternal exposure to lithium during the first trimester. In the normal heart, the mitral and tricuspid valves are offset so that the tricuspid valve is displaced up to 1.5 cm towards the right ventricular apex. In Ebstein's anomaly, the anterior leaflet usually inserts normally at the atrioventricular junction, but the attachments of the septal and sometimes mural (posterior) leaflets are apically displaced, causing atrialization of the proximal part of the right ventricle and reducing the size of the functional right ventricle. In addition the movement of the septal and mural leaflets is usually limited either by being thickened and fibrotic, or by being tethered by short chordae to the septum. The major haemodynamic effect is usually tricuspid regurgitation, but occasionally a muscular shelf or fused anteromedial commissure causes tricuspid stenosis.

Associated abnormalities

A patent foramen ovale or atrial septal defect is present in most cases. Left heart abnormalities occur as a consequence of alterations in left ventricular geometry due to leftwards displacement of the interventricular septum: for example, mitral valve prolapse may occur as a result of relatively long chordae in a left ventricle of reduced cavity size. Twenty per cent of patients have coexistent Wolff–Parkinson–White syndrome, usually with a right-sided or multiple pathway(s).

Clinical presentation and course

There is a broad spectrum of severity, ranging from intrauterine death to presentation in late adulthood. Mortality is influenced by age at presentation, the condition of the tricuspid valve, the cardiac rhythm, and the functional capacity of the right ventricle, including the severity of right ventricular outflow tract obstruction and the size of the right atrium in relation to the other cardiac chambers.

Cyanosis may develop in adulthood if there is an associated atrial septal defect or patent foramen ovale; as the right ventricular filling pressure increases there is a parallel rise in right atrial pressure, and a right to left interatrial shunt is established. These patients are at risk of paradoxical embolism. The risk of endocarditis is low, because the tricuspid regurgitant jet is of low velocity.

Heart failure may intervene as a result of the combination of severe tricuspid regurgitation and the onset of atrial fibrillation or flutter. These atrial arrhythmias may be particularly troublesome if a coexistent accessory pathway allows a rapid ventricular response rate. The onset of atrial fibrillation is a predictor of death within 5 years, and may account for the increased death rate in the fifth decade.

Physical signs

The patient may be acyanotic or cyanosed and clubbed. Even when tricuspid regurgitation is severe the jugular venous pressure may not be particularly high, nor the v wave prominent, because of the capacity of the right atrium and thin-walled atrialized right ventricle to accommodate the low pressure regurgitant volume. Once right ventricular failure develops the jugular venous pressure rises further and the a and v waves become more prominent. In the uncommon situation of tricuspid stenosis, the a wave is increased and may be giant. The first heart sound is widely split with a delayed tricuspid component, due to the extra distance that the large anterior leaflet has to travel to reach the limit of its systolic excursion. The second heart sound may be single because low pressure in the right ventricular outflow tract renders the pulmonary component inaudible, or it may be widely split reflecting right bundle branch block. The systolic murmur of tricuspid regurgitation varies from inaudible to loud enough to generate a thrill, but is classically decrescendo and scratchy.

Investigations

The chest radiograph is characteristic (Fig. 10). The electrocardiogram typically shows a superior axis and right atrial enlargement, with or without right bundle branch block. The p wave may be peaked and the P–R interval prolonged, reflecting the prolonged conduction in the large right atrium, or there may be evidence of pre-excitation. Right bundle branch block may occur due to abnormal activation and conduction in the atrialized right ventricle.

Two-dimensional echocardiography with colour flow Doppler establishes the diagnosis and severity of Ebstein's anomaly. The atrialized and functional portions of the right ventricle can be identified, as can the precise attachments and degree of tethering of the anterior leaflet of the tricuspid valve. Echocardiography is the investigation of choice in planning surgical intervention, tethering and restricted motion of the anterior leaflet and a small right ventricle being strong predictors of the need for tricuspid

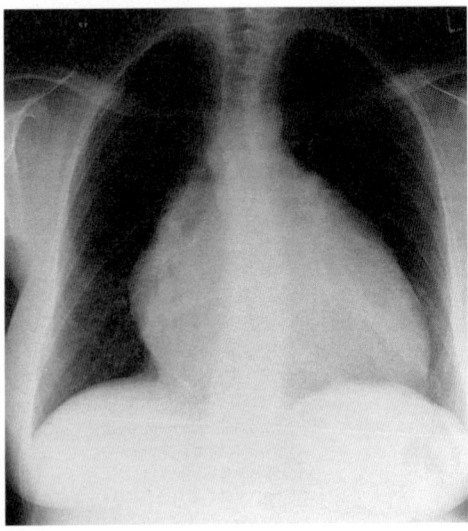

Fig. 10 Chest radiograph of a 43-year-old woman with classic cardiac silhouette of Ebstein's anomaly due to right atrial enlargement. The aortic knuckle and pulmonary arteries are inconspicuous and the lung fields oligaemic.

Table 8 Right ventricular dysplasia and Uhl's anomaly

	Arrhythmogenic right ventricular dysplasia	Uhl's anomaly 'Parchment heart'
Morphology	Patchy, localized fibrofatty replacement of parietal myocardium mostly affecting outflow tract. Other parts of right and occasionally left ventricle may be involved	Congenital absence of parietal ventricular myocardium with direct apposition of endocardium and epicardium. Normal interventricular septum and left ventricle
Sex ratio	2:1 male:female	Equal
Typical presentation	As young adult Exercise-induced ventricular tachycardia: palpitation, syncope, sudden death	In infancy Congestive cardiac failure

valve replacement rather than repair. Cardiac catheterization is only necessary if specific haemodynamic questions remain after non-invasive assessment.

Treatment

Once atrial arrhythmias develop, patients should be anticoagulated, particularly if there is an atrial septal defect. If re-entry tachycardias cannot be controlled with antiarrhythmic drugs, radiofrequency ablation of accessory pathways may be performed. However, ablation may be made difficult by the size and abnormal shape of the right atrium and abnormal position of the accessory pathway or pathways.

Surgery is indicated when the patient's clinical status deteriorates and aims to reduce the size of the right atrium and repair the tricuspid valve so that valve function and right ventricular geometry are improved. The best haemodynamic results are achieved if the valve can be repaired rather than replaced. The addition of a right-sided maze procedure may reduce the long-term risk of developing atrial fibrillation. In a subset of patients with a small right ventricle, the addition of a bidirectional Glenn anastomosis to offload the ventricle may facilitate repair.

Other right ventricular anomalies

Uhl's anomaly and arrhythmogenic right ventricular dysplasia (right ventricular cardiomyopathy) are rare sporadic or familial conditions affecting the right ventricle. Table 8 lists the key distinguishing features.

Ventricular septal defect

With the exceptions of bicuspid aortic valve and mitral valve prolapse, ventricular septal defect is the commonest congenital cardiac malformation, occurring in around 3 per 1000 live-born babies. Defects may exist in isolation, in association with other lesions such as coarctation of the aorta, or as an integral part of lesions such as tetralogy of Fallot. This section deals with isolated ventricular septal defects.

Morphology and classification

The ventricular septum is mostly muscular, with a small fibrous membranous portion. Ventricular septal defects are classified according to their borders, seen from the right ventricular aspect. There are three types: muscular, perimembranous, and doubly committed subarterial (Table 9). The position of muscular and perimembranous ventricular septal defects may be inlet, trabecular, or outlet, depending on which part of the right ventricle they open into.

Perimembranous ventricular septal defect is the commonest type of defect, only 5 to 7 per cent of ventricular septal defects in Europe and North America are doubly committed subarterial defects, whereas they account for up to 30 per cent of defects in Asian patients. Outlet perimembranous ventricular septal defects usually occur due to a malalignment between the outlet and trabecular septa with overriding of either the aortic or pulmonary valve. If the malalignment of the outlet septum is towards the right ventricle, the aorta overrides the defect and tends to cause subpulmonary obstruction; this is the type of defect typical of tetralogy of Fallot. Malalignment towards the left ventricle may cause subaortic obstruction and may be associated with hypoplasia of the aortic arch.

Clinical presentation and complications of unoperated ventricular septal defect

The grades of unoperated ventricular septal defect are shown in Table 10. Adults with unoperated restrictive ventricular septal defects are usually asymptomatic. There is a high risk of endocarditis in small ventricular septal defects due to the high velocity jet from left to right ventricle, particularly if the jet is directed on to the tricuspid valve. There is a small increased incidence of sudden death and ventricular tachycardia in unoperated small ventricular septal defect, but longevity is otherwise normal. The adult with an isolated unoperated restrictive ventricular septal defect is acyanotic with normal arterial and jugular venous pulses. There may be a thrill at the left sternal border, the left ventricular apex may be thrusting if the defect is large enough to cause volume overload, and a dilated pulmonary artery

Table 9 Types of ventricular septal defect

	Muscular	Perimembranous	Doubly committed subarterial
Border	Entirely muscular	Part muscle, posteroinferior border formed by fibrous tissue between valve leaflets, and by membranous septum	Roof formed by aortic and/or pulmonary valves in fibrous continuity owing to absence of subpulmonary infundibulum and outlet septum. Posteroinferior border may be muscular or fibrous
Conduction tissue	Remote from defect	Runs in posteroinferior border making it vulnerable to damage at operation	Vulnerable to damage if fibrous posteroinferior border, protected if muscular posteroinferior border
Spontaneous closure	Up to 50 per cent, usually by 3 years, but can close into adult life	Inlet defects may be closed by tricuspid valve tissue	May be closed by prolapse of aortic leaflet causing aortic regurgitation
Relation to aortic valve	No direct relation	If superior border formed by aortic valve, cusp may prolapse into defect causing aortic regurgitation	Aortic valve may prolapse into defect causing aortic regurgitation

Table 10 Grading of ventricular septal defects

	Small	Moderate	Large	Eisenmenger syndrome
Haemodynamic grading				
Pulmonary artery pressure:systemic pressure ratio	< 0.3	> 0.3	> 0.3	> 0.9
Qp:Qs	< 1.4:1	1.4–2.2:1	> 2.2:1	< 1.5:1
Clinical grading	Negligible haemodynamic changes, normal LV	LV enlargement and reversible pulmonary hypertension	Pulmonary vascular disease (Eisenmenger syndrome) will develop unless there is RVOTO.	
	Restrictive (RV pressure < LV pressure in absence of RVOTO)		Non-restrictive (equal RV and LV pressures in absence of RVOTO)	

LV, left ventricle; RV, right ventricle; RVOTO, right ventricular outflow tract obstruction.

may be palpable. The second heart sound is usually normally split. There is a loud harsh pansystolic murmur at the left sternal edge; the murmur being softer and shorter (early systolic) in very small defects.

Larger ventricular septal defects rarely present for repair in adulthood since the large left to right shunt is unlikely to allow unoperated survival unless pulmonary vascular disease developed. Non-restrictive defects are not associated with the classic ventricular septal defect murmur since left and right ventricular pressures are equal.

Investigations

Investigation should determine the type and number of ventricular septal defects, the size of the defect (restrictive or non-restrictive), estimate the size of the shunt (Qp:Qs), pulmonary artery pressure and resistance, and assess left and right ventricular function, and volume and pressure overload. Associated lesions that may alter management should be identified, especially aortic regurgitation, subaortic stenosis, and right ventricular outflow tract obstruction.

The chest radiograph is normal if the defect has been small from birth. If the ventricular septal defect is, or has been, larger, the left ventricle, left atrium, and pulmonary trunk may be dilated and there may be increased pulmonary vascularity. The electrocardiogram shows a normal QRS axis unless there are multiple defects, in which case there may be left axis deviation. In the presence of a large left to right shunt the p wave may be broad and there may be evidence of left ventricular hypertrophy. Two-dimensional echocardiography identifies the number and site of defects as well as describing the morphology and associated defects. Doppler is used to estimate the size and direction of the shunt, and right ventricle to left ventricle pressure difference, but this may not be accurate if there is an obliquely lying muscular ventricular septal defect. Cardiac catheterization is important to measure the size of shunt and pulmonary vascular resistance with reversibility studies if baseline resistance is high.

Indications for repair and postoperative sequelae

Repair of a ventricular septal defect is indicated in the presence of symptoms, if Qp:Qs is greater than 2:1, or if there is ventricular dysfunction with right ventricular pressure overload or left ventricular volume overload. Repair should also be undertaken if there are coexisting lesions such as significant right ventricular outflow tract obstruction, more than mild aortic regurgitation, or aortic valve prolapse in the presence of an outlet ventricular septal defect. A second episode of endocarditis may also be considered as an indication for ventricular septal defect closure. If the pulmonary artery pressure is greater than two-thirds systemic pressure, repair should only be considered if Qp:Qs is greater than 1.5:1 or if there is evidence of reversibility in response to pulmonary vasodilators such as oxygen and nitric oxide.

The surgical approach to repair aims at avoiding damage to important structures such as the conducting tissues that are especially vulnerable in perimembranous defects. Transatrial repair reduces the risk of postoperative ventricular arrhythmias by avoiding a right ventriculotomy. Transient postoperative complete heart block is associated with an

increased risk of late high-degree block. Permanent pacemaker implantation is indicated in the 1 to 2 per cent of patients in whom complete heart block persists, even if they are asymptomatic, because of the significant risk of sudden death. The prognosis after ventricular septal defect repair in the early years of life is good. However, left ventricular dilatation may persist and systolic function may be impaired if repair is delayed into late childhood. Long-term postoperative survival depends on the presence of pulmonary hypertension, left ventricular dysfunction, and complications such as aortic regurgitation and endocarditis.

Transcatheter device closure of ventricular septal defects is possible providing that valvar apparatus can be avoided. The approach is most suited to muscular ventricular septal defects, especially multiple defects that are difficult to close surgically and it may be combined with a surgical approach for inaccessible muscular defects.

Double-outlet right ventricle

In double-outlet right ventricle more than half the circumference of both great vessels arises from the morphological right ventricle. A complete or partial muscular infundibulum lies beneath each arterial valve. This definition includes variants of tetralogy of Fallot in which the aorta overrides the ventricular septal defect by more than 50 per cent.

The degree of pulmonary stenosis and the relation of the ventricular septal defect to the great vessels determine the haemodynamics. Eighty per cent of subaortic defects have pulmonary stenosis and Fallot-like physiology.

The Taussig–Bing anomaly accounts for less than 10 per cent of double-outlet right ventricle and describes a subpulmonary defect without pulmonary stenosis. There is transposition-like physiology with cyanosis and high pulmonary blood flow. As the pulmonary vascular resistance rises, pulmonary blood flow falls and cyanosis increases. Unoperated survival to adulthood is uncommon but occurs occasionally if the pulmonary vascular resistance establishes adequate, but not excessive, pulmonary blood flow. If such a survivor also has a patent arterial duct, there will be reversed differential cyanosis. Deoxygenated blood selectively enters the aorta to supply the arch vessels, whereas oxygenated blood enters the pulmonary artery and supplies the descending aorta via the duct: thus the fingers are more cyanosed and clubbed than the toes.

Tetralogy of Fallot

Tetralogy of Fallot is the commonest cyanotic defect, occurring in 1 per 3600 live-born babies. The four hallmarks of tetralogy of Fallot are:

- subvalvar pulmonary stenosis
- ventricular septal defect
- aortic valve overrides the ventricular septal defect
- right ventricular hypertrophy.

The fundamental abnormality is anterocephalad deviation of the outlet septum that both creates the subpulmonary stenosis and accounts for the aortic valve overriding the muscular septum. There is great anatomical variation, ranging from minimal aortic override to double-outlet right ventricle, and from minimal pulmonary stenosis to pulmonary atresia. The ventricular septal defect is perimembranous and there is usually additional pulmonary valvar stenosis.

Defects associated with tetralogy of Fallot include a right-sided aortic arch in 16 per cent, a left superior vena cava in around 15 per cent, additional ventricular septal defects in 5 per cent, and a secundum atrial septal defect ('pentalogy' of Fallot) in 8 per cent. The most important associated coronary anomaly is the crossing of the right ventricular outflow tract by a left anterior descending coronary artery arising anomalously from the right coronary sinus and vulnerable to damage during surgical repair via a right ventricular approach.

Unoperated natural history and management

Without surgical intervention, only 2 per cent of patients survive to their 40th year. Those that do survive may represent a select group in whom subpulmonary stenosis was not severe in early life, but progressed with advancing age. Such patients may rarely live into their eighth decade; one of our patients survived 77 years. Unoperated patients are at risk of the complications of cyanosis, endocarditis, atrial and ventricular arrhythmias, progressive ascending aortic dilatation, and aortic regurgitation which causes volume overload of both ventricles and subsequent biventricular failure. Systemic hypertension adds additional pressure overload to the work of both ventricles and further contributes to the onset of biventricular failure.

There is cyanosis and clubbing, a right ventricular heave, and sometimes a thrill over the right ventricular outflow tract. A right-sided aorta may be palpable to the right of the sternum. The second heart sound is usually single, and there is a loud pulmonary ejection murmur. There may be aortic regurgitation.

The electrocardiogram shows right axis deviation, right ventricular hypertrophy, and the QRS duration may be prolonged in older patients. The classic cardiac silhouette is a 'coeur en sabot', that is, a clog-shaped heart, but it is more likely to be seen in tetralogy with pulmonary atresia (see below). The heart size is usually normal and pulmonary vascularity reduced. There may be a right-sided aortic arch indenting the right of the trachea and also a prominent dilated ascending aorta. Two-dimensional echocardiography reveals infundibular stenosis with or without pulmonary valve stenosis, right ventricular hypertrophy, the typical ventricular septal defect, and varying degrees of aortic override. There may be evidence of left ventricular volume overload, aortic root dilatation, and aortic regurgitation. Cardiac catheterization should be performed prior to radical repair in adults. The anatomy of the right ventricular outflow tract obstruction (Fig. 11) and pulmonary arteries is defined, and pulmonary vascular resistance assessed. Selective coronary angiography demonstrates any anomalous origin and course as well as acquired coronary disease. Aortography shows aortic root dilatation and any aortopulmonary collaterals.

Palliated history

Helen Taussig first suggested palliative surgery in 1943, and the first Blalock–Taussig shunt was performed in 1945 (Fig. 12 and Table 11). Nowadays, palliative shunts are usually performed as a staging procedure in small infants; however, occasional patients reach the adult clinic having had palliation without subsequent radical repair. They are cyanosed and clubbed and have a continuous murmur under the clavicle and over the scapula on the side of the shunt. In a classic Blalock–Taussig shunt, the ipsilateral radial pulse is diminished or absent and the hand often small. Late complications of systemic to pulmonary artery shunts include infective endarteritis, acquired pulmonary atresia, aortic regurgitation, biventricular failure, increasing cyanosis, bronchopulmonary collateral development if the shunt blocks or is outgrown, and pulmonary vascular disease if the shunt is too big.

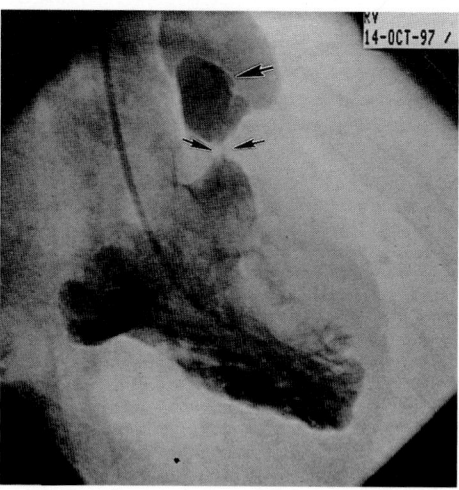

Fig. 11 Right ventricular angiogram (lateral projection) of a 45-year-old woman with unoperated tetralogy of Fallot. The right ventricle is entered via the aorta overriding the ventricular septal defect. There is severe muscular infundibular stenosis (small arrows), the pulmonary valve is thickened and doming (large arrow), and there is right ventricular hypertrophy.

Follow-up after radical repair

Radical repair involves patch closure of the ventricular septal defect with infundibular resection with or without pulmonary valvotomy or replacement. Eighty-six per cent of patients who undergo radical repair survive to 32 years of age, and these represent the majority of patients with tetralogy seen in the adult clinic. However, they remain at risk of late complications including pulmonary regurgitation and stenosis, arrhythmia, sudden death, endocarditis, and aortic regurgitation. Those repaired beyond late childhood have a higher morbidity and mortality than those repaired by the age of 12 years.

Free pulmonary regurgitation may be present since surgery if the valve was removed, or become progressively more severe, particularly if a monocusp valve or transannular patch was placed. Although well tolerated for

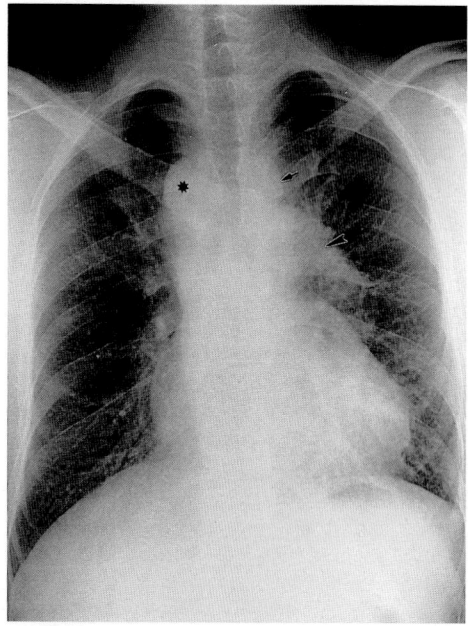

Fig. 12 Chest radiograph of a 36-year-old man with tetralogy of Fallot palliated by a classic left Blalock–Taussig shunt (small arrow). There is secondary dilatation of the left pulmonary artery (large arrow) and a right aortic arch (*).

Table 11 Systemic to pulmonary arterial shunts

Classic Blalock–Taussig shunt		Subclavian artery divided distally. Proximal subclavian artery anastomosed end-to-side to pulmonary artery
Modified Blalock–Taussig shunt		Prosthetic graft between subclavian and pulmonary arteries
Central shunt	Waterston shunt*	Side-to-side anastomosis between ascending aorta and (right) pulmonary artery
	Potts shunt*	Side-to-side anastomosis between descending aorta and (left) pulmonary artery
	Other	Prosthetic graft between aorta and pulmonary artery

*Now obsolete because not possible to control the size of the shunt adequately.

many years, pulmonary regurgitation may result in progressive right ventricular dilatation and increased risk of atrial and ventricular arrhythmias. A progressive prolongation of the QRS duration may reflect these changes and a QRS greater than 180 ms is a marker for patients at particular risk of ventricular arrhythmia. The timing of replacement of a regurgitant pulmonary valve remains difficult, but is indicated if there is dyspnoea, palpitation, and progressive right ventricular enlargement or dysfunction. Pulmonary regurgitation is worsened in the presence of pulmonary arterial stenosis that can occur at the site of a previous shunt. Right ventricular outflow tract obstruction may recur, especially if a valved right ventricular to pulmonary artery conduit was placed; this may be due to excessive formation of neointima (peel) in the conduit or to calcification of the valve. Valve calcification is readily seen on the lateral radiograph and can be followed as it encroaches on to the valve cusps to cause stenosis (Fig. 13).

The majority of patients have right bundle branch block after repair (Fig. 14). Bifasicular block and transient postoperative complete heart block carry a risk of developing late complete heart block. Atrial arrhythmias occur in 30 per cent of long-term survivors and are a major cause of morbidity. Those with left-sided volume overload and left atrial dilatation secondary to residual ventricular septal defect or previous shunts are at particular risk of atrial flutter and fibrillation. Rapidly conducted atrial flutter is particularly poorly tolerated and is likely to be responsible for a proportion of sudden deaths. Ventricular arrhythmias occur in up to 45 per cent of patients. However, the incidence of late sudden death is only 1 to

5 per cent, so not all patients with ventricular arrhythmias are at risk. Sustained monomorphic ventricular tachycardia is likely to be a significant risk factor for sudden death, as are atrial arrhythmias and heart block. Right ventricular risk factors may include right ventricular dilatation, outflow tract obstruction, hypertrophy, aneurysm, impaired myocardial blood flow, and pulmonary regurgitation. Surgical risk factors for late sudden death include transventricular as opposed to transatrial repair, large ventriculotomy scar, residual ventricular septal defect, previous complex or multiple operations, impaired left ventricular function, older age at operation, and length of follow-up.

Tetralogy of Fallot with pulmonary atresia (pulmonary atresia with ventricular septal defect)

This condition represents the extreme end of the spectrum of tetralogy. There is considerable anatomical variation, including acquired pulmonary atresia with well-developed confluent pulmonary arteries, hypoplastic confluent pulmonary arteries that may not supply all segments of the lungs, non-confluent pulmonary arteries, and complete absence of central pulmonary arteries. The right ventricular outflow tract is blind-ended and the pulmonary blood supply is derived entirely from three types of systemic vessels: a large muscular duct that resembles a collateral, a diffuse plexus of small 'bronchial' arteries arising from mediastinal and intercostal arteries, or from large tortuous systemic arterial collaterals. These large collaterals arise directly from the descending aorta, from its major branches (usually the subclavian artery), or from bronchial arteries. They may connect with central pulmonary arteries or supply whole segments or lobes of lung independently. This variation has also been termed complex pulmonary atresia.

Examination findings are similar to those of unoperated Fallot without pulmonary atresia, except that there are continuous collateral murmurs and often a collapsing pulse. Coexistent chromosome 22q11 deletion is more common than in tetralogy without pulmonary atresia. There may be dysmorphic facies, hypertelorism, narrow eye fissures, puffy eyelids, a small mouth, deformed earlobes, and sometimes a cleft palate.

The chest radiograph shows a right aortic arch in 25 per cent of cases and has a typical appearance (Fig. 15). The pulmonary collateral vessels may follow a bizarre pattern. Colour flow Doppler may identify collateral vessels, but conventional angiography is required to delineate precisely their origin, degree of ostial stenosis, and intrapulmonary course (Fig. 16). Coronary–pulmonary collaterals are a frequent finding (Fig. 17). Three-

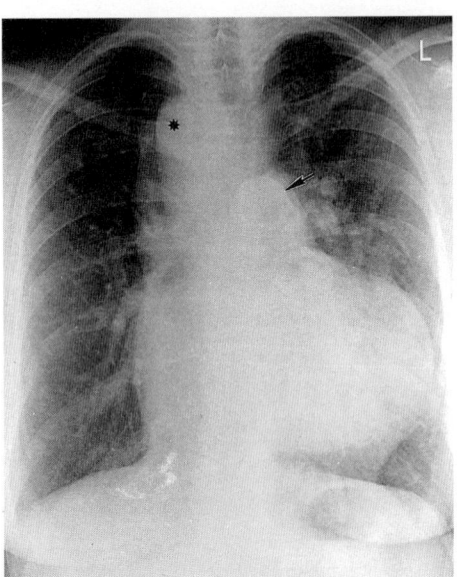

(a)

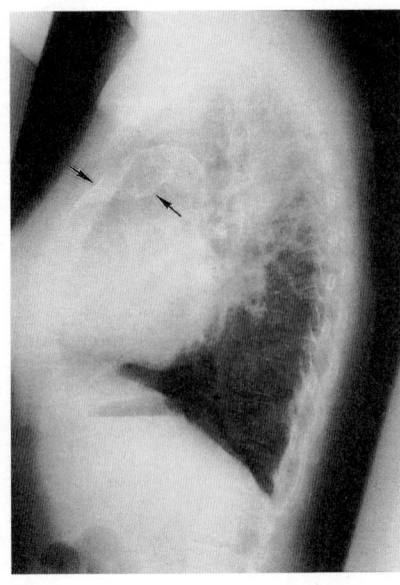

(b)

Fig. 13 Chest radiographs, (a) posteroanterior and (b) lateral, of a 30-year-old woman with tetralogy of Fallot and pulmonary atresia who underwent repair with a valved homograft conduit from right ventricle to pulmonary artery and ventricular septal defect closure 10 years previously. There is a right aortic arch (*) and a 'coeur en sabot' cardiac silhouette. The calcification in the homograft (arrows) is more clearly seen on the lateral radiograph. The abnormal pulmonary vasculature reflects persisting aortopulmonary collaterals.

dimensional magnetic resonance angiography is likely to prove a useful tool in imaging complex pulmonary vasculature.

Overall survival, including the effects of operation, is around 25 per cent at 20 years. Late complications in unoperated survivors include increasing cyanosis due either to the development of pulmonary vascular disease in lung segments perfused at systemic pressure through non-stenosed collaterals, or to the progressive stenosis of collateral vessels. In the latter, good symptomatic relief may be obtained from stenting the stenotic vessel. The aortic root may become markedly dilated and aortic regurgitation develop, resulting in biventricular volume overload and failure. Aortic valve endo-

carditis is a particular risk. Surgery to repair or replace the aortic valve in an unrepaired patient with pulmonary atresia is particularly hazardous because of the aortopulmonary collateral vessels. When cardiopulmonary bypass is instituted, aortic blood flows into the low resistance pulmonary collateral vessels so that it is not possible to maintain an adequate systemic perfusion pressure or to control pulmonary venous return to the left atrium.

Surgery to unifocalize collateral vessels (i.e. disconnect them from the aorta and anastomose them to the pulmonary artery, maintaining pulmonary blood supply by means of a shunt) may need to precede radical repair.

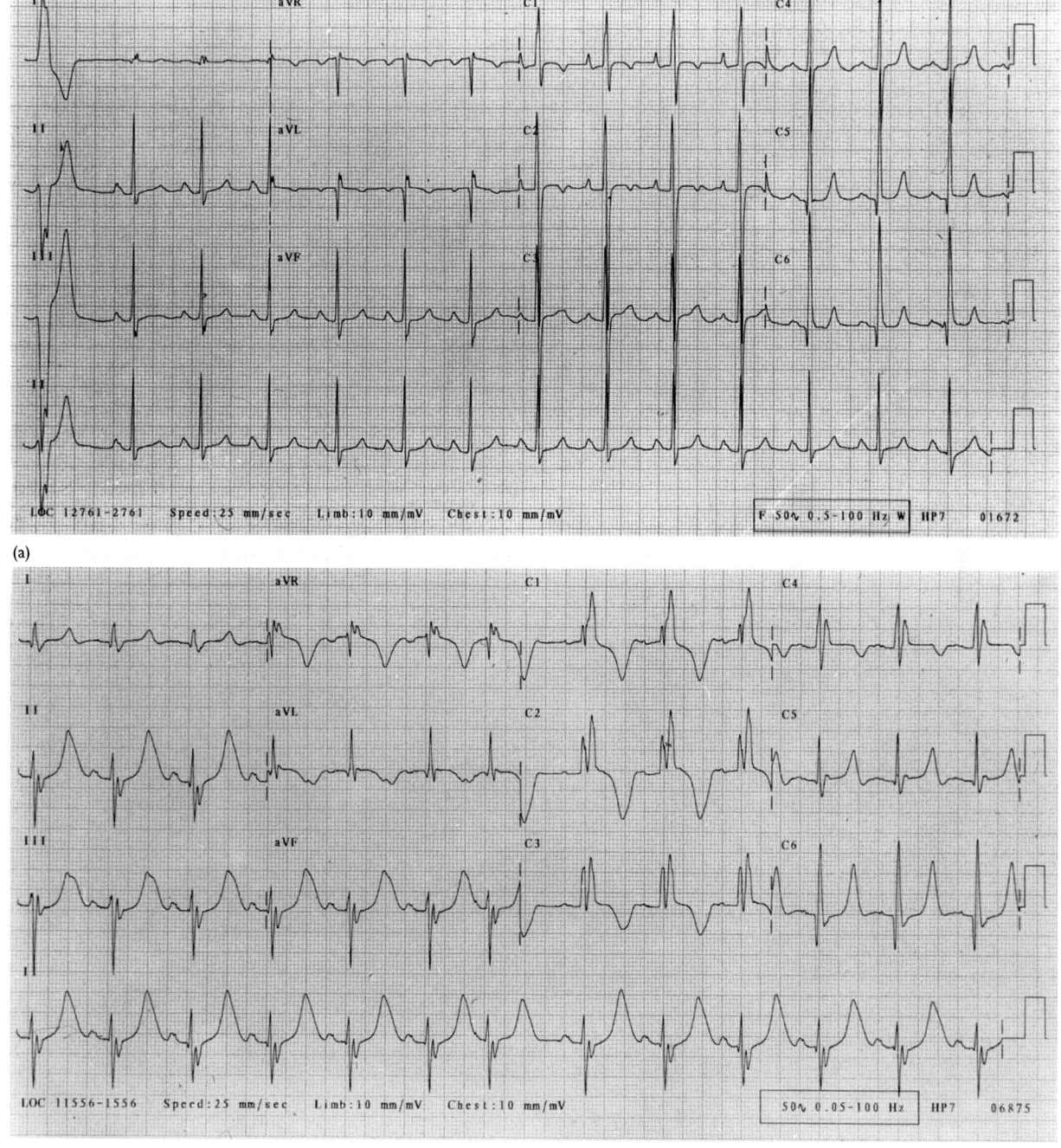

Fig. 14 Electrocardiograms of a 35-year-old woman who underwent radical repair of tetralogy of Fallot. Preoperatively (a) there is right ventricular hypertrophy, postoperatively (b) there is right bundle branch block, due to damage to the right bundle as it runs in the floor of the ventricular septal defect.

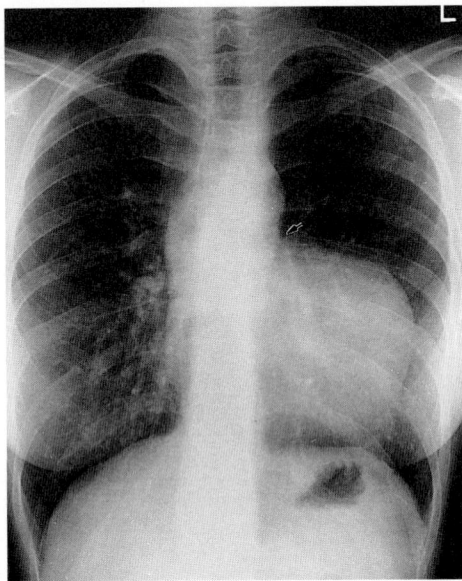

Fig. 15 Chest radiograph of a 21-year-old woman with tetralogy of Fallot and pulmonary atresia, no central pulmonary arteries, and multiple aortopulmonary collaterals which create an abnormal pulmonary vascular pattern. The typical 'coeur en sabot' silhouette is due to right ventricular hypertrophy and the pulmonary bay where the pulmonary artery should be (arrow).

Suitability for radical repair depends on the size of the pulmonary arteries and the proportion of lung they supply. The ventricular septal defect is closed and the right ventricular outflow tract connected to the pulmonary artery via a valved conduit. Right ventricular hypertension may follow surgery if the pulmonary arteries are small or distal pulmonary vessels inadequate. Both these factors and the number of aortopulmonary collaterals decrease long-term survival.

Tetralogy of Fallot with absent pulmonary valve syndrome

This variation accounts for around 3 per cent of cases of tetralogy. There is a ring-like malformation, usually stenotic, with failure of development of

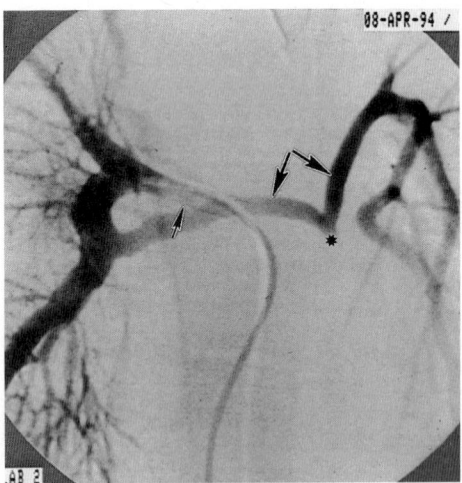

Fig. 16 Aortopulmonary collateral angiogram of a 24-year-old woman with tetralogy of Fallot and pulmonary atresia. There is a stent (small arrow) at the origin of the collateral from the descending aorta. Only after dilation and stenting of the collateral was its connection with confluent main pulmonary arteries (large arrows) apparent. The atretic main pulmonary artery is indicated (*).

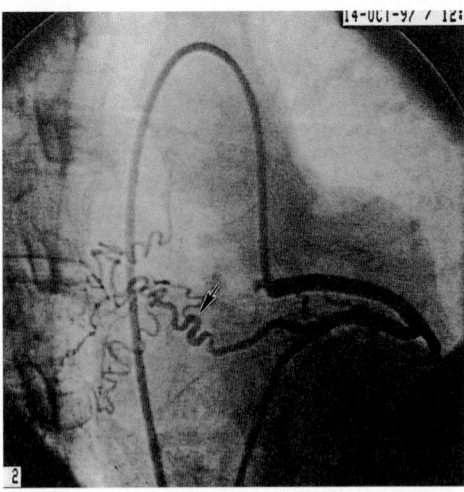

Fig. 17 Selective left coronary angiogram in same patient as Fig. 11

the pulmonary valve cusps. The central pulmonary arteries are usually hugely dilated or aneurysmal (Fig. 18).

Other right-sided obstructive lesions

Isolated pulmonary valve stenosis

Pulmonary stenosis is discussed in detail elsewhere. Cyanosis may be present if severe stenosis coexists with an atrial septal defect or patent foramen ovale. Noonan's syndrome is associated with valvar and infundibular stenosis as well as with hypertrophic cardiomyopathy.

Lone infundibular stenosis and double-chambered right ventricle

Abnormally placed muscle bands cause either infundibular obstruction, or if placed more inferiorly, subinfundibular obstruction and a double-chambered right ventricle. The degree of obstruction may be mild in childhood, but progress into adult life and cause symptoms as the right ventricle hypertrophies. A perimembranous ventricular septal defect usually coexists and may close spontaneously. Treatment is by surgical resection of the obstructing muscle bands.

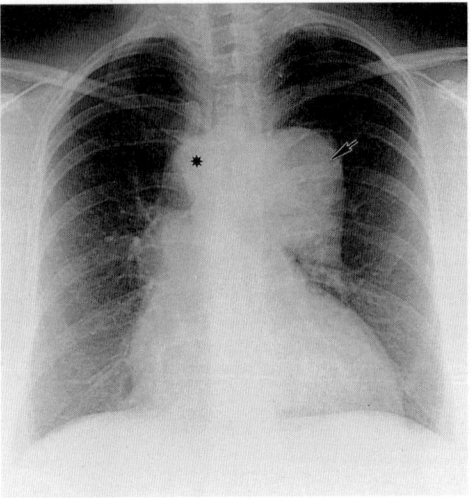

Fig. 18 Chest radiograph of a 54-year-old woman with repaired tetralogy of Fallot and absent pulmonary valve syndrome. The central pulmonary arteries are hugely dilated (arrow) and there is a right aortic arch (*).

Pulmonary atresia with intact septum

A full discussion of this complex lesion is beyond the scope of this chapter, since patients do not survive unoperated beyond infancy. Those currently in the adult clinics represent the mild end of the spectrum of this condition and are likely to have had a pulmonary valvotomy or valved right ventricular to pulmonary artery conduit.

Left ventricular outflow tract obstruction

Bicuspid aortic valve

The commonest congenital cardiac anomaly, occurring in 1 to 2 per cent of the population, bicuspid aortic valve is four times as common in males as females. In 20 per cent of cases it is associated with other lesions such as patent arterial duct and coarctation. There is also an association with aortic root dilatation and dissection. Aortic stenosis is discussed in detail elsewhere.

Supravalvar aortic stenosis

In this least common form of left ventricular outflow tract obstruction, there is a localized narrowing of the aorta immediately above the aortic sinuses. Fibromuscular thickening of the aortic wall at the site of obstruction may encroach into the coronary ostia or on to the aortic valve leaflets and adversely influence prognosis. Unlike other forms of left ventricular outflow obstruction, the coronary arteries lie proximal to the obstruction and so are exposed to high left ventricular pressures, resulting in premature atherosclerosis. The condition may be associated with Williams' syndrome, when the prognosis may be worse since there is diffuse arterial involvement that may involve the pulmonary and renal arteries.

Subaortic stenosis

Subaortic stenosis is due either to a discrete fibromuscular ridge or ring, or a long muscular tunnel. It may exist in isolation or as part of another lesion such as atrioventricular septal defect where the aorta is 'unwedged' and the left ventricular outflow tract elongated, or mitral valve anomalies where abnormal insertion of the mitral valve causes obstruction. Whether discrete or tunnel-like, subaortic stenosis tends to progress and may recur following surgical resection. It may result in functional disruption of the aortic valve and secondary aortic regurgitation, which may progress, even after resection of subaortic stenosis.

Coarctation of the aorta

One of the commonest congenital cardiac lesions, occurring in 1 per 12 000 live-born babies with a male to female ratio of 3:1, aortic coarctation is a narrowing of the aorta usually sited near the ligamentum arteriosum. There is considerable variation in anatomy and severity, ranging from a mild obstruction to interruption of the aorta, and from a discrete fibromuscular shelf to hypoplasia of the arch. Coarctation is most strongly associated with bicuspid aortic valve; other associations are ventricular septal defect, patent ductus arteriosus, subaortic ridge and mitral valve abnormalities. It is a frequent finding in Turner's syndrome and is also associated with congenital aneurysm of the circle of Willis.

Unoperated history

Most patients present in infancy, but some survive into adulthood before being diagnosed at routine examination or during investigation for hypertension, leg claudication (uncommon unless there is coexisting abdominal aortic coarctation), angina, heart failure, or cerebral haemorrhage. More than 75 per cent of patients with unoperated coarctation die by age 50 years, from coronary disease, stroke, or aortic dissection.

Clinical findings include upper body hypertension: the leg blood pressure is lower, as is that in the left arm if the subclavian artery is involved in the coarctation. If there is a good collateral supply, femoral arteries may be easily palpable, but they are usually reduced, with radiofemoral delay. Intercostal collaterals may be both visible and palpable over the patient's

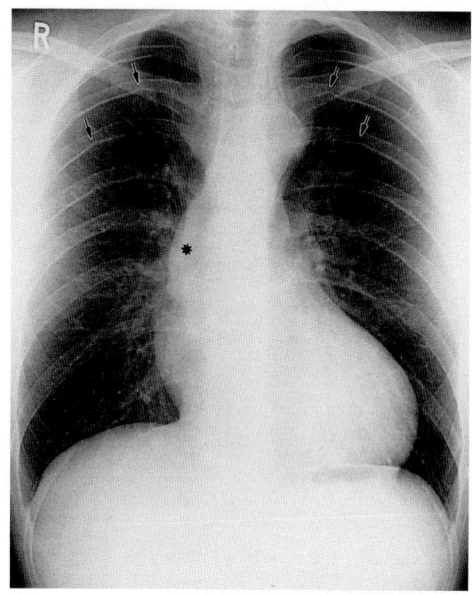

Fig. 19 Chest radiograph of an 18-year-old man with unoperated coarctation of the aorta and bicuspid aortic valve. There is bilateral rib notching (arrows), a dilated ascending aorta (*), and a prominent deformed aortic knuckle.

back. There is an ejection systolic murmur from the site of coarctation, and systolic collateral murmurs may be heard. Fundoscopy shows a typical corkscrew appearance of the retinal vessels and there may be evidence of hypertensive retinopathy.

There may be electrocardiographic evidence of left ventricular hypertrophy. The chest radiograph (Fig. 19) has a typical appearance. Transthoracic echocardiography may show left ventricular hypertrophy, but the coarctation site may not be visualized on two-dimensional imaging, although the severity of coarctation can be assessed using Doppler mode from the suprasternal notch. A peak gradient of gretaer than 20 mmHg is significant, especially if accompanied by a diastolic tail. Angiography allows full haemodynamic and anatomical data to be obtained from both the coarctation site and related vessels, as well as assessing secondary ischaemic myocardial disease. Magnetic resonance imaging provides excellent non-invasive haemodynamic data and two- and three-dimensional images of the coarctation site and related vessels. It may obviate the need for angiography unless coronary disease is suspected.

Repair of coarctation

Surgical repair is the conventional approach. There is a 0.4 per cent incidence of perioperative spinal cord ischaemia and paraplegia: patients without an abundant collateral circulation may be most at risk. Those with well-developed collaterals are at risk of significant intraoperative haemorrhage. Early postoperative hypertension is common and may be difficult to control, and postoperative intestinal ileus may persist for several days.

Transcatheter balloon dilatation and primary stenting of native coarctation in adults are reported, but data are limited and the procedures should still be considered experimental. Stenting has the hypothetical advantage of supporting the dilated segment of aorta which may sustain a significant intimal tear, and preventing aortic rupture or aneurysm formation.

Follow-up after coarctation repair

Follow-up after repair of coarctation should be life-long, since late complications are frequent: recoarctation, aneurysm formation, persistent hypertension despite adequate repair, premature atherosclerotic disease, and progression of associated lesions such as bicuspid aortic valve. Older age at repair is the main risk factor influencing longevity. Late survival is 92 per cent for patients repaired in infancy, 25-year survival is 75 per cent for

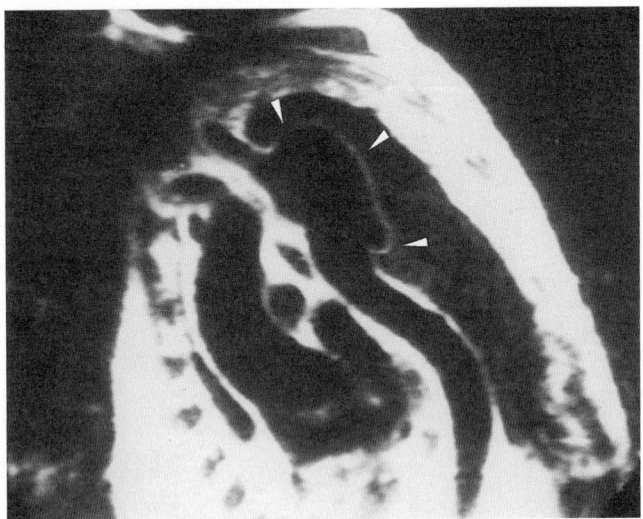

Fig. 20 Magnetic resonance spin echo image showing aneurysm of the descending aortic arch (arrows) following previous Dacron patch repair of coarctation

those repaired between the ages of 20 and 40 years, but 15-year survival is only 50 per cent for those repaired at age 40 years or more.

Recoarctation may be diagnosed when the resting arm–leg systolic blood pressure gradient is 20 mmHg at rest and 50 mmHg postexercise. It occurs most commonly in neonatal repair by end-to-end anastomosis. Recoarctation should be sought when there is new or persisting hypertension. Blood pressure should be recorded in both arms of all such patients; spuriously low readings may be obtained if one of the subclavian arteries (usually the left) is involved in the repair or recoarctation. Magnetic resonance imaging is the investigation of choice for both recoarctation and aneurysm formation after coarctation repair (Fig. 20). Balloon angioplasty with or without stent insertion is used to relieve the majority of recoarctations, but reoperation is required for some patients with complex anatomy.

Hypertension is a major risk factor for atherosclerotic disease and may persist despite an apparently good result from surgical repair. Continuing hypertension is thought to relate in part to older age at time of surgery. None the less, even if repaired in adulthood, systolic hypertension becomes less marked and easier to control, β-blocking agents being the antihypertensives of choice.

The 14-year incidence of aneurysm formation at the site of repair is up to 27 per cent, it occurs most commonly in adults and in those with Dacron patch repair (Fig. 20). The aneurysm may rupture into the bronchial tree: any patient with a history of coarctation who presents with haemoptysis should undergo emergency non-invasive diagnostic imaging (preferably MRI) and surgical repair. Bronchoscopy and conventional angiography are contraindicated since they may cause further damage to the ruptured area.

Congenitally corrected transposition of the great arteries (atrioventricular and ventriculoarterial discordance)

This rare condition accounts for less than 1 per cent of all congenital heart disease. Both atrial and arterial connections to the ventricles are discordant, so pulmonary venous blood passes through the left atrium, through the right ventricle, and into an anteriorly lying aorta. Similarly, systemic venous blood reaches the pulmonary trunk via the left ventricle. The circulation is therefore physiologically 'corrected', but the morphological right ventricle and tricuspid valve support the systemic circulation.

More than 95 per cent of cases have associated anomalies, most commonly ventricular septal defect and pulmonary stenosis, but also Ebstein anomaly of the systemic (tricuspid) atrioventricular valve, aortic stenosis,

atrioventricular septal defect, abnormalities of situs, and coarctation. Congenital complete heart block occurs in around 5 per cent of patients and may develop at any stage of life, particularly following surgery to the atrioventricular valve.

Presentation depends on associated lesions. Patients with isolated congenitally corrected transposition of the great arteries may remain asymptomatic and undiagnosed into old age, but failure of the systemic ventricle, systemic atrioventricular valve regurgitation, or the onset of complete heart block and atrial arrhythmias usually result in presentation with symptoms from the fourth decade onwards. Those with ventricular septal defect and pulmonary stenosis may be cyanosed, and those with ventricular septal defect alone may present with pulmonary hypertension.

A parasternal heave is usually palpable from the pressure-loaded anteriorly lying systemic right ventricle; this may be especially prominent if it is also volume-loaded by systemic (tricuspid) atrioventricular valve regurgitation. There may be a prominent aortic pulsation in the suprasternal notch and the aortic component of the second heart sound may be palpable and loud. The pulmonary component is soft or inaudible due to the posterior position of the pulmonary artery.

The electrocardiogram may show varying degrees of atrioventricular block or evidence of pre-excitation due to accessory pathways (associated with Ebstein-like anomalies of the systemic atrioventricular valve). There may be left axis deviation. The right and left bundles are inverted, so the initial septal activation is right-to-left, resulting in Q waves in V1 to 2 and an absent Q in V5 to 6; this pattern is often wrongly interpreted as a previous anterior myocardial infarction. The chest radiograph has a typical appearance (Fig. 21). Echocardiography confirms the discordant relations and assesses ventricular and systemic (tricuspid) atrioventricular valve function as well as other associated lesions. Ebstein's anomaly may be diagnosed if the tricuspid valve is apically displaced more than 8 mm. Cardiac catheterization is indicated to assess the haemodynamic importance of associated lesions.

ACE inhibitors may be useful when there is systemic ventricular dysfunction or atrioventricular valve regurgitation, but there are no trial data to support their use. Transvenous atrioventricular sequential pacing is indicated for complete heart block: active fixation ventricular leads are required because of the absence of coarse apical trabeculations in the morphologically left subpulmonary ventricle. If there are associated intracardiac shunts,

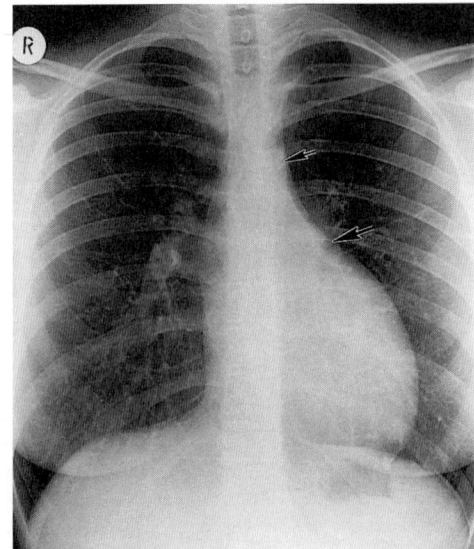

Fig. 21 Chest radiograph of a 23-year-old woman with congenitally corrected transposition of the great vessels. There is a narrow pedicle due to the abnormally related great arteries (small arrow) and the left heart border is straight (large arrow) due to the abnormal position of the left-lying anterior ascending aorta.

patients should be formally anticoagulated to reduce the risk of paradoxical embolism, or epicardial pacing should be considered.

The conventional surgical approach to systemic atrioventricular valve regurgitation is tricuspid valve replacement (repair is rarely successful), but if systemic ventricular function is poor (ejection fraction less than 40 per cent), transplantation may be the only option. Where there is coexistent ventricular septal defect and pulmonary stenosis, classic repair involves closure of the ventricular septal defect and insertion of a valved conduit between the left ventricle and pulmonary artery; the right ventricle continuing to support the systemic circulation.

Anatomical repair, so that the morphological left ventricle supports the systemic ventricle, has achieved short-term success in children with systemic atrioventricular valve regurgitation and systemic ventricular dysfunction. For patients with an associated non-restrictive ventricular septal defect the left ventricle is at systemic pressure and therefore 'pre-trained' to support the systemic circulation. If there is no pulmonary stenosis, a 'double switch' is performed, combining an intraatrial repair (usually Senning operation) with an arterial switch operation. If there is also pulmonary stenosis, the Senning operation is combined with a Rastelli-type repair, in which the ventricular septal defect is closed so that the left ventricle is tunnelled to the aorta, and a right ventricular to pulmonary artery conduit is placed. The regurgitant tricuspid valve and right ventricle are therefore placed in the pulmonary circulation. For children with corrected transposition whose left ventricle is at low pressure, a period of left ventricular 'training' is required before a double switch operation can be performed. Training is achieved by placing a pulmonary artery band to increase left ventricular pressure and induce hypertrophy. Pulmonary artery banding *per se* may improve symptoms, since the increased left ventricular pressure causes the interventricular septum to move towards the systemic ventricle, reducing systemic atrioventricular regurgitation. The long-term outcome of these anatomical approaches to corrected transposition is not yet known; complications relating to conduit replacement, neo-aortic valve regurgitation, and arrhythmia may become significant. There are reports of adults with ventricular septal defect and pulmonary stenosis having successfully undergone Mustard–Rastelli repair. However, whether it is possible to 'train' the adult left ventricle that has been at low pressure for many years remains to be seen, so this approach remains experimental in older patients.

Complete transposition of the great arteries (atrioventricular concordance, ventriculoarterial discordance)

Complete transposition of the great arteries accounts for around 5 per cent of congenital cardiac malformations and is four times more common in males than females. Associated anomalies such as ventricular septal defect and pulmonary stenosis occur in about one-third of patients. Desaturated systemic venous blood passes through the right atrium into the right ventricle and then to the aorta, and oxygenated pulmonary venous blood passes into the left atrium, through the left ventricle and back into the lungs. Once the arterial duct closes, survival depends on an intracardiac communication (non-restrictive patent foramen ovale or ventricular septal defect) allowing mixing of blood between the two separate circuits. Without intervention, 30 per cent of patients die within the first week and only 10 per cent survive their first year. A prostaglandin infusion maintains patency of the arterial duct until a balloon atrial septostomy is performed. The neonate remains cyanosed, but there is usually adequate mixing to allow him or her to thrive until definitive surgery.

Most patients in the adult clinic have survived intra-atrial repair (Senning or Mustard operation), or for those with associated ventricular septal defect and pulmonary stenosis, a Rastelli operation. Intra-atrial repair involves excision of the atrial septum and placement of a saddle-shaped patch ('baffle') to direct pulmonary venous blood into the right atrium, right ventricle and then to the aorta, and systemic venous blood into the left atrium, left ventricle and then into the pulmonary artery. The right ventricle supports the systemic circulation. In the Rastelli operation, the ventricular septal defect is closed so that the left ventricle carrying oxygenated blood empties into the aorta, and a conduit is placed between the right ventricle and pulmonary artery. The left ventricle supports the systemic circulation.

Since the late 1970s anatomical correction by the arterial switch operation began to supersede intraatrial repair as the operation of choice for most patients with transposition of the great arteries. Blood is redirected at arterial level by switching the aorta and pulmonary arteries so that the left ventricle becomes the subaortic ventricle supporting the systemic circulation. The coronary arteries are reimplanted into the neo-aortic root.

'Palliative' Mustard or Senning operations are performed for patients with transposition of the great arteries, ventricular septal defect, and pulmonary vascular disease to improve mixing of blood and oxygenation. The ventricular septal defect is left open. These patients should be treated as other patients with the Eisenmenger syndrome.

Follow-up

After intra-atrial repair of transposition of the great arteries, the systemic right ventricle causes a parasternal heave, the aortic component of the second heart sound may be palpable and loud, and the second sound single, due to the anterior-lying aorta. The presence of cyanosis suggests a baffle leak allowing right to left shunting between the systemic and pulmonary venous atria. Systemic venous pathway obstruction may be associated with elevation of the jugular venous pressure and hepatomegaly. The chest radiograph may show a dilated azygos vein indicative of systemic venous pathway obstruction, with run-off from the obstructed to the unobstructed pathway. Pulmonary interstitial fluid may reflect pulmonary venous pathway obstruction. Although late results of intraatrial repair are good, failure of the systemic right ventricle is exacerbated as the atrioventricular valve becomes regurgitant. In addition, baffle obstruction causing systemic or pulmonary venous obstruction may require transcatheter intervention or reoperation. Atrial arrhythmias, especially atrial flutter, occur in up to 10 per cent of patients 10 years postoperatively. They may be poorly tolerated and are associated with an increased risk of sudden death. Late sinus node dysfunction and complete heart block may also occur: active fixation leads are required to pace both the systemic venous atrium and left ventricle. As in congenitally corrected transposition of the great arteries, the conventional surgical approach for systemic atrioventricular valve regurgitation is tricuspid valve replacement. It is uncertain whether pulmonary artery banding to train the left ventricle and reduce regurgitation, followed by the arterial switch operation, will benefit adults in this situation.

The major late complication following the Rastelli operation is the need for conduit replacement. Late results from the arterial switch operation are awaited. It is likely to have long-term advantages over intra-atrial repair, since it restores normal connections so that the left ventricle supports the systemic circulation without the need for a conduit. Follow-up is needed to detect late pulmonary arterial stenosis, neo-aortic regurgitation, and coronary ostial stenoses.

Hearts with univentricular atrioventricular connection (double-inlet left ventricle and tricuspid atresia)

Also known as univentricular or single ventricle hearts, these hearts are defined by the connection of both atria to one ventricle, or by the absence of one of the atrioventricular connections. There is one dominant ventricle, with a second rudimentary and incomplete ventricle. When the rudimentary ventricle is of right morphology, it nearly always lies anteriorly. Less commonly, there is a posteriorly lying morphologically left rudimentary ventricle, and rarely there is solitary ventricle of indeterminate morphology.

This section considers double-inlet left ventricle and tricuspid atresia. Less common variants such as double-inlet right ventricle, mitral atresia, and more complex univentricular hearts are beyond the scope of this chapter. Hearts with a large ventricular septal defect and two fully formed ventricles are not correctly termed univentricular and are also excluded. None the less the pathophysiological principles are similar.

In double-inlet left ventricle, ventriculoarterial discordance (transposed great arteries) usually coexists; the aorta arises from the rudimentary right ventricle via the ventricular septal defect. Double-inlet left ventricle with concordant ventriculoarterial connection (Holmes heart) is rare. Tricuspid atresia has a number of morphological variations, but the different morphologies do not affect the basic haemodynamics: the only route out of the right atrium is via an atrial septal defect into the left atrium and then to the ventricular mass. The ventriculoarterial connection is most commonly concordant.

Pathophysiology

For all univentricular hearts, key factors determining the mode of presentation and survival are the presence and degree of pulmonary stenosis, presence and degree of subaortic stenosis, and the morphology of the dominant ventricle.

In hearts with concordant ventriculoarterial connections, pulmonary stenosis may be both valvar and subpulmonary, caused by a restrictive ventricular septal defect, since the pulmonary artery arises from the rudimentary ventricle. Absence of pulmonary stenosis results in high pulmonary blood flow and eventual pulmonary vascular disease. Severe pulmonary stenosis or atresia causes marked cyanosis but protects against pulmonary vascular disease. In hearts with ventriculoarterial discordance, a restrictive ventricular septal defect causes subaortic stenosis, since the aorta arises from the rudimentary ventricle. Subaortic stenosis may be acquired (see Introduction), resulting in preferential pulmonary blood flow and reduced cardiac output. If the dominant ventricle is of left morphology it is better able to adapt to its abnormal geometry and chronic volume overload than a right ventricle.

The outcome is most favourable for patients with left ventricular morphology, moderate pulmonary stenosis, and no subaortic stenosis. Unoperated survival into adulthood is uncommon, 50 per cent of patients with double-inlet left ventricle die before 14 years, 50 per cent with double-inlet right ventricle die by 4 years of age. None the less, rare patients with balanced circulation reach their sixth decade without surgical intervention.

Clinical signs in the unoperated adult

There is cyanosis and clubbing. A giant 'a' wave may be present in the jugular venous pulse in tricuspid atresia. An absent right ventricular impulse and prominent left ventricular impulse are characteristic of double-inlet left ventricle and tricuspid atresia. There may be a precordial thrill from pulmonary stenosis, particularly if the pulmonary artery lies anteriorly. If there are discordant ventriculoarterial connections, the aortic pulsation of the anteriorly lying aorta may be prominent in the suprasternal notch. The second heart sound is usually single and there may be a pulmonary ejection systolic murmur radiating laterally, also a pansystolic murmur of mitral regurgitation.

If pulmonary vascular disease has developed there will be additional signs of pulmonary hypertension. Signs of congestive heart failure may be present in the ageing patient, particularly with the onset of atrial arrhythmia: the venous pressure may be raised, with hepatomegaly and peripheral oedema.

Investigations

The chest radiograph shows cardiomegaly due to chronic ventricular volume overload. If ventriculoarterial connections are discordant, there is a narrow pedicle and the ascending aorta forms a straight edge along the left heart border. Pulmonary vascularity reflects the pulmonary blood flow. The main pulmonary arteries are small where there is significant pulmonary stenosis. Large main pulmonary arteries indicate high pulmonary blood flow, either past or present.

In tricuspid atresia the electrocardiogram usually shows right atrial hypertrophy, normal P–R interval, small or absent right ventricular forces, and left axis deviation. There is left axis deviation and large left ventricular forces in double-inlet left ventricle. If the rudimentary chamber lies to the right, the P–R interval is usually normal, but if it lies to the left, the P–R interval may be prolonged or there may be complete heart block.

Two-dimensional echocardiography and colour flow Doppler allow detailed assessment of the anatomy and physiology, including ventricular morphology and pulmonary and subaortic stenosis. Cardiac catheterization is required to assess pulmonary artery pressure and resistance and to detail pulmonary artery anatomy.

Operations for hearts with univentricular atrioventricular connections

All surgical approaches are palliative, since a biventricular repair is not possible. The aim of definitive surgery is to separate the systemic and pulmonary circulations. Early procedures such as the Glenn anastomosis partly achieved this aim, and it remains a useful staging procedure in children prior to definitive surgery, with the advantage of offloading the ventricle and perfusing the lung at low pressure. However, the relative contribution of the superior vena cava reduces as the child grows, so progressive cyanosis develops. It is therefore inadequate as the sole source of pulmonary blood supply in adults. Pulmonary arteriovenous fistulas are a late complication of Glenn anastomoses and are thought to relate to the exclusion of hepatic venous blood from the pulmonary circulation.

The Fontan operation creates an atriopulmonary connection so that systemic venous blood passes directly to the pulmonary artery, thus bypassing the ventricle, completely separating the systemic and pulmonary circulations and abolishing cyanosis. The ventricle supports the systemic circulation and systemic venous blood flows passively into the pulmonary arteries. The evolution of the Fontan operation and its successor, the total cavopulmonary connection is outlined in Fig. 22. Many variations of the Fontan operation have been developed that are beyond the scope of this chapter.

The Fontan-type circulation is one of a low cardiac output that can only be increased by increasing the heart rate. This lack of reserve and dependence on adequate systemic venous return both limits exercise tolerance and renders the patient susceptible to subsequent anaesthesia and surgery. Meticulous fluid balance and avoidance of hypovolaemia and excessive vasodilatation are required to prevent cardiovascular collapse.

Survival after Fontan-type surgery is dependent on patient selection and ranges from 81 per cent at 10 years for 'perfect candidates' to 60 to 70 per cent for all patients. Patients with preoperative adverse risk factors for Fontan-type surgery (Table 12) are also more likely to develop long-term complications (Table 13). Paroxysmal atrial flutter (intra-atrial re-entry tachycardia) is a major cause of morbidity in long-term survivors. Right atrial distension, high atrial pressures, atrial suture lines, and obstruction to the Fontan circuit contribute to the development of arrhythmias. Transoesophageal echocardiography and magnetic resonance imaging may visualize the Fontan connection, but cardiac catheterization is usually required to quantify the degree of obstruction. Since the velocities within the Fontan circuit are low (less than 1 m/s), a pressure drop of only 2 to 3 mmHg between the pulmonary artery and right atrium may indicate haemodynamically important obstruction. Atrial flutter is poorly tolerated so cardioversion should not be delayed. The arrhythmia may become increasingly difficult to control, and if ventricular function is impaired, amiodarone may be the most effective and best tolerated antiarrhythmic. However, amiodarone-induced thyrotoxicosis occurs in up to 40 per cent of Fontan survivors and may precipitate further tachyarrhythmias and heart failure, so thyroid function should be monitored carefully. Whether by excluding the atrium from the systemic venous–pulmonary artery circuit the total cavopulmonary connection will reduce atrial arrhythmia remains to be seen. There is early evidence that conversion of the Fontan to a total cavopulmonary connection, in combination with arrhythmia circuit cryoablation, may reduce the incidence of arrhythmia and improve functional class.

There is usually echocardiographic evidence of spontaneous contrast in Fontan survivors with a dilated right atrium, indicating sluggish flow and a high risk of thrombus formation. Patients with atrial arrhythmia are at particular risk and should be formally anticoagulated. A deficiency of anticoagulation factors in patients after Fontan procedures may also contribute towards thromboembolism.

Protein-losing enteropathy is one of the most debilitating complications of Fontan-type surgery, occurring in up to 13 per cent of late survivors, with a 5-year survival after its onset of less than 50 per cent. It is thought to result from the effects of chronically elevated systemic venous pressure on the lymphatic system causing gastrointestinal protein loss, with malnutrition, oedema, effusions, and ascites due to hypoalbuminaemia, as well as infections secondary to hypogammaglobulinaemia. The diagnosis is confirmed by a low serum albumin and high faecal α_1-antitrypsin. A high protein, low fat, high medium-chain triglyceride diet has been advocated, but is unpalatable. Treatment with corticosteroids, unfractionated heparin, or transcatheter fenestration of the atrial septum may be beneficial. Surgical relief of any Fontan obstruction may be successful, but carries a high mor-

tality and cardiac transplantation may be the only option, although protein-losing enteropathy may recur.

Most patients in the adult clinic have undergone Fontan-type surgery in childhood or adolescence. However, those patients with univentricular heart that survive to adulthood without an operation or with previous shunts are often considered for Fontan-type surgery. Such patients represent a highly selected group of survivors with a well-balanced circulation, and the long-term complications of cyanosis and ventricular volume overload should be weighed carefully against the risk of Fontan surgery in an adult and its long-term complications.

Other arterial anomalies

Persistent patent ductus arteriosus

The pathophysiological consequences of a patent arterial duct in adulthood depend on the size of the shunt. Small ducts are of no haemodynamic significance and are associated with a low risk of infective endarteritis. Moderate-sized ducts may cause left heart volume overload and late atrial fibrillation and ventricular dysfunction. A large non-restrictive duct may cause pulmonary vascular disease (see Eisenmenger syndrome).

If a duct is clinically detectable, that is there is a machinery murmur in the left subclavicular area, then closure is usually recommended to avoid

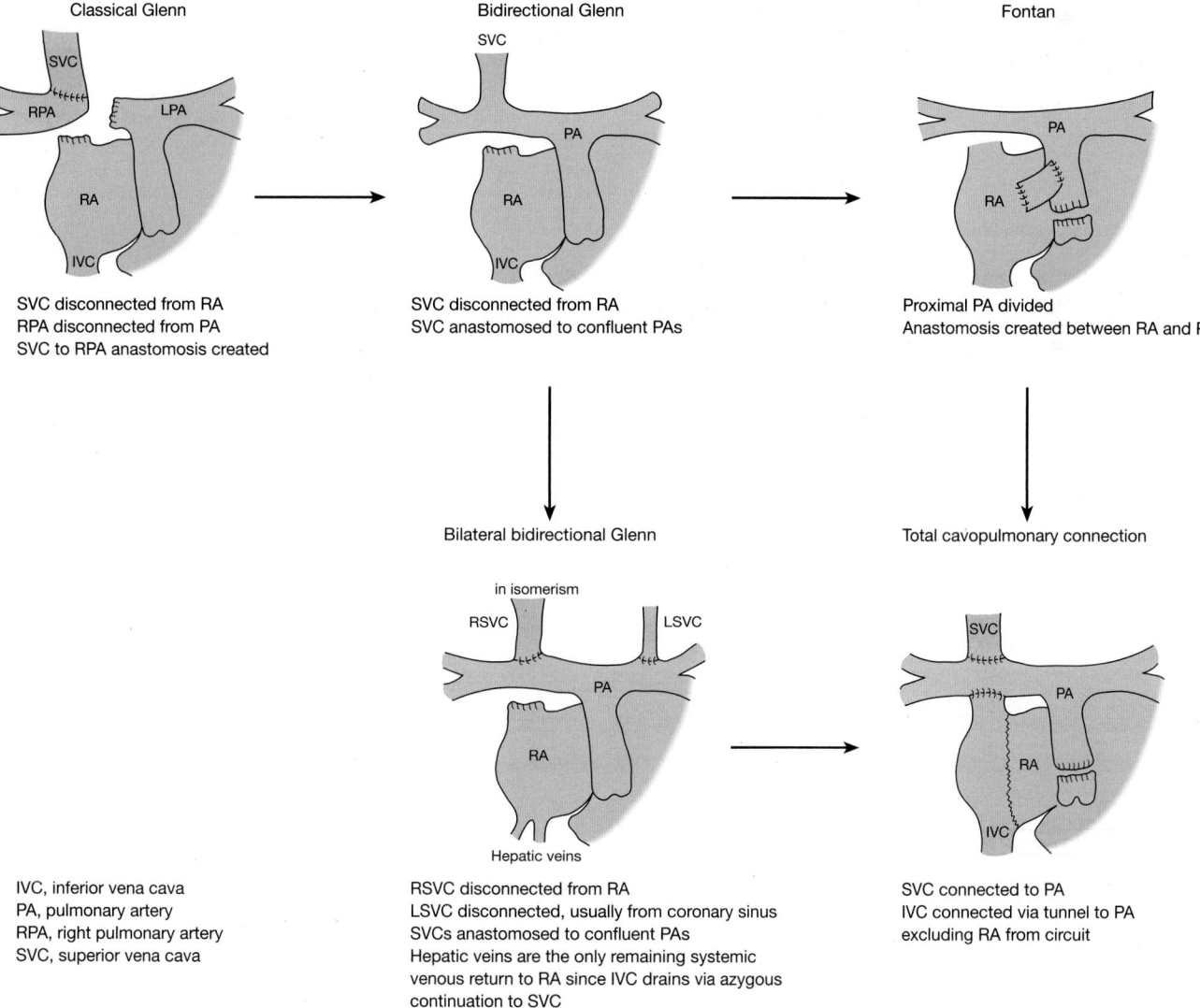

Classical Glenn

SVC disconnected from RA
RPA disconnected from PA
SVC to RPA anastomosis created

Bidirectional Glenn

SVC disconnected from RA
SVC anastomosed to confluent PAs

Fontan

Proximal PA divided
Anastomosis created between RA and PA

Bilateral bidirectional Glenn

in isomerism

RSVC disconnected from RA
LSVC disconnected, usually from coronary sinus
SVCs anastomosed to confluent PAs
Hepatic veins are the only remaining systemic
venous return to RA since IVC drains via azygous
continuation to SVC

Total cavopulmonary connection

SVC connected to PA
IVC connected via tunnel to PA
excluding RA from circuit

IVC, inferior vena cava
PA, pulmonary artery
RPA, right pulmonary artery
SVC, superior vena cava

Fig. 22 Evolution of the Fontan operation and total cavopulmonary connection.

Table 12 Adverse risk factors for Fontan-type surgery

Pulmonary vascular resistance > 4 Wood units
Mean pulmonary artery pressure > 15 mmHg
Ventricular hypertrophy
Impaired systolic ventricular function
Severe atrioventricular valve regurgitation
Aortic outflow obstruction
Age < 2 years and > 14 years
Small or distorted pulmonary arteries

long-term haemodynamic complications. Ducts up to about 8 mm in diameter are usually suitable for transcatheter device closure, but calcification and aneurysmal dilatation around the area of the duct may necessitate surgical repair. In large ducts, pulmonary vascular disease should be excluded before surgical repair is undertaken.

Truncus arteriosus

A single great artery arises from the heart and gives rise to the coronary arteries, aorta, and pulmonary arteries. There is a single semilunar 'truncal' valve that has three or more leaflets, and a subtruncal ventricular septal defect. Figure 23 shows the different patterns by which the pulmonary arteries arise, type 1 is the most common.

Most patients present in infancy with heart failure. If left unoperated, pulmonary vascular resistance rises, cyanosis becomes more marked, and the Eisenmenger reaction becomes established. Repair before pulmonary vascular disease develops involves closure of the ventricular septal defect, detachment of the pulmonary arteries from the common arterial trunk, and placement of a valved right ventricular to pulmonary artery conduit. The truncal valve then functions as the aortic valve. Late complications include truncal regurgitation and the need to replace stenotic conduits.

Table 13 Long-term complications of Fontan-type surgery

Atrial flutter/fibrillation
Progressive ventricular dysfunction
Atrioventricular valve regurgitation
Thromboembolism
Pathway obstruction
Protein-losing enteropathy
Recurrent effusions, ascites, peripheral oedema
Development of subaortic stenosis
Right lower pulmonary vein compression by dilated right atrium
Cyanosis (due to development of venous collaterals to the left atrium or
    pulmonary arteriovenous fistulas)

Aortopulmonary window

In this rare condition there is a direct communication between adjacent portions of the proximal ascending aorta and pulmonary artery. The communication is usually large and the physiological consequences are the same as for a patent arterial duct. Rare patients surviving without operation into adulthood are likely to have developed the Eisenmenger reaction. If pulmonary vascular resistance is low at the time of childhood repair, long-term postoperative survival is good.

Coronary artery anomalies

The importance of congenital coronary anomalies lies in their potential to impair myocardial blood flow and cause ischaemia and sudden death. Evidence of ischaemia is the main indication for repair. The major types of coronary anomaly are shown in Table 14.

Anomalous origin of the coronary arteries from an inappropriate aortic sinus

Ischaemia is particularly associated with an anomalous proximal coronary course between the aorta and pulmonary trunk, an intramural proximal segment of the coronary artery inside the aortic wall, and acute angulation between the origin of an anomalous coronary artery and the aortic wall.

Anomalous origin of the left coronary artery from the pulmonary artery

This rare condition usually presents in infancy with myocardial ischaemia and left ventricular failure when pulmonary vascular resistance decreases. However, 10 to 15 per cent survive into adulthood because an adequate intercoronary collateral circulation is established. Adults may be asymptomatic or present with myocardial ischaemia or mitral regurgitation due to papillary muscle dysfunction. Survival following surgical repair depends on the amount of ischaemic myocardial damage and degree of mitral regurgitation.

Congenital coronary arteriovenous fistulas

The coronary arteries arise normally from their aortic sinuses, but a fistulous branch communicates directly with the right ventricle in 40 per cent of cases (Fig. 24), the right atrium in 25 per cent, pulmonary artery in 15 per cent, or rarely the superior vena cava or pulmonary vein. Survival to adulthood is usual, but life expectancy is reduced and depends on the size of the fistulous connection and the presence of myocardial ischaemia resulting from any coronary steal phenomenon. Symptoms increase with age and there is a risk of endocarditis, heart failure, arrhythmia, myocardial ischaemia and infarction, and sudden death. Surgical repair is recommended unless there is a trivial isolated shunt. Some smaller fistulas are suitable for transcatheter device occlusion.

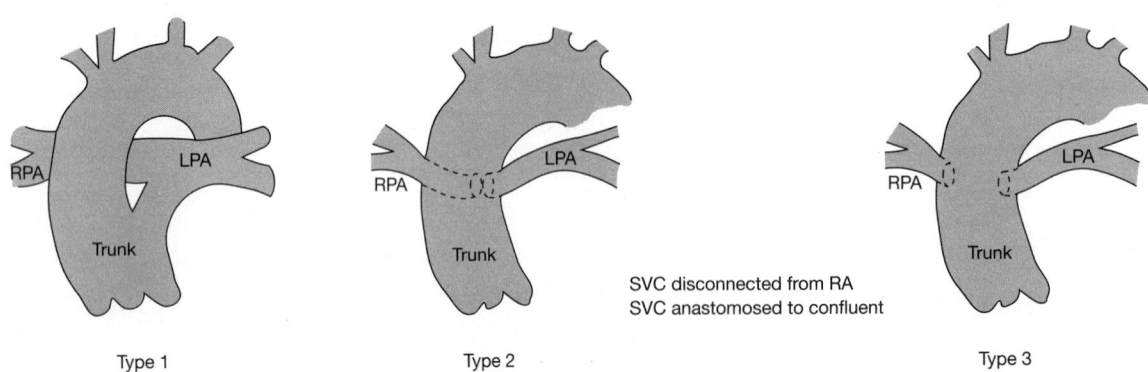

Fig. 23 Truncus arteriosus. Type 1 has a short main pulmonary artery arising from the common arterial trunk. Types 2 and 3 can be considered together, the pulmonary arteries have separate origins from the common trunk. LPA, left pulmonary artery; RPA, right pulmonary artery.

Table 14 Major types of coronary anomaly

Anomalous origin from inappropriate aortic sinus or coronary vessel	LAD from right aortic sinus or RCA
	Absent LMS (separate origins of LAD and Cx)
	Cx from right aortic sinus or RCA or absent Cx
	RCA from left aortic sinus, posterior sinus, or LAD
	Single coronary artery from right or left aortic sinus
Anomalous origin from other systemic artery (rare)	Innominate, subclavian, internal mammary, carotid, bronchial arteries, or descending aorta
Anomalous origin from pulmonary artery	
Coronary arteriovenous fistulas	

Cx, circumflex; LAD, left anterior descending; LMS, left main stem; RCA, right coronary artery.

Ruptured sinus of Valsalva aneurysm

Any of the three aortic sinuses of Valsalva may become aneurysmal and rupture. The right and non-coronary cusps are most often affected; rupture of the non-coronary sinus aneurysm is nearly always into the right atrium and of the right coronary sinus into the right ventricle or atrium. Involvement of the left coronary sinus is rare. Rupture usually occurs in early adulthood and may be precipitated by endocarditis. If sudden, it is accompanied by tearing chest pain, breathlessness, and congestive cardiac failure with a loud continuous murmur. Small perforations may remain asymptomatic for many years. The diagnosis and site of the rupture is confirmed angiographically prior to surgical repair. Transcatheter closure has also been reported.

Pregnancy in women with congenital heart disease

In general, the combined oral contraceptive pill is contraindicated in cyanosis, pulmonary hypertension, and following Fontan-type surgery. The progesterone-only pill and progesterone depot injections are safe alternatives, but the former is less reliable. Intrauterine devices are not ideal for many women because of the risk of endocarditis and menorrhagia. Women with pulmonary hypertension may wish to consider sterilization: although a delicate issue, sterilization of the male partner is not recommended as he is likely to outlive the patient and may wish to start a family later. Ven-

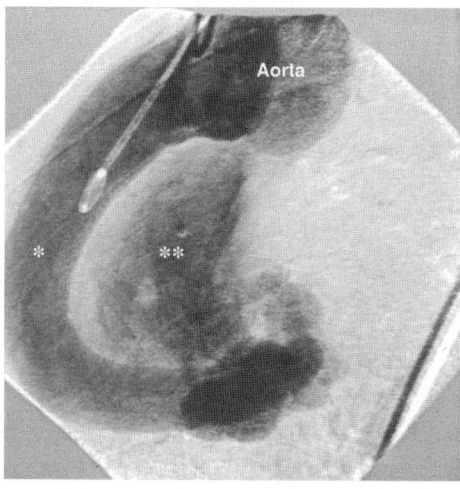

Fig. 24 Angiogram (left anterior oblique) of a 32-year-old man with a huge right coronary artery fistula (*) to the right ventricle (**).

tricular dysfunction and arrhythmias tend to deteriorate during pregnancy: regurgitant lesions are better tolerated than stenotic lesions. Pregnancy is contraindicated in pulmonary hypertension, severe systemic ventricular dysfunction (ejection fraction (EF) less than 20 per cent), and severe unoperated left-sided obstruction.

Unoperated atrial septal defect

Atrial septal defect is usually well tolerated in pregnancy; the major risk is of paradoxical embolism, so meticulous leg care and low-dose aspirin are important to avoid venous thrombosis. Haemorrhage may cause a significant increase in left to right shunting by reducing systemic venous return and increasing systemic vascular resistance. Women older than 30 years are at higher risk of developing atrial arrhythmias and right ventricular dysfunction as a result of the increased blood volume of pregnancy.

Tetralogy of Fallot after radical repair

Pregnancy is usually well tolerated after radical repair, provided there is little outflow tract gradient and ventricular function is good.

Ebstein anomaly

The risks relate to an inability of the functional right ventricle to accommodate the increased blood volume of pregnancy. Cyanosis and the risk of paradoxical embolism may present for the first time in pregnancy because of a rise in right ventricular pressure.

Systemic right ventricle

The ability of patients with congenitally corrected transposition of the great arteries or previous Mustard operation to tolerate pregnancy depends on the function of the systemic ventricle, systemic atrioventricular regurgitation, pulmonary venous baffle obstruction (patients with a Mustard procedure), and atrial tachyarrhythmias, all of which may worsen as pregnancy progresses. Patients with complete heart block may tolerate pregnancy better after the insertion of a permanent pacemaker.

Coarctation of the aorta

Pregnancy is a risk factor for aortic dissection and rupture, especially if there is an aneurysm at the site of repair or a coexisting bicuspid aortic valve. Histology of any dissected area shows cystic medial necrosis. Meticulous control of blood pressure is important and the second stage of labour should be kept short to reduce arterial wall stress.

After Fontan operation

Despite the limited ability to increase cardiac output, successful pregnancy is possible in patients with a good postoperative result who have not developed major late complications. There is a high incidence of early miscarriage.

Women with cyanosis but no pulmonary hypertension

Maternal mortality is considerably less in women with cyanosis but normal or low pulmonary artery pressures than in those with pulmonary hypertension. Maternal morbidity and fetal outcome are determined by ventricular function and cyanosis. The reduction in systemic vascular resistance and increase in cardiac output during pregnancy increases the right to left shunt, resulting in a fall in Sao_2. If resting Sao_2 is less than 85 per cent, the risk of miscarriage is around 80 per cent, with additional risks of low birth weight and prematurity. Heart failure may be precipitated by the increased blood volume, particularly if there is aortic regurgitation. The hypercoagulable state of pregnancy combined with a high haematocrit increases the risk of thrombosis and paradoxical embolism. Patients are also at risk of haemorrhage during delivery, particularly if a section is performed. Labour and

Table 15 Risks of infective endocarditis or endarteritis in congenital heart disease

Low risk: lesions with no or low velocity turbulence and no prosthetic material

Unoperated	Operated
Anomalous pulmonary venous drainage	Anomalous pulmonary venous drainage
Secundum atrial septal defect	Secundum atrial septal defect
Ebstein's anomaly	Ebstein's anomaly with repaired native valve
Mild pulmonary stenosis	Ventricular septal defect/tetralogy of Fallot
Isolated corrected transposition	without residual lesions
Pulmonary vascular disease with reversed shunt	Patent ductus arteriosus
Primary pulmonary hypertension	Glenn- or Fontan-type procedures
	Arterial switch for transposition

Moderate risk

Unoperated	Operated
Systemic atrioventricular valve regurgitation	Residual regurgitation of repaired native
Subaortic stenosis	aortic or systemic atrioventricular valve
Moderate to severe pulmonary stenosis	Non-valved conduits
Restrictive ventricular septal defect	
Tetralogy of Fallot	
Double-outlet right ventricle	
Univentricular heart with pulmonary stenosis	
Truncus arteriosus	
Coarctation	
Restrictive patent ductus arteriosus	

High risk

Unoperated	Operated
Bicuspid aortic valve	Prosthetic valves
Aortic regurgitation secondary to ventricular septal	Valved conduits
defect or subaortic stenosis	Aortopulmonary shunts, e.g. Gore-Tex, modified
	Blalock–Taussig

delivery must be managed carefully, avoiding hypovolaemia and vasodilatation which may precipitate intense cyanosis, syncope, and death.

Eisenmenger syndrome

Maternal mortality remains unchanged at about 40 per cent. Women should be counselled strongly against pregnancy, given adequate contraceptive advice, and be advised to undergo therapeutic termination if contraception fails.

Management of pregnant women with the Eisenmenger syndrome is difficult and requires expertise, not least because data to support treatment decisions are sparse. The fixed pulmonary vascular resistance and reduction in systemic vascular resistance enhance the right to left shunt, increasing maternal and fetal hypoxia. The patient should be admitted for bed rest during the second trimester and meticulous care given to avoid deep venous thrombosis, dehydration, and vasodilation. Oxygen therapy, nitric oxide, and heparin may be given, although there is no firm evidence that any are beneficial, and heparin increases the risk of haemorrhage. Abrupt changes in systemic vascular resistance or blood pressure during labour and delivery may induce intense cyanosis and death. Opinion is divided as to whether vaginal delivery with forceps assistance or caesarean section should be performed. Vaginal delivery may be safer, causing less rapid haemodynamic changes and less blood loss. The risk of sudden death continues for the first 2 weeks after delivery, either from deteriorating haemodynamics or pulmonary infarction.

Bacterial endocarditis

Endocarditis is discussed elsewhere; the risks for specific congenital lesions are outlined in Table 15.

Further reading

Reviews and books on congenital heart disease

Anderson RH, Becker AE (1997). *Controversies in the description of congenitally malformed hearts.* Imperial College Press, London.

Ho SY *et al.* (1995). *Colour atlas of congenital heart disease. Morphological and clinical correlations.* Times Mirror Publications Mosby-Wolfe, London.

Kirklin JW, Barratt-Boyes BG (1993). *Cardiac surgery,* 2nd edn. Churchill Livingstone, New York.

Perloff JK (1994). The clinical recognition of congenital heart disease. In: Perloff JK, ed. *Congenital heart disease in adults,* pp 293–380. WB Saunders, Philadelphia.

Perloff JK, Child JS (1998). *Congenital heart disease in adults.* WB Saunders, Philadelphia.

Stark J, de Leval MR, eds (1994). *Surgery for congenital heart defects.* WB Saunders, London.

Warnes CA (1997). Cyanotic congenital heart disease. In: Oakley C, ed. *Heart disease in pregnancy,* pp 83–96. British Medical Journal Publishing Group, London.

Introduction and genetics

Burn J *et al.* (1998). Recurrence risks in offspring of adults with major heart defects: results from first cohort of British collaborative study. *Lancet* **351**, 311–6.

Digilio MC *et al.* (1997). Recurrence risk figures for isolated tetralogy of Fallot after screening for 22q11 microdeletion. *Journal of Medical Genetics* **34**, 188–90.

Farrell MJ *et al.* (1999). HIRA, a di George syndrome candidate gene, is required for outflow tract septation. *Circulation Research* **84**, 127–35.

Kelly D *et al.* (1993). Confirmation that the velo-cardio-facial syndrome is associated with haplo-insufficiency of genes at chromosome 22q11. *American Journal of Medical Genetics* **45**, 308–12.

Li QY *et al.* (1997). Holt–Oram syndrome is caused by mutations in TBX5, a member of the Brachyury (T) gene family. *Nature Genetics* **15**, 21–9.

MacMahon B, McKeown T, Record RG (1953). The incidence and life expectation of children with congenital heart disease. *British Heart Journal* **15**, 121–9.

Nora JJ (1968). Multifactorial inheritance hypothesis for the etiology of congenital heart diseases: the genetic–environmental interaction. *Circulation* **38**, 604–17.

Trainer AH *et al.* (1996). Chromosome 22q11 microdeletion in tetralogy of Fallot. *Archives of Disease in Childhood* **74**, 62–3.

Eisenmenger syndrome

Ammash N, Warnes CA (1996). Cerebrovascular events in adult patients with cyanotic congenital heart disease. *Journal of the American College of Cardiology* **28**, 768–72.

Bowyer JJ *et al.* (1986). Effect of long term oxygen treatment at home in children with pulmonary vascular disease. *British Heart Journal* **55**, 385–90.

Harinck E *et al.* (1996). Air travel and adults with cyanotic congenital heart disease. *Circulation* **93**, 272–6.

Martínez-Lavín M (1997). Hypertrophic osteoarthopathy. *Current Opinion in Rheumatology* **9**, 83–6.

Maurer HM *et al.* (1975). Correction of platelet dysfunction and bleeding in cyanotic congenital heart disease by simple red cell volume reduction. *American Journal of Cardiology* **35**, 831–5.

Rosenzweig EB, Kerstein D, Barst RJ (1999). Long term prostacyclin for pulmonary hypertension with associated congenital heart defects. *Circulation* **99**, 1858–65.

Thorne SA (1998). Management of polycythaemia in adults with cyanotic congenital heart disease. *Heart* **79**, 315–16.

Wood P (1958). The Eisenmenger syndrome: or pulmonary hypertension with reversed central shunt. *British Medical Journal* **ii**, 701–9, 755–62.

Specific forms of congenital heart disease

Anomalies of venous drainage and atrial arrangement

Dupuis C *et al.* (1992). The 'adult' form of the scimitar syndrome. *American Journal of Cardiology* **70**, 502–7.

Van Mierop LHS, Eisen S, Schiebler GL (1970). The radiographic appearance of the tracheobronchial tree as an indicator of visceral situs. *American Journal of Cardiology* **26**, 432–5.

Van Mierop LHS, Gessner IH, Schiebler GL (1972). Asplenia and polysplenia syndromes. *Birth Defects* **8**, 36–44.

Atrial septal and atrioventricular canal defects

Campbell M (1970). Natural history of atrial septal defect. *British Heart Journal* **32**, 820–6.

Cherian G *et al.* (1983). Pulmonary hypertension in isolated atrial septal defect. *American Heart Journal* **105**, 952–7.

Clapp S *et al.* (1990). Down's syndrome, complete atrioventricular canal and pulmonary vascular obstructive disease. *Journal of Thoracic and Cardiovascular Surgery* **100**, 115–21.

Cooney TP, Thurlbeck WM (1982). Pulmonary hypoplasia in Down's syndrome. *New England Journal of Medicine* **307**, 1170–3.

Dalen JE, Bruce RA, Cobb LA (1962). Interaction of chronic hypoxia of moderate altitude on pulmonary hypertension complicating defect of the atrial septum. *New England Journal of Medicine* **266**, 272–7.

Gatzoulis MA *et al.* (1999). Atrial arrhythmia after surgical closure of atrial septal defects in adults. *New England Journal of Medicine* **340**, 839–46.

Helber U *et al.* (1997). Atrial septal defect in adults: cardiopulmonary exercise capacity before and 4 months and 10 years after defect closure. *Journal of the American College of Cardiology* **29**, 1345–50.

Konstanides S *et al.* (1995). A comparison of surgical and medical therapy for atrial septal defects in adults. *New England Journal of Medicine* **333**, 469–73.

Murphy JG *et al.* (1990). Long term outcome after surgical repair of isolated secundum atrial septal defect: follow up at 27–32 years. *New England Journal of Medicine* **323**, 1645–50.

Schamroth CL *et al.* (1987). Pulmonary arterial thrombosis in secundum atrial septal defect. *American Journal of Cardiology* **60**, 1152–6.

Lesions affecting ventricular inflow

Gentles TL *et al.* (1992). Predictors of longterm survival with Ebstein's anomaly of the tricuspid valve. *American Journal of Cardiology* **69**, 377–81.

Shiina A *et al.* (1983). Two-dimensional echocardiographic–surgical correlation in Ebstein's anomaly: preoperative determination of patients requiring tricuspid valve plication vs replacement. *Circulation* **68**, 534–44.

Theodoro DA *et al.* (1998). Right-sided maze procedure for right atrial arrhythmias in congenital heart disease. *Annals of Thoracic Surgery* **65**, 149–54.

Van Arsdell GS *et al.* (1996). Superior vena cava to pulmonary artery anastomosis: an adjunct to biventricular repair. *Journal of Thoracic and Cardiovascular Surgery* **112**, 1143–8.

Other right ventricular anomalies

Blake RS *et al.*(1982). Conduction defects, ventricular arrhythmias, and late death after surgical closure of ventricular septal defect. *British Heart Journal* **47**, 305–15.

Campbell M (1971). Natural history of ventricular septal defect. *British Heart Journal* **33**, 246–57.

Chaturvedi RR, Shore DS, Redington AN (1996). Intraoperative apical ventricular septal defect closure using a modified Rashkind double umbrella. *Heart* **76**, 367–9.

Kumar K, Lock JE, Geva T (1997). Apical muscular ventricular septal defects between the left ventricle and the right ventricle infundibulum: diagnostic and interventional considerations. *Circulation* **95**, 1207–13.

Lue HC (1986). Is subpulmonic ventricular septal defect an Oriental disease? In: Lue HC, Takao A, eds. *Subpulmonic ventricular septal defect*, 1st edn, pp 3–8. Springer-Verlag, Tokyo.

Moe DG, Guntheroth WG (1987). Spontaneous closure of uncomplicated ventricular septal defect. *American Journal of Cardiology* **60**, 674–8.

Tetralogy of Fallot

Blalock A, Taussig HB (1945). Surgical treatment of malformations of the heart in which there is pulmonary stenosis or pulmonary atresia. *Journal of the American Medical Association* **128**, 189–202.

Bricker JT (1995). Sudden death and tetralogy of Fallot. *Circulation* **92**, 162–3.

Bull K *et al.* (1995). Presentation and attrition in complex pulmonary atresia. *Journal of the American College of Cardiology* **25**, 491–9.

Gatzoulis MA *et al.* (1995). Mechanoelectrical interactions in tetralogy of Fallot. *Circulation* **92**, 231–7.

Kirklin JW *et al.* (1988). Survival functional status and reoperations after repair of tetralogy of Fallot with pulmonary atresia. *Journal of Thoracic and Cardiovascular Surgery* **96**, 102–16.

Murphy JG *et al.* (1993). Long-term outcome in patients undergoing surgical repair of tetralogy of Fallot. *New England Journal of Medicine* **329**, 593–9.

Redington AN, Somerville J (1996). Stenting of aortopulmonary collaterals in complex pulmonary atresia. *Circulation* **94**, 2479–84.

Left ventricular outflow tract obstruction and aortic coarctation

Campbell M (1999). Natural history of coarctation of the aorta. *British Heart Journal* **32**, 633–40.

Carvlho JS *et al.* (1990). Continuous wave Doppler echocardiography and coarctation of the aorta: gradients and flow patterns in the assessment of severity. *British Heart Journal* **64**, 133–7.

Koller M, Rothlin M, Senning Å (1987). Coarctation of the aorta: review of 362 operated patients. Long term follow up and assessment of prognostic variables. *European Heart Journal* **8**, 670–9.

Roberts CS, Roberts WC (1991). Dissection of the aorta associated with congenital malformation of the aortic valve. *Journal of the American College of Cardiology* **17**, 712–16.

Wells WJ *et al.* (1996). Repair of coarctation of the aorta in adults: the fate of systolic hypertension. *Annals of Thoracic Surgery* **61**, 1168–71.

Transposition of the great arteries

Cochrane AD, Karl TR, Mee RBB (1993). Arterial switch for late failure of the systemic right ventricle. *Annals of Thoracic Surgery* **56**, 854–61.

Imai Y *et al.* (1994). Ventricular function after anatomic repair in patients with atrioventricular discordance. *Journal of Thoracic and Cardiovascular Surgery* **107**, 1272–83.

Reddy VM *et al.* (1997). The double switch procedure for anatomical repair of congenitally corrected transposition of the great arteries in infants and children. *European Heart Journal* **18**, 1470–7.

Redington AN *et al.* (1998). *The right heart in congenital heart disease.* Greenwich Medical Media, London.

Yagihara T *et al.* (1994). Double switch operation in cardiac anomalies with atrioventricular and ventriculoarterial discordance. *Journal of Thoracic and Cardiovascular Surgery* **107**, 31–8.

Univentricular atrioventricular connection and the Fontan operation

Cromme-Dijkhuis AH *et al.* (1990). Coagulation factor abnormalities as possible thrombotic risk factors after Fontan operations. *Lancet* **336**, 1087–90.

de Leval M *et al.* (1988). Total cavopulmonary connection: a logical alternative to atriopulmonary connection for complex Fontan operations. *Journal of Thoracic and Cardiovascular Surgery* **96**, 682–5.

Driscoll DJ *et al.* (1992). Five to fifteen year follow-up after Fontan operation. *Circulation* **85**, 469–96.

Feldt RH *et al.* (1996). Protein-losing enteropathy after the Fontan operation. *Journal of Thoracic and Cardiovascular Surgery* **112**, 672–80.

Fontan F *et al.* (1990). Outcome after a 'perfect' Fontan operation. *Circulation* **81**, 1520–36.

Fontan F, Baudet E (1972) . Surgical repair of tricuspid atresia. *Thorax* **26**, 240–8.

Glenn WW (1958). Circulatory bypass of the right heart. IV. Shunt between superior vena cava and distal right pulmonary artery—report of clinical application. *New England Journal of Medicine* **259**, 117.

Mavroudis C *et al.* (1998). Fontan conversion to cavopulmonary connection and arrhythmia circuit cryoablation. *Journal of Thoracic and Cardiovascular Surgery* **115**, 547–56.

Moodie DS *et al.* (1984). Long term follow up in the unoperated univentricular heart. *American Journal of Cardiology* **53**, 1124–8.

Thorne SA *et al.* (1999). Amiodarone-associated thyroid dysfunction in adults with congenital heart disease. *Circulation* **100**, 149–54.

Coronary artery anomalies

Roberts WC (1986). Major anomalies of coronary arterial origin seen in adulthood. *American Heart Journal* **111**, 941–62.

Pregnancy and congenital heart disease

Canobbio MM *et al.* (1996). Pregnancy outcomes after Fontan repair. *Journal of the American College of Cardiology* **28**, 763–7.

Clarkson PM *et al.* (1994). Outcome of pregnancy after the Mustard operation for transposition of the great arteries with intact ventricular septum. *Journal of the American College of Cardiology* **24**, 190–3.

Connelly HM, Grogan M, Warnes CA (1999). Pregnancy among women with congenitally corrected transposition of the great arteries. *Journal of the American College of Cardiology* **33**, 1692–5.

Presbitero P *et al.* (1994). Pregnancy in cyanotic congenital heart disease. *Circulation* **89**, 2673–6.

Yentis SM, Steer P, Plaat F (1998). Eisenmenger's syndrome in pregnancy: maternal and fetal mortality in the 1990s. *British Journal of Obstetrics and Gynaecology* **105**, 921–2.

15.14 Disorders of the arteries

15.14.1 Thoracic aortic dissection

B. Gribbin and A. P. Banning

Introduction

Acute dissection of the thoracic aorta is uncommon: approximately 20 to 40 cases may be seen in a specialist cardiac unit each year. Unrecognized and untreated it carries a mortality of up to 2 per cent per hour and 90 per cent within the first few weeks. The catastrophic and potentially lethal nature of the dissection process means that quick recognition and treatment are fundamental. Non-invasive diagnostic imaging must be rapid, safe, and accurate. For patients with confirmed dissection of the ascending aorta, emergency surgery may be lifesaving, but when the ascending aorta is spared, aggressive control of blood pressure is the usual initial management, with surgery being considered if there is evidence of further progression of dissection or ischaemic complications.

Despite advances in aortic imaging, surgery, and anaesthesia, survivors of acute dissection have an uncertain long-term prognosis. Careful medical follow-up is recommended and serial aortic imaging can provide important prognostic information, but optimal management of survivors remains controversial.

Pathogenesis

The aortic wall is composed of three layers: a thin intimal lining; a thicker medial layer, largely composed of elastin fibres that provide strength; and a thinner adventitial outer layer from which small blood vessels, the vasa vasorum, arise to nourish the outer layers of the media. Dissection occurs when a breach in the integrity of the intima allows blood at high pressure to penetrate the media. Through this tear, pulsatile blood flow can then propagate distally, parallel to the lumen, often spiralling and splitting the arterial wall into an inner (intima–medial) and outer layer (media–adventitial). This process of tearing within the wall results in the formation of a false lumen, parallel to the original true lumen, and commonly of similar size (Fig. 1 and Plate 1). Further communication(s) between the lumens (or re-entry tears) can occur and may reduce the pressure within the false lumen thus limiting propagation of the dissection. However, the process often extends along the entire length of the aorta to the common iliac artery, threatening the origins of branch vessels which may be avulsed or narrowed by the mass effect of the false lumen, leading to ischaemia in the dependent vascular territories. When dissection extends retrogradely towards the heart it can cause occlusion of a coronary artery and distortion of the aortic valve causing aortic regurgitation. It may also rupture into the pericardial space causing tamponade. The weakened aortic wall can rupture at any point along its length: this is usually fatal.

Classification

The commonest sites for thoracic aortic dissection to begin are in the ascending aorta just above the sinuses of the aortic valve and in the upper descending aorta just beyond the origin of the left subclavian artery. Two classifications are used to describe the extent of aortic involvement. De Bakey and colleagues described a classification of dissection that is primarily anatomical and involves three groups: type 1—involving the ascending aorta and arch, with or without involvement of the descending aorta; type 2—involving the ascending aorta alone, without involvement of the arch or descending aorta; and type 3—involving only the descending aorta. When dissection involves the ascending aorta, emergency surgery is the usual treatment, whereas medical treatment is the initial treatment for patients with uncomplicated dissection sparing the ascending aorta. Therefore, using the De Bakey classification, types 1 and 2 dissection would be considered for surgery.

The Stanford group have subsequently proposed a classification that is directly linked to patient management. Dissection involving the ascending thoracic aorta is classified as type A and demands immediate surgery, whereas dissection which spares the ascending aorta is classified as type B and initial management is usually medical. This classification is recommended as it is unambiguous (Fig. 2).

Aetiology

The most common predisposing factor is hypertension, which is present in the great majority of patients with aortic dissection. Although the processes involved in the initiation of dissection remain incompletely understood,

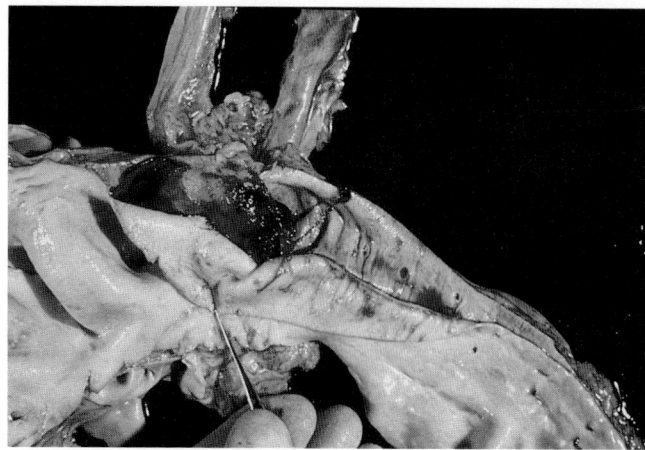

Fig. 1 Post-mortem specimen of aortic dissection. The intimal/medial flap is pulled back with a retractor to show the false lumen parallel to the true lumen. (See also Plate 1.)

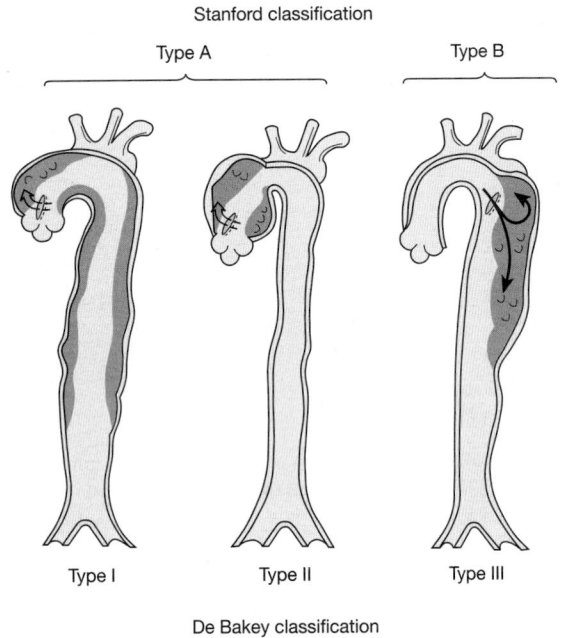

Stanford classification

Type A   Type B

Type I   Type II   Type III

De Bakey classification

Fig. 2 Diagram of the Stanford and De Bakey classifications of aortic dissection.

medial haemorrhage from rupture of vasa vasorum appears to be important. When this process is self-limiting and there is no expansion of the resultant haematoma by recurrent bleeding, healing may occur with reabsorption of the haemorrhage. Alternatively, and particularly when the bleeding is extensive or recurrent, a large intramural haematoma may form around the circumference of the aorta. This alters the distribution of tensile stresses within the aorta, with much of the redistributed stress affecting the intima/endothelium overlying the mass. An intimal tear may then result in splitting and separation of the media, propagation of a false lumen, and dissection.

Patients with the Marfan syndrome may present with aortic dissection or aortic root dilatation (see Chapter 15.12). It is proposed that abnormal fibrillin within the aortic media results in intimal instability, particularly when aortic dilation leads to increased wall stress. Although the absolute risk of dissection rises with increasing size of the ascending aorta, it is important to remember that all patients with Marfan syndrome are at risk, particularly when there is a family history of dissection. Patients with Ehlers–Danlos syndrome are also at risk of spontaneous dissection, not only of the aorta but of its principal branches, including the coronary arteries.

Patients with coarctation of the aorta and those with bicuspid aortic valves appear to be at increased risk of dissection: it is uncertain if this association is related to a defect in aortic wall composition. Dissection may also occur in patients with Turner syndrome, Noonan syndrome, and in the later stages of pregnancy, particularly in patients with Marfan syndrome. In high-risk patients with Marfan syndrome with dilated aortas or a family history of dissection, deferring pregnancy until after elective aortic root replacement may be advisable.

Clinical presentation

Most patients present with characteristic symptoms and clinical findings, in which case the diagnosis of dissection can be made with reasonable assurance. However, a minority present atypically and it is worth considering the possibility of aortic dissection in any patient who is haemodynamically unstable without satisfactory explanation.

The pain of acute dissection of the aorta can be described in terms of (i) its instantaneous onset, (ii) its cataclysmic severity, (iii) its pulsatile and

tearing quality, (iv) its location either in the anterior thorax or back, and (v) its migration as it follows the course of the dissection through the thorax. Careful interrogation about the presence of these five features will usually allow differentiation from other causes of chest pain. The instant onset, tearing/pulsatile quality, and migratory pattern contrasts particularly with the pain of cardiac ischaemia, which is usually gradual in onset, tight or crushing, and more unchanging in its distribution in the anterior chest. Syncope shortly after the onset of typical pain is not common but is another characteristic presentation of dissection, often caused by rupture of the false lumen into the pericardial cavity. Other uncommon modes of presentation include stroke and limb ischaemia with or without pain and very occasionally congestive heart failure resulting from severe aortic regurgitation.

Although patients with dissection usually appear shocked, their blood pressure may be normal or raised and their heart rate relatively slow. The distribution of the abnormalities detected by physical examination usually reflects the region of the aorta involved in the dissection and pressure on adjacent structures. Signs of aortic regurgitation or tamponade are likely to be found in a patient with dissection involving the ascending aorta, whereas absent upper limb pulses and cerebral abnormalities suggest involvement of the aortic arch. Expansion of the arch may compress venous return and cause engorgement of one or both jugular veins. Similarly, hoarseness and Horner's syndrome can follow pressure on the left recurrent laryngeal nerve and superior cervical ganglion, respectively. Tenderness over a carotid artery may be due to dissection extending up the artery from the arch. Involvement of the descending aorta can result in visceral and lower limb ischaemia.

Although traditional teaching emphasizes the relevance of blood pressure discrepancy between the arms, this is not a particularly sensitive sign, particularly when dissection spares the ascending aorta and arch. However, evidence of new aortic regurgitation or development of pulse deficits are specific signs of dissection and should be actively sought by the examining physician.

Abnormalities of the chest radiograph and electrocardiogram are not uncommon in patients with dissection, but neither investigation is diagnostic and further imaging is always necessary. Potential abnormalities on the chest radiograph include tracheal deviation, left pleural effusion, a widened mediastinum, and the 'calcium sign' (Fig. 3).

Non-specific ST-segment and T-wave changes on the electrocardiogram are often found, as are changes related to previous hypertension. Actual involvement of a coronary artery is relatively uncommon although the right coronary artery is more likely to be affected. An atypical distribution of ischaemic changes (i.e. generalized acute changes, not consistent with just one coronary territory) is more usual and should always alert the physician to the possibility of a diagnosis other than acute myocardial infarction

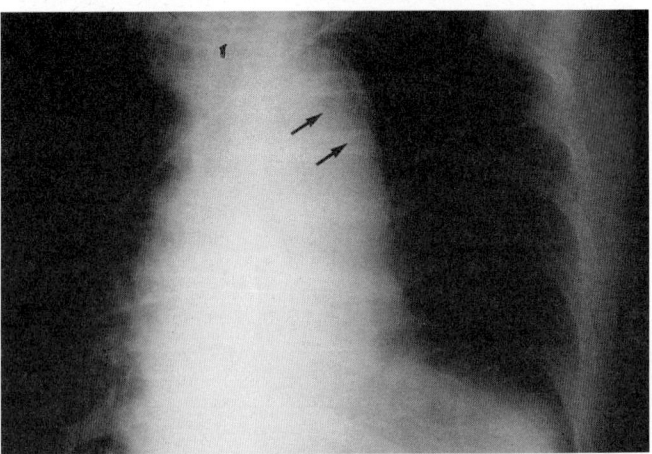

Fig. 3 Chest radiograph showing calcium in the aortic knuckle, which is displaced medially (arrows).

and the danger of the inadvertent administration of thrombolytic treatment.

Emergency management

Lowering systolic blood pressure and limiting shear stress reduces the likelihood of progression of dissection. Every patient with a clinical suspicion of dissection should therefore receive effective pain relief (intravenous morphine is usually required) and antihypertensive medication pending a definitive diagnosis by imaging. Patients should be cared for in a high dependency area with continuous monitoring of the electrocardiogram and regular blood pressure and urine output measurement. Ideally, systolic blood pressure should be maintained below 110 mmHg, using intravenous labetalol (initial dose 1 mg/min) or esmolol. Both of these agents produce a rapid and titratable reduction in blood pressure, with β-blockade particularly appropriate in this context as it reduces the force of cardiac contraction and the rate of rise of the arterial pressure. If blood pressure control remains suboptimal, an additional infusion of sodium nitroprusside may be used (0.5 to 8 μg/kg.min).

Optimal management of patients with dissection requires close liaison between district hospitals and cardiac surgical centres, using local guidelines for investigation that should reflect the available expertise and surgical opinion. Patients with a low clinical index of suspicion of dissection who are in a stable cardiovascular state should undergo prompt investigation in their local hospital, using a nominated non-invasive technique—usually CT scanning. Unless non-invasive imaging is available immediately, unstable patients with a high clinical index of suspicion should receive medical treatment and be transferred immediately to a surgical centre for both diagnostic imaging and management. This approach minimizes delay, a critical aspect of the management of acute aortic dissection.

Imaging

The priorities when imaging a patient with suspected dissection are to confirm the diagnosis and to decide if the ascending aorta is involved (Stanford type A) as this will determine whether or not surgery is required. The surgeon wants to know the entry site of the dissection, if the aortic valve is competent, if there is a pericardial effusion or tamponade, and if there is involvement of the coronary arteries. Several diagnostic techniques are available.

Historically, aortography was the investigation of choice, but it has several disadvantages. These include delay during the assembly of the catheter laboratory team, the risk of aortic rupture during catheter manipulation, and the nephrotoxicity of radiological contrast media when renal function may already be compromised by hypotension or renal artery involvement. Computed tomography (**CT**), magnetic resonance imaging (**MRI**), and echocardiography all have proven advantages over aortography.

Contrast-enhanced CT is non-invasive, but requires the use of radiological contrast medium. Its sensitivity and specificity is at least equivalent to aortography, but its accuracy is inferior to both MRI and transoesophageal echocardiography, although improved diagnostic accuracy has been demonstrated by ultrafast and spiral CT.

MRI is non-invasive and provides excellent images of the whole aorta. Its sensitivity and specificity for dissection is up to 100 per cent in some series, and the addition of cardiac gated and 'cine' techniques can give information on luminal blood flow and valvular regurgitation. MRI is therefore the investigation of choice for most diseases affecting the aorta, but it has several limitations in patients with suspected acute dissection of the aorta. These include the requirement for patient transfer to the scanner, with attendant delays, restricted access to the patient during scanning, and the high degree of patient co-operation required to obtain artefact-free images.

Transthoracic echocardiography cannot exclude aortic dissection as it has limited sensitivity and specificity. However, in some patients dissection of the ascending aorta can be confidently diagnosed using parasternal and suprasternal imaging, mandating urgent transfer to a surgical centre where additional information can be obtained by transoesophageal echocardiography in the anaesthetic room.

Transoesophageal echocardiography provides detailed anatomical information about the morphology of a dissection and can also demonstrate the consequences of proximal extension, including the presence of aortic regurgitation, pericardial effusion, and involvement of the coronary artery ostia, thus making complementary investigations such as angiography unnecessary. It can be performed rapidly by a single operator with nursing assistance, in an environment where the patient can be monitored and remains accessible to medical staff. This approach minimizes delay and allows rapid transfer to the operating theatre, making transoesophageal echocardiography the ideal diagnostic tool for the emergency situation (Fig. 4 and Plate 2).

Surgery for dissection of the ascending aorta

When the dissection involves the ascending aorta (Stanford type A), immediate surgery is required as there is a high risk of proximal extension causing dissection of the coronary arteries, incompetence of the aortic valve, and rupture into the pericardium. Surgery usually involves excision of the intimal tear in the ascending aorta and interposition of a dacron graft. This procedure protects the lower ascending aorta and valve from progressive dissection and prevents distal extension by reducing pressure within the false lumen. The false lumen may subsequently thrombose, or in cases with multiple intimal tears, may remain patent but decompressed.

Replacement of the aortic valve is usually performed only when resuspension of the valve is not possible. However, in patients with Marfan syndrome the ascending aorta and valve are usually replaced with a composite graft to prevent subsequent annular dilatation. In cases where dissection extends into the aortic arch, some surgeons advocate that the arch and great vessels should be included in the initial repair as arch involvement is a strong predictor of a requirement for repeat surgery. However, this extended surgery increases the duration of the operation and the risk of central nervous system damage, hence inclusion of the arch in dissection repair is generally restricted to centres with particular expertise.

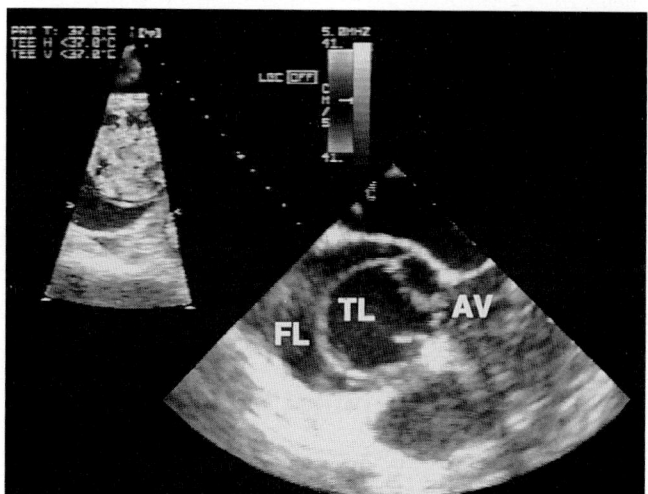

Fig. 4 Transoesophageal transverse two-dimensional and colour Doppler echo images of the ascending aorta showing a dissection membrane partitioning the true (TL) and false lumen (FL). Upper left panel shows systolic flow in the true but not the false lumen. (See also Plate 2.)

Management of descending aortic dissection

Proximal extension towards the heart is less likely when the dissection begins distal to the left subclavian artery (Stanford type B). These patients tend to be older than those with ascending aortic involvement and are more likely to have comorbidity. Diligent blood pressure management is the usual initial treatment as surgery upon the descending thoracic aorta carries significant mortality and morbidity, including impaired blood supply to the spinal cord and paraplegia.

This approach is not universally accepted, however, and some centres recommend elective surgery (after several weeks) in selected patients with Marfan syndrome, in younger patients with dissection associated with large aneurysms, and if thrombosis of the false lumen fails to occur. In addition, surgery for type B dissection should always be considered if there is evidence of proximal extension of the dissection, progressive aortic enlargement threatening external rupture, or ischaemic complications from involvement of major arteries. For example, the prognosis is extremely poor when ischaemia occurs in the territory of a major abdominal artery, in which case emergency surgical fenestration of the intimal flap can be life-saving.

Encouraging results have recently been achieved using endovascular stenting for patients with complicated dissection starting distal to the left subclavian artery. Using vascular access from a groin incision, a covered stent can be delivered to cover the intimal tear. In suitable cases this obliterates flow into the false lumen, relieving branch ischaemia and preventing further aneurysmal dilatation.

Follow-up of patients with aortic dissection

Strenuous efforts to control blood pressure are indicated for all patients who have survived aortic dissection. β-Blocking drugs are the agents of choice for most, with other agents added as required.

Despite advances in the medical and surgical management of patients with aortic dissection, their long-term prognosis remains uncertain, with several adverse risk factors identified. These include new or progressive dissection, aneurysm formation at the site of surgical anastomosis, and persistence of flow in the false lumen, the last seemingly related to the presence of multiple intimal tears that allow communication between the lumens. Management is controversial, but it has been suggested that in the chronic situation, endovascular stenting may have a role in sealing these communications, thus allowing thrombosis of the false lumen.

Imaging at least once a year is recommended, using the modality with which there is most local expertise. Increased frequency of imaging is recommended following any acute event, for example severe chest pain, and for some patients with Marfan syndrome.

Modern imaging techniques have shown that variants of acute aortic dissection occur. They present in much the same way as classic dissection and may be considered part of the acute aortic syndromes. They include spontaneous intramural haematoma and penetrating atherosclerotic ulcer.

Spontaneous intramural haematoma

Spontaneous intramural haematoma was described by pathologists in 1920. It occurs when the small arterioles (vasa vasorum) which run in the outer media of the aorta rupture and bleed. As it is a medial/adventitial event, the intima remains intact and there is no false lumen. The clinical presentation may mimic that of dissection and the diagnosis can only be made by exclusion of an intimal tear or a penetrating atherosclerotic ulcer. The intramural haematoma is not readily identifiable by aortography, but

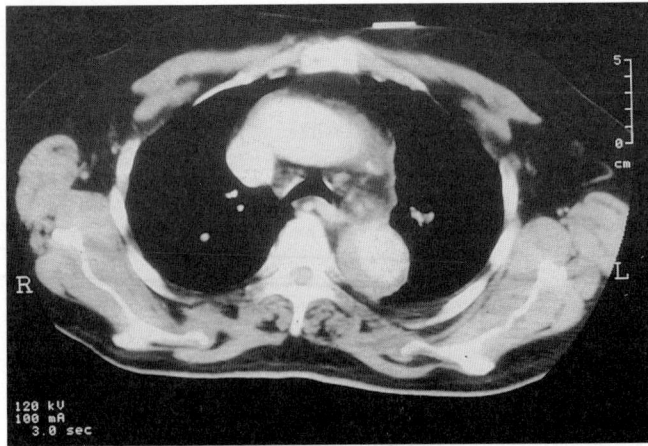

Fig. 5 CT of the thorax showing crescentric thickening of the posterior wall of the descending aorta (adjacent to the vertebra) without compromise of the aortic lumen. Transoesophageal echocardiography showed no intimal flap. The diagnosis is spontaneous haematoma of the aortic wall.

using non-invasive imaging, a circular or crescentic thickening of the aortic wall of more than 0.7 cm in depth associated with central displacement of any intimal calcification supports the diagnosis (Fig. 5).

As outlined earlier, there is increasing evidence that spontaneous intramural haematoma may be a precursor of aortic dissection. Clinical studies have supported this assertion: despite aggressive blood pressure control, up to 50 per cent of patients with an intramural haematoma develop dissection or aortic rupture and many now regard this condition as an indication for surgery when the ascending aorta is involved.

Penetrating atherosclerotic ulcer

Penetrating atherosclerotic ulcer presents with similar symptoms to aortic dissection, usually in patients with disseminated atheroma. Intimal disruption caused by atheroma results in perforation and secondary haemorrhage into the media. Imaging demonstrates an out-pouching from the lumen into the aortic wall with localized haemorrhage and evidence of diffuse atheroma.(Fig. 6). Rarely, this can cause a localized dissection, but the main threat is the high incidence of rupture. Treatment is currently surgical, but in the future endovascular stenting may be useful.

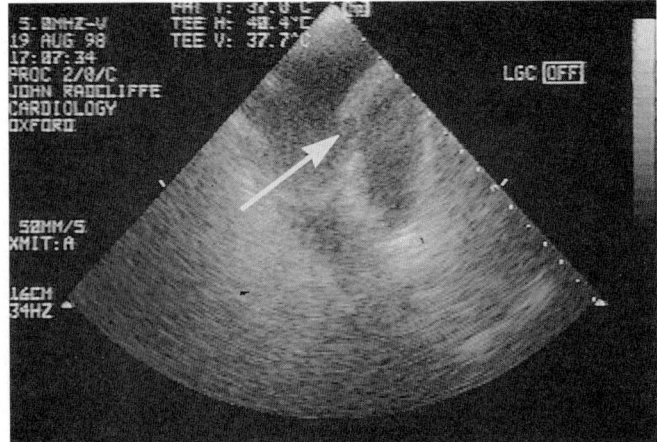

Fig. 6 Transoesophageal two-dimensional echo image of a penetrating ulcer (arrow).

Further reading

Dake MD *et al.* (1999). Endovascular stent graft placement for the treatment of acute aortic dissection. *New England Journal of Medicine* **340**, 1546–52. [Original paper describing this novel treatment for dissection.]

Davies MJ, Treasure T, Richardson PD (1996). The pathogenesis of spontaneous arterial dissection. *Heart* **75**, 434–5. [Review of the pathological processes which may result in arterial dissection.]

Erbel R *et al.* (1993). Effect of medical and surgical therapy on aortic dissection evaluated by transoesophageal echocardiography. *Circulation* **87**, 1604–15. [Original paper which outlines relationship between echocardiographic appearances and long-term prognosis.]

Khandheria BK (1993). Aortic dissection; the last frontier. *Circulation* **87**, 1765–8. [Editorial discussing imaging and management of dissection.]

Kouchoukos NT, Dougenis D (1997). Surgery of the thoracic aorta. *New England Journal of Medicine* **336**, 1876–88. [Authoritative surgical review of the literature.]

Miller DC (1993). The continuing dilemma concerning medical versus surgical management of patients with acute type B dissections. *Seminars in Thoracic and Cardiovascular Surgery* **5**, 33–46. [Editorial which outlines the principles and controversies of management of type B dissection.]

Nienaber CA *et al.* (1993). The diagnosis of thoracic aortic dissection by non-invasive imaging procedures. *New England Journal of Medicine* **328**, 1–9. [Original paper comparing different diagnostic imaging techniques in dissection.]

Robbins RC *et al.* (1993). Management of patients with intramural haematoma of the thoracic aorta. *Circulation* **88**, 1–10. [Original paper which describes the diagnosis of intramural haematoma and outlines management strategies.]

Vilacosta I *et al.* (1998). Penetrating atherosclerotic ulcer: documentation by transoesophageal echocardiography. *Journal of the American College of Cardiology* **32**, 83–9. [Original paper which describes the pathology, diagnosis, and treatment of atherosclerotic ulcer.]

Wooley CF, Sparks EH, Boudoulas H (1998). Aortic pain. *Progress in Cardiovascular Diseases* **40**, 563–89. [Detailed review of the clinical presentation and management of aortic pathology.]

15.14.2 Peripheral arterial disease

Janet Powell and Alun Davies

Introduction

Peripheral arterial disease, defined for the purpose of this chapter as diseases of the abdominal aorta and its branches, has risk factors and features that overlap with, but can be distinguished from, those of coronary artery disease. The two conditions often coexist, but patients with coronary disease are almost always referred directly to physicians, whilst those with peripheral arterial disease are referred directly to vascular surgeons, particularly in regions where angiology is a poorly developed specialty, since there are few effective medical therapies. Vascular surgeons also manage patients with arterial disease in the carotid vessels and upper limbs. These aspects will receive only passing mention in this chapter: for discussion regarding the clinical features and management of carotid artery disease, see Section 15.14.

The most common presentations of peripheral arterial disease are intermittent claudication and abdominal aortic aneurysm. Most peripheral arterial disease remains asymptomatic. It is not a new disease that results from a modern Westernized lifestyle. Atherosclerotic disease, partially occluding the peripheral arteries, has been described in the mummies of ancient Egypt. Life as a cavalry officer was associated with an increased risk of popliteal aneurysm, a condition treated by ligation by John Hunter, the pioneering eighteenth-century surgeon. Albert Einstein died of a ruptured abdominal aortic aneurysm.

Techniques for repairing abdominal aortic aneurysms were not developed until the middle of the twentieth century. This was the golden era for the development of vascular surgery as a specialty, with the increasing use of bypass surgery that has minimized the need for amputation. Today newer, less invasive approaches are being used—angioplasty and endovascular stenting—but few medical therapies are on the horizon.

Aetiology and epidemiology

Peripheral arterial disease may occur in the young but the prevalence increases sharply with age. Both young and old may suffer from occlusive (stenosing) disease of the peripheral arteries or dilating (aneurysmal) disease, while vasospastic disease is uncommon. However, the underlying causes of peripheral arterial disease in those below and above 50 years of age tend to be very different.

Peripheral arterial disease in patients less than 50 years old

In younger patients the cause of disease is most likely to be genetic, congenital, immunological, infectious, or traumatic. Patients with familial hypercholesterolaemia and related inherited disorders of lipid metabolism may present with peripheral limb ischaemia. There are also congenital causes of early-onset leg ischaemia. These include aortic hypoplasia, which occurs during the embryonic fusion of the distal aortas, and popliteal entrapment, where the popliteal artery takes an unusual course through the head of the gastrocnemius muscle, with exercise involving knee flexion causing intermittent occlusion of the artery and calf pain that resembles intermittent claudication. A fierce immunological inflammatory response to smoking causes Buerger's syndrome, which involves the artery, vein, and associated nerves in both the legs and the arms. This disease, seen principally in men, is particularly prevalent in the Indian subcontinent, and may resolve if the patient stops smoking. Sudden thrombotic occlusion of the iliac and distal arteries may occur in those below 50 years of age, suggesting the presence of an inherited thrombotic disorder. Embolic occlusion from a proximal source is also possible.

Marfan syndrome may sometimes be confirmed (mutation in the fibrillin-1 gene) only after a patient has presented with a ruptured abdominal aortic aneurysm. In some variants of Ehlers–Danlos syndrome, patients with mutations in type III collagen present with visceral artery aneurysms. In South Africa (and elsewhere) aneurysms of the abdominal, femoral, or popliteal arteries in those under 50 years have been attributed to infectious causes, from HIV to tuberculosis. Syphilitic aneurysms, which used to affect principally the thoracic aorta, are now rare.

Peripheral arterial disease in patients over 50 years old

For patients over 50 years of age, the principal risk factor for peripheral arterial disease—stenosing, aneurysmal, or vasospastic—is smoking. The pathology is atherosclerotic change with superimposed thrombosis. Of patients who present with peripheral arterial disease, less than 5 per cent have never smoked. For this reason, more men than women presented with peripheral arterial disease in the past, but recently more women have been presenting with the condition, perhaps a reflection of the increasing number of women who smoke. Nevertheless, unlike Buerger's disease, cessation of smoking is not associated with an immediate dramatic improvement in symptoms and it may take several years without smoking to improve prognosis.

Diabetes is another important risk factor for stenosing peripheral arterial disease. Other risk factors include hypertension, raised levels of plasma fibrinogen, and hyperlipidaemia, with elevated plasma triglycerides being a common finding. The risk factors for dilating arterial disease are similar, with the exception of diabetes, which is rare.

For aortic aneurysms, although strong familial clustering has been observed, no specific genetic mutations associated with aneurysmal disease have been identified and atherosclerotic change is commonplace. Caucasian and northern European populations appear to be at higher risk of aneurysmal disease than black populations. Stenosing and aneurysmal disease are associated with degenerative changes of the artery wall, the prevalence of both diseases increasing sharply with age (Table 1). Epidemiological studies also indicate a difference between stenosing and aneurysmal disease, with death from aneurysmal disease (aortic aneurysm) being more common amongst those of higher social classes and in affluent geographical areas.

Clinical features of leg ischaemia

The terms acute and chronic relate purely to the length of time that symptoms have been present and must not be confused with terms related to severity, such as critical limb ischaemia.

Critical leg ischaemia

Critical leg ischaemia is defined as gangrenous change, ulceration, or rest pain lasting for 2 weeks with an absolute ankle pressure of less than 50 mmHg, although patients with diabetes are difficult to include in this classification.

Acute leg ischaemia

The incidence of acute leg ischaemia, which presents as a painful, pale, and pulseless limb, is 1 in 12 000 patients per annum. It can be due either to an embolic event or thrombosis of an atherosclerotic stenosis. The commonest cause of a peripheral embolus used to be rheumatic heart disease in a patient with atrial fibrillation, but this is becoming less common, and other sources of emboli, such as an aortic aneurysm, must be considered. The development of a thrombosis at the site of an atherosclerotic stenosis, either in the superficial femoral artery or popliteal artery, is undoubtedly now the commonest cause of acute leg ischaemia. However, it should be stressed that, whatever the cause, there is no difference on clinical examination of the acutely ischaemic limb.

Arterial trauma, due to road traffic accidents and knife or gunshot wounds is becoming commoner, as is iatrogenic trauma following the insertion of intra-arterial catheters for diagnosis or therapy. A rare but dramatic cause of acute leg ischaemia is phlegmasia cerulea dolens, in which massive thrombosis of all the major veins of the limb occurs with gross swelling that obstructs the arterial supply.

Patients with a thrombosis of a popliteal aneurysm may present with classic symptoms of pain, paralysis, loss of power, paraesthesia, pallor, lack of pulse, and perishing cold. If the blood supply is not restored, fixed blue staining of the skin is a further sign of irreversible ischaemia, as is a tense calf with plantar flexion. However, the majority of patients presenting with acute ischaemia have symptoms that are less severe.

Chronic leg ischaemia

Chronic leg ischaemia is much more common than acute ischaemia (Table 1) and its main cause is atherosclerosis. In the young patient one should also consider cystic adventitial disease, entrapment of the popliteal artery, and occasionally fibromuscular hyperplasia of the iliac arteries, particularly in women.

Symptoms are pain on walking, claudication affecting the calf and thigh, rest pain, ulceration, and gangrenous change. Less commonly patients may present with buttock claudication and impotence (Leriche's syndrome). Whilst the differential diagnoses of the acutely ischaemic limb are few, in the chronically ischaemic limb pain may be due to nerve root compression or arthritis of the hip or knee. Classically the patient with claudication will complain of cramp-like pain in the calf, appearing after walking a particular distance, relieved by a few minutes rest, and recurring again at the same distance if the patient resumes walking. Failure of the pain to disappear on resting, or its reappearance after a shorter distance after each rest, suggest a possible musculoskeletal cause, particularly if distal pulses are present on examination. However, it should also be remembered that distal pulses may be felt at rest in the limbs of patients with claudication due to peripheral vascular disease, but disappear on exercise to the point of pain.

Investigation of the patient with an ischaemic leg

The main diagnostic method used to confirm the diagnosis of peripheral arterial disease is Doppler ultrasonography (duplex scanning), an example of which is shown in Fig. 1 and Plate 1. The ratio of systolic blood pressure at the ankle and in the arm, ankle–brachial pressure index (**ABPI**), provides a physiological measure of blood flow at the level of the ankle. At rest, in a normal leg, the ABPI lies between 1.0 and 1.4. As the blood flow in the leg is compromised, the ABPI falls sharply and values below 0.9 are considered abnormal and likely to confirm the diagnosis of peripheral vascular disease. To emphasize the important overlap between this condition and coronary artery disease, a reduction in ABPI nearly always signals the presence of coronary artery disease, which is the cause of death in the majority of patients with peripheral arterial disease.

Exercise testing provides an objective method of assessing walking distance and helps with the identification of disease processes such as angina that may be limiting. It only needs to be used in those people who have a

Table 1 The increasing prevalence of peripheral arterial disease with age in the populations of northern Europe

Population (age in years)		Asymptomatic peripheral arterial disease (ABPI < 0.9) (%)	Intermittent claudication (%)	Abdominal aortic aneurysm (> 3 cm) (%)
Men	55–64	8	1.2	5
Women	55–64	7	0.8	0.7
Men	65–74	16	2.5	7.5
Women	65–74	11	1.2	1.3
Men	75+	> 30	4.0	9
Women	75+	> 30	1.5	1.5

Most peripheral arterial disease, both stenosing and dilating, is asymptomatic. The data have been derived from several studies and geographical variation may occur. ABPI, ankle–brachial pressure index.

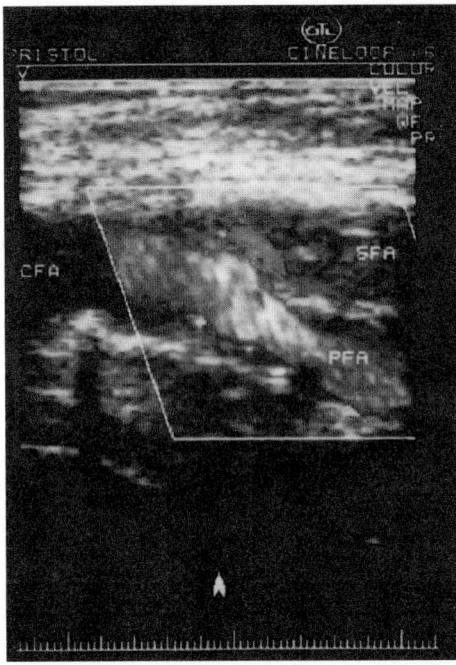

Fig. 1 Occlusion of the superficial femoral artery demonstrated by colour-coded duplex ultrasonography. On the left, the common femoral artery (CFA) lies outside the colour box. In the colour box antegrade flow through the profunda femoris artery (PFA) is shown in blue. The red flash represents rebound flow against the occluded origin of the superficial femoral artery (SFA). (See also Plate 1.)

history of claudication but have normal resting ankle–brachial pressure indices, and it can be used as a way of eliminating or suggesting other diagnoses.

In addition to establishing the diagnosis of peripheral arterial disease, duplex ultrasonography is able to determine the site of disease and to indicate the degree of stenosis or length of an occlusion and hence aid in the planning of interventional treatment. Angiography is only required as an adjuvant to endovascular treatment, for surgical planning in some circumstances, or in the management of the acutely ischaemic limb.

Attention to risk factors, in particular smoking and blood pressure, are important issues.

Management of critical and acute limb ischaemia

Critical limb ischaemia requires administration of analgesia and rapid surgical intervention. The severity of ischaemia will determine the treatment options considered. However, all patients with a severely ischaemic limb should be given adequate analgesia and 5000 units of heparin intravenously. Many will be old and frail, with significant medical comorbidities. These issues must be considered in deciding whether or not surgical intervention is appropriate for any individual case, with action taken to improve those aspects of the patient's medical condition that can be improved before surgery, or as part of continuing medical management.

For a patient with irreversible ischaemia (fixed skin staining and tense muscles), the main decision is whether a primary amputation or palliative care should be offered. If severe but potentially reversible ischaemia is present (white leg), surgery is usually the treatment of choice. Delay while thrombolytic therapy is tried is not advisable in this group. For patients with moderate limb ischaemia, where there is no paralysis and only mild sensory loss, arteriography with a view to thrombolysis should be performed. However, it should be remembered that thrombolysis is associated

with numerous potential complications, most notably gastrointestinal haemorrhage and stroke. If the limb is salvageable, it may be possible to offer the patient an endovascular procedure, such as an angioplasty (with or without stenting). Surgical treatment can involve simple embolectomy, but may require a bypass procedure or endarterectomy, and in the severely ischaemic limb fasciotomies may be needed to treat or prevent a compartment syndrome. For at least 10 per cent of patients, it will not be possible to offer revascularization. Such patients may benefit from the use of a prostacyclin analogue (Iloprost), which has been shown to reduce amputation rates and alleviate pain. Limb salvage rates for patients presenting with critical limb ischaemia are variable, probably 50 to 60 per cent at 2 years, dependent on the severity of disease.

In a patient presenting with acute leg ischaemia the outlook is poor with only about 60 per cent leaving hospital with an intact limb. The 30-day mortality for this group of patients can be as high as 30 per cent, the main cause of death being cardiac disease. The strategy for management is described in Fig. 2. The controversies that exist in the treatment of acute leg ischaemia are mainly related to the role of arteriography and which technique of thrombolysis is the safest and most cost effective.

In the patient who has had an embolic event, long-term anticoagulation should not be forgotten. Nor should a search for the source of embolus: if the patient is not in atrial fibrillation, has normal cardiac enzymes and 12-lead ECG, then they should have an echocardiogram to exclude any valvular lesion, a 24-h ECG to look for arrhythmia, an ultrasound to exclude abdominal aortic aneurysm, and a screen for thrombophilia.

Management of the chronically ischaemic leg

In chronic limb ischaemia management depends upon the severity of the disease. The vast majority of patients present with claudication, which is relatively benign. Only about 5 per cent of those who have claudication will go on to lose a limb, but claudication identifies patients with a threefold increased risk of death from either heart disease or cerebrovascular disease compared with age- and sex-matched controls. It is important when planning treatment that all the potential risk factors are covered. The general advice is to stop smoking and to exercise, with the use of structured exercise programmes shown to be of benefit. Surgical intervention is not usually required. Over 80 per cent of patients do not require any form of interventional procedure, and at least a third will have improvement of symptoms with simple medical treatment. The management of patients with chronic lower leg pain is shown in Fig. 3.

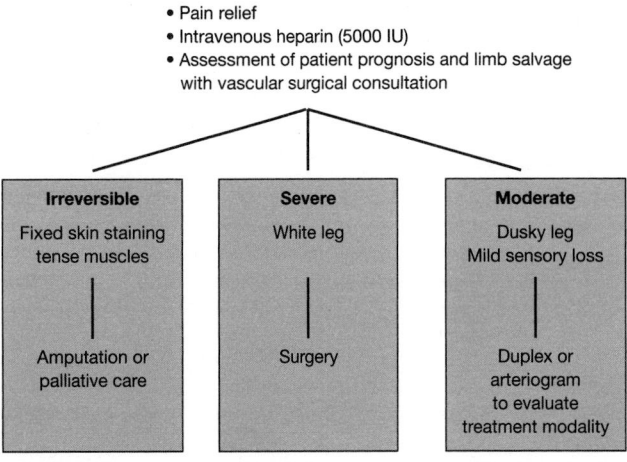

Fig. 2 Management of the acutely ischaemic leg.

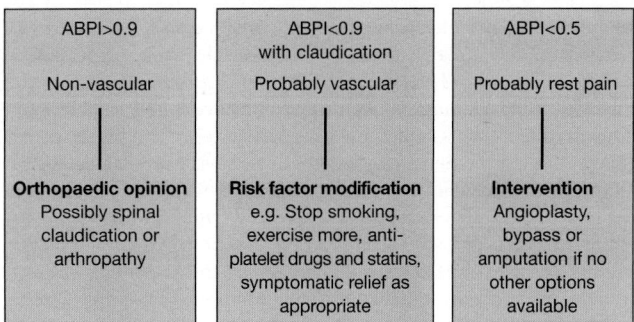

ABPI>0.9	ABPI<0.9 with claudication	ABPI<0.5
Non-vascular	Probably vascular	Probably rest pain
Orthopaedic opinion Possibly spinal claudication or arthropathy	**Risk factor modification** e.g. Stop smoking, exercise more, anti-platelet drugs and statins, symptomatic relief as appropriate	**Intervention** Angioplasty, bypass or amputation if no other options available

Fig. 3 Management of the patient with chronic lower leg pain.

General management

Careful attention must be paid to the cleanliness of ischaemic feet to avoid infection, and particular care should be given to the cutting of toe nails. In many patients this is best done by a careful younger relative or chiropodist, since apparently minor lacerations can lead to ulcers, infection, and gangrene. Walking to the point of claudication is not harmful, and may improve collateral circulation with beneficial results.

Smoking is by far the most significant risk factor for occlusive arterial disease and every effort should be made to encourage smokers to stop. If patients undergo surgical treatment, then the long-term patency rate following arterial reconstruction is four times greater in smokers who stop than in those who persist.

Medical treatment

Since coronary artery disease is the main cause of death in those with peripheral arterial disease, low-dose aspirin therapy (75 to 325 mg/day) should be recommended for all patients. If aspirin cannot be tolerated, ADP-receptor antagonists, such as clopidrogel, are equally effective in reducing the risk of cardiovascular events (stroke, myocardial infarction, and vascular deaths) and particularly effective for patients with peripheral arterial disease.

Secondary prevention trials have demonstrated the benefits of statin therapy following myocardial infarction. It is likely that similar benefits would be seen for patients with stenosing atherosclerotic disease of the peripheral arteries, particularly in those with elevated serum cholesterol concentrations. The new generation of fibrates, which lower both plasma fibrinogen and triglycerides, may also be effective in reducing cardiovascular events in patients with peripheral arterial disease, but randomized trials have not yet reported. Chelation therapy offers no benefits.

Few patients with peripheral arterial disease are prescribed β-blockers for control of hypertension or angina. However, when these patients require surgery, perioperative cover with a β-blocker is likely to minimize myocardial ischaemia and diminish postoperative morbidity and mortality associated with major vascular surgery.

Surgical treatment

In general, surgeons are becoming more conservative with respect to interventional treatment for patients with claudication, despite a possible early benefit for those having an endovascular procedure. However, in the patient who has severe claudication, with symptoms that significantly affect their quality of life, it is certainly possible and appropriate to offer interventional treatment.

Several issues in the management of chronic limb ischaemia are the subject of ongoing clinical trials. These include comparison of endovascular angioplasty and bypass surgery. For infrainguinal bypass, good-quality autologous vein is the conduit of choice. However, reasonable results can be obtained with synthetic grafts, particularly where the distal anastomosis is above the knee. Below the knee an adjuvant vein interposition in the form of either a Miller cuff or Taylor patch is used. The role of stenting in the leg vessels is contentious, and it may not be of value. The role of exercise therapy compared with angioplasty in the treatment of mild to moderate claudication continues to be debated.

Ischaemia of the arm

Ischaemia of the arm is usually a result of embolism from the heart. Occasionally the subclavian artery is diseased or has suffered traumatic injury or radiation damage following radiotherapy. The basic principles of investigation and management are the same as for the leg. However, it should be noted that the upper limb has multiple interconnection of collateral vessels, hence occlusion of the major arterial supply may still leave a viable limb. The other disease process that needs to be considered is the thoracic outlet syndrome, which gives rise to symptoms in the arm as a result of arterial, venous, or neurological compression caused by an additional cervical rib or by scalene bands. Management may require surgical intervention, either cervical rib excision or thoracic outlet decompression with the removal of the first rib.

Mesenteric ischaemia

Mesenteric ischaemia is uncommon. Over one-third of cases of acute mesenteric ischaemia are due to arterial embolism, with emboli lodging at the ostium of the superior mesenteric artery in many cases. Patients with acute mesenteric artery thrombosis have often had symptoms of mesenteric ischaemia prior to the acute episode. Chronic mesenteric ischaemia typically presents with weight loss and abdominal pain on ingestion of food, the classic story being that the patient is constantly hungry, but frightened to eat. Other causes of acute mesenteric ischaemia include venous thrombosis and non-occlusive ischaemia secondary to hypoperfusion.

Patients with acute mesenteric ischaemia will usually present with abdominal pain, but the abdominal physical signs may be much milder than would be anticipated from the subsequent clinical course. Suspicion of the diagnosis should be heightened in the presence of atrial fibrillation or widespread atheromatous vascular disease. Patients may deteriorate suddenly and present in shock.

The diagnosis of acute mesenteric ischaemia is difficult to make. In the acute situation clues to look for include leucocytosis, hyperamylasaemia, and unexplained acidosis. Liver function tests are usually normal. Radiological imaging is rarely able to make a positive diagnosis, although it can be very useful in excluding other possibilities. Angiography is not always accurate. CT scanning can be helpful in the diagnosis of mesenteric venous thrombosis.

Intensive resuscitation to replace fluids is essential. Surgery is usually necessary for the patient to survive, and the possibility of acute mesenteric ischaemia remains one of the dwindling number of reasons for requiring an emergency diagnostic laparotomy. Depending on the findings, resection of small bowel may suffice, but formal arterial surgery may be necessary, and in some unfortunate instances the extent of irreversible ischaemia can preclude an attempt at resection or revascularization. In cases where the surgeon is unsure of the viability of bowel remaining after resection, a second laparotomy may be planned to assess the situation a few days later. Repeat laparotomy may also be required to examine, and if necessary resect, more bowel in the patient who is not 'doing well' postoperatively. The prognosis for patients who present with acute mesenteric ischaemia is poor.

For patients who present with chronic mesenteric ischaemia, the aim of treatment is to improve blood flow and to act as a prophylactic procedure to prevent the catastrophic disaster of arterial occlusion. The potential options, having identified the site of the disease process by duplex scanning and angiography, include angioplasty, endarterectomy, reimplantation, or a surgical bypass procedure.

Abdominal aortic aneurysm

Definition

There is no fixed definition of an abdominal aortic aneurysm. It is a localized dilatation of the abdominal aorta, usually fusiform, with dilation starting distal to the renal arteries. One definition is when the maximum aortic diameter is more than 1.5 times the diameter of the undilated proximal aorta. Manual palpation to detect abdominal aortic aneurysms is unreliable, unless undertaken by a specialist on non-obese patients. The most convenient method of screening for the presence of these aneurysms is ultrasonography, measuring the anterior–posterior diameter. Since the reproducibility of ultrasound measurements of the suprarenal aorta is poor, a convenient working definition of an abdominal aortic aneurysm is when the maximum diameter exceeds 3 cm, which in most people is more than 1.5 times the diameter of the undilated proximal aorta. In practice, it is only aneurysms of 4 cm or greater in diameter that have been of clinical concern.

Epidemiology

Population screening studies in northern Europe have shown that the disease is usually without symptoms, much more common in men than in women (Table 1), and is strongly associated with smoking. The prevalence of large aneurysms (greater than 5 cm in diameter) detected by screening is only about 1 per cent in men and the large majority of these screen-detected aneurysms are 3 to 5 cm in diameter. The natural history of abdominal aortic aneurysms is progressive enlargement (with the diameter increasing by 2 to 5 mm each year) without symptoms, until the aortic wall is so weakened that it ruptures. Rupture is a catastrophic event.

The infrarenal aorta is by far the most common site of aneurysmal dilatation, and usually the abdominal aorta is the only site of dilatation. When patients present with aneurysms of the iliac, femoral, or popliteal arteries, abdominal aortic aneurysm is often present and screening for this is mandatory. This emphasizes the tendency of some patients to have a more generalized form of dilating arterial disease.

Ruptured aneurysms

The symptoms of a ruptured abdominal aortic aneurysm are collapse (shock) and severe back or abdominal pain.

Rarely a ruptured aneurysm will present with gastrointestinal bleeding from an aortoduodenal fistula or high-output cardiac failure from an aortocaval fistula.

Less than 20 per cent of patients with a ruptured abdominal aortic aneurysm reach hospital alive, and even among those that undergo emergency surgical repair almost half will die within 30 days of surgery. With this bleak prognosis and the very significant costs associated with emergency repair following rupture, it has been suggested that widespread screening to detect those with the largest aneurysms, at highest risk of rupture, would be cost-effective. A screening trial is in progress to assess the benefit of such a policy.

Management of ruptured aneurysms requires:

(1) access lines, cross-matched blood, and resuscitation;

(2) confirmation of diagnosis—ultrasound (to show aneurysm), CT scan or experienced vascular surgeon (to confirm diagnosis of rupture);

(3) rapid assessment of whether patient would benefit from emergency repair; and

(4) if yes, immediate surgical repair.

Aneurysms detected before rupture

Abdominal aortic aneurysms are commonly symptomless but rupture is catastrophic. However, elective repair of an abdominal aortic aneurysm, a major surgical procedure, is not without risk. Traditionally, larger aneur-

ysms have been repaired by cross-clamping of the aorta and insertion of a Dacron inlay graft at open surgery. This is a durable procedure and effectively 'cures' the patient. However, although some specialized surgical centres report an operative mortality of less than 2 per cent associated with this elective procedure, on a population basis the mortality is more likely to be 5 to 8 per cent. This very significant surgical mortality is an important reason for avoiding surgery in those with small aneurysms.

Recently, the United Kingdom Small Aneurysm Trial showed that for aneurysms of 4.0 to 5.5 cm in diameter the policy of early elective surgery conferred no long-term survival benefit, and surgery should not be recommended. For such patients surveillance, with measurement of ultrasound diameter every 6 months, is a safe policy which engenders little patient anxiety, and the risk of aneurysm rupture is very low—1 per cent per year. By contrast, for patients with aneurysms greater than 6 cm in diameter the risk of rupture may be as high as 25 per cent per year, and in most such cases elective repair is recommended.

Repair is recommended also when symptoms are attributed to the aneurysm, whatever its size, the commonest being back or abdominal pain, or tenderness to palpation. It is assumed that such aneurysms are at high risk of rupture and need early repair. As the aneurysm dilates, layers of laminated thrombus deposit in the lumen, like onion skins, leaving a blood flow channel of approximately normal aortic diameter. These layers of thrombus are very stable and only in rare circumstances are the source of emboli to the legs. The aneurysms which most often provoke symptoms have very thick, inflamed, fibrotic walls, which entrap nerves and may become adherent to other tissues. These are known as inflammatory aneurysms and the thickened wall can often be detected by CT scan or magnetic resonance imaging. They are technically demanding to repair. There is no convincing evidence that a course of preoperative corticosteroids is beneficial. In the Japanese population inflammatory aneurysms have been associated with active cytomegalovirus infection.

A strategy for the management of abdominal aortic aneurysms detected before rupture is shown in Fig. 4. Patients with small aneurysms should stop smoking and have their blood pressure controlled. Since screening detects mainly small aneurysms, it would clearly be beneficial if a treatment to limit aneurysm growth were available. Although propranolol has proved effective in limiting the dilation of the proximal aorta in patients with Marfan syndrome, as yet there is no evidence that it is effective for abdominal aortic aneurysms. Furthermore, many patients with abdominal aortic aneurysm have impaired lung function, perhaps through smoking, and β-blockers often are poorly tolerated. However, effective control of blood pressure and cessation of smoking are both likely to minimize the rate of aneurysm growth and the risk of rupture. Pathophysiological studies suggest that inflammation and proteolysis are important processes driving aneurysm growth, but there is no firm evidence that either anti-inflammatory or antiproteolytic therapy is effective. Surgery remains the only available treatment for aneurysms larger than 5.5 cm in diameter.

Recently a less invasive repair procedure has been developed, where an aortic graft is inserted via the femoral artery. This technique remains under

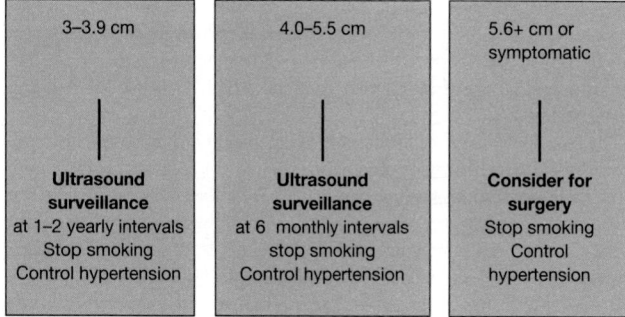

Fig. 4 Management of unruptured abdominal aortic aneurysms depending on their size as demonstrated by ultrasonography.

development, its durability is being investigated, and several randomized trials are comparing this new endovascular approach with the traditional surgical one.

Conventional surgical management

Preoperative evaluation requires CT or magnetic resonance imaging to define the anatomy and extent of the aneurysm. Cardiac, pulmonary, and renal function should always be assessed, poor renal and lung function being associated with an increased risk of postoperative morbidity and mortality.

The most common surgical approach to an abdominal aortic aneurysm is through a transperitoneal incision under general anaesthesia. The retroperitoneal approach, which avoids bowel manipulation and permits a more rapid return to oral diet, has similar cross-clamp, operating, and recovery times. The transperitoneal approach offers the advantage of exploring the abdominal cavity for other pathology. In this approach, after the bowel has been removed from the operative field, the aorta is exposed anteriorly from the left renal vein to the bifurcation. The infrarenal neck of the aneurysm is exposed anteriorly and laterally so that an occluding clamp may be applied. Both common iliac arteries are exposed for the placement of the distal occluding clamps. With the clamps in place, the aneurysm is opened longitudinally on the anterior surface and the remainder of the procedure performed from inside the aneurysm cavity, usually following a small dose of intravenous heparin. Clot and debris are evacuated and any back-bleeding lumbar or mesenteric arteries ligated. A Dacron prosthesis is then sutured, end to end, to the normal-diameter aorta above the aneurysm. This anastamosis is tested for leaks before the graft is trimmed to appropriate length and sutured in place above the aortic bifurcation. The aneurysm sac is closed over the prosthesis, before replacement of abdominal contents. Such tube grafts are the most common type, but when the iliac arteries are dilated or diseased a bifurcated prosthesis is used. The cross-clamp time should be less than an hour and the whole procedure completed within 2 to 4 h. The longest procedures involve inflammatory aneurysms and cases where the proximal aneurysm neck lies above the renal arteries. The patient should be ready to leave hospital 7 to 12 days after the operation, with a durable repair.

Endovascular aneurysm repair

The technique of endovascular repair was introduced in the early 1990s and the technology is still evolving. The procedure may be performed under general or epidural anaesthesia. This flexibility allows endovascular repair in patients where pulmonary or cardiac function is too poor to consider open repair, and the avoidance of aortic cross-clamping is an additional benefit for those with limited cardiac reserve.

Preoperative investigation to evaluate the extent and size of the aneurysm (spiral CT or magnetic resonance imaging) is of critical importance. The length of the aneurysm neck below the renal arteries, angulation of the aorta, and tortuosity of the iliac arteries must be evaluated precisely so that the correct size of graft can be placed via the femoral artery. The insertion of the graft is performed under fluoroscopic control. This requires the use of significant amounts of contrast material, which may underlie the unfavourable results reported in patients with high serum creatinine. The proximal end of the graft is held in place either by hooks or balloon-expandable stents.

The length of the procedure and the transfusion requirements are similar to those for open surgical repair, but the patient recovers rapidly and is ready to leave hospital within 2 to 5 days. The long-term success of the procedure depends on the successful exclusion of the aneurysm sac and the security of the proximal attachment to prevent graft migration. Endoleaks may develop when the aneurysm is not completely excluded or there is back-bleeding from lumbar vessels or the inferior mesenteric artery into the aneurysm sac. These are associated with an important risk of continued aneurysm expansion and rupture. For these reasons continued vigilance and repeated evaluation of the aneurysm with duplex or CT scanning is necessary at 6-monthly intervals. Currently, neither the durability of endovascular grafts nor their use in patients unfit for open repair has been properly evaluated in clinical trials.

Further reading

CAPRIE Steering Committee (1996). A randomised, blinded, trial of clopidogrel versus aspirin in patients at risk of ischaemic events. *Lancet* **348**, 1329–39.

Fowkes FGR (1988). The epidemiology of atherosclerotic arterial disease in the lower limbs. *European Journal of Vascular Surgery* **2**, 283–91.

Mangano DT *et al.* (1996). Effect of atenolol on mortality and morbidity after noncardiac surgery. *New England Journal of Medicine* **335**, 1713–20.

Meijer WT *et al.* (1998). Peripheral arterial disease in the elderly: The Rotterdam Study. *Arteriosclerosis, Thrombosis, and Vascular Biology* **18**, 185–92.

Perkins JMT *et al.* (1996). Exercise training versus angioplasty for stable claudication. Long and medium term results of a prospective, randomised trial. *European Journal of Vascular and Endovascular Surgery* **11**, 409–13.

Tetteroo E *et al.* (1998). Randomised comparison of primary stent placement versus primary angioplasty followed by selective stent placement in patients with iliac artery occlusive disease. Dutch Iliac Stent Trial Group. *Lancet* **351**, 1153–9.

UK Small Aneurysm Trial Participants (1998). Mortality results for randomised controlled trial of early elective surgery or ultrasonographic surveillance for small abdominal aortic aneurysm. *Lancet* **352**, 1649–55.

Whyman MR *et al.*(1996). Randomised controlled trial of percutaneous transluminal angioplasty for intermittent claudication. *European Journal of Vascular and Endovascular Surgery* **12**, 167–72.

15.14.3 Cholesterol embolism

C. R. K. Dudley

The clinical features of cholesterol embolism mimic a number of conditions, particularly systemic vasculitis, and if misdiagnosed can result in the inappropriate use of powerful immunosuppressive drugs.

Introduction

When atheromatous plaques ulcerate and become denuded of their endothelial covering, the underlying cholesterol-rich extracellular matrix can become detached and embolize. If the dislodged atheroma is sufficiently large, occlusion of a major systemic artery results in infarction of the organ or ischaemia of the limb supplied. This has been termed 'atheroembolism'. By contrast, cholesterol-crystal embolism occurs when much smaller and more numerous particles, composed principally of cholesterol crystals, lodge in a number of small arteries simultaneously. The presence of a collateral circulation usually prevents infarction and the event frequently passes unrecognized by the patient or their physician. However, tissue damage in a number of organs can result from multiple showers of emboli. Because severe ulcerative atherosclerosis is most frequently present in the abdominal aorta, cholesterol embolism commonly affects the lower limbs, gastrointestinal tract, and kidneys. The condition usually presents as a complication of vascular surgery or angiographic procedures, when mechanical dislodgement of crystals from ulcerated plaques occurs. Anticoagulant and thrombolytic use has also been implicated as a predisposing factor. The clinical features are those of a systemic disorder with renal failure that can mimic vasculitis.

Epidemiology

The incidence of cholesterol-crystal embolism found at postmortem is high: 77 per cent after aortic surgery, 30 per cent after aortography, and 25.5 per cent after cardiac catheterization. By contrast, the clinical syndrome of cholesterol-crystal embolism is rare, complicating less than 2 per cent of cardiac catheterizations.

Since the condition occurs in patients with severe atheromatous disease, it is most often seen in older male patients with obvious risk factors (hypertension, diabetes mellitus, smoking) and overt vascular disease (ischaemic heart disease, abdominal aortic aneurysm, cerebrovascular disease, etc.). Although spontaneous cholesterol embolism can occur, it is much more common after vascular surgery or invasive radiology including aortography, angiography, and angioplasty. Under these circumstances direct trauma to the vessel may result in detachment of atheromatous material from a ruptured plaque, or denude the endothelial lining of the vessel exposing the underlying atheroma for subsequent embolization. Anticoagulant use has been associated with cholesterol embolism, and it has been proposed that by preventing thrombosis of ulcerating atheromatous plaques, anticoagulants favour the dissemination of atheromatous material. However, a causal relationship is unproven and many patients with widespread atherosclerosis coincidentally receive anticoagulants for a variety of reasons. Cholesterol embolism following the use of thrombolytic agents has been rarely reported.

Clinical features

Symptoms are often non-specific with fever, weight loss, and myalgia. The clinical features are otherwise determined by the pattern of organ involvement and are usually referable to the gastrointestinal tract, kidneys, and lower limbs. Bilateral skin changes over the lower extremities are the commonest physical finding and include livedo reticularis, a purpuric rash, 'trash feet', blue toes (acral cyanosis), and focal digital necrosis (Figs 1 and 2 and Plates 1 and 2). Ulceration, nodules, and petechiae have also been described. Despite these skin changes and the presence of calf claudication (or frank myositis), pedal pulses may be felt easily, emphasizing that small vessels are occluded in this disorder. Carotid and femoral bruits are frequently heard, reflecting widespread and generalized atherosclerosis.

Abdominal pain, gastrointestinal bleeding, and pancreatitis may occur and embolism to the stomach, small bowel, colon, gallbladder, and spleen have all been reported. The most frequently involved of these sites is the colon.

Because of their large blood supply and proximity to the abdominal aorta, the kidneys are commonly affected. This usually manifests as a sub-

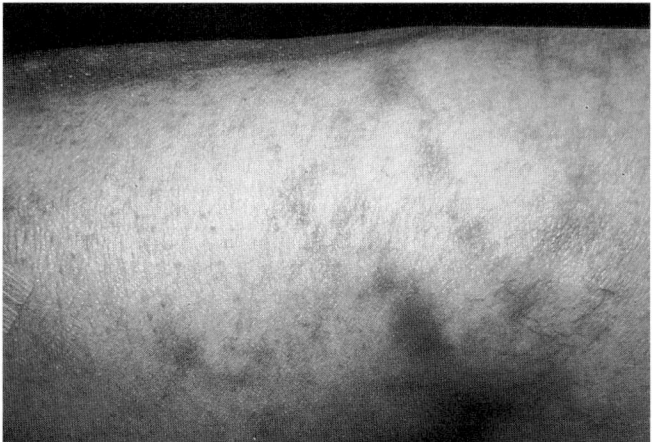

Fig. 1 Livedo reticularis and vasculitic-like erythematous nodules on the leg of a patient in whom cholesterol-crystal embolization occurred after coronary angiography. (See also Plate 1.)

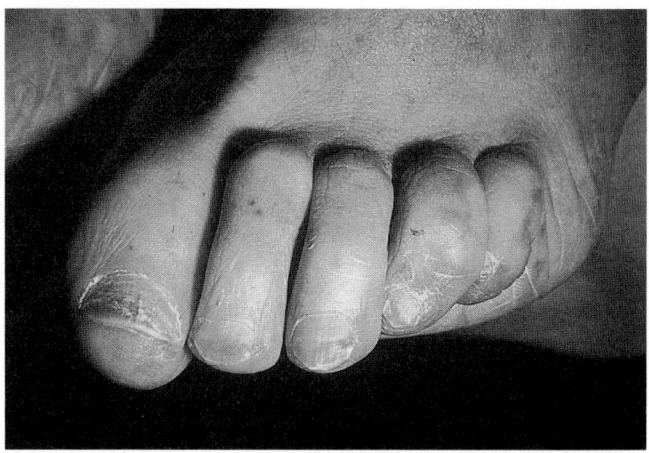

Fig. 2 Purpuric spots and acral cyanosis of the toes from cholesterol embolism after aortic aneurysm repair. (see also Plate 2.)

acute stepwise deterioration in renal function over 2 to 6 weeks, invariably accompanied by a worsening of pre-existing hypertension that can be labile and difficult to control. Cardiac failure with pulmonary oedema is a common accompaniment. Acute renal failure with necrotizing glomerulonephritis and crescent formation on renal biopsy has been described but is rare. Thus a typical case is an elderly man presenting after angiography with progressive renal failure accompanied by a low-grade fever, abdominal pain, livedo reticularis of the lower body, and purpura over the feet with focal digital ischaemia of the toes.

Transient ischaemic attacks, amaurosis fugax, and strokes can occur when embolism is from the carotid arteries or aortic arch. Retinal cholesterol-crystal emboli may be observed on ophthalmoscopy as bright refractile plaques within the retinal arterioles, especially at their bifurcation. Spinal cord infarction has also been reported.

Investigations

Laboratory findings are non-specific, but frequently include a raised erythrocyte sedimentation rate (**ESR**), plasma viscosity, and C-reactive protein (**CRP**). Leucocytosis and a transient eosinophilia are common and may be pronounced. Depending on the tissue involvement, an elevation in creatine phosphokinase, amylase, lactate dehydrogenase (**LDH**), serum aspartate aminotransferase (**AST**), and alkaline phosphatase may all be seen. Hypocomplementaemia is rare and usually mild. Antineutrophil cytoplasmic antibodies (**ANCA**) have been reported, and their presence may further confuse the diagnosis with a multisystem vasculitic process. Mild proteinuria is generally present and nephrotic-range proteinuria has been reported. Urine microscopy may be bland or reveal red cells, white cells (particularly eosinophils), and hyaline and granular casts. Renal failure is frequently non-oliguric.

Histology

The definitive histological diagnosis of cholesterol-crystal embolism can usually be made from biopsies of kidney, skin, or muscle (including clinically uninvolved areas), although sampling error may miss the lesion due to its patchy distribution. Antemortem histological diagnoses have also been made from other tissues, including a gastric biopsy, prostatic currettings, and a bone marrow biopsy.

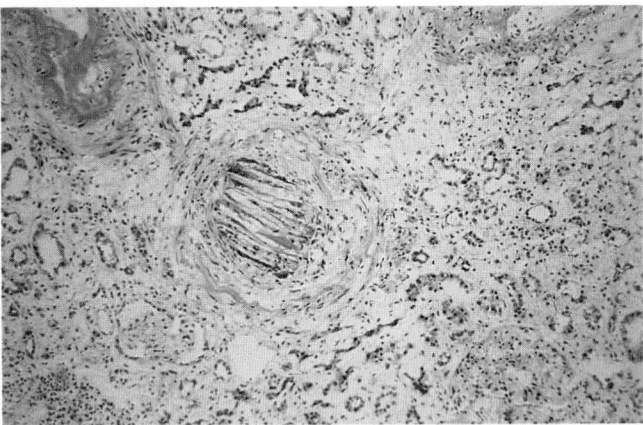

Fig. 3 Renal biopsy demonstrating the characteristic needle-shaped cholesterol clefts occluding a medium-sized renal arteriole with surrounding inflammatory cell infiltration, intimal proliferation, thickening, and concentric fibrosis. There is extensive autolysis (postmortem sample). (See also Plate 3.)

The diagnostic feature is of biconvex, needle-shaped cholesterol clefts within the lumen of arteries or arterioles that remain after the crystals have dissolved during routine histological preparation (Fig. 3 and Plate 3). In fresh samples, the crystals can be identified by birefringence under polarized light or by specific histochemical staining of cholesterol. In the kidneys, the typical finding is occlusion of small arteries and arterioles of between 150 and 200 μm in diameter, such as the arcuate and interlobular arteries, resulting in patchy areas of ischaemia and small areas of infarction. Crystals can also be seen within the glomeruli. In chronic cases, ischaemia produces a wedge-shaped lesion involving all components of the renal cortex radiating towards the capsule. The glomeruli appear ischaemic and sclerosed and the tubules become atrophic and separated by interstitial fibrosis. Grossly, the kidneys may be reduced in size with a rough granular surface and wedge-shaped scars.

Based on animal studies involving the injection of atheromatous material, the presence of cholesterol crystals in the vascular lumen is thought to trigger a localized inflammatory and endothelial vascular reaction. Inflammatory cells (mainly macrophages and eosinophils) infiltrate, and multinucleated giant cells engulf the cholesterol crystals, but these are resistant to the scavenger effects of macrophages and may persist for many months. The inflammatory phase is followed by marked intimal thickening with concentric fibrosis and occlusion of the vessel. Depending on the extent of organ involvement, these pathological changes result in ischaemia, infarction, or, rarely, necrosis of the distal tissue.

Differential diagnosis

The diagnosis is frequently missed during life. A high index of clinical suspicion is therefore required, particularly in elderly patients with evidence of atherosclerotic disease who develop renal failure after arteriography or following aortic or cardiac surgery; cholesterol embolism should also be considered in the differential diagnosis of a multisystem disease in elderly patients. Spontaneous cholesterol-crystal embolism associated with renal failure, fever, rash, and eosinophilia may not surprisingly be misdiagnosed as a vasculitic illness such as Wegener's granulomatosis, microscopic polyangiitis, Churg–Strauss syndrome, polyarteritis nodosa, or bacterial endocarditis (see Section xxxx, Rees). A false-positive ANCA test may further compound the diagnostic difficulty. Under these circumstances, renal biopsy is mandatory to make the correct diagnosis.

Clinical course and management

Mortality is high due to the coexistence of cardiac and vascular disease with renal failure in an elderly patient. Renal impairment may remain stable, but frequently progresses such that dialysis is required, although partial recovery has been reported, even after several months of dialysis. The mechanism of this recovery is uncertain.

There is no effective therapy. Steroids, aspirin, dipyridamole, and low molecular weight dextran have all been tried, but without any clear effect. There are anecdotal reports of a response to human menopausal gonadotrophin coenzyme A (**HMG CoA**)-reductase inhibitors (theoretically inducing plaque stabilization), but recovery may have been spontaneous. Anticoagulants are of no proven benefit and should be avoided given their potential role in the pathogenesis of the disorder. Encouraging results with iloprost have recently been reported although these observations require replication.

Computed tomography (**CT**) scanning of the aorta has been used to identify the precise source (for instance, aortic aneurysm, localized aortic plaque) of cholesterol emboli, and surgical replacement of the diseased vessel with a graft has been advocated. However, major surgery in elderly vasculopaths with renal impairment carries significant risks and is generally avoided.

Supportive therapy is directed at the control of hypertension and appropriate management of renal failure. Prevention is important, particularly with the increasing number of older patients submitted to invasive angiography. Non-invasive methods of arterial imaging such as CT or magnetic resonance (**MR**) angiography are to be preferred in patients with diffuse atherosclerosis. When invasive angiography is unavoidable, careful attention must be paid to the angiographic technique, including the arterial approach (brachial instead of femoral for cardiac catheterization), use of softer, more flexible catheters and reduced catheter manipulation.

Further reading

Belenfant X, Meyrier A, Jacquot C (1999). Supportive treatment improves survival in multivisceral cholesterol crystal embolism. *American Journal of Kidney Disease* 33, 840–50. [Recent study reporting good (87 per cent) 1-year patient survival with aggressive protocol-based supportive care.]

Case Records of the Massachusetts General Hospital (Case 34–1991). *New England Journal of Medicine* 325, 563–72. [Classic clinicopathological exercise in the best tradition.]

Elinav E, Chajek-Shaul T, Stern M (2002). Improvement in cholesterol emboli syndrome after iloprost therapy. *British Medical Journal* 324, 268–9. [New therapeutic approach requiring replication elsewhere.]

Fine MJ, Kapoor W, Falanga V (1987). Cholesterol crystal embolization: a review of 221 cases in the English literature. *Angiology* 38, 769–84. [Excellent review.]

Hyman BT, et al. (1987). Warfarin-related purple toes syndrome and cholesterol microembolization. *American Journal of Medicine* 82, 1233–7. [Association of cholesterol-crystal embolization with anticoagulant use.]

Keen RR, et al. (1995). Surgical management of atheroembolization. *Journal of Vascular Surgery* 21, 773–81. [Retrospective series of patients (45 per cent had cholesterol embolism alone) in whom the source of embolism was removed surgically.]

Mannesse CK (1991). Renal failure and cholesterol crystal embolization: a report of 4 surviving cases and a review of the literature. *Clinical Nephrology* 36, 240–5. [Excellent review.]

Moolenaar W, Lamers CBH (1996). Cholesterol crystal embolisation to the alimentary tract. *Gut* 38, 196–200. [Clinicopathological report of cholesterol crystal embolism to the gastrointestinal tract using the Dutch National Pathology database to identify cases.]

15.14.4 Takayasu arteritis

Fujio Numano

Introduction

Takayasu arteritis is a systemic chronic vasculitis that mainly involves the aorta and/or its major branches as well as the coronary and pulmonary arteries. Chronically progressive inflammation induces arterial stenosis and/or occlusion due to thrombus formation, resulting in the characteristic clinical picture of weak or absent arterial pulses (Fig. 1). By contrast, acute inflammation causes dilatation of vessel walls and/or aneurysm formation, which can lead to serious problems such as aneurysmal dissection, aortic regurgitation due to dilatation of the ascending aorta, or even aortic rupture. Clinical manifestations will clearly depend on which arteries are involved. The disease generally has a chronic progressive course, often presenting with non-specific inflammatory symptoms such as intermittent fever, fatigue, and malaise that may exist for months to years prior to the onset of full-blown vasculitis.

The first case of this disease was reported in 1908 at the Japan Ophthalmology Society Meeting by Mikito Takayasu who described interesting fundal findings in a 21-year-old woman suffering from pulmonary tuberculosis, characterized by coronary anastomosis of central retinal arteries (Fig. 2 and Plate 1). Similar ocular appearances were corroborated at the same meeting by K. Ohnishi and T. Kogoshima. Furthermore, both pointed out that they were associated with absence of one or both radial pulses. Today this condition is known to be a vasculitis and the characteristic ophthalmic condition thought to be the result of ischaemia of the retinal circulation due to stenosis or obstruction by arteritis of cervical arteries.

The first detailed pathological study was reported by K. Oota in 1940 of a 25-year-old woman with Takayasu arteritis who was admitted to hospital for visual loss and frequent syncopal attacks. He confirmed that this patient had systemic vasculitis involving the aorta, cervical arteries, and pulmonary arteries, and that inflammatory changes were seen not only in the media but in both intima and adventitia, thus calling this condition 'panarteritis'. In 1951, studying the clinical features of 31 cases, K. Shimizu and K. Sano applied the name 'pulseless disease' to the triad of clinical features comprising pulselessness, coronary anastomosis in the retinal vasculature, and accentuated carotid sinus reflex due to ischaemia of the cervical circulation.

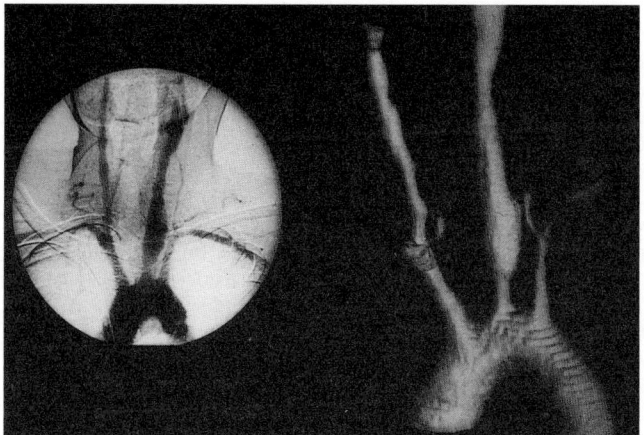

Fig. 1 Digital subtraction angiography and three-dimensional CT of the aortic arch and its branches in a patient with Takayasu arteritis.

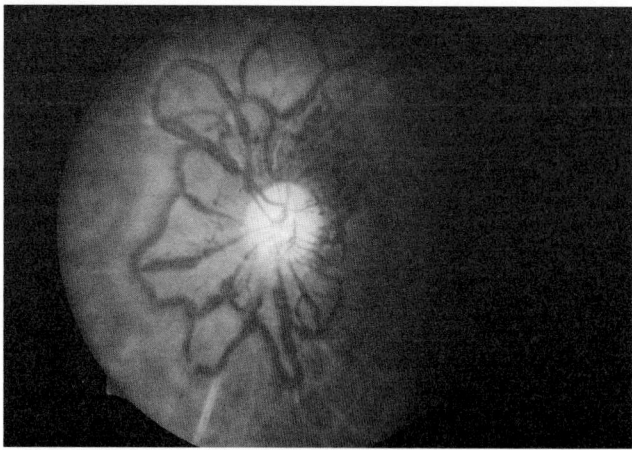

Fig. 2 Typical coronary anastomosis of retinal vessels in Takayasu arteritis. (See also Plate 1.)

Epidemiology

Takayasu arteritis is frequently encountered in Asian countries such as Japan, Korea, China, Singapore, Thailand, Vietnam, India, Israel, and Turkey; also on the American continent in countries such as Peru, Mexico, Brazil, and Colombia. The disease is rarely seen in Caucasian populations. There are geographical differences in sex-specific prevalence. In Japan more than 5000 patients have been treated, of which more than 80 per cent are women with a peak age in the twenties. A recent international comparative analysis revealed a decline of this female preponderance as one moves westwards from Japan; in Israel the sex ratio is almost equal.

Aetiology

The aetiology of Takayasu arteritis is still unknown. The suggestion that it might be due to tuberculosis is now discounted by most authorities, at least in Japan where tuberculosis has drastically decreased, whereas Takayasu arteritis is actually slightly increasing in number. Another hypothesis argues that vasa vasoritis due to virus infection may be the initiating phenomenon, and hyperoestrogenism is still discussed as one of the major causative factors because of the high prevalence of Takayasu arteritis in young women. However, clinical and laboratory findings together with a favourable response to steroid therapy strengthen the argument that autoimmune mechanisms are important.

HLA and other genetic factors

Familial occurrence of Takayasu arteritis has been reported, including three pairs of monozygotic twin sisters in Japan, India, and Brazil, strongly suggesting that some genetic factor(s) is involved in pathogenesis.

There is a close association of Takayasu arteritis with HLA B52 and DR2 in Japan, B5 in India, and B52, DR2, and DQ2 in Korea. In Japan, patients with Takayasu arteritis carrying haplotype A24-B52-DR2 show rapid progression and are resistant to steroid therapy when compared with patients of other haplotypes. Furthermore, patients carrying this haplotype sometimes have other coexisting autoimmune disorders such as Behçet's disease, systemic lupus erythematosus, or ulcerative colitis. Analysis of the MIC gene, which is located near the HLA B locus, also exhibits a close association with Takayasu arteritis. It may suggest that genes involved in pathogenesis may be located between the MIC and HLA B gene locus.

Pathology

Nasu classified Takayasu arteritis histologically into three types—granulomatous inflammation, diffuse productive inflammation, and fibrotic type—which chronologically characterize the progression of this disease. Hochi stressed elastophagia as an important characteristic feature of Takayasu arteritis, progressing segmentally and from the adventitial side towards intima. Inflammation originates around vasa vasorum in the outer side of the media and/or its neighbouring adventitia. The infiltrating cells are mainly T cells, which later are mixed with macrophages. Progression to vasculitis is characterized by destruction of medial smooth muscle cells, elastophagia, and fibrosis. Fibrocellular thickening of intima follows and atherosclerotic changes may accelerate intimal thickening, a complication that makes the diagnosis of Takayasu arteritis difficult in older patients. Skipped lesions composed of a mixture of involved and non-involved areas were once deemed to be a characteristic feature of Takayasu arteritis, but with early diagnosis and treatment this is no longer the case.

Clinical features

Some patients are totally free of symptoms and are diagnosed incidentally as having Takayasu arteritis during regular health examinations because of pulselessness, difference in blood pressure between the arms, or an elevated erythrocyte sedimentation rate. However, Takayasu arteritis can present with non-specific symptoms or, depending upon which vessels are involved, with a wide variety of symptoms, hence the diagnosis is sometimes very difficult to make.

Japanese patients usually have involvement of the ascending aorta and cervical vessels (Figs 1 and 3), with the main complaints relating to ischaemia of cerebral, ophthalmological, and/or upper extremity circulation—for example dizziness, syncope, visual disturbance, weak pulse, or pulselessness—as well as inflammatory symptoms such as general malaise, neck pain, and palpable cervical lymph nodes. These inflammatory signs in young women are sometimes misdiagnosed as tuberculosis, viral infection, or rheumatoid arthritis. A 'bird face' due to atrophy of facial muscles (Fig. 4), intermittent claudication of jaw muscles, and perforation of the nasal septum due to long-term cervical circulatory disturbance are helpful in establishing the diagnosis. Today it is becoming rare to find patients whose fundi show a typical retinal coronary anastomosis due to early diagnosis and early treatment; indeed the American College of Rheumatology Subcommittee has excluded this rarely seen ophthalmic condition from the diagnostic criteria of Takayasu arteritis.

Headaches and dizziness associated with hypertension are the most common symptoms of Takayasu arteritis in Asian countries except Japan.

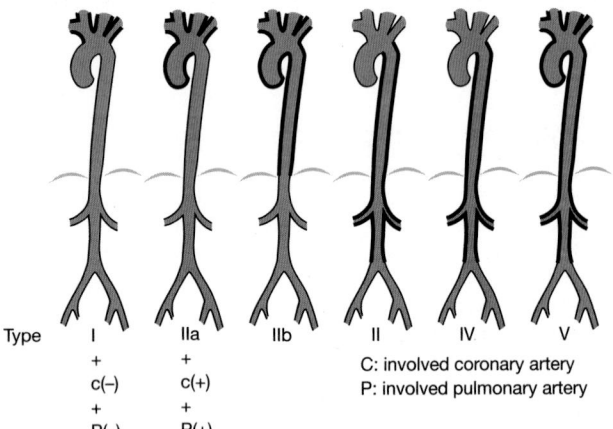

Fig. 3 New classification of the angiogram in Takayasu arteritis, according to the International Conference on Takayasu Arteritis, 1994. Type I involves branches of the aortic arch. Type IIa involves type I plus the ascending aorta and aortic arch. Type IIb involves type IIa plus the thoracic descending aorta. Type III involves the thoracic descending aorta, abdominal aorta, and/or renal arteries. Type IV involves only the abdominal aorta and/or renal arteries. Type V involves the whole aorta and its branches.

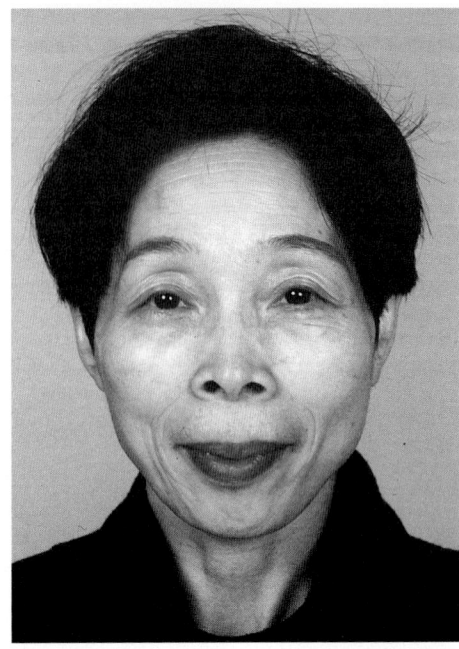

Fig. 4 'Bird face' of Takayasu arteritis: hollow cheeks and eye sockets.

These patients mainly have involvement of the abdominal aorta, inducing renovascular hypertension, and they show hypertensive retinal changes. Although rare in Japan, intermittent claudication is another characteristic symptom in China, India, and Thailand.

The commonest finding on physical examination is a weak or absent pulse in one or both brachial, radial, and/or ulnar arteries, which is noticed in almost 80 per cent of Japanese patients. These abnormalities are found more often in the left arm than the right, perhaps because the left axillary artery comes directly from the aortic arch whereas the right one arises from the brachiocephalic artery, thus making the left side more prone to inflammation.

Cardiac manifestations have become the most important cause of death in patients with Takayasu arteritis in Japan. Careful evaluation is required, particularly of aortic regurgitation due to a dilated ascending aorta, which can sometimes present as an emergency with congestive heart failure. The manifestations of ischaemic heart disease, including chest pain, arrhythmia, and/or congestive heart failure, have increased among patients with Takayasu arteritis. This may be due to involvement of the coronary arteries and/or complicated coronary atherosclerosis, which results from the increased longevity of many patients with Takayasu arteritis.

Respiratory symptoms such as dyspnoea, haemoptysis, and pleurisy due to involvement of the pulmonary artery or arteries are not uncommon. Easy thrombus formation predisposes to pulmonary infarction, but this may be clinically silent requiring a pulmonary scintigram in all patients diagnosed with Takayasu arteritis. More than 70 per cent of patients exhibited segmental and/or non-segmental pulmonary infarction in Japanese subjects.

Renal involvement in Takayasu arteritis is usually characterized by renovascular hypertension and renal dysfunction. In India, almost half of all patients with Takayasu arteritis exhibit renal artery involvement, including the ostia and a variable length of proximal renal artery. Severe proteinuria and hypercholesterolaemia (i.e. nephrotic syndrome) are characteristic of the renal dysfunction that arises in long-standing cases. It is believed that non-specific ischaemic glomerular lesions and mesangial deposition of immunoglobulin during the extended lifespan of patients receiving modern treatment have created this new renal complication of Takayasu arteritis and that it will become a major cause of death.

Hypertension and/or easy thrombus formation cause cerebral vascular accidents in many patients. Although these are no longer the dominant cause of death of patients with Takayasu arteritis in Japan, fatal stroke, hemiplegia, sensory disturbance, and aphasia are still frequently encountered despite well controlled blood pressure.

Laboratory findings and imaging modalities

The inflammatory process of Takayasu arteritis is expressed as an elevated erythrocyte sedimentation rate and C-reactive protein as well as hypergammaglobulinaemia and leucocytosis, as shown in Table 1. Changes of these indicators are well correlated with inflammatory activity and response to steroid therapy. Two national surveys in Japan conducted 10 years apart demonstrated almost equally high frequencies of accelerated erythrocyte sedimentation rate (greater than 20 mm/h) and positive C-reactive protein (greater than 20mg/l). Anaemia is often seen, probably due to chronic inflammation, and total T-cell count is significantly elevated. Other common findings are an increased antistreptolysin O titre and positive rheumatoid factor, which may suggest a common mechanism with rheumatic diseases.

There is a remarkable thrombogenic tendency during the acute inflammatory stage. Accelerated platelet aggregation, hyperfibrinogenaemia, expression of adhesion molecules, and accelerated coagulability give valuable information for assessing the clinical condition of these patients. HLA analysis also provides an additional clue to the diagnosis and is helpful in selecting patients for steroid treatment.

Calcification of the aorta on the chest radiograph in young women sometimes points to the diagnosis in patients free of subjective complaints. A definitive diagnosis can be established by angiography, which provides precise information about the vessels and sites involved, as well as about changes of the inner surface of blood vessels. For example, determining the affected site in the carotid artery is important, but not always straightforward, since it is possible that an easily palpable vessel is aneurysmal, whereas a poorly palpated one is normal. Digital subtraction angiography has become particularly popular because it does not require arterial puncture (Fig. 1). Imaging modalities such as CT, MRI, and /or magnetic resonance angiography (MRA) are also very useful in confirming Takayasu arteritis, even at an early stage, without seriously burdening the patient. Stenosis, dilatation, aneurysmal formation, and thrombosis can be well

Table 1 Findings of laboratory examinations in patients with Takayasu arteritis in Japan

Laboratory examination	Cases (%)	
	1973 to 1975 (at initial consultation)	1982 to 1984 (at deterioration)
Enhanced erythrocyte sedimentation rate	868/1193 (72.8)	997/1130 (88.2)
Increased white blood cell count	437/1249 (35.0)	506/1160 (43.6)
Anaemia	563/1175 (47.9)	629/1149 (54.7)
Increase in gammaglobulin	483/1008 (47.9)	502/ 972 (51.6)
Increase in antistreptolysin O titre	155/1067 (14.5)	142/ 920 (15.4).
C-reactive protein positive	666/1287 (51.7)	800/1153 (69.4)
Rheumatoid factor positive	108/1185 (9.1)	119/1010 (11.8)
Positive Wassermann reaction	23/1105 (2.1)	25/ 863 (2.9)
Positive tuberculin reaction	366/ 532 (68.8)	241/ 342 (70.5)
Increase in cardiothoracic ratio	413/1028 (40.2)	
Aortic calcification	239/1160 (20.6)	251/1142 (22.0)
Abnormal ECG	538/1221 (44.1)	578/1169 (49.4)

Table 2 Angiographic classification of Takayasu arteritis

Type	No. of cases (%)				
	Japan	Columbia	Brazil	India	Thailand
I	19 (24)	12 (35)	6 (21)	7 (7)	0
II a	9 (11)	4 (11)	1 (4)	1 (1)	0
II b	8 (10)	2 (6)	0	6 (6)	7 (11)
III	0	0	1 (4)	3 (3)	2 (3)
IV	1 (1)	7 (20)	4 (14)	29 (38)	12 (19)
V	42 (54)	10 (29)	16 (54)	56 (55)	42 (67)
Total	80	35	28	102	63

Source: International Conference on Takayasu Arteritis, 1994.

documented (Fig. 1). These procedures are also good for following the therapeutic effects of steroid treatment on the vasculature. In particular, as aortic regurgitation caused by dilatation of the ascending aorta is a serious complication that determines the prognosis, follow-up of the diameter of the ascending aorta by echocardiogram, MRI, or CT is critically important.

Figure 4 shows an angiographic classification of Takayasu arteritis. An international comparative study demonstrated that half of the patients in every country are type V; many Japanese patients show mainly involvement of cervical vessels and the aortic arch (type I, II); whilst many Indian and Thai patients have involvement of the abdominal aorta (type II, IV) (Table 2).

Diagnosis

Unless the physician is well aware of the disease, the diagnosis of Takayasu arteritis is frequently delayed due to its non-specific presentation. Table 3 includes the guidelines for clinical diagnosis of Takayasu arteritis summarized by the Committee of Takayasu Arteritis of the Ministry of Health and Welfare of Japan. Another set of criteria published by the American College of Rheumatology in 1990 lists six characteristics:

Table 3 Guidelines for making a clinical diagnosis of Takayasu arteritis in Japan

1. Symptoms
   (1) Cerebral ischaemia: vertigo (especially when looking upward), fainting spells, visual disturbance (especially at direct sunlight)
   (2) Ischaemia of the extremities: cold fingers, easy fatiguability of the upper extremities
   (3) Stenosis of the aorta or renal arteries: headache, vertigo, shortness of breath, which are considered to be due to hypertension
   (4) Generalized symptoms: slight fever may be recognized at the onset of the disease

2. Important findings for diagnosis
   (1) Abnormalities of the pulse of the upper extremities (weak or diminution and/or right/left difference of the radial pulse)
   (2) Abnormalities of the pulse of the lower extremities (accentuation or decrease of the pulse)
   (3) Vascular murmur in the arteries of the neck, back, or abdomen
   (4) Ophthalmological abnormalities

3. Abnormalities in laboratory examinations
   (1) Increased erythrocyte sedimentation rate
   (2) Positive C-reactive protein
   (3) Increase in gammaglobulin levels in the serum

4. Important diagnostic points
   (1) Prevalent in young women
   (2) Final clinical diagnosis can be made by an aortography

5. Differential diagnosis to be made
   Buerger's disease, arteriosclerosis, collagen disease, congenital vascular abnormalities

(1) age less than 40 years old;

(2) claudication of the arm;

(3) decreased brachial arterial pulse;

(4) greater than 10 mmHg difference in systolic blood pressure between the arms;

(5) bruit over subclavian arteries or aorta; and

(6) angiographic evidence of narrowing or occlusion of the aorta or its primary or proximal branches.

Presence of three out of six criteria is required for diagnosis, but by these criteria patients in several Asian countries whose abdominal aorta is predominantly involved would elude diagnosis. Although ophthalmological findings and/or symptoms are excluded, in Japan approximately 35 per cent of patients show abnormal ophthalmological findings including microaneurysm, retinal haemorrhage, cataract, or glaucoma.

Therapy

Steroid and antiplatelet therapies are essential in addition to symptomatic treatments such as antihypertensive and vasodilating drugs. The disease requires long-term observation, even after patients are completely free from symptoms, because vascular changes can progress silently and recurrence of vasculitis is not rare.

Steroids and immunosuppressants

Significant improvement can be achieved by steroid treatment, particularly when the disease is at an acute or active stage, starting with 0.5 to 1.0 mg/kg per day of prednisolone, then reducing by 5 mg/day every 2 to 3 weeks, depending upon the response of the erythrocyte sedimentation rate and C-reactive protein as well as symptoms. The target maintenance dose is 5 to 10 mg/day, gradually tapering before being discontinued, which in our experience is possible in 50 per cent of cases. If patients show a haplotype of HLA-B52-DR2 or B*3902, a larger dose (30 to 40 mg/day) of steroid and a longer tapering period may be necessary. Close observation is required because vasculitis can easily flare up during a common cold or other infection, requiring repeated steroid therapy or increased dose.

Immunosuppressive therapy is sometimes combined with steroid, allowing a lower dose and a shorter tapering period to be achieved, which is especially important for patients carrying an HLA B52-DR2 or B*3902 haplotype whose disease is relatively steroid resistant. Conventionally, 100 mg of cyclosporin is administered daily or every other day together with 10 to 20 mg/day of steroid.

Antithrombotic therapy

Antiplatelet therapy should be given to all patients for protection against subsequent thrombus formation. A small dose of acetylsalicylic acid (child bufferin) is the most popular drug used in Japan. Other antiplatelet drugs such as dipyridamole, ticlopidine, or cilostazol are sometimes employed, either alone in patients who cannot tolerate aspirin or combined with child bufferin. Thrombus formation is easily induced on the roughened surface of the arterial wall and active inflammation accelerates thrombus formation even more. Anticoagulant therapy with or without fibrinolytic therapy is necessary when thrombus formation is proceeding or already complete.

Percutaneous vascular intervention

Angioplasty and/or stenting can be effective procedures for some vascular complications of Takayasu arteritis, especially for coronary atherosclerosis. Several authors have reported successful percutaneous transluminal angioplasty (PTA) treatment of patients with renovascular hypertension, but this procedure seems most effective for atherosclerotic disorders involving mainly the intima and far less useful for Takayasu arteritis characterized by thickened adventitia and fibrous intima.

Surgery

The option of surgical treatment (usually bypass procedures) should always be considered for complications of Takayasu arteritis that are beyond medical treatment, for instance renovascular hypertension, coarctation of the aorta, severe ischaemia of the cerebral circulation, severe aortic regurgitation, progression of aneurysm, and dissecting aneurysm. Surgery should be performed, if possible, when inflammation is reasonably under control.

Prognosis

By early diagnosis and early initiation of treatment the prognosis of this disease has been improved. The clinical characteristics of 897 Japanese patients with Takayasu arteritis were studied in 1998: 71 per cent were well controlled and enjoyed an almost normal healthy lifestyle, many receiving no treatment. By contrast, 25 to 30 per cent suffered from severe complications such as aortic regurgitation, congestive heart failure, renal failure, or low visual acuity. In Japan the complications that determine prognosis are heart failure due to aortic regurgitation, thrombus formation leading to cerebrovascular accident, pulmonary infarction, and myocardial infarction. Cerebral haemorrhage due to hypertension is the main cause of death in Asian countries other than Japan.

Further reading

Arend WP et al. (1990). The American College of Rhematology: Criteria for the determination of Takayasu arteritis. Arthritis and Rheumatism 33, 1129–34.

Hashimoto Y et al. (1992). Aortic regurgitation in patients with Takayasu arteritis—assessment by color Doppler echocardiography. Heart Vessels Suppl 7, 111–15.

Hata A, Numano F (1995). Magnetic resonance imaging of vascular changes in Takayasu arteritis. Journal of Cardiology 52, 45–52.

Hochi M (1992). Pathological studies on Takayasu arteritis. Heart Vessels Suppl 7, 11–17.

Kimura A et al. (1996). Comprehensive analysis of HLA genes in Takayasu arteritis in Japan. International Journal of Cadiology 54, 61–9.

Kiyosawa M, Baba T (1998). Opthalmological findings in patients with Takayasu disease. International Journal of Cardiology 66(Suppl 1), 141–7.

Nagasawa T (1996). Current status of large and small vessel vasculitis in Japan. International Journal of Cardiology 54(Suppl), 75–82.

Numano F, Kakuta T (1996). Takayasu arteritis—five doctors in the history of Takayasu arteritis. International Journal of Cardiology 54(Suppl), 1–10.

Numano F, Kobayashi Y (1996). Takayasu arteritis: clinical characteristics and the role of genetic factors in its pathogenesis. Vascular Medicine 1, 227–33.

Numano F (1999). Takayasu arteritis beyond pulselessness. Journal of Internal Medicine 38, 226–32.

Numano F (2000). Vaso vasoritis, vasculitis and atherosclerosis. International Journal of Cardiology 75 (suppl.), 1–8.

Numano F (2001). Vascular manifestation in Takayasu arteritis. In: Asherson RA, Cervera R, eds. Vascular manifestations of systemic autoimmune disease, pp.251–72. CRC Press, Boca Raton.

Sekiguchi M, Suzuki J (1992). An overview on Takayasu arteritis. Heart Vessels Suppl 7, 6–10.

Takayasu M (1908). A case with peculiar changes of the retinal central vessels. Acta Societatis Ophthalmologicae Japonicae, 12, 554–5. [In Japanese.]

15.15 The pulmonary circulation

15.15.1 The pulmonary circulation and its influence on gas exchange

Tim Higenbottam, Eric Demoncheaux, and Tom Siddons

Introduction

The main functions of the lungs are the uptake of oxygen and elimination of carbon dioxide. These are driven by the respiratory demands of active cells in the body. The lungs also have important metabolic and endocrine functions. Gas exchange is achieved by a reciprocating cycle of airflow into and out of the lungs through a complex branching system of airways, the bronchi. The gas exchange takes place in the alveoli, the peripheral airspaces that are surrounded by circulating pulmonary capillary blood. This capillary blood is delivered continuously from the right ventricle and passes on to the left atrium. The total cardiac output circulates through the lungs, at flow rates that can vary from 5 litre/min at rest, to 24 litre/min during exercise. The functional anatomy of the airways and lungs are described in detail in Chapter 17.1.2; this section will focus on the pulmonary circulation.

The pulmonary circulation in health

Functional anatomy

The lungs receive blood from the pulmonary and bronchial arteries. The pulmonary arteries deliver the major blood flow, the bronchial blood supply normally being limited to a tiny fraction of the total, 1 to 2 per cent of the cardiac output, but in disease this can expand and disturb gas exchange.

The main pulmonary trunk and the large pulmonary arteries are responsible for connecting the right ventricle to the pulmonary circulation. They accompany the bronchi into the lungs and within the bronchovascular bundles branch dichotomously alongside the bronchi down to the level of the terminal bronchioles, before breaking up into the alveolar capillary bed. The close association of the dense capillary network containing deoxygenated blood to the alveoli offers an ideal environment for gas exchange to take place. Pulmonary venules collect the capillary blood and drain laterally to the periphery of the lung lobules, returning the blood to the left atrium by four branches of the pulmonary veins.

The vessels of the pulmonary circulation have thin walls and can be classified according to their calibre: those of greater than 1000 μm are considered as elastic arteries, those between 100 and 1000 μm as muscular arteries, and smaller ones with endothelial lining and a single elastic lamina but no muscular lining as pulmonary arterioles. The pulmonary capillaries form a dense network around the alveoli and are lined only by endothelial cells. Their diameter is about 7 μm and their walls fuse directly to the alveolar wall (in most places). There are rich anastomotic channels between pulmonary and bronchial vessels.

At rest the pulmonary capillary blood flow is about 5 litre/min. The pulmonary circulation has a pressure drop (from pulmonary artery to left atrium) of only 10 mmHg across it, as against 100 mmHg for the systemic circulation. The resistance of the pulmonary circulation is thus about 10 per cent of the systemic, making it a high-flow, low-resistance circuit. The pulmonary vascular bed has a high reserve capacity to adapt to increased blood flow, adaptation occurring in both large and small pulmonary arteries. The large vessels are dilated by a nitric oxide-dependent mechanism; blocking the production of endothelial nitric oxide limits adaptation. We as yet cannot explain the mechanism by which the precapillary arteries adapt to increased blood flow: these are responsible for the recruitment of previously unperfused capillaries, resulting in a change in gas exchange.

It has been suggested that the alveolar capillary bed is similar to a thin sheet of blood, interrupted in various places by posts, much akin to a large sprawling room with pillars. The oxygenated blood is collected from the capillary network by small pulmonary veins that anatomically run between the lobules of the lung, converge as four pulmonary veins (in humans), and drain back into the left atrium to be pumped by the left ventricle around the systemic circulation.

The lung also derives a very minor part of its circulation from bronchial arteries, which usually arise from the descending aorta and distribute oxygenated blood at systemic pressure to many different sites in the lungs, including the pleura, the nerves, walls of the pulmonary vessels, the intrapulmonary lymph node, and the bronchi down to the terminal bronchiole. Most of the blood supplied by the bronchial arteries drains in the pulmonary veins, thereby contributing to a limited degree of desaturation of arterial blood, a 'physiological shunt', which is present in normal healthy individuals. Small amounts of blood drain in the bronchial veins that enter the azygos and hemiazygous veins.

In pulmonary embolic disease blood flow from the bronchial arteries can sustain the lung tissue and prevent infarction of the lung. The bronchial arteries may undergo hypertrophy in chronic pulmonary inflammation and bronchial neoplasia. Major haemoptysis such as bronchiectasis or aspergilloma arises from hypertrophied bronchial rather than pulmonary arteries and may be treated with therapeutic bronchial artery embolization.

Physiology

The pulmonary circulation offers much lower resistance to flow and operates at lower perfusion pressure than the systemic circulation. The normal mean pulmonary artery pressure is in the region of 15 mmHg with a systolic of 25 mmHg and diastolic of 8 mmHg compared with the systemic pressures of 120/80 mmHg.

At the resting systolic pressure of the right ventricle, 15 mmHg, and in the upright position, gravity causes preferential flow to the basal regions of the lungs rather than the apices. Another mechanism that affects the distribution of blood flow is vasoconstriction of the resistance pulmonary arteries, which are localized just before the alveolar capillaries. Hypoxia in the alveoli and mixed venous blood (blood from the central veins) acts directly on smooth muscle cells in these vessels to cause vasoconstriction, leading to diversion of blood flow from regions of the lung with low oxygen levels towards those regions of higher oxygen tension. This acts to autoregulate the 'matching' of distribution of blood flow to distribution of ventilation.

The relationship between ventilation and perfusion

In the upright lung, after a full expiration at residual volume, the intrapleural pressure at the base of the lung (+3.5 cmH2O) is higher than the atmospheric pressure, but the apex (–4 cmH2O) still remains below atmospheric pressure. During tidal breathing, however, the region of the lung that experiences the greatest change in volume is the dependent part, the bases, when we are in an upright position. This is a result of the sigmoidal shape of the pressure-volume curve of the lung.

The effects of gravity mean that the rate of blood flow is not uniform throughout the lungs (Fig. 1), being higher in the basal regions than the apices. The different hydrostatic pressures within the blood vessels of the lung can explain this uneven distribution. An upright lung may be divided into three zones—1, 2, and 3. The blood flowing in the lung will also act like a continuous column due to the effect of gravity. In the uppermost parts, zone 1, alveolar air pressure (P_A) is usually greater than both arterial (Pa) and venous (Pv) pressures. This causes the 'squashing' of capillary beds and restriction of flow.

In the intermediate parts of the lung, zone 2, pulmonary artery pressures are increased due to the hydrostatic effect, but venous pressures (Pv) may still not be high enough to overcome alveolar pressures and blood flow is only slightly increased compared with the apex (zone 1) regions of the lung.

In the basal part of the lung, zone 3, the hydrostatic pressures generated in both the arterial and venous vessels due to the effect of gravity are greater than alveolar pressures. The flow here is chiefly determined by arterial–venous pressure difference and is therefore higher than in the intermediate and apical regions.

In summary, tidal ventilation is higher at the bases of the lung. Perfusion follows the same distribution to the bases. Ventilation–perfusion ratio (V/Q) values are high at the apex and diminish towards the base of the lung. In a normal healthy individual the overall V/Q ratio is closely matched to allow for efficient gas exchange to take place. Some small areas in the lung may still exist with good perfusion but poor ventilation (or vice versa). In many lung diseases it is likely that gross mismatch of V/Q ratios in many areas impair the process of gas exchange despite the individual having almost normal total ventilation and normal total pulmonary blood flow.

The three-compartment model of ventilation–perfusion and gas exchange

The lungs may be partitioned into a number of functional units in terms of ventilation–perfusion: these do not have discrete anatomical definitions but provide reference points for analysis of gas exchange.

In the absence of a diffusion barrier, the partial pressures of O_2 and CO_2 of the air in each alveolus are the same as those of the end-capillary blood draining it. For the lung as a whole this situation does not arise due to lack of uniformity of ventilation–perfusion within its various units, resulting predominantly from gravitational effects and pleural pressure gradients as described in the preceding section. To obtain the V/Q ratio of such units, the alveolar composition of O_2 and CO_2 would need to be known. Direct sampling of the alveoli is technically not feasible. Sampling at the mouth after deep maximal exhalation is flawed by the dependence of the technique on the speed of exhalation and the baseline state of lung inflation. Alveolar partial pressures of O_2 and CO_2 vary in different parts of the lungs and at different times in the respiratory cycle, hence samples obtained at the mouth are likely to be influenced by the rate and time of emptying of the various lung units.

The three-compartment model of Riley visualizes the lung perfusion as comprising (i) a physiological shunt (Qs), perfusing an area with no ventilation; (ii) alveolar capillary blood equilibrating with ideal alveolar air; and (iii) physiological deadspace (Vd). Detailed calculations are beyond the scope of this text, but in a resting man up to 70 per cent of the pulmonary ventilation is distributed to the well perfused areas of the lung and up to 95 per cent of the pulmonary capillary blood flow supplies lung units that are well ventilated. These areas are well matched for ventilation and perfusion and constitute the functional part of the lungs in terms of respiratory gas exchange. Approximately 30 per cent of the lung units are ventilated but unperfused, and this constitutes physiological deadspace. Similarly, at rest, 5 per cent of the lung units are well perfused but not ventilated and they constitute the physiological shunts.

There are methods by which the 'matching' between ventilation and perfusion can be assessed: these are still underdeveloped and need refinement, but are none the less providing improved understanding. One such method is the multiple inert gas excretion technique (MIGET). A physiological saline solution of the six inert gases is injected into a peripheral vein. The

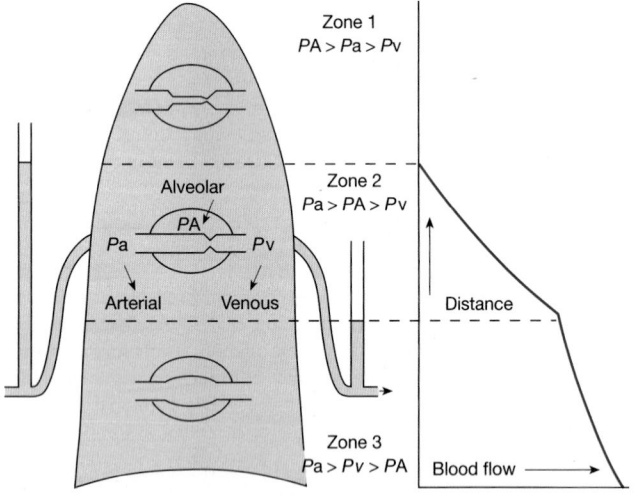

Fig. 1 Diagram of West showing the distribution of blood flow through the lung, which explains the uneven distribution of blood flow in different regions of the lung. Pa, arterial pressure; P_A, alveolar pressure; Pv, venous pressure. (Reproduced from West J (2000). *Respiratory physiology*, 6th edn. Lippincott Williams and Wilkins, with permission.)

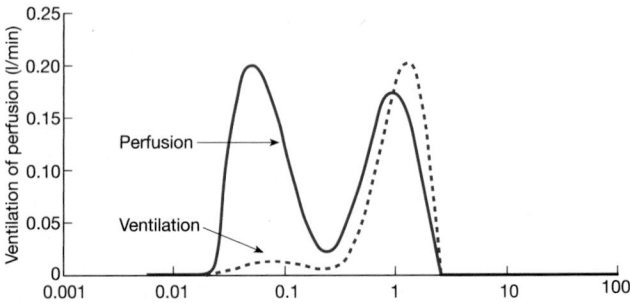

Fig. 2 A representative ventilation–perfusion distribution obtained from a patient with severe airways obstruction at rest. Large areas of perfusion are insufficiently ventilated resulting in hypoxaemia.

mixed arterial concentration of each of the gases is measured and taken as the blood-flow weighted mean for the various compartments of the lung. Mixed expired levels are measured and taken as the ventilation weighted mean of the compartmental values. Cardiac output and minute ventilation are also measured and used to calculate the corresponding mixed venous and alveolar concentrations. Based on mass balance considerations a lung ventilation–perfusion distribution is mathematically derived, which is compatible with the arterial and alveolar concentrations of all the inert gases concurrently (Fig. 2).

Further reading

Deffebach M *et al.* (1987). The bronchial circulation. Small but a vital attribute of the lung. *American Review of Respiratory Disease* **135**, 463–81.

Florence A, Attwood D (1998). *Physicochemical principles of pharmacy.* MacMillan Press, London.

Nunn J (1993). *Applied respiratory physiology.* Butterworth, London.

Silverman E, Gerritsen M, Collins T (1997). *Metabolic function of the pulmonary endothelium.* Raven Press, New York.

Singhal S, Henderson R, Horsfield K (1973). Morphometry of the human pulmonary arterial tree. *Circulation Research* **33**, 190–7.

Wagner P, Naumann P, Laravuso R (1974). Simultaneous measurement of eight foreign gases in blood by gas chromatography. *Journal of Applied Physiology* **36**, 600–5.

West J (1963). Distribution of gas and blood in the normal lungs. *British Medical Bulletin* **19**, 53–8.

West J (1977). Ventilation–perfusion relationships. *American Review of Respiratory Disease* **116**, 919–43.

West J, Wagner P, Derks C (1974). Gas exchange in distributions of VA/Q ratios: partial pressure–solubility diagram. *Journal of Applied Physiology* **37**, 533–40.

Williams S *et al.* (1979). Methods of studying lobar and segmental function of the lung in man. *British Journal of Disease of the Chest* **73**, 97–112.

15.15.2 Disorders of the pulmonary circulation

15.15.2.1 Primary pulmonary hypertension

Tim Higenbottam and Helen Marriott

Introduction

This chapter will consider the nature of primary pulmonary hypertension and how it relates to the other types of pulmonary hypertension. It will also consider the impact of pulmonary hypertension on survival in both primary pulmonary hypertension and that associated with other disease. The causes of the disease and effects of current treatments will be reviewed.

The publication of reports from the National Institutes of Health (**NIH**) sponsored registry of primary pulmonary hypertension provided a description of the clinical features and prognosis, also a clear diagnostic pathway for investigation. The introduction of heart–lung transplantation in 1981 by Bruce Rietz in Stanford University, California, offered the first real hope of long-term survival for those with primary pulmonary hypertension . However, the realization that transplant surgery could only be offered as a treatment for a tiny minority of patients provided the stimulus to consider alternative medical treatments. This led to the introduction of long-term

intravenous infusion of prostacyclin (prostaglandin I_2) in 1984, first considered as a bridge to lung transplantation, but subsequently demonstrated in controlled studies to improve survival and enhance quality of life. Inhaled nitric oxide was later recognized to act as a selective vasodilator of the pulmonary circulation (unlike prostacyclin) and has recently gained United States Food and Drug Administration approval as a therapy, specifically for neonatal pulmonary hypertension.

Finally, the quest to understand familial primary pulmonary hypertension has identified causal mutations of the gene for the bone morphogenetic protein receptor II. This is a member of the superfamily of transforming growth factor-β receptors, and mutations appear to increase the sensitivity of cellular responses to this important growth factor. The hope for new therapies that alter the structure rather than physiology of the pulmonary circulation could now be realized.

What is pulmonary hypertension?

In all its forms, pulmonary hypertension is characterized by fibromuscular intimal hypertrophy that results in narrowing and obliteration of the lumen of blood vessels, most commonly the precapillary arteries (Fig. 1 and Plate 1). By the time of presentation with primary pulmonary hypertension up to 80 per cent of lung vessels have been 'lost' (Fig. 2).

The physiological consequences of the dramatic loss of small arteries are that the pulmonary vascular resistance is increased, as is the ability of the pulmonary circulation to adapt to the increased blood flow associated with exercise. The resting pulmonary artery pressure is raised; by definition pulmonary hypertension is defined as a mean pulmonary artery pressure in excess of 25 mmHg at rest. More importantly, during exercise there is a rapid rise in pulmonary artery pressure as the pulmonary blood flow increases with cardiac output (Fig. 3).

Exercise limitation as a result of breathlessness is the most common symptom in primary pulmonary hypertension and probably caused by acute right ventricular failure. Because the cardiac output fails to rise appropriately with exercise, the mixed venous oxygen saturation (Svo_2 per cent) falls through increased tissue extraction of oxygen and the arterial oxygen saturation (Sao_2 per cent) also falls. In the later stages of disease the

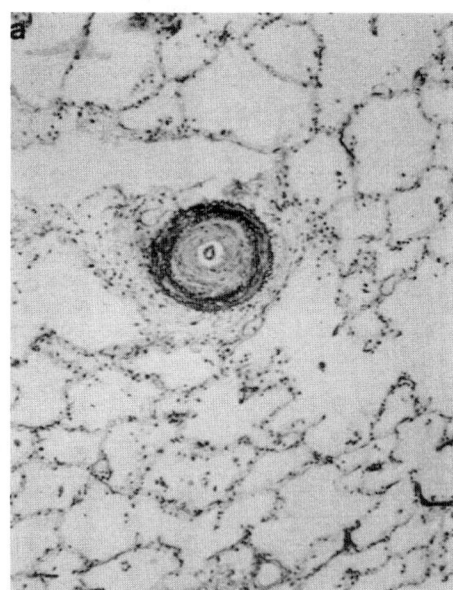

Fig. 1 Intimal thickening of a pulmonary artery in pulmonary hypertension (Chazova I *et al.*, 1995. Pulmonary artery adventitial changes and venous involvement in primary pulmonary hypertension. *American Journal of Pathology* **146**, 389–97). (See also Plate 1.)

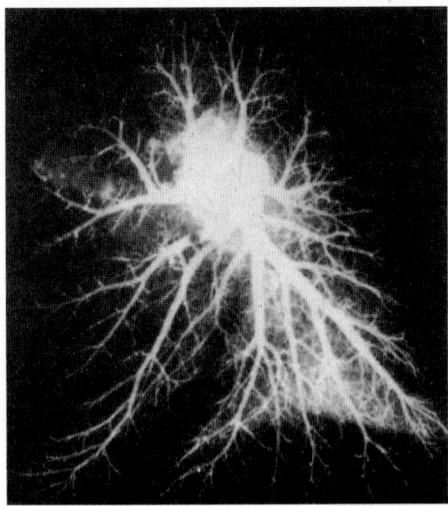

Fig. 2 Loss of precapillary arteries in the lung of a patient with primary pulmonary hypertension.

Sao_2 per cent falls even at rest. Right ventricular failure is the most common cause of death.

Clinical features

Pulmonary hypertension should be considered when there is unexplained breathlessness, with no obvious heart or lung disease. In the later stages of the disease symptoms of right ventricular failure become obvious, including syncope, angina-like chest pain, and peripheral oedema. General malaise and cachexia of cardiac failure are endstage symptoms.

In 85 per cent of patients a loud second heart sound is heard. The ECG shows right ventricular strain and RBBB pattern. Also in 85 per cent of patients chest radiography shows large pulmonary arteries.

The screening test is transthoracic echocardiography with Doppler estimation of the tricuspid valve regurgitant flow velocity, which allows the systolic pulmonary artery pressure to be estimated.

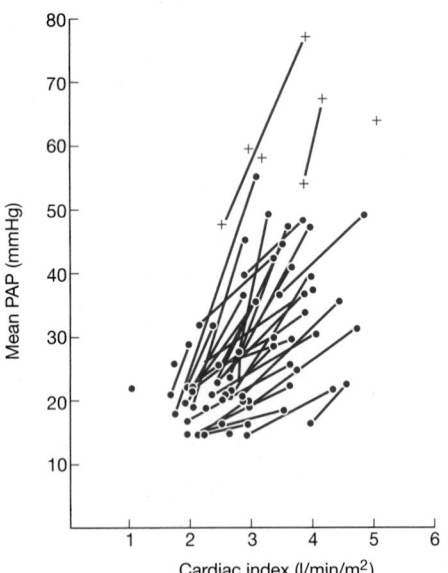

Fig. 3 The increase in pulmonary artery pressure (PAP) with increase in cardiac output (index).

At this point it is appropriate to refer all patients with severe pulmonary hypertension—where exercise limitation is a result of pulmonary hypertension—to a specialist centre because of the complexities of diagnosis and the difficulties in managing long-term treatments (Fig. 4). All require a ventilation and perfusion lung scintigraphy followed by a diagnostic right heart catheter. At this the right atrial pressure is measured along with the pulmonary artery pressure, the pulmonary wedge pressure, the cardiac output, and the Svo_2 per cent. A pulmonary angiogram is undertaken in those patients whose V/Q shows unventilated perfusion defects, although as an alternative investigation it is becoming common to use high-speed spiral CT with an injection of contrast media to assess proximal pulmonary artery obstruction in chronic thromboembolic pulmonary hypertension.

Classification of pulmonary hypertension

In 1973 the World Health Organization (**WHO**) sponsored the first meeting on pulmonary hypertension. This considered in detail the pathology of the condition and presented the first approach to the classification of the disorder. Unexplained or primary pulmonary hypertension was considered separately from secondary pulmonary hypertension, where an additional disease could be identified in association with pulmonary hypertension. Twenty-five years later the second WHO sponsored meeting focused more upon the common features of the different forms of pulmonary hypertension, in particular their response to treatments such as prostacyclin and the common histopathological changes. Five types of pulmonary hypertension were recognized (Fig. 5).

Pulmonary arterial hypertension

Pulmonary arterial hypertension was defined as the type of disease where the intimal proliferative changes are found in the arteries alone. In addition

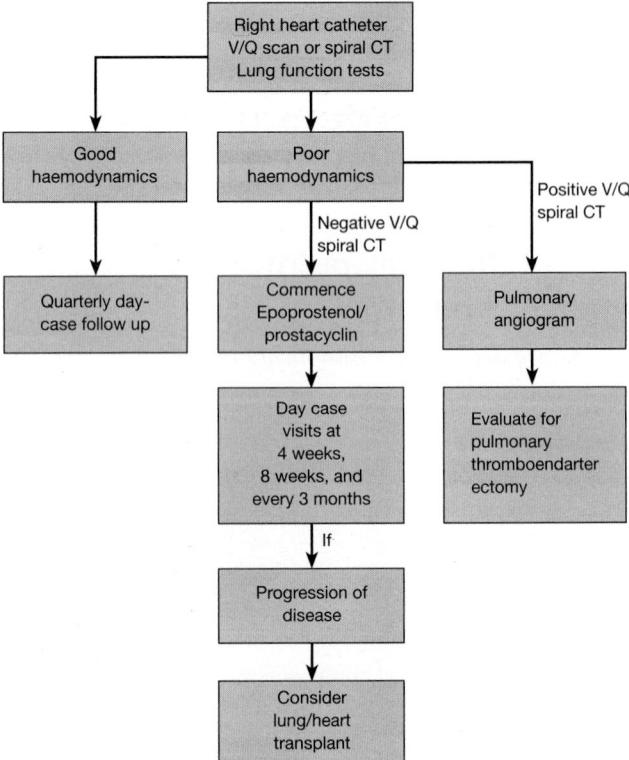

Fig. 4 The investigation and treatment pathway for a patient with pulmonary hypertension.

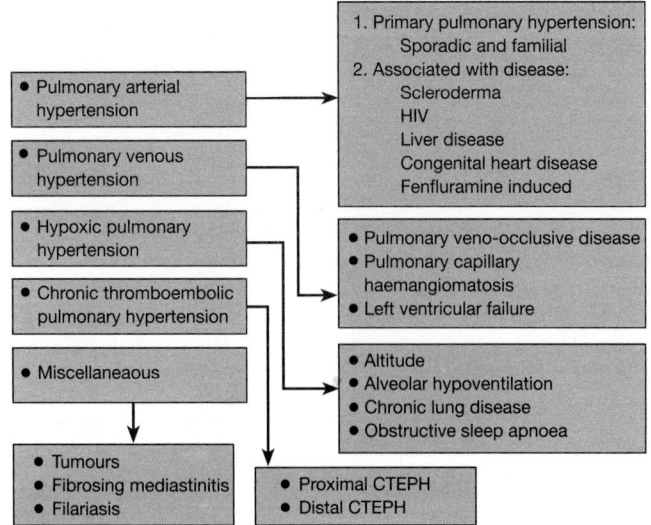

Fig. 5 Types of pulmonary hypertension. CTEPH, chronic thromboembolic pulmonary hypertension (Rich SE, 1998. Primary pulmonary hypertension: executive summary from the world symposium—Primary Pulmonary Hypertension. Available from the World Health Organization via the internet http://www.who.int/ncd/cvd/pph.thml).

there is medial hypertrophy of the muscular arteries and, in advanced disease, changes also include plexiform lesions that it has been suggested are neovascular structures which 'bypass' the obstructed precapillary arteries. Primary pulmonary hypertension is the exemplar and is divided into the sporadic and the familial forms. A necrotizing arteritis has also been described in primary pulmonary hypertension. Peripheral arterial thrombi are often present. Pulmonary arterial hypertension associated with other diseases includes that seen with HIV infection, liver disease, congenital heart disease (Eisenmenger's syndrome), scleroderma, and other connective tissue diseases. Up to 60 per cent of the pulmonary vascular bed can be obstructed before the symptoms of pulmonary hypertension develop.

The progressive reduction in number and narrowing of the lumen of precapillary arteries initially causes a loss of capacity of the pulmonary circulation to accommodate the increased pulmonary blood flow of exercise. Whilst the resting pulmonary artery pressure may not be raised initially, with exercise the pressure rises rapidly. Right ventricular failure, defined as an inability to sustain the required cardiac output, contributes to the exercise intolerance and the patient experiences breathlessness.

As the disorder advances the pulmonary artery pressure begins to rise, even at rest. The higher systolic and diastolic pressures in the right ventricle can limit diastolic filling of the right ventricular coronary arteries: angina can result, even in the absence of coronary artery disease. Sudden failure of the right ventricle accounts for the exercise-induced syncope seen in the late stages of the disorder. Palpitations on exercise are not uncommon and cardiac dysrhythmias are the cause of sudden death in advanced disease.

With failure of the right ventricle at rest the right atrial pressure rises and failing venous return results in the development of peripheral oedema and ascites. Gross hepatic engorgement may occur which impairs the liver's metabolic role.

In addition to these predominately vascular effects, many patients with primary pulmonary hypertension have impaired gas exchange. There is evidence of extensive ventilation/perfusion mismatch, in the main resulting from perfusion of regions of the lungs that are normally poorly ventilated, but also from ventilation of poorly perfused regions. Furthermore, as the cardiac output falls, the mixed venous oxygen level falls as a result of greater extraction of oxygen in the peripheries of the body. Selective flow of this profoundly deoxygenated blood through a limited number of perfused areas of the lungs leaves insufficient time for oxygen uptake to occur, par-

ticularly during exercise when the arterial oxygen level can fall profoundly.

In about 15 per cent of patients with primary pulmonary hypertension the foramen ovale of the atrial septum opens as a result of high right ventricular pressure, leading to a right-to-left intracardiac shunt of blood. This adaptation has been shown to prolong survival, as does the fashioning of an atrial septal defect in advanced primary pulmonary hypertension, particularly in infants. The mechanism of this effect is the opportunity for excessive right ventricular pressures during exercise to be released through the defect into the left side of the circulation. This means that the right ventricle does not fail acutely, but the cost is further reduction of arterial oxygen content. However, whilst being more hypoxic than their counterparts without septal defects, these patients can undertake more exercise and live longer.

Pulmonary venous hypertension

Pulmonary venous hypertension is where the intimal proliferation is found in the veins rather than the arteries. There are three main forms—two rare and one very common. Pulmonary veno-occlusive disease and pulmonary capillary haemangiomatosis are the rare conditions, whilst pulmonary venous hypertension from left ventricular failure and left-sided valvular heart disease are common. Any increase in left atrial pressure, pulmonary vascular resistance, and capillary blood flow can lead to a chronic increase in pulmonary venous pressure.

Distinction between pulmonary arterial and pulmonary venous hypertension can be clinically challenging. However, in pulmonary venous hypertension the pulmonary wedge pressure measured with a Swan/Ganz balloon catheter is elevated. On high-resolution computed tomography the lung fields show extensive interstitial lines in the interlobular septi, an appearance akin to left ventricular failure.

Hypoxic pulmonary hypertension

Acute pulmonary hypoxic vasoconstriction

The precapillary arteries of the lungs are sensitive to falls in both alveolar and capillary oxygen partial pressure. At values of oxygen partial pressure below 7.2 kPa, their vascular smooth muscle cells contract, dependent on the activity of voltage-dependent potassium channels, ensuring a matching of the distribution of perfusion of the capillaries to ventilation of the alveoli.

Chronic hypoxic pulmonary hypertension

Whilst transient pulmonary hypertension is often a feature of acute lung disease, normal distribution of perfusion is restored when the alveolar oxygen levels are returned to normal. However, in chronic lung disease (see Chapters 17.6 and 17.7) the structure of the walls of the precapillary arteries changes. As in pulmonary arterial hypertension the intima proliferates and there may be smooth muscle hypertrophy and adventitial fibrosis. These changes are extensive and not simply localized to those regions of the lungs that are predominantly under-ventilated. In other words the chronic changes in structure of the pulmonary arteries in hypoxic lung disease do not necessarily facilitate close matching between the distribution of ventilation and perfusion.

The increased pulmonary vascular resistance in patients with chronic hypoxic lung disease is usually less severe than in primary pulmonary hypertension, but it does contribute to ill health. There is evidence on echocardiographic studies that right ventricular function is impaired: this is exacerbated by exercise and could contribute to reduced exercise tolerance.

Chronic thromboembolic pulmonary hypertension

Chronic thromboembolic pulmonary hypertension is where the peripheral or proximal pulmonary arteries are occluded by thrombus and emboli, causing widespread segmental and subsegmental defects in lung perfusion.

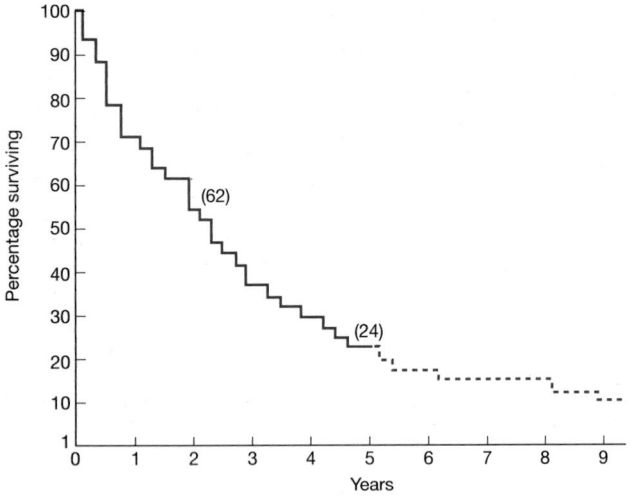

Fig. 6 Survival in primary pulmonary hypertension (Fuster V *et al.*, 1984. Primary pulmonary hypertension: natural history and the importance of thrombosis. *Circulation* **70**, 580–7).

These areas are usually normally ventilated and so gas exchange is impaired. Patients compensate with increased rates of ventilation: Pao_2 is often maintained with a lower than normal $Paco_2$ level. As in all forms of pulmonary hypertension, resting cardiac output may be reduced or is reduced when exercise is undertaken.

Miscellaneous

Finally there is the miscellaneous type of pulmonary hypertension. This includes pulmonary hypertension with fibrosing mediastinitis, pulmonary artery tumours, and obstructions associated with protozoal and nematode infestation, such as filariae and schistosomes.

Prognosis

The development of pulmonary hypertension shortens life. This is best seen in primary pulmonary hypertension, where the untreated 3-year post-diagnosis survival is less than 35 per cent (Fig. 6), but pulmonary hypertension also reduces survival when it is associated with other disease such as chronic obstructive bronchitis. This is a result of alveolar hypoxia, as sur-

vival is enhanced when the partial pressure of oxygen is restored to normal by long-term oxygen therapy (LTOT).

The cause of death in pulmonary hypertension depends on the severity of right ventricular failure. In patients with primary pulmonary hypertension it is possible to predict survival from haemodynamic measurements at right heart catheter studies: the presence of a cardiac output less than 2.5 litre/min, mean right atrial pressure more than 10 mmHg, and Svo_2 less than 63 per cent all being poor prognostic factors. For ease it is valuable to use the New York Heart Association Grade III or IV and pulmonary vascular resistance greater than 15 units to predict the chance of survival to be very low without treatment (Fig. 7). A very similar prediction can be made on the basis of haemodynamic measurements in patients with Eisenmenger's syndrome. Sudden death from right ventricular failure is responsible for 47 per cent of the deaths from primary pulmonary hypertension.

Treatment

All patients with pulmonary arterial hypertension should receive anticoagulation treatment as uncontrolled studies have shown overall survival to be improved by their use (Fig. 8). The treatment of chronic thromboembolic pulmonary hypertension with proximal obstructions is surgical thromboendarterectomy: for other types of pulmonary hypertension—with the exception of pulmonary venous hypertension—the use of vasodilators should be considered.

Early disease

In early/mild disease (cardiac output greater than 2.5 litre/min, mean right atrial pressure less than 10 mmHg, and Svo_2 greater than 63 per cent) decisions about other treatment are made following an acute vasodilator trial, most commonly using inhaled nitric oxide, intravenous prostacyclin, or adenosine. Only if there is evidence of a greater than 20 per cent drop in pulmonary vascular resistance are oral vasodilators considered. This response is found in less than 25 per cent of patients with primary pulmonary hypertension, and for these nifedipine, diltiazem, or amlodopine are used in therapeutic doses. Survival is improved, although the studies are uncontrolled (Fig. 9).

Severe disease

In patients with severe disease (cardiac output below 2.5 litre/min, right atrial pressure greater than 10 mmHg, or Svo_2 less than 63 per cent), long-term continuous infusions of prostacyclin improve survival and enhance the quality of life. Actuarial survival at 2 years has been increased to 80 per

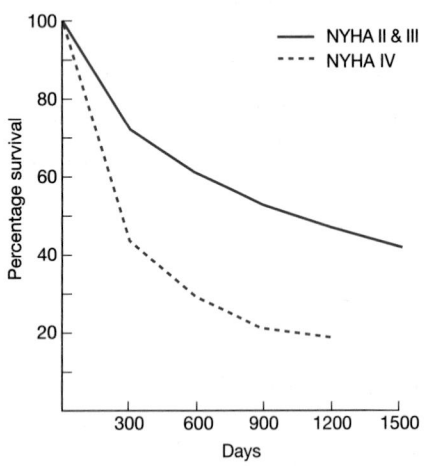

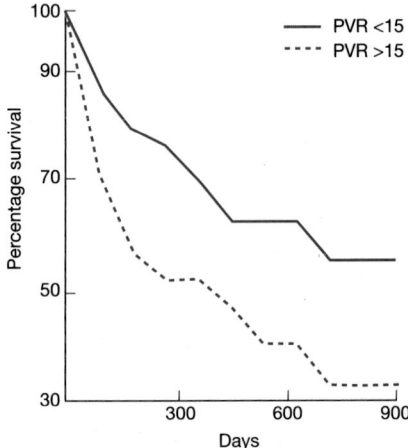

Fig. 7 Survival of patients with primary pulmonary hypertension in the NIH registry according to their New York Heart Association (NYHA) Grade and pulmonary vascular resistance (PVR) (D'Alonzo GE *et al.*, 1991. Survival in patients with primary pulmonary hypertension. Results from a national prospective registry. *Annals of Internal Medicine* **115**, 343–9).

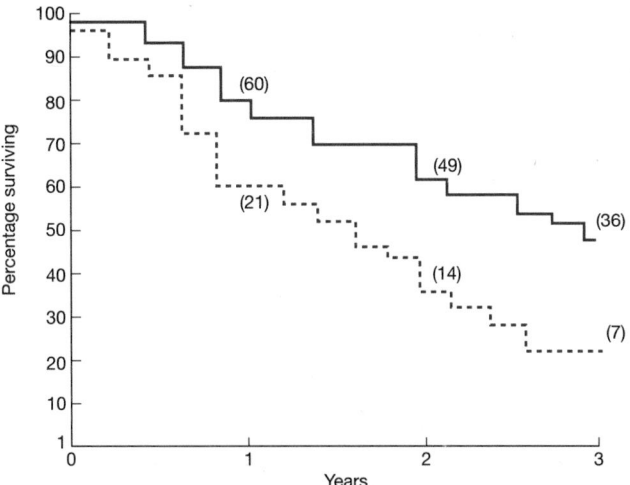

Fig. 8 Survival of patients with primary pulmonary hypertension treated (solid line) or not treated (broken line) with anticoagulation (Fuster V et al., 1984. Primary pulmonary hypertension: natural history and the importance of thrombosis. *Circulation* **70**: 580–7).

cent, which exceeds that of untreated patients and the survival following lung transplantation (Fig. 10). Of special interest is the recent report that prostacyclin may, when used long-term, reverse the disease to some extent, with pulmonary vascular resistance falling below the lowest level achieved during the initial right heart catheter study (Fig. 11). This has raised the hope that medical treatments may be able to reverse the disease process.

Primary pulmonary hypertension and Eisenmenger's syndrome have the poorest outcomes of any diseases after lung transplantation, the 3-year actuarial survival being only just in excess of the untreated patients. However, the introduction of prostacyclin has delayed the need for lung transplantation by on average 17.5 months and has improved the success of subsequent lung transplantation, with 1-year survival rate in excess of 80 per cent.

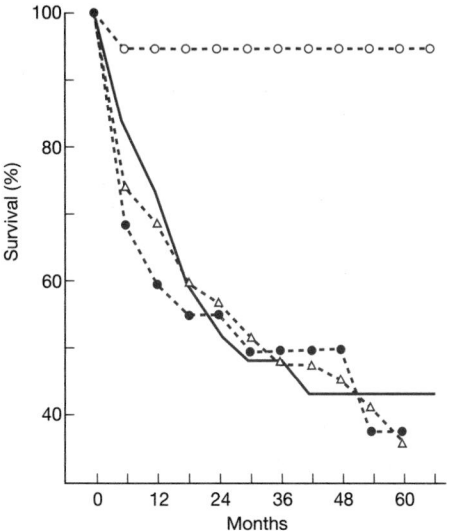

Fig. 9 Kaplan–Meier estimates of survival among patients who responded to treatment (open circles), those who did not respond (solid line), patients enrolled at the NIH registry who were treated at the University of Illinois (solid circles), and the NIH registry cohort (triangles).

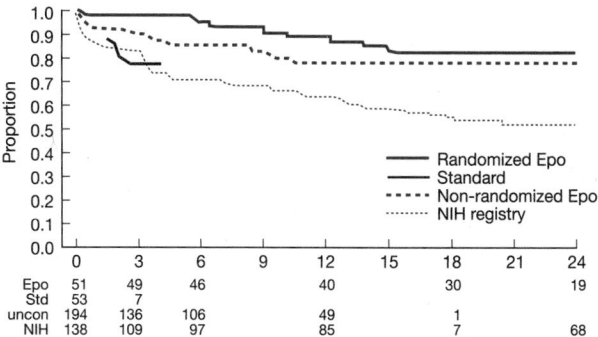

Fig. 10 Long-term continuous infusions of prostacyclin improve survival. Epo, epoprostanol; std, standard; uncon, uncontrolled non-randomized Epo; NIH, National Institute of Health Registry.

Use of vasodilators

Prostacyclin

In pulmonary hypertension the phenotypes of many cells that make up the blood vessels are changed: endothelium, the cells of the matrix tissues, and the vascular smooth muscle cells. In patients with primary pulmonary hypertension, urinary excretion of prostacyclin metabolites is reduced and endothelial cells from the pulmonary arteries express a reduced level of prostacyclin synthase, the enzyme that forms prostacyclin, hence it would seem appropriate to supplement the reduced endogenous production of prostacyclin with exogenous therapy.

The success of intravenous prostacyclin in primary pulmonary hypertension has led to its use in other forms of pulmonary arterial hypertension. In isolated pulmonary hypertension from scleroderma, prostacyclin also improves the quality of life, and in pulmonary arterial hypertension associated with congenital heart disease it improves survival. In those patients with chronic thromboembolic pulmonary hypertension who are not suitable for surgery, prostacyclin also achieves an equivalent improved survival chance to that seen in patients with primary pulmonary hypertension. By contrast, in pulmonary venous hypertension—that is, pulmonary veno-occlusive disease, pulmonary capillary haemangiomatosis, and left ventricular failure—long-term intravenous prostacyclin worsens the survival chances and should not be used. The increased perfusion leads to pulmonary oedema, respiratory failure, and death.

Analogues for prostacyclin have been developed. Iloprost, which is more stable, is of equivalent effect to prostacyclin when given intravenously and

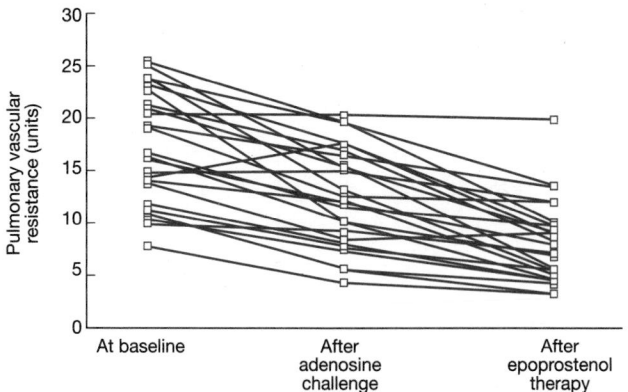

Fig. 11 Long-term prostacyclin may reverse pulmonary hypertension (McLaughlin VV et al. (1998). Reduction in pulmonary vascular resistance with long-term epoprostenol (prostacyclin) therapy in primary pulmonary hypertension. *New England Journal of Medicine* **338**, 273–7).

has also been used orally and by inhalation. Beroprost is another oral analogue, whilst UT-15 was introduced for continuous subcutaneous infusion. All are in clinical trials, with encouraging early results. There is evidence that inhaled iloprost achieves the same degree of 'reversal' of pulmonary hypertension as intravenous delivery when used long term.

Nitric oxide

As with prostacyclin synthase, expression of nitric oxide synthase and release of nitric oxide is also reduced in the pulmonary arteries in both primary and other types of pulmonary hypertension. Basal nitric oxide release seems normal from pulmonary hypertensive lungs, but stimulated release of the gas is reduced, particularly in hypoxic pulmonary hypertension. In advanced primary pulmonary hypertension there are clusters of new vessels, called plexiform lesions, branching from precapillary arteries. Nitric oxide synthase is overexpressed in these lesions, which develop in the region of the 'obstructed' precapillary pulmonary arteries, perhaps bypassing the obstruction and providing a route from pulmonary artery to the pulmonary veins.

In 1987 inhaled nitric oxide was shown to be a selective pulmonary vasodilator (Fig. 12). However, a problem of handling and using nitric oxide is its speed of oxidation to form nitrogen dioxide, which can injure the epithelial lung surfaces even at low concentrations of 5 parts per million (ppm). This rate of reaction is dependent on the concentration of the gas and the concentration of oxygen, hence it is necessary to mix the nitric oxide (which is stored in nitrogen) carefully with air or oxygen just before it is inhaled. This is straightforward when the patient is receiving mechanically assisted ventilation, but difficult when ventilation is spontaneous. It may be achieved, however, using a 'spiked' delivery system that adds nitric oxide as a small bolus of gas at the beginning of the breath using a patient triggered device. This can reduce the pulmonary vascular resistance by the same amount as when the breath is filled with 40 ppm of nitric oxide, but with only a fortieth of the dose with each breath.

Inhaled nitric oxide is about half as effective as a vasodilator as prostacyclin. It has not yet found a place in the treatment of primary pulmonary hypertension in general, although in some case reports it seems to 'reverse' established primary pulmonary hypertension when given long term. In chronic obstructive pulmonary disease, the pulmonary vascular resistance

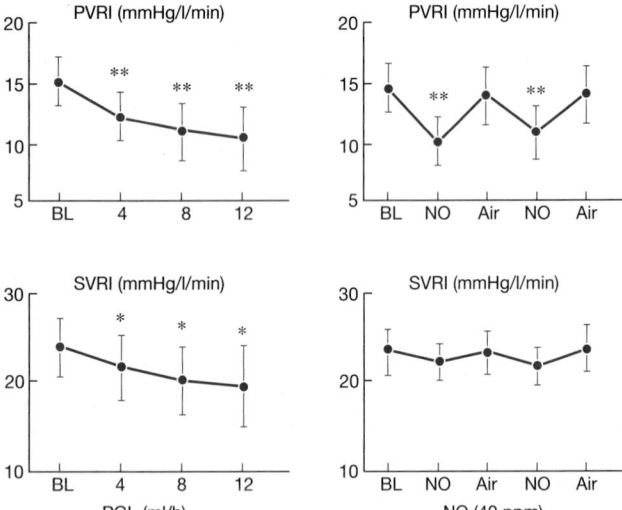

Fig. 12 Inhaled nitric oxide is a selective pulmonary vasodilator. PVRI, pulmonary vascular resistance index; SVRI, systemic vascular resistance index; ppm, parts per million (of inhaled nitric oxide); PGI$_2$, prostaglandin I$_2$; *, significantly different from baseline (Pepke Zaba J et al. (1991). Inhaled nitric-oxide as a cause of selective pulmonary vasodilatation in pulmonary-hypertension. *Lancet* **338**, 1173–4).

is reduced in patients receiving long-term oxygen therapy when nitric oxide is administered for 3 months, and in this group inhaled nitric oxide may have a part to play in reducing the pulmonary hypertension and right ventricular dysfunction seen during exercise. Long-term, randomized, controlled trials are awaited. As a therapy inhaled nitric oxide has recently been granted a licence for the treatment of pulmonary hypertension of the neonate, here avoiding the use of extracorporeal oxygenation.

Phosphodiesterase inhibitors

In the lungs the breakdown of cGMP, formed in vascular smooth muscle cells by nitric oxide, is predominately by the phosphodiesterase-5-enzyme that is especially expressed in lung and in the vascular cells of the corpus cavernosum. By use of the inhibitor sildenafil (Viagra) it is possible to induce pulmonary vasodilatation. Given orally long-term this reduces pulmonary vascular resistance and improves exercise tolerance in patients with pulmonary arterial hypertension.

Endothelin-1 antagonists

There have been numerous reports that endothelin-1 is expressed to a greater degree than normal in most types of pulmonary hypertension and that circulating levels of endothelin-1 are also elevated, especially in acute hypoxia of altitude and in chronic hypoxic lung disease. These findings have led to the suggestion that endothelin receptor antagonists might be effective treatments for pulmonary hypertension, and some 32 are in development. One agent, bosentan, has been shown to reverse structural abnormalities in experimental models of pulmonary hypertension. Anxieties about teratogenicity and liver injury have limited the widespread use of these compounds in clinical practice, but encouraging results have been observed in reports of series of patients with isolated pulmonary hypertension and scleroderma. Long-term, randomized, controlled trials have now reported improved exercise tolerance.

Particular causes of pulmonary arterial hypertension

Pulmonary hypertension in fenfluramine and dexfenfluramine users

In the late 1980s a physician in Paris, Francois Brenot, noticed an increasing number of patients with primary pulmonary hypertension being referred who had been treated with the anti-obesity drug fenfluramine or its isomer dexfenfluramine. This observation led to a case–control study of all patients with primary pulmonary hypertension diagnosed over a period of 18 months. For each of 192 patients with this condition three controls were found who were matches for gender, age, and district of residence. An independent panel of doctors checked the entry criteria for each patient with primary pulmonary hypertension. All had a detailed questionnaire administered on past and present therapies, including anti-obesity treatments. It was found that an excess number of patients had taken one of the two drugs, for at least 3 months. Indeed, 1 in 8000 was the calculated risk for developing primary pulmonary hypertension when either fenfluramine or dexfenfluramine was taken for more than 1 year, suggesting a causal relationship. By contrast, the appetite suppressant phentermine was not associated with pulmonary hypertension. Of note, in the 1960s a similar association had been found between the use of another anti-obesity drug, aminorex, and the development of primary pulmonary hypertension.

What is the mechanism by which fenfluramine/dexfenfluramine might cause primary pulmonary hypertension? Both accumulate in the lungs through uptake by the serotonin transporter for which they have a high substrate affinity, and both are metabolized by the cytochrome P450 enzyme CYP2D6 that is expressed in the liver, lungs, and right side of the heart. In part the susceptibility of certain individuals to develop primary pulmonary hypertension when taking fenfluramines can be accounted for by polymorphism of the CYP2D6 enzyme. About 8 per cent of Caucasian and 1 per cent of Asian people express little or no active enzyme, hence they will have little ability to metabolize these drugs within the lungs, with local lung toxicity a possible explanation for the development of pulmonary hypertension. Within the population of patients with primary pulmonary hypertension who have taken dexfenfluramine and fenfluramine there is a higher proportion of poor metabolizers compared with controls (20 per cent compared with 7 per cent). High concentrations of dexfenfluramine and fenfluramine are able to induce vascular smooth muscle contraction in humans as a result of inhibition of membrane potassium channels. In addition, fenfluramine at high concentration can inhibit expression of the 1.5Kv subunit of the voltage-dependent potassium channel of vascular smooth muscle cells.

Familial primary pulmonary hypertension

About 6 per cent of all patients with primary pulmonary hypertension have a family history of the condition, exhibiting an autosomal dominant pattern of inheritance with incomplete penetrance. The histopathology of the pulmonary vascular disease is identical to that found in sporadic primary pulmonary hypertension.

In 1998 two laboratories identified a region on chromosome two associated with familial primary pulmonary hypertension after detailed linkage analysis of extended families. Further work led to identification of mutations of a gene encoding for bone morphogenetic protein receptor II (*BMPR 2*) as the cause. This is a member of the superfamily of transforming growth factor-β receptors.

Transforming growth factor-β is an important cytokine regulator of pulmonary angiogenesis. It inhibits cell growth, cell differentiation, and stimulation of collagen deposition. In the inherited illness hereditary haemorrhagic teliangectasia, new vessels in the lungs and mucosa lead to bleeding. Mutations of the gene encoding endoglin, which is a transforming growth factor-β receptor-complex accessory protein, and of the transforming growth factor-β type 1 receptor ALK-1, have been identified in this disease. A 'failure' of signalling by transforming growth factor-β could account for the new vessel formation. By contrast, mutations of *BMPR 2* appear to enhance the effects of transforming growth factor-β, perhaps promoting vessel 'loss' and synthesis of collagen. Much needs to be learnt about the key ligands, receptors, and downstream signalling pathways. However, this lead from familial primary pulmonary hypertension could have identified a common mechanism for many different types of pulmonary hypertension. Overexpression of transforming growth factor-β is often found in both experimental and human forms of pulmonary hypertension. Lessons learnt from genetics could offer useful clues as to how we might 'fully' reverse pulmonary hypertension in the future.

Further reading

Abenhaim L *et al.* (1996). Appetite-suppressant drugs and the risk of primary pulmonary hypertension. *New England Journal of Medicine* **335**, 609–16.

Anderson E, Simon G, Reid L (1973). Primary and thromboembolic pulmonary hypertension: a quantitative pathological study. *Journal of Pathology* **110**, 273–93.

Barst RJ *et al.* (1996). A comparison of continuous intravenous epoprostenol (prostacyclin) with conventional therapy for primary pulmonary hypertension. The Primary Pulmonary Hypertension Study Group. *New England Journal of Medicine* **334**, 296–302.

Bourdillon P, Oakley C (1976). Regression of primary pulmonary hypertension. *British Heart Journal* **38**, 264–70.

Brenner O (1935). Pathology of the vessels of the pulmonary circulation. Part I. *Archives of Internal Medicine* **56**, 211–37.

Channick *et al.* (2001). Effects of the dual endothelin-receptor antagonist bosentan in patients with pulmonary hypertension: a randomised placebo-controlled study. *Lancet* **258**, 1119–23.

Chazova I *et al.* (1995). Pulmonary artery adventitial changes and venous involvement in primary pulmonary hypertension. *American Journal of Pathology* **146**, 389–97.

Conte JV *et al.* (1998). The influence of continuous intravenous prostacyclin therapy for primary pulmonary hypertension on the timing and outcome of transplantation. *Journal of Heart and Lung Transplantation* **17**, 679–85.

D'Alonzo GE *et al.* (1991). Survival in patients with primary pulmonary hypertension. Results from a national prospective registry. *Annals of Internal Medicine* **115**, 343–9.

Deng Z *et al.* (2000). Familial primary pulmonary hypertension (gene PPH1) is caused by mutations in the bone morphogenetic protein receptor-II gene. [In process citation.] *American Journal of Human Genetics* **67**, 737–44.

Fuster V *et al.*(1984). Primary pulmonary hypertension: natural history and the importance of thrombosis. *Circulation* **70**, 580–7.

Heath D, Whitaker W, Brown J (1957). Idiopathic pulmonary hypertension. *British Heart Journal* **19**, 83–92.

Heath D, Segel N, Bishop J (1966). Pulmonary veno-occlusive disease. *Circulation* **34**, 242–8.

Higenbottam T *et al.*(1984). Long-term treatment of primary pulmonary-hypertension with continuous intravenous epoprostenol (prostacyclin). *Lancet* **i**, 1046–7.

Higenbottam TW *et al.* (1999). Subjects deficient for CYP2D6 expression (poor metabolisers) are over-represented among patients with anorectic associated pulmonary hypertension. *American Journal of Respiratory and Critical Care Medicine* **159**(3 SS), A165.

Hoeper MM *et al.* (2000). Long-term treatment of primary pulmonary hypertension with aerosolized iloprost, a prostacyclin analogue. *New England Journal of Medicine* **342**, 1866–70.

Kay J, Smith P, Heath D (1971). Aminorex and the pulmonary circulation. *Thorax* **26**, 262–70.

Lane K *et al.* (2000). Heterozygous germline mutations in *BMPR2*, encoding a TGF-β receptor, cause familial primary pulmonary hypertension. *Nature Genetics* **26**, 81–4.

Lawson R., Higenbottam T (1999). Primary pulmonary hypertension. In: Grassi C *et al.* eds. *Pulmonary diseases*, pp 373–9. McGraw-Hill, London.

Loyd J, Primm R, Newman J (1984). Familial primary pulmonary hypertension: clinical patterns. *American Review of Respiratory Disease* **129**, 194–7.

Mosser K *et al.* (1983). Chronic thrombotic obstruction of major pulmonary arteries; results of thromboembolectomy in 15 patients. *Annals of Internal Medicine* **99**, 299–305.

Pepke Zaba J *et al.* (1991). Inhaled nitric-oxide as a cause of selective pulmonary vasodilatation in pulmonary-hypertension. *Lancet* **338**, 1173–4.

Rich S *et al.* (1987). Primary pulmonary hypertension. A national prospective study. *Annals of Internal Medicine* **107**, 216–23.

Rich SE (1998). Primary pulmonary hypertension: executive summary from the world symposium—Primary Pulmonary Hypertension. Available from the World Health Organization via the internet http://www.who.int/ncd/cvd/pph.thml

Rozkovec A, Montanes P, Oakley C (1986). Factors that influence the outcome of primary pulmonary hypertension. *British Heart Journal* **55**, 449–58.

Wagenvoort C, Wagenvoort N (1970). Primary pulmonary hypertension: a pathologic study of vessels in 156 clinically diagnosed cases. *Circulation* **42**, 1163–84.

Wang J *et al.* (1998). Action of fenfluramine on voltage-gated K+ channels in human pulmonary- artery smooth-muscle cells. [Letter.] *Lancet* **352**, 290.

15.15.2.2 Pulmonary oedema

J. S. Prichard* (revised by J. Firth)

Introduction

Acute fulminant pulmonary oedema is a terrifying event in which patients literally drown in their own body fluids. Much more commonly, the clinician is called to treat pulmonary oedema in its less acute form, for breathlessness disturbs the patient long before serious alveolar flooding has begun.

Because pulmonary oedema is very commonly seen as a manifestation of left-sided heart disease—where its relief by diuretics is so effective—there is a temptation to forget the very wide range of other causes. Indeed, it is prudent to make the diagnosis of hydrostatic pulmonary oedema of cardiac origin only when other manifestations of heart disease are present, and to consider wider possibilities in all other circumstances. Pulmonary oedema has many possible causes, which occur in combination more often than is usually recognized (see Table 1). Only by careful and clear analysis of clinical and pathophysiological data can the contributing factors be identified and the clinical situation fully understood.

Physiological and experimental aspects of pulmonary oedema

Fluid balance between the capillaries and the interstitial space

The continuous movement of water from the lung capillaries into the interstitium is regulated by the permeability of the endothelium to water and protein and by the imbalance of hydrostatic and osmotic forces across the membrane. The Starling hypothesis suggests that perturbation of any one of five factors could lead to oedema (Figs 1 and 2). These are capillary hydrostatic pressure (P_{cap}), interstitial tissue pressure (P_{int}), plasma colloid osmotic (oncotic) pressure (P_{cap}), endothelial permeability (expressed by k and s), and lymphatic function. Abnormalities in the first four will cause oedema by increasing water entry to the interstitial space, whilst impaired function of the last will diminish drainage. Interstitial colloid osmotic pressure (P_{int}) has not been included as an independent variable as it is determined by the plasma protein concentration and endothelial permeability.

Experimentally, the development of pulmonary oedema may be characterized by the relationship between tissue water and microvascular hydrostatic pressure (Fig. 3). In the normal lung, the water content rises only slowly until the capillary pressure reaches 25 to 30 mmHg: thereafter, the rise is rapid. The curve is shifted leftwards by decreased interstitial pressure, increased endothelial permeability, decreased plasma oncotic pressure, or impaired lymphatic drainage. Figure 3 illustrates the interactions between these factors: at low and normal hydrostatic pressures, changes in oncotic pressure, permeability, and lymphatic drainage do not readily cause oedema but, at higher hydrostatic pressures, their effect is much more dramatic. The fact that pulmonary capillary pressure may be raised to 25 to 30 mmHg before there is any significant accumulation of water in a normal lung is a considerable 'safety factor', due principally to the behaviour of the lymphatic system. In response to faster transcapillary water flux from whatever cause (see below), the lymphatic system can increase its activity so much that flow accelerates to between three and ten times the basal level before the drainage becomes overwhelmed. The situation in which the lung water content has increased only little whilst the transcapillary and lymph fluxes have increased considerably emphasizes that pulmonary oedema is a dynamic phenomenon, in which tissue swelling is but the endstage reached

---

* It is with regret that we report the death of Dr J. S. Prichard. Much of his chapter in the third edition has been retained here.

when lymphatic drainage capacity is exceeded. Only then does fluid accumulation begin—slowly at first in the interstitial space, but then rapidly as alveolar flooding begins.

Hydrostatic pulmonary oedema

Any increase in capillary hydrostatic pressure, whether from cardiac failure, fluid overload, or pulmonary venous occlusion, speeds the rate of water flow into the interstitium. Provided the increase in pressure is not too great, this process will be self-limiting. Thus, molecular sieving, by allowing water to enter the interstitial space more readily than macromolecular solutes, will reduce π_{int}. Increased interstitial water increases the interstitial hydrostatic pressure P_{int} and decreases the macromolecular exclusion volume—again increasing P_{int}. So, as long as lymphatic pumping can keep pace, the tissue water will expand only slightly. However, once the capacity of the lymphatic drainage is exceeded, accumulation of an oedema fluid with a

Table 1 Causes of pulmonary oedema

Hydrostatic pulmonary oedema

- Pulmonary venous hypertension—cardiogenic. Left ventricular failure; mitral stenosis and regurgitation; left atrial thrombosis; left atrial myxoma; cor triatriatum; loculated pericarditis
- Pulmonary venous hypertension—non-cardiogenic. Veno-occlusive disease; congenital pulmonary venous stenosis; mediastinal granulomas, fibrosis, masses; neurogenic
- Pulmonary arterial hypertension. Hyperkinetic states (extreme exercise, left–right shunts, hypoxia, anaemia, thyrotoxicosis); pulmonary emboli; high altitude

Permeability oedema

- Drugs and circulating toxic substances. Hydrochlorthiazide; phenylbutazone; aspirin; methylsalicylate; nitrofurantoin; hydralazine; bleomycin; heroin; morphine; methadone; dextropropoxyphene; paraquat; alloxan; α-naphthylthiourea; coral snake venom; silver nitrate; ammonium chloride; ammonium sulphate; chelating agents; oleic acid (fat embolus); diltiazem; iodine-containing contrast media; interleukin-2
- Immunological. Goodpasture's syndrome; antilung serum; Stevens–Johnson syndrome
- Radiation
- Viral infection
- Aspirated toxic substances. Fresh water; salt water; stomach contents
- Inhaled toxic substances. Smoke; nitrogen oxides; ozone; chlorine; cadmium oxide; oxides of sulphur; carbonyl chloride; phosgene; lewisite; oxygen
- Metabolic. Hepatic failure; renal failure
- Mechanical endothelial disruption. ?Neurogenic pulmonary oedema
- Mechanical epithelial disruption. ?Pulmonary hyperinflation
- Other causes of permeability oedema: adult respiratory distress syndrome. Particularly: shock lung; septicaemia; pancreatitis; burns; fat embolism; cardiopulmonary bypass; banked unfiltered blood; amniotic fluid embolism

Reduced alveolar septal tissue interstitial pressure

- Upper airway obstruction—acute. Laryngospasm; epiglottitis; laryngotracheobronchitis; spasmodic croup; foreign body; tumour; upper airway trauma; strangulation; peritonsillar abscess; Ludwig's angina; angio-oedema; near-drowning; ?asthma
- Upper airway obstruction—chronic. Obstructive sleep apnoea; adenoidal, tonsillar, or nasopharyngeal mass; thyroid goitre; acromegaly

Reduced plasma-colloid osmotic pressure

- Rare as sole cause. Contributes to oedemas of adult respiratory distress syndrome, hepatic and renal failure, fluid overload, myocardial infarction. Important when hypoproteinaemia occurs with other conditions predisposing to oedema

Failure of lymphatic clearance

- Lymphangitis carcinomatosa; mediastinal obstruction; lung transplant; contributes to oedema in adult respiratory distress syndrome, malaria, silicosis

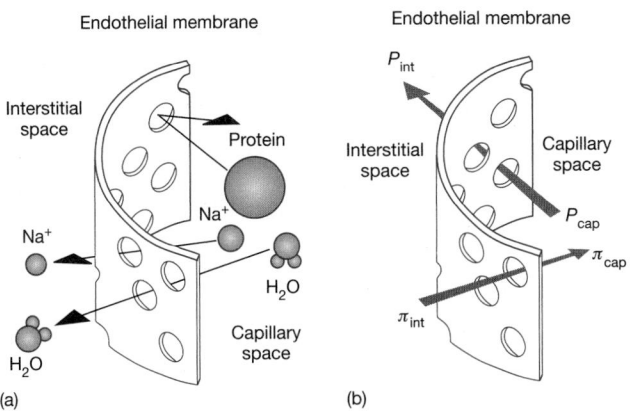

Fig. 1 (a) The lung endothelial membrane is permeable to water and electrolytes but less permeable to macromolecules. (b) The Starling equation: $Q_1 = K(P_{cap} - P_{int}) - Ks(\pi_{cap} - \pi_{int})$, where Q_1 is the net fluid filtration rate, K is the filtration coefficient, s is the reflection coefficient, $(P_{cap} - P_{int})$ is the hydrostatic pressure gradient from the capillary lumen to interstitial space, and $(\pi_{cap} - \pi_{int})$ is the oncotic pressure difference across the capillary membrane.

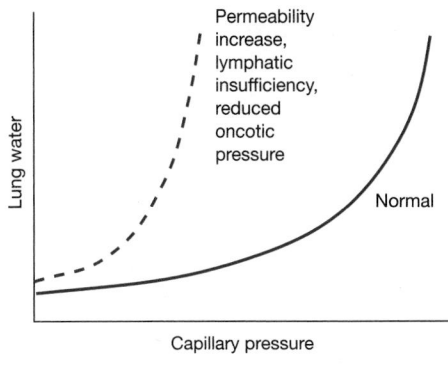

Fig. 3 Lung water content and capillary pressure. In the normal lung tissue, the water content does not begin to increase until the capillary pressure is approximately 30 mmHg. Where colloid osmotic pressure (e.g. plasma protein concentration) is reduced, endothelial permeability is increased or the lymphatic pump is impaired, the whole curve is shifted to the left. (Reproduced from Prichard JS (1982). *Edema of the lung*. Charles C. Thomas, Springfield, Illinois, with permission.)

low protein content begins. This starts in the lower parts of the lung (because it is here that hydrostatic pressures are greatest) and is associated with a characteristic redistribution of blood flow away from the lung bases.

The activity of lung lymphatics is critical in determining the onset and extent of hydrostatic oedema, and therefore it is not surprising to find that, in conditions where pulmonary vascular pressures are chronically elevated, the lymphatics undergo hypertrophy as a protective mechanism. Consequently, acute elevations of pulmonary vascular pressure will produce acute life-threatening oedema at levels that, when reached chronically, cause little distress and are registered clinically only by the characteristic radiological changes of lymphatic hypertrophy.

High permeability pulmonary oedema

Endothelial damage speeds water flux into the interstitial space. But, unlike hydrostatic oedema, there is also an increase in protein flux so that the oedema fluid has a high protein content. This has four consequences:

1. The oncotic pressure of the interstitial fluid increases and one of the major mechanisms for limiting the progress of oedema becomes unavailable.

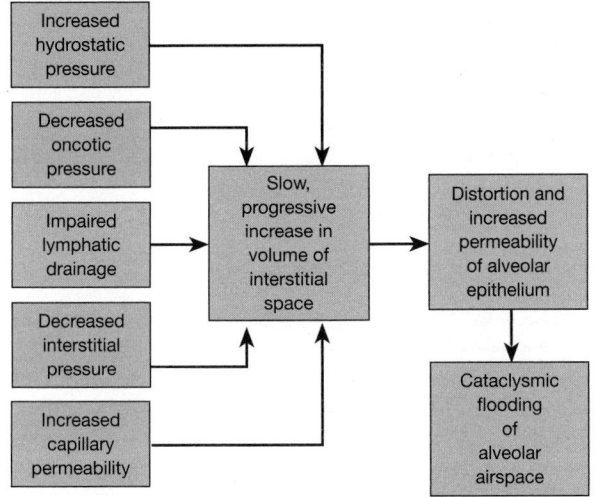

Fig. 2 The initiation of pulmonary oedema and the sequence of development.

2. Much of the protein reaching the tissue and alveoli is fibrinogen, which coagulates. Initially, the damage from interstitial coagulation is limited by fibrinolysis by plasminogen, but this defence is soon exhausted and mobilization of the coagulum ceases.

3. The residual coagulum impairs lymphatic drainage.

4. The residual coagulum becomes the skeleton on which lung fibrosis develops.

By far the most common cause of high permeability pulmonary oedema is the acute respiratory distress syndrome, which is discussed in Chapter 16.5.1. Less common causes include toxic gases and fumes (Chapter 17.11.17) and drugs (Chapter 17.11.19).

Pulmonary oedema and reduced plasma oncotic pressure

A reduction in plasma oncotic pressure increases fluid transudation into the lung and leads to pulmonary oedema at lower hydrostatic pressures than would otherwise be expected. Although this is readily demonstrable experimentally, it is frequently overlooked in clinical practice, where it may be of importance following myocardial infarction, after transfusion of crystalloids, and in adult respiratory distress syndrome. A useful clinical guide to the danger is the difference between pulmonary wedge pressure (measured by a Swann–Ganz catheter) and colloid osmotic pressure (the **COP–PAW** gradient). The normal lower limit of this index is about −12 mmHg, but at levels below −9 mmHg the risk of oedema is considerably enhanced. A practical problem in applying this method has been the difficulty in standardizing and maintaining protein oncometers. The alternative of using serum protein measurements is valuable but slower.

Lymphatic oedema and the role of the lung lymphatics

The lymphatic system provides the lung with its major 'safety factor'. It is capable of increasing the tissue clearance rate at least 10-fold before becoming overwhelmed. In chronic venous and capillary hypertension, as in mitral stenosis, even larger lymph flows occur because of lymphatic hypertrophy.

Oedema soon develops when lymphatic drainage is occluded experimentally. This has clinical relevance for patients with lung transplants, whose lung lymphatic pathways are severed and in whom initial alveolar flooding is common. Lymphatic oedema also plays a part in pulmonary oedema from lymphangitis carcinomatosa and in facilitating oedema in patients with silicosis and malaria.

Reduced interstitial pressure and pulmonary oedema

Tissue pressure within the interstitial space is one of the determinants of transendothelial fluid movement. It can be altered independently of intravascular events by changes in the intrapleural pressure. Thus, when extreme negative intrapleural pressures occur, the interstitial perialveolar tissue pressure can fall considerably below its normal subatmospheric level and accelerate the rate of fluid movement into the interstitium. Oedema will appear if the rate of fluid entry exceeds the rate at which it can move through the interstitium and be removed by the lymphatics.

The sequence of oedema accumulation

When oedema fluid begins to accumulate in lung tissue—irrespective of the underlying cause—it does so first around fissures, blood vessels, and airways because these tissues are 'loose' and swell easily without great change in tissue pressure. When this 'sump' has become near maximally dilated, swelling and thickening of the alveolar wall begin. Finally, after a phase of progressive alveolar wall thickening, fluid begins to accumulate in the alveoli themselves. This final phase begins at a point where total lung water has increased by about 30 per cent (Fig. 4).

At first, the fluid in the alveoli is confined to the alveolar angles. Subsequently, complete flooding of individual alveoli occurs. A striking feature of the microscopic appearance at this stage is the way in which alveoli are either completely filled with fluid or else have only minimal accumulation in the angles. There are no half-filled alveoli: flooding is a 'quantal' event, with flooded alveoli scattered at random throughout the affected area. Atelectasis is uncommon and air is rarely trapped, although the volume of each alveolus is smaller when fluid-filled than when air-filled.

The quantal nature of alveolar flooding arises from the interaction of surface and tissue forces (Fig. 5). The immediate precipitating factor is probably an increase in alveolar epithelial permeability caused by the distortion and swelling of the alveolar wall, which allows water to flood from the interstitium into the air space. An alternative, less likely, hypothesis is that fluid entry occurs via pores in the epithelium of the terminal airways. Irrespective of the route, the ease of fluid entry now makes the relationship between pressure and volume inverse and unstable, as explained in the legend to Fig. 5.

The resolution of pulmonary oedema

The extent and rapidity of resolution of pulmonary oedema depend upon its cause. Hydrostatic oedema and that due to low oncotic pressure can resolve completely and rapidly, but this is rarely the case with permeability oedema, where slow disappearance and permanent lung damage are the rule.

Resolution of hydrostatic oedema occurs in two phases: return of the capillary pressure towards normal, and then lymphatic and osmotic resorption of tissue and alveolar fluid. In cardiac failure, the shift of blood from the pulmonary to the systemic circulation by sitting up is the most powerful method of reducing capillary pressure, but other mechanisms have also been suggested, including:

(1) progressive hypovolaemia (from fluid extravasation into the lung);

(2) increasing plasma oncotic pressure from the relatively greater transendothelial loss of water than of plasma protein;

(3) hypoxic vasoconstriction of the muscular pulmonary arteries causing a fall in capillary pressure;

(4) exhaustion of sympathetic neurotransmitter in the systemic circulation with reduction in venomotor tone and left heart afterload.

The first three are all known to occur, but quantitatively their contributions are uncertain. The fourth is conjecture.

In hydrostatic oedema, once hydrostatic pressure has been reduced, fluid is removed from the interstitial space by lymphatic drainage, which can be increased for as long as 24 h after an acute episode in experimental models. Oncotic resorption into the circulation can also play a significant part. However, the mechanism of alveolar clearance is not well understood. Much fluid is removed by coughing and ciliary drainage and final resorption seems to occur as a result of active sodium ion transport, although it is uncertain whether this takes place in the alveolar or terminal airway epithelium.

The clearance mechanisms in high permeability oedema are considerably less efficient than in hydrostatic oedema because fibrin has coagulated

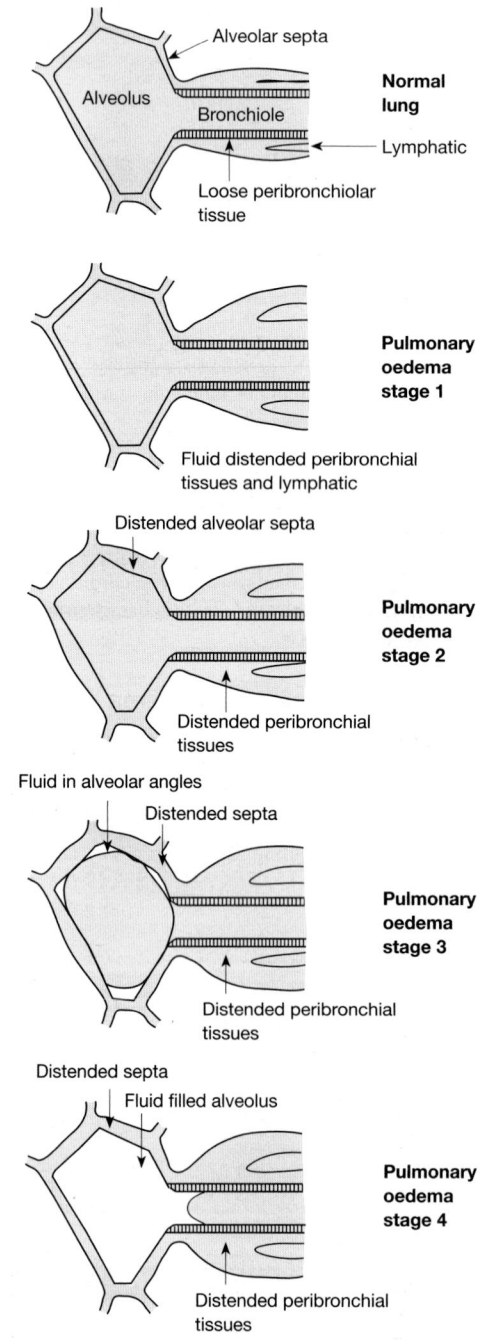

Fig. 4 Stages in the development of pulmonary oedema. Stage 1: peribronchial swelling; stage 2: distended alveolar septa; stage 3: limited accumulation of fluid in alveolar angles; stage 4: alveolar flooding. (Reproduced from Prichard JS (1982). *Edema of the lung.* Charles C. Thomas, Springfield, Illinois, with permission.)

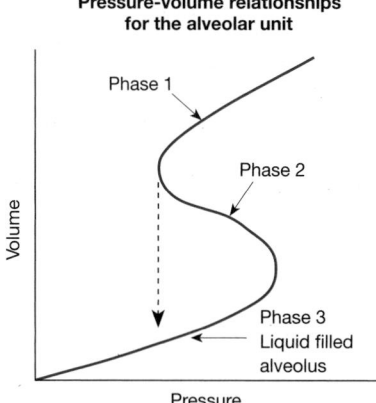

Pressure–volume relationships for the alveolar unit

Phase 1

Phase 2

Phase 3
Liquid filled
alveolus

Volume

Pressure

Fig. 5 Pressure–volume relationships in the alveolus. Phase 1 represents the normal alveolus lined by surfactant. Tissue elasticity, osmotic balance, and the presence of surfactant combine to produce a direct, mechanically stable relationship between pressure and volume. Phase 2 represents the situation in which alveolar permeability has increased. Any influx of fluid into the alveolus decreases the overall surface area. At these lower dimensions, surfactant is inoperative and surface tension is independent of area. The relationship between volume and pressure is that of an air bubble in liquid ($P = 2T/R$) and is unstable, a situation only resolved when the alveolus has flooded. The air volume therefore shrinks as air is expelled until phase 3 is reached. Here the remaining air is a 'bleb' at the bronchiolar orifice.

in the interstitium, lymphatics, and alveoli, and because the tissues have often been damaged. Regeneration of epithelium and endothelium is frequently necessary. In the case of the alveolar epithelium, cell replacement is by transdifferentiation from type II pneumocytes and this is rarely complete. Whether the transdifferentiated cells are able to play an efficient part in active transport and fluid removal is unknown.

Clinical aspects

Causes of pulmonary oedema

Table 1 lists the main causes of pulmonary oedema classified according to the predominant pathophysiological mechanism. However, the clinician should never forget that more than one cause may be operating (Table 2), and must not neglect one remediable factor at the expense of another, or

allow therapy itself to intensify the problem. For example, overvigorous fluid replacement following pulmonary endothelial damage may be the very factor that accelerates water and protein flow into the interstitium and provokes oedema.

Descriptions of the clinical manifestations and management of the more common diseases listed in Table 1 are provided elsewhere, but certain aspects need particular comment.

Pulmonary oedema in heart failure

Heart failure, discussed in detail in Chapter 15.2.2, is the cause of the commonest form of pulmonary oedema, but two features deserve comment. The first is the symptom of orthopnoea in which the oedema either first appears or, if already present, intensifies after a period of lying down. The cause is a shift of blood from the systemic to the pulmonary circulation, which occurs because of the change in posture. This leads to an increase in intracapillary hydrostatic pressure, which in turn triggers oedema. The symptom is at its most dramatic in paroxysmal nocturnal dyspnoea. The second feature—and one that frequently causes confusion because it is contrary to expectation—is the tendency of the blood pressure to rise as the patient progresses into left heart failure. The cause is probably increasing sympathetic activity and circulating catecholamines, which lead to intense systemic arterial and venous vasoconstriction, thereby increasing afterload and central venous pressure inappropriately and so intensifying the development of oedema.

Loculated constrictive pericarditis

Loculated constrictive pericarditis, predominantly involving the left ventricle, can occur in patients with chronic renal failure who are undergoing dialysis. Echocardiography is helpful in diagnosis, which may be difficult because the characteristic signs of pericardial tamponade may be missing. When located posteriorly, the fluid is difficult to aspirate percutaneously, but open drainage is rarely necessary because strict attention to fluid regulation during and between dialyses usually leads to resolution.

Pulmonary venous thrombosis

This is a rare condition that is difficult to diagnose. It may be idiopathic or may be a manifestation of conditions such as polyarteritis nodosa, other vasculitic disorders, and occult neoplastic disease. The idiopathic condition is most common in middle-aged women: symptoms of increasing lassitude and breathlessness, sometimes with a low-grade fever, are the presenting symptoms. Gross-effort dyspnoea and pulmonary oedema, usually with pleural effusions, develops later. Signs of pulmonary hypertension are present. Difficulty in obtaining a clear pulmonary artery wedge pressure tracing and normal left atrial pressure (measured directly by the trans-septal route)

Table 2 The multifactorial nature of pulmonary oedema

	Hydrostatic pressure increase	Oncotic pressure decrease	Endothelial permeability increase	Lymphatic drainage impairment	Reduced interstitial pressure	Reduced alveolar surfactant
Shock lung	From therapy	Yes	Yes	Yes		(Yes)
Hepatic failure		Yes	Yes			
Renal failure	Yes	(Yes)	Yes			
Neurogenic oedema	Yes		Yes			
Fluid overload	Yes	(Yes)				
Pulmonary emboli	Yes		Yes			
MI	Yes	(Yes)				
Carcinomatosis		Yes		Yes		
High altitude	Yes		Yes			
Re-expansion			(Yes)		Yes	(Yes)
Airway obstruction	(Yes)				Yes	

Parentheses indicate minor contributions.

MI, myocardial infarction.

should alert suspicion. Pulmonary artery angiography demonstrates poor segmental drainage in the regions affected by thrombosis. Open lung biopsy will confirm the diagnosis, but this is dangerous and should be undertaken only when there is real fear of missing an alternative cause of the oedema.

Left atrial myxoma, ball thrombus of the left atrium, and cor triatriatum

These are rare, but must not be missed as they are remediable by surgery. Their clinical presentation may be very similar to that of pulmonary venous thrombosis. All three conditions also enter into the differential diagnosis of tight mitral stenosis. Echocardiography is the key investigation.

High-altitude oedema

Some apparently normal people who ascend rapidly to high altitude experience acute pulmonary oedema. The condition develops only in that minority of individuals who have an exaggerated acute pulmonary arterial pressor response to hypoxia. These develop pulmonary hypertension at high altitude, with oedema possibly resulting from transarterial fluid leakage, but alternatively due to inhomogeneity of vasoconstriction and consequent extreme hyperperfusion of those areas not vasoconstricted. A further contribution may arise from the effects of vasoactive amines on the contractile filaments of endothelial cells leading to separation of endothelial junctions.

Pulmonary oedema with pulmonary arterial hypertension

Pulmonary arterial hypertension secondary to high output states, such as large shunts, can occasionally be associated with pulmonary oedema (possibly from transarterial leakage), especially following exercise. This is usually avoided because acute breathlessness is such a prominent early symptom.

Pulmonary oedema following acute intracranial lesions

A large variety of intracranial lesions may occasionally be associated with acute pulmonary oedema. It is probable that damage to the nucleus of the tractus solitarus and the hypothalamus lead to severe systemic vasoconstriction ('sympathetic storm'), which shifts blood to the pulmonary circulation, causing an extreme paroxysm of pulmonary hypertension. In addition, there is evidence to suggest that pulmonary venoconstriction also occurs, thus causing a rise in pulmonary capillary pressure even in excess of that predicted from the pulmonary arterial pressure measurements. The extreme high blood pressure in the capillaries first induces hydrostatic oedema and if sufficiently severe also damages the endothelium, leading to a less easily resolved permeability oedema.

Pulmonary thromboembolism

This may occasionally lead to florid pulmonary oedema, for which two hypotheses have been proposed: (1) local overperfusion caused by diversion of blood flow away from the occluded site; and (2) humoral alteration of permeability. It is possible that both mechanisms may play a part, and also that the causes may be different in micro- and macroemboli. Evidence for the overperfusion mechanism originates from experiments in which balloon occlusion of the major pulmonary vessels leads to oedema and increased flow of low protein lymph from other areas. As in high-altitude oedema, the site of fluid transudation is unclear: the arterial vessels have been proposed, but without strong evidence. In favour of permeability change is the observation that the lymphatic fluid following experimental microembolization is of high protein content, even when the microemboli are pharmacologically inert glass microspheres.

Expansion pulmonary oedema

Pulmonary oedema after expansion of a collapsed lung is rare, but more likely when the lung (or lobe) has been collapsed for some time. The likelihood may be reduced by ensuring that negative pressure in the pleural space during re-expansion does not exceed 10 cmH2O, that the procedure is terminated if cough develops, and that not more than 1500 ml of fluid is aspirated at any one time when collapse is related to an effusion. The mechanism is uncertain. Permeability change is likely as high protein oedemas have been found in both clinical and experimental situations. The mechanism of damage may be from toxic oxygen free radicals, as in cardiac reperfusion injury. Additional contributing factors could be loss of surfactant during the period of collapse and increased negativity of interstitial pressure during re-expansion.

Postobstructive pulmonary oedema

The initiating event is a markedly negative intrapleural pressure generated by forceful inspiratory effort against an obstructed upper airway, which is then transmitted to the pulmonary interstitial space. During normal breathing, intrapleural pressures rarely fall below -5 cmH2O, but in upper airway obstruction the value may be as low as -50 cmH2O. Postobstructive oedema should therefore be suspected wherever there is the rapid onset of dyspnoea, cyanosis, frothy pink sputum production, and radiological pulmonary infiltrates after the rapid relief of upper airway obstruction. The onset is usually immediate but, occasionally, delays of up to 2 h have been reported. The chronic form occurs in patients with obstructive sleep apnoea, in whom negative intrapleural pressures as low as -100 cmH2O have been recorded.

Lymphatic oedema and lymphatic obstruction

Although, in one sense, all pulmonary oedema can be thought of as lymphatic failure, surprisingly little is known of pulmonary lymphatic failure in clinical practice. Lymphatic occlusion underlies the oedema and dyspnoea of lymphangitis carcinomatosa. In cases where cardiac failure and pneumoconioses coexist it has been found that oedema develops at lower capillary pressures than would be expected, and this has been attributed to lymphatic blockage. Mechanical lymphatic disruption is probably a contributing factor to the ease with which lungs develop oedema immediately after transplantation.

Disorders of capillary permeability

Many of the conditions associated with adult respiratory distress syndrome (see Chapter 16.5.1) can also be associated with less dramatic degrees of oedema. It is a good rule always to consider the possibility that a permeability abnormality might exist as an associated cause in all cases of pulmonary oedema. The history can be particularly helpful, particularly with regard to possible infections, use of drugs, and occupational chemicals. The possibility of oxygen toxicity should be borne in mind in all patients in intensive care.

Unilateral oedema

This frequently causes diagnostic confusion. Unilateral oedema on the same side as pre-existing lung abnormalities (ipsilateral oedema) may arise from posture (lying on one side during oedema development), increased perfusion of one lung secondary to a systemic to pulmonary shunt, unilateral venous occlusion (either from unilateral veno-occlusive disease or from extrinsic compression), or unilateral lymphatic pathology such as lymphangitis carcinomatosa. Contralateral oedema is seen where the pre-existing pathology protects that lung. Instances include congenital unilateral pulmonary artery, Swyer–James–McLeod syndrome, unilateral thromboembolism, and unilateral fibrosis causing unilateral hypoxia and vasoconstriction.

The diagnosis of pulmonary oedema

The diagnosis of pulmonary oedema is by clinical observation and chest radiography.

Clinical features

The characteristic symptom of pulmonary oedema is breathlessness, probably generated by an awareness of inappropriate respiratory effort and by firing of 'J' (juxta-alveolar) receptors. This dyspnoea comes on more or less acutely in the first instance, often following exercise. Later, paroxysmal nocturnal dyspnoea develops because of postural hydrostatic factors. Only then are signs of diminished breath sounds at the bases and fine lung crepitations found. The crepitations (crackles) characteristic of pulmonary oedema are intermittent explosive sounds that each last for less than 20 ms. They are probably caused by the sudden opening of a succession of small airways, the acoustic wave being produced either by equalization of downstream and upstream pressures or by sudden alterations in the tension of the airway walls. They thus relate to the 'all-or-none' features of alveolar flooding observed physiologically. The rhonchi (musical sounds) that are sometimes heard, and which may cause considerable diagnostic confusion in the dyspnoeic patient, can arise either from bronchiolar wall oedema or from vagally mediated reflex bronchospasm.

Pulmonary oedema is never a static condition, but always either developing or regressing. The observations of Altschule, who over 40 years ago recorded the sequence of events as a patient progressed into ever greater left heart failure, are worth recalling.

(1) *premonitory*: anxiety, pallor, tachycardia, raised blood pressure, cold sweaty skin;

(2) *interstitial oedema*: dyspnoea, orthopnoea, cyanosis, congested neck veins, wheezing and rales;

(3) *intra-alveolar oedema*: crackling rales progressing to general bubbling; cough, sputum—becoming frothy then blood-stained;

(4) *shock*: clouding of consciousness;

(5) *terminal*: cardiac and respiratory arrhythmias.

The clinical features of the non-haemodynamic oedemas are not dissimilar but are generally less florid.

Chest radiography

The chest radiograph is a sensitive and easily available tool for spotting early pulmonary oedema (Figs 6 and 7). The majority of radiographical studies have been made during cardiogenic oedema where changes of oedema are necessarily superimposed on other circulatory alterations. Three successive and overlapping phases can be identified.

Preoedema

This reflects cardiac and circulatory changes and the increased flow of fluid that occurs through the lymphatics before swelling of the tissue takes place. Usually, the cardiothoracic ratio on a posteroanterior film is more than 0.5

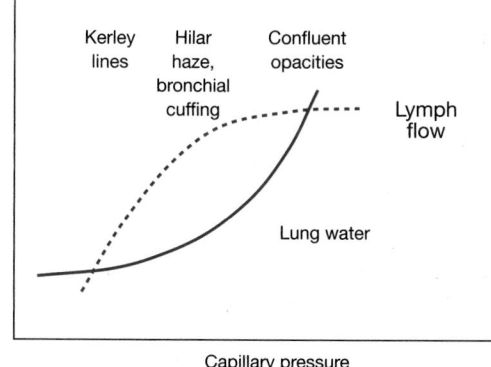

Fig. 6 Radiological signs and pulmonary pathophysiology. Kerley lines are a particularly useful radiological sign, as they occur at a stage where lymph flow and transinterstitial water flow have both increased but where appreciable tissue swelling has not yet appeared. (Reproduced from Prichard JS (1982). *Edema of the lung*. Charles C. Thomas, Springfield, Illinois, with permission.)

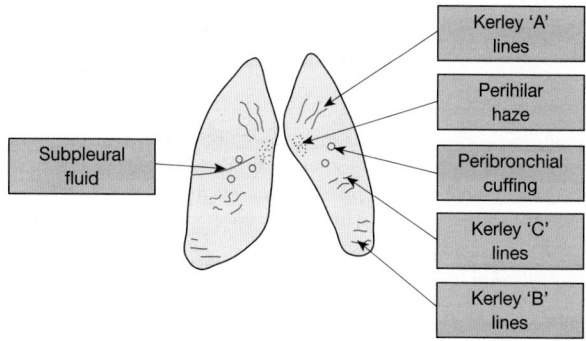

Fig. 7 Characteristic radiological appearances in interstitial oedema (see text). (Reproduced from Prichard JS (1982). *Edema of the lung*. Charles C. Thomas, Springfield, Illinois, with permission.)

(>0.57 for an anteroposterior film is standard when geometry is preserved). Distension and engorgement of blood vessels occur, particularly in the upper zone with inverse changes at the bases leading to reversal of the usual pattern. Distended lymphatics subsequently become identifiable as septal lines, perilobular lines, and rosettes. Septal lines were originally identified by Kerley: type A lines are ragged, unbranched, and run centripetally towards the hilum; type C lines are fine, interlacing, and seen most easily in the central and perihilar regions; type B lines are the best known and most commonly seen. They are short, sharp, horizontal, and found in the costophrenic angles. They occur most often in pulmonary oedema due to chronic pulmonary venous hypertension. Indeed, there is excellent correlation between the density of Kerley B lines and left atrial pressure in mitral stenosis. The lines are rarely seen below a mean left atrial pressure of 13.5 mmHg, are commonly found in the region of 22 mmHg, and are invariably present when the left atrial pressure exceeds 30 mmHg. Perilobular lines and rosettes are found on close inspection in about 3 per cent of radiographs and probably represent the lymphatics running around the respiratory acini.

Interstitial oedema

This first appears in areas of 'loose' connective tissue when wedge pressure begins to rise above 15 mmHg (see sequence of oedema accumulation, above). Visible interlobar and accessory lung fissures are the first manifestations. They are followed by perivascular and peribronchial cuffs, which contribute, respectively, to the homogeneous circular shadows formed by the already distended vessels and to the 'ring' shadows around bronchi seen close to the hilum. Micronoduli consist of small, round densities (<3 mm) arising from the accumulation of fluid around the smaller blood vessels. Blurring and hazing of the hilar regions represent the beginning of true alveolar septal interstitial oedema and, in hydrostatic oedema, begin at wedge pressures of around 20 mmHg. A diffuse increase in lung density (clouding) represents the final phase.

Alveolar oedema

This starts when wedge pressure reaches 25 to 28 mmHg. It is seen as a 'fluffy' loss of lucency, either around the hila in a 'butterfly' or 'batswing' pattern, or predominantly in the lower zones, usually reflecting a 'gravitational' distribution. Associated changes are the development of effusions and a loss of lung volume caused by a fall in lung compliance.

Radiologically, the permeability oedemas follow the pattern of the hydrostatic except that: (1) the distribution of alveolar oedema tends to be patchy; and (2) the characteristic vascular and cardiac changes are not present.

The presence of pre-existing lung disease—particularly chronic obstructive pulmonary disease—may modify the radiological appearance of pulmonary oedema considerably. Hyperinflation may render the silhouette of a large heart unremarkable; with the onset of interstitial oedema, a hyperinflated lung may shrink to normal size; the distribution of oedema shadowing may be patchy and only evident where parenchyma is sufficiently preserved; Kerley lines may be difficult or impossible to identify.

Other investigations

Computed tomography (**CT**) scanning is not necessary for the diagnosis of pulmonary oedema, but the appearances are characteristic, with thickening and increased visualization of interlobular septa and associated thickening of subpleural and peribronchial interstitial spaces. Alveolar oedema leads to varying degrees of alveolar consolidation. As in the plain radiograph, there may be associated heart and vascular changes and pleural effusions.

Pulmonary function in oedema of the lung

The oedematous lung shows a mixture of restrictive and obstructive defects, although the former dominate. The restrictive component arises from decreased compliance, which is a result of vascular congestion (in cardiogenic and fluid overload oedema), interstitial oedema, and surfactant washout. Of these, the interstitial oedema contributes surprisingly little, so that, to start with, restrictive changes are indicative of an engorged vascular system and later, of alveolar flooding.

Sometimes, airflow resistance may cause easily audible rhonchi and a reduction in forced expiratory volume in 1 s/forced vital capacity (**FEV1/FVC**), but, more usually, it is difficult to detect by simple methods because it occurs predominantly in the small airways of 1 to 2 mm diameter, which contribute relatively little to overall resistance. There could be a number of causes for such airflow obstruction. In the preoedematous phase of heart failure the smallest airways may be compressed by the distension of adjacent vessels in the bronchovascular bundle. In frank interstitial oedema it has been suggested that perivascular cuffing could do the same, but this has not been substantiated. However, submucosal oedema and vagally mediated reflex bronchoconstriction are proven and probably responsible for most of the effect. Restriction and obstruction may combine to reduce vital capacity, and serial measurements of this can be a good index of severity of and recovery from pulmonary oedema.

Tachypnoea is a prominent feature of all forms of pulmonary oedema. This is associated with a low tidal volume, but total ventilation (V_E)—both at rest and during exercise—is high relative to the prevailing level of carbon dioxide consumption. Most of this increase is accounted for by deadspace ventilation hence, unless the patient is progressing into severe alveolar oedema (see below), he or she remains normocapnic. The mechanism underlying this tachypnoea is uncertain. Hypoxic effects upon the central carbon dioxide chemostat do not appear to be an explanation, and recent evidence using perialveolar local anaesthetic suggests that the 'J' (juxta-alveolar) receptor—an unmyelinated nerve ending in the vicinity of the alveoli, which responds to interstitial swelling and distension—is only involved at more severe levels of oedema. Respiratory muscle fatigue is a possibility.

In acute, severe oedema the usual blood gas abnormalities are hypocapnia and hypoxia. The hypoxia is a result of ventilation/perfusion mismatching. The hypocapnia is accounted for by the reflex tachypnoea leading to an increased alveolar ventilation, which more than compensates for the increased pulmonary deadspace (volume of deadspace/volume of tidal air ratios, V_D/V_T ratio). However, in about 20 per cent of severe cases, hypercapnia (with respiratory acidosis) is seen, even when no chronic airflow disease coexists. A number of mechanisms have been proposed, including uncontrolled oxygen administration accompanied by low central carbon dioxide sensitivity, respiratory muscle fatigue, and severe ventilation perfusion imbalance. In acute oedema, blood gas abnormalities are usually accompanied by a mild metabolic acidosis, but occasionally the base excess may exceed −15 mmol/l. This frank metabolic acidosis is most likely in patients with severe oedema who already have carbon dioxide retention.

In the more chronic permeability oedemas—as in adult respiratory distress syndrome—the overwhelming problem is continuing severe hypox-

aemia. Three mechanisms have been proposed: (1) diffusion impairment; (2) low ventilation/perfusion₂ ($\dot{V}_A/\dot{Q}$) values; and (3) shunt ($\dot{V}_A/\dot{Q}$ <0.005). Using both the arterial oxygen response to changing fractional inspired oxygen concentration (**FiO2**) and the inert gas technique, it has been shown that diffusion impairment plays little part. Shunt and ventilation/perfusion mismatch are more important, but their contribution varies greatly from patient to patient.

Treatment of pulmonary oedema

Pulmonary oedema may result from increased microvascular hydrostatic pressure, decreased tissue interstitial pressure, decreased plasma colloid oncotic pressure, increased microvascular permeability, or impaired lymphatic drainage. Treatment of each form should include measures designed to reverse the specific cause. However, with the exception of a reduction of elevated hydrostatic pressure and relief of upper airway obstruction, these are rarely available and the clinician has to rely upon general supportive measures combined with meticulous attention to fluid balance and monitoring of plasma oncotic pressure. (See Chapters 16.1 and 16.5.2 for discussion of the clinical approach to the severely ill and breathless patient.)

Acute cardiogenic and fluid overload pulmonary oedema

By far the most common causes are acute and chronic left-sided heart disease, although the overenthusiastic use of intravenous fluid regimen containing normal saline are frequently an additional factor. The patient is most comfortable in the 'trunk up, legs down' position to help pool blood in the dependent parts and reduce central venous pressure. Oxygen, diuretics, intravenous nitrates, and morphine are the fundamentals of treatment. Thigh cuffs inflated to occlude venous return can help as a form of a bloodless phlebotomy and venesection, and removal of 200 to 500 ml of blood is an effective treatment when other measures are not available.

Hypoxia is relieved with a standard face mask, nasal prongs, or reservoir bag, delivering oxygen at high flow rates—up to 10 litres/min—providing an inspired concentration of up to 60 per cent. The fractional inspired oxygen concentration given should be as high as is necessary to keep the arterial partial pressure of oxygen near to the normal level—and no more—because, in permeability oedema: (1) high oxygen levels may lead to absorption atelectasis in areas of low ventilation/perfusion; (2) oxygen toxicity may become a problem where prolonged administration is necessary. If oxygen administration at normal airway pressure cannot maintain the arterial partial pressure of oxygen and/or hypercapnia develops, then application of a continuous positive airway pressure (**CPAP**) mask, non-invasive ventilation, or tracheal intubation and intermittent positive pressure ventilation will need to be considered (see Chapter 16.5.2).

A bolus dose of furosemide (frusemide) (or other loop diuretic), administered intravenously, is usually given. This acts both as a venous dilator, and as a diuretic. Diuretics are at their most valuable where pulmonary oedema is a component of congestive cardiac failure and where the volume of extracellular fluid is generally increased. By contrast, when left ventricular failure has come on acutely, significant fluid retention has not occurred and pulmonary oedema is a result of fluid shift from the systemic circulation, then overvigorous use of diuretics runs the risk of causing hypovolaemia. If the patient is *in extremis* or heavily sedated, it is wise to catheterize the bladder for, as a result of the diuresis, bladder distension may induce intense reflex systemic vasoconstriction leading, on occasion, to disastrous cardiac overload.

Intravenous nitrates, in particular isosorbide dinitrate at a dose between 2 and 20 mg/h, can effectively reduce venous pressure and alleviate pulmonary oedema. Arterial hypotension is the effect that usually limits dosage, the combination of heart failure with low blood pressure and pulmonary oedema being difficult to treat and of grave prognosis (see Chapter 16.2).

Morphine acts centrally to relieve the distress of dyspnoea and also dilates the systemic venous system. This reduces venous filling pressure to the heart and shifts blood from the pulmonary to the systemic circulation. It is best administered by slow intravenous injection in a total dose of 2 to 10 mg at a rate of 2 mg/min, together with an appropriate antiemetic.

Aminophylline has diuretic, bronchodilator, cardiac inotropic, and respiratory muscle inotropic effects. Its use would seem logical, but it is now scarcely ever given because of its capacity to induce arrhythmias and the availability of other effective treatments. If it is to be administered, a dose of 250 to 500 mg should be given intravenously in not less than 20 min.

Other types of pulmonary oedema

A reduction in oncotic pressure may contribute to pulmonary oedema, as in crystalloid fluid overload, hepatic failure, or nephrotic syndrome. In fluid overload, the most appropriate therapy is the use of diuretics, for these not only reduce the extracellular and blood volumes but also return osmotic pressure towards normal. It is more difficult to be certain about therapy in true hypo-oncotic states. Even where there is no evidence of endothelial damage, the effects of salt-free albumin and plasma concentrate are disappointing.

In high-permeability pulmonary oedema the best form of management would be to block the inappropriate activation and progress of the cascades that are responsible for the condition (see Chapter 16.5.1). Unfortunately, there is no therapy that allows this at present and management, aside from aiming to treat any precipitating disorder, is supportive (see Chapter 16.5.2).

Further reading

Anonymous (1986). Adult respiratory distress syndrome. *Lancet* **i**, 301–3.

Anonymous (1986). The enigma of breathlessness. *Lancet* **i**, 891–2.

Artigas A, *et al.* (1992). *The adult respiratory distress syndrome.* Churchill Livingstone, Edinburgh.

Egan EA (1983). Fluid balance in the air filled alveolar space. *American Review of Respiratory Disease* **127**, 37–9.

Guyton AO, Lindsey AW (1959). Effect of elevated left atrial pressure and decreased plasma protein concentration upon the development of pulmonary oedema. *Circulation Research* **7**, 649.

Kreiger BP, de la Hoz RE (1999). Altitude related pulmonary disorders. *Critical Care Clinics* **15**, 265–80.

Morgan PW, Goodman LR (1991). Imaging of diffuse lung diseases: pulmonary oedema and adult respiratory distress syndrome. *Radiologic Clinics of North America* **29**, 943–63.

O'Brodovich H (1990). When the alveolus is flooding, it is time to man the pumps. *American Review of Respiratory Disease* **142**, 1247–8.

Pang D, *et al.* (1998). The effects of positive pressure airway support on mortality and the need for intubation in cardiogenic pulmonary oedema: a systematic review. *Chest* **114**, 1185–92

Prichard JS (1982). *Edema of the lung.* Charles C. Thomas, Springfield, IL.

Sacchetti AD, Harris RH (1998). Acute cardiogenic pulmonary edema. What's the latest in emergency treatment? *Postgraduate Medicine* **103**, 145–7, 153–4, 160–2.

Simon RD (1993). Neurogenic pulmonary edema. *Neurologic Clinics* **11**, 309–23.

Szidon PS (1989). Pathophysiology of the congested lung. *Cardiology Clinics* **7**, 39–48.

Trimby J, *et al.* (1990). Mechanical causes of pulmonary oedema. *Chest* **98**, 973–9.

Veeraraghavan S, Koss MN, Sharma OP (1999). Pulmonary veno-occlusive disease. *Current Opinion in Pulmonary Medicine* **5**, 310–13.

Wiedemann HP, Matthay MA, eds (2000). Adult respiratory distress syndrome. *Clinics in Chest Medicine* **21**, 401–620.

15.15.3 Venous thromboembolism

15.15.3.1 Deep venous thrombosis and pulmonary embolism

Paul D. Stein and J. Firth

Introduction

Pulmonary embolism is a complication of deep venous thrombosis. Among patients with pulmonary embolism, the thrombi in 80 per cent or more originate in the legs. Deep venous thrombosis and pulmonary embolism are sometimes described together, using the term 'thromboembolism'. Strategies of management have been developed which are based on the diagnosis of either pulmonary embolism or deep venous thrombosis, provided the patient has good respiratory reserve. Treatment with anticoagulants is the same for both. Some believe, however, that patients can be managed better if it is known whether acute pulmonary embolism is present, even if a diagnosis of deep venous thrombosis is already established.

Mortality of untreated deep venous thrombosis and pulmonary embolism

The frequency of fatal pulmonary embolism in patients with untreated deep venous thrombosis has diminished as diagnostic tests have made it possible to diagnose deep venous thrombosis before it becomes extensive. In 1955, prior to the use of sensitive non-invasive tests for the early detection of deep venous thrombosis, the risk of fatal pulmonary embolism in untreated patients with clinically apparent deep venous thrombosis was 37 per cent. With the use of radioactive fibrinogen scintiscans, the risk of fatal pulmonary embolism in patients with untreated deep venous thrombosis, most of which was subclinical, was approximately 5 per cent.

Early diagnosis has also reduced the risk of death in those with pulmonary embolism. In the early 1960s, the mortality in untreated patients with acute pulmonary embolism, diagnosed on the basis of clinical features, was 26 to 37 per cent. An additional 36 per cent died of recurrent pulmonary embolism. In recent years, among patients with mild pulmonary embolism who inadvertently escaped treatment, the mortality was 5 per cent. The mortality of untreated patients with mild pulmonary embolism was comparable with the mortality from fatal pulmonary embolism in untreated patients with subtle deep venous thrombosis.

Deep venous thrombosis

Incidence and pathology

Deep venous thrombosis is often silent. In one study of those with deep venous thrombosis detected by screening with ^{125}I-labelled fibrinogen scans, clinical evidence was present in 49 per cent. The percentage of patients with acute pulmonary embolism who have clinically detectable deep venous thrombosis decreases with decreasing severity of pulmonary embolism, which implies more subtle disease. Of patients who died from acute pulmonary embolism, 53 per cent had clinically identified deep venous thrombosis. In patients with massive or submassive acute pulmonary embolism, most of whom survived, 34 per cent had clinically identifiable deep venous thrombosis. Among patients with mild as well as severe acute pulmonary embolism, only 15 per cent had clinically apparent deep venous thrombosis.

Proximal deep venous thrombosis was found at autopsy in 22 per cent of patients who died in a tertiary care hospital. Thrombosis of the leg veins usually occurs without inflammation. Inflammation of the walls of the veins, when it occurs, is usually secondary to the thrombus. No clear evidence indicates that inflammation of the veins prevents embolization, or that embolization is more frequent in those patients with thrombi not associated with venous inflammation.

In the past, patients who had thrombosed leg veins accompanied by signs of inflammation were diagnosed as having thrombophlebitis, based on the presumption that the primary event was inflammation of the walls of the veins. Patients with no clinical signs in the lower extremities who had thrombosis that resulted in pulmonary embolism were said to have phlebothrombosis. Histological investigations have not supported a distinction between the clinical diagnoses of thrombophlebitis and phlebothrombosis. Thrombus can induce inflammation in the underlying wall of the vein, and this inflammation in some patients is extensive enough to produce pain, tenderness, swelling, and fever.

The valve pockets are a frequent site of origin of thrombi. At autopsy, clinically unsuspected deep venous thrombosis is often extensive, causing collateral circulation around occlusions and dilatation of collateral veins. When the veins of the thigh and the calf are thrombosed in continuity, the thrombi in the calf are older than those in the thigh, which suggests that the thrombosis extended from the veins of the calves to the veins of the thighs.

Clinical diagnosis

Patients may complain of pain or swelling of the leg, but physical examination remains the means by which attention is usually drawn to the potential diagnosis of deep venous thrombosis.

Deep venous thrombosis sometimes, but not always, leads to swelling of the leg. If restricted to the popliteal and calf veins, swelling is confined to below the knee, but if thrombosis involves the femoral and pelvic veins (or inferior vena cava), then swelling of the thigh is also expected. A difference of circumference of the calves of greater than 1 cm, measured 10 cm below the tibial tuberosity, is abnormal. It is important to repeat the measurement of diameter of the calves and thighs at frequent intervals: proximal extension of a thrombus is likely to cause increased swelling. To allow repeated measurements to be made from a fixed point, it is good practice for the position of the first measurement to be marked indelibly on the patient's skin.

Homans' sign is positive when active and/or passive dorsiflexion of the foot is associated with any of the following: (i) pain, (ii) incomplete dorsiflexion (with equal pressure applied) to prevent pain, or (iii) flexion of the knee to release tension in the posterior muscles with dorsiflexion. This sign was present in 44 per cent of patients with deep venous thrombosis of the lower leg, and in 60 per cent of patients with femoral venous thrombosis. The elicitation of pain with inflation of a blood pressure cuff around the calf to 60 to 150 mmHg has been recommended as a test for deep venous thrombosis. This test, however, has not been shown to be more helpful than the assessment of direct tenderness or leg circumference.

In one study the sensitivity of oedema, erythema, calf tenderness, palpable cord, or Homans' sign alone, or greater than 1 cm calf asymmetry alone was 55 to 80 per cent, but the specificity only 49 per cent. The combination of one of these signs plus greater than 1 cm ipsilateral calf asymmetry increased the specificity to 87 per cent, but decreased the sensitivity to 15 to 33 per cent. The specificity increased to 91 per cent with one of these signs in combination with greater than 2 cm calf asymmetry. Only 3 to 10 per cent of patients had one or more qualitative signs plus greater than 3 cm ipsilateral calf asymmetry: in these, the specificity for deep venous thrombosis was 96 per cent.

Other clinical features of deep venous thrombosis, whose sensitivity and specificity have not been tested, include increased temperature on the affected side, cyanotic discoloration of the limb, and persistent engorgement of superficial veins. Superficial varicose veins almost always empty when the patient lies down: if they remain engorged, this suggests problems with drainage through the deep veins. In very rare cases, tense venous oedema can cause arterial compression and venous gangrene.

The clinical diagnosis of deep venous thrombosis is not always straightforward. Many of the findings described above can also be found in those with muscular strains and bruising, ruptured Baker's cyst or plantaris tendon, superficial thrombophlebitis, cellulitis, and other traumatic conditions. Given the sinister nature of untreated deep venous thrombosis, it is important to confirm or refute (so far as is possible) the diagnosis with appropriate investigations whenever clinical suspicion is aroused, unless the general condition of the patient makes this inappropriate.

Investigation

Detection of the physical presence of thrombus in leg veins

The 'gold standard' is contrast venography, but this can be unpleasant for patients, time consuming for radiology departments, and is expensive. This has driven the search for acceptable non-invasive methods of diagnosis. Among patients with deep venous thrombosis proven by contrast venography, B-mode ultrasonography using compression showed a 95 per cent sensitivity in symptomatic patients. In asymptomatic patients who were evaluated because of a high risk of deep venous thrombosis, venous compression ultrasound showed a sensitivity of only 67 per cent. Regarding veins of the calves, venous compression ultrasound was 93 per cent sensitive in symptomatic patients, but only 26 per cent sensitive in asymptomatic high-risk patients with deep venous thrombosis. In all instances, specificity was 97 to 99 per cent. Impedance plethysmography was 86 to 94 per cent sensitive for detection of deep venous thrombosis of the thighs, but the sensitivity was only 25 per cent for the veins of the calves. Specificity was high, 97 per cent. In most centres contrast venography and impedance plethysmography have been replaced by B-mode ultrasonography as the preferred first-line diagnostic technique.

Venous phase contrast enhanced spiral computed tomography (CT) appears promising for imaging the veins of the pelvis and thighs. Spiral CT imaging of the veins of the lower extremities and pelvis in combination with spiral CT imaging of the chest potentially offers a comprehensive study for thromboembolism. The sensitivity and specificity of contrast enhanced spiral CT, however, are still being evaluated.

Magnetic resonance imaging, tested in small numbers of patients, was 100 per cent sensitive for veins of the thighs and pelvis and somewhat less sensitive (85 per cent) for veins of the calves. Specificity in all regions was 95 to 100 per cent. Its problem is cost and availability.

Fibrinogen-uptake radionuclide scanning was used extensively in the 1960s. It is more sensitive for deep venous thrombosis in the calves than in the thighs. In view of the greater risk of pulmonary embolism with deep venous thrombosis of the thighs than of the calves, the value of fibrinogen-uptake scanning is limited.

Lately, technetium apcitide labelling of glycoprotein IIb/IIIa receptors expressed on activated platelets has permitted radionuclear imaging of acute proximal deep venous thrombosis and pelvic vein thrombosis. Its sensitivity has been incompletely evaluated.

Detection of evidence of thrombus within the circulation: D-dimer

D-Dimer is a specific degradation product released into the circulation by endogenous fibrinolysis of a cross-linked fibrin clot. A D-dimer measured by enzyme-linked immunosorbent assay (ELISA) below a cut-off of 300 to 540 ng/ml (the values differ slightly from one study to another) make the diagnosis of deep venous thrombosis (or pulmonary embolism) unlikely. A concentration of D-dimer above any particular cut-off level is not useful for making a positive diagnosis because of the large number of false positive tests. However, conventional ELISA assays are cumbersome and not suited for emergency use, which limited the practical utility of D-dimer measurements until the development of rapid ELISA assays. These provide the best balance of sensitivity and specificity among the various assays for the safe diagnostic handling of patients with suspected deep venous thrombosis and pulmonary embolism.

Strategy for diagnosis

For reasons given above, subjecting all patients who might have a deep venous thrombosis to contrast venography is not an attractive option for patients, physicians, radiologists or those who pay for health care. Much effort has therefore been expended in trying to develop management algorithms that will identify those at very low risk of deep venous thrombosis (or pulmonary embolism), who can then be spared invasive tests. These algorithms typically use scoring systems to stratify the clinical probability that the particular patient has a deep venous thrombosis (or pulmonary embolus), and then proceed to D-dimer testing of those with low probability. Patients with a low clinical probability and a negative D-dimer test are not investigated further. Patients with either a high clinical probability or a low clinical probability but elevated D-dimer proceed to tests for the presence of thrombus in the leg veins, typically by ultrasonography. Examples of a pre-test scoring system and management algorithm are shown in Table 1.

Prevention, treatment, and complications of deep venous thrombosis

The prevention of deep venous thrombosis is critical in the prevention of pulmonary embolism. Deep venous thrombosis itself carries extensive morbidity irrespective of pulmonary embolism. Severe postphlebitic syndrome (venous ulcer or combinations of pain, cramps, heaviness, pruritus, paraesthesia, pretibial oedema, induration, hyperpigmentation, venous ectasia, redness or pain with calf compression) occurs in 9 per cent of patients by 5 years after a 3-month course of treatment with anticoagulants. There is some evidence that the likelihood of this problem developing can be reduced by use of elastic stockings at the time of acute deep venous thrombosis and afterwards.

Proximal deep venous thrombosis leads to pulmonary embolism more frequently than deep venous thrombosis confined to the calf. Even so, symptomatic isolated calf vein thrombosis, limited to the calves and diagnosed by non-invasive testing, should be treated with anticoagulation for 3 months. If anticoagulation cannot be given, serial non-invasive studies of the leg veins should be performed over the next 7 to 14 days to assess for proximal extension of the thrombus.

Risk factors for deep venous thrombosis are almost certainly the same as those for pulmonary embolism (see later). Recommendations for the prevention of deep venous thrombosis are shown in Tables 2, 3, 4, and 5, and for treatment in Table 6.

Acute pulmonary embolism

Incidence

Acute pulmonary embolism is the third most common cardiovascular problem after coronary heart disease and stroke. The incidence of objectively diagnosed acute pulmonary embolism in a tertiary care hospital is probably higher than in most short-stay hospitals, but in one such centre a

Table 1 Pre-test clinical probability scoring system and care pathway for the patient with suspected deep venous thrombosis

(a) Pre-test probability score

Criteria	Score
Active cancer	+1
Paralysis, plaster cast	+1
Bed rest >3 days, surgery within 4 weeks	+1
Tenderness along veins	+1
Entire leg swollen	+1
Calf swollen >3 cm	+1
Pitting oedema	+1
Collateral veins	+1
Alternative diagnosis likely	-2

(b) Pre-test probability

Low	0
Moderate	1 or 2
High	3 or more

(c) Management algorithm

Pre-test probability score	Action	Result	Further action
0 or 1	Perform D-dimer	Negative	No further investigation
		Positive	Perform ultrasonography
2 or more	Do not perform D-dimer		
	Perform ultrasonography	Negative	Withhold treatment and repeat ultrasonography in 10–14 days. If serial ultrasonography is negative, pulmonary embolism rarely occurs.
		Positive	Diagnosis of venous thrombosis established

Notes

1 .Pre-test probability score from Wells et al. (1997).

2 .This management algorithm is typical of many used, but further prospective evaluation is warranted.

3 .If the physician's judgement is that deep venous thrombosis is very likely in a particular case, then they should proceed to investigations directed at detecting thrombus in leg veins whatever the scoring algorithm would suggest. If the result of ultrasonography is negative, and repeat ultrasonography in 10–14 days is also negative, pulmonary embolism rarely occurs.

4 .All patients who are discharged with 'deep venous thrombosis excluded' should be given written information describing how they can be reassessed if symptoms worsen or fail to settle over the next few days.

definitive diagnosis of pulmonary embolism was made in 0.3 to 0.4 per cent of patients. Inclusion of extrapolated data from autopsy studies and the estimated frequency of pulmonary embolism in patients with non-high probability lung scans increases the calculated incidence of acute pulmonary embolism to 1.0 per cent of patients admitted to hospital. Silent pulmonary embolism was not included in these calculations, and this has been reported in 38 to 51 per cent of patients with deep venous thrombosis.

In one major study, the incidence of acute pulmonary embolism was linearly related to age: more than half of patients were between 65 and 85 years of age, while fewer than 5 per cent were under age 24. Occasionally, however, young adults or adolescents had pulmonary embolism. In patients 50 years of age or older, the incidence of pulmonary embolism was higher among women. By contrast, the incidence was comparable in men and women under age 50 years, suggesting that childbirth and oral contraceptives had little impact.

In autopsy studies, when the pathologist judged that pulmonary embolism contributed to death or caused death, the diagnosis was unsuspected ante-mortem in 70 per cent. This was true in several series, encompassing university as well as non-university hospitals. Some of the unsuspected pulmonary embolism was in patients who died of malignancy, in whom a

diagnosis of pulmonary embolism may (appropriately) not have been actively pursued. But the time-honoured point remains as valid today as ever: a high index of suspicion is necessary to reduce the number of patients with unsuspected pulmonary embolism.

Table 2 Recommendations for prevention of deep venous thrombosis in patients undergoing general surgery

Indication	Recommendations
Low-risk general surgery patients	No specific prophylaxis other than early ambulation
• Undergoing minor procedures, <40 years of age, and with no additional risk factors	
Moderate-risk general surgery patients	LDUH, LMWH, ES, or IPC
• Undergoing minor procedures, but with additional thrombosis risk factors	
• Undergoing non-major surgery, between 40 and 60 years, no additional risk factors	
• Undergoing major operations, <40 years, no addtional clinical risk factors	
Higher-risk general surgery patients	LDUH, LMWH, or IPC
• Undergoing non-major surgery, >60 years or with additional risk factors	
• Undergoing major surgery, >60 years or with additional risk factors	
Higher-risk general surgery patients (see above) with a greater than usual risk of bleeding	Mechanical prophylaxis with IPC and ES at least initially
Very high-risk general surgery patients with multiple risk factors	LDUH or LMWH combined with IPC and ES
Selected very high-risk general surgery patients	Consider perioperative warfarin (INR 2.0–3.0) or postdischarge LMWH

DVT, deep venous thrombosis; ES, elastic stockings; INR, international normalized ratio; IPC, intermittent pneumatic compression; LDUH, low-dose unfractionated heparin; LMWH, low-molecular-weight heparin.
Adapted from Geerts et al. (2001). Further details of prophylactic anticoagulation regimes can be found in Chapter 15.15.3.2.

Table 3 Recommendations for prevention of deep venous thrombosis in patients undergoing major orthopaedic surgery

Indication	Recommendations
Elective hip replacement	Either SC LMWH therapy (started 12 h before surgery, 12–24 h after surgery, or 4–6 h after surgery at half the usual high-risk dose and then continuing with the usual high-risk dose the following day), or adjusted-dose warfarin (INR target = 2.5; range 2.0–3.0; started preoperatively or immediately after surgery) Adjusted dose heparin therapy (started preoperatively) is an acceptable but more complex alternative ES or IPC may provide additional efficacy (Not recommended: other agents, such as LDUH, aspirin, dextran, and IPC alone. These may reduce the overall incidence of VTE, but are less effective than the options outlined above.)
Elective knee replacement	LMWH or adjusted-dose warfarin IPC is an alternative option (Not recommended: LDUH)
Hip fracture surgery	LMWH or adjusted-dose warfarin LDUH is a possible alternative, but only limited data are available (Not recommended: aspirin alone, which is less efficacious than other approaches)
Other issues	The optimal duration of anticoagulant prophylaxis after THR or TKR surgery is uncertain, although at least 7-10 days is recommended Extended out-of-hospital LMWH prophylaxis (beyond 7–10 days after surgery) may reduce the incidence of clinically important thromboembolic events; this approach is recommended at least for high-risk patients (Not recommended: routine duplex ultrasonography screening at the time of hospital discharge or during outpatient follow-up in asymptomatic THR or TKR patients

DVT, deep venous thrombosis; ES, elastic stockings; INR, international normalized ratio; IPC, intermittent pneumatic compression; LDUH, low-dose unfractionated heparin; LMWH, low-molecular-weight heparin; SC, subcutaneous; THR, total hip replacement; TKR, total knee replacement; VTE, venous thromboembolism.
Tables 2,3, and 4 adapted from Geerts et al. (2001). Further details of prophylactic anticoagulation regimes can be found in Chapter 15.15.3.2.

Table 4 Recommendations for prevention of deep venous thrombosis in patients following neurosurgery

Indication	Recommendations
Patients undergoing intracranial neurosurgery	IPC with or without ES LDUH or postoperative LMWH are acceptable alternatives The combination of ES or IPC and LMWH or LDUH may be more effective than either modality alone

ES, elastic stockings; IPC, intermittent pneumatic compression; LDUH, low-dose unfractionated heparin; LMWH, low-molecular-weight heparin.

Table 5 Recommendations for prevention of deep venous thrombosis in medical patients

Indication	Recommendations
Acute myocardial infarction	Prophylactic or therapeutic anticoagulant therapy with SC, LDUH, or IV heparin in most patients
Ischaemic stroke with impaired mobility	LDUH, LMWH, or the heparinoid danaparoid If anticoagulant prophylaxis is contraindicated ES or IPC
Risk factors for VTE, e.g. cancer, bed rest, heart failure, severe lung disease	LDUH or LMWH

ES, elastic stockings; IPC, intermittent pneumatic compression; LDUH, low-dose unfractionated heparin; LMWH, low-molecular-weight heparin; VTE, venous thromboembolism.

Adapted from Geerts *et al.* (2001). Further details of prophylactic anticoagulation regimes can be found in Chapter 15.15.3.2.

Table 6 Recommendations for the treatment of deep venous thrombosis and/or pulmonary thromboembolism

1. Patients with deep vein thrombosis or pulmonary embolism should be treated with (i) intravenous or subcutaneous heparin sufficient to prolong the activated partial thromboplastin time to a range that corresponds to a plasma heparin level of 0.2 to 0.4 IU/ml by protein sulphate assay or 0.3 to 0.6 IU/ml by an amidolytic anti-Xa assay, or (ii) an appropriate dose of low-molecular-weight heparin.

2. Heparin or low-molecular-weight heparin and warfarin therapy can be started together. Among patients with deep venous thrombosis or stable submassive pulmonary embolism, heparin can be discontinued on day 5 or 6 if the INR has been therapeutic for 2 consecutive days. Among patients with massive pulmonary embolism or iliofemoral thrombosis, a longer period of heparin or low-molecular-weight heparin therapy of approximately 10 days may be considered.

In comparison to unfractionated heparin, LMW heparin offers the major benefits of convenient dosing and facilitation of outpatient treatment. LMW heparin treatment may result in slightly less recurrent VTE and may offer a survival benefit in patients with cancer. LMW heparin is recommended over unfractionated heparin.

3. Therapy should be continued for at least 3 months using oral anticoagulants to prolong the prothrombin time to an INR of 2.0 to 3.0. Unfractionated heparin should be administered in doses sufficient to prolong the activated partial thromboplastin time to a range that corresponds to a heparin level of 0.2 or 0.4 IU/ml by protamine sulphate assay. Low-molecular-weight heparin may be used when oral anticoagulants are either contraindicated (as in pregnancy) or inconvenient.

4. Patients with reversible or time-limited risk factors should be treated for at least 3 months. Patients with a first episode of idiopathic deep venous thrombosis should be treated for at least 6 months.

5. Patients with recurrent idiopathic venous thrombosis or a continuing risk factor should be treated for 12 months or longer.

6. Symptomatic isolated calf vein thrombosis should be treated with anticoagulation for 6 to 12 weeks. If for any reason anticoagulation cannot be given, serial non-invasive studies of the lower extremity should be performed over the next 10 to 14 days to assess for proximal extension of the thrombus.

Table 7 Predisposing factors for pulmonary embolism in all patients irrespective of previous cardiac or pulmonary disease (*n* = 383)

	Pulmonary embolism (%)
Immobilization	54
Surgery	42
Lung disease	27
Malignancy	18
Coronary heart disease	20
Thrombophlebitis—ever	19
Myocardial infarction	13
Trauma—lower extremities	12
Heart failure	12
Chronic obstructive pulmonary disease	10
Stroke	10
Asthma	7
Pneumonia—acute	7
Prior pulmonary embolism	6
Oestrogen	6
Collagen vascular disease	4
Postpartum—3 months or less	2
Interstitial lung disease	2

Unpublished data from PIOPED in Stein (1996), *Pulmonary embolism.*

Predisposing factors

Immobilization, irrespective of the cause, is the most frequent predisposing factor (Table 7). Immobilization of even 1 or 2 days may predispose to pulmonary embolism and most patients with pulmonary embolism are immobilized for less than 2 weeks.

Whether obesity is a predisposing factor is controversial. Most patients with pulmonary embolism had smoked at one time or continued to smoke at the time of their pulmonary embolism.

Thromboembolic events have been linked to high oestrogen content in oral contraceptives (greater than 50 μg), but this association has been questioned. Irrespective of whether the risk ratio is increased among women who take oral contraceptives, the absolute risk of venous thromboembolism is low. The United States Food and Drug Administration (**FDA**) in 1980 recommended the use of the lowest possible dose of oestrogen for birth control. Childbearing and oral contraceptives did not result in a higher incidence of pulmonary embolism among women under 50 years of age compared with men. The combination of surgery and oral contraceptives may increase the risk of thromboembolism. This is true even with oral contraceptives that have a low oestrogen content. For further discussion of these and other risks associated with oestrogen use, see Chapter 13.19 and 13.20.

There has been much recent interest in the subject of genetic predisposition to thromboembolism. Heterozygosity for the Factor V Leiden mutation increases susceptibility three- to eightfold in a variety of circumstances. Other genetic and acquired thrombophilic factors include protein C deficiency, protein S deficiency, antithrombin deficiency, prothrombin 20201A, high concentration of factor VIII, hyperhomocystinaemia, heparin cofactor II deficiency, dysfibrinogenaemia, decreased levels of plasminogen, decreased levels of plasminogen activators, antiphospholipid antibodies, heparin-induced thrombocytopenia, and myeloproliferative disorders. For full discussion of this and related issues, see Chapter 15.15.3.2.

Patients with the nephrotic syndrome are known to be at particularly high risk of deep venous thrombosis and pulmonary embolism.

Syndromes of acute pulmonary embolism

Pulmonary embolism can present in diverse ways. The syndrome of pleuritic pain or haemoptysis, in the absence of circulatory collapse, is the most frequent mode of presentation of acute pulmonary embolism. It occurred in 60 per cent of patients recruited in a collaborative investigation, the Prospective Investigation of Pulmonary Embolism Diagnosis (**PIOPED**). A syndrome of dyspnoea in the absence of haemoptysis or pleuritic pain or circulatory collapse occurred in 25 per cent. Circulatory collapse (systolic blood pressure less than 80 mmHg or loss of consciousness) was an uncommon mode of presentation, occurring in 15 per cent. Recognizing that patients with circulatory collapse may not be candidates for recruitment into trials of diagnostic investigations or therapies, and patients with circulatory collapse often die within the first few hours, it may be that the incidence of circulatory collapse as determined from such investigations is falsely low. Patients with pulmonary infarction have less severe pulmonary embolism than those with isolated dyspnoea, and those with circulatory collapse probably have the most severe of all. The clinical characteristics of patients with acute pulmonary embolism often reflect the severity of the syndrome.

Symptoms of acute pulmonary embolism

The clinical characteristics of acute pulmonary embolism have been derived from prospectively acquired data of patients recruited in trials of diagnostic investigations or therapies. Such trials clearly only include those in whom there was sufficient clinical suspicion to lead physicians to obtain diagnostic tests: whether subtle pulmonary embolism was overlooked is undetermined. The specificity of signs, symptoms, and ordinary clinical tests, among patients with suspected pulmonary embolism in whom the diagnosis was eventually excluded by pulmonary angiography, was low. The specificity of such tests when evaluated in a normal population, however, would be higher.

To characterize the diagnostic features of acute pulmonary embolism, it is useful to evaluate patients in whom the diagnosis is not confused by preexisting cardiac or pulmonary disease. When manifestations related to coexistent disease are excluded, dyspnoea is the most common symptom, occurring in 73 per cent (Table 8). Pleuritic chest pain (66 per cent of patients with pulmonary embolism) occurred much more often than haemoptysis (13 per cent of patients with pulmonary embolism).

Cough was common (37 per cent) among patients with pulmonary embolism and could be non-productive, or productive of purulent or bloody sputum. When haemoptysis occurred, the sputum typically was blood-streaked, but can be pure blood or blood-tinged. Purulent sputum was present in 7 per cent of cases.

The angina-like pain that occurred in a few (4 per cent) patients with pulmonary embolism did not radiate to either arm or to the jaw, which can assist in distinguishing it from true angina. It was usually located in the anterior chest and it was described as heavy.

Signs of acute pulmonary embolism

Tachypnoea (respiratory rate 20/min or greater) was the most common sign of acute pulmonary embolism among patients with no prior cardiac or pulmonary disease (70 per cent of patients) (Table 9). Tachycardia (heart rate greater than 100/min) occurred in 30 per cent; the pulmonary com

Table 8 Symptoms of acute pulmonary embolism in patients with no pre-existing cardiac or pulmonary disease (*n* = 117)

	Patients with symptom (%)
Dyspnoea	73
Pleuritic pain	66
Cough	37
Leg swelling	28
Leg pain	26
Haemoptysis	13
Palpitations	10
Wheezing	9
Angina-like pain	4

Data are modified from Stein *et al.* (1991) *Chest* and are reproduced with permission.

Table 9 Signs of acute pulmonary embolism in patients with no pre-existing cardiac or pulmonary disease (*n* = 117)

	Patients with sign (%)
Tachypnoea (≥ 2 0 /min)	70
Rales (crackles)	51
Tachycardia (> 100/min)	30
Fourth heart sound	24
Increased pulmonary component of second sound	23
Deep venous thrombosis	11
Diaphoresis	11
Temperature > 38.5°C	7
Wheezes	5
Homans' sign	4
Right ventricular lift	4
Pleural friction rub	3
Third heart sound	3
Cyanosis	1

Data are modified from Stein *et al.* (1991) *Chest* and are reproduced with permission.

ponent of the second sound was accentuated in 23 per cent; and deep venous thrombosis was clinically apparent in 11 per cent. A right ventricular lift, third heart sound, or pleural friction rub were uncommon, each occurring in 4 per cent or less of patients with pulmonary embolism.

Most patients with pulmonary embolism who had rales (crepitations) had pulmonary parenchymal abnormalities, atelectasis, or a pleural effusion on the chest radiograph. Rales, therefore, appeared to relate to the effects of pulmonary infarction or atelectasis.

Among patients with pulmonary embolism and no other source of fever, a temperature below 39.9°C was present in 12 per cent and fever of 39.9°C or higher occurred in 2 per cent. Fever in patients with pulmonary haemorrhage/infarction was not more frequent than among those with no pulmonary haemorrhage/infarction. Clinical evidence of deep venous thrombosis was often present in patients with pulmonary embolism and otherwise unexplained fever.

Combinations of signs and symptoms

Dyspnoea or tachypnoea (respiratory rate 20/min or greater) were present in 90 per cent of patients with acute pulmonary embolism. Dyspnoea or tachypnoea or pleuritic pain were present in 97 per cent. Dyspnoea or tachypnoea, pleuritic pain, radiographic evidence of atelectasis, or a parenchymal abnormality were present in 98 per cent of patients. The remaining 2 per cent had either deep venous thrombosis or an unexplained low Pao_2. In the absence of dyspnoea or tachypnoea or pleuritic pain, pulmonary embolism was rarely diagnosed.

Accuracy of clinical assessment

To emphasize the point that the diagnosis of pulmonary embolism is difficult to make, senior staff physicians and postgraduate fellows taking part in the PIOPED study were uncertain of the diagnosis in the majority of patients. Using individual clinical judgement without any specific predetermined criteria, senior staff were correct in the diagnosis in 88 per cent of cases when their clinical assessment indicated a high probability of pulmonary embolism. When their clinical assessment indicated a low probability of pulmonary embolism, senior staff correctly excluded pulmonary embolism in 86 per cent. Postgraduate fellows, on the basis of clinical assessment, were more accurate in excluding pulmonary embolism than they were in making the diagnosis.

Differential diagnosis of pulmonary embolism

The commonest presentation of acute pulmonary embolism is with dyspnoea and/or pleuritic chest pain. There are, however, several other possible causes of these symptoms, the commonest being musculoskeletal pain and pneumonia. Musculoskeletal chest pain can be very similar to that caused by pleurisy, and splinting of the chest can lead to a perception of breathlessness, which may be exacerbated by anxiety. If there is an obvious history of local trauma to the chest, then patients will rarely present to the physician, but it is worthwhile to ask specifically whether there has been any trauma or unaccustomed physical activity, whether the pain can be brought on by particular movements, and to examine carefully for local tenderness of ribs, muscles, or costal margins. Tenderness can sometimes be found in cases of pleurisy, but with appropriate history clearly supports a diagnosis of musculoskeletal pain. Pneumonia complicated by pleurisy can cause dyspnoea and chest pain. Important features to look for in the history include preceding systemic upset ('flu-like' symptoms), high fever, and rigors; and on examination, high fever, 'toxic' appearance, and chest signs of pneumonic consolidation. If a positive diagnosis of another cause of dyspnoea and/or pleuritic chest pain cannot be made, then the default position should be to assume that the patient has pulmonary embolism until proven otherwise.

Investigation

Simple laboratory tests

Among patients with pulmonary embolism in whom a possible or definite cause for leucocytosis was eliminated, 80 per cent had a normal white blood cell count, 6 per cent had a count of 10 100 to 11 900/mm^3, and 13 per cent had a count of 12 000/mm^3 or greater. None had a white blood cell count that was 20 000/mm^3 or greater. Leucocytosis was not more frequent in patients with the pulmonary haemorrhage/infarction syndrome than in other patients with acute pulmonary embolism.

Electrocardiogram

Electrocardiographic abnormalities are described among patients with pulmonary embolism who had no prior cardiopulmonary disease (Table 10). A normal electrocardiogram was shown in 30 per cent of patients with acute pulmonary embolism. Only 5 per cent of the patients with acute pulmonary embolism had atrial fibrillation or atrial flutter. Atrial flutter or atrial fibrillation in patients with acute pulmonary embolism is nearly always limited to individuals with prior heart disease.

Abnormalities of the ST segment and T wave are by far the most frequent electrocardiographic manifestation of acute pulmonary embolism. Non-

Table 10 Electrocardiographic manifestations: patients without prior cardiac or pulmonary disease (**n** = 89)

	Patients with electrocardiographic finding (%)
Rhythm disturbances	
Atrial flutter	1
Atrial fibrillation	4
Atrial premature contractions	4
Ventricular premature contractions	4
P Wave	
P pulmonale	2
QRS abnormalities	
Right axis deviation	2
Left axis deviation	13
Incomplete right bundle branch block	4
Complete right bundle branch block	6
Right ventricular hypertrophy	2
Pseudoinfarction	3
Low voltage (frontal plane)	3
ST segment and T wave	
Non-specific ST segment or T-wave abnormalities	49

Some patients had more than one abnormality.
Data are from Stein et al. (1991) Chest.

specific ST-segment or T-wave changes were observed in 49 per cent of patients in whom the severity of pulmonary embolism ranged from mild to severe.

Electrocardiographic manifestations of acute cor pulmonale (S1Q3T3, complete right bundle branch block, P pulmonale, or right axis deviation) were less common than ST-segment or T-wave changes. One or more of these abnormalities occurred in 26 per cent of patients with submassive or massive acute pulmonary embolism not associated with cardiac or pulmonary disease (32 per cent of patients with massive pulmonary embolism).

The electrocardiogram may simulate inferior infarction with Q waves and T-wave inversion in leads II, III, and aVF or anteroseptal infarction characterized by QS or QR waves in V1 and T-wave inversion in the right precordial leads. The development of Q waves and extensive T-wave inversion in the anterior and lateral leads has also been observed. A pseudoinfarction pattern, however, was seen in only 3 per cent of patients with no prior cardiopulmonary disease who had pulmonary embolism that ranged in severity from mild to massive.

New leftward shifts of the frontal plane axis in pulmonary embolism are frequent. Among patients with acute pulmonary embolism, left axis deviation was more frequent than right axis deviation. Low-voltage QRS complexes were observed in 3 per cent.

Inversion of the T waves was the most persistent electrocardiographic abnormality. Inversion of the T wave disappeared in only 22 per cent of patients 5 or 6 days after the pulmonary embolism was diagnosed, although it resolved in 49 per cent by 2 weeks. Depression of the ST segment tended to resolve somewhat faster. Abnormalities of depolarization resolved more quickly than abnormalities of repolarization. Well over half of the electrocardiograms that showed pseudoinfarction, S1S2S3, S1Q3T3, right ventricular hypertrophy, or right bundle branch block, no longer showed these abnormalities 5 or 6 days after the diagnosis was made.

Patients with ST-segment abnormalities, T-wave inversion, pseudoinfarction patterns, S1Q3T3 patterns, incomplete right bundle branch block, right axis deviation, right ventricular hypertrophy, or ventricular premature beats had larger perfusion defects on the lung scan or larger defects on the pulmonary arteriogram than those with normal electrocardiograms. Such patients had higher pulmonary arterial pressures and in general had low partial pressure of oxygen in arterial blood. Acute ventricular dilatation is speculated to be the most likely cause of the electrocardiographic changes.

Chest radiograph

The findings on the plain chest radiograph, when used together with the history, physical examination, electrocardiogram, and simple laboratory tests assist in identifying a syndrome of pulmonary embolism. The chest radiograph, when normal in a patient who is dyspnoeic, may hint that pulmonary embolism is a diagnostic possibility. Abnormalities on the plain chest radiograph may suggest a need for further diagnostic evaluation.

Among patients with pulmonary embolism who had no prior cardiopulmonary disease a normal chest radiograph was shown in 16 per cent (Table 11). Atelectasis or a pulmonary parenchymal abnormality were the most frequent abnormalities (68 per cent). When present, pleural effusions were usually small. The majority were limited to blunting of the costophrenic angle. In some studies, an elevated hemidiaphragm was the most frequent abnormality. The Westermark's sign (prominent central pulmonary artery and decreased pulmonary vascularity) was identified by radiologists in only 7 per cent of patients with pulmonary embolism.

In cases of pulmonary embolism, those with a normal plain chest radiograph had the lowest pulmonary artery mean pressures. The highest pulmonary artery mean pressures were in patients with a prominent central pulmonary artery or cardiomegaly.

Arterial blood gases and alveolar–arterial oxygen difference

A low partial pressure of oxygen in arterial blood (PaO$_2$) is typical of acute pulmonary embolism and supports the diagnosis, but patients with acute pulmonary embolism can have a normal Pao_2. Among patients with acute pulmonary embolism and no prior cardiopulmonary disease who had measurements of the Pao_2 while breathing room air, 24 per cent had a Pao_2 of 80 mmHg (10.5 kPa) or higher. Even among patients with submassive or massive acute pulmonary embolism, 12 per cent had a Pao_2 of 80 mmHg or higher. A normal alveolar–arterial oxygen difference (alveolar–arterial oxygen gradient) does not exclude acute pulmonary embolism. No value of the alveolar–arterial oxygen difference was diagnostic of pulmonary embolism, and no value excluded pulmonary embolism.

D-Dimer

As when considering the diagnosis of deep venous thrombosis, a 'negative' D-dimer test is useful for excluding pulmonary embolism in patients who are clinically thought to be at low risk, but a 'positive' result does not establish the diagnosis. Hence, when used in the appropriate clinical context, D-dimer testing is useful in defining a group of patients with suspected pulmonary embolism who do not require further investigation.

Table 11 Chest radiograph in pulmonary embolism: patients with no previous cardiac or pulmonary disease (*n* = 117)

	Patients with radiographic finding (%)
Atelectasis or pulmonary parenchymal abnormality	68
Pleural effusion	48
Pleural-based opacity	35
Elevated diaphragm	24
Decreased pulmonary vascularity	21
Prominent central pulmonary artery	15
Cardiomegaly	12
Westermark's sign*	7

Data are modified from Stein *et al.* (1991) *Chest* and are reproduced with permission.

* Prominent central pulmonary artery and decreased pulmonary vascularity.

Ventilation–perfusion lung scans

The ventilation–perfusion lung scan in pulmonary embolism, if high probability, indicates pulmonary embolism in 87 per cent of patients (Table 12 and Fig. 1). If normal, pulmonary embolism is excluded. If intermediate probability, the scan contributes no useful diagnostic information, pulmonary embolism being present in about 30 per cent. If low probability, pulmonary embolism is present in 14 per cent. A low probability ventilation–perfusion scan, therefore, by the criteria used in the Prospective Investigation of Pulmonary Embolism Diagnosis (PIOPED) does not exclude pulmonary embolism, and intermediate and low probability interpretations may be grouped as 'non-diagnostic'. Criteria for a very low probability lung scan (positive predictive value less than 10 per cent) have been developed since the conclusion of PIOPED.

Prior clinical assessment in combination with interpretation of the ventilation–perfusion scan improves the diagnostic validity (Table 12). If the ventilation–perfusion scan is interpreted as high probability for pulmonary embolism, and if the clinical impression is concordantly high, then the positive predictive value for pulmonary embolism is 96 per cent. If the ventilation–perfusion scan is low probability and the clinical suspicion is concordantly low, then pulmonary embolism is excluded in 96 per cent of patients.

The probability of pulmonary embolism can be determined based on the number of mismatched defects. A further refinement of probability can be made if the ventilation–perfusion scan is interpreted after being stratified according to prior cardiopulmonary disease. Fewer mismatched perfusion defects are required to diagnose pulmonary embolism among patients with no prior cardiopulmonary disease. Adding clinical assessment to the stratification results in a more accurate evaluation.

Repeat ventilation–perfusion lung scanning

A residual abnormality of perfusion 1 year after acute pulmonary embolism is more frequent among patients with prior cardiopulmonary disease than among patients with none. It is useful to obtain a post-therapy baseline ventilation–perfusion lung scan for use in the event of suspected recurrent pulmonary embolism. This will assist in determining if abnormalities

Table 12 Probability of pulmonary embolism using clinical assessment in combination with ventilation–perfusion lung scans

Scan category	Clinical probability, estimated prior to scanning (%)						All probabilities	
	80–100 PE+/*n*	(%)	20–79 PE+/*n*	(%)	0–19 PE+/*n*	(%)	PE+/*n*	(%)
High probability	28/29	96	70/80	88	5/9	56	103/118	87
Intermediate probability	27/41	66	66/236	28	11/68	16	104/345	30
Low probability	6/15	40	30/191	16	4/90	4	40/296	14
Near normal /normal	0/5	0	4/62	6	1/61	2	5/128	4
Total	61/90	68	170/569	30	21/228	9	252/887	28

* PE+ indicates angiogram reading that shows pulmonary embolism or determination of pulmonary embolism by the outcome classification committee on review. Pulmonary embolism status is based on angiogram interpretation for 713 patients, on angiogram interpretation and outcome classification committee reassignment for four patients, and on clinical information alone (without definitive angiography) for 170 patients.

Reproduced from A National Investigation by the PIOPED Investigators (1990). *Journal of the American Medical Association*.

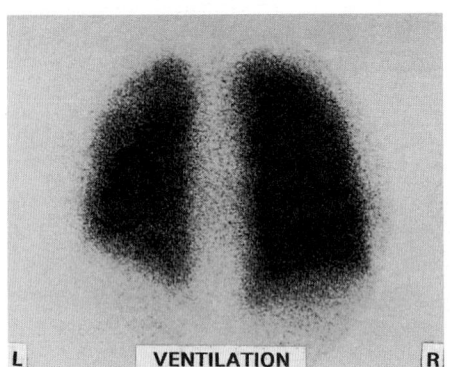

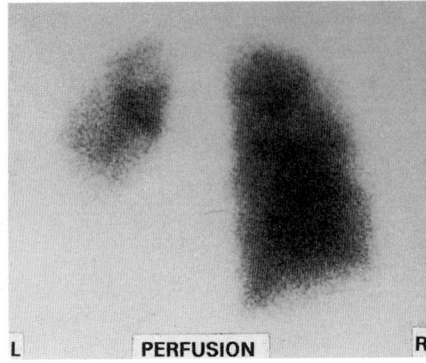

Fig. 1 Ventilation lung scan (left) and perfusion lung scan (right), posterior views. Left (L) and right (R) lungs are indicated. Ventilation scan, equilibrium phase, shows nearly normal ventilation. Perfusion scan shows absent perfusion in the left lower lobe and mismatched perfusion defects in the left upper lobe. Perfusion defects (grey areas) are also shown in the right lung. The ventilation–perfusion lung scan was interpreted as high probability for pulmonary embolism.

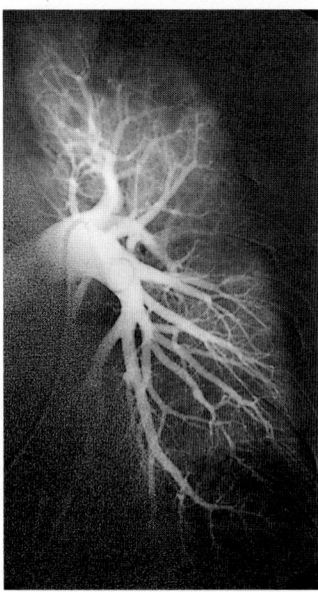

Fig. 2 Normal selective digital subtraction pulmonary angiogram of the left pulmonary artery. Vessels fill completely, taper gradually, and show numerous fine branches. This film and other pulmonary angiograms were supplied by Dr P.C. Shetty, Hurley Medical Center, Flint, Michigan, United States.

on a ventilation–perfusion scan are new or residual from prior pulmonary embolism.

Pulmonary angiography

Pulmonary angiography is associated with serious complications in about 1 per cent of patients. When needed, pulmonary angiography is useful and remains the diagnostic reference test for pulmonary embolism (Figs 2, 3, and 4). Patients in whom the risk of complications of pulmonary embolism are greatest are patients referred for angiography from the medical intensive care unit. Frequently such patients are on respiratory support and in an unstable condition. The presence or absence of pulmonary embolism and the magnitude of pulmonary hypertension did not relate to the frequency of morbidity from angiography. Elderly patients (70 years or older) are at greater risk of renal impairment than younger patients as a result of the

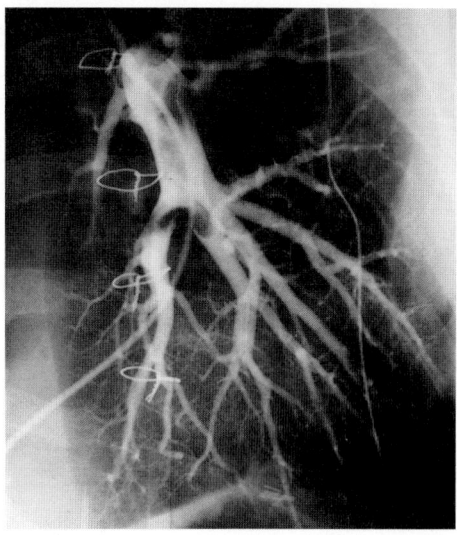

Fig. 4 Selective pulmonary angiogram of the left pulmonary artery showing a large intraluminal filling defect with a saddle embolus at the bifurcation.

injection of contrast material. A retrospective analysis of complications, among patients in whom angiography was performed with non-ionic low-osmolar contrast material, showed fewer (0.1 per cent) major complications.

Contrast-enhanced spiral computed tomography

The results of imaging with contrast-enhanced spiral computed tomography (**CT**) (Fig. 5) compared with pulmonary angiography or autopsy are sparse. Results of individual small case series varied widely, with reported sensitivities ranging from 50 to 93 per cent. These studies all utilized 5-mm CT sections. With newer equipment, thinner sections with less breathing artefact are available. The sensitivity and specificity should, therefore, improve. However, the sensitivity and specificity of contrast enhanced

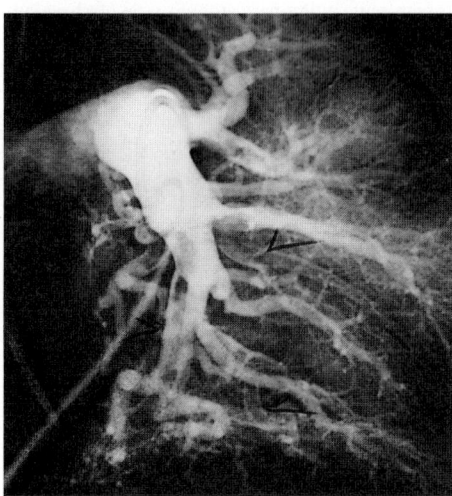

Fig. 3 Selective digital subtraction pulmonary angiogram of the left pulmonary artery showing multiple intraluminal filling defects indicative of pulmonary thromboemboli. Some of these have been identified by arrowheads.

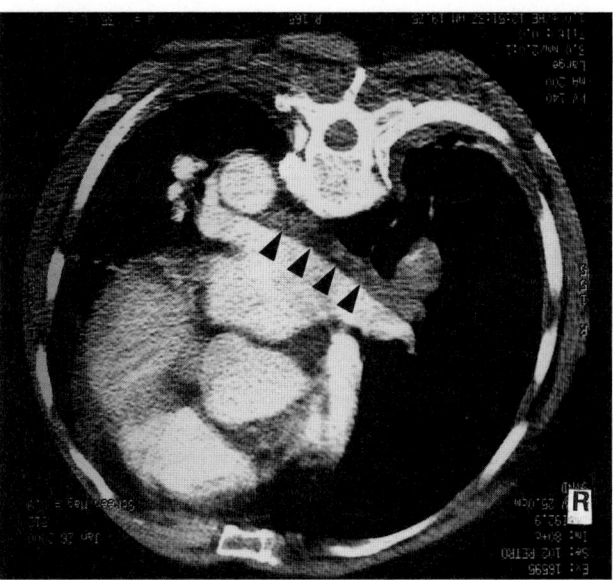

Fig. 5 Contrast-enhanced spiral computed tomogram showing a large intraluminal filling defect (arrowheads).

spiral CT with multidetector scanners have not yet been determined. Investigation is in progress.

Magnetic resonance imaging

Magnetic resonance imaging, including magnetic resonance angiography and gadolinium-enhanced magnetic resonance angiography for acute pulmonary embolism are 'evolving' techniques. Preliminary observations suggest that gadolinium-enhanced three-dimensional magnetic resonance angiography during a single breath hold shows promise as a potentially useful imaging technique. Among the potential advantages are rapidity, avoidance of nephrotoxic iodinated contrast agents, and minimal invasiveness. Potential disadvantages include lack of sensitivity in detecting subsegmental pulmonary embolism and the fact that some patients may have a contraindication to magnetic resonance imaging.

Echocardiography

Echocardiography may show right ventricular dilatation and evidence of pulmonary hypertension, which, in the proper clinical setting, may strengthen the clinical impression that pulmonary embolism has occurred. Transoesophageal echocardiography sometimes may show proximal pulmonary emboli, but it has limited value in this regard.

Clues for the diagnosis of pulmonary embolism

With increasing severity of pulmonary embolism, from pulmonary infarction to isolated dyspnoea to circulatory collapse, trends suggest that the prevalence of a high probability ventilation–perfusion lung scan increases, as does the pulmonary artery mean pressure, while the Pao_2 decreases. However, making the diagnosis of pulmonary embolism is difficult, and depends on consideration of clinical, laboratory, and imaging data. Clues that can assist the physician in assessing the possibility of pulmonary embolism and avoiding inadvertent exclusion of the diagnosis are as follows.

1. Some patients with pulmonary embolism and circulatory collapse do not have dyspnoea, tachypnoea, or pleuritic pain.

2. Rales (crepitations) are common among patients with pulmonary infarction, but less so in those with isolated dyspnoea or circulatory collapse. They occur in those with radiographic evidence of a parenchymal abnormality.

3. A normal electrocardiogram is frequent in patients with the pulmonary infarction syndrome, but uncommon in those with isolated dyspnoea.

4. Abnormalities on the chest radiograph, although more common among patients with pulmonary infarction, are often observed in those with isolated dyspnoea.

5. Patients with circulatory collapse may have a normal chest radiograph.

6. A high probability interpretation of the ventilation–perfusion scan occurs in a minority of patients with the pulmonary infarction syndrome, but it is found in the majority of patients with the isolated dyspnoea syndrome.

7. A low probability ventilation–perfusion scan can occur in patients with pulmonary embolism and circulatory collapse.

8. A Pao_2 higher than 80 mmHg (10.5 kPa) is not uncommon in patients with the pulmonary infarction syndrome, but such levels are uncommon in those with the isolated dyspnoea syndrome.

Strategy for diagnosis

There are clear parallels with the situation when the diagnosis of deep venous thrombosis is considered. Subjecting all patients who might have a pulmonary embolus to complex, expensive and/or invasive tests is best avoided, such that management algorithms have been developed to identify those at very low risk, who can then be spared invasive tests. These algorithms typically use scoring systems to stratify the clinical probability that the particular patient has a pulmonary embolus, proceeding to D-dimer testing of those with low probability. Patients with a low clinical probability and a negative D-dimer test are not investigated further. Patients with either a high clinical probability or a low clinical probability but elevated D-dimer proceed to tests for the presence pulmonary emboli, typically by ventilation-perfusion lung scanning or contrast-enhanced spiral computed tomography. Examples of a pre-test scoring system and management algorithm are shown in Table 13.

Management algorithms of the type described in Table 13 are now employed in many hospitals, but a note of caution is appropriate. Their use has not been well validated. When there is genuine clinical doubt and a ventilation perfusion lung scan is reported as of low or intermediate probability, then there is a considerable diagnostic problem. In many centres contrast-enhanced spiral CT has become the diagnostic method of choice for suspected pulmonary embolism, or is used as the next line of investigation if ventilation perfusion scanning does not produce a clear-cut result. However, some would argue that the method has not been tested sufficiently and the physician should weigh the value of angiography (if available) against its hazards in the context of the whole clinical situation. The finding that 57 per cent of positive angiograms in the PIOPED study occurred in those with intermediate and low probability scans strengthens the case for an angiogram. An alternative strategy is to image the veins in the legs if ventilation perfusion scanning does not allow confident exclusion of the diagnosis of pulmonary embolism. If imaging reveals thrombus, then treatment is given. If imaging is negative, then this does not exclude the diagnosis of venous thromboembolism (the thrombus may have gone into the lungs), but the patient can be followed safely with serial non-invasive imaging of the leg veins. The risk of pulmonary embolism is low in patients in whom serial investigations of the legs show no deep venous thrombosis.

Treatment

General measures

All patients who are hypoxic should be given supplementary oxygen at high concentration (enough to restore normal Po_2), excepting those few with coincident chronic chest disease where carbon dioxide retention is problematic. In the early stages, continuous monitoring of arterial oxygen tension by pulse oximetry is advised.

Resuscitation

Most patients with acute pulmonary embolism do not have substantial circulatory compromise, but those presenting with massive pulmonary embolism may have circulatory collapse. They may look as though they are about to die, with cool peripheries, cyanosis, profound hypotension, and marked elevation of the jugular venous pulse. Features typical of long-standing pulmonary hypertension (palpable right ventricular heave, right ventricular gallop, loud P2, hepatomegally, ascites, peripheral oedema) are unlikely to be present. This dramatic haemodynamic picture may not be simply due to the direct anatomical effects of occlusion of main pulmonary vessels (the same picture is not seen after pneumonectomy, when one pulmonary artery is tied off completely), but also secondary to pulmonary neurogenic reflexes and local release of vasoactive substances, including 5-hydroxytryptamine and thromboxane from activated platelets.

Even though the jugular venous pulse is markedly elevated in acute massive pulmonary embolism, volume expanders should be administered rapidly to increase right ventricular filling pressure still further. The aim is to support the circulation until measures designed to deal with the embolus (usually thrombolysis—see below) can be applied and take effect.

Antithrombotic treatment

Unless there are serious concerns about the potential side-effects of anticoagulation or imaging is immediately available, it is common and sensible practice to begin anticoagulant treatment as soon as the diagnosis of pulmonary embolism is suspected. The antithrombotic regimen is the same as for deep venous thrombosis: see Table 5 and Chapter 15.15.3.2. This treatment is effective: the mortality from acute pulmonary embolism or recurrent pulmonary embolism during the first 3 months among 297 patients treated only with anticoagulants in the PIOPED study was 1.7 per cent. An additional 2.0 per cent suffered non-fatal recurrent pulmonary embolism during the first 3 months. Among all patients, irrespective of the treatment, the mortality from pulmonary embolism during the first 3 months was 2.4 per cent and an additional 3.5 per cent suffered non-fatal recurrent pulmonary embolism.

Thrombolytic therapy

Thrombolytic therapy is not indicated for the routine treatment of pulmonary embolism. Hypotension and continuing hypoxemia while receiving high fractions of inspired oxygen (Fio_2) are indications for intervention. Right ventricular dysfunction on the echocardiogram may also be an indication.

Table 13 Pre-test clinical probability scoring system and care pathway for the patient with suspected pulmonary embolism

(a) Pre-test probability score

Criteria	Score
Clinical signs and symptoms of deep venous thrombosis (minimum of leg swelling and pain with palpation of deep vein region)	+3
No alternative diagnosis	+3
Heart rate >100/min	+1.5
Bed rest >3 days, surgery within 4 weeks	+1.5
Previous DVT or PE	+1.5
Haemoptysis	+1
Malignancy	+1

(b) Pre-test probability

Low (2–4% chance of PE)	0 or 1
Moderate (approximately 20% chance of PE)	2 to 6
High (approximately 60% chance of PE)	More than 6

(c) Management algorithm

Pre-test probability score	Action	Result	Action	Further action
0 or 1	Perform D-dimer	Negative	No further investigation	PE excluded
		Positive	Perform ventilation-perfusion lung scanning	Normal / low probability scan – no further investigation (PE excluded) Intermediate probability scan – perform bilateral venous ultrasonography. If negative, serial leg tests are unnecessary and PE can be considered to be excluded. High probability scan - diagnosis of PE established
2 or more	Do not perform D-dimer	Result would not alter	Perform ventilation-perfusion lung scanning	Normal scan - no further investigation (PE excluded)
		management -imaging is required		Low / Intermediate probability scan – action depends on patient's cardiorespiratory reserve and local availability / experience of further imaging tests: see notes
				High probability scan - diagnosis of PE established

Notes

1 .Pre-test probability score from Wells *et al.* (2000).

2 .This management algorithm is typical of many used, but further prospective evaluation is warranted. (a) If the pre-test probability is low (however determined) and there is a low probability ventilation-perfusion lung scan, there is a low likelihood of PE (4 per cent based on PIOPED). (b) If the pre-test probability is moderate or high and the ventilation-perfusion scan gives a low or intermediate probability result, further action should be determined by the patient's cardiorespiratory reserve. If this is adequate, serial ultrasonography of the leg veins over 10–14 days may be performed. If such serial testing is negative, pulmonary embolism rarely occurs. If cardiopulmonary reserve is inadequate, proceed to a definitive diagnostic test for pulmonary embolism (pulmonary angiography or perhaps spiral computed tomography).

3 . If the physician's judgement is that pulmonary embolism is very likely in a particular case, then he or she should proceed to investigations directed at detecting pulmonary embolism, whatever the scoring algorithm would suggest.

4 . All patients who are discharged with 'pulmonary embolism excluded' should be given written information describing how they can be reassessed if symptoms worsen or fail to settle over the next few days.

More rapid lysis of pulmonary thromboemboli occurs with thrombolytic agents than occurs spontaneously in patients treated only with anticoagulants. However, pulmonary reperfusion, as shown on perfusion lung scans, is similar after 2 weeks in patients treated with thrombolytic agents and those given anticoagulants.

A large prospective randomized trial in 1973 using urokinase showed no improvement of mortality and no difference of the rate of recurrence of pulmonary embolism among stable patients treated with thrombolytic therapy as opposed to anticoagulants. There have been no subsequent prospective randomized trials which contradict these results. A trend suggesting a lower rate of recurrent pulmonary embolism has been shown among patients with right ventricular dysfunction who were treated with tissue plasminogen activator.

Thrombolysis has risks. The frequency of major bleeding from tissue plasminogen activator among patients with pulmonary embolism diagnosed by angiography, based on pooled data, is 13 per cent. All investigations excluded patients at a high risk of bleeding, such as those with recent surgery, recent biopsy, peptic ulcer disease, blood dyscrasia, or severe hepatic or renal disease. The reported patients, therefore, had a low risk of bleeding. The risk of intracranial haemorrhage with tissue plasminogen activator (2 per cent) was higher among patients with pulmonary embolism than among patients who received tissue plasminogen activator for myocardial infarction.

Regimens of thrombolytic therapy

Regimens approved by the United States FDA for treatment of acute pulmonary embolism are:

(1) streptokinase, 250 000 IU over 30 min followed by 100 000 IU/h for 24 h;

(2) urokinase, 4400 IU/kg/h over 10 min followed by 4400 IU/kg/h for 12 to 24 h; or

(3) tissue plasminogen activator, 100 mg(50 million IU)/2 h.

Potentially advantageous regimens of thrombolytic therapy, not fully evaluated, are:

(1) urokinase, 15 000 IU/kg over 10 min; or

(2) tissue plasminogen activator, 0.6 mg/kg (max. 50 mg) over 2 min.

It is recommended that heparin be discontinued during thrombolytic therapy and reinstituted upon discontinuation of thrombolytic therapy. None of the FDA approved regimens utilize concomitant heparin.

Inferior vena cava occlusion

An inferior vena cava filter is recommended in a patient with proximal deep venous thrombosis or pulmonary embolism if:

(1) anticoagulants are contraindicated;

(2) pulmonary embolism has recurred while on adequate anticoagulant therapy; or

(3) pulmonary embolism is severe (right ventricular failure on physical examination, hypotension) and any recurrent pulmonary embolism may be fatal.

Insertion of an inferior vena cava filter is also strongly recommended in patients following pulmonary embolectomy.

Routine insertion of an inferior vena cava filter is not indicated only on the basis of a continuing predisposition for deep venous thrombosis. In special circumstances, however, this may be the best approach. Prophylactic insertion of vena cava filters may be considered for high-risk patients with deep venous thrombosis, severe pulmonary hypertension, and minimal cardiopulmonary reserve.

A number of vena cava filters have been designed for percutaneous insertion. They differ in outer diameter of the delivery system, maximal caval diameter into which they can be inserted, hook design, retrievability, biocompatability, and filtering efficiency. Filter migration, thrombosis, and cava wall perforation occur. Anticoagulant therapy after insertion of a filter is recommended. The filter alone, however, may be effective.

Symptomatic occlusion of the inferior vena cava is the most frequent complication, occurring in about 9 per cent of patients. Pulmonary embolism after insertion of an inferior vena cava filter is uncommon (1 per cent), and fatal pulmonary embolism is rare. Possible mechanisms that can explain pulmonary embolism after filter insertion are: (i) ineffective filtration, especially with tilting of the filter; (ii) growth of trapped thrombi through the filter; (iii) thrombosis on the proximal side of the filter; (iv) filter migration; (v) filter retraction from the caval wall; (vi) embolization through collaterals; (vii) embolization from sites other than the inferior vena cava; and (viii) incorrect position of the filter.

Complications of vena cava filters include filter deformation, filter fracture, insufficient opening of the filter, and improper anatomical placement of the filter. Filter-related complications include migration, angulation of the filter, caval stenosis, caval occlusion, erosion of the caval wall, and leg oedema. Complications at the site of insertion of the catheter do not differ from complications observed locally with other catheter techniques. Deep venous thrombosis at the puncture site generally has been reported in 8 to 25 per cent of cases.

Catheter interventions

Catheter-tip devices for the extraction or the fragmentation of embolus have the potential of producing immediate relief from massive pulmonary embolism. Such interventions may be particularly useful in patients in whom there is a contraindication to thrombolytic therapy. A suction-tip device for extraction of pulmonary embolism has been used in some patients. Thrombus fragmentation with a guide wire, angiographic catheter or balloon catheter, or specially designed devices have been reported in small case series or case reports. The release of fragmented thromboemboli into the distal pulmonary arterial branches is not a problem. A registry of management strategies used by hospitals throughout Germany showed use of thrombus fragmentation in 1.3 to 6.8 per cent of patients with pulmonary embolism, depending on the severity. Catheters also have been developed that deliver high-velocity jets in the region of the thrombus, causing the thrombus to be sucked into the adjacent low pressure zone and undergo fragmentation due to the powerful mixing forces.

Pulmonary embolectomy

Medical therapy is likely to give better results than embolectomy. The operative and perioperative mortality related to surgical pulmonary embolectomy ranges between 28 and 74 per cent. A candidate for pulmonary embolectomy should meet the following criteria: (i) massive pulmonary embolism, angiographically documented if possible; (ii) haemodynamic instability (shock) despite heparin therapy and resuscitative efforts; and (iii) failure of thrombolytic therapy or a contraindication to its use.

Chronic pulmonary thromboembolic hypertension

In a very few patients with extensive embolization, the emboli fail to resolve and undergo fibrovascular organization, causing chronic obstruction to pulmonary arterial blood flow. Subsequently this can result in chronic pulmonary thromboembolic hypertension. This occurs in about 0.1 to 0.2 per cent of survivors of acute pulmonary embolism. In most of these patients, a procoagulant abnormality or defect in the fibrinolytic system cannot be shown. In many patients, both acute and chronic emboli are simultaneously present. A proliferation of fibrous connective tissue and small blood vessels penetrate a variable distance into the thrombus and attach it to the intimal surface of the vessel wall. Pulmonary hypertension develops as the result of a critical reduction of cross-sectional area for blood flow. The relatively high flow through non-occluded vessels may cause secondary hypertensive changes in the resistive or precapillary vessels. Patients with mean pulmonary artery pressures over 30 mmHg had a 5-year survival of 30 per cent and if the mean pulmonary artery pressure was over 50 mmHg, the 5-year survival was 10 per cent.

Most patients do not have an obvious history of venous thrombosis or pulmonary embolism. Dyspnoea is present in virtually all, but in the early stages may occur only on exertion. Compensatory right ventricular hypertrophy develops, and there may be a period of months to years when symptoms remain stable, but ultimately right ventricular function deteriorates. Symptoms then include worsening dyspnoea, fatigue, presyncope, syncope (rarely), pleuritic pain, angina-like pain, abdominal swelling, and peripheral oedema. Signs of respiratory and right ventricular failure develop, with cyanosis, grossly elevated jugular venous pulse, palpable right ventricular heave, right ventricular gallop, loud P2, hepatomegaly, ascites, and peripheral oedema. Bruits may be heard over the pulmonary arteries.

Ventilation–perfusion lung scans typically show one or more mismatched segmental or larger perfusion defects, and most patients have several bilateral mismatched perfusion defects. Pulmonary angiography is the most definitive diagnostic test. It shows narrowed segmental pulmonary arteries, sometimes accompanied by post-stenotic dilatation, irregularity of the intima, luminal narrowing of the central arteries, and oddly shaped vessels. Pulmonary fibreoptic angioscopy is useful to define surgical accessibility.

Pulmonary thromboendarterectomy is the treatment of choice. The procedure is highly specialized and postoperative management is difficult and complex. Such surgery is performed only at a limited number of centres. At the most experienced centre, the operative mortality is 8.7 per cent.

Medical therapy is adjunctive and should not delay the assessment for surgery. Medical therapy fails to address the underlying problem of fixed pulmonary vascular obstruction. In patients awaiting surgery, it is important to prevent further emboli and to treat cor pulmonale. Anticoagulation should be initiated immediately and maintained for life. Insertion of an inferior vena cava filter is generally advisable. There is no role for thrombolytic therapy. Angioplasty has not been successful. The potential role of pulmonary vasodilator therapy is speculative.

For fuller discussion of the management of pulmonary hypertension see Chapter 15.15.2.

Further reading

Bates SM, Grand'Maison A, Johnston M, Naguit I, Kovacs MJ, Ginsberg JS (2001). A latex D-dimer reliably excludes venous thromboembolism. *Archives of Internal Medicine* **161**, 447–53.

Collaborative Study by the PIOPED Investigators (1990). Value of the ventilation/perfusion scan in acute pulmonary embolism—results of the prospective investigation of pulmonary embolism diagnosis (PIOPED). *Journal of the American Medical Association* **263**, 2753–9. [Landmark investigation of ventilation/perfusion lung scans.]

Geerts et al. (2001). Prevention of venous thromboembolism. *Chest* **119**(Suppl), 132S–75S. [Detailed and authoritative review of methods for prevention of venous thromboembolism.]

Hull RD et al.(1990).Noninvasive strategy for the treatment of patients with clinically suspected pulmonary embolism. *Archives of Internal Medicine* **154**, 289–97.

Hull RD, Raskob GE, Pineo GF, eds (1996). *Venous thromboembolism: an evidence-based atlas.* Futura Publishing, New York. [Comprehensive review of pulmonary embolism.]

Hyers TN et al. (2001). Antithrombotic therapy for venous thromboembolic disease. *Chest* **119**(Suppl), 176S–93S. [Authoritative and in-depth review of treatment with recommendations.]

Kearon C et al. (2001). Management of suspected deep venous thrombosis in outpatients by using clinical assessment and D-dimer testing. *Annals of Internal Medicine* **135**, 108–11.

National Cooperative Study (1973). The Urokinase Pulmonary Embolism Trial. *Circulation* **47**(Suppl II), II-1–II-108. [Basic investigation of thrombolytic therapy.]

Stein PD (1996). *Pulmonary embolism.* Williams & Wilkins, Media, Pennsylvania. [Detailed comprehensive review.]

Stein PD et al. (1991). Clinical, laboratory, roentgenographic and electrocardiographic findings in patients with acute pulmonary embolism and no pre-existing cardiac or pulmonary disease. *Chest* **100**, 598–603. [Shows detailed results of clinical findings in patients with pulmonary embolism.]

Stein PD, Hull RD, Pineo G (1995). Strategy that includes serial noninvasive leg tests for diagnosis of thromboembolic disease in patients with suspected acute pulmonary embolism based on data from PIOPED. *Archives of Internal Medicine* **155**, 2101–4. [Gives background for validity of strategy that includes serial non-invasive leg tests.]

Wells PS et al. (1997). Value of assessment of pretest probability of deep-vein thrombosis in clinical management. *Lancet* **350**, 1795–8.

Wells PS et al. (2000). Derivation of a simple clinical model to categorize patients probability of pulmonary embolism: increasing the models utility with the SimpliRED D-dimer. *Thrombosis and Haemostasis* **83**, 416–20.

Wells PS et al. (2001). Excluding pulmonary embolism at the bedside without diagnostic imaging: management of patients with suspected pulmonary embolism presenting to the emergency department using a simple clinical model and D-dimer. *Annals of Internal Medicine* **135**, 98–107.

Viner SM et al. (1994). The management of pulmonary hypertension secondary to chronic thromboembolic disease. *Progress in Cardiovascular Diseases* **37**, 79–92. [In-depth review of chronic pulmonary thromboembolic hypertension.]

15.15.3.2 Therapeutic anticoagulation in deep vein thrombosis and pulmonary embolism

David Keeling

Introduction

Deep vein thrombosis and pulmonary embolism are aspects of the same disease, venous thromboembolism. Forty per cent of patients with deep vein thrombosis without clinical evidence of pulmonary embolism have evidence of emboli on lung scanning. The principles of therapeutic anticoagulation are the same for both. In proximal deep vein thrombosis and pulmonary embolism this involves immediate anticoagulation with heparin followed by a period of anticoagulation with warfarin (or other oral vitamin K antagonist). Distal deep vein thrombosis can be managed in the same way, but an alternative strategy is to use serial non-invasive testing (e.g. ultrasound), which only reliably detects proximal thrombosis, to ensure that suspected distal thrombosis does not extend above the knee, withholding treatment if it does not.

There is clear evidence that heparin is needed in the initial phase and that anticoagulation with oral anticoagulants alone is inadequate. Warfarin can be commenced on the first day and heparin is continued for 5 days or until the international normalized ratio (**INR**) is greater than 2.0 for 2 consecutive days, whichever is the longer. Extending the period of heparinization from 5 to 10 days is not more effective and increases the risk of heparin-induced thrombocytopenia. However, for massive pulmonary embolism or severe ileofemoral thrombosis a longer period of heparin therapy may be considered.

Heparin

Heparin, a glycosaminoglycan, is composed of alternating uronic acid and glucosamine saccharides that are sulphated to a varying degree. Its mode of action is to potentiate the activity of the serine protease inhibitor (serpin) antithrombin, whose main mode of action is to inhibit thrombin, but which also inhibits several other coagulant proteases such as factor Xa. A specific pentasaccharide sequence determined by the sulphation pattern along the heparin chain binds to antithrombin and causes a conformational change, giving it full activation against factor Xa but only partial activation against thrombin. Heparins of 18 saccharides (MW 5400) or more can extend across the intermolecular gap and also bind to thrombin giving full antithrombin activity, which is lost if the chains are shorter. Unfractionated or standard heparins are a mixture of chains of different lengths (MW 5000 to 35 000, mean 13 000) and low-molecular-weight heparins (MW 2000 to 8000, mean 5000) are derived from them by enzymatic or physicochemical cleavage. Low-molecular-weight heparins have, with good reason, largely replaced unfractionated heparin for the treatment of venous thromboembolism, but the use of the latter will be discussed first.

Anticoagulation with unfractionated heparin

Unfractionated heparin has most often been given by continuous intravenous infusion, the rate of which has to be adjusted, usually by measuring the activated partial thromboplastin time (**APTT**). An inadequate APTT response in the first 24 h may increase the risk of recurrence of thromboembolism, though this does not seem to be critical if the starting infusion rate is at least 1250 IU/h. A validated regimen is to give a bolus dose of 80 IU/kg and to start the infusion at 18 IU/kg.h, performing the first APTT estimate after 6 h. The dose is then usually adjusted to maintain the APTT between 1.5 to 2.5 times the average laboratory control value. With older APTT reagents this corresponded to a therapeutic heparin level of 0.2 to 0.4 IU/ml by protamine titration or 0.3 to 0.6 IU/ml by anti-Xa assay. However, many current APTT reagents show an increased sensitivity to unfractionated heparin and with these higher ratios should be aimed for. The local laboratory should advise on the appropriate therapeutic range with its reagent. When the dose is therapeutic the APTT should be checked daily.

An alternative is to give unfractionated heparin subcutaneously once every 12 h, and a meta-analysis suggested that this might be more effective and at least as safe as continuous intravenous infusion. A reasonable starting dose is 250 IU/kg, adjusting the dose according to the mid-interval APTT.

Anticoagulation with low-molecular-weight heparin

Although much is made of the greater anti-Xa to antithrombin ratio of the low-molecular-weight heparins, their key clinical property is that they produce a much more predictable anticoagulant response than unfractionated heparin. This, combined with the fact that they have very high bioavailability after subcutaneous injection, means that the dose can be calculated by body weight and be given subcutaneously without any monitoring or dose adjustment. The actual dosage used differs slightly with the different low-molecular-weight heparins and the manufacturers' recommendations should be followed, but a typical dose is 200 IU/kg once a day. They are at least as effective and at least as safe as unfractionated heparin, even when given once a day. Their widespread use has enabled many patients with deep vein thrombosis to be managed as outpatients. Low-molecular-weight heparin is renally excreted so should be used with caution in renal failure (anti-Xa levels can be checked if necessary).

Complications of heparin treatment

If a patient on intravenous unfractionated heparin is excessively anticoagulated, it is usually sufficient simply to stop the infusion, the half-life being 1 to 2 h. If bleeding is severe the heparin can be neutralized with protamine sulphate, giving 1 mg for every 100 IU that have been infused over the previous hour. The reversal of low-molecular-weight heparin is more problematic. Although protamine sulphate may not neutralize the smaller chains it is often clinically effective, though estimating an appropriate dose is more difficult (the maximum dose is 50 mg, so this is often given if the subcutaneous injection was recent).

Heparin-induced thrombocytopenia is a feared complication, but much less common now short courses of low-molecular-weight heparin are used.

It is due to the development of an antibody to the heparin–platelet factor 4 complex and can be associated with serious venous and arterial thrombosis. Patients on heparin for 5 or more days should have their platelet count checked. If heparin-induced thrombocytopenia is suspected, then heparin must be stopped and an alternative substituted (danaparoid or hirudin being most suitable).

Long-term treatment, for example in pregnancy, is associated with osteopenia, but this may be less of a problem with low-molecular-weight heparin.

Warfarin

The oral vitamin K antagonists are the mainstay of long-term anticoagulant therapy. Warfarin is the commonest vitamin K antagonist given, though the shorter acting nicoumalone and the longer acting phenprocoumon are also used. Phenindione is used less commonly because of a high incidence of skin rashes. The procoagulant factors II, VII, IX, and X (and the anticoagulants protein C and protein S) need vitamin K for the γ-carboxylation of the glutamic acid residues that form their gla domains. Without this posttranslational modification they cannot bind calcium, and as a consequence cannot bind to anionic phospholipid surfaces, such that assembly of the key coagulation complexes is disrupted.

Warfarin takes about 4 days to become effective, during which period heparin is given. When warfarin is started the vitamin K-dependent factors fall according to their half-lives. Factor VII and protein C have the shortest half-lives, so that despite a prolongation of the INR due to factor VII deficiency, warfarin may initially be procoagulant. This is the mechanism for the rare problem of warfarin-induced skin necrosis, most often described in those with protein C deficiency.

Anticoagulation with warfarin

Initiation and monitoring

Monitoring of warfarin treatment is by the international normalized ratio (INR). This is a manipulation of the prothrombin time (**PT**) to allow for the different sensitivities of various laboratory reagents to the warfarin-induced coagulopathy. The INR equals $(PT/MNPT)^{ISI}$ where MNPT is the (mean normal) control PT and ISI is the international sensitivity index of the thromboplastin used in the assay. For the treatment of deep vein thrombosis and pulmonary embolism the target INR should be 2.5 (target range 2.0 to 3.0). If a recurrence occurs despite an INR of 2.0 to 3.0, then the dose is usually increased to a target INR of 3.5 (target range 3.0 to 4.0).

If the initial coagulation tests are not prolonged it is usual to give 10 mg of warfarin on the first evening and check the INR the following morning. Warfarin dose is adjusted according to the daily INR results until the patient is stable. Stable anticoagulation is more quickly and safely achieved if a dosing algorithm is followed (Table 1).

When patients are stable they may go for up to 8 weeks between INR checks. If the INR is unstable, patients are seen more frequently, but it should be noted that with warfarin it takes approximately 1 week (five times the half-life of 36 h) to reach a new steady state after dose adjustment and more frequent dosage alteration is inadvisable.

How long should the patient take warfarin?

It is a difficult clinical decision to decide how long to continue warfarin, a matter of balancing the risks of recurrence against the risks of warfarin. The latter are well known, 1 to 2 per cent of people on warfarin have a major bleed each year and 0.5 per cent suffer an intracranial bleed, of which 50 per cent die, giving a fatality rate of 0.25 per cent per annum. However, warfarin is highly (90 to 95 per cent) effective at preventing recurrence. The risk of a recurrent venous thromboembolism after a first deep vein thrombosis is approximately 5 per cent per year, when a case–fatality rate of 5 per cent (and some estimates for recurrent venous thromboembolism have been this high, though the overall rate for all venous thromboembolism is probably 1 to 2 per cent) would also give a fatality rate of 0.25 per cent per

Table 1 A warfarin induction regimen

Day 1 INR	Dose (mg)	Day 2 INR	Dose (mg)	Day 3 INR	Dose (mg)	Day 4 INR	Predicted maintenance dose (mg)
< 1.4	10	< 1.8	10	< 2.0	10	< 1.4	78
		1.8	1	2.0–2.1	5	1.4	8
		> 1.8	0.5	2.2–2.3	4.5	1.5	7.5
				2.4–2.5	4	1.6–1.7	7
				2.6–2.7	3.5	1.8	6.5
				2.8–2.9	3	1.9	6
				3.0–3.1	2.5	2.0–2.1	5.5
				3.2–3.3	2	2.2–2.3	5
				3.4	1.5	2.4–2.6	4.5
				3.5	1	2.7–3.0	4
				3.6–4.0	0.5	3.1–3.5	3.5
				> 4.0	0	3.6–4.0	3
						4.1–4.5	Miss out next day's dose then give 2 mg
						> 4.5	Miss out 2 days' doses then give 1 mg

From Fennerty et al. (1988) British Medical Journal **297**, 1285.

year. Other factors can be taken into account: the risk of recurrence is higher for the first 6 months, it is higher for proximal deep vein thrombosis and pulmonary embolism than for distal deep vein thrombosis, and it is lower if a transient risk factor was present (e.g. recent surgery, use of the contraceptive pill). Six months of anticoagulation has been shown to be more effective than 6 weeks of anticoagulation in all subgroups. Whether an inherited thrombophilia should influence the long-term management is not clear. Although they predict first events, the commoner defects (factor V Leiden and prothrombin G20210A) may not predict recurrence. Taking all this into account a reasonable approach is indicated in Table 2.

Complications of warfarin treatment

The only major complication of warfarin treatment is bleeding. Risk factors for bleeding are an age of 65 years or more, a history of stroke, a history of gastrointestinal bleeding, anaemia, renal impairment, diabetes, and recent myocardial infarction. A major problem in control is the starting and stopping of other medication. Many drugs interact with warfarin (see Table 3 for those with the most evidence) and patient education and constant vigilance is essential. Close monitoring of the INR is advised when concomitant medication is altered.

The approach taken to reverse over-anticoagulation with warfarin depends on the circumstances (see Table 4). Prothrombin complex concentrates, unlike fresh frozen plasma, reliably and rapidly correct the defect and should be used in life-threatening situations such as intracranial bleeding. Small doses of phytomenadione (vitamin K₁) can lower a high INR without making subsequent anticoagulation difficult, as is the case if high doses are given.

Fibrinolysis

Thrombolytic agents dissolve thrombi by directly or indirectly activating the zymogen plasminogen to plasmin. Plasmin then degrades fibrin to soluble peptides, but cannot distinguish fibrin in pathological thrombi from

Table 2 Duration of warfarin treatment

	Distal DVT	Proximal DVT/PE
Reversible risk factor	6 weeks	6 months*
Idiopathic	6 months*	6 months

*Consider shorter treatment (e.g. 3 months) if risk factors for bleeding (e.g. age).
Consider long-term treatment if recurrent or if associated with significant thrombophilic defect(s).
DVT, deep vein thrombosis; PE, pulmonary embolism.

fibrin in haemostatic plugs and it may also degrade and so deplete plasma fibrinogen. The use of thrombolytic agents for venous thromboembolism requires careful individual assessment. It is rarely given in deep vein thrombosis though its use can be considered in massive ileofemoral thrombosis. Although thrombolytic therapy for pulmonary embolism achieves more rapid resolution than heparin alone, there is no clear evidence of lasting benefit. Patients with pulmonary embolism who survive long enough to

Table 3 Many drugs interact with warfarin, the evidence is strongest for those listed

Potentiation	Inhibition
Amiodarone	Barbiturates
Cimetidine	Carbamazepine
Clofibrate	Chlordiazepoxide
Cotrimoxazole	Cholestyramine
Erythromycin	Griseofulvin
Fluconazole	Rifampicin
Isoniazid	Sucralfate
Metronidazole	
Miconazole	
Omeprazole	
Paracetamol	
Phenylbutazone	
Piroxicam	
Propafenone	
Propanolol	
Statins	
Sulphinpyrazone	

Table 4 Management of over-anticoagulation with warfarin

Major bleeding
Stop warfarin
Give PCC (50 IU/kg) or FFP (15 ml/kg)
Give vitamin K (5 mg intravenously)
No bleeding/minor bleeding
Stop warfarin until INR < 5
If: INR > 8 give phytomenadione
    INR 8–12 give 0.5 mg intravenously or 2.5 mg orally
    INR >12 give 1 mg intravenously or 5 mg orally

FFP, fresh frozen plasma; PCC, prothrombin complex concentrates. PCC should be used for life-threatening bleeding.

have the diagnosis made and treatment with heparin begun have an excellent prognosis, unless they have associated severe medical disease. Thrombolytic therapy, which carries a much greater risk of bleeding, is therefore reserved for those cases of massive pulmonary embolism with haemodynamic instability threatening the patient's life (see Chapter 15.15.3.1).

Streptokinase (which forms a complex with plasminogen that then activates free plasminogen), urokinase, and tissue plasminogen activator (**tPA**) have all been used. For pulmonary embolism, streptokinase is recommended as a 250 000 IU loading dose followed by an infusion for 24 h at 100 000 IU/h. Urokinase is given as a 4400 IU/kg loading dose followed by 2200 IU/kg.h for 12 h. Following the success of rapid fibrinolytic regimens in myocardial infarction, tPA given as 100 mg over 2 h has been used for pulmonary embolism, and the use of more rapid regimens with the other two agents has been suggested (see Chapter 15.15.3.1 for further discussion).

Treatment of venous thromboembolism in pregnancy

Heparin does not cross the placenta and can be used in pregnancy, as described above, but higher doses of unfractionated heparin are sometimes needed to achieve therapeutic levels. As pregnant women are excluded from clinical trials, experience with low-molecular-weight heparin is limited. However, the evidence seems to indicate that low-molecular-weight heparin, with all its logistical advantages, can be used effectively and safely in pregnancy.

The real problem is warfarin, which crosses the placenta and can cause an embryopathy if given between 6 and 12 weeks' gestation. At any time it can cause fetal bleeding and has been associated with central nervous system abnormalities. The usual treatment recommended for venous thromboembolism in pregnancy is to continue with full-dose heparin until term (long-term treatment with unfractionated heparin can be given by subcutaneous injection once every 12 h, and with low-molecular-weight heparin by injection once daily). As heparin may cause osteopenia (possibly less of a risk with low-molecular-weight heparin) some would consider the use of warfarin after the first trimester, switching back to heparin at 36 weeks. Warfarin can be used for the 6 weeks of the puerperium, and women taking warfarin can breast feed.

Further reading

Anonymous (1998). Guidelines on oral anticoagulation: third edition. *British Journal of Haematology* **101**, 374–87.

Anand S *et al.* (1996). The relation between the activated partial thromboplastin time response and recurrence in patients with venous thrombosis treated with continuous intravenous heparin. *Archives of Internal Medicine* **156**, 1677–81.

Leizorovicz A *et al.* (1994). Comparison of efficacy and safety of low molecular weight heparins and unfractionated heparin in initial treatment of deep venous thrombosis: a meta-analysis. *British Medical Journal* **309**, 299–304.

15.16 Hypertension

15.16.1 Essential hypertension

15.16.1.1 Prevalence, epidemiology, and pathophysiology of hypertension

C. G. Isles

Definitions of hypertension

The simplest and most widely accepted definition of hypertension in an adult is that hypertension is present when clinic systolic pressure exceeds 140 mmHg and/or clinic diastolic pressure exceeds 90 mmHg. The American and World Health Organization International Society of Hypertension definition of hypertension, reproduced in Table 1, gives a more detailed classification of blood pressure for adults aged over 18 years. Any definition of abnormality that is based on a measurement distributed within the population as a continuous variable, such as blood pressure, serum cholesterol, or height, must necessarily be somewhat arbitrary, and so it is with hypertension.

Prevalence

United Kingdom studies

Estimates of prevalence vary. The number of measurements made, the method used, and the circumstances in which measurements are made all influence prevalence. Also important here are age, gender, race, and socioeconomic status. In a representative population sample of 10 359 Scottish men and women aged 40 to 59 years between 1984 and 1986, and based on the average of two measurements at a single screening visit in a primary care setting, 1262 (25 per cent) men and 1061 (20 per cent) women were

Table 1 Classification of blood pressure for adults aged 18 years and older[a]

Category	Systolic	Diastolic
Optimal	< 120	< 80
Normal	< 130	< 85
High normal	130–139	85–89
Hypertension[b]		
Stage 1	140–159	90–99
Stage 2	160–179	100–109
Stage 3	≥ 180	≥ 110
Isolated systolic	≥ 140	< 90

[a] Based on the average of two or more readings taken at each of two or more visits after initial screening.

[b] When systolic and diastolic pressures fall into different categories, the higher category should be selected.

considered to be hypertensive, defined in this study as a blood pressure of 160/95 mmHg or higher or receiving antihypertensive drug treatment. A more recent survey of 12 116 English adults aged 16 years or more in 1994 yielded similar results. Based on the average of the second and third of three readings at a single screening visit in the respondent's home, 19 per cent of men and 20 per cent of women had a blood pressure of 160/95 mmHg or higher or were receiving antihypertensive drug treatment. Both surveys probably overestimate the prevalence of hypertension in the United Kingdom because they were based on the average of readings at a single screening session.

United States studies

The value of repeated measurements at different visits in determining prevalence of hypertension is apparent in a study of 158 906 mixed-race individuals aged 30 to 69 years examined in their homes or work places in the United States in the early 1970s. Twenty-five per cent had a diastolic blood pressure of 90 mmHg or higher at the first screen. When these subjects were rescreened in a clinic setting, there was a substantial fall in blood pressure such that only 25 per cent (6.4 per cent of the original cohort) remained hypertensive. The majority (75 per cent) were mildly hypertensive with a diastolic blood pressure in the range 90 to 104 mmHg. Put another way, in this large population survey most individuals with hypertension identified had a mild to moderate elevation of blood pressure, with less than 2 per cent of those screened having sustained hypertension with a diastolic blood pressure higher than 105 mmHg after two measurements.

The importance of age as a determinant of prevalence of hypertension is evident from data collected during the 1988 to 1991 National Health and Nutrition Examination Survey. The proportion of the United States population having a systolic blood pressure of 140 mmHg or higher, or a diastolic blood pressure of 90 mmHg or higher, based on the average of six measurements at two visits, or currently being treated with an antihypertensive drug, was 4 per cent for young adults aged 18 to 29 years, increasing to 65 per cent for those over 80 years (Fig. 1).

Recent data from Framingham, United States suggest that the increasing use of antihypertensive medication has resulted in a decline in the prevalence of hypertension. In an analysis of 10 333 subjects aged 45 to 74 years, examined over a 40-year period from 1950 to 1989, using definitions of 160 mmHg systolic or 100 mmHg diastolic on or off treatment, and based on an average of two separate measurements at each visit, the prevalence of hypertension decreased from 18.5 to 9.2 per cent for men, and from 28.0 to 7.7 per cent for women (Fig. 2).

Measuring blood pressure

If blood pressure is to be measured precisely, a device with validated accuracy that is properly maintained and calibrated must be used. For a long time the mercury sphygmomanometer has been the gold standard in clinical practice but—for health and safety reasons related to mercury—is likely to be replaced by aneroid, semi-automatic and automated devices in the near future. Information on the accuracy of the alternatives to mercury

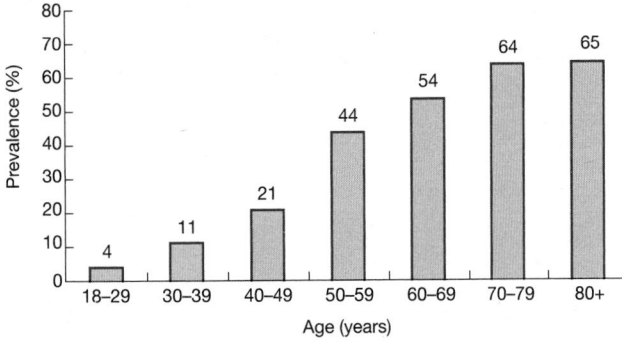

Fig. 1 Prevalence of hypertension, defined as a systolic blood pressure of 140 mmHg or higher, or a diastolic blood pressure of 90 mmHg or higher in the United States. Prevalence increases with advancing age. Adapted with permission from NHANES III.

sphygmomanometers can be obtained from the British Hypertension Society Information Services (e-mail: bhsis@sghms.ac.uk; website: www.hyp.a-c.uk/bhs/).

Cuff size

Whatever method is employed, a cuff with an appropriately sized bladder should be applied to the upper arm, leaving adequate space for the bell of a stethoscope to be positioned in the antecubital fossa. The arm should be supported at the level of the heart and unrestricted by tight clothing. For most patients an appropriately sized bladder is 14 by 35 cm, sometimes known as the alternative adult cuff. Smaller bladders will over-read blood pressure in fat arms, while larger bladders as used in thigh cuffs are too unwieldy for routine use. It is good practice to measure the blood pressure in both arms at the first visit and then to select the arm with the higher reading for future measurements; also to record pressure both seated and standing initially to exclude a significant postural fall, more likely in elderly and diabetic subjects.

Clinic/doctor's office (surgery)

If a mercury sphygmomanometer is being used, the correct procedure for measurement is to deflate the cuff at 2 mm/s and read blood pressure to the nearest 2 mmHg, recording diastolic pressure at the disappearance of the sounds (phase V). Patients in whom the sounds never disappear probably have arterial disease of their upper limb vessels causing turbulent flow and should have their pressure recorded as systolic/diastolic phase IV (muffling)/0 mmHg. At least two measurements should be made at each visit. Because blood pressure tends to fall with repeated measurements, patients whose pressure is found to be greater than 140/90 mmHg should be brought back for further measurements at intervals that may vary from 1 day to 1 month, according to the level of their pressure, before a diagnosis of sustained hypertension is made.

Home/ambulatory

Interest in home and ambulatory blood pressure measurement continues to grow. Both techniques permit the recording of numerous values in settings that are closer to daily life than the clinic or office. By averaging up to 60 readings taken at intervals of 20 to 30 min over the course of 24 h, ambulatory blood pressure measurement improves precision and reproducibility in blood pressure measurement. It also correlates more closely than clinic blood pressure with risk, as judged by evidence of target organ damage, but lacks the authority of an outcome trial, which means that it is not possible to recommend ambulatory blood pressure measurement over clinic pressure in routine practice.

White coat hypertension

Despite the reservations expressed above, ambulatory blood pressure measurement is widely used and can be valuable in a number of circumstances. Foremost among these is the evaluation of the patient with suspected white coat hypertension, also known as isolated clinic or office hypertension. White coat hypertension is present in up to 10 per cent of the hypertensive population and is usually defined as persistent clinic or office hypertension greater than 140/90 mmHg in the face of consistently normal readings less than 135/85 mmHg at home. Because white coat hypertension carries much less risk of cardiovascular disease, the decision to recommend or withhold drug treatment must be based on the overall risk profile. Subjects whose risk is low require continued monitoring only, whereas patients who already have vascular disease or are at high risk of developing vascular disease, for instance because they have diabetes or target organ damage, should be given antihypertensive drug therapy.

Other indications for ambulatory blood pressure measurement

Ambulatory blood pressure measurement may also be indicated in a number of other circumstances: when clinic blood pressure is unusually variable; when patients complain of postural symptoms related to their drug therapy; and in resistant hypertension, defined here as blood pressure greater than 150/90 mmHg despite lifestyle measures and three or more antihypertensive drugs. Whatever the indication for ambulatory blood pressure measurement, the average daytime pressure is recommended for decisions on treatment, rather than the average 24-h pressure or the percentage of readings that lie above a certain threshold. It must also be recognized that ambulatory blood pressure is systematically lower than clinic or office blood pressure by an average of at least 10/5 mmHg. This means that treatment thresholds and targets for achieved blood pressure should be adjusted downwards when using ambulatory blood pressure measurement. Pending the outcome of further prospective observational studies, average daytime ambulatory pressure of less than 135/85 mmHg should be regarded as probably normal, and average daytime ambulatory pressure of greater than 140/90 mmHg as probably abnormal and requiring drug treatment.

Epidemiology
Renfrew Paisley survey

Hypertension is an important contributor to morbidity and mortality from cardiovascular disease, particularly when present in combination with other cardiovascular risk factors. This is apparent from any one of a number of observational studies. The data shown in Fig. 3 are from the Renfrew and Paisley Survey in Scotland and show quite clearly that in this Western population, the relative risk of diastolic pressure for both coronary heart disease and stroke is approximately two to three in both sexes, when comparing high-risk with low-risk subjects; also that the rates of coronary heart disease are higher than those of stroke at all levels of blood pressure; and that coronary deaths are more common in men than in women, while gender differences in stroke mortality are much less apparent.

Framingham

Some authorities have suggested that the combined effects of risk factors are multiplicative rather than additive. Thus in Framingham, the probability of a 40-year-old male with a systolic pressure of 195 mmHg developing coronary heart disease over 6 years is said to be 10-fold greater if he smokes and has plasma cholesterol of 9 mmol/l with glucose intolerance and electrocardiographic left ventricular hypertrophy. The problem with data such as these is that very few subjects in Framingham (or elsewhere) possess so many risk factors. This means that the estimates of risk must necessarily be based on mathematical models rather than on actual numbers of events:

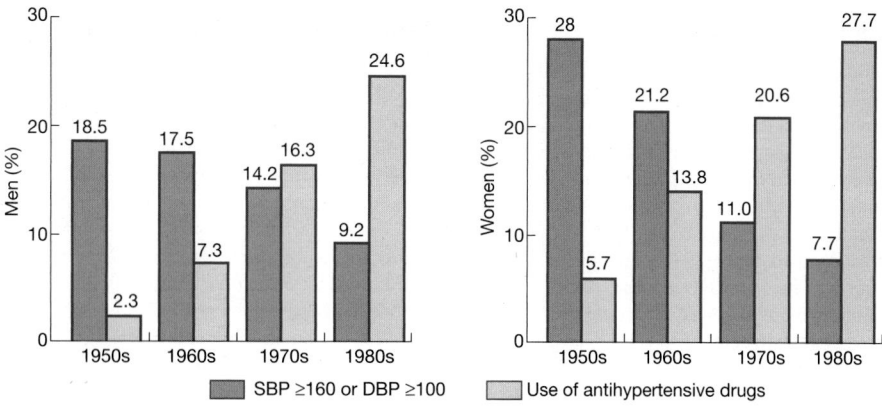

Fig. 2 Age-adjusted temporal trends in prevalence of raised blood pressure and use of antihypertensive drugs among men and women 45 to 74 years of age in Framingham, United States. Adapted with permission.

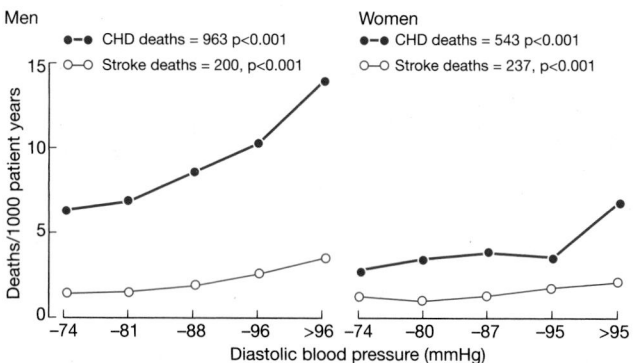

Fig. 3 Deaths per 1000 patient years among men and women aged 45 to 64 years after 17 years of follow-up in Renfrew and Paisley, Scotland. *P* value indicates significance of trend across quintiles of diastolic blood pressure. Reproduced with permission.

indeed the authors of the Framingham study concede that the models used assume a degree of non-linearity (Kannel WB, personal communication).

Oxford meta-analysis

The most powerful and persuasive study of the association between blood pressure and risk remains the Oxford meta-analysis of 843 strokes and 4856 coronary heart disease events in 420 000 individuals followed in nine major prospective observational studies for an average of 10 years (Fig. 4). The results of this meta-analysis were corrected for a phenomenon known as regression dilution bias by using repeated measurements to determine an individual's long-term average blood pressure, and showed that the relation between diastolic blood pressure, stroke, and coronary heart disease was at least 60 per cent stronger than had previously been thought. Within the range of diastolic blood pressure 70 to 110 mmHg, the risk of stroke and coronary heart disease was positive, continuous, and independent of other risk factors, even when diastolic pressure was supposedly normal, namely 70–90 mmHg. This raises the intriguing possibility, recently confirmed by the results of PROGRESS, that lowering blood pressure in 'normotensive' high-risk subjects might reduce their risk of vascular disease.

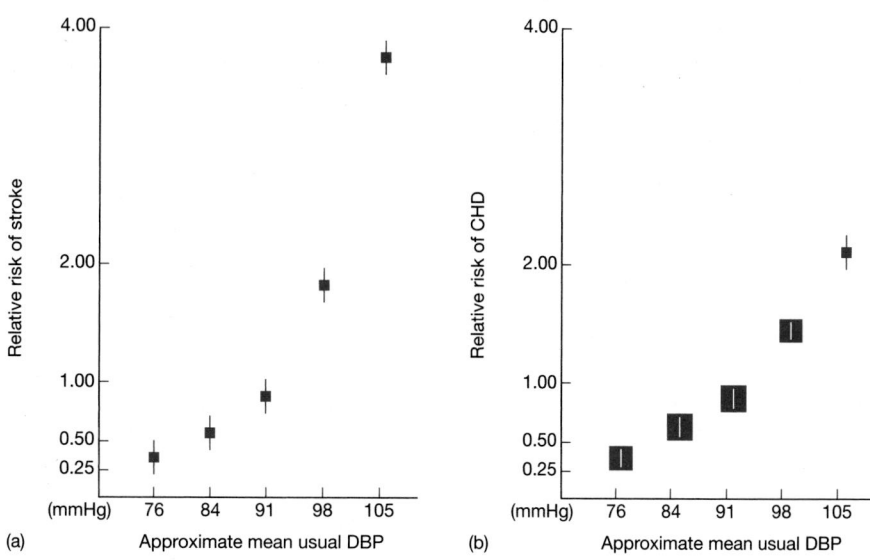

Fig. 4 Relation between diastolic blood pressure, stroke, and coronary heart disease during an average of 10 years follow-up. (a) Stroke and usual diastolic blood pressure. Seven prospective observational studies: 843 events. (b) Coronary heart disease and usual diastolic blood pressure. Nine prospective observational studies: 4856 events. (Reproduced with permission.)

Systolic hypertension and pulse pressure

Systolic blood pressure rises in a linear fashion with age, whereas diastolic pressure increases until the age of 50 then levels off and even begins to fall. This leads to an important transition in the form of hypertension with age. Isolated diastolic hypertension is more common in younger subjects, whilst isolated systolic hypertension emerges as the most common form of hypertension in the elderly. The underlying pathological process is loss of arterial elastic tissue, which means that the pressure wave created by left ventricular contraction can no longer be damped by the aorta and major vessels. Although clinicians have tended to focus on the diastolic component of blood pressure in the past, systolic blood pressure is a better predictor of cardiovascular risk and isolated systolic hypertension is now recognized to be an independent risk factor of cardiovascular disease. A wide pulse pressure has a similar influence on prognosis (Fig. 5).

Likely benefits of treatment

The relative risk of high blood pressure for heart attack and stroke is higher among younger subjects and decreases with age. Absolute risk, by contrast, increases with age. This means that attributable risk, which is the number of events that would be avoided if blood pressure were lower, is likely to be higher in the elderly. A similar logic can be applied to the likely impact of interventions that reduce mean blood pressure by even a few millimetres of mercury. The steepness of the slope relating diastolic blood pressure and stroke in the Oxford meta-analysis suggests that more strokes might be avoided than coronary heart disease events. However, the attributable risk of diastolic blood pressure for coronary heart disease, that is the number of coronary heart disease events that would be avoided if diastolic blood pressure were lower, is likely to be as great simply because coronary heart disease is more common than stroke in most Western populations.

Heart failure, renal disease, and recurrent events

Blood pressure is a powerful determinant not only of heart attack and stroke but also of heart failure and renal failure. A non-linear or J-shaped association between blood pressure and recurrent events has been reported for patients with previous myocardial infarction. Despite concerns that this might represent an adverse consequence of treatment, it is is now considered more likely to reflect the effect of disease on blood pressure—the bigger the myocardial infarction the bigger the fall in pressure—than the effect of blood pressure or its treatment on the disease.

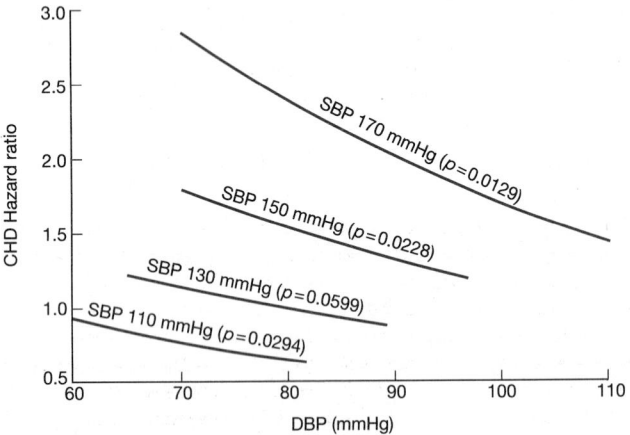

Fig. 5 Adjusted CHD risk in 1924 Framingham men and women between 50 and 79 years with no clinical evidence of CHD at baseline. At any given level of systolic pressure, risk was higher in those whose diastolic pressure was lower, highlighting the predictive power of pulse pressure..

Hypertension in black populations

Ethnic variations in the incidence, pathophysiology, and complications of hypertension are well described. Hypertension is more common in black than white populations, and more common in urban than rural black populations. Black individuals have a higher incidence of salt-sensitive hypertension than white individuals, and retain more sodium leading to expanded plasma volumes and lower plasma renin activity. The complications of hypertension also tend to be different in black populations with a higher incidence of left ventricular hypertrophy, stroke, and renal failure, and lower risk of coronary heart disease. The increased frequency of left ventricular hypertrophy, stroke, and renal failure may relate to the severity of hypertension in black individuals, and their relative lack of coronary heart disease may be due to more favourable lipid profiles.

Gender differences

Hypertension is an important risk factor for cardiovascular disease in women. Although premenopausal women have lower blood pressure than age-matched men, the prevalence of hypertension is higher in women than men after the age of 65. Obesity is significantly more common in middle-aged and older women, and is likely to contribute to the crossover in prevalence. Oral contraceptive use increases the risk of hypertension in younger women. Hormone replacement therapy (HRT) does not raise blood pressure in women who are normotensive at the start of treatment, but more research is required to determine whether blood pressure rises when hypertensive postmenopausal women are given HRT.

Pathophysiology

When asked to define hypertension, the clinician may reply 'that level of blood pressure above which treatment does more good than harm'. The response of the pathophysiologist is likely to be more complex, reflecting the fact that we don't fully understand the mechanisms involved. Most individuals with hypertension have essential hypertension, which is best thought of as a progressive rise in pressure with age, as a result of an interplay between genetic factors, environmental influences, and blood pressure control mechanisms. A much smaller number of patients (certainly less than 5 per cent of the hypertensive population) will have a renal or adrenal cause for their high blood pressure (see Chapter 20.10.2).

Genetic factors

The fact that high blood pressure runs in families does not tell us whether the genes or environment are responsible, because families usually share both. Helpful in sorting this out are studies of adopted children within a family, and of twins living apart. The twin studies suggest that approximately 50 per cent of the blood pressure variability between individuals is related to inheritable factors. The genetic component of the development of high blood pressure may not itself necessarily cause hypertension. Rather there may be a genetic predisposition to develop raised blood pressure in response to various environmental factors. For further information on the genetics of hypertension see Chapter 15.16.1.2.

Environmental influences

Environmental influences are more easily studied than genetic factors. Evidence of their importance comes from a number of sources, including studies of migrants, comparison between different communities, prospective population studies, and randomized trials of behaviour modification.

Migrant studies

Adults who migrate adopt the level of blood pressure, frequency of hypertension, and coronary heart disease risk of their destinations. Primitive Kenyan Luo tribespeople moving in search of work from their villages in rural Kenya to the urban slums of Nairobi show marked increases in blood pressure and body weight within a month of migration. Similar findings have been reported for Australian Aborigines migrating from the bush to Melbourne.

Comparison between different communities

In developed countries such as the United Kingdom, the rise in blood pressure that occurs with age is well recognized. The mechanisms responsible for this are not physiologically inevitable because primitive rural populations, most notably the Yanamamo Indians of Brazil and certain New Guinea tribes, show only a tiny rise in blood pressure with advancing age. These observations suggest that the rise in blood pressure seen with advancing age in urban societies must be due to some very powerful environmental factors.

Prospective population studies

A classic study compared Italian women entering a nunnery with a control group of women from the same town. In the control group, blood pressure rose normally with age whereas the nuns showed no rise in blood pressure over 20 years of follow-up. In another example, blood pressure did not rise as expected with age in long-term residents of a psychiatric hospital who entered with normal blood pressure. Studies such as these also provide evidence of which environmental influences might be important.

Specific environmental factors

The best known environmental influences on blood pressure are obesity, alcohol, and salt. Early nutritional deficiency may be important, and recent evidence suggests that psychosocial factors are likely to play a role in the development of essential hypertension. A small socio-economic gradient of blood pressure has been observed: inverse for developed and positive for developing countries. This probably reflects the higher prevalence of obesity, alcohol, and salt intake among those of lower socio-economic status in developed countries, and higher socio-economic status in developing countries. Recent evidence, to be discussed later, suggests that diets rich in fruit and vegetables with low total and saturated fats may protect against hypertension. Low calcium intake, although associated with hypertension in population studies, is now considered to play no part in pathogenesis.

Obesity

Fat people have higher blood pressures than thin people. This is not merely a consequence of cuff artefact, which is the tendency to overestimate blood pressure in fat arms when small cuffs are used, because the relation persists after correcting for arm circumference. Most studies have used body mass index (normal range 20 to 25 kg/m^2) as a measure of obesity, although it is probable that high blood pressure correlates more closely with an android (apple-shaped) rather than a gynoid (pear-shaped) fat distribution. This suggests that at least some of the association between blood pressure and obesity is due to sex hormones, which are an important determinant of these body features.

Epidemiologically there is an association between high blood pressure, obesity, impaired glucose tolerance, and dyslipidaemia (particularly low high-density lipoproteins with high triglycerides). The possibility that obesity causes insulin resistance which leads in turn to the other metabolic disturbances in the so-called insulin resistance syndrome is the subject of a great deal of research, and may explain why fat people are more prone to heart disease. The cause and effect relationship between obesity and hypertension has been confirmed in randomized trials, which show that blood pressure falls when hypertensive obese patients are given calorie restricted diets. The degree of blood pressure reduction is variable, but a 1 mmHg fall in diastolic blood pressure for each kilogram reduction in body weight might reasonably be anticipated from the data in these trials.

Alcohol

Epidemiological data have consistently shown an association between alcohol intake and blood pressure, while intervention trials confirm that blood pressure falls when alcohol is withdrawn from heavy drinkers. Moderate

drinking (2 to 3 units daily where 1 unit is equivalent to 8 to 10 g of ethanol) does not appear to exert a pressor effect, and is likely to be beneficial in coronary heart disease. The mechanism of the pressor effect in heavy drinkers is unknown. In a prospective study of 490 000 men and women in the United States, the relative risk of death from cardiovascular disease in moderate drinkers compared with non-drinkers was 0.7 for men and 0.6 for women.

Salt

The role of dietary sodium intake in the pathogenesis of essential hypertension, and of dietary sodium restriction in its treatment, is probably more controversial now than it was at the time of the last edition of this textbook. The failure to observe a rise in blood pressure with ageing and the absence of essential hypertension in some non-Westernised cultures has been attributed to very low sodium intake. However, there are other reasons why blood pressure in primitive societies may differ from blood pressure in the United Kingdom, United States, and Europe. Opinions on the merits or otherwise of sodium restriction are similarly polarized.

Those who favour the sodium hypothesis point to the results of randomized controlled trials of sodium restriction in hypertensive subjects. These suggest that sodium intake can be halved to less than 100 mmol/day with a fall in blood pressure of approximately 4/2 mmHg, leading to a worthwhile reduction in the number of individuals requiring antihypertensive therapy. By contrast, those who argue against the sodium hypothesis can claim that a systolic pressure reduction of less than 1 mmHg in normotensive subjects does not support a general recommendation to reduce sodium intake; and that a low sodium diet may have adverse effects on plasma renin, aldosterone, noradrenaline, total cholesterol, and low-density lipoprotein cholesterol.

Ultimately the health effects of a low sodium diet will only be resolved by trials relating nutrition to morbidity and mortality. Until such time as these have been completed, public policy recommendations regarding sodium intake for the general population should probably be withheld. Moderate salt restriction can still be recommended as a supplementary therapy in hypertensive individuals requiring drug treatment.

Fetal and infant growth

Babies who are small at birth have higher blood pressures during adolescence and are more likely to be hypertensive as adults. The relationship strengthens with advancing age such that subjects in their 60s show a decrease of approximately 5 mmHg for every 1 kg increase in birth weight. This has been interpreted as evidence that differences in blood pressure are initiated *in utero* and then amplified during adult life, and may explain a number of important clinical findings, including the higher prevalence of hypertension in black individuals, who are more likely to have small babies than white individuals, and also the increased risk of coronary heart disease seen in adults of low birth weight. For further discussion of this and similar issues see Chapter 15.4.1.1.

Psychosocial stress

It is well known that acute stress can raise blood pressure acutely—the act of taking blood pressure for example can increase systolic by up to 75 mmHg—and it has long been suspected that chronic stress may be a risk factor for hypertension. However, the role of chronic stress has been difficult to assess, partly because stress means different things to different people, and partly because stress is not easy to measure.

Recently, using sophisticated measures of assessment including ambulatory monitoring, it has been shown that in men, but not in women, job strain is associated with an elevated blood pressure, not only at work but also while at home and during sleep. Job strain is defined here as the result of a highly demanding job with low control, as in a shop-floor worker. Subjects in demanding jobs who are able to exert control over their work patterns (e.g. doctors !), do not show the same elevation of blood pressure.

The effect of job strain on blood pressure is independent of other environmental influences, and is as strong as that of obesity.

Blood pressure control mechanisms

The third components of the triad leading to essential hypertension are the blood pressure control mechanisms. Necessarily, these become involved as hypertension develops. The challenge for the researcher is to know whether abnormalities of the regulatory mechanisms are cause, consequence, confounder, or coincidental change. By comparison with our knowledge of environmental influences, this is an area fraught with difficulty.

Importance of the kidney

Transplantation experiments in genetically hypertensive rats, and observations following renal transplantation in humans, suggest that hypertension must result at least in part from renal mechanisms. For example, if a kidney from a genetically hypertensive rat is given to a control rat then that animal develops high blood pressure. Conversely, transplantation of a control kidney into a genetically hypertensive rat prevents the development of hypertension. Further studies have suggested that the genetic abnormality in the kidney expresses itself as a difficulty in handling sodium.

The resistance vessels

Blood pressure (BP) is a haemodynamic variable that depends on two other haemodynamic factors— cardiac output (CO) and total peripheral resistance (TPR), where BP = CO × TPR. The hallmark of essential hypertension is increased peripheral resistance with a normal cardiac output, and because of this any discussion on the pathogenesis of essential hypertension must centre on the resistance vessels. These are not the large arteries or capillaries, but the small arterioles.

The walls of small arterioles contain smooth muscle cells that respond to both circulatory and local hormonal influences, and to neural input through the sympathetic nervous system (Fig. 6). There is evidence that increased pressure within these small vessels leads to structural changes in vascular morphology, particularly an increase in the ratio of media thickness:lumen diameter. Recent data suggest this occurs mainly as a result of vascular remodelling (the rearrangement of existing material around a small lumen) and to a lesser extent by myocyte hypertrophy.

The possibility that these structural changes might act as vascular amplifiers in the hypertensive circulation, both contributing to and maintaining the rise in pressure, has been the subject of much debate. While undoubtedly attractive, the amplifier theory is not supported by results of studies that show no increase in pressor responsiveness when vasoconstrictor stimuli are infused into chronically hypertensive rats; or by restoration of normal pressure in rats when a pressor stimulus is withdrawn, before structural changes have reversed. The clinical significance of the structural changes in small blood vessels is therefore uncertain.

Atrial natriuretic peptides

A bewildering number of homeostatic mechanisms interact in a complex fashion to maintain blood pressure and adjust it in response to changing circumstances. Atrial natriuretic peptide (**ANP**) is one of a family of natriuretic peptides whose other members are brain natriuretic peptide (**BNP**) and C-type natriuretic peptide (**CNP**). ANP is secreted primarily by the right atrium when the atrial wall is stretched. BNP was identified initially in the brain but is also present in the ventricles and circulates in the blood at approximately one-fifth of the plasma level of ANP. CNP is produced by vascular endothelial cells and in the kidney.

The actions of ANP, which are mediated by its attachment to a specific receptor on the cell membrane, the natriuretic peptide receptor A, include natriuresis, diuresis, decreased secretion of renin and aldosterone, vasodilatation, and a modest fall in blood pressure. These effects raise the possibility that ANP may be involved in the development and maintenance of high blood pressure in essential hypertension. ANP is indeed implicated in the regulation of arterial pressure, but a lack of ANP is unlikely to be the cause of essential hypertension. From a therapeutic viewpoint, however, it is now possible to reduce blood pressure using a new class of drugs that combine neutral endopeptidase inhibition (which blocks the breakdown of ANP) and ACE inhibition.

Endothelial-based systems

The endothelium is known to play an important role in the regulation of vascular tone. Endothelial cells form nitric oxide from L-arginine via the activity of nitric oxide synthase. Nitric oxide, formally known as endothelium-derived relaxing factor or EDRF, is a powerful local vasodilator that also inhibits platelet aggregation and vascular smooth muscle cell proliferation. The action of nitric oxide is opposed by endothelin, a powerful vasoconstrictor peptide also secreted by endothelial cells, and a host of other vasoconstrictor influences. For further discussion see Chapter 15.1.1.2.

Using an analogue of arginine called L-NMMA which inhibits the action of nitric oxide synthase, it has been possible to show a decrease in nitric oxide production in the vasculature of patients with high blood pressure. However, the evidence suggests this is more likely to be a consequence than a cause of hypertension in humans. Equally, the demonstration that endothelin receptor antagonists reduce blood pressure does not prove that an excess of endothelin is the cause of hypertension.

Renin–angiotensin systems

Renin is an enzyme produced by the juxtaglomerular apparatus of the kidney in response to falls in renal perfusion pressure, sodium depletion, and increased sympathetic nerve activity. Renin acts on its substrate angiotensinogen to produce the decapeptide angiotensin I, which is in turn is cleaved by angiotensin-converting enzyme to give angiotensin II. Angiotension II is the effector component of the system, with a number of important actions on blood vessels (contraction), heart (hypertrophy), kidney (glomerulosclerosis), and adrenal cortex (release of aldosterone). In health, aldosterone feeds back on the kidney to cause sodium retention and potassium excretion, and in this way homeostasis is maintained (Fig. 7).

Recent interest in the renin–angiotensin system has focused on the demonstration that renin may be synthesized in a number of tissues apart from the kidney, including adrenal, heart, the blood vessel wall, and brain. Tissue renin–angiotensin systems have been implicated in the regulation of mineralocorticoid secretion by the adrenal cortex, left ventricular hypertrophy, resistance vessel hypertrophy, and central nervous control of blood pressure.

The role of the renin–angiotensin system in the pathogenesis of essential hypertension is unclear. Plasma renin levels vary widely in essential hypertension from low (30 per cent), to normal (50 per cent), to high (20 per

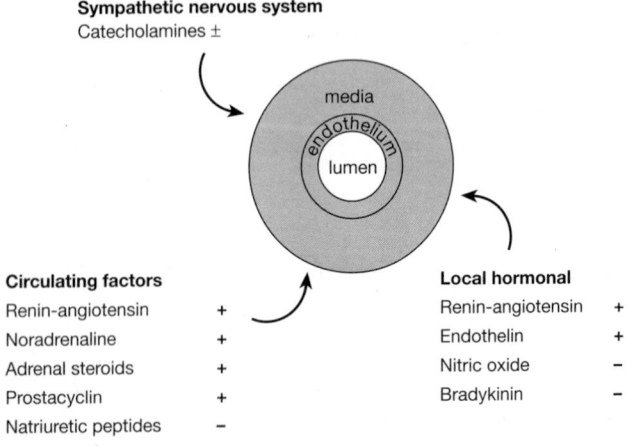

Sympathetic nervous system
Catecholamines ±

media
endothelium
lumen

Circulating factors

Renin-angiotensin	+
Noradrenaline	+
Adrenal steroids	+
Prostacyclin	+
Natriuretic peptides	−

Local hormonal

Renin-angiotensin	+
Endothelin	+
Nitric oxide	−
Bradykinin	−

Fig. 6 Arteriolar tone is determined by circulatory and local hormonal influences, also by neural input through the sympathetic nervous system. + vasoconstriction, - vasodilation.

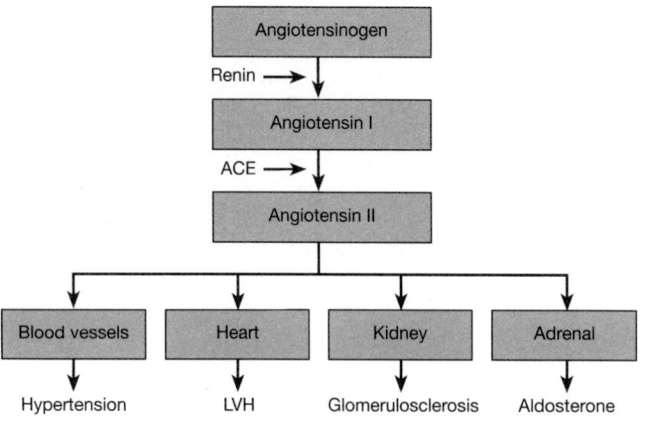

Fig. 7 The renin–angiotensin system.

cent). Hypertensive individuals with low renin are usually considered to have volume-dependent hypertension (that is their renin levels are suppressed), whereas high renin in hypertensive individuals may reflect increased levels of sympathetic nervous system activity. Black individuals and the elderly have a high prevalence of low renin hypertension, which may be the reason these groups respond best to diuretics. In everyday clinical practice, however, baseline renin measurements are hardly ever requested or needed.

Sympathetic nervous system

The sympathetic nervous system is known to be involved in the regulation of arteriolar resistance (Fig. 6), also of cardiac output, renin release by the kidney, and catecholamine and mineralocorticoid release by the adrenal gland, and as such might reasonably be expected to have a role in the pathophysiology of essential hypertension. There is no evidence however of sustained overactivity of the sympathetic nervous system in essential hypertension, and even though drugs that block the sympathetic nervous system can lower blood pressure, this does not prove that overactivity of the system is the cause of the disease. In summary, it seems unlikely that a defect in any one of the regulatory mechanisms is directly responsible for the rise in blood pressure in essential hypertension. More probably essential hypertension is a consequence of interactions between several mechanisms, the exact nature of which remain to be determined.

Further reading

Appel LG *et al.* (1997). A clinical trial of the effects of dietary patterns on blood pressure. DASH Collaborative Research Group. *New England Journal of Medicine* 336, 1117–24. [New evidence that diets rich in fruit and vegetables with low total unsaturated fats may protect against hypertension.]

August P, Oparil S (1999). Hypertension in women. *Journal of Clinical Endocrinology and Metabolism* 84, 1862–6. [Up-to-date review.]

Burt VL *et al.* (1995). Prevalence of hypertension in the US adult population. Results from the Third National Health and Nutrition Examination Survey 1988–1991. *Hypertension* 25, 305–13. [Large United States cross-sectional survey of hypertension prevalence, treatment, and control.]

Colhoun HM, Dong W, Poulter NR (1998). Blood pressure screening, management and control in England: results from the Health Survey for England 1994. *Journal of Hypertension* 16, 747–52. [Includes prevalence data for hypertension in a contemporary English population.]

Flack J *et al.* for the Multiple Risk Factor Intervention Trial Research Group (1995). Blood pressure and mortality among men with prior myocardial infarction. *Circulation* 92, 2437–45. [A J-curve analysis which supports the view that the main risk associated with blood pressure in survivors of myocardial infarction is due to high rather than low blood pressure.]

Franklin SS *et al.* (1999). Is pulse pressure useful in predicting risk for coronary heart disease? The Framingham Heart Study. *Circulation* 100, 353–60. [An analysis of Framingham data showing the predictive power of pulse pressure.]

Gibbons GH (1998). The pathophysiology of hypertension: the importance of angiotensin II in cardiovascular remodelling. *American Journal of Hypertension* 11, 177S–181S. [Emerging data on the role of the tissue renin–angiotensin system.]

Gibbs CR, Beevers DG, Lip GYH (1999). The management of hypertensive disease in black patients. *Quarterly Journal of Medicine* 92, 187–92. [Up-to-date review.]

Graudal NA, Galoe AM, Garred P (1998). Effects of sodium restriction on blood pressure, renin, aldosterone, catecholamines, cholesterols and triglyceride: a meta-analysis. *Journal of the American Medical Association* 279, 1383–91. [The results of this meta-analysis do not support a general recommendation to reduce sodium intake]

Guidelines Sub-Committee (1999). 1999 World Health Organization International Society of Hypertension Guidelines for the Management of Hypertension. *Journal of Hypertension* 17, 151–83. [The latest edition of the only international guideline.]

Heggarty AM (1997). Significance of structural changes in small arteries in hypertension. *Blood Pressure* 6(Supp 2), 31–3. [A review of the changes that occur in small blood vessels and their possible clinical significance.]

Isles C (1995). Blood pressure in males and females. *Journal of Hypertension* 13, 285–90. [An analysis of blood pressure in the Renfrew and Paisley Survey, one of the few United Kingdom population surveys to include both men and women.]

Joint National Committee on Prevention, Detection, Evaluation and Treatment of High Blood Pressure (1997). The sixth report of the Joint National Committee on Prevention, Detection, Evaluation and Treatment of High Blood Blood Pressure (JNC-VI). *Archives of Internal Medicine* 157, 2413–46. [The latest United States guideline.]

Klag MJ *et al.* (1996). Blood pressure and end stage renal disease in men. *New England Journal of Medicine* 334, 13–18. [An analysis of the MRFIT database showing that high blood pressure is a strong independent risk factor for renal failure.]

Law CM, Shiell AW (1996). Is blood pressure inversely related to birth weight? *Journal of Hypertension* 14, 935–41. [Strength of evidence from a systematic review of the literature.]

Levy D (1999). The role of systolic blood pressure in determining risk for cardiovascular disease. *Journal of Hypertension* 17(Supp 1), S15–S18. [All you ever wanted to know about systolic pressure in a single review.]

MacMahon S *et al.* (1990). Blood pressure, stroke and coronary heart disease. Part I, prolonged differences in blood pressure: prospective observational studies corrected for the regression dilution bias. *Lancet* 335, 765–74. [Important meta-analysis of studies showing relation between diastolic pressure and risk of vascular disease.]

Mancia G, Zanchetti A (1996). White coat hypertension: misnomers, misconceptions and misunderstandings: what should we do next? *Journal of Hypertension* 14, 1049–52. [Unravels the mysteries of ambulatory blood pressure monitoring.]

Mosterd A *et al.* (1999). Trends in the prevalence of hypertension, antihypertensive therapy and left ventricular hypertrophy from 1950–1989. *New England Journal of Medicine* 340, 1221–7. [A recent analysis from Framingham which supports the view that increasing use of antihypertensive medication has resulted in a reduced prevalence of high blood pressure and left ventricular hypertrophy.]

O'Brien E, Staessen JA (1999). What is 'hypertension'? *Lancet* 353, 1541–3. [Editorial which discusses the confusion still surrounding the definition of hypertension.]

O'Brien E *et al.* (2001). Blood pressure measuring devices: recommendations of the European Society of Hypertension. *British Medical Journal* 322, 531–636. [Includes alternatives to the mercury sphygmomanometer.]

Owens P *et al.* (1998). Ambulatory blood pressure in the hypertensive population: patterns and prevalence of hypertensive subforms. *Journal of Hypertension* 16, 1735–43. [Study confirming that isolated systolic hypertension is the most common form of hypertension in the elderly.]

PROGRESS Collaborative Group (2001). Randomised trial of a perindopril based blood pressure lowering regimen among 6105 individuals with previous stroke or transient ischaemic attack. *Lancet* **358**, 1033–41.

Ramsay LE *et al.* (1999). Guidelines for management of hypertension: report of the Third Working Party of the British Hypertension Society. *Journal of Human Hypertension* **13**, 569–92. [The latest British guideline.]

Schnall PL *et al.* (1998). A longitudinal study of job strain and ambulatory blood pressure: results from a three year follow up. *Psychosomatic Medicine* **60**, 697–706. [New evidence supporting the hypothesis that job strain is an occupational risk factor in the aetiology of essential hypertension.]

Thun MJ *et al.* (1997). Alcohol consumption and mortality among middle aged and elderly US adults. *New England Journal of Medicine* **337**, 1705–14. [The definitive meta-analysis of the protective effects of moderate alcohol intake.]

Van den Hoogen PCW *et al.* (2000). The relation between blood pressure and mortality due to coronary heart disease among men in different parts of the world. *New England Journal of Medicine* **342**, 1–8. [Prospective observational study showing similar relative risk but widely differing absolute risk of blood pressure for coronary heart disease in seven countries.]

15.16.1.2 Genetics of hypertension

N. J. Samani

Historical perspective

The concept that genetic factors may be involved in causing hypertension goes back more than two hundred years and predates the ability to measure blood pressure. In 1769, Morgagni observed that the father of a patient who had died of cerebral haemorrhage had himself died of 'apoplexy' (stroke). The history of the genetics of hypertension is marked by a celebrated debate in the 1950s and 1960s between Platt and Pickering, two doyens of British medicine. On the basis of a finding of a bimodal distribution of blood pressures in some families of patients with hypertension, and evidence of hypertension transmitted over three generations in a few pedigrees, Platt argued that hypertension was a distinct genetic disorder with a likely autosomal dominant mode of inheritance. By contrast, Pickering and colleagues showed that in the general population there was no obvious discontinuity of blood pressure distribution and that the familial resemblance of blood pressure spanned the whole range of blood pressures, and was not different for those with hypertension. Thus, Pickering argued that blood pressure, like height and weight, was a quantitative trait, and that although there was a significant genetic contribution, this was polygenic and that hypertension represented one extreme of the trait but was not a distinct disorder, except perhaps for rare monogenetic forms embedded in the blood pressure distribution curve. Today, the overwhelming mass of evidence supports the Pickering concept.

Genetic epidemiology of blood pressure

The extent of familial aggregation of blood pressure has been studied in diverse ethnic groups living in different places, ranging from Polynesians to Middle Americans. A remarkably consistent level of correlation of around 0.2 between first-degree relatives has been found, that is, if the blood pressure of one member of the family deviates from the norm by +10 mmHg, the first-degree relative will deviate +2 mmHg on average. Studies in children and infants suggest that the familial resemblance in blood pressure starts very early and is maintained throughout the rest of life.

Attempts to partition the familial resemblance of blood pressure between shared genes and shared environment have been made through studies of adoptees and twins. In the Montreal Adoption Study, correlations between natural siblings compared with adoptive siblings and between par-

ents and natural children compared with parents and adopted children were at least twice as great. Similarly, several studies have documented much higher correlations in blood pressure between monozygotic twins (0.55 to 0.85) compared with dizygotic twins (0.25 to 0.50), although the results from twin studies have to be viewed with some caution as there is substantial evidence of excess sharing of sociocultural environments by twin pairs, especially monozygotic twins.

However, taken together the epidemiological data suggest that genetic factors account for about 30 to 35 per cent of the population variability of blood pressure, common household environment for about 10 to 15 per cent, and non-familial factors for the remaining 50 to 55 per cent.

Genetic predisposition to hypertension

Although determination of familial correlations of blood pressure provides an overall view of the impact of heredity in determining blood pressure, a more relevant measure of the importance of genetic factors in determining susceptibility is relative risk. This is the ratio of the risk of an individual developing the condition given its presence in a first-degree relative compared with the overall population risk. For relatively rare monogenetic conditions such as cystic fibrosis, relative risk is as high as 500. For common and complex polygenic disorders, relative risk tends to be much lower. For hypertension, relative risk estimates vary between 2 and 5 depending on the criteria used to define family history. Values are highest when both parents have hypertension before the age of 55 years.

Apart from the increased familial risk, two other observations provide support for an important contribution of genetic factors in the pathogenesis of hypertension. First, spontaneous as well as salt-dependent hypertension can be inbred into animal strains. Second, there are a number of rare monogenetic forms of hypertension and hypotension, where the presence of a single defective gene is sufficient to cause altered blood pressure (Table 1). The molecular basis of several of these disorders has now been elucidated.

Mendelian forms of hypertension

Hypertension and hypokalaemia are features of 11β-hydroxylase and 17β-hydroxylase deficiency—two rare recessive gene disorders of adrenal steroid-synthesizing enzymes that, among others, cause congenital adrenal hyperplasia (see Chapter 12.7.2). 11β-Hydroxylase deficiency usually presents in infancy or early childhood with virilization of both sexes, while presentation of 17β-hydroxylase deficiency may be delayed until adolescence or adulthood. Hypertension due to a phaeochromocytoma may also

Table 1 Mendelian forms of blood pressure variation

Hypertension
Glucocorticoid-remediable aldosteronism
Syndrome of apparent mineralocorticoid excess
Liddle's syndrome
Gordon's syndrome (pseudohypoaldosteronism type II, PHA-II)
Hypertension exacerbated by pregnancy
Hypertension with brachydactyly
11β-hydroxylase deficiency
17β-hydroxylase deficiency
Multiple endocrine neoplasia Type 2 (Sipple's syndrome) with
    phaeochromocytoma

Hypotension
Aldosterone synthase deficiency
Pseudohypoaldosteronism type 1
Gitelman's syndrome
Bartter's syndrome
11β-hydroxylase deficiency

be a feature of multiple endocrine neoplasia type 2 (Sipple's syndrome), which when familial is inherited in an autosomal dominant pattern, or rarely be a feature of neurofibromatosis (von Recklinghausen's disease).

Apart from these conditions, several other mendelian disorders (glucocorticoid remediable aldosteronism, syndrome of apparent mineralocorticoid excess, Liddle's and Gordon's syndromes) where hypertension is the predominant manifestation have now been characterized at the molecular level. Although diverse in their molecular basis, all of them, interestingly, impact ultimately on the homeostatic role of the kidney in maintaining sodium balance.

Glucocorticoid-remediable aldosteronism (GRA)

GRA is a form of mineralocorticoid hypertension. It is inherited in an autosomal dominant fashion. The hypertension is accompanied by hypokalaemia (not invariably), a tendency to metabolic alkalosis, an elevated plasma aldosterone level, and a suppressed renin level. The hypertension often responds to thiazides or spironolactone. Patients are usually suspected of having primary aldosteronism (Conn's syndrome), although the age of onset, usually in the first two decades of life, is younger than typical of primary aldosteronism. The two hallmark features of GRA are the presence of large amounts of two abnormal steroids—18-hydroxycortisol and 18-oxocortisol—in the urine, and the paradoxical response of the hypertension, with return of plasma aldosterone to a normal level and disappearance of the abnormal steroids following treatment over a few days with a low dose of exogenous glucocorticoid, such as 0.5 to 1.0 mg of dexamethasone per day (hence the name).

The molecular basis of GRA was solved by Lifton and coworkers in 1992. Patients with GRA have a chimeric gene due to an unequal crossing-over event at meiosis between two adjacent and highly homologous genes involved in adrenocorticosteroid synthesis—aldosterone synthase (CYP11B2) (involved in aldosterone synthesis and normally regulated by angiotensin II) and 11β-hydroxylase (CYP11B1) (involved in glucocorticoid synthesis and normally regulated by ACTH). In the chimeric gene, the regulatory elements of CYP11B1 have become attached to the aldosterone synthase coding region of CYP11B2 (Fig. 1(a)). Thus, the gene produces aldosterone (and the other abnormal hormones), but under the control of ACTH and hence is suppressible by glucocorticoids, thereby explaining the clinical behaviour.

Syndrome of apparent mineralocorticoid excess (AME)

AME is an autosomal recessive disorder that usually presents in childhood with hypertension, hypokalaemia, and low renin activity. Despite the clinical features of mineralocorticoid excess, levels of all known mineralocorticoid hormones are low, yet the hypertension responds to spironolactone or amiloride. Patients with the disorder cannot metabolize cortisol to its inactive metabolite cortisone normally, resulting in a prolonged half-life of cortisol and a characteristic increase in urinary cortisol compared with cortisone metabolites.

Elucidating the defect causing AME first required the solution of another paradox—why cortisol, which circulates at a level several-fold greater than aldosterone, does not overwhelmingly activate the renal mineralocorticoid receptor *in vivo*, despite the two having equal affinity *in vitro* for the receptor. The reason relates to the enzyme 11β-hydroxysteroid dehydrogenase (**11β-HSD**), which has two isoforms. Type 1 11β-HSD is located in the liver, adipose tissue, and gonad and converts cortisone to cortisol. Type 2 11β-HSD is expressed in the mineralocorticoid target tissues—kidney, colon, and salivary gland—and inactivates cortisol to cortisone. In the kidney, the enzyme plays the crucial role of protecting the mineralocorticoid receptor on the distal tubule from activation by cortisol. In subjects with AME, a variety of disabling mutations in the type 2 11β-HSD gene cause a deficiency of the enzyme, allowing cortisol access to the mineralocorticoid receptor (Fig. 1(b)).

AME resembles the syndrome observed in subjects ingesting large amounts of liquorice or taking the now redundant antiulcer drug carbenoxolone. Both liquorice and carbenoxolone contain glycyrrhetinic acid, which inhibits type 2 11β-HSD. This, therefore, explains the hypertension and hypokalaemia observed with these compounds. Spillover access of cortisol to the mineralocorticoid receptor may also, at least in part, explain the

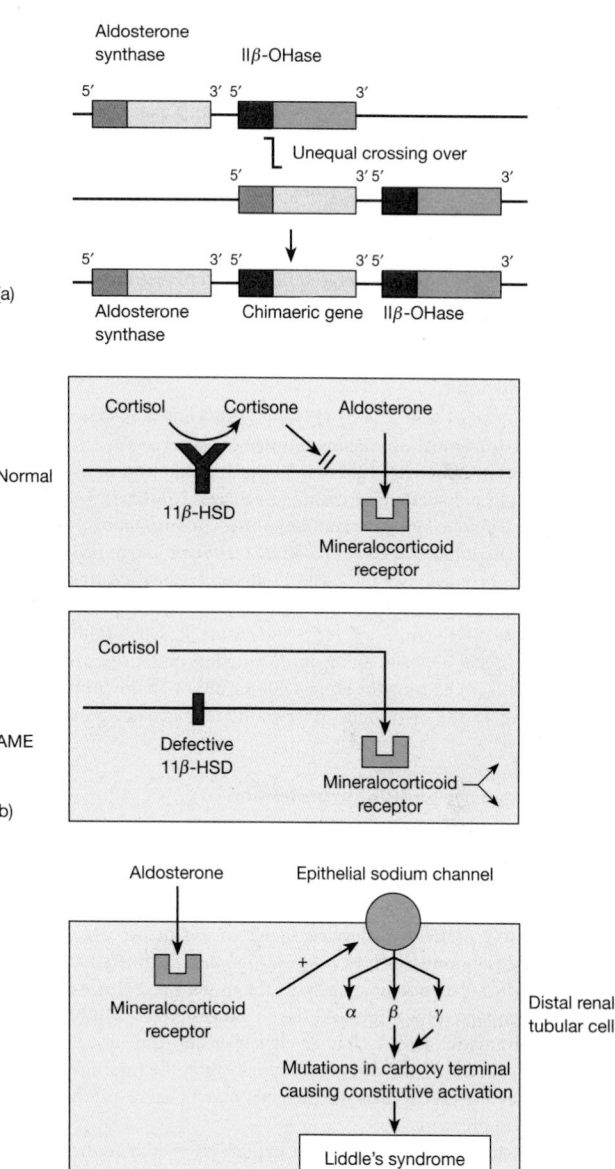

Fig. 1 Mechanisms underlying three forms of monogenetic hypertension. (a) Glucocorticoid-remediable aldosteronism—In GRA an unequal crossing-event leads to a chimeric gene where the coding region of aldosterone synthase (light pink bar) becomes attached to the regulatory region for 11β-hydroxylase (magenta bar). The chimeric gene produces excess amounts of aldosterone under the regulation of ACTH. (b) Syndrome of apparent mineralocorticoid excess—Normally, the mineralocorticoid receptor in the distal renal tubule is protected from stimulation by cortisol by the activity of the 11β-hydroxysteroid dehydrogenase enzyme. In AME, mutations in the enzyme allow cortisol to gain access to the receptor. (c) Liddle's syndrome—The trimeric epithelial sodium channel mediates sodium reuptake in the distal renal tubule under regulation by the mineralocorticoid receptor. In Liddle's syndrome, mutations in the β- and γ-subunits of the channel render the channel constitutively active.

hypertension accompanying some forms of Cushing's syndrome and gluco-corticoid resistance.

Liddle's syndrome

Liddle described a family in which the siblings were affected by early-onset hypertension and hypokalaemia, but with low renin and aldosterone levels. The clue to the nature of the molecular defect underlying this autosomal dominant disorder came from the observation that the hypertension does not respond to spironolactone, the mineralocorticoid receptor antagonist, but does respond to direct inhibitors (such as triamterene or amiloride) of the epithelial sodium channel which mediate the effects of activation of the mineralocorticoid receptor. This indicated that the defect lay downstream of the mineralocorticoid receptor, and Lifton and coworkers subsequently showed that the syndrome arises due to activating mutations in the β- or γ-subunits of this trimeric channel (Fig. 1(c)). All mutations identified so far cause an alteration or deletion of a proline-rich (PY) motif in the carboxy-terminal cytoplasmic tails of the subunits. This motif is necessary for regulatory proteins such as Nedd4 to bind and internalize the channel, and when its function is impaired the channel remains constitutively active at the cell surface.

Gordon's syndrome

Pseudohypoaldosteronism type II (PHA-II, also known as Gordon's syndrome), is an autosomal dominant disorder characterized by hyperkalaemia despite normal renal glomerular filtration, hypertension, and correction of physiological abnormalities by thiazide diuretics. Mild hyperchloraemia, metabolic acidosis, and suppressed plasma renin activity are variable associated findings. Genes for PHA-II have been mapped in different families to chromosomes 17, 1, and 12. Recently, the causative genes on chromosomes 12 and 17 have been identified as two members, WNK1 and WNK4, of the WNK family of serine-threonine kinases. Both proteins localize to the distal nephron and gain-of-function mutations are thought to be responsible for causing the abnormalities, although the precise mechanisms leading to the disturbance in electrolyte transport remain to be determined.

Other monogenetic forms of hypertension

A missense mutation in the ligand-binding domain of the mineralocorticoid receptor (MR) has been found to cause an autosomal dominant form of hypertension that is markedly accelerated in pregnancy. The mutation, MR S810L, causes partial, aldosterone-independent, activation of the receptor, causing carriers to develop hypertension before age 20. More interestingly, compounds such as progesterone that normally bind but do not activate MR are all potent agonists of the mutant receptor. Since pregnancy is accompanied by a 100-fold rise in progesterone, MR S810L carriers have dramatic acceleration of hypertension during pregnancy. Although the MR S810L mutation is extremely rare, the finding does raise the question of whether related mechanisms may underlie other forms of hypertension in pregnancy.

A gene causing autosomal dominant hypertension in conjunction with type E brachydactyly in a large Turkisk kindred has been mapped to chromosome 12p. The hypertension in this syndrome, unlike most of the disorders described above, closely resembles essential hypertension with no evidence of volume expansion or electrolyte imbalance. Elucidation of the genetic defect is keenly awaited.

Genetic defects causing hypotension

Just as single-gene disorders have been identified that cause hypertension, a number of mendelian syndromes where hypotension is a feature have recently been characterized at a molecular level (Table 1). Many are mirror images of the genetic abnormalities causing the mendelian forms of hypertension described above. Pseudohypoaldosteronism type 1 (PHA-I) occurs in two forms, autosomal recessive and autosomal dominant. Both are char-acterized by life-threatening dehydration in the neonatal period, hypotension, salt wasting, hyperkalemia, metabolic acidosis, and marked elevation of renin and aldosterone. The autosomal recessive form is due to inactivating mutations (compare with Liddle's syndrome) in any of the subunits of the epithelial sodium channel, while the autosomal dominant form is due to loss-of-function mutations in the mineralocorticoid receptor.

Gitelman's syndrome is also an autosomal recessive disorder. It is characterized by hypotension, neuromuscular abnormalities, hypokalaemia, metabolic alkalosis, and an activated renin–angiotensin system. It arises due to inactivating mutations in the gene encoding the renal thiazide-sensitive NaCl cotransporter.

Bartter's syndrome is distinguished from Gitelman's syndrome by hypercalciuria and presentation in the neonatal period with life-threatening hypotension. This disease is caused by mutations in one of several genes that are required for normal salt absorption in the thick ascending loop of Henle.

Does my patient have a recognized form of monogenetic hypertension?

Finding that a patient has GRA, AME, Liddle's syndrome, or Gordon's syndrome has important consequences for treatment (see above) and family screening. However, all of these syndromes are extremely rare and suspicion will usually go unrewarded. Phenotypic expression is highly variable. Features that may suggest a diagnosis of mendelian hypertension include a young age of onset, moderate to severe hypertension, strong family history, and electrolyte abnormalities, particularly of potassium (although this is not invariable). A good starting point is the measurement of plasma renin activity (suppressed in all three syndromes) and plasma aldosterone. If the aldosterone is significantly elevated then the differential diagnosis lies between the various forms of Conn's syndrome and GRA. Diagnosis of GRA would be supported by the finding of elevated 18-hydroxycortisol and 18-oxocortisol in the urine, and can now be relatively easily confirmed by finding a chimeric gene fragment with DNA testing. If the aldosterone level is suppressed, then finding an increased ratio of cortisol/cortisone metabolites in the urine would support a diagnosis of AME. The presence of hyperkalaemia, hyperchloraemia, and metabolic acidosis would suggest a diagnosis of Gordon's syndrome. No biochemical abnormalities specifically support a diagnosis of Liddle's syndrome. Ultimately, diagnosis of AME, Liddle's syndrome, and Gordon's syndrome also requires DNA confirmation, but this is not as straightforward as it is with GRA since several different mutations can give rise to each syndrome.

Progress towards identifying genes that increase susceptibility to essential hypertension

The genetic contribution to essential hypertension (and the population variability in blood pressure) is polygenic. However, little is known about the number of genes involved, their mode of transmission, their quantitative effect on blood pressure, their interaction with other genes, or their modulation by environmental factors. Further, the impact of genetic factors may be dependent on age, gender, and ethnicity, and may only influence specific blood pressure phenotypes such as systolic or diastolic blood pressure. Such complexities have contributed to the difficulty in elucidating the genetic basis of essential hypertension.

Despite evidence that the same genes that increase susceptibility to essential hypertension most likely also contribute to normal blood pressure variation, much of the work to date has focused on the former. Two main approaches have been used: (i) association studies in which the frequency of specific alleles are compared in hypertensive and normotensive subjects,

(ii) sibling-pair linkage studies, which test whether specific alleles or markers are shared more often by hypertensive sibling pairs than would be expected by chance. Association studies are most suited to study candidate genes, while with affected sibling pairs the whole genome can also be scanned using anonymous microsatellite markers to identify areas of linkage.

Association studies

Variants in over 30 candidate genes have been associated with hypertension (MEDLINE search under hypertension x genetics), although for the majority the findings are as yet far from robust. However, data for a number of genes are sufficiently persuasive, or otherwise interesting, to merit specific mention.

Angiotensinogen

Cleavage of angiotensinogen (**AGT**) by renin is the rate-limiting step in the generation of angiotensin II, the effector molecule of the renin–angiotensin system. Evidence for the involvement of the AGT gene comes from both linkage of the AGT locus to hypertension in Caucasian and Afro-Carribean hypertensive sibling pairs and association of a polymorphism (M235T) in the gene with hypertension. In a meta-analysis of 32 case–control studies corresponding to 13 760 patients, the TT genotype conferred a 31 per cent increased risk of hypertension compared with the MM genotype. Other estimates suggest that mutations in the AGT gene might be predisposing factors for hypertension in 3 to 6 per cent of subjects with onset before the age of 60. Data showing that the TT genotype is also associated with higher plasma and possibly tissue AGT levels, with its potential impact on angiotensin generation, provides a plausible explanation for the association of the AGT gene with hypertension.

Angiotensin- converting enzyme

Angiotensin converting enzyme (ACE) cleaves angiotensin I to form the vasoactive peptide angiotensin II. A common variant in the ACE gene, the insertion/deletion (I/D) polymorphism, is strongly associated with differences in plasma ACE levels. Although initial linkage and association studies were negative, recent analyses have shown significant association of the I/D polymorphism with blood pressure at least in males. Given the widespread and increasing use of ACE inhibitors and angiotensin receptor antagonists in treating hypertension and related cardiovascular diseases, these observations, if confirmed, could have pharmacological implications.

α-Adducin

Adducin is a ubiquitous α/β heterodimeric cytoskeletal protein that promotes the assembly of actin with spectrin. In the Milan hypertensive rat, point mutations in the adducin α- and β-subunits affect actin assembly and Na–K pump activity and possibly explain up to 50 per cent of the blood pressure difference compared with the Milan normotensive rat. In humans a polymorphism changing glycine for tryptophane at codon 460 in the α-adducin gene has been found to be more common in individuals with hypertension in Italian, French, and Japanese populations, although other studies have not shown an association. More persuasive are data showing a direct functional impact of the 460Trp variant. In an acute salt-sensitivity test, where change in blood pressure from a state of salt-loading to one of salt-depletion was measured, hypertensive individuals heterozygous for the 460Trp allele had a much greater decrease in mean arterial pressure than hypertensive individuals homozygous for the 460Gly allele (15.9 [SE 2.0] compared with 7.4 [SE 1.3] mmHg). Similarly, heterozygous hypertensive individuals showed a much greater fall in mean arterial pressure in response to 2 months' treatment with hydrochlorthiazide than did 460Gly homozygote individuals (14.7 [2.2] compared with 6.8 [1.4] mmHg). Consistent with these observations, the 460Trp variant was associated with a reduced-slope (more salt sensitive) pressure–natriuresis curve. Further

confirmation is required, but these findings suggest that variation at the adducin locus may contribute to salt sensitivity and through it to susceptibility to hypertension in some populations.

G protein β3 subunit

Increased activity of the pH-regulating transporter system, the sodium-proton exchanger, is seen in some patients with essential hypertension. Siffert and coworkers found that this was due to enhanced intracellular signal transduction via pertussis toxin-sensitive heterotrimeric G proteins. Sequencing revealed a polymorphism (C825T) in the gene encoding the β3 subunit (GNB3), which although itself silent, appears to cause a biologically active splice variant, Gβ3-s, missing 41 amino acids in those carrying the T allele. In an initial study of 426 hypertensive and 427 normotensive subjects, there was a significant association of carriage of the T allele with hypertension (53 compared with 44 per cent). In a further study, where hypertensive subjects were recruited on the basis of a very strong family history of premature hypertension affecting both parents, the association of hypertension with the T allele was even stronger. These early findings suggest that in some patients hypertension may be related to inherited dysfunction of G proteins.

Epithelial sodium channel

Attempts to show that less severe mutations in the genes responsible for monogenetic forms of hypertension (see above) may underlie essential hypertension have by and large met with disappointment. One exception may be the epithelial sodium channel involved in Liddle's syndrome, where a variant in the C-terminus of the β-subunit (T594M) was found to be four times more frequent in hypertensive black subjects resident in London compared with normotensive black subjects (8 compared with 2 per cent). Subjects carrying the mutation demonstrate increased activity of the nasal epithelial sodium channel (a possible surrogate marker of the renal channel) and lower plasma renin activity, supporting the notion of increased sodium reabsorption and volume-dependent hypertension. In turn, this could at least partly explain the generally poor response of black hypertensive subjects to angiotensin-converting enzyme inhibitors.

Epistatic interactions

Current findings (see above) suggest that individually, gene variants will, at best, only contribute a small amount to the risk of hypertension. Interest is therefore turning to additive and epistatic interactions. There are only a few publications, but in one recent study by Staessen and coworkers, possession in combination of the ACE DD genotype, the α-adducin Trp allele, and the aldosterone synthase CC genotype (at the −344C/T polymorphism), increased the risk of developing hypertension by 252 per cent compared with other genotypes. Over a median follow-up of 9.1 years the cumulative incidence rates for hypertension were 71.0 cases per 1000 person-years in those carrying the three risk genotypes compared with 20.2 cases per 1000 person-years in those without. If confirmed, the findings could have implications for prediction and primary prevention

Linkage studies

These have lagged behind association studies. However increasing numbers are being reported. The most consistent data have been found for a region on chromosome 17 where linkage has been found, not only to hypertension analysed as a qualitative trait in a panel of French and United Kingdom affected sib pairs (Julier and coworkers), but also to blood pressure analysed as a quantitative trait in subjects from the Framingham Heart Study (Levy and coworkers). Involvement of a gene in this region in blood pressure regulation is further supported by the fact that the syntenic interval is also linked to blood pressure in several strains of genetically hypertensive rats. Interestingly, the region overlaps with the chromosome 17 locus for Gordon's syndrome where a mutation in the WNK4 gene has recently been identified to be the cause. Whether other mutations in WNK4 are responsible for the reported linkage to essential hypertension and blood pressure variability remains to be determined.

Future perspectives

Recent progress suggests that in the next few years much more will be understood about the nature of individual genetic factors that influence susceptibility to hypertension and the environmental/genetic context in which they exert their effect on blood pressure. It may prove possible to sub-categorize patients with essential hypertension on the basis of molecular mechanisms. Although this information will not help with diagnosis (we already have an accurate tool– the sphygnomanometer), there could be several important applications. Preventive measures, such as salt restriction, could be better targeted if findings, for example with α-adducin, are confirmed. The information would almost certainly influence choice of antihypertensive medication (pharmacogenetics). Several studies have shown that individuals show significant variation in their response to different classes of antihypertensive agents. At present the choice of drug is largely empirical. The early findings with α-adducin and the epithelial sodium channel gene illustrate how the presence of a particular genetic variant could influence this choice. Finally, there is increasing experimetal as well as some clinical data to show that genetic factors not only contribute to the development of hypertension but also influence the development of end-organ damage. The ultimate goal of hypertension management is not just to lower blood pressure but to prevent complications, and strategies based on a more refined assessment of risk will undoubtedly be more cost-effective.

Further reading

Baker EH *et al.* (1998). Association of hypertension with the T594M mutation in the β subunit of epithelial sodium channel in black people resident in London. *Lancet* **351**, 1388–92. [The same gene as that involved in Liddle's syndrome may cause essential hypertension in some ethnic groups.]

Cusi D *et al.* (1997). Polymorphisms of α-adducin and salt sensitivity in patients with essential hypertension. *Lancet* **349**, 1353–7. [Key paper on the role of adducin.]

Geller DS *et al.* (2000). Activating mineralocorticoid receptor mutation in hypertension exacerbated by pregnancy. *Science* **289**, 119–23. [Describes an activating mutation in the mineralocorticoid receptor which makes it responsive to progesterone.]

Jeunemaitre X *et al.* (1992). Molecular basis of human hypertension: role of angiotensinogen. *Cell* **71**, 169–80. [Seminal paper describing involvement of the angiotensinogen gene in essential hypertension.]

Julier C *et al.* (1997). Genetic susceptibility for human essential hypertension in a region of homology with blood pressure linkage on rat chromosome 10. *Human Molecular Genetics* **6**, 2077–85. [Identification of the first locus for essential hypertension via methods not based on a candidate gene.]

Levy D *et al.* (2000). Evidence for a gene influencing blood pressure on chromosome 17. Genome scan linkage results for longitudinal blood pressure phenotypes in subjects from the Framingham Heart Study. *Hypertension* **36**, 477–83. [Findings from a quantitative trait approach supporting the presence of a gene on chromosome 17 that influences blood pressure.]

Lifton RP *et al.* (1992). A chimaeric 11 β-hydroxylase/aldosterone synthase gene causes glucocorticoid-remediable aldosteronism and human hypertension. *Nature* **355**, 262–5. [Describes the discovery of the molecular mechanism underlying glucocorticoid-remediable aldosteronism.]

Mune T *et al.* (1995). Human hypertension caused by mutations in the kidney isozyme of 11β-hydroxysteroid dehydrogenase. *Nature Genetics* **10**, 394–9. [Describes the discovery of the molecular mechanism underlying apparent mineralocorticoid excess.]

Shimkets RA *et al.* (1994). Liddle's syndrome: heritable human hypertension caused by mutations in the β subunit of the epithelial sodium channel. *Cell* **79**, 407–14. [Describes the discovery of the molecular mechanism underlying Liddle's syndrome.]

Siffert W *et al.* (1998). Association of a human G-protein β3 subunit variant with hypertension. *Nature Genetics* **18**, 45–8. [Findings suggesting that hypertension may be a G-protein related inherited disorder in some patients.]

Staessen JA *et al.* (2001). Effects of three candidate genes on prevalence and incidence of hypertension in a Caucasian population. *Journal of Hypertension* **19**, 1349–58. [One of the first studies demonstrating epistatic interactions between genes in increasing risk of hypertension.]

Swales JD (1985). *Platt verus Pickering: an episode in recent medical history.* Keynes Press, London. [Describes a celebrated debate about the nature of the genetic basis of essential hypertension.]

Ward R (1990). Familial aggregation and genetic epidemiology of blood pressure. In: Laragh JH, Brenner BM, eds. *Hypertension: pathophysiology, diagnosis and management*, pp 81–100. Raven Press, New York. [Comprehensive review of the evidence indicating a significant genetic contribution to hypertension.]

Wilson FH *et al.* (2001). Human hypertension caused by mutations in WNK kinases. *Science* **293**, 1107–12. [Describes the identification and characterisation of mutations at two loci causing Gordon's syndrome.]

15.16.1.3 Essential hypertension

*J. Swales**

Pathology

Introduction

High blood pressure induces changes in the heart and blood vessels. These are partly the direct effect of cyclic stress on the arterial wall and also due to indirect trophic effects. In addition, turbulence and shear stress influence endothelial function. Secondary changes may then occur in the organs served by these vessels, giving rise to the clinical features of hypertension. However, not all the pathological changes observed in the cardiovascular system are the result of pressure (Table 1). Hypertension is associated with risk factors for atheroma such as dyslipidaemia and insulin resistance. Smooth muscle growth is enhanced in some animal models of hypertension, probably as a result of genetic factors. There may be other cellular

Table 1 Pathological consequences of increased pressure and other features associated with essential hypertension

Feature	Location/pathology
Direct effect of pressure	
Disruption and collagen deposition	Aorta and large arteries (stiffness)
Necrosis and collagen deposition	Large arteries (malignant hypertension)
Trophic changes	Large and small arteries
Remodelling	Small vessels (resistance)
Impaired endothelial function	Large and small arteries
Associated features	
Dyslipidaemia	Aorta and large arteries (atheroma)
Insulin resistance	Aorta and large arteries (atheroma)
Increased angiotensin II	?Atheroma, trophic changes
Increased catecholamines	?Atheroma, trophic changes
Genetic regulation of cell function	?Contractility, trophic changes

---

* It is with regret that we report the death of Professor John Swales during the preparation of this edition of the *Oxford Textbook of Medicine*.

influences at work. Most of the powerful vasoconstrictors such as angiotensin II, catecholamines, vasopressin, and endothelins are also mitogens and may therefore have trophic effects.

Blood vessel changes

Aorta and large arteries

Recurrent pulsatile stress produces uncoiling, disruption and calcification of elastic fibres. At the same time, relatively inelastic collagen is increased. This is a result of ageing as well as hypertension: both processes therefore cause loss of the normal elastic reservoir function of the aorta and large arteries. The effects are additive, so that changes occur at an earlier age in hypertensive than in normotensive subjects. Another reason for the loss of arterial compliance in hypertensive patients is that, as pressure increases, the elastic fibres become fully stretched, causing the inelastic collagen fibres to bear the load. As a result of these changes, the pressure wave generated by left ventricular contraction is no longer buffered by the aorta and proximal arteries, but is transmitted into the arterial tree with greater amplitude. This is manifested clinically as increased pulse pressure, with higher systolic and lower diastolic pressures. In addition, loss of compliance produces increased pulse wave velocity. Pulse waves are reflected back from peripheral sites, normally returning in late diastole as a secondary wave visible on the aortic trace. When the arterial tree is stiffened the return of these waves amplifies the aortic late systolic wave. This is not demonstrable when brachial artery pressure is measured, but throws an additional load on the left ventricle. In addition, lower diastolic pressure reduces coronary artery perfusion.

Large artery changes in hypertension were ignored for many years. However, it is now clear that pulse pressure is an important risk factor in cardiovascular disease. This explains one curious feature of elderly hypertensive patients. Diastolic blood pressure in patients with isolated systolic hypertension is inversely related to prognosis, that is, for any given systolic blood pressure, the lower the diastolic, the worse the risk.

Decreased compliance of the large arteries also has an important effect on the carotid and aortic baroceptors which normally buffer rapid changes in blood pressure. These become less sensitive. As a result, circulatory adaptation to rapid changes in posture may be impaired. This rarely causes problems, except in elderly hypertensive subjects, when age and blood pressure have additive effects. The clinical manifestation is as postural hypotension or post-prandial hypotension in elderly patients whose blood pressure has been overtreated.

Medium-sized arteries

These arteries perform a conduit rather than reservoir function, reflected in their lower elastin content. The predominant pathological change is wall thickening caused by increased deposition of collagenous material.

Resistance vessels

The characteristic structural change in the smaller arteries and arterioles responsible for peripheral vascular resistance is an increase in wall:lumen ratio. This has important functional consequences. The vessels can still dilate in response to stimuli such as warmth or drugs, but maximal vasodilatation is reduced. This change is a response to pressure; it can be prevented by protecting vessels from the increased pressure load in hypertension by means of a mechanical constriction. There may be a genetic factor in hypertension which regulates the structural response, the evidence for which is largely based on animal studies.

In recent years it has become clear that what was thought to be a trophic response is largely if not entirely due to rearrangement of smooth muscle cells around a smaller lumen. There is little if any evidence of hypertrophy and no evidence of hyperplasia (i.e. increased number of cells). The mechanism of this is entirely unknown. Local growth factors, such as angiotensin II have been implicated. Thus lowering blood pressure by angiotensin-converting enzyme (**ACE**) inhibition is better at reversing remodelling than lowering it by β-blockade.

Atheroma in hypertension

The increased prevalence of atheroma in hypertensive patients reflects the cumulative effect of several contributory factors. The importance of local mechanical consequences of increased pressure and turbulence on the arterial wall are demonstrated by the distribution of lesions and the absence of atheroma in the pulmonary vessels of hypertensive patients. Endothelial dysfunction is probably the first stage in initiating a complex chain of local cellular processes leading to the formation of the atheromatous plaque. Increased adhesion molecule expression, increased permeability, and cell migration, accumulation, and proliferation are all involved. Most studies in patients with essential hypertension have shown impairment of endothelium-dependent vasodilatation, although animal studies have shown more complex changes in endothelial function.

Systemic factors are also of importance in the development of atheroma in hypertensive patients. Atheroma cannot usually be produced in hypertensive rabbits unless their lipid levels are raised by feeding them cholesterol. A combination of high perfusion pressure above induced aortic constriction and a high cholesterol diet induces atheroma above, but not below the constriction. A low cholesterol diet prevents it. This is analogous to the situation in humans, where the presence of insulin resistance or diabetes in a hypertensive patient further increases the risk of atheromatous complications.

It has also been postulated that the renin–angiotensin system plays a role in atherogenesis. Renin and angiotensin II levels are often raised in severe hypertension and in hypertension associated with increased sympathetic nervous system activity. In laboratory studies angiotensin II enhances the smooth muscle proliferative response observed in atheroma. High renin levels have been shown to be associated with a worse prognosis in some studies, although this finding is still controversial. Since drugs may either block or activate the renin–angiotensin system, this debate has important therapeutic implications which will only be resolved when the relevant trials report.

Vessels in malignant hypertension

The characteristic pathological lesion in malignant hypertension is fibrinoid necrosis (necrotizing arteriolitis). The normal structure of the vessel wall is lost and replaced with fibrin-like material. A variable cellular reaction takes place. Fibrinoid necrosis is usually associated with focal areas of vasodilatation and increased permeability. These changes are probably a primary mechanical effect. The endothelium of the dilated segments is disrupted and the vessel wall becomes permeable to particles as large as colloidal carbon. The increased permeability permits exudation of plasma into the media and local tissue destruction. The intima may become massively thickened by concentric collagenous rings as a result of locally released growth factors until the lumen is almost obliterated.

Specific organ changes in hypertension

The heart

Angina and myocardial infarction in the hypertensive patient are usually due to coronary atheroma. Coronary perfusion may also be lowered as a result of reduced diastolic pressures in patients with isolated systolic hypertension (see above). In a minority of patients, anginal pain occurs in the absence of significant coronary atheroma ('syndrome X'). A possible explanation is luminal narrowing of the coronary vessels associated with an increased wall:lumen ratio. Other explanations which have been put forward are increased vasomotor tone and increased pressure on the left ventricular wall causing subendocardial ischaemia. The most likely explanation for syndrome X in hypertensive patients is impairment of endothelial-dependent relaxation in the coronary vascular tree.

Left ventricular hypertrophy is demonstrable in about 50 per cent of untreated hypertensive patients when echocardiography is used, and in 5 to 10 per cent with electrocardiography using conventional criteria. Histologically, it is caused by an increase in size of cardiomyocytes with an increase in intercellular matrix. Its role as a powerful independent risk factor for cardiovascular disease and death has led to intensive research into its causes and reversal by treatment. Pressure load on the left ventricle is unquestionably important, as evidenced by the observation that ambulatory monitoring of blood pressure is much better correlated with left ventricular hypertrophy than clinic measurements of pressure. Furthermore, lowering blood pressure consistently produces regression of left ventricular hypertrophy. However, local trophic factors may also play a role. The sympathetic nervous system and renin–angiotensin–aldosterone system have been implicated by both clinical and experimental studies. Meta-analyses of clinical trials in which blood pressure was lowered by different classes of antihypertensive agent have suggested that ACE inhibitors have a greater effect in reversing left ventricular mass, even when other factors such as duration of therapy and degree of blood pressure reduction are taken into account. However, there have been no adequately sized trials in which agents have been formally compared, and this clinically very important possibility still remains to be demonstrated convincingly.

The bad prognosis carried by left ventricular hypertrophy in the hypertensive patient could have several explanations. These include:

(1) Arrhythmias—there is increased prevalence of simple and complex ventricular arrhythmias in hypertensive left ventricular hypertrophy;

(2) Relative ischaemia produced by increased muscle mass;

(3) Decrease in ventricular compliance causing pulmonary oedema; and

(4) Ventricular hypertrophy is also a marker for integrated exposure of the circulation to high blood pressure over a prolonged period.

Central nervous system

Cerebral (atherothrombotic) infarction in a hypertensive patient is usually attributable to atheroma of one of the larger cerebral arteries (usually the middle cerebral artery) and accounts for about 80 per cent of the strokes which these patients suffer. Intracerebral haemorrhage accounts for 10 to 15 per cent, usually the result of rupture of a small intracerebral degenerative microaneurysm (Charcot–Bouchard aneurysm). These lesions develop in the small (less than 200 µm diameter) perforating arteries in the region of the basal ganglia, thalamus, and internal capsule. Hyaline degeneration (lipohyalinosis) occurs in the aneurysmal wall with a defect in the media at the neck of the aneurysm. The incidence of Charcot–Bouchard aneurysms is closely correlated with age and blood pressure, the two factors acting additively so that lesions are rarely if ever seen in younger normotensive people. The remaining strokes in hypertensive patients are due to subarachnoid haemorrhage. Transient ischaemic attacks due to disease of extracranial vessels are also more frequent in hypertensive subjects.

More diffuse changes account for the cognitive decline that may occur, particularly in untreated hypertension and in older patients. Functional imaging studies have shown relative reductions in blood flow in parietal and forebrain areas in hypertensive patients during memory tasks and areas of cortical and subcortical hypometabolism. More advanced vascular disease gives rise to multiple, punctate, hyperintense white matter lesions on MRI. These are due to focal ischaemia, either as a result of lipohyalinosis or microatheromatous disease, tortuosity, and narrowing of the perforating arteries. All degrees of impairment of cognitive performance may occur as a result of these lesions, ranging from effects only detectable with sensitive psychometric testing to lacunar strokes and Binswanger's disease.

Hypertensive encephalopathy

The cerebral vessels usually constrict in the face of increased pressure and dilate in the face of decreased pressure to maintain a constant flow (autoregulation). Resistance vessel remodelling and hypertrophy seem to have a protective function in this respect, so that the autoregulatory range is raised in long-standing hypertension. When blood pressure rises above the autoregulatory range, however, focal areas of vasodilatation and localized perivascular oedema and fibrinoid necrosis occur. Focal haemorrhages, ischaemia, and infarction may result, giving rise to the clinical picture of encephalopathy.

The kidney

In non-malignant hypertension, glomerular filtration rate is well preserved. However, filtration fraction is increased since efferent glomerular arteriolar resistance increases more than afferent resistance, causing a rise in intraglomerular capillary pressure. The long-term renal damage produced by glomerular hypertension probably accounts for progressive glomerulosclerosis in essential hypertension. Thus, the decline in glomerular filtration rate with age is more rapid in hypertensive than normotensive subjects. This phenomenon is not usually significant in mild to moderate essential hypertension where endstage renal disease in the absence of any other lesion is unusual.

Hypertension-induced glomerulosclerosis is much more important, however, in severe and malignant hypertension and in the presence of intrinsic renal disease due to (for instance) diabetes or glomerulonephritis. Effective control of blood pressure arrests or retards the process, and acute hypertension-induced renal failure can be partially or completely reversed by early treatment in many cases. Hyaline degeneration is particularly observed in the afferent arterioles of the kidney in association with ageing and hypertension. Involvement of the juxtaglomerular baroceptor may account for the decline in renin secretion which is demonstrable in elderly and hypertensive populations. In malignant hypertension, glomerular hypertension and vascular necrosis produce proteinuria, haematuria, and progressive renal failure.

Atheromatous renal vascular disease much more commonly causes renal impairment in elderly hypertensive subjects than younger patients with treated mild to moderate hypertension.

Clinical features

Symptoms

Elevated blood pressure is usually asymptomatic until organ damage occurs. However, most patients labour under the illusion that any concurrent symptom is attributable to high blood pressure or its treatment. In some cases, the knowledge that a patient has high blood pressure creates a fertile soil for the growth of functional symptoms. Thus, patients who have been told that they are hypertensive have a much higher incidence of headache than hypertensive patients who are unaware of the fact. In some studies, 'labelling' a patient as hypertensive has led to an increased absenteeism from work, although no target organ damage had occurred. It is a common lay fallacy that a patient can recognize when their blood pressure is elevated, usually on the basis of such symptoms as plethoric features, palpitations, dizziness, or a feeling of tension. A screening survey in the United States examined the frequency of such symptoms as headache, epistaxis, tinnitus, dizziness, and fainting in healthy subjects. None of these symptoms was more prevalent in subjects with diastolic blood pressures over 100 mmHg.

In spite of such evidence, it should be borne in mind that target organ damage can occur and may not be clinically obvious. This may be particularly relevant in the elderly patient with diffuse cerebrovascular disease, whose fairly non-specific symptoms may be dismissed. Functional imaging has shown this to be much more frequent than was once believed (see above). Additionally, higher blood pressure levels may be responsible for some symptoms, such as headache.

Headache

The classic hypertensive headache is present on waking in the morning, situated in the occipital region of the head, radiating to the frontal area, throbbing in quality, and wears off during the course of the day. Most headaches in hypertensive patients are tension headaches not directly related to blood pressure at all. The incidence of such symptoms rises when patients become aware of the diagnosis. Nevertheless, effective treatment of hypertension reduces the incidence of headache. How far this is a specific consequence of blood pressure lowering and how far it is due to reassurance is uncertain. Morning headaches in obese hypertensive patients may be due to sleep apnoea.

Epistaxis

Whilst epistaxis is not associated with mild hypertension, it is much more common in moderate to severe hypertension. When patients present with epistaxis and high blood pressure, it is particularly important to dissociate hypertension as a cause of epistaxis from a pressor response to an alarming episode.

Nocturia

This is one of the most frequent clinically apparent consequences of blood pressure elevation resulting from reduction in urine-concentrating capacity.

Impotence

Erectile dysfunction occurs frequently in hypertension, but is usually not spontaneously mentioned by the patient or enquired about by the physician. It is often attributed by both patient and doctor to drug therapy. Although this may be the case with some classes of drug, untreated hypertension has been associated with an increased incidence of erectile dysfunction in the few studies that have specifically addressed this issue. It is probably a consequence of structural change in the peripheral vasculature limiting the capacity for acute increase in penile perfusion.

Symptoms associated with target organ damage

Cardiovascular system

Effort dyspnoea and orthopnoea suggest cardiac failure. Increased left ventricular mass is associated with decreased compliance and impaired cardiac output response to exercise. This is more likely in elderly patients whose cardiac reserves are less. Claudication suggests peripheral atheromatous vascular disease and is usually associated with atheroma elsewhere, such as the renal or carotid arteries. Angina of effort is also usually due to atheroma, although the coronary vascular tree may be free of plaques in a few cases.

Central nervous system

Scotomas suggest fundal haemorrhages or exudates, whilst blurring of vision is associated with papilloedema. These symptoms therefore deserve particular attention. Decline in cognitive performance detectable only by formal psychometric testing is more common than was once believed. It occurs particularly in long-standing untreated hypertension and in the elderly. More clinically apparent failure in concentration and memory may be due to more advanced cerebrovascular disease, depression, or centrally acting antihypertensive drugs. Extensive disease of the perforating arteries may give rise to a lacunar state characterized by progressive pseudobulbar palsy and dementia. The presence or absence of diffuse cerebrovascular disease can have important consequences for the development of dementia in Alzheimer's disease. Patients without such vascular lesions are less likely to show cognitive impairment than those with vascular lesions in the presence of the characteristic pathology of Alzheimer's disease.

Renal system

Haematuria or haematospermia suggest the malignant phase of hypertension in the absence of any other cause. Advanced renal failure in the absence of malignant hypertension suggests bilateral atheromatous renovascular or other forms of renal disease.

Clinical examination

The objectives of clinical examination are to assess blood pressure, any consequences of its elevation, and any associated disease which might modify its treatment.

Blood pressure measurement

Direct blood pressure measurement

The most accurate way to measure blood pressure is by direct arterial cannulation. Portable recording devices enable continuous arterial blood pressure measurements to be made with this technique, which antedates the modern indirect ambulatory devices. The advantages are precision, independence of arterial wall changes, the absence of any 'white coat effect' as a result of cuff inflation, and the ability to observe beat by beat variability in blood pressure and pulse. Until recently, this was not possible with indirect instruments. However, the inconvenience and morbidity caused by indwelling arterial catheters have prevented their use in routine clinical practice. The only role for direct blood pressure measurement by arterial cannulation in essential hypertension is when calcification of the arterial wall in elderly patients is suspected of causing spuriously high systolic blood pressure measurements. It is also used to monitor blood pressure in severely hypertensive patients during parenteral therapy.

Indirect manual measurement

The 'gold standard' for clinical measurement is still the mercury sphygmomanometer, using the Korotkoff sounds. However, concerns about the toxicity of mercury and the greater reliability of more recent electronic devices is now leading to their increasing usage.

The manual auscultatory technique is based upon the sounds described by Korotkoff in 1905 and uses the inflatable air-filled cuff constructed by Riva-Rocci in 1897. The brachial artery is occluded by inflating the cuff above the pressure at which the radial pulse disappears to palpation. Pressure in the cuff is estimated by a mercury or aneroid manometer. The pressure is then slowly lowered through the valve on the inflating bulb, whilst listening for the Korotkoff sounds.

Although frequently employed, auscultatory measurement of blood pressure is often carried out badly: inter- and intraobserver variability is often unacceptably high. Training videos and CDs are available for doctors and nurses and have been shown to improve measurement technique. Important points to note include the following.

Bladder and cuff If the cuff is too small (usually as a result of an obese arm) inadequate pressure will be applied and blood pressure will be overestimated. The length of the bladder should be at least 80 per cent and the width of the bladder 40 per cent of the arm circumference. The optimal size is 26×12 cm for normal-sized arms and 40×12 cm for obese arms. Minor overlap of the ends of the bladder on thinner arms does not significantly influence readings.

Manometers Mercury manometers should be vertical and should read zero when no pressure is applied to the cuff. Aneroid manometers require calibration every few months.

Bulb and tubing These require checking for significant leaks (i.e. more than 1 mmHg/s) and for smooth working of the valve and inflation systems.

Technique of blood pressure measurement The patient should be seated or supine and allowed a minimum of 2 to 3 min rest. On initial assessment or when excessive postural falls are suspected, standing pressures should be measured as well. The patient should be relaxed and the arm supported in the horizontal position with the cuff at heart level. The arm should not be constricted by tight clothing. The bladder mid-point should be placed over the brachial artery. Blood pressure should be recorded in both arms on initial examination and the arm found to have the higher pressure subsequently used. Systolic blood pressure is initially determined by palpation and then the stethoscope is lightly placed over the brachial artery and the cuff pressure raised to approximately 30 mmHg above the point at which the radial pulse disappears and then released at the rate of 2 to 3 mm/s. Both systolic and diastolic pressures should be read to the nearest 2 mm mark. The point of disappearance of sounds (Korotkoff phase V) is preferable to the point of muffling (phase IV). The reasons for this are as follows.

1. Direct arterial blood pressure measurements indicate that the phase of muffling is 5 to 10 mmHg higher than actual diastolic pressure. Korotkoff phase V is 3 to 7 mmHg higher.

2. There are fewer observer errors in identifying the disappearance of sounds.

3. Most of the epidemiological data and multicentre trials of treatment used phase V as the criterion for diastolic blood pressure.

In some clinical situations where blood flow through the brachial artery is high (immediately after exercise, in hyperthyroidism, pregnancy, and anaemia), sounds can be detected down to zero cuff pressure. Under these circumstances, the fourth phase should be recorded, with a note of the fact. Blood pressure in infants and neonates should be measured using a small cuff and Doppler ultrasound as a detection device.

Pseudohypertension in elderly people is due to an incompressible brachial artery wall. Suspicions should be raised when a high systolic pressure is associated with little in the way of target organ damage (particularly echocardiographic left ventricular hypertrophy), postural symptoms on treatment, and a firm radial artery despite cuff occlusion (Osler's phenomenon). Proof depends upon measurement of blood pressure by a method which does not depend upon arterial compression, such as arterial cannulation, finger volumetric, or automatic oscillometric devices.

Home blood pressure monitoring

Patients can usually be taught to measure their own blood pressure by electronic devices which use the Korotkoff sounds or oscillometry. A large range of cheap devices is now available. These are of varying reliability. Only those tested by specialist or consumer bodies and approved should be used. They should also be checked against manual blood pressure measurements. Home blood pressure monitoring has three advantages:

(1) Blood pressure can be measured at the end of a dosing interval of an antihypertensive drug, even when this occurs in the evening or early morning.

(2) 'White coat effects' as a result of measurement by a doctor or nurse are avoided, although occasional patients find measurement stressful even when carried out by themselves.

(3) By encouraging participation in treatment, self-recorded blood pressures are useful both for encouraging compliance and giving reassurance.

Readings should be taken at a consistent time each day. After work in the evening is usually optimal. Blood pressures measured during stressful work are difficult to interpret and provide no useful guidance for treatment. Home blood pressure monitoring gives somewhat higher readings than 24-h ambulatory monitoring, which includes blood pressures during sleep. However, they are usually substantially lower than clinic or office blood pressures. Current evidence suggests that readings of 135/85 mmHg or higher should be considered elevated.

Indirect ambulatory blood pressure monitoring

These devices automatically inflate a cuff at set intervals during the day and night. A recording device is suspended on a belt or sling and the record subjected to computer analysis and print-out at the end of the recording period. One device ('Portapress') measures volumetric change in the finger with each heart beat and therefore offers a means to measure beat to beat variability without requiring large artery compression. At present its use is confined to research, but potentially it offers a novel approach to blood pressure evaluation.

Blood pressure falls during sleep, hence it is preferable to analyse daytime and night-time readings separately using fixed times. Alternatively, an activity meter can detect when the patient is actually asleep. The patient should keep a diary during the day so that blood pressures can be correlated with activity. Night-shift workers rapidly reverse their diurnal rhythm. A reduced or absent nocturnal fall in pressure is associated with a worse cardiovascular prognosis. Pooled analysis of population studies has yielded a figure of 138/87 mmHg for the upper 95 percentile level for daytime

Table 2 Suggested criteria for hypertension using ambulatory indirect blood pressure measurements

	Normal	Abnormal
Daytime	< 135/85	≥ 140/90
Night-time	120/70	≥ 125/75
24 Hour	< 130/80	≥ 135/85

blood pressures. The difference between ambulatory daytime pressures and clinic blood pressures is, on average 12/7 mmHg, but individual variability is great. Suggested criteria for abnormality are shown in Table 2.

Ambulatory blood pressures have been shown repeatedly to be more closely correlated with target organ damage than clinic blood pressures. This is true of left ventricular hypertrophy, carotid wall thickness, fundal vessel changes, and microalbuminuria. There is also increasing evidence that ambulatory blood pressure monitoring is better at predicting cardiovascular events when clinic and ambulatory blood pressures diverge. However, this may partly be due to the fact that many more readings contribute to the calculated average. Multiple measurements of blood pressure have more prognostic value than a few.

Indirect ambulatory blood pressure monitoring is labour intensive and costly. Its place in routine practice therefore lies in situations where it adds information to clinic blood pressures which influences treatment. Where the decision to treat is based upon cardiovascular complications or target organ damage, or where the overall cardiovascular risk is below the level for drug treatment, there is no indication for carrying it out. On the other hand, where clinic blood pressures are sustained at high levels (such as 160/100 mmHg or higher) and treatment is not justified by high cardiovascular risk, ambulatory monitoring may be useful in confirming the presence of blood pressure elevation meriting therapy in its own right. Normal readings suggest 'white coat hypertension' under these circumstances. Other indications for ambulatory monitoring are to confirm resistance to antihypertensive medication in the absence of target organ damage, to assess 24-h control of blood pressure and episodic hypertension, and to investigate hypotensive symptoms in treated patients with no supporting evidence from clinic blood pressures.

'White coat hypertension'

Some patients have consistently elevated clinic blood pressures in the treatment range but unequivocally normal ambulatory blood pressure readings. Clearly the proportion depends critically on the criteria used. However, it is probable that about 20 per cent of patients who would be treated on the basis of high clinic blood pressures have normal ambulatory blood pressures. Almost all patients show blood pressure falls with repeated clinic measurement, so the need for sustained elevation of clinic blood pressures is critical. The prognostic significance of 'white coat hypertension' (some authorities use the term 'isolated office hypertension') is uncertain. Some of the cardiovascular changes observed in hypertension have been described in some studies and not others. There is little in the way of end-point data. Such as there is suggests that the cardiovascular risk is low compared with patients who have elevated ambulatory and clinic blood pressures. Where 'white coat hypertension' is diagnosed, the best advice is to monitor blood pressure and target organ damage and not treat unless ambulatory blood pressures become elevated.

Fundal examination

Fundal appearances provide vital information on vascular pathology and prognosis in hypertension. The Keith Wagener classification is still frequently used, although it has serious shortcomings. Chief amongst these is that grade I and II changes are produced by arterial wall thickening as a result of ageing as well as high blood pressure. Clinically, the main requirement is to differentiate between malignant and non-malignant hypertension on fundal appearances.

Non-malignant hypertension

The earliest effects of blood pressure elevation are generalized reduction in arterial calibre with consequent reduction in arteriovenous ratio. Focal arterial narrowing is seen less often, usually when an acute rise in blood pressure has occurred. The remaining changes are frequently seen in older patients with arteriosclerosis, where their value in assessing hypertensive organ damage is small. They only have significance when seen in younger patients. The light reflex from the arterial wall is increased as a result of thickening. Nipping of the retinal veins occurs largely as a result of the optical effect of the thickened arterial walls preventing visualization of the columns of blood within the veins. Thus the veins appear to taper until they disappear before actually being crossed by the arteries. The veins may also be displaced laterally or posteriorly. Venous obstruction is much less common.

Malignant hypertension

Flame-shaped haemorrhages are superficial and owe their character to constraints imposed by nerve fibres. Dot and blot haemorrhages are deep to nerve fibres and so are not limited in the same way. Haemorrhages usually disappear after a few weeks of effective blood pressure control. There are two types of exudates. Hard or waxy exudates represent the end result of fluid leakage into the fibre layers of the retina from damaged vessels. Fluid is resorbed leaving a protein–lipid residue that is slowly removed by macrophages. Soft exudates or cotton-wool patches are aetiologically and ophthalmoscopically quite different. They are usually larger than hard exudates and have a woolly, ill-defined edge. They are not true exudates, but nerve fibre infarcts caused by hypertensive vascular occlusion. Unlike hard exudates, these lesions disappear within a few weeks of establishing adequate antihypertensive therapy.

Papilloedema is associated with raised pressure in the disc head secondary to severe vascular damage and increased permeability. Venous distention is followed by increased vascularity of the optic disc, which has a pink appearance with blurring of the disc margins and loss of the optic cup. Raising of the optic disc with anterior displacement of the vessels occurs later. The surrounding retina often shows oedema, small radial haemorrhages, and cotton-wool exudates.

The presence of haemorrhages and exudates (grade III), or papilloedema (grade IV) in essential hypertension all carry the same prognosis and the terms 'accelerated' and 'malignant' hypertension should therefore be considered synonymous.

Other physical signs

Clinical evidence of left ventricular hypertrophy and a loud aortic second sound indicate moderate or severe hypertension. Other physical signs indicate target organ damage to the cardiovascular, renal, or central nervous systems.

Investigations

Concentrations of urea, electrolytes, creatinine, and uric acid are usually normal in essential hypertension unless renal damage has occurred. Severe hypertension may be associated with elevated plasma renin and aldosterone levels, which can give rise to a modest hypokalaemic alkalosis. Serum sodium is usually low normal or low under these circumstances. This is an important differentiating point from primary aldosteronism, in which hypokalaemic alkalosis is usually associated with a high or high normal serum sodium concentration.

Microalbuminuria (20 to 200 μg/min or 30 to 300 mg/24 h) in hypertensive patients is prognostic of target organ damage. Other urinary changes, such as urinary casts, haematuria, and proteinuria, usually indicate that hypertension has entered the malignant phase or reflect primary renal disease.

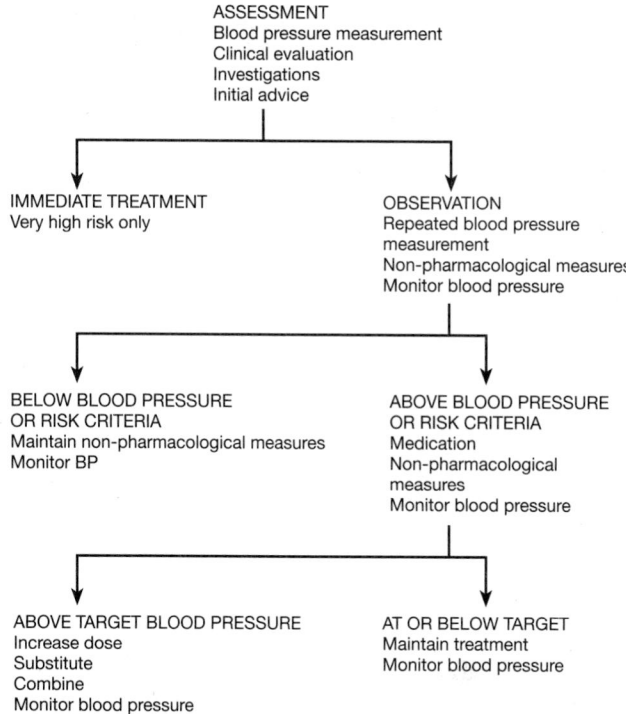

Fig. 1 Treatment plan for hypertension.

Electrocardiographic left ventricular hypertrophy in the absence of any other cause indicates moderate or severe hypertension and is a valuable independent risk factor in hypertension. Echocardiography is much more sensitive in detecting early changes of left ventricular hypertrophy and provides the best independent evidence of severity in mild to moderate hypertension. Chest radiography is insufficiently sensitive as a measure of left ventricular hypertrophy. 'Unfolding of the aorta' is often observed in moderate and severe hypertension.

Management of essential hypertension

A number of national and international expert bodies have drawn up guidelines for the management of hypertension. Although these differ in detail, the overall structure of the recommendations is similar (Fig. 1). Initial clinical assessment is followed by a period of observation and monitoring depending upon the level of cardiovascular risk. During this period treatment of other cardiovascular risk factors and non-pharmacological measures are undertaken. If, at the end of this period, the patient is still at sufficient risk, antihypertensive drugs are recommended.

Assessment

The patient with essential hypertension may present in one of three ways:

(1) As an asymptomatic individual whose blood pressure has been measured at routine examination for employment, insurance, or as a result of screening or preoperatively;

(2) As a patient presenting with an unrelated disorder; or

(3) Much less commonly, as a result of symptoms produced by hypertension or by the complications of hypertension.

Clinicians who deal with hypertension are at a great disadvantage. Whilst treatment of most symptomatic conditions leads to subjective improvement, drug treatment of hypertension may create unpleasant symptoms in an individual who was previously, to the best of their knowledge, perfectly well. It is imperative, therefore, to explain the significance of high blood pressure at the earliest opportunity. It is important to point out that in most cases it does not have a single cause. Many patients find difficulty in grasping the concept of blood pressure variability. Often they are alarmed by the inevitable occasional high reading. Discussion of the rationale for evaluation and treatment and an explanation of the nature of high blood pressure and its very high prevalence serves to reassure patients and improve compliance. Much literature is now available to help.

Establishing the diagnosis

History and examination usually provide few positive features in the uncomplicated hypertensive patient. The usually quoted range for age of onset is 35 to 55 years, but this of course reflects the arbitrary criteria for diagnosis, and many patients who subsequently develop unequivocal hypertension have a blood pressure in the upper part of the 'normal range' below the age of 35. Moderate or severe hypertension first occurring outside the 35 to 55 age range suggests a secondary cause. The presence of hypertension in parents or siblings is of modest value in making the diagnosis. Often a negative family history simply reflects ignorance or failure to diagnose hypertension, particularly in the previous generation when health checks were less common. In addition, a positive family history can often be obtained fortuitously for a condition of very high prevalence such as essential hypertension. Positive indications of a cause for hypertension are of more value, for example a history of oestrogen-containing contraceptive pill exposure or exposure to other medications which elevate blood pressure, previous renal disease or clinical features suggestive of phaeochromocytoma, renal disease, or primary aldosteronism. Specific enquiries should be made regarding heavy alcohol intake.

Clinical evaluation

This provides essential information in the decision to treat. A history of smoking, diabetes, dyslipidaemia, or cardiovascular disease should always be sought. The presence of cardiovascular target organ damage in the form of coronary artery, cerebrovascular, or peripheral vascular disease, generalized or focal fundal arterial narrowing, or clinical left ventricular hypertrophy, all place the patient in a high-risk category. Fundal changes of malignant hypertension, left ventricular failure, encephalopathy, and hypertensive renal failure place the patient in a very high-risk category. Obesity is important as a factor in hypertension and is an independent cardiovascular risk factor.

The presence of conditions such as obstructive airways disease, diabetes, or gout may play a role in the selection of antihypertensive drug.

Investigations

When there is no clinical suspicion of secondary hypertension, extensive investigation for a primary cause is unnecessary, because the prevalence of secondary hypertension is so low. Measurement of serum urea, sodium, potassium, and creatinine, urinary microscopy, and dip-stick testing for protein are sufficient. Risk factor assessment should include an ECG, which is an important but insensitive indicator of left ventricular hypertrophy. Echocardiography is preferable as a more sensitive but expensive alternative. Where left ventricular hypertrophy is present, it offers an excellent means of excluding white coat hypertension. Fasting glucose and total cholesterol (preferably together with high-density lipoprotein cholesterol) should always be measured to define the patient's cardiovascular risk profile.

Initial advice

Except for patients who are at very high risk, or present as hypertensive emergencies, repeated measurements of blood pressure on several occasions should be carried out. The plan should be explained to the patient and advice given to improve cardiovascular risk and lower blood pressure before antihypertensive medication is considered. Cessation of smoking is probably the most important feature of advice at this stage. Other advice is directed at non-pharmacological blood pressure lowering by lifestyle modification, including dietary and behavioural measures. Dietary methods

Table 3 Non-pharmacological therapy in hypertensive patients

	Fall in blood pressure:	
	Systolic	Diastolic
5 kg weight loss	6.0	5.0
50 mmol sodium reduction	1.9	0.5
Fruit and vegetable diet	7.2	2.8
80 mmol potassium supplements	8.2	4.5
Alcohol withdrawal in heavy drinkers	5.0	3.0
More than 3 g fish oil per day	3.0	1.5
Regular moderate exercise	11.0	6.0

Values are taken from meta-analyses of controlled trials in each case, apart from the fruit and vegetable diet.

include weight reduction, sodium restriction, reduced alcohol intake in heavy drinkers, and increased fruit and vegetable intake. Behavioural methods include physical training, biofeedback, and relaxation. Successful non-pharmacological treatment may allow patients with milder degrees of hypertension to avoid drug treatment and enable lower doses of antihypertensive medication to be used in others.

Weight reduction

The epidemiological relationship between weight and blood pressure is reflected in a number of trials which have shown that dietary weight reduction produces a useful fall in blood pressure (Table 3). The mechanism for the fall in blood pressure is debated, but the most likely explanation is a fall in sympathetic efferent output to the cardiovascular system.

Sodium restriction

The average intake of sodium in Westernized cultures is 120 to180 mmol/day. Severe salt restriction (less than 10 mmol/day) produces substantial blood pressure lowering and, together with increased potassium intake, was probably responsible for the efficacy of the Kempner rice–fruit diet, used in the treatment of severe hypertension before the modern drug era. Long-term sodium restriction of this degree is not feasible and carries significant risks. More moderate sodium restriction (70 to 80 mmol/day) can be achieved by abstaining from adding salt at the table, avoiding salt in cooking, and avoiding heavily salted processed foods. As sole therapy, such moderate salt restriction produces a modest reduction in blood pressure, particularly in older subjects and black individuals (Table 3). The individual response is variable: patients showing a more substantial blood pressure fall have been classified as 'salt sensitive'. The reproducibility of 'salt sensitivity' is poor, however, and although a genetic factor has been postulated, the only way of identifying such individuals is by empirically testing the blood pressure response to salt restriction. Salt restriction enhances the blood pressure-lowering action of ACE inhibitors, angiotensin receptor blockers, β-blockers, and diuretics. Curiously, it is ineffective in patients treated with calcium antagonists.

Increased fruit and vegetable intake

Adoption of a vegetarian diet produces a modest fall in blood pressure and increased fruit and vegetable intake has been part of combined regimens of non-pharmacological blood pressure control involving reduction in weight and sodium restriction. However, a recent large trial (DASH—Dietary Approaches to Stop Hypertension) has shown that increased intake of fruit and vegetables can have an important blood pressure-lowering action, equivalent to the effect of a single antihypertensive drug. This was independent of any change in weight or salt intake (Table 3). These effects were produced by doubling the average American intake of 4.3 servings of fruit and vegetables a day. Larger effects were observed when this diet was combined with reduction in total and saturated fats. One contributory factor was probably the increase in potassium intake which occurred. Potassium supplementation has a significant blood pressure-lowering effect, partly at least through natriuresis. There is, however, no justification for potassium supplementation as an independent form of treatment unless the patient is potassium depleted. Although other features of the high fruit and vegetable diet, such as increased fibre and magnesium content, have been claimed to have a blood pressure-lowering action, these actions have not been persuasively demonstrated.

Reduced alcohol intake

The elevated blood pressures shown by heavy drinkers (more than 6 units of alcohol a day) are lowered by withdrawal. This is not related to changes in weight or electrolyte intake. This useful clinical effect has to be differentiated from the pressor response sometimes exhibited by chronic alcoholics on abstention from alcohol, which is mediated by sympathetic overactivity. The optimal intake is 2 to 3 units/day (2 units/day in women). Although some epidemiological studies have shown slightly lower blood pressures in moderate drinkers compared with total abstainers, the individual effect is likely to be small, has not been tested by intervention studies, and it would seem undesirable to advise moderate alcohol intake to teetotal hypertensive patients.

Fish oil and other dietary manoeuvres

Large increases in dietary fish oil (more than 3 g/day of omega-3 fatty acids) lower blood pressure modestly. The effect is only seen in those whose consumption of fish is low. Many patients find the ingestion of such amounts unacceptable, either in the form of oily fish or capsules. Olive oil has been shown to have a very small blood pressure-lowering action in some studies, but there is little evidence to support a therapeutic effect of other unsaturated fatty acids. Claims have also been made for calcium, garlic, protein, and vitamin C, but these are not persuasive.

Physical exercise

Regular aerobic exercise lowers blood pressure independently of any weight loss. Although the overall reduction in blood pressure is impressive, the figures quoted in Table 3 may reflect design flaws in some of the trials, since proper controls are difficult to achieve and the true effect is usually less. Moderate physical activity equivalent to 40 to 60 per cent of maximal oxygen consumption is optimal. This may take the form of, for instance, 30 to 45 min of brisk walking daily. This is also often associated with an improvement in well being attributable to endorphin release.

Other behavioural manoeuvres

Theoretically, interventions which reduce sympathetic efferent output and the alerting response should lower blood pressure. Although superficially attractive as a means of avoiding drug therapy, training in these procedures is labour intensive for professionals and carrying them out is time consuming for patients. A number of controlled trials have claimed such effects, but most have been flawed in design and there is no consistent evidence of efficacy.

Use of non-pharmacological therapy

All patients should receive relevant lifestyle advice. A diet high in fruit and vegetables, and low in salt and saturated fats, together with a recommendation of regular exercise, provide a core management strategy additional to medication, where that is necessary. Weight reduction, even in only marginally overweight patients, is probably the most efficacious manoeuvre of all. Some patients may find it feasible to increase their intake of oily fish. Patients should be advised to reduce heavy alcohol intake.

Although clinical trials have now demonstrated that these various manoeuvres can produce significant blood pressure lowering under rigorous conditions, the effects are often quite small in clinical practice, except perhaps in the case of weight reduction. Some of the dietary advice is expensive for patients (if not for drug budgets), and it is important that those asked to modify their lifestyle substantially are not disappointed by the outcome, or that the uncritical medical enthusiasm which occasionally invests this field does not imply that an aberrant life style is to blame for the development of essential hypertension.

Observation period

A period of observation extending from 1 to 2 weeks up to 1 year before antihypertensive drugs are prescribed is imperative in most patients. There are three reasons for this:

(1) Multiple readings on a number of occasions provide a much better estimate of overall risk than readings on one occasion only;

(2) Blood pressure usually falls owing to diminution in the alerting response as a result of repeated measurement; and

(3) Non-pharmacological management may produce additional blood pressure falls.

The latter two effects may enable substantial numbers of patients with mild hypertension to avoid drug treatment. The observation period is omitted or shortened only if the patient is at high risk. The level of overall cardiovascular risk also determines whether a patient requires antihypertensive medication or not. It is therefore central to the management of essential hypertension.

Cardiovascular risk profile

The epidemiological risks associated with hypertension are not only correlated with sustained systolic and diastolic pressures, but also with:

(1) Irreversible factors such as age, race, male gender, family history, and ethnicity;

(2) Associated, potentially reversible factors, such as smoking, dyslipidaemia, diabetes, and obesity;

(3) The presence of asymptomatic target organ damage such as left ventricular hypertrophy, atheromatous plaques on imaging, or microalbuminuria; and

(4) Clinical complications such as ischaemic heart disease, heart failure, cerebrovascular disease, symptomatic peripheral arterial disease, renal disease, and malignant hypertensive fundal changes.

Higher absolute risk conferred by these other factors is translated to greater potential benefit from blood pressure lowering. The blood pressure levels at which drug treatment is initiated should therefore be lower in the presence of additional risk factors.

It is possible to calculate risk using the Framingham epidemiological data. Some guidelines, such as those issued in Britain and New Zealand, recommend this using a printed risk chart (Fig. 2) or computer program. The complexity of the data requires access either to a computer or printed table. Other guidelines—such as those issued by the American Joint National Committee (**JNC**), World Health Organization (**WHO**), and International Society of Hypertension (**ISH**)—use summary tables to assign risk to a limited number of categories (Table 4). The disadvantage of this approach is that it takes no account of differential weighting of risk factors. Age, for instance, becomes a dominant risk factor in the elderly compared with, say, dyslipidaemia.

All guidance suggests that the uncomplicated hypertensive patients with no other risk factors above a sustained threshold value for systolic and diastolic pressure should be treated with antihypertensive medication. The British Hypertension Society guidelines recommend values of 160 and 100 mmHg, respectively. The WHO–ISH thresholds are 150 and 95 mmHg, whilst the JNC thresholds are 140 and 90 mmHg.

The presence of added risks modifies both the period of observation and, in some cases, the blood pressure threshold for drug treatment. The British Hypertension Society guidelines reduce the thresholds to 140 and 90 mmHg in the presence of a 15 per cent or more 10-year risk of coronary heart disease (approximately equal to a 20 per cent 10-year risk of coronary heart disease and stroke). Patients with target organ damage, complications, or diabetes associated with hypertension reach this level without further risk-factor calculation. These higher-risk patients and those with high sustained levels (200/110 mmHg or higher) should be observed for shorter periods of 1 to 4 weeks, whilst lower-risk patients should be observed for 12 weeks according to these criteria. The WHO–ISH recommend treating medium-risk patients after observation for 3 to 6 months if blood pressures

NO DIABETES

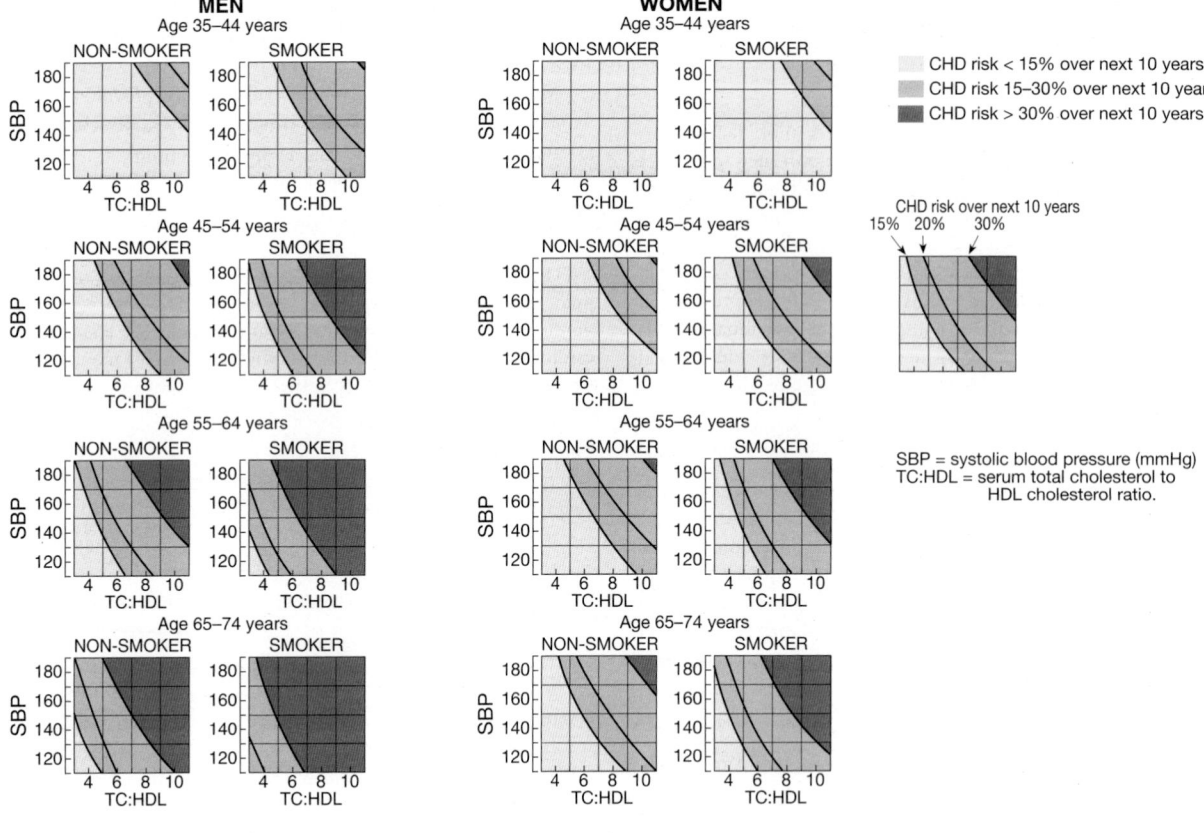

DIABETES

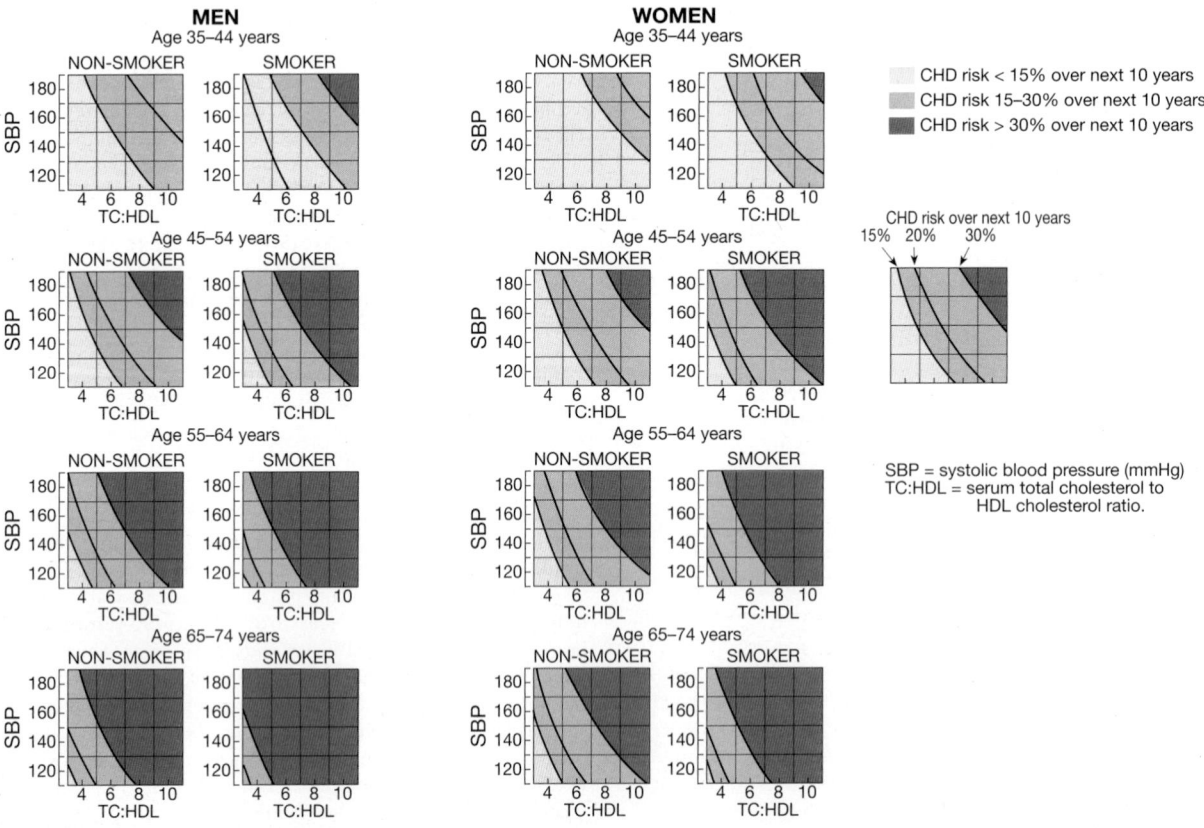

Fig. 2

How to use the Coronary Risk Prediction Chart for Primary Prevention

These charts are for estimating coronary heart disease (CDH) risk (non fatal MI and coronary death) for individuals who have not developed symptomatic CHD or other major atherosclerotic disease.

The use of these charts is not appropriate for patients who have existing disease which already puts them at high risk. Such diseases are:

- CHD or other major atherosclerotic disease.
- Familial hypercholesterolaemia or other inherited dyslipidaemia.
- Established hypertension (systolic BP > 160 mmHg and/or diastolic BP > 100 mmHg) or associated target organ damage.
- Diabetes mellitus with associated target organ damage.
- Renal dysfunction.

- To estimate an individual's absolute 10 year risk of developing CHD find the table for their gender, diabetes (yes/no), smoking status (smoker/non smoker) and age. Within this square define the level of risk according to systolic blood pressure and the ratio of total cholesterol to high density lipoprotein (HDL) cholesterol. If there is no HDL cholesterol result then assume this is 1.0mmol/l and then the lipid scale can be used for total cholesterol alone.
- High risk individuals are defined as those whose 10 year CHD risk exceeds 15% (equivalent to a *cardiovascular* risk of 20% over the same period). As a minimum those at highest risk (≥ 30% red) should be targeted and treated now, and as resources allow others with risk of >15% (orange) should be progressively targeted.
- Smoking status should reflect lifetime exposure to tobacco and not simply tobacco use at the time of risk assessment.
- The initial blood pressure and the first random (non fasting) total cholesterol and HDL cholesterol can be used to estimate an individuals risk. However, the decision on using drug therapy should be based on repeat risk factor measurements over a period of time. The chart should not be used to estimate risk after treatment of hyperlipidaemia or blood pressure has been initiated.
- CHD risk is higher than indicated in the charts for:
- Those with a family history of premature CHD (men <55 years and women <65 years) which increases the risk by a factor of approximately 1.5.
- Those with raised triglyceride levels.
- Those who are not diabetic but have impaired glucose tolerance.
- Women with premature menopause.
- As the person approaches the next age category. As risk increases exponentially with age the risk will be closer to the higher decennium for the last four years of each decade.
- In ethnic minorities the risk chart should be used wth caution as it has not been validated in these populations.
- The estimates of CHD risk from the chart are based on groups of people and in managing an *individual* the physician also has to use clinical judgement in deciding how intensively to intervene on lifestyle and whether or not to use drug therapies.
- An individual can be shown on the chart the direction on which the risk of CHD can be reduced by changing smoking status, blood pressure or cholesterol.

Fig. 2 Coronary risk prevention chart recommended for risk assessment in the British Hypertension Society guidelines. (Reproduced from British National Formulary (2001), **42**, with permission.)

Table 4 Risk factor profiling as suggested in the WHO–International Society of Hypertension guidelines (slightly modified)

Grade 1: SBP 140–159 or DBP 90–99	Grade 2: SBP 160–179 or DBP 100–109	Grade 3: ≥ 180 or DBP ≥ 110
I. No other risk factors		
Low	Medium	High
II. One or two risk factors		
Medium	Medium	Very high
III. Three or more risk factors or target organ damage or diabetes		
High	High	Very high
IV. Complications		
Very high	Very high	Very high

DBP, diastolic blood pressure; SBP, systolic blood pressure.

are 140/90 mmHg or higher, while low-risk patients should be observed for 6 to 12 months before treatment. The JNC risk advice suggests observation periods of up to 12 months in low-risk individuals (most of whom would not be treated on the basis of the other recommendations); other non-urgent patients are treated after two follow-up visits (Table 5).

Patients at the highest risk should be treated more promptly. Accelerated hypertension and hypertension associated with acute complications such as left ventricular failure require immediate treatment. The WHO–ISH recommends treating patients in the 'high' and 'very high' risk groups within a few days, after repeated measurement of blood pressure. The JNC guidelines imply a similar policy.

Adoption of the JNC or WHO–ISH recommendations will result in many more patients receiving drug treatment than the British guidelines. The 10-year level of cardiovascular risk in those who would be given drug treatment according to both sets of recommendations falls below 15 per cent. This is not an issue which clinical trials can resolve. It reflects a balanced judgement of the benefits of treatment set against the cost and inconvenience of life-long therapy, both to the individual and to society. The final decision depends upon the values of both. Often the language of guidelines in the treatment of hypertension has a prescriptive tone. It should not be forgotten that their only objective is to inform the professional so that appropriate options can be presented to the patient.

Treatment of hypertension

Target blood pressure

The one clinical trial which has addressed the issue of target blood pressure suggested no significant differences in outcome when blood pressure control was aimed at different strata below 140/90 mmHg, although the lowest number of events occurred around pressures of 138/83 mmHg. There was no indication of a worse outcome when pressures were reduced to lower levels than this (the so-called 'J-shaped curve'). Rigorous blood pressure control is particularly important in diabetic hypertensive patients, where pressures should be kept below 140/80 mmHg.

Impact of drug treatment

A number of important, large multicentre trials have demonstrated the impact of antihypertensive treatment on cardiovascular disease. Patients recruited have differed, and in particular some trials have been confined to elderly subjects. In addition, drug regimens and protocols have been widely disparate. Nevertheless, the conclusions have shown an impressive degree of concordance. Meta-analysis of the data has demonstrated that in these trials, for a drug-induced fall in systolic blood pressure of 12 to 13 mmHg, coronary heart disease is reduced by 21 per cent, stroke by 37 per cent, and cardiovascular mortality by 25 per cent. A fall in diastolic pressure of 5 to 6 mmHg produced figures of 16, 38, and 21 per cent, respectively. The benefits of treatment were seen in patients with isolated elevation of systolic or diastolic blood pressure. The epidemiological risk of stroke associated with these blood pressure differences was almost identical, so that, at least over the period of the trials, the risk of stroke attributable to hypertension was totally reversed. This does not imply that drug treatment abolishes the life-long risk of stroke, but it does indicate that pharmacological lowering of blood pressure reduces the short-term risks both of atherothrombotic and haemorrhagic strokes. The impact of treatment on coronary events is also significant, but probably falls short of complete reversibility. The reasons for this are still controversial.

Selection of therapy

A number of different classes of hypertensive drug are available and widely used.

Thiazide and related diuretics

Diuretics were used in several of the end-point trials which demonstrated efficacy in treating hypertension. Thiazides are ineffective in patients with a glomerular filtration rate below 40 ml/min. The more potent short-acting

Table 5 JNC guidelines for treatment of hypertension

Blood pressure stages (mmHg)	Risk group A (No risk factors, target organ damage, or complications)	Risk group B (At least one risk factor, not including diabetes; no target organ damage or complications)	Risk group C (Target organ damage/complications and/or diabetes, with or without other risk factors)
130–139/85–89	Lifestyle modification	Lifestyle modification	Drug therapy*
140–159/90–99	Lifestyle modification (up to 12 months)	Lifestyle modification (up to 6 months)	Drug therapy
≥ 160/≥ 100	Drug therapy	Drug therapy	Drug therapy

* For those with heart failure, renal insufficiency, or diabetes.

loop diuretics have less antihypertensive efficacy over 24 h since rebound sodium retention occurs at the end of the diuretic and natriuretic effect. They are more inconvenient for patients and should not be used except where sodium balance has to be controlled. Their major indication is to control sodium retention associated with hypertension, for example due to renal or cardiac failure. Potassium-retaining diuretics are commonly used in combination with thiazides or, in larger doses, in the treatment of primary aldosteronism. A recent study showing the beneficial effect of spironolactone on morbidity and mortality in heart failure is likely to increase use of this agent. If it, or other potassium-retaining agents, are given to patients with renal impairment, then close monitoring is required because of the danger of hyperkalaemia. This may also occur in patients who are receiving treatment which blocks the renin–angiotensin–aldosterone system. An incidental advantage of thiazides may be reduction in osteoporosis as a result of calcium retention.

Only low doses of diuretics should now be used for uncomplicated hypertension. These have a degree of patient acceptability similar to placebo in more recent studies. The dose–response curve is flat and dose titration is not required. The adverse metabolic effects on potassium balance, plasma lipids, and insulin resistance have attracted attention, since these worsen the cardiovascular risk profile. They are minimal on low-dosage regimens, even in patients with diabetes. Urate retention may precipitate gout in predisposed patients. The incidence of erectile dysfunction (which is elevated in untreated hypertension) is increased. In long-term cohort studies the risk of renal cell carcinoma has been reported as doubled, although the absolute incidence remains very low. Sodium and fluid depletion with prerenal failure is very unusual with low-dose thiazide therapy, but is much more common with loop diuretics, particularly in elderly subjects.

Dosage regimens of selected diuretics are shown in Table 6.

β-Blockers

β-Blockers have also been shown to reduce cardiovascular events in trials of the treatment of hypertension.

There are clinically important differences between the pharmacological properties of different members of the class. β_1-Selective blocking agents have less action upon bronchial and vascular β_2-adrenergic receptors, and so are less likely to cause bronchospasm or vasoconstriction in susceptible patients (for example patients with chronic obstructive airways disease or Raynaud's phenomenon). There is, however, still significant risk as tissues have mixed populations of receptors. Some β-blockers have partial agonist action at the β_1-receptor (intrinsic sympathomimetic activity) so that there is less slowing of the heart, although the heart rate response to exercise is still blunted. The clinical significance of this is uncertain. Heart rate is a risk factor for cardiac mortality and slowing might therefore be thought to be advantageous. However, bradycardia is associated with increased stroke volume and pulse pressure, which constitutes an adverse risk factor. There have been no comparative trials to address this issue in hypertension, although prevention of secondary infarction has been observed only in trials of agents without intrinsic sympathetic activity.

β-Blockers are contraindicated in hypertensive patients with asthma, chronic obstructive airways disease, heart block greater than grade 1, and sick sinus syndrome. They should be used with great caution in cardiac failure, although low-dose β-blockade with carvedilol or metoprolol has reduced morbidity and mortality in end-point trials. The combination of β-blockade with the calcium-channel blockers verapamil and diltiazem may have additional depressant actions on the sinatrial and atrioventricular node and have negative inotropic effects in patients with cardiac disease, and therefore should be avoided.

β-Blockers can have a large number of side-effects. Exercise capacity is decreased and fatiguability increased, most frequently causing problems in athletes and enthusiasts for regular physical training. They probably cause erectile dysfunction, although the incidence is not as high as that reported with diuretics where this has been recorded in trials. Non-selective β-adrenergic blockers inhibit β_2-induced vasodilatation. This may cause cold extremities and worsening of symptoms in peripheral vascular disease and Raynaud's disease. This action may also become important when there are high circulating concentrations of noradrenaline, for instance in patients with phaeochromocytoma, or after clonidine withdrawal, or in patients treated with sympathomimetic medication. Under these circumstances, non-selective β-blockade worsens hypertension. Serum triglycerides are slightly elevated and high-density lipoprotein cholesterol is reduced. This effect is not seen with drugs having intrinsic sympathomimetic activity and is less marked with cardioselective agents. β-Blockade delays the recovery from hypoglycaemia in diabetic patients and may worsen glucose intolerance. These effects are less with cardioselective drugs. β-Blockade may also mask symptoms of hypoglycaemia due to adrenaline. These are relative disadvantages in patients with diabetes and glucose intolerance that have to be balanced against benefits, for example in patients with ischaemic heart disease.

Table 6 Dosage regimens of selected diuretics for the treatment of hypertension

	Dosage (mg/day)	Doses/day
Thiazide diuretics*		
Chlortalidone (chlorthalidone)	12.5–50	1
Hydrochlorothiazide	12.5–50	1
Bendrofluazide	2.5–5.0	1
Indapamide	1.25–5.0	1
Metolazone†	0.5–10	1
Loop diuretics		
Bumetanide	0.5–4.0	2–3
Ethacrynic acid	25–100	2–3
Frusemide	40–240	2–3
Torasemide	5–100	1–2
Potassium-retaining diuretics		
Amiloride	5–10	1
Spironolactone	25–100	1
Triamterene	25–100	1

* Lowest doses should be used in uncomplicated hypertension.

† Metolazone is a thiazide but acts at several sites along the nephron and can induce profound diuresis and volume depletion. It should only be used to treat hypertension when this is associated with refractory oedema.

Table 7 Pharmacological properties and dosage regimens of β-adrenergic blocking drugs for the treatment of hypertension

	ISA	Cardio-selectivity	Dose (mg/day)	Doses/day
Acebutolol	+	+	400–800	1–2
Atenolol	0	++	25–100	1
Betaxolol	0	++	10–40	1
Bisoprolol	0	++	2.5–20	1
Carteolol	+	0	5–10	1
Carvedilol*	0	0	12.5–50	2
Celiprolol*	0	++	200–400	1
Labetolol*	+	0	200–2400	2
Metoprolol	0	++	100–200	1–2
Nadolol	0	0	80–240	1
Oxprenolol	+	0	80–320	2–3
Penbutolol	++	0	10–60	2–3
Pindolol	+	0	10–45	1
Propranolol	0	0	160–320	2
Timolol	0	0	10–60	2

ISA, intrinsic sympathomimetic activity.

* Additional vasodilatory action.

Table 8 Dosage regimens of calcium-channel blockers for the treatment of hypertension

	Dosage (mg/day)	Doses/day
Dihydropyridines		
Amlodipine	5–10	1
Felodipine	2.5–10	1
Isradipine	2.5–10	1–2
Lacidipine	2–6	1
Lercanidipine	10–20	1
Nicardipine*	60–120	2
Nifedipine*	20–90	1
Nisoldipine*	10–40	1
Phenylalkylamines		
Verapamil*	120–480	1–2
Benzothiazepines		
Diltiazem*	120–360	1–2

* Modified release preparations. These vary in pharmacokinetics and the brand should therefore be specified.

Some members of the class—such as propranolol, metoprolol, and timolol—are lipid soluble: entry into the brain appears to be associated with nightmares and sleep disturbances. These effects are unusual with water-soluble agents such as atenolol, nadolol, celiprolol, and betaxolol. Sudden discontinuation of β-adrenergic blockers in patients with cardiac disease has been associated with sudden death and it is preferable to tail off treatment in such patients over a week or two.

Pharmacological properties and dosage regimens of β-adrenergic blocking drugs are shown in Table 7.

Calcium antagonists

This class of drugs has been extensively used in treating hypertension since the 1970s. There is evidence of reduction in cardiovascular disease in end-point trials of systolic hypertension in elderly patients.

The dihydropyridine channel blockers act mainly upon vascular smooth muscle, causing vasodilatation. The non-dihydropyridines include diltiazem, a benzothiazepine, and verapamil, a phenylalkylamine. These cause less marked vasodilatation but have more pronounced effects upon cardiac contractility and atrioventricular conduction. Short-acting dihydropyridines (such as nifedipine) cause reflex baroreceptor-mediated tachycardia. If vasodilatation is not maintained, the baroreceptors do not reset, and so there may be a sustained increase in pulse rate, with other features of sympathetic activity such as sweating, palpitations, and headache. These side-effects occur in a substantial number of patients. Sustained release preparations, or dihydropyridines with prolonged action (such as amlodipine), do not usually produce these effects. Flushing and ankle oedema occur frequently with all dihydropyridines. Oedema reflects local increase in pressure distal to dilated precapillary resistance vessels causing transudation of fluid into the tissues.

Considerable controversy was generated in 1995 by a case–control study and a meta-analysis of clinical trials which suggested that calcium-channel blockade in hypertension was associated with an increased incidence of coronary events. Although this finding was hotly disputed, it does seem likely that the first-generation, short-acting dihydropyridines were producing an adverse outcome through repeated sympathetic activation. For this reason they are best avoided in treating hypertension. Other associations with increased incidence of cancer have not been confirmed, and an association with gastrointestinal haemorrhage is still debated.

Verapamil may precipitate cardiac failure in predisposed patients and exacerbate conduction disorders. It should therefore be avoided in patients with sick sinus syndrome and atrioventricular block. Although these dangers are less with diltiazem, it is also best avoided in such patients. An action upon colonic smooth muscle causes constipation with verapamil: this is usually the only adverse effect that interferes with the quality of life with this drug. This side-effect is less commonly seen with diltiazem, although headache is more frequent.

Dosage regimens of calcium-channel blockers are shown in Table 8.

Angiotensin-converting enzyme (ACE) inhibitors

These agents have been used since the late 1970s in treating hypertension. Only one rather inconclusive end-point trial in hypertension has so far been reported, but there has been impressive evidence for reduction of morbidity and mortality in cardiac failure. Their major advantage is that they are very well tolerated with the exception of dry, unproductive cough, observed in about 20 per cent of patients. Since this does not occur with angiotensin-receptor blockers, it is probably due to bradykinin potentiation. Where patients find it unacceptable, there is no alternative to discontinuing ACE inhibitors and substituting another class of drug.

There are two serious side-effects, which are uncommon and avoidable in most cases. First, angiotensin II maintains renal glomerular hydrostatic pressure and filtration fraction by efferent arteriolar constriction. Blockade may therefore reduce glomerular filtration rate, although renal blood flow is increased. This is clinically important when renal blood flow is critically reduced, as for instance in bilateral renal artery stenosis or stenosis of the artery supplying a single kidney. It may also occur when renal perfusion is reduced through salt and water depletion, congestive cardiac failure, or renal microvascular disease. In all these situations, ACE inhibitors may precipitate acute renal failure. When glomerular filtration rate is reduced in the ischaemic kidney in patients with unilateral renal artery stenosis, the effect may not be diagnosed without imaging studies since routine tests of renal function may not be affected. Second, administration of ACE inhibitors to patients with high circulating renin levels due to salt and water depletion may precipitate severe hypotension. Where there is this clinical possibility, a small dose, preferably of a short duration agent such as captopril (6.25 mg), should be administered under supervision.

A small elevation of plasma potassium consistently occurs as a result of reduction in aldosterone secretion. This may be clinically important in those with renal failure. For this reason, ACE inhibitors should not normally be combined with potassium-sparing diuretics. Angioneurotic oedema has occurred rarely.

Dosage regimens of ACE inhibitors are shown in Table 9.

Angiotensin II receptor antagonists

The newest major class of drugs used in treating hypertension are the angiotensin II subtype 1 receptor (AT(1)) antagonists. No hard end-point

Table 9 Dosage regimens of ACE inhibitors for the treatment of hypertension

	Dosage (mg/day)	Doses/day
Benazepril	5–40	1–2
Captopril	25–150	2–3
Cilazapril	1–5	1
Enalapril	2.5–40	1–2
Fosinopril	10–40	1–2
Imidapril	2.5–20	1
Lisinopril	2.5–40	1
Moexipril	3.75–30	1–2
Perindopril	2–8	1
Quinapril	2.5–80	1–2
Ramipril	1.25–10	1–2
Trandolapril	0.5–4	1

trials in hypertension have so far been reported. Experience to date indicates a very low incidence of side-effects and very good patient acceptability.

Although, like ACE inhibitors, their prime target is the renin–angiotensin system, they are different in potentially important ways. Thus, while blocking the AT(1) receptor, they stimulate the angiotensin II subtype 2 (AT(2)) and other receptors as a result of high angiotensin II levels. The role of these other receptors is uncertain, and the major actions of angiotensin receptor antagonists reflect inhibition of the 'classic' effects of the renin–angiotensin system mediated by the AT(1) receptor on the blood vessels, heart, adrenal gland, kidneys, brain, and sympathetic nervous system. The actions are in this respect identical with those of ACE inhibitors. The same adverse effects in sodium-depleted patients and in patients with critical reduction of renal blood flow are therefore seen.

Addition of an AT(1) receptor antagonist to an ACE inhibitor has, in some trials, produced additional blood pressure lowering, perhaps due to more complete blockade of the renin–angiotensin system. They have no bradykinin-potentiating activity, accounting for the absence of drug-induced cough and giving these agents an important place as substitutes for ACE inhibitors when unacceptable cough occurs. Losartan is unique in this class of drugs in having a uricosuric effect.

Dosage regimens of AT(1) receptor antagonists are shown in Table 10.

α-Adrenergic blocking drugs

These drugs have been available for over 40 years, but early members of the class were never used routinely in the treatment of hypertension because of severe postural hypotension and the development of tolerance. Prazosin was initially introduced as a direct-acting vasodilator in 1976, but subsequently found specifically to inhibit post-synaptic α_1-receptors. Initially, the recommended dosage was too high and postural hypotension and syncope proved serious problems which retarded the acceptance of this class of drugs, although the use of lower doses and the development of longer-acting agents has largely overcome this problem. Blockade of sphincteric receptors produces improvement in symptoms in patients with benign prostatic hyperplasia. Occasionally, the sphincteric effects worsen symptoms in patients with stress incontinence. Improvement in penile blood

Table 10 Dosage regimens of angiotension II subtype 1 (AT(1)) receptor antagonists for the treatment of hypertension

	Dosage (mg/day)	Doses/day
Candesartan	2–16	1
Eprosartan	300–800	1
Irbesartan	75–300	1
Losartan	25–100	1–2
Telmisartan	20–80	1
Valsartan	40–160	1

Table 11 Dosage and regimens of α_1-adrenoceptor blocking drugs for the treatment of hypertension

	Dosage (mg/day)	Doses/day
Doxazosin	1–16	1
Indoramin	50–200	2–3
Prazosin	0.5–20	2–3
Terazosin	1–20	1
Phenoxybenzamine*	10–150	2
Phentolamine*	2–5, intravenous bolus	

* Only used in the management of phaeochromocytoma.

flow is associated with some benefit in patients with erectile dysfunction. Priapism has been reported rarely. Indoramin has additional central effects, causing dry mouth, nasal congestion, and extrapyramidal syndromes. Uniquely amongst antihypertensive drugs, the α_1-antagonists produce favourable changes in plasma lipids, with a reduction in total and low-density lipoprotein cholesterol and triglycerides, and an increase in high-density lipoprotein cholesterol.

Dosage regimens of α_1-adrenoreceptor blocking drugs are shown in Table 11.

Centrally acting sympatholytic drugs

Methyldopa was originally developed in the late 1950s and for many years it was one of the mainstays of antihypertensive therapy. However, it frequently causes sedation, impaired psychomotor performance, dry mouth, and erectile dysfunction. Its unfavourable impact upon quality of life caused it to be replaced by equally effective drugs in the 1970s, although it is still used extensively in the management of hypertension of pregnancy.

The withdrawal syndrome is an occasional but potentially dangerous feature of these drugs. It is most common with clonidine, when discontinuation results in a rebound rise in catecholamines with features that may resemble phaeochromocytoma, such as severe hypertension, tachycardia, and sweating. This is exacerbated when patients are also receiving non-selective β-blockers such as propranolol, which inactivates peripheral β-vasodilator adrenoceptors. The syndrome is treated by readministering the drug and then gradually discontinuing. A combined adrenoceptor inhibitor such as labetolol can be used to control blood pressure in an emergency situation. These central side-effects are shared by guanabenz, guanfacine, and clonidine. Recently, more specific agents such as moxonidine, directed at the imidazoline receptor, have been developed. These have a lower incidence of central side-effects.

Dosage regimens of centrally acting drugs are shown in Table 12.

Direct vasodilators

Hydralazine was extensively used as part of a stepped care regimen. The main disadvantages were sympathetic activation and the development of a lupus-like syndrome, particularly in patients with the slow acetylator genotype. These disadvantages, together with the need for multiple daily dosage, have resulted in the replacement of hydralazine by other agents, except for occasional use in severe hypertension and hypertension associated with pregnancy. No end-point trials have been carried out.

Table 12 Dosage regimens of centrally acting drugs for the treatment of hypertension

	Dosage (mg/day)	Doses/day
Clonidine	0.15–1.2	2–3
Guanabenz	8–32	2
Guanfacine	1–3	1
Methyldopa	500–3000	2–3
Moxonidine	0.2–0.6	1–2

Usage of the more potent vasodilator minoxidil is confined to severe, resistant hypertension because of its side-effects, which include hypertrichosis and severe fluid retention. For this reason, combination with a potent loop diuretic is almost always necessary. T-wave changes and S–T depression may occur in the early phases of treatment with minoxidil due to increased cardiac work as a result of generalized vasodilatation. On these grounds, it is preferable to combine minoxidil with a β-blocker unless contraindicated.

Dosage regimens of oral vasodilators are shown in Table 13.

Drug regimens

Indications and contraindications for specific classes of drugs are shown in Table 14.

Monotherapy on average reduces systolic pressure by 7 to 13 mmHg and diastolic pressure by 4 to 8 mmHg. There is, however, marked heterogeneity in response among individuals to particular drugs. Treatment should normally commence with a low dose of the drug selected. If an adequate response is not obtained, which certainly applies if the blood pressure remains above the level at which treatment was deemed to be indicated in the individual (Tables 4 and 5), then a number of strategies can be pursued. Firstly, the dose of the initial drug can be titrated upwards against blood pressure, except in the case of diuretics, where a single dose is used. Secondly, a small dose of a second drug can be used either separately or as a combination tablet as a means of limiting dose-related side-effects. Thirdly, the initial drug can be stopped and another class of antihypertensive agent started in the hope of greater efficacy. One study found that a rotational policy of four agents tried sequentially increased the chance of successful control of blood pressure (defined as < 140/90 mmHg) with monotherapy from 39 per cent to 73 per cent. This study also found that the responses to ACE inhibitor (A) and β-blocker (B) were correlated, as were those to calcium-channel blocker (C) and diuretic (D), hence an 'AB/CD' rule was proposed. If the initial drug used did not produce a satisfactory response, it could be substituted with one of the drugs in the other pair of treatments, thus abbreviating the rotation for use in routine practice.

In any situation a drug that is poorly tolerated must be substituted, and when a satisfactory response cannot be produced by a single agent, another class of drug must be added. Three or even four classes of drug may be needed to control more resistant hypertension. However, some combinations of drugs, which share mechanisms of antihypertensive action, have less than additive effects and are best avoided, unless the drugs are indicated on other grounds. Such combinations include a β-blocker and ACE inhibitor or angiotensin receptor antagonist, and a calcium antagonist and diuretic. Effective combinations include:

(1) diuretic and β-blocker;

(2) diuretic and ACE inhibitor or angiotensin receptor antagonist;

(3) dihydropyridine calcium antagonist and β-blocker;

(4) α-blocker and β-blocker; and

(5) α-blocker with any other class of agent as third-line treatment.

Drug selection

The strong end-point trial data, patient acceptability, and low cost make diuretics or β-blockers the preferred first-line therapy in hypertensive patients who do not have indications for other drugs. The Medical Research Council Trial of Treatment in Hypertension in the Elderly suggested that diuretics were associated with a better outcome in terms of ischaemic heart disease and they should therefore normally be the first-line therapy in elderly patients. There are powerful reasons for using other drugs in the presence of comorbidity, for instance ACE inhibitors in the patient with cardiac failure and β-blockers in the patient with angina. Diuretics or dihydropyridine calcium antagonists are recommended for isolated systolic hypertension on the basis of end-point trials, but it is probable that benefit is common to most classes of drug. The only possible exception to this are rate-limiting β-blockers and calcium antagonists, where cardiac filling and stroke volume may be increased with a consequent rise in pulse pressure.

Follow-up

It is essential that patients are monitored regularly. It is important that they understand the need for this, or default is more likely. The interval between clinic visits may be short initially, usually varying between 1 and 4 weeks.

Table 13 Dosage regimens of oral vasodilators for the treatment of hypertension

	Dosage (mg/day)	Doses/day
Hydralazine	50–100*	2
Minoxidil	2.5–50	1–2

* 100 mg/day is the usual maximal dose in the treatment of hypertension. There is a risk of SLE-like syndrome after long-term treatment with over 100 mg daily (or less in women and slow acetylator individuals).

Table 14 Indications and contraindications to specific classes of drugs in the treatment of essential hypertension

	Indications	Contraindications
Diuretics	Cardiac failure	
	Elderly patients	
	Systolic hypertension in the elderly	
β-Blockers	Angina	Asthma and chronic obstructive airways disease
	After myocardial infarction	Peripheral vascular disease
	Tachyarrhythmias	
	Cardiac failure*	
Calcium antagonists	Systolic hypertension in the elderly	Heart block (verapamil and diltiazem)
ACE inhibitors	Cardiac failure	Pregnancy
	Left ventricular dysfunction	Renovascular disease
	After myocardial infarction (higher-risk patients)	Sodium and fluid depletion
	Diabetic nephropathy and other proteinuric renal disease	Hyperkalaemia
Angiotensin receptor antagonists	As for ACE inhibitors in presence of ACE inhibitor-induced cough or intolerance	As for ACE inhibitors
α-Blockers	Prostatism	Urinary incontinence

* With care.

When blood pressure is controlled, it is probably not necessary to see patients more often than once every 6 months.

Other treatment

Other risk factors may need control, such as serum lipids, obesity, and glucose intolerance, all of which are more prevalent in hypertensive patients. Advice about smoking is of paramount importance, since the risks of this habit exceed those of mild hypertension in many patients. Low-dose aspirin (75 mg/day) has been shown to reduce the incidence of myocardial infarction in higher-risk patients over 50 years old and this should be offered routinely to patients who fall in this category and who do not have contraindications. In view of the increased incidence of haemorrhage, it is probably not indicated in lower-risk hypertensive patients.

Resistant hypertension

In the absence of evidence of target organ damage, 'white coat hypertension' should be excluded by 24-h ambulatory monitoring. However, in some cases, blood pressures measured in the clinic, at home, or by ambulatory monitoring may remain high despite therapy with four, or occasionally five, classes of drug in optimal dosage. Minoxidil, in combination with a diuretic and preferably a β-blocker, should be reserved for such cases, titrating the dose against blood pressure, and adjusting the dose of diuretic to control oedema. Possible explanations of resistance should be sought if such measures fail to control blood pressure. These are:

(1) Secondary hypertension (e.g. renovascular or endocrine);

(2) Ingestion of drugs which may raise blood pressure (e.g. non-steroidal anti-inflammatory agents);

(3) Heavy alcohol intake;

(4) Sodium and fluid retention as a result of inadequate diuretic therapy; and

(5) Poor patient compliance.

Poor compliance is often difficult to detect in hypertensive patients. Clues are provided by an initial reluctance to take medication, absence of expected pharmacological effects (such as bradycardia with some β-blockers, oedema with minoxidil), or evidence of failure to consume tablets, as revealed by tablet counts or prescription frequency. Other forms of poor compliance, such as incorrect dosing intervals, are more frequent but only detectable by electronic pill counting. In some cases it may be necessary to admit a patient to hospital and supervise administration of treatment. Where compliance is obviously poor, a number of manoeuvres can help to improve it. The regimen should be kept as simple as possible, using once daily drugs and combination tablets. A carer needs to be involved in administering medication to those who are confused. Whenever possible, effective communication with full information and involvement of the patient in his or her treatment is essential. Nurses, pharmacists, and other health professionals can play a vital role in this process.

Hypertension in specific groups of patients

Hypertension in Afro-Caribbean patients

Hypertension is more prevalent in black Afro-Caribbean patients and carries a worse prognosis. Meticulous blood pressure control therefore assumes greater importance than normal. Black patients as a group tend to respond better to diuretics, calcium antagonists, and dietary salt restriction than white patients. ACE inhibitors, angiotensin receptor antagonists, and β-blockers are, as a rule, less effective, although there is substantial patient variability in responsiveness. Activation of the renin–angiotensin system by diuretics may restore blood pressure responsiveness to ACE inhibitors or angiotensin receptor antagonists.

Hypertension in the elderly

The elderly are a very high-risk group. Inevitably, therefore, more elderly patients will meet the criteria for antihypertensive medication than will those in younger age groups. A number of surveys have shown that doctors consistently underestimate the risks of hypertension in the elderly and therefore under-treat. However, the elderly present some particular problems as a result of the changed physiology of ageing. Thus:

1. Arterial wall stiffness gives rise to systolic hypertension and increased pulse pressure (isolated systolic hypertension). This also causes impaired baroreflex sensitivity with increased risk of orthostatic hypotension.

2. Renal conservation of sodium and fluid in the face of depletion is impaired. Elderly patients are therefore more subject to dehydration as a result of diuretic therapy or dietary restriction.

3. Clearance of drugs and their active metabolites is decreased as a result of declining hepatic and renal function.

4. Cardiac compliance and reserve are reduced and patients are therefore much more likely to develop cardiac failure. End-point trials of hypertension treatment have consistently shown reductions in morbidity and mortality from cardiac failure.

5. Comorbidity is much more common.

6. Communication and compliance may be difficult with decline in cognitive function. Some evidence from clinical trials suggests that this decline may be retarded by antihypertensive treatment.

Despite these important considerations, there is no fundamental difference in the approach to treating hypertension in the elderly patient. As a general rule, drug regimens should be as simple as possible and dosages increased more gradually. The greatest danger results from lowering pressure too much and too rapidly. Although trial evidence is limited in the very old (i.e. those over 80), there is no reason to manage these patients any differently from those who are not as old. Biological rather than chronological age should be the deciding factor in initiating antihypertensive treatment.

Essential hypertension in children

Although secondary hypertension is more common in children than in adults, no specific cause is found for hypertension in the majority of adolescents. The criteria for drug treatment, however, have to be modified because of the lower blood pressure range. The American Joint National Committee guidelines recommend that blood pressures above the 95th percentile taking into account age, height, and sex should be considered elevated. In principle, regimens are the same as those recommended for adults, with appropriate dose adjustment.

Further reading

Appel LJ *et al.* (1997). A clinical trial of the effects of dietary patterns on blood pressure. *New England Journal of Medicine* **336**, 1117–24. [The DASH trial of increased fruit and vegetable intake producing substantial blood pressure lowering.]

British Cardiac Society, British Hyperlipidaemia Association, British Hypertension Society (1998). Joint British recommendations on prevention of coronary heart disease in clinical practice. *Heart*, **80**(Suppl 2), S1–S29. [Contains important risk chart for multiple risk factor profiling.]

Dickerson JE *et al.*(1999). Optimisation of antihypertensive treatment by crossover rotation of four major classes. *Lancet* **353**, 2008–13.

Fagard RH (1993). Physical fitness and blood pressure. *Journal of Hypertension* **11**(Suppl 5), S47–S52. [A meta-analysis of the effects of training on blood pressure.]

Graudal NA, Galoe AM, Garred P (1998). Effects of sodium restriction on blood pressure, renin, aldosterone, catecholamines, cholesterols and triglyceride: a meta-analysis. *Journal of the American Medical Association* **279**, 1383–91. [Important meta-analysis of the effects of salt restriction in hypertensive and normotensive subjects.]

Hansson I *et al.* (1998). Effect of intensive blood pressure lowering and low-dose aspirin in patients with hypertension: principal results of the Hypertension Optimal Treatment (HOT) trial. *Lancet* **351**, 1755–62. [The only trial specifically to address the question of optimal target blood pressure for treatment.]

Joint National Committee on Detection, Evaluation and Treatment of High Blood Pressure (1997). Sixth Report (JNC VI). *Archives of Internal Medicine* **157**, 2413–46. [The latest United States guidelines.]

Kaplan NM (1998). *Clinical hypertension*, 7th edn. Williams & Wilkins, Baltimore. [One of the most comprehensive recent texts from the United States perspective, fully referenced.]

Keil U *et al.* (1998). Alcohol, blood pressure and hypertension. In: *Alcohol and cardiovascular disease, Novartis Foundation Symposium* **216**, pp 125–51.Wiley, Chichester. [Systematic review of alcohol and hypertension.]

Medical Research Council Working Party (1985). MRC trial of treatment of mild hypertension: principal results. *British Medical Journal* **291**, 97–104. [One of the major and most influential trials.]

Medical Research Council Working Party (1992). MRC trial of treatment of hypertension in older adults: principal results. *British Medical Journal* **304**, 405–12. [A major trial of treatment in elderly patients which compares β-blockers and diuretics.]

Packer M *et al.* (2001). Effect of carvedilol on survival in severe chronic heart failure. *New England Journal of Medicine* **344**, 1651–8.

Peto R, Collins R (1994). Anti-hypertensive drug therapy: effects on stroke and coronary heart disease. In: Swales JD, ed. *Textbook of hypertension*, pp 1156–64. Blackwells, Oxford. [Important meta-analysis of the effects of antihypertensive medication in the large end-point trials.]

Pitt B *et al.* (1999). The effect of spironolactone on morbidity and mortality in patients with severe heart failure. Randomized Aldactone Evaulation Study Investigators. *New England Journal of Medicine* **341**, 709–17.

Psaty BM *et al.* (1997). Health outcomes associated with anti-hypertensive therapies used as first line agents: a systematic review and meta-analysis. *Journal of the American Medical Association* **277**, 739–45. [Comparison of different medications used in the large end-point trials.]

Ramsay LE *et al.* (1999). Guidelines for management of hypertension: report of the third working party of the British Hypertension Society. *Journal of Human Hypertension* **13**, 569–92. [The most recent British guidelines.]

Ramsay LE *et al.* (1999). British Hypertension Society guidelines for hypertension management 1999: summary. *British Medical Journal* **319**, 630–5.

SHEP Cooperative Research Group (1991). Prevention of stroke by antihypertensive drug treatment in older persons with isolated systolic hypertension. Final results of the Systolic Hypertension in the Elderly Program (SHEP). *Journal of the American Medical Association* **265**, 3255–64. [An important trial showing the benefits of treating isolated systolic hypertension.]

Staessen J, Fagard R, Amery A (1988). The relationship between body weight and blood pressure. *Journal of Human Hypertension* **2**, 207–17. [Meta-analysis of weight reduction trials and blood pressure.]

Swales JD (2000). *Manual of hypertension*. Blackwells, Oxford. [British textbook with emphasis on clinical aspects of hypertension.]

Vasan RS *et al.* (2001). Assessment of frequency of progression to hypertension in non-hypertensive participants of the Framlingham Heart Study: a cohort study. *Lancet* **358**, 1682–6.

World Health Organization–International Society of Hypertension (1999). Guidelines for the management of hypertension. *Journal of Hypertension* **17**, 151–83. [The only international guidelines. Comprehensive and with a good literature review.]

15.16.2 Secondary hypertension

15.16.2.1 Hypertension—indications for investigation

Lawrence E. Ramsay

Introduction

Sustained hypertension is very common in the general population, with a prevalence of 10 to 20 per cent of adults depending on the definition used. Most of these people will have their hypertension managed entirely in primary care, without referral for specialist investigation or treatment. About 90 per cent have idiopathic or essential hypertension, meaning that no specific cause can be identified. Perhaps 5 per cent of hypertension may be caused by drug therapy (Table 1), particularly non-steroidal anti-inflammatory drugs or oestrogen-containing oral contraceptive preparations; a further 5 per cent may be caused by renal or renovascular disease; while phaeochromocytoma, Conn's and Cushing's syndromes, coarctation, acromegaly, and other even rarer conditions together account for less than 1 per cent of all hypertension.

Note that an identifiable cause does not equate with 'curable' hypertension. In many cases, for example those with bilateral parenchymal renal disease, the cause cannot be rectified. Even when the underlying cause can be corrected, hypertension persists in about 30 per cent of cases regardless of whether the original aetiology was renal, renovascular, or endocrine. Thus, curable hypertension is very uncommon, so much so that routine extensive investigation of all patients with hypertension is unjustifiable. National and international guidelines for hypertension management agree that the investigations for all patients with hypertension should be limited in number and simple, so that they can be done readily in primary care. Detailed investigation should be reserved for patients who have specific indications in the clinical evaluation, and these patients should generally be referred for specialist opinion. This policy for investigation is logical but often not followed: a proportion of patients with hypertension do not receive even very basic tests such as creatinine and electrolyte measurement, while in hospital practice investigations are often done that are unnecessary, costly, inconvenient, and even invasive or potentially harmful.

Clinical evaluation

One consequence of reserving detailed investigation for selected patients is that the detection of uncommon but important cases of curable hypertension relies heavily on thoroughness and clinical acumen in the initial

Table 1 Drugs that cause hypertension or affect the control of hypertension

Oestrogen-containing oral contraceptives
Non-steroidal anti-inflammatory drugs
Sympathomimetics (e.g. phenylpropanolamine, ephedrine) in cold cures or nasal decongestants
Corticosteroids
Cyclosporin A
Carbenoxolone
Sodium bicarbonate
Erythropoietin
Ergotamine
Monoamine oxidase inhibitors (with tyramine-containing foods)

Table 2 Features in the initial evaluation of the patient with hypertension that may suggest an underlying cause for hypertension

Paroxysmal features such as palpitation, perspiration, pallor, panic, pain in head or chest—*phaeochromocytoma*

Present, past, or family history of *renal disease*

Drug history—*drug-induced hypertension* (Table 1)

Tetany, muscle weakness, polyuria—*Conn's syndrome*

General appearance—*Cushing's syndrome, acromegaly*

Palpable kidney(s) suggesting *polycystic kidneys*, rarely *hydronephrosis* or *neoplasm*

Abdominal or loin bruit—*renovascular disease*

Delayed or weak femoral pulses—*coarctation*

Proteinuria, haematuria, elevated creatinine—*renal or renovascular disease*

Hypokalaemia—*Conn's syndrome, liquorice ingestion*

clinical evaluation. The aims of clinical evaluation are to elicit and document:

(1) causes of hypertension, such as renal disease and endocrine causes;

(2) contributory factors, such as obesity, high salt intake, and excess alcohol;

(3) complications of hypertension, such as previous stroke and left ventricular hypertrophy;

(4) cardiovascular risk factors, such as smoking, family history, sex, and age; and

(5) contraindications to specific drugs, such as asthma (β-blockers) and gout (thiazides).

Those aspects of the clinical evaluation pertinent to detecting possible causes of hypertension are described in more detail in Table 2.

Routine investigations

There is agreement in recent guidelines that routine investigation should be limited to:

* urine strip test for protein and blood

* serum creatinine and electrolytes

* blood glucose

* serum total:HDL cholesterol

* electrocardiogram.

Some guidelines, such as the World Health Organization/International Society of Hypertension and the United States JNC VI guidelines, add 'optional' investigations to those above, implying that these are at the discretion of individual doctors. The British Hypertension Society guidelines do not endorse 'optional' investigations, because any additional investigations performed should be justifiable by evidence that there is some useful influence on clinical management or outcome.

Note that only two of these routine investigations are aimed primarily at detecting underlying causes for hypertension, namely urinalysis (renal causes) and creatinine and electrolytes (for renal causes and for mineralocorticoid excess such as Conn's syndrome). The other routine tests, namely glucose, total:HDL cholesterol, and electrocardiogram for left ventricular hypertrophy, are performed to assess cardiovascular risk, and are combined with other major risk factors (age, sex, smoking, and family history) to estimate cardiovascular or coronary risk formally using a chart, table, or computer program based on the Framingham risk function. Formal cardiovascular or coronary risk assessment is central to decisions on antihypertensive treatment for people with mild hypertension who have no cardiovascular complications, and also central to decisions on aspirin or lipid-lowering drug therapy.

Indications for further investigation

Common indications for more detailed investigation in hypertension are:

(1) any evidence of an underlying cause in the history or examination (Table 2);

(2) proteinuria, haematuria, or elevated serum creatinine;

(3) hypokalaemia not caused by diuretics;

(4) accelerated (malignant) hypertension;

(5) documented recent onset or recent worsening of hypertension;

(6) resistant hypertension (uncontrolled by a regimen of three antihypertensive drugs); or

(7) young age, meaning any hypertension in patients less than 20 years old, or hypertension needing treatment in patients aged 20 to 35 years.

In those with accelerated hypertension, a recent onset or worsening of hypertension, or resistant hypertension, the prevalence of secondary hypertension is about 25 per cent, and all should have screening tests for phaeochromocytoma, renal disease, and renovascular disease. Investigation is readily justified in these patients because their hypertension is more difficult to manage, and they often have an impaired prognosis. The chance of curing hypertension is relatively small, but underlying conditions such as phaeochromocytoma, obstructive uropathy, or some parenchymal renal diseases may require treatment in their own right. The 'enrichment' of the patient population that is investigated so as to yield positive findings in about 25 per cent is important for the performance of the screening tests widely used. Tests to screen for renovascular disease and phaeochromocytoma are imperfect, meaning that their sensitivity and specificity are less than 100 per cent. Sensitivity and specificity do not depend on the prevalence of the abnormality sought, but the predictive values of the tests are highly dependent on the underlying prevalence. Screening tests that are valuable in this selected 'enriched' population of patients are often misleading if used to screen all patients with hypertension indiscriminately.

Hypertension at a young age is generally accepted as an indication for detailed investigation, but note that the yield of underlying causes for hypertension and curable hypertension is disappointingly small when young age is the only indication for investigation. The main justification for more aggressive investigation in young patients is that detection of curable hypertension is more valuable when the alternative is many decades of antihypertensive treatment.

Positive screening investigations will often prompt more definitive tests. These are summarized in Table 3, and discussed in more detail in the chapters dealing with renal and renovascular hypertension (Chapter 15.16.2.2), phaeochromocytoma (Chapter 15.16.2.4), Conn's syndrome (Chapter 15.16.2.3), Cushing's syndrome (Chapter 12.2), and coarctation of the aorta (Chapter 15.16.2.5).

Individual investigations

Renal and renovascular disease

Investigations for renal and renovascular disease are discussed in more detail elsewhere (Chapter 15.16.2.2), but some difficulties surrounding this topic are mentioned here. Policies for renal investigation in hypertension are not uniform, and indeed few institutions or even individual clinicians seem to agree as regards the use of (for example) renal ultrasound, intravenous urogram, isotope renogram (with or without captopril), intravenous digital subtraction angiography, renal artery Doppler, magnetic resonance angiography, or renal arteriography. This unfortunate situation has arisen because those who evaluate different diagnostic methods are not always aware of, or do not address, the diagnostic problem facing clinicians. Investigation of appropriately selected patients with hypertension turns up a wide range of renal problems, among which the most common are renovascular disease, renal scarring (previously called chronic pyelonephritis), and obstructive uropathy. The clinical evaluation does not usually indicate

Table 3 Summary of investigation plans for different causes of secondary hypertension

Cushingoid appearance	Paroxysmal features	Reduced or delayed femoral pulses	Proteinuria, raised creatinine, renal bruit	Hypokalaemia
↓	↓	↓	↓	↓
Cushings syndrome?	Phaeochromocytoma?	Coarctation of aorta?	Renal/renovascular disease?	Conn's syndrome?
↓	↓	↓	↓	↓
Urinary free cortisol	Urinary catecholamines	Doppler ankle–brachial pressure index	Renal ultrasound	Plasma aldosterone: renin ratio
	↓	↓	↓	↓
Single-dose dexamethasone suppression test	CT scan abdomen MIBG scan	Magnetic resonance angiography	Magnetic resonance angiography	CT scan adrenals Postural aldosterone response
		Aortography	Renal angiography	

which of these renal pathologies is present, although there are exceptions to this. For example a young patient with hypertension and a family history of polycystic kidney disease is likely to have polycystic kidneys, and the investigation of choice is clearly ultrasound. However, patients with resistant or accelerated hypertension may have any of the renal abnormalities mentioned above. The clinician does not want a test that is specific and highly accurate for renovascular disease, or for scarring, or for obstructive uropathy, but rather needs a screening test or sequence of tests that is general purpose, that is, capable of detecting all the renal abnormalities commonly found in hypertension. Used singly some tests are clearly unsuitable for this purpose, for example the isotope renogram. The best imaging policy now is renal ultrasound, followed by magnetic resonance angiography with gadolinium enhancement where this is available; when magnetic resonance angiography is not available, ultrasound followed by arteriography; and where resources are limited the rapid-sequence intravenous urogram remains a valuable general purpose investigation.

Routine measurement of creatinine clearance is not useful, but is indicated when serum creatinine is elevated and there is uncertainty whether this is related to large muscle mass or a renal abnormality. Measurement of microalbuminuria has no proven value in non-diabetic patients.

Tests for primary aldosteronism

Measurement of the aldosterone:renin ratio to screen for primary aldosteronism (Conn's syndrome) is usually triggered by finding hypokalaemia. However, patients with primary aldosteronism may have intermittent hypokalaemia or even persistent normokalaemia, and primary aldosteronism may be more common than is generally believed. The question arises whether the aldosterone:renin ratio should be measured more often, or even routinely, even without hypokalaemia. From a practical point of view the priority is to detect primary aldosteronism caused by an aldosterone-secreting adrenal adenoma, because surgical removal of the tumour may cure the hypertension and biochemical disturbance. Patients with adrenal hyperplasia causing aldosterone excess are managed medically, and have no prospect of cure of hypertension. The severity of biochemical disturbance relates to the adrenal pathology, so that patients with adrenal adenomas have more marked hypokalaemia. From a pragmatic point of view investigation only of those patients who have hypokalaemia is likely to detect those with surgically curable Conn's syndrome. However, there may be a case for measuring the aldosterone:renin ratio in patients with resistant hypertension, even when hypokalaemia is absent, or for trying the effect of spironolactone in such patients. These issues are discussed in more detail elsewhere (Chapter 15.16.2.3).

Other blood tests

Routine measurement of full blood count is sometimes advocated because of the link between hypertension and polycythaemia, but its value is doubtful. The relation between primary hyperparathyroidism and hypertension might suggest that serum calcium should be measured routinely, but treatment of the primary hyperparathyroidism does not influence the blood pressure or cardiovascular risk. Serum uric acid is often elevated in untreated hypertension, and related to male sex, obesity, alcohol use, and renal impairment. Might routine measurement allow avoidance of diuretic treatment and reduce the risk of precipitating gout? In fact there is little relation between pretreatment uric acid and the risk of gout, and most hyperuricaemic patients do not develop gout on diuretics. Many patients would be denied these valuable drugs unnecessarily with this policy, and routine measurement of serum uric acid is not recommended. Fasting serum triglycerides make no important contribution to cardiovascular risk assessment provided HDL-cholesterol is measured, and need not be measured routinely.

Ambulatory blood pressure measurement

Ambulatory blood pressure measurement should not be used routinely or indiscriminately in the management of hypertension according to current guidelines. Specific indications for ambulatory blood pressure measurement (**ABPM**) are:

(1) extreme variability of blood pressure at different visits or in different situations;

(2) symptoms suggesting hypotensive episodes;

(3) hypertension resistant to a three-drug regimen; or

(4) sustained clinic, surgery, or office hypertension in people otherwise at low cardiovascular risk.

The last category is most important because it concerns the phenomenon termed white-coat hypertension (or isolated clinic hypertension). It is not necessary or feasible to perform ABPM to exclude white-coat hypertension in all patients with hypertension. It is not indicated in those who are at high cardiovascular or coronary risk, including patients who already have target organ damage or cardiovascular complications, and those who have an estimated coronary risk of 15 per cent or higher over 10 years. In these patients treatment decisions should be based on clinic pressures rather than ABPM, as was the case in outcome trials of hypertension treatment. ABPM is also unnecessary in patients with mild hypertension (140 to 159/90 to 99 mmHg) who have no target organ damage, no cardiovascular complications, and an estimated 10-year coronary risk of less than 15 per cent. These patients can be left untreated without using ABPM, but should be followed up. ABPM is indicated when the average clinic blood pressure is 160/100 mmHg or higher, but there is no target organ damage or cardiovascular complication, and the estimated 10-year coronary risk is less than 15 per cent. Here elevated blood pressure is the only indication of high cardiovascular risk and for antihypertensive treatment, and normal blood pressure by ABPM may alter the treatment decision. However, any decision to withhold treatment in such patients should be based on appropriately adjusted normal values for ambulatory measurement, and should be confirmed by a second ABPM record because of within-patient variability and limited reproducibility.

Echocardiography

Echocardiography is more 'sensitive' than the electrocardiogram for detecting left ventricular hypertrophy, but this does not mean that it is better or useful. Left ventricular hypertrophy is used to estimate cardiovascular risk, and the relevant question is whether echocardiography is superior to the electrocardiogram for estimating cardiovascular risk. In fact it does enhance the accuracy of risk estimation, but only very slightly, and the gain does not justify routine echocardiography. It is indicated in patients who have 'voltage criteria' for left ventricular hypertrophy, but no T-wave abnormalities. Voltage criteria alone are very unreliable, particularly in young men, and should not be used to diagnose left ventricular hypertrophy without confirmation by echocardiography.

Further reading

British Cardiac Society, British Hyperlipidaemia Association, British Hypertension Society, endorsed by the British Diabetic Association (1998). Joint British Recommendations on prevention of coronary heart disease in clinical practice. *Heart* **80**(Suppl 2), S1–S29. [British guidelines including policy for investigation and method of coronary risk assessment.]

Cameron HA *et al.* (1992). Investigation of selected patients with hypertension by the rapid-sequence intravenous urogram. *Lancet* **339**, 658–61. [Detailed outcome of investigating selected patients with hypertension related to different indications for investigation.]

Guidelines Subcommittee (1999). 1999 World Health Organization–International Society of Hypertension guidelines for the management of hypertension. *Journal of Hypertension* **17**, 151–83. [International guidelines including policy for investigation.]

Haq IU *et al.* (1995). Resistant hypertension. In: Kendall MJ, Kaplan NM, Horton RC, eds. *Difficult hypertension*, pp 97–115. Martin Dunitz, London. [Review of clinical assessment, investigation, and treatment of resistant hypertension.]

Joint National Committee (1997). The sixth report of the Joint National Committee on prevention, detection, evaluation, and treatment of high blood pressure. *Archives of Internal Medicine* **157**, 2413–46. [United States guidelines including policy for investigation.]

Lever AF, Swales JD (1994). Investigating the hypertensive patient: an overview. In: Swales JD, ed. *Textbook of hypertension*, pp 1026–30. Blackwell, Oxford. [Rationale for policy of selective investigation in hypertension.]

Ramsay LE *et al.* (1999). Guidelines for management of hypertension: report of the third working party of the British Hypertension Society. *Journal of Human Hypertension* **13**, 569–92. [British guidelines including policy for investigation.]

Wallace EJ *et al.* (2000). Coronary and cardiovascular risk estimation for primary prevention: validation of a new Sheffield table in the 1995 Scottish health survey population. *British Medical Journal* **320**, 671–6. [Principles, practice, and accuracy of cardiovascular risk assessment in mild hypertension.]

15.16.2.2 Renal and renovascular hypertension

Lawrence E. Ramsay

Introduction

Renal or renovascular abnormalities are present in about 5 per cent of all hypertensives, and 25 per cent of those selected appropriately for detailed investigation (see Chapter 15.16.2.1). Some renal lesions are incidental to hypertension, some cause the hypertension but are uncorrectable, some cause the hypertension and are correctable, but without cure of the hypertension, and finally a few cause the hypertension, and are correctable with cure of hypertension. Unfortunately this last category, curable hypertension, is very uncommon. Fibromuscular renal artery stenosis is the only form of renal hypertension that is 'usually' curable, meaning that more than 50 per cent of patients are cured.

Investigation of hypertension often uncovers renal diseases that need management or monitoring in their own right, such as polycystic kidneys, glomerulonephritis, chronic pyelonephritis, or obstructive uropathy. However, policies for investigation and particularly for intervention should be tempered by the knowledge that renal or renovascular hypertension can rarely be cured. Intervention should generally be reserved for patients with a compelling indication, for example severe and resistant hypertension, declining renal function, or 'flash' pulmonary oedema. The outcome is generally best with younger age (under 60 years), normal renal function, and a short history of hypertension.

Causes and mechanisms

Renal abnormalities that may be found in hypertensive patients are shown in Table 1, but note that the relation between hypertension and the renal lesion differs among these. In bilateral parenchymal disorders such as glomerulonephritis, interstitial nephropathy, or polycystic kidneys the prevalence of hypertension in the early stages is about 30 per cent, although it

Table 1 Renal and renovascular abnormalities that may be found in hypertensive patients

Bilateral: glomerular	**Primary GN**
	Minimal lesion
	Proliferative
	Membranous
	Membranoproliferative
	Focal proliferative
	Focal segmental
	Secondary GN
	Diabetes mellitus
	SLE
	Microscopic polyangiitis
	Wegener's granulomatosis
	Henoch–Schonlein purpura
	Infective endocarditis
	Goodpasture's syndrome
Bilateral: other	Renovascular disease
	Polycystic kidneys
	Chronic pyelonephritis
	Obstructive nephropathy
	Analgesic nephropathy
	Sarcoidosis
	Sickle cell disease
	Myeloma
	Systemic sclerosis
	Radiation nephropathy,
	Toxic nephropathy (e.g. lead, drugs)
Unilateral	Renal artery stenosis
	Chronic pyelonephritis
	Hydronephrosis
	Simple cyst
	Segmental infarction
	Traumatic renal artery stenosis/ thrombosis
	Arteriovenous fistula
	Tuberculosis
	Radiation nephritis
	Renal carcinoma
	Nephroblastoma
	Renin-secreting tumour
	Ask–Upmark kidney

varies with the pathology. For example, hypertension is more common in mesangiocapillary type 1 glomerulonephritis (40 per cent) than in minimal change nephropathy (16 per cent). Again, hypertension is three times more likely in the common form of polycystic kidneys associated with mutations at the *PKD1* locus than in non-*PKD1* disease. The hypertension early in these conditions is probably renin dependent. With progression to renal failure the prevalence of hypertension increases to 80 to 90 per cent, and hypertension then reflects imbalance between volume and vasoconstriction, with the emphasis on volume dependence. Volume-dependent hypertension that is usually curable also occurs in bilateral obstructive uropathy, caused for example by bladder neck obstruction.

The relation of unilateral renal and renovascular abnormalities (Table 1) to hypertension also varies for different entities. Unilateral chronic hydronephrosis is no more common in hypertensive than normotensive subjects and relief of obstruction does not cure the hypertension. It is therefore an incidental finding and should be managed entirely on its own merits. Simple renal cysts or neoplasms are also generally incidental, but very rarely they can cause curable renin-dependent hypertension, either through renin production or by compression of renal tissue leading to renin release. Unilateral chronic pyelonephritis (renal scarring, reflux nephropathy) commonly causes hypertension, yet nephrectomy rarely cures the hypertension. The reason is that the contralateral kidney is usually abnormal also, due either to scarring or to the effects of hypertension itself. Fibromuscular renal artery stenosis is the most convincing cause of reversible hypertension, because correction by angioplasty cures hypertension in at least 50 per cent of cases. The relation of atherosclerotic renal artery stenosis to hypertension is complex. Correction of the stenosis cures hypertension in fewer than 10 per cent of cases, but it is significantly 'treatment sparing'. Thus intervention sometimes improves but rarely cures hypertension. The relation of atherosclerotic renal artery stenosis to hypertension probably differs between patients: in some, renal artery stenosis may be coincidental to, or even a complication of, hypertension; in others, renal artery stenosis may have caused hypertension, which has then become irreversible because of ischaemia or atheroembolic disease (cholesterol embolism); and in a minority (less than 10 per cent) renal artery stenosis is the cause of reversible hypertension. Unfortunately, no tests can distinguish between these. Investigations such as renal vein renin or split function measurements having no useful predictive value.

Clinical evaluation

Pointers to a possible renal abnormality include documented recent onset or worsening of hypertension, onset before 35 years of age, accelerated phase hypertension, resistance to drug therapy, or renal failure precipitated by ACE inhibitor treatment. The physician should enquire about present or past urinary symptoms or loin pain, a family history of renal disease or polycystic kidneys, clues to systemic conditions that may cause renal disease, such as diabetes or vasculitis, and ingestion of drugs that may be nephrotoxic. Examine for palpable kidneys (polycystic kidneys, neoplasm) or bladder (obstructive uropathy), and auscultate the epigastrium and renal angles for a vascular bruit. Systolic bruits are common and have low specificity, whereas continuous or systolic–diastolic bruits are rare but highly suggestive of renovascular disease.

Investigation

Routine investigation for renal disease is limited to serum creatinine and glucose (to exclude diabetes), and a urine stick test for protein and blood. When clinical evaluation and these routine tests are normal, further investigation is not indicated. If they suggest renal abnormality, further investigation may include:

- microscopy and culture of midstream urine; but note that absence of proteinuria, red cells, and casts does not exclude glomerular or interstitial disease with certainty

- quantitation of proteinuria over 24 h to help distinguish between glomerular and interstital disease; proteinuria of more than 1 g/24 h also signals the need for a lower blood pressure target and ACE inhibitor treatment

- renal ultrasound.

Depending on the results of these tests, additional investigation might include tests for systemic causes of renal disease ((for example antinuclear factor (ANF), DNA antibodies, antineutrophil cytoplasmic antibodies (ANCA)), renal biopsy if glomerulonephritis or interstitial nephropathy is suspected, or imaging for renovascular disease (see below). However, it is often appropriate to watch rather than investigate further at this stage. For example, a patient with severe hypertension, proteinuria less than 1 g/day, mild renal impairment, and normal renal ultrasound most likely has renal damage caused by previous accelerated hypertension. It is entirely reasonable to control the hypertension, monitor the renal function closely, and investigate further only if the renal function declines.

Unilateral renal disease

Unilateral renal abnormalities should generally be treated on their own merits because nephrectomy rarely cures hypertension. However, lesions such as renal cysts or radiation nephropathy very rarely do cause curable hypertension, and patients therefore have to be considered individually. Nephrectomy should be considered only when:

- hypertension is severe and difficult to control

- hypertension is of recent onset

- the affected kidney has no or very little function

- the contralateral kidney is completely normal on detailed investigation

- serum creatinine is normal

- the patient is young and generally fit

- the patient is willing to accept a small chance of cure or improvement from operation.

In practice these criteria are rarely satisfied, and hypertension is managed medically in almost all patients with unilateral renal disease. Lateralizing tests such as renal vein renin measurements have no useful predictive value in this situation.

Renovascular disease
Aetiology

Only 20 per cent of patients with renovascular disease have fibromuscular dysplasia, but it is important that cases are recognized because patients are often young and hypertension is often curable. The most common dysplastic pathology is medial fibroplasia, in about 70 per cent (Fig. 1), with stenotic lesions that are generally distal, multifocal, rarely cause occlusion, and may affect other vessels such as the carotid or mesenteric arteries. Other forms of medial dysplasia, and perimedial fibroplasia or adventitial fibroplasia, are uncommon. Some of these are unifocal, proximal, and can cause occlusion, and are therefore readily mistaken for atherosclerotic renovascular disease. Fibromuscular dysplasia is five times more common in women than men, bilateral in about 25 per cent of cases, and much more common on the right.

About 80 per cent of renovascular disease is atherosclerotic (Fig. 2). This is strongly associated with vascular disease elsewhere, particularly peripheral vascular disease, and with major risk factors for atherosclerosis including male sex, old age, diabetes, hyperlipidaemia, hypertension itself, and, particularly, cigarette smoking. Atherosclerotic stenotic lesions are usually proximal, often at the ostium of the renal artery, and bilateral in 25 per cent of cases. Atherosclerotic renovascular disease is progressive, leading to arterial occlusion in about 2 per cent of patients per year, and progression

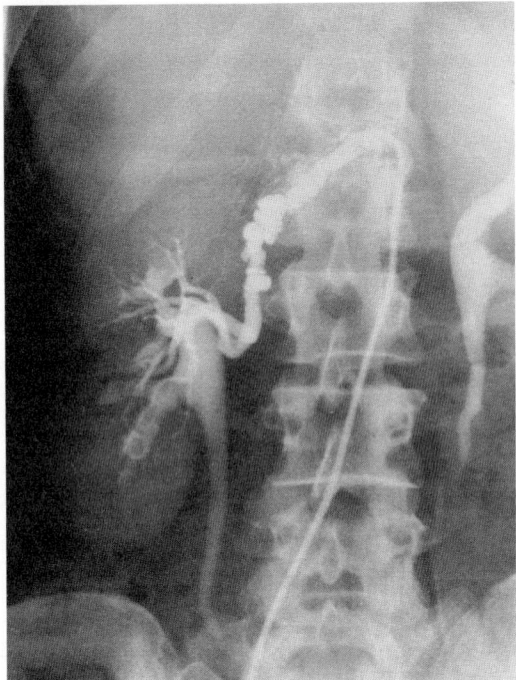

Fig. 1 Selective right renal angiography in a patient with hypertension caused by fibromuscular dysplasia of the common medial fibroplasia type. Note that the lesions involve the distal part of the renal artery, are multifocal, and show the 'string of beads' appearance of alternating stenoses and poststenotic dilatations.

to high-grade stenosis in about 10 per cent of patients per year. Loss of about 70 per cent of the artery lumen is necessary for haemodynamic significance, but radiological assessment of the degree of stenosis is imprecise.

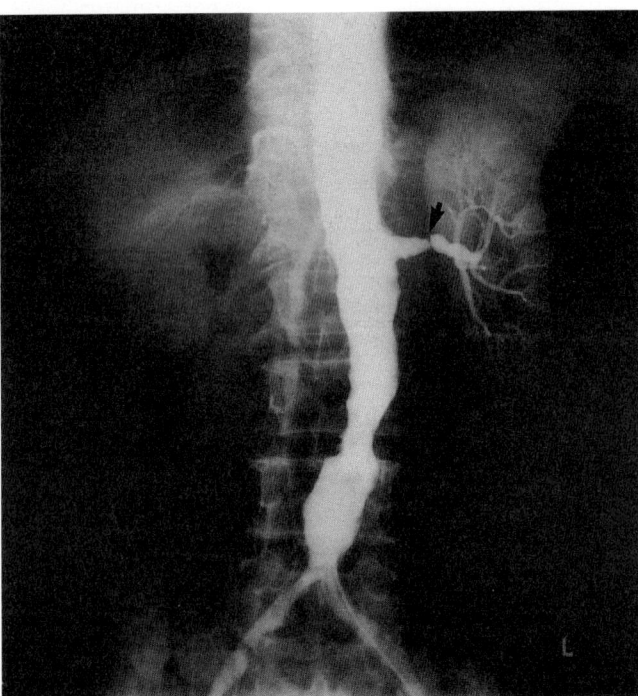

Fig. 2 Aortography in a 65-year-old man with severe atherosclerotic renovascular disease. There is total occlusion of the right renal artery, tight stenosis of the left renal artery (arrow), and extensive aortic atheroma.

Less common causes of renovascular disease include neurofibromatosis, transplant renal artery stenosis, aortic or renal artery dissection, embolism, Takayasu's arteritis, arteriovenous fistula, and radiation.

Diagnosis

Patients who have treatment-resistant hypertension or a decline in renal function with ACE inhibitor treatment should be assessed by a clinical prediction method that uses nine simple variables and estimates the probability that renovascular disease is present (Table 2, Fig. 3). This is at least as accurate as many of the non-invasive screening tests in wide use, such as renin measurements or isotope renography with or without an ACE inhibitor. The probability estimate should be considered together with the clinical circumstances to decide on further investigation. For example, a young patient with severe hypertension that is difficult to control, and with side-effects from drugs, would certainly be considered for investigation even if the probability of renovascular disease was only 10 per cent. By contrast, an elderly patient who was well controlled by three drugs, entirely comfortable on treatment, and had normal renal function, would be managed conservatively even if the probability of renovascular disease was much higher.

When the probability of renovascular disease and clinical circumstances warrant further investigation, renal ultrasound is done first to exclude other abnormalities. The non-invasive investigation of choice then is magnetic resonance angiography of the renal arteries with gadolinium enhancement. Spiral computed tomography angiography is equally accurate but needs contrast medium and ionizing radiation. Doppler ultrasound examination of the renal arteries is also accurate, but highly operator dependent. Intra-arterial digital subtraction angiography is the gold standard, but is invasive. Magnetic resonance angiography, spiral computed tomography, or Doppler are all valuable methods when they are available:

Table 2 Prediction rule for quantifying the probability of renal artery stenosis. (From Krijnen *et al.* (1998) with permission)

Predictor	Score*	
	Persons who never smoked	Former or current smokers
Age†		
20 years	0	3
30 years	1	4
40 years	2	4
50 years	3	5
60 years	4	5
70 years	5	6
Female sex	2	2
Signs and symptoms of atherosclerotic vascular disease‡	1	1
Onset of hypertension within 2 years	1	1
Body mass index < 25 kg/m²	2	2
Presence of abdominal bruit	3	3
Serum creatinine concentration†		
40 µmol/l	0	0
60 µmol/l	1	1
80 µmol/l	2	2
100 µmol/l	3	3
150 µmol/l	6	6
200 µmol/l	9	9
Serum cholesterol level > 6.5 mmol/l or cholesterol-lowering therapy	1	1

* The sum score is obtained by adding all relevant scores. The sum score can be used to obtain the predicted probability of renal artery stenosis from Fig. 3.

† For intermediate values, the score can be linearly interpolated.

‡ Femoral or carotid bruit, angina pectoris, claudication, myocardial infarction, cerebrovascular accident, or vascular surgery.

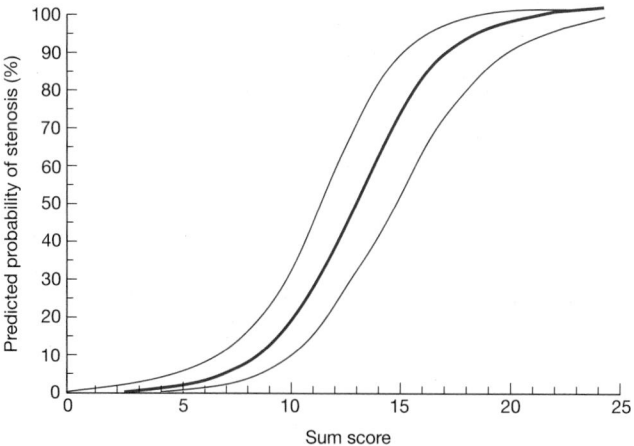

Fig. 3 Predicted probability of renal artery stenosis in patients with drug-resistant hypertension as a function of the sum score. The sum score is derived from the prediction rule in Table 2. The thin lines represent 95 per cent confidence intervals. From Krijnen *et al.* (1998) with permission.

when they are not, ultrasound should be followed by intra-arterial digital subtraction angiography.

Management

Interventional

Stenosis caused by fibromuscular renovascular disease can be corrected completely by angioplasty in 90 per cent of cases, and does not usually require stent insertion. Hypertension is cured completely in around 50 per cent of patients and complications are uncommon. Patients who are not suitable for angioplasty should be considered for surgical bypass or reconstruction in a centre experienced in these techniques.

Atherosclerotic renovascular disease often cannot be corrected completely by angioplasty alone, but stent insertion has greatly increased the technical success and long-term patency rates. However, stenting has not improved the disappointing outcome, with hypertension cured in less than 10 per cent of patients. Complications of the procedure are common and sometimes serious. The effect of angioplasty with stent insertion on renal function in atherosclerotic renovascular disease is unclear, and currently being studied in controlled trials. Limited evidence suggests that renal function improves in one-third, declines in one-third, and remains stable in one-third, and that angioplasty with stent insertion may slow the decline in renal function in some cases. Many patients with atherosclerotic renovascular disease have a very limited prognosis because of their widespread vascular disease. Given these considerations, angioplasty with stent insertion should be considered for atherosclerotic renovascular disease in the following circumstances:

- Hypertension that is severe and uncontrollable by several drugs in combination, including high doses of a loop diuretic.

- 'Flash' pulmonary oedema—patients with critical renovascular disease, meaning severe bilateral stenosis or tight stenosis to a single functioning kidney, may develop fulminant pulmonary oedema even when left ventricular function is normal or near normal. This condition can respond dramatically to correction of atherosclerotic renovascular disease.

- Progressing renal failure in a patient with bilateral renovascular disease, despite adequate blood pressure control, and with no other cause. Intervention hoping to prevent progression is justified pending the outcome of controlled trials in progress.

Surgical correction of renovascular disease should be considered for these same indications when angioplasty with stent insertion is technically impossible, although morbidity and mortality are daunting because of extensive cardiovascular disease.

The combination of hypertension, renal impairment, and one small kidney is a common presentation in elderly patients, and is caused by renal artery thrombosis with stenosis in the contralateral renal artery. This is usually best managed medically. However, in appropriate cases revascularization of a kidney with renal artery thrombosis can restore renal function, and should be considered if the kidney length is more than about 8 cm, the thrombosis is fairly recent, and renal biopsy shows no irreversible fibrosis or glomerular loss.

Medical

Patients with hypertension and atherosclerotic renovascular disease or renal failure usually have severe hypertension that is resistant to drug therapy. As a rule they will need several antihypertensive drugs in combination. Thiazide diuretics are ineffective or insufficiently effective in patients with resistant hypertension or renal impairment, and a loop diuretic is needed, often at high dosage. ACE inhibitors are a two-edged sword in patients with hypertension and renal disease. In critical renovascular disease, defined as severe bilateral renal artery stenosis or tight stenosis to a single functioning kidney, glomerular filtration is entirely dependent on increased efferent arteriolar tone, which is maintained by angiotensin II. Treatment with ACE inhibitors or angiotensin II antagonists abolishes the increased efferent arteriolar tone, stops glomerular filtration entirely, and causes acute renal failure. ACE inhibitors and angiotensin II antagonists should be avoided, or used with extreme caution and close monitoring of renal function, in patients known to have renovascular disease or who may have renovascular disease, for example those with peripheral vascular disease or unexplained renal impairment. On the other hand, ACE inhibitors are renoprotective and positively indicated in patients who have hypertension, renal impairment, and proteinuria over 1 g/day.

Hypertensive patients who have atherosclerotic renovascular disease or renal impairment are at very high cardiovascular and coronary risk. In addition to good blood pressure control they often need treatment with low-dose aspirin, and with a statin if the serum cholesterol is equal to or more than 5 mmol/litre.

Further reading

Aitchison F, Page A (1999). Diagnostic imaging of renal artery stenosis. *Journal of Human Hypertension* **13**, 595–603. [Review of non-invasive methods for diagnosing renovascular disease.]

Cameron HA *et al.* (1992). Investigation of selected patients with hypertension by the rapid-sequence intravenous urogram. *Lancet* **339**, 658–61. [Renal abnormalities in consecutive hypertensive patients investigated appropriately related to indication for investigation.]

Caps MT *et al.* (1998). [Prospective study of atherosclerotic disease progression in the renal artery. *Circulation* **98**, 2866–72. Natural history of atherosclerotic renovascular disease.]

Harden PN *et al.* (1997). Effect of renal-artery stenting on progression of renovascular renal failure. *Lancet* **349**, 1133–6. [Effect of angioplasty and stent insertion on renal function in atherosclerotic renovascular disease.]

van Jaarsveld BC *et al.* (2000). The effect of balloon angioplasty on hypertension in atherosclerotic renal-artery stenosis. *New England Journal of Medicine* **342**, 1007–14. [Largest and best randomized controlled trial of angioplasty for atherosclerotic renovascular disease.]

Krijnen P *et al.* (1998). A clinical prediction rule for renal artery stenosis. *Annals of Internal Medicine* **129**, 705–11. [Probability of renovascular disease predicted from simple clinical and biochemical variables.]

Pickering TG *et al.* (1988). Recurrent pulmonary oedema in hypertension due to bilateral renal artery stenosis: treatment by angioplasty or surgical revascularisation. *Lancet* **1**, 551–2. [First description of 'flash' pulmonary oedema related to critical renovascular disease.]

Ramsay LE, Waller PC (1990). Blood pressure response to percutaneous transluminal angioplasty for renovascular hypertension: an overview of published series. *British Medical Journal* **300**, 569–72. [Overview of outcome of angioplasty in fibromuscular and atherosclerotic renovascular disease.]

Robertson JIS (1992). Unilateral renal disease in hypertension. In Robertson JIS, ed. *Handbook of hypertension, Vol. 15: Clinical hypertension*, pp 266–325. Elsevier, Amsterdam. [Excellent review of unilateral renal and renovascular disease and hypertension.]

van de Ven PJG *et al.* (1999). Arterial stenting and balloon angioplasty in ostial atherosclerotic renovascular disease: a randomised trial. *Lancet* **353**, 282–6. [Controlled trial showing increased arterial patency with stent insertion, but no advantage on blood pressure control.]

Whitworth JA (1992). Renal parenchymal disease and hypertension. In Robertson JIS, ed. *Handbook of hypertension, Vol. 15: Clinical hypertension*, pp 326–56. Elsevier, Amsterdam. [Excellent review of bilateral renal disease and hypertension.]

15.16.2.3 Primary hyperaldosteronism (Conn's syndrome)

M. J. Brown

Introduction

Conn's syndrome is the eponymous term that embraces the various causes of primary aldosteronism. Although the current trend in medicine is away from eponymous nomenclature and towards names that reveal more of a disease's pathogenesis, there are good arguments for retaining the eponym when there is a need to ensure much wider recognition, and diagnosis, of the syndrome. All drugs receive two names, a generic and brand name: the former is more informative but often forgettable (or unpronounceable), encouraging the use of the memorable brand name after patent life expires. 'Patent life' on Conn's description of primary hyperaldosteronism as a cause of hypertension, in 1966, long since expired, but controversy remains regarding many aspects of the syndrome—prevalence, pathogenesis, treatment—and look-alikes continue to appear.

Within the continuum of hypertension are a number of so-called secondary syndromes, meaning that the hypertension is due to a specific, recognizable cause. The search for secondary causes is sometimes motivated by the aim of finding a curable cause, but it is better to think of the aim as finding the optimal treatment.

The three different types of Conn's syndrome embrace, and illustrate, the spectrum of hypertension. Firstly, adrenal adenoma is the only curable type, but the overlap with hyperplasia contributes to the hazards of predicting cure. Secondly, bilateral hyperplasia can be hard to differentiate from the low-renin end of the spectrum of essential hypertension and on recognition is not curable, but diagnosis is still rewarding because of the usually excellent blood pressure response to spironolactone. Thirdly, the only definite genetic cause of Conn's syndrome identified to date, glucocorticoid remediable aldosteronism, is clearly incurable, but the genetic test provides an infallible diagnosis and predicts a reversal of the hypertension by an otherwise ineffective treatment.

Physiological background

The zona glomerulosa, where aldosterone—the principal salt-retaining hormone—is synthesized, is the outermost of the three secretory zones of the adrenal cortex and the usual site of the tumours or hyperplasia in Conn's syndrome. The zonas glomerulosa and fasciculata, where cortisol is synthesized, are distinguished by their respective expression of the closely related genes, *CYP11B1* encoding 11β-hydroxylase, and *CYP11B2* encoding aldosterone synthase. The secretion of aldosterone is regulated by angiotensin II, whose concentration is determined by that of circulating renin. However, aldosterone secretion also responds in some degree to ACTH, acting both directly on zona glomerulosa cells and through release of endothelin from adrenal endothelial cells and of 5-HT from mast cells. It is these alternative stimuli that may be responsible for aldosterone-dependent hypertension in low-renin patients.

The main receptor for aldosterone, the mineralocorticoid receptor, is a nuclear hormone receptor in the distal tubules and collecting duct of the kidney. Stimulation of the receptor leads to activation of the epithelial sodium channel on the apical (luminal) surface of the tubular cells, through the action of a serine/threonine kinase called serum glucocorticoid kinase, which disappears from the renal tubules after adrenalectomy. As an apparently passive consequence of the increased apical Na^+ flux into the cells, there is also enhanced activity of the basolateral Na^+,K^+-ATPase, which pumps Na^+ into the peritubular interstitium and thereby into the blood.

Of the two main adrenal steroids, cortisol is much the more abundant, by 100- to 1000-fold. Since both steroids have a similar affinity for the mineralocorticoid receptor, it used to be a mystery why aldosterone is the physiological agonist. The explanation became clear with the discovery, in the same distribution as mineralocorticoid receptors, of the enzyme 11-hydroxysteroid dehydrogenase: this enzyme inactivates cortisol to cortisone, preventing access to the receptor. The enzyme is inhibited by liquorice, or the old antiulcer drug carbenoxolone, and is congenitally deficient in homozygotes with the rare syndrome of apparent mineralocorticoid excess (see Chapter 15.16.1.2). The enzyme is also inhibited (or, rather, saturated) by very high plasma concentrations of cortisol, such as occur in patients with the ectopic ACTH syndrome (see Chapter 12.7.1). These patients develop the clinical and biochemical features of Conn's syndrome before (or without) becoming floridly cushingoid. Indeed, the lowest levels of plasma K^+ (less than 2.5 mmol/litre) in the presence of plasma Na^+ over 145 mmol/litre should suggest the diagnosis of ectopic ACTH rather than primary hyperaldosteronism.

Incidence

This is contentious. Until recently, the figure was considered to be 1 to 2 per cent of hypertensives, but this is based on the incidence in patients with the typical electrolyte pattern described below, which is now recognized to be absent in many patients. Selected series of hospital patients have suggested figures as high as 15 per cent of hypertensives. Our own survey of plasma aldosterone to renin ratios in 800 unselected hypertensive patients suggests that the true prevalence is at least 5 per cent, most of whom do not have adenomas. The increased recognition of Conn's syndrome is mainly among patients with plasma K^+ levels within the normal range. Previous algorithms designed to distinguish adenomas from bilateral hyperplasia have emphasized the absolute level of aldosterone as a guide to adenoma: it seems likely that patients with adenomas will therefore have more instantly recognizable plasma electrolyte abnormalities, unless these have been masked by treatment with a calcium-channel blocker.

Clinical characteristics

Adenomas are said to occur more commonly in women and bilateral hyperplasia more often in men, but the differences are too slight to be helpful diagnostically. Except for the rare monogenic syndrome of glucocorticoid remediable aldosteronism, Conn's syndrome is not a cause of childhood hypertension. The main, and essential, clinical feature of Conn's syndrome is hypertension, any other clinical features being secondary to hypertension or hypokalaemia, but the majority of patients are asymptomatic.

Two important features differentiate patients with Conn's syndrome from those with secondary hyperaldosteronism, in which increased aldosterone secretion is driven by elevated levels of renin and angiotensin. First, patients with Conn's do not develop oedema; it is assumed that secretion of a natriuretic hormone, such as atrial natriuretic hormone, leads to escape from the salt-retaining effect of aldosterone (the 'escape phenomenon'). Secondly, and of diagnostic value, the plasma Na⁺ concentration is within—or just above—the upper part of the normal range, usually more than 140 mmol/litre, whereas in secondary hyperaldosteronism the reduced free water clearance caused by angiotensin II results in some dilution of the plasma Na⁺, whose concentration is therefore less than 140 mmol/litre. Very rarely, primary hyperaldosteronism is associated with phaeochromocytoma, primary hyperparathyroidism, or acromegaly.

Investigation

Who requires investigation?

In patients with hypertension the diagnosis of Conn's syndrome should be suspected in two main circumstances. The conventional one is the presence of hypokalaemia and high normal plasma sodium concentration. Because in general practice K⁺ measurements can be unreliable if samples have stood for some hours before separation, routine measurement of bicarbonate is recommended in the initial sample from a hypertensive patient. Conn's patients typically have hypokalaemic alkalosis because stimulation of the epithelial sodium channel by aldosterone causes exchange of Na⁺ for both K⁺ and H⁺ ions. It is important to have increased suspicion when the plasma K⁺ falls (or the bicarbonate rises) substantially on diuretic treatment: the low doses of thiazide diuretics commonly used nowadays in the treatment of hypertension do not usually lower K⁺ by more than 0.5 mmol/litre.

The second circumstance under which Conn's syndrome should be suspected is when patients appear resistant to conventional antihypertensive treatment and the electrolytes are 'in the direction' of Conn's, without necessarily being outside the normal range (plasma Na⁺ more than 140, K⁺ less than 4.0 mmol/litre).

Establishing the diagnosis of Conn's syndrome

When the diagnosis of Conn's syndrome is suspected, it should be pursued by estimation of plasma aldosterone and renin, seeking evidence of elevated aldosterone secretion in the absence of elevated renin production. An aldosterone to renin ratio of over 850 is usually diagnostic, and should at least trigger a trial of spironolactone therapy and an adrenal scan. Application of the ratio, rather than consideration of the absolute level of aldosterone, is useful in encouraging measurement of the hormones under more everyday conditions than is recommended for either hormone alone. Thus, a patient whose aldosterone secretion is elevated by physical activity will have a similar elevation in plasma renin activity. A further important practical point is that most antihypertensive drugs can be continued, provided that the clinician is aware of some potential for interference.

Effects of antihypertensive drugs on plasma renin and aldosterone

ACE inhibitors and angiotensin receptor antagonists markedly reduce the aldosterone to renin ratio in most non-Conn's patients by interrupting the negative feedback inhibition of renin secretion by angiotensin II, but do not prevent detection of an elevated ratio in low-renin patients with autonomous aldosterone secretion (i.e. Conn's). β-Blockers elevate the ratio by suppressing renin secretion more than aldosterone; in patients whose ratio but not absolute level of aldosterone is elevated, a repeat estimation of β-blockade may be worthwhile. Calcium blockers cause variable suppression of aldosterone and renin secretion, sometimes sufficiently to mask the diagnosis of Conn's syndrome. It is not necessary to stop a calcium blocker in order to measure aldosterone except in patients whose electrolyte abnormalities have been corrected by the calcium blocker. Diuretics increase renin and aldosterone in parallel, and the measurement of the aldosterone to renin ratio therefore readily distinguishes Conn's from diuretic induced hypokalaemia.

Further investigations in patients with an elevated aldosterone to renin ratio

Once the probable diagnosis is established, the next question is whether the patient has a unilateral adenoma or a bilateral hyperplasia. The answer clearly has a major influence on the choice of long-term treatment, although it is important to remember that Conn's adenomas are always benign and that some patients will opt for long-term medication in preference to surgery. A number of algorithms have been devised to help distinguish the two conditions. Some of these are based on the relatively greater response of aldosterone secretion from adenomas and hyperplasia to ACTH and angiotensin II, respectively. Thus, there is a greater diurnal rhythm in aldosterone levels in patients with adenomas, but greater response to posture in hyperplasia. The problem with these algorithms is that they usually depend on multiple measurements, requiring admission of patients to hospital, and the result is still only a probability of one or other diagnosis, insufficiently strong to make a decision about surgery. The practicalities of outpatient investigation, coupled with the quality of modern imaging techniques, dictate a more empirical approach. The clinician wants to know the following:

- Is there an operable adenoma?
- Is the contralateral adrenal anatomically normal (i.e. no adenoma)?
- Is aldosterone secretion unilateral and from the side with the adenoma?

A good magnetic resonance or computed tomography scan will usually answer the first two questions, and where imaging reveals an adrenal mass 1–2 cm in size, the probability of adenoma is high enough to justify surgery without further troublesome investigations (Fig. 1). Above this size, the possibility of an adrenal carcinoma should be considered. Below 1 cm, the anatomical scan cannot with certainty exclude non-functioning myelolipomas ('incidentalomas') or large nodules within a hyperplastic gland. Magnetic resonance imaging has the slight edge over computed tomography on specificity, but the choice between the two scans can reasonably depend on local availability.

There are two tests for lateralization, neither of which is ideal. The better is measurement of the aldosterone to cortisol ratio in samples from the adrenal veins, with a reference sample from the vena cava. A 'perfect' result is a ratio in blood from the adenoma that is ten times greater than the reference sample, with the suppressed contralateral adrenal having a ratio lower than reference. However, suppression is not always demonstrable, and a serious problem with the test is that cannulation of both adrenal veins is technically demanding; few radiologists can claim a greater than

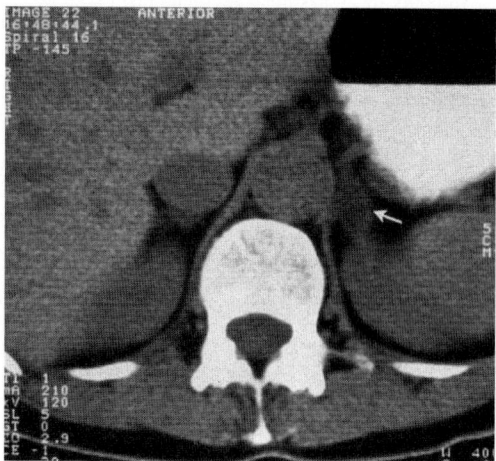

Fig. 1 Computed tomography scan of a 2 × 1 cm left adrenal adenoma (arrowed) in a patient with Conn's syndrome.

75 per cent success at cannulating the right adrenal vein, which drains directly into the back of the inferior vena cava. A hooked catheter with side holes should be used.

The alternative test is the radio-isotope scan using selenium cholestenol as a precursor for adrenal steroids. This is less invasive than venous sampling, but in practice can inflict more discomfort and is less accurate. Because most steroid synthesis takes place in the zona fasciculata of the adrenal, this needs to be blocked by pretreatment with dexamethasone for at least a week. In addition, several of the main antihypertensives, including those most likely to be effective in Conn's syndrome, can interfere with the scan and need to be stopped. Scanning is usually performed at 3, 7, and sometimes 14 days after radionuclide administration. For reasons that are not clear, the scan is often misleading, failing to detect any uptake in some patients, and failing to lateralize in some patients with adenomas.

Treatment

Medical

The medical treatment of choice is spironolactone, which is a competitive antagonist of the aldosterone receptor. It can be started once the diagnosis is suspected from the biochemical results, and the blood pressure response is valuable in confirming the presence of increased aldosterone secretion. Most patients will have a substantial fall in blood pressure, and normalization of plasma electrolytes after a month's treatment at a dose of 50 mg daily. This relatively low dose has the advantage of reducing the risk of adverse reactions, of which dyspepsia is the main short-term and gynaecomastia the main long-term problem. However, 50 mg is too small a dose for larger patients, and it is worth prescribing as near as possible to 1 mg/kg (using the available 50 mg and 25 mg size tablets). The dose can sometimes be reduced after prolonged administration.

Not all patients with Conn's syndrome tolerate or respond adequately to spironolactone alone. Usually a dose is tolerated sufficient to permit control of hypokalaemia; if not, high doses (20–40 mg) of amiloride may be required. As mentioned above, the calcium blockers can suppress aldosterone secretion and are a logical addition. However, patients with Conn's syndrome can develop quite resistant hypertension, which is a reason for trying harder to make the diagnosis at an early stage in the development of hypertension. Spironolactone should be stopped a week before any lateralization tests, because of the risk that suppression of the contralateral adrenal is removed.

Surgical

This is the treatment of choice for patients with the unilateral adenomas. Because the tumours are always small, they lend themselves well to laparoscopic surgery, although patients should always be warned about the possible need to proceed to an open operation. Patients should be on spironolactone (if tolerated) in the period running up to surgery, but there are few risks of uncontrolled hypertension or postoperative hypotension in the surgery of Conn's syndrome.

No steroid replacement is required after surgery, when most patients are able to discontinue all antihypertensive therapy. This may not be possible in older patients, perhaps because the adenoma arose on a background of essential hypertension. There is no need for long-term follow-up.

It seems likely that Conn's is familial more often than has been recognized, or can be currently explained by any known genetic variant, and it is therefore worth considering whether siblings with hypertension should have their plasma renin and aldosterone measured.

Further reading

Barzon L *et al.* (1999). Risk factors and long-term follow-up of adrenal incidentalomas. *Journal of Clinical Endocrinology and Metabolism* **84**, 520–6.

Brown MJ, Hopper RV (1999). Calcium-channel blockade can mask the diagnosis of Conn's syndrome. *Postgraduate Medical Journal* **75**, 235–6.

Dluhy RG, Lifton RP (1999). Glucocorticoid-remediable aldosteronism. *Journal of Clinical Endocrinology and Metabolism* **84**, 4341–4.

Ganguly A (1998). Primary aldosteronism. *New England Journal of Medicine* **339**, 1828–34.

Gordon RD *et al.* (1994). High incidence of primary aldosteronism in 199 patients referred with hypertension. *Clinical and Experimental Pharmacology and Physiology* **21**, 315–18.

Nomura K *et al.* (1992). Plasma aldosterone response to upright posture and angiotensin II infusion in aldosterone-producing adenoma. *Journal of Clinical Endocrinology and Metabolism* **75**, 323–7.

Stewart PM (1999). Mineralocorticoid hypertension. *The Lancet* **1353**, 1341–7.

Stewart PM *et al.* (1996). Hypertension in the syndrome of apparent mineralocorticoid excess due to mutation of the 11 beta-hydroxysteroid dehydrogenase type 2 gene. *The Lancet* **347**, 88–91.

Stowasser M *et al.* (1995). Plasma aldosterone response to ACTH in subtypes of primary aldosteronism. *Clinical and Experimental Pharmacology and Physiology* **22**, 460–2.

15.16.2.4 Phaeochromocytoma

M. J. Brown

Introduction

Phaeochromocytoma is a rare tumour. Estimates of incidence are unreliable because none has been undertaken in an unselected group of patients, but it is probably in the range 0.1–1 per cent of hypertensives. During a study of prevalence of hypertension, we measured blood pressure in 30 000 healthy subjects in general practice, selected only for the absence of known hypertension or vascular disease: 8 per cent were found to have a systolic blood pressure of more than 150 mmHg, and two were subsequently found to have a phaeochromocytoma, giving an incidence of about 0.1 per cent of hypertensives. This fits our parallel experience in 750 patients referred over 10 years by general practitioners following their own diagnosis of hypertension and before initiation of treatment; only one of these patients was found to have a phaeochromocytoma. Both these series will have missed those cases in whom typical symptoms led to correct diagnosis soon after presentation with hypertension, but it is reassuring to know that for a potentially malignant tumour (unlike the situation in Conn's syndrome, see Chapter 15.16.2.3) the typical picture is unlikely to be just the tip of an iceberg.

Despite its rarity, phaeochromocytoma justifies the disproportionate interest and awareness of the condition that exists among physicians. Like a few other rare conditions which share this position, such as infective endocarditis or Addison's disease, phaeochromocytoma combines the potential for being lethal if not diagnosed and treated, and for cure in most patients if diagnosed. The diagnosis of phaeochromocytoma offers the best chance of a cure of all the secondary causes of hypertension (especially those presenting in the second half of life), and avoidance of the need for lifelong antihypertensive therapy.

The need for maintaining a high awareness of the condition is emphasized by the small number of deaths each year, in both anaesthetic and obstetric practice, due to undiagnosed phaeochromocytoma.

Catecholamine biochemistry

An understanding of the tests used to diagnose phaeochromocytoma requires reference to an outline of both the synthetic and degradative pathways of catecholamine metabolism. The term catechol refers to a phenyl ring with hydroxyl groups at adjacent carbons (conventionally, the 3′ and 4′ positions). The precursor essential amino acid, phenylalanine, is not itself a catechol; neither is tyrosine which has only the 3′ hydroxyl. This amino acid is the substrate for the rate-limiting step in the biosynthetic pathway, tyrosine hydroxylase, which yields L-dopa, the first catechol and still an amino acid. Decarboxylation of L-dopa yields the first catecholamine in the pathway, dopamine. This can occasionally be the principal catecholamine secreted by phaeochromocytomas, or more often by childhood neuroblastomas, but in the chromaffin tissue from which phaeochromocytomas originate dopamine is usually further hydroxylated, in the sidechain bearing the amine group, to noradrenaline. The final step in the biosynthetic pathway is the N-methylation of noradrenaline to adrenaline, the prefix 'nor' being used for substances that are N-demethylated, a common step in degradative metabolism.

N-methylation usually occurs in only two sites in the body: the adrenal medulla and certain hindbrain nuclei involved in blood pressure control. The enzyme responsible, phenylethanolamine-N-methyltransferase, may differ between these sites, as outside the central nervous system it is dependent for induction on glucocorticoids, which are provided in the adrenal through the portocapillary circulation. The clinical importance of this is threefold. First, extra-adrenal phaeochromocytomas rarely produce adrenaline, most of the reports to the contrary being in older literature when the methodology was less satisfactory for separating adrenaline and noradrenaline. Secondly, the normal adrenal produces mainly adrenaline, and accounts for less than 2 per cent of circulating noradrenaline concentrations. Thirdly, when a tumour is present in the adrenal, the disruption of the portocapillary circulation causes a reversal of the normal adrenaline to noradrenaline ratio. The relevance of these to the clinical features and diagnosis of phaeochromocytoma will become apparent.

The metabolic breakdown of catecholamines is due to two principal enzymes, monoamine oxidase and catechol-O-methyltransferase. The metabolism of catecholamines is different from normal in phaeochromocytoma in that adrenaline and noradrenaline are liberated directly into the bloodstream rather than mainly into the synaptic gap around sympathetic nerve endings. Noradrenaline released into these gaps is largely recaptured by neuronal and extraneuronal uptake, being metabolized before any free amine escapes into the bloodstream. Consequently, the proportion of parent amine to metabolite is usually higher in blood and urine in the presence of a phaeochromocytoma than in any other cause of elevated catecholamine production.

The most abundant product of the action of monoamine oxidase and catechol-O-methyltransferase (acting in sequence, in either order) is vanillylmandelic acid. Normetanephrine and metanephrine are produced by catechol-O-methyltransferase from noradrenaline and adrenaline, respectively. The products of monoamine oxidase alone are less often used in diagnosis, but in specialized laboratories the ratio of one of these, dihydroxyphenylglycol, to noradrenaline is a useful clue to the origin of noradrenaline, as dihydroxyphenylglycol arises mainly intraneuronally, and relatively little is therefore formed from noradrenaline liberated directly into the bloodstream as in phaeochromocytoma.

Laboratory diagnosis of phaeochromocytoma

Measurements of catecholamine metabolites in 24-h urine samples are the most appropriate screening tests because they offer an integrated measure of total catecholamine release over this period and can be performed in most routine laboratories. Vanillylmandelic acid is the product least prone to interference, L-dopa being the only drug that can crossreact in measurement through its equivalent metabolite, homovanillic acid. Although, for the reasons discussed, quantitation of vanillylmandelic acid is less sensitive than other measures, it remains very rare that a patient with a secreting phaeochromocytoma has a 24-h vanillylmandelic acid result that is normal. High doses of α-methyldopa reduce, and occasionally normalize, vanillylmandelic acid levels by competitively inhibiting catechol-O-methyltransferase. However, there is a problem of distinguishing the true positive from the relatively large number of hypertensive patients with results in the 'grey zone'. Metanephrines are arguably more sensitive than vanillylmande-

lic acid, but their assay is more prone to interference by drugs, especially by β-blockers.

The measurement of free catecholamines is a more specialized procedure. Assays can be made in plasma or urine, the former generally being more accurate and also allowing variation in secretion to be assessed because of the very short half-life in plasma (around 1 min) of catecholamines. The assay generally used is based on high-performance liquid chromatography separation of the catecholamines, followed by electrochemical or fluorometric detection. However, this technique does not eliminate the possibility of interference, especially in the adrenaline peak, and it is necessary to be particularly suspicious of any result showing a higher adrenaline than noradrenaline concentration. A few centres still undertake the gold-standard radioenzymatic assay in which the catecholamines are converted to their [³H]-methylated derivative in the presence of catechol-O-methyltransferase and a [³H]-methyl donor, a double-isotope technique usually being used to ensure accurate quantification.

Pathology

Phaeochromocytomas arise in chromaffin tissue, and their anatomical distribution closely parallels the sites where this tissue is present at the time of birth. These tumours, like the normal sympathoadrenal tissue, are of neuroectodermal origin. The term phaeochromocytoma reflects the dusky colour of the cut surface of the tumour, whereas the term chromaffin refers to the brownish colour caused by contact with dichromate salts, which oxidize the catecholamines. Much has been written about pathological differences between extra-adrenal phaeochromocytomas at various sites, but this is not relevant to clinical practice except as a possible explanation for the failure of some head and neck phaeochromocytomas to accumulate the noradrenaline analogue used as a radionuclide in scanning, as discussed later.

The pathogenesis of most phaeochromocytomas is unknown. However, at least 10 per cent of patients have inherited, as an autosomal dominant, their susceptibility to phaeochromocytoma. Two syndromes are recognized, both with germline mutations in a tumour suppressor gene. In multiple endocrine neoplasia type 2 syndrome, phaeochromocytoma is most commonly associated (not necessarily at the same time) with medullary carcinoma of the thyroid. In von Hippel–Lindau syndrome, multiple other tumours can occur, most commonly retinal angiomas, but also hypernephroma and central nervous system haemangioblastomas. There is evidence of somatic mutations in the same genes as responsible for these syndromes in some of the sporadic phaeochromocytomas. Given the large size of the von Hippel–Lindau gene, it is likely that many more sporadic phaeochromocytomas have such mutations than have been identified. Familial phaeochromocytoma without other tumours can be caused by mutations in the succinate dehydrogenase complex.

Most phaeochromocytomas are benign. However, the pathologist can rarely provide a clear distinction between benign and malignant phaeochromocytomas: benign tumours can appear to be invading the capsule of the tumour, which is often ill defined, and malignant tumours may show no mitoses because of their slow rate of division.

Clinical features

Hypertension is the most common presentation of phaeochromocytoma in clinical practice; other rare presentations include unexplained heart failure or paroxysmal arrhythmias. Increasingly, small and asymptomatic phaeochromocytomas are detected through regular screening of patients with a genetic diagnosis of multiple endocrine neoplasia or von Hippel–Lindau syndrome.

In the hypertensive patients, a spontaneous history or direct enquiry will usually reveal at least one of a group of characteristic symptoms. The most common are headache, sweating, and palpitations. Less frequent are episodes of pallor, a feeling of 'impending doom', and paraesthesiae. Examination rarely reveals useful signs, but an exception is a Raynaud's-type of discoloration over the extremities and the larger joints in the limbs. This is due to ischaemia and occasionally progresses to atrophic ulceration over pressure points.

A rare initial presentation, pathognomonic of phaeochromocytoma, is with wildly swinging blood pressure, between extremes of hypertension and hypotension, in combination with other signs of retroperitoneal haemorrhage. Even prompt recognition of the diagnosis, spontaneous haemorrhage and infarction of the tumour, is not always sufficient to save patients presenting in this way. By contrast, it is important to emphasize that some patients with large tumours, causing significant hypertension, may be asymptomatic.

Many of the symptoms of phaeochromocytoma can be readily ascribed to the expected effects of the excess catecholamine, and disappear rapidly on initiation of appropriate treatment. Some remain more difficult to explain, including the sweating whose control in healthy subjects is usually ascribed to cholinergic sympathetic innervation. Because large tumours secrete principally noradrenaline, even when arising within the adrenal gland, tachycardia is usually only modest, and can be replaced altogether by reflex bradycardia when episodes of hypertension are triggered by release of noradrenaline alone. The author once treated a 'cardiac arrest' with phentolamine when the arrest call was for an episode of apparent asystole that was in reality a vagal reaction to an arterial pressure of 300/160. Severe bradycardia is also recorded in response to the paradoxical rise in blood pressure when a patient with a phaeochromocytoma is inadvertently given a non-selective β-blocker such as propranolol. In a few patients, excess catecholamine can cause myocardial necrosis, which is probably due to a mixture of α-receptor mediated vasoconstriction and a β-receptor direct toxic effect on the cardiomyocytes. These are rare presentations and it is important to recognize that clinical features are usually less impressive than expected, possibly because the adrenoceptors have been downregulated by years of exposure before the diagnosis is first entertained. Indeed, hypertensive patients who complain of symptoms suggestive of excess catecholamines are more likely to be found to be suffering from side-effects of a vasodilator drug activating the baroreflex than to have a phaeochromocytoma.

Establishing the diagnosis

The diagnosis is not usually difficult once the possibility of phaeochromocytoma has been entertained, and it is important to exclude the diagnosis in patients who have clinical and/or biochemical features of catecholamine excess due to sympathetic overactivity rather than phaeochromocytoma. There are two distinct questions to ask: 'Does the patient have a phaeochromocytoma?' and 'Where is it?'. The tests required to answer the first question are mainly biochemical, as described above, whereas the second is answered by radiological investigation. A golden rule, which saves false positives and negatives, and therefore a large number of unnecessary investigations and sometimes operations, is that the first question should be answered before proceeding to the second. No single radiological investigation is sufficiently accurate to detect more than 80 to 90 per cent of phaeochromocytomas, whilst computed tomography scanning of the adrenal glands can detect non-functional myoleiomas that should not lead to further investigation in the absence of biochemical abnormalities.

The symptoms of a functioning phaeochromocytoma are remarkably variable and may be absent. To avoid missing the diagnosis, therefore, an average size general hospital might expect each year to screen several hundred patients with hypertension, tens of patients with unexplained heart failure, and all their known patients with multiple endocrine neoplasia or von Hippel–Lindau syndromes. Although the diagnosis is often postulated in other patients with isolated features of catecholamine excess, for example patients without hypertension but complaining of palpitation, headaches,

sweating, or panic attacks, the chance of such patients having a phaeochromocytoma is very, very small. In a 15-year period during which the author investigated more than 100 phaeochromocytomas and more than 1000 patients referred with a possible phaeochromocytoma, none has proven to have phaeochromocytoma in the absence of hypertension, heart failure, or a genetic syndrome.

The next question is how should screening be performed? There is no single perfect or 'best' test. It is important to recognize the diversity of analyses in use, quite different from the position for most standard endocrine analyses, and reflecting the difficulty of achieving an entirely reliable method in routine laboratories. Our own practice is to use 24-h urine vanillylmandelic acid as the initial screen in most patients, supplemented when necessary with the specialized catecholamine analyses. An entirely normal 24-h urine vanillylmandelic acid measured in a good hospital laboratory is most unlikely in the presence of a phaeochromocytoma. Conventionally, patients are asked to avoid vanilla-containing foods during the collection for assay of vanillylmandelic acid and to undertake three collections in order to exclude the diagnosis of phaeochromocytoma. Both of these precautions are unnecessary in the majority of cases: those with phaeochromocytoma have become relatively insensitive to the effects of catecholamines, hence a patient with 'significant' hypertension (diastolic blood pressure over 100 mmHg) must have a several-fold elevation of catecholamine secretion. Although the urinary vanillylmandelic acid is not proportionally elevated, for the reasons discussed earlier, the elevation is still sufficient to ensure an abnormal result provided that this is correctly measured. A vanilla-free diet is unnecessary because the dietary contribution to vanillylmandelic acid excretion is small compared with that derived from noradrenaline, and is unlikely to push the vanillylmandelic acid excretion into an abnormal range.

Most patients whose vanillylmandelic acid excretion is more than twofold above the upper limit of normal will prove to have a phaeochromocytoma, and a threefold elevation is almost always diagnostic. Patients who need further biochemical analyses are those with a less than twofold elevation of vanillylmandelic acid excretion, of whom only a very small proportion (less than 5 per cent) will have a phaeochromocytoma. Here, the single most helpful investigation is measurement of plasma noradrenaline, which will be at least twofold elevated in those with a phaeochromocytoma, whereas a single resting plasma noradrenaline will often be normal in those without.

Suppression tests

If the urinary vanillylmandelic acid analysis and assay of resting plasma noradrenaline does not resolve whether or not a patient has a phaeochromocytoma, there are two further useful investigations. The most widely used is a pharmacological suppression test, in which physiological elevations of noradrenaline release are temporarily suppressed by administration of either the ganglion-blocking drug pentolinium, or centrally acting α₂-agonist, clonidine. The former is more widely used in the United Kingdom and has three advantages:

1. It is most effective at suppressing noradrenaline release in the problem patients—namely those with elevated sympathetic nervous activity but without a phaeochromocytoma.

2. It also suppresses release of adrenaline from the adrenal medulla.

3. It has a short half-life (of approximately 20 min) so that the test can be completed in the outpatient clinic.

Clonidine has the supposed advantage of suppressing release of noradrenaline even when the basal level is normal, but when this is the case a suppression test is rarely necessary. An exception is in patients with von Hippel–Lindau syndrome found to have a small adrenal mass on their annual abdominal computed tomography (**CT**) or magnetic resonance scan: they may have a normal plasma noradrenaline concentration and, unlike the multiple endocrine neoplasia patients with phaeochromocytoma, the tumour secretes little adrenaline. In the multiple endocrine neoplasia patients, by contrast, an elevated plasma adrenaline concentration is the first biochemical abnormality, and biochemical diagnosis is likely to precede radiological diagnosis in multiple endocrine neoplasia, where annual scans are not indicated.

Only patients with normal or near normal renal function (serum creatinine less than 150 μmol/litre) are suitable for the pentolinium test, as this agent is entirely excreted by the kidneys. After the patient has rested supine for 15 to 30 min, plasma catecholamines are measured in two samples taken 5 min apart from an intravenous cannula, and in two further samples taken 10 and 20 min after an intravenous bolus of pentolinium 2.5 mg. They should remain supine for a further 60 min, and their erect arterial pressure should be checked before they are allowed to leave the clinic. A normal response to pentolinium is a fall of both plasma noradrenaline and adrenaline concentrations into the normal range or by 50 per cent from baseline. It should be noted that since ganglion-blocking drugs are less effective at low rates of sympathetic nerve discharge there may be little fall in plasma catecholamine values when the basal levels are already within the normal range.

Another test that can sometimes be helpful is to assay a plasma sample for dihydroxyphenyl glycol, the deaminated metabolite synthesized principally in sympathetic nerve endings. The ratio of dihydroxyphenyl glycol to noradrenaline is reversed from normal (more dihydroxyphenyl glycol than noradrenaline) in patients with phaeochromocytoma, allowing an alternative method to a suppression test for distinguishing patients with borderline noradrenaline results.

Localization of phaeochromocytomas

It is helpful to measure plasma catecholamines even in patients with unequivocal elevation of their 24-h urine vanillylmandelic acid as the adrenaline level is a most useful clue to the location of a phaeochromocytoma. Most adrenal phaeochromocytomas do secrete adrenaline, although the proportion of noradrenaline to adrenaline is reversed from that in normal subjects, whilst it is exceptional for extra-adrenal phaeochromocytomas to secrete adrenaline because of the lack of cortisol stimulation.

Although a major clue to localization can be provided by measurement of plasma adrenaline, CT scanning is the method of choice. The adrenal gland, where 90 per cent of phaeochromocytomas arise (Fig. 1), is easy to visualize, and imaging is able to distinguish cortical tumours such as a Conn's tumour from medullary tumours. These differences should, however, not be used as a basis for diagnosis: mistakes will be made if the differentiation between these tumours is attempted radiologically rather than biochemically. It should also be emphasized that both of these tumours account for a minority of adrenal tumours identified by CT, the majority of which are non-functional adenomas of no significance.

While modern CT is capable of whole body imaging at high resolution, it is preferable to withhold CT for extra-adrenal phaeochromocytomas until the radiologist can be given some clue as to where to direct their activities. In about 85 per cent of patients, this can be achieved by radio-isotope scanning, using the iodinated analogue of noradrenaline, m-iodobenzylguanidine. There is a case for undertaking such scanning in addition to CT, even for patients found to have an adrenal phaeochromocytoma, to identify extra-adrenal secondary deposits when tumours are malignant, and because there may be coexisting adrenal and extra-adrenal phaeochromocytomas.

If these investigations fail to localize a phaeochromocytoma diagnosed by biochemical assays, the next step is to undertake selective venous sampling. In this procedure, about 25 samples of blood for estimation of catecholamine concentration are collected under fluoroscopic guidance from various sites in the vena cava and the veins that drain into it. An arterial sample taken at the end of the procedure is invaluable for interpretation of

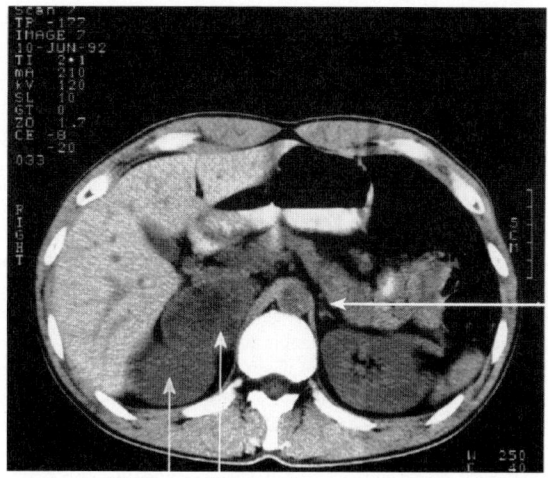

Normal adrenal

Kidney Phaeochromocytoma

Fig. 1 CT scan of a right adrenal phaeochromocytoma. The phaeochromocytoma has the typical non-homogeneous appearance due to areas of haemorrhage and infarction. The normal left adrenal has the typical tricornuate appearance with concave borders.

data, as it enables sites with a positive venoarterial difference to be readily detected. Although invasive, venous sampling is free of significant hazard, but it is important that the radiologist is not tempted to undertake a venogram of the phaeochromocytoma, since this can cause immediate infarction of the tumour with release of the stored catecholamines and catastrophic consequences. The procedure is more helpful in the diagnosis of phaeochromocytoma than of other endocrine tumours because of the very short half-life of catecholamines in the circulation (about 1 min), such that most is removed during one passage round the circulation, hence the concentration at the tumour site is usually several fold greater than concentrations elsewhere. This procedure should not usually be used for adrenal phaeochromocytomas because the concentration of catecholamines is much higher than elsewhere in veins draining normal adrenals, and because CT scanning should have already rendered their imaging unnecessary. An exception, once again, is in patients with von Hippel–Lindau syndrome with small adrenal masses. As discussed above, these are the patients in whom all other biochemical tests may be normal, and the diagnosis of phaeochromocytoma is suggested by a reversal of the normal excess of adrenaline to noradrenaline in the adrenal vein. Because in von Hippel–Lindau syndrome the adrenal phaeochromocytomas are frequently bilateral, but asymmetrical, venous sampling may be required to determine whether one or both adrenals need to be removed.

The place of angiography has been much diminished but not entirely removed by the advent of CT scanning. As phaeochromocytomas are vascular tumours, they provide a good tumour blush, and angiography should resolve equivocal CT scans. However, by contrast to venous sampling, this procedure can provoke an outpouring of catechols. Patients must be fully α- and preferably also β-blocked prior to angiography, and their blood pressure, pulse rate, and ECG must be monitored during the procedure with phentolamine and atenolol readily available to treat arterial hypertension or tachycardia.

In some centres, magnetic resonance imaging may be tried before angiography to determine the nature of lesions of doubtful significance on CT. However, the semi-infarcted nature of some phaeochromocytomas can make it difficult to interpret magnetic resonance scans, and in our experience such imaging has only helped with a few head and neck phaeochromocytomas that were not detected by m-iodobenzylguanidine or CT scanning.

Other investigations

It is important to check blood glucose in every patient as there may be α mediated inhibition of insulin release prior to effective treatment. All patients should be screened for an associated medullary carcinoma of the thyroid by plasma calcitonin estimation.

Apart from the catecholamines, most phaeochromocytomas also secrete one or more neuropeptides, especially neuropeptide Y (NPY), which is a normal cotransmitter of noradrenaline and adrenaline. There is no need routinely to measure other neurotransmitters that may be cosecreted with the catecholamines, but unusual symptoms may indicate that a gut peptide screen should be undertaken. Although very rare, it is essential to detect (especially preoperatively) coexisting ectopic adrenocorticotropic hormone syndrome that manifests as gross hypokalaemia. A particular catch is that the excess secretion of catecholamines may suppress release of other peptides until treatment with α-blockade is initiated, hence it is important to recheck the electrolytes after a few days of α-blocking treatment.

Even where there is no suggestive family history, routine slit-lamp examination of the fundi has resulted in a more frequent diagnosis of von Hippel–Lindau syndrome, sometimes as a *de novo* occurrence.

Treatment

The definitive treatment is surgical removal of the tumour or tumours. Even the small number of phaeochromocytomas that can be recognized to be malignant preoperatively (e.g. by the presence of bone or liver metastases) may still benefit from resection of the primary tumour. The task for the physician is to make the surgery safe. The mainstay of medical treatment is α-blockade, but not all patients—especially those without elevated plasma adrenaline levels—require β-blockade. The objective of this treatment is not solely control of blood pressure but also the expansion of blood volume, which is always reduced in those with a phaeochromocytoma. The α-blocker of choice is phenoxybenzamine, the principal reason for this being that it is irreversible, actually destroying the α-receptor by alkylation. More modern α-blockers, such as prazosin, doxazosin, and the mixed α- and β-blocker, labetalol, cause competitive blockade, which can be overcome by a surge of noradrenaline release from the tumour. An additional advantage of phenoxybenzamine is that it will block both α_1- and α_2-receptors. Blockade of the latter is considered disadvantageous in essential hypertension since the main α_2-receptors outside the central nervous system are presynaptic and may serve a useful role in damping neuronal release of noradrenaline, whereas in phaeochromocytoma patients α_2-receptor blockade may be advantageous because a small population of extrasynaptic α_2-receptors mediate direct vasoconstriction by circulating (non-neuronal) catecholamines. The diabetogenic effect of catecholamines is also an α_2-mediated response.

The starting dose of phenoxybenzamine depends on the degree of catecholamine excess, but is usually 10 mg twice daily. The effect of irreversible antagonists is cumulative, and the effect of the drug—and each subsequent dose increment—takes several days to reach maximum. It is reasonable to aim for a diastolic blood pressure of between 90 and 100 mmHg during outpatient treatment, and to admit patients for 5 days preoperatively, during which time the dose is increased until there is at least a 10 mmHg postural fall in blood pressure and little if any variability in arterial pressure. An important objective of preoperative α-blockade is expansion of intravascular volume. Surgery should not take place until a new steady-state weight has been achieved, which usually requires about a month.

The need for β-blockade is indicated by tachycardia, which may become apparent only after treatment with phenoxybenzamine. Lower doses of β-blocking drugs are necessary than used generally in the treatment of hypertension, and it is usually better to use a selective β_1-selective agent so that the peripheral vasodilatation mediated by β_2-receptors is not affected. The reason for using as low a dose as possible is that immediately upon removal of the phaeochromocytoma there may be a period of hypotension despite the preoperative preparation that has been outlined. This is due to

the withdrawal of any α-mediated vasoconstriction, and should normally be offset by the ability to mount a tachycardia. It is important to note that if hypotension does occur, it should not be treated with pressor agents; the correct treatment is by volume replacement, supplemented if necessary by β-agonists. Most vasoconstrictor drugs are unlikely to be effective, because of the previous treatment with phenoxybenzamine. Angiotensin is no longer available as a pharmaceutical preparation.

The treatment of malignant phaeochromocytomas remains uncertain and unsatisfactory. As is the case for many endocrine cancers, the rate of growth is usually slow, but outcome can vary from local recurrence at intervals of many years to rapid demise, sometimes precipitated by surgery. These tumours are not particularly sensitive to either chemotherapy or radiotherapy. There has been interest in the use of therapeutic doses of *m*-iodobenzylguanidine, as a means of targeting high doses of radioactivity to the tumour, and some patients show considerable regression after such treatment. Long-term results are less certain. If the primary tumour has been removed or debulked, it is rare for the pharmacological effects of the tumour to be the principal problem. However, if this is the case, then high doses of phenoxybenzamine are greatly preferable to α-methyltyrosine, occasionally used as an inhibitor of noradrenaline synthesis, but which also depletes noradrenaline in the brain, causing sedation and depression.

Prognosis

Ninety per cent of phaeochromocytomas are benign. For adrenal phaeochromocytomas, the proportion is probably even higher, whereas extraadrenal phaeochromocytomas have a greater than 10 per cent likelihood of proving malignant. However, because of the difficulties already described in ascertaining malignancy, all patients with a phaeochromocytoma should be followed indefinitely with at least an annual measurement of arterial pressure and analysis of one of the indices of catecholamine secretion.

The removal of a phaeochromocytoma cures most patients of their hypertension, especially the younger ones. In only 13 out of a personal series of 76 patients with phaeochromocytoma was the blood pressure greater than 140/85 at 6 and 12 months postoperatively (compared with an average 172/114 at presentation), and these 13 were all aged over 50 (compared with an average age of 37 for all 76 patients).

Further reading

Allison DJ *et al.* (1983). Role of venous sampling in locating a phaeochromocytoma. *British Medical Journal* **286**, 1122–4.

Brown MJ *et al.* (1981). Increased sensitivity and accuracy of phaeochromocytoma diagnosis achieved by use of plasma adrenaline estimations and a pentolinium suppression test. *The Lancet* **i**, 174–7.

Col V *et al.* (1999). Laparoscopic adrenalectomy for phaeochromocytoma: endocrinological and surgical aspects of a new therapeutic approach. *Clinical Endocrinology* **50**, 121–5.

Manger WM (1997). *Pheochromocytoma*. Springer, Berlin.

Richards FM *et al.* (1998). Molecular genetic analysis of von Hippel–Lindau disease. *Journal of Internal Medicine* **243**, 527–33.

Sisson JC, Shulkin BL (1999). Nuclear medicine imaging of pheochromocytoma and neuroblastoma. *Quarterly Journal of Nuclear Medicine* **43**, 217–23.

15.16.2.5 Aortic coarctation

Lawrence E. Ramsay

Coarctation is a congenital narrowing of the aorta near the junction with the ligamentum arteriosum and usually distal to the left subclavian artery. About 20 per cent of coarctations present in adolescent or adult years, often with hypertension, but coarctation is very rare in unselected hypertensive

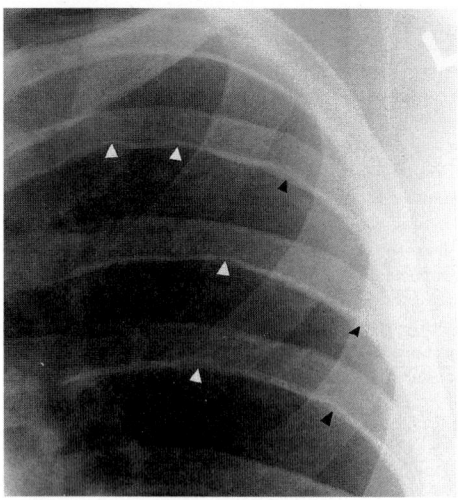

Fig. 1 Chest radiographic appearances of rib notching in a patient with coarctation of the aorta. (By courtesy of Dr N. Boon.)

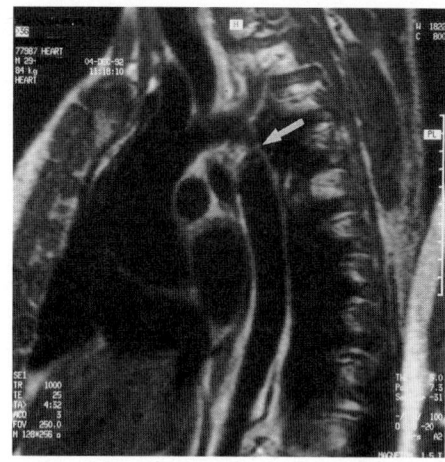

Fig. 3 Sagittal spin echo magnetic resonance image scan showing a well defined coarctation (arrow) in the typical position. (By courtesy of Dr N. Boon.)

patients. It is very easy to overlook, but should come to mind in hypertensive patients who are young, male (four times commoner than in females), have isolated or disproportionate systolic hypertension, have a prominent murmur over the precordium or back, have disproportionate left ventricular hypertrophy, or have Turner's syndrome. About 70 per cent have other congenital abnormalities, most commonly a bicuspid aortic valve, but also ventricular septal defect or patent ductus arteriosus. Palpate routinely for delayed or weak femoral pulses in all hypertensive patients. When coarctation is suspected, seek other clinical features which include palpable collaterals in the back, displaced apex beat and systolic thrill, systolic murmurs over the coarctation, collaterals, or aortic valve, and an ejection click or loud aortic valve closure. Measuring blood pressure in the legs with a sphygmomanometer is a nightmare, and Doppler measurement of the ankle–brachial pressure index is much more accurate. A chest radiograph may show rib notching (Fig. 1), cardiomegaly, and abnormal aortic configuration. The diagnosis is confirmed by aortography (Fig. 2) or magnetic resonance imaging (Fig. 3). Echocardiography reveals the state of the aortic valve and left ventricle, and aortography is done before intervention to define the anatomy and haemodynamics.

Untreated coarctation has a bad prognosis because of heart failure, aortic rupture or dissection, cerebral haemorrhage related to berry aneurysms, bacterial endocarditis or endarteritis, and other complications of hyper-

tension. Correction of coarctation improves survival, but not to a normal life expectancy. The prognosis after correction is affected adversely by correction at an older age, and persistent hypertension after correction. Coarctation should therefore be dealt with as soon as it is diagnosed, provided that this is technically possible and the patient is otherwise fit. Surgical repair may be complicated by postoperative paradoxical hypertension, and mesenteric or spinal ischaemia. Balloon angioplasty has lower immediate morbidity and mortality, and is possible as a primary procedure in about 90 per cent of cases, and also for recoarctation. There is uncertainty about the long-term outcome after angioplasty, particularly as regards development of aneurysms, but data to 5–10 years postangioplasty are reassuring. Nevertheless, indefinite follow-up and monitoring with repeat magnetic resonance scans are needed to detect possible recurrence or aneurysm development. About 30 per cent of patients still need treatment for hypertension after correction, with a higher probability as the age at correction increases. Patients need advice on prophylaxis against bacterial endocarditis before and after correction.

Further reading

Fawzy ME *et al.* (1997). 1–10 year follow-up results of balloon angioplasty of native coarctation of the aorta in adolescents and adults. *Journal American College of Cardiology* **30**, 1542–6.

Jenkins MP, Ward C (1999). Coarctation of the aorta: natural history and outcome after surgical treatment. *Quarterly Journal of Medicine* **92**, 365–71.

de Leeuw PW, Birkenhäger WH (1992) Coarctation of the aorta. In: Robertson JIS, ed. *Handbook of hypertension, Vol.15: Clinical hypertension*, pp 236–65. Elsevier, Amsterdam.

15.16.2.6 Other rare causes of hypertension

Lawrence E. Ramsay

Identifiable causes of hypertension are commonly renal, renovascular, drug-induced, primary aldosteronism, or a phaeochromocytoma. There are numerous other causes of, or associations with, hypertension (Table 1). Some are rare conditions that usually cause hypertension (for example, liquorice excess, renin-secreting tumour); some are rare conditions that rarely cause hypertension (for example, carcinoid syndrome); some are

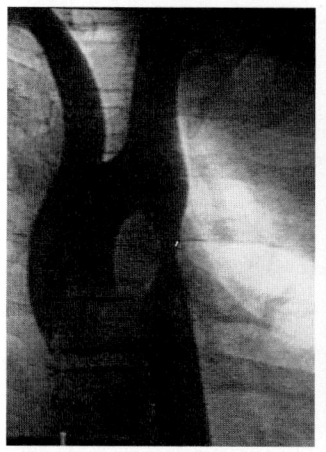
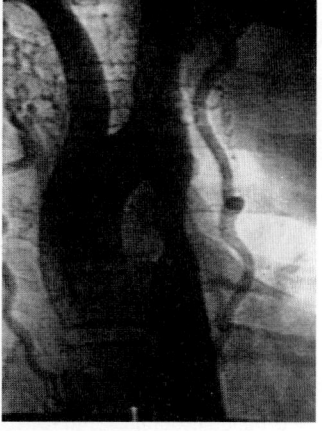

Fig. 2 (a) Digital aortogram showing typical appearances of a coarctation of the aorta. (b) A later frame showing marked dilatation of the internal mammary arteries due to increased collateral flow. (By courtesy of Dr N. Boon.)

(a)

(b)

Table 1 Uncommon causes of, or associations with, hypertension

Mineralocorticoid excess	Endocrine
Liquorice excess	Cushing's disease
11-Dehydrogenase deficiency	Pseudocushings (alcohol)
Ectopic ACTH	Primary hyperparathyroidism
DOC excess	Renin-secreting tumours
Liddle's syndrome	Acromegaly
	Thyrotoxicosis
	Hypothyroidism
Metabolic	
Acute intermittent porphyria*	**Neurogenic**
Lead poisoning*	Increased intracranial pressure
Carcinoid syndrome*	Posterior fossa tumour*
Gordon's syndrome	Spinal cord lesion*
Alcohol withdrawal	Autonomic neuropathy*
	Panic attacks*
Cardiovascular	Diencephalic epilepsy*
Hyperdynamic circulatory states**	Page's syndrome*
Acute left ventricular failure	**Pregnancy**
	Pre-eclampsia

DOC, deoxycorticosterone.
* May cause paroxysmal hypertension.
** May cause systolic hypertension

common conditions that rarely present as hypertension (for example, pregnancy presenting as pre-eclampsia); and some are associations that may not be causal (such as hypothyroidism, acromegaly).

Mineralocorticoid excess is suggested by hypertension, hypokalaemia, and high or high-normal serum sodium levels. Primary aldosteronism (Conn's syndrome, see Chapter 15.16.2.3) is the commonest cause, but rare causes should be suspected (Table 1) if the aldosterone level is low or normal rather than high. Most important among these is excess liquorice ingestion, because asking one simple question may avoid complex and costly investigations and rapidly resolve the hypertension and biochemical abnormalities. Liquorice excess causes hypertension, hypokalaemia, and increased levels of free cortisol in urine through an acquired 11-dehydrogenase deficiency.

Table 1 includes several conditions that can cause paroxysmal hypertension, sometimes with additional symptoms that may closely mimic a phaeochromocytoma. Some also show excess urinary or plasma catecholamines, particularly posterior fossa tumours near the fourth ventricle, which may be tiny and virtually undiagnosable. These causes of paroxysmal hypertension should be considered when investigation of a patient with features suggesting phaeochromocytoma fails to localize a phaeochromocytoma or other catecholamine-secreting tumour.

Further reading

Laragh JH, Brenner BM, eds (1990). *Hypertension. Pathophysiology, diagnosis and management*. Raven Press, New York.
Swales JD, ed (1994). *Textbook of hypertension*. Blackwell Scientific, Oxford.

15.16.3 Hypertensive emergencies and urgencies

Gregory Y. H. Lip and D. Gareth Beevers

Introduction

Hypertensive emergencies occur when severe hypertension is associated with acute end-organ damage. These can take a variety of forms and can

Table 1 Hypertensive emergencies and urgencies

Hypertensive emergencies
Hypertensive encephalopathy
Hypertensive left ventricular failure
Hypertension with myocardial infarction or unstable angina
Hypertension with aortic dissection
Severe hypertension with subarachnoid haemorrhage or stroke
Phaeochromocytoma crisis
Recreational drugs (amphetamines, LSD, cocaine, Ecstasy)
Perioperative hypertension
Severe pre-eclampsia or eclampsia
Hypertensive urgencies
Malignant hypertension
Chronic renal failure
Pre-eclampsia
Severe non-malignant hypertension

LSD, lysergic acid diethylamide.

occur at any age. They may be acute life-threatening medical conditions, and are associated with either severe hypertension or sudden marked increases in blood pressure (Table 1). Symptomatic patients with complications such as aortic dissection and hypertensive encephalopathy require parenteral antihypertensive therapy to reduce the blood pressure promptly, but in a controlled manner and with careful monitoring. However, over-rapid treatment may itself be hazardous, leading on occasions to ischaemic complications such as stroke, myocardial infarction, or blindness. Thus, in patients who have severe hypertension but are asymptomatic, slower controlled reduction in blood pressure should be achieved with oral antihypertensive agents, making such situations hypertensive 'urgencies' rather than 'emergencies'.

In general, there has been a decline in the incidence of hypertensive emergencies over the past 20 years in the Western world, which may possibly be the result of the more effective detection, diagnosis, and treatment of mild to moderate hypertension.

If patients with hypertensive emergencies are not recognized or treated appropriately, the mortality and morbidity can be very high, with the 1-year mortality being 70 to 90 per cent, and the 5 year mortality 100 per cent. With adequate blood pressure control, the 1-year and 5-year mortality rates decrease to 25 and 50 per cent, respectively. The mortality of untreated malignant phase hypertension (a hypertensive urgency rather than emergency) is around 80 per cent at 2 years, and if managed inappropriately there is also a high rate of progression to renal dysfunction, necessitating long-term dialysis, in addition to strokes and heart failure.

Clinical presentations

Hypertensive emergencies occur most commonly in patients with previous hypertension, especially if inadequately managed. Nevertheless, some patients can present with hypertensive emergencies *de novo*, without any previous history of hypertension.

Very severe and malignant hypertension are more likely to be associated with underlying causes such as renovascular disease, primary renal diseases, phaeochromocytoma, and connective tissue disorders, but malignant hypertension complicating primary hyperaldosteronism (Conn's syndrome) is very rare. Approximately 50 per cent of patients with malignant hypertension have an underlying cause.

Pathophysiology

The common denominator in hypertensive emergencies is intense peripheral vasoconstriction, resulting in a rapid rise in blood pressure and a vicious circle of events, including ischaemia of the brain and peripheral organs. This ischaemia stimulates neurohormone and cytokine release, exacerbating vasoconstriction and ischaemia, further increasing blood pressure and resulting in target organ damage. In addition, myointimal proliferation in the vasculature may exacerbate the situation, as can disseminated intravascular coagulation. Also, renal ischaemia leads to activation of the renin–angiotensin system, causing further rise in blood pressure and microvascular damage.

With mild to moderate elevation of blood pressure, the initial response of the vasculature is arterial and arteriolar vasoconstriction. Thus autoregulation maintains tissue perfusion at a relatively constant level and prevents the raised blood pressure from damaging the smaller, more distal blood vessels. Later, arteriolar hypertrophy also minimizes the transmission of pressure to the capillary circulation. In chronic hypertension, the lower limit of autoregulation of cerebral blood flow is shifted towards higher blood pressures, with impairment of the tolerance to acute hypotension. In normotensive subjects, the upper limit of autoregulation can be a mean arterial pressure of 120 mmHg (equivalent to 160/100 mmHg), but in individuals whose vessels are hypertrophied by long-standing hypertension, this upper limit is substantially higher (Fig. 1 and Plate 1). However, with rapid and severe rises in blood pressure, this process of autoregulation fails, leading to a rise in pressure in the arterioles and capillaries, causing vascular damage. Disruption of the endothelium allows plasma constituents (including fibrinoid material) to enter the vessel wall, narrowing or obliterating the lumen in many tissue beds. The level at which fibrinoid necrosis occurs is dependent upon the baseline blood pressure. In the cerebral circulation this can lead to the development of cerebral oedema and the clinical picture of hypertensive encephalopathy.

In addition to protecting the tissues against the effects of hypertension, autoregulation maintains perfusion during the treatment of hypertension via arterial and arteriolar vasodilatation. However, falls in blood pressure below the autoregulatory range can lead to organ ischaemia, and the arteriolar hypertrophy induced by chronic hypertension means that target organ ischaemia will occur at a higher pressure than in previously normotensive subjects.

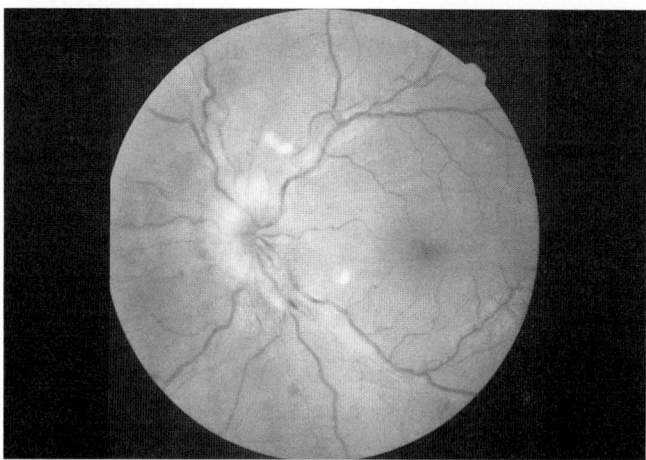

Fig. 2 Ocular fundus in hypertension, showing papilloedema, exudates, and a few haemorrhages. (See also Plate 1.)

Malignant hypertension

The malignant phase of hypertension is a rare condition characterized by very high blood pressures, with bilateral retinal haemorrhages and/or exudates or cotton wool spots, without the added requirement for papilloedema (Fig. 2). This clinical definition of malignant hypertension includes both Keith, Wagener, and Barker grades 3 and 4 retinopathy, previously designated as 'accelerated' and 'malignant' hypertension, respectively. Differentiation between Keith, Wagener, and Barker grades 3 and 4 retinopathy has been shown to be unhelpful, as the presence of papilloedema is an unreliable sign. Furthermore, both categories carry an equally bad prognosis and should therefore be considered the same disease—'malignant' hypertension.

The pathophysiological definition of malignant hypertension is based on the histological hallmark of fibrinoid necrosis of arterioles in many tissues, particularly the kidney. The histological changes are broadly similar to those seen in the haemolytic–uraemic syndrome or scleroderma. Mucoid intimal proliferation in renal interlobular arteries and ischaemic collapse of the glomerular tufts may also be seen. In black patients, myointimal hyperplasia is a common finding. The consequent intrarenal vascular disease leads to ischaemia of the juxtaglomerular apparatus and activation of the renin–angiotensin system with further vasoconstriction and wall damage, as well as exacerbation of the hypertension.

Epidemiology

Malignant hypertension has been reported to be becoming rarer in some countries, particularly amongst white populations. However, malignant hypertension still remains a common problem in the Third World and in other populations with health and social deprivation, where it is an important cause of endstage renal failure. Furthermore, in west Birmingham in the United Kingdom, the incidence of malignant hypertension was found to be around 1 to 2 per 100 000 population per year, with no clear reduction between 1970 and 1993 in the number of new cases seen, the mean duration of known hypertension before presentation, presenting blood pressures, or the number of antihypertensive drugs that were being used.

Whilst essential hypertension is usually the most common underlying cause of malignant hypertension in adults, secondary causes are more prevalent among younger patients. In children (aged less than 16 years) with malignant hypertension, parenchymal renal disease is the commonest cause (63 per cent), with 33 per cent having renovascular hypertension (aortoarteritis and fibromuscular dysplasia), and only 5 per cent with essential hypertension.

There is an association between cigarette smoking and malignant hypertension, which remains unexplained. Very rarely, the oral contraceptive pill

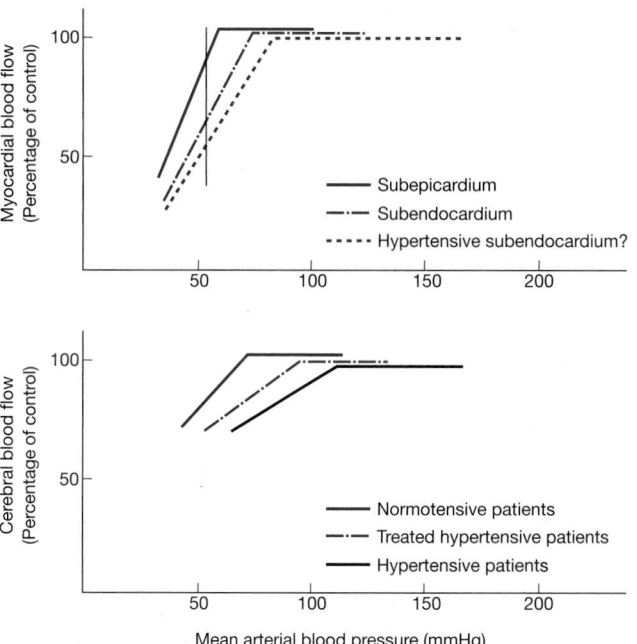

Fig. 1 Autoregulation of myocardial and cerebral blood flow in normotensive and hypertensive patients. (Reproduced from Strandgaard S, Haunsø S (1987). Why does antihypertensive treatment prevent stroke but not myocardial infarction? *Lancet* **ii**, 658–60, with permission.)

may be implicated, consistent with the well-recognized increase in blood pressure in some women taking the 'combined' oestrogen/progesterone oral contraceptive pill. It is uncertain whether oral contraceptives directly cause hypertension, or whether they simply exaggerate a tendency in women who already have a propensity to raised blood pressure. Malignant hypertension may also occur in the elderly, and is more common in Afro-Caribbean than white Caucasian and Indo-Asian populations. Possible reasons for the higher proportions of black and Asian people include the relative resistance of black patients to some antihypertensive therapies and perhaps poorer drug compliance.

One reason for the failure of malignant hypertension to decline in some centres may be inadequate medical screening facilities among poorly educated people with a limited understanding of the nature of the disease and the need to comply with antihypertensive therapy. Any reduction in the incidence of malignant hypertension may be because of the increasing use of drug therapy in the milder grades of hypertension preventing progression to the malignant phase. Nevertheless, it is possible that there has been no real decline in malignant hypertension, but merely a failure to recognize this life-threatening condition.

Clinical features

Some patients with malignant hypertension remain asymptomatic, but others present at a late stage of their disease. This proportion ranged from 10 to 75 per cent in one series from Nigeria. The predominant presenting symptom is visual disturbance with or without headaches. In the west Birmingham series, the presenting mean systolic and diastolic blood pressures have remained surprisingly similar over the 24 years surveyed (average blood pressure 228/142 mmHg), despite improvements in antihypertensive therapy. Heart failure, angina, or myocardial infarction are complicating features in approximately 20 per cent of patients with malignant hypertension, and ECG shows a high proportion of patients to have cardiomegaly and left ventricular hypertrophy. Nevertheless, some patients do have normal chest radiographs, ECGs, or echocardiograms despite very high blood pressure, suggesting that hypertension may have been of acute onset.

Investigation of malignant hypertension

All patients with malignant hypertension need a detailed clinical history and examination and investigation with blood tests (full blood count, serum biochemistry—including electrolytes and renal function), 12-lead ECG, chest radiography, and urinalysis. Fundoscopy and retinal photography are mandatory. The kidneys should be imaged by abdominal ultrasound to assess renal size and appearance, with a low threshold for proceeding to renal angiography to look for renal artery stenosis if the kidneys are asymmetric. A 24-h urine collection is necessary for urine catecholamines and protein excretion in all patients. These initial screening tests serve to identify patients in whom additional investigations may be appropriate to detect a secondary cause of hypertension.

The full blood count and film may reveal the anaemia of chronic renal failure or occasionally a microangiopathic haemolytic anaemia, with red cell fragmentation and intravascular coagulation, possibly related to the degree of arteriolar fibrinoid necrosis. Serum urea or creatinine should initially be measured daily, and if stable, creatinine clearance may be measured to give a more precise estimate of renal function. Raised serum creatinine or urea, indicating renal impairment, may have significant prognostic implications. Mild hypokalaemia may be present, due to secondary hyperaldosteronism. This usually resolves after control of the hypertension. Only very rarely does hypokalaemia indicate primary hyperaldosteronism (Conn's syndrome), but if it is extreme or persists despite good blood pressure control, then the characteristic findings of low renin levels but high aldosterone concentrations may be present. More commonly, both plasma renin and aldosterone levels are high in malignant hypertension, usually attributed to juxtaglomerular ischaemia. Urinalysis may demonstrate proteinuria and haematuria, even in the absence of primary renal disease, but the presence of proteinuria is a poor prognostic sign. Inflammatory markers (erythrocyte sedimentation rate and C-reactive protein) are often modestly elevated in malignant hypertension, but measurement of autoantibodies (antinuclear antibodies and antineutrophil cytoplasmic antibodies) can be used to discern uncommon cases due to vasculitis. Renal biopsy is required to make a specific diagnosis in some instances, but should not be performed until after blood pressure is controlled. The chest radiograph may show cardiomegaly and the presence of pulmonary oedema. Cardiomegaly and the presence of left ventricular hypertrophy can also be assessed using echocardiography.

Retinopathy in malignant hypertension

The most widely used classification of hypertensive changes in the fundus is that of Keith, Wagener, and Barker (Table 2). The strength of this classification was the correlation between clinical findings and prognosis, where grades 3 and 4 had a poor prognosis compared with grades 1 and 2. Although widely used, this grading system has some limitations, and has been made obsolete by advances in the understanding of the pathophysiology of arterial hypertension and the availability of effective antihypertensive therapy. This and other traditional grading systems have therefore become less applicable to clinical practice than previously. The ophthalmoscopic grading can be simplified into two workable groups: grade A (nonmalignant)—arteriolar narrowing and focal constriction, which also correlate with age and general cardiovascular status as well as blood pressure;

Table 2 The Keith, Wagener, Barker Classification and Prognosis

	Grade 1 (benign hypertension)	Grade 2 (more marked hypertension retinopathy)	Grade 3 (mild angiospastic retinopathy)	Grade 4 (malignant hypertension)
Retinal findings	Mild narrowing or sclerosis of the retinal arterioles	Moderate to marked sclerosis of the retinal arterioles Exaggerated arterial light reflex Venous compression at arterio-venous crossings ('nipping')	Retinal oedema, cotton wool spots and haemorrhages Sclerosis and spastic lesions of retinal arterioles Macular star	All the above and optic disc oedema
Percentage surviving in original series				
1 year	90	88	65	21
3 years	70	62	22	6
5 years	70	54	20	1

NB. Grades 1 and 2 are broadly similar and are related to age and general cardiovascular status as well as blood pressure. Grades 3 and 4 are much more alike and both are now considered to be 'malignant'.

and grade B (malignant)—linear flame-shaped haemorrhages, and/or exudates, and/or cotton wool spots with or without disc swelling.

Similar retinal appearances with haemorrhages and papilloedema can occur in severe anaemia, connective tissue disease, and infective endocarditis. Benign intracranial hypertension may cause bilateral papilloedema, but is usually self-limiting and minimally symptomatic. Nevertheless, severe hypertension and lone bilateral papilloedema may be a variant of malignant hypertension, with similar clinical features and prognosis. The retinal features of malignant hypertension regress over a period of 2 to 3 months if good blood pressure control is achieved.

The kidney in malignant hypertension

Renal involvement in malignant hypertension has been referred to as malignant nephrosclerosis, manifest as haematuria, proteinuria, and (sometimes) acute renal failure. Renal failure was the commonest cause of death in the west Birmingham series, and presenting urea and creatinine levels were independent predictors of survival. The Aberdeen Hypertension Clinic also found that serum creatinine at referral was an independant predictor of survival.

When antihypertensive therapy is initiated and blood pressure control achieved, the effect on renal function is variable. In the short term, renal function stabilizes in 10 per cent of cases, deteriorates progressively in 30 per cent, and deteriorates transiently before improving over a matter of weeks in the remainder. Isles and coworkers have suggested that the renal outcome of patients with malignant hypertension can be considered in three groups, each with a different renal prognosis: (i) patients whose serum creatinine is less than 300 µmol/l at presentation, who do well with effective antihypertensive therapy; (ii) patients with chronic renal failure (serum creatinine greater than 300 µmol/l) who do not require renal dialysis immediately, but are unlikely to maintain or recover renal function, except possibly in the short term, and commonly progress to endstage renal failure; and (iii) a small group with acute renal failure. Some of these patients may have post-streptococcal acute nephritic syndrome, characterized by retinopathy, fluid retention, and usually complete renal recovery. Thus, in the long term, some patients with mild renal impairment at first presentation may improve or even regain normal renal function as fibrinoid necrosis heals, especially with good blood pressure control. This is unlikely to occur in patients with more severe renal impairment at presentation.

There are varying reports of the frequency of renovascular disease in malignant hypertension, and this variation may be due to the frequency of renal angiography. In older patients, renal artery stenosis is more likely to be due to atheromatous disease which itself may be a consequence of chronic hypertension and chronic hyperlipidaemia, as well as cigarette smoking. In younger patients and particularly in women, renal artery stenosis may be due to fibromuscular dysplasia of the renal arteries with the characteristic 'string of beads' appearance on renal angiography. The value of surgical or angioplastic correction of atheromatous disease is debatable, possibly producing no better results than effective blood pressure control with antihypertensive drugs. In patients with fibromuscular dysplasia, however, renal angioplasty is worthwhile and may sometimes lead to a normal blood pressure level.

Practical guidelines for management of malignant hypertension

All patients with malignant hypertension should be admitted for assessment, investigation, and commencement of therapy under supervision. The initial aim of treatment is to lower the diastolic pressure to about 100 to 105 mmHg over a period of 2 to 3 days, with oral therapy and dose escalation at daily intervals if necessary. The maximum initial fall in blood pressure should not exceed 25 per cent of the presenting value. Blood pressure should be measured 4 hourly. Gradual reduction will allow adaptation of disordered tissue autoregulation and avoid target organ ischaemia. More

aggressive antihypertensive therapy is both unnecessary and dangerous as it may reduce the blood pressure to below the autoregulatory range, leading to ischaemic events such as strokes, heart attack, or renal failure.

The first-line oral antihypertensive agent is either a short-acting calcium antagonist (such as nifedipine) or a β-blocker (such as atenolol). An appropriate dose of nifedipine is 10 to 20 mg of the tablet formulation, which can be repeated or increased as necessary to bring about gradual reduction in blood pressure. Nifedipine is not absorbed from the oral mucosa, and there have been reports of complications including visual loss, cerebral infarction, and myocardial infarction with nifedipine therapy using the short-acting sublingual capsules. Sublingual nifedipine produces unpredictable falls in blood pressure and should never be used. β-Blockers are useful alternatives, but should be avoided in patients with asthma or where there is a high suspicion of an underlying phaeochromocytoma. It is sensible to start with small doses, such as 25 mg of atenolol, increasing as necessary. The combination of oral atenolol and nifedipine is often a well tolerated and effective regime.

Diuretics should be restricted to those with evidence of fluid overload. Some patients are volume depleted, presumably secondary to a pressure-related diuresis and activation of the renin–angiotensin system. Captopril and the other ACE inhibitors can produce rapid and dangerous falls in blood pressure, particularly in patients with hypokalaemic secondary hyperaldosteronism and hyponatraemia secondary to juxtaglomerular ischaemia or renovascular disease, which may be unrecognized in the acute situation. Over a period of about 1 to 2 weeks, further antihypertensive drugs should be added in to achieve a gradual reduction of blood pressure to less than 140/85 mmHg. Triple or quadruple drug regimens are invariably necessary in the long term.

Prognosis

If malignant hypertension is left untreated, around 80 per cent of patients die within 2 years, hence the name. The importance of early diagnosis is emphasized as patients tend to develop clinical symptoms only at a late stage of their disease. Black male patients with malignant hypertension have a poor prognosis when compared with other ethnic groups or women. These patients also present with more severe hypertension and greater renal damage, which represent independent predictors of outcome and explain the poorer prognosis.

The advent of effective and tolerable antihypertensive drug therapy has meant that this prognosis is greatly improved. For example, in the west Birmingham malignant hypertension series, median survival times for the patients presenting before 1970, between 1970 and 1979, and between 1980 and 1989 were 39.2, 68.6, and 144.0+ months, respectively, suggesting an improvement in prognosis with more recently diagnosed patients (Fig. 3). The series by Scarpelli and coworkers reported a 12-year survival rate of about 69 per cent, although patients with malignant hypertension diagnosed after 1980 had a 100 per cent survival rate. Whatever the cause, progressive renal impairment is still a common complicating factor in malignant hypertension, with many patients needing dialysis in the long term.

Hypertensive left ventricular failure

Hypertension causes heart failure by a number of mechanisms: these include pressure overload on the heart due to the raised peripheral vascular resistance, reduced left ventricular compliance (for example, in left ventricular hypertrophy), an increased risk for coronary artery disease and the precipitation of cardiac arrhythmias (such as atrial fibrillation). Severe hypertension results in a significant increase in afterload and may result in decompensation of the failing heart.

In addition to the conventional management with opioids and loop diuretics, in very severe hypertension with marked pulmonary oedema, intravenous sodium nitroprusside may be necessary to reduce preload and

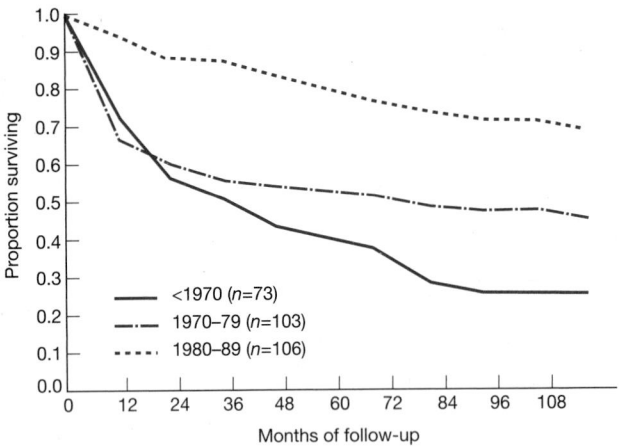

Fig. 3 Prognosis in 282 patients with malignant hypertension, divided into cohorts depending on year of presentation. (Reproduced from Lip GYH, Beevers M, Beevers DC (1995). Complications and survival of 315 patients with malignant-phase hypertension. *Journal of Hypertension* **13**, 915–24, with permission.)

afterload. Nitrates may also be used, but are less potent than sodium nitroprusside. ACE inhibitors should be considered in these patients only after stabilisation. These drugs are well-established to be life-saving in patients with left ventricular systolic impairment, and in addition they lead to long-term regression of LVH, which may also improve heart failure secondary to diastolic dysfunction.

Hypertensive encephalopathy

Hypertensive encephalopathy refers to the presence of signs of cerebral oedema caused by breakthrough hyperperfusion following severe and sudden rises in blood pressure. There is failure of autoregulatory vasoconstriction with focal or generalized dilatation of small arteries and arterioles. This leads to high cerebral blood flow, dysfunction of the blood–brain barrier, and the formation of brain oedema, which is thought to cause the clinical symptoms. The condition is very rare, and it is essential to ensure that this hypertensive emergency is distinguished from other neurological syndromes associated with high blood pressure, including intracerebral or subarachnoid haemorrhage, ischaemic stroke, or lacunar infarction.

Hypertensive encephalopathy is usually associated with a history of hypertension which has been inadequately treated, or where previous treatment has been discontinued. The condition is characterized by the insidious onset of headache, nausea, and vomiting, followed by visual disturbances and fluctuating non-localizing neurological symptoms such as restlessness, confusion, and, if the hypertension is not treated, seizures and coma. Severe retinopathy is frequently present, but not always.

The cerebrospinal fluid is usually normal but is at an increased pressure. The electroencephalogram may show variable transient, focal, or bilateral abnormalities. The CT scan or MRI may demonstrate white matter oedema: one of these tests is mandatory to exclude cerebral haemorrhage or infarction. Indeed, the increased use of CT scanning has demonstrated that almost all patients who appear to have hypertensive encephalopathy have cerebral infarction or haemorrhage with surrounding oedema and space-occupying cerebral symptoms.

Sodium nitroprusside is the drug of choice for genuine hypertensive encephalopathy but is not usually given if there is a cerebral infarct or haemorrhage. Parenteral labetalol and nitrates have also been used successfully. Rarely, diazoxide and hydralazine have been used, but they can cause precipitate and life-threatening acute falls in blood pressure. Sublingual nifedipine capsules should never be used (see above).

Severe pre-eclampsia and eclampsia are discussed in detail elsewhere. They may present with clinical features similar to hypertensive encephal-

opathy and treatment is broadly similar with antihypertensive drugs, magnesium sulphate, and early delivery of the fetus.

Hypertension with unstable angina or acute myocardial infarction

In a patient presenting with unstable angina or acute myocardial infarction and severe hypertension, a 'true' hypertensive emergency, such as aortic dissection, must first be ruled out. The risk of bleeding and stroke is significantly increased if anticoagulation with heparin or thrombolytic therapy is administered.

The appropriate initial treatment of patients with severe hypertension (greater than 180/110 mmHg) and an acute coronary syndrome should include the initiation of intravenous nitrates, with intravenous labetalol, sodium nitroprusside, or nicardipine as alternatives. The reduction of blood pressure should not be too abrupt, and (as with malignant hypertension) a gradual reduction is recommended, so that further myocardial or brain ischaemia is avoided. Sublingual nifedipine, which was once considered as a first-line drug, should not be used, in view of the negligible oral absorption and unpredictable hypotensive effects from later gastric absorption. Once the blood pressure is adequately controlled (less than 180/110 mmHg), anticoagulation or thrombolytic therapy can then be administered.

Hypertension with acute stroke

It is common to find modestly elevated blood pressure in patients admitted to hospital following an acute stroke. Cerebral autoregulation is commonly disturbed in this situation and excessive antihypertensive treatment may only serve to worsen the cerebral damage resulting from intracerebral infarction or haemorrhage. Such treatment should only be administered for severe elevation of blood pressure (diastolic blood pressure greater than 130 mmHg). In these cases, oral therapy with small doses of nifedipine or atenolol may be required. Parenteral treatment or sublingual nifedipine is almost always contraindicated. The calcium antagonist nimodipine has beneficial effects on cerebral vasospasm following subarachnoid haemorrhage, but these effects are not related to the small fall in blood pressure with this drug.

Severe hypertension after a stroke is a risk factor for further stokes and long-term treatment is worthwhile. It is unclear whether the immediate treatment of mild hypertension is of benefit. The role of antihypertensive medication before, during, and after a stroke can therefore be summarized as follows.

1. Before a stroke: it is of benefit to have blood pressure reduced to below 140/85 mmHg, as stroke prevention can be achieved.

2. During a stroke: it is detrimental to have hypertension treated aggressively, in view of the disordered cerebral autoregulation.

3. After a stroke: the role of antihypertensive medication remains unanswered, as the value of long-term antihypertensive therapy in mildly hypertensive patients following a stroke remains uncertain. Ongoing trials will answer this question. Nevertheless, drug therapy should be prescribed if blood pressure exceeds 160/100 mmHg.

The management of blood pressure in a patient with aortic dissection

The detailed presentation, diagnosis, and treatment of aortic dissection is discussed elsewhere. On suspicion of the diagnosis, whether or not surgery is indicated, all patients should be treated pharmacologically to reduce the systolic blood pressure to around 110 mmHg and the heart rate to 60 to 70 beats/min, thus reducing the force of systolic ejection to reduce aortic shear stress and limit the size of the dissection. Labetalol is an effective agent, or

Table 3 Oral drugs for hypertensive emergencies and urgencies

Category	Example	Comment
β-Blockers	Atenolol 25–50 mg	Safe unless contraindicated
Calcium channel blockers	Nifedipine capsules	Dangerous
	Nifedipine tablets 10–20 mg	Safe
	Amlodipine	Onset of action is slow (~5 days)
	Verapamil	Useful if tachycardia or associated supraventricular arrhythmia
	Nicardipine	Not better than nifedipine by mouth
α-Blockers	Prazosin	Little experience
	Doxazosin	Little experience
	Phenoxybenzamine	Phaeochromocytoma
Diuretics	Thiazides	Slow onset
	Loop diuretics	Only if heart failure
ACE inhibitors	Captopril 6.25–50 mg, three times a day	If patient on diuretic, may cause rapid falls in blood pressure and acute renal failure
		If renal artery stenosis undiagnosed, may cause rapid falls in blood pressure and acute renal failure

alternatively, sodium nitroprusside in conjunction with a β-blocker may be used. Patients should have haemodynamic monitoring with an arterial line and a Swan–Ganz catheter in position. Diagnostic tests are then performed on an urgent basis to confirm the dissection, identifying whether the ascending aorta is involved and defining any vascular abnormalities resulting from the dissection.

Summary of drug treatment options for hypertensive urgencies and emergencies

In uncomplicated malignant hypertension, where acute target organ damage is absent, and in uncomplicated severe hypertension, immediate blood pressure reduction with parenteral drugs is not indicated and blood pressure should be gradually reduced with oral agents (Table 3). Thus malignant hypertension, pre-eclampsia, and very severe hypertension without end-organ damage can be classified as hypertensive 'urgencies' rather than emergencies. Parenteral drugs to lower blood pressure may be dangerous and sublingual or capsular nifedipine should never be used.

In hypertensive crises the high blood pressure is directly responsible for a pressing clinical problem (hypertensive encephalopathy, left ventricular failure, or aortic dissection) and controlled reduction with parenteral treatment over a matter of hours is needed (Table 4). All such patients should be admitted to a high dependency or intensive care unit for monitoring. Blood pressure should be reduced by 25 per cent over several hours, depending on the clinical situation, usually with a target diastolic blood pressure of less than 100 to 110 mmHg. Thus, the goal of blood pressure reduction in those with hypertensive emergencies as well as urgencies is not to return blood pressure to a normal value immediately.

While nitroprusside is used in most hypertensive emergencies, its metabolism to cyanide, possibly leading to the development of cyanide or rarely thiocyanate toxicity, may be a limitation, especially in children. Toxicity is manifest by clinical deterioration, altered mental status, and lactic acidosis, and can be fatal; the risk of toxicity is increased with prolonged treatment (more than 24 to 48 h), underlying renal insufficiency, and high doses (greater than 2 µg/kg.min). An infusion of sodium thiosulphate can be used in affected patients to provide a sulphur donor to detoxify cyanide into thiocyanate.

Other parenteral agents such as labetolol, hydralazine, and diazoxide are alternatives. Phentolamine is used only in patients with severe hypertension due to increased catecholamine activity, such as that seen in phaeochromocytoma, or after tyramine ingestion in a patient being treated with a monoamine oxidase inhibitor. Direct vasodilators such as diazoxide or hydralazine require concurrent β-blocker administration to minimize reflex sympathetic stimulation and are rarely used. ACE inhibitors are best avoided in the early stage as they may, even in very low dose, cause precipitate falls in blood pressure and life-threatening reduction in cerebral perfusion. These rapid falls occur when patients are fluid depleted due to diuretic therapy or in renal artery stenosis.

Final summary

Hypertensive emergencies and urgencies carry a poor short- and long-term prognosis unless adequately managed. Initially, reduction of blood pressure to a normal value is dangerous, but in the long term, blood pressure should be reduced to 140/85 mmHg.

Further reading

Ahmed MEK *et al.* (1986). Lack of difference betwen malignant and accelerated hypertension. *British Medical Journal* **292**, 235–7.

Bloxham CA, Beevers DG, Walker JM (1979). Malignant hypertension and cigarette smoking. *British Medical Journal* **i**: 581–3.

Clough CG, Beevers DG, Beevers M (1990). The survival of malignant hypertension in blacks, whites and Asians in Britain. *Journal of Human Hypertensionn* **4**, 94–6.

Elliot JM, Simpson FO (1980). Cigarettes and accelerated hypertension. *New Zealand Journal of Medicine* **91**, 447–9.

Gudbrandsson T *et al.* (1979). Malignant hypertension. Improving prognosis in a rare disease. *Acta Medica Scandinavica* **206**, 495–9.

Harvey JM *et al.* (1992). Renal biopsy findings in hypertensive patients with proteinuria. *Lancet* **340**, 1435–6.

Isles C *et al.* (1979). Excess smoking in malignant-phase hypertension. *British Medical Journal* **i**: 579–81.

Isles CG, McLay A, Boulton Jones JM (1984). Recovery in malignant hypertension presenting as acute renal failure. *Quarterly Journal of Medicine* **212**, 439–52.

Islim IF *et al.* (1993). Prevalence of electrocardiographic left ventricular hypertrophy in malignant hypertension and its correlation with renal function. *Journal of Hypertension* **11** (Suppl 5), S106–S107.

Jhetam D *et al.* (1982). The malignant phase of essential hypertension in Johannesburg blacks. *South African Medical Journal* **61**, 899–902.

Kadiri S, Olutade BO (1991). The clinical presentation of malignant hypertension in Nigerians. *Journal of Human Hypertension* **5**, 339–43.

Keith NM, Wagener HP, Barker NW (1939). Some different types of essential hypertension: their course and prognosis. *American Journal of the Medical Sciences* **196**, 332–43.

Table 4 Parenteral drugs for the treatment of hypertensive emergencies

	Action	Administration	Use and adverse effects	Comment
Sodium nitroprusside	Dilates both arterioles and veins via generation of cyclic GMP which then activates calcium-sensitive potassium channels in the cell membrane	Intravenous infusion; rapid onset and offset of action, minimizing the risk of hypotension Recommended starting dose is 0.25–0.5 µg/kg per minute, increased as necessary to a maximum dose of 8–10 µg/kg per minute, for up to 10 min Nitroprusside should not be given to pregnant women	Can cause intrapulmonary shunting and coronary 'steal' Thiocynate and cyanide toxicity manifest by clinical deterioration, muscle twitching, altered mental status, and lactic acidosis, and can be fatal	The most effective parenteral drug for most hypertensive emergencies Easy to control on a minute-to-minute basis
Nitroglycerin (glyceryl trinitrate)	Similar action to nitroprusside, but greater venodilation	Intravenous infusion, 5–100 µg/min Onset of action is 2–5 min, while the duration of action is 5–10 min	Headache (due to direct vasodilation) and tachycardia (reflex sympathetic activation) Vomiting Methaemoglobinaemia	Most useful in patients with symptomatic coronary disease and in those with hypertension following surgery
Labetalol	Combined β-adrenergic and α-adrenergic blocker	Rapid onset of action (5 min or less) Bolus of 20 mg initially, followed by 20–80 mg every 10 min to a total dose of 300 mg The infusion rate is 0.5–2 mg/min	Avoid in patients with contraindications to β-blockers	Safe in patients with active coronary disease since it does not increase the heart rate Also useful in the perioperative care of patients with severe hypertension
Esmolol	β-Adrenergic blocker	Rapid onset and offset of action Intravenous infusion, titrated to heart rate and blood pressure response	Reduces myocardial ischaemia Avoid in patients with contraindications to β-blockers	Useful in tachycardias, hyperdynamic heart, arrhythmias (e.g. atrial fibrillation), perioperative hypertension, aortic dissection
Nicardipine	Dihydropyridine calcium channel blocker	Intravenous infusion at 5–15 mg/h	Headache and flushing Tachycardia	Becoming more popular Useful for most hypertensive emergencies except acute heart failure
Diazoxide	Arteriolar vasodilator that has little effect on the venous circulation	Intravenous bolus 50–150 mg or infusion 2–10 mg/h Peak effect seen within 15 min, lasts for 4–24 h	Do not use in patients with angina pectoris, myocardial infarction, pulmonary oedema, or a dissecting aortic aneurysm Can cause marked fluid retention and a diuretic may be needed	Give β-blocker to block reflex activation of the sympathetic nervous system Rarely used nowadays as may cause excessive blood pressure reduction which is difficult to reverse
Hydralazine	Direct arteriolar vasodilator	Intravenous bolus Initial dose is 10–20 mg The fall in blood pressure begins within 10–30 min and lasts 2–4 h.	Tachycardia, flushing, headache, vomiting Aggravation of angina Hypotensive response to hydralazine is less predictable	Used in pregnant women
Phentolamine	α-Adrenergic blocker	Intravenous bolus, 5–10 mg every 5–15 min as necessary	Severe hypertension due to phaeochromocytoma and other syndromes of increased catecholamine activity, such as drug abuse, MAO-induced hypertension, etc.	Tachyphylaxis means that doses need to be escalated

MAO, monoamine oxidase.

Kincaid Smith P (1985). What has happened to malignant hypertension? In: Bulpitt CJ, ed. *Handbook of hypertension*, Vol 6, *Epidemiology of hypertension*, pp 255–65. Elsevier, Amsterdam.

Kincaid-Smith P (1991). Malignant hypertension. *Journal of Hypertension* **9**, 893–9.

Kumar P *et al.* (1996). Malignant hypertension in children in India. *Nephrology, Dialysis, Transplantation* **11**, 1261–6.

Ledingham JGG, Rajagopalan B (1979). Cerebral complications in the treatment of accelerated hypertension. *Quarterly Journal of Medicine* **189**, 25–41.

Leishman AWD (1959). Hypertension—treated and untreated: a study of 400 cases. *British Medical Journal* **i**: 1361–3.

Lim KG *et al.* (1987). Malignant hypertension in women of childbearing age and its relation to the contraceptive pill. *British Medical Journal* **294**, 1057–9.

Lip GYH *et al.* (1995). Severe hypertension and lone bilateral papilloedema: a variant of malignant phase hypertension. *Blood Pressure* **4**, 339–42.

Lip GYH *et al.* (1995). Malignant hypertension in the elderly. *Quarterly Journal of Medicine* **88**, 641–7.

Lip GYH, Beevers M, Beevers DG (1997). Does renal function improve following diagnosis of malignant phase hypertension? *Journal of Hypertension* **15**, 1309–15.

Mamdani BH *et al.* (1974). Recovery from prolonged renal failure in patients with accelerated hypertension. *New England Journal of Medicine* **291**, 1343–4.

McGregor E *et al.* (1986). Retinal changes in malignant hypertension. *British Medical Journal* **292**, 233–4.

Pitcock JA *et al.* (1976). Malignant hypertension in blacks. Malignant intrarenal arterial disease as observed by light and electron microscopy. *Human Pathology* **7**, 333–46.

Scarpelli PT *et al.* (1997). Accelerated (malignant) hypertension: a study of 121 cases between 1974 and 1996. *Nephrology* **10**, 207–15.

Shapiro LM, Mackinnon J, Beevers DG (1981). Echocardiographic features of malignant hypertension. *British Heart Journal* **46**, 374–9.

Strandgaard S, Paulson OB (1996). Antihypertensive drugs and cerebral circulation. *European Journal of Clinical Investigation* **26**, 625–30.

Veriava Y *et al.* (1990). Hypertension as a cause of end-stage renal failure in South Africa. *Journal of Human Hypertension* **4**, 379–83.

Webster J *et al.* (1993). Accelerated hypertension—patterns of mortality and clinical factors affecting outcome in treated patients. *Quarterly Journal of Medicine* **86**, 485–93.

Zampaglione P *et al.* (1996). Hypertensive urgencies and emergencies. Prevalence and clinical presentation. *Hypertension* **27**, 144–7.

15.17 Lymphoedema

Peter S. Mortimer

Introduction

Lymphoedema is swelling due to the accumulation of lymph within the tissues and results from a failure of lymphatic drainage. Lymphoedema differs clinically from other forms of chronic oedema by its altered skin texture and the brawny quality of the subcutaneous tissues, which limit pitting. There may be no distinguishing clinical features, particularly in the early stages of swelling.

It is the essential function of the lymphatic system to return to the plasma any proteins which escape from the blood circulation. Impairment of lymph drainage therefore causes the accumulation of protein as well as fluid since both enter the tissues in substantial amounts. The lymphatics act as a safety valve or buffer in the event of fluid overload in the tissues. Therefore, theoretically, oedema should not arise as long as lymph flow can respond to the increased 'lymph load'.

In addition, the lymph drainage pathways are responsible for the removal and processing of foreign organic material, such as microbes, as well as for the trafficking of immunologically active cells such as lymphocytes. Consequently, a predisposition to infection, which can be relapsing, is a common occurrence with lymphoedema. The elimination of dying and mutant cells is via the lymphatic system, but the mechanism by which lymph vessels attract and channel cancer cells is not understood.

Aetiology/pathophysiology

In practice, the clinician is faced with a problem of oedema, usually a swollen limb, for which the cause may not be obvious. Rather than assemble a list of specific medical conditions, such as heart failure and venous oedema, as differential diagnosis, it is more sensible to consider causes of oedema from physiological principles as there may be more than one reason for the swelling.

Oedema

Oedema is swelling due to the excessive accumulation of fluid within tissues. Interstitial fluid volume must increase by over 100 per cent before oedema is clinically detectable. Oedema develops when the capillary filtration rate exceeds the lymph drainage rate for a sufficient period. All oedema, whatever the cause, results from an imbalance between capillary filtration and lymph drainage. Therefore it follows that the pathogenesis of any oedema results from either a high filtration rate or a low lymph flow or a combination of the two.

Elevation of capillary pressure is usually secondary to chronic elevation of venous pressure caused by heart failure, fluid overload, or deep vein thrombosis. A rise in blood (arterial) pressure alone should not raise capillary pressure sufficiently to cause oedema. Reduced plasma colloid osmotic pressure, for example in hypoproteinaemia, raises net filtration rate. Changes in capillary permeability, for example due to inflammation, increase the escape of proteins into the interstitium and water follows osmotically. Any change to the Starling forces governing fluid exchange can influence oedema formation (Box 1).

Most oedemas arise from increased capillary filtration overwhelming lymph drainage. To some extent any oedema incriminates the lymphatic system through its failure to keep up with demand (capillary filtration). Lymphoedema, however, is strictly oedema arising principally from a failure of lymph drainage.

Lymphoedema

Lymph drainage may fail either because of a defect intrinsic to the lymph conducting pathways (primary lymphoedema, Box 2(a)) or because of irreversible damage from some factor(s) originating from outside the lymphatic system (secondary lymphoedema, Box 2(b)).

Physiologically there are only a limited number of ways that lymphatics can fail. They may be reduced in number (aplasia/hypoplasia), obliterated (lymphangitis), obstructed, lose contractility (pump failure), or become incompetent (valvular reflux). A lack of sensitive methods for investigation makes it difficult to distinguish between these mechanisms.

Primary lymphoedema

True congenital lymphoedema, which presents at or soon after birth, is rare. Milroy's disease is both congenital and familial: both features are required for the diagnosis. The fault is a hypoplasia of peripheral lymphatic vessels. The gene for Milroy's disease is vascular endothelial growth factor C receptor, which is known to be involved with lymphangiogenesis.

Congenital lymphoedema may present as a result of a developmental malformation either in pure form, such as lymphangiectasia, or in combination with a congenital vascular syndrome. Lymphoedema may coexist with cardiovascular malformations in other genetic syndromes such as Turner's and Noonan's.

Most forms of primary lymphoedema present at or after puberty with distal lower limb swelling, usually bilateral. Familial forms frequently occur (Meige's syndrome) in which lymphangiograms usually demonstrate a reduction in size and number of peripheral leg lymphatic (main collecting) vessels. Familial post-pubertal lymphoedema, associated with an extra row of ingrowing eyelashes (distichiasis–lymphoedema syndrome), seems to be associated with hypertrophy of leg lymphatics (increase in number and size of vessels). Mutations in *FOXC2*, a forkhead family transcription factor, have been found responsible.

Genetic forms of lymphoedema are usually (ultimately) symmetrical with predominantly distal limb swelling. Lymphoedema of the proximal obstructive type with unilateral whole leg swelling is sporadic in type. Lymphangiograms of this form of lymphoedema demonstrate obstruction at the iliac nodes, but no cause can be identified. It is of paramount importance to exclude serious pathology such as tumour or thrombosis. Whole leg swelling can sometimes be bilateral due to megalymphatics. Grossly dilated (varicose) lymphatics with valvular incompetence give rise to lymph and sometimes chylous reflux, indicating the primary fault lies with abdominal lymphatics.

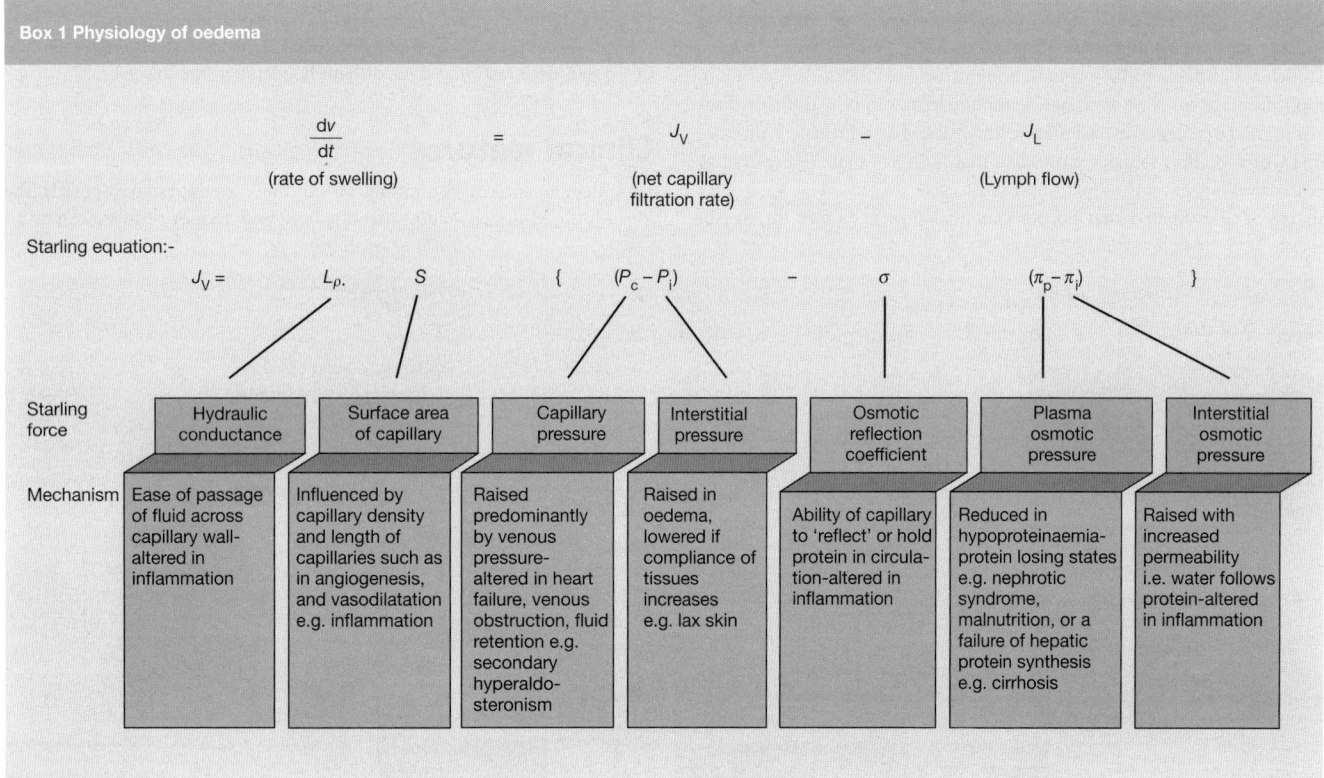

Box 1 Physiology of oedema

$$\frac{dv}{dt} \qquad = \qquad J_V \qquad - \qquad J_L$$

(rate of swelling)   (net capillary filtration rate)   (Lymph flow)

Starling equation:-

$$J_V = \quad L_\rho . \quad S \quad \{ \quad (P_c - P_i) \quad - \quad \sigma \quad (\pi_p - \pi_i) \quad \}$$

Starling force	Hydraulic conductance	Surface area of capillary	Capillary pressure	Interstitial pressure	Osmotic reflection coefficient	Plasma osmotic pressure	Interstitial osmotic pressure
Mechanism	Ease of passage of fluid across capillary wall-altered in inflammation	Influenced by capillary density and length of capillaries such as in angiogenesis, and vasodilatation e.g. inflammation	Raised predominantly by venous pressure-altered in heart failure, venous obstruction, fluid retention e.g. secondary hyperaldosteronism	Raised in oedema, lowered if compliance of tissues increases e.g. lax skin	Ability of capillary to 'reflect' or hold protein in circulation-altered in inflammation	Reduced in hypoproteinaemia-protein losing states e.g. nephrotic syndrome, malnutrition, or a failure of hepatic protein synthesis e.g. cirrhosis	Raised with increased permeability i.e. water follows protein-altered in inflammation

Protein-losing enteropathy and hypogammaglobulinaemia may arise from intestinal lymphangiectasia. The yellow nail syndrome is characterized by yellow, non-growing, over-curved nails, pleural effusions, bronchiectasis, chronic sinusitis, and peripheral oedema, but the mechanism is unknown.

Secondary lymphoedema

Damage to lymph-conducting pathways may be secondary to outside influences. In developed countries, surgical removal or radiation (or both) of lymph nodes as a necessary part of cancer treatment probably represents the largest group. Trauma to lymphatics either from elective surgery or by accident usually needs to be extensive to induce lymphoedema. The experimental production of lymphoedema is extremely difficult owing to the efficient regenerative powers of lymphatics. It is probably the failure of lymphatics to regenerate or regrow through scarred or irradiated tissue which is responsible for lymphoedema following cancer therapy. Cancer rarely presents with lymphoedema, except in advanced disease, but relapsed tumour (after first-line treatment) frequently produces swelling because of infiltration of collateral lymphatic routes which hitherto have prevented oedema.

Filariasis is probably the most common cause of lymphoedema worldwide. Microfilariae are introduced into the skin by mosquitoes and migrate to the lymphatics. Adult worms develop within the main lymphatic vessels proximal to the nodes. Animal studies have shown that within days of infection, vigorous movement by adult worms directly impacts on the endothelial lining of the lymphatic trunks and indirectly distorts the local lymph-node architecture. The result is enlarged lymph nodes and lymphatics with thickened walls and valves, thrombus formation, and perilymphangitis.

Lymphangitis or cellulitis probably only cause lymphoedema when the lymphatics are perilously vulnerable. Any patient suffering recurrent lymphangitis/cellulitis in the same region is likely to have impaired lymph drainage. Proving which came first—the cellulitis or the lymphatic insufficiency—is difficult. Recurrent acute inflammatory episodes frequently lead to a stepwise deterioration in swelling.

Podoconiosis is a form of endemic non-filarial lymphoedema caused by particles of silica dust which penetrate the feet during barefoot walking. The microparticles are taken up by lymphatics and result in fibrosis.

Cellulitis (acute inflammatory episodes)

Evidence supporting the role of the lymphatic route in immunosurveillance was provided during the early days of organ transplantation. Lymphatics convey antigens to lymph nodes. Without intact lymphatics a primary immune response cannot develop. T lymphocytes constantly recirculate between central organs, blood, and tissues for the purpose of immunosurveillance. Disturbances in host defence mechanisms within the lymph drainage area in lymphoedema probably predispose to infections such as cellulitis. However, in some patients even prophylactic antibiotics fail to control recurrent attacks, thus questioning infection as the sole explanation.

Epidemiology

Filarial lymphoedema is a major health problem in tropical and subtropical areas where the disease is endemic. The number of infected people worldwide is estimated to be 750 million. Morbidity is high. Fever ('mumu' attacks) is the earliest symptom followed by enlarged lymph nodes. Damage to central abdominal nodes results in reflux of lymph or chyle into lower limbs and genitalia with swelling and seepage of lymph on to this skin surface (lymphorrhoea). Chyluria may also occur.

The cumulative prevalence of arm swelling following curative treatment for breast cancer has been reported at 28 per cent. Similar values are quoted for incidence in hospital series if surgery and radiotherapy are combined.

Primary lymphoedema is perceived as uncommon, yet chronic ankle oedema—particularly in the elderly—is considered common. Lymphatic insufficiency is likely to be a contributing cause because of the decline in lymph drainage function with age. Lymphoedema can be a difficult diagnosis in mild or early cases and may be underdiagnosed. Primary lymphoedema tends to affect females more than males. In less than 10 per cent of cases is swelling present at birth and most cases present at or soon after puberty. It is estimated that 80 per cent will present before the age of

35 years (lymphoedema praecox) and 10 per cent after the age of 35 years (lymphoedema tarda). In a study of 1000 normal young adults, 8 per cent of women demonstrated signs of lymphoedema in the lower limb.

Clinical features

Lymphoedema most commonly affects the extremities, particularly the lower limb. Midline swelling affecting head and neck or genitalia can be an

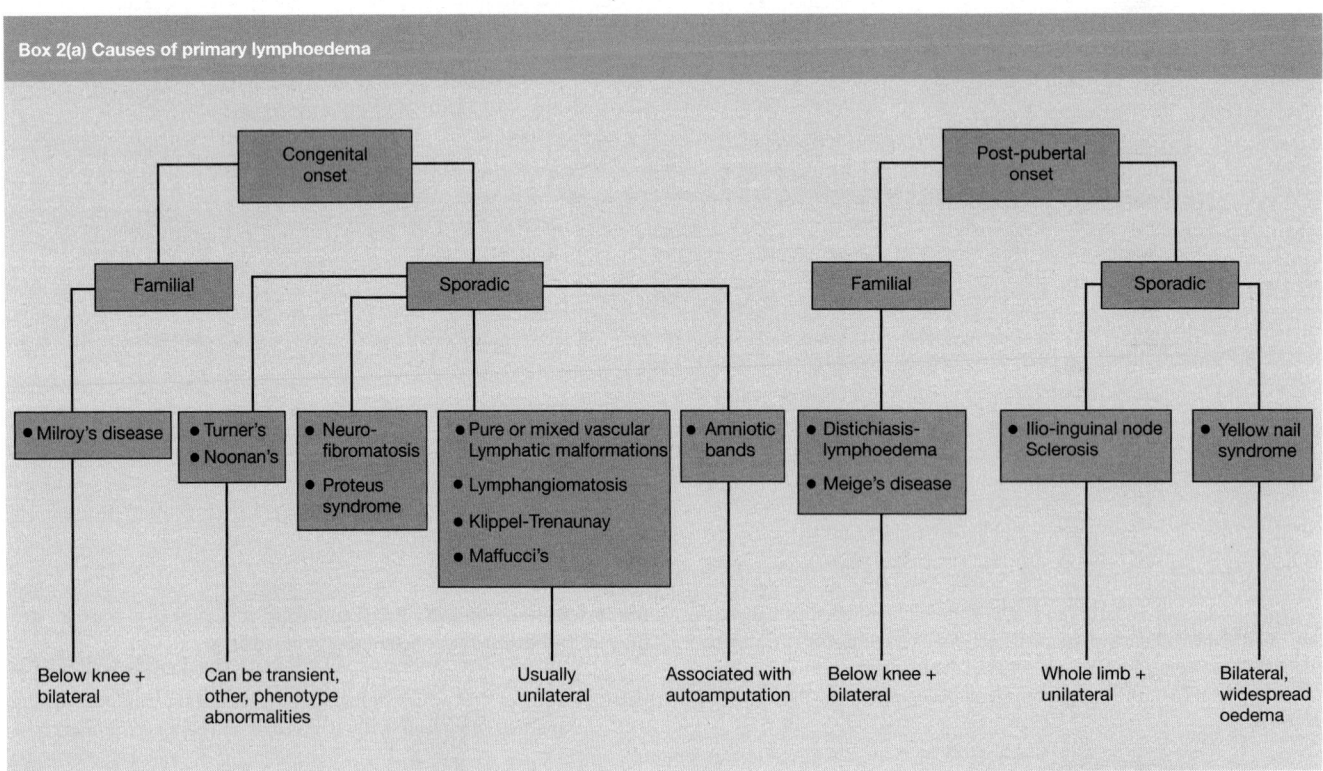

Box 2(a) Causes of primary lymphoedema

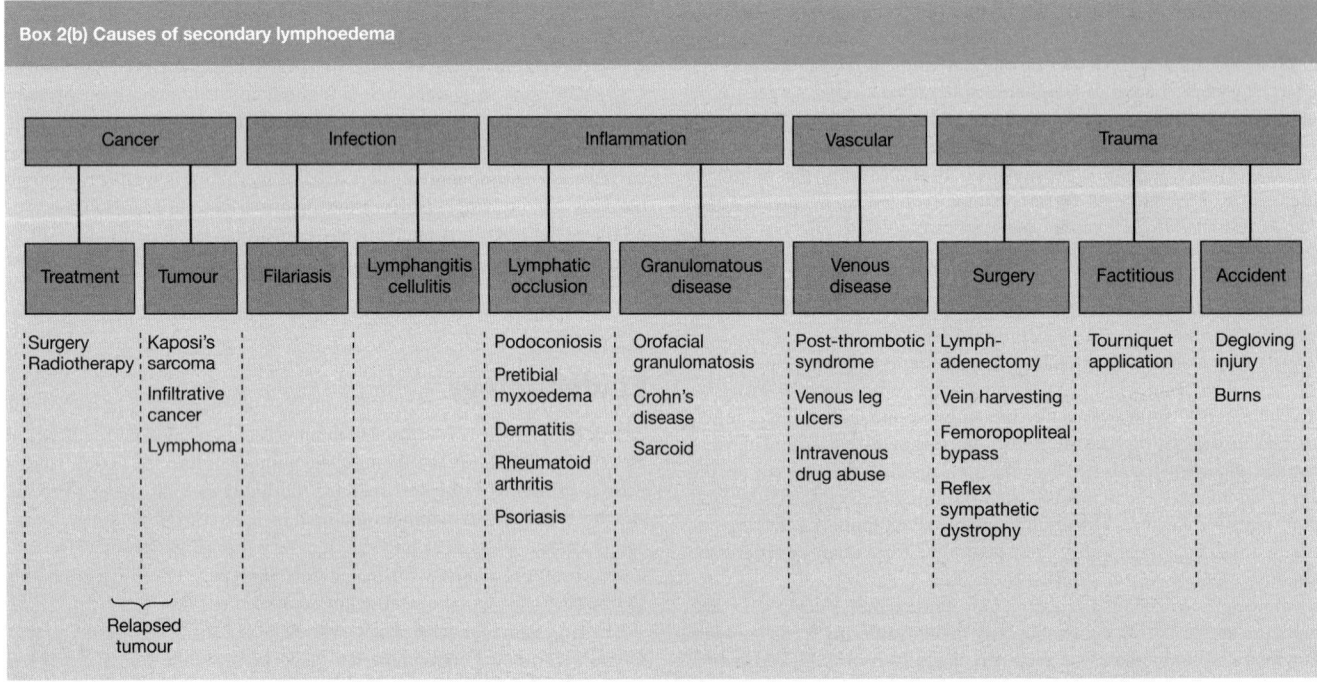

Box 2(b) Causes of secondary lymphoedema

isolated finding. Truncal oedema is often observed in the adjoining quadrant of the trunk to an affected limb because of the shared lymph drainage route.

Cells, proteins, lipids, and debris accumulate giving a 'solid' as well as a 'fluid' component to the swelling, hence the brawny texture to lymphoedema. Pitting occurs in most patients and many early cases will pit readily.

History

Swelling frequently develops rapidly—overnight—but may be mild and intermittent at first. Pain may feature initially, prompting diagnoses such as deep vein thrombosis and soft tissue injury. With time, oedema becomes more permanent and painless, although discomfort, aching, and heaviness are common symptoms. Functional impairment is slight until swelling becomes more severe. The major problem is disfigurement (Fig. 1).

Lymphoedema does not usually respond to elevation or diuretics, except in the early stages or when it is compounded by increased capillary filtration. Chronic oedema that does not reduce significantly overnight is likely to be lymphatic in origin.

Clinical signs

Most swelling occurs in the subcutaneous layer, but it is the skin which exhibits most changes. It becomes thicker, as demonstrated by the Kaposi–Stemmer sign (a failure to pick up or pinch a fold of skin). Skin creases become enhanced and a warty texture develops (hyperkeratosis). Accumulation of stagnant lymph in the dermis can produce surface bulges resembling cobblestones that feel firm to the touch (papillomatosis). The resemblance of the skin texture to elephant hide explains the term elephantiasis. Dilated lymphatics (lymphangiectasia) can also bulge on the surface like a blister from which lymph can leak.

Lymphatic insufficiency has three major consequences: (i) swelling (oedema); (ii) a predisposition to infection, in particular cellulitis; and (iii) the uncommon complication of malignancy arising with the lymphoedema (Stewart–Treves syndrome).

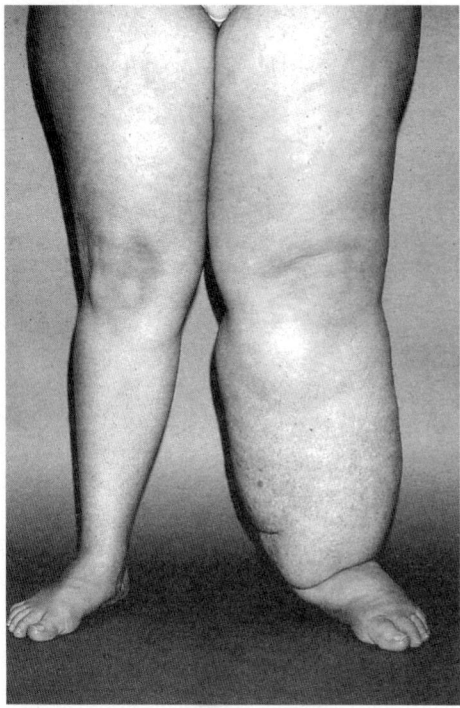

Fig. 1 Lymphoedema of the left lower limb exhibiting characteristic skin changes and loss of shape with folds developing around the ankle.

Oedema

Most cases of primary lymphoedema present with bilateral but asymmetrical oedema of the feet, ankles, and lower legs (distal hypoplastic type). However, it may take months to years before oedema manifests in the contralateral limb. Whole limb swelling usually indicates a problem at the level of the regional lymph nodes such as following cancer treatment or in filariasis. Oedema that begins proximally and spreads distally suggests an obstructive process (proximal obstructive type). Abnormalities of central abdominal and thoracic lymphatics may produce lower limb swelling, often bilateral, with lymph or chyle reflux. Lymph and chyle effusions can be observed in the pleural, peritoneal, and pericardial cavities and rarely in joints.

Cellulitis (acute inflammatory episodes)

Acute inflammatory episodes describe the attacks of apparent infection, simulating cellulitis, which afflict patients with lymphoedema. A typical attack starts rapidly, often without warning. Fever, rigors, headache, and vomiting can occur, but patients usually feel as if influenza is starting. A feeling of heat, redness, and increased swelling occurs within the lymphoedematous area. Pain may precede the rash. Areas of clearly demarcated erythema with a migrating border, as seen in classic cellulitis, may not be observed, presumably because of rapid dissemination throughout the oedematous tissue. Sometimes the condition may 'grumble' in a rather chronic manner for days or weeks and only on complete recovery after prolonged antibiotics and rest can the diagnosis be made. A characteristic of lymphoedema is for acute inflammatory episodes to recur. Intervals may be more than 12 months or as short as 3 weeks.

Lymphangiosarcoma

Lymphangiosarcoma (Stewart–Treves syndrome) is the most serious but rarest complication of lymphoedema. Chronic lymphoedema is a major predisposing factor in the development of malignant vascular tumours irrespective of the cause of the lymphoedema. The clinical appearance is usually of a fixed purple or bruise-like discoloration within the lymphoedematous skin. Infiltrated plaques and nodules later appear.

Differential diagnosis of the swollen limb (Box 3)

Both excessive capillary filtration and compromised lymph drainage frequent coexist.

'Venous' oedema

Most cases of chronic venous disease do not manifest oedema because of increased lymph flow in response to increased capillary filtration. This suggests that the development of oedema in post-thrombotic syndrome and venous ulceration is as much a failure of lymph drainage to compensate as it is due solely to overwhelming filtration. The expansion of the venous pool in the leg due to dilatation of veins will also contribute to an increase in limb girth independent of oedema.

'Armchair' legs

This syndrome refers to those patients who sit in a chair night and day with their legs dependent. Immobility results in minimal lymph drainage and 'functional lymphoedema' ensues, compounded by increased capillary filtration from gravitational forces. Predisposed are those patients suffering cardiac or respiratory failure who cannot lie flat, those paralysed from strokes or spinal damage including spina bifida, and those with arthritis, particularly rheumatoid arthritis.

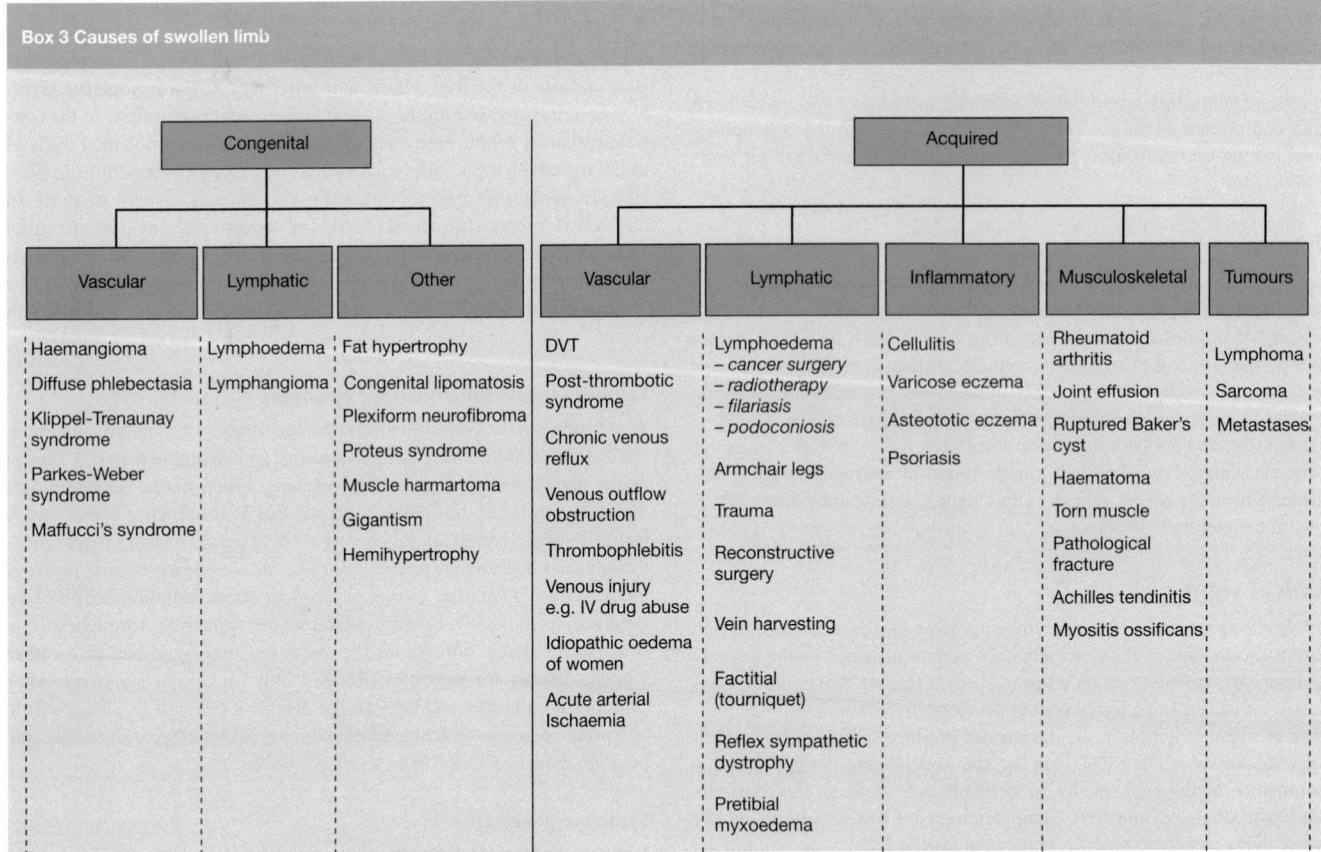

Box 3 Causes of swollen limb

Congenital
- **Vascular**
  - Haemangioma
  - Diffuse phlebectasia
  - Klippel-Trenaunay syndrome
  - Parkes-Weber syndrome
  - Maffucci's syndrome
- **Lymphatic**
  - Lymphoedema
  - Lymphangioma
- **Other**
  - Fat hypertrophy
  - Congenital lipomatosis
  - Plexiform neurofibroma
  - Proteus syndrome
  - Muscle harmartoma
  - Gigantism
  - Hemihypertrophy

Acquired
- **Vascular**
  - DVT
  - Post-thrombotic syndrome
  - Chronic venous reflux
  - Venous outflow obstruction
  - Thrombophlebitis
  - Venous injury e.g. IV drug abuse
  - Idiopathic oedema of women
  - Acute arterial Ischaemia
- **Lymphatic**
  - Lymphoedema
    - – cancer surgery
    - – radiotherapy
    - – filariasis
    - – podoconiosis
  - Armchair legs
  - Trauma
  - Reconstructive surgery
  - Vein harvesting
  - Factitial (tourniquet)
  - Reflex sympathetic dystrophy
  - Pretibial myxoedema
- **Inflammatory**
  - Cellulitis
  - Varicose eczema
  - Asteototic eczema
  - Psoriasis
- **Musculoskeletal**
  - Rheumatoid arthritis
  - Joint effusion
  - Ruptured Baker's cyst
  - Haematoma
  - Torn muscle
  - Pathological fracture
  - Achilles tendinitis
  - Myositis ossificans
- **Tumours**
  - Lymphoma
  - Sarcoma
  - Metastases

Lipoedema (lipidosis, lipodystrophy)

Frequently misdiagnosed as lymphoedema, lipoedema is peculiar to females with onset at or after puberty. A 'fatty', non-pitting swelling affects legs, thighs, and hips. Characteristic inverse shouldering occurs above the ankle because of sparing of the foot. The skin is soft, tender, and bruises easily. Pain may feature. Lipoedema is not influenced by dieting and is distinct from morbid obesity.

Investigation

The investigation of choice for confirming that oedema is primarily of lymphatic origin is lymphoscintigraphy (isotope lymphography). Conventional direct-contrast X-ray lymphography is now rarely undertaken to investigate lymphoedema. MRI, in preference to CT, is of value in identifying a cause for lymphatic obstruction.

Lymphoscintigraphy

A radiolabelled protein or colloid is administered via a subcutaneous injection and its movement through lymphatic vessels to nodes is monitored. The dynamics of lymph flow, as depicted by tracer removal from injection site and/or trapping in regional nodes, can be captured using a scintiscanner or γ-camera. Off-line calculation of time–activity curves from regions of interest permit quantitative analysis of lymph drainage. A normal lymphoscintigram is shown in Fig. 2 and an abnormal one in Fig. 3.

Direct-contrast X-ray lymphography (lymphangiography)

The technique requires the identification of a peripheral lymphatic (usually in the foot) by subcutaneous injection of a vital dye, such as patent blue.

The oily contract medium Lipiodol is then administered into the canulated lymphatic, with subsequent imaging by X-ray as the contrast passes through the main limb lymphatics. The failure to identify a lymphatic with vital dye suggests lymphoedema with distal hypoplasia of vessels, particularly if the dye persists in the tissues for days. Lymphography is an invasive procedure which provides little functional information, but it remains the gold standard for delineating lymph vessel and node anatomy.

Magnetic resonance imaging

MRI (and CT) demonstrates a thicker skin and a characteristic 'honeycomb' pattern in the subcutaneous compartment. Following deep vein thrombosis in the leg the muscle compartment is enlarged, but this remains unchanged in lymphoedema.

Treatment

Physical therapy

This first-line approach is designed to stimulate lymph drainage within main or collateral lymph routes. Intermittent changes in tissue pressure are normally responsible for moving materials and fluid from tissue spaces into initial lymphatics. Lymphatic collecting vessels that possess smooth muscle then actively pump the lymph downstream. In lymphoedema, exercise, through dynamic muscle contractions undertaken while compression is applied to the skin surface, encourages movement of lymph through lymph vessels in a matter akin to external cardiac massage. In practice, this means fitting of compression hosiery or bandages and instruction on exercise. Overexertion and excessive static exercises, such as gripping, increase blood flow and can therefore increase oedema. Compression has the added benefit of opposing excessive capillary filtration should it coexist. Manual lymph drainage, a specific form of lymphatic massage, is added to stimulate lymph flow and redirect the lymph towards the functioning lymph nodes in an unaffected lymphatic basin.

In moderate to severe lymphoedema an intensive period of treatment using multilayer bandaging, exercise, and manual lymph drainage is used to reduce swollen limbs so that subsequent maintenance treatment with hosiery and exercise is more effective at controlling the condition.

Pneumatic compression therapy, such as Flowtron, softens and reduces limb volume during treatment but it is doubtful that there is any long-term benefit compared with hosiery (and exercise) alone.

Infection

Prevention of acute inflammatory episodes (cellulitis) is crucial to the control of lymphoedema. Care of the skin, good hygiene, treatment of any dermatitis or fungal infection, and antisepsis following minor wounds are important. Prompt administration of antibiotics, such as co-amoxiclav in a dose of 625 mg three times daily at the onset of an attack, is mandatory (Box 4). For relapsing cellulitis, prophylactic antibiotics, preferably phenoxymethylpenicillin in a dose of 500 mg twice daily, are indicated for an indefinite period. Control of the oedema may help to reduce antibiotic requirements.

Drug therapy

Diuretics remain the most commonly used treatment but have very little benefit in established lymphoedema because their main action is to reduce

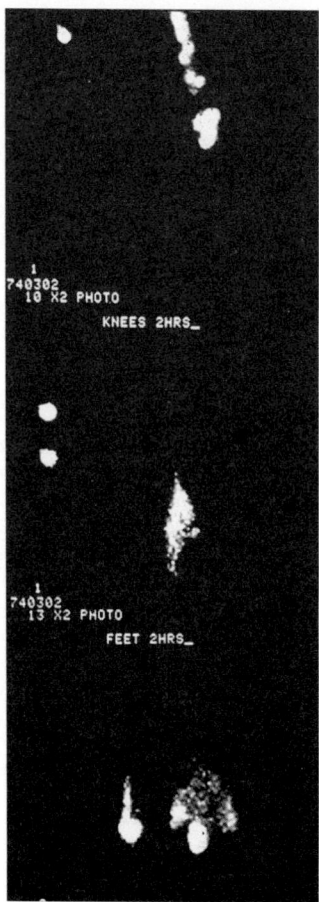

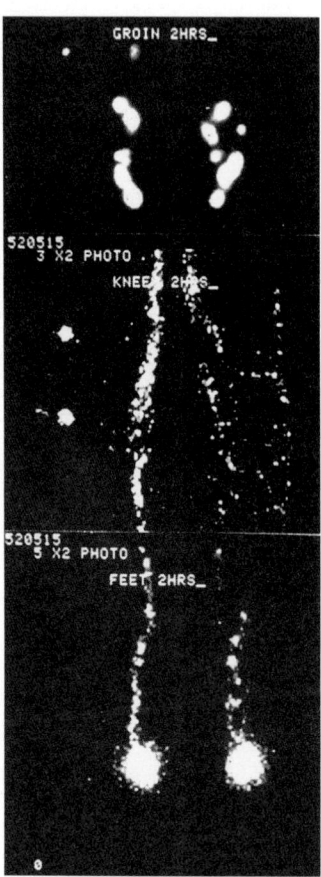

Fig. 2 A normal lymphoscintigram apart from some collateral lymph drainage in the left thigh. Following a web space injection of radiolabelled colloid (^{99m}Tc–antimony sulphide colloid) the transport of radioactivity is imaged by a γ-camera. Measurement of radioactivity over the ilio-inguinal nodes for a given time interval can quantify lymph drainage function.

Fig. 3 A lymphoscintigram in a patient with Milroy's disease (congenital familial lymphoedema) demonstrates no migration of tracer in the affected right leg. The left leg (clinically normal) shows normal ilio-inguinal nodal uptake but extravasation of tracer where lymphatics are abnormal.

capillary filtration. Improvement with diuretics suggests that the predominant cause of the oedema is not lymphatic. Diuretics, such as spironolactone, may be necessary in circumstances where there is substantial truncal lymphoedema, particularly if venous hypertension coexists.

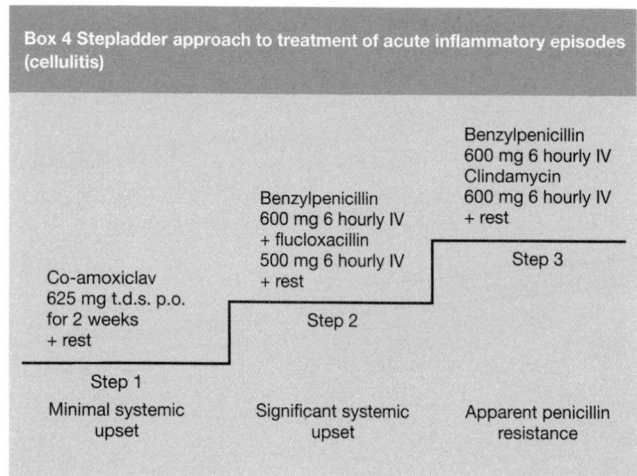

Box 4 Stepladder approach to treatment of acute inflammatory episodes (cellulitis)

Co-amoxiclav
625 mg t.d.s. p.o.
for 2 weeks
+ rest

Step 1
Minimal systemic
upset

Benzylpenicillin
600 mg 6 hourly IV
+ flucloxacillin
500 mg 6 hourly IV
+ rest

Step 2
Significant systemic
upset

Benzylpenicillin
600 mg 6 hourly IV
Clindamycin
600 mg 6 hourly IV
+ rest

Step 3
Apparent penicillin
resistance

The benzopyrone group of drugs, for instance rutosides and coumarin, have been advocated, but the clinical effect is minimal.

Surgery

Surgery can involve removal of excess tissue (reducing/debulking operations or liposuction) or bypassing of local lymphatic defects. The defective region may be bridged with omentum or an isolated segment of gut. Microsurgery such as lymphovenous anastomoses remains experimental. All surgery is followed by continued compression therapy, such as hosiery.

Prevention

Primary lymphoedema usually develops spontaneously without warning. A diagnosis of lymphoedema should be entertained if oedema is persistent. Lymphoscintigraphy is the investigation of choice at this stage as clinical signs are few in the early stages. In the future, identification of the genes programming for inherited lymphoedema may help predict those at risk.

Secondary lymphoedema can, in theory, be prevented by avoiding the cause or limiting the damage. Less intervention to lymph nodes for staging and treatment of cancer would help. Patients at significant risk of lymphoedema should receive advice from the appropriate professional, such as a breast-care nurse, and any oedema should be treated early, at a stage when it is more responsive to intervention and when it may even be reversible.

Further reading

Kaipainen A *et al.* (1995). Expression of the fms-like tyrosine kinase 4 gene becomes restricted to lymphatic endothelium during development. *Proceedings of the National Academy of Sciences, USA* **92**, 3566–70. [The first indication of the genetic basis of lymphangiogenesis.]

Karkkainen MJ *et al.* (2000). Missense mutations interfere with VEGFR-3 signalling in primary lymphoedema. *Nature Genetics* **25**, 153–9. [The first gene mutation found for lymphoedema.]

Kinmonth JB (1982). *Lymphatics, lymphology and disease of the chyle and lymph systems*, 2nd edn. Edward Arnold, London. [The original definitive clinical reference book.]

Ko DSC (1998). Effective treatment of lymphedema of the extremities. *Archives of Surgery* **133**, 452–8. [Open study but with robust data on physical therapy for lymphoedema.]

Levick JR (1995). *An introduction to cardiovascular physiology*, 2nd edn. Butterworth-Heinemann, Oxford. [Physiology made simple and meaningful.]

Roddie IC (1990). Lymph transport mechanisms in peripheral lymphatics. *News in Physiological Science* **5**, 85–9. [Understanding how lymph drainage operates.]

Stewart G *et al.* (1985). Isotope lymphography: a new method of investigating the role of lymphatics. *British Journal of Surgery* **72**, 906–9.

Yoffey JM, Courtice JM (1970). *Lymphatics, lymph and the lymphomyeloid complex*. Academic Press, New York. [A classic scientific review.]

15.18 Idiopathic oedema of women

J. Firth

Definition and diagnosis

In some women fluid retention occurs in the absence of any clear explanation and is termed idiopathic oedema. Since the condition typically fluctuates in severity from one time to another it is sometimes called cyclical or periodic oedema, but these terms mislead; first, because there is rarely any recognizable periodicity, and second, because the condition is not related to menstrual periods. Most women retain fluid just before the menses and lose this fluid immediately afterwards. Idiopathic oedema occurs most commonly in women aged 20 to 40 years, but has no clear relationship with the menstrual cycle and can persist after the menopause or oophorectomy.

The diagnosis of idiopathic oedema depends on the exclusion of other causes of oedema, including cardiac, hepatic, renal, allergic, or hypoproteinaemic disease, venous or lymphatic obstruction, and use of some medications. The role of diuretics, causally or in treatment, is contentious, as discussed below. However, it is always unsatisfactory when a diagnosis is made by exclusion of other conditions rather than on the basis of 'positive' criteria. Such criteria for the diagnosis of idiopathic oedema have not been universally agreed, although both Thorn and McKendry (see Kay *et al.* for discussion) have made proposals. These require evidence of substantial weight gain during the course of the day from morning to evening, with a figure of more than 1.4 kg often quoted, although this does not provide a clear-cut separation from normal. They also demand the presence of emotional or psychological factors. Many authors comment on the aggravation of swelling by prolonged sitting or standing, but this does not feature in the diagnostic criteria mentioned.

Clinical features

The patient's complaint is of swelling, which usually waxes and wanes but can be constant. In the morning the face and eyelids feel swollen and heavy. By the end of the day the areas worst affected are the hands, breasts, trunk, abdomen, thighs, ankles, and feet. Rings no longer fit the swollen fingers and undergarments and clothes can feel uncomfortably tight such that they have to be removed or replaced with something larger. The feet and ankles may be relatively spared, hence the disposition of oedema tends to be different from that in most other oedematous states, where it begins distally in the feet and ankles and progresses proximally.

Episodes or exacerbations of fluid retention often occur unpredictably, but obesity, emotional stress, and consumption of high-carbohydrate food are thought to be triggers in some. Sufferers are often mentally and physically lethargic during periods of fluid retention, frequently expressing the view that they feel bloated and ugly, even though this may not be apparent to the observer. Many appear to be emotionally labile or anxious and some are depressed, invariably (and perhaps correctly) claiming that this is secondary to the fluid retention. Other common symptoms include carpal tunnel syndrome, non-articular rheumatism, palpitations, non-ulcer dyspepsia, and headaches.

Aside from oedema, which may or may not be present at the time of medical assessment, examination is unremarkable, as are routine investigations for the cause of oedema. Those patients that have used diuretics may have a hypokalaemic hypochloraemic metabolic alkalosis.

Pathophysiology

The cause of idiopathic oedema is not known (by definition). Diurnal weight fluctuation of more than 1.4 kg is required for diagnosis, but weight may fluctuate from day to day by up to 4 or 5 kg. During periods of weight gain the patient may be oliguric, passing low volumes of urine in which there is little sodium (less than 20 mmol/l). The blood vessels of women with idiopathic oedema are more permeable to albumin, the fractional catabolic rate of albumin is increased, both intravascular and total body albumin pools are smaller, and the plasma volume decreases by more on standing than in normal controls. Activation of the sympathetic nervous system, renin–angiotensin–aldosterone system, and high levels of ADH in the plasma that are consistent with intravascular volume depletion have all been reported, as has reduction in dopaminergic activity. These changes provide a plausible explanation for why the kidney retains salt and water in idiopathic oedema, but the prime mover remains uncertain. They also form the background to postural water-loading or sodium-loading tests that have been advoated as diagnostic tools, although these are not used routinely in clinical practice. After similar loading on two separate occasions, patients with idiopathic oedema who remain upright throughout the test excrete less water or sodium than they do if they remain supine.

Many patients seen in hospital practice will already be taking diuretics or have taken them in the past, and some will be consuming large doses of loop agents every day. One influential study reported 10 such patients who started to take diuretics because of concern about swelling or their body weight and who continued to take them because cessation provoked rapid weight gain, facial bloating, and abdominal distension. When prevailed upon to stop diuretics they each gained weight (up to 5 kg), reaching a maximum in 4 to 10 days, but by 20 days 7 of the 10 had fallen to below their previous weight, and 9 of the 10 remained free of oedema over a long period of follow-up without taking diuretics. This led the authors to suggest that diuretic abuse might be the cause of all cases of idiopathic oedema. This view is not held by most with experience in the field, but rebound oedema on diuretic withdrawal can undoubtedly be an exacerbating feature, and it is appropriate to look for evidence of diuretic abuse if the patient denies taking such drugs and yet routine biochemical testing of blood and urine suggests the possibility (see Chapter 20.2.2 for further discussion).

Management

Women with idiopathic oedema frequently complain that doctors have not taken their condition seriously, and there is no doubt that it is a frustrating disorder for both patients and their physicians. Sympathetic explanation of the nature of the problem helps management.

If the patient is obese, then they should be given advice as to how to lose weight, and—independent of any effect on weight—some find that reducing dietary carbohydrate helps. They should be advised to avoid long periods of standing or sitting and to wear loose-fitting clothing, although most will have discovered these things for themselves. Avoidance of an excessive dietary intake of sodium is a sensible recommendation. On theoretical grounds the use of elastic stockings would also seem appropriate, since these might reduce the postural reduction in plasma volume seen in idiopathic oedema. However, few find that their benefits outweigh their disadvantages and it is difficult to get most patients to persist with them for long enough to see whether or not they really would be of help.

Diuretics are a real problem. It seems intuitively obvious to most patients and to many doctors that someone who is retaining fluid would benefit from a diuretic, hence many patients with idiopathic oedema end up on very large doses of loop agents, often combined with amiloride or spironolactone. Rather than helping, these may worsen symptoms of tiredness, lethargy, weakness, and dizziness by exacerbating intravascular volume depletion, and attempts to stop typically lead to rebound oedema. Explanation is the key here in that if patients recognize rebound oedema for what it is and relieve oedema with supine rest rather than renewed consumption of high doses of diuretics, then there is a reasonable chance that they can be weaned off diuretics with benefit.

Levodopa, carbidopa, bromocriptine, captopril, and a variety of other agents have been tried in idiopathic oedema, but none is of proven benefit.

Further reading

Kay A, Davis CL (1999). Idiopathic edema. *American Journal of Kidney Diseases* **34**, 405–23.

MacGregor GA, *et al.* (1979). Is 'idiopathic' edema idiopathic? *Lancet* **i**, 397–400.

Marks AD (1983). Intermittent fluid retention in women. Is it idiopathic edema? *Postgraduate Medicine* **73**, 75–83.

Sabatini S (2001). Hormonal insights into the pathogenesis of cyclic idiopathic edema. *Seminars in Nephrology* **21**, 244–50.

Streeten DH (1995). Idiopathic edema. Pathogenesis, clinical features, and treatment. *Endocrinology and Metabolism Clinics of North America* **24**, 531–47.

16

Critical care medicine

16.1 The clinical approach to the patient who is very ill

J. Firth

Introduction—recognizing the problem

As a young doctor, I vividly remember watching a senior physician at a teaching hospital endeavouring to take a history from a middle-aged man who looked grey and very unwell. The man was not giving lucid answers and the conversation seemed increasingly unlikely to lead to a useful conclusion. After a period of silence his breathing became extremely laboured, and within a minute he suffered a cardiac arrest from which he could not be resuscitated.

The first priority in the management of patients who are very ill is to recognize that this is the situation. It is a sensible discipline when dealing with emergency admissions (and sometimes in other contexts) to ask yourself the question: Is this patient well, ill, very ill, or nearly dead? Some physicians will recognize this intuitively, others will have to make a conscious effort, lest they make the sort of error described in the previous paragraph. In general the approach to the patient begins with the history, followed by the examination, and sometimes the ordering and appraisal of the results of investigations, before a diagnosis is reached and treatment commences. This approach can be fatal in those who are very ill or nearly dead at the start.

Key features—summarized as airway, breathing, circulation (ABC)—to assess immediately in the patient who is very ill or worse are shown in Table 1. If in any doubt, the most important of the questions to answer is: 'Do you think that this patient can keep breathing like this for the next 10 min?' If the answer is no, then you need to get help immediately: this will usually involve summoning someone directly from the intensive care unit, or putting out a 'cardiac arrest' call. It is better to do this 10 min before the heart stops than 2 min afterwards, a strategy emphasized by replacing the 'cardiac arrest team' with a 'medical emergency team' in one

Table 1 Key questions to ask when assessing someone with cardiorespiratory collapse

Airway and breathing
- Is the airway patent?
- Is the patient making a respiratory effort, and is the chest expanding with it?
- Is the chest expanding symmetrically? Could there be a tension pneumothorax? (trachea deviated, mediastinum shifted, absent breath sounds on hyperinflated side of the chest)
- Does the patient look as though they could keep this breathing up for the next 10 min?

Circulation
- Do the peripheries feel cold or hot?
- Can you feel the pulse, and what is the rate and rhythm?
- What is the blood pressure?
- Is there a postural drop if the patient is moved from lying to being propped up?
- What is the jugular venous pressure? If you can't see it: is it too high or too low?

study. One doctor, with or without one nurse, is not enough to deal optimally with the patient who is *in extremis*.

Immediate management of airway and breathing

The immediate treatment priorities for the patient with cardiorespiratory collapse are shown in Table 2.

Airway and oxygen

If a patient is having problems breathing, then is there a difficulty in maintaining the upper airway? If a head tilt/chin lift manoeuvre is beneficial, then a gentle attempt to insert an oropharyngeal airway should be made. This should not be done against resistance—a fight is much more likely to do harm than good—and if the patient spits the airway out it almost certainly means that it is not necessary.

All patients who are extremely ill should be given oxygen in as high a concentration as possible by face mask. A fraction of inspired oxygen (Fio_2) of around 60 per cent can be obtained using a standard face mask with a reservoir bag and an oxygen flow rate of 10 litre/min. An obvious concern about this recommendation is that it may induce carbon dioxide retention in those who are prone to this (usually patients with chronic obstructive pulmonary disease), but the downside of denying someone oxygen can be substantial: hypoxia kills, hypercarbia merely intoxicates. If blood gas analysis shows that the patient is retaining carbon dioxide, the Fio_2 can gradually be reduced or elective ventilation can be used.

If a patient with respiratory difficulty has received opioids within the past 48 h, or could have done so, then give intravenous naloxone (0.2 to 0.4 mg in those who have received opioids; 0.8 to 2.0 mg repeated to a maximum of 10 mg in case of overdosage). This sometimes produces a dramatic response.

Table 2 Immediate treatment priorities for the patient with cardiorespiratory collapse

Airway and breathing
- Give high-flow oxygen (10 l/min) via face mask with reservoir bag
- Consider oropharyngeal airway
- Give intravenous naloxone if any suspicion that patient has received opioids
- Consider elective intubation and ventilation
- If tension pneumothorax, decompress immediately

Circulation
- Obtain intravenous access using a safe technique (see text)
- See Table 4 for further discussion.

Elective ventilation

The patient should be electively intubated and ventilated if breathing seems to be failing despite the measures indicated above, although in some circumstances non-invasive ventilation may be an appropriate alternative. There is no substitute for wise clinical judgement in deciding when this should be done, and it is easy for the inexperienced to be led astray. Too soon is better than too late. A 'normal' respiratory rate of, say, 12 breaths/min may indicate normality, but is also compatible with near death in the patient with a severe respiratory problem who is becoming exhausted. A blood gas level that 'doesn't seem too bad', meaning perhaps a P_{O_2} of 9 kPa and P_{CO_2} of 5.5 kPa, which may not be a cause for any concern at all in a patient who is comfortable and breathing room air, is not at all reassuring if the patient is breathing 60 per cent oxygen and looks very tired.

The work of breathing accounts for up to one-third of the body's oxygen consumption, hence taking this burden from patients by sedating, paralysing, and ventilating them can have a dramatically beneficial effect, whatever the reason for their predicament. However, one note of caution: whilst being ventilated can be very helpful, the minute or two when the patient is being sedated, paralysed, and intubated is a time of very high risk, since the pharmacological agents used can, to varying degrees, induce profound hypotension culminating in a 'crash'. The chances of this happening can be reduced by giving the patient a bolus of fluid (a rapid infusion of 500 ml of 0.9 per cent saline or colloid) immediately before induction, with dilute adrenaline (1:10 000; not 1:1000) given as 1-ml intravenous pushes (up to one push/min) in the event of a dramatic fall in blood pressure. Whilst the anaesthetist is attending to the airway, the match-hardened physician will stand by a site of intravenous access with such a syringe in their hand and not skulk off into a corner.

Tension pneumothorax

If the patient has a tension pneumothorax, then this should be decompressed immediately by inserting a large-bore venous cannula into the chest in the second intercostal space in the mid-clavicular line and then withdrawing the stylet. The response to this is dramatic and satisfying. A chest drain with underwater seal can then be inserted at (relative) leisure.

The prospect of performing chest decompression is daunting for many junior physicians, and even more so for most of their senior colleagues. Remember that the physical signs are not subtle, the patient with '? minor shift of the trachea' as the only relevant sign does not have a tension pneumothorax. If the patient is blue and can't breathe, one side of the chest looks blown up and there are no breath sounds over it, then (after attending to the airway and oxygen and calling the cardiac arrest team) stick in the cannula. There is much to be gained from doing so, and little to be lost if it does not lead to improvement.

Immediate management of the circulation

The patient who is volume depleted

In a patient who is very ill, if the pulse rate is less than about 60 to 70/min, or above 120/min other than with a sinus tachycardia, then manoeuvres to speed it up (atropine, isoprenaline, pacing) or slow it down (DC cardioversion or antiarrhythmics, but avoiding any of the latter that are negatively inotropic excepting in rare circumstances) are likely to improve the circulation. (See Chapters 16.3 and 15.6 for further information.)

Most patients who are very ill will have a sinus tachycardia, when there is no advantage in attempting to alter pulse rate and rhythm, indeed there is much to be lost from ill-advised attempts to do so. The key question then becomes: Is the filling pressure optimal? Does the patient need to be given fluid, or is there too much fluid on board? Those who do not see many very ill patients might think that it should be easy to tell the difference, but the answer is not always obvious, and yet the physician must decide rapidly, often without anything other than clinical judgement to guide them. Although they may yearn for a measurement of central venous or pulmon-

Table 3 Clinical evaluation of volume status

Clinical signs of intravascular volume depletion[a]
- Low jugular venous pressure[b]
- Hypotension, particularly postural hypotension with a drop in systolic pressure of more than 10 mmHg (lying and sitting if lying and standing not possible)
- Cool peripheries (nose, fingers, toes) and collapsed peripheral veins

Clinical signs of volume overload
- High jugular venous pressure[b]
- Gallop rhythm
- Hypertension, basal crepitations, liver congestion, peripheral oedema

[a]Reduced skin turgor, dry mouth and tongue, and sunken eyes are not reliable indicators of intravascular volume depletion. All may be present in patients who are dehydrated, meaning deficient in body water, which is not the same as having intravascular volume depletion. Many elderly patients have low skin turgor; nasal blockage and tachypnoea causes a dry mouth and tongue; and to wait until the eyes sink is to leave things much too late.

[b]Absolute values are deliberately not given. The normal right atrial pressure is in the range +4 to +8 mmHg (measured from the mid-axillary line), that is, the jugular venous pressure can range from not being visible when the patient is lying with their torso at 45° to elevated a few centimetres above the angle of Louis. In some circumstances the optimal jugular venous pressure may be considerably outside this normal range, for example much higher if there is pulmonary hypertension.

ary capillary wedge pressure, or for a chest radiograph to see whether or not there is pulmonary oedema, to delay management might be fatal. The clinical features to look for are listed in Table 3, and the appropriate responses discussed in Table 4.

Obtaining venous access

The need is to insert a cannula into a decent-sized vein quickly, and with as low a risk of complication as possible. Try initially for a peripheral vein in the forearm or antecubital fossa, but if these are constricted and cannot be cannulated and the patient is *in extremis*, then go for the femoral vein, which lies medial to the artery in the groin (NAVY, nerve artery vein Y-fronts). The procedure is easiest if the patient can lie flat, but can be performed with the patient propped up if respiratory difficulty means that lying down is impossible. Feel for the femoral pulse just below the crease of the groin and, after giving local anaesthetic, insert the needle (with the bevel pointing forwards) one finger breadth medial to the point of maximum pulsation at an angle of about 60° to the skin and parallel to the long axis of the leg. The only significant complication of this procedure is inadvertent arterial puncture (Table 5), the consequences of which are much less likely to be severe in the groin than in the neck or below the clavicle.

An attempt to insert a central venous cannula into the internal jugular or subclavian vein of a patient who is *in extremis* has led to more deaths than such catheters have prevented. If the patient's intravascular volume is depleted, then the veins are constricted and small, cannulation is very difficult, and the procedure tends to degenerate into what is known in the trade as the 'sewing machine technique', where multiple stabs culminate in something being hit, often not the vein that was being (increasingly loosely) targeted. If patients are volume overloaded and in respiratory difficulty, then they will not tolerate being laid flat for the cannulation attempt: if you try to make them do so, they won't lie still for long, and if they do become still it might be because they have died.

When the patient who is volume depleted has had intravascular volume restored, or when the situation of the patient who is volume overloaded and breathless has been rendered safe (perhaps by intubation and ventilation), then the insertion of a central venous catheter can be helpful in diagnosis (for example to allow passage of a right heart catheter for measurement of the pulmonary capillary wedge pressure), monitoring (for example fall in the central venous pressure indicating further gastrointestinal haemorrhage), and treatment (for example infusion of inotropes, other drugs, or parenteral nutrition). The approaches for internal jugular and subclavian vein cannulation are shown in Figs 1 and 2, with details of safety and reliability in Table 5.

Table 4 Immediate clinical response to determination of volume status

Main problem	Key clinical signs	Immediate management
Hypotension	Peripheries cool and shut down Postural hypotension Low jugular venous pressure	Intravenous fluid given rapidly until clear evidence that physical signs are being restored to normal, then slower infusion
Breathing difficulty	High jugular venous pressure Gallop rhythm Basal crepitations	Do not give fluid Sit up Consider intravenous loop diuretic and/or venodilator Consider need for ventilation
Hypotension and breathing difficulty	Peripheries cool and shut down Jugular venous pressure likely to be high May be gallop rhythm Likely to be basal crepitations	Likely to need urgent ventilation, preferably before suffering cardiorespiratory arrest (see text for details of medical management of this process) Trial of fluid infusion may be appropriate: give 200 ml of plasma expander, keeping patient under continuous observation and terminating infusion immediately in the event of clinical deterioration

All patients should be given high-flow oxygen.

Vigorous attempts should be made to diagnose and treat the underlying condition concurrent with efforts to resuscitate.

If the patient remains hypotensive despite 'optimization' of intravascular volume, then consideration can be given to the use of inotropes and vasoactive agents: see Chapter 16.2 for further discussion.

What fluid should you give, and how much?

A great deal of heat, but little light, has been generated in the literature on the subject of when to replace fluid, what to give, and how much. For patients with penetrating trauma to the torso it has been shown that delayed resuscitation, where venous access is established but fluid is not given until the patient is in the operating theatre, is preferable to immediate resuscitation, but there is no obvious analogy between this situation and that of the vast majority of patients with circulatory collapse and the rule, in general, remains that resuscitation should start as soon as possible.

It is logical that the fluid given to the patient whose intravascular volume is depleted should be one that remains substantially within the intravascular compartment. Solutions based on dextrose (with zero or low concentration of sodium) are most certainly not appropriate, since they partition throughout the body water and relatively little remains in the intravascular compartment, but beyond this it is not possible to make any firm recommendation. If the patient has lost blood, then it would seem sensible to give blood, and most physicians would recommend this. Whether isotonic crystalloid (usually 0.9 per cent saline), hypertonic crystalloid (usually saline), or various types of colloid are best in other situations is not clear. Cochrane reviews have failed to find significant differences between the use in critically ill patients of crystalloid or colloid, between isotonic or hypertonic fluids, and between different types of colloid solution, although there is evidence that albumin infusion may increase the risk of death in this situation.

At the outset it is not possible to judge precisely how much fluid will be needed to resuscitate a patient. The only way to determine this is by frequent clinical examination as fluid is given. In the patient who is very unwell and clearly volume depleted, standard practice is to give 500 ml of blood or plasma expander (as appropriate and as available) as fast as the giving set and venous cannula will allow (applying pressure to the bag by manual or mechanical compression if the patient is *in extremis*). A second 500 ml infusion is commenced whilst checking peripheral perfusion, pulse rate, blood pressure, and the jugular venous pressure. Rapid infusion is continued until there is clear evidence that the situation is beginning to improve, as manifest by warming of the peripheries, slowing of the pulse rate, and rise in blood pressure. Interpretation of change in the height of the jugular venous pressure requires some care. It rises as fluid starts to be given, but may then fall for two reasons: first, if there is further fluid loss,

Table 5 Complications during insertion of 5465 central venous catheters

Approach	Number of procedures	Complication					
		Pneumothorax (%)	Arterial puncture (%)	Repeated puncture, meaning two or more consecutive attempts to puncture a vein using the same approach (%)	Necessity to shift to another approach (%)	Failure to cannulate central vein, even after shifting to another approach (%)	Malposition of catheter (%)
Femoral vein	1014	Not relevant	9	5	4	0.1	0.1
High approach to internal jugular	460	0	7.7	9	22	0.5	4.5
Low lateral approach to internal jugular	1767	0	1.2	3.3	12	0.1	0.8
Axial approach to internal jugular	104	1	7	12	20	1	2
Infraclavicular approach to subclavian vein	1273	2.5	2.8	6.5	8.6	0.4	2.6
Supraclavicular approach to subclavian vein	847	1.1	3.6	4	8	0.2	1.4

Data from Pittiruti *et al.*, 2000, *Journal of Vascular Access* **1**, 100–7.

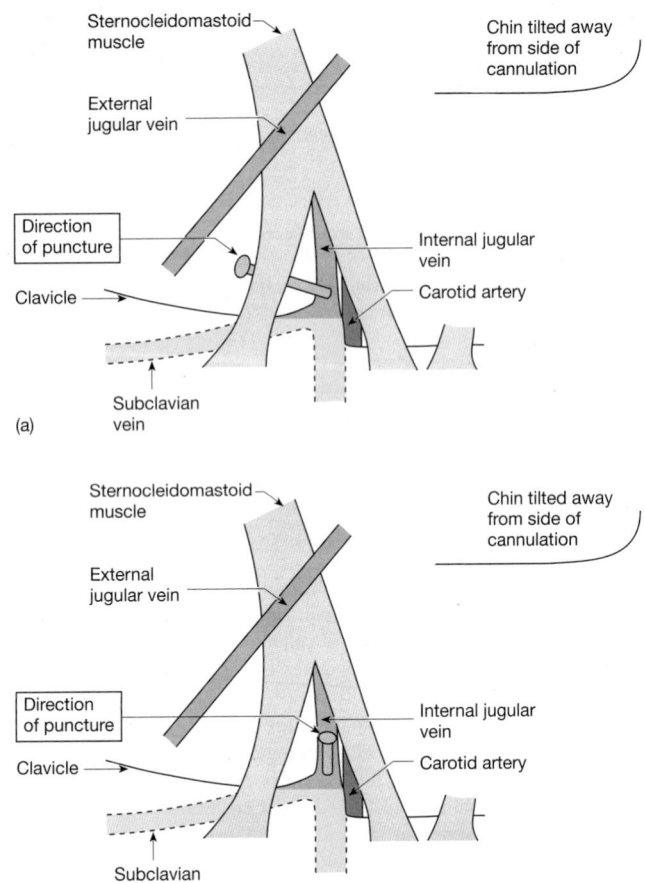

(a)

(b)

Fig. 1 The low lateral (a) and axial (b) approaches to the internal jugular vein. (a) The patient is supine with the head turned away from the side of the puncture. A towel may be placed under both shoulders to extend the neck. After preparation of the skin and drapes, and insertion of local anaesthetic, the bed is tilted to a 25° head down position. The needle is inserted just lateral to the posterior border of the clavicular head of the sternocleidomastoid muscle, about one finger breadth above the clavicle. It is then advanced parallel to the line of the clavicle and just behind the sternocleidomastoid muscle. The internal jugular vein, which lies superficially at this point, is cannulated close to its junction with the subclavian vein. As soon as the vein is entered the needle is angulated caudally to ease cannulation, the guidewire passing directly into the innominate vein. The risk of complications was lower with this technique than for any other method of central venous cannulation used in one large series (see Table 5

most typically haemorrhage; and second, as venoconstrictor tone diminishes in the patient who is 'warming up' with adequate resuscitation. Their different effects on peripheral perfusion, pulse rate, and blood pressure easily distinguish these two eventualities.

As soon as it is clear that the patient's circulation is beginning to improve, the rate of fluid infusion should be slowed so as not to risk precipitating pulmonary oedema by forcing very high hydrostatic pressures in a circulation that is still 'tight' due to the effect of endogenous vasoconstrictors. Hence the patient who has lost, say, 2 litres of blood, may be optimally treated by receiving the first litre as quickly as possible, followed by the second litre over the next 2 h or so as the circulation 'relaxes'.

When resuscitation is complete—meaning that peripheral perfusion, pulse rate, blood pressure, and jugular venous pressure have all returned to acceptable levels—fluid input should then be given with regard to fluid output. At this stage it is good practice to insert a urinary catheter into any patient who has presented with severe cardiorespiratory disturbance. Urinary flow rate reflects renal perfusion, which is a marker of the overall state

of the circulation, and accurate measurement of urinary output is essential to judge continuing fluid requirement. If patients have developed acute tubular necrosis with oliguria as a result of hypotension, they will not be well served by a 'standard' prescription of 3 litres of fluid per day to follow on from that given to resuscitate. This will inevitably lead to pulmonary oedema if continued in the face of diminished urinary output. A daily input equal to the last 24-hours' output plus 500 to 1000 ml for insensible losses is appropriate in these circumstances.

The patient who is volume overloaded

Acute volume overload manifests as pulmonary oedema, which can be a most terrifying condition. When severe, patients cannot get their breath and, with good reason, think they are going to die. As for patients in extreme respiratory difficulty, they sit up and use their accessory muscles. They are sweaty, cool peripherally, tachycardic, hypertensive (usually), centrally cyanosed, the jugular venous pressure is raised, and there is a gallop rhythm, although this may be hard to appreciate amidst the widespread

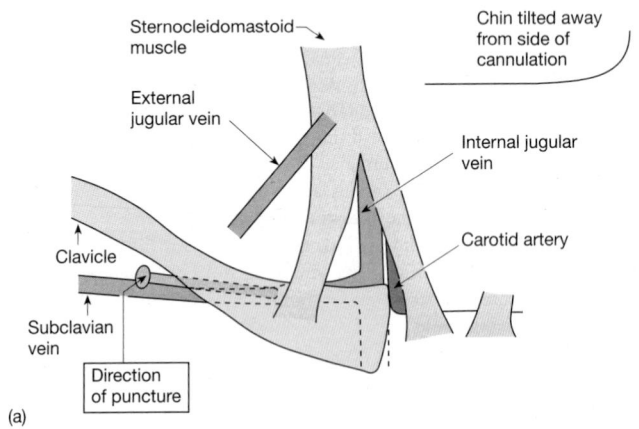

(a)

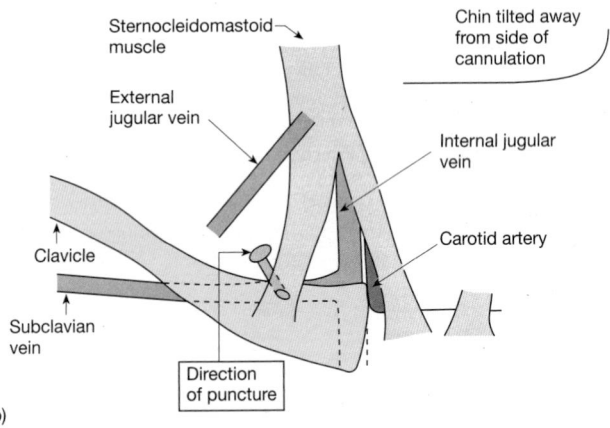

(b)

Fig. 2 The infraclavicular (a) and supraclavicular (b) approaches to the subclavian vein. (a) The patient is positioned as described for the low lateral approach to the internal jugular vein (Fig. 1, (a)), excepting that instead of a towel being placed under both shoulders it should be positioned under the spine, allowing the shoulders to retract to reduce the risk of pneumothorax. The needle enters the skin below the mid-point of the lower border of the clavicle and is advanced under the clavicle towards the upper edge of the junction of the clavicle with the manubrium. See Table 5 for details of complications using this approach. (b) The patient is positioned as described for the infraclavicular approach to the subclavian vein. The needle is inserted into the angle between the superior border of the clavicle and the posterior border of the clavicular head of the sternocleidomastoid and advanced caudally, medially, and ventrally. See Table 5 for details of complications using this approach.

Table 6 Examination and investigation of the patient with cardiorespiratory collapse

Diagnosis		Key finding on examination	Key initial investigation	Definitive investigations
Cardiovascular	Myocardial infarction	No specific findings likely	ECG	ECG, cardiac enzymes
	Arrhythmia	Pulse rate and rhythm	ECG	ECG
	Aortic dissection	Absence or reduction in one or more peripheral pulses, especially left radial. Blood pressure lower in left arm than right	Chest radiograph showing widened mediastinum	Imaging of aorta, usually by CT scan or trans-oesophageal echocardiography
	Cardiac tamponade	Raised jugular venous pressure. Pulsus paradoxus (pulse becomes impalpable on inspiration in extreme cases)	Chest radiograph may show globular heart. ECG may show low-voltage complexes or electrical alternans	Echocardiography
Cardiorespiratory	Pulmonary embolus	Raised jugular venous pressure. Right ventricular heave. Loud P2. Right ventricular gallop rhythm. Signs of deep vein thrombosis in leg	ECG may show features of acute right heart strain	Ventilation/perfusion scan. Imaging of pulmonary vessels by CT scan or pulmonary angiography
	Pulmonary oedema	Gallop rhythm. Crackles (see text)	Chest radiograph	Usually cardiac—ECG, echocardiography
Respiratory	Tension pneumothorax	Tracheal deviation. Hyperexpansion of one side of chest. Mediastinal shift. Absent breath sounds on one side of chest	Chest radiograph—but should be treated on basis of clinical diagnosis (see text)	Chest radiograph— but should be treated on basis of clinical diagnosis (see text)
	Pneumonia	May have high fever. Signs of consolidation or pleurisy	Chest radiograph	Chest radiograph. Blood culture. Serological tests
	Asthma	Wheezes, but beware of silent chest	Response to treatment (β-agonist), but chest radiograph excludes other respiratory diagnoses	Peak flow measurements before and after β-agonist
	Exacerbation of chronic obstructive pulmonary disease	Features of chronic obstructive pulmonary disease	A clinical diagnosis, but chest radiograph excludes other respiratory diagnoses	See Chapter 17.6
Abdominal	Gastrointestinal haemorrhage	Usually obvious, but don't forget rectal examination for blood/melaena in the patient with unexplained hypotension	A clinical diagnosis	Endoscopy
	Perforated viscus	Peritonism	Erect abdominal radiograph to look for free air	CT scan or laparotomy, depending on clinical situation
	Pancreatitis	Peritonism. Bruising in flanks	Serum amylase	Imaging of pancreas, usually by CT scan
	Ruptured abdominal aortic aneurysm	Peritonism. Palpable aneurysm. Bruising in flanks	A clinical diagnosis	CT scan or laparotomy, depending on clinical situation
Sepsis		May have high fever. May have warm peripheries and bounding pulse, but could be cold and shut down. No specific findings likely, but look for rash or localized infection, such as abscess	A clinical diagnosis	Blood culture
Metabolic	Many possible causes, such as renal failure, hepatic failure, profound acidosis, but collectively these are rare causes of presentation with cardiorespiratory collapse	May have evidence of organ failure, or of drug overdose. May have no specific findings	Electrolytes, renal and liver function tests. Blood gases	As indicated following initial tests
Anaphylaxis		Facial, tongue, and throat swelling. Stridor. Wheeze. Urticarial rash. Skin erythema or extreme pallor	A clinical diagnosis	Serum mast cell tryptase. Specific IgE for suspect allergens. See Chapter 16.4 for further information

Primarily neurological disorders may compromise the airway or ventilation, but rarely cause cardiovascular collapse. If a patient with cardiovascular collapse has a severely depressed conscious level (Glasgow coma scale less than 8) or focal neurological signs, then the assumption—until proven otherwise—should be that the neurological impairment is secondary to the cardiovascular collapse and not the cause of it.

crackles and wheezes in the chest. In extreme forms, frothy pink oedema fluid may come from the mouth. For further information see Chapter 15.15.2.2. The main features of treatment are shown in Table 4.

The underlying condition

The initial management of patients who are desperately ill does not depend on making a precise diagnosis of the cause of their predicament. However, as soon as resuscitation is underway, attention must turn towards making a diagnosis. Although the naive might think that the more severe the illness, the more obvious the cause should be, the opposite is often the case. When dead, all patients look identical, and the same is true just before they die. Patients who are *in extremis*, whether due to profound hypoxia or with next to no blood pressure, are not lucid historians, and it may be that the only question that they can usefully answer is: 'Do you have any pain?' If they indicate their chest or their abdomen, this might be a helpful clue.

The pragmatic approach to making a diagnosis in the patient with cardiorespiratory collapse is to use a 'surgical sieve' technique, looking systematically for features on examination and investigation to nail the diagnosis of conditions that can kill (Table 6). Details of the management of the many specific disorders listed in Table 6 can be found in the relevant sections of this book, but there is one general point: if initial investigations do not give any clear diagnostic lead, then do not be afraid to start treatment 'on suspicion', especially for those disorders that cannot reliably be diagnosed or excluded by clinical examination or with those tests that are rapidly available. In particular, consider pulmonary embolism and sepsis.

If the clinical context makes pulmonary embolism likely, for instance the patient has collapsed after an operation a week or so ago, then—in the absence of other explanation for the problem—it would not be unreasonable to start anticoagulation with intravenous heparin (which can be reversed if necessary) pending definitive imaging, but it would be unwise to give thrombolytic agents until the diagnosis was established. I began this chapter with a paragraph describing a failing of another doctor, so it is fair and reasonable that I also include details of one of my own. When I was a medical registrar 'on call' 15 years ago, I was asked to see a woman in her 60s from a long-stay psychiatric ward because the nurse looking after her thought that 'she wasn't her usual self'. She would not speak to me, but this was not abnormal since she had not spoken to anyone for many years. I examined her with some difficulty, because she did not co-operate, and could find nothing wrong, except that her systolic blood pressure was 60 mmHg. ECG and chest radiography were unremarkable, blood tests were taken, and I arranged to 'review with the results'. She died 4 h later. The next day the microbiologist phoned to say that streptococci had been grown from all blood cultures. Even awkward patients should have a blood pressure, and serious disease is likely if they don't. Give broad-spectrum parenteral antibiotics as soon as blood cultures have been taken if the cause of cardiorespiratory collapse is not apparent. And with regard to sepsis, ask if patients have travelled recently: if they have, the diagnosis may be malaria.

Communication

Once resuscitation and diagnostic endeavours are underway, and certainly when you have a clear idea what the diagnosis is, do not forget to speak to the patient's relatives and record in the medical notes what you have told them.

Further reading

Alderson P *et al.* (2000). Colloids versus crystalloids for fluid resuscitation in critically ill patients. *Cochrane Database System Review* CD000567.

Bickell WH *et al.* (1994). Immediate versus delayed fluid resuscitation for hypotensive patients with penetrating torso injuries. *New England Journal of Medicine* **331**, 1105–9.

Bristow PJ *et al.* (2000). Rates of in-hospital arrests, deaths and intensive care admissions: the effect of a medical emergency team. *Medical Journal of Australia* **173**, 236–40.

Bunn F *et al.* (2000). Colloid solutions for fluid resuscitation. *Cochrane Database System Review* CDOO1319.

Bunn F *et al.* (2000). Human albumin solution for resuscitation and volume expansion in critically ill patients. The Albumin Reviewers. *Cochrane Database System Review* CDOO1208.

Bunn F *et al.* (2000). Hypertonic versus isotonic crystalloid for fluid resuscitation in critically ill patients (Cochrane Review). *Cochrane Database System Review* **4**, CD002045.

Pittiruti M *et al.* (2000). Which is the easiest and safest technique for central venous access? A retrospective survey of more than 5400 cases. *Journal of Vascular Access* **1**, 100

16.2 The circulation and circulatory support of the critically ill

David F. Treacher

Introduction

This section considers global and regional oxygen delivery, the concept of shock, assessment and monitoring of the circulation, and the use of vaso-active drugs and in the critically ill patient.

The aphorism 'prevention is better than cure' should guide the management of the circulation, since early identification of circulatory derangement and the prompt diagnosis and treatment of underlying pathology provides the best chance for the rapid and complete recovery of the patient. However, with the limited monitoring and supervision available outside critical care units, early detection may be difficult. Hypotension is widely considered to be the cardinal sign of circulatory dysfunction, but other global features such as poor peripheral perfusion, persistent tachycardia, restlessness, confusion, tachypnoea, respiratory distress, hypoxaemia, and progressive metabolic acidaemia frequently occur earlier. These reflect the activation of powerful homeostatic mechanisms that maintain pressure at the expense of flow.

Features of regional circulatory failure include:

- oliguria with deteriorating renal function;
- confusion and impaired conscious level;
- chest pain, dysrhythmias, and ischaemic changes on electrocardiography (**ECG**);
- nausea, vomiting, and impaired gastrointestinal function: these symptoms of splanchnic ischaemia are often an early manifestation, but their significance is frequently overlooked.

Recent studies have demonstrated that evidence of an impending critical illness is often present—but not acted upon—for over 24 h in many of those patients on general wards who are subsequently admitted to intensive care units (**ICU**) following a cardiorespiratory arrest or with progressive organ failure. Such delay results in mortality rising almost exponentially as the number of organs that fail increases, leading to recommendations that 'rapid-response' or 'patient-at-risk' teams should be created with the aim of ensuring that experienced evaluation is rapidly available and timely admission to a critical care unit is arranged.

In high-risk surgical patients, preoperative 'optimization' of the circulation that ensures an oxygen delivery greater than 600 ml/min per m² through fluid resuscitation and, if necessary, inotrope/vasodilator therapy, has reduced mortality in controlled studies from over 20 per cent to less than 5 per cent, and the length of hospital stay by over 30 per cent.

Oxygen delivery and shock

Circulatory problems prompting a patient's admission to an ICU are cardiac arrest, pulmonary oedema, systemic hypotension, metabolic acidaemia, and organ failure, all situations that either threaten or have resulted from a failure of global or regional oxygen delivery. These patients are frequently described as suffering from 'shock'. The term has the advantage of brevity but little else, since it is imprecise and is applied to circulatory states that differ profoundly when analysed pathophysiologically. It can therefore guide neither management nor prognosis, but is irreversibly part of critical care terminology. Shock may be defined as inadequate cellular perfusion and oxygen uptake with consequent tissue hypoxia and organ failure. The terms 'early' and 'late' shock reflect the association between the duration and severity of the circulatory derangement and the prospect for recovery.

The major categories of shock, with examples, are:

- *Hypovolaemic*: haemorrhage, burns, gastrointestinal fluid loss;
- *Cardiogenic*: myocardial infarction, myocarditis, valve dysfunction;
- *Obstructive*: pulmonary embolus, cardiac tamponade, tension pneumothorax;
- *Anaphylactic*: drugs, blood transfusion, insect sting;
- *Septic*: bacterial infection, non-infective inflammatory conditions, e.g. pancreatitis, burns, trauma.

The primary problem in hypovolaemic, cardiogenic, and obstructive shock is a progressive decline in cardiac output and global oxygen delivery (Do_2), which—if not corrected—leads to secondary failure of the peripheral circulation and progressive organ dysfunction. By contrast, in sepsis and anaphylaxis, the primary problem is a failure of control of the peripheral circulation with disruption of the regional distribution of cardiac output, hence the alternative description of peripheral or distributive shock.

The initial physiological goal in the circulatory resuscitation of the critically ill patient is to restore global oxygen delivery while appropriate specific treatment is instituted.

Oxygen delivery

The delivery of oxygen from the external environment via the lungs to the mitochondria within individual cells is summarized in Fig. 1, with typical values quoted for normal activity in a 70-kg individual. Global oxygen delivery (Do_2) is calculated from the cardiac output, the oxygen saturation, and the haemoglobin concentration of arterial blood (Table 1).

Apart from the adequacy of overall Do_2, the regional distribution both between and within organs is important in maintaining normal organ function. If the myocutaneous bed receives a disproportionately high blood flow, but the flow to the splanchnic bed is poor, then the gastrointestinal tract and liver will become ischaemic despite a high Do_2.

The final parts of the oxygen cascade depend on diffusion, determined by the Po_2 gradient and the distance from capillary to cell, and also upon the integrity of cellular metabolic function. Increased levels of Do_2 cannot compensate for either the disruption of regional distribution or impaired diffusion between capillary and cell, or for primary metabolic failure within the cell as occurs in cyanide poisoning and sepsis. This explains why strategies that improve global oxygen delivery may even adversely affect cellular oxygen status—for example: (1) vasoactive agents altering the distribution of Do_2 between and within organs; (2) excessive volume loading producing tissue oedema and impairment of diffusion; (3) inotropes that increase cellular oxygen requirements (for instance, epinephrine (adrenaline) and dobutamine) may increase cellular oxygen debt.

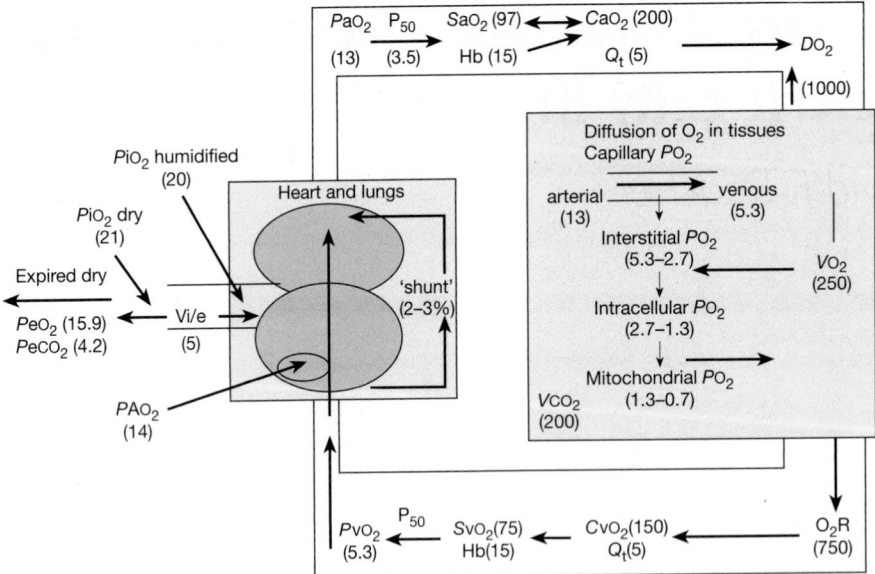

Fig. 1 Oxygen transport from the atmosphere to the mitochondria. Values in parentheses are for a normal 70-kg individual (body surface area (BSA), 1.67 m²) breathing air (fractional inspiratory oxygen concentration (Fio_2), 0.21) at standard atmospheric pressure (PB), 101 kPa. Partial pressures of O_2, CO_2 in kPa; saturation in per cent; contents (Cao_2, Cvo_2) in ml/litre; Hb in g/100 ml; blood/gas flows (Qt, Vi/e) in litres/min; oxygen transport (Do_2, o_2R), Vo_2, and Vco_2 in ml/min. Abbreviations: So_2, oxygen saturation (%); Po_2, partial pressure of oxygen (kPa); Pio_2, partial pressure of inspired O_2; Peo_2, partial pressure of mixed expired O_2; $Peco_2$, partial pressure of mixed expired CO_2; PAo_2, partial pressure of alveolar O_2; Pao_2, partial pressure of arterial O_2; Sao_2, arterial So_2; Svo_2, mixed venous So_2; Qt, cardiac output; Hb, haemoglobin; Cao_2, arterial O_2 content; Cvo_2, mixed venous O_2 content; Vo_2, oxygen consumption; Vco_2, CO_2 production; o_2R, oxygen return; Do_2, oxygen delivery; Vi/e, minute volume-inspiration/expiration.

Although achieving and maintaining an adequate global Do_2 is undoubtedly important, particularly in early resuscitation, the ability to measure and control regional distribution is now the challenge in the circulatory management of the critically ill patient.

Relationship between oxygen delivery and consumption

The oxygen extraction ratio (**OER**) is the percentage of the oxygen delivered that is extracted by the tissues, which is normally approximately 25 per cent. As metabolic demand (Vo_2) increases or supply diminishes, the OER increases to maintain aerobic metabolism. However, as demonstrated by point B in Fig. 2, there is a maximum extraction ratio (slope AB) that can be achieved. This is around 60 to 70 per cent for most tissues, beyond

which a further increase in Vo_2 or decline in Do_2 must lead to an inadequate availability of oxygen, at least in certain tissue beds, thus leading to anaerobic metabolism and increased lactic acid production. The dotted line, DEF, represents the altered relationship that may exist during critical illness. The slope of maximum OER falls, reflecting the reduced tissue extraction of oxygen, but the relationship does not plateau as in the normal relationship, that is to say oxygen consumption continues to rise with increasing delivery.

An enthusiasm for achieving supranormal levels of Do_2, so called 'goal-directed' therapy, arose from the concept of shock as a failure of adequate global oxygen delivery and the belief that oxygen consumption had become 'supply-dependent'. Observations of postoperative patients in the early 1980s led to a decade of ICU practice that focused on such goal-directed therapy. Based on studies relevant to postoperative patients, many critically ill patients with established 'shock' in ICU were managed with the aim of

Table 1 *Calculations used to assess the circulation, oxygen delivery and consumption*

Systemic vascular resistance (SVR)	=	[(MAP – RAP)/Qt] × 79.9 dyn s cm⁻⁵
Pulmonary vascular resistance (PVR)	=	[(PAP – LAP)/Qt] × 79.9 dyn s cm⁻⁵
Ventricular stroke work (VSW)	=	SV × ('afterload' – 'preload')
LVSW	=	SV × (MAP – LAP) × 0.0136 g m
RVSW	=	SV × (PAP – RAP) × 0.0136 g m
Arterial O_2 content (Cao_2)	=	[(Hb × Sao_2 × 1.36) + (Pao_2 × 0.023)] × 10 ml/l
Oxygen delivery (Do_2)	=	Qt × Cao_2 ml/min
Oxygen consumption (Vo_2)	=	Qt × (Cao_2–Cvo_2)
Oxygen extraction ratio (OER)	=	Vo_2 ÷ Do_2

SV, stroke volume; MAP, mean arterial pressure; PAP, pulmonary artery pressure; RAP/LAP, right/left atrial pressure; Ca, arterial content; Cv, venous content.

Pressures are measured in mmHg, cardiac output (Qt) in litres/min, and haemoglobin (Hb) in g/dl.

Values for resistance, stroke work, oxygen delivery, and consumption are frequently indexed by dividing by the patient's body surface area derived from the patient's height and weight.

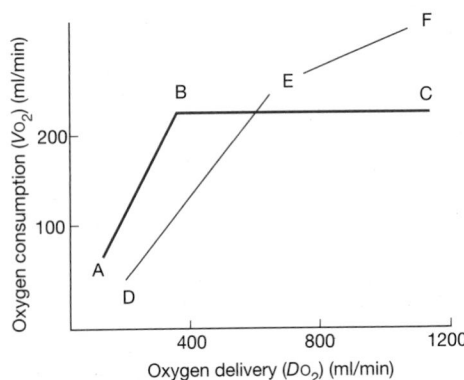

Fig. 2 Relationship between oxygen delivery and consumption. The effects of changing oxygen delivery on consumption. The solid line, ABC, represents the normal relationship and the fine line, DEF, the relationship believed to exist in critically ill patients.

achieving oxygen deliveries *above* 600 ml/min per m² using vigorous volume loading and inotropic support, frequently with dobutamine, in the belief that this would increase V_{O_2}, relieve tissue hypoxia, prevent multiorgan failure, and improve prognosis. Several major studies have now failed to demonstrate any benefit from this approach in the treatment of established shock, where such aggressive volume loading can be detrimental. In these studies, the patients who failed to achieve the desired D_{O_2} levels despite volume loading and dobutamine had a poorer outcome than those with a higher D_{O_2}, whether achieved spontaneously or following intervention, as did patients with low levels of D_{O_2} in the control group. This 'physiological reserve' or ability to increase D_{O_2} in response to the stress of critical illness is an important prognostic marker, which progressively diminishes with the length of time that the state of shock persists and as the circulatory state changes from early to late or 'irreversible/unresponsive' shock.

Although the relationship DEF of Fig. 2 may be unproven for established or late shock, the concept that a point B exists beyond which a further reduction in D_{O_2} causes progressive tissue hypoxaemia is valid early in the evolution of shock. This is particularly so for the low cardiac output/high vascular resistance causes (hypovolaemia, cardiogenic, obstructive) and also in early septic shock with intravascular depletion and low flows. In these situations the appropriate treatment is to increase D_{O_2} promptly by restoring the intravascular volume, relieving obstruction, or augmenting cardiac function. However, in the later stages of established shock from any cause the problem becomes peripheral at the microcirculatory level, with failure of autoregulation, abnormal regional distribution of flow within the organs, and direct cellular toxicity preventing oxygen uptake and utilization despite high levels of global D_{O_2}.

Aside from variations in D_{O_2}, tissue oxygenation may also be improved and aerobic metabolism sustained by reducing oxygen demand—achieved by controlling those factors that increase metabolic rate, such as: sympathetic activation from pain, agitation, shivering, and various interventions (nursing procedures, physiotherapy, visitors), drugs, and pyrexia. For each degree Celsius rise in temperature, oxygen consumption increases by 10 to 15 per cent.

Assessment of global circulatory performance

Cardiac output (Qt) depends upon:

(1) ventricular 'preload', i.e. atrial filling pressures (right atrial pressure (**RAP**), left atrial pressure (**LAP**));

(2) ventricular 'afterload', i.e. mean pulmonary and systemic arterial pressures (**PAP**, **SAP**);

(3) ventricular contractility;

(4) heart rate and rhythm.

Preload

Ventricular preload, traditionally assessed from the atrial filling pressures (RAP, LAP), determines the end-diastolic ventricular volume. This, according to Starling's law and depending on ventricular contractility, will in turn determine the work generated by the next cardiac contraction, the resulting stroke volume depending on the afterload.

Both ventricular contractility and afterload will affect the atrial filling pressures, but the predominant factor influencing preload is venous return, which is determined by the intravascular volume and the venous 'tone'. The systemic venous 'tone' or compliance is controlled by the autonomic nervous system and circulating catecholamines and can vary from 30 to over 300 ml/mmHg, such that the normal 70-kg person can compensate through venoconstriction for an intravascular volume loss of up to 1.5 litres without developing overt circulatory disturbance.

If the preload is low and either blood pressure or cardiac output is inadequate, the treatment priority is volume loading to restore the intravascular volume and venous return.

A high preload reflects one or more of the following: (1) high intravascular volume; (2) impaired myocardial contractility; or (3) increased 'afterload'. If treatment to reduce the preload is warranted, the options are therefore: to remove volume from the circulation (diuretics, venesection, haemofiltration) or to increase the capacity of the vascular bed with venodilator therapy (e.g. glyceryl trinitrate, morphine); to improve contractility; or to reduce the resistance of the relevant arterial bed.

In interpreting atrial pressures as measures of preload, two points must be considered. First, if the intrathoracic pressure (**Pt**) is raised, the intravascular pressure (**Pv**) may be misleading as a measure of preload since the true ventricular distending pressure is the transmural pressure (Pv – Pt). This is particularly relevant in situations where there is significant alveolar gas trapping, as in asthma or ventilation with high end-expiratory pressure and an increased ratio of inspiratory to expiratory time. Second, when the ventricle is dilated and poorly compliant the end-diastolic pressure-volume relationship is not necessarily linear, and ideally volume rather than pressure preload should be measured.

Afterload

Afterload influences the tension developed in the ventricular wall during systole, and is determined by the resistance to ventricular outflow from valvular abnormalities and the peripheral vascular resistance. The systemic and pulmonary vascular resistances (**SVR**, **PVR**) are calculated by analogy with Ohm's law as the pressure drop across the resistance bed divided by the flow, making the considerable assumption that flow in the circulation is linear and non-pulsatile.

Appropriate circulatory management requires an appreciation of the relationship between pressure, resistance, and flow: for a constant ventricular stroke work, the cardiac output will be inversely related to arterial pressure and resistance. The drugs used to manipulate pulmonary and systemic resistances are listed in Table 2.

Myocardial contractility

The ventricular stroke work is the external work performed by the ventricle with each beat and is calculated from the stroke volume and the pre- and afterload pressures (Table 1). The relationship between filling pressure, stroke work, and the resulting stroke volume for a constant afterload defines myocardial contractility. Consideration of ventricular work is important since circulatory management involves achieving the necessary pressures and flows to maintain satisfactory perfusion and oxygen delivery to all organs at maximum cardiac efficiency, that is for the least ventricular work, so that myocardial ischaemia is avoided.

Myocardial contractility is frequently reduced in critically ill patients due either to pre-existing cardiac disease, most often ischaemic heart disease, or as a consequence of the disease process, particularly sepsis. If the cardiac output is inadequate and myocardial contractility is poor, as defined by a 'flattened' stroke work/filling pressure equation, the available options are to:

* *reduce afterload* using an arteriolar dilator (nitrates, α-receptor blocker, angiotensin-converting enzyme (**ACE**) inhibitor). However, this may be limited by the consequent fall in systemic pressure.

* *increase preload*. Although appropriate if the preload is low or the intrathoracic pressure is high, the filling pressure will often already be raised and any further increase may not only fail to augment stroke volume but could increase ventricular wall tension, compromise ventricular blood supply, particularly to the endocardium, and potentially cause further impairment of contractility as well as pulmonary oedema.

* *increase myocardial contractility*, either by removing negatively inotropic influences (acidaemia, hyperkalaemia, drugs (for example,

Table 2 Circulatory effects of commonly used vasoactive drug infusions

Drug	Receptors	Cardiac contractility	HR	BP	Cardiac output	Splanchnic blood flow	SVR	PVR
Dopamine (<5 µg/kg per min)	DA_1, β_1, α	+	0/+	0/+	+	0/+	0/+	0/+
Dopamine (>5 µg/kg per min)	β_1, α, DA_1, β_2	++	+	+	++	0	+	+
Epinephrine (adrenaline)	β_1, α, β_2	++	+	++	+++	−	+	+
Norepinephrine (noradrenaline)	α, β_1	0/+	0	++	−	−−	++	++
Isoprenaline	β_1, β_2	+	++	+/0	+	0/+	0/−	−
Dobutamine	β_1, β_2	+	+	+/0	++	0	−	−
Dopexamine	β_2, DA_1, DA_2	+	+	0	+	+	−	−
Glyceryl trinitrate	via NO	0	+	−	+	+	−	−
Nitroprusside	via NO	0	+	−−	+	+	−−	−
Milrinone	PDE	+	+	−	++	0/+	−−	−
Nitric oxide (inhaled)	via NO	0	0	0	0/+	0	0	−−
Prostacyclin		0	+	−−	+	+	−	−−

'+' increases; '0' no change; '−' decreases.

These effects are guidelines only—the response will depend on the circulatory state of the patient when the drug is started, as well as the differential effects on α-adrenergic, β-adrenergic, dopamine, and phosphodiesterase (PDE) receptors and nitric oxide (NO)/cyclic guanosine monophosphate (cGMP) with increasing dose.

β-receptor blockers), or by using an inotrope (Table 2). The possible adverse effects of vasoactive agents on regional distribution of flow must also be considered.

Heart rate and rhythm

If the heart rate is low (<65 beats/min) with a low cardiac output, then increasing the rate either with a β_1-receptor agonist (for example, isoprenaline) or by pacing should be considered. Atrial pacing, or atrioventricular sequential pacing, has the advantage of maintaining co-ordinated atrial contraction that increases ventricular end-diastolic volume and hence stroke volume without increasing myocardial irritability.

Heart rates above 120 beats/min, other than sinus tachycardia, should be controlled either by drugs and/or DC cardioversion after ensuring that low plasma potassium and magnesium levels have been corrected.

Monitoring

The purpose of monitoring the critically ill patient is both to alert staff if a physiological variable is not maintained within preset limits and to guide therapy. Critically ill patients require the following investigations: continuous monitoring of heart rate and rhythm; intravascularly measured blood pressure and RAP; arterial oxygen saturation by oximetry; intermittent blood gas analysis, which usually also provides electrolyte, glucose, and lactate concentrations; and hourly fluid balance measurements.

Pulmonary artery catheterization

Of the six primary circulatory variables measured in an intensive care unit, three (RAP, mean arterial pressure (**MAP**), and heart rate) are routinely available even outside an ICU. Conventionally, the other three (PAP, LAP, and Qt) are measured by the insertion of a pulmonary artery catheter. Apart from the derivation of vascular resistances, ventricular work, and oxygen delivery, the mixed venous oxygen saturation can be measured and used to calculate oxygen consumption (Table 1).

Sampling from the pulmonary artery is necessary to ensure good mixing of the venous blood, since the saturation of venous blood from different organs does vary considerably. Hepatic venous saturation may only be 40 per cent, whereas renal venous saturation may exceed 80 per cent, reflecting the considerable difference between these organs in oxygen delivery compared to their metabolic requirements. Provided the peripheral distribution of Do_2 and cellular metabolic function are normal, a value of Svo_2 above 65 per cent indicates that oxygen delivery is satisfying tissue oxygen requirements.

The focus on 'goal-directed therapy' led to the widespread use of pulmonary artery (**PA**) catheters, with an annual consumption of over 2 million in the United States. However, their indiscriminate use has been challenged by:

(1) evidence that goal-directed therapy, although probably appropriate for under-resuscitated perioperative patients, may be harmful for other critically ill patients;

(2) a multicentre case-controlled study of the use of the PA catheter, which suggested that those patients managed with a PA catheter had a poorer prognosis than those managed without such an intervention;

(3) doubts about the appropriateness of using pressure preload as reflected by the pulmonary artery occlusion pressure as a surrogate for the volume preload of the left ventricle.

Although the PA catheter is undoubtedly associated with complications, particularly infection (see Table 3), and the measurements subject to significant error, the results of this study probably reflected poor training in the use of the catheter and a failure to respond appropriately to the data obtained. Insertion of a PA catheter should still be considered:

• if the RAP is raised and the relationship with the LAP is uncertain due to a recent myocardial infarction, valvular abnormalities, or high pulmonary vascular resistance—the most useful finding is a low 'wedge' pressure, demonstrating that further volume is indicated, but a high value does not necessarily exclude the need for further volume;

Table 3 Complications of central venous and pulmonary artery cannulation

Insertion
- Pneumothorax—more likely with subclavian than internal jugular approach
- Haematoma from arterial puncture
- Air embolism
- Dysrhythmia
- Damage to thoracic duct with left internal jugular approach
- Knotting of catheter*
- Pulmonary vessel rupture causing haemoptysis*

In situ
- Sepsis
- Thrombosis
- Pulmonary infarct*
- Erroneous information
- Inappropriate response to information

*Risk associated specifically with PA catheterization.

- if the patient's condition fails to improve with initial management;

- to measure cardiac output to guide the appropriate choice of vasoactive drug, particularly when high doses are being used;

- if continuous monitoring of PA pressures and evaluation of right ventricular (**RV**) function is indicated

The PA catheter debate has, however, led to considerable interest in alternative, less invasive methods of assessing cardiac output and the adequacy of left ventricular preload.

Measurement of global cardiac output

Table 4 summarizes the features of the alternative methods available for measuring cardiac output, with an assessment of those aspects other than accuracy that should be considered. Any additional information that is provided, such as continuous mixed venous oxygen saturation with a PA catheter, should be considered when selecting the most appropriate monitor.

The most widely used method for measuring cardiac output remains the thermodilution technique using a PA catheter. Although generally viewed as the 'gold standard', the error is at least 10 per cent and there are potentially serious complications, particularly infection.

Clinical assessment of systemic vascular resistance and pulse volume allows cardiac output to be estimated with sufficient accuracy to direct initial management. This approach is rapid, requires no invasive monitoring, may be performed outside the intensive care unit, and is relevant for use in less-well resourced countries. If the patient does not improve with management based on this initial assessment, more invasive monitoring is indicated.

With the oesophageal Doppler technique an ultrasound transducer probe is positioned in front of the descending aorta and blood flow velocity measured, from which cardiac output is derived using an estimate of the aortic cross-sectional area calculated from the patient's height, weight, and age. Intravascular volume status can also be assessed from changes in the size and shape of the aortic velocity waveform. It can be inserted rapidly and left *in situ* for up to a week without serious complication and is notionally non-invasive. However it is expensive, operator-dependent, and cannot easily be used in patients who are not intubated.

The recently reported technique of lithium dilution cardiac output can be performed with a peripheral venous and arterial line and compares favourably with the thermodilution method.

Pulse contour analysis relies on analysis of the arterial pressure waveform to provide a beat-by-beat estimation of the stroke volume. Regular calibration by thermal or lithium dilution is necessary but only requires a central venous injection of the indicator, and from this both intrathoracic blood volume and lung water can also be derived to provide an assessment of the adequacy of intravascular fluid resuscitation.

Measurement of regional blood flow

Appropriate management of the circulation requires information about regional as well as global flow. Urine output is sensitive to changes in renal perfusion, provided the kidneys have not developed acute tubular necrosis (**ATN**) or been poisoned with drugs, particularly diuretics. The lower limit is 0.5 ml/kg per min, but twice this rate is appropriate in the catabolic patient.

Peripheral perfusion and changes in cardiac output and its distribution can be assessed from the gradient between the peripheral temperature, usually measured over the dorsum of the foot, and the central or core temperature (rectal, oesophageal, or possibly tympanic).

Splanchnic blood flow, which is particularly sensitive to hypovolaemia and vasoconstricting inotropes and which is important in the aetiology of multiple organ failure, can be assessed by tonometry. The gastric tonometer is a nasogastric tube with a second channel connected to a balloon that can be inflated with saline or air. When the P_{CO_2} within the gastric mucosal cells ($P_{CO_{2i}}$), stomach lumen, and the balloon have equilibrated, a sample is withdrawn from the balloon to measure P_{CO_2}. From this measurement and the arterial bicarbonate concentration, the intracellular pH (pHi) can be calculated. Some perioperative studies in patients have shown that pHi is valuable both prognostically and in guiding treatment. Its role in the established critically ill patient is less clear. The gastric mucosal and alveolar P_{CO_2} gradient is probably a more appropriate measure. However, problems remain with obtaining useful data when the patient is being enterally fed, and there is also uncertainty whether gastric $P_{CO_{2i}}$ reflects the energy and oxygen status of other parts of the bowel. Although tonometers can be placed in the small bowel and sigmoid colon, the technique remains predominantly a research tool.

The new technologies of magnetic resonance spectroscopy and positron emission tomography allow more detailed study of the regional circulation, tissue oxygenation, and cellular bioenergetics and will soon become available for clinically based studies in the critically ill patient.

Echocardiography is useful in assessing ventricular volume preload and will also provide information about cardiac function and structure. It is particularly valuable in the diagnosis of obstructive shock and aortic dissection. The transthoracic approach may be difficult in ventilated patients

Table 4 Comparison of features and the available techniques for measuring cardiac output

Method	Invasion/risk	Discomfort	Complexity	Measurement error	Cost
Indicator dilution					
Thermodilution	+++	++	++	+ (?)	++
Fick	+++	++	+++	+ (?)	++
Indocyanine Green	+++	++	++	+	++
Lithium	++	+	+	+	+
Respired gas					
Modified Fick	+	+	++	++	+
Inert gas rebreathing	+	+	+++	++	+
Doppler					
Transoesophageal	+	++	++	++	+++
Echocardiography	0	0	++	+++	+
Impedance cardiography	0	0	++	++	+
Pulse contour analysis	+	0	+	++	+
Clinical assessment	0	0	+	++	0

due to a poor 'echo window', but the transoesophageal approach has been a major advance.

Acid–base balance and serum lactate are useful metabolic indices of the circulation and both are sensitive to intravascular volume depletion, particularly in the presence of inotropic support. Progressive metabolic acidaemia requires diagnosis and effective treatment. The serum lactate level reflects the balance between increased production in hypoxic tissues and metabolic clearance, which is predominantly hepatic. High lactate levels often indicate splanchnic ischaemia when there is both increased production and reduced clearance due to hepatic ischaemia. A single measurement is difficult to interpret, but the trend is valuable in assessing the response to treatment.

Key points in monitoring the circulation

- Regular clinical examination should never be forgotten: the symptoms and signs already discussed are as important as impressively displayed numbers on expensive monitors.

- Trends are more useful than a single observation.

- Pressure is no guarantee of flow.

- Although the jugular venous pressure (**JVP**) is traditionally measured from the sternal angle, in ICU pressures are measured from the mid-axillary line in the 5th intercostal space. From this reference point, in the supine position, the normal RAP is between +4 and +8 mmHg and the LAP or 'wedge' between +10 and +14 mmHg.

- If monitor data and clinical judgement conflict, check for common sources of error in the monitoring such as catheter blockage or malposition, failure to re-zero after postural change.

- Critical care monitoring is invasive, potentially hazardous (Table 3), expensive, and mostly of no proven benefit. The device should be used while *in situ*, but it should be removed as soon as the information obtained is no longer required.

- Outcome benefit from the use of any monitor depends on the data being displayed accurately (zero and calibration), observed promptly, and interpreted appropriately and on an effective intervention being available and rapidly instituted.

Management of the circulation in the critically ill

General principles

The circulation should be assessed as shown in Table 5, which provides examples of the circulatory abnormalities in various conditions. The severity of the condition and pre-existing cardiorespiratory disease will affect the precise figures obtained in individual cases. It is not always necessary to use invasive monitoring to obtain precise measurements, but the discipline of estimating the key variables commits the clinician to a logical analysis of the problem and an awareness of which measurements need to be confirmed, invasively if necessary, if the patient's condition fails to improve.

The six key questions in managing the circulation are:

1. *What are the appropriate targets for blood pressure and cardiac output?*—Despite the emphasis placed on blood flow to the tissues, adequate perfusion pressure is also necessary to achieve the appropriate distribution of cardiac output and oxygen supply. The target for mean arterial pressure should be 65 mmHg but adequate splanchnic and renal perfusion may require higher pressures, particularly in the elderly patient with pre-existing hypertension or widespread atheroma. In treating a patient with cerebral oedema the target pressure should be 65 mmHg *above* the intracranial pressure.

   A minimum cardiac output of 2.8 litres/min per m² should ensure that tissue hypoxia is not due to inadequate global oxygen supply. Thereafter, management of organ dysfunction should concentrate on the regional distribution.

2. *Has sufficient fluid been given?*—Conventionally this is based on measurement of the atrial filling pressures (RAP and LAP, or pulmonary artery occlusion/'wedge' pressure). Before starting inotropic support, fluid should be given to achieve an RAP up to 12 mmHg or a 'wedge' pressure of 18 mmHg. This assumes that the relationship between the atrial filling pressures, the permeability of the pulmonary capillary membranes, and the intrathoracic pressure are all normal, but none of these assumptions is necessarily valid in the critically ill patient. A low value (RAP <10 mmHg, LAP <14 mmHg) is helpful since further volume will improve cardiac work. Higher levels are more difficult to

Table 5 Circulatory measurements in a normal adult and in various cardiorespiratory conditions causing shock

| | RAP | LAP | PAP | MAP | HR/ min | Cardiac output | SVR* | PVR* | Stroke work g m | | Venous compliance | Cao2 ml/100 ml | Do2 |
	mmHg	mmHg	mmHg	mmHg		l/min			LV	RV	ml/mmHg		ml/min
Normal	5	10	15	90	70	5.0	17	1.0	78	10.0	300	20	1000
Major haemorrhage	0	3	10	80	100	3.2	25	2.2	34	4.4	40	16	510
Left ventricular failure	7	19	23	90	100	3.6	23	1.1	35	8.0	80	18	650
Cardiac tamponade	14	16	19	65	110	2.3	22	1.3	14	1.4	50	20	460
Major PE	10	6	35	70	110	2.6	23	11.0	21	8.0	40	16	420
Exacerbation of COAD	10	9	35	80	100	6.5	11	4.0	63	22.0	150	13	850
Septic shock:													
(i) prevolume	2	7	17	49	130	4.2	11	2.4	18	7.0	340	15	630
(ii) postvolume	10	14	25	68	120	8.0	7	1.4	49	14.0	200	14	1120

RAP/LAP, right/left atrial pressure; PAP/MAP, mean pulmonary artery/arterial pressure; HR, heart rate; SVR/PVR, systemic/pulmonary vascular resistance; LV/RV, left/right ventricle; Cao2, arterial oxygen content; Do2, global oxygen delivery; PE, pulmonary embolism; COAD, chronic obstructive airways disease.
The severity of the condition and pre-existing cardiorespiratory disease will affect the precise figures obtained in individual cases. See Table 1 for the calculation of resistance, stroke work, and Do2.
Pressures referenced to zero at the mid-axillary line in a supine patient. Subtract the vertical distance from the mid-axilla to the sternal angle (approx. 5–7 mmHg) if the sternal angle is used as the reference point.
*Multiply by 79.9 to give SI units: dyn s cm⁻⁵.

interpret, particularly in the ventilated patient, since, although an inadequate volume preload is not necessarily excluded, further fluid may result in pulmonary oedema.

Intravascular volume depletion is suggested by hypotension precipitated by sedation, analgesia, postural change, or during the inspiratory phase of positive-pressure ventilation. Brief disconnection from the ventilator causes the blood pressure to rise and venous pressure to fall: the measurement 'off' the ventilator more accurately reflects the ventricular end-diastolic transmural pressure. This manoeuvre is relatively contraindicated in patients with acute respiratory distress syndrome (**ARDS**), since loss of positive end-expiratory pressure may cause widespread alveolar collapse.

The difficulty in interpreting the absolute levels of RAP/LAP can be resolved by a fluid challenge: 200 ml of colloid is administered and the impact on blood pressure, flow, and preload observed. In the volume-depleted patient, blood pressure and flow will increase with only a small, transient increase in filling pressures. While pulmonary gas exchange remains satisfactory there is less anxiety about giving further colloid. Sufficient volume will have been given when either the target pressures are achieved and the evidence of poor peripheral perfusion and organ dysfunction has resolved, or when there is a sustained rise in filling pressures to a level above which there is a risk of pulmonary oedema developing.

3. *Which fluids should be used?*—The previous day's crystalloid and colloid balance should be reviewed, both intravascular and extravascular compartments should be assessed, and the volume of fluid to be given over the following 24 h should be decided. The crystalloid balance should include the planned enteral intake, fluid for central lines and drug infusions, urine output, and correction for both 'insensible' losses (sweat, diarrhoea) and the state of hydration of the extravascular tissue space. A daily target balance ranging from −1.5 to >+3 litres may be appropriate, but typically it will be between −0.5 and +1.5 litres.

If the intravascular space is underfilled, the rate of infusion of normal saline should be increased by up to 100 ml/h, but, acutely, the extra volume required to reach the preload target should be given as colloid. With an active haemorrhage or if the haemoglobin concentration is less than 8 g/dl, blood should be used. Traditionally, the target haemoglobin has been 10 g/dl, since this was believed to represent the balance between oxygen content and viscosity that achieved optimum tissue oxygen delivery. However, a prospective randomized study to assess the impact of the haemoglobin level on outcome demonstrated that, for patients without significant coronary artery disease, survival was improved if the haemoglobin was maintained between 7 and 9 g/dl rather than between 10 and 12 g/dl.

After appropriate blood transfusion, synthetic colloid rather than albumin should be used. A much-debated meta-analysis comparing the use of albumin with crystalloid or synthetic colloid concluded that, in the critically ill, albumin was associated with an increased mortality. Certainly, attempting to correct a low serum albumin level in such patients exhibiting a significant inflammatory response is futile, since their vascular endothelium will be freely permeable to albumin. There is relatively little evidence on which to base the choice of synthetic colloid (starch or gelatin) but the increase in intravascular volume is sustained for longer with the starch solutions, which also provide a wider range of molecular weight products and a sodium-free option.

4. *Are there metabolic factors that require correction?*—Metabolic acidaemia with a pH below 7.20 or a base deficit above 10 mmol/l should be corrected, as myocardial contractility increases linearly with rising pH to values above 7.40. The suggestion that sodium bicarbonate will produce a damaging paradoxical intracellular acidosis is misleading, since the experiments demonstrating this effect were performed *in vitro* with unphysiological solutions, within a 'closed system' that allowed no correction for any rise in carbon dioxide concentration, and the sodium

bicarbonate was given by bolus injection rather than infusion. Sodium bicarbonate, given as a physiological infusion at between 1 and 2 mmol/min, improves myocardial contractility and cardiac output, as demonstrated by several clinical studies and shown by the benefits of bicarbonate haemofiltration in lactate-intolerant, critically ill patients.

Hyperkalaemia, hypocalcaemia, and hypophosphataemia also impair myocardial contractility and should be corrected.

5. *Is ventilatory support indicated?*—Hypoxaemia should be corrected promptly to ensure that oxygen saturation is at least 92 per cent, both to prevent myocardial ischaemia and to ensure maximum oxygen delivery. The work of breathing may account for up to one-third of oxygen consumption and, if provided mechanically, circulatory demands will be reduced significantly. Non-invasive ventilatory support should first be considered: both continuous positive airway pressure (**CPAP**) and pressure support ventilation can be provided by a face or nasal mask. If formal mechanical ventilation with intubation becomes necessary, colloid volume should be given and a vasoconstricting inotrope infusion should be available to prevent the potentially catastrophic hypotension that may result from the use of sedative anaesthetic drugs in the volume-depleted patient with high endogenous catecholamine levels and raised SVR.

6. *Which vasoactive agents should be used?*—If the target systemic pressure and cardiac output/oxygen delivery are not achieved with appropriate intravascular filling, a suitable vasoactive agent or combination must be selected (Table 2). The impact of such treatment in individual patients will be influenced by their baseline circulation state (that is, if it is either intensely constricted or dilated the same drug will potentially produce different effects on pressure, flow, and its distribution). The initial choice of vasoactive agent will depend on the mean arterial pressure (**MAP**), cardiac output, and derived systemic vascular resistance (**SVR**). If, for example:

- cardiac output and MAP are both low with a high SVR, an inotropic and dilating (inodilator) effect is required and epinephrine (adrenaline) with glyceryl trinitrate or dobutamine would be appropriate. If cardiac output rises but MAP falls, as may happen when dobutamine is given, a constricting agent such as norepinephrine (noradrenaline) is required.

- MAP and SVR are low with a high cardiac output, as frequently occurs in sepsis after volume resuscitation, then arteriolar constriction with norepinephrine is needed.

- MAP is at or above target but the cardiac output is low with a raised SVR, a dilating agent (glyceryl trinitrate) or an inodilator is appropriate treatment.

When the PVR and RAP are acutely raised, a pulmonary vasodilator to 'offload' the right ventricle and maintain cardiac output is required. A nitrate or β-receptor agonist, such as isoprenaline, would be appropriate, but hypotension may result from arteriolar dilatation and hypoxaemia due to increased ventilation–perfusion mismatch.

A vasoactive drug that could influence regional flow would be valuable. The belief that low-dose dopamine selectively improves renal blood flow has resulted in its widespread use. However, the evidence to support this belief is scanty, and a study of its use in perioperative patients suggested that it may even be harmful. Its undoubted effect in increasing urine output is probably due to an improvement in MAP and cardiac output together with a natriuretic effect, rather than to any specific effect on renal blood flow. When these effects are required, provided it is not used as a substitute for adequate volume replacement, it remains useful. Dopexamine, with both dopamine (DA1, DA2)- and β-receptor effects, is used to improve splanchnic blood flow. However, despite reported benefits when used with volume loading in perioperative patients, there is little evidence of outcome benefit in the treatment of established shock.

Phosphodiesterase inhibitors, such as milrinone, offer a theoretically attractive approach to improving myocardial contractility by increasing intracellular cAMP when there is reduced responsiveness to β-agonists. Useful increases in cardiac output can be achieved, but these agents are powerful vasodilators and hypotension may limit their use and results in the need for a norepinephrine infusion.

Management in specific conditions

Myocardial infarction/pulmonary oedema

The aim should be a dilated circulation to achieve the target cardiac output for the minimum cardiac work, but with a diastolic pressure above 50 mmHg to protect coronary artery perfusion. The preload should be reduced with nitrate therapy, both to reverse pulmonary oedema and to avoid ventricular overdistension and increased wall tension that reduces epicardial to endocardial flow. An ACE inhibitor should be started early, although hypotension and impairment of renal function may cause delay. The intra-aortic balloon pump has the advantage of augmenting cardiac work, improving coronary artery perfusion, and reducing the left ventricular afterload and hence the need for inotropic drugs.

Haemorrhage

During a major haemorrhage, sympathetic activation with intense venoconstriction prevents hypotension developing until 30 per cent of the circulating blood volume is lost, which explains the response to subsequent transfusion. As volume is lost, venous 'tone' increases to maintain venous return and only late is there a marked fall in venous pressure, cardiac output, and finally arterial pressure. If the rate of fluid replacement does not exceed the speed of resolution of the reflex increase in sympathetic tone, the atrial filling pressures will not rise excessively. However, rapid transfusion may produce very high atrial pressures and even pulmonary oedema, even though the volume replaced is less than the volume lost from the circulation.

Major pulmonary embolism

Oxygen delivery should be maintained by oxygen administration, volume expansion, and inotropic stimulation, while the obstruction is relieved by heparinization with thrombolysis or embolectomy.

The RAP should be raised to at least 15 mmHg using colloid to increase right ventricular work, and the resulting expansion of the pulmonary vascular bed may reduce the pulmonary vascular resistance by up to 50 per cent. Hydraulic pulmonary oedema does not occur since the atrial pressure relationship is reversed. An initial intravenous bolus of heparin (15 000 units) should be given to initiate anticoagulation and to reverse the reflex pulmonary vasoconstriction that occurs in the unobstructed pulmonary vascular bed. Digitalization improves right ventricular contractility and is sensible prophylaxis against supraventricular tachycardias.

Sedation, diuretics, haemorrhage, induction of anaesthesia, vena caval ligation, and the administration of contrast material during angiography may produce a disastrous fall in RAP and cardiac output. To prevent such changes, venous return must be maintained with volume expanders and by venoconstriction with α-agonists such as norepinephrine or phenylephrine.

Septic shock

In septic shock the circulatory changes are primarily peripheral, with cytokine release and activated white cells producing both direct cellular toxicity and microcirculatory chaos. As a result of the 'shunting' of blood through the tissues and the failure of cellular oxygen utilization, the tissues remain hypoxic despite high Do_2. This results in a low oxygen extraction ratio, a raised lactate level, and a reduced arteriovenous oxygen difference with a paradoxically high Svo_2. Secondary failure of the global circulation is caused by:

- volume depletion due to the increased leakiness of the vascular endothelium and sequestration secondary to venodilatation; and

- toxic effects on the myocardium impairing both systolic contraction and diastolic relaxation.

The typical circulatory profiles before and after volume resuscitation are shown in Table 5.

Despite a low SVR, the patient may feel cold peripherally and present as having unexplained hypotension with a speed of onset that suggests a major pulmonary embolus or myocardial infarction. However, palpation of a surprisingly large volume yet a rapid central pulse reveals that the cardiac output must be high, effectively ruling out these other causes of shock and indicating the true diagnosis.

Deciding on the 'appropriate' fluid volume to give in sepsis can be difficult. Frequently, the decision represents a balance between giving sufficient volume to prevent the use of excessive doses of constricting inotropes and giving excessive amounts with consequent tissue oedema and deterioration in pulmonary gas exchange.

Norepinephrine and epinephrine infusions will often be necessary, with doses adjusted as previously described to achieve pressure and flow targets. If high doses (>0.15 μg/kg per min) are required, splanchnic ischaemia is a major concern and should be suspected if the patient develops abdominal tenderness, large nasogastric aspirates, and a lactic acidosis. Patients with severe sepsis develop β-receptor desensitization with reduced intracellular cAMP levels, which makes the use of phosphodiesterase inhibitors such as milrinone logical. However, their use may exacerbate hypotension and result in the dose of vasoconstrictor drugs being increased.

Earlier studies suggested there was no role for steroids in the treatment of septic shock. However, there is now evidence that, at a lower dose (100 mg hydrocortisone, three times per day) than previously used, they can reduce the marked vasodilatation associated with a persistent and excessive inflammatory response, so that the doses of constricting inotropes can be reduced with potential benefit for regional perfusion.

Several large studies of anticytokine therapy and of antithrombin III supplementation in patients with severe sepsis have all failed to improve outcome. Similarly, a trial of N-monomethyl-L-arginine (L-NMMA)—an antagonist of the effects of inducible nitric oxide synthase, an enzyme responsible for the excess production of nitric oxide that is central to the severe peripheral vasodilatation associated with septic shock—had to be stopped prematurely because of an adverse outcome in the treatment group. However, a study in which activated protein C was given as an infusion over 4 days to patients with severe sepsis has now shown a significant reduction in mortality at 28 days.

Further reading

Bernard GR, *et al.* (2001). Recombinant human protein C. Worldwide Evaluation in Severe Sepsis (PROWESS) Study Group. *New England Journal of Medicine* **344**, 699–709.

Bradley RD (1977). *Studies in acute heart failure.* Edward Arnold, London.

Cochrane Injuries Group Albumin Reviewers (1998). Human albumin administration in critically ill patients: systematic review of randomised controlled trials. *British Medical Journal* **317**, 235–40.

Connors A, *et al.* (1996). The effectiveness of right heart catheterisation in the initial care of critically ill patients. *Journal of the American Medical Association* **276**, 889–97.

Consensus Conference (1996). Tissue hypoxia: how to detect, how to correct, how to prevent. *American Journal of Respiratory and Critical Care Medicine* **154**, 1573–8.

Gutierrez G, *et al.* (1992). Gastric intramucosal pH as a therapeutic index of tissue oxygenation in critically ill patients. *Lancet* **339**, 195–9.

Hayes MA, *et al.* (1994). Elevation of systemic oxygen delivery in the treatment of critically ill patients. *New England Journal of Medicine* **330**, 1717–22.

Hebert PC, *et al.* (1999). A multicenter, randomized, controlled clinical trial of transfusion requirements in critical care. *New England Journal of Medicine* **340**, 409–17.

Iberti TJ, *et al.* (1990). A multi-centre study of physicians' knowledge of the pulmonary artery catheter. *Journal of the American Medical Journal* **264**, 2928–32.

Leach RM, Treacher DF (1992). Oxygen transport: the relation between oxygen delivery and consumption. *Thorax* **47**, 971–8.

Schierhout G, Roberts I (1998). Fluid resuscitation with colloid or crystalloid solutions in critically ill patients: a systematic review of randomised trials. *British Medical Journal* **316**, 961–4.

Shippy CR, *et al.* (1984). Reliability of clinical monitoring to assess blood volume in critically ill patients. *Critical Care Medicine* **12**, 107–12.

Shoemaker WC, *et al.* (1988). Prospective trial of supranormal values of survivors as therapeutic goals in high-risk surgical patients. *Chest* **94**, 1176–87.

Wilson J, *et al.* (1999). Reducing the risk of major elective surgery: randomized, controlled trial of preoperative optimisation of oxygen delivery. *British Medical Journal* **318**, 1099–103.

16.3 Cardiac arrest

C. A. Eynon

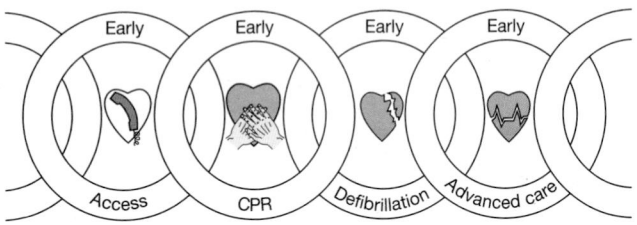

Fig. 1 The sequence of events in emergency cardiac care is displayed schematically by the 'chain of survival' metaphor. (From Cummins RO *et al.*, 1991. Improving survival from sudden cardiac arrest: the 'chain of survival' concept. *Circulation* **83**, 1832–47.)

Introduction

Cardiac arrest is a clinical syndrome consisting of unresponsiveness, absence of a detectable pulse, and either apnoea or agonal respiration. Cessation of cardiac activity is common to all causes of death and it is important to remember that cardiopulmonary resuscitation (**CPR**) was only developed to treat potentially reversible causes.

From the earliest recorded times it has been recognized that there is a period in which it is possible to reverse the transition from life to death. In Ancient Egyptian mythology, Isis, the goddess of healing, revived her husband Osiris by breathing into his mouth. In the Old Testament, Elijah successfully resuscitated an apparently dead child. The techniques that comprise modern CPR were all described before the end of the 19th century. Accounts of mouth-to-mouth ventilation appeared in the recommendations of the Dutch Humane Society in 1767, and in 1775 Abildgaard described the effects of electricity in first killing, and then resuscitating chickens. The earliest reports of closed-chest compression were in the late 1800s. It was only from the mid-1950s, however, that these individual modalities were combined and evolved into the concept of the 'chain of survival' (Fig. 1).

Aetiology

In the adult population, sudden cardiac arrest commonly results from ischaemic heart disease, 30 per cent of victims having evidence of recent myocardial infarction at autopsy. Other cardiac causes include primary arrhythmias, cardiomyopathies, and structural abnormalities. A wide range of non-cardiac conditions can precipitate a secondary cardiac arrest.

Three cardiac arrest rhythms are recognized: ventricular fibrillation (**VF**) or pulseless ventricular tachycardia (**VT**), asystole, and pulseless electrical activity (**PEA**). VF is characterized by a chaotic, uncoordinated waveform on the electrocardiogram (**ECG**). Asystole occurs when no ventricular electrical activity is present. Although atrial and ventricular asystole usually coexist, ventricular asystole may precede atrial asystole by a short time, producing an ECG in which there are isolated p waves. PEA occurs when

there are clinical features of cardiac arrest despite an ECG rhythm that would normally be associated with a palpable pulse. Outside hospital, up to 75 per cent of cardiac arrests are due to VF/VT. In hospital, asystole and PEA are more common. This may reflect the greater prevalence of comorbid conditions in the hospital population.

Epidemiology

Sudden cardiac arrest remains the leading cause of unexpected death in the Western world, with 500 000 cases annually in the United States. With resuscitation the rate of return of spontaneous circulation is approximately 30 per cent for patients suffering an in-hospital cardiac arrest, but only around 15 per cent survive to discharge. Patients who suffer an out-of-hospital cardiac arrest have a worse outcome, with 8 to 22 per cent surviving to admission and 2 to 8 per cent being discharged. This variation in outcomes results from differences in emergency medical systems and study methodology. The main determinant of outcome is the initially documented cardiac rhythm. The survival rate for patients in VF/VT is 10 to 15 times that for asystole or PEA.

Pathophysiology

During cardiac arrest there is global ischaemia. Therapy is directed at maintaining perfusion of vital organs and re-establishing organized myocardial activity. Release of endogenous catecholamines and other vasoactive peptides causes redistribution of blood flow to the brain and heart and away from other organs. The brain is the organ most susceptible to ischaemia, and the rate of neurologically intact survival decreases rapidly to virtually zero at 20 min following cardiac arrest.

Myocardial ischaemia causes maximal coronary vasodilatation and myocardial blood flow becomes dependent on the coronary perfusion pressure: the pressure gradient between the aorta and right atrium during diastole. A coronary perfusion pressure of 15 mmHg during resuscitation appears to be the threshold for successful return of spontaneous circulation. Under normal conditions, coronary blood flow is autoregulated and coronary artery stenoses of up to 70 per cent do not compromise flow. However, during cardiac arrest autoregulation is lost and relatively insignificant lesions may reduce distal perfusion.

Following resuscitation there is a period of reversible organ dysfunction. Neurological impairment often persists for 12 to 24 h. Thereafter, two patterns emerge: progressive improvement, or persisting coma and stable neurological deficit. Myocardial dysfunction contributes to the high mortality from arrhythmias and heart failure in the hours and days after resuscitation. Other organ systems are relatively resistant to periods of ischaemia compatible with successful resuscitation. Although multiple organ support may be necessary, permanent damage of organs other than the brain is uncommon in survivors.

Management

The current European Resuscitation Guidelines for adult basic and advanced life support are shown in Figs 2 and 3. The most important factors affecting outcome are the times before institution of CPR, defibrillation, and advanced care. For VF/VT, survival rates correlate with the time to defibrillation. For asystole and PEA, the aim of treatment is to maintain organ perfusion until remediable causes for cardiac arrest can be identified and treated.

Early access/assessment

Immediate activation of the emergency medical systems is essential once it has been determined that the patient is unresponsive. Campaigns have highlighted the need for witnesses of cardiac arrest to notify the emergency services correctly. Awareness of the appropriate telephone number is impaired by the use of different numbers in different countries. The Council of the European Communities has recommended that the number '112' should be used throughout Europe, but this has not been widely implemented, and telephone codes to summon the cardiac arrest team within hospitals have also not been standardized.

After activation of the emergency medical systems, assessment of the patient continues with **ABC** (airway, breathing, and circulation). Airway obstruction commonly results from loss of muscle tone in the tongue and jaw muscles, allowing the tongue and epiglottis to occlude the airway. In the absence of head or neck trauma, the airway should be opened using the

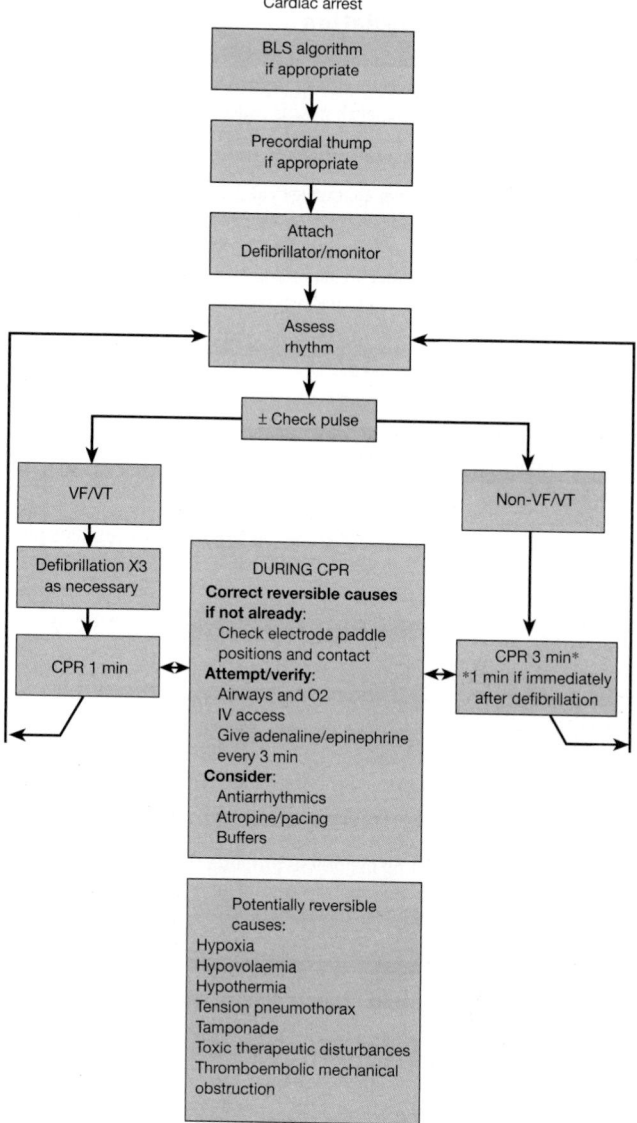

Fig. 3 European Resuscitation Council guidelines for adult advanced life support. (From Robertson C *et al.*, 1998. The 1998 European Resuscitation Council guidelines for adult advanced life support. A statement from the Working Group on Advanced Life Support, and approved by the executive committee of the European Resuscitation Council. *Resuscitation* **37**, 81–90. © ERC. Published by Elsevier Science Ireland Ltd.)

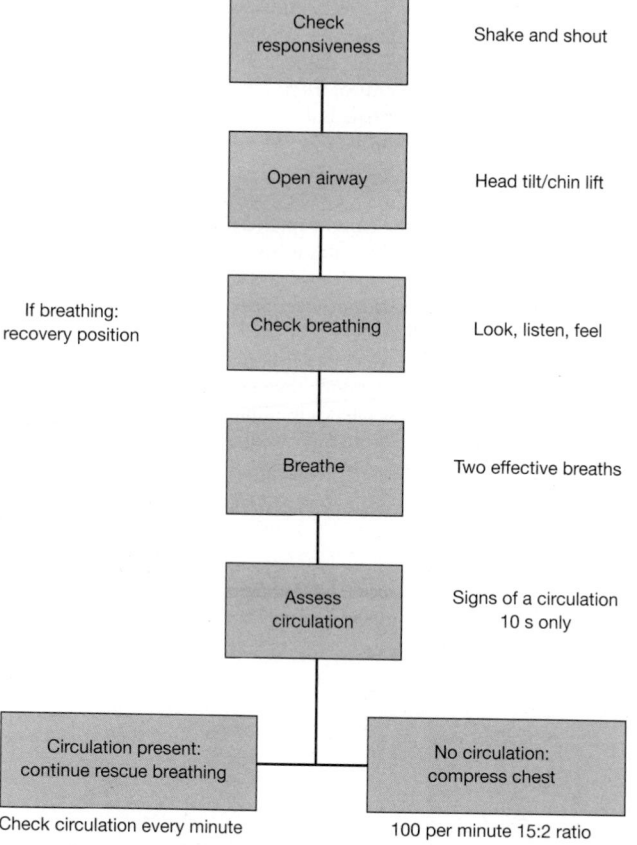

Fig. 2 European Resuscitation Council guidelines for adult basic life support. (From Handley AJ *et al.*, 1998. The 1998 European Resuscitation Council guidelines for adult single rescuer basic life support. A statement from the Working Group on Basic Life Support, and approved by the executive committee of the European Resuscitation Council. *Resuscitation* **37**, 67–80. © ERC. Published by Elsevier Science Ireland Ltd.)

head-tilt, chin-lift manoeuvre. The rescuer should then look for chest movement, listen for breath sounds, and feel for air movement on their cheek. Absence of breathing should be confirmed over 10 s. The patient should then be examined for signs of circulation for up to 10 s.

Basic life support

The objective of basic life support is to generate sufficient flow of oxygenated blood to the heart and brain until definitive therapy can be applied and spontaneous circulation re-established. Basic life support at least doubles the chances of survival if applied between the time of collapse and first defibrillation.

Mouth-to-mouth ventilation

Maintenance of the airway and ventilation may be performed concurrently using the mouth-to-mouth method. The rescuer's lips are placed around the patient's mouth and the patient's nose is sealed by pinching the nostrils together. The recommended tidal volume is 400 to 600 ml. Current recommendations are for two ventilations to 15 chest compressions. Normal expired air contains 15 to 17 per cent oxygen and 4 per cent carbon dioxide. Hyperventilation increases the oxygen concentration to 18 per cent and reduces the carbon dioxide concentration to 2 per cent. Enough oxygen can be administered in this manner to maintain an adequate arterial oxygen saturation in the early stages of cardiac arrest.

Closed-chest compression

Closed-chest compressions are performed by placing the heel of one hand over the lower sternum, two fingerbreadths from the xiphisternal junction. The heel of the second hand is placed over the first. The sternum is compressed 4 to 5 cm in the adult, maintaining compression for 50 per cent of the compression–relaxation cycle. The rate should be 100 compressions per minute. Properly performed closed-chest compressions can produce peak systolic arterial pressures of 60 to 80 mmHg, but diastolic arterial pressure and coronary perfusion pressure fall rapidly after the first few minutes. Cardiac output during closed-chest compression ranges from a quarter to a third of normal.

The mechanism leading to blood flow during closed-chest compressions is still debated. The cardiac pump hypothesis proposes that direct compression of the heart between the sternum and the paraspinal structures results in ejection of blood. The aortic and pulmonary valves open during compression, whilst closure of the mitral and tricuspid valves prevents regurgitation of blood. As compression is released, intracardiac pressures fall and the mitral and tricuspid valves open, promoting ventricular filling. In contrast, the thoracic pump hypothesis proposes that the entire thorax is the pump, with the heart being a passive conduit and the pulmonary vascular bed acting as a reservoir for blood. This theory is supported by the finding that patients in cardiac arrest can maintain prolonged consciousness by forceful coughing. Coughing increases intrathoracic pressure which results in antegrade blood flow. Also favouring this theory are studies showing no significant reduction in left ventricular dimensions and patent heart valves, during closed-chest compression.

The major complication from closed-chest compression is trauma. Rib and sternal fractures occur in up to 30 per cent of patients, even with well-trained rescuers. Incorrectly performed compressions may injure the thoracic or abdominal contents.

Adjuncts to standard CPR

The airway may be maintained using either nasopharyngeal or oropharangeal airways. These hold the base of the tongue away from the posterior pharynx. Pocket masks for mouth-to-mask ventilation reduce possible spread of pathogens and can incorporate supplementary oxygen. Bag–valve–mask devices with a reservoir bag can deliver an inspired oxygen concentration of over 90 per cent.

Alternative methods of closed-chest compression

The poor survival rate following closed-chest compression has driven the search for more effective methods. Interposed abdominal counterpulsation aims to increase venous return to the heart prior to chest compression. Active compression–decompression CPR uses a device applied to the chest wall to reduce intrathoracic pressure and increase venous return during decompression. Vest CPR uses a circumferential vest around the thorax. Sequential inflation and deflation alters intrathoracic pressure resulting in blood flow. Although promising in animal trials and limited human studies, no survival benefit has been seen in larger studies for any of these methods.

Open-chest cardiac massage

The ease of closed-chest compression led to it quickly supplanting open-chest cardiac massage without trials to demonstrate its superiority. Experimental evidence, coupled with reports of patient survival using open-chest cardiac massage after prolonged periods of unsuccessful closed-chest compression, have led to a resurgence of interest in the open-chest method. The American Heart Association recommends open-chest cardiac massage for cardiac arrest associated with penetrating trauma, hypothermia, pulmonary embolus, pericardial tamponade, abdominal haemorrhage, or where chest or vertebral anomalies prevent effective closed-chest compression.

Advanced life support

Defibrillation

The majority of survivors of cardiac arrest are in VF/VT. Defibrillation is the only effective method of terminating these rhythms and its effectiveness falls rapidly with time (Fig. 4). Over 80 per cent of patients successfully resuscitated from VF/VT are resuscitated by one of the first three shocks. A precordial thump may terminate VF/VT and should be considered for witnessed arrests when a defibrillator is not immediately available.

Mechanism of defibrillation

The mechanism of defibrillation is unknown. The critical mass hypothesis suggests that defibrillation occurs when sufficient current passes through the heart to depolarize approximately 75 per cent of the myocardium. This causes arrest of the activating wave and allows a normal rhythm to be re-established. The upper limit of vulnerability theory proposes that fibrillation terminates only when the strength of shock is greater than the threshold limit for the whole myocardium. Sub-threshold shocks induce refractoriness in susceptible tissue but lead to new activation waveforms from regions excited by the shock. This second theory is supported by the finding of a period of electrical silence after a countershock, followed by resumption of fibrillation with a different morphology.

As little as 4 per cent of the current applied using external defibrillation actually crosses the heart. The current applied depends on the energy selected and the impedance of the thorax. Transthoracic impedance is altered by electrode size, the use of couplants (usually preformed gel pads) between electrodes and chest wall, multiple shocks, the phase of respiration, and the pressure with which the electrodes are applied.

The recommended energy level for the initial shock is 200 joules. This aims to produce a high success rate whilst minimizing the risk of damage to the heart. If a second shock is required it should also be 200 J. Transthoracic

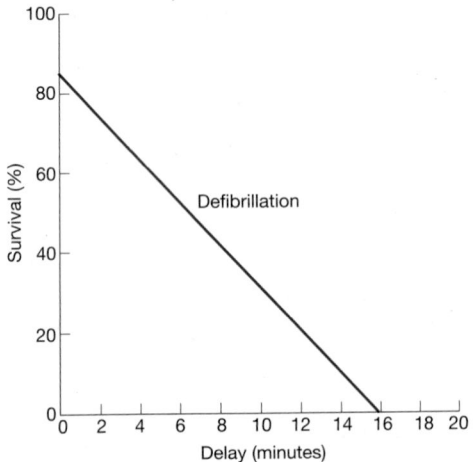

Fig. 4 Effect of time on success of defibrillation. (From Colquhoun MC, Handley AJ, Evans TR, 1998. *ABC of resuscitation*, 3rd edn. © BMJ Books.)

impedance reduces with successive shocks and each shock should deliver more energy to the myocardium. Subsequent shocks are delivered at 360 J, which is the maximum available on most defibrillators. The most commonly used electrode placement is apex–anterior with one placed to the right of the upper sternum below the clavicle, and the other over the apex of the heart. Alternative placements may result in successful defibrillation in some patients.

Current-based defibrillation uses a microprocessor to measure transthoracic impedance. The operator selects the required current and the defibrillator charges a capacitor to the energy required to deliver that current. Using biphasic waveforms rather than the standard damped sinusoidal waveform may reduce energy requirements. Both of these methods have shown promise in early clinical trials.

Automated external defibrillators

It is important that the first responder at a cardiac arrest can defibrillate. Even small reductions in the time to first shock can dramatically improve survival. Interpretation of ECG rhythms is difficult even for medical professionals and can delay defibrillation. Automated external defibrillators are capable of analysing the ECG rhythm and advise that a countershock be given if VF is present. Fully automated machines deliver the shock after offering an audible warning. By simplifying the training required, they may be used by a wide range of non-medical personnel.

Early advanced care

Advanced care is required if CPR and defibrillation fail to achieve or sustain a spontaneous circulation.

Advanced airway support

Endotracheal intubation remains the gold standard of airway management. Intubation maintains and protects the airway, permits administration of additional oxygen and certain drugs, and allows adjustment of ventilation. Successful intubation requires a high level of skill and regular practice. Laryngeal mask airways are commonly used in anaesthesia and increasingly for airway management during cardiac arrest. Their use requires a lower level of training than does intubation.

Drug therapy

Peripheral venous cannulation is the quickest method of administering medication during cardiac arrest. Peak drug levels are lower and circulation times are longer using peripheral rather than central routes. If there is delay in obtaining venous access, adrenaline, atropine, and lignocaine may be administered via the endotracheal tube. They should be given at 2 to 3 times the normal intravenous dose and diluted in 10 ml of normal saline. Drug absorption and pharmacodynamics are less predictable when given via the endotracheal route.

Vasopressors

Adrenaline has not been proved to improve survival from cardiac arrest. The standard dose of 1 mg originates from studies using 0.1 mg/kg in 10 kg dogs. This was translated into human use without evidence of comparable efficacy. In a dose range of 0.045 to 0.2 mg/kg (3 to 14 mg in a 70 kg man), adrenaline improves the arterial pressures generated during CPR and increases myocardial and cerebral blood flow. High-dose adrenaline has failed to show any survival benefit compared with standard dosage. Currently, the majority of studies support the use of adrenaline for patients who remain in cardiac arrest after CPR and defibrillation.

No other adrenergic agonist has been shown to have advantages over adrenaline in the treatment of cardiac arrest. The vasoconstrictor vasopressin has been used in limited clinical trials with encouraging results.

Antiarrhythmics

The advantage of routine use of antiarrhythmics in cardiac arrest is unproved. Although bretylium and lignocaine are effective in suppressing arrhythmias after myocardial infarction, they have not shown clear benefit in the setting of cardiac arrest. Amiodarone has been used in trials of persistent ventricular arrhythmias with reported improvement. Magnesium sulphate is the treatment of choice for torsade de pointes. Empirical magnesium supplementation has not, however, been shown to be of benefit in cardiac arrest.

Atropine is of value in haemodynamically compromising bradycardia, but the recommendation for its use in asystole is based on limited data. It is hypothesized that excessive vagal tone may inhibit cardiac action. Small-scale studies suggest that atropine has a favourable effect on cardiac rhythm.

Buffers

Cardiac arrest causes a mixed respiratory and metabolic acidosis due to retention of carbon dioxide and lactic acid. Low blood flow during CPR often causes differences between venous and arterial samples with a mixed venous acidosis despite arterial hypocarbic alkalosis. No clinical data support correction of the acidosis by means other than adequate ventilation and tissue perfusion. Addition of bicarbonate causes further increases in venous carbon dioxide and venous respiratory acidosis. Sodium bicarbonate also has the theoretical disadvantages of hyperosmolarity and hypernatraemia. Alternative buffering agents have shown no benefit. Buffers remain of use in cases of cardiac arrest associated with tricyclic antidepressant overdose and pre-existing metabolic acidosis.

Pacing

External pacing of asystole may be beneficial in the small group of patients who arrest shortly before pacing is instituted. For the majority, application of external pacing is too late.

Post-resuscitation care

Following return of spontaneous circulation the cause of the cardiac arrest should be ascertained and tissue perfusion optimized. Emergency thrombolysis or angioplasty may offer benefit for patients with acute myocardial infarction. Prolonged coma following resuscitation is associated with poor outcome. Neurological assessment after 72 h can predict the likelihood of long-term survival. Trials to evaluate treatment that might reduce cerebral damage have been disappointing. Myocardial dysfunction accounts for the majority of early deaths after return of spontaneous circulation. The only method of minimizing post-resuscitation sequelae is to strengthen the chain of survival.

Training in life support measures

Most sudden cardiac arrests occur in the community. For these patients, the highest rates of survival have been achieved when CPR is initiated within 4 min. Well-performed basic life support is more successful than poorly performed basic life support, and some basic life support is better than none. Training in the technique is well established in many communities. The use of automated external defibrillators is now included in the American Heart Association basic life support programme.

Ethics of resuscitation

When resuscitation is not attempted, death is virtually inevitable. Only with evidence that resuscitation is not indicated should it be omitted.

Advanced directives or living wills are becoming more common, especially in the United States. These convey the patients' wishes with respect to specific treatments when they are unconscious or incapacitated. If possible, decisions not to attempt resuscitation (DNR orders) should be made after discussion with the patient. If the patient is not competent to make the decision, factors to be considered include the quality of life prior to the illness, the expected quality of life assuming recovery, and the likelihood of successful resuscitation.

Although doctors are not required to offer a treatment if it is deemed futile, determinations of futility vary greatly between physicians. Resuscitation has been deemed futile for the following reasons.

1. An adequate trial of basic and advanced life support has already been attempted without return of spontaneous circulation.

2. No physiological benefit from basic or advanced life support can be expected because the patient's vital functions are deteriorating despite maximum therapy.

3. No survivors after cardiopulmonary resuscitation have been reported under the given circumstances.

The presence of sepsis, disseminated cancer, or major organ failure is associated with very poor outcome. Lower survival rates in the elderly result from a higher presence of comorbidity rather than from age itself. In practice, doctors must determine the merit of attempting CPR for each patient. If resuscitation is attempted but return of spontaneous circulation does not occur promptly, consideration must be given to termination of the attempt. This decision depends on a number of factors in addition to those cited above.

1. Time intervals to initiation of basic life support and defibrillation—delays of over 5 min to basic life support or 30 min to defibrillation are associated with extremely poor prognosis.

2. Evidence of cardiac activity—termination of resuscitation effort after 15 to 20 min has been suggested for non-VF/VT arrests.

3. Protective factors—hypothermia or ingestion of sedatives, hypnotics, or narcotics confer a measure of protection from the sequelae of cardiac arrest.

Relatives and resuscitation

The presence of relatives in the resuscitation room remains controversial. Whilst common in paediatric practice it is not routine in adult cardiac arrest. However, if properly managed witnessing resuscitation does no harm and probably aids the grieving process should the patient not survive.

Practical skill training using the recently dead

Mannikins have largely replaced the use of the recently dead for training in the practical skills used in resuscitation.

Future developments

End-tidal carbon dioxide levels (ET_{CO_2})

ET_{CO_2} meters are widely used to confirm correct endotracheal tube placement. During cardiac arrest, ET_{CO_2} levels depend primarily on the cardiac output generated by resuscitation. A value of 10 mmHg at 20 min can distinguish patients who may survive from ones who will not. Use of ET_{CO_2} may clarify when resuscitation attempts can be deemed futile.

Invasive support

Cardiopulmonary bypass

Whilst cardiopulmonary bypass is a proven treatment for cardiac arrest associated with hypothermia, its role in routine arrests is likely to be limited by cost as well as the time required to achieve bypass.

Minimally invasive direct cardiac massage

In this technique a plunger device is placed directly on to the pericardium via a small thoracotomy. Manual compression of the ventricles provides an artificial circulation.

Anstadt cup

This is a biventricular assist device placed around the heart. Its role is limited by the requirement for significant surgical skill and equipment.

Retroaortic perfusion

This involves insertion of an aortic occlusion balloon into the descending aorta and infusion of oxygenated blood or blood substitutes into the proximal aorta.

Further reading

Advanced Life Support Working Group of the International Liaison Committee on Resuscitation (1997). Early defibrillation. An advisory statement by the Advanced Life Support Working Group of the International Liaison Committee on Resuscitation. *Resuscitation* **34**, 113–15.

Becker LB (1996). The epidemiology of sudden death. In: Paradis NA, Halperin HR, Nowak RM, eds. *Cardiac arrest: the science and practice of resuscitation medicine*, pp 28–47. Williams & Wilkins, Baltimore.

British Medical Association (1993). Decisions related to cardiopulmonary resuscitation. A statement from the BMA and RCN in association with the Resuscitation Council (UK). BMA, London.

Handley AJ *et al.* (1998). The 1998 European Resuscitation Council guidelines for adult single rescuer basic life support. A statement from the Working Group on Basic Life Support, and approved by the executive committee of the European Resuscitation Council. *Resuscitation* **37**, 67–80.

Paradis NA *et al.* (1989). Simultaneous aortic, jugular bulb, and right atrial pressures during cardiopulmonary resuscitation in humans: insights into mechanisms. *Circulation* **80**, 361–8.

Paradis NA *et al.* (1990). Coronary perfusion pressure and the return of spontaneous circulation in human cardiopulmonary resuscitation. *Journal of the American Medical Association* **263**, 1106–13.

Robertson C *et al.* (1998). The 1998 European Resuscitation Council guidelines for adult advanced life support. A statement from the Working Group on Advanced Life Support, and approved by the executive committee of the European Resuscitation Council. *Resuscitation* **37**, 81–90.

16.4 Anaphylaxis

Anthony F. T. Brown

Introduction

The term anaphylaxis was introduced by Richet and Portier in 1902, literally meaning 'against protection'. It is currently used to describe the rapid, generalized, and often unheralded IgE immunologically mediated events that follow exposure to some foreign substances in those who have previously been sensitized. An identical clinical syndrome involving release of similar potent mediators but not triggered by IgE, and thus not necessarily requiring previous exposure, is termed an anaphylactoid reaction. Despite aetiological differences of vital importance to subsequent follow-up and prevention, the clinical term anaphylaxis is often used to describe both of these syndromes (as in this chapter).

Anaphylaxis is potentially the most severe of the immediate-type hypersensitivity reactions. It is the quintessential medical emergency that may be mild or severe, gradual in onset or fulminant, involve multiple organ systems or cause isolated wheeze or shock. It often occurs without warning in otherwise healthy people, and since there is no immediate confirmatory laboratory test it mandates prompt clinical recognition and treatment to prevent death from hypoxia or hypotension in severe cases.

Epidemiology

The true incidence and prevalence of anaphylaxis are unknown. The literature is heterogeneous, retrospective, and utilizes variable definitions. Emergency department presentations range from 1 in 440 to 1 in 1500 attendances, representing an incidence from 1 per 3400 to 1 per 10 000 catchment population per year. Hospital discharge data suggest 10 per 100 000 admissions are due to anaphylaxis. No age, sex, race, or locality is exempt, with cases occurring from infancy to old age.

Atopy increases the risk of idiopathic anaphylaxis and that caused by ingested antigens, latex, radiocontrast media, and exercise. Asthma increases the risk of dying from anaphylaxis. Patients taking β-blocking drugs develop more severe reactions which may be resistant to therapy, and those taking angiotensin-converting enzyme (ACE) inhibitor drugs are particularly prone to angioedema that can be life threatening. The newer angiotensin-II receptor antagonists cause fewer reactions but are also implicated.

Deaths from anaphylaxis are rare, although penicillins, hymenopteran stings, and radiocontrast media account for the majority.

Aetiology

IgE-mediated anaphylaxis

A vast array of IgE immune-mediated triggers are recognized (Table 1), the most important being β-lactam antibiotics including the penicillins and cephalosporins, hymenopteran stings such as wasps and bees, and foods.

Antibiotics

Penicillins are the most common cause of anaphylaxis in adults, occurring after 1 in 5000 parenteral doses, and are the most frequent cause of death. True cross-sensitivity to the cephalosporins is considerably less than 10 per cent and largely confined to the first-generation cephalosporins. Fatalities to oral penicillins are exceedingly rare.

Hymenoptera

Reactions to hymenopteran venom, such as from wasps, bees, hornets, and fire ants, are second only to antibiotics in frequency, occurring in up to 3 per cent of the population. Large local reactions, toxic reactions, and late serum sickness-like, non-IgE reactions may also occur following a sting.

Foods

Peanuts, other legumes, true nuts, shellfish, milk, and eggs cause the largest number of food-related cases, particularly in children. Reactions occur rapidly and may recur several hours later (biphasic reaction). Cross-reactivity to seemingly unrelated plants is seen. Mislabelling and contamination at the manufacturing stage or in the home cause inadvertent exposure.

Latex

Allergy to latex (rubber) is seen particularly in hospital personnel, children with spina bifida and genitourinary abnormalities, and in workers with occupational exposure. It may occur by contact, parenteral administration, and aerosol transmission and is one cause of perioperative anaphylaxis,

Table 1 Causes of IgE antibody formation

Drugs:	
Proteins	Insulin (bovine > porcine > human), vasopressin, parathormone
Non-protein (haptens)	Penicillins, cephalosporins, sulphonamides, muscle relaxants, local anaesthetics, thiamine, folic acid
Foods	Peanuts, other legumes, true nuts, fish, shellfish, milk, eggs, chocolate
Venoms	Wasp, hornet, bee, fire ant, ticks, reduvid bugs, snakes, scorpions
Vaccine and foreign protein agents	Influenza, yellow fever, tetanus toxoid, gammaglobulin, protamine, venom antitoxin, semen
Enzymes and chemicals	Trypsin, chymopapain, streptokinase, penicillinase, formaldehyde, ethylene oxide
Environmental	Pollen, mould, animal dander, hydatid cyst rupture
Latex	

Note: Cross-reactivity may occur, such as to egg protein in avian-based vaccines, or to certain foods with latex allergy.

Table 2 Causes of anaphylactoid reactions

Complement activation—classic pathway or alternate pathway	Blood transfusion including IgG anti-IgA immune complex formation, albumin, radiocontrast media, dialysis membranes, protamine, hereditary and acquired angioedema
Kinin production or potentiation; coagulation/fibrinolysis system activation	ACE inhibitors, radiocontrast media, plasma protein fraction
Direct pharmacological release of mediators:	
Histamine release	Opiates, radiocontrast media, Haemaccel, N-acetylcysteine, muscle relaxants, fluorescein, mannitol, protamine, vancomycin, progesterone
Modulators of arachidonic acid metabolism	Aspirin, NSAIDs
Sulphiting agents	Metabisulphite
Exercise induced	With or without prior foods or NSAIDs
Idiopathic	

Note: Multiple mechanisms may coexist, such as with radiocontrast media and protamine.

along with thiopentone, neuromuscular blocking drugs, antibiotics, protamine, and anaphylactoid reactions to opiates, colloids, or blood.

Non-immune, anaphylactoid reactions

Various less well understood, non-immunological mechanisms lead to the release of similar inflammatory mediators in anaphylactoid reactions. Agents responsible include aspirin, non-steroidal anti-inflammatory drugs (**NSAIDs**), radiocontrast media, and opiates, and in the case of infusions may relate to their rate, concentration, and volume delivered (see Table 2).

Radiocontrast media

These were the most common cause of anaphylactoid reactions, but the incidence has declined to less than 1 in 200 patients receiving the newer low osmolality, non-ionic agents. Asthma, atopy, and patients on β-blockers or with prior reactions are at greatest risk.

Aspirin and NSAIDs

Bronchospasm following these is common in patients with nasal polyps and reactive airway disease, but systemic anaphylactoid reactions may occur in their absence following cyclo-oxygenase inhibition. Cross-reactivity occurs between different NSAIDs and rare reactions have occurred to the newer COX-II (cyclo-oxygenase II) inhibitors.

Pathogenesis

Irrespective of the triggering event, two main groups of mediators are released by mast cells and basophils. These groups include the preformed, granule-associated mediators histamine, neutrophil and eosinophil chemotactic factors, enzymes such as tryptase and β-glucuronidase, and proteoglycans such as heparin. They also include newly synthesized mediators from arachidonic acid metabolism via the cyclo-oxygenase pathway, such as prostaglandin D_2 and thromboxane A_2, and via the lipoxygenase pathway, such as the leukotrienes. In addition, platelet-activating factor and cytokines such as the interleukins are also rapidly formed.

All these mediators act by inducing vasodilatation, increasing capillary permeability and glandular secretion, causing smooth muscle spasm (including bronchoconstriction), and by attracting new cells to the area (see Chapter 5.2 for further discussion).

Clinical features

Anaphylaxis is typically a disease of those who are fit and is rarely seen or described in patients who are critically ill or shocked other than those suffering from asthma. The speed of onset of symptoms and signs is related to the severity of the process, with life-threatening reactions occurring in minutes to parenteral antigen exposure, although deaths have been associated with oral, topical, or cutaneous triggers. Most symptoms occur within 30 min, but may be delayed for some hours, particularly following oral or topical exposure.

Over half the deaths from anaphylaxis occur within the first hour of onset. Seventy five per cent result from asphyxia due to upper airway oedema and hypoxia from severe bronchospasm. The remaining 25 per cent are due to circulatory failure with shock related to vasodilatation and hypovolaemia from plasma volume losses, cardiac arrhythmias, pulmonary hypertension, and (possibly) decreased myocardial activity in the absence of cardiac disease.

Ninety five per cent of patients have cutaneous features, but these can sometimes be absent, particularly in cases presenting with the rapid onset of laryngeal oedema or circulatory shock, or resolve spontaneously or in response to prehospital treatment.

Cutaneous features

A premonitory aura, tingling, or warm sensation may precede generalized erythema, urticaria with pruritus, local oedema or angioedema, and occasionally pallor. Rhinitis and conjunctivitis are also seen.

Respiratory system features

Sudden cough, hoarseness, throat tightness, or the sensation of a 'lump' may precede shortness of breath, dyspnoea, stridor, wheeze, and cyanosis due to oropharyngeal or laryngeal oedema and bronchospasm.

Cardiovascular and neurological features

Apprehension, light-headedness, dizziness, or syncope may precede or accompany cardiovascular collapse with tachycardia, hypotension, and cardiac arrhythmias. Hypoxia, hypoperfusion, and the direct effect of mediators lead to incontinence, confusion or coma, and myocardial or cerebral ischaemia or infarction.

Gastrointestinal and miscellaneous features

Cramping abdominal pain, nausea, vomiting, and diarrhoea are common, but the more obviously life-threatening features described above usually overshadow these gastrointestinal manifestations. In rare instances there may be back pain, watery vaginal discharge, pulmonary oedema, and even disseminated intravascular coagulation.

Differential diagnosis

The protean manifestations of anaphylaxis allow a potentially vast differential diagnosis, although the rapid onset, accompanying cutaneous feature, and relationship to a potential trigger suggest the diagnosis of anaphylaxis in most cases. However, the following alternative diagnoses may be considered.

Facial swelling or oedema

These may result from bacterial or viral infection, although fever and pain should predominate. Traumatic or spontaneous bleeding, particularly in patients on warfarin, usually causes recognizable bruising.

Wheeze and difficulty breathing

Bronchial asthma, cardiogenic pulmonary oedema, foreign body inhalation, irritant chemical exposure, and tension pneumothorax should be distinguished on the basis of associated presenting features.

Light-headedness and syncope

A vasovagal reaction must be considered in the context of a painful procedure such as an injection or local anaesthetic infiltration: bradycardia, pallor, and rapid response to a recumbent position are usual. Panic attacks are common in allergic patients confronted by an unexpected, potential allergen exposure.

Angioedema

Angioedema in the absence of urticaria may be caused by actual or functional C_1 esterase inhibitor deficiency. This may be hereditary with autosomal dominant inheritance or acquired related to lymphoproliferative disorders. A family history, the absence of pruritus, prominence of abdominal symptoms, and recurrent attacks suggest the hereditary cause. C_1 esterase inhibitor concentrate or fresh frozen plasma is used to treat recalcitrant cases.

Investigation

The diagnosis of anaphylaxis is clinical. No immediate laboratory or radiological tests confirm the process and investigation must not delay immediate management.

Disease progress may be monitored by pulse oximetry, arterial blood gases (looking for metabolic or respiratory acidosis), haematocrit level (may rise with extravasation of fluid), and measurement of electrolytes and renal function. These tests together with blood glucose level, chest radiograph, and ECG are necessary if there is a slow response to therapy or when there is doubt about the diagnosis.

Mast cell tryptase

The only direct marker of mast cell activation is an elevated serum tryptase level. Tryptase is released in both anaphylactic and anaphylactoid reactions, beginning to rise within 30 min and remaining high for up to 6 h. It is of value when the diagnosis of anaphylaxis is uncertain clinically, particularly during anaesthesia, and may also be useful after death. Frozen serum specimens must be sent to a specialist laboratory.

Management

Patients with anaphylaxis may present directly to their family doctor or to the emergency department, or the reaction may start in hospital in the radiology department, theatre, on the ward, or even in the outpatient department. Cutaneous features of generalized mediator release may be the first signal, followed by more serious systemic symptoms or signs.

Any causative agent, such as an intravenous drug or infusion, must be stopped immediately. The patient should initially be managed in a monitored resuscitation area, or equipment including at least a pulse oximeter, non-invasive blood pressure device, and ECG monitor brought to them.

After a brief history of possible allergen exposure is obtained, a rapid assessment of the extent and severity of the reaction must be made, particularly looking for upper and lower respiratory tract involvement and the early signs of shock.

Oxygen, adrenaline, and fluids are the mainstay of treatment, with antihistamines and steroids only utilized as second-line agents once the cardiorespiratory status has been stabilized (see Tables 3 and 4). A more detailed exposure history may be taken at this time.

Table 3 First-line therapy for anaphylaxis

Oxygen:	Via face mask with reservoir bag; rarely endotracheal intubation or surgical airway
Adrenaline:	
Early, mild, or progressing slowly, difficult venous access, or unmonitored patient:	0.3 to 0.5 mg (0.3 to 0.5 ml of 1:1000) adrenaline intramuscularly, repeated every 5 to 10 min according to the response
Stridor or severe wheeze, whilst preparing intravenous dose:	1 to 4 mg (1 to 4 ml of 1:1000) adrenaline nebulized with oxygen
Shock, severe dyspnoea, airway compromise, or deteriorating patient:	0.75 to 1.5 µg/kg of 1:100 000 adrenaline intravenously * at 10 to 20 µg/min (1 to 2 ml/min) initially, repeated as necessary (must have ECG monitored)
Colloid:	10 to 20 ml/kg for shock

* 1:100 000 adrenaline preparation: Draw up 1 mg of adrenaline (1 ml of 1:1000) in a 20 ml syringe and add 9 ml of saline to give a total volume of 10 ml. Discard all but 2 ml (leaving 200 µg of adrenaline in the syringe), then draw up further saline to a total volume of 20 ml, giving a final concentration of 10 µg/ml.

First-line treatment

Oxygen and airway patency

Oxygen by face mask should be given to all patients, aiming to maintain an oxygen saturation above 92 per cent. Allow the patient to remain upright unless shocked, and call urgently for experienced anaesthetic help if there are signs of impending airway obstruction such as worsening hoarseness or stridor, or rapidly progressive respiratory failure with tachypnoea and wheeze. Cyanosis and exhaustion indicate imminent respiratory arrest, but sedative or muscle relaxant drugs should not be given unless the physician is competent in the management of a difficult airway, since endotracheal intubation and mechanical ventilation may be extremely difficult. As a last resort, a surgical airway via the cricothyroid membrane should be established before hypoxic cardiac arrest occurs.

Adrenaline

Adrenaline is the drug of choice and should be given in all but the most trivial cases, particularly to patients with airway swelling, bronchospasm,

Table 4 Second-line therapy for anaphylaxis (restore cardiorespiratory stability first with oxygen, adrenaline, and fluids)

Antihistamines:
H_1-blocker, such as chlorpheniramine at 10 to 20 mg intravenously (maximum 40 mg/day) or promethazine at 12.5 to 25 mg intravenously 8-hourly
plus
H_2-blocker, such as ranitidine at 50 mg intravenously 8-hourly
Change to orally when patient tolerates it (chlorpheniramine at 4 mg 6-hourly or promethazine at 10 mg 8-hourly *plus* ranitidine at 150 mg 12-hourly)
Steroids (definitely for severe bronchospasm):
Hydrocortisone at 5 mg/kg intravenously, then 2.5 mg/kg intravenously 6-hourly
Change to orally when patient tolerates it (prednisolone at 40 to 50 mg/day)
Salbutamol (bronchospasm):
5 mg via oxygen-driven nebulizer
Glucagon (if patient on β-blocker):
1 mg intravenously every 5 min, then infusion at 5 to 15 µg/min
Aminophylline (refractory bronchospasm):
5 mg/kg intravenously over 30 min as loading dose, then infusion at 0.5 mg/kg per hour

Note: On discharge, give oral H_1- plus H_2-blockers and steroids as above for 2 to 3 days.

or hypotension. It has beneficial α-, β₁-, and β₂-adrenergic effects, including a rise in intracellular cyclic AMP that inhibits further mast cell and basophil mediator release.

When anaphylaxis is treated early, is mild or progressing slowly, if venous access is difficult or delayed, or in an unmonitored patient, give 0.3 to 0.5 ml of 1:1000 adrenaline (0.3 to 0.5 mg) intramuscularly in adults. This has advantages in terms of safety and is usually rapidly effective. The dose may be repeated every 5 to 10 min or longer according to response, and is preferred to the subcutaneous route.

However, in serious or quickly progressing cases, particularly in the presence of vascular collapse and shock, marked airway compromise, or severe bronchospasm, intravenous adrenaline is essential to achieve more rapid and reliable delivery. Although 1:10 000 adrenaline containing 100 µg/ml is readily available, for instance as the Min-I-Jet preparation, it is difficult to give this slowly in small quantities titrated to response. An alternative is to prepare a 1:100 000 dilution containing 10 µg/ml, and to give 1 to 2 ml (10 to 20 µg) per minute at an initial dose of 0.75 to 1.5 µg/kg (see Table 3). Intravenous adrenaline must only be given under ECG control in a monitored resuscitation area by doctors experienced in its use.

Whilst parenteral adrenaline is being prepared, patients may be given nebulized 1:1000 adrenaline from 1 to 4 ml (1 to 4 mg) via an oxygen-driven system. This may dramatically improve upper airway oedema or bronchospam.

Fluids

A large-bore intravenous cannula should be inserted as soon as possible in patients with shock to administer a 10 to 20 ml/kg fluid bolus. Gelatin preparations such as Haemaccel or Gelofusine are best, although normal saline in larger quantities is suitable and there are no outcome data favouring one infusion over another. Further fluid boluses are indicated by the clinical response, although it is important to give adrenaline in addition.

Second-line treatment

Once the cardiorespiratory status and tissue oxygenation have been improved with oxygen, adrenaline, and fluids, other drugs may be given in a supporting role.

Antihistamines

Although popular, antihistamines must never be relied upon as sole therapy. They are only indicated: when the reaction is not life threatening; when it is progressing slowly with predominant cutaneous features such as angioedema and urticaria; to prevent later recrudescence of symptoms or signs; as pretreatment to prevent reactions to radiocontrast media or volume expanders; and finally as prophylaxis during anaesthesia.

Newer, second-generation 'non-sedating' H₁-antihistamines such as loratadine and cetirizine are available orally, but still may cross the blood–brain barrier to cause drowsiness, particularly with alcohol. H₂-antihistamines have been used successfully in protracted anaphylaxis with shock, and increasingly now in combination with H₁-antihistamines. H₁- and H₂-antihistamines given together are supported by improved outcome in both prevention and treatment of acute anaphylaxis, combined with steroids in some instances.

Steroids

Steroids are of limited value despite many theoretical beneficial effects on mediator release and tissue responsiveness. They may prevent or shorten protracted reactions, particularly those associated with bronchospasm, and may reduce the likelihood of relapse of symptoms, particularly after discharge. They are, however, essential in the management of recurrent idiopathic anaphylaxis.

Salbutamol, aminophylline, and glucagon

Nebulized salbutamol may be given for bronchospasm and has the advantage of familiarity. Aminophylline intravenously has additive effects to adrenaline in refractory bronchospasm. Glucagon may be used, particularly in patients already taking β-blockers, who at the same time may be both therapeutically resistant yet overly sensitive to unopposed α-mediated effects of adrenaline.

Admission, observation, and follow-up

Patients with cutaneous features alone who remain well may be discharged after a short 3- to 4-h period of observation, dependent on the nature and time of the suspected allergen exposure and their response to treatment.

Patients with significant systemic anaphylactic reactions, including all those receiving adrenaline, must be observed for a minimum of 6 to 8 h after apparent full recovery, as late deterioration may occur in 1 to 5 per cent of cases (biphasic response).

Those patients with unstable vital signs or with protracted or resistant anaphylaxis should remain monitored and be admitted to an intensive care area. An adrenaline infusion at 1 to 10 µg/min may be needed as a temporizing measure, and can be given by adding 1 ml of 1:1000 adrenaline to 100 ml of normal saline and infusing this at 6 to 60 ml/h.

Discharge medication

Following a successful period of observation, patients discharged from the emergency or outpatient department should be given combined oral H₁-and H₂-antihistamines and steroids for 2 to 3 days, such as chlorphenir-amine at 4 mg 6-hourly, ranitidine at 150 mg 12-hourly, and prednisolone at 50 mg once daily in adults.

Patients who have had a life-threatening reaction, particularly to a food or insect sting, should also be prescribed a self-administered adrenaline syringe. Several devices are available, including the EpiPen that delivers 300 µg intramuscularly via a pressure-activated, spring-loaded needle, or the EpiPen Jr delivering 150 µg. It is essential that the patient and their immediate family are taught how and when to use the device before they are discharged from hospital, and appropriate early follow-up with an allergy specialist must be arranged.

Allergy referral

All patients who have suffered a severe anaphylactic reaction and those with significant attacks, particularly if they are recurrent or the stimulus is unknown or unavoidable, should be referred to an allergy specialist. This must include all those prescribed an EpiPen, and patients suitable for immunotherapy following a wasp or bee sting. Expert knowledge is required to determine whether skin testing, *in vitro* IgE tests, and/or challenge tests should be used to confirm the suspected cause.

A detailed letter of the nature and circumstances of the anaphylactic reaction, the treatment given, and the suspected causative agent(s) should accompany the patient home. If the cause of the reaction was unclear, ask the patient to write a brief diary of events of the immediate 6 to 12 h preceding the reaction, including all foods ingested, drugs taken (including non-proprietary), cosmetics used, and so on, and all activities performed outside as well as indoors. Later recall of events will be flawed unless documented.

Prevention

Education

Patient education about the nature and cause of the reaction and the relevance of carrying an EpiPen is fundamental. Individualized antigen elimination measures must be carefully explained, including hymenopteran avoidance, and recognizing hidden or unexpected sources of antigen such as salicylate in over-the-counter preparations and trace food elements such as nuts, plus possible cross-reactions to unrelated antigens. Latex-sensitive patients may require all future medical care in a latex-controlled environment.

An alert bracelet such as Medic-Alert should be worn, particularly following a severe reaction that may recur and render the patient unable to give a history. This should highlight drug or vaccine allergy to avoid inadvertent iatrogenic exposure.

Pretreatment

Pretreatment is only helpful in limited situations, for example prednisolone at 50 mg orally, with or without an antihistamine, 12 and 2 h prior to radiocontrast media in patients with asthma or those with previous reactions, and 1:1000 adrenaline at 0.25 ml subcutaneously prior to polyvalent snake antivenom. In the latter situation antihistamines are of no proven value.

Skin testing and short-term desensitization

In some clinical circumstances, such as when a penicillin is considered essential and there is a history of possible penicillin allergy, skin testing followed—if positive—by short-term desensitization over several hours with increasing doses at 15-min intervals may be instituted under strict medical control in a monitored area.

Long-term desensitization (immunotherapy)

Hyposensitization immunotherapy is principally reserved for wasp and bee allergy, as these preventable reactions may become life threatening. β-Blockade is a contraindication, and asthma or ACE inhibitor use require careful risk–benefit evaluation. Therapy needs to be continued for at least 3 to 5 years.

Drug avoidance

Wherever possible give therapy orally, and if intravenous use is chosen, always administer a drug slowly. Avoid drugs known to predispose to reactions, particularly aspirin and NSAIDs, as well as β-blockers and ACE inhibitors. Patients at risk of anaphylaxis with hypertension or ischaemic heart disease should ideally be taken off β-blockers, and care taken not to substitute an ACE inhibitor.

Conclusion

Anaphylaxis is a common clinical and diagnostic challenge for physicians. Prompt treatment with oxygen, adrenaline, and fluids to restore cardiorespiratory stability is followed with second-line therapy such as antihistamines and steroids. Proactive discharge planning with allergy referral when appropriate protects against further unheralded or potentially avoidable attacks.

Further reading

Bochner BS, Lichtenstein LM (1991). Anaphylaxis. *New England Journal of Medicine* **324**, 1785–91.

Brown AFT (1998). Therapeutic controversies in the management of acute anaphylaxis. *Journal of Accident and Emergency Medicine* **15**, 89–95.

Fan HW *et al.* (1999). Sequential randomised and double blind trial of promethazine prophylaxis against early anaphylactic reactions to antivenom for bothrops snake bites. *British Medical Journal* **318**, 1451–3.

Hollingsworth HM, Giansiracusa DF, Upchurch KS (1991). Anaphylaxis. *Journal of Intensive Care Medicine* **6**, 55–70.

Joint Task Force on Practice Parameters (1998). The diagnosis and management of anaphylaxis. *Journal of Allergy and Clinical Immunology* **101**, S465–S528.

Krause RS. Anaphylaxis. http://www.emedicine.com/emerg/topic25.htm (accessed Aug 7th, 2001).

Lin RY *et al.* (2000). Improved outcomes in patients with acute allergic syndromes who are treated with combined H$_1$ and H$_2$ antagonists. *Annals of Emergency Medicine* **36**, 462–8.

O'Brien J, Howell JM (2000). Allergic emergencies and anaphylaxis: How to avoid getting stung. *Emergency Medicine Practice: An Evidence-Based Approach to Emergency Medicine* **2**(4), 1–20.

Premawardhena AP *et al.* (1999). Low dose subcutaneous adrenaline to prevent acute adverse reactions to antivenom serum in people bitten by snakes: randomised, placebo controlled trial. *British Medical Journal* **318**, 1041–3.

Project Team of the Resuscitation Council (UK) (1999). The emergency medical treatment of anaphylactic reactions. *Resuscitation* **41**, 93–9.

Project Team of the Resuscitation Council (UK) (2000). Update on the emergency medical treatment of anaphylactic reactions for first medical responders. *Resuscitation* **48**, 241–3.

Simons FER *et al.* (1998). Epinephrine absorption in children with a history of anaphylaxis. *Journal of Allergy and Clinical Immunology* **101**, 33–7.

16.5 Respiratory support of the critically ill

16.5.1 Pathophysiology and pathogenesis of acute respiratory distress syndrome

C. Haslett

Introduction

The acute respiratory distress syndrome (**ARDS**) is a form of acute inflammatory lung injury, initiated as part of an injurious, generalized, systemic inflammatory microvasculature response that may also result in failure of other organs (multiple organ failure). It occurs in an unpredictable fashion after a 'latent' period of several hours or days following a wide range of predisposing events, which may injure the lung directly (for instance, severe pneumonia, acid inhalation, toxic gas inhalation, near-drowning), or indirectly (for example, multiple trauma, sepsis, pancreatitis). Despite the varied causes, there appears to result a common clinical picture of non-cardiogenic alveolar oedema and a common histopathological picture of 'diffuse alveolar damage'.

Although subclinical forms of ARDS are likely to be common, many patients require mechanical ventilation. Mortality is high in this group, with around 50 per cent of patients dying, usually as a result of multiple organ failure, nosocomial infection in the injured lung, and episodes of septicaemia. The only treatment available is supportive. Recent advances in the understanding of pathophysiology, particularly in the role of inflammatory processes, leads to the hope that we will soon see novel mechanism-driven therapies that could perhaps be applied in the early stages of disease, before the full complexity of lung injury has evolved.

Pathophysiology

Oedema

Gas-dilution studies have shown that only one-third to one-half of the total lung volume is gas-filled in patients with acute lung injury. The use of computed tomography (**CT**) scanning has revealed that most of the alveolar oedema fluid is distributed to the dependent parts of the lungs. Sometimes changing the position of the patients to the prone position can improve gas exchange. Other studies have demonstrated that oedema distribution is more uniform in patients who are ventilated by high-frequency jet ventilation, suggesting that the mode of ventilation may also have an important influence on how oedema fluid is distributed.

Changes in surfactant

Other pathophysiological consequences may result from disturbance of surfactant production in acute lung injury, which is disordered both in volume and quality, perhaps the result of dysfunction of type II alveolar epithelial cells. Qualitative changes in surfactant may be sensitive markers of early alveolar injury, and in some studies surfactant alterations during the risk period and early stages of ARDS correlate with the severity of lung function changes in full-blown disease. Progressive alterations in the percentage composition of certain phospholipids during the later stages of the natural history of ARDS have been observed, but their functional significance is uncertain. Surfactant function may also be detrimentally influenced by reactive oxygen intermediates and phospholipases that are released locally by neutrophils and other inflammatory cells, and it is also likely that the high protein concentration in the inflammatory exudate markedly impairs surfactant function. These qualitative and quantitative changes in surfactant composition and adverse influences on its function undoubtedly make a major contribution to the evolution of atelactasis, the reduced functional residual capacity, reduced compliance, and increased shunt found in established ARDS.

Other changes in surfactant function may relate to other aspects of lung disease in ARDS. Little is known about alterations in the protein composition and function of surfactant in patients with ARDS. These surfactant proteins (SpA, B, C, and D) have recently been subjected to detailed study (see Chapter 17.1.3) and have been found to possess a number of properties, including bacterial opsonization, and to exert effects on inflammatory cells including macrophages. It is possible that changes in these proteins could have secondary influences, particularly on host defence in the damaged lung, which we know is particularly prone to secondary and often devastating infections with Gram-negative and other bacteria.

Pulmonary hypertension

Pulmonary hypertension is a common complication of the early stages of ARDS, contributes to the generation of alveolar oedema, and is associated with increased mortality. It probably arises as the result of the release of vasoconstrictor mediators, but in the late stages of ARDS it may occur as a result of pulmonary thromboembolism or remodelling of the injured lung. Pulmonary hypertension may contribute to right ventricular dysfunction, although poorly characterized circulating factors also directly depress the contractility of both the right and left ventricles.

At different stages of ARDS both augmented hypoxic pulmonary vasoconstriction and loss of the normal hypoxic vasoconstrictor response are thought to play a role in the development of pulmonary hypertension and increased right to left shunting, respectively.

Decreased cardiac output in patients with ARDS may lead to impaired oxygen delivery to tissues, even in the presence of the normal arterial Po_2. This problem may be compounded by impaired tissue oxygen uptake that is particularly common in patients with sepsis, and which may occur as a result of tissue oedema, microembolization of capillaries, or loss of local microvascular control mechanisms. Finally, to make matters worse, in many of these patients there is an increased tissue oxygen demand as a result of fever, inflammation, and repair processes.

Pathology

The non-specific acute alveolar injury that characterizes ARDS was first described in detail by Liebow and given the term 'diffuse alveolar damage' (**DAD**). Like the clinical situations in which diverse predisposing conditions appear to result in the common clinical picture described by Asbaugh *et al.*, diffuse alveolar damage can be induced by a wide variety of noxious stimuli. In its early stages the alveoli may show atelactasis and the lung microvessels may appear engorged. The alveolar septa are oedematous with inflammatory exudate and extravasated erythrocytes, and a proteinaceous inflammatory exudate may flood the alveoli in some areas of the lung.

The initiation of lung injury is likely to occur within the pulmonary capillaries (see below). Increased numbers of neutrophils may be seen in these and in the interstitial spaces and, if obtained at the earliest stages, bronchoalveolar lavage fluid shows large numbers of neutrophils. Neutrophil numbers in bronchoalveolar lavage and the concentration of neutrophil secreted products therein appear to correlate with ARDS and its severity. These observations draw attention to the likely role of neutrophils early in ARDS pathogenesis. On ultrastructural examination there is clear evidence of endothelial and epithelial injury: this may be extensive. Hyaline membranes, which are the light-microscopical hallmark of diffuse alveolar damage, are likely to be derived from layers of necrotic epithelial cells.

It is important to recognize that these pathological events do not occur in a strictly ordered sequence, and may appear to have reached different stages in different parts of the lungs at the same time. It is not unusual to find evidence of continued inflammatory injury concurrent with alveolar type II cell proliferation or other evidence of attempts at repair. In those patients who die after just a few days of mechanical ventilation there is often evidence of a pronounced fibroproliferative response, including fibroblast migration into injured alveoli, and fibroblast proliferation and collagen deposition that within 2 weeks can achieve quite remarkable proportions. Nevertheless, in those patients who survive the initiating condition and who are mechanically ventilated, death is not usually due to progressive respiratory failure. Most patients die from the failure of other organs involved in multiple organ failure that are less easy to support than the lung, septicaemia, or secondary nosocomial infections in the injured lung, although barotrauma from mechanical ventilation of poorly compliant lungs can be a major problem in some patients.

Since case reports describing lung biopsies that have been repeated for clinical indications are extremely rare, very little is known about the pathology of the recovery phase of ARDS. Those that have been done suggest that some pulmonary remodelling had occurred. The remarkable examples of patients with severe ARDS, yet who nevertheless appear to regain virtually normal lung function, suggest that some forms of inflammatory lung injury, and perhaps even fibrosis, have the capacity to resolve and/or become significantly remodelled.

Pathogenesis—cellular and humoral mechanisms

Neutrophils and other inflammatory cells

Neutrophils have long been recognized in the lung tissues of necropsy specimens obtained early in the course of ARDS, and bronchoalveolar lavage cytology shows a high percentage of neutrophils and their products, such as myeloperoxidase, which correlate with the development and severity of ARDS. Other potentially injurious neutrophil products including neutrophil elastase and collagenase are also found; and, of importance, peripheral blood levels of neutrophil elastase in patients at risk of ARDS correlate with subsequent ARDS development. External imaging of radiolabelled neutrophils has demonstrated neutrophil accumulation in the lungs of patients with ARDS. Recent studies have suggested that the neutrophil chemokine interleukin-8 (**IL-8**) may be specifically related to the development of this

condition. Studies in animal models of acute lung injury, using stimuli of relevance to the pathogenesis of ARDS, critically implicate the neutrophil.

This is not to suggest that other inflammatory cells are unimportant in the pathogenesis of ARDS. Although this condition has been described in neutropenic patients, histology does show the presence of some neutrophils in the lungs, and it is uncertain how much of a neutrophil 'load' may be required: neutrophil replenishment experiments in neutropenic animals replace only a small proportion of the total neutrophil complement. Nevertheless, studies of neutropenic patients raise the possibility that other cells, perhaps monocytes, play an important ancillary role or may even substitute for granulocytes under some circumstances: these cells possess most (if not all) of the potentially injurious mechanisms and capacity of neutrophils.

It is now generally believed that one of the earliest initiation mechanisms in ARDS is damage to the capillary endothelial cells and the airway epithelial cells that form the delicate alveolar gas-exchange membrane. This is caused by toxic products of inflammatory cells that have become sequestered and activated as a result of inflammatory mediators generated as a consequence of the initiating insult (see Fig. 1). It is uncertain why lung injury is so prominent and often the first clinically obvious event in the multisystem microvascular injury of multiple organ failure. However, this may partly be due to the fact that most of the 'marginating pool' of neutrophils resides in lung capillaries, and even in the healthy state neutrophils (average diameter 7.5 μm) have to squeeze through lung capillaries (mean diameter 5.5 μm), thus presenting a massive surface area of contact between this potentially injurious cell and the at-risk gas-exchange membrane (see below). With regard to this interaction, neutrophils cannot injure cells or degrade matrix proteins without extremely close apposition, and it is essential for us to understand the kinetics and adhesion mechanisms that relate to this critical interaction to gain a full appreciation of the pathogenesis of acute lung injury. Finally, neutrophil secretion is not necessarily an all-or-nothing phenomenon: for maximum release of reactive oxygen intermediates or granule enzymes the neutrophil needs to be exposed to agents that 'prime' the cell, together with those that trigger it.

Mediators

A very large number of mediators, indeed several mediator cascades, have been implicated in the pathogenesis of ARDS.

Endotoxin

Endotoxic lipopolysaccharide (**LPS**) is the main 'active' ingredient of the cell walls of *Escherichia coli* and other Gram-negative organisms that cause sepsis syndrome, septic shock, and ARDS. When injected into animals, LPS

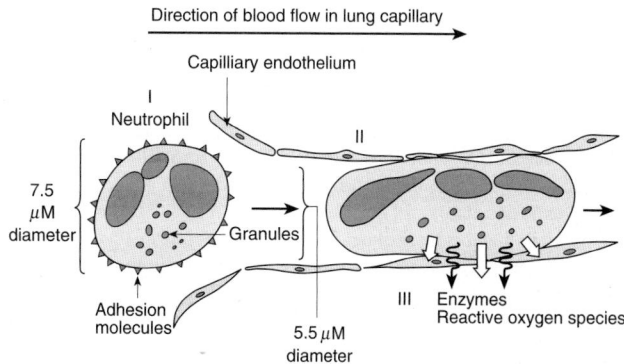

Fig. 1 Initiating insults and toxic products of inflammatory cells that are involved in ARDS. I: Neutrophils became 'primed' by circulating mediators (lipopolysaccharide (**LPS**), platelet-activating factor (**PAF**)) to become 'stiff', 'sticky', and very responsive to secretagogues. II: Primed neutrophils sequester abnormally in the pulmonary capillaries. III: Sequestered primed neutrophils are acted upon by circulating secretagogues (e.g. IL-8) to release injurious reactive oxygen species (**ROS**) and enzymes.

causes many of the pathophysiological features of septic shock. Low concentrations of LPS may enter the circulation of patients with circulatory shock by the process of 'translocation' through the compromised gut lining. LPS exerts a number of direct influences on neutrophils. In the presence of serum, very low concentrations of LPS (pg/ml) are required to cause enhanced expression of neutrophil surface adhesion molecules that bind the activated endothelium (see Chapters 4.4 and 5.1) and cause a direct reduction in neutrophil deformability, both of which promote excessive and prolonged neutrophil sequestration in pulmonary microvessels. LPS also causes macrophages to release cytokines, including IL-1 and tumour necrosis factor-α (**TNF-α**), which play key roles in the initiation of inflammation and activate other cascades, including the complement, coagulation, and kinin cascades, as well as generating systemic cytokines including IL-6 that regulate the acute-phase response.

Peptide mediators

The complement peptide C5a is an effective neutrophil chemotaxin and secretagogue *in vitro*, and is found in the blood of patients at risk of ARDS as well as in those with established disease. However, most workers in this field believe that chemokines, especially IL-8, play a more important role in neutrophil chemoattraction to the lung in ARDS. There has been much less study of the role of the contact system, which activates bradykinin, and the clotting and fibrinolytic cascades, but these are also likely to be important in the pathogenesis of ARDS. Activated kinins are vasoactive and cause increased vascular permeability: they can also act as secretagogues for neutrophils and other inflammatory cells.

Cytokines

Cytokines are a diverse group of soluble, hormone-like polypeptides produced by leucocytes and also by some constitutive tissue cells, especially macrophages, endothelial cells, epithelial cells, and fibroblasts. It is likely that cytokines (see Chapters 4.4 and 5.1) play key roles at all stages of the evolution of ARDS. TNF-α and IL-1 are generated by alveolar macrophages on exposure to LPS and other stimuli of relevance to ARDS pathogenesis, and are likely to play key initiator roles by stimulating other resident cells, particularly epithelial and microvascular endothelial cells, to release IL-8 and other potent neutrophil chemokines. They also act on capillary endothelial cells to induce the expression and activation of adhesion molecules necessary for neutrophil sequestration and for the creation of an 'injury-promoting' microenvironment. Other cytokines—for example, platelet-derived growth factor (**PDGF**), fibroblast growth factor (**FGF**), transforming growth factor-β (**TGF-β**)—are likely to play an important part in the vascular remodelling, fibroblast chemotaxis, and fibroblast proliferation and collagen synthesis that characterize the poorly understood fibroproliferative or 'chronic' phase of ARDS.

Chemokines

This expanding family of small molecular weight peptides has received much recent attention. Depending on the position of cysteine in the molecule they have been subdivided into the 'C–X–C' and 'C–C' chemokines. The C–X–C subgroup contains a variety of peptides that are powerful neutrophil chemoattractants and activators, whereas the C–C group exert their chemotactic influences on monocytes and/or eosinophils.

It is now generally agreed that IL-8 and its family members are responsible for neutrophil attraction to the lung in ARDS. IL-8 is an 8.0 kDa polypeptide that is a potent neutrophil chemoattractant and a powerful stimulus for angiogenesis. IL-8, of a plethora of candidates, was the only mediator to correlate with subsequent ARDS development in studies of patients at the earliest stage of the risk period for ARDS. Other chemokines are likely to play important roles in subsequent monocyte emigration, but these are less well characterized.

Membrane phospholipid derivatives

Membrane-derived phospholipid products, including platelet-activating factor (PAF), leukotrienes, prostaglandins, and prostacyclin, may influence inflammatory cells (PAF is an important neutrophil priming agent, for example), but they also exert major influences on local blood vessels and promote the generation of oedema fluid. Thromboxanes can cause marked pulmonary vasoconstriction and may be partly responsible for the pulmonary hypertension that characterizes the early stages of ARDS.

An injury-promoting microenvironment between abnormally sequestered neutrophils and pulmonary capillary endothelial cells

Neutrophils do not injure endothelial cells *in vitro* without there being direct contact. It is likely that stimulated neutrophils interact with endothelium in a fashion that leads to the formation of a specialized intercellular microenvironment, within which concentrations of histotoxic agents (such as enzymes and reactive oxygen intermediates) would reach high levels, whereas their high molecular weight inhibitors would be relatively excluded (Fig. 2). Furthermore, many potent neutrophil enzymes, such as elastase, are preferentially located on the 'leading surface of the cell' and would need close apposition in order to cause effects. Finally, some of the most potent reactive oxygen intermediates are so labile that they are likely to have a very short distance of activity in tissues. This concept, of a restricted intercellular microenvironment necessary for neutrophil-mediated injury, is supported by experiments showing that matrix degradation occurs only in areas where stimulated neutrophils are tightly adherent and continues in the presence of the large molecular weight antiproteinase, α-1 proteinase inhibitor. The creation of such a microenvironment between neutrophils and endothelial cells in lung capillaries is likely to occur by a combination of adhesion mechanisms and a reduction in the ability of neutrophils to deform.

Neutrophil–endothelial surface adhesive molecules

Adhesion between neutrophils and endothelial cells *in vitro* is greatly enhanced within minutes of the addition of inflammatory mediators. Much of this enhanced adhesion can be abolished by monoclonal antibodies directed against the CD11/CD18 group of adhesive leucoproteins on the neutrophil surface. Similarly, endothelial cells that have been activated by LPS or cytokines express adhesion molecules on their surface, and others that are already expressed become activated. *In vivo*, it is likely that neutrophil adhesion to endothelial cells in microvessels occurs by a complex process that involves at least two phases. In the first transient phase of adhesion, which is nevertheless necessary for the second phase, interactions between molecules of the selectin family on neutrophils and endothelial cells are particularly important. In the second phase of 'tight' adhesion,

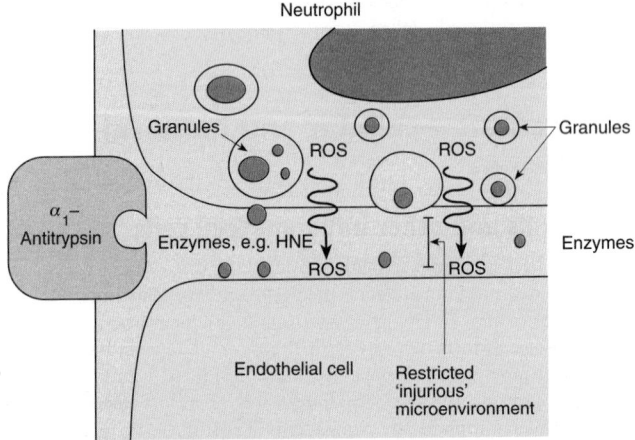

ROS = Reactive oxygen species
HNE = Human neutrophil elastase

Fig. 2 The neutrophil and the injurious microenvironment in ARDS.

which is necessary for the creation of an injurious microenvironment and also for capillary transmigration of neutrophils, integrin molecules play the central role.

Reduced neutrophil deformability

As described previously, neutrophils are normally required to 'squeeze' through the narrow lung capillaries. Hence, any factors that reduce neutrophil deformability would significantly increase their time of sequestration, and thereby increase the time of contact between activated neutrophils and the delicate gas-exchange membranes. Although it was generally believed that abnormal sequestration occurs mainly by upregulation of neutrophil and endothelial surface adhesive molecules, alteration in neutrophil deformability is also likely to play an important role in the pulmonary circulation. Neutrophils treated with relevant inflammatory mediators demonstrate markedly reduced deformability *in vitro*, and when injected intravenously have prolonged residence time in the pulmonary microcirculation. The molecular mechanisms controlling neutrophil deformability are much less well understood than those governing the expression of surface adhesion molecules.

Neutrophil priming, triggering, and secretion of injurious products

Even when neutrophils are tightly apposed to matrix proteins or 'target' endothelial cells *in vitro*, the induction of neutrophil-mediated injury is not an all-or-nothing phenomenon. When neutrophils are prepared by stringent methods that avoid their exposure to ubiquitous LPS or other agents that might influence their function, stimulation with secretagogues causes little or no release of reactive oxygen intermediates or enzymes unless they are previously exposed to low concentrations of priming agents such as LPS. These priming and triggering phenomena have a number of implications for tissue injury. First, the presence *per se* of neutrophils in tissue does not equate with injury—it is likely that they need to be primed and triggered to achieve a maximal secretory state. Second, when examined in this context, many of the mediators implicated in ARDS pathogenesis exert different effects: for instance, LPS, TNF-α, and PAF are poor secretagogues but highly effective priming agents, whereas C5a, IL-8, and leukotriene-4 (LTB₄), together with other neutrophil chemotaxins, are potent secretagogues for primed cells. Therefore, rather than seeking a 'single common mediator' it is perhaps more important to define how certain key mediators act together to influence neutrophil secretion and other critical mechanistic events.

The vast array of potentially injurious neutrophil products represents another example of the remarkable redundancy of the inflammatory response. Most of these products have probably evolved to assist the neutrophil in its rapid passage to the inflamed/infected site, and in its effective killing of bacteria, but in neutrophil-mediated tissue injury and disease processes the difficulty of identifying centrally important toxic agents cannot be exaggerated. Over the years, much circumstantial evidence has accrued to support a role for neutrophil-generated reactive oxygen intermediates in ARDS. However, studies in the early risk period for ARDS suggest that neutrophil elastase is also an important agent.

Lung scarring in ARDS

Whether or not there has been a critical level of epithelial injury in the primary inflammatory damage to the lung seems to be a key factor in determining whether excessive scarring occurs. Most pathologists now believe that the lung can tolerate a certain degree and extent of injury to type I alveolar epithelial cells without the necessity for excessive scarring. In these circumstances it is thought that gaps in the epithelium are repaired by the division of type II epithelial pneumocytes to form a new monolayer of type I cells. However, if there is extensive disruption of the epithelium, and particularly if the basement membrane is severely damaged and loses its archi-

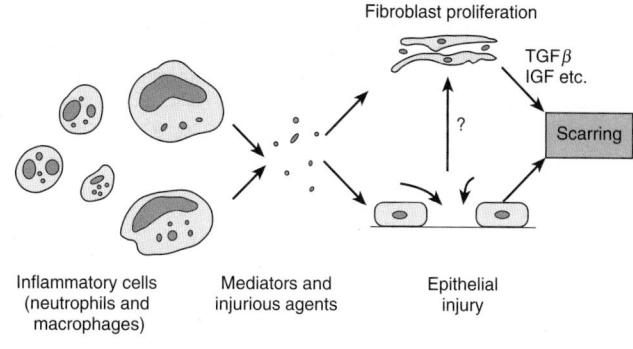

TGFβ = Transforming growth factor beta
IGF   = Insulin-like growth factor

Fig. 3 Inflammation and scarring in ARDS.

tectural integrity, it appears that a scarring response is more likely to result. The inflammatory response can impinge at two levels on the scarring process (Fig. 3). First, on the degree of epithelial injury caused by the inflammatory process; second, by inflammatory cells producing agents that can induce fibroblasts to proliferate and deposit scar-tissue matrix proteins.

Granulation tissue (the precursor of scar tissue) is a very cellular and dynamic tissue, particularly in the lung. It is composed of proliferating fibroblasts that lay down scar-tissue matrix proteins such as collagen. Collagen production by fibroblasts is normally a highly regulated process, with controls being exerted at several levels. All but 30 per cent of the extracellularly secreted collagen is normally degraded, mainly by the effect of fibroblast-derived collagenase. The effect of collagenase is under a further internal control mechanism whereby it is kept in check by inhibitors, for example by tissue inhibitors of metalloproteinases (**TIMPs**). Fibroblast activity is also under the control of external factors including cytokines and growth factors, many of which can be secreted in large quantities by local cells, particularly inflammatory macrophages. Most of these factors, including PDGF, TGF-β, FGF, and insulin-like growth factor (**IGF**), have been shown to exert permissive or stimulatory effects on fibroblast growth and secretion. External factors exerting negative influences must also exist. Although these have received less attention, prostaglandin E₂ represents a good example of a factor with mainly inhibitory effects on fibroblast function.

Further reading

Baggiolini M, Walz A, Kunkel SL (1989). Neutrophil-activating peptide-1/interleukin-8, a novel cytokine that activates neutrophils. *Journal of Clinical Investigation* **84**, 1045–9.

Biondi JW, et al. (1990). Mechanical heart–lung interaction in the adult respiratory distress syndrome. *Clinics in Chest Medicine* **11**, 691–714.

Donnelly SC, et al. (1993). Interleukin-8 and development of adult respiratory distress syndrome in at-risk patient groups. *Lancet* **341**, 643–7.

Donnelly SC, et al. (1994). Role of selectins in development of adult respiratory distress syndrome. *Lancet* **344**, 215–19.

Erzurum S, et al. (1992). Cell mechanics of neutrophils: induction of stiffness and actin by lipopolysaccharide. *Journal of Immunology* **149**, 154–62.

Fowler AA, et al. (1983). Adult respiratory distress syndrome: risk with common predispositions. *Annals of Internal Medicine* **98**, 593–7.

Guthrie LA, et al. (1984). The priming of neutrophils for enhanced release of oxygen metabolites by bacterial lipopolysaccharide: evidence for increased activity of the superoxide-producing enzyme. *Journal of Experimental Medicine* **160**, 1656–71.

Haslett C, et al. (1985). Modulation of multiple neutrophil functions by preparative methods or trace concentrations of bacterial lipopolysaccharide. *American Journal of Pathology* **119**, 101–10.

Snow RL, *et al.* (1982). Pulmonary vascular remodelling in adult respiratory distress syndrome. *American Review of Respiratory Disease* **126**, 887–92.

Warshawski F, *et al.* (1986). Abnormal neutrophil–pulmonary interaction in the adult respiratory distress syndrome: qualitative and quantitative assessment of pulmonary-neutrophil kinetics in humans with *in vivo* indium-111 neutrophil scintigraphy. *American Review of Respiratory Disease* **133**, 792–804.

16.5.2 The management of respiratory failure

Christopher S. Garrard

Acute respiratory failure: intensive care

Respiration is a complex process involving ventilation, pulmonary gas exchange, oxygen delivery by the circulation, and oxygen utilization by the tissues for the production of cellular high-energy phosphate. By convention, respiratory failure is used in a clinical context to mean failure of ventilation and/or pulmonary gas exchange. Accordingly, the treatment of acute respiratory failure is directed at:

(1) establishing and maintaining the airway;

(2) administering oxygen;

(3) maintaining adequate ventilation, using mechanical ventilation if necessary;

(4) enhancing oxygen 'on-loading' by the lungs, that is, improving the efficiency of getting oxygen into the blood for any given concentration of inspired oxygen;

(5) identifying and treating the underlying cause (not the subject of this chapter);

(6) monitoring Sao_2 (the oxygen saturation of arterial blood—pulse oximetry), ECG, and vital signs; and

(7) staged withdrawal of respiratory support (weaning) as the underlying disease process resolves.

Establishing and maintaining the airway

Simple manoeuvres to re-establish and clear the airway must always be followed. These include positioning and maintaining the head and neck in the 'sniff position', inspection of the oropharynx, suctioning, and if necessary, the insertion of an oral or pharyngeal airway.

Endotracheal intubation

If a reliable or adequate airway cannot be established by the above means, endotracheal intubation must be performed. Orotracheal intubation is particularly suited to the emergency situation. Nasotracheal intubation requires a little extra time and should be avoided in those with coagulation defects or thrombocytopenia because of the risk of serious haemorrhage. Whatever technique is selected, intubation should be performed in a safe and expeditious manner by the most experienced clinician available. Neuromuscular relaxant drugs to facilitate intubation should only be used by experienced personnel.

The complications of endotracheal intubation are due to occlusion or displacement of the tube, and airway trauma. The appropriate endotracheal tube size for most adult men is 8 to 9 mm in internal diameter, and for women 7 to 8 mm. For children, a rough calculation using the child's age in years divided by 4, plus 4.0 will provide the tube internal diameter in millimetres.

It is essential that the endotracheal tube be securely anchored and the cuff inflation pressure restricted to less than 30 cmH$_2$O. High-volume, low-pressure cuffed tubes are generally recommended and cuff inflation pressures should be checked periodically using an aneroid manometer and adjusted accordingly. Using higher cuff pressures does not improve airway protection against aspiration but may damage the tracheal mucosa and risk later subglottic stenosis. Smaller tubes, as used for children, are typically uncuffed.

Difficulties with endotracheal intubation can be encountered in those with a short 'bull' neck or receding lower jaw. Any patient with restricted neck and jaw movements (rheumatoid arthritis or cervical spine injury) or who has abnormal oropharyngeal anatomy (tumour or trauma) should also be regarded as a potential problem. Several options can be considered in these situations. Inhalational anaesthesia by face mask can facilitate intubation, but under no circumstances must muscle relaxants be given unless satisfactory airway access can be ensured. Awake intubation can be performed with topical anaesthesia. Blind nasal intubation or intubation using a fibreoptic bronchoscope or laryngoscope requires considerable skill and training but may be the safest option.

Tracheostomy

Tracheostomy should only replace endotracheal intubation for specific indications and not merely after the elapse of a predefined time interval. Using modern endotracheal tubes and techniques, endotracheal intubation can be tolerated without permanent harm to the airway for months if necessary: the greater part of mucosal damage is done in the first week of intubation with little additional change thereafter.

The common indications for replacement of endotracheal intubation by tracheostomy include the need for chronic or permanent ventilation, to help weaning after previously failed attempts at extubation, to facilitate oral nutrition, or the presence of upper airway complications of endotracheal intubation.

Most tracheostomies for patients in intensive care units are now performed by a percutaneous Seldinger technique: this can be done at the bedside, avoiding the need for moving the patient to the operating theatre. Although percutaneous tracheostomy 'kits' have made the procedure rapid and safe, the clinician needs to be aware of serious complications such as the formation of false tracks and perforation of structures adjacent to the trachea.

The same principles of cuff pressure management apply to tracheostomy tubes as to endotracheal tubes. Tracheostomy is associated with fewer but more serious complications than endotracheal intubation. These include tube displacement, pneumothorax, severe haemorrhage, and wound infection.

Minitracheostomy

Some patients with an ineffective cough or neurological impairment require continued suctioning of airway secretions without the need for formal endotracheal intubation or tracheostomy. In such cases a 3.5- to 4.0-mm diameter, cuffless minitracheostomy tube can be inserted percutaneously, under local anaesthesia, through the cricothyroid membrane. These tubes cannot be used for conventional ventilation, may result in local haemorrhagic complications, and can be the source of infection.

Cricothyroidotomy

A cricothyroidotomy may be needed in life-threatening, upper airway obstruction where endotracheal intubation is not feasible and there is insufficient time to perform tracheostomy. A full-sized tracheostomy tube (6 to 8 mm internal diameter) can be inserted under local anaesthesia to allow mechanical ventilation.

Table 1 Oxygen delivery systems

Method of delivery	FiO_2 achieved
Nasal cannula (1 to 2 litre/min)	0.24 to 0.30
Venturi mask	0.24 to 0.50
Partial rebreathing mask	0.60 to 0.80
Non-rebreathing reservoir mask	Up to 0.90
Anaesthetic face mask or endotracheal tube	Up to 1.0

FiO_2, inspired oxygen concentration.

The administration of oxygen

Hypoxia should never be tolerated through a concern over oxygen toxicity; although this is a recognized complication of prolonged administration of a high concentration of oxygen, the use of 50 or 100 per cent oxygen for less than 24 h is usually considered acceptable. Oxygen can be delivered by a variety of means depending upon the concentration desired and the patient's minute ventilation (Table 1).

Oxygen should be given in such concentrations as to prevent hypoxia with the caveat that controlled (limited) oxygen concentrations should be administered, usually by a 'Venturi type' of face mask, to patients with chronic obstructive lung disease. The response to oxygen therapy can best be measured continuously by pulse oximetry (SaO_2) or by intermittent gas sampling of arterial blood. Once oxygen therapy has been initiated, sudden or abrupt removal of oxygen supplementation runs the risk of severe hypoxia, with the risk of neurological impairment, arrhythmias, or even cardiac arrest.

Mechanical ventilation

Indications for intubation and mechanical ventilation

Failure to intervene promptly can clearly have catastrophic consequences for the patient, but mechanical ventilation is not to be undertaken lightly since it is associated with much morbidity and some mortality.

The indications for mechanical ventilation fall into two broad categories: (i) inadequate alveolar ventilation with increasing PCO_2 and (ii) inadequate gas exchange with increasing $D(A\text{-}a)O_2$ and arterial hypoxaemia. Guidelines for mechanical ventilation in acute respiratory failure are shown in Table 2: the physician should exercise clinical judgement in the interpretation of these and anticipate problems before they arise. For example, one of the simplest criteria for mechanical ventilation is a respiratory rate of 35 breaths/min or more. If, with a respiratory rate of 30 breaths/min a patient is clearly fatiguing, then early elective intubation is clearly preferable to an emergency procedure an hour or so later. Similarly, a progressive fall in vital capacity in a patient with myasthenia gravis receiving full medication may need ventilatory support although the critical value of less than 15 ml/kg is not reached.

The treatment of hypoventilatory respiratory failure consists of assisting ventilatory function, usually by mechanical external means. Figure 1 shows a flow diagram outlining the decision process involved in the assessment of patients who may require mechanical ventilation.

Features and applications of a mechanical ventilator

The principles of mechanical ventilation using simple mechanical ventilators need to be understood before moving on to consideration of the complex and sophisticated mechanical ventilators that offer a bewildering range of features. Those not familiar with the field run the risk of being overwhelmed by an overabundance of studies claiming superiority of certain techniques over others. Fortunately, the application of common sense

and sound physiological principles will serve better than devotion to attractive technical innovation.

Most adult patients are supported on volume/time-cycled, pressure-limited ventilators (volume ventilator or flow generator). These deliver pre-set tidal volumes regardless of changes in lung compliance or impedance. The price paid for this desirable characteristic is that the inflation pressure will rise to overcome any mechanical load. A limit must be set to protect the

Table 2 Guidelines for introduction of endotracheal intubation and mechanical ventilation

General indications in acute respiratory failure
Inadequate ventilation, indicated by:
    Apnoea, upper airway obstruction, unprotected airway
    Respiratory rate > 35 breaths/min (normal range 10–20)
    Vital capacity < 15 ml/kg (normal range 65–75)
    Tidal volume < 5 ml/kg (normal range 5–7)
    Negative inspiratory force < 25 cmH_2O (normal range 75–100)
    $PaCO_2$ > 8 kPa (60 mmHg) (normal range 4.7–6.3 kPa (35–47 mmHg))
    V_D/V_T ratio > 0.6 (normal range < 0.3)
Inadequate gas exchange oxygenation, indicated by:
    PaO_2 < 8 kPa, (60 mmHg) on FiO_2 > 0.6
    $D(A\text{-}a)O_2$ on FiO_2 1.0 > 47 kPa (350 mmHg), (normal range 3.3–8.7 kPa
    (25–65 mmHg))

Specific indications, with or without previous respiratory pathology
Chronic obstructive lung disease
    Failure of conservative measures
    Inability to co-operate with care
    Decreased consciousness
    Cardiac instability
    Apnoea
    Severe respiratory acidosis
    Acute management of nocturnal obstructive hypoventilation
Chronic restrictive lung disease
    Severe hypoxaemia
    Fatigue and impending exhaustion
Severe acute asthma
    Failure of conservative measures
    Obtundation
    Cardiac instability
    Increasing $PaCO_2$
    Fatigue and impending exhaustion
Head trauma
    Unconscious
    Unprotected airway
    Cerebral oedema
    Apnoea or global hypoventilation
Chest trauma
    Flail chest with hypoventilation and hypoxaemia
    Pulmonary contusion with hypoxaemia
Neuromuscular weakness
    Apnoea or progressive hypoventilation (see above)
    Airway protection, nocturnal hypoventilation/hypoxaemia
    Organophosphate poisoning
Other neurological disorders
    Status epilepticus
    Tetanus
    High cervical spine injury
Upper airway protection
    Loss of consciousness
    Neck and oropharyngeal trauma
    Epiglottitis
    Acute neuromuscular event
Drug overdose
    Apnoea, hypoventilation, airway protection, seizures

(After Pontoppidan *et al.*, also Garrard CS, *Oxford Textbook Of Surgery*, 2nd edn, Oxford University Press.)

patient from inappropriately high pressure: when this limit is reached the ventilator terminates inspiration regardless of the volume delivered and triggers an alarm.

Neonates and infants can be satisfactorily ventilated using time-cycled, pressure-limited devices (pressure ventilator or pressure generator). The pressure-limited paediatric ventilator offers simplicity and reliable ventilation, although the delivered tidal volume is difficult to measure. In the premature neonate this is not a serious limitation and pressure-limited ventilation is the preferred technique.

Specifically designed, compact, lightweight ventilators, driven by cylinder oxygen and utilizing fluid logic circuits are available for transporting ventilator-dependent patients. These are pressure generators and can be used for both adults and children. By entraining air, a choice of either 60 or 100 per cent oxygen is available.

Modes of ventilation

Depending upon the underlying pathophysiology, the clinician must select the mode of ventilation, choose the ventilation parameters, and set the ventilator alarms. The most commonly available ventilator modes include:

(1) control mechanical ventilation (**CMV**);

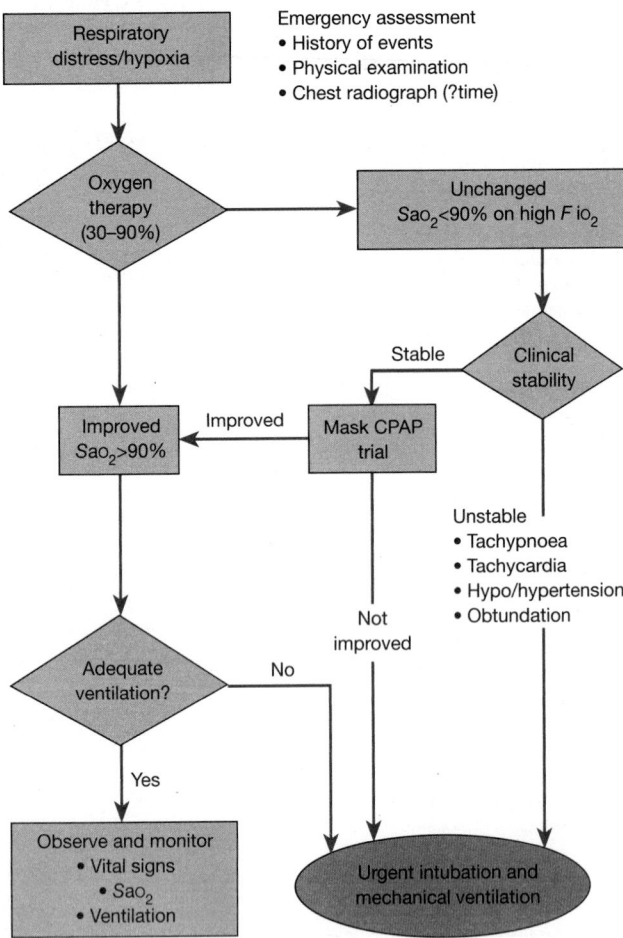

Fig. 1 Respiratory failure algorithm.

(2) assist control (triggered ventilation, volume cycled);

(3) pressure support (triggered ventilation, pressure cycled);

(4) intermittent mandatory ventilation (**IMV**, or if synchronized, **SIMV**)—volume or pressure controlled;

(5) bi-level positive airway pressure (**BiPAP**); and

(6) others.

Control mechanical ventilation (CMV)

This provides time- and volume-cycled, pressure-limited breaths at a preset rate, but does not allow the patient to breathe spontaneously. This mode is suitable for the paralysed or heavily sedated patient.

Assist control

Assist control or triggered ventilation synchronizes the ventilator to the patient's own respiratory rhythm, delivering a volume-preset, pressure-limited tidal volume. A trigger sensitivity is selected, usually −0.5 to −2.0 cmH$_2$O, by which the patient can initiate volume-preset breaths. As a safety requirement, a high respiratory rate alarm is needed and a 'back-up' ventilation rate must be set in the event of apnoea. Assist control is better tolerated than CMV and the patient requires less sedation, but does have a tendency to hyperventilate.

Pressure support

Pressure support uses a triggering facility to deliver, not a volume-preset breath as in assist control, but a pressure-limited breath (i.e. as with paediatric pressure ventilation). The inspiratory flow rate is usually high so as to minimize phase lag and the work of breathing. Pressure support may be used alone or in conjunction with SIMV when it assists spontaneous breaths. Pressure support provides an efficient maintenance and weaning mode that is well tolerated by the patient. The trigger mechanism is usually a negative pressure threshold, but some ventilators trigger on changes in circuit gas flow that potentially could be more sensitive and reduce the work of breathing.

Intermittent mandatory ventilation (IMV)

This was originally devised for weaning but is now widely adopted as a maintenance mode. It provides the opportunity for the patient to breathe spontaneously and supplement the positive-pressure minute ventilation. In the standard IMV mode there is a theoretical risk of stacking a ventilator breath on top of a spontaneous breath. More modern ventilators utilize the triggering or assist facility to synchronize the IMV breaths with the patient's own spontaneous breathing pattern (synchronized IMV, SIMV). The IMV mode can provide complete or partial ventilation support and, with the patient taking spontaneous breaths, IMV is better tolerated than CMV. Compared with CMV, SIMV results in lower mean airway pressures, has less effect on the cardiovascular system, and allows patients to regulate their own Pco$_2$ to at least some degree.

Bi-level positive airway pressure (BiPAP)

This is a form of pressure-controlled ventilation based upon raising airway pressure from a lower setting (equivalent to constant positive airway pressure/positive end-expiratory pressure, **CPAP/PEEP**) to a higher setting (equivalent to the peak airway pressure). The lower pressure level should be set at a point above the inflection point in the respiratory pressure–volume curve. A potential advantage of this mode is that it allows spontaneous ventilation to occur at both the lower and higher positive airway pressures, which may be better tolerated by the patient. BiPAP has been successfully adopted as a method of delivering non-invasive positive-pressure ventilation via a nasal or full face mask.

High frequency ventilation

This may have potential advantages in supporting patients with acute respiratory distress syndrome. In randomized studies, peak airway pressures are lower but mean airway pressure and mortality are unchanged.

High frequency ventilation can be delivered by several techniques including 'jet' ventilation and high frequency oscillation: both are capable of sustaining adequate oxygenation and carbon dioxide clearance. These techniques have been promoted by enthusiasts for over three decades and yet have failed to establish themselves in routine management of respiratory failure. However, high frequency ventilation may be useful following reconstructive laryngeal, tracheal, or bronchial surgery, or for patients with bronchopleural or bronchocutaneous fistulas, but even in these applications the advantage, if any, over conventional modes of ventilation seems marginal.

Mandatory minute ventilation (MMV)

This is an innovative mode whereby the combined spontaneous and mechanical ventilation must reach a minimum preset level. As the patient's spontaneous ventilation increases the mechanically assisted breaths become fewer. Individual ventilators vary in their ability to achieve successful MMV.

Setting ventilator parameters

Once a ventilation mode has been selected (at least temporarily), ventilatory parameters must be set before attaching the patient to the ventilator. The ventilator parameters include:

(1) tidal volume;

(2) ventilation rate;

(3) inspiratory/expiratory (**I:E**) ratio;

(4) flow waveform;

(5) inspired oxygen concentration (Fio_2, 0.21 to 1.0);

(6) pressure limit (if using volume cycling);

(7) trigger threshold (if triggered mode selected)—-pressure trigger (–0.5 to –5 cmH2O) or flow trigger (3 to 5 l/min); and

(8) positive end-expiratory pressure (PEEP) or constant positive airway pressure (CPAP) (0 to 20 cmH2O).

Tidal volume and respiratory rate

The delivered, inspiratory tidal volume may be set at 10 to 12 ml/kg body weight. This should be reduced if the patient has restrictive lung disease or has undergone lobectomy or pneumonectomy. Using respiratory rates of more than 10 breaths/min with such tidal volumes will provide full ventilatory support. If the patient is breathing spontaneously, an IMV mode will be preferred at rates of between 4 and 8 breaths/min. If assist control or pressure support is chosen, the respiratory rate will be the patient's spontaneous rate.

Respiratory rate, I:E ratio, inspiratory flow rate

These variables are linked and often affect one another. The ratio of inspiratory to expiratory time (I:E ratio) generally ranges from 1:2 to 1:4, allowing sufficient time for full passive exhalation. The higher the set respiratory rate the shorter expiration becomes and the I:E ratio falls. In patients with obstructive lung disease, failing to allow adequate time for exhalation results in air-trapping and hyperinflation, the extra pressure remaining in the alveoli at end-expiration being referred to as auto- or intrinsic-PEEP. This can lead to the paradoxical situation in the patient with chronic obstructive pulmonary disease where the Pco_2 rises as the ventilator rate is increased (usually at rates higher than 20 breaths/min).

The I:E ratio can be adjusted is several ways depending upon the make of ventilator: in some a ratio can be selected directly, whilst in others the inspiratory flow rate determines the duration of inspiration. An acceptable range for inspiratory flow rates is between 30 and 60 litre/min (0.5 to 1.0 litre/s)

Minute ventilation

Some ventilators require the minute ventilation to be set as a primary variable (e.g. Servo 900C). Setting the respiratory rate then effectively determines the tidal volume.

Inspiratory waveforms

Many volume- and time-cycled (flow generator) ventilators allow the choice of several waveforms. Although there is little evidence to favour one over another, a square waveform delivers the tidal volume in the least time and with higher peak pressures. A decelerating flow pattern results in lower peak pressures, longer inspiratory intervals, and lower I:E ratios.

Inspired oxygen concentration (Fio_2)

This should be constantly adjusted to provide adequate arterial oxygenation without hyperoxia. Too high a Fio_2 may risk oxygen toxicity and is frequently the cause of failure to wean patients with chronic obstructive pulmonary disease from a mechanical ventilator (by depressing 'hypoxic respiratory drive').

Pressure limit

In volume-cycled modes, a pressure limit about 10 cmH2O above the peak pressure reached during each ventilator cycle protects the patients against inadvertently high pressures experienced during coughing or straining. Hitting the pressure limit terminates inspiration and triggers an audible alarm.

PEEP/CPAP

Maintaining airway pressure above barometric pressure in a spontaneously breathing patient is called constant positive airway pressure (CPAP, Fig. 2). The same pressure applied to a patient on intermittent positive-pressure ventilation is called positive end-expiratory pressure (PEEP). PEEP/CPAP is used to increase lung volume (functional residual capacity) in conditions where this is reduced, for example acute respiratory distress syndrome or cardiogenic pulmonary oedema. It may also be beneficial in patients with flail chest segments by splinting the chest wall. The terms PEEP and CPAP can be used interchangeably provided that the differences regarding spontaneous and assisted ventilation are recognized.

PEEP/CPAP is achieved by the inclusion of a resistance at the expiratory end of the breathing circuit. Ideally this resistance should be as close to a threshold resistor as possible, such as an underwater column. In practice most of the valves produce some flow-dependent retardation of expiration that increases the work of breathing in spontaneously breathing patients.

Sighs

Before the advent of high tidal-volume ventilation and PEEP/CPAP, sighs were added to ventilation protocols to prevent progressive atelectasis. Each sigh was delivered 2 to 6 times/h and was equivalent to about twice the conventional tidal volume. The risks of barotrauma probably outweigh the theoretical benefits.

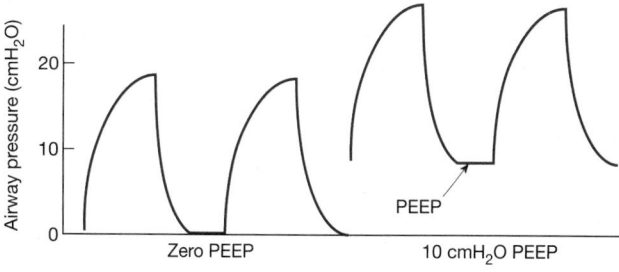

Fig. 2 Schematic of airway pressure measured without PEEP and following the addition of 10 cmH2O PEEP. By preventing end-expiratory pressure from falling to zero, reinflation and recruitment of alveolar units is encouraged.

Ventilator-induced lung injury and permissive hypercapnia

Animal and human studies indicate inhomogeneous reinflation of the lung in patients ventilated for acute respiratory distress syndrome. Some parts of the lung are therefore exposed to excessive shear stresses, resulting in a process known as 'volutrauma' that may lead to permanent fibrocystic changes. In the early 1990s evidence from randomized studies suggested that survival from acute respiratory distress syndrome could be improved if inflation pressures were kept below 40 mmHg. As a consequence there was an inevitable degree of hypoventilation and CO_2 retention ($Paco_2$ 8 to 12 kPa). This technique of 'permissive hypercapnia' has been widely adopted and may reduce the incidence of ventilator-induced lung injury.

Ventilator monitors and alarms

The ventilation monitors and high/low alarms that must be set and maintained include the following:

- exhaled tidal volume (V_T)
- exhaled minute ventilation
- spontaneous respiratory rate
- airway pressure and circuit disconnect
- peak airway pressure
- inspired oxygen concentration (Fio_2)
- inhaled gas temperature

The importance of ventilator alarms cannot be overemphasized. The modern, microprocessor-based ventilator is not only more efficient but is significantly safer than its predecessors. An audible alarm alerts the nurse or doctor to an adverse event, while an alarm section of the ventilator control panel indicates the exact event. Some ventilators have progressive alarms that change in character, sounding more urgent, until the alarm is cancelled or the alarm condition rectified.

Clinical monitoring of mechanical ventilation

An essential aspect of monitoring is regular clinical examination of the patient, and inspection of the ventilator and ventilator circuit. Expansion of the chest should be symmetrical with each ventilator-cycled breath (CMV, SIMV), assisted breath (assist control or pressure support), or unassisted spontaneous breath (SIMV). Auscultation should confirm air entry and detect any added sounds. The patient should be sat up or rolled side to side to allow inspection of the whole of the chest. The endotracheal tube should be secure and as comfortable as possible for the patient, and the endotracheal cuff pressure should be adjusted to less than 30 mmHg or so that a small air leak becomes audible with a stethoscope on the side of the neck with each ventilator cycle. The ventilator circuit should feel warm but be free of significant amounts of condensed water. The humidifier temperature and water level should be checked.

The pulse oximeter has contributed significantly to the monitoring and safety of patients on mechanical ventilation. Not only does it provide a continuous measurement of oxygenation but it also reduces the need for arterial blood gas sampling.

Much can be appreciated from watching the ventilator pressure gauge with each cycle. In addition to evaluating peak inspiratory pressure the clinician will be able to judge whether the patient is 'fighting' the ventilator. Comparing inspiratory and expiratory tidal volumes may indicate a leak in the circuit, either at circuit connections or at the endotracheal tube cuff. When peak pressures are high, the internal compliance of the ventilator and circuit (about 2 to 2.5 ml/cmH2O) may account for much of the volume loss. An assessment of the compliance of the respiratory system can be made from the peak inflation pressures and the resulting exhaled tidal vol-

ume during SIMV-delivered breaths. Normal values approximate 50 to 60 ml/cmH2O, while in severe acute respiratory distress syndrome, effective static respiratory system compliance may fall to 10 ml/cmH2O.

Methods of enhancing oxygen on-loading

Positive end-expiratory pressure/constant positive airway pressure (PEEP/CPAP)

PEEP/CPAP is the most commonly adopted method of enhancing oxygen on-loading (other than oxygen administration) and is often used in the presence of refractory hypoxaemia due to acute lung injury. Trends in the application of PEEP/CPAP in patients with respiratory failure have changed over the years. The use of maximum tolerated levels of PEEP ('super-PEEP') and 'best' PEEP have generally been replaced by the employment of 'least' or 'enough' PEEP to allow adequate arterial oxygenation with an Fio_2 less than 0.6. However, it is still not uncommon to have to consider levels of PEEP greater than 10 or 15 cmH2O, particularly in patients with acute respiratory distress syndrome.

An indication of the optimal PEEP level can be determined from the pressure–volume curve during lung inflation. An inflection point at the lower end of the curve suggests that areas of the lung are being allowed to collapse and therefore require higher pressures for their re-expansion. PEEP should be set above the inflection point to prevent collapse/re-expansion stresses.

Care must be exercised to ensure that oxygen delivery is not impaired in the unbridled pursuit of a higher level of arterial oxygenation. Monitoring continuous cardiac output or Svo_2 using a specially developed pulmonary artery catheter is particularly useful in detecting adverse effects of PEEP. If oxygenation is considered inadequate or the Fio_2 is greater than 0.6, increases in PEEP above 10 cmH2O can be attempted in increments of 2.5 to 5 cmH2O. If there are adverse effects, such as hypotension or reduced cardiac output (or Svo_2), then intravenous volume loading or circulatory support with an inotrope or pressor agent such as adrenaline may stabilize the patient.

Mask CPAP

CPAP can be applied without resorting to endotracheal intubation in the treatment of selected patients with acute respiratory failure. Close-fitting CPAP masks, which are very similar to standard anaesthetic masks, are widely available together with disposable circuitry and gas supply/pressure regulator mechanisms to ensure the safe delivery of air/oxygen mixtures.

The patient must be fully alert and co-operative since there is a major risk of aspiration should vomiting occur. Mask CPAP is particularly suited to patients with diffuse, reversible, interstitial processes such as cardiogenic pulmonary oedema or interstitial pneumonia (e.g. *Pneumocystis carinii* pneumonia). Recovery should be expected within 1 or 2 days since it is difficult for the patient to tolerate a tight-fitting CPAP mask for much longer periods, and CPAP levels above 10 to 15 cmH20 should not be employed. In general, patients with established acute respiratory distress syndrome are unsuitable if a long or protracted period of treatment is envisaged.

Suitable patients must be carefully selected and managed in a clinical area where appropriate observation and monitoring can be assured, usually an intensive care, high dependency, or respiratory unit. Continuous assessment by the clinical team is essential so that endotracheal intubation can be substituted for the mask system if necessary.

PEEP/CPAP in unilateral lung disease

The use of PEEP/CPAP in patients with unilateral or irregularly distributed lung disease may not result in improved oxygenation. Indeed, paradoxical falls in oxygenation may occur as a result of the shunting of blood from areas of well matched V/Q to parts of the lung that are poorly ventilated. Unilateral lung consolidation, lung collapse, massive pleural effusion, and pulmonary infarction may therefore not benefit from PEEP/CPAP. Treatment should be directed at correction of the specific lung pathology whenever possible.

Weaning of PEEP

Reduction or weaning of PEEP/CPAP should be conducted carefully and gradually once the underlying pathology (e.g. sepsis) has resolved. Ideally, the Fio_2 should have been reduced to 0.4 or less to maintain a Pao_2 of 10 kPa (80 mmHg) and the PEEP/CPAP level should not have changed for at least 12 h. Even when these criteria are satisfied, a significant proportion of patients will require the return of PEEP/CPAP to previous or even higher levels. Reduction of PEEP/CPAP in 2.5 or 5.0 cmH$_2$O decrements should be carried out at 10- to 15-min intervals after clinical, pulse oximeter, and blood gas assessment. Even after resolution of lung pathology the retention of low levels of PEEP/CPAP of 3 to 5 cmH$_2$O ('physiological PEEP') up to the time of extubation may help maintain normal lung volumes and improve gas exchange.

Prone positioning

A feature of the patient with acute respiratory distress syndrome is the extensive gravity-dependent lung collapse that is best visualized by CT scan. To a large degree this is a consequence of nursing the patient for prolonged periods in the supine position. Sitting the patient as upright as possible minimizes the volume of dependent lung. In recognition that dependent regions of the lung exhibit severe atelectasis and loss of volume, it is logical to alternate the patient between prone and supine positions every 8 to 12 h. Up to half of patients with severe acute respiratory distress syndrome show improved oxygenation with such manoeuvres. The major drawback is that vascular access sites and airway access can be dislodged during the process of turning the patient over. However, of all the methods of enhancing oxygen on-loading, only prone positioning actively addresses the issue of dependent lung atelectasis.

Nitric oxide therapy

The addition of low concentrations of nitric oxide (2 to 10 parts per million NO) to the inspired gas mixture will improve oxygenation in about 50 per cent of patients with acute respiratory distress syndrome, but there is no evidence from randomized studies that survival is better. Care must be exercised with delivery systems to ensure correct doses and avoid excessive production of toxic metabolites (nitrogen dioxide and methaemoglobin).

Extracorporeal membrane oxygenation

Extracorporeal membrane oxygenation in premature infants with persistent respiratory distress significantly improves survival. Its use for respiratory failure in adults was largely abandoned over two decades ago following controlled, randomized investigation. With the availability of improved oxygenators there has been renewed interest in combining extracorporeal partial CO$_2$ removal and low frequency conventional ventilation. Whether this approach offers significant advantages over techniques of permissive hypercapnia remains unproven, although there are enthusiasts who promote the use of extracorporeal membrane oxygenation in adults. Both techniques are aimed at reducing the deleterious effect of positive pressure upon the alveolar epithelium and may therefore hasten recovery from acute respiratory distress syndrome.

Surfactant

Following the dramatic benefit from the use of surfactant in neonatal respiratory distress, attempts to achieve similar effects in adults have been explored. Despite encouraging anecdotal reports, surfactant has not produced consistent improvement in acute respiratory distress syndrome, particularly when resulting from sepsis syndrome. This failure may stem in part from uncertainty regarding the type of surfactant (synthetic or animal derived) and the dose of surfactant required.

Liquid ventilation

Alveolar instability and collapse in acute respiratory distress syndrome stems, in part, from the high surface tensions at the alveolar air/liquid interface. Von Neerguard demonstrated in the 1920s that a liquid to liquid interface in the lung would remove surface tension effects. Application of this observation can be found in liquid lung ventilation, using a liquid with a high carrying capacity for both oxygen and carbon dioxide instead of air/oxygen mixtures. Perfluorocarbons (carbohydrate molecules with the hydrogen elements replaced by fluorine) are inert liquids that are capable of sustaining gas exchange when instilled into the lung. By partially filling the lungs with perfluorocarbon a conventional ventilator can be used to oxygenate the liquid, which in turn transfers the oxygen to the alveolar membrane (partial liquid ventilation). Most experience has been gained in infants initially sustained by extracorporeal membrane oxygenation. Much greater experience with this technique is required before more widespread use can be justified.

Weaning of mechanical ventilation

More than 80 per cent of patients who are ventilated postoperatively can be weaned simply by clinically evaluating their spontaneous ventilation on a 'T-piece' or similar circuit. The remainder require a progressive reduction in ventilatory support until measurement of ventilation parameters can be made, including the negative inspiratory force and vital capacity. A negative inspiratory force greater than –25 cmH$_2$O or a vital capacity greater than 10 ml/kg usually indicates sufficient ventilatory reserve for spontaneous ventilation. However, these parameters cannot be applied reliably to patients with severe chronic obstructive pulmonary disease, when blood gases have to be followed with each reduction in ventilation support. Modes of ventilation such as SIMV, IMV, BiPAP, and pressure support are very suitable for weaning since they allow gradual and progressive reduction in support. Regular clinical and physiological assessment after each reduction in ventilation support is essential. Failure to wean a patient successfully from mechanical ventilation should prompt the questions addressed in Table 3.

Complications of mechanical ventilation

Several complications of mechanical ventilation can be attributed to the local effects of the endotracheal tube upon the airway. These include airway obstruction due to tube displacement and pressure necrosis leading to vocal cord injury and subglottic stenosis. The risk of nosocomial pneumonia is increased in the intubated patient.

Table 3 Questions to ask when weaning is difficult

1. Is the endotracheal tube of optimal size? Small endotracheal tubes of less than 7 mm internal diameter have a high resistance.
2. Has the patient been seated upright to aid lung mechanics?
3. Is there evidence of airway obstruction that would improve with bronchodilator or steroid therapy?
4. Are respiratory depressant drugs being administered?
5. Is there evidence of occult neuromuscular disease? Exclude interactions with aminoglycosides.
6. Is there evidence of hypothyroidism, hypophosphataemia, or hypomagnesaemia?
7. Is there a metabolic alkalosis? If so this should be corrected with potassium, chloride, and volume replacement as appropriate.
8. Is there evidence of malnourishment on history or simple laboratory test such as serum albumin?
9. In patients with chronic obstructive pulmonary disease, are the target blood gases similar to the premorbid values?
10. Is there evidence of diaphragmatic dysfunction due to phrenic nerve injury?
11. Is tracheostomy indicated?

Many complications are the direct consequence of positive-pressure ventilation. Haemodynamic effects such as reduced cardiac output, reduced renal perfusion, salt and water retention are primarily the result of mechanical, neuroreflex, and humoral factors. The greatest concern relates to the risk of pneumothorax, pneumomediastinum, pneumopericardium, or subcutaneous emphysema (barotrauma). Pneumothorax is the most feared of these because it is associated with rapid deterioration unless dealt with quickly. Signs of tension pneumothorax include arterial desaturation (pulse oximeter), sudden rise in peak airway pressure, asymmetry of chest wall movement, hypotension and tachycardia, and finally circulatory collapse.

Tube thoracostomy is mandatory for pneumothorax in the ventilated patient since progression to a tension pneumothorax is very likely. However, prophylactic thoracostomy tubes are not recommended, even in the presence of pneumomediastinum. Emergency decompression with a 14-gauge cannula is essential in tension pneumothorax, can produce temporary relief of a pneumothorax not under tension, and may have a diagnostic role, but tube thoracostomy should be performed without delay and without radiographic confirmation if necessary. Blunt dissection through the parietal pleura with forceps and digital exploration of the pleural space prior to insertion of the thoracostomy tube is essential if lung damage is to be avoided. Thoracostomy tubes with rigid metal stylets must not be used under any circumstances.

Non-invasive methods of ventilation support

Positive pressure non-invasive ventilation

Non-invasive assisted ventilation may offer an alternative to endotracheal intubation in selected patients with acute respiratory failure. Current evidence suggests that positive pressure non-invasive techniques support the respiratory muscles and avoid upper airway obstruction better than negative pressure techniques. Non-invasive positive pressure ventilation can be applied with volume cycled ventilation, bi-level positive airway pressure (BiPAP), and pressure support modes delivered via face and nasal masks.

Although the principle of the treatment is straightforward, with the application of positive pressure being used to assist ventilation, the practice can sometimes be difficult. Masks must fit tightly or else leakage prevents the generation of adequate positive pressure, and they can be uncomfortable, particularly if not expertly fitted. Indeed, failure to tolerate the mask, sometimes with the development of pressure damage to the face or nose (up to and including necrosis), often prevents effective treatment. If patients are going to respond well to non-invasive ventilation, benefit is apparent within the first 60 min. The maximal duration of successful ventilatory support using non-invasive positive pressure ventilation is usually less than 7 days. A specialist unit with expertly trained nursing care is essential for best results.

Although suitable for those with a variety of causes of respiratory failure, the main use of non-invasive ventilation is in the management of patients with acute exacerbation of chronic obstructive pulmonary disease, and an increasing number of studies testify to its efficacy in this disorder. A prospective randomized study compared non-invasive pressure support ventilation delivered through a face mask with standard treatment in selected patients with acute exacerbation of chronic obstructive pulmonary disease admitted to five intensive care units. This found that non-invasive ventilation reduced the need for endotracheal intubation (11 of 43 (26 per cent) versus 31 of 42 (74 per cent)), the frequency of complications (16 versus 48 per cent), the mean hospital stay (23 days versus 35 days), and the in-hospital mortality rate (9 versus 29 per cent). In a similar population non-invasive ventilation has also been shown to be better than continued invasive pressure support ventilation by an endotracheal tube in a randomized study of weaning from mechanical ventilation, both reducing the duration of mechanical ventilation (from 17 to 10 days) and the time spent in

the intensive care unit (15 versus 24 days), and improving survival at 60 days (92 versus 72 per cent).

The use of non-invasive ventilation has also been examined in a general respiratory ward setting. A prospective randomized controlled study in 14 United Kingdom hospitals compared this treatment with standard therapy in patients with acute exacerbation of chronic obstructive pulmonary disease and mild to moderate acidosis. The use of non-invasive ventilation reduced the need for intubation as defined by objective criteria from 27 per cent (32/118) to 15 per cent (18/118) and reduced in-hospital mortality from 20 per cent to 10 per cent.

Negative-pressure ventilation (NPV)

Negative-pressure ventilation is achieved by applying subatmospheric pressures to the surface of the thorax during inspiration and provides an alternative means of assisting ventilation without intubation. Expiration is usually accomplished passively by the elastic recoil pressure of the lungs and chest wall. Negative pressures at predetermined frequencies and depths can be applied to the whole body (iron lung), chest wall, or chest and abdominal wall (cuirass). Some devices can maintain a negative pressure at end-expiration to maintain lung recruitment in a negative-pressure equivalent of PEEP. The haemodynamic effects of NPV are variable and depend on whether negative pressure is applied to the whole body or only to the thorax.

NPV using 'iron lungs' has been used mostly in patients with neuromuscular disorders, such as poliomyelitis or muscular dystrophy, and in those with chronic obstructive pulmonary disease. NPV with negative end-expiratory pressure (NEEP) has been used in patients during hypoxaemic respiratory failure due to acute respiratory distress syndrome and Pneumocystis carinii pneumonia.

The negative intratracheal pressures generated during NPV may adduct the vocal cords producing laryngeal obstruction. As a result NPV is not ideal for diseases that may be complicated by upper airway obstruction, such as Guillain–Barré syndrome and myasthenia gravis. For similar reasons, NPV may be ineffective in patients with sleep apnoea. By contrast, the application of nasal CPAP (positive pressure) to such patients is recognized as reliably preventing upper airway obstruction (see Chapter 17.8.1).

Recent developments of the cuirass type of negative-pressure ventilator (Hayek®) permit high frequency oscillations to be used, resulting in enhanced gas exchange.

Specific strategies in ventilator management

Restrictive lung disease

Patients with restrictive lung diseases such as sarcoidosis or fibrosing alveolitis should be ventilated with small tidal volumes of between 5 to 8 ml/kg at rates of 15 to 20 breaths/min. Oxygen need not be restricted in the manner recommended for patients with chronic obstructive pulmonary disease.

Chronic obstructive pulmonary disease

Low rate SIMV (6 to 8 breaths/min) or low pressure levels of pressure support are ideal for patients suffering from chronic obstructive pulmonary disease with acute or chronic respiratory failure. The $Paco_2$ should be reduced very slowly towards—but not to—normal levels. The Fio_2 rarely needs to be higher than 0.35. High ventilator rates (more than 16/min) are associated with incomplete expiration and air trapping, and the $Paco_2$ may rise paradoxically if ventilator rates are increased in an attempt to increase minute ventilation. To avoid this, the I:E ratio should be maintained at 1:2 or more.

Weaning can begin as soon as the precipitating cause of respiratory failure has been corrected. Weaning will be unsuccessful if there is any underlying metabolic alkalosis or the patient receives sedative or analgesic agents. The Pa_{CO_2} can be allowed to rise slowly to above normal levels provided sufficient time is given for the blood pH to correct and the FI_{O_2} is kept below 0.35. Carbon dioxide production can be minimized by providing balanced nutrition with calories from both lipid and carbohydrate.

Asthma

Probably less than 1 per cent of acute severe asthma attacks require mechanical ventilation. However, some patients suffer cardiac arrest and die every year because intubation and mechanical ventilation was not performed in time. Hypercarbia alone is generally insufficient as an indication for ventilation, but a combination of a rising Pa_{CO_2}, fatigue, failure of conservative measures, or arrhythmias does call for elective intubation and mechanical ventilation. Adequate oxygenation must be ensured by the administration of unrestricted and high concentrations of oxygen, in contrast to the patient with CO_2-retaining chronic obstructive pulmonary disease for whom controlled oxygen (24 to 28 per cent) is generally indicated.

Patients with asthma may be difficult to ventilate initially and often require high inflation pressures. Hypoxia may persist despite the use of high concentrations of oxygen and is probably the result of mucus plugging of the airways. A philosophy of 'permissive hypercapnia' or 'controlled hypoventilation' should be adopted with the Pa_{CO_2} remaining at elevated levels (7 to 8 kPa, 50 to 60 mmHg). This allows lower tidal volumes and respiratory rates; lower inspiratory flow rates result in lower peak pressures and reduced risk of barotrauma. Deaths in ventilated asthmatic patients are rare but are usually the result of barotrauma, hypotension in volume-depleted patients, arrhythmias, or lung infection.

Maximal bronchodilator therapy including corticosteroids should be continued throughout the period of mechanical ventilation, supplemented if necessary with inhalational anaesthetics such as isoflurane or the intravenous anaesthetic ketamine. Both of these agents are potent bronchodilators. Rehydration and adequate humidification of inspired gases will ordinarily mobilize secretions and mucous plugs; if not, bronchoalveolar lavage may be indicated.

The use of extracorporeal membrane oxygenation and CO_2 removal has been reported in acute asthma. These must be considered exceptional cases and such techniques cannot be generally recommended.

Further reading

Brochard L, et al. (1995). Noninvasive ventilation for acute exacerbations of chronic obstructive pulmonary disease. New England Journal of Medicine 333, 817–22.

Cameron PD, Oh TE (1986). Newer modes of mechanical ventilatory support. Anaesthesia and Intensive Care 14, 258–66.

Downs JB et al. (1973). IMV: A new approach to weaning patients from mechanical ventilators. Chest 64, 331–5.

Downs JB, Block AJ, Vennum KB (1974). Intermittent mandatory ventilation in the treatment of patients with chronic obstructive pulmonary disease. Anesthesia and Analgesia 53, 437–43.

Dreyfuss D, Saumon G (1998). Ventilator-induced lung injury: lessons from experimental studies. American Journal of Respiratory and Critical Care Medicine 157, 294–323.

Garrard CS (1992). Mechanical ventilation support in severe asthma. Care of the Critically Ill 8, 201–11.

Gattinoni L et al. (1980). Treatment of acute respiratory failure with low frequency positive-pressure ventilation and extracorporeal removal of CO_2. Lancet ii, 292–4.

Hess DR (1999). Noninvasive positive pressure ventilation for acute respiratory failure. International Anesthesiology Clinics 37(3), 85–102.

Hickling KG, Henderson SJ, Jackson R (1990). Low mortality associated with low volume pressure limited ventilation with permissive hypercapnia in severe adult respiratory distress syndrome. Intensive Care Medicine 16, 372–7.

Hill NS (1993). Noninvasive ventilation: does it work, for whom, and how? American Review of Respiratory Disease 147, 1050–5.

Kirby RR et al. (1975). High level PEEP in acute respiratory insufficiency. Chest 67, 156–63.

Kumar A et al. (1970). Continuous positive-pressure ventilation in acute respiratory failure. New England Journal of Medicine 283, 1430–6.

Nava S, et al. (1998). Noninvasive mechanical ventilation in the weaning of patients with respiratory failure due to chronic obstructive pulmonary disease. A randomized, controlled trial. Annals of Internal Medicine 128, 721–8.

Patel RG, Petrini MF (1998). Respiratory muscle performance, pulmonary mechanics, and gas exchange between the BiPAP S/T-D system and the Servo Ventilator 900C with bilevel positive airway pressure ventilation following gradual pressure support weaning. Chest 114, 1390–6.

Plant PK, et al. (2000). Early use of non-invasive ventilation for acute exacerbations of chronic obstructive pulmonary disease on general respiratory wards: a multicentre randomised controlled trial. Lancet 355, 1931–5.

Rabatin JT, Gay PC (1999). Noninvasive ventilation. Mayo Clinic Proceedings 74, 817–20.

Slutsky AS (1999). Lung injury caused by mechanical ventilation. Chest 116(Suppl), 9S–15S.

Smith RA, Desautels DA, Kirby RR (1985). Mechanical ventilators. In: Kirby RR, Smith RA, Desautels DA. Mechanical ventilation, pp 327–474. Churchill Livingstone, New York.

Suter PM, Fairley HB, Isenberg MD (1975). Optimum end-expiratory pressure in patients with acute pulmonary failure. New England Journal of Medicine 292, 284–9.

Sykes MK (1985). High frequency ventilation. Thorax 40, 161–5.

Tobin MJ (1988). Predicting weaning outcome (Editorial). Chest 94, 227.

Tuxen DV (1989). Detrimental effects of positive end-expiratory pressure during controlled mechanical ventilation of patients with severe airflow obstruction. American Review of Respiratory Disease 140, 5–9.

Wood LH, Prewitt RM (1981). Cardiovascular management in acute hypoxemic respiratory failure. American Journal of Cardiology 47, 963–72.

16.6 Other medical issues on the ICU

16.6.1 Sedation and analgesia in the critically ill

G. R. Park and B. Ward

Sedation and analgesia are used to increase patient comfort by minimizing the pain and anxiety produced by illness and its treatment. Factors contributing to patient discomfort are shown in Fig. 1.

The relief of pain is an obvious part of being comfortable, but the role of sedation is more complex. The term sedation covers a broad range of conscious states, from almost wide awake to deeply unresponsive. The 'ideal' level of sedation for most patients is at ease, without signs of anxiety or agitation and easily rousable from light sleep. Sedation is needed for a variety of reasons, including:

(1) reduction of anxiety caused by fear, inability to communicate, loss of control, or unfamiliar environment;

(2) allowing patients to tolerate treatment—e.g. stops them pulling out the tracheal tube;

(3) allowing patterns of ventilation to be imposed which do not synchronize with a normal breathing pattern;

(4) prevention of awareness when neuromuscular paralysis is used;

(5) minimizing distress during uncomfortable procedures;

(6) allowing sleep; and

(7) control of fits.

Patients will usually tolerate a tracheal tube without the need for paralysis if the ventilator is properly set and they are properly sedated. The

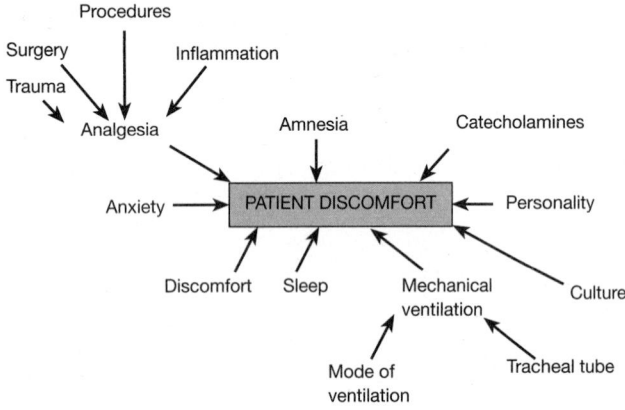

Fig. 1 Factors contributing to patient discomfort.

indications for neuromuscular relaxation in the critically ill are listed below: the use of muscle relaxants is otherwise avoided.

(1) Acute respiratory distress syndrome (ARDS)—paralysis allows the patient to tolerate unusual ventilatory modes, e.g. reverse ratio ventilation;

(2) raised intracranial pressure—paralysis prevents coughing and straining; and

(3) status asthmaticus—paralysis can reduce risks of barotrauma to lungs.

The intravenous route is used almost exclusively for the administration of analgesia and sedation in the critically ill, as it is faster and more reliable than other routes. Drugs can be given either as repeated bolus doses, or as a continuous infusion. Although a continuous infusion has the advantage of avoiding peaks and troughs associated with bolus doses, there is also an increased risk of inadvertent overdose or accumulation.

The analgesic needs of most patients can best be met with regular bolus doses of analgesic titrated against repeated assessment of the pain. A patient- or nurse-controlled syringe pump driver will deliver a bolus of a predetermined amount of drug when triggered to do so. There is usually a predetermined 'lockout' safety period during which further requests for bolus doses will be ignored. Morphine is the drug most commonly given in this manner, but diamorphine, pethidine, and fentanyl can also be used. A loading dose may be needed before starting.

Hazards of sedation and analgesia

The use of drugs for sedation and analgesia involves risks to the patient. These include:

(1) over-sedation or a prolonged sedative effect caused by poor elimination in the critically ill;

(2) hypotension/myocardial depression;

(3) antitussive effects leading to failure to clear pulmonary secretions;

(4) hypoventilation, delaying weaning;

(5) toxic effects due to accumulation of sedative/analgesic agents or their metabolites; and

(6) expense, both of the drugs and their adverse effects.

There are many reasons why the behaviour of drugs administered to the critically ill patient may be abnormal. These include:

(1) hepatic failure leading to poor metabolism or biliary excretion of the drug;

(2) renal failure leading to decreased excretion of the drug or its metabolites;

(3) haemofiltration/dialysis may have unpredictable effects on clearance of the drug or its metabolites;

(4) reduced plasma protein levels (e.g. albumin) may lead to increased free (active) drug levels;

(5) volume of distribution may be affected by oedema, ascites, or hyper/hypovolaemia;

(6) interactions between drugs; and

(7) solvent toxicity.

The risks of using drugs can me minimized by a knowledge of their routes of breakdown and excretion. Agents that are unlikely to accumulate should be chosen when possible. Drugs with more than one site of metabolism, or those which can undergo non-organ-based breakdown are preferred. The risk of accumulation of a sedative drug can be reduced by stopping it every 24 h whenever possible and letting the patient recover from its effects. If the patient wakes or becomes restless, the drug can be restarted knowing that accumulation has not occurred.

To avoid under- or over-sedation, drugs need some assessment of their effects. Because of the many components which are involved in sedation, no simple method exists. Although work is progressing on physical methods of assessing the level of sedation (e.g. spectral analysis of electroencephalogram waveforms), the most commonly used methods rely on bedside observations. We use a scoring system comprising several different elements (Fig. 2) (see below). The key to avoiding under- or over-sedation is regular assessment of the patient and adjustment of the sedation regimen accordingly.

Psychological disturbances

Severe illness, the intensive care environment, and drugs usually prevent patients from sleeping normally. Deprivation of sleep, especially if prolonged, combined with the fear of dying may make some patients psychotic. Close attention to environment (e.g. normal day/night light levels, noise etc.) may help. Drugs may be of some benefit, but can cause prolonged sedation. If the patient has a prolonged recovery phase then depression is common. Antidepressants are rarely of value and can have toxic effects.

Drug treatment

Before using drugs, causes of pain and agitation such as a full bladder or rectum should be excluded.

Sedative drugs

There are two main types of drugs, those principally sedative and those mostly analgesic. The agents most commonly used for sedation are the benzodiazepine midazolam and the anaesthetic agent propofol. These, and other agents commonly used for sedation in the intensive care unit, are described below.

	Element	Date/time	1	2	3	4	5
	Agitated						
	Awake			X			
Sedation score	Roused by voice		X		X	X	
	Roused by tracheal suction						X
	Unrousable						
	Paralysed						
	Asleep						
	Pain YES/NO		N	Y	N	N	N
	Comfortable on ventilator YES/NO		Y	Y	Y	Y	Y

Fig. 2 The Addenbrooke's Sedation Score.

Midazolam

Midazolam is a water-soluble benzodiazepine, which can be given peripherally without causing thrombophlebitis or pain. Like all benzodiazepines it has sedative, amnesic, anxiolytic, and anticonvulsive properties. It has a rapid onset, short half-life (approximately 2 h), and is commonly used in combination with morphine in order to achieve both analgesia and sedation. Midazolam is primarily metabolized by the liver, and accumulation occurs in liver failure. The (phase I) metabolic product, l-hydroxymidazolam has around 10 per cent of the activity of the parent drug. In renal failure, accumulation of l-hydroxymidazolam glucuronide (the phase II metabolic product) can cause prolonged sedation or coma.

Lorazepam

This has been used as an alternative to midazolam. It undergoes metabolism only by glucuronidation to render it water soluble. This makes it less likely for the parent drug to accumulate. It is dissolved in propylene glycol.

Diazepam

Diazepam is rarely used in the critically ill, having been replaced by midazolam. It has a much longer duration of action and has many metabolites with significant activity of their own. This increases the risk of accumulation.

Propofol

Propofol (2,6-di-isopropylphenol) was introduced as an anaesthetic agent but is widely used for sedation in the critically ill as a continuous infusion. Emergence from sedation is rapid and without hangover effect. Propofol is a respiratory depressant, and prolonged apnoea can occur after bolus doses. Hypotension associated with propofol use is common in the critically ill and is dose related. Although metabolized primarily in the liver, extrahepatic breakdown does occur. There are no active metabolites and propofol does not accumulate in hepatic or renal failure to a significant extent. However, because it is formulated in soya bean extract, prolonged infusion (more than 48 h) can lead to hyperlipidaemia. Propofol is expensive, and its use is often limited to those patients who require short-term sedation only.

Dexmedetomidine

Dexmedetomidine is a potent, highly selective, α_2-adrenoceptor agonist. It has sedative, anxiolytic, amnesic, and sympatholytic effects. In addition, dexmedetomidine appears to reduce requirements for opioid analgesia. These effects are mediated centrally at post-synaptic α_2-receptors. In contrast to the agents already discussed, dexmedetomidine does not seem to cause respiratory depression, and exhibits remarkable cardiovascular stability. Because of these features, there is currently great interest in the use of this agent.

Thiopentone

The intravenous anaesthetic agent thiopentone retains certain specialized indications, for example use in status epilepticus or to reduce raised intracerebral pressure. Thiopentone has a half-life of 11 h, and prolonged infusion (i.e. > 24 h) is usually associated with extremely prolonged action.

Combinations of agents

Sedative drugs often act via differing mechanisms and so have slightly different actions. This difference can be used to advantage. For example propofol is mostly an hypnotic, whilst midazolam is a good anxiolytic and amnesic agent as well as producing hypnosis. In combination they are synergistic.

Table 1 Properties of opioid drugs

Opioid	Onset of action	Suitable* for PCAS/ NCAS	Liable to accumulate in hepatic failure	Liable to accumulate in renal failure
Morphine	Slow	Yes	Yes	Yes
Diamorphine	Moderate	Yes	Yes	Yes
Pethidine	Moderate	Yes	Yes	Yes
Fentanyl	Fast	Yes	Yes	Yes
Alfentanil	Very fast	No*	Yes	No
Remifentanil	Very fast	No*	No	No

PCAS, patient-controlled analgesia system; NCAS, Nurse-controlled analgesia system.

*Except with special supervision.

Analgesic drugs

Opioid drugs remain the mainstay of analgesic treatment in the critically ill, and morphine is the most common choice. Some properties of the opioid drugs used in the critically ill are listed in Table 1.

Morphine

Morphine is a cheap and effective analgesic agent and is the opioid against which others are judged. It has both analgesic and sedative effects, although an excessive dose would be required to produce adequate sedation by its use alone. It is often given with a benzodiazepine, such as midazolam, to achieve analgesia and sedation. It is the standard agent for use in patient- and nurse-controlled syringe pumps. Morphine is metabolized in the liver, forming two major metabolites—morphine 3-glucuronide (**M3G**) and morphine 6-glucuronide (**M6G**), both of which are active. M6G is a potent analgesic, whilst M3G is thought to be antianalgesic.

Pethidine

Pethidine is a synthetic compound and was originally developed as an anticholinergic agent. It does tend to cause anticholinergic effects, such as dry mouth, blurred vision, and tachycardia. It is claimed that pethidine induces less constriction of the biliary sphincter than morphine, and perhaps the only indication for its use is in patients with biliary pathology. It is metabolized in the liver to form norpethidine, pethidinic acid, and pethidine-N-oxide. These metabolites are excreted by the kidneys, and in renal failure significant amounts of norpethidine may accumulate, leading to grand mal convulsions.

Fentanyl

Fentanyl is approximately 100 times as potent as morphine, and has a rapid onset of action (3 min). In low doses the analgesic effect of fentanyl ends after about 20 min by its rapid redistribution around the body. With larger doses, tissues may become saturated and drug action is prolonged, termination depending on the slow process of N-demethylation in the liver. The major metabolite, norfentanyl, is excreted by the kidneys, and its accumulation may cause toxic delirium in patients with renal failure. Accumulation of fentanyl itself may occur in hepatic failure, causing prolonged effect. Fentanyl has a potent apnoeic effect, and in large doses, fentanyl can produce muscle rigidity, particularly of the chest wall.

Alfentanil

Alfentanil is approximately 10 to 20 times as potent as morphine, and has a very fast onset time (1 min). The effects of alfentanil are short lived (approximately 10 to 15 min), ending by redistribution to tissues. Because of this, alfentanil is unsuitable for use in patient-controlled syringe pumps, and it is administered by continuous infusion. Elimination takes place almost exclusively in the liver, and alfentanil is the current drug of choice in severe renal impairment. It can accumulate in hepatic failure, cirrhosis, or when hepatic enzyme inhibitors such as cimetidine are used.

Remifentanil

Remifentanil is a relatively new agent which may prove to have pharmacological properties useful in critically ill patients. It has a fast onset of action and a very short half-life (10 to 21 min). Remifentanil has an ester linkage within its structure, which is broken down by a non-specific, non-saturable enzyme system present in plasma. This breakdown pathway means that accumulation does not occur, and the drug wears off rapidly even after prolonged infusions and in renal or hepatic failure. Remifentanil must be given by constant infusion, indeed the effects wear off so rapidly that even small delays, such as the time taken to make up a new syringe, can leave the patient without analgesia.

Sedative and analgesic antagonists

When accumulation of a drug or its metabolite is suspected as the cause of prolonged sedation, the diagnosis can be confirmed with the use of antagonists. Naloxone will quickly (but temporarily) reverse the effects of opiates, whilst flumazenil is a benzodiazepine antagonist. Their use is not recommended in patients suffering from head injury. Large doses of either antagonist given quickly can produce sudden arousal, causing agitation. When using naloxone, the sudden reversal of analgesia can cause a massive outpouring of catecholamines and precipitate arrhythmias.

Regional and epidural anaesthesia

For analgesia after certain surgical procedures or trauma, regional and epidural techniques can be extremely effective. Lumbar or thoracic epidurals can prevent hypoventilation and diaphragmatic splinting caused by pain after abdominal or thoracic procedures and fractured ribs, whilst avoiding the side-effects of high-dose opioids. The problem of correct placement of regional blocks in critically ill patients is a considerable one, and complications (such as pneumothorax following intercostal block) must be carefully considered. Epidural analgesia, although desirable, may be contraindicated in the critically ill patient because of coagulopathy or sepsis.

Further reading

Bion JF, Oh TE (1997). Sedation in intensive care. In: Oh TE, ed. *Intensive care manual*, pp 672–8. Butterworth Heineman, Oxford. [An overview of the principles and practice of sedation in intensive care.]

Burns AM, Shelly MP, Park GR (1992). The use of sedative agents in critically ill patients. *Drugs* **43**, 507–15. [A full review of the drugs used to sedate critically ill patients.]

Carrupt PA *et al.* (1991). Morphine 6-glucuronide and morphine 3-glucuronide as molecular chameleons with unexpected lipophilicity. *Journal of Medical Chemistry* **34**, 1272–5. [An important paper that describes how metabolites that should be inactive change their configuration to become active.]

Park GR (1996). Molecular mechanisms of drug metabolism in the critically ill. *British Journal of Anaesthesia* **77**, 32–49. [Describes the problems of drug elimination, solvent toxicity, and makes brief mention of protein binding in the critically ill.]

Park GR, Sladen RN, eds (1995). *Sedation and analgesia in the critically ill*, pp 18–50. Blackwell Science, Oxford. [A multinational book that describes sedation in various diseases, rather than looking at the use of individual drugs.]

Shapiro BA *et al.* (1995). Practice parameters for intravenous analgesia and sedation for adult patients in the intensive care unit: an executive summary. *Critical Care Medicine* **23**, 1596–600. [An American consensus document on how to provide sedation and analgesia in the critically ill.]

Shelly MP, Pomfrett CJD (1999). Assessment of sedation and analgesia and muscle relaxation in the intensive care unit. *Current Opinion in Critical Care* **5**, 269–73. [A paper reviewing clinical as well as experimental methods of assessing sedation and analgesia.]

Tryba M, Kulka PJ (1993). Critical care pharmacotherapy. *Drugs* **45**, 338–52. [Interesting review looking at propofol, isoflurane, clonidine, and sufentanil for sedation. Also reviews H_2-receptor antagonists and sucralfate against gastrointestinal bleeding.]

Venn R *et al.* (1999). Monitoring the depth of sedation. *Clinical Intensive Care* **10**, 81–9. [A review on how to measure sedation and analgesia in the critically ill.]

16.6.2 Management of raised intracranial pressure

David K. Menon

Introduction

The normal intracranial pressure (**ICP**), measured at the level of the foramen of Monro, is between 5 and 15 mmHg in supine subjects. Intracranial hypertension (ICP >20 mmHg) is a common accompaniment of many central nervous system (**CNS**) diseases, when it is often the most important cause of symptoms and modulator of outcome, and—in fatal cases—frequently the immediate cause of death.

Pathophysiology

The cranial cavity contains brain (80 per cent), blood (10 per cent), and cerebrospinal fluid (10 per cent). These incompressible contents are contained in a rigid skull with a fixed capacity, hence an increase in volume of any of these contents, or the presence of any space-occupying pathology, results in an increase in ICP unless one of the other constituents can be displaced or its volume decreased (Fig. 1). This principle is referred to as the Monroe–Kelley doctrine. Increases in intracranial volume may be caused by:

1. *Brain oedema*, which may have different pathogenic mechanisms:
   - cytotoxic oedema occurs as a result of cell swelling, most commonly due to ischaemic energy depletion and rises in intracellular sodium and water;
   - vasogenic oedema results from an increased permeability of the blood–brain barrier with an expansion of the extracellular fluid compartment;
   - interstitial oedema occurs in the context of hydrocephalus, where increased intraventricular cerebrospinal fluid (**CSF**) pressures result in permeation of CSF into adjacent brain, typically in the frontal periventricular regions.

2. *Vascular engorgement*, which results from an increased cerebral blood volume. This may be due to the vasodilatation that accompanies normal or abnormal (for example, epileptiform) neuronal activity. In other situations vasodilatation may be due to the loss of vasoregulation, either due to disease (vasoparalysis), or to the effect of potent physiological (carbon dioxide) or pharmacological (nitrates and other nitric oxide donors) cerebral vasodilators.

3. *Hydrocephalus*, which may be non-communicating (where an obstruction prevents the ventricular system communicating with the subarachnoid space), or communicating (where there is a defect in CSF reabsorption).

4. *Space-occupying lesions* (**SOLs**), which may be chronic (for example, intracranial tumours) or acute (for example, intracranial haematomas associated with trauma).

Temporal patterns of ICP change

Initial increases in intracranial volume are buffered by the displacement or reduction in volume of other contents. Thus, cerebral oedema may result in compression of the ventricles, with translocation of CSF to the spinal subarachnoid space, and compression of cerebral vasculature. Over longer

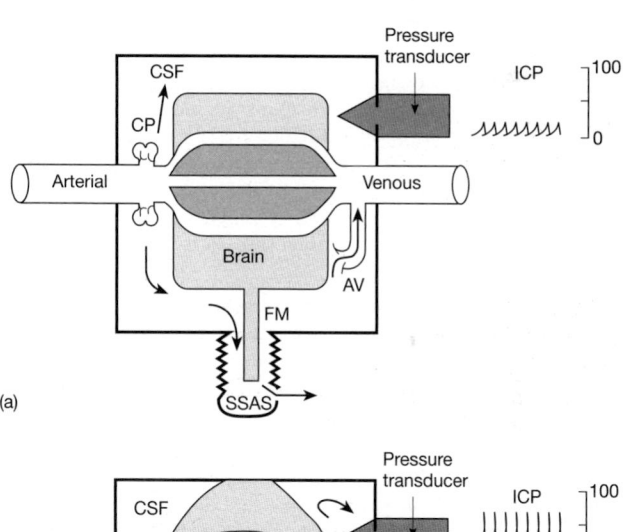

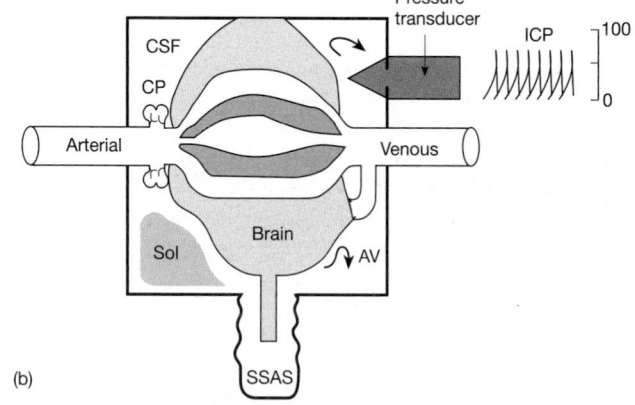

Fig. 1 Schematic diagram showing intracranial contents in the normal brain (a) and with elevated intracranial pressure (b). Note that cerebrospinal fluid (CSF) produced by the choroids plexus (CP), circulates freely, passing through the foramen magnum (FM) into the spinal subarachnoid space (SSAS), before absorption by arachnoid villi (AV) in the cerebral venous sinuses. Increases in ICP may be due to brain oedema, vascular engorgement, space-occupying lesions (SOL), or impaired CSF circulation or absorption. Compensatory mechanisms include translocation of CSF to the SSAS, and compression of cerebral vascular beds. The ICP trace shows a higher mean value, and the inability of the non-compliant brain to cope with increased blood during each systole results in an increased pulsatility of the ICP waveform.

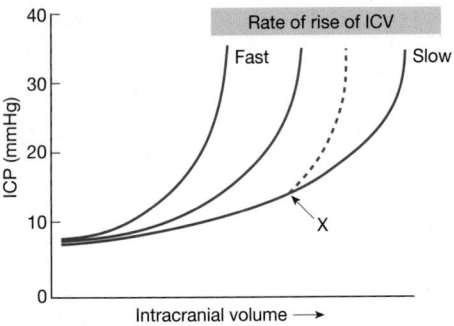

Fig. 2 Intracranial volume/pressure curves. Increases in intracranial volume (ICV) are initially buffered by compensatory mechanisms, but eventually result in elevation of intracranial pressure (ICP). The ability to buffer increases in ICV depends on the speed at which pathology develops. Gradually progressive ICV increases (such as those produced by a slow growing tumour) may be well compensated, until a precipitating factor (e.g. the development of hydrocephalus, denoted by X in the diagram) shifts the relationship to a steeper curve.

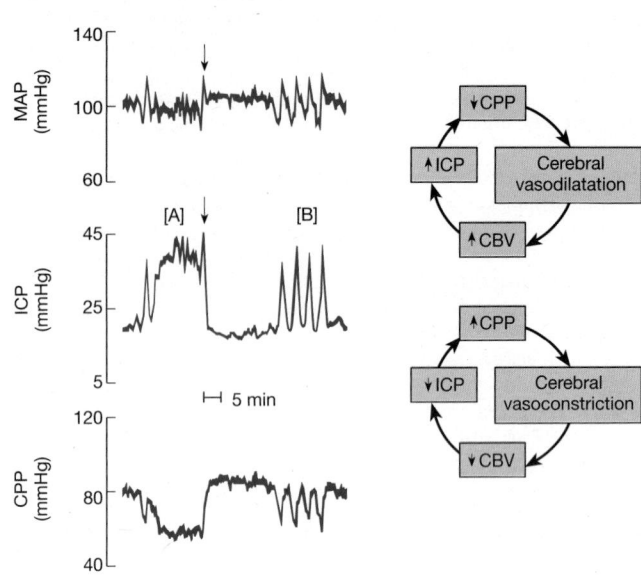

Fig. 3 Intracranial pressure (ICP) traces show phasic variations that may last several minutes (Lundberg A waves (A)) or be more transient (Lundberg B waves (B)). Elevations of ICP are often initiated by reductions in mean arterial pressure (MAP), which reduce cerebral perfusion pressure (CPP) and thereby trigger compensatory vasodilatation and increase cerebral blood volume (CBV) and ICP. This vicious cycle may be terminated by spontaneous hypertension associated with a Cushing response (arrow in MAP and ICP traces), or by therapeutic elevation of MAP, which triggers compensatory cerebral vasoconstriction and reductions in ICP. Note that a period of stable MAP greater than 100 mmHg is associated with a low, stable ICP. (Figure modified with permission from Rosner MJ (1993). Pathophysiology and management of increased intracranial pressure. In: Andrews BT, ed. *Neurosurgical intensive care*, p 75. McGraw-Hill, New York.)

periods, normal brain may be compressed and CSF production diminished. The relationship between intracranial volume (**ICV**) and ICP is commonly depicted as a hyperbolic curve, with an initial flat part during which compensatory mechanisms are effective, moving after their progressive exhaustion to a steep phase when even small increases in intracranial volume produce large increases in ICP. However, the extent and efficiency with which these mechanisms buffer increases in volume depend on the speed of disease progression, and given these considerations it is more appropriate to depict the evolution of pathophysiology as a family of curves, with variable rates of progression (Fig. 2). It is important to make three further points in this context:

1. A precipitating factor may suddenly increase the speed of progression of a relatively slow pathophysiological process, and be the proximate cause of symptomatic decompensation.

2. Acute changes in cerebrovascular physiology are an important cause of such deterioration. Both hypoxia and hypercarbia can cause cerebral vasodilatation and elevate ICP, and whilst *severe* hypertension may result in cerebral oedema, it is far more common to find that relatively minor reductions in mean arterial pressure compromise cerebral perfusion and trigger reflex vasodilatation and a secondary increase in ICP. Such haemodynamic instability may be the underlying cause of phasic increases in ICP (Fig. 3).

3. Finally, since patients with significant intracranial hypertension operate on the steep part of the ICV/ICP curve, even small decreases in intracranial volume (for example, a 5-ml decrease in cerebral blood volume produced by mild hyperventilation) can have a gratifyingly large effect on ICP.

Why treat intracranial hypertension?

Brain perfusion depends on the difference between mean arterial pressure (**MAP**) and ICP, termed 'cerebral perfusion pressure' (**CPP**). While the normal brain autoregulates cerebral blood flow across a large range of CPP values, the lower limit of such autoregulation is about 50 mmHg in healthy subjects, but may be significantly higher (60–70 mmHg) in disease. CPP reductions below the lower limit of autoregulation result in cerebral ischaemia, and even minor reductions in CPP may trigger reflex vasodilatation and increase ICP in a non-compliant intracranial cavity.

An expanding focal mass can generate pressure gradients within the intracranial cavity. Moreover, the resulting displacement of brain against rigid structures and protrusion (herniation) of brain through narrow openings between intracranial compartments can press on vital structures and result in death (Fig. 4).

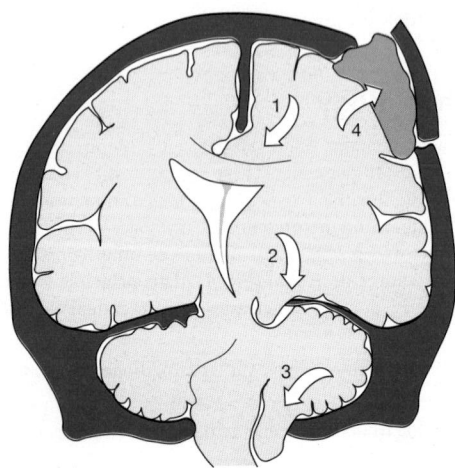

Fig. 4 Cerebral herniation may be: (1) subfalcine (beneath the falx cerebri); (2) transtentorial (through the tentorial hiatus with compression of the midbrain and posterior cerebral artery); (3) tonsillar (where the cerebellar tonsils herniate through the foramen magnum and compress the lower brainstem upper and cervical cord); or (4) transcalvarial (through a traumatic or surgical defect in the roof of the cranial cavity). (Modified with permission from Fishman RA (1975). *New England Journal of Medicine* **293**, 706.)

Prolonged intracranial hypertension may result in permanent damage to critical structures. Thus, benign intracranial hypertension rarely results in herniation syndromes, but frequently causes optic atrophy if left untreated.

Diagnosis

Symptoms

The symptoms that accompany ICP elevation are non-specific and insensitive. The cardinal feature is headache, which may be described as severe ('worst ever') and explosive in its onset in the setting of intracranial haemorrhage. By contrast, the headache of an intracranial tumour is often progressive, worst on awakening (possibly due to ICP elevations associated with the supine position and Pa_{CO_2} elevation during sleep), and exacerbated by coughing and straining. However, it may be indistinguishable from a common tension headache, and dangerous intracranial hypertension may occur without headache. The headache is often accompanied by vomiting, which is classically described as projectile and not preceded by nausea. Visual disturbances are common and may be attributable to optic or ocular motor nerve compression, with accompanying visual failure or diplopia, respectively. There may be alterations in mental function or conscious state, ranging from impaired concentration, through increased irritability, impaired cognition and memory, and altered personality to increased somnolence and deep coma.

Signs

Papilloedema is the classical sign associated with ICP elevation, but is not seen with acute intracranial hypertension and may be absent even where there are large intracranial masses. Pressure on the cranial nerves may result in weakness of ocular movement. The abducens nerve is often involved in such a process due to its long intracranial course; the resultant diplopia provides the classical example of a false localizing sign. Lesions that irritate the meninges of the posterior fossa can produce neck stiffness.

Progressive rises in ICP result in bradycardia and hypertension, which constitute the Cushing response, and signify stimulation of brainstem autonomic nuclei. Worsening brainstem compression and/or ischaemia result progressively in Cheyne–Stokes respiration, central neurogenic hyperventilation, and irregular respiratory patterns ('ataxia of breathing'). Both neurogenic pulmonary oedema and the adult respiratory distress syndrome have been associated with intracranial hypertension.

Severe ICP elevation may result in herniation of the temporal lobe through the tentorial notch (Fig. 4). This produces clinical features due to pressure on the ipsilateral oculomotor nerve (ipsilateral pupillary dilatation), pyramidal tract (contralateral weakness), and brainstem (Cushing response and abnormal respiratory patterns followed by circulatory collapse and respiratory arrest). The posterior cerebral artery is frequently compressed by the herniating temporal lobe, and successful resuscitation from threatened or early transtentorial herniation may leave a patient with an ipsilateral occipital infarction and cortical blindness.

Imaging

Tomographic imaging now provides most diagnostic information in intracranial hypertension. Computed tomographic scanning may reveal subarachnoid or intracerebral blood, contusions, or a tumour. In addition, cerebral oedema may be manifest by a loss of sulci, compression of the third and lateral ventricles, and effacement of the perimesencephalic and suprasellar cisterns. Unilateral lesions may result in a midline shift, compression of the ipsilateral lateral ventricle, and, in some cases, dilatation of the contralateral ventricle due to obstruction of the foramen of Monro. It is important to recognize that overt ventricular dilatation may be absent when hydrocephalus coexists with cerebral oedema. Indeed, the presence of normal-sized ventricles in the context of intracranial hypertension should suggest the possibility of coexisting hydrocephalus and trigger the consideration of CSF drainage as a means of therapy.

Magnetic resonance imaging may provide better definition of underlying pathology, particularly in the posterior fossa, and its multiplanar capability may allow a better appreciation of the extent of space-occupying lesions. Modern imaging methods can also detect patients who may have relatively normal ICP but are at high risk of severe intracranial hypertension, for example a patient with a middle cerebral artery territory infarction is at high risk of severe brain swelling if more than 50 per cent of the middle cerebral artery territory is hypodense.

Lumbar puncture

A lumbar puncture offers the opportunity to directly measure CSF pressure, and can be the defining investigation in meningitis, subarachnoid haemorrhage, or benign intracranial hypertension. However, in the context of clinical features that suggest intracranial hypertension, a lumbar puncture **must be preceded** by CT scanning, and **avoided** if the basal cisterns are effaced by cerebral oedema. Removal of CSF from the lumbar subarachnoid space under these circumstances can markedly increase the pressure differential in the supratentorial compartment, and precipitate transtentorial herniation.

Monitoring intracranial pressure

The clinical evaluation of intracranial hypertension is difficult due to its non-specific clinical picture and phasic variations. Management may therefore be greatly facilitated by direct monitoring of ICP using intraparenchymal or ventricular monitoring devices. Such monitoring is mandatory in patients with severe intracranial hypertension and in those who are sedated or deeply unconscious, in whom changes in clinical signs do not provide an alternative means of assessing progress and response to therapy.

Management

Management focuses on four areas.

Monitoring disease progression and response to therapy

The approach to monitoring will depend on the clinical context. Repeated clinical examination with regular charting of the Glasgow Coma Scale may suffice in many cases. Patients with benign intracranial hypertension may require a regular visual field assessment, whilst those with head injury, intracranial haemorrhage, or severe cerebral oedema may benefit from direct ICP monitoring. The value of ICP monitoring may be substantially enhanced by the use of other monitoring modalities such as jugular bulb oximetry.

Maintenance of stable physiology and removal of precipitating factors

Hyponatraemia and low plasma osmolality will tend to worsen cerebral oedema by favouring water entry into the brain: they should be corrected vigorously. Maintenance of cerebral perfusion pressure with fluid resuscitation and vasoactive agents will prevent cerebral ischaemia. Comatose patients should have their arterial blood gas levels measured, with intubation and ventilatory support provided if airway protection is required or gas exchange is impaired. Whilst hyperventilation has been widely used to control ICP in the past, there is increasing concern regarding the induction of critical cerebral ischaemia by hypocapnic vasoconstriction. Current recommendations suggest that near-normal Pa_{CO_2} levels (4.5–5 kPa) should be maintained, with moderate hyperventilation (Pa_{CO_2} 4.0–4.5 kPa) guided by jugular bulb oximetry, and reserved for the control of acute episodes of severe intracranial hypertension. Attention should also be paid to treating epilepsy and significant pyrexia, both of which can precipitate rises in ICP, and to discontinuing or reversing the action of drugs such as opiates, which may be responsible for physiological derangements that precipitate ICP elevation.

Table 1 Treatment of intracranial hypertension

CPP augmentation by increasing MAP	Maintenance of CPP >60–70 mmHg prevents ischaemia, and further increases(90–100 mmHg) may reduce ICP by autoregulatory cerebral vasoconstriction. Efficacy demonstrated in the treatment of head injury.
Corticosteroids	Reduce vasogenic oedema by restoring blood–brain barrier integrity. Particularly effective in peritumoral oedema and benign intracranial hypertension. Probably ineffective in trauma. Prophylactic use *may* reduce the incidence of hydrocephalus in bacterial meningitis.
Diuretics	Frusemide (furosemide) used to potentiate mannitol. Acetazolamide and thiazide diuretics used in the treatment of benign intracranial hypertension.
Osmotic agents	Glycerol now rarely used. Mannitol is effective in emergencies and can be used repeatedly if effective and plasma osmolality ≤325 mOsm/l. Hypertonic NaCl (3–30 per cent) may reduce ICP when mannitol is ineffective and tends to cause fewer problems with major fluid shifts.
Reduction of cerebral blood volume	Sedation and the treatment of epilepsy can produce reductions in CBF and CBV that are coupled to a reduction of neuronal metabolism. Hyperventilation has been commonly used to reduce CBV by inducing cerebral vasoconstriction, but it can produce critical reductions in CBF. Needs to be used with care and with monitoring of cerebral oxygenation, usually with jugular bulb oximetry.
Hypothermia	Mild to moderate hypothermia (33–36 °C) may be directly neuroprotective but is also effective at controlling refractory intracranial hypertension by multiple mechanisms, including metabolic suppression and anti-inflammatory effects.
CSF drainage	Ventriculostomy provides emergency drainage of CSF in trauma, acute hydocephalus (subarachnoid haemorrhage, tumours). Ventriculoperitoneal, ventriculoatrial, and lumboperitoneal shunts provide chronic CSF diversion in idiopathic or secondary hydrocephalus. Endoscopic third ventriculostomy provides communication between ventricular and cisternal CSF in non-communicating hydrocephalus. May remove the need for shunts and the associated risk of shunt malfunction and sepsis
Surgical decompression	Large decompressive craniectomies are useful for refractory intracranial hypertension in cases of head injury if used early. There is increasing interest in the decompression of non-dominant MCA stroke with severe cerebral oedema, but this is not an established treatment. Optic nerve decompression may prevent visual deterioration in benign intracranial hypertension.

CPP, cerebral perfusion pressure; MAP, mean arterial pressure; ICP, intracranial pressure; CBF, cerebral blood flow; CBV, cerebral blood volume; CSF, cerebrospinal fluid; MCA, middle cerebral artery.

Table 2 Management of the unconscious patient with intracranial hypertension

Suspect the diagnosis
- Considering the possibility of intracranial hypertension may modify management(e.g. may trigger CT scanning/postpone lumbar puncture)

Clinical findings
- History from family and witnesses may be useful in making a diagnosis
- Deep coma, deterioration on the Glasgow Coma Scale, or pupillary dilatation may prompt intubation and ventilatory support and more aggressive management

CT imaging
- Look for the cause of coma and evidence of raised ICP or findings that denote a high risk of developing intracranial hypertension

Maintain physiology
- Ensure normoxia and normocapnia (Pao_2 >11 kPa, $Paco_2$ 4.5–5 kPa), with tracheal intubation and ventilatory support where required
- Use fluid loading and vasoactive agents to maintain CPP >70 mmHg, or MAP at 90–100 mmHg if ICP not monitored

Treat precipitating factors
- Fits; pyrexia; blood glucose, electrolyte, and osmolality abnormalities

Treat ICP elevation
- 200 ml of 20 per cent mannitol over 15–30 min
- Dexamethasone 8–16 mg at once and 4–8 mg, IV, 6 hourly for tumours
- Hyperventilation ($Paco_2$ ~ 4 kPa) if pupillary dilatation/clinical picture merits
- Consider IV anaesthetics, hypothermia, surgical decompression/CSF drainage

Monitor ICP if appropriate
- ICP monitoring is particularly relevant in trauma, intracranial haemorrhage, major non-dominant hemispheric infarction, sedated patients

Treat underlying condition—*this may need to be an early intervention*

CT, computed tomography; ICP, intracranial pressure; CPP, cerebral perfusion pressure; MAP, mean arterial pressure; IV, intravenous.

Treatment of the underlying condition

Early neurosurgical evaluation and operative therapy may be lifesaving if a patient has an acute intracranial haematoma, a large tumour, or established hydrocephalus. Specific antimicrobial therapy may be required for meningitis, encephalitis, or a brain abscess. Systemic arterial hypertension commonly accompanies intracranial hypertension: it should generally not be treated since it may be needed to preserve cerebral perfusion. It is best to avoid nitric oxide donors such as nitrates if therapy is needed for extreme hypertension or for hypertensive encephalopathy: these can cause cerebral vasodilatation and further increase ICP.

Specific treatment of intracranial hypertension

Several therapies can be used to reduce intracranial pressure: their application will depend on the cause and severity of ICP elevation. Commonly used interventions and their indications are outlined in Table 1, but it must be pointed out that few of these have been assessed by good-quality outcome studies.

Treatment pathways for the emergency management of an unconscious patient with suspected intracranial hypertension are outlined in Table 2.

Further reading

Brain Trauma Foundation. The American Association of Neurological Surgeons. The Joint Section on Neurotrauma and Critical Care (2000). Guidelines for the treatment of severe head injury. *Journal of Neurotrauma* **17**(6–7), 449–554. [Series of articles in a special issue.] Also on http://www.braintrauma.org/index.nsf/Pages/Guidelines-main

Kimelberg HK (1995). Current concepts of brain edema: review of laboratory investigations. *Journal of Neurosurgery* **83**, 1051–9.

Maas AIR, *et al.* (1997). EBIC guidelines for management of severe head injury in adults. *Acta Neurochirugica (Wien)* **139**, 286–94.

Menon DK (1999). Cerebral protection in severe brain injury. Physiological determinants of outcome and their optimisation. *British Medical Bulletin* **55**, 226–58.

Menon DK (2000). Cerebral circulation. In: Priebe H-J, Skarvan K, eds. *Cardiovascular physiology*, pp 240–77. BMJ Books, London.

Plum F, Posner JB (1992). *Diagnosis of stupor and coma*, 3rd edn. FA Davis, Philadelphia.

Roberts I, Schierhout G, Alderson P (1998). Absence of evidence for the effectiveness of five interventions routinely used in the intensive care management of severe head injury: a systematic review. *Journal of Neurology, Neurosurgery, Psychiatry* **65**, 729–33.

Rosner MJ (1993). Pathophysiology and management of increased intracranial pressure. In: Andrews BT, ed. *Neurosurgical intensive care*, pp 57–112. McGraw-Hill, New York.

16.6.3 Brainstem death and organ donation

M. J. Lindop

Introduction

The statement by the Conference of Royal Medical Colleges and their Faculties in 1976 led to the establishment of the concept of brainstem death in British practice. Similar procedures took place in many other countries, such as The President's Guidelines in the United States in 1981. Although the motive was to clarify the practice of organ donation for transplantation, the concept has proved useful in determining appropriate care for many patients in intensive care who are certainly not suitable as organ donors.

The concept of brainstem death

Brain death in the United States is defined as the 'irreversible cessation of all functions of the entire brain, including the brainstem … that are clinically ascertainable'. In the United Kingdom the focus has been on brainstem function since it is argued that, in the absence of brainstem function, there will be no activity of the reticular formation and the capacity for consciousness is lost. Deep unconsciousness results from damage bilaterally to a circumscribed area in the tegmentum of the mesencephalon and the rostral pons. In the determination of brainstem death, there is no testing of the function of other areas of the brain, such as electroencephalography of the cerebral cortex. The diagnosis can be made on clinical signs alone, and half of those who fulfil the necessary clinical criteria will have a cardiac arrest despite intensive treatment within 24 h, and this happens to almost all within 72 h.

Managing the patient who is potentially brainstem dead (Fig. 1)

The patient with severe brain damage will be unconscious and on a ventilator. There will have been testing to chart progress showing that it is likely that the clinical signs of brainstem death will be present. The admitting consultant or the intensive care consultant should see the family to discuss the severity of the brain damage. They are told that there will be formal clinical testing of brainstem reflexes that will determine whether there is any prospect of recovering consciousness. A timetable for this testing is proposed. This interview is an opportunity to discuss the option for organ donation with the family. Organ donation when brainstem death occurs is now well known to the public, and often the family will be the first to raise the matter. In the United Kingdom there is no legal obligation for the doctor to raise the subject, but many families will feel cheated if they have had no chance to offer organ donation: they feel comfort when donation is seen as the only good that can come out of the disaster of an unexpected death. A transplant co-ordinator will be available to meet the family and discuss the process of organ donation. This is the time to check whether the patient fulfils the criteria for acting as an organ donor. The family may decide which organs should be available for donation, but they may not influence or make conditions regarding the choice of recipient.

Diagnosis of brainstem death

Planning the tests (Fig. 2)

The diagnosis must be confirmed by two medical practitioners that are competent in neurological examination and have been registered with the General Medical Council for more than 5 years. At least one should be a consultant, and neither can be a member of the transplant team. They can conduct the tests either separately or jointly. A second testing is done at a later time to remove the risk of observer error. The interval between the tests is not fixed, but usually between 1 and 6 h: it should be based on clinical judgement that will reassure all those concerned with the care of the patient that there has been a measured assessment. The legal time of death is the completion of the first set of tests that reveals no brainstem function. The declaration of death and, if organs will not be donated, the stopping of the ventilator take place after the second testing. Most intensive care units now have a proforma which guides the process of testing.

Performance of the tests

There are three essential components to the clinical testing of brainstem function prior to the declaration of brainstem death—preconditions, exclusions, and clinical criteria.

Preconditions

1. The diagnosis must give an aetiology that confirms that the damage is irreversible.

2. The patient must be in unresponsive coma, though spinal reflexes do not exclude the diagnosis.

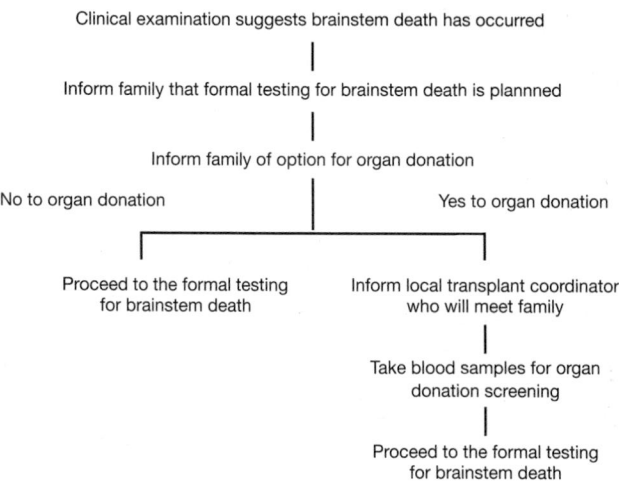

Fig. 1 Management of brainstem death diagnosis.

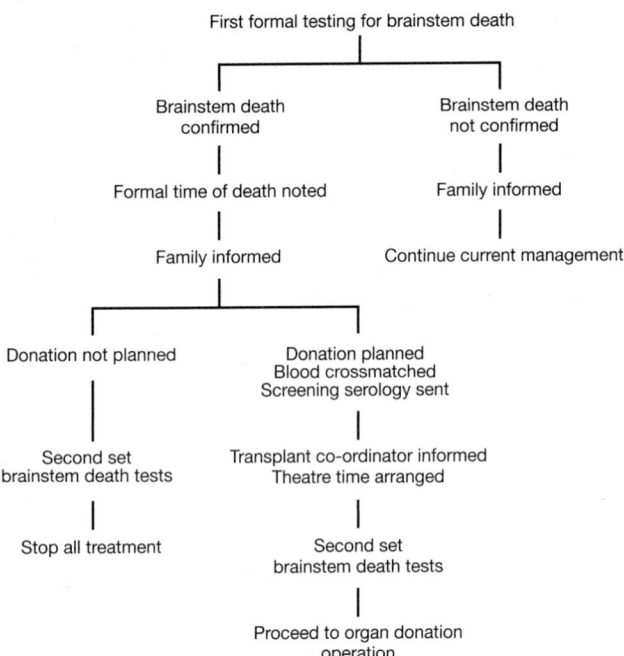

Fig. 2 Organization of brainstem death testing after first family interviews.

Exclusions

Reversible causes of coma must be excluded with certainty.

1. Drug activity, such as narcotics, muscle relaxants, or hypnotics. Due attention must be made to the possibility of prolonged action from previous overdosage, or from metabolism that could be impaired by hepatic or renal failure.

2. Metabolic or endocrine causes of coma—such as hypoglycaemia, hyperglycaemia, hyponatraemia, hepatic failure, uraemia, myxoedema, or Reye's syndrome.

3. Hypothermia—there is no fixed recommendation, but testing should be done at higher than 35°C.

Clinical criteria

These tests show absence of brainstem reflexes, and absence of spontaneous respiration. It is helpful to remember them by relating them to the relevant cranial nerves.

1. No pupillary response to light (II, III).

2. Absent corneal reflexes (V, VII).

3. Absent vestibulo-ocular reflex (VIII)—no nystagmus with installation of 20 ml of cold fluid into the unblocked ears.

4. No motor response within cranial nerve distribution with pain stimulus to face, trunk, or limbs. No limb response to painful pressure over supraorbital notch (V, VII).

5. Absent gag reflex (IX).

6. Absent cough reflex (X).

7. Absence of spontaneous respiration—the apnoea test. At the beginning of reflex testing, the ventilator should be set to deliver 100 per cent oxygen to denitrogenate the lungs (for more than 10 min). A blood gas may be taken. The patient is disconnected from the ventilator and oxygen is insufflated via a catheter into the tracheal tube. Although less than 1 litre/min is absorbed, a flow of 6 litre/min is usually recommended. In apnoea the $Paco_2$ rises at between only 0.5 and 1 kPa/min. Careful observation of the patient for respiratory movements during the disconnection continues until a blood gas shows that the $Paco_2$ has risen to more than 7 kPa (just over 50 mmHg). Oxygenation is usually

well maintained. An alternative arrangement is to connect the patient to an anaesthetic breathing circuit with a reservoir bag. Respiratory movements may be seen more easily, but small cardiac pulsations can be transmitted and these can be mistaken for breathing activity by inexperienced staff. The patient is usually reconnected to the ventilator once the target $Paco_2$ is reached if this is the first testing, or if organ donation is planned.

The patient who is brainstem dead and will not become an organ donor

After the completion of the apnoea test in the second testing, the oxygen catheter is removed from the tracheal tube, the patient is not reconnected to the ventilator and death is pronounced. The heart will stop over the next 15 min.

The patient who is brainstem dead and will become an organ donor

Acceptability as an organ donor

Transplant co-ordinators will ensure that the criteria in Table 1 are met.

Clinical management of the organ donor on the intensive care unit

The management of the patient now changes dramatically. Previously all therapy has been directed at maintaining cerebral perfusion to preserve brain function. Now the emphasis changes to care of the potential donor organs. The transplant co-ordinator is informed that the tests have now been completed and have confirmed brainstem death, and the donor operation is arranged as soon as possible.

Table 1 Criteria for organ donation

(1)	**General**	
	(a)	Age up to 75—upper age limit varies with organ
	(b)	Brainstem death is confirmed
	(c)	Currently on a ventilator
	(d)	No known malignant disease, unless group 1 primary brain tumour (Council of Europe Consensus document 1997)
	(e)	No systemic sepsis
	(f)	No known social or medical high risk factors for HIV
(2)	**Registration with the United Kingdom Transplant Support Services Authority (UKTSSA)**	
(3)	**Consent from the coroner or fiscal may be required because of the circumstances of the death, but is not specifically required for organ donation. Nevertheless the coroner or fiscal is usually informed about a death leading to organ donation.**	
(4)	**Family confirmation that contraindications to transplantation do not exist. The donor should not:**	
	(a)	have been positive for HIV, hepatitis B, or C
	(b)	have been treated for haemophilia or clotting disorders
	(c)	have injected themselves with drugs
	(d)	have had sexual relationships with special risk of virus transmission
	(e)	have had Creutzfeld–Jacob disease (CJD), nor be related to a sufferer of CJD, nor have had any neurological disease of unknown cause
	(f)	have had malaria, rabies, or tuberculosis
	(g)	have had a previous malignant disease

Table 2 Causes of hypotension in brainstem death

(1) Hypovolaemia
    Drug- or hyperglycaemia-induced diuresis
    Diabetes insipidus
    Previous therapeutic fluid restriction
    Blood loss
(2) Peripheral vasodilatation from loss of vasomotor tone
(3) Myocardial depression
    Ischaemic damage
    Impaired oxidative metabolism and low energy stores
        from hormonal changes
    Previous contusion (or tamponade)
    Acute electrolyte disturbances

The common problems of the organ donor are hypotension, cardiac arrhythmias, diabetes insipidus, pulmonary oedema, and disseminated intravascular coagulation.

Cardiovascular problems

Cardiovascular instability is the commonest problem in the organ donor. Brainstem death leads to high catecholamine levels that may increase heart rate, blood pressure, cardiac output, and systemic vascular resistance. Widespread myocardial ischaemic damage can occur associated with defective oxidative metabolism. These changes in autonomic tone, combined with myocardial ischaemia and metabolic and electrolyte instability, all lead to a high incidence of cardiac rhythm disturbance. The ECG may show atrial and ventricular arrhythmias, atrioventricular conduction blocks, and widespread ST-segment and T-wave changes.

An initial hypertensive phase is followed by hypotension in 80 per cent of patients, the common causes of which are shown in Table 2.

Cardiovascular management

Instability is so common that direct arterial and central venous pressure monitoring are essential. A pulmonary artery catheter often proves useful. Targets for management are:

(1) mean arterial pressure at least 70 mmHg;

(2) central venous pressure about 10 mmHg; and

(3) urine output at least 1 ml/kg per hour.

Fluid replacement should be with blood or colloid, though urinary losses should be replaced with electrolyte solutions (nasogastric water or intravenous 5 per cent dextrose in uncontrolled diabetes insipidus). Likely electrolyte imbalance such as hypokalaemia must be sought by regular blood electrolyte measurements. Anti-arrhythmic drugs, inotropic agents, and vasopressors may be required. Inotropes and vasopressors are used as sparingly as possible since the direct action of large doses will threaten perfusion and function of the donor organs. Their use should only be considered when cardiac output studies confirm an indication; for example, when a profound fall in systemic vascular resistance with high cardiac output may justify use of noradrenaline in a minimal dose of 0.02 µg/kg per min. Some protocols use dopamine at 2 µg/kg per min routinely to improve renal, mesenteric, and coronary blood flow. Dopexamine at 1 µg/kg per min may give similar benefit. Use of a hormone replacement regimen may improve cardiovascular stability (see below).

Tight control of fluid balance is important as overload can impair organ function, particularly in lung transplantation.

Endocrine problems

Pituitary damage leads to failure of endocrine homeostasis. Tri-iodothyronine (T_3) and thyroxine (T_4) levels fall. Loss of antidiuretic hormone (ADH) leads to diabetes insipidus in up to 65 per cent of donors: Table 3 shows the characteristics of this condition. Cortisol production may fall, though this does not seem to correlate with cardiovascular changes. Blood sugar control is often defective and an insulin infusion is commonly required.

Endocrine management

The routine use of endocrine supplements is not established. Animal studies show no correlation between hormone deficiencies and cardiovascular instability, but endocrine supplements should be used where there is significant cardiovascular instability with substantial inotrope requirements. A suitable regimen is:

(1) tri-iodothryonine as a 4 µg bolus with infusion of 3 mµg/h;

(2) desmopressin or vasopressin (see Table 3);

(3) insulin at 1 unit/ml, with continuous infusion of 1 to 10 ml/h titrated to keep blood sugar at 6–8 mmol/l; and

(4) hydrocortisone supplements at 100 mg every 2 h (there is no risk of toxicity during the short period prior to donation).

Respiratory problems

The organ donor commonly has some pulmonary dysfunction. Possible causes are pneumonia, aspiration of gastric contents, neurogenic pulmonary oedema, and direct contusion.

Respiratory management

Controlled ventilation is used to achieve $Paco_2$ in the normal range (4.5 to 5.5 kPa) to avoid hypocapnic reduction of peripheral oxygenation and disruption of regional blood flows. Sufficient oxygen is given to achieve a Pao_2 of 11 to 13 kPa. A large tidal volume (12 to 15 ml/kg) delivered at a low ventilatory rate promotes gas exchange and reduces atelectasis. Modest positive end-expired pressure (**PEEP**), about 5 cmH$_2$O, is useful, but higher levels may impair cardiac output , and hepatic and renal blood flow.

'Neurogenic' pulmonary oedema occurs in about 20 per cent of donors. The causes of this are not known and there is no specific therapy. The usual approach is to monitor the circulation closely and endeavour to optimize left ventricular function. PEEP often helps, but even at high levels (up to 15 or 20 cmH$_2$O) is not always effective.

Unless there is pulmonary oedema, regular tracheal toilet to prevent accumulation of secretions and atelectasis is important. Strict asepsis must be maintained as the lungs may be implanted into a recipient prone to infection. If PEEP is being used, then tracheal suction should be used sparingly and via a closed system.

Coagulation abnormalities

Disseminated intravascular coagulation can be precipitated in 30 per cent of donors by release of tissue thromboplastin, fibrinolytic substances, and plasminogen activators in severe head injury. Characteristic changes are thrombocytopenia with fall in fibrinogen levels and the appearance of D-dimer fibrin degradation products. Effective haemostasis is needed during the donor operation to reduce blood loss and maintain cardiovascular stability. Fresh frozen plasma and platelets should be given to correct the deficiencies. Antifibrinolytics such as epsilon aminocaproic acid must be avoided in case they provoke microvascular thrombosis in donor organs.

Temperature control

Temperature regulation is impaired. Heat production falls with low metabolic rate and muscle inactivity. Vasodilatation promotes heat loss. Cooling can lead to impaired oxygen delivery to tissues, aggravation of cardiac arrhythmias, increased diuresis, and impaired platelet function. There

Table 3 Diabetes insipidus

Urine flow > 4 ml/kg.h
Urine osmolality < 300 mosmol/kg
Urine sodium < 10 mmol/l
Treatment to achieve urine flow of 1 ml/kg.h:
    desmopressin as a 1–4 µg intravenous bolus up to hourly,
    or vasopressin at 2 units/h by continuous infusion

should be active warming (higher than 35°C) by use of limitation of exposure to the environment, warming blankets, fluid warming, and proper humidification of inspired gases.

Clinical management of the organ donor operation

The operation lasts 3 to 6 h. Four units of blood should be cross-matched to compensate for blood loss. Although anaesthesia is not required, an anaesthetist will be required to supervise cardiovascular monitoring and maintenance of a stable circulation. Reflex hypertension can be a problem and small doses of vasodilating isoflurane or intravenous vasodilators are often required.

Further reading

Chase TN, Moretti L, Prensky AL (1968). Clinical and electroencephalographic manifestations of vascular lesions of the pons. *Neurology* **18**, 357–68. [Consequences of loss of function of brainstem.]

Council of Europe (1997). Standardisation of organ donor screening to prevent transmission of neoplastic diseases. ISBN 92-871-3485-5. [Detailed recommendations where organ donors have neoplastic disease.]

Honorary Secretary of the Conference of Royal Medical Colleges and their Faculties in the United Kingdom (1976). Diagnosis of brain death. *British Medical Journal* **ii**, 1187–8. [The initial formal statement in the United Kingdom.]

Mackersie RC, Bronsther OL, Shackford SR (1991). Organ procurement in patients with fatal head injuries. The fate of the potential donor. *Annals of Surgery* **213**, 143–50. [Survival of patients with head injuries who fulfil brain death criteria.]

Mollaret P *et al.* (1959). Coma dépassé et nécroses nerveuses centrales massives. *Revue Neurologique* **101**, 116–39. [Original description of catastrophic brain damage with loss of autonomic control which led to concept of brain death.]

Morgan G, Morgan V, Smith M (1999). *Donation of organs for transplantation.* Intensive Care Society, Tavistock House, London WC1H 9HR. [A clear comprehensive account of current practice.]

Wheeldon DR *et al.* (1993). Transplantation of unsuitable organs. *Transplantation Proceedings* **25**, 3014–15. [Argument for use of endocrine supplements in unstable patients.]

16.6.4 The patient without hope

M. J. Lindop

The nature of the problem

A long-standing dilemma for doctors has been to judge the appropriateness of further treatment for patients who are already gravely ill. There has commonly been a reluctance to embark on major treatment, such as mechanical ventilation, for fear that it will be more difficult to withdraw this treatment than to avoid its introduction in the first place. Decisions are made on a constantly changing background—the views of society on the ethics of medical management, and the efficacy of new medical techniques are two prime factors.

Who is the patient without hope?

The public finds increasing difficulty with the concept that death is inevitable. There can be a pressure to prolong life for its own sake. Most people would cite as abilities that were important features for an adequate quality of life:

(1) an ability to interact with others;

(2) an awareness of his or her own existence with a pleasure in the fact of that existence; and

(3) an ability to achieve some purposeful or self-directed action, or some self-set goal.

Where it is possible to know the patient's own wishes and values, it may be possible to infer whether he or she would consider life-prolonging treatment to be beneficial.

How certain is the outcome of a medical treatment?

Many treatments in intensive care will prolong life (mechanical ventilation or haemofiltration) but may not have a high likelihood of allowing complete recovery. Scoring systems, such as **APACHE** (Acute Physiology And Chronic Health Evaluation), and later APACHE II and III, have been developed to describe the severity of initial illness and have had some success in predicting hospital mortality. However, they have proved of little value in making decisions on individual patients.

Is the decision to withdraw treatment different from the decision not to institute therapy?

Although it is emotionally easier for the doctor to avoid embarking on treatment than to withdraw it once started, there are no legal or moral differences between these options. The patient will never have the chance of benefit if the treatment is untried. Precedent is not useful in determining the appropriateness of treatment. A treatment is reviewed by looking forward to whether the patient will gain benefit from it. Prolongation of life itself is not necessarily a benefit unless it is associated with the aforementioned qualities. If no benefit can be argued, a treatment should be withdrawn. Knowing that it is possible to withdraw a treatment can give the confidence to embark on that treatment where its outcome is uncertain.

Ways of tackling the problem

How is the decision to withhold or to withdraw treatment made?

The patient

Some patients, such as those with particular types of advanced neurological disease, will be able to participate in decision making. This may be in the form of an advance directive made before the moment of decision about life-prolonging treatment. In this situation the patient's view is paramount and limits the need for further discussion, but it is important that a full account of treatment options and their implications is given and that the patient is judged to understand the issues involved. The challenge for the physician is to embark on these discussions: they must not be avoided, but must take place at a time that has been chosen with the advice of family and nursing staff.

The family

Much time may need to be spent with the family to gain information about the quality of previous lifestyle, and the likelihood that the patient will see life-prolonging treatment as a benefit. They should understand and support any discontinuation of treatment, but should not be asked to make the decision to stop treatment, or be put in a position where they think that they are being asked to do so. This is rarely a problem if full discussions have taken place throughout the course of the illness. In rare instances, families can have complex structures and it will be clear that they are not able to put the interest of the patient first. In this situation further discussions may be required and the help of social workers and religious advisers can be useful in orchestrating dialogue. Neither the next of kin nor those with enduring power of attorney have any legal right to determine treatment. This responsibility remains with the doctor assisted by the health-care team, and, very rarely, by the courts of law.

The medical, nursing, and paramedical team

Much important information can be gained by talking to the patient's own doctor (general practitioner). The nurses caring for a patient over a prolonged period will be able to provide much useful information and should be consulted. Several physicians may have cared for patients with complex problems. In an intensive care unit there will be a team of consultants, and a formal arrangement should be made to consult all these doctors in the process of making the decision. Their opinions should be carefully documented. Their help will be needed to answer the essential questions:

1. Is the diagnosis secure? Are further investigations required before a decision can be made?

2. Is the benefit of further treatment to the patient clear?

3. Is the invasiveness of any treatment justified in the circumstances?

How can treatment be withdrawn?

Once a decision is made a drug or a feeding regimen can simply be stopped. An intermittent therapy such as haemofiltration can be omitted. However, patients who are mechanically ventilated need more careful management. Despite the discussions about terminal weaning of patients in the 1980s, a survey of critical care physicians in 1994 revealed widespread disparity of practice.

Terminal weaning is a protocol that allows death with dignity as mechanical ventilation is discontinued without causing distress to the patient or his family and carers. This is conducted as follows:

1. Stop vasoactive and antibiotic drugs.

2. Stop any paralysing drugs.

3. Continue sedatives and analgesics to avoid distress.

4. Continue physiological monitoring and recording of observations and medical actions.

5. Change the mode of ventilation to synchronized intermittent mandatory ventilation (**SIMV**), which allows the patient to breathe but superimposes a defined number of breaths per minute.

6. Halve the SIMV rate every 30 min until less than 6. Then discontinue SIMV.

7. Use morphine to control dyspnoea and benzodiazepines to control restlessness.

8. If breathing has become stable, allow the patient to breathe spontaneously, and consider lying the patient on the side for extubation.

9. Usually the patient will have died by this stage, but it may be necessary to transfer them to a general ward area for basic care. This can be very disruptive for the family and should be avoided if possible.

Decisions not to escalate treatment, and not to resuscitate a patient

Careful discussions as described above, which should be clearly documented in the medical notes, are a prerequisite of making decisions not to escalate treatment, or not to resuscitate a patient. The decisions must be reviewed each day by the consultant in charge of the patient to ensure their continuing relevance.

Do not escalate

If further complications supervene it can be decided that new treatment is unlikely to give the patient real benefit. A 'do not escalate' order is made so that no therapies will be added. Typically it may be decided not to increase the inotrope dose, not to use haemofiltration, not to transfuse blood or blood products, or not to implement or to increase ventilatory support. In summary, treatment continues only whilst the patient continues to show a beneficial response.

Do not resuscitate

In similar circumstances it may be appropriate to decide that in the event of unexpected circulatory arrest no resuscitation will be attempted. If the documentation is not clear, a resuscitation attempt will be necessary and this can be very distressing to the family at the bedside if it seems inappropriate. Where circulatory arrest has occurred as a result of a drug administration error, a tension pneumothorax, or a complication of therapy, it may be appropriate that a limited (5 min) attempt at resuscitation is made despite the existence of a 'do not resuscitate' order.

Does basic care include provision of fluids and nutrition?

Basic care provides warmth, shelter, hygiene, and comfort to the patient by relieving pain and distress. It includes the regular offer of oral fluid and nutrition. Fluid and nutrition provided 'artificially' by intravenous infusion, or by tube (whether nasogastric or percutaneous endoscopic gastrostomy—PEG), is considered a form of treatment and as such can be withdrawn (although in the specific instance of the persistent vegetative state in England and Wales, review by a court of law is needed).

Summary

Key points in the management of patients who are severely ill and in whom escalation of treatment may not be kind or sensible are:

(1) early anticipation of possible outcomes;

(2) continuing review of whether treatments remain beneficial;

(3) establishment of local guidelines for limiting or withdrawing treatment;

(4) good communication skills within the health team;

(5) good communication skills with the patient and the family; and

(6) clear documentation of decisions.

Case report

An 80-year-old patient with many severe chronic health problems is admitted shocked with acute abdominal pain. A laparotomy is required to establish the diagnosis. The patient may be admitted to an intensive care unit for stabilization prior to surgery.

1. The bowel is extensively infarcted with no hope of survival. The patient is extubated at the end of surgery, and is allowed to die peacefully with appropriate analgesia and sedation, perhaps in the post-anaesthesia care unit or the general ward.

2. There is extensive peritoneal sepsis that could respond to definitive surgery and antibiotic therapy. The patient is admitted to an intensive care unit where monitoring and initial treatment is aggressive. Limits are set beyond which treatment will not escalate. These may be a maximum dose of adrenaline of, say, 0.25 μg/kg per min, no haemofiltration in the event of renal failure, and no resuscitation and no continuing mechanical ventilation after 48 h if there has been no improvement.

Further reading

British Medical Association (1999). *Withholding and withdrawing life-prolonging medical treatment*. BMJ Publishing Group, London. [A guidance for decision making—the outcome of widespread consultation through the British Medical Association's Medical Ethics Committee in 1998.]

Faber-Langendoen K (1994). The clinical management of dying patients receiving mechanical ventilation. *Chest* **106**, 880–8. [A survey of problems of inconsistent intensive care practice persisting over 10 years.]

Grenvik A (1983). Terminal weaning: discontinuance of life-support therapy in the terminally ill patient (Editorial). *Critical Care Medicine* **11**, 394–5. [An influential editorial for intensive care practice.]

Knaus WA *et al.* (1991). The APACHE III prognostic system. *Chest* **100**, 1619–36. [An example of a physiological scoring system.]

17

Respiratory medicine

17.1 Structure and function

17.1.1 The upper respiratory tract

J. R. Stradling

The upper respiratory tract extends from the anterior nares to the larynx. This part of the respiratory tract has to cope with specific problems: it is exposed to incoming air and has to double as the entry to the digestive system. This has led to specific evolutionary adaptations which are not always perfect.

The nose

The anterior nares, which includes the nasal valve just inside the nose, is usually the narrowest part of the respiratory tract and accounts for about 40 to 50 per cent of the total respiratory resistance. In normal subjects the resistance in the lower airways is small (less than 25 per cent) compared with the larynx and nose. This anterior nasal resistance is actively controlled by the levator alae nasi and procerus muscles, which flare the nostrils, and the compressor naris muscle, which narrows the nasal valve further. During mild exercise these muscles (combined with sympathetic nasal mucosal vasoconstriction) can halve the nasal resistance and allow minute ventilations up to 30 litre/min before conversion to oral breathing is necessary. These muscles receive a phasic inspiratory signal, to brace open the nares with each breath, just in advance of diaphragmatic activity.

Occasionally, owing to deformity of the anterior nasal cartilages, the anterior nares are very narrow and limit inspiration, particularly during sleep when the dilator muscle activity is reduced. This is one of the rarer causes of snoring which is amenable to treatment.

The main function of the nose is as first-line defence against problems with the incoming air. In this respect it acts as a coarse particle filter and a conditioner (temperature and humidity) of the air, and with the sense of smell helping to detect noxious substances that are best avoided. The turbinates in the nose present a surface on to which large inhaled particles, such as pollen grains and house dust mite faecal particles, will be retained, with the potential for an allergic response producing allergic rhinitis. Debris arriving on the mucosal surfaces is wafted backwards to be swallowed eventually. Without this so-called 'mucociliary carpet' there is decreased resistance to infections (usually a generalized respiratory problem and not just in the nose) with pooling of mucopurulent material, and recurrent sinus infections. This mucociliary function can be tested by placing a saccharine tablet on the anterior floor of the nasal cavity and timing the period that elapses before it can be tasted in the oral cavity. The normal interval is about 15 to 20 min, but when ciliary defects exist this can extend to an hour or more.

The turbinates fill such a large proportion of the nasal cavity that minor swelling produces large changes in nasal airflow resistance (Fig. 1). There are several rich vascular beds at different depths in the nasal mucosa, pro-viding a large surface area to warm and humidify incoming air. These are supplied by the sphenopalatine branch of the maxillary artery, with venous drainage passing back into the cavernous sinus around the carotid artery. The volume of fluid in these vascular beds is controlled via the vidian nerve (containing sympathetic vasoconstriction and parasympathetic vasodilation) acting on both arterioles and venules. The overall blood flow and total volume of blood in the sinusoids determines the degree of mucosal congestion, which undergoes a cyclical reciprocal change across the two sides of the nose over 2 to 4 h, that is, as the mucosa on one side is congesting, that on the other side is shrinking. This cycle, usually only obvious to individuals with already narrowed nasal passages (when blockage can occur intermittently), can be interrupted by a reflex mediated by pressure on the side of the thorax or in the axilla. Thus, in the decubitus position, the upper nostril becomes clearer and the lower more congested, with the two sides swapping within a minute or two of turning on to the other side. The purpose of this nasal cycle is not known, but using the upper rather than the lower nostril when lying on one's side may lessen the chance of inhaling particulate matter. In addition to this effect, there is a general increase in nasal congestion on lying down due to a hydrostatic rise in capillary pressure.

The volume of fluid needed to humidify the incoming air is considerable, but is reduced by condensation of some of this moisture back on to the cooler nasal mucosa during exhalation. Of course, this conditioning is lost during oral breathing, which has important implications for exercise-induced asthma, which is due to cooling and drying of intrathoracic airways.

Nasal secretions come mainly from submucosal glands that are stimulated by parasympathetic (cholinergic) fibres. There is some evidence that sympathetic activity can also stimulate secretions, but of higher viscosity.

The sensory fibres from the nose travel in the maxillary nerve (mainly the ophthalmic branch) and are the afferent limb of some interesting

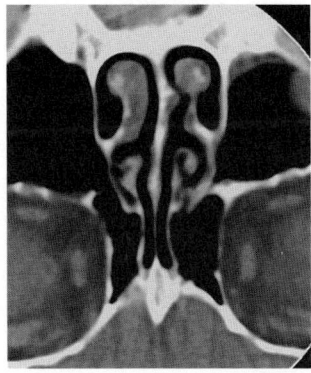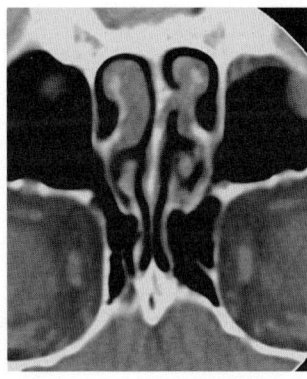

Fig. 1 Coronal sections of human maxillary sinuses and the turbinates in the nose. The view in the panel on the left is taken after ephedrine drops and shows mucosal shrinkage. The consequent small increase in the size of the lumina was attended by a large increase in maximum nasal airflow. (By courtesy of Dr F. Gleeson.)

reflexes. Airflow is sensed and can itself influence breathing pattern. Nerves containing substance P in the epithelium seem to be responsible for sensations leading to sneezing. Sneezing is like coughing in that an explosive expiration is generated in an attempt to expel foreign matter. Coughing involves closure of the larynx until pressure builds up, whereas sneezing involves closure of the pharynx. Unlike coughing, sneezing is never voluntary. Sensory fibres from much of the upper airway, nose, and face are also involved in the diving reflex. This reflex is of great importance to diving mammals when the combination of facial stimulation by cold water, apnoea, and hypoxaemia produce intense peripheral, splanchnic, renal, and muscular vasoconstriction. This diverts blood to the brain and conserves oxygen (producing a heart–lung–brain circulation that prolongs diving time), with the rise in blood pressure limited by a marked vagally induced bradycardia. This vestigial reflex in humans can be utilized in the control of some cardiac arrhythmias, when a brisk increase in vagal tone can be produced by applying ice-cold water to the face.

Nasal irritation can lead to either bronchoconstriction or bronchodilation. The bronchoconstriction can be prevented by atropine and is presumably vagally mediated. This reflex may be important in provoking bronchospasm in some asthmatics. Negative pressure in the nasal cavities can also be sensed, producing a reflex increase in upper airway dilator action (see the following section on the pharynx).

Olfaction depends on recognition of molecules by mucosal receptors at the very top of the nose. These olfactory cells have central axons that pass through multiple tiny holes in the skull (cribriform plate) to the brain. At this point they are very vulnerable to shearing forces during a blow to the head, leading to anosmia (loss of ability to smell).

The pharynx

The pharynx is divided into the nasopharynx, oropharynx, and laryngopharynx or hypopharynx—behind the soft palate, the back of the oral cavity down to the tip of the epiglottis, and the tip of the epiglottis down to the cricoid cartilage, respectively. Thus the top end is level with the base of the skull and the bottom end is about level with the sixth cervical vertebrae, giving an overall length of about 12 cm. When being used to breathe through, the pharynx has to be a rigid tube (like the trachea), but during swallowing it has to be a collapsed tube capable of peristalsis (like the oesophagus). This combination of functions is achieved by having a mus-

cular tube that can constrict to propel food, but also has external muscles whose function is to brace open the pharynx when required. Figure 2 shows the enormous complexity of the pharyngeal musculature, supplied mainly by the hypoglossal nerve (XII). The pharyngeal constrictors (superior, middle, and lower) are the main peristaltic muscles; the lower part of the inferior constrictor also functions as a sphincter to the top of the oesophagus, preventing air entry during inspiration. Most of the other pharyngeal muscles work in concert to hold open the pharynx. For example, the genioglossus pulls forward the tongue, the geniohyoid together with the strap muscles (sternothyroid, thyrohyoid, etc.) pulls forward the hyoid (enlarging the oropharynx), and the stylopharyngeus probably pulls sideways on the lateral pharyngeal walls. The palatopharyngeus will hold open the pharynx if supported by the levator palati, but will also pull forward the palate to open the nasopharynx. The upper pharyngeal muscles (tensor palati and levator palati) also close off the nasal cavity during swallowing to prevent regurgitation of fluids into the nose. To prevent aspiration, closure of the larynx and the false cords above is co-ordinated with swallowing. Some of these actions require sensory information about the exact location and consistency of any food being swallowed, carried via the glossopharyngeal and vagus nerves (IX and X). Sensory branches of these nerves also supply the ear, which explains why pharyngeal lesions may present with pain in the ear.

Given the complexities of pharyngeal function, it is not surprising that severe swallowing difficulties with aspiration of food and drink are often seen following cerebrovascular accidents in the brainstem involving the control of pharyngeal muscles and the sensory pathways.

Powerful mechanisms are available to maintain patency of the pharyngeal airway during breathing. As with the alae nasi, the pharyngeal dilator muscles receive a respiratory input in time with diaphragm activation. The diaphragm receives a gradually increasing level of phrenic activity to overcome elastic recoil as tidal volume increases, whereas the pharyngeal activation follows more of a 'square wave'. This makes teleogical sense, since the collapsing force is dependent on inspiratory flow and this is roughly constant throughout inspiration. In addition, if pharyngeal patency is threatened, the dilator activity increases. Figure 3 shows the increase in genioglossus tone in response to a fall in intrapharyngeal pressure. This negative pressure will pull in the pharyngeal walls, and there are thought to be 'distortion' receptors of some kind mediating this reflex. Snoring occurs when the pharynx narrows enough to vibrate, and there is some evidence that this vibration itself can also activate pharyngeal dilators, thus warding

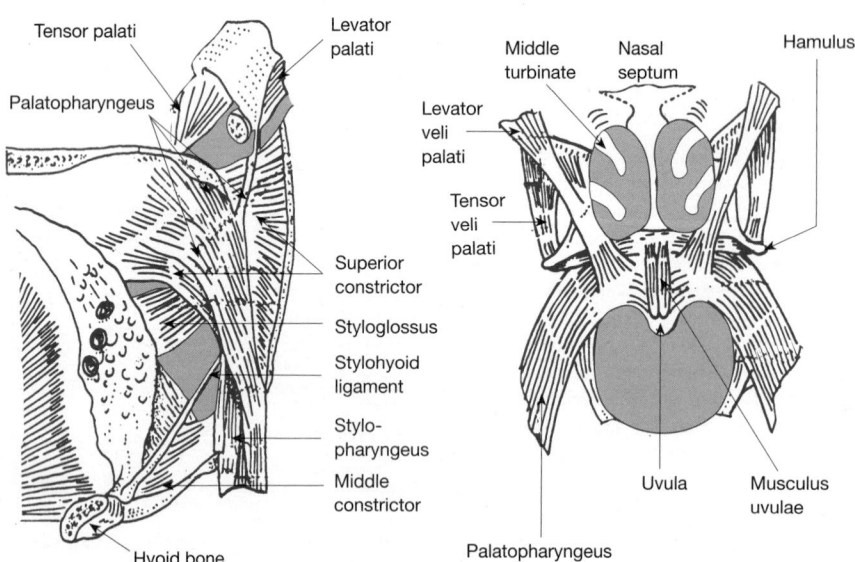

Fig. 2 Two views of the pharyngeal muscles: from inside the pharynx looking laterally, and from high up on the posterior pharyngeal wall looking anteriorly. These muscles act in concert and the physical effect of their contraction depends on which other muscles are simultaneously activated.

off full collapse. The factors predisposing to pharyngeal collapse during sleep are discussed in Chapter 17.8.2.

Sets of lymphoid tissue (Waldeyer's ring), comprising the adenoids, the palatine tonsils, and the lingual tonsils (back of tongue), are situated in the pharynx. These subepithelial collections of lymphoid tissue are ideally suited to process inhaled and swallowed antigens. Unfortunately, if they hypertrophy too much in response to recurrent infections, they are also positioned such that they obstruct the airway, particularly in small children. This is usually first apparent during sleep, but may become severe enough to provoke inspiratory stridor, even while awake. Adenoidal enlargement, by blocking nasal airflow, will force mouth breathing which, if it occurs early enough (perhaps under 18 months of age), retards development of the lower jaw (the so-called 'adenoidal facies'). This probably leads to overcrowding of the teeth and a narrower retroglossal space (this is further discussed in Chapter 17.8.2).

The larynx

The larynx (Fig. 4) has three important functions: communication, protection of the airway, and dynamic control of lung volume.

A minority of the intrinsic and extrinsic muscles of the larynx (e.g. cricothyroid, posterior cricoarytenoid) open (abduct) or brace the vocal cords, whereas the majority (e.g. thyroarytenoid, transverse and oblique arytenoids) close (adduct) the cords. The recurrent laryngeal nerve (from the vagus) supplies all the muscles apart from the cricothyroid (supplied from the superior laryngeal nerve, which is also a branch of the vagus). The left recurrent laryngeal nerve comes off the vagus and passes under the aortic arch before running up close to the thyroid gland to the larynx. This

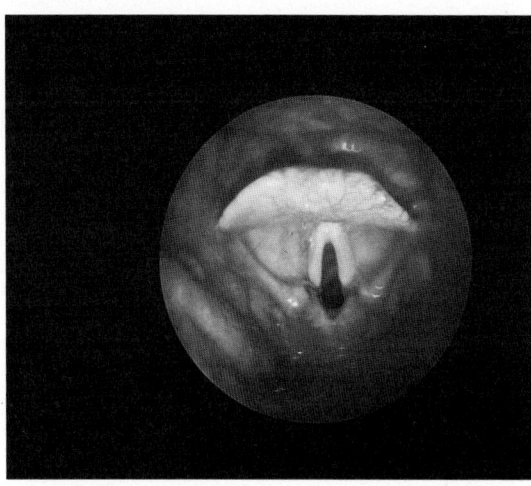

Fig. 4 Bronchoscopic view of the larynx from above. The top of the picture is the anterior. (By courtesy of Dr P. Stradling.)

means that it can be damaged by a tumour at the left hilum and surgically during a thyroidectomy. The right recurrent laryngeal nerve passes under the right subclavian artery where it can be damaged by a right-sided apical lung tumour.

Complete paralysis of the recurrent laryngeal nerve gives permanent hoarseness of the voice, and the affected cord assumes a position midway between full abduction and adduction. The cord is floppy and can be moved passively very easily, being 'sucked' towards the mid-line during inspiration and blown open during expiration. The unparalysed cord may eventually compensate to some degree and move nearer the paralysed cord, improving the voice. If paralysis of the recurrent laryngeal nerve is incomplete, the affected cord may take up the adducted position, presumably because fibres running to the abductors are damaged first. When there is bilateral damage to the recurrent laryngeal nerves, loss of adequate abduction causes inspiratory stridor as the cords are passively drawn together.

As mentioned earlier, there are reflexes initiated by supralaryngeal sensory fibres (mainly via the internal branch of the superior laryngeal nerve) designed to protect the airway. Fluid or food landing on or near the vocal cords will provoke coughing and/or laryngeal closure. During sleep, irritation of the cords tends to produce apnoea and laryngeal adduction, and coughing occurs only when wakefulness supervenes.

One of the less well-known functions of the larynx is to brake expiratory flow and thereby control lung volume. In some species, and in neonates, laryngeal expiratory braking is very important, acting rather like positive end-expiratory pressure to maintain end-expiratory lung volume above the passive functional residual capacity, thus preventing atelectasis. In adults there is no good evidence that the rate of expiration is under active laryngeal control, but this mechanism may come into action during respiratory illnesses (such as pneumonia), especially if there is marked hypoxaemia. If the upper airway is bypassed, for instance by tracheostomy or intubation, then other mechanisms come into play to maintain end-expiratory lung volume, such as postinspiratory contraction of the diaphragm (thus delaying expiration) and shortening of expiratory time (thus starting inspiration again before lung volume has fallen too far). Figure 5 is from a tracheotomized dog with areas of atelectasis. This shows how once laryngeal braking is denied to the animal, expiration proceeds faster, lung volume falls, and expiratory time is shortened to produce tachypnoea. This reflex was not present when the areas of atelectasis had resolved. The clinical correlate of this is sometimes seen as an expiratory grunt in babies who have a respiratory illness. Intubation may worsen gas exchange in this situation unless positive end-expiratory pressure is also applied.

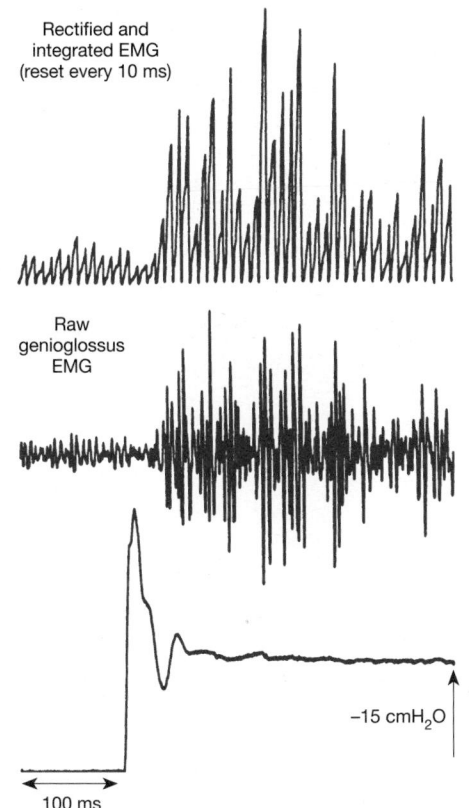

Rectified and integrated EMG (reset every 10 ms)

Raw genioglossus EMG

−15 cmH$_2$O

100 ms

Fig. 3 Response of the genioglossus muscle in a conscious human to a sudden fall in intrapharyngeal pressure. The time delay (about 50 ms) is too short to be due to a cortical response and is presumably a spinal cord reflex. (Reproduced from Horner 1991, with permission.)

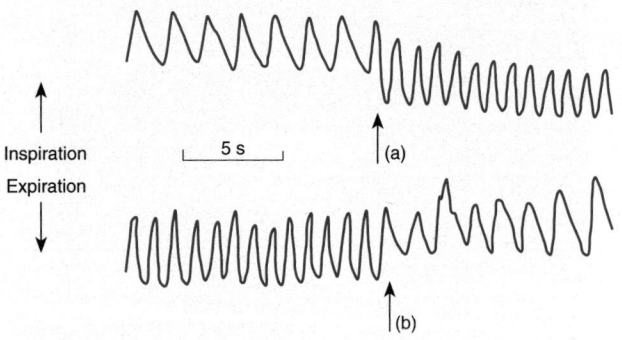

Inspiration
Expiration

5 s

(a)

(b)

Fig. 5 Recorder tracings in a dog with atelectasis showing the effect of switching from upper airway to tracheostomy breathing (arrow at (a)) and from tracheostomy to upper airway breathing (arrow at (b)). The signal is from an inductive plethysmograph measuring movement of both the rib cage and abdomen which represents lung expansion and contraction.

Further reading

Brouillette RT, Thach BT (1979). A neuromuscular mechanism maintaining extrathoracic airway patency. *Journal of Applied Physiology* **46**, 722–9.

Gautier H (1973). Control of the duration of expiration. *Respiration Physiology* **18**, 205–21.

Horner RL (1991). Evidence for reflex upper airway dilator muscle activation by sudden negative airway pressure in man. *Journal of Physiology* **436**, 15–29.

Matthew OP, Sant 'Ambrogio GS (1988). Respiratory function of the upper airway. In: *Lung biology in health and disease*, Vol. 35. Marcel Dekker, New York.

Remmers JE, Bartlett D (1977). Reflex control of expiratory airflow and duration. *Journal of Applied Physiology* **42**, 80–7.

17.1.2 Structure and function of the airways and alveoli

Peter D. Wagner

The organ of gas exchange

The lung is the organ of gas exchange, providing the means of transferring oxygen (O_2) from the air to the blood for subsequent distribution to the tissues. At the same time it enables removal of metabolically produced carbon dioxide (CO_2) from the blood, which is then exhaled to the atmosphere. Not just in health, but also in lung disease, the volumes of O_2 taken up and CO_2 removed by the lung per minute must equal the rate of O_2 consumption and CO_2 production by the aggregate tissues of the body.

The lung will also exchange any other gas that is presented to it, but the principles involved—passive diffusion—mirror those for O_2 and CO_2. Quantitative but not qualitative differences occur in how such gases (e.g. anaesthetic agents, carbon monoxide, toxic gases inhaled by accident) are handled by the lung. These differences stem from the means by which any particular gas is transported in the blood; whether in simple physical solution alone, or also in some chemical combination with molecules such as haemoglobin.

The principles are similar for gas uptake into blood and elimination from the blood. In fact, because gas exchange occurs by passive diffusion, whether a gas is taken up from the air into the blood or eliminated from the

blood into the air depends simply on the partial pressures of the gas on each side of the blood–gas barrier, the 0.3-μm thick tissue layer separating alveolar gas from pulmonary capillary blood.

For transfer of a gas from the environment to the blood to occur, the gas in question must first be brought to the alveolar blood–gas barrier by the process of ventilation. Diffusion across this barrier then occurs at a rate proportional to: (i) the alveolar surface area available, (ii) the partial pressure difference between alveoli and blood, and inversely proportional to the thickness of the barrier, in concordance with the rules of simple passive diffusion. The gas molecules, now present dissolved physically in plasma, also distribute into the red cells. Depending on the gas, chemical associations may occur—with haemoglobin in the case of O_2, CO_2, carbon monoxide (CO) and nitric oxide (NO), and through transformation to bicarbonate ion for CO_2. The last element of the exchange process now occurs—the transport of the gas in blood pumped by the heart through the systemic circulation to the tissues of the body.

This chapter focuses on the first two of these three steps in gas exchange—ventilation and diffusion. A separate chapter deals with the third step—the pulmonary circulation (see Chapter 15.15.1). The structural basis of ventilation and diffusion, and the associated functional consequences, will be presented with particular emphasis on implications for disease. Lung diseases of many types commonly affect each of the steps involved in gas exchange, and the clinical consequences can usually be readily understood if the structure–function relationships are known.

Basic airway and alveolar design

In essence, the lung is a balloon undergoing cyclical inflation and deflation (ventilation, or tidal breathing) around some partially inflated state; the main anatomical elements are shown in Fig. 1. The gas-filled interior of the balloon corresponds to the alveolar gas spaces of the lung. The thin wall of the balloon may be likened to the blood–gas barrier, with the pulmonary capillary network imagined as covering the balloon's surface, separated from the interior gas by the elastic material making up the balloon's wall.

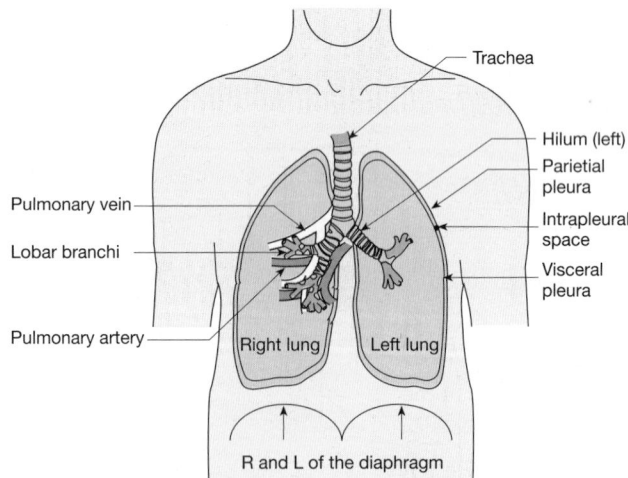

Fig. 1 The right and left lungs are separately encased within the thorax, and each is covered by a visceral pleural membrane. This is continuous with the parietal pleural membrane which lines the interior thoracic cavity, and the thin fluid-filled space between the visceral and parietal pleuras constitutes the intrapleural space. The hila of the two lungs contain the main stem bronchi, and accompanying pulmonary arteries and veins. The main stem bronchi join at the carina to form the trachea. The pulmonary arteries emanate from the right ventricle; the pulmonary veins empty into the left atrium. Within the lungs, the airways and blood vessels continue branching for approximately 20 generations. The major muscle of inspiration, the diaphragm, consists of two domes upon which the right and left lungs sit, and which separate the thoracic and abdominal contents.

The balloon is inflated through its neck (trachea) with each inspiration, thus bringing fresh air (21 per cent O_2, no CO_2) to the balloon's interior. This fresh gas is rapidly mixed with resident gas already present. This resident gas is partially depleted of O_2 by ongoing diffusion of O_2 into the capillaries, whilst at the same time, CO_2 is evolved into the gas from the capillary blood. Each inflation, by bringing fresh air into the alveoli, slightly increases alveolar PO_2 and decreases alveolar PCO_2. Each deflation moves some of this alveolar gas back to the environment. This rids the lung of some CO_2, but also removes some O_2, albeit at lower concentrations than in room air. In normal quiet breathing, alveolar O_2 concentration averages about 16 per cent over a respiratory cycle, whilst that of CO_2 is about 5 per cent, and a long-term steady-state of gas exchange is achieved.

Because the process of gas exchange depends on simple, passive diffusion, a large area of contact between alveolar gas and capillary blood is required to ensure sufficient gas flux across the blood–gas barrier to meet metabolic demand. The balloon analogy, while useful as an initial concept, thus exhibits a major difference from how the real lung is configured. The real lung has its total gas volume constituted not as a single balloon-like gas chamber, but as a very large number (about 300 million) of very small (radius, r, about 150 µm) almost spherical balloons or alveoli. Since the volume (V) of a sphere is $V = (4/3) \times \pi \times r^3$, while its surface area (A) is $A = 4 \times \pi \times r^2$, dividing a lung of a given volume (given because the lung must fit within the thoracic cage no matter whether as one large alveolus or 300 million small alveoli) into many small alveoli allows a much larger total surface area than if the lung were indeed a single large chamber, as seen from dividing the expression for surface area by that for volume: $A/V = 3/r$. Since total volume V is fixed by the thoracic cage, total surface area A increases as the number of alveoli is increased because radius of each alveolus must be reduced if volume is to remain constant. A typical value for V is 4000 ml. A single sphere of this volume would thus have a radius of about 10 cm, and a surface area of about 1200 cm², only slightly more than 1 square foot. By contrast, 300 million alveoli, each with a radius of 150 µm, would by the above formulae have the same total volume, thereby fitting equally as well inside the chest, but have a total surface area of about 800 000 cm². This approximates the area of a tennis court, and is about 650 times larger than the 1200 cm² area were the lung a single chamber. Since the laws of diffusion state that diffusive gas transport is proportional to surface area, and since the maximal rate of O_2 uptake in a normal man is about 4000 ml/min in heavy exercise, maximal pulmonary O_2 exchange would be insufficient for life were the lung a single chamber, at 4000/650 or 6 ml/min. Normal resting O_2 utilization by the tissues is about 300 ml/min. These calculations serve to highlight the critical importance of dividing the lung into a large number of small alveoli, and set the stage for discussing the structural configuration of a lung that must find a way to ventilate simultaneously 300 million separate, miniscule units of gas exchange.

The lungs inside the thoracic cavity

As with a balloon, the lung cannot inflate itself (although, as an elastic structure, once inflated it is capable of unassisted deflation just like a balloon). Inflation requires creation of a pressure difference between the outside and inside of the lung, pressure being higher inside. This may be accomplished in one of only two ways. One is by positive pressure inflation, typical of most clinical ventilators that are connected to the trachea and produce inflation by mechanically increasing intratracheal airway pressure. Spontaneous breathing throughout normal life does not happen in this way, and so the only possibility of normally achieving lung inflation is by the second option—that of decreasing the pressure around the lungs below that of the surrounding air. This is accomplished by encasing the lungs within the closed thoracic cavity, and having the muscles in the wall of this cavity (the intercostal muscles and the diaphragm) contract when inflation is desired. Contraction of these muscles moves the diaphragm caudally and expands the rib cage in both anteroposterior and lateral dimensions. As a result, the pressure inside the thoracic cavity but external to the lungs (that is, within the intrapleural space) is reduced to below that of the air. Since

the alveolar tissue is extremely thin and easily deformable, the pressure within the alveolar gas spaces is also reduced to below that of the air, and thus inflation occurs as a result of a hydrostatic pressure gradient from the mouth to the alveoli.

Inflation in the course of normal tidal breathing usually commences from a state of partial lung inflation that reflects that particular volume of the lung at which its own elastic recoil tendency to collapse is exactly balanced by the opposite, natural tendency of the rib cage to expand outwards. This volume is known as the functional residual capacity (**FRC**) and because it reflects recoil balance between lung and chest wall, it is the only volume which can be maintained without muscular effort. Thus, to inhale above FRC or to exhale below FRC both require respiratory muscle contraction, but the return to FRC from either higher or lower volumes can be passive, stored elastic energy provided by respiratory muscle contraction from the preceding active volume change being used to reverse the transpulmonary pressure difference and enable gas flow from the alveoli to the mouth.

Clinical significance

Elastic properties and lung volume

If the elastic properties of either the lungs or the chest wall are altered by disease, FRC will change. Should the lungs become less elastic, typically seen in emphysema due to disorganization of the elastin and collagen fibres making up much of the alveolar wall structure, the tendency for the lung to collapse is less, and the lung/chest wall recoil balance shifts to a higher lung volume, thus increasing FRC. By contrast, diseases characterized by proliferation of alveolar wall elements, collagen in particular, render the lung more elastic and thus collapsible, shifting FRC to lower values. These changes in FRC may be used to aid in diagnosis and in following the natural history and response to treatment of such diseases, since FRC is readily measured in the pulmonary function laboratory by either plethysmography or helium dilution methods. Changes in FRC also have important implications for lung function, discussed later in this chapter.

Whilst FRC is a key volume upon which to focus, the lung can normally be inflated to well above FRC, and also deflated to considerably below FRC. At maximal inflation, lung volume is referred to as the total lung capacity (**TLC**), while at maximal deflation, lung volume is called the residual volume (**RV**). Of major significance, RV is well above zero volume. As will be apparent, if all alveoli could be fully emptied of gas, they would be very difficult to reinflate to allow resumption of gas exchange, due to surface tension. The difference between TLC and RV is called the vital capacity (**VC**). As with FRC, each of these volumes is readily measured during routine pulmonary function testing, and together they provide a simple yet informative profile useful in characterizing many lung diseases and their progress. Unlike some physiological variables such as arterial pH or haemoglobin concentration, all of the above volumes depend to a major extent on body size. They also depend to a lesser degree on gender (smaller in females), age (deterioration with ageing), bodily habitus (often smaller in the obese), and ethnicity. Many tables of normal values have been published, and interpretation must allow for all of the determinants mentioned above.

Trachea, main bronchi, and pleura

For all 300 million alveoli to participate in the gas exchange process, each must be connected to the environment by an air pathway. The analogy now changes from a balloon to a tree. Imagining an upside-down tree, the main trunk represents the trachea, the single common airway segment through which inhaled and exhaled gas from all alveoli must pass. The upper end of the trachea begins at the lower margin of the larynx. The trachea lies anteriorly in the neck and chest, passing caudally in the midline retrosternally to the level of about the sternal attachment of the second rib. There it divides into left and right mainstem bronchi, each smaller and shorter than the trachea. These two airways angle caudally and laterally within the upper mediastinum to enter the left and right lungs at the left and right hilar regions, respectively, and they divide into the lobar bronchi, three on the right to feed the right upper, middle, and lower lobes, and two on the left to feed the two left lobes, upper and lower.

Note that the two hilar regions are the only normal points of actual connection of the left and right lungs to any thoracic structures, and also contain the large pulmonary arteries and veins, lymphatics, and nerves. The entire remaining lungs, while opposed against the chest wall, are not connected to it and are able to slide easily over the inner chest wall surface. This inner surface is covered by the parietal pleural membrane, and the outer surface of the lungs is similarly covered by the visceral pleural membrane. These two pleural membranes are joined at the hilar regions to form a fully enclosed sac that separates the lung and chest wall. The left and right pleural sacs do not communicate with each other, and normally contain only a very thin layer of plasma-like fluid and no gas at all. This arrangement may be pictured by imagining a sealed, but empty, plastic sandwich bag from which all air has been expelled and which contains a very small volume of water. If one's right hand is balled into a fist and invaginates this bilayered bag against the cupped left hand, we have the analogy to the right (or left) lung and chest wall. The balled right fist is the lung; the right wrist and forearm represent the hilar structures. The cupped left hand is the chest wall, and the two layers of the closed sandwich bag form the pleural membranes.

Clinical significance

Mainstem bronchial branching angles

The mainstem bronchial branching from the trachea is not quite symmetrical. The right mainstem bronchus continues caudally a little more directly in line with the trachea above it than does the left, which angles laterally more sharply. As a result, accidentally inhaled foreign bodies more frequently lodge in the right than left lungs. For similar reasons, advancing an endotracheal tube too deeply may cause it to lodge in the right mainstem bronchus rather than where intended—the trachea. This will result in lack of ventilation of the left lung, and if not recognized, hypoxaemia from continued perfusion of this unventilated lung with venous blood, and ultimately left lung collapse (over minutes to hours).

The intrapleural space and pneumothorax

The pressure within the pleural space (i.e. between visceral and parietal pleural surfaces) is normally subatmospheric because of the above-mentioned counterbalancing inward lung and outward chest wall recoil forces. This prevents lung collapse. Disruption of either the visceral or parietal pleura (i.e. pneumothorax) allows air to enter the pleural space, increasing the intrapleural pressure back to atmospheric. This results in collapse of the lung, with abolition of ventilation even if chest wall muscle contraction continues. Gas exchange therefore ceases, with life threatened. In humans, since the right and left lungs are encased in separate pleural sacs, if one side suffers pneumothorax, gas exchange can usually be maintained by the other. Pneumothorax can occur from rupture of lung surface alveoli in predisposed individuals, or from chest wall trauma in anyone. Whether the source of the intrapleural air is alveolar gas as in the former case or room air in the latter makes no difference. However, depending on conditions, intrapleural air pressure may actually rise above that of room air. This situation, the tension pneumothorax, can arise whenever air enters the pleural space via a valve-like mechanism, when the patient's respiratory effort or that of a mechanical ventilator can lead to intrapleural pressure rising well above atmospheric. The lung collapses, but the (increasingly desperate) respiratory effort or mechanical ventilator keeps pumping air into the

pleural space via the torn lung surface. This is a true emergency requiring immediate needle puncture of the chest wall of the affected side to relieve the built-up pressure. If this is not done, the high intrathoracic pressure compresses and distorts the mediastinum and vena cavae, impeding venous return. Both pulmonary gas exchange and the circulation fail, and death follows rapidly.

Mediastinal shifts

The separation of the right from left pleural spaces provides for lateral movement of the mediastinum should there be a difference in mechanical properties of the right and left lungs or their associated pleural spaces or chest wall structures. For example, fibrosis of the right lung, or alternatively its collapse from complete airway obstruction, will reduce the volume of intrathoracic contents and therefore pressure on that side, and mediastinal contents will shift towards the right, visible on chest radiography. In fact, the trachea may also be shifted from its normal midline location in this direction, evident on clinical examination of tracheal position just above the suprasternal notch. Conversely, a pleural effusion on the right or a right pneumothorax (see below) may raise intrathoracic pressure above that on the left, and have the opposite effects on mediastinal and tracheal position.

The bronchi and bronchioles

After the mainstem bronchi have arisen from the trachea, the airways continue an essentially dichotomous branching pattern until the alveoli are reached. Thus, successive branching yields of the order of 50 000 to 100 000 airways (called terminal bronchioles) that constitute the 16th generation ($2^{16} = 65\ 536$). The entire collection of airways from the trachea to these last bronchioles before alveoli begin forms a system of connected conducting pipes needed to deliver gas between the alveoli and the environment during ventilation (Fig. 2).

As with the branching of a tree, both the diameter and the length of each successive branch falls. The trachea typically is 12 cm long and 2 cm in diameter. By contrast, the typical terminal bronchiole is just 1 to 2 mm long and 0.6 mm in diameter. Airflow is normally mostly laminar (except for that in the upper airways) and therefore is governed by Poiseuille's law of fluid dynamics. The essence of this law is that resistance to airflow depends inversely on the fourth power of the airway radius, but varies only in direct proportion to airway length. As airways become both narrower and shorter with increasing branching, it is evident that resistance of a single airway increases dramatically because of the dominating effect of the fourth power of the radius. However, if one asks how the entire system behaves by plotting how airway pressure must fall from trachea to generation 16 during, for example, steady inspiratory flow, one must allow for the fact that all airways of any single generation are arranged in parallel with one another. Because branching is essentially dichotomous, there are twice as many airways in any given generation as in the one before. Thus, total airway resistance of any one generation is diminished in proportion to the exponentially increasing number of airways as branching continues. This actually overcomes the fourth power disadvantage of Poiseuille's law, such that most of the pressure drop, or put another way, most of the system airway resistance, is associated with the first few generations despite their large individual airway size.

Another way to understand this somewhat counterintuitive result is to consider the sum total of the cross-sectional areas of all airways in a single generation. This is of course the area of a typical airway multiplied by the number of airways in that generation. That number is low for the first few generations, but then rises dramatically because of the exponentially increasing number of airways in each generation. Airway resistance of a generation therefore falls from the first few generations to the terminal

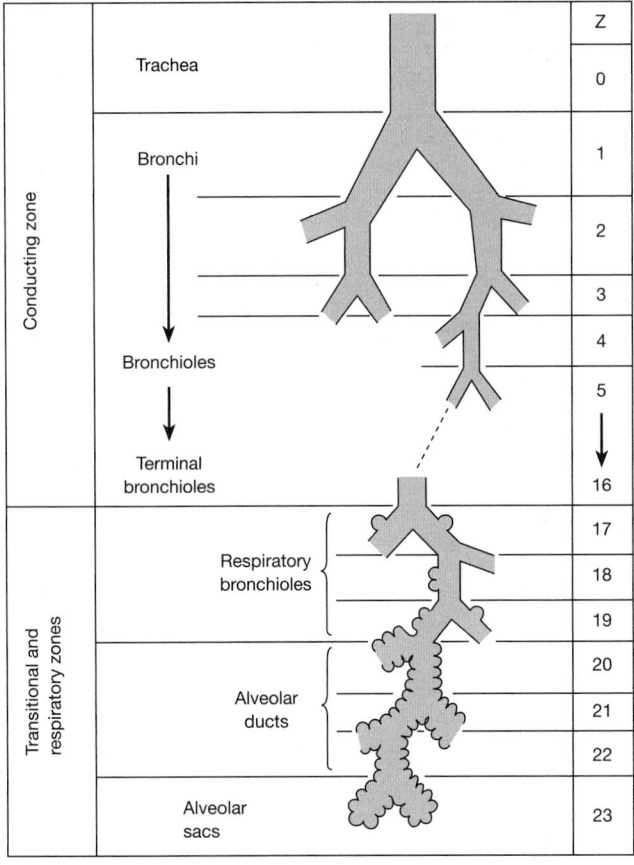

(a)

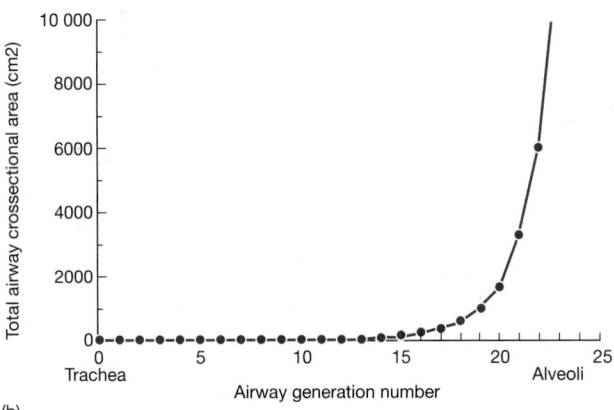

(b)

Fig. 2 (a) This shows a stylized model of the branching of the airways from trachea to alveoli encompassing some 23 generations of branching. The first 16 generations contain no alveoli and are purely conducting airways, but the next 7 generations contain progressively more alveoli in the airway walls and serve the dual -purpose of conducting air to the alveolar sacs and also providing gas exchange. (b) Total cross-sectional area of each generation shown in (a). This is obtained by multiplying the average cross-sectional area of a single airway by the number of airways in the particular generation. Cross-sectional area is small throughout the conducting zone (first 16 generations), but then increases exponentially in the respiratory zone. The implications are that the forward velocity of inspired gas falls dramatically in the respiratory zone such that diffusion becomes the faster mode of molecular movement. In addition, this diagram implies that during flow between the mouth and alveoli, most of the airways resistance resides in the first 15 generations. (Adapted from Weibel ER, 1984, with permission.)

bronchioles. The summed total volume of gas contained within all 16 generations of these conducting airways is only about 150 ml despite their prodigious number.

Clinical significance

Dead space

The interposition of airways between the mouth and the alveoli creates a volume of gas (about 150 ml as mentioned) called the anatomical dead space. The gas in this dead space simply passes back and forth during inspiration and expiration without contributing to gas exchange since the conducting airways contain no alveoli in their walls. It constitutes a penalty since it adds an obligatory 150 ml volume requirement to every breath taken. This is of no importance in health, but in patients with severe lung disease such as chronic obstructive lung disease or fibrosis, the energy cost of overcoming either high resistance in obstructed airways or low compliance of fibrotic lung tissue, and of thus mounting adequate ventilation, may be greatly increased. Then, the need to breathe some 150 ml more per breath than actually required for alveolar gas exchange can be clinically important as a factor contributing to respiratory failure. Recognition of this has led to the use of transtracheal insufflation of air, which permits the anatomical dead space of at least the upper airways to be circumvented and reduces the ventilation necessary for any given activity.

Particle deposition

Ventilation involves breathing some 6 to 10 litres of air every minute of our lives. Air contains much particulate matter of very small size. Depending on particle size, rate of gas flow in the airways, and airway geometry, such particles may move harmlessly in and out with the next breath or they may be deposited somewhere on the epithelial surface in the bronchial tree. To the extent that they do deposit and are chemically or physically harmful to tissue, they can be responsible for disease. Pneumoconioses, chronic obstructive pulmonary disease, bacterial and viral infections, asthma, and other diseases may all be initiated and/or afftected by such mechanisms. The dividing airway structure described above combines ever-diminishing individual airway diameter with ever-diminishing gas velocity (due to increasing summed cross-sectional airway area of all airways in a generation) as branching continues. As airways narrow and flow velocity falls, the chance of airborne particles being deposited on airway walls increases. It is for this reason that coal dust, for example, settles mostly in the terminal bronchiolar region deep within the branching system. Thus, the basic nature of gas exchange, demanding the branching network of airways described, leads to intrinsic vulnerability to disease from airborne particulate matter.

Mucociliary function

As seen commonly in evolutionary responses to deleterious phenomena, a protective system has been developed to mitigate the consequences of particle deposition in the airways. This is the mucociliary apparatus. It has several components. There are submucosal glands in the walls of the conducting airways that secrete mucus into the airway lumen when stimulated by irritant signals. These glands are supported by other secretory cells in the epithelium of the airways such as goblet cells. The epithelial cells that line the entire conducting airway system are ciliated, and they function in a co-ordinated manner, beating rhythmically to move the secreted mucus upward from smaller to larger airways. The primary purpose of the mucus is to trap inhaled particulates before they can reach and damage the airway and lung tissues themselves. This upwardly transported mucus is clinically evident as sputum.

The volumes of sputum produced normally are so small as to be unnoticeable, and are usually swallowed. However, inhalation of toxic irritants, infectious agents, and other particles will rapidly increase the volume of sputum to noticeable levels, and chronic airway inflammation from, for example, cigarette smoking will produce chronically increased amounts of mucus that give rise to the syndrome of chronic bronchitis. It is especially noteworthy that in asthma, not only is the volume of mucus increased, probably from airway inflammation, but its composition is altered, rendering it much more tenacious and difficult to eliminate by the ciliary system. Mucus thus accumulates in the airway lumina, particularly those of the smaller conducting bronchioles, creating mucus plugs that cause obstruction to airflow and marked reduction in ventilation of alveoli lying distal to them. When this occurs, asthma is often refractory to usual pharmacological therapy, and patients dying from asthma universally exhibit widespread airway mucus plugging.

Dynamic airway compression

Another intrinsic physiological problem of the branching airway system within the chest is related to the mechanical nature of respiration—the need for inflating and deflating the lung by altering the pressure around it—combined with the fact that the airways are not rigid tubes. The airways are thus susceptible to expansion and compression (and therefore to collapse) on inspiration and expiration, respectively. The intrapleural pressure may be transmitted to the conducting airways, and while reduction in this pressure on inspiration will only distend the airways, allowing air to flow more freely, opposite effects during expiration may not be innocuous. Passive expiration, that is, expiration fuelled only by the elastic energy stored in the lung tissue from the previous inspiration, without active expiratory muscle effort, does not compress the airways because the intrapleural pressure remains subatmospheric. However, active expiratory muscle contraction as occurs during a forced expiratory manoeuvre and during heavy exercise leads to compression of the airways because intrapleural pressure is raised to above atmospheric. In fact, the greater the expiratory effort made, the greater the increase in intrapleural pressure and the degree of airway compression. Because of this, flow rates during forced expiration cannot be increased by making a greater muscular effort: any greater driving pressure for expiratory flow is balanced by the increased resistance resulting from more compression. As a result, even in normal subjects, expiratory flow of air under these conditions is limited by this phenomenon, known as dynamic compression, which is illustrated in Fig. 3.

The loss of elastic recoil in emphysema, mentioned above in the context of its effects on FRC, also has a major influence on dynamic compression. The airways are much more susceptible to dynamic compression (discussed below), such that even breathing at rest with just small increases in intrapleural pressure from active expiratory muscle contraction may be subject to flow limitation by this mechanism. When this problem is compounded by the separate phenomenon of increased airway luminal mucus from chronic inflammation induced by cigarette smoking, it is easy to understand how chronic obstructive lung disease (emphysema and chronic bronchitis) has airway obstruction as its major disturbance.

In the consideration of dynamic compression it is important to note that the alveoli are not physically independent of one another or of the conducting airways, which run within the lung parenchyma from the lobar bronchi all the way out to the terminal bronchioles. The alveoli share walls in their mutual attachments, and the alveoli beside any intrapulmonary conducting airway are physically connected to the outside of that airway wall. A good analogy for how the alveolar parenchyma is configured comes from examining the cut surface of a sponge where the myriad air cells are surrounded by thin tissue walls. Every wall serves two adjacent air cells, and the overall structure is solid (rather than like the leaves of the tree which are physically independent of each other even while being connected to the same dividing network of branches). The net result of this matrix of alveolar and airway connections is that when the lung is inflated, the elastic tension in the parenchyma exerts radial traction on the conducting airways, increasingly so as the lung is further inflated. This stiffens the airway walls and acts to oppose dynamic compression during active expiration. That maximal expiratory flows are greater at high than low lung volumes is explained by the greater radial traction at high volumes as the alveoli are stretched more.

The walls of the larger conducting airways (the trachea and first few generations of bronchi) are reinforced with cartilage rings that further help

to counter the forces favouring dynamic compression. However, the smaller conducting airways do not enjoy this protection, and it is in the smaller airways that dynamic compression usually has its major effects.

Airway smooth muscle

All generations of conducting airways contain smooth muscle cells. When stimulated to contract, their concentric arrangement leads to reduction in airway lumen size, and airway obstruction results. While not a significant effect in normal individuals, patients with asthma have hyperresponsive airway smooth muscle that contracts in response to the inflammatory reaction usually present in the asthmatic airway walls. This is a major mechanism of airway obstruction in asthma, and is the basis of the mainstay therapy in this disease—bronchodilators. For reasons that remain unclear, smooth muscle contraction does not occur to the same degree in all airways of the asthmatic lung: there are different degrees of obstruction both with respect to airway generation number and among airways of a given generation. Ventilation of alveoli is thus very uneven, with many alveoli being very poorly supplied with air, yet others well-supplied. Gas exchange becomes inefficient as a result, and arterial hypoxaemia is seen.

Airway smooth muscle also contracts when local CO_2 concentrations fall. This happens commonly in pulmonary thromboembolism, when vascular obstruction results in focal areas of hypoperfusion that remain relatively overventilated, such that their local alveolar CO_2 tension falls. This, possibly in concert with bronchoactive inflammatory mediators released in

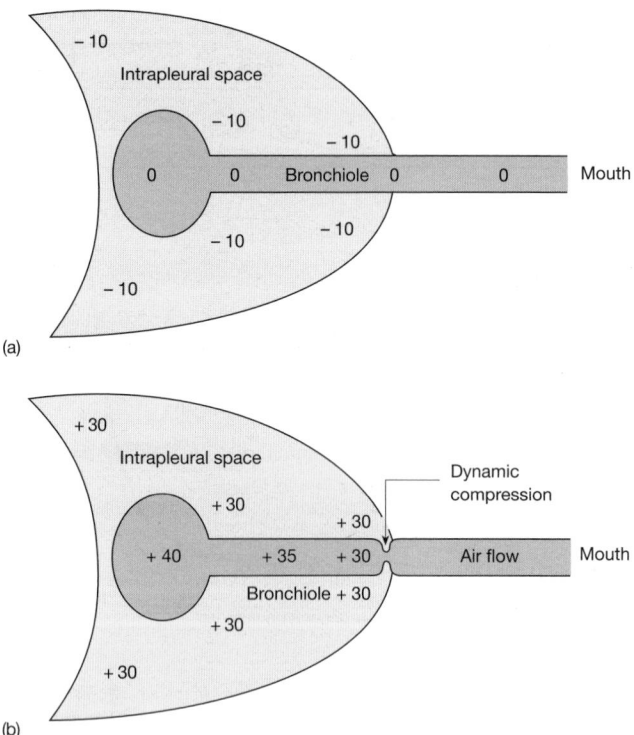

Fig. 3 Diagram to explain dynamic compression during expiration. (a) This depicts intrapleural, alveolar, and airway pressures while breath holding with an open glottis at total lung capacity. Due to lung elasticity, intrapleural pressure is negative (−10 cmH2O), but because of breath holding there is no flow, and pressure in the airways and alveoli equals that at the mouth, 0 cmH2O. Immediately after commencing a forced expiration from total lung capacity (b), intrapleural pressure is high due to expiratory muscle contraction (+30 cmH2O). Alveolar pressure is even higher due to 10 cmH2O of lung elastic recoil pressure. However, due to flow resistance, pressure falls from +40 gradually to +30 as shown. At this point, intrapleural pressure equals intraluminal pressure and immediately downstream dynamic compression occurs as airway pressure falls even further and is now less than intrapleural pressure.

association with the embolic event, can produce local airway smooth muscle contraction and airway obstruction. This might tend to better matching of local ventilation with blood flow, but the benefit is generally small, and local bronchoconstriction can manifest as wheezing, which should not be mistaken for asthma.

Dynamic tests of airflow

All of the consequences of the branched structure of the airways and their interconnectedness need to be integrated if one is to understand common pulmonary function tests. How the 'static' lung volumes (FRC, TLC, VC, and RV) are affected by changes in elastic recoil are discussed above, but such measures form only a part of standard pulmonary function testing. Usually included are 'dynamic' tests that measure expiratory and inspiratory gas flow rates, conventionally during manoeuvres wherein the patient is asked to make a maximal inspiratory or expiratory muscle effort. These are discussed in Chapter 17.3.2.

Distribution of ventilation

The extremely large number of very small respiratory bronchioles creates an environment in which alveoli distal to each bronchiole become susceptible to impaired ventilation. Small intrinsic or pathological reductions in airway diameter of such bronchioles can impair distal ventilation substantially. When the effects of variation in mucus secretion, bronchial smooth muscle tone, and radial traction are added to this inherently vulnerable system, it is surprising that the distribution of ventilation to the 300 million alveoli is as uniform as it is. Were it not, there would probably be considerable hypoxaemia, even in health. This topic is discussed further below.

The parenchyma distal to the terminal bronchioles

The terminal bronchioles (16th generation airways) are the final divisions of the wholly conducting airways. They are completely lined with ciliated epithelium, and function primarily as simple conduits for gas, linking the air around us to the alveoli where gas exchange occurs. The next few divisions of the airways result in transitional airways called respiratory bronchioles, so named because they serve a dual role—as continued gas conduits and as the first locations for gas exchange. Respiratory bronchioles are partly lined with ciliated epithelium, but also have small alveolar outpouchings opening directly into the airway lumen. With continued branching of these bronchioles, more and more of the luminal surface is given to the alveolar outpouchings, and less and less to ciliated epithelium. After about three generations of respiratory bronchioles, the airways, whilst still essentially tubular in shape, are made up entirely of alveolar tissue capable of gas exchange, and are called alveolar ducts. These alveolar ducts branch even further into collections of alveoli whose distal end is blind, known as alveolar sacs, the end of the line of the airway branching system. A diagram of the functional lung unit is shown in Fig. 4. With some 7 orders (or division points) of branching between the terminal bronchioles and the final alveoli, together with 16 orders of branching in the conducting airway segment, the whole airway tree consists of about 23 orders or branch points. Because, after the final branch point, the alveolar sacs are blind, the process of ventilation must occur as a tidal (back and forth) event, alternately adding air to, and removing alveolar gas from, each alveolus with each breath.

The transport of gas in either direction between the trachea and the last conducting airway takes place principally by convective flow, much as water flowing in a pipe depends on the pressure difference between the two ends of the pipe and the flow resistance of the pipe. Since flow is mostly laminar, velocity profiles are largely parabolic, flow being highest in the centre of the lumen and lowest at the airway wall, just as is the velocity profile across a quietly flowing river. There are, however, minor additional influences of diffusive movement at the interface between the convective front of each inspiration and residual gas from the previous breath. These interactions,

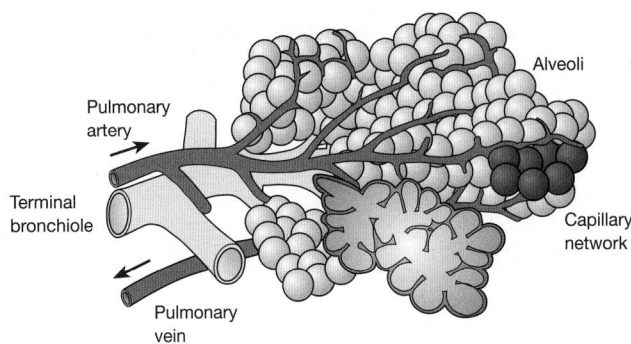

Fig. 4 Diagram of the functional lung unit. The collection of alveoli and associated pulmonary arteries and veins distal to the terminal bronchiole constitutes a functionally homogeneous unit of gas exchange. Mixing of gas amongst alveoli and of blood in the capillary networks of the alveoli in the unit is sufficiently rapid that gas concentrations are in effect uniform throughout. This unit, also called the acinus, corresponds approximately to generations 17 to 23 of Fig. 2

and eddies that develop at each branch point, may assist gas mixing, but their effects are physiologically small. Of much more significance is the fact that the total luminal cross-sectional area of each generation increases exponentially as the airways divide. Since total volumetric flow of gas is the same in each generation, average gas velocity falls reciprocally with the increase in area.

By the time inspired gas reaches the first alveoli, forward velocity has dropped to such a low level that random, thermally fuelled molecular motion (i.e. diffusion) becomes a more important mechanism of gas transport than convection. The small size of the alveoli, about 150 μm in radius, means that diffusive mixing of each new breath with gas resident in the alveoli from prior breaths is nearly instantaneous. Although careful physiological studies can show that low-molecular-weight gases mix slightly faster than those of high molecular weight, this turns out to be of essentially no quantitative significance to gas exchange. Even in emphysema, where many alveolar spaces are enlarged, there is evidence that diffusive mixing in alveolar gas is functionally complete and does not pose a gas exchange threat.

Of more concern for gas exchange is whether all alveoli receive a similar share of each breath. It was pointed out above that the intrinsic structure of the lungs makes it vulnerable to ventilatory inequality, and that this has the potential to disrupt gas exchange. Indeed, recent studies of the structural influence on gas distribution reveals that there are sometimes substantial differences in the ventilation of different alveoli. One property of the system that lessens the negative effects of such inhomogeneity on gas exchange is the finding that individual alveoli do not maintain gas exchange differences from closely adjacent alveoli. In fact, a fairly large number of connected alveoli are normally able to function as a single homogeneous unit of gas exchange. This is no doubt due partly to the rapid diffusive movement of molecules throughout the alveolar gas mentioned above, but it is also facilitated by the rich capillary network lying in the wall of each alveolus. The density of capillaries is so great that should flow fall in one, its neighbour can seamlessly take over its gas exchange role without any resultant inefficiency. It turns out that the functional unit of gas exchange, known as the acinus, corresponds approximately to all the alveoli distal to the last terminal bronchiole.

Clinical significance

The functional lung unit

Pathological events, in either the alveoli or the capillaries, occurring at a scale smaller than that of the functional lung unit will not *per se* have much impact on gas exchange. Thus, a large number of tiny pulmonary emboli each lodging in one capillary of different functional lung units will not impair gas exchange function, whilst a single large embolus of the same total mass obstructing one much larger vessel may. However, if enough microvessels within functional units become obstructed, their summed effects may become considerable.

Surface tension and mechanical instability of the lung

Another consequence of the branched nature of the lungs resulting in so many very small alveoli is inherent mechanical instability. The alveolar wall, where it interfaces with alveolar gas, forms a roughly spherical air–liquid interface. In this context, the alveoli may be likened to a mass of soap bubbles lying together. All air–liquid interfaces are subject to surface tension, which in this case will act to minimize the surface area of each bubble. For an enclosed bubble, this tension increases the pressure inside the bubble, with the relationship between the tension and the interior pressure given by the law of Laplace: pressure = 2 × surface tension/radius. Thus, pressure inside a small bubble exceeds that inside a larger bubble, and if two such unequal bubbles are in contact and their interiors become connected, the small bubble will collapse into the larger. This process of bubble accretion may continue until the many small soap bubbles have collapsed into a single large one. Based on the opening premise of this chapter, if small alveoli had this tendency to collapse into larger neighbours due to surface tension effects, the end result would be disaster for gas exchange. There would be massive alveolar collapse, and with loss of surface area, sufficient O_2 exchange to support metabolic needs would not be possible. Only if all alveoli were identical in both size and surface tension would this problem be avoided, but when 300 million alveoli exist, it is impossible to imagine them all being identical, and indeed they are not.

The lung avoids this dilemma through two quite separate but complementary mechanisms of stabilization. The first, already mentioned above in a different context, is the interconnected nature of the whole alveolar structure. Any tendency for one alveolus to collapse would have to increase the tension on all its immediately connected neighbours. This tension from surrounding alveoli will automatically serve to splint open the alveolus in question, thus opposing its tendency to collapse. This concept, termed alveolar interdependence, is felt to be of considerable importance in maintaining alveolar stability. The second mechanism is the presence of phospholipid molecules that reduce surface tension in the alveolar air–liquid interface. Termed surfactant, and produced in conjunction with proteins from alveolar type II epithelial cells lying free in the alveolar spaces against alveolar walls, this material reduces surface tension severalfold (Fig. 5). Thus, whilst that of water is some 75 dyn/cm, surface tension of the alveolar lining fluid is only about 10 dyn/cm. Moreover, probably due to molecular realignment of surfactant molecules, surface tension is even lower when lung volume is reduced. Based on the law of Laplace given above, this can be seen to be even more advantageous for evening out surface tension differences among alveoli of different size.

Surfactant is thought to have another crucial role that promotes efficient gas exchange between alveolar gas and capillary blood. Given that adjacent alveoli share a common wall, the tendency for surface reduction in each alveolus will create a force that tends to reduce the interstitial tissue pressure around capillaries in the alveolar wall between the adjacent alveoli. From the Starling relationship that governs water escape out of capillaries in any tissue (based on the transcapillary differences in both hydrostatic and oncotic pressures), reducing pressure around the capillary will lead to increased water escape into the alveolar wall. This could have several deleterious consequences. First, the affected alveolar walls would become stiffer and harder to inflate, tending to reduce lung volume. Second, the tissue separating gas from capillary blood would become thicker, directly impairing diffusive transport between gas and blood. Third, this water would find its way into the pulmonary lymphatics, which begin in the alveolar interstitium and run along the large airways and vessels to the hilar regions, before exiting the lungs and emptying into the superior vena cava. Extra water frequently accumulates in the peribronchial and perivascular spaces

and results in their partial compression, reducing distal ventilation and/or blood flow of subtended alveoli, causing maldistribution of either or both, and rendering gas exchange inefficient. The presence of surfactant is thought to reduce the rate of transcapillary water exchange, and therefore to contribute to efficient gas exchange.

Clinical significance

Impaired surfactant activity

When surfactant is not present, when its rate of renewal is insufficient, or when it is inactivated rapidly, pathological changes can be severe. Best known is the infant respiratory distress syndrome, occurring in otherwise normal premature infants born before the late-maturing surfactant system is functional. Without exogenous surfactant replacement therapy the condition may be fatal because of alveolar collapse and pulmonary oedema. Surfactant activity is also compromised in the adult respiratory distress syndrome and may compound the disturbances of pulmonary function arising from the primary cause of the pulmonary disease.

Gravity and lung function

Causes of potential unequal distribution of ventilation or blood flow to the alveoli extend beyond those associated with the intrinsic branching structure of the lungs discussed above. In particular, the presence of gravity influences lung function because key components of the lungs have significant weight. The weight of the parenchyma itself, plus the blood within the alveolar capillaries, feeding arteries and draining veins, together cause the lungs to sag toward the diaphragm in the upright lung sitting at FRC. The

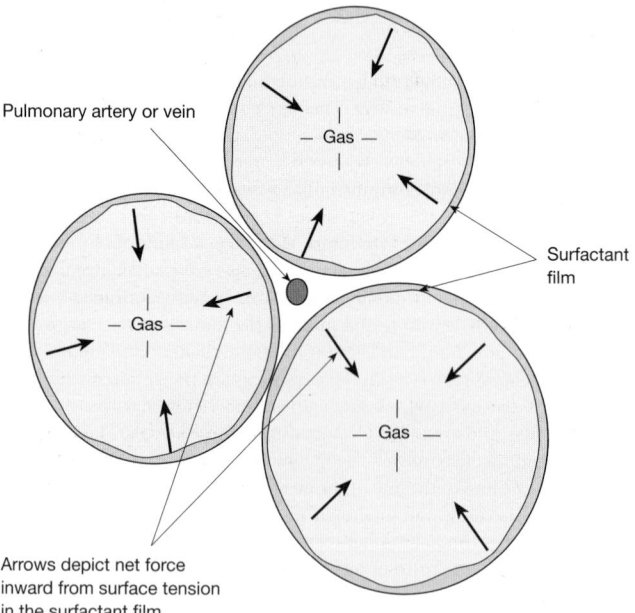

Pulmonary artery or vein

Surfactant film

Arrows depict net force inward from surface tension in the surfactant film

Fig. 5 Diagram to indicate potential effects of surface tension on lung structure and function. Three gas-filled alveoli are shown, each lined by a thin film of surfactant. A pulmonary artery or vein is shown in the corner formed where the three alveoli come together. Arrows show the net inward force produced by surface tension, tending to reduce alveolar gas volume and promote atelectasis. In addition, the pressure in the perivascular space around the corner vessel shown will be reduced by these inward surface forces, increasing the pressure difference from inside to outside the vessel lumen and thereby promoting fluid movement from plasma to interstitial space. The presence of surfactant reduces the magnitude of surface tension forces and therefore stabilizes the alveoli against atelectasis and reduces the transmural pressure difference, attenuating transvascular fluid movement.

upper pole of the lungs is still applied to the parietal pleural surface of the chest wall—there is no pleural airspace created by this gravitational stress. Rather, the rest of the lung is displaced caudally, sagging much like a heavy sweater pegged to a clothes line. As expected, this creates stress in the alveolar walls, more in the uppermost than lowermost alveoli. A good analogy is the toy Slinky—a coiled spring that when hanging vertically under its own weight shows wider separation between adjacent coils at its top than at its bottom. Correspondingly, the uppermost alveoli in the upright lung are larger than the lowermost alveoli. The lowermost alveoli are thus more compliant—that is, able to be further inflated more per unit transpulmonary pressure—than the uppermost alveoli, because the latter are stretched almost to their limit. Accordingly, normal ventilation from FRC results in greater ventilation of the lung bases than of the lung apices. Much the same effect is seen for blood flow: apical blood flow is less than that at the base of the upright lung. In this case it is the weight of the blood itself that is responsible: perfusion depends on pulmonary arterial pressure, which falls linearly with height up the lung.

The apex to base differences in perfusion exceed those of ventilation, such that the ratio of ventilation to blood flow is higher at the apex than at the base. The local ventilation/perfusion ($\dot{V}A/\dot{Q}$) ratio determines local alveolar P_{O_2} and P_{CO_2}, P_{O_2} increasing and P_{CO_2} falling as the $\dot{V}A/\dot{Q}$ ratio increases. Thus, P_{O_2} at the apex is higher, and P_{CO_2} lower than at the base. If the $\dot{V}A/\dot{Q}$ ratio everywhere was the same, so too would be P_{O_2} and P_{CO_2}, and the exchange of O_2 and CO_2 would be maximally efficient. However, the presence of a range of $\dot{V}A/\dot{Q}$ ratios (no matter what its cause) results in gas exchange inefficiency and arterial hypoxaemia.

Clinical significance

Effects of gravity on lung function in disease

Although gravity creates $\dot{V}A/\dot{Q}$ maldistribution, common disease processes are in large part randomly distributed in the lungs, and their effects on $\dot{V}A/\dot{Q}$ matching generally much greater than those of gravity. Thus, whilst the effect of gravity on $\dot{V}A/\dot{Q}$ mismatching in normal lungs is barely measurable, $\dot{V}A/\dot{Q}$ mismatching based on non-gravitational influences in many diseases leads to profound gas exchange disturbances. However, the presence of gravity must not be discounted in several disease states.

Emphysema, and even the normal ageing process, often causes tissue breakdown in the apical lung regions because, as in the Slinky analogy, the alveolar wall stresses are largest there. When mechanical failure occurs, it is most likely to happen in the regions of greatest stress, and as a result the alveolar wall breakdown so typical of emphysema, and to a much lesser extent normal ageing, is often exaggerated in the apices. An important gravitational influence occurs in patients in intensive care with severe lung disease. In any body position, both blood flow and alveolar fluid collection tend to be concentrated in dependent regions (e.g. posteriorly in the supine patient). Those regions with high blood flow may also have little or no ventilation if their alveoli are filled with fluid and cell debris. The blood flowing through such regions can therefore pick up little or no O_2, and hypoxaemia may be severe. This has led some intensive care staff to rotate their patients from supine to lateral to prone and back. The argument being that the gravitational influences on blood flow are essentially instantaneous, whilst those on alveolar fluid collection may take hours to respond to body positional changes. Thus, for a time after rotating a patient, the dependent region may enjoy high flow but not yet be fluid filled and thus still be well ventilated. Gas exchange is therefore enhanced, and arterial hypoxaemia is mitigated. Such behaviour may also explain positional influences on gas exchange in patients with unilateral lung disease such as pneumonia, effusion, or atelectasis.

Further reading

Crystal R, West JB (1994). *The lung: scientific foundations*. Raven Press, New York.

Weibel ER (1963). *Morphometry of human lung*. Springer-Verlag, Berlin.

Weibel ER (1984). *Pathway for oxygen: structure and function in the mammalian respiratory system*. Harvard University Press, Cambridge, Massachusetts.

West JB (1990). *Respiratory physiology, the essentials*, 4th edn. Williams & Wilkins, Baltimore, Maryland.

17.1.3 'First-line' defence mechanisms of the lung

C. Haslett

Introduction

In their critically important service as our central gas exchange organs the lungs are continuously exposed to more than 7000 litres of air per day, but their membranes are delicate and require to be kept moist and protected from the daily bombardment of particles including dust, pollen, and pollutants, together with viruses and bacteria. These agents have the potential to cause lung injury or to invade the lung and generate potentially life-threatening infections. That these problems rarely occur is because the lung possesses very effective local 'primary' protective mechanisms, which are the focus of this chapter. If an infectious agent is able to penetrate these defences and set up a 'bridge-head', highly effective and complex 'secondary' responses, including the inflammatory and classic immune responses, can be recruited rapidly. In the event that immune or inflammatory responses should be initiated, the lung also has mechanisms by which it can protect itself from their potentially detrimental local side-effects. The inflammatory and immune responses themselves will only briefly be alluded to; detailed treatment of these processes is beyond the scope of this chapter (see Chapter 16.5.1 for further discussion).

The respiratory tract is protected by different mechanisms at its various levels. In general terms, physical mechanisms, including cough, are particularly important in the large airways; the lower airways are protected by complex mucociliary clearance mechanisms; and the gas exchange units at the alveolar level are protected by surfactant and by 'patrolling' alveolar macrophages. The lung lining fluids (mucus in the airways and surfactant in the gas exchange units) contain a variety of proteins that are particularly important in host defence. In this section we will therefore consider physical defences, mucociliary clearance mechanisms, surfactant and important defensive proteins in the lining fluid of the lung, and how the 'second-line defences'—the classic inflammatory and immune responses—can be initiated in the lungs.

Physical defences

The nose makes an important contribution to the physical defences of the upper airway. It comprises a stack of fine aerodynamic filters of respiratory epithelium arranged over the turbinate bones. These remove most large particles from inspired air. Their filtering effect is greatly enhanced by fine hairs in the anterior nares and by mucociliary action that, apart from a small area anterior to the inferior turbinates, is directed posteriorly such that trapped particles are swallowed or expectorated. The larynx acts as a sphincter during cough and expectoration and is an essential protective mechanism for the lower airways during swallowing and vomiting.

Particles with a size greater than 0.5 μm that survive passage through the nose will be trapped by the lining fluid of the trachea and bronchi, to be cleared by the mucociliary clearance mechanism, which has been called the 'mucociliary escalator'.

Mucociliary clearance

Cilia

The mucociliary escalator works by a complex interaction between cilia, which are a series of projections on the bronchial epithelial cells, and mucus, forming a 'raft' on top of the cilia, which then sweep this raft in a cephalad direction. The combined effect of this interaction can readily be appreciated by scanning electron microscopy (Fig. 1). There are about 200 cilia on each of the pseudostratified columnar epithelial cells lining the bronchi and it has been calculated that these can carry weights of up to 10 g/cm without slowing, working with a ciliary beat frequency of 12 to 14 beats/s. Their motility depends upon the contraction of longitudinal fibrils that contain the contractile protein tubilin arranged as nine outer and two central microtubular pairs, and their effectiveness in sweeping mucus in the cephalic direction is enhanced by small 'claws' in their tips, which penetrate the overlying mucus sheet. The actual driving mechanism of the cilia is

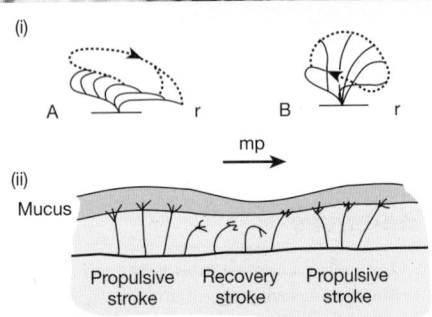

(a)

(b)

Fig. 1 (a) Scanning electron micrograph (× 14 000) of the 'mucociliary escalator' of the bronchial epithelium. The cilia and the overlying 'raft' of mucus (mu) are clearly seen. (By courtesy of Dr P.K. Jeffery.) (b) Beat cycle of a tracheal cilium seen from the side: (i) In a single cilium during the recovery stroke (A) the cilium starts from its rest position r and unrolls backwards; in the propulsive stroke it remains extended to reach its rest position (B). Mucus is propelled to the right (mp). (ii) Groups of cilia move in co-ordinated waves with clusters in their propulsive phase bordered by those in recovery. (Adapted from Sleigh MA, Blake JR, Liron N (1988). The propulsion of mucus by cilia. *American Review of Respiratory Disease* **137**, 726.)

uncertain, but involves dynein, an ATPase protein that forms a major part of the cilium. This appears to derive energy from ATP along the cilium and convert it into the forces that are generated by the contractile proteins.

It is generally believed that ciliary beating occurs by the microtubules, which provide the 'skeleton' of the cilia, sliding over each other, much like the sliding fibre theory of muscle contraction. Since not all microtubular pairs move at the same time, their co-ordinated shortening leads to reduction in length of some microtubules relative to those at the opposite side of the cilium, and with the skeletal rigidity that is provided by the radial pairs of the microcilial 'spokes' and their basal anchoring system, this causes the cilium to bend in the direction of shortening. The ciliary beat itself can be divided into two phases: the forward mucus-propulsive stroke, and a slower recovery stroke (much like the forward and recovery actions of a whip, Fig. 1(b)). Where this occurs in a co-ordinated fashion in the ciliated epithelium, the wave-like motion of numerous cilia effected through their terminal claws propels the mucus raft in a cephalad direction.

Ciliary function can be assessed in a number of ways, facilitated by the fact that cilia can survive freezing for up to a month and may beat for several hours after death of the host. Thus, it is possible to assess their motility directly in cytological specimens from nasal and bronchial brushings and to perform detailed photometry and determine ciliary beat frequency in epithelial specimens sampled by biopsy. Cilial structure can also be assessed by electron microscopy. In a simple and practical clinical test, the time taken for saccharine placed in the anterior nares to cause a sweet taste in the mouth (around 11 min normally) can be used as a convenient clinical measure of ciliary function, which is informative because in most examples of ciliary disease the nasal cilia are also affected. Other more complex methods of assessing mucociliary clearance *in vivo* include cinebronchography and assessment of the rate of clearance of radio-aerosols.

Mucus

Mucus is secreted by the goblet cells and submucosal glands of the first few bronchial generations. Secretion is under the control of a variety of chemical mediators: neuropeptides including substance P, vasoactive intestinal polypeptide, and bombesin, in addition to vagal stimulation and acetylcholine, will cause discharge. In health, mucus is composed of 95 per cent water, the mucus glycoproteins or mucins, and a variety of other proteins (see below), which although present in low concentration, probably play an important part in defence of the bronchial tree. The function of mucus is to trap and clear particles, to dilute noxious influences, to lubricate the airways, and to humidify respired air. The viscoelastic or rheological properties of mucus are likely to be controlled by the concentration of different mucins and are probably critical in determining adequate mucociliary transport.

Factors that affect mucociliary clearance

A number of external factors may reduce mucociliary clearance by interfering with ciliary function or by causing direct ciliary damage. These include pollutants, cigarette smoke, local and general anaesthetic agents, bacterial products, and viral infection. In severe asthma it is thought that eosinophil products including major basic protein may have detrimental effects on ciliary function. Thus there are a number of diseases in which mucociliary clearance may be adversely affected in a secondary fashion. There is also an autosomal recessive condition (occurring with a frequency of about 1 in 30 000 population), called primary ciliary dyskinesia, in which defects in cilial dynein may be associated with male infertility and situs inversus (Kartagener's syndrome). Primary ciliary dyskinesia is associated with repeated sinusitis and respiratory infections that often progress to persistent lung suppuration and severe bronchiectasis, thus underlining the importance of cilia in antibacterial lung defences.

There is now a great deal of interest in abnormal properties of mucus and deranged mucociliary clearance in cystic fibrosis. In this condition, mucus is abnormally viscous with grossly altered rheological properties resulting in markedly retarded mucociliary clearance (see Chapter 17.10).

Surfactant and surfactant 'collectins'

As is discussed in more detail elsewhere (Chapter 17.1.2), surfactant is a complex surface-active material that lines the alveolar surface to reduce surface tension and prevent the lung from collapsing at resting transpulmonary pressures. It also provides a simple mechanism for alveolar clearance since, at end expiration, surface tension decreases and the surface film moves from the alveolus towards the bronchioles, thus carrying small particles and damaged cells towards the mucociliary transport system.

Surfactant is synthesized and secreted by the alveolar type II pneumocytes. It comprises phospholipids, neutral lipids, and at least four different specific proteins, termed surfactant proteins A, B, C, and D (**SP-A**, **SP-B**, **SP-C**, and **SP-D**). It is now recognized that in addition to promoting the surface-active properties of surfactant these proteins have important roles in host defence. SP-B and SP-C are likely to have the major surface-active roles, since both accelerate the adsorption of lipids to an air–liquid interface. Although SP-A can act co-operatively with SP-B in the formation of a surface film, there is no significant derangement of surfactant function or metabolism in SP-A gene-targeted ('knockout') mice, whereas genetically engineered SP-D deficient mice demonstrate abnormal accumulation of surfactant, suggesting a previously unsuspected role for SP-D in surfactant homeostasis.

While it has been recognized for decades that, in addition to its surface-active properties, surfactant can modulate host defence responses, interest in this area has recently intensified with the discovery that SP-A and SP-D, which are secreted by Clara cells in the epithelial lining of the lungs, are members of the collectin (collagen-like lectins) family of proteins. Members of this family in the serum are known to possess important bacterial binding and opsonization properties, and also to influence inflammatory cell function, including stimulation of chemotaxis and the production of reactive oxygen species and cytokines by immune cells. Moreover, mutations of the serum collectin mannose-binding lectin are linked to repeated infections in neonates and children. The collectin family now includes mannose-binding lectin, conglutinin, and CL-44 in blood, and SP-A and SP-D in lung secretions. The collectins are also known as the group II C-type lectins, since their binding to carbohydrate requires calcium.

SP-A and SP-D have been shown to bind to a wide variety of pathogenic microbes (Table 1) and *in vitro* will stimulate the uptake of many of these by macrophages. More recently SP-A, which has been better studied than SP-D, has been shown to possess a number of other properties to suggest that it represents an important component of the lungs armamentarium in the first line of defence against infection (Table 2). Gene-targeted mice deficient in SP-A show marked reduction in the ability to clear *Streptococcus pneumoniae*, *Pseudomonas aeruginosa*, and respiratory syncytial virus from their lungs. The relevance of these observations to human disease remains to be clearly defined.

Table 1 Some microbial targets of surfactant collectins

SP-A	SP-D
Streptococcus pneumoniae	*Haemophilus influenzae*
Staphylococcus aureus	*Klebsiella pneumoniae*
Group A streptococci	*Pseudomonas aeruginosa*
Group B streptococci	*Pneumocystis carinii*
Haemophilus influenzae type A	*Escherichia coli*
Escherichia coli	*Salmonella minnesota*
Klebsiella pneumoniae	*Aspergillus fumigatus*
Pseudomonas aeruginosa	*Cryptococcus neoformans*
Mycobacterium tuberculosis	Influenza A
Pneumocystis carinii	Respiratory syncytial virus
Cryptococcus neoformans	
Aspergillius fumigatus	
Influenza A	
Herpes simplex virus	
Respiratory syncytial virus	

Table 2 Some potential first-line defence roles of SP-A

- Interacts with a variety of micro-organisms (see Table 1), enhances the phagocytosis of some, both by acting as an opsonin and by acting as an activation ligand
- Enhances directed migration of alveolar macrophages
- Stimulates production of reactive oxygen species by alveolar macrophages
- Stimulates IgM, IgA, and IgG production by splenocytes
- Stimulates cytokine (tumour necrosis factor-α, interleukin 1α, IL-1β, IL-6) production by peripheral blood monocytes and alveolar macrophages
- Enhances concanavalin A-dependent lymphocyte proliferation

It has long been recognized that surfactant lipids suppress a variety of immune cell functions, including lymphocyte proliferation, whereas SP-A (and probably SP-D) mainly enhance immune cell functions, suggesting the intriguing possibility of counter-regulatory effects of changes in lipid/protein ratios that might be important in regulating the immune status of the lung. Levels of SP-A (and SP-D) can vary greatly in human disease, with reduced concentrations in HIV-positive patients and markedly reduced concentrations in adult respiratory distress syndrome (**ARDS**) and severe pneumonias. While it is tempting to speculate that low levels of SP-A predispose to infection and immune dysfunction in these settings, it is not certain whether these changes are 'cause' or 'effect' (for example simply reflecting local consumption). There has been less study of SP-D, but it may well possess many of the immune modulatory functions as well as the bacterial-binding properties of SP-A; studies in SP-D ' knockout mice' suggest an important role in influenza neutralization *in vivo*.

Other protective proteins of the lining fluid of the respiratory tract

These may be derived from plasma (e.g. albumin, transferrin, α₂-antiplasmin, α₂-macrogrobulin), by secretion from local epithelial cells, macrophages, or inflammatory cells (e.g. lysozyme, lactoferrin, and defensins), or by selective epithelial transport (e.g. IgA). Clearly the local availability of plasma-derived proteins increases greatly during the exudative phase of any inflammatory process, thus adding more complement, antiproteinases, immunoglobulins, and proteins, including cytokines derived from inflammatory cell secretion.

Defensins and other antibacterial proteins and peptides

Some of the principal antimicrobial molecules isolated from human pulmonary secretions are outlined in Table 3.

Lactoferrin

Lactoferrin was first recognized as a high-affinity iron chelator in human milk, but in the 1960s it was found to possess bacteriostatic properties that were thought to be exerted by deprivation of iron, which is essential for bacterial growth. It occurs in the primary granules of neutrophils and

Table 3 Antibacterial proteins and peptides in the lung

Lysozyme
Lactoferrin
Bactericidal/permeability-increasing protein (BPI)
α-Defensins
    Human neutrophil peptides (HNP) 1–4
β-Defensins
    Human β-defensin (HBD) 1, 2
Cathelicidins
    LL-37/hCAP-18
Small-molecular-weight antiproteinases (SLPI, elafin)

mammalian exocrine secretions, including lung fluids. More recently it has been shown to exert direct membrane effects on some bacteria and to have important modulatory effects on the inflammatory process. Some of these effects may be mediated by its high-affinity binding to bacterial lipopolysaccharide and include the inhibition of cytokine release from cells of the monocyte/macrophage series and modulation of the proliferation and differentiation of immune cells.

Lysozyme

Lysozyme is a 1,4-β-N-acetylmuraminidase that enzymatically degrades a glycosidic linkage of bacterial membrane peptidoglycan. Acting alone, human lysozyme can lyse and kill a variety of Gram-positive micro-organisms, but most Gram-negative organisms are resistant to its direct effects. Like lactoferrin, lysozyme is a major component of the specific granules of neutrophils and is found in the mucosal secretions of the respiratory tract; it has recently been suggested that they may collaborate in killing Gram-negative bacteria such as *Escherichia coli* by disrupting the cell membrane.

Defensins

Defensins are small-molecular-weight, cationic, cysteine-rich peptides that are able to kill a wide range of micro-organisms. They are membrane active and are believed to aggregate in order to 'punch' pores or channels in microbial cell membranes. The α-defensins are major constituents of the neutrophil α granule and are also found in airway secretions. In humans, the α-defensins HNP 1 to 4 account for about 5 per cent of the total cellular protein of neutrophils and are active against staphylococci, *E. coli, Pseudomonas aeruginosa, Cryptococcus neoformans,* and some enveloped viruses such as herpes simplex virus 1 and vesicular stomatitis virus. The β-defensins are derived from the epithelial lining and were first discovered in cattle as antimicrobial peptides of airway cells, for instance tracheal antimicrobial peptide. At least three human β-defensins have been identified. HBD-1 and HBD-2 are expressed in airway epithelial cells from patients with and without cystic fibrosis. HBD-2 protein is found in lung secretions from patients with cystic fibrosis, patients with inflammatory lung disease, and also from healthy volunteers, whereas HBD-1 protein is not detected in healthy controls but is found in lung secretions from patients with cystic fibrosis and inflammatory lung diseases. Together with the observation that the pro-inflammatory mediator interleukin 1β stimulates epithelial generation of HBD-2 but not HBD-1 *in vitro*, these observations suggest that in the lung HBD-2 is induced by inflammation whereas HBD-1 may serve as a lung defence in the absence of lung inflammation. HBD-1 has also recently been implicated in the pathogenesis of cystic fibrosis where it appears to be inactivated by the high salt milieu.

Cathelicidins

Cathelicidin peptides contain a highly conserved signal sequence ('cathelin') but show substantial heterogeneity in the C-terminal domain. The first human cathelicidin to be characterized—LL-37/hCAP-18—is expressed in airway epithelium and displays antibiotic activity against a range of Gram-negative and -positive organisms.

Small-molecular-weight antiproteinases

Agents such as secretory leukoproteinase inhibitor and elafin, previously thought to exist in lung secretions solely as part of the 'antiproteinase protective shield', have now been shown to possess important additional antibacterial properties. Both secretory leukoproteinase inhibitor and elafin display major activity against *Pseudomonas aeruginosa* and *Staphylococcus aureus*, which resides in a molecular position distinct from their powerful antineutrophil elastase activities.

In summary, a growing number of antibiotic peptides are now shown to demonstrate a marked selectivity for prokaryotic and eukaryotic micro-organisms, thus providing an effective but simple method whereby diverse classes of micro-organisms can be recognized and destroyed as 'non-self'. Many more peptides and proteins like these are likely to emerge, displaying properties that combine antibacterial actions with important roles in

modulating the key cells responsible for our host defences, perhaps providing important links between primary 'innate' defence mechanism and the generation of secondary inflammatory and immune responses. Some of these agents may be of value in future therapeutic regimes, particularly in situations where the lungs are injured and at risk of secondary infection, such as cystic fibrosis and the adult respiratory distress syndrome.

Immunoglobulins

Normal lung secretions contain all the immunoglobulins present in plasma, but in different proportions. In the absence of disease, immunoglobulins are produced locally, with IgA greatly in excess and only small contributions from IgG and IgM. It is thought that B lymphocytes and plasma cells are particularly important in producing secretory IgA in the upper airways by a collaborative mechanism involving the epithelial cells as follows. Dimeric IgA is assembled in the plasma cells from two monomeric IgA molecules and joined by another protein, the J chain. Dimeric IgA then binds to the secretory component on the surface of epithelial cells, forming a dimeric IgA–secretory component complex that is pinocytosed, transported through the epithelial cell, and released from its luminal surface into the airways. The secretory component appears to protect IgA from enzymic attack during bacterial infection and inflammation in the host. IgA is produced in very high concentrations in the upper airways and is therefore likely to serve a number of important roles, but these are not fully understood. IgA deficiency is associated with local defects in immunity.

IgG concentrations in lung secretions are quantitatively similar to plasma IgG concentrations and may be particularly important in the lower airways where IgG may act as a very effective opsonin and activator of complement. IgG deficiency is associated with recurrent respiratory tract infection, suggesting that it provides an important local defence mechanism.

Complement proteins, proteinase inhibitors, etc.

Most of the proteins involved in the complement system have been identified in lung secretions. Most are probably derived by plasma exudation during inflammation, and C3a, C3b, and C5a may be secreted by alveolar macrophages. Patients with C3 deficiency have recurrent upper and lower respiratory tract infections, particularly with *Streptococcus pneumoniae* and *Haemophilus influenzae*. C3 is likely to play a key role in opsonization (via C3bi) of bacteria.

Lung secretions also contain a variety of antiproteinases, including the large molecules α_2-macroglobulin and α_1-proteinase inhibitor as well as moieties of lower molecular weight, such as secretory leukoproteinase inhibitor and elafin. Antiproteinases are probably secreted in higher concentrations by local epithelial cells and alveolar macrophages during inflammatory and injurious processes, at which time there will be additional contribution to local defences from leakage of plasma protein-derived antiproteinases. It is likely that these antiproteinases play an important part in the antiproteinase 'shield' which is necessary to protect the healthy local tissues against damage from the release of proteinases by inflammatory cells.

The alveolar macrophage and other alveolar cells

Alveolar macrophages are highly differentiated cells that have matured in the lung from bloodborne, bone marrow-derived monocytes. They normally 'patrol' the alveoli (Fig. 2), where they exist with a half-life of several weeks. The technique of bronchoalveolar lavage, whereby fluid is instilled into the small airways via a fibreoptic bronchoscope and fluid and harvested cells (normally greater than 95 per cent alveolar macrophages in

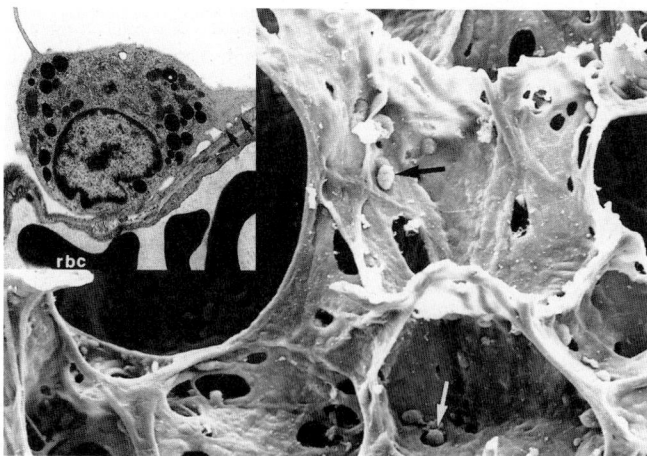

Fig. 2 Scanning electron micrograph (× 350) showing alveolar macrophages (arrows) 'patrolling' the alveolar airspaces. A high power view of a single alveolar macrophage adhering to the alveolar lining (arrows illustrate points of adhesion) is shown in section on the inserted (top left) transmission electron micrograph. (By courtesy of Dr P.K. Jeffery.)

healthy individuals) are returned by suction, has greatly facilitated the *ex vivo* study of the various functions of these versatile cells. It was quickly recognized that alveolar macrophages possessed marked phagocytic ability, with the capacity to ingest and destroy pathogenic bacteria, but only recently has their capacity to generate mediators of central importance in the initiation of inflammation and to present antigen in the initiation of the immune response been fully recognized. The alveolar macrophage could therefore be considered as a 'microcomputer', sampling and sensing via a vast array of receptors (Table 4) the external environment in the alveolar spaces and subsequently determining whether inflammatory or immune responses should be generated. It is also likely to assist the inflammatory monocyte-derived macrophages in the scavenging roles required during the aftermath of infections and the resolution of inflammation, and may play a further important role in the processes whereby inflammatory tissue injury

Table 4 Some receptors on and molecules binding to macrophages

Complement components
C1q, C3b, C3bi, C3d, C5a
Immunoglobulins
IgG, IgA, IgE
Growth factors and cytokines
IFN-α/β/γ, CSF-1, GM-CSF, TNF-α
IL-1, IL-2, IL-3, IL-4, IL-6
Adhesion molecules and phagocytic receptors
LFA-1, MAC-1, p150/95, ICAM-1, $\alpha_v\beta_3$ (VnR), CR1, CR3, FcR
Glycoproteins and carbohydrates
Mannosyl fucosyl receptor
Mannose-6-phosphate
Heparin
Advanced glycosylation end-products
Protein and hormones
Fibronectin, laminin, transferrin, fibrin, lactoferrin, calcitonin
Oestrogen, insulin, parathormone, progesterone
Peptides and small molecules
Adenosine, bombesin, bradykinin, adrenaline
Dexamethasone, glucagon, histamine
Tachykinins, PAF, serotonin, substance P
VIP
Lipids and lipoproteins
Leukotrienes C, D$_4$, B$_4$, E$_2$
LDL, β-VLDL, modified LDL

Table 5 Some secretory products of macrophages

Cytokines and growth factors
IFN-α/β/γ, IL-1, IL-6, TNF-α
IL-8, GRO-α, MCP-1
TGF-β, PDGF, FGF, IGF, GM-CSF, G-CSF
Erythropoietin, lactoferrin
Enzymes
Elastase, collagenase, lysozyme
Phospholipase A$_2$, amylase
Hyaluronidase, acid hydrolases
β-galactosidase, β-glucuronidase
Nucleases, ribonucleases, acid phosphatases
Sulphatases, cathepsins
Enzyme inhibitors
α$_1$-proteinase inhibitor, α$_2$-macroglobulin
Lipomodulin, α$_1$-antichymotrypsin
Inhibitors of plasminogen and plasminogen activator
Reactive oxygen intermediates
O$_2^-$, H$_2$O$_2$, OH$^-$, hypohalous acid
Reactive nitogen intermediates
NO, NO$_2$, NO$_3$
Complement components etc.
C1, C4, C2, C3, C5, factor B, factor D, properdin
Lipids
Leukotrienes B, C, D, E, PGE, PGF$_{2\alpha}$
PAF, prostacyclin, thomboxane A$_2$
Matrix proteins
Fibronectin, thrombospondin, proteoglycans
Coagulation factors
Factor X, IX, V, and VII, tissue factor, prothrombin, thromboplastin

is repaired, since it can produce a number of proteins involved in tissue repair processes and can generate a variety of cytokines that influence fibroblast function (Table 5).

Phagocytosis and bacterial killing

Macrophages can recognize and ingest opsonized (via their surface CR3 or FcR) or non-opsonized particles by a variety of receptors (Table 4). Within the phagolysosome, ingested particles are subjected to the combined destructive forces of reactive oxygen intermediates generated via the metabolic burst and a wide range of degradative enzymes that have the capacity to digest proteins, lipids, and carbohydrates. It appears that the local generation of nitric oxide is an important defence mechanism against a variety of micro-organisms. Activated macrophages form nitrite (NO$_2$), nitrate (NO$_3$), and nitric oxide (NO). *In vitro* experiments suggest that these products, particularly NO and the peroxynitrite anion, contribute to antifungal, antiparasitic, and tumoricidal activity of macrophages. Macrophages may 'call in antibacterial reinforcements' of other phagocytic cells including neutrophils, monocytes (which mature into inflammatory macrophages), and eosinophils by the generation of specific chemotaxins (see below). They may also generate a local immune response by presenting antigen and producing a variety of lymphokines.

Despite the availability of such powerful mechanisms, it is clear that not all phagocytosed particles are effectively destroyed. For example, asbestos, silica, and a number of micro-organisms including tuberculosis, some strains of *H. influenzae*, and trypanosomes at various stages of their lifecycle are able to resist destruction within macrophages.

Generation of the inflammatory response

Macrophages can secrete a number of chemotactic proteins in the chemokine family as well as mediators in the 5-lipoxygenase and cyclo-oxygenase pathways, all of which can exert profound pro-inflammatory effects. Neutrophil chemotaxins include interleukin 8, leukotriene B$_4$, and NAP-2. Peptides chemotactic for monocytes include MCP-1 and MIP-1. Other macrophage-derived cytokines may have important secondary pro-inflammatory effects through their influences on other cells. For example, tumour necrosis factor and interleukin 1 act not only on endothelium to stimulate the expression of adhesion molecules necessary for inflammatory cell emigration, but may also act on local fibroblasts to produce interleukin 8 that exerts neutrophil chemotactic effects. Thus, macrophages not only generate chemoattractants for inflammatory cells, but they can also recruit other local cells such as fibroblasts to help in the initiation of inflammation, thereby governing graded levels of amplification of the inflammatory response.

Generation of the immune response

Alveolar macrophages are effective antigen-presenting cells and can display partially degraded antigens on their surface to interact with recirculating T and B cells, generating clonal expansion and initiating the immune response.

Tissue remodelling and repair

Alveolar macrophages can secrete proteins, including fibronectin, vitronectin, and laminin, which are important in tissue repair. Macrophages can also produce a number of cytokines including PDGF, TGF-β, and interleukin-1 that can influence the behaviour of other cells, particularly fibroblasts that are critically involved in the repair process (see Chapter 16.5.1).

The pulmonary marginated pool of neutrophils

The neutrophil is the archetypal acute inflammatory cell, equipped with a variety of mechanisms that make it a very effective agent in host defences against bacteria such as streptococci. After release from the bone marrow, mature neutrophils exist in the vascular compartment with a half-life of about 6 h. Unlike red blood cells, up to half of the neutrophils in the vascular compartment do not circulate at any given time, but form a 'marginated pool', which is in dynamic equilibrium with the 'circulating pool' of vascular neutrophils. The marginated pool can be released into the circulating pool by exercise or adrenaline. The vascular beds of the lung and spleen appear to make the most important contribution to the marginated pool, which may serve as a source of rapidly releasable neutrophils in times of stress or injury. The presence of large numbers of neutrophils in the pulmonary microvascular bed is likely to increase the mobilization and effectiveness of local lung defences in response to their inevitable exposure to inhaled micro-organisms or toxins. The mechanisms underlying the formation of the lung marginated pool are uncertain. It could be formed as the result of low-grade adhesive interactions between neutrophils and lung capillary endothelial cells, but it is likely that the rheological properties of neutrophils in pulmonary capillaries are more important in the physiological margination of neutrophils in the lung. The mean diameter of the pulmonary capillary is 5.5 μm, whereas that of the neutrophil is 7.5 μm, hence neutrophils are normally required to squeeze through the pulmonary capillaries and minor changes in their deformability or alterations in the fluid pressure gradient across the lung capillary bed would be expected to influence markedly the size of the pulmonary marginated pool. The presence of this pool of neutrophils in the lung may have advantages for host defence, but, paradoxically, it could also partly explain why the lung appears to be such an important target in conditions such as the adult respiratory distress syndrome, which may result from systemic or distant insults, such as Gram-negative septicaemia, multiple trauma, or pancreatitis (see Chapter 16.5.1).

Further reading

Clark HW, Reid KBM, Sim RB (2000). Collective and innate immunity in the lung. *Microbes and Infection* **2**, 273–8.

Ganz T *et al.* (1985). Defensins. Natural peptide antibiotics of human neutrophils. *Journal of Clinical Investigation* **78**, 1427–35.

Hancock RE (1997). Peptide antibiotics. *Lancet* **349**, 418–22.

Singh PK *et al.* (1998). Production of β-defensins by human airway epithelia. *Proceedings of the National Academy of Sciences, USA* **95**, 14961–6.

Sleigh MA, Blake JR, Liron H (1988). The propulsion of mucus by cilia. *American Review of Respiratory Disease* **137**, 726–41.

Van Wetering S *et al.* (1999). Defensins: key players or bystanders in infection, injury, and repair in the lung? *Journal of Allergy and Clinical Immunology* **104**, 1131–8.

Wright JR (1997). Immunomodulatory functions of surfactant. *Physiological Reviews* **77**, 931–62.

17.2 The clinical presentation of chest diseases

D. J. Lane

The presenting symptoms of chest diseases are few, but the structural and functional disturbances that these symptoms reflect are numerous and the underlying disease entities are many. The symptoms of lower respiratory tract disease can be grouped under just three headings: cough, breathlessness, and chest pain.

Cough may or may not produce sputum. Patients occasionally report the expectoration of sputum while denying they have a cough. This seems to be a socially determined separation of the act of 'clearing the throat' to expel sputum, from a non-productive cough which, perhaps because it appears to have no purpose, is regarded as more sinister. Breathlessness itself is a complex symptom. Wheezing and stridor, which are audible accompaniments to the act of breathing, are rarely reported without breathlessness and so they will all be considered together. Discussion of chest pain will include mention of chest tightness.

In the analysis of symptoms it is important to recognize and differentiate between the pathology or disordered physiology likely to be responsible for the symptoms, and the clinical diagnoses associated with that symptom. The investigation of mechanism, although superficially of little clinical relevance, can be the key to symptomatic treatment, creating opportunities for relief when the underlying condition is untreatable. Knowledge of the clinical significance of symptoms is largely empirical, but forms the essential diagnostic base of clinical medicine. Thus research into the mechanisms of breathlessness, for example, will continue to be a proper concern of clinicians as long as disabling and irreversible conditions such as chronic airways obstruction exist. By contrast, knowing the mechanism of dyspnoea in pleural effusion is unimportant compared with knowing how to relieve the symptom by draining the effusion, and being able to diagnose the underlying clinical condition.

Cough

Coughing is a defensive reflex designed to clear and protect the lower respiratory tract. The act of coughing is essentially a forced expiratory effort against a transitorily closed glottis, which then opens allowing a sudden expulsion of air from the lungs. Except when the cough arises from laryngeal irritation, there is an initial deep inspiration which allows the respiratory muscles to act to greater mechanical advantage, although this could draw any offending material deeper into the bronchial tree. The pressure that builds up behind the closed glottis can reach as much as 40 kPa and, if often repeated in a sequence of coughs, can seriously impede venous filling of the heart. The consequent drop in cardiac output is responsible for the well-described 'cough syncope'.

Mechanism

The cough reflex can be initiated by the stimulation of irritant receptors in the pharynx, larynx, trachea, and major bronchi. These receptors respond to mechanical irritation by mucus, dust, or foreign bodies, and to chemical irritation by fumes and toxic gases. Mechanical events within the thorax, such as sudden and large changes in airway calibre or lung collapse, can also stimulate cough receptors. The afferent fibres run in the branches of the superior laryngeal nerve and the vagus to the medulla, where the resultant efferent activity of virtually the whole of the respiratory musculature is co-ordinated. The explosive action of the respiratory muscles produces laryngeal air velocities that can approach the speed of sound and is accompanied by bronchial constriction, mucus secretion, and a transient systemic hypertension.

Causes of cough

An epidemiological analysis of cough would reveal an acute, viral, upper respiratory tract infection affecting the pharynx, larynx, or postnasal space as the most common cause of short-lived cough at all ages, with smoking being the main cause of chronic cough in adults. Half of those smoking 20 or more cigarettes a day can expect to have a persistent cough. Children exposed to passive smoking from their parents are twice as likely to cough as children in non-smoking families. Asthma is the next commonest cause at all ages, with chronic upper or lower respiratory tract infection also important. Tuberculosis heads the list in the developing world. Of the more sinister causes, carcinoma of the lung is the most important. It remains the commonest neoplasm in men and is second only to carcinoma of the breast in women, and must feature high in the differential diagnosis of a new presentation of cough or a change in the character of cough in a middle-aged smoker. Less usual causes are endobronchial sarcoidosis and pulmonary fibrotic conditions. Both beta-blockers and angiotensin-converting enzyme (**ACE**) inhibitors can cause an irritating and persistent cough. Although rare, an inhaled foreign body must not be forgotten.

Clinical features

The clinical description of cough relies on its sound, its timing, and whether or not there is expectoration. A dry cough with an irritative barking quality, short and often repeated, is heard in pharyngitis, tracheobronchitis, and early pneumonia. With laryngitis the sound is harsh and hoarse ('croup'). The long inspiratory sound that gives whooping cough its name is also produced by tracheal and laryngeal inflammation. Abductor paralysis of the vocal cords creates a cough that is prolonged and lowing like the sound of cattle, and hence is described as 'bovine'. The usual cause is pressure on the left recurrent laryngeal nerve by lesions in the thorax: carcinoma of the bronchus or oesophagus, enlarged (usually neoplastic) hilar nodes, or (now very rarely) aortic aneurysm. If similar lesions press on the trachea but spare the nerve, the cough has a hard metallic quality described as 'brassy'. Unilateral abductor palsy of the larynx does not affect the voice, and even with additional abductor palsy the voice often remains good. Complete paralysis of both cords gives aphonia and a weak ineffectual cough. Weakness of the thoracic muscles, as in polyneuritis or the muscular dystrophies, will lessen the expulsive force in coughing, as will the general weakness of prostration, toxaemia, or the deeper states of unconsciousness. Cough may be suppressed when there is severe thoracic or upper abdominal pain.

Certain aspects of the timing of coughing may give useful diagnostic clues. A cough that awakens the patient in the small hours of the night suggests asthma; wheezing need not be evident. Cough with expectoration on rising in the morning is characteristic of chronic bronchitis, although it may also be reported by asthmatics. A bout of coughing with food or when lying down after a meal points to oesophageal, pharyngeal, or neuromuscular disease, causing aspiration into the lungs. Changes of posture can also set off coughing in the bronchiectatic; and free expectoration of sputum at any time of day is common in these patients. A dry cough that persists over many weeks can signify a neoplasm, but a non-productive barking cough that has lasted for years is more likely to be a nervous habit often perpetuated by psychogenic factors.

A cough may fail to produce expectoration because there is nothing to produce, because secretions are swallowed (as is almost universal in children), because there is severe airways obstruction, because of weakness (as outlined above), or because the secretions are too viscid. In the last four instances the sound quality of the cough differs from that of a dry cough, in the sense that secretions can be heard moving in the major airways. This type of cough and the cough productive of sputum can be described as 'moist' or 'loose'.

Phlegm and sputum

Phlegm, the secretions of the lower respiratory tract, is admixed with nasal and pharyngeal secretions as well as saliva to give expectorated sputum. It has been very difficult to study the natural secretions of the healthy tracheobronchial tree in man, for only about 100 ml is produced daily and most of this is swallowed. In disease the quantity of secretions is often sufficient to swamp contamination from the upper respiratory tract, so that valid observations can be made, but it may be necessary to obtain lung secretions by induced coughing or by bronchoscopy.

Mucus is viscoelastic. Its viscosity or stickiness influences the effect of forces applied to it in coughing. Initially it resists flow, but then as increasing force is applied it becomes more and more liquid, returning to its original state when the flow stops. The elasticity of sputum appears to alter with the rate of application of stress to it, and this may be important in relation to the rate of beating of the bronchial epithelial cilia. Intrabronchial mucus exists in two layers: one of low viscosity and high elasticity touching the cilia, and above this a more viscous layer which, in disease, carries globules of mucus.

Airway mucus is 95 per cent water and derives its distinctive physical characteristics from the glycoprotein content. Two components of these glycoproteins, sialic acid and sulphate, enable airway mucus to be chemically analysed and identified *in situ* in histological sections. At least four glycoproteins have been identified in human bronchial mucus, produced in various combinations by different mucous-cell types. Serous fluid is produced from other cells in the bronchial glands, and with water, lipids, and proteins makes up a transudate component. Although bronchial secretions do not show diagnostically distinctive changes in disease, there is, for example, a shift towards greater glycoprotein production in chronic bronchitis and greater transudate formation in asthma. In infection both components increase, and the breakdown of leucocytes and of bronchial mucus increases the DNA content of sputum, making it less viscid. The accumulated debris of cells and micro-organisms imparts a yellow colour to infected sputum, and the subsequent action of verdoperoxidase derived from leucocytes gives a green colour.

The distinction between infected and non-infected is one of the most obvious descriptive features of sputum that is relevant in clinical medicine. Non-infected mucoid sputum is variously described as clear, white, or like jelly. Viscid mucoid sputum is sometimes seen in asthma, and the patient may report seeing pellets or even branching plugs of mucus that are presumed to be casts of small bronchi. In bronchopulmonary aspergillosis, similar pellets or casts have a dark brown colour. In city dwellers, and those in dusty occupations, mucoid sputum can be various shades of grey. Coal miners may produce jet-black sputum (melanoptysis) if an area of fibrosis breaks down and is expectorated.

In most lower respiratory tract infections pus is admixed with mucus to produce mucopurulent sputum. Pure pus can be expectorated from a lung abscess or from stagnant bronchiectatic cavities. An offensive smell to the sputum, particularly in these last two conditions, often comes from infection with anaerobic organisms. A rarely seen but distinctive brown discoloration ('anchovy sauce') is seen with pus from an amoebic lung abscess, usually secondary to hepatic amoebiasis.

Apart from its appearance, the only other macroscopic attribute to sputum is its quantity. Excessively large quantities of sputum are found in bronchiectasis, particularly where this is widespread, as in cystic fibrosis, and in alveolar-cell carcinoma where large quantities of watery mucus can occasionally be produced. The amount of sputum in both chronic bronchitis and asthma is very variable, but can be excessive. Briefly, severe pulmonary oedema leads to the production of a large quantity of frothy sputum.

Haemoptysis

Patients rightly regard the presence of blood in the sputum as sinister. Despite this, a definite cause of haemoptysis is only found in about half of cases in most series. In the assessment of haemoptysis it is important to establish first that the blood-stained material has come from the chest and not from the gastrointestinal tract. Some patients find this difficult. Haemoptysis is produced with a 'cough' not a 'retch'. Accompanying features of an appropriate disease are usually present, but it is worth remembering that in haemoptysis there is usually froth due to admixed air, and the blood is bright red, not dark brown. Gastric contents should be acid; bronchial contents should be alkaline. Another trap for the unwary is contamination with blood from the nose or upper respiratory tract.

It is unwise to attribute haemoptysis simply to 'bronchitis' or infection. In bronchiectasis, however, haemoptysis not uncommonly mixes with mucopurulent sputum. In the early stages of pneumococcal pneumonia a 'rusty' staining of mucoid sputum is quite characteristic. In tuberculosis, frank blood in otherwise mucoid sputum is well recognized. Sudden haemoptysis is a hallmark of pulmonary embolism with infarction. In bronchial neoplasia there may be streaking of the sputum with blood or more substantial bleeding with clots, often observed daily. Recurrent bloodstaining of the sputum is seen in idiopathic pulmonary haemosiderosis and also, although usually over a shorter time span, in Goodpasture's syndrome, which are both uncommon conditions. Cardiac conditions associated with blood in the sputum are pulmonary oedema, with pink frothy sputum, and mitral stenosis. The recurrent haemoptyses of the latter condition are infrequently seen today. In a general context, it may be necessary to consider thoracic trauma, endometriosis, or a blood coagulation disorder as causes of haemoptysis.

In the investigation of haemoptysis the chest radiograph will often indicate a probable diagnosis, for example an apical tuberculous infiltrate or a neoplastic hilar mass, but this must be backed up by appropriate microbiological or cytological examination of the sputum. Old, presumably healed and calcified, tuberculous lesions may be reactivated and may be a sufficient cause for haemoptysis simply due to local bronchiectasis, and invasion by mycetoma must be considered. Bronchiectasis and pulmonary infarction may not be evident on a plain radiograph, but both should give a suggestive history. High-resolution computed tomography (HRCT) will diagnose bronchiectasis, and ventilation–perfusion scanning or spiral CT will diagnose a pulmonary embolism.

If examination of the sputum and radiology (plain or specialized) yields no obvious cause for haemoptysis, then bronchoscopy must be considered. After a single haemoptysis in a young person with a normal chest radiograph, this can be deferred for a month. A recurrence of haemoptysis or a single episode in an older person, particularly a smoker, are indications for early bronchoscopy.

Laboratory examination of sputum

Expectorated sputum should be subjected to microscopic and microbiological investigation as appropriate (see Chapter 17.3.3). Sputum eosinophilia is a good guide to airway allergy. The cytological examination of sputum for malignant cells can only be done by an expert, but in skilled hands it is invaluable and time-saving.

Investigating cough

The cause of a cough of recent onset will usually be obvious enough. Infection tops the list. Carcinoma must be excluded in the smoker and radiology will detect parenchymal disease. In the case of persistent cough without apparent cause in a non-smoker, occult asthma should first be eliminated. Assessment of airflow variability using either diurnal peak flows or a histamine reactivity test are first-line investigations (see Chapter 17.4.1.1). It is worth looking for a chronic sinonasal infection or allergy and then for gastro-oesophageal reflux before proceeding to bronchoscopy, which statistically is not very rewarding in the context of cough as a lone symptom.

Treatment

Once diagnosed, the cause may well be treatable, even if the only appropriate advice is to stop smoking. If the condition is not treatable or if no cause can be found, symptomatic measures need to be considered. Two lines of approach are open: to suppress the cough or, accepting the cough as inevitable, to make expectoration easier.

All cough suppressants in common use act centrally. Most are opiate derivatives. Codeine and pholcodine have a weak antitussive action, but when made into a sweet syrup they seem to have a soothing effect. Methadone and the stronger opiates are more powerful in suppressing cough, but they depress respiration and also cause constipation. In terminal bronchial carcinoma they are invaluable. Attempts to suppress cough by a peripheral action on bronchial afferent receptors have not been successful. Inhaled local anaesthetic can be helpful, and its effect on cough may long outlast its anaesthetic action. Drugs that act on the production of bronchial mucus will lessen cough if its purpose is the expectoration of that mucus. Atropine is used to this end preoperatively, but rarely in disease. Corticosteroids can diminish mucus production in asthma and in alveolar-cell carcinoma.

Agents claimed to increase sputum quantity or accelerate expectoration include the volatile oils such as menthol and inorganic salts such as potassium iodide. The movement of particles up the mucociliary escalator of the bronchial tree has been charted using radioisotope techniques and shown to increase under the influence of ingested guaifenesin (present in several 'cough medicines'), inhaled beta-adrenergic agonists, and hypertonic (1.2 M) saline.

Attempts to decrease the viscosity of sputum using mucolytic agents have been clinically disappointing, despite definite in vitro evidence of activity. Inhaled acetylcysteine works more convincingly as a mucolytic but has the great disadvantage of inducing bronchoconstriction. In cystic fibrosis, DNase has been used with modest success.

Most patients with haemoptysis require no more than treatment appropriate to their underlying condition, but occasionally haemoptysis is massive and life-threatening. The recorded mortality of 50 per cent with haemoptysis of 200 ml or more includes patients with initially poor respiratory reserve, as well as those who asphyxiate. At bronchoscopy it may be difficult to locate the source of bleeding, but local endoscopic measures may be applicable (topical epinephrine (adrenaline) application, balloon tamponade, and cold saline lavage). An open surgical approach (lobectomy or pneumonectomy) carries a mortality of up to one-third, and if operative intervention is contemplated, bronchial arteriography should be considered. The source of bleeding is from the bronchial arteries, so that embolization of the appropriate bronchial artery has successfully been used to control massive haemoptysis in a high proportion of patients who are actively bleeding.

Breathlessness

This major symptom of pulmonary, cardiovascular, and other systemic diseases suffers much because it is so frequently referred to by physicians as dyspnoea. Whilst patients sometimes speak of difficulty in breathing, they more frequently use the terms 'breathlessness', 'short of breath', or 'out of breath'. It is usually only on direct questioning that specific features reveal clues that are likely to be useful clinically. Despite the often quoted statement of Comroe that dyspnoea is not tachypnoea, hyperpnoea, or hyperventilation, but difficult, laboured, or uncomfortable breathing, patients are quite unaware of these fine distinctions. Rapid breathing, the necessary increase in ventilation in response to exercise, and ventilation in excess of metabolic requirements are all at times described by patients as breathlessness. Just what degree or quality of awareness of respiratory movement deserves to be called breathlessness is probably indefinable; awareness undoubtedly varies from patient to patient and even within the same subject from time to time. However, the implication of most terms used by patients to describe this type of pulmonary sensation is that in some way the performance of the respiratory apparatus ('breath-') is not meeting ('-less') a demand placed on it.

Pathophysiology

The respiratory muscles are supplied by motor nerve fibres from cervical and thoracic anterior horn cells, from C3 to T12. Like all other anterior horn cells, the respiratory motor nerve cells are served by pyramidal fibres from the motor cortex in the precentral gyrus. Directives from the cortex enable respiratory movement to be modulated to serve such functions as talking, holding the breath, voluntary hyperventilation, and the performance of lung function tests. This pathway will also be responsible for the conscious, and perhaps unconscious, transmission of anxiety or a calming influence on respiratory performance. However, to an extent that is unparalleled in other mammalian skeletal muscle, the respiratory motor neurones are under dual control, the second component being the motor output from the brainstem respiratory centre responsible for involuntary or automatic respiratory movement. This is the movement necessary to satisfy metabolic requirements for oxygen supply and carbon dioxide removal.

For the purposes of understanding breathlessness, respiratory centre activity can be seen as being under the influence of chemical and neurogenic stimuli. The chemical stimuli of hypoxia and acidaemia are relevant to the breathlessness of high altitude and diabetic coma. The general traffic of neurogenic stimuli impinging on the reticular formation from all sources maintains a certain level of activity in the medullary respiratory neurones irrespective of more specific stimuli. The modest quietening of this activity in sleep is associated with a small drop in minute ventilation, and the dramatic curtailment of spinal ascending information that sometimes occurs following high spinal tractotomy (usually for intractable pain) can completely abolish automatic medullary respiratory activity. There is no clear-cut association between increased reticular formation activity causing hyperventilation and states of breathlessness, but the increase in ventilation at the very onset of exercise is thought to be neurogenic in origin, possibly originating from the exercising muscles.

The respiratory centre receives information from the lungs through the vagus nerve. This originates in bronchial epithelial irritant receptors, stretch receptors, and interstitial J receptors within the alveolar/capillary interface. Stimulation of all these receptors will produce reflex effects, amongst which (for example) tachypnoea will make up a component of breathlessness in an appropriate setting. Whether the afferent information travelling up the vagus itself reaches the sensorium, or whether it merely modulates some other afferent pathway, is not clear. Afferent information that undoubtedly reaches consciousness is that concerning the rate and degree of thoracic cage movement and, quite accurately, a sense of lung volume (degree of lung inflation/deflation). This information comes from joint, tendon, and muscle receptors in the chest wall, and for sense of movement (of air) perhaps also from the oropharyngeal mucosa. It seems evident that information from these latter sources is part of natural and healthy sensation; it also seems likely that the same channels will signal an increased rate or depth of movement which, if excessive, will be described as breathlessness. In exercise the description 'breathless' often comes at the point where the smooth linear relation between ventilation and oxygen consumption is disturbed. Ventilation becomes excessive for metabolic requirements. How this becomes described as a shortness or loss of breath is not clear.

Two 'unnatural' respiratory sensations that can only be inadequately mimicked in a healthy individual are those associated with abnormal lung mechanics (for example in airways narrowing) and muscle paralysis. An obvious parallel for the first is breathing through an external resistance, and this technique has been widely used by those investigating dyspnoea. The useful finding that may have some bearing on the clinical situation is that in resistance breathing the ability to detect an increased load depends not on the absolute magnitude of the load, but on the ratio of that load to pre-existing loading of the system. Thus, a given absolute increase in airways resistance will be much more obvious to an individual with near-normal airways function than to one already suffering from pathological airways narrowing. The sensations of those few normal individuals who have undergone muscle paralysis for experimental purposes include phrases such as 'choking' and 'I would give anything to be able to take one deep breath'. These are similar to the reported symptoms of patients with paralytic diseases affecting the respiratory muscles. The element of inadequate performance is stressed. Whether this sensation can be simulated by the voluntary withholding of respiratory movement, as in breath-holding, is very doubtful. This much studied experimental model undoubtedly gives sensations, most of which probably arise from the diaphragm twitching ineffectually, and it is difficult to see where this fits into a clinical setting.

If any common thread can be drawn between these examples, it is at the level of an interaction between the drive to breathing and achievement—a drive that fails to achieve because of poor performance or mechanical loading of the respiratory system. The neurophysiological implications of this hypothesis are that there should be monitoring systems for both drive and performance. It is obviously feasible for the brain to assess and summate the various drives to breathing, and so monitor motor output. The muscle spindle has been proposed as the probable detector of achievement, but several objections exist to this proposal, not least that there are relatively few muscle spindles in the diaphragm, which is the most important muscle of respiration.

When it comes to the application of these principles to disease, some parallels are obvious, but an example from one common condition—acute bronchial asthma—will illustrate that the situation is not straightforward, and frequently multifactorial. In acute asthma there may be excessive drive from bronchial irritant receptors, and often cortical drive expressing itself in anxiety, even panic, as well as hyperventilation. There is clearly poor performance because of the increased resistance of narrowed airways, but in addition it seems likely that the respiratory muscles will act at a mechanical disadvantage because of lung hyperinflation.

The clinical analysis of breathlessness

Whilst bearing these neurophysiological points in mind, when it comes to devising symptomatic measures for the relief of breathlessness the clinician must still largely rely on an empirical approach to the analysis of this symptom. Such an analysis will rely on four characteristics of breathlessness: its quality, its timing, its severity, and the circumstances that precipitate or relieve it.

Quality

Breathlessness is difficult to describe. Most patients can go no further than saying that they are 'short of breath'. The asthmatic will generally recognize the quality of wheeze and, contrary to the opinion of physiologists, usually finds it more difficult to breathe in than out. An asthmatic who develops more persistent breathlessness between attacks often recognizes this as 'different from my asthma'. A sense of suffocation is a feature of massive pleural effusions and of pulmonary oedema. Phrases such as 'I can't fill my lungs properly' and 'I need to take a big breath' suggest the possibility of psychogenic breathlessness, but muscle weakness must be carefully excluded.

Timing

Of the greatest value in separating out conditions likely to be associated with breathlessness is noting its rate of onset. There are five categories. Breathlessness may be of dramatic onset (over minutes), acute onset (over hours), subacute onset (over weeks), or chronic onset (over months or years), or it may be intermittent. Table 1 gives a guide to conditions falling into these categories. The subdivisions are not rigid. Asthma again provides an example. About half of all acute attacks of asthma build up in less than 24 h, but some asthmatics slowly deteriorate over a week or so and, occasionally, they can be transformed from being asymptomatic to having desperate breathlessness and unconsciousness within 15 min; in addition, asthma is also intermittent. Likewise, left ventricular failure, although usually developing over hours, may be dramatic in, for example, aortic valve rupture, or more persistent in long-standing hypertension. Pulmonary embolism can also present in a very variable manner, ranging from the dramatically sudden to the chronic.

The pattern of breathlessness in certain disorders depends on the stage of the disease and the structural or functional changes that it causes. Thus in early sarcoidosis, diffuse infiltration of the lungs can cause the quite rapid development of breathlessness over a week or so; by contrast, the late fibrotic stage of sarcoid will be associated with relentlessly progressive breathlessness as pulmonary reserve diminishes. Breathlessness in a condition such as carcinoma of the lung will be determined by the pattern of structural change—whether there is, for example, bronchial stenosis, collapse, or pleural effusion.

Severity

The severity of breathlessness is traditionally gauged on scales relating to activity. Many scales have been devised. All have two faults. The first is that there is a temptation to assume that the grading system with which one is

Table 1 Conditions causing breathlessness classified by rate of onset

1.	**Dramatically sudden: over minutes**
	upper airway obstruction
	pneumothorax
	pulmonary embolism
2.	**Acute: over hours**
	pneumonia
	asthma
	left ventricular failure/pulmonary oedema
	acute pulmonary infiltrations, e.g. allergic alveolitis
3.	**Subacute: over days**
	pleural effusion
	bronchogenic carcinoma
	subacute pulmonary infiltrations, e.g. sarcoidosis
4.	**Chronic: over months or years**
	chronic airflow obstruction
	diffuse fibrosing conditions
	chronic non-pulmonary causes, e.g. anaemia, hyperthyroidism
5.	**Intermittent: episodic breathlessness**
	asthma
	left ventricular failure/pulmonary oedema

Note: The subdivisions are not rigid, e.g. pulmonary embolism can cause dramatically sudden, acute, subacute, or chronic breathlessness.

Table 2 The Borg Visual Analogue

Scale for exertional breathlessness

0	not at all
0.5	very, very slightly
1	very slightly
2	slightly
3	moderately
4	quite severely
5	severely
6	
7	very severely
8	
9	very, very severely
10	maximally

familiar is universally known. It is not. Thus it is preferable to describe the amount of exercise limitation on an individual patient basis. Second, no scale suggests a convention for dealing with variable breathlessness. Very few patients have a consistent level of severity of breathlessness, but any attempt to introduce a range of severity will have to be accompanied by some assessment of the time extent of each grade, which is an almost impossible task.

A refinement of the scaling technique can be used to record the degree of breathlessness during exercise. During a standard exercise test a record is made of breathlessness on a visual analogue scale concurrently with minute ventilation. The sort of data produced can be used to assess the benefits of therapeutic intervention. The Borg scale (Table 2) can be similarly adapted and has been used with simple exercise tests. Tests such as the distance walked in a specified time (for example, a 6- or 12-min walk), are influenced by training and motivation. Patients may differ in their approach to a treatment benefit. One might walk no further and be relieved to achieve the same distance with less breathlessness, whereas another might extend the walking distance by being prepared to become just as breathless as before.

Occurrence

The circumstances under which breathlessness is experienced can give important diagnostic clues. Only psychogenic breathlessness bears no relation to exertion or is experienced only at rest. Many patients with organic diseases are breathless at rest as well as on exertion, this being an expression of severity. Breathlessness made worse by lying flat (orthopnoea) is characteristic of left ventricular failure and is also experienced by patients with diaphragmatic paralysis. Nocturnal awakening with suffocating breathlessness and frothy sputum production (paroxysmal nocturnal dyspnoea) is a more serious manifestation of left ventricular failure and can be relieved by sitting or standing up. The asthmatic also awakens in the small hours of the night with breathlessness accompanied by coughing and wheezing, or these symptoms may be delayed until the normal waking hours. Any sputum produced by the asthmatic under these circumstances is likely to be sticky and mucoid. Postexertional breathlessness and the immediate triggering of an episode of wheezing breathlessness by non-specific irritants (dust and fumes) or specific allergic stimuli (pollen, animal danders, etc.) also characterize the asthmatic. In occupational asthmas, breathlessness will bear a temporal and circumstantial relation to the working environment. In byssinosis the first day at work is characteristically troublesome (Monday morning tightness). Patients with type III hypersensitivity reactions such as bronchopulmonary aspergillosis or extrinsic allergic alveolitis (Chapter 17.11.11) will notice breathlessness 4 to 6 h after exposure. An intercurrent respiratory tract infection will worsen breathlessness in patients with any form of diffuse airway or parenchymatous lung disease.

Spontaneous improvement occurs in most breathless patients with rest or the removal of trigger factors. The postexertional breathlessness of the asthmatic is an important, though temporary, exception. Patients with pulmonary hypertension, even with severe exertional breathlessness, improve dramatically quickly as soon as they sit down.

The investigation of the breathless patient

The clinical history may immediately suggest a probable cause. Beyond this the two most helpful pointers are simple lung function tests and chest radiology. Spirometric testing will define three groups: normal, an obstructive pattern, and a restrictive pattern (see Chapter 17.3.2). The chest radiograph will be of most value in furthering the diagnosis in conditions giving a restrictive pattern. The further investigation of the patient with airflow obstruction is dealt with in Section 17.4.

Breathlessness in a patient with normal spirometric testing and a clear chest radiograph presents special problems. In this situation four categories should be considered. Is there intermittent disease? Are the tests being used too crude to pick up significant abnormalities? Is there extrathoracic disease? Is this psychogenic breathlessness?

Many asthmatics reviewed in a clinic will have normal lung function. The value of serial recordings of lung function over several days in these patients cannot be overemphasized. Conditions affecting the heart and pulmonary circulation can also be intermittent, but more often the problem is that conventional tests of lung function do not seem to demonstrate significant abnormalities when there is quite considerable dyspnoea. Pulmonary embolism is a good example of this: imaging to assess the integrity of the pulmonary vascular bed is required. Tests of muscle power will pick up neuromuscular conditions weakening respiratory movement. The hyperventilation of acidosis, as in uraemia or diabetic coma, is not often described by patients as breathlessness and is otherwise easily diagnosed. However, hyperthyroidism and anaemia should not be forgotten as causes of breathlessness. Some 60 per cent of patients with a haemoglobin level of less than 8 g/dl will have this symptom.

Psychogenic breathlessness is diagnosed by exclusion, although there may be clues in the history and examination. The quality of the breathlessness has been described above. The sighing and irregular breathing will be readily noticeable to a keen observer. Associated complaints directly related to the hyperventilation are paraesthesiae in the hands and perhaps feet, dizziness, and collapse. Apparently non-specific features such as fatigue, insomnia, weakness, or chest pains may all be part of the syndrome. Depression and anxiety may both be aspects of the underlying psychiatric state. By definition, in pure psychogenic breathlessness, the chest radiograph and lung function are normal. However, some patients may develop breathlessness because they have been told they have a 'shadow on the lung' or through anxiety exhibit a degree of breathlessness disproportionate to a mild functional abnormality. The latter patients tend to have an obsessional personality or may be looking for compensation for supposed 'lung damage' due to injury or occupation.

Treatment

The relief of breathlessness is best achieved by treating the underlying condition. This may mean the removal of 'mass' lesions (pneumothorax, pleural effusion), or the treatment of pneumonia, airflow obstruction, or alveolitis. Loss of muscle power is occasionally treatable, as in myasthenia gravis, or may recover spontaneously. An attempt to relieve breathlessness should not be neglected, even when the underlying condition is untreatable (pleural effusion in carcinoma of the bronchus, or a reversible steroid-responsive component in a patient with chronic airflow obstruction).

The symptomatic treatment of breathlessness is far from satisfactory, but can usefully be considered in terms of the physiological disorder(s) that can be responsible for the symptom. Excessive respiratory drive may be dampened, for example by oxygen for the hypoxic. A direct approach to the vagal afferent system has met with little success: local anaesthetic to the airways gives a short-lived effect but may itself be irritant. In a select few with intense breathlessness due to diffuse infiltrative disease, vagotomy in the thorax has given some relief. Psychogenic breathlessness may be helped with β-blockers (but asthma must be excluded with absolute certainty). Dihydrocodeine reduces breathlessness in chronic obstructive lung disease but is very constipating and, like the more powerful opiate sedatives, can dangerously depress respiration. There has been a sad failure to find opiate derivatives with more selective action on breathlessness. Diazepam and promethazine have given subjective relief to some patients disabled by breathlessness from severe emphysema. The use of rehabilitation measures is considered elsewhere (Chapter 17.7).

Chest pain

The greater part of the lower respiratory tract is insensitive to pain and most parenchymal lung disorders proceed to an advanced state without becoming painful. However, the parietal pleura is exquisitely sensitive to painful stimuli and unpleasant sensations can arise from the tracheobronchial tree.

Pleurisy

Typical pleural pain has a sharp, stabbing, and knife-like character; is aggravated by respiration and coughing; and leads to rapid, shallow breathing and a suppressed cough. The pain is likely to be due to stretching of the inflamed parietal pleura and can be relieved by splinting the chest wall.

Afferent pain fibres from the parietal pleura pass through the intercostal nerves. Those from the central portion of the diaphragm run in the phrenic nerve to the cervical cord (C3/4). Central diaphragmatic pleurisy is thus referred to the lateral side of the neck and shoulder tip; indeed, local anaesthesia to the shoulder trigger area can relieve diaphragmatic pleurisy. The outer portions of the diaphragm are served by intercostal nerves (T7–12), causing referred pain to be felt in the lower thorax, lumbar region, and upper abdomen.

Most conditions giving rise to pleuritic pain are acute and inflammatory, either infective (usually pneumonia) or infarctive, as in pulmonary embolism. The immunologically based pleurisies (as in systemic lupus erythematosus or rheumatoid disease) give pain less frequently. Recurrent pleurisy at the same site should suggest bronchiectasis; at different sites it suggests embolism or bronchopulmonary aspergillosis. Sudden chest pain occurs at the onset of a pneumothorax. It is pleural in origin, due to the inrush of air from the lungs and, sometimes, the tearing of adhesions.

If pleurisy progresses to pleural effusion, the sharp pain largely disappears and is replaced by a dull and more constant ache or heaviness. Pleural fibrotic disease is rarely painful, but pleural neoplasia frequently is. The severity and quality of pain depends on the extent of the tumour, and particularly on spread into the chest wall. A superior sulcus tumour of bronchial origin (Pancoast's tumour) infiltrating the brachial plexus gives very severe and persistent pain in the shoulder and in the distribution of C8, T1, and T2.

Pain from the chest wall

Chest-wall pain can mimic pleurisy, and conditions in the chest wall provide its most important differentials. Pain due to strain or tearing of thoracic muscles can be quite sharp, and since it is likely to be caused or exacerbated by coughing and lead to shallow respiration, it can easily be confused with pleurisy. However, there is always local tenderness over the affected muscle and none of the ancillary investigations for pleurisy prove positive. Patients with persistent cough or distressing breathlessness, particularly due to asthma, may complain of muscular pain around the lower rib cage.

Epidemic myalgia or Bornholm's disease is a bothersome manifestation of Coxsackie B infection giving fever and recurrent muscle pain. If the intercostal muscles are involved (pleurodynia), the associated breathlessness and tachypnoea can exactly mimic pleurisy, as can the pre-eruptive stage of thoracic herpes zoster, which gives a stabbing pain in the distribution of the affected nerve. Costal cartilage pain is generally not inflammatory. In Tietze's disease there is a painful protuberance of one or more costal cartilages, usually the second to fourth, probably due to asymmetrical growth of the rib cage. Osteoarthritis and dislocation of the costo-

sternal joints can give chronic pain. Rib fractures rarely present diagnostic problems, but cough fracture in osteoporotic bone should not be forgotten. Thrombophlebitis of chest-wall vessels after surgery or trauma gives anterior chest pain and a tender palpable vascular cord. Most primary chest-wall tumours are not painful, but the more common metastatic disease of bone frequently is, and may be symptomatic before radiological change is evident.

Fleeting transient chest pains are often part of chronic somatized anxiety states, and when this is the case tend to be accompanied by tachycardia, palpitations, and features indicating hyperventilation. Perhaps the commonest chest pain of all is left inframammary pain. This is a transitory sharp but quite severe pain, felt over the apex of the heart at rest or on mild activity. It lasts up to a few minutes and may cause a catching of the breath or shallow breathing. Its cause is unknown but it seems to be totally benign.

Central chest pain

Sensations arising from the tracheobronchial tree are less easy to characterize as painful, although some are exceedingly unpleasant. Instrumentation of the trachea causes pain referred to the anterior chest wall. This is usually abolished by vagotomy and is most likely to be perceived from irritant receptor discharge. Tracheal inflammation, as in infective tracheobronchitis or following the inhalation of toxic vapours, causes a raw painful retrosternal sensation. It is difficult to say how much or how often sensations arising from the main airways are describable as pain. There is often a component described as tightness, and this is a common complaint of patients with generalized airflow obstruction, although it is probably naïve to think that the sensation is a direct appreciation of airways narrowing. Further complicating the interpretation of sensation in these conditions is the almost universal association with coughing which, if persistent, can itself lead to soreness in the upper airways and trachea.

Finally, the mediastinal structures of the thorax are responsible for a multitude of pains, the majority of which are dealt with elsewhere in the chapters on cardiology and gastrointestinal disease. Few central pulmonary lesions give mediastinal pain. Only neoplasia is a common culprit. A central bronchial carcinoma or hilar nodes associated with it can be responsible for a deep dull aching pain in the centre of the chest. Similar pain can sometimes occur in the early stages of sarcoidosis with hilar lymphadenopathy and in lymphoma.

Other symptoms in pulmonary diseases

Patients or their relatives on their behalf may complain of noisy breathing, generally using the word 'wheeze'. A harsh inspiratory wheezing sound arising from obstruction in the larynx or major airways is termed stridor. There may be accompanying hoarseness or features of intrathoracic disease. Wheeze is the externally audible counterpart of the sounds heard with the stethoscope in asthma and obstructive bronchitis. It is a term frequently used by asthmatic patients to describe their respiratory symptoms.

When airflow obstruction is suspected, specific enquiries should be made for the features of bronchial irritability. In response to changes in atmospheric conditions (particularly temperature) or to the inhalation of dusts, fumes, or vapours, the patient with irritable bronchi will respond with a variety of symptoms: cough, tightness in the chest, wheeze, or breathlessness.

Rarely, patients may complain that they are blue (cyanosed), although their carers may do so more often. This and finger clubbing are more often elicited as physical signs (see below).

General history

A full history is essential, emphasizing the following features:

(1) cardiac disease as a cause or aggravating factor in breathlessness;

(2) the legs for ankle oedema as a result of lung disease or deep venous thrombosis;

(3) the upper respiratory tract for infectious, allergic, or vasculitic disorders;

(4) the skin for eczema, urticaria, erythema nodosum, or vasculitis;

(5) features of rheumatoid or collagen-vascular disease;

(6) the nervous system for disease that might impair ventilatory control; and

(7) pointers to metastatic spread or the non-metastatic manifestations of malignant disease.

The past history may reveal atopy, tuberculosis, or other serious infectious disease, particularly in childhood. It is always worth asking about previous chest radiographs which may be obtainable for comparison.

A full smoking history is essential. A detailed drug history is essential because of potential toxic effects on the lungs (see Chapter 17.11.19).

A complete occupational and environmental history is of the utmost importance. Whilst the mining industries will be obvious, many other occupations that create dusts of both inorganic and organic materials are now recognized as presenting hazards to the chest (see Chapter 17.11.7). Certain working environments may lead to exposure to organisms likely to cause pulmonary infection: *Chlamydia psittaci* from contact with domestic or wild birds, *Coxiella burnetti* in slaughterhouses, and tuberculosis through working with susceptible groups.

Finally, certain disorders have a familial predisposition. These include asthma and other atopic diseases (see Chapter 17.4.1), cystic fibrosis (see Chapter 17.10), Kartagener's syndrome, familial fibrocystic pulmonary dysplasia (a form of fibrosing alveolitis) (see Chapter 17.11.2), pulmonary lymphangiomyomatosis (see Chapter 17.11.10), and alveolar microlithiasis (see Chapter 17.11.16). A family or personal contact history of tuberculosis should be noted, as should any record of previous tuberculin testing or bacille Calmette–Guérin (**BCG**) vaccination.

Physical signs in pulmonary disease

Inspection of the chest

The pattern of breathing and the configuration of the chest must be observed. The normal respiratory rate when the subject believes him or herself to be unobserved is around 10 to 14 per min. Higher rates than this are commonly recorded in the healthy, but a rate above 20 per min is abnormal. Pneumonia, many interstitial lung disorders, and abnormal drives to breathing, including anxiety, will increase the rate. If the chest is free to move, the tidal volume will also increase, but this is not the case with restrictive disease or painful conditions of the thoracic cage or upper abdomen. An abrupt stop to inspiration when there is pain can be seen. The frequency of deep sighs, normally 8 to 10 per hour in quiet breathing, is greatly increased in psychogenic breathlessness, when there may be an irregular pattern including phases of rapid breathing and relative apnoea. A regular alternation of apnoeic periods of 5 to 30 s with a period of increasing and then decreasing ventilation characterizes Cheyne–Stokes respiration. This and several other irregular breathing patterns are usually associated with brainstem or cerebral lesions, but they can also be a feature of severe heart failure.

In observing respiratory movement, particular attention must be paid to expansion. Poor movement of the chest on one side only always indicates pathology on that side. Generally poor expansion is seen in the hyperinflated chest of the patient with severe airflow obstruction and in the fixed thoracic cage of advanced ankylosing spondylitis. In airflow obstruction two other features may be observed: an indrawing of intercostal spaces during inspiration (reflecting the negative intrapleural pressure necessary to draw air into the lungs) and abnormal movement of the lower chest. Normally, the lower chest moves outwards during inspiration, but in gross hyperinflation the diaphragm is flat and its contraction merely causes the lower thoracic cage to move inwards. In the same patients the anterior abdominal wall may also move inwards during inspiration instead of outwards, and this asynchrony of movement carries a poor prognosis.

Abnormalities of the shape of the chest are well recognized. An increased anteroposterior diameter to give a 'barrel chest' is as often a sign of the kyphosis that accompanies senile osteoporosis as it is of the hyperinflation of emphysema and chronic airflow obstruction. Pectus carinatum (pigeon chest), an outward protuberance of the sternum, may reflect severe attacks of asthma in childhood when it may be accompanied by bilateral indrawing of the anterior portions of the lower ribs (Harrison's sulci); it is now rarely due to rickets. The opposite, pectus excavatum (depressed sternum), is a congenital anomaly. Scoliosis is important because of the severe impairment of respiratory movement that it causes, and it can lead to respiratory failure (see Chapter 17.13). Localized collapse and fibrosis may draw in the adjacent rib cage (which will also move poorly) and, if severe, unilateral fibrosis of the whole lung can cause a scoliosis with its curvature towards the affected lung.

Palpation of the chest

Palpation is used to confirm the observed patterns of chest expansion and to identify the position of the trachea and apex beat. The trachea should be localized in the suprasternal notch with the index finger. With the patient looking directly forwards, any deviation of the trachea from the mid-line should be assessed using a combination of touch and vision. Aside from tension pneumothorax, deviation of the trachea to one side is due to either apical fibrosis pulling it to the affected side or a mass in the neck (for example, goitre) or upper mediastinum pushing it to the opposite side. As with the trachea, the position of the apex beat can reflect pressure against or traction on mediastinal structures, but due consideration must be given to displacement of the apex beat due to intrinsic cardiac disease.

The detection of the transmission of vocal sounds by the placing the palm of the hand on the chest (vocal fremitus) should be abandoned in favour of vocal resonance (listening with the stethoscope for voice sounds), except for a simultaneous comparison of the two sides of the chest.

Percussion of the chest

In properly performed percussion, the examiner listens for the pitch and loudness of the percussive note, and both listens and feels for the postpercussive vibrations that give the note its resonance. The sides of the chest must be compared from identical sites. A dull note lacks resonance and is higher in pitch and softer than a normal percussion note; it signifies the presence of solid tissue or fluid underneath the percussed area. 'Stony' dullness with a complete lack of any vibrations coming back from the lung is heard and felt over pleural effusions. It is important to delineate the surface markings of any dullness: pneumonic consolidation and collapse will follow the distribution of the affected lobe, whereas the upper limit of a pleural effusion will be determined by the effects of gravity. It requires a fine ear to pick up Ellis's S-shaped line—a slightly higher level of dullness in the axilla when the patient is in the sitting position. Large effusions which displace mediastinal contents may produce an area of dullness at the opposite base close to the mid-line (Grocco's sign).

A hyper-resonant note is lower in pitch and louder than normal, and occurs over hyperinflated lung as in emphysema or an air-filled space, that is to say a large bulla or a pneumothorax. It is more difficult to be certain about hyper-resonance than dullness, particularly in thin subjects.

Auscultation of the chest

There are three types of sound that can be heard coming from the lung: breath sounds, adventitious sounds, and voice sounds.

Breath sounds

Normal breath sounds are better termed 'normal' rather than 'vesicular'. They are certainly not generated in the vesicles or alveoli of the lung where air flow is too low, but probably reflect turbulent flow in major bronchi. The pattern and intensity of breath sounds reflects regional ventilation. Thus, in the normal upright lung, breath sounds are loudest at the apex in early inspiration and at the bases in mid-inspiration. Breath sounds are quietened over areas of atelectasis. During expiration normal breath sounds rapidly fade out, probably due to the decreasing air-flow rate.

Bronchial breathing is heard over airless lung as in consolidation, atelectasis, or dense fibrosis. There is some resemblance to the sounds heard over the normal trachea, but, by comparison with normal breath sounds, bronchial breathing is higher in pitch and more blowing in quality. It does not have to be loud. Bronchial breath sounds are classically heard throughout both inspiration and expiration. Very quiet breath sounds are heard over hyperinflated lungs as in emphysema or when breath sounds are prevented from reaching the chest wall by a layer of air, fluid, or fibrosis.

Adventitious sounds

The terminology of adventitious sounds is confused. This arises because, whereas Laennec originally used the term rales (rattle) to embrace all added sounds, Latham, introducing the classification dry and moist sounds in 1876, applied rale exclusively to the former and rhonchi to the latter. Until recently the established convention in the United Kingdom was to drop rale altogether and to call interrupted non-musical sounds crepitations and continuous musical sounds rhonchi. The move to replace the term crepitations with crackles and the term rhonchi with wheezes has now gained widespread acceptance. Crackles may be coarse or moist when they are due to the movement of sputum in large airways, or fine when they are probably created by small airways snapping open as pressure equalizes in the distal lung compartment. Coarse early inspiratory and expiratory crackles are often heard in respiratory tract infection, particularly in patients with chronic obstructive lung disease, whilst fine late inspiratory crackles are characteristic of pulmonary oedema and fibrosing alveolitis. Occasionally a single mid to late inspiratory 'squawk' is heard in patients with a variety of pulmonary fibroses.

Wheezes signify obstruction in airways. A sound of single pitch (monophonic) in inspiration and/or expiration, which cannot be altered by coughing to shift mucus, signifies a localized obstruction in a major airway. Several sounds of varying pitch (polyphonic) heard randomly in inspiration and expiration are typical of the widespread airways obstruction of asthma and chronic obstructive bronchitis. A polyphonic wheeze on forced expiration signifies diffuse airflow obstruction and can be a useful sign when tidal breathing is free of added sounds.

A pleural rub is the diagnostic added sound of pleurisy. It is a superficial grating or rasping sound synchronous with late inspiration and early expiration, best heard at the bases and rarely at the apices. A soft friction rub may be mistaken for crepitations, but is not altered by coughing and can be made louder by pressure with the stethoscope. Inflammation of the pleura close to the heart can give a friction rub that synchronizes with the heart beat but will cease if the breath is held.

Voice sounds

A long sound such as 'ninety-nine' is favoured for detecting voice sounds that are transmitted by normal lung, but not by air space or fluid, and pass through solid lung with undue clarity, even allowing whispered sounds to be heard (whispering pectoriloquy). Certain physical characteristics of a solid lung allow low frequency sounds to be filtered out, leaving a sound of bleating or nasal quality (aegophony); this is particularly noticeable over a collapsed lung adjacent to a pleural effusion.

The relevance of the general examination in respiratory disease

Clues to the diagnosis of respiratory disease and critical extrathoracic manifestations of primary lung conditions must be sought in the general examination.

Overall appearance

Obesity places an added burden on the respiratory system, sometimes sufficient in itself to cause a degree of exertional breathlessness and potentially a cause of obstructive sleep apnoea (see Chapter 17.8.2). Truncal obesity with moon facies and skin bruising is an unfortunate complication of oral corticosteroid therapy which may have to be given for several pulmonary diseases.

Weight loss is a feature of emphysematous obstructive lung disease and, of course, malignancy, with the late stages of bronchial carcinoma and pleural mesothelioma often being characterized by a distressing cachexia. Malabsorption can result in weight loss in cystic fibrosis if inadequately managed.

Body habitus can alert to possible respiratory complications, particularly the more severe degrees of kyphoscoliosis, which can lead to hypoventilation, and also rarer disorders such as Marfan's syndrome (associated with pneumothorax) or ankylosing spondylitis.

Cyanosis

Cyanosis is the blue discoloration imparted to the nailbeds, lips, and tongue by hypoxaemic blood. Peripheral cyanosis due to a sluggish peripheral circulation, as in cold weather, will leave the tongue still pink, whereas in central cyanosis the tongue will be blue and the peripheries blue yet often warm. The frequently repeated statement that 5 g of reduced haemoglobin is required before cyanosis can be detected is false. Most patients with a saturation of 90 per cent or less will appear cyanosed. This represents just 1.5 g of reduced haemoglobin if the total haemoglobin is 15 g. Cyanosis is less marked in severe anaemia and more obvious in polycythaemia. The curious phenomenon of orthocyanosis (hypoxia occurring only in the upright position) is generally associated with pulmonary arteriovenous malformations.

Clubbing of the fingers

Loss of the natural angle between the nail and the nailbed in a properly manicured finger, and a boggy fluctuation of the nailbed are cardinal signs of clubbing (Fig. 1). An increased curvature of the nail and enlargement of the end of the finger develop later. The toes may also be affected. The differential diagnosis of clubbing of the fingers includes many extrathoracic conditions but, as far as the lungs are concerned, three categories deserve consideration: (1) suppurative disease, particularly bronchiectasis of longstanding but also acute lung abscess and empyema, but not uncomplicated bronchitis; (2) fibrosing alveolitis and asbestosis, but rarely other diffuse fibrotic diseases; (3) malignant disease, particularly carcinoma of the bronchus and also pleural malignancy. If finger clubbing is associated with hypertrophic pulmonary osteoarthropathy, a painful osteitis of the distal ends of the long bones of the lower arms and legs, malignancy is associated in 95 per cent of cases.

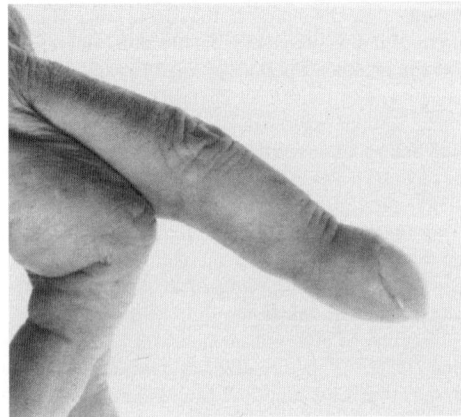

Fig. 1 Clubbing of the fingers.

There is no satisfactory explanation for clubbing and hypertrophic pulmonary osteoarthropathy. Pathologically, there is abnormal vascularity and new bone formation in the peripheries, and evidence of abnormal bronchopulmonary anastomoses in the lungs. The latter may be under vagal control since vagotomy has sometimes abolished clubbing in lung cancer patients. These intrathoracic channels may allow substances normally detoxified by the lungs, which could be responsible for the peripheral changes, to enter the systemic circulation.

The skin and eyes

Eczema and urticaria point to an atopic diathesis and hence possible asthma. Erythema multiforme can accompany mycoplasma pneumonia, rarely other pneumonias, and pulmonary blastomycosis. Erythema nodosum, tender nodules fading to a bruised purple on the shins and occasionally the forearms, is a classical presentation of sarcoidosis, frequently associated with hilar lymphadenopathy and less often with pulmonary infiltrates. It may also be found in primary tuberculosis and rarely in other chest infections.

Several other dermatological, ocular, arthritic, and internal manifestations may also alert to the diagnosis of sarcoid. Skin and eyes are also the site of lesions in Wegener's granulomatosis, systemic lupus erythematosus, systemic sclerosis, and dermatomyositis, each of which has potential pulmonary manifestations.

Patients with diffuse neurofibromatosis and tuberous sclerosis can both develop a severe pulmonary fibrosis with late-stage destructive emphysema. Rarely, hereditary haemorrhagic telangiectasia, with its characteristic lesions on the lips, face, and mouth, can extend to the lungs with pulmonary haemangiomas which give haemoptysis as well as the more commonly found gastrointestinal lesions. The latter give anaemia, and this, whatever its cause, can cause breathlessness and so must be checked for, as must jaundice by looking at the eyes.

The skin is the site of secondary deposits from carcinoma of the lung in a small percentage of cases, although usually late in the disease when the diagnosis is all too obvious. Other carcinomas may spread to skin and lungs, and Kaposi's sarcoma is a cutaneous manifestation of disseminated HIV infection (see Chapter 7.10.21).

Head and neck

Signs of upper respiratory tract disease are relevant in pointing to a site and source of infection that could track down to the lungs, and for the ways in which they signify allergy. Furthermore, neurological disease of the pharynx or structural abnormalities of the larynx encourage aspiration and repeated respiratory tract infection. A short thick neck, retrognathia, and a large uvula can all predispose to sleep apnoea. A goitre may be large enough to compress the trachea and cause stridor. It could be associated with hyperthyroidism and so breathlessness; or hypothyroidism and hence hypoventilation; or even be a source of a carcinoma that could metastasize to the lungs. Even more important are signs in the neck that represent primary intrathoracic malignancy. Hard enlarged cervical lymph nodes are a well-recognized metastatic site for carcinoma of the lung, but can signify lymphoma or primary cancer from elsewhere (stomach, breast). The local extension of central bronchogenic carcinoma gives superior vena caval thrombosis. There is fixed elevation of jugular venous pressure, a large neck, a congested face and head, and, in severe cases, exophthalmos and impaired vision.

Cardiovascular system

The pulse is of poor volume in pulmonary hypertension, bounding and full in hypercapnic respiratory failure, and waxes and wanes in acute severe airflow obstruction (pulsus paradoxus). In the last of these the pulse can actually disappear at the height of the negative intrapleural pressure swing (mid to late inspiration).

The pulmonary hypertension that accompanies severe hypoxic cor pulmonale is manifested on physical examination by a raised jugular venous pressure with a prominent A wave, peripheral pitting oedema, and cardiac signs of right ventricular heave, a loud P2 wave, and, in failure, a gallop rhythm. Oedema alone should add differential diagnoses such as liver or renal disease, both of which can have pulmonary manifestations.

17.3 Clinical investigation of respiratory disease

17.3.1 Thoracic imaging

Susan Copley and David M. Hansell

Despite recent technological advances, chest radiography remains the cornerstone of thoracic imaging. The chest radiograph is justifiably regarded as an integral part of the examination of the patient in respiratory medicine. Because of the wealth of information available from chest radiography, careful interpretation of the chest radiograph remains a necessary clinical skill. Advances in cross-sectional imaging have had a great impact in improving the diagnosis of thoracic pathology, not only for the assessment of mediastinal disease but also in the evaluation of patients with suspected diffuse lung disease. Nevertheless, a chest radiograph should always be obtained and looked at carefully before submitting a patient to more sophisticated imaging techniques. The expense and radiation burden, in the case of computed tomography, is an important consideration.

Techniques in thoracic imaging

Chest radiography

The first chest radiograph was taken over 100 years ago and chest radiography is now the most frequently requested radiological investigation worldwide. The technique has changed surprisingly little over the years, although digital technology has recently been used to overcome some of the shortcomings of conventional film-based radiography.

Technical considerations

An ideal chest radiograph is taken with the patient standing erect, suspending respiration at total lung capacity, and with the X-ray beam traversing the thorax from back to front (the posteroanterior (**PA**) or frontal view). Because of the wide range of densities within the chest (soft tissues of the mediastinum through to aerated lung), perfect exposure of every part of the chest radiograph is impossible. The resulting suboptimal exposure of the denser part of the chest can be partially overcome with a high-kilovoltage technique (120 to 150 kVp). With this technique there is greater penetration of the mediastinum, which improves visualization of the trachea and main bronchi. A disadvantage of high-kilovoltage radiography is the relatively poor demonstration of calcified structures so that rib fractures and calcified pulmonary nodules or pleural plaques are less conspicuous. Even with an optimal technique, nearly a third of the lungs are partially obscured by overlying mediastinum, diaphragm, and ribs.

Automatic exposure devices have been developed to expose accurately the various parts of the chest. One of these, the Advanced Multiple Beam Equalisation Radiography (**AMBER**) system, produces chest radiographs which greatly improve the demonstration of both mediastinal anatomy and pulmonary abnormalities (see Fig. 16). Another approach to this problem is phosphor-plate computed radiography, which uses digital technology.

This is ultimately expected to replace conventional film radiography, and has already done so in some centres. A phosphor plate is handled in a conventional cassette (which does not contain film) and is exposed in the normal way. The energy of the incident X-ray beam is stored as a latent image. The phosphor plate is then scanned with a laser beam and the light emitted from the excited latent image is detected by a photomultiplier. Thereafter this signal is processed in digital form, and the image may either be viewed on a television monitor or laser-printed on to film. The advantage of phosphor-plate computed radiography is that it can retrieve an image of diagnostic quality from an imperfect exposure, which would otherwise result in a non-diagnostic conventional film radiograph. Manipulation or processing of the digital image data can enhance certain features of the radiograph to improve diagnosis.

Standard radiographic views of the chest

The posteroanterior projection is the standard view (see Fig. 11(a)). The patient is positioned with his anterior chest wall against the film cassette and his arms are abducted to rotate the scapulas away from the posterior chest. Chest films taken in the anteroposterior (**AP**) projection are usually taken when the patient is too ill to stand for a formal PA radiograph. A consequence of this view is that the heart is magnified because it lies further from the film. Moreover, the shorter X-ray tube-to-film distance, which is inevitable when a portable AP radiograph is taken, causes further magnification that must be taken into account when assessing the heart size on an AP chest radiograph.

The lateral radiograph is obtained by placing the patient at right angles to the film cassette (see Fig. 11(b)). The lateral projection provides the third dimension and helps to determine the site of a lesion identified on the PA projection (although it is surprising how often an opacity clearly seen on the PA radiograph is invisible on the lateral radiograph). As well as allowing accurate localization of lesions, the lateral radiograph may reveal concealed abnormalities that lie behind the heart or diaphragm. Furthermore, with some experience, evaluation of the hilar structures and major airways is aided by the lateral radiograph (see later section on the anatomy on the lateral chest radiograph).

Over the years, a number of supplementary projections have been developed to provide information about areas that are not easily seen on the standard PA and lateral radiograph. With the advent of cross-sectional imaging, notably computed tomography (**CT**), many of these extra views have become obsolete. However, even with access to CT, some of these views supply extra anatomical detail readily and inexpensively and these will be considered briefly.

The lateral decubitus projection is sometimes useful for the demonstration of small pleural effusions. For this view the patient lies on his side, with the side in question downwards; the film is positioned behind the patient and the X-ray beam traverses the patient horizontally. Small quantities of pleural fluid (50 to 100 ml), which are not detectable on a PA chest radiograph, can be demonstrated tracking up the lateral chest wall, but ultrasonography is increasingly being used as a reliable technique for demonstrating small pleural effusions. Other supplementary projections, for example apical and lordotic views, improve visualization of the lung at the extreme apices. These are now rarely performed, CT being much more effective at showing pathology in these difficult areas.

The technique of screening the patient with fluoroscopy has the advantage of allowing 'real time' radiographic examination. It allows localization of lesions by the use of unusual oblique projections, for example to distinguish a small pleural plaque from an intrapulmonary nodule. Fluoroscopy is also the quickest method of evaluating diaphragmatic movement and diagnosing air-trapping in a child who is suspected of inhaling a foreign body.

Ultrasonography

High-frequency sound waves do not traverse air and are completely reflected at interfaces between soft tissue and air. The use of this technique in the chest is therefore limited by normally aerated lung. However, fluid can be readily detected and the main use of ultrasound is for the localization of small or loculated pleural effusions. Furthermore, ultrasound can differentiate between pleural fluid and pleural thickening in cases in which radiography cannot make this distinction. Ultrasonography is an extremely useful technique for guiding percutaneous needle biopsy of masses arising from the chest wall or pleura, or peripheral pulmonary masses or consolidation, and for aiding the accurate placement of a chest drain within a pleural collection. Ultrasonography may show numerous septations within an exudative pleural effusion (Fig. 1), but thoracocentesis may be required to distinguish between a parapneumonic effusion and an empyema.

Computed tomography

Computed tomography (CT) depends on the same basic principle as conventional radiography, namely the differential absorption of X-rays by tissues of disparate densities. However, CT is much more sensitive to differences in attenuation of X-rays by various tissues. A CT machine consists of an X-ray source and an array of detectors which surround the patient. The X-ray source rotates around the patient and the resulting attenuated beam is measured by the detectors. The signals from the detectors are used to construct an image by a mathematical technique. The reconstructed images are transverse (axial) cross-sections of the patient and are viewed as if from the patient's feet (i.e. on the image, the patient's right side is to the viewer's left). Each CT section is a matrix of three-dimensional elements (voxels) containing a measurement of X-ray attenuation, arbitrarily expressed as Hounsfield Units (**HU**): water measures 0 HU, air – 1000 HU (so that lung parenchyma is approximately –600 HU), fat –80

HU, soft tissue 40–80 HU, and bone 800 HU. If a voxel is completely occupied by a tissue of uniform density (most frequently the case with narrow sections) then the HU will be truly representative of that tissue. If the section contains tissues of two different densities (more likely with thicker sections), for example half lung and half dome of diaphragm, then the attenuation value will be a weighted average of the two components: the so-called 'partial volume' effect.

Because of the cross-sectional nature of CT it can accurately localize lesions seen on only one view on chest radiography. The superior contrast resolution of CT gives exquisite detail of the various components of mediastinal anatomy (for example, lymph nodes and vessels) and density differences (for example, calcifications within a pulmonary nodule). Different image settings are needed to view the soft tissue structures of the mediastinum and the aerated lung parenchyma (Fig. 2).

Spiral (helical) CT

The principle of spiral CT involves the continuous rotation of the X-ray beam and detectors around the patient while the table moves into the gantry. Markedly reduced scan times are possible with the introduction of spiral CT, allowing the entire thorax to be imaged in a single breath-hold. An examination of sufficient diagnostic quality can be obtained in dyspnoeic patients and young children during quiet respiration. It also allows an intravenous injection of contrast medium to be accurately timed to give

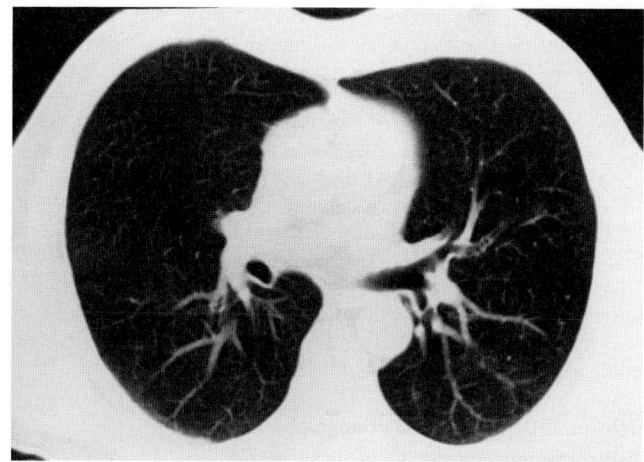

(a)

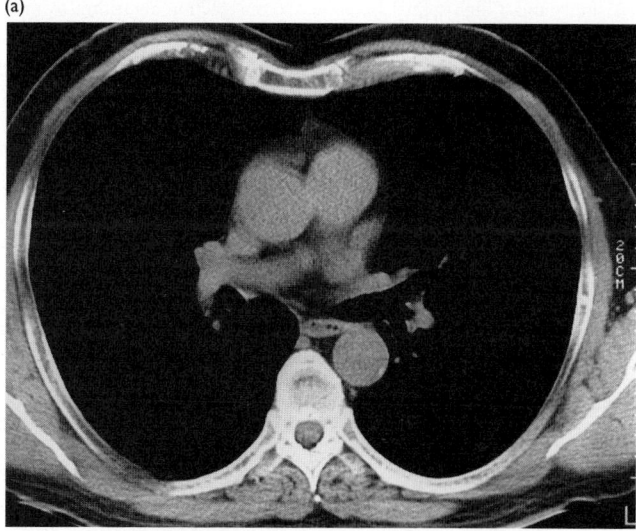

(b)

Fig. 2 Computed tomography section through the mid-thorax. The window settings have been adjusted to show details of (a) the lungs and (b) the soft tissues of the mediastinum.

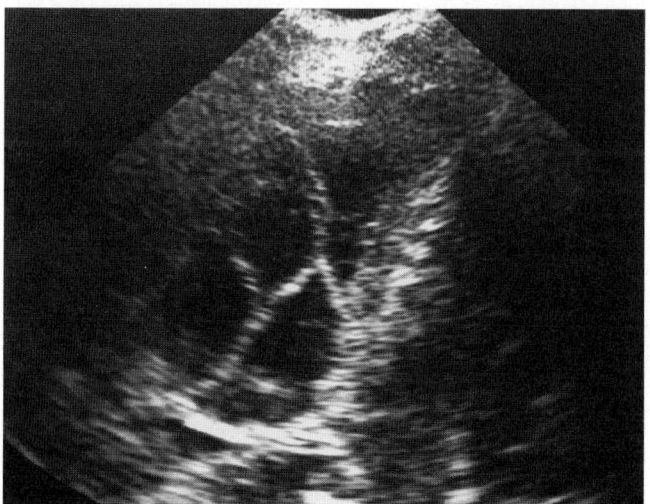

Fig. 1 Ultrasonography showing a pleural effusion. Fibrinous septations traverse the pleural space.

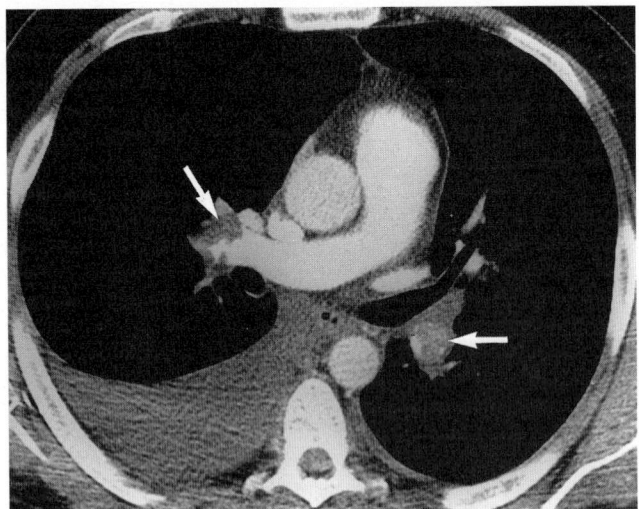

Fig. 3 Computed tomography of a patient with acute bilateral pulmonary emboli. Filling defects in contrast media opacification are seen within the right main pulmonary artery and the left interlobar pulmonary artery (arrows). Note the right-sided pleural effusion.

the optimum opacification of, for example, the pulmonary arteries, thus enabling the detection of pulmonary emboli (Fig. 3). In many centres, spiral CT has supplanted ventilation–perfusion radionuclide imaging in the investigation of patients with suspected pulmonary embolism and, with optimum technique, the accuracy approaches that of pulmonary arteriography for the diagnosis of central, lobar, and segmental pulmonary emboli. However, radiation dose and availability are important considerations. The technique is most useful in patients with coexisting lung disease which would result in an inconclusive ventilation–perfusion radionuclide study.

Computer software can perform multiplanar two- and three-dimensional image reconstructions of spiral CT images, which provide novel views of the bronchial tree that can aid interventional techniques such as bronchial stent placement (Fig. 4).

High-resolution computed tomography

High-resolution computed tomography (**HRCT**) uses very thin sections (1–3 mm) and a high spatial frequency reconstruction algorithm to produce highly detailed sections of the lung parenchyma. Both conventional and spiral CT scanners can produce thin sections, and the terms 'spiral CT'

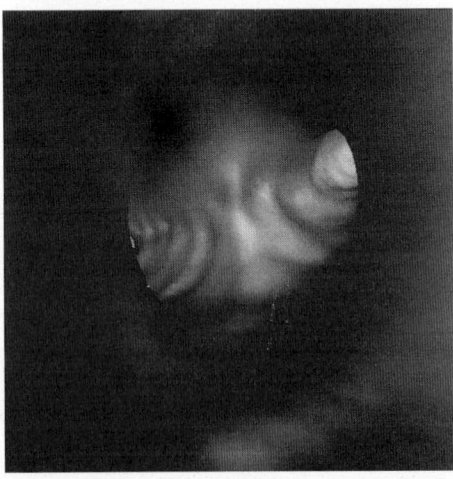

Fig. 4 Reconstructed three-dimensional image from spiral CT showing the carina and the right and left main bronchi viewed from above.

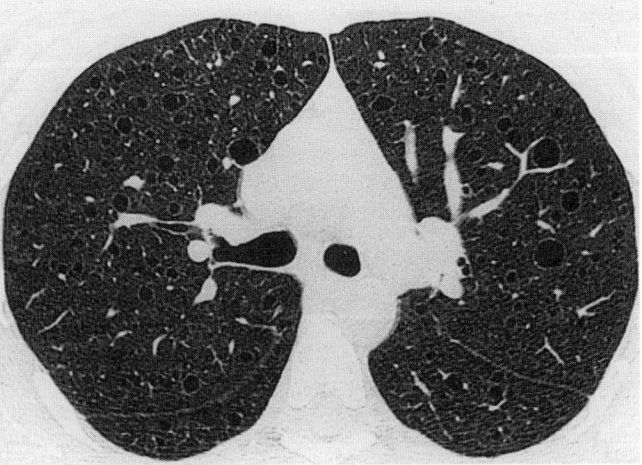

Fig. 5 High-resolution computed tomography of a patient with lymphangioleiomyomatosis showing thin-walled cysts throughout the lungs. These cysts were not apparent on chest radiography.

and 'high-resolution CT' should not be confused. Submillimetre structures can be resolved with this technique, and the subtle and sometimes complex morphology of interstitial lung diseases can be shown with great clarity (Fig. 5). Since the mid-1980s, the development of high-resolution computed tomography has changed the radiological approach to the diagnosis of diffuse lung disease. High-resolution CT images of the lung correlate closely with the macroscopic appearances of pathological specimens, so that HRCT represents a substantial improvement over chest radiography in terms of sensitivity, specificity, and diagnostic accuracy. Furthermore, CT samples a far greater volume of lung than even the most generous lung biopsy, making it less prone to sampling errors.

High-resolution CT has also been shown to provide useful information regarding prognosis and response to treatment in some diffuse lung diseases. Nevertheless, despite the increased confidence with which a specific diagnosis of diffuse lung disease can be made with HRCT, open lung biopsy is still required to achieve a definitive histological diagnosis in difficult cases. The extent of diffuse lung disease can be estimated precisely on HRCT and, when a biopsy is indicated, the distribution of disease will indicate whether a transbronchial biopsy or an open lung biopsy is more likely to obtain a representative specimen.

The disadvantages of CT are its relatively high cost and increased radiation exposure to the patient, particularly in comparison with chest radiography. For these reasons, CT should not be regarded as a routine investigation and examinations should always be tailored to solve questions not answered by less sophisticated investigations. The commonest indications for thoracic CT are summarized in Table 1.

Magnetic resonance imaging

The physical principles of magnetic resonance imaging (**MRI**) are very different to those governing CT scanning. An MR image is obtained by placing an individual in a strong magnetic field which polarizes some of the ubiquitous hydrogen protons (which can be thought of as behaving like randomly oriented bar magnets) in the body so that they have the same alignment. The application of radiofrequency wave pulses of specified lengths and repetition (pulse sequences) displace the protons and some of this transmitted energy is absorbed by them. With the cessation of the radiofrequency pulse, the protons return to their initial alignment and in so doing they emit, as a weak signal, some of the energy they have absorbed; this signal is received and then amplified and handled in digital form, and is subsequently reconstructed into an image.

The advantages of MRI include its ability to obtain sections in any plane (Fig. 6), the improved contrast resolution between different soft tissues

Table 1 Indications for CT of the thorax

1. Elucidation of an abnormal mediastinal or hilar contour on chest radiography
2. As part of the staging procedure in the evaluation of a patient with known lung cancer (the findings on CT must be interpreted in conjunction with other investigations)
3. Detection of pulmonary disease in the face of a questionably abnormal chest radiograph (notably diffuse interstitial disease and bronchiectasis)
4. Investigation of a patient with haemoptysis in whom chest radiography and bronchoscopy are normal
5. Detection of pulmonary embolism
6. Assessment of complex pleural or chest wall pathology when chest radiography does not adequately show the extent of disease
7. As a means of guiding the percutaneous needle biopsy of centrally placed pulmonary lesions, mediastinal masses, or chest wall pathology

compared with CT scanning, and the use of special sequences which give functional information, for instance the velocity of blood flow. Another important advantage of MRI is the lack of any known hazard to the patient, in contrast to CT scanning with its small attendant risk from ionizing radiation. Disadvantages of MRI include the long scan time (although this is continually being shortened), reduced spatial resolution compared with CT, the inability to image calcium, its reduced acceptability to patients because of the claustrophobic bore of the magnet, and important contraindications such as permanent cardiac pacemaker devices and ferromagnetic intraocular foreign bodies.

In many respects the imaging of the mediastinum by CT scanning and MRI are comparable. However, MR images of the lungs are currently markedly inferior to CT scanning. This is because of the very low water (and therefore proton) content of the lungs: the signal produced by a normal lung is therefore small and not visualized by conventional sequences.

Radionuclide imaging

Ventilation–perfusion radionuclide scanning is an effective non-invasive method of providing both anatomical and physiological information about the lung. It is the commonest radionuclide study of the lungs, and is most

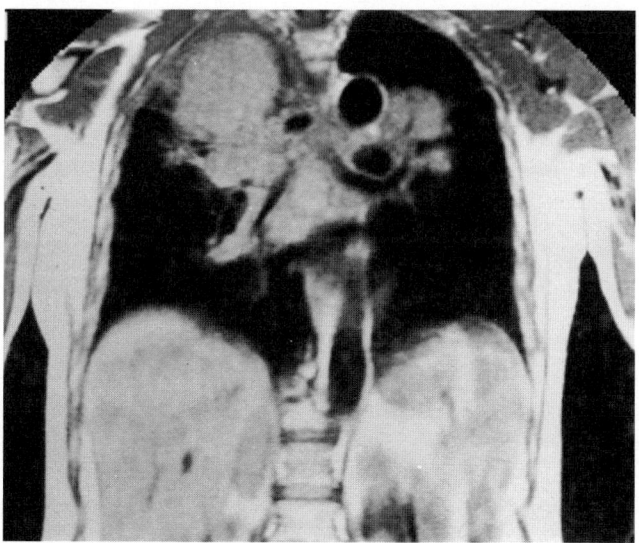

Fig. 6 Magnetic resonance image (coronal section) showing the relationship of an apical bronchial carcinoma to the chest wall and adjacent mediastinum. There are enlarged subcarinal lymph nodes and a metastatic deposit in the right adrenal gland.

frequently used to confirm or exclude the diagnosis of suspected pulmonary embolism.

Regional pulmonary capillary perfusion can be assessed following the intravenous injection of a bolus of particles which have been labelled with technetium-99m. The minute particles are microspheres or macroaggregates of human albumin (between 15 μm to 70 μm in diameter). These particles are evenly dispersed by the time they reach the pulmonary circulation and become temporarily lodged in a very small fraction (less than 0.5 per cent) of the precapillary arterioles and capillaries of the lungs. There is a small theoretical risk of compromising the pulmonary vascular bed in patients with severe pulmonary hypertension, but this is not an absolute contraindication to the examination. The distribution of gamma-ray emission from the technetium-labelled particles is directly proportional to the regional pulmonary flow, and a significant defect in perfusion is usually readily detected. It is important to appreciate that such defects may be due to a variety of conditions other than a pulmonary embolism, including any cause of hypoxic vasoconstriction such as an area of subsegmental collapse or space-occupying lesions not supplied by the pulmonary circulation. However, in these cases the affected area of lung will be neither ventilated nor perfused, in contrast to acute pulmonary embolism in which there is no corresponding defect of ventilation. Thus, to improve the specificity of the diagnosis of a pulmonary embolism, ventilation scintigraphy is usually performed at the same time as perfusion scanning.

Evaluation of ventilation of the lungs depends on filling the distal air spaces with a gamma-ray emitting radionuclide. The radionuclides suitable for inhalation are the inert gases xenon-133 and krypton-81m or a technetium-99m aerosol (Technegas). While krypton-81m gives the highest quality images, Technegas is being increasingly used because of its ready availability. The characteristic abnormality of pulmonary embolism is the so-called mismatched defect in which a regional defect in perfusion is not matched by a defect in ventilation (Figs 7(a) and (b)). However, the picture in pulmonary embolism may not always be clear-cut, particularly when pulmonary infarction has occurred, when there will be a matched defect of both ventilation and perfusion. Because of the importance of establishing a correct diagnosis of pulmonary embolism, ventilation–perfusion scans should always be interpreted in the light of current chest radiographs and clinical information. Even then a proportion of ventilation–perfusion scans remain indeterminate, hence the increasing use of CT angiography in the management of these patients. Due to the decreased radiation burden, V/Q scanning remains a reasonable first-line investigation in young patients with no pre-existing lung disease and a low pretest probability for pulmonary embolism.

Positron emission tomography

Positron emission tomography (**PET**) relies on the tissue uptake of radioisotopes which decay by positron emission. Detectors located around the patient map the site of origin of the two resultant photons emitted at 180 degrees from each other. The most widely used isotope for the detection of pulmonary malignancy is [^{18}F]fluorodeoxyglucose (**FDG**), a D-glucose analogue. The increased uptake and retention of glucose by malignant cells allows differentiation of benign from malignant pulmonary masses, detection of lymph node involvement by tumour, and identification of distant metastases (Fig. 8). Limitations of the technique include false-positive results caused by granulomatous infection or acute inflammation, and false-negative results with certain tumours (e.g. bronchioloalveolar carcinomas and carcinoid tumours). The technique is not widely available at present.

Pulmonary and bronchial arteriography; superior vena cavography

The 'gold standard' for identifying emboli within the pulmonary arteries has traditionally been pulmonary arteriography (Fig. 9). This requires the puncture of an antecubital, jugular, or femoral vein, with the catheter

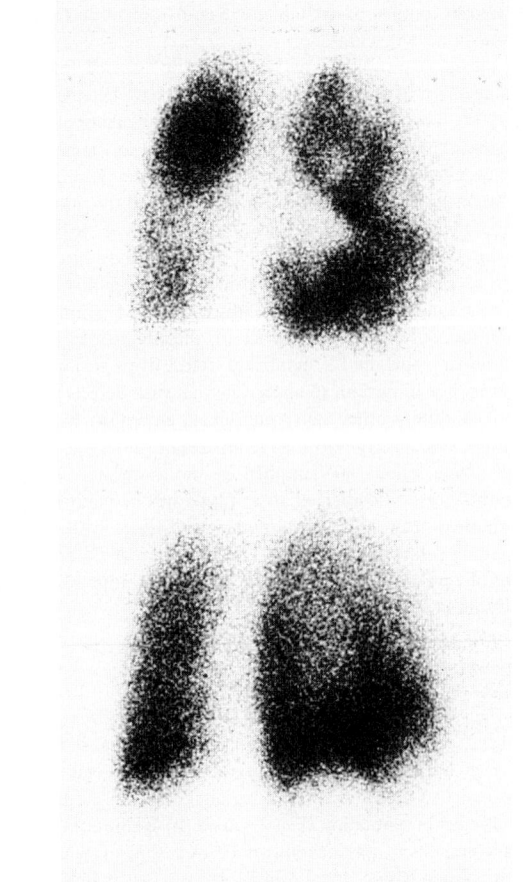

(a)

(b)

Fig. 7 A ventilation–perfusion radionuclide study (oblique views). The perfusion scan (a) shows a defect in the left mid-zone which is not matched on the corresponding view of the ventilation scan (b). The so-called mismatched defect is characteristic of a pulmonary embolus.

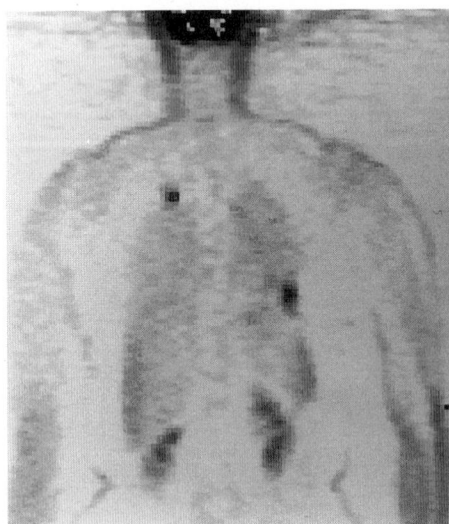

Fig. 8 Positron emission tomography image showing increased uptake of [^{18}F]fluorodeoxyglucose (FDG) in the left lower zone corresponding to a primary bronchial carcinoma. Note the pulmonary metastasis at the right apex.

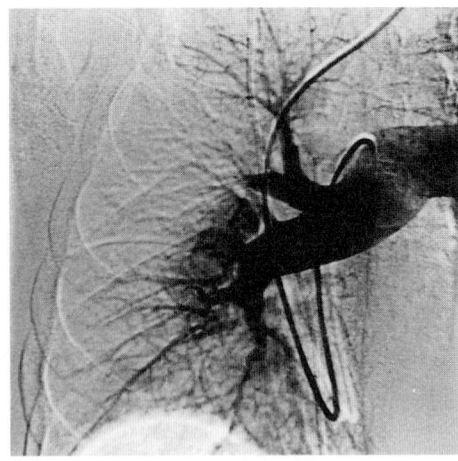

Fig. 9 A digital subtraction pulmonary arteriogram showing abrupt termination of the vessels supplying the right upper lobe caused by a pulmonary embolus.

guided through the right heart under fluoroscopic control. While the complication rate is low, it is a time-consuming procedure requiring an experienced angiographer.

The bronchial arteries which supply the airways become hypertrophied in chronic inflammatory pulmonary disease, notably in bronchiectasis. Rupture of these vessels can cause severe and life-threatening haemoptysis. The bronchial arteries can be selectively catheterized by the passage of a catheter via the femoral artery and aorta. Having identified the abnormally hypertrophied bronchial arteries (Fig. 10), they can be therapeutically embolized. This technique is usually successful in abating massive haemoptysis in patients unable to undergo immediate surgical treatment.

Superior vena cavography is usually performed to evaluate the exact site of narrowing in patients with symptoms of obstruction of the superior vena cava: it is not generally required to confirm the diagnosis, which is usually evident from the clinical signs alone. Patients with symptoms of superior vena cava obstruction, most frequently due to neoplastic involvement of mediastinal lymph nodes, can be successfully palliated by radiotherapy or the insertion of an expandable metallic wire stent at the site of the narrowing.

Percutaneous lung biopsy

Percutaneous needle biopsy of a pulmonary lesion or mediastinal mass is usually performed in patients in whom a bronchoscopic biopsy has failed to produce a histological specimen, or if a thoracotomy to resect the lesion

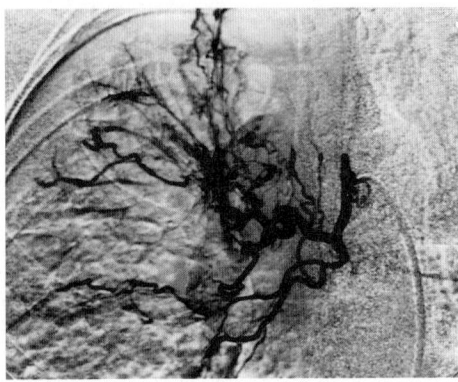

Fig. 10 Abnormally hypertrophied bronchial arteries supplying the right upper lobe shown on a selective digital subtraction bronchial arteriogram. The patient had cystic fibrosis and had had a massive haemoptysis; these bronchial arteries were subsequently embolized.

is deemed inappropriate. It should not be regarded as a routine procedure in the investigation of all solitary pulmonary nodules, and should only be performed after considering the risks to the patient and whether the information forthcoming from the procedure will direct management.

Many different types of needles have been developed, and the frequency of complications, mainly pneumothorax and haemoptysis, is partly related to the diameter of the needle and the depth of the lesion. Percutaneous biopsy is performed under local anaesthesia with CT guidance: ultrasound guidance can be used if the mass abuts the pleura. Contraindications to the procedure include any patient with poor respiratory reserve who would be unable to withstand a pneumothorax, and pulmonary arterial hypertension.

Normal radiographic anatomy

The mediastinum

On a PA chest radiograph (Fig. 11(a)) the mediastinal structures are superimposed on one another and thus cannot be distinguished individually. The mediastinum is conventionally divided into superior, anterior, middle, and posterior compartments. The practical use of these arbitrary divisions is that specific mediastinal pathologies show a definite predilection for individual compartments (for example, a superior mediastinal mass is most frequently due to intrathoracic extension of the thyroid gland, a middle mediastinal mass is usually due to enlarged lymph nodes). However, it should be borne in mind that the position of a mass within one of these compartments is no guarantee of a specific diagnosis, nor do these boundaries preclude disease from spreading from one compartment to the next.

Because only the outline of the mediastinum and the air-containing trachea and bronchi are clearly seen on a PA chest radiograph, the mediastinal anatomy will be considered in more detail in the description of CT anatomy. On a chest radiograph, the right superior mediastinal border is formed by the right brachiocephalic vein and superior vena cava. The mediastinal border to the left of the trachea above the aortic arch represents the sum of the left carotid and left subclavian arteries together with the left brachiocephalic and jugular veins. The left cardiac border comprises the left atrial appendage which merges inferiorly with the left ventricle. The cardiac silhouette is always sharply outlined: any blurring of the border denotes replacement of the aerated lung immediately adjacent to the heart, usually by collapse or consolidation (see Silhouette sign in Common radiological signs of disease).

The density of the cardiac shadow to the left and right of the vertebral column should be identical, and any difference signals pulmonary pathology (for example, consolidation in a lower lobe). A density with a convex lateral border is often seen through the right heart border on a well-penetrated film: this apparent mass is due to the confluence of the pulmonary veins as they enter the left atrium and is of no pathological significance.

The trachea and main bronchi are visible through the upper and middle mediastinum. The trachea is rarely straight and is often to the right of the mid-line at its mid-point. In elderly patients, the trachea may appear dramatically displaced by a dilated aortic arch. The angle of the carina is usually somewhat less than 80 degrees. Splaying of the carina is a sign of gross disease, either in the form of massive subcarinal lymphadenopathy, or a markedly enlarged left atrium. A more sensitive sign of a subcarinal mass is obliteration of the azygo-oesophageal line which is usually visible on a well-penetrated chest radiograph. The origins of the lobar bronchi, where they are projected over the mediastinal shadow, can usually be made out, but the segmental bronchi within the lungs are not generally seen on plain radiography.

The hilar structures

The hilar shadows on a chest radiograph are a complex summation of the pulmonary arteries and veins, with virtually no contribution from the overlying bronchial walls or normal-sized lymph nodes. The hila are approximately the same size, with the left hilum always lying between 0.5 cm and 1.5 cm above the level of the right hilum. The size and shape of the hila in normal individuals show remarkable variation so that subtle abnormalities are difficult to detect. In detecting a mass at the hilum, at least as important as an abnormal contour is a discrepancy in density between the two hila. Both hilar shadows, at equivalent points, will be of equal density, and a mass at the hilum (or an intrapulmonary mass projected over the hilum) will be evident as increased density of that hilum.

The pulmonary fissures, vessels, and bronchi

The lobes of each lung are surrounded by visceral pleura: the upper and lower lobes of the left lung are separated by the major (or oblique) fissure. The upper, middle, and lower lobes of the right lung are separated by the major (or oblique) and minor (horizontal or transverse) fissures. The

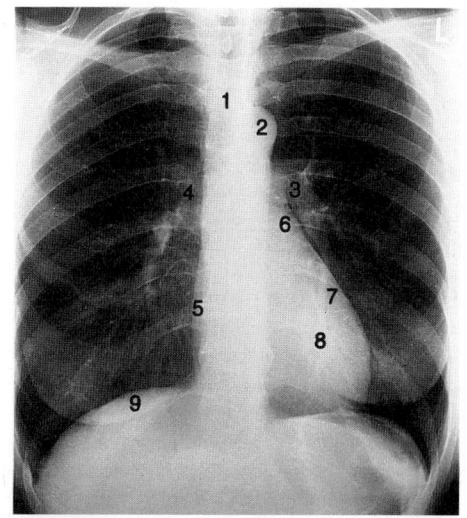

(a)

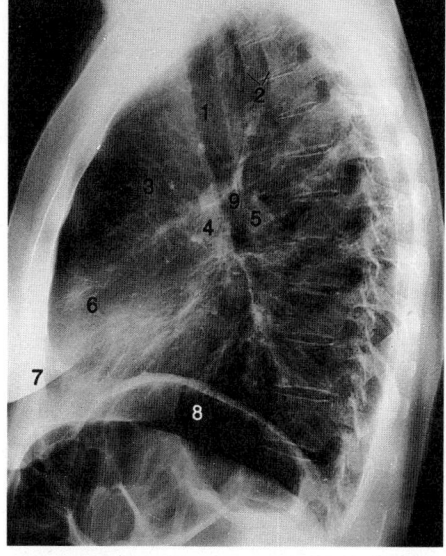

(b)

Fig. 11 Normal radiographic anatomy on (a) PA and (b) lateral chest radiographs. (a) 1, Trachea; 2 aortic arch; 3, left main pulmonary artery; 4, right main pulmonary artery; 5, right atrial border; 6, left atrial appendage; 7, left ventricular border; 8, right ventricle; 9, right dome of the diaphragm. (b) 1, Trachea; 2, scapulas; 3, anterior aortic arch; 4, right pulmonary artery; 5, left pulmonary artery; 6, right ventricle; 7, breast shadows; 8, gastric bubble under the left hemidiaphragm; 9, left main bronchus.

minor fissure is visible in about 60 per cent of normal PA chest radiographs. In normal individuals, this fissure runs horizontally and any deviation from this course represents a loss of volume of a lobe. The major fissures are inconstantly identifiable on lateral radiographs. Other fissures are occasionally seen, for example in the left lung a minor fissure can occur which separates the lingula from the remainder of the upper lobe.

All the branching structures seen within the lungs on a chest radiograph represent either pulmonary arteries or veins. The larger pulmonary vessels can be traced back to the hila and mediastinum. The pulmonary veins can sometimes be differentiated from the pulmonary arteries: the superior pulmonary veins have a distinctly vertical course, but in practice it is often impossible to distinguish arteries from veins in the outer two-thirds of the lung. On a chest radiograph taken in the erect position, there is a gradual increase in the diameter of the vessels, at equidistant points from the hilum, travelling from lung apex to base: this is a gravity-dependent effect and is abolished if the patient is supine or in cardiac failure.

The lobes of the lung are divided into segments, each of which is supplied by its own segmental bronchi. The walls of the segmental bronchi are rarely seen on the chest radiograph, except when lying parallel with the X-ray beam when they are seen end-on as ring shadows measuring up to 8 mm in diameter.

The diaphragm and thoracic cage

The interface between aerated lung and the domes of the diaphragm is sharp, and in general the highest point of each dome is medial to the mid-clavicular line. The right dome of the diaphragm is higher than the left by up to 2 cm in the erect position, unless the left dome is temporarily elevated by air in the stomach. Laterally, the diaphragm dips steeply downwards to form an acute angle with the chest wall. Filling in or blunting of these costophrenic angles usually represents pleural disease, either pleural thickening or an effusion.

Localized humps on the dome of the diaphragm are common and represent minor weaknesses or defects. Similarly, interposition of the colon in front of the right lobe of the liver is a frequently seen normal variant.

Deformities of the thoracic cage may cause distortion of the normal mediastinum and so simulate disease. One of the commonest deformities is pectus excavatum, which, by compressing the heart between the depressed sternum and vertebral column, causes displacement of the apparently enlarged heart to the left and causes blurring of the right heart border.

High-kilovoltage chest radiographs often allow the vertebral bodies to be seen through the cardiac shadow. However, the ribs, particularly their posterior parts, are often rendered invisible by this technique.

Anatomy on the lateral chest radiograph

It is useful to get accustomed to viewing a lateral film (Fig. 11(b)) in the same orientation, whether it is a right or left lateral projection. Familiarity with the same orientation improves the viewer's ability to detect deviations from normal.

The trachea is angled slightly posteriorly as it runs towards the carina and the posterior wall of the trachea is always visible as a fine stripe. Furthermore, the posterior walls of the right main bronchus and the right intermediate bronchus are outlined by air and are also seen as a continuous stripe on the lateral radiograph. The spines of the scapulas are invariably seen running almost vertically in the upper part of the lateral radiograph and they should not be confused with intrathoracic structures. Further spurious shadows are formed by the soft tissues of the outstretched arms which are projected over the anterior and superior mediastinum. Although the carina is not visible on the lateral radiograph, the two transradiancies projected over the lower trachea represent the right main bronchus (superiorly) and the left main bronchus (inferiorly).

More lung is obscured by overlying structures on a lateral radiograph than on the PA view. The unobscured lung in the retrosternal and retrocardiac regions should be of the same transradiancy. Furthermore, as the eye travels down the dorsal spine, the viewer should be aware of a gradual increase in transradiancy. The loss of this phenomenon suggests the presence of disease in the posterobasal segments of the lower lobes (sometimes not visible on the frontal radiograph).

The two major fissures are seen as diagonal lines, often incomplete and of a hair's breadth, running from the upper dorsal spine to the anterior surface of the diaphragm. Care must be taken not to confuse the obliquely running edges of ribs with fissures. The minor fissure extends horizontally from the mid right major fissure. It is often impossible to distinguish the right from the left major fissures with confidence. Similarly, although the two hemidiaphragms may be identified individually (especially if the gastric bubble is visible under the left dome of the diaphragm), the distinction between the right and the left is often impossible. A helpful sign is the relative heights of the two domes: the dome furthest from the film is usually higher because of magnification.

The summation of both hila on the lateral radiograph generates a complex shadow. However, there are some generalizations which aid the interpretation of this difficult area. The right pulmonary artery lies anterior to the trachea and right main bronchus, whereas the left pulmonary artery hooks over the left main bronchus so that a large part of it lies posterior to the major bronchi. As a result, any mass identified on a PA and lateral radiograph that lies anterior to the left hilum or posterior to the right hilum is not vascular in origin and is most likely to represent enlarged hilar lymph nodes.

A band-like opacity is often seen along the lower third of the anterior chest wall behind the sternum. This represents a normal density and occurs because there is less aerated lung in contact with the chest wall because the space is occupied by the heart: it should not be confused with pleural disease.

Normal CT anatomy of the mediastinum

As computed tomography provides unique information about the anatomy of the mediastinum, it is often used to provide further information about abnormalities which are seen merely as a deformity of the mediastinal contour on chest radiography. The normal structures that are always identified on a CT of the mediastinum are the blood vessels (which make up the bulk of the superior mediastinum), the major airways, the oesophagus, and mediastinal fat. An appreciation of the relationship of these structures to each other is crucial for the correct interpretation of CT scans: four important levels are shown in Figs 12(a)–(d)).

Normal lymph nodes surrounded by fat may be identified throughout the mediastinum. Many schemes have been devised to map their precise locations, but they can be broadly divided into: (1) anterior mediastinal; (2) posterior mediastinal; and (3) tracheobronchial. The latter can be further subdivided into the following regions: (a) right and left paratracheal; (b) subaortic; (c) pretracheal; (d) subcarinal. It is important to appreciate that the absolute size of lymph nodes identified on CT (or by direct inspection at mediastinoscopy) should not be regarded as a foolproof criterion for significant disease, particularly in the context of lung cancer. Although markedly enlarged lymph nodes, greater than 2 cm in diameter, almost invariably signify important pathology, moderate enlargement of mediastinal lymph nodes may represent reactive hyperplasia of little clinical significance. Conversely, small-volume lymph nodes or lymph nodes not identified by CT may sometimes contain micrometastases from a distant primary neoplasm.

The thymus gland occupies a large part of the anterior mediastinum in children. In adult life the remnants of the normal thymus are normally inconspicuous on CT.

Points in the interpretation of a chest radiograph

Even when there is an obvious radiographic abnormality, there is much to recommend a careful and systematic method in reviewing a chest radiograph. Such an approach will allow an appreciation of normal variations of anatomy to be built up with time. With increasing experience an appreciation of a deviation from normal appearances becomes more rapid, which leads quickly to a directed search for related abnormalities.

Before interpreting a chest radiograph, it is vital to establish whether there are any previous radiographs for comparison: the sequence and pattern of change is often as important as the identification of a radiographic abnormality. Information gained from preceding radiographs, particularly the lack of serial change, will often prevent needless further investigation. Demographic details, particularly the age and racial origin of the patient,

should be noted, since this information may increase the probability of a differential diagnosis which is based on the radiographic findings alone.

A quick check that the radiograph is of satisfactory quality includes an estimation of the radiographic exposure, depth of inspiration, and position of the patient. As a general rule, the intervertebral disc spaces of the entire dorsal spine should be visible on a correctly exposed radiograph, with the mid-point of the right hemidiaphragm lying at the level of the anterior end of the sixth rib if the patient has taken a satisfactory breath in. The patient is axially rotated if the medial ends of the clavicles are not equidistant from the spinous process of the thoracic vertebral body at that level.

The order in which the structures on a chest radiograph are analysed is unimportant. A suggested sequence is to start with a scrutiny of the position of the trachea, mediastinal contour (which should be sharply outlined in its entirety), and then the position, outline, and density of the hilar shadows. Only then are the lungs examined, taking into account their size, the relative transradiancy of each zone, and the position of the horizontal

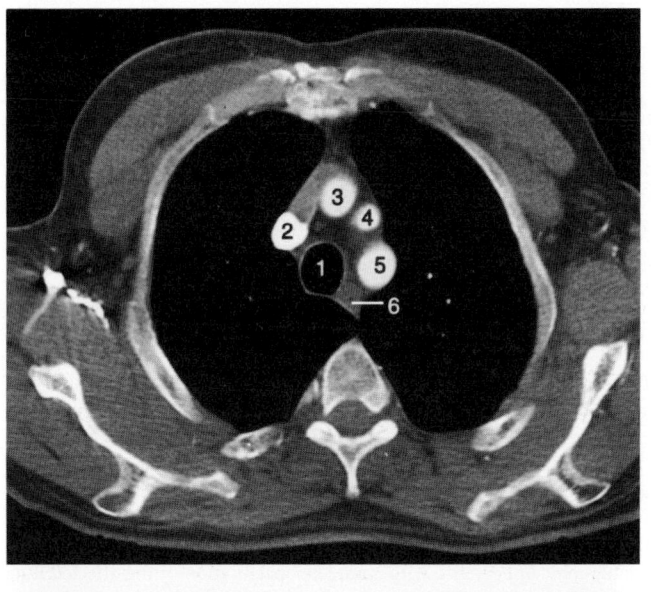
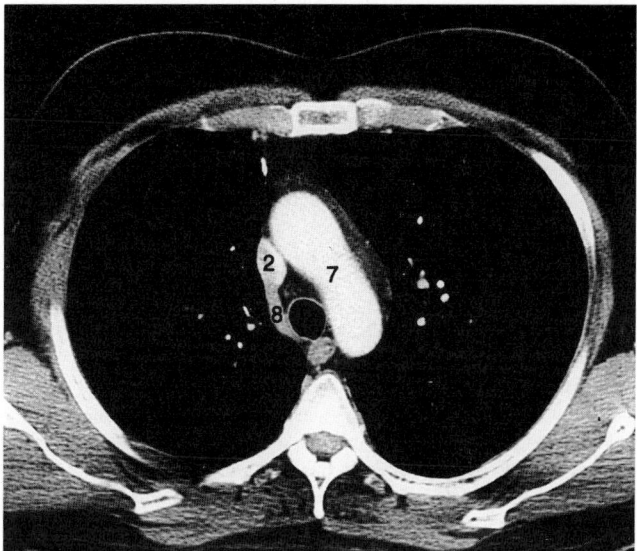
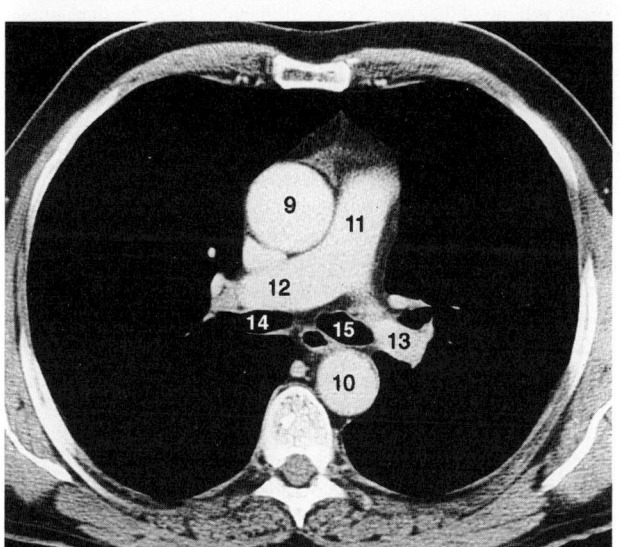
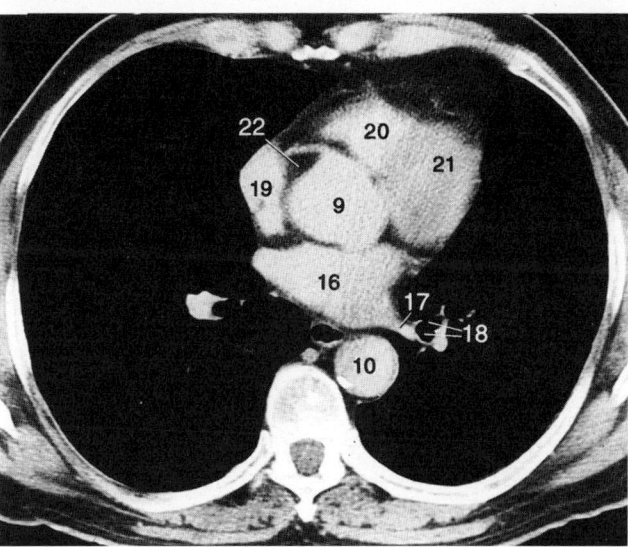

Fig. 12 (a–d) Computed tomography with contrast enhancement to show the normal anatomy at four levels through the mediastinum. 1, Trachea; 2, superior vena cava; 3, brachiocephalic artery; 4, left common carotid artery; 5, left subclavian artery; 6, oesophagus; 7, aortic arch; 8, azygos vein; 9, ascending aorta; 10, descending aorta; 11, main pulmonary artery; 12, right pulmonary artery; 13, left pulmonary artery; 14, right main bronchus; 15, left main bronchus; 16, left atrium; 17, left inferior pulmonary vein; 18, segmental bronchi of the left lower lobe; 19, right atrium; 20, right ventricular outflow; 21, left ventricle.

fissure (and any other indirect signs of volume loss—see later section on lobar collapse). Pulmonary vessels are seen as far as the outer third of the lung and the number of vessels should be roughly symmetrical on the two sides. Next, the position and clarity of the hemidiaphragms should be noted, followed by an assessment of the ribs and soft tissues of the chest wall. Special care should be taken to look for pleural thickening along the lateral chest walls which can easily be overlooked.

Before saying that a chest radiograph is normal, it is worth reviewing areas which are either poorly demonstrated or often misinterpreted. These include: (1) the central mediastinum, where even a large mass may be barely visible on the PA view; (2) the areas behind the heart and hemidiaphragms; (3) the lung apices, often obscured by overlying clavicle and ribs; and (4) the lung and pleura just inside the chest wall.

Once a radiographic abnormality has been detected it should be considered in terms of gross pathology. Both the site and the radiographic characteristics of the lesion will allow the observer to proceed to, at the very least, a generic diagnosis. A precise (unique) diagnosis can only rarely be achieved from the radiographic appearances alone without knowledge of the clinical context.

Common radiological signs of disease

Pulmonary consolidation

Consolidation is a pathological description of the state of the lungs when the normal air-filled spaces, distal to the bronchi, are occupied by the products of disease (for example, water, pus, or blood). The most important radiographic signs of pulmonary consolidation are: (1) an area of increased opacification in the lungs which obscures the underlying blood vessels and has a poorly defined margin—unless it is bounded by a fissure; (2) an 'air bronchogram'; and (3) the 'silhouette sign' (Fig. 13). The air bronchogram is a distinctive and certain sign of intrapulmonary pathology and is seen as a radiolucent (grey) branching structure of the bronchi against a more opaque (white) background of an air-less lung. Although an air bronchogram is seen almost invariably in consolidation, a lung which has become collapsed and air-less, for example due to a large surrounding pleural effusion, may also show an air bronchogram. The silhouette sign is seen when the normally clear border of a structure is lost because the air-filled lung outlining the border is replaced by fluid or a mass. Recognition of this sign can help to localize the area of abnormality within the lungs, for example consolidation in the lingula will make the left heart border indistinct. As with the air bronchogram sign, the silhouette sign may be seen in either pulmonary consolidation or collapse, for example loss of a clear right heart

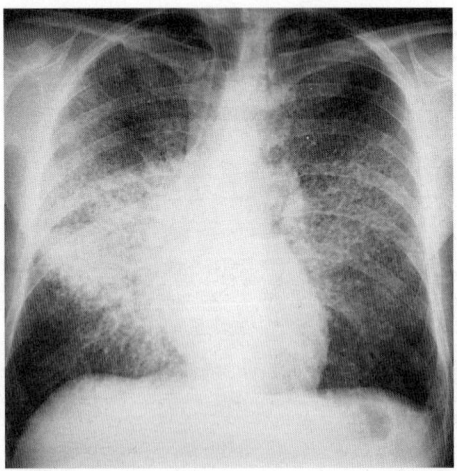

Fig. 13 Widespread pulmonary consolidation in a patient with alveolar proteinosis. The right heart border is obscured, confirming that a large part of the consolidation is in the right middle lobe (the silhouette sign).

Table 2 Causes of widespread pulmonary consolidation

Pulmonary oedema	Cardiogenic/fluid overload
	Acute respiratory distress syndrome
	Inhalational injury (noxious gases)
	Drug abuse
	Neurogenic (raised intracranial pressure or head injury)
	Renal disease
	Traumatic (fat embolism)
Exudate	Infective consolidation
	Eosinophilic lung disease
	Collagen vascular disease
	Cryptogenic organizing pneumonia
	Radiation pneumonitis
Neoplasm	Bronchioloalveolar cell carcinoma
	Lymphoproliferative disorders
Blood	Contusion
	Infarction
	Idiopathic pulmonary haemorrhage (Goodpasture's syndrome)
Other	Alveolar proteinosis
	Sarcoidosis

border may be due to right middle lobe consolidation with or without lobar collapse: the common feature is loss of normal aeration of the affected lung. The causes of widespread pulmonary consolidation are numerous but may be broadly divided into five categories shown in Table 2.

Pulmonary collapse

This is the term used to describe the loss of aeration and therefore inflation in part or all of a lung. Depending on the cause, collapse may occur at any level from small, subsegmental areas of lung through to an entire lung. Small areas of subsegmental collapse occur very commonly in debilitated and postoperative patients, where they are seen as linear, usually horizontal, opacities. At the other end of the spectrum, collapse of an entire lung, usually due to an endobronchial lesion or inhaled foreign body, has a dramatic radiographic appearance with complete opacification of the affected lung and loss of volume of that hemithorax. At the lobar level, the signs of collapse of an individual lobe are characteristic, but, depending on the lobe, may be very subtle. Recognition of the collapse of individual lobes is important and these are described in detail.

Collapse of individual lobes

Right upper lobe: on the frontal radiograph there is elevation of the minor fissure and of the right hilum. If the collapse is complete the non-aerated lobe is seen as a density alongside the superior mediastinum (Fig. 14). On the lateral view the minor fissure moves upwards and the major fissure moves forwards. The retrosternal area becomes progressively more opaque and the anterior margin of the ascending aorta becomes obscured.

Right middle lobe: on the frontal radiograph the lateral part of the minor fissure moves down. There is blurring of the normally sharp right heart border, which may be a subtle abnormality that is easily overlooked (Fig. 15). On the lateral view the minor fissure moves downwards and the lower half of the major fissure moves forwards, giving rise to a triangular shadow with its apex at the hilum and its base behind the lower sternum.

Right lower lobe: there is an increase in density overlying and obscuring the medial portion of the right hemidiaphragm, and the right hilum is displaced inferiorly on the frontal radiograph (Fig. 16). By contrast to right middle lobe collapse, the right heart border usually remains sharply defined since this is in contact with the aerated right middle lobe. On the lateral view the major fissure moves backwards and downwards; with increasing

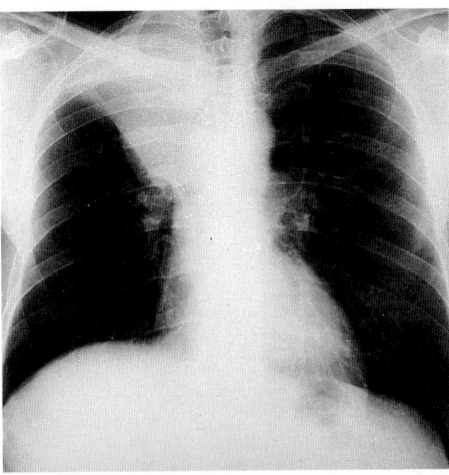

Fig. 14 Right upper lobe collapse.

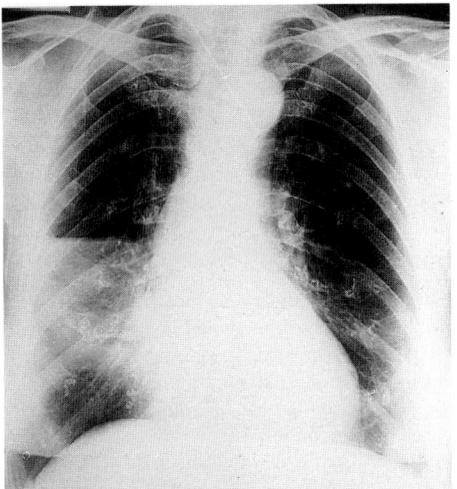

Fig. 15 Right middle lobe collapse.

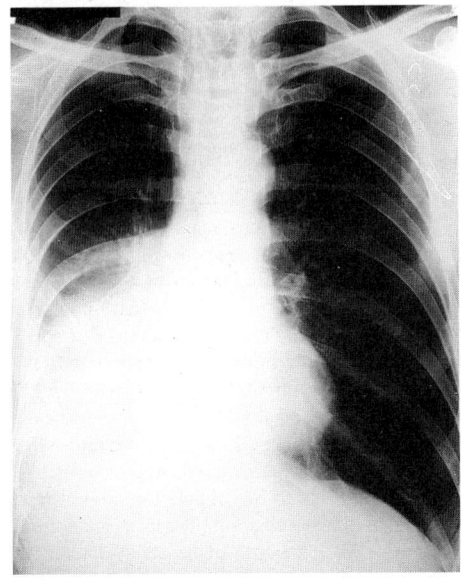

Fig. 16 Right lower lobe collapse.

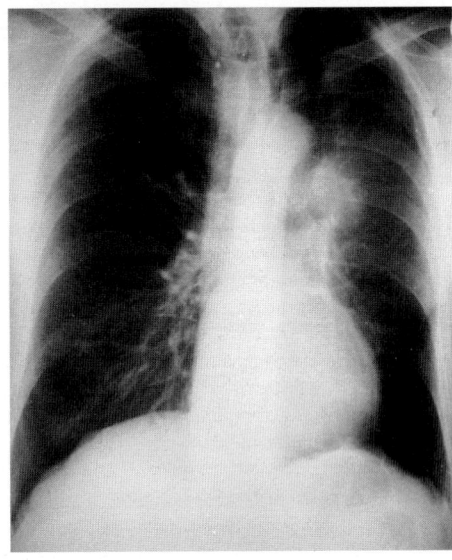

Fig. 17 Left upper lobe collapse.

collapse there is a loss of definition of the posterior part of the right hemidiaphragm as well as increased density overlying the lower dorsal vertebral column.

Left upper lobe: the main finding on the frontal radiograph is a veil-like increase in density, without a sharp margin (quite unlike right upper lobe collapse), spreading outwards and upwards from the elevated left hilum (Fig. 17). The outlines of the aortic knuckle, left hilum, and left heart border become ill-defined. As the collapse increases, the lobe moves centrally and the apical segment of the left lower lobe expands to fill the space left by the collapsed upper lobe: this is the cause of the relatively transradiant lung apex. With complete left upper lobe collapse, a sharp border may return to the aortic arch because it is surrounded by the hyperinflated apical segment of the lower lobe. On the lateral view the major fissure moves superiorly and anteriorly while remaining relatively vertical and roughly parallel to the anterior chest wall.

Left lower lobe: on the frontal radiograph there is a triangular density behind the heart with loss of the medial part of the left hemidiaphragm (Fig. 18). Even on a properly exposed radiograph it may be difficult to appreciate the collapsed lobe behind the heart. Supplementary signs include inferior displacement of the left hilum, loss of volume and increased transradiancy of the left hemithorax. On the lateral view there is

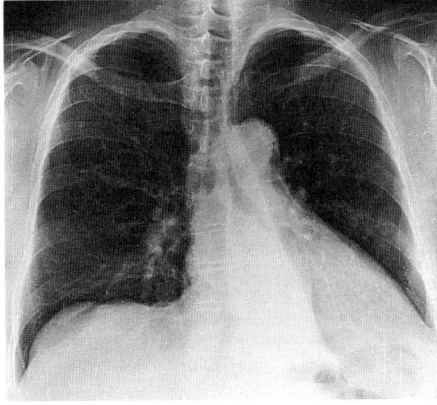

Fig. 18 Left lower lobe collapse (an AMBER chest radiograph which improves exposure in the mediastinal region).

posterior displacement of the major fissure. As with right lower lobe collapse, there is increased density over the lower dorsal vertebral column and the posterior part of the left hemidiaphragm is effaced.

Complete opacification (or a white-out) of a hemithorax is generally due to either collapse of a lung or a large pleural effusion or tumour. Shift of the mediastinum to the affected side implies that volume loss, that is to say collapse of the lung, has occurred. By contrast, a pleural effusion or soft tissue mass which is large enough to cause complete opacification of a hemithorax will almost invariably displace the mediastinum away from the side that is opacified. An important exception is an advanced mesothelioma which may encase one lung and 'freeze' the mediastinum and prevent a contralateral mediastinal shift. Occasionally, when there is no obvious shift of the mediastinum, it is surprisingly difficult to differentiate between these two completely different causes of an opacified hemithorax. In these instances, ultrasonography and computed tomography allow the distinction to be made with confidence and may give further information about the underlying disease.

Increased transradiancy of a hemithorax

There are many causes of an increased transradiancy (darkening) of one lung, ranging from a loss of soft tissues of the chest wall (for example, a mastectomy) through to reduced perfusion of one lung due to hypoxic vasoconstriction resulting from underventilation of the lung because of an inhaled foreign body, or a tumour in a main bronchus. It is surprisingly easy to overlook this important radiographic abnormality, especially when the density difference between the two lungs is slight. A subtle discrepancy in density between the two hemithoraces is more readily appreciated by viewing the radiograph from a distance of at least 1.5 metres. The commonest causes of a relatively transradiant hemithorax are shown in Table 3. Close scrutiny of the chest radiograph will usually indicate which one of the categories of causes is responsible for this radiographic sign. If there is any clinical suggestion that the cause of the increased transradiancy is due to an obstructing lesion in a central airway, a chest radiograph taken in full expiration will accentuate the increased transradiancy and will show that the lung fails to empty.

Once it has been established that the difference in density of the lungs is not due to a technical problem, for example rotation of the patient, points to look for are: (1) loss of symmetry of the soft tissues of the chest wall; (2) discrepancy in the volumes and vascular pattern between the two lungs; (3) a visceral pleural edge (denoting a pneumothorax). The identification of a pneumothorax on an erect chest radiograph is usually straightforward because of the appearance of the collapsed lung which is clearly demarcated by the fine edge of the visceral pleura. However, in the supine patient, such an edge is often not seen because air in the pleural space drifts anteriorly to the least dependent part of the chest. In this situation, a pneumothorax is only seen as a vague area of increased transradiancy over the lower zone of the chest. It is vital to recognize when the pressure of the air trapped in the

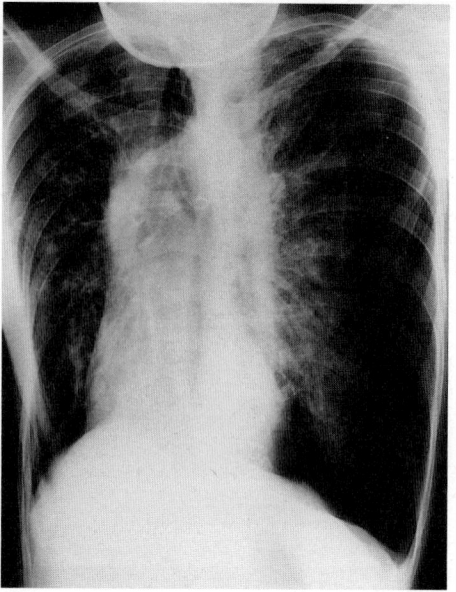

Fig. 19 A left-sided tension pneumothorax in a patient with cystic fibrosis. Note the mediastinal shift and straightening of the left hemidiaphragm.

pleural space exceeds alveolar pressure, a so-called tension pneumothorax. The typical signs are of a contralateral mediastinal shift with straightening and flattening of the ipsilateral dome of the diaphragm (Fig. 19).

The pulmonary mass

Many pulmonary masses are discovered incidentally on a chest radiograph. Whenever possible, previous films should be obtained so that the growth rate of the lesion can be estimated. The growth rate is a more reliable indicator of the likely nature of a pulmonary mass than any one of its radiographic features: if a lesion doubles in volume (increases in diameter by approximately 25 per cent on serial chest radiographs) in less than 1 week or more than 18 months, it is very unlikely to be malignant. The doubling time of most malignant lesions is between 1 and 6 months.

Over the years much importance has been attached to the radiological characteristics of a solitary pulmonary mass in an attempt to make the crucial distinction between benign and malignant lesions. With the possible exception of heavy calcification within the lesion (most commonly seen in ancient granulomas), no radiological appearance will reliably differentiate a benign from a malignant mass. Although generalizations can be made (for example, that bronchial carcinomas have irregular and spiculated margins, whereas benign lesions are more likely to have smooth outlines), in the individual patient it is not safe to rely on these radiographic features alone to make the distinction between a benign and malignant lesion.

After the discovery of a pulmonary mass on chest radiography, further imaging and other investigations of a patient will depend on the symptomatology, age, and smoking history of the patient. Computed tomography is valuable in evaluating extension of a central mass into the mediastinum (Fig. 20); for demonstrating the presence or absence of enlarged mediastinal lymph nodes, which may (but not invariably) indicate local tumour spread; and also for the detection of distant metastases, for example to the contralateral lung, adrenal glands, and liver. It is usually the overall pattern and extent of disease on a staging CT examination, rather than any single abnormality, which indicates whether a patient with bronchial carcinoma, who is otherwise fit, is likely to be suitable for surgical resection. Local invasion of the chest wall by an adjacent bronchial carcinoma is not always demonstrated by CT: MRI, because of its ability to image in different planes, may be useful. When surgery is not indicated and a histological diagnosis is needed, percutaneous needle biopsy of central lesions can be

Table 3 Causes of increased transradiancy of one hemithorax

Technical	Rotation of the patient
Chest wall	Loss of soft tissues, most commonly due to a mastectomy
Pneumothorax	Particularly in supine patients
Compensatory overinflation	Postlobectomy Overlooked lobar collapse (e.g. left lower lobe)
Reduced pulmonary perfusion	Hypoxic vasoconstriction due to underventilation caused by an inhaled foreign body or endobronchial tumour Following childhood viral infection (MacLeod's syndrome) Recurrent pulmonary emboli (rarely unilateral)

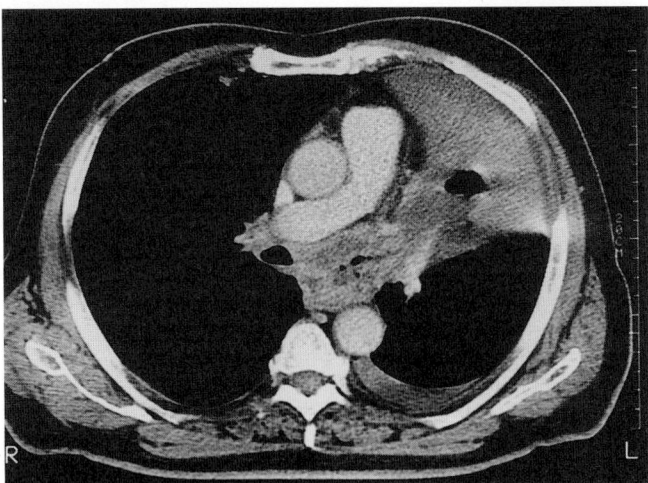

Fig. 20 Computed tomography of a central cavitating bronchial carcinoma showing direct extension of the tumour into the subcarinal region of the mediastinum.

performed safely under CT guidance. Similarly, smaller peripheral lesions that are not accessible by bronchoscopy may be biopsied under CT or, if abutting the pleura, ultrasound guidance.

Cavitating pulmonary lesions

The radiological definition of cavitation is a lucency, representing air, within a mass or area of consolidation. The cavity may or may not contain a fluid level or an intracavitary body, and is surrounded by a wall of variable thickness. The two most likely diagnoses in an adult presenting with a cavitating pulmonary mass on chest radiography are bronchial carcinoma (central, large, and often squamous in type) (Fig. 21) or a lung abscess (usually peripheral and sometimes multiple). Cavitation is recognized in a variety of bacterial pneumonias, particularly those due to tuberculosis, staphylococcus, anaerobes, and klebsiella infections. Less commonly, cavitation is seen within pulmonary infarcts and in areas of pulmonary contusion due to trauma. Long-standing cavities in lungs scarred by previous tuberculosis infection predispose to the formation of mycetomas; once these fungus balls occupy most of the cavity, a characteristic translucent 'air-crescent sign' may be seen between the upper surface of the fungus ball and the margin of the cavity on chest radiography (Fig. 22).

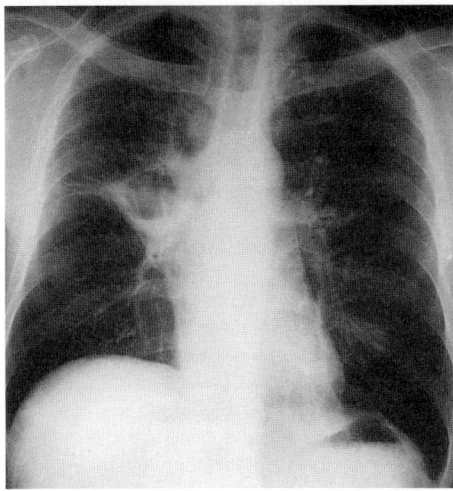

Fig. 21 Chest radiograph of a large cavitating squamous-cell bronchial carcinoma adjacent to the right hilum. The right hemidiaphragm is raised because of phrenic nerve invasion by the tumour.

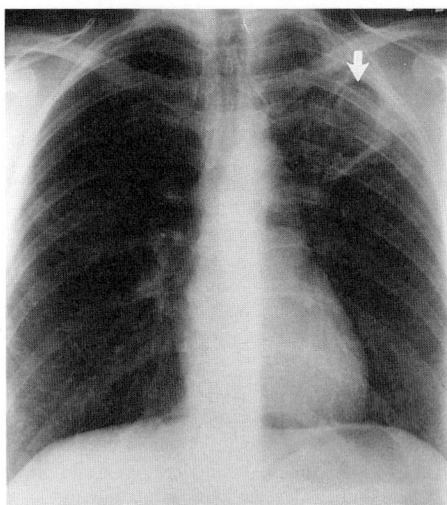

Fig. 22 An air crescent (arrow) around a fungus ball at the left apex. This had developed in a tuberculous fibrotic cavity.

Multiple pulmonary nodules

Many conditions are characterized by multiple small pulmonary nodules (Fig. 23). Only by combining the relevant clinical information with a precise description of the size and distribution of the nodules can the differential diagnosis be narrowed. In the United Kingdom, metastatic deposits are by far the commonest cause of multiple pulmonary nodules of varying sizes in an adult. In some parts of the southern United States, histoplasmosis is endemic and multiple granulomatous nodules are commoner than those due to disseminated malignancy. In the absence of a known malignancy and when clinical findings and laboratory investigations are inconclusive, biopsy of one of the nodules may be the only means of establishing a diagnosis.

A myriad of small nodules, less than 5 mm in diameter, produces a pattern which is often described as miliary. A list of causes of miliary shadowing is given in Table 4. An important diagnosis to consider in any patient with this radiographic pattern is miliary tuberculosis. Other differential diagnoses in an asymptomatic patient with numerous pulmonary nodules include sarcoidosis, metastatic disease, or, if there is a relevant occupational history, a pneumoconiosis. As always, comparison with previous radiographs will give invaluable information about the rate of progression and thus the likely nature of the pulmonary nodules. To a lesser extent the distribution of nodules is a consideration in refining the differential diagnosis

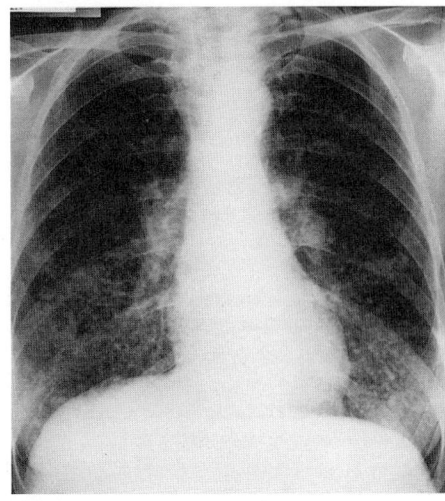

Fig. 23 Multiple pulmonary nodules of varying sizes typical of metastatic disease.

Table 4 Differential diagnosis of widespread fine nodular (0.5–3 mm diameter) shadowing

Miliary tuberculosis
Fungal diseases
Metastatic disease
Pneumoconiosis
Sarcoidosis
Extrinsic allergic alveolitis
Idiopathic pulmonary haemorrhage

of multiple pulmonary nodules: for example, the small nodules of pulmonary sarcoidosis tend to be mid-zone and perihilar, whereas haematogenous metastases are generally of varying sizes and have a predilection for the lower lobes (probably because of increased blood flow to these regions).

The density of nodules sometimes provides conclusive evidence that the nodules are of benign aetiology, for example the heavily calcified nodules which are seen following histoplasmosis or chickenpox (varicella) pneumonia. The majority of multiple pulmonary nodules are of soft tissue density, and it may be extremely difficult to judge whether small nodules are of calcific or soft tissue density because their apparent density depends so critically on the radiographic technique used.

Numerous poorly defined nodules of low density of approximately 8 mm in diameter may be seen around areas of pulmonary consolidation. In other areas they may be confluent and so make up a larger poorly defined opacity; occasionally these nodules will be uniformly distributed through out the lungs. At a pathological level these nodules correspond to individual acini which are full of the products of disease, such as pulmonary oedema, an inflammatory exudate, or haemorrhage.

Further reading

Armstrong P, *et al.* (2000). *Imaging of diseases of the chest*, 3rd edn. Mosby Year Book, St Louis.

Austin JHM, *et al.* (1996). Glossary of terms for CT of the lungs: recommendations of the Nomenclature Committee of the Fleischner Society. *Radiology* **200**, 327–31.

Engeler CE (200q). Interpreting the chest radiograph. In: Grainger RG, Allison DJ, Adam A, Dixon AK, eds. *Diagnostic radiology: a textbook of medical imaging*, 4th edn, pp. 303–14. Churchill Livingstone, Edinburgh.

Fleischner Society (1984). Glossary of terms for thoracic radiology: recommendations of the Nomenclature Committee of the Fleischner Society. *American Journal of Roentgenology* **143**, 509–17.

Goodman LR (1999). *Felson's principles of chest roentgenology*, 2nd edn. WB Saunders, Philadelphia.

Heitzmann ER (1988). *The mediastinum: radiologic correlations with anatomy and pathology*, 2nd edn. Springer-Verlag, Berlin.

Lowe VJ, Naunheim KS (1998). Current role of positron emission tomography in thoracic oncology. *Thorax* **53**, 703–12.

Mathieson JR, *et al.* (1989). Chronic diffuse infiltrative lung disease: comparison of diagnostic accuracy of CT and chest radiography. *Radiology* **171**, 111–16.

Müller NL (1991). Clinical value of high resolution CT in chronic diffuse lung disease. *American Journal of Roentgenology* **157**, 1163–70.

Naidich DP, *et al.* (1999). *Computed tomography and magnetic resonance of the thorax*, 3rd edn. Lippincott-Raven, Philadelphia.

Proto AV, Speckman JM (1979). *The left lateral radiograph of the chest. Medical Radiography and Photography* **56**, 38–64.

Rémy-Jardin M, Rémy J (1996). *Spiral CT of the chest*. Springer-Verlag, Berlin.

Webb RW, Müller NL, Naidich DP (2001). *High-resolution CT of the lung*, 3rd edn. Lippincott Williams and Wilkins, Philadelphia.

17.3.2 Respiratory function tests

G. J. Gibson

Scope of respiratory function tests

The clinical roles of respiratory function tests include diagnosis, assessment of severity, monitoring the effects of treatment, and assessing prognosis of various respiratory conditions. In the diagnosis of specific diseases, respiratory function tests, like functional tests of other organs, inevitably have limitations. Their use as a diagnostic tool is in recognizing that different patterns of abnormality characterize particular types of disease. More often they are used to quantify the severity of functional disturbance or to locate the likely anatomical site(s) of disease, such as airways, alveoli, or chest wall. The results should be compared with reference values obtained in healthy populations (see Appendix) and should always be evaluated in the light of clinical and radiographic information. The commonly applied tests are most conveniently classified as tests of (1) respiratory mechanics, (2) pulmonary gas exchange (and acid–base balance), and (3) exercise. Measurements made during sleep are described elsewhere (see Chapter 17.8.2).

Tests of respiratory mechanics

The volume of air in the lungs at the end of tidal expiration (functional residual capacity—**FRC**) represents the 'neutral' volume of the thorax, that is, the volume pertaining when the respiratory muscles are inactive (as during anaesthesia with muscle paralysis). Expansion of the lungs above FRC is achieved by contraction of the inspiratory muscles (predominantly the diaphragm), which results in a negative (subatmospheric) alveolar pressure. Normal resting tidal expiration is essentially passive with the driving force provided by elastic recoil of the lungs. The main expiratory muscles are those of the abdominal wall, contraction of which increases abdominal pressure which in turn is transmitted to the thorax. In health these muscles become active when ventilation is increased markedly, as on exercise, or during coughing, when a high intrathoracic pressure aids the clearance of airway secretions.

Measurements of tidal breathing (tidal volume, respiratory frequency) are rarely made in the resting awake subject, other than conventional recording of respiratory rate, which is part of clinical examination. Measurement of ventilation is of more importance in patients receiving ventilatory support (such as in intensive care units), during detailed exercise testing, and during sleep investigations. During exercise testing, ventilation is usually obtained by electrical integration of airflow measured at the mouth, but this approach is impracticable for prolonged monitoring (such as during sleep) and the application of a mouthpiece and nose clip may itself disturb the pattern of resting breathing. An alternative, less intrusive method is to measure external movement of the chest wall (rib cage and abdomen), but the estimates of ventilation obtained are at best semiquantitative.

In principle, the mechanical function of the respiratory system can be characterized by the compliance of the lungs and chest wall and the resistance of the airway. In practice, however, neither of these is commonly measured directly in clinical testing. Measurement of pulmonary compliance (an index of the 'stiffness' of the lungs) requires measurement of oesophageal pressure, which equates to pleural pressure and allows calculation of the pressure required to distend the lungs. In clinical investigation, the elastic properties of the lungs are usually inferred from measurements of lung volumes, because lungs which are unusually stiff and poorly compliant (as in pulmonary fibrosis) are usually shrunken and reduced in volume, while lungs with abnormally high compliance are easily distensible

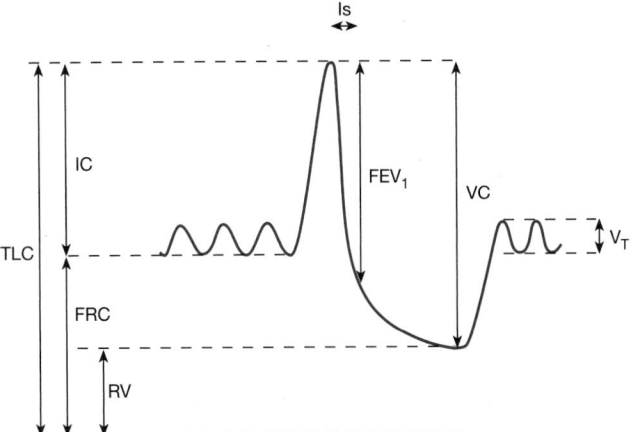

Fig. 1 Subdivisions of lung volume illustrated by spirometric recording of volume against time during tidal breathing for three breaths, followed my maximal inspiration and then maximal forced expiration, before returning to tidal breathing in a normal subject. RV, residual volume; FRC, functional residual capacity; IC, inspiratory capacity; TLC, total lung capacity; FEV_1, forced expiratory volume in 1 s; VC, vital capacity; V_T, tidal volume. Note that TLC = FRC + IC = VC + RV.

and are associated with increased total lung capacity (as in emphysema). The traditional subdivisions of lung volume are illustrated in Fig. 1.

Measurement of airway resistance requires estimation of the pressure difference along the airway—between the alveoli and mouth. The various techniques available for obtaining alveolar pressure include oesophageal pressure monitoring, body plethysmography, and transient interruption of airflow, with mouth pressure during occlusion taken to equal alveolar pressure. None of these is widely used in clinical testing. An alternative method, which has recently gained popularity, involves superimposition of a small oscillating pressure at the mouth during tidal breathing; the resulting pressure and flow information is used to calculate airway resistance. In practice, however, airway function is most commonly assessed by tests based on forced expiration.

Measurements of lung volume

A spirometer measures only the air which can be displaced from the lungs and does not give an indication of their absolute volume because the unmeasured residual volume (**RV**) remains in the lungs after full expiration. The vital capacity (**VC**) is the maximum volume expired after a full inspiration (or inspired after a full expiration) and the total lung capacity (**TLC**) represents the volume of air in the lungs after full inspiration— the sum of VC and RV (Fig. 1).

Two main clinical methods are used for measurement of absolute lung volume: inert gas dilution and whole body plethysmography. With the former, the subject breathes from a closed circuit a gas mixture containing an inert marker gas, usually helium. The helium equilibrates gradually with the gas in the lungs so that its concentration falls progressively and stabilizes once mixing is complete. In a healthy individual this occurs in 5 to 10 min, but in patients with diffuse airway disease such as asthma or chronic obstructive pulmonary disease (**COPD**), equilibration is much slower due to unequal ventilation, and the end point may be much less definite. The lung volume measured is that in the lungs when the subject was connected to the circuit (usually FRC). After disconnection from the rebreathing circuit the subject inspires fully and the volume inspired (inspiratory capacity, **IC**) added to FRC gives TLC (Fig. 1). With moderate or severe airway disease the uneven distribution of the inspired gas and poor mixing in the lungs results in underestimation of lung volumes.

In the alternative plethysmographic technique, the subject sits within a large air-tight chamber and makes gentle breathing efforts against a shutter, which closes the airway at the mouth. Since the pressure within the rigid

plethysmograph changes as lung volume changes according to Boyle's law (pressure × volume = a constant), this allows calculation of thoracic gas volume, from which total lung capacity and residual volume are derived by full inspiration and expiration immediately on opening the shutter. This method measures the volume of any air spaces within or without the lung which share pressure changes during breathing efforts, so that poorly ventilated (or even totally unventilated, such as a bulla) areas of lung are included.

Some increase in TLC occurs in most patients with symptomatic diffuse airway obstruction. A large increase is characteristic of emphysema but is not specific for this condition. Increases are seen in asthma, even when the condition is in relative remission. A pathological reduction in TLC occurs in several conditions (Table 1), not only lung diseases such as pulmonary fibrosis, but also extrapulmonary diseases affecting the pleura, thoracic skeleton, or respiratory muscles, conditions which all potentially impede full lung expansion.

Tests of forced expiration

The strengths of tests of forced expiration include the simplicity of both the manoeuvre and equipment required, and also the relative independence of the measurements on the effort applied by the patient. Forced expiratory tests are effort dependent to the extent that a preceding full inspiration is required, but during forced expiration the larger intrathoracic airways are subject to dynamic compression by the surrounding pleural pressure. The net result is that, provided a modest effort is applied, increasing the effort merely compresses the airway further and produces no increase in flow. This effort independence is more marked as forced expiration proceeds and is also more marked in patients with airway obstruction than in healthy subjects. At higher lung volumes (i.e. closer to full inflation), maximum expiratory flow is more dependent on effort. Since peak expiratory flow (**PEF**) is attained very rapidly at the start of forced expiration, it is more effort dependent than the forced expiratory volume in 1 s (**FEV1**), which effectively integrates flow over a large proportion of the volume range. PEF is measurable with a very simple peak flow meter which has the advantage of portability and is used routinely, particularly in asthma, to monitor respiratory function at home. Although more effort dependent, PEF is reproducible by most patients after a few practice efforts.

The most commonly used index of mechanical function of the lungs in hospital is the 1 s forced expiratory volume (FEV_1)—the volume expired forcefully in 1 s following complete inspiration (Fig. 1). This is usually obtained together with the forced vital capacity (**FVC**). In healthy subjects the FVC is effectively the same as VC, but in patients with airway disease the FVC is often appreciably less than the true ('relaxed') VC obtained when the subject is encouraged to expire completely without excessive initial effort.

The characteristic feature of diffuse airway obstruction is slowing of the rate of expiration so that the ratio of FEV_1 to FVC (or FEV_1 to VC) is reduced. This defines an 'obstructive' ventilatory defect as opposed to the 'restrictive' pattern in which both FEV_1 and FVC are reduced in approximate proportion. Although in patients with diffuse airway obstruction the FVC and VC are reduced, at least in patients with symptomatic disease, the

Table 1 Causes of reduced total lung capacity

Intrapulmonary	Surgical removal
	Pulmonary collapse
	Consolidation
	Pulmonary oedema
	Interstitial fibrosis
Extrapulmonary	Pleural effusion
	Pleural thickening
	Pneumothorax
	Rib cage deformity, e.g. scoliosis
	Respiratory muscle weakness
	Gross obesity

reduction is proportionally less than the reduction in FEV_1. The ratio of FEV_1 to FVC indicates the presence of airway obstruction but is a poor guide to severity, which is better assessed by comparing the FEV_1 alone with its predicted value. An obstructive spirometric pattern is seen in asthma, COPD, and bronchiectasis, while a restrictive spirometric pattern is seen in all those conditions which are also associated with a reduced TLC (Table 1). A further feature of diffuse airway obstruction is an increase in RV and in the ratio RV/TLC, but this is less specific than the spirometric pattern as it also occurs in some patients with cardiac disease or with respiratory muscle weakness. With dual pathology, combined obstructive (low FEV_1/VC) and restrictive (low TLC) defects are seen. Sometimes in this situation total lung capacity may be within the normal range due to opposing influences with, for example, lung fibrosis tending to shrink the lungs and airway obstruction tending to produce hyperinflation.

Spirometric measurements such as FEV_1 are less sensitive to localized narrowing of the central airway than to the diffuse airway narrowing of COPD or asthma. If upper airway obstruction is suspected, it is helpful to visualize the information obtained during forced expiration (and also inspiration) in a different manner as the maximum flow–volume curves, which relate instantaneous flow to volume expired and inspired (Fig. 2). The expiratory curve has a characteristic shape with an early peak (equivalent to the PEF obtained with a peak flow meter). Maximum expiratory flow then declines progressively as volume is expired. In young healthy subjects (Fig. 2(a)), the descending limb of the curve approximates a straight line, whilst in older normal subjects (Fig. 2(b)), maximum expiratory flow decreases, particularly at lower lung volumes so that the curve appears concave. In patients with diffuse intrathoracic airway obstruction (such as COPD or asthma) this ageing appearance is greatly exaggerated so that expiratory flow is reduced more markedly as lung volume declines (Fig. 2(d)). The shape of the flow–volume curve does not distinguish between different causes of diffuse airway narrowing, that is, it does not allow the distinction of asthma from COPD or emphysema.

The maximum inspiratory flow–volume curve has a more symmetrical appearance than the expiratory curve. In patients with diffuse airway narrowing there is an overall reduction in inspiratory flow, but little change in

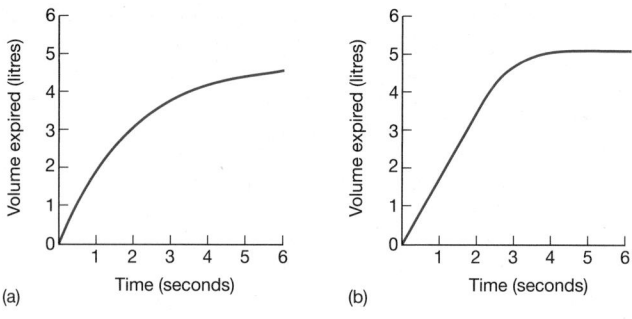

Fig. 3 Spirograms of two patients with airway obstruction and similar FEV_1. (a) Diffuse intrathoracic airway narrowing (COPD or asthma). Note that forced expiration is continuing after 6 s. (b) Upper airway narrowing with 'straight' spirogram which corresponds to plateau of flow in earlier part of expiration.

shape (Fig. 2(d)). In patients with a restrictive ventilatory defect caused, for example, by pulmonary fibrosis, the volume displaced (FVC) is reduced but absolute flows are little affected (Fig. 2(c)).

Characteristic flow–volume curves are seen in patients with localized narrowing of the proximal airway, with the pattern depending on whether the narrowing is extra- or intrathoracic. Extrathoracic narrowing (Fig. 2(e)), such as occurs with subglottic tracheal stenosis or tracheal tumours, has a relatively greater effect on inspiratory than expiratory flow (which corresponds to the predominantly inspiratory timing of the stridor of upper airway narrowing). It also affects maximum expiratory flow but (unlike COPD or asthma) the effects are most marked at higher lung volumes, often producing a virtual 'plateau' of expiratory flow in the first part of forced expiration. If, on the other hand, the central airway is narrowed within the thorax (for example the lower trachea, carina) a similar plateau of expiratory flow, often with a small initial peak, may be seen, but maximum inspiratory flow is less affected than with narrowing of the extrathoracic airway (Fig. 2(f)). These patterns of abnormality of maximum flow can be quantified in terms of various ratios, such as the ratio of maximum expiratory to inspiratory flow at 50 per cent VC, or the ratio of PEF (markedly reduced with upper airway obstruction) to FEV_1 (proportionally less reduced). Usually, however, it is essential to visualize the curves and interpret such derived indices in the light of the overall contour.

The 'plateau' of maximum expiratory flow over a significant proportion of the FVC which occurs with upper airway obstruction has implications for the shape of the more commonly recorded forced expiratory spirogram in this situation. Since flow on the spirogram (relation of volume to time) is given by the instantaneous gradient of the curve, a plateau on the flow–volume curve implies a 'straight' (rectilinear) spirogram over the same volume range. This appearance should therefore alert the investigator to the likelihood of narrowing of the central airway rather than the more common diffuse airway obstruction seen with asthma and COPD (Fig. 3).

Respiratory muscle function

The simplest method of measuring respiratory muscle strength is for the subject to perform forcible static inspiratory and expiratory efforts against a closed airway. This provides values of maximum expiratory and inspiratory pressures (*P*Emax, *P*Imax). In general the expiratory (predominantly abdominal) muscles perform most effectively at high lung volumes and the inspiratory muscles (predominantly the diaphragm) at lower volumes. $P_E$max is therefore usually measured after full inspiration and $P_I$max at either FRC or RV. Unfortunately the normal ranges for these tests are wide and some subjects find difficulty in performing the manoeuvres (which are, of course, by definition completely effort dependent). An alternative method for assessing inspiratory muscle strength is by making the measurement during a forceful sniff, with the pressure measured in the nose via an occluded nostril (sniff nasal inspiratory pressure—SNIP). Many

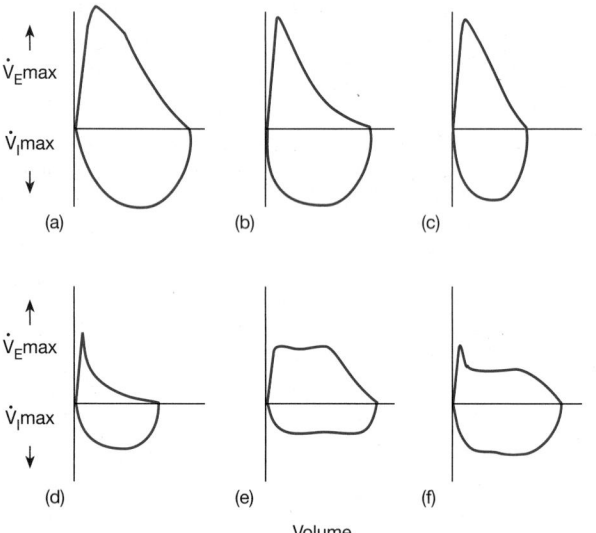

Fig. 2 Schematic maximum expiratory and inspiratory flow–volume curves in: (a) normal young adult; (b) normal older adult; (c) patient with fibrosing alveolitis and reduced FVC; (d) patient with moderately severe COPD showing markedly reduced V̇Emax, particularly at lower lung volumes; (e) patient with subglottic (extrathoracic) tracheal stenosis showing markedly reduced V̇Imax at all volumes and reduced V̇Emax at higher volumes; (f) patient with central intrathoracic (carinal) tracheal narrowing showing similar plateaus of flow to (e) but greater reduction of V̇Emax than of V̇Imax.

patients find this easier than performing maximum static manoeuvres so that the sniff technique tends to give more reproducible results.

These measurements all assess the global strength of the inspiratory or expiratory muscles. More specific information on diaphragmatic function requires measurement of transdiaphragmatic pressure using pressure sensing devices in both oesophagus and stomach, a specialized investigation available in only a few centres. A simple indirect index of disproportionate diaphragmatic weakness or paralysis is a large (more than 25 per cent) reduction in VC in the supine compared with the erect posture. However, isolated bilateral diaphragmatic paralysis or severe weakness is very unusual and most patients with respiratory muscle weakness have disease affecting all the muscles. The causes include not only primary neuromuscular diseases such as myopathies, muscular dystrophy, motor neurone disease, and myasthenia gravis, but also drug treatment (corticosteroids), several endocrine and connective tissue disorders, and cachexia from whatever cause. Respiratory muscle weakness is often an important factor preventing weaning from assisted ventilation.

Measurements of respiratory muscle function are indicated in evaluation of patients with various neuromuscular diseases. They are also helpful in confirming or excluding muscle problems in those with otherwise unexplained dyspnoea and in patients with a restrictive ventilatory defect in whom the cause of the lung volume reduction is not apparent on clinical and radiographic grounds. Interpretation of results may be complicated in patients with airway obstruction (such as COPD or asthma) because the associated hyperinflation of the lungs (increased FRC) itself impairs inspiratory muscle function simply because of the distorted thoracic mechanics. Consequently an apparently impaired maximum inspiratory pressure in such patients may not necessarily reflect true muscle weakness. Maximum expiratory pressure is not significantly affected by hyperinflation, however, and can be used as a guide to the presence of true muscle weakness in this situation.

Tests of pulmonary gas exchange

Carbon monoxide uptake

Carbon monoxide (CO) diffusing capacity or transfer factor (TL_{CO}) is used widely as a simple test of the integrity of the alveolar capillary membrane and of the overall gas exchanging function of the lungs. It has good sensitivity but poor specificity, as impairment can result from a variety of pathological processes (Table 2). The subject takes a full inspiration of a gas mixture containing a very low concentration of CO and the rate of uptake

Table 2 Causes of reduced carbon monoxide (CO) transfer factor

Pulmonary diseases	COPD/emphysema*
	Asthma (severe airway obstruction)
	Pneumonectomy
Systemic diseases	Pulmonary fibrosis*
	Sarcoidosis
	Pulmonary vascular disease*
Extrapulmonary conditions	Pleural disease
	Rib cage deformity
	Respiratory muscle weakness
Cardiac diseases	Pulmonary oedema*
	Mitral valve disease*
	Congenital right to left shunts*
Systemic diseases	Anaemia*
	Renal failure*
	Hepatic cirrhosis*
	Rheumatoid disease
	Systemic sclerosis*
	Systemic lupus*

COPD, chronic obstructive pulmonary disease.

* K_{CO} usually also reduced.

Table 3 Conditions producing increased TL_{CO} and K_{CO}

	↑ TL_{CO}	↑ K_{CO}
Asthma	Sometimes	+
Pneumonectomy	–	+
Extrapulmonary restriction:		
pleural disease	–	+
rib cage deformity	–	+
respiratory muscle weakness	–	+
Left to right shunts	+	+
Polycythaemia	+	+
Lung haemorrhage	+*	+*

*May be an increase from an initially reduced value (e.g. Goodpasture's syndrome).

of gas is measured during breath holding for 10 s. The test was introduced originally as a method of assessing diffusion of gas across the alveolar capillary membrane, but thickening of the diffusion pathway for carbon monoxide in disease is quantitatively less important than other mechanisms, the most important factor being the effective surface area of alveoli available for gas exchange. Consequently TL_{CO} is reduced when this area is diminished, for example after resection of lung or with widespread emphysema, in which normal alveoli are replaced by much larger air spaces. TL_{CO} is also reduced when there is loss of the 'effective' alveolar volume (V_A). The latter is measured simultaneously from the dilution of helium which is also included in the test breath. The 'effective' V_A is reduced if there is maldistribution of ventilation as this causes some alveoli to receive little or none of the inspired gas. Other factors affecting the TL_{CO} include the availability of haemoglobin and disease of the pulmonary capillaries.

The transfer coefficient (K_{CO}), which is obtained along with the TL_{CO}, represents the uptake of CO per litre of 'effective' alveolar volume, that is, $K_{CO} = TL_{CO} / V_A$. To a large extent, K_{CO} allows correction for any real or effective reduction of alveolar volume, tending to be normal after lung resection, when both TL_{CO} and V_A are reduced approximately to the same degree. K_{CO} is usually normal (or even mildly increased) in asthma, where any reduction in TL_{CO} is due only to maldistribution of ventilation secondary to airway narrowing. By contrast, in widespread emphysema, TL_{CO} is reduced due not only to maldistribution of inspired gas, but also because the gas exchanging surface area is diminished even in the relatively better ventilated parts of the lung. Consequently, there is an associated reduction in K_{CO}. Diseases associated with reductions in TL_{CO} and K_{CO} are listed in Table 2.

In some conditions K_{CO} and, less commonly, TL_{CO} may increase (Table 3). The latter usually results from an increase in red blood cells in the lungs due to greater blood flow, haemorrhage, or polycythaemia. K_{CO} is similarly increased in these conditions, as it is if, at full inflation, the density of pulmonary capillaries per unit alveolar volume is greater than normal. This occurs most commonly in patients with extrapulmonary volume restriction, when the density of pulmonary capillaries is unusually high in relation to the (restricted) lung volume at which the measurement is made.

Arterial blood gases

The primary measurements made by modern blood gas analysers are the arterial partial pressures of oxygen (Pa_{O_2}) and carbon dioxide (Pa_{CO_2}), and pH. The alternative commonly used method of assessing oxygenation is by pulse oximetry, which estimates arterial oxygen saturation (Sa_{O_2}). An oximeter has the advantage of allowing continuous monitoring but it provides no information on P_{CO_2}. The general relation between oxygen pressure and saturation is defined by the oxygen–haemoglobin dissociation curve (Fig. 4). The position of this curve is influenced by the prevailing pH, temperature, and P_{CO_2}. In addition, several rare abnormal variants of the haemoglobin molecule cause the curve to shift either to the right (reduced oxygen affinity) or the left (increased affinity). Approximate values for normal arterial and resting mixed venous P_{O_2} and saturation are shown in

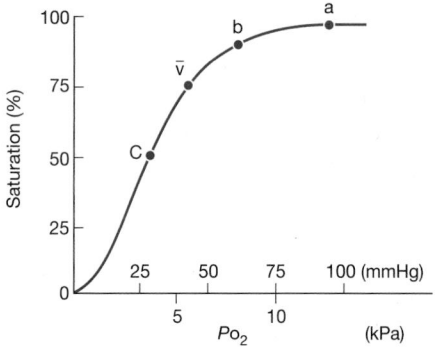

Fig. 4 Normal haemoglobin–oxygen dissociation curve relating saturation to P_{O_2}. Point a represents normal arterial values (P_{O_2} 90 mmHg, 12 kPa; S_{aO_2} 98 per cent) and v̄ normal resting mixed venous values ($P_{\bar{v}O_2}$ 40 mmHg, 5.3 kPa; S_{aO_2} 75 per cent). Also shown are the P_{O_2} (~ 60 mmHg, 8 kPa) corresponding to 90 per cent saturation (point b) and the P_{50} (point c), i.e. P_{O_2} corresponding to 50 per cent saturation (~ 27 mmHg, 3.5 kPa).

Fig. 4. Another clinically useful 'landmark' is a saturation of 90 per cent which, with a normally positioned curve, represents a P_{O_2} of approximately 8 kPa (60 mmHg). Also shown in Fig. 4 is the P_{50}, that is, the P_{O_2} at a saturation of 50 per cent, which for normal adult haemoglobin is approximately 3.5 kPa (27 mmHg). This is essentially an *in vitro* measurement which is used to characterize abnormal haemoglobin molecules associated with increased (low P_{50}) or decreased (high P_{50}) affinity for oxygen.

A reduction in P_{aO_2} can occur by various mechanisms (Table 4). In disease, the commonest is mismatching of alveolar ventilation ($\dot{V}_A$) and perfusion ($\dot{Q}$). Even in healthy lungs, distribution of both ventilation and perfusion is uneven. In normal subjects this results mainly from the effects of gravity. In the upright posture, both ventilation and perfusion increase towards the lung bases, but the effects on perfusion are relatively greater, so that the ratio of ventilation to perfusion ($\dot{V}_A/\dot{Q}$) is higher towards the apices and lower towards the bases. In disease, these relatively small gravitational effects are outweighed by unevenly distributed pathological changes affecting the distribution of ventilation or perfusion or both. Alveoli with greater than average $\dot{V}_A/\dot{Q}$ have higher than average local P_{O_2} and lower P_{CO_2}, that is, closer to those of inspired air. Conversely, those with lower than average $\dot{V}_A/\dot{Q}$ have lower P_{O_2} and higher P_{CO_2}, that is, closer to the values in mixed venous (pulmonary arterial) blood. The gas tensions in the draining pulmonary capillaries essentially reflect those of the alveoli which they subtend as, within a single alveolus, complete equilibration of local gas tensions usually occurs. For CO_2 the effects of high $\dot{V}_A/\dot{Q}$ and low $\dot{V}_A/\dot{Q}$ areas on the final arterial value approximately cancel each other out, that is, the P_{aCO_2} is close to the average value in all the capillaries draining the alveoli with a variety of local P_{CO_2} values. However, for oxygen the situation is different as blood draining alveoli with high $\dot{V}_A/\dot{Q}$ (and relatively high local P_{O_2}) cannot compensate for the areas with low $\dot{V}_A/\dot{Q}$ (and low P_{O_2}) because of the shape of the oxygen dissociation curve. The relatively flat upper part of the curve means that increasing P_{O_2} adds very little to oxygen saturation and therefore to oxygen concentration. Consequently, mixed pulmonary ven-

ous (and therefore systemic arterial) blood has an appreciably lower P_{O_2} than would be found in mixed alveolar air.

An approximate assessment of the overall effects of $\dot{V}_A/\dot{Q}$ mismatching on arterial oxygenation and P_{aO_2} is given by calculation of the alveolar to arterial oxygen pressure gradient ($P(A-a)_{O_2} = P_{AO_2} - P_{aO_2}$). This requires estimation of the average alveolar P_{O_2} (P_{AO_2}) which is determined by the inspired P_{O_2} (P_{IO_2}) and the average alveolar P_{CO_2} (P_{ACO_2}). For the reasons discussed above, alveolar and arterial P_{CO_2} (unlike P_{O_2}) are virtually the same and the alveolar P_{O_2} is given simply by:

$$P_{AO_2} = P_{IO_2} - P_{aCO_2}/0.8$$

The P_{IO_2} breathing room air at sea level is 20 kPa (150 mmHg). In normal young subjects the upper limit for $P(A-a)_{O_2}$ is 2.5 kPa. It rises with age and in healthy subjects aged 60 to 70 years may be up to 4.7 kPa (35 mmHg). Unfortunately interpretation of the $P(A-a)_{O_2}$ is complicated by the fact that its relation to the severity of $\dot{V}_A/\dot{Q}$ mismatching is not constant. For a given degree of $\dot{V}_A/\dot{Q}$ mismatching, the $P(A-a)_{O_2}$ increases as the alveolar P_{O_2} increases. It therefore increases if the inspired oxygen is increased or if P_{aCO_2} falls (see Equation 1).

Alternative indices which relate more predictably to the degree of $\dot{V}_A/\dot{Q}$ mismatching are the ratios of arterial to alveolar P_{O_2} (a/A P_{O_2}) and of arterial P_{O_2} to the inspired oxygen fraction (P_{aO_2}/F_{IO_2}). The former is normally greater than 0.75 and changes little as F_{IO_2} increases, whereas the more traditional $P(A-a)_{O_2}$ difference increases. The ratio of P_{aO_2}/F_{IO_2} is widely used in assessment of patients with severe problems of oxygenation. For example, in acute lung injury a value greater than 300 (P_{aO_2} in mmHg, F_{IO_2} as a fraction) indicates relatively mild hypoxaemia, whilst a value of less than 100 represents very severe disturbance of gas exchange.

The dependence of $P(A-a)_{O_2}$ on inspired oxygen is exemplified by the effects of breathing pure oxygen. This is used as a test for the presence of anatomical right to left shunting, since the effects of $\dot{V}_A/\dot{Q}$ mismatching on P_{aO_2} are effectively eliminated by breathing pure oxygen. Even in diseased lungs, nitrogen is gradually 'washed out' of all the alveoli and the only remaining cause of arterial hypoxaemia is the anatomical shunt via channels which bypass the lungs, or through the capillaries supplying any alveoli which are totally unventilated. Although prolonged breathing of 100 per cent oxygen may itself encourage alveolar atelectasis which would exaggerate the shunt, in practice the technique is useful in investigation of causes of hypoxaemia. The usually quoted normal upper limit for the 'anatomical' shunt measured in this way is 5 per cent of the cardiac output. In terms of the P_{aO_2}, a value greater than 500 mmHg (more than 73 kPa) is usually achieved, representing a $P(A-a)_{O_2}$ of more than 100 mmHg, which greatly exceeds the normal upper limit when breathing room air. At these levels of P_{aO_2} haemoglobin is virtually fully saturated with oxygen and increasing the P_{aO_2} above 200 to 300 mmHg results in greater oxygen carriage by simple solution only. Consequently, increases in oxygen content and P_{O_2} become linearly related on the 'flat' part of the dissociation curve. As a rule of thumb, with a P_{aO_2} greater than 300 mmHg, each 20 mmHg of $P(A-a)_{O_2}$ represents an anatomical shunt of 1 per cent.

Respiratory failure

Respiratory failure is defined conventionally in terms of the arterial blood gas tensions as a reduction in P_{aO_2} below 8 kPa (60 mmHg) at sea level, either without ('type I') or with ('type II') CO_2 retention. Hypercapnic (type II) respiratory failure is also known as ventilatory failure. The causes of type I respiratory failure are legion and include virtually all diseases which can affect the alveoli or the airways, either primarily or secondarily (as in cardiac failure). Hypercapnic (type II) respiratory failure is most commonly due to severe chronic airway disease and less often to reduced ventilation as, for example, with severe respiratory muscle weakness or scoliosis. The mechanisms of elevation of P_{aCO_2} in type II respiratory failure are twofold. Sustained 'pure' hypoventilation, that is, a reduction in overall ventilation resulting in hypercapnia, is rare. It is seen with inadequate performance of the respiratory 'bellows', for example in neuromuscular disease or because of reduced drive to breathe in the unconscious

Table 4 Mechanisms of arterial hypoxaemia

Mechanism	Cause
Low inspired P_{O_2}	Altitude (including air travel)
Hypoventilation	Neuromuscular diseases
	Drugs depressing ventilatory drive
$\dot{V}_A/\dot{Q}$ mismatching	All pulmonary diseases
Anatomical shunt	Intracardiac right to left shunt
	Pulmonary arteriovenous malformations
Limitation of oxygen diffusion	Pulmonary fibrosis (on exercise)

Table 5 Acid–base disturbances

Arterial	pH	Pa_{CO_2}	$[HCO_3^-]$
Respiratory acidosis:			
acute	↓↓	↑	↑
chronic	↓	↑	↑↑
Respiratory alkalosis	↑	↓	↓
Metabolic acidosis	↓	↓	↓
Metabolic alkalosis	↑	↑ or →	↑

subject. Much more commonly in chronic airway disease, the 'effective' alveolar ventilation is reduced as a consequence of mismatching of ventilation and perfusion. In this situation there is often a considerable amount of ineffectual or wasted ventilation ('physiological dead space') and consequently in such patients the total ventilation is often greater than normal, even in the presence of hypercapnia.

Acid–base balance

The carriage of CO_2 by the blood and its excretion by the lungs constitute one of the two homeostatic mechanisms for regulating the acid–base status of the body. Because of the ease with which CO_2 excretion can normally be increased, the lungs are able to adjust acid–base balance much more rapidly than the kidneys.

The concentrations of hydrogen ions, bicarbonate, and carbonic acid in the blood are linked inevitably by the carbonic acid association/dissociation equation:

$$CO_2 + H_2O \leftrightharpoons H_2CO_3 \rightleftharpoons H^+ + HCO_3^-$$

This defines the chemical relation between the three variables, pH, Pco_2, and $[HCO_3^-]$ and if two are measured, the third is readily calculated. Abnormal acid–base disturbances are classified in terms of these variables as one of four classic types (Table 5 and Fig. 5), but combined disturbances are frequently seen. The commoner causes of acid–base disturbance are given in Table 6.

Respiratory acidosis and alkalosis

In respiratory acidosis the prime event is accumulation of CO_2 due to inadequate or ineffective ventilation. This causes the equilibrium of Equation 2 to shift to the right, generating both hydrogen and bicarbonate ions. The immediate increase in bicarbonate concentration is dictated by this chemical relationship and not by the physiological response, which occurs later. The vast majority of hydrogen ions produced are buffered by proteins with the result that the measured rise in $[HCO_3^-]$ is actually very much greater than the measured increase in hydrogen ion concentration. (The logarithmic pH scale is deceptive in that both the hydrogen ion concentration in the blood and the changes which occur in disease are extremely small. For example, a normal pH of 7.4 represents a $[H^+]$ of 40×10^{-9} mol, whereas $[HCO_3^-]$ is measured to 10^{-3} mol, i.e. the hydrogen ion concentration is approximately 1 millionth of the concentration of bicarbonate). Conventionally the effects of acute respiratory acidosis are distinguished from the 'chronic' respiratory acidosis which results after several hours or days. This follows renal retention of even more bicarbonate, which in turn tends to correct the pH towards normal (Fig. 5).

In respiratory alkalosis the primary event is an increase in CO_2 excretion resulting from increased ventilation, so that both $[HCO_3^-]$ and hydrogen ion concentrations fall (pH rises). Again, most of the reduction in hydrogen ion concentration is buffered. It is less useful to distinguish acute and chronic respiratory alkalosis than it is to distinguish acute and chronic forms of respiratory acidosis.

Metabolic acidosis and alkalosis

In metabolic acidosis, $[H^+]$ rises (pH falls) and $[HCO_3^-]$ falls. The physiological response is so rapid that acute and chronic phases are not distin-

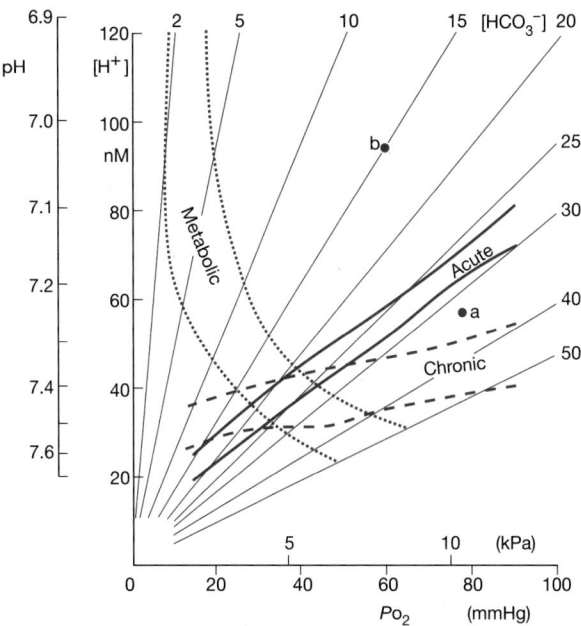

Fig. 5 Relations of pH and $[H^+]$ to Pco_2 in acid–base disorders. Bands indicate the expected ranges in uncomplicated respiratory disorders (acute and chronic) and in metabolic acidosis and alkalosis. Isopleths represent corresponding estimates of arterial $[HCO_3^-]$ (mmol/l). Values outside these bands indicate intermediate or combined disturbances. For example: patient a with an acute exacerbation of COPD has an 'acute on chronic' respiratory acidosis (Pco_2 10.6 kPa, pH 7.24, $[HCO_3^-]$ 34 mmol); patient b with both respiratory and circulatory failure has a combined respiratory and metabolic acidosis (Pco_2 8 kPa, pH 7.04, $[HCO_3^-]$ 15 mmol).

guishable. Any tendency for Pco_2 to rise (equilibrium of Equation 2 shifted to the left) is more than offset by the increased drive to breathe resulting from production of acid, and the measured effect is a reduction in Pco_2.

In metabolic alkalosis there is an increase in $[HCO_3^-]$ and a reduction in $[H^+]$ (pH increases). The measured result is somewhat variable as opposing influences are involved; any increase in Pco_2 tends to stimulate breathing but the reduced acidity tends to inhibit it. In subjects with healthy lungs, the net effect is often maintenance of Pco_2 in the high normal range, unless the alkalosis is profound (as, for example, is seen with pyloric stenosis and severe depletion of acid). However, in patients with chronic airway disease and either pre-existing or incipient hypercapnia, a more marked increase in Pco_2 is frequently seen. This is particularly relevant to patients with COPD receiving treatment with diuretics and corticosteroids, both of which tend to produce a metabolic alkalosis.

Several other indices of acid–base status have their advocates. Standard bicarbonate, base excess and deficit, and total buffer base are often derived when blood gases are measured by automated equipment. They are obtained by titration of the blood *in vitro* to specified standard values of pH and/or Pco_2. As such, they are open to the very real objection that the results differ from those which would be obtained if the same titration could be performed *in vivo*, where the extracellular fluid, and not just the blood, participates in buffering. Indices such as standard bicarbonate and base excess are used mainly to distinguish 'respiratory' and 'metabolic' components of an acid–base disturbance, but in this context the 'metabolic' component includes renal compensation for a primary respiratory disturbance. Consequently, in a respiratory acidosis an increased standard bicarbonate indicates some degree of chronicity.

Table 6 Commoner causes of acid–base disturbances

Disturbance	Cause
Respiratory acidosis	
Cerebral	Drugs (sedatives, hypnotics, anaesthetics)
	Raised intracranial pressure
	Primary alveolar hypoventilation (very rare)
Spinal cord	Trauma
Motor neurones	Motor neurone disease, poliomyelitis
Peripheral nerves	Guillain–Barré syndrome etc.
Motor end plate	Myasthenia gravis, neuromuscular blocking agents
Respiratory muscles	Myopathies, dystrophies etc.
Rib cage	Scoliosis, trauma, thoracoplasty
Lung parenchyma	ARDS, pulmonary oedema (severe), interstitial fibrosis (very advanced)
Airways	COPD, asthma (severe), upper airway obstruction (very severe)
Respiratory alkalosis	
Cerebral	Anxiety, central neurogenic hyperventilation (very rare), drugs (aspirin)
Pulmonary	Pulmonary fibrosis etc., pneumonia, pulmonary embolism, asthma, pulmonary oedema
Iatrogenic	Mechanical overventilation
Metabolic acidosis	
Increased anion gap	Ketoacidosis, uraemia, lactic acidosis, drugs (aspirin)
Normal anion gap	Renal tubular acidosis, severe diarrhoea
Metabolic alkalosis	
Severe vomiting	Pyloric stenosis etc
Iatrogenic	Diuretics, corticosteroids, bicarbonate infusion

ARDS, adult respiratory distress syndrome; COPD, chronic obstructive pulmonary disease.

One further frequently available index of acid–base status is the venous 'bicarbonate' (strictly total CO_2 content) which is often obtained routinely when electrolytes are measured. A raised value is seen with primary metabolic alkalosis, but in patients with respiratory disease it may be a useful clue to unsuspected ventilatory failure.

Exercise testing

Exercise tests allow observation of patients and their performance at a time when symptoms are present. This can be useful in assessing breathlessness as the meaning of the term varies among patients: to some it means excessive ventilation, to others difficulty in breathing because of airway narrowing, while some interpret the sensation of myocardial ischaemia as breathlessness. Formal quantification of exercise performance also provides objective assessment of disability and an exercise test may give useful information on the likely factors limiting exercise in that individual.

In healthy subjects, ventilation and cardiac output increase progressively with oxygen consumption. Oxygen uptake ($\dot{V}O_2$) increases with work rate, but at high levels of exercise anaerobic respiration increases with generation of lactate. Initially, CO_2 output increases in proportion to oxygen consumption until increasing anaerobic metabolism results in disproportionate production of CO_2. Measurement of an 'anaerobic threshold' is favoured by some investigators, but the criteria used for its identification are not universally agreed.

The maximum oxygen consumption or maximum aerobic capacity of a healthy subject is determined by the ability of the circulation to supply oxygen to exercising muscle, rather than by the maximum ventilation which can be achieved. In patients with pulmonary disease, particularly airway disease, the maximum attainable ventilation is reduced, approximately in proportion to the abnormality of pulmonary mechanics. This may then determine exercise capacity, although circulatory factors and deconditioning also contribute in many patients and dominate in some.

Exercise tests vary considerably in complexity and in the number and types of measurements made. Simple self-paced tests of walking distance, most commonly in 6 min, aim to mimic the real life situation and are widely used for global assessment of disability. However, such tests are insensitive to mild disease and there is a significant learning effect, as well as dependence on motivation and encouragement. In the shuttle walk test the subject increases his walking speed each minute, giving results which are more reproducible and closer to laboratory-based tests of maximum performance. More formal testing involves exercise on a bicycle ergometer or treadmill. Usually the workload is increased by a constant amount, with periods of 1 to 3 min at each level. Measurements include heart rate, ventilation, and gas exchange ($\dot{V}O_2$ and $\dot{V}CO_2$) and oxygen saturation by pulse oximetry. The subject exercises at increasing loads until no longer able to continue because of discomfort, or until stopped by the investigator. The maximum oxygen consumption (symptom limited $\dot{V}O_2$max) is a useful indicator of overall exercise capacity. Comparison of the maximum ventilation and heart rate at the end of progressive exercise with those predicted from spirometric measurements and age, respectively, gives some indication of the likely factor(s) limiting performance. The level of breathlessness at each workload in an incremental test can also be usefully assessed using simple self-rating scales (visual analogue scale or Borg scale). Arterial oxygen desaturation is seen particularly in interstitial lung disease and pulmonary vascular disease and this may be helpful in predicting which patients are likely to benefit from use of ambulatory oxygen.

A common reason for performing an exercise test is to evaluate the main cause of breathlessness and, in particular, to determine whether this is due predominantly to cardiac or ventilatory abnormalities. If a patient achieves the predicted maximum heart rate during a progressive test (as is seen in normal subjects), it is reasonable to conclude that the limit to further exercise is set by the cardiovascular system. In most respiratory diseases, patients cease exercise with a lower heart rate as more often the limit is set by the maximum ventilation achievable.

The identification of exercise-induced asthma has rather different requirements. During exercise, most subjects with asthma show some degree of bronchodilatation, and in those who develop exercise-induced asthma, bronchoconstriction develops after exercise. Many patients with asthma, of course, become breathless during exercise, but this is not necessarily due to bronchoconstriction. The intensity of exercise necessary to provoke asthma is relatively high and for this reason exercise-induced asthma is relevant mainly to children and young adults. Optimally it is demonstrated after exercise for at least 5 min at a constant rate, chosen to increase ventilation to around 50 per cent maximal or to increase heart rate to around 80 per cent maximal. FEV_1 or peak flow should be measured beforehand and for up to 30 min afterwards.

Miscellaneous tests

Analysis of expired air has traditionally been limited to oxygen and carbon dioxide, but recently attention has turned to other gases which are present in very low concentrations. The concentration of exhaled carbon monoxide has been used for some years as a guide to its inhalation and as a valuable method for confirming non-smoking claims. The measurement can now be made very simply with a portable analyser. Breath carbon monoxide is also increased in non-smoking subjects with asthma, where it appears to be released as a result of airway inflammation. In similar fashion, expired nitric oxide concentration is increased as a consequence of airway inflammation and it has been proposed as a non-invasive way of assessing airway inflammation and its treatment, particularly in those with asthma. Care needs to be taken to avoid contamination of expired air from the bronchial

Table 7

Variable	Unit	Regression equation	RSD	1.64RSD
		Men		
FVC	l	$5.76H - 0.026A - 4.34$	0.61	1.00
TLC	l	$7.99 - 7.08$	0.70	1.15
RV	l	$1.31H + 0.022A - 1.23$	0.41	0.67
FRC	l	$2.34H + 0.009A - 1.09$	0.6	0.99
RV/TLC	%	$0.39A + 13.96$	5.46	9.0
FRC/TLC	%	$0.21A + 43.8$	6.74	11.1
FEV_1	l s^{-1}	$4.30H - 0.029A - 2.49$	0.51	0.84
FEV_1/VC	%	$-0.18A + 87.21$	7.17	11.8
		Women		
FVC	l	$4.43H - 0.026A - 2.89$	0.43	0.71
TLC	l	$6.60H - 5.79$	0.60	0.99
RV	l	$1.81H + 0.016A - 2.00$	0.35	0.58
FRC	l	$2.24H + 0.001A - 1.00$	0.50	0.82
RV/TLC	%	$0.34A + 18.96$	5.83	9.6
FRC/TLC	%	$0.16A + 45.1$	5.93	9.8
FEV_1	l	$3.95H - 0.025A - 2.60$	0.38	0.62
FEV_1/FVC	%	$-0.19A + 89.10$	6.51	10.7

H, standing height (m); A, age (year); RSD, residual standard deviation.

*Between 18 and 25 years substitute 25 years in the equations.

tree with that from the nose and nasal sinuses, which contain higher concentrations.

Further reading

American Thoracic Society and European Respiratory Society (2001). Statement on standardization of respiratory muscle tests. *American Journal of Respiratory and Critical Care Medicine*, in press.

Clark JS *et al.* (1992). Non-invasive assessment of blood gases. *American Review of Respiratory Disease* **145**, 220–32.

Gibson GJ (1996). *Clinical tests of respiratory function*, 2nd edn. Chapman & Hall, London.

Hughes JMB, Pride NB, eds (1999). *Lung function tests: physiological principles and clinical applications.* Saunders, London.

Kharitonov S, Alving K, Barnes PJ (1997). ERS Task Force Report: Exhaled and nasal nitric oxide measurements: recommendations. *European Respiratory Journal* **10**, 1683–93.

Roca J, Whipp BJ, eds (1997). Clinical exercise resting. *European Respiratory Monograph* **2**(6).

West JB, Wagner PD (1997). Ventilation–perfusion relationships. In: Crystal RG, West JB, eds. *The lung: scientific foundations*, 2nd edn, pp 1693–709. Lippincott-Raven, Philadelphia.

Sources of normal reference values

Cerveri I *et al.* (1995). Reference values of arterial oxygen tension in middle-aged and elderly. *American Journal of Respiratory and Critical Care Medicine* **152**, 934–41

Cotes JE (1993). *Lung function: assessment and application in medicine*, 5th edn. Blackwell, Oxford.

European Respiratory Society (1993). Standardised lung function testing. *European Respiratory Journal* **6**(Suppl 16).

Jones NL, Summers E, Killian KJ (1989). Influence of age and stature on exercise capacity during incremental cycle ergometry in men and women. *American Review of Respiratory Disease* **140**, 1373–80

Appendix

Normal values of lung volumes and ventilatory flows vary considerably with age and height. Table 7 is modified from that produced by the European Respiratory Society (1993). Standardised lung function testing. *European Respiratory Journal* **6**, Suppl 16.

Summary equation for lung volumes and ventilatory flows for Caucasian adults aged 18 to 70 years*. The lower 5 or upper 95 percentiles are obtained by substracting or adding the figure in the last column from the predicted mean.

17.3.3 Microbiological methods in the diagnosis of respiratory infections

*Robert Wilson**

Microbiological investigations in clinical practice

Microbiological investigations are an important part of the management of infected patients, since few aetiological agents produce diagnostic clinical features and other investigations are not specific. However, treatment of a severe infection should not be delayed while awaiting the results of laboratory tests because this can be fatal. Clinicians need to know the types of respiratory infection that are prevalent and the likelihood of antibiotic resistance to enable them to select appropriate empirical treatment. However, the level of microbiological investigation needed to provide this information for surveillance purposes usually exceeds that required in clinical practice.

Once the clinical diagnosis of a respiratory infection has been made the physician must decide whether to perform any investigations before starting treatment. The type of patient and the severity of the illness will guide this decision. However, even with extensive testing, it is recognized that the causal pathogen may not be identified in over 50 per cent of patients with community-acquired pneumonia, a condition in which a bacterial aetiology is most likely. The proportion of negative results rises steeply if the patient has received an antibiotic before the microbiological samples are

*I thank Maureen Chadwick and Paul Taylor from the Microbiology Department at Royal Brompton Hospital for their helpful comments on the manuscript.

taken. Other explanations for negative bacteriology results include a viral infection being the cause, the presence of non-infectious conditions mimicking pneumonia, the presence of unusual pathogens that go unrecognized (for example, fungi), and the presence of pathogens that are currently not identified or recognized.

This chapter describes the available microbiological methods, and Table 1 indicates the clinical conditions for which they should be used. Some patients should receive more intensive investigation. These include those patients with more serious illness; those with underlying medical problems that put them at higher risk of serious illness (for example, those who are immunocompromised); those at risk of exposure to more unusual pathogens (for instance, nursing-home residents), or of nosocomial infections; and those not responding to treatment. Decisions regarding more invasive investigations, which might have a greater likelihood of giving a positive result, need to be balanced against the risks of any procedure.

Interpretation of results

The interpretation of positive microbiological results may call for fine judgement, and careful consultation between the clinician and medical microbiologist. There are two situations that commonly cause difficulty: the isolation of a species which is part of the commensal flora, and the isolation of an opportunistic pathogen. In these circumstances particularly, but true always, the microbiological results should be considered together with the clinical information and the results of non-microbiological investigations.

The mucosal surfaces of the mouth, nose, pharynx, larynx, and trachea are colonized by a complex variety of bacterial species that make up the commensal flora, whereas the middle ear cavity, the paranasal sinuses, and the lower airways distal to the first bronchial division are usually sterile. The commensal flora confer a level of protection against infection by occupying a niche within the body that might otherwise be colonized by species with greater pathogenicity, and by providing non-specific and specific (via crossreactive antigens) stimulation to the immune system. Some of the commensal species, for example *Streptococcus pneumoniae* and unencapsulated non-typable *Haemophilus influenzae*, may, under permissive conditions, be pathogenic and are amongst the most common causes of respiratory infection.

Many respiratory samples are obtained via routes that are naturally colonized by commensal flora (for example, expectorated sputum), so there is always some uncertainty whether the bacterium has been cultured from the

Table 1 Common microbial causes of respiratory infections and recommended routine clinical investigations

Condition	Common microbial causes	Recommended investigations
Common cold and acute bronchiolitis	Viruses: rhinovirus, coronavirus, adenovirus, myxoviruses (respiratory syncytial, influenza, parainfluenza)	Adults: none Paediatric: acute bronchiolitis (respiratory syncytial most common) immunofluorescent- labelled antibody examination of exfoliated cells in nasopharyngeal secretions
Pharyngitis/tonsillitis	Bacteria: Group A β-haemolytic streptococci, *M. pneumoniae*, *C. pneumoniae* Viruses: as above for common cold and infectious mononucleosis	None unless complications of streptococcal pharyngitis: throat swab and group A streptococcal antibody titres
Otitis media	Bacteria: *S. pneumoniae*, non- typable, *H. influenzae* Viruses: as above for common cold	None unless complications: culture of needle aspiration through tympanic membrane
Sinusitis	Bacteria: *S. pneumoniae*, *S. aureus*, non-typable *H. influenzae* Viruses: as above for common cold	None unless via ENT examination
Acute tracheobronchitis	Bacteria: *M. pneumoniae*, *C. pneumoniae*, secondary infections following primary viral illness due to *S. pneumoniae*, non-typable *H. influenzae* Viruses: as above for common cold.	None
Chronic obstructive pulmonary disease	Bacteria: non-typable *H. influenzae*, *S. pneumoniae*, *Moraxella catarrhalis* Viruses: as above for common cold	None unless empirical treatment fails: sputum culture
Community-acquired pneumonia	Bacteria: *S. pneumoniae*, *M. pneumoniae*, *C. pneumoniae* Viruses: incidence variable in different studies, influenza, adenovirus	Managed in community: none Admitted to hospital: sputum culture, blood cultures, pleural aspirate if effusion present (but see Chapter 17.5.2.1 for further discussion)
Nosocomial/ventilator-associated pneumonia	Bacteria: Gram-negative bacilli, e.g. *Enterobacter* spp, *Klebsiella* spp, *Proteus* spp, *Serratia marcescens*, *P. aeruginosa* *Acinetobacter* spp, *Haemophilus* spp; Gram-positive, e.g. *S. aureus*, *S. pneumoniae*	As for community-acquired pneumonia plus cultures of aspirate via endotracheal tube; in selected patients bronchoscopy to obtain samples for Gram stain and culture
Pneumonia in the immunocompromised	Bacteria: Gram-negative bacilli as above, *S. pneumoniae*, *S. aureus*, *Nocardia* spp., *Mycobacteria* spp. Mycoses: *P. carinii*, *Aspergillus* spp, *Candida* spp. Viruses: cytomegalovirus	As for nosocomial/ventilator- associated pneumonia; invasive procedures more commonly used and extra tests on sample tests for unusual pathogens (see text)
Empyema	Bacteria: *S. pneumoniae*, *S. aureus*, anaerobes, Gram-negative bacilli as above, *M. tuberculosis*	Percutaneous aspiration of pleural fluid for aerobic and anaerobic culture, and smear and culture for acid-fast bacilli
Lung abscess	Bacteria: *S. aureus*, *Klebsiella pneumoniae*, anaerobic species	Sputum culture, blood cultures; in selected patients bronchoscopy or percutaneous aspiration

putative site of infection in the bronchial tree or has contaminated the sample during its passage through the oropharynx. A significant proportion of exacerbations of chronic bronchitis have a non-bacterial aetiology, but clinical information can be used as a guide, since patients who have an increased sputum volume which is purulent and increased breathlessness are more likely to have a bacterial infection.

Opportunistic pathogens do not infect patients with intact normal host defences, but do so if the host defences are impaired, either by a humoral or cellular defect, or when the defences are breached artificially, for example by an endotracheal tube. Opportunistic pathogens, for example *Pseudomonas aeruginosa*, have relatively low pathogenicity. However, chronic infection commonly occurs for many years in conditions such as cystic fibrosis and other forms of bronchiectasis. Patients have acute exacerbations intermittently when their symptoms increase and the level of lung inflammation is greater. The sputum bacteriology during these exacerbations is usually the same as when the patient is in a stable state, although bacterial numbers may be greater. Other features, such as the white cell count and C-reactive protein level are helpful in differentiating an acute exacerbation. *P. aeruginosa* can also colonize the bronchial tree of patients who are being ventilated, without causing a significant deterioration in their condition, but this bacterium is also a major cause of ventilator-associated pneumonia, a condition with high mortality. An increase in temperature and the appearance of a new infiltrate on the chest radiograph, as well as a rise in the inflammatory markers, signal the onset of pneumonia.

Direct investigations

Non-invasive tests

Upper respiratory tract samples

Nose and throat swabs provide no useful information about the likely pathogen in patients with sinusitis and otitis media. Throat swabs should be performed during investigation of suspected complications of group A β-haemolytic streptococcal pharyngitis (acute rheumatic fever or glomerulonephritis). Virus isolation is dependent on the presence of an adequate number of infected epithelial cells and high-quality samples are imperative; nasopharyngeal washes or aspirates may provide a better sample than swabs in paediatric cases.

Sputum culture

The information gained from this frequently performed test is limited, unless careful steps are taken to improve specificity. Often, the patient cannot produce a sample to order, which limits its usefulness for outpatients or when empirical treatment is to be commenced quickly. The sample should be transported to the laboratory within 2 h to avoid overgrowth by rapidly growing species. The yield of positive cultures is higher if the sample is purulent; a good sample should have fewer than 10 squamous epithelial cells, indicating the lack of significant contamination from the upper respiratory tract, and more than 25 neutrophils per low-power field (at 100 × magnification). As bacteria are unevenly distributed in sputum, the sample is first homogenized by vigorous agitation in Ringer's solution or by the addition of a commercially available digestion agent, and then is diluted so that a quantitative assessment can be made of the bacteria present.

Gram stain of sputum has been advocated as a rapid diagnostic test, such as when Gram-positive diplococci are seen indicating a pneumococcal pneumonia. However, interpretation of the stain can be subjective and this test should not be performed by an inexperienced observer. In addition, it has to be kept in mind that respiratory infections can be mixed, so focused therapy based on the result of a Gram stain might not cover co-infection with an atypical pathogen such as *Mycoplasma pneumoniae*.

Sputum culture is an important non-invasive investigation in patients with pneumonia of sufficient severity to lead to hospital admission. However, it is rarely useful in the community; nor is it usually helpful in chronic bronchitis, when the results are predictable and unlikely to influence the choice of antibiotic. It might be considered if a patient fails empirical therapy, when culture may reveal a β-lactamase-producing strain, or occasionally in severe chronic obstructive pulmonary disease an unexpected pathogen such as *P. aeruginosa*. Results of routine sputum culture performed in a cystic fibrosis outpatient clinic (and in other patients with chronic infection, for example bronchiectasis) may be used to guide empirical treatment when the patient presents with an acute exacerbation; sensitivity testing is also useful in these situations to monitor the development of resistance. A new pathogen that would alter management, for example *Burkholderia cepacia*, might also be identified by routine screening of this type of patient.

A range of culture media are inoculated: blood agar, chocolate (heated blood) agar to aid the isolation of *Haemophilus* species, and MacConkey's agar for some Gram-negative bacilli and coliforms. Special culture medium can be used for other bacteria, for example *Legionella* species, various fungi, and acid-fast bacilli. Although many species can be identified to guide the choice of antibiotic after overnight culture, full identification and determination of antibiotic sensitivities take a further 24 h. For some patients (for example, cystic fibrosis with mixed infections), a range of selective media can be used to encourage the growth of some species whilst suppressing others. Additional special staining techniques can be used in appropriate clinical circumstances, for example for acid-fast bacilli and *Pneumocystis carinii*. Culture of *Mycobacterium tuberculosis* on standard media such as Lowenstein–Jensen used to take 6 to 8 weeks before antibiotic sensitivities were available, but nowadays more rapid automated liquid cultures, for example BACTEC®, provide a result in 2 to 4 weeks.

A considerable proportion of patients cannot produce a sample of sputum even with the help of a physiotherapist. This difficulty led to the development of a technique to induce sputum, which has been particularly useful in human immunodeficiency virus (**HIV**)-infected patients with suspected *P. carinii* or mycobacterial infection. The patients brush their teeth and gums, gargle with water, and hydrate themselves with a couple of glasses of water. They then inhale nebulized 3 per cent saline for 20 min, and every 5 min are encouraged to cough. A β2-agonist can be given before the procedure, but the technique has been limited in its application because of the severity of coughing and bronchospasm that may be produced. The procedure should not be performed in an open ward or an area where there are other immunocompromised patients, because of the danger of spreading pathogens.

Several new diagnostic tools have been developed or are in development to examine sputum and other specimens. Broadly speaking, these detect antigens or other products of micro-organisms directly by immunological techniques based on monoclonal antibodies; or they use molecular techniques to identify the organism's DNA or RNA, either directly using a probe or following amplification by the polymerase chain reaction (**PCR**). At the present time, molecular techniques are most commonly used in selected patients to identify *M. tuberculosis*, and in particular isolates carrying the antibiotic-resistance gene for rifampicin. Probes for other resistance genes will follow in time and provide a powerful tool in the diagnosis of multidrug-resistant tuberculosis. Molecular techniques are also being introduced for the detection of cytomegalovirus from cases of pneumonia in immunodeficient patients. It is in this area that new microbiological methods in the diagnosis of respiratory infections are likely to appear, and they will be particularly useful if problems of sensitivity and specificity can be solved so that they can be applied to readily obtained samples such as sputum.

Other non-invasive investigations

In patients with pneumonia two sets of blood cultures should be taken before antibiotics are started. Bacteraemia is intermittent, so ideally samples for culture should be taken at least 1 h apart using the inoculum volume recommended by the supplier, but treatment should not be delayed unless the patient's condition allows it. The presence of bacteraemia increases the risk of complications from pneumonia, so a positive result has prognostic as well as diagnostic implications. However, the sensitivity of the investigation is only 10 to 20 per cent overall, with *S. pneumoniae* being the most common pathogen identified by this method.

A significant pleural effusion should always be aspirated and the following investigations requested: white cell count and differential; measurement of protein, glucose, lactate dehydrogenase, and pH; Gram stain and staining for acid-fast bacilli; culture for bacteria, mycobacteria, and fungi.

Pneumococcal antigen detected in the urine by counter-immunoelectrophoresis has an acceptable sensitivity, which is even higher in pleural fluid, but this is a cumbersome test to perform in the laboratory and is rarely used. *L. pneumophila* antigen in the urine is now used routinely and identifies serotype-1 infection, which is the most common serotype causing pneumonia.

The isolation of respiratory viruses requires sensitive cell-culture systems. Incubation time is very variable from 24 h with herpes simplex to 14 days for cytomegalovirus, but in most cases it is too long for the test to be clinically useful. Viral infection of exfoliated cells can be diagnosed rapidly using immunofluorescent techniques incorporating monoclonal antibodies. Conjugated monoclonal antibodies are available for a range of viruses including respiratory syncytial, influenza, parainfluenza, adeno- and cytomegaloviruses, as well as other microbes (for example *L. pneumophila* and *P. carinii*). Other viruses may require an indirect method using unlabelled mouse antibody and a second step with anti-mouse conjugated antibody.

Invasive tests

A number of invasive diagnostic techniques have been developed to obtain specimens directly from the lower airways that are relatively uncontaminated by oropharyngeal flora. In all cases, the yield is greater if antibiotics have not been commenced prior to the procedure; if the patient is already receiving antibiotics they should not have been changed for several days before the test is performed.

Transtracheal aspiration

Although still performed in some centres this approach is not recommended due to poor patient tolerance and low specificity.

Bronchoscopic protected brush catheter (PBC)

This technique employs a double-catheter brush system which is inserted via the bronchoscope. A distal wax plug in the catheter is dislodged by advancing the inner catheter only when the bronchoscope is in the correct position to take a sample from the identified area. The brush is advanced to take the specimen and then retracted before withdrawing the whole catheter from the bronchoscope. The brush is aseptically cut into a vial containing Ringer's solution, or its equivalent, and agitated to ensure all bacteria are removed, then quickly transported to the laboratory where quantitative cultures are performed. Care should be taken when interpreting the results obtained from patients with chronic obstructive pulmonary disease who can have lower airway bacterial colonization without parenchymal infection.

Bronchoscopic bronchoalveolar lavage (BAL)

This technique also uses the bronchoscope to obtain samples from distal airways and the alveolar space, but it is more likely to be contaminated by nasopharyngeal commensals during insertion of the bronchoscope in the non-ventilated patient. The bronchoscope is wedged into a distal segment of the identified area and sterile normal saline (about 50 to 100 ml) is instilled and aspirated to provide about 10 ml for investigation. The fluid from an initial aliquot may be discarded to try to reduce any contamination with bacteria from the upper airways. Squamous epithelial cells signify upper airway contamination, while the presence of intracellular organisms in phagocytic cells indicates true bacterial infection. Quantitative cultures are again recommended. A certain level of bacterial growth is required to be regarded as significant in both PBC and BAL, usually 10^3 colony-forming units/ml for the former and 10^4 colony-forming units/ml for the latter.

However, detection of some microbial species should be considered significant whatever their concentration—for example, *P. carinii*, *Toxoplasma gondii*, *Legionella* species, *M. tuberculosis*, respiratory syncytial virus—whereas isolation of fungi and environmental *Mycobacteria* species need to be correlated with clinical and radiographic findings.

Percutaneous fine-needle aspiration

This may be guided by computed tomography (**CT**) scanning. Complications are infrequent in centres experienced in this technique.

These invasive procedures are rarely used in patients with community-acquired pneumonia, particularly since retrospective data has shown that outcome is not improved by establishing a specific aetiology in those patients with a severe illness. However, bronchoscopy is useful in patients who have failed empirical therapy. This may reveal resistant or unusual pathogens or a mechanical factor delaying resolution, for example an obstructing endobronchial lesion.

Invasive procedures are used more commonly in the immunocompromised patient with pneumonia, when the range of pathogens is much larger, and consequently the choice of empirical therapy much more difficult. In addition, the likelihood of a non-infectious cause of 'pneumonia' is greater. The bronchoscopic techniques have reasonable sensitivity and specificity when performed correctly, carry less risk of complications, and are usually more acceptable to patients. A transbronchial biopsy can be taken during the bronchoscopy to obtain lung tissue for histology and culture. Direct histological examination of the lung or pleura is important in several situations: detection of herpes simplex virus or cytomegalovirus is not an accurate indicator of pneumonitis without histological confirmation; cytomegalovirus pneumonitis is clinically very similar to acute rejection in transplant patients; granulomas suggest mycobacterial or fungal infection and acid-fast bacilli or fungi with characteristic features may be seen.

In ventilated patients there is less agreement about the role of invasive tests. Culture of endotracheal aspirates should be performed routinely. Failure to culture bacteria from a patient not being given antibiotics has a high negative predictive value for ventilator-associated pneumonia. There may be a higher percentage of false-positive results compared to bronchoscopic techniques, due to bacterial colonization; but quantitative cultures taken together with clinical information and the results of other investigations usually indicate the significance of a positive culture. In ventilator-associated pneumonia this approach is simpler than bronchoscopy; moreover, studies have failed to demonstrate that the information obtained from invasive techniques reduces mortality. Also, bronchoscopy may not be readily available in some hospitals, and by sampling a limited area of the lung it may be less sensitive.

Indirect investigations

Respiratory infections caused by a range of pathogens can be detected late in the infection or retrospectively by serological tests. The delay required until the antibody response occurs means that the results are rarely clinically relevant and these investigations therefore do not need to be performed routinely.

Serological methods are commonly used for viral infections and the atypical bacterial pathogens that are difficult to culture: *L. pneumophila*, *M. pneumoniae*, and *Chlamydia pneumoniae*. Seroconversion takes 3 to 6 weeks, but in elderly patients legionella can take up to 14 weeks. In several rarer infections (for example, histoplasmosis, coccidiomycosis, filariasis), a positive antibody result suggests the presence of active infection. Several serologic methods are available. For many years the most widely used, because of its flexibility, was the complement fixation assay. This detects primarily IgG antibody and, therefore, requires a fourfold rise in antibody levels between acute and convalescent serum samples to demonstrate a new infection. The complement fixation assay has now been replaced for some species by enzyme-linked immunosorbent assays (**ELISA**) that detect specific IgM, which is predictive of a recent or active infection in a sample collected 10 days or more after the onset of symptoms.

Further reading

American Thoracic Society (2001). Guidelines for the management of adults with community-acquired pneumonia: diagnosis, assessment of severity, antimicrobial therapy, and prevention. *American Journal of Respiratory and Critical Care Medicine* **163**, 1730–54

Blasi F, Costentini R (1997). Non-invasive methods for the diagnosis of pneumonia. In: Torres A, Woodhead M, eds. *Pneumonia. European Respiratory Monograph*, pp. 157–74. European Respiratory Society Journals, Sheffield.

Davidson M, Tempest B, Palmer DL (1976). Bacteriologic diagnosis of acute pneumonia. *Journal of the American Medical Association* **235**, 158–63.

Roberts DE, Cole PJ (1980). Use of selective media in bacteriological investigation of patients with chronic suppurative respiratory infection. *Lancet* **i**, 796–7.

Sanchez-Nieto JM, *et al.* (1997). Impact of invasive and noninvasive quantitative culture sampling on outcome of ventilator-associated pneumonia. *American Journal of Respiratory and Critical Care Medicine* **156**, 1–6.

Wilson R (1999). Bacterial infection and chronic obstructive pulmonary disease. *European Respiratory Journal* **13**, 233–5.

Wimberley N, Faling SJ, Bartlett JG (1979). A fibreoptic bronchoscopy technique to obtain uncontaminated lower airway secretions for bacterial culture. *American Review of Respiratory Diseases* **119**, 337–43.

17.3.4 Diagnostic bronchoscopy, thoracoscopy, and tissue biopsy

M. F. Muers

Introduction

Diagnostic bronchoscopy, thoracoscopy, and tissue biopsy are an integral part of the investigation of respiratory disease. They should be regarded as complementary to, rather than substitutes for, simpler and cheaper tests.

The introduction of the flexible fibreoptic bronchoscope by Ikeda in 1974 and the subsequent improvements in instrumentation, together with a widening number of applications, have revolutionized the practice of respiratory medicine worldwide. By contrast, rigid bronchoscopy—although essential in some circumstances—has become much less common. Thoracoscopy, the examination of the pleural cavity by a percutaneously introduced instrument, was first performed in 1913 by the Swedish physician, Jacobaeus. The technique has remained similar ever since, but has in recent years been substantially improved with the introduction of video-assisted equipment—the **VATS** (video-assisted thoracoscopic surgery) approach. With respect to other methods of tissue sampling, the major change in recent years has been the improved accuracy and safety of percutaneous needle-biopsy techniques by the simultaneous use of cross-sectional imaging or ultrasound.

Table 1 Indications for bronchoscopy

Diagnosis	Suspected malignancy
	Unexplained localized or diffuse radiographic opacity (e.g. 'persistent pneumonia')
	Unexplained respiratory symptoms (especially haemoptysis, wheezing)
	Microbiological sampling (e.g. ?TB but no sputum; ?PCP in AIDS)
	Bronchoscopic bronchogram
Therapy	Removal of secretions—foreign body
	Palliation of carcinoma symptoms by laser, diathermy, cryotherapy, endobronchial radiotherapy

TB, tuberculosis; PCP, *Pneumocystis carinii* pneumonia; AIDS, acquired immunodeficiency syndrome.

Bronchoscopy

Indications (Table 1)

Bronchoscopy is mainly used to investigate or confirm the possibility of carcinoma, and/or to obtain histological and cytological confirmation of a clinical diagnosis, and to provide evidence about operability. A diagnosis at bronchoscopy does not just depend on tissue sampling as many abnormal appearances are characteristic. It is particularly useful in excluding endobronchial abnormalities as a cause for persistent symptoms in the presence of a normal radiograph. The use at bronchoscopy of imaging and flexible instruments allows sampling of distal bronchi or lung parenchyma that cannot be seen directly.

Techniques

Fibreoptic bronchoscopy

Fibreoptic bronchoscopy is usually an outpatient procedure, done with local anaesthesia and sedation. The list of preoperative requirements is shown in Table 2. The procedure causes a fall in Pao_2 of about 2.5 kPa. For this reason, and particularly because many patients have impaired lung function, oxygen supplementation by nasal cannulation to maintain the Sao_2 at 90 per cent or greater is recommended, with oxygen saturation monitored by pulse oximetry and oxygen supplementation continued postoperatively.

The bronchoscope is best inserted through the nose, but if the nasal passages are too narrow, the instrument can be inserted through the mouth with an appropriate guard. The nose, oropharynx, vocal cords, and bronchial tree are anaesthetized with lidocaine (lignocaine) aerosol or gel. Care must be taken not to over use lidocaine: a maximum total dose <7 mg/kg should be ensured.

There have been four large retrospective studies of the safety of fibreoptic bronchoscopy involving between 4000 and 48 000 patients. Reported mortality rates have ranged between 0 and 0.04 per cent and major complication rates between 0.08 per cent and 0.5 per cent. It is accepted that the risk of complications is greater when transbronchial biopsy is performed, in the presence of coagulopathies, and in patients who are frail or very ill.

Postprocedure infection is very rare, occurring in one in 2500 procedures in a large study. There have been no reported cases of the human

Table 2 Preparations for fibreoptic bronchoscopy

Posteroanterior and lateral chest radiograph
Spirometry: measurement of arterial blood gases if FEV_1 <40 per cent
Coagulation studies if transbronchial lung biopsy
Bronchodilators for asthmatics

Nil by mouth, 4 h food, 2 h liquids
Intravenous access for all
Verbal and written patient information and informed consent

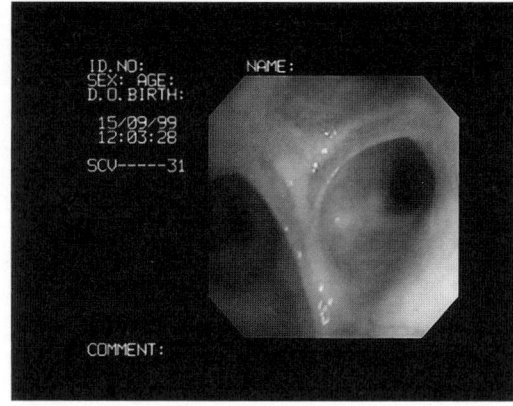

(a)

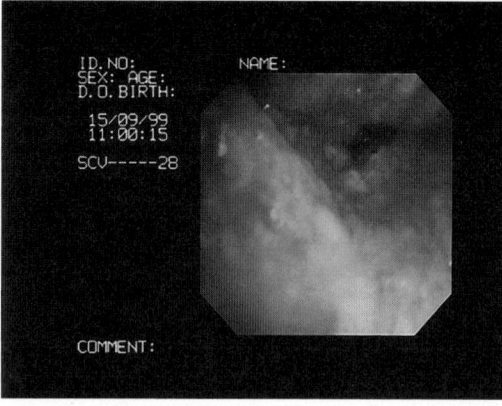

(b)

Fig. 1 Appearances at bronchoscopy. The normal thin mucosa and sharp interlobar carinae of the normal left side (a) are in contrast to the irregular exophytic appearance of an advanced non-small cell tumour of the right main bronchus (b) in the same 73-year-old patient. (See also Plate 1.)

immunodeficiency virus (**HIV**) being transmitted by bronchoscopy. However, contamination of bronchoscopes is important for another reason, namely that organisms introduced into the lungs and sampled may give a false impression of infection. This is a particular difficulty with non-tuberculous mycobacteria, which can grow in contaminated rinse water and be resistant to some disinfectants. The most common disinfecting agent is gluteraldehyde. This has to be handled with care: it is a potent sensitizer of the respiratory tract and aerosol contamination of the working environment can put staff at risk of contracting occupational asthma.

Rigid bronchoscopy

Rigid bronchoscopy is performed under general anaesthesia with oxygen Venturi ventilation. The procedure is indicated if previous fibreoptic bronchoscopy has failed to make a diagnosis and there is still a suspicion of pathology, if there is anxiety about uncontrolled bleeding, or when foreign body removal is being contemplated. Most surgeons will re-inspect the bronchial tree before a planned resection to reassess operability, and rigid bronchoscopy offers better conditions for some difficult therapeutic procedures such as laser therapy and the insertion of stents—although both of these can be performed with the fibreoptic instrument. Rigid bronchoscopy is preferable for children.

Diagnosis at bronchoscopy

The standard 5-mm diameter fibreoptic bronchoscope allows inspection of all the lobes to subsegmental level; smaller 3-mm diameter paediatric bronchoscopes extend this range of vision but cannot be used for biopsies. Approximately 70 per cent of bronchial carcinomas are within visible and sampling range. Many diagnoses can be made without biopsy: for example, paralysis of the left recurrent laryngeal nerve causing vocal cord paresis; endobronchial pus from infected segments; distortion due to lung collapse or metastatic carcinoma; or a large endobronchial tumour (Fig. 1 and Plate 1). Although the appearance of many tumours is quite characteristic, it must be borne in mind that the differential diagnosis of primary lung cancer at bronchoscopy includes adenomas, endobronchial metastatic deposits, for example from breast cancer, or more rarely endobronchial tuberculosis or sarcoidosis.

Endobronchial brushing, biopsy, and 'washing'

The majority of endobronchial lesions are carcinomas and best sampled by a combination of brushing of the surface for cytology, forceps biopsy for histology, and (where sampling has been difficult) bronchial 'wash' for cytology. Sheathed disposable nylon brushes can safely be applied to most tumours and the resulting specimens rubbed on to slides and air- or ethanol-fixed for cytology. Flexible biopsy forceps provide adequate samples from most endobronchial tumours, but it is advisable to take up to four or five biopsies of each lesion. For a diagnostic bronchial wash, 20 to 40 ml of normal saline is injected over the endobronchial lesion into the peripheral

lung and the residual fluid rapidly aspirated in to a trap. A combination of brushing, biopsy, and washing gives the highest yield for malignancy, and this should be well over 80 per cent. If the tumour appears vascular, it is wise to brush first, and proceed to biopsy if significant bleeding does not occur.

A bronchial wash is also useful for microbiological tests particularly for mycobacteria or fungi—for example, if there is a suspicion of tuberculosis in an upper lobe, but no sputum.

Bronchoalveolar lavage

This technique provides a sample of cells from the peripheral airways and alveoli of a lung segment or lobe. It is occasionally useful for the diagnosis of diffuse lung disease, and has been used extensively as a research tool. A bronchoscope is wedged into a segment of lung, either guided by a radiographic abnormality or if not, usually the right middle lobe. Between 150 and 300 ml of buffered normal saline at 37 °C are instilled by syringe pressure in 50 to 60 ml aliquots. Low-pressure suction is continuously applied after each aliquot and the aspirated fluid collected in a trap, the average return being approximately 60 per cent of the injected volume. Particular care has to be taken when the procedure is undertaken in patients with an FEV_1 of less than 1.5 litres (FEV_1, forced expiratory volume in 1 second). Supplementary oxygen is nearly always necessary, and after 10 per cent of lavages there is transient pyrexia lasting for between 4 and 8 h.

The lavage specimen is centrifuged down and subjected to cytological examination, when absolute yields and differential cell counts as well as functional studies can be made (Table 3). Lavage in normal non-smoking

Table 3 Bronchoalveolar lavage

(a) Normal cellular constituents

Cells	Non-smoker	Smoker
Total ($\times 10^4$/ml)	13	42
PAM (%)	80–95	85–98
Lymphocytes (%)	<15	10
Neutrophils (%)	<3	<5
Eosinophils	>0.5	<3

(b) Pathognomonic appearances

Cells	Diagnosis
Haemosiderin-laden PAMs	Idiopathic pulmonary haemosiderosis
	Pulmonary haemorrhage
PAS-positive PAMs	Alveolar proteinosis
Lamellar structures on EM	
Intracellular X bodies (OKT6 staining)	Langerhans' cell histiocytosis
Multinucleated PAMs containing tungsten	Hard metal disease

PAM, pulmonary alveolar macrophages; EM, electron microscopy.

subjects shows a preponderance of alveolar macrophages with less than 20 per cent of the cells being lymphocytes, polymorphonuclear neutrophils, and eosinophils. Cell counts are increased approximately threefold in smokers and altered in many diffuse lung diseases, particularly sarcoidosis and allergic alveolitis. Although characteristic profiles can be recognized, lack of specificity is a major problem, and in routine clinical practice they provide only supportive evidence for most diagnoses. There are, however, a few pathognomonic appearances (see Table 3). Lavage specimens are particularly useful in the investigation of diffuse lung shadowing in patients who are immunocompromised (see below).

Transbronchial biopsy

This technique enables specimens of lung parenchyma (namely small bronchi, bronchioles, alveoli, and their associated vessels) to be examined. It may be useful in the diagnosis of diffuse parenchymal lung disease (**DPLD**) and occasionally in the diagnosis of localized lesions, for example persistent consolidation.

Closed, flexible, bronchial biopsy forceps are advanced to within about 1 cm of the pleura and then opened, next they are moved gently backwards and forwards two or three times to ensure full opening, before being firmly advanced more peripherally, whilst the patient is asked to breathe out (Fig. 2). The forceps are then closed and withdrawn, usually with a perceptible 'tug'. The bronchoscope is left in position to check there is no appreciable bleeding. The specimens, which are approximately 1 to 2 mm^3, are put in formal saline for histology, or in normal saline for microbiological culture. The diagnosis of diffuse lung disease needs two or three specimens, and more are required for the accurate diagnosis of focal lesions. The diagnostic rate depends very much on the lung pathology being sampled. In fibrosing alveolitis biopsies are often unsatisfactory, but in a condition such as lymphangitis carcinomatosa or sarcoidosis, diagnostic rates may approach 80 per cent or more. For peripheral tumours, the diagnostic rate depends upon the size, but it is characteristically about 50 per cent. An alternative procedure here is a percutaneous lung biopsy.

Complications are more common in immunocompromised patients or in the presence of coagulopathies. Mild haemorrhage occurs in 5 to 10 per cent of patients, and pneumothorax in 1 to 5 per cent, with a mortality rate of approximately 0.1 per cent. Bleeding can be reduced by the broncho-

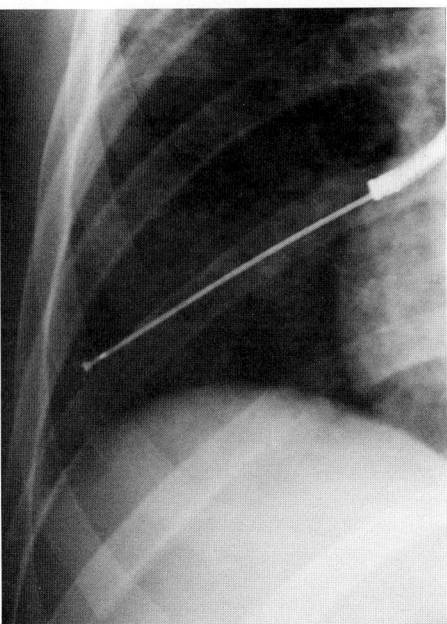

Fig. 2 Transbronchial biopsy through the fibreoptic bronchoscope. The bronchoscope is wedged in the right lower lobe bronchus. Flexible biopsy forceps have been advanced to within 1 cm of the chest wall under screening. The diagnosis: miliary tuberculosis in a renal transplant recipient.

scopic injection of 1 to 5 ml of 1:10 000 epinephrine (adrenaline). Because of the risk of pneumothorax, transbronchial biopsy is usually restricted to one lung, although bilateral samples are taken in cases of heart lung transplantation for the surveillance of transplant rejection. A postprocedure radiograph is usual: if pneumothorax is not present 1 h afterwards, it is very unlikely to develop later. There is debate as to whether fluoroscopic screening is required routinely: it is certainly an advantage when the technique is being learned, but in skilled hands the yield and complication rate is similar whether or not screening is used. It is possible to take transbronchial biopsies from patients on intermittent positive-pressure ventilation, but under these circumstances bronchoalveolar lavage alone or an open lung biopsy is probably safer and the latter has a far higher chance, usually, of achieving an accurate diagnosis.

Transbronchial needle aspiration

This technique can be used to sample abnormal bronchial mucosa, peripheral lesions, and occasionally peribronchial lymph nodes. A sampling needle, in a flexible sheath, is passed through the bronchoscope and the needle advanced into lung tissue. Suction is applied to obtain a cell sample.

The technique can be used in addition to, but not usually as a substitute for, the assessment of endobronchial tumours by forceps biopsy, brush, and wash. It is likely to be more useful if a carcinoma has spread submucosally, when bronchial biopsies are often difficult. In this instance the needle is inserted at an angle to the bronchial wall.

Transbronchial needle aspiration is an alternative to transbronchial forceps biopsy for the assessment of peripheral lesions under fluoroscopic guidance. For small peripheral lesions less than 2 cm in diameter, the sensitivity is similar to that of forceps biopsy, about 35 per cent, but may be up to 75 per cent for larger lesions.

Transbronchial needle aspiration can be used to stage lung cancer by obtaining samples from peribronchial nodes. The technique used is similar to that for submucosal sampling, but the needle has to be inserted more perpendicular to the bronchial wall, between bronchial cartilage rings. There is good evidence that directing sampling in the light of a previous thoracic computed tomography (**CT**) scan improves the yield. Under these circumstances about 65 per cent of true-positive nodes may be sampled. The technique is relatively easy when subcarinal nodes are sampled but is much more difficult if the nodes are paratracheal. Probably for this reason, most centres still prefer mediastinoscopy or mediastinotomy.

Bronchoscopic bronchography

High-resolution CT (**HRCT**) is now the diagnostic methods of choice for the investigation of possible bronchiectasis. Bronchography is reserved for the uncommon indication of a focal lung lesion in which HRCT has given equivocal results.

Percutaneous needle biopsy

In 1883 Leyden made a diagnosis of pneumonia by needle aspiration, and in 1886 it was used by Menetier to diagnose lung cancer. The development of fine-bore needles and screening techniques means that this is a very widely used method of obtaining lung tissue. The indications for needle biopsy are usually to confirm a diagnosis of lung cancer, particularly where there is a peripheral lesion not easily accessible to bronchoscopy; occasionally to prove that a lesion is benign; to obtain micro-organisms from an area of consolidation or abscess; and to diagnose a mediastinal mass.

Percutaneous fine-needle aspiration biopsy (FNAB)

This produces samples for cytological examination, but lung architecture is not preserved. Screening is required: fluoroscopic, CT, or (if the lesion abuts the pleura) real-time ultrasonography. A fine spinal 22- to 25-gauge needle is advanced perpendicular to the skin under local anaesthesia until the tip lies within the lesion (Fig. 3). Suction is applied and the needle tip is moved slightly to increase the tissue yield. Aspirated material is expressed on to slides for cytology, or sent for culture. The procedure can be repeated, but multiple passes increase the chance of a pneumothorax. A postprocedure radiograph is mandatory.

There are no absolute contraindications to needle biopsy, but an uncooperative patient, severe emphysema or pulmonary hypertension, a coagulopathy, or a contralateral pneumonectomy can substantially increase the risk. A positive diagnosis can be obtained in patients with cancer in about 90 per cent of cases. The rate is influenced by the size and depth of the lesion and the experience of the operator. False-positive rates (namely a diagnosis of cancer where none is present) are extremely low at well under 2 per cent, but the false-negative rate is much higher, probably 30 per cent to 40 per cent. This means that it is wiser to attempt a specific histological diagnosis of a benign lesion rather than rely on the reported absence of malignant cells. Cell typing of a carcinoma is more difficult from needle aspirates than from histological specimens. The most common complications of FNAB are pneumothorax and minor haemoptysis (about 10 per cent). A large haemoptysis, haemothorax, and implantation of tumour in to the needle track are rarer complications.

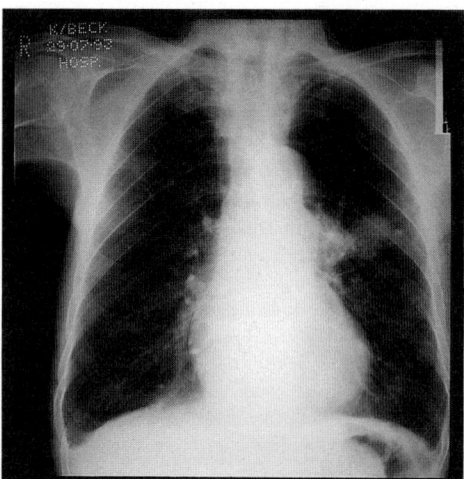

(a)

(b)

Fig. 3 Chest radiograph (a) showing a mass in the left upper lobe with hilar node enlargement; (b) fine-needle aspiration biopsy under CT guidance. The diagnosis: squamous-cell lung cancer.

Percutaneous cutting-needle biopsy

This technique uses larger gauge needles to obtain a specimen suitable for histology. A 20-gauge or more Trucut biopsy needle or a spring-loaded instrument such as the Biopty are used. The sampling technique is similar to FNAB, but multiple biopsies are accompanied by a much higher complication rate. The indications for using a cutting needle are usually when there is an area of pleural thickening or mass, or when an accessible lesion is thought, prebiopsy, to be benign and requires a specific diagnosis. Theoretically cutting needles can sample diffuse lung disease, but because of the high complication rate transbronchial biopsy or a thoracoscopic biopsy are probably safer.

Pleura and pleural fluid sampling

Most unilateral and some bilateral pleural effusions need samples to be taken for diagnosis. Larger effusions can be sampled by needle aspiration using the physical signs on the chest radiograph to direct the needle into the intercostal space above the area of maximum dullness to percussion. Smaller effusions require fluoroscopic or ultrasound guidance. A 21-gauge venepuncture needle fitted to a 20 to 50 ml syringe can be used in the clinic or on the ward, usually without local anaesthesia. Diagnostic information is obtained from the appearance of the fluid, for example whether it is blood-stained, pus, or chylous, and from various microbiological, cytological, and biochemical tests, as indicated in Table 4. Measurement of pleural fluid atrial natriuretic factor (ANF) is very occasionally helpful in making the diagnosis of systemic lupus erythematosus (SLE). For malignancy, simple aspiration cytology has a diagnostic sensitivity of about 60 per cent, rising to about 75 per cent after repeated aspirations.

Pleural biopsy

Percutaneous pleural biopsy using an Abram's needle is usually done at the same time as a first or repeat aspiration of pleural fluid, when local pleural disease (as opposed to organ failure) is suspected as the cause, and when the diagnosis has not been obtained by simple aspiration. It is necessary to use an aseptic technique, to give adequate local anaesthesia down to the pleural surface (commonly 20 ml of 2 per cent lidocaine (lignocaine)), and to verify the presence of an effusion by prebiopsy aspiration of fluid. A deep incision is made above a rib so that the puncture biopsy needle can be introduced without undue effort in to the pleural space. Multiple samples should be taken, avoiding the inferior surface of the rib above. These should be sent for histological examination and for microbiological culture, particularly if tuberculosis is suspected. The technique is not easy, although samples are highly specific for tuberculosis and malignancy. Routine biopsy after repeatedly negative fluid cytology increases the diagnostic yield for neoplasia by about 10 per cent. False-negative biopsies are common, particularly in mesothelioma. If there is a prebiopsy suspicion of localized pleural tumour, particularly mesothelioma, cutting-needle biopsy under screening is a preferred technique.

Thoracosopy and diagnostic thoracotomy

Thoracoscopy allows direct inspection and biopsy of the pleural cavity. The use of video-assisted equipment in recent years has allowed the expansion of this technique to include more complex procedures (Table 5).

Thoracoscopy

This is indicated if a pleural effusion remains undiagnosed after percutaneous aspiration and needle biopsy. It can be done under sedation and local anaesthesia, but more commonly a general anaesthetic is employed. The patient lies on the contralateral side, a small stab wound is made in the mid-axillary line in the 6th or 7th interspace, and after blunt dissection a

Table 4 Diagnostic information obtained from the appearance of pleural fluid

(a) Pleural fluid: examinations

Features	Examined for	Comment
Appearance	Pus, blood, chyle	
Cytology	Cell differential	Rarely diagnostic alone
	Neoplasia	Repeat if negative and suspicion high
Microbiology	Bacteria (micro and culture)	+ve cultures in empyema
	AAFB (micro and culture)	+ pleural biopsy if TB likely
Biochemistry	Adenosine deaminase	>45 U/ml+ lymphocytosis suggestive of TB
	Glucose	Parallels blood glucose; many causes of low value
	Amylase	High in pancreatitis and oesophageal rupture
	pH	<7.1 in empyema
	LDH	High in exudates
		>1000 U/l in empyema

(b) Pleural fluid: transudate or exudate?

Light's criteria		Transudate	Exudate
(1)	*Pleural protein*: serum protein	<0.5	≥0.5
(2)	*Pleural LDH*: serum LDH	<0.6	≥0.6
(3)	*Pleural LDH*: ULN serum LDH	<0.7	≥0.7
Traditional			
Pleural protein		<0.3 g/l	≥0.3 g/l
Additional			
Pleural cholesterol		<60 mg/dl	≥60 mg/dl

AAFB, Acid alcohol-fast bacilli; TB, tuberculosis; LDH, lactate dehydrogenase; ULN, upper limit of normal.

rigid 9-mm thoracoscope is used to enter the pleural space. A flexible fibre-optic thoracoscope has been developed, but its use is not widespread.

Pleural fluid is drained, then 200 ml of air is introduced to collapse the lung and allow the pleural surface to separate. The thoracoscope is manipulated to allow inspection of the whole of the pleural surface, and biopsies of abnormal pleura can then be done under direct vision. Adhesions can be broken down, and, if needed, a pleurodesis can be achieved either by using talc powder or a slurry of talc in saline. A chest drain is placed postoperatively. Complications are rare and death from the procedure extremely uncommon. The sensitivity of thoracoscopy for the diagnosis of malignant pleural effusion or tuberculosis is more than 90 per cent.

Video-assisted thoracic surgery (VATS)

In recent years the technique of video-assisted minimally invasive surgery has been applied to the thorax. This avoids the postoperative pain and morbidity associated with many thoracotomies. It allows lung biopsy or resection in patients who might be at high risk because of poor lung function for an open procedure, but the technique is difficult and adequate training is mandatory. Under general anaesthesia the ipsilateral lung is collapsed with the use of a standard double-lumen endotracheal tube, and a stab incision with adjacent instrumentation ports is made in the 6th or 7th intercostal space in the mid-axillary line (Fig. 4). In other respects the technique is

Table 5 VATS procedures

Procedure	Typical indication
Pleural biopsy	Diagnosis of pleural thickening
Wedge lung biopsy	Diagnosis of DPLD
Pleurodesis	Malignant pleural effusion
Pleurectomy	Recurrent pneumothorax
Bullectomy	Large peripheral bullae
Assessment of mediastinum	Staging of lung cancer
Mediastinal node sampling	
Wedge resection	Diagnosis of solitary pulmonary nodule
Lobectomy	Carcinoma stages I or II
(Pneumonectomy)	Carcinoma stages I or II
Pericardiectomy	Malignant pericardial effusion
(Lung volume reduction surgery)	Severe COPD

VATS, video-assisted thoracoscopic surgery; DPLD, diffuse parenchymal lung disease; COPD, chronic obstructive pulmonary disease. Terms in parentheses indicate unusual indications.

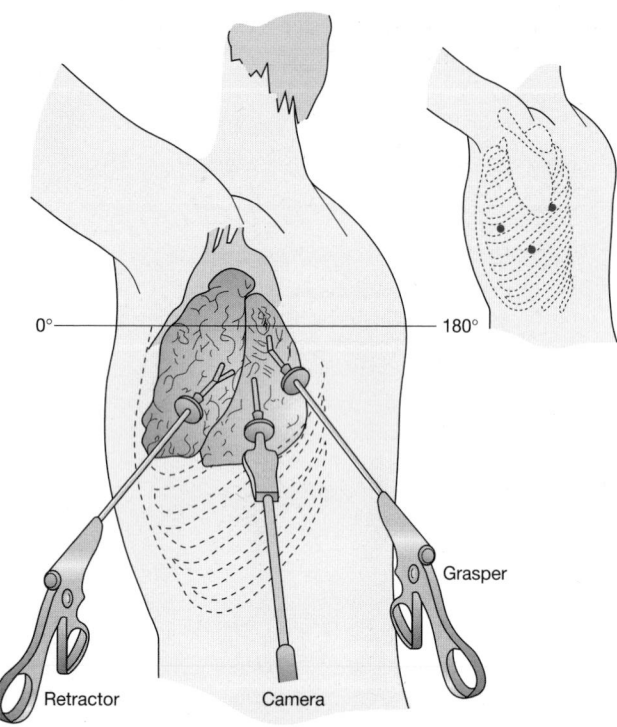

Fig. 4 The arrangement of ports for video-assisted thoracic surgery (VATS). Note the principal access is in the mid-axillary line. (Taken with permission from Landreneau RJ, *et al.* (1992). *Annals of Thoracic Surgery* **54**, 425.)

similar to standard thoracoscopy, and postprocedure pulmonary tube drainage is required. Patients require a shorter hospital stay than after a standard thoracotomy.

VATS can be used for diagnosis and treatment. Control of malignant pleural effusions can be achieved by simple talc pleurodesis, providing the lung remains flexible and the visceral and pleural surfaces can be apposed. Alternatives are mechanical pleurodesis by abrading the visceral pleural surface, or total or partial pleurectomy. However, effusions accompanied by contraction and trapping of the lung by tumour or fibrous tissue cannot be effectively pleurodesed. Although small peripheral lesions up to 3 cm in diameter and in the outer third of the lung parenchyma can be relatively easily removed at VATS, greater skill is needed to achieve lobectomy. VATS is an excellent technique for the treatment of persistent pneumothorax, since peripheral bullae can be recognized and excised and a pleurodesis undertaken. Rarer indications include mediastinal sampling—an alternative to percutaneous techniques—and the treatment of malignant or benign pericardial disease by pericardiectomy.

Open lung biopsy

Introduced by Klassen in 1949, the sampling of lung tissue under direct vision through a small 7- to 10-cm thoracotomy under general anaesthesia was the final arbiter in difficult cases, particularly of diffuse lung disease. It has largely been superseded by VATS biopsy. Bilateral diffuse lung disease is best sampled by a right submammary incision allowing samples to be taken from the right upper, middle, and lower lobe. Sampling from an upper lobe lesion, particularly the apical segments, requires a much larger incision. Surgeons are advised not to simply sample the most visibly affected areas, but also the less abnormal, where active pathology rather than fibrosis is more often to be found. As with VATS it is important that CT scanning is obtained to direct the biopsy.

Adequate material for histology is nearly always obtained and a specific diagnosis achieved in more than 90 per cent of cases. However, indications

for open lung biopsy, particularly for the confirmation of fibrosing alveolitis, are decreasing due to the combination of high-resolution CT scanning and transbronchial biopsy.

Mediastinal sampling

Mediastinal sampling is required when the clinical problem is either the diagnosis of a mediastinal mass or the assessment of operability of lung cancer.

Needle biopsy of the mediastinum

Mediastinal masses can be diagnosed by percutaneous needle biopsy. The techniques used are similar to those described above for pulmonary sampling by a cutting needle. Biopsy under fluoroscopy was introduced in the late 1970s but has now been largely superseded by real-time ultrasound, which allows sampling of anterior and posterior mediastinal masses that abut the chest wall, or CT scanning which allows anterior middle and posterior mediastinal compartment masses to be sampled.

As with pulmonary lesions, fine-needle aspiration biopsy is both sensitive and highly specific for a diagnosis of cancer, but much less satisfactory if the prebiopsy diagnosis is considered likely to be a benign lesion, a cyst, lymphoma, or a thymic tumour. If this is the case, a cutting-needle biopsy is required. Thus, fine-needle aspiration biopsy has a sensitivity of approximately 85 per cent for any malignancy, but allows an accurate histological diagnosis in only about 60 per cent of cases. Diagnostic sensitivity of a cutting-needle biopsy approaches 90 per cent.

Complications are rare, but include pneumothorax and bleeding, which should occur in much less than 10 per cent of cases.

Surgical mediastinal sampling

The usual indication is for the staging of lung cancer. It is also used when needle biopsy has failed to produce an accurate diagnosis of a mediastinal mass.

Mediastinoscopy

This was introduced by Karlens in 1959, who developed a rigid cervical mediastinoscope. Under general anaesthesia a small 3- to 4-cm transverse excision is made 1 to 2 cm above the suprasternal notch. Blunt dissection approaches the pretracheal fascia and the trachea is followed downwards, again by blunt dissection. The mediastinoscope is inserted and the anterior mediastinum can be dissected and sampled. Complications occur in less than 2 per cent of cases. Hilar nodes, and on the left side the aortic nodes, are best reached by anterior mediastinotomy, using a 6 cm incision in the 2nd intercostal space to allow direct inspection of the mediastinal and hilar structures below.

Special cases
Children

General anaesthesia is needed for both rigid and fibreoptic bronchoscopy. The 3.5-mm diameter paediatric fibreoptic bronchoscopes do not easily allow biopsy, although small forceps are now available. Other sample techniques are similar to those for adults.

The elderly

With appropriate attention to sedation and oxygenation, fibreoptic bronchoscopy and other biopsy techniques are safe and effective in the elderly.

The intensive care unit

Fibreoptic bronchoscopy is easily performed through an endotracheal tube with appropriate attention to oxygenation. Transbronchial biopsy is also possible, although pneumothorax is more likely. In difficult cases it is often better to request an urgent open lung biopsy through a mini-thoracotomy if non-invasive tests, including bronchoalveolar lavage, are non-diagnostic.

Diagnostic clinical applications

This section discusses the use of the techniques described above to assist in the diagnosis and management of different, common respiratory conditions.

Perihilar lesions

In modern adult practice the most common and important diagnosis is lung cancer. Usually, if simple investigations are inconclusive, fibreoptic bronchoscopy should be considered unless there are technical contraindications or good clinical reasons why further information is not needed. The advantage of bronchoscopy over information derived from further imaging is that tissue diagnosis may be obtained and some aspects of operability can be assessed—such as the proximity of a tumour to the carina. However, recent evidence has suggested that if facilities exist, a better algorithm may be to request a spiral CT scan with contrast before bronchoscopy. This has been shown to reduce the number of negative bronchoscopies as the technique allows some benign diagnoses, can demonstrate that needle biopsy would be better for some patients, and it can direct bronchoscopy to a particular area of interest. This approach depends on having rapid access to scanning, and for most units bronchoscopy is much more easily available.

If plain radiology shows a perihilar lesion but the bronchoscopy is entirely normal, then most physicians would proceed to a conventional CT scan followed by appropriate sampling, usually by percutaneous needle aspiration biopsy or surgical approach. If an endobronchial lesion is seen, a biopsy is unhelpful, but then the options are a repeat bronchoscopy with more biopsies and transbronchial needle aspiration or rigid bronchoscopy.

Solitary pulmonary nodule

When these are detected on plain radiographs, the immediate concern is usually whether or not the nodule represents an early (therefore curable) primary lung cancer. Whether the policy should be one of immediate removal, biopsy, or observation depends upon a careful assessment of the probabilities of a particular diagnosis in any one case. For example, the probability of cancer would be very high in a heavily smoking elderly man with a recent haemoptysis, and it would be lower if the lesion appeared to be calcified or, for example, it had a very smooth edge and was growing slowly. Algorithms exist to assist physicians in what can be a complex decision. It is sensible in most cases to request a thoracic CT scan. This usually gives much helpful additional information such as the density of the lesion, whether it is truly solitary or multiple, whether there is associated lymphadenopathy, and it allows very precise localization. At the same time, if the probability of tumour is high and immediate resection is not planned, the scan can be combined with a fine-needle aspiration biopsy. The majority of nodules are probably better sampled by this technique than by directed bronchoscopy using screening, since the diagnostic sensitivity of bronchoscopic sampling of peripheral lesions that are not visible is only about 50 per cent. This might be an appropriate approach, however, if the patient was not thought to be able to tolerate a pneumothorax or percutaneous biopsy was not available.

An alternative in some cases might be a VATS procedure or a mini-thoracotomy and removal of the nodule, with immediate frozen-section examination to determine whether it is malignant. If so, a decision can be made by the surgeon as to whether to limit the resection to segmentectomy or to proceed to formal thoracotomy and lobectomy. Needle biopsy is not appropriate if the prebiopsy diagnosis is likely to be a vasculitis or other complex

disease. A larger sample is required for an accurate diagnosis and a VATS or mini-thoracotomy biopsy should be obtained.

Diffuse parenchymal lung disease

Under this heading are both widespread bilateral interstitial alveolar shadows and also similar shadows confined to one lobe or segment of the lung, for instance a persistent 'pneumonia'. The role of tissue biopsy in the diagnosis and management of patients with these shadows is difficult to clarify, because published series do not necessarily give adequate answers to the questions of when and how the lung should be biopsied.

Practical points are as follows:

1. Biopsies should not be considered until an adequate history has been taken and there has been a careful physical examination, looking particularly for evidence of systemic disease, and the patient has had a full set of pulmonary function tests and a high-resolution CT scan. After these investigations there will be a high probability of a particular diagnosis in many cases, and in some the HRCT scan will show pathognomonic appearances, such as lymphangitis carcinomatosa or bronchiectasis, rendering a tissue diagnosis unnecessary.

2. Biopsy should not be considered if the tissue diagnosis is almost certain not to result in any change of management, increased precision of diagnosis, or a more accurate prognosis.

3. Any biopsy should be performed by an experienced operator, or under their immediate supervision, and the possible complications should be explained beforehand to the patient.

4. Biopsy should not be performed if the occurrence of such a complication, particularly a pneumothorax in the presence of poor lung function, would endanger the patient.

For a fuller discussion of the diagnostic approach to the patient with diffuse parenchymal lung disease, see Section 17.11.

Pleural disease

Most pleural effusions can be diagnosed confidently with a combination of basic clinical information and needle aspiration. This should always be the first approach. For the remainder the usual problem is to decide whether a persistent exudative effusion is or is not due to malignancy. If a first aspiration fails to provide a diagnosis then it should normally be repeated with closed punch biopsies and at least one of these sent for microbacterial culture and the others for histology. This approach is reasonable if there is no evidence from the plain radiographs that diffuse pleural thickening is present. If this is the case it is probably wiser to obtain a CT scan, and consider the next step in the light of the findings. The CT scan has a large advantage over plain radiology in that it can indicate the most appropriate point for pleural biopsy. Localized pleural thickening can be guided by this information and a percutaneous cutting-needle biopsy (for example, a Trucut or Biopty needle) is then superior to bedside biopsy with the Abram's punch.

An increasingly common problem in industrialized countries is the appearance of a pleural effusion due to mesothelioma in a previously well patient. This is notoriously difficult to diagnose. Early scanning is required, and if there is no obvious target for percutaneous needle biopsy, early thoracoscopy is recommended. This has the advantage that multiple samples can be taken, and if a frozen section demonstrates a malignancy, an immediate pleurodesis can be performed. However, some mesotheliomas have a florid fibrous stroma and all biopsies are negative, so that in a small proportion of cases confirmation of the diagnosis remains elusive and observation has to be advised.

There is a small risk that percutaneous procedures will be followed by tumour nodules as a result of seeding along the biopsy-needle tract. Trials have shown that this possibility is much reduced by a postprocedural, localized, short course of radiotherapy. It is the author's opinion that the advantages to the patient of a precise diagnosis and the possibility of better management of his/her effusion outweighs this risk. Bronchoscopy is usually unrewarding if the only radiographic abnormality is a small to moderate effusion.

Tuberculosis

Further sampling is often required in cases where tuberculosis is suspected on clinical grounds, but where conventional sputum specimens are negative or absent, and further information is thought necessary before treatment begins. Samples can be obtained either by induced sputum or at bronchoscopy. The former technique uses 3 per cent (hypertonic) saline, usually in volumes of 70 to 100 ml in an ultrasonic nebulizer, to induce coughing and sputum. At bronchoscopy a 40- to 60-ml wash of the affected segment is usually combined with brushing for microscopy, and occasionally with transbronchial biopsy. Comparative studies have shown that the diagnostic yield in patients with focal radiographic abnormalities is similar. Where miliary tuberculosis seems likely and sputum is absent, bronchoscopy is the preferred technique, with a diagnostic sensitivity of about 80 per cent. Florid endobronchial tuberculosis is a comparatively rare disease, but it can be mistaken for tumour. Biopsy shows profuse organisms.

Tuberculosis is often an important differential diagnosis of large pleural effusions, not only in younger patients where primary disease is likely, but also in the elderly where reactivation may have occurred. Pleural fluid sampling alone is much less satisfactory than combining this with closed pleural biopsies. Multiple samples should be sent both for histological examination and for culture. In parts of the world where tuberculosis is common, a high level of pleural fluid adenosine deaminase can be a strong indication that this is the underlying diagnosis, but false-positives occur in empyemas and sometimes in cancer.

Mediastinal disease

For details of the preoperative assessment of the patient with lung cancer, see Chapter 17.14.1.

A tissue diagnosis is required for most mediastinal masses. Sampling under CT guidance is best. Ultrasound is equally good if the mass is anterior or posterior and abuts the chest wall. If the prior working diagnosis is carcinoma, then fine-needle aspiration biopsy is recommended. If this test is negative (no malignant cells) or there is an indication on the smear that the diagnosis may be thymoma or lymphoma, or if the prior working diagnosis is either of these, then a cutting-needle biopsy should be preferred. It is unwise to diagnose thymoma or lymphoma on the results of a fine-needle aspiration. In all other cases, open surgical biopsy is required usually at mediastinotomy or mediastinoscopy.

Biopsy outside the thorax

It is always important to look at the whole patient, and not just the thorax or chest radiograph. Abnormal tissue outside the thorax may be considerably easier to biopsy than tissue within it. A good example would be enlarged supraclavicular nodes, easily accessible to fine-needle aspiration biopsy in cases of suspected cancer. On occasion, putative liver metastases may be easier to sample than a small thoracic primary.

Therapeutic clinical applications

Bronchoscopic suction and saline lavage through either a fibreoptic bronchoscope or a rigid bronchoscope can be used to relieve obstruction due to viscid secretions. Rigid bronchoscopy is necessary if these are inspissated or very tenacious, as in many cases of non-asthmatic mucus impaction in the

elderly. Bronchoscopy should be considered for this reason in cases of 'resistant asthma' in this age group.

Carcinoma

Impressive palliation of distressing symptoms due to endobronchial tumour, such as stridor, breathlessness, or cough, can be obtained in a number of ways. Immediate relief can be produced by deploying endobronchial stents, or using diathermy, cryotherapy, or laser therapy to obliterate tumours. Insertion of stents usually requires rigid bronchoscopy, although techniques have been described allowing placement by physicians using fibreoptic bronchoscopes. In laser therapy, a plastic catheter containing an optical fibre is passed through the instrument channel of the bronchoscope and directed at a tumour. Pulses of high-energy light, usually from a neodynium–YAG laser, cause superficial vaporization and charring of tumour tissue whilst small blood vessels are sealed, providing a relatively dry field. Treatment of haemoptysis in this way is easy, but tumour ablation is a longer and more difficult procedure. Nevertheless, palliation is provided in about 60 to 80 per cent of cases.

Brachytherapy (endobronchial radiotherapy) can complement external beam radiation and has been shown to produce adequate palliation either as initial treatment or if further external beam treatment cannot be given. At fibreoptic bronchoscopy, a catheter is inserted into the narrowed bronchus and the tip passed peripherally. Under fluoroscopic guidance a marker wire is inserted to allow the prescription of treatment, the bronchoscope is withdrawn, and using a remote control device a radioactive source is advanced through the catheter, delivering a high dose of radiotherapy endobronchially, for example 10 Gy at a distance of 1 cm. A single treatment suffices. Relief is not immediate. Combining brachytherapy with other techniques appears to predispose patients to severe haemoptysis.

Photodynamic therapy utilizes the fact that previously injected haematoporphyrins are selectively taken up by tumour cells and, when activated by appropriate laser light, release active oxygen radicals which destroy these cells. There have been reports of treatment of early tumours by this technique, and in skilled hands it can be used to palliate, in a similar fashion to laser therapy. Disadvantages are that repeat bronchoscopy may be needed to remove tumour debris, and the requirement for the patient to remain out of bright light for a period after treatment.

New developments

Early cancer

It is difficult for even an experienced bronchoscopist to detect early tumours such as carcinoma *in situ*. Bronchial epithelium passes through a number of malignant stages before invasive carcinoma develops—these are metaplasia, dysplasia, and then carcinoma *in situ*. It is known that when the bronchial epithelium is illuminated with laser light 405 to 442 nm in wavelength, there is progressive reduction in fluorescence intensity as tissue becomes more abnormal. Thus, if at bronchoscopy the bronchial walls are illuminated with laser light, endoscopists are able to detect and biopsy areas that may be abnormal. Experience with this technique is limited at the moment, but it is likely that with greater refinement it will have an important role in the surveillance of those at very high risk, or in the investigation of 'difficult cases', for example repeated minor haemoptyses with a normal routine white light examination.

Different degrees of epithelial abnormality are accompanied by an increase in number and a change in the nature of chromosomal abnormalities in exfoliated cells. Examples are loss of heterozygosity or the presence of DNA adducts, or the amplification of proto-oncogenes. With the ability of induced sputum techniques to obtain representative samples of bronchial epithelial cells, even in patients who do not routinely produce sputum, there is considerable interest in the possibility of using such techniques in screening programmes. At present, however, there is insufficient discrimination between minor abnormalities unlikely to develop in to cancer and those that are more likely to.

Tuberculosis

At present, if a sample is smear-negative, confirmation of a diagnosis of tuberculosis may wait upon a culture result taking up to 6 to 8 weeks to mature. Accelerated culture methods are now available, and in addition the introduction of the polymerase chain reaction (**PCR**), although beset by the problems of false-positives, does allow a more confident diagnosis to be made quickly in such cases.

Further reading

Abolhoda A, Keller SM (2000). Surgical staging of the mediastinum. In: Pass HI, *et al.*, eds. *Lung cancer: principles and practice*, 2nd edn, pp. 628–48. Lippincott-Raven, Philadelphia.

Anderson C, Inhaber N, Menzies D (1995). Comparison of sputum induction with fibreoptic bronchoscopy in the diagnosis of tuberculosis. *American Journal of Respiratory and Critical Care Medicine* **152**, 1570–4.

British Thoracic Society Guidelines (1998) The diagnosis, assessment and treatment of diffuse parenchymal disease in adults. *Thorax* **54**, S1.

British Thoracic Society Guidelines on Diagnostic Flexible Bronchoscopy (2000) *Thorax* **56 Suppl.**, 1–21.

Burgess CJ, *et al.* (1995). Use of adenosine deaminase as a diagnostic tool for tuberculous pleurisy. *Thorax* **50**, 672–4.

Flower CDR, Schneerson JM (1984). Bronchography via the fibreoptic bronchoscope. *Thorax* **39**, 260–3.

Hansell DM (1995). Interventional techniques. In: Armstrong P, Wilson AG, Hansell DM, eds. *Imaging of diseases of the chest*, 2nd edn, pp. 894–912. Mosby, St Louis. (Includes a general account of needle biopsy.)

Haplin DMG, Colins J (1995) Bronchoscopy and lavage. In: Brewis RAL, *et al.* eds. *Respiratory medicine*, 2nd edn, pp. 362–74. WB Saunders, London. (A general account of bronchoscopy.)

Hernandez P, *et al.* (1995). High dose rate brachytherapy for the local control of endobronchial carcinoma following external irradiation. *Thorax* **51**, 354–8.

Hetzel MR, Smith SGT (1991). Palliation of tracheobronchial malignancies. *Thorax* **46**, 325–33.

Klech H, Hunter C, eds. (1990) Clinical guidelines and indications for bronchoalveolar lavage (BAL): Report for the European Society of Pneumonology Task group on BAL. *European Respiratory Journal* **3**, 937–74.

Lamb S, MacAuley CE (1998). Endoscopic localisation of pre-neoplastic lung lesions. In: Martinet Y, *et al.*, eds. *Clinical and biological basis of lung cancer prevention*, pp. 231–8. Birkhauser Verlag, Berlin.

Muers MF (1994). How much investigation? In: Thatcher N, Spiro S, eds. *New perspectives in lung cancer*, pp. 77–104. BMJ Publishing Group, London. (An account of the application of bronchoscopy and biopsy techniques for the diagnosis of lung cancer.)

Simpson, FG, *et al.* (1986). Postal survey of bronchoscopic practice by physicians in the United Kingdom. *Thorax* **41**, 311–17.

Vansteenkiste J, *et al.* (1994). Transcarinal needle aspiration biopsy in the staging of lung cancer. *European Respiratory Journal* **7**, 265–8.

Wilcox PA, *et al.* (1986). Rapid diagnosis of sputum negative miliary tuberculosis using the fibreoptic bronchoscope. *Thorax* **41**, 681–4.

17.4 Allergic rhinitis and asthma

17.4.1 Asthma: genetic effects

J. M. Hopkin

Introduction

Asthma is a heterogeneous syndrome characterized clinically by labile airflow obstruction. There are distinct pathological features of prominent eosinophilic inflammation, additional T-lymphocyte infiltration, mucous gland hypertrophy and hypersecretion, smooth muscle hypertrophy and hyper-reactivity, and, in a long-established case, epithelial basement membrane thickening. Asthma's closest correlate is atopy, the state of allergic response to common environmental antigens mediated by the antibody IgE, and both conditions are characterized by exuberant **TH2** (subset 2 of T-helper cells) immune mechanisms. Atopy is present in more than 90 per cent of people between 5 and 30 years of age with asthma, but only 30 per cent of those with atopy develop asthma. In older life asthma may arise in non-atopics exposed to isocyanates and other substances at work. Some develop the syndrome as a result of aspirin sensitivity. In others no 'trigger' is demonstrable—so-called intrinsic asthma, arising as a result of both environmental and genetic influences.

Environment and genetics

Besides the clear involvement of reaction to the extrinsic agents noted above, there has been a surge in the prevalence of atopic disorder, and with it asthma, in recent decades. This is centred on developed communities, pointing to important environmental determinants of atopy and asthma that relate to socioeconomic development.

Epidemiological and experimental findings suggest that the rise of atopy and asthma in developed countries may be due to changing patterns of microbial exposure in early childhood. Natural exposure to *Mycobacterium tuberculosis*, measles, *Helicobacter pylori*, *Toxocara carnis*, and hepatitis A all predict less subsequent atopy. Oral antibiotic receipt in early childhood predicts more subsequent atopy, perhaps because of the deletion of gut microflora. Hence it has been proposed that exposure to certain microbes in early childhood may strongly promote natural immune restraint mechanisms and that these, through the actions of TH3 and TR1 cells (and IL-10 and TGF-β), cause repression of TH2 mechanisms against allergens. Inoculations of mycobacteria do effectively prevent experimental allergy in mice.

Despite the evident importance of environmental factors, there are also clear indications of important genetic determinants. Both atopy and asthma aggregate in families, though there is no consistent pattern of inheritance. Twin studies, comparing concordance rates for asthma and IgE sensitization in monozygotic and dizygotic twins, indicate that genetic variables have accounted for approximately 50 per cent of atopy and asthma syndromes in recent decades.

Genome screening studies

The recognition of the genetic contribution to atopy and asthma has resulted in a clutch of genome screening studies over the past decade. The results have been predictably complex. The use of affected sibling-pairs and microsatellite DNA markers has identified linkages at a number of chromosomal locations, with a significant impression that the linkages may vary between racial groups. To date the following chromosomes have shown repeatable linkages—2q, 5q, 6p, 11q, 12q, 13q, 14q, and 16p—with either asthma *per se* or IgE levels.

However, the complex mix of heterogeneous genetic factors and environmental input places important limitations on exact gene mapping. Direct candidate gene approaches, based on the pathophysiology of asthma and allergy and allied to chromosomal approaches, are providing advance.

HLA

Genetic linkage studies and direct genetic association studies demonstrate a clear relationship between HLA variants on the long arm of chromosome 6 (that is, chromosome 6q) and clinical atopy or asthma. HLA variants relate to allergic responses to distinct antigens or epitopes, e.g. HLA-DR2 and one component of the ragweed antigen (Amb a V) and HLA-DR3 and acid-anhydride sensitization asthma. DR variants have also been associated with allergic aspergillosis.

Interleukin (IL)-4 and IL-13 signalling

Because of the prominent involvement of these cytokines in bronchial inflammation and IgE production they have been targets for direct genetic investigation, and a number of important relationships are emerging. Figure 1 illustrates the signalling pathways of IL-4 and IL-13 and emphasizes that the receptors for both include IL-4Rα, and that IL-13 in comparison with IL-4 has the greater actions in promoting bronchial mucosal pathology.

A number of coding variants of IL-4Rα (encoded on the short arm of chromosome 16; namely chromosome 16p) have been identified, and these relate to atopic disorder in genetic association studies. For instance, an extracellular variant—ILe50Val—is substantially more prevalent in its homozygous state in young Japanese asthmatics compared with controls. In transfection experiments it appears to upregulate receptor response to IL-4, with enhanced signalling transduction (through STAT 6 activation (**STAT**, signal transducers and activators of transcription)), increased TH2-cell growth and increased cellular IgE production. Intracellular variants of IL-4Rα, for example Gln551Arg, associate with total serum IgE

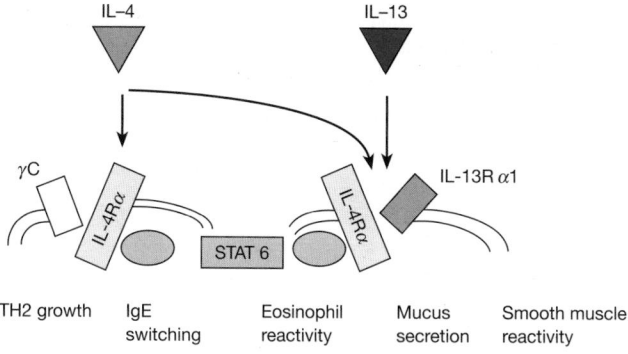

Fig. 1 Interaction between IL-4 and IL-13 signalling in overactive TH2 immunity in bronchial asthma. IL-4Rα is common to the receptors for both IL-4 and IL-13.

levels, atopic eczema, asthma, and the rare hyper-IgE syndrome. Gln576Arg may also have an action on STAT-6 binding. Thus variants at the IL-4Rα locus enhance atopy *per se*, and have an important effect on predicting disease, including asthma, in the diverse populations.

A charge-changing variant (Gln110Arg) in the helical tail portion of IL-13 ligand (encoded on chromosome 5q) associates with asthma, both allergic and non-allergic, in Caucasian and Asian populations. Molecular modelling studies indicate that position 110 of IL-13 plays a crucial role in ligand receptor interaction (Fig. 2) and suggest that the amino acid substitution results in increased affinity between ligand and receptor.

One relatively common variant of IL-13Rα1 shows association with both high IgE levels and asthma. Of note, IL-13Rα1 is encoded on the X chromosome and the risk of atopic disorder and asthma for this variant is confined to young males.

In summary, relatively common variants of IL-4 and IL-13 signalling have been recognized which relate significantly to atopy and asthma in epidemiological and experimental studies. The existence of such TH2-promoting variants in human populations may relate to their potential to enhance protective TH2 mechanisms against certain phases of helminthic infestation—a regular threat to mankind in certain environments now, and almost ubiquitously in the past.

The IgE receptor

One of the first linkages noted for atopy was on chromosome 11q, a linkage that is variably present in different Caucasian and Asian populations. The principal candidate locus here is the β-subunit of the high-affinity IgE

receptor. This is an important amplifier of signals through the receptor, and any genetic variants that would enhance its expression or its activity might have important effects on the allergen–IgE interaction and the triggering of mast cells in the bronchial mucosa to release proinflammatory mediators. A number of variants of FCεR1-β, both coding and non-coding, show association with high IgE levels and asthma. No functional effect has been demonstrated as yet, and studies continue.

Effector mechanisms

Although IL-4 and IL-13 signalling, and the secretion of IgE, are primary mediators of the asthma and atopy syndromes, their actions require the adjunctive activity of a whole set of effector molecules. Genetic variants also play some role here in predisposing to disease. A variant within the promoter of the 5-lipoxygenase gene (encoding for the synthesis of inflammatory leukotriene mediators) associates with the response to the antileukotriene, anti-asthma pharmacological agents. Variants of the leukotriene C4 synthase promoter associate with the increased risk of aspirin-sensitivity asthma. Variants of the β2-adrenergic receptor, involved in smooth muscle activity and other inflammatory mechanisms, modulate receptor activity and associate with adverse clinical response to long-acting β-adrenergic bronchodilators seen in people with asthma.

Conclusion

Genetic and environmental factors play equally important parts in the development of asthma. Genetic factors are complex and heterogeneous. In keeping with the TH2-driven bronchial pathology typical of asthma, common variants pertinent to these mechanisms have an important impact on the risk of disease—including those in IL-4 and IL-13 signalling, and IgE binding to mast cells.

Further reading

Collaborative Study on the Genetics of Asthma (1997). A genome wide search for asthma susceptibility loci in ethically diverse populations. *Nature Genetics* **15**, 389–92.

Renauld JC (2000). New insights into the role of cytokines in asthma. *Journal of Clinical Pathology* **54**, 577–89.

Shirakawa T, *et al.* (2000). Atopy and asthma: genetic variants of IL-4 and IL-13 signalling. *Immunology Today* **21**, 60–4.

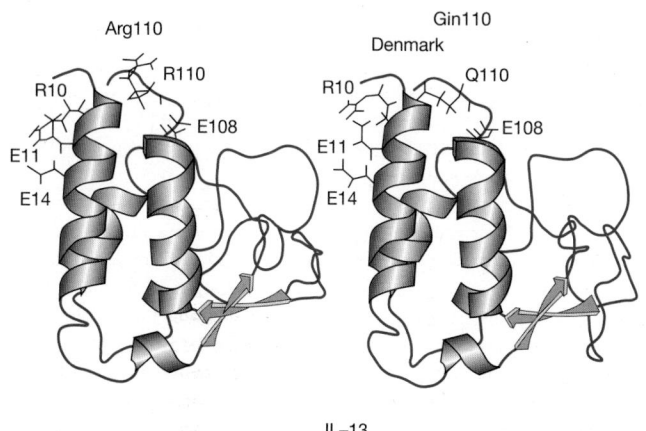

Fig. 2 The Gln110Arg variant of IL-13 is in the helical tail of the ligand, a position that critically mediates receptor binding.

17.4.2 Allergic rhinitis ('hay fever')

S. R. Durham

Introduction

Rhinitis refers to inflammation of the nasal mucosa. In clinical terms it may be defined as symptoms of nasal itching, sneezing, discharge, or blockage, which occur for more than 1 h on most days. Although frequently trivialized, allergic rhinitis remains a common cause of morbidity and social embarrassment. Estimates have suggested that 10 to 15 per cent of the population of the United Kingdom have perennial and/or seasonal rhinitis. Furthermore, the prevalence of hay fever appears to be increasing: in the United Kingdom: in 1955–56 there were 5.1 consultations with general practitioners for hay fever per 1000 population; in 1981–82 there were 19.8.

The lining of the nose and paranasal sinuses is in continuity with the lower respiratory tract and diseases of the upper and lower airways frequently coexist. The nose provides an accessible 'window' for studying allergic disorders and other diseases that can affect the lower airways. Nasal disease may also be the presenting feature of systemic disorders. The aetiology and pathogenesis of allergic rhinitis are described in this chapter, followed by practical guidelines for the diagnosis and management of allergic rhinitis.

Aetiology

Seasonal allergic rhinitis

Pollens of importance include tree pollens in the spring and grass pollens during the summer (Fig. 1). Weed pollens and mould spores predominate in the latter part of the summer and early autumn. Grass pollen counts above 50/m³ are considered high and represent the threshold level at which most hay fever sufferers experience symptoms.

Perennial allergic rhinitis

By far the commonest cause of perennial allergic symptoms is the house dust mite (*Dermatophagoides pteronyssinus*, *Dermatophagoides farinae*, and *Euroglyphus maynei*). Mites are found in almost every home, where they live in the dust that accumulates in carpets, bedding, fabrics, and furniture. They live on shed human skin scales and thrive in temperatures of between 15 and 20 °C and a relative humidity of 45 to 65 per cent, which are typical of many modern centrally heated homes. The major allergen of the house dust mite (Der p1) is a digestive enzyme present in the gut and excreted in high concentrations in the mite faeces.

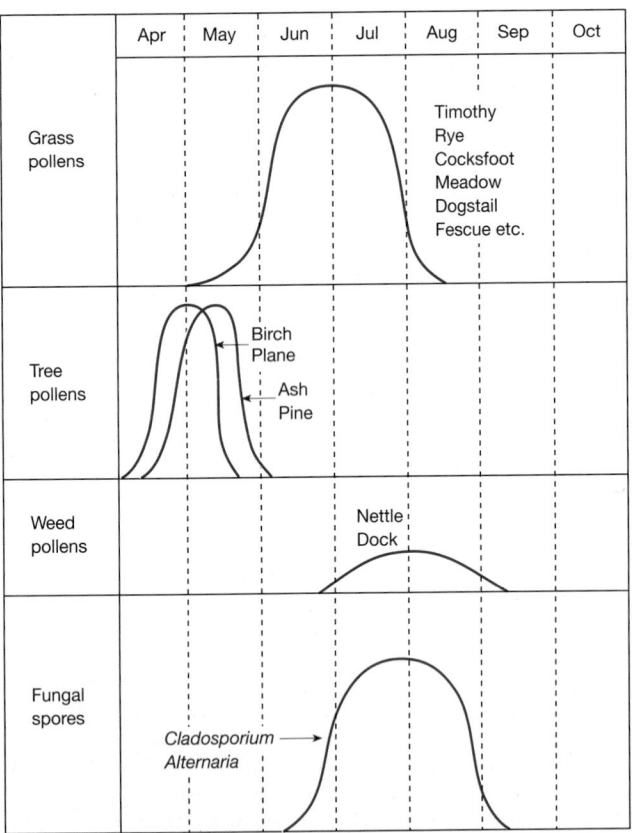

Fig. 1 Calendar of common seasonal aeroallergens (by courtesy of Professor A. B. Kay, Imperial College School of Medicine, London).

Domestic pets are the second important cause of perennial allergy, identifiable in up to 40 per cent of children with asthma and/or rhinitis. The major allergen (Fel d1) is a salivary protein, which is preened on to the fur and released on very small particles (less than 2.5 μm diameter) which remain airborne for many hours, explaining why a sensitized person can experience symptoms almost immediately upon entering a home containing a cat without being directly exposed to the animal. Dog allergens are less well characterized (Can F1). Recently, cockroaches have been described as a cause of perennial allergic symptoms, particularly in inner-city areas.

Food allergy is unusual as a cause of rhinitis in the absence of other organ involvement. However, rhinitis may be one component of IgE-mediated food-induced symptoms commonly due to egg, milk, and nuts in children; nuts, fish, shellfish, and fruit in adults. Preservatives such as tartrazine, benzoates, and sulphites may provoke symptoms of rhinitis. Important drugs that can trigger rhinitis include beta-blockers, aspirin, and (occasionally) angiotensin-converting enzyme (**ACE**) inhibitors.

Occupational rhinitis

Occupational rhinitis refers to rhinitis caused by an agent inhaled in the workplace. Like other causes of seasonal and perennial rhinitis, occupational rhinitis may also be associated with bronchial asthma. Occupations at risk include laboratory animal workers (rats, guinea-pigs, mice), bakers (flour, grain mites), agricultural workers (cows, pollens, fungal spores), electronic solderers (colophony), and health workers and users of rubber gloves (latex).

Pathophysiology

Immediate symptoms of allergic rhinitis occur as a consequence of allergen crosslinking adjacent IgE molecules on the surface of mast cells in the nasal mucosa (Coombs' classification type-1 immediate hypersensitivity). This results in the release of a range of granule-derived mediators, including histamine and tryptase, and the generation of bradykinin. IgE-dependent activation of mast cells also results in the release of newly formed membrane-associated mediators derived from arachidonic acid associated with the membrane lipid. These include leukotriene C4 (LTC4), LTD4 and LTE4 and prostaglandin D2.

In patients with allergic rhinitis, eosinophils are prominent in nasal washings and in biopsies of the nasal mucosa. The mechanism of this tissue eosinophilia is largely unknown. Chemotactic factors released following mast-cell activation may play a role. Recent evidence suggests that peptide messengers (cytokines) released predominantly from T lymphocytes—but also from mast cells, eosinophils and other cell types—may be important.

A hypothesis for the pathogenesis of allergic rhinitis is shown in Fig. 2. Helper (CD4+) T lymphocytes may be subdivided according to their profile of cytokine release: 'TH₁-type' cells producing predominantly interleukin-2 (**IL-2**) and interferon-γ (**IFN-γ**) and 'TH₂-type' cells producing mainly IL-4 and IL-5. The biological properties of TH₂-type cytokines suggest their involvement in allergic rhinitis, and increases in cells expressing these cytokines have been detected in the nasal mucosa during the 'late' nasal responses that occur in sensitized subjects between 6 and 24 h following experimental nasal provocation with allergen. IL-4 is the major cytokine responsible for switching B-cell immunoglobulin production from IgM and IgG to predominantly IgE. IL-3 is a growth factor for mast cells. IL-3, IL-5, and granulocyte-macrophage colony-stimulating (**GM-CSF**) factor are important in the proliferation of eosinophils from bone marrow precursors and their maturation, activation, and prolonged survival in tissues. IL-5 promotes the selective adhesion of eosinophils to vascular endothelium prior to diapedesis. **VCAM-1** (vascular cell-adhesion molecule-1) is selective for the ligand **VLA-4** (very late activation antigen-4; an integrin) expressed on eosinophils, and is upregulated by IL-4 and IL-13, an alternative pathway of eosinophil recruitment.

Mechanism of effect of treatments

Topical nasal corticosteroids and allergen injection immunotherapy (desensitization) are highly effective treatments for allergic rhinitis (see later). They appear to act by distinct mechanisms. Topical corticosteroids have multiple anti-inflammatory effects. They reduce the number of antigen-presenting cells (**APCs**; Langerhan's cells) within the nasal mucosa during natural pollen exposure. They also inhibit the recruitment of basophils and mast cells to the nasal epithelium and inhibit the production of TH2-type cytokines such as IL-4 and IL-5 from T lymphocytes and possibly other cell sources, including basophils. By contrast, immunotherapy acts by altering the TH2/TH1 balance in favour of the production of inhibitory cytokines such as IFN-γ, which downregulate IL-4-induced B-cell switching in favour of IgE and IgG production. This shift may occur either as a consequence of immune deviation of TH2 responses (TH2→TH1) or induction of T-cell unresponsiveness (anergy) of TH0/TH2-type responses to aeroallergens (Fig. 2).

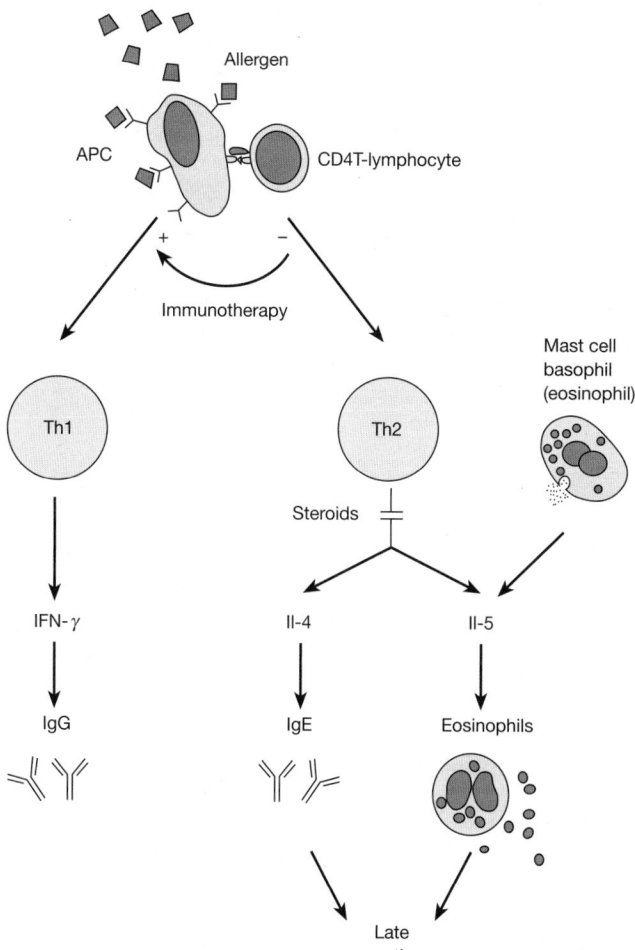

Fig. 2 Hypothesis: pathogenesis of allergic rhinitis and influence of treatment. TH2 cells are predominantly T lymphocytes, although mast cells, basophils, and eosinophils represent alternative sources of TH2-type cytokines. Topical corticosteroids downregulate the production of TH2-type cytokines from T lymphocytes and other cells. Allergen-immunotherapy alters the TH2/TH1 T lymphocyte balance, either by inducing immune deviation, TH2→TH1 responses and/or by inducing T-cell unresponsiveness (anergy) of TH0/TH2-type responses to specific allergens.

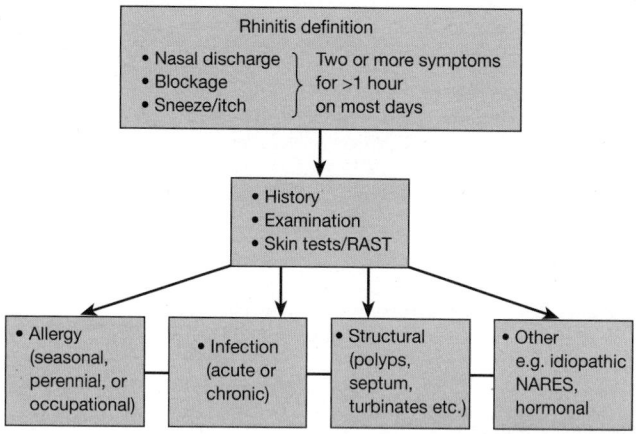

Fig. 3 Diagnostic approach to patients presenting with nasal symptoms. A careful history, clinical examination, and skin-prick tests and/or measurement of serum allergen-specific IgE (RAST or ELISA) should be performed in every case. More than one cause may be present. 'Other' causes include hormonal (pregnancy, premenstrual), drugs (aspirin, β-blockers, ACE inhibitors, cocaine abuse, and atrophic, postsurgical, and ageing). Idiopathic rhinitis refers to nasal hyper-reactivity of unknown cause, manifest as an exaggerated response to non-specific stimuli such as changes in temperature, tobacco smoke, domestic sprays, etc. The differential diagnosis includes vasculitis (Churg-Strauss syndrome), granulomatous conditions (Wegener's, sarcoidosis), atrophic (old age, surgical), and, rarely, tumours of the nose and paranasal sinuses.

Clinical diagnosis

An approach to the diagnosis of patients presenting with nasal symptoms is summarized in Fig. 3. The diagnosis of allergic rhinitis is usually straightforward. However, the differential diagnosis should be considered in every case: frequently more than one cause coexists.

History

A careful history is essential both to establish the diagnosis of rhinitis and to assess the severity of symptoms. An allergic aetiology is suggested by dominant itching, sneezing, and watery nasal discharge. Associated eye or chest symptoms (asthma) also point to an allergic cause, and a history of potential allergic triggers should always be sought. However, in addition to provoking immediate nasal symptoms, allergen may also cause late symptoms several hours after exposure, and these may not be recognized as being related. A history of potential allergic triggers includes enquiry into the seasonality of symptoms and whether symptoms are work-related (in other words, do they occur at work or in the evening following work, with improvement at weekends and during holiday periods). The home environment, including the presence of domestic pets, birds, fitted carpets, central heating, and the use of blankets on beds should be established. A personal or family history of atopy is extremely common in patients with allergic rhinitis.

There are many alternative causes of rhinitic symptoms. It is common for there to be more than one cause, and important to consider the differential diagnosis (Table 1). The presence of facial pain, fever, systemic upset, and mucopurulent discharge suggests infection. Nasal obstruction, which alternates with the nasal cycle, is common to both allergic and infective causes. Nasal crusting and/or bleeding may occur in granulomatous disorders, atrophic rhinitis, or, rarely, tumours (particularly if associated with persistent unilateral symptoms). Impaired taste and/or smell may occur with many forms of rhinitis. It is particularly common with nasal polyposis and may occasionally follow trauma (olfactory nerve damage).

The presence of infertility and recurrent respiratory infections (including bronchiectasis) should raise the possibility of mucus abnormalities (Young's syndrome or cystic fibrosis) or ciliary dysfunction (primary ciliary

Table 1 Causes of rhinitis

Allergic
Seasonal (tree, grass pollens)
Perennial (house dust mite, domestic pets)
Occupational (latex, laboratory animals, antibiotics etc.)

Non-allergic
Infective (acute, chronic)
Autonomic
Hormonal (premenstrual, pregnancy, hypothyroidism)
Drugs (aspirin, β-blockers)
Mucociliary abnormalities (Kartagener's, Young's syndromes)
Immunodeficiency syndromes (congenital and acquired, including HIV)
Atrophic
Idiopathic

Differential diagnosis
Structural (polyps, deflected nasal septum, etc.)
Connective tissue disorders
Granulomatous disorders (sarcoid, Wegener's)
Tumours (benign, malignant)
CSF rhinorrhoea (secondary to trauma or surgery)

Table 2 Advantages of skin-prick tests

- They diagnose atopy—the underlying predisposition to develop allergic disorders
- They provide helpful supportive evidence (positive or negative) for the clinical history
- They are essential when potentially expensive and time-consuming environmental control measures, the removal of a family pet, or a change of occupation are involved
- They have educational value, providing a clear illustration to the patient and reinforcing verbal advice

urement of serum IgE antibodies by radioallergosorbent test (**RAST**) or enzyme-linked immunosorbent assay (**ELISA**) is indicated. A useful basic skin-prick testing kit should include the following:

(1) a positive control (histamine 10 mg/ml);
(2) negative control (allergen diluent solution);
(3) house dust mite (*D. pteronyssinus*);
(4) grass pollen;
(5) cat fur;
(6) *Aspergillus fumigatus*.

Skin-prick tests should be performed with a sterile 23-gauge needle or lancet, which is lightly inserted through the epidermis without inducing bleeding. Responses are recorded as the mean weal diameter at 15 min. A positive prick test is defined as a weal diameter 3 mm or more greater than that of the negative control test.

Treatment

Treatment for allergic rhinitis involves the avoidance of provoking allergens where possible and the use of topical corticosteroids and H1 selective antihistamines. Allergen immunotherapy has a place in patients who do not respond to these measures. The approach is summarized in Table 3.

Allergen avoidance

It is impossible to avoid pollens, although sensible advice includes wearing sunglasses and keeping car windows tightly shut. All windows should be kept closed, particularly in high buildings. Walking in parks and wide open spaces should be avoided, particularly during the late afternoon or evening when pollen counts are highest. A holiday by the sea or abroad during the peak pollen season may be helpful.

House dust mite control and avoidance measures should be undertaken in the homes of sensitive individuals with disease. Precise advice concerning the bedroom can be provided, with avoidance of non-synthetic bedding, restriction of soft toys, which should be washable, the use of mattress covers, changes to vinyl or cork flooring, and thorough vacuum cleaning and damp-dusting at least once weekly. A leaflet entitled *House dust mites: avoidance measures for allergy sufferers* is available from the British Allergy Foundation, Deepdene House, 30 Bellgrove Road, Welling, Kent DA16 3BY.

Table 3 Treatment of allergic rhinitis

- Allergen avoidance (house dust mite, animal danders, occupational causes)
- Non-sedative antihistamines, either alone or in combination with topical corticosteroids
- Topical corticosteroids; check technique and place emphasis on regular use even when symptoms are absent
- Sodium cromoglycate or nedocromil are useful for allergic eye symptoms
- Immunotherapy is helpful in pollen-sensitive patients unresponsive to the above measures
- If the patient fails to respond, review the diagnosis and treat any associated conditions (e.g. antibiotics for infection, surgery for structural problems)

dyskinesia, Kartagener's syndrome). Recurrent respiratory infections or a history of chronic rhinosinusitis should also raise the possibility of immune deficiency disorders including hypogammaglobulinaemia and acquired immune deficiency syndrome (AIDS).

Hormonal imbalance (premenstrual symptoms, pregnancy, hypothyroidism, or acromegaly) may be associated with rhinitis. A history of trauma or previous nasal surgery should be sought.

Enquiry regarding associated chest disease is important. Rhinitis and asthma frequently coexist and recognition and appropriate treatment of rhinitis may improve asthma control. The efficacy, frequency, and regularity of previous treatments should also be considered, as should the patient's perception of possible side-effects of treatment, a frequently missed cause of poor compliance.

Examination

Local examination may be performed with a head mirror and speculum or an auroscope. Allergic rhinitis is accompanied by a pale bluish 'boggy' appearance of the nasal mucosa only if the patient has current symptoms. A red inflamed appearance with pus suggests an infective cause. A granular appearance with fine pale nodules is diagnostic of sarcoidosis. Enlarged turbinates may be confused with polyps by the unwary. If doubt exists, further examination with a rigid and/or flexible endoscope should be performed. The identification of structural abnormalities such as polyps, deflected nasal septum, or enlarged turbinates is important: surgical treatment may be indicated (a major advance has been the development of minimally invasive endoscopic sinus surgery).

Examination of the nose should also include tests of smell and examination of the ears, eyes, mouth, and throat. Examination of the chest and a general examination should be performed when indicated, in view of the common association of nasal disease with lower respiratory and systemic conditions.

Investigations

Skin-prick tests

In the presence of a clear history, particularly of seasonal hay fever symptoms, skin-prick testing is not essential. However, skin-prick tests are useful for several reasons (Table 2). They should only be interpreted in conjunction with the clinical history, and not performed when the patient is taking antihistamines, if 'dermographism' (wealing in response to pressure) is present, or in the presence of severe eczema. In these circumstances meas-

Treatment for adults should be concentrated on the bedroom and living room, while measures for mite-sensitive children should be extended to all parts of the home. Measures to eradicate mites and allergens should be undertaken only following proper diagnosis and with appropriate medical supervision. There is no firm evidence to recommend the additional use of air conditioners, air ionizers, or acaracides. A recent meta-analysis has questioned the value of avoidance measures in mite-allergic patients. Where animal exposure is relevant, there is frequent resistance to advice to remove a family pet. However, patients can be advised to avoid replacing animals, to confine them to the kitchen or outdoors where possible, and to avoid contact with them or contaminated clothing. Recent evidence suggests that washing both cats and dogs may be effective in reducing pet allergen exposure.

Pharmacotherapy

The availability of potent specific histamine H1 receptor antagonists with a low potential for anticholinergic side-effects and a low sedative profile has been a major advance. Antihistamines are particularly effective for sneezing, itching, and rhinorrhoea, but unlike topical corticosteroids they have less effect on nasal blockage. They are also effective for eye and throat symptoms.

A rare but important complication of terfenadine is prolongation of the QT interval on the electrocardiogram (**ECG**). This only occurs when doses in excess of those recommended are employed, or in the presence of hepatic impairment or concomitant use of ketoconazole or erythromycin, both of which modify the hepatic metabolism of terfenadine. Astemizole may have the same effect in overdose. Acrivastine, loratadine, des-loratidine, cetirizine, ebastine, fexofenadine, and mizolastine are effective second-generation H1 antihistamines with an extremely low (or absent) potential for cardiac side-effects. H1-selective antihistamines can also be given as a topical nasal spray (levocabastine, azelastine). Antihistamines should be avoided during pregnancy.

Topical corticosteroids are highly effective in the majority of hay fever sufferers. Preparations include beclometasone, budesonide, fluticasone, triamcinolone, and mometasone. Aqueous formulations are better tolerated and have a better local distribution in the nose. Treatment should begin before the hay fever season for maximal effect, and the importance of regular treatment, even when symptoms are absent, should be emphasized. Side-effects are minor. Systemic effects are virtually absent at conventional doses, but caution should be exercised in children, particularly those receiving additional corticosteroids by other routes (for example, for associated asthma and/or eczema).

The topical anticholinergic agent ipratropium bromide is a potent inhibitor of glandular secretion and may be effective where watery nasal discharge is the dominant symptom, uncontrolled by the measures described above.

Sodium cromoglycate is available as a topical nasal spray for use four times daily. It is less effective than topical corticosteroids. Topical cromoglycate eye drops are effective for allergic eye symptoms in the majority of patients. Topical nedocromil sodium eyedrops have the advantage of a longer duration of action, allowing twice daily administration.

In the small proportion of patients whose symptoms are not otherwise controlled, there is a place for a short course of prednisolone (20 mg daily for 5 days). This approach may unblock the nose, thereby improving access for topical corticosteroids, which may then be more effective.

Topical decongestants (oxymetazoline) are effective in treating nasal blockage, although they should only be used for short periods (no more than 2 weeks) in view of the risk of tachyphylaxis and rebound persistent nasal blockage (so-called rhinitis medicamentosa).

Allergen immunotherapy

In patients with severe summer hay fever unresponsive to topical corticosteroids and antihistamines and in those reluctant to take long-term medication, immunotherapy (desensitization) is an alternative treatment option. Immunotherapy involves the subcutaneous injection of increasing concentrations of allergen (standardized pollen extract) at weekly intervals for 6 to 12 weeks, followed by monthly injections of a maintenance dose for 3 to 5 years. It should only be given by those who are properly trained, and with epinephrine (adrenaline) and facilities for cardiopulmonary resuscitation immediately available. Patients should be kept under medical observation for at least 60 min following injections.

Recent controlled studies have confirmed the efficacy of immunotherapy, particularly for patients with grass pollen-induced summer hay fever (WHO guidelines). It is less effective in those with perennial rhinitis and asthma, where the disease is frequently heterogeneous with multiple allergic sensitivities and/or other causes of ongoing symptoms. The risk/benefit is less favourable in patients with chronic bronchial asthma in whom the risks of systemic adverse reactions are greater. Recent data suggests that pollen immunotherapy may confer long-term benefit. In patients who had received 3 to 4 years' treatment, clinical improvement was maintained for at least 3 years following discontinuation. This suggests that allergen immunotherapy, unlike pharmacotherapy, confers long-term benefit and has the potential to modify the course of the disease.

Future prospects for immunotherapy include the use of alternative safer routes such as local nasal or sublingual immunotherapy. Low molecular weight allergen peptides represent an alternative strategy for vaccine development, with the potential to modify T-cell responses with clinical benefit without the potential for IgE crosslinking and attendant risk of serious IgE-mediated side-effects.

Further reading

Abramson M, Puy R, Weiner J. (1999). Immunotherapy in asthma: an updated systematic review. *Allergy* **54**, 1022–41.

Akdis CA, Blaser K (1999). IL-10-induced anergy in peripheral T cell and reactivation by microenvironmental cytokines: two key steps in specific immunotherapy. *FASEB Journal* **13**, 603–9.

Bousquet J, Lockey RF, Malling HJ (1998). WHO position paper: allergen immunotherapy: therapeutic vaccination for allergic diseases. *Allergy* **53**, Supplement 44.

Colloff MJ, *et al.* (1992). The control of allergens of dust mites and domestic pets: a position paper. *Clinical and Experimental Allergy* **22**(Suppl. 2), 1–28.

Durham SR, Till SJ (1998). Immunologic mechanisms associated with allergen immunotherapy. *Journal of Allergy and Clinical Immunology* **102**(2), 157–64.

Durham SR, *et al.* (1999). Long term clinical efficacy of grass pollen immunotherapy. *New England Journal of Medicine* **341**, 468–75.

Fleming DM, Crombie DL (1987). Prevalence of asthma and hayfever in England and Wales. *British Medical Journal* **294**, 279–83.

Gotzsche PC, Hammarquist C, Burr M (1998). House dust mite control measures in the management of asthma: meta-analysis. *British Medical Journal* **317**, 1105–10.

Lund V, *et al.* (1994). International consensus report on the diagnosis and management of rhinitis. *Allergy* **49**(Suppl. 19), 1–34.

17.4.3 Basic mechanisms and pathophysiology of asthma

Tak H. Lee

Introduction

Bronchial asthma is characterized by episodic wheezing, airways obstruction that is reversible, either spontaneously or with therapy, bronchial hyper-responsiveness to non-specific stimuli, and airways inflammation.

Risk factors for the development of asthma

Atopy is the strongest risk factor for the development of asthma. The most important mechanism by which IgE determines the expression of atopy is through its binding to high-affinity receptors (Fcε-RI) expressed on the surface of tissue mast cells and basophils, and to lower-affinity receptors (Fcε-RII or CD23) on macrophages, eosinophils, and platelets. Cross-linkage of IgE with a specific allergen results in the non-cytotoxic release of an array of preformed and newly generated mediators of inflammation.

The domestic house dust mite (**HDM**, *Dermatophagoides pteronyssinus*) is the major allergenic cause of perennial asthma. To date, seven groups of HDM allergens have been identified, the first four of which are known to exhibit proteolytic or other enzymatic activities. For example, Der p1, the major allergen of *D. pteronyssinus*, is a cysteine protease derived from the mite's gastrointestinal tract, whereas Der p2 is a lysozyme and Der p3 a chymotryptic enzyme. The potent biological activities of other allergens might explain why these particular proteins are able to penetrate epithelial surfaces so easily and lead to specific sensitization.

Maternal smoking, both before and after birth, is a risk factor for developing respiratory disease early in life. Exposure to environmental tobacco smoke has been shown to increase IgE in adults, and some studies have suggested that maternal smoking in pregnancy increases cord-blood IgE and the subsequent risk of atopic disease.

Other factors implicated in the early-life origins of asthma include respiratory-tract virus infections, particularly with the respiratory syncytial virus (**RSV**), possibly through damage to the bronchial epithelium, thereby augmenting the penetration of the airway mucosa by inhaled allergens. Exposure to environmental air pollutants, such as ozone, sulphur dioxide, and oxides of nitrogen, has recently been shown to enhance allergen sensitization of the lower respiratory tract.

Pathology

Histological examination of the airway tissue in an asthmatic lung shows the presence of an inflammatory reaction, with extensive remodelling of the airway wall. The inflammation is a multicellular process; even in the mildest of asthmatic individuals there is *in vivo* evidence of infiltration of the bronchial mucosa with mast cells, mononuclear cells, and granulocytes, of which the eosinophil is prominent. The tenacious plugs that fill the lumen are an exudate of plasma and inflammatory cells, particularly eosinophils, which have migrated into the lumen, as well as epithelial cells that have sloughed from the airway surface, often leaving the basement membrane denuded. The basement membrane appears thickened when viewed under the light microscope, which is due to an increase in the amount of collagen deposition at this site, but the lamina densa, which forms the true basement membrane, is normal when observed with the electron microscope.

The changes in the lumen and wall of the airways of asthmatic lungs are reflected in the cytological examination of sputum from patients with the disease. Early studies of the sputum showed the presence of Creola bodies (sloughed epithelial clumps), Charcot-Leyden crystals (remnants of eosinophils), and Curschmann spirals (casts of the airway formed by the exudate). More recent studies have established that the eosinophil is the prominent cell found in the sputum of asthmatic patients.

There is a clear increase in wall thickness throughout the bronchial tree in patients with asthma, and all the tissue layers participate in this generalized increase in airway wall thickness. The volume of the bronchial microvasculature is also increased in both the submucosa and the adventitia of the airways. It has been calculated that the thickening of the airway wall caused by asthma has only a minor effect on the lumen of a fully dilated airway, but when a modest increase in wall thickness is associated with smooth-muscle shortening, the two factors acting together produce markedly increased airway resistance.

Inflammatory cells

Bronchial inflammation is orchestrated by a network of cytokines and growth factors, including those encoded by the **GM-CSF/IL-4/IL-5** (granulocyte–macrophage colony-stimulating factor/interleukin-4/-5) gene cluster on chromosome 5, derived from both inflammatory and structural cells in the airways.

Mast cells

Mast cells are clearly important in initiating the acute bronchoconstrictor responses to allergen, and probably to other indirect stimuli such as exercise and hyperventilation (via osmolarity or thermal changes). When sensitized subjects inhale specific allergen it causes both early (5–15 min—early airway response, **EAR**) and late (2–6 h—late airway response, **LAR**) bronchoconstrictor responses, which last approximately 60 min and between 12 and 24 h, respectively. The LAR is accompanied by an acquired increase in bronchial responsiveness to such stimuli as inhaled histamine and methacholine (Fig. 1).

Measurement of mediators in the peripheral blood and bronchoalveolar lavage fluid together with their metabolites in urine has shown that the EAR is a mast cell-dependent response resulting from the IgE-dependent secretion of constrictor substances. The type of mast cell involved in this reaction contains predominantly tryptase as its neutral protease. Among its biological actions, tryptase is able to produce a prolonged increase in microvascular permeability, upregulate adhesion molecules, attract and activate eosinophils, and augment epithelial and fibroblast proliferation. Histamine exerts most of its airway effects via H1 receptors, which are present both on airway smooth muscle and on the microvasculature, whilst prostaglandin D2 (**PGD2**) contracts airway smooth muscle by interacting with thromboxane (TP1) receptors. Once released from mast cells, LTC_4 is rapidly metabolized to LTD_4 and subsequently to LTE_4, the three cysteinyl leukotrienes responsible for the smooth-muscle contractile and vasoactive properties of the biological activity previously described as **SRS-A** (slow-reacting substance of anaphylaxis) (Fig. 2).

Eosinophils

The late airway response has an inflammatory basis. During this response there is an increased bronchoalveolar lavage eosinophilia, suggesting the selective recruitment of these cells into airway tissue from the microvasculature. Eosinophil infiltration is a characteristic feature of asthmatic airways and differentiates asthma from other inflammatory airway conditions. There is a close relationship between eosinophil counts in peripheral blood or bronchoalveolar lavage (**BAL**) fluid and airway hyperresponsiveness.

Eosinophil migration may be due to the effects of lipid mediators, such as leukotrienes, or to the effects of cytokines such as GM-CSF, IL-5, RANTES, and eotaxin (**RANTES**, regulated upon activation, normal T-cell

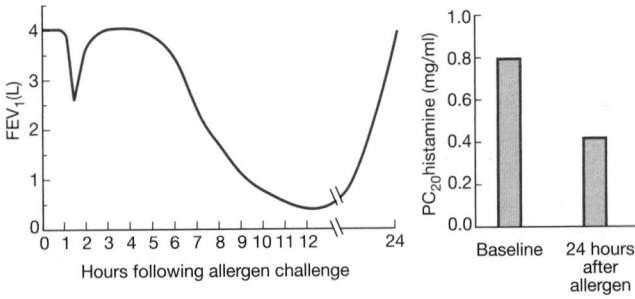

Fig. 1 Changes in **FEV₁** (forced expiratory volume in 1 second) and histamine airway responsiveness after allergen inhalation challenge in an asthmatic subject. PC_{20} histamine is the concentration of histamine producing a 20 per cent decrease in FEV₁. It is a measure of 'non-specific' airway responsiveness.

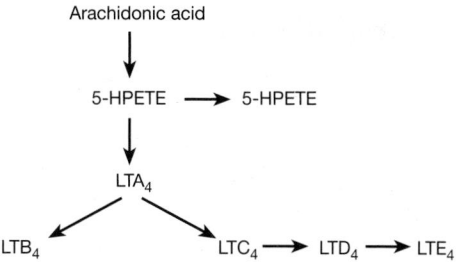

Fig. 2 The 5-lipoxygenase pathway. 5-HPETE = 5-hydroperoxy-eicosatetraenoic acid, 5-HETE = 5-hydroxy-eicosatetraenoic acid. LT = leukotriene.

expressed and secreted chemokine). Several of these molecules might also be very important for the survival of eosinophils in the airways and may 'prime' eosinophils to exhibit enhanced responsiveness. There appears to be a co-operative interaction between IL-5 and chemokines, so that both cytokines are necessary for the eosinophilic response in airways. Once recruited to the airways, eosinophils require the presence of various growth factors, of which GM-CSF and IL-5 appear to be the most important. In the absence of these growth factors eosinophils undergo programmed cell death (apoptosis).

Within the airways, active eosinophils secrete a wide array of preformed and newly generated inflammatory products. These compromise the toxic granule components of the eosinophil (major basic protein, eosinophil cationic protein, and eosinophil-derived neurotoxin) and a range of lipid products, including leukotrienes and platelet activating factor (**PAF**). The administration of LTD_4 antagonists prior to allergen provocation of sensitized airways produces marked inhibition of both the EAR and LAR and attenuation of the acquired increase in bronchial hyper-responsiveness. Although PAF was at one time regarded as a prime mediator of the late-phase inflammatory response and bronchial hyper-responsiveness, investigation of the orally active PAF receptor antagonist WEB 2086 has failed to reveal any inhibitory effect on either early- or late-phase, allergen-induced airway events. Eosinophils are also involved in the generation of oxygen-derived free radicals.

Other leucocytes

The mechanism(s) by which leucocytes move into the airway and become activated have attracted considerable interest. At 6 h following allergen challenge, there is marked upregulation of E-selectin, whose ligand on neutrophils and other leucocytes is sialyl-Lewis × and intercellular adhesion molecule-1 (**ICAM-1**), a member of the immunoglobulin superfamily. One ligand for ICAM-1 is lymphocyte function-associated antigen-1 (**LFA-1**) (an integrin heterodimer CD11a–CD18) expressed on a large number of leucocytes, but especially on lymphocytes, neutrophils, and eosinophils. Another member of the immunoglobulin superfamily, vascular cell-adhesion molecule-1 (**VCAM-1**), is expressed in the airway microvasculature at a low level, but this is not increased within the time frame of 6 h following allergen provocation. A positive correlation has been observed between the extent of ICAM-1 expression and leucocyte infiltration, and more specifically between E-selectin and the increase in neutrophil numbers, suggesting an important role for these molecules in the allergic inflammatory process.

The initial expression of P-, L-, and E-selectins, which contain lectin binding regions that interact with carbohydrate ligands and leucocytes (e.g. sialyl-Lewis ×) results in the rolling of leucocytes along the endothelial cell, whereas upregulation of ICAM-1 and VCAM-1 arrests the leucocytes, thereby facilitating transendothelial migration. In non-human primates naturally sensitized to *Ascaris* antigen, blocking antibodies directed to E-selectin and ICAM-1 abrogate the LAR and the resultant bronchial hyper-responsiveness following allergen challenge, in parallel with a reduction in neutrophils and eosinophils.

The role of neutrophils in human asthma is less clear. They are found in the airways of patients with chronic bronchitis and bronchiectasis who do not have the degree of airway hyper-responsiveness found in patients with asthma. Neutrophils are rarely seen in the airways of patients with chronic asthma, but large numbers are seen in those who die suddenly of asthma. This may reflect the rapid kinetics of neutrophil recruitment compared with eosinophil inflammation.

Macrophages, which are derived from blood monocytes, traffic into the airways and may orchestrate the inflammatory response. Macrophages may both increase and decrease inflammation, depending on the stimulus. Alveolar macrophages normally have a suppressive effect on lymphocyte function and may play an important role in preventing the development of allergic inflammation, but this may be impaired in asthma after allergen exposure. Macrophages can also act as antigen-presenting cells (**APCs**), processing allergen for presentation to T-lymphocytes, but alveolar macrophages are far less effective in this respect than macrophages from other sites. By contrast, dendritic cells, which are specialized macrophage-like cells in the airway epithelium, are very effective antigen-presenting cells and might play a very important role in the initiation of allergen-induced responses in asthma.

T lymphocytes play a very important role in co-ordinating the inflammatory response in asthma through the release of specific patterns of cytokines, resulting in the recruitment and survival of eosinophils and the maintenance of mast cells in the airways. T lymphocytes are coded to express a distinctive pattern of cytokines, which may be similar to that described in the murine TH2 type of T lymphocyte that characteristically express IL-4, IL-5, and IL-13. There appears to be an imbalance of TH cells in asthma, with the balance in favour of TH2 cells. The balance between TH1 cells and TH2 cells may be determined by locally released cytokines such as IL-12, favouring the expression of TH1 cells, and IL-4, favouring TH2 cells. There is a suggestion that early infections might encourage TH1-mediated responses to predominate and that a lack of infection in childhood may favour TH2-cell expression and thus atopic diseases.

Structural cells

Structural cells of the airways, including epithelial cells, fibroblasts, and airway smooth muscle cells, are also important sources of inflammatory mediators, such as cytokines and lipid mediators, in asthma. In addition, epithelial cells may play a key role in translating inhaled environmental signals into an airway inflammatory response and are probably a major target cell for inhaled glucocorticoids.

Inflammatory mediators

Many different mediators have been implicated in asthma. Those such as histamine, prostaglandins, and leukotrienes contract airway smooth muscle, increase microvascular leakage, increase airway mucus secretion, and attract other inflammatory cells. The availability of specific receptor antagonists has defined the critical role of certain mediators. For instance, the cysteinyl leukotrienes LTC_4, LTD_4, and LTE_4, are potent constrictors of human airways and have been reported to increase airway hyper-responsiveness, recruit eosinophils, and possibly play an important role in asthma. Potent LTD_4 antagonists protect against exercise-, aspirin-, and allergen-induced bronchoconstriction, suggesting that cysteinyl leukotrienes contribute to bronchoconstrictor responses. Chronic treatment with cysteinyl leukotriene antagonists improves lung function and symptoms in asthmatic patients.

Cytokines

Cytokines play a central role in orchestrating the type of inflammatory response. Many inflammatory cells (macrophages, mast cells, eosinophils, and lymphocytes) are capable of synthesizing and releasing these proteins, and structural cells such as epithelial cells and endothelial cells may also release a variety of cytokines and therefore participate in the chronic inflammatory response. While inflammatory mediators like histamine and leukotrienes may be important in the acute and subacute inflammatory responses and in exacerbations of asthma, it is likely that cytokines play a dominant role in chronic inflammation.

As atopy is a major risk factor for the development of asthma, it is essential to understand how IgE synthesis is regulated. IL-4 interacts with B cells via specific cell-surface receptors, and is a key cytokine involved in the isotype-switching of B cells from synthesizing IgM and IgG to IgE. An important accessory signal for IgE-switching is provided by CD40 on T cells signalling through the CD40 ligand on B cells. IL-13, which exhibits 30 per cent homology with IL-4, has also been shown to mediate IgE isotype-switching through its own specific receptors but, unlike IL-4, it is also a differentiation factor for dendritic cells. Switching of B cells to IgE synthesis is potently inhibited by interferon-gamma (IFN-γ) from TH₁ cells and monocytes/macrophages.

In vivo evidence for cytokine involvement in asthma

Bronchoalveolar lavage (BAL)

Increased proportions of cells positive for IL-4 and IL-5 mRNA are found using the technique of in situ hybridization in atopic asthmatic subjects. Symptomatic asthmatic subjects have greater proportions of cells positive for IL-3, IL-4, IL-5, and GM-CSF mRNA in BAL fluid than asymptomatic asthmatics. No differences between the groups in the numbers of cells expressing IL-2 and IFN-γ mRNA are detected. In addition, there are significant associations between the number of cells expressing mRNA for IL-4, IL-5, and GM-CSF and baseline airflow obstruction, airway hyper-responsiveness, and asthmatic symptoms. Increased levels of tumour-necrosis factor-α (**TNF-a**), GM-CSF, and IL-6 have been found in BAL fluid of symptomatic as compared to asymptomatic asthmatic subjects.

Studies on alveolar macrophages of asthmatic subjects showed that IL-1β expression is upregulated and that the level of IL-1β in BAL fluid of subjects with symptomatic asthma is higher than that of normal subjects or subjects with asymptomatic asthma. Additionally, bronchoalveolar lavage fluid from symptomatic non-allergic asthmatic subjects contains elevated levels of IL-1.

Evidence from challenge models further supports cytokine involvement in asthma. Increases have been shown in the number of cells expressing mRNA for the TH2 cytokines IL-4, IL-5, and GM-CSF but not IL-3, IL-2, or IFN-α after allergen challenge. Furthermore, IL-4 and IL-5 mRNAs transcripts were associated with activated CD4+ T cells.

Bronchial biopsies

Immunohistochemical analysis of bronchial biopsies from symptomatic and asymptomatic atopic and non-atopic asthmatics reveals increased immunoreactivity with IL-1/2/3/4/5, GM-CSF, **MCP-1** (monocyte chemotaxis protein-1), and TNF-α as opposed to asymptomatic control subjects.

Mucosal biopsies obtained from atopic asthmatics after allergen challenge demonstrate an increased influx of activated eosinophils and activated CD4+ T cells, and an increase in the number of cells expressing mRNA for IL-5 and GM-CSF. There is a significant inverse correlation between the numbers of cells expressing mRNA for IL-4 and IFN-α. This supports the hypothesis that allergen-induced late asthmatic responses are accompanied by T-cell activation, cytokine mRNA expression for IL-5 and GM-CSF, and local recruitment and activation of the eosinophils in the bronchial mucosa.

Effects of inflammation

The chronic inflammatory response may alter the structure and function of critical target cells in the airways.

Airway epithelium

Airway epithelial shedding may be important in contributing to airway hyper-responsiveness, and may explain how several different mechanisms (for example, ozone exposure, certain virus infections, chemical sensitizers, and allergen exposure) can lead to the development of this condition. All these stimuli may lead to epithelial disruption, which may contribute to airway hyper-responsiveness by the loss of barrier function to allow penetration of allergens, loss of enzymes (such as neutral endopeptidase) that normally degrade inflammatory mediators, and exposure of sensory nerves, which might lead to reflex neural effects on the airway.

Airway smooth muscle

An abnormality in smooth muscle function is thought to be the basis of the bronchial hyper-responsiveness in asthma, but studies of isolated human bronchi from asthmatic subjects have failed to demonstrate a clear consensus for the presence of a functional abnormality. Of eight reports of individuals who are hyper-responsive to histamine and methacholine in vivo, half have shown increased force generation by asthmatic airways in vitro, compared to control airway preparations; the remainder report no difference in force generation by asthmatic or normal isolated airway preparations. The reasons for this anomaly are unclear. In general, studies have been carried out using airways from mild asthmatics and differences in optimal length for maximum force generation and smooth muscle content have not been accounted for. Similarly, passive sensitization studies have produced conflicting data. In three of four studies, exposure of airways removed from non-atopic patients to serum from patients with high IgE levels confers increased responsiveness to specific allergen and hyper-responsiveness to non-specific stimuli such as histamine and neuropeptides.

Other functional changes may be important. Reduced responsiveness to β₂-adrenoceptor agonists has been reported in both postmortem and surgically removed bronchi from asthmatic patients, although the number of β-adrenoceptors is not reduced, suggesting that these receptors have in some way become functionally uncoupled. This aspect of altered airway smooth muscle function can be modelled in vitro, where treatment of airway smooth muscle cells with cytokines induces a similar refractoriness to β₂-adrenoceptor agonists.

Changes in compliance of the extracellular connective tissue components between individual muscle cells and in the stiffness of parallel elastic elements in the extracellular compartment may reduce the tethering loads of the muscle and allow greater shortening. Indeed, treatment of human airway smooth muscle preparations with the matrix degrading enzyme collagenase enhances force generation and shortening.

It seems likely that the involvement of the smooth muscle in excessive airway narrowing in asthma involves several mechanisms. These include an increased content of smooth muscle in the airway wall, or a combination of increased content and altered function. It is now recognized that, in addition to contractile function, airway smooth muscle can undergo hyperplasia and/or hypertrophy, leading to apparently irreversible changes in wall structure and contributing to the development of persistent airway obstruction and non-specific airway hyper-responsiveness. Numerous studies have characterized some of the proinflammatory mediators and growth factors that elicit proliferation of smooth muscle. Other trophic factors such as altered mechanical stress and reactive oxygen species have also been identified. Components of the extracellular matrix that are increased in asthma may also impact on the proliferation of airway smooth muscle.

Proliferating airway smooth muscle cells undergo phenotypic modulation from a contractile to synthetic–proliferative state, where additional

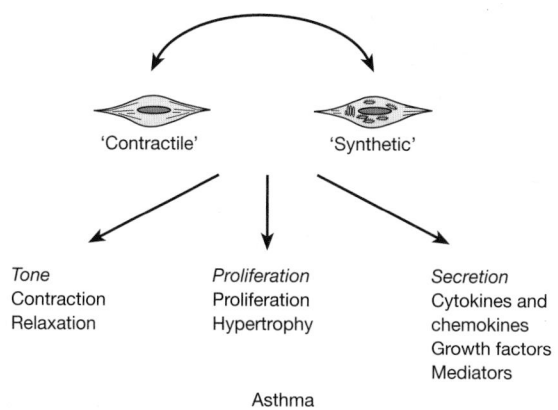

Fig. 3 The role of airway smooth muscle in chronic severe asthma (by courtesy of S. Hirst).

functions of airway smooth muscle such as cytokine/chemokine and extracellular matrix secretion become more apparent. This is likely to be of particular relevance in the diseased asthmatic lung where the content of airway smooth muscle as a fraction of the total cells in the airway wall is already increased. Human airway smooth muscle releases several chemokines important for the activation of eosinophils. These include chemotaxins such as RANTES and eotaxin, as well as GM-CSF. Airway smooth muscle cells also interact by direct contact with immunocytes such as T lymphocytes through the expression of cell-adhesion molecules and the induction of myocyte DNA synthesis. T lymphocytes derived from bronchoalveolar lavage fluid following antigen challenge of atopic subjects adhere to human airway smooth muscle cells in culture, inducing ICAM-1 and HLA-DR expression on the smooth muscle cells.

As additional functions of airway smooth muscle are described, a view (Fig. 3) is emerging that airway smooth muscle cells may adopt an immunoeffector role in chronic asthma by proliferating, secreting cytokines, expressing adhesion molecules, and by interacting with various immunocytes. This may involve changes in the phenotypic status of airway smooth muscle, and, as a result, these cells may play an active role in perpetuating and orchestrating airway inflammation in the remodelled airway. These novel insights question previously held paradigms of altered neural activity and inflammation in asthma, and emphasize the importance of the response of the end-organ, namely the smooth muscle cell.

Vascular responses

Vasodilatation occurs in inflammation, yet little is known about the role of the airway circulation in asthma, partly because of the difficulties involved in measuring airway blood flow. The bronchial circulation may play an important role in regulating airway calibre, since an increase in the vascular volume may contribute to airway narrowing. Increased airway blood flow may be important in removing inflammatory mediators from the airway, and may play a role in the development of exercise-induced asthma.

Microvascular leakage is also an essential component of the inflammatory response. It may increase airway secretions, impair mucociliary clearance and enhance mucosal oedema, thereby contributing to airway narrowing and increased airway hyper-responsiveness.

Neural effects

Non-adrenergic, non-cholinergic (**NANC**) nerves and several neuropeptides have been identified in the respiratory tract, in addition to those involved in classical cholinergic and adrenergic mechanisms. It is unclear whether abnormalities of autonomic function in asthma are secondary to the disease or primary defects. It is recognized that inflammation may interact with autonomic control by several mechanisms. For instance, neuropeptides such as substance P, neurokinin A, and calcitonin gene-related

peptide may be released from sensitized inflammatory nerves in the airways and may amplify the inflammatory response. There is evidence for an increase in substance P-immunoreactive nerves in the airways of patients with severe asthma, although this has not been confirmed in patients with mild disease. There may also be a reduction in the activity of enzymes such as neutral endopeptidase which degrade neuropeptides such as substance P. There may also be increased expression of the receptor that mediates the inflammatory effects of substance P.

Further reading

Arm JP, Lee TH (1993). Chemical mediators II: Leukotrienes and eicosanoids. In: Weiss EB, Stein M, eds. *Bronchial asthma: mechanisms and therapeutics*, 3rd edn., pp. 112–34. Little, Brown Co.

Cockcroft DW, Murdock KY (1987). Changes in bronchial responsiveness to histamine at intervals after allergen challenge. *Thorax* **42**, 302–8.

Israel E, et al. (1993). The pivotal role of 5-lipoxygenase products in the reaction of aspirin-sensitive asthmatics to aspirin. *American Review of Respiratory Disease* **148**, 1447–51.

Jeffery PK, et al. (1989). Bronchial biopsies in asthma: an ultrastructural quantification study and correlation with hyperreactivity. *American Review of Respiratory Disease* **140**, 1745–53.

Johnson SR, Knox AJ (1997). Synthetic functions of airway smooth muscle in asthma. *Trends in Pharmacological Science* **18**, 288–92.

Lambert RK, et al. (1993). Functional significance of increased airway smooth muscle in asthma and COPD. *Journal of Applied Physiology* **74**, 2771–81.

Lee TH (1998). Cytokine networks in the pathogenesis of bronchial asthma: implications for therapy. *Journal of the Royal College of Physicians of London* **32**, 56–64.

Moreno RH, Hogg JC, Pare PD (1986). Mechanisms of airway narrowing. *American Review of Respiratory Disease* **133**, 1171–80.

Panettieri RA (1998). Cellular and molecular mechanisms regulating airway smooth muscle proliferation and cell adhesion molecule expression. *American Journal of Respiratory and Critical Care Medicine* **158**, S133–S140.

Rabe KF (1998). Mechanisms of immune sensitisation of human bronchus. *American Journal of Respiratory and Critical Care Medicine* **158**, S161–S170.

Reiss TF, et al. (1998). Montelukast, a once-daily leukotriene receptor antagonist, in the treatment of chronic asthma: a multicenter randomized, double-blind trial. *Archives of Internal Medicine* **158**, 1213–20.

Robinson DS, et al. (1992). Evidence for a predominant Th 2-type bronchoalveolar T-lymphocyte population in atopic asthma. *New England Journal of Medicine* **326**, 298–304.

Seow CY, Schellenberg RR, Pare PD (1998). Structural and functional changes in the airway smooth muscle of asthmatic subjects. *American Journal of Respiratory and Critical Care Medicine* **158**, S179–S186.

Shirakawa T, et al. (1997). The inverse association between tuberculin responses and atopic disorder. *Science* **275**, 77–9.

Stewart GA (1994). The molecular biology of allergens. In: Holgate ST, Busse W, eds. *The mechanisms of asthma and rhinitis*, pp. 898–932. Blackwell Science, Boston.

Wegner CD, et al. (1996). ICAM-1 in the pathogenesis of asthma. *Science* **247**, 416–18.

17.4.4 Asthma

A. J. Newman Taylor

Introduction

Asthma is a chronic inflammatory disease of the bronchial airways, which is characterized by a desquamative eosinophilic bronchitis (Fig. 1). The defining clinical characteristics of asthma—reversible airway narrowing and increased airway responsiveness to non-specific provocative stimuli—are manifestations of the underlying chronic inflammatory process. Definitions of asthma that have focused on these clinical characteristics, to distinguish it from diseases associated with predominantly irreversible airway narrowing, have emphasized the intermittent nature of asthma rather than the persistence of the underlying inflammation, with potentially inappropriate implications for treatment.

Table 1 Inducers and provokers of asthma

Inducers of asthma		
Allergens		Increased airway inflammation
Viral respiratory tract infections	→	Increased airway responsiveness
Low molecular weight chemicals		Increased severity of asthma
Provokers of asthma		
Exercise		
Cold dry air		
Respiratory irritants (e.g. sulphur dioxide)	→	Acute transient airway narrowing in individuals with
Histamine		hyperresponsive airways
Methacholine		

The recognition that asthma is a chronic inflammatory disease implies that, in addition to identifying and avoiding inducing causes, such as domestic pets and occupational sensitizers, disease control is likely to require long-term anti-inflammatory treatment. Appreciation of the inflammatory nature of asthma has also led to recognition of the associated injury and damage to the airway wall—airway remodelling—which may lead to irreversible loss of function, and be preventable by the early institution of anti-inflammatory treatment.

Asthma and airway hyperresponsiveness: inducers and provokers

The distinguishing abnormalities of lung function in bronchial asthma are: (i) reversible airway narrowing and (ii) airway hyperresponsiveness to non-specific provocative stimuli.

Airway responsiveness describes the ease with which acute airway narrowing can be provoked by a variety of stimuli. Non-specific provocative stimuli include exercise, inhalation of cold dry air, inhaled respiratory irritants such as sulphur dioxide, and pharmacological agents such as histamine and methacholine (Table 1). Provocation of asthma by specific allergens can induce hyperresponsiveness to non-specific stimuli, when smaller doses of such stimuli provoke acute airway narrowing. Inhaled non-specific provocative stimuli, such as histamine or methacholine, incite airway narrowing that usually resolves within minutes; exercise provokes asthma within minutes that resolves within 1 h.

The degree of airway responsiveness can be expressed as the dose or concentration of the stimulus which provokes a specified fall in the forced expiratory volume in 1 s (FEV_1), commonly the dose or concentration of histamine or methacholine which provokes a 20 per cent fall in FEV_1—**PD20** or **PC20**, histamine or methacholine.

While provokers of asthma incite acute airway narrowing in individuals with hyperresponsive airways, inducers of asthma increase the magnitude of airway hyperresponsiveness and the clinical manifestations of asthma by increasing the severity of the underlying airway inflammation, which can persist for days or weeks. The principal inducers of asthma are inhaled allergens, low molecular weight chemicals encountered at work, and viral respiratory tract infections (Table 1).

Allergen inhalation tests are a good model of the airway response to an inducer and demonstrate the interrelationship between airway inflammation, airway narrowing, and airway hyperresponsiveness. Inhalation of an allergen by an individual allergic to it with asthma will provoke:

(1) an immediate fall in FEV_1, which develops within minutes and usually resolves spontaneously within 1 to 1.5 h; and

(2) a subsequent late fall in FEV_1, which develops in about 50 per cent of cases 1 h or more after the inhalation test and persists for several hours, on occasions for days.

The immediate fall in FEV_1 is IgE dependent and is due to airway smooth muscle contraction and airway wall oedema provoked by mediators, such as histamine, released from mast cells resident in the airways. It

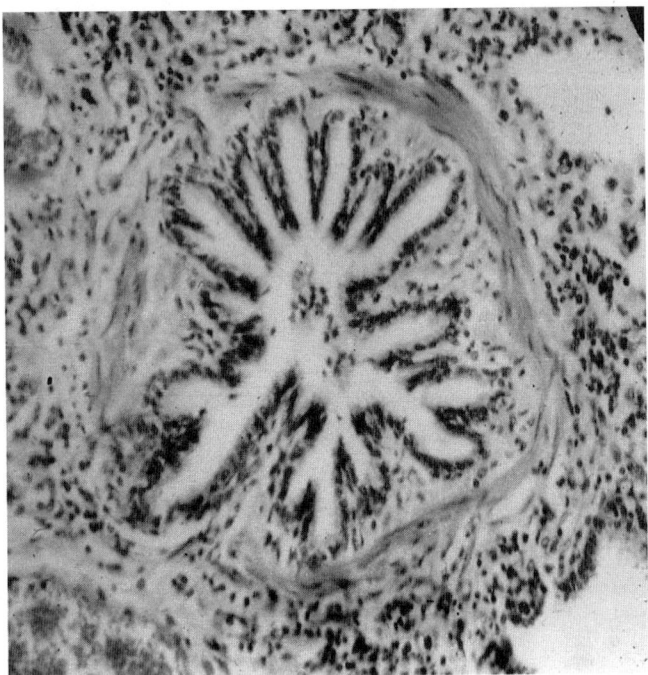

(a)

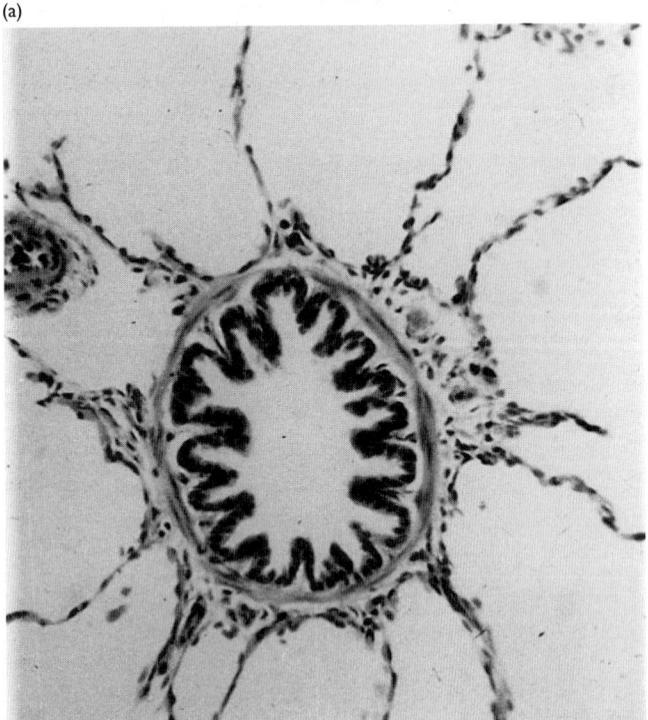

(b)

Fig. 1 The defining pathology of asthma: (a) desquamative eosinophilic bronchitis in patient with asthma, in comparison with (b) normal histological appearances.

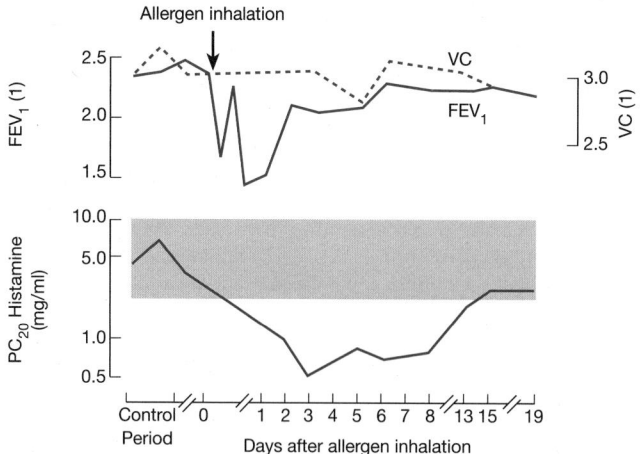

Fig. 2 Increased airway responsiveness associated with late asthmatic reaction provoked by inhalation of ragweed pollen.

is not associated with an increase in airway responsiveness. The late fall in FEV_1 is the outcome of recruitment to the airways of inflammatory cells, particularly T_{H2} lymphocytes and eosinophils, reducing airway calibre. It is associated with an increase in airway responsiveness (manifest as a reduction in PC_{20}) that can persist, with associated increased diurnal variation in airway calibre, for several days after resolution of airway narrowing (Fig. 2).

Prevalence of asthma

Asthma is a common disease, frequently disabling and, uncommonly, the cause of death. In the Western world it now has an estimated prevalence of more than 10 per cent in children and more than 5 per cent in adults. In the United Kingdom in 1999 it was the cause of 86 000 hospital admissions and the certified cause of death of 1520 people.

The prevalence of asthma in children and young adults has increased markedly in the Western world during the past 20 to 30 years (Fig. 3). Although in part this increase may reflect a greater awareness of and tendency to diagnose asthma, repeat cross-sectional studies of children in the United Kingdom, using identical methods of ascertainment at different time points, have shown a definite increase in disease prevalence. A study of Aberdeen school children found the prevalence of wheeze and of diagnosed asthma had increased 2.5-fold between 1964 and 1989. A similar study in South Wales, made at two time points 15 years apart, found a history of reported asthma to have doubled from 6 to 12 per cent. This study also reported a similar increase of reported hay fever and eczema, and in the proportion of children in whom exercise provoked asthma.

Comparison of the prevalence of asthma in different parts of the world suggests that the high and increasing prevalence in the Western world is

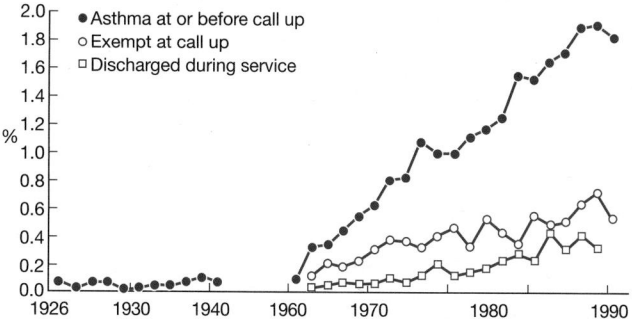

Fig. 3 Increasing prevalence of asthma in Finnish military recruits.

associated with urbanization and material prosperity. A study of school children in Zimbabwe found asthma to be uncommon in those living in a rural area, more common in poor urban dwellers, and most common in affluent urban dwellers, equally in the black and white population, in Harare. In Europe the reunification of Germany allowed comparison of the prevalence of asthma and associated conditions in cities in former East and West Germany. The prevalence of asthma, hay fever, eczema, and atopy (identified as immediate skin test responses to common inhalant allergens) was greater in school age children living in the West German city of Munich than in the East German cities of Leipzig and Halle. This greater prevalence of asthma, atopy, and atopic diseases in Western compared with Eastern Europe has been replicated in comparison studies between other countries (such as Finland compared with Estonia). Interestingly, the prevalence of atopy (particularly skin test responses to pollens) and hay fever, but not asthma, has subsequently increased in children now living in reunified Germany who had lived the first 5 years of their lives in Leipzig.

Many explanations have been advanced to explain these observations. These include increased indoor allergen exposure (particularly house dust mite and cat), increased exposure to vehicle exhaust pollution, increased tobacco smoking by women of childbearing age, changing diet, and reduced infection rates in childhood. Of these, outdoor air pollution has, until recently, attracted most public attention, although there is no substantive evidence in its support: the prevalence of asthma in urban parts of the United Kingdom is no greater (and possibly less) than in rural parts, including Skye, where measured levels of air pollutants are the lowest in the United Kingdom. Similarly, there is little evidence that the increased prevalence of asthma and other atopic disease has been caused by increased indoor allergen exposure or tobacco smoking, although the increase in asthma has been paralleled by an increase in cigarette smoking by women of childbearing age. Several dietary explanations have also been advanced, including increased salt and reduced antioxidant intake. The most plausible explanation advanced to date is that the increase in atopy and asthma is a consequence of a reduction in rates of infection during childhood. The evidence is both indirect and direct, although not yet conclusive. The most consistent observation, now from several studies, is of an inverse relationship between family size, and birth order, and the risk of atopy and hay fever. This has been interpreted as being consistent with the age at which a child encounters infectious agents having a decisive influence on the development of atopy and associated diseases: children in large families and those with older siblings are more likely to encounter infections earlier in life, reducing their risk of becoming atopic. Several, although not all, subsequent studies of the relationship of atopy and atopic disease to childhood infection have supported this hypothesis. In a group of children studied in Guinea-Bissau, West Africa the risk of being atopic (and in particular having specific IgE to *Dermatophagoides pternonyssinus*) was inversely related to having had measles in early childhood. Similarly, the risk of atopy, hay fever, and asthma was inversely related to having been infected with *Mycobacterium tuberculosis* in Japanese school children, and to having serum antibodies to hepatitis A, considered an indicator of hygiene in early life, in Italian military recruits.

Risk factors for asthma

The geographical variation and considerable increase in recent decades in the prevalence of asthma indicate important environmental influences on the development of the disease. There is also evidence for genetic susceptibility. The risk of asthma is associated with atopy, for which genetic influences are strong. As with many common complex diseases, such as diabetes mellitus, asthma is probably the outcome of multiple genes and their interaction with the environment.

Atopy

Atopy is defined as the production of specific IgE antibody to common inhalant allergens, such as grass pollen, house dust mite, and cat. Atopy may be identified by the presence of immediate skin prick test responses (or of specific IgE in serum) to extracts of common inhalant allergens and has a prevalence of some 40 per cent in the adult United Kingdom population. The risk of developing asthma as well as eczema and hay fever is increased in atopic individuals. In a random population sample in the south-west United States, a close relationship was found at all ages between skin test responses to local inhalant allergens and the prevalence of asthma and allergic rhinitis. Similarly, in Canadian university students the prevalence of airway hyperresponsiveness to inhaled histamine correlated significantly with the degree of atopy. For further discussion see Chapters 17.4.1.1 and 17.4.1.2.

Genetic susceptibility

Asthma and atopy show clear indications of genetic susceptibility: the frequency of disease in family members is greater than in the population as a whole and is greater in identical than non-identical twins.

In one study the population prevalence of asthma was estimated at between 5 and 10 per cent; the risk for the child of a parent with asthma and atopy was 14 per cent when one parent was affected and 29 per cent when both parents were affected. The risk for the child of a parent with asthma but not atopy was little more than the population frequency of asthma; whereas atopy increased the risk of a child developing asthma some threefold. The reasons for genetic susceptibility are discussed in section 17.4.1.1, but it is important to recognize that genetic influences alone cannot explain the striking geographical variation and recent secular change in the prevalence of asthma.

Allergen exposure

In people with asthma, natural allergen exposure induces asthma and airway hyperresponsiveness. Both the severity of asthma and airway responsiveness increased in patients with asthma who were allergic to ragweed pollen during the ragweed pollen season. Similarly, avoidance of relevant allergen exposure is associated with an improvement or resolution of asthmatic symptoms, improved lung function, and decreased airway responsiveness. Patients with asthma who were allergic to house dust mite have shown considerable symptomatic and objective improvement when avoiding house dust mite for several months at altitude in Davos in the Swiss Alps; also for several weeks in a London hospital. In south-east United States, asthma deaths in patients allergic to the mould *Alternaria alternata* increase during the months of the year when *Alternaria* spore counts are highest.

Although there is clear evidence that natural exposure to allergens to which they are allergic can induce asthma in patients (and avoidance can improve it), the influence of allergen exposure on the development of asthma is less clear. Studies comparing populations born and living in different environments and climates, and therefore exposed to different allergens in childhood, demonstrate allergy and associated disease in relation to allergens present in the particular environment. Comparison of children born and living in Marseilles (humid and at sea level, encouraging the growth of house dust mite) and in Briancon, the highest town in the French Alps (not conducive to the growth of house dust mite, but encouraging to the growth of many flowering plants), showed that allergy to house dust mite was considerably more prevalent in Marseilles than in Briancon, whereas allergy to pollens was considerably more prevalent in Briancon than Marseilles. The prevalence of asthma was similar in both environments, although the associated allergies differed. The introduction of a new allergen into an environment can cause the development of allergy and asthma, particularly among adults. Unloading soya beans in Barcelona harbour caused 'epidemic days', when the number of hospital admissions with asthma increased several-fold: these continued for 7 years until the cause was identified and a filter placed on the silos to prevent the release and dissemination of soya bean during unloading.

Respiratory virus infections

While respiratory virus infections have long been suspected to be the major cause of exacerbations of asthma, it is only with the development and use of polymerase chain reaction in controlled studies that the true proportion of virus-induced exacerbations of asthma has become clear. In studies of asthma in the community, 85 per cent of asthma attacks in children and 44 per cent in adults were induced by upper respiratory tract infections, of which the great majority were caused by rhinoviruses. Seasonal patterns of respiratory infections are strongly correlated with hospital admissions for asthma. In school children the major determinant of paediatric admission is school attendance, with the peaks of respiratory infections and asthma admissions both occurring at the start of the school term.

Exacerbations of asthma provoked by respiratory infections are often severe and can be prolonged and associated with increased airway responsiveness. In school children, peak flow measurements can remain abnormal for several weeks after a respiratory tract infection.

Drugs

Relatively few drugs exacerbate asthma. Of those which do, β-blockers and non-steroidal anti-inflammatory drugs (**NSAIDs**) are the most important.

β-Blockers

Precipitation or worsening of asthma was first reported with propanolol, but subsequently found to occur with all non-selective β-adrenoceptor antagonists, implying adrenergic bronchodilator tone in asthmatic airways. The severity of the airway narrowing provoked by β-blockers is not predictable, nor is it closely related to the severity of airway hyperresponsiveness. The dose provoking asthma can be low: severe asthma can be precipitated by timolol eye drops, a non-selective β-blocker used to treat glaucoma. Selective β-antagonists, such as atenolol, acebutalol, and metoprolol, provoke less severe reactions than non-selective β-blockers. However, although the fall in lung function provoked by a β-blocker may be reversed by an inhaled β$_2$-agonist, the severity of airway narrowing is unpredictable; alternative drugs are available for their indications (such as hypertension and angina), and patients with asthma should avoid β-blockers including β$_1$-selective antagonists. Although ACE inhibitors can cause cough and occasionally rhinitis, they have not been associated with the provocation of asthma and are not contraindicated in asthma.

Aspirin and NSAIDs

Aspirin and other NSAIDs which inhibit cyclo-oxygenase 1, can provoke severe attacks of asthma in some 10 per cent adults with asthma, more frequently in women than men. Aspirin-induced asthma may be part of a well-recognized association of aspirin intolerance, asthma, and rhinitis with nasal polyps (Samter's triad), which is characterized by severe mucosal eosinophilic inflammation of the nose and airways. The onset is usually in the third or fourth decade, with chronic nasal congestion, discharge, and nasal polyps, followed by development of asthma and aspirin-induced asthma. Ingestion of aspirin or a NSAID then characteristically provokes acute severe asthma within 1 h, accompanied by profuse nasal discharge, peri-orbital oedema, conjunctival infection, in some cases with flushing of the head and neck and, on occasions, with vomiting and diarrhoea. Aspirin-induced asthma can provoke life-threatening asthma resistant to bronchodilators: in one survey, 25 per cent of 145 patients requiring mechanical ventilation for acute severe asthma had aspirin-induced asthma although aspirin ingestion had not necessarily provoked this attack.

Despite avoidance of aspirin and NSAIDs, severe asthma and rhinitis with nasal polyps usually persist, associated with a raised blood eosinophil count and intense eosinophil infiltration of the nasal and airway mucosa. The most plausible explanation of aspirin-induced asthma is that it occurs as a consequence of specific inhibition in respiratory cells of intracellular cyclo-oxygenase enzymes. NSAIDs which inhibit cyclo-oxygenase activity provoke asthma in patients with aspirin-induced asthma; NSAIDs which do not inhibit cyclo-oxygenase activity do not provoke asthma. The potency of NSAIDs to inhibit cyclo-oxygenases correlates with their ability to provoke asthma in individuals with aspirin-induced asthma; and cross-tolerance to NSAIDs that inhibit cyclo-oxygenase occurs after desensitization to aspirin. Cross-tolerance involving such chemically distinct moieties argues strongly against aspirin-induced asthma being an immunological reaction.

The intense tissue eosinophilia is accompanied by overproduction of cysteinyl leukotrienes. In aspirin-induced asthma, cyclo-oxygenase inhibition is associated with release of cysteinyl leukotrienes that are important mediators of nasal inflammation and asthma. Cysteinyl leukotrienes, continuously synthesized in patients with aspirin-induced asthma, even in the absence of aspirin ingestion, are released into nasal and bronchial secretions and can be collected in urine. Aspirin-provoked nasal and asthmatic reactions are attenuated by leukotriene antagonists, both cysteinyl leukotriene receptor antagonists (zafirlukast, montelukast, and pranlukast) and 5-lipoxygenase inhibitors (zileuton).

Patients with aspirin-induced asthma should avoid all aspirin-containing products and other analgesics that inhibit cyclo-oxygenase (Table 2). Patients with aspirin-induced asthma can usually, although not always, take paracetamol. Selective inhibitors of cyclo-oxygenase 2 (celecoxib and rofecoxib) should theoretically be safe, but have not yet been investigated for cross-reactions with aspirin.

Tolerance to aspirin and NSAIDs can be induced in patients with aspirin-induced asthma by the ingestion of increasing doses of aspirin over 2 to 3 days, until 400 to 650 mg of aspirin can be tolerated. Daily doses of between 80 and 325 mg of aspirin can maintain tolerance, allowing aspirin and other cyclo-oxygenase inhibitors to be taken safely. A dose of aspirin of 650 mg twice daily can provide improvement in asthma and particularly nasal inflammation. One report has suggested that regular aspirin treatment after sinus surgery for polypectomy may delay recurrence of nasal polyps, on average by 6 years. However, aspirin desensitization requires daily maintenance of high-dose aspirin, which may not be well tolerated. Furthermore, omission of aspirin for 2 to 3 days can result in complete loss of tolerance, in which case the initial desensitization protocol needs to be repeated. It is also not clear whether aspirin desensitization has the potential to modify the long-term course of asthma. For these reasons, aspirin desensitization has not been widely adopted.

Clinical features of asthma

The development of asthma

Knowledge of the way that asthma develops has been hindered by the lack of a clear workable definition that includes all cases (sensitive) and excludes non-cases (specific), and by the relative paucity of longitudinal data on well-defined community cohorts, which include a representative group of cases of asthma and are not limited to those coming to medical attention. None the less, there is now sufficient information to allow a reasonable view of the situation.

The relationship between wheezing in preschool children and asthma in school-age children has been clarified by a number of overlapping studies. Wheezing and cough in children aged less than 2 to 3 years is common and typically associated with viral respiratory infections. The important risk factors are reduced lung function at birth, prematurity or low birth weight, and maternal smoking during pregnancy. The prognosis for such children is good, with remission in the majority by school age and normal lung function in adult life. 'Wheezy bronchitis' in preschool years does not occur more frequently in school-age children with asthma, whose risk factors are different, suggesting the two disorders are independent. The peak prevalence of asthma occurs between the ages of 5 and 10 years, is associated with eczema in infancy, and evidence of sensitization to common inhalant allergens (identified either by skin test responses or by increased total IgE).

The outcome for children who develop asthma has been the subject of several general-practice and hospital-based reports, which of necessity will describe the prognosis of more severe cases. The outcome for cases identified in random population samples has been reported from Australia and the United Kingdom. The Australian study found that the risk of asthma persisting at ages 21 and 28 years was associated with the frequency of wheezing at ages 7 and 14 years. Children who wheezed infrequently in childhood and adolescence were least likely to have continuing asthma as young adults: more than half of those with asthma before the age of 7 years that had remitted by the age of 14 years remained symptom free aged 21 years. However, less than 20 per cent of those with persistent symptoms in childhood were symptom free in adolescence, and frequent attacks in this group continued to the age of 28 years. Some two-thirds of those without symptoms in adolescence remained free of asthma at the age of 28 years. The United Kingdom study described the incidence of wheezing from birth to age 33 years. The incidence of wheezy illness at all ages was related to a history of eczema and hay fever. One-quarter of children with a history of asthma or wheezy bronchitis by the age of 7 years continued to have symptoms when aged 33 years. Asthma developing in adult life was strongly associated with cigarette smoking and a history of hay fever.

In both the United Kingdom and Australian studies, asthma recurred in adult life after a period of remission in adolescence. More than one-half of those in the United Kingdom study who had wheezed before the age of 7 years and reported wheezing aged 33 years had been free of symptoms for 7 years between the age of 16 and 23 years. Similarly, in the Australian study, wheezing had recurred in 30 per cent of those who were free of wheezing aged 21 years. In both studies asthma recurred in some individuals with mild symptoms in childhood, which were frequently not recalled, and who would otherwise have been labelled as having 'adult-onset' asthma.

Symptoms and signs

The symptoms of asthma are non-specific: shortness of breath, wheezing, chest tightness, and cough. These are manifestations of airway narrowing, which is usually variable in severity over short periods of time, but can be persistent, and of airway hyperresponsiveness. Asthma as the cause of these

Table 2 NSAIDs that cross-react with aspirin in respiratory reactions

	NSAID
1. Inhibitors of both cyclo-oxygenase 1 and 2: On first exposure to the drug, cross-reactions with low provoking doses	Piroxicam
	Indomethacin
	Sulindac
	Tolmetin
	Ibuprofen
	Naproxen
	Naproxen sodium
	Fenoprofen
	Meclofenamate
	Mefenamic acid
	Flurbiprofen
	Diflunisal
	Ketoprofen
	Diclofenac
	Ketoralac
	Etodolac
	Nabumetone
2. Poor inhibitors of cyclo-oxygenase 1 and 2: A small percentage of patients with aspirin-induced asthma cross-react with high dose of these drugs	Oxaprozin
	Paracetamol
	Salsalate
3. Selective inhibitors of cyclo-oxygenase 2: In theory should not cross-react but have not been studied	Celecoxib
	Rifecoxib

symptoms is suggested by the variability in their severity and distinguished by their periodicity (such as daily, weekly, monthly, or seasonal), their provocation by specific (such as allergen) and non-specific stimuli, and their reversibility with bronchodilators or corticosteroids.

Patients with asthma can be categorized, at any one time, by whether their symptoms are intermittent or persistent, and by the severity of their symptoms and underlying airway narrowing (measured by lung function tests. Even those with mild asthma–intermittent or persistent–can develop severe asthma.

1. Mild intermittent asthma—symptoms occur less than weekly with normal or near normal lung function between episodes.

2. Mild persistent asthma—symptoms occur more than weekly but less than daily with normal or near normal lung function between episodes.

3. Moderate persistent asthma—symptoms occur daily with mild to moderate variable airflow limitation.

4. Severe persistent asthma—symptoms occur daily and interfere with normal activities. There is frequent nocturnal waking and moderate to severe variable airflow limitation.

5. Severe asthma—severe distressing symptoms prevent sleep. Severe airflow limitation responds poorly to inhaled bronchodilators and can be life-threatening.

Symptoms of asthma are typically worse at night, waking the affected individual in the early hours of the morning (on occasion several times), and on first waking in the morning, when chest tightness may be the dominant symptom. Asthmatic symptoms may also be provoked by non-specific stimuli such as exercise and cold air, and by specific allergens such as domestic animals, particularly cats.

Respiratory viral infections that occur predominantly in the winter months are the most important precipitating causes of exacerbations of asthma. In patients allergic to pollens or moulds, asthmatic symptoms occur or worsen during the relevant season (in the United Kingdom—late spring: tree pollen; May and June: grass pollen; late summer months: mould spores). In those with asthma induced by occupational sensitizers, symptoms characteristically increase in severity during the working week and improve when away from work on holidays of 1 week or more, if not at weekends (see Chapter 17.4.1.5). In some women asthma has a monthly periodicity, becoming increasingly severe during the days before menstruation, improving with its onset.

Although breathlessness and wheeze are often considered the most characteristic symptoms of asthma, cough can be the dominant and on occasions, particularly in children, the only symptom of asthma. Nocturnal cough suggests asthma, although in community studies isolated nocturnal cough has been found to be a poor predictor of the condition. 'Cough-variant asthma' is occasionally seen in adults who do not have airway narrowing and in whom cough and eosinophil-rich sputum are the only manifestations of the disease.

The characteristic symptoms of asthma are manifestations of variable airway narrowing and airway hyperresponsiveness. Patients with chronic severe asthma have more persistent airway narrowing and are limited in their day to day activities by breathlessness. They may have less symptomatic evidence of spontaneous variability of airway narrowing, although they can be awoken by asthma at night as well as having symptoms provoked by inhalation of cold air or by laughter.

Patients with acute severe asthma are usually distressed by severe shortness of breath with wheezing, unable to sleep and to complete sentences in one breath because of the severity of the airway narrowing.

The physical signs of mild or moderate asthma may be limited to expiratory wheezes audible over the lungs. Because of the variable nature of the airway narrowing, some patients have normal lung sounds, although expiratory wheezes would be anticipated in patients with persistent symptomatic asthma. Patients with chronic persistent asthma can develop hyperinflated lungs.

In acute severe asthma, patients are usually severely short of breath, sitting up or leaning forward using their accessory muscles of respiration. With increasingly severe airway narrowing, expiration becomes increasingly prolonged and alternates with short inspiratory gasps, impairing speech. Tachycardia and pulsus paradoxus often accompany acute severe asthma, but pulsus paradoxus is not a reliable indicator of severity. Airway narrowing may become sufficiently severe for no wheeze to be audible (the 'silent chest') and gas exchange sufficiently impaired to cause detectable cyanosis. Patients with asthma of this severity are usually distressed, hyperventilating, anxious, apprehensive, and can be confused because of hypoxia. Exhaustion ultimately leads to inadequate ventilation and a rising PCO_2, the two cardinal features that indicate the need for transfer to an intensive care unit in the event that assisted ventilation is required.

Diagnosis of asthma

Although asthma is now defined by characteristic pathological changes in the airways, it is usually identified by its pathophysiological manifestations, variable or reversible airway narrowing and airway hyperresponsiveness. In some patients the presence of eosinophils in sputum or a raised eosinophil count in the blood can be a valuable diagnostic pointer.

Asthma is usually diagnosed by the demonstration of airflow limitation that varies spontaneously over short periods of time, or which reverses after inhalation of short-acting β-agonists or, over a more prolonged period, in response to inhaled or oral corticosteroid. In a small minority of patients, provocation tests using exercise, or pharmacological agents such as histamine or methacholine can be valuable. In suspected cases of occupational asthma, inhalation tests with the specific agent may be indicated (see Chapter 17.4.1.4); inhalation tests with common inhalant allergens are rarely indicated in clinical practice.

Airflow limitation

The most clinically useful measurements of airflow limitation are: (i) forced expiratory volume in 1 s (FEV_1), which may be expressed as a proportion of the forced vital capacity (**FVC**) as FEV_1/FVC per cent, and (ii) peak expiratory flow rate (**PEFR**). Both tests require the patient to provide a reproducible maximal forced expiratory manoeuvre using tested and validated equipment. FEV_1 has the advantage of a visible tracing of the expelled volume of air over time, which allows the observer to determine whether reproducible maximal forced expiratory manoeuvres have been made. PEFR testing does not provide this opportunity. However, peak flow meters employed to measure PEFR, unlike spirometers required to measure FEV_1, can be used regularly by patients to monitor their lung function, indicating the need for altered treatment at an early stage. Whether abnormality of FEV_1 and PEFR should be expressed in absolute or proportional terms remains undecided. Expression as an absolute difference from the average value anticipated for an individual of given age, gender, and height has more physiological validity, but the majority of lung function laboratories in the United Kingdom continue to define as abnormal, values of FEV_1 or PEFR of 20 per cent or more below the mean predicted value.

The difference of the measured from the predicted mean value for an individual can be conveniently expressed as a Z value, which is the number of standard deviations the measured value is from the predicted mean:

$$Z = \frac{\text{predicted mean value} - \text{measured value}}{\text{standard deviation (c.0.5)}}$$

The distribution of FEV_1 around the mean predicted value is similar at all ages (from 25 to 70 years) with a standard deviation of some 0.5 litres. The disadvantage of using a proportional rather than an absolute difference can best be appreciated by comparing a patient whose predicted FEV_1 is 5 litres with one whose predicted FEV_1 is 2.5 litres. In the first patient a 20 per cent reduction equates to a loss of 1 litre (2 standard deviations); in the second

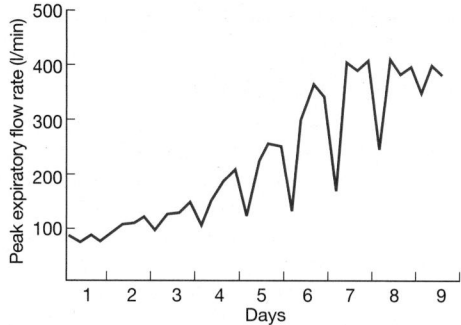

Fig. 4 Circadian rhythm in peak expiratory flow rate in a patient with asthma recovering from an acute attack.

a 20 per cent reduction equates to a loss of 0.5 litres (1 standard deviation).

Variability and reversibility of airflow limitation

Serial measurements of PEFR in most patients with asthma show spontaneous variability. The most characteristic pattern is of a circadian variation, with airflow limitation most severe on waking in the morning (and during the night if awoken) with improvement occurring during the morning after waking (Fig. 4). A small circadian variation in PEFR or FEV$_1$ is seen in normal individuals; in asthma a difference of 20 per cent or more between the highest and lowest values may be found. Other patterns of variation in severity of airflow limitation may be imposed on this circadian rhythm, such as falls in PEFR provoked by exercise or exposure to an allergen or occupational sensitizer, which resolve after avoidance of the stimulus. While variations of 20 per cent or more in FEV$_1$ or PEFR are commonly regarded as indicating asthma, in patients with severe airflow limitation, with an FEV$_1$ of 1 litre, 20 per cent variability equates to 200 ml, a level of spontaneous variation observed in people without asthma.

The most commonly used means to identify asthma in clinical practice is an improvement after 15 to 20 min in airflow limitation, identified by FEV$_1$ or PEFR, after inhalation of a bronchodilator, usually a short-acting β-agonist such as salbutamol in a dose of 200 μg—evidence of asthma is usually regarded as an improvement in FEV$_1$ or PEFR of 20 per cent or greater. However, it is important to appreciate that the absence of a significant improvement in lung function after inhalation of a bronchodilator does not exclude a diagnosis of asthma (that is, it is a more specific test than it is sensitive). Rapid reversibility of airflow limitation is more readily seen in young adults with mild or moderate asthma than in older patients with more severe airflow limitation. Reversibility cannot be tested in a patient whose lung function is normal at the time of testing.

An increase of 20 per cent or more from baseline FEV$_1$ or PEFR is generally accepted as diagnostic of asthma. Expressing change as a proportion of baseline will exaggerate the degree of improvement in those with a low initial FEV$_1$ or PEFR. A 20 per cent increase in FEV$_1$ in a patient with a baseline FEV$_1$ of 4 litres is 800 ml, but only 200 ml in a patient whose baseline FEV$_1$ is 1 litre. Studies of short-term (20 min) variability in FEV$_1$ in patients with airflow limitation have found that the increase in FEV$_1$ needed to exclude natural variability with 95 per cent confidence was 160 ml. This value did not differ significantly from the value in normal individuals, in whom an absolute increase in FEV$_1$ of 190 ml was needed to exclude a chance increase with 95 per cent confidence. In both normal individuals and those with an airflow limitation, expression of variability as an absolute difference was similar at all levels of FEV$_1$, whereas when expressed as a percentage change, the degree of variability decreased with increasing FEV$_1$. Selecting a specific percentage change in FEV$_1$ (or PEFR) to define asthma will necessarily include a greater proportion of patients with lower prebronchodilator FEV$_1$. Equally, patients with a higher baseline FEV$_1$ need to achieve a greater absolute increase to fulfil the defined criterion. Expres-

sion of variability as an absolute change has more biological and statistical validity, and an increase of more than 200 ml in FEV$_1$ has a probability of less than 5 per cent of occurring by chance. As with expression of lung function, it is unlikely that the use of results based on absolute values, although biologically more valid, will be adopted. It should be appreciated, however, that in patients with a low FEV$_1$ a 20 per cent increase in FEV$_1$ may have occurred by chance, and in those with a high FEV$_1$ an increase of more than 200 ml is unlikely to have occurred by chance.

In some patients with asthma, particularly those with severe airflow limitation, inhalation of a short-acting bronchodilator does not provide significant improvement in FEV$_1$ or PEFR. In these circumstances the diagnosis of asthma and differentiation from less reversible causes of airflow limitation, such as chronic bronchitis and emphysema, can be made with a 'trial' of treatment with corticosteroids. Significant improvement in airflow limitation both implies a diagnosis of asthma and demonstrates that corticosteroids (inhaled or oral) are effective treatment. However, corticosteroids can also improve exercise tolerance by enhancing mood and outlook, hence the benefit of a trial of steroids has to be judged by its effect on lung function. Although there is no formally agreed protocol for a steroid trial, a generally acceptable trial would be oral prednisolone taken in a dose of 0.6 mg/kg, (40 mg/day in a 70 kg male) for 3 weeks, with measurement of spirometry made on at least two separate occasions, once before and once at the end of the trial supplemented by three times daily home peak flow measurements. Symptomatic improvement with an increase in FEV$_1$ or PEFR of 20 per cent or more during the trial is generally considered as evidence of asthma and an indication for treatment with corticosteroids, inhaled or oral.

Tests of airway hyperresponsiveness

Airway hyperresponsiveness—an exaggerated response to non-specific provocative stimuli—is a cardinal feature of asthma. Tests of airway responsiveness to exercise and to inhaled histamine or methacholine, which can provoke acute airway narrowing in a dose-dependent fashion, can be of value in the diagnosis of asthma, particularly in patients with symptoms suggestive of the condition but in whom measured lung function is normal or, if abnormal, shows no reversibility with inhaled bronchodilators. These tests are required in only a few patients and each has its limitations: exercise testing can be insensitive (false negatives) and tests of airway reactivity to inhaled histamine or methacholine non-specific (false positives), although the provocation of a 20 per cent fall in FEV$_1$ by histamine at 4 mg/ml or less (or equivalent) occurs uncommonly in those without asthma.

Exercise testing

Acute airway narrowing provoked by exercise is a common feature of asthma, particularly in children. Testing for exercise-provoked asthma requires continuous exertion for 5 min. This is most conveniently undertaken in a lung function laboratory by running on a treadmill or exercising on a cycle ergometer, although free running is more likely to provoke an asthmatic reaction. Measurements are made of FEV$_1$ or PEFR 5 min before, during, and at 5 min intervals for 30 min after the test. A normal individual will have a less than 5 per cent increase in FEV$_1$ or PEFR during and a less than 10 per cent fall after exercise. Depending on the level of baseline, patients with asthma can have a greater than 5 per cent increase during exercise and greater than 10 per cent fall from pretest value afterwards. Exercise is a valid and reproducible test for asthma, although it can have false negatives, particularly when undertaken by methods other than free running.

Airway reactivity to inhaled histamine or methacholine

Acute airway narrowing can be provoked in a dose-dependent manner by the inhalation of increasing doses of a bronchoconstrictor, of which histamine or methacholine are the most commonly used. The test as described by Cockcroft and colleagues consists of tidal breathing of doubling doses of histamine, with measurement of FEV$_1$ 6 min after each inhaled dose. The percentage change in FEV_1 from a post-saline baseline after each concentration of inhaled (histamine) can be plotted, the test being terminated when either a 20 per cent or greater fall in FEV_1 is provoked or the maximum concentration (usually 16 or 32 mg/ml) is reached. The level of airway reactivity is usually expressed as the concentration of histamine that provokes a 20 per cent fall in FEV_1 (PC_{20} histamine), which can be identified by linear interpolation. The lower the PC_{20}, the more reactive the airways. The test is usually repeatable within one doubling dose, but may not be consistent in any individual, PC_{20} falling, for instance, after exposure to allergen or occupational sensitizer.

In population studies the major determinants of airway reactivity have been atopy (in children and young adults) and smoking in older adults (probably reflecting reduced FEV_1). Airway responsiveness can be increased in atopic children with rhinitis and in healthy adults after a viral respiratory tract infection. Hence, evidence of measurable airway reactivity is not necessarily evidence of asthma, but it is uncommon for individuals without asthma to have a PC_{20} histamine of methacholine of less than 8 mg/ml. Measurement of airway reactivity to histamine or methacholine is more sensitive than exercise testing, although a less specific test for asthma. Like exercise testing its value in clinical practice is primarily in symptomatic patients with normal or near normal FEV_1 and without evidence of spontaneous variability or reversibility. A negative test in a symptomatic patient suggests that current asthma is unlikely to be the cause of their symptoms.

Imaging in asthma

Imaging of the chest is not commonly of diagnostic value in asthma, but can be important in identifying its complications. In patients in whom asthma develops over the age of 30 years, the chest radiograph is usually normal. However, about one-quarter of children and one-fifth of adults show changes of hyperinflation on the chest radiograph. These changes include a low diaphragm (below the sixth intercostal space anteriorly) and an increased retrosternal space. In some children with chronic persistent asthma, the length of the lung becomes greater than the width of the thorax, with the posterior ends of the ribs becoming more horizontal.

The most commonly observed radiographic sign in asthma is of thickened bronchial walls due to eosinophilic infiltration of the airways: these are visible on the chest radiograph as parallel lines ('tram lines') or as a thick-walled ring shadow when seen end on.

Complications of asthma that can be seen on the chest radiograph include pneumothorax, pneumomediastinum, pulmonary collapse, and eosinophilic pneumonia. The physical signs of pneumothorax can be difficult to detect in an asthmatic attack, but its detection can be lifesaving. Pneumomediastinum is of less clinical importance. Plugging of the airways by a mucus plug characteristically occurs in allergic bronchopulmonary aspergillosis, but also in asthmatic patients without this condition: in both it can cause atelectasis, which is usually lobar or segmental. Eosinophilic pneumonia is characterized by consolidation on the chest radiograph accompanied by a raised blood eosinophil count. This can be a manifestation of several conditions that include allergic bronchopulmonary aspergillosis, helminth infections, and drug reactions, as well as being of unknown cause—acute and chronic eosinophilic pneumonia. Of these, allergic bronchopulmonary aspergillosis and chronic eosinophilic pneumonia (which can be a manifestation of Churg–Strauss syndrome—allergic granulomatosis) are the most common causes of eosinophilic pneumonia in patients with asthma. (See Chapters 17.11.5, 17.11.9 and 17.11.11 for further discussion of these conditions.)

Differential diagnosis of asthma

Asthma needs to be differentiated from:

(1) localized airways obstruction;

(2) other causes of generalized airways obstruction; and

(3) other causes of intermittent breathlessness.

Localized airways obstruction

Upper airways obstruction, of the larynx or trachea, causes a monophonic inspiratory wheeze (stridor) audible over the trachea with a characteristic abnormality of the flow volume loop—decreased inspiratory flow rates. In a child, wheezing can be caused by an inhaled foreign body (classically a peanut), which should be particularly suspected when the problem develops suddenly in a previously healthy individual. The chest radiograph may show the foreign body if it is opaque, or distal atelectasis, consolidation, or air trapping on an expiratory film (which may not be possible to obtain in small children). However, it can be normal and, if foreign body inhalation is suspected, bronchoscopy should be undertaken to identify and remove it or to exclude the possibility. In adults, localized airway narrowing is more likely to be due to a tumour—benign or malignant—which may occasionally cause a unilateral monophonic wheeze. The tumour may be visible on the chest radiograph, but definitive diagnosis will require bronchoscopy and biopsy.

Generalized airways obstruction

The major causes of generalized airways obstruction from which asthma needs to be distinguished are chronic bronchitis and emphysema, although in some cases these may coexist with asthma. Other causes such as obliterative bronchiolitis are less common. In general, chronic bronchitis and emphysema cause breathlessness on exertion that increases slowly in severity over years and only uncommonly causes breathlessness before the age of 40 years. Nocturnal waking by respiratory symptoms is uncommon in chronic bronchitis and emphysema, although not universal in asthma. Chronic severe asthma responsive to corticosteroids, but without significant reversibility to inhaled bronchodilators, may have similar radiographic and spirometric abnormalities. In both, the lungs may be hyperinflated on the chest radiograph, but in asthma, unlike emphysema, there is no associated loss of vascular markings. Lung function tests in both asthma and emphysema can show airflow limitation with reduced FEV_1, reduced FEV_1/FVC ratio, and hyperinflated lungs with increased total lung capacity. However, while factor transfer (TL_{CO}) and gas transfer coefficient (K_{CO}) are reduced in emphysema, in asthma K_{CO} is normal or increased. Differentiation from chronic bronchitis can be difficult because, like asthma, there is no loss of vascular markings on the chest radiograph or reduction of K_{CO}. If present, sputum (and blood) eosinophilia suggests asthma, but differentiation in these circumstances often depends on the outcome of a trial of steroids.

In young children asthma needs to be differentiated from wheezing episodes associated with viral respiratory tract infections, and in children and adolescents from cystic fibrosis. Cystic fibrosis is suggested by disproportionate production of (usually discoloured) sputum, weight loss, and an abnormal chest radiograph. The presence of staphylococci in sputum and development of nasal polyps in childhood is very suggestive of cystic fibrosis.

Other causes of intermittent breathlessness

The most important causes of intermittent breathlessness from which asthma should be differentiated are left ventricular failure, pulmonary emboli, extrinsic allergic alveolitis, hyperventilation, and vocal cord dysfunction.

Left heart failure sufficient to cause breathlessness will usually be apparent on clinical examination, chest radiograph, ECG, and echocardiogram. The heart is clinically and radiographically enlarged, with the exception of pulmonary venous hypertension caused by mitral stenosis. Inspiratory crackles are usually audible at the lung bases and the jugular venous pressure may be elevated. In addition to an enlarged heart the chest radiograph may show upper lobe venous distension, Kerley 'B' lines, and pleural effusion. Echocardiography will usually show evidence of left ventricular disease, or in the case of mitral stenosis, left atrial enlargement. Identification of the cause of breathlessness can be difficult when left heart failure is provoked by an intermittent arrhythmia.

Pulmonary embolism causes breathlessness that can occasionally be associated with wheezing; the diagnosis is suggested by associated pleuritic pain and haemoptysis. The chest radiograph and CT scan may show pleural-based 'humpback' opacities and pleural effusion. The diagnosis is most securely made angiographically, but more usually from a ventilation perfusion scan or spiral CT scan. A normal ventilation perfusion scan makes all but the smallest emboli unlikely, although interpretation can be difficult in patients with widespread ventilatory disease. A normal spiral CT scan excludes pulmonary emboli to subsegmental level.

Extrinsic allergic alveolitis

Extrinsic allergic alveolitis can provoke recurrent episodes of breathlessness which characteristically develop 4 to 8 h after exposure to the cause (usually mouldy hay or birds—pigeons or budgerigars). Breathlessness in extrinsic allergic alveolitis is usually not accompanied by wheeze but with fever, flu-like symptoms, and a neutrophil leucocytosis. The chest radiograph often shows widespread nodular or groundglass shadowing and the CT scan discrete areas of groundglass opacification. Lung function tests show a proportionate reduction in FEV_1 and FVC, which may be accompanied by a reduced TLco and Kco. (See Chapter 17.11.11 for further discussion.)

Hyperventilation

Episodes of hyperventilation may be difficult to distinguish symptomatically from asthma, and can in some cases complicate asthma. The diagnosis should be suspected in a patient who complains of breathlessness that occurs without identifiable cause (for example while sitting reading), may be associated with pins and needles in the fingers and dizziness (attributable to hypocapnia), and does not disturb sleep. The symptoms complained of can often be reproduced by a short period of voluntary overbreathing; 20 deep breaths is usually sufficient. The reason why some patients present with hyperventilation is unknown: Howell has suggested that it develops in obsessional (perfectionist) personalities and is usually precipitated by one of three events: bereavement, resentment, or concern about illness. However, it is important to recognize that asthma is characteristically a variable condition and a diagnosis of hyperventilation should not be made on the basis of absent physical signs or normal lung function at the time of consultation, but based on the characteristics described above.

Vocal cord dysfunction

Vocal cord dysfunction is easily misdiagnosed as asthma and may coexist with asthma. Wheezing, in vocal cord dysfunction, is caused by paradoxical adduction of the anterior two-thirds of the vocal cords on inspiration, and does not occur during sleep. The diagnosis is best made by direct examination of the cords during an attack. Management can be difficult, but recognition of the condition can allow high-dose oral corticosteroid treatment for 'uncontrolled asthma' to be avoided.

Hyperventilation and vocal cord dysfunction can each occur in patients with underlying asthma, frequently in association with underlying psychosocial problems. A critical point can be to determine the relevant life events associated in time with the onset of deterioration in the patient, who has often had previously well-controlled asthma. Vocal cord dysfunction is more common in women and in those engaged in health care provision.

Management of asthma

Objectives

The objectives of treating patients with intermittent or persistent asthma are:

(1) to prevent troublesome symptoms (such as cough, shortness of breath) at night or with exercise;

(2) to enable patients to achieve normal levels of activity;

(3) to maintain normal or near normal lung function; and

(4) to prevent recurrent episodes of acute severe asthma and minimize the need for emergency hospital treatment.

These objectives are most likely to be achieved by treatment that reduces airway inflammation, either by avoidance of its inducing cause or by drugs with anti-inflammatory activity. The risk of side-effects of asthma treatment should be appreciated and minimized, patients' concerns about the potential side-effects of long-term treatment should be recognized, and relevant information provided to them.

Treatment selection

Randomized controlled trials of asthma treatments published in the past decade have shown the magnitude of benefit of different treatment interventions in patients with asthma of varying severity. This information has provided a secure basis for deciding which treatment is likely to be most effective in individual patients. Of particular importance has been the broadening of the indications for the use of inhaled corticosteroids. Inferences from these studies on the optimal treatment for asthma of differing degrees of severity has informed the published guidelines for asthma management in the United Kingdom, United States, and elsewhere.

The targets for effective asthma treatment in individual patients are:

(1) normal daytime activities, such as going to work and to school, as well as the ability to enjoy physically demanding activities (such as sport);

(2) sleeping through the night without awakening by respiratory symptoms;

(3) use of 'rescue' medication with inhaled β_2-agonists needed less than once per day;

(4) normal or near normal PEFR and FEV_1, with less than 20 per cent variability between best and worst values; and

(5) avoidance of drug side-effects.

Targets 1, 2, and 5 are of the most interest to the patients, who will primarily be seeking improvement in their quality of life from treatment. Zealous pursuit of restoration of normal lung function in a patient whose quality of life has already been restored by treatment is of questionable value.

Asthma, except where caused by a dominant and avoidable agent (such as a domestic pet or occupational sensitizers), is not usually curable, but current treatment offers the great majority of patients the opportunity to enjoy a normal life. Most asthma is mild: in one community survey only 15 per cent of patients had persistent asthma of moderate severity (step 3 of British Thoracic Society (**BTS**) guidelines or worse—see below). However, some 5 per cent of patients have severe asthma that responds poorly to conventional treatment. These patients suffer most, both from their disease and from the side-effects of its treatment, and are at highest risk of admission to hospital and death from asthma.

Treatments for asthma

Allergen avoidance

The identification and, where feasible, the avoidance of relevant allergens at home or at work should be considered an essential part of the management of asthma. It enables patients to recognize important causes of their asthma and to take responsibility for their avoidance. Allergen avoidance should be regarded as complimentary to drug treatment of asthma, with the advantage in some cases (where a single allergen is the dominant cause) of providing a cure with avoidance of the possible side-effects of drugs. Complete avoidance of exposure to house dust mite, domestic pets, and occupational causes of asthma has been associated with marked improvement in respiratory symptoms, lung function, and airway hyperresponsiveness. Avoidance of exposure is most clearly indicated and usually most feasible when the cause of asthma is an agent inhaled at work (see Chapter 17.11.1.5). Removal of a pet, particularly a cat from the home, is most effective when accompanied by thorough cleaning and washing of the house to remove residual allergen, which can otherwise persist in concentrations sufficient to provoke asthma for many months. Avoidance of exposure to the house dust mite, *D. pternonyssinus*, by spending several months in the Alps or in a hospital, has been shown to provide symptomatic and functional improvement. However, house dust mites are ubiquitous in many environments, including much of the United States, United Kingdom, and Europe, and it can be difficult to eliminate mites sufficiently from the home so that exposure to the relevant allergens (such as Der p1) is reduced to concentrations which do not continue to induce airway inflammation. The issue with house dust mite avoidance is the feasibility of securing an effective intervention.

Drug treatment

The drugs primarily used to treat asthma are the progeny of two hormones secreted by the adrenal glands: cortisol and adrenaline. Pharmaceutical research in the past 50 years has led to the development of selective β_2-agonists, both short and long acting, and lipid-soluble topically active inhaled corticosteroids. β_2-Agonists and corticosteroids account for nearly 90 per cent of prescriptions for asthma in the United Kingdom. Other drugs used include sodium cromoglycate and nedocromil sodium amongst the prophylactic agents, and ipratropium bromide and theophyllines amongst the bronchodilators. The core treatment for mild and moderately severe persistent asthma is inhaled corticosteroids and inhaled β_2-agonists. Other agents are used as additional treatments when these alone are not sufficient to provide control. Leukotriene receptor antagonists and 5-lipoxygenase inhibitors have been introduced recently; their place in the treatment of asthma is currently being assessed.

Corticosteroids

Corticosteroids are the most effective treatment for asthma. Systemic corticosteroids were introduced for this purpose in the 1950s, but their use was limited by serious unwanted side-effects, which stimulated research into the development of equally effective but safer alternatives. The introduction of topically active corticosteroids that can be administered by inhalation and are free of the systemic side-effects of oral corticosteroids at therapeutically effective doses has revolutionized the treatment of asthma.

Corticosteroids suppress airway inflammation, with improvement in airway hyperresponsiveness, lung function, and associated respiratory symptoms. Although the mechanism of action of steroids in asthma continues to be debated, they inhibit the formation of cytokines relevant to asthmatic inflammation, such as interleukin 4 (**IL-4**), IL-5, IL-13, and granulocyte–macrophage colony-stimulating factor, by lymphocytes and macrophages, by inhibition of transcription of cytokine genes.

Corticosteroids suppress the chronic inflammation in the asthmatic airways, but do not cure the disease. To be effective they must therefore be taken continuously—oral steroids usually daily and inhaled steroids usually twice daily.

Oral corticosteroids Oral corticosteroids—prednisolone and prednisone—are rapidly absorbed from the gut, achieving peak plasma levels at 1 to 2 h. Prednisone is biologically inactive but rapidly and completely converted in the liver to the active form, prednisolone. Some 20 per cent of prednisolone is inactivated in the liver by first-pass metabolism leaving 80 per cent of the oral dose bioavailable. The plasma half-life of prednisolone is usually 2 to 3 h. Corticosteroids are inactivated in the liver by conjugation. Hepatic enzyme inducers such as rifampicin, barbiturates, and phenytoin can reduce the half-life of prednisolone by 50 per cent. To counter the consequent reduction in anti-inflammatory activity, the dose of oral prednisolone should be doubled in patients concurrently receiving these treatments.

Oral corticosteroids effect detectable improvement in airflow limitation in patients with asthma within 6 to 12 h of administration. In cases of

severe asthma, maximum improvement can take several days, probably reflecting the time to reverse the inflammatory changes in the airways.

The early use of oral corticosteroids in the treatment of asthma was severely limited by the high risk of unwanted effects, which include osteoporosis, hypertension, diabetes mellitus, cataract formation, and (in children) growth suppression. The introduction in the 1970s of inhaled corticosteroids revolutionized the treatment of asthma by providing local anti-inflammatory activity in doses that did not cause these limiting systemic side-effects.

Inhaled corticosteroids Inhaled corticosteroids are highly lipophilic and rapidly enter cells within the airways. They combine high topical potency with low systemic bioavailablity of the swallowed dose and rapid metabolic clearance of any corticosteroid reaching the systemic circulation, conferring a high benefit:risk ratio. Although 80 to 90 per cent of a dose from a metered dose inhaler is deposited in the oropharynx, swallowed, and absorbed, more than 80 per cent of beclomethasone, 90 per cent of budesonide, and 99 per cent of fluticasone is inactivated by first-pass metabolism in the liver. The 10 to 20 per cent of the inhaled dose deposited in the airways is available for absorption into the systemic circulation. For fluticasone and budesonide, devices that increase lung deposition (such as large volume spacer and Turbohaler) therefore increase the dose available for systemic absorption.

At present, three inhaled corticosteroids are generally available: beclamethasone diproprionate, budesonide, and fluticasone proprionate. Beclomethasone and budesonide are equipotent; fluticasone is twice as potent, requiring half the dose to achieve the same benefit. In general, most of the benefit of inhaled corticosteroids in the treatment of asthma is effected at low doses, where there is little evidence of adverse effects. By contrast, adverse effects develop at higher inhaled doses, where there is little evidence of greater benefit.

The clinical effects and side-effects of inhaled corticosteroids have been the subject of considerable clinical investigation. A systematic review of five randomized controlled trials comprising 141 adults with mild, persistent asthma that compared inhaled steroids with β_2-agonists found significant improvement in lung function in those receiving inhaled steroids. A randomized controlled trial that compared inhaled budesonide at 1200 µg/day with regular inhaled terbutaline in adults found improvement in the budesonide group during the 2 years of the study in respiratory symptoms, morning peak flow rates, airway hyperresponsiveness to inhaled histamine, and requirement for symptomatic β_2-agonists. In a subsequent study of the same population, no deterioration in symptoms or lung function, including airway responsiveness to inhaled histamine, occurred in three-quarters of those randomly assigned to reduce their dose of budesonide from 1200 to 400 µg/day, whereas deterioration in symptoms and lung function occurred in two-thirds of those assigned to discontinue budesonide and take placebo. Symptoms and lung function improved in those patients who had received terbutaline during the initial study and were subsequently assigned to budesonide at 1200 µg/day. However, the extent of improvement was less than in those originally assigned budesonide 2 years earlier, suggesting possible benefit from the earlier institution of inhaled corticosteroid treatment.

Several recent studies have compared the benefit of increasing the dose of inhaled steroid with the addition of a long-acting β_2-agonist (salmeterol or formoterol) in patients whose asthma was not controlled by conventional doses of inhaled steroids. Two randomized controlled trials found that the addition of twice daily inhaled salmeterol provided more benefit in terms of symptom-free days and nights, improvement in FEV_1 and PEFR, and need for rescue β_2-agonists than doubling the dose of inhaled steroids (Fig. 5). A third randomized controlled trial of 852 patients with moderately severe asthma investigated (i) the addition of formoterol 12 µg twice daily to budesonide 100 µg, (ii) increasing the dose of budesonide to 400 µg twice daily, and (iii) the addition of formoterol 12 µg twice daily to budesonide 400 µg twice daily. Symptoms of asthma and lung function were

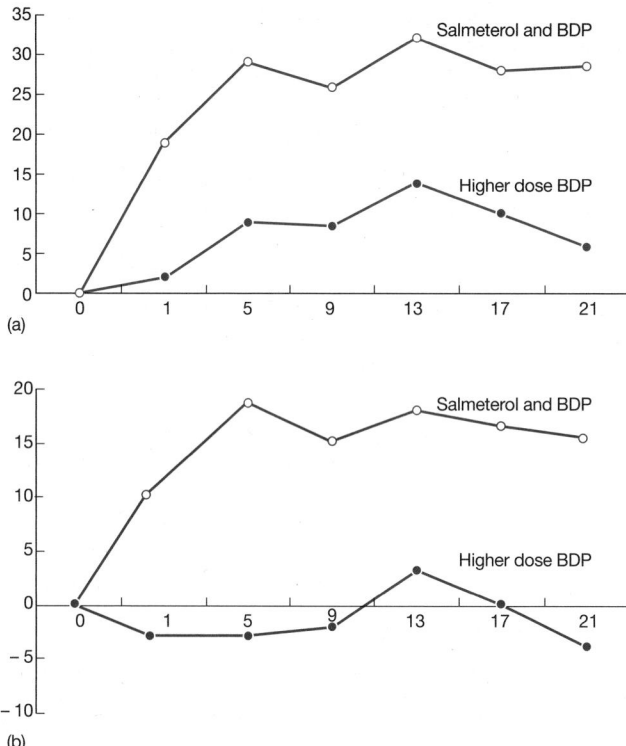

(a)

(b)

Fig. 5 Comparison of addition of salmeterol compared with doubling dose of inhaled steroid (BDP).

improved with both higher dose budesonide and with formoterol, but greater improvements were obtained with the additions of formoterol.

Inhaled corticosteroids are as effective in the treatment of asthma in children as in adults. Comparison in a randomized controlled trial of inhaled budesonide (600 µg/day) with an inhaled placebo for an average of 22 months in 116 children aged between 7 and 16 years also taking inhaled salbutamol at 200 µg/day showed marked benefit in the group taking inhaled budesonide: 26 children (45 per cent) in the placebo group withdrew from the study compared with only 3 (5 per cent) in the budesonide group. Symptoms and lung function (FEV$_1$, PEFR, and airway response to inhaled histamine) improved significantly in the budesonide group. Cessation of inhaled budesonide treatment in a randomized controlled trial in children aged 11 to 18 years previously treated for 28 to 36 months was associated with: recurrence of symptoms, in some of sufficient severity to need treatment with prednisolone; increased use of inhaled β$_2$-agonists; and deterioration in lung function, both FEV$_1$ and airway response to inhaled histamine. Such deterioration did not occur in the group continuing to take budesonide at 600 µg/day.

Side-effects of inhaled corticosteroids

Local side-effects The severe adverse effects of systemic steroids and the widening indications for the use of inhaled corticosteroids has led to close scrutiny of the side-effects of inhaled corticosteroids. Local side-effects are well recognized and are dose dependent. These are oropharyngeal candidiasis (thrush) and dysphonia. Oropharyngeal candidiasis occurs in about 5 per cent of patients and can be a problem, particularly in the elderly. The risk of its development can be reduced by the use of a large volume spacer and rinsing the mouth out after each inhaled dose. Dysphonia occurs in at least one-third of patients and can cause particular problems for public speakers and professional singers. It is believed to be due to a myopathy of the laryngeal muscles and reverses when treatment is stopped. Inhaled corticosteroids do not cause atrophy of the airway epithelium after 10 years of

treatment and are not associated with an increased risk of pulmonary infection, including tuberculosis.

Systemic side-effects Concern about systemic side-effects of inhaled steroids stems from the need for their regular use for prolonged periods (years or decades) both in adults and children. Because many patients who take inhaled corticosteroids have also required oral corticosteroids, distinguishing the adverse systemic effects of inhaled corticosteroids can be difficult. In general, current evidence indicates that inhaled corticosteroids do not cause important side-effects in doses of up to 400 µg/day in children and 800 µg/day in adults. There is some evidence of side-effects at higher doses, more with beclomethasone than with budesonide or fluticasone. However, systemic absorption and the risk of systemic side-effects can be reduced by the use of a spacer with metered dose inhalers and by rinsing the mouth after inhalation of a dry powder inhaler, which should be recommended when doses of 400 µg/day or more in children and 800 µg/day or more in adults are prescribed.

Two important risks of inhaled corticosteroids that have been the subject of recent concern are osteoporosis in adults and growth suppression in children. A cross-sectional study of 81 patients with asthma aged between 20 and 40 years compared bone mineral density in 47 (19 men) who had taken inhaled steroids in doses of between 100 and 3000 µg/day (mean dose 620 µg/day) for at least 5 years with 34 (19 men) who had never taken inhaled or oral corticosteroids. Bone mineral density was not different in the two groups, but cumulative inhaled steroid dose was associated with a reduction of bone mineral density in the lumbar spine of 0.1 standard deviations per 1000 µg inhaled corticosteroid per year. In a subsequent study of adults aged between 20 and 40 years, who had taken inhaled steroids on average for 6 years, bone mineral density of the lumbar spine and femoral neck was inversely correlated with cumulative inhaled corticosteroid dose: doubling of inhaled corticosteroid dose was associated with an estimated decrease in bone mineral density of 0.16 standard deviations. Although unlikely to be associated with fracture in this age group, these results imply that bone mineral density would become significantly decreased in adults taking inhaled corticosteroids by their fifth and sixth decades, potentially increasing the risk of osteoporotic fracture substantially in later life.

Inhaled corticosteroids also increase the risk of posterior subcapsular cataract, glaucoma, and easy skin bruising.

Both asthma and oral corticosteroids can impair growth in children, but longitudinal studies have found no evidence of growth impairment in children taking inhaled corticosteroids in doses of up to 800 µg/day. A meta-analysis of 21 studies, including more than 800 children, found no effect of inhaled beclamethasone on height. None the less, the potential of inhaled corticosteroids taken in high doses for prolonged periods to impair growth remains, and regular monitoring of the growth of children taking inhaled steroids should be undertaken.

Beclomethasone and budesonide in doses of more than 160 µg/day taken by a metered dose inhaler cause a dose-dependent reduction in morning plasma cortisol and 24-h urinary cortisol excretion. However, 2000 µg/day of these inhaled corticosteroids when taken via a spacer has no effect on 24-h urinary cortisol. In children, beclomethasone in daily doses of 800 µg had no effect on 24-h urinary cortisol excretion.

The evidence of side-effects caused by inhaled corticosteroids, particularly osteoporosis, is now sufficient to mean that the lowest dose of inhaled corticosteroid which is clinically effective should be prescribed in both children and adults, and particularly in patients taking topical corticosteroids by other routes (such as nose or skin), and the dose tapered to the minimum necessary when symptomatic and functional improvement is achieved.

β$_2$-Adrenoreceptor agonists

β-Agonists are sympathomimetic amines that include catecholamines—both naturally occurring adrenaline, noradrenaline, and dopamine and synthetic isoprenaline—and non-catecholamines, both short-acting, such as salbutamol and terbutaline, and long-acting, such as salmeterol and formoterol. Catecholamines have been replaced in the treatment of asthma by

β_2-selective non-catecholamines, which have a longer half-life than catecholamines because they are not subject to catecholamine uptake mechanisms and not broken down by catechol-O-methyl transferase. The duration of bronchodilatation after inhalation of non-catecholamines is longer; the effects of salbutamol and terbutaline persisting for 3 to 6 h and of salmeterol and formoterol for up to 12 h.

The actions of β-agonists in asthma are the result of stimulation of β-adrenoreceptors that are located in the airways, on airway epithelium, submucosal glands, airway and vascular smooth muscle. β-Receptors in the airways are entirely β_2, with the exception of some β_1-receptors on submucosal glands.

β_2-Agonists can influence airways function through several mechanisms:

(1) relaxation of bronchial smooth muscle by direct effect on β_2-receptors;

(2) inhibition of mast cell mediator release; and

(3) enhanced mucociliary clearance.

Inhalation of a β_2-agonist by a patient with asthma increases airway calibre and reduces airway hyperresponsiveness. β_2-Agonists also cause tachycardia and increased cardiac output, systemic vasodilatation, and increased muscle blood flow. The tachycardia and increased cardiac output are the results of both stimulation of cardiac β-adrenoreceptors and a reflex response to peripheral vasodilatation. In addition β_2-agonists cause tremor and have metabolic actions, of which hypokalaemia is probably the only potentially important clinical effect.

Inhaled, selective, short-acting β_2-agonists reverse mild acute airway narrowing and are sufficient treatment, alone, for mild intermittent asthma causing occasional symptoms. (Step 1 of BTS guidelines: Table 3.)

Studies comparing regular with as-needed inhaled β_2-agonists in patients with asthma not taking inhaled corticosteroids have shown that regular treatment confers no benefit over as-needed inhalation and can have adverse consequences. A randomized controlled trial in 255 patients with mild intermittent asthma, comparing salbutamol taken as-needed with regular treatment, found no difference at 16 weeks in respiratory symptoms, airway function, or frequency of exacerbations. However, those taking regular salbutamol took more salbutamol, showed more variability in peak flow rates, and had increased airway responsiveness to inhaled methacholine. Short-acting β_2-agonists should, in general, be reserved to provide reversal of acute airway narrowing, taken as-needed or prior to exercise in patients with exercise-provoked asthma, except in cases of severe asthma not controlled with maximal doses of inhaled corticosteroids and additional long-acting β_2-agonist (step 4 BTS guidelines), when regular inhaled short-acting β_2-agonists can be added.

By contrast, long-acting β_2-agonists—salmeterol and formoterol—are taken regularly and their addition to inhaled corticosteroids has been shown to be more effective than doubling the dose of the inhaled corticosteroids in improving symptoms and lung function in patients not controlled by low-dose inhaled corticosteroids. Regular treatment with long-acting β_2-agonists, when taken with inhaled corticosteroids, has not been associated with deterioration in asthma control.

Two epidemics of asthma deaths, the first in the 1960s in six countries which followed the introduction of Isoprenaline Forte, the second in the mid-1970s in New Zealand after the introduction of fenoterol, have led to concerns about the safety of inhaled β-agonists. Case–control studies have also identified an association between asthma deaths and overuse of inhaled β_2-agonists. However, the evidence for cause and effect is confounded because overuse of β_2-agonists to treat frequent symptoms is more likely to occur in patients with severe uncontrolled asthma who are at high risk of a fatal attack. The evidence for cause and effect in the asthma epidemics is stronger: the increased death rates that followed the introduction of the particular inhaled β-agonists fell rapidly after recognition of the association and no other plausible explanation has been advanced. Isoprenaline is a non-selective β-agonist and fenoterol is less selective than salbutamol and terbutaline. Both drugs were marketed in high dose and are cardiotoxic in the presence of hypoxia, hence both epidemics may have been due to the acute cardiac effects of β-agonists inhaled in high dose by hypoxic patients with acute severe asthma. The evidence that selective β_2-agonists formulated in lower doses have a similar cardiotoxic effect and cause asthma deaths outside these epidemics is limited to associations in case–control studies, from which it is not possible to infer cause and effect. However, a small effect can be difficult to detect and, as pointed out by Tattersfield, if a fatal arrhythmia occurred in 1 in 8000 patients treated with β-agonists each year this would account for 50 per cent of asthma deaths in patients under 65 years, but its detection would require observation of many thousands of patients.

Methylxanthines

Theophylline is the pharmacologically active methylxanine most usually employed in clinical medicine, because of its greater bronchodilator activity, less erratic absorption, and longer half-life. More predictable theophylline absorption can be obtained by slow-release formulations and the addition of ethylene diamine to theophylline (aminophylline) provides the increased solubility required for intravenous administration. None the less, theophylline has a relatively narrow 'therapeutic window' for a safe and effective dose, with wide differences among individuals in its metabolism, which can also be adversely affected by several extrinsic factors to cause clinically important side-effects. The most common side-effects are 'caffeine-like': anorexia, nausea, and vomiting, followed by headache and insomnia. At higher concentrations, potentially fatal fits and arrhythmias can occur.

Theophylline relaxes bronchial smooth muscle and, like β-agonists, is a functional antagonist that causes bronchial muscle relaxation irrespective of the constrictor stimulus. Its action was thought to be mediated via phosphodiesterase inhibition increasing intracellular cyclic AMP. However, the intracellular concentration necessary for theophylline to achieve this is some 20 times greater than its therapeutic plasma levels. More recently,

Table 3 Steps in the British Thoracic Society guidelines on the management of chronic asthma

Step	Treatment
Step 1	Inhaled short-acting β_2-agonist as required
Step 2	Add inhaled steroid: 200–800 μg/day BDP or equivalent adults (<400 μg/day children) If inhaled steroid cannot be used, use other preventative medicine If control on 800 μg/day inadequate–go to Step 3

Step 3	Add long-acting β_2-agonist
	If no benefit–stop long-acting β_2-agonist
	Consider trial of :
	    SR theophylline
	    β_2-agonist tablet
	    leucotriene receptor antagonist
	If there is benefit but control is inadequate–go to Step 4

Step 4	Increase inhaled steroid to 800 μg/day (if not already at this dose)
	Consider trials of:
	    increased inhaled steroid to 800–2000 μg/day
	    SR theophylline) if not
	    β_2-agonist tablet) already
	    leucotriene receptor agonist) tried in Step 3

Step 5	Add daily steroid tablet in lowest dose providing adequate control Maintain inhaled steroid at 2000 μg/day Consider trial of a steroid sparing agent

BDP, beclomethasone dipropionate

Table 4 Factors influencing the half-life of theophylline

Increase half-life	Decrease half-life
Liver disease	Cigarette smoking
Heart failure	Alcohol
Virus infection	
Drugs:	Drugs:
Cimetidine	Rifampicin
Erythromycin	Barbiturates
Clarithomycin	Phenytoin
Ciprofloxacin	Carbamazepine
Oral contraceptives	

anti-inflammatory activity in 'subtherapeutic' concentrations has been suggested as a possible mechanism of action in asthma.

In addition to bronchodilatation, theophylline increases the force and rate of heart contraction and causes vasodilatation. In toxic doses it can cause arrhythmias, which may be fatal. It is also a central nervous system stimulant, causing increased alertness and, in toxic doses, confusion, irritability, and fits.

Theophylline is metabolized to inactive products by cytochrome P-450 enzyme-dependent pathways in the liver. The variation in its metabolism among individuals is large, and the half-life of theophylline can vary between 4 and 24 h. This may in part reflect the wide range of exogenous factors that influence hepatic metabolism of the drug: its half-life is increased by several drugs—cimetidine (but not ranitidine), erythromycin, ciprofloxacin, and oral contraceptives—and decreased by rifampicin, barbiturates, and carbamazepine (Table 4).

Bronchodilatation increases linearly with increase in serum theophylline concentration. Toxic effects also show a similar linear relationship, but at higher concentrations, although there are considerable differences between individuals in the serum concentration at which side-effects occur, in some occurring at low serum concentrations. Serum concentrations of between 10 and 20 $\mu g/ml^{-1}$ combine substantial bronchodilatation with a low risk of side-effects.

Safe and effective theophylline treatment requires monitoring of plasma concentration at the start of treatment to ensure a concentration within the therapeutic window, and subsequently to ensure its maintenance. This can be measured by immunoassay, when in patients on regular, twice daily, maintenance treatment the difference between peak and trough levels is usually between 5 and 10 $\mu g/ml^{-1}$, although greater in smokers, who may require treatment three times daily.

Theophyllines are now most commonly used as an additional treatment in asthma that is inadequately controlled by inhaled corticosteroids. Comparison in a randomized controlled trial of budesonide at 400 μg twice daily plus theophylline (250 or 375 mg twice daily) with budesonide at 800 μg twice daily for 3 months in 62 patients, whose asthma was not controlled by the lower dose of inhaled steroid, found the combination of low-dose inhaled corticosteroid and theophylline provided the greater improvement in lung function, peak flow variability, and β_2-agonist use. In those receiving it, median theophylline concentration was 8.7 $\mu g/ml$, hence this additive effect was achieved at doses lower than those conventionally considered therapeutic (10 to 20 $\mu g/ml$) and similar to that provided by inhaled salmeterol. This suggests that oral theophylline may therefore be an appropriate alternative to inhaled salmeterol at stage 3 of BTS guidelines.

Sodium cromoglycate

Sodium cromoglycate is a bischromone that has prophylactic but not bronchodilator activity in asthma. Originally available as a dry powder (mixed with lactose), it is now also formulated as a metered dose inhaler and as a nebulizer solution for children.

In inhalation tests, sodium cromoglycate inhibits asthmatic reactions provoked by inhaled allergen, exercise, and other provocative stimuli including sulphur dioxide and adenosine, although it is less effective in a dose of 20 mg than salbutamol at 200 μg in preventing asthma provoked by

exercise. The major benefit of sodium cromoglycate is its safety. However, it is less effective than inhaled corticosteroids, needs to be taken four times daily, and its use is now generally reserved for children with mild asthma and taken immediately prior to exercise to prevent exercise-induced asthma. Sodium cromoglycate is no longer recommended in the new BTS Guidelines.

Nedocromil sodium

Nedocromil sodium has a similar activity profile to sodium cromoglycate. It is available as a metered dose inhaler and needs to be taken four times a day.

Its activity is equivalent to low-dose inhaled corticosteroid and it can be used either in place of inhaled corticosteroid or to reduce the dose of inhaled corticosteroid. Nedocromil sodium is an alternative to inhaled corticosteroids if inhaled steroids cannot be used in step 2 of BTS guidelines.

The 'stepped' approach to treatment of asthma

The purpose of treatment of asthma varies from the reversal of occasional mild symptoms to the restoration of normal life in a patient with severe disabling ill health. Treatment needs will vary greatly among different patients and underlie the 'stepped' approach to treatment, which is the basis of current guidelines for asthma management, including the British Thoracic Society (BTS) guidelines published in 1997. In the stepped approach, asthma severity is defined by the treatment step (1 to 5) needed to achieve and maintain good control. Inhaled corticosteroids form the mainstay of maintenance treatment for the majority of patients. In deciding the starting treatment step, a 'start high–go low' policy has been recommended, recognizing that initial control of airway inflammation is likely to need a higher dose of inhaled corticosteroid than will subsequent maintenance of disease control. Sodium cromoglycate or nedocromil sodium may be used as alternative inhaled anti-inflammatory drugs, but are less efficacious than inhaled corticosteroids and are now primarily used for the treatment of mild asthma in children.

Inhaled β_2-agonists are used primarily for symptomatic relief. There is good evidence that regular treatment with short-acting β_2-agonists alone is less effective than regular inhaled corticosteroids, and provides less good control of asthma—both symptomatically and of lung function—when taken regularly than as-needed.

Steps 1 to 5 of the BTS guidelines identify the treatment requirements for asthma of increasing severity (Table 3). Failure to achieve treatment targets at any step implies the need to increase treatment to a step that provides good control. Figure 6 shows the proportion of patients on each of the BTS guideline steps.

Step 1

This comprises patients with mild intermittent asthma whose asthma is controlled by the use of an inhaled shorter-acting β_2-agonist (such as salbutamol or terbutaline) less than once a day. Requirement for more regular

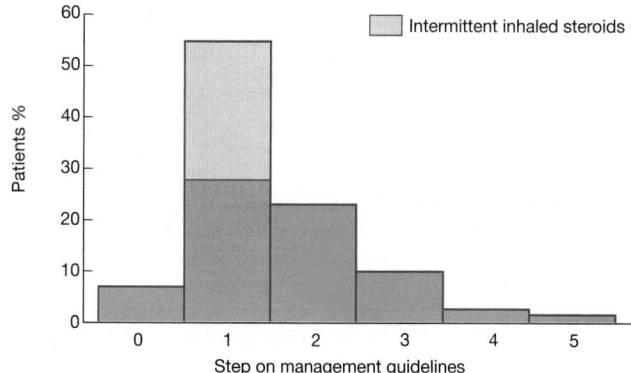

Fig. 6 Proportion (per cent) of 3372 patients with asthma on each of the BTS guideline steps.

treatment implies the need for regular anti-inflammatory treatment (that is, a higher step).

Step 2

This comprises patients with mild persistent or intermittent asthma that is of sufficient frequency to require regular anti-inflammatory treatment. Inhaled corticosteroids are the most effective and commonly used anti-inflammatory drugs, with sodium cromoglycate and nedocromil sodium as alternatives. Treatment with an inhaled corticosteroid should be started at a dose of 400 µg of beclomethasone twice daily or equivalent. This dose should be continued for at least 3 months, the period when most benefit of the inhaled steroid is obtained, before reducing the dose to the minimum required for maintenance of good control. This can be achieved by reducing the dose by 25 to 50 per cent every 1 to 3 months. Short-acting β_2-agonists are used as required for symptomatic relief.

Step 3

This comprises patients with moderate persistent asthma that is not controlled despite adherence to inhaled steroid (or equivalent prevention) treatment and correct inhaler technique. The recommended treatment is a regular long-acting β_2-agonist (salmeterol or formoterol) added to low-dose beclomethasone (less than 800 µg/day) or equivalent.

Two randomized controlled trials have shown that the addition of salmeterol to a low-dose inhaled corticosteroid was more effective than doubling the dose of inhaled corticosteroid in improving symptoms and lung function. In a third randomized controlled trial the addition of formoterol increased the benefit provided by both low-dose and high-dose budesonide. These studies suggest that the addition of a long-acting β_2-agonist to low-dose inhaled corticosteroid is the preferred option for improvement of day to day control of asthma that is not controlled by low-dose inhaled corticosteroid, whereas reducing the frequency of exacerbations of asthma was best achieved by increasing the dose of inhaled steroid and additional long-acting β_2-agonist.

If there is no benefit, stop long-acting β_2-agonist and consider:

(a) trial of: slow-release theophylline added to low-dose inhaled corticosteroid. (One randomized controlled trial of 133 patients found the addition of oral slow-release theophylline to beclomethasone at 400 µg/day for 6 weeks was as effective in improving symptoms and lung function as doubling the dose of beclomethasone to 800 µg/day.)

or (b) β_2-agonist tablet

or (c) leucotriene receptor antagonist.

Step 4

This involves a combination of the alternatives in step 3—high-dose inhaled corticosteroid (up to 2000 µg/day of beclomethasone or equivalent) together with a long-acting β_2-agonist or alternative bronchodilators, such as an oral β_2-agonist or slow-release theophylline or leucotriene receptor antagonist, if these were not tried at Step 3.

Step 5

Patients who fail to respond to these combinations of step 4 treatments will require the addition of an oral corticosteroid. This is an important decision, which should be made in consultation with a respiratory physician and requires continuous monitoring to identify, and where possible avoid, the associated side-effects. The risk of osteoporosis can be reduced by taking regular exercise, and by not smoking. Bone density should be monitored regularly and where appropriate calcium, vitamin D, and bisphosphonates given. Postmenopausal women can benefit from hormone replacement therapy.

Most patients with asthma in the community have disease of severity indicated for steps 1 and 2 of the BTS guidelines; 'difficult' asthma, requiring treatment equivalent to step 5, constitutes less than 5 per cent of patients. A recent community study of five large general practices in south Nottinghamshire (a population of 38 865) found a prevalence of asthma of 9 per cent, with a peak of 17 per cent in 10 to 14 year olds, falling to less than 6 per cent in adults aged over 70 years. Most of those diagnosed with asthma were either not receiving treatment (8 per cent) or receiving treatment equivalent to steps 1 and 2 (76 per cent); 11 per cent were on step 3, and some 5 per cent on steps 4 and 5. The authors endeavoured to assess the effectiveness of asthma treatment in this population by measuring the proportion of patients who during a 1-year period required oral corticosteroid courses or were prescribed 10 or more short-acting β_2-agonist inhalers: 12.5 per cent of patients not taking them regularly had been prescribed one or more courses of oral corticosteroids, 1.6 per cent on three or more occasions; 13.6 per cent of patients had been prescribed 10 or more short-acting β_2-agonist inhalers. Both were increasingly more frequent in patients on steps 3 or higher of the BTS guidelines. However, because only a minority of patients (15 per cent) were in these categories, more than half of the patients who required either oral corticosteroids or 10 or more β_2-agonist inhalers were on steps 1 or 2, indicating continuing significant morbidity among some patients with asthma receiving either low-dose or no anti-inflammatory treatment.

Difficult asthma

Difficult asthma is asthma not controlled by maximum doses of inhaled treatment, including inhaled corticosteroids in doses of beclomethasone of up to 2000 µg/day or equivalent, with additional treatment such as long-acting β_2-agonists. It occurs uncommonly, probably in less than 5 per cent of patients with asthma, but is important. The severity of disease and associated disability is considerable, the risk of near fatal and fatal asthma is high, and the adverse consequences of treatment are severe, and only worthwhile if treatment is demonstrably effective.

Failure to respond to maximal inhaled treatment can result from several causes (Table 5). It is clearly important to confirm the diagnosis of asthma and exclude other diseases that may be mistaken for it. Demonstration of spontaneous variability or reversibility of airflow limitation is important to avoid treatment of irreversible airflow limitation, due either to localized obstruction or chronic obstructive pulmonary disease, with ever increasing doses of oral corticosteroids. Assessment of reversibility may require a formal trial of oral prednisolone in a dose of 30 to 40 mg taken each morning

Table 5 Difficult asthma: failure to respond to maximal inhaled treatment

Wrong diagnosis
COPD (irreversible airflow limitation)
Localized obstruction
Left heart failure
Pulmonary thromboembolic disease
Vocal cord dysfunction
Poor adherence to treatment or inhaler technique
Unidentified provoking factors:
Allergens
Occupational sensitizers
Upper airway disease—rhinitis/sinusitis
Gastro-oesophageal reflux
Drugs—β-blockers
NSAIDs
Vasculitis—Churg–Strauss syndrome
Psychological factors
Unstable asthma:
Nocturnal asthma
Premenstrual asthma
Brittle asthma:
Type I
Type II
Corticosteroid-dependent asthma
Corticosteroid-resistant asthma

COPD, chronic obstructive pulmonary disease; NSAIDs, non-steroidal anti-inflammatory drugs.

for 1 month to determine whether this provides a significant improvement in airway function.

The conditions most easily mistaken for asthma were considered earlier (see differential diagnosis). Once the diagnosis of asthma has been confirmed, it is important to ensure good inhaler technique and adherence to prescribed treatment: failure to take treatment properly is a common reason for failure to respond. This may reflect lack of understanding that preventive treatment needs to be taken regularly and not 'as needed', or poor inhaler technique. Patients may take preventive treatment irregularly because, unlike short-acting β₂-agonists, it does not provide immediate symptomatic relief. Others may be inappropriately concerned about potential side-effects or resent the need to take regular treatment. In patients taking oral corticosteroids, blood eosinophil count is markedly reduced and often reported as zero, hence a blood eosinophil count above 0.3 in a patient prescribed oral steroids suggests that these are not to being taken regularly, or alternatively another disease, particularly Churg–Strauss syndrome, may accompany the asthma.

One study, using a computerized timing device in a dry powder inhaler, found that only 18 per cent of patients took inhaled steroids as prescribed. Adherence to inhaled treatment is difficult to monitor, and poor adherence to treatment may be suspected as a cause of difficult asthma in patients whose asthma improves when treatment, although unchanged, is supervised. Patient understanding of the effectiveness of regular treatment may also be reinforced by this means.

Unidentified provoking factors include allergens, commonly domestic pets, in particular cats, whose allergens can be present in sufficient concentrations to cause asthma for several months after cats have left the home. Sensitizing agents encountered at work can also cause asthma that is poorly controlled by inhaled treatment. Early identification and avoidance of the cause is important to minimize the risk of development of chronic asthma. Aspirin, NSAIDs, and β-blockers can also be important provoking factors.

Rhinitis commonly accompanies asthma and its treatment can be assocaited with improvement in asthma and airway hyperresponsiveness. The explanation for this association is unclear, but may be a consequence of inflammatory mediators in post-nasal drip increasing airway responsiveness and provoking cough. Similarly gastro-oesophageal reflux can provoke cough and worsen asthma; where this is suspected a trial with a proton pump inhibitor such as omeprazole should be instituted, but objective improvement in asthma with such treatment is uncommon.

Uncommonly asthma may be a manifestation of systemic disease, particularly a systemic vasculitis, Churg–Strauss syndrome, when asthma, which can be difficult to control, is accompanied by a high blood eosinophil count (usually more than 1.5). Other manifestations including eosinophilic pneumonia, pleural and pericardial effusions, and mononeuritis multiplex. Effective treatment requires high-dose oral corticosteroids and in some cases immunosuppressant treatment, initially with cyclophosphamide and subsequently azathioprine (see Chapter 17.11.5).

Nocturnal asthma can persist in some patients despite treatment with inhaled corticosteroids, which provides good daytime control. This may be improved by the addition of a long-acting β₂-agonist or slow-release theophylline.

Premenstrual deterioration of asthma is not uncommon, and can in some patients be severe and unresponsive to corticosteroid treatment. Symptoms characteristically increase, and PEFR falls, 2 to 5 days before the menstrual period, improving with the onset of menstruation. This coincides with the fall in progesterone secretion and increase in oestrogen:progesterone ratio. Asthma in some patients is improved by treatment with intramuscular, but not oral, progestogen during the week before menstruation. Patients with severe premenstrual exacerbations can require hospital admission, in some cases ventilation, and may (very rarely) experience improvement only by surgical removal of the ovaries.

Brittle asthma is characterized by widely varying peak flow rates uncontrolled by maximum inhaled treatment. Two patterns of brittle asthma have been distinguished:

(1) type I—persistent daily chaotic variability in peak flow (usually greater than 40 per cent diurnal variation in PEFR more than 50 per cent of the time); and

(2) type II—sporadic sudden falls in PEFR against a background of usually well-controlled asthma with normal or near normal lung function.

Treatment of brittle asthma of both types is difficult. Type I brittle asthma, not responding to inhaled long-acting β₂-agonists, can be improved by subcutaneous terbutaline administered via an insulin infusion pump, usually in a dose of between 3 and 12 mg in 24 h: this treatment is limited by side-effects, of which the most important is muscle cramp associated with increased levels of serum creatinine kinase.

Type II brittle asthma requires immediately available treatment for what can be catastrophic falls in peak flow. The speed of onset of attacks requires immediately injected bronchodilator and such patients should have preloaded adrenaline syringes (such as Epi-pen) available at all times and wear a Medic-alert bracelet. Potential provoking factors, such as foods, should be sought and avoided.

Asthma in a very few patients is only controlled with continuous oral corticosteroids, often in high doses; reduction in dose is followed by worsening of asthma. The term corticosteroid-dependent asthma has been used for the condition in these patients. They differ from those with corticosteroid-resistant asthma in their response to oral corticosteroids. Patients with corticosteroid-resistant asthma show no response to oral corticosteroids, even in high dose, but do show spontaneous variability of peak flow and reversibility with inhaled bronchodilators. Corticosteroid-resistant asthma is very uncommon, estimated at between 1 in 1000 and 1 in 10 000 patients. It probably forms the end of a spectrum of resistance to the anti-inflammatory activity of corticosteroids, to which corticosteroid-dependent asthma also belongs. Treatment of corticosteroid-resistant asthma is difficult, but should include stopping oral corticosteroids, which still cause side-effects, and relying on other forms of treatment, including long-acting β₂-agonists.

Treatment of acute exacerbations of asthma

Asthma exacerbations are episodes of progressively worsening airway narrowing, associated with increasing shortness of breath, cough, wheezing, chest tightness, or some combination of these. Exacerbations can vary in severity from episodes which patients are able to manage themselves by following an agreed treatment plan, to severe and potentially life-threatening episodes that require medical attention and hospital admission. Severe attacks also vary in their speed of onset, ranging from deterioration over days to episodes that progress rapidly and can become life-threatening within minutes or hours. In about one-half of cases of fatal asthma the attack lasted more than 24 h, in one-quarter less than 1 h. Fatal or near fatal attacks of asthma are associated with the following.

1. Attacks may occur in patients who have previously required hospital admission for severe asthma and who require regular oral steroid treatment.

2. The doctor may fail to recognize the severity of the asthma. This can be minimized by making appropriate objective measurements of respiratory, heart, and peak flow rates to assess severity.

3. Patients may fail to recognize the severity of their asthma. Those with long-standing asthma can become accustomed to their symptoms and not appreciate an important increase in their severity, which may persist for days or weeks. This may also be associated with psychosocial problems and poor adherence to treatment.

4. The asthma attack may have been undertreated or given inappropriate treatment. Failure to use oral corticosteroids in adequate doses early in an exacerbation is probably the single most remediable factor. The use of sedatives or anxiolytics to reduce the anxiety or agitation that can often accompany acute severe asthma is absolutely contraindicated.

Many of these problems can be overcome by improved patient understanding, allowing them to have control over their illness supported by a jointly agreed management plan. A systematic review of 22 studies comparing self management education for asthma with usual care found that self management reduced hospital admissions and days off work by nearly one-half and emergency room visits by one-quarter. Results were best when self management included a written action plan.

Moderate exacerbations

Exacerbations of asthma with increased symptoms, both during the daytime and at night, frequently follow an upper respiratory tract infection, allergen exposure in allergic individuals, or a reduction in anti-inflammatory treatment. Increase in symptoms associated with deterioration in peak flow can often be treated adequately by the patient increasing their frequency of inhaled short-acting bronchodilators, doubling the dose of inhaled steroids, or taking a short course of oral steroids. Several studies have shown that a short course of oral steroids taken at the start of an acute exacerbation reduces the need for hospital admission, the frequency of relapse, and the need for β_2-agonists. One recent overview of seven randomized controlled trials in 320 persons found that systemic corticosteroids, taken at the onset of an acute exacerbation, reduced hospital admissions in both children and adults by 65 per cent in the first week compared with placebo, an effect maintained for 21 days. No difference was observed between the use of oral and intramuscular corticosteroids.

Acute severe asthma

Acute severe asthma is a potentially life-threatening increase in the severity of asthma that can develop over minutes, hours, or usually days and which has often failed to respond to conventional, inhaled bronchodilator treatment. It is usually the outcome of airways increasingly narrowed by the consequences of chronic inflammation, resulting in increasing resistance to airflow identified as a reduction in PEFR and FEV_1, hyperinflated lungs, ventilation–perfusion inequality, and hypoxia, which is the most serious consequence of severe asthma. Initially this stimulates alveolar hyperventilation, but with increasing airway narrowing and exhaustion, arterial Po_2 continues to fall while arterial Pco_2 rises to normal, and subsequently increases steeply, due to alveolar hypoventilation: Pco_2 rises into the normal range when FEV_1 is some 25 per cent and PEFR 30 per cent of predicted normal values.

The clinical features of importance in identifying acute severe asthma and assessing its severity are shown in Table 6. Patients are usually extremely breathless and unable to complete sentences in one breath. A rapid respiratory rate and heart rate are good markers of severity of asthma and hypoxia. Although anxiety and increased use of β_2-agonists can increase heart rate, tachycardia should not be ignored by attributing it to these factors. An objective measure of airflow limitation should be made because severity is difficult to assess clinically with accuracy. Although PEFR is an effort-dependent measurement, it can usually be obtained from patients with severe asthma: a value of less than 50 per cent of predicted or

Table 6 Acute severe asthma: assessment of severity

Features of acute severe asthma:
Unable to complete sentences in one breath
Respiration rate more than 25 breaths/min
Pulse rate higher than 110 beats/min
PEFR less than 50 per cent of predicted or best

Life-threatening features:
PEFR less than 33 per cent of predicted or best
Silent chest
Bradycardia or hypotension
Exhaustion, confusion, or coma

Markers of very severe life-threatening attack:
Normal (5 to 6 kPa or 36 to 44 mmHg) or high Pco_2
Severe hypoxia: Po_2 less than 8 kPa (60 mmHg)
Low pH or high H^+

of the recent best value in an adult aged less than 50 years indicates severe asthma, a value of less than 33 per cent, a potentially life-threatening attack.

Blood gas measurements should be made in adults seen in hospital as an important guide to the severity of asthma; children can often safely be managed by measurement of Sao_2 alone. Most patients admitted to hospital with acute severe asthma are hypoxic, of whom about one-third will have a Po_2 of less than 8 kPa (60 mmHg). Pco_2 is reduced in patients with moderately severe asthma, but with increasingly severe airways obstruction and fatigue, Pco_2 falls and subsequently rises in parallel with a falling Po_2. A normal Pco_2 in a hypoxic patient with acute severe asthma indicates impending hypoventilation, with a rapidly increasing Pco_2, falling Po_2, acidosis, narcosis, and death.

Treatment of acute severe asthma

The aims of the treatment of acute severe asthma are to reverse the hypoxia, airflow limitation, and airway inflammation with oxygen, bronchodilators, and corticosteroids (Table 7).

Oxygen Oxygen relieves the hypoxia present in most patients with acute severe asthma. High concentrations of inspired oxygen are safe in patients with asthma, and certainly in those aged less than 50 years; a high $Paco_2$ in acute severe asthma reflects fatigue and the severity of airways obstruction and is not a contraindication for a high concentration of inspired oxygen. Oxygen can be administered by nasal cannulas or by facemask in the highest available concentration (usually Fio_2 between 40 and 60 per cent). The aim is to increase Sao_2 to above 92 per cent or Pao_2 to above 9 kPa (80 mmHg).

Bronchodilators The purpose of bronchodilator treatment in acute severe asthma is to reverse airway narrowing due to smooth muscle contraction, before the onset of the anti-inflammatory action of corticosteroids, which usually takes 6 to 12 h from administration.

Inhaled high-dose β_2-agonists, salbutamol and terbutaline, are now used as initial treatment, usually from a nebulizer. The benefit of the nebulizer is that it allows inhalation of bronchodilator to be driven by a high flow of oxygen. This can be important in severe asthma as β_2-agonists may increase ventilation–perfusion inequality and consequently arterial hypoxia, hence in hypoxic patients β_2-agonists should not be administered without oxygen. Nebulized salbutamol in a dose of 5 mg, or terbutaline in a dose of 10 mg, driven by 6 litre/min oxygen can be given safely by trained ambulance crews during transfer to hospital. However, nebulizers are inefficient and widely variable in their performance, which has led to the suggestion of large volume spacers as alternative delivery systems. In adults and children

Table 7 Treatment of acute severe asthma

Initial treatment:
- Oxygen (60 per cent Fio_2)
- Nebulized salbutamol, 2.5 to 5 mg via nebulizer driven by O_2
or terbutaline, 5 to 10 mg via nebulizer driven by O_2
- Oral prednisolone, 30 to 60 mg
or intravenous hydrocortisone, 200 mg
If poor response after 30 min to initial treatment:
- Continue O_2
- Repeat nebulized salbutamol or terbutaline at 30-min intervals
- Add ipatropium, 0.5 mg to nebulized β-agonist
- Hydrocortisone, 200 mg intravenously 4 hourly
- Aminophylline,* 250 mg intravenously over 20 min
or salbutamol, 250 µg intravenously over 10 min
or terbutaline, 250 µg intravenously over 10 min
- Investigations :
Chest radiograph to exclude pneumothorax
Monitor serum K^+ (with high-dose β-agonist)
If poor response within 1 h:
Admit to intensive care for possible intubation and ventilation

* Do not give bolus intravenous aminophylline to patients taking theophyllines regularly.

with severe but not life-threatening asthma treated outside hospital, inhalation of β_2- agonist by nebulizer has not been found to provide additional bronchodilatation compared with use of a metered dose inhaler via a spacer, but it is important to note that the studies on which this is based are of patients without life-threatening asthma who did not require hospital admission. Spacers do not easily allow concurrent administration of oxygen and require patient co-operation, which can be difficult in severely breathless patients.

The available intravenous bronchodilators are β_2-agonists and theophylline. The theoretical advantage of intravenous β_2-agonists is access to peripheral airways so narrowed that they cannot be reached by inhalation. However, inhaled salbutamol is rapidly absorbed from the lungs, reaching a peak concentration within 10 min of inhalation. The major disadvantage of intravenous β_2-agonists, by comparison with inhalation, is the greater frequency of systemic side-effects. What is relevant is whether intravenous β_2-agonists provide additional improvement in bronchodilator response to inhaled β_2-agonists and corticosteroids. In adults with acute asthma, intravenous salbutamol at 12 μg/min given 4 hourly after an initial dose of 5 mg of nebulized salbutamol and intravenous hydrocortisone provided greater bronchodilation compared with three further doses of nebulized salbutamol given during 2 h, although the patients receiving intravenous salbutamol had a greater increase in heart rate. Similarly, in a study of children with acute severe asthma, the addition of salbutamol (15 μg/kg) in a 10-min infusion to nebulized salbutamol and intravenous hydrocortisone was associated with a reduced period of need for inhaled salbutamol, a decreased requirement for oxygen, and earlier discharge from the emergency department.

The use of intravenous aminophylline in the treatment of asthma has decreased with the recognition that it does not provide additional benefit to repeated nebulized β_2-agonist bronchodilators in the initial hour of emergency treatment. This, together with its narrow therapeutic window, need for drug monitoring, and interactions with other drugs has led to its replacement as first-line bronchodilator treatment of asthma by inhaled β_2-agonists. However, it is recommended as additional therapy for patients not responding to initial treatment with inhaled β_2-agonists and corticosteroids, and as initial treatment in the very severely ill patient with a normal or high Pco$_2$. In those who have not been taking theophylline prior to admission, a loading dose of 5 mg/kg body weight over 20 min should be followed by a maintenance dose of 0.5 to 0.9 mg/kg body weight per hour until a serum level of 10 to 20 μg/ml is obtained. The loading dose should be omitted in patients currently taking theophyllines, in whom the serum concentration should be measured. The infusion rate should be decreased in patients with liver or heart failure or those taking cimetidine, macrolide antibiotics, or ciprofloxacin (Table 4). Toxic side-effects are increasingly common in patients with serum levels exceeding 25 μg/ml, ranging from gastrointestinal symptoms to fits and cardiac arrhythmias.

The BTS guidelines for the treatment of acute severe asthma recommend the administration of intravenous β_2-agonist or aminophylline to patients not responding to oxygen, inhaled β_2-agonists, and corticosteroids after the addition of inhaled ipratropium, or as initial treatment for those with life-threatening features.

Antimuscarinics The purpose of antimuscarinic treatment is to reverse airway narrowing caused by increased vagal tone and not responsive to high-dose inhaled β_2-agonists. Several studies have suggested the addition of an inhaled antimuscarinic provides additional benefit in the treatment of acute severe asthma. One multicentre study found the addition of inhaled ipratropium to inhaled salbutamol increased bronchodilation by 10 to 20 per cent compared with inhaled salbutamol alone. However, other studies have failed to demonstrate additional benefit from the addition of ipratropium to inhaled high-dose β_2- agonist. The evidence is consistent with considerable individual variation in response to inhaled antimuscarinics, maximal response occurring in those with exaggerated cholinergic tone. Inhaled antimuscarinics have few side-effects, can provide benefit in some patients, and are recommended in the guidelines as additional treatment in

a dose of 0.25 to 0.5 mg for patients not responding to initial high-dose inhaled β_2-agonists.

Corticosteroids Systemic corticosteroids are given in acute severe asthma to reverse the underlying airway inflammation. The anti-inflammatory action requires 6 to 12 h from administration for demonstrable bronchodilatation to occur. Steroids may also reverse β_2-receptor desensitization induced by regular β_2- inhalation within 1 h of their administration. The value of corticosteroid treatment in acute severe asthma was first demonstrated in a randomized controlled trial in 1956 and their value in the treatment of acute severe asthma has since been generally accepted. They are usually given by intravenous administration, but other than in life-threatening asthma and in patients vomiting or unable to swallow, there is no demonstrable advantage of intravenous over oral administration. When indicated, intravenous doses initially of 200 mg every 4 to 6 h can be followed by oral prednisolone in a dose of 40 to 60 mg/day. The duration of treatment with oral prednisolone will depend on the severity and rate of recovery of the acute episode. In general, oral prednisolone should be continued until resolution of the acute episode with return to usual daytime activities, resolution of nocturnal symptoms, and PEFR within 80 per cent of the patient's predicted or best values. Short courses of oral corticosteroids (taken for less than 3 weeks) do not need to be tapered, provided patients are taking an appropriate dose of inhaled corticosteroid. Although some studies in patients with relatively mild exacerbations of asthma (PEFR greater than 60 per cent of predicted or best) have suggested that high-dose inhaled steroids are an effective alternative to oral corticosteroids, these results should not be extrapolated to acute severe asthma where the recommended guideline is that all patients should be treated with systemic corticosteroids.

Intensive care and intermittent positive-pressure ventilation Most attacks of acute severe asthma respond to treatment with high-concentration inspired oxygen, systemic corticosteroids, and inhaled β_2-agonists. However, this treatment is insufficient in a few patients who require intensive care and, on occasion, intermittent positive-pressure ventilation (**IPPV**). This occurs in two particular situations: patients who have a catastrophic hyperacute attack, and patients whose asthma progressively increases in severity despite maximal bronchodilator and corticosteroid treatment. The indications for intensive care and IPPV are given in Table 8. Patients with increasing drowsiness or who lose consciousness with hypoxia and worsening hypercapnia require IPPV, as do those who suffer a respiratory arrest. However, because of the high inflation pressures needed to overcome the high airway resistance and poorly compliant hyperinflated lungs and chest wall, IPPV in acute severe asthma can be difficult and hazardous. High inflation pressures can cause barotrauma with pneumomediastinum and, on occasion, pneumothorax. In addition up to one-third of patients can develop clinically significant hypotension, requiring inotropic support.

Table 8 Acute severe asthma: indications for intensive care and for mechanical ventilation

Indications for intensive care:
    Hypoxia (Pao$_2$ less than 8 kPa) despite Fio$_2$ 60%
    Hypercapnoea (PaCo$_2$ greater than 6 kPa)
    Exhaustion, feeble respiration
    Confusion or drowsiness
    Unconsciousness
    Respiratory arrest
Indications for intermittent positive-pressure ventilation (IPPV):
    Hypoxia (Pao$_2$ less than 8 kPa) despite Fio$_2$ 60%
    Increasing hypercapnia
    Drowsiness, unconsciousness
    Respiratory arrest

Further reading

Barnes PB (1998). Current issues for establishing inhaled corticosteroids as the anti-inflammatory agents of choice in asthma. *Journal of Allergy and Clinical Immunology* **101**, 5427–33.

Barnes PJ, Pederson S, Busse WW (1998). Efficiency and safety of inhaled corticosteroids. *American Journal of Respiratory and Critical Care Medicine* **157**, S1–S53.

British Thoracic Society (1997). The British guidelines on asthma management. *Thorax* **52**(Suppl 1), S1–21.

Drazen JM *et al.* (1996). Comparison of regularly scheduled with as needed use of albuterol in mild asthma. Asthma clinical research network. *New England Journal of Medicine* **335**, 841–7.

Evans DJ *et al.* (1997). A comparison of low dose inhaled budesonide plus theophylline and high dose inhaled budesonide for moderate asthma. *New England Journal of Medicine* **337**, 1412–18.

Garbelt JF *et al.* (1997). Nebulised salbutamol with and without ipratropium bromide in the treatment of acute asthma. *Journal of Allergy and Clinical Immunology* **100**, 165–70.

Greening AP *et al.* (1994). Added salmeterol versus higher dose corticosteroid in asthma patients with symptoms on existing inhaled corticosteroid. *Lancet* **344**, 219–24.

Haahtela T *et al.* (1991). Comparison of a β₂ agonist terbutaline with an inhaled corticosteroid budesonide in newly detected asthma. *New England Journal of Medicine* **325**, 388–92.

Haahtela T *et al.* (1994). Effects of reducing or discontinuing inhaled budesonide in patients with mild asthma. *New England Journal of Medicine* **331**, 700–5.

Marquette CH *et al.* (1992). A 6 year follow up study of 145 asthmatic patients who underwent mechanical ventilation for near-fatal attack of asthma. *American Review of Respiratory Diseases* **146**, 76–81

Newman Taylor AJ (1995). Environmental determinants of asthma. *Lancet* **345**, 296–9.

Pauwels RA *et al.* (1997). Effect of inhaled formoterol and budesonide on exacerbations of asthma. *New England Journal of Medicine* **337**, 1405–11.

Walsh LJ *et al.* (1999). Morbidity from asthma in relation to regular treatment: a community based study. *Thorax* **54**, 296–300.

Woolcock AJ *et al.* (1996). Comparison of addition of salmeterol to inhaled steroids with doubling of the dose of inhaled steroids. *American Journal of Respiratory and Critical Care Medicine* **153**, 1481–8.

17.4.5 Occupational asthma

A. J. Newman Taylor

Occupational asthma is asthma induced by an agent inhaled at work. Agents inhaled at work can aggravate pre-existing asthma, but the term occupational asthma is usually restricted to asthma initiated or induced by such agents.

Asthma may be initiated or 'switched on' either by respiratory irritants inhaled in toxic concentrations—irritant-induced asthma—or as the outcome of an acquired specific hypersensitivity response. Hypersensitivity-induced occupational asthma is considerably more common than irritant-induced asthma and is important to recognize because in the majority of cases it improves or resolves with the avoidance of further exposure. Furthermore, the earlier further exposure is avoided, the more probable is complete resolution of the asthma. Identification and avoidance of the specific occupational cause therefore provides one of the few opportunities to cure asthma in adult life.

Causes of occupational asthma

The known causes of irritant-induced asthma are relatively few and include well-recognized respiratory irritants such as chlorine and ammonia, as well as others such as toluene di-isocyanate inhaled in toxic concentrations. However, any respiratory irritant inhaled in concentrations toxic to the epithelial cells in the airways is a potential cause of reactive airways dysfunction syndrome.

By contrast, the number of reported causes of hypersensitivity-induced occupational asthma is considerable, and with the rapid development of biotechnology and the continuous introduction of newly synthesized organic chemicals is likely to increase. The causes described include proteins of animal, vegetable, and microbiological origin, naturally occurring organic chemicals, synthetic chemicals, and inorganic chemicals, particularly metal salts. Some of the more important are listed in Table 1.

Agents and occupations associated with occupational asthma

The proportion of cases of asthma in the general population that are attributable to an occupational cause is not known, although estimates have varied between 2 and 15 per cent. A recent community-based study in Spain of adults aged between 20 and 44 years estimated that the risk of asthma attributable to occupation was between 1 in 20 (5 per cent) and 1 in 15 (6.7 per cent). The highest risks occurred in spray painters, bakers, and laboratory technicians. During the past 10 years a voluntary reporting scheme for registering new cases of occupational lung disease seen by respiratory and occupational physicians in the United Kingdom (SWORD) has estimated the incidence of occupational asthma in different occupations and provided information about the relative importance of its causes. Both have remained remarkably stable during 10 years of reporting to the scheme. Organic agents, such as flour/grain, colophony, wood dust, and laboratory animals, and chemicals, isocyanates, and glutaraldehyde, account for some two-thirds of the reported cases (Table 2). The relative frequency of the different causes has also remained similar during this period, with the exception of some reduction in the proportion of cases attributed to isocyanates and an increase in the number of cases attributed to latex (Fig. 1).

The estimated annual incidence by occupation varied from 1380 per million per year in coach and other spray painters to 12 per million per year in transport and storage workers (i.e. a range of two orders of magnitude).

Table 1 Some important causes of occupational asthma

Origin	Proteins	Low-molecular-weight chemicals
Animal	Excreta of rats, mice, etc.	
	Locusts	
	Grain mites	
Vegetable	Grain, flour	Plicatic acid (western red cedar)
	Green coffee bean	Colophony (pinewood resin)
	Castor bean	
	Latex	
	Ispaghula	
Microbial	Harvest moulds (*Alternaria, Cladosporium*)	Antibiotics (e.g. penicillin, cephalosporins)
	Enzymes (protease, amylase, etc.)	
Minerals		Isocyanates
		Acid anhydrides
		Complex platinum salts
		Reactive dyes
		Glutaraldehyde

Table 2 Agents most frequently reported to SWORD as causes of occupational asthma (1989–97) (after McDonald *et al.*, 2000)

Agent		1989–91	1992–4	1995–7
Organic	**Total**	**468 (31%)**	**793 (28%)**	**1126 (38%)**
	Flour/grain	101 (7%)	229 (8%)	280 (9%)
	Solder/colophony	85 (6%)	101 (4%)	118 (4%)
	Wood dust	63 (4%)	119 (4%)	186 (6%)
	Laboratory animals	87 (6%)	131 (5%)	117 (4%)
	Crustaceans/fish	34 (2%)	20 (1%)	82 (3%)
Chemical	**Total**	**551 (36%)**	**1003 (35%)**	**890 (30%)**
	Isocyanate	336 (22%)	413 (14%)	410 (14%)
	Glutaraldehyde	30 (2%)	128 (4%)	113 (4%)
Metals	**Total**	**60 (4%)**	**153 (5%)**	**89 (3%)**
Miscellaneous	**Total**	**328 (21%)**	**619 (22%)**	**700 (23%)**
	Grand total	**1528**	**2857***	**2991***

* Estimates based on sampling.

The estimated annual incidence in high-risk occupations between 1992 and 1997 is shown in Table 3.

Determinants of occupational asthma

Four major determinants of occupational asthma have been identified, which vary in their importance in relation to different causes: exposure intensity, atopy, smoking, and HLA genotype. Intensity of exposure is the single most important determinant of irritant-induced occupational asthma. Evidence for exposure–response relationships has also been found for many of the causes of hypersensitivity-induced occupational asthma, both for proteins, including laboratory animal proteins and enzymes, and for low-molecular-weight chemicals, including acid anhydrides and complex platinum salts. The risk of asthma is increased in atopics exposed to many of the protein causes of occupational asthma such as enzymes, latex, and laboratory animals, and in cigarette smokers exposed to low-molecular-weight chemicals that induce IgE production, such as complex platinum salts and acid anhydrides. HLA DR3 has been associated with an increased risk of developing specific IgE and asthma in those exposed to acid anhydrides and complex platinum salts. It should be appreciated, however, that the prevention of occupational asthma is more effectively achieved by reducing the intensity of exposure to its causes in the workplace than by exclusion of 'susceptible' individuals who are atopic, cigarette smokers, or HLA DR3 positive.

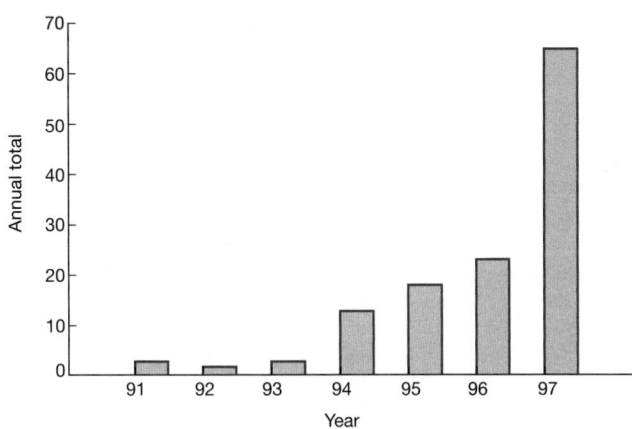

Fig. 1 Annual reports to SWORD of occupational asthma attributable to latex (1991–7).

Table 3 Estimated annual incidence rates (1992–7) of occupational asthma per million persons employed in high-risk occupations (after McDonald *et al.*, 2000)

Occupational group	Incidence (per 10⁶ per year)
Coach and spray painters	1367
Bakers	958
Metal treatment workers	643
Chemical processors	641
Plastics workers	447
Welding, soldering, electronic assembly	279
Food processing (excluding bakers)	256
Laboratory technicians and assistants	214
Woodworkers	147

Pathology and pathogenesis

The pathological changes in the airways of patients with asthma of occupational cause are no different in any important way from those in patients with asthma of other or unknown cause: a desquamative eosinophilic bronchitis with infiltration of the airway wall by eosinophils and lymphocytes, accompanied by desquamation of bronchial epithelial cells.

In common with asthma caused by allergy to proteins encountered in the general environment, hypersensitivity-induced occupational asthma is probably the outcome of T_{H2} lymphocyte stimulation, and the pathological features observed are primarily the consequence of T_{H2} lymphocyte–eosinophil interaction. The evidence for T_{H2} lymphocyte stimulation is in part direct, but primarily comes from evidence of specific IgE antibody to many, although not all, of the causes of occupational asthma. In a few cases specific IgG antibodies can also be detected. These seem to reflect exposure, whereas IgE is more closely associated with disease. In general, specific IgE has been identified with the protein causes of occupational asthma, but only with a minority of the non-protein causes. Whilst it is likely that the majority of the low-molecular-weight chemicals that cause occupational asthma do so by binding to body proteins and acting as haptens, the difficulties of preparing the relevant hapten–protein conjugate *in vitro* have limited demonstration of this process, other than with chemicals such as acid anhydrides and reactive dyes that form stable conjugates with human serum albumin.

Clinical features

Irritant-induced asthma

Asthma caused by the inhalation of an irritant chemical in toxic concentrations is usually one manifestation of general tissue injury to exposed mucosal surfaces—eyes, nose, throat, and bronchial airways. The onset of symptoms follows a single identifiable exposure to a toxic chemical. Running, swelling, and discomfort of the eyes, running and obstruction of the nose, and painful throat usually occur within minutes of the exposure, and symptoms of asthma (shortness of breath, wheezing, chest tightness, and cough) develop within a few hours—certainly within 24 h—of inhalation of the chemical in toxic concentrations. Respiratory symptoms often have the characteristic circadian pattern characteristic of asthma: they are more severe during the night and on waking than during the daytime. In most cases asthma resolves spontaneously within a few weeks, but can occasionally persist for several years, if not indefinitely.

Hypersensitivity-induced asthma

In the commoner cases of hypersensitivity-induced occupational asthma respiratory symptoms develop insidiously and do not follow a single identifiable exposure to its cause. Asthma develops after an initial symptom-free period of exposure, commonly within 1 year of starting a new job or changing duties at work, although in some cases asthma may not develop until there have been several years of exposure. The onset of asthma may have been preceded or be accompanied by 'hay fever'-like symptoms of the nose and eyes. Characteristically, symptoms become increasingly severe during the working week and improve during absences from work during holidays and at weekends. However, the patient may not appreciate the relationship of respiratory symptoms to work, particularly when symptoms develop during the second half of the day and are most severe, as is characteristic of asthma, in the evenings, during the night, and on waking in the morning. Asthmatic symptoms can also persist for several days after avoidance of exposure, in which case appreciable symptomatic improvement at weekends does not occur, but improvement is usually sufficient to be appreciated by the end of a 2-week holiday or deterioration to be recognized on return to work. With continuing exposure asthma can become chronic and the relationship between symptoms and periods at work less clear, although even in these circumstances it is usual for some symptomatic improvement to occur on avoidance of exposure, although this may take several weeks.

The findings on clinical examination depend upon the severity of the asthma at the time of the examination. There may be no abnormal findings if seen when away from exposure. During a period of symptomatic exposure the patient will have typical signs of airflow limitation with breathlessness and wheeze, and depending on severity, other signs described in Section 17.4.

Diagnosis

The diagnosis of occupational asthma should be considered in any adult who develops asthma or whose asthma has deteriorated in working life. In the case of irritant-induced asthma the association of the onset of asthma with inhalation of a toxic chemical is usually clear. The association of asthma caused by a specific hypersensitivity reaction is often less apparent, and the diagnosis is based on the following:

1. Exposure to a sensitizing agent at work.

2. Characteristic history of:

   (a) onset of asthma after an initial symptom-free period of exposure;

   (b) deterioration in symptoms during periods at work and improvements during absence from work.

3. Results of objective investigations:

   (a) lung function tests

   (b) immunological tests

   (c) inhalation tests.

Objective investigations

Lung function tests

The most commonly used criterion for diagnosing asthma—improvement in airflow limitation (usually measured as forced expiratory volume in 1 s (**FEV1**) or peak expiratory flow (**PEF**)) after inhalation of bronchodilator—is often absent in cases of occupational asthma because lung function may be normal when the patient is seen away from work and, if present, does not identify a work relationship.

The measure of lung function most commonly used to identify work-related asthma is serial self-recorded PEF. A patient with suspected occupational asthma is asked to record his or her PEF at intervals of 2 to 3 h for a month from waking to sleeping, and at night if awoken, both during periods at and absences from work. The results can be summarized in a graphical display that records the best, worst, and average values for each day, allowing comparison of PEF during days at work with days away from work (Fig. 2). The diagnostic value of the test depends on the reproducibility of the patient's forced expiratory manoeuvres and their honesty and compliance. Concurrent treatment can influence the results, particularly when treatment is systematically increased during periods at work and reduced during absences from work. When possible treatment should be kept constant during the period of testing, or at least recorded. Comparisons with the results of inhalation testing as the 'gold standard' have shown that serial self-recorded PEF measurements are a sensitive and specific index of work-related asthma. Patients with evidence of work-related asthma on PEF records reacted on inhalation testing to a specific agent inhaled at work and had occupational asthma; patients who did not show evidence of asthma on PEF records (i.e. less than 20 per cent within-day variability) did not react in inhalation tests. The major diagnostic difficulties were patients with evidence of asthma on PEF records without a work relationship, of whom a proportion were eventually shown to have occupational asthma; the commonest reason for this false-negative response was insufficient time away from work for significant improvement to have occurred.

Immunological tests

The presence of specific IgE antibody, identified either by immediate skin test response to a soluble protein extract or a hapten–protein conjugate or by immunoassay in serum (usually radio-allergosorbent testing) is evidence of sensitization to a specific agent. The diagnostic value of a positive test depends upon its predictive value in cases of asthma among those exposed to the specific agent. Specific IgE can be identified in most, if not all, protein causes of occupational asthma, and in a small number of low-

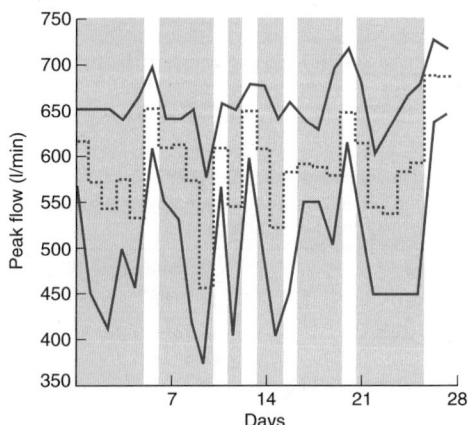

Fig. 2 Serial peak expiratory flow results in a baker sensitive to flour. The best, worst, and average values are plotted for each day. Shaded areas are periods at work; unshaded areas are periods away from work. Peak flows are consistently worse in each work period and improve during each period away from work.

molecular-weight chemical causes of asthma, notably complex platinum salts, acid anhydrides, and reactive dyes. No reliable immunological test has been developed for sensitivity to the other important causes of asthma such as isocyanates and colophony. The diagnostic value of a positive test has been formally examined for few of the causes of occupational asthma, and in these cases has been found to be significantly associated with asthma caused by both proteins and low-molecular-weight chemicals inhaled at work.

Inhalation testing

The objective of an inhalation test is to expose the individual under single-blind conditions to the putative cause of their asthma in circumstances that resemble as closely as possible the conditions of exposure at work. The different test methods used depend upon the physical state of the test material, which can be water soluble (most proteins) and inhaled in solution, a volatile organic liquid inhaled as a vapour, or a dust. Any change in lung function in both airways calibre (usually measured as FEV_1 or PEF) and airways responsiveness to inhaled histamine or methacholine, measured as PC_{20}, (concentration of inhaled histamine or methacholine which provokes a 20 per cent fall in FEV_1) is compared with results on appropriate control days. The patterns of airways response provoked by specific inhalation tests have been distinguished by their time of onset and duration. Immediate asthmatic responses occur within minutes of the test exposure and usually resolve spontaneously within 1 to 2 h (Fig. 3). Late asthmatic responses develop 1 h or more after the test exposure and can persist for 24 to 36 h (Fig. 4). Late asthmatic (but usually not immediate) responses are accompanied by an increase in non-specific airways responsiveness 3 h and, less reliably, 24 h after the test inhalation. An immediate response followed by a late response has been called a dual response.

Inhalation testing allows the identification of specific causes of asthma in individuals exposed to them. Provided that the agent being tested is not a non-specific mucosal irritant and does not provoke an immediate asthmatic response in patients with hyper-responsive airways, for example sulphur dioxide, histamine, or exercise, the provocation of an asthmatic response by an occupational agent implies that it is a cause of asthma. This causal relationship is strengthened if the agent reproducibly provokes a late asthmatic response and increases non-specific airways responsiveness.

There are four major indications for inhalation testing in the diagnosis of occupational asthma:

(1) Where the agent considered responsible for causing asthma has not previously been reliably shown to do so.

(2) Where an individual with occupational asthma is exposed at work to more than one potential cause that cannot be distinguished by other means.

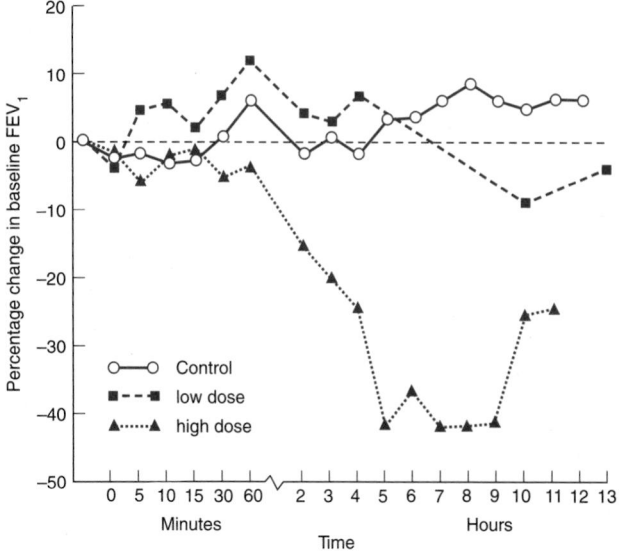

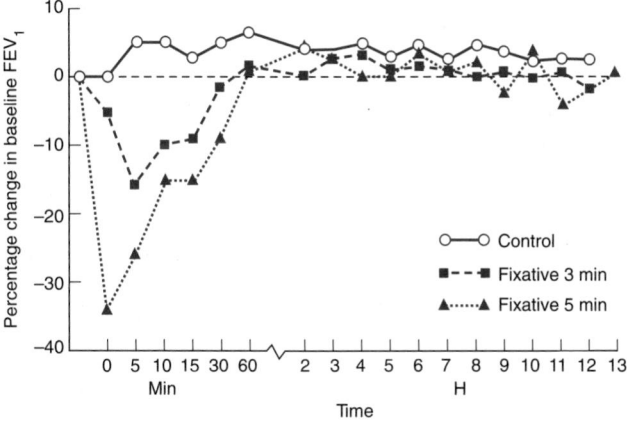

Fig. 3 Immediate asthmatic reactions in a radiographer provoked in inhalation tests of 3 and 5 min with X-ray fixative material, but not by the control test.

Fig. 4 Late asthmatic reaction in a platinum refiner provoked by exposure to the complex platinum salt ammonium hexachloroplatinate in a concentration of 10 mg (high dose) but not 1 mg (low dose) in 250 g of lactose (the control material).

(3) Where asthma is of such severity that further uncontrolled exposure at work is unjustifiable.

(4) Where the diagnosis or cause of occupational asthma remains in doubt after other investigations, including serial PEF and immunological tests where applicable, have been completed.

Inhalation tests should be undertaken only for clinical purposes, to provide information important for future management advice. Inhalation tests undertaken solely for medicolegal purposes are not justified.

Differential diagnoses

The diagnosis of occupational asthma requires differentiation:

(1) from other causes of similar respiratory symptoms, in particular chronic airflow limitation and hyperventilation;

(2) of occupational from non-occupational cause;

(3) of asthma initiated by an agent inhaled at work from pre-existing or incidental asthma aggravated by non-specific provocative stimuli encountered at work, such as sulphur dioxide, exercise, and cold air.

Prognosis

Asthma initiated by an agent inhaled at work and caused by toxic damage to the airway epithelium (irritant-induced asthma) or as the outcome of a hypersensitivity response may become chronic and persist for several years, if not indefinitely. Chronic asthma induced by a hypersensitivity response has been reported most frequently in cases caused by low-molecular-weight chemicals such as isocyanates, colophony, plicatic acid from western red cedar, and acid anhydrides. Continuing asthmatic symptoms and airways hyper-responsiveness have been reported in 50 per cent or more of patients several years after avoidance of exposure to the initiating cause. Chronic asthma has also been reported in snow crab process workers in Canada in whom airways responsiveness improved during the first 2 years of avoidance of exposure but subsequently reached a plateau.

The only important determinant for developing chronic asthma identified to date has been the duration of symptomatic exposure to the initiating cause after the onset of asthma: those who remain exposed to the cause are more likely to develop chronic asthma.

Management

Patients who develop occupational asthma in whom a specific cause is identified should be advised to avoid further exposure to that cause. This seems particularly important where low-molecular-weight chemicals such as isocyanates, plicatic acid, or anhydrides are the cause, as continuing symptomatic exposure to these is particularly associated with the development of chronic asthma and airways hyper-responsiveness.

Avoidance of further exposure may require a change or loss of job that, for social or financial reasons, may not be possible. A change of occupation can be particularly difficult for those who are highly trained, such as experimental scientists whose livelihood depends on their knowledge and experience of working with laboratory animals. Such individuals and others sensitized to biological dusts who are unable to change their job, at least in the short term, should be advised to minimize exposure to the cause of their asthma and to wear adequate respiratory protection, most conveniently laminar-flow equipment, when in contact with the organic dust. In addition, background prophylaxis such as sodium cromoglycate can minimize the risk of the provocation of asthma by indirect allergen contact, such as dust on colleagues' clothing. None the less, it should be emphasized that such measures are temporary, and in the long term means should be sought to avoid exposure to the cause of asthma.

When individuals remain in employment exposed to the cause of their asthma, either directly or indirectly, the effectiveness of relocation or of respiratory protection needs to be monitored. This can be conveniently done by serial self-recordings of PEF to determine whether or not asthma is continuing and, if so, whether it is work related.

Compensation

Statutory compensation in the United Kingdom

Occupational asthma is a prescribed disease for 'employed earners'. The terms of prescription have recently been broadened considerably. They now include asthma caused by exposure to 22 specified groups of agents (listed below) as well as a 'z' category, which specifies 'any other sensitizing agent inhaled at work':

(a) isocyanates

(b) platinum salts

(c) acid anhydride and amine hardening agents

(d) fumes arising from the use of rosin as a soldering flux

(e) proteolytic enzymes

(f) animals including insects and other arthropods or their larval forms used for the purposes of research, education, in laboratories, pest control, or fruit cultivation

(g) dusts arising from barley, oats, rye, wheat or maize, or meal or flour made from such grain

(h) antibiotics

(i) cimetidine

(j) wood dusts

(k) ispaghula

(l) castor bean dust

(m) ipecacuanha

(n) azodicarbonamide

(o) glutaraldehyde

(p) persulphate salts or henna arising from their use in the hairdressing trade

(q) crustaceans or fish or products arising from these in the food processing industry

(r) reactive dyes

(s) soya bean

(t) tea dust

(u) green coffee bean dust

(v) fumes from stainless steel welding

and

(z) any other sensitizing agent inhaled at work.

Byssinosis

In the United Kingdom byssinosis occurs most commonly in cotton mill workers, usually after some 20 to 25 years of exposure to cotton dust. It is probably a response to agents inhaled in the cotton bract and is characterized by chest tightness on the first day of the working week, which usually develops some 3 to 4 h after the start of a work shift. Typically, the chest tightness improves on subsequent working days, despite continuing exposure to cotton dust. The symptoms are often, although not always, accompanied by changes in lung function and the majority of cases of byssinosis have hyper-responsive airways. Cotton dust also provokes acute airway narrowing in about one-third of persons exposed to an extract of cotton bract for the first time; this reaction is probably an important contributory factory in the high turnover in the early months of employment in cotton mills. Whether byssinosis causes long-term respiratory impairment and disability remains controversial. Several studies have failed to find an increase in mortality from respiratory causes, which has been interpreted as suggesting that exposure to cotton dust does not cause chronic lung disease. However, in one survey of a community which included ex-cotton workers, a reduction in FEV_1 of between 2 and 8 per cent was observed in the ex-cotton textile workers and a loss of lung function in those with 15 years' heavy exposure to cotton dust that was equivalent to that observed in light and ex-smokers.

Byssinosis should probably be considered as a form of occupational asthma: the characteristic symptoms are associated with acute reductions in FEV_1 and patients with byssinosis commonly have hyper-responsive airways.

Further reading

Bernstein IL *et al.*, eds (1999). *Asthma in the workplace*, 2nd edn. Marcel Dekker, New York.

Fishwick D and Pickering CAL (1992). Byssinosis—a form of occupational asthma. *Thorax* **47**, 401–3.

McDonald JC, Keynes H, Meredith S (2000). Reported incidence of occupational asthma in the United Kingdom 1989–1997. *Occupational and Environmental Medicine* **57**, 823–9.

Newman Taylor AJ (2000). Asthma. In: McDonald JC, ed. *Epidemiology of work related diseases*, 2nd edn, pp 149–74. BMJ Books, London.

17.5 Respiratory infection

17.5.1 Upper respiratory tract infections

P. Little

Introduction

Acute upper respiratory tract infections (URTIs) include acute pharyngitis/tonsillitis and acute rhinitis. Acute sinusitis, acute otitis media, and influenza also come under the umbrella of infections of the upper respiratory tract. Otitis media and influenza will be discussed elsewhere: this chapter will concentrate on acute pharyngitis/tonsillitis, acute rhinitis, and acute sinusitis.

Acute URTIs are the commonest reason for patients to seek medical advice in the United Kingdom, and nearly all cases are managed in primary care. Respiratory tract infections are also the commonest reason for antibiotics to be prescribed. A serious concern is that the inappropriate use of antibiotics for predominantly self-limiting conditions will foster the development of antibiotic resistance, with the danger that serious infections will become untreatable. Thus it is currently a national priority in the United Kingdom, and should be in other countries, to discourage the use of antibiotics unless there is good evidence of their efficacy. The evidence for the effectiveness of treatments for URTI in this chapter comes from a search of the Cochrane Library databases of systematic reviews and randomized controlled trials.

Pharyngitis/tonsillitis

Clinical presentation

Pharyngitis is caused by both bacterial and viral organisms, and has been somewhat arbitrarily divided into nasopharyngitis (with nasal symptoms, that is to say rhinitis), and pharyngitis or tonsillopharyngitis (without nasal symptoms). Causal organisms include group A beta-haemolytic streptococcus (**GABHS**); adenoviruses; influenza A and B; parainfluenza 1,2,3; Epstein–Barr virus (**EBV**); enteroviruses; *Mycoplasma pneumoniae*; and *Chlamydia pneumoniae*. In addition to a sore throat, pharyngitis is often accompanied by fever, headache, nausea, vomiting, anorexia, and sometimes abdominal pain, with or without enlarged and tender cervical lymph nodes, tonsillar erythema and exudate. Scarlet fever has a characteristic 'scarlatiform' rash caused by GABHS exotoxins. Infectious mononucleosis due to the Epstein–Barr virus may present with or without exudative tonsillitis, cervical or general lymphadenopathy, palatal petechiae, splenomegaly, rhinitis, and cough.

Throat swabs, rapid tests, and clinical algorithms

Antibiotics can be targeted to those patients who have positive throat swabs for group A streptococcus, a positive rapid streptococcal test, or clinical characteristics associated with a positive throat swab (for example, the 'Centor' criteria of fever, tonsillar exudate, anterior cervical adenopathy, and absence of cough). However, the throat swab is not a very good test: in both unselected and clinically selected populations in primary care practice it is neither particularly sensitive nor specific when compared to a rise in Anti Streptolysin O Titres (**ASOT**) or Anti DNAse B titres. A rise in ASOT or Anti DNAase B are better indicators of true infection and predict complications, but are not suitable for clinical diagnosis. The results of throat swabs take days to return to the clinic, and they greatly increase the costs of managing what is mostly a self-limiting condition. Furthermore, evidence suggests that in practice clinicians do not use the results, even of rapid tests, and that the overall accuracy of decision-making is little changed when they are used.

Attempts to derive algorithms or clinical-decision rules based on the throat swab have the same limitations of validity as the throat swab itself. Although clinical scoring methods may provide a crude method of identifying patients at a higher risk of complications (see below), better evidence is needed about how well each clinical sign correlates with proof of infection.

Treatment

Antibiotics for symptoms

The Cochrane review of the efficacy of antibiotics for the treatment of sore throat indicates that antibiotics have modest benefit in reducing the duration of symptoms—by a few hours to half a day—but may have a role in preventing complications (acute otitis media, sinusitis, rheumatic fever, and quinsy). This marginal benefit of antibiotics in resolving symptoms suggests that, for patients who are not unwell systemically, the physician should either not prescribe, or use a delayed prescribing approach, advising the patient to wait for several days before collecting or using their prescription. Both these approaches have been shown in a large randomized controlled trial to be acceptable, change attitudes and behaviour, and not to delay symptom resolution appreciably.

In the context of a likely streptococcal infection, trial evidence suggests that delaying the prescription results in 20 per cent fewer recurrences than the immediate prescriptions of antibiotics, presumably because antibiotics modify local or systemic immune mechanisms. Thus, any marginal symptomatic benefit from an immediate prescription of antibiotics for the current illness must be weighed against the disadvantage that the patient is more likely to suffer symptoms from a recurrence.

Antibiotics to prevent complications

The Cochrane review of antibiotics for treating a sore throat supports the use of antibiotics to prevent complications, but the evidence is limited by both clinical importance and generalizability. For the commoner complications, for example otitis media, 30 children and 140 adults would have to be treated to prevent one case of a self-limiting illness, in other words it is not important clinically. For the rarer complications the evidence is not generalizable; for instance, evidence of efficacy in rheumatic fever is based largely on trials where intramuscular penicillin was used in barracked military personnel after the Second World War. This evidence cannot be sensibly applied to healthier modern settings where the attack rate is much lower, and oral antibiotics are used.

The commonest complication of practical importance to the health service is quinsy; this is relatively uncommon, about 1 in 400 following presentation in primary care with sore throat. The Cochrane systematic review, which demonstrates that antibiotics prevent quinsy, relies on data from patients with tonsillitis who were systemically unwell enough to be admitted to hospital shortly after the Second World War, when the prevalence of quinsy in untreated patients was very high (1:18). Clearly, this data cannot be extrapolated to patients presenting from healthier modern populations who are not systemically unwell, treated with oral antibiotics, and where the prevalence of quinsy is much lower. Quinsy following sore throat is possibly slightly more common (1:60) in those who are unwell, with three out of four Centor criteria, most of whom have fever. Rigorously conducted placebo-controlled trials in patients with these criteria suggest quinsy may be prevented by oral penicillin. However, in routine clinical practice, where compliance is not assessed, the preventive benefit of penicillin is not likely to be 100 per cent, as reported in the trials where compliance was assured. Limited routine data suggests that many patients who develop quinsy after being seen in primary care do this despite being given penicillin. Whether using the clinical Centor criteria is better than the primary care physician's assessment of how unwell patients are is unclear: 20 per cent of those considered 'not to be very unwell systemically' by the physician will still have three out of four of the Centor criteria, and the criteria do not necessarily predict the very few individuals who will develop quinsy. Thus, where the primary care physician judges the patient to be both systemically unwell and/or have three out of four of the Centor criteria, it would be reasonable to treat with penicillin or at least discuss with patients the likely risks of non-treatment.

Which antibiotic and for how long?

If an antibiotic is to be prescribed, then it is probably preferable to use one of the narrow-spectrum agents (for example, penicillin V) to minimize both side-effects and the risk of resistance. There are arguments for using a large dose, given the variable absorption of penicillin V (e.g. 2 g per day for adults and 1 g per day for children). The length of course is debatable: 10 days may better eradicate streptococcus microbiologically, but the clinical significance of this in affluent western populations is unclear. Longer courses also have the theoretical disadvantage of poorer compliance, and concerns about antibiotic resistance. There is preliminary evidence that a twice-daily dosing of penicillin V, compared to the same amount spread over four doses, results in better compliance, and also better clinical and microbiological outcomes. Amoxicillin and ampicillin are effective against streptococcus but cause a rash in patients with glandular fever: this can be very severe, such that amoxicillin or ampicillin should not be used to treat sore throat, and erythromycin used where penicillin allergy has been documented.

Treatment of patients with rheumatic fever

Patients who have had one attack of rheumatic fever are at a higher risk from new infections since they are likely to develop recurrent attacks of rheumatic fever and complications. Although most of the evidence for the prevention of rheumatic fever comes from old trials in unusual settings, it seems reasonable to treat patients with a past history who are at a high risk of recurrence and secondary complications, since what evidence there is suggests penicillin prevents rheumatic fever. (See Chapter 15.10.1 for further discussion of the issues involved.)

Other medical treatments

Treatment with aspirin in children is contraindicated due to the small but avoidable risk of Reye's syndrome. There are several trials of the use of non-steroidal anti-inflammatory drugs (**NSAIDs**) in providing effective relief of pain and fever in tonsillitis and pharyngitis. However, only one trial has made a key clinical comparison of NSAIDs with standard treatment (paracetamol), demonstrating no superiority of NSAIDs. Limited trial data suggests that other useful analgesic adjuncts include caffeine, and benzydamine hydrochloride gargle.

Recurrent attacks

A Cochrane review identified only one published randomized trial of tonsillectomy in children (with serious methodological problems) and none in adults. Further evidence is needed before surgery can be advocated firmly for recurrent tonsillitis. There is preliminary trial evidence for the use of α-streptococci spray, immune stimulants, and pneumococcal vaccination, but further confirmation is required.

Nasal congestion and rhinorrhoea

Nasal symptoms are a common reason for attending the doctor. They may be due to a variety of causes, commonly acute viral infection (common cold), allergic rhinitis and sinusitis, vasomotor rhinitis and rhinitis medicamentosa, and less commonly atrophic rhinitis, hormonal rhinitis, and mechanical/obstructive rhinitis. Colds are responsible for significant morbidity: on average there are 0.4 episodes and 1.2 days of restricted activity per person per year for the common cold.

Acute rhinitis

Symptoms are acute nasal congestion and rhinorrhoea, mild malaise, sneezing, sore throat, variable loss of taste and smell, and usually last from 1 to 2 weeks unless sinusitis is present. Examination reveals a hyperaemic and oedematous mucosa, with or without purulent secretions.

Treatment

Symptomatic treatment

Trial evidence supports the use of both oral and topical decongestants for the symptoms of rhinitis. Intranasal ipratropium bromide is also effective symptomatic treatment, but is only available (in the United Kingdom) on prescription. However, topical decongestants should probably not be used for more than a maximum of 7 days: rhinitis medicamentosa starts to develop at 10 days. Due to their moderate systemic effects, care should be taken with oral decongestants in patients with heart disease and hypertension. Saline drops are commonly advocated, but saline or medicated nose drops have been shown to be ineffective in trials in both children and adults. A Cochrane review suggests that steam may provide some relief of symptoms.

Antibiotics

The use of antibiotics for the common cold has been assessed in a Cochrane systematic review and shown not to be helpful.

Other treatments

Reviews of trials indicate little benefit from antihistamines, nor from zinc lozenges. A Cochrane review of the herb echinacea demonstrated positive results in most studies, but there was not enough evidence to recommend the use of a specific product. Trials in adult volunteers with URTI indicate that intranasal sodium cromoglycate may help to relieve symptoms, and limited evidence suggests that NSAIDs may improve both symptoms and mucociliary clearance. There is also preliminary evidence of promise for the use of immune stimulants in preventing recurrent URTIs.

Acute sinusitis

Diagnosis

Acute sinusitis, usually defined as an infection that lasts for less than 3 weeks, is an uncommon complication of coryzal illness and pharyngitis. There is no absolute standard against which symptoms and signs can be compared for accuracy of diagnosis: aspiration by sinus puncture is probably the definitive investigation, since it indicates the presence of infecting organisms, but for obvious reasons this is rarely performed, and contamination by commensal organisms can occur.

The four-view radiographs show acceptable agreement with aspiration and culture, although only moderate interobserver agreement. The US Agency for Health Care and Policy Research (**AHCPR**) has reviewed the diagnosis and treatment of sinusitis: combining all studies comparing sinus radiographs with sinus puncture demonstrated a sensitivity of 73 per cent and specificity of 80 per cent. A history of purulent nasal discharge, maxillary toothache, purulent secretions on examination, poor response to decongestants, and abnormal illumination of the sinuses, are all predictive of sinusitis defined using four-view radiographs as the standard: four or more symptoms or signs giving a likelihood ratio of a positive test of six. A problem with sinus illumination as a diagnostic tool in primary care is that it performs differently in different settings, probably due to operator sensitivity. There is preliminary evidence comparing symptoms with computed tomography (**CT**) as the 'standard', which is justified since the presence of fluid and total opacification of the sinuses on CT predicts antibiotic response. Purulent rhinorrhoea, purulent secretion in the cavum nasae, a history of 'double sickening' (getting better, then getting worse again), and an erythrocyte sedimentation rate (**ESR**) of greater than 10 are predictive of a CT diagnosis of sinusitis—three of these features giving a likelihood ratio of a positive test of 1.8.

However, using a four-item clinical risk score—of purulent rhinorrhoea with unilateral predominance, local pain with unilateral predominance, bilateral purulent rhinorrhoea, and presence of pus in the nasal cavity—is as sensitive and specific as any other method in predicting the results of sinus puncture. Thus, for acute sinusitis, diagnostic tests are not currently indicated, and until valid near-patient tests are available clinical targeting probably performs as well as any other method.

Treatment

Antibiotics

A Cochrane review of all controlled trials suggests that the absolute benefit for symptom resolution is moderate, and must be balanced against the disadvantages of prescribing antibiotics. Furthermore, this review does not include all the trials from primary care, which show moderate or no effect, and thus both the effectiveness and cost-effectiveness of antibiotic treatment of acute sinusitis in primary care is questionable for most patients.

Other treatments

Preliminary trial evidence shows that decongestants are unlikely to be helpful. There is limited evidence that antihistamines may be helpful for patients with a history of allergic rhinitis who develop sinusitis, and some evidence that proteolytics (e.g. bromelain) and mucolytics may help.

There is mixed trial evidence for the benefit of topical steroids. Although trials of NSAIDs suggest they are helpful, they may not be significantly more effective than paracetamol.

Further reading

Cochrane database of systematic reviews. Cochrane Library, January 2000. (sore throat: antibiotics, tonsillectomy; colds: antihistamines, zinc, echinacea, steam, antibiotics; sinusitis: antibiotics)

Cochrane database of randomised controlled trials. Cochrane Library, January 2000.

Systematic review of diagnosis of sore throat

Del Mar C (1992). Managing sore throat: a literature review. I: Making the diagnosis. *Medical Journal of Australia* 156, 572–5.

Antibiotics and recurrent sore throat, the 'medicalizing' effect of prescribing antibiotics, and the use of delayed prescriptions

Little PS, *et al.* (1997). An open randomised trial of prescribing strategies for sore throat. *British Medical Journal* 314, 722–7.

Little PS, *et al.* (1997). Reattendance and complications in a randomised trial of prescribing strategies for sore throat: the medicalising effect of prescribing antibiotics. *British Medical Journal* 315, 350–2.

Use of the 'Centor' criteria to target antibiotic prescribing for sore throat

Zwart S, *et al.* (2000). Penicillin for acute sore throat: randomised double blind trial of seven days versus three days treatment or placebo in adults. *British Medical Journal* 320, 150–4.

Diagnosis and treatment of sinusitis

US Department of Health and Human Services (1999). *Evidence report/technology assessment number 9: diagnosis and treatment of acute bacterial rhinosinusitis.* AHCPR, Rockville, MD.

Diagnosis of rhinitis

Canadian Rhinitis Symposium (1994). Proceedings of the Canadian Rhinitis Symposium 1994. Assessing and treating rhinitis: a practical guide for Canadian physicians. *Canadian Medical Journal* 15(Suppl. 4), 1–27.

17.5.2 Infection of the lung

17.5.2.1 Pneumonia—normal host

John G. Bartlett

Introduction

Pneumonia is an acute or chronic infection involving the pulmonary parenchyma. Most cases are caused by microbial pathogens, including bacteria, viruses, fungi, and parasites. Pneumonia may also refer to inflammation involving the pulmonary parenchyma due to non-microbial causes such as chemical pneumonia. Other modifying terms are used as follows: pneumonia may be acute, subacute, or chronic, depending on the duration of symptoms; it may be described as bronchopneumonia, consolidated (lobar) pneumonia, or interstitial pneumonia based on chest radiography changes; or it may be named after the putative agent, for example pneumococcal pneumonia, mycoplasma pneumonia, *Pneumocystis carinii* pneumonia, etc. Pneumonia is also identified by the place of acquisition—as community-acquired, nursing home-acquired, or hospital-acquired. This chapter will be restricted to community-acquired pneumonia in the adult immunocompetent host.

Aetiology

Although the list of microbes that can cause pneumonia is legion, only a relatively small number are frequent pathogens, for example: *Streptococcus*

Table 1 Microbiology of community-acquired pneumonia

Microbial agent	British Thoracic Society* (%)	Meta-analysis** (%)
Bacteria		
Streptococcus pneumoniae	60–75	65
Haemophilus influenzae	4–5	12
Staphylococcus aureus	1–5	2
Gram-negative bacilli	rare	1
Miscellaneous agents***	(not included)	3
Atypical agents	–	12
Legionella spp.	2–5	4
Mycoplasma pneumoniae	5–18	7
Chlamydia pneumoniae	(not included)	1
Viral	8–16	3
No diagnosis	–	–

* Estimates based on analysis of 453 adults in a prospective study of community-acquired pneumonia in 25 British hospitals.

** Meta-analysis of 122 reports in the English-language literature, 1966–1995; the analysis is restricted to 7079 cases in which a suspected pathogen was reported.

*** Includes *Moraxella catarrhalis*, group A streptococcus, *Neisseria meningitides*, *Acinetobacter*, *Coxiella burnetii*, and *Chlamydia psittaci*.

pneumoniae, *Haemophilus influenzae*, *Mycoplasma pneumoniae*, *Chlamydia pneumoniae*, *Legionella* spp., anaerobic bacteria, and viruses. Less common pathogens are *Moraxella catarrhalis*, *Streptococcus pyogenes*, *Acinetobacter* spp., *Chlamydia psittaci*, *Coxiella burnetii*, *Neisseria meningitidis*, *Staphylococcus aureus*, and enteric Gram-negative rods. In most reported series, each of these generally accounts for less than 1 to 2 per cent of cases. The relative frequencies of different pathogens causing community-acquired pneumonia in two large studies are summarized in Table 1. However, important limitations of these studies should be acknowledged: all the cases in the review conducted by the British Thoracic Society were inpatients, as were the great majority of those reviewed in the meta-analysis. Most studies

of pneumonia show that only 20 to 30 per cent of patients are sufficiently sick to require hospitalization. Furthermore, nearly all studies, including those that use extensive diagnostic resources, only identify a likely aetiological agent in 40 to 60 per cent of cases. This suggests that fastidious microbes are under-represented and that many cases of pneumonia may be caused by, as yet, unidentified organisms.

Epidemiology

Pneumonia is the most important infectious disease in terms of morbidity and mortality. It is estimated that in the United States there are four million cases of pneumonia per year (45 000 deaths), and worldwide there are 4400 million cases per year (4 million deaths). In the United States, data suggest that between 20 and 30 per cent of all patients with a diagnosis of pneumonia are hospitalized, and that the mortality rate for this subpopulation is about 14 per cent. The crude death rate from influenza and pneumonia in the United States for 1994 was 31.8 deaths per 100 000 of the population; this represents a 59 per cent increase over the 20.0 deaths per 100 000 recorded in 1979, suggesting that the frequency of lethal pneumonia in the United States is increasing. Those aged 65 or older accounted for 89 per cent of the deaths in 1994, suggesting that increases in longevity account for most of this increase in mortality rate.

Those pathogens associated with specific epidemiological and underlying conditions are summarized in Table 2.

When an aetiological agent is identified, just three microbial agents account for the majority of lethal cases of community-acquired pneumonia. Influenza accounts for an average of 20 000 deaths per year in the United States: the majority involve influenza A, occur in patients over 65 years of age, and most deaths are due to complications of influenza rather than influenza *per se*. The second common cause of lethal pneumonia is pneumococcal pneumonia; risk factors for a fatal outcome include: bacteraemia, advanced age, and concurrent alcoholism. Legionella is the third agent, with associated mortality rates generally reported

Table 2 Epidemiological conditions related to specific pathogens in patients with selected community-acquired pneumonia*

Condition	Commonly encountered pathogens
Alcoholism	*Streptococcus pneumoniae*, anaerobes, Gram-negative bacilli
COPD/smoker	*S. pneumoniae*, *H. influenzae*, *Moraxella catarrhalis*, *Legionella* spp.
Nursing-home residency	*S. pneumoniae*, Gram-negative bacilli, *H. influenzae*, *S. aureus*, anaerobes, *C. pneumoniae*
Poor dental hygiene	Anaerobes
Epidemic Legionnaire's disease	*Legionella* spp.
Exposure to bats or soil enriched with bird droppings	*Histoplasma capsulatum*
Exposure to birds	*Chlamydia psittaci*
Exposure to rabbits	*Francisella tularensis*
HIV infection	*S. pneumoniae*, *Pneumocystis carinii*, *H. influenzae*, *Mycobacterium tuberculosis*
Exposure to farm animals or parturient cats	*Coxiella burnetii* (Q fever)
Influenza active in community	Influenza, *S. pneumoniae*, *S. aureus*, *S. pyogenes*, *H. influenzae*
Suspected large volume aspiration	Anaerobes, chemical pneumonitis, obstruction
Structural lung disease (bronch-iectasis, cystic fibrosis, etc.)	*P. aeruginosa*, *Burkholderia* (*Pseudomonas*) *cepacia*, or *S. aureus*
Injection drug use	*S. aureus*, anaerobes, tuberculosis, *S. pneumoniae*
Airway obstruction	Anaerobes

* Adapted with permission from Bartlett *et al.* (2000).

COPD, chronic obstructive pulmonary disease.

between 15 and 25 per cent for patients with community-acquired infections.

Nearly all studies show that the risk of death with pneumonia is strongly associated with age extremes. Concurrent conditions that contribute to increased mortality rates include neoplastic disease, hepatic failure, congestive heart failure, cerebrovascular disease, and renal disease.

Pathogenesis

As with nearly all infectious diseases, the probability of disease depends on the virulence of the organism, the inoculum size, and the status of host defences. The normal tracheobronchial tree and lung parenchyma is sterile below the level of the larynx, so that agents of pneumonia must reach this site from external or adjacent sources, usually either by aspiration or inhalation. Organisms may also reach the lung by haematogenous seeding, direct extension from infection in a contiguous structure, or by activation of dormant organisms in the lung. These mechanisms are pathogen-specific, as summarized in Table 3.

Most pneumonias are probably caused by aspiration, which is defined as the abnormal entry of endogenous secretions or exogenous substances into the lower airways. There is a problem here with semantics because most cases of pneumonia are probably due to aspiration as classically described, but 'aspiration pneumonia' probably accounts for only 5 to 10 per cent of cases. The explanation is presumably quantitative, 'aspiration' generally referring to the abnormal entry of relatively large volumes in patients who are so predisposed due to dysphagia or a compromised level of consciousness. The alternative form is presumed to be 'microaspiration', involving the aspiration of very small numbers of microbes, a process that commonly takes place in healthy patients during sleep and with no apparent sequelae.

Clinical features

The classic presentation of pneumonia is of a cough and fever with the variable presence of sputum production, dyspnoea, and pleurisy. Most patients have constitutional symptoms such as malaise, fatigue, and asthenia, and many also have gastrointestinal symptoms. Although patients with pneumonia usually possess these characteristic clinical features, there can be major differences in presentation based on the host and the aetiological agent, as summarized below.

Pneumococcal pneumonia

Streptococcus pneumoniae is nearly always the most commonly identified pathogen in patients hospitalized with a community-acquired pneumonia. A meta-analysis of 122 reports of community-acquired pneumonia by Fine *et al.* for the period 1966 to 1995 showed that *S. pneumoniae* accounted for

65 per cent of all cases where a microbial pathogen was defined and 66 per cent of all bacteraemic cases (referenced in the Further reading list). Studies using transtracheal aspiration or transthoracic aspiration, methods that avoid the problem of expectorated sputum contamination, show the presence of *S. pneumoniae* in 50 to 80 per cent of cases.

The classic presentation is of a previously healthy adult with an upper respiratory tract infection who then develops a rigor followed by fever, dyspnoea, pleurisy, and a cough that usually becomes productive with a purulent, blood-streaked or 'rusty' sputum. However, many patients show variations in this pattern, including one of a more subtle onset. Moreover, atypical presentations are particularly common in elderly patients. Chest radiography invariably shows an infiltrate, and lobar consolidation specifically suggests this diagnosis (Fig. 1). A pleural effusion is present in about 25 per cent of patients, but only 1 to 2 per cent have an empyema.

Important observations over the past decade include the declining frequency of cases where this organism is identified and the increasing resistance of *S. pneumoniae* to penicillin and a variety of other antibiotics. The declining frequency is commonly ascribed to a general decline in the quality of microbiological testing currently performed in cases of pneumonia in general, and decreased antibiotic susceptibility is thought to reflect antibiotic abuse. The question still remains as to why, when these drugs were introduced in the 1940s but penicillin resistance was not really encountered until the 1990s, has there been such a long delay in the development of resistance?

Poor prognostic findings in patients with pneumococcal pneumonia include advanced age, bacteraemia, alcoholism, and multiple lobe involvement.

The preferred antibiotics are amoxicillin for oral treatment and ceftriaxone or cefotaxime for parenteral treatment; penicillin-resistant strains may be treated with fluoroquinolones, vancomycin, or linazolide.

Haemophilus influenzae

This organism was originally described in 1892 by Pfeiffer who erroneously thought it was the agent of influenza; it was sometimes referred to as 'Pfeiffer's bacillus'. *H. influenzae* is always the second most common agent (behind *S. pneumoniae*) when an identified bacterial pathogen is found in community-acquired pneumonia. However, the diagnosis is difficult owing to problems with its recognition by direct Gram stain, the fastidious growth requirements of the organism, and with interpretation—even when it is recovered—because it commonly colonizes the upper airways, leading to contamination of expectorated specimens. Type-B *H. influenzae* is a well-

Table 3 Predominant mechanisms of pneumonia

Pathogen	Usual mechanisms
S. pneumoniae	Microaspiration
H. influenzae	Microaspiration
Gram-negative bacilli	Microaspiration
Anaerobic bacteria	Aspiration
Mycobacterium tuberculosis	Inhalation—patient source
Influenza	Inhalation—patient source
Legionella spp.	Inhalation—environmental source
Aspergillus spp.	Inhalation—environmental source
Pathogenic fungi	Inhalation—environmental source
Mycoplasma pneumoniae	Inhalation—patient source
S. aureus	Embolic or inhalation or aspiration
Pneumocystis carinii	Endogenous in lung
Cytomegalovirus	Endogenous in host white cells

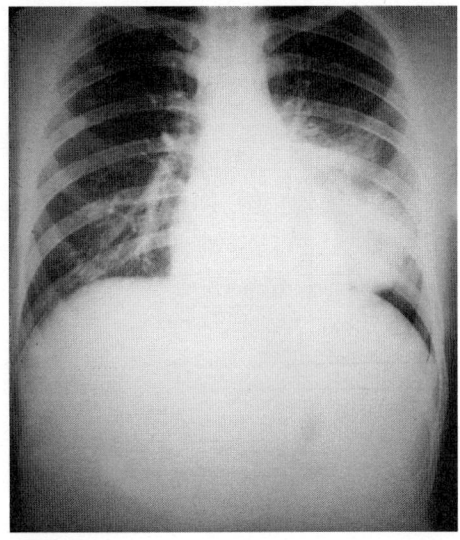

Fig. 1 Chest radiograph showing a left lower lobe pneumonia. Blood cultures grew *S. pneumoniae*.

established pathogen primarily in infants and young children, but is a relatively rare cause of disease in adults or anyone who has received *H. influenzae* vaccine. *H. influenzae* strains causing pneumonia in adults are usually non-typable.

The clinical features are rather non-specific and include fever, cough, purulent sputum, leucocytosis, and radiographic evidence of pneumonia—usually in a bronchopneumonic pattern, but it may occasionally be lobar. Patients with chronic obstructive lung disease often harbour *H. influenzae* in their lower airways and, allegedly, are prone to pneumonia caused by this organism, although supporting data for the association are not strong. Bacteraemia with *H. influenzae* in adults is infrequent. Most patients simply have a non-specific pneumonia, with *H. influenzae* as the only potential pathogen identified in expectorated sputum.

About 30 to 45 per cent of strains produce β-lactamase so that penicillin and amoxicillin are often ineffective. When *H. influenzae* is suspected or established the preferred agents are second- and third-generation cephalosporins, any combination of a β-lactam–β-lactamase inhibitor, azithromycin, or a fluoroquinolone.

Anaerobic bacteria

These organisms are the dominant components of the microbial flora in the upper airways and average 10^{12}/ml in the gingival crevice. Anaerobes are the major pathogens identified in aspiration pneumonia and its sequelae, lung abscess and empyema. The major pathogens in this group are *Peptostreptcocci* spp., *Bacteroides* spp. (other than *B. fragilis*), *Prevotella* spp., and *Fusobacterium nucleatum*.

The typical patient has gingival crevice disease combined with a predisposition for aspiration that is usually due to a suppressed level of consciousness or dysphasia. The clinical presentation is usually more subtle than that for pneumococcal pneumonia in that the infection evolves over a period of many days, weeks, or even months. Chest radiographs usually show infection in a dependent segment (usually the superior segments of the lower lobes or posterior segments of the upper lobes since these are dependent in the recumbent position), fever, sputum that is often putrid, and evidence of chronic disease with weight loss or anaemia. Putrid discharge is very characteristic and diagnostic of anaerobic bacterial infection (Fig. 2).

Aspiration pneumonia may also be due to chemical insults from gastric acid or other toxins, or may reflect the aspiration of foreign bodies or fluids (victims of drowning). However, the most common sequel to aspiration is bacterial infection involving the anaerobes that normally colonize the upper airways, and such bacteria account for 60 to 80 per cent of cases of aspiration pneumonia, lung abscess, and, in many case series, empyemas. Although the bacterial aetiology can be identified from anaerobic cultures of uncontaminated specimens, these are generally not obtained except in the case of pleural fluid in the presence of empyema; even then the cultures are often falsely negative due to inadequate techniques used to recover oxygen-sensitive bacteria. Thus, the aetiological diagnosis is usually based on the clinical features—where key clues are the chronicity of the infection, associated conditions suggesting aspiration, tissue necrosis with abscess formation, or a bronchopleural fistula leading to empyema and/or putrid discharge.

The preferred drugs are clindamycin or a β-lactam–β-lactamase inhibitor.

Mycoplasma pneumoniae

This organism is one of the most common causes of lower airways' infection in young adults, and it is now more frequently recognized in older adults. The original appellation was 'primary atypical pneumonia', a term applied in the 1930s to a relatively benign form of pneumonia to distinguish it from pneumococcal pneumonia. Early work showed that it was associated with a serum factor that agglutinated erythrocytes in the cold; furthermore, Eaton reported that the infection was transmissible from person to person by intracheal inoculations. Thus, atypical pneumonia, cold-agglutinin pneumonia, and Eaton-agent pneumonia were found to be synonymous.

The typical patient is usually a young adult who experiences a respiratory tract infection accompanied by headache, myalgia, cough, and fever and with a chest radiograph that shows bronchopneumonia. The cough is often non-productive, but when sputum is obtained it is mucoid, shows predominantly mononuclear cells, and no dominant organism. A characteristic feature is the relatively high frequency of extrapulmonary complications such as rash, neurological syndromes (aseptic meningitis, encephalitis, neuropathies), myocarditis, pericarditis, and haemolytic anaemia. The diagnosis should be suspected in those patients with a relatively mild form of pneumonia, particularly in previously healthy young adults.

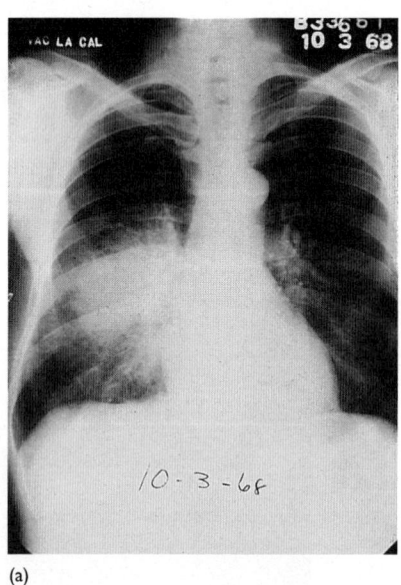

(a)

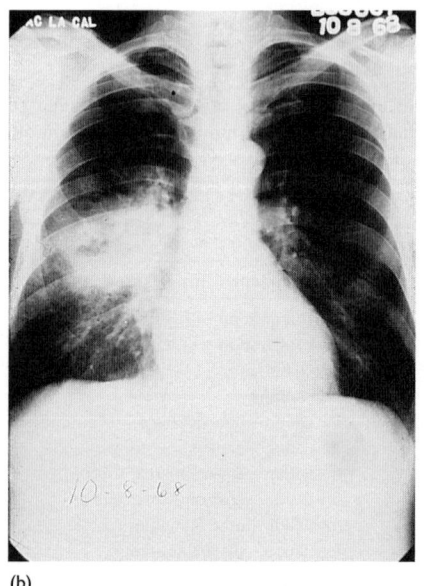

(b)

Fig. 2 (a) Consolidated pneumonia in the superior segment of the right lower lobe in a 56-year-old alcoholic. A transtracheal aspirate showed numerous anaerobic bacteria including *Prevotella melaninogenicus* and *Peptostreptococcus* spp. (b) A follow-up radiograph five days later showing cavitation.

Most laboratories do not cultivate mycoplasma due to the effort needed to recover the organism, the long time required, and the ease of empirical treatment. Serological tests may be used, but their merits are disputed. Polymerase chain reaction (**PCR**) and other rapid diagnostic tests are under development.

With regard to treatment, the pathogen lacks a cell wall and hence is not susceptible to penicillin, cephalosporins, or other cell-wall active antibiotics. The usual therapeutic agents are macrolides (such as erythromycin, clarithromycin, or azithromycin) or doxycycline; fluoroquinolones are also active.

Chlamydia pneumoniae

This relatively recently identified pathogen is now thought to account for about 5 to 10 per cent of all community-acquired cases of pneumonia, often in young adults who present in a fashion quite similar to that of patients with a mycoplasma pneumonia. *C. pneumoniae* continues to be regarded as a relatively benign agent of pneumonia: most patients have an upper airways' infection with this organism, laryngitis is relatively common, bronchitis is less common, and pneumonitis is an infrequent complication. *C. pneumoniae* plays a role in exacerbations of asthma, and the organism may also be involved in some chronic conditions such as cardiovascular disease.

The diagnosis of chlamydia pneumonia is difficult. The organism is cultivated like a virus using tissue cultures, but few laboratories offer this test. Serology is difficult to interpret; the usual titres for IgM or serial changes with acute and convalescent sera are arbitrary. Like mycoplasma, this is an organism that is often suspected, infrequently proven, and easily treated empirically.

The usual treatment is doxycycline, a macrolide (erythromycin, clarithromycin, or azithromycin), or a fluoroquinolone.

Legionella spp.

Legionnaires' disease was originally described during the American Legion Convention in Philadelphia in 1976, with the putative agent reported the following year. Legionella cause two major syndromes: the pneumonic form or legionnaires' disease, referring to the American Legion Convention epidemic, and a benign influenza-like illness called 'Pontiac fever' in reference to an outbreak in 1967 in Pontiac, Michigan. Although legionnaires' disease is often grouped with mycoplasma and chlamydia infection as being an 'atypical pneumonia', it is quite different pulmonary infection because it occurs primarily in older adults, is a serious and often lethal form of pneumonia, and most hospital laboratories have diagnostic resources to establish the aetiology. Legionnaires' disease is defined as pneumonia caused by any species of the genera *Legionella*, but the great majority of cases are caused either by *L. pneumophila* (80 to 90 per cent of cases) or *L. mcdadei* (5 to 10 per cent). This disease may be epidemic or sporadic. Epidemics usually occur in buildings, especially hotels and hospitals, and they reflect legionella contamination of the potable water or cooling systems of air conditioners. Predisposing factors include exposure to environmental sources of legionella (there is no patient-to-patient transmission), age over 40 years, smoking, or reduced cell-mediated immune responses as with organ transplantation, cancer chemotherapy, or chronic corticosteroid usage; patients with AIDS do not seem to be uniquely susceptible.

There are no remarkable features of the clinical presentation, except that patients are almost invariably quite sick and may be critically ill. In addition to the typical symptoms of pneumonia with cough and dyspnoea, most present with a profound systemic illness with high fever and myalgias, often with gastrointestinal and neurological symptoms.

The diagnosis can be established with a urinary antigen assay for the detection of *L. pneumophila* serogroup I, culture of respiratory secretions on selective media, serology, or direct fluorescent stain (**DFA**) of sputum. All these tests are quite specific, but none are sufficiently sensitive to exclude the diagnosis when they are negative.

The drugs of choice are fluoroquinolone or a macrolide, or one of these given with rifampicin. However, the mortality rate is generally reported to be 5 to 15 per cent even with proper therapy.

Staphylococcus aureus

Staphylococcus pneumonia was classically described as a complication of influenza during the 1918 epidemic of 'Spanish Flu'. This organism continues to be a potentially important superinfecting pathogen in influenza, and is the most common form of embolic pulmonary infection with injection-drug use and tricuspid valve endocarditis. Staphylococcal pneumonia may be acute or chronic and, despite common impressions to the contrary, pulmonary abscess is a relatively unusual complication. Most patients simply have bronchopneumonia; lobar pneumonia is rare. Those patients with embolic pneumonia show multiple embolic infiltrates that are diffusely scattered and which often cavitate.

The organism can usually be recovered in blood cultures and in respiratory secretions. However, care must be exercised when interpreting respiratory secretion cultures that yield *S. aureus* since this may be a contaminant, and it is particularly common as a contaminant in those patients who have received previous antibiotic treatment.

The treatment should be based on *in vitro* susceptibility tests, usually an antistaphylococcal penicillin (flucloxacillin, oxacillin, or nafcillin), a first-generation cephalosporin (cefazolin), or vancomycin (for methicillin-resistant strains and for patients with severe penicillin allergy).

Gram-negative bacilli

Klebsiella pneumoniae was originally described in 1882 by Friedlander, who believed it was the cause of pneumococcal pneumonia. This organism has continued to be a rare but important cause of community-acquired pneumonia, accounting for about 0.5 to 1.5 per cent of all cases. The classic presentation of 'Friedlander's pneumonia' was a serious pneumonia in an alcoholic patient with a chest radiograph that showed upper lobe involvement and the 'bulging fissure sign' (indicating abscess formation) and sputum that resembled currant jelly. This form of klebsiella pulmonary infection is rarely encountered now, although klebsiella infection is occasionally implicated in community-acquired pneumonia.

Other Gram-negative bacilli may also cause pneumonia, but the frequency in immunocompetent hosts is very low. A possible exception is *Acinetobacter* spp., which may cause pneumonia in otherwise healthy adults. *Pseudomonas aeruginosa* is a rare pulmonary pathogen, but should be suspected when recovered in respiratory secretions from patients with specific predisposing conditions including structural lung disease, neutropenia, cystic fibrosis, or advanced AIDS. Gram-negative bacteria are commonly encountered in cultures of respiratory secretions, but care must be exercised in interpretation because they are often contaminants reflecting upper airway colonization, especially in patients who have previously received antibiotics.

Treatment should be based on *in vitro* sensitivity tests.

Viruses

Viral infections of the lower airways account for pneumonia in 10 to 15 per cent of inpatients, and probably a substantially larger number of those managed as outpatients. The most frequent pathogens are influenza, parainfluenza, and respiratory syncytial virus (**RSV**). Influenza infections with bronchitis occur in epidemics, but influenza pneumonia is rare. More common in influenza patients with chest radiographs showing infiltrates is bacterial superinfection, most frequently with *S. pneumoniae* or *S. aureus*; less common superinfecting pathogens in this setting are *N. meningitidis* and group A streptococcus. The diagnosis of influenza can be made by the combination of an established epidemic and typical influenza symptoms, especially fever. The alternative is to establish the presence of the organism by one of several rapid tests for influenza-A or influenza-B antigen. These rapid tests provide results that are available in about 20 minutes and have a sensitivity of about 70 to 80 per cent.

Clinical features of influenza are generally well known and include cough, fever, purulent sputum, and myalgias. Patients with bacterial super-infections will usually have typical flu-like symptoms, improve, and then deteriorate after 1 to 2 weeks.

Infections involving influenza A may be treated with amantidine or rimantadine; influenza A or B may be treated with these agents, or the neuraminidase inhibitors Relenza (zanamivir) or oseltamivir. If given within 48 h of the onset of symptoms, these anti-influenza drugs reduce the duration of typical symptoms by 1 to 1.5 days and are more effective in seriously ill patients. However, their role in primary influenza pneumonia or in patients with complications of influenza is unknown.

RSV has usually been considered a pathogen in paediatric patients, but is now recognized with increasing frequency in adults, especially the elderly. The diagnosis is easily established with a DFA stain of respiratory secretions for RSV. Ribivirin is active against RSV and is sometimes used by inhalation therapy in children, but there is no treatment with established merit for adult cases.

Laboratory diagnosis

Laboratory tests are used to establish the diagnosis, evaluate the severity, and identify the aetiological agent (Table 4).

Tests to establish the diagnosis and evaluate severity

Chest radiography

The chest radiograph is a pivotal test for the confirmation of pneumonia. It is impossible to make this diagnosis in the absence of a new infiltrate, with four possible exceptions:

1. Although severe dehydration allegedly accounts for a false-negative chest radiograph, animal studies do not support this contention and clinical evidence is weak.

2. Severe neutropenia may give rise to a false-negative radiograph due to the patient's inability to generate an acute inflammatory response. While this is theoretically possible, data suggest that the frequency is low.

3. Some patients have a normal radiograph early in the course of disease, and physicians in the pre-penicillin era claimed they could detect rales

Table 4 Recommended laboratory tests in suspected community-acquired pneumonia

Outpatients:
Sputum Gram stain and culture or sputum on heat-fixed slide for later reference (optimal)

Inpatients:
- Chest radiography
- Blood culture
- Full blood count
- Chemistry panel including glucose, sodium, liver function tests, renal function tests, electrolytes
- Blood gases or pulse oximetry
- HIV serology for patients aged 15–54 years (with informed consent)
- Gram stain and culture of expectorated sputum that is physician procured, processed within 2–5 h of collection, and subjected to cytological screening as a contingency for culture
- Specialized tests for selected patients
  - legionella: urinary antigen and/or legionella culture
  - acid-fast bacteria: sputum for acid-fast stain and culture, in triplicate
  - pleural fluid pH, cell count, Gram stain, and culture

before the radiograph showed an infiltrate. This appears to be true, but it applies only to the first 24 h and even then is uncommon.

4. *Pneumocystis carinii* pneumonia may present with a completely normal chest radiograph in 20 to 30 per cent of cases, and probably represents the only form of pneumonia commonly seen nowadays where false-negative routine chest radiographs are common.

Most patients with symptoms of pneumonia and a negative chest radiograph have acute bronchitis, which is generally caused by viral pathogens that do not respond to antibiotic treatment. Thus, the importance of the chest radiograph is in confirming pneumonia, which is a critical feature in avoiding antibiotic abuse. Additional advantages of the chest radiograph is that it provides assistance in identifying the aetiological agent, establishes a baseline for subsequent evaluation, provides prognostic information, and permits the detection of underlying or associated conditions such as a neoplasm.

Other laboratory tests

The most useful additional laboratory tests to determine the severity of illness and need for hospitalization are evaluation of blood oxygenation with pulse oximetry or arterial blood gas determination, blood chemistries (glucose, blood urea nitrogen, and serum sodium levels), and a full blood count. Patients who are hospitalized should generally undergo HIV serology, provided their informed consent is given.

Studies to determine microbial aetiology

Laboratory studies for identifying pulmonary pathogens are among the most controversial issues in pneumonia management. The American Thoracic Society guidelines endorse a nihilistic approach, with the conclusion that microbial studies in pneumonia cases are usually negative, are not cost-effective, and are largely unnecessary since empirical treatment is generally successful. The guidelines from the Infectious Diseases Society of America emphasize the conduct of studies to identify the microbial pathogen(s) in order to promote pathogen-specific treatment and reduce antibiotic abuse, and to identify epidemiologically important organisms such as penicillin-resistant *S. pneumoniae*, *Legionella* spp., influenza, or Hantavirus. It is acknowledged that many recent reports show a low yield of such organisms and fail to document a benefit in terms of cost or outcome; nevertheless, this is attributed to the serious decline in the quality of microbiological standards in recent years.

While empirical therapy is generally advocated for outpatients, routine microbiological testing to identify the aetiological agent of pneumonia is generally only recommended for inpatients. Such tests include blood cultures (from blood samples taken prior to the initiation of antibiotic treatment), which yield a pathogen in about 12 per cent of cases. In general, the only additional test commonly performed to identify an aetiological agent is an expectorated sputum Gram stain and culture. Practice standards for this process include the following:

- The specimen should be obtained by deep cough and should be grossly purulent. It should be collected before antibiotic therapy, preferably in the presence of a physician or nurse.

- The specimen should be promptly transported to the laboratory for processing and incubation within 2 to 5 h.

- A qualified technician should select a purulent portion for Gram stain and culture.

- Cytological screening should be done under low-power magnification ($\times$ 100) to determine cellular composition as a contingency for culture.

- The sample should be cultured using standard techniques, with results reported by semiquantitative assessment; most pathogens are recovered in 3 to 4 plus growth, indicating more than five colonies in the second streak.

- Interpretation should be based on the correlation of the Gram stain, semiquantitative culture results, and clinical observations.

The aetiological agent of pneumonia is considered to be clearly established if a likely pulmonary pathogen is recovered from an uncontaminated specimen such as blood culture, pleural fluid, transtracheal aspiration, or transthoracic aspirate. Alternatively, the very presence of a likely pathogen recovered from respiratory secretions is tantamount to a diagnosis; organisms in this category include *Legionella* species, *Mycobacterium tuberculosis*, most viruses other than the herpesvirus group (influenza virus, respiratory syncytial virus, Hantavirus, parainfluenza virus, and adenovirus), and certain fungi (*Histoplasma capsulatum*, *Coccidioides immitis*, *Blastomyces dermatitidis*, and *P. carinii*). Organisms such as *S. pneumoniae*, *M. catarrhalis*, *H. influenzae*, and *S. aureus* may be pulmonary pathogens, but interpretation is problematic due to possible contamination with specimens from the upper airway flora. Organisms that virtually never represent pulmonary pathogens include *S. epidermidis*, *Enterococcus* spp., *Neisseria* spp. other than *N. meningitidis*, *Candida* spp., and Gram-positive bacilli other than *Nocardia* spp. or actinomyces.

Transtracheal aspiration was once a popular method of obtaining specimens from the lower airways that avoided upper airway contamination, but the technique requires a skilled clinician and is generally thought to be too invasive for routine use. Transthoracic aspiration has the same limitations, and furthermore seems to give a relatively large number of false-negative results. Bronchoscopy is an attractive method for obtaining respiratory secretions directly from the lower airways; however, the procedure is complicated by contamination with instrument passage through the upper airways so that routine cultures of bronchoscopic aspirates are no better than expectorated sputum. These results may be substantially improved with quantitative cultures of bronchoalveolar lavage specimens or quantitative brush specimens, but many laboratories do not offer this type of analysis, and many pulmonary services cannot provide the samples in a timely fashion.

Most hospital laboratories offer diagnostic tests for detecting the atypical causative agents of pneumonia, for instance of *Legionella* spp. The preferred tests for legionella detection are the urinary antigen assay and culture. Urinary antigen testing is advocated because it is rapid, simply performed, and highly specific; disadvantages include the fact that it only detects *L. pneumophila* serogroup 1, although this accounts for 70 per cent of cases. The alternative test for detecting *Legionella* spp. is culture, which has the advantage of detecting all species of *Legionella*; but the disadvantage is that it requires three days, requires specialized media, and is technically demanding. Most laboratories do not offer diagnostic tests to detect *M. pneumoniae* or *C. pneumoniae*, despite their presumed frequency. This reflects the lack of an acceptable test that is easily performed, provides adequate sensitivity and specificity, and can provide results in a timely fashion.

Treatment

Critical components of initial treatment may include intravenous hydration, oxygenation, and/or intubation and mechanical ventilatory support. Pleural effusions should be sampled to exclude empyema and, when the effusions are large, drained to improve oxygenation. Most authorities feel that expectorants, cough suppressants, and chest physiotherapy are of little value.

Antibiotic therapy

Antibiotics are the mainstay of therapy. Suggestions for specific agents according to microbial pathogen are summarized in Table 5. Most of these are relatively non-controversial and demonstrate the advantage of establishing an aetiological agent. However, as noted above, no pathogen can be detected in 40 to 60 per cent of cases despite arduous attempts to do so; even when an agent is found, this information is usually not available when initial therapeutic decisions are needed. For this reason, most patients are treated empirically, at least initially, whilst microbiological results are pending. Recommendations for empirical treatment are summarized in Table 6. These options are selected on the basis of predicted activity against the most likely pathogens and extensive clinical trials. Nevertheless, this is one of the most controversial areas in medicine based on concerns for antibiotic abuse, increasing resistance of *S. pneumoniae* to many antimicrobials, and sharp geographical differences in the rates of *S. pneumoniae* resistance.

Of major concern in recent years is *S. pneumoniae*, the most common identified agent of pneumonia, because it shows escalating rates of resistance to penicillin, other β-lactams, macrolides, trimethoprim–sulfamethoxazole (**TMP–SMX**), clindamycin, and tetracycline. The only drug that is virtually always active is vancomycin, but the use of this agent in pulmonary infections is discouraged due to a somewhat limited published experience of using vancomycin to treat pneumonia, and concern for the possible promotion of vancomycin-resistant enterococci. Fluoroquinolones with enhanced activity against *S. pneumoniae* include levofloxacin, moxifloxacin, clinafloxacin, trovafloxacin, and gatifloxacin. Most strains of *S. pneumoniae* are susceptible, although some laboratories are reporting increasing resistance to the fluoroquinolones as well as the other antibiotics noted. Multiple large therapeutic trials are underway of patients randomized to receive macrolides, fluoroquinolones, or β-lactams, nearly all of which show therapeutic equivalence. However, there are also reports of anecdotal cases of failure correlating with *in vitro* resistance to β-lactams, macrolides, and fluoroquinolones.

Timing of antibiotic therapy

A large retrospective trial showed that mortality increased with a progressive delay in the time taken to initiate antibiotic therapy after patients had been evaluated. The increase in mortality became statistically significant when the delay exceeded 8 hours. This observation is not surprising since pneumonia is a potentially lethal infection that usually responds to antibiotics, so any delay in treatment would be expected to have deleterious effects. As a result of these observations, many hospitals in the United States are now audited to determine their compliance with antibiotic administration, where necessary, within 8 hours of a patient's admission to the emergency room or admission to the hospital.

Monitoring response to therapy

Subjective responses are usually noted within 3 to 5 days of initiating treatment. Objective parameters to monitor include fever, oxygen saturation, peripheral leucocyte count, and changes on serial chest radiographs. The most carefully documented responses are mortality rates, time to defervescence, and duration of hospital stay. With regard to fever, the temperature in young adults with pneumococcal pneumonia usually drops within 2 to 3 days, patients with bacteraemic pneumococcal pneumonia usually require 6 to 7 days, and elderly patients often respond more slowly. Blood cultures in bacteraemic patients are usually negative within 24 to 48 h. Cultures of sputum will usually show eradication of bacterial pathogens within 24 to 48 h, a major exception being *P. aeruginosa*. Radiographic appearances are slow to improve and much less useful than clinical observations for evaluating response. Follow-up radiographs are generally not recommended, except for patients who are over 40 years of age or are smokers, and the suggested time to do this is 7 to 12 weeks after initiating treatment. Patients who are initially treated with intravenous antibiotics can usually be changed to receive oral agents when they are able to take oral medications and show clinical improvement, such as a temperature below 38 °C for 24 h, a respiratory rate of less than 24/min, and when the Po_2 has returned to normal.

Failure to respond

The major considerations in patients who fail to respond according to the guidelines noted above are:

Table 5 Treatment of pneumonia by pathogen

Agent	Preferred antimicrobial	Alternative antimicrobial
Streptococcus pneumoniae Penicillin-susceptible (MIC <2 µg/ml)*	Penicillin G Amoxicillin	Cephalosporins: cefazolin, cefuroxime, cefotaxime, ceftriaxone, cefepime Oral cephalosporins: cefpodoxime, cefprozil, cefuroxime Imipenem or meropenem Macrolides,* clindamycin Fluoroquinolones** Doxycycline Penicillins: ampicillin ± sulbactam, piperacillin ± tazobactam
Penicillin-resistant*** (MIC >2 µg/ml)	Agents based on *in vitro* sensitivity tests, including cephalosporins Fluoroquinolone** Vancomycin	Linezolid
Haemophilus influenzae	Cephalosporin—2nd or 3rd generation Doxycycline β-Lactam–β-lactamase inhibitors	Azithromycin; TMP–SMX; Fluoroquinolone**
Moraxella catarrhalis	Cephalosporin—2nd or 3rd generation TMP–SMX Amoxicillin–clavulanate	Macrolides Fluoroquinolone** β-Lactam–β-lactamase inhibitors
Anaerobes	β-Lactam–β-lactamase inhibitors Clindamycin	
*Staphylococcus aureus*** Methicillin-sensitive	Nafcillin/oxacillin ± rifampicin or gentamicin***	Cefazolin or cefuroxime Vancomycin, clindamycin, TMP–SMX, fluoroquinolone**
Methicillin-resistant	Vancomycin ± rifampicin or gentamicin	Requires *in vitro* testing; TMP–SMX
Enterobacteriaceae (coliforms: *E. coli*, *Klebsiella*, *Proteus*, *Enterobacter* spp., etc.)***	Cephalosporin—3rd generation ± aminoglycoside Carbapenem	Aztreonam β-Lactam–β-lactamase inhibitors Fluoroquinolone**
*Pseudomonas aeruginosa***	Aminoglycoside + antipseudomonal β-lactam: ticarcillin, piperacillin, mezlocillin, ceftazidime, cefepime, aztreonam or carbapenem	Aminoglycoside + ciprofloxacin, ciprofloxacin + antipseudomonal β-lactam
Legionella spp.	Macrolide* ± rifampicin Fluoroquinolone** (including ciprofloxacin)	Doxycycline ± rifampicin
Mycoplasma pneumoniae	Doxycycline Macrolide*	Fluoroquinolone**
Chlamydia pneumoniae	Doxycycline Macrolide*	Fluoroquinolone**
Chlamydia psittaci	Doxycycline	Erythromycin, chloramphenicol
Nocardia spp.	TMP–SMX Sulphonamide ± minocycline or amikacin	Imipenem ± amikacin Doxycycline or minocycline
Coxiella burnetii (Q fever)	Tetracycline	Chloramphenicol

Table 5 continued

Agent	Preferred antimicrobial	Alternative antimicrobial
Influenza	Amantadine or rimantadine (Influenza A) Zanamavir or oseltamivir (influenza A or B)	
Hantavirus	Supportive care	

* Macrolide: erythromycin, clarithromycin, azithromycin, dirithromycin.

** Fluoroquinolone: levofloxacin, sparfloxacin, gatifloxacin, moxifloxacin, or other fluoroquinolone with enhanced activity against *S. pneumoniae*; ciprofloxacin is appropriate for *Legionella* spp., *C. pneumoniae*, *M. pneumoniae*, fluoroquinolone-sensitive *S. aureus*, and most Gram-negative bacilli.

*** *In vitro* sensitivity tests are required for optimal treatment; for *Enterobacter* spp. the preferred antibiotics are the fluoroquinolones and carbapenems.

MIC, minimum inhibitory concentration; TMP–SMX, trimethoprim and sulfamethoxazole.

- The disease is too far advanced at the time of treatment, or treatment is delayed for too long: this is most commonly seen with pneumonia caused by *Streptococcus pneumoniae* or *Legionella* spp.
- The wrong antibiotic was selected: but this is uncommon.
- An inadequate antibiotic dosage is given: this is most common with the aminoglycosides
- The wrong diagnosis is made: for example, a non-infectious disease such as pulmonary embolism with infarction, congestive failure, Wegener's granulomatosis, sarcoidosis, atelectasis, chemical pneumonitis.
- The wrong microbial diagnosis is made.
- The patient may be debilitated, have a severe associated disease, or be immunosuppressed: or there may be other host inadequacies.
- There may be a complicated pneumonia with undrained empyema, metastatic site of infection (meningitis), or bronchial obstruction (foreign body, carcinoma).
- There may be a pulmonary superinfection: most patients in this category respond and then deteriorate with a new fever.

Prognosis

The overall mortality for patients who are hospitalized with community-acquired pneumonia, according to a meta-analysis of 122 reports, is 14 per cent. Risk factors for lethal outcome were well described in the pre-penicillin era, when extremes of age were probably the most important factor. Other risks included bacteraemia, the concentration of bacteria according to quantitative blood cultures in those who were bacteraemic, the extent of changes on chest radiography, alcohol consumption, and the extent of leucocytosis. More recent studies have continued to show that these factors, especially age, are major risk factors for morbidity and mortality. Investigators from the Pneumonia Patient Outcomes Research Team (**PORT**) have developed a prediction rule using a cumulative point score obtained from five categories comprising 19 variables (Table 7). This prediction rule was

applied retrospectively to 38 039 inpatients and showed a direct correlation between numerical score and mortality, the authors concluding that these factors predict outcome and can also be used to determine the need for hospitalization.

With regard to specific pathogens, the major agents of community-acquired pneumonia associated with high mortality rates are bacteraemic pneumococcal pneumonia and Legionnaires' disease. Influenza is directly or indirectly implicated in about 20 000 deaths per year in the United States, but primary influenza pneumonia is relatively rare and most of the influenza-associated deaths are of elderly patients who succumb to complications of influenza. It should also be noted that pneumonia is an extremely common terminal event in patients who die of other conditions, presumably because of aspiration in the terminal stages. Thus, pneumonia is a common autopsy finding when other medical conditions are actually the major cause of death.

Prevention and control

The major preventive measures are influenza and *S. pneumoniae* vaccines. The components selected for the influenza vaccine each year are based on the anticipated strains for the forthcoming season, a prediction that has been quite accurate in 10 of the 11 influenza seasons from 1988 to 99 through 1999 to 2000. Protective efficacy is generally 60 to 70 per cent in the general population when there is a good match between the vaccine strains and the epidemic strain; it is less in elderly vaccinees, but those who develop influenza after vaccination usually have attenuated courses with significant reductions in mortality. The current recommendation is for vaccination between October and November of patients living in the Northern hemisphere. Targeted populations are summarized in Table 8. Amantadine, rimantadine, zanamivir, and oseltamivir may be used to prevent influenza in unvaccinated patients who are so exposed.

The 23-valent vaccine for *S. pneumoniae* contains capsular polysaccharide from 23 serogroups that are responsible for 80 to 85 per cent of bacteraemic pneumococcal infections. Studies of this vaccine suggest a 60 per cent efficacy in preventing bacteraemic pneumococcal infection in immunocompetent adults in the United States, but efficacy is reduced or negligible in immunosuppressed hosts. There is a newly developed 7-valent protein-conjugated pneumococcal vaccine that has the advantage of stimulating a good antibody response in children under 2 years of age, but this vaccine has not been extensively tested in adults.

Controversies

There are probably few diseases in medicine that have been better studied than pneumonia, but with such extraordinary controversy in management guidelines. The major controversies are the utility of microbiology studies,

Table 6 Empirical treatment of community-acquired pneumonia

Outpatients	Doxycycline, macrolide*, or fluoroquinolone**
Inpatients–general hospital	β-Lactam*** + macrolide* or fluoroquinolone** alone
Intensive-care unit	β-Lactam*** + macrolide* or β-lactam*** + fluoroquinolone**
Special circumstances	Aspiration pneumonia: clindamycin or β-lactam–β-lactamase inhibitor Structural disease of lung: treat with regimen that includes activity against *P. aeruginosa*

* Macrolide: erythromycin, clarithromycin, azithromycin

** Fluoroquinolone: levofloxacin, gatifloxacin, moxifloxacin, or other fluoroquinolone with enhanced activity against *S. pneumoniae*.

*** β-Lactam: cefotaxime or ceftriaxone.

Table 7 Prediction rule for outcome

(a) Scoring system[*]

Variable		Points
Age	male	Age in years
	female	Age in years – 10
Nursing home:		+10
Comorbidity:		Neoplasm, +20; liver disease, +20; congestive failure, +10; cerebrovascular disease, +10; renal disease, +10
Physical examination:		Altered mental status, +20; respiratory rate >30/min, +20; SBP <90 mmHg, +20, temperature, <35 °C or >40 °C, +15, pulse >125/min, +10
Laboratory:		Arterial pH <7.35, +30; BUN >30 mg/dl (>5 mmol/l), +20; sodium <130 mEq/l, + 20; glucose >250 mg/dl (>15 mmol/l), +10; haematocrit <30%, +10; arterial P_{O_2} <60 mmHg, +10; pleural effusion, +10

(b) Risk class validation[*]

Risk class	Points	No. patients	Mortality (%)	Recommended site of care
I	No predictors	3034	0.1	Outpatient
II	≤70	5778	0.6	Outpatient
III	71–90	6790	2.8	Outpatient or brief hospitalization
IV	91–130	13104	8.2	Hospital
V	>130	9333	29.2	Hospital

[*] Adapted with permission from Fine MJ *et al.* (1997). A prediction rule to identify low-risk patients with community-acquired pneumonia. *New England Journal of Medicine* **336**, 243.

SBP, systolic blood pressure; BUN, blood urea nitrogen.

the empirical selection of antibiotics, and the use of pneumococcal vaccine.

Studies of microbial aetiology

Culture and Gram stain of expectorated sputum is the time-honoured method for determining the microbiology of community-acquired pneumonia. Nevertheless, there is substantial controversy regarding the worth of this exercise and a wealth of medical reports with highly divergent findings that simply fuel the debate. In general, the optimal results were achieved in the pre-penicillin era when sputum bacteriology was an art and many patients underwent transthoracic needle aspiration. The reason being that the only available therapy was type-specific antisera for *S. pneumoniae*, thus requiring retrieval of the specific strain. High-quality laboratory technology persisted through the mid-1980s, when the yield of *S. pneumoniae* in expectorated sputum samples for inpatients with community-acquired pneumonia was generally reported at 40 to 70 per cent. The more recent experience is much different, in that the yield of *S. pneumoniae* in expectorated sputum by either Gram stain or culture is only 10 to 20 per cent in most series. Occasional investigators report a higher yield, but they generally employ an antigen-detection method using blood, urine, or respiratory secretions for pneumococcal polysaccharide, which is controversial based on disagreements about specificity. An additional concern is that antigen detection fails to identify other microbial agents of pneumonia, so that culture is generally required to determine *in vitro* sensitivity test results in an era of escalating resistance. Arguments favouring sputum microbiology are the benefits of pathogen-directed therapy that restrains antibiotic abuse, limits side-effects, and reduces cost. In addition, this permits the identification of epidemiologically important organisms, knowledge of which provides the database for empirical therapy recommendations. Arguments against microbiological studies include the facts that: this procedure, as currently performed in most laboratories, shows a low yield; the information is infrequently available when therapeutic decisions are made; empirical treatment usually works (Fig. 3); and, even if a pathogen is recovered, there is no good way to exclude the presence of a copathogen.

Antibiotic selection

Recommendations for the empirical selection of antibiotics include drugs that are active against the major pathogens, including *S. pneumoniae*, *H. influenzae*, and the atypical agents. The favoured classes are tetracyclines, macrolides, and fluoroquinolones. When *S. pneumoniae* is identified or strongly suspected, many authorities conclude that β-lactams are the preferred drugs, despite the fact that β-lactam resistance is 10 to 20 per cent, is substantially higher in some regions, and is increasing in virtually all areas. *S. pneumoniae* is also increasingly resistant to tetracyclines and macrolides, and to a lesser extent, fluoroquinolones. As noted above, large therapeutic trials comparing these four categories of drugs have shown no differences, but there are multiple reports of anecdotal cases with failures involving resistant strains. The controversy regarding empirical therapy is largely explained by geographical differences in resistance patterns, and the concern for fluoroquinolone abuse. With regard to geography, the rates of resistance to the various categories of drugs are highly variable in different parts of the world and within different parts of individual countries. Thus, doxycycline or a macrolide may be rational options in one area, but not another. With regard to the fluoroquinolones, these drugs are active *in vitro* against more than 98 per cent of *S. pneumoniae* strains as well as virtually all atypical organisms, but there is concern that extensive use will result in increasing resistance, a concern that is already being witnessed in some parts of the world. The attractive feature of the fluoroquinolones is the nearly uniform activity against *S. pneumoniae*, the ease of once-daily administration, the availability of both parenteral and oral forms, extensive therapeutic trials to confirm efficacy, and good *in vitro* activity against virtually all treatable pulmonary pathogens.

Pneumococcal vaccine

The polysaccharide vaccine has established merit in young adult African men, but some retrospective analyses and most prospective, randomized, controlled trials have failed to show a significant benefit in terms of reducing the rates of pneumonia, rates of pneumococcal pneumonia, or rates of bacteraemic pneumococcal pneumonia. Most reports of a beneficial effect of vaccination have been based on statistical analyses of the serotype of patients with pneumococcal infection, which demonstrated higher rates of vaccine strains in unvaccinated patients. Even these studies failed to show a benefit in the highest risk group, namely the elderly and the immunosuppressed. The need for a pneumococcal vaccine is widely appreciated due to the extent of morbidity and mortality caused by *S. pneumoniae* and the increasing difficulty caused by resistance in treating these infections. Many authorities feel that the best solution to the dilemma is a better pneumococcal vaccine.

Further reading

Bartlett JG, Mundy L (1995). Community-acquired pneumonia. *New England Journal of Medicine* **333**, 1618–24.

Bartlett JG, *et al.* (2000). Community-acquired pneumonia in adults: guidelines for management. *Clinical Infectious Diseases* **31**, 347–82.

British Thoracic Society (1993). Guidelines for the management of community-acquired pneumonia in adults admitted to hospital. *British Journal of Hospital Medicine* **49**, 346–50.

Chen DK, *et al.* (1999). Decreased susceptibility of *Streptococcus pneumoniae* to fluoroquinolones in Canada. *New England Journal of Medicine* **341**, 233–9.

File TM, *et al.* (1997). A multicenter, randomized study comparing the efficacy and safety of intravenous and/or oral levofloxacin versus ceftriaxone and/or cefuroxime axetil in treatment of adults with community-acquired pneumonia. *Antimicrobial Agents and Chemotherapy* **41**, 1965–72.

Fine MJ, *et al.* (1996). Prognosis and outcomes of patients with community-acquired pneumonia. *Journal of the American Medical Association* **275**, 134–41.

Table 8 Recommendation for influenza vaccination[*]

Groups at increased risk for influenza-related complications
1. Persons ≥ 65 years
2. Residents of nursing homes and other chronic-care facilities housing persons of any age with chronic medical conditions
3. Persons with chronic disorders of the pulmonary or cardiovascular system, including those with asthma
4. Adults and children who required regular medical follow-up or hospitalization during the previous year for chronic metabolic diseases (diabetes), renal dysfunction, haemoglobinopathies, or immunosuppression
5. Children and teenagers who are receiving long-term aspirin therapy (risk of Reye's syndrome)
6. Women who will be in the second or third trimester of pregnancy during the influenza season

Groups that can transmit influenza to high-risk patients
1. Physicians, nurses, and other personnel who have contact with high-risk patients
2. Employees of nursing homes and chronic-care facilities who have contact with patients or residents
3. Employees of assisted living and other residences for those at high risk
4. Providers of home care to high-risk persons
5. Household family members of high-risk persons

Other groups to consider
1. Persons who desire it
2. Persons who provide essential community services
3. Persons in institutional settings, including students
4. Persons with HIV infection. One study showed an increased risk of complications;[a] patients with low CD4 counts show reduced antibody response,[b] and vaccination may cause a transient increase in HIV viral load[c]
5. Elderly and other high-risk persons embarking on international travel: tropics, all year; Southern hemisphere, April–September

[*] Recommendations of the Advisory Council on Immunization Practices. *Morbidity and Mortality Weekly Reports* 1999, **48**, R-4.

[a] *Journal of the American Medical Association* 1999, **281**, 901; [b] *AIDS* 1994, **8**, 469; [c] *Lancet* 1992, **339**, 1549.

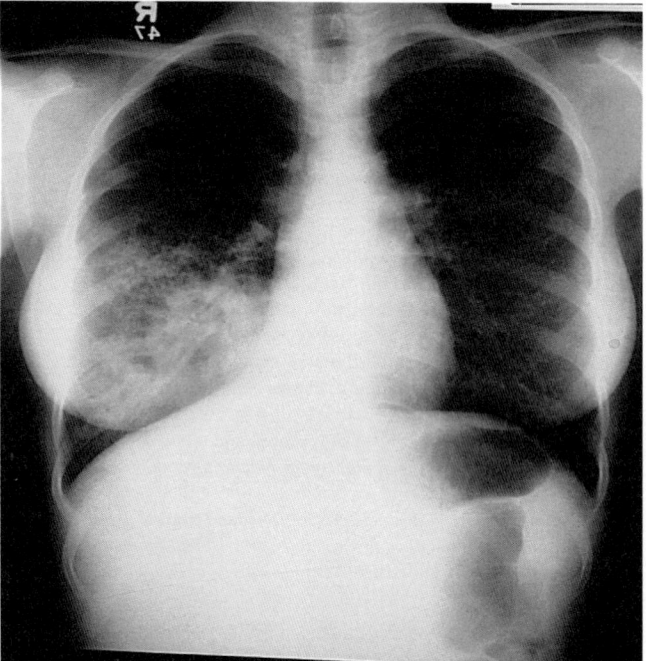

(a)

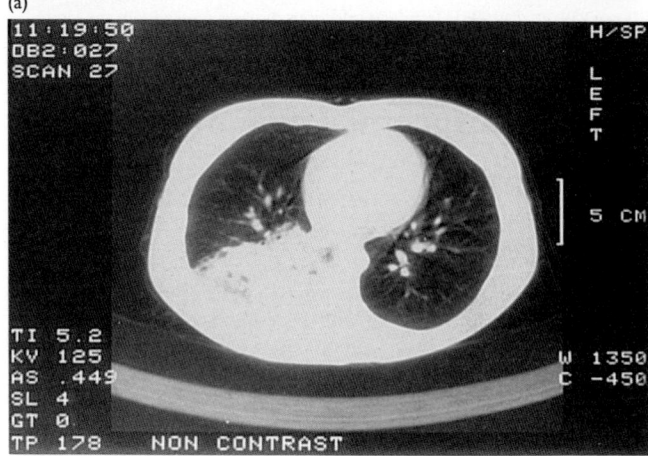

(b)

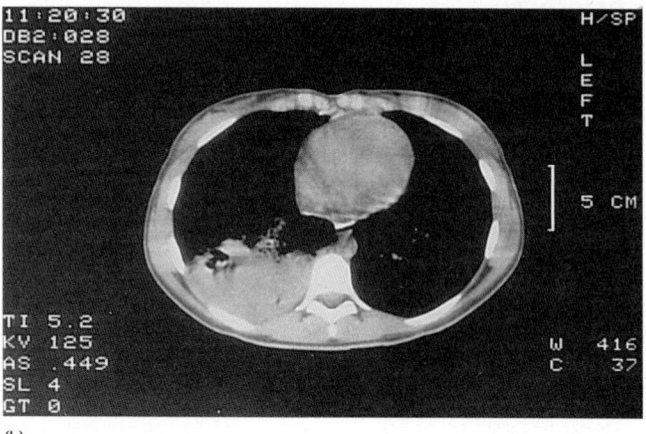

Fig. 3 Chest radiograph (a) and CT scan (b) showing pneumonitis in the right lower lobe of an 18-year-old college student. The patient responded to empirical antibiotic treatment.

Fine MJ, *et al.* (1997). A prediction rule to identify low-risk patients with community-acquired pneumonia. *New England Journal of Medicine* **336**, 243–50.

Gleason PP, *et al.* (1999). Associations between initial antimicrobial regimens and medical outcomes for elderly patients with pneumonia. *Archives of Internal Medicine* **159**, 2562–72.

Heffelfinger JD, *et al.* (2000). Management of community-acquired pneumonia in the era of pneumococcal resistance. *Archives of Internal Medicine* **160**, 1399–408.

Heffron R. (1939). *Pneumonia: with special reference to pneumococcus lobar pneumonia. A Commonwealth Fund Book.* Copyright 1939. The Commonwealth Fund. (Reprinted by Harvard University Press, Cambridge, MA in 1979.)

Marrie TJ, *et al.* (2000). A controlled trial of a critical pathway for treatment of community acquired pneumonia. *Journal of the American Medical Association* **283**, 749–55.

Meehan TP, *et al.* (1997). Quality of care, process and outcomes in elderly patients with pneumonia. *Journal of the American Medical Association* **278**, 2080–4.

Niederman MS, *et al.* (1993). Guidelines for the initial empiric therapy of community-acquired pneumonia: Proceedings of an American Thoracic Society Consensus Conference. *American Review of Respiratory Disease* **148**, 1418–26.

Pallares R, *et al.* (1995). Resistance to penicillin and cephalosporin and mortality from severe pneumococcal pneumonia in Barcelona, Spain. *New England Journal of Medicine* **333**, 474–80.

Pinner RW, *et al.* (1996). Trends in infectious diseases mortality in the United States. *Journal of the American Medical Association* **275**, 189–93.

17.5.2.2 Nosocomial pneumonia

John G. Bartlett

Introduction

Nosocomial pneumonia is generally defined as a new pulmonary infiltrate on chest radiography, combined with evidence of infection expressed as fever, purulent respiratory secretions, and/or leucocytosis, with onset at least 72 h after admission. These infections account for only about 15 per cent of all nosocomial infections, but they are the most frequent, lethal, nosocomial infection. The bacteriology and management are different than that of community-acquired infections of the lung (see Chapter 17.5.2.1).

Aetiology

The microbiology of nosocomial pneumonia shows that Gram-negative bacteria account for 50 to 70 per cent of cases; other common pathogens include *Staph. aureus*, anaerobic bacteria, *H. influenzae*, and *Streptococcus pneumoniae* (Table 1). Legionella accounts for about 4 per cent of all nosocomial pneumonia, but the frequency may be much higher when it is epidemic or endemic within a hospital. Viruses are implicated in 10 to 20 per cent, primarily influenza and respiratory syncytial virus and, in the immunocompromised host, cytomegalovirus. Tuberculosis is rare, but important to remember. Fungi are also rare, with the exception of *Aspergillus* in selected immunocompromised patients.

Epidemiology

Most reports indicate that 0.5 to 1 per cent of all hospitalized patients develop nosocomial pneumonia. The rates in intensive care units are generally reported at 15 to 20 per cent, and among patients who are mechanically ventilated, the rate is 20 to 50 per cent. However, it should be noted that some of these incidence statistics are disputed due to the lack of precision in the diagnosis of nosocomial pneumonia: other processes that may cause pulmonary infiltrates with variable presence of fever, purulent respiratory secretions, and/or leucocytosis include congestive heart failure, pulmonary embolism, atelectasis, adverse drug reactions, pulmonary haemorrhage, and the acute respiratory distress syndrome.

The epidemiology of the pathogens in nosocomial pneumonia is highly variable. Some organisms become endemic, especially in intensive care units; the major pathogens in this setting being *Acinetobacter*, *Serratia*, *Xanthomonas*, *Pseudomonas*, *Enterobacter*, and methicillin-resistant *S. aureus*. Another important nosocomial pathogen is *Legionella*, which may cause outbreaks of Legionnaire's disease in hospitals that can sometimes be traced to water supplies with distribution via air conditioning cooling systems or showerheads. In these cases, the same species and serogroup found in the nosocomial cases should be found in the epidemiologically-linked water supply. Aspergillosis may occur as epidemics among vulnerable patients with compromised cell-mediated immunity, neutropenia, or both. Influenza is highly contagious, and patients with influenza are commonly hospitalized, hence it is now recommended that all patients with suspected influenza have confirmation of this diagnosis by rapid influenza testing, and the preference is for a single room when this is feasible.

Pathogenesis

The relatively high rates of pulmonary infections among patients who are hospitalized reflects (Table 2):

(1) clustering of highly vulnerable patients;

(2) patients rendered particularly vulnerable by violations of the integrity of the upper airways by intubation or tracheostomy;

(3) many patients who are prone to aspiration due to compromised consciousness caused by associated medical conditions and anaesthesia;

(4) patients rendered susceptible due to organ transplantation, cancer chemotherapy, and AIDS.

The dominant pathogen in nosocomial pneumonia are Gram-negative bacteria, which reach the lung by aspiration of gastric contents or by micro-aspiration of upper airway secretions. The best explanation for this association between bacteriology and pathogenesis is the observation that patients with serious illness commonly have abnormal colonization of the

Table 1 Microbiology of nosocomial pneumonia

Microbe	Frequency
Bacteria	80–90%
Gram-negative bacteria	50–70%
Staph. aureus	15–30%
Anaerobic bacteria	10–30%
Haemophilus influenzae	10–20%
Streptococcus pneumoniae	10–20%
Legionella	4%
Viral	10–20%
Fungi	<1%

Table 2 Risks for nosocomial pneumonia

Endotracheal intubation and tracheostomy
Associated conditions
   age >70 years
   chronic lung disease
   poor nutritional status
Risk of aspiration
   decreased consciousness
   intubation, tracheostomy, nasogastric intubation
Thoracic or upper abdominal surgery
Altered host defenses
   immunosuppressive disorders

upper airways by Gram-negative bacteria. Thus, throat cultures show that Gram-negative bacteria are found in only 2 to 3 per cent of healthy persons, psychiatric patients, physicians, and medical students, whereas the rate of colonization in patients who are moderately ill is 30 to 40 per cent, and in intensive care units the rate is 60 to 70 per cent. These colonization rates are independent of antibiotic administration. It can also be shown that buccal epithelial cells from patients who are seriously ill have enhanced attachment by Gram-negative bacteria *in vitro*. The frequency of positive throat cultures for Gram-negative bacteria and the number that attach to respiratory cells is directly correlated with the severity of the associated disease. The usual mechanism of Gram-negative bacillary pneumonia in most hospitalized patients is aspiration of these organisms in the upper airways, or aspiration of these organisms from gastric contents after they are swallowed.

Pathogenesis of other organisms is quite different. *Legionella*, tuberculosis, influenza, and *Aspergillus* are inhaled, the usual source being environmental (*Legionella* or *Aspergillus*) or another patient (influenza or tuberculosis).

Clinical features

The classic presentation for pneumonia is cough and fever, usually with purulent respiratory secretions. The diagnosis of pneumonia requires the demonstration of a pulmonary infiltrate on chest radiography. These same symptoms may be present in patients with acute bronchitis, which is virtually always a viral infection that does not merit antibacterial treatment. A notable exception is patients who have violation of the airways with endotracheal tubes or tracheostomies who may have 'febrile tracheobronchitis' due to bacterial infection, most frequently at the tip of the tube, the site of the cuff, or the site of insertion. As noted previously, many patients who satisfy the definition for nosocomial pneumonia based on a pulmonary infiltrate accompanied by fever and purulent respiratory secretions have alternative diagnoses when studied by reliable microbiological techniques using bronchoscopy with quantitative cultures of a bronchial-protected brush or bronchoalveolar lavage (BAL).

Laboratory diagnosis

Tests to establish diagnosis and evaluate severity

The chest radiograph is critical for the confirmation of pneumonia. Major causes of false-negative radiographs in the presence of nosocomial pneumonia are severe neutropenia and pneumonia caused by *P. carinii*. CT scans may reveal infiltrates that are not present on plain films, but it is not clear that this distinguishes a group that requires antibiotic treatment. Thus, the chest radiograph is generally viewed as adequately sensitive for detection of nosocomial pneumonia.

It is important to monitor blood gases to determine severity of illness and to monitor respiratory support.

Studies to determine microbial aetiology

Blood cultures are positive in 2 to 6 per cent of patients with nosocomial pneumonia and clearly identify the causative agent. Some patients will have empyemas, and thoracentesis is necessary for both diagnosis and treatment. Again, this represents an uncontaminated source for culture, providing definitive evidence of the responsible pathogen. Empyema is an infrequent complication of nosocomial pneumonia, excepting in patients who have undergone thoracotomy who often have an empyema as a complication of chest tube placement.

Legionella, *M. tuberculosis*, and respiratory viruses (influenza, parainfluenza, and respiratory syncytial virus) represent definitive pathogens when recovered in respiratory specimens since these organisms do not colonize the normal respiratory tract.

The majority of patients with nosocomial pneumonia do not have bacteraemia, empyema, or the pathogens that do not colonize the normal airway. In these cases, the physician usually must rely on routine bacterial cultures of respiratory secretions or resort to invasive diagnostic tests using bronchoscopy with quantitative cultures of BAL specimens or of the protected brush. Multiple studies have tested the validity of these techniques for distinguishing contaminants and pathogens. The results are somewhat variable, but often dependent on the precision of methodology. The use of these techniques has also resulted in substantial controversy in the management of nosocomial pneumonia, especially in intensive care units where the stakes are high due to high mortality rates. Arguments in favour of invasive diagnostic studies with bronchoscopy are the facts that the technology is well studied, about one-half of patients with suspected pneumonia have negative results and antibiotics can be avoided in this population, and the clear definition of pathogens permits pathogen-specific antibiotic treatment. Others argue that the invasive methods are unrealistic or unnecessary because many hospital laboratories do not provide an adequate microbiology service, patients with the characteristic clinical features will be treated with antibiotics regardless of the bronchoscopy results, or because of the perception that semiquantitative cultures of tracheal aspirates are cheap, easy, and provide information that is equally valid.

Regardless of the method to obtain respiratory secretions for microbiology studies, it is usually beneficial to examine the specimen cytologically. Cultures should be reported with either quantitative or semiquantitative results. For quantitative results, the usual threshold for significance with the protected brush is 10^3/ml, and for BAL specimens it is usually 10^3 or 10^4/ml. With semiquantitative techniques, moderate or heavy growth usually indicates 'significant concentrations.' The major pathogens are summarized in Table 1: *S. epidermidis*, diphtheroids, *H. parainfluenza*, *Enterococcus*, and α-haemolytic *Streptococcus* are generally regarded as contaminants, regardless of concentrations. Anaerobic bacteria are frequently neglected pulmonary pathogens, but it is difficult to obtain specimens valid for anaerobic cultures, and many laboratories struggle with anaerobic microbiology even when the right specimens are obtained. The diagnosis of anaerobic pneumonia should be suspected when Gram stains show mixed bacteria, especially when there are morphotypes suggesting anaerobes, and specimens obtained by tracheal aspirate or bronchoscopy should be examined for these organisms. Putrid drainage always indicates anaerobic infection.

Treatment

The major management issues are antibiotic selection and respiratory support. The optimal method to select antibiotics is to base this decision on results of Gram stains and cultures (Table 3). When empiric decisions are necessary in seriously ill patients, agents are directed against Gram-negative bacteria, and the favoured drugs in this context are ceftazidime, cefepime, imipenem/meropenem, piperacillin/piperacillin–tazobactam, ticarcillin/ticarcillin–sulbactam, or ciprofloxacin. For *S. aureus*, vancomycin is often added on the basis of Gram stain results or the perceived need to cover this pathogen. Treatment for *P. aeruginosa*, the predominant Gram-negative bacillus in nosocomial pneumonia in intensive care units, should be based on *in vitro* sensitivity tests. Anaerobic bacteria are well treated with imipenem/meropenem or any β-lactam–β-lactamase inhibitor; clindamycin can be used if these organisms are suspected and the alternatives are not used for other pathogens. The role of aminoglycosides in pulmonary infections involving Gram-negative bacilli is controversial because these agents appear to have a marginal activity at the concentrations achieved in the lung and at the pH of pulmonary secretions. Nevertheless, they appear to work well in animal experiments. The recommendation is that if they are used, they are always combined with a second agent that should have activity against Gram-negative bacilli as summarized above, and that there is assurance of adequate levels with either once-daily dosing or with monitoring of levels with thrice-daily dosing.

Table 3 Treatment of nosocomial pneumonia

Pathogen	Antibiotic
Bacteria	
Gram-negative bacilli	
P. aeruginosa*	Ceftazidime, imipenem, piperacillin/ticarcillin, cefepime, aztreonam, ciprofloxacin ± tobramycin
Xanthomonas*	Trimethoprim-sulfa
Entero-bacteriaceae*	Cephalosporin (2nd or 3rd generation), β-lactams–β-lactamase inhibitor, aztreonam, imipenem, fluoroquinolone ± aminoglycoside
Anaerobes	Imipenem, β-lactam–β-lactamase inhibitor, clindamycin
S. aureus*	Vancomycin
Legionella	Gatifloxacin, levofloxacin, or azithromycin + rifampin
Viruses	
Influenza	Rimantadine, zanamivir, oseltamivir
Fungi	
Aspergillus	Amphotericin

* Need *in vitro* susceptibility data.

It should be emphasized that cultures of respiratory secretions obtained after the inception of antibiotic treatment have substantially reduced validity. This observation emphasizes the importance of pretreatment cultures and caution with therapeutic decisions based on post-treatment cultures other than those of blood and plural fluid.

Outcome

Nosocomial pneumonia is associated with a mortality rate reported at 8 to 20 per cent for all cases. The mortality rate for infections acquired in the intensive care unit is 20 to 40 per cent, with a mean of 25 per cent. In the latter group the attributable mortality is 30 to 33 per cent, meaning that associated conditions are the major factors in causing death.

Prevention

The frequency of nosocomial pneumonia and high mortality rate, especially in intensive care units, has prompted extensive studies of prevention. The methods that have withstood the test of time and have proven meritorious are the use of the semiupright position to reduce the risk of aspiration, and hand washing between patients to prevent transmission of nosocomial pathogens.

The concern for patient positioning is based on marker studies showing that stomach contents are displaced to the lower respiratory tract with high frequency in patients in the recumbent position, and this can be easily corrected by use of an upright or semiupright position. The assumption is that nosocomial pneumonia is frequently due to bacteria that reside in the stomach as a result of oral colonization. With regard to hand washing, this is a time-honoured method to reduce nosocomial infection that is commonly neglected by hospital personnel. It appears to be particularly important in the transmission of *S. aureus*, and is often important in organisms that are endemic or epidemic within hospital units such as *Acinetobacter*, *Serratia*, *Xanthomonas*, *Pseudomonas*, and *Enterobacter*.

A common practice in intensive care units is prophylaxis to prevent peptic ulceration of the stomach, but neutralization of gastric acid eliminates the gastric barrier, the defence mechanism that prevents colonization of the stomach by bacteria, including Gram-negative bacteria from the upper airways. As a result, sucralfate is commonly advocated in place of H2 agonists or antacids. Another approach to dealing with colonization of the upper airways and stomach is 'selective decontamination' to interrupt the cycle of colonization of the colon by Gram-negative bacteria followed by coloniza-

tion of the upper airways by the same organisms. The goal of selective decontamination is elimination or reduction in Gram-negative bacteria in the gastrointestinal tract with antibiotics that also preserve the anaerobic bacteria in the flora, since these are largely responsible for population control in the colon. Drugs that are commonly used are oral preparations of polymyxin, aminoglycosides, poorly absorbed fluoroquinolones, aztreonam, trimethoprim–sulfamethoxazole, or cephalosporins. These drugs are given orally with the expectation that they will have a major impact on the colonic flora, and they are sometimes also incorporated into paste formulations for application to the upper airways as well. Extensive trials with selective decontamination show that they achieve a substantial reduction in nosocomial pneumonia, but do not seem to influence mortality due to nosocomial pneumonia. Major concerns are:

(1) the failure to reduce mortality rates;

(2) excessive costs of the regimens; and

(3) the perception of antibiotic abuse with encouragement of resistance.

Topical antibiotics have also been tested for utility in prophylaxis. The method is installation of drugs (usually polymyxin or aminoglycosides) through tracheostomies, endotracheal tubes, or by aerosolization. Extensive therapeutic trials with this tactic have shown that they are sometimes successful in interrupting epidemics due to susceptible bacteria, especially *P. aeruginosa*, but mortality rates have generally remained unchanged, and there is concern about the evolution of resistant bacteria. Topical antibiotics are generally not recommended, excepting for some patients with cystic fibrosis.

Interruption of epidemics involving *Legionella* and *Aspergillus* requires different tactics because these organisms are inhaled. For *Legionella* and *Aspergillus*, the goal is to eliminate the environmental source. Influenza is transmitted from person-to-person, so the goal is to eliminate this type of contact, which must include removal of health-care workers with influenza from jobs that require patient contact. All hospital personnel should have influenza vaccine as a method to protect patients, and hospital personnel with jobs that require patient contact must be furloughed if they have suspected or established influenza.

Further reading

American Thoracic Society (1995). Hospital-acquired pneumonia in adults: diagnosis, assessment of severity, initial antimicrobial therapy and preventative strategies. A consensus statement. *American Journal of Respiratory and Critical Care Medicine* **153**, 1711–25. [Guidelines for managing nosocomial pneumonia, including diagnostic studies and antibiotic selection.]

Fagon J-Y, Chastre J, Wolff M, *et al.* (2000). Invasive and noninvasive strategies for management of suspected ventilator-associated pneumonia. *Annals of Internal Medicine* **132**, 621–30. [A multicenter, randomized trial; there were significantly fewer deaths at 14 days in the group that had invasive bacteriological methods.]

Fagon JY, Chastre J, Hance AJ, *et al.* (1988). Detection of nosocomial lung infection in ventilated patients: use of a protected specimen brush and quantitative culture techniques in 147 patients. *American Review of Respiratory Disease* **138**, 110–16. [Over half of the patients who had standard criteria for ventilator-associated pneumonia actually had an alternative diagnosis.]

Fagon JY, Chastre J, Vuagnat A, Trouillet JL, Novara A, Gibert C (1996). Nosocomial pneumonia and mortality among patients in intensive care units. *Journal of the American Medical Association* **275**, 866–9. [A review of mortality data for nosocomial pneumonia.]

Johanson WG Jr, Woods DE, Chaudhuri T (1979). Association of respiratory tract colonization with adherence of gram-negative bacilli to epithelial cells. *Journal of Infectious Diseases* **139**, 667–73. [Gram-negative bacilli stuck to buccal epithelial cells better if the source was seriously ill. This is thought to be the explanation for high rates of pharyngeal colonization in these patients.]

Johanson WG, Pierce AK, Sanford JP (1969). Changing pharyngeal bacterial flora of hospitalized patients: emergence of gram-negative bacilli. *New England Journal of Medicine* **281**, 1137–40. [Colonization of the pharynx by Gram-negative bacilli correlates with severity of associated illness. These strains are thought to be the precursor of Gram-negative bacillary pneumonia due to aspiration.]

Morehead RS, Pinto SJ (2000). Ventilator-associated pneumonia. *Archives of Internal Medicine* **160**, 1926–36. [A review of the topic. The authors claim that invasive diagnostic methods require extensive resources, but may save costs. Prompt use of antibiotics is stressed. Prevention is reviewed without endorsement of selective decontamination.]

17.5.2.3 Pulmonary complications of HIV infection

Mark J. Rosen

Since 1995, the relentless increase in death rates from AIDS in developed nations has reversed due to the use of highly active antiretroviral therapy (HAART), and there is now hope that AIDS may not be uniformly fatal. Nevertheless, thousands of people are infected with HIV each year, and thousands more still develop opportunistic infections and HIV-associated neoplasms because they do not know they are infected, have limited access to these treatments, choose not to use them, or the treatments are unsuccessful. Antiretroviral therapy is too expensive to be available to millions of people with AIDS worldwide, and the AIDS epidemic will be devastating in Africa, Asia, and South America.

Spectrum of pulmonary disorders

Lung diseases have been important causes of illness and death in AIDS since the beginning of the epidemic. The first cases of AIDS were described in homosexual men in Los Angeles who had *Pneumocystis carinii* pneumonia, without a known reason for immunodeficiency. The incidence of *Pneumocystis carinii* pneumonia is declining because of the widespread use of prophylaxis and HAART, but it is still the most common AIDS-defining opportunistic infection in the United States and Western Europe. Despite the importance of *Pneumocystis carinii* pneumonia as an AIDS-defining disorder, clinicians should not assume that most HIV-infected persons with pulmonary disease have *Pneumocystis carinii* pneumonia, because there is a wide range of pulmonary infections, neoplasms, and inflammatory disorders associated with HIV infection (Table 1). These range from mild abnormalities in pulmonary function unaccompanied by respiratory symptoms to fatal opportunistic infections.

Early investigations of the types of pulmonary disorders that occur in patients with HIV infection were limited by analysis of data from single sites, and by restricting the scope of analysis to patients who had an opportunistic infection or neoplasm. This approach systematically underestimated the incidence and importance of pulmonary disorders that occur in early HIV infection. In the Pulmonary Complications of HIV Infection Study, 1353 subjects were followed prospectively in six American cities to determine the prevalence, incidence, and types of lung diseases that occur in persons in selected HIV transmission categories. After 18 months of follow-up, the most frequent respiratory diagnoses in the HIV-seropositive subjects were upper respiratory infection (33.4 per cent), acute bronchitis (16 per cent), and acute sinusitis (5.3 per cent). Although these disorders were also common in a control group of HIV-seronegative gay men and injecting drug users, bronchitis and sinusitis were reported more frequently in the HIV-infected subjects. The types and frequencies of lower respiratory tract disorders diagnosed in the first 18 months of follow-up are listed in Table 2. After 64 months of follow-up, the incidence of bacterial pneumonia remained higher than that of *Pneumocystis carinii* pneumonia.

Table 1 Pulmonary complications of HIV infection

Bacteria
Streptococcus pneumoniae
Haemophilus influenzae
Staphylococcus aureus
Moraxella catarrhalis
Pseudomonas aeruginosa
Rhodococcus equii
Nocardia asteroides
Mycobacterium tuberculosis
Mycobacterium avium-intracellulare
Other non-tuberculous mycobacteria

Fungi
Pneumocystis carinii
Aspergillus fumigatus
Cryptococcus neoformans
Blastomyces dermatitides
Coccicioides immitis
Histoplasma capsulatum
Penicillium marneffei

Protozoa
Strongyloides stercoralis
Toxoplasma gondii

Viruses
Cytomegalovirus
Adenovirus
Herpes simplex

Malignancies
Kaposi's sarcoma
Non-Hodgkin's lymphoma
Carcinoma of the lung

Other pulmonary disorders
Lymphocytic interstitial pneumonitis
Non-specific interstitial pneumonitis
Bronchiolitis obliterans organizing pneumonia
Primary pulmonary hypertension
Emphysema

Table 2 Eighteen-month incidence rates of lower respiratory disorders in 1116 HIV-seropositive people[*]

Disorder	No of patients	%
Bacterial pneumonia	53	4.8
Pneumocystis carinii	43	3.9
Non-tuberculous mycobacteria	12	1.1
Mycobacterium tuberculosis	10	0.9
Non-specific pneumonitis	8	0.7
Cryptococcus neoformans	5	0.5
Cytomegalovirus	3	0.3
Carcinoma	3	0.3
Kaposi's sarcoma	2	0.2
Congestive heart failure	2	0.2
Herpes simplex	1	0.1
Toxoplasma gondii	1	0.1
Histoplasma capsulatum	1	0.1
Lung abscess	1	0.1
Pulmonary embolism	1	0.1
Pneumothorax	1	0.1

[*] Adapted from Wallace *et al.* (1993).

Pulmonary tuberculosis and fungal infections are also common in patients with AIDS, and are addressed in other sections of this textbook. Non-infectious disorders may also involve the lung in HIV-infected individuals: these include neoplasms (especially Kaposi's sarcoma), non-specific and lymphocytic interstitial pneumonitis, primary pulmonary hypertension, and bronchiolitis obliterans organizing pneumonia. These disorders may vary in severity from asymptomatic to life threatening.

Diagnostic approach

When a homosexual man or an injecting drug user presents with a respiratory illness, most clinicians will suspect an HIV-related disorder. However, the incidence and prevalence of HIV infection is increasing rapidly among patients who acquired HIV infection by heterosexual contact, and should be considered in all patients with pneumonia, especially in communities where the prevalence of HIV infection is high. Conversely, many patients with known HIV infection have disorders that are common in the community.

The initial approach to patients with suspected HIV-related pulmonary disorders is the same as for any other patient: the clinician will take a careful history, perform a physical examination, and determine whether or not to perform diagnostic tests. In HIV-infected patients, careful consideration of risk factors for specific pulmonary diseases and the chest radiograph are especially important in formulating a differential diagnosis.

Patients with HIV-associated pulmonary disorders typically present with non-specific symptoms such as cough, dyspnoea, sputum production, and wheezing. Pulmonary symptoms are more common in HIV-infected people than in the general population; in the Pulmonary Complications of HIV Infection Study, 15 per cent of 1171 HIV-infected persons who did not have a diagnosed pulmonary disorder or an AIDS diagnosis complained of cough and dyspnoea at the time of enrolment. Both dyspnoea and cough were more prevalent in injecting drug users than others, and were strongly associated with cigarette smoking. Respiratory symptoms may be unrelated to the HIV infection, and disorders that are common in the general population, such as asthma or bronchitis, must be considered.

Risk factors for specific pulmonary disorders

The risk of developing particular HIV-associated disorders is strongly influenced by the patient's immune status, demographic characteristics, current or prior place of residence, use of antiretroviral agents, and prophylaxis against common HIV-associated infections. Genetic factors are undoubtedly important, but are less precisely defined.

Immune status

The severity of immunosuppression probably has the strongest influence on the risk of specific AIDS-associated disorders, and the CD4+ lymphocyte count is the best surrogate marker for immune function and predictor of the probability of developing specific diseases. In early HIV infection, when the immune system is not severely compromised, respiratory disorders are similar to those that affect the general population, while opportunistic infections occur only with severe immunodeficiency. The CD4+ lymphocyte count, together with quantitative assay of plasma HIV RNA (a surrogate marker of HIV replication), provides the best predictor for disease progression and death.

The association between the CD4+ lymphocyte count and the risk of developing specific diseases was explored in a survey of more than 18 000 HIV-infected subjects who received care in 10 American cities as part of the Adult/Adolescent Spectrum of HIV Disease surveillance system (Table 3). Common problems like sinusitis, bronchitis, and pharyngitis occurred at all strata of CD4+ cell counts. With lower counts, different pulmonary infections occurred with increasing frequency. Bacterial pneumonia and pulmonary tuberculosis occur with relatively intact CD4+ lymphocyte counts, while opportunistic infections like *Pneumocystis carinii* pneumonia and disseminated *Mycobacterium avium* complex and fungi are likely to

occur only with severe immunosuppression. Conversely, if the CD4+ lymphocyte count has a sustained increase to more than 200 cells/µl following HAART, the risks of developing *Pneumocystis carinii* pneumonia and other opportunistic infections decline to the point that prophylaxis can be discontinued. Hence knowing the CD4+ count is very helpful in formulating a differential diagnosis in a patient with known or suspected HIV infection. Respiratory problems like sinusitis and bronchitis may occur at any level of CD4+, and bacterial pneumonia and tuberculosis often occur before AIDS-defining opportunistic infections and neoplasms. Declining immune function increases the risk for all HIV-associated respiratory disease, except perhaps for mild upper respiratory tract infections.

Demographic factors

The demographic characteristics of those infected with HIV influence the incidence of specific pulmonary disorders, and the changing demographics of HIV infection in the United States and Europe are accompanied by a changing spectrum of disease. Injecting drug users are at increased risk of developing bacterial pneumonia and pulmonary tuberculosis, and HIV-infected drug users are at especially high risk.

Race and ethnicity may also influence the risk of developing bacterial pneumonia and tuberculosis, but these associations are confounded by differences in access to health care, the higher prevalence of tuberculosis in minority communities, and disproportionately high numbers of injecting drug users who are Black or Hispanic. Nevertheless, the risk of tuberculosis is higher in Blacks and Hispanics than Whites, while Whites have a higher risk of HIV-associated malignancies and cytomegalovirus disease.

Residence

Geographical considerations influence the types of diseases that HIV-infected individuals are at risk of developing. In the United States, the incidence of HIV-associated tuberculosis is highest in the northeast. The high incidence of *Pneumocystis carinii* pneumonia in the United States and Europe contrasts sharply with most regions in Africa, where it is much less common. It is still unknown whether inherited differences in susceptibility

Table 3 Incidence of selected disease conditions, listed by CD4+ count, from a study of 18 000 HIV-infected people (number of cases, per cent reported during follow-up)*

CD4+ < 100 cells/µl		
Disseminated *Mycobacterium avium* complex	1144	6.5%
Cytomegalovirus disease	513	2.9%
Extrapulmonary cryptococcosis	280	1.6%
Disseminated histoplasmosis	57	0.3%
Pulmonary candidiasis	35	0.2%
Disseminated coccidioidomycosis	14	0.1%
CD4+ 100–199 cells/µl		
Pneumocystis carinii pneumonia	1097	7.3%
Kaposi's sarcoma	695	4.0%
Bacterial sepsis	557	3.1%
Disseminated *Mycobacterium tuberculosis*	153	0.9%
CD4+ 200–299 cells/µl		
Pulmonary *Mycobacterium* (excludes tuberculosis)	464	2.6%
Recurrent pneumonia	375	2.1%
CD4+ 300–399 cells/µl		
Pneumonia (one episode)	1418	8.4%
Pulmonary *Mycobacterium tuberculosis*	149	0.8%
Cardiomyopathy	158	0.9%
CD4+ > 500 cells/µl		
Infectious sinusitis/mastoiditis/otitis	2350	14.2%
Bronchitis	2037	12.2%
Pharyngitis	1613	9.5%
Lung cancer	17	0.1%

* Adapted from Hanson *et al.* (1995).

to *Pneumocystis carinii* or environmental factors account for the lower incidence of *Pneumocystis carinii* pneumonia in Africa.

The geographical distribution of endemic fungi is also a strong determinant of risk of those infections; disseminated histoplasmosis and coccidioidomycosis are common in patients with AIDS who live in endemic areas. These infections may also occur as reactivation disease after HIV-infected persons move to other areas and develop immunocompromise. For example, cases of disseminated histoplasmosis were reported in New York in patients with AIDS who had relocated from Puerto Rico years before.

Antiretroviral therapy

The availability of potent drugs that inhibit HIV replication led to the development of combination regimens that can accomplish prolonged and near complete suppression of viral replication, with improvement in immune function and clinical outcomes. The standard care of those infected with HIV now includes use of combination antiretroviral therapy with a goal of suppressing HIV replication below the limits of detection, guided by monitoring plasma HIV RNA levels and CD4+ lymphocyte counts. Since the introduction of HAART into clinical practice, death rates from AIDS and AIDS-related opportunistic disorders have fallen dramatically. In a study of 1255 patients with severe immune deficiency, defined by at least one CD4+ count of less than 100 cells/μl, morbidity, mortality, and the incidence of opportunistic infections declined as the use of combination antiretroviral therapy including protease inhibitors increased. These trends were not explained by patient characteristics (sex, age, race/ethnicity, HIV risk) or increasing use of prophylaxis against opportunistic infections. Rather, improving outcomes were attributable to the intensity of antiretroviral therapy, especially with protease inhibitors.

The new antiretroviral agents, and especially the protease inhibitors, interact with many other drugs, and clinicians must investigate possible drug interactions when prescribing new medications for patients taking antiretrovirals. These drug interactions have particular importance in the treatment of tuberculosis in patients with HIV infection, discussed in Chapters 7.10.21 and 7.11.22.

Pneumocystis carinii prophylaxis

Even before the introduction of HAART, anti-*Pneumocystis* prophylaxis had a profound impact on the spectrum of HIV-associated pulmonary diseases by reducing the incidence and mortality rate due to that infection, and the prognosis for survival after developing immunosuppression or an AIDS-defining diagnosis also improved, largely attributable to that treatment. However, mortality from non-tuberculous mycobacterioses, cytomegalovirus disease, bacterial infections, non-Hodgkin's lymphoma, tuberculosis, and other opportunistic infections increased.

Chest radiography

The chest radiograph is extremely useful in evaluating symptomatic HIV-infected patients, because different radiographic patterns are associated with specific disorders. These are shown in Table 4. A normal radiograph may be seen with common disorders like bronchitis or asthma, but also with *Pneumocystis carinii* pneumonia or tuberculosis. Patients with normal films who are suspected of having one of these infections should proceed to CT scan or pulmonary function tests with carbon monoxide diffusing capacity: if either of these studies is normal, the diagnosis of *Pneumocystis carinii* pneumonia is extremely unlikely. An abnormal film will prompt a diagnostic evaluation based on the pattern of the abnormality, and influenced by the clinician's perception of the relative risk of different disorders. For example, focal infiltrates are usually caused by bacterial pneumonia or tuberculosis, but fungal infection is possible in endemic areas. Diffuse opacities are usually associated with *Pneumocystis carinii* pneumonia, but may also be seen with other disorders. Diagnostic algorithms based on the radiographic findings in patients with suspected HIV-associated pulmonary disorders are summarized in Table 5.

Table 4 HIV Infection: Chest radiographic patterns and common aetiologies

Radiographic pattern	Aetiology
Focal infiltrates	Bacteria
	Mycobacterium tuberculosis
	Pneumocystis carinii
Diffuse infiltrates	*Pneumocystis carinii*
	Mycobacterium tuberculosis
	Kaposi's sarcoma
	Bacteria
	Fungi
	Cytomegalovirus
Diffuse nodular infiltrates	Kaposi's sarcoma (large nodules)
	Mycobacterium tuberculosis (miliary)
	Fungi (small nodules)
Pneumothorax	*Pneumocystis carinii*
Mediastinal lymphadenopathy	*Mycobacterium tuberculosis*
	Mycobacterium avium-intracellulare
	Kaposi's sarcoma
	Lymphoma
	Fungi
Pleural effusion	Bacteria
	Mycobacterium tuberculosis
	Kaposi's sarcoma
	Lymphoma
	Fungi
	Cardiomyopathy
	Hypoproteinemia
Cavitation	*Mycobacterium tuberculosis* (high CD4+)
	Pneumocystis carinii (low CD4+)
	Pseudomonas aeruginosa (low CD4+)
	Rhodococcus equii
	Fungi

Table 5 Diagnostic algorithms

Diffuse pulmonary disease

Step 1:
- Start empirical therapy for *Pneumocystis carinii*
- Nodules, lymphadenopathy or pleural effusion make *Pneumocystis* less likely
- Sputum induction for *Pneumocystis* and mycobacteria (spontaneous sputum, if produced, is best for acid-fast bacilli)

Step 2:
- If no diagnosis, bronchoscopy with bronchoalveolar lavage and transbronchial biopsy*

Focal pulmonary disease

Step 1:
- Blood cultures, pleural fluid studies if effusion present
- Empiric therapy for bacterial pneumonia
- Stain and culture sputum for mycobacteria

Step 2:
- If not improving, no diagnosis: sputum induction for *Pneumocystis carinii* and mycobacteria is an option before bronchoscopy

Step 3:
- If not improving, no diagnosis: bronchoscopy with bronchoalveolar lavage and transbronchial biopsy
- Gram's stain, sputum culture, or invasive techniques (quantitative bronchoalveolar lavage, protected catheter brushing) to diagnose bacterial pneumonia may be performed

Adapted from Salzman (1999).

* Some practitioners perform bronchoscopy only if the patient fails to improve on empirical anti-*Pneumocystis* therapy; some do bronchoalveolar lavage without transbronchial biopsy on an initial bronchoscopy.

Specific pulmonary diseases

Bacterial pneumonia

HIV infection impairs humoral as well as cellular immunity, increasing the risk of developing bacterial infections, including sinusitis and pneumonia. Although a first episode of bacterial pneumonia usually occurs before the diagnosis of AIDS, the risk of developing pneumonia increases as the CD4+ lymphocyte count declines. Drug users are at higher risk than other groups, and neutropenia is an independent risk factor. Patients who use trimethoprim-sulfamethoxazole to prevent *Pneumocystis carinii* pneumonia have a reduced risk of developing bacterial pneumonia.

Streptococcus pneumoniae, *Haemophilus influenzae*, and *Staphylococcus aureus* are the most common bacterial pathogens, but disturbing patterns of antimicrobial resistance are emerging, and new aetiologies of pneumonia are recognized more commonly, especially in patients with advanced HIV disease. For example, pneumonia caused by *Pseudomonas aeruginosa*, which was rarely diagnosed in the 1980s, is a relatively common pathogen in severely immunocompromised patients, typically with CD4+ counts of less than 50 cells/μl, and especially following another opportunistic infection. Although pneumonia due to 'atypical' pathogens like *Mycoplasma*, *Chlamydia*, and *Legionella* is reported, these pathogens are relatively uncommon. *Rhodococcus equii*, an aerobic Gram-positive acid-fast bacillus, may cause focal consolidation, endobronchial disease, and cavitation, usually in patients with advanced HIV disease. *Nocardia asteroides* may cause nodules, consolidation, cavitation, pleural effusions, empyema, and intrathoracic lymphadenopathy in patients with HIV infection.

Bacterial pneumonia usually presents with the same symptoms as those who are HIV seronegative, with fever, chills, productive cough, and localized areas of consolidation on chest radiography. While this clinical picture strongly suggests bacterial pneumonia, it may also occur with tuberculosis and fungal infection, and patients with bacterial pneumonia sometimes have diffuse pulmonary opacities that resemble *Pneumocystis carinii* pneumonia.

The approach to diagnosis and treatment is the same as that for HIV-seronegative patients (see section 17.5.2.1). Polyvalent pneumococcal vaccine is recommended for all HIV-infected people, although they may not mount an adequate antibody response. The vaccine against *Haemophilus influenzae* type b is not used in patients with HIV infection because most *Haemophilus* infections are with strains not covered by this vaccine. Although annual influenza vaccine is recommended, there are no data indicating that patients with HIV infection are at increased risk of contracting influenza, or that the illness is more severe than in the general population.

Pneumocystis carinii pneumonia

Clinical features

Pneumocystis carinii pneumonia typically presents with gradually increasing dyspnoea and cough over weeks, but sometimes as an acute illness with rapid deterioration over a few days. The chest radiograph usually has diffuse ground glass opacities, which strongly suggests the diagnosis, but sometimes shows nodular opacities, lobar consolidation, or a normal film. All of these radiographic patterns may also occur with other infections and neoplasms. Cystic abnormalities and spontaneous pneumothoraces in patients with known or suspected HIV infection are usually caused by *Pneumocystis carinii* pneumonia.

The diagnosis of *Pneumocystis carinii* pneumonia may be supported by adjunctive tests. *Pneumocystis carinii* pneumonia is unlikely in a patient who had a CD4+ cell count above 200 cells/μl in the preceding 2 months in the absence of other HIV-associated symptoms. Approximately 90 per cent of patients with *Pneumocystis carinii* pneumonia have an elevated serum lactic dehydrogenase, but this may occur with other pulmonary diseases. Oxygen desaturation with exercise is a relatively sensitive and specific test in patients suspected to have *Pneumocystis carinii* pneumonia, but is not diag-

nostic. Gallium-67 and indium-111 lung scans are highly sensitive indicators of *Pneumocystis carinii* pneumonia, but isotope uptake also occurs in other pulmonary infections, so they are seldom useful in a diagnostic evaluation.

Microbiological diagnosis

Pneumocystis carinii cannot yet be cultured *in vitro*, so the diagnosis of *Pneumocystis carinii* pneumonia can be confirmed only by demonstrating organisms in a lung-derived specimen. The least invasive diagnostic test is the analysis of sputum induced with 3 per cent saline delivered by ultrasonic nebulization. Using modified Giemsa, methenamine silver, or immunofluorescent staining, and depending on the experience of the laboratory, *Pneumocystis carinii* can be identified in up to 80 per cent of cases. Other pathogens, particularly *Mycobacterium tuberculosis* and fungi, may also be found using appropriate staining and culture techniques.

It is controversial whether to routinely proceed with fibreoptic bronchoscopy to confirm the diagnosis of *Pneumocystis carinii* pneumonia in patients suspected of having the disease, but who have non-diagnostic sputum specimens. Some prefer to treat empirically for *Pneumocystis carinii* pneumonia, and establish a diagnosis only if there is no clinical response within 5 days. Proponents of this approach hold that a presumptive diagnosis of *Pneumocystis carinii* pneumonia is usually accurate, and that the procedure carries unnecessary inconvenience, risk, discomfort to patients, and expense. Proponents of early bronchoscopy maintain that using an empirical approach will subject many patients to treatment and its attendant toxicity for a disease that they do not have, and non-responders may be too ill to undergo bronchoscopy after several days of inappropriate therapy. Furthermore, coinfection with other pathogens is common, may not be diagnosed in patients treated empirically, and adjunctive corticosteroid therapy may transiently improve symptoms in patients with other pulmonary disorders, contributing to the emergence of other opportunistic infections such as aspergillosis and cytomegalovirus.

Patients with suspected *Pneumocystis carinii* pneumonia who have non-diagnostic sputum studies should have fibreoptic bronchoscopy with bronchoalveolar lavage as the next procedure in the diagnostic evaluation. The complication rate is very low, and the yield is over 90 per cent in most centres. This yield is optimized by performing lavage in more than one lobe, and is higher in the upper lobes than the lower. All lavage specimens should be examined for the presence of acid-fast bacilli, fungi, and viral cellular inclusions, since patients with suspected *Pneumocystis carinii* pneumonia may have another infection, or may be coinfected with other pathogens. The role of bronchoalveolar lavage in the diagnosis of bacterial pneumonia in HIV-infected persons is not established. Some clinicians also perform bronchoscopic lung biopsies routinely during bronchoscopy, as this procedure increases the diagnostic yield for *Pneumocystis carinii* and other disorders. Others reserve biopsy for patients who have no diagnosis after bronchoalveolar lavage. Bronchoscopic biopsy is contraindicated in the presence of bleeding disorders, and the high risk of pneumothorax usually precludes biopsy in patients undergoing mechanical ventilation. Diagnosing *Pneumocystis carinii* pneumonia by video-assisted thoracoscopy or an open procedure is rarely necessary.

Respiratory failure caused by *Pneumocystis carinii* pneumonia

Despite HAART, antipneumocystis prophylaxis, and declining mortality rates from *Pneumocystis carinii* pneumonia, it is still the most common cause of respiratory failure and admission to intensive care units in patients with AIDS. When treatment of *Pneumocystis carinii* pneumonia is postponed or ineffective, a clinical syndrome develops that resembles the acute respiratory distress syndrome, with severe hypoxaemia, intrapulmonary shunt, reduced pulmonary compliance, and the appearance of diffuse radiographic opacities. Just as severe *Pneumocystis carinii* pneumonia clinically resembles acute respiratory distress syndrome, the supportive treatment, including intubation, mechanical ventilation, and application of positive end-expiratory pressure, is similar. Continuous positive airway pressure delivered by mask may improve gas exchange without endotracheal intubation, but its usefulness is limited in patients with severe disease. However, it may afford the patient and physician more time to consider whether mechanical ventilation is desirable.

As changes in therapy have modified the prognosis, three distinct 'eras' of critical care for patients with *Pneumocystis carinii* pneumonia and respiratory failure can be identified. Initially, the outlook for survival was dismal, at around 15 per cent, and in some centres admissions to intensive care units declined because physicians did not recommend aggressive interventions, and patients were more likely to decline them. After 1986, mortality rates seemed to improve to around 50 per cent, attributed to selection of patients with a better prognosis and to the benefits of adjunctive corticosteroid therapy. We are now in a third 'era' of outcomes, when patients who require mechanical ventilation for *Pneumocystis carinii* pneumonia again have a high mortality rate since they are more likely to have failed prophylaxis, anti-*Pneumocystis* treatment, or adjunctive corticosteroid therapy, and therefore are expected to have a poor prognosis. Recent studies show that when respiratory failure follows several days of appropriate therapy for *Pneumocystis carinii* pneumonia, the probability of survival is only around 20 per cent.

The prospects for long-term survival following *Pneumocystis carinii* pneumonia and respiratory failure are more hopeful than earlier in the epidemic. Prolonged survival is probably related to the selection of patients with a better prognosis for mechanical ventilation, and to the use of HAART and prophylaxis against subsequent infections.

Airway diseases

For unknown reasons, patients with advanced HIV infection may have chronic bronchitis and bronchiectasis, even if they do not smoke. These patients usually have severe immunodeficiency, with CD4+ counts of less than 100 cells/μl. Standard antimicrobial agents are usually effective, but symptoms are likely to recur, especially when *Pseudomonas aeruginosa* is isolated from the sputum. The role and efficacy of bronchodilators and antiinflammatory agents in HIV-associated airway diseases have not been studied systematically. HIV infection also predisposes to early emphysema, possibly related to enhanced pulmonary cytotoxic T-lymphocyte activity.

Kaposi's sarcoma

Kaposi's sarcoma, probably caused by human herpevirus 8, is the commonest malignancy in people with HIV infection, and the skin is the major site of involvement. This virus infects many healthy adults, and may be isolated commonly in saliva, prostatic tissue, and semen. It is probably transmitted by sexual contact, and causes disease when activated by HIV-associated immunosuppression. This hypothesis helps to explain why Kaposi's sarcoma is much more common among HIV-infected gay men than in other transmission groups.

Kaposi's sarcoma may involve many organs, including the lung. Patients with pulmonary Kaposi's sarcoma usually have obvious mucocutaneous lesions, but the lung may be the only site of disease in up to 15 per cent of cases. Involvement of the airways, parenchyma, pleura, and intrathoracic lymph nodes causes a diverse range of symptoms and radiographic findings. The majority of patients with pulmonary Kaposi's sarcoma diagnosed antemortem have cough, dyspnoea, and fever.

Kaposi's sarcoma lesions in the airways do not usually cause symptoms, but sometimes lead to obstruction or haemoptysis. The finding of typical lesions on inspection of the airways is usually considered diagnostic. Histological diagnosis may be difficult because the yield of forceps biopsy is low, and some authors believe that forceps biopsy of Kaposi's sarcoma lesions places the patient at significant risk of bleeding, but this is controversial.

Parenchymal involvement with Kaposi's sarcoma is suggested by bronchial wall thickening, nodules, Kerley B lines, and coexisting pleural effusions, especially in patients with cutaneous disease. Patients may be bronchoscoped to determine whether diffuse radiographic opacities are caused by Kaposi's sarcoma or an opportunistic infection. The yield of

bronchoscopic lung biopsies in the diagnosis of Kaposi's sarcoma is low, and even open lung biopsy is non-diagnostic in approximately 10 per cent of cases because of the focal distribution of lesions. The diagnosis of pulmonary parenchymal Kaposi's sarcoma is therefore usually inferred in patients with cutaneous disease, chest radiographs that suggest this disorder, visual confirmation of airway lesions, and no evidence of opportunistic infection on bronchoalveolar lavage or bronchoscopic lung biopsy. Patients with parenchymal opacities who have typical lesions in the airways and no identified pulmonary infection are assumed to have parenchymal Kaposi's sarcoma.

When Kaposi's sarcoma involves the pleura, effusions are usually exudative and sanguinous, but cytological examination is non-diagnostic. Closed pleural biopsy is rarely positive due to the focal nature of pleural lesions and predominant involvement of the visceral rather than parietal pleura. Since establishing a diagnosis usually necessitates a thoracoscopic or open pleural biopsy, the presence of pleural involvement with Kaposi's sarcoma is usually inferred in a patient with cutaneous disease and a serosanguinous effusion without a reasonable alternative explanation.

Lymphoma

Non-Hodgkin's B-cell lymphoma is associated with HIV infection. Although pulmonary involvement is usually clinically innocuous, the lung is a common site of extranodal disease. Even in patients with an established diagnosis of lymphoma, lung involvement is usually a late feature of disease. If symptoms occur, they are usually late in the course of HIV disease, and simulate common opportunistic infections, presenting with lobar consolidation, nodules, reticular opacities, and masses. Intrathoracic lymphoma usually presents with lymphadenopathy, pleural effusions, or pleural thickening. Airway involvement may cause atelectasis, and pulmonary involvement may be seen in the form of nodules or consolidation. The diagnosis is established by lung or lymph node biopsy, or by cytological analysis of pleural fluid.

Carcinoma of the lung

A few series report an increased incidence of lung cancer in those infected with HIV, and that these cancers are more aggressive, diagnosed at a more advanced stage, and are associated with shorter survival than lung cancer in HIV-negative individuals. The link between HIV infection and lung cancer is supported by genomic differences between lung cancers in patients with and without HIV infection. However, lung cancer is still very rare compared with opportunistic infections and Kaposi's sarcoma.

Further reading

Afessa B, Green B (2000). Bacterial pneumonia in hospitalized patients with HIV infection. *Chest* 117, 1017– 22. [Shows that *Pseudomonas aeruginosa* is a common cause of pneumonia in persons with AIDS.]

Batungwanayo J *et al.* (1994). Pulmonary disease associated with human immunodeficiency virus in Kigali, Rwanda: a fiberoptic bronchoscopic study of 111 cases of undetermined etiology. *Amercian Review of Respiratory and Critical Care Medicine* 149,1591– 6. [Shows that *Pneumocystis carinii* pneumonia is uncommon in Central Africa, even among patients with severe immunocompromise.]

Burack JH *et al.* (1994). Microbiology of community-acquired bacterial pneumonia in persons with and at risk for human immunodeficiency virus type 1 infection. *Archives of Internal Medicine* 154, 2589– 96. [Documents the pathogens that cause bacterial pneumonia in HIV infection, showing that resistant organisms are becoming more common.]

Carpenter CCJ *et al.* (2000). Antiretroviral therapy in adults. Updated recommendations of the International AIDS Society—USA Panel. *Journal of the American Medical Association* 283, 381– 90. [Latest recommendations.]

Centers for Disease Control (1980). *Pneumocystis pneumonia*—Los Angeles. *Morbidity and Mortality Weekly Review* **30**, 250– 2. [First report of patients with AIDS.]

Centers for Disease Control and Prevention (1999). 1999 USPHS/IDSA guidelines for the prevention of opportunistic infections in persons infected with human immunodeficiency virus: U.S. Public Health Service (USPHS) and Infectious Diseases Society of America (IDSA). *Morbidity and Mortality Weekly Review* **48**, (No RR-10), 5– 6. [Latest recommendations.]

Diaz PT *et al.* (2000). Increased susceptibility to pulmonary emphysema among HIV-seropositive smokers. *Annals of Internal Medicine* **132**, 369– 72. [Demonstrates that emphysema is common in HIV-infected persons, and possibly related to enhanced cytotoxic T-lymphocyte activity.]

Fauci AS (1999). The AIDS Epidemic. Considerations for the 21st century. *New England Journal of Medicine* **341**, 1046–50.

Hanson DL *et al.* (1995). Distribution of CD4+ T lymphocytes at diagnosis of acquired immunodeficiency syndrome-defining and other human immunodeficiency virus-related illnesses. *Archives of Internal Medicine* **155**, 1537– 42.

Hirschtick RE *et al.* (1995). Bacterial pneumonia in patients infected with human immunodeficiency virus. *New England Journal of Medicine* **333**, 845– 51. [Elucidates the risk factors for developing bacterial pneumonia and the pathogens identified.]

Hoover DR *et al.* (1993). Clinical manifestations of AIDS in the era of *Pneumocystis* prophylaxis. *New England Journal of Medicine* **329**, 922– 1926. [As the incidence of *Pneumocystis carinii* pneumonia declined due to prophylaxis, the rates of other opportunistic infections increased.]

Huang L *et al.* (1996). Presentation of AIDS-related Kaposi's sarcoma diagnosed by bronchoscopy. *American Journal of Respiratory and Critical Care Medicine* **153**, 1385– 90. [Describes the clinical features of Kaposi's sarcoma involving the lung.]

Jones JL *et al.* (1999). Surveillance for AIDS-defining opportunistic illnesses, 1992– 1997. *Morbidity and Mortality Weekly Review* **48**, (No SS-2), 1– 22. [Documents the declining incidence of *Pneumocystis carinii* pneumonia since 1994.]

Markowitz N *et al.* (1997). Incidence of tuberculosis in the United States among HIV-infected persons. *Annals of Internal Medicine* **126**,123– 32. [Relates the risk of tuberculosis with CD4+ lymphocyte count and place of residence.]

Mocroft A *et al.* (1998). The incidence of AIDS-defining illnesses in 4883 patients with human immunodeficiency virus infection. *Archives of Internal Medicine* **158**, 491– 7. [These studies relate the risk of developing specific HIV-associated disorders with CD4+ lymphocyte counts.]

Palella FJ *et al.* (1998). Declining morbidity and mortality among patients with advanced human immunodeficiency virus infection. *New England Journal of Medicine* **338**, 853– 60. [Improving survival and reduced incidence of opportunistic infections are related to the increased use of HAART.]

Rosen MJ (1999). Intensive care of patients with HIV infection. *Seminars in Respiratory Infection* **14**, 366– 71. [Comprehensive review.]

Salzman SH (1999). Bronchoscopic techniques for the diagnosis of pulmonary complications HIV infection. *Seminars in Respiratory Infections* **14**, 318– 26. [Detailed review.]

Verghese A *et al.* (1994). Bacterial bronchitis and bronchiectasis in human immunodeficiency virus infection. *Archives of Internal Medicine* **154**, 2086– 90. [Describes the clinical features of airways disease in patients with advanced HIV infection.]

Wallace JM *et al.* (1993). Respiratory illness in persons with human immunodeficiency virus infection. *American Review of Respiratory Diseases* **148**, 1523– 9. [Eighteen-month follow-up of a multicenter prospective study of HIV-seropositive persons, showing that bacterial pneumonia is more common than *Pneumocystis carinii* pneumonia.]

White DA, Matthay RA (1989). Noninfectious pulmonary complication of infection with the human immunodeficiency virus. *American Review of Respiratory Diseases* **140**, 1763– 87. [Comprehensive review.]

Wistuba II *et al.* (1998). Comparison of molecular changes in lung cancers in HIV-positive and HIV-indeterminate subjects. *Journal of the American Medical Association* **279**, 1554– 9. [Supports the hypothesis that HIV infection increases the risk of developing lung cancer.]

17.6 Chronic obstructive pulmonary disease

William MacNee

Introduction

Chronic obstructive pulmonary disease (**COPD**) produces considerable morbidity and mortality: it is the sixth commonest case of death worldwide, and set to become the third commonest cause by the year 2020. It is a slowly progressive condition characterized by airflow limitation that is largely irreversible.

Definitions

The group of conditions characterized by airways obstruction that is incompletely reversible have no universally accepted definition. The term COPD has become accepted in recent years, but is not truly a disease, rather a group of diseases. A major problem in defining COPD is the difficulty in differentiating this condition from asthma, particularly the persistent airways obstruction of older chronic asthma sufferers that is often difficult or even impossible to distinguish clinically from that in COPD, although a history of heavy cigarette smoking, evidence of emphysema by imaging techniques, decreased diffusing capacity for carbon monoxide, and chronic hypoxaemia favour a diagnosis of COPD.

Chronic bronchitis is defined clinically as the presence of a chronic productive cough on most days for 3 months, in each of two consecutive years, in a patient in whom other causes of chronic cough have been excluded. Chronic bronchitis can be classified into three forms: simple bronchitis, defined as mucus hypersecretion; chronic or recurrent mucopurulent bronchitis in the presence of persistent or intermittent mucopurulent sputum; and chronic obstructive bronchitis when chronic sputum production is associated with airflow obstruction.

Emphysema is defined as abnormal, permanent enlargement of the distal airspaces, distal to the terminal bronchioles, accompanied by destruction of their walls and without obvious fibrosis. As with chronic bronchitis the definition of emphysema does not require the presence of airflow obstruction. Thus emphysema is defined pathologically.

Bronchiolitis or small airways disease results from inflammation, squamous cell metaplasia, and/or fibrosis in airways less than 2 mm in diameter. These changes are amongst the earliest to appear in cigarette smokers but are difficult to detect by physiological measurements. Although relatively little is known of the natural history of this condition, it is considered to contribute increasingly, as it progresses, to the airways obstruction of COPD.

The relative contribution made by airway abnormalities or distal airspace enlargement to the airways obstruction in an individual patient with COPD is difficult to determine. Thus in the United States the term COPD was introduced in the early 1960s to describe patients with largely irreversible airways obstruction, due to a combination of airways disease and emphysema, without defining the contribution of these conditions to the airways obstruction.

In their statement on the Standards for Diagnosis and Care of Patients with COPD, the American Thoracic Society defined COPD as 'a disease state characterized by the presence of airflow obstruction due to chronic bronchitis or emphysema; the airflow obstruction is generally progressive, may be accompanied by airway reactivity, and may be partially reversible'. The European Respiratory Society has adopted a similar definition—'a disorder characterized by reduced maximum expiratory flow and slow forced emptying of the lungs, features which do not change markedly over several months'. The definition produced by the British Thoracic Society is similar— 'a slowly progressive disorder characterized by airways obstruction (reduced FEV_1 and FEV_1/VC ratio), which does not change markedly over several months. Most of the lung function impairment is fixed, although some reversibility can be produced by bronchodilator (or other) therapy'. Recently, the global initiative on obstructive lung disease introduced the concept of COPD as an inflammatory disease by suggesting in their definition that COPD was characterized by 'an abnormal inflammatory response in the lungs to inhaled particles or gases'.

In clinical practice a diagnosis of COPD is usually associated with:

(1) a history of chronic progressive symptoms (cough, wheeze, and/or breathlessness), with little variation;

(2) usually a cigarette smoking history of more than 20 pack years (1 pack year is 20 cigarettes per day for 1 year); and

(3) objective evidence of airways obstruction, ideally by spirometry, that does not return to normal with treatment.

The term COPD excludes a number of specific causes of chronic airways obstruction, such as cystic fibrosis, bronchiectasis, and bronchiolitis obliterans (for example associated with lung transplantation or chemical inhalation). The differentiation of COPD from asthma remains a problem, particularly as a large proportion of patients with COPD show some reversibility of their airflow obstruction with bronchodilators.

Aetiology

Chronic mucus hypersecretion

Population studies of respiratory symptoms show a much higher prevalence of cough and sputum among smokers than among non-smokers. A survey in urban and rural populations in the United Kingdom found that a history of chronic bronchitis was present in 17.6 per cent of males aged 55 to 64 years who were heavy smokers, in 0.9 per cent of light smokers, 4.4 per cent of ex-smokers, and was absent in non-smokers. Stopping smoking produces cessation of the sputum production in 90 per cent of cases. Pipe and cigar smokers have a much lower prevalence of chronic bronchitis and less impairment of respiratory function, possibly reflecting lower rates of smoke inhalation.

The 'British hypothesis' suggested that chronic airflow obstruction resulted from the development of chronic mucus hypersecretion as a result of recurrent bronchial infection. This hypothesis was tested in the landmark studies of Fletcher and Peto in working men in London followed up between 1961 and 1969, which showed that smoking accelerated the decline in forced expiratory volume in 1 s (**FEV1**), but failed to show a correlation between the degree of mucus hypersecretion and an accelerated decline in FEV$_1$ or mortality. By contrast, mortality was strongly related to the development of low FEV$_1$.

More recent data, from a study of 15 000 adults from the general population in Copenhagen followed up between 1976 and 1994, suggested that mucus hypersecretion was not such an innocent phenomenon, since it was associated with increased risk of hospital admission and accelerated decline in FEV$_1$. Moreover, as the FEV$_1$ decreases, the association between mucus hypersecretion and mortality becomes stronger. Differences in the degree of airflow obstruction between the populations in these two studies may explain the different findings.

Cigarette smoking

Cigarette smoking is the single most important identifiable aetiological factor in COPD. However, only 10 to 20 per cent of smokers develop clinically significant COPD, whilst approximately half will never develop a clinically significant physiological deficit. In general, the greater the total tobacco exposure, the greater the risk of developing COPD. However, for any exposure there are clearly individual variations in susceptibility to the effects of tobacco smoke (Fig. 1). Although smoking is the dominant risk factor, COPD does occur in non-smokers, such as in patients with α$_1$-antitrypsin deficiency.

The most important evidence linking smoking and mortality from bronchitis comes from a study of 40 000 medical practitioners in the United Kingdom who recorded their smoking habits. In male doctors, mortality from chronic bronchitis fell between 1953 and 1967 by 24 per cent, compared with a fall of only 4 per cent in other men in the United Kingdom of the same age. This difference was attributed to the decrease in smoking in doctors compared with an overall increase in smoking in the general population.

Passive smoking

There is a trend to an increased relative risk of the development of chronic airflow obstruction from passive smoking, but not powerful enough to demonstrate statistical significance. Cumulative lifetime exposure to environmental tobacco smoke during childhood is associated with significantly lower peak levels of FEV$_1$ in adulthood. Maternal smoking is associated with low birth weight, and smoking by either parent is associated with an increased incidence of respiratory illnesses in the first 3 years of life.

Air pollution

The introduction of the clean air acts (1956, 1965) led to a reduction in smoke and sulphur dioxide levels during the 1960s, which produced less discernible peaks of pollution related to morbidity and mortality, compared with the 1950s. More recent studies show an association between respiratory symptoms in patients with airways disease, general practitioner consultations, and hospital admissions in patients with airways diseases at levels of particulate air pollution below 100 μg/m^3, levels that are currently experienced in many urban areas in Europe and the United Kingdom. Furthermore, levels of particulate air pollution are associated with deaths from all causes, particularly cardiorespiratory deaths.

Although there have been associations between exacerbations of airways diseases and photochemical air pollutants, such as nitrogen dioxide and ozone, this association has been largely confined to patients with asthma. There are a few longitudinal studies on the effects of air pollution on decline in lung function, but the data are conflicting. Indoor air pollution, for example as a result of the use of biomass fuel for cooking is associated with the development of COPD in low income countries, particularly in women.

Protease inhibitor deficiency

α$_1$-Antitrypsin or α$_1$-protease inhibitor is a polymorphic glycoprotein that is responsible for most of the antiprotease activity in the serum. Laurell and

Eriksson in 1963 were the first to describe the association between α$_1$-antitrypsin deficiency and the development of early onset emphysema, and that the abnormality was transmitted as an autosomal recessive gene. Since the discovery of the deficiency, over 75 biochemical variants have been described relating to their electrophoretic properties, giving rise to the phase inhibitor (**Pi**) nomenclature. The commonest allele in all populations is PiM and the most common genotype is PiMM, which occurs in

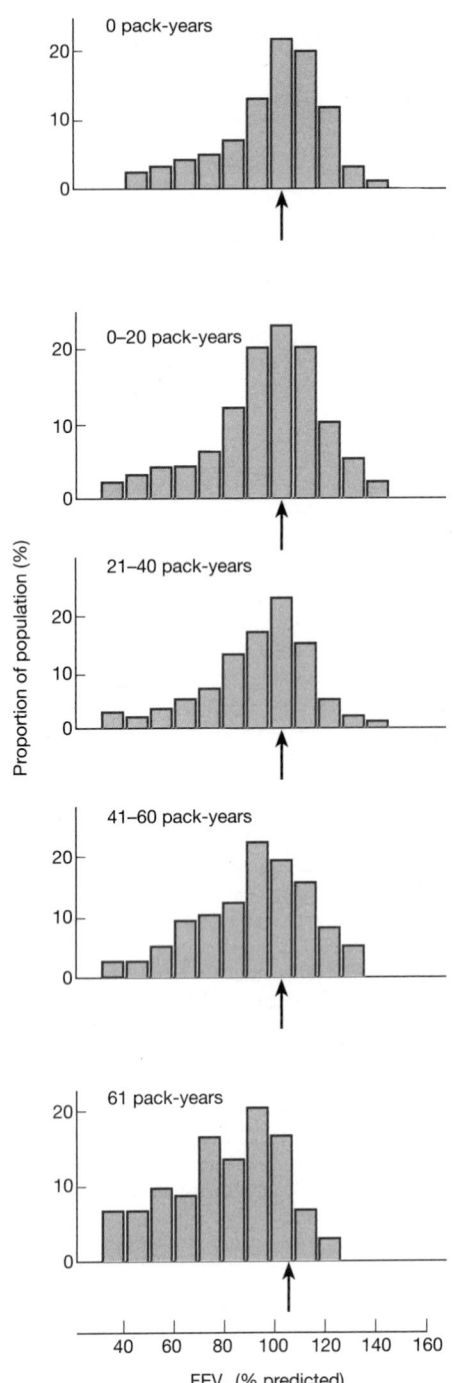

Fig. 1 Effect of increasing cigarette smoke consumption on FEV$_1$. Although the mean FEV$_1$ falls as smoking consumption increases, there is a wide variation in this effect, suggesting variable susceptibility to the effects of tobacco smoke. (Adapted from Burrows B et al., 1977, *American Journal of Respiratory and Critical Care Medicine* **115**, 195–205.)

around 86 per cent of the United Kingdom population. PiMZ and PiMS are the next two commonest genotypes and are associated with α_1-protease inhibitor levels of between 50 and 75 per cent of mean levels of PiMM subjects, as is the much less common PiSS type. The homozygous PiZZ type, in which serum levels are 10 to 20 per cent of the average normal value, is the strongest genetic risk factor for the development of emphysema. The most important other type is PiSZ, where basal levels are 35 to 50 per cent of normal values. A few rare variants that result in complete functional absence of α_1-protease inhibitor account for the remainder of the severely deficient patients.

In the United States, screening of adult blood donors identified a 1 in 2700 prevalence of PiZZ subjects, of which most had normal spirometry. Around 1 in 5000 children in the United Kingdom are born with the homozygous deficiency (PiZZ). However, the number of subjects identified with disease is much less than predicted from the known prevalence of the deficiency. Therefore it is by no means inevitable that all individuals with a homozygous deficiency develop respiratory disease. Indeed a few PiZZ individuals live beyond their sixth decade and escape the development of progressive airways obstruction. Prospective follow-up of PiZZ subjects has shown a greatly accelerated decline in FEV_1, but with large variations among individuals. There is a clear interaction with cigarette smoking, but this cannot entirely account for the variation in the decline in FEV_1 observed. Life expectancy of subjects deficient in α_1-protease inhibitor is significantly reduced, especially if they smoke.

Occupation

It is generally accepted that there is a causal link between occupational dust exposure and the development of mucus hypersecretion. Cigarette smoke has been a confounding feature since the prevalence of smoking remains disproportionately high in many workers who are exposed to dust. Longitudinal studies on workforces exposed to dusts show an association with dust exposure and a more rapid decline in FEV_1 and increased mortality.

The accumulating evidence for an association between coal dust exposure and the development of COPD led recently to the establishment of COPD as a disease that is considered for compensation in miners in the United Kingdom. A small, but significant effect of exposure to welding fumes on the development of COPD was shown in a study of shipyard workers. Workers exposed to cadmium have an increased risk of emphysema.

Chronic bronchopulmonary infection

Studies in the 1960s and 1970s in men with chronic bronchitis demonstrated that prophylactic antibiotics to prevent recurrent infective exacerbations did not slow the decline in lung function. However, acute bronchopulmonary infection was associated with an acute decline in lung function that may persist for several weeks, but which usually recovers completely.

Cough and sputum production between the ages of 20 and 36 years is more commonly reported in those with a history of chest illness in childhood. The association between childhood respiratory illness and ventilatory impairment in adulthood is probably multifactorial. Several factors such as low economic status, greater exposure to passive smoking, poor diet and housing, and residence in areas of high pollution may all contribute to this finding.

Growth and nutrition

Several recent studies have suggested that mortality from chronic respiratory diseases and adult ventilatory function correlate inversely with birth weight and weight at 1 year of age. Thus, impaired growth *in utero* may be a risk factor for the development of chronic respiratory diseases.

One study of British adults has shown that there is a correlation between consumption of fresh fruit in the diet and ventilatory function, a relationship that held both in smokers and in those who had never smoked. Dietary factors, particularly a low intake of vitamin C and low plasma levels of ascorbic acid, were related to a diagnosis of bronchitis in the United States National Health and Nutrition Examination Survey.

Atopy and airway hyperresponsiveness

In the 1960s Dutch workers proposed that smokers with chronic, largely irreversible airways obstruction and subjects with asthma shared a common constitutional predisposition to allergy, airway hyperresponsiveness, and eosinophilia—the 'Dutch hypothesis'. Numerous studies have shown that smokers tend to have higher levels of IgE and higher eosinophil counts than non-smokers, but the levels are not as high as those in individuals with asthma. Studies in middle-aged smokers with a degree of impairment of lung function show a positive correlation between accelerated decline in FEV_1 and increased airway responsiveness to either methacholine or histamine. However, atopic status, as defined by positive skin tests, does not differ between smokers and those who have never smoked.

Whether airway hyperresponsiveness is a cause or consequence of COPD is still a matter of debate.

Epidemiology

Prevalence

The symptom of mucus hypersecretion has been extensively studied in general population surveys over the last 40 years. In these studies, usually in middle-aged men, the prevalence of chronic cough and sputum production ranges between 15 and 53 per cent, with a lower prevalence of between 8 and 22 per cent in women, being more prevalent in urban than in rural areas. A study in the late 1980s showed a decline in the prevalence of chronic cough and phlegm in middle-aged men to 15 to 20 per cent, with little change in women.

Prevalence studies of COPD are normally based on values of percentage of predicted FEV_1, which defines individuals with and without airways obstruction. In a survey in 1987 of a representative sample of 2484 men and 3063 women in the United Kingdom, in the age range 18 to 64 years, 10 per cent of men and 11 per cent of women had an FEV_1 that was greater than 2 standard deviations below their predicted values, the numbers increasing with age, particularly in smokers. In current smokers in the age range 40 to 65 years, 18 per cent of men had an FEV_1 greater than 2 standard deviations below normal and 14 per cent of women, compared with 7 and 6 per cent of male and female non-smokers, respectively.

Studies from the United States, which used a lower limit of normal for FEV_1 of less than 65 per cent of the predicted value, show the prevalence of COPD in men falling from 8 per cent in the 1960s to 6 per cent in the late 1970s, whereas in women the prevalence of 3 per cent did not change over a similar period. National surveys of consultations in British general practices have shown a modest decline in the number of middle-aged men consulting their doctor with symptoms suggestive of COPD and a slight increase among middle-aged women. These trends are confounded by changes over the years in the application of the diagnostic labels for this condition, particularly the overlap between COPD and asthma.

Mortality

There are large international variations in the death rate for COPD, which cannot be entirely explained by differences in diagnostic patterns, labels, or by differences in smoking habits (Fig. 2). COPD is often a contributory factor to the cause of death, and thus figures from death certification underestimate the mortality from COPD. Most of the mortality from this condition occurs in the over 65 years age group. Within the United Kingdom, age-adjusted death rates from chronic respiratory diseases vary by a factor of 5 to 10 in different geographical locations. Mortality rates tend to be higher in urban areas than in rural areas.

Mortality from chronic respiratory disease (ICD 9 490–493 and 496) in males aged 55 to 84 years has been falling, except in the group over 75 years

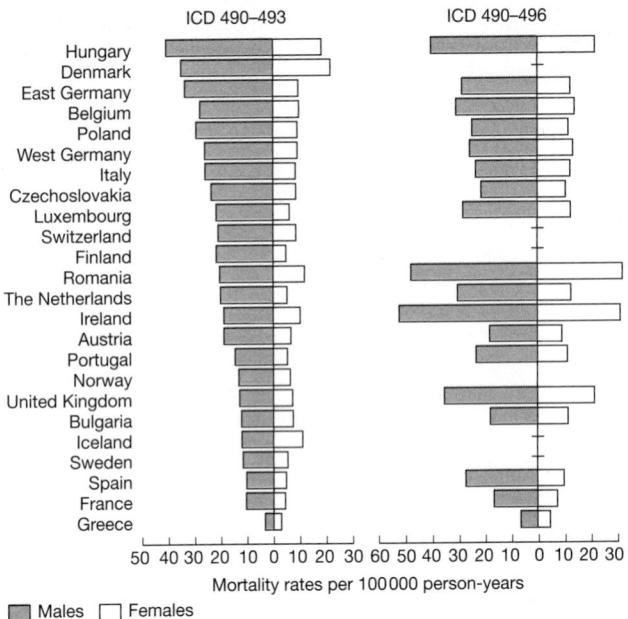

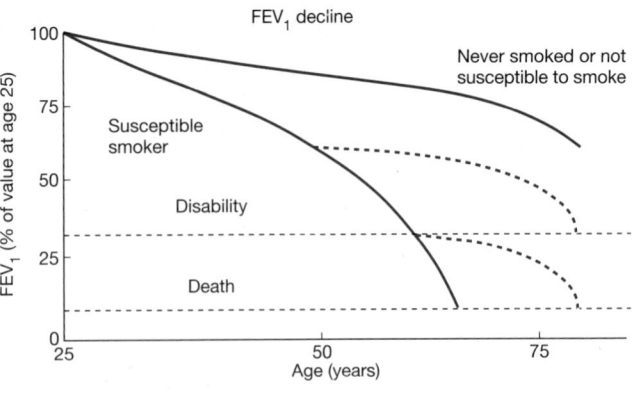

Fig. 3 The effect of age upon airflow obstruction in normal subjects and susceptible cigarette smokers. Cessation of smoking (dotted curved lines) returns the rate of decline to normal.

Fig. 2 Age standardized mortality rates in Europe, 1988 to 1991, for chronic obstructive pulmonary disease (COPD). ICD 490–496 = COPD and similar conditions. Closed bars to the left indicate mortality rates in males; open bars to the right in females. (Adapted from Siafakas NM et al., 1995, European Respiratory Journal **8**, 1398–420.)

of age. Similar trends have been recorded in American men, whereas in women (whose mortality is one-third that of men) the decline in mortality which was recorded until 1975 has since shown a slight increase in those over the age of 65 years. These trends presumably relate to the later time of the peak prevalence of cigarette smoking in women compared with men.

In the United Kingdom there are around 30 000 deaths per year from COPD. These accounted for 6.4 per cent of all male deaths and 3.9 per cent of all deaths in females in 1994.

Morbidity/use of health resources

COPD places an enormous burden on health-care resources. An estimate of the annual workload in primary and secondary care attributable to COPD and its associated conditions in an average United Kingdom health district is shown in Table 1. It has been calculated that airways diseases (chronic bronchitis and emphysema, COPD, and asthma) account for 24.4 million lost working days per year in the United Kingdom, which represents 9 per cent of all certified sickness absence among men, and 3.5 per cent of the total among women. Respiratory diseases in the United Kingdom rank as

Table 1 Estimated annual health service workload due to chronic respiratory disease in an average United Kingdom health district serving 250 000 persons

	Hospital admissions	Inpatient bed-days	General practice consultations
Chronic bronchitis	100	1500	4400
Emphysema and COPD	240	3300	2700
Asthma	410	1800	11900
Chronic bronchitis, emphysema, asthma, and COPD	750	6600	19000

Modified from Anderson et al. (1994). Epidemiologically based needs assessment: lower respiratory disease. Department of Health, London.

the third commonest cause of days of certified incapacity; COPD accounting for 56 per cent of these days lost in males and 24 per cent in females.

History and prognosis

Severe airways obstruction occurs in susceptible smokers as a result of years of an accelerated decline in FEV_1. In non-smokers the FEV_1 declines at a rate of 20 to 30 ml/year (Fig. 3); this occurs at a faster rate in smokers, reported changes in FEV_1 in patients with COPD being more than 50 ml/year. Fletcher and colleagues found a relationship between the initial level of FEV_1 and the annual rate of decline in FEV_1 over a follow-up period of 8 years in working men in London. From these data they suggested that susceptible cigarette smokers could be identified in early middle age by a reduction in the FEV_1 (Fig. 3). They also suggested that there was a tracking effect, whereby individuals in the highest or lowest FEV_1 percentiles remained in the same percentiles over subsequent years. Support for the tracking effect comes from a study of 2718 working men, whose pulmonary function was assessed in the 1950s and subsequently followed up over 20 years. In those whose initial FEV_1 was more than 2 standard deviations below predicted values, the risk of death from chronic airways obstruction was 50 times greater than those whose initial FEV_1 was above average. There is a tendency for annual rates of decline in FEV_1 to be slower in advanced than in mild disease.

The strongest predictors of survival in patients with COPD are age and baseline FEV_1. Less than 50 per cent of patients whose FEV_1 has fallen to 30 per cent of predicted are alive 5 years later. There is an even stronger relationship between survival and the post-, rather than prebronchodilator FEV_1. Other unfavourable prognostic factors include severe hypoxaemia, raised pulmonary arterial pressure, and low carbon monoxide transfer, which become apparent in patients with severe disease. Factors favouring improved survival are stopping smoking and a large bronchodilator response. A reduced FEV_1 is also an important additional risk factor for lung cancer, independent of age or cigarette smoking.

Pathology

The pathological changes in patients with COPD are complex and occur in both the large and small airways, and in the alveolar compartment. The relative contributions that the pathological changes in the airways and those of emphysema make to airways obstruction have been the subject of considerable study. In general, pathological changes correlate rather poorly with both clinical and functional patterns of the disease. As a result there is still no clear consensus on whether the fixed airway obstruction in COPD is largely due to inflammation and scarring in the small airways, resulting in narrowing of the airway lumen, or to loss of support for the airways due to loss of alveolar walls, as in emphysema. Although the pathology of COPD is complex, it can be simplified by considering separately the three sites described above in which pathological changes could, in smokers, produce a clinical pattern of largely fixed airways obstruction. The clinicopathological picture is complicated by the fact that these three entities, or any combination of the three, may exist in an individual patient.

Chronic bronchitis

The pathological basis of hypersecretion of mucus is an increase in the volume of the submucosal glands, and an increase in the number and a change in the distribution of goblet cells in the surface epithelium. Submucosal glands are confined to the bronchi, decrease in number and in size in the smaller, more peripheral bronchi, and are not present in the bronchioles.

In healthy subjects who have never smoked, goblet cells are predominantly seen in the proximal airways, and decrease in number in more distal airways, being normally absent in terminal or respiratory bronchioles. By contrast, in smokers, goblet cells not only increase in number, but extend more peripherally.

The use of bronchoscopy to obtain airway cells by bronchoalveolar lavage and bronchial tissue samples by biopsy has added new insights into the role of inflammation in COPD. Bronchial biopsy studies confirm those of resected lung material, which show bronchial wall inflammation in this condition. As in asthma, bronchial biopsies in patients with chronic bronchitis reveal that activated T lymphocytes are prominent in the proximal airway walls. However, in contrast to asthma, macrophages are also a prominent feature and the CD8 suppresser T-lymphocyte subset, rather than the CD4 subset, predominates.

Bronchial biopsies from limited studies in patients during exacerbations of chronic bronchitis show increased numbers of eosinophils in the bronchial walls, although their numbers are small compared with exacerbations of asthma and, by contrast to those in asthma, these cells do not appear to have degranulated.

Bronchoalveolar lavage, or more recently studies of spontaneously produced or induced sputum, have shown increased intraluminal airspace inflammation in patients with chronic bronchitis, with or without airways obstruction, and predominantly neutrophils and macrophages in bronchoalveolar lavage studies. There is also evidence that airspace inflammation in patients with chronic bronchitis persists following smoking cessation if the production of sputum persists.

These studies of sputum and bronchial biopsies in chronic bronchitis have mainly sampled the proximal airways. Recent studies suggest that inflammatory changes present in the large airways may reflect those present in the small airways, and perhaps even in the alveolar walls.

Emphysema

Airspace enlargement can be identified macroscopically on the cut surface of an inflated lung when the airspace size reaches 1 mm. Two major types of emphysema are recognized, according to the distribution of enlarged airspaces within the acinar unit (Fig. 4):

(1) centriacinar (or centrilobular) emphysema, in which enlarged airspaces are initially clustered around the terminal bronchiole; and

(2) panacinar (or panlobular) emphysema, where the enlarged airspaces are distributed throughout the acinar unit.

Centriacinar emphysema is more common in the upper zones of the upper and lower lobes: panacinar emphysema may be found anywhere in the lungs, but is more prominent at the bases, and is associated with α_1-protease inhibitor deficiency. Both types of emphysema can occur alone or in combination in a patient with emphysema. There is still debate over whether centriacinar and panacinar emphysema represent different disease processes, and hence have different aetiologies, or whether panacinar emphysema is a progression from centriacinar emphysema. There is a

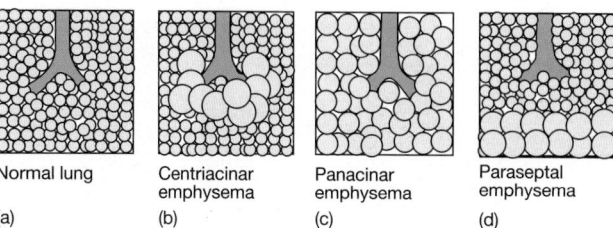

| Normal lung | Centriacinar emphysema | Panacinar emphysema | Paraseptal emphysema |
| (a) | (b) | (c) | (d) |

Fig. 4 Diagramatic representation of the distribution of abnormal airspaces within the acinar unit in different types of emphysema. (a) This represents the acinar unit in a normal lung, (b) shows the focal enlargement airspaces around the respiratory bronchioles in centriacinar emphysema, (c) shows the confluent even involvement of the acinar unit in panacinar emphysema, and (d) shows the peripherally distributed enlarged airspaces abutting the pleura in paraseptal emphysema. (Adapted from Lamb (1995). In: Calverley P, Pride N, eds. *Chronic obstructive pulmonary disease*, pp.9–34. Chapman and Hall, London.)

clearer association between centriacinar emphysema and cigarette smoking than with panacinar emphysema. Smokers with centriacinar emphysema have more small airways disease than those patients with predominantly panacinar emphysema.

Periacinar (or paraseptal or distal acinar) emphysema describes enlarged airspaces along the edge of the acinar unit, but only where it abuts against a fixed structure such as the pleura or a vessel. This is less common and usually of little clinical significance except when extensive in a subpleural position and may be associated with pneumothorax.

Scar or irregular emphysema is used to describe enlarged airspaces around the margins of a scar, unrelated to the structure of the acinus. This lesion is excluded from the current definition of emphysema.

A bulla represents a localized area of emphysema that has locally overdistended; conventionally greater than 1 cm in size.

Absence of fibrosis is a prerequisite in the most recent definition of emphysema. However, fibrosis occurs in the terminal or respiratory bronchioles as part of a respiratory bronchiolitis in asymptomatic cigarette smokers. Furthermore, there is an increase in collagen in the lung parenchyma in smokers compared with non-smokers.

The bronchioles and small bronchi are supported by attachment to the outer aspect of their walls of adjacent alveolar walls. This arrangement maintains the tubular integrity of the airways. It has been suggested that loss of these attachments may lead to distortion and irregularity of airways, which results in airflow limitation (Fig. 5).

Bronchiolitis/small airways disease

Hogg, Macklem, and Thurlbeck introduced the concept of 'small airways disease' in studies using a retrograde catheter in which they showed that the increased flow resistance in the lungs in patients with COPD largely occurred in the small airways at the periphery of the lungs. Several pathological changes are found in small airways (Fig. 6):

- inflammatory infiltrate in the airway wall

- mucus and cells in lumen

- goblet cell hyperplasia

- fibrosis in the airway wall

- squamous cell metaplasia

- mucosal ulceration

- increased amount of muscle

- pigmentation.

The pathological changes in the pulmonary vasculature and the right ventricle are described in Section 15.15.2.

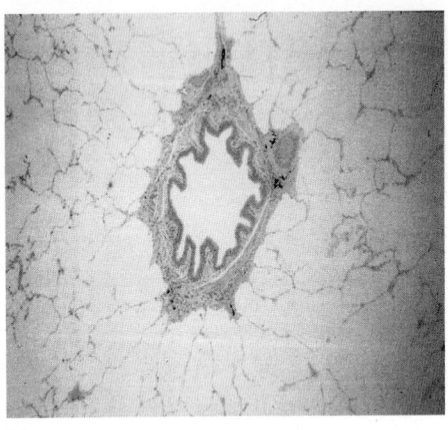
(a)

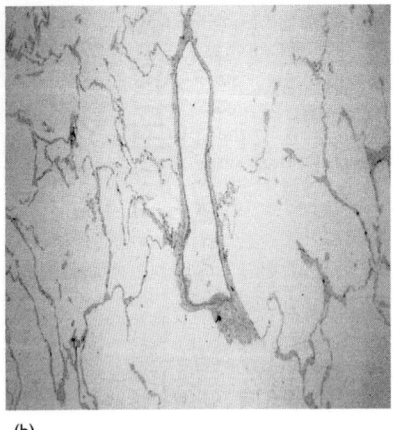
(b)

Fig. 5 (a) Cross-section of a normal small peripheral bronchiole, showing a circular outline supported by adjacent alveolar walls. (b) A small bronchiole at the same magnification in a patient with emphysema. The loss of alveolar supporting walls results in an eliptical airway.

Pathogenesis of COPD

Important to the pathogenesis of COPD were the observations of an association between α_1-antitrypsin deficiency and the development of early onset emphysema, and the development of emphysema following instillation of the proteolytic enzyme papain into rat lungs. These two important observations form the basis of the protease/antiprotease theory of the pathogenesis of emphysema. This hypothesis states that under normal circumstances the release of proteolytic enzymes from inflammatory cells that migrate to the lungs to fight infection does not cause lung damage because of inactivation of these proteolytic enzymes by an excess of inhibitors. However, in conditions of excessive enzyme load, or where there is an absolute or a functional deficiency of antiproteases, an imbalance develops between proteases and antiproteases in favour of proteases, leading to uncontrolled enzyme activity and degradation of lung connective tissue in alveolar walls, resulting in emphysema (Fig. 7).

α_1-Antitrypsin/α_1-protease inhibitor

α_1-Antitrypsin is a potent inhibitor of serine proteases, and has greatest affinity for the enzyme neutrophil elastase. It is synthesized in the liver and increases from its usual plasma concentration of approximately 2 g/l as part of the acute-phase response. The activity of the protein is critically dependent on the methionine–serine sequence at its active site.

The average α_1-antitrypsin plasma levels for the more common phenotypes are shown in Table 2. The Z deficiency state (PiZ) is associated with periodic acid–Schiff (PAS)-positive inclusion bodies in the liver, which represent accumulations of the α_1-antitrypsin protein. Although liver and mononuclear cells from PiZ patients can manufacture normal amounts of mRNA, and the protein can be translated, there is little secretion of the protein. It is now recognized that the Z α_1-antitrypsin gene is normal except for a single point mutation, resulting from substitution of a glycine nucleotide for adenine in the DNA sequence that codes for the amino acid at position 342 on the molecule. This results in spontaneous polymerization of the protein. Large polymers of α_1-antitrypsin accumulate in the liver and are unable to pass through the rough endoplasmic reticulum. Their accumulation impairs α_1-antitrypsin secretion.

Pathogenesis of emphysema in patients without α_1-antitrypsin

The pathogenic mechanisms of emphysema and also of the small airways disease in COPD are clearly more complex than in patients with α_1-antitrypsin. In this case the clearest association is with cigarette smoking, but since only 15 to 20 per cent of cigarette smokers develop COPD, the question of susceptibility has to be considered. The development of pulmonary emphysema in smokers is thought to occur as a result of several mechanisms:

- increased protease burden
- oxidant/antioxidant imbalance
- decreased antiprotease function
- decreased synthesis of elastin.

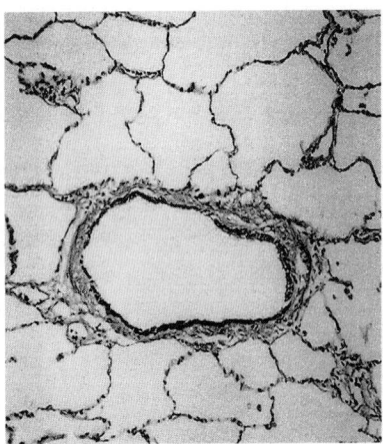

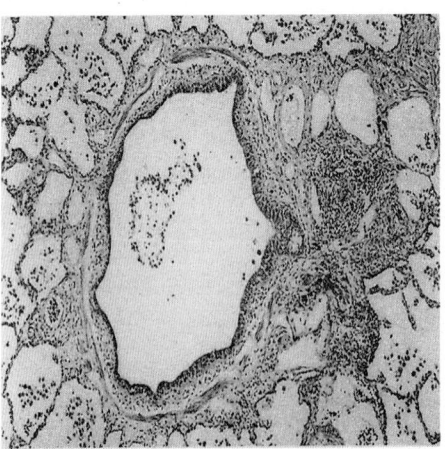

Fig. 6 Normal bronchiole (left) and a bronchiole of a patient with small airways disease/bronchiolitis (right), showing marked increase in inflammatory cells in the walls and in the airway lumen.

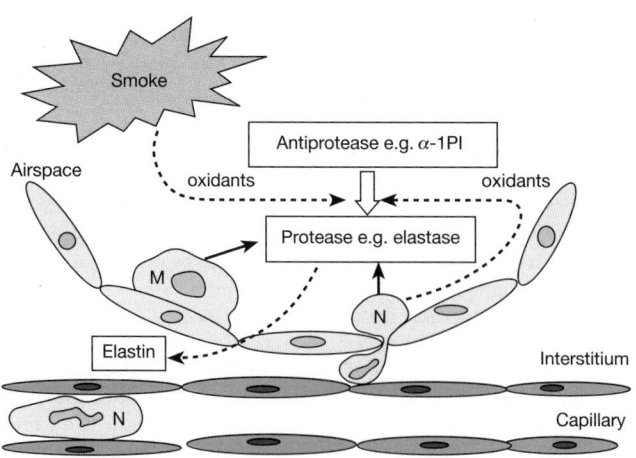

Fig. 7 Simplified protease/antiprotease theory of the pathogenesis of emphysema. Neutrophils (N) sequester in the pulmonary capillaries, initially as a result of the oxidant effect of cigarette smoke that decreases neutrophil deformability. Activated neutrophils adhere to the endothelial cells and subsequently migrate into the airspaces. Oxidants either directly from cigarette smoke or released from activated airspace neutrophils inactivate antiproteases such as α_1-protease inhibitor (α_1-PI) reducing its ability to bind to and hence inactivate proteases, particularly elastase. This allows active elastase to enter the lung interstitium and bind to and destroy elastin, causing destruction and enlargement of the distal airspace walls. This simplified protease/antiprotease theory is complicated by the presence of other antiproteases such as antileucoprotease, and other proteases such as metalloproteases released from macrophages (M). There is also the potential for neutrophils to be activated and release elastase while sequestered in the pulmonary capillaries without the need to migrate.

Proteases other than neutrophil elastase and antiproteases other than α_1-protease inhibitor may be involved in the protease–antiprotease imbalance in emphysema (Fig. 7).

Pathophysiology

Lung mechanics

The characteristic physiological abnormality in COPD is a decrease in maximum expiratory flow. Two major factors can reduce forced expiratory flow:

(1) loss of lung elasticity; and

(2) an increase in airways resistance in small and/or large airways.

In healthy young subjects significant airway closure only occurs below functional residual capacity (**FRC**). However, enhanced airway closure occurs in the early stages of COPD, which can be measured by plotting the nitrogen concentrations against expired volume following a single vital capacity breath of 100 per cent oxygen. The 'closing volume' measures the

lung volume at which expired nitrogen concentrations increase abruptly during slow deflation from total lung capacity (**TLC**) and is determined by the lung volume at which some lung units close their airways and hence stop emptying. In healthy young non-smokers, closing volume is about 5 to 10 per cent of vital capacity (**VC**), rising to 25 to 35 per cent of VC in old age. Compared with non-smokers, young asymptomatic adult smokers have an increase in closing volume. As airways disease progresses the ability to define a closing volume decreases and therefore the test is not useful in established disease. Asymptomatic smokers who develop a reduced FEV_1, initially had an abnormal single-breath nitrogen washout test. Conversely, many subjects who have an abnormal single-breath nitrogen washout test do not develop an abnormal FEV_1.

In comparison with non-smokers, asymptomatic smokers also show frequency dependence of lung compliance, implying increased inequality of time constants in the lungs, resulting from changes in the compliance and resistance of parallel lung compartments. The pathological changes that occur in the peripheral airways in COPD are thought to be reflected in changes in maximum flow at lung volumes below 50 per cent of VC.

Tests of overall lung mechanics such as the FEV_1 and airways resistance are usually abnormal in patients with COPD when breathlessness develops. Residual volume, FRC, and (in some cases) TLC increase. Maximum expiratory flow–volume curves (MEFV) show a characteristic convexity towards the volume axis, initially with preservation of peak expiratory flow (Fig. 8).

The uneven distribution of ventilation in advanced COPD causes a reduction in 'ventilated' lung volume and thus the carbon monoxide transfer factor (TL_{CO}) is almost always reduced, although the TL_{CO} normalized to ventilated alveolar volume (K_{CO}) may remain relatively well preserved in those without emphysema.

The characteristic changes in the static pressure/volume (P/V) curve of the lungs in COPD are an increase in static compliance and a reduction in static transpulmonary pressure at a standard lung volume (Fig. 9). These changes are generally thought to indicate emphysema.

The major site of the fixed airway narrowing in COPD is in the peripheral airways less than 2 to 3 mm in diameter. In addition, loss of lung elastic recoil pressure is also important in terms of airways obstruction, particularly in those with severe emphysema, as a result of a reduction in the distending force on all of the intrathoracic airways. Dynamic expiratory compression of the airways is enhanced by loss of lung recoil and by atrophic changes in the airways and loss of support from the surrounding alveolar walls, allowing flow limitation at lower driving pressures and flows.

Table 2 α_1-Antitrypsin phenotypes: frequency in United Kingdom population, concentration of serum α_1-protease inhibitor, and the risk for emphysema

Phenotype	Frequency (%)	Average concentration (g/l)	Risk factor for emphysema
MM	86	2	No
MS	9	1.6	No
MZ	3	1.2	No
SS	0.25	1.2	No
SZ	0.2	0.8	Yes
ZZ	0.03	0.4	Yes

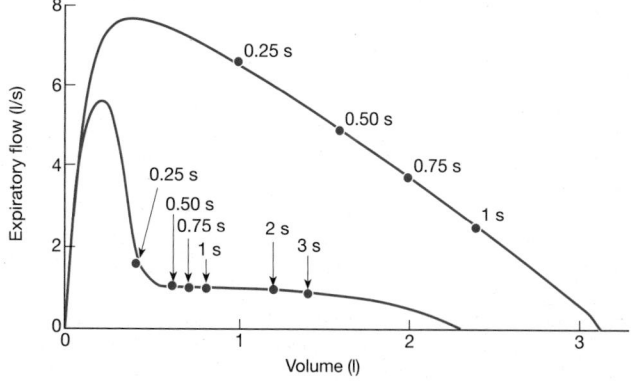

Fig. 8 Maximum flow–volume curves in a healthy subject (FEV_1 2.4 litres) and a subject with COPD and airways obstruction (FEV_1 0.8 litres). The development of convexity of the expiratory curve in mild obstruction is characteristic, as is the relative preservation of peak expiratory flow in the patient with COPD compared to the FEV_1. The figures on the flow–volume curve represent time in seconds for both curves.

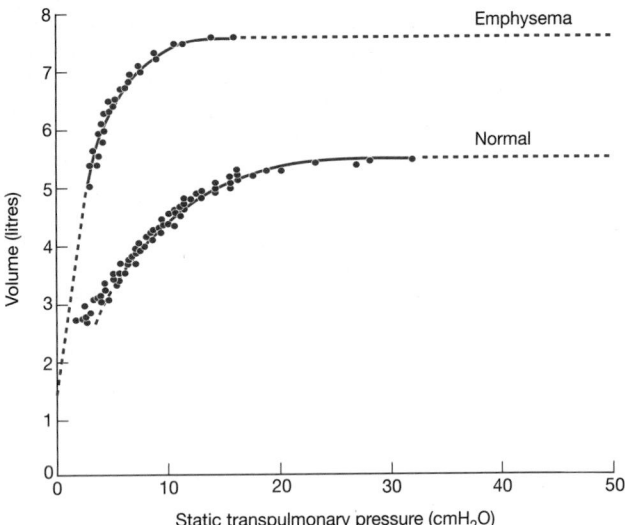

Fig. 9 Static expiratory pressure–volume curves of lungs in a subject with severe emphysema compared with a normal subject. The broken lines represent extrapolation of the curve to infinite pressure and to the volume axis at zero pressure.

Pulmonary gas exchange

Ventilation–perfusion (V/Q) mismatching is the most important cause of impaired pulmonary gas exchange in COPD. Other causes such as alveolar hypoventilation, impaired alveolar–capillary diffusion to oxygen, and increased shunt are of much less importance. The distribution of ventilation is very uneven in patients with COPD. A reduction of blood flow is produced by several mechanisms including local destruction of vessels in alveolar walls as a result of emphysema, hypoxic vasoconstriction in areas of severe alveolar hypoxaemia, and passive vascular obstruction as a result of increased alveolar pressure and distension.

Respiratory muscles

In patients with severe COPD a combination of pulmonary overinflation and malnutrition, resulting in muscle weakness, reduces the capacity of the respiratory muscles to generate pressure over the range of tidal breathing. In addition, the load against which the respiratory muscles need to act is increased, due to the increase in airways resistance. Overinflation of the lungs leads to shortening and flattening of the diaphragm, thus impairing its ability to generate pressure in order to lower pleural pressure. During quiet tidal breathing in normal subjects, expiration is largely passive and depends on the elastic recoil of the lungs and the chest wall. Patients with COPD increasingly need to use their rib cage muscles and inspiratory accessory muscles, such as the sternomastoids, even during quiet breathing. During exercise, this pattern may be even more distorted and result in paradoxical motion of the rib cage.

Patients with COPD have impaired values of global function of the respiratory muscles such as maximum inspiratory mouth pressures (Pe_{max}), although these measurements are very effort dependent. Diaphragmatic function can be assessed during inspiration by measurement of transdiaphragmatic pressure (Pdi), using balloon-tipped catheters with small transducers placed in the oesophagus and stomach. Measurements of Pdi are reduced in patients with COPD.

Cor pulmonale

Pulmonary arterial hypertension occurs late in the course of COPD with the development of hypoxaemia (Pao_2 less than 8 kPa) and usually also hypercapnia. It is the major cardiovascular complication of COPD and is associated with the development of right ventricular hypertrophy ('cor pul-

monale') and poor prognosis. Further details can be found in Section 15.15.2.

Clinical features

Symptoms

Patients with COPD characteristically complain of the symptoms of breathlessness on exertion, sometimes accompanied by wheeze and cough, which is often, but not invariably, productive. Breathlessness is the symptom that commonly causes the patient to seek medical attention and is usually the most disabling problem. Patients often date the onset of their illness to an acute exacerbation of cough with sputum production, which leaves them with a degree of chronic breathlessness. However, close questioning will usually reveal the presence of a 'smoker's cough', with the production of small amounts of mucoid sputum, often predominating in the morning, for many years.

A smoking history of at least 20 pack years is usual before symptoms develop, commonly in the fifth decade, following which there is progression through the clinical stages of mild, moderate, and severe disease. Breathlessness, usually first noticed on climbing hills or stairs, or hurrying on level ground, heralds the development of moderate impairment of airway function and patients may adapt their breathing pattern and their behaviour to minimize the sensation of breathlessness. The perception of breathlessness varies greatly for individuals with the same impairment of ventilatory capacity. However, when the FEV_1 has fallen to 30 per cent or less of the predicted values, breathlessness is usually present on minimal exertion. Severe breathlessness is often affected by changes in temperature and occupational exposure to dust and fumes. Some patients have severe orthopnoea, relieved by leaning forward, whereas others find greatest ease when lying flat. Breathlessness can be assessed on the Medical Research Council, Borg, and Visual Analogue scales.

A productive cough occurs in up to 50 per cent of cigarette smokers, may precede the onset of breathlessness, and many patients may dismiss this as simply a 'smoker's cough'. The frequency of nocturnal cough does not appear to be increased in stable COPD. Paroxysms of coughing in the presence of severe airway obstruction generate high intrathoracic pressures, which can produce syncope and 'cough fractures' of the ribs. Wheeze is common, but not specific to COPD, since it is due to turbulent airflow in large airways from any cause.

Chest pain is common in patients with COPD, but is often unrelated to the disease itself, and may be due to underlying ischaemic heart disease or gastro-oesophageal reflux. Chest tightness is a common complaint during exacerbations of breathlessness, particularly during exercise, and this is sometimes difficult to distinguish from ischaemic cardiac pain. Pleuritic chest pain may suggest an intercurrent pneumothorax, pneumonia, or pulmonary infarction.

Haemoptysis can be associated with purulent sputum and may be due to inflammation or infection. However, this symptom should be treated seriously and the need for investigations for bronchial carcinoma should be considered.

Weight loss and anorexia are features of severe COPD and thought to result from both decreased calorie intake and hypermetabolism. Psychiatric morbidity, particularly depression, is common in patients with severe COPD, reflecting social isolation and the chronicity of the disease. Sleep quality is impaired in advanced COPD, which may contribute to the impaired neuropsychiatric performance.

Occupation/smoking history

A detailed smoking history is important in patients with COPD since the disease is rare in lifelong non-smokers. Although there is, in general, a dose–response relating the number of cigarettes smoked and the level of the FEV_1, there are huge individual variations, reflecting variations in the susceptibility to cigarette smoke (Fig. 1). Occupational exposure to dusts has an additive effect on the decline in lung function, as has been shown in coal miners, where both smoking and years of dust exposure contribute to the decline in FEV$_1$, although the contribution of smoking was three times as great as that of the dust exposure.

Clinical signs

General examination

The physical signs in patients with COPD are not specific, and depend on the degree of airflow limitation and pulmonary overinflation. The sensitivity of physical signs to detect or exclude moderately severe COPD is poor. Tachypnoea may be present in patients with severe COPD and prolonged forced expiratory time (more than 5 s) can be a useful indicator of airway obstruction. The breathing pattern in COPD is often characteristic, with a prolonged expiratory phase, some patients adopting pursed lipped breathing on expiration, which reduces expiratory airway collapse. Use of the accessory muscles of respiration, particularly the steromastoids, is often seen in advanced disease and these patients often adopt the position of leaning forward, supporting themselves with their arms to fix the shoulder girdle, allowing the use of the pectorals and the latissimus dorsi to increase chest wall movement.

Tar-stained fingers emphasize the smoking habit. In advanced disease cyanosis may be present, indicating hypoxaemia, but may be diminished by anaemia or accentuated by polycythaemia, and is a fairly subjective sign. The flapping tremor, associated with hypercapnia, is neither sensitive nor specific, and papilloedema associated with severe hypercapnia is rarely seen. Weight loss may also be apparent in advanced disease, as well as a reduction in muscle mass. Finger clubbing is not a feature of COPD and should suggest the possibility of complicating bronchial neoplasm or bronchiectasis.

Examination of the chest

In the later stages of COPD the chest is often barrel-shaped with a kyphosis and an apparent increased anterior/posterior diameter, horizontal ribs, prominence of the sternal angle, and a wide subcostal angle. Due to the elevation of the sternum, the distance between the suprasternal notch and the cricoid cartilage (normally three finger-breadths) may be reduced. These are all signs of overinflation. An inspiratory tracheal tug may be detected, which has been attributed to the contraction of the low flat diaphragm. The horizontal position of the diaphragm also acts to pull in the lower ribs during inspiration—Hoover's sign. Widening of the xiphisternal angle and abdominal protuberance occur, the latter due to forward displacement of the abdominal contents, giving the appearance of apparent weight gain. Increased intrathoracic pressure swings may result in indrawing of the suprasternal and supraclavicular fossas and of the intercostal muscles.

On percussion of the chest there is decreased hepatic and cardiac dullness, indicating overinflation. A useful sign of gross overinflation is the absence of a dull percussion note, normally due to the underlying heart, over the lower end of the sternum. Breath sounds may have a prolonged expiratory phase, or may be uniformly diminished, particularly in the advanced stages of the disease. Wheeze may be present both on inspiration and expiration, but is not an invariable clinical sign. Crackles may be heard particularly at the lung bases, but are usually scanty and vary with coughing.

Cardiovascular examination

The presence of emphysema or overinflation of the chest produces difficulty in localizing the apex beat and reduces the cardiac dullness. The characteristic signs that indicate the presence or consequences of pulmonary arterial hypertension may be detected in advanced cases. The heave of right ventricular hypertrophy may be palpable at the lower left sternal edge. Heart sounds are generally soft, although the pulmonary component of the second heart sound may be exaggerated in the second left intercostal space. A gallop rhythm may be detectable, with a third sound audible in the fourth intercostal space to the left of the sternum. The jugular venous pressure can be difficult to see in patients with COPD as it swings widely with respiration and is difficult to discern if there is prominent accessory muscle activity. When the fluid retention of cor pulmonale occurs there may be evidence of functional tricuspid incompetence, producing a pansystolic murmur at the left sternal edge. The liver may be tender, pulsatile, and a prominent 'v' wave may be visible in the jugular venous pulse. The liver may also be palpable below the right costal margin as a result of overinflation of the lungs.

Peripheral vasodilatation accompanies hypercapnia, producing warm peripheries with a high-volume pulse. Pitting peripheral oedema may also be present as a result of fluid retention.

Investigation

Physiological assessment

The most important disturbance of respiratory function in COPD is obstruction to forced expiratory airflow. The degree of airflow obstruction cannot be predicted from the symptoms and signs and therefore an assessment of the degree and the progression of airways obstruction should be made. At an early stage of the disease conventional spirometry may reveal no abnormality, since the earliest changes in COPD affect the alveolar walls and small airways, producing a modest increase in peripheral airway resistance that is not reflected in spirometry measurements. Tests of small airway function, such as the frequency dependency of compliance and closing volume may be abnormal. These tests are difficult to perform, have high coefficients of variation, and are only valid when lung elastic recoil is normal and there is no increase in large airway resistance. They are therefore not recommended in normal clinical practice.

Spirometry

Spirometry is the most robust test of airflow limitation in patients with COPD. A low FEV$_1$ with an FEV$_1$/VC ratio below the normal range is a diagnostic criterion for COPD. The rate of decline of the FEV$_1$ can be used to assess susceptibility in cigarette smokers, progression of the disease, and to test reversibility of the airways obstruction. It is important that a volume plateau is reached when performing the FEV$_1$, which can take 15 s or more in patients with severe airways obstruction. If this manoeuvre is not carried out the FVC can be underestimated. The FEV$_1$ as a percentage of the predicted value can be used to assess the severity of the disease (Table 3).

Flow volume loops

Expiratory flows at 75 or 50 per cent of vital capacity have been used as a measure of airflow limitation. These measurements are less reproducible than spirometry, so that abnormal values must fall to below 50 per cent of the predicted values. Flows at lung volumes less than 50 per cent of vital capacity were previously considered to be an indicator of small airways function, but probably provide no more clinically useful information than measurements of FEV$_1$.

Peak expiratory flow

Peak expiratory flow can either be read directly from the flow volume loop or measured with a hand-held peak flow meter; the latter are relatively easy to use and are particularly useful in subjects with asthma for revealing variations in serial measurements. However, in COPD many variations are often within the error of the measurement. The peak expiratory flow may underestimate the degree of airflow obstruction in COPD (Fig. 8).

Lung volumes

Static lung volumes such as total lung capacity (TLC), residual volume (RV), and functional residual capacity (FRC) are measured in patients with COPD to assess the degree of overinflation and gas trapping. Dynamic overinflation occurs particularly during exercise and may be an important determinant of the symptom of breathlessness.

Table 3 Assessment of severity of COPD (from BTS (1997). Guidelines for the management of chronic obstructive pulmonary disease. *Thorax* **52**, Supplement 5.)

	Clinical state	Results of measurements	Use of health-care resources
Mild	Smoker's cough, but little or no breathlessness. No abnormal signs	FEV_1 60–79 per cent of predicted value. FEV_1/VC and other indices of expiratory flow mildly reduced	Unknown—presymptomatic within the community
Moderate	Breathlessness (± wheeze) on exertion, cough (± sputum) and some abnormal signs	FEV_1 40–59 per cent of predicted value, often with increased FRC and reduced $TLco$. Some patients are hypoxaemic, but not hypercapnic	Known to general practitioner with intermittent complaints
Severe	Breathlessness on any exertion. Wheeze, cough prominent. Clinical overinflation usual, plus cyanosis, peripheral oedema, and polycythaemia in some	FEV_1 less than 40 per cent of predicted value, with marked overinflation. $TLco$ variable, but often low. Hypoxaemia usual and hypercapnia in some	Likely to be known to hospital and by general practitioner, with frequent problems and hospital admissions

The standard method of measuring static lung volumes, using the helium dilution technique during rebreathing, may underestimate lung volumes in COPD, particularly in those patients with bullous disease, where the inspired helium does not have time to equilibrate properly in the airspaces. Body plethysmography uses Boyle's law to calculate lung volumes from changes in mouth and plethysmographic pressures. This technique measures trapped air within the thorax, including poorly ventilated areas, and therefore gives higher readings than the helium dilution technique.

Reversibility to bronchodilators

Assessment of reversibility to bronchodilators is recognized as an essential part of the investigation and management of patients with COPD. Reversibility tests are important:

(1) to help distinguish those patients with marked reversibility who have underlying asthma;

(2) to aid with future management; and

(3) since the post-bronchodilator FEV_1 is the best predictor of survival.

There is, however, no agreement on a standardized method of assessing reversibility, which is usually recorded as change in FEV_1 or peak expiratory flow. However, there may be changes in other lung volumes after bronchodilators, such as inspiratory capacity: this may explain why symptoms improve in some patients following a bronchodilator without change in spirometry. An improvement in FEV_1 in response to a bronchodilator does not necessarily predict a symptomatic response.

The European Respiratory Society and the British Thoracic Society guidelines both recommend that changes should only be considered significant if they exceed 200 ml and represent a 15 per cent improvement over the baseline value. A change over baseline of greater than 12 per cent of the predicted normal value is regarded as a significant bronchodilator response by the American Thoracic Society. A third approach, which has received less support, is to express the change in FEV_1 as a percentage of the potential possible change, which is the predicted value minus the baseline value. Daily variations in airway smooth muscle tone may affect the response to bronchodilators in patients with COPD. Thus, when airway smooth muscle tone is higher, and thus FEV_1 is lower, a response to bronchodilators may be more likely to be achieved than when muscle tone is lower and FEV_1 is higher.

It is usually recommended that the response to a bronchodilator be assessed with a large dose, either using repeated doses from a metered dose inhaler, or by the nebulized route, since this produces a larger number of patients with a significant response. In some cases the addition of a second drug, such as an anticholinergic drug to a β-agonist, will produce a further increase in FEV_1.

Reversibility to corticosteroids

Whether all patients with symptomatic COPD should have a formal assessment of steroid reversibility remains controversial. The commonest regimen is the administration of 30 mg of prednisolone for a period of 2 weeks. Those patients who have previously shown a response to nebulized bronchodilators are more likely to show a response to steroids. However, it is not possible to predict the response to corticosteroids in an individual patient.

An alternative approach is to assess the response to inhaled steroids, usually over a 6-week period, measuring the FEV_1 before and after the average of the first 5 days and the last 5 days measurements of peak expiratory flow.

Gas transfer for carbon monoxide ($TLco$)

A low $TLco$ is present in many patients with COPD. Although there is a relationship between the $TLco$ and the extent of microscopic emphysema, the severity of the emphysema in an individual patient cannot be predicted from the $TLco$, nor is a low $TLco$ specific for emphysema. The commonly used method is the single-breath technique, which uses alveolar volume calculated from helium dilution during the single-breath test. This will underestimate alveolar volume in patients with severe COPD, producing a lower value for the $TLco$.

Arterial blood gases

Arterial blood gases are needed to confirm the degree of hypoxaemia and hypercapnia in patients with COPD. It is essential to record the inspired oxygen concentration when reporting blood gases. It is also important to note that it may take at least 30 min for a change in inspired oxygen concentration to have its full effect on the Pao_2, because of long time constants for alveolar gas equilibration in COPD, particularly during exacerbations. Pulse oximetry is increasingly used to measure the level of oxygenation, but should not replace an assessment of blood gas tensions, since measurements of $Paco_2$ are often required. Acid–base status can also be assessed from the arterial pH (hydrogen ion concentration) and the bicarbonate. Increases in $Paco_2$, which can occur rapidly, can be compensated by renal conservation of bicarbonate ions, which is a relatively slow process. Acid–base status, particularly mixed respiratory and metabolic disturbances, can be characterized by plotting values on an acid–base diagram (Fig. 10).

Exercise tests

Exercise increases oxygen consumption and carbon dioxide production from skeletal muscle. Patients with COPD have the same oxygen consumption for a given workload as normal subjects, but because their dead-space ventilation is higher, a larger minute ventilation is needed to maintain a constant carbon dioxide level. Since in many patients expiratory airflow is limited within the tidal volume range, the only way to increase minute ventilation is to increase inspiratory flow and/or shift the end expiratory position. Both of these manoeuvres are problematic in patients with COPD and require more work from already compromised inspiratory muscles, or result in progressive overinflation, which increases both the work of breathing and symptoms. Metabolic acidosis develops at lower work rates in patients with severe COPD. In patients with COPD, progressive cycle exercise is limited by dyspnoea in 40 per cent and by leg fatigue in 25 per cent, probably reflecting general debility.

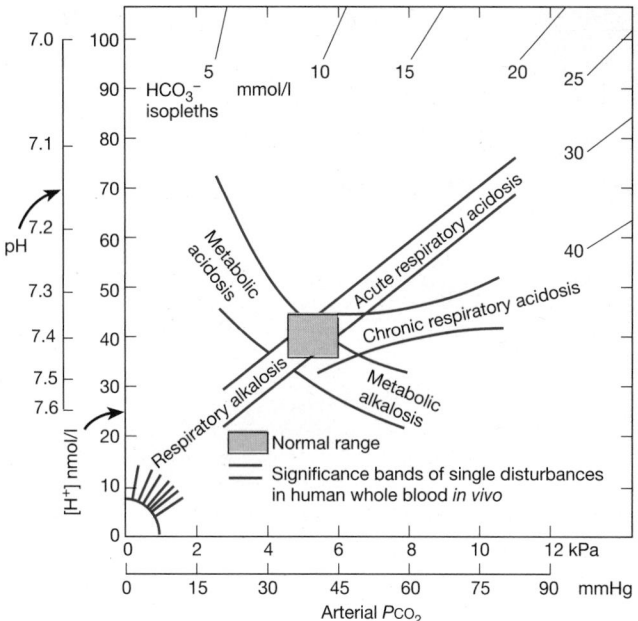

Fig. 10 A non-logarithmic acid–base diagram derived from the measured acid–base status of patients within the five abnormal bands illustrated and of normal subjects (hatched box). This plot of carbon dioxide tension against hydrogen ion concentration (pH) allows the likely acid–base disturbance and calculated bicarbonate value (obtained from the relevant isopleth) to be determined, whilst changes during treatment can be plotted serially for each patient. (Adapted from Flenley DC, 1971, *Lancet* **i**, 961–5.)

Three forms of exercise test can be performed, which provide useful information.

Progressive symptom-limited exercise

In this test the patient is encouraged to maintain exercise, on a treadmill or a cycle, until symptoms prevent them from continuing. A maximum test is usually defined as a heart rate of greater than 85 per cent of predicted or ventilation greater than 90 per cent predicted. The results are useful to assess whether coexisting cardiac or psychological factors contribute to exercise limitation.

Self-paced exercise

These tests are easy to perform. The 6-min walk is the most commonly used test and has a coefficient of variation of around 8 per cent. Shortening the walk to 2 min decreases the reproducibility. The test is only useful in patients with moderately severe COPD (FEV_1 less than 1.5 litres) who would be expected to have an exercise tolerance of less than 600 m in 6 min. There is a weak relationship between walking distance and FEV_1.

Steady-state exercise

This involves exercise at a sustainable percentage of maximum capacity for 3 to 6 min, during which blood gases are measured, enabling calculation of dead space:tidal volume ratio (VD/VT) and shunt. This assessment is seldom required in patients with COPD.

Sleep studies

Hypoxaemia occurs during sleep, particularly rapid eye movement sleep, in patients with COPD. However, measurement of nocturnal hypoxaemia does not provide any further prognostic or clinically useful information in the assessment of patients with COPD, unless coexisting sleep apnoea syndrome is suspected.

Non-physiological assessments

Identifying polycythaemia is important in patients with severe COPD since it predisposes to vascular events. Polycythaemia should be suspected when the haematcrit is greater than 47 per cent in women and 52 per cent in men, and/or the haemoglobin is greater than 16 g/dl in women and 18 g/dl in men, provided other causes of spurious polycythaemia, due to decreased plasma volume, such as caused by dehydration or diuretics, can be excluded.

There is no indication for measuring blood biochemistry routinely in patients with clinically stable COPD. α_1-Antitrypsin levels and phenotype should be measured in all patients under the age of 40 years, and in those with a family history of emphysema at an early age.

Routine electrocardiography is not required in the assessment of patients with COPD and is an insensitive technique in the diagnosis of cor pulmonale.

Radiology

Plain chest radiography

The features on a plain posterior–anterior chest radiograph are not specific for COPD and are usually those of severe emphysema. There may be no abnormalities, even in patients with very appreciable disability. Bronchial wall thickening, shown as parallel line opacities on plain chest radiography, has been described, but this finding may relate to coincidental bronchiectasis. The most reliable radiographic signs of emphysema can be divided into those due to overinflation, vascular changes, and bullae.

Overinflation of the lungs results in the following.

1. There is a low flattened diaphragm (Fig. 11). Low means that the border of the diaphragm in the mid-clavicular line is at or below the anterior end of the sixth or seventh rib. In a flattened diaphragm the maximum perpendicular height from a line drawn between the costal and cardiophrenic angles to the border of the diaphragm is less than 1.5 cm.

2. An increased retrosternal airspace occurs when the horizontal distance from the anterior surface of the aorta to the sternum exceeds 4.5 cm on the lateral film at a point 3 cm below the manubrium.

3. There is an obtuse costophrenic angle on the posterior–anterior or lateral chest radiograph.

4. The inferior margin of the retrosternal airspace is 3 cm or less from the anterior aspect of the diaphragm.

The vascular changes associated with emphysema result from loss of alveolar walls and appear as:

(1) a reduction in size and number of pulmonary vessels, particularly at the periphery of the lung;

(2) vessel distortion, producing increased branching angles, excess straightening, or bowing of vessels; and

(3) areas of transradiency.

A general increased transradiency may be due to an overexposed chest radiograph. Focal areas of transradiency surrounded by hairline walls represent bullae. These may be multiple, as part of a generalized emphysematous process, or localized. An 'increase in lung markings' rather than areas of increased transradiency has often been described in patients with COPD: the cause of these changes is unknown, but may at least be contributed to by non-vascular linear opacities due to scarring.

The accuracy of diagnosing emphysema on the plain chest radiograph increases with the severity of the disease and has been reported as being 50 to 80 per cent accurate in patients with moderate to severe disease. However, the sensitivity has been reported as being as low as 24 per cent in patients with mild to moderate disease.

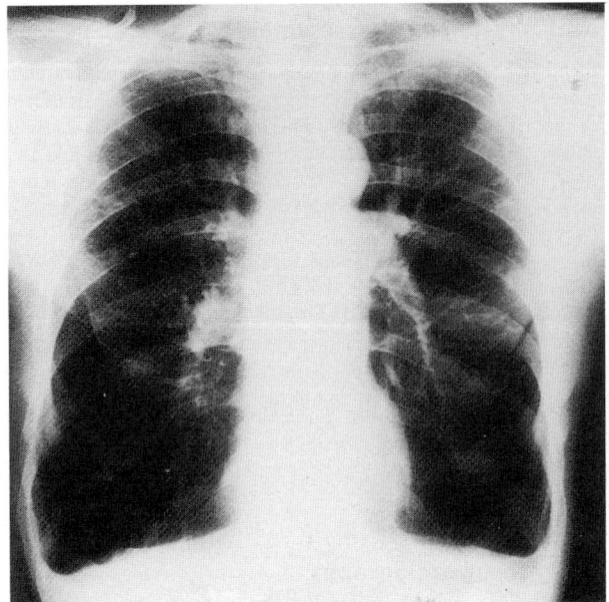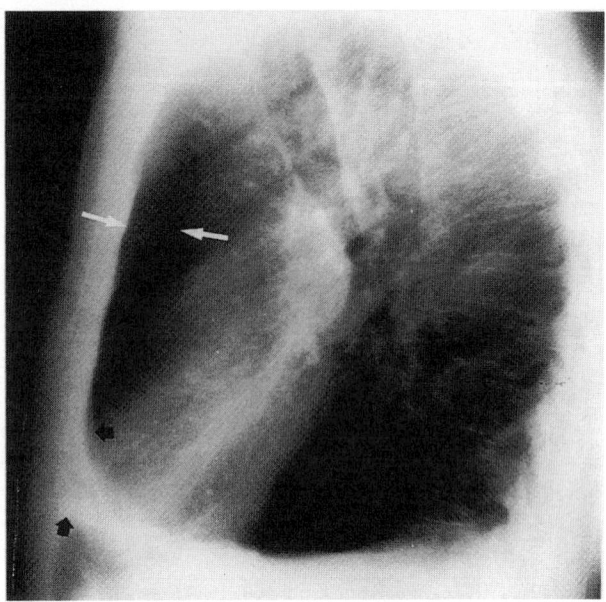

Fig. 11 Generalized (panacinar) emphysema on plain chest radiograph. The diaphragm is low (below the anterior ends of the seventh ribs) and flat. The lower zones are transradient because of oligaemia and there are obtuse costophrenic angles. On the lateral chest radiograph the diaphragm is mildly inverted, the retrosternal transradiency is wide (white arrows) and inferiorly it closely approaches the diaphragm (black arrow).

Computed tomography (CT)

CT scanning has been used since the early 1980s to detect and quantify emphysema. Studies using CT scanning can be divided into those that use visual assessment of low-density areas of the CT scan, which can be either semiquantitative or quantitative, and those that use CT lung density to quantify areas of low x-ray attenuation. These studies roughly divide into those that measure macroscopic or microscopic emphysema, respectively.

A visual assessment of emphysema on CT scan (Fig. 12(a and b)) reveals:

(1) areas of low attenuation without obvious margins or walls;

(2) attenuation and pruning of the vascular tree; and

(3) abnormal vascular configurations.

The sign that correlates best with areas of macroscopic emphysema is an area of low attenuation. However, visual assessment of the extent of macroscopic emphysema by CT scanning is insensitive, subjective, and has a high intra- and interobserver variability. Thus, in most of this type of study CT scanning tends to underestimate the severity of the disease, with centrilobular lesions smaller than 5 mm particularly likely to be missed.

It is possible using high-resolution CT to distinguish the various types of emphysema, particularly when the changes are not severe, depending on the distribution of the lesions.

A more quantitative approach of assessing macroscopic emphysema is by highlighting pixels within the lung fields in a predetermined low-density range, between −910 and −1000 Houndsfield units, the so-called 'density mask' technique. The choice of the density range is fairly arbitrary. A good correlation has been shown between pathological emphysema scores and CT 'density mask' score, but this technique may still miss areas of mild emphysema.

Microscopic emphysema can be quantified by measuring CT lung density. CT density is expressed on a linear scale in Houndsfield units (water = 0; air = −1000). In this range, CT lung density is a direct measure of physical density and is determined by the relative mix of air, blood, and interstitial fluid in tissue. Thus, as emphysema develops, a decrease in alveolar surface area would occur as alveolar walls are lost, associated with an increase in distal airspace size, which would decrease lung CT density in association with a decrease in lung function.

More studies are required before CT lung density can be used as a standardized technique to quantify microscopic emphysema. It is particularly important to define the range of normality, and to standardize the calibration of CT scanners and the lung volume at which scans should be performed. However, at present, CT scanning is the most sensitive and specific imaging technique for assessing emphysema in life and can detect mild emphysema in symptomatic patients with a normal chest radiograph.

Pulmonary hypertension/cor pulmonale

Right ventricular hypertrophy or enlargement produces non-specific cardiac enlargement on the plain chest radiograph, the most widely used measurement to assess the presence of pulmonary hypertension being the width of the right descending pulmonary artery, measured just below the right hilum, where the borders of the artery are delineated against air in the lungs laterally and the right main-stem bronchus medially. The upper limit of the normal range of the width of the artery in this area is taken as 16 mm in males and 15 mm in females. Other studies have suggested an upper limit of normal ranging between 16 and 20 mm, which gives a sensitivity of detecting a pulmonary arterial pressure greater than 20 mmHg of 68 to 95 per cent, with a specificity of 65 to 88 per cent. Although these measurements can be used to detect the presence or absence of pulmonary arterial hypertension, they cannot accurately predict the level of the pulmonary artery pressure, and can therefore only be used as a screening test.

Emphysematous bullae

A bulla has been defined arbitrarily as an emphysematous space greater than 1 cm in diameter. On the plain chest radiograph a bulla appears as a localized avascular area of transradiency, usually separated from the rest of the lung by a curvilinear hairline wall. Marked compression of the surrounding lung may be seen, and bullae may also depress the diaphragm. CT scanning is much more sensitive than plain chest radiography at detecting bullae and can be used to determine their number, size, and position. Ventilation of the bullae can also be assessed using inspiratory/expiratory images. It is also possible to estimate the volume of bullae by measuring the area of the bullae in each CT lung slice.

Prevention

Since tobacco smoking is the major aetiological factor in COPD, the disease is theoretically preventable, with cessation of cigarette smoking the single most important way of affecting the outcome. Other important aetiological factors such as atmospheric pollution are also preventable. In the United Kingdom around 31 per cent of men and 29 per cent of women are current cigarette smokers, and around 80 to 90 per cent of patients with COPD have been regular smokers at sometime in their life. At least 90 per cent of smokers are aware of the adverse health effects of cigarette smoking, 70 per cent wish to give up smoking, and the majority of these have made a serious attempt to quit. However, only 40 per cent of regular smokers have succeeded in quitting cigarette smoking by age 60. Nicotine in tobacco smoke is addictive and regular smokers who reduce or cease their nicotine intake

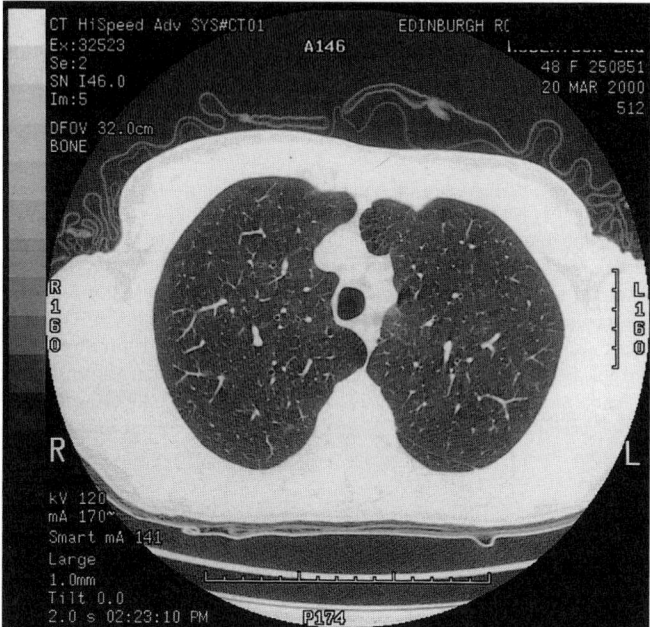

(a)

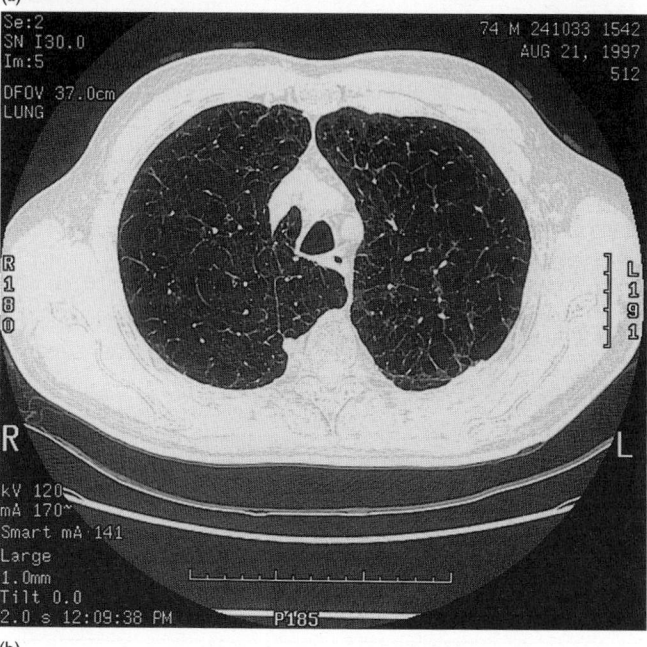

(b)

Fig. 12 High resolution CT scan of (a) normal lung, (b) panacinar emphysema.

experience the characteristic withdrawal syndrome resulting from nicotine craving, manifest as anxiety, lack of concentration, irritability, restlessness, and increased appetite. Nicotine addiction develops rapidly and withdrawal symptoms can be shown to occur even in adolescent smokers. Thus a critical preventive measure is to reduce the number of children starting smoking.

Smoking cessation

Smoking cessation reduces the subsequent decline in lung function (Fig. 3), therefore smoking cessation is the single most important step that can be taken to prevent the progression of the disease. This is particularly true during the early stages of COPD, where both symptoms and lung function may improve. In advanced disease, quitting smoking may not improve pulmonary function, but symptoms such as cough may still improve.

Every patient who smokes should have a discussion of the implications for their future health. Asking about smoking habit in every patient may have a positive reinforcing effect against starting smoking in non-smokers. The reported success rates of smoking cessation interventions come mainly from studies conducted in a primary care setting, and vary between 10 and 30 per cent. A recent review of the literature suggests that in those who request extra help to stop smoking, and when this is given in the form of nicotine replacement or even contact with a support group, the success rate can be up to 25 per cent.

Although it would seem logical, as in other addictions, to suggest a reduction in nicotine levels by a gradual reduction in the number of cigarettes smoked, so as to reduce the severity of withdrawal symptoms, it has been shown that patients who gradually cut down the number of cigarettes smoked tend to inhale more to maintain their usual blood nicotine levels. It has also been shown that those who are unable to quit abruptly are not successful in reducing their consumption of cigarettes over the long term.

The intensity of the strategy employed in a cessation programme should depend on the motivation of the patient to give up smoking. There is no difference in the success rates between regimes involving brief intervention and those with more prolonged intervention in unselected smokers, whereas it is clear that those who are motivated to attend smoking cessation clinics have a better chance of long-term cessation than those who have a brief intervention by the general practitioner. It is therefore better to put time and effort only into those patients who are motivated to give up, and offer only a brief intervention in those with less motivation.

It is important that patients are given a clear strategy for smoking cessation and that the success rates are measured by corroboration with carbon monoxide measurements in breath, or urinary cotinine levels. Meta-analysis of randomized controlled trials of nicotine gum found a clear benefit in terms of abstinence rates at 1 year (23 compared with 13 per cent) in a smoking cessation clinic, but no effect in a general practice setting (11 compared with 12 per cent). Similar abstinence rates at 1 year have been quoted in a general hospital study in the United Kingdom.

Nicotine skin patches allow a slow infusion of nicotine, which creates plasma nicotine levels up to half of those produced by smoking. Trials carried out with nicotine patches indicate that similar success rates to nicotine chewing gum can be achieved. Recent studies using the antidepressant drug bupropion have also shown quit rates similar to those of nicotine replacement therapy in smokers. Based on a recent review of the literature, a strategy for smoking cessation has been suggested (Table 4).

Management of stable COPD

Bronchodilators

Bronchodilator therapy is the cornerstone of treatment in patients with COPD to reduce symptoms and increase exercise tolerance. By contrast with bronchial asthma, the effects are small in patients with COPD, due to structural changes within the airways. The principal bronchodilators—β_2-agonists, anticholinergic drugs, and theophylline derivatives—relax airway

Table 4 Smoking prevention and cessation strategy for medical outpatients

Intervention	To whom?	Time per patient	Success rate[a]
Ask about smoking, record in notes	All attenders	10 s	Prevention?
Measure CO, give advice + leaflet	Smokers (no extra help requested)	4 min	4 per cent
Prescribe nicotine replacement, arrange quit-date + follow-up	Smokers who ask for extra help	15 min	10 per cent
Group treatment with nicotine replacement (5 × 1 h per group)	Smokers who ask for more support	22.5 min	25 per cent
Overall strategy	All patients	Mean = 2.3 min	5.8 per cent of smokers

[a]A 'success' is a patient who stops smoking immediately following the intervention and maintains abstinence for at least 1 year. CO, Carbon monoxide

Modifed from Foulds J, Jarvis MJ (1995). Smoking cessation and prevention. In: Cavlerley P, Pride N, eds. *Chronic obstructive pulmonary disease*, pp.374–90. Chapman and Hall, London.

smooth muscle as their primary action and hence decrease airway resistance. However, these drugs may also reduce overinflation of the lungs, allowing the lungs to empty more completely. It should be emphasized that relatively small changes in airway dimensions can have major effects on respiratory mechanics, which may be translated into improvement in symptoms and exercise capacity.

β-Agonists

Inhaled β_2-agonists are preferred to oral preparations, since they are as efficacious in much smaller doses and have fewer side-effects. They have a relatively rapid onset of action and are therefore used for symptomatic relief, and can also increase exercise tolerance in patients with COPD. There is no evidence that the response to a β-agonist diminishes with time and patients with COPD should be told to take them as required, although those with severe disease may prefer to take regular doses three to four times daily to obtain symptomatic relief.

There is limited information on the effects of long-acting β_2-agonists in patients with COPD. In randomized placebo-controlled studies there was an improvement in symptoms and a small improvement in spirometry, without any significant change in exercise capacity but with an improvement in symptoms and quality of life. There is little evidence to support the use of sustained-release oral β_2-agonists in patients with COPD.

Anticholinergics

Like β_2-agonists, anticholinergics affect both central and peripheral airways and also reduce functional residual capacity (FRC). They have a 30- to 60-min time to peak effect in most patients with COPD, which is slower than β_2-agonists, but act for longer than β_2-agonists (6 to 10 h).

Optimal bronchodilatation occurs with 80 μg of ipratropium and 200 μg of oxitropium bromide, and studies comparing these treatments suggest no difference in the peak or duration of bronchodilatation. Thus 80 μg of ipratropium should be used in patients with COPD, rather than the customary 40 μg, to produce maximum effect. Tiotropium bromide is a newly developed anticholinergic agent that appears to have a longer time course of action than ipratropium.

Some studies found an increase in maximum exercise and a reduction in oxygen consumption at any given workload with both ipratropium bromide and oxitropium bromide. In a large group of patients with COPD the Lung Health Study showed that treatment with ipratropium bromide produced a small but significant beneficial effect on FEV_1 during treatment, but had no other effect on the decline in FEV_1 over a 5-year period.

Clinical studies of anticholinergic drugs show that they are at least as efficacious as β_2-agonists in patients with COPD and some report a more prolonged bronchodilator response.

Theophyllines

Theophyllines, or methylxanthine derivatives, produce a modest bronchodilator effect in patients with COPD. Their effect on symptoms and on exercise tolerance is variable and often occurs at the top of the therapeutic range. Long-term treatment with theophyllines is limited to the oral route, resulting in a slower onset of action compared with inhaled bronchodilators. Improvement in the phamacokinetics of oral theophyllines has occurred with the production of long-acting formulations.

The bronchodilator action of theophyllines is relatively limited in patients with COPD. Exercise tolerance in patients with COPD changes little with theophylline treatment, showing no or little improvement. Any improvement in exercise tolerance has been thought to result from an effect on respiratory muscles or a fall in trapped gas volume, but these mechanisms are still the subject of debate. Other non-bronchodilator effects of theophylline, such as improving right ventricular performance or anti-inflammatory actions, are of questionable clinical significance.

Theophyllines have a narrow therapeutic index and patients often experience side-effects within the therapeutic range. Other factors that are common in COPD, such as smoking, hypoxaemia, and infection, all alter theophylline clearance and make the control of theophylline dosage difficult, requiring measurement of plasma theophylline levels (Table 5). The possible beneficial effects of theophyllines have to be balanced against their potential side-effects and the fact that a similar benefit may be achievable with inhaled bronchodilators, hence theophyllines are reserved for patients in whom other treatments have failed to control symptoms adequately.

Combination therapy

Studies of combination therapy are difficult to assess owing to problems of suboptimal dosing. Some studies suggest that drug combinations such as salbutamol and ipratropium or salbutamol and aminophylline produce improvement in exercise tolerance in the face of trivial changes in spirometry. It is unclear whether higher doses of salbutamol could have achieved a similar effect. Thus, combinations of bronchodilator drugs should only be used if single drugs have been tried and have failed to give adequate symptomatic relief. Combination therapy should only be continued if there is good subjective or objective benefit.

Drug delivery devices

Compliance with inhaled treatment is poor. In the Lung Health Study the overall compliance with therapy was 65 per cent. Since many patients with COPD are elderly, the difficulties encountered with standard metered dose inhalers (MDI) are exaggerated. These problems can often be overcome by dry powdered formulations or by a spacer device. However, patients with

Table 5 Theophylline metabolism in COPD

Increased	Decreased
Cigarette smoking**	Arterial hypoxaemia (< 6.0 kPa)**
Anticonvulsant drugs	Respiratory acidosis *
Rifampicin	Congestive cardiac failure
	Liver cirrhosis
	Erythromycin **
	Ciprofloxacin (not ofloxacin)
	Cimetidine (not ranitidine)
	Viral infections
	Old age*

Many factors influence theophylline metabolism and those posing particular problems in COPD are indicated by asterisks, the number depending upon the likely hazards.

severe COPD are only able to achieve low inspiratory flow rates, and rates as low as 40 litre/min may cause failure of the one-way valve in a spacer device to open.

Home nebulizer therapy

There is controversy over the use of home nebulizer therapy in patients with COPD. Using end-points such as spirometry and corridor walking exercise, it has been shown that nebulized salbutamol is no more effective in patients with COPD than lower doses of the same drug given through a spacer device. However, patients appear to prefer nebulized bronchodilator therapy. This may be because the total dose of the drug delivered by nebulizer therapy is higher, and the facial cooling that occurs with the nebulized solution itself may have an effect on dyspnoea, independent of any effect on airway calibre.

Acute improvement in spirometry with nebulized bronchodilator therapy does not necessarily predict a long-term response and only a minority of patients are likely to obtain benefit from high-dose bronchodilator therapy. Patients should only be supplied with a nebulizer if they have been fully assessed by a respiratory physician who is able to assess the risk/cost benefit. This assessment should include ensuring that optimal use is made of a simple metered dose inhaler or dry powdered device and that some assessment is made of the patient's response to nebulizer therapy, including a home trial with peak expiratory flow measurements. Dosage regimes must be tailored to individual patient's needs and their side-effects monitored.

Corticosteroids

The chronic inflammation that occurs in the large and small airways provides a rationale for the use of corticosteroids in COPD. However, the use of corticosteroids in patients with COPD remains contentious, particularly the prediction of which patients will respond to this treatment.

Oral corticosteroids

A subgroup of patients respond to corticosteroids. A meta-analysis of trials of oral corticosteroids indicates that a significant improvement in FEV_1 (over 15 per cent and greater than 200 ml improvement) occurs in 10 to 20 per cent of patients with clinically stable COPD. There are no reliable predictors of which patients will respond. Furthermore, the response to high doses of oral prednisolone in short-term studies does not necessarily predict continued FEV_1 response to long-term inhaled steroids. Data from uncontrolled retrospective studies of oral corticosteroids suggest that long-term treatment may slow the decline in FEV_1, although 10 mg of prednisolone per day was required to prevent the decline in FEV_1 and patients with asthma may have been included. This treatment cannot be recommended in view of adverse side-effects.

Inhaled corticosteroids

Two large controlled trials of the effects of inhaled corticosteroids in patients with mild COPD have now been published. Both the Copenhagen City Lung study and the EUROSCOP study showed no effect of budesonide at a dose of 800 μg twice daily on the rate of decline in FEV_1 over a follow-up period of 3 years. In patients with a mean FEV_1 of 77 per cent of predicted (i.e. mild airways obstruction) who continued to smoke, the EUROSCOP study showed an initial improvement in FEV_1 over the first 6 months (at a rate of 17 ml/year—Fig. 13), which was maintained over the 3-year follow-up period. This was not the case in the Copenhagen study. A third trial in moderate COPD (FEV_1 50 per cent of predicted) in a mixed group of smokers and ex-smokers also showed a similar small improvement in FEV_1 over 3 months in a group treated with fluticasone at a dose of 1000 μg/day, but no significant effect on the rate of decline in FEV_1. However, there was a significant benefit in health status, and a reduction in exacerbation rates by 25 per cent. Since exacerbations of COPD have an adverse effect on health status, these two effects may be linked.

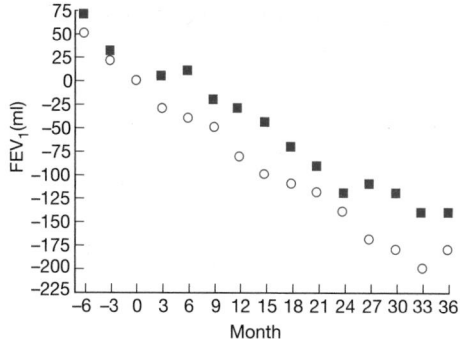

Fig. 13 Effects of budesonide at 800 μg twice daily (closed squares) or placebo (open circles) on the rate of decline in FEV_1 in patients with COPD and mild airways obstruction. There is a small decrease in the rate of decline in FEV_1 over the first 3 months of treatment in the budesonide but not in the placebo group, but no subsequent difference in the rate of decline in either group.

Based on the results of these large-scale trials there appears to be no effect of inhaled corticosteroids on the prognosis of mild to moderate COPD as assessed by the decline in FEV_1. However, there may be an effect on health status and exacerbation rates in moderate COPD. Inhaled corticosteroids may therefore be of benefit to patients with moderate to severe COPD who have frequent exacerbations, as well as those who show reversibility of their airway obstruction. Further studies are required to distinguish the subpopulation of patients with COPD who show a response to inhaled corticosteroids.

Other therapeutic agents

There is no evidence for the use of anti-inflammatory drugs such as sodium cromoglycate, nedocromil sodium, or antihistamines in patients with COPD. Although used widely in continental Europe, mucolytic drugs are rarely used in the United Kingdom. There is no evidence to support the use of continuous or intermittent prophylactic antibiotics in patients with COPD.

British Thoracic Society guidelines suggest an approach to management of patients with COPD based on the severity of disease (Fig. 14).

Domiciliary oxygen therapy

The only treatment that improves the long-term prognosis in patients with COPD is long-term domiciliary oxygen therapy, given for at least 15 h per day, as shown by two multicentre trials, one conducted by the Medical Research Council (**MRC**) in the United Kingdom, and the other by the

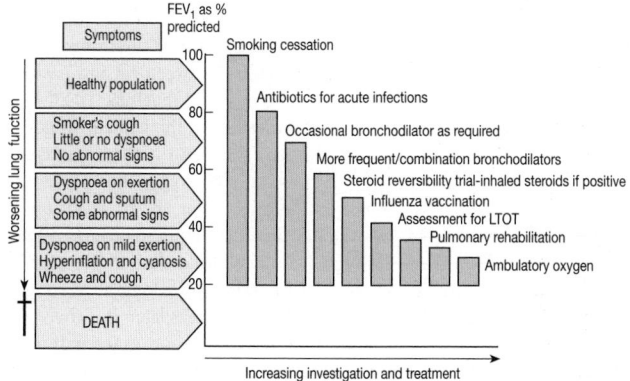

Fig. 14 The chronic obstructive pulmonary disease escalator: as lung function declines the treatments need to be increased. LTOT, long-term oxygen therapy. (Adapted from BTS Guidelines, 1997, *Thorax* **52**, S1–S18.)

nocturnal oxygen therapy trial (**NOTT**). These are discussed in Chapter 17.7.

The reasons for the improvement in survival with oxygen therapy in patients with COPD are still uncertain, but are not clearly related to improvements in pulmonary haemodynamics. As usual, survival is related to the level of pulmonary arterial hypertension in patients who receive long-term oxygen therapy. In the MRC trial, there was no significant improvement in pulmonary arterial pressure following oxygen therapy, but the increase of 3 mmHg per year in pulmonary arterial pressure in the control group did not occur in those who were treated. Overnight oxygen therapy, which abolishes nocturnal desaturation, also decreases pulmonary arterial pressure. However, since the changes in pulmonary haemodynamics produced by long-term oxygen therapy are small, it seems unlikely that these have a major influence on survival.

In addition to the improvement in survival, a number of studies have examined other effects of supplementary oxygen therapy. The effects of oxygen therapy on breathlessness remain unclear, but several studies have shown that oxygen therapy can lead to an improvement in exercise endurance in patients with COPD, associated with a reduction in ventilation at a given submaximal work rate, and an improvement in walking distance and in ability to perform daily activities. Assessment of patients taking part in the NOTT study showed that they have marked disturbances in mood and quality of life: after 6 months of oxygen therapy, 42 per cent showed evidence of an improvement in cognitive function, but little change in mood or quality of life. As in all studies of patients with COPD, the FEV_1 is the strongest predictor of survival in patients receiving long-term oxygen therapy, but this does not influence the decline in FEV_1.

Long-term oxygen therapy has been shown to affect the polycythaemia that occurs in patients with chronic hypoxaemia, by reducing both the haematocrit and the red cell mass. The clinical relevance of these haematological changes produced by oxygen therapy remains unclear. Continued cigarette smoking should be a relative contraindication to long-term oxygen therapy.

Criteria for the prescription of domiciliary oxygen therapy

There are three forms of domiciliary supplemental oxygen therapy:

(1) long-term controlled oxygen therapy for at least 15 h per day in patients with chronic respiratory failure;

(2) portable oxygen therapy for exercise-related hypoxaemia; and

(3) short-burst oxygen therapy, as a palliative treatment for the temporary relief of symptoms.

The criteria for the prescription of long-term oxygen therapy are based on the clinical parameters of those patients with COPD who showed an improved survival in the two controlled trials of long-term oxygen therapy. Central to the prescription criteria is the demonstration of significant hypoxaemia in a patient with COPD breathing room air, measured when clinically stable (Table 6).

In the United States, long-term oxygen therapy can be prescribed based on pulse oximetry and in patients whose Pao_2 lies between 7.3 and 7.9 kPa, provided there is evidence of cor pulmonale or polycythaemia.

Long-term oxygen therapy is usually prescribed in the United Kingdom in the form of oxygen concentrators, although the majority of home oxygen therapy is given to patients with COPD as cylinder oxygen therapy for the relief of breathlessness. Adherence to the criteria for the prescription of long-term oxygen therapy is less than optimal, applying to around 40 per cent of patients. Data from the NOTT study showed that 43 per cent of patients who were initially shown to fit the criteria for long-term oxygen therapy were no longer eligible when reassessed 4 weeks later. It is therefore essential that clinical stability is demonstrated, with no exacerbation of COPD for at least 4 weeks, before a decision is made to prescribe long-term oxygen therapy, and that other treatments such as bronchodilators and inhaled steroids are optimized before the prescription of long-term oxygen therapy. Furthermore, reassessment is recommended to ensure that the patient remains significantly hypoxaemic and still fits the criteria for long-

Table 6 Prescribing criteria for long-term oxygen therapy

United Kingdom: DHSS Drug Tariff, 1985

1. Absolute indications: COPD, hypoxaemia, oedema
   FEV_1 < 1.5 litre; FVC < 2.0 litre
   Pao_2 < 55 mmHg; $Paco_2$ > 45 mmHg
   Stability demonstrated over 3 weeks
2. Relative indications: as above but without oedema or $Paco_2$ > 45 mmHg
3. Palliative

Europe: Report of a SEP Task Group, 1989

1. Pao_2 < 55 mmHg, 'steady-state COPD'
2. Pao_2 55–65 mmHg with additional features as in the United States (Group 2)
3. Restrictive disease with Pao_2 < 55 mmHg

United States of America:

1. Pao_2 = 55 mmHg (room air)
   Sao_2 = 88%
2. Pao_2 = 59 mmHg with evidence of at least one of the following:
   P pulmonale (> 3 mm in leads II, III)
   (pulmonary hypertension ? right ventricular hypertrophy?)
   Dependent oedema (cor pulmonale?)
   Erythrocytosis (haematocrit > 56%)
   CMN—Certificate of Medical Necessity
   For Group 1—Annual update of CMN required
   For Group 2—Revised CMN required after 3 months

Australia: Thoracic Society of Australia, 1985

1. Pao_2 < 56 mmHg. COPD, right ventricular hypertrophy, polycythaemia, oedema
2. Desaturation < 90% on exercise
3. Refractory dyspnoea associated with cardiac failure

Modifed from Cooper CB (1995). Domiciliary oxygen therapy. In: Cavlerley P, Pride N, eds. *Chronic obstructive pulmonary disease*, pp.495–526. Chapman and Hall, London.

term oxygen therapy and to ensure that adequate oxygenation is achieved while breathing oxygen. A Pao_2 of 8 kPa is desirable, and this can usually be achieved by nasal prongs at flow rates between 1 and 3 litre/min. Precipitation of increasing hypercapnia with long-term oxygen therapy is seldom a problem in clinically stable patients. Long-term oxygen therapy should be prescribed continuously during sleeping hours, which prevents episodes of oxygen desaturation at night, and improves sleep quality.

Portable oxygen therapy

There are no established criteria for the prescription of portable oxygen in the form of small light-weight cylinders or liquid oxygen therapy (available in the United States and continental Europe, but not currently in the United Kingdom). Patients who desaturate during exercise by 5 per cent or more may be suitable for this treatment, although exercise capability may improve irrespective of arterial oxygen desatuation. The use of portable oxygen therapy to enhance mobility should be encouraged in patients to help to prevent the downward spiral of immobility and physical deconditioning.

Controlled oxygen is typically delivered by means of nasal prongs, or by mask in patients who are intolerant of nasal cannulas owing to local irritation and dermatitis. Patient compliance with masks is generally less than with nasal prongs. In patients in whom there is refractory hypoxaemia, oxygen can be delivered by the trans-tracheal route. This can reduce the resting flow rate requirements by 25 to 50 per cent compared with nasal cannulas, resulting in considerable savings, particularly if liquid oxygen is the supply mode. However, there are complications, including the formation of mucus balls in 25 per cent of cases, cough, infection, and catheter dislodgement. Reservoir devices have also been developed to reduce total oxygen requirement and cost: these work on the basis that the reservoir fills during the patient's exhalation and supplies oxygen only during inspiration.

Travel

Commercial aircraft cabins are pressurized to the equivalent of an altitude of no greater than 2600 m, producing a cabin oxygen tension of around 100 mmHg. Worsening hypoxaemia may exacerbate the symptoms of breathlessness, particularly in patients who are already hypoxaemic with a Pao_2 less than 8 kPa, in which case the airline should be contacted by letter by the patient's respiratory physician, recommending the use of oxygen: most will provide oxygen throughout the flight.

Pulmonary rehabilitation

The aim of pulmonary rehabilitation is to prevent or reverse the deconditioning that occurs with lack of exercise and immobility due to dyspnoea, thereby allowing the patient to cope with his/her disease. Before considering rehabilitation, it is vital that investigations and therapy are directed towards any reversible component of the airflow limitation and that this treatment is optimized. Patients with moderate to severe COPD should be considered for pulmonary rehabilitation programmes and each rehabilitation programme should be tailored to fit individual patient's needs, depending on the factors that are deemed to limit exercise.

Pulmonary rehabilitation programmes

Establishing a pulmonary rehabilitation programme requires a multidisciplinary approach and appropriate health-care resources. Exercise training programmes have taken two approaches. The first is to attempt to improve cardiorespiratory fitness by aerobic exercises of 20 to 30 min duration at least three times per week. However, patients with COPD may be unable to achieve the necessary increase in oxygen uptake to produce the required 'training effect' because of breathlessness, hence this approach is usually restricted to those with mild to moderate exercise limitation. The second approach, used in patients unable to sustain sufficient exercise to improve anaerobic fitness, aims to improve mobility. This can be achieved by providing regular exercise sessions so that the patient works to his/her maximum tolerable ventilatory limit. In patients with very severe COPD there are no established guidelines for pulmonary rehabilitation programmes, but carefully supervised exercise conditioning in the hospital setting, with oxygen supplementation, should be considered in those who develop hypoxaemia during exercise.

Respiratory muscle training

A meta-analysis of 17 randomized trials of respiratory muscle training in patients with COPD showed that although training, using either resistance breathing or isocapnic hyperventilation, improved respiratory muscle strength and endurance, there was no overall improvement in exercise tolerance.

Numerous *in vitro* studies have shown that methylxanthines, such as theophyllines (in doses not possible in humans), potentiate the response of fresh and fatigued muscle strips to an electrical stimulus. Studies *in vivo* in humans have been less convincing, reporting either little or no improvement in the transdiaphragmatic pressure (Pdi) generated during maximal voluntary effort.

Some uncontrolled studies have suggested that resting the respiratory muscles, by long-term nocturnal use of either negative pressure, applied to the chest wall, or intermittent positive pressure ventilation (IPPV) using a nasal mask, results in some improvement in respiratory muscle function. However, a large controlled study failed to show any benefit on respiratory muscle function in patients with COPD.

The results of controlled trials on the effects of nutritional supplementation on respiratory muscle function in malnourished patients with COPD have shown no consistent benefit. Those studies that have achieved positive results have done so in association with an increase in weight.

Controlled breathing techniques have been used as part of a pulmonary rehabilitation programme to diminish breathlessness by training patients to breathe efficiently. This treatment aims to:

(1) restore the diaphragm to a more normal position and function;

(2) decrease the respiratory rate by using a breathing pattern that diminishes air trapping;

(3) diminish the work of breathing; and

(4) reduce dyspnoea and patient anxiety.

Techniques such as pursed lip breathing have been employed and some studies have shown an improvement in blood gases.

The outcome of a pulmonary rehabilitation programme is usually assessed by measuring improvement in lung function or exercise tolerance, but benefit may not always be apparent in these variables. In general, studies show a favourable effect on exercise tolerance and a reduction in symptoms such as breathlessness during exercise. Since social factors contribute to the disability in COPD, assessment of quality of life should be included in a rehabilitation programme (measured by a health profile questionnaire), as should that of compliance, longevity, and cost–benefit.

Other aspects

Nutrition

Weight loss is common in patients with COPD, particularly those with severe airways obstruction, and is associated with high mortality. However, studies that have addressed this issue have produced variable results, although those who do show weight gain may have improved survival. Obesity should be discouraged by appropriate dietary advice in patients with COPD to avoid additional strain on the cardiorespiratory system.

Depression

Mood disturbances, particularly depression, are very common in patients with advanced disease and often contribute to an enhanced perception of symptoms, particularly breathlessness, and to social isolation. Antidepressant drugs can often produce encouraging results in these patients.

Vaccination

Influenza vaccination is recommended for patients with COPD, although specific evidence is lacking. The rationale relates to other studies in elderly patients, not specifically with COPD, where a 70 per cent reduction in mortality from influenza can be demonstrated.

Management of acute exacerbations of COPD

Exacerbations of COPD occur on a background of established disease and are amongst the commonest acute respiratory problems presenting to either primary or secondary care. Many patients can be managed in the community.

Antibiotics

Infection is a common precipitating feature in exacerbations of COPD, although only 50 per cent of patients with severe exacerbations with associated respiratory failure will have a positive sputum culture for a bacterium. The commonest organisms are *Haemophilus influenzae*, *Streptococcus pneumoniae*, and *Moraxella catarrhalis*. However, patients with COPD are often chronically colonized with common bacterial pathogens, hence culture of one of these organisms during an acute exacerbation does not imply that this organism is responsible for the exacerbation. Viral infections have been shown to be responsible for up to 30 per cent of all exacerbations of COPD.

There is limited information from controlled trials on the effects of antibiotics in exacerbations of COPD. In a trial of 173 patients with 362 exacerbations of COPD, patients received either a 10-day course of sulphamethoxazole, amoxycillin, doxycycline, or placebo: relief of symptoms within 21 days was achieved in 68 per cent of the antibiotic-treated group and in 55 per cent of the placebo-treated exacerbations. Peak expiratory flow recovered faster with antibiotics, although the differences were small, and treatment failures were twice as common with placebo. The difference in successful outcome between antibiotic and placebo were significant if two of the following symptoms were present—increase in dyspnoea, increase in sputum volume, and increase in sputum purulence: antibiotics are recommended if two of these symptoms are present.

In view of the limited range of bacteria present in the sputum of these patients, broad-spectrum antibiotics such as amoxycillin at a dose of 250 mg three times daily or clarithromycin at 250 to 500 mg twice daily—as an alternative in patients with penicillin allergy—are recommended. Prescription of antibiotics should take into account local bacteriological sensitivity patterns, particularly the prevalence of β-lactamase-positive *H. influenzae*, which is around 20 per cent in most areas, and *Moraxella catarralis*, of which 90 per cent are β-lactamase positive. If the patient is known to have had β-lactamase-positive organisms previously in sputum, or fails to respond to amoxycillin, then co-amoxiclav should be considered. Antibiotics should be given orally unless there is a specific indication for intravenous treatment.

Bronchodilators

The use of nebulized bronchodilators in acute exacerbations of COPD is recommended. These should be given as soon as possible on admission and at 4- to 6-hourly intervals thereafter, or more frequently if required. In patients with COPD, particularly in those with an elevated Pa_{CO_2}, the nebulizer should be driven by compressed air and not by oxygen, to avoid a further rise in Pa_{CO_2}. Oxygen can be given by nasal prongs at 1 to 2 litre/min during nebulization. β-Agonists (salbutamol at 2.5 to 5 mg, or terbutaline at 5 to 10 mg) or an anticholinergic drug (ipratropium bromide at 0.5 mg) are the drugs commonly used. In acute exacerbations of COPD, no difference has been shown between these drugs given alone or in combination in nebulized form.

A response to a nebulized bronchodilator in an acute exacerbation does not imply long-term benefit and assessment for a home nebulizer should be made when the patient is in a stable condition. Several studies have shown no difference in the degree of bronchodilatation achieved when the same dose of bronchodilator is given by a metered dose inhaler, with or without a spacer device, or via a nebulizer, even in patients with an acute exacerbation of airways obstruction. However, patients with respiratory failure have been excluded from these studies and hence nebulized bronchodilators are still recommended, but in most cases these should only be necessary for 24 to 48 h and a change to a metered dose inhaler, or a dry powder device should be made 24 to 48 h before discharge.

If a patient is not responding to nebulized bronchodilators during an exacerbation, then intravenous methylxanthines should be considered. However, a small randomized placebo-controlled trial of intravenous aminophylline showed no differences in spirometry, arterial blood gases, or the sensation of dyspnoea between the aminophylline and placebo groups over a period of 72 h following admission with exacerbation of COPD. Thus, the prescription of theophyllines has no clear role in management of acute exacerbations of COPD and the possible benefits should be weighed against the side-effects, particularly in patients with COPD who have hypoxaemia, infection, and are receiving antibiotics, all of which can affect theophylline clearance. Thus the dose must be carefully individualized and the serum level maintained within a narrow therapeutic range (10 to 20 mg/l). The usual loading dose is 6 mg/kg of aminophylline with maintenance dosage of 0.5 mg/kg.h.

Corticosteroids

There are now several controlled trials showing benefit of oral corticosteroids in patients with acute exacerbations of COPD. A placebo-controlled study in hospital patients without hypercapnic respiratory failure showed improvement in FEV_1 and reduction in days in hospital in those treated with 30 mg prednisolone daily. A further study of exacerbations treated with prednisolone in the community also showed a positive result.

There is therefore good evidence that corticosteroids are beneficial in exacerbations of COPD, the usual regime being 30 mg prednisolone daily for 2 weeks. The lowest dose that produces benefit requires further study.

Diuretics

In patients with fluid retention as a result of respiratory failure and cor pulmonale, diuretics should be used judicially, as they have the potential to reduce right ventricular end-diastolic volume considerably and hence cardiac output.

Anticoagulants

Pulmonary emboli are probably are under-recognized in severe COPD. It is difficult to diagnose pulmonary emboli in such patients: ventilation/perfusion abnormalities are often present and can lead to false-positive reports of pulmonary thromboembolic disease. Prophylactic subcutaneous heparin is often given to patients with exacerbations of COPD, particularly those who have respiratory failure.

Physiotherapy

There is very little evidence to support the use of physiotherapy to improve expectoration in patients with acute exacerbations of COPD, although some studies suggest that there is some benefit in patients producing large amounts of sputum.

Assessment of recovery from acute exacerbations of COPD

Arterial blood gases should be checked while breathing air, which gives a guide to the need for later formal reassessment for long-term oxygen therapy. Antibiotics need not usually be given for more than 7 days. Respiratory failure in COPD is dealt with in Chapter 17.7.

Surgical treatment in COPD

Bullous emphysema

Exertional dyspnoea is the usual presenting feature in patients with bullous disease, although a single bulla of moderate size is unlikely to produce symptoms when the remaining lung is normal. Bullae may present as a chance finding on a chest radiograph or as a pneumothorax. Occasionally they become infected, in which case there may be a fluid level, sometimes with surrounding consolidation. Such infection may result in closure of the bronchial connection, shrinkage, or even obliteration of the bulla.

Respiratory function tests may be non-specific and simply reflect COPD. Almost always there is some degree of airway obstruction, which may result from concomitant diffuse emphysema or airways disease, or as a result of the loss of lung elastic recoil that accompanies large bullae. Overinflation is typically present, but is underestimated if measured by the helium dilution technique rather than by plethysmography. Gas exchange is usually impaired as shown by a reduced TL_{CO}. The K_{CO} may reflect the quality of the non-bullous lung if the bullae are non-ventilating, which may be helpful in making a decision concerning surgery.

Treatment

The only treatment that is considered for large bullae is surgical obliteration. This should not be offered to patients who are asymptomatic, since the operation does have an appreciable risk. The principal indication is progressive dyspnoea, but in those with airflow limitation it has been difficult to determine which patients benefit from bullectomy. Many techniques have been used in the past to assess patient's suitability for this procedure, such as bronchography and pulmonary angiography, which have now been essentially replaced by CT scanning. A critical feature is the quality of the non-bullous lung: airflow limitation is determined by the degree of emphysema in the non-bullous lung rather than the extent of the bullous disease. Quantitative perfusion scanning may demonstrate retained perfusion in collapsed peribullous lung, which may improve after operation. Patients with bullae occupying less than 50 per cent of the hemithorax, with an FEV_1 of less than 1 litre, or hypercapnia carry a high risk of a poor response to surgery.

The aims of surgery are to obliterate the bullous space and restore the elastic integrity of the lung. Several techniques have been described, including excision, plication, marsupialization, and intracavity drainage. Most operations are performed by a conventional lateral thoracotomy, but superficial bullae have also recently been dealt with using thoracoscopic and laser techniques. The perioperative mortality in published series ranges from 0 to 20 per cent in patients with a wide range of disability and hence operative risk.

The best functional results occur in younger patients with mild symptoms, with large bullae, relatively well-preserved pulmonary function, and normal surrounding lung. Those with small bullae (less than 1 litre or less than 50 per cent of the hemithorax), poor overall lung function (FEV_1 less than 1 litre), and diffuse emphysema have least functional improvement and in these the improvement has to be weighed against the risk of surgery. Studies of the long-term follow-up of patients after surgery indicate that giant bullae do not recur.

Lung transplantation

It was originally considered that patients with endstage COPD were not suitable for a single lung transplant since perfusion would be preferentially directed towards the transplanted lung because of its lower pulmonary vascular resistance, producing profound ventilation/perfusion mismatch. The current success of a single lung transplant, despite the presence of abnormal mechanics in the native lung, is due in part to improved patient selection, lung preservation, and anaesthetic management. There are problems if residual infection is present in the native lung, and large bullae in the native lung may show gross hyperinflation in the early postoperative period, causing mediastinal shift and compression of the transplanted lung. Hence those patients with recurrent pulmonary infection or bilateral large bullae are considered for heart–lung transplantation or bilateral sequential lung transplantation. For detailed discussion of lung transplantation, see Chapter 17.16.

Lung volume reduction surgery

The growing number of patients with emphysema on waiting lists for lung transplantation has led to a recent re-examination of previous surgical techniques that might give symptomatic relief, particularly the technique of lung volume reduction surgery (pneumonectomy or pneumoplasty). The rationale for this technique is to reduce the volume of overinflated emphysematous lung by 20 to 30 per cent, with the aim of improving the elastic recoil of the lungs, diaphragm configuration, chest wall mechanics, and gas exchange. Persistent postoperative air leaks were overcome by the use of strips of bovine pericardium to buttress the stapling line. The technique is usually performed via a median sternotomy, without the need for cardiopulmonary bypass. Thoracoscopic laser pneumoplasty has been developed as an alternative technique to the more conventional excisional surgery. Careful patient selection is necessary on the basis of a distended thorax, predominantly upper lobe disease demonstrated by CT scanning, and severe functional disability in spite of a programme of pulmonary rehabilitation.

The early results are encouraging: improvements in lung function that have occurred up to 6 months after surgery are impressive and better than can be produced by conventional medical treatment with bronchodilators or corticosteriods. Controlled trials of this technique are underway but have not yet been published.

A recent study compared lung volume reduction surgery with single lung transplant for emphysema: disease severity was greater in the lung transplant group, and their increase in FEV_1 and FVC was greater, but the increase in 6-min walking distant was similar in both groups.

Many questions concerning this technique require answers from future studies, particularly knowledge of the duration of the benefit, the best selection criteria for patients, and the mechanism of the improvement.

Further reading

American Thoracic Society (1995). Standards for the diagnosis and care of patients with chronic obstructive pulmonary disease. *American Journal of Respiratory and Critical Care Medicine* **152**, S77–S120.

Anthonisen NR (1994). The Lung Health Study; effects of smoking intervention and the use of an inhaled anticholinergic bronchodilator on the rate of decline of FEV_1. *Journal of the American Medical Association* **272**, 1497–505.

British Thoracic Society (1997). British Thoracic Society guidelines for the management of chronic obstructive pulmonary disease. *Thorax* **52**(Suppl 5), S1–S28.

Burrows B (1991). Predictors of loss of lung function and mortality in obstructive lung disease. *European Respiratory Journal* **1**, 340–5.

Calverley P, Pride N (1996). *Chronic obstructive pulmonary disease.* Chapman & Hall, London.

Davies L, Calverley PMA (1996). Lung volume reduction surgery in chronic obstructive pulmonary disease. *Thorax* **51**(Suppl 2), S29–S34.

Jeffrey PK (1996). Bronchial biopsies and airway inflammation. *European Respiratory Journal* **9**, 1583–7.

Lange P *et al.* (1990). The relation of ventilatory impairment and of chronic mucus hypersecretion to mortality from obstructive lung disease and from all causes. *Thorax* **45**, 579–85.

MacNee W (1994). State of the Art: pathophysiology of cor pulmonale in chronic obstructive pulmonary disease. *American Journal of Respiratory and Critical Care Medicine* **150**, Part I—833–52, Part II—1158–68.

MacNee W (2000). Chronic bronchitis and emphysema. In: Seaton A, Seaton D, Leitch AG, eds. *Crofton and Douglas's respiratory diseases*, 5th edn, pp.616–95. Blackwell Science, Oxford.

MacNee W (2000). Respiratory failure. In: Seaton A, Seaton D, Leitch AG, eds. *Crofton and Douglas's respiratory diseases*, 5th edn, pp.696–717. Blackwell Science, Oxford.

Medical Research Council Working Party (1981). Long term domiciliary oxygen therapy in chronic cor pulmonale complicating chronic bronchitis and emphysema. *Lancet* **i**, 681–6.

Nagai A *et al.* (1985). The National Institutes of Health Positive-Pressure Breathing Trial: Pathology Studies. I. Inter relationship between morphologic lesions. *American Review of Respiratory Diseases* **132**, 937–45.

Nagai A, West WM, Thurlbeck WM (1985). The National Institutes of Health Intermittent Positive-Pressure Breathing Trial: Pathology Studies. II. Correlations between morphologic findings, clinical findings and evidence of expiratory airflow obstruction. *American Review of Respiratory Diseases* **132**, 946–53.

Nocturnal Oxygen Therapy Trial Group (1980). Continuous or nocturnal oxygen therapy in hypoxemic chronic obstructive pulmonary disease: a clinical trial. *Annals of Internal Medicine* **93**, 391.

Pauwels RA *et al.* for the European Respiratory Society Study on Chronic Obstructive Pulmonary Disease (1999). Long-term treatment with inhaled budesonide in persons with mild chronic obstructive pulmonary disease who continue smoking. *New England Journal of Medicine* **340**, 1948–53.

Saetta M (1997). Airway pathology compared with asthma. *European Respiratory Review* **45**, 211–15.

Siafakas NM *et al.* (1995). ERS Consensus Statement. Optimal assessment and management of chronic obstructive pulmonary disease (COPD). *European Respiratory Journal* **8**, 1398–420.

Vestbo J, Prescott E, Lange P and the Copenhagen City Heart Study Group (1996). Association of chronic mucus hypersecretion with FEV_1 decline and chronic obstructive pulmonary disease morbidity. *American Journal of Respiratory and Critical Care Medicine* **153**, 1530–5.

Vestbo J *et al.* (1999). Long-term effect of inhaled budesonide in mild and moderate chronic obstructive pulmonary disease: a randomised controlled trial. *Lancet* **353**, 1819–23.

17.7 Chronic respiratory failure

P. M. A. Calverley

Introduction

Although respiration is ultimately a biochemical process involving the generation of ATP, the term respiratory failure is used more loosely to describe the failure of gas exchange within the lung to maintain arterial blood gas homeostasis. Defining normal blood gas tensions is harder than it may appear initially as Pa_{O_2} falls with age and the extent of this is debated. The most commonly applied formula to describe this is:

$$Pa_{O_2} \text{ (kPa)} = 13.86 - [0.036 \times \text{age (years)}]$$

Thus a Pa_{O_2} of 10.6 kPa may be abnormal in a man of 24 years but a 'normal' value in a woman of 80. Subnormal levels of arterial oxygenation are described as hypoxaemia, whilst arterial CO_2 tensions, which do not show similar age dependence, are considered to be hypercapnic when they exceed 6.0 kPa (45 mmHg).

Respiratory failure is defined primarily in terms of hypoxaemia and is arbitrarily considered to be present when the arterial P_{O_2} (at sea level) is less than 8.0 kPa (60 mmHg). It need not be accompanied by hypercapnia, but when this develops it leads to acidosis due to the accumulation of carbonic acid by the Henderson–Hasselbalch equilibrium. If the acidosis is not rapidly progressive, and in the presence of intact renal compensatory mechanisms that generate bicarbonate ions, it becomes 'chronic'—a compensated state where the arterial pH returns to normal.

In summary, chronic respiratory failure describes a clinical state when the arterial P_{O_2} breathing air is less than 8.0 kPa, which may or may not be associated with hypercapnia, but is accompanied by a normal arterial pH and has been present for several days or more. This definition emphasizes the physiological determinants of gas exchange that characterize the problem.

Unlike other forms of organ system failure, such as cardiac or hepatic failure, the clinical symptoms and signs of chronic respiratory failure are relatively undramatic, but its development is equally significant, both as a marker of disease progression and in producing serious complications beyond those normally seen with the underlying disease. This chapter will review the causes, clinical features, and assessment of chronic respiratory failure as well as specific means of treatment. However, to do so logically requires some understanding of the principles underlying the development of this condition, as well as the factors relevant to the selection of the threshold values used in defining this state.

Physiological determinants of blood gas tensions

In health there is a predictable fall in the partial pressure of oxygen from that in the room air to that in mixed venous blood. This reflects the effect of diluting room air with resident gas in the alveoli, the efficiency of pulmonary oxygen exchange, and the consumption of oxygen by metabolizing tissues. Conversely, there is a predictable increase in the amount of CO_2 added to the circulation and subsequently removed from the lungs during expiration. This simple system is reliant on a range of physical processes that

differ somewhat for O_2 and CO_2. Within the lungs gas transport is largely by convective bulk transport and in the alveoli by diffusion. In the blood oxygen combines with haemoglobin, which augments transportation to the tissues where diffusion is the final process involved. By contrast, CO_2 transport begins with diffusion from relatively high tissue concentrations and is buffered in solution in the blood. This complex mechanism can be deranged in a number of predictable ways that are discussed below.

In the last 20 years the analysis of pulmonary gas exchange has been revolutionized by the use of the complex multiple inert gas elimination technique in research laboratories around the world. This gives a relatively complete description of the distribution of gas exchange abnormalities within the lungs. However, for an understanding of the general principles involved in disease states the traditional three-compartment model is easier to follow. This assumes that alveolar air within the lungs is either ideally matched to pulmonary arterial blood flow within the pulmonary capillary bed or is totally mismatched, meaning that either the ventilation–perfusion ratio is unity, that is, ventilation without perfusion (physiological dead space, V_D), or this ratio is zero, that is, perfusion without ventilation (venous admixture effect). The physiological dead space includes a component due to dilution of the resident gas in the airways, the anatomical dead space, while the shunt fraction incorporates the very small amount of cardiac output (less than 1 per cent) not passing through the pulmonary capillary bed.

Hypoxaemia

The principal mechanisms leading to arterial hypoxaemia are shown in Table 1. Individuals resident at altitude, for example the high Andes and Himalayas, experience significantly lower inspired oxygen tensions than those at sea level and even individuals with normal lungs can develop clinically significant hypoxaemia, especially during sleep. Even minor degrees of respiratory impairment in these circumstances can produce dramatic changes in blood gas tensions and the early onset of cor pulmonale. Conversely, people with established hypoxaemia at sea level can occasionally experience worsening symptoms when travelling by air where cabin pressurization is 75 per cent of atmospheric. However, in clinical practice, this is relatively infrequent.

Table 1 Determinants of a reduced arterial oxygen tension

Inspired oxygen concentration	Reduced at altitude and iatrogenically
Pulmonary factors	
V/Q mismatching	
Alveolar hypoventilation	
Diffusion limitation	
Arteriovenous shunts	
Extrapulmonary factors	
Increased oxygen uptake	Reduced mixed venous P_{O_2}
Low cardiac output	Reduced mixed venous P_{O_2}
Reduced pulmonary capillary transit time	Reduced end-capillary P_{O_2}

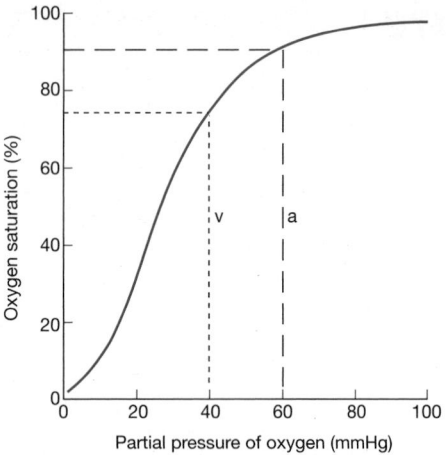

Fig. 1 The haemoglobin–oxygen dissociation curve. a, partial pressure of oxygen of 8 kPa (60 mmHg), which is the definition of arterial hypoxia. v, partial pressure of oxygen of 5.3 kPa (40 mmHg), which is typical of mixed venous blood. Note that once the Pao_2 falls below 8 kPa small further falls dramatically decrease the arterial oxygen saturation.

Four processes cause arterial hypoxaemia due to inefficient pulmonary gas exchange:

- ventilation–perfusion (V/Q) mismatch
- hypoventilation
- diffusion limitation
- true shunt.

Much the most important of these is ventilation–perfusion mismatching. In many diseases where minute ventilation is increased, the additional inspired gas is distributed to well-perfused areas of the lungs, but when the opposite occurs and perfusion exceeds effective ventilation (low V/Q states), arterial Pao_2 falls. At first this might seem surprising as most diseases associated with ventilation–perfusion imbalance are of patchy distribution and compensation from areas of high V/Q ratios might be expected. However, this does not occur owing to an important feature of the oxyhaemoglobin dissociation curve (Fig. 1), whose sigmoid shape means that well-perfused parts of the lung cannot increase the arterial oxygen saturation of the blood leaving them beyond 100 per cent, hence the saturation of the pulmonary venous blood must fall as long as low V/Q areas are present.

The second important mechanism contributing to arterial hypoxaemia is alveolar hypoventilation, where the supply of fresh oxygen is globally reduced because of generally inadequate minute ventilation. This process often coexists with ventilation–perfusion mismatching and tends to exacerbate it. In some situations, such as during exercise, total minute ventilation may lie within the normal range but can still be inappropriately low for the subject's metabolic requirements, thereby leading to hypoxaemia.

Two less important mechanisms are anatomical shunting and diffusion limitation. The former occurs predominantly with intrapulmonary arteriovenous malformations. Congenital cardiac anomalies such as ventricular septal defects with reversed flow are often lumped in with this problem, although technically they are extrapulmonary in origin. The failure to increase Pao_2 to greater than 40 kPa (300 mmHg), even when exposed to 100 per cent oxygen, is diagnostic. Diffusion limitation was initially believed to be important in many diseases, the assumption being that passive diffusion of oxygen was reduced to the point where equilibration with haemoglobin during red cell transit of the pulmonary capillaries was incomplete. Detailed studies with modern techniques of gas exchange analysis have largely discredited this, except for small falls in arterial oxygen tension at maximum levels of performance in elderly athletes and possibly during exercise in some forms of interstitial lung disease.

Although not the sole explanation of arterial hypoxaemia, the degree of hypoxaemia can be worsened when the mixed venous arterial oxygen tension is significantly reduced as occurs in low cardiac output states or conditions where peripheral oxygen consumption is increased.

Hypercapnia

Analysis of the pulmonary causes for changes in arterial CO_2 tension is much simpler, the relevant relationship being:

$$Paco_2 = K \times Vco_2/V_A$$

where Vco_2 is the CO_2 production by the body, V_A is the alveolar ventilation, and K is a constant.

It is easy to see that inadequate alveolar ventilation, due to either low total alveolar ventilation or an inability to increase V_A in response to an increase in metabolic CO_2 production, will increase the arterial CO_2. Alveolar ventilation is influenced by a range of factors, reflecting the balance of the intrinsic capacity of the ventilatory pump and the demands placed on it (Fig. 2).

The second important mechanism is ventilation–perfusion abnormality, although here the important component is the increased physiological dead space. This can be seen by a rearrangement of the equation above as shown below:

$$Paco_2 = K \times Vco_2/\ V(1-V_D/V_T)$$

where V_D/V_T is the ratio of the physiological dead space to the tidal volume and V is the total minute ventilation.

An increase in V_D occurring when ventilation–perfusion ratios are high can lead to an increase in CO_2 tension. Rather surprisingly, low ventilation–perfusion units are much less important in producing CO_2 retention than they are in producing hypoxia since CO_2 transport from the blood to the alveolar gas is linear (Fig. 3). This means that in areas of normal ventilation–perfusion ratios an increase in overall minute ventilation will increase CO_2 elimination and compensate for the CO_2 that is not excreted from areas of reduced perfusion.

In most cases of chronic respiratory failure with CO_2 retention, both of these processes operate and the patient is unable to sustain the high overall levels of ventilation needed to maintain CO_2 tensions within the normal range. An important compensatory mechanism in the trade-off between the increased chemical drive to breathing and the mechanical limitations on ventilation is the breathing pattern. In both chronic obstructive and restrictive lung disease a rapid shallow breathing pattern is adopted to minimize respiratory discomfort whilst maintaining minute ventilation. However, the relative fall in tidal volume further worsens the V_D/V_T ratio and can itself contribute to CO_2 retention. Some of these problems are resolved

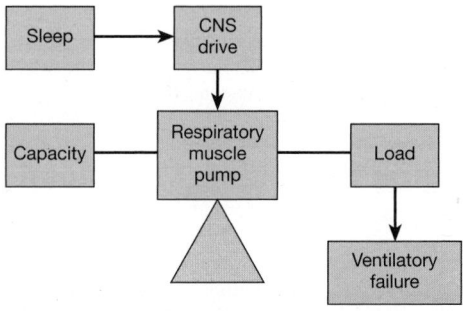

Fig. 2 Alveolar ventilation reflects the balance of the intrinsic capacity of the ventilatory pump and the demands placed on it. A reduced respiratory drive, particularly during sleep, reduces alveolar ventilation but does not produce significant hypercapnia.

when the buffering capacity of the blood rises as compensation for respiratory acidosis occurs.

Special circumstances

As already noted, residence at altitude and exercise pose particular problems for gas exchange and may induce temporary respiratory failure. There is now a wealth of data indicating that similar changes can occur during sleep. All healthy people show an approximately 15 per cent reduction in minute ventilation in the transition from wakefulness to stable non-REM (rapid eye movement) sleep, and this may be greater still in phasic REM sleep. The ventilatory responses to both hypoxia and hypercapnia decline as sleep deepens and upper airway resistance rises, especially in those who snore. Despite this the blood gas tensions vary little in health during sleep, but dramatic abnormalities can develop during periods of repetitive upper airway obstruction (see Chapter 17.8.2) or when coexisting neuromuscular weakness leads to excessive dependence on muscle groups whose activity declines with sleep (see below).

Gas transport to the tissues

Oxygen delivered to the tissues depends on the oxygen saturation of arterial blood (Sao_2), the haemoglobin concentration (**Hb**), and the cardiac output (**C.O.**), related as follows:

$$\text{Oxygen delivery } (Do_2) = \text{C.O.} \times (\text{Hb} \times 1.34) \times (Sao_2/100)$$

This is influenced only indirectly by the effectiveness of gas exchange. Since oxygen delivery is the clinically relevant outcome of oxygenation, decisions about when and how much to intervene therapeutically will be influenced by this variable. Small changes in saturation become clinically more important in individuals with impaired cardiac function and/or reduced haemoglobin concentration, and a higher Sao_2 should be maintained. In general, there is little to be gained by increasing Sao_2 to the high 90s, especially as this may cause secondary carbon dioxide retention in some diseases. As is clear from Fig. 1, desaturations below 90 per cent only occur when the arterial oxygen tension is below 8.0 kPa (60 mmHg) and this is also influenced by a number of other factors that determine the position of the dissociation curve (see Table 2). This provides the rationale for the choice of 8.0 kPa as the cut-off point for the onset of respiratory failure.

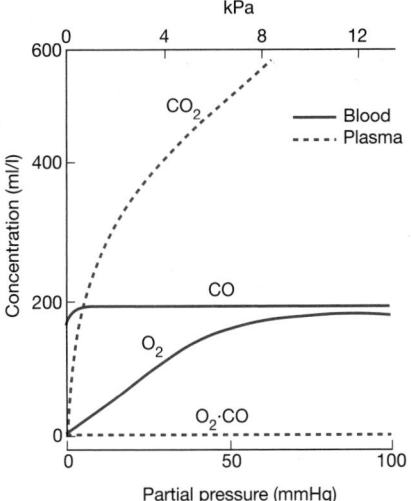

Fig. 3 Concentration of oxygen (O_2), carbon monoxide (CO), and carbon dioxide (CO_2) in blood and plasma at differing partial pressures of these gases.

Table 2 Important facts about the oxygen dissociation curve

$Pao_2 = 100$ (13.3), $Sao_2 = 97.5\%$	Arterial blood values
$Pao_2 = 80$ (10.7), $Sao_2 = 96\%$	Lower limit of normal
$Pao_2 = 60$ (8.0), $Sao_2 = 89\%$	Dissociation curve changes shape
$Pao_2 = 40$ (5.3), $Sao_2 = 75\%$	Mixed venous blood, or severe arterial hypoxaemia
Increased temperature, Pco_2, acidosis, 2-3 DPG shifts the curve to the right and vice versa	Reduces O_2 uptake from pulmonary venous blood but increases O_2 delivery in the tissues

2-3 DPG is 2,3 diphosphoglycerate in the red cells. Figures for Pao_2 are mmHg (kPa), Sao_2 is oxygen saturation.

Causes of chronic respiratory failure

The principal causes of chronic respiratory failure are summarized in Table 3. This list is extensive, but the commonest causes are discussed below.

Chronic airflow limitation

This term covers the most important cause of chronic respiratory failure, chronic obstructive pulmonary disease (**COPD**), but is also relevant to diseases such as chronic bronchial asthma, which is now excluded from the definition of COPD, and bronchiectasis, where airflow obstruction is a frequent finding as the disease advances. In all these cases there is a reduction in the forced expiratory volume in 1 s (FEV_1) to forced vital capacity (**FVC**) ratio below 70 per cent and a reduction in the FEV_1, which is commonly below 35 per cent predicted before chronic respiratory failure is noted clinically.

In all these cases, hypoxaemia is the first abnormality, which is largely due to ventilation–perfusion mismatching. Early attempts at relating these changes to structural patterns of airway and alveolar disease in COPD have proved unsuccessful. As lung mechanics worsen (commonly when FEV_1 falls below 1.5 litres or 35 per cent of the predicted value), arterial CO_2 increases. This has been related to the development of inspiratory threshold loading (PEEPi) with the onset of chronic hyperinflation, but the degree of CO_2 retention varies between subjects suggesting that individual variations in chemoresponsiveness/perception of ventilatory load contribute to this process. There is no predictable relationship between the severity of impaired lung mechanics below the thresholds indicated and the degree of hypoxaemia or hypercapnia, and many patients who maintain arterial CO_2 tensions within the normal range develop acute CO_2 retention during exacerbations of their disease. These changes can be relatively short lived and the hypercapnia resolves by the time of discharge. Coexisting left ventricular impairment reduces cardiac output and increases venous admixture, which can cause severe hypercapnia and acidosis, which none the less respond rapidly to appropriate treatment.

Patients with COPD in association with persistent hypercapnic respiratory failure have a worse prognosis than those with intermittent hypercapnia during exacerbations (Fig. 4). The pattern in chronic asthma and bronchiectasis appears similar to COPD indicating that lung mechanics rather than individual pathology dictates the severity of the gas exchange disorder.

Interstitial lung disease

Despite the wide range of primary pathologies covered by the term interstitial lung disease they present with a relatively stereotyped physiological picture. A restrictive physiological disorder (FEV_1/FVC greater than 75 per cent with a reduced absolute FEV_1 and FVC) is usual, although patients with sarcoidosis commonly show airways involvement and can present with severe airflow limitation or a mixed physiological pattern. Near normal spirometry can be seen with significant exercise limitation and exercise-induced oxygen desaturation in some patients where COPD and interstitial lung disease coexist. Typically, resting gas exchange is relatively preserved in interstitial lung disease until late in the course of disease, whereas exercise-induced desaturation is an early finding, often seen when spirometric changes are unimpressive. Studies using the multiple inert gas technique have described a bimodal pattern of ventilation–perfusion distribution, with some areas of lung having normal V/Q relationships and others relatively little ventilation, that is, increased physiological shunting. This situation worsens during exercise. A small number of patients with severe interstitial lung disease develop CO_2 retention in the terminal phase of their illness and cor pulmonale. The physiological mechanisms underlying this are poorly studied but are probably similar to those in COPD.

Table 3 Causes of chronic hypoxaemia alone or with hypercapnia

With normal or low Pa_{O_2}
Pulmonary diseases
Obstructive ventilatory disorders
   COPD
   Chronic asthma
Mixed ventilatory disorders
   Bronchiectasis
   Sequelae of tuberculosis
Interstitial lung disorders
   Idiopathic pulmonary fibrosis
   Pneumoconiosis
   Sarcoidosis
   Extrinsic allergic alveolitis
Pulmonary vascular diseases
   Pulmonary vascular hypertension
   Chronic pulmonary thrombosis
   Arteriovenous malformations
Non-pulmonary diseases
   Severe heart failure
   Hepatopulmonary syndrome

With hypercapnia
Pulmonary diseases
Obstructive ventilatory disorders
   COPD
Mixed ventilatory disorders
   Bronchiectasis
   Sequelae of tuberculosis
Non-pulmonary diseases
Dysfunction of respiratory centres
Primary alveolar hypoventilation
Obesity hypoventilation syndrome
Depressant drugs
Myxoedema
Lesion of brainstem
Neuromuscular diseases
   Poliomyelitis
   Amyotrophic lateral sclerosis
   Myasthenia gravis
   Muscular dystrophies, polymyositis
Chest wall deformities
   Kyphoscoliosis
   Ankylosing spondylitis
   Chest trauma
   Thoracoplasty
Pleural thickening
Obstruction of upper respiratory tract

COPD, chronic obstructive pulmonary disease.

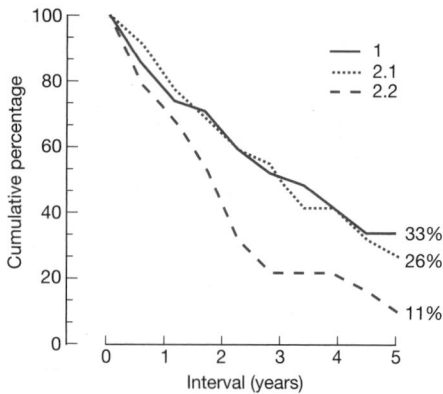

Fig. 4 Survival after index admission in three groups of COPD patients with similar initial spirometry. Group 1 never exhibited CO_2 retention, group 2.1 retained CO_2 during the admission but this resolved, while group 2.2 had persistent arterial hypercapnia. (Based on data from Costello *et al.* 1997.)

Chest wall and neuromuscular disease

Here the underlying lung structure and potential for gas exchange are unimpaired, but the ability to maintain adequate alveolar ventilation is reduced. This can be due to increased chest wall stiffness as in kyphoscoliosis, or reduced inspiratory muscle force as in neuromuscular disease. In this latter group the reduction in maximum inspiratory pressure can be global, such as in Duchenne muscular dystrophy, or more specific, such as isolated diaphragmatic weakness, where gas exchange abnormalities may only be present during specific sleep stages. Significant abnormalities of gas exchange at rest only occur with advanced disease and not in every patient. Alveolar hypoventilation is the dominant mechanism of both hypoxaemia and hypercapnia, although secondary changes such as pulmonary microatelectasis may contribute an element of V/Q mismatching. Assessing exercise hypoxaemia is difficult in these patients due to their generalized muscle weakness. However, sleep-related oxygen desaturation, particularly during REM sleep when the inspiratory system is most dependent on diaphragm function, is a common finding in patients with mild daytime hypoxaemia due to chest wall problems or neuromuscular diseases. Occasionally these changes are dramatic, but in boys with muscular dystrophy the presence of transient hypoxaemic episodes was no better guide to prognosis than was measurement of the vital capacity (Fig. 5). Arterial CO_2 tensions often lie in the high normal range, daytime hypercapnia only being seen in advanced disease.

Non-pulmonary disorders

Patients with stable congestive cardiac failure often show mild reductions in Pa_{O_2} and a normal or low Pa_{CO_2} due to premature airway closure secondary to pulmonary oedema. Some patients with severe liver cirrhosis develop the so-called hepatorenal syndrome, with otherwise unexplained hypoxaemia

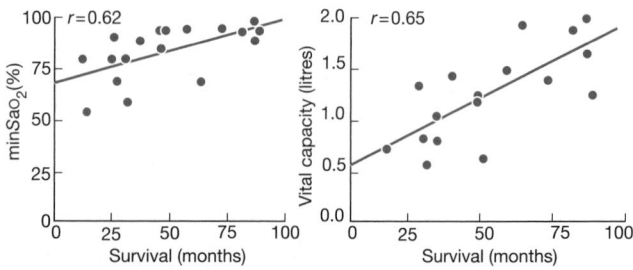

Fig. 5 Survival of boys with respiratory failure due to neuromuscular disease plotted against minimum arterial oxygen saturation recorded during sleep and vital capacity. (Based on data from Phillips *et al.* 1999.)

due to V/Q mismatching and true anatomical shunting through arteriovenous communications in the pulmonary circulation. Morbidly obese individuals can develop hypoxaemia and hypercapnia due to profound nocturnal hypoventilation and chemoreceptor resetting. Rather more common are the problems of patients with severe obstructive sleep apnoea who develop daytime hypoxaemia and hypercapnia secondary to recurrent nocturnal upper airway obstruction and oxygen desaturation. Careful review of these 'Pickwickian' patients often shows coexisting hypothyroidism or obstructive lung disease. This diagnosis should be suspected in any patient with COPD with significant respiratory failure and an FEV_1 greater than 1.5 litres. Correction of the sleep apnoea by nasal continuous positive airway pressure can produce significant improvement in daytime blood gases, but in the great majority of patients with obstructive sleep apnoea no significant abnormalities of waking gas exchange are seen.

Pulmonary vascular disease

This is an uncommon cause of hypoxaemia and at the time of diagnosis CO_2 retention is rare. Rather variable changes in D_LCO are reported, but as pulmonary hypertension becomes more advanced, exercise and resting hypoxaemia develops, a significant component being secondary to the reduced cardiac output and increase in mixed venous oxygen tension.

Assessment of chronic respiratory failure

This is relatively straightforward. The diagnosis of mild/moderate hypoxaemia rests on an awareness of the possibility rather than any specific clinical finding. When the arterial Po_2 is below 8.0 kPa, impairment of concentration and memory can be demonstrated, but these features are extremely non-specific. Although tempting to ascribe to hypoxaemia, the principal cause of breathlessness in these patients is usually the underlying disease. Reduction of peripheral chemoreceptor activity by supplementary oxygen can be beneficial, but this is usually secondary to a fall in minute ventilation rather that to any specific 'dyspnogenic' effect of hypoxia itself.

Hypercapnia is equally non-specific, with headache the most commonly attributed symptom. There are no good data to support this in compensated respiratory failure, although a generalized degree of vasodilation is seen in some patients with CO_2 retention, which may be accompanied by a large volume pulse and warm peripheral extremities.

On examination central cyanosis may be apparent as a bluish discoloration of the mucous membranes associated with an increase in the reduced circulating haemoglobin to approximately 5 g/dl. It is an unreliable clinical sign in some ethnic groups and in the presence of artificial illumination. An increased facial colouring due to secondary polycythaemia can occur, whilst the jugular venous pressure may be elevated and ankle swelling can develop in the face of worsening CO_2 retention.

The principal diagnostic steps are listed in Table 4. Measurement of arterial blood gases, preferably breathing air, is the most reliable way of diagnosing chronic respiratory failure. It is essential to know whether the patient was using oxygen when the sample was taken, and if so, at what inspired concentration. Patients with chronic airflow limitation treated with bronchodilators nebulized in oxygen may show unexpectedly high

Table 4 Diagnostic steps in detecting respiratory failure

1. Consider the possibility—see Table 3
2. Look for central cyanosis and other clinical signs
3. If the probability is high or unanticipated signs are present, measure arterial blood gases while breathing air
4. If it is not possible to measure arterial blood gases on air, note the inspired oxygen concentration
5. Blood gas tensions can change with the clinical state of the patient and measurements need to be repeated when this happens
6. Non-invasive pulse oximetry is useful for monitoring progress but cannot diagnose hypercapnia or its acidosis

Pao_2 for some time after this treatment. Non-invasive measurement of arterial oxygen saturation using pulse oximetry can be used to screen individuals at risk of chronic respiratory failure and to monitor patients in hospital or overnight, but it is no substitute for assessing blood gas tensions to make the diagnosis correctly.

Treatment of chronic respiratory failure

Managing stable chronic respiratory failure involves several steps:

(1) making a firm diagnosis;
(2) correction of the underlying disorder;
(3) increasing the inspired oxygen concentration; and
(4) increasing alveolar ventilation.

Making a firm diagnosis

This is essential for rational management. It is important to remember that more than one process may contribute to the development of chronic respiratory failure; for example, poor left ventricular function due to cardiac disease and chronic obstructive pulmonary disease together. The relative importance of each factor should be determined.

Correction of the underlying disorder

In general, treatment of the primary pathology improves both V/Q relationships and hence oxygenation, and respiratory system mechanics, which increases ventilatory capacity and lowers the $Paco_2$. In patients with COPD this usually involves administration of inhaled bronchodilators and corticosteroids (see Chapter 17.6), but marked improvement is the exception rather than the rule in patients where chronic respiratory failure has developed. Medical therapy tends to be ineffective by the time chronic respiratory failure has developed in interstitial lung disease and the neuromuscular disorders.

Specific pulmonary vasodilator treatment has been used to treat pulmonary hypertension, with most evidence of improvement seen after infusion of prostacyclin in primary pulmonary hypertension. Attempts to improve gas exchange in secondary pulmonary hypertension by the use of inhaled nitric oxide, a specific pulmonary arterial vasodilator, have been disappointing and in general, resting gas exchange has deteriorated after this treatment rather than improved.

Increasing the inspired oxygen concentration

Hypoxaemia secondary to V/Q mismatch or global hypoventilation is relatively easily corrected by supplementary oxygen. In chronic airflow limitation and especially COPD, where respiratory time constants for gas exchange are long, it may take 30 minutes before a new steady state is reached when breathing relatively low concentrations of oxygen. Monitoring of blood gases should be adjusted accordingly.

In the chronic stable state, treatment with oxygen is given to prevent or reverse the chronic consequences of hypoxaemia. The benefits of regular oxygen treatment on breathlessness are marginal and there are no data to suggest that the severity or subsequent progression of breathlessness is influenced by chronic oxygen treatment. Almost all data about oxygen therapy in chronic respiratory failure are based on observations in hypoxaemic COPD, treatment in other conditions being offered by analogy with this more common problem.

Two well-performed randomized clinical trials have shown that regular treatment of patients with COPD and stable hypoxaemia (Pao_2 less than 55 mmHg) prolongs life (Fig. 6(a)). These data suggest that patients using more oxygen (the 'continuous' limb of the Nocturnal Oxygen Therapy Trial Group) do better than either the United Kingdom Medical Research Council treatment group or the North American patients using oxygen only at night. A more recent Polish study found no benefit when patients with

COPD with a Pao_2 of 7.3 to 8.8 kPa were treated with oxygen at home for 15 h/day (Fig. 6(b)), emphasizing that chronic oxygen therapy is only of value when the oxygen saturation falls below 90 per cent.

These studies showed that progression of secondary pulmonary hypertension can be halted by regular oxygen treatment and secondary polycythaemia can be corrected. However, secondary polycythaemia in COPD is influenced by the amount of carboxyhaemoglobin from cigarettes and patients who continue to smoke do not show a fall in red cell mass or packed cell volumes with oxygen treatment. Neuropsychological effects of chronic hypoxaemia have been described and may be improved by regular oxygen treatment, although the evidence for this is limited.

Giving oxygen during exercise increases performance and particularly endurance in patients with COPD who are relatively normoxaemic, as well as those with resting hypoxaemia. Again carbon monoxide from cigarette smoking reduces this response, and whether oxygen desaturation during exercise is necessary for the benefit to occur has not been conclusively established, although it is used as a reimbursement criterion for portable oxygen in North America.

Oxygen concentrators are the most cost-effective way of delivering oxygen for near continuous use. These devices have proved reliable and safe and use the ability of zeolite cells to separate nitrogen from room air and so generate an oxygen-enriched inspirate. Liquid oxygen has the advantage of allowing refilling of portable oxygen units relatively easily for use during exercise. Oxygen masks are the most accurate way of delivering oxygen and a range of inspired concentrations (24, 28, 35 per cent) are available. However, they are easily dislodged during sleep and plastic oxygen nasal prongs with a long extension pipe offer an easier system for use in the home. Occasional patients, especially those with severe interstitial lung disease, may

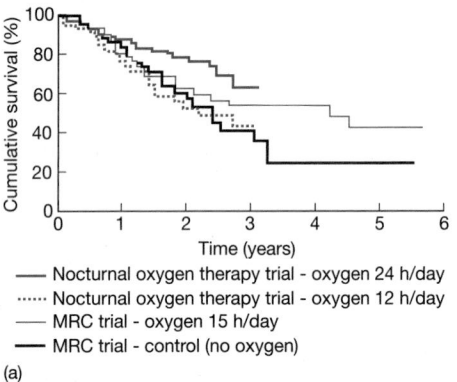

(a)

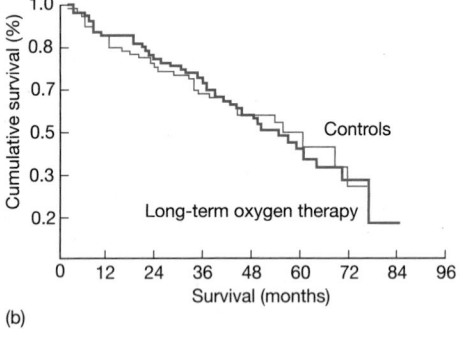

(b)

Fig. 6 The effect of regular domicilliary oxygen on survival in COPD. Panel (a) combines data from the MRC and NIH oxygen trial in the United States. Survival is greatest in those receiving oxygen for the whole 24-h day. Panel (b) is based on the study of Gorecka et al. for COPD patients with a Pao_2 between 7.3 and 8.5 kPa who were treated with oxygen or normal medical therapy. There was no survival benefit in the oxygen treated group, confirming the importance of the 7.3 kPa threshold in selecting patients for this therapy.

have difficulties obtaining a Pao_2 greater than 8.0 kPa with these systems. Transtracheal oxygen delivery may have a role here, but early enthusiasm for this has been tempered by problems with cannula occlusion, infection, and bleeding. A variety of oxygen-conserving devices that deliver oxygen only during inspiration have been developed which increase the time between refills of portable oxygen equipment as well as having financial advantages in some health-care systems.

Improving alveolar ventilation

Mechanical

This is a valuable way of reducing arterial CO_2 in disorders like COPD and can increase arterial oxygen tension as well, especially in conditions such as neuromuscular disease where hypoventilation predominates. The use of tank respirators in neuromuscular weakness has now been superseded by the development of non-invasive nasal positive-pressure ventilation (**NIPPV**), which is normally only needed at night. This therapy is used increasingly in the management of acute on chronic respiratory failure in patients where the primary problem is ventilatory without coexisting pneumonia/acute lung injury. Its chronic use arose from the belief that respiratory muscle fatigue was an important cause of CO_2 retention in COPD and the empirical observation that gas exchange and survival were better in patients with kyphoscoliosis treated with night-time cuirass ventilation. Newer studies have shown that respiratory muscle function is well preserved in COPD when allowance in made for the muscle shortening secondary to pulmonary hyperinflation. Several trials of NIPPV in stable hypoxaemic but normacapnic COPD have reported relatively unimpressive results. By contrast, NIPPV mainly given at night improved blood gases in patients with hypercapnic COPD, as well as leading to benefits in health status. No good randomized trial of this therapy has yet been reported and the role of NIPPV in the treatment of hypercapnic COPD is still controversial.

By contrast, significant symptomatic and blood gas improvements have been demonstrated in patients with kyphoscoliosis, but again no randomized clinical trial data are available. At present, it appears unlikely that these will be performed given the significant and sustained symptomatic benefits seen clinically. The only study to report prospective data on muscular dystrophy found no effect of regular NIPPV on survival in normocapnic patients, but use of this therapy as supportive treatment in the terminal phases of advanced muscular dystrophy appears to be associated with prolonged survival. It is always important in the face of progressive disease such as muscular dystrophy or motor neurone disease that the patient should be fully informed of the complications of NIPPV and the fact that it is unlikely to influence the underlying progression of the condition. Provided a good dialogue between patient, carer, and physician is established, then reasonable decisions about the use of this ethically difficult treatment are still possible.

Although volume-cycled ventilation was initially preferred, most patients are now managed with a bilevel pressure-cycled patient triggered device. This may have some advantages in obstructive lung disease where small amounts of PEEP can be added to reduce static PEEPi. Adequate peak inspiratory pressure generation, preferably in excess of 20 cmH2O, is needed in both COPD and kyphoscoliosis, where total respiratory system compliance is reduced. Patient–mask interfaces remain a major problem, especially in patients with unusual craniofacial structure where getting a comfortable mask fit without excessive tightness can be difficult. Progress should be assessed by regular blood gas measurements, and overnight monitoring of oxygenation and CO_2 tensions is useful at the start of therapy. Patience and trained respiratory therapists are the best way of ensuring long-term compliance with treatment.

Specific pharmacological therapy

Whilst mechanical ventilatory support is effective it is also cumbersome, uncomfortable, and restricting, hence a simple drug treatment would be invaluable. Although medroxyprogestrone acetate has non-specific ventilatory stimulant effects and can produce small falls in CO_2 tension in patients with COPD, its oestrogen-like side-effects limit its use. Methylxanthines like theophylline have some chemoreceptor stimulant effects, but are mainly of use for their bronchodilator and anti-inflammatory properties. Almitrine bismethylate is an interesting specific peripheral chemoreceptor stimulant drug, which also modifies intrapulmonary V/Q matching and increases arterial oxygen while reducing CO_2 tensions in patients with resting hypoxaemia. These properties have led to its use in parts of Europe, but it is associated with the development of peripheral neuropathy and possibly increasing pulmonary artery pressure during exercise, which has limited its more widespread application.

Despite the attractions of a pharmacological approach, concerns over the precipitation of inspiratory muscle fatigue and the recognition that, in most diseases, the central drive to breath is already high, mean that treatment with respiratory stimulant therapy is likely to have only limited clinical application.

Further reading

Anonymous (1980). Continuous or nocturnal oxygen therapy in hypoxemic chronic obstructive lung disease: a clinical trial. Nocturnal Oxygen Therapy Trial Group. *Annals of Internal Medicine* **93**, 391–8.

Anonymous (1981). Long term domiciliary oxygen therapy in chronic hypoxic cor pulmonale complicating chronic bronchitis and emphysema. Report of the Medical Research Council Working Party. *Lancet* **i**, 681–6.

Calverley PM, Leggett RJ, Flenley DC (1981). Carbon monoxide and exercise tolerance in chronic bronchitis and emphysema. *British Medical Journal* **283**, 878–80.

Calverley PM et al. (1982). Cigarette smoking and secondary polycythemia in hypoxic cor pulmonale. *American Review of Respiratory Disease* **125**, 507–10.

Costello R et al. (1997). Reversible hypercapnia in chronic obstructive pulmonary disease: a distinct pattern of respiratory failure with a favorable prognosis. *American Journal of Medicine* **102**, 239–44.

Doherty MJ et al. (1997). Cryptogenic fibrosing alveolitis with preserved lung volumes. *Thorax* **52**, 998–1002.

Gorecka D et al. (1997). Effect of long-term oxygen therapy on survival in patients with chronic obstructive pulmonary disease with moderate hypoxaemia. *Thorax* **52**, 674–9.

Haluszka J et al. (1990). Intrinsic PEEP and arterial P_{CO_2} in stable patients with chronic obstructive pulmonary disease. *American Review of Respiratory Disease* **141**, 1194–7.

Meecham JD et al. (1995). Nasal pressure support ventilation plus oxygen compared with oxygen therapy alone in hypercapnic COPD. *American Journal of Respiratory and Critical Care Medicine* **152**, 538–44.

Phillips MF et al. (1999). Nocturnal oxygenation and prognosis in Duchenne muscular dystrophy. *American Journal of Respiratory and Critical Care Medicine* **160**, 198–202.

Raphael JC et al. (1994). Randomised trial of preventive nasal ventilation in Duchenne muscular dystrophy. French Multicentre Cooperative Group on Home Mechanical Ventilation Assistance in Duchenne de Boulogne Muscular Dystrophy. *Lancet* **343**, 1600–4.

17.8 The upper respiratory tract

17.8.1 Upper airways obstruction

J. R. Stradling

Definition

The trachea and carina are usually included in discussions of upper airways obstruction because many of the conditions that can completely block off the main airway can affect the trachea, presenting in a similar way to those affecting the larynx and pharynx. For convenience, the causes of upper airways obstruction are divided into acute (within minutes or hours) and non-acute, although there is not quite such a clear distinction in clinical practice. Many of the causes of upper airways obstruction (particularly infection) are more common in children, but this section deals with the problem mainly from an adults' physician's perspective.

At resting levels of minute ventilation, the main airway can be reduced to a diameter of 3 mm or so before respiratory distress and stridor occur. Little more narrowing is required to precipitate complete asphyxia. Hence, when upper airways obstruction is suspected, assessment of severity, diagnosis, and treatment must be regarded as a medical emergency. The causes are listed in Table 1 and discussed in more detail below.

Diagnosis

Diagnosis of upper airways obstruction requires a high degree of clinical suspicion. Not all that wheezes is asthma. If upper airways obstruction develops gradually, then it is most likely to be misdiagnosed as asthma or

Table 1 Causes of upper airways obstruction

Acute	Non-acute
Inhaled foreign body	Tumours
Oedema	Tracheal stenosis
allergy	postintubation
angioneurotic oedema	post-tracheostomy
smoke burns	Tracheal compression
Infections	tumour
pharyngitis	thyroid
tonsillitis	aneurysm
epiglottitis	Tracheal abnormalities
retropharyngeal abscess	tracheomalacia
croup	tracheobronchiomegaly
	tracheobronchopathia-osteochondroplastica
	Recurrent laryngeal nerve palsy
	Laryngeal dysfunction

chronic airways obstruction, particularly if, for example, a carcinoma of the trachea coexists with chronic airways obstruction. This is not uncommon, since both are usually caused by smoking. Clues in the history will be a more rapid onset than might be expected for chronic airways obstruction and no previous history of a similar problem. The progression is usually relentless, without fluctuations, although a course of steroids prescribed for 'asthma' may produce temporary tumour shrinkage. At first, stridor or noisy breathing will only be heard on exercise, but it will gradually appear at lower and lower levels of activity. Sometimes the patient is well aware that the blockage is 'somewhere in the neck' and such a complaint should be taken seriously, as should associated haemoptysis. A non-productive cough is often present. A change in the voice in association with shortness of breath indicates the possibility of laryngeal obstruction. Upper airways obstruction is sometimes more symptomatic on lying down.

Examination

In pure upper airways obstruction, the noisy breathing will localize to the airway and tends to be monophonic and stridulous. Stridor may be absent if there is a long segment of obstruction. The only sound at the periphery on auscultation of the chest will be the transmitted noise of the stridor. However, as mentioned above, some patients will have coincidental lower airways obstruction, which should not discourage further investigation of a suggestive history. If upper airways obstruction is extrathoracic, stridor will tend to be worse on inspiration, and the converse may be true when the lesion is intrathoracic. The reasons for this are discussed below.

Tests of lung function

During a forced expiration from total lung volume down to residual volume there is a progressive fall in expiratory flow rate. This is largely due to the fact that the airways become narrower as the lungs become smaller, and this progressively restricts maximum flow rate regardless of the effort made. This can be displayed graphically as a plot of expiratory flow against the volume exhaled from total lung capacity down to residual volume, the so called 'flow–volume' plot or loop (Fig. 1(a)). This fall-off in maximal flow rates with falling lung volume is called 'volume dependence of flow'. However, if a fixed resistance is introduced (such as tracheal stenosis), then the maximal flow rate possible is independent of the lung volume. High flow rates, usually seen at larger lung volumes, cannot be generated and, instead of the normal triangular appearance of the flow–volume plot, it has a squared appearance. At lower lung volumes the normal intrinsic airways resistance may again exceed the abnormal upper airways resistance so that the flow–volume plot may once again follow the normal path (Fig. 1(a)).

If the apparatus required to measure flow–volume plots or loops is not available, a peak expiratory flow (PEF) meter and spirometry plot may be useful. Because the fixed extra expiratory resistance clips the high flow rates predominantly, then the PEF rate will be reduced disproportionately to the

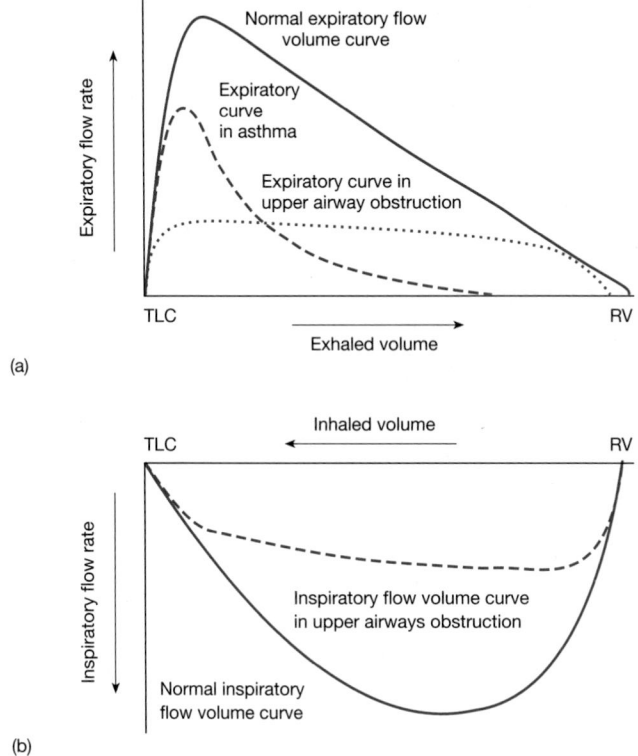

(a)

(b)

Fig. 1 (a) Expiratory flow–volume loop. The subject exhales with maximum effort from total lung capacity (TLC) until residual volume (RV) is reached. Normally, maximum flow (vertical axis) is reached early on and the flow falls almost linearly with lung volumes thereafter. In lower airways obstruction (e.g. asthma), all flows are reduced, but particularly at lower lung volumes. In upper airways obstruction, the maximum flow is clipped and roughly constant across most of the manoeuvre. (b) Inspiratory volume loop. The subject inhales maximally from residual volume (RV) up to total lung capacity (TLC). Normally, maximum flow is reached at about half-way when there is the best combination of airways size and muscle strength (see text). In upper airways obstruction, maximum flow is determined by the size of the remaining orifice and is roughly constant across the manoeuvre.

forced expiratory volume in 1 s (FEV_1). This is because the FEV_1 is a measure over a longer time period, which includes lower flow rates because of the falling lung volume. This gives rise to a simple index of upper airways obstruction; FEV_1 (ml) divided by the PEF rate (l/min). Normally the value will be less than 10, but as the PEF rate is preferentially clipped (which does not happen when there is increased diffuse airways obstruction such as asthma) it may rise above 10 in upper airway obstruction. However, an index of less than 10 does not exclude upper airways obstruction because the lesion may not be rigid and, if it is intrathoracic, it may also narrow a little as lung volume falls. Another spirometric clue to upper airway obstruction is the shape of the FEV_1 curve. Normally this is curved because flow rate falls with time, but it becomes straighter if flow rate is fixed (Fig. 2(a)).

If flow–volume plotting apparatus is available, inspiratory patterns can also be examined. The normal inspiratory limb of the flow–volume loop is almost semicircular (Fig. 1(b)). This is because at residual volume the airways are small and limit flow; towards total lung capacity the inspiratory muscles are reaching their full contraction and power is falling off. Hence maximum flows are achieved in the midrange of lung volume (Fig. 1(b)). Again, if upper airways obstruction is present, this pattern may be replaced by a squarer shape owing to the imposition of a lower maximum flow rate by the fixed resistance (Fig. 1(b)).

Comparison of the inspiratory and expiratory limbs of the flow–volume loop may give a clue as to the location of an upper airways obstruction. If

the lesion is extrathoracic and has any variability to its lumen, it will tend to be narrowest during inspiration (walls sucked together) and widest during expiration (blown apart). Conversely, an intrathoracic lesion will tend to be squashed on expiration by the raised intrathoracic pressures, thus presenting a higher resistance than during inspiration when it will tend to be pulled open. Although in theory these statements are correct, in practice flow–volume loops are not always sufficiently characteristic to allow a confident diagnosis about the exact site and presence of an upper airways obstruction. They may be more useful as a tool to follow changes, such as in response to treatment.

Vocal cord paresis due to bilateral recurrent laryngeal nerve damage is often very much worse on inspiration. Simple spirometry can be diagnostic here. The expiratory tracing will be normal as the cords are blown apart. If the patient immediately inhales back from the spirometer (make sure that a new in-line filter is present first) the inspiratory rate will be tortuously slow (Fig. 2(b)). The forced inspiratory volume in 1 s (FIV_1) will often be much smaller than the FEV_1, whereas normally the reverse is true (Fig. 2(b)).

The effect of breathing a low-density gas mixture, such as 21 per cent oxygen in helium (Heliox), on airways resistance has also been used to try

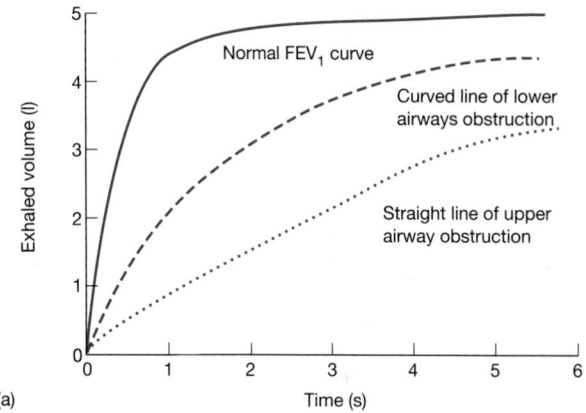

(a)

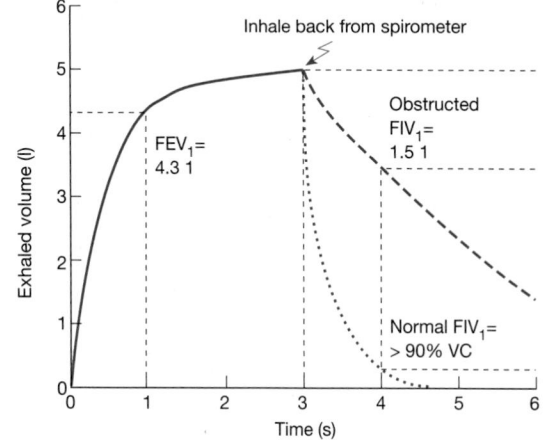

(b)

Fig. 2 (a) Curves of forced expiratory volume (FEV) against time. Normally exhalation is rapid, and more than 75 per cent of the final volume (vital capacity (VC)) is exhaled in 1 s (FEV_1). In lower airways obstruction, flows are slower and thus less air is exhaled in 1 s; the line is still curved because flows are falling. In upper airways obstruction, because flows are roughly constant at a low level set by the remaining orifice, the line is nearly straight and FEV_1 is also low. (b) Following a forced exhalation manoeuvre into a spirometer, a forced inhalation can be made. Normally inspiration is fast and the forced inspiratory volume in 1 s (FIV_1) is almost the vital capacity (VC). If there is upper airways obstruction, particularly extrathoracic such as at the vocal cords, then inspiration will be very limited and FIV_1 will be small.

to differentiate lower from upper airways obstruction. Flow in small airways is largely laminar and not affected by the density of the intraluminal gas. However, flow at a tight stenosis will be turbulent, and then it becomes dependent on the gas density. Thus airflow resistance will fall on breathing Heliox if the obstruction is in the upper airways, but will remain unchanged when the increased resistance is due to peripheral airways narrowing. This test may be particularly useful when there is evidence of both lower and upper airways obstruction, but proof of a significant contribution from an upper airways lesion is required before considering any further intervention.

For simple monitoring of progress of a patient with known upper airways obstruction on the ward, for example during treatment, sophisticated tests are not required, and measurement of the PEF rate is probably adequate for most purposes.

Specific causes

Acute causes of upper airway obstruction

Aspiration

Upper airways obstruction due to aspiration is usually due to the object lodging in the larynx, since this is the narrowest portion of the airway until two or three divisions down the bronchial tree. The usual culprit is a piece of food, and thus this condition has been colourfully called the 'café coronary'. The patient suddenly becomes distressed, is unable to talk, and apparently unable to breathe. He may point to his throat trying to indicate the problem. Inspiration to provide the air necessary for a good expulsive cough may not be possible. Indeed, lung volume may 'ratchet' down to residual volume.

The Heimlich manoeuvre was invented for this circumstance and its principles should be taught to first-aid workers. If the patient is still upright, then the helper stands behind with his arms clasped around the upper abdomen. A very forceful pull, backwards and upwards, will drive the diaphragm upwards and should provide enough expired air to shift the aspirated food from the cords (Fig. 3). The manoeuvre can be repeated, of course, but a forceful first try is likely to be the most successful. If the Heimlich manoeuvre fails, then it may be possible to dislodge the lump of food with a finger once the patient has become unconscious. The only alternative is an emergency cricothyrotomy which requires a hole to be made in

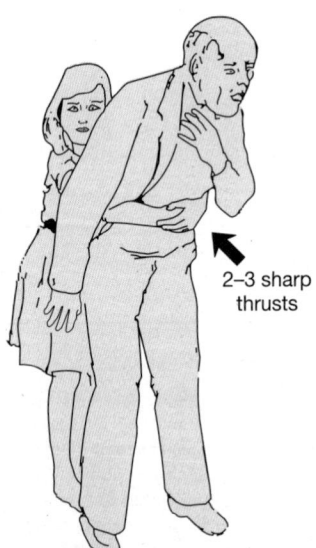

Fig. 3 The Heimlich manoeuvre for the emergency treatment of acute pharyngeal or laryngeal obstruction due to a bolus of food. Two or three sharp thrusts in the direction of the arrow may cause the food to be ejected. (Reproduced with permission from Flenley, 1990.)

the cricothyroid membrane just below the Adam's apple of the thyroid cartilage and above the cricoid cartilage. Even a small hole (2 mm or so) will allow sufficient ventilation to keep the patient alive. Emergency cricothyroidotomies have been attempted with everything from penknives to ballpoint pens: special large-bore curved-needle kits are available for the purpose and are safer than an unskilled attempt at a tracheostomy.

Oedema

Acute oedema of the larynx or pharynx is usually either due to allergy (atopic or non-atopic), a hereditary abnormality in the complement pathway, or inhalation of noxious gases.

Allergic oedema

Episodes of upper airways and facial oedema sometimes have no known cause and appear without warning. Often there will be an atopic history with a specific allergy. Some allergic reactions are not based on atopy and IgE, but may occur through IgG or direct activation of other inflammatory pathways. Allergies to nuts, strawberries, etc. may involve this latter mechanism rather than IgE. Insect stings usually produce pharyngeal and glottic oedema via IgE mechanisms.

Treatment of these allergic causes of upper airways obstruction consists of subcutaneous (or intramuscular) adrenaline (1 ml of 1:1000) with antihistamines and steroids (see Section xxx on acute anaphylaxis). Aerosolized adrenaline may also be useful, using 10 ml of 1:10 000 in an ordinary nebulizer.

Hereditary and acquired angioedema

Hereditary and acquired angioedema are due to deficiency of plasma C1 esterase inhibitor. This defect may be caused by impaired synthesis, due to a genetic defect causing failure of protein production, or production of inactive protein (hereditary angioedema), or by increased catabolism (acquired angioedema). The absence of C1 esterase inhibitor means that the enzyme activating the first component of the complement pathway is unchecked, allowing abnormal increase in activity of the whole pathway and production of vasoactive products.

Hereditary angioedema typically presents in infancy. An episode of oral and facial swelling is often precipitated by local trauma, such as a tooth extraction or a blow to the face, and lasts about 48 to 72 h. The skin manifestations do not itch in the way that allergic oedema does. Colicky abdominal pain due to intestinal oedema is an alternative presentation, when pooling of fluid in oedematous bowel can be sufficient to cause hypotension and shock. Diagnosis hinges on the clinical presentation, a positive family history (autosomal dominant), and low levels of C1 esterase inhibitor. In the form where normal amounts of inactive C1 esterase inhibitor are present, it is necessary to demonstrate low C4 levels during an attack.

Acquired angioedema presents in adult life. It is not familial. It may be associated with lymphoproliferative or other malignant diseases (type I) or more commonly with the presence of autoantibodies to C1 inhibitor (type II).

The disease is serious: 25 to 30 per cent of sufferers of hereditary angioedema die from asphyxia. As for cases of allergic upper airway oedema, treatment of the acute attack consists of adrenaline and steroids, but the response is much less satisfactory. Emergency tracheostomy or cricothyrotomy may be necessary. C1 esterase inhibitor plasma concentrate can be used for severe attacks, but very large doses are frequently needed for those with an acquired defect. Fresh-frozen plasma has been reported to work sometimes, but it contains larger amounts of the substrates C4 and C2 which might theoretically provoke worsening oedema.

Attenuated androgens, for example danazol, raise C1 esterase inhibitor levels within a few weeks, probably by increasing hepatic synthesis, and can usually prevent attacks in hereditary angioedema. Acquired angioedema generally fails to respond to this treatment, but can be treated prophylactically with antifibrinolytic agents. If episodes such as tooth extractions are triggers, then C1 esterase inhibitor can be given beforehand.

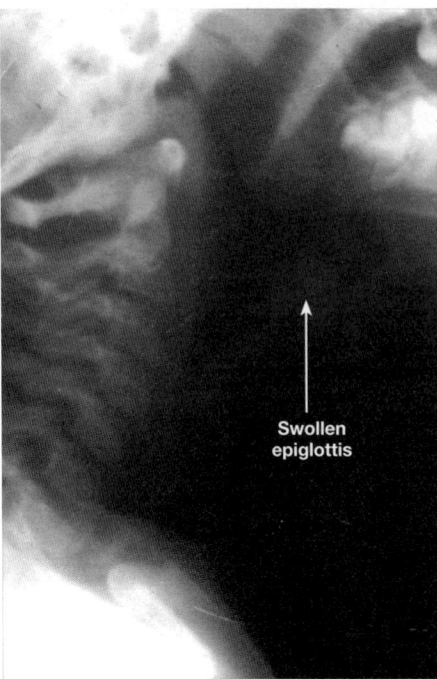

Fig. 4 Lateral neck radiograph of a child with epiglottitis. Note the swollen epiglottis overlying the glottis.

Swollen
epiglottis

Smoke inhalation

Inhalation of hot smoke can burn the upper airways and contributes significantly to deaths due to fires. Upper airways obstruction due to heat injury and mucosal swelling usually develops within 24 h of exposure, but stenosis due to scarring can develop later. A hoarse voice, stridor, severe conjunctivitis, burnt nasal hairs, and falling peak flow all suggest significant upper airways damage. Bronchoscopy is then the best tool to establish whether there is significant oedema or mucosal ulceration obstructing the airways.

Management usually consists of simple measures such as elevating the head of the bed and inhaling cool moist air with added oxygen. If peak flow continues to fall, then transfer to an intensive care unit and bronchoscopy with the capability to perform an intubation, guided by direct vision, is the correct approach.

Infections

Upper airway infections rarely cause obstruction in adults, but can do so in infants and young children. Whilst they can present dramatically with upper airways obstruction, prodromal symptoms usually occur. Streptococcal pharyngitis, tonsillitis, and retropharyngeal abscesses are amongst the most important. Croup (due to respiratory syncytial, parainfluenza, and other viruses) is very common, with narrowing of the subglottic trachea, sometimes with a thick purulent coating over the larynx and trachea. Treatment consists of cool mist and supplemental oxygen, with careful monitoring of upper airways function.

Although again more common in children, acute epiglottitis, usually due to *Haemophilus influenzae*, can affect adults. Pyrexia, drooling, hoarse voice, difficulty in breathing, intense sore throat, and stridor are the usual presenting symptoms. Compared with croup, there is usually a faster onset and course. The diagnosis may be missed initially but lateral neck radiographs show swelling of the epiglottis (Fig. 4). Attempts to examine the back of the throat may precipitate further obstruction, particularly in children. Even tipping the head back for a lateral neck radiograph can provoke complete obstruction and be disastrous. Thus, if there is evidence of breathing difficulty with stridor and the clinical diagnosis is epiglottitis, then the correct management for children is immediate transfer to inten-

sive care and intubation for 48 to 72 h whilst the infection is controlled by ampicillin or chloramphenicol. In adults, close monitoring in intensive care is probably adequate and prophylactic intubation is not routinely practised. General use of *H. influenzae* vaccines should make this problem increasingly rare.

Non-acute causes of upper airway obstruction

Tumours

Laryngeal, and less commonly tracheal, tumours are usually seen in smokers. The dominant cell type is squamous. Spread of a primary bronchial carcinoma into the base of the trachea is probably the commonest cause of upper airways obstruction in pulmonology practice.

Laryngeal tumours nearly always present with hoarseness, or voice change, and cough. Large airways tumours are commonly not diagnosed until far advanced. This is because they mimic lower airways obstruction, as mentioned earlier, and chest radiography is often normal. Tumours may also respond to asthma therapy, showing temporary shrinkage with steroids, which may further mask the real diagnosis.

If history, examination, and lung function tests suggest an upper airways obstruction, then some form of imaging is required. CT is the least invasive approach and therefore least likely to disturb the airway and make matters worse, but will provide no histology. Plain films (posteroanterior and lateral) may show tracheal narrowing but can be very deceptive. Direct visualization is usually necessary for diagnosis, biopsy, and to aid future therapy.

There is some disagreement as to whether fibreoptic or rigid bronchoscopy should be the investigation of first choice. Rigid bronchoscopy requires anaesthesia and sometimes this precipitates acute obstruction, when the bronchoscope then has to be passed quickly and forced through the obstructing tumour. This 'core-out' can reduce tumour bulk, with control of haemorrhage possible under direct vision, and improvement in the airway may buy time while other treatments such as radiotherapy are employed. Flexible fibreoptic bronchoscopy may be possible without disturbing the tumour, although coughing and increased secretions can precipitate complete occlusion. Direct application of adrenaline may help as an initial emergency treatment, and in theory cocaine (a vasoconstrictor) would be preferable to lignocaine as a local anaesthetic. If stenosis reduces tracheal diameter to less than 4 mm or so, it is best left alone during flexible bronchoscopy and should certainly not be biopsied (Fig. 5). In cases that are likely to be difficult, it can be helpful to pass an endotracheal tube over the flexible bronchoscope before it is introduced. This allows a guided intubation in an emergency, using the bronchoscope as a guidewire.

Aside from intubation or tracheostomy (when appropriate), emergency treatment of tumours compromising the upper airway consists of dexamethasone (12 mg daily), nebulized adrenaline (10 ml of 1:10 000 up to six

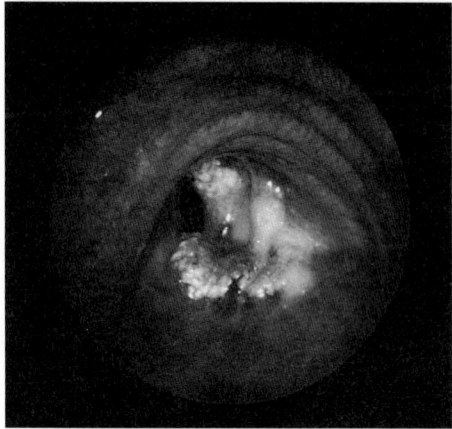

Fig. 5 Bronchoscopic view of a tracheal carcinoma blocking most of the lumen. (By courtesy of Dr P. Stradling.)

times daily), humidification of inspired air, and breathing Heliox (21 per cent oxygen in helium). Improvement in the airway may then be achieved by treatment of the tumour with chemotherapy or radiotherapy. Sometimes, however, these can initially provoke swelling of the tumour, so that steroids are usually prescribed first, with emergency treatments kept close to the hand (Heliox, adrenaline). If these therapies do not help, then palliation can be achieved with the use of bronchoscopically guided laser therapy or cryotherapy, which literally either burn or freeze away tumour tissue with a low incidence of serious haemorrhage. Laser therapy is a laborious procedure, currently only available in a few specialist centres. Cryotherapy is quicker and safer, and can be performed down a flexible bronchoscope. These techniques are only of use with intraluminal tumours and cannot be applied when the narrowing is due to external compression. Another approach is the use of silicon or metal endobronchial stents. Some of these can be inserted via a flexible bronchoscope; others require surgery. They are particularly useful when external compression is present, and can produce dramatic resolution of symptoms. It is rarely appropriate to 'debulk' a malignant tumour at thoracotomy in an attempt to improve large airway patency.

Unfortunately, upper airways obstruction from a tumour becomes a terminal event in many cases. Powerful sedation is indicated to make the patient unaware that he or she is asphyxiating and choking to death.

Some rare, non-malignant tumours can obstruct the trachea, and rarely granulomatous conditions such as sarcoid and Wegener's granulomatosis may mimic tumour.

Tracheal stenosis

Tracheal stenosis usually develops following prolonged intubation or after a tracheostomy has been allowed to close following tube removal (Fig. 6). This scarring may appear some time after the initiating event. Again, radiology or bronchoscopy will usually confirm the diagnosis, already strongly suspected from the history. Temporary relief may be obtained by dilating the stricture at rigid bronchoscopy. Definitive treatment involves resection of the stenosed portion and reanastomosis.

Tracheal compression

Tracheal compression (Fig. 7) may be due to malignant or non-malignant conditions. External compression by malignant tumour (primary or secondary) has been covered in the previous section. Non-malignant causes include thyroid enlargement, aortic aneurysm, sclerosing mediastinitis, mediastinal neurofibroma, and Castleman's disease. If definitive treatment is not possible, then stenting the airway is the only option available. When thyroid enlargement leads to tracheal obstruction, surgical removal may not solve the problem completely. Prolonged pressure on the trachea can

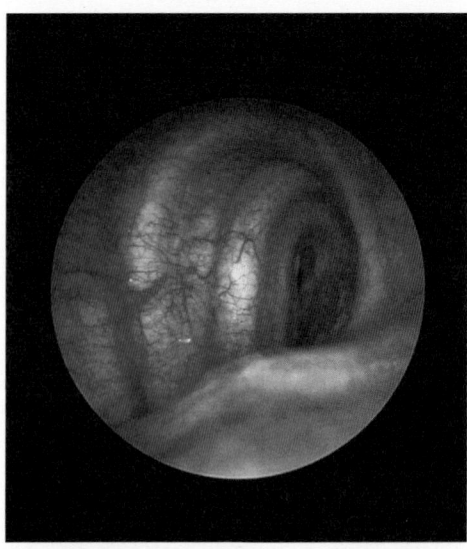

Fig. 7 Bronchoscopic view of external tracheal compression by right-sided paratracheal malignant nodes. (By courtesy of Dr P. Stradling.)

lead to tracheomalacia, so that the tracheal wall collapses when unsupported by the thyroid. Temporary use of an endotracheal stent is then appropriate.

Tracheal abnormalities

Tracheomalacia may be secondary to prolonged external compression (see above) or a primary abnormality that presents in childhood. It is essentially a weakness or deficiency of the supporting cartilages. It is sometimes seen secondary to a long history of chronic airways obstruction. Normally the anteroposterior diameter of the trachea decreases by up to about 10 per cent during a cough. In tracheomalacia, collapse during coughing is over 50 per cent and sometimes is complete. The symptoms of this are usually stridor, shortness of breath, and paroxysms of coughing. In addition, inefficient coughing can lead to recurrent pneumonia and bronchiectasis.

A 'scabbard trachea' is said to be present when the lateral dimensions of the trachea are significantly narrower than the anteroposterior dimensions. This deformity, usually present along the whole intrathoracic trachea, is normally associated with chronic airways obstruction. It rarely causes severe upper airways obstruction and on a plain chest radiograph there is obvious tracheal ring calcification.

Tracheobronchiomegaly (or Mounier–Kuhn disease) is probably an inherited structural abnormality of the trachea presenting in adult life as apparent chronic airways obstruction. The trachea is dilated from the larynx to the second- or third-generation airways. There is atrophy of both cartilage and muscle. It is usually misdiagnosed as chronic airways obstruction, but the presence of prolonged but ineffectual coughing and harsh upper airway sounds should lead to lung function tests which then show evidence of an expiratory (intrathoracic) upper airway resistance. Radiological examination will show the dilated airways.

Tracheobronchopathia osteochondroplastica is a very rare condition characterized by cartilaginous and bony excrescences growing into the large airway lumina. This can lead to significant upper airways obstruction, but is more often a post mortem finding which is unsuspected in life.

Relapsing polychondritis is an 'autoimmune' systemic disorder affecting cartilage all over the body (ribs, trachea, ear lobes, nose, joints) and may be associated with systemic lupus erythematosus, Wegener's granulomatosis, and cryptogenic liver cirrhosis. Large airways involvement is a frequent cause of death in this condition. There is irregular narrowing of the trachea and main airways, with flaccidity of the tissues sometimes allowing marked collapse on expiration. The diagnosis can be hard to make: involvement of other cartilaginous sites is the critical feature to look for. The condition is

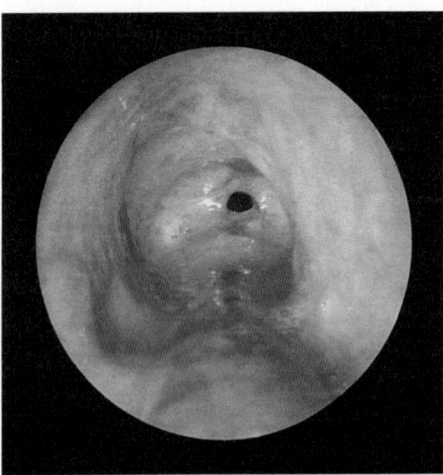

Fig. 6 Bronchoscopic view of a post-tracheostomy tracheal stricture. The remaining hole is about 2 to 3 mm in diameter. (By courtesy of Dr P. Stradling.)

often difficult to treat. Aside from local surgical or stenting procedures, steroids and other immunosuppressive therapies are usually given.

Laryngeal dysfunction

Damage to one recurrent laryngeal nerve usually causes a weak voice that improves a little with time as the opposite cord 'learns' to compensate by moving slightly across the midline to improve apposition. As the recurrent laryngeal nerve is invaded or compressed (usually by tumour at the left hilum), differential effects on abductors and adductors may be seen. For example unopposed adduction may occur prior to complete paralysis.

Bilateral recurrent laryngeal nerve paralysis produces flaccid cords that lie passively midway between full abduction and adduction. Abduction is very poor, such that rapid inspiration will draw the cords together and produce stridor, thus limiting exercise tolerance. Inspiratory stridor may initially be present only during sleep, when general decrease in muscle tone reduces any residual laryngeal abductor activity. Although this may be labelled as snoring, careful questioning of a witness will identify whether snoring or the machinery-like screech of inspiratory stridor is present (particularly if the physician can imitate the two noises!).

The usual clinical history is of voice change following thyroidectomy some years before. This may have been quite subtle, such as difficulty in singing, but with speech relatively unaffected. Nocturnal stridor and reduction in exercise tolerance then develop over a period of years. Eventually the obstruction at night can be sufficient to produce obstructive apnoea and respiratory failure. These events may be due to involvement of the previously damaged recurrent laryngeal nerves in scarring at the thyroidectomy site. Sometimes bilateral paralysis can occur for no apparent reason, and it is assumed that the aetiology is similar to Bell's palsy or the diaphragmatic palsy of neuralgic amyotrophy. A very rare differential diagnosis is an Arnold–Chiari malformation causing brain stem compression and presenting with sleep-related stridor in association with ventilatory failure.

Laryngeal surgery could prevent inspiratory cord closure, but would do so at the expense of the voice. Thus a tracheostomy with a speaking tube is the usual approach. However, if the night-time obstruction is the main problem (with sleep disruption and daytime sleepiness), nasal continuous positive airway pressure therapy will usually keep the cords apart during sleep.

Damage to the superior laryngeal nerves supplying the cricothyroid (a vocal cord tensor) causes only a weak voice. Speech is still possible because the main adductors still function

Apart from laryngeal paralysis, laryngeal destructive conditions such as rheumatoid arthritis can lead to poor abduction with inspiratory stridor, particularly at night. In Parkinson's disease with autonomic involvement (Shy–Drager syndrome) or more generalized brain atrophy (multisystem atrophy) there can be a fairly specific wasting of the laryngeal abductors. This also presents with inspiratory stridor (or apnoea) at night and can progress to respiratory failure.

Functional laryngeal abnormalities, with narrowing during inspiration and/or expiration, can occur. These may be due to psychological problems, but the syndrome blends with reflex laryngeal dysfunction in patients with asthma. Expiratory laryngeal wheezing can occur in response to emotional pressure even in well-controlled asthma. In this situation, the laryngeal component of the increased airways resistance can be considerable. Inhalations of histamine can sometimes mimic this, which might therefore be due to a reflex originating from afferent receptors. Why this should happen is not clear, but it may be activation of the laryngeal braking mechanism to help raise functional residual capacity.

Functional inspiratory stridor is not particularly related to asthma, but may follow a respiratory tract infection. There is some evidence that techniques used by speech therapists can help with this problem.

Further reading

Cicardi M, Bergamaschini L, Cugno et al. (1998). Pathogenetic and clinical aspects of C1 inhibitor deficiency. *Immunobiology* **199**, 366–76.

Empey DW (1972). Assessment of upper airways obstruction. *British Medical Journal* 3, 503–5.

Flenley DC (1990). *Respiratory medicine.* Baillière Tindall, London.

Fraser RG, Paré JAP, Paré PD, Fraser FS, Genereux GP (1990). *Diagnosis of diseases of the chest*, Vol. 3. W.B. Saunders, Philadelphia, PA.

Goldman J and Muers M (1991). Vocal cord dysfunction and wheezing. *Thorax* **46**, 401–4.

Valsecchi R, Reseghetti A, Pansera B, Di Landro A (1997). Autoimmune C1 inhibitor deficiency and angioedema. *Dermatology* **195**, 169–72.

17.8.2 Sleep-related disorders of breathing

J. R. Stradling

Introduction

This chapter discusses the disorders of breathing that appear only during sleep. This rapidly expanding subspecialty within respiratory medicine now provides about 10 to 15 per cent of the speciality's referrals. Following its first proper description in 1967 as a medical curiosity, obstructive sleep apnoea and its variants are now thought to significantly impair the functioning of about 0.5 to 1 per cent of the population. Most general hospitals will have some form of monitoring system for the diagnosis of sleep apnoea syndromes, although tertiary centres tend to provide most of the treatment. The diversity of symptoms produced by these disorders means that all physicians need to have an understanding of them and are likely to come across many cases during their professional life.

Normal physiology of breathing during sleep (Table 1)

Sleep can be divided into two very different states. The dominant sleep stage is non-rapid eye movement (NREM) sleep (Figs 1 and 2). This phase of sleep, which is preferentially reclaimed following sleep deprivation, appears to be when the brain shuts down and is necessary for maximum daytime alertness and continuing cognitive function. NREM sleep shows a continuum from drowsy down to very deep sleep, arbitrarily subdivided into stages 1, 2, 3, and 4. The awake electroencephalogram (EEG) is characterized by low voltage, high frequency activity, with the only dominant frequency being the so-called alpha activity (approximately 10 Hz), present when the eyes are closed. As sleep supervenes, the alpha activity disappears, overall EEG frequency falls, muscle tone (usually measured from a chin electromyogram (EMG)) falls, and the eyes begin to roll from side to side. This transition phase is called stage 1. Stage 2 is defined by the appearance of K complexes (isolated large waves) and sleep spindles (bursts of about 13 Hz activity). As sleep deepens further, increasing amounts of large, slow waves (approximately 1 Hz) appear. These stages are called 3 and 4, or slow-wave sleep.

The other main phase of sleep is rapid eye movement (REM) sleep or dreaming sleep. This stage is characterized by a return of the EEG to a pattern resembling wakefulness. The EMG tone falls to very low levels and there are bursts of rapid eye movements, mainly from side to side, under closed eyelids. Effectively the cortex is 'awake' again, processing images and able to integrate outside noises or other stimuli into complex dreams. The fall in EMG tone is because the rest of the body's muscles have been 'cut off' from the brain and paralysed, hence the fall in EMG tone. This paralysis (or atonia) is under active control from a centre in the pons that hyperpolarises the lower motor neurones via inhibitory reticulospinal pathways. Cats in

Table 1 Sleep and breathing

	NREM	REM
Electroencephalogram	Progressively slower frequency and higher amplitude	Similar to the awake pattern
Eye movements	Initially slow and pendular, then none	Bursts of rapid binocular movements
Postural muscle tone	Reduced from wakefulness	Very much reduced or absent
Factors controlling breathing	Loss of wakefulness input Brain-stem and classical stimuli dominate, but reduced compared with wakefulness	Cortical over-riding and apparent reduction in responses to classical stimuli
Arousal response	Small changes in Pao_2 and $Paco_2$, with the consequent ventilatory response, are required for arousal	Larger changes in Pao_2 and $Paco_2$ required before arousal occurs
Potential effect on breathing	Fall in minute ventilation Rise in pharyngeal resistance Fall in Pao_2	Further rise in pharyngeal resistance Loss of use of accessory muscles of respiration Further falls in Pao_2 tolerated longer before rescued by arousal

NREM, non-rapid eye movement: REM, rapid eye movement.

whom this centre has been destroyed no longer show atonia during REM sleep, and as a consequence they may get up and walk around or appear to chase phantom birds, presumably reflecting their dream content. The function of this atonia centre may therefore be to prevent the dreaming brain from influencing the rest of the body. Paralysis during REM sleep occurs dominantly in muscles that normally have a tonic postural activity; thus the diaphragm is spared although pharyngeal, intercostal, and accessory muscles are all affected to differing extents.

The normal pattern of the oscillation between NREM and REM sleep is shown in Fig. 2. This 'hypnogram', as it is called, is constructed by classify-ing successive 30-s epochs from tracings of EEG, EMG, and eye movement data into either awake, movement, REM sleep, or stages 1–4; thus 960 epochs are obtained in an 8-h night.

During wakefulness breathing is influenced by a variety of pathways, some conscious and voluntary, others entirely automatic and involuntary. Classic responses to hypoxia, hypercapnia, and vagal afferents (integrated in the brainstem) can be overruled by cortical signals to subserve functions such as talking. These two types of control are separate and can be damaged separately by disease processes. The presence of wakefulness itself provides an input to the respiratory centre, almost equivalent to the amount of ventilation seen at rest. Thus, following a period of hyperventilation, a normal subject will go on breathing at just below normal levels, despite hypocapnia and hyperoxia, until the carbon dioxide rises, when normal ventilation is re-established. This is not true during NREM sleep, when hypocapnia will produce apnoea until the $Paco_2$ rises back to a critical threshold level.

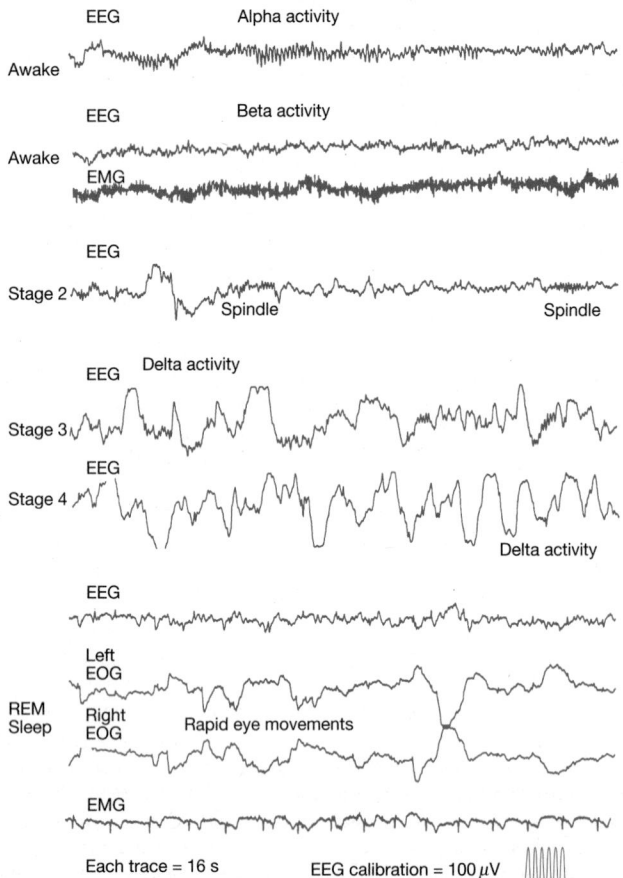

Fig. 1 Examples of electrical brain activity (EEG), eye movements (EOG), and chin muscle tone (EMG) during wakefulness and the different sleep stages.

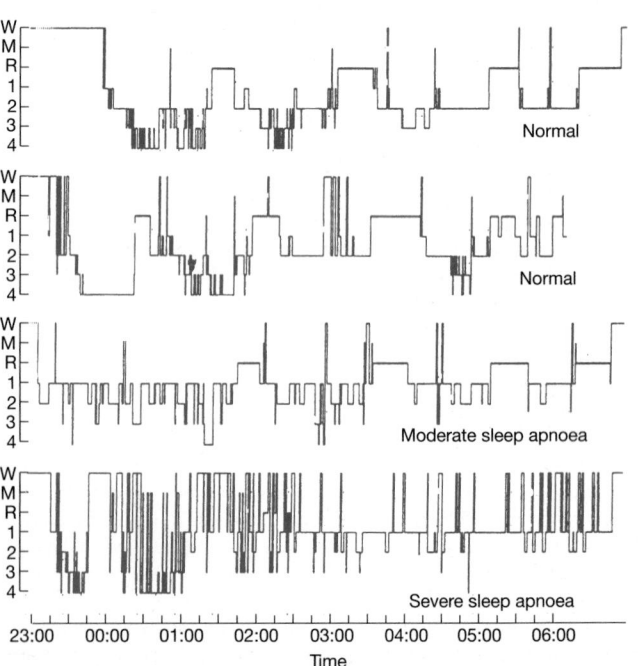

Fig. 2 Examples of all-night hypnograms (based on 20-s epochs) in two normal subjects and two patients with sleep apnoea. Note the reduced deep sleep (stages 3 and 4) in the patients, but no indication that they are waking up hundreds of times a night. W, awake; M, movement (awake); R, REM sleep; 1 to 4, stages 1, 2, 3, 4 of non-REM sleep.

Another component of wakefulness is the high muscle tone that holds the body in the required posture. This 'awake' input into the anterior horn cells means that other inputs, such as those from the respiratory centre, can further activate muscles, including the intercostals and pharyngeal. The withdrawal of this 'awake' tone with the onset of sleep means that a certain respiratory centre output to the relevant anterior horn cells is less able to raise membrane potentials to firing threshold, such that respiratory muscle activity falls with sleep onset, minute volume typically reduces by about 10 to 15 per cent, and $Paco_2$ rises by 3 to 8 mmHg. Reduction of pharyngeal muscle tone narrows the lumen, and thus there is normally a rise in upper airway resistance. This reduction in ventilation has trivial effect on the arterial oxygen saturation (Sao_2) in the normal circumstance when Sao_2 is on the flat part of the haemoglobin dissociation curve, but dramatic falls in saturation will be apparent when Sao_2 starts below 92 per cent, the steep part of the curve. If ventilatory responses to carbon dioxide or hypoxia are measured during NREM sleep, the slopes are flatter and right shifted, indicating a reduced overall sensitivity. Exactly why this occurs is not known, but reduced tone of the respiratory muscles, the withdrawal of awake drive, increased upper airway resistance, and (probably) true reduction in central sensitivity to carbon dioxide or [H$^+$] could all contribute. If, as a consequence of respiratory disease, compensatory mechanisms are already employed to cope with the extra work of breathing, then these seem to be particularly reduced during sleep as well.

During REM sleep, overall ventilation stays much the same as in NREM sleep, but the breath-to-breath variability increases considerably, sometimes with apnoeas during the actual periods of eye movements, and compensatory increases in between. Sensitivities to carbon dioxide and hypoxia were originally thought to be further reduced, but they are hard to measure in the presence of spontaneously variable breathing and more recent evidence suggests they may not change much at all. What is far more important is the atonia of postural muscles. The hyperpolarization of the anterior horn cells greatly reduces the efficacy of respiratory signals to the intercostal, accessory, and pharyngeal muscles. This will not matter in a normal subject with an efficient diaphragm and a non-compromised pharynx. However, if the subject is dependent on muscles other than the diaphragm for breathing, or has a narrow compromised pharynx, then REM sleep may powerfully interfere with ventilation with consequent hypoxaemia and hypercapnia.

Also of relevance to breathing during REM sleep are the reduced arousal responses to respiratory stimuli compared with non-REM sleep. The arousal responses to some ventilatory stimuli (hypoxia, hypercapnia, extra resistive load) are believed to be mediated mainly by the perception of the ventilatory effort made in response, rather than the specific ventilatory stimulus itself. If a ventilatory response to hypoxia is measured during REM sleep, then the subject will usually tolerate a much lower Sao_2 before arousing compared to NREM sleep. Furthermore, if the drive to sleep is high, such as after sleep deprivation, arousal will be delayed still further.

It can be seen from the above that, although sleep is not a problem for those with normal respiratory systems, once abnormalities are present there is potential for a damaging interaction between sleep and breathing, particularly during REM sleep.

Obstructive sleep apnoea

Definition

Sleep apnoea was first properly documented in neurophysiological sleep laboratories using techniques that had been developed for the investigation of conditions such as insomnia, narcolepsy, and depression. It was realized that hundreds of episodes of breath cessation, or apnoea, usually due to upper airway obstruction with associated snoring, were related to marked sleep disturbance. Because simple oronasal flow detectors were used, the critical event was defined as an episode of apnoea. Because it was easy to measure, an arbitrary definition was made, and breath cessation for longer than 10 s became an official apnoea. Early work suggested that normal,

Table 2 Causes of obstructive sleep apnoea

Anatomical
Central (neck) obesity
Micro- or retrognathia
Maxillary underdevelopment (e.g. cranial dysostoses, such as Aperts and Treacher Collins syndromes)
Pharyngeal encroachment (e.g. tonsillar hypertrophy, acromegaly, tumours, mucopolysaccharidoses, oedema)
Neuromuscular
Bulbar palsies
Neurological degenerative disorders (e.g. multisystem atrophy)
Myopathies (e.g. Duchenne dystrophy)
Other provoking factors
Alcohol
Sedative drugs
Sleep deprivation
Increased nasal resistance
Hypothyroidism

young people rarely had more than about 30 apnoeas per night, so that the standard definition of 'sleep apnoea syndrome' became more than 35 apnoeas per night, or more than five per hour of sleep, each lasting for 10 s or longer. This definition has existed long beyond its clinical usefulness: it is quite clear that recurrent partial obstruction to the upper airway can fragment sleep just as severely with no actual apnoeas or hypopnoeas developing at all. A more pragmatic and clinically useful definition might now be 'a sleep disruption syndrome that is due to a respiratory problem engendered by sleep itself, sufficient to cause symptoms when awake. Usually this is upper airway incompetence during sleep, but may also be due to problems of respiratory drive'. As the pathogenesis of sleep apnoea is explained, this shift in emphasis, with the inclusion of symptoms, will become clear.

Aetiology (Table 2)

The upper pharyngeal airway has to serve two functions, swallowing and breathing, which require different design features. When used for swallowing the pharynx has to behave like the oesophagus, and when used for breathing it has to remain an open tube like the trachea. These dual functions are achieved by having a floppy and collapsible muscular tube that is also capable of being held open rigidly by dilator muscles. The muscles responsible for this dilator function are discussed in the section on the structure and function of the upper respiratory tract (see Chapter 17.1.1). All these muscles have reduced activation during sleep, so that some pharyngeal narrowing occurs normally. There are, then, additional factors that determine whether this reduction leads to significant upper airflow obstruction in a particular individual. There are various theories as to these additional factors, but essentially they divide into two groups. Firstly, there may be abnormalities of the activation of the pharyngeal dilator muscles, perhaps due to defective or unstable central control. Secondly, there may be anatomical abnormalities that allow significant obstruction to occur even with the normal sleep-related reduction in muscle tone.

Neuromuscular function

Early investigations of EMG activity in pharyngeal muscles found reductions in tone with sleep during obstructive apnoeas. However, it was very difficult to show that these reductions were truly abnormal. Recent evidence shows that there is in fact an increase in activity of these muscles, both awake and asleep, in response to factors provoking pharyngeal collapse. In some patients with primary neuromuscular problems (from brainstem lesions to myopathies) there can be associated obstructive sleep apnoea, and pharyngeal muscle involvement seems a probable explanation. However, the majority of patients with obstructive sleep apnoea do not show evidence of any other neuromuscular problems.

During inspiration, pharyngeal dilator activity has to be synchronized with diaphragmatic activity and be adequate to overcome negative intrapharyngeal pressure. It has been suggested that a lack of co-ordination between diaphragmatic and pharyngeal activation may allow the pharynx to collapse. For example normal subjects breathing against an inspiratory resistance can be made to have a few obstructive apnoeas by artificially inducing periodic breathing during sleep. The gradual return of respiratory drive, following the nadir of ventilation, seems to activate the diaphragm first, leaving the pharynx unbraced. The presence of an inspiratory resistance then 'challenges' the pharynx and allows collapse for a few breaths before pharyngeal tone returns and restores patency.

Although instability of respiratory control during sleep has been postulated as a cause of obstructive sleep apnoea, following treatment with nasal continuous positive airway pressure therapy (see later) there is no evidence of a premorbid underlying respiratory instability, nor does altering respiratory drive have a useful effect. More convincing is the suggestion that there may be failure of normal reflex protective mechanisms in the pharynx, whereby receptors in the pharynx detect falls in pressure that distort the airway and provoke protective increases in pharyngeal dilator tone (see Section 17.1.1). Snoring itself may also be one of the stimuli that activate this dilator reflex, and it is conceivable that interruption of this reflex arc can occur, perhaps through years of pharyngeal trauma from snoring, mucosal oedema, or toxic agents such as cigarette smoke and alcohol.

Anatomical causes

Anatomical abnormalities influence pharyngeal function in a variety of ways. Simple encroachment of the pharyngeal lumen, for example with tonsillar hypertrophy, means that the normal fall in pharyngeal dilator tone with sleep can lead to critical narrowing and obstruction. Alternatively, there are abnormalities which 'load' the upper airway, requiring increased dilator muscle action that is then lost during sleep (for example high nasal resistance or increased external compression from neck obesity). Finally, there may be mechanical problems such that muscular activity fails to dilate the pharyngeal lumen effectively.

There are many case reports of obvious anatomical abnormalities provoking obstructive sleep apnoea, for example tonsillar hypertrophy, pharyngeal oedema, tumours, acromegaly, mucopolysaccharidoses, and mandibular or maxillary underdevelopment. These reports show that pharyngeal narrowing (asymptomatic whilst awake) can provoke obstructive sleep apnoea, but such diagnoses represent only a small proportion of cases.

The majority of patients with obstructive sleep apnoea are overweight. In many clinics the average obesity index is well over 30 kg/m², equivalent to being about 30 per cent overweight, for example 95 kg (15 stone) at a height of 1.78 m (5 ft 10 in). Weight loss can certainly cure obstructive sleep apnoea, and all studies identifying risk factors have found obesity to be dominant, accounting for up to 40 per cent of the variance in severity.

Most groups have found neck circumference to be a better predictor of severity of obstructive sleep apnoea than obesity itself, suggesting that it is neck obesity and external pharyngeal loading that is important. Animal studies have shown that only a small amount of extra external pressure over the pharynx is required to collapse it during sleep, and recent imaging studies have suggested that quite small amounts of extra fat do occur either side of the pharynx in patients with obstructive sleep apnoea, together with larger amounts subcutaneously.

Although general obesity is related to neck obesity, the overall correlation is only about 0.75. This is because fat distribution varies considerably between individuals. The 'female' distribution tends to be in the lower body and the 'male' distribution is more central. Thus a man who is not particularly overweight can have a large neck and vice versa.

As mentioned earlier, there is evidence that some of the upper airway dilator muscles (e.g. genioglossus) of obese patients with obstructive sleep apnoea are actually working harder than normal, perhaps as compensation for the added external loading from neck obesity. Compensations by the

respiratory system for other types of extra loading have been shown to be much less active during sleep.

In summary, overall the evidence suggests that most obstructive sleep apnoea in adults is due to loading of the upper airway caused by obesity. This external loading can be fended off during wakefulness but not during sleep, when the withdrawal of postural muscle tone allows the pharyngeal dilators to be overwhelmed, leading to excessive narrowing or collapse of the airway, with consequent apnoea.

However, not all adult sleep apnoea can be explained by obesity or intrapharyngeal anatomical abnormalities. The significance of marked retro- or micrognathia for obstructive sleep apnoea was recognized early on, particularly in children (Pierre–Robin syndrome). Careful cephalometric studies of facial and skull morphology have revealed that some patients with obstructive sleep apnoea have longer faces, retropositioning of the mandible (measured as a more acute angle between the sella to nasion and nasion to supramentale planes), a downward movement of the hyoid, elongation of the soft palate, and a narrower anteroposterior distance behind the tongue. Some, or all, of these changes may be secondary to many years of sleep apnoea rather than part of the cause. However, the retropositioning of the mandible may be contributory, and surgery to advance the mandible may be curative in carefully selected cases.

Retropositioning of the mandible may be a legacy from childhood. There is good evidence that nasal blockage and mouth breathing very early in life alter facial development (the so-called 'adenoidal facies'), and one feature of this is mandibular retropositioning. Following early adenoidectomy and resumption of nasal breathing, the mandible can return to its normal position. One theory is that mandibular underdevelopment and obesity are two relatively common independent risk factors for obstructive sleep apnoea that together may be synergistic.

Other factors provoking obstructive sleep apnoea

Alcohol is a potent reducer of muscle tone, and can further reduce pharyngeal dilator muscle tone during sleep. It is well known that alcohol worsens snoring, but it can also convert snoring to full apnoea. Other sedatives, such as the benzodiazepines, barbiturates, and opiates, can do the same, and this has important consequences for anaesthesia in such patients. Sleep deprivation itself can reduce upper airway muscle tone during subsequent sleep, provoking a vicious circle, whereby apnoea causes sleep disruption, causing worsening apnoea.

Nasal blockage can contribute to the tendency of the pharynx to collapse by lowering intrapharyngeal pressure. If extra effort has to be made to inspire through a high nasal resistance, there will be a greater vacuum effect in the pharynx, increasing its tendency to collapse. Once collapse occurs, flow ceases, pharyngeal pressure returns to atmospheric, the lumen opens, and the cycle repeats. This certainly leads to snoring, but may no longer be very important when there is full apnoea. However, nasal obstruction may contribute long term to sleep apnoea by damaging the pharynx through years of snoring, making it more collapsible, but improving nasal patency rarely cures obstructive sleep apnoea.

Hypothyroidism is associated with obstructive sleep apnoea, but the mechanism is not clear. It may be through weight gain or through tissue or fluid deposition in the pharynx. Alternatively, a low thyroxine level may interference directly with muscle function.

Immediate consequences of sleep apnoea

Upper airway narrowing, sometimes with complete apnoea, usually commences as sleep passes from awake to stage 2. Once significant obstruction occurs there will be increasing respiratory effort to try and overcome it. The length of such events is highly variable, ranging from only a few seconds to well over a minute. At some point arousal occurs, with an improvement in upper airway resistance, resolution of any asphyxia, and then a return to sleep, whereupon the cycle repeats (Figs 3, 4, and 5). Hypoxaemia and mild hypercapnia usually accompany these periods of obstructed breathing. If there is complete apnoea, the rate of fall of Sao_2 will depend mainly on the amount of oxygen stored in the lungs. This depends on the functional residual capacity since apnoeas occur at end-expiration, preventing inspiration. The length of the apnoea also determines how low the Sao_2 will fall, and varies considerably between patients. The consequences of such hypoxaemia and hypercapnia are not clear. Because the blood gas derangements are so transient they may do little harm, unless there is already ischaemic heart disease, for example.

Hypoxaemia was believed to play an important part in the arousal response that saves the patient from continuing asphyxia. In animal models, removal of the carotid body abolishes significant ventilatory response to hypoxaemia during sleep and there is no arousal. Giving extra added oxygen does prolong apnoeas to a small extent and delay arousal. However, recent evidence suggests that the main arousal stimulus is the actual respiratory effort being made in response to asphyxia, rather than the asphyxia per se. Normal subjects tend to wake when they have to make respiratory efforts about three times above the normal (10–20 cmH_2O

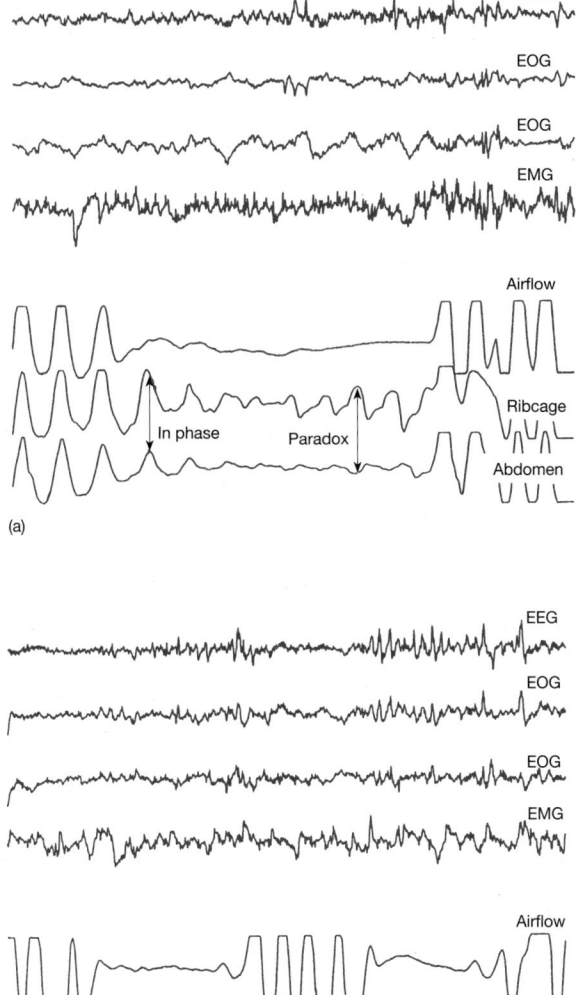

(a)

(b)

Fig. 3 Obstructive (a) and central (b) apnoeas (16-s traces): (a) airflow ceases, but rib-cage and abdominal movements persist and become paradoxical; (b) rib-cage and abdominal movements cease as well as airflow.

pleural pressure swings). This degree of effort is easily reached in obstructive sleep apnoea, when pressures down to –80 cmH_2O can be recorded during the frustrated inspiratory efforts. Such pressures can also be reached by heavy snorers, even if they do not develop hypoxaemia, and this also leads to arousals.

In terms of symptoms, the most important consequence of sleep-induced upper airway narrowing is sleep fragmentation. The original methodology of sleep analysis, using coarse 30-s epochs to stage sleep, effectively glossed over the multitude of transient arousals that are the main consequence of obstructive sleep apnoea. Superficially, a sleep hypnogram in a moderately severe case (Fig. 2) could look almost normal despite hundreds of arousals. The importance of trying to measure these has recently been appreciated, and technology to measure arousals automatically is being developed. However, the level of sleep disruption (number and 'size' of arousals) necessary to cause daytime symptoms is not known. There is a clear, but variable, relationship between increasing sleep disruption and deteriorating daytime function, meaning that there is no clear cut off between normality and abnormality.

In addition to blood gas disturbances and sleep disruption, there are many other consequences of obstructive sleep apnoea. During the apnoea there is activation of the diving reflex that produces bradycardia, particularly when there is associated hypoxaemia. Upon arousal there is a sudden pulse rate and blood pressure rise, probably due to activation of the sympathetic nervous system as part of the arousal process itself. During the actual frustrated inspiratory efforts, blood pressure falls with each reduction in intrathoracic pressure (pulsus paradoxus) and, in conjunction with the blood pressure rise on arousal, produces a very characteristic trace (Fig. 4). As well as increased nocturnal catecholamine secretion in patients with obstructive sleep apnoea, there is also a suppression of growth hormone and testosterone levels. There is marked polyuria during sleep (a reversal of the normal relative oliguria), but the mechanism is not clear. It may be related to the recurrent arousals, or to increased atrial natriuretic peptide (ANP) production following right atrial distension due to large inspiratory efforts.

It will be clear from this account that there are grey areas of uncertainty regarding definition and measurement of significant aspects of sleep apnoea. We discussed earlier that original definitions centred on the actual obstructive event. There has now been a shift towards trying to look more closely at the most important result—sleep fragmentation. This is particularly necessary now we know that 10-s apnoeas are not the only result of upper airway narrowing during sleep that can provoke multiple arousals and daytime sleepiness. Since heavy snorers can have considerable sleep fragmentation without significant falls in Sao_2, examining blood gas abnormalities (for example with an oximeter) is not always good enough either. The implications for this in terms of investigations are discussed later. A considerable amount of effort is being put into establishing which variable, measured during a sleep study, best defines the severity of the disorder. At present there is no clear answer and therefore there remain many different approaches to diagnosis and management.

Symptoms and presentation

The main symptom of obstructive sleep apnoea is daytime hypersomnolence, and this correlates broadly with the degree of sleep disruption. Early in the development of the disorder the daytime sleepiness is little more than often experienced by normal people after a few disturbed nights. Whilst occupied there is little difficulty in concentrating and staying awake, but once activities become more boring, unwanted sleepiness intervenes. Initially this may be viewed as normal, such as falling asleep in front of the television every evening. As the sleep disruption worsens there will be interference with an increasing number of activities. Of particular importance is sleepiness whilst driving. Sleepiness can be devastating, particularly on long motorway journeys after dark, when sensory stimulation is low. Initially there will be lane wandering with sudden arousal and correction. Accidents involving driving off the road, or driving into vehicles in front,

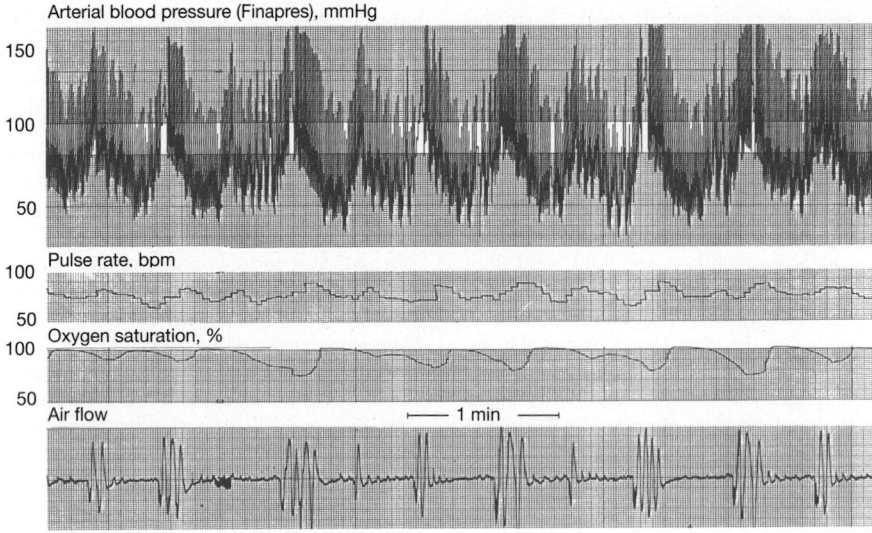

Fig. 4 Five-min tracing from a patient with obstructive sleep apnoea. The rises in blood pressure (top trace) and heart rate (second trace) coincide with the cessation of each apnoea and an arousal. During each apnoea (evident from the bottom airflow trace) each frustrated inspiratory effort is accompanied by a fall in blood pressure (pulsus paradoxus).

are more common in patients with obstructive sleep apnoea. Sleepiness also impinges greatly on work performance and home life. The patient will develop a reputation for slothfulness and lack of interest.

It is important to ask the right questions to assess sleepiness. It is not the same as tiredness, which is a lack of energy or desire to get up and do anything, without a desire to sleep. Because of the insidious onset of obstructive sleep apnoea, any sleepiness may be regarded as normal by the patient, and thus situational questions need to be asked such as 'how often do you have to pull off the road whilst driving owing to sleepiness?' rather than just 'are you sleepy?' A well validated and simple way to do this is with the Epworth Sleepiness Scale (Fig. 6). Objective sleepiness can be assessed in the sleep laboratory by measuring how long the patient takes to fall asleep on a number of occasions across the day. This is useful for research purposes but adds little to the clinical management of such patients. A list of other symptoms seen in obstructive sleep apnoea is given in Table 3. It is sad to say, but the corrosive effect of sleepiness on all aspects of a patient's life has often been present for years before someone (usually not a doctor) tumbles to the diagnosis.

A typical case history would be that of a middle-aged man complaining of increasing daytime sleepiness. It is usually some specific event that prompts initial consultation, such as falling asleep whilst driving, operating machinery, or during an important board meeting. There will be a long history of gradually worsening snoring with apnoeas, possibly witnessed by the spouse, who will probably have moved out of the bedroom owing to the noise. There is likely to have been a weight gain over the last few years with an obesity index of greater than 30 kg/m^2 and a collar size of 17 inches or more. There is usually a history of fairly high alcohol intake and smoking. On examination there may be nasal stuffiness, evidence of a small lower jaw (such as teeth crowding or several extractions for this problem), and a small pharynx with mucosal bogginess and wrinkling. Of course, it should be stressed that not all these features are likely to be present in one individual.

Part of the history and examination of patients with possible obstructive sleep apnoea should be directed towards precipitating factors such as hypothyroidism and acromegaly. Other diagnoses such as mucopolysaccharidosis, pharyngeal tumours, tonsillar hypertrophy, neurological disorders, and significant retrognathia will be more obvious.

Diagnosis

Following the history and examination, further outpatient tests may be appropriate, for example thyroxine or growth hormone estimations. Blood gases and simple lung function tests may be necessary if associated diurnal respiratory failure is suspected. A raised haemoglobin may also signify diurnal respiratory failure, as will a raised venous bicarbonate. Obstructive sleep apnoea tends to go with the findings that constitute the so-called 'syndrome X', namely hypertension, obesity, and insulin resistance. Blood pressure and blood sugar should be measured.

Unless the presenting problem turns out not to be sleep related, some form of sleep study will be required. In the past, the usual procedure was to employ full polysomnography, which measured sleep state and respiratory variables (Figs 2 and 3). This investigation and its analysis is expensive and time consuming, particularly if all recurrent arousals are documented. The primary requirement is to assess sleep fragmentation, establish if a respiratory problem is responsible, and decide if upper airway obstruction is the primary cause. Full polysomnography, properly interpreted, will usually allow this, with the EEG and EMG giving good information on sleep disruption, and aspects of respiration deduced from rib-cage/abdominal movement transducers, oronasal airflow, and snoring and continuous oximeter recordings. However, there is considerable signal redundancy in such recordings, and the essential derivatives—sleep disruption and respiration—can be assessed in much simpler ways (Fig. 5). Most clinical respiratory sleep laboratories have abandoned routine, conventional polysomnography because of its unnecessary expense.

Sleep fragmentation can be inferred from a variety of signals. The most sensitive appears to be autonomic markers of brainstem activation, such as blood pressure and pulse rate rises. In addition, since most abnormal respiratory events will end in some form of arousal, counting body movements provides some guide to the degree of sleep fragmentation, and may be most predictive of daytime symptoms. Upper airway obstruction can be inferred from snoring, a particular inspiratory pattern on a nasal flow tracing (flow limitation), paradoxical ribcage/abdominal movements, and from pulsus paradoxus visible on a beat to beat blood pressure tracing (now easily obtainable non-invasively, Fig. 4). Many simple, commercial monitoring systems can be used to record these signals and to assess the extent of the sleep fragmentation and whether upper airways obstruction is the likely cause. Recent work suggests that these simpler measures can predict sleepiness in obstructive sleep apnoea, and its response to treatment, at least as well as EEG-based approaches, which are clearly not the gold standard they were once thought to be. The attention paid to each signal, and perhaps the exact sleep study system used, will depend to some extent on the condition under investigation. Figure 5 shows data provided by the system in routine use in our laboratory, designed primarily to identify obstructive sleep apnoea and its variants, but it will also identify central sleep apnoea (see below) and non-respiratory problems such as periodic movements of the legs during sleep.

Because of the imprecise relationship between the number of abnormalities on a sleep study and the severity of symptoms, trying to count them exactly is pointless, particularly given that there can be considerable night to night variation. Hence, the reporting of sleep studies tends to be more qualitative than previously, with divisions simply into mild, moderate, and severe. The reporter is essentially trying to see if there is an adequate and understandable explanation for the patient's symptoms.

Treatment

Once it is established that the patient's symptoms are likely to be due to sleep disruption from sleep-induced upper airway obstruction, then therapy has to be tailored to symptom severity.

Mild symptoms may resolve with simple treatments and advice (Table 4). Weight loss is undoubtedly effective, but often very difficult to achieve. If sleep disruption only occurs whilst supine, when upper airway obstruction tends to be worst, then learning to lie on one's side may be helpful. Stopping sedatives and evening alcohol can help. Initial enthusiasm for the tricyclic antidepressants has waned, although they may slightly improve mild cases. They are believed to work through REM sleep suppression and by improving upper airway tone. No other drug has shown any consistent effect.

If symptoms are severe, there is one effective therapy—nasal continuous positive airway pressure (NCPAP). This treatment involves wearing a small mask (Fig. 7) over the nose whilst asleep, kept above atmospheric pressure by a pump. Pressures in the region of 10 cmH$_2$O are enough to splint open the pharynx and resist collapse, allowing unobstructed breathing and undisturbed sleep (Fig. 8). The response is dramatic, in terms of both physiology and daytime symptoms. These resolve rapidly, even after one night of treatment. There are several randomized, placebo-controlled trials proving beyond doubt the symptomatic benefit. The unpleasantness and unaesthetic appearance of this treatment initially repels patients, but once the benefits have been experienced, acceptance is high. Off-the-shelf systems, with comfortable soft masks, are now available for home use at about £300 each. Such equipment will last for years and represents extraordinary value for money given the enormous improvement in patient functioning that they produce. NCPAP machines have recently been introduced that

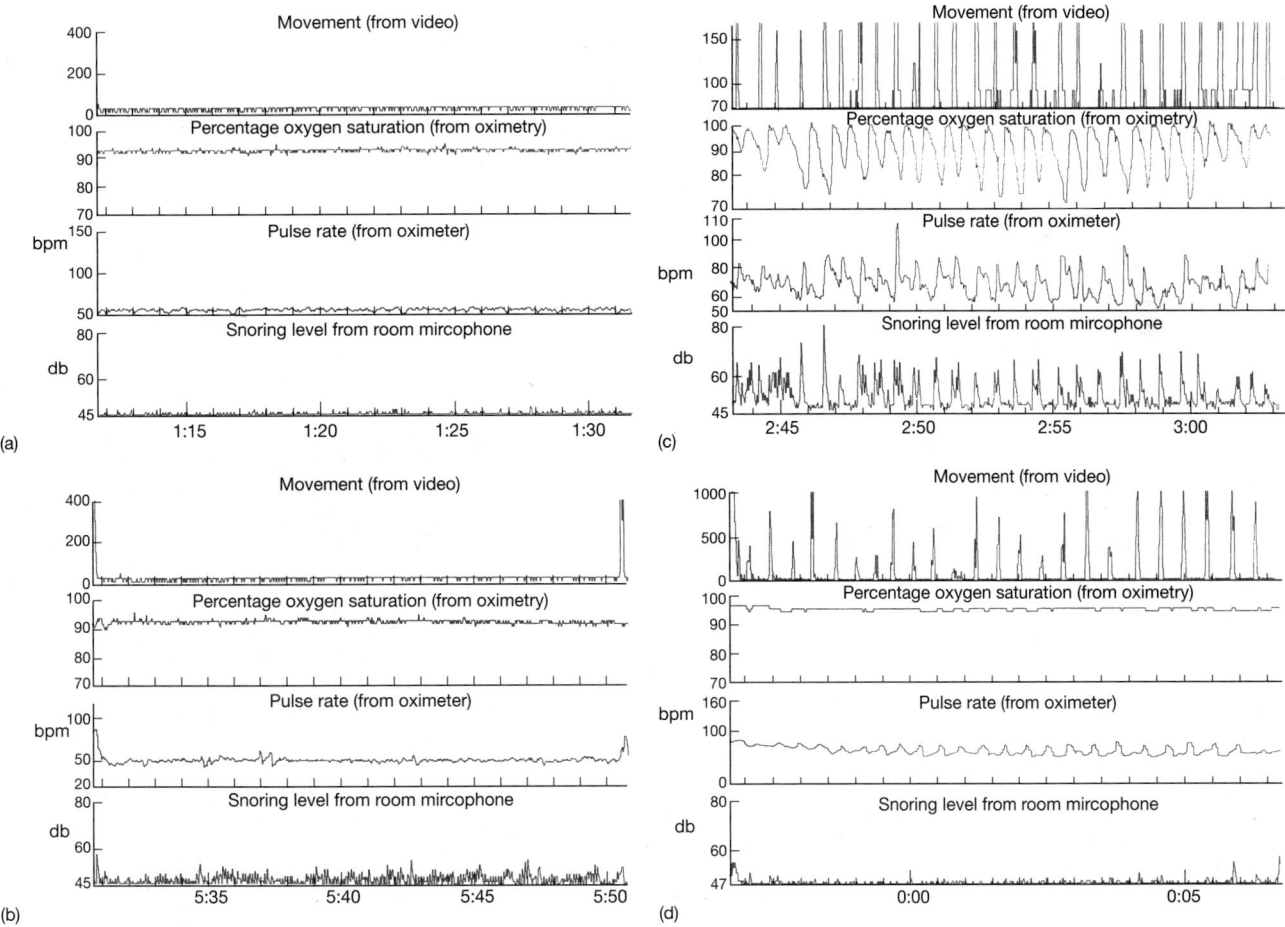

Fig. 5 Short sleep tracings of body movement, Sao$_2$, pulse rate, and snoring level in four different subjects. (a) Normal subject (no fluctuations in any signals), 20 min. (b) Patient with continual low level snoring and almost no arousals, 20 min. (c) Patient with classical obstructive apnoeas, evident from the snoring–silence–snoring pattern together with movements and oscillations in the pulse and Sao$_2$, 20 min. (d) Patient with periodic movements of the legs during sleep, recurrent arousal (oscillations in pulse and body movements), but no evidence of a respiratory cause (no snoring or Sao$_2$ dips), 10 min. A video recording of the whole night is always available and can be viewed when the exact cause of abnormal signals is not immediately obvious.

hunt automatically the pressure required by the patient to overcome their obstructive sleep apnoea. These are mainly used in the sleep laboratory as there is no evidence to support their more general use.

Much effort is put into helping patients to become established on NCPAP, through attentive education and comfort-improving measures such as humidification. Once established on NCPAP, a patient with obstructive sleep apnoea is likely to require it for life unless he can lose a significant amount of weight. This may only be achieved through gastric surgery, such as silastic ring gastroplasty to reduce food consumption. Another surgical treatment, whose popularity is decreasing, is uvulopalato-pharyngoplasty, which consists of removing part of the soft palate and any residual tonsils, and 'tightening up' the sidewalls of the pharynx. Although it can reduce snoring, its success rate at treating obstructive sleep apnoea is not good: approximately 50 per cent of patients experience a 50 per cent

EPWORTH SLEEPINESS SCALE

Name: .... Hospital number ....

Date: .... Your age (Yrs) .... Your sex (Male = M/Female = F) ....

How likely are you to doze off or fall asleep in the situations described in the box below, in contrast to feeling tired?

This refers to your usual way of life in recent times.

Even if you haven't done some of these things recently try to work out how they would have affected you.

Use the following scale to choose the *most appropriate number* for each situation:-

0 = would *never* doze

1 = *Slight* chance of dozing

2 = *Moderate* chance of dozing

3 = *High* chance of dozing

Situation	Chance of dozing
Sitting and reading	
Watching TV	
Sitting, inactive in a public place (eg a theatre or a meeting)	
As a passenger in a car for an hour without a break	
Lying down to rest in the afternoon when circumstances permit	
Sitting and talking to someone	
Sitting quietly after a lunch without alcohol	
In a car, while stopped for a few minutes in the traffic	

Thank you for your cooperation

Fig. 6 Questionnaire scale to assess subjective sleepiness. The scores for each answer (0–3) are summed to give a range from 0 (no sleepiness at all) to 24 (maximally sleepy). The upper limit of normal is about 9, and most patients with symptomatic obstructive sleep apnoea are in the middle teens.

Table 3 Symptoms of obstructive sleep apnoea

Most common (>60%)
Loud snoring
Excessive daytime sleepiness
Restless sleep
Unrefreshing sleep
Nocturia
Apparent personality changes
Witnessed apnoeas
Less common (10–60%)
Choking or shortness of breath sensations at night
Reduced libido
Nocturnal sweating
Morning headaches
Rare ('10%)
Enuresis
Complaint of recurrent arousals and insomnia
Nocturnal cough
Symptomatic oesophageal reflux

improvement in the number of apnoeas per hour. Attempts to improve the selection of patients have had very limited success, although thin patients with large soft palates, residual tonsils, and milder disease do the best. The operation may have a more significant role in the treatment of snoring-induced arousals than full apnoeas, although this is not established.

Other operative techniques involving advancement of the mandible (and sometimes the maxilla) may be appropriate in highly selected cases. Tracheostomy was the first therapy ever tried and was (of course) very effective. It may still be appropriate in occasional patients.

Table 4 Advice for patients with snoring or mild to moderate obstructive sleep apnoea usually due to postural dependence

1. Learn to sleep on your side and avoid sleeping on your back
2. No alcohol after 18.00 hours
3. No sedatives
4. Lose weight
5. Stop smoking
6. Keep the nose as clear as possible

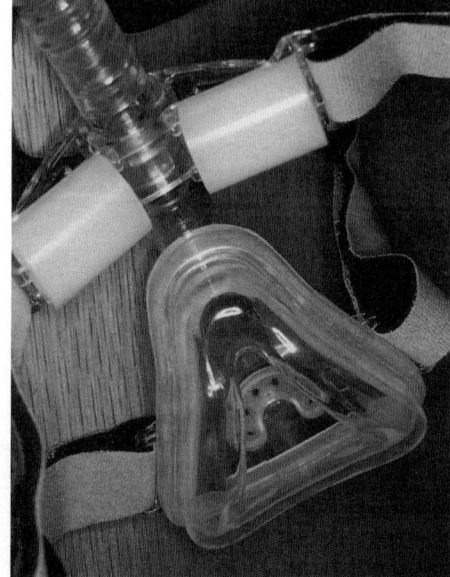

Fig. 7 A soft silicone nasal mask and its head gear, used in the treatment of obstructive sleep apnoea.

A newer approach has been the use of mandibular advancement devices, worn in the mouth at night (Fig. 9). These hold the lower jaw closed and forward, thus increasing the space behind the tongue and hence pharyngeal volume. They are undergoing extensive trials in a variety of situations, but the situation is complicated by the plethora of such devices available. The current conclusion is that they do work, but less so as the severity of the obstructive sleep apnoea (and usually therefore the obesity) increase. Their main use currently is in the control of unacceptable snoring.

Epidemiology

Given difficulties over definition, the prevalence of symptomatic obstructive sleep apnoea is hard to establish, and will depend on where an arbitrary cut-off is drawn. In an early study, about 0.3 per cent of men aged 35 to 65 years clearly had severe, symptomatic obstructive sleep apnoea, requiring nasal continuous positive airway pressure (NCPAP) therapy and responsive to such treatment. However, about 5 per cent had more than five dips of more than 4 per cent SaO_2 per hour, one suggested threshold for normality. However, most of these subjects were not obviously symptomatic and would not have wanted a treatment such a NCPAP. Overall in this study, sleepiness correlated with snoring, and more sleepiness seemed to be due to snoring than classical sleep apnoea. Other studies in Israel, the United States, and Italy have found prevalences of 'significant' sleep apnoea in the 0.5 to 2 per cent range.

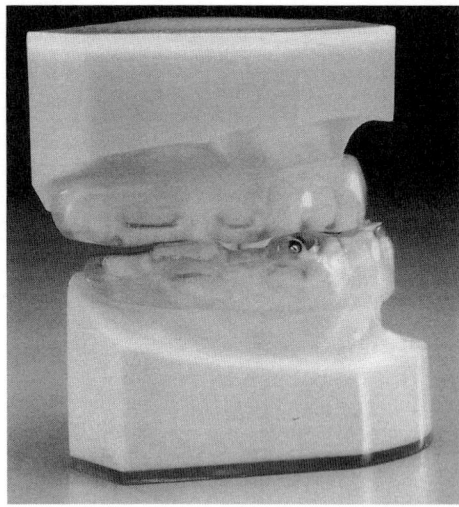

Fig. 9 Example of a mandibular advancement device, worn in the mouth at night. These hold the lower jaw forward and closed, thus increasing pharyngeal dimensions. They are used extensively for the control of snoring but they are not very effective in any more than mild obstructive sleep apnoea.

Predictors of sleep apnoea in these prevalence studies have been obesity, snoring, age, self-reported sleepiness, and alcohol consumption. Snoring is more common in men than women, and obstructive sleep apnoea syndrome itself is about five to ten times more common in men. The prevalence in women probably increases after the menopause with redistribution of body fat to a more male-like, upper body, distribution.

If these prevalence studies are correct, then obstructive sleep apnoea is more common than sarcoidosis and fibrosing alveolitis combined; and every chest physician in the United Kingdom should have about 100 patients on NCPAP.

Prognosis and long-term complications

Although the main reason for treating obstructive sleep apnoea is to relieve the daytime symptoms, mainly sleepiness, there is also limited evidence that these patients have an increased cardiovascular mortality (Fig. 10). Two studies have looked at the long-term survival of patients with treated obstructive sleep apnoea and compared them with some form of untreated control patients. Both found an increased mortality due to cardiovascular

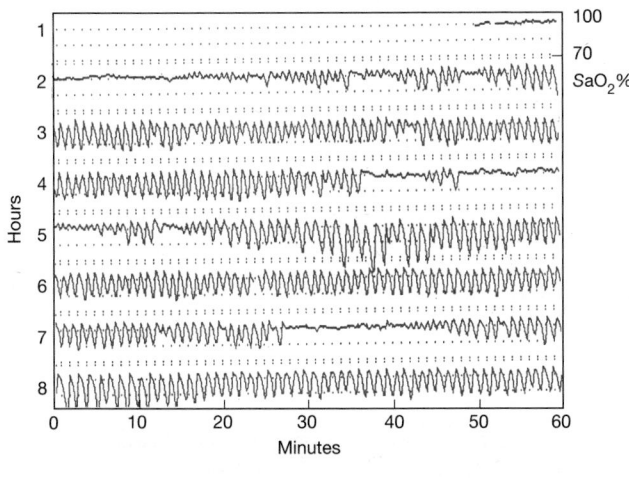

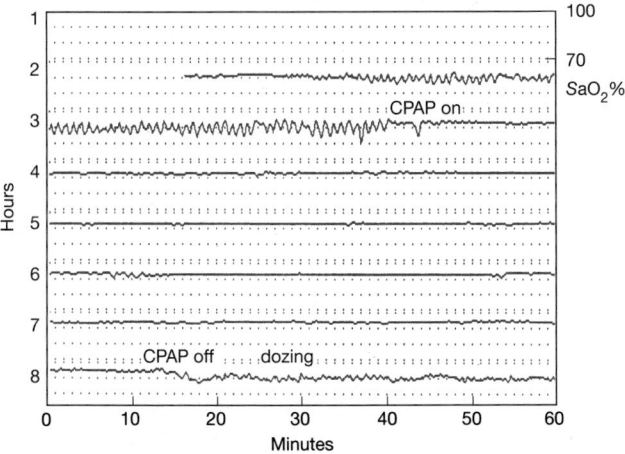

Fig. 8 Two all-night oximetry tracings from a patient with obstructive sleep apnoea, before treatment and during his first night on nasal CPAP. Each tracing starts top left and finishes bottom right. Each tracing is continuous for 8 h with the vertical axis for each individual line scaled 70–100 per cent SaO_2.

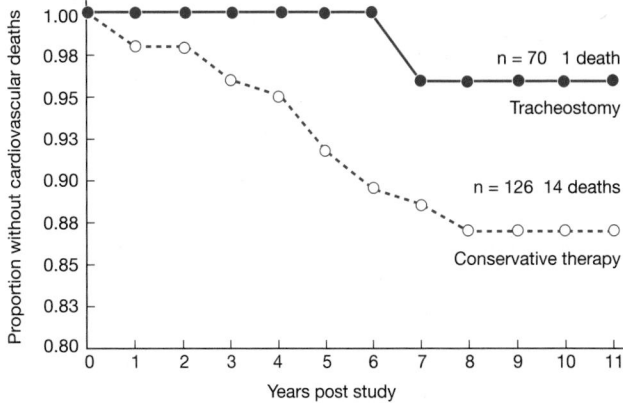

Fig. 10 Long-term survival without a cardiovascular death of 196 patients with obstructive sleep apnoea. The two groups consisted of one with 70 patients who accepted the definitive treatment then available of tracheostomy, and one with 126 patients who declined such therapy and merely attempted weight loss. (Reproduced with permission from C. Guilleminault and M. Partinen (1990). *Obstructive sleep apnoea syndrome.* Raven Press, New York.)

events such as myocardial infarction and stroke in the untreated group. The cause of this is not clear and a variety of hypotheses have been advanced. The main problem is that, because a variety of cardiovascular risk factors also contribute to the production of obstructive sleep apnoea (central obesity, smoking, alcohol), it is difficult to identify the real contribution made independently by obstructive sleep apnoea to cardiovascular deaths. Possibilities include sustained hypertension, intermittent nocturnal hypertension, increased catecholamine release, hypoxia-induced cardiac arrhythmias, insulin resistance, hyperlipidaemia, and left ventricular hypertrophy. As yet, most of these risk factors have not been shown to differ between patients with obstructive sleep apnoea and well-matched controls. The exception are the episodic blood pressure rises that occur with each apnoea, a very small increase in diastolic blood pressure (about 2 mmHg), and a small carryover of the raised systolic nocturnal blood pressure into the first few hours of wakefulness (Figs 4 and 11). These nocturnal surges in blood pressure may be harmful to the vascular system, and absence of the usual nocturnal fall in blood pressure is said to be a marker of cardiovascular morbidity. Treatment with nasal NCPAP prevents these surges in blood pressure by abolishing the apnoea-induced arousals, and this may be the mechanism by which NCPAP improves mortality in obstructive sleep apnoea, although there are many other possible explanations.

Nasal CPAP produces a demonstrable improvement in vigilance and sleepiness, which in a randomized, controlled trial was reflected in improved performance on a driving simulator. There is also some evidence that the higher car accident rate in patients falls after treatment. In the 3 years prior to diagnosis, health care utilization by patients with obstructive sleep apnoea, compared to matched controls, is about twice as high. Recent data suggest that this too falls following treatment.

Conclusions

There has been a move away from considering obstructive sleep apnoea to be a condition that one either has or does not have. There is a continuum from light intermittent snoring through to severe, all-night, obstructive sleep apnoea. An analogy can be drawn with hypertension, where there is also a continuum of severity, variability in the measurement, only moderate correlation between the measured abnormality and the physiological consequences, uncertainty over the most relevant way to measure it (one-off versus 24-h blood pressure monitoring), and the target organ damage (e.g. atheroma) may not just be due to the blood pressure. In addition, benefits of treatment have to be weighed against any side-effects. Sleep-

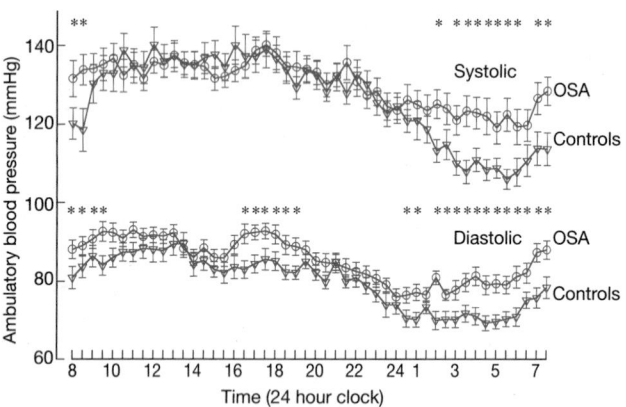

Fig. 11 Twenty-four-h blood pressure records (half hourly) from a group of patients with obstructive sleep apnoea, and individually matched control subjects. The asterisks indicate the times when there were significant differences between the groups. Note the higher systolic and diastolic pressures at night in the patients with obstructive sleep apnoea, with persistence of this into the early morning after awakening, and a generally higher diastolic for much of the day. (Reproduced from Davies C, et al (2000). Thorax, 55, 736–40, with permission.)

induced upper airway obstruction should really be viewed in a similar way.

Sleep-induced hypoventilation and central sleep apnoea

So far we have discussed the sleep-related disorders of breathing that are due to sleep-induced narrowing of the upper airway. Breathing during sleep may also decrease, not because of upper airway obstruction, but because of a reduction in central output to the respiratory muscles—so-called central, rather than obstructive, apnoea (Fig. 3). There are many causes for central sleep apnoea or hypoventilation, and Table 5 shows one way of classifying them. Some of the central apnoeas disturb sleep and present with daytime sleepiness, whereas others tend to present with symptoms of respiratory failure, such as morning headaches with cyanosis and confusion, ankle oedema, and shortness of breath on exertion.

Absent ventilatory drive

Brainstem abnormalities may damage the areas responsible for automatic chemical control of ventilation. Whilst awake, the wakefulness-related ventilatory drive may be adequate to maintain Pao_2 and $Paco_2$ levels, but on falling asleep, drive falls or even disappears with marked hypoventilation (or apnoea) and hypoxaemia. Arousal is then necessary to restore the blood gases. This failure of brainstem automatic control (known as Ondine's curse) can be congenital, or may be acquired as the result of a stroke, infection, surgical damage, multiple sclerosis, or compression by a tumour or syrinx.

Reduction of chemical drive can occur as a secondary problem when ventilation is reduced by mechanical problems such as chronic airways obstruction or weak respiratory muscles. It appears that chronic underventilation can lead to blunting of ventilatory drive, perhaps through alteration in acid–base buffering in the brainstem, and can also lead to marked falls in ventilation during sleep.

Unstable ventilatory drive

The wakefulness-related ventilatory drive stabilizes ventilation and prevents it from falling below a certain level. If reasons for ventilatory instability exist then, by removing this stabilizing effect, sleep will allow periodic respiration to develop. The usual provoker of instability is an increased drive to breathe. Control theory shows that increasing the gain in any feedback system causes instability through overshoot and undershoot. A good example of this is the hypoxaemia of altitude, which accentuates the response to change in arterial carbon dioxide tension, promoting instability. When sleep occurs there is the usual fall in ventilation. This leads to increased hypoxaemia and a rise in carbon dioxide tension, causing increased ventilation, both provoking arousal. This provides extra awake ventilatory drive, which restores the blood gases, and the cycle repeats. Thus, periodic breathing with recurrent arousals is very common at altitude, with the expected daytime consequence of sleepiness and complaints of insomnia. Acetazolamide produces a metabolic acidosis and increases ventilation overall, the hypoxaemia is relieved, and thus the ventilatory response to carbon dioxide becomes less steep. Both these factors restore stability and reduce periodic respiration.

In left ventricular failure there is also extra ventilatory drive, mainly due to stimulation of interstitial lung receptors by the raised pulmonary venous pressure. In conjunction with the longer circulation time seen in heart failure, this also provokes instability with waxing and waning of the ventilation. This periodic breathing, or Cheyne–Stokes respiration, is quite common in heart failure, and through sleep disruption produces daytime sleepiness and complaints of nocturnal dyspnoea (Fig. 12). The patient is usually aware that on arousal the dyspnoea disappears within a few seconds, unlike the paroxysmal nocturnal dyspnoea of pulmonary oedema which usually takes at least 15 min or so to abate following getting out of

Table 5 Suggested breakdown of causes of central apnoea

Type of central apnoea	Examples	Daytime arterial CO_2 level
1. Absent or reduced ventilatory drive (Ondine's curse)	Brain-stem damage or congenital abnormality Acquired blunting, e.g. secondary to lung disease	Raised
2. Unstable respiratory drive	Sleep onset, hypoxaemia, altitude, heart failure	Normal or low
3. REM-related oscillations	Normal in REM sleep Due to neuromuscular disorders and respiratory muscle weakness	Normal or raised
4. Reflex central apnoea	Pharyngeal collapse inhibits inspiration	Normal
5. Apparent central apnoea (wrongly diagnosed)	Respiratory muscle weakness or gross obesity cause chest-wall movement transducers to fail to demonstrate any ventilatory effort during obstructive apnoeas	Normal or raised

bed. Treatment with either overnight oxygen or acetazolamide can sometimes reduce the periodicity and improve both sleep quality and symptoms. There has been some recent interest in NCPAP as a treatment for left ventricular failure and periodic breathing. The mechanism of any action is unknown, and at present the evidence does not justify its general use.

Instability of respiratory control can also occur in normal subjects in the early stages of sleep or if sleep is disturbed for other reasons. This is because sleep depth is oscillating back and forth between drowsy wakefulness and light sleep, with the ventilatory drive oscillating as well.

REM sleep apnoeas

During normal REM sleep the phasic bursts of eye movements are associated with transient falls in ventilation, and even the occurrence of apnoeas. The rib-cage muscles are affected most, but diaphragmatic excursion can also fall. Such periodicities are entirely normal.

As discussed earlier, the REM sleep inhibition of most muscles (apart from the diaphragm) can greatly reduce overall ventilation when the accessory muscles of respiration are needed for breathing. Thus on entering REM sleep there can be profound falls in ventilation and Sao_2 in patients with neuromuscular diseases, chest-wall abnormalities, and chronic airways obstruction.

Generalized neuromuscular diseases tend to involve the respiratory muscles in concert with other muscles. However, in some disorders the respiratory muscles, particularly the diaphragm, may be involved very early on, at a time when other muscles are virtually normal. A particular example of this is adult-type acid maltase deficiency, where patients may present in respiratory failure whilst still able to walk normally. REM-sleep-related hypoxaemia may be the first sign that there are problems, and it is not known whether this actually accelerates the onset of eventual diurnal respiratory failure, or is merely a marker that respiratory failure will soon

follow. Sometimes there may be associated upper airway obstruction during REM sleep, leading to even larger falls in Sao_2. Overnight oximetry studies will indicate the degree of hypoxaemia but will not establish if there is additional upper airway obstruction.

There has been great interest in the REM-sleep-related hypoxaemia seen in chronic airways obstruction. It was thought possible that these hypoxic episodes might be the reason why some patients developed respiratory failure but others did not. However, it appears that REM sleep hypoventilation and a fall in Pao_2 is fairly universal in this group of patients. If the patient is initially well oxygenated and on the flat part of the haemoglobin dissociation curve, the fall in Sao_2 (which is usually what is monitored) is not particularly dramatic; however, if the patient is initially poorly oxygenated and on the steep part of the curve, similar hypoventilation will produce dramatic falls in Sao_2. As yet there is no evidence that these REM sleep falls in Sao_2 contribute to the morbidity and mortality of patients with chronic airflow obstruction, although some centres have shown that overnight oxygen therapy reduces arousals, thus improving sleep quality. The main problem is that the falls in Sao_2 can look superficially like obstructive sleep apnoea leading to an erroneous diagnosis and the inappropriate use of NCPAP.

Reflex apnoea

Central respiratory output can be modified by a number of reflexes from receptors in the upper airway. There is a reflex from the pharynx that inhibits inspiratory flow when the pharynx is being sucked in and collapsed. This makes teleological sense, as a slowing of inspiratory flow would reduce the tendency to collapse. There are some patients with pharyngeal collapse who, instead of struggling to inspire against the blocked airway, simply stop breathing until they finally arouse, presumably due to the fall in Pao_2 and rise in $Paco_2$. This then appears as a central apnoea, despite the

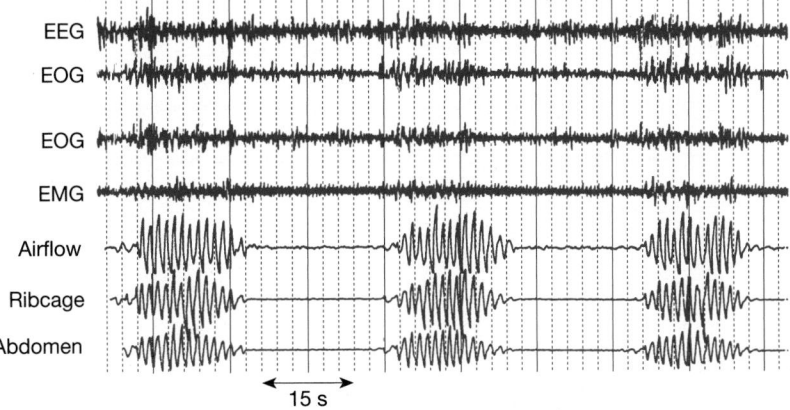

Fig. 12 Tracing of Cheyne–Stokes respiration from a patient with poor left ventricular function but no radiological or clinical evidence of current pulmonary oedema. With each return of respiration there is arousal from sleep (not clearly visible with this compressed EEG tracing).

aetiology being pharyngeal collapse. This tends to happen when the patient is supine, with snoring or ordinary obstructive apnoeas when decubitus. If the pharynx is anaesthetized experimentally, then inspiratory attempts return, suggesting that superficial receptors are responsible. These patients usually present with typical histories of obstructive sleep apnoea, respond to NCPAP, and can be managed in the same way.

Apparent central apnoea

The diagnosis of central apnoea depends on demonstrating the absence of respiratory effort when airflow at the nose and mouth stops. Surface measurements of rib-cage and abdominal movement are usually employed as evidence of continuing respiratory effort. However, in two circumstances, marked obesity and muscular weakness, the surface transducers may fail to register that inspiratory efforts are still being made (although more sensitive measures of inspiratory effort, such as oesophageal pressure tracings, will usually do so). Obesity lessens the sensitivity of surface transducers, and with muscle weakness the inspiratory muscles may not be able to move the chest wall detectably against a closed upper airway.

Overnight ventilation for central sleep apnoea or hypoventilation

The chronic ventilatory failure associated with some neurological disorders (e.g. acid maltase deficiency, postpoliomyelitis syndrome, motor neurone disease, Duchenne dystrophy) usually progress rapidly to death, even when quality of life is otherwise very good. The same is true of chest-wall restrictive disorders such as scoliosis, as well as the ventilatory failure that can develop many years after extensive thoracoplasty. However, supporting breathing overnight can fully reverse ventilatory failure, and the response to treatment can be dramatic, with resolution of all symptoms and restoration of normal blood gases, even when off the ventilator during the day. The mechanism by which supporting breathing at night corrects ventilatory failure is not clear and there are various possibilities. Firstly, it may simply be that the respiratory muscles are rested so that they can respond better to the demands of the respiratory centre during the day. Secondly, it may be that improving the blood gases at night, and preventing the marked REM sleep deteriorations, leads to resetting of the respiratory centre back towards normal, that reverses an acquired blunting of drive. Tricyclic antidepressants such as protriptyline can virtually abolish REM sleep periods and their associated hypoxaemia and have been shown to improve daytime blood gases temporarily, suggesting that simply abolishing these periods of particular hypoxia can help. Thirdly, by increasing chest-wall and lung excursion (tidal volumes in excess of the voluntary vital capacity are sometimes obtained) overall respiratory compliance may improve, allowing the muscles to work more efficiently. Whatever the explanation, there is no doubt that this is a life-saving therapy that in certain conditions can add decades of active life.

Most of the original techniques to support ventilation overnight evolved from the iron lung that was developed to support poliomyelitis victims. Evacuating the air from around the chest expands the lungs, recreating the normal way of breathing. A range of devices involving airtight jackets and shells over the chest were developed, but required much attention to detail

and often individual, tailor-made systems. Unfortunately a specific complication, resulted from the abolition of spontaneous ventilatory drive to the diaphragm and pharyngeal muscles, upper airway collapse can occur during the mechanical inspiratory phase and greatly limit efficacy. The recent development of comfortable nasal and face masks has revolutionized the overnight ventilation of these patients. Positive pressure ventilation can be used via a face mask, or more comfortably via the nasal masks used for NCPAP (Fig. 7). Although there are still many problems to be overcome when establishing patients on such equipment (particularly mask comfort and air leaks through the mouth when using nasal masks), the systems can be bought off the shelf ready to use (current cost approximately £3500). Most units now use positive pressure ventilation in preference to the negative pressure systems.

Electrical pacing of the diaphragm is occasionally used for supporting ventilation in conditions where the phrenic nerve and diaphragm are intact and the problem is central. This involves the implantation of bilateral phrenic electrodes and induction coils under the skin that are activated by external induction coils.

Conclusions

Ventilatory failure should not be viewed as a diagnosis. It is a finding that requires a specific explanation. Many of the causes become most obvious at night, when they produce dramatic falls in the level of Sao_2 due to further failure of ventilatory drive mechanisms. Specific treatments aimed at reversing these sleep-related failures of ventilatory drive can produce rapid and satisfactory resolution of symptoms, as well as prolongation of life.

Further reading

Gastaut H, Tassinari CA, Duron B (1966). Polygraphic study of the episodic diurnal and nocturnal (hypnic and respiratory) manifestations of the Pickwick syndrome. *Brain Research* **2**, 167–86.

Guilleminault C, Stoohs R, Duncan S (1991). Snoring (1). Daytime sleepiness in regular heavy snorers. *Chest* **99**, 40–8.

Jenkinson C, Davies RJO, Mullins R, Stradling JR (1999). Randomised prospective parallel trial of therapeutic nasal continuous positive airway pressure (NCPAP) against sub-therapeutic NCPAP for obstructive sleep apnoea. *Lancet* **353**, 2100–5.

Remmers JE, de Broot WJ, Sauerland EK, Anch AM (1978). Pathogenesis of upper airway occlusion during sleep. *Journal of Applied Physiology* **44**, 931–8.

Stradling JR (1995). Obstructive sleep apnoea: definitions, epidemiology and natural history. *Thorax* **50**, 683–9.

Stradling JR (1997). Practical approach to sleep disordered breathing. In: Farthing M, ed. *Horizons in medicine*. Royal College of Physicians, London.

Sullivan CE, Issa FG, Berthon-Jones MCHR, Eves L (1981). Reversal of obstructive sleep apnoea by continuous positive airway pressure applied through the nares. *Lancet* **i**, 862–5.

Weiss JW, Remsburg S, Garpestad E, Ringler J, Sparrow D, Parker JA (1996). Hemodynamic consequences of obstructive sleep apnea. *Sleep* **19**, 388–97.

17.9 Bronchiectasis

D. Bilton

Introduction

The definition of bronchiectasis is based on morbid anatomy first described by Laennec, who in 1819 found abnormal chronic dilatation of the bronchi in an infant who died following whooping cough. The word itself is from the Greek *bronchion* (wind pipe or tube) and *ektasis* (stretched out or extension). By 1891 it was recognized in a textbook of medicine that bronchiectasis was 'not a separate disease' but 'a result of various affectations of the bronchi', hence bronchiectasis is not a final diagnosis but a final pathology of a number of causes which may require their own specific treatment.

Prevalence

Up to 1953, estimates of the prevalence of bronchiectasis in the United Kingdom varied from 0.77 to 1.3 per 1000 population, but it seems that the prevalence has since fallen, at least of severe disease, as judged by a reduction in hospital admissions and deaths. This follows the introduction of antibiotic therapy for pulmonary infection, the control of tuberculosis, and effective vaccination for whooping cough and measles. However, the figures quoted may be an underestimate of the true prevalence of bronchiectasis: the diagnosis depends on demonstrating the cardinal feature of abnormal chronic dilatation of one or more bronchi, and it is likely that many people with chronic sputum production are mislabelled as 'bronchitic'. Indeed, recent CT scanning studies of patients with so-called 'chronic bronchitis' suggest that this is the case, and only the application of non-invasive imaging in large community surveys would tell us the true prevalence of the disorder. Bronchiectasis is regarded as a common problem in less developed countries where antibiotics are less readily available, socio-economic conditions are poor, and the prevalence of both tuberculosis and HIV are high.

Pathology

Macroscopic inspection of bronchiectatic lung reveals permanent dilatation of subsegmental airways that are inflamed, tortuous, and often partially or totally obstructed with secretions. The process also includes bronchioles, and at endstage there may be marked fibrosis of small airways. In allergic bronchopulmonary aspergillosis the changes are predominantly in proximal airways. Bronchiectasis caused by cystic fibrosis is likely to be more marked in the upper lobes. There is a spectrum of disease that ranges from cylindrical, where there is uniform dilatation, to saccular, where there may be gross terminal dilatation of the bronchi (saccules or cyst). An intermediate form is termed varicose bronchiectasis.

Microscopic features

The overall appearance is of chronic inflammation in the bronchial wall with inflammatory cells and mucus in the lumen. There is destruction of the elastin layer of the bronchial wall with a variable amount of fibrosis.

Neutrophils are the main cell population in the bronchial lumen, whereas the commonest cells in the bronchial wall are mononuclear. The label follicular is applied when there is lymphoid follicle formation as part of extensive mural inflammation, which in subepithelial sites may cause finger projections blocking the bronchial lumen.

Aetiology and pathogenesis

There is a broad spectrum of causes and underlying conditions associated with bronchiectasis. These are summarized in Table 1.

Table 1 Causes of bronchiectasis and associated conditions

Type of cause	Examples
Developmental defects	Deficiency of bronchial wall—Williams–Campbell syndrome
	Structural:
	Pulmonary sequestration
	Tracheobronchomegaly—Mounier–Kuhn syndrome
	Biochemical:
	α_1-Antitrypsin deficiency
Immune deficiency	Primary:
	Panhypogammaglobulinaemia
	Selective immunoglobulin deficiency
	Secondary:
	HIV infection
	Malignancy (CLL)
Excessive immune response	Allergic bronchopulmonary aspergillosis
	After lung transplantation
Mucociliary clearance defects	Primary ciliary dyskinesia
	Cystic fibrosis
	Young's syndrome
Toxic insult	Aspiration of gastric contents
	Inhalation of toxic gases or chemicals, such as ammonia
Mechanical obstruction	Intrinsic—tumour or foreign body
	Extrinsic—such as tuberculous lymph node
Postinfective	*Bordetella pertussis*
	Measles
	Tuberculosis
Associated conditions	Chronic rhinosinusitis
	Rheumatoid arthritis
	Inflammatory bowel disease—ulcerative colitis, Crohn's disease
	Coeliac disease
	Yellow nail syndrome
	Connective tissue disorders and vasculitides
Idiopathic	

CLL, chronic lymphatic leukaemia.

The pathogenesis of bronchiectasis requires the combination of an infective insult with impaired clearance mechanisms that may result from local obstruction, impaired local structural defences, or defective immune defences. This is supported by work in animal models, which also show that the infection must be active, with damage to the airway wall occurring as a result of direct microbial insult or the secondary effects of the host inflammatory response.

The term 'vicious cycle' has been proposed to explain the development of bronchiectasis in a predisposed individual following a trigger insult, as shown in Fig. 1, which also demonstrates the key role played by neutrophil elastase. Neutrophils are recruited as part of the natural defences, but the inflammation is not self-limiting and in patients with bronchiectasis neutrophils persist in the airway secretions, with free neutrophil elastase activity usually present. Elastase, a neutrophil-derived serine proteinase, is known to inhibit ciliary beating, damage epithelia, act as a mucus secretagogue, and inhibit opsonophagocytosis via cleavage of immunoglobulins. All these actions contribute to persistence of bacteria in the respiratory tract and long-term tissue damage. Figure 1 illustrates that whenever a patient enters the pathway, for example in primary ciliary dyskinesia (which inhibits mucociliary clearance), or with immunoglobulin deficiency (which favours persistence of microbes in the bronchial tree), the vicious cycle becomes self-perpetuating with the final outcome of airway damage.

Developmental defects

The congenital forms of bronchiectasis frequently show deficiency of elements of the bronchial wall that are necessary to prevent collapse and hence 'obstruction' of the airway. In Williams–Campbell syndrome there is deficiency of the bronchial cartilage. The Mounier–Kuhn syndrome or tracheobronchomegaly is the 'adult equivalent' of congenital deficiency of bronchial cartilage. Pulmonary sequestration predisposes to bronchiectasis because of decreased pulmonary clearance of the affected segment.

Mechanical obstruction

Bronchiectasis confined to a single lobe may be the result of local mechanical obstruction, either in the lumen (intrinsic), for example by a tumour or foreign body, or originating outside the lumen (extrinsic), for example by lymph node enlargement from tuberculosis or a tumour.

Disorders of mucociliary clearance

The disease cystic fibrosis provides the archetypal model of a genetic predisposition for the development of bronchiectasis. In this disorder (described in Chapter 17.10) there is dysfunction of the cystic fibrosis transmembrane regulator, a transmembrane chloride channel and ion transport regulatory protein. The resulting abnormal salt and water transport across respiratory epithelia predisposes to respiratory infection and the effects of the vicious cycle are clearly demonstrated as a structurally normal lung suffers progressive airway damage and the development of bronchiectasis.

Primary ciliary dyskinesia describes a group of inherited disorders in which mutation of several different genes may give rise to non-functional cilia. It is generally considered to be an autosomal recessive disorder with variable penetrance. The diagnosis is made by demonstrating abnormality of the cilia on electron microscopy. In the largest subgroup of this syndrome, and the form first described, the cilia lack dynein arms, which are the structures responsible for movement of cilia or spermatozoa. Subsequently it has been appreciated that a variety of components of the cilia are affected.

The intriguing observation that about 50 per cent of all subjects with immotile cilia syndrome have situs inversus is true for most subgroups, apart from those who have absent cilia or those whose main characteristic is lack of the two central microtubules. When ciliary dyskinesia is associated with abnormal situs the condition is labelled Kartagener's syndrome after the paediatrician who described four patients with the association of dextrocardia, sinusitis, and bronchiectasis in 1933.

Young's syndrome seems to represent an acquired defect of mucociliary clearance in which obstructive azoospermia is associated with sinusitis and bronchiectasis. The condition may occur after a man has successfully fathered a child, and may be associated with mercury poisoning from 'tooth powders' used in infancy (Pink's disease).

Secondary ciliary dyskinesia refers to the situation in which cilia are intrinsically normal but ciliary beating is reduced because of toxic damage

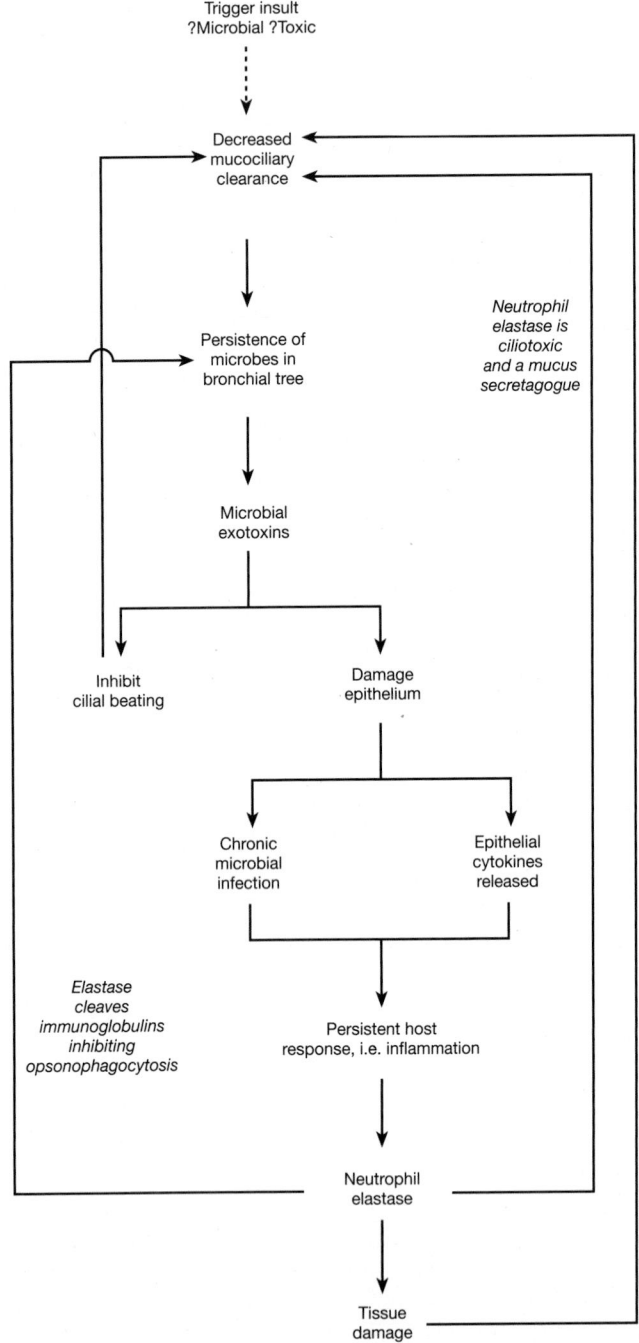

Fig. 1 The vicious cycle of infection and inflammation leading to progressive tissue damage in bronchiectasis.

from neutrophil or bacterial products. Tobacco smoke and other environmental pollutants have also been implicated in reducing ciliary beat frequency.

Postinfective bronchiectasis

The true incidence of postinfective bronchiectasis is difficult to establish because studies have been retrospective, relying on histories obtained 'second hand' from parents. The micro-organisms known to cause infection likely to progress to bronchiectasis are *Bordetella pertussis*, measles virus, adenoviruses, *Trypanosoma cruzi*, and *Mycobacterium tuberculosis*.

As mentioned above, the pattern of bronchiectasis has changed since the introduction of vaccinations and widespread availability of antibiotics in the developed world. A population with cylindrical bronchiectasis has superseded the gross saccular bronchiectasis associated with severe repeated childhood respiratory infections in the pre-antibiotic era. This may be associated with a childhood history of a chesty cough, with a long period of remission of symptoms through the teens and twenties, followed by the onset of symptoms of productive cough of purulent sputum and/or sinusitis in the third or fourth decade of life. Some of these patients may report having whooping cough or measles in childhood, but it is not appropriate to label them as postinfective unless symptoms have been persistent, without remission since childhood.

Immune deficiency

Immune deficiency is an important cause of bronchiectasis because treatment with intravenous immunoglobulin (where appropriate) will correct the defect and should prevent progression of disease.

Bronchiectasis presenting in childhood should trigger an extensive assessment of phagocytic and cellular immune defences. The rare disorder, X-linked hypogammaglobulinaemia, presents early in life and bronchiectasis is a frequent complication if untreated.

Adult-onset acquired panhypogammaglobulinaemia frequently presents with recurrent respiratory infection and is complicated by bronchiectasis if untreated. Selective deficiencies of IgG and IgM, and of IgG subclasses, are also treatable causes of bronchiectasis. Moreover, functional antibody deficiencies and failure to mount and maintain adequate responses to antigen challenge (for example pneumococcal vaccine) may be present despite normal total immunoglobulins, hence subtle humoral deficiency, a treatable cause of bronchiectasis, can be easily missed.

Immune defects may be secondary to malignancy or be related to treatment with immunosuppressive agents. Bronchiectasis is now a recognized complication of HIV disease.

Excessive immune response

Figure 1 illustrates the mechanism by which damage may occur as a result of the host response to chronic airway infection. Allergic bronchopulmonary aspergillosis is a condition in which the excessive reaction to a 'non-infecting' organism seems to be the major factor in producing the associated characteristic proximal upper lobe bronchiectasis. The appearance of obliterative bronchiolitis and subsequent bronchiectasis in lung transplant rejection further highlights the role of a damaging immune response in the development of bronchiectasis.

Toxic insult

In some patients there is a clear history of an inhalation accident or exposure to hot gases, for example in a fire victim. Aspiration of gastric contents is another important cause of bronchiectasis insomuch as treatment to prevent aspiration will prevent further airway damage.

Associated conditions

The association of rheumatoid arthritis with bronchiectasis is well recognized. Treatment of bronchiectasis in patients with rheumatoid arthritis

can be difficult, reflecting the need to achieve the right balance of immunosuppression, which helps the underlying inflammatory disease process but can simultaneously impair antimicrobial defences. The association of inflammatory bowel disease with bronchiectasis also highlights the issue of immunosuppression: some patients with both conditions report an improvement in chest symptoms when they take systemic corticosteroids for flares of inflammatory bowel symptoms.

Rhinosinusitis

About 80 per cent of patients with bronchiectasis have upper respiratory tract symptoms, with postnasal drip being the most common problem. Some 30 per cent of patients have chronic sinus sepsis, with fewer having recurrent ear infections. In ciliary dyskinesia, however, ear infections are almost invariably present.

Idiopathic bronchiectasis

The underlying cause of bronchiectasis remains unknown in 40 to 60 per cent of patients, even in specialist bronchiectasis clinics.

Clinical features

History

Bronchiectasis should be suspected when there is a history of persistent cough productive of mucopurulent or purulent sputum throughout the year. Patients have frequently been treated for recurrent chest infections and labelled as 'bronchitic', often despite the absence of a history of smoking.

Patients may produce mucoid sputum early in their disease, developing purulent sputum when they suffer an exacerbation associated with viral upper respiratory tract infection. Such exacerbations may be associated with pleuritic chest pain, haemoptysis, fever, and sometimes wheeze. Those presenting as adults often recall a 'chesty cough' or 'wheezy bronchitis' associated with upper respiratory tract infections in childhood, followed by complete resolution of symptoms in the teens and early adult life before these return after a viral trigger. Upper respiratory tract symptoms such as postnasal drip are common, and in about 30 per cent of cases there is a history of chronic sinusitis.

Patients with bronchiectasis also suffer from undue tiredness, which many find more troublesome than the productive cough.

Examination

Severe 'classic' cases of bronchiectasis seen in the pre-antibiotic era or in less developed countries are associated with obvious clinical signs including finger clubbing and widespread course crackles. Nowadays it is much more likely for clinical examination to be normal. The absence of clubbing or lung crackles does not exclude bronchiectasis.

Investigation

Radiological imaging

The chest radiograph may be normal in at least 50 per cent of patients with CT or bronchographic evidence of bronchiectasis. If it is abnormal the findings relate to thickened and dilated bronchi, which produce tram-line opacities and ring shadows. Retained mucus may be seen as tubular opacities, and there may be associated volume loss of the affected lobe.

The gold standard for the diagnosis of bronchiectasis is thin section, high-resolution CT (**HRCT**) of the chest, which has replaced the more

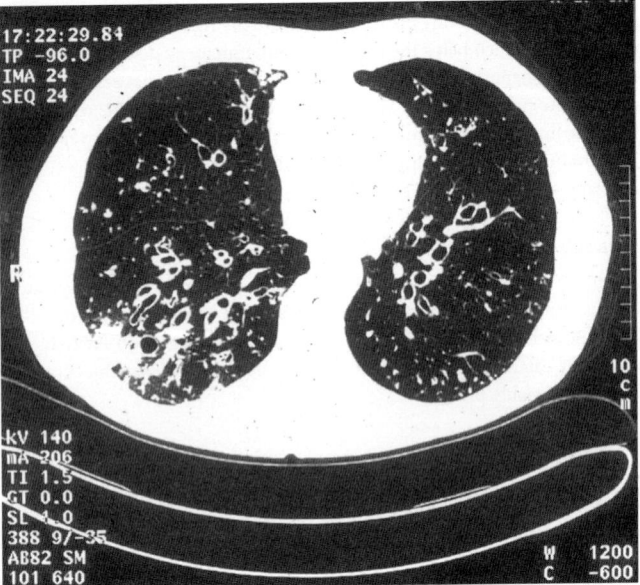

Fig. 2 CT scan of patient with bronchiectasis showing characteristic signet-ring sign.

Table 2 Investigations to assess current disease status

HRCT scan
Assess extent of bronchiectasis—single or multilobular involvement?
Lung function tests
To assess extent of loss of airway function
Include assessment of reversibility to β₂-agonists and anticholinergic agents
Sputum culture
To assess colonizing micro-organisms, including culture for acid-fast bacilli and aspergillus
Haematology
Differential white count, erythrocyte sedimentation rate, and C-reactive protein

invasive investigation of bronchography. The diagnostic criteria for bronchiectasis on HRCT depend on finding both dilatation and thickening of the affected bronchi, dilatation being present if the internal diameter of the bronchus is greater than the diameter of its accompanying pulmonary artery. The classic appearance of a cross-section of a thick-walled dilated bronchus next to the accompanying pulmonary artery is the 'signet ring' sign, as shown in Fig. 2. Bronchial dilatation is also recognized when airways are seen in longitudinal section on CT and there is a failure of tapering as the bronchus courses towards the periphery.

There is a morphological spectrum of bronchiectasis, with cylindrical bronchiectasis forming one group, cystic or saccular bronchiectasis at the other end of the spectrum, and an intermediate group termed 'varicose' bronchiectasis. The CT appearances of this spectrum are well described. In cylindrical bronchiectasis there is uniform dilatation of the bronchi as they extend towards the periphery. By contrast, varicose bronchiectasis produces a beaded appearance, best shown when bronchi are imaged in the plane of the scan. Cystic bronchiectasis is recognized by rings representing markedly dilated bronchi, which may be clustered together and may contain air–fluid levels.

In addition to defining the extent of bronchiectasis, CT scanning may suggest the need for a bronchoscopy; for example if there is a bronchial obstruction, perhaps due to a foreign body or tumour.

Other tests

Once HRCT has proved the presence of bronchiectasis, investigations are directed towards defining the status of the disease and at attempting to establish an underlying cause. Table 2 highlights the minimum required to assess the current state of disease. Examination of a sputum specimen is crucial, it being important to document its character—mucoid or purulent—and to determine the colonizing organism, typical organisms being non-typeable *Haemophilus influenzae*, *Moraxella iatarrhalis*, *Streptococcus pneumoniae*, and *Pseudomonas aeruginosa*. *H. influenzae* is the most common (40 to 60 per cent). *P. aeruginosa* is usually associated with worsening symptoms and more severe lung disease. (See Chapter 17.3.3 for further information on the microbiological investigation of patients with lung disease.)

As the sputum microbiology may alter over time it is helpful to obtain repeated samples to ensure that an appropriate antibiotic management plan is in place. Measurement of inflammatory markers allows an assess-

ment of the patient's current 'inflammatory burden'. Many have come to accept persistent purulent sputum over a period of time and may not complain of being particularly unwell. A raised erythrocyte sedimentation rate and/or C-reactive protein would weight the argument in favour of early antibiotic intervention.

Table 3 outlines the investigations required to tie down a cause of bronchiectasis, some of which will then require specific treatment, for example immunodeficiency. Allergic bronchopulmonary aspergillosis is an important treatable cause: corticosteroid therapy produces substantial improvements in symptoms and well being, restores lung function, and prevents the development of further bronchiectasis. Similarly, the appreciation that chronic aspiration is the precipitant of lung damage can lead to appropriate therapeutic manoeuvres aimed at prevention of further damage.

Cystic fibrosis/bronchiectasis overlap

The diagnosis of cystic fibrosis should be considered in any patient with unexplained bronchiectasis, but particularly in the presence of upper lobe bronchiectasis, colonization with *Staphylococcus aureus* and *Pseudomonas aeruginosa*, or male infertility. A normal sweat test no longer excludes a diagnosis of cystic fibrosis as mutations occur which produce mild disease and a normal sweat test. If doubt exists, then the patient should be referred to specialist centre for further investigation (see Chapter 17.10).

Table 3 Investigations to assess underlying causes of bronchiectasis

Bronchoscopy	If CT suggests bronchial obstruction—to establish whether tumour or foreign body
Saccharin test	As screening test of nasal mucociliary clearance
Nasal brushing/biopsy	To establish ciliary beat frequency and obtain electron microscopic appearances of cilia
Nasal nitric oxide	As evidence of primary ciliary dyskinesia
Seminal analysis	If primary ciliary dyskinesia or cystic fibrosis is suspected
Cystic fibrosis genetics and sweat test	To exclude cystic fibrosis
Immunoglobulins and IgG subclasses, vaccine responses to pneumovax, tetanus, and flu	To identify immunodeficiency
Barium swallow ± oesophageal physiology studies	If aspiration is suspected
Measure α₁-antitrypsin	To identify α₁-antitrypsin deficiency
Autoantibody screen	To identify associated connective tissue disorders or vasculitis
Aspergillus skin testing and IgE and RAST to aspergillus	To identify allergic bronchopulmonary aspergillosis (ABPA)

Table 4 Principles of management of bronchiectasis*

Medical treatment of bronchiectasis
Sputum clearance:
Physiotherapy
Mucolytic therapy
Antimicrobial therapy:
Chronic prophylactic therapy
Acute exacerbation
Anti-inflammatory therapy
Bronchodilator therapy
Surgical treatment
To resect 'single' lobe bronchiectasis
Lung transplantation for endstage disease

*In addition to specific treatment of underlying cause (whenever possible).

Management

The principles of management of bronchiectasis are outlined in Table 4. The medical approach is two-pronged, with close attention given to treatment of any underlying cause whilst also treating the established bronchiectasis.

Sputum clearance

Since mucociliary clearance is reduced in bronchiectasis it seems sensible to aid sputum clearance by employing physiotherapy. Physiotherapy does not simply prevent mucus retention, but also allows a patient to expectorate sputum at a chosen convenient time rather than coughing throughout the day or night. There are no controlled trials to prove or disprove its usefulness in terms of disease modification or survival.

The use of mucolytics in bronchiectasis is controversial. The success of recombinant human DNAase in cystic fibrosis was not repeated in bronchiectasis that was not due to cystic fibrosis, when patients did not derive benefit in terms of lung function. A recent Cochrane review concluded that there is insufficient evidence to evaluate the routine use of mucolytics for bronchiectasis.

Antimicrobial therapy

There are two approaches to the use of antimicrobial therapy in bronchiectasis. The first involves the treatment of acute exacerbations. The second is based on the vicious cycle hypothesis, suggesting that chronic targeted antimicrobial therapy should reduce bacterial numbers, thereby reducing the host response and hence the potential for further lung damage. Whilst the latter approach has theoretical merits it has not been proved to be better than the former in randomized controlled trials.

In practice, the modern approach to antimicrobial treatment in bronchiectasis has been derived from regimens used in cystic fibrosis, which have yielded impressive improvements in survival (see Chapter 17.10). This depends on knowledge of a patient's colonizing organism, but there are some issues that apply regardless of the bacterial species. First, high doses of antibiotics are often required. These are necessary to penetrate scarred, thickened bronchial walls and the tenacious secretions that act as a physical barrier to antibiotic penetration to the microbes, which may also be harbouring drug-inactivating enzymes such as β-lactamases. Second, to avoid a high oral dose of an antibiotic that may result in unacceptable side-effects, the nebulized or parenteral route may be employed to achieve high levels of drug in the bronchial wall and secretions. Third, to determine the best treatment regimen for a patient it is worth assessing their initial response to an agent appropriate for the colonizing organism and then assessing the rapidity of return of purulent sputum. If purulent sputum becomes mucoid after a 14-day course of oral antibiotics and remains mucoid until the next viral trigger, then one is likely to recommend 'exacerbation only' treatment. However, if sputum returns to purulent within a few days of treatment finishing, then it is likely that chronic suppressive therapy will be required.

Figure 3 suggests an approach to the treatment patients with bronchiectasis depending on the characteristics of their sputum and the colonizing organism, but it must be pointed out that there has not been a systematic study of the benefits of this approach in the management of this condition.

Bronchodilator therapy

Patients with bronchiectasis can have a restrictive or an obstructive picture. Some may have significant reversibility, and it is therefore worth assessing each individual for their response to β$_2$-agonists and anticholinergic agents.

Anti-inflammatory therapy

The vicious cycle hypothesis would suggest that the addition of anti-inflammatory therapy to antibiotics should be of benefit in patients with bronchiectasis. In cystic fibrosis, trials of oral corticosteroids have shown significant benefit in terms of lung function. Short-term trials of inhaled corticosteroids have been carried out in bronchiectasis, but evidence supporting long-term use (summarized in a Cochrane review) is limited and further trials are required. However, a trial of oral steroids is warranted whenever there is reversible airflow obstruction: if there is a documented improvement in lung function after a 2-week course, then introduction of inhaled steroids is justified.

Monitoring response to treatment

As each patient requires a tailored management plan it is critical that both the patient and physician agree defined criteria for assessing response. Measurement of lung function clearly produces an objective measure of response to corticosteroids, whereas the introduction of antibiotics may not alter lung function to a great degree but does improve sputum colour, volume, and consistency, and may also produce improvement in general well being. Studies have confirmed the validity of grading sputum colour as a marker of the microbial and inflammatory load in these patients, and diary cards documenting these parameters have proved helpful. This approach also facilitates patient education and self-management plans.

Surgery

Surgery represents the only 'curative' treatment for a select group of patients and should be carefully considered. Resection of bronchiectatic areas of lung was common in the pre-antibiotic era and provided a successful treatment at the time. Physicians' judgment regarding surgery may be unduly coloured by the bias of patients returning to chest clinics with a recurrence of symptoms some years after resection, and the finding of bronchiectasis in other areas of the lung on CT scanning. These patients highlight the need for full assessment of the extent of bronchiectasis and a careful search for an underlying cause. If bronchiectasis is isolated to a single lobe and is the result of a localized obstruction, then surgery provides a cure and removes the need for lifelong treatment. However, surgery is unlikely to effect a cure if bronchiectasis is present in several lobes, and lobar resection is only indicated in two instances. First, if there is uncontrolled bleeding unresponsive to bronchial artery embolization. Second, if it is felt—after failure of aggressive antimicrobial therapy—that a particular

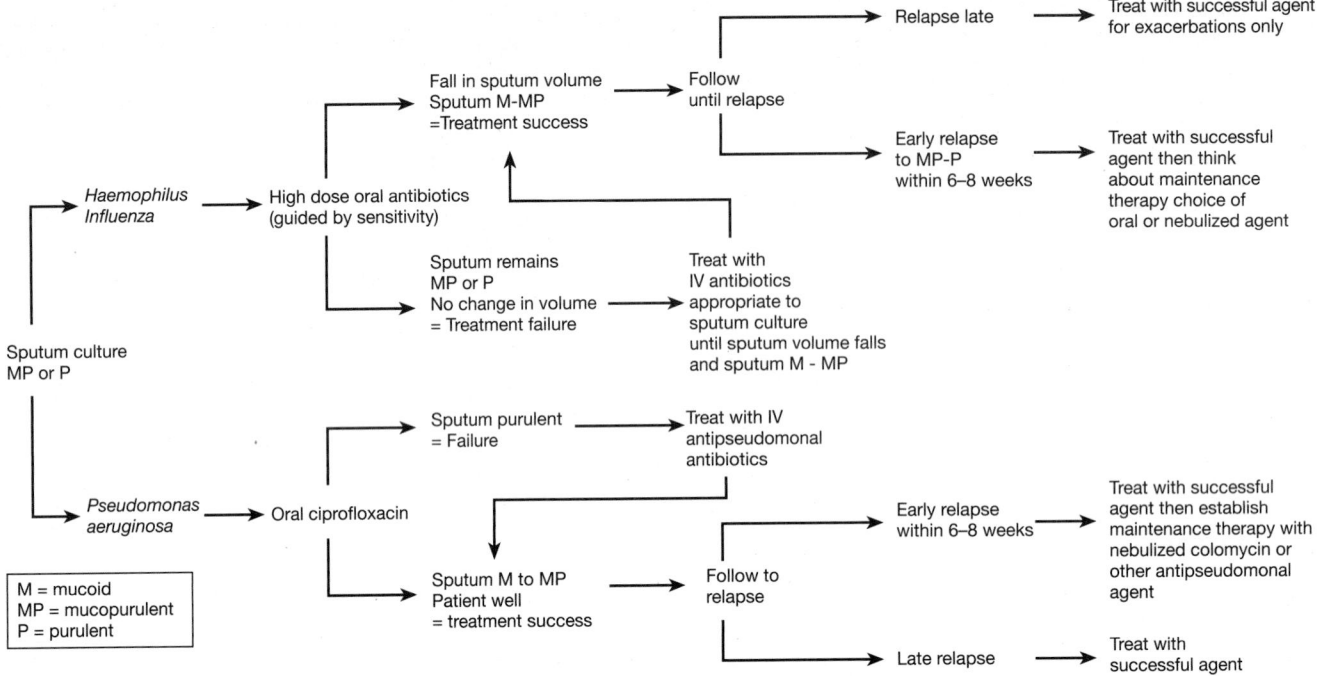

Fig. 3 Guide to therapy for patients with bronchiectasis.

lobe is acting as a 'sump' of infection which prevents good control of symptoms with medical therapy.

Lung transplantation

Lung transplantation provides an effective treatment for endstage bronchiectasis providing an underlying cause has been carefully assessed, treated, and is unlikely to jeopardize the transplanted organs. Patients with immunoglobulin deficiencies are not discounted from transplant assessment providing they are receiving adequate immunoglobulin replacement therapy. (See Chapter 17.16 for further discussion.)

Complications

Infective exacerbations are the most common complications to precipitate hospital admissions in patients with bronchiectasis. It is not common for patients to experience chest pain localized over an area of bronchiectasis, which may become pleuritic in nature during an infective exacerbation. Massive haemoptysis is rare nowadays: it is managed by embolization or, if that fails, by resection of the affected lobe. Minor haemoptysis is a common occurrence associated with infective exacerbations. Metastatic spread of infection rarely occurs in the developed world with good control of pulmonary infection with antibiotics. For similar reasons empyema is now very rare. Amyloidosis is often quoted as a classic complication of bronchiectasis, but is now extremely rare in the United Kingdom. Arthropathy is seen as a complication of bronchiectasis: this seems to flare in association with the chest disease, when active antimicrobial treatment will often result in remission of joint pain. Some patients may suffer vasculitic skin lesions in association with flares of bronchiectasis.

Prognosis

It was reported in 1940 that 70 per cent of 400 patients with bronchiectasis were dead before the age of 40. The situation is clearly different now: in the developed world we do not see the florid postinfective saccular type of bronchiectasis, but more commonly see patients presenting in their fourth and fifth decade of life with symptoms developing after a trigger illness and CT findings of cylindrical bronchiectasis. In 1981 a study following 116 patients for 14 years revealed that 20 per cent of patients treated medically and 17 per cent of surgically treated patients died at a mean age of 53 years. A Finnish study published in 1997 used the national hospital discharge register from 1982 to 1986 to identify newly diagnosed cases of bronchiectasis: 842 such patients were age and sex matched with individuals with chronic obstructive pulmonary disease or asthma discharged at the same time. Over a 10-year follow-up the prognosis for those with bronchiectasis was better than for those patients with chronic obstructive pulmonary disease, but poorer than that for patients with asthma. Bronchiectasis was the main cause of death in 13 per cent of the patients with this condition.

Further research

Further studies are required to identify the major factors that affect prognosis. For example, chronic colonization with *Pseudomonas* sp. may be a bad prognostic factor, but this may be negated by aggressive antimicrobial therapy. Study of homogeneous groups of patients (with respect to aetiology and colonizing organisms) should help assess various management regimens with regard to their effect on decline in lung function and survival. It is likely that a careful search for genetic factors that affect lung defences will yield new causes of bronchiectasis and allow the current so-called idiopathic group to be assigned a cause. We may then be able to define an at-risk population and aim to prevent development of bronchiectasis.

Further reading

Afzelius BA (1998). Immotile cilia syndrome: past, present, and prospects for the future. *Thorax* **53**, 894–7. [An overview of cilial disorders.]

Crockett AJ *et al.* (2000). Mucolytics for bronchiectasis. *Cochrane Database System Reviews (England)* (2) pCD001289. [Review of therapy for bronchiectasis.]

Jeffrey J, Swigris DO, Stoller JK (2000). A review of bronchiectasis. *Clinics in Pulmonary Medicine* 7, 223–30. [This is a comprehensive review of bronchiectasis.]

Jones AP, Rowe BH (2000). Bronchopulmonary hygiene physical therapy for chronic obstructive pulmonary disease and bronchiectasis. *Cochrane Database System Reviews (England)* (2) pCD00045. [Review of therapy for bronchiectasis.]

Keistinen T *et al.* (1997). Bronchiectasis: an orphan disease with a poorly-understood prognosis. *European Respiratory Journal* 10, 2784–7. [A recent paper describing the prognosis of bronchiectasis compared with asthma and chronic obstructive pulmonary disease.]

Kolbe J, Wells A, Ram FS (2000). Inhaled steroids for bronchiectasis. *Cochrane Database System Reviews (England)* (2) pCD000996. [Review of therapy for bronchiectasis.]

Pasteur MC *et al.* (2000). An investigation into causative factors in patients with bronchiectasis. *American Journal of Respiratory and Critical Care Medicine* 162, 1277–84. [A paper covering large series of patients demonstrating the variety of aetiology of bronchiectasis.]

Smith IE, Flower CDR (1996). Review article: Imaging in bronchiectasis. *British Journal of Radiology* 69, 589–93. [A description of HRCT scanning as the gold standard for diagnosis of bronchiectasis with a useful discussion of association between clinical features and radiological appearances.]

Stockley RA (1987). Bronchiectasis—new therapeutic approaches based on pathogenesis. *Clinics in Chest Medicine* 8, 481–94. [A review of the approach to therapy based on the vicious cycle hypothesis.]

17.10 Cystic fibrosis

Duncan Geddes and Andy Bush

Definition

Cystic fibrosis is a recessively inherited disease caused by mutations in the cystic fibrosis gene located on the long arm of chromosome 7. The classical clinical picture is a combination of pancreatic insufficiency, suppurative lung disease, and high sweat sodium concentration, presenting in childhood and progressing to early death from respiratory failure. However, genetic analysis has identified many patients with less severe disease and cystic fibrosis mutations are also associated with male infertility and idiopathic pancreatitis, so expanding the clinical spectrum of cystic fibrosis lung disease. In general, carriers are healthy.

The genetic defect

The cystic fibrosis gene codes for a 168-kDa membrane protein named the cystic fibrosis transmembrane regulator protein (CFTR). CFTR is primarily an ATP responsive chloride channel but it also influences other cellular functions such as sodium transport across the respiratory epithelium, cell surface glycoprotein composition, and normal antibacterial defences. The protein is expressed in organs involved in cystic fibrosis disease—lungs, pancreas, sweat gland, etc.—but also in some places that do not seem to be affected clinically, such as the choroid plexus, heart, and renal tubules.

More than 900 disease-related mutations of the cystic fibrosis gene have been described. Their distribution in relation to the cystic fibrosis gene and its related protein are shown in Fig. 1. The mutations have been classified according to their impact at a cellular level—type 1: no protein; type 2:

disordered trafficking; type 3: defective regulation; type 4: defective channel function; type 5: reduced protein synthesis. The understanding of these abnormalities is valuable as a basis for the design of new potentially corrective treatments, as illustrated in Fig. 2.

Most mutations are very rare; the commonest in European populations is δF508 which is found on 70 per cent of affected chromosomes. Most genetic laboratories restrict routine testing to the commonest six to eight mutations which account for over 90 per cent within a given population. Genotype–phenotype correlations have shown linkage of so called severe mutations, such as δF508, to pancreatic insufficiency and a tendency to more severe lung disease, while mild mutations go with pancreatic sufficiency and a tendency to less severe lung disease. However, in general, the correlation between genotype and the severity of lung disease is poor. All disease-associated mutations are linked with congenital absence of the vas deferens, resulting in male infertility, while rarer mutations are linked with isolated male infertility with no other evidence of cystic fibrosis disease.

Pathogenesis

Sweat duct

The primary secretion of the sweat duct is normal in volume and electrolyte concentration. However, as this secretion passes along the sweat duct mutant CFTR fails to absorb chloride ions, which therefore remain in the lumen and secondarily impair sodium absorption. The resultant sweat has

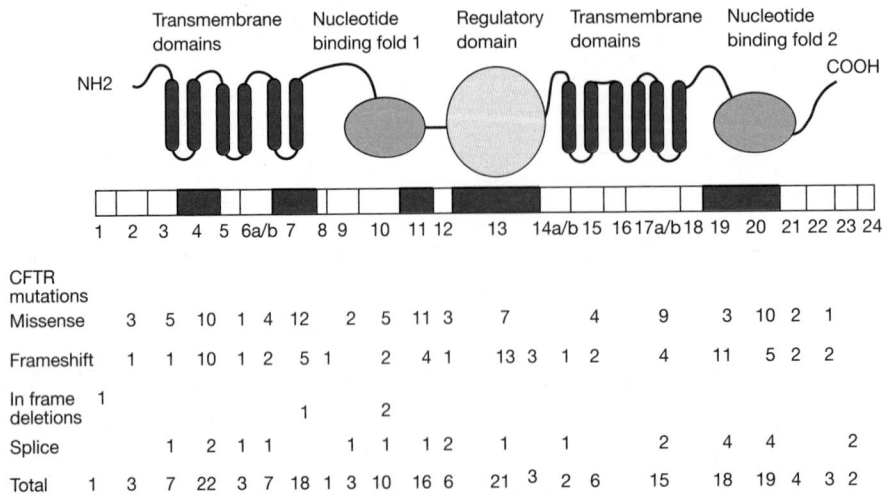

Fig. 1 Distribution of mutations within different regions of the CFTR gene. (Reproduced from Santis G. Basic molecular genetics. In: *Cystic fibrosis* (ed. Hodson ME, Geddes DM), p. 25. Chapman and Hall, London, with permission.)

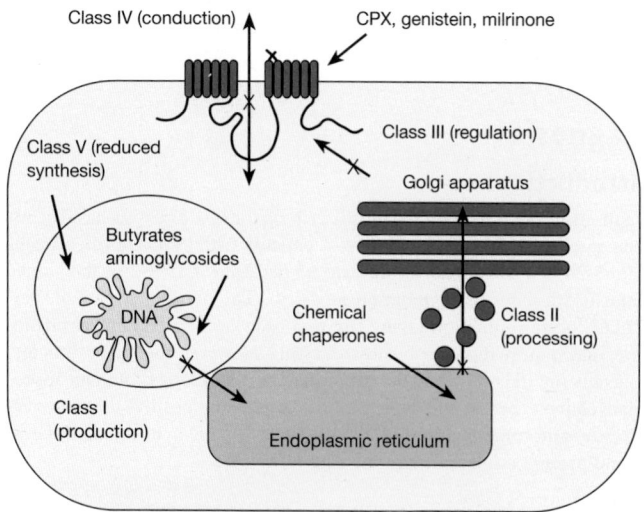

Fig. 2 Five categories of cystic fibrosis mutation with possible corrective treatments. (Reproduced from Rosenstein BJ, Zeitlin PL (1998). Seminar on cystic fibrosis. *Lancet*, **351**, 278, with permission.)

high concentrations of both sodium and chloride which is useful for diagnosis but can lead to salt depletion in hot weather.

Pancreas

The synthesis and secretion of pancreatic enzymes in the acinus is normal, but disordered ion transport—primarily chloride and secondarily bicarbonate—results in relative dehydration of pancreatic secretions. This in turn leads to low flow and stagnation of secretions in the pancreatic ducts with subsequent autodigestion. The clinical consequences are that low volumes of bicarbonate-depleted pancreatic secretions reach the duodenum, with consequent malabsorption and progressive destruction of the pancreas with cyst formation. Although the islet cells are relatively unaffected at first, they too are progressively destroyed leading to insulin deficiency.

Biliary tract

Intrahepatic biliary secretions are probably normal in cystic fibrosis, but disordered electrolyte transport across the bile duct results in reduced water movement into the lumen. The bile is therefore concentrated, and the volume depleted, leading to plugging and chronic local damage. This eventually causes biliary cirrhosis and associated extrahepatic biliary stenoses. There are secondary changes in bile acids.

Gut

Gastric secretions have decreased volume with increased viscosity and sodium levels. The chloride transport defect similarly leads to altered fluid movement across large and small intestine. These changes are worsened by the addition of dehydrated biliary and pancreatic secretions, as well as by alterations in the osmotic load in the lumen secondary to pancreatic exocrine failure. The resulting deficiency of intraluminal water contributes to meconium ileus in neonates and the distal intestinal obstruction syndrome in adults.

Respiratory tract

The epithelium in the nose, paranasal sinuses, and intrapulmonary conducting airways is disordered in cystic fibrosis, while alveolar function is normal. Defective chloride transport is associated with increased sodium absorption from the lumen. This has two important consequences. Firstly, net surface electrical charge is altered from a normal of –20 mV to cystic

fibrosis levels of –40 mV, which can be used for diagnosis. Secondly, increased sodium absorption takes water with it and dehydrates the airway surface liquid, reducing mucociliary clearance and favouring bacterial colonization. In addition, local antibacterial defences—including lactoferrin, lysozyme, and the cationic antibacterial peptides such as the β-defensins—may be impaired by local changes in salt concentration, and bacterial adherence to epithelial cells is increased by changes in cell surface glycoproteins. The net effect is to promote bacterial colonization and to reduce bacterial clearance, with subsequent inflammatory lung damage.

One consequence of bacterial colonization of the lower respiratory tract is an exuberant neutrophilic inflammatory response involving especially interleukin-8 (IL-8) and neutrophil elastase. The combination of elastase and other inflammatory mediators, while initially providing a useful antibacterial defence, is thought to contribute to lung damage and speed the progression of bronchiectasis and small airway narrowing.

Heterozygote advantage

The high frequency of the carrier rate in European populations (1:25) has led to a number of suggested advantages for the carrier, none of which are proven. These range from reduced susceptibility to infections such as cholera (reduced gut chloride secretion) and typhoid (reduced ingestion of bacteria by gut epithelium) to increased fertility among cystic fibrosis carriers.

Epidemiology

Genotype

The prevalence and distribution of the 900 disease-related mutations in the cystic fibrosis gene vary with ethnic origin. δF508 is commonest in northern European populations, accounting for 82 per cent of cystic fibrosis chromosomes in Denmark but only 32 per cent in Turkey. The W1282X mutation is common in Ashkanazi Jews (48 per cent of cystic fibrosis chromosomes) but rare in other populations. All disease-associated mutations are rare in African and almost unknown in Chinese populations.

Phenotype

Birth incidence varies with country of origin from 1:2000 to 1:100 000 as listed in Table 1. Prevalence figures are few and less reliable. In the third world, cystic fibrosis is likely to be under-diagnosed since early childhood malnutrition, diarrhoea, and chest infections are so common. There are at least 6000 people in the United Kingdom and 30 000 in the United States with cystic fibrosis and numbers are increasing along with life expectancy.

Survival

From 1938 to 1960, most children with cystic fibrosis died before the age of 10. Since 1968, the first year mortality (chiefly from meconium ileus) has fallen from 18 per cent to 4 per cent and survival curves are linear thereafter, showing progressive improvement over succeeding decades. In 1986,

Table 1 Frequency of cystic fibrosis in different populations

Country	Incidence	Calculated carrier frequency
United Kingdom	1:2500	1:25
Turkey	1:3000	1:27
United States	1:2000–1:4000	1:22–1:32
Israel	1:5000	1:35
Italy	1:15 000	1:60
African Americans	1:17 000	1:65
Finland	1:40 000	1:100
China	?1:100 000	?1:160

the median survival was 25 years and in 1999 about 30 years. Cohort survival analysis shows continuing improvement and estimated survival for a child born with cystic fibrosis in the late 1990s is 40 to 50 years. Age specific mortality rates for females are a little worse then males, although this difference is narrowing and the world record for both sexes is now over 70 years.

Microbiology

People with cystic fibrosis have no detectable immune deficiency and, except for the respiratory tract, have no increased susceptibility to infection. The lungs show evidence of inflammation very early in childhood and thereafter become chronically colonized, characteristically by *Staphylococcus aureus* and *Haemophilus influenzae*, followed some years later by *Pseudomonas aeruginosa*. Many other organisms have been implicated, especially in advanced disease, including *Burkholderia cepacia* and *Stenotrophomonas maltophilia*. *Aspergillus fumigatus* is frequently isolated, but is associated with allergic rather than invasive disease, and atypical mycobateria are occasionally found. Viral, chlamydial, pneumococcal, and other respiratory infections are not more common or severe in cystic fibrosis, but the consequences of these infections may be more important in the damaged and permanently colonized cystic fibrosis lung. The microbiology of the nose and sinuses is the same as for the lung, but the clinical consequences are usually less important.

Staphylococcus aureus

This is the commonest colonizing organism in childhood, with a prevalence of over 50 per cent in children aged 0 to 9. The predeliction of *Staph. aureus* for cystic fibrosis lungs has been ascribed to high electrolyte content of airway surface liquid or enhanced retention in the airways. No phage type predominates and the organism usually remains sensitive to flucloxacillin in spite of prolonged antibiotic treatment. Resistance to tetracycline or erythromycin is relatively common but multiple antibiotic resistance is rare. The prevalence falls in adult life when *Pseudomonas aeruginosa* colonization predominates.

Pseudomonas aeruginosa

This is the commonest colonizing organism after the age of 10 years, with reported prevalence varying between 40 and 80 per cent. Enhanced adherence to cystic fibrosis airways promotes colonization but prior antibiotic treatment may play a part. No particular phage type predominates, but siblings with cystic fibrosis often carry the same type, and environmental sources have been identified in cystic fibrosis centres, dentistry equipment, hydrotherapy pools, and nebulizers. After some months or years of colonization, *Pseudomonas aeruginosa* produces mucoid alginate as a protective biofilm and the organisms live in mucoid microcolonies. This mucoid variant is associated with a worse prognosis and greater antibiotic resistance. Most colonizing *Pseudomonas aeruginosa* are sensitive to antibiotics at first but over the years and in associated with antibiotic treatment multiple resistance to most antibiotics (except colomycin) develops.

Haemophilus influenzae

Non-capsulated *H. influenzae* is a relatively frequent colonizing organism with prevalence of up to 30 per cent, although it may not be isolated due to over-growth of *Staph.* or *Pseudomonas*. Antibiotic resistance is seldom a problem.

Burkholderia cepacia

The overall prevalence of this organism is low, at 3 to 5 per cent, but it poses a particular problem due to occasional cross-infection with a virulent epidemic form that can cause rapid deterioration in patients previously only mildly affected. More usual is chronic asymptomatic carriage or progressive deterioration in the late stage of lung disease. Multiple antibiotic resistance is characteristic.

Diagnosis

Introduction

A consensus document on diagnostic criteria for cystic fibrosis has recently been published. The vast majority of patients with cystic fibrosis can be diagnosed by a sweat test (more than 98 per cent of 19 992 in the United States Cystic Fibrosis Foundation Registry). The occasional patient, particularly with a mutation giving rise to a mild or atypical clinical phenotype, may require more sophisticated testing. However, the major difficulty is usually not in confirming the diagnosis but in thinking of it in an appropriate context (below, and Table 2). Conversely, false positive diagnoses are not rare, and a new referral of a cystic fibrosis patient to the adult clinic should prompt a full review of the diagnosis.

Presenting features

The various age-related problems that can lead to a diagnosis of cystic fibrosis are given in Table 2. Paediatric presentations are relevant to adult life in that if an adult with atypical respiratory disease turns out to have a family history of a child with cystic fibrosis or an illness shown in Table 2, then cystic fibrosis should be considered in the adult. The new diagnosis of cystic fibrosis in a younger relative will also prompt cascade screening (below), usually aiming to discover carriers, but occasionally someone with a clinically mild cystic fibrosis phenotype is discovered. The United States Cystic Fibrosis Foundation Registry data show that as many as 10 per cent of cystic fibrosis patients are not diagnosed until adult life.

Less than 5 per cent pancreatic function is necessary for normal digestive function, and those presenting with cystic fibrosis in adult life are clinically pancreatic sufficient. The main presentation is with respiratory problems, usually recurrent lower respiratory infections with chronic sputum production. Some patients have prior a diagnosis of bronchiectasis, atypical asthma, nasal polyposis, or allergic bronchopulmonary aspergillosis. A new cystic fibrosis diagnosis has been described even in adults in their seventh decade. Depletion of sodium, chloride, and potassium due to excessive sweating, and secondary renal chloride retention, may result in presentation with dehydration and heat exhaustion in an otherwise apparently completely fit adult.

Another important mode of presentation is male infertility due to azoospermia because of congenital bilateral absence of the vas deferens (CABVD). CABVD exists in different forms: firstly, in association with congenital malformations of the upper urinary tract, in which case there is no increased incidence of cystic fibrosis mutations; secondly, as part of classical cystic fibrosis; and thirdly, as a truly isolated forme fruste of cystic fibrosis, with only a single cystic fibrosis mutation and ion transport abnormalities overlapping with, but different from, true cystic fibrosis. Portal hypertension secondary to macronodular cirrhosis in adult life may also be the first presentation of cystic fibrosis.

There is considerable debate as to the status of adults with single organ manifestations characteristic of, but not confined to, cystic fibrosis—for example pancreatitis or allergic bronchopulmonary aspergillosis. Some series report a higher than expected incidence of cystic fibrosis mutations, and the occasional unsuspected cystic fibrosis compound heterozygote. In practice, although cystic fibrosis should be excluded as far as possible by appropriate investigations in the patient with a possible single organ disease, most will not have the traditional clinical cystic fibrosis disease as it is currently defined.

Sweat testing

The test must be performed by someone who is experienced. Techniques include the classical pilocarpine iontopheresis of Gibson and Cooke, and more recently the macroduct collection. For the diagnosis to be established, tests should be performed in duplicate. The normal concentrations of sweat sodium and chloride increase with age. To diagnose cystic fibrosis in a child, the sweat chloride concentration should be greater than 60 mmol/l, and the sweat sodium concentration less than that of chloride. A sweat chloride of less than 40 mmol is normal in older children and adults, and intermediate concentrations are equivocal. However, there are undoubted cases of cystic fibrosis with normal sweat electrolytes, and the sweat test should always be interpreted in the light of the whole clinical picture. If the sweat test is equivocal, consider repeating it the day after giving fludrocortisone 3 mg/m^2 for 2 days. In cystic fibrosis patients, sweat electrolyte concentrations fail to suppress into the normal range. There are a few rare conditions which also cause elevation in sweat electrolyte concentration, but these are rarely a serious diagnostic consideration in practice (Table 3).

Nasal electrical potential difference

The abnormal potential difference across mucosal surfaces can be measured by passing a soft catheter under the inferior turbinate, referencing it to an electrode placed on the abraded skin of the forearm. Normal values are −10 to −30 mV, the cystic fibrosis range −34 to −60 mV. The test is unreliable if the patient has an upper respiratory tract infection. The diagnosis can be further refined by perfusing the nose with solutions of amiloride to block sodium transport, and isoprenaline/low chloride to stimulate CFTR. Nasal potentials require extensive experience if results are to be accurate.

Ion transport can be measured directly from intestinal biopsies in an Ussing chamber, but this remains a research technique only.

Cystic fibrosis genotype

More than 900 different mutations causing cystic fibrosis have been reported. Testing for all is not currently practical. Thus DNA analysis can confirm the diagnosis if two mutations are found, but not exclude it. Linkage analysis can be used for antenatal diagnosis if a couple have already had an affected child, even if the actual mutations are not known.

Other investigations

In doubtful cases, evidence of subclinical organ dysfunction may be sought. Pancreatic dysfunction may be manifest by elevation in 3 day faecal fat excretion, low stool elastase, or abnormal results of pancreatic stimulation tests. CT scan of the chest or bronchoscopy may be used to discover minor bronchiectatic changes or infection with typical cystic fibrosis organisms. Azoospermia is strongly supportive of the diagnosis of cystic fibrosis. But note that it is important not to place too much diagnostic weight on clinically minor changes.

Conclusions

The diagnosis of cystic fibrosis is usually easy to confirm with a properly performed sweat test. There remain a few atypical cases which defy a firm diagnosis. In that event, clinical organ dysfunction should be treated appropriately, and the patient followed up very carefully: often time will clarify the diagnosis.

Table 2 Presentation of cystic fibrosis by age group

Age group	Presenting complaint
Antenatal	Chorionic villus sampling
	Ultrasound diagnosis of bowel perforation[1]
	Fetal hyperechogenic bowel[2]
At or soon after birth	Bowel obstruction (meconium ileus[1], bowel atresia)
	Haemorrhagic disease of the newborn
	Prolonged jaundice
	Screening (population based or previous affected sibling)
Infancy and childhood	Recurrent respiratory infections
	Diarrhoea and failure to thrive[3]
	Rectal prolapse[4]
	Nasal polyps[5]
	Acute pancreatitis
	Portal hypertension and variceal haemorrhage[6]
	Pseudo-Bartter's syndrome, electrolyte abnormality
	Hypoproteinaemia and oedema
	Screening as a result of cystic fibrosis diagnosis in a sibling/ relative
Adolescence and adult life	Recurrent respiratory infections
	Atypical asthma
	Bronchiectasis
	Male infertility (congenital bilateral absence of the vas deferens)
	Electrolyte disturbance/heat exhaustion
	Screening as a result of diagnosis in affected relative
	Portal hypertension and variceal haemorrhage

[1]Note that meconium ileus may be seen in pancreatic sufficient infants with cystic fibrosis, as well as rarely in those without cystic fibrosis.
[2]Most fetuses with hyperechogenic bowel are normal; around 6% have a trisomy, and 4% cystic fibrosis.
[3]Note that up to 15% may be pancreatic sufficient, at least at diagnosis; thriving does not exclude cystic fibrosis.
[4]One in six cases of rectal prolapse are due to cystic fibrosis, if obvious anatomical abnormalities are excluded.
[5]Unlike in adults, where aspirin-sensitive asthma is commonly associated with polyps, children with polyps almost invariably have cystic fibrosis.
[6]Presentation with hepatocellular failure is very rare.

Table 3 Conditions which are characterized by elevated sweat electrolyte concentrations; in most cases, confusion with cystic fibrosis is very unlikely

Cystic fibrosis
Untreated adrenal insufficiency
Type 1 glycogen storage disease
Nephrogenic diabetes insipidus
Malnutrition
Panhypopituitarism
Acquired immunodeficiency syndrome
Artefact (incorrectly performed sweat test, eczema)
Fucoscidosis
Hypothyroidism
Ectodermal dysplasia
Mucopolysaccharidosis

Screening

Introduction

Screening tests can be used to make an early diagnosis of cystic fibrosis in populations in order for early treatment to be instituted, and to detect cystic fibrosis carriers to allow antenatal diagnosis and the option of termination of affected pregnancies. In both areas there is controversy as to the indications and methods to be used. Currently neither is routinely available.

Methods

In the past, crude tests on meconium have been used, but these lacked accuracy and have been superseded by tests carried out on the routine heel prick blood sample collected from all babies in the first few days of life. These include immunoreactive trypsin, often combined with PCR for one or more common abnormal genes, or pancreatitis-related protein. If routine neonatal screening is to be instituted, it will probably be with immunoreactive trypsin and PCR. Pancreatitis-related protein screening may perform equally well, and obviates the need for genetic testing, which may be an advantage in some cultures.

Carrier screening is by PCR for several of the common cystic fibrosis genes on a blood or mouthwash sample. In principle, this sort of screening may be offered to relatives of known cystic fibrosis patients (cascade screening), by written invitation to the general population, or opportunistically at routine antenatal clinic visits or the GP surgery. It is generally considered that carrier testing at birth will not be useful because of the time lag between obtaining and utilizing the information.

Results

The evidence for the value of screening for the disease has come from a number of retrospective trials, all showing benefit, but with the disadvantage of using historical controls. There has been one prospective, randomized trial of neonatal screening from Wisconsin, United States in which 650 341 babies were screened. Of those in whom the diagnosis of cystic fibrosis was made, in 56 the diagnosis was communicated to the parents, and in 40 the diagnosis was suppressed until it emerged on clinical grounds. There were small but clear-cut nutritional benefits in the group in which the screening diagnosis was communicated, persisting to 10 years of age. The benefits were clearest early in life, at the time when growth is at its most rapid.

In general, carrier screening is poorly taken up when done by invitation, and at antenatal clinics it may be difficult to obtain a sample from the putative father. Cascade screening is generally better utilized, and should be offered at the time of making a new diagnosis.

Conclusions

Any screening test has false positives, which engender unnecessary anxiety, and false negatives, which may result in complacency. The balance of evidence is clearly in favour of neonatal screening so that early treatment can be given, and antenatal diagnosis offered for future pregnancies. The anxiety about false positives seems transient and deemed by the parents to be an acceptable price for subsequent reassurance. Carrier screening other than by cascade is more difficult, and, unless combined with wider public education, is unlikely to have a major impact.

Respiratory management

Introduction

Most of the morbidity and mortality of cystic fibrosis is due to respiratory disease. Much of the treatment is therefore devoted to preventing chronic infection and inflammation, which lead to bronchiectasis, progressive airflow obstruction, cor pulmonale, and ultimately death.

Typical physical findings are finger clubbing, cough with purulent sputum, together with crackles and occasional wheezes, chiefly in the upper lobes. Clinical scoring systems include the comprehensive Schwachman and simpler Taussig scores. The chest radiograph shows thickened bronchial walls and small areas of consolidation which start in the upper lobes and may progress to involve the whole lung (Fig. 3(a)). A variety of radiographic scoring systems have been proposed, for example Crispin–Norman or Brasfield score. Lung function tests show obstruction with relatively well preserved gas transfer. The forced expiratory volume in 1 s (FEV1) is conventionally used to assess the extent and progression of lung disease. Exercise tolerance and arterial blood gases are well maintained until there is extensive lung damage, when hypoxaemic respiratory failure supervenes. Carbon dioxide retention occurs late.

Infection

Oral antibiotics

The use of prophylactic antistaphylococcal antibiotics is controversial: most would use continuous twice daily oral flucloxacillin if there is evidence of chronic colonization. Minor exacerbations of respiratory symptoms in the patient not colonized with *Pseudomonas* should be treated with a 1-month course of a high-dose antibiotic which will cover *Staph. aureus* and *Haemophilus influenza*.

Ciprofloxacin is used at the time of first isolation of *Pseudomonas aeruginosa*, combined with nebulized antibiotics (below) to try to prevent chronic colonization: the duration of therapy is controversial. Ciprofloxacin is also used to cover exacerbations of symptoms in the *Pseudomonas* colonized patient; however, ciprofloxacin resistance soon becomes common.

Nebulized antibiotics

Nebulized colomycin combined with oral ciprofloxacin is indicated at the time of first isolation of *Pseudomonas aeruginosa*. This approach has been shown in a randomized trial to delay chronic colonization. Once *Pseudomonas aeruginosa* colonization is established, randomized controlled trials have shown benefit from long-term nebulized antibiotics. In Europe, colomycin is the drug most often used. In the United States, nebulized tobramycin is preferred. No comparision of the two has been reported. Occasional patients bronchoconstrict with nebulized antibiotics: a test dose should therefore be given, and if necessary pretreatment with a bronchodilator prescribed.

Intravenous antibiotics

Infective exacerbations not responding to oral antibiotics, particularly those of *Pseudomonas aeruginosa*, are usually treated with a combination of an intravenous aminoglycoside and a semisynthetic antipseudomonal penicillin or cephalosporin. These are frequently given at home. Unlike the circumstance of the febrile patient with neutropenia, there is no evidence to support the use of single daily doses of aminoglycoside in the patient with cystic fibrosis. Drug metabolism in the cystic fibrosis patient is very different from normals and other patient groups. Some centres recommend 3-monthly courses of intravenous antibiotics, irrespective of symptoms, for all cystic fibrosis patients colonized with *Pseudomonas aeruginosa*. A randomized trial in the United Kingdom, although underpowered, did not support this approach.

Cross-infection issues

Fear of nosocomial acquisition of resistant organisms is widespread in the cystic fibrosis community. The apparent increase in prevalence of *Pseudomonas aeruginosa* in specialized clinics probably reflects more assiduous bacterial culture techniques. However, some centres advocate separate clinics for cystic fibrosis patients with and without *Pseudomonas aeruginosa*. Strict cohorting has also been advocated with regard to more resistant organisms such as *Burkholderia cepacia*, but it has subsequently been realized that not all of these organisms are of equal virulence, and cohorting has actually resulted in cystic fibrosis patients acquiring a virulent organism.

Sensible guidelines should be applied to all cystic fibrosis patients: these include diligent handwashing, no sharing of physiotherapy equipment, and the use of single cubicles for inpatients with difficult organisms. Communal physiotherapy and keep fit sessions should be discouraged, and there is no doubt that conferences for cystic fibrosis patients can result in transmission of infection. Careful microbiological surveillance is essential, and special measures may be needed if there is a true epidemic strain within a particular clinic.

Importance of viral infections

Viral infections, trivial in themselves, have been implicated in causing transient reduction in airway defences and an increased risk of *Pseudomonas aeruginosa* acquisition. Most physicians would at least give oral antibiotics (above) to cover viral exacerbations. Annual influenza immunization is advisable.

Atypical mycobacteria

These organisms are often harmless commensals: unlike *M. tuberculosis*, evidence of tissue invasion is generally held to be required to diagnose infection. This evidence cannot often be sought in cystic fibrosis, and decisions as to whether to treat are difficult. Evidence from autopsy studies suggests that atypical mycobacteria should they be treated only if they are repeatedly found in sputum.

Airway clearance

Chest physiotherapy should be performed twice daily as a routine, increasing at times of infective exacerbation. Different groups advocate different techniques (for example active cycle of breathing, autogenic drainage; and mechanical devices, such as the positive expiratory pressure (PEP) mask, flutter, and external oscillation jacket). There are no good comparisons between these approaches, and none has emerged as best. Physical exercise such as swimming supplements, but should not replace formal airway clearance sessions.

Reduction of mucus viscosity

Mucolytics have their advocates but, in general, are not useful. Human recombinant DNase *in vitro* reduces sputum viscosity. In the largest, randomized, controlled trial in the literature, once daily nebulized human recombinant DNase resulted in small but sustained improvement in lung function and reduction in infective exacerbations. Individual responses are very variable, and the treatment is expensive. A carefully monitored n=1 trial is recommended before long-term therapy.

Oxygen and other respiratory support

By analogy with the Medical Research Council and Nocturnal Oxygen Treatment Trial (NOTT) trials of oxygen in COPD, one would anticipate that long-term oxygen would be beneficial to the chronically hypoxic cystic fibrosis patient. The only trial of this approach was underpowered and thus

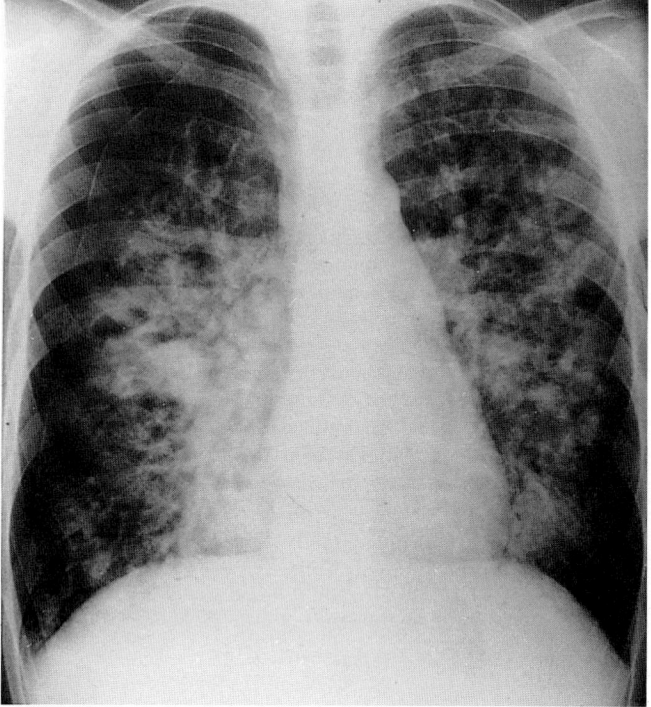

(a)

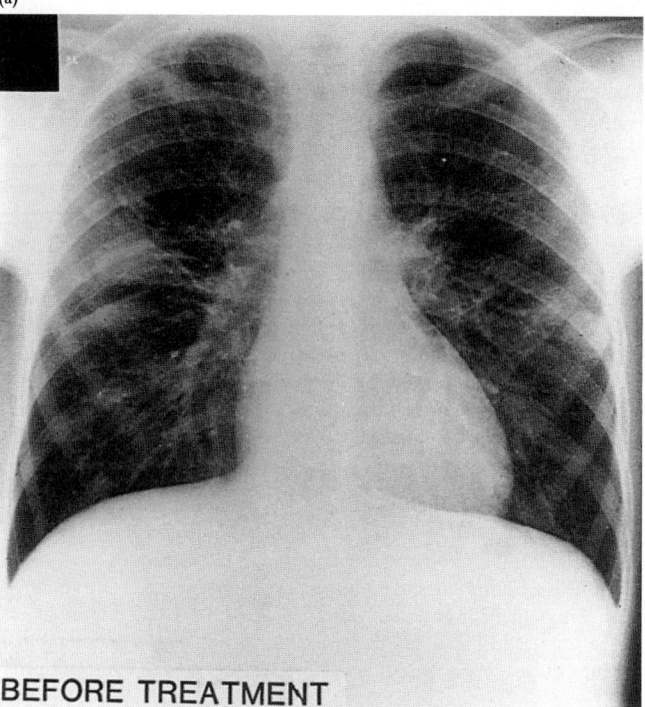

BEFORE TREATMENT

(b)

Fig. 3 (a) The typical chest radiograph appearances of advanced cystic fibrosis lung disease. There is also a right pneumothorax. (b) The chest radiograph in an adolescent child with cystic fibrosis complicated by allergic bronchopulmonary aspergillosis. Note the large wedge-shaped shadow.

inconclusive. Oxygen is usually prescribed for symptoms only. Nasal ventilation may be a useful short-term expedient while transplantation is awaited.

Bronchodilatation

Bronchial hyper-reactivity is common. Troublesome wheeze may need treatment with short-acting bronchodilators. However, β_2-agonists may cause paradoxical bronchoconstriction, and should be used cautiously. Long-acting β_2-agonists should only be given if there is clear-cut evidence of benefit. Persistent recurrent wheeze, particularly in the atopic cystic fibrosis patient, may be treated with inhaled or oral corticosteroids.

Aspergillus, including allergic bronchopulmonary aspergillosis

Evidence of exposure to *Aspergillus fumigatus* is common in cystic fibrosis (e.g. positive skin prick test, RAST, IgG precipitins, and sputum culture) but clinical disease is relatively rare. The prevalence of allergic bronchopulmonary aspergillosis is disputed, but is probably around 10 per cent. The major diagnostic criteria for this condition are also common features of cystic fibrosis. Sophisticated immunological testing has been used to try to refine the diagnosis, but an abrupt four-fold rise in total IgE, often in association with IgG precipitins to aspergillus, is the simplest and most reliable investigation. By contrast to typical infective exacerbations of cystic fibrosis, large fleeting radiographic shadows are typical (Fig. 3(b)). Treatment is with oral corticosteroids; the role of itraconazole is controversial.

Anti-inflammatory therapy

The pathogenesis of cystic fibrosis lung disease includes an exuberant IL-8 driven, neutrophil mediated, inflammatory response (see above), which, via the release of neutrophil elastase, may cause much of the tissue damage in the airways. This has lead to the seemingly paradoxical proposal that patients with chronic bronchopulmonary sepsis should be iatrogenically immunosuppressed. Various approaches have been tried, although none are in wide clinical use.

Oral corticosteroids

Usage in severe airway obstruction and allergic bronchopulmonary aspergillosis are discussed above. Long-term routine use was assessed in a multicentre, double-blind trial comparing prednisolone 2 mg/kg on alternate days, 1 mg/kg on alternate days, and placebo. This showed: (a) no benefit, except in patients colonized with *Ps. aeruginosa*; (b) sustained improvement in lung function in colonized patients; (c) unacceptable side-effects (growth failure, cataract, glucose intolerance), necessitating stopping the higher dose after 2 years and the lower dose after 4 years. Although in some patients, regular alternate-day steroids may be considered for up to 2 years, their routine use cannot be justified.

Inhaled corticosteroids

Since oral steroids are beneficial, but at the cost of unacceptable side-effects, it would seem logical to use long-term inhaled corticosteroids. Unfortunately there is no satisfactory trial confirming benefit: only small, relatively short-term studies have been done. Currently, inhaled corticosteroids can only be recommended for persistent wheeze, particularly in the atopic cystic fibrosis patient.

Ibuprofen

A multicentre, double-blind, placebo-controlled trial of ibuprofen showed a slowing of the rate of decline of lung function, particularly in young patients. However, ibuprofen is not widely used. This may be because: (a) not all age groups benefited; (b) there are theoretical reasons for believing that lower doses may actually be harmful, meaning that ibuprofen levels need to be measured and a high dose given; and (c) if intravenous aminoglycosides have to be administered for an acute exacerbation of chest disease, there is a significant risk of nephrotoxicity.

Other anti-inflammatory approaches

Although anti-inflammatory defences are normal in cystic fibrosis, they are overwhelmed by the burden of neutrophil elastase. Boosting the natural defences (α_1-antitrypsin, secretory leukoprotease inhibitor) by nebulizer has been the subject of small and inconclusive trials. Further safety and efficacy data are awaited.

Cytotoxics

There are anecdotal reports of the successful use of methotrexate, cyclosporin, and intravenous immunoglobulin in cystic fibrosis, particularly in those with severe, non-bronchiectatic airflow obstruction. There are no large trials of these approaches.

Haemoptysis

Blood streaking of sputum is common in cystic fibrosis and requires no special treatment. Massive haemoptysis is variously defined, usually as the expectoration of more than 250 ml of blood in 24 h, and is a frightening emergency which does require active management. It is usually a complication of quite severe lung disease, and the source is from hypertrophied bronchial arteries. The patient should be admitted, given antipseudomonal intravenous antibiotics, and any clotting abnormalities corrected. Careful chest physiotherapy should be continued. Trasylol and vasopressin are sometimes used to try to control haemorrhage. If bleeding does not settle, or recurs, then bronchial artery embolism should be considered. All sizeable bronchial arteries should be occluded. Preoperative bronchoscopy does not influence management, and often fails to define the side of bleeding in any case. The major risk of embolization is inadvertent occlusion of a major spinal artery, resulting in paraplegia. Lobectomy is rarely necessary, and carries a high risk in these patients, who are often very compromised.

Pneumothorax

This is usually a complication of late-stage lung disease. Shallow pneumothoraces require no special measures; more severe air leaks are initially treated with tube drainage. Careful physiotherapy must be continued, and intravenous antibiotics given. If there is a continued air leak, pleurodesis should be undertaken. However, it is important to consult with the local transplant service before doing this, because aggressive pleurectomy is seen by some to be a contraindication to subsequent transplantation.

Upper airway disease

Nasal polyps are seen in up to 50 per cent of adults with cystic fibrosis. Treatment is with nasal steroids in the first instance. If medical management fails, surgical polypectomy is indicated, but 50 per cent will require a second procedure within 2 years. Abnormal sinus radiographs are universal, but symptomatic sinusitis relatively rare. If present, sinusitis should be treated medically with prolonged antibiotics, nasal steroids, and possibly decongestants in the first instance; surgery is rarely needed. Rarely, surgery is needed for mucocele of the frontal sinuses.

Gastrointestinal management

Pancreatic insufficiency needs to be treated in 85 per cent of cases; meconium ileus or distal intestinal obstruction syndrome affects up to 30 per cent; symptomatic liver disease occurs in about 5 per cent, but in general the gastrointestinal manifestations of cystic fibrosis are less important than the lung disease. For a few patients, however, they are the dominant problem.

Pancreatic insufficiency

This is usually present from birth with low levels of bicarbonate and lipolytic and proteolytic enzymes in pancreatic secretions. Those with clinical pancreatic sufficiency secrete low but adequate levels of enzymes. Some develop pancreatic insufficiency later in life. The usual presentations are neonatal meconium ileus or failure to thrive with associated steatorrhoea and malnutrition. Consequences can include anaemia, vitamin deficiency, and occasionally oedema; complications include rectal prolapse, intussusception, volvulus, and distant intestinal obstruction.

The diagnosis is confirmed by estimation of stool elastase, demonstration of unsplit fat globules in the stool, or increased faecal fat on a 2 or 3-day stool collection. Formal testing of pancreatic function is seldom required.

Treatment with pancreatic enzyme and vitamin supplementation is usually straightforward and successful. Enteric coated enzyme preparations are taken before meals and the quantity adjusted to achieve normal stools. Most adults need four to eight capsules with main meals and two to four with snacks and learn to adjust the dose according to the fat content of the meal. The commonest cause of failure is poor compliance, although occasionally lactose intolerance, inflammatory bowel disease, coeliac disease, or bowel infection/infestation may coexist. A few patients need to take H_2 blockers, proton pump inhibitors, or antacids to achieve complete control of symptoms. Large bowel strictures have developed in some patients (usually children) taking high-strength enzyme preparations, probably as a toxic effect of the coating rather than the enzymes themselves.

Nutrition

Vitamin supplementation should be given to all patients to cover fat soluble vitamin deficiency. Multivitamin tablets contain vitamins A and D, but vitamin E needs to be given separately to maintain adequate intake. The diet should otherwise be normal, with a high calorie intake, usually 130 per cent of recommended daily allowance. Patients unable to maintain weight in spite of optimal dietary advice can be helped by enteral feeding, which is better tolerated by gastrostomy than by a nasogastric tube in the long term.

Distal intestine obstruction syndrome

Constipation and a loaded colon are relatively common in cystic fibrosis and usually respond to modification of the diet, pancreatic supplements, and a high fluid and roughage intake; occasionally lactulose or cisapride are helpful. Severe constipation merges into the distal intestine obstruction syndrome with pain, palpable faecal masses, and complete obstruction with faecal material in the distal ileum or ascending colon. The cause is multifactorial with imbalance of pancreatic enzymes and diet, disturbed fluid and electrolyte transport, faecal dehydration, and abnormal intestinal mobility all playing a part.

Patients present with chronic intermittent pain or episodes of complete obstruction. Although the differential diagnosis is wide and includes common conditions such as appendicitis, most patients improve with medical treatment and surgery should be avoided unless there is clear evidence of another diagnosis. Treatment with a balanced intestinal lavage solution, 500 to 1000 ml/h by nasogastric tube, usually moves the faecal blockage within 4 to 6 h. Alternatives are gastrograffin by mouth or enema, or oral n-acetylcysteine. Occasionally, removal of inspissated faeces at colonoscopy is needed.

Other gastrointestinal complications

Pancreatitis is rare but should be excluded in cases of abdominal pain. It usually affects those who are clinically pancreatic sufficient. Treatment is conventional, with special attention to pulmonary infections, because the pain of pancreatitis may interfere with physiotherapy. Gastro-oesophageal reflux is common, sometimes with overt vomiting, and may be associated with coughing, physiotherapy, and bronchodilators which may relax the oesophageal sphincter. Aspiration of stomach contents is seldom a clinical problem. Although peptic ulcer disease might be expected in view of the low pancreatic bicarbonate secretion, there is only one report of an increased frequency of ulceration. *Helicobacter pylori* infection is uncom-

mon, perhaps because of antibiotic treatment. Lactose intolerance, coeliac disease, and inflammatory bowel disease occur with the expected or slightly increased frequency in the cystic fibrosis population, but symptoms may be misattributed to cystic fibrosis and diagnosis therefore delayed. Both giardiasis and *Clostridium difficile* gut infection have been reported as being more frequent in cystic fibrosis but are not common clinical problems.

Liver disease

Liver disease causes problems in 5 per cent and death in 2 per cent of people with cystic fibrosis, but abnormal liver function tests are very common and up to 50 per cent have biliary cirrhosis demonstrable at post mortem. With increasing survival, liver disease may become more important.

Although liver enlargement and jaundice occasionally occur in early childhood, liver disease is usually signalled by hepatosplenomegaly or abnormal liver function on routine testing. Decompensation with jaundice, ascites, or encephalopathy are rare and occur late. Variceal bleeding only occurs in a minority of those with established chronic liver disease. Minor or modest elevations of aminotransferase, gamma glutamyl transpeptidase, or alkaline phosphatase levels are very common but do not correlate with established liver disease unless the enzyme levels are greater than four times normal. Routine ultrasound detects fatty change or multilobular cirrhosis: the finding of portal vein dilatation, splenomegaly, or colateral vessels indicating portal hypertension. Cholangiography is occasionally needed for treatment of gall stones: this may reveal irregularities of the intrahepatic ducts, suggesting chronic liver disease, and significant strictures of the common bile duct may also be seen. Liver biopsy is seldom needed.

No treatment has been shown to modify the course of chronic liver disease in cystic fibrosis, although clinical and biochemical improvements have been shown following treatment with ursodeoxycholic acid. This bile acid stimulates bile flow, may protect the hepatocyte from toxicity of bile acids, and is helpful in primary biliary cirrhosis. Many hepatologists therefore recommend its use in cystic fibrosis.

Jaundice must be investigated to exclude drug hepatotoxicity or treatable obstructive cause, but is otherwise a late event with poor prognosis. Variceal bleeding is treated with injection sclerotherapy or banding ligation, and in the short-term balloon tamponade or vasoconstrictor drugs may buy a little time. Surgical treatment is hazardous due to lung disease and in a few patients the insertion of a transjugular intrahepatic portal systemic shunt may be an alternative. Prophylactic treatment of varices has not been shown to help and may be detrimental. Ascites and encephalopathy are rare and are usually preterminal events to be managed conventionally.

In most cases of complicated chronic liver disease, management is made more difficult by the presence of lung infection that must be aggressively treated. Respiratory failure may develop concurrently. When this occurs, intubation and ventilation are seldom successful.

Diabetes

Glucose intolerance in cystic fibrosis increases with age, being rare under 10 years, affecting 14 per cent by 15 years, and over 65 per cent at 25 years, by which age 32 per cent are frankly diabetic. Even when glucose tolerance is normal, reduced insulin secretion is frequent. This is caused by gradual and progressive loss of beta cell mass in line with pancreatic fibrosis. Peripheral insulin sensitivity is normal and autoimmune factors are not involved.

Diagnosis is based on conventional WHO recommendations. Some recommend annual oral glucose tolerance tests, but screening for diabetes in a cystic fibrosis clinic is usually done by measurement of HBA1c, together with random or fasting blood sugar levels. Diabetes is usually diagnosed at such screening, but a few patients present with weight loss and increased frequency and severity of chest infections, although polyuria and polydipsia occasionally develop first. It has been suggested that the onset of diabetes is a marker of general deterioration, but many patients return to their previous level of health when diabetes is controlled. Oral hypoglycaemic agents provide control in a minority of patients for a limited time: insulin replacement is usually necessary. Control of blood sugar is relatively simple, with slow release preparations given twice daily. Ketoacidosis and insulin resistance are almost unknown.

The dietary management of diabetes in cystic fibrosis differs from that of other forms of diabetes: high dietary intake is maintained and insulin adjusted to fit the diet rather than the other way round. The usual recommendations are an energy intake of 150 per cent of normal with frequent balanced meals.

Early microangiopathy has been shown in cystic fibrosis patients with diabetes, but retinopathy, neuropathy, and nephropathy are very rare. This is due in part to the mildness of the diabetes and in part to short survival. Nevertheless, cystic fibrosis patients with diabetes tend to have excess morbidity and slightly increased rate of decline in weight and lung function.

Other organ systems

Reproduction

Almost all cystic fibrosis males have obstructive azoospermia with otherwise normal sexual function. This is due to absence of the vas deferens, and although there are no sperm in the ejaculate there is normal spermatogenesis and Leydig cell function. Counselling about infertility should be done by the time of puberty, ideally before permanent relationships develop. Most men opt to confirm the azoospermia by a sperm count. *In vitro* fertilization using aspirated sperm has been successful and there are now many cystic fibrosis fathers.

Early reports of reduced fertility in cystic fibrosis women have not been confirmed and most can conceive normally. The child must carry one mutation from the mother: the risk of cystic fibrosis is therefore 1 in 50 in a Caucasian populations with a carrier frequency of 1 in 25. Counselling and paternal genotyping allows reassurance for the majority of cystic fibrosis pregnancies and identifies a 1 in 2 risk when the father is a carrier. Successful pregnancies have been completed by many hundreds of cystic fibrosis women, but women with severe lung disease may not be able to complete a pregnancy safely, the risks rising with impaired lung function and especially when the 1 s FEV1 is less than 30 per cent predicted. Children born have been healthy, without an increased frequency of birth defects despite the mothers' extensive drug treatment. Lactation is normal.

Vaginal candidiasis secondary to antibiotic treatment is relatively common in cystic fibrosis, but otherwise there are no specific gynaecological problems. Sexual behaviour in both genders may be inhibited by low weight, delayed puberty, cough, sputum, haemoptysis, breathlessness, and indwelling catheters, but most people adapt well and persistent problems are few.

Skin and joints

Clubbing is almost universal in those with significant lung disease and regresses after successful lung transplantation. Hypertropic osteoarthropathy is rare. Episodic arthritis, predominantly affecting the large joints, is quite common and is associated with chest infections. Erosive arthritis is rare. Pain responds to non-steroidal anti-inflammatory drugs and steroids or immunosuppression are seldom needed. Systemic vasculitis has occasionally been reported but is surprisingly rare considering the extent of immune activation, the frequency of circulating immune complexes, and the number of drugs taken.

Kidneys

Glomerulonephritis has been reported but is probably no more frequent than in the normal population. Drug-induced renal damage is rare and is usually associated with higher than recommended aminoglycoside levels. Very large numbers of aminoglycoside treatments appear to be safe when serum levels are well controlled. Renal stones are commoner in cystic fibrosis, probably due to excess oxylate absorption secondary to altered bowel bacterial flora. Systemic amyloidosis has occasionally been reported secondary to prolonged pulmonary infection.

Central nervous system

Ototoxicity occasionally results from aminoglycoside treatment but is not seen when serum levels are well controlled. Cerebral abscess rarely complicates lung sepsis. Vitamin E deficiency leads to a cerebellar syndrome combined with peripheral neuropathy.

Osteoporosis

Reduced bone mineral density is common in cystic fibrosis, with a prevalence among adults of up to 60 per cent. This is partly due to general malnutrition as well as vitamin D malabsorption, but relative immobility is sometimes a factor. An increased rate of fractures has been reported and rib fractures from coughing can interfere with adequate physiotherapy. Vertebral compression fractures are fortunately rare. Regular bone mineral density measurements are recommended with extra vitamin D and calcium supplementation when low. Bisphosphonates can cause bone pain and have not yet been fully evaluated.

Management of respiratory failure

Recurrent and persistent chest infection leads to progressive decline in lung function with eventual respiratory failure in the vast majority of patients; in about 2 per cent the liver fails first. At this stage palliation of symptoms should replace aggressive treatment unless there is a realistic prospect of a lung or liver transplant. If this is feasible, then preoperative work-up, counselling, surgical assessment, and placement on the waiting list should take place 2 years before the predicted date of death.

Lung transplantation (see also Chapter 17.16)

Selection criteria are listed in Table 4. The timing of assessment is judged on the level and rate of decline of lung function, arterial blood gases, and the frequency and severity of chest infections. Patients on the waiting list must be managed optimally to maintain lung function and nutrition, usually with gastrostomy feeding. Non-invasive ventilatory support can provide a bridge to transplantation for patients with progressive respiratory failure but intubation and conventional ventilation are not recommended. Donor organs are scarce and at least 50 per cent of listed cystic fibrosis patients never receive a transplant. The results for lung transplantation are

Table 4 Selection criteria for lung transplantation

Indications	Severe respiratory failure in spite of optimal treatment
	Severely impaired quality of life
	Patient positively wants a transplant
Strong contraindications	Active aspergillus or mycobacterial infection
	Non-compliance with treatment
	Other end organ failure
	Gross malnutrition
Risk factors	Preoperative ventilation
	Previous thoracic surgery
	Chemical pleurodesis

the same as for other lung diseases with a survival of 70 per cent at 1 year and 50 per cent at 3 years.

Liver transplantation is appropriate for the occasional patient dying of liver failure with relatively good lung function: survival at 1 year is 40 per cent. For patients with respiratory failure and severe liver disease combined lung and liver transplantation is a possibility but with poor survival and with limited organ availability the operation is difficult to justify.

Terminal care

The timing of the decision to switch to palliative care is difficult and should be made in conjunction with the patient and relatives. The most distressing symptoms are cough, sputum retention, breathlessness, and exhaustion. Small doses of morphine are usually well tolerated and only seldom worsen respiratory failure.

The cystic fibrosis team

As with many chronic diseases, the purely medical care of cystic fibrosis is relatively straightforward. Proper holistic care requires a team approach, and without such a team, care will be second rate. Typically, the core of the team is formed by a specialist nurse, a physiotherapist, a dietician, a psychologist, and a social worker, together with a specialist doctor. It is unrealistic to expect every hospital to provide this, and so close contact with a tertiary centre is advisable. Many of the physical issues (airway clearance, nutritional management) have been discussed above. Equally important are many of the psychological problems springing from the presence of a chronic disease.

The normal tasks of adolescence include rebelling and breaking free of parental care. In those with cystic fibrosis this may never have been achieved, because the parents have wanted to keep control of treatment regimens, and have been reluctant to allow independence. Although the paediatric clinics should have established a pattern of the adolescent coming into the consulting room alone, frequently this does not happen, and the adult physician is confronted with parents who resent the idea that their now grown-up child should be seen on their own. Conversely, the consequences of a full-blown adolescent revolt (no treatment done, abuse of cigarettes, alcohol, and soft and hard drugs) may be particularly catastrophic in the cystic fibrosis patient. The authors know of no easy answer to adolescence and its aftermath.

Knowledge of fertility issues is notoriously poor amongst adult men with cystic fibrosis: these may need to be tackled tactfully. The issues surrounding pregnancy in the cystic fibrosis girl, who may herself be severely breathless, but desperately wishing for a child, also require sensitive handling. Further education and employment are also difficult issues in the setting of chronic physical disability, but skilled help may allow the cystic fibrosis patient to maximize their potential. A fuller account of the many and complex psychosocial issues surrounding care can be found elsewhere: appreciation of these issues is just as important as knowing the correct management of the physical problems of cystic fibrosis.

Future prospects

The growth in basic scientific understanding of cystic fibrosis will lead to a number of new treatments directed at the mutant CFTR gene or protein. These include gene therapy, which has already reached preliminary clinical trials, protein replacement therapy, and drug therapy to correct the molecular defect (as illustrated in Fig. 2). Research into correction of the disordered electrophysiology with sodium channel blockers, such as amiloride, or promoters of chloride transport, such as UTP, is already well advanced. There is, therefore, a real prospect of new fundamental treatments to prevent the development of cystic fibrosis disease and lead to improved health, prolonged survival, and reduction in life-long supportive therapy.

Further reading

Anguiano A, Oates RD, Amos JA, *et al.* (1992). Congenital bilateral absence of the vas deferens. A primary genital form of cystic fibrosis. *Journal of the American Medical Association* **267**, 1794–7. [Report setting out a new form of CF mutation associated disease.]

Armstrong DS, Grimwood K, Carlin JB, *et al.* (1997). Lower airway inflammation in infants and young children with cystic fibrosis. *American Journal of Respiratory and Critical Care Medicine* **156**, 1197–204. [The other side of the controversy as to whether infection is a necessary prerequisite for inflammation in CF.]

Cantin A (1995). Cystic fibrosis lung inflammation: early, sustained and severe. *American Journal of Respiratory and Critical Care Medicine* **151**, 939–41. [Brief review of lung inflammation.]

Caplen NJ, Geddes DM, Alton EWFW (1998). Gene therapy for respiratory disease. *Clinics in Pulmonary Medicine* **5**, 250–9. Overview relevant to the development of CF gene therapy.

Cleghorn GJ, Stringer DA, Forstner GG, Durie PR (1986). Treatment of distal intestinal obstruction in cystic fibrosis with balanced intestinal lavage solution. *Lancet* **1**, 8–11. [Establishment of modern management of obstruction in CF.]

Cohn JA, Friedman KJ, Noone PG, Knowles MR, Silverman LM, Jowell PS (1998). Relations between mutations of the cystic fibrosis gene and idiopathic pancreatitis. *New England Journal of Medicine* **339**, 653–8. [A paper illustrating the expanding spectrum of cystic fibrosis and the related diseases in which there may be a higher than normal prevalence of cystic fibrosis mutations.]

Cox KL, Ward RE, Furguiele TL, Cannon RA, Sanders KD, Kurland G (1987). Orthoptic liver transplantation in patients with cystic fibrosis. *Pediatrics* **80**, 571–4. [Key paper establishing the success of liver transplantation in CF.]

Cystic Fibrosis Foundation, Patient Registry 1996 (1997). *Annual data report.* Bethesda, Maryland. [Consensus group on diagnosis of atypical cases of cystic fibrosis in particular. Valuable source of epidemiological data from the United States.]

Cystic Fibrosis Genotype-Phenotype Consortium (1993). Correlation between genotype and phenotype in patients with cystic fibrosis. *New England Journal of Medicine* **329**, 1308–13.

Davidson TM, Murphy C, Mitchell M, Smith C, Light M (1995). Management of chronic sinusitis in cystic fibrosis. *Laryngoscope* **105**, 354–8. [Practical paper on clinical management.]

Davis PB, Drumm M, Konstan W (1996). Cystic fibrosis. *American Journal of Respiratory and Critical Care Medicine* **154**, 1229–56. [Comprehensive review article with emphasis on basic science and pathogenesis.]

Eigen H, Rosenstein BJ, Fitzsimmons S, *et al.* (1995). A multicenter study of alternate-day prednisone therapy in patients with cystic fibrosis. *Journal of Pediatrics* **126**, 515–23. [Disappointing full stop to the prednisolone story—an excellent study which failed to confirm previous results.]

Farrell PM, Kosorok MR, Laxova A, *et al.* (1997). Nutritional benefits of neonatal screening for cystic fibrosis. *New England Journal of Medicine* **337**, 963–9. [The only large randomized controlled trial of screening in CF.]

FitzSimmons SC (1993). The changing face epidemiology of cystic fibrosis. *Journal of Paediatrics* **122**, 1–9. [Survey of improvements from the United States registry.]

Frederiksen B, Koch C, Hoiby N (1997). Antibiotic treatment of initial colonization with *Pseudomonas aeruginosa* postpones chronic infection and prevents deterioration of pulmonary function in cystic fibrosis. *Pediatric Pulmonology* **23**, 330–5. [Review of the Danish clinic infection and antibiotic policies.]

Fuchs HJ, Borowitz DS, Christiansen DH, *et al.* (1994). Effect of aerosolized recombinant human DNase on exacerbations of respiratory symptoms and on pulmonary function in patients with cystic fibrosis. *New England Journal of Medicine* **331**, 637–42. [The largest randomized trial ever performed in CF establishing pulmonary function changes with DNase treatment.]

Hodson ME (1992). Vasculitis and arthropathy in cystic fibrosis. *Journal of the Royal Society of Medicine* **85** (Suppl. 19), 38–40. [Report of systemic manifestations of inflammation in CF.]

Hodson ME, Geddes DM, eds (1995). *Cystic fibrosis*. Chapman and Hall, London. [Comprehensive textbook with a clinical slant.]

Hodson ME, Madden BP, Steven MH, Tsang VT, Yacoub MH (1991). Non-invasive mechanical ventilation for cystic fibrosis patients: a potential bridge to transplantation. *European Respiratory Journal* **4**, 524–7. [A practical contribution to pretransplant care.]

Khan TZ, Wagener JS, Boat T, Martinez J, Accurso FJ, Riches DWH (1995). Early pulmonary inflammation in infants with cystic fibrosis. *American Journal of Respiratory and Critical Care Medicine* **151**, 1075–82. [Important study showing early onset of bronchial inflammation even in infants diagnosed by screening.]

Konstan MW, Byard PJ, Hoppel CL, Davis PB (1995). Effect of high-dose ibuprofen in patients with cystic fibrosis. *New England Journal of Medicine* **332**, 848–54. [Large multicentre study of non-steroidal anti-inflammatory medication in CF.]

Marchant JL, Warner JO, Bush A (1994). Rise in total IgE as an indicator of allergic broncho-pulmonary aspergillosis in cystic fibrosis. *Thorax* **49**, 1002–5. [References criteria for diagnosis of ABPA, and a simple laboratory test for diagnosis and following treatment.]

Middleton PG, Geddes DM, Alton EWFW (1994). Protocols for in vivo measurement of the ion transport defects in cystic fibrosis nasal epithelium. *European Respiratory Journal* **7**, 2050–6. [Methods for using nasal potentials in diagnosis which is also applicable to monitoring new treatments.]

Mukhopadhyay S, Singh M, Cater JI, Ogston S, Franklin M, Olver RE (1996). Nebulised antipseudomonal antibiotic therapy in cystic fibrosis: a meta-analysis of benefits and risks. *Thorax* **51**, 364–8. [Meta-analysis of randomised controlled clinical trials of nebulized antibiotics.]

Ramsey BW, Pepe MS, Quan JM, *et al.* (1999). Intermittent administration of inhaled tobramycin in patients with cystic fibrosis. *New England Journal of Medicine* **340**, 23–30. [Large, randomized trial of nebulized tobramycin in CF.]

Rosenstein BJ, Cutting GR, for the Cystic Fibrosis Foundation Consensus Panel (1998). The diagnosis of cystic fibrosis: a consensus statement. *Journal of Pediatrics* **132**, 589–95.

Rosenstein B, Zeitlin PL (1998). Cystic fibrosis. *Lancet* **351**, 277–82. [Brief but balanced review with selective list for further reading.]

Smyth RL, Van Velzen D, Smyth AR, Lloyd DA, Heaf DP (1994). Strictures of the ascending colon in cystic fibrosis and high strength pancreatic enzymes. *Lancet* **343**, 35–6. [Important report of a new side-effect.]

Tomashefski JF, Stern RC, Demko CA, Doershuk CF (1990). Non-tuberculous mycobacteria in cystic fibrosis: an autopsy study. *American Journal of Respiratory and Critical Care Medicine* **142**, 940–53. [Good autopsy study of atypical mycobacteria in CF.]

Tsang V, Hodson ME, Yacoub MH (1992). Lung transplantation for cystic fibrosis. *British Medical Bulletin* **48**, 949–71. [Details report of early and successful experience with lung transplantation for CF.]

Tsui LC (1995). The cystic fibrosis transmembrane conductance regulator gene. *American Journal of Respiratory and Critical Care Medicine* **151**, S47–53.

Valerius NH, Koch C, Hoiby NM (1991). Prevention of chronic *Pseudomonas aeruginosa* colonisation in cystic fibrosis by early treatment. *Lancet* **338**, 725–6. [Important trial of early and aggressive therapy to eradicate *Pseudomonas aeruginosa* and the results of treatment.]

Wallis C, Leung T, Cubitt D, Reynolds A (1997). Stool elastase as a diagnostic test for pancreatic function in children with cystic fibrosis. *Lancet* **350**, 1001. [Stool elastase has recently been described as a sensitive and specific test for pancreatic insufficiency, requiring only a spot sample; clinically extremely valuable.]

Weaver LT, Green MR, Nicholson K, *et al.* (1994). Prognosis in cystic fibrosis treated with continuous flucloxacillin from the neonatal period. *Archives of Disease in Childhood* **70**, 84–9. [Randomized trial of prophylactic flucloxacillin in CF.]

Webb AK, Govan J (1998). *Burkholderia cepacia*: another twist and a further threat. *Thorax* **53**, 333–4. [Important review of the biology of this increasingly important pathogen.]

Welsh MJ, Smith AE (1993). Molecular mechanisms of CFTR chloride channel dysfunction in cystic fibrosis. *Cell* **73**, 1251–4. [Summary of the molecular pathology of CF.]

17.11 Diffuse parenchymal lung disease

17.11.1 Diffuse parenchymal lung disease: an introduction

R. M. du Bois

Definition

The definition of diffuse parenchymal lung disease has become confused. This is due to a combination of muddled nomenclature, the overuse of synonyms, and a lack of precision in defining the individual diseases that come under this 'umbrella' term.

Diffuse parenchymal lung disease used to be known as interstitial lung disease. The change of terminology recognized that it was not just the parenchyma but also the airspace components of the acini that are involved in the diffuse parenchymal lung diseases. Infective pneumonias and some malignancies involve the acinar regions of the lung but are excluded from the classification by convention, although they must be considered as part of a differential diagnosis when diffuse parenchymal lung diseases are being considered.

Each specific disease will be considered in subsequent chapters and this introduction will focus on the approach to the classification of the diffuse lung diseases and their diagnosis and management.

Classification

Diffuse parenchymal lung diseases can be subdivided into five major groupings:

- associated with systemic diseases including rheumatological disease;
- diseases caused by environmental triggers or drug-ingestion;
- granulomatous diseases;
- idiopathic interstitial pneumonias;
- other diffuse lung diseases.

The majority of the environmentally and drug-induced lung diseases and granulomatous lung diseases are of known cause. Diffuse parenchymal lung diseases occurring in the context of systemic disease have known associations but are generally of unknown cause. The majority of the heterogeneous group of 'other' diffuse parenchymal lung diseases is of unknown cause as are, by definition, the idiopathic interstitial pneumonias. Table 1 and Fig. 1 illustrate the diseases of known and unknown cause that fall within each of the above broad headings, and Table 2 illustrates disorders that present more acutely, an important distinguishing feature.

Idiopathic interstitial pneumonias

The group of diseases known together as the 'idiopathic interstitial pneumonias' are those that have produced most confusion in terms of nomenclature and understanding. This is largely because pathological pattern descriptions have been used interchangeably with disease 'labels' without consistency. Over the last five decades, two parallel processes—clinical and histopathological—were used to define diseases that are now included within the idiopathic interstitial pneumonias.

Clinical

In 1944, Hamman and Rich described four patients who died of a rapidly progressive process; the histopathological appearances showed interstitial pneumonia and fibrosis. Subsequently, similar disease patterns occurring over a more chronic time frame were identified. All of these were characterized by the presence of progressive breathlessness, crackles heard on auscultation of the chest, chest radiography which showed reticulonodular patterns of abnormality in the periphery and the bases of the lung fields, and a restrictive ventilatory defect on lung function testing. Similar but less acute disorders were subsequently described. Together all of these disorders have been loosely labelled as 'cryptogenic fibrosing alveolitis' or 'idiopathic pulmonary fibrosis' in the United States and elsewhere. Bronchoalveolar lavage was later introduced as an investigative tool and the presence of excess neutrophils and/or eosinophils helped to confirm this diagnosis. More recently, high resolution computed tomography has been used to define patterns of disease, helping to identify a number of quite distinct patterns that had previously been included under the single diagnostic 'label' of 'cryptogenic fibrosing alveolitis'.

Histopathological

In 1975, Liebow described five interstitial pneumonias that could be associated with clinical disease that mimics 'cryptogenic fibrosing alveolitis':

- usual interstitial pneumonia (UIP);
- desquamative interstitial pneumonia (DIP);
- bronchiolitis obliterans with usual interstitial pneumonia (BIP);
- lymphoid interstitial pneumonia;
- giant cell interstitial pneumonia.

Over subsequent years it became clear that not all of these interstitial pneumonias were idiopathic. Lymphocytic interstitial pneumonia was generally due to lymphoproliferative disorders, rheumatological disease, or AIDS-related disease. Giant cell interstitial pneumonia was found to be due to the exposure to the alloy hard metal (cobalt, tungsten carbide, titanium salts).

This resulted in a revision of the classification such that the interstitial pneumonias, defined histopathologically, of known cause, were removed. The idiopathic group now included UIP and DIP from the original classification. To these were added respiratory bronchiolitis–interstitial lung disease (RB-ILD), diffuse alveolar damage (DAD), and non-specific interstitial pneumonia (NSIP). BIP was renamed 'organizing pneumonia.'

Usual interstitial pneumonia

Usual interstitial pneumonia is by definition, the pattern seen in cryptogenic fibrosing alveolitis. The hallmark of usual interstitial pneumonia is a

Table 1 Diffuse parenchymal lung disease

Associated with systemic diseases

Rheumatological
  Systemic sclerosis
  Rheumatoid arthritis
  Systemic lupus erythematosus
  Sjögren's syndrome
  Ankylosing spondylitis
  Polymyositis/ dermatomyositis
  Mixed connective tissue disease

Vasculitis
  Giant cell arteritis
  Takayasu's arteritis
  Microscopic polyangiitis
  Wegener's granulomatosis
  Churg– Strauss granulomatosis
  Behçet's syndrome
  Pulmonary–renal syndrome (including Goodpasture's syndrome)
  Capillaritis

Vascular
  Antiphospholipid syndrome
  Coagulopathies
  A–V malformations
  Primary pulmonary hypertension
  Idiopathic pulmonary haemosiderosis
  Pulmonary veno-occlusive disease

Diseases caused by environmental triggers or drug ingestion

Environmental—organic causes
  Extrinsic allergic alveolitis
    Fungal
    Bacterial
    Avian
    Chemical
Environmental—inorganic causes
  Fibrogenic inorganic dusts
    Asbestos
    Silica
    Hard metal alloy
    Beryllium
    Coal
    Aluminium
  Non-fibrogenic
    Siderosis
    Stannosis
    Baritosis
    Antimony
Drugs*
  Chemotherapeutic
  Cardiovascular
  Antibiotics
  Anti-inflammatory
  Illicit
  Psychotropic
  Radiation
  Pesticides
  Oxygen

Granulomatous diseases

  Sarcoidosis
  Berylliosis
  Extrinsic allergic alveolitis
  Langerhans cell histiocytosis
  Wegener's granulomatosis
  Churg–Strauss syndrome
  Lymphomatoid granulomatosis
  Bronchocentric granulomatosis

Table 1 Continued

Idiopathic interstitial pneumonias

  Cryptogenic fibrosing alveolitis (idiopathic pulmonary fibrosis; UIP or NSIP variants)
  Non-specific interstitial pneumonia
  Desquamative interstitial pneumonia
  Respiratory bronchiolitis–interstitial lung disease
  Acute interstitial pneumonia
  Cryptogenic organizing pneumonia
  Lymphocytic interstitial pneumonia

Other diffuse lung diseases

Inherited disorders
  Tuberous sclerosis
  Neurofibromatosis
  Hermansky–Pudlak syndrome
  Lipid storage disorders
  Familial fibrosing alveolitis
Pulmonary eosinophilia
  known causes e.g. fungi, parasites, drugs
  unknown causes e.g. acute and chronic idiopathic
Lymphangioleiomyomatosis
Alveolar proteinosis
Alveolar microlithiasis
Amyloidosis
Chronic aspiration

*see www.pneumotox.com for full listing.
UIP, usual interstitial pneumonia; NSIP, non-specific interstitial pneumonia.

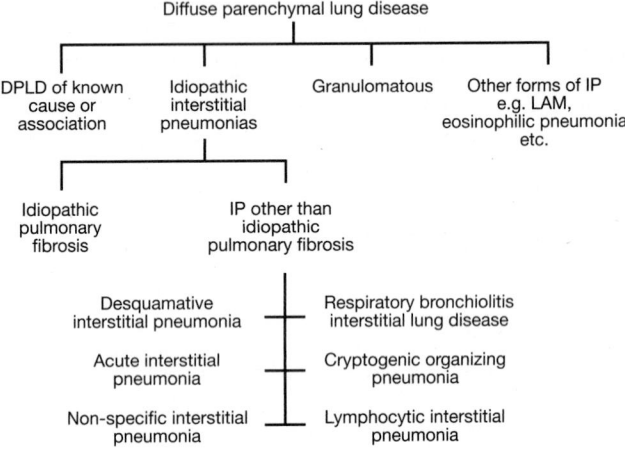

Fig. 1 Classification of diffuse parenchymal lung disease. DPLD, diffuse parenchymal lung disease; IP, interstitial pneumonia; LAM, lymphangioleiomyomatosis.

Table 2 Diffuse parenchymal lung disease of acute onset

Acute interstitial pneumonia
Diffuse alveolar haemorrhage
  (vasculitis or coagulopathy most common causes)
Acute pneumonitis due to rheumatological disease
Extrinsic allergic alveolitis
Drugs (selected)
Pulmonary eosinophilia, acute or chronic
Cryptogenic and known causes of organizing pneumonia
Mimics
  Pulmonary oedema of any cause
  Infection, especially opportunistic with *Pneumocystis carinii*

patchy distribution of interstitial fibrosis, chronic inflammatory cells, cystic airspaces (honeycomb lung), and areas of relatively normal lung. This pattern of pathology has a non-uniform appearance, best visible under low microscopic power, suggesting that the pathological process is at different stages of evolution throughout the biopsy (i.e. temporally heterogeneous), a feature that distinguishes usual interstitial pneumonia from other interstitial pneumonias. Another key feature is abundant fibroblastic foci.

Desquamative interstitial pneumonia

The characteristic feature of desquamative interstitial pneumonia is the diffuse accumulation of alveolar macrophages within the airspace in a rather monotonous, uniform pattern. There may be some interstitial inflammation and fibrosis but this is minor by comparison with the intra-alveolar inflammation. This pattern of disease is found almost exclusively in cigarette smokers.

Respiratory bronchiolitis–interstitial lung disease

The histopathological features of respiratory bronchiolitis–interstitial lung disease are very similar to those of desquamative interstitial pneumonia. They are differentiated by being less profuse, with pigmented macrophages accumulating in the airspaces around the bronchioles, which are themselves inflamed. The similarity of alveolar macrophage accumulation between desquamative interstitial pneumonia and respiratory bronchiolitis–interstitial lung disease (which also occurs almost exclusively in cigarette smokers) has led some to believe that these histopathological patterns are both part of the same spectrum of disease, but this view is not held unequivocally.

Diffuse alveolar damage

Diffuse alveolar damage is uncommon and the histopathological changes suggest an acute insult. This is the pattern of disease seen in both the adult respiratory distress syndrome and acute interstitial pneumonia (effectively, the adult respiratory distress syndrome of unknown cause). It is characterized by the presence of hyaline membranes lining damaged alveoli and, in more subacute states, the presence of buds of organization in the alveoli of those acini that have been damaged and are undergoing the healing process.

Non-specific interstitial pneumonia

This is arguably the least satisfactory histopathological entity and 'label'. Despite its name, there are specific features that define this histopathological pattern. There are varying degrees of interstitial inflammation and fibrosis within the interstitium but, unlike usual interstitial pneumonia, with which it is most likely to be confused (see Table 3), the appearances are uniform with none of the temporal heterogeneity of usual interstitial pneumonia and significantly less of the fibroblastic foci that are hallmarks of usual interstitial pneumonia.

American Thoracic Society and European Respiratory Society consensus statements on the nomenclature

Over the last few years these parallel clinical and histopathological approaches to the differentiation of the idiopathic interstitial pneumonia subgroup of the diffuse parenchymal lung diseases have become more integrated. The American Thoracic Society and European Respiratory Society have met to provide a consensus statement on the nomenclature of these

Table 3 Key differences between the histopathological appearances of idiopathic usual interstitial pneumonia (UIP) and non-specific interstitial pneumonia (NSIP).

UIP	NSIP
Dense fibrosis and honeycombing	Preserved architecture; variable fibrosis and cellularity
Fibroblastic foci prominent	Few fibroblastic foci
Patchy, heterogeneous pattern	Temporally homogenous
Subpleural, paraseptal distribution	Inconsistent distribution

Table 4 American Thoracic Society/European Respiratory Society nomenclature of idiopathic interstitial pneumonias

Clinical diagnosis	Pathology pattern
Cryptogenic fibrosing alveolitis (idiopathic pulmonary fibrosis)	Usual interstitial pneumonia
Desquamative interstitial pneumonia (alternative name: alveolar macrophage pneumonia)	Desquamative interstitial pneumonia
Respiratory bronchiolitis–interstitial lung disease	Respiratory bronchiolitis–interstitial lung disease
Acute interstitial pneumonia	Diffuse alveolar damage
Cryptogenic organizing pneumonia	Organizing pneumonia
Lymphocytic interstitial pneumonia	Lymphocytic interstitial pneumonia

diseases, which is summarized in Table 4. This classification attempts to provide a disease nomenclature that incorporates clinical, radiological, and histopathological patterns and to separate this from a pure histopathological classification that describes only the pattern of disease down the microscope without taking into account the clinical pathway that the disease has taken to reach that pathology. This is an important point because different insults could result in similar histopathological patterns. For example asbestos exposure can produce a usual interstitial pneumonia pattern of disease but, because it is of known cause, it is not included within the idiopathic interstitial pneumonias. Similarly, exposure to environmental agents to produce extrinsic allergic alveolitis can result in a non-specific interstitial pneumonia pattern, but this is clearly a distinct disease from that of a patient who presents with features similar to cryptogenic fibrosing alveolitis, who may have a similar histopathological pattern on lung biopsy.

The key issue that has emerged from the idiopathic interstitial pneumonias nomenclature debate, therefore, is that all clinical, radiological, and histopathological data must be taken into account before a diagnostic 'label' is applied to an individual patient. This new approach now allows a more precise definition of those diseases that are included within the idiopathic interstitial pneumonias.

Cryptogenic fibrosing alveolitis

The American Thoracic Society and European Respiratory Society consensus statement on this disease now recommends that cryptogenic fibrosing alveolitis (synonymous with idiopathic pulmonary fibrosis in the United States and elsewhere) must have the usual interstitial pneumonia pattern of pathology, or the appropriate clinical features, high resolution computed tomography pattern, and a bronchoalveolar lavage or transbronchial biopsy that excludes other disease (Table 5).

This is arguably the most contentious of the disease definitions in that there is a distinct subgroup of individuals who have all of the clinical, radiological, and bronchoalveolar lavage features of cryptogenic fibrosing alveolitis but who are found to have the non-specific interstitial pneumonia pattern of histopathology. At present it would be best to define these as the non-specific interstitial pneumonia variant of cryptogenic fibrosing alveolitis.

Desquamative interstitial pneumonia and respiratory bronchiolitis–interstitial lung disease

These diseases bear the same name as the histopathological classification because the idiopathic variants appear to be fairly uniform in their clinical and radiological features. Both are rare and it is possible that idiopathic variants may emerge.

Acute interstitial pneumonia

This disease resembles the adult respiratory distress syndrome in mode of onset, radiological and histopathological features, sharing the diffuse alveolar damage pattern of histopathology. Acute interstitial pneumonia is distinguished from adult respiratory distress syndrome by the absence of a known trigger. This nomenclature should not be used in the context of the

Table 5 American Thoracic Society/European Respiratory Society 2000 consensus statement on idiopathic pulmonary fibrosis/cryptogenic fibrozing alveolitis

IN PRESENCE OF A SURGICAL BIOPSY SHOWING UIP:
Exclusion of other causes of diffuse lung disease
Restrictive lung volumes; increased FEV_1/FVC ratio; and/or isolated impairment of gas exchange
Typical abnormalities on imaging
    chest radiograph
    high resolution computed tomography

IN ABSENCE OF A SURGICAL BIOPSY SHOWING UIP:
Major criteria (all needed)
Exclusion of other causes of diffuse lung disease
Restrictive lung volumes; increased FEV_1/FVC ratio; and/or isolated impairment of gas exchange
Bibasilar reticular change with honeycombing and little or no ground glass change on high resolution computed tomography
Transbronchial lung biopsy suggests no alternate diagnosis and/or the presence of excess granulocytes (neutrophils ± eosinophils) in bronchoalveolar lavage

Minor criteria (3/4 needed)
Age >50 years
Insidious onset of dyspnoea
Duration of illness >3 months
Bibasilar fine crackles

UIP, usual interstitial pneumonia.

rheumatological diseases in which a similar pattern of pathology can be seen.

Non-specific interstitial pneumonia

There are a number of clinical and radiological pathways that lead to a similar pattern of histopathology. However, once known causes and associated diseases have been excluded there appear at present to be no disease entities that have this histopathological variant other than the cryptogenic fibrosing alveolitis variant described above. Future studies are needed to validate this conclusion.

Cryptogenic organizing pneumonia

This disease was first defined in 1983 and was then redesignated 'bronchiolitis obliterans organizing pneumonia' in the United States in 1985. This nomenclature was so similar to 'bronchiolitis obliterans' that confusion ensued. Bronchiolitis obliterans organizing pneumonia is a pneumonic-like illness whereas bronchiolitis obliterans is an airway disease with distinct clinical, radiological, physiological, and histopathological appearances. It has therefore been decided to rename this disease cryptogenic organizing pneumonia to make the distinction between bronchiolitis obliterans quite clear and to define this disease as having the histopathological pattern of organizing pneumonia.

Lymphocytic interstitial pneumonia

This is included for completeness because this histopathological pattern can be seen in patients with rheumatological disease that can mimic the idiopathic interstitial pneumonias. It is likely that this will be included in the future within the non-specific interstitial pneumonia classification because the majority of diseases that have this pattern on biopsy are either lymphoproliferative or AIDS-associated.

Diagnostic approach

There are more than 200 entities included within the diffuse parenchymal lung disease group. A logical approach to diagnosis and management helps to avoid the major pitfalls that can be encountered in making a firm diagnosis. This approach can be considered in two phases:

Phase 1
- clinical history
- clinical examination
- chest radiography
- pulmonary function tests
- selective blood tests

Phase 2
- high resolution computed tomography
- bronchoalveolar lavage
- lung biopsy

This two-phase approach to diagnosis is summarized in Fig. 2.

Clinical history

Most patients present with slowly progressive breathlessness, with or without a cough that is usually dry and non-productive. Duration and speed of onset are important: disease presenting acutely narrows down the differential diagnosis considerably (see Table 2).

The presence of wheeze is discriminatory as this implies that the diffuse lung disease process has an airway component that narrows the differential diagnosis. Examples of this include lymphangioleiomyomatosis or Langerhans cell histiocytosis. Other respiratory symptoms are uncommon and when present may also help to focus diagnosis. Pleurisy may occur in the

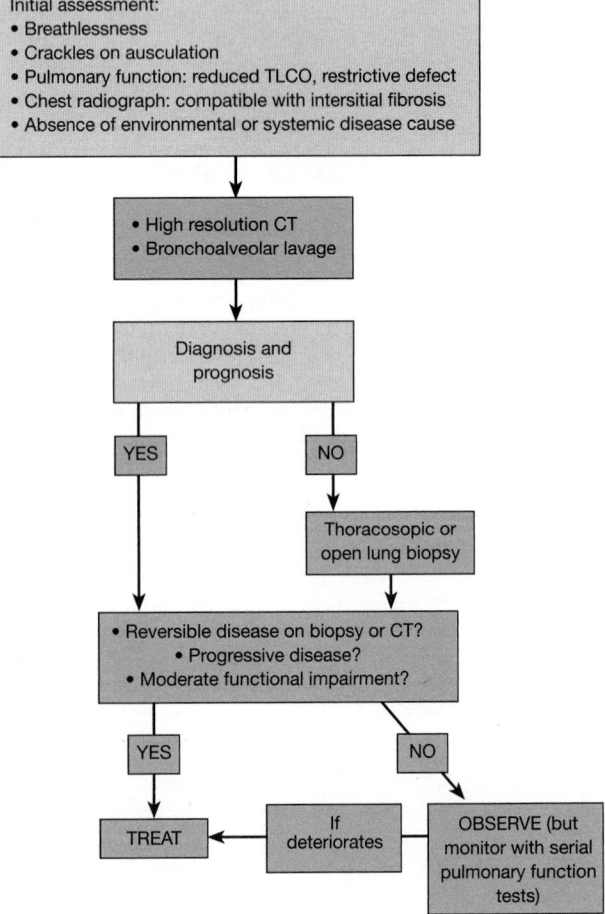

Fig. 2 Algorithm for the diagnosis, assessment, and management of suspected idiopathic interstitial pneumonia.

rheumatological diseases and drug-induced disease, but never in cryptogenic fibrosing alveolitis or extrinsic allergic alveolitis. Haemoptysis may suggest alveolar haemorrhage that can be due to a variety of causes. A history of pneumothorax suggests peripheral lung cysts, which occur most commonly in Langerhans cell histiocytosis and lymphangioleiomyomatosis.

The past medical history can provide crucial information, particularly if there is a history of rheumatological disease, other systemic disease such as systemic vasculitis, or previous diseases that have required long-term drug therapy.

A complete occupational and domestic environmental history is necessary. The occupational history should include all occupations from school-leaving because many diseases caused by occupational environmental exposure occur after a lag period. The environmental dusts that are of relevance are those that are respirable, that is can penetrate the acinar regions of the lungs. The environmental conditions in which such dusts are found involve most commonly the sawing, grinding, drilling, or other working of materials that produce dusts of the appropriate size. A comprehensive occupational history therefore requires knowledge of the materials that are processed in particular job definitions and also of materials that can produce chronic lung inflammation. Organic dusts that provoke disease are most commonly those that occur in the context of fungal contamination of materials such as hay (as in farmers lung) or avian proteins found on the bloom and in the excreta of domestic birds such as budgerigars, pigeons, and hens (producing extrinsic allergic alveolitis). Table 1 includes diseases that need to be considered.

A history of foreign travel is also important because this may suggest the possibility of parasitic infection that can produce pulmonary eosinophilia.

A history of cigarette smoking will help to define predisposition to Langerhans cell histiocytosis, desquamative interstitial pneumonia, respiratory bronchiolitis–interstitial lung disease, and can provoke acute exacerbations of lung vasculitis as in Goodpasture's syndrome. By contrast, smoking appears to 'protect' patients from sarcoidosis and extrinsic allergic alveolitis.

A drug ingestion history also needs to be comprehensive. The list of drugs that can produce a diffuse parenchymal lung disease is increasing rapidly. A good source of drug-induced pulmonary adverse effects can be found on the web site listed at the end of this chapter.

Clinical examination

This is often unrewarding in the respiratory tract. Digital clubbing is common in cryptogenic fibrosing alveolitis but much less so in the other diffuse parenchymal lung diseases. Showers of fine end inspiratory crackles are typical of fibrosing alveolitis but more sporadic crackles can be found in many diffuse parenchymal lung diseases. Expiratory wheeze helps to define associated airway disease, which can be discriminatory.

More helpful is the examination of the rest of the systems to identify ocular disease (suggesting sarcoidosis or vasculitis), skin disease (that might support a diagnosis of sarcoidosis or rheumatological disease), musculoskeletal signs suggesting rheumatological disease, neurological disease (such as mononeuritis multiplex in vasculitis), or a variety of central and peripheral neuropathies (in sarcoidosis).

Chest radiography

Chest radiography is one of the key components in the process of diagnosis of diffuse parenchymal lung disease. Five features should be noted:

* lung size;

* distribution of abnormalities;

* size and nature of nodular and/or reticular abnormalities;

* presence of confluent shadows;

* presence of pleural disease or lymphadenopathy.

Lung size

Patients with fibrosing lung diseases will generally have small lungs on chest radiography. Pitfalls include patients who have failed to take a full inspiration and patients with neuromuscular and other extrathoracic lesions that preclude full inspiration. This can mimic a fibrosing lung disease and needs to be considered if the small lungs appear to have normal parenchyma.

If other clinical features have suggested a diagnosis of fibrosing alveolitis, normal or large-size lungs indicate the coexistence of emphysema and fibrosing alveolitis: this admixture of disease processes is not uncommon as both are associated with cigarette smoking.

Other causes of large or normal sized lungs on chest radiography occurring together with nodular or reticular shadowing include Langerhans cell histiocytosis, lymphangioleiomyomatosis (a disorder involving smooth muscle proliferation that occurs only in women of childbearing age), tuberous sclerosis, of which lymphangioleiomyomatosis is believed by some to be a *forme fruste*. Chronic sarcoidosis can also feature large lungs, but this is usually associated with severe upper zone fibrosis causing a retraction of the hilar shadows towards the apices. Idiopathic bronchiectasis or cystic fibrosis can also be mistaken for diffuse parenchymal lung disease but the history of regular purulent sputum production will discriminate.

Distribution of abnormalities

The distribution of the abnormalities is always helpful. Fibrosing alveolitis occurring alone, in association with rheumatological diseases, or due to asbestos exposure produces reticular or reticulonodular abnormality predominantly in the basal zones, but also visible in the periphery of the lung, obscuring the diaphragm and the right and left heart borders. Predominantly upper zone disease, particularly involving loss of lung volume with an upward shift of the hilar shadows denoting upper zone fibrosis, occurs in chronic sarcoidosis and tuberculosis, extrinsic allergic alveolitis in its chronic stage, bronchopulmonary aspergillosis (almost always in the presence of asthma), and occasionally in Langerhans cell histiocytosis.

Predominant mid-zone abnormalities occur in sarcoidosis, extrinsic allergic alveolitis in its acute and chronic forms, and Langerhans cell histiocytosis.

Size and nature of nodular and reticular abnormalities

The size and shape of the abnormalities are helpful pointers to diagnosis. Very small 'granular' nodules less than 1 mm in size are seen in conditions such as idiopathic pulmonary hemosiderosis, miliary tuberculosis, and alveolar microlithiasis. Nodules up to 5 mm in diameter are seen in sarcoidosis, extrinsic allergic alveolitis, and silicosis. Shadows greater than 5 mm in size are present in Wegener's granulomatosis, rheumatoid arthritis, lymphoma, and other malignancies. Nodules of differing size and shape are highly suggestive of metastatic malignancy, and nodules that cavitate raise suspicion of Wegener's granulomatosis, other necrotizing granulomas, and rheumatoid nodules. Necrotizing squamous cell carcinomas and multiple staphylococcal abscesses need to be excluded. Lower zone reticulonodular shadowing is the pattern in fibrosing alveolitis of whatever cause.

Confluent shadowing

Confluent shadowing denotes airspace opacification. The presence of air bronchograms is very helpful in defining consolidation. All conditions that have predominant alveolar-filling histopathology will produce this pattern of radiographic change. These disorders include pulmonary alveolar proteinosis, diffuse alveolar haemorrhage, pulmonary eosinophilia (in which the confluent shadowing is often peripheral, as it frequently is in cryptogenic organizing pneumonia). Infection, particularly opportunistic infection in the immunosuppressed patient, alveolar cell carcinoma, and lymphoma must be differentiated, particularly as all of these can be complications of diffuse lung disease or its treatment.

Pleural disease and lymphadenopathy

The presence of pleural disease (with or without effusion) helps to exclude certain diagnoses such as extrinsic allergic alveolitis and cryptogenic fibrosing alveolitis. It is a common feature of the rheumatological diseases, particularly rheumatoid arthritis and systemic lupus erythematosus. It is also a feature of drug-induced lung disease, may occur in sarcoidosis, and is relatively common in Churg–Strauss granulomatosis and Wegener's granulomatosis.

Symmetrical hilar lymphadenopathy is usually due to sarcoidosis. Tuberculosis and lymphoma (and other malignancies) must always be considered, and these are more likely if the changes are unilateral. Lymphadenopathy is rarely observed on chest radiography in other diffuse lung diseases, with the notable exception of silicosis. Hilar calcification occurs in sarcoidosis and silicosis in addition to tuberculosis.

Radionuclide imaging

Gallium scanning has now fallen out of favour as a diagnostic tool for diffuse lung disease. Ventilation perfusion scanning as a means of identifying thromboembolic disease produces frequent false positives in the presence of diffuse lung disease and should not be used in this circumstance, spiral computed tomography being preferred. 99^mTc-DTPA clearance from the lungs has been used in some centres as a tool for early detection of diffuse lung disease and as a predictor of outcome. In patients with fibrosing alveolitis occurring alone or in the context of rheumatological disease, sarcoidosis and other diffuse lung diseases, rapid clearance predicts disease that is more likely to be progressive.

Pulmonary function testing

In the majority of patients with diffuse parenchymal lung disease, lung function tests reveal a restrictive pattern of ventilatory defect with reduced gas transfer (DL_{CO}). Arterial oxygen tensions (Pao_2) may be normal or low and $Paco_2$ may also be normal or low. In more subtle disease with normal gas transfer at rest, exercise tests can unmask abnormality: Pao_2 falls and the alveolar–arterial oxygen gradient (A–a gradient) widens, indicating abnormalities of gas exchange usually due to ventilation–perfusion mismatch, but with an increased diffusion component on exercise. The anatomical dead space to tidal volume ratio (V_D/V_T) falls on exercise in the normal individual but remains the same or increases in restrictive lung disease. These investigations of pulmonary function can confirm the presence of disease but cannot discriminate between the different causes.

In disorders in which an airway component is associated with the diffuse parenchymal lung disease, a mixed obstructive–restrictive ventilatory defect is observed. This occurs in Langerhans' cell histiocytosis and more advanced sarcoidosis, both of which are bronchocentric disease processes. Evidence of subtle airway disease can sometimes be seen in less chronic sarcoidosis and also in early extrinsic allergic alveolitis. Combined pathologies may coexist; in patients with fibrosing alveolitis who have been cigarette smokers, a mixed obstructive–restrictive process is present due to a combination of emphysema and fibrosing alveolitis.

Blood tests

Routine haematology and biochemical tests are not of any discriminatory value in the diffuse lung diseases. Peripheral blood eosinophilia (above 1.5 $\times 10^9$/l) is a prerequisite for diagnosis of pulmonary eosinophilia. This is particularly helpful in the chronic forms of pulmonary eosinophilia, when total IgE levels are low, as this can discriminate between the allergic forms of disease that can affect the lung in which IgE levels match eosinophil levels.

Angiotensin converting enzyme concentrations are helpful in sarcoidosis but are not diagnostic. Their main value is in monitoring the burden of disease if found to be elevated at presentation. Routine immunoglobulin estimates are of no diagnostic value.

By contrast, autoantibody testing is important. The finding of a positive antinuclear antibody, with particular specific extractable nuclear antigen profiles, or of rheumatoid factor, may indicate that lung disease is the first manifestation of a systemic rheumatological condition. This form of presentation is reported increasingly and has important implications in terms of the precise diagnosis of the diffuse parenchymal lung disease and prognosis. Good examples of this include: the anti-DNA topoisomerase autoantibody, which is associated with fibrosing alveolitis in systemic sclerosis; the anticentromere antibody, which is associated with pulmonary vascular disease in systemic sclerosis; the anti-t-RNA synthetase autoantibodies, which occur when polymyositis is found in association with diffuse parenchymal lung disease; anti-Sm in systemic lupus erythematosus; SS-A and SS-B in Sjögrens syndrome; and the anti-RNP autoantibody in mixed connective tissue disease.

Antineutrophil cytoplasmic antibody (ANCA) is particularly helpful if the pattern is cytoplasmic, suggesting that the diffuse parenchymal lung disease is a manifestation of Wegener's granulomatosis or microscopic polyangiitis. The perinuclear (pANCA) pattern is much less discriminatory and is found in elevated titre in a wide variety of disorders, including rheumatological disease.

Bronchoalveolar lavage

When this technique was first employed, roughly 20 years ago, it was hoped that it could replace surgical biopsy in providing precise diagnostic information. This has proved not to be the case. It was also hoped that serial bronchoalveolar lavage might be a better monitoring tool than other indices of change. This has also been disproved. Nonetheless, bronchoalveolar lavage does still have a role in the diagnosis of diffuse lung diseases. It provides very helpful confirmatory evidence of diffuse lung disease in patients who cannot (for reasons of comorbidity or disease severity) or will not consent to a surgical biopsy following initial investigations. It is also helpful in excluding infection or malignancy.

The pattern of inflammatory cell infiltrate will differentiate the fibrosing lung conditions (characterized by neutrophils and/or eosinophils) from the granulomatous or drug-induced lug diseases (characterized by an excess of lymphocytes with or without granulocytes). Furthermore, the patterns of bronchoalveolar lavage are beginning to become helpful in differentiating the different idiopathic interstitial pneumonias: granulocytes in cryptogenic fibrosing alveolitis; granulocytes and lymphocytes together with 'smoker's inclusions' in macrophages in desquamative interstitial pneumonia; neutrophils, often in very high numbers, in acute interstitial pneumonia; granulocytes and lymphocytes in non-specific interstitial pneumonia and organizing pneumonia; and lymphocytes in lymphocytic interstitial pneumonia.

Bronchoalveolar lavage can provide diagnostic material in some of the rarer lung disorders, such as: pulmonary alveolar proteinosis (milky effluent; PAS-positive material; phospholipid, membrane-like structures under electronmicroscopy; biochemistry); Langerhans cell histiocytosis (increased numbers of Langerhans cells identified by CD1a staining); mineral dust exposure (energy dispersive analysis by X-rays, asbestos bodies); iron-laden macrophages (alveolar haemorrhage). Other very helpful appearances include the bizarre multinuclear giant cells obtained from patients exposed to the alloy hard metal and the proliferative response of T-cells obtained from the lungs of patients with beryllium exposure, confirming a diagnosis of chronic berylliosis.

High resolution computed tomography

High resolution computed tomography provides a three dimensional anatomical reconstruction of the whole of both lungs. This provides a number of significant advantages over plain chest radiography in the diagnosis and discrimination of the different parenchymal lung diseases, and some patterns are pathognomonic (Table 6).

Table 6 Diffuse parenchymal lung disease with characteristic high resolution computed tomography features

Cryptogenic fibrosing alveolitis
Extrinsic allergic alveolitis
Sarcoidosis
Langerhans cell histiocytosis
Lymphangioleiomyomatosis
Alveolar proteinosis

Table 7 Recommended biopsy approaches for individual diffuse parenchymal lung disease

Transbronchial biopsy
Sarcoidosis
Extrinsic allergic alveolitis (but may need to be surgical if pretest probability of this disease is low)
Cryptogenic organizing pneumonia (only if pretest probability of this disease is high; otherwise surgical biopsy)
Chronic berylliosis
Alveolar proteinosis
Lymphangitis carcinomatosa

Surgical biopsy
Pulmonary vasculitis
Lymphangioleiomyomatosis (if CT features atypical)
Langerhans cell histiocytosis (if CT features atypical)
All idiopathic interstitial pneumonias:
    Cryptogenic fibrosing alveolitis
    Desquamative interstitial pneumonia
    Respiratory bronchiolitis–interstitial lung disease
    Acute interstitial pneumonia
    Lymphocytic interstitial pneumonia
    Non-specific interstitial pneumonia

The major advances that computed tomography has provided is in the earlier detection of suspected lung disease, when chest radiography is often normal; the differentiation of one diffuse lung disease from another; an estimate of the likely reversibility of the disease process—in general a 'ground glass' appearance favours reversibility in response to therapy, or sometimes spontaneously, whereas a coarse reticular pattern of abnormality is generally irreversible and indicates fixed fibrosis. Other irreversible features include the thin cystic structures seen in Langerhans cell histiocytosis and lymphangioleiomyomatosis. Less definitive patterns include variably sized nodules of varying density, linear opacification, and more subtle reticular change. Thickening of the interlobular septa or around the bronchovascular bundles imply a lymphatic component of the disease process. This degree of anatomic precision is the reason why high resolution computed tomography increases sensitivity, specificity, predictive value and, most importantly, confidence of diagnosis in the diffuse lung diseases. An assessment of the degree of reversibility also allows a better estimate of prognosis.

In patchy disease, the location of the best site for a surgical biopsy can be identified using high resolution computed tomography and more subtle pleural disease and airway disease can be identified. These additional features, in the context of the features of diffuse parenchymal lung disease, also help in the differential diagnosis. Good examples include the combination of airway and diffuse disease in rheumatological disorders such as rheumatoid arthritis and the subtle combination of patchy parenchymal disease together with pleural tags in drug-induced disease.

Computed tomography provides a better correlation with functional abnormalities than any other index, including surgical biopsy. In this regard, the extent of disease on computed tomography best matches measures of gas exchange and survival. The availability of high resolution imaging has therefore reduced the need for surgical biopsy in patients with diffuse lung disease considerably, but not removed it entirely.

Lung biopsy

It is imperative that a precise diagnosis is made from the large number of potential causes of diffuse parenchymal lung disease. The advantage of having a firm diagnosis is that the appropriate treatment can be instituted, treatment changed if that which has been started is inappropriate, a balance of cost–benefit to the patient can be better established, and, most importantly, the patient can be better informed about outcome, both with and without treatment. The oft used empirical approach of a trial of treatment—and if that fails then biopsy—is flawed. The major flaws being firstly that treatment will modify the disease process, making diagnosis more difficult with a subsequent biopsy, and secondly, the patient may have deteriorated during this waiting period, making biopsy more risky, and side-effects consequent upon treatment may also complicate the process. It is therefore recommended that, if there is any doubt about diagnosis after using all investigative tools other than biopsy, biopsy should be advised.

There are two types of biopsy. Transbronchial biopsy is used where the disease process is centred around the small airways, allowing access to the transbronchial approach, and when the diagnosis can be made on small biopsies, meaning that the pathological appearances must be so characteristic on small biopsies that there is no doubt. The best examples of this are the granulomatous diseases such as sarcoidosis or malignant diseases such as lymphangitis carcinomatosa.

For the more difficult diffuse lung diseases, particularly the idiopathic interstitial pneumonias, a surgical biopsy is necessary so that the overall pattern of disease can be appreciated. This does require a larger sample. The surgeon is also able to take samples from more than one site, thereby increasing the likelihood of obtaining representative tissue. Two approaches have been used: the limited thoracotomy approach or the more recently introduced video-assisted thoracoscopic surgical technique. The latter is a less invasive approach that is now preferred, providing equivalent sized samples to the more open technique but with some evidence of lessened morbidity. For choice of biopsy procedure in particular diseases see Table 7.

Further reading

Classification

Bjoraker JA, Ryu JH, Edwin MK, *et al* (1998). Prognostic significance of histopathologic subsets in idiopathic pulmonary fibrosis. *American Journal of Respiratory and Critical Care Medicine* **157**, 199–203.

Bouros D, Nicholson AC, Polychronopoulos V, du Bois RM (2000). Acute interstitial pneumonia. *European Respiratory Journal* **15**, 412–8.

Daniil ZD, Gilchrist FC, Nicholson AG, *et al.* (1999). A histologic pattern of nonspecific interstitial pneumonia is associated with a better prognosis than usual interstitial pneumonia in patients with cryptogenic fibrosing alveolitis. *American Journal of Respiratory and Critical Care Medicine* **160**, 899–905.

Diffuse Parenchymal Lung Disease Group (1999). The diagnosis, assessment and treatment of diffuse parenchymal lung disease in adults. *Thorax* **54** (Suppl. 1).

Katzenstein AL, Myers JL (1998). Idiopathic pulmonary fibrosis: clinical relevance of pathologic classification. [Review] [66 refs]. *American Journal of Respiratory and Critical Care Medicine* **157**, 1301–15.

Liebow AA (1975). Definition and classification of interstitial pneumonias in human pathology. In: Basset F, Georges R, eds. *Progress in respiration research*, pp. 1–33. Karger, New York.

Joint American Thoracic Society and European Respiratory Society Group (2000). Idiopathic pulmonary fibrosis: diagnosis and treatment. International consensus statement. *American Journal of Respiratory and Critical Care Medicine* **161**, 646–64.

Drug-induced disease

www.pneumotox.com

Imaging

Hansell DM. High resolution computed tomography and diffuse lung disease (1999). *Royal College of Physicians of London* **33**, 525–31.

Mathieson JR, Mayo JR, Staples CA, Muller NL (1989). Chronic diffuse infiltrative lung disease: comparison of diagnostic accuracy of CT and chest radiography. *Radiology* **171**, 111–6.

Muller NL, Colby TV (1997). Idiopathic interstitial pneumonias: high-resolution CT and histologic findings. *Radiographics* **17**, 1016–22.

Wells AU, Rubens MB, du Bois RM, Hansell DM (1997). Functional impairment in fibrosing alveolitis: relationship to reversible disease on thin section computed tomography. *European Respiratory Journal* **10**, 280–5.

Bronchoalveolar lavage

BAL Co-operative Group Steering Committee (1990). Bronchoalveolar lavage constituents in healthy individuals, idiopathic pulmonary fibrosis, and selected comparison groups. *American Review of Respiratory Diseases* **141**, S169–S202.

Drent M, Mulder PG, Wagenaar SS, Hoogsteden HC, van Velzen-Blad H, van den Bosch JM (1993). Differences in BAL fluid variables in interstitial lung diseases evaluated by discriminant analysis. *European Respiratory Journal* **6**, 803–10.

17.11.2 Cryptogenic fibrosing alveolitis

R. M. du Bois

Introduction

The first description of what we currently recognize as fibrosing alveolitis was in 1907. Since then nomenclature has been confused; multiple synonyms have been used, including Hamman–Rich syndrome. With the advent of a new histopathological classification and the recognition of particular patterns of disease on high resolution computed tomography, it is now possible to define cryptogenic fibrosing alveolitis very specifically

Definition

The International Consensus Statement on cryptogenic fibrosing alveolitis (idiopathic pulmonary fibrosis in the United States) has defined the disease as a specific form of chronic fibrosing interstitial pneumonia, requiring, in the presence of a surgical biopsy showing the usual interstitial pneumonia pattern of pathology (see Chapter 17.11.1):

- the exclusion of other known causes of interstitial lung disease such as drug toxicities, environmental exposures, and rheumatological disease;
- abnormal pulmonary function studies that include evidence of restriction (reduced vital capacity (VC) often with an increased FEV_1/FVC ratio) and/or impaired gas exchange (increased alveolar–arterial oxygen gradient ($P(A–a)O_2$) at rest or on exercise or decreased carbon monoxide transfer factor (DL_{CO}));
- typical features on chest radiography or high resolution computed tomography scans.

In the absence of a surgical lung biopsy, the diagnosis of cryptogenic fibrosing alveolitis is less certain. However, in the immunocompetent adult, the presence of all of the following major diagnostic criteria as well as at least three of the four minor criteria increases the likelihood of a correct clinical diagnosis of cryptogenic fibrosing alveolitis:

Major criteria

- exclusion of other known causes of diffuse lung disease such as certain drug toxicities, environmental exposures, and rheumatological diseases;
- abnormal pulmonary function studies that include evidence of restriction (reduced VC often with an increased FEV_1/FVC ratio) and impaired gas exchange (increased $P(A–a)O_2$ at rest or on exercise or decreased DL_{CO});
- bibasilar reticular abnormalities with honeycombing and minimal or no ground glass opacities on high resolution computed tomography scans;
- transbronchial lung biopsy or bronchoalveolar lavage showing no features to support an alternate diagnosis, such as granulomas on biopsy or an excess of lymphocytes on bronchoalveolar lavage.

Minor criteria

- age more than 50 years;
- insidious onset of otherwise unexplained dyspnoea on exertion;
- duration of illness more than 3 to 6 months;
- bibasilar, inspiratory crackles on chest auscultation.

Aetiology

Epidemiology

Cryptogenic fibrosing alveolitis may occur in any decade of life but is most commonly seen between the ages 50 to 60 years; children do not get the disease, although they can develop a diffuse lung disease that mimics the condition but does not have the usual interstitial pneumonia pathology. Cryptogenic fibrosing alveolitis occurs in males slightly more frequently than females. There is no geographic variation. Prevalence and incidence rates (approximately 5 per 100 000) are only estimates in the United Kingdom and elsewhere, but are increasing based on evidence from mortality statistics for England and Wales. A registry-based study from the United States estimated a prevalence of 20.2 cases per 100 000 for males and 13.2 cases per 100 000 for females and an incidence of 10.7 cases per 100 000 per year for males and 7.4 cases per 100 000 per year for females.

Possible trigger factors

By definition there is no known aetiology. Multiple factors are likely to be involved. The disease is more common in patients who have a history of cigarette smoking. Viruses, particularly Epstein–Barr virus, have been implicated as trigger factors but this is not proven. More recently, an increased occupational exposure to metal dusts, wood fires, and antidepressant medication has been associated with excess cryptogenic fibrosing alveolitis by comparison with control populations.

In most patients, there is no family history of fibrosing alveolitis but, in a small subgroup a familial pattern is observed. The inheritance pattern is unpredictable and it is likely therefore that transmission involves variable penetrance. The clinical features of the familial and sporadic variants are identical. There are, as yet, no known predisposing immunogenetic factors, unlike other diffuse lung diseases that can produce lung fibrosis such as the Hermansky–Pudlak syndrome (a condition characterized by oculocutaneous albinism and abnormal platelets), the diffuse lung disease of systemic sclerosis (associated with the anti-DNA topoisomerase I autoantibody, in turn highly associated with an excess of the HLA DRB1*II and DPB1*1301 class II MHC alleles), and sarcoidosis.

Pathogenesis

The pathogenetic processes that give rise to cryptogenic fibrosing alveolitis involve lung injury, an immunological and inflammatory response, and fibrogenesis. All four components appear to be occurring in parallel and this is reflected in the heterogeneity of the histopathological appearances. The various trigger agents implicated in the disease are likely to be the causes of injury, complemented by an adverse imbalance in the oxidant–antioxidant profile within the lung, together with the release of tissue-damaging enzymes from macrophages and granulocytes.

The inflammatory response is variable and its relationship to fibrogenesis is unclear. In brief, all of the cellular and molecular biological mechanisms that determine immune and inflammatory cell recruitment and activation have been shown to operate in the lungs of patients with cryptogenic fibrosing alveolitis. Key components appear to be the up-regulation of tumour necrosis factor-α, chemokines, notably interleukin 8, and growth factors, most notably transforming growth factor-β and connective tissue growth factor. Whether up-regulation of the mechanisms that result in inflammatory cell traffic is pathological or a physiological response to injury is not clear.

The evidence that the fibrogenetic response has become autonomous (i.e. not a simple tissue repair mechanism) is strong. In gene over-expression animal models, the transient over-expression of transforming growth factor-β resulted in a progressive fibrosing lung disease that mimicked cryptogenic fibrosing alveolitis, with a histopathological appearance that was indistinguishable from usual interstitial pneumonia.

Pathology

Usual interstitial pneumonia is the pattern seen in patients with cryptogenic fibrosing alveolitis. The hallmark of usual interstitial pneumonia is a patchy distribution of interstitial fibrosis, chronic inflammatory cell infiltrate, enlarged cystic air spaces (honeycomb lung), and normal lung (Fig. 1 and Plate 1). Inflammation is often mild and the fibrosis characterized by acellular collagen bundles with foci of proliferating fibroblasts. This non-uniform appearance, which is often visible under low microscopic power, suggests the pathological processes are at different stages of development (temporal heterogeneity), a feature that distinguishes usual interstitial pneumonia from other interstitial pneumonias.

Clinicopathological correlations

Correlations between clinical and physiological indices of disease and lung biopsy appearances have, in general, proved to be disappointing. This is probably a reflection of the fact that biopsy samples a small area of the peripheral (and most involved) part of the lung, whereas other indices reflect the function of the whole of both lungs. Despite this, it has been shown that the degree of lung involvement can be correlated with lung function indices. More recent studies have utilized high resolution computed tomography (that 'samples' the anatomy of the whole of both lungs) instead of biopsy and have shown better correlations with lung function indices, especially gas transfer, and have concluded that high resolution computed tomography provides a more accurate prediction of outcome.

Clinical features

History

A history of progressive breathlessness on exertion in the absence of wheeze is typical. A dry cough may be present, but sputum production is unusual until the later stages of the disease. Haemoptysis is uncommon and should suggest the development of lung malignancy that occurs with a 7 to 14-fold

relative risk in cryptogenic fibrosing alveolitis. Chest pain is uncommon. Constitutional symptoms such as weight loss and lethargy are recognized.

A full occupational and domestic environmental exposure (from school leaving), and drug ingestion history, are necessary to identify diseases that can mimic cryptogenic fibrosing alveolitis (see Table 1). A history of other diseases, particularly the rheumatological disorders, is important because the diffuse lung disease in this context can mimic, but is quite different from, cryptogenic fibrosing alveolitis.

Examination

Digital clubbing is present in 70 to 80 per cent of patients. On auscultation, very fine crackles are heard at the lung bases and in the midaxillary line, occurring at the end of inspiration in early cases but becoming paninspiratory in more advanced disease. In the presence of more subtle disease, the crackles may disappear as the patient leans forward, but usually they persist in the midaxillary line.

At more advanced stages of disease, central cyanosis may be evident, also signs of pulmonary hypertension and right ventricular failure. In addition,

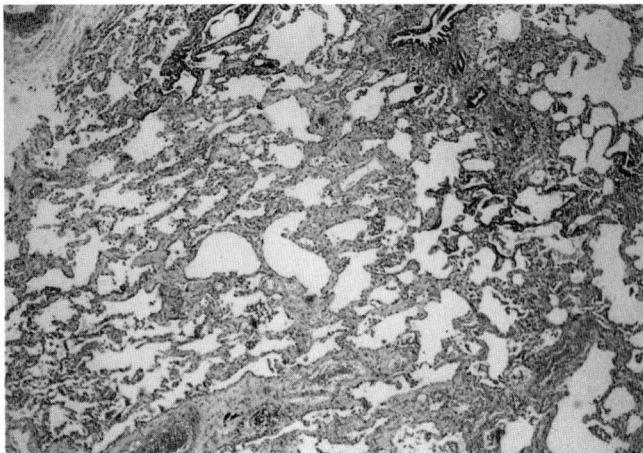

(a)

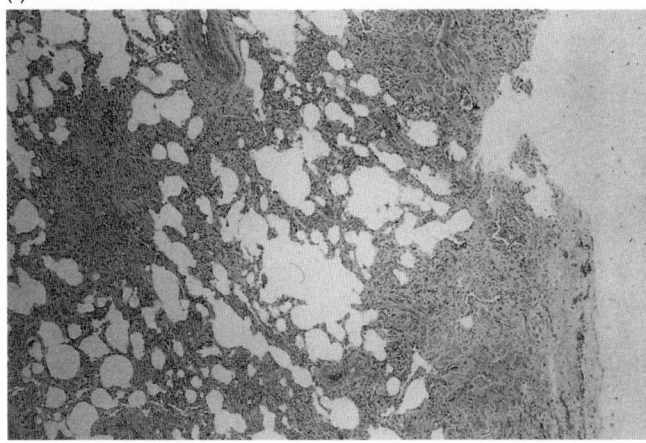

(b)

Fig. 1 Histopathological appearance of cryptogenic fibrosing alveolitis and the non-specific interstitial pneumonia 'mimic'. (a) Usual interstitial pneumonia, the histopathological pattern seen in cryptogenic fibrosing alveolitis. Note the pale, fibroblast foci that are the hallmark of usual interstitial pneumonia. (b) The non-specific interstitial pneumonia 'mimic' of cryptogenic fibrosing alveolitis. This is much less common than usual interstitial pneumonia. Note the uniformity of the pathology throughout the section. (See also Plate 1.)

Table 1 Known causes of diffuse lung disease which may mimic cryptogenic fibrosing alveolitis[a]

Rheumatological diffuse lung disease
Extrinsic allergic alveolitis (chronic stage)
Sarcoidosis (chronic stage if pattern unusually basal)
Occupational lung disease
asbestosis
hard metal disease
Drug therapy
cytotoxic e.g. bleomycin, busulfan, carmustine, methotrexate
antibacterial e.g. nitrofurantoin, sulfasalazine
cardiological e.g. amiodarone, tocainide
rheumatological e.g. gold, d-penicillamine
analgesics e.g. heroin
anticoagulants e.g. diphenylhydantoin
Inhaled agents
mercury vapour
nitrogen dioxide
Ingested agents
paraquat
Irradiation

[a]See also Chapter 17.11.1.

general examination may reveal non-pulmonary features that would suggest alternative, systemic diseases, such as arthropathy, vasculitis, skin disorders, and peripheral lymphadenopathy.

Investigations

Imaging

Chest radiography

A typical chest radiograph of a patient with cryptogenic fibrosing alveolitis is characterized by small lung fields and reticulonodular shadowing, particularly at the periphery of the lung and at the bases, obscuring the right and left heart borders and making the diaphragmatic surfaces irregular (Fig. 2). Even in more subtle examples of fibrosing alveolitis, this distribution of radiographic abnormality should suggest the diagnosis. In more advanced cases, all lung zones are involved, at which point evidence of honeycomb shadowing may be present.

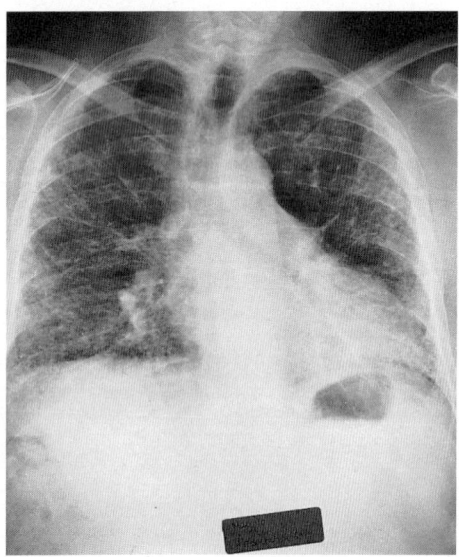

Fig. 2 Chest radiograph of a patient with cryptogenic fibrosing alveolitis. This shows the typical features of the disease with peripheral, predominantly basal, reticulonodular changes obscuring the heart borders and diaphragms.

Lymphadenopathy is rarely observed on chest radiography and the presence of pleural disease should suggest an alternative diagnosis. Cardiomegaly and prominent pulmonary arteries indicate secondary pulmonary hypertension.

High resolution computed tomography

The use of high resolution computed tomography over the last 10 years has revolutionized the approach to diffuse lung disease. The pattern of abnormality may be characteristic in a number of diffuse lung diseases (see Chapter 17.11.1) and is virtually pathognomonic in cryptogenic fibrosing alveolitis. Typical early changes are of a peripheral rim of reticular change at the bases, posteriorly (Fig. 3). As disease becomes more extensive, these changes are observed in the other lung zones and more centrally. Computed tomography confirms that pleural disease is not present in cryptogenic fibrosing alveolitis but, by contrast to the observation on plain chest radiography, mediastinal lymphadenopathy is commonly present. In more subtle cases, it is important to perform prone as well as supine scans to exclude the contribution of gravity to the radiographic appearances due to vascular and interstitial pooling in the dependent areas.

Radionuclide imaging

Ventilation–perfusion scans

Ventilation–perfusion scans show mismatching of perfusion to ventilation in cryptogenic fibrosing alveolitis, making the test unreliable in excluding thromboembolic disease in this situation. This is important because there is an increased incidence of pulmonary embolus in this disease and the diagnosis of pulmonary embolus will therefore rely on the clinical features, identification of the venous source of emboli, and, in some instances, spiral computed tomography to identify vascular occlusion in the more proximal arteries.

Gallium scanning

Gallium scanning is a highly sensitive but non-specific test, being positive in a wide range of diffuse processes that involve macrophage activation. It has no role in the diagnosis or management of cryptogenic fibrosing alveolitis.

^{99m}Tc-diethylinetriamine pentacetate (DTPA) clearance

Clearance from the lung of inhaled ^{99m}Tc-diethylinetriamine pentacetate (DTPA) is of value in identifying early disease and is a helpful test in prognosis; patients with a persistently normal clearance run a more stable, nonprogressive course. Cigarette smoking will produce increased clearance rates and the test is therefore only of value in non-smokers or those who have given up smoking for at least 1 month prior to assessment. The role of DTPA clearance studies in routine clinical management is not yet clear.

Lung function tests

Fibrosing alveolitis is characterized by a restrictive ventilatory defect of mechanical function resulting in reduced pulmonary compliance, vital capacity, and total lung capacity. Residual volume is usually decreased unless there is coincident airflow obstruction due to cigarette smoking and lung recoil pressure is increased.

Carbon monoxide transfer factor ($DLco$, a measure of diffusion capacity) is reduced and may be the only abnormality in early disease. In most patients the gas transfer measurement adjusted for alveolar volume (Kco) is also reduced, but less than $DLco$, indicating that the capacity to exchange gas is impaired in lung that has not been destroyed. If there is significant coexisting emphysema, lung volumes will be well preserved in the face of a disproportionately depressed gas transfer measurement in both $DLco$ and Kco. Gas transfer is reduced by both the emphysematous and the fibrosing processes, whereas lung volumes will tend to be increased by emphysema but reduced by fibrosis and these two opposing influences result in relatively normal-sized lungs radiographically and physiologically.

Typical blood gas measurements will reveal a reduced Pao_2 value with a normal or low $Paco_2$ measurement. In more advanced cases, the $Paco_2$ will

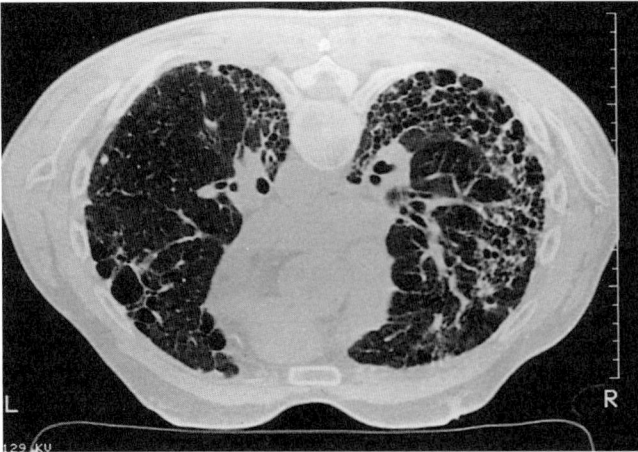

(a)

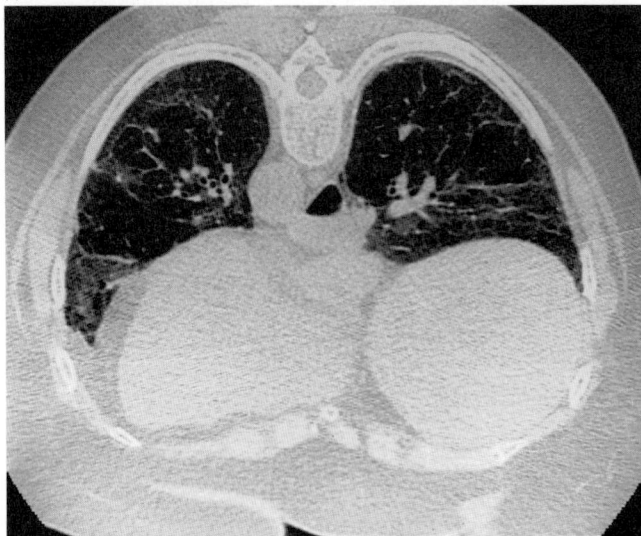

(b)

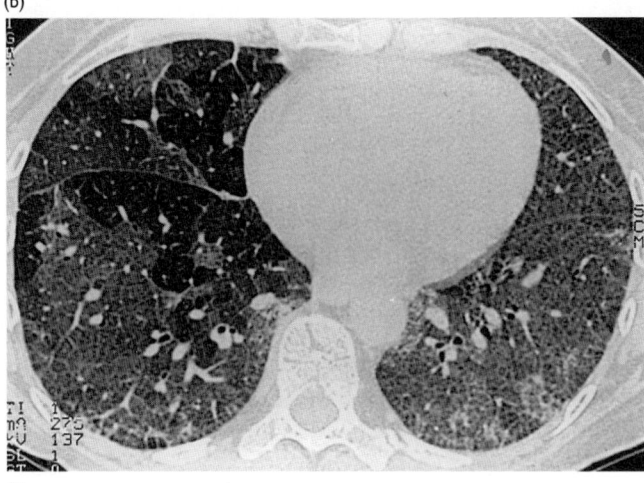

(c)

Fig. 3 High resolution computed tomography of patients with diffuse lung diseases that can mimic cryptogenic fibrosing alveolitis. (a) The predominantly peripheral, coarse honeycombing is characteristic of cryptogenic fibrosing alveolitis. (b) More fine fibrotic change is seen in non-specific interstitial pneumonia. Note the absence of honeycombing and the less clear-cut peripheral distribution of disease. (c) Desquamative interstitial pneumonia showing widespread, ground glass opacification with maintenance of the fine architecture of the lung and no evidence of fibrosis.

be reduced because of the increase in ventilatory drive in a patient with more severe lung stiffening due to fibrosis, but in terminal stages CO_2 may rise. The low Pao_2 is largely attributable to ventilation–perfusion mismatching. On exercise, hypoxaemia is exacerbated and a widening of the alveolar–arterial (A–a) gradient is observed. Infrequently, these abnormalities on exercise testing are the only physiological abnormalities, but usually by the time the patient seeks advice there is already some abnormality in the gas transfer measurement at rest.

Lung function measurements (to include gas transfer) should be made sequentially to assess the progression of the disease process. Spirometry alone or, worse, peak flow measurements, are inadequate. It is sensible to plot out serial lung function studies to visualize more gradual change that may be missed if results are compared only with the previous set of measurements.

Blood tests

Blood tests are of little value in the diagnosis of cryptogenic fibrosing alveolitis. In severe cases, secondary polycythaemia may be observed and a high neutrophil count may indicate superadded infection. Corticosteroid therapy will elevate total white count to around 13 to $14 \times 10^9/l$, sometimes even higher.

Elevations in one or more classes of immunoglobulins, particularly IgG and IgM, may be seen and rheumatoid factor or antinuclear antibody may be present in abnormal titres in approximately 45 per cent of patients, but none of these immunological assessments is specific. The titres of autoantibodies do not approach those seen in the rheumatological diseases. In cases where there is a history of significant antigen exposure, or when there is doubt about relevant exposures, it is helpful to perform precipitin tests against the fungal antigens which produce diseases such as farmer's lung or the avian antigens which can provoke budgerigar or pigeon fancier's lung.

Bronchoalveolar lavage

Bronchoalveolar lavage is valuable in excluding infection and as confirmation that the histopathological pattern is likely to be the usual interstitial pneumonia pattern in patients who cannot or will not tolerate surgical biopsy. In a typical patient with cryptogenic fibrosing alveolitis, bronchoalveolar lavage would produce an increase in total cell returns of three to six fold (up to $6 \times 10^5/ml$ of fluid return), and of these up to 20 per cent may be neutrophils or eosinophils. A large excess of lymphocytes suggests an alternative diagnosis such as granulomatous or drug-induced causes of lung disease. Serial bronchoalveolar lavage is of no value in monitoring disease.

Lung biopsy

The only lung biopsy technique that provides useful information is surgical lung biopsy, either through minithoracotomy or video-assisted thoracoscopic biopsy (the most common procedure). The surgeon will biopsy at least two sites to ensure representative sampling and the biopsy can be divided into parts that will be stored, if necessary, for immunohistochemical, molecular, and electron microscopical analysis in addition to the more routine histopathological evaluation.

Transbronchial biopsy cannot be used for diagnosis of cryptogenic fibrosing alveolitis and is only helpful in excluding other conditions such as granulomatous disease. The specimens produced are small, and do not allow an assessment to be made of the individual patterns that are important in differentiating the different idiopathic interstitial pneumonias.

Treatment

Established drug regimens

There have been no prospective, placebo-controlled, randomized trials of treatment in this condition. Most information on drug efficacy is derived

Table 2 Treatment of cryptogenic fibrosing alveolitis

Drug(s)dosage	Length of initial treatment	Taper regimen
First-line options		
prednisolone 20 mg alternate days AND	6–12 months	Azathioprine 25 mg/ 2–3 months
azathioprine 2.5mg/kg per day (max 150 mg) OR		
prednisolone 20 mg alternate days AND	6–12 months	Cyclophosph-amide 25 mg/ 2–3 months
cyclophosphamide 100 mg/day (<65 kg) or 125 mg/day (>65 kg)		
Second-line options		
colchicine 0.5–1 mg/day		

from individual comparative series. Many of these have been retrospective. Assessment of efficacy is further complicated by recent knowledge that historic series probably included patients whose disease had the histopathological appearances of interstitial pneumonias other than usual interstitial pneumonia. These qualifications mean that the level of evidence base on which recommendations are made is low. However, world-wide experience, coupled with the recently published American Thoracic Society/ European Respiratory Society statement on cryptogenic fibrosing alveolitis, suggests that a combination of low-dose prednisolone (dosage varies between centres internationally but 20 mg on alternate days is the author's preference) together with azathioprine at 2.5 mg/kg per day up to a maximum of 150 mg/day should be the first-line treatment (Table 2). Azathioprine treatment should be commenced at 50 mg/day for 1 month with weekly full blood count monitoring to ensure that the individual does not have the methyltransferase deficiency that predisposes to enhanced toxicity. Provided blood counts are stable at 4 weeks, dosage can be increased to the maximum. Full blood count and liver function tests need to be performed 6 to 8-weekly .

An alternative to azathioprine is cyclophosphamide at 2 mg/kg per day up to a maximum of 150 mg per day. In addition to the potential bone marrow toxicity, haemorrhagic cystitis and bladder neoplasm are complications. Regular dipstick analysis for blood is recommended by some, ideally at weekly intervals. There is no place for high-dose corticosteroid treatment in the routine management of cryptogenic fibrosing alveolitis.

Other treatment regimens

Other drugs that have been used to treat this disease are colchicine (which has a similar efficacy to corticosteroids alone but with less side-effects), cyclosporin (very little data and no justification for use of this agent), penicillamine (no evidence of efficacy), pirfenidone (possible disease stabilization during corticosteroid reduction in a small subset of patients, but not commercially available), and interferon-γ (small study with reservations that the subgroup studied was not representative of cryptogenic fibrosing alveolitis as defined above). None of the approaches other than colchicine are recommended for the reasons indicated.

Acute exacerbations or accelerated disease

Sudden deterioration can occur. Supervening infection, heart failure, and thromboembolism must be excluded. If accelerated disease is believed to be the cause of the deterioration, intravenous corticosteroids (1 g/day methylprednisolone for 3 days) together with intravenous cyclophosphamide (600 mg/m² as a single dose, repeated at roughly 2-week intervals if blood counts are satisfactory) should be considered.

Transplantation

Single lung transplantation is now the organ replacement therapy of choice for end-stage fibrosing alveolitis. The procedure has not been used for a sufficiently long period to provide information about long-term survival, but approximately 60 per cent are alive at 3 years.

Supportive therapy

When all treatment options have failed, supportive therapy is necessary. Supplemental oxygen may be required and this can be provided in the home through oxygen concentrators. Diuretics may be necessary and infection should be treated promptly. In the terminal phases, small dosages of opiates have been shown to suppress the sensation of extreme breathlessness that occurs as the lungs become much less compliant.

This chronic, often relentlessly progressive, disease has a disabling affect on the patient and their close family. Full support by medical and non-medical health-care professionals should be involved in the patient's care; medical social workers, physiotherapists, occupational therapists, and rehabilitation programmes for patients form an important part of supportive management.

Monitoring of treatment

Immunosuppression can take 3 to 6 months, and sometimes longer, to produce a maximal effect. Patient monitoring with full lung function tests at 3-monthly intervals during the first year is recommended. If the disease becomes stable or improvement is seen, treatment should be continued until the disease has stabilised for a total of 1 year. A tapering, with a view to complete withdrawal of immunosuppression, should be tried at this point. If function deteriorates, alternative drug therapies need to be tried. Once lung function is less than 30 per cent predicted, consideration for transplantation is required. The age limit imposed by some transplantation centres needs to be taken into account when planning management.

Prognosis

Historically, survival was thought to be roughly 50 per cent at 4 years. More recent studies comparing survival of incident cases as opposed to prevalent cases, and with a more rigid definition of cryptogenic fibrosing alveolitis as outlined above, have shown the prognosis is even more desperate, with median survival being less than 3 years and 10-year survival of 5 to 10 per cent. These appalling survival figures highlight the need for early detection, early introduction of treatment, and early consideration of transplantation in patients who fail to respond to therapy.

Areas of uncertainty

What is the cause?

It is unlikely that a single aetiology will be identified and, even if it were, removal of that cause is unlikely to be curative. Multiple trigger factors are likely to operate in conjunction with some form of genetic predisposition resulting in disease. Patients often expect clinicians to be able to identify a cause that results in a cure and they need to be told that this will not happen.

Should all patients undergo surgical biopsy?

Decisions about biopsy need to take into account the degree of certainty of diagnosis using all of the investigations outlined above, particularly high resolution computed tomography and bronchoalveolar lavage. If there is any doubt about diagnosis, then surgical biopsy is needed to confirm the diagnosis. These decisions must always take into account the individual patient and need to be made in the context of other potentially complicating, comorbid conditions and whether there is a likelihood of an increased complication rate. Chronological age should not be a factor but clearly biological age is.

When should treatment be commenced?

It is a mistake to wait until a patient has limiting breathlessness before commencing treatment. At this stage at least 50 per cent of lung function is likely to have been lost and the patient will have little reserve. Many studies have shown that treatment is more likely to be successful if commenced early. The key issue is the likelihood of improving or stabilizing disease against the likelihood of side-effects. This has to be related to the individual. Factors that predict likely response to therapy are ground glass appearances (indicating cellularity) on high resolution computed tomography and comorbid conditions such as hypertension and diabetes mellitus that will increase the risk of corticosteroid-induced side-effect.

It is also important to remember that functional deficit caused by lung damage and scarring cannot be reversed; it is only the more recent, inflammatory pathological response that is responsive to currently used treatment. Improvement in lung function is seen in only 5 to 10 per cent of cases. Therapeutic response, if it occurs, more probably results in disease stability. The patient, and some clinical colleagues, need to be told this. This emphasizes the importance of attempting to stabilize disease at a level of function that is acceptable to the patient.

How long should treatment continue?

Optimal duration of therapy is not known. An approach to the management of immunosuppressant drugs is described above under 'Treatment'. The issue with regard to corticosteroids is less clear-cut. There is anecdotal evidence that complete corticosteroid withdrawal can result in a rebound of disease activity, which cannot then be controlled. It is therefore reasonable to attempt to reduce corticosteroids to approximately 10 mg every other day and, if disease remains stable at this level, then this dosage of drug should be continued indefinitely. The likelihood of significant side-effects on such a small dosage is low set against the possibility of disease flare-up on complete withdrawal of treatment.

Areas for future research

The major areas of future research involve a clarification of epidemiological issues and a resolution of the issue of possible immunogenetic predisposition and the relationship between environmental exposures and immunogenetic predisposition. Differences in the evolution of fibrogenesis in different patterns of idiopathic interstitial pneumonia need to be studied and this will probably involve a better appreciation of different functional phenotypes of fibroblasts, with particular regard to their connective tissue matrix products. Prospective, properly controlled, double-blind studies of treatment efficacy, using cohorts of patients with the usual interstitial pneumonia histopathological pattern, are of paramount importance to identify optimal treatment. This will require an international collaborative effort.

Further reading

Clinical

Joint Authors Group (2000). Idiopathic pulmonary fibrosis: diagnosis and treatment. International consensus statement. *American Journal of Respiratory and Critical Care Medicine* **161**, 646–64.

Carrington CB, Gaensler EA, Coutu RE (1978). Natural history and treated course of usual and desquamative interstitial pneumonia. *New England Journal of Medicine* **298**, 801–9.

Diffuse Parenchymal Lung Disease Group (1999). The diagnosis, assessment and treatment of diffuse parenchymal lung disease in adults. *Thorax* **54** (Suppl. 1).

Liebow AA (1975). Definition and classification of interstitial pneumonias in human pathology. In: Basset F, Georges R, eds. *Progress in respiratory research, 8. Alveolar interstitium of the lung*, pp. 1–33. Karger, New York.

Scadding JG, Hinson KFW (1967). Diffuse fibrosing alveolitis (diffuse interstitial fibrosis of the lungs). *Thorax* **22**, 291–304.

Pathology

Katzenstein AL, Myers JL (1998). Idiopathic pulmonary fibrosis: clinical relevance of pathologic classification. *American Journal of Respiratory and Critical Care Medicine* **157**, 1301–15. Review with 66 references.

Pathogenesis

Agostini C, Semenzato G (1996). Immunology of idiopathic pulmonary fibrosis. *Current Opinions in Pulmonary Medicine* **2**, 364–9.

Gauldie J, Sime PJ, Xing Z, Marr B, Tremblay GM (1999). Transforming growth factor-beta gene transfer to the lung induces myofibroblast presence and pulmonary fibrosis. *Current Topics in Pathology* **93**, 35–45.

Sime PJ, Xing Z, Graham FL, Csaky KG, Gauldie J (1997). Adenovector-mediated gene transfer of active transforming growth factor- beta1 induces prolonged severe fibrosis in rat lung. *Journal of Clinical Investigation* **100**, 768–76.

Imaging

Howling SJ, Hansell DM (2000). Spiral computed tomography for pulmonary embolism. *Hospital Medicine*, **61**, 41–5.

Wells A (1998). Clinical usefulness of high resolution computed tomography in cryptogenic fibrosing alveolitis. *Thorax* **53**, 1080–7. Review with 67 references.

Bronchoalveolar lavage

Haslam PL, Turton CWG, Lukoszek A, *et al.* (1980). Bronchoalveolar lavage fluid cell counts and cryptogenic fibrosing alveolitis and their relation to therapy. *Thorax* **35**, 328–9.

Weinberger SE, Kelman JA, Elson NA (1978). Bronchoalveolar lavage in interstitial lung disease. *Annals of Internal Medicine* **89**, 459–66.

Treatment

Johnson MA, Kwan S, Snell NJC, *et al.* (1989). Randomised controlled trial comparing prednisolone alone with cyclophosphamide and low dose prednisolone in combination in cryptogenic fibrosing alveolitis. *Thorax* **44**, 280–8.

Lynch JP, McCune WJ (1997). Immunosuppressive and cytotoxic pharmacotherapy for pulmonary disorders. *American Journal of Respiratory and Critical Care Medicine* **155**, 395–420. Review with 353 references.

Mason RJ, Schwarz MI, Hunninghake GW, Musson RA (1999). NHLBI workshop summary. Pharmacological therapy for idiopathic pulmonary fibrosis. Past, present, and future. *American Journal of Respiratory and Critical Care Medicine* **160**, 1771–7.

Raghu G, DePaso WJ, Cain K, *et al.* (1991). Azathioprine combined with prednisolone in the treatment of idiopathic pulmonary fibrosis: A prospective double blind randomised placebo controlled clinical trial. *American Review of Respiratory Diseases* **144**, 291–6.

Selman M, Carrillo G, Salas J, *et al.* (1998). Colchicine, D-penicillamine, and prednisone in the treatment of idiopathic pulmonary fibrosis: a controlled clinical trial. *Chest* **114**, 507–12.

Ziesche R, Hofbauer E, Wittmann K, Petkov V, Block LH (1999). A preliminary study of long-term treatment with interferon gamma-1b and low-dose prednisolone in patients with idiopathic pulmonary fibrosis [see comments]. *New England Journal of Medicine* **341**, 1264–9.

Prognosis

du Bois RM (1997). Management of idiopathic pulmonary fibrosis: prognostic indicators. *Monaldi Archives for Chest Disease* **52**, 547–51. Review with 61 references.

Turner-Warwick M, Burrows B, Johnson A (1980). Cryptogenic fibrosing alveolitis: response to corticosteroid treatment and its effect on survival. *Thorax* **35**, 593–9.

Watters LC, King TE, Schwartz MI (1986). A clinical, radiographic and physiologic scoring system for the longitudinal assessment of patients with idiopathic pulmonary fibrosis. *American Review of Respiratory Diseases* **133**, 97–103.

17.11.3 Bronchiolitis obliterans and organizing pneumonia

R. M. du Bois

Introduction

The bronchioles are defined as airways that have no cartilaginous support and comprise the terminal bronchioles and the respiratory bronchioles leading to the alveolar ducts. In many diffuse parenchymal lung disorders, the small bronchioles are involved in the histopathological process and bronchiolar disorders are often included in the classification of diffuse parenchymal lung diseases. The nomenclature of bronchiolitis has become confused. This is because pathological and clinical descriptions have been used interchangeably. There are three main histopathological patterns (Fig. 1 and Table 1):

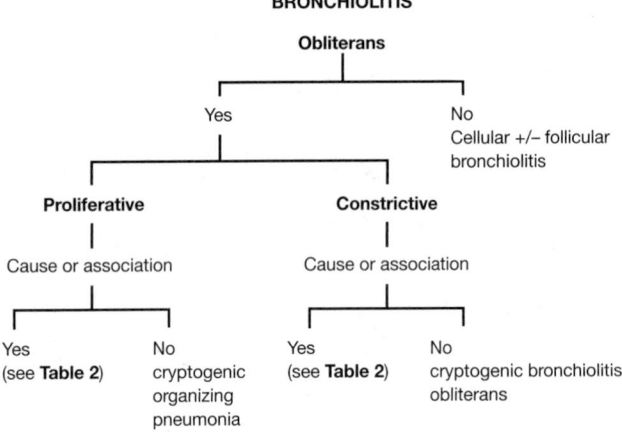

Fig. 1 Algorithm for the classification of bronchiolitis.

- proliferative bronchiolitis;
- constrictive bronchiolitis;
- cellular/ follicular bronchiolitis.

Proliferative and constrictive bronchiolitis patterns both cause obliteration of the bronchioles—'bronchiolitis obliterans'—but are associated with distinct clinical patterns of disease. Both may be the result of a known or unknown cause or association (see Table 2).

Nomenclature

Bronchiolitis obliterans is a term that has been used for many years to denote a relentless fibrosis of the bronchioles that results in severe, generally irreversible, airflow obstruction, and is characterized by obliteration of the terminal bronchioles by fixed fibrosis. In 1983, Davison *et al.* described a group of patients who presented with pneumonic-like features, but without evidence of infection, and in whom histopathological appearances were those of intra-alveolar organization spreading proximally to the terminal bronchiole. This disorder also obliterated the bronchioles, but with intraluminal loose, fibrous tissue, quite different from that seen in bronchiolitis obliterans. No cause was found for this condition and it was termed cryptogenic organizing pneumonitis. In 1985, Epler *et al.* rediscovered the entity, reporting the results of analysis of a large number of histopathological specimens, and gave the disease the name bronchiolitis obliterans organizing pneumonia. This confusion of nomenclature resulted in bronchiolitis obliterans and organizing pneumonia being regarded as synonyms.

An American Thoracic Society/ European Respiratory Society nomenclature committee has now redefined the diffuse lung diseases, including organizing pneumonia. It recommended that the idiopathic (or cryptogenic) variant of organizing pneumonia should be known as cryptogenic organizing pneumonia, with the histopathological features of organizing pneumonia. It must be noted that this disease and these pathological features are synonymous with idiopathic bronchiolitis obliterans organizing pneumonia, a term that will undoubtedly still appear in the literature. Bronchiolitis obliterans should be the term for the irreversible airway disease.

Bronchiolitis obliterans

Introduction

As with every form of bronchiolitis, attempts should be made to identify a potential trigger (see Table 2). Once all known triggers and associations have been excluded, the disease can be considered cryptogenic. Occasionally, the initial presentation of rheumatological disease is with the pulmonary manifestation, and it is therefore important to exclude this as far as possible through a full clinical history and examination, and also by testing for autoantibodies.

This disease is the result of progressive obliteration of the terminal bronchioles with connective tissue matrix. It is a relentless condition that is usually non-responsive to therapy. The pathogenesis is unknown.

Table 1 Histopathological classification of bronchiolitis

Constrictive bronchiolitis (see Fig. 2)	Proliferative bronchiolitis (see Fig. 2)	Cellular/ follicular bronchiolitis
Obliteration of airways	Terminal airways filled with granulation tissue	Airways compressed by prominent lymphoid follicles
Fibrosis in walls and lumens	Alveoli filling with buds of granulation tissue	Chronic inflammatory cells in walls
Alveoli and alveolar ducts spared	Chronic inflammatory cells in alveolar walls and surrounding alveoli	Fibrosis minor
	Foamy macrophages	
	Minimal scarring	

Table 2 Causes of bronchiolitis obliterans and organizing pneumonia

Bronchiolitis obliterans	Organizing pneumonia
Infection	Infection
viral, mycoplasma	viral, bacterial, fungal, parasites
Inhaled gases	
Rheumatological disease[a]	Rheumatological disease[a]
especially rheumatoid arthritis, Sjögren's syndrome	especially dermato/polymyositis, rheumatoid arthritis
Transplantation[a]	Transplantation
bone marrow, heart/lung, lung	bone marrow, lung
Drugs[b]	Drugs
e.g. penicillamine	e.g. amiodarone, sulphasalazine, gold, minocycline
Cryptogenic	Cryptogenic

Histopathology

The terminal bronchioles are predominantly involved with some extension into the proximal respiratory bronchioles. The lumens are significantly narrowed and often obliterated by a mixture of cellular inflammation and fibrosis–constrictive bronchiolitis (Fig. 2 and Plate 1). In advanced stages, the airways are occluded by dense, relatively acellular connective tissue matrix.

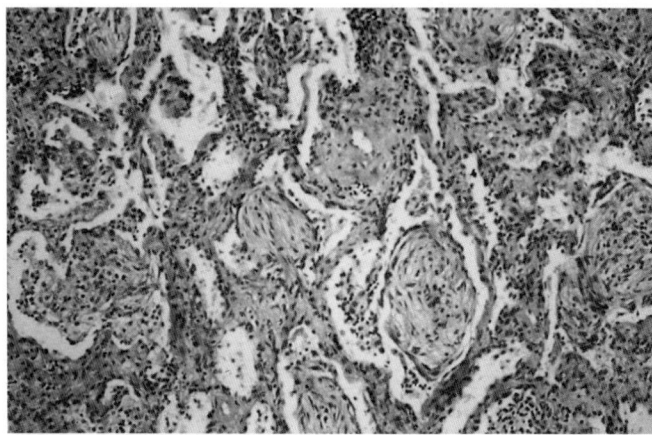

(a)

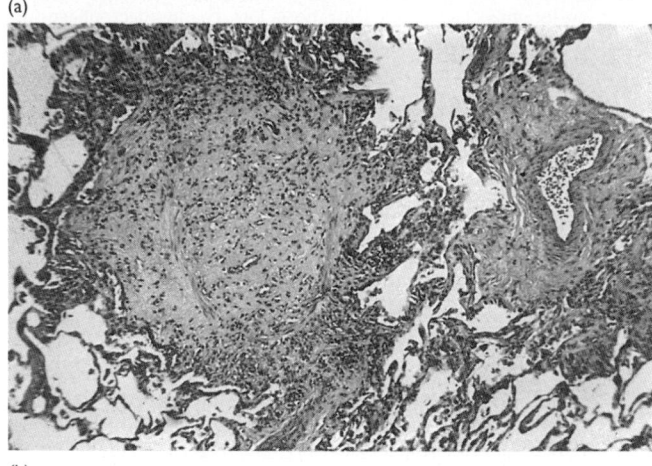

(b)

Fig. 2 Histopathology. (a) Proliferative bronchiolitis. (b) Constrictive bronchiolitis. Note the loosely packed granulation tissue in (a) in contrast to the more established scarring in (b). (See also Plate 1.)

Clinical features

The most striking clinical feature is progressive breathlessness, often with little wheeze despite this being predominantly an airway disease. Cough may occur, but is rarely productive, and haemoptysis is not a feature. Chest pain is uncommon but chest tightness may be described. Clinical examination of the respiratory system is unremarkable. Occasionally an inspiratory 'squeak' is heard, which is very characteristic of small airway disease. Examination of other systems may identify subtle rheumatological disease.

Investigations

Imaging

Chest radiography shows large lung fields with some loss of vascular markings but no evidence of infiltration.

High resolution computed tomography is more informative (Fig. 3). There is a patchiness of attenuation, described as 'mosaicism'. This represents variable degrees of lung perfusion caused by patchy vasoconstriction in affected

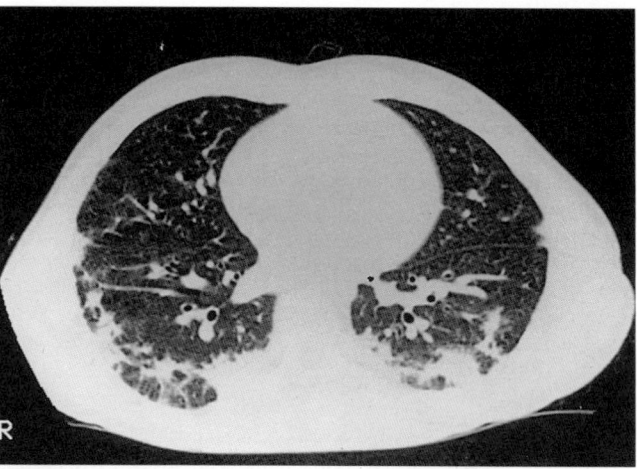

(a)

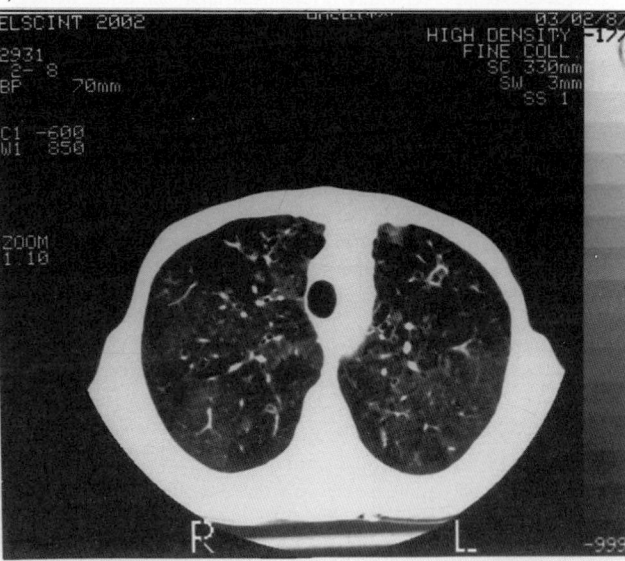

(b)

Fig. 3 High resolution computed tomography. (a) Organizing pneumonia. Peripheral consolidation is the classic feature. Histopathology is proliferative. (b) Bronchiolitis obliterans. The attenuation of the lung fields varies from grey (normal perfusion) to black (reduced perfusion due to hypoxic vasoconstriction resulting from airway obliteration). Histopathology is constrictive.

areas, this being due to reflex hypoxic vasospasm in response to airway obliteration. The mosaic pattern is enhanced on expiratory CT because gas trapping enhances the differences between perfused and non-perfused lung.

Lung function tests

Lung function tests show fixed airflow obstruction with an increase in residual volume and total lung capacity measured by plethysmography. Total gas transfer for carbon monoxide (DLco) is reduced, but the gas transfer index (total gas transfer corrected for alveolar volume) is preserved. This is an important distinguishing feature from airway diseases that cause obliteration of the vascular bed, such as emphysema. The arterial partial pressure of oxygen (Pao$_2$) is relatively well preserved until disease is severe.

Other investigations

Blood tests are unhelpful, with the exception of assays for autoantibodies that might suggest rheumatological disease. Bronchoalveolar lavage is not normally indicated and may be dangerous if disease is severe. However, when performed, an excess of neutrophils is characteristic.

Differential diagnosis

Cryptogenic bronchiolitis obliterans should be distinguished from other forms of chronic airflow obstruction, such as asthma, chronic obstructive pulmonary disease (COPD), and known causes or associations that result in bronchiolitis obliterans. The relatively well-preserved gas transfer index is an important feature distinguishing this condition from emphysema. The appearances on high resolution computed tomography (particularly the expiratory scan) are characteristic of obliterated small airways. In exceptional circumstances, surgical biopsy is needed to confirm the diagnosis. If this is undertaken, the characteristic airway abnormalities can sometimes be elusive. Multiple sectioning throughout the whole block is required to obtain regions that would allow a correct diagnosis to be made.

Treatment

Treatment response is generally poor. It is important to give a trial of corticosteroids to exclude reversibility. A reasonable approach would be to give 40 mg of prednisolone per day for 4 weeks, measuring pulmonary function before and after, paying particular attention to changes in residual volume and gas transfer. If there is significant objective response, steroid dosage should be tapered and maintenance inhaler therapy given. This should consist of inhaled corticosteroids and, possibly, a long-acting β_2-adrenoceptor agonist such as salmeterol or eformoterol. Immunosuppressants, typically azathioprine, have been tried but with limited success.

In the younger patient, lung transplantation should be considered. However, the most common long-term problem encountered with lung transplantation is an obliterative bronchiolitis. Counselling of the patient is particularly important in this situation.

Organizing pneumonia

Introduction

Known causes of, and associations with, organizing pneumonia should be identified (see Table 2). In the absence of these, the term cryptogenic organizing pneumonia is used. Clinical features are very similar for the cryptogenic and non-cryptogenic disease.

Histopathology

The most striking abnormality is the filling of the airways distal to the terminal bronchiole and the alveoli with granulation tissue in a peribronchiolar distribution, comprising buds of loose collagen and connective tissue matrix cells with a uniform appearance (Fig. 2). There may be some sur-

rounding chronic inflammation. The intra-alveolar granulation tissue may spread from one alveolus to another thorough the pores of Kohn.

Clinical features

The disease presents subacutely with a history of, usually, 2 to 3 months' non-productive cough, shortness of breath, and the systemic features of fever, weight loss, and malaise. It affects men and women equally and occurs predominantly in the fifth and sixth decades. Digital clubbing is rare. A few crackles may be heard on auscultation, but this is not invariable. Features of systemic disease may suggest that the lung problems are secondary.

Investigations

Imaging

Chest radiography shows, most commonly, a bilateral, predominantly peripheral, and often basal, pattern of consolidation. Very occasionally there is an interstitial pattern reminiscent of fibrosing alveolitis, and even more rarely the pattern is of a single nodule. Cavitation can occur but is uncommon. Pleural disease is rare.

High resolution computed tomography defines the pattern more clearly and often shows the disease as more extensive than would be suspected from plain chest radiography (Fig. 3). The predominantly peripheral pattern of confluent disease with air bronchograms may be confirmed. A rarer variant, with a very marked peribronchovascular bundle distribution, can be associated with changes suggestive of fibrosis. This more interstitial variant is less likely to resolve.

Lung function tests

Lung function tests show a restrictive ventilatory defect with reduced gas transfer. Pao$_2$ is well maintained unless disease is severe.

Other tests

Blood tests are non-specific, suggesting an inflammatory process with a leucocytosis, elevated erythrocyte sedimentation rate, and C-reactive protein. A seasonal variant of disease (occurring between February and May) has been reported in one series and this was associated with abnormal liver function tests.

Bronchoalveolar lavage

Typical features are in increase in lymphocytes together with neutrophils and/or eosinophils. The CD4:CD8 ratio is low. Foamy macrophages are characteristic. Occasionally, mast cells and plasma cells may be seen.

Differential diagnosis

All other causes of consolidation visible on imaging need to be considered. These include infection, eosinophilic pneumonia, alveolar haemorrhage, alveolar proteinosis, alveolar cell carcinoma, vasculitis, and lymphoma. Patients who have atypical features or who have not responded to treatment as completely as would be expected should have the alternative diagnoses considered.

Diagnosis is most cases will require a surgical biopsy. In exceptional circumstances, the diagnosis may be made in the context of the classical (consolidation) form of disease on the basis of typical bronchoalveolar lavage findings, together with a transbronchial biopsy that is consistent. It is noteworthy, however, that areas of organization are seen on histopathological examination of biopsies from a variety of disorders such as vasculitis, eosinophilic pneumonia, and malignancy, but in these circumstances they are minor features and not the dominant pathology. Unfortunately, a transbronchial biopsy may only sample these minor features, thereby resulting in misdiagnosis.

Treatment

Corticosteroids usually work extremely well. It is usual to commence with a dosage of 0.75 mg/kg per day orally for a month and then gradually taper whilst monitoring symptomatic, radiological, and physiological improvement. It is usually possible to discontinue corticosteroids after 6 to 12 months. Relapses can occur at any time but usually respond to a reintroduction of corticosteroids. Rarely, immunosuppressants, such as azathioprine or cyclophosphamide, need to be used as steroid-sparing agents or in more resistant disease.

Occasionally patients present with respiratory failure due to very extensive disease and in this situation pulsed intravenous methylprednisolone at 500 to 1000 mg daily for 3 days can be life saving. It is very unusual to have to use mechanical ventilation.

Prognosis

The prognosis is generally very good. Indices of a poor prognosis include organizing pneumonia that is secondary to rheumatological or other systemic disease, an imaging pattern that shows an interstitial or mixed pattern of disease, and a bronchoalveolar lavage that has no lymphocytes. Estimates of 5-year survival are 73 per cent for primary disease compared to 44 per cent for disease that occurs secondary to other disorders. Deaths due to organizing pneumonia are uncommon and in various series range from 3 to 13 per cent of cases.

Further reading

Wells AU, du Bois RM (1993). Bronchiolitis in association with connective tissue disorders. In: King TE, ed. *Clinics in chest medicine*, pp. 655–66. WB Saunders , Philadelphia.

Cordier J-F (2000). Organising pneumonia. Thorax rare disease series 8. *Thorax* 55, 318–28.

King TE Jr (2000). Bronchiolitis. In: du Bois R M and Olivieri D, eds. *European Respiratory Monograph* 14, 244–66.

Lynch JP, Belperio J, Flint A, Martinez F (1999). Bronchiolar complications of connective tissue disorders. *Seminars in Respiratory and Critical Care Medicine* 20, 149–67.

Wright JL, Cagle T, Churg A, Colby TV, Myers J (1992). Diseases of the small airways. *American Review of Respiratory Diseases* 146, 240–62.

17.11.4 The lungs and rheumatological diseases

R. M. du Bois and A. K. Wells

Introduction

Lung involvement can occur in all rheumatological diseases, with different patterns of respiratory pathology predominant in different diseases. The frequency and best management of these problems is often uncertain because, although common, they have been less well documented than the more obvious rheumatological features. Respiratory involvement may be subclinical, symptoms often being masked by exercise limitation due to musculoskeletal factors.

In some patients, diffuse lung disease is the presenting feature of the rheumatological disease, when typical computed tomography appearances together with autoantibody studies will point to the correct diagnosis.

Imaging

Chest radiography will identify the predominantly reticulonodular pattern of the diseases that mimic fibrosing alveolitis (see Chapters 17.11.1 and 17.11.2), the consolidation of organizing pneumonia and alveolar haemorrhage, the ground glass pattern of acute pneumonitis, the hyperinflation of bronchiolitis obliterans, and the presence of pleural disease.

High resolution computed tomography will enhance the sensitivity, precision, and accuracy of diagnosis. It will also reveal combinations of patterns that suggest specific rheumatological diseases. In fibrosing alveolitis, there is a reticular pattern that is initially basal and peripheral with honeycombing. More extensive disease progresses upwards and anteriorly. Ground glass changes are found in more cellular disease; mosaicism (alternating regions of increased and decreased attenuation) is typical of small airway disease. Bronchiectasis and pleural changes are seen more clearly than on chest radiography. Prediction of reversibility is much more precise than with chest radiography.

Lung function

Lung function testing does not discriminate in terms of precise pulmonary diagnosis but will differentiate obstructive ventilatory defects, characteristic of airways disease, from the restrictive pattern with reduction in gas transfer that is seen in all forms of diffuse lung disease. Lung function testing is the gold standard measure of extent of disease. Exercise tests will unmask more subtle disease, often subclinical, but are not routine requirements. A measure of gas transfer, however, is always needed.

Clinical features of lung disease in particular autoimmune rheumatic disorders

Systemic sclerosis

The criteria for classification of systemic sclerosis are described in Chapter 18.11.3. Pulmonary involvement has emerged as the major cause of excess morbidity and mortality in this disorder. The patterns of lung disease with which systemic sclerosis may present are variable and are shown in Table 1.

Fibrosing alveolitis

Clinical features

Lung disease may be the first manifestation of systemic sclerosis, and dyspnoea occurs in roughly 55 per cent of patients with this condition. Cough is a less frequently reported symptom, but when it occurs is dry and nonproductive; haemoptysis indicates complicating carcinoma or bronchial telangiectasia. Pleuritic chest pain is uncommon. A history of Raynaud's phenomenon is often present. Digital clubbing is rare because of the poor vasculature of the digits. Fine crackles are heard at the bases and are of 'velcro' character. Capillaroscopy , digital thermography, and a positive antinuclear antibody can be helpful in suggesting the correct diagnosis. Lung fibrosis occurs more commonly in patients with the Scl 70, anti-DNA topoisomerase autoantibody. Chest radiographic series have identified diffuse lung disease in up to 67 per cent of patients. Oesophageal dilatation may be seen on chest radiography and is almost universally present on high resolution computed tomography. ^{99m}Tc-diethylinetriamine pentacetate clearance has been used in some centres to identify early disease and to predict prognosis—persistently normal clearance predicts lung function stability. Lung function abnormalities are found in up to 90 per cent of patients; scleroderma of the chest wall may rarely cause extrathoracic restriction. Bronchoalveolar lavage is of value in excluding complicating infection and malignancy and in suggesting the most likely histopathological pattern, but it is of no value in monitoring disease. In non-specific interstitial pneumonia (NSIP, see Chapter 17.11.1), the most common histopathological pattern, granulocytes and lymphocytes may be present in excess; usual interstitial pneumonia is less common, associated with excess of neutrophils with or without eosinophils on lavage.

Table 1 Lung manifestations of rheumatological diseases

Systemic sclerosis	Polymyositis/dermato-myositis	Rheumatoid arthritis	Sjögren's syndrome	Systemic lupus erythematosus
Fibrosing alveolitis	**Diffuse lung disease**	**Fibrosing alveolitis**	**Airways inflammation**	**Atelectasis**
Isolated pulmonary vascular disease	**Organizing pneumonia**	**Bronchiectasis**	**Lymphocytic interstitial pneumonia**	**Pleural disease**
Organizing pneumonia	Acute pneumonitis	**Pleural disease**	Diffuse lung disease	Acute pneumonitis
Aspiration pneumonia	Aspiration pneumonia	Organizing pneumonia	Lymphoproliferation	Diffuse lung disease
Chest wall restriction	Pulmonary vasculitis	Obliterative bronchiolitis	Organizing pneumonia	Alveolar haemorrhage
	Respiratory muscle weakness	Follicular bronchiolitis		Pulmonary hypertension
		Vasculitis		Shrinking lung syndrome
		Nodules		
		Lymphocytic interstitial pneumonia		

Most common manifestation(s) for each rheumatological disease are shown in bold type.

Prognosis

The prognosis of fibrosing alveolitis in systemic sclerosis is dependent upon the extent of disease at presentation, but it is much better than in cryptogenic fibrosing alveolitis. Significant improvements can be achieved in response to therapy, despite the prevalent view held by many (Fig. 1). Worse lung function, particularly vital capacity and gas transfer (DLco),

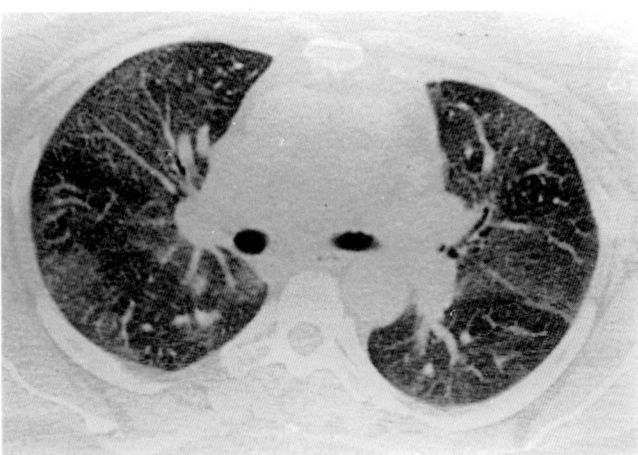

(a)

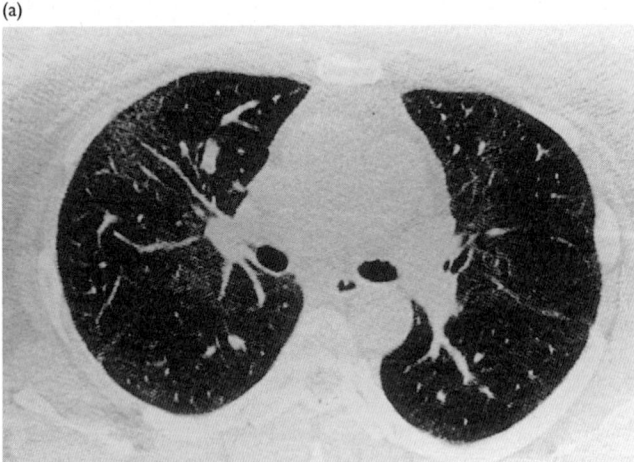

(b)

Fig. 1 CT scans of a patient with the fibrosing alveolitis of systemic sclerosis, demonstrating a non-specific interstitial pneumonia pattern of disease. (a) Before treatment. Note the widespread ground glass pattern of disease, with some areas in which the airways have been distracted demonstrating fine fibrosis. (b) After treatment. The residual, more fibrotic areas remain, but much of the abnormality has cleared.

indicates a poorer outcome, and similar observations have been made using extent of disease on computed tomography as the criterion. Crude mortality rates are 3.9 per cent per year for males and 2.6 per cent per year for females with systemic sclerosis, with lung disease the commonest cause of death. There is also an increased risk of lung cancer.

Pulmonary vascular disease in systemic sclerosis

Unlike the other rheumatological diseases, vascular involvement in systemic sclerosis is caused not by vasculitis but by concentric fibrosis replacing the normal intima and media of small arterioles. Isolated pulmonary vascular disease occurs mainly in the limited form of systemic sclerosis (including the CREST syndrome—calcinosis, Raynaud's phenomenon, oesophageal dysmotility, sclerodactyly, telangiectasiae) and in individuals with the anticentromere autoantibody. Chest radiography, high resolution computed tomography, and bronchoalveolar lavage are all normal. Lung function studies show an isolated fall in DLco and gas transfer index (Kco). When damage to the pulmonary vascular bed is extensive (gas transfer <50 per cent predicted) the risk of pulmonary hypertension increases. Mortality rates are increased with increasing pulmonary hypertension, for which Doppler echocardiography is a good screening test.

Other pulmonary complications

Aspiration pneumonia is uncommon, particularly considering the prevalence of oesophageal dysfunction in systemic sclerosis. Pleural disease is also uncommon. Rarely, the extent of skin tightness over the chest wall produces an extrinsic restriction of ventilation. Occasionally, the first manifestation of pulmonary parenchymal disease is organizing pneumonia

Polymyositis/dermatomyositis

The defining criteria for polymyositis and dermatomyositis are described in Chapter 18.11.7.

Pulmonary complications occur in up to 64 per cent of patients in combined series and are the most frequent cause of death. The main manifestations of lung disease are summarized in Table 1.

Diffuse lung disease

Diffuse lung disease is the commonest problem encountered in the context of dermatomyositis/ polymyositis. The pattern of diffuse lung disease often mimics that of fibrosing alveolitis, but a rapidly progressive form of acute pneumonitis can occur. Organizing pneumonia may also be the presenting feature. A recent report has described an acute presentation of pulmonary capillaritis with alveolar haemorrhage in association with polymyositis.

Clinical features depend upon the nature of the lung process. Breathlessness on exertion without wheeze is a common presenting symptom and, if the myopathy is severe, orthopnoea can be striking. Haemoptysis may occur if there is capillaritis. Pleural disease is uncommon. Computed tomography can be particularly helpful; a combination of patchy consolidation with a peripheral reticular pattern being highly characteristic. In recent alveolar haemorrhage or marked myopathy, there may be a disproportionate preservation of gas transfer index (Kco). It must be remembered, however, that acute haemorrhage can occur in the context of previous chronic disease and so the Kco may be normal or subnormal, but elevated from the baseline level. Autoantibodies to aminoacyl-tRNA synthetases are often found when inflammatory myopathies coexist with diffuse lung disease—Jo-1 (antihistidyl tRNA synthetase) is the most common. This occurs in 20 to 30 per cent of patients with inflammatory myopathy, but in 50 to 100 per cent of cases of inflammatory myopathy and diffuse lung disease, in contrast to less than 5 per cent of patients without diffuse lung disease.

Other pulmonary manifestations

Aspiration pneumonia needs to be considered if there is upper airway/pharyngeal muscle weakness. The predilection for the posterior lung segments may suggest this diagnosis. Respiratory muscle weakness may be present in the absence of parenchymal lung disease and requires studies of muscle function for confirmation.

Rheumatoid arthritis

The American Rheumatism Association revised criteria for the classification of rheumatoid arthritis (rheumatoid arthritis) are described in Chapter 18.8. Pleuropulmonary manifestations are summarized in Table 1.

Fibrosing alveolitis

The fibrosing alveolitis of rheumatoid arthritis has a male predominance (male:female 3:1), is associated with HLA-B8 and HLA-Dw3 positivity, and is histologically similar to cryptogenic fibrosing alveolitis, but some patients may have non-specific interstitial pneumonia rather than usual interstitial pneumonia. Minor pulmonary fibrosis is common; in one open lung biopsy series pulmonary fibrosis was seen in 60 per cent of patients. Smoking is a risk factor for the development of overt pulmonary fibrosis and has also been associated with subclinical disease. High titres of rheumatoid factor and the presence of rheumatoid nodules are also associated with an increased prevalence of diffuse lung disease.

The most frequent symptom is exertional dyspnoea, although this may be masked by a general loss of mobility due to systemic disease. The clinical picture is usually identical to cryptogenic fibrosing alveolitis with bilateral, predominantly basal crackles and tachypnoea. Digital clubbing is more prevalent than in other rheumatological diseases. Reductions in carbon monoxide diffusing capacity are found in up to 40 per cent of unselected rheumatoid arthritis patients, but radiologically overt pulmonary fibrosis is found in only 1 to 5 per cent of cases (based on three large chest radiographic series).

Organizing pneumonia

The clinical presentation of organizing pneumonia is similar to infective pneumonia with systemic features of fever and weight loss, multifocal consolidation on chest radiograph and computed tomography, a restrictive functional defect, and generally a good response to corticosteroids. Histopathology shows acini filled with loose connective tissue and a variable inflammatory infiltrate. Organizing pneumonia is more common in rheumatoid arthritis than in other rheumatological diseases, with the possible exception of polymyositis.

Bronchiolitis obliterans

The clinical presentation is of progressive breathlessness. Clinical signs reveal hyperinflation of the chest, often with an inspiratory 'squeak'. Chest radiography confirms hyperinflation with no infiltration. High resolution computed tomography shows a 'mosaic' pattern of variable perfusion as a result of the hypoxic vasoconstriction that results from the airway occlusion. Lung function is often a mixed obstructive/restrictive pattern, with obstruction predominating; gas transfer index (Kco) is preserved. Bronchiolitis obliterans is characterized histologically by destruction of the ter-

minal bronchiolar wall by granulation tissue, effacement of the lumen, and eventual replacement of the bronchiole by fibrous tissue. There is great heterogeneity in the speed of progression, with some patients having indolent disease.

The association of the use of penicillamine with obliterative bronchiolitis was first reported in the late 1970s. Following a number of case reports and small series, obliterative bronchiolitis was identified in a large cohort study in 3/133 rheumatoid arthritis patients using penicillamine, compared to 0/469 who were not using this drug. Obliterative bronchiolitis has, however, been reported in many rheumatoid arthritis patients not using penicillamine, and the relationship of the drug to this airways obliteration is unclear.

Bronchiectasis

The prevalence of bronchiectasis is higher in rheumatoid arthritis than in other rheumatological diseases. A recent literature review identified 289 patients with bronchiectasis associated with rheumatoid arthritis reported since 1928. Although associated with long-standing rheumatoid arthritis in one study, bronchiectasis was found on computed tomography in 30 per cent of 50 rheumatoid arthritis patients with normal chest radiographs on prospective evaluation. Bronchiectatic changes (often subtle) are easily visualized on computed tomography, and a combination of diffuse lung disease and airway disease on computed tomography should raise the suspicion of rheumatological disease, especially rheumatoid arthritis or Sjögren's syndrome, in patients whose lung disease may be the first manifestation of their rheumatological disorder (Fig. 2).

Pulmonary vasculitis

Pulmonary vasculitis is a potential but uncommon complication of rheumatoid arthritis, given the relatively high prevalence of systemic vasculitis in the disease. Similarly, diffuse alveolar haemorrhage is a rare complication of rheumatoid arthritis.

Pulmonary rheumatoid nodules

These may be single (when distinguishing from malignancy can be impossible, especially in the cigarette smoker) or multiple, and are found on chest radiography in less than 1 per cent of patients with rheumatoid arthritis,

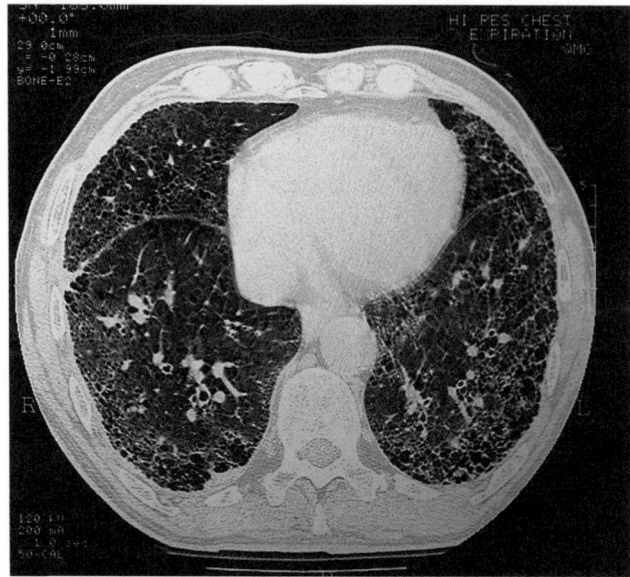

Fig. 2 High resolution computed tomography of a patient with rheumatoid arthritis. There are areas showing reticular changes consistent with fibrosing alveolitis. In addition, in areas where there is no fibrosis, there is evidence of bronchial wall thickening and bronchiectasis. This combination of computed tomographic features is highly characteristic of rheumatoid arthritis.

usually in association with rheumatoid nodules elsewhere in the body. They may vary in size according to underlying rheumatoid activity, and can be as much as 7 cm in diameter. Nodule cavitation occasionally causes haemoptysis, and pneumothorax can result from the rupture of subpleural nodules, but generally these are found as asymptomatic abnormalities on chest radiography. Caplan's syndrome is the association of single or multiple nodules with coal-miner's pneumoconiosis.

Pleural disease

Pleural disease is seen at autopsy in approximately 50 per cent of patients with rheumatoid arthritis and 20 per cent give a history of pleuritic chest pain. Pleural effusions are found in less than 5 per cent, usually in males, and are frequently asymptomatic, often being identified on routine chest radiography. In a minority, pleuritic pain and fever are prominent and the exclusion of empyema (which may be more prevalent in rheumatoid arthritis) is required. Occasionally, effusions may develop acutely in association with pericarditis or exacerbations of arthritis; more typically, radiographic abnormalities are chronic, often remaining unchanged for years. The fluid is an exudate, with a low glucose level (correlating poorly with serum glucose), a low pH, and, usually, a predominant lymphocytosis (although a neutrophilia is occasionally found).

Other pulmonary manifestations

Other pulmonary complications of rheumatoid arthritis are rare. Lower respiratory tract infection is increased in frequency, bronchopneumonia is a common terminal event, accounting for 15 to 20 per cent of deaths.

Sjögren's syndrome

The defining features of Sjögren's syndrome are described in Chapter 18.11.6. Pulmonary involvement is common, with objective evidence of pulmonary abnormalities in approximately a quarter of cases. This usually consists of lymphocytic infiltration producing diffuse lung disease and tracheobronchial disease.

Diffuse lung disease

Although often asymptomatic, diffuse lung disease in Sjögren's syndrome may present with cough, dyspnoea, crackles on auscultation, reticular or reticulonodular abnormalities on chest radiography, and a restrictive pattern of functional impairment. Interstitial involvement can be classified as fibrosing alveolitis or lymphocytic interstitial pneumonia in up to 10 per cent of patients with primary Sjögren's syndrome. Lymphoma may be a complicating problem and can mimic organizing pneumonia. Organizing pneumonia (bronchiolitis obliterans organizing pneumonia, BOOP) has been reported in Sjögren's syndrome, but occurs less frequently than in rheumatoid arthritis or polymyositis.

Tracheobronchial disease

Tracheobronchial disease may take the form of loss of mucus secretion in the trachea (xerotrachea), chronic bronchitis, or small airways disease. Xerotrachea occurs in up to 25 per cent of patients with primary Sjögren's syndrome and consists of atrophy of tracheobronchial mucous glands in association with a lymphoplasmocytic infiltrate, manifesting clinically as a relentless dry cough and endobronchial inflammation at bronchoscopy. It is likely that similar histological abnormalities in bronchi and bronchioles account for an increased prevalence of bronchial hyper-responsiveness, reported in 40 to 60 per cent of patients with primary and secondary Sjögren's syndrome. The evaluation of airflow at low lung volumes in unselected patients with primary and secondary Sjögren's syndrome has demonstrated a high prevalence of small disease.

Systemic lupus erythematosus (SLE)

The 1982 revised ACR criteria for the diagnosis of systemic lupus erythematosus are described in Chapter 18.11.2. Pleuropulmonary manifestations of this condition are shown in Table 1.

Diffuse lung disease

The prevalence of diffuse lung disease on lung biopsy or at autopsy is highly variable (4–70 per cent). Only 3 per cent of systemic lupus erythematosus patients have clinical evidence of diffuse lung disease at the onset of systemic disease, and a disease resembling fibrosing alveolitis develops during follow-up in less than 5 per cent. The clinical presentation (dyspnoea, cough, predominantly basal crackles, a restrictive lung function defect or isolated reduction in carbon monoxide diffusing capacity, basal infiltrates on chest radiography) is typical of rheumatological fibrosing alveolitis. However, features not typical of cryptogenic fibrosing alveolitis include variably associated pleuritic pain, a paucity of patients with morphologically extensive or functionally severe lung fibrosis, and the frequent presence of enlarged peribronchiolar lymphoid follicles at lung biopsy (although other histological findings are indistinguishable from cryptogenic fibrosing alveolitis).

Acute lupus pneumonitis, seen in less than 2 per cent of systemic lupus erythematosus patients, is life-threatening with a mortality rate despite treatment of over 50 per cent once respiratory failure has developed. It must be distinguished from organizing pneumonia.

Extrapulmonary restriction

Extrapulmonary restriction is a well-recognized complication of systemic lupus erythematosus that results in exertional dyspnoea, a restrictive functional defect, and marked elevation of K_{CO}. The 'shrinking lung syndrome' was first described in patients with severe restriction and a marked reduction in lung volume on chest radiography, and is generally ascribed to respiratory muscle weakness. There is no treatment of proven efficacy, although some patients have improved with corticosteroid or immunosuppressive therapy.

Diffuse alveolar haemorrhage

Although seen more frequently than in other rheumatological disorders, diffuse alveolar haemorrhage is rare in systemic lupus erythematosus. The typical presentation of acute dyspnoea and extensive pulmonary infiltrates on chest radiography may mimic acute lupus pneumonitis, especially in the absence of haemoptysis. Diffuse alveolar haemorrhage is often life-threatening, with a mortality similar to acute lupus pneumonitis.

Pulmonary hypertension

Pulmonary hypertension was once considered rare in systemic lupus erythematosus, but is now reported with increasing frequency, and has a 2-year survival of less than 50 per cent in severe disease. Abnormalities indicative of subclinical pulmonary hypertension are found on echocardiography in 10 per cent of patients, usually in association with Raynaud's phenomenon, and thus it is likely that pulmonary hypertension results from vasoconstriction, rather than pulmonary vasculitis (which is seldom identified in systemic lupus erythematosus even at autopsy). An important alternative mechanism for pulmonary hypertension is thromboembolism, which has a high prevalence in systemic lupus erythematosus, especially in patients with antiphospholipid antibodies.

Pleural disease

Pleural disease is the most common pulmonary manifestation of systemic lupus erythematosus. Clinical or radiographic evidence of pleural involvement is seen in 20 per cent of patients at the onset of systemic disease and occurs in at least 50 per cent at some time (with pleural abnormalities at autopsy in 50–100 per cent). Pleural disease is often asymptomatic, but pleuritic pain may be recurrent or intractable. Pleural fluid is usually serosanguinous (but occasionally haemorrhagic) and exudative, with a neutrophilia in patients with pleurisy but a predominant lymphocytosis in chronic effusions.

Relapsing polychondritis

Relapsing polychondritis is described in Chapter 17.8.1. Respiratory involvement probably accounts for around 10 per cent of deaths in this condition. Pulmonary parenchymal disease is rare, but vasculitis may occur. Destruction and obstruction of the glottis, trachea, and bronchi lead to airway stricture, collapse, and distal infection. Lung function testing shows diminution in maximal inspiratory (large, extrathoracic airways) and expiratory flow (smaller, intrathoracic airways) rates, suggesting airway collapse while static recoil pressures are preserved. Chest radiography may suggest bronchiectasis, with airway thickening and dilatation being confirmed on high resolution computed tomography. Dynamic computed tomography scanning showing collapse of the larger airways on inspiratory manoeuvres can help to localize disease. Treatment is by mechanical stenting. Immunosuppression may be helpful.

Ankylosing spondylitis

Ankylosing spondylitis is described in Chapter 18.7. Fibrotic lung disease on chest radiography, largely or entirely confined to the upper zones, is the main pulmonary complication of this condition; diffuse reticulonodular infiltrates in the upper zones are usually symmetrical and are seldom extensive, except in patients with severe spinal disease or a long history of the disorder. This is uncommon, seen in only 1 to 2 per cent of a series of 2080 patients with ankylosing spondylitis. However, on high resolution computed tomography, limited interstitial lung disease, bronchiectasis, or paraseptal emphysema are present in the majority of patients, even when chest radiographic appearances are normal. There is no proven treatment to prevent the development of apical fibrosis; resistance to corticosteroid therapy being the rule. Cavities may develop within distorted fibrotic apical tissue and are sometimes colonized by mycobacteria or fungi, especially *Aspergillus fumigatus* that are isolated in up to 60 per cent of patients with apical cavitation. Life-threatening haemoptysis is an occasional complication of mycetoma formation within cavities; this may be controllable by bronchial artery embolization, the resection of a mycetoma being a treatment of last resort, due to the high prevalence of postoperative bronchopleural fistula or empyema.

Extrapulmonary restriction due to immobilization of the chest wall (costovertebral ankylosis) is an occasional complication of ankylosing spondylitis, associated with surprisingly little impairment in pulmonary function, perhaps because the diaphragm is able to make a major contribution in the presence of a high resting volume.

Mixed connective tissue disease

This syndrome is defined by the presence of features of systemic lupus erythematosus, systemic sclerosis, and polymyositis (Sjögren's syndrome may also be seen) in association with high titres (>1:1600) of autoantibody directed against the extractable nuclear antigen U1-RNP (see Chapter 18.11.2 for discussion). Pleuropulmonary complications occur in 20 to 85 per cent of patients, most commonly diffuse lung disease. Pulmonary involvement, investigations, and treatment are as for the individual rheumatological disease.

Treatment of lung disease in particular autoimmune rheumatic disorders

Treatment is directed at the type of lung disease, irrespective of the rheumatological disease in which it is found (Table 2). Opportunistic infection and pulmonary side-effects caused by treatment of the rheumatological disease can mimic pulmonary complications of the rheumatological disease and must be excluded. Similarly, carcinoma and lymphoma are complications of diffuse lung disease in rheumatological lung disease that must be differentiated.

Table 2 Drugs used in the treatment of the major pulmonary complications of rheumatological diseases

Drug	Dose	Duration	Comments	Monitoring
Azathioprine	2.5 mg/kg per day max. 150 mg/day	Continuous	Maximal effect may not be evident for 6–9 months but has better adverse effect profile than cyclophosphamide. May be used long term. Starting dose 50 mg daily with monitoring FBC in case of thiopurine methyltransferase deficiency, maintenance dose from 1 month.	Full blood count Liver function tests
Cyclophosphamide	oral: 2 mg/kg per day to 150 mg/day IV: 600 mg/m² monthly for 1–6 months	Continuous Variable	Intravenous therapy for rapid induction of remission at 2–4 mg/kg per day for 3–4 days for vasculitis. For other indications, pulsed IV cyclophosphamide may be given at 1–3 monthly intervals with better adverse effect profile and lower long-term cumulative dose, particularly in non-vasculitic disease. Oral cyclophosphamide may be used continuously or substituted at 3 months for azathioprine because of more favourable adverse effect profile in DLD.	Full blood count Liver function tests Urinalysis for blood
Cyclosporin A	5 mg/kg per day	Continuous	Bioavailability variable thus blood monitoring necessary. May be used in combination with prednisolone.	Blood pressure Urea and creatinine Cyclosporin level
Methotrexate	7.5–20 mg/week	Continuous	Little information to support use except as second line therapy after first line treatment. Pulmonary toxicity may be limiting.	Full blood count Liver function tests
Prednisolone	1 mg/kg per day or 20 mg alternate days	Continuous	Prednisolone used alone in high dose for cellular DLD and then titrated to control. In conjunction with immunosuppressants for more fibrotic disease, the low-dose regimen is used.	Blood pressure Blood glucose Weight
Methylprednisolone	IV 500–1000 mg daily	3–5 days	Used for aggressive induction of remission particularly for vasculitis or acute pneumonitis, then followed by maintenance therapy of prednisolone or prednisolone plus immunosuppressive agent.	

IV, intravenous; DLD, diffuse lung disease.

Further reading

General reading

du Bois RM, Stirling RG (1999). Connective tissue disorders. In: Albert R, Spiro S, Jett J, eds. *Principles of respiratory medicine*, pp. 53.2–53.14. Mosby International, Barcelona.

du Bois RM, Wells AU (2000). Pulmonary involvement of connective tissue disease. In: Murray JF and Nadel JA, eds. *Respiratory medicine*, pp. 1691–715. WB Saunders, Philadelphia.

Specific reading

Cervera R, Khamashta MA, Font J, *et al.* (1993). Systemic lupus erythematosus: clinical and immunologic patterns of disease expression in a cohort of 1000 patients. The European working party on systemic lupus erythematosus. *Medicine* **72**, 113–24.

Friedman AW, Targoff IN, Arnett FC (1996). Interstitial lung disease with autoantibodies against aminoacyl-tRNA synthetases in the absence of clinically apparent myositis. *Seminars in Arthritis and Rheumatism* **26**, 459–67.

Haupt HM, Moore GW, Hutchins G (1981). The lung in systemic lupus erythematosus. Analysis of the pathologic changes in 120 patients. *American Journal of Medicine* **71**, 791–8.

Hyland RH, Gordon DA, Broder I, *et al.* (1983). A systematic controlled study of pulmonary abnormalities in rheumatoid arthritis. *Journal of Rheumatology* **10**, 395–405.

Marie I, Hatron PY, Hachulla E, Wallaert B, Michon-Pasturel U, Devulder B (1998). Pulmonary involvement in polymyositis and dermatomyositis. *Journal of Rheumatology* **25**, 1336–43.

Papiris SA, Maniati M, Constantopoulos SH, Roussos C, Moutsopoulos HM, Skopouli FN (1999). Lung involvement in primary Sjögren's syndrome is mainly related to the small airways disease. *Annals of the Rheumatic Diseases* **58**, 61–4.

Tanoue LT (1998). Pulmonary manifestations of rheumatoid arthritis. *Clinics in Chest Medicine* **19**, 667–85.

Wells AU, Cullinan P, Hansell DM, *et al.* (1994). Fibrosing alveolitis associated with systemic sclerosis has a better prognosis than lone cryptogenic fibrosing alveolitis. *American Journal of Respiratory and Critical Care Medicine* **149**, 1583–90.

17.11.5 The lung in vasculitis

R. M. du Bois

Introduction

The nomenclature of vasculitis has been confused. This is because there is overlap between clinical and histopathological features in a group of disorders of unknown aetiology. It is useful to subdivide pulmonary vasculitides into primary systemic or secondary, and to differentiate them from non-vasculitic disorders that can affect the pulmonary circulation (Table 1). The secondary and non-vasculitic diseases are discussed in other chapters: Table 2 summarizes the primary vasculitides, indicating those in which the lung is involved.

Clinical manifestations of pulmonary vasculitis

Lung involvement in vasculitic disease can manifest as:

(1) diffuse alveolar haemorrhage or

Table 1 Pulmonary vascular disease

Vasculitic	Non-vasculitic
Primary systemic	Thromboembolic
Secondary	Primary pulmonary hypertension
Rheumatological	Secondary pulmonary hypertension
Pulmonary–renal	Systemic sclerosis
Behçet's syndrome	Idiopathic pulmonary haemosiderosis
Chronic infection	Arteriovenous malformations
Lymphoma	
Drugs	
Penicillamine	
Hydralazine	
Propylthiouracil	
Nitrofurantoin	

(2) isolated gas transfer for carbon monoxide (DL_{CO}) deficit with or without pulmonary hypertension.

Other features of the underlying or associated disease may be present, and the pulmonary disorder may present as part of a pulmonary–renal syndrome, of which Goodpasture's disease is the best-known example.

Diffuse alveolar haemorrhage

The presenting features of diffuse alveolar haemorrhage often mimic infective pneumonia. The patient may give a history of fever, weight loss, and other systemic symptoms pointing towards the underlying diagnosis, but cough, breathlessness, and clinical signs suggestive of pneumonia are the main respiratory features. Indeed, if pneumonia is suspected on clinical and radiological grounds, but no organism is found, then other explanations need to be considered, including alveolar haemorrhage. A history of previous haemoptysis is helpful but not invariable: the first manifestation of diffuse alveolar haemorrhage can be acute.

Chest radiography shows consolidation, typically resolving within a matter of days, quite unlike the pattern seen in infective pneumonia, a point that can be helpful retrospectively if alveolar haemorrhage is not suspected at presentation. High-resolution computed tomography may reveal more subtle ground-glass partial alveolar filling. An acute fall in haemoglobin can occur; chronic iron-deficient anaemia suggests chronicity.

In the absence of a history of haemoptysis, confirmation of alveolar haemorrhage can be obtained by bronchoalveolar lavage that will reveal frank blood-staining in sequential lavage in the acute presentation, or the presence of numerous macrophages containing iron, identified by Perl's stain, in more chronic disease. The gas transfer corrected for alveolar volume (K_{CO}) is elevated in acute haemorrhage, but where this has occurred on a background of small, previously undetected, haemorrhage, the interstitial fibrosis consequent upon this chronic haemorrhage may have

Table 2 Chapel Hill International Consensus nomenclature of systemic vasculitis (1992)

	Lung disease
Large vessel	
Giant-cell arteritis	Rare
Takayasu's arteritis	Frequent
Medium size vessel	
Polyarteritis nodosa	Rare
Kawasaki disease	No
Small vessel (medium size vessel involvement may be present)	
Wegener's granulomatosis	Frequent
Churg–Strauss syndrome	Frequent
Microscopic polyangiitis	Frequent
Henoch–Schönlein purpura	No
Essential cryoglobulinaemia	No

Table 3 Investigations for suspected pulmonary vascular disease

Imaging
  Chest radiography with or without high-resolution computed tomography
Lung function tests
  Kco
Renal function
  Urine dipstick testing and microscopy for proteinuria, haematuria, and
    cellular casts; estimation of renal function; consider renal biopsy (if
    evidence of nephritis)
Immunology
  Antineutrophil cytoplasmic antibodies (ANCA), antiglomerular basement
    membrane (anti-GBM), immune complexes, rheumatoid factor,
    antinuclear antibodies (ANA), antiphospholipid antibodies
Bronchoalveolar lavage
  Iron-laden macrophages
Biopsy
  Renal
  Skin
  Lung (surgical)

reduced gas transfer such that an elevation above normal is not observed. If diagnosis remains elusive, surgical biopsy may be necessary to make the diagnosis and reveal the aetiology if vasculitis is responsible.

If a diagnosis of alveolar haemorrhage is suspected, investigations shown in Table 3 should be considered. Diffuse pulmonary haemorrhage occurring without identifiable cause or association is known as idiopathic pulmonary haemosiderosis (see Chapter 17.11.8). Pulmonary vasculitis can be primary or secondary.

Treatment is for the underlying cause. Prognosis can be poor in certain situations, most notably alveolar haemorrhage in rheumatological disease.

Isolated gas transfer deficit with or without pulmonary hypertension

A patient with an abnormality of the pulmonary vasculature, but in the absence of alveolar haemorrhage, will present with breathlessness on exertion. Clinical examination of the respiratory system will be normal, as will routine lung imaging. Lung function tests will show relatively well-preserved lung volumes, but with a reduced gas transfer factor (DLco and Kco). Exercise testing will demonstrate a fall in Pao$_2$, a drop in oxygen saturation, and widening of the alveolar–arterial (A–a) gradient, with a high ventilatory reserve. In severe pulmonary vascular disease, clinical features of pulmonary hypertension may be observed. This is most easily confirmed by echocardiography, particularly if tricuspid regurgitation is present, when a Doppler estimate of pulmonary artery pressures can be obtained. Right heart catheterization may be required to confirm the diagnosis. Other causes of vascular compartment abnormality such as systemic sclerosis, primary pulmonary hypertension, or coagulation abnormalities must be excluded.

Specific disorders

Churg–Strauss syndrome

This disease, first described by Churg and Strauss in 1951, is defined by the presence of numerous eosinophils and granulomatous inflammation in the respiratory tract, together with a necrotizing vasculitis affecting small to medium-sized vessels, and associated with asthma and eosinophilia. It is a rare disorder, mainly affecting adults around the age of 40 years, but has been reported in individuals from ages 7 to 74 years. In combined series

there is roughly a 2:1 prevalence for males to females. There is little information about geographical variation.

Aetiology and pathogenesis

This is not known, but thought to be an eosinophilic granulomatous response to a foreign antigen, akin to the eosinophilic granulomatosis seen in schistosomiasis. In this regard, immunological stimuli in the form of vaccination or immunotherapy have been reported as a trigger for the disease, but the pauci-immune nature of the histopathology raises doubts about this trigger mechanism.

More recently the introduction of antileukotriene therapy for asthma has resulted in an apparent increased incidence of Churg–Strauss syndrome. Two possible reasons have been advanced for this finding. First, that the drug has been a trigger for Churg–Strauss syndrome in predisposed individuals. Second, that the withdrawal or reduction of corticosteroids that has been possible with the introduction of non-steroid therapy has 'unmasked' the underlying condition. However, some individuals who have never been on corticosteroids have developed Churg–Strauss syndrome with the introduction of one of these drugs.

The relationship of antineutrophil cytoplasmic antibodies (**ANCA**) to disease pathogenesis is unclear. There have been studies demonstrating an up-regulation of the receptor for ANCA on the surface of neutrophils at disease sites, and ANCA can also interact with endothelial cells, causing injury and coagulation.

Clinical

Two sets of criteria have been used to define the disease clinically: Lanham's criteria and the criteria of the American College of Rheumatology. In addition to systemic features such as fever and weight loss, Lanham defined the disease as requiring the presence of the following:

(1) asthma;

(2) eosinophilia greater than 1.5×10^9/l in the peripheral blood; and

(3) evidence of systemic vasculitis in two or more non-lung organs.

The American College of Rheumatology defined Churg–Strauss syndrome as requiring four of the following six criteria:

(1) the presence of asthma;

(2) eosinophilia greater than 10 per cent in the peripheral blood;

(3) evidence of a neuropathy in a vasculitic pattern (e.g. mononeuritis multiplex);

(4) transient pulmonary infiltrates;

(5) a history of sinus disease; and

(6) evidence of extravascular eosinophilia on biopsy.

The disease is considered to evolve in three phases, the first (prodromal) consisting of a long history of rhinitis with nasal polyps that slowly progresses (often over years) to late-onset asthma, which is frequently difficult to treat. The second phase is of increasing peripheral blood and tissue eosinophilia that can wax and wane. The third and final phase is the manifestation of systemic vasculitis. This pattern of disease evolution has been shown in studies to be greater than 95 per cent specific and sensitive for Churg–Strauss syndrome. Table 4 illustrates the major pulmonary manifestations.

Other organ involvement

Skin lesions

These are seen in about 60 per cent of patients, generally manifesting as palpable purpura or subcutaneous nodules. Skin infarcts may also been seen.

Cardiac involvement

The heart may be involved diffusely, producing congestive cardiac failure or restrictive cardiomyopathy. Coronary artery inflammation may also be

Table 4 Distinguishing thoracic imaging features in primary vasculitis

	Churg–Strauss syndrome	Wegener's granulomatosis	Microscopic polyangiitis
Subglottic stenosis		+	+
Multiple nodules	+	+	
Solitary nodules		+	
Cavities		+	
Localized infiltrates		+	+
Transient infiltrates	+		+
Pleural involvement	+	+	
Cardiac involvement	+		

Adapted from Specks U (1998).

present, as can pericardial effusion. Cardiac disease is the most common cause of death in Churg–Strauss syndrome.

Renal disease

This is much less common than in Wegener's granulomatosis or microscopic polyangiitis, but the histopathology is very similar, consisting of a focal segmental necrotizing glomerulonephritis. Renal disease is generally mild, but endstage renal failure is reported.

Central nervous system

Mononeuritis multiplex is the most common manifestation, occurring in up to 75 per cent of patients. Cranial nerve involvement is less common, but cerebrovascular disease may occur.

Gastrointestinal involvement

Vasculitis of the mesenteric vessels may produce bowel abnormality, including perforation. Less commonly, eosinophilic infiltration may cause obstruction.

Musculoskeletal system

Arthritis is relatively common, as are myalgias.

Pathology

Lung biopsy shows a necrotizing angiitis, granulomas, and tissue eosinophilia. Giant cells and fibrinoid necrosis are present. It is not unusual to find only some of these features in a single biopsy and there can be overlap with the histopathological appearances of Wegener's granulomatosis and microscopic polyangiitis.

Investigations

Chest radiography shows areas of infiltration in the lung in up to 77 per cent of patients; pleural disease is seen in up to 50 per cent, and pericardial disease may occur with effusions sufficiently severe to cause tamponade. Computed tomography adds greater resolution to the imaging: nodules are uncommon and the main abnormalities are areas of ground-glass infiltrate, particularly if there is alveolar haemorrhage, which may also produce areas of consolidation.

There is a peripheral blood eosinophilia, matched by a marked eosinophilia on bronchoalveolar lavage. Antineutrophil cytoplasmic antibodies are found in roughly two-thirds of cases and are usually of the p-ANCA pattern.

Treatment

Initial treatment depends upon severity of presentation and the organs involved. In isolated pulmonary disease, the first-line treatment of choice is prednisolone at 1 mg/kg per day (up to a total of 60 mg/day) orally or, in more urgent situations such as alveolar haemorrhage, up to 1 g of methylprednisolone intravenously on each of three successive days. Response is usually good.

In more severe disease, particularly life-threatening situations when mechanical organ support is required, cyclophosphamide is added. This is

given either orally at 2 mg/kg per day up to a maximum usually of 150 mg/day, or intravenously as a bolus of 600 mg/m² as frequently as weekly in more severe disease. It is thought that intravenous administration of cyclophosphamide is less likely to provoke the major complication of cyclophosphamide therapy—haemorrhagic cystitis and subsequent malignancy—that are seen with prolonged oral use of this drug. Other immunosuppressive approaches have been tried, including azathioprine, methotrexate, and mycophenolate mofetil: the evidence in support of these treatments is less firm.

Because of the long-term side-effect profile of cyclophosphamide, especially bladder tumours, arguably the best approach to therapy would be to induce remission with either prednisolone alone or, in more severe presentations, prednisolone and pulsed intravenous cyclophosphamide, before maintaining that remission with prednisolone and one of the other immunosuppressant drugs. There is strong evidence that plasma exchange has no place in this or any other pauci-immune pulmonary vasculitis. Prophylactic co-trimoxazole (trimethoprim 160 mg/sulphamethoxazole 800 mg) three times a week is often used to reduce the risk of *Pneumocystis carinii* opportunistic infection.

Prognosis

Prognosis is generally good for those with isolated intrathoracic disease, but worsens with two or more extrapulmonary complications, particularly proteinuria greater than 1 g/day, renal insufficiency (creatinine greater than 140 μmol/l), cardiomyopathy, gastrointestinal disease, or central nervous system involvement. Five-year mortality for two or more of these complicating factors is 46 per cent, compared with 26 per cent with one and 12 per cent with none of the extrapulmonary features: recognition of this is useful in helping to determine initial therapy. Main causes of death are cardiac disease followed by renal failure, cerebrovascular involvement, and gastrointestinal disease. Lung disease accounts for 10 per cent of deaths.

Wegener's granulomatosis

The main description of Wegener's granulomatosis occurs elsewhere (see Chapter 20.10.3). It is a granulomatous inflammation due to necrotizing vasculitis affecting small to medium-sized vessels, typically involving the respiratory tract (both upper and lower) and often causing necrotizing glomerulonephritis.

Incidence

Wegener's granulomatosis is the third most common systemic vasculitis after giant-cell arteritis and rheumatoid arthritis. In 90 per cent of cases involvement of the upper and/or lower respiratory tract is the first manifestation, and in various series up to 85 per cent of patients have lung involvement at some stage of the disease. Males and females are affected equally.

Pulmonary presentation

In 34 per cent of cases lung involvement is asymptomatic. The main manifestations in the lung are (see Table 4):

(1) one or more nodules which can cavitate;

(2) localized or diffuse infiltrates (pleural effusions may be seen);

(3) alveolar haemorrhage that may be part of a pulmonary–renal syndrome; and

(4) large and small airway disease.

There is often a history of rhinosinusitis, often pre-dating other manifestations but seen at some stage of the disease in up to 92 per cent of cases. Presentations of lower respiratory tract involvement include the non-specific symptom of cough, with or without purulent sputum and haemoptysis. There is often fever, weight loss, and the systemic features of non-respiratory disease.

Chest radiography will show the presence of nodules or consolidation, the latter possibly due to inflammatory infiltrate or alveolar haemorrhage.

Pleural effusion may be present. High-resolution computed tomography will show these features with greater resolution and is the better modality to identify the number of nodules and determine whether they are cavitating. It is also very helpful in identifying tracheal and bronchial abnormality, including frank bronchiectasis. Characteristic airway involvement includes subglottic stenosis and stenosis of the main airways. Subtle parenchymal fibrosis may be seen as a reticular subpleural process mimicking fibrosing alveolitis.

Fibre-optic bronchoscopy may confirm airway disease, showing evidence of tracheobronchitis including ulceration and 'cobble-stoning' of the mucosa with, in more chronic situations, cicatricial narrowing of the airways with scar tissue. Bronchoalveolar lavage returns an excess of neutrophils and usually of eosinophils (with diffuse infiltrates) or lymphocytes (more interstitial disease), but the most important use of this procedure is to exclude an infective complication of the disease or its treatment, or alveolar haemorrhage. Transbronchial biopsy can be hazardous, resulting in major haemorrhage, and should be avoided. If lung biopsy is necessary to confirm the diagnosis, a surgical approach should be used, but usually it is possible to obtain a histological diagnosis from other tissue, particularly skin or kidney.

Haematological and biochemical investigations reflect the inflammatory process. The presence of c-ANCA is highly specific for this disease (up to 95 per cent in some series) and can be diagnostic in the right clinical context.

Pathology

The histopathological appearances of Wegener's granulomatosis include a necrotizing vasculitis, granuloma formation, necrosis, and surrounding inflammation with a combination of acute and chronic inflammatory cells. This and other non-pulmonary features are discussed in Chapter 20.10.3.

Treatment

First-line treatment is a combination of prednisolone at 1 mg/kg per day (usually up to a maximum of 60 mg), together with cyclophosphamide given either orally up to 150 mg/day or intravenously at 600 mg/m^2 at intervals dependent on disease severity. The hazards of cyclophosphamide given long-term and the alternative treatments are as for Churg–Strauss syndrome (see above). Co-trimoxazole therapy has been efficacious in this disease for localized upper respiratory tract or minor lower respiratory tract disease, but is not recommended for more systemic disease, although it appears to have a role in the maintenance of remission.

Prognosis

Since the introduction of combination immunosuppression the mortality from this disease has improved from a mean survival of 5 months to a 75 per cent complete remission. However, relapse occurs in up to 50 per cent of cases: long-term follow-up is needed.

Microscopic polyangiitis

The main description of microscopic polyangiitis occurs elsewhere (see Chapter 20.10.3). It is a necrotizing vasculitis that affects small vessels, with few or no immune complex deposits. Lung disease is said to occur in between 34 and 55 per cent of cases.

Pulmonary presentation (see Table 4)

The major presentation in the lung is diffuse alveolar haemorrhage, which can have a poor prognosis. Pulmonary capillaritis may be associated with evidence of disease outside the lung, particularly necrotizing glomerulonephritis, mononeuritis multiplex, and skin lesions. It may be difficult to distinguish microscopic polyangiitis from Wegener's granulomatosis without a biopsy, but if this is performed then the key issue is whether or not granulomas are present. Granulomas are not found in microscopic polyangiitis, whilst they are characteristic of Wegener's granulomatosis. Renal biopsies can be identical in the two conditions. Microscopic polyangiitis also needs

to be distinguished from polyarteritis nodosa that, by definition, only affects arteries, rarely arterioles, and never small vessels. Renal vasculitis with microaneurysm formation occurs in polyarteritis nodosa but not microscopic polyangiitis, and diffuse alveolar haemorrhage does not occur in polyarteritis nodosa.

Other diseases

Other primary systemic vasculitides may occasionally present with respiratory features.

Takayasu's arteritis

This arteritis affects predominantly the aorta and its main branches but can involve the pulmonary arteries in up to 50 per cent of patients, presenting with features of pulmonary vascular occlusion.

Giant-cell arteritis

There is rarely objective evidence of lung involvement, but 25 per cent of patients with giant-cell arteritis have associated cough, hoarseness, and sore throat at presentation.

The other systemic vasculitides that feature in the Chapel Hill International consensus nomenclature, but which rarely if ever present with lung disease, are Henoch–Schönlein purpura and essential cryoglobulinaemia.

Behçet's disease

This occurs predominantly in Mediterranean countries and can produce pulmonary vascular inflammation affecting all sizes of vessels and resulting in pulmonary arterial aneurysms, arterial and venous thrombosis, pulmonary infarcts, and pulmonary haemorrhage. It is crucial to differentiate haemorrhage from thrombosis because of the treatment implications.

Pulmonary veno-occlusive disease

This is a disorder of unknown cause that manifests with progressive occlusion of the post-capillary venules, resulting in features similar to those of pulmonary oedema. There is no known effective treatment. Differentiation from cardiogenic causes of raised pulmonary venous pressure must be made.

Lymphomatoid granulomatosis

This has been included historically within the category of pulmonary vasculitis but is now believed to be a lymphoproliferative disease.

Further reading

Conron M, Beynon HLC (2000). Churg–Strauss syndrome. In: du Bois RM, Tattersfield A, eds. *Thorax Rare Disease Series. Thorax*, **55**, 870–7.

Fauci AS *et al.* (1983). Wegener's granulomatosis: prospective clinical and therapeutic experience with 85 patients for 21 years. *Annals of Internal Medicine* **98**, 76–85.

Guillevin L *et al.* (1996). Prognostic factors in polyarteritis nodosa and Churg–Strauss syndrome. A prospective study in 342 patients. *Medicine* **75**, 17–28.

Jennette JC *et al.* (1994). Nomenclature of systemic vasculitides. Proposal of an International consensus conference. *Arthritis and Rheumatism* **37**, 187–92.

Langford CA, Hoffman GS (1999). Wegener's granulomatosis. In: du Bois RM, Tattersfield A, eds. *Thorax Rare Disease Series. Thorax* **54**, 629–37.

Lanham JG *et al.* (1984). Systemic vasculitis with asthma and eosinophilia: the clinical approach to the Churg–Strauss syndrome. *Medicine (Baltimore)* **63**, 65–81.

Lhote F, Guillevin L (1998). Polyarteritis nodosa, microscopic polyangiitis and Churg–Strauss syndrome. *Seminars in Respiratory and Critical Care Medicine* **19**, 27–46.

Specks U (1998). Pulmonary vasculitis. In: Schwarz MI, King TE Jr, eds. *Interstitial lung disease*, pp 507–34. BC Dekker, Hamilton, Canada.

17.11.6 Sarcoidosis

Robert P. Baughman and Elyse E. Lower

The aetiology of sarcoidosis is unknown. It is characterized by the presence of non-caseating granulomas in at least two organs. Patients may experience a variable course ranging from spontaneous remission to severe chronic disease and occasionally death.

Historical introduction

The disease was first recognized in 1869 by Jonathan Hutchinson, who treated a man with skin lesions that appeared unrelated to tuberculosis or any other process that he had encountered. Initially, most reports described patients with skin lesions. Since the disease is often self-limiting, pathological information was scarce. Schaumann in Sweden was one of the first to recognize the multiorgan nature of the disease, with the common pathological feature of granulomas. His original thesis was written in 1914, but not published until 1936.

After the Second World War, the use of routine screening radiography identified asymptomatic patients with abnormal chest radiographs. Lofgren described a group of patients with erythema nodosum, uveitis, and hilar adenopathy. Others began to appreciate the unique aspects of sarcoidosis compared with tuberculosis. Interestingly, as tuberculosis becomes less frequent in a country, sarcoidosis becomes more obvious. The observation that sarcoidosis is a disease of industrial nations and temperate climates may reflect this phenomenon. However, several groups have reported series of patients with sarcoidosis in India, Thailand, and China.

Pulmonary sarcoidosis can be evaluated by chest radiography. Scadding in Scotland and Wurm in Germany described a staging system based on the appearances seen on the chest radiograph, and this became a useful method of describing the extent of lung involvement. It also has prognostic significance and has been used for 40 years as the method of choice for characterizing lung involvement with sarcoidosis.

Newer radiological techniques have been evaluated in sarcoidosis. The chest CT scan provides more detailed information regarding adenopathy, but has not replaced the prognostic information available from the chest radiograph. A gallium scan will reveal increased uptake in areas of inflammation, such as lung and mediastinum. Magnetic resonance imaging (**MRI**) and positron emission tomography (PET) have brought new methods for evaluating extrapulmonary disease.

Bronchoalveolar lavage has provided a new method for sampling lower airway secretions, and it soon became apparent that the lavage findings from patients with sarcoidosis are distinctly different from normal subjects, providing insights into the true inflammatory response of the lung.

The definition of sarcoidosis had been the subject of much debate. An international sarcoidosis group began meeting in 1958. Currently this group, the World Association of Sarcoidosis and Other Granulomatous Diseases (WASOG), is chaired by D. Geraint James and tries to provide order from what was chaos. By consensus, the definition of sarcoidosis has been established and further refined over the years. The group now meets every 2 years and stresses the international aspects of the disease.

Aetiology

The cause of sarcoidosis remains obscure. One hypothesis is that sarcoidosis is an inflammatory response to an environmental agent (including infectious) which occurs in a susceptible host. Susceptibility is determined on the basis of genetic predisposition.

Several potential infectious agents have been proposed as causes of sarcoidosis. The granulomatous reaction reminds many of tuberculosis, and much effort has been expended trying to identify a mycobacterial cause. Several studies using polymerase chain reaction (PCR) and similar molecular biological techniques have been employed, but there is still no convincing evidence that *Mycobacterium tuberculosis* causes most cases of sarcoidosis. It may lead to an occasional case of sarcoid-like reaction. Other mycobacteria have been identified in some cases. Cell wall-deficient mycobacteria have been grown from the blood of patients with sarcoidosis. However, a recently completed control trial failed to demonstrate a difference in the incidence of cell wall-deficient mycobacteria between those with sarcoidosis and controls.

Epidemiology

Sarcoidosis is a worldwide disease. It has been reported to have a higher prevalence in Scandinavian countries as well as in Ireland. Table 1 summarizes the relative frequency of sarcoidosis per 100 000 people around the world. In the United States, a higher incidence of sarcoidosis has been reported in African-American people.

The disease presentation varies in different parts of the world. Table 1 also lists some of the more frequent patterns seen with various ethnic groups. For example, lupus pernio is common among African-American and West Indian people who have migrated to Great Britain, while erythema nodosum is common among Scandinavians. Cardiac disease has been reported at a higher frequency in Japanese patients with sarcoidosis than for other groups. HLA studies have suggested that there may be certain genetic patterns associated with particular manifestations of the disease.

Table 1 Sarcoidosis around the world

| | Scandinavia | Ireland | Japan | United States | | West Indies |
				African-American	Caucasian	
Prevalence per 100 000	1200	213	20	90	20	180
Female predominant	No	Yes	No	Yes	No	No
Erythema nodosum	+3 *	+3	Rare	Rare	+2	Rare
Lupus pernio	Rare	Rare	Rare	+1	Rare	+1
Hypercalcaemia	+3	+2	Rare	Rare	+2	Rare
Cardiac	Rare	Rare	+3	+1	+1	+1
Neurological	+1	+1	+1	+1	+1	+1
Hypergamma-globulinaemia	+1	+1	+1	+4	Rare	+1

* Scale from rare (< 1 per cent), +1 (1–5 per cent), +2 (5–10 per cent), +3 (10–30 per cent), +4 (>30 per cent).

Occupational exposures have been studied as a possible cause of sarcoidosis. Beryllium is a metal used in certain industries (ceramics, nuclear processing) which can cause a reaction in the lung and skin indistinguishable from sarcoidosis. Besides clinical history, the distinguishing feature about berylliosis is that lymphocytes are stimulated to replicate when exposed to beryllium salts. The lymphocyte stimulation test of blood, or the more sensitive bronchoalveolar lavage, is a reliable way of detecting which patients are reacting to beryllium.

There are other occupations associated with sarcoidosis. These include health-care workers, who have been found to be at increased risk. In one study, the odds ratio of a health-care worker acquiring sarcoidosis was 64 times the rate of the general population. Such a high rate could be due to work-related exposures (medications, disinfectants), or be due to an infectious agent. Clusters of sarcoidosis have been reported among firemen and aircraft-carrier personnel.

Obviously, none of these occupational exposures encompass all cases of sarcoidosis. One possible cause of sarcoidosis is that it is the common reaction to several possible agents.

Pathogenesis

Sarcoidosis is defined by its immunological reaction, the granuloma. Original immunological studies stressed a lack of systemic immune response by the patient with sarcoidosis. This includes anergy, which is a common feature of active sarcoidosis. A reduction in circulating leucocytes, especially lymphocytes, is an important feature of the disease.

In the 1970s, new techniques helped us understand sarcoidosis better. The most important tool introduced at the time was bronchoalveolar lavage, which provided a sample of the inflammatory cells in the lower respiratory tract. In normal lavage fluid, alveolar macrophages are the usual resident inflammatory cell retrieved; lymphocytes and neutrophils are found much less frequently. In lavage fluid from patients with active sarcoidosis, the preponderance of T lymphocytes is usually increased. These lymphocytes are often T-helper/inducer cells (CD4+), and the ratio of CD4

to CD8 lymphocytes is increased from that normally found in the blood, often to greater than 3.5.

The CD4 lymphocyte is a crucial cell in cell-mediated immunity. The CD4 lymphocytes are activated and release several cytokines, including interleukin 2 (**IL-2**) and γ-interferon. The T lymphocyte can mount either a T_{H1} or T_{H2} response. The T_{H1} response is associated with granuloma formation, while T_{H2} is associated with an eosinophilic response and fibrosis. The initial response of sarcoidosis follows a T_{H1} pattern. The lymphocytes release IL-2 spontaneously, and γ-interferon is released by both lymphocytes and macrophages. An increase in IL-12 and lower levels of IL-10 have also recently been described, consistent with a T_{H1} response.

The alveolar macrophage is also activated in sarcoidosis, and increased levels of IL-1, tumour necrosis factor, and oxygen free radicals are released by macrophages retrieved by bronchoalveolar lavage. During the evolution of the disease, the macrophages and other resident cells may release factors associated with fibrosis. For example, IL-8 is found in the bronchoalveolar lavage fluid of some patients with sarcoidosis, and this increase in IL-8 is associated with the finding of fibrosis in the lung.

The resolution of sarcoidosis has also been studied with serial lavages. The T lymphocytes remain elevated for some time, but the proportion of CD4 to CD8 decreases to the ratio in blood (0.8 to 2.2). The amount of cytokines released also decreases. This return to normal of the inflammatory response has been shown to occur during treatment of sarcoidosis with corticosteroids or methotrexate.

Clinical features

Patients with sarcoidosis may have a variety of presentations. Commonly affected organs include the lung, skin, and eyes. Less commonly, the liver, heart, and brain are affected by the disease. Individual organ involvement by sarcoidosis can be proved by a biopsy showing non-caseating granuloma. Presumed organ involvement is assumed if certain criteria are met. Table 2

Table 2 Organ involvement in patients with biopsy-confirmed sarcoidosis

Organ	Definite	Probable
Lung	Positive biopsy of lung	Lymphocytic alveolitis by bronchoalveolar lavage
	Chest radiograph characteristic for sarcoidosis (hilar adenopathy, diffuse infiltrates, or upper lobe fibrosis)	Any other pulmonary infiltrate
	Pulmonary function tests showing restriction	Isolated reduction of DLCO
Skin	Positive biopsy of skin	Macular/papular lesion
	Lupus pernio	New nodules (including subcutaneous)
	Erythema nodosum	
	Annular lesion	
Eyes	Positive biopsy of eye	Blindness
	Lacrimal gland swelling	
	Uveitis	
	Optic neuritis	
Liver	Positive biopsy of liver	Compatible CT scan
	Liver function tests more than 3 times normal	Elevated alkaline phosphatase
Neurological	Positive biopsy of nerve tissue	Other abnormalities on MRI
	MRI with gadolinium uptake in meninges, brainstem, or mass lesion	Unexplained neuropathy
	Cerebral spinal fluid with increased lymphocytes or protein	Positive electromyogram
	Diabetes insipidus	
	Cranial seventh nerve paralysis	
	Other cranial nerve dysfunction	
Cardiac	Positive cardiac biopsy	Cardiomyopathy or ventricular arrhythmias and no
	Treatment-responsive cardiomyopathy	other cardiac problems
	ECG showing intraventricular or nodal block	Positive thallium scan
	Positive gallium scan of heart	

Patients with documented sarcoidosis and no other explanation for organ-specific abnormality.

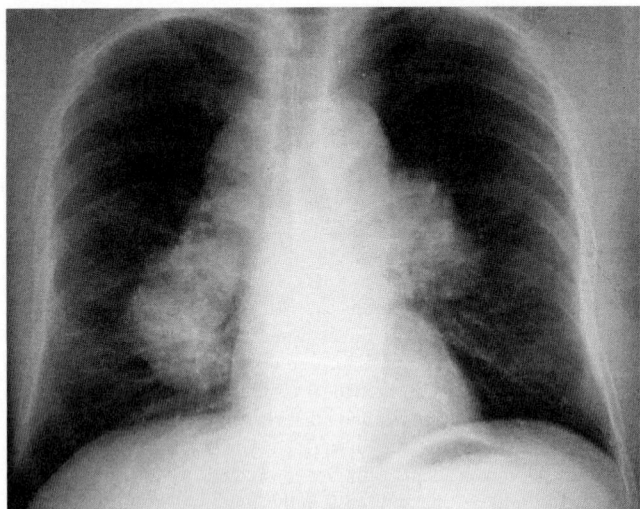

Fig. 1 Chest radiograph showing stage 1 sarcoid.

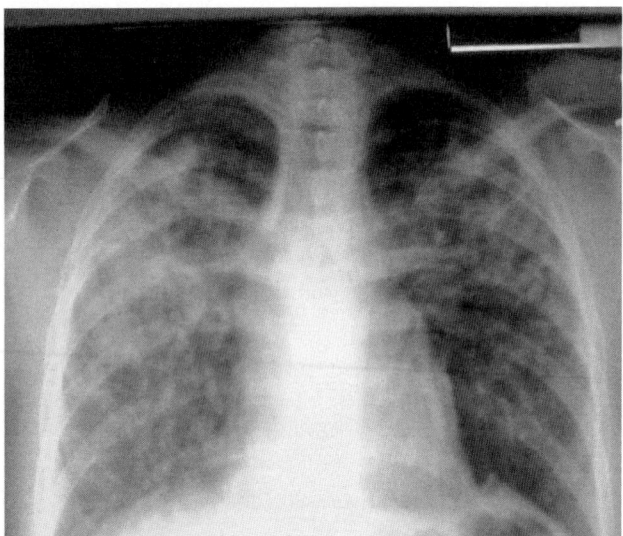

Fig. 2 Chest radiograph showing stage 3 sarcoid.

lists some of the criteria suggested for definite or probable organ involvement for some of the more commonly affected organs in sarcoidosis.

Lung

Respiratory involvement has been described in more than 90 per cent of patients. The lung involvement includes both the lymph nodes and the lung parenchyma. Scadding and Wurm independently described four stages of the chest radiograph: stage 1 is hilar adenopathy alone (Fig. 1), stage 2 is adenopathy and parenchymal disease, stage 3 is parenchymal disease alone (Fig. 2), and stage 4 is fibrosis. The interstitial disease usually has a diffuse reticulonodular appearance, but confluent patches of disease (alveolar sarcoidosis) have been described. Fibrotic changes due to sarcoidosis are usually in the upper lobe, with retraction. The staging system has proved useful in standardizing reports of pulmonary level of involvement. It has also proved a useful prognostic measure. Patients with stage 1 disease have a 90 per cent rate of resolution within 2 to 3 years, while patients with stage 3 disease possess only a 30 per cent chance of resolution. However, it does not predict the degree of extrapulmonary disease. The choice of the term 'stage'

is therefore unfortunate. However, it is so standard that it will not be easily replaced.

Table 3 lists the other diseases to be considered in the differential diagnosis based on the chest radiograph pattern. The presence of mediastinal adenopathy alone (stage 1 disease) is certainly consistent with lymphoma or metastatic cancer. It has been pointed out that symmetrical bilateral adenopathy with right paratracheal adenopathy in an asymptomatic individual is almost always sarcoidosis. Asymmetrical adenopathy raises the question of lymphoma, and a tissue diagnosis is usually required. For patients with diffuse infiltrates, adenopathy points one toward sarcoidosis. However, several other conditions may have some adenopathy, including hypersensitivity pneumonitis and idiopathic pulmonary fibrosis. The larger the adenopathy, the more likely is sarcoidosis.

The use of the CT scan has changed our evaluation of many interstitial lung diseases. In sarcoidosis, peribronchial thickening is often seen in the upper lobe. Adenopathy is usually seen in sarcoidosis, making the staging system only applicable for plain radiographs. The CT scan may identify adenopathy in a patient with possible extrapulmonary sarcoidosis. This may help in deciding where to proceed with a tissue diagnosis (brain biopsy or mediastinoscopy).

Pulmonary function studies in patients with sarcoidosis classically demonstrate a restrictive pattern, with reduction of lung volumes. The transfer factor is usually reduced out of proportion to the loss of lung volume, as one would expect in an interstitial lung disease. In advanced cases, the oxygen level will be reduced, especially during exercise. Obstructive disease can also occur in sarcoidosis. This can be due to airway involvement by the sarcoidosis or associated with cough, a common complaint in the condition.

Skin

The skin is the second most commonly affected organ in sarcoidosis. There are six major manifestations. Hyperpigmentation, hypopigmentation, and keloid reaction may demonstrate granulomas on biopsy. However, their appearance is not always specific. Waxy, maculopapular lesions, which occur on the extremities, back, and face, are usually raised, with the majority less than 2 cm in diameter. When these occur on the face, especially on the cheeks and nose, they are called lupus pernio. Erythema nodosum—red nodular lesions on the extremities—usually involves the legs. The constellation of erythema nodosum, arthritis (in the ankles), hilar adenopathy, and uveitis is referred to as Lofgren's syndrome and is a diagnostic manifestation of sarcoidosis. It is associated with a good prognosis. Interestingly, the skin lesions from erythema nodosum do not contain granulomas, but are felt to be due to circulating immune complexes from the disease.

Eye

The eye can be affected in more than 20 per cent of patients with sarcoidosis. The most common findings are uveitis and lacrimal gland involvement. Anterior uveitis is often self-limiting, and can be treated topically; however, posterior uveitis is a more chronic form of the disease and may require injections of corticosteroids or systemic therapy. Sicca (dry eyes) and glaucoma are long-term complications which are encountered in patients often years after other sarcoidosis symptoms have resolved. They are consequences of the fibrotic changes in the lacrimal glands and eye. They do not respond to anti-inflammatory therapy. Optic nerve involvement can be seen with sarcoidosis, with idiopathic disease and multiple sclerosis being the other major causes of this sight-threatening complication. Retinal disease has also been reported. Fortunately, blindness from sarcoidosis is rare, and usually a consequence of untreated uveitis, retinitis, or optic neuritis.

Neurological

Neurological disease from sarcoidosis includes cranial nerve, central nervous system, and peripheral nerve involvement. Bell's palsy (seventh cranial nerve) is a common complaint in neurosarcoidosis. Central nervous system lesions can lead to a lymphocytic meningitis. Hypothalamic involvement is

Table 3 Stage of chest radiograph and differential diagnosis

Stage 1 Hilar adenopathy	Stage 2 Adenopathy plus lung infiltrates	Stage 3 Lung infiltrates alone	Stage 4 Fibrosis
Other common diseases with similar radiographic pattern			
Tuberculosis	Lymphangitic carcinoma	Lymphangitic carcinoma	Lymphangitic carcinoma
Lymphoma	Pneumocystis carinii	Pneumocystis carinii	Pneumoconiosis
Enlarged pulmonary arteries	Pneumoconiosis	Pneumoconiosis	Histoplasmosis
Metastatic carcinoma	Histoplasmosis	Histoplasmosis	Idiopathic pulmonary fibrosis
Histoplasmosis	Berylliosis	Idiopathic pulmonary fibrosis	Berylliosis
		Berylliosis	Hypersensitivity pneumonitis
		Hypersensitivity pneumonitis	Bronchoalveolar cell carcinoma
		Bronchoalveolar cell carcinoma	Pneumonia
		Pneumonia	Congestive heart failure
		Congestive heart failure	Collagen vascular disease associated lung disease
		Collagen vascular disease associated lung disease	Eosinophilic granuloma
		Eosinophilic granuloma	
Other rare diseases with similar radiographic pattern			
Leukaemia	Alveolar proteinosis	Sjögren's syndrome	Sjögren's syndrome
Infectious mononucleosis	Idiopathic haemosiderosis	Haemosiderosis	Haemosiderosis
	α_1-Antitrypsin disease	Alveolar proteinosis	Alveolar proteinosis
	Bronchoalveolar cell carcinoma		

a characteristic finding, with diabetes insipidus as a resulting complaint. The use of contrast-enhanced magnetic resonance imaging is the most sensitive method for detecting central nervous system disease. The lumbar puncture is complementary, with increased protein and lymphocytes often seen in active disease. Detection of angiotensin-converting enzyme in the spinal fluid is suggestive but not diagnostic of neurosarcoidosis.

Other manifestations

Liver and spleen involvement may be found in over half of patients with sarcoidosis. However, symptomatic disease occurs in less than 10 per cent of patients. Often, elevated liver function tests (especially the alkaline phosphatase and γ-glutamyl transferase) are seen, suggesting an obstructive pattern. Hyperbilirubinaemia is relatively rare, but implies extensive disease and is usually an indication for therapy. Massive splenomegaly can occur, and occasionally splenectomy is performed to avoid rupture.

Hypercalcaemia and hypercalcinuria are seen with sarcoidosis. The mechanism is related to the effect of the granuloma on vitamin D_3. The granuloma itself converts the vitamin D_3 to the biologically active form $1,25-D_3$. This form of the vitamin has immunological activity as well as enhancing calcium absorption from the gastrointestinal tract. In some patients with sarcoidosis, the $1,25-D_3$ can leak into the bloodstream and produce a systemic effect. Increased sunlight exposure also increases the levels of $1,25-D_3$. In America, hypercalcaemia is far more common in Caucasian than African-American individuals. Because of the effect of increased calcium absorption, urolithiasis may also be seen in patients with sarcoidosis. Recently, it has been appreciated as a marker for chronic disease.

A less common, but serious complication of sarcoidosis is cardiac involvement. Direct involvement of the heart can lead to arrhythmias such as heart block and ventricular ectopy. This can lead to sudden death. If the problem is recognized, the use of an implanted defibrillator may reduce this risk. Cardiomyopathy is also seen, and cardiac sarcoidosis should be considered in a young patient who presents with unexpected heart failure. Endomyocardial biopsy rarely makes a diagnosis, since the granulomas are patchy. The technetium scan showing non-segmental fixed defects is the most sensitive test. Gallium uptake of the heart is more specific than a thallium scan.

Sarcoidosis granulomas can involve virtually any organ of the body. Rare manifestations include bone cysts, usually in the distal portion of the

fingers, sinus invasion, pleural disease, breast disease, and ovarian or testicular masses.

The multiorgan involvement of sarcoidosis distinguishes it from other diseases. Lymphoma and tuberculosis are two diseases often considered in the differential diagnosis of patients with possible sarcoidosis. Table 4 summarizes the common features in all three of these diseases and points out those features that can be used to separate them.

Pathology

The non-caseating granuloma is the characteristic pathological feature of sarcoidosis (Fig. 3). The centre of the granuloma includes macrophages and giant cells which are of the Langerhans type and can contain over 10 nuclei. This core of cells is surrounded by two rings of lymphocytes, the larger inner component of CD4 helper cells, while the outer ring can be CD8

Table 4 Comparison of features of sarcoidosis, tuberculosis, and lymphoma

Feature	Sarcoidosis	Tuberculosis	Hodgkin's lymphoma
Bilateral hilar adenopathy	Very common	Rare, except in patients with HIV	Common
Skin lesions	Common	Rare	Rare
Lupus pernio	Diagnostic	None	None
Erythema nodosum	Common	Rare	Very rare
Hypercalcaemia	Can occur	Very rare	Rare
Eye disease	Common	Rare	Very rare
Pleural disease	Very rare	Common	Common
Bell's palsy	Common	Very rare	Very rare
Elevated ACE	Very common	Rare	None
Tuberculin skin test	Anergic	Positive	Anergic
Bronchoalveolar lavage lymphocytes	Very common	Common	Very rare

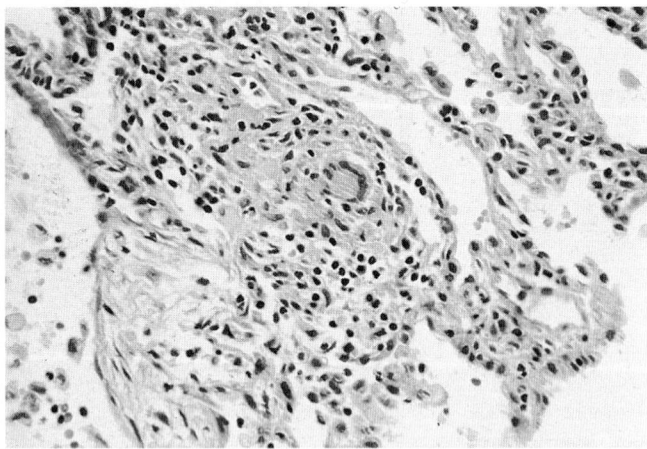

Fig. 3 Transbronchial biopsy demonstrating a non-caseating granuloma in the centre of the field. A multinuclear giant cell is seen within the granuloma. (Haematoxylin and eosin stain, original magnification ×40.)

suppressor cells. The granulomas tend to be well formed, and in lung biopsies are often well demarcated from normal tissue. The central area will occasionally contain a Schaumann body, formed of crystallized material (calcium phosphate). This is different in appearance from foreign bodies or caseation, which can be seen in other granulomatous diseases. Occasionally the granuloma will have a necrotic area, but the majority of the granulomas do not.

Because the cause of sarcoidosis is unknown, one can never be absolutely confident of the diagnosis, which is always one of exclusion. However, the finding of non-caseating granulomas in two or more organs is considered diagnostic. Cultures and special stains for tuberculosis and deep-seated fungal infections should be taken to rule out infection as the cause of granulomas. Close examination should also be made for foreign bodies and malignancy, both of which can lead to a granulomatous reaction.

Laboratory diagnosis

Serum angiotensin-converting enzyme (ACE) levels

In 1976, Lieberman reported that ACE level was elevated in the blood of some patients with sarcoidosis. Mild elevations have also been reported in diabetes mellitus and osteoarthritis. High levels have been detected in patients with infectious granulomatous diseases such as tuberculosis, histoplasmosis, and coccidioidomycosis; but also in Gaucher's disease, leprosy, and hyperthyroidism. Because ACE is measured using a biological assay, patients on ACE inhibitors may have low levels.

In those with granulomatous disease, the source of the ACE is not the lung (the usual source), but the granulomas themselves. It appears that ACE has immunoregulatory properties.

Determining the significance of the ACE level in sarcoidosis can be difficult for a variety of reasons. Sixty per cent of patients with acute disease will have elevated values, whilst only 10 per cent of patients with disease for more than 2 years will continue to have an elevated level. The ACE level will decrease in response to treatment or disease resolution, and it has therefore been proposed as a marker for disease activity. However, corticosteroids independently suppress ACE levels, and reducing the dose of corticosteroids may lead to a rise in ACE level without a clinical worsening of disease. Furthermore, since ACE levels are elevated in only a small proportion of those with chronic disease, decreases observed with serial measurement may simply reflect the long-standing nature of the disease.

There is a genetic polymorphism for ACE, with an insertion (I) or deletion (D) of a genomic DNA fragment. There appears to be no difference in the distribution of the alleles in patients with sarcoidosis compared with the general population. Interestingly, ACE levels are higher in DD patients,

and this needs to be considered when one is measuring the serum ACE level. There is some evidence that the DD allele is associated with a worse prognosis in patients with sarcoidosis, and it is interesting to note that DD alleles have also been associated with a worse outcome in patients with coronary artery disease.

The serum lysozyme can also be elevated in sarcoidosis in the same way as ACE. However, it is elevated in a smaller proportion of patients and not routinely used in clinical practice.

Tests of the lung

Bronchoalveolar lavage findings can be characteristic in sarcoidosis. The finding of increased lymphocytes, especially an increased CD4 to CD8 ratio, has been interpreted by some groups as enough to make the diagnosis of sarcoidosis, and in a patient with a compatible clinical history and no evidence for infection or malignancy, the lavage findings may be considered sufficient. A more definitive answer from bronchoscopy includes a transbronchial biopsy showing non-caseating granulomas. In over 60 per cent of patients with a stage 1 chest radiograph the biopsy should be positive, rising to 80 per cent in patients with stage 2 or 3 disease. Transbronchial needle aspiration has recently been used to sample hilar lymph nodes, but raises the problem of incomplete sampling in patients with a malignancy and granulomatous response to the lesion. Mediastinoscopy and videoassisted thoracoscopy provide a minimally invasive method to obtain more tissue.

The gallium scan can reveal increased activity in patients with sarcoidosis. The activated macrophage has increased levels of transferrin receptors on its surface and this results in an increase in gallium uptake. Unfortunately, interpreting the uptake in the lung may be difficult as it is non-specific and occurs with other inflammatory lung diseases. It also rapidly returns to normal with corticosteroid therapy. On the other hand, the uptake in the parotid and conjunctiva (the 'panda' sign) and the uptake in the hilar nodes (the 'lambda' sign) are fairly characteristic for sarcoidosis and are useful confirmation in difficult cases.

Other tests

The Kveim–Siltzbach agent is a suspension of spleen tissue from a patient with confirmed sarcoidosis. Six weeks after an intradermal injection of the agent, the site is inspected for a reaction, which will occur in over 60 per cent of patients with acute sarcoidosis. On biopsy, the reaction will show non-caseating granulomas, consistent with sarcoidosis. Properly prepared Kveim–Siltzbach agent has a less than 1 in 500 chance of causing a false positive. However, because of the difficulties in preparing the agent and concerns regarding the risk of transmission of an infectious agent, the test is rarely used except in those centres with a well established reagent.

Other laboratory tests may support the diagnosis of sarcoidosis or be useful in monitoring the level of disease activity. The erythrocyte sedimentation rate can be elevated in sarcoidosis and fall with remission of the disease, but one-third of patients will have a normal sedimentation rate, so it is not specific or sensitive.

Serum calcium is elevated in 10 per cent of cases and is supportive of the diagnosis, but hypercalcaemia can be seen in other conditions which mimic sarcoidosis, such as malignancy. Hypercalcaemia due to sarcoidosis should be associated with a normal to low serum phosphorus. In patients with significant hypercalcaemia, renal failure may occur, reversible in many cases with lowering of the serum calcium.

Hypergammaglobulinaemia is also a feature of sarcoidosis. Activated T lymphocytes in the lung are capable of stimulating circulating peripheral blood B cells, leading to the polyclonal gammaglobulin response. As a result of this non-specific reaction, serological markers for some diseases may be falsely elevated. This includes antifungal antibodies and antinuclear antibodies. Hypergammaglobulinaemia is more common in African-American than Caucasian individuals.

Liver involvement occurs in over half of patients with sarcoidosis. In some cases the liver blood tests are entirely normal, but the majority of patients with liver involvement have elevated serum enzymes. Usually the pattern is obstructive, with a rise in the serum alkaline phosphatase, but in some an elevation of the transaminases is seen. Elevation of the serum bilirubin is less frequent and associated with more extensive liver involvement. Rarely, lymphadenopathy at the porta hepatis can lead to biliary obstruction.

Haematological abnormalities are common in sarcoidosis. Lymphopenia is frequently seen, and is probably due to sequestration of lymphocytes into the area of inflammation, such as the lung. Anaemia has been reported in about 20 per cent of patients. The mechanism is multifactorial, including a high proportion of patients with iron deficiency. Other causes include direct bone marrow invasion by granulomas. Cytokines such as IL-2 may also result in suppression of the bone marrow.

Treatment

The natural course of sarcoidosis is unclear, since corticosteroids are normally used to treat symptomatic patients. For the patient with no symptoms on presentation, the prognosis is often good. Spontaneous resolution commonly occurs within a year or two of diagnosis, but the disease can also take a chronic form, with symptoms for many years. The concept of acute disease, which lasts for less than 2 years, as opposed to chronic disease has been a useful method for considering patients, especially in terms of therapy. Table 5 lists several factors associated with resolution within 2 to 5 years as well as those predicting chronic disease. Acute disease is associated with erythema nodosum, hilar adenopathy, anterior uveitis, and Bell's palsy. Whereas chronic disease includes such manifestations as lupus pernio, stage 4 chest radiograph, posterior uveitis, and bone cysts. Most chronic disease is controllable by therapy, but there is a refractory form of the disease which often involves the cardiac and central nervous systems. Mortality from sarcoidosis occurs, but is less than 5 per cent in most series.

The major indication for therapy in sarcoidosis is symptoms. Hypercalcaemia should be treated, even if the patient is asymptomatic. An eye examination should be performed in all patients with sarcoidosis. Uveitis may be misdiagnosed as sicca (dry eyes). The former will require anti-inflammatory agents, while the latter will only need a wetting agent.

If possible, treatment should be topical. Corticosteroid creams and eye drops are effective if inflammation is superficial. The effectiveness of inhaled steroids is less clear-cut. The higher-potency steroids such as budesonide appear to have a role in reducing the dosage of systemic corticosteroids. Several randomized trials have indicated a role for this drug as maintenance therapy for a patient who has received systemic therapy for 3 months to induce remission.

It is not clear whether corticosteroids change the natural course of the disease. Early randomized trials found no difference in the long-term outcome of patients who received corticosteroids compared with controls. A British Thoracic Society randomized study did demonstrate a small benefit for corticosteroids over placebo for patients with persistent, but not severe, disease. One of the difficulties in assessing this and other trials is that the

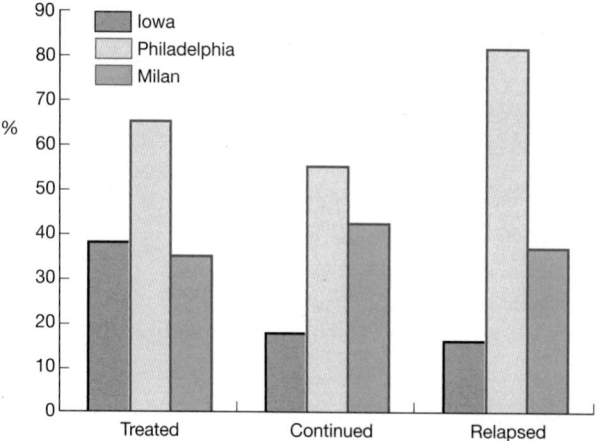

Fig. 4 The results of corticosteroid therapy from three medical centres. The first set of columns demonstrates the percentage of patients treated. The second set of columns represents the percentage of patients who required therapy to be continued beyond 2 years. The last set of columns reports the subgroup of people initially treated with corticosteroids and tapered off treatment who subsequently required reinstitution of therapy.

more severely affected patients were treated with corticosteroids and excluded from the study.

Figure 4 summarizes the use of systemic corticosteroid therapy at three large centres over a period of several years. The genetic background of each group varies, with the Iowa group being mostly of Scandinavian descent, Philadelphia being African-American, and Milan being Italian. In general, 30 to 60 per cent of patients never required therapy. However, once therapy was instituted, in 18 to 53 per cent of the patients it could not be withdrawn. In patients who were tapered off corticosteroids, one group found that 80 per cent eventually relapsed and required reinstitution of therapy. The differences in rate of continued therapy and relapse between the centres could be due to either the genetic background of the patients or the bias of the treating physicians.

Once systemic steroids are initiated, one has to remember that a prolonged course is usually necessary. In the beginning, doses may be changed every 1 to 3 months, but after a patient tolerates a lower dose (equivalent to less than 10 mg of prednisolone per day), tapering may be prolonged. The use of alternate-day corticosteroids is strongly advocated by some, but others are less enthusiastic. Rarely will alternate-day therapy be sufficient for initial control of the disease.

The toxicity of corticosteroids is well known. These include weight gain, diabetes mellitus, hypertension, and mood swings. Avascular necrosis and osteopenia are significant problems with prolonged use. Some patients with sarcoidosis will have lost weight as part of their disease. However, the weight gain with treatment often surpasses the amount of weight loss. The longer a patient is on corticosteroids, the greater the risk of problems. Unfortunately, most patients will require more than a year of treatment.

Several alternatives to systemic corticosteroids have been proposed over the years. These are summarized and compared with corticosteroids in Table 6. We include the usual doses, commonly encountered toxicities, an estimate of response rate, and the usual indications for use.

The commonly prescribed antimalarial agents chloroquine and hydroxychloroquine possess anti-inflammatory activity with their major toxicities being eye and gastrointestinal. Because hydroxychloroquine, especially at 400 mg a day or less, is unlikely to cause eye toxicity, it is more frequently prescribed. However, some experts feel chloroquine is a more effective agent. These drugs concentrate in the skin and are most efficacious for skin disease and hypercalcaemia. They are less successful in the treatment of pulmonary disease. A recent report described some utility in patients with neurological disease.

Table 5 Features predictive of clinical course of sarcoidosis

Organ	Acute	Chronic
Chest radiograph	Stage 1	Stage 4
Skin	Erythema nodosum	Lupus pernio
Eyes	Anterior uveitis	Posterior uveitis
		Pars planitis
Joint involvement		Bone cysts
Calcium metabolism	Hypercalcaemia	Renal stones
Cardiac		Cardiomyopathy
Neurological	Cranial seventh nerve palsy	Central nervous system mass
Sinus		Sinus involvement

Table 6 Treatment for sarcoidosis

Drug	Dosage	Efficacy (%)	Toxicity	Usage
Prednisone/prednisolone	5–40 mg/day	90	Weight gain, diabetes, hypertension, osteoporosis, psychiatric	Acute, chronic, refractory
Methotrexate	10–25 mg once a week	60–80	Haematological, gastrointestinal, lung, hepatic, mutagenic	Chronic, refractory
Hydroxychloroquine	200–400 mg/day	30–50	Gastrointestinal, retinal	Acute, chronic
Azathioprine	50–200 mg/day	50–80	Haematological, gastrointestinal, carcinogenic, mutagenic	Chronic, refractory
Pentoxifylline	400 mg three times a day	50	Gastrointestinal	Acute
Cyclophosphamide	50–150 mg/day orally, 500–2000 mg every 2 weeks intravenously	80	Gastrointestinal, haematological, carcinogenic, bladder, teratogenic	Chronic, refractory
Thalidomide	50–100 mg/day	80	Teratogenic, somnolence, peripheral neuropathy	Chronic, refractory

Methotrexate is an antimetabolite chemotherapy used for various solid tumours. Over 30 years ago it was first noted as an immunosuppressant for the treatment of rheumatoid arthritis. In that disease, it prevents joint destruction and is often used to avoid steroid toxicity. In sarcoidosis, methotrexate has been most studied as a treatment for chronic disease. This probably reflects the fact that it may require 6 months for the drug to become effective. The usual dose is 10 to 15 mg orally each week, adjusted if this proves toxic. Acute toxicity including mucositis and nausea can be minimized with supplements of folic acid at 1 mg/day. Leucopenia can also occur, but is usually insignificant unless the patient is already leucopenic from sarcoidosis or the patient has renal insufficiency. We have successfully treated patients with doses as small as 2.5 mg of methotrexate a week. The long-term toxicity of methotrexate can include hypersensitivity pneumonitis and cirrhosis. The latter is a concern, because 50 per cent of patients with chronic disease will have sarcoid granulomas in a liver biopsy, and we recommend liver biopsies every 2 years for patients requiring the drug long term. Methotrexate is teratogenic, but current data suggest it is not carcinogenic.

The response rate to methotrexate in chronic sarcoidosis is 60 to 80 per cent. Most patients who respond can be treated with methotrexate alone. Approximately 20 per cent of patients will require additional low-dose corticosteroids. In most patients skin lesions can be easily controlled with methotrexate, but studies have also reported benefit for disease in the lungs, eyes, and nervous system.

Azathioprine has been used for many years as an immunosuppressant for patients receiving solid-organ transplants and those with idiopathic pulmonary fibrosis. However, its use in sarcoidosis has been more sporadic, usually reserved for chronic cases. Its major side-effects are gastrointestinal and haematological.

Other drugs have been used for refractory sarcoidosis. Cyclophosphamide is used in the treatment of many vasculitic diseases and has been reported as very useful in neurological and cardiac sarcoidosis, but it has more gastrointestinal, haematological, and bladder toxicity than methotrexate or azathioprine.

Case reports suggest that thalidomide may be useful in treating sarcoidosis. It has severe teratogenic effects and may cause peripheral neuropathy and drowsiness. Cyclosporin has been used with limited success in some neurological cases. A recent randomized trial failed to show additional benefit over corticosteroids alone in patients with pulmonary sarcoidosis. The drug is relatively expensive, causes hypertension and renal failure, and requires blood levels to be monitored. Pentoxyfylline has been shown by one centre to provide some benefit in acute sarcoidosis. It is associated with significant gastrointestinal toxicity, which is dose dependent.

There is no single treatment for all patients with sarcoidosis. Figure 5 summarizes our clinical approach. The first step is to determine whether the patient requires treatment. The decision to treat is usually based on the patient's symptoms. The clinician needs to determine the extent of the symptomatic disease and whether the disease is acute or chronic. Asymp-

tomatic or minimally symptomatic patients with hypercalcaemia, cardiac, or central nervous system disease may require therapy to prevent life-threatening complications. The use of systemic therapy usually means corticosteroids first. However, over time, the patient and the physician may need to seek alternatives.

Prognosis

Sarcoidosis will resolve within 2 to 5 years in the majority of cases. Approximately 25 per cent of patients will develop residual fibrosis. In a minority of patients, the disease will become chronic and persist for more than 5 years.

For the patient with chronic disease, treatment can usually palliate the symptoms. However, organ failure—including eye, liver, cardiac, or respiratory—can occur as a result of disease.

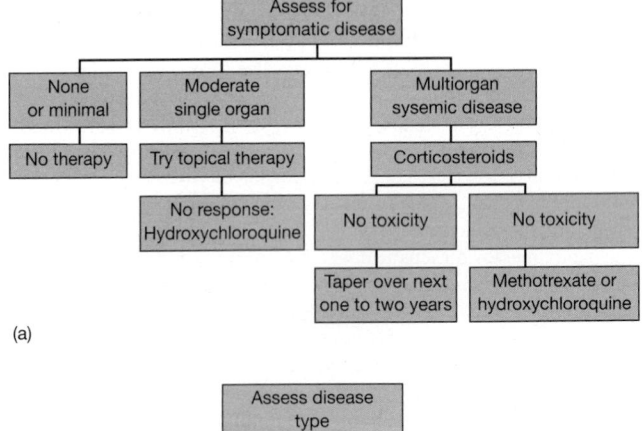

(a)

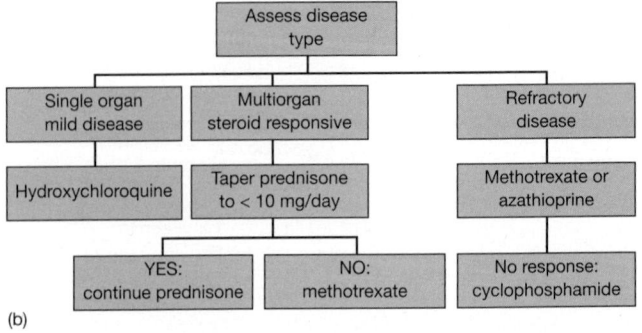

(b)

Fig. 5 The approach to treatment of patients with sarcoidosis at the Interstitial Lung Disease Clinic at the University of Cincinnati. Patients are initially classified as having either acute (a) or chronic (b) disease. Further evaluation depends on their symptoms and response to therapy.

Most series from referral centres report a 5 per cent mortality from sarcoidosis, most commonly due to respiratory failure, but with cardiac, neurological, and hepatic failure as other causes. Respiratory failure leading to death can be predicted from pulmonary function tests. For example, one study found that of those with a vital capacity persistently less than 1 litre, a third died of respiratory failure, whereas no patient with a vital capacity of over 1.5 litres did so. The 5 per cent mortality reported from referral centres is higher than that encountered in a non-referral setting, where the mortality approximates 1 per cent. Organ transplantation has been performed successfully in patients with sarcoidosis. Although sarcoidosis lesions can occur in the new organ, organ failure due to recurrent sarcoidosis is unlikely.

Special problems

Endstage lung disease is the most common problem for patients with severe sarcoidosis. The fibrotic disease leads to cor pulmonale and respiratory distress. In addition, cavitary lesions can lead to bronchiectasis or become colonized with aspergillus. Aspergillomas can cause fatal haemoptysis. Their treatment can be difficult because most patients are not good surgical candidates. Embolization has been used for life-threatening bleeding.

Steroid-induced osteopenia is a significant problem with long-term corticosteroid therapy. Because of the risk of hypercalcaemia, patients are often not given calcium supplements, but this should be considered if a patient requires long-term systemic steroids. Monitoring serum calcium during therapy is usually sufficient to avoid complications. The use of nasal calcitonin or oral bisphosphonates should also be considered.

Areas of uncertainty/controversy

Some clinicians have proposed the use of bronchoalveolar lavage as the exclusive diagnostic test for sarcoidosis. This is based on the rationale that in the appropriate clinical setting, bronchoalveolar lavage findings of increased lymphocytes and a CD4 to CD8 ratio of greater than 3.5 represents a granulomatous process. In patients with cultures negative for tuberculosis and fungal infection, sarcoidosis is most likely and no further diagnostic testing may be needed. The percentage of patients with increased lymphocytes and CD4 to CD8 ratio varies from centre to centre. In our institution, at least 50 per cent of patients with sarcoidosis will meet these criteria. However, the use of bronchoalveolar lavage does not provide an absolute diagnosis of sarcoidosis. As previously noted, transbronchial needle aspirate may also be useful in making a diagnosis; however, the finding of a granuloma does not guarantee the diagnosis. One way to interpret the bronchoalveolar lavage or tissue results is to consider each as complementary in making the diagnosis of sarcoidosis.

The use of corticosteroids for the treatment of sarcoidosis remains controversial. In the patient with minimal symptoms, treatment can be withheld or topical agents used. If the disease spontaneously resolves, no therapy is indicated. However, if the patient becomes symptomatic, corticosteroids will probably be useful. The treatment of the patient with persistent, mild disease is unclear. The British Thoracic study suggests that these patients should receive corticosteroids, but others argue that the benefits are small and do not justify the use of these agents.

Areas needing further research

The cause of sarcoidosis remains unknown. The newer techniques of molecular biology may provide additional insight into a causative agent or the underlying genetic predisposition for the disease.

Patients with chronic disease represent a disproportionate number of cases with increased morbidity and need for medical services. The use of corticosteroids alone is not adequate for many of these patients. Research into whether other agents are truly steroid sparing and associated with a good clinical outcome are still necessary.

Further reading

Agbogu BN *et al.* (1995). Therapeutic considerations in patients with refractory neurosarcoidosis. *Archives of Neurology* **52**, 875–9.

Agostini C, Semenzato G (1998). Cytokines in sarcoidosis. *Seminars in Respiratory Infections* **13**, 184–96.

Bardelli AM *et al.* (1993). Eye involvement in sarcoidosis: survey of 197 patients. *Sarcoidosis* **10**, 158–9.

Baughman RP, Lower EE (1997). Steroid-sparing alternative treatments for sarcoidosis. *Clinics in Chest Medicine* **18**, 853–64.

Baughman RP *et al.* (1997). Predicting respiratory failure in sarcoidosis patients. *Sarcoidosis Vasculitis and Diffuse Lung Diseases* **14**, 154–8.

Crystal RG *et al.* (1981). Pulmonary sarcoidosis: a disease characterized and perpetuated by activated lung T-lymphocytes. *Annals of Internal Medicine* **94**, 73–94.

Gibson GJ *et al.* (1996). British Thoracic Society Sarcoidosis study: effects of long term corticosteroid treatment. *Thorax* **51**, 238–47.

Gottlieb JE *et al.* (1997). Outcome in sarcoidosis. The relationship of relapse to corticosteroid therapy. *Chest* **111**, 623–31.

Hance AJ (1998). The role of mycobacteria in the pathogenesis of sarcoidosis. *Seminars in Respiratory Infection* **13**, 197–205.

Hirose Y *et al.* (1994). Myocardial involvement in patients with sarcoidosis. An analysis of 75 patients. *Clinics in Nuclear Medicine* **19**, 522–6.

Hunninghake GW *et al.* (1994). Outcome of the treatment for sarcoidosis. *American Journal of Respiratory and Critical Care Medicine* **149**, 893–8.

Izumi T (1988). Sarcoidosis in Kyoto (1963–1986). *Sarcoidosis* **5**, 142–6.

James DG, ed. (1994). *Sarcoidosis and other granulomatous disorders.* Marcel Decker, New York.

Johns CJ, Zachary JB, Ball WC (1974). A ten year study of corticosteroid treatment of pulmonary sarcoidosis. *The Johns Hopkins Medical Journal* **134**, 271–83.

Judson MA *et al.* (1999). Defining organ involvement in sarcoidosis: the ACCESS proposed instrument. *Sarcoidosis Vasculitis and Diffuse Lung Diseases* **16**, 75–86.

Lower EE, Baughman RP (1995). Prolonged use of methotrexate for sarcoidosis. *Archives of Internal Medicine* **155**, 846–51.

Lower EE *et al.* (1997). Diagnosis and management of neurologic sarcoidosis. *Archives of Internal Medicine* **157**, 1864–8.

Lower EE *et al.* (1988). The anemia of sarcoidosis. *Sarcoidosis* **5**, 51–5.

Lynch JPI, McCune WJ (1997). Immunosuppressive and cytotoxic pharmacotherapy for pulmonary disorders. *American Journal of Respiratory and Critical Care Medicine* **155**, 395–420.

Lynch JP, Kazerooni EA, Gay SE (1997). Pulmonary sarcoidosis. *Clinics in Chest Medicine* **18**, 755–85.

Lynch JP, Sharma OP, Baughman RP (1998). Extrapulmonary sarcoidosis. *Seminars in Respiratory Infection* **13**, 229–54.

Maliarik MJ *et al.* (1998). Angiotensin-converting enzyme gene polymorphism and risk of sarcoidosis. *American Journal of Respiratory and Critical Care Medicine* **158**, 1566–70.

Neville E, Walker AN, James DG (1983). Prognostic factors predicting the outcome of sarcoidosis: an analysis of 818 patients. *Quarterly Journal of Medicine* **208**, 525–33.

Newman LS, Rose CS, Maier LA (1997). Sarcoidosis. *New England Journal of Medicine* **336**, 1224–34.

Parkes SA *et al.* (1987). Epidemiology of sarcoidosis in the Isle of Man—1: A case controlled study. *Thorax* **42**, 420–6.

Pietinalho A *et al.* (1999). Oral prednisolone followed by inhaled budesonide in newly diagnosed pulmonary sarcoidosis: a double-blind, placebo-controlled, multicenter study. *Chest* **116**, 424–31.

Rizzato G, Montemurro L (1993). Reversibility of exogenous corticosteroid-induced bone loss. *European Respiratory Journal* **6**, 116–19.

Rizzato G, Montemurro L, Colombo P (1998). The late follow-up of chronic sarcoid patients previously treated with corticosteroids. *Sarcoidosis Vasculitis and Diffuse Lung Diseases* **15**, 52–8.

Selroos O (1969). The frequency, clinical picture and prognosis of pulmonary sarcoidosis in Finland. *Acta Medica Scandinavica Supplementum* **503**, 3–73.

Selroos O, Sellergren TL (1979). Corticosteroid therapy of pulmonary sarcoidosis. *Scandinavian Journal of Respiratory Diseases* **60**, 215.

The Committee on Sarcoidosis of the American Thoracic Society (1999). Statement on sarcoidosis. *American Journal of Respiratory and Critical Care Medicine* **160**, 736–55.

Thomas PD, Hunninghake GW (1987). Current concepts of the pathogenesis of sarcoidosis. *American Review of Respiratory Disease* **135**, 747–60.

17.11.7 Pneumoconioses

A. Seaton

Most lung diseases are caused or provoked at least in part by the inhalation of harmful material. A wide range of lung conditions, including cancer (exposure to asbestos, radon daughters in mines, polycyclic aromatic hydrocarbons, nickel refining, chloromethyl ethers), pneumonia (legionnaire's disease in hospitals), asthma (flour, isocyanates, epoxy resins), allergic alveolitis (farmer's lung, maltworker's lung), and toxic pneumonitis (silo-filler's disease, chlorine poisoning, cadmium poisoning), may occur as a result of workplace exposure. When exposure to mineral dust in the workplace results in a diffuse, usually fibrotic, reaction in the lung acinus, the condition is called a pneumoconiosis.

The distinction between tuberculosis and a specific effect of dust in the causation of respiratory disease was made in the mid-nineteenth century. By this time silicosis, often complicated by tuberculosis, was widespread amongst metal miners, tunnellers, potters, and cutlers. The Industrial Revolution stimulated the need for coal, and the production of this fuel resulted in increasing numbers of sufferers from coal-worker's pneumoconiosis. This in turn was not distinguished from silicosis until the late 1940s, and in some countries the two conditions are still referred to by the one name.

In the United Kingdom, and generally in the West, dust control in mines and decline of traditional industries have resulted in a reduction in the numbers of workers suffering from these two diseases. By contrast, industrialization of developing countries has stimulated the need for indigenous coal and minerals, and in China, South America, and India several million workers are employed in mining, often in conditions which ensure a high incidence of pneumoconiosis. At the same time, the rise of the asbestos and chemical industries has added new problems for society in weighing the benefits of the product against the cost in terms of human morbidity. Fortunately, these problems are potentially soluble by application of preventive measures, as emphasized in the following sections.

Coal-worker's pneumoconiosis

Coal-worker's pneumoconiosis is caused by inhalation of coal-mine dust, a complex mixture of coal, kaolin, mica, silica, and other clay minerals. It is now uncommon in the United Kingdom, and good dust control together with reductions in the workforce imply that the disease may disappear in the next few years. Nevertheless, the strategic importance of coal as a long-term source of fuel supply and as a chemical feedstock means that it will continue to be needed, and any relaxation of dust control in mines will be followed by the reappearance of pneumoconiosis. There has also been a reduction in the incidence of coal-worker's pneumoconiosis in other West-ern countries, but in China the disease is widespread and in India it afflicts about 1 to 2 per cent of the current workforce of 800 000.

Aetiology and pathology

The pathogenicity of coal dust differs in different areas. If lung damage is to occur, the dust must be inhalable to acinar level within the lung. Thus the particles must have aerodynamic characteristics that make them equivalent to a sphere of unit density between 0.5 and 7 μm in diameter. Once inhaled, the particles must be able to overcome the lung's defences. Some, containing a high proportion of quartz (crystalline silicon dioxide), are toxic to macrophages and cause their disruption after phagocytosis. Such particles are cleared predominantly to the lymph nodes where they remain and set up a fibrotic reaction that ultimately destroys the node. However, some remain in the peribronchiolar and perivascular parts of the acinus, where whorled fibrosis occurs leading to the typical silicotic nodule. The mechanisms of quartz-induced fibrosis are discussed further in the silicosis section. However, since most coal dust contains relatively little quartz and is not particularly toxic to macrophages *in vitro*, some other explanation for its harmfulness must be sought. *In vivo* studies in rats have shown that inhalation of relatively low concentrations of coal dust, comparable with those occurring in United Kingdom mines in the recent past, cause inhibition of macrophage migration and provoke an inflammatory response, mediated *inter alia* by interleukin 1 (**IL-1**) and tumour necrosis factor, resulting in the release of elastase and the degradation of fibronectin. It seems likely that these toxic effects *in vivo* on macrophages are fundamental to the pathological processes in coal-worker's pneumoconiosis, including the concomitant centriacinar emphysema.

The total amount of dust inhaled is also a critical factor in the development of pneumoconiosis. Epidemiological studies have shown clear relationships between cumulative dust exposure and radiological evidence of disease. However, this is not straightforward, as some coal dusts are clearly more toxic than others, and it is not always possible to characterize this toxicity by the relative mineralogical composition of the coal dust. There is evidence that the different minerals in coal dust interact and that some clays may reduce its overall toxicity, perhaps by blocking the surface activity of the toxic fraction. As a general rule, the higher the combustibility (rank) of the coal, the more likely is its dust to cause pneumoconiosis (Fig. 1).

Pathologically, coal-worker's pneumoconiosis is characterized by the presence of multiple centriacinar and interlobular foci of dust, inflammatory cells, macrophages, and reticulin or collagen—the coal macule (Fig. 2). In miners exposed to relatively high proportions of quartz, the lesions have a greater resemblance to the silicotic nodule. The presence of small discrete nodules is known as simple pneumoconiosis, and when sufficient numbers of these lesions are present they become visible on a radiograph. Complicated pneumoconiosis, or progressive massive fibrosis, is present by definition when one or more of these lesions is greater than 1 cm in diameter

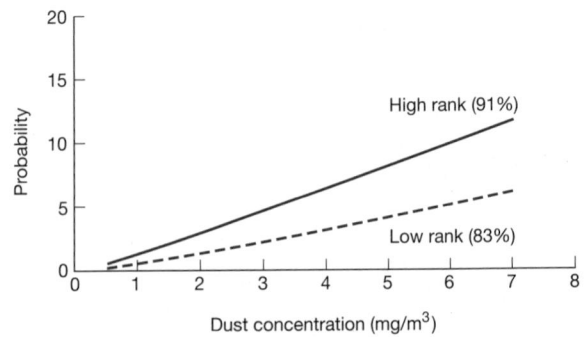

Fig. 1 Relationship between risk of category 2 or 3 radiological simple pneumoconiosis and daily exposure over a working lifetime to different concentrations of coal dust. The greater risk in association with exposure to dust from coals of higher combustibility (rank) should be noted.

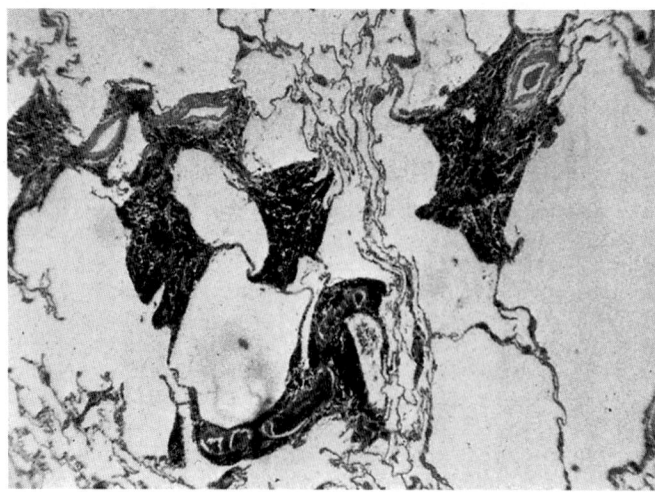

Fig. 2 Simple coal macules, showing accumulations of dust and cells around centre of lobule with associated emphysema.

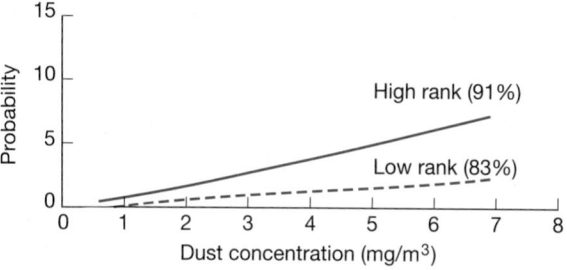

Fig. 4 Relationship between risk of progressive massive fibrosis and exposure to dust over a working lifetime. Again, greater risk in association with exposure to dust from coals of higher combustibility (rank) should be noted.

(Fig. 3). This occurs either by aggregation of several, usually collagenous, smaller nodules or by a more diffuse accumulation of dust associated with dead cells and ischaemic necrosis of lung tissue. The former, less common, mechanism occurs particularly in relation to relatively high quartz exposures, while the latter seems more frequent with exposure to high carbon dusts. With either type, and with intermediate types, there is a tendency for the lesions to grow and to be associated with surrounding bullous emphysema, ultimately being responsible for destruction of large volumes of the lung.

The aetiology of progressive massive fibrosis is not completely understood. It is more common in the upper lung zones and in taller men, suggesting a relationship to failure of lung clearance. High carbon or high quartz dusts are particularly liable to cause progressive massive fibrosis, and the higher the dust exposure, the greater is the risk (Fig. 4). Tuberculous infection is no longer an important factor in the developed world, although it may have been in the past. The rheumatoid diathesis is responsible for initiating a rare type of progressive massive fibrosis (Caplan's syndrome),

but this is not an important factor overall. For further discussion of the aetiology of progressive massive fibrosis, see the section on silicosis below.

Clinical features

The people most at risk of coal-worker's pneumoconiosis are those working in the dustiest areas, such as face-workers cutting coal, drilling for shot-firing, developing headings, and drilling bolts into the roof to prevent it falling. Open-cast miners rarely work in such dusty circumstances, except in hot dry countries such as India where loading operations may be extremely dusty. Simple coal-worker's pneumoconiosis causes no symptoms or physical signs, nor any important physiological abnormality. This fact is of importance, as symptoms of respiratory disease in a miner with this condition are due to some other cause, such as bronchitis, heart failure, or asthma, which may be treatable. Radiological progression or regression of simple pneumoconiosis occurs only very rarely after dust exposure ceases, apparent regression sometimes being associated with the development of emphysema.

The danger associated with simple pneumoconiosis is that it predisposes to progressive massive fibrosis, a risk directly related to the profusion of simple pneumoconiosis on the radiograph. Progressive massive fibrosis may occur during working life or appear for the first time after (sometimes many years after) dust exposure ceases, even when there is no apparent simple pneumoconiosis on the radiograph. Progressive massive fibrosis usually progresses and causes a mixture of restriction of lung volumes and, owing to associated emphysema, airflow obstruction. Ultimately it may lead to cor pulmonale and death. However, the rate of progression is very variable. In general, the earlier progressive massive fibrosis develops in a person's life, the more rapidly progressive and thus the greater a threat to health it is.

The patient with progressive massive fibrosis may complain of shortness of breath and symptoms of cor pulmonale. An unusual, but pathognomonic, symptom is melanoptysis—the expectoration of the black contents of a cavitated lesion. Haemoptysis and finger clubbing suggest lung cancer and should not be attributed to pneumoconiosis. Abnormal signs in the chest, if present, relate to the presence of bullae, although sometimes lobar collapse can occur.

Coal-worker's pneumoconiosis is not associated with an increased risk of tuberculosis or lung cancer, although obviously these diseases can occur in coal miners and should be suspected if unusual progression of radiological changes occurs. The association between pneumoconiosis and emphysema has been controversial, but there is now clear evidence of a parallel association between dust exposure and two effects—pneumoconiosis and airflow obstruction. The more dust that a miner has been exposed to, the greater are his risks of pneumoconiosis on the one hand, and productive cough, reduction in forced expiratory volume in 1 s (FEV_1), and presence of centriacinar emphysema on the other. Of course, the latter risks are also related to cigarette smoking, and the effect of dust exposure is additive.

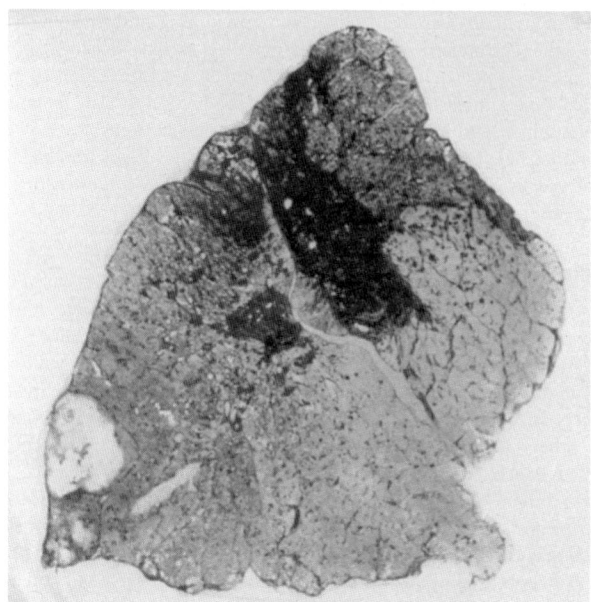

Fig. 3 Whole-lung section of a coal-miner's lung showing progressive massive fibrosis.

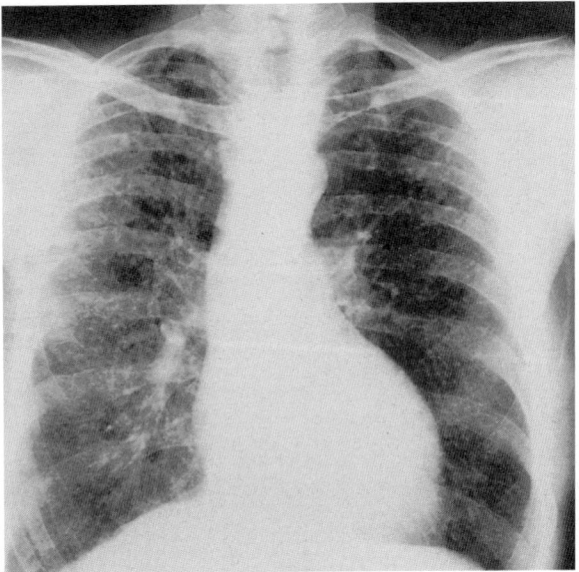

Fig. 5 Radiograph of a coal miner showing small round lesions of simple pneumoconiosis. Some irregular shadows are also present in the lower zones.

The radiological lesions in simple pneumoconiosis are predominantly rounded opacities between 1 and 5 mm in diameter, although small irregular and linear opacities and Kerley B lines are frequently present also. The round opacities tend to be more profuse in the upper and middle zones, whereas the irregular lesions predominate in the lower zone (Fig. 5). Progressive massive fibrosis almost always starts in an upper zone, gradually increasing in size until it may occupy up to a third of the lung. Such lesions are frequently multiple. They are often shaped like short fat sausages, with their outer border curved with the chest wall and separated from the pleura by bullous emphysema (Fig. 6). Calcification is not a feature, but cavitation of progressive massive fibrosis may occur. Caplan's syndrome is the name given to the combination of rheumatoid disease and several round nodules (usually 1 to 5 cm in diameter) in the lungs of a coal miner. The lesions have a rheumatoid histology and rarely cause any serious pulmonary impairment; they often cavitate and disappear. The radiological features of all pneumoconioses are properly described in terms of a set of standard radiographs produced by the International Labour Organization, and use of these standards is mandatory for epidemiological studies.

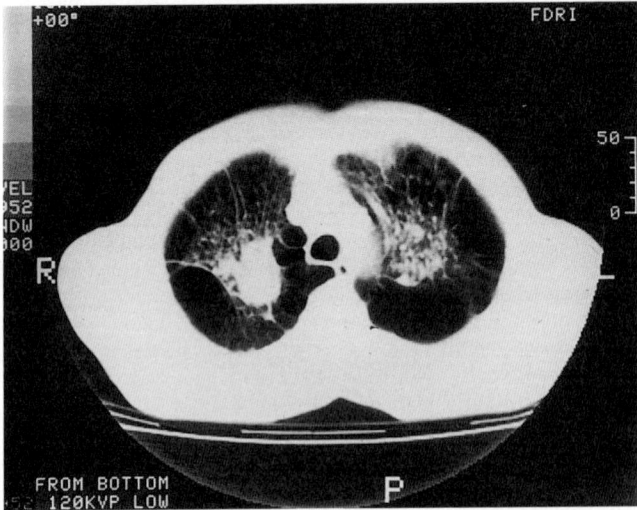

Fig. 6 CT scan of miner, showing central progressive massive fibrosis and surrounding bullous emphysema.

Prevention and management

Epidemiology has shown an exposure–response relationship between the total mass of respirable coal dust to which miners have been exposed and their risks of developing simple pneumoconiosis. This has allowed standards to be set for coal-mine dust levels, which have resulted in falls in the prevalence of the disease in coal mines in the West. Their success depends on regular monitoring of the respirable dust by gravimetric sampler, constant attention to dust suppression by ventilation and the use of water at points of dust production, and regular radiography of the workforce to detect early signs of dust retention. The incidence of progressive massive fibrosis is largely controlled by preventing miners from contracting simple pneumoconiosis, and working conditions in British mines are currently such that this disease is now very rare indeed. The present British standard is 7 mg/m³, measured in the air returning from the coalface.

If a miner develops simple pneumoconiosis late in his career, no action normally needs to be taken, apart from (in the United Kingdom) advising him to apply to the Respiratory Diseases Board via the Benefits Agency for assessment of disablement and possible benefit payments. A younger man, with several years of further dust exposure ahead, should be advised to work in an area of approved low dust conditions. This advice should be given in the United Kingdom by the employer's occupational health service. Men with more than the earliest stages of radiological change are entitled to disablement benefits from the Benefits Agency, the value of these depending on the extent of disability. Since simple pneumoconiosis *per se* does not disable, these benefits are often small. Payment of benefits for airflow obstruction as an associated effect of coal dust exposure are also made in the United Kingdom if the miner has worked underground for a minimum of 20 years and his FEV_1 is a litre below that predicted. The presence of associated radiological change is no longer necessary.

Silicosis

Silicosis is a fibrotic disease of the lungs due to inhalation of crystalline silicon dioxide, usually in the form of quartz. Such a disease has occurred in metal miners and masons since ancient times, but assumed particular importance in the cutlery and pottery trades in the nineteenth century. Silicosis may affect anyone involved in quarrying, carving, mining, tunnelling, grinding, or sandblasting, if the dust generated contains quartz. In the United Kingdom the traditional trades that caused the disease (pottery, cutlery, flint knapping, sandblasting, tin and iron mining, and slate quarrying) have either introduced safe substitute materials or have declined, so that true silicosis is now quite rare. Between 50 and 60 cases are diagnosed in the United Kingdom each year, usually in the production of slate or granite, among miners cutting through rock, and in fettlers in foundries. However, the author has seen a series of severe cases in British workers who had been employed in circumstances where the risks had been forgotten or were being ignored.

Aetiology and pathology

Crystalline silica is present in the earth's crust usually as quartz, although other forms such as crystobalite and tridymite occur occasionally. All are extremely toxic to macrophages. quartz seems to be most toxic when freshly fractured, suggesting that surface properties are important in toxicity. This concept is supported by experimental evidence that various clay minerals and other chemicals which occlude the surface reduce the toxicity of inhaled quartz when inhaled simultaneously in mixtures of dust. The quartz content of dust from different types of stone may vary considerably from some sandstones which are 100 per cent quartz to shales and slates which may contain less than 10 per cent.

Inhaled particles of quartz small enough (generally less than 7 μm aerodynamic diameter) to reach the acinus are engulfed by macrophages and cause disruption of the phagosome, probably by peroxidation of membrane lipids. Before macrophage death, other reactions occur leading to release of inflammatory mediators, including IL-1, various growth factors, tumour necrosis factor, and fibronectin, largely from interstitial rather than alveolar macrophages. Silica is probably transported across the alveolar epithelium by migrating macrophages and by endocytosis by type 1 alveolar cells, and it is clear from the distribution of pathological lesions that quartz is transported widely in the lung via lymphatics, much of it ultimately being deposited in hilar nodes, which it destroys. This destruction of the nodes is very likely to be responsible for blockage of the exit route for further inhaled dust, and therefore for its retention in the lung and the development of progressive massive fibrosis or, rarely, accelerated or even acute silicosis.

Macroscopic inspection of silicotic lungs shows fibrous pleural adhesions, enlarged lymph nodes that contain fibrotic, often calcified, nodules, and grey nodules throughout the lung. These nodules vary from a few millimetres to several centimetres in diameter and are more profuse in the upper zones (Fig. 7). They may be calcified, and they have a typical whorled appearance when cut across (Fig. 8). The largest lesions consist of many such nodules that have become confluent, and, as in coal-worker's pneumoconiosis, this progressive massive fibrosis may undergo ischaemic necrosis and cavitate. Under the microscope the silicotic nodule consists of concentric layers of collagen surrounded by a zone of doubly refractile silica particles, macrophages, and fibroblasts. The nodule may contain the remnants of the respiratory bronchiole and arteriole, destroyed by fibrosis. The mechanisms responsible are destruction of macrophages leading to inflammation and laying down of collagen, release of the quartz, further macrophage attraction, and repetition of the cycle. This presumably occurs first in nodes on the drainage pathway, and as these become progressively blocked the process is repeated in the lung. As the quartz never gets removed thereafter, the process continues indefinitely and severity of disease depends on the mass inhaled and retained.

Macroscopically, acute silicosis appears like pulmonary oedema. Under the microscope, the alveoli are filled with eosinophilic fluid and the alveolar walls contain plasma cells, lymphocytes, fibroblasts, and silica. In the

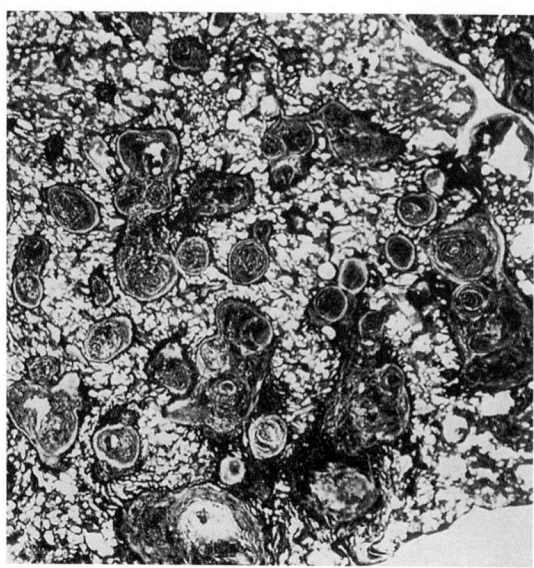

Fig. 8 Silicotic nodules, showing the typical whorled appearance.

author's experience, this condition first requires hilar node destruction by the inhaled quartz.

Clinical features

Silicosis presents a spectrum of clinical appearances depending on the circumstances in which it is contracted. The most severe, acute silicosis, may be acquired after very heavy exposure over only months, such as may occur in sandblasting without respiratory protection. Such patients become intensely breathless and die within months. The radiograph shows appearances resembling pulmonary oedema. Less heavy exposure causes progressively less dramatic symptoms, ranging from a progressive upper lobe fibrosis with slowly increasing exertional dyspnoea over several years (accelerated silicosis) to radiographic nodular change similar to coal-worker's pneumoconiosis unassociated with any symptoms or physical signs. The latter type of silicosis is the most common, and is usually associated with exposure to dust containing 10 to 30 per cent silica over a prolonged period. Simple nodular silicosis differs from coal-worker's pneumoconiosis in that the lesions tend to be larger (3 to 5 mm) and that it is progressive even after dust exposure ceases. Lesions increase in size and become more profuse. Moreover, extensive simple silicosis may be associated with some restriction of lung volumes. Simple silicosis rarely seems to be associated with emphysema, unlike coal-worker's pneumoconiosis, but silicotic progressive massive fibrosis is commonly associated with bullous disease. Curiously, it has only recently been recognized that acute enlargement of hilar nodes mimicking sarcoidosis may be an early feature of silicosis. Accelerated silicosis and progressive massive fibrosis cause lung restriction and lead to cor pulmonale and cardiorespiratory failure.

Apart from evidence of cardiac failure or distortion of lung architecture by extreme degrees of massive fibrosis, physical signs are not prominent. Clubbing and crackles are not seen. Diagnosis depends on a history of exposure and the radiographic appearances. The most characteristic of these are nodules between 3 and 5 mm in diameter, predominantly in the upper zones, and eggshell calcification in the hilar nodes (Fig. 9). The latter is virtually a pathognomonic feature, only occurring otherwise, very rarely, in sarcoidosis. All forms of silicosis are liable to be complicated by tuberculosis, usually due to reactivation of a quiescent lesion.

Other mycobacterial diseases (*Mycobacterium kansasii* and *Mycobacterium avium-intracellulare*) also occur more frequently than would be expected in those with silicosis. There is now evidence of a weak association between silicosis and lung cancer, even when exposures to cigarette smoke and other occupational carcinogens have been accounted for. The evidence

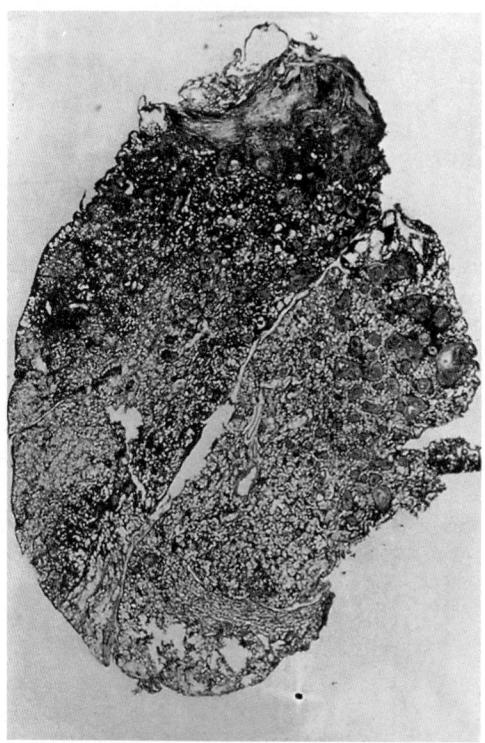

Fig. 7 Whole-lung section from a coal miner whose work had been predominantly in hard rock, showing silicotic nodules in upper parts of upper and lower lobes.

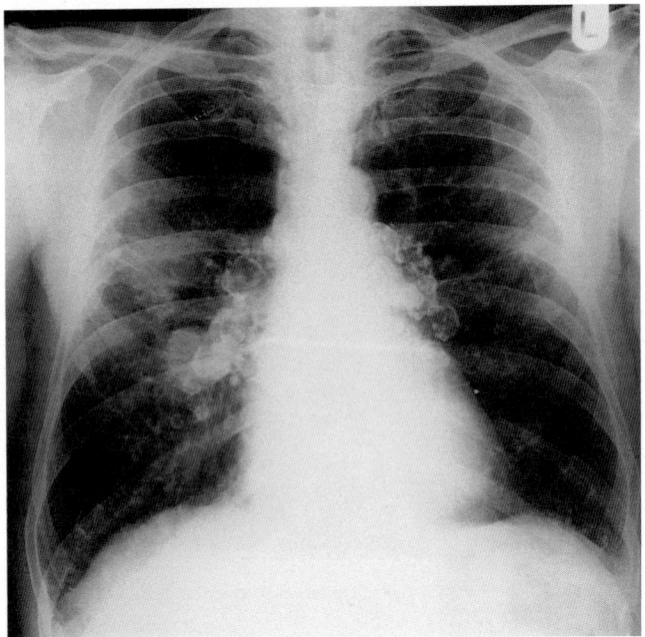

Fig. 9 Radiograph of a hard rock miner, showing massive fibrosis in right mid-zone and eggshell calcification of hilar nodes.

is sufficient for lung cancer to have been recognized as an occupational disease in patients with silicosis in the United Kingdom. Pneumothorax is an occasional complication of silicosis, as it is of any disease associated with lung fibrosis.

Subjects with silicosis, particularly of the accelerated type, seem to be at increased risk of the development of autoantibodies and of rheumatoid disease, scleroderma, and systemic lupus erythematosus; these conditions have been described in about 10 per cent of some series of patients with silicosis. Focal glomerulonephritis has also been described in silicosis, but the cause of this is unknown.

Prevention and management

The epidemiological evidence suggests that workers exposed to levels of respirable silica in excess of 1 mg/m³ have a high risk of silicosis, and that a risk may still exist even at levels of around 0.1 mg/m³. The United Kingdom maximum exposure limit is 0.3 mg/m³, and industry is obliged to keep exposures of workers below this level as far as practicable, by appropriate ventilation, extraction, and other dust suppression measures. For historic reasons, quartz exposures in coal mining are controlled by total dust levels rather than the silica component of the dust. If higher levels are inevitable, the worker should wear appropriate respiratory protection, although this must be regarded as a second-best and potentially risky procedure. Once a worker has developed the disease, he should be prevented from working with silica again. The only medical management necessary is regular sputum examination for tubercle bacilli, as tuberculosis accelerates the lung damage but responds normally to modern chemotherapy. Acute silicosis would nowadays be an indication for consideration of transplantation. In the United Kingdom, workers with silicosis (whether or not complicated by lung cancer) should apply to the Respiratory Diseases Board of the Benefits Agency for industrial injuries benefits.

Asbestosis

Asbestosis is pulmonary fibrosis caused by exposure to fibres of asbestos. It was originally described in the 1900s and its importance as an occupational disease was recognized by epidemiological studies in the 1930s. However, in the first century AD, Pliny recorded that the weavers of wicks for the lamps

of the vestal virgins wore masks for respiratory protection, and so some recognition of its hazards goes back to antiquity.

Asbestos is mined principally in Canada, South Africa, and the former Soviet Union. It is a generic term for a group of fibrous silicates, the most important being chrysotile (white), crocidolite (blue), and amosite (brown). Chrysotile has a serpentine configuration and breaks up into microfibrils, while the other types (amphiboles) are straight and less liable to longitudinal fracture (Fig. 10). All types are resistant to physical and chemical destruction, which gives them their commercial value in fireproofing, insulation, reinforcement of cement, weaving into cloth, bonding in brake linings and plastics, and so on. The asbestos is obtained by crushing the rock to release the fibres, which are then carded and transported in non-porous bags to the user industry.

Asbestos causes several separate pleuropulmonary lesions. The commonest are benign pleural plaques, but acute effusion and diffuse fibrosis also occur. Mesothelioma, discussed in Chapter 17.14.1), is the most important. It now occurs in over 1000 people in Britain annually and the incidence is predicted to rise further in relation to exposures some 30 years previously. It is most frequent in people who have worked in construction, ship repair, and such trades as electrician, plumber, and insulator, where regular direct or indirect exposure to asbestos has occurred. The pulmonary disease asbestosis occurs in about 100 people annually in the United Kingdom; all have worked regularly with asbestos for many years. Risk of lung carcinoma is also related to asbestos exposure, interacting multiplicatively with smoking. All these risks appear to have been greater with exposure to amphiboles than with exposure to chrysotile, but most workers

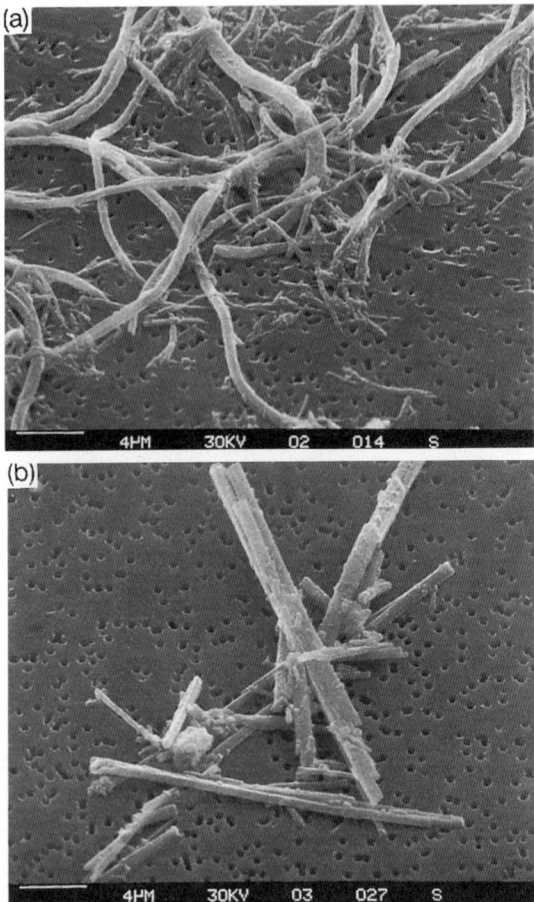

Fig. 10 Scanning electron micrographs of (a) chrysotile and (b) amosite on Millipore filters. The curly configuration and microfibrils of chrysotile should be noted. Scale bar, 4 µm.

(except in specific mining/production industries) have usually been exposed to a mixture of the different types.

Aetiology and pathology

The harmful asbestos fibres are those less than 3 μm in transverse diameter and greater than 10 μm in length, that is, sufficiently narrow to be inhaled to the acinus, yet too long to be removed by macrophages. Their toxicity depends on their dimensions and their persistence in lung tissue once inhaled. All types of asbestos of these dimensions can cause fibrosis and carcinoma when inhaled by rats. Moreover, injection of any asbestos type (and indeed many non-asbestos fibres) into the peritoneum of rats causes mesothelioma in a dose-related manner. The lower risk of mesothelioma in association with pure chrysotile exposure in humans is related to this fibre's curly configuration, which reduces the number penetrating the acinus, and its propensity to break up into minute short fibrils that can eventually be removed from the lung by the action of macrophages. As with coal and silica, the fibrogenicity of asbestos is probably related to damage to macrophages which are unable to cope with fibres much longer than themselves and the liberation of substances that activate fibroblasts to produce collagen. Among the substances shown to result from experimental challenge of rats with asbestos are tumour necrosis factor and macrophage- and platelet-derived growth factors.

The macroscopic appearance of an asbestotic lung is of grey fibrosis more marked peripherally and in the lower zones. In severe cases the fibrosis appears like a honeycomb. Yellow shiny parietal pleural plaques are also usually seen in the thoracic cavity, although these frequently also occur in the absence of pulmonary fibrosis. Microscopically there is diffuse alveolar wall fibrosis with minimal cellular infiltrate or desquamation of type 2 pneumocytes, initially around the centre of the acinus and later spreading to destroy the acinar structure, leading to the appearance of honeycombing. Larger asbestos fibres may be seen coated with a protein–ferritin complex (the asbestos or ferruginous bodies), while smaller fibres remain uncoated but may still just be visible with the light microscope (Fig. 11). However, for every fibre visible by light microscopy, several hundred uncoated fine fibres can always be found on electron microscopy. Pleural plaques have the appearance of basket-weave collagen, and fibres are almost never seen within them.

Clinical features

Asbestosis occurs in people exposed regularly over years to airborne asbestos as a result of the material being used or removed, and not as a result of occasional exposure. It is more likely to be seen in trades involving the application or removal of asbestos in lagging and insulation than in asbestos mining, preparation, or weaving, where control of fibre levels is more

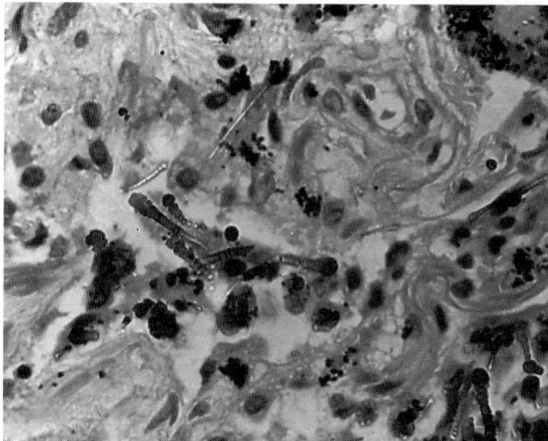

Fig. 11 Histological appearance of asbestosis, with interstitial fibrosis, asbestos bodies, and several uncoated fibres.

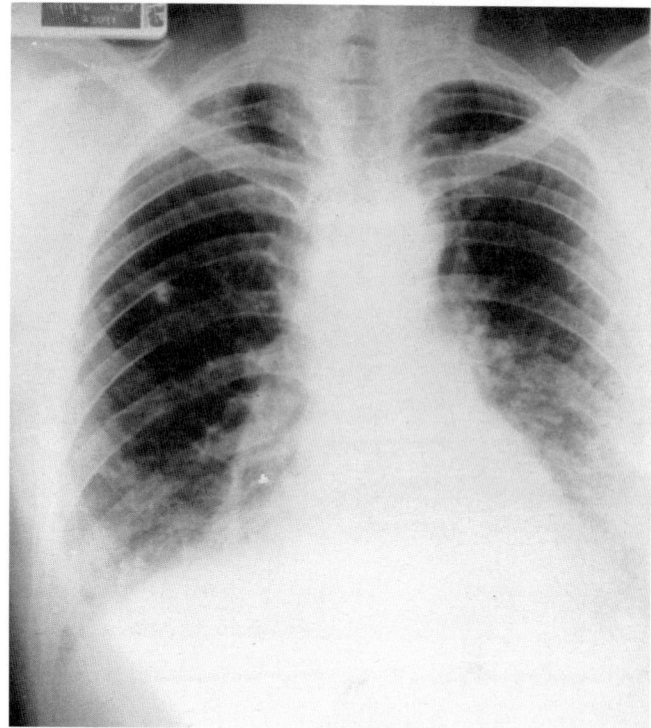

Fig. 12 Radiograph of a lagger with asbestosis. The irregular basal and middle zone fibrosis should be noted.

careful. The disease may first become apparent and progress after exposure has ceased.

The symptoms are shortness of breath, initially on exertion, and dry cough. Repetitive end-inspiratory basal crackles commonly precede symptoms, and finger clubbing may occur later. The disease is usually progressive, the speed of progression being related to the dose of asbestos to which the lungs have been subjected, and results in increasing disability and death from cardiorespiratory failure. Forty to fifty per cent of smokers with asbestosis die of bronchial carcinoma, but there is no increased risk of tuberculosis.

The radiological appearance of asbestosis is identical to that of cryptogenic pulmonary fibrosis —predominantly basal and peripheral irregular linear shadowing progressing to honeycombing (Fig. 12). The presence of pleural plaques, which frequently calcify, is an indication of asbestos exposure and may help in the differential diagnosis (Fig. 13). In advanced asbestosis the fibrosis obscures the cardiac border, giving a shaggy appearance. The radiological appearances are best described by comparison with the International Labour Organization standard radiographs. CT scans are useful in differentiating asbestosis from diffuse pleural fibrosis, which may mimic it clinically and radiologically (Fig. 14).

Asbestosis causes a restrictive pattern of lung function, with reduced volumes and transfer factor. These measurements are the most suitable for screening for the disease and following its progress. Pulmonary compliance is reduced in relation to the extent of the fibrosis, and arterial oxygen desaturation occurs in the later stages.

Pleural plaques cause no symptoms and are usually a coincidental finding on chest radiography. Diffuse bilateral pleural thickening, often calcified, which can cause breathlessness and restricted lung volumes, occurs infrequently. Inspiratory crackles may be heard over this in the absence of significant asbestosis. Very uncommonly, benign pleural effusion may occur. This develops within the first two decades after exposure as a transient haemorrhagic effusion and is diagnosed by the exclusion of infective

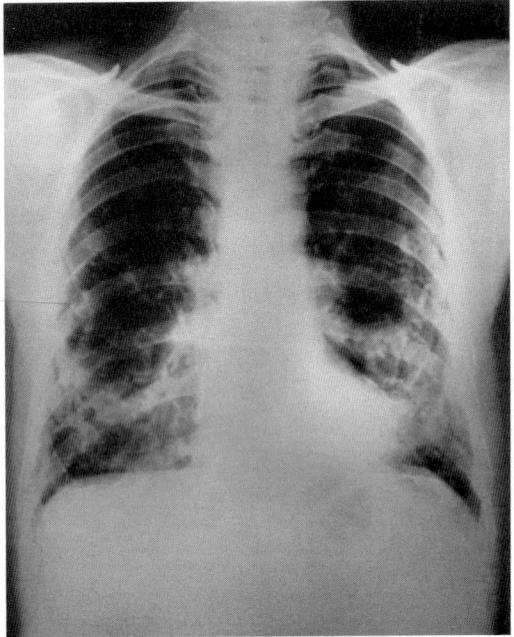

Fig. 13 Radiograph of a lagger, showing extensive calcified pleural plaques.

and malignant causes. There is no evidence that any of these benign disorders predisposes to pleural mesothelioma, the risk of which relates to the prior extent of asbestos exposure.

Prevention and management

The prevention of asbestosis, as of other pneumoconioses, depends on reducing the exposure of individuals to fibre levels that have been shown to be insufficient to cause the disease in a lifetime of exposure. Unfortunately, the difficulties of making valid measurements of airborne fibres and the uncertainties attached to the early diagnosis of asbestosis have prevented the formulation of really reliable evidence on which to base a standard. The present British standard for chrysotile of 0.5 respirable fibres/ml has been based on work that suggests such levels would, when breathed over a working lifetime, result in asbestosis in fewer than 1 per cent of those exposed. The corresponding standard for amphiboles is 0.2 fibres/ml. Many indus-

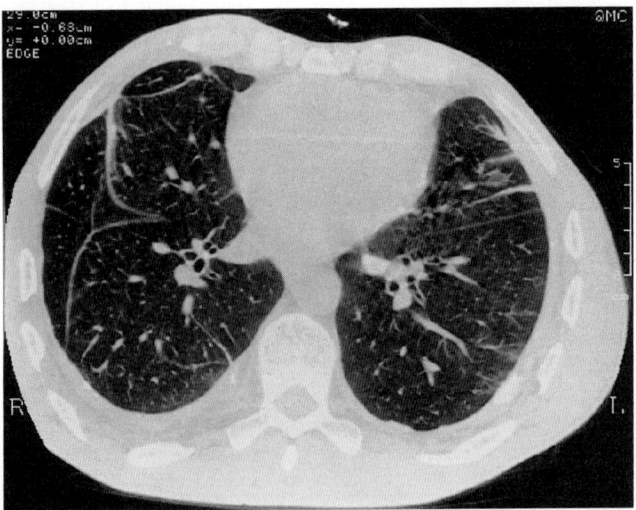

Fig. 14 CT scan of a thermal insulator, showing bilateral pleural fibrosis with areas of calcification and fibrous strands extending into peripheral lung. This does not imply the same functional effects or prognosis as asbestosis.

tries have now introduced other fibrous or crystalline minerals in place of asbestos. The potential of such new materials to cause similar diseases depends on their fibre dimensions, solubility in tissue, and the concentrations achieved in the workplace air. It is important that they should be handled with appropriate care by industry.

Regular medical and radiological examination of asbestos workers is essential for the early detection of asbestosis, and there is some evidence that removal of the worker from exposure at this stage is associated with slower progression. Workers should also be advised not to smoke in view of the interaction between cigarettes and asbestos in causing lung cancer. Once asbestosis is suspected, the British worker should apply to the Benefits Agency for assessment for industrial injuries benefit. Diffuse pleural fibrosis also attracts benefits, as does lung cancer in the presence of asbestosis or pleural fibrosis, but pleural plaques do not.

Risks of asbestos-related disease in the non-occupationally exposed population

Much anxiety has been engendered amongst the general public by media interest in asbestos, and doctors may find themselves being asked about, for example, the risks to children of asbestos wall panelling in houses or asbestos inserts in ironing boards. In general it can be stated that asbestosis only occurs in people working regularly with asbestos for years. However, this has included, at least in the past, wives washing the dusty clothes of asbestos workers and people who have lived or worked near polluting asbestos factories. Occasional or incidental exposure to asbestos can be dismissed as a significant cause of asbestosis. Similarly, lung cancer risks seem to be significantly increased only with the doses of asbestos that lead to asbestosis, and individuals who do not smoke and who only have asbestos fittings in their houses can be reassured that their risks of this disease are negligible. Mesothelioma however, while also dose-related, occurs after smaller exposures and it is well established that a sufficient dose of crocidolite or amosite can be inhaled in a period of intense exposure of a few months. Of the 1000 cases occurring in the United Kingdom each year, almost all individuals give a history of having worked in a trade known to have been associated with asbestos use and have large numbers of fibres in their lungs, suggesting that employment rather than incidental exposure has been responsible. Small and occasional exposures to asbestos are highly unlikely to entail an important risk, but if regular exposures are thought to be occurring in the domestic or general environment, steps should be taken to eliminate them.

Other silicate pneumoconioses

Several silicates apart from asbestos are of commercial importance, and some of these have been shown to cause pneumoconiosis. Talc (hydrated magnesium silicate) is mined as soapstone in the United States, China, and the Pyrenees. It is milled and has many uses including in cosmetics, the rubber industry, paints, ceramics, and pharmaceuticals. Kaolin (hydrated aluminium silicate) is quarried in south-west England, Georgia in the United States, Japan, Egypt, Germany, and former Czechoslovakia. It is used mainly in the manufacture of ceramics, paper and paint, and in pharmaceuticals. Fuller's earth (calcium montmorillonite) is an absorbent clay quarried in England, the United States, and Germany. It was originally used in fulling or removing grease from wool, and is now used in oil refining and bonding foundry moulds. Mica is a complex aluminium silicate occurring in two forms—muscovite and phlogopite. The former is mined in the United States and India and used in fire-resistant windows and the manufacture of paper and paint. Phlogopite, mined in Canada, is used in the electrical industry because of its resistance to heat and electricity.

Two widely used silicate materials—cement and vitreous fibres—are not established as causes of pulmonary disease. Although cement exposure has occasionally been reported to be associated with pneumoconiosis, the evidence for this is flimsy. It is often mixed with asbestos, and asbestosis may occur in its production. Artificial vitreous fibres (glass wool and rock wool) have not so far been shown to cause pulmonary fibrosis or neoplasia in humans exposed to them, although mesothelioma has been produced by intraperitoneal injection in rats.

Other pneumoconioses

Talc pneumoconiosis

Talc is commonly contaminated with tremolite, a non-commercially exploited amphibole asbestos, and with silica. It has been difficult to disentangle the effects of these components. The disease appears clinically to resemble asbestosis, with finger clubbing and basal crackles, although radiological descriptions emphasize lesions predominantly in the middle zones with nodular as well as reticular components. Progressive massive fibrosis has been described.

Talc has also been shown to be associated with pulmonary disease in a number of other circumstances. Bronchoconstriction may occur in children exposed to high concentrations and drug users may have granulomatous reactions in the lungs as a result of either intravenous injection or inhalation of ground-up tablets. Fortunately, the widespread use of talc for producing pleurodesis has not been shown to be associated with the later development of mesothelioma, probably because the grades of talc used have not been contaminated with tremolite.

Kaolin pneumoconiosis

Kaolin causes a pneumoconiosis similar to coal-worker's pneumoconiosis with small discrete nodular lesions initially and a tendency to produce massive fibrosis. It has been described in workers involved in the drying and milling processes in the production of china clay. Kaolin may also have been the component of the dust responsible for pneumoconiosis in the now defunct Scottish shale oil industry. There is no evidence linking kaolin pneumoconiosis with carcinoma or tuberculosis.

Fuller's earth pneumoconiosis

This condition has been described in workers extracting this clay mineral. It is a benign nodular pneumoconiosis similar in pathological and radiological appearance to simple coal-worker's pneumoconiosis; progressive massive fibrosis has not been described.

Mica pneumoconiosis

A few reports of radiological change in those exposed to ground mica have been recorded, but there is no recent publication describing pathological or clinical features.

Fibrous erionite

Exposure to this fibrous hydrated aluminium silicate occurs in certain areas of Turkey and probably elsewhere in the Middle East. The populations of several villages have been exposed for many generations as they use local erionite rock as stucco and whitewash in their homes. Pleural plaques, pulmonary fibrosis, and both lung cancer and mesothelioma are endemic in these villages. Fibrous erionite has no general commercial use, but this episode illustrates the potential dangers of inhaling fine fibrous material, whether asbestos or some other mineral.

Berylliosis

Beryllium is a metal that is used in alloys for the nuclear industry and in the production of X-ray tubes. It was used in ceramics, metallic alloys, and fluorescent lights until its toxicity was recognized and it was replaced by other materials. It is mined as an ore mostly in South America and extracted by chemical processes.

Beryllium is highly toxic when inhaled, and may also cause granulomatous ulcers on contact with the skin. Inhalation of high concentrations

causes an acute pneumonitis and tracheobronchitis, which can be fatal. Chronic berylliosis, which may occur as a sequel to acute exposure, usually follows more prolonged exposure to lower levels. It is not common in the United Kingdom, where no more than about 50 cases have been diagnosed, but it has been recorded much more frequently in the United States. Reported cases have occurred in beryllium workers, in wives exposed to dust from their husbands' clothes, and in people living near the factories.

The patient with chronic berylliosis presents with cough and shortness of breath. The features mimic those of sarcoidosis: bilateral pulmonary mottling with upper lobe fibrosis is the usual radiographic feature initially, with bilateral hilar lymphadenopathy being less common. The disease typically progresses to diffuse fibrosis (Fig. 15), but the rate of progression is very variable. The functional lesion is a restrictive pattern with a low transfer factor. The progress of the disease can be controlled with corticosteroid therapy, but this needs to be continued indefinitely in most cases.

The pathological lesion is identical with that of sarcoidosis, with non-caseating granulomas and varying amounts of interstitial fibrosis. The diagnosis is made on the basis of a history of exposure, compatible clinical and histological features, and a negative Kveim test. A skin-patch test is inadvisable as it can cause sensitization.

Berylliosis is prevented by keeping exposures below the threshold limit value (2 ng/m³), although as it is a hypersensitivity disease even this will not prevent all cases. Efficient respiratory protection should also be provided.

Less common pneumoconioses

Many other pneumoconioses have been described, although most are of very limited prevalence and are relatively benign. Haematite lung, occurring in iron ore miners, used to be seen in Cumbria in the United Kingdom; it is a fibrotic reaction to a mixed dust containing silica and iron. Radiographically it resembles silicosis and pathologically only differs from it in that the lungs are coloured red. There was an increased risk of lung cancer, probably due to radiation in the mines. Closely related to haematite lung is siderosis, a benign iron oxide pneumoconiosis occurring in welders and other workers in iron foundries. The radiological lesions often regress after exposure ceases. Barium processing and tin refining may be associated with the development of dramatic radiological nodular shadowing—baritosis and stannosis, respectively. These are also benign conditions, the radiological appearances reflecting radio-opaque dust in macrophages. Pneumoconiosis associated with diffuse lung fibrosis has been described in work with aluminium oxide (Shaver's disease) and tungsten carbide (hard metal disease). This latter condition, which is probably a hypersensitivity reaction

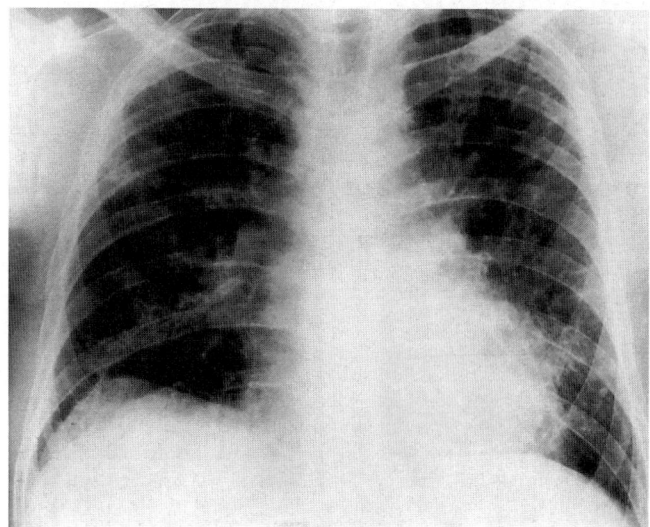

Fig. 15 Radiograph of a beryllium refiner worker, showing the diffuse fibrosis of berylliosis.

to cobalt in cooling liquids, may also present with features of asthma or allergic alveolitis. A pneumoconiosis resembling that in coal miners has been described in workers with graphite and other forms of carbon, and in shale miners. A benign pneumoconiosis, consisting of simple accumulations of dust and macrophages with minimal nodular radiological shadowing, has also been described in workers producing polyvinyl chloride.

Further reading

Henderson VL, Enterline PE (1979). Asbestos exposure: factors associated with excess cancer and respiratory disease mortality. *Annals of the New York Academy of Sciences* **330**, 117–26.

Hurley JF *et al.* (1982). Coalworkers' simple pneumoconiosis and exposure to dust at 10 British coalmines. *British Journal of Industrial Medicine* **39**, 120–7.

International Labour Organization (1980). *Guidelines for the use of ILO International classification of radiographs of pneumoconioses.* Occupational Safety and Health Series No. 22 (rev. 87), International Labour Organization, Geneva.

Marine WM, Gurr D, Jacobsen M (1988). Clinically important respiratory effects of dust exposure and smoking in British coal miners. *American Review of Respiratory Disease* **137**, 106–12.

Morgan WKC, Seaton A (1995). *Occupational lung diseases*, 3rd edn. WB Saunders, Philadelphia.

Mossman BT *et al.* (1990). Asbestos: scientific developments and implications for public policy. *Science* **247**, 294–301.

Peto J *et al.* (1995). Continuing increase in mesothelioma mortality in Britain. *Lancet* **345**, 535–9.

Seaton A (1990). Coalmining, emphysema and compensation. *British Journal of Industrial Medicine* **47**, 433–5.

Seaton A (1998). The new prescription: industrial injuries benefit for smokers? *Thorax* **53**, 335–6.

Seaton A, Cherrie JW (1998). Quartz exposure and severe silicosis: a role for the hilar nodes. *Occupational and Environmental Medicine* **55**, 383–6.

Seaton A *et al.* (1991). Accelerated silicosis in Scottish stonemasons. *Lancet* **337**, 341–4.

17.11.8 Pulmonary haemorrhagic disorders

*D. J. Hendrick and G. P. Spickett**

Bleeding within the lung and subsequent haemoptysis is common in clinical practice and may be the consequence of many unrelated disorders. What then is the value of the term 'pulmonary haemorrhagic disorder'? The answer lies with its use in special circumstances only—bleeding arising diffusely from pulmonary alveolar capillaries. A preferable and more explicit diagnostic term is therefore pulmonary capillary (or alveolar) haemorrhage. This is not a disease entity of itself, merely a feature of several diseases, but most notable in two conditions, Goodpasture's syndrome and idiopathic pulmonary haemosiderosis.

While the lung can accommodate only small quantities of blood in the major airways without threatening life from asphyxiation, it can sequester surprisingly large amounts (litres) at alveolar level. This leads to a curious characteristic, unique among diffuse parenchymal diseases of the lung and of considerable diagnostic value; the carbon monoxide gas transfer (*TL*co)

*Dr D. J. Lane wrote on this subject in the third edition of the *Oxford Textbook of Medicine*. Much of his text has been retained in this revision and we acknowledge his contribution with grateful thanks.

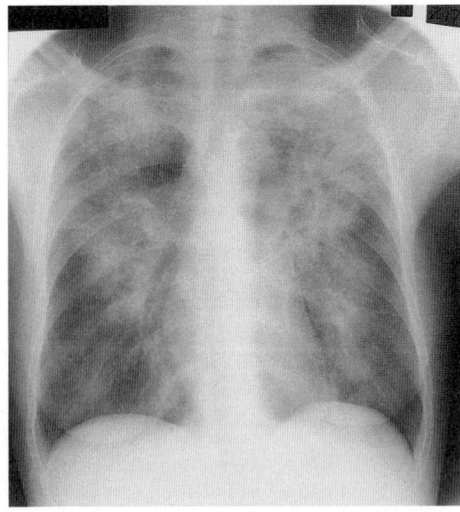

Fig. 1 Radiograph showing gross alveolar shadowing following major pulmonary haemorrhage in a 60-year-old man with systemic vasculitis.

is raised significantly above normal. Not only are physiologically useful red cells within the alveolar capillaries able to absorb the inhaled carbon monoxide, but so too are those lost from the circulation into the alveolar spaces.

Pulmonary capillary haemorrhage is thus characterized by haemoptysis, breathlessness, diffuse air space shadowing on the chest radiograph (Fig. 1), anaemia (normochromic normocytic if acute, iron deficient with chronicity), and an elevated *TL*co (see Chapter 17.3.2). The extravasated red cells are not readily expectorated, although enough generally escape to cause haemoptysis, and so haemosiderin accumulates within alveolar macrophages as the red cells and their debris are engulfed. When haemosiderin-laden macrophages are identified in sputum, the diagnosis of pulmonary capillary haemorrhage is largely confirmed, but if sputum is not expectorated or haemoptysis is absent, minimal, or otherwise explained, then bronchoalveolar lavage and/or lung biopsy are often necessary to establish the diagnosis. An alternative approach is CT and MRI, which may alone provide convincing evidence of blood sited diffusely within the alveoli.

While diffuse alveolar capillary haemorrhage may characterize or complicate a wide variety of specific diseases or disease settings (each associated with its particular range of clinical, diagnostic, and mechanistic features, and management options), the direct effects of the haemorrhage itself are not influenced by the cause, nor are the means by which it can be recognized. There may, nevertheless, be substantial differences at presentation from case to case according to severity and chronicity.

Goodpasture's syndrome

Goodpasture described a man with renal failure, glomerulonephritis, and pulmonary haemorrhage. A number of conditions can cause such a 'pulmonary–renal syndrome', the best characterized of which (although almost certainly not the illness suffered by the patient in the original report) is now termed Goodpasture's disease, which consists of diffuse pulmonary haemorrhage and glomerulonephritis with linear deposition of antibody (90 per cent of which are directed against the α-3 chain of type IV collagen) along the glomerular basement membrane. Goodpasture's disease is described in Chapter 20.7.9 and other causes of pulmonary–renal syndrome in Chapter 20.10.3.

Clinical features

In practice, glomerulonephritis proves to be a much commoner threat to survival than lung haemorrhage, and the diagnosis of Goodpasture's disease is reached more conveniently by serological testing (for anti-GBM antibodies) and from kidney rather than lung biopsy. In some cases, however, lung disease dominates the clinical picture, when the majority of patients are male smokers and some have recent exposure to volatile hydrocarbons; case reports have additionally identified recent exposure to chlorine and smoked cocaine. This suggests that when there is susceptibility, inhaled toxic agents enhance pulmonary endothelial damage and thus allow the initiation of autoimmunity or the ready access of existing autoantibody to basement membrane. Respiratory presentation is with cough, breathlessness, and haemoptysis, which is intermittent and ranges from occasional streaks to massive fatal bleeding. Systemic symptoms of fever, joint pains, or weight loss are unusual. The chest radiograph shows patchy or diffuse shadowing due to intra-alveolar blood, usually resolving over the course of 2 weeks unless there is further bleeding. At the time of bleeding there may be arterial hypoxaemia and reduced lung volumes. Serial measurement of TL_{CO} can be used to monitor progression, and prolonged bleeding may lead to iron-deficiency anaemia. Renal function may be normal initially and then deteriorate over days to weeks. Steroids, other immunosuppressant drugs (cyclophosphamide in particular), and plasmapheresis are all used (in some circumstances) to control renal disease, and are additionally helpful in treating pulmonary haemorrhage. Patients should not smoke and should avoid hydrocarbon exposure.

Idiopathic pulmonary haemosiderosis

This is a rare disorder of children and young adults in which there is recurrent alveolar bleeding in the absence of kidney disease. Anti-basement membrane antibody has not been detected, and nor have any other substantial immunological clues to the causal mechanism, although serum IgA is commonly elevated. The electron microscopic appearance of the basement membrane shows no consistent abnormality. The alveolar blood may provoke a fibrogenic stimulus and the development of diffuse pulmonary fibrosis, as may recurrent alveolar bleeding from mitral stenosis and chronic severe left ventricular failure.

Although termed idiopathic pulmonary haemosiderosis, the condition is associated with premature birth and an increasing number of environmental exposures. One such that has incited particular interest is to the mould, *Stachybotrys*, which may contaminate wet or damp accommodation, and which releases a particularly potent toxin with haemorrhagic properties. This is now thought to have aetiological significance in some childhood cases, perhaps in synergy with environmental tobacco smoke. Associations with cow's milk allergy, rheumatoid arthritis, and coeliac disease are also recognized, but the latter might be a consequence of cow's milk allergy also rather than gluten intolerance. A number of other environmental causes have been suggested; but the stronger the evidence for their causal roles, the less appropriate is the diagnostic rubric, idiopathic pulmonary haemosiderosis. They are consequently identified below under the heading 'other causes'.

Clinical features

Recurrent alveolar haemorrhage is generally manifested by cough with haemoptysis and breathlessness, but haemoptysis is not invariably present, and in children a failure to thrive may be prominent, together with the effects of severe chronic iron-deficiency anaemia. Acute bleeds are more common in childhood and may be life threatening. Physical examination is unhelpful. The chest radiograph and CT scan show the non-specific appearances of intra-alveolar blood, which usually clear spontaneously over 1 to 3 weeks. With chronicity, the appearances of diffuse pulmonary fibrosis with honeycombing may supervene. Lung function tests then show a progressive loss of volume and reduction of gas transfer; an obstructive pulmonary defect occurs occasionally, which is unexplained.

Treatment and prognosis

Supportive treatment is required during acute bleeding, and artificial ventilation is occasionally necessary. There are case reports recording responses to the avoidance of milk and gluten, and to the use of immunosuppressive agents including corticosteroids and cyclophosphamide. Some patients recover spontaneously with or without residual pulmonary damage.

Other causes of diffuse alveolar haemorrhage

Although diffuse alveolar haemorrhage is not a principal pulmonary feature of disorders other than Goodpasture's syndrome and idiopathic pulmonary haemosiderosis, it may occur with or complicate a wide variety of disorders with immunological, vasculitic, vascular, haemostatic, toxic, or unknown origins. In many of the cases that have been reported, several different disorders, their complications, and their various treatments could all have played a contributory role.

Vasculitic disorders can occasionally cause prominent diffuse alveolar haemorrhage, particularly Wegener's granulomatosis. This may simulate Goodpasture's disease, since it commonly causes acute necrotizing glomerulonephritis, but is distinguished from it clinically by the common involvement of upper respiratory tract structures (and because diffuse alveolar haemorrhage is an uncommon respiratory manifestation); histologically by the appearances of a granulomatous vasculitis; and immunologically by the presence of circulating anti-neutrophil cytoplasmic antibodies (**ANCA**), directed against proteinase-3, in about 90 per cent of cases. Other vasculitic disorders involving the lung are very rare causes of diffuse alveolar haemorrhage; they include Henoch–Schönlein purpura and Churg–Strauss syndrome. The latter may be associated with ANCA directed against myeloperoxidase and against eosinophil granule enzymes.

Diffuse alveolar haemorrhage may also arise as an unusual respiratory feature of several non-vasculitic immunological disorders. Most prominent is systemic lupus erythematosus (in which lupus anticoagulant, thrombcytopenia, and active nephritis may all play a role), but there are reports also of diffuse alveolar haemorrhage complicating antiphospholipid antibody syndrome, IgA nephropathy, idiopathic membranous nephropathy, scleroderma, renal and bone marrow transplantation, and chronic active hepatitis.

Other reports have implicated hymenopteran stings, moulds other than *Stachybotrys* and their mycotoxins, infections (group A streptococcal, leptospirosis, strongyloidiasis, *Stenotrophomonas*, dengue fever, cytomegalovirus, AIDS, varicella), occupational exposure to tri- and pyro-mellitic anhydride, lymphangiography contrast media, and several medications (valproate, nitrofurantoin, mitomycin C, azathioprine, D-penicillamine, surfactant therapy, anaesthetic agents). The list is completed by causes of chronic pulmonary venous congestion (mitral stenosis, chronic left ventricular failure, pulmonary veno-occlusive disease), malignant hypertension, and disorders that disrupt bleeding and coagulation mechanisms (thrombocytopenia, leukaemia, thrombinolytic therapy, platelet glycoprotein IIb/IIIa inhibitor, anticoagulant poisoning, factor V deficiency). Combinations of such factors are commonly found in individual cases, and it may be that important interactions occur, without which the probability of diffuse haemorrhage is remote. Although capillary stress from high pressure gradients is thought to be a major factor underlying diffuse pulmonary haemorrhage in exercizing horses (and camels), it appears a rare or unheard cause in most other species. Nevertheless, the use of negative pressure ventilation in humans has been reported to have a similar effect.

Further reading

Anonymous (2000). From the Centers for Disease Control and Prevention. Update: pulmonary hemorrhage/hemosiderosis among infants—

Cleveland, Ohio, 1993–1996. *Journal of the American Medical Association* **283**, 1951–3.

Bhandari V *et al.*(1999). Pulmonary hemorrhage in neonates of early and late gestation. *Journal of Perinatal Medicine* **7**, 369–75.

Colombo JL, Stolz SM (1992). Treatment of life threatening pulmonary hemosiderosis with cyclophosphamide. *Chest* **102**, 959–60.

Leatherman JW, Davies SF, Hoidal JR (1984). Alveolar haemorrhage syndromes; diffuse and microvascular lung haemorrhage in immune and idiopathic disorders. *Medicine, Baltimore* **63**, 343–61.

Pacheco A *et al.* (1991). Long term follow-up of adult idiopathic pulmonary hemosiderosis. *Chest* **99**, 1525–6.

Peters DK *et al.* (1982). Treatment and prognosis of anti-basement membrane antibody mediated nephritis. *Transplant Proceedings* **14**, 513–21.

Ryan JJ *et al.* (1998). Recombinant alpha-chains of type IV collagen demonstrate that the amino terminal of the Goodpasture autoantigen is crucial for antibody recognition. *Clinical and Experimental Immunology* **113**, 17–27.

Vats KR *et al* (1999). Henoch–Schönlein purpura and pulmonary hemorrhage: a report and literature review. *Pediatric Nephrology* **13**, 530–4.

Weishaupt D *et al.* (1999). Pulmonary hemorrhage: imaging with a new magnetic resonance blood pool agent in conjunction with breathheld three-dimensional magnetic resonance angiography. *Cardiovascular and Interventional Radiology* **22**, 321–5.

17.11.9 Eosinophilic pneumonia

*D. J. Hendrick and G. P. Spickett**

When alveolar spaces are consolidated because of eosinophil inflammation/infiltration, there is said to be eosinophilic pneumonia. This is not meant to imply that there is microbial infection, and most commonly there is not. There is characteristically an accompanying eosinophilia of peripheral blood, hence the alternative terms, pulmonary eosinophilia and pulmonary infiltrates with eosinophilia (PIE syndrome). Eosinophilic pneumonia is the preferred term, however, since eosinophilia of peripheral blood may be present coincidently when eosinophils are not relevant to a pulmonary infiltrate, and conversely true eosinophilic pneumonia is occasionally not associated with blood eosinophilia. To avoid further confusion, it should be noted that eosinophilic granuloma is a distinct disease unrelated to eosinophilic pneumonia: it is a disorder of Langerhans (dendritic) cells and not characterized by eosinophil infiltration of the alveolar spaces.

The plethora of diagnostic terms is exceeded by the multitude of causes, and evenly matched by the systems of classification that have been suggested. In essence they reflect the following points concerning eosinophilic pneumonia.

1. It may arise acutely and resolve quickly (acute eosinophilic pneumonia, Löffler's syndrome, simple pulmonary eosinophilia).

2. It may arise gradually and persist for many months, leading sometimes to pulmonary fibrosis (chronic eosinophilic pneumonia, prolonged pulmonary eosinophilia).

3. It may be a consequence of allergy, particularly to bloodborne parasites (tropical eosinophilia), moulds (allergic bronchopulmonary mycosis), or other common environmental allergens.

*Dr D. J. Lane wrote on this subject in the third edition of the *Oxford Textbook of Medicine*. Much of his text has been retained in this revision and we acknowledge his contribution with grateful thanks.

4. It is often associated with asthma (asthmatic eosinophilia).

5. It is often due to drugs (whether through allergy, idiosyncrasy, or toxicity).

6. It may be associated with pulmonary vasculitis (Churg–Strauss syndrome, polyarteritis nodosa, Wegener's granulomatosis).

7. It may be a component of the hypereosinophilic syndrome.

8. It may be associated with a variety of other distinct disease entities (rheumatoid disease, sarcoidosis, T-cell lymphoma, Hodgkin's disease, shock, and the adult respiratory distress syndrome).

9. It may seem to be idiopathic.

Since there is often overlap—to give a recent example, the affected subject may have asthma, be taking a relevant drug (a leukotriene receptor antagonist), have prolonged manifestations, and have a pulmonary vasculitis (Churg–Strauss syndrome)—there is limited benefit from using any classification. The important issue is to identify any potentially remediable cause.

Diagnosis

In practice the finding of a blood eosinophilia in association with a radiographic pulmonary infiltrate provides a valuable clue that pneumonia of infectious origin may not be the explanation. Since such a disorder is not likely to respond to conventional antibiotic medication, the need to confirm or exclude the possibility of eosinophilic pneumonia will soon arise. Equally, if an apparent pneumonia fails to respond to antibiotics, a blood eosinophil count should be obtained. Once suspected, eosinophilic pneumonia is most conveniently confirmed by demonstrating an excess of eosinophils in bronchoalveolar lavage fluid in the absence of pathogenic micro-organisms. Sometimes sputum alone is sufficient, whether expectorated spontaneously or induced. Alternatively, an excess of alveolar eosinophils is revealed in lung biopsy tissue. The use of CT scanning has shown that episodes of recurrent pulmonary infiltration occur, not surprisingly, more frequently than can be detected from plain chest radiographs in subjects with confirmed eosinophilic pneumonia.

Once eosinophilic pneumonia is confirmed, a variety of possible causes should be considered before it is assumed to be idiopathic in origin and before empirical treatment with corticosteroids is administered.

1. Is there parasitic infestation?

2. Have any drugs been administered?

3. Is there asthma?

4. Is there evidence of allergy to parasites or drugs?

5. Is there evidence of allergic bronchopulmonary mycosis (particularly aspergillosis)?

6. Is there evidence of vasculitis?

7. Is there evidence of the hypereosinophilic syndrome?

8. Is there evidence of other disorders known to be associated with eosinophilic pneumonia?

Treatment

Eosinophilic pneumonia itself often responds well to corticosteroid medication, though treatment may need to be prolonged (6 months or more) in the chronic forms of the disorder. The importance of identifying whether it is associated with the causal factors listed above lies with the additional need to treat these also. Otherwise eosinophilic pneumonia may not respond adequately to steroid therapy and the associated diseases may produce other manifestations.

Particular varieties of eosinophilic pneumonia

Löffler's syndrome (acute eosinophilic pneumonia, simple pulmonary eosinophilia)

The essential features of the syndrome are transitory migratory pulmonary shadows with associated modest peripheral eosinophilia in patients with a mild self-limiting illness. Some cases are asymptomatic and discovered incidentally. Most patients present with cough, sometimes with oddly yellowish sputum containing an abundance of eosinophils, and a few have general malaise and a mild fever. The pulmonary shadows reflect fanshaped areas of consolidation, often peripheral and sometimes rather nodular, which last a few days only and appear haphazardly in various lobes, seldom following a truly segmental pattern. In some cases they are single and in others they are multiple. The peripheral eosinophilia is obviously but rarely gross; a differential of more than 20 per cent in a modestly raised total white cell count is unusual and more often the absolute eosinophil count ranges between 1×10^9 and 2×10^9/l (normal: $< 0.4 \times 10^9$/l).

Patients who develop Löffler's syndrome are often atopic and may have other manifestations of an atopic diathesis such as asthma, urticaria, and angio-oedema. Allergy has been shown since Löffler's original description to play an important role, and cases can be seen to fall into two broad aetiological groups with a third miscellaneous group of unexplained aetiology.

In the first group eosinophilic pneumonia represents an allergic reaction to bloodborne parasites migrating through the lung, particularly larvae of *Ascaris lumbricoides* and occasionally *A. suum*. *Ancylostoma*, *Trichuris*, *Trichinella*, *Taenia*, and *Strongyloides* species provide further examples.

Drugs form the second major aetiological group. Löffler's syndrome is well described after administration of *p*-amino salicylic acid, aspirin, sulphonamides (including the antimalarial combination sulphadiazine and pyrimethamine or Fansidar), penicillin, and imipramine. It may also occur with nitrofurantoin (although this can also give a diffuse reticulonodular radiological picture and is a cause of the more chronic type of eosinophilic pneumonia), toxic smoke, and lymphangiography contrast medium.

Successful management requires the irradication of any parasites or the cessation of relevant medication, as well as the administration (if necessary) of oral corticosteroids.

Tropical eosinophilia

Eosinophilic pneumonia in tropical climates is often a consequence of migrating larvae of the filarial worms *Wucheria bancrofti* and *Brugia malayi*. The effects are fundamentally similar to those of Löffler's syndrome, but tend to be more persistent and more serious, are more often associated with asthma, and may be associated with systemic symptoms of weight loss, persistent fever, and lymphadenopathy. Also the peripheral eosinophil count tends to be greater than in Löffler's syndrome ($> 3 \times 10^9$/l), and the total serum IgE level is markedly elevated. With chronicity, pulmonary fibrosis is characteristic. A cure is to be expected with antifilariasis medication (diethylcarbamazine).

Chronic eosinophilic pneumonia (prolonged pulmonary eosinophilia)

Eosinophilic pneumonia persisting for more than a month is distinguished from the more transitory Löffler's syndrome, although its clinical characteristics are fundamentally similar. As with eosinophilic pneumonia associated with tropical filariasis, it tends to be more persistent and more serious than Löffler's syndrome (it is sometimes life threatening), and to be associated with systemic symptoms (particularly fever), progressive pulmonary fibrosis, and fixed airway obstruction. It may last for several months and be associated additionally with eosinophilic pleural effusion, focal skin lesions, atopic manifestations such as rhinitis, sinusitis, and angio-oedema, hepatosplenomegaly, and even hepatic necrosis. The pulmonary disease is often extensive, causing dyspnoea and hypoxia, and is characterized radiologically by a curious peripheral distribution dubbed a 'negative photographic image of pulmonary oedema'. The radiological abnormalities tend to recur and last for weeks or months, and like the shadows of Löffler's syndrome may vary in site during the course of the illness.

Chronic eosinophilic pneumonia is more commonly idiopathic (cryptogenic) than Löffler's syndrome, but may also be a consequence of parasite infestation (e.g. tropical filariasis) or drug hypersensitivity. Case reports over recent years have identified aminoglutethimide, bicalutamide, chlorpropamide, clomipramine, dapsone, diflunisal, ethambutol, mesalazine, minocycline, nitrofurantoin, sertraline, sotalol, sulphonamides, and venlafaxine as possible causes. Peripheral blood eosinophilia is less consistent with chronic compared with acute forms of eosinophilic pneumonia, although is often of greater level ($> 1 \times 10^9$/l). When a definitive cause is identified, appropriate specific management should follow, but often no cause is evident and oral corticosteroid therapy should be given. Responses are often dramatic, but recurrences are common if treatment is discontinued within 6 to 12 months. There may be a persistent mixed obstructive and restrictive loss of ventilatory function, and radiographic evidence of persistent pulmonary fibrosis.

Eosinophilic pneumonia with asthma

Eosinophilic pneumonia is commonly associated with asthma, even in the absence of parasite infestation or drug hypersensitivity. Two particular associations are noteworthy.

Allergic bronchopulmonary mycosis

When fungal hypersensitivity develops in atopic subjects with asthma, additional manifestations may occur in the lung: these include eosinophilic pneumonia, mucoid impaction, bronchiectasis, and pulmonary fibrosis. The ensuing syndrome of allergic bronchopulmonary mycosis occurs most commonly with *Aspergillus fumigatus*, though has been reported with other *Aspergillus*, *Candida*, *Curvularia*, and *Helminthosporium* species. It accounts for most cases of eosinophilic pneumonia with asthma in the United Kingdom and is best considered a complication of atopic asthma, appearing to result from airway colonization by the relevant mould. The mechanism, however, is clearly one of hypersensitivity, not infection/invasion, and both IgE and IgG antibodies are necessary to support its diagnosis.

In acute phases, there is patchy obstruction of bronchi with inspissated mucus that, if expectorated, appears as brown rubbery lumps in the sputum (plugs). Fungal hyphae may be recovered from them, indicating fungal growth has occurred within the airway. This impaction of mucus in one or more bronchi leads to patchy atelectasis within, or of, segments (even lobes) and is often associated with eosinophilic pneumonia. The radiographic appearances are of fleeting pulmonary infiltrates (Fig. 1). It usually responds well to corticosteroids, a useful diagnostic feature being the expectoration of plugs during this period of resolution. In the medium term the involved bronchi (generally proximal) may become bronchiectatic, leading in turn to the characteristic features of bronchiectasis (productive cough, intermittent haemoptysis). In the longer term, pulmonary fibrosis may ensue, particularly in the upper lobes and apices, so that the radiographic appearances resemble tuberculosis, and if mucoid impaction and/or eosinophilic pneumonia become superimposed, the radiographic appearances may simulate active tuberculosis very closely. Suspicion of tuberculosis in an individual with atopic asthma should always prompt consideration of allergic bronchopulmonary mycosis.

Churg–Strauss syndrome

A much rarer association of eosinophilic pneumonia with asthma is that involving Churg–Strauss syndrome, a vasculitic and granulomatous disorder that commonly involves lungs, gut, peripheral nerves, skin, and kidneys. It is characterized typically by asthma, eosinophilic pneumonia, and very high numbers of circulating eosinophils ($> 5 \times 10^9$/l), but the pulmonary manifestations may additionally include localized haemorrhage and haemoptysis. Serological investigation may also demonstrate raised serum levels of IgE and eosinophil cationic protein, P-ANCA (peripheral antineutrophil cytoplasmic antibodies) with myeloperoxidase activity (in 60 per cent of cases), and C-ANCA with proteinase-3 specificity (in 10 per cent). Other autoantibodies against eosinophil granule enzymes have also been described. Pathologically there is vasculitis of small arteries and veins with necrotizing extravascular granulomas. Biopsy tissue is needed to confirm the diagnosis.

The clinical syndrome and the histological features resemble those of polyarteritis nodosa, but the differences are sufficiently clear to establish Churg–Strauss syndrome as a separate entity. Although idiopathic in most cases, a minority appear to be a consequence of drug hypersensitivity, a recent example of particular interest being allergic granulomatosis and angiitis (the nomenclature of Churg and Strauss) complicating the use for asthma of newly introduced oral leukotriene receptor antagonists. It has

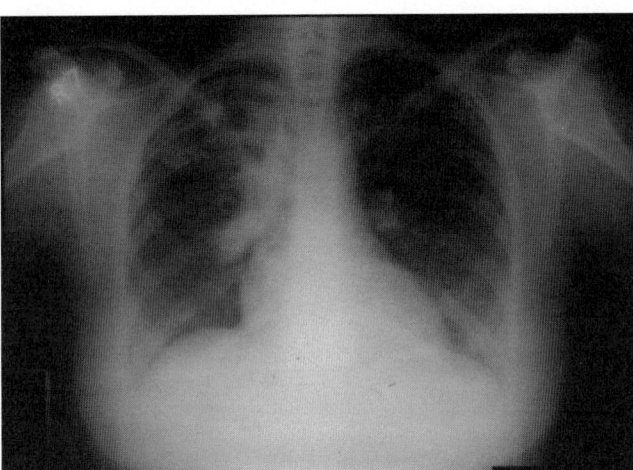

(a)

(b)

Fig. 1 Allergic bronchopulmonary aspergillosis: two radiographs taken 6 months apart from an East African woman with asthma, peripheral eosinophilia, and high titres of IgE and precipitating IgG antibodies to *Aspergillus fumigatus*.

been suggested, however, that the drugs themselves do not cause the disease, but merely lead to it being uncovered as the beneficial effect of leukotriene receptor antagonism allows a reduction (or withdrawal) of chronic steroid therapy. The disease may become life threatening if there is extensive vasculitic involvement of several organs, though generally responds satisfactorily to immunosuppressive therapy with corticosteroids. Other immunosuppressive or steroid sparing agents, such as azathioprine and cyclophosphamide, are usually required in addition.

Hypereosinophilic syndrome

The hypereosinophilic syndrome completes what might be described as a spectrum of overlapping disorders in which eosinophilic pneumonia is a prominent feature. The eosinophils appear mature, and infiltrate a number of organs by increasing degrees to cause progressive dysfunction, even death. The bone marrow is particularly densely infiltrated, raising the possibility that the disorder is primarily leukaemic in nature. Although the clinical picture does resemble that of eosinophilic leukaemia, the apparent maturity of the cells argues against this; current wisdom favours the hypereosinophilic syndrome as a distinct disorder, though one of unknown cause.

The clinical manifestations vary according to the organ(s) of principal involvement, and the extent of eosinophil infiltration. At the benign end of the spectrum the respiratory effects may be confined to an irritant cough, mild asthma, and minor episodes of eosinophilic pneumonia. When the disorder becomes life threatening, eosinophilic pneumonia may be extensive and associated with pleural effusion, but the chief threat to survival comes from myocardial and central nervous system infiltration. In most cases corticosteroids control progression, but when this fails, there may be progressive cardiac failure, or progressive functional impairment of central and peripheral nervous systems. This is often accompanied by weight loss, muscle weakness, enlargement of spleen and lymph nodes, gut and renal dysfunction, and venous thromboembolism. When corticosteroid therapy is ineffective, the use of antileukaemic agents may provide benefit.

Further reading

Churg J, Strauss (1951). Allergic granulomatosis, allergic angiitis and periarteritis nodosa. *American Journal of Pathology* **27**, 277–301.

Franco J, Artes MJ (1999). Pulmonary eosinophilia associated with montelukast. *Thorax* **54**, 558–60.

Kim Y *et al.* (1997). The spectrum of eosinophilic lung disease: radiologic findings. *Journal of Computer Assisted Tomography* **21**, 920–30.

Marchand E *et al.* (1998). Idiopathic chronic eosinophilic pneumonia. A clinical and follow-up study of 62 cases. *Medicine* **77**, 299–312.

Middleton WG *et al.* (1977). Asthmatic pulmonary eosinophilia. A review of 65 cases. *British Journal of Diseases of the Chest* **71**, 115–22.

Ong RK, Doyle RL (1998). Tropical pulmonary eosinophilia. *Chest* **113**, 1673–9.

Pearson DJ, Rosenow EC, III (1978). Chronic eosinophilic pneumonia (Carrington's): a follow up study. *Mayo Clinic Proceedings* **53**, 73.

17.11.10 Lymphocytic infiltrations of the lung

D. J. Hendrick

Introduction

A number of disorders are characterized by lymphocytic infiltration of the lung. Several are rare and poorly understood, while others are relatively common and possess additional distinctive characteristics. For the latter group, classification poses few problems and individual diseases are readily distinguishable. These include, for example, Sjögren's syndrome, sarcoidosis, Wegener's granulomatosis, extrinsic allergic alveolitis, cryptogenic organizing pneumonia, bronchiolitis obliterans with organizing pneumonia, and cryptogenic fibrosing alveolitis, all of which are described separately in other chapters. However, for the first group, which constitutes the subject of this chapter, classification poses a continuing challenge: precise mechanisms and full natural histories are yet to be defined.

Disorders of lymphocytic infiltration are often considered as a spectrum of overlapping conditions, ranging from relatively benign infiltration of apparently normal lymphocytes without involvement of other cellular lines, through vasculitic and granulomatous inflammation, to frank malignancy. Apparent progression from disorder to disorder within the spectrum is not uncommon, but it is not always clear whether individuals affected in this way truly progress from one disease to another, or have a single disease whose early manifestations are similar to (and mistaken for) those of less serious neighbours in the disease spectrum. This has given rise to an alternative view that one end of the spectrum comprises a group of inflammatory disorders whose vasculitic and granulomatous features link more appropriately with diseases such as Wegener's granulomatosis and sarcoidosis; while the other end comprises the various malignant lymphomas.

Dominant lymphocytic infiltration is, nevertheless, a convenient definitive feature from which to consider the small group of uncommon pulmonary diseases that are described in this section. There is often paraprotein production, implying that a lymphocyte clone is involved. Depending on severity, these disorders are characterized clinically by cough (usually dry) and progressive undue exertional breathlessness; though systemic features of fever, malaise, and weight loss may also be prominent. Clubbing is not common, but there are frequently inspiratory crackles at the lung bases. The chest radiograph shows a diffuse interstitial pattern or patchy 'pneumonic' (i.e. air space) infiltrates with the more benign disorders, but nodular shadows at the more malignant end of the disease spectrum. Lung function tests show a non-specific pattern of ventilatory restriction with impaired parenchymal function.

Lymphocytic (and plasma cell) interstitial pneumonitis (pneumonia)

At the most benign end of the spectrum of lymphocytic infiltrations, lymphocytic (or lymphoid) interstitial pneumonitis is characterized by diffuse infiltration of the lung interstitium and alveolar walls with small mature lymphocytes, immunoblasts (activated lymphocytes), and plasma cells. Occasionally plasma cells dominate the lymphoid cell infiltrate, and in these circumstances the term plasma cell interstitial pneumonitis is preferred.

Lymphocytic pulmonary infiltration may occur in isolation without obvious cause; it may also be a non-specific feature of underlying pulmonary or systemic disease, such as HIV or Epstein–Barr virus (**EBV**) infection, drug hypersensitivity (sometimes toxicity), Castleman's disease (giant follicular lymph node hyperplasia), and (like Castleman's disease) a variety of autoimmune disorders, of which rheumatoid disease, Sjögren's syndrome, and systemic lupus erythematosus are most prominent. It may also be a consequence of a graft-versus-host reaction, and of common variable immunodeficiency—a primary antibody deficiency syndrome. When it occurs in children with AIDS it is thought to be largely a consequence of EBV infection. It may progress to (or be complicated by) the development of lymphoma, or be a feature of it. This too is particularly associated with Sjögren's syndrome.

The infiltrating lymphocytes show various levels of activation, and excess circulating immunoglobulins, whether monoclonal or polyclonal, are commonly observed. Occasionally there is hypo- rather than hyper-gammaglobulinaemia. When plasma cells rather than lymphocytes are dominant, the immunoglobulins are much less likely to be of the IgM class, though later complications may still include Waldenstrom's macroglobulinaemia or multiple myeloma. Bronchoalveolar lavage shows an excess of CD8+ T cells when lymphocytic interstitial pneumonitis is associated with HIV, whilst in Sjögren's syndrome the recovered lymphocytes are of the CD4+ phenotype.

The radiographic features, best seen with high resolution CT scans, are those of diffuse interstitial shadowing similar to cryptogenic fibrosing alveolitis, or (less commonly) air space filling. Cysts are often present, the mechanism being uncertain, and occasionally there are large nodules (> 10 mm in diameter). Effusion is not characteristic. The overall appearances are not specific, and since the disorder is rare, open biopsy is generally required for definitive diagnosis. It is seen in both sexes, usually in middle age, though children are not uncommonly represented. Slow progression is characteristic, though lymphocytic interstitial pneumonitis is rather more responsive to corticosteroid or other immunosuppressive therapy than is cryptogenic fibrosing alveolitis, and it sometimes remits spontaneously. There may, however, be complicating (even fatal) sepsis. The ultimate prognosis depends most on that of any underlying disease.

Benign lymphocytic angiitis

Lymphocytic infiltration in this condition is centred in small arteries and arterioles, necrosis is characteristically absent, and not infrequently there is granuloma formation. It therefore has both vasculitic and granulomatous features. It is rare, relatively benign, and usually affects the lungs or the skin. Most often there is no obvious provoking cause, but there have been reports of it emerging as a consequence of drug administration (streptokinase), HIV infection, or intrathoracic malignancy (thymoma).

Pulmonary lesions are usually single and most commonly present as asymptomatic nodules on a chance chest radiograph, the diagnosis being made following biopsy or resection. There may be systemic symptoms, however, and treatment with corticosteroids or cytotoxic agents may be necessary. The disease may progress to produce the more characteristic features of lymphomatoid granulomatosis, but more typically there is spontaneous remission. This suggests that benign lymphocytic angiitis is primarily a benign reactive vasculitis rather than a malignant lymphoma. It may be that similar histological features sometimes occur early in the course of lymphomatoid granulomatosis.

Immunoblastic (angio-immunoblastic) lymphadenopathy

This is a systemic and often febrile disorder characterized by widespread reactive lymphadenopathy and the infiltration of various organs by activated lymphoid cells, usually but not uniformly T lymphocytes. CD8+ cells, often clonal, are observed more commonly than CD4+ cells in affected organs, but in peripheral blood active disease is characterized by decreased numbers of T cells and an increase in B lymphocytes. The latter are possibly released from T-cell control and this might explain the frequency of paraprotein production. Infiltration of blood vessels may be prominent, hence the original term, angio-immunoblastic lymphadenopathy.

It occurs most commonly in the elderly and frequently in isolation, but it is often a consequence of infection (prominently HIV infection in recent years in younger subjects) or drug administration (often antibiotics), and it may be associated with autoimmunity.

Respiratory involvement is not common, usually comprising mediastinal or hilar lymphadenopathy, though diffuse interstitial infiltration and pleural effusion may occur. The involvement and enlargement of other lymphoid organs, particularly lymph nodes, liver, and spleen, usually offers a ready biopsy site for definitive diagnosis.

Management requires treatment of any provoking cause and, if necessary, the use of corticosteroids or other immunosuppressive agents. Occasionally there is spontaneous remission, but more commonly a T-cell lymphoma evolves. Indeed, the view is strengthening that most cases are due to peripheral (i.e. post-thymic) T-cell lymphoma.

Lymphomatoid granulomatosis (angiocentric lymphoma)

Lymphomatoid granulomatosis is now widely considered to be a low-grade lymphoma, though the typical histological appearances of prominent infiltration of blood vessel walls and granuloma formation have, until recently, suggested a disease of more benign nature. The infiltrating cells comprise a mixture of lymphocytes, plasma cells, histiocytes, and atypical (usually malignant) lymphoid cells. The latter are derived from B lymphocytes, in some cases probably because of infection with EBV, but activated T cells are also prominent in focal lesions. Proliferation and vascular infiltration were initially assumed to cause luminal obstruction followed by ischaemic necrosis, but there are now doubts whether true vasculitis and true granuloma formation actually occur. As a consequence it has been proposed that angiocentric lymphoma is a more appropriate descriptive term.

The disease is uncommon in childhood but occurs throughout adult life with a slight predilection for males. It may arise on a background of an immunocompromised state. The lungs are almost invariably affected, but skin, central nervous system, and renal involvement is frequently seen, and there is often peripheral neuropathy. The disease is typically multifocal, affecting several organs, and may simulate disseminated carcinoma. Pulmonary lesions are usually discrete and nodular, whether single or multiple, but may vary in size from less than a centimetre in diameter to several centimetres across. Occasionally outlines are irregular and indistinct, suggesting patchy consolidation. Cavitation may occur, when an inflammatory cause may consequently be suspected, the radiographic appearances simulating those of Wegener's granulomatosis.

Symptoms are commonly dominated by systemic upset (fever, malaise, and weight loss), but respiratory involvement is likely to cause cough (sometimes with haemoptysis) or undue breathlessness. The involvement of other organs may provide valuable diagnostic insight, but biopsy is necessary for definitive diagnosis. Temporary improvement sometimes follows treatment with corticosteroids alone, but a realistic chance of cure requires cytotoxic therapy for lymphoma.

Lymphoma

Unquestionably at the malignant end of the disease spectrum lies lymphomatous infiltration of the lung. All lymphoma types may present with intrathoracic disease, and all may involve the thorax later if they present elsewhere. Lymph nodes, lymphatics, and lung parenchyma may all become infiltrated, but the pattern may vary between tumour types.

A comprehensive review of lymphomas is beyond the scope of this section, and the reader is referred to Section 22 for full details. To the chest physician the distinction of Hodgkin's disease and low-grade non-Hodgkin's disease from high-grade non-Hodgkin's disease is of particular value, since the former are now generally curable—or at least highly responsive to treatment.

Hodgkin's disease is generally a disease of adults and adolescents. When it involves the thorax it usually does so by infiltrating hilar or mediastinal lymph nodes, though patchy or even diffuse parenchymal infiltration does rarely occur, with or without lymphadenopathy. Asymmetrical nodal enlargement favours lymphoma over sarcoidosis, the other disorder (apart from tuberculosis in endemic areas) that commonly produces hilar and mediastinal adenopathy. Hodgkin's disease frequently involves other nodal sites at presentation, but may be confined to the thorax. Pleural effusion is not uncommon, and occasionally there is infiltration of the chest wall.

Biopsy and staging are essential to diagnosis and management, though the advent of computed tomographic scanning has greatly simplified the latter by eliminating the need for laparotomy. Radiotherapy is normally curative for localized nodal disease and is invaluable as an adjunct in reducing local 'bulk' when the disease is disseminated. It carries much less risk than chemotherapy, which is required for parenchymal or disseminated disease, and for the small proportion of patients with localized nodal disease who show features of poor prognostic significance (e.g. high 'bulk', systemic symptoms, and anaemia).

Non-Hodgkin's lymphoma is more common than Hodgkin's disease and tends to affect a rather older population. Its thoracic manifestations are similar to those of Hodgkin's disease, but it is the more likely malignant 'complication' of the other lymphocytic pulmonary infiltrations discussed in this section. It also has a greater tendency to be disseminated at presentation, to have more 'high grade' features histologically and clinically, and (not surprisingly) to be less responsive to therapy. Nevertheless, localized and low-grade tumours are often curable, and useful palliation is generally achieved for all but the most high-grade tumours.

High resolution CT scanning shows that both types of lymphoma are most commonly characterized by an air space filling pattern rather than interstitial shadowing, and by large nodules and pleural effusions.

Chemotherapeutic regimens for the treatment of lymphoma continue to develop rapidly and have properly become the responsibility of specialist haemato-oncologists. Chemotherapy is, of course, attended by the familiar risks of bone marrow suppression and an immunocompromised state, but with regard to those with lung disease it is noteworthy that many of the chemotherapeutic agents can themselves cause interstitial lung disease—including lymphocytic infiltration. The supervising physician may consequently face a classic diagnostic dilemma when, following an initial satisfactory remission, the patient's radiographs show pulmonary shadows consistent with infection, drug hypersensitivity/toxicity, or recurrent lymphomatous infiltration. A prompt and accurate diagnosis is essential since each possibility requires fundamentally different management. Expectorated secretions may provide adequate evidence of infection to justify a trial of antibiotic therapy, but if immediate progress is unsatisfactory, fibreoptic bronchoscopy with lavage and/or transbronchial biopsy is generally needed. It may be that with increasing use of the polymerase chain reaction to amplify fragments of genetically specific microbial material, sputum or even oropharyngeal secretions will prove adequate to identify the infecting organisms. However, the cause of pulmonary shadows in this situation is often complex, and any combination of these three diagnostic groups may develop (perhaps with more than one infecting micro-organism). A multi-disciplinary approach to management has consequently become essential, involving chest physicians, radiologists, microbiologists, and histopathologists under the expertise of supervising oncologists or haematologists.

Further reading

Calabrese LH *et al.* (1989). Systemic vasculitis in association with human immunodeficiency virus infection. *Arthritis and Rheumatism* **32**, 569–76.

Churg A (1983). Pulmonary angiitis and granulomatosis revisited. *Human Pathology* **14**, 868–83.

Donnelly TJ, Tuder RM, Vendegna TR (1998). A 48-year-old woman with peripheral neuropathy, hypercalcaemia, and pulmonary infiltrates. *Chest* **114**, 1205–9.

Frizzera G, Moran EM, Rappaport H (1974). Angio-immunoblastic lymphadenopathy with dysproteinaemia. *Lancet* **ii**, 1070–3.

Glickstein M *et al.*(1986). Non lymphomatous lymphoid disorders of the lung. *American Journal of Roentgenology* **147**, 227–37.

Guinee DR *et al.* (1998). Proliferation and cellular phenotype in lymphomatoid granulomatosis: implications of a higher proliferation index in B cells. *American Journal of Surgical Pathology* **22**, 1093–100.

Haque AK *et al.* (1998). Pulmonary lymphomatoid granulomatosis in acquired immunodeficiency syndrome: lesions with Epstein–Barr virus. Modern Pathology **11**, 347–56.

Honda O *et al.* (1999). Differential diagnosis of lymphocytic interstitial pneumonia and malignant lymphoma on high-resolution CT. *American Journal of Roentgenology* **173**, 71–4.

Katzenstein A-LA, Carrington CB, Liebow AA (1979). Lymphomatoid granulomatosis. A clinicopathologic study of 152 cases. *Cancer* **43**, 360–73.

Liebow AA (1973). Pulmonary angiitis and granulomatosis. *American Review of Respiratory Disease* **108**, 1–18.

O'Connor NT *et al.* (1986). Evidence for monoclonal T lymphocyte proliferation in angioimmunoblastic lymphadenopathy. *Journal of Clinical Pathology* **39**, 1229–32.

Watanabe S *et al.* (1986). Immunoblastic lymphadenopathy, angioimmunoblastic lymphadenopathy, and IBL-like T-cell lymphoma. A spectrum of T-cell neoplasia. *Cancer* **58**, 2224–32.

Weiss LM *et al.* (1986). Clonal T-cell populations in angioimmunoblastic lymphadenopathy and angioimmunoblastic lymphadenopathy-like lymphoma. *American Journal of Pathology* **122**, 392–7.

17.11.11 Extrinsic allergic alveolitis

D. J. Hendrick and G. P. Spickett

Historical background

Farmer's lung is often regarded as the prototype of the alveolar and bronchiolar disorders that result from hypersensitivity to inhaled organic dusts. These occur worldwide and are known collectively by the term extrinsic allergic alveolitis, although it is recognized that the underlying inflammatory response occurs diffusely throughout the gas exchanging tissues and is not confined to the alveoli. For this reason many prefer the term hypersensitivity pneumonitis. These alveolar disorders were not clearly distinguished from asthma until 1932 when Campbell published his celebrated report describing three affected English farm workers, the appellation 'farmer's lung' being suggested in 1944. However, the disease had been recognized in Iceland in the nineteenth century, and probably contributed to the occupational ailments of grain workers so graphically described by Ramazzini in the eighteenth century.

Part of the eminence of farmer's lung itself stems from its industrial importance, and part from its historical role in the understanding of extrinsic allergic alveolitis. Its relation to the inhalation of dust from mouldy hay, straw, or grain had been recognized from the outset, but it was not until 1961 when Pepys and colleagues demonstrated the presence of precipitins to antigens of mouldy hay in patients suffering from the disease that the idea of an allergic aetiology gained general acceptance. These and other investigators showed that the main sources of antigen were contaminating thermophilic actinomycetes, particularly *Micropolyspora faeni* (now known as *Saccharopolyspora rectivirgula*) and *Thermoactinomyces vulgaris*. These thermophilic microbes (which are actually bacteria not fungi) colonize fermenting damp vegetable produce as it heats up. When it eventually dries, a respirable dust laden with antigenic microbial spores is left. Symptoms are consequently most common during winters following wet summer harvests, when hay or grain is used for feeding stock, and astonishing numbers of spores (thousands of millions per cubic metre) are released into the air.

For deposition of the dust to occur predominantly in the gas exchanging tissues, particle size must be largely confined to the range 0.5 to 5 µm. This encompasses the diameters of many antigenic bacterial and fungal spores, and a large number of microbial species are now recognized as causes of extrinsic allergic alveolitis. In addition, the disease has been described following respiratory exposure to a variety of antigens derived from animal, vegetable, and even chemical sources, both in the workplace and in the home. It may also occur because of allergy to ingested agents, chiefly medications, but only inhalant causes will be addressed in this chapter. Drug-induced examples of the disease are discussed in Chapter 17.11.19.

Causative agents

Table 1 lists the various agents, principally organic proteins, reported to cause extrinsic allergic alveolitis. Most are encountered in working environments and so the disease is usually occupational, but some are encountered in the home or in recreational environments. Most are micro-organisms that are found contaminating a variety of vegetable products, but some are derived directly from animal or vegetable sources, and a few are reactive chemicals. The latter are thought to act as haptens, combining with body proteins to produce a larger and now antigenic molecule. Although the micro-organisms associated with the more celebrated disorders—farmer's lung, mushroom worker's lung, and bagassosis—are usually thermophilic, the majority causing extrinsic allergic alveolitis are not. Even with mouldy hay and farmer's lung there is evidence that non-thermophilic organisms (e.g. *Aspergillus* spp.) may occasionally be involved.

Some microbial contamination may occur during growth of the vegetable host, but most of the antigenic load is usually acquired after harvest. Prolonged storage under damp conditions increases the risk of extrinsic allergic alveolitis substantially, whilst drying to reduce the water content below 30 per cent greatly lessens the risks. Farmer's lung and bagassosis are not therefore primary disorders of hay, grain, or sugar cane harvest. They usually arise months or even years later when the stored product is used or moved. In the interim, moulding is likely to have involved a series of different micro-organisms that colonize the forage material sequentially. As the exothermic process increases the ambient temperature, so thermophilic microbes come to dominate.

Inevitably there are situations where contamination arises with a number of different microbes, and affected subjects show antibodies to several of them. Unless time-consuming inhalation challenge tests are carried out with extracts of the individual microbial species, it is not possible to identify a single responsible agent in a given case or cases, and it is conceivable that several could be relevant in these circumstances. This is a characteristic feature of contaminated water reservoirs in humidifiers and air conditioners, and a great variety of agents have been suggested as possible causes of humidifier lung, including bacteria, mycobacteria, fungi, protozoa (amoebae), and metazoa (nematode debris). Some authors prefer to distinguish extrinsic allergic alveolitis attributable in such circumstances to micro-organisms growing in cool or cold water (humidifier lung) from that arising from heated water (ventilation pneumonitis). Additional sources of causal organisms include hot tubs and saunas, containing both thermophilic and non-thermophilic organisms (including non-tuberculous mycobacteria), and water-based metal working fluids. The latter, often contaminated with oil, are recycled during use to lubricate and cool rotating or cutting equipment in the metal working industry, and may therefore be dispersed as respirable aerosols. The chief microbial contaminants are generally environmental non-tuberculous mycobacteria or fungi, but a variety of other organisms may be involved. Since granulomatous responses might be expected from mycobacterial infection, the mechanism of diffuse pneumonitis when mycobacteria are involved may not be one of hypersensitivity.

Curiously, contamination with multiple microbial species does not seem to be a feature of Japanese summer-type pneumonitis, which arises seasonally in the hot and humid regions in the south and west of Japan and neighbouring countries. This is the result of the excessive growth of *Trichosporon* spp. in unsanitary and poorly ventilated homes.

Table 1 Agents reported to cause extrinsic allergic alveolitis

Agent	Source	Appellation
Micro-organisms		
Acinetobacter iwoffii	Metal working fluid	Machine worker's lung
Alternaria	Paper mill wood pulp	Wood pulp worker's lung
Aspergillus clavatus	Whisky maltings	Malt worker's lung
Aspergillus fumigatus	Vegetable compost	Farmer's lung
Aspergillus versicolor	Dog bedding (straw)	Dog house disease
Aureobasidium pullulans	Redwood	Sequoiosis
Bacillus subtilis	Domestic wood	
Cephalosporium	Sewage	Sewage worker's lung
Cryptostroma corticale	Maple	Maple bark stripper's lung
Graphium	Redwood	Sequoiosis
Lentinus edodes	Mushrooms	Mushroom worker's lung
Lycoperdon	Puffballs	Lycoperdonosis
Merulius lacrymans	Domestic wood	
Mucor stolonifer	Paprika	Paprika splitter's lung
Mycobacterium sp.	Metal working fluid	Machine worker's lung
Penicillium camembertii[1]	Salami production	
Penicillium casei	Cheese	Cheese washer's lung
Penicillium chrysogenum/	Domestic wood	
Penicillium cyclopium		
Penicillium frequentens	Cork	Suberosis
Pezizia domiciliana	Flooded basement	El Niño lung
Pleurotus osteatus	Mushrooms	Mushroom worker's lung
Rhodotorula sp.	Ultrasonic humidifier	
Saccharomonspora viridis	Logging plant	
Sporobolomyces	Horse barn straw	
Streptomyces albus	Soil/peat	
Thermophilic actinomycetes	Hay/straw/grain/	Farmer's lung
(*Saccharopolyspora rectivirgula*,	mushroom compost/	Mushroom worker's lung
Thermoactinomyces	bagasse/heated water	Bagassosis
sacchari/vulgaris)		
Trichosporon cutaneum/	Japanese summer air	Summer-type hypersensitivity
Trichosporon ovoides		pneumonitis
Miscellaneous bacteria/mycobacteria/fungi/	Air conditioners/humidifiers/	Humidifier lung, ventilation
amoebae/nematode debris	tap water/heated pools	pneumonitis, sauner taker's lung
Unknown	Roof thatch	New Guinea lung
Animals		
Arthropods (*Sitophilus granarius*)	Grain dust	Wheat weevil disease
Birds	?Bloom / ?excreta	Bird fancier's lung
Fish	Fish meal	Fish meal worker's lung
Mammals		
Pituitary (cattle, pig)	Pituitary extracts	Pituitary snuff taker's lung
Hair	Fur	Furrier's lung
Mollusc shell	Nacre-button manufacture	
Urine (rodents)	Urinary protein	Rodent handler's lung
Vegetation		
Coffee	Coffee bean dust	Coffee worker's lung
Esparto grass[2]	Plaster	
Peat moss[3]	Peat moss packaging plant	
Shimeji[4]	Shimeji cultivators	
Tiger nut	Tiger nut dust	
Wood (*Gonystylus bacanus*)	Wood dust	Wood worker's lung
Chemicals		
Bordeaux mixture (fungicide)	Vineyards	Vineyard sprayer's lung
Cobalt dissolved in solvents	Tungsten carbide grinding	
Diphenyl methane diisocyanate	Plastics industry	
Formaldehyde[5]	Laboratory	
Hexamethylene diisocyanate	Plastics industry	
Pauli's reagent	Laboratory	
Phthalic (or trimellitic) anhydride	Epoxy polyester powder paint	
Pyrethrum	Insecticide spray	
Toluene diisocyanate	Plastics industry	
Trimellitic anhydride	Plastics industry	

[1]Alternative possible causes, *Penicillium notatum*, *Aspergillus fumigatus*.

[2]Possibly due to microbial contamination (*Aspergillus* sp.).

[3]Possibly due to microbial contamination (*Monocillium* sp., *Penicillium citreonigrum*).

[4]Possibly due to microbial contamination (*Cladosporium sphaerospermum*, *Penicillium frequentens*, or *Scopulariopsis* sp.).

[5]One subject, possibly toxic not allergic response.

Epidemiology

Extrinsic allergic alveolitis is an uncommon but not rare disease. Its comparative scarcity limits epidemiological knowledge, as does the use of different methods of investigation. For every case there may be 100 cases of 'extrinsic allergic' asthma, but there is even greater geographical variation than with asthma reflecting the much larger dependence of extrinsic allergic alveolitis on occupational causes and climate. As a consequence, its incidence and its principal causes vary considerably from country to country, and from region to region.

Incidence

Experience over 3 years with the **SWORD** project (Surveillance of Work-related and Occupational Respiratory Disease) indicated that extrinsic allergic alveolitis of occupational origin accounted for 2 per cent of occupational lung diseases in the United Kingdom. Asthma, the most common, accounted for 26 per cent. This does, of course, ignore extrinsic allergic alveolitis of non-occupational origin, which is much less easily assessed. It also disguises the absolute risk since few workers encounter relevant occupational exposures. Almost 50 per cent of reported cases involved farmers or farm workers, followed by 15 per cent affecting workers in material, metal, or electrical processing trades. Among the farmers, the average incidence was 41 per million per year, though this approached 100 in some regions, and has been estimated at 3000 in Quebec, Canada. However, the estimated incidences are crude and must vary considerably according to the prevailing weather. They may be compared with 200 to 700 per million per year among working groups at greatest risk of developing occupational asthma in the United Kingdom. Contaminating micro-organisms underlie over 50 per cent of the cases of extrinsic allergic alveolitis reported to SWORD, followed in order of importance by animal antigens in 6 per cent and chemicals in 5 per cent. In 27 per cent of reports a suspected agent was not specified.

Prevalence

Figures for prevalence (the proportion affected among a given population at a given point of time) are more readily available than those for incidence, and demonstrate quite marked national differences. In developed countries, humidifier lung is being recognized with increasing frequency in both the workplace and the home, and remarkable prevalences of 15 to 70 per cent have been suggested in populations from contaminated offices in North America. Bird fancier's lung may be more prevalent at present over the whole of the United Kingdom, simply because of the great popularity of keeping budgerigars and pigeons. Budgerigars are kept in some 12 per cent of British homes, and it has been estimated that 0.5 to 7.5 per cent of the population involved are likely to have extrinsic allergic alveolitis as a consequence, albeit mildly in most cases. Pigeon keeping is 40 times less common, and the measured prevalence of pigeon fancier's lung among pigeon keepers has been a good deal more varied (0 to 21 per cent). This may reflect both true differences between groups of pigeon breeders as exposure levels vary, for instance, according to number of birds, duration of exposure, loft ventilation, and cleaning habits, and artefactual differences arising as a result of selection bias and the notorious lack of compliance shown by pigeon fanciers in epidemiological studies. The avian antigen responsible and its precise source have yet to be identified, but bloom from the feathers containing oil, saliva, and secretory IgA is currently favoured over dust emanating from dried droppings.

In areas of high rainfall where 'traditional' farming methods are used, the prevalence of farmer's lung may reach 10 per cent. This is likely to be the commonest cause of extrinsic allergic alveolitis in developing countries. In developed countries, where modern farming methods are used, prevalences rarely exceed 2 to 3 per cent and are usually a good deal less. Furthermore, the farming population at risk represents a mere 1 to 2 per cent of the population at large, although there are marked regional variations. Even smaller populations are employed making whisky from germinating barley (maltings), raising mushrooms on a variety of antigenic composts, or handling bagasse (the fibrous stem that remains when sugar is extracted from sugar cane), but within some of these populations extrinsic allergic alveolitis was a common problem until excessive exposure levels were controlled. Extrinsic allergic alveolitis associated with animals other than birds is extremely uncommon, as is the case with chemical-induced extrinsic allergic alveolitis.

In Japan, the seasonal summer growth of *T. cutaneum* in the home is by far the commonest cause of extrinsic allergic alveolitis where the remarkable 'summer-type hypersensitivity pneumonitis' accounts for about 75 per cent of all cases of extrinsic allergic alveolitis. It is approximately 10 times as common as farmer's lung and 20 times as common as bird fancier's lung. Occasionally other subspecies of *Tricosporon* are responsible.

Pathogenic mechanisms

Histology

There has been little opportunity to characterize the acute form of extrinsic allergic alveolitis histologically because biopsies are very rarely taken within 24 to 48 h of a provoking exposure, and because death leading to autopsy is even less common. Initially there is a non-specific diffuse pneumonitis with inflammatory cellular infiltration of the bronchioles, alveoli, and interstitium, accompanied by oedema and luminal exudation. With ongoing exposure, whether continuous or intermittent, the more familiar appearances of the subacute forms of extrinsic allergic alveolitis evolve. The most characteristic feature is the formation of epithelioid non-caseating granulomas. These are generally less well formed than in sarcoidosis, less profuse, and often evanescent. They can be recognized within 3 weeks of the initiating exposure, and generally resolve within 6 to 12 months. In parallel, fibrosis evolves alongside cellular infiltration of the interstitium with histiocytes, lymphocytes, and plasma cells. Macrophages with foamy cytoplasm may be prominent in the alveolar spaces, and organization of the inflammatory exudate may lead to intra-alveolar fibrosis. Obstruction or obliteration of bronchioles is common. Foreign body giant cells may reflect the dependence of extrinsic allergic alveolitis on antigens derived from inhaled foreign material, as does a peribronchial predominance of the inflammatory response. Vasculitis is notable by its absence. The typical histological appearance of subacute extrinsic allergic alveolitis is illustrated in Fig. 1.

With continued exposure, progressive, widespread, and irreversible fibrosis may occur, leading to disruption of the normal architecture of the lung. In advanced cases honeycombing may develop. Granulomas are no longer characteristic, and the overall appearances may differ little from other causes of progressive interstitial pulmonary fibrosis. With extrinsic

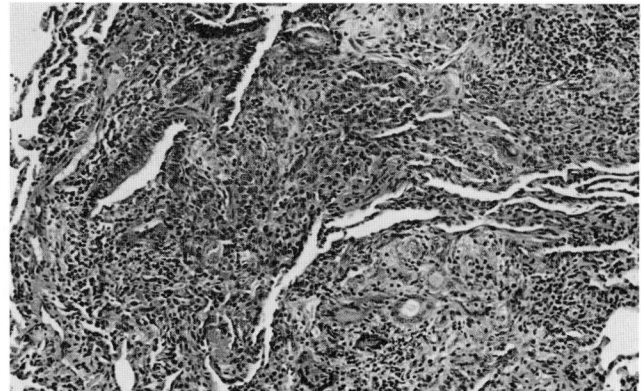

Fig. 1 Histological appearance: subacute disease (by courtesy of Dr T. Ashcroft). Haematoxylin and eosin stain. Medium magnification. There is bronchocentric interstitial fibrosis and chronic inflammation, with poorly formed interstitial granulomas including giant cells.

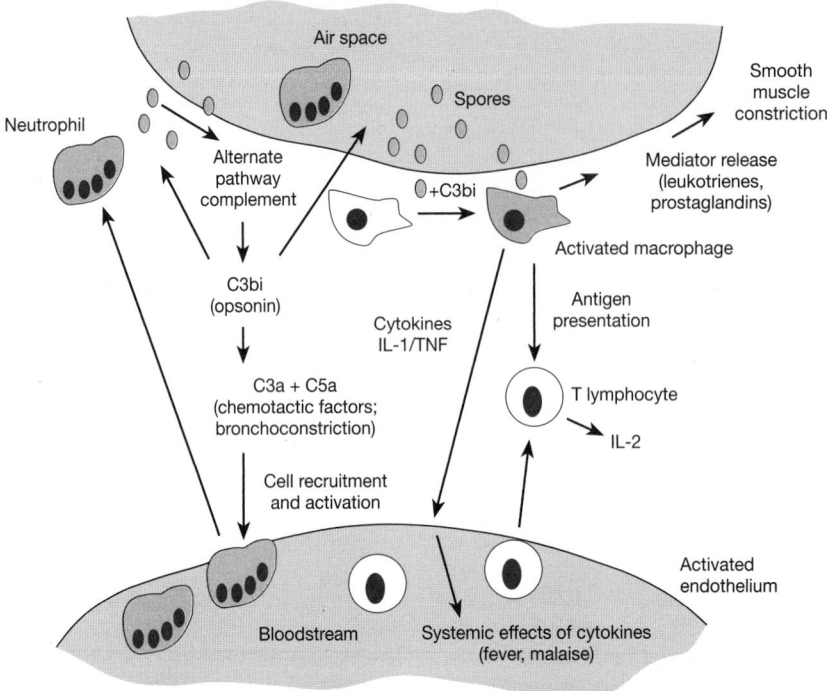

Fig. 2 Possible immunopathogenesis: acute phase.

allergic alveolitis, however, there may be disproportionate fibrosis of the upper lobes.

Immune mechanisms

An outline of the possible immunopathology of extrinsic allergic alveolitis through acute, subacute, and chronic phases is illustrated in Figs 2 and 3. The presumption that complexes of antigen and complement-activating antibodies are primarily responsible for extrinsic allergic alveolitis is now largely discarded. The evidence for deposition of immune complexes is not convincing, and neither IgG nor IgM antibodies are uniformly demonstrated in the sera of affected subjects unless sensitive detection techniques such as the enzyme-linked immunosorbent assay or radioimmunoassays

are used. More importantly, these antibodies are frequently found in subjects who are similarly exposed but clinically unaffected, irrespective of the method of detection. A closer association of disease with the IgG4 antibody subclass has been suggested, but the significance of this is not yet apparent. It is clear, however, that vasculitis—a cardinal feature of the experimental Arthus reaction—is not a characteristic; the inflammatory reaction is dominantly lymphocytic or mononuclear rather than polymorphonuclear. However, a transitory polymorphonuclear leucocyte response is typical immediately following exposure. Lung tissue is most commonly examined during subacute phases of the disease, at which time a non-caseating granulomatous response suggesting cell-mediated hypersensitivity is the usual finding.

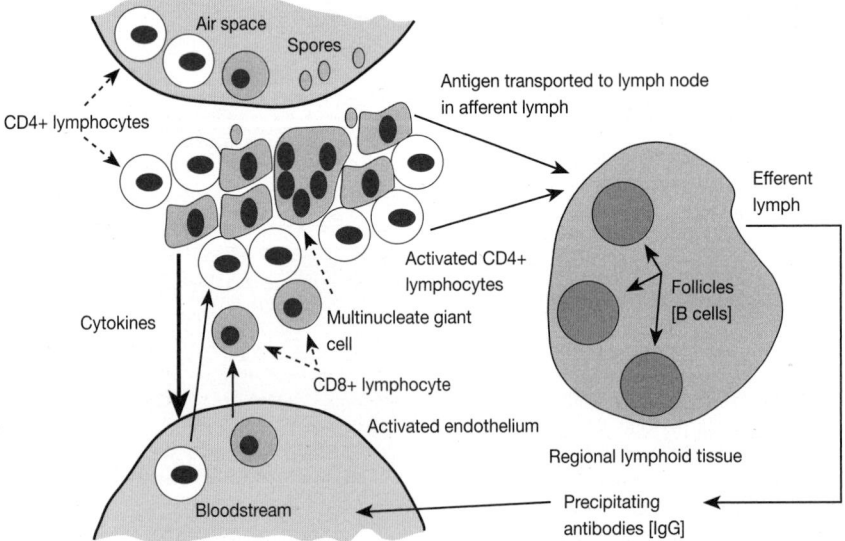

Fig. 3 Possible immunopathogenesis: subacute/chronic phase.

It could be argued that these histological appearances merely represent a healing reaction, but the consistent finding of an acute T-lymphocyte response in fluid obtained at bronchoalveolar lavage supports the current consensus that cell-mediated hypersensitivity plays the dominant pathogenic role in extrinsic allergic alveolitis. The results from animal models of the disease are consistent with this, disease being transferred from animal to animal only with sensitized T lymphocytes. This is not to say that other mechanisms play no role, nor that all inflammatory diseases of the gas exchanging tissues induced by organic dusts share a common mechanism. Indeed, the onset of symptoms within a few hours of exposure, coupled with polymorphonuclear leucocytosis in bronchoalveolar lavage fluid and peripheral blood, favours the participation of an additional (perhaps priming) immunological or toxic process, and B-lymphocyte aggregates have been noted in transbronchial biopsies obtained during the acute phase. Components of a number of organic dusts associated with extrinsic allergic alveolitis are known to activate complement by the alternative pathway and this, with or without humoral hypersensitivity, might also prove to be relevant.

In fact, bronchoalveolar lavage in similarly exposed subjects has shown excess numbers of T lymphocytes whether they were clinically affected or not, though the proportions of T-cell subpopulations has varied according to disease activity and the circumstances of exposure. Most investigators have detected a relative excess of CD8+ T cells in exposed but asymptomatic subjects, thereby 'inverting' the normal CD4+ to CD8+ ratio. The balance appears to be less disturbed in those with disease, and in one sequential study the ratio changed from 0.43 to 1.47 with disease progression. In an intriguing study of an animal model of extrinsic allergic alveolitis, monkeys that developed characteristic reactions to inhalation challenge showed a helper CD4+ cell lymphocytosis in bronchoalveolar fluid and a relative deficiency of suppressor CD8+ cells, compared with the monkeys giving no clinical reaction who showed responses with both CD4+ and CD8+ cells. When the non-reactors were challenged again after low doses of whole-body irradiation had impaired suppressor more than helper cell function, characteristic reactions were noted. These observations suggest that a relative impairment of suppressor cell function, or of its activation following antigenic exposure, is fundamental to the development of extrinsic allergic alveolitis—a situation that has interesting parallels with sarcoidosis. It is also interesting that lymphopenia in peripheral blood is a typical feature of acute exacerbations of the disease, the T lymphocytes migrating from blood to lungs within hours of the provoking exposure. It is small wonder that studies of systemic and local immune responses have given discordant results, and clear that continuing research should address both aspects of the immune response.

It is known that different antigenic determinants from a given inducing microbial source may lead to different immunological responses, and it seems likely that cytotoxic activity and released cytokines (e.g. interleukin 6 and tumour necrosis factor-α) play some role, possibly by activating the vascular endothelium and thereby recruiting and activating further macrophages and inflammatory cells. In experimental models interferon-γ has been shown to play a major role (an excess of interferon-γ-producing T cells is present in the lungs), and interleukin 10 ameliorates the disease. This indicates that extrinsic allergic alveolitis is a T_{H1}-type disease. Interleukin 8, a chemotactic factor for neutrophils, and monocyte chemotactic protein-1 are both elevated in some types of the disease, perhaps accounting for the increase in macrophage and neutrophil recruitment and activation. Serum levels of interleukin 6 and intercell adhesion molecule 1 (ICAM-1) are also raised. Bronchoalveolar lavage has shown that natural killer cells (CD57+) and mast cells may be prominent additional players in pathogenesis, and there is evidence that the capacity of macrophages to present antigen is enhanced by viral infection. It is diminished by cigarette smoking, which is known to decrease the severity of clinical symptoms as well as the immunological abnormalities.

Cytokines, possibly together with anaphylotoxins from the degradation of complement components (C4, C3, C5), are likely to be responsible for the systemic influenza-like symptoms that are so characteristic of the acute form of extrinsic allergic alveolitis. These symptoms are indistinguishable from those of grain fever in grain workers, 'Monday fever' in cotton workers, humidifier fever in subjects exposed to microbially contaminated humidifiers, and metal fume fever in welders. In these situations, the febrile disorder is not characteristically associated with clinical alveolitis, raising the possibility that its occurrence with the acute form of extrinsic allergic alveolitis is an independent phenomenon, not an integral part of extrinsic allergic alveolitis itself. In favour of this hypothesis has been the finding of high levels of endotoxin from Gram-negative bacteria (which are known to provoke these symptoms) in grain dust, cotton dust, contaminated humidifiers, and many of the 'mouldy' vegetable dusts that cause extrinsic allergic alveolitis. However, neither metal fume nor several other causative agents of extrinsic allergic alveolitis are likely to be contaminated with endotoxin, and so endotoxin-induced release of inflammatory mediators is not an entirely satisfactory explanation. For example, inhalation provocation tests with uncontaminated bird serum in subjects with bird fancier's lung reproduce both alveolar and influenza-like responses. Evidently the influenza-like response is an integral feature of the acute form of extrinsic allergic alveolitis, but it is relatively non-specific and can occur in many other situations.

Extrinsic allergic alveolitis occurs in families only sporadically, and few associations with HLA phenotypes have been demonstrated. However, a number of recent studies have suggested associations between HLA D alleles and pigeon fancier's lung and Japanese summer-type hypersensitivity pneumonitis. Such alleles may exert effects on immune suppression, and offer one mechanism by which a genetic predisposition could play a role in the development of extrinsic allergic alveolitis. It has also been suggested that an acute inflammatory episode (from viral infection or the inhalation of microbial toxins or chemicals) may be necessary to disrupt the normal defence equilibrium of surface membrane and local immune responses, and thereby permit antigen to be presented in a fashion that leads to hypersensitivity. Undue 'leakiness' of the alveolar membrane can be demonstrated by an increased clearance of inhaled $^{99}Tc^m$-DTPA, and this has been reported in both the early and continuing phases of extrinsic allergic alveolitis.

Relation to smoking

The disruptive effect of smoking on the alveolar membrane does not appear to augment the risk for extrinsic allergic alveolitis or to increase its severity. Rather, the reverse is true. Although smoking enhances acute-phase reactions and IgE production, it diminishes IgA, IgG, and IgM antibody responses, increases circulating CD8+ T-lymphocyte numbers, and probably reduces the incidence and severity of extrinsic allergic alveolitis. However, the smoker without IgG antibodies is particularly liable to find his respiratory symptoms attributed to other diseases, and so this negative association between extrinsic allergic alveolitis and smoking may have been exaggerated. That it is real is supported by evidence that smoking may also reduce the risk for other T-cell-mediated immunological disorders such as sarcoidosis, ulcerative colitis, and some types of occupational asthma (generally those associated with low molecular weight chemicals). The key cell in a complex series of interactions is probably the alveolar macrophage, which is critical in presenting antigen to CD4+ T lymphocytes and so to activating cellular immune mechanisms. Although smoking increases macrophage numbers and their metabolic activity, the activated cells show impairment of both the expression of surface major histocompatibility class 2 antigens and the production or release of interleukin 1 and inflammatory mediators derived from arachidonic acid metabolism (leukotriene B4, prostaglandin E_2, thromboxane B_2). It is also argued that the increased macrophage numbers down-regulate pulmonary immune responses in a purely non-specific fashion by impairing antigen access to more effective blood monocytes.

Relation to coeliac disease

Reports that cryptogenic fibrosing alveolitis and extrinsic allergic alveolitis (and particularly bird fancier's lung) might be associated with coeliac disease led to the interesting hypothesis that in some cases absorbed food antigens from the disrupted bowel mucosa might play a role in the pathogenesis of the lung disorder; that is, the lung disorder might be a 'metastatic' complication of the bowel disease. Alternatively, systemic hypersensitivity to a common inhaled and ingested avian antigen might give rise to similar immune reactions and diseases in the relevant target organs. The avian IgG antibody response seen in coeliac disease is, however, distinct from that associated with bird fancier's lung and seems to be a response to dietary egg. It is not related to environmental exposure to birds but does correlate with the activity of the bowel disorder. Subsequent experience suggests a much less strong association between these bowel and lung disorders that, if real, is probably a consequence of their dependence on similar immunological mechanisms and host susceptibility to them.

Clinical features

Acute form

The acute form of extrinsic allergic alveolitis is the most easily recognized, because symptoms are often distressing and incapacitating, and have a high degree of specificity. Following a sensitizing period of exposure, which may vary from weeks to years, the affected subject experiences repeated episodes of an influenza-like illness accompanied by cough and undue breathlessness some hours (usually 3 to 9) after commencing exposure to the relevant organic dust. The systemic influenza-like symptoms generally dominate those that are respiratory, and the affected subject complains most of malaise, fever, chills, widespread aches and pains (particularly headache), anorexia, and tiredness. He is unlikely to feel like exercising and may well put himself to bed, therefore remaining unaware of undue shortness of breath, though he is likely to develop a dry cough without wheeze and to have some difficulty taking deep, satisfying breaths. Occasionally there is an asthmatic or bronchitic response and wheezing or productive cough becomes an additional feature.

Despite the delay in onset after exposure begins, affected subjects soon learn to associate symptoms with the causative environment, especially if they follow a period away from work or the causal exposure. Recognition is particularly easy for groups such as farmers and pigeon fanciers for whom these risks are well known. However, in some cases there may be a tendency to deny such a relationship for fear of compromising the ability to pursue livelihood or hobby, and the clinical history may appear much less convincing than it should.

The severity and duration of symptoms depend critically on exposure dose and individual susceptibility. With low levels of acute exposure, symptoms are mild and persist for a few hours only. When occupation is responsible, the affected worker may feel unwell only at home during the following evening or night, and be fully recovered by the next morning, hence obscuring the relevance of the workplace. When severe responses follow particularly heavy exposures the relation of the one to the other will be more obvious, and complete remission may require several days or even weeks.

In exceptionally severe cases, life-threatening respiratory failure may develop and emergency admission to hospital becomes necessary. Death is not unknown. Respiratory distress at rest with fever and gravity-dependent crackles comprise the major physical signs, with breathing being fast but shallow. Clubbing is very rarely seen. Hypoxaemia is typically accompanied by hypocapnia, and the chest radiograph shows a diffuse alveolar filling and interstitial pattern. Supplemental oxygen may be required, and in rare cases there may be a brief need for mechanical ventilatory support. Spontaneous recovery can be expected to begin within 12 to 24 h, and can be accelerated with corticosteroids.

Most subjects recover fully from each acute exacerbation, and if the cause is recognized and further exposure avoided, there is little risk of persisting pulmonary dysfunction. However, it is not always realistic to expect affected individuals to avoid further exposure, particularly among farming communities, and there is some risk that continuing exposure and repeated acute exacerbations will eventually lead to permanent impairment of lung function.

Chronic form

In some subjects extrinsic allergic alveolitis presents in a much less dramatic but potentially more serious way. Exercise tolerance is gradually lost due to shortness of breath, but without systemic upset aside from (in some cases only) prominent loss of weight. This is the result of diffuse pulmonary fibrosis, which has often been progressing for years before the affected subject seeks advice: the slower the progression, the longer the delay, and the greater the likely degree of permanent fibrotic damage. Eventually hypoxaemia and pulmonary hypertension may supervene, and the right heart fails. There are no acute exacerbations, and each day and each month are much like any other. The clinical features are similar to those of other varieties of pulmonary fibrosis, although clubbing is uncommon, and it may prove extremely difficult to distinguish this form of extrinsic allergic alveolitis from cryptogenic fibrosing alveolitis, sarcoidosis, or other slowly progressive forms of pulmonary fibrosis. There may also be asthmatic or bronchitic symptoms, but these are best regarded as independent airway manifestations of hypersensitivity to the causal agent.

The chronic form of extrinsic allergic alveolitis is typically seen in the subject who keeps a single budgerigar (known as a parakeet in North America) in the home. The level of antigenic exposure to avian dust is comparatively trivial (compared with the farm worker forking bales of heavily contaminated hay in a poorly ventilated barn), but it is encountered almost continuously, particularly if the affected subject is someone confined to the home. Differing exposure patterns are largely responsible for these distinct forms of extrinsic allergic alveolitis, although differences in host responsiveness must exert an important additional influence. There may consequently be considerable variability in clinical features among individuals affected by the same source of antigenic exposure.

Intermediate forms

The fact that the acute form of extrinsic allergic alveolitis can be produced by inhalation provocation tests in subjects with the chronic form of the disease emphasizes the major role that dose exerts in determining the clinical nature of the response that occurs. Depending on exposure dose and host responsiveness a variety of intermediate forms of extrinsic allergic alveolitis are recognized, and some subjects will experience different patterns of response at different times. Hence it is possible for acute exacerbations to occur in subjects manifesting predominantly the chronic form of the disease, and for a limited degree of recovery to follow cessation of exposure. In general, however, the individual affected by the chronic form of extrinsic allergic alveolitis should be satisfied if no further progression occurs following cessation of exposure, because in some cases fibrotic damage continues regardless.

Investigation

Establishing a diagnosis of extrinsic allergic alveolitis involves three areas of investigation: the lungs, the exposure, and the evidence for hypersensitivity.

Pulmonary

In many cases extrinsic allergic alveolitis is first suspected after the presence of diffuse alveolitis or progressive pulmonary fibrosis is established. With the acute form of the disease the chest radiograph commonly shows no abnormality unless symptoms are moderately severe. Normal radiographic appearances are particularly common with humidifier lung, possibly because antigen is largely presented in soluble rather than particulate form. When the radiograph is abnormal, there is a widespread ground-glass appearance or an alveolar filling pattern, particularly in the lower and mid-zones. This may resolve within a mere 24 to 48 h once exposure has ceased. In more subacute forms small reticular opacities, simulating asbestosis, are seen within the same distribution: these may persist for several weeks despite cessation of exposure and, if exposure continues, honeycombing may develop. Occasionally a more nodular pattern occurs. In contrast to the distribution of acute and subacute radiological abnormalities, the upper zones are predominantly affected by the irreversible fibrotic process that characterizes the chronic form of disease. This may simulate sarcoidosis or even tuberculosis, and may lead to considerable shrinkage and distortion. In practice, the radiographic appearances vary considerably from patient to patient, and correlate poorly with the clinical severity of the disease.

Computed tomographic (CT) scans provide a much clearer picture of the type of radiographic abnormality and of its extent, particularly when thin-section high-resolution techniques are used, but they have shown that no single feature or pattern is pathognomonic (Fig. 4). Again, investigation within hours of exposure has been limited and experience is largely confined to patients with subacute and chronic disease. Increased ground-glass density of the lung parenchyma is the most prominent finding in the subacute form, followed almost equally by reticular or nodular infiltration. At end expiration a mosaic pattern is characteristic, reflecting patchy bronchiolar involvement and the different degrees by which residual gas can be expelled from distal lobules. The attenuated areas may then be normal, the translucent areas indicating gas retention. Neither lymph node enlargement nor pleural involvement are characteristic. The CT scan is appreciably more sensitive than the plain chest radiograph, and shows a more uniform involvement of the lung fields in subacute disease than is obvious from plain radiographs. With chronic forms, the CT scan shows a similar pattern of fibrosis and disruption to the plain radiograph, but again is considerably more sensitive.

Lung function studies vary according to severity and recent activity. As with asthma, they may be unremarkable in the acute form of the disease when there has been little recent exposure. When lung function is impaired, the pattern suggests parenchymal and interstitial disease but is otherwise non-specific. There is impaired carbon monoxide gas transfer (diminished TLco and Kco) with restricted ventilation (i.e. forced vital capacity, FVC, is diminished as much as forced expiratory volume, FEV1, or more so, with respect to predicted values), decreased compliance, and (in more severe cases) arterial hypoxaemia and hypocapnia, particularly on exercise. Although total lung capacity is reduced, residual volume is often increased, suggesting air trapping as a result of bronchiolar involvement. Occasionally there is also obstruction of the large airways, but this implies a coincidental asthmatic or bronchitic effect. Serial measurements of lung function may be particularly useful in demonstrating that impairment is closely related to the relevant exposure.

Bronchoscopy and bronchoalveolar lavage are useful in demonstrating that there is no macroscopic abnormality, apart from the occasional presence of mucosal inflammation, and that no microbial growth occurs on culture. If lavage fluid is obtained within a matter of hours of exposure, a polymorphonuclear leucocyte response may dominate, simulating cryptogenic fibrosing alveolitis, but this is followed by an accumulation of lymphocytes over the following 24 to 48 h. In the subacute and chronic forms of the disease, T lymphocytes represent 10 to 20 per cent or more of recovered cells, though the absolute numbers of macrophages are generally increased also. This characteristic cellular picture is not specific for extrinsic allergic alveolitis, but it strongly supports the diagnosis if other suggestive features are present. Other granulomatous disorders, such as sarcoidosis and tuberculosis, hypersensitivity reactions to drugs, and a number of rare lymphoid infiltrative disorders are also associated with a lymphocytosis in lavage fluid, but in practice sarcoidosis is generally the most plausible alternative diagnosis.

In sarcoidosis, B-lymphocyte numbers are decreased and the excess T lymphocytes are typically CD4+ helper cells. The CD4+ to CD8+ ratio normally exceeds 1, and so is exaggerated. By contrast, the ratio is typically reversed in extrinsic allergic alveolitis, CD8+ cells outnumbering CD4+ cells, and B-lymphocyte numbers are not decreased. Lymphocyte markers may therefore help distinguish sarcoidosis from extrinsic allergic alveolitis. Unfortunately, the pattern favouring extrinsic allergic alveolitis does not distinguish so readily between subjects with exposure and symptoms and those with exposure but no symptoms. Both T-cell types show increased numbers if there is exposure, and the number of CD8+ cells tends to show a relatively greater, not lesser, increase in asymptomatic subjects, as described above. The absolute value of the CD4+ to CD8+ ratio therefore provides limited diagnostic benefit in identifying active disease, but this is rarely a relevant issue outside a research setting. A number of cytokines can also be recovered from the lavage fluid, but these are of research rather than diagnostic interest.

Transbronchial or open lung biopsy may occasionally be indicated when other diagnostic procedures do not distinguish extrinsic allergic alveolitis from cryptogenic fibrosing alveolitis or other diffuse infiltrative or fibrotic disorders of the lung. Biopsy is more likely to be needed in the subacute or chronic forms of the disease when hypersensitivity is less obvious, or acutely when there has been an unduly heavy exposure to microbial spores and there is suspicion of microbial invasion.

Environmental exposure

In many cases the history alone provides the evidence of relevant exposure, but this is not always reliable and an independent account of the exposures involved can be invaluable. Ideally, industrial hygiene measurements are made (particularly from personal samplers) so that respirable agents can be recognized and quantified, and microbiological techniques are used to identify specific microbial contaminants. These are sophisticated investigations and usually indicated only when extrinsic allergic alveolitis is first suspected in an environment not previously associated with the disease, particularly in industries where many individuals may be at risk and where

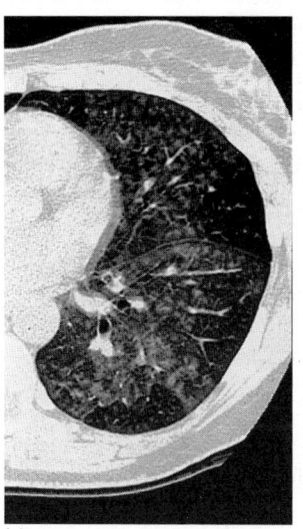 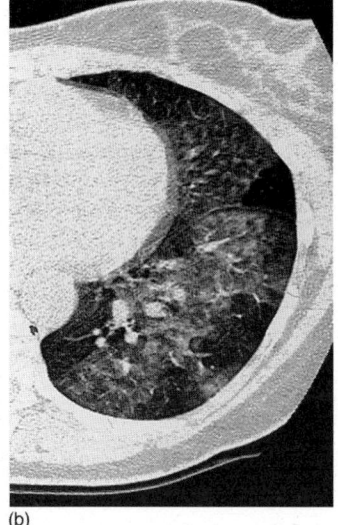

(a)　　　　　　　　　　　(b)

Fig. 4 (a) CT scan of a never-smoking woman aged 44 years whose lung biopsy showed the typical appearances of subacute EAA. She kept two budgerigars in her home and had serum precipitins to avian antigens. The scan shows marked groundglass attenuation of the lung parenchyma, which is nodular in some areas due to characteristic peribronchiolar (and centrilobular) foci. In other areas there is increased translucency because of bronchiolar obstruction and air trapping. Both the groundglass attenuation and the increases in translucency are exaggerated in the expiratory film (b), giving a 'mosaic' pattern. She recovered fully after the birds left her home..

modification of the plant and its respirable environment may be a costly matter.

Hypersensitivity

The demonstration of a serum IgG antibody response to the inducing organic dust is the most widely used method of 'confirming' hypersensitivity (saliva may be used more conveniently in children), but this has proved to be unsatisfactory. Although affected subjects tend to have higher antibody levels than those who are exposed but unaffected, the antibody response tends to correlate more closely with exposure than with disease. If the more sensitive enzyme-linked immunosorbent assay (ELISA) is used, rather than the traditional Ouchterlony double-gel diffusion test, even higher rates of false-positive results are obtained. However, this produces greater specificity and in practice the absence of an IgG precipitin response is extremely uncommon in subjects eventually proved to have extrinsic allergic alveolitis, providing they are non-smokers. This is of considerable value in that a negative test generally excludes the diagnosis. The limited value of a positive test is to be expected in view of the current belief that cellular, not humoral, immunity provides the principal mechanism underlying the disease. It is unfortunate that practicable tests for cellular hypersensitivity are not readily available.

When the diagnosis remains in doubt, some form of inhalation challenge test may be necessary. The simplest method involves comparison of experimental periods spent away from the suspected causative environment with similar periods of continuing exposure. The acute form of the disease is likely to be recognized in this way, though the procedure can be time consuming and there may be practical problems of compliance. When a definitive diagnosis is particularly important, laboratory-based inhalation challenge tests can be used. These employ a variety of techniques, ranging from nebulizing soluble extracts to recreating natural environmental exposures in an exposure chamber. The influenza-like component of positive reactions is often uncomfortable, and if excessive doses are administered these tests can be hazardous. What is more, objective evidence for positive reactions may be difficult to obtain from conventional lung function tests. Tests of this nature should therefore be restricted to centres with special expertise. Personal experience of evaluating objective changes in body temperature, circulating neutrophil and lymphocyte numbers, forced vital capacity, and exercise tests from 144 tests is summarized in Table 2. Together they provide high specificity and high sensitivity. Auscultation, chest radiography, measurements of gas transfer, and arterial blood gas analyses are often too insensitive to provide useful diagnostic information.

Differential diagnosis

Acute extrinsic allergic alveolitis is not the only disorder characterized by systemic influenza-like symptoms and respiratory distress to follow an unusually heavy exposure to microbially contaminated vegetable produce. In 1986 an international symposium considered a further disorder that occurs within hours of heavy respiratory exposure to dusts containing fungal toxins, especially those released on decapping silos. It is the result of direct toxicity rather than hypersensitivity and the term organic dust toxic syndrome was recommended to describe it. Its effects are usually mild and self-limiting, but severe respiratory embarrassment can occur and there is a small risk of ongoing, and potentially fatal, fungal invasion of the lungs. This risk could be enhanced if corticosteroid treatment is given, and death has occurred in subjects who appear to have been fully immunocompetent. Not only does organic dust toxic syndrome occur in circumstances which favour the occurrence of extrinsic allergic alveolitis (particularly silos and swine/poultry confinement buildings), but its clinical features have much in common with extrinsic allergic alveolitis, and to a lesser extent with nitrogen dioxide toxicity, which may also affect silo workers. Indeed, there is so much overlap that it can be very difficult indeed to distinguish one disorder from the others (Table 3).

The acute form of extrinsic allergic alveolitis can only be the result of an acute and recent (a matter of hours) exposure to the relevant causal antigen. This limits the opportunity for diagnostic error, though the circumstances of an unusually heavy exposure may be subtle. For example, a pigeon fancier might spend rather less time than usual with his birds, but much more time than usual in the more hazardous dusty car he uses regularly to transport racing birds for training exercises.

Just as acute and heavy exposures to organic dusts may cause disorders other than extrinsic allergic alveolitis, they may also be quite irrelevant and purely coincidental to the acute respiratory disorder with which the patient presents. Consequently the differential diagnosis should include consideration of other acute disorders of the lung parenchyma and interstitium, such as infections, other immunological disorders, drug reactions, and even paraquat poisoning, which sometimes occurs accidentally in farm workers. In bird keepers the diagnosis of viral, mycoplasmal, and chlamydial infection may itself be confounded by false-positive microbial antibody tests. This is the result of pre-existing avian antibodies cross-reacting with egg protein in the microbial cultures used to provide the test agents.

When subacute or chronic forms of extrinsic allergic alveolitis are encountered, the differential diagnosis lies with other diffuse infiltrative and fibrotic disorders of the lung. Those most frequently resembling extrinsic allergic alveolitis include cryptogenic fibrosing alveolitis, sarcoidosis, pneumoconiosis, tuberculosis, and metastatic cancer, although a huge variety of less common disorders may also need to be considered.

Management

Management of the individual

Management centres on reducing any further exposure to a minimum, though first demands that the diagnosis is secure. There is no place for desensitization. Ideally, the affected individual changes the relevant working, domestic, or recreational environment completely, but this may mean a profound loss in income or great expense, and is often unrealistic. Nor is it fully justified on purely medical grounds since continued exposure does not lead inevitably to progressive disease.

The affected individual who continues to work in the occupation responsible for his disease can often reduce his exposure substantially by changing the pattern of his particular duties. An alternative is the use of industrial respirators, which filter out 98 to 99 per cent of respirable dust

Table 2 Diagnostic features of positive inhalation challenge tests

Diagnostic changes within 36 h of challenge exposure	Sensitivity (%)
1. Increase in body temperature to > 37.2°C	78
2. Increase in circulating neutrophils by ≥ 2.5×10⁹/litre	68
3. Decrease in circulating lymphocytes by ≥ 0.5×10⁹/litre with lymphopenia (< 1.5×10⁹/l)	52
4. Decrease in forced vital capacity by ≥ 15 per cent	48
5. Increase in exercise minute volume by ≥ 15 per cent	85
6. Increase in exercise respiratory frequency by ≥ 25 per cent	64

The data were taken from a series of 144 antigen and control challenge tests in 31 subjects. Diagnostic end-points were chosen to produce specificities of approximately 95 per cent, after mean changes associated with positive challenge tests were shown to be highly significant. When each monitoring parameter was given a score of 1 for a significant result, a total score of 2/6 or more was associated with a specificity of 100 per cent and a sensitivity of 78 per cent for the 144 challenge tests.

Table 3 Characteristics of nitrogen dioxide toxicity (silo filler's disease), organic dust toxic syndrome, and acute farmer's lung

	Nitrogen dioxide toxicity	Organic dust toxic syndrome	Acute farmer's lung
Susceptibility in smokers	Unknown	Unknown	Decreased
Relation to time of harvest	Days	Months to years	Months to years
Microbial decomposition of harvest product	Little	Marked	Variable
Confined exposure space	+++	+	+
Previous episodes	–	+	++
Symptoms			
Dry cough	++	++	++
Breathlessness	++	++	++
Wheeze	–	–	–
Systemic upset	+	+	++
Signs			
Basal crackles	+	+	+
Fever	+	+	+
Time of onset after beginning exposure	1–10 h	1–10 h	1–10 h
Duration	Hours to days	Hours to days	Hours to days
Investigations			
Leucocytosis	+	+	+
Radiograph—small irregular opacities, alveolar shadows	+	-/+	+
Restricted ventilation	+	-/+	+
Reduced gas transfer	+	-/+	+
Hypoxaemia	+	-/+	+
Fungi from secretions/biopsy	–	++	+
Methaemoglobinaemia	+	–	–
Serum precipitins	–	–	+ (?- in smokers)
Response to steroids	+	–	++
Life threatening	Not uncommonly	Rarely	Rarely

from the ambient air. They are especially valuable when exposures are intermittent and short, but may be uncomfortably hot when worn for long periods or when there is heavy work, and so compliance with their use may be poor.

Whatever course is followed, continuing exposure should be accompanied by regular medical surveillance. If there is no progression, it is reasonable for some exposure to continue. When there is progressive disease, exposure should cease. This may involve a loss of earnings, and may entitle the affected worker to compensation. Rarely, the individual with progressive disease will refuse to change his occupation or hobby, and the physician must weigh the possible advantages of long-term corticosteroid therapy against the risks.

Management of the environment

Once extrinsic allergic alveolitis is recognized in one individual, the environment concerned should be assessed for the risk it poses to others. In many circumstances this will be well known already, and exposure levels will be within the range considered acceptable. In others, neither the risk nor the precise causative agent (nor its level of exposure) will be known, and in such unfamiliar circumstances there may be a need to survey the exposed population at risk. Questionnaires and serological tests are most convenient for this, at least as a screening procedure. When large populations are involved, comprehensive investigation is sensible before major modifications are considered to the working environment.

Modifications can always be made to the environment to lessen the level of exposure, but their extent will be limited by expense and should be justified by need. Dry storage and adequate ventilation are the two most important factors when vegetable produce is involved, and in some farming areas there is benefit in drying produce artificially after harvest. An alternative is some form of 'pickling', so that the produce is preserved chemically. With silage, for example, newly cut grass is kept under impervious covering in relatively sealed conditions. Initial enzymic and moulding processes use up available oxygen, and produce aldehydes and other preserva-

tive chemicals. These create nearly anaerobic conditions which protect the produce until it is used. Similarly, hay may be sealed in plastic bags, or grain or bagasse may be treated with propionic acid.

When ventilation and humidification systems are themselves responsible for extrinsic allergic alveolitis, major mechanical alterations may be necessary and the methods of humidification and temperature control may need to be changed. The crucial need is to reduce the ease with which normal airborne microbial contaminants are able to proliferate in stagnant collections of water. For this there may be a role for 'biocide' sterilizing agents, but these are also likely to become airborne and respirable and so must have low intrinsic toxicity and sensitizing potency. For one such biocide (isothiazolinone) there have been reports of occupational dermatitis and asthma, though not of extrinsic allergic alveolitis.

The need for rapid air changes coupled with close control of humidity and temperature poses formidable problems. The use of recirculated filtered air is the most economical, but effective filters are expensive and can become contaminated themselves, increasing rather than decreasing the load of respirable microbial antigens. The use of heat exchangers minimizes the cost of temperature control if contaminated exhaust air is not recirculated but does not conserve water.

Outcome

No further exposure

As with occupational asthma, the risk of continuing symptoms following cessation of exposure increases with the duration of exposure. With the acute form of extrinsic allergic alveolitis the exposure period is generally short and the disorder usually resolves without sequelae once the diagnosis is made and exposure ceases. However, one study using bronchoalveolar lavage and DTPA clearance has indicated continuing inflammation and membrane leakiness after a follow up period of 2 to 15 years. The significance of this is unclear, since all subjects were asymptomatic and gave normal results on radiographic and lung function studies.

Continuing exposure

There is greater concern when exposure continues. This may lead not only to recurrent acute attacks but to progressive and permanent fibrotic damage—that is, to the chronic form of the disease. While concern for the risk of progressive fibrosis is undoubtedly justified, this happens in only a minority of affected subjects. A 2- to 40-year follow-up survey of 92 farm workers presenting with the acute form of farmer's lung showed that while most continued to live on farms, only some developed radiographic evidence of pulmonary fibrosis (39 per cent) or impairment of carbon monoxide gas transfer (30 per cent). As many as 28 per cent gave histories of chronic productive cough and 25 per cent had airway obstruction. A similar 10-year outcome has been reported in pigeon fanciers with acute extrinsic allergic alveolitis; again the majority elected to continue their antigenic exposures despite medical advice to the contrary.

Therefore, in some cases—perhaps the majority—important protective mechanisms emerge that lead to tolerance of the effects of further acute exposures, or at least prevent the development of damaging fibrosis. A history of similar increasing tolerance is occasionally noted with occupational asthma, and tolerance not progressive disease is the rule rather than the exception in most animal models of extrinsic allergic alveolitis. However, with both asthma and extrinsic allergic alveolitis some affected subjects give clear accounts of increased responsiveness to a given level of exposure months or years after initial antigen exclusion, which suggests that protective mechanisms may be down-graded more quickly than the causal mechanisms.

As with sarcoidosis, there is debate as to whether the use of corticosteroids for acute episodes confers any long-term benefit. The answer is not clear, but one recent investigation failed to demonstrate any long-term functional differences between groups treated randomly with corticosteroids or placebo for the initial acute episode of farmer's lung. Whilst the corticosteroid group recovered more quickly from the acute episode, there was the suspicion, already voiced by other investigators, that early steroid therapy carries a greater risk of long-term recurrence. It is possible that the initial response to steroids encouraged less care over subsequent exposures. Alternatively steroid therapy may have induced a different equilibrium between immunological responses, perhaps interfering disproportionately with the development of protective mechanisms.

Compensation of industrial causes

In the United Kingdom, industrial injuries legislation provides compensation from central government for disability in employees (but not employers) from extrinsic allergic alveolitis of occupational origin. The level of disability, and hence compensation, is assessed following examination by a 'Medical Board'. If disability arose before 1991, the affected worker may also be entitled to a 'reduced earnings allowance' if ongoing employment (or lack of it) has resulted in a loss of earned income. Both benefits are limited to a joint maximum figure, which is adjusted from time to time according to inflation. Reduced earnings allowance for new cases was discontinued in 1991.

Acceptance of state compensation in the United Kingdom no longer debars the recipient from seeking redress additionally in the civil courts, which is the primary mechanism of compensation in many countries.

Further reading

Banaszak EF, Thiede WH, Fink JN (1970). Hypersensitivity pneumonia due to contamination of an air conditioner. *New England Journal of Medicine* **283**, 271–6.

Braun SR *et al.* (1979). Farmer's lung disease: long-term clinical and physiologic outcome. *American Review of Respiratory Disease* **119**, 185–91.

Grammar LC (1999). Occupational allergic alveolitis. *Annals of Allergy, Asthma, and Immunology* **83**, 602–6.

Hansell DM, Moskovic E (1991). High-resolution computed tomography in extrinsic allergic alveolitis. *Clinical Radiology* **43**, 8–12.

Hendrick DJ *et al.* (1980). Positive 'alveolar' responses to antigen inhalation provocation tests: their validity and recognition. *Thorax* **35**, 415–27.

Hendrick DJ, Faux JA, Marshall R (1978). Budgerigar fancier's lung: the commonest variety of allergic alveolitis in Britain. *British Medical Journal* **ii**: 81–4.

Kokkarinen JI, Tukiainen HO, Terho EO (1992). Effect of corticosteroid treatment on the recovery of pulmonary function in farmer's lung. *American Review of Respiratory Disease* **145**, 3–5.

Kreiss K, Cox-Ganser J (1997). Metalworking fluid-associated hypersensitivity pneumonitis: a workshop summary. *American Journal of Industrial Medicine* **32**, 423–32.

Leatherman HP *et al.* (1984). Lung T cells in hypersensitivity pneumonitis. *Annals of Internal Medicine* **100**, 390–2.

Meredith SK, Taylor VM, McDonald JC (1991). Occupational respiratory disease in the United Kingdom 1989: a report to the British Thoracic Society and the Society of Occupational Medicine by the SWORD project group. *British Journal of Industrial Medicine* **48**, 292–8.

Morgan DC *et al.* (1973). Chest symptoms and farmer's lung: a community survey. *British Journal of Industrial Medicine* **30**, 259–65.

Ohtani Y *et al.* (1999). Sequential changes in bronchoalveolar lavage cells and cytokines in a patient progressing from acute to chronic bird fancier's lung disease. *Internal Medicine* **38**, 896–9.

Pepys J *et al.* (1963). Farmer's lung. Thermophilic actinomycetes as a source of 'farmer's lung hay' antigens. *Lancet* **ii**: 607–11.

Peterson LB *et al.* (1977). An animal model of hypersensitivity pneumonitis in the rabbit. Induction of cellular hypersensitivity to inhaled antigens using Carageenan and BCG. *American Review of Respiratory Disease* **116**, 1007–12.

Ramirez-Venegas A *et al.* (1998). Utility of a provocation test for diagnosis of chronic pigeon breeder's disease. *American Journal of Respiratory and Critical Care Medicine* **158**, 862–9.

Von Essen S, Donham K (1999). Illness and injury in animal confinement workers. *Occupational Medicine* **14**, 337–50.

Yoshizawa Y *et al.* (1999). Chronic hypersensitivity pneumonitis in Japan: a nationwide epidemiologic survey. *Journal of Allergy and Clinical Immunology* **103**, 315–20.

17.11.12 Eosinophilic granuloma of the lung and pulmonary lymphangiomyomatosis

D. J. Hendrick*

Pulmonary histiocytosis X

Eosinophilic granuloma is a disorder of dendritic (Langerhans) cells that arise from CD34+ progenitors and have special function in presenting antigen to T cells. In this context, however, an abnormal proliferation of these cells is associated with eosinophils (though not peripheral eosinophilia) and granulomatous damage of the lung. Lesions characteristically show

* Dr R. J. Shaw wrote on this subject in the third edition of the *Oxford Textbook of Medicine*. Much of his text has been retained in this revision and we acknowledge his contribution with grateful thanks.

cavitation and fibrotic healing, which results in foci of 'stellate' scars, alveolar wall deformation, honeycombing, and the formation of small cysts.

Langerhans cell granulomatosis is the currently favoured generic term rather than histiocytosis X, which was used previously to describe eosinophilic granuloma, Letterer–Siwe disease, and Hand–Schüller–Christian disease. The latter term is used to describe Langerhans granulomas in organs other than the lung (principally bone and the posterior pituitary), and so can be considered a multifocal form of Langerhans cell granulomatosis (eosinophilic granuloma). It is not clear whether Letterer–Siwe disease is truly related to the other two, or whether it is even primarily a disease of Langerhans cells. It is best considered separately. For further discussion, see Section 22.

Eosinophilic granuloma generally affects men and women between the ages of 20 and 40 who are almost exclusively smokers. The main clinical manifestations reflect its chief pathological features—diffuse interstitial fibrosis and cyst formation. The cysts may rupture causing spontaneous pneumothorax, and the fibrosis may progress causing exertional dyspnoea. Cough is common also, and cyst rupture may be associated with pleuritic pain. Because cysts occur bilaterally there is the potential for devastating and immediately life-threatening pneumothoraces to occur on both sides concurrently. One report indicates that occasionally a single pulmonary granuloma may occur, closely simulating carcinoma.

The chest radiograph typically shows diffuse micronodular and reticular changes in the early stages (Fig. 1), which progress with the development of honeycombing. Appearances on high-resolution CT scanning are characteristic (Fig. 1). Pulmonary physiological tests reveal a mixed obstructive and restrictive pattern (decreased vital capacity and total lung capacity, increased residual volume, and decreased carbon monoxide transfer). Bronchoalveolar lavage may reveal Langerhans cells or 'atypical histiocytes', which are most readily identified by immunohistochemical staining of the S100 protein. The major histological characteristics are not readily identified from transbronchial biopsy, and so open biopsy or video-assisted thoracoscopic biopsy is generally required. The major identifying feature of the Langerhans cell is an X body or Birbeck granule, which appears as a pentalaminar rod-like structure in the cytoplasm under the electron microscope.

Eosinophilic granuloma of the lung usually occurs in isolation, but may be associated with wider manifestations of multifocal Langerhans cell granulomatosis, particularly skin rashes, bone pain, and diabetes insipidus from granulomas in skin, bone, and pituitary. The clinical course is variable, and treatment in general is supportive rather than specific. In many cases the disease ceases to progress at some point, leaving residual impairment of variable degree. In one case where lung transplantation became necessary, the disease recurred in the transplanted lung, though responded to cyclosphosphamide therapy.

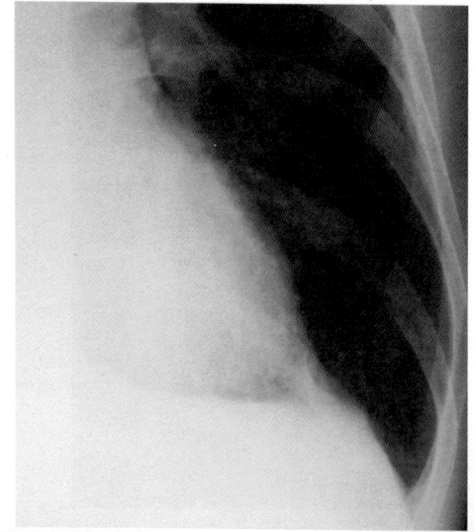

(a)

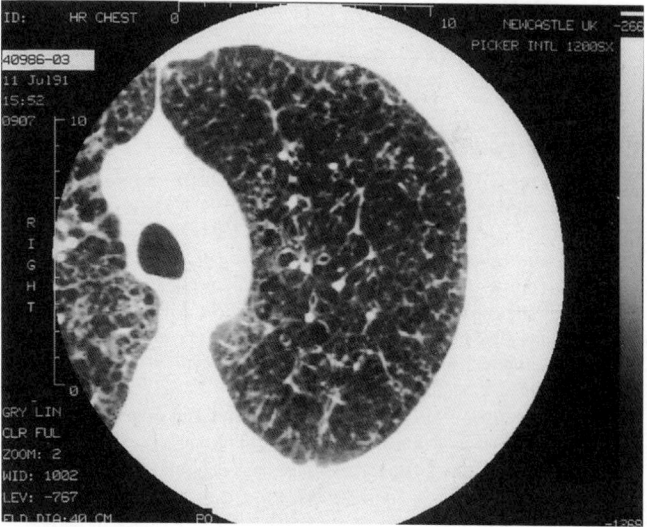

(b)

Fig. 1 Chest radiograph (a) and CT scan (b) of a 45-year-old smoking man with biopsy proven (S100 positive) eosinophilic granuloma. The plain film shows a mixed micronodular and reticular pattern which is due principally to multiple small cysts that make the surrounding interstitium more prominent. This is more readily evident from the CT image.

Lymphangiomyomatosis

Lymphangio(leio)myomatosis of the lung is a rare disorder characterized clinically by progressive interstitial disease causing breathlessness and cough, and cyst formation causing spontaneous pneumothorax. Further features are chylous pleural effusion and haemoptysis. It occurs almost exclusively in women of reproductive age, and appears to be a 'forme fruste' of tuberous sclerosis. However, only a minority of patients with tuberous sclerosis show evidence of lymphangiomyomatosis in the lung, and most patients presenting with pulmonary lymphangiomyomatosis do not show other manifestations of tuberous sclerosis. Nor do they appear to pass on the disorder to the next generation. The pulmonary disorder is characterized pathologically by hamartomatous proliferation of smooth-muscle cells in pulmonary lymphatics, venules, and airways. It is often associated with angiomyolipomas of the kidney (and bleeding into the renal tract), and this has been linked with a shared cell surface marker, premelansosome glycoprotein (HMB-45), that can be recognized by immunohistochemical staining.

The typical clinical picture is of progressive loss of exercise capacity associated with a dominantly obstructive loss of ventilatory function and reduced gas transfer. This is interrupted by intermittent episodes of chylous pleural effusion, spontaneous pneumothorax, and haemoptysis. The early chest radiographic appearances are of reticular shadowing and Kerley B lines because of obstructed lymphatics, small nodules due to hamartomatous smooth-muscle aggregates, and pleural effusions. Honeycombing and cystic dilation occur later when pneumothorax becomes increasingly common. These abnormalities are most readily seen by CT scanning (Fig. 2). The diagnosis generally follows lung biopsy, but can been made from cytological examination of aspirated pleural fluid if this contains clusters of immature smooth muscle cells.

Progesterone therapy or bilateral oophorectomy is sometimes effective in limiting disease progression, and may also help to control pleural effusions. If untreated, most patients die within 10 years, and so lung transplantation becomes the principal option if anti-oestrogen therapy is ineffective. In one case this was associated with recurrent disease in the allograft.

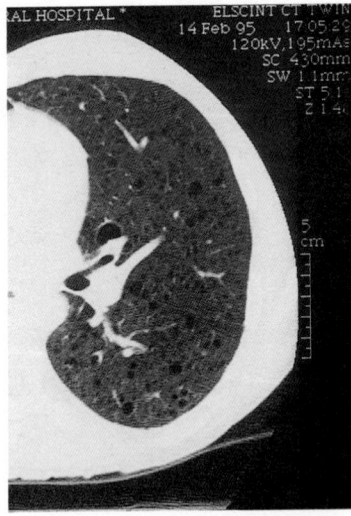

Fig. 2 CT scan of a 37-year-old woman with tuberous sclerosis and pulmonary lymphangiomyomatosis. She had experienced sequential spontaneous pneumothoraces affecting each side. The scan shows multiple thin-walled cysts throughout the lung. (By courtesy of Dr S. J. Bourke.)

Further reading

Anonymous (1994). Case records of the Massachusetts General Hospital. Weekly clinicopathological exercises. Case 5–1994. A 34-year-old woman with mild exertional dyspnea and interstitial pulmonary lesions [clinical conference]. *New England Journal of Medicine* 330, 347–53.

Anonymous (1994). Case records of the Massachusetts General Hospital. Weekly clinicopathological exercises. Case 1–1994. A 37-year-old woman with interstitial lung disease, renal masses, and a previous spontaneous pneumothorax [clinical conference]. *New England Journal of Medicine* 330, 1300–6.

Bonelli FS *et al.* (1998). Accuracy of high-resolution CT in diagnosing lung diseases. *American Journal of Roentgenology* 170, 1507–12.

Brauner MW *et al.* (1997). Pulmonary Langerhans cell histiocytosis: evolution of lesions on CT scans. *Radiology* 204, 497–502.

Chan JK *et al.* (1993). Lymphangiomyomatosis and angiomyolipoma: closely related entities characterized by hamartomatous proliferation of HMB-45-positive smooth muscle. *Histopathology* 22, 445–55.

Costello LC, Hartman TE, Ryu JH (2000). High frequency of pulmonary lymphangioleiomyomatosis in women with tuberous sclerosis complex. *Mayo Clinic Proceedings* 75, 591–4.

Gabbay E *et al.* (1998). Recurrence of Langerhans' cell granulomatosis following lung transplantation. *Thorax* 53, 326–7.

Lieberman PH *et al.* (1996). Langerhans cell (eosinophilic) granulomatosis. A clinicopathologic study encompassing 50 years. *American Journal of Surgical Pathology* 20, 519–52.

Taylor JR *et al.* (1990). Lymphangioleiomyomatosis: clinical course in 32 patients. *New England Journal of Medicine* 323, 1254–60.

17.11.13 Pulmonary alveolar proteinosis

D. J. Hendrick

First described in 1958, pulmonary alveolar proteinosis is a rare but interesting disorder that exerts its primary effects in the alveolar spaces. Over a period ranging from months to years, these become filled with an amorph-ous, largely cell-free, lipoproteinaceous material that is not readily expectorated. Inflammation and fibrosis are conspicuously absent and there are two major consequences. First, depending on the number of alveoli involved, the lungs become stiff, ventilatory function becomes restricted, and shunting occurs at the alveolar capillary level, causing hypoxaemia. The outcome is breathlessness, reduced exercise tolerance, and in some cases death from respiratory failure. Second, and a not uncommon cause of death, is secondary infection. The responsible organisms are generally those that are associated with intracellular infection and impaired T-lymphocyte function, nocardia being particularly prominent. In many cases, however, extensive involvement does not occur, there being little or no progression, or even spontaneous remission. Epidemiological data are scarce but one estimate suggests an annual incidence of the order 2 to 5 per million worldwide.

Pathogenesis

Men appear to be affected more commonly than women: all age groups may be involved, and smoking may enhance the risk. The cause in most cases is unknown, but an apparently identical (though relentlessly progressive) disorder can arise within months of massive exposure to respirable mineral dust, especially silica—both in the unfortunate worker exposed negligently without adequate respiratory protection and in experimental animal models. This has been called acute silicoproteinosis or silicolipoproteinosis. Less commonly aluminium dust may be responsible, and there have been reports implicating titanium and insecticides. A few reports describe affected siblings, implying a possible hereditary factor, and some associate pulmonary alveolar proteinosis with haematological disorders (usually malignant and often after the use of cytotoxic agents) or immunodeficiency disorders.

The secreted material is rich in protein and phospholipid, and stains strongly with periodic acid–Schiff (**PAS**) and eosin. It also contains structures resembling tubular myelin, which are derived from lamellar bodies of surfactant-producing type II pneumocytes. The secretions themselves are chiefly the product of these cells, and the chief phospholipid is dipalmitoyl phosphatidylcholine—the dominant phospholipid of normal surfactant. It is unclear, however, whether the accumulation of these secretions results from an abnormality of the type II pneumocytes (excessive or abnormal production), or from impaired resorption by alveolar macrophages. Recent research suggests that both mechanisms may be relevant, also that the pulmonary alveolar proteinosis phenotype can arise through a number of different processes. In most cases the PAS stain is taken up uniformly, as is peroxidase-labelled immunoglobulin raised against the apolipoproteins of surfactant. In others, particularly those associated with haematological or immunological disorders, uptake is heterogeneous, and it has been suggested that fundamentally different processes underlie this 'secondary' form of pulmonary alveolar proteinosis.

Mice deficient in granulocyte-macrophage colony-stimulating factor (**GM-CSF**), or with a disrupted GM-CSF receptor, develop alveolar accumulations of surfactant material, simulating pulmonary alveolar proteinosis. Benefit occurs when GM-CSF is administered locally, when normal bone marrow is transplanted, or when the faulty gene is replaced by some other method. This suggests that pulmonary alveolar proteinosis could arise because of impaired macrophage differentiation and function as a consequence of an inherited genetic defect, or an acquired defective bone marrow clone. The vulnerability to infection with opportunistic organisms and the *in vitro* demonstration of a number of abnormalities of macrophage function additionally incriminate the macrophage more than the pneumocyte. This is also consistent with pulmonary alveolar proteinosis arising after macrophage function has been disrupted by massive exposure to silica, and with pulmonary alveolar proteinosis being associated with impaired T-cell immunity (and hence diminished macrophage activation).

It has been shown, however, that ingestion of material produced in pulmonary alveolar proteinosis may itself cause impairment of phagocytic function in macrophages harvested from normal controls, and so in some cases the primary abnormality could still lie with the type II pneumocyte and its alveolar secretions. This would be consistent with the belief that chemotherapeutic agents associated with the development of pulmonary alveolar proteinosis (e.g. bleomycin) are more likely to damage pneumocytes than macrophages. Strong support for this view comes from the recent demonstration of a GM-CSF inhibitory factor within the bronchoalveolar secretions of pulmonary alveolar proteinosis, to which GM-CSF binds more avidly than it does to the cells it should stimulate. Its source of origin, however, has not yet been shown to be the type II pneumocyte.

Clinical features

The patient usually presents with progressive shortness of breath due to the disease itself or with a pneumonic illness due to superimposed infection. Occasionally, the disease is without symptoms and is first recognized from the appearances of an incidental chest radiograph, when it may be mistaken for sarcoidosis. Cough is common and may be productive, particularly if there is infection. Low-grade fever, haemoptysis, and pleuritic pain occur infrequently, though some authors report an initial febrile incident. There may be crackles and clubbing in advanced stages, and fever becomes typical when infection supervenes. When nocardia is not responsible for this, aspergillus, candida, cryptococcus, cytomegalovirus, histoplasma, HIV, mucor, mycobacteria, pneumocystis, and viruses are the most common culprits.

Diagnosis

The chest radiograph characteristically shows an alveolar filling pattern, which radiates from the hila and simulates pulmonary oedema. There is no associated evidence of heart failure, however, and the appearances may be somewhat patchy and asymmetrical. Diffuse pulmonary fibrosis is very rare, unless provoked by complicating infection. A micronodular infiltration is occasionally seen, particularly in children, but lymphadenopathy is usually absent. CT scanning, particularly with high resolution, shows the non-specific features of air space filling (ground-glass attenuation), and commonly a patchiness which distinguishes affected from unaffected lobules. There may also be septal thickening and hence the 'crazy paving' appearance typical of combined alveolar and interstitial disease.

Pneumonia or aspiration is often suspected initially, but the cough produces little or no sputum and no organisms are isolated if the disease remains uncomplicated. Occasionally, white gelatinous material is expectorated, and bronchoalveolar lavage fluid is typically milky in colour. Gallium scanning may be useful in showing negligible pulmonary uptake in contrast to the findings in pneumonia. In established pulmonary alveolar proteinosis, a positive gallium scan (or a CT scan) may be invaluable in suggesting the development of superimposed infection.

The key to the diagnosis of uncomplicated pulmonary alveolar proteinosis rests with the demonstration that the alveolar secretions are strongly PAS-positive but contain no organisms and no excessive cellular response. Indeed, the macrophages appear to be deficient in numbers as well as function. Biochemical and immunochemical tests may be used to show that phospholipids and specific surfactant proteins are present in excess. Occasionally the sputum provides diagnostic material, identification of lamellar bodies or their debris by electron microscopy being particularly useful. These may be found within macrophages or pneumocytes, or may lie free within the secretions. More commonly, bronchoalveolar lavage or transbronchial lung biopsy is required, though the former should suffice since PAS-positive amorphous globules demonstrated by cytological smears have high diagnostic specificity. Ultrastructural examination shows that these also generally contain multilaminated structures derived from lamellar bodies. The characteristic histological features are shown in Fig. 1.

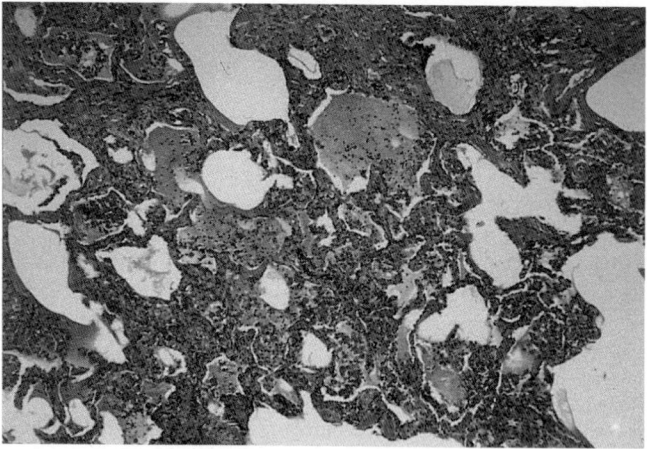

Fig. 1 Pulmonary alveolar proteinosis arising acutely following massive exposure to silica (by courtesy of Dr D.E. Banks). Some alveoli are filled with a non-inflammatory proteinaceous exudate, characteristic of pulmonary alveolar proteinosis. The lung interstitium shows fibrosis and inflammation which can be attributed to acute silicosis (haematoxylin and eosin, medium magnification).

Raised serum levels of surfactant proteins and lactic dehydrogenase are to be expected, but these occur in a number of other diffuse disorders of the lung and so are of no value in diagnosis. Serum levels of the mucin-like glycoprotein KL-6, which is released from type II pneumocytes, are also raised in pulmonary alveolar proteinosis. Although not specific, it has been suggested that these provide a good biochemical correlate for disease activity, and may therefore be a useful marker in assessing when treatment becomes necessary.

Management

In a third to a half of cases, no appreciable disability develops and the disease remits spontaneously or fails to progress. The choice of treatment, when necessary, is strictly limited. Corticosteroids are of no value and may increase the risk of infection. Prolonged periods of inhalation therapy with expectorants (potassium iodide) or proteolytic enzymes (trypsin) have been claimed to offer benefit, but frequently cause irritative responses in the airways. Furthermore, trypsin does not digest *in vitro* the material produced in pulmonary alveolar proteinosis. Neither form of treatment is currently recommended, although the addition of trypsin to therapeutic bronchalveolar lavage fluid has been reported to be both effective and well tolerated.

The most effective measure is physical removal of secretions by bronchoalveolar lavage, usually performed under general anaesthesia using a double-lumen endotracheal tube. The treatment is repeatedly carried out on one lung with a total of 20 to 50 litres of warm sterile buffered saline while the other is mechanically ventilated. The procedure is then reversed so that the other lung is treated. The practice of adding heparin and acetyl cysteine to the lavage fluid has not been shown to be beneficial, but chest percussion during the procedure does seem to enhance the yield. When severe respiratory failure has already supervened despite ventilatory support, cardiopulmonary bypass has been used successfully to maintain gas exchange during the lavage procedure. An alternative is sequential lobar lavage using a fibreoptic bronchoscope and a cuffed catheter. Further lavage is usually necessary every few weeks or months, but the activity of the disease may lessen and the need for frequent treatment may diminish.

Sometimes there is fatal progression with marked loss of weight despite repeated lavage. It may be that current experimental use of GM-CSF might lead to an improved outlook for such patients in the future. In one prominent case treatment involved bilateral lung transplantation, but this was followed by recurrent pulmonary alveolar proteinosis, raising the question of whether bone marrow transplantation might be more appropriate.

The risk of premature death in most series has been low (mostly less than 10 per cent), but a considerable threat to life is associated with complicating infection. This should be recognized and treated promptly. An accelerated clinical course together with the development of fever, increased (and productive) cough, malaise, evidence of systemic illness, and the radiographic demonstration of cavitation or pleural effusion all provide pointers to its development. Blood cultures together with smear and culture studies of sputum may identify the organism or organisms responsible, but often bronchoscopy with brushings and diagnostic lavage is needed. Sometimes a biopsy procedure is considered necessary, particularly when the underlying presence of alveolar proteinosis is not clearly established. When opportunistic organisms are involved, the eradication of infection may prove to be unduly difficult, perhaps reflecting an underlying impairment of macrophage (or GM-CSF) function. It has therefore been argued that regular bronchoalveolar lavage, even in the absence of impaired exercise tolerance, may limit the degree of immunosuppression and provide valuable prophylaxis against such life-theatening infections. A recent study did indeed demonstrate improved macrophage function following lavage, which slowly diminished over 18 months as clinical relapse occurred. If the argument is followed fully, lavage may also play a role in eradicating the acute infection.

Further reading

Burkhalter A *et al.* (1996). Bronchoalveolar lavage cytology in pulmonary alveolar proteinosis. *American Journal of Clinical Pathology* **106**, 504–10.

Claypool WD, Rogers RM, Matuschak GM (1984). Update on the clinical diagnosis, management, and pathogenesis of pulmonary alveolar proteinosis (phospholipidosis). *Chest* **85**, 550–8.

Gaine SP, O'Marcaigh AS (1998). Pulmonary alveolar proteinosis: lung transplant or bone marrow transplant. *Chest* **113**, 563–4.

Goldstein LS *et al.* (1998). Pulmonary alveolar proteinosis: clinical features and outcomes. *Chest* **114**, 1357–62.

Huffman JA *et al.* (1996). Pulmonary epithelial cell expression of GM-CSF corrects the alveolar proteinosis in GM-CSF-deficient mice. *Journal of Clinical Investigation* **97**, 649–55.

Mikami T *et al.* (1997). Pulmonary alveolar proteinosis: diagnosis using routinely processed smears of bronchoalveolar lavage fluid. *Journal of Clinical Pathology* **50**, 981–4.

Reed JA *et al.* (1999). Aerosolized GM-CSF ameliorates pulmonary alveolar proteinosis in GM-CSF-deficient mice. *American Journal of Physiology* **276**, L556–63.

Selecky PA *et al.* (1977). The clinical and physiological effect of whole lung lavage pulmonary alveolar proteinosis: A 10 year experience. *Annals of Thoracic Surgery* **24**, 451–61.

Seymour JF *et al.* (1996). Efficacy of granulocyte-macrophage colony-stimulating factor in acquired alveolar proteinosis. *New England Journal of Medicine* **335**, 1924–5.

Tanaka N *et al.* (1999). Lungs of patients with idiopathic pulmonary alveolar proteinosis express a factor which neutralizes granulocyte-macrophage stimulating factor. *FEBS Letters* **442**, 246–50.

Wang BM *et al.* (1997). Diagnosing pulmonary alveolar proteinosis: a review and an update. *Chest* **111**, 460–6.

17.11.14 Pulmonary amyloidosis

D. J. Hendrick

Clinically important involvement of the lungs in amyloidosis is extremely uncommon, only a few dozen cases having been reported over recent dec-

ades, but lung infiltration is said to occur in the majority of cases of primary (**AL**) amyloid, less commonly in secondary (**AA**) amyloid. The proteinaceous material which is responsible for amyloid infiltration is composed of a fibrillar polypeptide and a non-fibrillar glycoprotein. They produce a unique β-pleated structure which may be deposited progressively and widely, eventually interfering with organ function. The glycoprotein (amyloid P or AP protein) comprises a mere 10 per cent of amyloid tissue. It is derived from a parent serum protein (SAP) made in the liver and is common to all types of amyloid tissue. The fibrillar polypeptide on the other hand is of two distinct types (Fig 1).

The type seen with 'primary' amyloidosis and amyloidosis associated with myeloma is derived from the variable region of immunoglobulin light chains and is known as AL protein. It is the product of a plasma cell clone, whether benign or malignant. Monoclonal immunoglobulin (M-component) may sometimes be detected in the serum by electrophoresis, and free light chains (Bence Jones protein) may be detected in the urine. The type of fibrillar polypeptide (AA protein) seen with 'secondary' amyloidosis and most of the familial forms of amyloidosis (such as Mediterranean fever) is derived from an acute phase serum component (SAA). The chronic inflammatory diseases associated with persistently raised levels of SAA (and C reactive protein and interleukin-6) are those that are most commonly associated with secondary amyloidosis, but only a small minority of subjects affected by these chronic inflammatory disorders show evidence of complicating amyloidosis.

Clinical features

Those affected are usually middle aged or elderly, and the sexes are equally represented. Hilar or mediastinal lymphadenopathy is rarely demonstrated on plain chest radiographs, but mild nodal enlargement is commonly seen on CT scanning. The pleura are rarely involved, but recurrent pleural effusion may occur.

Symptomatic pulmonary involvement is generally a consequence of localized disease affecting the upper and central airways, or systemic disease at alveolar–interstitial level. Localized disease is usually due to deposition of amyloid containing the light chain derived AL protein, and is

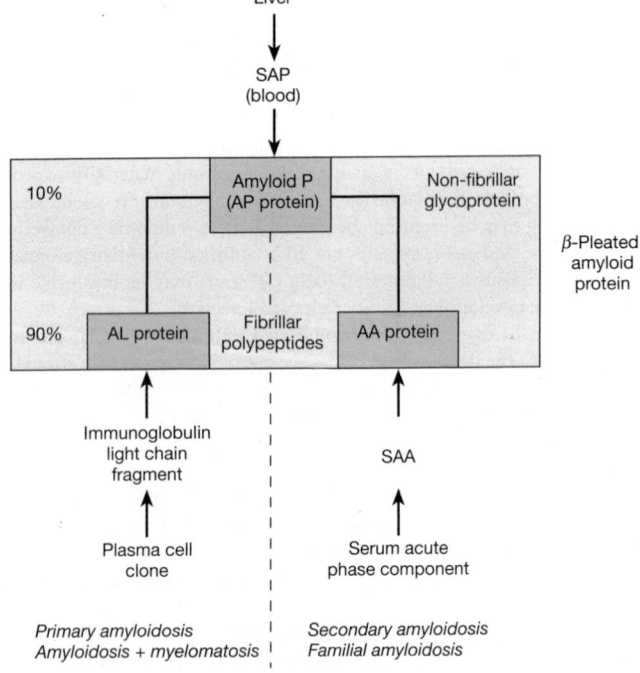

Fig. 1 Pathogenic pathways underlying primary and secondary amyloidosis.

essentially benign in nature. Its effects depend on the site of deposition. Diffuse alveolar–interstitial disease is usually associated with systemic disease and may be the consequence of either AL or AA protein deposition. It carries a poor prognosis, though death is usually due to the involvement of organs other than the lung.

The following varieties of pulmonary amyloidosis, in descending order of epidemiological importance, are the most clearly recognized.

1. Localized laryngotracheobronchial: discrete, and often multiple, masses of amyloid protein enlarge in the walls of the airways or the peribronchial tissues causing cough, obstruction, and sometimes bleeding. Obstruction of airways may lead to wheeze, stridor, breathlessness, atelectasis, and infection, and may eventually give rise to bronchiectasis. When a single lesion is involved it may simulate the effects of a bronchial adenoma, appearing as a polypoid mass on endoscopic inspection.

2. Localized parenchymal nodule(s): discrete nodules or masses, which may be single or multiple and may occasionally reach the size of a tennis ball, are seen within the lung parenchyma on the chest radiograph. They rarely cause symptoms or disrupt lung function and may eventually calcify, cavitate, or even ossify. They are likely to simulate bronchial neoplasms if single and so be resected; if multiple they often lead to biopsy. Biopsy in one unusual case (that of an HIV-positive intravenous drug abuser) showed no evidence of AL protein, but there was focal birefringency and a foreign body giant cell reaction reflecting deposition of the carrier material of the illicit drug. This implies that focal inflammation within the lung may occasionally lead to localized 'secondary' amyloid (i.e. AA protein) deposition. In the future it may be that CT and MRI will offer a useful means of distinguishing amyloid tissue from tumour, so obviating the need for biopsy.

3. Diffuse alveolar–interstitial: amyloid tissue is deposited diffusely throughout the alveolar walls and interstitium of the lung, and is usually a feature of systemic amyloidosis (Figs 2 and 3). There is progressive breathlessness and dry cough. Scattered crackles are characteristic and there may be pleural effusions. Eventually respiratory failure may supervene as ventilation becomes increasingly restricted and gas transfer impaired, though death more commonly results from cardiac or renal involvement.

Histological examination may also show evidence of amyloid infiltration of the pulmonary vasculature. This is usually of no clinical consequence, but has been reported to cause pulmonary hypertension and undue bleeding after biopsy, although other reports suggest that biopsy,

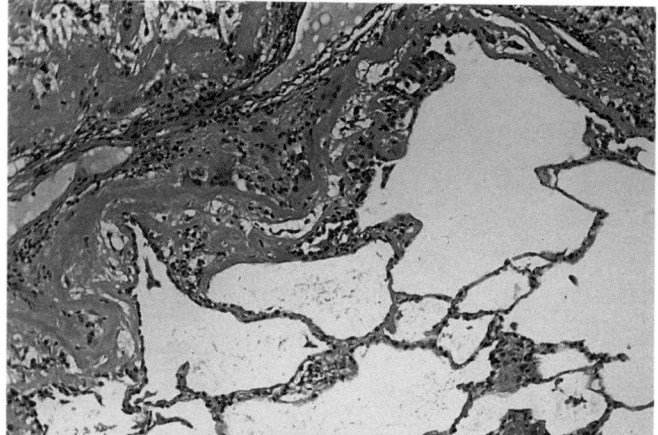

Fig. 2 Amyloidosis of the lung: alveolar-interstitial type [i] (by courtesy of Dr T. Ashcroft). There are interstital deposits of hyaline eosinophilic material with a foreign body type giant cell response in adjacent tissue. This is an almost unique feature of amyloidosis affecting the lung (haematoxylin and eosin, medium magnification).

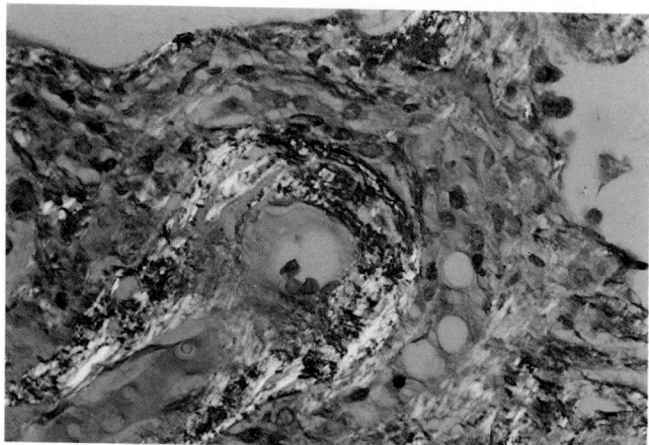

Fig. 3 Amyloidosis of the lung: alveolar-interstitial type [ii] (by courtesy of Dr T. Ashcroft). Amyloid gives a characteristic dichroic birefringence (Congo red stain under polarized light. High magnification).

particularly transbronchial biopsy, is generally both safe and effective. Another rare effect of amyloidosis on respiratory function is enlargement of the tongue, which can cause or exacerbate obstructive sleep apnoea.

Diagnosis

The diagnosis rests on the demonstration of amyloid tissue in an affected organ. When the protein is derived from plasma cells or lymphocytes, it may be possible to demonstrate light chains in the urine or M-component in the serum, and a plasma cell or lymphocyte dyscrasia may be clinically evident. When systemic reactive amyloidosis is the diagnosis, a provoking chronic inflammatory disease should be obvious, and high levels of SAA will be present in the serum. Measurement of SAA is rarely routinely available, but C-reactive protein is a useful surrogate. Immunohistochemical studies should, in any event, identify the specific biochemical nature of the protein sampled at biopsy, as should the ultrastructural appearances at electron microscopy.

Management

For discussion of the treatment of systemic amyloidosis, which is often unrewarding, see Section 11.12. Ultimately, organ transplantation may become the only hope of survival, and when renal failure or cardiac failure is the only immediate threat to life, this is often carried out. A need for lung transplantation has not yet been reported.

With the local forms of the disease of whatever aetiology, the outlook is a good deal brighter. Progression may be slow, and the disease may become quiescent. The laryngotracheobronchial deposits can sometimes be resected or depleted piecemeal endoscopically, perhaps using laser therapy, but there is some risk of serious bleeding from this. Corticosteroids have been reported to have a beneficial effect when there is critical airway stenosis. Parenchymal nodules in the lung rarely need to be removed, providing their histological nature is not in doubt.

Further reading

Ihling C *et al.* (1996). Amyloid tumors of the lung—an immunocytoma? *Pathology, Research and Practice* **192**, 446–52.

Kavuru MS *et al.* (1990). Amyloidosis and pleural disease. *Chest* **98**, 21–3.

Matsumoto K *et al.* (1997). Primary solitary amyloidoma of the lung: finding on CT and MRI. *European Radiology* **7**, 586–8.

Miyamoto T *et al.* (1999). Monoclonality of infiltrating plasma cells in primary pulmonary nodular amyloidosis: detection with polymerase chain reaction. *Journal of Clinical Pathology* **52**, 464–7.

Pickford HA, Swensen SJ, Utz JP (1997). Thoracic cross-sectional imaging of amyloidosis. *American Journal of Roentgenology* **168**, 353–5.

Rubinow A *et al.* (1978). Localized amyloidosis of the lower respiratory tract. *American Review of Respiratory Disease* **118**, 603–11.

Shah SP *et al.* (1998). Nodular amyloidosis of the lung from intravenous drug abuse: an uncommon cause of multiple pulmonary nodules. *Southern Medical Journal* **91**, 402–4.

Shiue ST, McNally DP (1988). Pulmonary hypertension from prominent vascular involvement in diffuse amyloidosis. *Archives of Internal Medicine* **148**, 687–9.

Utz JP, Swensen SJ, Gertz MA. Pulmonary amyloidosis. The Mayo Clinic experience from 1980 to 1993. *Annals of Internal Medicine* **124**, 407–13.

17.11.15 Lipoid (lipid) pneumonia

D. J. Hendrick

Exogenous

When mineral or vegetable lipids are deposited in the lung, they usually prove to be relatively inert but difficult to remove. Lung lipases have little effect, and the macrophages are slow to transport the free or emulsified material into the lymphatics. The result is often a chronic low-grade inflammatory response that may lead to secondary infection and/or local fibrosis. It is known as lipoid, or lipid, pneumonia. It should be suspected whenever a 'pneumonic' illness is slow to resolve or is recurrent, especially if there is the possibility of impaired swallowing and recurrent aspiration. Some animal lipids are more readily degraded by lung lipases, thus releasing irritating fatty acids. In these circumstances a brisk pneumonitis may occur.

Pathogenesis

Aspiration of vegetable or mineral oil is not common in the population at large, but is seen not infrequently within certain subgroups—particularly those with impaired swallowing mechanisms. Most affected are the very young and the elderly, and the regular nasal instillation of vegetable oils (e.g. olive oil) or paraffin to relieve congestion, or their ingestion to relieve constipation, are often responsible. A portion of any nasal dose is likely to enter the trachea, as may part of an ingested dose if the subject then reclines in bed or has any disturbance of swallowing. The critical point is that paraffin and many vegetable oils are not irritating to the tracheal mucosa, and so coughing is rarely excited and aspiration occurs without immediate sequelae.

The reluctant child forced to swallow cod liver oil is said to have encountered similar risks during the 1940s and 1950s, though infants are likely to face much greater hazard by virtue of less well developed deglutition. Patients fed by nasogastric tube are particularly vulnerable, as are those fed regularly with high lipid diets (for example with milk fat, ghee). A recent case report indicates a rather less obvious risk in an infant—that of lipid embolism from repeated mineral oil enemas. Lipoid pneumonia from embolism may also occur because of intravenous infusion, whether accidental or wilful.

Adults with unimpaired swallowing are affected only sporadically. Shipwrecked sailors have occasionally aspirated floating oil, and lipoid pneumonia has been recognized in workers exposed to oil mists and burning fats. In an exceptional case associated with recurrent tuberculosis, the spontaneous rupture of a longstanding oleothorax (oil plombage) led to a widespread iatrogenic lipoid pneumonia. Aspirated petroleum products such as kerosene may be absorbed from the lung and give rise to toxic responses in other organs (particularly the heart), and this may prove to be life threatening. The potential risk from oil aerosols has been highlighted recently in a diver breathing unfiltered air from an oil-contaminated surface compressor. Less unwilling inhalers of mineral oil and vaseline have been the blackfat tobacco smokers of Guyana, who obtain more satisfaction when these additives are mixed to native tobacco leaf. A distinctive geographical picture of progressive and often fatal pulmonary fibrosis complicates this habit in some 20 per cent of blackfat users, but has not been observed among non-smoking residents.

Clinical features

If there is little or no pulmonary response, there may be no symptoms, and the affected subject presents by chance with an abnormal chest radiograph. In about 50 per cent of cases there is a chronic 'pneumonic' illness with productive cough, low-grade fever, and (occasionally) haemoptysis. Often there is a cyclical course with intermittent symptoms. Repeated aspiration may lead to fibrotic shrinkage of the affected segment or segments (usually in the lower lobes or the middle lobe), bronchiectasis, or persistent consolidation. The radiographic appearances may closely simulate bronchial carcinoma, and many resections have been carried for this reason, sometimes revealing a characteristic granulomatous mass (paraffinoma). When more substantial quantities are aspirated the radiographic abnormalities are necessarily more diffuse, and when the lipid material is more reactive an acute 'pneumonic' illness occurs.

Diagnosis

The key to diagnosis is the demonstration of lipid material within pulmonary secretions or alveolar macrophages, whether obtained from sputum or bronchoalveolar lavage. If lung tissue is resected or a biopsy is taken, there may be fibrosis, evidence of chronic inflammation, and foreign body granulomas/giant cells in addition to lipid material retained within alveoli and macrophages (Fig. 1). An innovative use of computed tomography has recently identified excess deposits of lipid from its X-ray absorption characteristics, a technique that could offer a valuable alternative to biopsy or

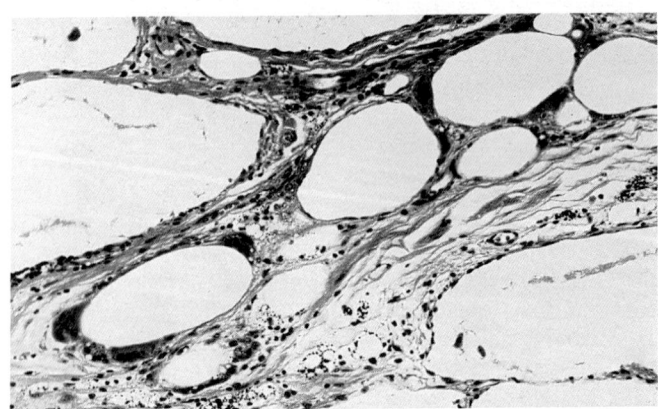

Fig. 1 Lipoid pneumonia (by courtesy of Dr T. Ashcroft). Exogenous lipoid pneumonia due to aspirated paraffin. There is interstitial fibrosis containing oil vacuoles which are enclosed within multinucleated giant cells (haematoxylin and eosin stain, medium magnification).

bronchoalveolar lavage in the diagnosis of atypical pneumonias. More generally, computed tomography shows patchy areas of ground-glass attenuation and interstitial thickening, thereby producing a 'crazy paving' pattern. This may be seen more readily with high resolution scans, which may additionally show interspersed poorly defined small nodules. Nuclear magnetic resonance scanning appears less effective, though a loss of signal intensity has been reported to have diagnostic specificity.

Management

Prophylactic management centres on minimizing any tendency to aspiration associated with impaired swallowing, and in persuading the misuser (or abuser) of vegetable and mineral oils to adopt alternative habits. Once aspiration has occurred there may be a role for therapeutic bronchoalveolar lavage, since this may remove substantial quantities of lipid from the alveoli. During episodes of secondary bacterial infection, there is an obvious role for antibiotics, and when there is acute inflammation corticosteroids are sometimes used.

Endogenous

The body may itself produce and retain lipid (mainly cholesterol) within the lungs, though this is not a common phenomenon. It occurs chiefly at sites of chronic inflammation, obstruction, or tissue necrosis, and is derived from the necrotic cells. This lipid will also be ingested by macrophages and may be recovered in the sputum. Sputum macrophages laden with lipid are not therefore pathognomonic of aspiration from an exogenous source, though chemical tests can distinguish the two varieties and histological examination of affected lung does not show a granulomatous response to endogenous lipid. Endogenous lipid is most commonly deposited when chronic inflammation accompanies bronchiectasis, bronchial carcinoma, or some other cause of persisting localized bronchial obstruction, and appears to depend on cigarette smoking. The radiological appearances are of a persisting pneumonia, which may also stimulate resection for fear a carcinoma is present. Very recently endogenous lipid pneumonia in a more diffuse form has been associated with the use of amiodarone in patients dying with adult respiratory distress syndrome.

Further reading

Annobil SH *et al.* (1991). Lipoid pneumonia on children following aspiration of animal fat (ghee). *Annals of Tropical Paediatrics* **11**, 87–94.

Corrin B, Soliman SS (1978). Cholesterol in the lungs of heavy smokers. *Thorax* **33**, 565–68.

Cox JE, Choplin RH, Chiles C (1996). Case report. Chemical-shift MRI of exogenous lipoid pneumonia. *Journal of Computer Assisted Tomography* **20**, 465–7.

Donaldson L *et al.* (1999). Acute amiodarone-induced lung toxicity. *Intensive Care Medicine* **25**, 242–3.

Gondouin A *et al.* (1996). Exogenous lipid pneumonia: a retrospective multicentre study. *European Respiratory Journal* **9**, 1463–9.

Laurent J *et al.* (1999). Exogenous lipoid pneumonia: HRCT, MR, and pathologic findings. *European Radiology* **9**, 1190–6.

Lee JS *et al.* (1999). Exogenous lipoid pneumonia: high-resolution CT findings. *European Radiology* **9**, 287–91.

Miller GJ *et al.* (1971). The lipoid pneumonia of blackfat tobacco smokers in Guyana. *Quarterly Journal of Medicine* **40**, 457–70.

Oldenburger D *et al.* (1972). Inhalation lipoid pneumonia from burning fats. *Journal of the American Medical Association* **222**, 1288–9.

Silverman JF *et al.* (1989). Bronchoalveolar lavage in the diagnosis of lipoid pneumonia. *Diagnostic Cytopathology* **5**, 3–8.

17.11.16 Pulmonary alveolar microlithiasis
D. J. Hendrick

This is a very rare disorder, with only 200 to 300 cases reported since its initial description in 1918. It is remarkable for a number of unusual if not unique features. Tiny 0.2- to 5-mm calcified concretions, which may be concentrically laminated, form progressively in the alveolar spaces, usually with some degree of interstitial fibrosis. As their profusion slowly increases in the lung, they produce a striking 'white-out' appearance on the chest radiograph as the border of one intensely radio-opaque microlith overlaps that of another, even if the two are not immediately adjacent. There are few clues to the cause of this curious disorder and, apart from transplantation, there is no effective means of therapy.

Pathogenesis

No abnormality of calcium metabolism has been demonstrated, but a disproportionate number of cases (almost half) occurs in siblings and in countries bordering the eastern Mediterranean. This points to a genetic rather than environmental basis, perhaps autosomal recessive inheritance. One hypothesis suggests that the calcific response is directed to an alveolar exudate (whether induced by inhaled particles or microbes) that cannot be reabsorbed adequately. The primary explanation could thus lie with an unusual inhalant stimulus, a deranged alveolar exudative response, or a failure of the usual mechanisms of reabsorption.

That similar concretions are not generally noted in other sites of membrane reabsorption possibly diminishes the probability of the last of these, though microliths have been noted in seminal vesicles in some cases, and azoospermia in others. Analytical studies, including X-ray energy spectroscopy and microscopic infrared spectroscopy, have showed no evidence of mineral dust deposition, and no microbial cause has been confirmed. The possibility of a deranged alveolar response has consequently attracted particular interest, perhaps an abnormality of surfactant function following oxidant stress. The calcified microliths (salts of calcium and phosphorus, and calcium carboxyapatite) are formed in the alveolar spaces, and some can be flushed out by bronchoalveolar lavage or even expectorated in sputum.

Clinical features

The disease usually presents in middle age, but the whole age spectrum may be involved and both sexes are equally represented. Almost invariably the patient is symptom free when an initial film is taken for incidental reasons, and there may be wonder that this can be possible when the radiograph is grossly abnormal. This is a consequence of there being no associated cellular, exudative, fibrotic, or vascular disruption of normal physiological processes in the early stages of the disease. Physical signs are conspicuous by their absence for most of its long course, though crackles, clubbing (even hypertrophic pulmonary osteoarthropathy), and signs of respiratory failure may be observed ultimately as the alveolar spaces are progressively filled with microliths and fibrosis of the interstitium advances. Shunting occurs at alveolar-capillary level causing hypoxaemia, and the bronchial circulation contributes increasingly to pulmonary venous return. In some cases subpleural cysts give rise to spontaneous pneumothoraces, and pleural adhesions may become prominent.

Although death supervened rapidly in the reported cases of two newborn infants, survival of 10 to 20 years is characteristic, and may be much longer. In most cases there is slowly progressive undue breathlessness with dry cough. Haemoptysis occurs occasionally. The lungs stiffen, ventilation becomes restricted, and gas transfer is impaired. Eventually respiratory failure and cor pulmonale supervene. At death, extensive areas of the chest radiograph show a dense 'white-out' appearance due to the considerable accumulation of calcium, the lungs are difficult to cut, and they sink in water.

Diagnosis

The radiographic appearances of profuse small calcified nodules are almost specific, particularly in moderately advanced cases when the dense 'white-out' picture is seen but symptoms are still absent or unimpressive. One case of sarcoidosis has been reported with similar appearances. With less advanced disease, biopsy, bronchoalveolar lavage, or expectorated sputum should provide diagnostic material, but with transbronchial biopsy it may prove difficult to close the forceps and extract them through the fibreoptic bronchoscope. Initially the chest radiograph shows a mere haziness of the lower zones, and computed tomography may be invaluable in demonstrating the nodular shadows and their calcific nature. It may also confirm an early predominance for the basal and posterior segments. High resolution images may also demonstrate the presence of interstitial fibrosis. As profusion and size of the calcified concretions increase, the lung fields become diffusely and densely opaque. Measurement of lung function during the asymptomatic stage reveals little or no abnormality, the affected subject remaining well for many years, but eventually ventilatory restriction, impairment of gas transfer, and arterial hypoxaemia are to be expected.

Management

Corticosteroids, calcium chelating agents, bisphosphonates, and bronchoalveolar lavage have not proved to be effective therapies, and in the absence of lung transplantation, treatment is merely supportive. A detailed description of a 37-year-old man presenting in respiratory failure, recorded severe hypoxia and pulmonary hypertension. Considerable intrapulmonary shunting was demonstrated, which was greatly improved by nasal continuous positive airway pressure, but not by conventional supplemental oxygen therapy. This presumably reflects the dominant effect of the disease in restricting alveolar ventilation over impairing gas diffusion. Although lung transplantation experience is necessarily limited in such a rare disorder, it clearly provides the most optimistic outlook for advanced disease. The dilemma is that the natural history is characteristically one of very slow progression, implying that duration of survival may not be greatly improved unless transplantation is left until the terminal phase. At such a time the probability of success is much reduced.

Further reading

Edelman JD *et al.* (1997). Bilateral sequential lung transplantation for pulmonary alveolar microlithiasis. *Chest* **112**, 1140–4.

Freiberg DB *et al.* (1992). Improvement in gas exchange with nasal continuous positive airway pressure in pulmonary alveolar microlithiasis. *American Review of Respiratory Disease* **145**, 1215–6.

Helbich TH *et al.* (1997). Pulmonary alveolar microlithiasis in children: radiographic and high-resolution CT findings. *American Journal of Roentgenology* **168**, 63–5.

Mariotta S *et al.* (1997). Pulmonary alveolar microlithiasis: review of Italian reports. *European Journal of Epidemiology* **13**, 587–90.

Moran CA *et al.* (1997). Pulmonary alveolar microlithiasis. A clinicopathologic and chemical analysis of seven cases. *Archives of Pathology and Laboratory Medicine* **121**, 607–11.

Nouh MS (1989). Is the desert lung syndrome (non-occupational dust pneumoconiosis) a variant of pulmonary alveolar microlithiasis? Report of four cases with review of the literature. *Respiration* **55**, 122–6.

Volle E, Kaufmann HJ (1987). Pulmonary alveolar microlithiasis in pediatric patients. A review of the world literature and two new observations. *Pediatric Radiology* **17**, 439–42.

Weinstein DS (1999). Pulmonary sarcoidosis: calcified micronodular pattern simulating pulmonary alveolar microlithiasis. *Journal of Thoracic Imaging* **14**, 218–20.

17.11.17 Toxic gases and fumes

D. J. Hendrick*

Noxious substances may be delivered airborne to the respiratory tract in molecular (gases and vapours) or particulate form. A vapour is the gaseous form of a substance that is liquid (occasionally solid) at ambient temperature and pressure. The effects of noxious gases and vapours are determined mainly by their solubility in water; those with high solubility are largely dissolved in the secretions lining the upper respiratory tract, those with low solubilities penetrate to the gas-exchanging tissues and exert their dominant effects there. However, with overwhelming exposures adverse effects will occur at all levels of the respiratory tract, and dose becomes a more important determinant of outcome than solubility.

Particulates that are dispersed in air (aerosols) may be solid (dusts) or liquid (mists), and may carry toxic chemicals through surface adsorption or solution, even if the carrier agent itself is harmless. If the particles are large (diameter > 10 μm), they become trapped in the nose, throat, or major airways. If they are small (diameter < 5 μm), they are deemed 'respirable' and may readily penetrate deeply to become retained in the gas-exchanging tissue and (through macrophage transport) the lung interstitium. Fume is a dispersion of fine (readily respirable) particles that form as vaporized metal condenses at ambient temperature and oxidizes to produce the metal oxide.

Many adverse effects may follow the inhalation of irritant or toxic gases and aerosols. Most are manifested in the lung itself, but some are manifested in other organs after the lung provides a route for absorption (e.g. poisoning from carbon monoxide or hydrogen cyanide). Not only do the respiratory effects occur at different levels, but they may appear at different times. It is useful, therefore, to consider acute and chronic (and sometimes subacute) effects separately, and to recognize that some are dominantly airway effects while others are dominantly parenchymal effects. The chronic effects, such as chronic bronchitis, emphysema, pneumoconiosis, pleural thickening, and lung cancer, generally require months or years of exposure, and arise only after a latency of 10 to 20 years or more. Although 'toxic' or 'irritant' in nature, rather than a consequence of allergy or infection, they are usually considered separately from the disorders attributable to 'toxic gases and fumes', and are described in other chapters.

In general, the acute effects of toxic gases and aerosols are the result of industrial or farming accidents, since the potential for toxic exposure is rare outside occupational environments. However, train or tanker crashes have occasionally caused the rupture of chemical containers and the release of toxic gases into non-occupational environments, and the tragic events at Bhopal illustrate the alarming potential for an industrial accident to have profound effects well beyond the work place.

*Professor J. M. Hopkin wrote on this subject in the third edition of the *Oxford Textbook of Medicine*. Much of his text has been retained in this revision and we acknowledge his contribution with grateful thanks.

Site of respiratory injury

Acute upper airway toxicity

If gases or vapours of high solubility (e.g. ammonia, hydrogen chloride, or sulphur dioxide) are involved, or aerosols comprising particles of large average diameter, the adverse effects will dominate in the upper respiratory tract and large airways. Laryngeal oedema, severe enough to cause airflow obstruction and require intubation, is the most important effect, but oedema is to be expected also in the conjunctivae, nose, mouth, and throat, together with inflammatory secretions, even bleeding. One breath is usually sufficient to provoke an immediate withdrawal from further exposure, if this is possible, and so protects against further damage.

Acute tracheobronchitis

If withdrawal from exposure is not possible, or less soluble gases are involved at less pungent levels of exposure (e.g. chlorine), there will be greater penetration beyond the larynx and an acute tracheobronchitis results. This too may become life threatening, and may predispose to secondary infection. If there is survival, full recovery is the rule, but a minority of patients are left with asthma that persists for weeks, months, or even indefinitely. Such an outcome has been called the reactive airways dysfunction syndrome.

Acute pneumonitis

Gases of low solubility (e.g. oxides of nitrogen, ozone, or phosgene) penetrate readily to the gas-exchanging tissues. In the absence of immediate toxicity to the upper respiratory tract they may be encountered in an increasing cumulative and hence dangerous dose. The outcome is an acute pneumonitis and pulmonary oedema some hours later, and is exemplified by nitrogen dioxide toxicity. This gas may be encountered in hazardous concentrations in unventilated silos, particularly when they are decapped (silo filler's disease), when welding is carried out in poorly ventilated sites, and with the combustion of nitrogen-containing substances, such as nitrocellulose. One notorious episode involved a fire of stored radiographs. When grain is stored in silos (or silage is preserved under impervious coverings) microbial contamination leads to the release of nitrogen dioxide along with other toxic gases (principally aldehydes) and asphyxiants (carbon dioxide, methane) and the removal of oxygen. Such processes have the beneficial effect of 'pickling' and preserving the vegetable produce, but they create a dangerous environment for the unwary farm worker. Moulding vegetable produce can similarly provoke a toxic pneumonitis through releasing microbial toxins, and it may be difficult to distinguish this (pulmonary mycotoxicosis or organic dust toxic syndrome, see Chapter 17.11.11) from nitrogen dioxide toxicity.

A curious observation with nitrogen dioxide toxicity has been a recurrent episode of pulmonary oedema 1 to 3 weeks after the initial exposure. The explanation is not clear, though possibly represents the well recognized complication of adult respiratory distress syndrome (**ARDS**) that may follow any cause of toxic pneumonitis. The prophylactic use of oral steroid is said to reduce this risk. Once ARDS occurs, additional risks of pneumothorax and secondary infection arise, sometimes with fatal result. Otherwise recovery is usually full, though rarely bronchiolitis obliterans (or bronchiolitis obliterans with organizing pneumonia) complicates the picture (Chapter 17.11.3).

Illustrative causal agents

Fire smoke

Smoke from fires is a complex mixture of gases and particulates released during combustion and pyrolysis. Its nature can vary greatly with the severity of the fire, the availability of oxygen, and the nature of the burning materials. It may contain toxic concentrations of carbon monoxide, hydrogen cyanide, ammonia, sulphur dioxide, chlorine, phosgene, nitrogen dioxide, aldehydes, and other gases, together with particulates derived from the burning material and surface absorbed gases. Thus, its effects may be diverse, and include suffocation or metabolic poisoning as well as direct toxic injury throughout the respiratory tract.

Metal fume fever

Metal fume fever is an acute and self-limiting febrile illness that characteristically occurs after unusually heavy exposures to metal fume, and recurs on re-exposure after a brief absence from work. It closely simulates other occupational fevers, such as Monday fever in cotton workers (see byssinosis, Chapter 17.4.1.5), polymer fever in chemical workers, and the fevers associated with humidifier lung and allergic alveolitis (see Chapter 17.11.11). It can occur on the first day of exposure. It results from alveolar deposition of very fine particulate metal oxides (fumes) produced in processes such as welding, burning (oxyacetylene cutting), and smelting of metal. It particularly, but not exclusively, involves zinc, copper, and magnesium. Within some 6 h of exposure, there is thirst, a metallic taste in the mouth, cough, tightness in the chest, and chills, with fever, headache, myalgia, and leucocytosis. Resolution follows within 24 h without permanent sequelae. This benign course is dramatically distinguished from that associated with heavy exposure to fume released from heating cadmium. Cadmium is an anticorrosive metal used in electroplating and the production of alloys. Cadmium fumes may be encountered during extraction, soldering, burning, and welding in poorly ventilated conditions, and may lead to an acute toxic reaction in both lungs and kidneys. It is associated with high mortality.

Simple asphyxiants

Some inhaled gases have no toxic effects, but may severely threaten life through asphyxiation by displacing oxygen from inhaled air. Most common are carbon dioxide and methane, which replace oxygen when vegetable produce decomposes through microbial contamination. A less common source is the slow combustion of coal in disused mines or cellars. Oxygen-deficient air in working mines (blackdamp) has been long recognized as a cause of asphyxiation in miners, but careful monitoring and high levels of ventilation provide effective prevention. Occasionally, however, disused mines accumulate blackdamp during periods of high barometric pressure, only to release the asphyxiant gas when the barometric pressure falls. Most escapes harmlessly to the atmosphere from mine shafts but some may be trapped in the ground under impervious layers of rock or clay. This may find an escape route through faults in the strata and so be emitted at high flow rates into surface buildings. Cellars that breach a layer of clay in coal mining areas may provide a particularly dangerous environment for the unsuspecting. Decaying vegetable matter in the soil may also provide the mechanism for carbon dioxide to replace oxygen, and entry of this oxygen-deficient air into wells during periods of low barometric pressure has also led to asphyxiation.

Management

The management of toxic and asphyxiant insults is essentially supportive. Prompt removal from the source of exposure is followed by attention to the airway, and the administration of specific antidotes when, rarely, this is indicated (for example with cyanide poisoning or methaemoglobinaemia). Because of the risk of laryngeal obstruction or pulmonary oedema following toxic insults, a minimum period of 24 h of hospital care is needed for subjects presenting with hoarseness, stridor, wheeze, or hypoxaemia, and those with a history indicative of heavy exposure to a poorly soluble toxic gas. Humidified air, oxygen supplementation, and bronchodilators may be required. Bronchoscopy may be needed to remove excessive secretions and clear the airway. Laryngeal obstruction demands intubation, and tracheostomy may be necessary if there is extensive upper airway inflammation. Severe pulmonary oedema should be managed as for the adult respiratory distress syndrome (see section 16.04.02). The role of corticosteroids in limiting inflammation is unclear; these drugs add to the risk of secondary infection but have been claimed to prevent the development of late pulmonary oedema after nitrogen dioxide exposure.

Further reading

Ainslie G (1993). Inhalational injuries produced by smoke and nitrogen dioxide. *Respiratory Medicine* **87**, 169–74.

Brooks SM, Weiss MA, Bernstein IL (1985). Reactive airways dysfunction syndrome (RADS). Persistent asthma syndrome after high level irritant exposures. *Chest* **88**, 376–84.

Charan NB *et al.* (1979). Pulmonary injuries associated with acute sulfur dioxide inhalation. *American Review of Respiratory Disease* **119**, 555–60.

Hjortso E *et al.* (1988). ARDS after accidental inhalation of zinc chloride smoke. *Intensive Care Medicine* **14**, 17–24.

Horvarth EP, do Pico GA, Barbee RA (1978). Nitrogen dioxide-induced pulmonary disease. *Journal of Occupational Medicine* **20**, 103–10.

Kanluen S, Gottlieb CA (1991). A clinical pathologic study of four adult cases of acute mercury inhalation toxicity. *Archives of Pathology and Laboratory Medicine* **115**, 56–60.

Schwartz DA. (2002). Toxic tracheitis, bronchitis, and bronchiolitis. In: Hendrick DJ *et al.* eds. *Occupational disorders of the lung: their recognition, management, and prevention* pp.93–103. WB Saunders, London.

Schwartz D, Smith D, Lakshminarayan S (1990). The pulmonary sequelae associated with accidental inhalation of chlorine gas. *Chest* **97**, 820–5.

Smith TJ, Petty TL, Ridding JC (1976). Pulmonary effects of exposure to airborne cadmium. *American Review of Respiratory Disease* **114**, 161.

17.11.18 Radiation pneumonitis

*D. J. Hendrick**

Local therapeutic irradiation of malignancies of the breast, oesophagus, mediastinum (including lymphoma), and lung may damage normal pulmonary tissue. Normal lung is also damaged by the total body irradiation used in preparation for bone marrow transplantation, and by any pulmonary shunting of therapeutic radioactive agents administered via the arterial route to other organs (e.g. yttrium-90 microspheres to the liver). Effects are compounded by the use of chemotherapeutic agents such as methotrexate. However, the risks appear to differ between the various chemotherapeutic agents, for instance that for adriamycin exceeds that for cisplatin. Furthermore, segments of irradiated lung may prove to be unduly susceptible to drug toxicity if chemotherapeutic agents are administered subsequently. Knowledge of the radiation port is therefore important in distinguishing localized toxic pneumonitis from infection.

*Professor J. M. Hopkin wrote on this subject in the third edition of the *Oxford Textbook of Medicine*. Much of his text has been retained in this revision and we acknowledge his contribution with grateful thanks.

The scale of pulmonary damage is strongly dependent on the volume of lung exposed, and the dose and fractionation of irradiation. Clinical manifestations range from asymptomatic radiographic opacification to fatal respiratory failure. The latter is fortunately vanishingly rare as radiotherapy techniques are better refined. The dose administered by each fraction is possibly the most important determinant, with values exceeding 2.67 Gy reported to carry most risk. If the same total dose is administered by two fractions during the same day, the risk appears to diminish. Pre-existing fibrotic damage and coincident infection additionally augment the risk.

Radiation releases toxic and mutagenic free radicals within tissue. The resultant DNA damage causes mitotic cell death as tissue cells pass through the first two or three cell divisions after irradiation. The principal cells injured in the lung (the capillary endothelium and type 2 alveolar pneumocyte) have turnover times ranging from 2 to 6 weeks under different circumstances, which explains why the maximum pulmonary effect occurs at about 2 months after injury. The capillary endothelium leaks protein and fluid, and the interalveolar septae become thickened, thereby leading to air space filling (consolidation) and interstitial fibrosis.

The pathogenic pathways appear to involve T lymphocytes. If thymectomy is performed before whole-body irradiation for bone marrow transplantation, the risk of radiation pneumonitis is reduced. When unilateral pneumonitis complicates the irradiation of only one lung in the treatment of breast cancer, a marked but equal increase in lymphocyte numbers from bronchoalveolar lavage in both lungs 4 to 6 weeks later is correlated with a decrease in vital capacity. Animal models suggest that the release of nitric oxide from alveolar macrophages and alveolar epithelial cells also plays a role, as does the recruitment of neutrophils.

The pathological changes can be categorized as (i) acute (up to 3 months), when there is vascular damage with thrombosis and packing of alveoli with surfactant (released from type 2 pneumocytes) and protein-rich fluid; (ii) subacute (2 to 6 months), when there is type 2 pneumocyte renewal and proliferation with macrophage and fibroblast infiltration into the alveoli and interstitium; and (iii) chronic (up to 24 months), when there is alveolar and interstitial fibrosis with capillary sclerosis.

Clinical features

Symptoms begin within a few weeks and may persist for weeks or months. They occur in 10 to 30 per cent of patients following radiotherapy for lung cancer. A rise of the plasma concentrations of transforming growth factor-β_1 and soluble intercellular adhesion molecule-1 have been shown to be markers for those at higher than average risk, thereby providing insights to possible mechanisms, and pointers to identifying subjects who are most suited to escalating radiotherapy treatment.

The severity of symptoms is dependent upon the extent of lung damage, and minor degrees may only be detected incidentally from routine chest radiographs. Cough, which can be severe and may produce thick sputum, and breathlessness are the principal symptoms, but may be accompanied by fever of variable degree. On examination there may be tachypnoea, cyanosis in severe disease, and local crepitations. Telangiectases, the result of cutaneous radiation damage, are often observed in the overlying skin.

The most characteristic radiographic feature is an area of hazy consolidation demarcated by a sharp margin (crossing anatomical pulmonary planes) that corresponds to the limits of the irradiation field, though additional effects are usually detectable beyond these boundaries. Radioisotope scanning shows marked perfusion impairment within the affected portion of lung. In extensive disease, the clinical and radiographic features may be typical of adult respiratory distress syndrome (Chapter 16.04.02). Computed tomography provides the best means of early identification, ground-glass attenuation and interalveolar septal thickening being the early characteristic features.

Up to a year or two after the radiation insult, dense local fibrosis may develop, and magnetic resonance imaging may be required to allow differentiation from tumour recurrence. This can also arise in the apparent absence of earlier pneumonitis, and it may be complicated by pleural effusion, pneumothorax, or fungal colonization (e.g. *Aspergillus* sp.). Fractures resulting from irradiation-induced bone necrosis may occur in nearby ribs.

Treatment

In cases where symptoms are slight, no specific treatment is needed. In more severe disease, corticosteroids produce relief during the acute phase in most patients. Any response to corticosteroids occurs within 3 to 4 days, with clinical and radiographic improvement, and treatment should be continued for 3 to 4 weeks before tapering and stopping. Corticosteroids do not, however, influence the extent of subsequent pulmonary fibrosis. Symptomatic relief of cough and hypoxaemia by an opioid antitussive and oxygen supplementation may also be needed. Prevention offers the best means of control, and further development of methods to detect undue susceptibility and early disease may prove to be valuable in developing safer fractioning protocols.

In laboratory animals, interferon-γ has reduced neutrophil recruitment and protein leakage in the early phase of radiation pneumonitis, angiotensin-converting enzyme (ACE) inhibitors have prevented or limited increases in central venous and pulmonary artery pressure (and diminished exudation and oedema), and nitric oxide synthase inhibitors have reduced disease progression. Such observations may provide direction for additional measures of prevention and control in humans, though one study has already noted no significant benefit in those who by chance had used ACE inhibitor medication. A further experimental approach has involved the prophylactic use of selenium-enriched spiruline, which appeared to reduce the development of fibrosis by impairing the synthesis of hydroxyproline and type III collagen.

Further reading

Anscher MS *et al.* (1998). Plasma transforming growth factor-β_1 as a predictor of radiation pneumonitis. *International Journal of Radiation Oncology, Biology, Physics* **41**, 1029–35.

Ishii Y, Kitamura S (1999). Soluble intercellular adhesion molecule-1 as an early detection marker for radiation pneumonitis. *European Respiration Journal* **13**, 733–8.

Kwa SL *et al.* (1998). Radiation pneumonitis as a function of mean lung dose: an analysis of pooled data of 540 patients. *International Journal of Radiation Oncology, Biology, Physics* **42**, 1–9.

McBride WH, Vegesna V (2000). The role of T-cells in radiation pneumonitis after bone marrow transplantation. *International Journal of Radiation Biology* **76**, 517–21.

Roach M, III *et al.* (1995). Radiation pneumonitis following combined modality therapy for lung cancer: analysis of prognostic factors. *Journal of Clinical Oncology* **13**, 2606–12.

Roberts CM *et al.* (1993). Radiation pneumonitis: a possible lymphocyte-mediated hypersensitivity reaction. *Annals of Internal Medicine* **118**, 696–700.

Rosiello RA *et al.* (1993). Radiation pneumonitis. Bronchoalveolar lavage assessment and modulation by a recombinant cytokine. *American Review of Respiratory Disease* **148**, 1671–6.

Salinas FV, Winterbauer RH (1995). Radiation pneumonitis: a mimic of infectious pneumonitis. *Seminars in Respiratory Infections* **10**, 143–53.

Sigmund G, Slanina J, Hinkelbein W (1993). Diagnosis of radiation-pneumonitis. *Recent Results in Cancer Research* **130**, 123–31.

17.11.19 Drug-induced lung disease

*D. J. Hendrick and G. P. Spickett**

Adverse effects of drugs on the lungs frequently present diagnostic problems. This chapter is centred on direct effects of drugs in usual therapeutic doses on the airways, alveoli and interstitium, pulmonary vasculature, pleura, and mediastinal structures. Respiratory disorders arising through occupational exposure (manufacture, transport, dispensing, administration) are considered only briefly. Excluded are indirect effects, such as the predisposition to opportunistic lung infection resulting from cytotoxic agents, the worsening of respiratory failure after sedatives, and the consequences of overdosage or inadequate control of dosage (e.g. pulmonary haemorrhage with anticoagulants).

Asthma

The underlying pathophysiological basis of asthma is an unusually high level of airway responsiveness—the tendency of the airways to constrict following a variety of stimuli, whether specific (e.g. allergens) or non-specific (e.g cold dry air). Airway responsiveness is distributed unimodally in the population at large, individuals with asthma being those in the tail with the highest levels. In theory, drugs (like other environmental agents) may produce asthmatic symptoms either by elevating the pre-existing level of airway responsiveness into the asthma range, or by acting as a specific or non-specific stimulus when airway responsiveness lies already within the asthmatic range. By the first mechanism, the drug acts as a cause of asthma (an asthma inducer), by the second it acts as a cause of asthmatic reactions (an asthma trigger). Some drugs doubtless act through both mechanisms. The mechanism is of limited consequence in the drug setting (though not in the occupational setting), since treatment cessation and future avoidance is the way forward in both circumstances. If, nevertheless, a given drug is known to be a potential trigger but not an inducer, concern over its use need arise only for individuals who are already asthmatic.

In practice, airway obstruction provoked by drugs usually presents as an exacerbation of pre-existing asthma, and the drug acts as a trigger not inducer. In some cases asthma has not previously been recognized until it is exacerbated by the adverse effect of a drug and thus 'uncovered'. In such instances clues to pre-existing asthma are usually elicited when the appropriate history is taken. Drugs that exacerbate symptoms in subjects with pre-existing asthma may conveniently be classified as those that produce a more or less predictable effect, related to their pharmacological properties, and those which produce bronchoconstriction due to an idiosyncratic effect (Table 1). Less commonly, asthma develops *de novo*, probably because immunological hypersensitivity has developed.

Asthmatic symptoms can also be a consequence of the particular formulation of a drug or its method of delivery. For example, nebulized solutions of low osmolality can trigger asthmatic reactions if there is a high level of airway responsiveness. This appears to have been the main mechanism of bronchoconstriction induced paradoxically by nebulized ipratropium bromide. Since the drug was reformulated in isotonic solution the problem has largely disappeared. A further cause of bronchconstriction from nebulized drugs has been the presence of certain preservatives or stabilizers (e.g. benzalkonium chloride, edetate disodium) in the excipient solution. If the administered drug is used for asthma, the effect is particularly unexpected. A further paradox is associated with the evolving use of hydrofluoroalkane

*Professor G. J. Gibson wrote on this subject in the third edition of the *Oxford Textbook of Medicine*. Much of his text has been retained in this revision and we acknowledge his contribution with grateful thanks.

Table 1 Drugs that may cause or exacerbate asthma

Pharmacological effects
Cholinergic agents (e.g. carbachol, pilocarpine)
Cholinesterase inhibitors (e.g. pyridostigmine)
Prostaglandin F
Histamine-releasing agents (e.g. curare derivatives)
β-Sympathetic antagonists
ACE inhibitors (cough without asthma more common)
Sensitizing and idiosyncratic effects
Oral
　　　Aspirin and other NSAIDs
　　　Tartrazine-containing preparations
　　　Nitrofurantoin (alveolar reaction more common)
　　　Carbamazepine
　　　Propafenone
Parenteral
　　　Penicillin
　　　Iron–dextran complex
　　　Aminophylline
　　　Hydrocortisone sodium succinate
　　　N-Acetylcysteine
Inhaled
　　　Nebulized pentamidine
Eye drops
　　　NSAIDs

ACE, angiotensin-converting enzyme; NSAIDs, non-steroidal anti-inflammatory drugs

propellants (rather than ozone-depleting chlorofluorocarbons) in pressurized aerosol inhalers used to treat asthma. These may have a minor non-specific irritant effect on hyperresponsive airways, which is masked if they are used as the vehicle to administer short-acting β-agonist bronchodilators. However, with the long-acting β-agonist salmeterol (though not eformoterol), the bronchodilator effect is less speedy and hydrofluoroalkane may trigger brief symptoms. The epidemiological importance of this adverse effect is at present unclear.

Pharmacological effects

Cholinergic drugs, such as carbachol, given systemically occasionally produce bronchoconstriction, and in very sensitive asthmatic patients exacerbations have occurred after use of pilocarpine as eye drops. An inhaled anticholinergic agent would seem a logical approach to this problem and has been shown to be effective in reversing occasional untoward effects of cholinesterase inhibitors in asthmatic patients with myasthenia gravis.

The bronchoconstrictor prostaglandin $F_{2\alpha}$, if used to induce abortion, may be hazardous in asthmatic patients. The occurrence of bronchoconstriction after thiopentone, opiates, and muscle relaxants (tubocurarine, suxamethonium, and pancuronium) is probably due to their capacity to release histamine.

A more common problem is worsening of airway obstruction by β-adrenergic antagonist agents. Although these have been increasingly refined to select agents with the least β_2-antagonism, thus minimizing effects on the airways, none is completely specific for β_1-receptors. The degree of selectivity varies, with propranolol the least and practolol probably the most selective agents used so far. Unfortunately, practolol causes its own distinctive side-effects (see below) and is no longer available. Of the β-blockers currently available, atenolol and metoprolol seem to have the least adverse effects on airway function, but many patients with asthma will show a reduction in forced expiratory volume in 1 s (FEV_1) or peak flow on therapeutic doses of these agents and considerable caution is necessary. The problem of β-blockers in patients with clear-cut asthma is relatively straightforward, but the situation with chronic airway obstruction is less clear. Adverse reactions in such patients are less common and usually less severe, which possibly reflects the coincidental presence of mild asthma rather than a true adverse effect on chronic obstructive pulmonary disease

attributable to emphysema or obstructive bronchiolitis. Many patients who develop symptoms and worsening airway obstruction after use of β-blockers are subsequently thought to have had 'latent' asthma.

Although the adverse effects of oral or systemic β-blockers are well recognized, those of ophthalmic preparations are easily overlooked. Timolol, which is used commonly in eye drops for the treatment of glaucoma, is a potent non-selective β-blocker. Its use has frequently been associated with worsening asthma. The ophthalmic formulation of the newer β-blocker betaxolol appears to be less dangerous, but should be avoided in patients with asthma unless no suitable alternative is available.

Effects from sensitization and idiosyncrasy

The mechanism by which drugs lead to asthmatic symptoms when there is no obvious pharmacological effect is often unclear, though immunological sensitization and idiosyncrasy are likely to provide the major pathways.

The most dramatic presentation of drug-related asthma is as part of an acute anaphylactic reaction, and penicillin and intravenously administered iron–dextran are particularly noteworthy among the causal agents. Other drug hypersensitivity reactions that include asthma among the manifestations are often associated with blood eosinophilia and/or eosinophilic pneumonia, and are discussed more fully in Chapter 17.11.9.

Immunological hypersensitivity is presumed to underlie most causes of occupational asthma, some of which involve pharmaceutical agents. Most prominent are certain antibiotics (e.g. cephalosporins, isoniazid, penicillins, piperazine, spiramycin, tetracycline,), the H_2-receptor antagonist cimetidine, the laxative psyllium (ispaghula), pancreatic enzymes, and certain hormones (adrenocorticotrophic hormone, gonadotrophin, pituitary snuff). If a sensitized worker subsequently uses the relevant drug therapeutically, the potential arises for an asthmatic reaction (Fig. 1). The history, when symptoms suggest asthma, should always include details of occupation and medication, and if the patient has ever worked in the pharmaceutical industry the possibility of occupationally induced hypersensitivity to a current medication should be considered.

Idiosyncrasy probably underlies many asthmatic symptoms related to medication, and is the likely explanation for exacerbations following use of intravenous N-acetylcysteine in severe paracetamol poisoning. Its use in asthmatic patients requires caution. Idiosyncrasy more obviously underlies asthmatic reactions to aspirin and other non-steroidal anti-inflammatory drugs (**NSAIDs**). Exacerbation of asthma after ingestion of aspirin was described as long ago as 1910, but its precise mechanism remains elusive. Most patients who are sensitive to aspirin also react to other NSAIDs, their widely differing chemical structures making an immunological hypersensitivity reaction unlikely. As with cholinergic drugs and β-blockers, asthmatic reactions to NSAIDs may rarely follow ocular administration, and so eye drops deserve careful attention when asthma worsens unexpectedly.

NSAIDs are inhibitors of prostaglandin synthesis via the cyclo-oxygenase pathway, and it is presumed that their adverse effects are mediated in this way. It is possible that metabolism of arachidonic acid is diverted to the production of bronchoconstrictor leukotrienes, but why only a proportion of patients with asthma should be affected is not clear (hence the idiosyncrasy). Deaths have been reported with both aspirin and indomethacin. Of the commonly used analgesic agents, paracetamol is the least likely to provoke a significant response, although occasional adverse reactions are well documented. A further interesting feature is that aspirin-sensitive individuals can be made tolerant to further aspirin by ingesting graded doses over a couple of days. This state of tolerance can then be maintained by daily treatment with aspirin, but sensitivity returns within a few days of discontinuing regular treatment. Any attempt at inducing tolerance in this way requires very careful supervision.

Many patients with analgesic-induced asthma are also sensitive to the azo dye tartrazine (and often to alcoholic beverages). Tartrazine has hitherto been a commonly used colouring agent in medications (particularly those coloured orange or red) and foodstuffs, and since it is an approved food and drug additive, its presence is not always declared and the extent of the problems it may cause is not clear. In the past tartrazine was present, ironically, in some medications used to treat asthma, but most pharmaceutical companies no longer use it in their formulations. Other dyes may, however, have similar adverse effects and some of these still occur in drug formulations. Patients with aspirin and tartrazine sensitivity may also develop troublesome nasal polyposis, as well as asthma. Such patients may benefit from a low salicylate and azo-dye free diet, in addition to strict avoidance of NSAIDs.

The potential exacerbation of asthma by drugs used to treat it presents an acute dilemma, as a drug effect may be difficult to dissociate from spontaneous deterioration. There are well documented reports of worsening asthma after both intravenous aminophylline and hydrocortisone. Sensitivity to hydrocortisone is a particular problem in asthmatic patients who also show adverse reactions to aspirin and NSAIDs. The sensitivity to hydrocortisone of these individuals does not extend to other steroids; it appears to be related to the succinate moiety of the hydrocortisone sodium succinate molecule as it is not seen with the alternative phosphate salt.

The frequent use of nebulized pentamidine for treatment or prophylaxis of pneumocystis infection in patients with HIV infection has been associated with bronchoconstriction in many individuals. The mechanism is unclear. Although patients with asthma show larger responses, others with no previous evidence of asthma may also be affected. The adverse effect is inhibited by prior use of a nebulized bronchodilator, an approach that has become standard in many centres.

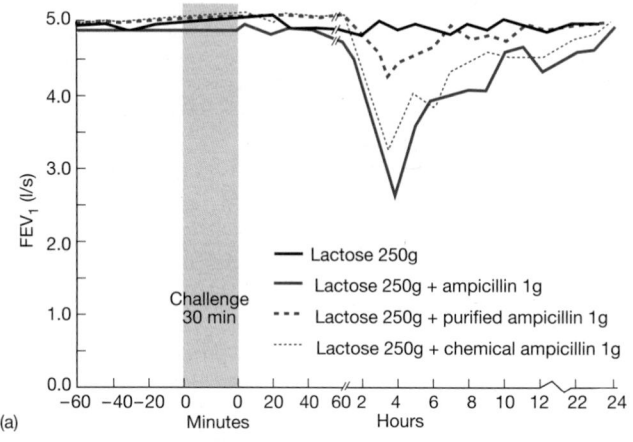

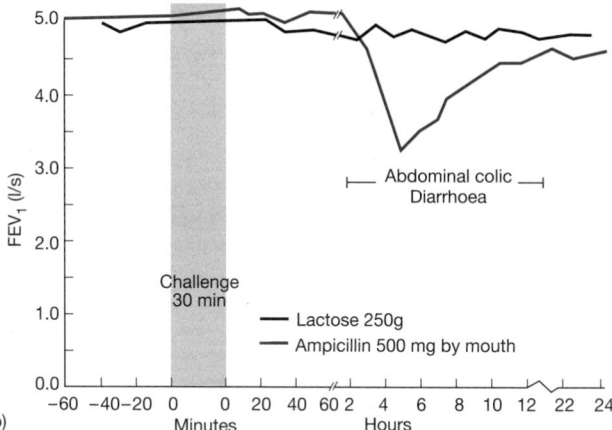

Fig. 1 Results of inhalation and ingestion challenge tests with ampicillin. The inhalation test confirmed that the patient had become sensitized to ampicillin as a consequence of respiratory exposure at work, and the ingestion test showed that asthmatic reactions would be provoked also by oral ingestion at therapeutic dose levels. (Data taken from Davies et al.(1974).)

Cough

Cough in the absence of asthma is a well-recognized side-effect of treatment with inhibitors of angiotensin-converting enzyme. It develops in 10 to 20 per cent of individuals so treated and is an effect of the class of drug rather than of specific agents. The cough is non-productive. There appears to be a weak relation to dose such that dose reduction may result in some improvement, but in many individuals the symptom is sufficiently troublesome to necessitate drug withdrawal. Deterioration of pre-existing asthma has also been reported occasionally, but in most individuals with cough related to angiotensin-converting enzyme inhibition, features of asthma are not present. The mechanism is unclear; angiotensin-converting enzyme catalyses not only the conversion of angiotensin I to angiotension II, but also the breakdown of bradykinin and substance P. Since these agents are cough stimulants, their accumulation offers a possible mechanism for this unusual adverse effect. The cough disappears on withdrawal of the drug.

Alveolar reactions

There is no generally accepted classification of alveolar reactions to drugs. They range from acute non-cardiogenic pulmonary oedema (e.g. from cremaphor, the agent used to provide soluble cyclosporin A for intravenous use) or the adult respiratory distress syndrome at one extreme to insidiously developing pulmonary fibrosis at the other. The reactions are conveniently considered under three main headings: alveolar capillary leakage, alveolar and interstitial inflammation/fibrosis, and eosinophilia (Table 2). Some overlap is inevitable: inflammatory reactions (whether toxic or allergic) may cause capillary leakage and hence radiographic air space filling; allergic reactions may or may not be characterized by inflammation and eosinophil infiltration.

Of the drugs that may produce the picture of adult respiratory distress syndrome, hydrochlorothiazide and salicylates are the commonest. The reaction to hydrochlorothiazide is idiosyncratic and is not shared by other thiazide drugs. In the case of salicylates there is a clearer relation to dose, with reactions usually occurring with frank overdose (as also occurs with opiates) or, occasionally, with chronic high-level ingestion. Infused β_2-adrenergic agonists are sometimes used as uterine relaxants (tocolytics) to inhibit premature labour. Several, in particular isoxsuprine, ritodrine, and terbutaline, have been associated with florid pulmonary oedema. This reaction is occasionally life threatening and caution is required over the rate of infusion.

Several drugs produce widespread alveolar damage ('pneumonitis' or 'alveolitis'), which may or may not be followed by fibrosis (Table 2). Patients can present acutely with cough, fever, shortness of breath, and occasionally systemic upset. Alternatively, there is slowly progressive fibrosis with gradually worsening dyspnoea and widespread shadowing on the chest radiograph. The mechanism(s) of such reactions are uncertain, but may include toxicity, hypersensitivity, and possibly idiosyncrasy. In some cases, including bleomycin, carmustine, amiodarone, and nitrofurantoin, there is evidence of a relation to dose or duration of treatment. Recent evidence in the cases of nitrofurantoin and bleomycin suggests a role for the production of toxic oxygen radicals in the lungs, perhaps providing a link with the known pulmonary toxicity of oxygen itself and with the synergistic adverse effects of high oxygen concentrations and some cytotoxic agents.

Much recent interest has centred on the cardiac antiarrhythmic drug, amiodarone. It has been estimated that approximately 6 per cent of patients taking 400 mg or more per day for 2 months or more will develop overt pulmonary toxicity. There have also been several well-documented cases involving smaller doses. The mechanism may include both immunologically mediated and direct toxic effects. Histologically the lung shows features of chronic inflammation together with interstitial and intra-alveolar fibrosis (Fig. 2). Characteristic 'foamy' macrophages are seen, but they are not specific for serious toxic reactions as they are also demonstrable in the majority of patients taking the drug without adverse clinical effects. Occasionally, the histological picture is of bronchiolitis obliterans organizing pneumonia (**BOOP**), which is also known as cryptogenic organizing pneumonia. Symptoms include progressive dyspnoea, a troublesome cough, and (occasionally) pleuritic chest pain. Radiographic appearances are varied: most frequently there is a diffuse nodular or alveolar filling pattern, sometimes with upper lobe predominance (Fig. 3); occasionally a pleural effusion is present.

Differential diagnoses in the population of patients likely to be taking this drug include left ventricular failure and pneumonia. Further investigation, including measurement of pulmonary wedge pressure and lung biopsy, is often necessary. Bronchoalveolar lavage in some (but not all) patients shows a lymphocytic pattern. This investigation is also of value for the exclusion of infection, but the finding of 'foamy' macrophages in lavage fluid is, for the reasons discussed above, insufficient to confirm the diagnosis. If amiodarone lung toxicity is suspected, cessation of treatment is desirable, but the very long half-life of drug metabolites (many weeks) means that elimination will be very slow. Corticosteroids probably suppress the reaction and sometimes allow treatment to be continued or recommended in cases of 'malignant' dysrhythmias unresponsive to other agents.

Table 2 Alveolar reactions

Acute pulmonary oedema/adult respiratory distress syndrome
Cytosine arabinoside
Hydrochlorothiazide
Low-molecular-weight dextran
Naloxone
Salicylates
Tocolytic agents (e.g. isoxsuprine, ritodrine, terbutaline)
Diffuse lung injury (alveolitis) and/or fibrosis
Oxygen
Nitrofurantoin
Amiodarone
Tocainide
Cytotoxic agents
     Azathioprine
     Bleomycin
     Busulphan
     Carmustine (BCNU)
     Chlorambucil
     Cyclophosphamide
     Cytosine arabinoside
     Lomustine (CCNU)
     Melphalan
     6-Mercaptopurine
     Mitomycin C
Eosinophilic reactions
Aspirin
Carbamazepine
Chlorpropamide
Chlorpromazine
Gold salts*
Imipramine
Methotrexate*
Naproxen
Nitrofurantoin*
Penicillamine*
Penicillins
Phenytoin
Procarbazine*
Sulphasalazine
Sulphonamides
Tetracycline

*Eosinophilia not consistent.

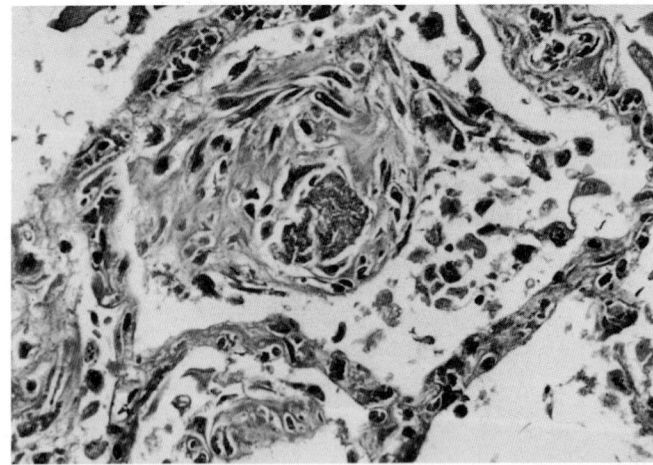

(a)

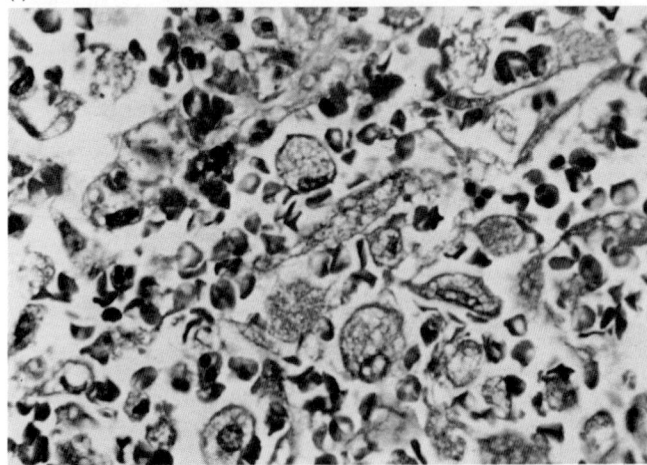

(b)

Fig. 2 Histological specimen of the lung of a patient who died from amiodarone pulmonary toxicity: (a) alveolar wall thickening and organizing intra-alveolar exudates; (b) higher power view of alveolar exudate showing characteristic 'foamy' macrophages. (Reproduced from Adams *et al.* (1986). *Quarterly Journal of Medicine* **59**, 449–71, with permission.)

BOOP is a rare manifestation of drug-induced lung disease, but is increasingly recognized in complex settings where drug therapy may have played a dominant or contributory role. In addition to amiodarone, associations have been reported with carbamazepine, nitrofurantoin, phenytoin, sotalol, tacrolimus, ticlopidine, and a number of herbal medications. One of particular interest is a presumed (but unproven) anorectic agent derived from the leaf of an Asian shrub of the *Euphoriaceae* family, *Sauropus androgynus*. In a remarkable period of a few months, more than 60 people who had ingested juice containing uncooked leaf extract of *S. androgynus* presented to hospital in Taiwan with progressive undue breathlessness. In 23 of these patients whose breathlessness was severe, responses to corticosteroid therapy were poor. Plain radiographs were essentially normal, but CT scanning and biopsies demonstrated BOOP with (in a few cases) bronchiectasis in the segmental and subsegmental bronchi.

Cytotoxic and immunosuppressive drugs pose an increasing problem for the lung parenchyma, with the majority reported to cause pulmonary complications. Bleomycin causes problems most frequently, followed by busulphan and methotrexate. Cyclophosphamide and azathioprine are the most widely used drugs in this group, because of their roles in non-malignant disease, but produce adverse pulmonary reactions only occasionally. In

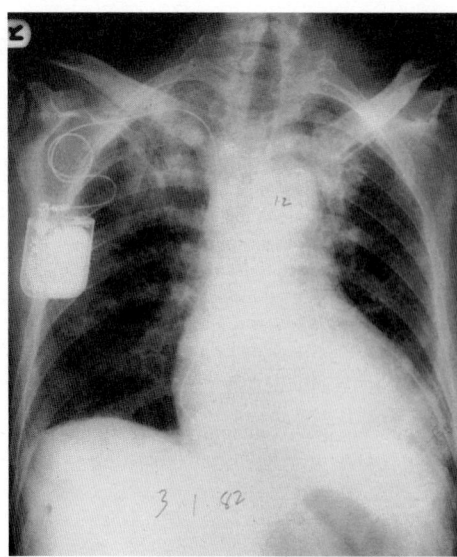

Fig. 3 Chest radiograph of a second patient with amiodarone pulmonary toxicity showing confluent alveolar shadowing in both upper lobes. (Reproduced from Adams *et al.* (1986). *Quarterly Journal of Medicine* **59**, 449–71, with permission.)

most cases it is not clear whether the effects are due to direct toxicity or to hypersensitivity. With bleomycin, however, there is evidence of a dose–response relationship: cumulative doses of less than 150 mg are less likely to cause serious reactions, whereas death due to respiratory failure consequent upon severe fibrosis has occurred in about 10 per cent of patients receiving more than 500 mg.

The recorded frequency of adverse reactions varies with the means by which they are detected; for example, on clinical and functional criteria, fibrosis occurs in 5 to 10 per cent of patients treated with busulphan, but pathological and cytological evidence suggest lung toxicity in much higher proportions. Similarly, the increasing use of CT scanning shows an appreciably higher prevalence than found in surveys that employ plain chest radiography. The frequency of overt lung involvement may also be related to length of survival, as determined by the primary disease. With busulphan, the average interval between starting treatment and the appearance of toxic effects can be as long as 4 years, and in some cases the lung changes appear to progress after the drug has been discontinued. With carmustine (BCNU) it has been shown that pulmonary fibrosis may first be recognized several years after treatment has finished. Other factors that may increase the toxicity of a given drug include advanced patient age and synergism with other drugs, lung radiation, or the subsequent inhalation of high concentrations of oxygen.

Histologically, most cytotoxic drugs produce evidence of diffuse alveolar damage with destruction of lining cells, formation of hyaline membranes, and variable degrees of inflammatory infiltration and fibrosis. Fibrosis is particularly common with busulphan and bleomycin, but rare with methotrexate. With methotrexate and procarbazine (and very occasionally with bleomycin) there may be blood and tissue eosinophilia and correspondingly a good therapeutic response to steroids.

Eosinophilic reactions in the lung include conditions that would be classified as Löffler's syndrome, simple or prolonged pulmonary eosinophilia, and eosinophilic pneumonia (see Chapter 17.11.9). Tissue eosinophilia is a more consistent feature than peripheral blood eosinophilia. Historically, sulphonamides have been the drugs most frequently reported as causes of pulmonary eosinophilia; such reactions have even occurred to a vaginal cream containing sulphonamide. Sulphonamide sensitivity may also explain some of the reactions to sulphasalazine and to chlorpropamide,

which is chemically related. The pulmonary eosinophilia recorded with aspirin appears to be distinct from aspirin-induced asthma. Nitrofurantoin may produce an acute eosinophilic reaction in addition to more insidious fibrosis.

The roles of gold salts and penicillamine in eosinophilic reactions have been a matter of some debate, but the evidence suggests that both are involved. It seems unlikely, however, that drugs are responsible for many of the cases of fibrosing alveolitis associated with rheumatoid arthritis. Penicillamine has been incriminated in two other types of adverse pulmonary reaction: first, Goodpasture's syndrome with pulmonary haemorrhage when used in high doses in treatment of Wilson's disease, and second, obliterative bronchiolitis, an unusual form of airway obstruction which is seen occasionally in patients with rheumatoid arthritis. The evidence against penicillamine in the latter is not conclusive.

The clinical severity of eosinophilic reactions is very variable, ranging from a transient and asymptomatic radiographic opacity to a severe illness with dyspnoea, cough, fever, and hypoxaemia due to widespread eosinophilic pneumonia. Concomitant asthma is not uncommon. The chest radiograph shows fluffy opacities, frequently with peripheral or predominantly upper-lobe distribution. The prognosis is usually good: the changes often subside spontaneously on withdrawal of the drug, and in more severely ill patients there is usually a dramatic improvement on instituting treatment with corticosteroids. Although repeated exposure to the offending agents continues to produce reactions, the severity of these may progressively decrease.

Pulmonary vascular reactions

Pulmonary thromboembolism related to use of the contraceptive pill is well established; its frequency correlates with the oestrogen content and has been reduced since the introduction of low oestrogen preparations. (See Chapters 13.19 and 13.20 for further discussion.)

The statistical association between pulmonary hypertension and the use of the anorectic agent aminorex in Switzerland, Germany, and Austria in the 1960s was of great theoretical interest. When the drug was withdrawn, the epidemic of pulmonary hypertension subsided and no similar rise was seen in countries that did not introduce this agent. Occasional cases of pulmonary hypertension have been reported also in patients taking various amphetamine-like drugs, but the evidence is not conclusive. (See Section 15.15.2 for further discussion.)

Analgesics given during labour have been implicated in the development of pulmonary hypertension in the newborn; drugs such as aspirin, indomethacin, and naproxen delay premature labour but, by their inhibitory effects on prostaglandin synthesis, may also cause constriction of the ductus arteriosus leading to pulmonary hypertension *in utero* that persists into the postpartum period and causes respiratory distress.

Pleura and mediastinum

Hilar and mediastinal adenopathy are occasionally seen as part of the generalized lymphadenopathy produced by the anticonvulsant phenytoin, and mediastinal lipomatosis has been reported in patients receiving large doses of corticosteroids.

Drugs that have been associated with pleural reactions (effusion or thickening) are shown in Table 3. Several have been reported to produce a syndrome like systemic lupus: the anti-arrhythmic procainamide is most often implicated, but other agents include gold, hydralazine, isoniazid, penicillamine, and sulphonamides. The main respiratory target of this syndrome is the pleura, but (as with pleural disease induced by methysergide and bromocriptine) there is often some fibrosis of underlying lung.

The now obsolete selective β-sympathetic antagonist, practolol, produced a characteristic 'oculomucocutaneous' syndrome. This syndrome

Table 3 Drugs associated with pleural reactions

Drug-induced lupus	Procainamide, gold, hydralazine, isoniazid, penicillamine, sulphonamides
Oculomucocutaneous syndrome	Practolol
Isolated	Methysergide, bromocriptine, methotrexate, dantrolene, acebutalol

differed from systemic lupus erythematosus in that autoantibodies to histones were not usually present, and ocular symptoms are not usually a feature of drug-induced systemic lupus erythematosus. Pleural effusions and subsequent pleural thickening occurred in association with characteristic corneal ulceration, discoid rash, and fibrinous peritonitis. Affected patients sometimes developed effusions months or years after discontinuing the drug. In some the chronic changes led to significant respiratory disability. Minor degrees of pulmonary involvement were reported in some patients, but the predominant abnormality was related to the pleural surface. Other β-sympathetic antagonists, in particular acebutolol, have been reported occasionally to cause an alveolar or pleural reaction, but it seems unlikely that other β-blockers are associated with the full-blown and severe 'oculomucocutaneous' syndrome.

Methysergide, which is used in treatment of the carcinoid syndrome and occasionally for migraine, may induce mediastinal or pleural fibrosis with or without retroperitoneal fibrosis. Improvement follows early withdrawal of the drug. Bromocriptine has some structural similarities to methysergide and can also produce chronic pleural effusions and thickening. The pleural fluid characteristically contains a high proportion of lymphocytes. The frequency of this reaction is uncertain, but it may be relatively common. Methotrexate has been associated with pleurisy, independent of its alveolar effects. The smooth-muscle relaxant, dantrolene, which is used for relief of spasticity, has been reported to produce an unusual type of pleurisy with effusion in which fluid and blood eosinophilia are prominent. There is no evidence of any parenchymal abnormality, and although the changes gradually resolve on withdrawing the drug, some residual pleural fibrosis may remain.

Complications of radiographic and other procedures

Lipoid pneumonia may follow bronchography with oily media. There is an oleogranulomatous reaction that can progress to fibrosis and may sometimes produce a localized mass simulating a neoplasm. Similar reactions can follow aspiration of oily medicines (e.g. laxatives) into the lungs. (See Chapter 17.11.15 for further discussion.)

Lymphangiographic media that drain through the thoracic duct, and so into the venous circulation, enter and can impact in the pulmonary circulation. This is often symptomless, but may cause dyspnoea and cough with the expectoration of fat globules or haemoptysis. Occasional deaths have been recorded. The chest radiograph characteristically shows a fine stippling.

Pleural effusion and, less commonly, mediastinitis occur following endoscopic sclerotherapy of oesophageal varices. The symptoms usually subside within a few days.

Further reading

Beasley R *et al.* (1998). Preservatives in nebulizer solutions: risks without benefit. *Pharmacotherapy* **18**, 130–9.

Camus PH, Gibson GJ (1995). Adverse pulmonary effects of drugs and radiation. In: Brewis RAL *et al.*, eds. *Respiratory medicine*, 2nd edn, pp 630–57. WB Saunders, London.

Cooper JAD (1990). Drug-induced pulmonary disease. *Clinics in Chest Medicine* **11**, 1–194.

Davies RJ, Hendrick DJ, Pepys J (1974). Asthma due to inhaled chemical agents: ampicillin, benzyl penicillin, 6-amino-penicillanic acid and related substances. *Clinical Allergy* **4**, 227–47.

Lai R-S *et al.* (1996). Outbreak of bronchiolitis obliterans associated with consumption of *Sauropus androgynus*. *Lancet* **348**, 83–5.

Rosenow EC *et al.* (1992). Drug-induced pulmonary disease. An update. *Chest* **102**, 239–50.

Ryrfeldt A (2000). Drug-induced inflammatory responses to the lung. *Toxicology Letters* **112–13**, 171–6.

17.12 Pleural disease

M. K. Benson

Introduction

The pleural surfaces form the interface between the lung parenchyma and chest wall. The parietal pleura is applied to the chest wall and the surfaces of the ribs, with a thin layer of connective tissue separating it from the periosteum. At the hilum, the pleura form a sleeve-like structure encompassing the major vessels and bronchi. The visceral pleura covers the surface of the lungs and extends into the major fissures which separate the lobes of the lung. The pleura is a membranous structure, the surface of which is covered with a single layer of mesothelial cells. These cells have microvilli over their surface that facilitate the absorption of pleural fluid.

The pleura is not essential for adequate functioning of the lungs, although the smooth surfaces do permit movement of the lungs within the thorax with minimal energy loss. Obliteration of the pleural space following surgery or as a result of inflammatory disease does not result in significant respiratory impairment. Between the two layers of pleura there is a potential space, the surfaces of which are lubricated by a thin layer of fluid. The pressures within the pleural cavity are generated by the difference between the elastic forces of the lungs and the chest wall. At functional residual capacity the outward recoil of the chest wall is equal to the inward recoil of the lung parenchyma (see Chapter 17.1.2).

A number of pathological processes can affect the pleura. Inflammation results in characteristic pleuritic pain, aggravated by deep inspiration, coughing or sneezing, and often accompanied by a pleural rub. The accumulation of fluid in the pleural space results in a pleural effusion. Air can also enter the pleural space resulting in a pneumothorax. Primary tumours of the pleura are relatively uncommon. Involvement by metastatic malignant disease or by lymphoma is much more frequent.

Pleural fluid formation

Normal lubrication of the pleura is provided by a thin layer of fluid, an ultrafiltrate of plasma, although surfactant may also be present and plays a role. Although the turnover of pleural fluid is probably in the order of 1 litre per day, the volume of fluid present at any one time is only 20 to 30 ml. Under normal circumstances two factors operate to prevent the accumulation of fluid in the pleural space: the pleura itself acts as a semipermeable membrane, and the flux of fluid across the pleural space is accounted for by the forces involved in Starling's law of transcapillary exchange. The hydrostatic gradient from the capillaries of the parietal pleura favours fluid efflux into the pleural space. Pressure in the capillaries in the visceral pleura is close to that of the pulmonary capillaries, and this lower pressure favours reabsorption of fluid. The lymphatic system provides a second important method of preventing excess fluid accumulation. In addition, it enables proteins to be recovered from the pleural space and return to the circulating plasma. Factors likely to result in excess fluid accumulation in the pleural space can be identified, including the following:

(1) imbalance between the hydrostatic and oncotic forces as defined in Starling's equation, such fluid is usually a transudate;

(2) alteration in the permeability of pleural capillaries;

(3) impaired lymphatic drainage;

(4) abnormal sites of entry (e.g. transdiaphragmatic passage of fluid in patients with ascites).

Pleural effusion

A pleural effusion is an abnormal accumulation of fluid in the pleural space. It is traditional to divide effusions into transudates and exudates, although blood, pus, or chyle can also form collections in the pleural space. The main causes are listed in Table 1.

Clinical features

The clinical history and examination play an important part in diagnosing the presence of pleural fluid and may yield significant clues as to the pathogenesis. Symptoms related to pleural disease are pain and breathlessness. The extent to which these occur is likely to vary and clinical presentation will, at least in part, be determined by the underlying pathogenesis. Pleuritic pain is relatively easy to recognize and causes severe discomfort on deep inspiration or coughing and is most often associated with an inflamed pleural surface or the presence of a pneumothorax. There can, however, be

Table 1 Causes of pleural fluid collections

	Common	Less common
Transudates	Cardiac failure	Nephrotic syndrome
		Cirrhosis
		Peritoneal dialysis
		Myxoedema
Exudates		
inflammatory (infective)	Parapneumonic	Subphrenic abscess
	Tuberculosis	Viral
		Fungal
inflammatory (non-infective)	Pulmonary emboli	Collagen vascular disease
		Pancreatitis
		Drug reactions
		Asbestos exposure
		Dressler's syndrome
		Yellow nail syndrome
Neoplastic	Metastatic carcinoma	Meigs' syndrome
	Lymphoma	
	Mesothelioma	
Haemothorax	Trauma	Spontaneous
		Bleeding disorders
		Aortic aneurysm
Chylothorax	Lymphoma	Lymphangio-myomatosis
	Carcinoma	
	Trauma	

significant collections of pleural fluid without pain. The other major symptom is breathlessness, which only becomes apparent if there is a large effusion or in patients who already have impaired respiratory reserve.

There may be no abnormal physical signs if the effusion is relatively small, but these are often diagnostic if the effusion is large. Chest wall movement may be normal, although it will tend to be limited, particularly if there is pain, and there can also be a lag of chest wall motion on the affected side. The percussion note is very dull and breath sounds are diminished or absent, as are vocal resonance and tactile vocal fremitus. Compression of the lung above the effusion can result in signs of consolidation with bronchial breathing and increased vocal resonance. The position of the mediastinum, as judged by the trachea and apex beat, will help in distinguishing between a large effusion and a collapsed lung. In the former, the mediastinum is central or displaced away from the side of the effusion, whereas in the latter deviation is towards the affected side.

Given the diversity of pathologies that may result in pleural fluid, systemic symptoms and signs often yield important diagnostic information.

Investigation of pleural effusion

The presence of a pleural effusion should be suspected on clinical examination and can be confirmed by using radiographic imaging or ultrasound. Whilst clinical features play an important part in identifying the pathogenesis, examination of the pleural fluid or pleural biopsy material is most likely to lead to a definitive diagnosis.

Radiographic techniques

Radiographic techniques are helpful in identifying the presence of an effusion but are of limited value in determining the pathogenesis. A conventional posteroanterior chest radiograph is usually adequate to confirm the presence of a clinically significant effusion. Fluid tends to accumulate in dependent parts of the thorax and small effusions in the order of 200 ml will result in blunting of the costophrenic angle. Larger effusions produced increased opacification and mediastinal shift (Fig. 1). Variations from the normal appearance will result if the fluid is loculated, a situation more likely to occur with an empyema or if there are pleural adhesions (Fig. 2).

Ultrasound can be helpful in confirming the presence and site of an effusion. Pleural fluid is identified as an echo-free space between chest wall and lung. The presence of echoes within the fluid may indicate an empyema or haemothorax, and ultrasound can also demonstrate the presence of septation and loculi (Fig. 3).

CT scan can complement ultrasound examination in demonstrating the site of a pleural collection and has the additional advantage of imaging the underlying lung. The appearance of the pleural surface can be useful in helping to differentiate between benign and malignant pleural disease. In addition, CT-guided percutaneous biopsy techniques can increase the diag-

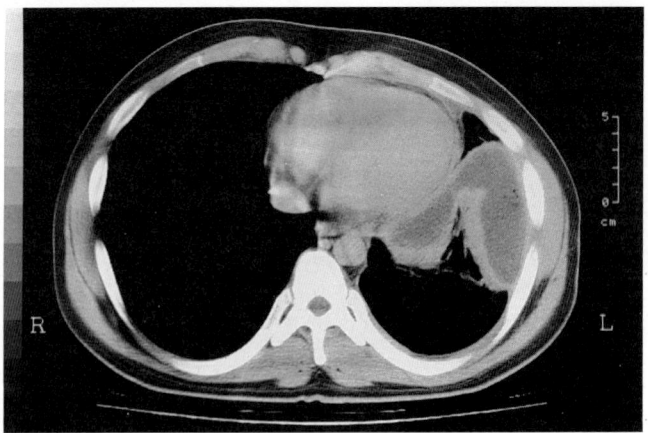

Fig. 2 CT scan demonstrating a loculated effusion due to an empyema.

nostic yield if taken from areas of gross pleural thickening, visualized on the CT scan.

Examination of pleural fluid

Thoracentesis, whereby pleural fluid is aspirated percutaneously, is a relatively simple procedure that can be undertaken for diagnostic purposes and, in the case of larger effusions, can relieve breathlessness. It is usually performed with the patient upright in a comfortable position with the arms and head supported on a pillow. Unless the fluid is loculated, a conventional site for aspiration is posteriorly about 10 cm lateral to the spine and one intercostal space below the upper level of the fluid as detected by percussion. A common error is to attempt aspiration as low as possible, but this often yields a dry tap since it is impossible on clinical grounds to determine the level of the diaphragm. The procedure is performed with strict aseptic technique. The skin and underlying tissues are infiltrated with local anaesthetic, taking care to avoid the intercostal nerves and vessels that run immediately beneath the rib. For diagnostic purposes it is usually adequate to remove 50 to 100 ml of fluid. If therapeutic aspiration of large amounts of fluid is being undertaken, it is best to introduce a small plastic cannula into the pleural space to minimize the risk of damage to the underlying lung.

Failure to obtain fluid can arise for a number of reasons, including misdiagnosis of the presence of fluid, incorrect site of aspiration, and the presence of viscid fluid. Ultrasound examination can help to identify the reason for a failed tap and guide further attempts if fluid is present. Biochemical, cytological, and microbiological examination of pleural fluid can help to establish a diagnosis if this is not apparent on clinical grounds (Table 2).

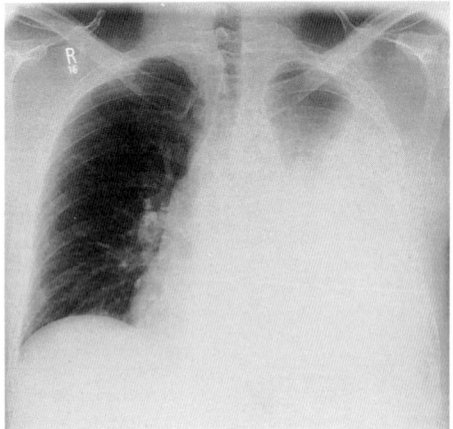

Fig. 1 Chest radiograph showing opacification of the left hemithorax and mediastinal shift indicating a large pleural effusion.

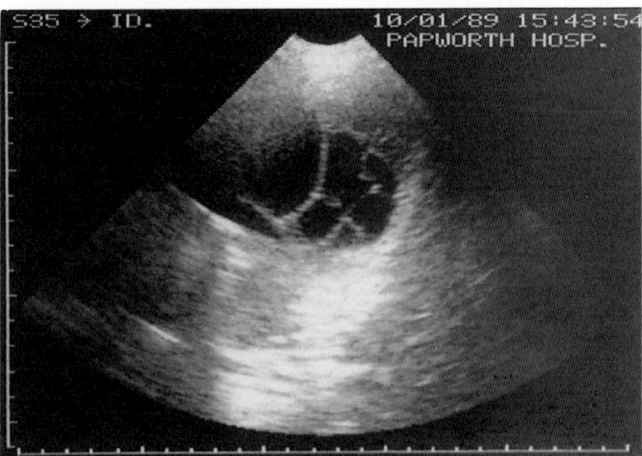

Fig. 3 Chest ultrasound showing pleural effusion with septation.

Table 2 Tests to evaluate cause of pleural effusion

Cell type		
Red blood cells	>100 000/mm³	Trauma, malignancy
		Pulmonary embolism
White blood cells	>10 000/mm³	Pyogenic infection
neutrophils	>50%	Pyogenic infection
lymphocytes	>90%	Tuberculosis, lymphoma
		Malignancy
eosinophils	>10%	Not diagnostic, usually benign
mesothelial cells	Absent	Tuberculosis
Malignant cells	Present	Malignancy
Biochemistry		
Protein concentration	>30 g/l	Exudate
Protein F:S ratio	>0.5	Exudate
LDH	>200 IU	Exudate
LDH F:S ratio	>0.6	Exudate
Glucose	<4 mmol/l	Rheumatoid arthritis, infection,
		malignancy
Amylase F:S ratio	>1	Pancreatitis
pH	<7.2	Malignancy, infection
Microbiology	Positive	Infection

F:S ratio, fluid-to-serum ratio; LDH, lactic dehydrogenase.

Macroscopic appearance

The appearance of the pleural fluid and its odour may provide diagnostic information. Transudates are clear, straw-coloured fluids that do not clot on standing. Many exudates have a similar appearance but they can be turbid due to the presence of cells. Blood-tinged fluid is of little diagnostic significance, but a uniformly bloody effusion is likely to be associated with malignancy. Pus can be very viscid and difficult to aspirate. It is turbid in appearance, yellow in colour, and often foul smelling. Chyle is odourless and milky in appearance.

Biochemistry

Exudates will generally have a higher protein content than transudates, but although a level of 30 g/l has traditionally been used to differentiate between the two, there is significant overlap and values should be interpreted with caution. Better differentiation may be obtained by comparing concentrations of protein and lactic dehydrogenase (LDH) in the pleural fluid with those in blood. The criteria that can prove helpful in identifying an exudate are as follows:

(1) fluid to serum ratio of total protein above 0.5;

(2) fluid to serum ratio of LDH above 0.6;

(3) fluid LDH concentration above 200 international units.

The concentration of glucose in pleural fluid is normally equal to that in serum, but in effusions associated with rheumatoid arthritis the glucose concentration in the pleural fluid is rarely above 1.6 mmol/l. Reduced concentrations are also found in association with tuberculosis, empyema, malignancy, and lupus. Measurement of pleural fluid amylase may be diagnostically useful if the pleural effusion is associated with acute pancreatitis, a pancreatic pseudocyst, or oesophageal rupture. Pleural fluid with a pH less than 7.3 in the presence of a normal blood pH occurs in a number of conditions including empyema and parapneumonic effusions, malignancy, tuberculosis, and collagen vascular diseases. Thus as a diagnostic investigation its use is limited. It may have some prognostic significance in patients with malignant disease in that a low pH is associated with more extensive disease. When associated with infection, a pH of less than 7.2 is one of the criteria indicating the need for tube drainage.

Microscopic and cytological examination

Most transudates have cell counts of less than 1000/mm³, with the cells being a mixture of lymphocytes, polymorphs, and mesothelial cells. Exudates tend to have higher white counts, although this in itself is of little diag-

nostic value. A polymorphonuclear leucocytosis is indicative of a bacterial infection but can also be seen in association with a pulmonary infarct or pancreatitis. A predominance of lymphocytes raises the possibility of tuberculosis but can also occur in association with malignancies, including lymphoma, and also is seen after coronary artery by-pass surgery. The presence of excess eosinophils is not in itself diagnostic but tends to be associated with benign inflammation.

Cytological examination of pleural fluid for suspected malignancy is a rapid and efficient diagnostic procedure. Fifty ml of fluid should be sent for immediate examination. The finding of malignant cells is likely to be diagnostic, although actively dividing mesothelial cells can mimic an adenocarcinoma. A positive diagnosis is made in approximately 60 per cent of malignant effusions. The diagnosis of a malignant mesothelioma presents particular difficulties but the use of monoclonal antibodies CEA, B72.3, and Leu-M1 can help distinguish an adenocarcinoma from mesothelioma.

Microbiology

Gram stain and culture of the pleural fluid are of diagnostic value if an infective aetiology is suspected. Identification of an organism confirms the diagnosis and sensitivity testing will assist in the appropriate choice of antibiotics. Tuberculous pleurisy is difficult to diagnose and acid fast smears are positive in only about 10 per cent of cases. Cultures are more likely to be positive if a reasonable volume of fluid is concentrated and then examined.

Pleural biopsy

Pleural biopsy may be indicated if initial analysis of pleural fluid fails to establish a diagnosis. It is most likely to give diagnostic information if there is an underlying malignancy or tuberculosis. The diagnostic yield is likely to be greatest when used in conjunction with CT scanning to identify areas of particular thickening or nodularity. Blind percutaneous biopsies are usually performed using an Abraham's or Cope's needle. Both of these are large blunt-tipped needles with a hook to catch a sample of parietal pleura. The technique is similar to that used for pleural aspiration except that a small incision is made in the skin and subcutaneous tissue to enable ease of insertion of the needle. The Abraham's needle consists of an outer trocar with a side hole and an inner cannula with a cutting edge. Once in the pleural space, confirmed by aspiration of fluid, the side hole is opened by rotating and slightly withdrawing the inner cannula. The needle is then withdrawn at an angle to the chest wall such that the side hole gently catches on to the parietal pleura, and at this point the inner cannula is advanced to obtain a biopsy. Several samples can be taken using this technique, but care is needed to avoid damage to the intercostal nerves and vessels. Samples for histological examination should be placed in 10 per cent formaldehyde and those for culture for mycobacteria should be put into saline.

Thoracoscopy

Direct visualization of the pleura is possible using a thoracoscope, and this should be considered as a diagnostic procedure when less invasive procedures have failed to yield a definitive diagnosis. It is particularly useful in suspected malignancy or tuberculosis. For further details regarding this technique, see Chapter 17.3.4.

The relative diagnostic yields of thoracocentesis, pleural biopsy, and thoracoscopy with respect to tuberculosis and malignancy are given in Table 3. Pleural aspiration is easy to perform, requires limited expertise,

Table 3 Diagnostic yield of thoracentesis, pleural biopsy, and thoracoscopy

	Pleural fluid	Blind biopsy	Thoracoscopy
Malignancy	60%	55%	90%
Tuberculosis	20%[1]	90%[2]	95%

[1] Direct stain and culture.

[2] Histology and culture.

and has only minor risks. Pleural biopsy requires more expertise and complications include pain, pneumothorax, haemothorax, and vasovagal reactions. Thoracoscopy is only available in specialist centres and, in addition to the risks associated with pleural biopsy, may result in subcutaneous emphysema. The diagnostic yield and choice of technique will depend on the medical indications and local expertise.

Chest drain insertion

Chest drainage is used therapeutically in a number of clinical situations, including the management of malignant pleural effusions, empyemas, pneumothoraces, postoperatively, and when there has been bleeding into the pleural cavity. Doctors working in a variety of specialties should therefore be capable of inserting an intercostal drain. It is potentially a painful procedure and the patient needs reassurance, comfortable positioning, and adequate analgesia and local anaesthesia. Ideally, narcotic medication should be given prior to the procedure unless medically contraindicated. The position of the patient will depend on the site of insertion. For the axilla, the patient is usually lying at 45° with the arm behind their head such that the axillary area is exposed.

The site of insertion will depend on the clinical and radiological findings. In patients with a large pleural effusion or a pneumothorax, the most usual site is in the axilla, in a triangle bounded by the anterior axillary line, the lateral margin of the pectoralis major, and a horizontal line at the level of the nipple. An alternative site for an apical pneumothorax is in the second intercostal space in the mid clavicular line. Where there are loculated collections of air or fluid, real-time ultrasonography can ensure optimum placement of the catheter.

The appropriate drain size remains a subject of debate. Large bore tubes (28–30 French) are used postoperatively and in the management of haemothorax. Whilst some authorities advocate their use in other clinical situations, such as management of pneumothoraces and empyemas, small bore catheters (10–14 French) are as effective, easier to insert, and better tolerated by patients.

Insertion of a chest drain with aseptic technique is important to minimize the risk of infection. The site for tube insertion is infiltrated with local anaesthetic (1 per cent lignocaine—maximum dose 3 mg/kg) to achieve satisfactory anaesthesia of skin, subcutaneous tissues, and pleura, care being taken to avoid intercostal vessels that run beneath each rib. The infiltrating needle should also be used to aspirate air or fluid from the pleural space once the pleura has been punctured, and a chest tube should not be inserted until this has been achieved. An incision is made in the skin parallel to the ribs and slightly larger than the catheter to be inserted. Blunt dissection of subcutaneous tissue and muscle is achieved by opening and closing a curved clamp: this separates the muscle fibres and can also be used to penetrate the pleura. If a large tube is to be inserted, the track can be explored with a gloved finger to ensure that there are no organs that might be penetrated. However for smaller catheters, an inappropriately large track can result in leakage around the catheter. The central trocar can be used to support the catheter, but forcible insertion should be avoided because of potential for damage to lung and mediastinal structures. Alternative techniques include the use of pigtail catheters after insertion of a guide-wire and dilatation of the track.

Although traditionally the catheter is inserted towards the apex for pneumothoraces and towards the base for pleural effusions, precise positioning is relatively unimportant. There should, however, be sufficient catheter within the thorax to minimize the risk of displacement. A strong non-absorbable suture, such as 1–0 silk, should be used to secure the drain, which should also be supported with a small square of gauze and a bioclusive dressing over the insertion site. Tape can be wrapped around the drain at the point of ligature to help prevent the suture from slipping on the tube. Once the tube has been inserted and anchored, it is attached to an underwater-seal bottle, allowing one-way flow of air or fluid. This has the disadvantage of restricting mobility, but enables observations to be made about tube patency—judged by inspiratory pressure swings—and allows the continued drainage of air or fluid to be monitored. Good nursing care

with regular 4-hourly observations are necessary to ensure that the tube has not become kinked or blocked and that it has not become displaced. Uni-jet directional flutter valves permit greater mobility and can be used in ambulant patients for the management of pneumothoraces, but they are inappropriate for use when there are fluid collections.

Specific pleural fluid collections

Transudates

A transudate is characterized by low concentration of protein and other large molecules. Excess fluid forms when there is an increase in capillary hydrostatic pressure or reduction in colloid osmotic pressure. The former occurs predominantly in congestive cardiac failure, and the latter when there is hypoalbuminaemia associated with nephrotic syndrome or hepatic disease.

Cardiac failure

Small effusions are common in congestive cardiac failure or constrictive pericarditis. Right-sided failure results in increased pressures in the systemic capillaries and thus an increased efflux of fluid from the parietal pleura. Elevated left heart pressures will be reflected in the pulmonary circulation with a consequent diminution in fluid reabsorption from the visceral pleura. The clinical features of cardiac failure are usually sufficient to make a diagnosis. Thus cardiomegaly, elevated jugular venous pressure, and third or fourth heart sounds may all be present. The effusions are frequently bilateral. Unilateral effusions are more common on the right side and may cause diagnostic uncertainty. Pleural aspiration can help to confirm the diagnosis by demonstrating the presence of a transudate. Resolution with treatment of heart failure offers further confirmation of the diagnosis.

Hepatic cirrhosis

Hypoalbuminaemia, which may occur in patients with chronic liver disease, is a major contributory factor to the development of generalized oedema. Ascites and pleural effusions are both common, with effusions more often seen on the right than on the left. In some patients, ascitic fluid seems to pass directly into the pleural space, either through a defect in the diaphragm or via lymphatics.

Exudates

Neoplastic pleural effusions

Malignant involvement of the pleura is the commonest cause of a large pleural effusion. Lung cancer may spread directly or via lymphatics and is the commonest metastatic cancer (40 per cent). Breast cancer also spreads via the lymphatic system and is the commonest cause of a malignant effusion in women. Metastatic spread from gastrointestinal or genitourinary tumours is less common. Lymphomas can occur at any age and account for approximately 10 per cent of malignant effusions. Extensive investigation for an asymptomatic primary is of limited value, although it may be appropriate to exclude disease originating in breast or ovary because of the potential response to hormonal treatment or chemotherapy.

Symptoms directly attributable to the effusion are most commonly breathlessness or chest discomfort. The degree of breathlessness depends on the size of the effusion and the presence of pre-existing lung disease. Specific symptoms attributable to the primary tumour are often absent. Non-specific symptoms include malaise, anorexia, weight loss, and sweats.

Appropriate investigations have already been outlined above. They include imaging with a posteroanterior chest radiograph and chest CT scan. Aspirated fluid is usually an exudate and is blood stained in approximately 50 per cent of cases. Malignant cells can be identified in approximately 60 per cent of cases. CT-guided pleural biopsy may be justified where aspiration has proved diagnostically unhelpful. If the diagnosis remains in doubt, the options are either to await events, since the diagnosis may become obvious with the passage of time, or to obtain further biopsy material at thoracoscopy.

Once cancer has metastasized to the pleura, treatment is essentially palliative, although chemotherapy or hormonal treatment may be appropriate depending on the primary, the cell type, and the functional status of the patients. Removal of the pleural fluid and measures to prevent reoccurrence are only necessary if the size of the effusion results in significant breathlessness. If the patient is comfortable, no action may be necessary. Percutaneous needle aspiration of 1 to 2 l of fluid is a simple outpatient procedure and often results in considerable symptomatic benefit. The fluid is likely to recur, but repeated aspiration may be an appropriate therapeutic option. Intercostal tube drainage can be used to remove the bulk of the fluid, but this is also likely to be of temporary benefit unless combined with pleurodesis. If the effusion is large, it should be drained gradually over 24 h to reduce the risk of re-expansion pulmonary oedema. A number of sclerosing agents have been used with varying degrees of success. Unfortunately there is a marked paucity of comparative data. Sclerosing agents include antibiotics (tetracycline, doxycycline, minocycline), antineoplastic agents (bleomycin), and non-specific irritants (sterile talc, *Corynebacterium parvum*, mepacrine). Until recently, tetracycline (1 g/50 ml saline) has been the most widely used sclerosant, but production of the intravenous preparation has been discontinued. Of the remaining sclerosants, talc slurry (2–5 g in 100 ml) achieves success rates of about 90 per cent and is likely to be the most effective. The pleural space is drained to dryness and after adequate local and systemic analgesia, the sclerosant is injected and the tube clamped for 2 to 4 h. Any residual fluid is then drained and the tube removed after 24 h. An alternative approach is to insufflate iodized talc into the pleural space at thoracoscopy. Surgical pleurectomy or pleural abrasion is also very effective at preventing recurrence, although rarely regarded as an appropriate option because of its invasive nature and unacceptably high morbidity and mortality.

Meigs' syndrome

This rare syndrome describes an association between pleural effusions, ascites, and a benign ovarian tumour. Surgical removal of the tumour results in disappearance of the pleural and peritoneal fluid. The mechanism of pleural effusion is uncertain, but it is generally assumed that ascitic fluid reaches the pleura through diaphragmatic channels or lymphatics. There is no evidence of spread of the tumour, and the syndrome should not be confused with effusions that can result from metastatic spread of ovarian cancer.

Endometriosis of the pleura

This rare condition is one in which endometrial tissue is implanted on visceral or parietal pleura. Catamenial pleural chest pain or a pneumothorax can be presenting features. More commonly, there is an associated effusion that on aspiration reveals blood or chocolate brown fluid. Thoracotomy will reveal multiple cystic structures, but surgical ablation is unsuccessful because of the nature of the disease. Treatment is directed at suppressing ovulation using progesterones or androgens.

Infection

Inflammation of the pleura associated with infection is usually due to pneumonia or lung abscess. Other possible sources of pleural infection include subdiaphragmatic pathology, mediastinitis, oesophageal perforation, or direct contamination following penetrating trauma or surgery. Inflammation can result in pleurisy without significant fluid production, a non-infective exudate (a parapneumonic effusion), or infected fluid (an empyema). Distinction between a parapneumonic effusion and an empyema is somewhat arbitrary since there can be a transition from one to the other. A parapneumonic effusion may be slightly turbid, contains an excess of polymorphs, but has no organisms: by contrast, an empyema contains increased numbers of polymorphs and is frankly turbid. pH measurement of the pleural fluid can assist in management: a pH below 7.2 is generally

Table 4 Organisms resulting in empyema thoracis

Single organisms (75%)	
Gram-positive aerobes	*Strep. milleri* +++
	Strep. pneumoniae ++
	Staph. aureus +
Gram-negative aerobes	*E. coli* +
	H. influenzae +
	Proteus +
Anaerobic bacteria	*B. melaninogenicus* ++
	Streptococci+
	Fusobacterium +
Fungi	*Candida spp.* +
Multiple organisms (25%)	*Strep. milleri* plus anaerobes

+++, common; +, rare.

regarded as an indication for pleural drainage. Organisms are likely to be present when there is frank pus, although isolation and identification may be difficult if antibiotics have already been administered. The spectrum of organisms most frequently encountered in the United Kingdom is listed in Table 4.

The presentation will vary depending on the pathogenesis. In a patient with pneumonia, an empyema should be suspected if there is persisting fever and elevated white count despite appropriate use of antibiotics. Pleuritic chest pain may be present but is not invariable. Classical signs of effusion can be difficult to detect, particularly if the pleural collection is loculated. Anaerobic organisms are commonly encountered; these may be secondary to aspiration from the oropharynx or upper respiratory tract.

A chest radiograph that shows apparent loculation of pleural fluid should alert the clinician to the possibility of an empyema. Gas may be present, revealed by a fluid level. Ultrasound examination or CT scan can be useful for identifying the most appropriate approach for attempted aspiration, and also demonstrate the presence of loculi.

Treatment is discussed elsewhere.

Tuberculous pleurisy

Pleural involvement with tuberculosis is a common manifestation of primary infection with direct extension from a subpleural focus. Gross parenchymal disease is rare and the primary site often cannot be identified clinically or radiologically. It is more common in younger patients and in those of Asian origin.

The presenting features are usually acute or subacute with fever, pleuritic pain, and breathlessness, but some patients may give a longer history of malaise, sweats, and weight loss. The effusion is often large (in excess of 2 l) and tends to recur after initial aspiration. The fluid is a serous exudates, often with an excess of lymphocytes whose presence should alert the clinician to the possibility of tuberculosis. Bacilli are rarely identified on pleural aspirate. Culture is more likely to be positive, but even so the diagnostic yield is low, and pleural biopsy is more likely to give a diagnostic result, showing granulomatous inflammation in approximately two-thirds of patients. Thoracoscopic biopsy is most likely to give a definitive diagnosis, but this is not universally available and often it may be appropriate to commence treatment on clinical grounds alone.

A tuberculous empyema with pus in the pleural space is rare, but occasionally complicates cavitating parenchymal disease. A bronchopleural fistula can result, and in advanced disease the empyema can present with a draining sinus through the chest wall. Other bacterial pathogens may be present in the pleural fluid.

Treatment involves the use of standard antituberculous chemotherapy together with adequate drainage if there is frank pus. Steroids have been shown to promote rapid resolution of the effusion and improve symptoms in the short term, but may have no long-term benefits. Rarely, surgical closure of a bronchopleural fistula or decortication is required.

Subdiaphragmatic infection

Inflammation or infection below the diaphragm should always been considered if there is an unexplained effusion with features suggesting infection. A subphrenic abscess is frequently associated with an effusion, usually on the right side. This may follow abdominal surgery, but can also be caused by perforated peptic ulcer, appendicitis, diverticular disease, or cholecystitis. Hepatic abscesses can also cause a right-sided effusion. Even without infection, upper abdominal surgery can result in pleural effusion, but such effusions are usually small and transient.

If there is evidence of sepsis, the source needs to be identified, and if pus is present it must be drained. Ultrasound examination or CT scanning are both effective ways of diagnosing a subphrenic abscess and guiding percutaneous aspiration. The pleural fluid is usually an exudate and although turbid with a polymorphonuclear leucocytosis, it rarely becomes infected.

Pancreatitis is associated with a pleural effusion in approximately 20 per cent of patients. In the majority, the effusion is on the left side and results from inflammation caused by enzyme-rich pancreatic fluid. Whilst the classical symptoms of abdominal pain, nausea, and vomiting usually predominate, pleurisy and breathlessness can occasionally be presenting features. The pleural fluid is often blood stained and contains abnormally high levels of amylase.

Pulmonary emboli

Pleurisy, often associated with a pleural effusion, is a common presenting feature of pulmonary emboli, particularly if there is associated pulmonary infarction. The effusion is usually small and in itself does not require specific treatment. The fluid is often blood stained but the cellular content is variable and there are no specific diagnostic features. The diagnosis of pulmonary emboli is based on clinical features supplemented by appropriate radiographic or isotopic imaging techniques.

Rheumatoid arthritis

Pleural effusions are the commonest pulmonary manifestation of rheumatoid arthritis. They occur in approximately 3 per cent of patients with active rheumatoid disease and are more common in men than in women. The development of an effusion can antedate the onset of joint symptoms in a small proportion of patients. There is no relationship to the severity of the arthritis, but effusions are more likely to occur in patients with subcutaneous nodules and those who have high titres of rheumatoid factor.

The effusions are usually small but can enlarge to a size that results in breathlessness. Although usually unilateral they may be bilateral in about 20 per cent of patients. The fluid is an exudate and may appear turbid due to cholesterol crystals. The cellular content is not diagnostic, but polymorphonuclear cells usually predominate. Although not specific to rheumatoid effusions, a diagnostic clue is the presence of a low glucose concentration (usually below 1.5 mmol/l). The pH is also low and the lactic dehydrogenase concentration elevated. Whilst these findings may also be present in infective and malignant effusions, the associated clinical features rarely lead to diagnostic uncertainty. Pleural biopsy is non-specific although it can reveal the epithelioid cells and multinucleate giant cells found in rheumatoid nodules.

Symptomatic treatment with anti-inflammatory analgesics is indicated if pleuritic pain is a feature. Systemic steroids can speed resolution of the pleural fluid although they are rarely necessary. The majority of effusions resolve spontaneously within a few months but there may be some residual fibrosis.

Systemic lupus erythematosus

Pleural involvement is common in patients with this condition. Approximately 50 per cent of patients will have pleurisy at some stage and the majority of these will have an associated effusion, usually small. Aspiration of the fluid is rarely necessary for either diagnostic or therapeutic purposes.

The fluid is an exudate and has high concentrations of antinuclear antibodies. Lupus erythematosus cells can also be identified. There is a good therapeutic response to oral corticosteroids.

Haemothorax

A haemothorax is the result of bleeding into the pleural space and is arbitrarily diagnosed on the basis of having a haematocrit more than half that of peripheral blood. This distinguishes it from a blood stained effusion, which can be associated with a number of different pathological processes. The vast majority of haemothoraces are associated with penetrating or non-penetrating trauma, including iatrogenic procedures such as central venous catheterization. Bleeding usually results from parenchymal laceration or damage to intercostal vessels. A pneumothorax is present in a high proportion of patients.

The treatment of choice is to insert a large intercostal drain (28–32 French), allowing evacuation of blood and reducing the incidence of subsequent fibrothorax. If this reveals continued bleeding, thoracotomy may be required. Surgery is not indicated simply to remove any residual blood clots since in a majority of patients there is spontaneous lysis with no residual damage.

Spontaneous bleeding into the pleural space can occur in association with a pneumothorax (a haemopneumothorax) and presumably results from the tearing of pleural adhesions. Other rare causes of a haemothorax include bleeding disorders, or excess anticoagulants and rupture of the thoracic aorta.

Chylothorax

A chylothorax results from leakage of chylous fluid from the thoracic duct. Absorbed fat is transported as chylomicrons in the intestinal lymphatics and, together with lymph originating in the lower limbs and abdomen, reaches the blood stream via the thoracic duct. The flow of lymph in the thoracic duct is approximately 100 ml/h under basal conditions but can increase five-fold after a fatty meal.

Congenital absence of the thoracic duct is a rare cause of a chylothorax, but the majority of cases are acquired either as a result of trauma or neoplastic invasion. Surgery is the commonest cause of traumatic damage, particularly those operations that involve mobilization of the aortic arch or oesophageal resection. Penetrating trauma occasionally results in damage to the thoracic duct but rupture can also occur from non-penetrating injuries. The commonest single cause of rupture of the thoracic duct is damage caused by neoplastic infiltration, including lymphomas and carcinomas. Other rare associations include pulmonary lymphangioliomyomatosis, the yellow nail syndrome, and filariasis.

There are no specific clinical features and the diagnosis of a chylothorax is usually made after pleural aspiration. The fat is typically milky and opalescent due to the presence of fat globules, and needs to be distinguished from an empyema or from pseudochyle. In empyema, any discoloration is due to a cellular deposit and after centrifugation the supernatant is clear. Pseudochyle is due to high lipid levels, usually cholesterol crystals, which occur in chronic effusions, particularly following tuberculosis. Cholesterol crystals can be recognized on smears of the sediment, and the addition of ethyl alcohol to the fluid results in clearing if high concentrations of cholesterol are responsible for the opalescence.

Spontaneous resolution can occur if the chyle is removed by thoracocentesis and the subsequent flow of chyle reduced by the use of medium chain triglyceride diets or parenteral nutrition. If there is known malignancy, mediastinal irradiation may also assist resolution. Malnutrition and lymphopenia are likely to occur if large volumes of chyle continue to be drained, and under such circumstances surgical ligation of the thoracic duct above the diaphragm can be combined with pleurodesis.

Pneumothorax

A pneumothorax results from gas entering the potential space between visceral and parietal pleura. A spontaneous pneumothorax is a consequence of rupture of a bulla or cyst on the surface of the lung, allowing air to escape from the alveoli into the pleural space. Following penetrating trauma, atmospheric air may enter the pleural space through the wound or the visceral pleura may be punctured allowing entry of alveolar gas. An iatrogenic pneumothorax can occur as a result of damage inflicted during catheterization of a subclavian vein or following percutaneous or transbronchial lung biopsy.

Pathophysiology

At functional residual capacity the inward elastic recoil of the lung and the outward recoil of the chest wall results in a negative pressure in the potential space between visceral and parietal pleura. Pressures with respect to atmosphere become more negative during inspiration and only become positive during forced expiration. Because of the elastic recoil of the lung, pleural pressure is always less than alveolar pressure. Thus, if there is a breach of the visceral pleura due to rupture of a surface bulla, gas moves from lung to pleural space. As the lung collapses down, the pressures equilibrate and net flow of gas ceases.

The functional effect of a pneumothorax is to reduce the vital capacity and the total lung capacity as the lung collapses. Ventilation of the affected side is reduced, although perfusion may also fall such that the anticipated alveolar–arterial oxygen gradient and consequent hypoxia are less than might be anticipated. Ventilatory failure with a rise in arterial $P\mathrm{CO_2}$ is rare, except in patients with pre-existing lung disease.

Once the original leak has sealed, reabsorption of pleural gas occurs and re-expansion of the lung takes place at approximately 1.25 per cent of the volume of the hemithorax per day. Pleural gas is absorbed because the total gas pressure, which is similar to that of arterial gas, is greater than that of venous blood.

Tension pneumothorax

Occasionally, and with devastating consequences, the site of air leak acts as a valve, allowing air to enter the pleural space during inspiration but preventing return flow during expiration. If this happens, then pleural pressure rises and a tension pneumothorax results, with compromise of the circulation, mediastinal shift, and impaired function of the opposite lung.

Clinical syndromes

A spontaneous pneumothorax usually occurs without any warning or obvious precipitating factor. A primary pneumothorax occurs in individuals with apparently normal lungs. A secondary pneumothorax is a consequence of pre-existing lung disease.

Primary pneumothorax

A primary pneumothorax is a relatively common condition with an annual incidence of about 9/100 000. It is particularly common in young men, with a male to female ratio of approximately 4 to 1. It is commoner in smokers. Patients are often tall with a marfanoid appearance. The cause of the pneumothorax is assumed to be rupture of a surface bulla or cyst, often near the lung apex. Only rarely can these be visualized radiologically. Approximately 50 per cent of patients suffer from a recurrence within 4 years. Whilst this is usually on the same side as the initial event, there is also an increased chance of contralateral pneumothorax.

Secondary pneumothorax

Older patients presenting with a spontaneous pneumothorax are likely to have underlying lung disease as a predisposing factor, most commonly chronic obstructive pulmonary disease. Rarely, acute exacerbations of asthma may be complicated by a spontaneous pneumothorax, presumably due to high alveolar pressures associated with gas trapping. Some pulmonary infections can result in rupture of necrotic lung with subsequent air leak into the pleura. Staphylococcal pneumonia, anaerobic lung abscesses, and tuberculosis are among the most likely infecting organisms. A secondary pneumothorax can also be caused by lung malignancy. There are also a number of parenchymal and connective tissue disorders in which pneumothorax is a recognized complication; these include cystic fibrosis, lymphangiomyomatosis, pulmonary neurofibromatosis, Langerhan's cell histiocytosis, Marfan's syndrome, and Ehlers–Danlos syndrome.

Iatrogenic pneumothorax

A number of diagnostic and therapeutic procedures can cause pneumothorax. Percutaneous needle aspiration or biopsy of the lung carries the greatest risk, with estimates ranging from 5 to 50 per cent. The risk is related to the presence of underlying lung disease, the size of the needle, and the depth of penetration. Bronchoscopy rarely causes problems, but a transbronchial biopsy carries a small risk, particularly if undertaken in the absence of screening. Intermittent positive pressure ventilation, especially when used with positive end-expiratory pressures, can result in pneumothorax, which can present under tension. Attempted catheterization of subclavian veins can result in puncture of the lung, particularly when carried out by inexperienced personnel.

Clinical features

Symptomatically, a spontaneous pneumothorax will present with chest pain and breathlessness. The pain is usually of sudden onset and typically pleuritic, being localized to the affected side. Inspiration is often painful and breathing is shallow to minimize discomfort. Dyspnoea is partly engendered by the difficulty in taking a deep breath, but is also dependent on the size of the pneumothorax and the presence of underlying lung disease. The initial sensation of breathlessness can improve rapidly before the resolution of the pneumothorax and may be due to reflex changes from receptors in the lung and airways. A significant proportion of patients do not tend to seek medical advice for several days.

Abnormal physical signs may be difficult to detect if the pneumothorax is small or the underlying lung is emphysematous. The most consistent finding is a reduction in breath sounds on the affected side. Movement of the chest wall may be reduced, particularly if there is pain. The percussion note will be resonant, and although hyper-resonance is a recorded feature, it may be difficult to detect any difference from the non-affected side. Vocal fremitus and tactile vocal resonance are diminished. A left sided pneumothorax is occasionally associated with a clicking noise synchronous with the heart beat (Hamman's sign), probably due to contact and separation of the pleural surfaces in time with the heart beat.

Tension pneumothorax

Pneumothorax rarely causes severe respiratory distress and hypoxia unless associated with pre-existing lung disease, or the pneumothorax is under tension. Tension pneumothorax is rare, but a medical emergency. The patient looks as though they are about to die, with severe breathlessness, cyanosis, tachycardia, hypotension, grossly elevated jugular venous pulse, and evidence of mediastinal shift (trachea and apex displaced away from the side of the chest under tension, which may appear unduly prominent).

Associated conditions

Pneumomediastinum

A pneumomediastinum can present in isolation or together with a pneumothorax. Air tracks along the bronchovascular sheath to the hilum and mediastinum. It can be associated with sudden rises in alveolar pressure during sneezing or straining, and be found in patients undergoing intermittent positive pressure ventilation. Precordial chest discomfort may be a presenting symptom and subcutaneous emphysema can usually be detected in the neck and supraclavicular fossae. No specific treatment is indicated since the condition is benign and self-limiting.

Haemothorax

The presence of blood and air in the pleural space is most commonly the result of trauma. A spontaneous pneumothorax can occasionally have associated bleeding into the pleural space, presumably due to tearing of pleural adhesions.

Pyopneumothorax

A pyopneumothorax usually results from rupture of necrotic lung, but can also be due to oesophageal perforation. The clinical picture is one of a combined empyema and pneumothorax.

Investigations

Confirmation of a pneumothorax is best made by chest radiograph. An erect posteroanterior film is adequate. Although a film during expiration increases the radiodensity of the lung and enhances the contrast between lung and pleural gas, it is rarely necessary. The cardinal radiological features are illustrated in Fig. 4. The outer margin of the lung can be seen as a thin line with the space between it and the chest wall devoid of any lung markings. Pleural adhesions can result in part of the lung being tethered to the chest wall with some distortion of the normal radiographic appearance. A large emphysematous bulla can sometimes be mistaken for a pneumothorax on both clinical and radiological grounds, although the inner margins are usually concave. A CT scan may help to resolve the diagnostic uncertainty.

Lung function tests are inappropriate in the presence of a suspected pneumothorax, although oximetry or arterial blood gases may provide information that will influence decisions regarding treatment.

Management

The diversity of therapeutic options listed in Table 5 is a manifestation of uncertainty as to what is best. Two principal therapeutic objectives are to achieve rapid resolution of the pneumothorax, particularly if there is evidence of respiratory distress, and to reduce the likelihood of recurrence.

Natural resolution

A small pneumothorax with a radiological rim of air of less than 2 cm in an otherwise healthy patient may require no treatment other than reassurance and relief of pain. Non-steroidal anti-inflammatory drugs are usually effective in this respect. Admission to hospital is unnecessary provided the patient has ready access to medical care and is advised to return if symptoms worsen.

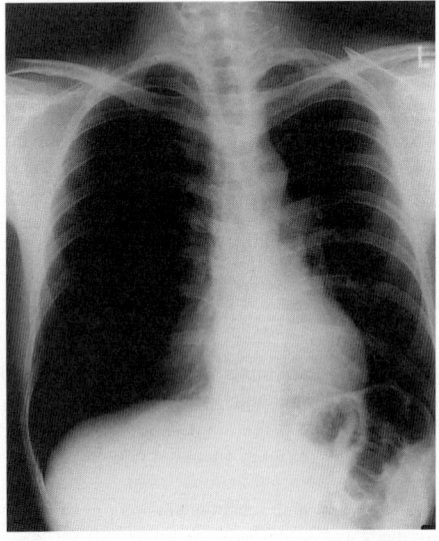

Fig. 4 Chest radiograph demonstrating a tension pneumothorax.

Table 5 Treatment options for a pneumothorax

Option	Indication
Natural resolution	Small primary pneumothorax
Aspiration	Large primary pneumothorax, particularly if the patient is breathless
Intercostal drain (± pleurodesis)	Failed aspiration, secondary pneumothorax
Thorascopy + pleurodesis	Recurrent pneumothorax, failed intercostal drainage
Thoracotomy	Recurrent pneumothorax
Limited pleurectomy	Failed intercostal drainage
Pleurodesis	
Ligation of bullae	

Simple aspiration

Simple aspiration is the treatment of choice for a patient with a large primary pneumothorax and is also the initial emergency treatment in patients with a tension pneumothorax. If successful, it will not only speed resolution but also relieve associated breathlessness or chest discomfort. It is simple to perform and has negligible morbidity, even in relatively inexperienced hands. The site for aspiration is usually the second intercostal space in the mid clavicular line. After infiltrating with local anaesthetic, a 16 to 18 gauge intravenous cannula attached to a syringe containing a small amount of sterile water is inserted through the chest wall gently aspirating until bubbling seen in the syringe confirms that the pleural space has been entered. The internal needle is then removed (in tension pneumothorax allowing immediate release of pleural pressure) and a 50-ml syringe with three-way tap is connected to the cannula to allow aspiration of air, which should stop if resistance is encountered or if the patient experiences undue discomfort or coughing. If more than 2 to 3 l of air has been evacuated, it is likely that there is a persisting air leak, and aspiration should be abandoned and a decision made as to whether an intercostal drain should be inserted. This is likely to be necessary if the patient is breathless, but conservative management with repeated aspiration after an interval of a day or two may be more appropriate for those who are relatively asymptomatic. Simple aspiration has been shown to be less painful and require a shorter duration of hospital stay than treatment with an intercostal drain. There are no significant differences in recurrence rate.

Intercostal tube drain

This approach may be indicated if simple aspiration has failed. It is more likely to be needed in patients with underlying lung disease, when even a small pneumothorax can result in severe respiratory failure. The technique for insertion has already been described. Bubbling will cease once the air leak has ceased and the lung fully expanded. A check radiograph should be undertaken before the catheter is removed since drainage of air will also cease if the tube is blocked or has become dislodged. Clamping of the tube prior to removal is unnecessary. The value of additional suction is unproven and may serve to maintain the patency of the original air leak. It can be tried if the lung fails to re-expand, with the aim of evacuating the pleural air and allowing apposition of the pleural surfaces.

Medical pleurodesis

This is undertaken in an attempt to obliterate the pleural space and reduce the likelihood of recurrent pneumothorax. There is a marked paucity of information as to who might benefit and as to the best approach (see previous discussion). It should be considered in those with recurrent pneumothoraces whose underlying condition makes a surgical operation unduly hazardous.

Surgical intervention

Referral rates for surgery vary considerably. The main indications include persisting air leak after prolonged intubation (usually 1–2 weeks) and recurrent pneumothoraces. In the latter group, referral is most commonly made after the second or third ipsilateral recurrence, or if there have been bilateral pneumothoraces. The preferred surgical options include over-sewing or excision of any large bullae, combined with apicolateral pleurectomy or pleural abrasion. Surgical morbidity in otherwise healthy patients is very low. Risks are greater in those with underlying lung disease, but this must be balanced against the life-threatening potential of further pneumothorax.

Video-assisted thoracoscopic surgery (VATS) offers a less invasive approach to the surgical management of pneumothoraces, but experience is limited. The morbidity does not seem to be significantly different from that of thoracotomy, and there is a significant chance of recurrence (5–10 per cent). Its role may be limited to those who would be regarded as otherwise unfit for an open procedure.

Further reading

Pleural effusions—diagnosis

Ansai T (1998). Management of undiagnosed persistent pleural effusions. *Clinics in Chest Medicine* **19**, 407–17. Useful clinical review with respect to diagnostic approach to the diagnosis of pleural effusions.

Heffner JE (1997). Diagnostic value of tests that discriminate between exudative and transudate pleural effusions. *Chest* **111**, 970–80. Systematic review of tests used to discriminate between transudates and exudates.

Hsu C (1987). Cytological detection of malignancy in pleural effusions: a review of 5,255 samples from 3,811 patients. *Diagnostic Cytopathology* **3**, 8–12. Review of the diagnostic yield from cytological examination of pleural fluid.

Light RW (1995). *Pleural diseases*, 3rd edn. Williams and Wilkins, Baltimore. Authoritative textbook of pleural disease.

Page R (1989). Thoracoscopy: a review of 121 consecutive surgical procedures. *Annals of Thoracic Surgery* **48**, 66–8. Retrospective review of the value of diagnostic thoracoscopy.

Prakash UBS, Reiman HM (1985). Comparison of needle biopsy with cytological analysis for the evaluation of pleural effusion: analysis of 414 cases. *Mayo Clinic Proceedings* **60**, 158–63. Retrospective study comparing results of thoracentesis and needle biopsy in malignant and non-malignant pleural disease.

Sahn S (1988). State of the art. The pleura. *American Review of Respiratory Diseases* **138**, 184–234. Comprehensive review of normal anatomy and physiology, pathology, and clinical features of pleural disease.

Thoracostomy—techniques

American College of Surgeons Committee on Trauma (1993). Thoracic trauma. In: *Advanced trauma life support program for physicians: instructor manual*. Chicago. Practical guidelines regarding indications for and technique of tube thoracostomy.

Hyde J, Sykes T, Graham T (1997). Reducing morbidity from chest drains. *British Medical Journal* **314**, 914–15. Editorial emphasizing importance of not using a trocar to penetrate chest wall.

Kline JS, Schultz S, Heffner JE (1995). Interventional radiology of the chest; image-guided percutaneous drainage of pleural effusions, lung abscess and pneumothorax. *American Journal of Radiology* **164**, 581–8. Descriptive review of image-guided drainage techniques.

Tomlinson MA, Treasure T (1997). Insertion of a chest drain; how to do it. *British Journal of Hospital Medicine* **58**, 248–52. Step by step guide to insertion of chest drain concentrating specifically on large bore tubes.

Malignant effusions

Lynch J Jnr (1993). Management of malignant pleural effusions. *Chest* **103** (Suppl.), 385S–9S. Review of different therapeutic approaches to management of malignant pleural effusions.

Patz ER *et al.* (1998). Sclerotherapy for malignant pleural effusions; a prospective randomised trail of bleomycin vs. doxycycline with small-bore catheter drainage. *Chest* **113**, 1305–11. Prospective study in 106 patients comparing bleomycin and doxycycline sclerotherapy.

Zimmer PW *et al.* (1997). Prospective randomised trial of talc slurry vs. bleomycin in pleurodesis for symptomatic malignant pleural effusions. *Chest* **112**, 430–4. Comparative study in 29 patients with 90 per cent success rate of pleurodesis.

Empyema

Alfageme I *et al.* (1993). Empyema of the thorax in adults. Etiology, microbiologic findings and management. *Chest* **103**, 839–43. Retrospective clinical review of 80 patients with empyema.

Ferguson AD *et al.* Empyema Subcommittee of the Research Committee of the British Thoracic Society (1996). The clinical course and management of thoracic empyema. *Quarterly Journal of Medicine* **89**, 285–9. A multicentre review of clinical features and management of thoracic empyema.

Tuberculosis

Berger HW, Magier E (1973). Tuberculous pleurisy. *Chest* **63**, 88–92. Critical review of clinical presentation and diagnosis of tuberculous pleurisy.

Epstein DM *et al.* (1967). Tuberculous pleural effusions. *Chest* **91**, 107–9. Retrospective review of clinical presentation and treatment.

Miscellaneous

Bynum LJ, Wilson JE (1976). Characteristics of pleural effusions associated with pulmonary embolism. *Archives of Internal Medicine* **136**, 159–62. Features of pleural fluid associated with pulmonary embolism.

Emerson PA (1966). Yellow nails, lymphoedema and pleural effusions. *Thorax* **21**, 247–50. Classical description of yellow nail syndrome.

Eppler GR, McLeod TC, Gaensler EA (1982). Prevalence and incidence of benign asbestos pleural effusion in a working population. *Journal of the American Medical Association* **247**, 617–22. Review of asbestos-related pleural effusions.

Fairfax AJ, McNabb WR, Spiro SG (1986). Chylothorax: A review of 18 cases. *Thorax* **41**, 880–5. A retrospective review of patients presenting with a chylothorax.

Hunninghake GW, Fauci AS (1979). Pulmonary involvement in the collagen vascular diseases. *American Review of Respiratory Disease* **119**, 471–503. State of the art review.

Kay MD (1968). Pleural pulmonary complications of pancreatitis. *Thorax* **23**, 297–306. Description of pleural complications associated with pancreatitis.

Meigs IV (1954). Meigs' syndrome. *American Journal of Obstetrics and Gynaecology* **67**, 962–6. Meigs' original description of the eponymous syndrome.

Pneumothorax

Allmind M, Lange P, Viscum K (1989). Spontaneous pneumothorax: comparison of simple drainage, talc pleurodesis and tetracycline pleurodesis. *Thorax* **44**, 627–30. Randomized study comparing three treatment options with subsequent rates of relapse.

Harvey JE (1993). Comparison of a simple aspiration with intercostal drainage in the management of spontaneous pneumothorax. *Thorax* **48**, 430–1. Randomized study of aspiration versus intercostal tube drainage. No subsequent difference in rate of recurrence.

Massard G, Thomas P, Wihlm J-M (1998). Minimally invasive management for first and recurrent pneumothorax. *Annals of Thoracic Surgery* **66**, 592–9. Review of treatment options in the management of pneumothoraces.

Miller AC, Harvey JE (for Standards of Care Committee, British Thoracic Society) (1993). Guidelines for the management of spontaneous pneumothorax. *British Medical Journal* **307**, 114–6. British consensus-based guidelines for the management of pneumothoraces.

Parry GN, Juniper ME, Dussek JE (1992). Surgical intervention in spontaneous pneumothorax. *Respiratory Medicine* **86**, 1–2. Editorial review of role of thoracoscopic surgery for pneumothorax.

So SY, Yu DYC (1982). Catheter drainage of spontaneous pneumothorax, suction or no suction, early or late removal?. *Thorax* **37**, 46–8. Randomized study on use of suction or no suction drainage in the management of pneumothoraces.

17.13 Disorders of the thoracic cage and diaphragm

J. M. Shneerson

Introduction

Skeletal disorders of the thorax are an important group of conditions that frequently impair ventilation. They are often associated with respiratory muscle weakness due to neuromuscular disorders, which are described elsewhere. Most of these conditions restrict the development and/or the expansion of the lungs so that alveolar ventilation rather than intrapulmonary gas exchange is primarily impaired.

Disorders of the spine

Scoliosis

Scoliosis is defined as a lateral curvature of the spine, but it is invariably also associated with rotation of the vertebral bodies. This results in an unstable lordosis rather than a kyphosis, and hence the frequently used term kyphoscoliosis is inaccurate. A mild degree of scoliosis is very common. Angles of curvature of 5° or 10° have been used to define when it becomes pathological, but these are arbitrary figures. Postural scoliosis can be distinguished from a structural scoliosis by its temporary nature and because it disappears on bending forward.

The age of onset and natural history of scoliosis vary according to its cause (Table 1). When it is due to a neuromuscular disorder ('paralytic' scoliosis) it usually arises during childhood or adolescence, or in poliomyelitis within about 2 years of the acute infection. Typically, the curve has a long C shape and may be severe. The scoliosis is due to asymmetrical weakness of the axial muscles so that the spine rotates and moves to one side. Weakness of chest wall muscles is almost invariable, occurs in a pattern which is characteristic of each disorder, and may have a profound influence on the clinical features.

Table 1 Causes of scoliosis

Idiopathic
Infantile, adolescent
Osteopathic
Congenital (e.g. hemivertebrae)
Thoracoplasty
Neuromuscular
Syringomyelia
Friedreich's ataxia
Poliomyelitis
Duchenne's muscular dystrophy
Connective tissue disorders
Marfan's syndrome
Neurofibromatosis
Osteogenesis imperfecta
Pleuropulmonary
Empyema
Pneumonectomy
Unilateral lung fibrosis

When the scoliosis is due to a congenital abnormality, such as a hemivertebra or a segmentation defect, it usually becomes apparent early in childhood. The scoliosis of neurofibromatosis and Marfan's syndrome is probably due to an abnormality of connective tissue. Scoliosis due to pleural or pulmonary disease is less common than in the past, now that chronic infections are less frequent and more successfully treated.

The commonest type is adolescent idiopathic scoliosis, where the spinal deformity develops at the time of the pubertal growth spurt. It is around four times as common in girls as in boys, and the convexity of the deformity is on the right in 80 per cent of cases. The scoliosis may continue to worsen slightly even after growth of the spine stops. An infantile form of idiopathic scoliosis is less common, and, although it often resolves spontaneously, it can progress to a severe deformity.

Pathophysiology

The most important organic consequence of scoliosis is the respiratory abnormality. A direct result is that the compliance of the chest wall is reduced. This is more marked in older subjects, possibly owing to degenerative changes in the costovertebral joints. The compliance of the lungs is also reduced, largely because of their small volume. In addition, the distortion of the rib cage puts the inspiratory muscles at a mechanical disadvantage; those on the side of the convexity of the scoliosis are shortened and those on the side of the concavity lengthened. The vital capacity falls when changing from the sitting to the supine position, implying that diaphragmatic function is impaired. A restrictive defect and reduction of the maximum inspiratory and expiratory pressures develops even in the absence of any muscle weakness, but is more marked if this is present.

In adults with severe scoliosis, exercise capacity is linked to the degree of reduction of the vital capacity and the forced expiratory volume in 1 s (FEV_1). The tidal volume increases initially and then remains constant, whilst respiratory rate rises as exercise becomes more intense. Ventilation at any given oxygen uptake is greater than normal, and maximal exercise ventilation, which limits exercise capability, is often severely curtailed. The cardiac output may increase normally during exercise, but pulmonary artery pressure rises rapidly, and its rate of increase is linearly related to oxygen uptake and inversely related to the vital capacity.

In mild scoliosis, the arterial blood gases are often normal, but the first abnormality is a fall in the partial pressure of oxygen (Po_2). This is due to suboptimal ventilation and perfusion matching, particularly at the bases of the lungs. Even when the anatomical distortion of the two lungs is gross, there is usually rather less difference in function between the two lungs than might be expected. Acute ventilatory failure may be precipitated by, for instance, a chest infection or asthma, but chronic hypoventilation initially occurs during sleep. Sleep is associated with loss of the voluntary respiratory drive and a reduction in the reflex drive in response to hypoxia, hypercapnia, and other stimuli. Muscle activity is reduced, and whereas in non-rapid eye movement sleep (NREM) this affects all the respiratory muscles to an equal extent, in rapid eye movement sleep (REM) diaphragmatic activity is selectively retained. Relaxation of the other respiratory muscles is more intense than during NREM and loss of activity in the upper airway dilator muscles increases the upper airway resistance and the work of the chest wall muscles.

These changes during sleep are particularly important in scoliosis, where the diaphragm is attached to an asymmetrical rib cage and where the respiratory pump often has little reserve. The effects of sleep are accentuated when the scoliosis is the result of neuromuscular disorders, because the presence of muscle weakness in addition to the skeletal deformity reduces tidal volume and increases respiratory frequency, leading to alveolar hypoventilation. Arousals from sleep initially occur in REM, which becomes fragmented, and at a later stage in NREM, with loss particularly of stages 3 and 4. Sleep fragmentation itself reduces the respiratory drive and impairs the strength and probably the endurance of the respiratory muscles, promoting a vicious circle in which there are progressively more respiratory-induced arousals and a deterioration in respiratory drive and muscle function. Central apnoeas and hypopnoeas develop; hypercapnia then appears during wakefulness as well as in sleep.

Chronic hypercapnia during the day is uncommon in childhood and is determined by the following:

1. Age of onset: if the scoliosis appears before the age of about 8 years it may prevent normal alveolar multiplication so that the lungs fail to develop fully. The capillary surface area is reduced and there is an increased risk of developing respiratory and right heart failure later in life. The later onset of adolescent idiopathic scoliosis is probably the major reason why these complications only rarely occur in this condition.

2. Level of the scoliosis: in general, the higher the curve in the thoracic spine, the more marked are the cardiac and respiratory problems. Thoracolumbar or lumbar scoliosis has virtually no effect on respiration.

3. Severity of scoliosis: the angle of scoliosis is closely related to the reduction in lung volume. This association is seen with the residual volume, total lung capacity, and functional residual capacity, as well as with vital capacity, except in patients with neuromuscular disorders, where the changes in lung volumes are due to the weakness of the respiratory muscles as well as the degree of deformity. The changes in lung volumes become significant when the angle of scoliosis is greater than about 100°.

4. Presence of muscle weakness: the functioning of the respiratory muscles is impaired in scoliosis, and any further loss of strength or endurance due to neuromuscular disorders may precipitate respiratory failure. Conversely, respiratory function often worsens in neuromuscular disorders when scoliosis develops as the strength of the axial muscle becomes asymmetrical.

5. Small lung volumes: respiratory failure usually occurs when lung volumes have been reduced to a degree such that vital capacity is less than 1.0 to 1.5 1.

Hypoxia causes pulmonary vasoconstriction which increases the pulmonary vascular resistance and leads to pulmonary hypertension. If this is prolonged, right ventricular and atrial hypertrophy develop. Significant pulmonary hypertension is rarely seen unless the arterial Po_2 is less than around 8 kPa. Pulmonary hypertension by itself rarely causes right heart failure, and the exact mechanisms underlying this are uncertain. The increase in sympathetic activity and circulating catecholamines associated with hypoxia cause renal vasoconstriction and a reduction in renal blood flow. This activates the renin–angiotensin–aldosterone system leading to sodium and water retention. Hypercapnia is associated with an increase in renal tubular hydrogen ion excretion with sodium reabsorption in exchange for hydrogen. This leads to fluid retention, which is accentuated by an increase in antidiuretic hormone secretion. Hypercapnia probably also increases capillary permeability, which contributes to the appearance of oedema.

Polycythaemia occasionally occurs as a result of erythropoietin release from the kidneys in response to hypoxia. This adaptive mechanism increases the oxygen content of the blood, but also increases blood viscosity, which increases the work of the right and left ventricles and predisposes to arterial and venous thrombosis.

Symptoms and physical signs

The earliest symptom of scoliosis is usually a change in the appearance of the patient, such as asymmetry of the shoulders or prominence of the posterior rib hump. Backache is a late and uncommon symptom. With mild curvatures there may be no respiratory symptoms, but mild shortness of breath on exertion is common. A change in this often signifies the development of complications such as respiratory failure. Orthopnoea suggests that diaphragmatic function is impaired. When respiratory failure develops, fatigue, ankle swelling, and even syncope may indicate that pulmonary hypertension and right heart failure are present. Frequent awakenings during sleep, associated with excessive daytime somnolence, indicate sleep fragmentation due to apnoeas and hypopnoeas, and are important symptoms that warn of impending respiratory failure.

Physical examination may reveal the cause of the scoliosis, such as Marfan's syndrome or neurofibromatosis, and other congenital abnormalities. Any associated muscle weakness or congenital heart disease may be apparent. Rib cage expansion may be predominantly lateral or anterior, or achieved by extension of the spine. In some subjects, chest expansion is mainly oblique because of the rotation of the spine, and some areas of the chest wall may move paradoxically. Accessory muscle action is usually prominent. The presence of central cyanosis indicates that the arterial oxygen saturation is below around 80 per cent. Signs of hypercapnia may also be present. These include tachycardia, large volume pulse, peripheral venous dilatation, papilloedema, a flapping tremor, reduction in tendon reflexes, small pupils and, if severe, confusion and coma (CO_2 'narcosis').

Investigations

The severity of scoliosis can be demonstrated radiologically, but chest radiography is often unhelpful in thoracic scoliosis because rotation of the spine obscures much of the lung fields. This can be overcome by obtaining an oblique view of the chest which, by aligning the spine behind the heart, simulates a posteroanterior view. Lung function testing reveals a restrictive defect with reduction in all lung volumes, although the change in residual volume is least marked and, therefore, the ratio of residual volume to total lung capacity is increased. Kco is raised, as in other chest wall disorders that cause a restrictive defect and in which the lung tissue is normal. Maximum inspiratory and expiratory pressures and trans-diaphragmatic pressure are reduced. Chest wall and lung compliance are less than normal, and exercise tolerance is impaired. Arterial blood gas analysis reveals a slightly low Pco_2 in mildly affected subjects, but later in the course of disease a rise in Pco_2 and a proportional fall in Po_2 develop. Sleep studies show a variable degree of hypoxia and hypercapnia which are usually most marked in REM sleep. Electrocardiography and echocardiography may be required to establish whether congenital heart disease is present and, if so, to identify the abnormality.

Prognosis

The prognosis in adolescent idiopathic scoliosis is virtually normal, but life expectancy is reduced in many of the other forms of scoliosis. This is particularly so in scoliosis of early onset, when it is both severe and high in the thorax and associated with respiratory muscle weakness, low vital capacity, and abnormal blood gases.

In most subjects the cause of death is either cardiac or respiratory. Pneumonia and respiratory failure are particularly common in neuromuscular disorders, but hypoxic dysrhythmias during sleep are probably responsible for some deaths. Congenital heart defects, which have an increased prevalence in subjects with scoliosis, particularly when this is due to a congenital abnormality or of the idiopathic type, also contribute to mortality.

Treatment

Mild scoliosis does not need any specific treatment. The prognosis is normal and there is minimal respiratory deficit. However, as the scoliosis becomes more severe, spinal fusion or a costectomy, in which the parts of the ribs comprising the posterior hump are removed, may be of cosmetic value. Spinal fusion may also be required to prevent progression of the scoliosis, to stabilize the spine, particularly in neuromuscular disorders, and in selected cases to try to improve cardiac or respiratory function or to prevent its deterioration.

The value of spinal fusion to prevent cardiorespiratory deterioration in adolescent idiopathic scoliosis is still under debate. A large number of studies of respiratory function before and after surgery have shown remarkably little change in lung volumes, blood gases, or exercise ability. However, in some patients with muscle weakness, particularly Duchenne's muscular dystrophy, the rate of fall of the vital capacity can be slowed considerably, and it can even be improved in patients who have had poliomyelitis. Despite these short-term improvements, there have been no studies which indicate whether or not spinal fusion performed in childhood or adolescence prevents respiratory failure from appearing later in life. If respiratory failure does develop, any acute illness which may have precipitated it should be actively treated. This is most commonly an infection or bronchial asthma. Non-invasive ventilation or endotracheal intubation and ventilation may be required during the acute illness. If the latter is needed, the patient is then weaned from this either completely or onto a non-invasive method of long-term respiratory support.

Chronic ventilatory failure usually responds to long-term mechanical respiratory support. Administration of oxygen at night and/or during the day may be dangerous because of the risk of hypercapnia. Nasal or face mask positive pressure ventilation is the treatment of choice, but a negative pressure system, such as a cuirass or jacket, is an alternative. Non-invasive ventilation is usually only required during sleep, but some patients benefit from 1 or 2 h treatment during the day as well. A tracheostomy is rarely required to provide ventilatory support, but in complex neuromuscular disorders it may be indicated to bypass upper airway obstruction, for instance due to vocal cord adduction, or to gain access to the tracheobronchial tree to aspirate secretions, or to protect the airway from aspiration of material from the pharynx.

Non-invasive ventilatory support can considerably improve the quality of life, arterial blood gases, maximum inspiratory and expiratory pressures, and the quality of sleep, as well as reducing the number of visits required by general practitioners and the quantity of drugs prescribed. Survival once treatment has been instituted is around 75 per cent at 5 years and 60 per cent at 10 years (Fig. 1).

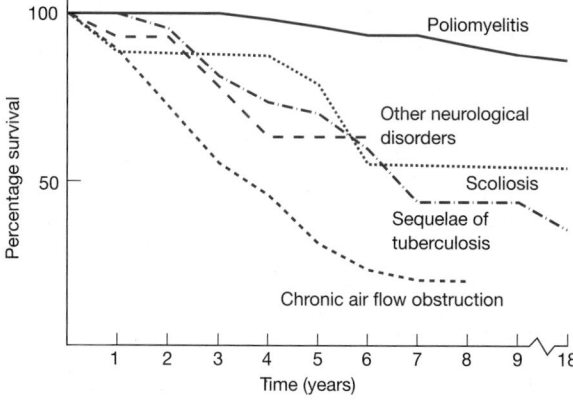

Fig. 1 Actuarial survival during treatment with ventilatory assistance for respiratory failure. (Reproduced with permission from Shneerson JM (1988). *Disorders of ventilation*, Blackwell, Oxford.)

Kyphosis

Exaggeration of the normal thoracic kyphosis is most commonly due to osteoporosis and is not usually associated with any significant changes in respiratory function. The exception to this is when a very sharp kyphosis (gibbus) develops. This is usually caused by tuberculous osteomyelitis of the spine (Pott's disease), although other conditions such as radiotherapy can cause a similar picture.

The spine becomes rigid in the region of the gibbus, and when tuberculosis is the cause the costovertebral joints also become ankylosed and limit the expansion of the rib cage. A restrictive defect in which the total lung capacity is reduced more than the residual volume is characteristic, but respiratory problems are uncommon unless the gibbus is high in the thoracic spine and develops in early childhood. This is probably because the thoracic deformity prevents the normal development of the lungs in a similar way to early-onset scoliosis. Hypoxia and hypercapnia appear during sleep before they become apparent during wakefulness, but may be severe. Pulmonary hypertension and right heart failure frequently develop once chronic hypercapnia has become established.

Slight breathlessness on exertion is common in the presence of a gibbus, but is rare in other types of kyphosis. Physical examination reveals the spinal deformity and limitation of rib cage expansion.

The posteroanterior chest radiograph shows superimposition of the spinal deformity on the lung fields and heart, which makes it difficult to interpret. The extent and severity of the kyphosis is usually well seen on a lateral projection. The typical changes in lung volumes have been described above. The arterial Po_2 and Pco_2 are usually normal, and, as in scoliosis, the earliest abnormalities are revealed by sleep studies.

Treatment of the acute tuberculous infection with chemotherapy often prevents a gibbus from developing. Once it has been established and respiratory failure has developed, the only effective treatment is long-term respiratory support. This is best provided non-invasively by a nasal positive pressure ventilator, rather than a negative pressure system, since the sharp kyphosis makes it difficult to lie in the supine position required for negative pressure ventilation.

Straight-back syndrome

In this disorder the normal thoracic kyphosis is absent or greatly reduced. This may result in a mild restrictive ventilatory defect, but cardiac problems are more prominent. The heart and great vessels may be compressed between the anterior rib cage and the spine with results similar to those seen in pectus excavatum. The right ventricular outflow tract or pulmonary artery may be narrowed, causing a systolic murmur, and occasionally right ventricular filling is impaired.

Ankylosing spondylitis

The initial manifestation of ankylosing spondylitis is usually painful inflammation of the sacroiliac joints, but this may spread to affect almost any joint including the intervertebral, costovertebral, manubriosternal, costochondral, and chondrosternal joints. When the inflammatory phase of the disease subsides, the joints become ankylosed and the spinal ligaments calcify.

The effect of ankylosing spondylitis on the thorax is that the rib cage becomes rigid. There is little spinal mobility, and a pronounced kyphosis often develops. The changes in lung volumes are characteristic in that, unlike all other skeletal disorders affecting the thorax, functional residual capacity increases. This is because the rib cage becomes fixed at its own relaxation volume. This is greater than the normal functional residual capacity which is influenced by the inward pull of the elastic recoil of the lungs. Total lung capacity and vital capacity are slightly reduced, and residual volume often increases.

The immobility of the rib cage leads to atrophy of the intercostal muscles and both maximal inspiratory and expiratory pressures are reduced. However, there is no impairment of diaphragmatic function and this largely compensates for the restriction of rib cage expansion. The ventilatory responses to exercise are virtually normal and exercise is usually limited by circulatory rather than respiratory factors. Respiratory failure is extremely uncommon in ankylosing spondylitis, probably as a result of the normal diaphragmatic function, unless another complication develops, which may be one of the following:

1. Air flow obstruction: cricoarytenoid arthritis is a feature of ankylosing spondylitis and may present with stridor, hoarseness of the voice, breathlessness, obstructive sleep apnoeas, or respiratory failure.

2. Pleural thickening and effusion: these rare complications of ankylosing spondylitis may precipitate respiratory failure.

3. Aspiration pneumonia: oesophageal motility is often impaired in ankylosing spondylitis and aspiration pneumonia may develop.

4. Bullae: apical fibrobullous lung disease is a feature of ankylosing spondylitis and may be complicated by opportunist infections such as *Aspergillus fumigatus* or saprophytic Mycobacteria, and occasionally pulmonary tuberculosis.

5. Abdominal surgery: this restricts diaphragmatic function on which adequate respiration depends. Conversely, thoracic surgery has relatively little effect on respiration because of the small contribution that rib cage expansion plays.

Chest pain during sudden movements such as coughing and laughing is common if the active phase of inflammation affects the thorax. These symptoms, which originate in either the joints or the muscles, become less prominent as the disease advances. Breathlessness and other respiratory symptoms are uncommon. Occasionally, cricoarytenoid arthritis may present with hoarseness, stridor, or breathlessness, and extensive fibrobullous disease may also cause breathlessness.

The most obvious physical sign is restriction of rib cage movement associated with prominent accessory muscle activity and abdominal respiratory movements.

Chest radiography may show calcification of the paraspinal ligaments (bamboo spine) and reveal evidence of complications of ankylosing spondylitis such as pleural thickening, aspiration pneumonia, and apical fibrobullous disease. The changes in lung volumes have been described above. Chest wall compliance is reduced but lung compliance is normal. The Kco is increased and arterial blood gases are normal during both rest and exertion.

Physiotherapy and non-steroidal anti-inflammatory drugs may improve vital capacity and chest expansion, particularly in the early phase of the disease or during acute exacerbations.

Disorders of the sternum and ribs

Congenital abnormalities

Congenital abnormalities of the ribs and sternum rarely cause any important respiratory problems. Occasionally, multiple congenital rib abnormalities may lead to paradoxical movement of the chest wall or impair diaphragmatic function if they occur in the region of the insertion of this muscle. Severe congenital defects of the sternum, such as agenesis or a bifid sternum, are rare, but may require surgery in the neonatal period in order to stabilize the anterior chest wall.

Pectus excavatum

Pectus excavatum is a depression deformity of the sternum which is often present at birth but may worsen during the adolescent growth spurt. It is occasionally familial and may be associated with other abnormalities such as the straight-back syndrome or scoliosis. It appears to result either from an increased inward pull on the sternum by the sternal diaphragmatic fibres or from an abnormally compliant chest wall.

Transient paradoxical movement of the sternum during respiration is seen in neonates, particularly in the presence of upper airway obstruction

or pneumonia. The sternal depression may become permanent even if the cause, such as enlarged tonsils, resolves completely.

In adults pectus excavatum rarely causes any symptoms. Lung volumes are normal or only slightly diminished, and chest wall mobility appears to be normal. Arterial blood gases are normal both at rest and during exercise. Right ventricular filling can be impaired if the heart is compressed between the depressed sternum and the spine, and compression of the pulmonary outflow tract may cause a systolic murmur. These problems are most marked in the erect position and during exercise. Occasionally atrial arrhythmias develop. Surgery is sometimes indicated for cosmetic reasons, although the result can be disappointing. It has little or no effect on the mild restrictive defect or exercise ability, except in the rare situation when right ventricular filling is impaired or atrial arrhythmias have developed.

Pectus carinatum

Pectus carinatum is a protrusion deformity of the sternum in which the chest is often narrowed transversely as well. It becomes most marked during the pubertal growth spurt, although it may be present from birth and is occasionally associated with severe childhood asthma or ventricular septal defects. It is probably the result of excessive growth of the ribs or costal cartilages, and if this is asymmetrical the sternum becomes oblique.

The respiratory consequences of pectus carinatum have hardly been investigated. Chest pain may arise at the insertions of the intercostal muscles anteriorly, or in the costal cartilages and anterior ribs. Lung volumes appear to be normal, and surgery is indicated only for cosmetic reasons and not in order to improve respiratory function or exercise ability.

Asphyxiating thoracic dystrophy (Jeune's disease)

Asphyxiating thoracic dystrophy is a generalized disorder of cartilage in which the radiological changes are most prominent in the pelvis, phalanges, and other limb bones. Like the other long bones, the ribs are shortened so that the rib cage becomes narrowed. Lung development may be impaired as a result, and respiratory failure often appears during infancy or childhood. Surgical reconstruction of the rib cage with splitting of the sternum to enable lung growth to occur has been largely unsuccessful.

Acquired abnormalities

Flail chest

A flail chest is one in which multiple rib fractures cause paradoxical movement of the chest wall during respiration. It may be associated with other injuries, such as rupture of the aortic arch or spleen, and with fractures of the skull and long bones. It is frequently associated with pulmonary contusion, pneumothorax, or haemothorax.

Surgical stabilization of the chest wall is rarely required. In milder cases, sufficient analgesia to enable the patient to cough adequately may be all that is required, as long as the paradoxical movement does not impair alveolar ventilation. If it is more severe, positive pressure ventilation achieves 'pneumatic splinting' of the flail segment. The effectiveness of this has not been definitely established, but it appears that positive end expiratory pressure or continuous positive airway pressure is beneficial by preventing any negative pressure swings within the pleura.

Thoracoplasty

The operation of thoracoplasty was developed for the treatment of pulmonary tuberculosis. Varying lengths of up to 11 ribs were removed in order to collapse the chest on the affected side. It has been superseded by antituberculous chemotherapy, but is still occasionally required to treat chronic infections, particularly when there is a problem in obliterating the pleural space after pulmonary resection. It is estimated that as many as 30 000 operations were carried out in the United Kingdom between 1951 and 1960, and many of these patients still survive. Increasing numbers of this important cohort are being seen by chest physicians because of the late complications of the surgical procedure.

The consequences of thoracoplasty on respiratory function have been hard to elucidate because they are often combined with the effects of the underlying lung disease for which the surgery was carried out, and those of other treatments such as lung resection. However, the removal of the ribs has the direct result of flattening the chest and reducing the volume of the thorax. The normal movements of the rib cage may be impaired and paradoxical movement at the site of the thoracoplasty is common. The compliance of the chest wall is reduced, and it may fall further because the small range of movements of the costovertebral joints after surgery probably induces soft tissue changes which further limit the mobility of these joints. Chest wall compliance is also reduced by the almost invariable development of a thoracic scoliosis. This is convex to the side of the thoracoplasty and may progress for several years after the surgery. The severity of the scoliosis correlates with the number of ribs removed, but also depends on the details of the surgical technique.

Respiratory muscle function is impaired by a thoracoplasty. The intercostal and shoulder girdle muscles are directly damaged by the surgery, and distortion of the rib cage and the development of a scoliosis put the inspiratory muscles at an additional mechanical disadvantage. Diaphragmatic excursion is reduced, particularly on the side of the thoracoplasty, but also occasionally contralaterally.

The combination of reduced chest wall compliance and impaired respiratory muscle function accounts for the restrictive defect. All lung volumes are reduced, and in general the severity of the restrictive defect is proportional to the number of ribs that have been resected. A rapid respiratory rate with a small tidal volume is the characteristic respiratory pattern, particularly during exertion. Exercise is limited by ventilatory factors rather than by the cardiovascular system. In some patients, chronic air flow obstruction, which may be due to either tuberculous endobronchitis or the effects of tobacco smoking, may be significant, resulting in a progressive fall in exercise ability and contributing to the development of respiratory failure.

Ventilation and perfusion of the lung on the side of the thoracoplasty are usually reduced equally, so that the arterial P_{O_2} often remains virtually normal. The function of the contralateral lung is much more important in determining the blood gases. Hypoxaemia usually first appears during sleep, as in scoliosis, and may be associated with hypercapnia. The presence of daytime hypercapnia correlates with the reduction in maximal inspiratory and transdiaphragmatic pressures.

The symptoms of patients with a thoracoplasty are similar to those with a scoliosis, but if a productive cough develops, recurrence of pulmonary tuberculosis should be suspected and investigated. Right heart failure often develops insidiously, either when respiratory failure appears or subsequently. It may be manifested by progressively worsening ankle swelling and fatigue. Physical examination reveals a thoracotomy scar and a flattened area of chest in the region of the thoracoplasty which may move paradoxically. Accessory muscle activity, particularly on the side of the thoracoplasty, is often marked.

The chest radiograph shows the extent of the thoracoplasty, other features which indicate the site and extent of previous tuberculous infection, and the sequelae of treatment such as a previous phrenic nerve crush or an artificial pneumothorax. This often causes extensive, calcified pleural thickening. The characteristic physiological defect is restrictive, but airflow obstruction may also be significant. Maximum inspiratory and expiratory pressures and transdiaphragmatic pressures are reduced. Most patients are mildly hypoxic, but later in the clinical course the arterial P_{CO_2} may rise, particularly during sleep.

Life expectancy is reduced after a thoracoplasty for pulmonary tuberculosis: death occurs particularly from respiratory but also from cardiac causes. These complications are related to the extent of the tuberculosis and to whether or not an artificial pneumothorax was induced on the contralateral side to the thoracoplasty, since this often leads to pleural thickening and may indicate extensive tuberculous damage of the underlying lung. Respiratory failure can develop quite suddenly after a long period of stability, even when an acute illness such as a chest infection is not responsible.

Conventional treatment of airflow obstruction with, for instance, bronchodilators may be effective and right heart failure may respond to diuretics and angiotensin-converting enzyme inhibitors

Chronic ventilatory failure usually responds well to nocturnal, noninvasive respiratory support. Some patients can be managed adequately with oxygen during the day and/or at night as long as the P_{CO_2} remains normal or only slightly raised. When respiratory support is required, a nasal positive pressure ventilation or a negative pressure system such as a cuirass or jacket used at night is usually adequate initially. Some patients gradually require more intensive support, so that treatment is needed during the day as well as at night. This deterioration may be due to progressive worsening of small airway obstruction or respiratory muscle function, or to a fall in oxygen delivery to the tissues caused by a deteriorating cardiac output associated with advancing pulmonary hypertension.

Disorders of the diaphragm

Aetiology

Diaphragmatic paralysis or paresis may be due to lesions affecting either the diaphragm itself or the phrenic nerve, its nucleus, or higher control centres or pathways. The most common causes of diaphragmatic weakness are shown in Table 2. Often no cause is found in unilateral weakness, and it is presumed to be due to a cryptogenic phrenic neuropathy, either as part of a widespread peripheral neuropathy or isolated to the phrenic nerves.

Pathophysiology

Unilateral weakness of the diaphragm causes it to move upwards (paradoxically) into the thorax during inspiration, instead of descending. This decreases the tidal volume and the mechanical efficiency of breathing. It is worse in the supine position when the weight of the abdominal contents pushes the paralysed diaphragm further into the thorax and decreases the functional residual capacity. The diaphragm is splinted in an expiratory position so that it moves relatively little even though it is paralysed. When the subject lies on one side, the lower half of the diaphragm behaves in this way if it is paralysed, but if the upper half is paralysed it moves paradoxically.

The loss of inspiratory muscle strength is partially compensated by recruitment of intercostal and accessory muscles, but the maximum inspiratory and transdiaphragmatic pressures are reduced. The vital capacity in the upright position is approximately 20 to 25 per cent less than normal and a further fall of about 15 per cent occurs when lying supine. Similar changes in the total lung capacity and functional residual capacity occur. The residual volume is unchanged and expiratory muscle strength is largely preserved.

The distribution of ventilation and perfusion is affected by unilateral diaphragm weakness. Ventilation is slightly diminished, particularly at the base on the side of the diaphragmatic paralysis in the sitting position, but this is more marked when supine. Similar changes occur with perfusion on a regional basis, but ventilation–perfusion matching is impaired and hypoxia results. Hypercapnia does not occur during wakefulness or sleep.

Table 2 Main causes of diaphragmatic weakness

Unilateral	Bilateral
Congenital (e.g. agenesis, eventration)	Trauma
Trauma	High cervical cord lesions
Adjacent mass (e.g. neoplasm, aneurysm)	Motor neurone disease
Herpes zoster	Poliomyelitis
Poliomyelitis	Peripheral neuropathy
Peripheral neuropathy	Acute idiopathic polyneuropathy
Neuralgic amyotrophy	Myopathies
Open-heart surgery	Muscular dystrophies

The physiological abnormalities seen with bilateral diaphragmatic weakness in adults are much more marked than in unilateral diaphragmatic disorders. The diaphragm moves paradoxically during inspiration and expiration, and intrapleural pressure changes are transmitted across it so that abdominal pressure falls during inspiration and the anterior abdominal wall moves paradoxically. The maximum transdiaphragmatic pressure falls in proportion to the degree of diaphragm weakness, and since the diaphragm is the main inspiratory muscle, the maximum inspiratory pressure is correspondingly reduced. The vital capacity in the sitting position is about 50 per cent of that predicted and may fall by a further 50 per cent when supine. The influence of the supine position is greater than with unilateral diaphragmatic weakness because the weight of the abdominal contents pushes both halves of the diaphragm into the thorax. Ventilation is particularly reduced at the bases in the supine position, with less change in perfusion so that the arterial Po_2 falls. This postural change is partly responsible for the hypoxia that has been observed during sleep, but the rapid respiratory rate, small tidal volume, and short inspiratory time contribute to this and to hypercapnia.

Symptoms and physical signs

Unilateral diaphragmatic paralysis in adults rarely causes symptoms unless there is coexisting pulmonary disease or weakness of other respiratory muscles. In contrast, bilateral weakness can cause severe breathlessness. This may occur during exertion, but a specific feature is orthopnoea. This occurs within a few seconds of lying flat and is relieved promptly by sitting up, in contrast to left ventricular failure and nocturnal asthma with which it is frequently confused. Breathlessness may also occur when standing in water since the passive inspiratory descent of the diaphragm due to gravity is prevented by the raised extra abdominal pressure.

The physical signs of unilateral diaphragm weakness can be subtle. Dullness to percussion over the lower part of the thorax may be present and the level of dullness may rise paradoxically on the paralysed side during inspiration. The normal inspiratory outward movement of the abdomen may be reduced or absent on the side of diaphragmatic paralysis, and expansion of the lower chest may lag behind the normal expansion of the other side.

The physical signs of bilateral diaphragmatic paralysis are much more clear cut. Orthopnoea is usually readily apparent and the abdomen moves paradoxically inwards as the diaphragm ascends during inspiration. A maximum transdiaphragmatic pressure of less than 30 cmH$_2$0 is necessary for this sign to be detected. The accessory muscles are active, particularly in the supine position. The quality of sleep is often poor and as a result excessive daytime somnolence may be a problem. Bilateral, basal dullness due to the high diaphragms is characteristic, but can be mimicked by bilateral pleural effusions.

Investigations

The chest radiograph in unilateral diaphragmatic paralysis shows whether the affected diaphragm is elevated and usually reveals any adjacent mass that may be responsible. If there is bilateral paralysis, both the diaphragms are raised. There is often some basal linear shadowing due to subsegmental lung collapse. Diaphragmatic screening or ultrasound examination reveals that the diaphragm moves paradoxically, particularly during sniffing. This test should be carried out in the supine position with a weight on the abdomen. These precautions prevent abdominal muscle contraction during expiration from mimicking diaphragmatic activity by reducing the end expiratory volume below functional residual capacity, so that inspiration then occurs through the elastic recoil of the lungs and chest wall. In the upright position, the effect of gravity on the abdominal contents can lead to inspiration without any diaphragmatic activity.

A low vital capacity, which falls further in the supine position, is the hallmark of diaphragmatic weakness, particularly when this is severe and bilateral. All lung volumes are reduced except for the residual volume since expiratory muscle strength is largely preserved. Maximum inspiratory pressure is also reduced, but diaphragmatic weakness can be more specifically

diagnosed by estimating the transdiaphragmatic pressure. This can be carried out by asking the patient to sniff or to take a maximum inspiratory effort, or by magnetic or percutaneous electrical stimulation of the phrenic nerve in the neck. Care is required to carry out these investigations using a standardized method in order to obtain repeatable results. The function of the phrenic nerve can be estimated by measuring its conduction time. This is normally less than about 9.5 ms, but is prolonged if the nerves are diseased.

The arterial Po_2 is characteristically slightly reduced, with a normal Pco_2 during the daytime and in sleep as long as pulmonary function is normal and there is no other muscle weakness. If either of these are present, however, bilateral diaphragmatic weakness can cause hypercapnia with profound hypoxia during sleep.

Treatment

Plication for hemidiaphragmatic paralysis is rarely required in adults unless coexistent pulmonary disease is severe enough to cause breathlessness. Bilateral plication is not effective and mechanical respiratory support is often required if there is bilateral weakness. Treatment with nasal positive pressure ventilation or a negative pressure ventilator, such as a cuirass or jacket is usually required, although rocking beds have also been found to be effective in the past. Ventilatory support is usually needed only at night and until the function of the diaphragm or phrenic nerve improves. Phrenic nerve pacemakers are only indicated when diaphragmatic weakness is due to lesions above the phrenic nerve nucleus in C3 to 5 or 6. The commonest cause of this is a high cervical spinal cord injury. Breathlessness on exertion often remains a problem, but may lessen as other inspiratory muscles partially compensate for diaphragmatic weakness.

Further reading

Bredin CP (1989). Pulmonary function in long-term survivors of thoracoplasty. *Chest* **95**, 18–20.

Dolmage TE, Avendano MA, Goldstein RS (1992). Respiratory function during wakefulness and sleep among survivors of respiratory and non-respiratory poliomyelitis. *European Respiratory Journal* **5**, 864–70.

Elliott CG, Hill TR, Adams TE, Crapo R, Nietrzeba RM, Gardner RM (1985). Exercise performance of subjects with ankylosing spondylitis and limited chest expansion. *Bulletin Eurropeen de Physiopathologie Respiratoire* **21**, 363–8.

Franssen MJAM, van Herwaarden CLA, van de Putte LBA, Gribnau FWJ (1986). Lung function in patients with ankylosing spondylitis. A study of the influence of disease activity and treatment with non-steroidal antiinflammatory drugs. *Journal of Rheumatology* **13**, 936–40.

Gibson GJ (1989). Diaphragmatic paresis: pathophysiology, clinical features, and investigations. *Thorax* **44**, 960–70.

Haller JA Jr, Colombani PM, Humphries CT, *et al.* (1996). Chest wall constriction after too extensive and too early operations for pectus excavatum. *Annals of Thoracic Surgery* **61**, 1618–25.

Kafer ER (1975). Idiopathic scoliosis. Mechanical properties of the respiratory system and the ventilatory response to carbon dioxide. *Journal of Clinical Investigation* **55**, 1153–63.

Kinnear WJM, Hockley S, Harvey J, Shneerson JM (1988). The effects of one year of nocturnal cuirass-assisted ventilation in chest wall disease. *European Respiratory Journal* **1**, 204–6.

Laroche CM, Moxham J, Green M (1989). Respiratory muscle weakness and fatigue. *Quarterly Journal of Medicine, New Series* **71** (265), 373–97.

Lindahl T (1954). Spirometric and bronchospirometric studies in five-rib thoracoplasties. *Thorax* **9**, 285–90.

Midgren B, Petersson K, Hansson L, Eriksson L, Airikkala P, Elmqvist D (1988). Nocturnal hypoxaemia in severe scoliosis. *British Journal of Diseases of the Chest* **82**, 226–36.

Mier-Jedrzejowicz A, Brophy C, Moxham J, Green M (1988). Assessment of diaphragm weakness. *American Review of Respiratory Disease* **137**, 877–83.

Newsom-Davis J, Goldman M, Loh L, Casson M (1976). Diaphragm function and alveolar hypoventilation. *Quarterly Journal of Medicine* **145**, 87–100.

O'Brien JW, Johnson SH, Van Steyn SJ, *et al.* (1991). Effects of internal mammary artery dissection on phrenic nerve perfusion and function. *Annals of Thoracic Surgery* **52**, 182–8.

Pehrsson K, Bake B, Larsson S, Nachemson A (1991). Lung function in adult idiopathic scoliosis: a 20 year follow up. *Thorax* **46**, 474–8.

Phillips MS, Kinnear WJM, Shneerson JM (1987). Late sequelae of pulmonary tuberculosis treated by thoracoplasty. *Thorax* **42**, 445–51.

Phillips MS, Kinnear WJM, Shaw D, Shneerson JM (1989). Exercise responses in patients treated for pulmonary tuberculosis by thoracoplasty. *Thorax* **44**, 268–74.

Ras GJ, van Staden M, Schultz C, *et al.* (1994). Respiratory manifestations of rigid spine syndrome. *American Journal of Respiratory and Critical Care Medicine* **150**, 540–6.

Robert D, Gerard M, Leger P, *et al.* (1983). La ventilation mechanique a domicile definitive par tracheostomie de l'insuffisant respiratoire chronique. *Revue Francaise des Maladies Respiratoires* **11**, 923–6.

Sawicka EH, Branthwaite MA, Spencer GT (1983). Respiratory failure after thoracoplasty: treatment by intermittent negative-pressure ventilation. *Thorax* **28**, 433–5.

Shneerson JM (1978). The cardiorespiratory response to exercise in thoracic scoliosis. *Thorax* **33**, 457–63.

Shneerson J (1998). Sleep in neuromuscular thoracic cage disorders. *European Respiratory Monograph* **10**, 324–44.

Smith IE, Laroche CM, Jamieson SA, Shneerson JM (1996). Kyphosis secondary to tuberculous osteomyelitis as a cause of ventilatory failure: Clinical features, mechanisms and management. *Chest* **110**, 1105–10.

Tzelepis GE, McCool FD, Hoppin FG Jr (1989). Chest wall distortion in patients with flail chest. *American Review of Respiratory Disease* **140**, 31–7.

17.14 Neoplastic disorders

17.14.1 Lung cancer

S. G. Spiro

General epidemiology

Lung cancer is the most common malignant disease in the Western world. It has shown the greatest relative and absolute rise in mortality of any tumour this century in England and Wales, and particularly in Scotland. It causes 38 000 deaths per year in England and Wales, with 80 per cent of these occurring in men. In the European Community, there were 1.35 million deaths per annum in men (the highest death rate from any tumour) and 229 000 deaths per annum in women during the period 1978 to 1982. In the United States, it has been increasing in incidence by up to 10 per cent per year since the 1930s, but over the last decade this trend has levelled off, particularly in men. Nevertheless, approximately 120 000 American men die of lung cancer each year; the figure for women being 34 000, similar to that for breast cancer.

Age-standardized mortality rates for cancer for 1985 to 1989 show that in the European Community lung cancer in men was by far the commonest cause of death. Belgium has the highest mortality (77.16 deaths per 100 000 population) with Scotland (75.9) second, and England and Wales (60.9) fifth. The figures for Central and Eastern Europe are worse in that the death rates for lung cancer are rising exponentially, particularly in men—75.8/100 000 in the Czeck Republic, 74.0 in Hungary, 69.4 in Poland, and 68.7 in Slovakia. For females, Scotland has the highest incidence (27.2, equal to the rate of breast cancer in Scottish women), with England and Wales (20.4) third. Age-adjusted lung cancer death rates in Eastern Europe are still considerably less than in the Western countries, ranging from 14.4 in Hungary to 6.8 in Slovakia. Perhaps the worst epidemic is in China where 0.8 million men will die in the year 2000 from smoking-related diseases. The relative risk of dying from lung cancer is about 3.0 in male smokers compared to non-smokers, and 2.0 for female smokers. Of all deaths attributed to tobacco in China, 15 per cent were due to lung cancer.

Aetiological factors

Tobacco

In every country, the increase in mortality from lung cancer has appeared to coincide with an increase in tobacco usage, particularly cigarette smoking, after what seemed to be an appropriate latent interval. Early retrospective studies showed that, amongst patients with carcinoma of the bronchus, there were many fewer non-smokers and many more heavy smokers than among the controls, and that there was an association between the amount smoked and the risk of lung cancer. Prospective studies, amongst which the long-term study of British doctors was particularly informative, confirmed the increased risk of death from lung cancer from any tobacco use, but most specifically that of cigarettes. There was a strong dose–response relationship with the number of cigarettes smoked, illustrated in Table 1. The most important variable in smoking intensity is the number of cigarettes smoked, but other variables include the depth of inhalation, number of puffs, butt length, use of a filter, and the type of tobacco smoked. Further evidence that the relationship was causal came from a study which documented reduction in mortality after stopping smoking: 15 years after cessation the risk of death fell from 15.8 times to twice that in non-smokers, equivalent to 11 per cent of that pertaining in those who continued to smoke.

Globally, there has been a huge change in cigarette consumption. While there has been a drop of 25 per cent and 9 per cent in consumption in the United Kingdom and the United States, respectively, between 1970 and 1985, the overall world consumption has risen by 7 per cent. This is due to huge increases in Asia (22 per cent), Latin America (24 per cent), and Africa (42 per cent). The current epidemic of smoking in China lags behind Western society by 20 years. Thus in China in 1996, the average number of cigarettes smoked per adult male was 11 per day, a figure that that peaked in the West at 10 a day in 1980.

Wide differences in smoking habits in the United Kingdom are seen between social classes, with 57 per cent of unskilled manual workers smoking compared with only 21 per cent of professional workers. During the last 5 years the number of adult men smoking in England and Wales has fallen from 64 to 36 per cent, but has remained at 35 per cent for adult women. The effect of the lower-tar cigarettes has not yet had time to become established.

Passive smoking

Evidence that passive smoking predisposes to lung cancer is far from certain. Approximately 15 per cent of lung cancers occur in non-smokers, and 5 per cent of these have been attributed to passive smoking.

Table 1 Death rate from lung cancer in males by smoking habits when last asked (British doctors' study)

Tobacco use category	Death rate (age standardized per 100 000)
Non-smokers	10
Ex-smokers	43
Continuing smokers	
Any tobacco	104
Pipe and/or cigar only	58
Mixed	82
Cigarette smokers only	140
Number smoked per day	
1–14	78
15–24	127
25 or more	251

Occupation

A number of different factors have now been identified as associated with lung cancer; subjects who develop this disease as a result of their occupation represent a small but important group. The association of asbestos with lung cancer is now firmly established; various studies have identified that those exposed are at 4.9 to 7.3 times greater risk than those who are not. This risk is much enhanced if the asbestos industry worker smokes cigarettes; one study estimating this at 93 times that for non-smokers not exposed to asbestos. In Norway, it is illegal to employ a smoker in an asbestos-related job. Exposure to radioactive isotopes, mainly radon daughters, is associated with a higher risk of lung cancer and occurs among various groups of miners, particularly those involved in extraction of pitchblende and uranium. Polycyclic aromatic hydrocarbons are believed to be responsible for the increased risk in workers in gas and coke ovens and in foundry workers. Nickel refining, chromate manufacture, and arsenical industrial workers are also exposed to a higher risk of lung cancer. The amount of lung cancer caused by occupational exposure may well have been underestimated in the past, and a summary of the importance industrial products and processes involved appears in Table 2.

Air pollution

The decline in male mortality is occurring earlier than would be expected from changes in smoking habits. The high mortality figures in the United Kingdom and Germany compared with France and Italy, for example, seem likely to be due in part to heavy industry and coal burning. Analysis by county in the United States shows an association between lung cancer deaths and counties with chemical, petroleum, ship-building, and paper industries. Legislation for cleaner air has caused both environmental and occupational pollution to fall dramatically in the past 30 years, and this has preceded changes in smoking habits.

Pathology

A detailed understanding of the natural history, pathology, and pathogenesis of bronchial carcinoma is becoming increasingly important as the assessment, management, and prognosis of the disease depends largely upon the cell type and the presence or absence of metastases at the time of presentation. It has been estimated that about seven-eighths of a tumour's life will have passed when it is diagnosed and that the vast majority will be disseminated at the time of diagnosis.

Bronchogenic carcinomas seem to arise most commonly in segmental and subsegmental bronchi in response to repetitive carcinogenic stimuli or inflammation and irritation. The mucosal lining is most susceptible to injury at the bifurcation of bronchial structures. Dysplasia is followed by

Table 2 Industrial products and processes known to cause or suspected of causing lung cancer

Fibre exposure (asbestos)
Nickel refining
Aluminium industry
Arsenic and arsenic compounds
Benzoyl chloride
Beryllium
Cadmium
Chloromethyl ether
Chromates
The electronics industry
Irradiation
Soots, tar, oils
Mustard gas

Reproduced from Coggan and Acheson (1983), with permission.

carcinoma *in situ* when the entire thickness of the mucosa may be replaced by proliferating neoplastic cells. These changes may be strictly localized or multicentric. Tumour infiltration follows loss of the basal membrane. The precise origins of small-cell carcinomas remain an enigma, and those of adenocarcinomas are not precisely defined. The latter may arise from the mucosal lining or from the submucosal bronchial mucous glands. A significant number of lung tumours arise in the periphery of the lung, perhaps three-quarters of adenocarcinomas and large-cell anaplastic malignancies, one-third of squamous (or epidermoid) carcinomas, and one-fifth of small-cell carcinomas.

The WHO classification of lung cancer according to cell type and the approximate distribution of each type as a percentage of all lung cancers is shown in Table 3. The squamous-cell tumour has a relatively slow growth rate (volume doubling time, 90 days) and the lowest incidence of distant haematogenous metastasis. Small-cell tumours grow rapidly (volume doubling time, 30 days) and there is very early dissemination by both the haematogenous and the lymphatic routes, with metastasis being present in more than 90 per cent of patients at the time of diagnosis. Adenocarcinomas and anaplastic large-cell tumours occupy an intermediate position. It is now recognized that significant heterogeneity of cell morphology can be visualized within individual tumours. Squamous-cell tumours, adenocarcinomas, and large-cell tumours are often collectively called non-small-cell lung cancers, and the approach to their management differs from that for small-cell lung cancer.

Squamous (epidermoid) carcinoma

These tumours are composed predominantly of flattened to polygonal neoplastic cells that tend to stratify, form intercellular bridges, and elaborate keratin. About 60 per cent present as obstructive lesions in lobar and mainstem bronchi. The tumours tend to be bulky and to produce intraluminar granular or polypoid masses. As a result, distal pneumonia and abscess formation is common, and cavitation is seen in about 10 per cent. The cells are usually well differentiated, but in some cases differentiation is poor and the appearances are those of predominantly anaplastic cells, frequently arranged in the classical pattern of stratifying sheets.

Small-cell (oat-cell) anaplastic carcinoma

This is now recognized as a pathologically and clinically distinct form of lung cancer. Small-cell lung cancer may originate from the amine precursor uptake and decarboxylation (APUD) series of cells. The tumour is composed of neoplastic cells with dark oval to round spindled nuclei and scanty, indistinct cytoplasm arranged in ribbons, nests, and sheets. The cells tend to crush easily on biopsy, and extensive areas may be necrotic. This type of tumour presents as a proximal lesion in 75 per cent of cases and may arise anywhere in the tracheobronchial tree and rapidly invade vessels and lymph nodes, disseminating widely even before symptoms arise from the primary tumour. Extensive, advanced disease exists in more than half the patients at presentation. The cells secrete peptides which cause clinical syndromes in 10 per cent of cases.

Adenocarcinoma

This tumour forms acinar or granular structures, having prominent papillary processes, and may be mucin-provoking. About 70 per cent appear to originate peripherally in the lung and are frequently fairly circumscribed; in about 10 per cent, the initial presentation is a pleural effusion. If related to bronchi, they tend to cuff and stenose the lumen. They occasionally arise in old tuberculous scars.

Large-cell carcinoma

These tumours, which have been described as an unclassified category, include all tumours that show no evidence of maturation or differentiation. They are composed of pleomorphic cells with variable enlarged nuclei, prominent nucleoli, and nuclear inclusions, and abundant cytoplasm; they

Table 3 Classification of epithelial tumours of the lung (based on revised WHO classification)

	Frequency (%)		Frequency (%)
Main			
Epidermoid carcinoma (squamous cell)	35–45	Adenocarcinoma	35–40
		Acinar	
		Papillary	
		Bronchiolar alveolar	
Small-cell carcinoma	20–24	Large-cell carcinoma	6–10
Oat-cell		With stratification	
Fusiform		With mucin-production	
Others		Giant-cell	
		Clear-cell	
Less common			
Tumours showing mixed differentiation		Bronchial gland	
		Adenoid cystic	
		Mucoepidermoid	
		Others	
Carcinoid tumours			
Carcinoma *in situ*			

are mucin-producing in many instances. The tumours tend to be bulky and are often necrotic; they are frequently peripheral, they invade locally, and disseminate widely, with about half the patients having disseminated disease on presentation. Although they are highly malignant and undifferentiated, the cure rate after surgery is surprisingly high, but radiotherapy is ineffective in controlling the disease. Large-cell carcinoma is a smoking-related disease in over 90 per cent of patients.

Bronchioloalveolar carcinoma

There has been considerable controversy as to whether this tumour, which has the least association with tobacco smoking, arises from alveolar or bronchial epithelium, but derivation from the alveolar type II cell has been suggested. The tumour tends to spread as cuboidal or columnar 'epithelium' along the lining of the alveoli, with single or multiple rows of cells and often papillary formation (Fig. 1). There is production of a large amount of mucus in 20 per cent of cases and it is believed that malignant cells shed into the mucus may carry over into the contralateral lung. The tumour can spread within a lobe and occupy it fully. Sometimes, however, the tumour is multicentric in origin, and diffuse nodular lesions are to be found on radiographic examination. Invasion of neighbouring tissue and lymph nodes is common, but extrathoracic spread is unusual. There is some resemblance to metastases from adenocarcinomas emanating from other organs, and this sometimes leads to confusion. The tumour tends to grow along alveolar septae as a framework, and it may be difficult to distinguish from metastatic tumours from colon, breast, or pancreas.

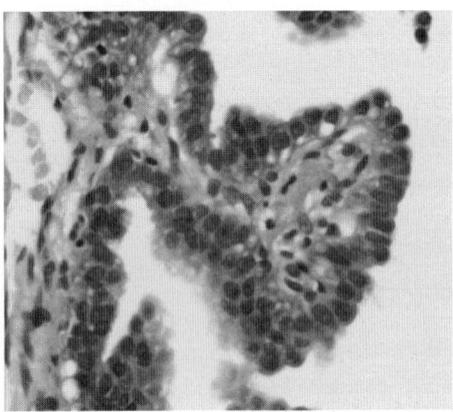

Fig. 1 Bronchoalveolar cell carcinoma: malignant cuboidal epithelium spreads along alveolar walls.

Carcinoid tumours

Carcinoid tumours are described in Chapter 14.8.

Carcinoma *in situ*

Many investigators have suggested that cells undergoing malignant change do not necessarily invade the lungs at the onset of this biological mutation, but continue to exist at a particular location (cancer *in situ*). Exfoliated cancer cells sloughed from such a location may be seen fortuitously by the cytologist; even more rarely, such a site may be biopsied at bronchoscopy.

Genetics and biology

Genetic influences may play a role in the development of lung cancers, particularly in patients under 50. In one study, lung cancers were attributable to a mendelian dominant inheritance pattern in 27 per cent of patients under 50, but only 9 per cent of those over 70.

Both small-cell and non-small-cell lung cancer can be cultured as cell lines which can be transplanted into nude mice. The resultant tumours are morphologically and histologically similar to the original human tumour. Two major categories of cell lines are established for small-cell lung cancer—classic and variant. Classic cell lines account for 70 per cent of the total and are characterized by high expression of neuroendocrine markers such as L-dopa decarboxylase and bombesin/gastrin-releasing peptide, neurone-specific enolase, and creatine kinase-BB. The variant cell lines have selective loss of some of these neuroendocrine markers, and many have substituted amplification of the c-*myc* oncogene. These neuroendocrine and proto-oncogenic properties are thought to be of prognostic significance, playing an important role in regulation of tumourigenesis. In non-small cell lung cancer, approximately 8 per cent of tumours and 20 per cent of tumour cell lines have myc family amplification, and overexpression of these proteins is associated with poorer prognosis.

The ras family of oncogenes (H, K, and N) was the first to be described in association with lung cancer. Ras gene mutations occur in 20 to 40 per cent of non-small cell lung cancer, especially adenocarcinomas, and the presence of K-*ras* mutations is linked with significantly shortened survival.

Lung cancer cells not only show mutations that activate dominant cellular proto-oncogenes, but also genetic mechanisms that inactivate recessive tumour suppressors. The commonest abnormality is a deletion in the short arm of chromosome 3, which is found in over 90 per cent of small-cell lung cancer and 50 per cent of non-small-cell lung cancer patients. Other sites of loss of heterozygosity include 11p, 13q, and 17p. Tumour suppressor genes have been identified in inherited cancers, mainly in studies of familial retinoblastoma. Mutations in P53 occur in 75 per cent of small cell lung cancer and 50 per cent of non-small cell lung cancer. The gene is located on the short arm of chromosome 13q14, and it is thought that it may normally protect cells against accumulation of mutations. Depletions and mutations of P53 are linked with metastatic disease. Alterations of P53 protein have been found in early bronchial neoplasia, and may be a useful marker for the early detection of lung cancer. Other markers, including heterogenous nuclear ribonuclear protein A2/B1 overexpression in sputum, may allow earlier detection of tumours.

Several monoclonal antibodies have been generated against lung-cancer-associated antigens. Thirty-six monoclonal antibodies raised against small-cell lung cancer have been grouped into eight clusters. No antigen is specific for small-cell lung cancer. Antibodies belonging to the major cluster (cluster 1) are directed against the neural-cell adhesion molecule (NCAM), whilst the nature of the other antigens remains unclear. Studies of both small-cell and non-small-cell lung cancer cell lines show that NCAM expression is associated with a neuroendocrine phenotype irrespective of the histological type of lung cancer. Monoclonal antibodies may have a therapeutic value when coupled with a radionuclide or a toxin. Radiolabelled antibodies can be used to detect minimal disease in bone marrow aspirates or biopsy specimens.

The growth factors bombesin/gastrin-releasing peptide, insulin-like growth factor 1, and transferrin stimulate can all stimulate tumour growth. There is much interest in attempts to retard or disrupt these processes.

Clinical features

The clinical features of lung cancer are very variable. In about 5 per cent of patients the presentation is a radiographic abnormality found on routine examination and unassociated with symptoms, but patients may present with extremely advanced disease and die rapidly.

Clinical manifestations may be due to: local presence of the tumour in the lung, including bronchial obstruction or invasion of contiguous structures in the thorax and mediastinum; metastasis through blood or lymph vessels; and endocrine, metabolic, and neurological syndromes.

Cough is the most common initial presenting symptom (Table 4), but because it is a symptom of so many respiratory disorders, the possibility of tumour may be overlooked and cough may be attributed to some other cause, particularly in smokers who have had chronic bronchitis for many years. Patients who have a persistent cough should have a chest radiograph, particularly if they are smokers over 40 years of age. A change in the cough habit is significant and also requires investigation. If the trachea or main bronchi are involved, the cough may be brassy in character and may be accompanied by wheezing or stridor. If cough is manifestly ineffective, involvement of the recurrent laryngeal nerve should be suspected.

Table 4 Frequency of initial symptoms and signs of lung cancer

Symptom/sign	Frequency (%)
Cough	75
Weight loss	60–70
Dyspnoea	50–60
Chest pain	45–50
Haemoptysis	25–35
Bone pain	25
Fever	15
Weakness	10
Superior vena cava obstruction	4
Dysphagia	2
Wheeze	2

Studies summarized by Scagliotti GV (1995). Symptoms and signs and staging of lung cancer. In: SG Spiro, ed. *Carcinoma of the lung*, European Respiratory Monograph Vol 1, No.1, 91–137.

Expectoration of sputum may be due to spread of the tumour itself or to infection occurring distal to partial bronchial obstruction. In the early stages of the disease the sputum is often grey and viscid; it is usually purulent in the presence of infection distal to a tumour and in cavitated tumours. The value of sputum cytology in diagnosis is described below.

Haemoptysis, which occurs as a sole presenting symptom in about 5 per cent of cases and at some stage in the disease in 50 per cent of patients, is a symptom not easily ignored by patient or physician. The degree varies from streaking of the sputum with blood to larger amounts, but massive haemoptysis (>200 ml) is rare, except as a terminal event. The most significant description given by patients is that of coughing up blood every morning for several days in succession.

Wheeze may be observed in a few patients. Localized persistent wheeze even after coughing is a significant observation indicating obstruction of a larger or central airway.

Stridor is a feature which is poorly recognized and is often confused with wheeze. It is due to narrowing of the glottis, trachea, or major bronchi, and is best heard after the patient coughs and then breathes in deeply with the mouth open.

Dyspnoea is a presenting symptom in only a small number of patients. As the disease progresses dyspnoea is inevitable, being proportional to the amount of lung involved, either directly by tumour replacement or indirectly by endobronchial disease causing airway narrowing or obstruction. Progressive breathlessness is also a salient feature of malignant pleural and, rarely, pericardial effusion, superior vena caval obstruction, and lymphangitis carcinomatosis.

Chest discomfort is a common symptom, occurring in up to 40 per cent of patients at diagnosis. The discomfort is often of an ill-defined nature and may be described in terms of intermittent aching somewhere in the chest. Definite pleural pain may occur in the presence of infection, but invasion of the pleura by tumour is often painless. However, invasion of the ribs or vertebrae causes continuous, gnawing, localized pain. A tumour in the superior pulmonary sulcus (Pancoast tumour) can cause progressive constant pain in the shoulder, upper anterior chest, or interscapular region, soon spreading to the arm once the brachial plexus is invaded. Other symptoms of this type of tumour include weakness and atrophy of the muscles of the hand, Horner's syndrome, hoarseness, and spinal cord compression at levels D1 and D2.

Lack of energy and, more particularly, loss of interest in normal pursuits are symptoms of great importance; a sensation of vague ill health commonly occurs.

Fever, chills, and night sweats may occur due to chest infection, but fever may very rarely be present in rapidly progressive tumours without evidence of infection, particularly if there are hepatic metastases.

Invasion of adjacent intrathoracic structures gives rise to certain specific clinical features. Involvement of the last cervical and first thoracic segment of the sympathetic trunk by cancer produces Horner's syndrome. Malignant infiltration of the recurrent laryngeal nerve—almost always the left branch because of its course adjacent to the left hilum—gives rise to vocal chord paralysis. The right recurrent laryngeal nerve is occasionally affected in the base of the neck. Recurrent aspiration pneumonias may follow vocal chord paralysis. Extension of the tumour with invasion or compression of the superior vena cava or by paratracheal lymphadenopathy results in the characteristic features of superior vena caval obstruction—awareness of tightness of the collar, fullness of the head, and suffusion of the face, particularly after bending down, blackouts, breathlessness, and engorgement of veins with a downward venous flow in the neck, the upper half of the thorax, and arms, often accompanied by oedema of the face.

Dysphagia is due to compression of the oesophagus from without by tumour masses and only rarely to direct invasion. Cardiac metastases usually occur late in the disease and are manifested clinically by tachycardia, arrhythmias, pericardial effusion, breathlessness, and cardiac failure. Invasion of the phrenic nerve results in elevation and paralysis of the hemidiaphragm.

The clinical features associated with involvement of the ribs, spine, and pleura are described elsewhere. Very rarely bronchogenic carcinoma causes spontaneous pneumothorax. It must not be forgotten that spread of tumour to the other lung may occur or that synchronous primaries may coexist.

Metastatic lesions from lung cancer may occur in any organ of the body and produce symptoms which form the presenting complaint. Metastases to nodes are frequent and should be sought with great care, particularly those in the scalene area, which are usually the first to be involved and can be palpated. The best position for examination is from behind with the patient seated relaxed in a chair. The side affected usually corresponds to the side of the lung lesion, the exception being that tumours from the left lower lobe may metastasize to the nodes in the right scalene area. Involvement of the nodes in the floor of the supraclavicular fossa is equally common.

Bony metastases are common, particularly in small-cell tumours, and occur predominantly in the ribs, vertebrae, humeri, and femora. Early involvement may be detected by a rise in alkaline phosphatase of bony origin, isotope scanning, or biopsy. Conventional skeletal surveys are often unhelpful and misleading. Liver secondaries are common and may be silent, although a rise in liver enzymes, particularly alkaline phosphatase of liver origin, may be an early sign. Isotope liver scans and ultrasound may detect involvement in a liver which is not clinically enlarged, but as the metastases develop the liver becomes grossly enlarged with an irregular outline. Friction rubs may sometimes be heard over a grossly involved liver. Metastases to brain may account for the presenting symptom in lung cancer in 4 per cent of patients and may be encountered at some time in the illness in 30 per cent. The symptoms simulate those of any expanding brain tumour. The adrenal glands are involved in 15 to 20 per cent of patients, rarely producing symptoms. The skin should be examined for the presence of the typical, slightly bluish, umbilicated lesions of tumour spread. Subcutaneous metastases may be found at almost any site.

Endocrine and metabolic manifestations

It is becoming more apparent that many of the hitherto unexplained and often unusual manifestations of malignant disease are the result of endocrine and metabolic manifestations of the cancer itself. Cancer cells appear to be able to synthesize polypeptides that mimic virtually all the hormones produced by conventional endocrine organs—hence the term 'ectopic hormones'. From time to time the clinical features resulting from ectopic hormone secretion precede those of the pulmonary tumour, emphasizing the importance of a high index of suspicion in such circumstances. Ectopic hormone measurement cannot, however, be used for screening purposes.

Syndrome of inappropriate secretion of antidiuretic hormone (SIADH)

The continued secretion of vasopressin (ADH) in an amount in excess of the body's needs leads to overhydration in both the intracellular and extracellular compartments. The cerebral oedema resulting from water intoxication causes drowsiness, lethargy, irritability, mental confusion, and disorientation, with fits and coma being the most profound features. Peripheral oedema is remarkably rare. The patient is usually asymptomatic until the sodium falls below 120 mmol/l and the hyponatraemia is dilutional in type with a low serum osmolality. Urine osmolality usually exceeds 300 mosmol/kg. The commonest cancer causing this syndrome is small-cell cancer, where it is clinically obvious in 10 per cent of cases, with subclinical involvement detectable by a water-loading test in more than 50 per cent. Restriction of fluid to a daily intake of 700 to 1000 ml may redress the hyponatraemia, but demethylchlortetracycline (demeclocycline) 600 to 1200 mg daily is often highly effective, making water restriction unnecessary. Azotaemia may occur as a result of increased urea production and a mild drug-induced nephrotoxicity so that adjustment of dosage may be necessary. Infusion of hypertonic saline is hazardous, often precipitating cardiac failure or cerebral oedema.

Ectopic ACTH syndrome

Secretion of an adrenocorticotrophic substance by a small-cell carcinoma or bronchial carcinoid leads to bilateral adrenal hyperplasia and to secretion of large amounts of cortisol. The onset of symptoms may be so acute that death may occur within a few weeks, and the typical features of Cushing's syndrome do not have time to develop. Chief clinical features are thirst and polyuria, oedema, pigmentation, and hypokalaemia. Hypertension and profound myopathy may also be present. Serum cortisol is often grossly elevated, with loss of the normal diurnal rhythm; the level is not suppressed by dexamethasone; and hypokalaemic alkalosis can be severe, with plasma potassium frequently below 3.0 mmol/l and HCO_3 above 30 mmol/l. Drugs which block adrenocortical steroid biosynthesis may produce partial and reversible medical adrenalectomy, and metyrapone in doses from 250 mg thrice daily to 1 g four times daily may cause temporary relief of symptoms. Removal of the tumour, if practicable, will cause remission.

Hypercalcaemia (see also Chapter 12.6)

Hypercalcaemia may be associated with ectopic secretion of parathormone by squamous-cell cancers but is more commonly due directly to the presence of multiple bone metastases. The primary tumour may also produce a cyclic-AMP-stimulating factor or a prostaglandin causing hypercalcaemia. Hypercalcaemia is unlikely to cause symptoms unless the serum calcium exceeds 2.8 mmol/l, and levels much higher than this are sometimes encountered. The main clinical features are nausea, vomiting, abdominal pain and constipation, polyuria, thirst and dehydration, muscular weakness, psychosis, drowsiness, and eventually coma. Immediate treatment is to relieve fluid depletion, and large volumes of intravenous saline (up to 5 litres in 24 h) may be required. Corticosteroids (400 mg hydrocortisone or 40 mg prednisolone in 24 h initially) are effective in about half of the cases. However, intravenous diphosphonates followed by oral maintenance therapy is now the treatment of choice. Other treatments which are sometimes effective are calcitonin 200 to 400 units every 8 h, mithramycin 10 to 15 µg/kg by infusion over 4 h every 21 days, aspirin 2 to 4 g/day, and indomethacin 50 to 100 mg/day. The calcium level drops dramatically within 48 h if the tumour is removed.

Gynaecomastia

Swelling of the breasts, which may be painful, occurs mainly in the subareolar area, and there may be atrophy of the testes. The association is chiefly with large-cell carcinomas. Increased gonadatrophin production is the cause.

Other endocrine manifestations

Hyperthyroidism occurs rarely, but neither goitre nor eye signs are prominent features. Spontaneous hypoglycaemia, the masculinizing syndrome in young women, and hyperglycaemia are very rarely encountered. Pigmentation associated with α- and β-melanocyte-stimulating hormone may occur. The carcinoid syndromes are described elsewhere.

Neuromyopathies

The term carcinomatous neuropathy is used to describe those abnormalities of the central nervous system, the peripheral nerves, the muscles, and the autonomic nervous system that occur in association with malignancy. These disorders can be subdivided as follows: myopathies (polymyositis, myasthenia, and dermatomyositis), neuropathies (sensory and mixed sensorimotor, encephalopathy, and myelopathy). Toxic, infective, nutritional, and autoimmune causes have been suggested, but none has been fully substantiated. Neuromyopathies respond variably following treatment of the primary tumour by surgery, radiotherapy, or chemotherapy.

Most neuromyopathies are not tumour-cell-type specific, except for the Lambert–Eaton syndrome seen occasionally in small-cell lung cancer patients. This often precedes the appearance of the tumour by up to 15 months, and is characterized by proximal muscle weakness, depressed tendon reflexes (which often return following repetitive exercise), autonomic features, and difficulty with swallowing. There appears to be an association with HLA-B8 and the IgG heavy-chain allotype GM2. Prednisolone and 3–4 amidopyridine 10 to 20 mg four times daily are used for treatment.

Finger clubbing and hypertrophic pulmonary osteoarthropathy

Finger clubbing accompanies a variety of intrathoracic disorders. Gross clubbing is readily recognizable; its early presence may best be demonstrated by the ability to rock the nail on its abnormally spongy bed. Clubbing of the toes is usually present also. Its incidence in lung cancer has variously been reported as being between 10 and 30 per cent. Clubbing may disappear after resection of tumour.

Hypertrophic pulmonary osteoarthropathy, which may be preceded by finger clubbing alone, consists of periostitis, arthropathy, and usually gross finger clubbing. It is most commonly associated with lung tumours but is also very common in pleural tumours, preceding the diagnosis of tumour in about one-third of patients. It is much commoner in peripheral lesions and squamous tumours.

The long bones of the extremities are affected by a periosteal reaction resembling elm bark; the changes are symmetrical and affect mainly the distal ends of the bones of the forearms and shins, with the knees and elbows being involved less commonly. Synovial thickening and joint effusions are rare. The typical radiographic appearances are shown in Fig. 2. The affected areas are hot and painful and sometimes oedematous, making walking difficult. Removal of the tumour is followed by immediate regression, but symptoms recur if the tumour recurs. Vagotomy alone is sometimes effective, supporting the theory of a vagal mediation of increased blood flow as an aetiological factor in hypertrophic pulmonary osteoarthropathy.

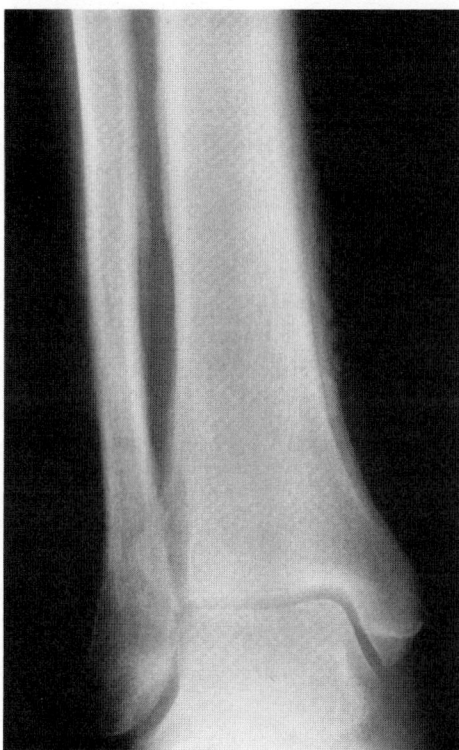

Fig. 2 Hypertrophic pulmonary osteoarthropathy showing persistent new bone formation.

Miscellaneous

The haematological effects of lung cancer are normally non-specific. Normocytic normochromic anaemia is the most common finding. Leucoerythroblastic anaemia denotes bone marrow infiltration and is particularly likely in small-cell lung cancer. Venous thrombosis and thrombophlebitis due to hypercoagulability are common complications of malignancy and may precede the detection of the underlying cancer; recurrent migratory phlebitis resistant to anticoagulation is an ominous feature. Marantic endocarditis is extremely rare, as are skin lesions such as acanthosis nigricans, dermatomyositis, hypertrichosis languinosa, and erythema gyratum repens. Rarely, the nephrotic syndrome due to membranous glomerulonephritis is encountered.

Staging and investigations

The investigations used to make the diagnosis and assess the stage of lung cancer will vary according to the presentation, the cell type, and the age and general condition of the patient.

The very rapid doubling time of small-cell lung cancer causes it to disseminate rapidly and widely, and at diagnosis is very rarely considered operable. However, the slower doubling times for squamous-cell cancers and adenocarcinomas, together with the relatively lesser tendency for the former to disseminate, makes surgery the best option whenever possible for the non-small-cell lung cancers. A precise anatomical staging classification was only applied to lung cancer in 1973 and immediately demonstrated that the prognosis of non-small-cell lung cancer depended strongly on the extent (or stage) of the disease. The introduction of the TNM staging system (T describing the primary tumour, N the extent of regional lymph node involvement, and M the absence or presence of metastases) encouraged an ordered assessment of investigations and selection of cases for surgery. On the basis of this experience, the system was modified in 1997 (Table 5).

Investigations

The following investigations form the basis for the diagnosis and staging of patients with lung cancer.

Radiological assessment

The value of the chest radiograph in the diagnosis and management of pulmonary neoplasm needs no emphasis. No initial examination is complete without a lateral film. Coned views of the ribs may help where rib invasion is suspected clinically.

The finding of a normal radiograph of the chest does not exclude bronchial carcinoma as patients presenting with haemoptysis and a normal chest radiograph are sometimes found to have a central tumour on bronchoscopy. The rounded or ovoid shadow of a peripheral tumour is described in greater detail below; these are sometimes cavitated (Fig. 3). The common appearance of a tumour arising from the main central airways (70 per cent of all cases) is enlargement of one or other hilum (Fig. 4). Even experienced observers sometimes have difficulty in deciding whether or not a hilar shadow is enlarged, and if there is any suspicion, investigation by bronchoscopy and/or CT should be pursued. Consolidation and collapse distal to the tumour may have occurred by the time that the patient presents, with the tumour itself often being obscured in the process. Collapse of the left lower lobe is often hard to identify (Fig. 5), as is a tumour situated behind the heart (Fig. 6). Apically located masses or superior sulcus tumours (Pancoast tumours) may be misdiagnosed as pleural caps, and often have a long history of pain in the distribution of the brachial nerve roots. Loss of the head of the first, second, or third rib is not unusual (Fig. 7).

The mediastinum may be widened by enlarged nodes. Involvement of the phrenic nerve may lead to paralysis and elevation of the hemidiaphragm, which then moves paradoxically on sniffing. Tumour spreading to

Table 5 Definitions for staging lung cancer (American Joint Committee on Cancer Staging, 1997)

Primary tumour (T)

T 0	No evidence of primary tumour
T X	Primary tumour cannot be assessed, or tumour proven by the presence of malignant cells in sputum or bronchial washings but not visualized by imaging or bronchoscopy
TIS	Carcinoma *in situ*
T 1	Tumour <3 cm in greatest dimension, surrounded by lung or visceral pleura, without bronchoscopic evidence of invasion more proximal than the lobar bronchus
T 2	Tumour with any of the following features of size and extent: >3 cm in greatest dimension, involves the main bronchus, ≥ 2 cm distal to the carina, invades the visceral pleura, associated with atelectasis or obstructive pneumonitis that extends to the hilar region but does not involve the entire lung
T 3	Tumour of any size that directly invades any of the following: chest wall (including superior sulcus tumours), diaphragm, mediastinal pleura, parietal pericardium; or tumour in the main bronchus <2 cm distal to the carina, but without involvement of the carina; or associated atelectasis or obstructive pneumonitis of the entire lung
T 4	Tumour of any size that invades any of the following: mediastinum, heart, great vessels, trachea, oesophagus, vertebral body carina; or tumour with a malignant pleural or pericardial effusion; or with satellite tumour nodule(s) within the ipsilateral primary-tumour lobe of the lung

Regional lymph nodes (N)

N 0	No regional lymph node metastasis
N 1	Metastasis to ipsilateral peribronchial and/or ipsilateral hilar lymph nodes, and intrapulmonary nodes involved by direct extension of the primary tumour
N 2	Metastasis to ipsilateral mediastinal and/or subcarinal lymph nodes
N 3	Metastasis to contralateral mediastinal, contralateral hilar, ipsilateral or contralateral scalene or supraclavicular lymph nodes

Distant metastasis (M)

M 0	No distant metastasis
M 1	Distant metastasis present

Staging summary

Operable	
Stage IA	T1 N0 M0
Stage IB	T2 N0 M0
Stage IIA	T1 N1 M0
Stage IIB	T2 N1 M0
	T3 N0 M0
Stage IIIA	T3 N1 M0
Usually inoperable	T1–3 N2 M0
Inoperable	
Stage IIIB	T4 any N M0
	Any T N3 M0
Stage IV	Any T any N M1

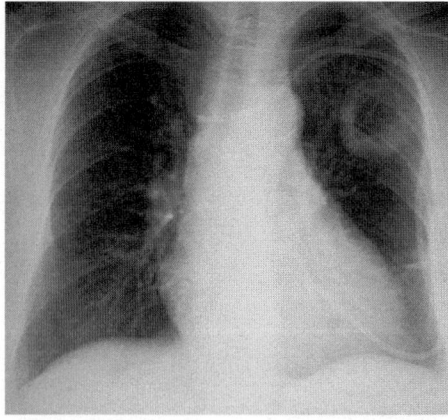

Fig. 3 Cavitating peripheral squamous-cell carcinoma.

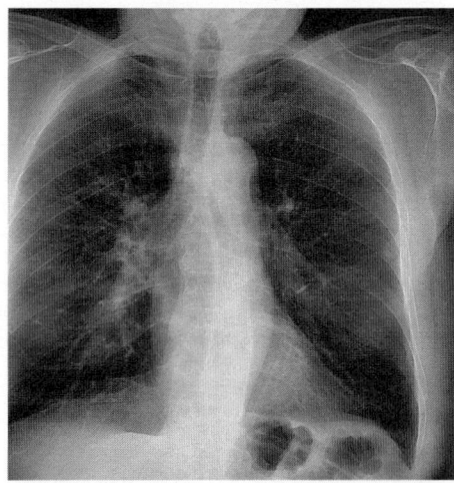

Fig. 4 Enlarged right hilum. Bronchoscopy revealed a tumour in the right intermediate bronchus.

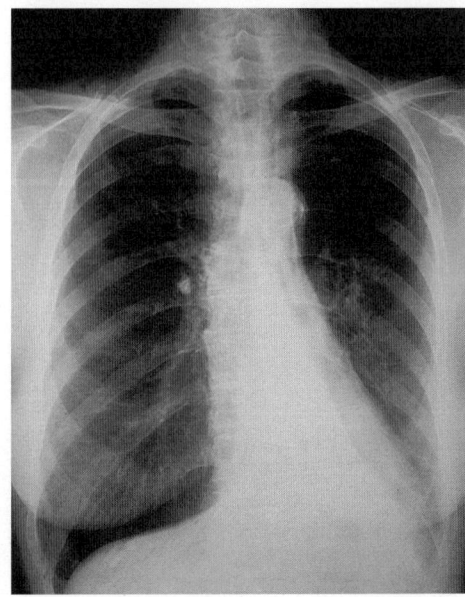

Fig. 5 Collapsed left lower lobe showing loss of the medial third of the left diaphragm.

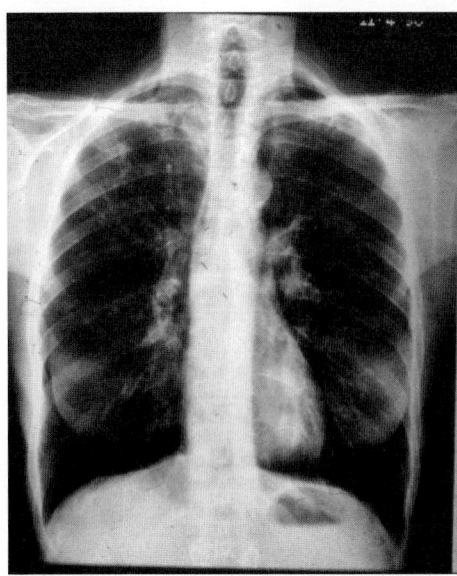

Fig. 6 Squamous-cell carcinoma lying behind the heart in the left lower lobe.

the pleura causes effusion, but such an abnormality may be secondary to infection beyond obstruction caused by a central tumour. The ribs and spine should be carefully examined for the presence of metastasis. Spread of tumour from mediastinal nodes peripherally along the lymphatics gives the appearance characteristic of lymphangitis carcinomatosa—bilateral hilar enlargement with streaky shadows fanning out into the lung fields on either side. Rarely, localized obstructive emphysema may be observed.

Sputum cytology

Cytological examination of sputum is a very useful, non-invasive test for the diagnosis of malignant pulmonary disease. The yield increases according to the number of specimens examined, and three consecutive morning specimens should be submitted in the first instance. The yield increases with the number of specimens examined, rising to 85 per cent after four samples in a study of those in whom a diagnosis of lung cancer was made. The positive incidence is lower with tumours less than 2 cm in diameter (40 per cent) and higher with larger masses (60 per cent). Central tumour

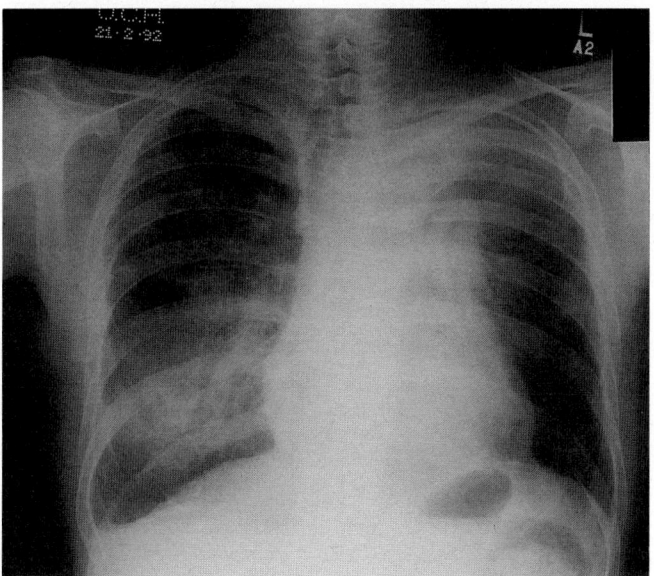

Fig. 7 Huge apical tumour with destruction of posterior parts of the second and third ribs.

yields a higher proportion of positive results (60 per cent) than peripheral lesions (48 per cent).

Bronchoscopy

Bronchoscopy, which is described in detail in Chapter xxx , is frequently the definitive diagnostic method in lung cancer. About 70 per cent of all lung cancers arise in a main bronchus, lobar, first, or second generation subsequent division, and will be visible and within biopsy or cytology brush range. Bronchoscopy also yields valuable information regarding suitability for surgical resection. Attempts to resect are ill-advised if the main carina is obviously involved, or unequivocally broad with splaying of the main bronchi and immobility on respiration, or where there is involvement of the trachea, unless confined to the right lateral wall. Histological confirmation is now obtainable in 85 to 90 per cent of bronchoscopically visible lesions.

Transbronchial biopsy

Transbronchial biopsy via the fibreoptic bronchoscope is rarely used for peripheral tumours. It remains useful for more diffuse lesions such as may be seen in adenocarcinoma, bronchoalveolar-cell carcinoma, and lymphangitis carcinomatosis. However, transthoracic needle biopsy under imaging guidance has largely replaced this technique.

Percutaneous needle biopsy

Percutaneous needle biopsy may be carried out using a variety of cutting needles to obtain a core of tissue for both histology and cytology. The procedure should be performed under fluoroscopic, CT, or ultrasound control, and is best avoided in patients with poor respiratory function or with bleeding diatheses. Positive yields as high as 90 per cent have been reported. Cytological samples remain the least satisfactory for cell type specificity. It is a useful diagnostic method in patients for whom exploratory thoracotomy may be hazardous, or in attempts to determine whether a solid mass is a primary, secondary, or benign tumour. Pneumothorax occurs following about 25 per cent of procedures, with some 5 per cent requiring a chest drain. Small haemoptyses are a common complication.

Thoracoscopy

Visualization of the parietal and visceral pleura plays an important part in the diagnosis of effusions and pleural tumours. Biopsy of lesions can be carried out under direct vision, and absence of pleural tumour is important in decisions about resectability of a lung tumour. Thoracoscopy is inadvisable in the absence of effusion or pneumothorax, and is unsatisfactory in the presence of empyema or gross haemothorax. However, in otherwise operable tumours with a pleural effusion that is not bloodstained and without positive cytology or pleural biopsy, thoracoscopy may be a useful next step in determining operability. Video-assisted thoracoscopy (VATS) has extended this technique and will also permit inspection and sampling of suspicious mediastinal lymph nodes.

Computed axial tomography (CT)

Thoracic CT scanning is important in the staging of lung cancer. It can identify the site, size, and extension of the primary tumour far more clearly than conventional radiology. It also frequently identifies mediastinal lymphadenopathy when posteroanterior and lateral chest radiographs fail to show any abnormality. Mediastinal lymphadenopathy on CT is arbitrarily taken to be pathological by most centres if the glands are greater than 1.0 cm in transverse diameter. However, previous infective conditions such as tuberculosis or an associated distal pneumonia can cause appearances identical with that of malignant enlargement. Thus positive CT scans of the mediastinum must be confirmed preoperatively by mediastinal lymph node biopsy (mediastinoscopy) to confirm tumour involvement.

Another potential advantage of CT is its ability to detect tumour invasion of the surrounding pleura and chest wall, in addition to the mediastinum itself. However, not all tumours with CT evidence of invasion prove unresectable, and if possible invasion of the mediastinum or chest wall appears the only contraindication to resection, then thoracotomy should be performed.

The predictive value of a negative CT is of the order of 90 to 95 per cent, and in such cases a mediastinoscopy can be omitted before thoracotomy. However, microscopic invasion of normal-sized mediastinal nodes is increasingly reported in patients with adenocarcinoma of the lung. Perhaps patients with this cell type should undergo mediastinoscopy routinely, irrespective of whether the mediastinal lymph nodes appear normal in size on a staging CT scan.

Positron emission tomography (PET) scanning

PET scanning shows promise, particularly in identifying the nature of a solitary pulmonary nodule, showing uptake in mediastinal nodes involved by tumour, and in assessing extrathoracic spread. When used in addition to CT, unsuspected metastases have been identified in up to 30 per cent of cases, changing management in up to 40 per cent of cases. The procedure is expensive and has limited availability but might become the final staging test where CT scans fail to show evidence of metastatic disease.

Lung function testing

The ability to climb one flight of stairs without breathlessness has been claimed to be a very good indication of fitness for resection, but formal evaluation of lung function is essential in all patients for whom surgery is being considered. Simple spirometry is usually adequate, but it may be necessary to evaluate exercise capability in a more sophisticated manner. Pneumonectomy should probably not be undertaken if the patient cannot sustain a forced expiratory volume in 1 s (FEV1) of more than 1.2 litres, bearing in mind that patients who have coexistent chronic obstructive airflow disease may not sustain their usual value during exacerbations. In borderline cases, the risk of resection is a matter requiring careful judgement based on estimation of maximum tolerable resection and assessment of the functional integrity of the non-tumour-bearing lung. A combination of pulmonary function tests, including the 6-min walking test and regional function studies using xenon-133, may be used in patients with borderline function. However, as lung cancer is such a serious disease, consideration may sometimes have to be given to carrying out resection in patients whose physical performance defies the results of pulmonary function tests.

Other investigations

In general, the ability to identify small metastatic deposits is as unsatisfactory for lung carcinomas as for other solid tumours. The available techniques are relatively crude, and this partially explains the high extrathoracic relapse rate following so-called 'curative' resections for non-small-cell lung cancer. In patients with no symptoms other than those caused by their primary tumour, imaging scans of brain, liver, and bones are unhelpful if there is no clinical evidence of neurological, hepatic, or bony disease and normal biochemistry. CT brain scans have a high accuracy in detailing cerebral metastases in patients with neurological symptoms. In patients with a palpable liver and/or abnormal liver function tests, a liver CT scan or ultrasound should be performed. CT scan of the upper abdomen identifies abnormalities of one or both adrenal glands in up to 10 per cent of patients considered for surgery. Fine-needle aspiration of the adrenal gland should be performed if this remains the only contraindication to pulmonary resection. Bone scans have a high false-positive rate due to Paget's disease, active arthritis, healing fractures, renal disease, and hyperparathyroidism. However, a bone scan should be ordered in patients with bone pain, local tenderness, or non-specific symptoms of weight loss or malaise.

Biopsy or cytology aspiration of enlarged lymph nodes and skin metastases should be carried out whenever indicated. If an isolated hepatic or bony lesion identified with isotope or CT scanning appears to be the only

contraindication to surgery, this should be biopsied under radiological control.

The staging investigations for non-small-cell lung cancer are summarized in Fig. 8. The final procedure before thoracotomy is assessment of the mediastinum, since this may be involved in up to 50 per cent of patients with a peripheral, poorly differentiated tumour and in a much greater percentage of centrally occurring lesions. If CT scanning is normal, the surgeon can proceed directly to thoracotomy. If the CT scan is abnormal or is not available, mediastinal exploration should be performed first. Cervical mediastinoscopy in patients who appear radiologically operable on conventional films will demonstrate mediastinal lymph node involvement in 10 to 15 per cent of cases considered for surgery. Left anterior mediastinotomy can provide further information. This involves an approach through the bed of the second left costal cartilage to palpate glands draining tumours from the left upper lobe.

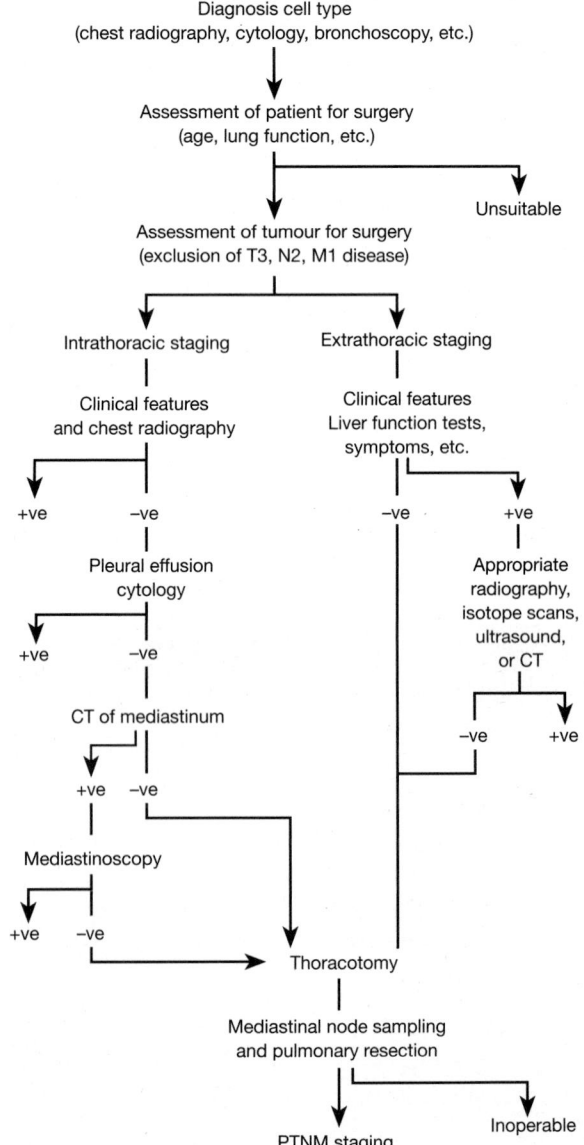

Fig. 8 Preoperative staging of non-small-cell lung cancer: +ve, positive; –ve negative; PTNM staging, postsurgical pathological staging. (Reproduced with permission from Spiro and Goldstraw, 1984.)

Treatment and prognosis of non-small cell lung cancer

Surgery

Surgery remains the single modality most likely to be curative in non-small-cell lung cancer. Prior to surgery the patient should have been carefully staged (Fig. 8), and the chances of long-term survival will be greatly influenced by this. All patients with stage IIIB disease (Table 5) should be rejected for thoracotomy, but those with stage I, II, and some with IIIA disease can be resected. In general, patients with squamous-cell carcinomas have higher 5 and 10-year survival rates than those with adenocarcinoma and large-cell carcinomas, and the more differentiated the tumour the better is the prognosis. Table 6 summarizes survival data at 5 years for preoperatively staged non-small-cell lung cancer. Clearly, small peripheral lesions with no nodal disease fare best (up to 70 per cent survival at 5 years), but the survival rate decreases with both size of tumour and increasing involvement of hilar nodes.

In all, approximately 20 per cent of patients who present with non-small-cell lung cancer eventually come to thoracotomy. Most of the others are excluded almost immediately because of clinically evident metastatic disease, radiological or bronchoscopic evidence of inoperability, too advanced an age to withstand surgery, significant associated other illnesses, or inadequate lung function. Of those having a 'curative' resection, the overall survival rate at 5 years is approximately 25 per cent and at 10 years is 16 to 18 per cent. Death from local or distant recurrence of the tumour is equally probable, highlighting the inadequacies of current staging techniques. However, the careful application of the TNM system and the advent of more sophisticated scanning equipment may lead to improvement.

Only very rarely is there an indication for palliative surgery, and resection should not be considered in the presence of intrathoracic or distant metastasis. There are diametrically opposed views as to whether surgery should be undertaken in Pancoast tumours.

Advanced age is not a contraindication to surgery. Patients over 70 years of age appear to tolerate lobectomy as well as younger patients, although the mortality for pneumonectomy (8–10 per cent) is double that of those under 70. There is no evidence that tumours grow more slowly in the elderly, and therefore the disease is as likely to be the terminal event in the aged as in younger patients. Hence resection should be encouraged in fit patients. Smokers should be persuaded to stop smoking before thoracotomy; continued smoking increases perioperative complications.

Thoracoscopic resection of peripheral masses is currently reserved for those with inadequate lung function for lobectomy, as hilar and mediastinal node evaluation and dissection is not always possible. The cure rates for segmentectomy by video-assisted thoracic surgery is less good than by open thoracotomy and lobectomy with lymph node dissection.

Radiotherapy

Patients who are excluded from surgery because of adverse prognostic factors, advanced stage of tumour, or other coincidental disease constitute the largest group treated with radiotherapy. Although the usual aim of radiotherapy will be palliative, there will be a small group of patients in whom more aggressive therapy will be used in the hope of cure, or at least long-term survival, particularly in those who have refused surgery. Radiotherapy for lung cancer is limited by the comparative radiosensitivity of three critical normal tissues likely to be included in the radiation beam: normal lung, spinal cord, and heart, each of which has a critical tolerance dose. Increased radiation dose leads to greater killing of tumour cells but may produce unwanted damage to normal cells. Radiation dose must be expressed not only in terms of total dose but also numbers of fractions and overall time. There is no clear evidence for an optimum radiation dose, but doses of 5000 to 6000 rad (50–60 Gy) in 5 to 6 weeks are appropriate; higher doses will be associated with unacceptable morbidity.

The role of radiotherapy

Alternative to surgery

In some patients with a technically resectable tumour, there may be medical contraindications for resection or the patient may refuse surgery. In general, the results of radical radiotherapy in these patients are inferior to the 5-year survival following surgery. The best result for radiotherapy was a 5-year survival rate of 22 per cent for peripheral squamous-cell cancers, but other series post a 5-year survival rate of 6 per cent.

Preoperative radiotherapy

Preoperative radiotherapy has been attempted in a few uncontrolled studies, but there is no evidence that this approach improves survival.

Postoperative radiotherapy

A recent meta-analysis has shown no benefit from postoperative radiotherapy for stage I and II disease. Any value in stage IIIA disease with nodal involvement is not as clear, but benefit is likely to be small.

Radical radiotherapy for locally inoperable disease

In otherwise fit patients with small-volume intrathoracic disease which is not resectable, usually because of mediastinal involvement, it is common practice to attempt to cure with radiotherapy. Results with daily single fractions are disappointing, even with doses of up to 60 Gy, with 5-year survival rates ranging from 5 to 17 per cent.

Recently, continuous hyperfractionated accelerated radiotherapy (CHART), with three fractions a day for 12 consecutive days to a total of 54 Gy have been compared to conventional radiotherapy in non-small cell lung cancer. CHART gave an absolute improvement in 2-year survival from 20 per cent to 29 per cent, with the greatest benefit (14 per cent absolute improvement) in squamous cell cancers. This appears a real advance in the provision of radiotherapy for locally advanced, inoperable tumours.

Palliation

The value of radiotherapy in palliating certain symptoms is beyond dispute. Haemoptysis and cough, two of the most distressing symptoms, can

Table 6 Cumulative percentage surviving 5 years and median survival by clinical and surgical TNM subsets

TNM subset	Clinical			Surgical		
	No.	Percentage surviving	Median survival (months)	No	Percentage surviving	Median survival (months)
T1 N0 M0	591	61.9	60	429	68.5	60
T2 N0 M0	1012	35.8	26	436	59.0	60
T1 N1 M0	19	33.6	20	67	54.1	60
T2 N1 M0	176	22.7	17	250	40.0	29
T3 N0 M0	221	7.6	8	57	44.2	26
T3 N1 M0	71	7.7	8	29	17.6	16
Any N2 M0	497	4.9	11	168	28.8	22

be controlled by radiotherapy in up to 80 per cent of cases. Administration of single fractions (each of 8.5 Gy, 1 week apart) appears adequate. Dyspnoea from bronchial obstruction and dysphagia are relieved in the majority of cases. The syndrome of superior vena caval obstruction is relieved in about 80 per cent of sufferers, but usually requires a more conventional course of five to ten fractions of radiotherapy. Pain from bone secondaries can be relieved in more than 50 per cent of sufferers by a single fraction of 8 Gy, often given at the same time as a clinic visit. Brain metastases generally respond poorly to radiotherapy. A 48-h trial of dexamethasone, 4 mg orally four times daily, is recommended as initial management. If a worthwhile response follows the resolution of the oedema surrounding the metastases, then radiotherapy will consolidate this gain. The steroids should then be rapidly withdrawn on completion of radiotherapy. Spinal cord compression is a relatively common occurrence associated with vertebral body metastatic disease. Pain and bony tenderness often precede it and may be helpful in localizing the lesion. Responses to radiotherapy are usually incomplete and disappointing, often because of interruption of the vascular supply to the spinal cord by the tumour.

Chemotherapy

Several cytotoxic agents show activity against non-small cell lung cancer, but much less frequently than with small-cell tumours (Table 7). However, combination chemotherapy can achieve impressive response rates; partial responses in 50 per cent of patients with locally advanced disease and in 35 per cent of those with advanced extrathoracic disease have been reported. The most active regimens include: cisplatin, ifosfamide, and mitomycin; or cisplatin, mitomycin, and vindesine. A meta-analysis of all controlled studies randomizing patients to receive or not receive chemotherapy in addition to surgery, radiotherapy, or to best supportive care was published in 1995. This suggested a 5 per cent advantage for the addition of chemotherapy to surgery (confidence intervals −1 to 7 per cent), a smaller non-significant advantage for the addition of chemotherapy to radiotherapy, and a 10 per cent improvement in survival at 1 year for the addition of chemotherapy to best supportive care. Many institutions are attempting to confirm these encouraging data. In advanced disease, chemotherapy only confers a survival advantage of 6 to 8 weeks compared to best supportive care alone, making evaluation of effects on quality of life important. Thus chemotherapy in non-small cell lung cancer is still recommended to be given within clinical trials. The place of the newer agents such as carboplatin, vinorelbine, gemcitabine, the taxols, and campotethecins are being evaluated.

Table 7 Objective average response to single-agent chemotherapy in lung cancer

Drug	Response (%)	
	Small cell	Non-small cell
Ifosfamide	63	23–36
Vincristine	42	0–23
Epipodophyllotoxin	40	0–40
Cyclophosphamide	33	20–33
Methotrexate	30	12–30
Adriamycin	30	15–25
Cisplatin	35	13–20
Topotecan	40	13–40
Irinotecan	–	20–41
Paclitaxol	40	21–25
Docetaxol	–	21–25
Vinorelbine	–	14–33
Gemcitabine	35	21–25

Treatment and prognosis of small-cell lung cancer

Small cell lung cancer is separated from the other types of lung cancer because of its very different biological and clinical features. It has an explosive growth pattern so that the TNM staging classification makes no impact on prognosis or survival, almost certainly because careful staging puts most patients into the inoperable category and because small metastases remain undetected for a few months. However, simple staging has some prognostic impact and those with limited disease (tumour confined to one hemithorax and the ipsilateral supraclavicular fossa) fare better than those with extensive disease (involvement of any site outside the hemithorax). The life expectancy of those with untreated small-cell lung cancer is about 3.5 months for limited disease and 6 weeks for extensive disease.

Prognostic factors

Multivariate analyses of large patient populations show that routine biochemical values such as serum sodium, albumin, and alkaline phosphatase allow separation of prognostic subgroups. In addition, performance status and extent of disease are important influences. For instance a good performance status and normal biochemical values (i.e. a good prognostic category) has a 2-year survival rate of 20 per cent, yet a correspondingly low performance status with one or more abnormal biochemical parameters (poor prognosis) has virtually no 2 year survivors (Fig. 9). Women tend to do better than men and those under 60 better than those over 60 years of age. These factors are helpful both for stratification within clinical studies and for identifying those patients likely to do well with chemotherapy and those for whom intensive toxic chemotherapy would appear inappropriate. Survival beyond 5 years (cure) is achieved in 4 to 12 per cent of patients with limited disease and in hardly anyone with extensive disease at diagnosis. Most studies of long-term survival report late deaths due to other cancers, including non-small-cell lung cancers in up to 30 per cent of these long-term survivors.

Surgery

In small-cell lung cancer the very occasional patient can be surgically cured, usually those presenting with a peripheral tumour and no evidence of local spread or metastasis despite extensive staging investigations. These patients are rare, but nevertheless have a 5-year survival rate in the region of 30 to 40 per cent.

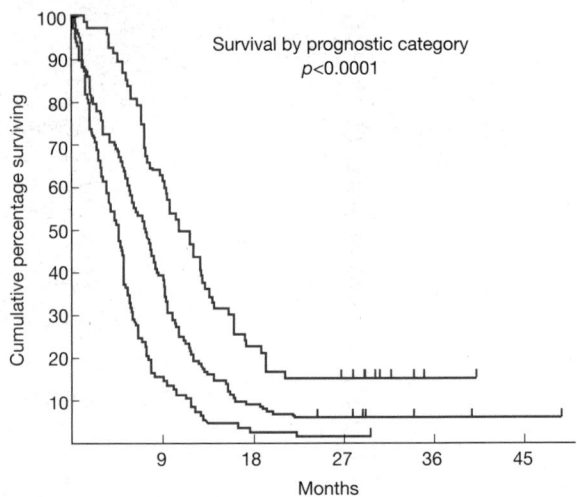

Fig. 9 The effect of prognostic grouping in survival in small-cell lung cancer. The upper curve represents good prognosis patients; the lower two curves are intermediate and poor prognosis groups respectively.

Radiotherapy

Radiotherapy has an important role in palliation of symptoms that may develop after relapse following chemotherapy. However, in approximately 15 per cent of patients with limited disease, there is a small but definite benefit when thoracic irradiation is added to combination chemotherapy. Chest irradiation also significantly decreases the rate of recurrence at the primary tumour site and in the mediastinum. A total dose of 40 to 50 Gy is usually given. The optimal timing of radiotherapy in relation to chemotherapy is not clear, but the trend is in favour of early radiotherapy given concurrently with chemotherapy. However, acute and late toxicity are both increased when radiotherapy and chemotherapy are given in combination.

Cranial irradiation

Cranial metastases are common. Ten per cent of patients in remission develop brain metastases as their first site of relapse. Prophylactic cranial irradiation given at the end of chemotherapy will delay the presentation of cerebral metastases and also reduce their overall incidence. However, there is no evidence of prolonged survival, and those who receive prophylactic cranial irradiation are at greater risk of late neurological complications—particularly psychometric and psychological impairment. However, the morbidity of cerebral metastases is so great that it seems helpful to attempt to prevent this socially disastrous form of relapse.

Chemotherapy

Small-cell lung cancer is much more sensitive to cytotoxic chemotherapy than the non-small-cell lung cancer tumours, with a much higher response rate for several cytotoxic drugs (Table 7). In the late 1970s, there was a very rapid improvement in median survival using combinations of three and four drugs, but responses have subsequently reached a plateau. Nevertheless, with modern combination cytotoxic treatment, which is usually given on an outpatient basis every 3 weeks, the median survival has been extended to 14 to 18 months for limited disease and to 9 to 12 months for extensive disease. Most combinations include etoposide, cisplatin, cyclophosphamide, doxorubicin, and vincristine. Modern regimens would be expected to achieve a complete response rate (i.e. disappearance of all measurable disease) in 40 to 50 per cent of cases and a partial response rate (greater than 50 per cent reduction in tumour bulk) in a further 40 per cent, giving a total response rate of 80 to 85 per cent. All these regimens have side-effects. Most patients will experience some nausea and vomiting, and alopecia is practically universal. Life-threatening septicaemia occurs in 1 to 4 per cent, but treatment-related deaths are uncommon.

Much effort has been applied during the last 5 years to improve the median and long-term survival of patients with small-cell lung cancer. In general, those patients in whom further progress is to be made are those who present with limited disease and a good performance status. Patients with extensive disease tend to have a universally bad prognosis and very few survive beyond 2 years. However, it seems that some metastatic sites (bone and bone marrow) are not as sinister as others (brain or liver) and the occasional patient with extensive disease does well with chemotherapy, but in general treatment is offered in this circumstance for palliation and not in the hope of cure. Studies assessing the quality of life in patients presenting with small-cell lung cancer have shown that over 70 per cent have important symptoms such as weight loss, malaise, bone pain, dyspnoea, and haemoptysis. The majority of these patients have extensive disease, but after 3 months of chemotherapy symptoms can be relieved in 60 to 70 per cent of sufferers, making chemotherapy worthwhile, with symptomatic benefits far outweighing the potential side-effects. Ten per cent of small-cell lung cancer patients present with superior vena caval obstruction: this responds as well as any presentation to chemotherapy.

Intensity of treatment

Intensifying the dosage or the frequency of administration of cytotoxic agents has been thoroughly explored without real benefit on median survival. Small advantages are occasionally seen, but these have to be balanced by the increased toxicity resulting from a more aggressive approach. Attempts to overcome or delay the emergence of cell resistance to chemotherapy have involved alternating combinations of drugs, but these more complicated regimens have not been rewarding either.

Duration of treatment

Toxicity of chemotherapy increases with the number of courses given. It is now apparent that most of the tumour response to chemotherapy occurs within the first two or three cycles. Studies attempting to minimize the duration of chemotherapy without adversely affecting survival have shown that six courses of combination chemotherapy, that is a course every 3 weeks, is optimal, with no benefit from maintenance regimens.

General management of patients with lung cancer

There are certain complications which require specific measures to alleviate symptoms.

Patients who seem likely to survive for 6 months or more and who have vocal chord paralysis find considerable help from an injection of Teflon into the affected chord which restores voice production in a high percentage of cases and reduces the risk of aspiration. Occurrence of upper airway obstruction causing stridor, or obstruction of the lower major airways, in non-small-cell lung cancer patients is usually initially treated with radiotherapy. Should this complication recur or be unsuitable for radiotherapy, it can sometimes be treated by laser photocoagulation administered either via a fibreoptic bronchoscope or under general anaesthetic via a rigid instrument. Laser therapy for carcinoma of the bronchus is most suitable as a palliative treatment in central tumours occluding large airways. There are technical limitations to its application via the flexible bronchoscope, but removal of considerable quantities of tumour can be achieved in a single treatment session with the rigid instrument. Laser therapy is used predominantly for recurrence of tumour in the central airways, usually after radiotherapy has failed. Trials are in progress assessing the additional benefits of endobronchial radiotherapy (brachytherapy) using iridium or caesium wires delivered via the fibre optic bronchoscope. This procedure irradiates endobronchial tumour to a circumferential depth of about 1 cm, and will often produce a further remission. It is used where further external beam radiotherapy cannot be given because of the risk of exceeding normal tissue tolerance.

Infection distal to tumour requires antibiotic therapy and, where appropriate, oxygen therapy and bronchodilators. Severe, recurrent haemoptysis may be controlled by radiotherapy or laser.

Malignant pleural effusion recurs after aspiration unless the pleural space is obliterated. Chemical pleurodesis can be induced by intrapleural instillation of a number of agents or by the more invasive procedure of talc pleurodesis. Intrapleural tetracycline is most commonly used, giving successful pleurodesis in 50 to 70 per cent of patients. However, the increasing availability of thoracoscopy makes a talc pleurodesis preferable in all reasonably fit patients who can undergo a general anaesthetic.

Dexamethasone, 4 to 16 mg orally daily, may control the symptoms of brain metastasis and, if so, this should be consolidated with radiotherapy to prevent severe steroid-induced myopathy. Prednisolone, 20 mg orally daily, is often used to improve the sense of well-being, as are blood transfusion or hyperalimentation.

Terminal care is described in Section 30 , but the importance of the combined support to the patient and the family given by the family doctor, palliative care medical and nursing staff, and hospice organizations, and the hospital team cannot be overemphasized.

Prevention

Lung cancer is an almost totally preventable disease and is very largely due to smoking, particularly of cigarettes. The strategy of any preventive measures must be based on the following observations. Firstly, that lung cancer is extremely rare in non-smokers. Secondly, that there is no threshold limit below which no effect is produced, although the risk increases proportionately to the amount smoked. Thirdly, that the benefit from stopping smoking is evident within 5 years. Fourthly, that the risk for an exsmoker at any given time after stopping is determined by the length of time he or she had smoked before stopping. Thus strenuous efforts must be made to persuade people not to start smoking, to establish more effective methods of enabling people to stop smoking, and to promote further research into effective methods of health education. The promotion of cigarettes with low tar, nicotine, and carbon monoxide contents may have made a small contribution to prevention, but low-tar cigarettes are not a substitute for giving up smoking. Penal taxation by governments may also help.

The identification of occupational hazards and implementation of appropriate measures to safeguard the health of employees are clearly important preventive measures, even although the number at risk is very small.

Prospective lung cancer screening programmes in males aged 45 years and above who smoke at least 20 cigarettes per day have been carried out using both chest radiography and pooled 3-day sputum analysis every 4 months. They are unlikely to form the basis of standard practice as there is no evidence that early detection is translated into increased cure rate.

Carcinoid tumours

The slow-growing intrabronchial lesions previously grouped under the heading of bronchial adenoma have now been reclassified into bronchial carcinoids, adenoid cystic tumours, and mucoepidermoid tumours. They are not related to cigarette smoking, and tend to be diagnosed at a younger age than carcinoma of the bronchus. True bronchial adenomas derived from bronchial glands are rare. These tumours were once thought to be benign, but they are potentially and often frankly malignant, being capable not only of destructive local growth but also of metastasis to regional lymph nodes in about one-third of patients and to distant organs, particularly liver and brain, in about 10 per cent. They are occasionally located in the trachea.

The most common symptoms are cough, haemoptysis, and recurrent pneumonia, although not infrequently the lesion is discovered on routine radiographic examination before symptoms develop. In the few cases that have extensive liver secondaries, there may be the classical symptom pattern of intermittent cyanotic flushings, intestinal cramps and diarrhoea, bronchoconstriction, and cardiovascular lesions. The radiographic appearances are those of a solitary nodule, pulmonary collapse, or obstructive hyperinflation. As the majority of the tumours occur in main stem or proximal portions of lobar bronchi, bronchoscopy is usually the definitive diagnostic measure. The tumour appears as a white or pink polypoid or lobulated mass, with the bronchial mucosa appearing to be intact. Biopsy may be followed by brisk haemoptysis.

Surgical resection is the treatment of choice. In the absence of regional spread or distant metastases 5-year survival prospects are excellent, but if there is involvement of regional nodes, survival rates fall to 70 per cent. Some aggressive carcinoid tumours carry a much worse prognosis. The mechanism and management of the general symptoms of the carcinoid syndrome are described in Chapter 14.8.

Further reading

Ahrendt SA, Chow JT, Xu LH, Yang SC, Eisenberger CF, *et al.* (1999). Molecular detection of tumor cells in bronchoalveolar lavage fluid from patients with early stage lung cancer. *Journal of the National Cancer Institute* **91**, 332–9.

Bruske-Hohlfeld I *et al.* (2000). Occupational lung cancer risk for men in Germany: results from a proband case-control study. *American Journal of Epidemiology* **151**, 384–95.

Carney DN (1992). Biology of small-cell lung cancer. *Lancet* **339**, 843–6.

Coggon D, Acheson ED (1983). Trends in lung cancer mortality. *Thorax* **38**, 721–3.

Goldstraw P (1992). The practice of cardiothoracic surgeons in the perioperative staging of lung cancer. *Thorax* **47**, 1–2.

Hansen HH (1992). Management of small-cell lung cancer. *Lancet* **339**, 846–9.

Izbicki JR *et al.* (1992). Accuracy of computed tomographic scan and surgical assessment for staging of bronchial carcinoma. A prospective study. *Journal of Thoracic and Cardiovascular Surgery* **104**, 413–20.

Kaplan DK (1992). Mediastinal lymph node metastases in lung cancer: is size a valid criterion. *Thorax* **47**, 332–3.

Landreneau RJ *et al.* (1992). Thoracoscopic resection of 85 pulmonary lesions. *Annals of Thoracic Surgery* **54**, 415–19.

Mountain CF (1997). Revisions in the international system for staging lung cancer. *Chest* **111**, 1710–17.

Muers MF, Round CE (1993). Palliation of symptoms in non-small cell lung cancer. *Thorax* **48**, 339–43.

Pless-Mulloli T *et al.* (1998). Lung cancer, proximity to industry, and poverty in northeast England. *Environmental Health Perspectives* **106**, 189–96.

Saunders M *et al.* on behalf of the CHART Steering Committee (1997). Continuous hyperfractionated accelerated radiotherapy (CHART) versus conventional radiotherapy in non-small-cell lung cancer: a randomised multicentre trial. *Lancet* **350**, 161–5.

Scagliotti GV (1995). Symptoms and signs and staging of lung cancer. In: SG Spiro, ed. *Carcinoma of the lung*, European Respiratory Monograph, Vol. 1, No.1, pp. 91–137. European Respiratory Society Journals, Sheffield, UK.

Spiro SG, Goldstraw P (1984). The staging of lung cancer. *Thorax* **39**, 401–7.

Thatcher N, Ranson M, Lee SM, Niven R, Anderson A (1995). Chemotherapy in non-small cell lung cancer. *Annals of Oncology* **6** (Suppl. 1), S83–95.

Tockman MS *et al.* (1997). Prospective detection of preclinical lung cancer: results from two studies of heterogeneous nuclear riboprotein A2/B1 overexpression. *Clinical Cancer Research* **3**, 2237–46.

Wells FC, Kendall SWH (1992). Thoracoscopy: the dawn of a new age. *Respiratory Medicine* **86**, 365–6.

17.14.2 Pulmonary metastases

S. G. Spiro

Malignant metastasis to the lung may present as a solitary enlarging nodule, as multiple nodules, or with diffuse lymphatic involvement.

Solitary metastasis represents some 10 per cent of round lesions in general, but some 70 per cent of round lesions in patients with a known malignancy. Colorectal cancer is reported to be the commonest tumour of origin. Diagnosis can usually be secured by percutaneous CT-guided biopsy. In rare cases, surgical excision may prolong survival or result in cure, depending on the state of the primary tumour and the likelihood of other occult metastases. In general, the longer the interval between resection of the primary tumour and the appearance of the metastases the better the prognosis.

Multiple metastases range enormously in size and number from 'cannon balls' to miliary shadowing, and may be accompanied by hilar lymphadenopathy or pleural effusion. Breast, colon, renal, and lung primaries are probably the commonest underlying tumours, but other tumours amenable to chemotherapy, such as testicular cancer and choriocarcinoma, and also sarcomas, occur. Diagnosis may be achieved by cytology or histology on various samples from the pleura or lung and can occasionally be made from cytology on expectoration or induced sputum. Tumours that are suitable for chemotherapy (e.g. choriocarcinoma) or endocrine manipulation (e.g. breast) need to be recognized. Solitary or multiple Kaposi's sarcoma is a feature of AIDS, and can involve the bronchi and pleura as well as lung tissue.

Lymphangitis carcinomatosa is most commonly due to breast and primary lung tumours (usually adenocarcinomas). Patients can be asymptomatic when the disease is first suspected on the basis of a radiograph showing diffusely increased interstitial markings accompanied by Kerley B lines, hilar lymphadenopathy, or pleural effusion. Diagnosis may be established by cytology from sputum or pleural fluid, but often requires bronchoscopic or transbronchial lung biopsy. Later, progressive and severe breathlessness with hypoxaemia often develops, and requires vigorous palliative relief with opiate and oxygen administration.

Occasionally metastasis, presenting as haemoptysis, may be confined to a bronchus and not visible on a plain chest radiograph. Renal carcinoma and malignant melanoma are recorded causes. Diagnosis requires bronchoscopy, and radiotherapy is usually effective in controlling the haemoptysis.

Further reading

Gephardt GN (1981). Malignant melanoma of the bronchus. *Human Pathology* **12**, 671–3.

Ishida T *et al.* (1992). Metastatic lung tumours and extended indications for surgery. *International Surgery* **77**, 173–7.

Lower EE, Baughman RP (1992). Pulmonary lymphangitis metastasis from breast cancer. Lymphocytic alveolitis is associated with favourable prognosis. *Chest* **103**, 1113–17.

Ognibene FP, Masur H, Rogers P (1985). Kaposi's carcinoma causing pulmonary infiltrates and respiratory failure in AIDS. *Annals of Internal Medicine* **102**, 471–5.

Stewart JR *et al.* (1992). Twenty years' experience with pulmonary metastasectomy. *American Surgeon* **58**, 100–3.

17.14.3 Pleural tumours

M. K. Benson

Primary pleural tumours are relatively rare, although malignant mesothelioma has received much attention because of its increasing incidence and association with asbestos exposure. Pleural plaques are also associated with asbestos exposure but should not be regarded as tumours since they simply represent local areas of fibrocollagenous thickening. The classical benign tumour of the pleura is a fibrous mesothelioma (pleural fibroma).

By contrast, pleural involvement by metastatic disease is very common. It can occur with most carcinomas, but is particularly associated with primary tumours arising in the lung, breast, colon, and ovary. Malignant lymphomas can also present with pleural involvement. Tumours arising in adjacent structures, such as diaphragm and chest wall, may also involve the pleura, and both benign and malignant tumours can originate from muscle, adipose tissue, nerves, blood vessels, and bony thorax. All are rare, and the diversity of sites and types of tumour results in a variety of clinical presentations. Radiographic techniques can help to demonstrate the site and nature of the tumour, but diagnosis is usually established on biopsy.

Benign tumours

Benign fibrous mesothelioma

These tumours are rare but can occur in virtually any age group. They bear no relationship to the development of malignant mesothelioma and are not associated with exposure to asbestos or other industrial pollutant. They originate from a pedicle, usually from the visceral pleura. Macroscopically they are firm, lobulated, and well encapsulated. The cut surface is white or grey and can have a whorled appearance. They vary in size, but can on occasions be very large, weighing up to 2 or 3 kg.

The tumours are often discovered on routine chest radiology in otherwise asymptomatic individuals (Fig. 1). Large tumours can cause chest discomfort and breathlessness, presumably due to compression of adjacent lung. Spontaneous hypoglycaemia is an associated feature in a small proportion of patients.

Radiologically, it can be difficult to decide whether a nodule arises from the pleura or within adjacent lung. The differential diagnosis includes a localized area of pleural thickening, a whorled nodule, although this generally has a less clearly defined outline. The diagnosis is usually established only after surgical excision. Although a fibrous mesothelioma is benign, with no potential for metastatic spread, there is a possibility of local recurrence if the pedicle has not been completely excised.

Pleural plaques

These are areas of fibrocollagenous thickening. They produce no clinical symptoms and are usually detected on routine chest radiographs. They can be single or multiple and are best seen in oblique projection or using tomography. Although associated with asbestos exposure, they are entirely benign and should not be regarded as precursors to the development of a malignant mesothelioma.

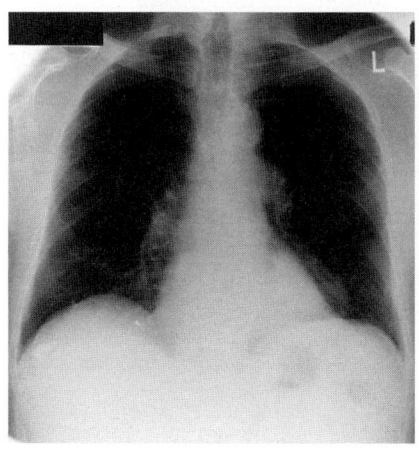
(a)

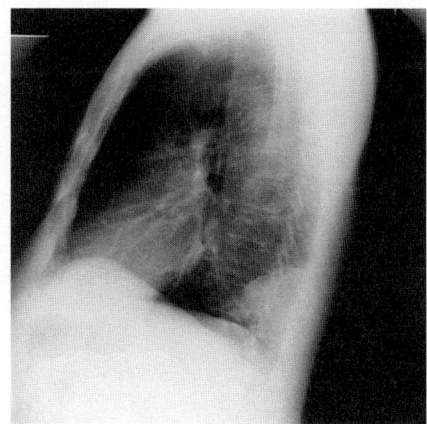
(b)

Fig. 1 Chest radiographs, posteroanterior (a) and lateral (b), showing a pleural-based nodule at the left base. The patient had no respiratory symptoms and resection confirmed this to be a benign fibrous mesothelioma.

Malignant tumours

Malignant mesothelioma

Malignant mesothelioma derives from mesothelial cells, most commonly in the pleura, but also in the peritoneum or (rarely) pericardium. Malignant mesothelioma arising from the pleura was first recognized in the 1950s, and during the 1960s much evidence accumulated indicating a strong link between the condition and exposure to asbestos. Asbestos is a collective term given to a group of silicate minerals, commercially useful because of their heat resistant properties, and widely used in industry for the past 100 years. In addition to asbestos exposure, there has been recent interest in the possible role of Simian virus 40 (SV40) in the aetiology of mesothelioma. This oncogenic virus was a contaminant of polio vaccines used in the 1950s, and SV40-like DNA sequences have been found in pleural mesotheliomas, although it is not clear what this means.

Epidemiology

There is overwhelming evidence that mesotheliomas are caused by asbestos, and the higher incidence in men indicates that most exposure is occupational rather than environmental. The risk is a function of the concentration of fibres and duration of exposure. Fibre type is also of relevance, since although most asbestos workers have been exposed to a mixture of fibres, there is good evidence that crocidolite (blue asbestos) is more hazardous than chrysotile (white asbestos). Exposure is greatest in those involved in mining or quarrying the material and those who handle the raw fibres. Significant exposure has also occurred in individuals employed in the manufacture and use of asbestos-containing products. Many workers engaged in the ship-building industry in the 1940s and 50s were exposed to asbestos, and more recently there has been widespread use in the building industry.

The increasing incidence of mesothelioma is a reflection of the long latent interval between exposure and the development of disease. It is rare for mesotheliomas to develop within 20 years of exposure and most patients were initially exposed 30 or more years before clinical presentation. In the United Kingdom, although the risk was first recognized in the 1960s, it was not until the mid-1970s that there was a significant reduction in exposure to asbestos. Current mesothelioma rates are a quantitive indication of previous population exposure. The increasing rates in the United Kingdom are predicted to continue for the next 20 years, with annual deaths increasing from the current levels of approximately 1100 to 2000 per annum. Men born between 1945 and 50 are those at greatest risk. Similar trends are also being seen in much of Western Europe, although in North America mortality rates may have already peaked because of earlier measures to limit asbestos exposure.

Low levels of environmental contamination have been shown to result in a slightly increased risk of mesothelioma, although it has been estimated that the annual incidence in subjects with no clear history of asbestos exposure is about 1 per million. Endemic pleural mesothelioma has been reported from certain areas of central Turkey, Cyprus, and Greece. Locally mined zeolite and other environmental asbestos minerals are regarded as responsible.

Pathology

A mesothelioma can arise from either the visceral or parietal pleura, initially as a local mass, often associated with pleural effusion. As it progresses, there is gradual encasement of the lung and extension into adjacent structures including the chest wall, mediastinum, and pericardium. Macroscopically, the tumour is usually white and fibrous in texture, sometimes with areas of necrosis. Metastatic disease is relatively uncommon, but involvement of the contralateral lung and pleura, liver, and bone are recognized sites for secondary spread.

The histological diagnosis can be difficult as there are a variety of appearances, ranging from well-differentiated epithelial or sarcomatous patterns to undifferentiated forms. Even after biopsy there can be difficulty in distinguishing between a malignant mesothelioma and benign pleural disease on purely morphological grounds. A second problem is differentiation between mesothelioma and secondary adenocarcinoma. Histochemistry, immunohistochemistry, and electron microscopy can also provide useful information when there is diagnostic uncertainty.

Clinical presentation

The age of presentation is usually between 50 and 70, although incidence is increasing in older patients. There is a male predominance, reflecting the greater likelihood of previous occupational exposure, which should be sought with a careful lifetime occupational history. Symptoms due to local disease are mainly those of pain and breathlessness. Pain may be pleuritic in nature, but is often a dull ache due to direct involvement of the chest wall. Shortness of breath is usually associated with a pleural effusion, although as the tumour progresses is gradually encases the lung. Systemic symptoms include tiredness, anorexia, weight loss, fever, and occasionally drenching sweats. Finger clubbing has been recorded but is rare. Physical findings in the chest are those of a pleural effusion, but with advanced disease there is progressive reduction in chest wall movement. Direct extension through the chest wall can result in a palpable mass, and this may develop at the site of previous biopsy.

Investigations

A chest radiograph often demonstrates a pleural effusion, with tumour suspected if there is pleural thickening with a lobulated outline (Fig. 2). This can be more easily identified on CT scanning, which can also be used as a staging procedure. Magnetic resonance imaging gives similar information. The presence of benign pleural plaques offers evidence of previous asbestos exposure, although they are not in themselves precursors of malignant change.

Pleural aspiration with cytological examination of pleural fluid yields a definitive diagnosis in up to a third of patients. There is further modest diagnostic yield from percutaneous needle biopsy. Samples obtained under direct vision, either at thoracoscopy or thoracotomy, have the highest diagnostic yield, with thoracoscopy being the investigation of choice. In some instances, it may be appropriate to make a diagnosis solely on the basis of clinical and radiological features, since even with histological confirmation there is unlikely to be any alteration in management. However, it is important to note that malignant mesothelioma is an industrially notifiable disease for which the patient and family can receive financial compensation.

Treatment and prognosis

A variety of treatments have been used for patients with mesothelioma, but rates of cure are uniformly disappointing. Surgical resection employing extrapleural pneumonectomy has its advocates, but reports are of highly

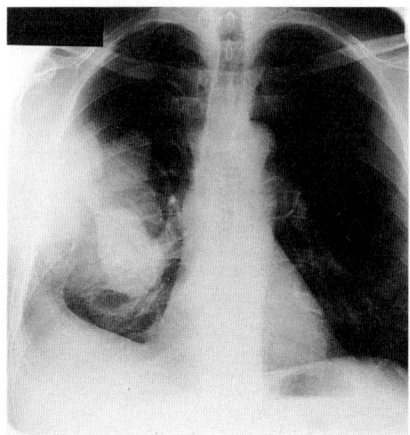

Fig. 2 Chest radiograph showing lobulated pleural thickening due to mesothelioma.

selected patients with no satisfactory control group. There is significant perioperative morbidity and mortality, with median survival figures in the range of 10 to 20 months. Response to radiotherapy is also disappointing, although occasionally palliative relief of pain can be achieved when there has been direct extension into the chest wall. It may also prevent seeding along a biopsy tract. A variety of cytotoxic agents have been tried, either as single agents or in combination, but so far without any convincing success.

Relief of pain usually requires regular opiates, although nerve blocks may also be helpful for localized pain. Pleural aspiration and pleurodesis is of benefit for the relief of breathlessness due to recurrent pleural effusions.

The prognosis is poor with the median survival of approximately 12 months. A few patients seem to have fairly indolent disease and may survive for periods of up to 5 years.

Further reading

Aisner J (1995). Current approach to malignant mesothelioma of the pleura. *Chest* **107**, 332S–44S. Review of treatment options for malignant mesothelioma.

Anthony VB *et al.* (1992). NHLBI workshop summaries, pleural cell biology in health and disease. *American Review of Respiratory Disease* **145**, 1236–9. Workshop overview of pleural cell biology and responses to injury and repair.

Curran D *et al.* (1998). Prognostic factors in patients with pleural mesothelioma; the European Organisation for Research and Treatment of Cancer experience. *Journal of Clinical Oncology* **16**, 145–52. Prospective study of 204 patients with mesothelioma identifying factors influencing prognosis.

Hubbard R (1997). The aetiology of mesothelioma: are risk factors other than asbestos exposure important? *Thorax* **52**, 496–7. Brief review of possible factors in non-asbestos-related mesotheliomas.

Ong ST, Vogelzang NJ (1996). Chemotherapy in malignant pleural mesothelioma: a review. *Journal of Clinical Oncology* **14**, 1007–17. Review of 55 phase two clinical studies using both single agent and combination chemotherapy for the treatment of malignant mesothelioma.

Peto J *et al.* (1999). The European mesothelioma epidemic. *British Journal of Cancer* **79**, 666–72. Elegant analysis linking current and future trends in mesothelioma mortality to prior asbestos exposure.

Rebak J, Selikoff IJ (1992). Survival of asbestos insulation workers with mesothelioma. *British Journal of Industrial Medicine* **49**, 732–5. Epidemiological study in individuals working in the asbestos industry.

17.14.4 Mediastinal tumours and cysts

M. K. Benson

The mediastinum encompasses those structures within the thorax, excluding the lungs. The superior boundary is the thoracic inlet represented by a plane at the level of the first rib. The inferior boundary is the diaphragm. Traditionally, the mediastinum is subdivided into a number of compartments: superior and inferior, with the latter being subdivided into anterior, middle, and posterior divisions. However, there are no true anatomical boundaries, and structures in the superior mediastinum are in general contiguous with those inferiorly. Thus a more logical subdivision is simply into anterior, middle, and posterior compartments (Figs 1 and 2). Such a division can help to compartmentalize complex anatomical arrangements and give some guide as to the most likely pathology occurring in any particular area.

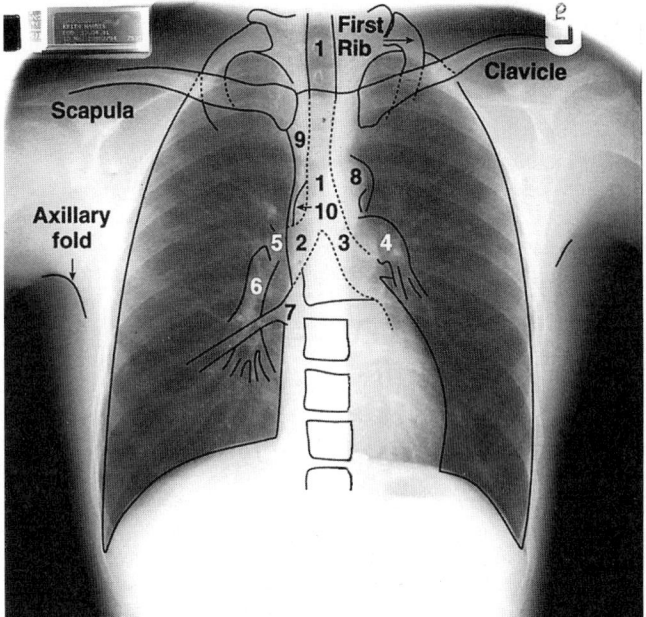

Fig. 1 Posteroanterior chest radiograph with diagrammatic overlay to illustrate normal mediastinal structures: (1) trachea, (2) right main bronchus, (3) left main bronchus, (4) left main pulmonary artery, (5) right upper lobe pulmonary vein, (6) right interlobar artery, (7) right lower and middle lobe vein, (8) aortic knuckle, (9) superior vena cava, (10) azygos vein.

The anterior mediastinum is bounded anteriorly by the sternum and posteriorly by the pericardium, aorta, and brachiocephalic vessels. It contains the remnant of the thymus gland, branches of the internal mammary artery, veins, and associated lymph nodes. The middle mediastinum contains the pericardium, ascending aorta and aortic arch, the vena cavae, the brachiocephalic vessels, and the pulmonary arteries and veins. It also

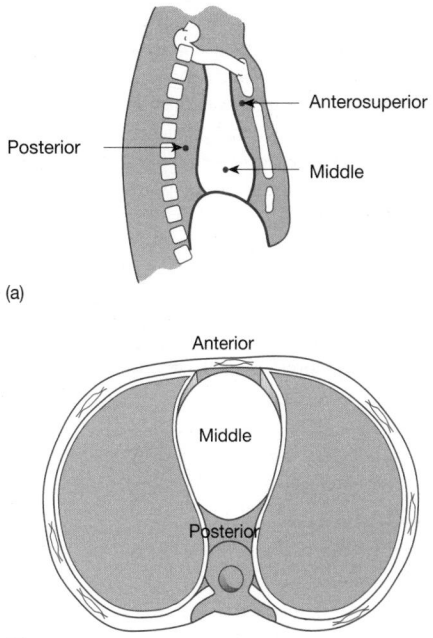

Fig. 2 A schematic representation of the mediastinal compartments: (a) lateral projection showing division into anterior (or anterosuperior), middle, and posterior compartments, (b) cross-sectional depiction.

encompasses the trachea and major bronchi with their associated lymph nodes, the phrenic nerves, and the vagus nerve. The posterior mediastinum is bounded anteriorly by the pericardium, laterally by the mediastinal pleura, and posteriorly by the vertebral bodies, including structures in the paravertebral gutter. It contains the descending thoracic aorta, oesophagus, azygos veins, thoracic duct, lymph nodes, and autonomic nerves.

Lymph nodes are common to all three compartments and knowledge of their anatomical relationships, together with sites of drainage, is helpful in interpreting an abnormal chest radiograph with mediastinal enlargement. The most important group of visceral nodes lie in the middle mediastinum and are predominantly subcarinal and paratracheal. Bronchopulmonary or hilar nodes are numerous but are not visible radiographically unless pathologically enlarged.

Diagnostic approach

The finding of a mediastinal abnormality on chest radiograph, whether or not accompanied by specific clinical features, is usually an indication for further investigation. Computed tomography (CT) provides accurate localization of mediastinal masses. It can define their relationship to and displacement of normal structures, and may be able to define lines of demarcation, particularly if there is adjacent fatty tissue. It is not ideal for determining the composition of any particular mass, although it can demonstrate heterogeneity or the presence of calcification. Contrast enhancement can be used to identify vascularity. Magnetic resonance imaging has relatively little to offer over and above CT scanning, the one exception being in the assessment of spinal tumours.

Fine-needle aspiration biopsy is valuable in the investigation of pulmonary masses, but is of more limited use in assessing those in the mediastinum. The presence of a cyst can be confirmed by aspiration of clear fluid. Anterior mediastinal masses can easily be approached percutaneously, although cytological examination alone may be insufficient for diagnosis. Anterior mediastinotomy allows open biopsy of such lesions. This is performed through an incision in the neck and allows inspection of structures surrounding the superior vena cava and trachea as far as the carina. It is particularly useful for obtaining lymph node biopsies when surgery for lung cancer is contemplated. Bronchoscopy is of limited value in the evaluation of mediastinal masses, except when there is a suspicion of a bronchial neoplasm or possible lymphadenopathy due to sarcoidosis. Neural tumours arising in the posterior mediastinum usually require surgical resection and there is little to be gained by preceding this with fine-needle aspiration.

Clinical features

General considerations

It is not surprising that the diversity of anatomical structures in the mediastinum is reflected in an equally diverse range of neoplastic, developmental, and inflammatory masses (Table 1). Whilst clinical symptoms and signs may give diagnostic clues, a significant proportion of mediastinal masses, particularly those which are benign, tend to be asymptomatic and are usually detected on routine chest radiography.

Mediastinal masses in children are more likely to be malignant than those in adults. There have been a large number of studies documenting the relative frequency of different causes of primary mediastinal tumours and cysts: neurogenic and thymic tumours are the commonest (approximately 20 per cent each), followed by lymphoma, reduplication cysts, germ cell tumours, and thyroid masses.

Non-specific, constitutional symptoms such as fever or weight loss are more likely to occur with malignant tumours such as lymphomas or thymomas. The commonest symptoms are cough and chest pain, arising as a consequence of distortion of normal mediastinal anatomy. Compression of vital structures can also result in specific symptoms. Thus, tracheal or bronchial compression leads to breathlessness with stridor or wheeze; oesophageal narrowing results in dysphagia; and superior vena caval compression produces the characteristic features of facial and periorbital oedema, chemosis, and distended veins. Involvement of the recurrent laryngeal nerve results in hoarseness and a bovine cough; whilst this usually results from a malignant tumour, it can also occur with benign lesions such as aneurysm of the aortic arch. Involvement of the sympathetic chain as it emerges in the upper mediastinum is also likely to be due to malignant infiltration and results in Horner's syndrome with enophthalmos, miosis, ptosis, and unilateral facial anhidrosis. Compression of intercostal nerves can produce neuralgia, and intraspinal extension of tumours lead to long tract signs.

Anterior mediastinal masses

Thymus

The normal thymus is located in the superior portion of the anterior mediastinum. Its main function is the production of T lymphocytes. Radiographically, the normal thymus can only be seen in infancy and regression occurs during adolescence. Enlargement of the thymus is the commonest single cause of an anterior mediastinal mass. It can be due to the development of a thymoma, thymic hyperplasia, or a thymic cyst. In addition, the thymus can be a site of involvement by lymphoma, particularly Hodgkin's disease.

Table 1 Mediastinal masses

Anterior compartment	Middle compartment	Posterior compartment
Thyroid	Pericardium	Oesophagus
goitre	cysts	gastroenteric cyst
carcinoma	Vascular	leimyoma
Thymus	aneurysm	Vascular
thymoma	anomalous vessels	aneurysm
hypoplasia	Bronchogenic cysts	Neural tumours
cyst	Lymph nodes[1]	neurilemmoma
lymphoma	sarcoidosis	neurofibroma
Germ cell tumours	infections	malignant shwannoma
dermoid cyst	(tuberculosis)	ganglioneuroma
seminoma	lymphoma	neuroblastoma
non-seminoma	metastatic cancer	phaechromocytoma
Parathyroid adenoma	Castleman's disease	

[1]May be present in more than one compartment.

Thymomas are neoplastic proliferations of the thymus gland, with peak incidence in middle age. They are often benign, but can behave in a malignant fashion, with invasion of adjacent structures and distant metastases, in which case localized symptoms of chest pain and cough are more common. Systemic symptoms that can occur in association with thymic tumours are of particular interest. Myasthenia gravis is the commonest, occurring in some 30 per cent of patients. Other rare associations include red cell aplasia, hypogamma–globulinaemia, systemic lupus erythematosus, and polymyositis.

The majority of thymomas are slowly growing, lobulated masses that are well encapsulated. In these patients surgical resection can be expected to be curative. Local invasion is not common, but often precludes complete resection and recurrence is the rule. Adjuvant radiotherapy or chemotherapy has been used in such patients with debatable benefit.

Thymic cysts are uncommon. They can be unilocular or multilocular and usually contain straw-coloured fluid. The majority of patients are asymptomatic, but since cystic change can occur in some thymomas and in Hodgkin's disease, thorough cytological examination of the cyst's contents and wall must be carried out to exclude malignant disease.

Thymic lymphoma is fairly frequent, particularly in patients with Hodgkin's disease. The histological picture is usually of the nodular sclerosing variety, and the presence of mediastinal or hilar nodes should alert the clinician to the possibility of a lymphoma.

Germ cell tumours

This group of neoplasms includes tumours that are identical to certain testicular and ovarian neoplasms, and thought to be derived from primitive germ cells which have migrated to the mediastinum during oncogenesis.

Benign teratomas (dermoid cysts) consist of a disorganized mixture of ectodermal, mesodermal, and endodermal tissues, which can include skin, hair, cartilage, bone, epithelium, and neural tissue. They often contain cystic areas and CT appearances give a strong clue to the diagnosis. Unless there is a substantial contraindication to surgery, they should be excised to prevent further expansion and to exclude malignant change.

Malignant germ cell tumours are classically divided into seminomas and teratomas, although biopsy often reveals a spectrum of malignant tissue. Non-seminomatous germ cell tumours (malignant teratoma) can range from well-differentiated to trophoblastic. They are associated with elevated serum levels of β-human chorionic gonadotropin and α-fetoprotein, which can be used both diagnostically and to monitor response to treatment. Seminomas tend to be non-secretory. Both types of tumour are very malignant and invade adjacent mediastinal structures. They are not curable by surgery, but both are responsive to chemotherapy using cisplatin-based regimes, although results are disappointing when compared with their testicular counterparts, with response rates ranging from 30 to 70 per cent.

Thyroid masses

Retrosternal extension of an enlarged thyroid represents one the commoner causes of a mass in the superior mediastinum. The majority are multinodular benign goitres, arising in the neck and extending into the mediastinum through the thoracic inlet. They may contain cystic areas, sometimes with haemorrhage and areas of calcification. Radiographically, they have a sharply defined and often lobulated outline. Whilst they rarely cause symptoms, compression of the trachea at the thoracic inlet can result in respiratory distress and is an indication for surgical resection. Thyroid cancer can also involve the mediastinum, either by direct extension or by metastases to intrathoracic nodes.

Middle mediastinal masses

Lymphadenopathy

Enlarged nodes are not confined the middle mediastinum although this represents the commonest site of intrathoracic lymphadenopathy. Reactive changes occur in association with many pulmonary infections, although nodes are not grossly enlarged and are often undetected on plain chest radiograph. Gross lymphadenopathy is a feature of tuberculosis and also occurs in histoplasmosis. Other common causes of significant lymph node enlargement include metastatic carcinoma, lymphomas, and sarcoidosis.

Giant follicular lymph node hyperplasia (Castleman's disease) is rare but merits specific mention (Fig. 3). Its aetiology is unknown and it is not clear whether it represents a focus of lymphoid hyperplasia or has an infectious origin. The lesion consists of a vascular tumour with satellite lymphadenopathy. Two histological subgroups are described, (1) a more common hyaline vascular picture with lymphoid follicles and penetrating capillaries, and (2) a plasma cell type characterized by sheets of plasma cells between germinal centres. Both types can result in symptoms from local pressure, but the plasma cell type also causes systemic symptoms with fever, anaemia, and weight loss. There are no diagnostic radiographic features. The picture is simply one of a solitary mass and the diagnosis is usually made after surgical resection or biopsy. The condition is regarded as benign, but a small group of patients with multicentric disease have progressive hyperplasia, recurrent infections, and subsequently develop a frank lymphoma.

Mediastinal cysts

Cysts within the mediastinum are a relatively common cause of a mediastinal mass. They can arise in association with the pericardium, bronchi, gut, or thoracic duct. The majority of patients are asymptomatic.

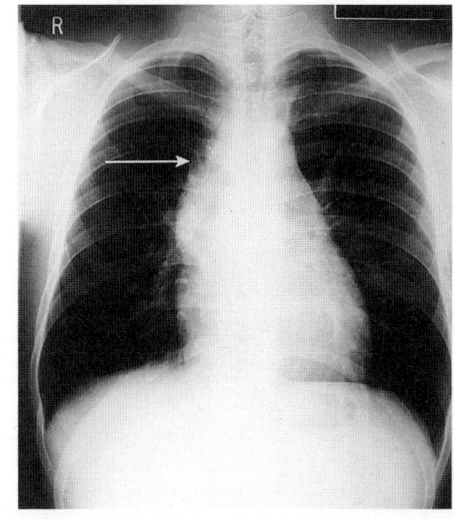

(a)

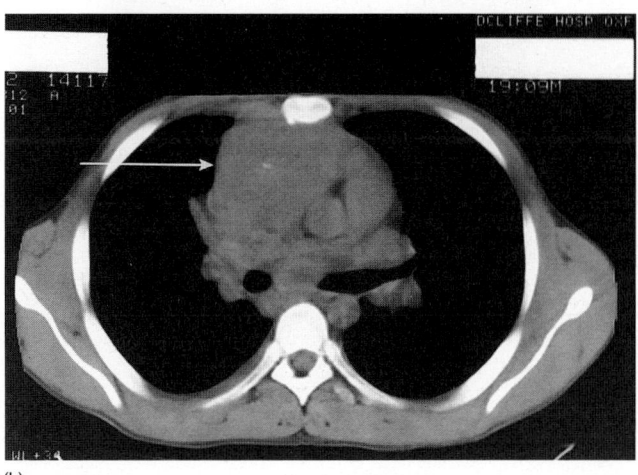

(b)

Fig. 3 Chest radiograph and CT scan showing large anterior mediastinal mass which on histology showed features of Castleman's disease.

Pericardial cysts develop embryologically in relationship to the pericardium, although direct communication with the pericardial sac is rare. Radiographically they appear as smooth, clear, demarcated densities that can be mistaken for a pericardial fat pad or a hernia through the foramen of Morgagni. Aspiration reveals clear fluid. Surgical excision is not recommended.

Bronchogenic cysts arise in association with the major airways and are lined by respiratory epithelium. They may contain inspissated mucus. Local pressure on the trachea or bronchi can result in cough or wheezing. Occasionally the cysts communicate with the trachea, and when this is the case there is an increased tendency to recurrent infections. Surgical excision is recommended, particularly if there are associated symptoms (Fig. 4).

Reduplication cysts may also be associated with the oesophagus and can be lined by gastric or oesophageal mucosa.

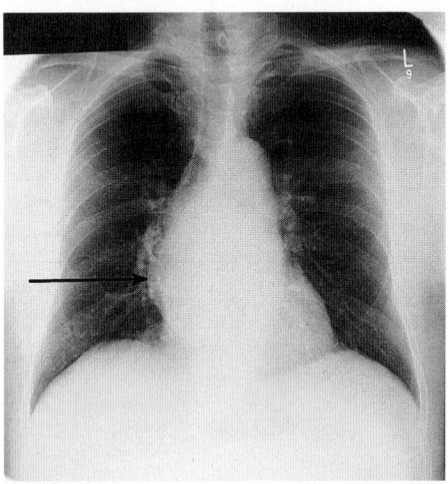

(a)

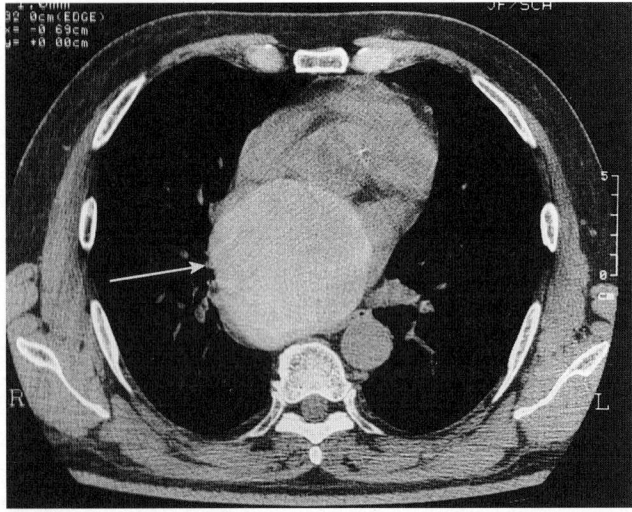

(b)

Fig. 4 Chest radiograph and CT scan showing a large mass in the mediastinum. This is a large bronchogenic cyst, present for 20 years, and finally removed when compression of the oesophagus resulted in dysphagia.

Posterior mediastinal masses

Oesophageal lesions and aneurysms of the descending thoracic aorta can both result in abnormal shadows in the posterior mediastinum. Tumours, particularly those found in the paravertebral gutters, are likely to be neural in origin. Benign tumours tend to be asymptomatic, whilst malignant tumours cause pressure effects. Occasionally, spinal cord compression results from direct extension into the intravertebral foramen. Tumours arising from peripheral nerve cell sheaths include neurilemmoma (Schwannoma) and neurofibroma together with their malignant counterparts. Tumours of the autonomic chain include ganglioneuroma and neuroblastoma.

A neurilemmoma is the commonest neural tumour arising in the mediastinum. These are more common in middle age and can extend into the intravertebral foramen producing a dumb-bell appearance. Radiographically they can erode adjacent bone and CT scanning or MRI should be undertaken prior to surgical excision. Neurofibromata are also common. They may be solitary and the clinical and radiological features are very similar to those of a neurilemmoma. A significant proportion of patients will have neurofibromatosis. Surgical resection is recommended, in part because of the small risk of developing a malignant neurosarcoma. These tumours have a poor prognosis.

Ganglioneuroma arise from the autonomic plexus and are usually found close to the spine. Associated endocrine symptoms include hypertension, flushing, sweating, and diarrhoea. These tumours are often very large before they become clinically apparent. Prognosis is good after surgical resection. Ganglioneuroblastoma and neuroblastoma represent the malignant end of the spectrum and are predominantly tumours of infants and children. Neuroblastoma in particular is very invasive, with metastatic spread often established by the time of presentation.

Further reading

Adkins RB, Maples MD, Ainsworth J (1994). Primary malignant mediastinal tumours. *Annals of Thoracic Surgery* **38**, 648–59. Authors' experience of 38 patients presenting with mediastinal tumours together with a review of the literature.

Bower RJ, Kiesewetter WB (1977). Mediastinal masses in infants and children. *Archives of Surgery* **112**, 1003–9. Experience based on review of 93 infants and children presenting with mediastinal masses.

Davies RD Jr, Oldham HM Jr, Sabiston DC Jr (1987). Primary cysts and neoplasms of the mediastinum: recent changes in clinical presentation, methods of diagnosis, management and results. *Annals of Thoracic Surgery* **44**, 229–35. Report on series of 400 patients presenting with mediastinal tumours and cysts.

Hejna M, Haberl I, Raderer M (1999). Non surgical management of malignant thymoma. *Cancer* **85**, 1871–84. Systematic review of radiotherapy and chemotherapy in treatment of malignant thymoma.

Morrissey B *et al.* (1993). Percutaneous needle biopsy of the mediastinum: review of 94 procedures. *Thorax* **48**, 632–7. Sensitivity and specificity of percutaneous biopsy techniques in the diagnosis of mediastinal tumours.

Shields TW, Reynolds M (1988). Neurogenic tumours of the thorax. *Surgical Clinics of North America* **68**, 645–68. Systematic review of clinical presentation, treatment, and prognosis in patients with intrathoracic neurogenic tumours.

Thomas CR Jr, Wright CD, Loehrer PJ Sr (1999). Thymoma: state of the art. *Journal of Clinical Oncology* **17**, 2280–9. Review article on clinical presentation, pathology, and treatment of thymoma.

17.15 The genetics of lung diseases

J. M. Hopkin

Genetic factors are important in lung biology and disease, ranging from monogenic disorders, for example cystic fibrosis, to multifactorial effects, for example those underlying the syndrome of asthma, in which there are crucial interactions between heterogeneous genetic effects and environmental factors. Subtle genetic factors are being steadily uncovered, for example those that modulate the risk of respiratory infection such as tuberculosis.

The bronchial tree

Cystic fibrosis

Cystic fibrosis is the most common fatal, autosomal recessive disease in Caucasians, with an incidence of 1/1500 and carrier frequency of 1/22. This condition is discussed in detail in Chapter 17.10.

Immotile ciliary syndrome

The immotile ciliary syndrome, or primary ciliary dyskinesia, is a rare (incidence 1/30 000), genetically heterogeneous disorder in which inheritance is usually autosomal recessive. The ciliary abnormality, especially lack of dynein arms, can normally be observed on electron microscopy of a ciliated mucosal biopsy or in spermatozoa. Impaired ciliary function results in impaired mucus clearance and leads to bronchiectasis, sinusitis (often with absence of the frontal sinuses and ear disease), and infertility in males. Kartegener's syndrome is one clinical subgroup of the immotile cilia syndrome where there is also dextracardia or situs inversus as the result of impaired organ rotation in development. Multiple linkages have been found. Loss of function mutations in dyneia chain is one cause

Atopy and asthma

Atopy is an immune disorder in which there is allergy or hypersensitivity to common antigens, such as the house dust mite and pollens, and which results in muocsal inflammation. It is one leading cause of the asthma syndrome and is characterized by exuberant Th-2 immune mechanisms and excessive production of IgE to such common antigens (see Chapter 17.4.1).

Twin studies demonstrate the shared input of genetic and environmental factors. For example the concordance in monozygotic twins for allergy to any common inhaled antigen is 71 per cent, compared with 36 per cent in dizygotic twins. Genetic searches for linkage to either high IgE levels or clinical asthma have identified a whole set of linkages on many chromosomes, thus confirming the heterogeneous genetic input. The first genetic variant shown to have both epidemiological and functional links to atopy and asthma is within the cellular receptor for the Th-2 cytokine IL-4 (IL4Rα). Substitution of isoleucine for valine in the extracellular domain of the receptor (position 50, Ile50Val) associates strongly with atopic asthma in Japanese children. In transfection experiments, Ile50Val up-regulated cellular response to IL-4 challenge and increased secretion of IgE. An amino acid charge-changing variant of another key Th-2 signalling cytokine,

IL-13, also predicts asthma and atopy in different populations. One possible benefit of unravelling the heterogeneous genetics of atopy and asthma is the tailoring of novel therapies to patients with genetic variants of specific proteins or pathways.

The pulmonary parenchyma

α_1-Antitrypsin deficiency

Emphysema is mainly the consequence of cigarette smoking, but α_1-antitrypsin deficiency is a substantial risk factor for the development of accelerated emphysema in cigarette smokers. This leads to the proteolysis hypothesis for emphysema in smokers, which proposes that proteases such as elastase are released from pulmonary neutrophils and macrophages 'excited' by cigarette smoke. The actions of elastase on supportive tissue in the lung are opposed by the serine protease inhibitor (serpin) α_1-antitrypsin. When α_1-antitrypsin is deficient, or when smoking is very heavy, then the balance falls in favour of tissue destruction and the development of emphysema. This condition is discussed elsewhere.

In deficient individuals, the most important practical point in management is absolute avoidance of cigarette smoking. Replacement of α_1-antitrypsin protein, now available as a molecular engineered product, can increase lung levels when administered by infusion or by aerosol inhalation—but trials showing major clinical impact are still awaited. In a family with an affected individual, the risk of α_1-antitrypsin deficiency in a further sibling is one-quarter: molecular prenatal diagnosis is possible. The risk to the children of carrier siblings is very small since the incidence of severe α_1-antitrypsin deficiency alleles in the population is low.

Miscellaneous rare disorders

Pulmonary alveolar proteinosis is a rare heterogeneous disorder, characterized by the accumulation of PAS positive proteinaceous material in the alveoli. It can be secondary to malignancy or infection, for example histoplasmosis. The infant form is usually fatal and in some cases is probably a genetic disease. In one family with two affected siblings there was absence of surfactant protein B and its mRNA in the alveoli but markedly increased amounts of surfactant protein C.

Rare, but striking, reports of familial aggregation of early-onset diffuse alveolitis and pulmonary fibrosis are recorded, but their molecular genetic origins are obscure. In pulmonary alveolar microlithiasis, there are multiple, minute calcifications in the alveoli producing a typical radiographic appearance. Affected sib-pairs are well described and the observation of consanguinity suggests a very rare autosomal recessive disorder of obscure molecular genetic origin.

General genetic syndromes with parenchymal lung involvement

A number of well-described genetic syndromes may display a pulmonary component.

Diffuse interstitial pulmonary infiltrates on chest radiograph are recorded in a number of 'in-born errors of metabolism'—such as Farber's lipogranulomatosis, Niemann–Pick's disease type A and Gaucher's disease types I and III. Lethal pulmonary involvement may occur in lysinuric protein intolerance. Niemann–Pick's disease is caused by mutations in the gene for acid sphingomyelinase and results in the development of abnormal 'Niemann–Pick cells' that are histocytes whose cytoplasm is filled with lipid droplets or particles. Particularly severe pulmonary involvement in Niemann–Pick type B is accompanied by infiltration of these abnormal cells into the substance of the lung and also its lymphatics and vessels. In Gaucher's disease, a lysosomal glycolipid storage disorder characterized by the accumulation of glucosyl ceramide (glucocerebroside), there are mutations in the gene on chromosome 1 encoding the enzyme β-glucosidase. Although pulmonary involvement is rare, it is severe and progressive when present; pathology shows infiltration by Gaucher monocytes/macrophage cells with their characteristic tubular cytoplasmic inclusions.

In the phakomatoses, for example neurofibromatosis or tuberose sclerosis, pulmonary involvement may be observed with pulmonary fibrosis, bulla formation, or lyomyomatosis.

In Marfan's syndrome there is an increased risk of spontaneous pneumothorax. In some subjects, apical bullae are present; more rarely, congenital cystic lung disease may be found. There is also a clear clinical impression that many young individuals presenting with spontaneous pneumothorax are rather tall and thin, whilst not having Marfan's syndrome. They may ultimately prove to have some genetically determined, mild connective tissue disorder.

The immune system

The lung is constantly exposed to the risk of infection and there are well-recognized genetic syndromes that predispose to chest infection. Many genetic variants with subtle effects on the risk of infection, for example tuberculosis, are being discovered.

Antibody deficiency may be secondary (for example to protein loss in renal or bowel disorder) or primary. X-linked and autosomal recessive forms of the latter are described and make infection with encapsulated bacteria and mycoplasmas common and severe. Variable combinations of IgA and IgG subclass and IgM deficiency are recognized. The clinical picture may be of repeated pneumonias, with typical systemic upset, or of bronchiectasis with chronic sepsis.

Severe combined immunodeficiency is a genetically heterogeneous syndrome with profound functional deficiency of both cellular (T cell) and humeral (B cell) immunity. In the X-linked form of disease, most of the mutations are in the gamma chain of the cellular receptor for the cytokine interleukin-2. Recessive disease in most cases is due to mutations in the purine catabolic enzyme, adenosine deaminase, and genotherapy may become possible in this condition. In severe combined immunodeficiency, symptoms start in infancy with failure to thrive, diarrhoea due to parasitic and viral infections, and pneumonia due to *Pneumocystis carinii*, an organism that typically requires effective T-lymphocyte function for its control.

Loss of function mutations in the receptors for Il-12 and IFN-γ signalling leads to impaired Th-1 immunity and predispose to disseminated BCG infection, and disease due to environmental mycobacteria of low pathogenicity.

Ataxia telangiectasia is a complex autosomal recessive disorder that includes variable immune deficiency, cerebellar ataxia, and a propensity to develop leukaemias; it results from mutations in ATM kinase. The Wiskcott–Aldrich syndrome includes combined immune deficiency, haemorrhage due to thrombocytopenia, autoimmune disorder, and a tendency to malignancy. The locus X-chromosome encodes for a protein (WASP) that is important in the actin-based cytosketon.

Chronic granulomatous disease is associated with recurrent pyogenic infection of the respiratory tract, skin, and lymphoid tissue by catalase-positive bacteria and fungi. It is genetically heterogeneous. Oxygen-dependent microbial killing is crucial in phagocytes and the process is mediated by a multicomponent NADPH oxidase; the four major oxidase components being encoded at different chromosome locations—1q, 7q, 16p, and Xp. The most frequent form is X-linked and due to mutation in the gene for the large subunit of cytochrome b. Another important property of the phagocyte is accumulation at the site of infection, which is dependent upon the cell's adhesive properties and mobility. In leucocyte adhesion deficiency, an autosomal recessive condition, there are mutations in the CD18 gene, which codes for the β2 integrin subunit.

The complement system plays an essential role in the propagation of inflammation and host defence. Deficiencies have been described for many of its components. Deficiency of C3, an autosomal recessive, increases susceptibility to encapsulated bacteria because of the deficiency of C3b-dependent opsonization.

The vascular system

Pulmonary embolism

Pulmonary embolism, from venous thrombosis, is a common and important pulmonary syndrome. Genetic deficiencies, causing thrombophilia underlie the disorder in some individuals, particularly those with early-onset of disease, unusual sites of venous thrombosis, and recurrent disease.

Miscellaneous rare syndromes

Pulmonary arterial venous fistulas can be single or multiple and may be sporadic or genetic disorders. They can occur as part of the Osler–Rendu–Weber (hereditary haemorrhagic telangiectasia) syndrome. This is a genetically heterogeneous autosomal dominant in which the pulmonary lesions are usually multiple and asymptomatic but can bleed and cause haemoptysis, breathlessness, and chest pain. There are a number of reports of primary pulmonary hypertension clustering in families. This is rare and its mechanism, if distinct from a thrombotic tendency, is unknown.

Neuromuscular disorders affecting pulmonary function

Many genetic syndromes of the neuromuscular system can cause secondary respiratory insufficiency or failure, with a tendency to recurring chest infection because of impaired coughing. The most notable are the muscular dystrophies (for example the X-linked recessive Duchenne muscular dystrophy), dominantly inherited myotonic dystrophy, and autosomal recessive acid maltase deficiency (type II glycogenosis). In acid maltase deficiency, diaphragmatic involvement is common and patients sometimes present with respiratory failure.

Pharmacogenetics

Idiosyncratic reactions to various therapeutic drugs are well recognized and cause a great range of pulmonary disorders. The response of patients to therapeutic agents administered for lung disease also varies in terms of both therapeutic benefit and toxicity. A number of factors underlie such behaviour—including age, state of nutrition, hepatic function, and renal function. In a significant proportion, there may be discrete underlying genetic causes, but relatively few have been well characterized.

The cytochromes P450 are a large family of haemoproteins that metabolize foreign chemicals, including therapeutic drugs and some carcinogens, as well as some endogenous compounds such as steroids. Genetic polymorphisms influence their function and hence the response to drugs; debrisoquine and phenytoin are well described. Genetic polymorphism is also recognized at the locus for NAT2 encoding *N*-acetyltransferase. These polymorphisms or variants of NAT2 influence the rate of acetylation and therefore detoxification of isoniazid; slow acetylators are at risk of drug-related neuropathy (due to accumulated isoniazid) or hepatitis (thought to be due to production of a toxic isoniazid metabolite through an alternative biochemical pathway). Slow acetylators therefore need lower doses of medication to achieve a therapeutic effect and to avoid toxicity. The genetic variants of NAT2 can now be recognized by direct and simple PCR based assays; they are most commonly found in Asian populations.

Tumour genetics

Many potent carcinogens are also potent mutagens, suggesting that malignant transformation is based on heritable mutations in somatic cells. Cigarette smoke is a particularly powerful mutagen, containing a great range of chemical mutagens including aromatic hydrocarbons, nitrosamines, and pyrrholized amino acids.

There are varying sites and types of somatic mutation underlying malignancy, including visible chromosomal rearrangements and discrete mutations at 'oncogene' loci encoding cellular growth factors and their receptors, and growth regulators. For example in both small-cell and non small-cell carcinomas of the bronchus somatic mutations in the gene for P53, an important growth regulator, are well described. Mutations in the cellular oncogene K-*ras* are found in adenocarcinomas of the lung.

Germline mutations are also important in influencing risk of tumour development in a number of ways—for example through pre-existent mutations in an oncogene or through variant metabolism of carcinogens. Thus polymorphisms of P4501A1 (which metabolizes polycyclic aromatic hydrocarbons) and of P4502E1 (which metabolizes nitrosamines) are associated with increased risk of lung cancer in smokers.

Microbial genetics

Respiratory infection is of massive, world-wide importance. The molecular genetics of the diverse organisms are being defined and the essential genetic foundations for pathogenicity and response to antimicrobial drugs are being clarified.

In antibiotic resistance, a number of genetic mechanisms have been identified. Antibiotic inactivating enzymes are an important mechanism and involve β-lactams, macrolides, and chloramphenicol, for example β-lactamase production by *Haemophilus influenzae*. This kind of resistance can be transferred between bacteria by gene transfer on plasmids.

Change of target is another mechanism, for example mutation in bacterial cell wall peptidoglycans inhibits penicillin binding in *Streptococcus pneumoniae*. In one form of resistance of *M. tuberculosis* to isoniazid, there are mutations in the *InhA* gene (whose protein mediates mycolic acid metabolism and hence cell wall structure), resulting in impaired binding of isoniazid to the target enzyme.

A third mechanism involves bacterial mutations that limit antibiotic penetration through the cell wall; this is thought to occur in the lipoproteins of the cell wall of pseudomonas species and causes reduced permeability and hence resistance to β-lactams and aminoglycosides.

Detailing the molecular genetics of respiratory pathogens offers important practical gains. For example organism-specific DNA sequences can be used as powerful diagnostic tools whose specificity and sensitivity are impressive when linked to *in vitro* DNA amplification. Successful PCR diagnostic assays have been developed for a number of pulmonary pathogens, including *Pneumocystis carinii*. Rapid DNA diagnostics can be used also to identify specific mutations that predict antibiotic resistance. DNA vaccines may become very effective immunizers for intracellular pathogens such as the influenza virus or *M. tuberculosis*, since the microbial DNA is taken up by cells and, following incorporation and expression, presented 'more naturally' to the immune system.

Further reading

Bartsch H *et al.* (2000). Genetic polymorphism of CYP genes, alone or in combination risk modifier of tobacco-related cancers. *Cancer Epidemiology, Biomarkers and Prevention* **9**, 3–28.

Ciba Foundation (1997). *Antibiotic resistance: origins, evolution, selection and spread*. John Wiley and Sons, Chichester.

Shirakawa T *et al.* (2000). Atopy and asthma: genetic variants of Il-4 and Il-13 signalling. *Immunology Today* **21**, 60–4.

Stevenson FK, Rosenberg W (2001). DNA vaccination: a potential weapon against infection and cancer. *Vox Sanguis* **80**, 12–18.

Toloza EM, Roth JA, Swisher SG (2000). Molecular events in bronchogenic carcinoma and their implications for therapy. *Seminars in Surgery and Oncology* **18**, 91–9.

Winf C (2001). Do delta F508 have a selective advantage? *Genetic Research* **78**, 41–7.

17.16 Lung and heart–lung transplantation

K. McNeil

Introduction

The first successful heart–lung transplant in 1981 heralded lung transplantation as a viable therapeutic option for endstage cardiopulmonary and pulmonary lung disease. The successful introduction of single and bilateral lung transplantation in the late 1980s led to greater availability of donor organs, with a consequent expansion in the number of potential recipients. Over 12 000 lung and heart–lung procedures have been performed over the past 18 years, with steadily improving results. Patients can now realistically expect a survival of 5 or more years and there is every prospect that these results will continue to improve.

The lung allograft is unique in that it remains in contact with the external environment, exposing it directly to numerous potential infections and allergens, which predispose to many of the problems encountered immediately post-transplant and in the longer term.

The major obstacles faced by lung transplant programmes are the shortage of suitable donor organs, the need to find more selective (less toxic) methods of immunosuppression, and the means to either prevent or reduce the impact of chronic allograft dysfunction.

The transplant process

The five factors which constitute the transplant process are recipient selection, donor selection, donor/recipient matching and the surgical procedure, immediate post-operative care, and long term follow-up.

Recipient selection

From the 'pulmonary' point of view, recipient suitability is determined by two factors—the underlying disease indication and the severity of that disease. Virtually any endstage pulmonary disease is amenable to transplantation. Most suitable diseases are confined to the thorax, although there are a number of systemic diseases with pulmonary manifestations where carefully selected patients can be transplanted successfully.

The diseases fall into four main categories: septic lung diseases (cystic fibrosis, bronchiectasis), obstructive lung diseases (emphysema/chronic obstructive pulmonary disease, asthma, obliterative bronchiolitis), fibrotic lung diseases (cryptogenic fibrosing alveolitis, sarcoidosis, fibrosis related to drug reactions, occupational exposures, acute lung injury, etc.), and pulmonary vascular diseases (primary pulmonary hypertension, Eisenmenger's syndrome). In addition, a number of other conditions such as lymphangioleiomyomatosis, histiocytosis, and even bronchoalveolar cell carcinoma have been treated successfully with transplantation.

Patients are usually listed for transplantation when their survival is estimated to be less than 2 years and there are no further medical or alternative therapies available. For patients with cystic fibrosis, primary pulmonary hypertension, and cryptogenic fibrosing alveolitis, prognostic indices are available to guide appropriate timing for referral and listing for transplantation. By contrast, it has become apparent that the survival of patients with Eisenmenger's syndrome and emphysema is the same on the waiting list as following transplantation. In this setting, transplantation is performed primarily for quality of life issues. Table 1 summarizes referral recommendations based on the guidelines used at Papworth Hospital, United Kingdom.

Contraindications are well defined. Most are relative, and considered in the context of the patient's overall status. Older patients have a poorer outcome, particularly with the more extensive surgical procedures. Thus, for heart–lung transplantation the upper age limit is usually 55 years, whereas for single and bilateral transplants the limit is usually set at 60 years. Recipients well above these limits have, however, been transplanted successfully.

Well-controlled diabetes and low-dose steroid therapy are no longer considered exclusion criteria. Significant coexisting kidney or liver disease precludes isolated thoracic organ transplantation, but selected patients can be considered for combined thoracic and abdominal organ transplants. Pleural disease (previous pleurectomy, infection, etc.) must be considered carefully because of the increased risk of bleeding. Patients with antibiotic-resistant organisms such as *Burkholderia cepacia* are at increased risk of perioperative sepsis and death, and different units will have individual policies on their suitability for transplantation.

Active malignancy (excluding localized squamous and basal cell carcinomas of the skin), major psychosis, extrapulmonary infection, severe malnutrition, and significant extrathoracic organ dysfunction are considered absolute exclusion criteria. Mechanical ventilation is an absolute contraindication in some units, but this does not generally include non-invasive or ambulatory support.

Donor selection

As the shortage of donor organs increases, criteria for acceptance of donor organs has liberalized. All donors are brainstem dead and should be free of systemic infection or disease. Lung allograft donors are generally less than 55 years of age, although there is an increasing trend to accept organs from older donors with acceptable results. Lung allograft suitability is based on function (gas exchange and compliance) and appearance (macroscopic, bronchoscopic, and radiographic). Haemodynamic performance and the macroscopic appearance of the coronary arteries determine the cardiac status of the heart–lung donor. Echocardiography and angiography are sometimes used but are not routinely available at every donor hospital.

Following acceptance of the allograft, matching of the donor organ with a suitable recipient is based on ABO blood group and size. Size matching is determined by comparing predicted donor total lung capacity (based on height, age, and sex) with measured and/or predicted recipient total lung capacity. Perfect size matching is rarely achieved but significant (more than 10 per cent) oversizing should be avoided because of the resultant lung compression and atelectasis. Conversely, undersizing of 10 to 20 per cent is easily accommodated by the natural compliance of the lung(s).

Surgery

There are three basic options when replacing diseased lung tissue—single-lung transplantation, bilateral sequential single (double) lung transplantation, and heart–lung transplantation. The choice of procedure is determined by the recipient's underlying disease. Diseases involving both the heart and lungs such as Eisenmenger's syndrome and endstage primary pulmonary hypertension are usually treated with heart–lung transplantation. Septic lung diseases such as cystic fibrosis and bronchiectasis require replacement of both lungs (bilateral lung transplantation or heart–lung transplantation). Most other diseases can be treated with single-lung transplantation.

Single-lung transplantation involves a pneumonectomy followed by implantation of the allograft with anastomoses of the main bronchus, pulmonary vein, and pulmonary artery. Bilateral lung transplantation is performed as two sequential single-lung transplants. These are performed via either a sternotomy or bilateral thoracotomy, with or without cardiopulmonary bypass. Heart–lung transplantation mandates cardiopulmonary

bypass and is performed via a sternotomy. Implantation is performed with tracheal, aortic, and atrial anastomoses.

The surgery must be performed meticulously. Careful dissection avoids damage to important structures such as the phrenic and recurrent laryngeal nerves and minimizes the chance of bleeding. Careful implantation reduces the risks of anastomotic complications. Ideally, implantation and reperfusion should be completed within 6 h.

Postoperative care

The first 24 to 48 h are critical to the long-term outcome of the transplant as well as for the survival of the recipient, and a principal aim of immediate postoperative care is to reduce allograft injury during this critical period.

The allograft inevitably sustains endothelial injury because of ischaemia and preservation, causing a breakdown of the capillary–endothelial barrier, resulting in leakage of fluid into alveoli. Increasing damage leads to a progressive impairment in gas exchange. This may necessitate prolonged mechanical ventilatory support, with an increased risk of infection and barotrauma often resulting in irreversible damage to the allograft.

The main principles of postoperative care of the lung transplant recipient are detailed below.

Early extubation

In the majority of patients, extubation is possible within 12 h of the procedure (in many cases much earlier than this). Extubation permits active coughing and clearance of secretions, institution of enteral nutrition, and early commencement of rehabilitation.

Fluid (crystalloid) restriction and diuresis

During the first 24 to 48 h, restriction of crystalloid intake and promotion of diuresis minimize the development of the pulmonary oedema characteristic of ischaemia-reperfusion injury. Crystalloid intake is limited to 1500 ml/day during this time. Colloid solutions are used for haemodynamic requirements.

Early mobilization

Patients with endstage lung disease are usually debilitated and in poor condition. It is therefore vitally important they are mobilized as early as possible. This improves appetite and sleep, and prevents complications such as basal atelectasis and deep venous thrombosis. Most patients are able to sit out of bed within 24 h and can participate in a gymnasium program by day 3. Adequate analgaesia is imperative for effective rehabilitation at this early stage.

Nutrition

The early institution of adequate calorie intake is necessary to overcome the severe catabolism stimulated by surgery. This is particularly important in patients with a poor pretransplant nutritional state. In most cases, enteral feeding can be started within 24 h (orally or via a nasogastric or percutaneous gastrostomy tube). If the gut is not functioning, parenteral nutrition should be used.

Prevention of infection

Bacterial infection remains the most significant early problem and is responsible for most deaths during the perioperative period. In most cases the organism is recipient derived. Antibiotic prophylaxis is administered until the patient is mobile, all drains have been removed, and respiratory secretions are clear. The underlying disease and/or pretransplant microbiology results dictate the choice of antibiotic. In cystic fibrosis and other septic lung diseases the antibiotics used cover *Pseudomonas aeruginosa* and *Staphylococcus aureus*. In other patients, community acquired respiratory pathogens (pneumococcus, haemophilus, etc.) and *Staphylococcus aureus* are targeted.

Fungal infection in the form of oropharyngeal candidiasis is common post-transplant and prophylaxis with topical nystatin or amphotericin is

Table 1 Disease-specific indications for lung transplantation

Underlying disease	Characteristics for referral for transplant assessment
Obstructive lung disease/non-cystic fibrosis bronchiectasis	FEV_1 < 25% predicted without reversibility Respiratory failure Cor pulmonale Severely limited quality of life (NYHA class III–IV dyspnoea)
Cystic fibrosis	The following parameters are associated with a 2-year survival on the waiting list of 20%. Adolescent females with rapidly declining lung function should be referred early FEV_1 < 25% predicted Respiratory failure Severely reduced exercise capacity: ≤ 500 m on a 12 min walk Compromised nutrition: BMI ≤ 17
Primary pulmonary hypertension	The following parameters are associated with a median survival of only 12 months, and an overall survival of < 20% at 3 years. Patients requiring increasing doses of prostacyclin should also be referred for assessment Mean right atrial pressure > 15 mmHg Mixed venous oxygen saturation < 60% Cardiac index < 2.0 l/min/m²
Eisenmenger's syndrome	Severely compromised quality of life Refractory right heart failure Frequent presyncopal or syncopal events Poorly controlled arrhythmia
Cryptogenic fibrosing alveolitis	These patients often deteriorate rapidly, with up to a 50% death rate on the waiting list. Consequently, they should be referred early. Gas transfer values < 60% predicted are indicative of advanced disease Progressive disease/failure of immunosuppression Respiratory failure NYHA class III dyspnoea

Abbreviations: FEV_1, forced expiratory volume in 1 s; BMI, body mass index; NYHA, New York Heart Association.

effective. Systemic prophylaxis against candida is not generally necessary. Aspergillus is the commonest cause of invasive fungal disease, and in single and bilateral lung transplantation, nebulized amphotericin (5 mg three times a day) given for the first month post-transplant is effective in reducing aspergillus-related problems. Routine use of itraconazole prophylaxis is dependent on local policy and experience. It is very uncommon for heart–lung transplantation recipients to have problems with aspergillus in this period as the tracheal anastomosis is not ischaemic, and all diseased lung tissue is removed. Routine prophylactic strategies are therefore not required.

Viral infections (specifically herpesviruses) tend to occur later in the recovery period but prophylaxis must be administered from the early stages to be effective. Ganciclovir is very effective in reducing both the incidence and severity of cytomegalovirus and other herpesvirus related illness, but there is no consensus on the optimal prophylaxis regimen. Most units opt for a combination of intravenous and oral therapy for 1 to 3 months, given to any recipient who is serologically cytomegalovirus-positive or who receives an allograft from a cytomegalovirus-positive donor. Herpes simplex virus commonly causes mucocutaneous infection. In the occasional cytomegalovirus-negative donor/recipient match (where ganciclovir is unnecessary) aciclovir is used for herpes simplex prophylaxis.

Cotrimoxazole prophylaxis is used to prevent both pneumocystis infection and toxoplasma reactivation. Standard therapy is 480 mg daily or 960 mg three times a week. Therapy is given for a minimum of 12 months or until corticosteroid therapy has been reduced to physiological replacement doses. If cotrimoxazole is not tolerated, nebulized pentamidine (300 mg per month) is an effective alternative.

Prevention of rejection

In lung transplantation, there are three basic phases of immunosuppression—induction, consolidation, and maintenance. The details of the exact combinations and doses of agents used vary from unit to unit. Table 2 shows a typical regimen.

Induction phase

Typically, antithymocyte globulin, azathioprine, and corticosteroids are used. Therapy commences immediately pretransplant. The use and length of induction with antithymocyte globulin is not standardized and varies with local unit policy.

Consolidation phase

This phase covers the period when stabilization of the immunosuppressive regimen is achieved. The aim is to achieve optimal immunosuppression (prevention of acute rejection) with tolerable side-effects. It is important to remember that the primary goal is to minimize acute rejection. Inevitably

side-effects do occur, but these should not determine immunosuppression levels at the expense of acute rejection. Cyclosporin is introduced and dosing modified to achieve whole blood trough levels above 350 ng/litre. This is usually achieved with doses around 10 mg/kg/day (given in two divided doses). Drug absorption in the perioperative period can be very variable, especially in cystic fibrosis patients where dosing three times a day is usually necessary to achieve satisfactory levels. Azathioprine is continued at a dose of 1 to 2 mg/kg/day, aiming for a white blood cell count of 4×10^9 to 6×10^9/litre. Prednisolone doses are gradually reduced to a maintenance level of 0.2 mg/kg/day.

Maintenance phase

This phase continues for the life of the recipient and is discussed below.

Follow-up

The thrust of management in the longer term is to maintain allograft function, and to minimize the side-effects of immunosuppression. Best lung function is usually established by 6 to 9 months post-transplant. The incidences of acute rejection and infection are highest in the first 3 months. Immunosuppression can be slowly reduced, aiming to stop prednisolone after 12 months and achieving target cyclosporin levels at this time of 150 to 250 ng/litre. Immunosuppression must, however, be tailored to individual requirements and prevention of acute rejection remains the primary goal.

Monitoring of symptoms, chest radiography, and spirometry are the basis of allograft surveillance. Small handheld spirometers enable daily home monitoring of lung function. A 10 per cent or greater fall in the forced expiratory volume in 1 s (FEV_1) prompts review and investigation of the cause.

When allograft dysfunction occurs, transbronchial biopsies are performed to diagnose the cause. Acute rejection and infection cannot be distinguished clinically, and may occur simultaneously. Histopathological diagnosis of the cause of dysfunction is therefore mandatory. Some units perform regular surveillance transbronchial biopsies, but there is no evidence that there is any advantage to this approach in terms of outcomes.

Specific complications

Lung transplantation is rarely an uncomplicated endeavour. All recipients will suffer at some stage either a complication of the process or a side-effect of medication. Surprisingly, however, most patients do not experience life-threatening or major complications until the inevitable onset of chronic allograft dysfunction.

Table 2 Immunosuppression regimen based on protocol from Papworth Hospital

Timing	Drug	Dosage
Arrival	Azathioprine	2 mg/kg orally or IV
Induction of anaesthesia	Methylprednisolone	500 mg IV infusion over 30 mins
Commencement of cardiopulmonary bypass	RATG	1–2 mg/kg. Dilute in 250 ml 0.9% saline. Run over 10 h. Premedicate with 10 mg IV chlorpheniramine
Reperfusion	Methylprednisolone	500 mg IV infusion over 30 min
Immediate postoperative period	Methylprednisolone	125 mg IV bolus. Three doses given 8, 16 and 24 h postoperatively
	RATG days 1 and 2 (premedicate with paracetamol and chlorpheniramine)	1–2 mg/kg aiming for T cells < 20% lymphocyte count
Maintenance therapy	Prednisolone	1 mg/kg/day in two divided doses, reducing by 5 mg/day to 0.2 mg/kg/day
	Azathioprine	1–2 mg/kg single daily dose. Titrate to WCC $(4–6) \times 10^9$/l
	Cyclosporin	First dose day 3. Commence 50 mg, increase 50 mg per dose to total 10 mg/kg/day in two divided doses (three times a day for CF patients). Aim for cyclosporin level of ≥ 400 ng/l (EMIT assay) by day 7

Abbreviations: IV, intravenous; RATG, rabbit antithymocyte globulin; WCC, white cell count; CF, cystic fibrosis; EMIT, enzyme multiplied immunoassay technology.

Many of the complications experienced by lung transplant recipients are common to all forms of solid organ transplantation and relate to drug side-effects (hypertension, renal dysfunction, osteoporosis, hypercholesterolaemia, etc.). The following problems relate specifically to lung transplantation.

Rejection

Rejection occurs in three distinct forms, defined by the underlying immunological events and the histological changes. Acute and chronic rejection are not defined by the timing of occurrence after transplant. Acute rejection can occur at any time, and 'chronic rejection' can occur after only 3 months. The two processes can coexist and probably have distinct immunological aetiologies.

Hyperacute rejection

This occurs within 24 to 48 h of transplantation and is caused by the presence of preformed antibodies in the recipient directed against donor HLA. Complement activation and widespread endothelial damage with vascular thrombosis result in rapid and severe allograft dysfunction, which is usually fatal. Removal of the antibodies with plasma exchange, and institution of an anti-B-cell therapy such as cyclophosphamide is the usual treatment.

Acute rejection

Almost all patients will experience at least one episode of acute rejection defined by the strict histological criteria listed in Table 3. The essential findings are a perivascular lymphocytic (predominantly T cell) infiltrate. Clinically, the patient often complains of 'flu-like' symptoms with dyspnoea and low-grade fever. In the early stages the chest radiograph may be normal or show pleural effusion and/or subtle alveolar shadowing. Left untreated, widespread alveolar shadowing and hypoxaemia occur. The diagnosis should be confirmed histologically (via transbronchial biopsy), as it is common for infection to occur simultaneously. These problems cannot be distinguished clinically.

Acute rejection is treated with intravenous methylprednisolone (0.5–1 g daily for 3 days). This is effective in the majority of cases. Steroid-resistant rejection is usually treated with either a polyclonal (ATG) or monoclonal (OKT3) antilymphocytic agent. In addition, it is also now usual to change the background immunosuppression by substituting either tacrolimus for cyclosporin or mycophenolate for azathioprine (or both).

Chronic rejection (obliterative bronchiolitis)

In lung transplantation, the term 'chronic rejection' denotes the presence of obliterative bronchiolitis. It is defined histologically (airway fibrosis and/or vascular sclerosis), not by the time of occurrence after transplant. The term 'chronic rejection' is something of a misnomer in this setting, as there are many processes (both alloimmune and non-alloimmune) that result in fibrotic obliteration of the airway lumen. The term 'chronic allograft dysfunction' is preferred: this implies the presence of obliterative bronchiolitis but does not imply an exclusively alloimmune aetiolgy.

Pathology

Obliterative bronchiolitis is a fibroproliferative scarring process, resulting in either total or subtotal obliteration of the airway lumen. In some cases, there is accompanying vascular sclerosis. Rarely, vascular sclerosis exists without airway changes

Physiology

The airway pathology translates into fixed airflow obstruction. This has enabled a non-invasive marker of the presence and severity of obliterative bronchiolitis to be developed, namely the bronchiolitis obliterans syndrome. Bronchiolitis obliterans syndrome is functionally defined by a fall in the FEV_1, as measured from a baseline average of the two best FEV_1 measurements achieved post-transplant taken at least 1 month apart. No reversible cause of the fall in lung function should be present. Table 4 summarizes the bronchiolitis obliterans syndrome grading system. It has been confirmed in a number of large series that bronchiolitis obliterans syndrome accurately reflects the presence and severity of obliterative bronchiolitis, and is widely used in clinical practice for this purpose.

Aetiology

Obliterative bronchiolitis is undoubtedly multifactorial in aetiology. Any discrete insult resulting in significant damage (e.g. aspiration, viral pneumonitis) will inevitably lead to scarring. The precise alloimmune mechanisms involved remain unknown.

There are two risk factors identified as being strongly predictive of the development of obliterative bronchiolitis—the frequency of early acute rejection and cytomegalovirus serological status. Recipients with more than two episodes of acute rejection in the first 3 months post-transplant have a threefold or higher risk of developing obliterative bronchiolitis than those with no acute rejection. Any cytomegalovirus serological positivity

Table 3 Working formulation for the classification and grading of pulmonary allograft rejection (adapted from International Society of Heart and Lung Transplantation guidelines)

A: Acute rejection. Diagnosed on transbronchial lung biopsy. At least five alveolated pieces of lung are required for confident diagnosis	**Grade 0:** no infiltrates
	Grade 1 minimal: scattered perivascular mononuclear cell infiltrates, not obvious at low magnification
	Grade 2 mild: frequent perivascular mononuclear cell infiltrates recognizable at low magnification
	Grade 3 moderate: dense perivascular mononuclear cell infiltrates usually associated with endothelialitis. Extension of inflammation into surrounding tissue
	Grade 4 severe: diffuse lymphocytic, eosinophilic, and neutrophil infiltrates with pneumocyte damage, hyaline membranes, and haemorrhage
B: Airway inflammation. Deleted in this revised classifaction	
C: Chronic airway rejection: obliterative bronchiolitis	**a: active** **b: inactive**
D: Chronic vascular rejection	Accelerated graft vascular sclerosis

Table 4 Classification of bronchiolitis obliterans syndrome (BOS)

BOS grade 0	FEV_1 > 80% baseline*
BOS grade 1	FEV_1 66–79% baseline
BOS grade 2	FEV_1 51–65% baseline
BOS grade 3	FEV_1 < 50% baseline
Histopathology	a = no obliterative bronchiolitis or no biopsy
	b = obliterative bronchiolitis demonstrated

* Baseline = average of two best FEV_1 measurements achieved post-transplant, taken at least 1 month apart.

FEV_1 = forced expiratory volume in 1 s.

confers an increased risk of developing obliterative bronchiolitis, with cytomegalovirus-negative recipients who receive organs from a cytomegalovirus-positive donor being at greatest risk.

Natural history

Obliterative bronchiolitis confers an increased risk of death, with the hazard ratio increasing with worsening bronchiolitis obliterans syndrome status. Patients in bronchiolitis obliterans syndrome grade 3 have a risk of dying six times higher than those in bronchiolitis obliterans syndrome 0. Once acquired, bronchiolitis obliterans syndrome usually progresses quickly, with a mean time for progression to the next stage or death of only 150 days. This is more pronounced in patients with frequent early acute rejection who are at risk of an even greater acceleration of their disease. The main cause of death in patients with obliterative bronchiolitis is infection. Inevitably, bronchiectasis develops in association with the obliterative bronchiolitis, with organisms such as pseudomonas and aspergillus becoming problematic.

Treatment

There are no controlled trials to guide treatment of this condition. In some cases, the disease arrests spontaneously. Augmented immunosuppression increases the risk of infection and is not usually effective. Most units now change immunosuppression early in the disease, substituting tacrolimus for cyclosporin, or mycophenolate for azathioprine. In advanced disease, numerous treatments such as methotrexate, phototherapy, and total lymphoid irradiation have been tried, but no consensus exists regarding the best course of action. If the disease progresses despite the above changes, immunosuppression is reduced in an attempt to minimize the impact of infections.

Specific infections

Cytomegalovirus

Before the introduction of ganciclovir, cytomegalovirus pneumonitis had a mortality rate of 50 per cent in cytomegalovirus-naive lung transplant recipients. This led to the matching of cytomegalovirus-negative recipients with cytomegalovirus-negative donors to prevent primary (donor acquired) infection. Ganciclovir therapy (both treatment and prophylaxis) has proven very effective in reducing both the morbidity and mortality associated with this infection.

Prophylaxis is effective in both delaying the onset of clinical infection and reducing the severity of subsequent infective episodes. In lung transplant recipients, cytomegalovirus most commonly causes pneumonitis. Cytomegalovirus syndrome describes an illness characterized by fever, malaise, and leucopenia, and may accompany target organ infections such as pneumonitis or hepatitis. Treatment is with intravenous ganciclovir (10 mg/kg/day). In cases of ganciclovir intolerance or resistance, foscarnet is used. Many patients will have cyclosporin related renal dysfunction and appropriate dose adjustments are necessary. Ganciclovir causes bone marrow suppression and severe leucopenia can occur in association with the low white cell count caused by cytomegalovirus. Antiviral therapy should be continued, and in this setting the addition of granulocyte colony stimulating factor is usually effective. Cytomegalovirus retinitis is uncommon in

lung transplant recipients and requires specialist ophthalmology review and follow-up.

Aspergillus

Aspergillus infection occurs in pulmonary and extrapulmonary forms. Extrapulmonary disease is always invasive. There are several forms of pulmonary infection, and significant differences in the timing and pattern of aspergillus infection related to the type of transplant. In single and bilateral lung transplants where the bronchial anastomosis is relatively ischaemic, aspergillus related problems tend to occur early (most within the first 3 months). In addition, there is a very high risk of developing an airway problem if aspergillus is present in this setting. By contrast, in heart–lung transplantation, the tracheal anastomosis is not ischaemic (due to a collateral blood supply from the coronary arteries), and most aspergillus related problems occur later with the onset of obliterative bronchiolitis.

Aspergillus infection of any sort must be diagnosed and treated early. Airway manifestations and early invasive parenchymal disease have a good prognosis. Late-stage or disseminated disease is usually fatal. Treatment with systemic amphotericin in high doses is used. Liposomal amphotericin B is the preferred therapy because of its much improved side-effect profile compared with the conventional preparation (CAB). This is very evident in the setting of cyclosporin induced renal dysfunction which severely limits therapy with CAB. Treatment starts at a single dose of 5 mg/kg/day. It is well tolerated and can be given via a peripheral line.

The role of azoles (primarily itraconazole) as primary treatment of aspergillus infection in this population is not established. Itraconazole is generally reserved for prolonged treatment following a course of liposomal amphotericin B, or where long-term prophylaxis is required. The latter situation usually arises when aspergillus is repeatedly isolated in the setting of an airway complication, or in the presence of obliterative bronchiolitis.

Pneumocystis

Pneumocystis infection is now an uncommon occurrence following the introduction of specific (cotrimoxazole) prophylaxis. Pneumocystis pneumonia in lung transplant recipients presents in a very different manner from pneumocystis pneumonia in AIDS patients, and if not recognized can be fatal. The onset is often insidious, with a low-grade febrile illness and mild to moderate dyspnoea, often only on exertion. Chest radiograph may be normal or show subtle alveolar shadowing, usually in the upper lobes. High-resolution computed tomography scanning shows a ground-glass pattern. Severe hypoxaemia and gross radiographic changes are uncommon. Transbronchial biopsies typically show a granulomatous pneumonitis. On occasions, the histology mimics acute rejection and if special staining is not performed the organisms will be missed. In addition, in distinct contrast to pneumocystis pneumonia in AIDS, the organism load in lung transplant recipients is very low. Pneumocysts are not usually recovered from bronchoalveolar lavage fluid, and can be very difficult indeed to find in biopsy tissue. Repeated transbronchial biopsies may be necessary to diagnose the condition. Treatment is the same as that employed in HIV infected patients, although very high-dose therapy is usually not required with the low organism loads.

Mycobacterial infection

Tuberculous mycobacterial and non-tuberculous mycobacterial disease occur at an increased frequency in lung transplant recipients when compared with the general population. Occult and old mycobacterial disease is sometimes found unexpectedly in explanted organs. In single lung transplantation, disease may remain in the native lung.

With previous inadequately or untreated tuberculous mycobacterial infection, prophylaxis with isoniazid should be considered. The use of rifampicin as a chemoprophylactic agent is not advisable because of the profound interaction with cyclosporin. If full treatment is required, standard robust antituberculous regimens are indicated, and since rifampicin has the profound effect of inducing hepatic metabolism, cyclosporin doses must be adjusted accordingly (dose increases of four- to fivefold are usually required).

Non-tuberculous mycobacterial infections tend to occur later in the post-transplant course than tuberculous mycobacterial disease. Treatment is based on ethambutol and rifampicin with the addition of a macrolide (clarithromycin or azithromycin) and ciprofloxacin. There are no data to guide the choice or length of treatment, but a minimum of 12 months' therapy is usually required, depending on the organism. Intolerance of medication is a significant problem that often limits treatment options in the longer term.

Gastrointestinal complications

Gastrointestinal problems are common after lung transplantation. They often relate to the side-effects of medication and are usually limited to upper gastrointestinal symptoms and/or diarrhoea. All patients receive antibiotics post-transplant and *Clostridium difficile* should be considered in the differential diagnosis of any case of diarrhoea or large bowel problems. Cytomegalovirus (discussed above) is the only other common infective gastrointestinal complication.

Upper gastrointestinal motility problems are common in recipients with cystic fibrosis and are exacerbated by vagus nerve damage during the procedure. All patients are prone to constipation because of immobility and drug therapy such as narcotic analgaesia. Regular laxative therapy should be used throughout the perioperative period. Cystic fibrosis patients are particularly prone to this complication, manifesting as distal intestinal obstruction syndrome. This life-threatening complication is managed aggressively with oral gastrograffin.

Bowel perforations are a catastrophe requiring urgent laparotomy for diagnosis and treatment. The signs of acute abdomen may be modified or absent in patients on steroids, and a high index of suspicion is needed to ensure rapid diagnosis and appropriate intervention. Gastrointestinal lymphoma often presents with small bowel perforation.

Pancreatitis affects a small number of patients and, unless related to gallstones, is usually fatal. Drugs such as azathioprine and prednisolone, and cardiopulmonary bypass are recognized risk factors. α_1-antitrypsin-deficient and cystic fibrosis recipients are also at increased risk. Treatment is along standard lines but there is usually rapid progression to multiorgan failure and death.

Neurological complications

Most of the neurological problems encountered post-transplant are related to cyclosporin toxicity and respond to dose reduction. Tremor and headache are very common, peripheral neuropathy less so. Diffuse cerebral oedema has occurred in a number of patients and been attributed to an idiosyncratic reaction to cyclosporin. Recipients with cystic fibrosis are particularly prone to seizures, particularly in the setting of high cyclosporin levels and/or hypertension (also a side-effect of cyclosporin). Infection of the central nervous system and lymphoma should always be considered in the differential diagnosis of central neurological symptoms.

Malignancy

Solid organ and lymphoid malignancies occur at an increased frequency, affecting up to 4 per cent of recipients. Lymphoproliferative disorders are related to the intensity of immunosuppression, and are driven by replication of Epstein–Barr virus. Most cases are focused in the allograft and most occur in the first 12 to 18 months post-transplant. Classification of these disorders is problematic. Some are clearly a polyclonal lymphocyte proliferation that usually respond to a reduction in immunosuppression and aciclovir therapy. Other cases present as lymphoma (non-Hodgkin's) and are treated with standard chemotherapy regimens. There are many cases where the disorder falls between these two extremes and treatment decisions are often very difficult. In these cases, histology is not a reliable guide to clinical behaviour or response to treatment. Patients are usually given a 1 to 2 month trial of aciclovir and reduced immunosuppression, with either non-response or progression indicating the need for chemotherapy. Reduction of immunosuppression involves decreasing cyclosporin levels by 30 to 50 per cent, stopping azathioprine, and reducing prednisolone to 10 mg or less per day. There are, however, no evidence-based data to support these recommendations, which are based on clinical experience. The prognosis of these disorders is surprisingly good, especially if confined to a single organ system. Most respond to reducing immunosuppression. In those requiring chemotherapy, complications of the treatment are largely responsible for the morbidity and mortality seen. Patients diagnosed with advanced disease invariably have a poor outcome.

The commonest solid organ tumours seen are cutaneous malignancies (squamous or basal cell carcinoma). With early diagnosis and treatment they carry a very good prognosis. By contrast, other solid organ malignancies (lung, gastrointestinal tract, etc.) carry a very poor prognosis, usually resulting in death within 3 to 6 months of diagnosis.

Airway complications

The bronchial anastomosis is prone to problems, with most units experiencing an airway complication rate of around 10 per cent. The bronchial anastomosis is devoid of its normal bronchial arterial supply, relies on retrograde perfusion from the pulmonary arteries, and is therefore relatively ischaemic. Bronchial artery revascularization procedures are time-consuming, technically demanding, and not widely performed. Complications range from minor narrowing of the bronchus, to severe narrowing requiring surgical intervention, to dehiscence and death. Bronchial stenoses are treated with dilatation and/or stenting.

The situation in heart–lung transplantation is completely different. The tracheal anastomosis has a collateral blood supply derived from the coronary arteries. The airway is well vascularized and serious airway/anastomotic problems are rare.

Outcome

Many studies have shown that lung transplantation confers significant survival and quality of life benefits to the majority of recipients. In experienced units, survival figures of better than 80 per cent at 1 year and 50 per cent at 5 years are now achieved for all types of transplant and underlying disease category. For those surviving the first year, the adjusted 5-year survival figure is 60 to 70 per cent.

The main cause of death in the first 12 months is infection (predominantly bacterial). Acute rejection rarely causes death directly. Its main impact is as a risk for the development of obliterative bronchiolitis, which is the main factor determining long-term survival in the majority of lung transplant recipients.

Survival is usually associated with markedly improved lung function and this translates into an improved functional capacity. As an example, in our own cystic fibrosis recipient group, FEV_1 improved from a mean of only 21 per cent predicted pretransplant, to 88 per cent predicted at 1 year post-transplant. Many patients are able to return to work and live a near normal life. Several female lung transplant recipients have undergone normal pregnancies without specific transplant related complications.

Conclusion

Lung and heart–lung transplantation offer the only therapeutic option for many patients with a variety of endstage pulmonary and cardiopulmonary diseases. With increasing experience and the development of more effective immunosuppression, survival figures continue to improve. The limiting factor in providing transplants is the critical shortage of donor organs.

Further reading

Barr ML *et al.* (1998). Recipient and donor outcomes in living related and unrelated lobar transplantation. *Transplantation Proceedings* **30**, 915–22.

Dennis CM *et al.* (1993). Heart–lung transplantation for end-stage respiratory disease in patients with cystic fibrosis at Papworth Hospital. *Journal of Heart and Lung Transplantation* **12**, 893–902. Series highlighting the outcome in terms of both survival and quality of life of cystic fibrosis patients receiving heart–lung transplants.

Dennis CM *et al.* (1996). Heart–lung–liver transplantation. *Journal of Heart and Lung Transplantation* **15,** 536–8. Report of the outcome of a unique series of patients receiving combined abdominal and thoracic transplants.

Gross CR *et al.* (1995). Long-term health status and quality of life outcomes of lung transplant recipients. *Chest* **108**, 1587–93.

Heng D *et al.* (1998). Bronchiolitis obliterans syndrome: incidence, natural history, prognosis, and risk factors. *Journal of Heart and Lung Transplantation* **17**, 1255–63. Largest series dealing with the clinical behaviour of bronchiolitis obliterans syndrome.

Higgins R *et al.* (1994). Airway stenosis after lung transplantation: management with expanding metal stents. *Journal of Heart and Lung Transplantation* **13**, 774–8. Large series detailing the management of airway complications after lung transplantation.

Hosenpud JD *et al.* (1999). The Registry of the International Society for Heart and Lung Transplantation: Sixteenth Official Report—1999. *Journal of Heart and Lung Transplantation* **18**, 611–26. Summary of the worldwide experience and outcome of all forms of pulmonary transplantation.

Joint Statement of the American Society for Transplant Physicians/American Thoracic Society/European Respiratory Society/International Society for Heart and Lung Transplantation (1998). International guidelines for the selection of lung transplant candidates. *American Journal of Respiratory and Critical Care Medicine* **158**, 335–9. Outline of the key criteria used for judging the timing of referral and listing for lung transplantation.

Jonas M, Oduro A (1997). Management of the multi-organ donor. In: Higgins RSD *et al.*, eds. *The multi-organ donor. Selection and management*, pp 123–9. Blackwell Scientific Publications, Oxford. Detailed account of optimal donor resuscitation and management.

McNeil K, Dennis CM (1998). Heart–lung transplantation: intensive care. In: Klinck JR, Lindop MJ, eds. *Anaesthesia and intensive care for organ transplantation*, pp 115–20. Chapman and Hall, London. A detailed account of the principles involved in the intensive care management of these patients.

McNeil K, Wallwork J (1997). Principles of lung allocation. In: Collins GM *et al.*, eds. *Procurement, preservation and allocation of vascularised organs*, pp 223–6. Kluwer Academic Publishers, Dordrecht.

Meester JD *et al.* (1999). Lung transplant waiting list: differential outcome of type of end-stage lung disease, one year after registration. *Journal of Heart and Lung Transplantation* **18**, 563–71. Highlights the importance of the underlying disease in determining death on the waiting list.

Yeatman M *et al.* (1996). Lung transplantation in patients with systemic diseases: an eleven year experience at Papworth Hospital. *Journal of Heart and Lung Transplantation* **15**, 144–9.

Yousem SA *et al.* (1996). Revision of the 1990 Working Formulation for the Classification of Pulmonary Allograft Rejection: Lung Rejection Study Group. *Journal of Heart and Lung Transplantation* **15**, 1–15. Describes the pathological changes and grading of rejection in lung transplants.

Index

Note: Numbers 1., 2. and 3. preceding the page numbers denote the volume. Numbers in italic refer to tables and/or illustrations separate from the text.